W9-APU-378

Luckmann and Sorensen's

Medical-Surgical Nursing

A Psychophysiologic Approach

Fourth Edition

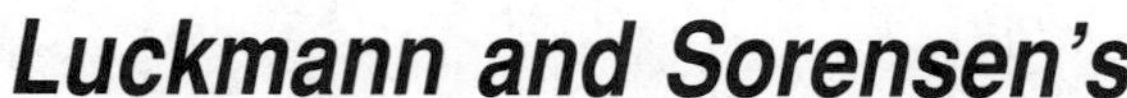

Luckmann and Sorensen's

Medical-Surgical Nursing

A Psychophysiologic Approach

Fourth Edition

JOYCE M. BLACK, M.S.N., R.N.,C.
Assistant Professor
College of Nursing
University of Nebraska Medical Center
Omaha, Nebraska

ESTHER MATASSARIN-JACOBS, Ph.D., R.N., O.C.N.
Associate Professor
Niehoff School of Nursing
Loyola University of Chicago
Chicago, Illinois

W.B. SAUNDERS COMPANY
A Division of Harcourt Brace & Company
Philadelphia London Toronto Montreal Sydney Tokyo

W.B. SAUNDERS COMPANY
A Division of Harcourt Brace & Company

The Curtis Center
Independence Square West
Philadelphia, Pennsylvania 19106

Library of Congress Cataloging-in-Publication Data

Luckmann and Sorensen's medical-surgical nursing : a psychophysiologic approach. — 4th ed. / [edited by] Joyce M. Black, Esther Matassarin-Jacobs.
p. cm.
Rev. ed. of: Medical-surgical nursing / Joan Luckmann, Karen Creason Sorensen. 3rd ed. 1987.
Includes bibliographical references and index.
ISBN 0-7216-3506-7
1. Nursing. 2. Surgical nursing. 3. Psychophysiology. I. Black, Joyce M. II. Matassarin-Jacobs, Esther. III. Luckmann, Joan. Medical-surgical nursing. IV. Title: Medical-surgical nursing.
[DNLM: 1. Nursing Care. 2. Surgical Nursing. WY 150 L9412 1993]
RT41.L87 1993
610.73 — dc20
DNLM/DLC
for Library of Congress 93-15131

Luckmann and Sorensen's Medical-Surgical Nursing:
A Psychophysiologic Approach, 4th Edition ISBN 0-7216-3506-7

International Edition ISBN 0-7216-4808-8

Printed in the United States of America.

Last digit is the print number: 9 8 7 6 5 4 3 2 1

Dedication

To Steve, Jon, Katy, and Tricia. Sometimes I work far too hard and forget to enjoy you: the most wonderful people in my life.

J.M.B.

To my parents, F. W. Matassarin, MD, and Grace Matassarin, RN. Thank you both for all your love and understanding. You must have done something right.

To my husband, Philip, who is the reason for all this hard work. Without his love and support, I would never have taken on or completed this mammoth task.

E.M.J.

About the Authors

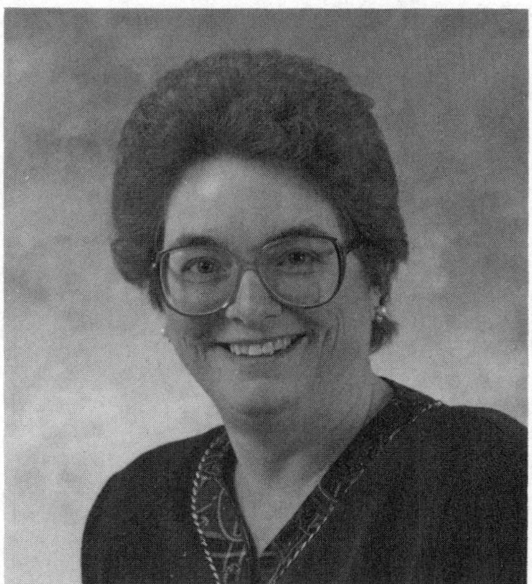

Joyce M. Black, M.S.N, R.N.,C. is an Assistant Professor with the University of Nebraska Medical Center in the Adult Health and Illness Department. Ms. Black received her Master's Degree from the University of Nebraska Medical Center and her undergraduate degrees from Winona State University in Winona, Minnesota, and Rochester Community College in Rochester, Minnesota.

Joyce Black has also had several years experience as a medical-surgical nurse at Saint Mary's Hospital, which is affiliated with the Mayo Clinic in Rochester, Minnesota. Her nursing practice included critical care, burns, respiratory disorders, orthopedics, and plastic surgery. Ms. Black is certified by the ANA in medical-surgical nursing and by the American Society of Plastic and Reconstructive Surgical Nurses. She currently serves as editor of *Plastic Surgical Nursing*.

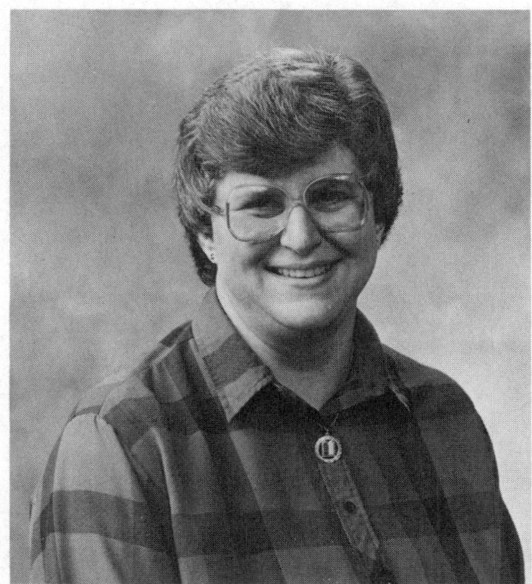

Esther Matassarin-Jacobs, Ph.D., R.N., O.C.N., is an Associate Professor of Medical/Surgical Nursing at the Niehoff School of Nursing, Loyola University Chicago. She is an oncology certified nurse and currently is in charge of the oncology major in the graduate program at Loyola. She has taught nursing for 20 years in diploma and baccalaureate programs including the last 14 years at Loyola. She has been very active in preparing graduate nurses nationwide for the licensure examination for the past 15 years, including publishing two successful NCLEX review books. Her areas of research include success on the NCLEX, critical thinking in undergraduates, and assessment and management of pain.

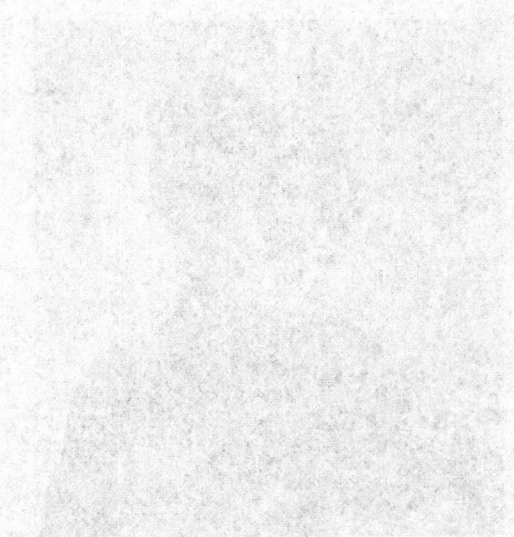

Contributors

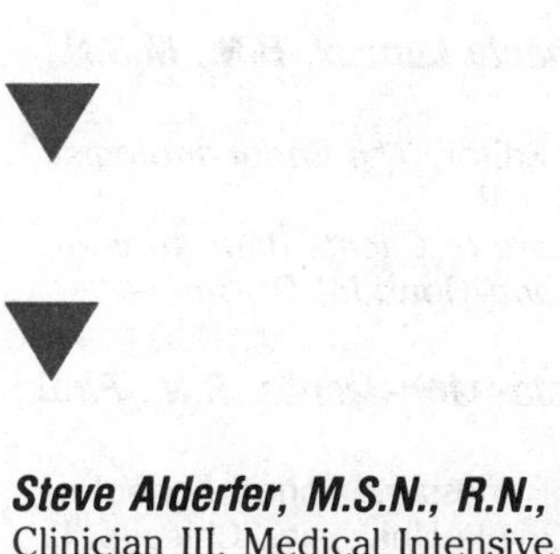

Steve Alderfer, M.S.N., R.N., C.C.R.N.
Clinician III, Medical Intensive Care Unit, University of Virginia Health Sciences Center, Charlottesville, VA
Common Respiratory Interventions

Helen A. Andrews, B.S.N.
Staff Nurse, Bergan Mercy Medical Center, Omaha, NE
Common Musculoskeletal Interventions; Nursing Care of Clients with Musculoskeletal Trauma or Overuse

Bonnie Angel, Diploma, B.S.N., M.S.N.
Clinical Assistant Professor, University of North Carolina, School of Nursing, Chapel Hill, NC
The Family

Minerva I. Applegate, Ed.D., R.N.
Nursing Consultant and Project Coordinator, H.C.A., L.W. Blake Hospital, Bradenton, FL
Ethics

Ellen Barker, M.S.N., R.N., C.N.R.N.
President, Neuroscience Nursing Consultants, Newark, DE
Assessment of Clients with Neurologic Disorders; Nursing Care of Clients with Loss of Protective Function

Maureen B. Barrett, M.S., R.N., C.
Assistant Professor, Loyola University of Chicago, Chicago, IL
Perioperative Nursing

Carol Birch, M.S., R.N., C.C.R.N.
Instructor, College of Nursing, South Dakota State University, Rapid City, SD
Nursing Care of Clients with Thyroid and Parathyroid Disorders

Joyce M. Black, M.S.N., R.N.,C.
Assistant Professor, College of Nursing, University of Nebraska Medical Center, Omaha, NE
Nursing Process; Theories of Health and Illness; Cross-Cultural Nursing; The Cell; Wound Healing; Assessment of Clients with Neurologic Disorders; Nursing Care of Clients with Loss of Protective Function; Nursing Care of Clients with Peripheral Vascular Disorders; Structure and Function; Assessment of Clients with Metabolic Disorders; Nursing Care of Clients with Endocrine Disorders of the Pancreas; Nursing Care of Clients with Musculoskeletal Trauma or Overuse

Barbara J. Boss, Ph.D.
Professor of Nursing, University of Mississippi Medical Center, School of Nursing, Jackson, MS
Structure and Function of the Nervous System

Carol Bova, M.S., R.N., C.
Nurse Practitioner, HIV Clinical Center, and Instructor, Graduate School of Nursing, University of Massachusetts Medical Center, Worcester, MA
Nursing Care of Clients with Altered Immune Systems

Evelyn Butera, M.S., R.N., C.N.N.
Manager, Education Services, Northwest Kidney Centers, Seattle, WA
Nursing Care of Clients with Renal Disorders

Diane Butts-Krakoff, M.S.N., C.D.E.
Diabetes Nurse Educator, St. Vincent Hospitals, Indianapolis, IN
Structure and Function; Assessment of Clients with Metabolic Disorders; Nursing Care of Clients with Endocrine Disorders of the Pancreas

Lynne C. Carpenter, R.N., M.S., Ph.D.C., O.C.N.
Clinical Nurse Specialist, University of Michigan Breast Care Center, Ann Arbor, MI
Structure and Function of the Female and Male Reproductive Systems; Assessment of Clients with Reproductive Disorders; Nursing Care of the Client with Breast Disorders

Gretchen J. Carrougher, R.N., M.N.
Clinical Nurse Specialist, Medical-Surgical Nursing, Medical Center Hospital, San Antonio, TX; Clinical Instructor, University of Texas Health Science Center, School of Nursing, San Antonio, TX
Nursing Care of Clients with Burn Injury

Ann J. Clark, Ph.D., R.N.
Director, Center for Nursing Research, University of Alabama at Birmingham, Birmingham, AL
Structure and Function of the Female and Male Reproductive Systems; Assessment of Clients with Reproductive Disorders; Nursing Care of Women with Gynecologic Disorders

Sherill Nones Cronin, Ph.D., R.N., C.
Assistant Professor of Nursing, Bellarmine College, Louisville, KY; Nurse Researcher, Jewish Hospital, Louisville, KY
Nursing Care of Clients with Lower Airway Disorders

Pamela D. Dennison, R.N., B.S.N., M.S.N.
Assistant Professor of Nursing, University of Virginia, Charlottesville, VA; Practitioner Teacher, University of Virginia Health Sciences Center, Charlottesville, VA
Nursing Care of Clients with Peripheral Vascular Disorders

Patricia E. Downing, M.N., R.N.
Formerly of School of Nursing University of California San Francisco, CA
Nursing Care of Clients with Sexually Transmitted Diseases

Mary Elizabeth Egloff, M.S.N., R.N., C.C.R.N.
Pulmonary Clinical Nurse Specialist, Sharp Memorial Hospital, San Diego, CA
Assessment of Clients with Respiratory Disorders

Darrell A. Follman, M.S., B.S., R.N., O.N.C.
Independent Consultant in Orthopedic Nursing and Quality Assurance Consultant, Health Connections, Inc., Skokie, IL
Structure and Function of the Musculoskeletal System; Assessment of Clients with Musculoskeletal Disorders

Mary Jane Garrett, B.S.N., M.S.N., Ph.D.
Assistant Professor, University of Nebraska at Omaha, College of Nursing, Omaha, NE
Chronic Conditions

Terri Goodman, M.A.E.D., B.S.N., C.N.O.R.
Clinical Educator for Surgical Services, Shady Grove Adventist Hospital, Rockville, MD
Nursing Care of Clients Having Plastic Surgery

Deanna E. Grimes, Dr.P.H., R.N., M.S.N.
Associate Professor, University of Texas at Houston, Health Science Center, School of Nursing, Houston, TX
Nursing Care of Clients with Infectious Diseases

Margie J. Hansen, Ph.D., R.N.
Assistant Professor of Pharmaceutical Science, North Dakota State University, Fargo, ND
Acid-Base Imbalances

Jane H. Hawks, R.N., C., M.S.N., D.N.Sc., C.
Assistant Professor, Midland Lutheran College, Fremont, NE
Human Sexuality

Susan Hockenberger, M.S.N., Ed.D., R.N.
Dean, Lansing School of Nursing, Bellarmine College, Louisville, KY
Wound Healing

Laura Haynes Jacobson, B.S., M.S.N., C.C.R.N.
Staff Nurse IV, Coronary Care, Emory University Hospital, Atlanta, GA
Assessment of Clients with Cardiovascular Disorders

Linda Janusek, R.N., Ph.D.
Associate Professor, Loyola University School of Nursing, Chicago, IL
Structure and Function of the Immune System

Patricia F. Jassak, M.S., R.N., C.S., O.C.N.
Oncology Clinical Nurse Specialist, Loyola University Medical Center, Maywood, IL
Treatment Modalities for Neoplastic Disorders

Cindy Kallsen, R.N., B.S.N.
Assistant Unit Director, University of Nebraska Medical Center, Omaha, NE
Nursing Care of Clients with Biliary and Exocrine Pancreatic Disorders

Joyce Kee, R.N., M.S.
Associate Professor Emerita, University of Delaware, Newark, DE
Fluid and Electrolyte Balance

Lynn Keegan, R.N., Ph.D.
"Consultant," University of Texas Health Science Center at San Antonio, San Antonio, TX; Director, Bodymind Systems, Temple, TX
Spirituality; Health Promotion

Annabelle Keene, B.S.N., M.S.N., R.N., C.
Assistant Professor, University of Nebraska at Omaha, College of Nursing, Omaha, NE
Health Assessment; Physical Examination

Carol Ren Kneisl, M.S., R.N., C.S.
President and Education Director, Nursing Transitions, Inc., Williamsville, NY
Nursing Care of Clients with Substance Abuse

Mary Ann Krol, R.N., M.S.N.
Clinical Nurse Specialist, Surgery, Loyola University Medical Center, Maywood, IL
Treatment Modalities for Neoplastic Disorders

Teresa Choate Loriaux, R.N., M.S.N., CDE
Managing Editor, *The Endocrinologist*, West Linn, OR
Nursing Care of Clients with Adrenal, Pituitary, and Gonadal Disorders

Esther Matassarin-Jacobs, R.N., Ph.D., O.C.N.
Associate Professor, Neihoff School of Nursing, Loyola University, Chicago, IL
Nursing Process; Pain Assessment and Intervention; Basic Concepts of Neoplastic Disorders; Nursing Care of Clients with Altered Immune Systems; Nursing Care of Clients with Connective Tissue Disorders; Structure and Function of the Urinary System; Assessment of Clients with Urinary Disorders; Nursing Care of Clients with Disorders of the Ureters, Bladder, and Urethra; Nursing Care of Clients with Intestinal Disorders; Structure and Function of the Liver, Biliary System, and Exocrine Pancreas; Assessment of Clients with Hepatic, Biliary, and Pancreatic Disorders; Nursing Care of Clients with Hepatic Disorders; Structure and Function of the Female and Male Reproductive Systems; Assessment of Clients with Reproductive Disorders; Nursing Care of Men with Reproductive and Urinary Disorders; Nursing Care of Women with Gynecologic Disorders

Louise Nelson, M.S.N., R.N.
Assistant Professor, University of Nebraska College of Nursing, Omaha, NE
Shock

Noreen Heer Nicol, M.S., R.N., E.N.C.
Dermatology Clinical Specialist/Nurse Practitioner, National Jewish Center for Immunology and Respiratory Medicine, Denver, CO; Clinical Senior Instructor,

University of Colorado Health Sciences Center, School of Nursing, Denver, CO
Structure and Function; Assessment of Clients with Integumentary Disorders; Nursing Care of Clients with Integumentary Disorders

Margaret Nield, Ph.D., R.N.
Critical Researcher, Sharp Memorial Hospital, San Diego, CA; Adjunct Professor, San Diego State University, San Diego, CA
Structure and Function of the Respiratory System

Barbara Ott, R.N., Ph.D., C.C.R.N.
Assistant Professor, Wichita State University, Wichita, KS
Structure and Function of the Cardiovascular System; Nursing Care of Clients with Cardiac Structure Disorders

Judy Ozuna, B.S.N., M.N.
Clinical Nurse Specialist in Neurology, Veterans Affairs Medical Center, Seattle, WA
Nursing Care of Clients with Degenerative Neurologic Disorders

Janet Pavel, R.N.
Chief Nurse, Blood Services, National Institutes of Health, Bethesda, MD
Basic Concepts of Hematology; Nursing Care of Clients with Hematologic Disorders

Lynn Allchin Petardi, M.S.N., R.N.
Doctoral Student, Loyola University at Chicago, Chicago, IL
Basic Concepts of Neoplastic Disorders

Joann Petty, M.S.N., R.N.
Nursing Staff Educator, Foster G. McGaw Hospital, Loyola University Medical Center, Maywood, IL
Treatment Modalities for Neoplastic Disorders

Bonita Ann Pilon, D.S.N., R.N., CNAA
Assistant Professor and Specialty Director of Nursing Administration Graduate Program, Vanderbilt University, Nashville, TN
Nursing Practice

Ann Plunkett, R.N.
Apheresis Supervisor, Blood Services, National Institutes of Health, Bethesda, MD
Basic Concepts of Hematology; Nursing Care of Clients with Hematologic Disorders

Nina A. Rauscher, R.N., C., O.N.C.
Consultant, North Andover, MA
Nursing Care of Clients with Musculoskeletal Disorders

Juanita Reigle, R.N., M.S.N., C.C.R.N.
Practitioner/Teacher, University of Virginia, Charlottesville, VA
Nursing Care of Clients with Disorders of Cardiac Function

Marlene Reimer, R.N., M.N., C.N.N.(C).
Associate Professor, Faculty of Nursing, Val University of Calgary, Calgary, Alberta, Canada
Sleep and Sensory Disorders

Kathleen A. Ringel, D.N.S., R.N., C.
Assistant Professor, University of Nebraska Medical Center, College of Nursing, Omaha, NE
Nursing Care of Clients with Disorders of Cardiac Function

Shirley M. Ruder, B.S.N., M.S., M.S.N., Ed.D.
Coordinator of Nursing, Edison Community College, Ft. Myers, FL
Structure and Function of the Gastrointestinal System; Assessment of Clients with Gastrointestinal Disorders; Nursing Care of Clients with Ingestive Disorders; Nursing Care of Clients with Gastric Disorders; Nursing Care of Clients with Intestinal Disorders

Linda T. Schuring, M.S.N., R.N.
Director of the Balance Disorder Clinic, Warren Otologic Group, Warren, OH
Structure and Function; Assessment and Nursing Care of Clients with Ear Disorders

Sally Strong Schnell, R.N., M.S.N.
Clinical Nurse Specialist, Loyola University Medical Center, Maywood, IL; Clinical Instructor, Department of Medical-Surgical Nursing, Loyola University at Chicago, Chicago, IL
Nursing Care of Clients with Cerebral Disorders; Nursing Care of Clients with Disorders of the Spinal Cord, Cranial Nerves, and Peripheral Nerves

Barbara Sigler, R.N., M.N.Ed.
Clinical Nurse Specialist, Otolaryngology, Head and Neck Surgery Department, Eye and Ear Institute, University of Pittsburgh Medical Center, Pittsburgh, PA
Nursing Care of Clients with Upper Airway Disorders

Bonnie Sink, R.N., B.S.N.
Clinical Nurse, Blood Services, National Institutes of Health, Bethesda, MD
Basic Concepts of Hematology; Nursing Care of Clients with Hematologic Disorders

Kris Strasburg, R.N., C.C.T.C.
Heart and Lung Transplant Coordinator, University of Minnesota Transplant Center, Minneapolis, MN
Structure and Function of the Liver, Biliary System, and Exocrine Pancreas; Assessment of Clients with Hepatic, Biliary, and Pancreatic Disorders; Nursing Care of Clients with Hepatic Disorders

Lisa L. Strohmyer, M.S.N., R.N.
Medical-Surgical Clinical Nurse Specialist, University of Nebraska Medical Center, University Hospital, Omaha, NE
Nursing Care of Clients During Medical-Surgical Emergencies

Michele J. Upvall, Ph.D., R.N.
Assistant Professor of Nursing, Northern Arizona University, Flagstaff, AZ
Cross-Cultural Nursing

Linda A. Vader, B.S., R.N., CRNO
Head Nurse, University of Michigan, Kellogg Eye Center, Ann Arbor, MI
Structure and Function; Assessment and Nursing Care of Clients with Eye Disorders

The assessment portions of chapters throughout the book were written by Annabelle Keene, B.S.N., M.S.N., R.N., C.

All of the ETHICAL ISSUES IN NURSING features *except* those for Chapters 21 and 39 (Tuberculosis Testing) were written by Lisa Anderson-Shaw, R.N., C., M.S.N., M.A., Clinical Nurse Specialist, Eye and Ear Infirmary, University of Illinois at Chicago.

The following BRIDGE TO HOME HEALTH CARE features were coordinated by Karen Martin, R.N., M.S.N., F.A.A.N., Director of Research at The Visiting Nurse Association, Omaha, NE. Individual BRIDGE TO HOME HEALTH CARE boxes were written by the following people, all of The Visiting Nurse Association, Omaha, NE:
Karen M. Martin, R.N., M.S.N., F.A.A.N. (Chap. 2, p. 33); Bridget Young, R.N., B.S.N. (Chap. 8); Cindi Leo-Gofta, R.N., B.S.N., and June McAtee, B.S., C.S.W., M.S.W. (Chap. 9); Kathy Moritz Byrnes, B.S. (Chap. 10); Joanie Kush, R.N., B.S.N. (Chap. 16); Barbara Michaud,

R.N., B.S.N. (Chap. 22); Patricia Hann, R.N., M.P.H. (Chap. 25); Linda Svatora, O.T.R./L., B.S. (Chap. 26); Judy Porter, R.P.T. (Chap. 32); Bernadette Mruz, R.N. (Chap. 33); Bernice Belik, R.N., B.S.N. (Chap. 34); Terri Brown, R.N., B.S.N. (Chap. 37); Mary Murphy, R.N., B.S.N. (Chap. 39); Sandra Nimmo, R.N., B.S.N. (Chap. 42); Jody Hooi, R.N., B.S.N. (Chap. 44); Kaye Feilen, R.N. (Chap. 46); Colette McVaney, R.N., B.S.N. (Chap. 54, p. 1600); Peg Neumann, R.N., M.P.H. (Chap. 61); Mary McQuin, B.S.P.T (Chap. 66); Iva Mueller, R.N., B.S.N., M.Min. (Chap. 70); Karen Martin, R.N., M.S.N., F.A.A.N., and Mary McQuin, B.S.P.T. (Chap. 71, p. 2009); Sandra Elsea, R.N., M.N. (Chap. 77); Catherine Alexander, R.N., B.S.N. (Chap. 78); Jane Allen, R.N., B.S.N. (Chap. 79).

BRIDGE TO HOME HEALTH CARE boxes for Chapters 30, 31, and 38 were written by Kerrie Greear, R.N., B.S.N., South Dakota State College of Nursing.

Contributions to previous editions of *Luckmann and Sorensen's Medical-Surgical Nursing: A Psychophysiologic Approach* by the following people are gratefully acknowledged: Jeanette Anders; Patricia L. Baum; Deanna Bland; Heather Boyd-Monk; Charles Cleeland; Kathleen Dietz; Linda Felver; Marie Elizabeth Folk-Lighty; Barbara A. Given; George Heidrich, III: Colleen F. Johnson; David Johnson; Mary Lou Johnson; Winnifred H. Kataoka; Rosemary Craig Kelly; Christine A. Kessler; Diane Kizer; Eileen Enny Leach; Mary Pat Lovely; Margaret M. McMahon; John Sanders; Kathleen Smith-DiJulio; Helene A. Stith; Janice M. Swanson; Irene T. Takemori; Barbara Wittman; Linda C. Yergey; Kerry Cavanaugh Zellers; and Constance E. Ziegfeld.

Reviewers

Cynthia Amerson, R.N., B.S.N., M.S.
Staff Nurse, ICU, Titus County Memorial Hospital, Mt. Pleasant, TX

Lisa K. Anderson-Shaw, R.N., C., M.S.N., M.A.
Eye and Ear Infirmary, University of Illinois, Chicago, IL

Helen A. Andrews, R.N., B.S.N.
Bergan Mercy Hospital, Omaha, NE

Margaret M. Andrews, Ph.D., R.N., C.T.N.
Nazareth College, Rochester, NY

Cecilia R. Barron, Ph.D., R.N.
College of Nursing, University of Nebraska Medical Center, Omaha, NE

Roberta P. Bartee, M.S., R.N.
Tulane University Medical Center, New Orleans, LA

Patricia Bates, R.N., B.S.N., C.U.R.N.
Oregon Urology Clinic, Portland, OR

Pamela Baker, M.S., R.N.
Clarkson Centre for Wound Healing, Omaha, NE

Barbara Bires, R.N., M.S.N., C.C.R.N., C.E.N.
University of California at San Francisco, San Francisco, CA

Steven B. Black, M.D.
Plastic Surgeon, Private Practice, Omaha, NE

Suzanne Smith Blancett, Ed.D., R.N.
Journal of Nursing Administration, Bradenton, FL

Janice Strom Borman, R.N., M.S.
University of Illinois at Chicago, Chicago, IL

Ellen K. Boyda, R.N., B.S.N., M.S.
Taylor Hospital, Ridley Park, PA

Patricia Broten, R.N., M.N., Ed.D.
Nazareth College, Kalamazoo, MI

Sally A. Brozenec, R.N., Ph.D.
Rush Medical Center, Chicago, IL

Valerie Miller Capallo, R.N., M.S.
The Union Memorial Hospital School of Nursing, Baltimore, MD

Kathryn Carlson, R.N., B.S.N., C.P.A.N.
Abbott-Northwestern Hospital, Minneapolis, MN

Marcia Chorba, R.N., M.S.N.
Mercy Hospital School of Nursing, Pittsburgh, PA

Imelda Clements, R.N., M.S.N., M.P.H., M.A., Ph.D.
Bellarmine College School of Nursing, Louisville, KY

Bonnie Leigh Closson, R.N., M.S., M.S.N., M.R.C.
Mayo Clinic, Rochester, MN

Shirley E. Coleman-Aikin, M.A., R.N.
Pacific Lutheran University, Tacoma, WA

Janet Ann Coors, R.N.
Ear Medical Center, Cincinnati, OH

Sherrill Nones Cronin, Ph.D., R.N., C.
Jewish Hospital, Louisville, KY

Carolyn A. Cunningham, R.N., M.S., C.S., C.C.R.N.
Frazier Rehabilization Center, Louisville, KY

Victora A. Fahey, R.N., M.S.N.
Northwestern Memorial Hospital, Chicago, IL

Darrell A. Follman, M.S., B.S., R.N., O.N.C.
Independent Consultant, Skokie, IL

Benjamin R. Gelber, M.D.
Neurosurgeon, Private Practice, Lincoln, NE

Mary Jo Gerlach, R.N., M.S.N.Ed.
Medical College of Georgia at Athens, Athens, GA

Terri Goodman, M.A.E.D., B.S.N., C.N.O.R.
Shady Grove Adventist Hospital, Rockville, MD

Debra Suzanne Goodwin, R.N., B.S.N., M.S.
Bellair SurgiCenter, Clearwater, FL

Marcia D. Gragert, Ph.D., R.N.
Montana State University, Bozeman, MT

Edythe Lyn Greenberg, R.N., M.S., Ph.D.
School of Nursing, University of Texas at Houston, Houston, TX

Barbara P. Harrison, R.N., C., M.Ed., M.S.N.
Bellarmine College, Louisville, KY

Jane Hokanson Hawks, R.N., C.
Formerly, Bishop Clarkson College, Omaha, NE

Diane M. Hayko, B.S.N., R.N., C.
St. Joseph Hospital at Creighton University Medical Center, Omaha, NE

Penny Hergenroeder, R.N., B.S.N., C.E.T.N.
William Beaumont Hospital, Royal Oak, MI

Marcia J. Hill, R.N., M.S.N.
The Methodist Hospital, Houston, TX

Gloria A. Hinderer, M.S., R.N., C.C.R.N., C.S.
Rush Presbyterian St. Luke's Medical Center, Chicago, IL

Renee J. Hinojosa, M.S., R.N.
University Hospital and Clinics, Columbia, MO

Ann Noreen Hotter, R.N., M.S.N., C.C.R.N., C.S.
Orlando Regional Medical Center, Orlando, FL

Patricia W. Iyer, R.N., M.S.N., C.N.A.
Patricia Iyer Associates, Stockton, NJ

Ellen H. Janosik, M.S.
Alfred University, Alfred, NY

Patricia A. Johnson, R.N.
Tri County Hospital, Wadena, MN

Shayna J. Johnson, M.S., R.N.
Mayo Medical Center, Rochester, MN

Cindy Kallsen, R.N., B.S.N.
University of Nebraska Medical Center, Omaha, NE

Karen A. Karlowicz, R.N., M.S.N.
Urologic Nurse Consultant, Virginia Beach, VA

Lon W. Keim, M.D.
Pulmonary Medicine Services, Bishop Clarkson Memorial Hospital, Omaha, NE

Karen M. Kleeman, Ph.D., R.N., C.S.
School of Nursing, University of Maryland at Baltimore, Baltimore, MD

Carol L. Kohn, D.N.Sc., R.N.
Rush University College of Nursing, Chicago, IL

Diane Butts Krakoff, M.S.N., R.N., C.D.E.
Mount Carmel Medical Center, Columbus, OH

Ronnie E. Leibowitz, R.N., M.A., C.I.C.
Veterans Affairs Medical Center, New York, NY

Charles E. Martin, Ph.D.
Rutgers University, New Brunswick, NJ

Madeleine T. Martin, R.N., Ed.D.
College of Nursing and Health, University of Cincinnati, Cincinnati, OH

Susan K. Masten, R.N., B.S.N.
University of Michigan Medical Center, Ann Arbor, MI

Ruth McCorkle, Ph.D., F.A.A.N.
University of Pennsylvania, Philadelphia, PA

Kay McCoy, R.N., C.R.N.O.
ASORN's INSIGHT, Drake, CO

Deborah Prenger Meis, B.A., M.Ed.
Charity-Delgado School of Nursing, New Orleans, LA

Joyce Mendenhall, R.N., M.S., C.D.E.
University of Nebraska Medical Center, Omaha, NE

Terry R. Misener, R.N., F.N.P., Ph.D., F.A.A.N.
College of Nursing, University of South Carolina, Columbia, SC

Georgia A. Moncada, R.N., C.P.S.N.
Specialties of Plastic, Hand & Microsurgery, P.C., Pittsburgh, PA

Martha J. Morrow, R.N., M.S.N.
Shenandoah University, Winchester, VA

Phyllis Anne Luers Naumann, R.N., M.A., C.E.N.
School of Nursing, The Union Memorial Hospital, Baltimore, MD

Marian Newton, R.N., B.S.N., M.N., Ph.D.
Albany Veteran Affairs Medical Center, Albany, NY

Noreen Heer Nicol, M.S., R.N., F.N.C.
National Jewish Center for Immunology and Respiratory Medicine, Denver, CO

Mary Palandri, R.N., B.S.N.
University of Nebraska Hospital, Omaha, NE

Betty J. Paulanka, R.N., E.E.D.
University of Delaware, Newark, DE

Mary Ellen Pike, R.N., M.S.N.
Bellarmine College, Louisville, KY

Tim Porter-O'Grady, Ed.D., R.N., C.S., C.N.A.A. F.A.A.N.
Tim Porter-O'Grady, Inc., Atlanta, GA

Barbara Ann Preib, R.N., C., M.S.N.
University of Illinois Hospital and College of Nursing, Chicago, IL

Betty J. Pugh, Ph.D., R.N.
The Pennsylvania State University, University Park, PA

Priscilla W. Ramsey, R.N., Ph.D.
East Tennessee State University, Johnson City, TN

Ginger Renkiewicz, R.N., B.S.N., M.S.A.
William Beaumont Hospital, Royal Oak, MI

Nancy J. Reilly, R.N., M.S.N., C.U.R.N.
Hospital of the University of Pennsylvania, Philadelphia, PA

Kathleen A. Ringel, D.N.Sc., R.N., C.
College of Nursing, University of Nebraska Medical Center, Omaha, NE

Rev. Daniel R. Ritter, B.S., M.DIV.
Trinity Lutheran Church, Blair, NE

Brenda Roberts, R.N., B.S.N., M.S.N., D.S.N.
Jacksonville State University, Jacksonville, AL

Diane Roberts, R.N., M.S.N.
Eden Hospital Trauma Center, Castro Valley, CA

Rosemary Ann Roth, R.N., M.S.N., C.N.O.R.
The Genesee Hospital, Rochester, NY

Mary Patricia Ryan, R.N., Ph.D.
Hospice Care of Broward County, Inc., Ft. Lauderdale, FL

Mary E. Sampel, R.N., M.S.N.
St. Louis University School of Nursing, St. Louis, MO

Olive A. Santavenere, R.N., M.S.
Southern Connecticut State University, New Haven, CT

Stanley H. Schack, M.D.
Otolaryngologist, Private Practice, Omaha, NE

Nancy Warren Schneckloth, M.S.N., R.N., C.N.O.R.
University of Nebraska Medical Center, Omaha, NE

Sally Strong Schnell, R.N., M.S.N.
Loyola University Medical Center, Maywood, IL

Linda T. Schuring, M.S.N., R.N.
Warren Otologic Group, Warren, OH

Deborah Wright Shpritz, M.S., R.N., C.C.R.N.
University of Maryland School of Nursing, Baltimore, MD

DuAnne Foster Smith, R.N., M.N., C.C.R.N., C.S.
St. Mary's Hospital, Rochester, MN

Stephen B. Smith, M.D.
Pulmonary Medicine Services, Bishop Clarkson Memorial Hospital, Omaha, NE

Donna Ayers Snelson, M.S.N., R.N.
College Misericordia, Dallas, TX

Martha A. Spies, R.N., B.S.N., M.S.N.
Deaconess College of Nursing, St. Louis, MO

Judith A. Spross, M.S., R.N., O.N.C.
Massachusetts General Hospital Institute of Health Professions, Boston, MA

Lisa Bacon Strohmyer, R.N., M.S.N., C.C.R.N.
University of Nebraska Medical Center, Omaha, NE

Mary Helene Sunderman, R.N., Ph.D.
College of Nursing, University of Nebraska Medical Center, Omaha, NE

Mary Ann Thompson, R.N., C., M.S.N.
St. Joseph College, West Hartford, CT

Janice J. Twiss, Ph.D., R.N.
College of Nursing, University of Nebraska Medical Center, Omaha, NE

Peter J. Ungvarski, M.S., R.N.C.
Home Care, Visiting Nurse Service of New York, New York, NY

Linda A. Vader, B.S., R.N., C.R.N.O.
University of Michigan, Kellogg Eye Center, Ann Arbor, MI

Rita DeSciscio Van Fleet, R.N.
Bishop Clarkson Memorial Hospital, Omaha, NE

Nancy E. Vangieson, R.N., C.N. III
University of Michigan Medical Center, Ann Arbor, MI

Sharon Wahl, R.N., M.S., Ed.Dc.
San Jose State University, San Jose, CA

Kathleen C. Walsh, M.S.N., R.N., C.S.
William Beaumont Hospital, Royal Oak, MI

Bernadette A. White, R.N., M.S.N.
College of Nursing, University of Nebraska Medical Center, Omaha, NE

Valorie D. White, M.A., C.C.C.-A.
Boystown Research Hospital, Omaha, NE

Marlene K. Wilken, R.N., M.N., M.A.
College of Nursing, University of Nebraska Medical Center, Omaha, NE

Marianne Zelewsky, M.S.N., R.N., C.
Loyola University at Chicago, Chicago, IL

Foreword

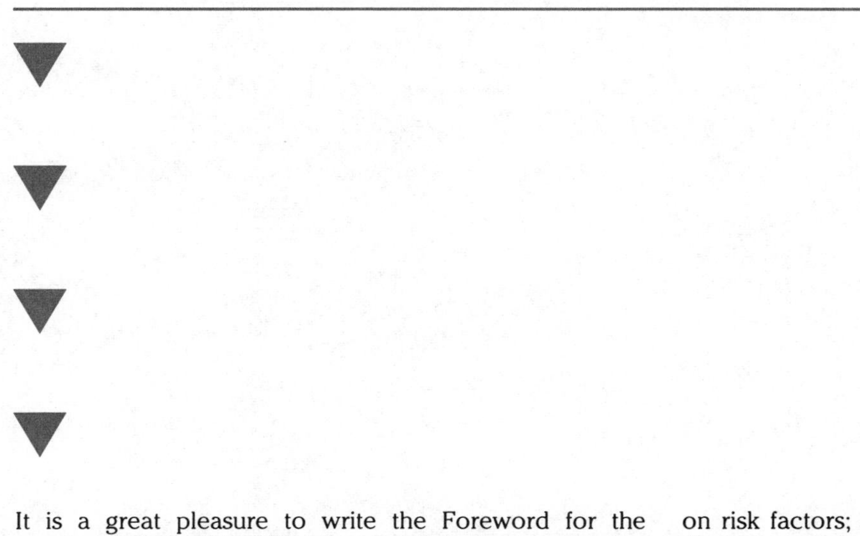

It is a great pleasure to write the Foreword for the fourth edition of *Medical-Surgical Nursing: A Psychophysiologic Approach*. For me, the publication of this new edition is a major landmark. Twenty-five years ago, Karen Sorensen and I began working on the proposal for the first edition of *Luckmann and Sorensen*. During the years that followed acceptance of our proposal, we worked hard to produce a book that would meet the educational needs of nursing students, nursing faculty, and the thousands of nurses providing health care throughout the world. I am pleased that Joyce Black and Esther Matassarin-Jacobs have undertaken the enormous responsibility of revising *Luckmann and Sorensen,* and have produced a book that will continue to serve the nursing profession.

Although the new authors have retained the features that made earlier editions of *Luckmann and Sorensen* so successful, they have also added a great deal of important new information, and they have developed many exciting new features. Thus, the fourth edition of *Luckmann and Sorensen* continues to be comprehensive, and it still offers the in-depth coverage of physiology, pathophysiology, medical-surgical disorders, nursing and medical interventions, and the nursing process that has been its hallmark in earlier editions. To these basic strengths, Black and Matassarin-Jacobs have added the following: cross-cultural nursing; a greater emphasis on psychosocial aspects of nursing, including the family, spirituality, and ethics; integrated sections on risk factors; and more learning materials on chronic disease, care of the elderly, and discharge planning. The authors have also developed helpful boxed materials on ethical issues, critical care, home health care, nursing research, and client education.

By combining the best features of prior editions of *Luckmann and Sorensen* with numerous up-to-date and enlightening new features, the fourth edition of *Luckmann and Sorensen* has evolved into a truly holistic nursing textbook. It is a book that nursing students and practicing nurses can rely on as they care for clients in the complex clinical settings of today.

In closing, I want to thank Joyce Black and Esther Matassarin-Jacobs for undertaking and carefully preparing the revision of *Medical-Surgical Nursing: A Psychophysiologic Approach*. I also wish to thank the book's many contributors, revisers, and reviewers, who have given so generously of their knowledge and expertise over the years. I also appreciate the support and encouragement given by the editors at W.B. Saunders Company who believed in the book, and who endeavored to ensure its successful publication. Finally, I especially want to thank the thousands of loyal nursing students and graduates who still turn to *Luckmann and Sorensen*—for the information, inspiration, and clear answers they need to meet the challenge of nursing!

Joan Luckmann, R.N., M.A.

Preface

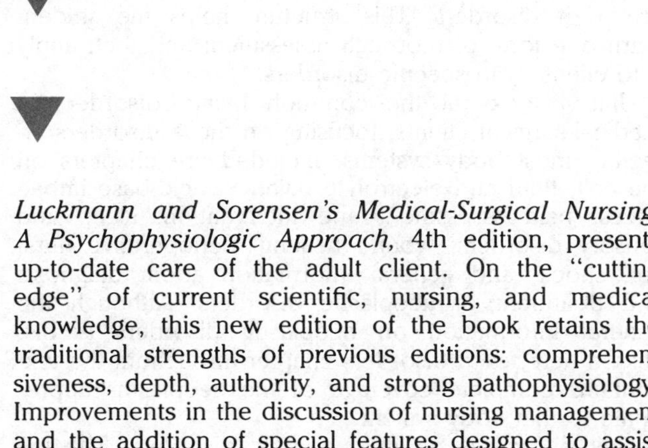

Luckmann and Sorensen's Medical-Surgical Nursing: A Psychophysiologic Approach, 4th edition, presents up-to-date care of the adult client. On the "cutting edge" of current scientific, nursing, and medical knowledge, this new edition of the book retains the traditional strengths of previous editions: comprehensiveness, depth, authority, and strong pathophysiology. Improvements in the discussion of nursing management and the addition of special features designed to assist the nurse in the clinical setting allow a clear transition from the book to the bedside.

PHILOSOPHY AND APPROACH

This book portrays the reality of nursing care, where often there is a clear differentiation between nursing management and medical management. The text represents our belief that although nurses and physicians do not compete with each other but collaborate for the benefit of the client, still, nursing and medicine are separate disciplines. In the text, Nursing Management and Medical Management are separate headings and are not intermingled with general management of clients. Because nursing and medicine are collaborative efforts, however, it is often difficult for nursing students to understand one without the other.

We used the nursing process to illuminate nursing care, but did not apply the nursing process to every disorder, electing instead to use the nursing process for prototypical disorders. Within the nursing process for a disorder, we developed nursing diagnoses and, as appropriate, collaborative problems, each with its own expected outcomes and implementation. Expected outcomes and implementation have been written for each nursing diagnosis because we have found, from our teaching experience, that lists of diagnoses followed by lists of expected outcomes and implementations cannot easily be teased apart and rebuilt into a care plan by the student. Collaborative problems define those areas of nursing practice that are not resolvable through independent nursing actions. Collaborative problems are potential complications that a client may develop due to the disorder, surgery, or other treatments. They complete the picture of nursing care and eliminate the need of force-fitting the various nursing diagnoses to each client problem that may be encountered.

A head-to-toe body systems approach is used in this edition. This is more easily adapted to a variety of conceptual frameworks than the use of a conceptual framework of our own. Concepts prevalent in medical-surgical practice, such as pain, perioperative care, shock, and chronic conditions, are found in the first quarter of the book.

Because a significant portion of medical-surgical disorders occur in the elderly, we added content on normal aging of individual body systems. Then, to help the student to modify care accordingly, there is a section at the end of each processed disorder called "Modification of Plan of Care for the Elderly."

The strong psychosocial underpinning of past editions of *Luckmann and Sorensen's Medical-Surgical Nursing: A Psychophysiologic Approach* has been reinforced by doubling the number of chapters on psychosocial content. There are chapters on ethics, cross-cultural nursing, spiritual needs, human sexuality, the family, and chronic conditions. This text focuses on not only the client's individual response to illness but also the effect of illness on a client's family. With shortened hospital stays, the family has become an extension of the medical-surgical nurse, who often works in tandem with the family to prepare them for their part in continued assessment and provision of care. This planning for home care is highlighted in the text in a section called "Discharge Teaching."

SPECIAL FEATURES

Bridging the distance from the theoretical to the practical, and from the medical-surgical setting to the home, is essential in nursing. To that end, we have included several such "bridges" to clinical care.

In addition to a separate chapter on "Ethics" (Chap. 4), a feature called "Ethical Issues in Nursing" was written by a nurse ethicist and appears frequently throughout the book. An ethical dilemma is presented, not necessarily for resolution but for reflection.

The "Bridge to Home Health Care" feature also appears throughout the text, and gives practical suggestions on how to help clients in the home setting. These bridges were written by practicing home health care nurses.

Another feature, the "Bridge to Critical Care," highlights common modalities of treatment or assessment in critical care. Although there is no attempt to discuss all of critical care nursing, we present a basic understanding of hospital-based critical care treatments as they are used in post-hospital care. Some examples are pulmonary pressure monitors, ventilators, and arterial lines.

"Nursing Research" boxes provide illustrative examples to show students how nursing research may be used in client care.

Finally, in recognition of the need to make the client a collaborator in the care plan, we include "Client Education Guides."

ORGANIZATION

The first four units of the text are devoted to material common to all medical-surgical clients, including the client's significant others. The material in this first portion of the book helps the nurse provide comprehensive care regardless of the specific diagnosis or problem the client is experiencing.

The remainder of the text is divided by body systems. Each unit includes sections on structure and function of the involved system, assessment of the client with disorders of that system, and nursing care of clients with disorders specific to that system.

Unit 1 covers nursing and health care. Chapter 1 focuses on the nursing process including current NANDA-approved nursing diagnoses and an explanation of the use of nursing diagnosis. The role of research in relation to the nursing process is covered. A brief overview of the major models/theories of nursing is included so the student can be introduced to this. Finally, the models/theories are applied to the same case situation so the student can see the differences among them. Chapter 2 examines the "stakeholders" in health care delivery. Medical-surgical nurses in all areas of practice, not just managers, must be aware of health care financing. The chapter also considers the roles of nurses in service to a wide variety of clients.

Unit 2 looks at the holistic aspects of health care. This unit is designed to help the nurse look at the client in a holistic manner. The focus of this unit is the psychosocial factors that affect and direct individualized client care. This unit contains chapters on the theories of health and illness, ethics in the practice of nursing, cross-cultural nursing, spirituality, sexuality, the family, and chronic conditions.

Unit 3 covers health assessment and promotion, addressing the broad topics of health promotion, health assessment, and the physical examination of all adult clients. The format for health assessment and physical examination set up in these chapters is then carried through in an "Assessment" chapter for every major group of disorders. This structure helps the student learn one form of thorough assessment and then apply it to clients with specific disorders.

Unit 4 looks at the common health disorders in medical-surgical clients, focusing on those disorders affecting most body systems. Included are chapters on the cell, fluid and electrolyte balance, acid-base imbalances, pain assessment and intervention, sleep and sensory disorders, wound healing, perioperative nursing, shock, and general information about diagnosis and treatment of neoplastic disorders. Although the general information on neoplastic disorders is discussed here, each disorders chapter throughout the text contains complete coverage of the neoplasms appropriate to that body system.

Unit 5 focuses on immunologic disorders. The immune system is discussed in general in Chapter 23, whereas Chapter 24 is devoted to the care of clients with altered immune systems, focusing primarily on the care of clients with human immunodeficiency virus infection. The information on human immunodeficiency virus infection includes all the current information from the Centers for Disease Control, including the new definitions of the disease and universal precautions. Hypersensitivity and organ transplantation, from the standpoint of immunity, are also covered in this unit. An overview of infectious disorders and infection control is also included.

Unit 6 covers neurologic disorders, focusing first on the common problems associated with disorders of the nervous system. Alterations in consciousness, confusion, increased intracranial pressure, seizures, and alterations in body thermal regulation are discussed. This is followed by an extensive coverage of the care of clients with cerebral disorders, degenerative neurologic disorders, and disorders of the spinal cord, peripheral nerves, and cranial nerves. Complete and up-to-date information on dementia of the Alzheimer's type (DAT) is included.

Unit 7 looks at sensory disorders, covering disorders

of the eye and ear. Ocular changes related to aging, such as age-related macular degeneration, as well as those secondary to disease processes, such as diabetic retinopathy, are discussed.

Unit 8 presents respiratory disorders, providing information on common respiratory interventions, pharmacologic agents, oxygen administration, and ventilation. A section on respiratory care in the home is also included. Upper and lower airway disorders are discussed, including parenchymal disorders and disorders of the pleura, pleural space, diaphragm, and pulmonary vasculature. Tuberculosis is covered in depth, reflecting its resurgence as a common condition. Cystic fibrosis in the adult is also included because many children with cystic fibrosis now survive well into adulthood.

Unit 9 examines cardiovascular disorders, including disorders of the heart and peripheral vascular system. Cardiac arrest and resuscitation are also covered. The cardiac problems are covered as problems in cardiac function or cardiac structure. Cardiac surgery, including bypass surgery and cardiac transplantation, is discussed. Expanded content on new diagnostic tests and cardiomyopathy is presented. Peripheral vascular disorders, such as arteriosclerosis, hypertension, aneurysms, and venous occlusive conditions are discussed in depth. Care of clients having arterial bypass is discussed, along with amputations.

Unit 10 centers on hematologic disorders. Clients experiencing disorders of the red blood cells, white blood cells, and the lymphatic system are discussed. Sickle cell anemia and hemophilia, congenital conditions in which the client survives to adulthood, are also covered. Transfusions are discussed in detail, including client preparation, the transfusion itself, and nursing management of reactions.

Unit 11 presents urinary disorders. The care of clients with bladder disorders includes a discussion of cystitis and the newer treatments for cancer, such as the Indiana pouch. Care of clients with renal disorders is discussed, including renal failure, dialysis, and the current information on transplantation.

Unit 12 covers gastrointestinal disorders, including care of clients with ingestive, gastric, and lower intestinal disorders. Nutritional support covering both enteral and parenteral nutrition is discussed. Care of clients with eating disorders such as bulimia, anorexia, and obesity is presented. Care of clients with stomas, including the continent ileostomies, is discussed as is care of clients with common intestinal disorders such as diarrhea, constipation, and hemorrhoids.

Unit 13 looks at the care of clients with liver, biliary tract, and exocrine pancreatic disorders. Care of clients with hepatitis is presented, including current information on the types and vaccines. Care of the client with cirrhosis and its complications is covered, as well as commonly occurring problems, including cholecystitis, cholelithiasis, and cholecystectomy.

Unit 14 focuses on metabolic disorders, including endocrine disorders. Care of the client with diabetes is extensively covered, and care of clients with thyroid, parathyroid, adrenal, pituitary, and gonadal disorders is presented.

Unit 15 covers the care of clients with musculoskeletal conditions. Common musculoskeletal interventions such as rest, traction, casts, surgical procedures, exercise, and assistive devices are presented. Care of clients with metabolic bone disease, including osteoporosis, an important topic, is discussed; and care of clients with bone tumors and disorders of the hand and foot, and muscular disorders is presented. Trauma to the musculoskeletal system is covered separately.

Unit 16 covers care of clients with integumentary disorders. Nursing care of clients with dermatologic disorders is presented, and a separate chapter on care of clients with burns is included. Care of clients having plastic surgery is presented, including rejuvenating as well as reconstructive and replantation surgeries. Current information available on breast implants is also included in this section.

Unit 17 is devoted to the care of men and women with reproductive disorders and men with urinary disorders. Care of clients with benign prostatic hypertrophy and prostatic cancer is discussed along with newer treatment modalities, such as balloon dilation, new screening tests, and recently approved medications. Care of clients with female reproductive conditions, including menstrual disorders and menopause, along with common problems such as fibroids and cervical cancer, is presented in depth. Ovarian cancer is also presented. A separate chapter is devoted to the care of women with breast disorders. Sexually transmitted diseases are discussed in a separate chapter. The importance of prevention is stressed along with guidelines for appropriate treatment.

Unit 18 presents care of clients with substance abuse and during emergency situations. The effects of substance abuse on the major body systems is also discussed. Populations at risk for substance abuse are identified, and strategies for care are covered. Care of clients during a variety of medical-surgical emergencies are discussed. Chapter 80 clearly illuminates the nurse's role in all settings. Finally, it also includes a section on death and dying in emergency care situations.

SUPPLEMENTAL PACKAGE

This text comes with a complete learning package of ancillary learning materials to support the content.

Pocket Companion

A pocket companion is available for this text. This conveniently sized paperback, fully referenced to the text, is perfect for the student to use in the clinical setting. The alphabetically listed diseases and disorders outline essential content, including risk factors, clinical assessments, medical-surgical management, and specific nursing interventions, including discharge and client teaching.

Student Study Guide

This guide helps the student better understand each chapter. Learning objectives are provided to help the student focus on critical content. Learning activities, such as case studies, study questions, terminology quizzes, and nursing diagnosis/nursing intervention exercises are included.

Instructor's Manual

The *Instructor's Manual* is designed to help faculty develop lectures, assignments, and clinical assignments based on the content of this text. Included for each chapter are learning objectives that match the ones in the student study guide and suggestions for

- Classroom assignments
- Lecture/discussion (including suggested transparencies)
- Guest speakers
- Group activities

This manual also includes

- Skills laboratory, suggested activities
- Clinical site activities
- Clinical conference activities

Transparencies

Transparency masters and two-color transparencies are provided to support the presentation of the content. Faculty will find these very helpful. The *Instructor's Manual* suggests appropriate transparencies for each lecture.

Testbank

A computerized testbank is cross-referenced by both objectives and text page number.

The new *Luckmann and Sorensen's Medical-Surgical Nursing: A Psychophysiologic Approach, 4th edition,* offers the best of the traditional book with a new level of excellence.

Acknowledgments

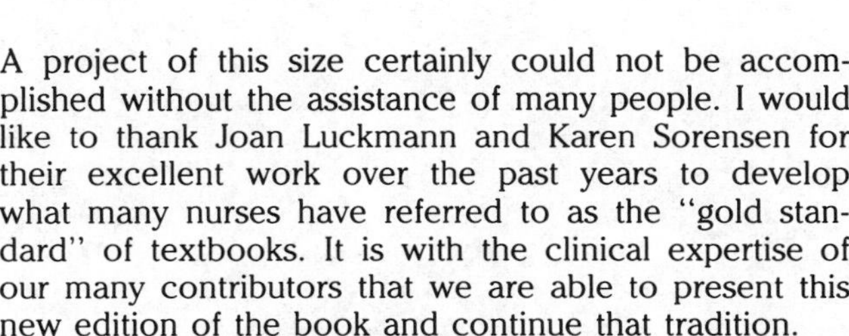

A project of this size certainly could not be accomplished without the assistance of many people. I would like to thank Joan Luckmann and Karen Sorensen for their excellent work over the past years to develop what many nurses have referred to as the "gold standard" of textbooks. It is with the clinical expertise of our many contributors that we are able to present this new edition of the book and continue that tradition.

There are several people at W.B. Saunders Company who have made this monumental task a "do-able" project and who deserve mention. Thank you, Michael Brown, former Editor in Chief of Nursing Books, for having faith in me to ask me to edit this new edition. Thank you, Thomas Eoyang, current Editor in Chief of Nursing Books, for the ongoing words of encouragement and help when I needed it. Robin Richman, Developmental Editor, without your help and day-to-day management, I would still be behind on the deadlines. Thank you for keeping me on track. Thank you, Alison Kieber, Illustration Coordinator, and Sharon Iwanczuk, Medical Illustrator, for providing stunning new artwork; I know the students will learn better from your efforts. Thanks to Karen O'Keefe, Designer, for giving us the means to present a lot of complex information clearly and attractively. Thank you, Carol DiBerardino, my Copy Editor, for finding just the right words when I couldn't. Peter Faber, Production Manager, made it possible to get the book out in record time. Thanks; I know it was a big job. To David Nazaruk, Marketing Manager, go my thanks for developing a classic marketing campaign for this edition.

There are also several people at the University of Nebraska who lifted me up and made my workload lighter while this project went on. Thank you, Dr. Lani Zimmerman, Bernadette White, and Annabelle Keene.

Finally, I must thank my family for their ongoing understanding of considerable strain on "Mom's" time and energy.

—Joyce M. Black, M.S.N., R.N.,C.

Acknowledgments

I would like to acknowledge all the help provided by W.B. Saunders Company in the preparation of this book, especially Robin Richman, Thomas Eoyang, and Ilze Rader (who helped by not calling). I would like to thank Michael Brown for putting the team together. I would like to acknowledge the support of Loyola University Chicago for granting me a supported leave of absence to work on this project. I would also like to acknowledge the assistance and support of Dr. Eileen Dvorak, Dean, Niehoff School of Nursing, Loyola University Chicago. I want to thank all my friends and coworkers who have accepted my status as a "hermit" while this *huge* project was being completed, especially Beverly Kopala, Ph.D., R.N. and Marybeth Young, Ph.D., R.N.C.

—Esther Matassarin-Jacobs, Ph.D., R.N., O.C.N.

Contents in Brief

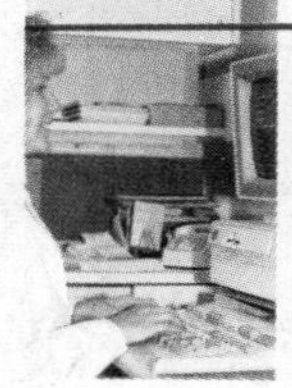

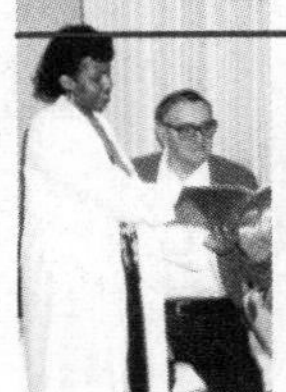

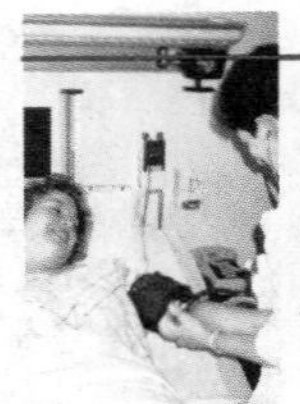

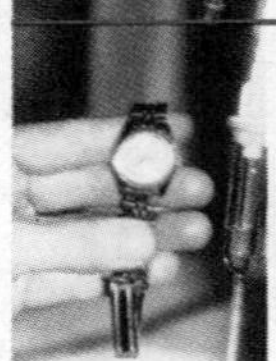

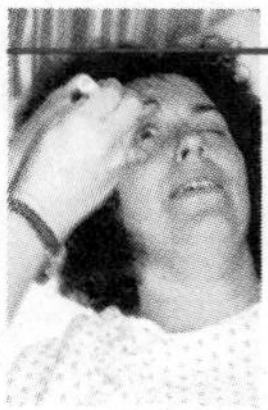

Contents in Detail

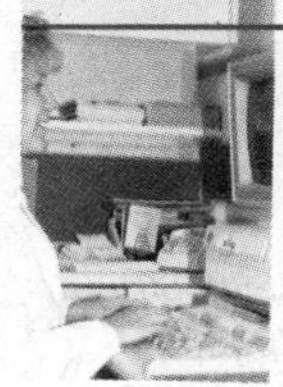

*Disorders that follow the nursing process in entirety are marked with an asterisk (*) and may have the following subheads: Definition; Incidence; Etiology; Risk Factors; Pathophysiology; Clinical Manifestations; Medical Management; Nursing Management (Assessment, Nursing Intervention, Nursing Diagnosis/Collaborative Problem, Planning: Expected Outcomes, Implementation, Evaluation); Modification of Plan of Care for the Elderly; Post-hospital Care (Discharge Teaching, Home Care Needs, Follow-up Care).

Chapter 7
Human Sexuality 103

Chapter 8
The Family 113

Chapter 9
Chronic Conditions 127

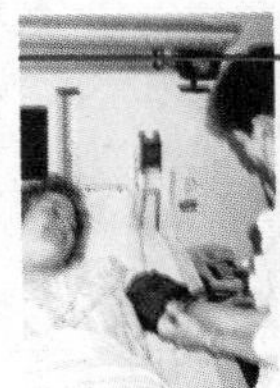

Unit 3
Health Promotion and Assessment 145

Chapter 10
Health Promotion 147

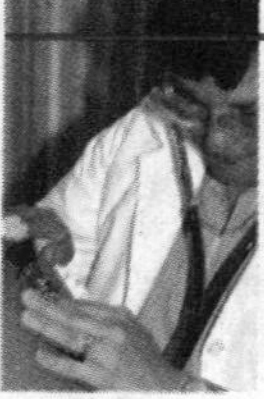

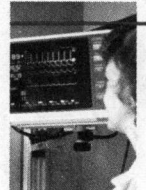

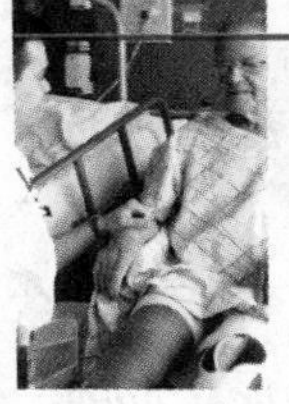

Unit 15 Musculoskeletal Disorders 1863

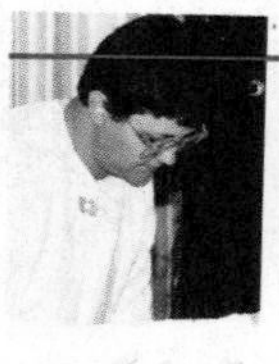

Special Features

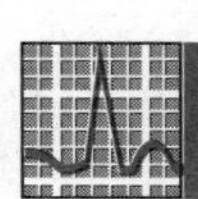

BRIDGES TO CRITICAL CARE

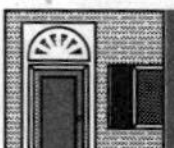

BRIDGES TO HOME HEALTH CARE

BRIDGES TO HOME HEALTH CARE

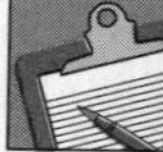

CARE PLANS

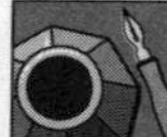

CLIENT EDUCATION GUIDES

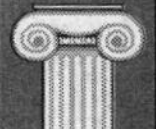

ETHICAL ISSUES IN NURSING

NURSING RESEARCH

Unit 1

Nursing and Health Care

Nursing is a unique profession. Theory and interpersonal skills are applied to people, who are often much less predictable than the focus of other professions. For example, engineering is a very exact science because the mathematical calculations used in constructing buildings and bridges must be precise, and the laws of physics make the construction fairly predictable. Nursing science is equally precise, for example, in the administration of medications. The difference is that there are no laws governing human behavior in the same way the world is governed by gravity and physics. Even though everyone's heart beats in the same way and their eyes focus in the same way, each person has a very unique health background and expectations of health care.

This human side of nursing has been called nursing "art." Early textbooks of nursing were concerned with the art of nursing. Usual content included material on hygiene, preparation of the environment, sterilizing equipment, and preparing meal trays. Disorders of the body were not discussed, except through principles of sciences, such as bacteriology. Obviously, nursing care has changed. Medical advancements have developed, clients have gotten sicker, and nurses are now considered front-line providers. Today, understanding the art of nursing is still important, but it is not enough. Nurses must know what to assess, when data indicate a problem, and the usual treatment for that problem.

Nursing process and nursing practice are the foci of the first unit of this textbook. Nursing process, the problem-solving technique used by nurses in education and practice, has become the common denominator to identify problems. Once the process is learned, it becomes an integral part of problem solving and is actualized in each nurse. Nursing process is used in every practice setting, of which there are many. Nurses practice in hospitals, clinics, homes, offices, and colleges. The opportunities for practice abound.

Chapter 1

Nursing Process

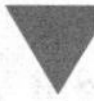
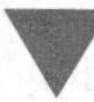

Nursing process is a method of problem solving in client care. Almost all people use some form of problem solving in order to do their work—the auto mechanic may test drive a car to determine what is wrong with it, and the hairdresser washes the hair and combs it to analyze its condition. In both of these examples, the person (the mechanic or the hairdresser) uses some type of process to determine what is wrong and then decides what to do to fix the problem. Nursing, as you can imagine, is no different. But owing to the complexity of situations on which nurses focus, the process is more involved. This chapter describes the use of nursing process, its future, and the use of nursing theorists within the process.

HISTORY OF NURSING PROCESS

Nursing process can be seen throughout the history of nursing. Since the beginning of the human species, each individual needed nurturing, which was provided primarily by the mother of the family. During the time of Hippocrates, when the profession of medicine evolved, the profession of nursing evolved simultaneously because every ill person needed someone to nurture him or her back to health. In time, the role of the nurse-mother evolved from the nurturing of ill family members to the care of other ill people outside of the home. Most of these "nurses" were women and men from various religious orders. These people volunteered to help other needy people. Up to the time of Florence Nightingale, the "training" of nurses was performed in a happenstance method of telling and showing another new nurse what to do for various clients. Thus, the trial and error method was the most common form of early problem solving in client care. During the time of Florence Nightingale, actual training of nurses began and nurses were required to "learn" about the needs of the client. Each of the nurses, whether the nurse-mother, volunteer nurse, or trained nurse used some form of process to provide care for clients. The problem was assessed, and a treatment was chosen based on previous experience or knowledge gained from other nurses or education. The nurses of the past served in many capacities. They were often social workers, dieticians, and physical therapists as well as nurses.

Today, the role of the nurse has evolved, and many of the previous tasks of dietician, social worker, and physical therapist are completed by professionals trained in those areas. With these new disciplines providing some care, the role of the nurse focuses on the coordination of these other services. But most important, the nurse focuses on the total needs of the client. The nurse is one of the few health care professionals educated to evaluate the client's response to health and illness, response of the family, social implications of the illness, psychological adjustment, and teaching needs and to monitor the physical response to the disorder and medications used in treatment. It does sound like a lot. The use of the nursing process is one method to be sure that all aspects of care are included.

Years ago, nursing students were taught a little bit of medicine and a true science of nursing did not exist. By the early 20th century, there was a need to distinguish nursing from medicine for licensing and educational purposes. But it was not until the 1950s that nursing curricula were designed to analyze patient problems and needs rather than medical diagnoses. This separation of nursing from medicine continues today with the development of various models to examine nursing and nursing care. These models and the theorists who developed them are presented later in this chapter.

Today's nursing process, as we know it, has evolved over many years. In 1955, Hall first described nursing as a process. Then over the next few years, the actual steps of the process were identified by other nurses. In 1967, Yura and Walsh identified four steps in the process—assessment, planning, implementation, and evaluation. During the mid-1970s, many other nurses added a fifth step, that of diagnosis. The steps of the process have not changed much from that time. For teaching purposes, the inclusion of rationale for interventions may be included. This step is not an actual step of the process, but it is used to validate that care given is based on scientific principles.

Since that time, the nursing process has been clearly recognized as the guiding framework for nursing practice. The American Nurses' Association and the various state nursing associations have used the process in development of Standards of Nursing Practice. Most nursing curricula have incorporated these standards as a method of teaching and describing the functions of nursing. Recently, the state boards of nursing examinations have begun to test the various steps of the nursing process.

DEFINITION

The nursing process is a problem-solving approach used by nurses to meet the needs of the client. It is a deliberative method that relies on the use of cognitive, interpersonal, and psychomotor skills.

Yura and Walsh[27] describe the nursing process as a set of actions to assist clients in maintaining optimal wellness. For the client who cannot attain wellness, nursing process is used to assist the client in attaining the highest quality of life for as long a time as possible.

Nursing process is just that, a process. Even though the steps of the process are followed in an systematic order, the process itself is not a static or fixed method of providing care. The process is flexible, and at times, the various steps of the process may take place concurrently. For example, the nurse may assess one problem while implementing a plan of care for a different problem. It is not a recipe for the care of clients. Clients may have exactly the same medical diagnoses and require similar nursing care, but their response to the care will not be identical. Since nursing process is focused on the client, the individual needs of the client can be addressed and individual goals set.

Consider these two clients:

John is a 19-year-old college freshman who injured his back while water skiing. He is hospitalized during August and may require surgery. His parents' insurance is paying for the medical care but he has lost his summer job and may not be able to afford his tuition and book payments this Fall.

Jack is a 42-year-old man who slipped a disc while lifting boxes at work. He also may need surgery on his back. He has had multiple back injuries and is aware that he may lose his job after this incident. But he says he is not worried because he and his family can live off of his worker's compensation payments.

Both John and Jack have the same medical diagnosis and may have the same operation to repair the damage. But consider the variations in their responses—John may not be able to afford to go back to school but Jack thinks he will be able to manage finances while he is not working. Treating John and Jack in the same manner after surgery may not encourage them to discuss the issues in their lives. The use of the nursing process would individualize their care and provide opportunities for exploration of feelings.

In order to use the nursing process to its fullest potential, the nurse must have a broad base of knowledge. Client assessment takes place on many levels, such as psychology, sociology, nutrition, and teaching.

The term "nursing process" is sometimes used interchangeably with "nursing care plans." However, nursing care plans are actually different: The process is the mental work that goes on to assess, plan, deliver, and evaluate care. Processes of any kind are fluid and dynamic. The care plan is the written document, which usually follows the nursing process format. It is a static item; once it is written, it is usually outdated, as the client's situation changes. Most nursing students write care plans using a nursing process system. Writing down the process helps to teach a nursing student how to think in a nursing process format. The written nursing care plan allows the instructor to analyze the students' thoughts and offer alternatives.

▼ STEPS OF NURSING PROCESS

ASSESSMENT

The first step of nursing process is assessment. Assessment is the collection of data about the client from a variety of sources.

Prerequisites to Assessment

BELIEFS

The nurse's beliefs encompass a caring philosophy about the client's rights, responsibilities, and health and illness, and the role of nursing in health care. These philosophies do not blossom overnight but are molded during the course of nursing education by nurses, other students, instructors, and clients.

Consider this client: Martha L. is a 96-year-old woman who was admitted from a nursing home with a broken hip and head injury after a fall. She is semiconscious on admission. The family is notified and asked to give permission for surgery to repair the hip. The daughter states that a few weeks before the fall her mother had asked that nothing be done "to keep her alive." The family gives permission for the surgery because the hip is painful and Mrs. L.'s mobility is limited but asks that nothing extraordinary be done for Mrs. L. During the assessment phase, the nurse records what positions are most comfortable for Mrs. L. as well as other routine assessments. The nurse communicates the family's desires to other health care professionals. It is the nurse's beliefs about caring for Mrs. L., the client's right to make decisions about her own care, and the nurse's role to support the decision that provided a foundation for practice.

KNOWLEDGE

The knowledge base for nurses is extensive, and nurses are required to use information from sciences such as nursing, anatomy, physiology, psychology, microbiology, pharmacology, chemistry, and nutrition. Using all of these sciences as guidelines, the nurse can analyze data collected about the client.

For example, the nurse is caring for a client with an infection. The client has a fever and is being treated with antibiotics. The nurse uses knowledge from all the sciences to assess the client's response to the infection, monitor the fever, administer the antibiotic at a time when it would be most effective, provide adequate nutrition and fluids, and prevent the spread of the infection to others.

SKILL

A variety of skills are required to perform a complete assessment of the client. They include psychomotor and interpersonal skills.

Psychomotor skills are the technical skills required in many phases of nursing process. During the assessment phase, the most common skills are those of physical assessment, such as inspection, palpation, and auscultation. These techniques are discussed in Chapter 12. For example, the use of a stethoscope allows the nurse to assess blood pressure, lung sounds, and bowel sounds. During the intervention phase, many other psychomotor skills are used to provide care.

Interpersonal skills are important in all phases of nursing process but are a critical component of the assessment phase. Use of interpersonal skills allows the nurse to assess the client's perception of the disorder or current complaint and to recognize the client's priorities. The term *therapeutic relationship* is often used to describe the communication techniques that allow the client and family to share views and feelings openly.

Obviously, the nurse needs excellent communication skills, which include listening skills, in order to accurately assess the client. Attentive listening creates a therapeutic relationship with the client and family. Listening skills convey to the client that the nurse feels she or he is important and shows respect. Attentive listening also allows the client to feel comfortable and express concerns. Attentive listening is a difficult skill to learn. Most people tend to concentrate on their next response to the client rather than listen to what the client is saying. Some elements of active listening are listed in Box 1–1.

For example, the nurse who sits at eye level with the client, provides privacy by pulling the curtain, and turns down the volume of the television conveys genuine concern to the client. In contrast, the nurse who stands at the bedside and looks out into the hall conveys a

Box 1–1. Elements of Attentive Listening

Focus your attention on the client and concentrate on what is being said

Stay quiet inside yourself; do not formulate your next response while the client is still talking

Remove physical barriers to talking, such as turning down the volume of the television set

Be attentive to barriers within the client that reduce communication ability, such as pain or anxiety

Maintain eye-to-eye contact with the client

Validate what the client said by restating it. This procedure will assure you and the client that you are listening

Reduce the influence of your own biases to attentive listening, such as if the client is telling you something you do not want to hear, you feel dislike toward the client, or the client has different views than you have

Avoid being interrupted

sense of hurriedness and not much concern. Research has shown that clients perceive much more time was spent with them when the nurse sits down alongside of them rather than when he or she stands at the bedside.

The nurse also needs to be aware of nonverbal cues from the client and follow up on these cues. For example, if the client is admitted following a fall and is noted to be rubbing the leg, the nurse would ask if the client has pain in the leg from the nonverbal cue.

Finally, communication needs to be flexible, creative, and based in common sense. The nurse would need to use different techniques in order to obtain the needed data concerning a client who is experiencing difficulty with hearing, or who is blind, young, or in pain.

The process of assessment begins with taking the client's history. On admission to an agency, this step of history taking can be lengthy because all areas are explored. After that time, the client is generally asked about a specific problem through a symptom analysis, rather than reviewing the entire history, before physical examination is performed.

The Initial History

When a client is initially assessed (for example on admission to an agency), a complete history is obtained. In some agencies, the client can begin the process by filling out a questionnaire; in other agencies, the client is asked for the information. Most agencies have specific forms to guide assessment in order to have a complete and systematic assessment. The data collected in this step usually include the historical data (past illnesses), current data (the current complaint), and demographic data (date of birth, address).

It is helpful to address the client's chief complaint early in the interview process. This method assures the client that the nurse is aware of the problem. It will also help guide the nurse in exploring the impact of the primary problem on the other body systems. A complete discussion of history taking is presented in Chapter 11.

Symptom Analysis

When a client expresses a problem, the nurse conducts a complete analysis of the symptom. This process begins with symptoms analysis, which is the collection of subjective data about the problem. Symptoms analysis requires the client to identify the location of the symptoms, describe the symptoms, severity of the pain, timing of the symptoms (including onset, duration, and frequency), aggravating and relieving symptoms, and any associated symptoms. It is crucial that the nurse be able to perform a complete symptoms analysis. The data obtained can guide the nurse in deciding what the problem is and what degree of priority it should be given.

For example, the nurse is caring for two clients with reports of chest pain. Through symptoms analysis, the nurse is able to identify the following data: one client's pain is a burning sensation in the midlower chest that begins about 2 hours after eating. It is relieved by taking milk, food, and antacids. The client has had this type of pain for 3 to 4 months since losing his job.

The other client reports crushing chest pain, which is described "like someone is squeezing my chest." It is located on the left side of the chest, jaw, and arm. He has had the pain constantly for about 30 minutes and nothing relieves it. His skin is pale, and he is diaphoretic (sweating).

Without symptoms analysis, the nurse only knows that the each client has chest pain. But is it apparent that the second client has a much more serious problem; he is having a heart attack and requires emergency care. The first client has had this pain for months and knows what relieves it. He can be cared for later without suffering harm.

More information on symptoms analysis in located in Chapter 11.

Approaches to History Taking

There are various approaches that can be used to provide a systematic guide to assessment. Gordon has devised functional health patterns (see Box 1-2), and the North American Nursing Diagnosis Association (NANDA) has devised human response patterns based on patterns of unitary persons (see Box 1-3). A body systems approach, such as heart, lung, and abdomen, may also be used to collect data, although this approach is being phased out in favor of nursing models. The nurse must be certain to add the psychosocial aspects of care when using a body systems approach in order to collect all data. For example, information on how the client is responding to hospitalization would not be collected in the typical body systems approach.

Physical Examination

Physical examination of the client is the second portion of assessment. Examination allows the nurse to gain objective data through the use of inspection, percussion, palpation, and auscultation. These data further define the client's response to the disorder, provide a baseline of data for further comparison, and elaborate on the subjective data provided in the client's history.

Once data are collected from the client, either by history or physical examination, the nurse can use secondary sources of information to expand the data base. Secondary sources of data include the previous medical record, family members, and other health care team members. The client should always be used as the primary data source, but there are instances when this is not possible. For example, when a client is admitted to the emergency department in a coma, the client can only be examined for objective data, and secondary sources would be needed to gain a full data base.

Box 1–2. Standardized Nursing Diagnoses According to Gordon's Functional Health Patterns

1. Health Perception–Management

-Altered growth and development in health
-Altered health maintenance
-Ineffective management of therapeutic regimen (individual)
-High risk for injury
-High risk for poisoning
-High risk for suffocation
-High risk for trauma
-High risk for self-mutilation
-High risk for infection
-Noncompliance
-High risk for disuse syndrome
-Health seeking behaviors (specify)
-Impaired home maintenance management

2. Nutritional–Metabolic

-High risk altered body temperature
-Breastfeeding, ineffective
-Interrupted breastfeeding
-Ineffective infant feeding pattern
-Fluid volume altered: excess
-Fluid volume altered: deficit (1)
-Fluid volume altered: deficit (2)
-Hyperthermia
-Hypothermia
-High risk for infection
-Altered nutrition: less than body requirements
-Altered nutrition: more than body requirements
-Altered nutrition: potential for more than body requirements
-Altered oral mucous membrane
-Impaired skin integrity
-High risk for impaired skin integrity
-Impaired swallowing
-Ineffective thermoregulation
-Impaired tissue integrity

3. Elimination Pattern

-Constipation
-Diarrhea
-Bowel incontinence
-Colonic constipation
-Perceived constipation
-Functional urinary incontinence
-Reflex incontinence
-Stress incontinence
-Total incontinence
-Urge incontinence
-Altered patterns of urinary elimination
-Urinary retention

4. Activity-Exercise

-Activity intolerance
-High risk for activity intolerance
-Ineffective airway clearance
-High risk for aspiration
-Ineffective breathing pattern
-Dysfunctional ventilatory weaning response
-Inability to sustain spontaneous ventilation
-Decreased cardiac output
-Diversional activity deficit
-Impaired gas exchange
-Fatigue
-Impaired physical mobility
-Altered (specify) tissue perfusion (cerebral, cardiopulmonary, renal, gastrointestinal, peripheral)
-High risk for peripheral neurovascular dysfunction
-Bathing/hygiene self-care deficit
-Dressing/grooming self-care deficit
-Feeding self-care deficit
-Toileting self-care deficit
-Disuse syndrome
-Dysreflexia
-Growth and development, altered

5. Cognitive-Perceptual

-Decisional conflict (specify)
-Pain (chronic pain)
-Knowledge deficit (specify)
-Neglect, unilateral
-Sensory-perceptual alterations (specify) (visual, auditory, kinesthetic, gustatory, tactile, olfactory)
-Thought process, altered
-Unilateral neglect

6. Sleep–Rest

-Sleep pattern disturbance

7. Self-Perception–Self-Concept

-Anxiety
-Fear
-Hopelessness
-Powerlessness
-Self-concept disturbance
  -Body image disturbance
  -Personal identity disturbance
  -Self-esteem disturbance

8. Role–Relationship

-Impaired verbal communication
-Impaired adjustment
-Altered family process
-Anticipatory grieving
-Dysfunctional grieving
-Altered parenting
-High risk for altered parenting
-Parental role conflict
-Impaired social interaction
-Social isolation
-Potential for violence: self-directed or directed at others
-Altered role performance
-Relocation stress syndrome
-High risk for care giver role strain
-Care giver role strain

9. Sexuality–Reproductive

-Rape-trauma syndrome
-Sexual dysfunction
-Altered sexuality patterns

10. Coping–Stress Tolerance

-Adjustment, impaired
-Family coping: potential for growth
-Ineffective family coping: compromised
-Ineffective family coping: disabling
-Ineffective individual coping
-Defensive coping
-Post-trauma response

11. Value–Belief

-Spiritual distress

Box 1–3. North American Nursing Diagnosis Association (NANDA) Taxonomy I: Approved Nursing Diagnoses

Pattern 1: Exchanging

1.1.2.1. Altered nutrition: More than body requirements
1.1.2.2. Altered nutrition: Less than body requirements
1.1.2.3. Altered nutrition: High risk for more than body requirements
1.2.1.1. High risk for infection
1.2.2.1. High risk for altered body temperature
1.2.2.2. Hypothermia
1.2.2.3. Hyperthermia
1.2.2.4. Ineffective thermoregulation
1.2.3.1. Dysreflexia
1.3.1.1. Constipation
1.3.1.1.1. Perceived constipation
1.3.1.1.2. Colonic constipation
1.3.1.2. Diarrhea
1.3.1.3. Bowel incontinence
1.3.2. Altered patterns of urinary elimination
1.3.2.1.1. Stress incontinence
1.3.2.1.2. Reflex incontinence
1.3.2.1.3. Urge incontinence
1.3.2.1.4. Functional incontinence
1.3.2.1.5. Total incontinence
1.3.2.2. Urinary retention
1.4.1.1. Altered (specify) tissue perfusion (renal, cerebral, cardiopulmonary, gastrointestinal, peripheral)
1.4.1.2.1. Fluid volume excess
1.4.1.2.2.1. Fluid volume deficit (1)
1.4.1.2.2.1. Fluid volume deficit (2)
1.4.1.2.2.2. Potential fluid volume deficit
1.4.2.1. Decreased cardiac output
1.5.1.1. Impaired gas exchange
1.5.1.2. Ineffective airway clearance
1.5.1.3. Ineffective breathing pattern
1.6.1. High risk for injury
1.6.1.1. High risk for suffocation
1.6.1.2. High risk for poisoning
1.6.1.3. High risk for trauma
1.6.1.4. High risk for aspiration
1.6.1.5. High risk for disuse syndrome
1.6.2.1. Impaired tissue integrity
1.6.2.1.1. Altered oral mucous membrane
1.6.2.1.2.1. Impaired skin integrity
1.6.2.1.2.2. High risk for impaired skin integrity
*Dysfunctional ventilatory weaning response
*Inability to sustain spontaneous ventilation
*High risk for self-multilation
*High risk for peripheral neurovascular dysfunction

Pattern 2: Communicating

2.1.1.1. Impaired verbal communication

Pattern 3: Relating

3.1.1. Impaired social interaction
3.1.2. Social isolation
3.2.1. Altered role performance
3.2.1.1.1. Altered parenting
3.2.1.1.2. High risk for altered parenting
3.2.1.2.1. Sexual dysfunction
3.2.2. Altered family processes
3.2.3.1. Parental role conflict
3.3. Altered sexuality patterns
*Relocation stress syndrome

Pattern 4: Valuing

4.1.1. Spiritual distress (distress of the human spirit)

Pattern 5: Choosing

5.1.1.1. Ineffective individual coping
5.1.1.1.1. Impaired adjustment
5.1.1.1.2. Defensive coping
5.1.1.1.3. Ineffective denial
5.1.2.1.1. Ineffective family coping: Disabling
5.1.2.1.2. Ineffective family coping: Compromised
5.1.2.2. Family coping: Potential for growth
5.2.1.1. Noncompliance (specify)
5.3.1.1. Decisional conflict (specify)
5.4. Health-seeking behaviors (specify)
*Care giver role strain
*High risk for care giver role strain
*Ineffective management of therapeutic regimen (individual)

Pattern 6: Moving

6.1.1.1. Impaired physical mobility
6.1.1.2. Activity intolerance
6.1.1.2.1. Fatigue
6.1.1.3. High risk for activity intolerance
6.2.1. Sleep pattern disturbance
6.3.1.1. Diversional activity deficit
6.4.1.1. Impaired home maintenance management
6.4.2. Altered health maintenance
6.5.1. Feeding self-care deficit
6.5.1.1. Impaired swallowing
6.5.1.2. Ineffective breastfeeding
6.5.1.3. Effective breastfeeding
6.5.2. Bathing/hygiene self-care deficit
6.5.3. Dressing/grooming self-care deficit
6.5.4. Toileting self-care deficit
6.6. Altered growth and development
*Ineffective infant feeding pattern
*Interrupted breastfeeding

Pattern 7: Perceiving

7.1.1. Body image disturbance
7.1.2. Self-esteem disturbance
7.1.2.1. Chronic low self-esteem
7.1.2.2. Situational low self-esteem
7.1.3. Personal identity disturbance
7.2. Sensory/perceptual alterations (specify: visual, auditory, kinesthetic, gustatory, tactile, olfactory)
7.2.1.1. Unilateral neglect
7.3.1. Hopelessness
7.3.2. Powerlessness

Pattern 8: Knowing

8.1.1. Knowledge deficit (specify)
8.3. Altered thought processes

Pattern 9: Feeling

9.1.1. Pain
9.1.1.1. Chronic pain
9.2.1.1. Dysfunctional grieving
9.2.1.2. Anticipatory grieving
9.2.2. High risk for violence: Self-directed or directed at others
9.2.3. Post-trauma response
9.2.3.1. Rape-trauma syndrome
9.2.3.1.1. Rape-trauma syndrome: Compound reaction
9.2.3.1.2. Rape-trauma syndrome: Silent reaction
9.3.1. Anxiety
9.3.2. Fear

▼▼▼

Used by permission of North American Nursing Diagnosis Association, 1992.

*Accepted in 1992 but unnumbered at press time.

Diagnostic Studies

Other components to the data collection phase include the review of diagnostic studies. The results of laboratory studies and other diagnostic tests should be reviewed in light of the client's disorders. For example, it would be common for a client with renal failure to have a low hemoglobin level.

NURSING DIAGNOSIS

Diagnostic Reasoning

CLASSIFICATION

The initial step of data analysis is classification of the data. Data need to be organized in order to be clearly analyzed, and the most logical means to organize data is to classify them. The body systems approach and functional health pattern approach are two convenient methods of classification. When these methods are used for taking a history and performing a physical examination, the data are already classified. Once classified, data can be searched for missing pieces. Some data may be obviously missing, such as the client's age. Other missing data may not be as easily recognized.

For example, a 45-year-old female client tells the nurse that her mother died of breast cancer and that she had a breast biopsy last year. When the data are classified, it becomes apparent that the current status of the client's breast disease is not clear. Therefore, the nurse would ask about the outcome of the biopsy and the frequency of the client's breast self-examination. The nurse pays particular attention to breast palpation during the physical examination and assesses the client's potential reaction to her risk of breast cancer (Iyer et al.).[12]

VALIDATION

The next step of data analysis is validation. In this step, the nurse verifies the diagnosis by speaking to the client. The nurse can easily say to the client "You have a fever this morning, do you feel feverish?" This allows the client to verify the findings, be aware of the problem, and comply with the treatment. If the nurse entered the client's room with medications and treatment for fever reduction without telling the client a fever was present, the client could become startled and less likely to trust the nurse because the client was given no input into his or her own care.

At times, the nurse gathers conflicting data from the client and is unable to draw a firm conclusion. For example, the client is noted to be sitting in a dark room. He is difficult to converse with and is holding his head. From these data the nurse can imply that the client has pain, perhaps a headache. But if the client says he has no pain when asked, the nurse cannot conclude that pain is present. At this point, the nurse should confront the client with the data present. "I see that you are holding your head and sitting in the dark. It would appear that you are in pain. Is something else the matter?" By confronting the client, the nurse may find out that the client's wife called with bad news. The client may need help finding the appropriate resources, not pain medication.

The nurse can validate findings with the family, especially if the client is unable to communicate. For example, the nurse could ask about scars or wounds and, therefore, expand the data base on the client. The nurse can also validate the diagnosis by comparing it to textbook material or by talking to other nurses.

INTERPRETATION

The final step of data analysis is interpretation of the data. This involves identification of abnormal data, comparing it with standards from a textbook, and recognizing patterns of data that indicate potential problems. Each piece of data should be examined, and the nurse asks "Is this normal?" If the answer is "yes," then the data can be stored for future reference. If the answer is "no," the nurse needs to determine if it is expected (such as fever with infection) or unexpected (such as calf pain and the presence of Homans' sign). If the response is unexpected, the nurse needs to further analyze it to determine the significance. A client with calf pain and a Homans' sign may have thrombophlebitis, a serious complication that may lead to fatal pulmonary emboli.

Sometimes, a single piece of data cannot be interpreted. This single piece of data is called a *cue*. Further cues must be collected and then combined for analysis. Consider the two situations presented in Table 1–1 and examine how the single cue of "loose stools" was examined to find two different diagnoses.

INDUCTIVE VERSUS DEDUCTIVE REASONING

The nurse may use inductive or deductive reasoning to interpret data. Inductive reasoning begins with a set of facts from which a conclusion is drawn. Inductive reasoning is the use of cues, as listed in Table 1–1, to draw a conclusion of constipation.

Again, considering the above-mentioned cues, the process of deductive reasoning begins with the facts that the client is on bed rest and taking narcotics and concludes (deduces) that the client is at an increased risk of constipation.

ERRORS IN DIAGNOSIS

There are two basic areas of potential errors in making a diagnosis: (1) having incomplete data and (2) drawing an inaccurate interpretation.

Incomplete Data. Common causes of incomplete data occur during the interview phase of assessment. Communication barriers and biased questions may discourage the client from giving the nurse complete answers. Some clients withhold information intentionally because they feel embarrassed or are unsure how the nurse would react to the information. HIV-positive clients

TABLE 1–1. Data Collection: Cues and Nursing Diagnoses

Cue	Nursing Diagnosis
History of exposure to the flu 8 small liquid BMs this morning Abdominal cramps Nausea Slight fever Flat abdomen Loose stools	Diarrhea R/T a viral infection
History of surgery one week ago No formed BM for the past 6 days Distended abdomen Mass in left lower quadrant On strict bed rest Taking narcotics	Constipation with impaction

may feel this way. Finally, if the nurse allows distractions during the interview, the client or the nurse may lose the train of thought and fail to complete the data base.

Inaccurate Interpretation. Data from the client can be misinterpreted in several ways. The problem can be diagnosed before the data are completely collected. For example, a confused and combative 85-year-old client was restrained based on the diagnosis of senility. This diagnosis was based on one visit to the client when the nurse noticed the behavior. The nurse failed to examine the client's history to realize that the client was diabetic and had not been eating properly for the past 3 days because of the flu. When all of the data were examined, the client's diabetic status was reassessed and it was found that the client's blood sugar was very low, and he was not senile after all.

Sometimes, the nurse can have a personal prejudice about the client. This situation can resemble the story about the boy who cried wolf. Consider this problem: Mrs. R. is a 60-year-old widow who is admitted with a respiratory infection. She frequently develops shortness of breath and calls the staff into her room often. The nurses have become exasperated with her frequent requests for help when they believe she is not really in dire distress. After a while, they spend less time assessing her and assume she is not having trouble at all but "just wants attention." It is obvious that if this client develops a serious problem, it will be difficult to draw anyone's attention.

Lack of Knowledge or Experience. The lack of clinical experience and knowledge may result in inaccurate data processing. Failure to recognize a problem is a common experience for most nurses. The inexperienced nurse may overlook important data or fail to realize the significance of the data. Sometimes the client requires so much care in one area that other areas are overlooked. Because it is not possible to be given clinical experience, the nurse's best approach to these situations is to have another more experienced nurse assist in problem solving. This situation does not occur only with the student nurse or the new graduate. Whenever a nurse is moved to a new area and exposed to the problems of a new client, the lack of clinical experience in that area would increase the risk of inaccurate interpretation of data.

Using a Nursing Diagnosis

After data have been interpreted, a diagnosis can be made about the client's condition. The diagnosis is anything abnormal or that concerns the client, or strengths of the client. Diagnoses within the realm of nursing are the responses of the client to a state of health or illness and include physical, psychosocial, spiritual, and educational areas. These diagnoses and their treatment are within the legal scope of nursing practice. The actual conditions that nurses are educated to handle and licensed to treat are called *nursing diagnoses.*

There are other conditions, resulting from the medical condition, in which the nurse cannot resolve the problem but is instrumental in the monitoring of the disorder. These situations are called *collaborative problems* and are discussed later in this chapter.

Because the role of nurses can vary greatly between settings, there has always been difficulty in describing the work of nursing. Over the past decade, NANDA has addressed this need to describe, organize, and communicate the work of nursing. NANDA has provided national leadership in the development of standardized statements, or nursing diagnoses, to describe human responses to actual or potential health problems nurses treat. To date, NANDA has approved over 100 nursing diagnoses. The approval process requires review by other nurses, and each diagnosis must be treated by nursing action. The current list of NANDA approved diagnoses are listed in Boxes 1–2 and 1–3. In this book, NANDA's list of nursing diagnoses have been used to describe the problems seen in clients.

Writing a Nursing Diagnosis

A nursing diagnosis should be written in three parts, indicating the human response, related factors, and defining characteristics. The human response is the client's problem stated as a nursing diagnosis. The related factors are the possible causes or etiology of the problem, and the defining characteristics are the data indicating the problem is present. The phrase "related to" should be used to link the human response and related factors and the phrase "as manifested by" or "as evidenced by" should be used to link the related factors to the defining characteristics. In some agencies, the defining characteristics are not recorded on the problem sheet or care plan, because these data are located in the chart.

Examples of nursing diagnoses statements written in the three parts are

Ineffective airway clearance related to retained secretions as manifested by rales, rhonchi, productive cough, and decreased activity tolerance

Anxiety related to upcoming surgery as manifested by client statement "I have never been to surgery before, what is going to happen to me?"

Clients at high risk for specific human responses do not have defining characteristics until the problem actually occurs. In these cases, the nurse can record a two-part nursing diagnosis statement, such as

High risk for infection related to decreased immune response

or the nurse can record the risk factors in place of defining characteristics, such as

High risk for impairment of skin integrity related to immobility, as evidenced by reddened sacrum.

One-part statements are used to label wellness diagnoses, such as

Family coping: potential for growth

Health-seeking behaviors

THE HUMAN RESPONSE

Most nurses use NANDA nursing diagnosis as the human response statement, but other forms of problem statements are possible. In fact, if there does not appear to be a nursing diagnosis that describes the client's problem accurately, the nurse is encouraged to use another statement that does describe it more accurately. The nurse must be certain to describe the client's response to health or illness in this problem statement rather than redescribe pathophysiology or a medical diagnosis.

There are times when the medical diagnosis is clear to the nurse, and the nurse could easily diagnose the client. The nurse must remember that although a medical diagnosis can be made, the nurse is not legally licensed to make the diagnosis and to prescribe treatment. In fact, the physician's diagnosis focuses on the cure and treatment of the problem. Nurses' diagnoses focus on the response by the client to the problem of the treatment. Consider the examples given in Table 1-2.

The human response should always be stated as a response to care rather than as a need for care. Needs for care, such as needs to be fed or needs to be turned every 2 hours, describe a nursing intervention rather than a client problem. Other rules for writing a correct nursing diagnosis are presented in Box 1-4.

Modifiers. The words "high risk for" or "possible" are modifiers that can be used with the problem statement. When the client has known risk factors that may lead to a problem, the phrase "high risk for" is used as a modifier. The word "possible" precedes problems when not enough data are accumulated to make the diagnosis. These modifiers are used because they alert other nurses to the problem and speed future diagnosis.

TABLE 1-2. Comparison of Medical Diagnoses and Nursing Diagnoses

Medical Diagnosis	Nursing Diagnosis
AIDS	Social isolation R/T decreased support systems as evidenced by avoidance of family and friends
Adenocarcinoma of the breast	Decisional conflict R/T fear of disfiguring surgery as evidenced by asking many questions
Pneumococcal pneumonia	Ineffective breathing pattern R/T pain with respiration as evidenced by shallow breathing and rales

THE RELATED FACTORS

The related factors is the second component of the nursing diagnosis. This section of the statement describes the factors associated with the problem. These factors may be environmental, psychological, physiologic, sociocultural, or spiritual.[12] Because these factors direct nursing actions aimed at resolving, preventing, or reducing the problem, the related factor should be directed at an aspect of the client response on which the nurse can have an impact. Therefore, the related factor should not be written as a medical diagnosis, because the nurse legally cannot resolve the problem.

For example, "Constipation related to colon surgery" does not list a related factor on which a nurse can have an impact. In contrast, if the diagnosis were written as "constipation related to incisional pain with defecation," there is a clearly related factor. The nurse cannot take any action to reduce, eliminate, or prevent "colon surgery," but nursing action could be taken to reduce, eliminate, or prevent "pain with defecation."

The nurse should clarify the human response by indicating the related factors. Therefore, the related factors statement should not repeat the problem. For example, "Self-care deficit: feeding related to feeding problems" is not a clear statement. No further description of the client's problem is given. It would be clearer if written as "Self-care deficit: feeding related to casted right arm as evidenced by uneaten food," because the nurse now knows what interventions may assist this client.

Caution should be used to avoid value-laden statements about the client. The use of the words "inadequate," "poor," and "unhealthy" may imply a personal judgement. For example, the diagnosis "impaired skin integrity related to poor hygiene and laziness" implies a personal value judgement by the nurse, when in fact the client may have been unable to perform personal care for another reason.

Box 1–4. Ten Rules for Writing a Nursing Diagnosis

1. *Write the diagnosis in terms of the client's response rather than nursing need*
   Avoid beginning the diagnosis with the word "needs," such as "needs turning" or "needs feeding." Instead begin with a nursing diagnosis, because it focuses on the client's response.
2. *Use "related to" rather than "due to" or "caused by" to connect the first two parts of the statement*
   The use of the phase "related to" shows the connection between the client's response and the related factors. It also implies that if one factor changes, another one may also.
3. *Write the diagnosis in legally advisable terms*
   Statements that imply guilt or blame others or the client are not legally advisable and may not be accurate. The interventions planned are based upon the client's response, and only these responses should be listed.
4. *Write the diagnosis without value judgements*
   Words such as inadequate, poor, lazy, inept, and unhealthy imply that the client was judged according to the nurse's personal standards.
5. *Avoid reversing the parts of the statement*
   Begin each nursing diagnosis by using a human response. If the parts are reversed, the outcomes will be difficult to set and communication about the problem will be hampered.
6. *Avoid using single cues as the first part of the statement*
   The first part of the statement, the nursing diagnosis, is derived from conclusions made from many cues. Seldom does one cue allow an accurate diagnosis to be made. For example, diagnosing a client with anxiety from the single cue of restlessness may not be accurate. The restlessness may be a result of decreased oxygen levels.
7. *The two parts of the statement should not mean the same thing*
   For example, the diagnosis "Impaired swallowing related to swallowing difficulties" is not clear. The diagnosis is more clearly written as "Potential for aspiration related to swallowing difficulties."
8. *Express the related factor in terms that can be changed*
   The related factor should be an aspect of human response that the nurse can reduce or eliminate. At times, this is a difficult component to identify. Nurses should avoid restating the disease state in its pathophysiologic process in the related factors. Instead the nurse should focus on nursing's role in the client's response. If no nursing oriented related factor can be identified, the nurse should reconsider if the problem is within the domain of nursing, or if it could be more clearly stated as a collaborative problem.
9. *Do not include the medical diagnosis in the nursing diagnosis*
   The use of medical diagnoses within the nursing diagnostic statement reduces the essence of nursing. Some practitioners will insert the medical diagnosis into the nursing diagnostic statement with the connector of "secondary to" or "2°." For example "Impaired gas exchange related to retained secretions 2° to pneumonia."
10. *State the diagnosis clearly and concisely*
   The nurse needs to condense and summarize the related factors and defining characteristics into a clear statement. Wordy statements can be confusing and time consuming to read.

▼▼▼

From Iyer, P., Taptich, B., & Bernocchi-Losey, D. (1991). *Nursing process and nursing diagnosis* (2nd ed.) Philadelphia, W. B. Saunders.

DEFINING CHARACTERISTICS

This last step of the three-part diagnosis is the listing of data indicating that the problem existed. Defining characteristics are the most common data seen with a nursing diagnosis. Many textbooks of nursing diagnosis list these data to facilitate diagnosing. Major and minor defining characteristics approved by NANDA are listed as well as related factors. When the client is at risk of developing a problem, the risk factors are identified, rather than defining characteristics.

Collaborative Problems

As nurses have continued to work with nursing diagnosis, shortcomings of the system have been identified. A major weakness is the inability to express client conditions clearly when using the new language. This is especially true when previous labels worked well. For example, the word "hemorrhage" is clearer than "altered tissue perfusion." Another aspect of this problem is also seen in the relationship of nursing care to medical care. Nurses do not exist in a vacuum. They provide more than the nursing care that is within their realm to prescribe. In fact, most nursing care entails monitoring the client's response to or complications from the treatment or disorder. This monitoring function is performed in collaboration with the physician. The problems being assessed are called *collaborative problems.* Carpenito[4] defines collaborative problems as the physiologic complications that have resulted or may result from the pathophysiologic and treatment-related conditions, and from other situations. Nurses monitor to detect the onset and status of complications, and collaborate with physicians in treatment.

Examples of collaborative problems are

Thrombophlebitis with bed rest
Hemorrhage following surgery
Maintainance of breathing by mechanical ventilation

It is clear that the nurse cannot treat the above-mentioned problems independently but is instrumental in the continued monitoring of the condition as well as proper notification of the physician. This text lists collaborative problems along with the nursing diagnosis under each medical or surgical condition. The relationship of nursing diagnosis and collaborative problems for the client with pneumonia is shown in Box 1-5.

PLANNING

The next step in the nursing process is planning activities to promote healthy client responses or prevent, correct, or reduce unhealthy client responses. Planning and setting expected outcomes begins by determining the priority of the human responses. This step is followed by setting expected outcomes and nursing interventions that will move the client toward the outcome.

Setting Priorities

The process of setting priorities is becoming an everyday issue for nurses. Clients are staying in the hospital for shorter periods of time and, therefore, nurses must make the most use of the time given. The use of a hierarchy can assist in prioritizing.

Box 1-5. Nursing Diagnoses and Collaborative Problems for the Client with Pneumonia

Nursing Diagnoses

Ineffective airway clearance R/T chest pain with coughing and difficulty clearing secretions

Altered nutrition: less than body requirements R/T anorexia and dyspnea as evidenced by consuming less than 1000 calories in 24 hours

Pain R/T pleuritic inflammation as evidenced by verbal reports

Activity intolerance R/T impaired oxygen/carbon dioxide exchange as evidenced by shortness of breath

Altered health maintenance R/T insufficient knowledge of pneumococcal vaccine as evidenced by not having vaccination

High risk for hyperthermia R/T infectious process

High risk for altered oral mucous membranes R/T mouth breathing and frequent expectoration

High risk for fluid volume deficit R/T increased insensible fluid loss secondary to fever, hyperventilation, and mouth breathing

Collaborative Problems

Bacteremia

Septic shock

Respiratory insufficiency

Paralytic ileus

Meningitis

Pericarditis

Pleural effusion

▼▼▼

Data from Carpenito, L. (1991). *Nursing diagnosis: Application to clinical practice.* Philadelphia; J. B. Lippincott.

Consider these examples: The nurse has two clients with low hemoglobin levels. One client had surgery yesterday, and the hemoglobin is expected to be lower as a result of blood loss in surgery. No immediate interventions are required for this client except ongoing monitoring of the hemoglobin level. The nurse's other client was admitted with abdominal pain and had blood in the stool this morning. The nurse assessed the client and found increased abdominal tenderness and a decrease in blood pressure. The nurse notified the physician quickly about the second client's condition. The client was taken for emergency surgery to repair a bleeding ulcer.

In these two situations, the nurse analyzed data (hemoglobin levels) against the normal levels and then considered what the expected response might be for each client. The nurse also validated the data through physical examination regarding the client's response to the low hemoglobin level. Both clients had low hemoglobin levels, but only the second client required prompt treatment. In this case, the nurse's accurate assessment and analysis of the data allowed the client to get the needed emergency treatment.

KALISH'S HIERARCHY

Kalish[13] developed a hierarchy from earlier work by Maslow. In 1943, Maslow described a five-layer hierarchy that had physical needs on the bottom, and therefore, these needs had to met first. The top of Maslow's hierarchy contained physiologic needs. Maslow's theory was that lower level needs (physical) must be met before higher level needs will surface.

Survival. Kalish adapted Maslow's hierarchy into one that is more relevant to nurses (Fig. 1-1). The first level centers on survival needs and includes the need for food, air, water, temperature control, elimination, rest, and the avoidance of pain. When the client has needs on this level, these needs are a priority. For example, the client who has difficulty breathing is not concerned about his or her appearance. Likewise, the client who is experiencing severe pain is not going to be concerned about other people's feelings (a need within the level focusing on love, belonging, and closeness).

Stimulation. The second level focuses on stimulation needs. These needs are related to activity, exploration, manipulation, novelty, and sex. When the client's survival needs are met, the client attempts to meet these stimulation needs. In the hospital setting, the nurse can recognize this level of need by noting when the client becomes interested in the surroundings and getting out of bed. Likewise, if a client cannot ambulate to meet stimulation needs, diversional activities may be used.

Safety. Within the safety level are the needs for safety, security, and protection. The safety portion of this level is met, in a general way, by providing a safe environment for the client within the hospital setting. The proper use of oxygen, handwashing, and restraints, and correct administration of medications prevent thermal,

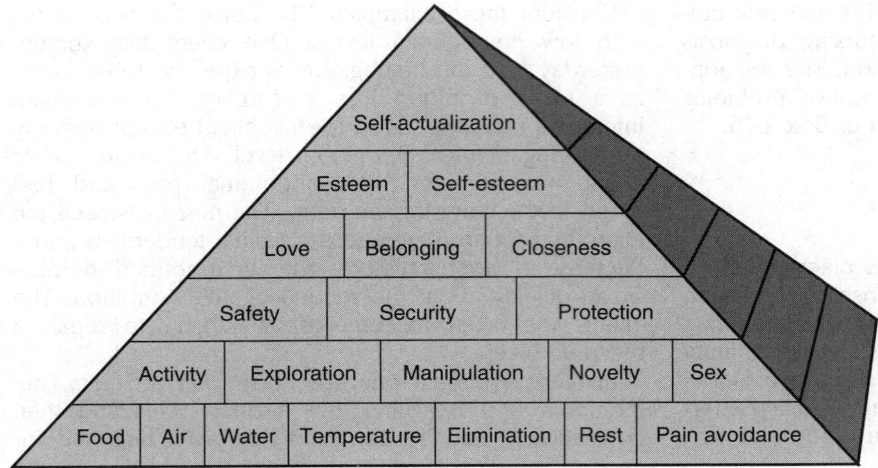

▲ *Figure 1–1*

Kalish's refinement of Maslow's model. (From Kalish, R. [1983]. *The psychology of human behavior* [5th ed.]. Monterey, CA: Brooks/Cole [division of Wadsworth Publishing Co.].)

bacteriologic, mechanical, and chemical injury. This component of safety is provided by the nurse. There is another aspect of safety—it is the client's need to feel safe and secure. The client may request familiar items from home. For example, an elderly client may use a homemade afghan on the bed, or a child may sleep with a teddy bear. The client may also have a need to be taught a safe method to use a cane or crutches to ambulate. Likewise, the elderly client may need the home assessed for safety to reduce the risk of falls.

Love and Belonging. Love and belonging needs center around a need to be a part of a group and close to others. The nurse may identify these needs when visiting is restricted, as is the case in critical care settings, if hospitalization is prolonged, or when the client is hospitalized away from home and family.

Esteem. The fifth level of Kalish's model features the need for recognition, usefulness, independence, dignity, and freedom. Clients may be made to feel helpless in the hospital, when in fact, they can perform a part of their bathing and grooming. Other clients may have a sense of loss after an operation that has altered their appearance.

Self-actualization. The top of the model is the need "to make the most of your physical, mental, emotional, and social competencies in order to feel that you are the sort of person you wish to be."[13] It is unlikely that clients within the hospital setting focus on self-actualization needs. But clients in long-term care settings, especially rehabilitation units, may grapple with these concerns frequently. Issues such as alcohol and drug abuse and violent behavior toward self and others may be symptoms of an underlying inability to reach this level. These types of problems are best acted on by a group of health care professionals, such as psychiatrists, social workers, and drug abuse counselors.

When the nurse has developed a list of nursing diagnoses, the list can be compared with the model and priority given to the problems. Table 1–3 lists various nursing diagnoses within each of the levels of Kalish's model.

TABLE 1–3. Nursing Diagnoses Organized by Kalish's Model*

Category of Need: SURVIVAL
Nursing Diagnoses:

Air:
- Airway clearance, ineffective
- Aspiration, high risk for
- Breathing pattern, ineffective
- Cardiac output, decreased
- Gas exchange, impaired
- Suffocation, high risk for
- Tissue perfusion, altered

Water:
- Fluid volume deficit
- Fluid volume deficit, high risk for
- Fluid volume excess

Temperature:
- Body temperature, altered: high risk for
- Dysreflexia
- Hyperthermia
- Hypothermia
- Skin integrity, impaired
- Skin integrity, high risk for
- Thermoregulation, ineffective
- Tissue integrity, impaired

Food:
- Nutrition, altered: less than body requirements
- Nutrition, altered: more than body requirements
- Nutrition, altered: high risk for
- Oral mucous membrane, altered
- Swallowing, impaired

Elimination:
- Constipation
- Constipation, colonic
- Constipation, perceived
- Diarrhea

TABLE 1–3. Nursing Diagnoses Organized by Kalish's Model* Continued

Incontinence, bowel
Incontinence, functional
Incontinence, reflex
Incontinence, stress
Incontinence, total
Incontinence, urge
Urinary elimination, altered patterns of
Urinary retention

Rest:
Sleep pattern disturbance

Pain Avoidance:
Pain
Chronic pain

Category of Need: STIMULATION
Nursing Diagnoses

Activity:
Activity intolerance
Activity intolerance, high risk for
Diversional activity deficit

Exploration:
Mobility, impaired physical
Fatigue

Manipulation:
Breastfeeding, effective
Breastfeeding, ineffective
Disuse syndrome
Self-care deficit

Novelty:
Sensory/perceptual alterations

Sex:
Sexual dysfunction
Sexuality patterns, altered

Category of Need: SAFETY
Nursing Diagnoses

Security:
Anxiety
Fear
Growth and development, altered
Home maintenance management, impaired

Safety:
Infection, high risk for
Injury, high risk for
Poisoning, high risk for
Trauma, high risk for
Thought process, altered
Unilateral neglect
Violence, high risk for

Protection:
Protection, altered

Category of Need: LOVE AND BELONGING
Nursing Diagnoses

Love:
Parenting, altered
Parenting, altered, high risk for

Belonging:
Coping, family, ineffective, compromised
Coping, family, ineffective, disabled
Coping, defensive
Coping, individual, ineffective
Denial, ineffective
Family processes, altered
Grieving, anticipatory
Grieving, dysfunctional
Post-trauma response
Role performance, altered
Spiritual distress

Closeness:
Adjustment, impaired
Conflict, decisional
Conflict, parental role
Social interaction, impaired
Social isolation

Catetory of Need: ESTEEM
Nursing Diagnoses

Body image disturbance
Denial, ineffective
Dysfunctional grieving
Hopelessness
Personal identity disturbance
Powerlessness
Rape-trauma response
Rape-trauma syndrome: compound reaction
Rape-trauma syndrome: silent reaction
Self-esteem: chronic low
Self-esteem disturbance
Self-esteem: situational, low

Category of Need: SELF-ACTUALIZATION
Nursing Diagnoses

Family coping: potential for growth
Health-seeking behaviors
Knowledge deficit
Noncompliance

*Note: This listing cannot be used as a guarantee that a specific nursing diagnosis will be ranked in priority as shown. Each client's situation should be considered individually.

In addition to using the model, the nurse should consider if the problem is an actual or high risk problem. Most of the time, actual problems rank higher in priority than do high risk ones. There are exceptions to this rule of thumb though—for example, the client at risk for choking related to difficulty swallowing.

It is important to recognize that many client responses may be identified through the assessment process, but owing to time constraints some responses may not be resolved during acute care. The nurse should not hesitate to refer these responses to other health care providers, such as visiting nurses, or plan their resolution through ongoing education, such as through a local community resource group (e.g., the American Cancer Society).

Planning Expected Outcomes

Expected outcomes (also called goals) are objectives of care and are designed to reduce, eliminate, or alleviate the problem identified in the nursing diagnosis. Most outcome statements include the overall goal and specific objectives to measure the degree of goal attainment.

WRITING AN OUTCOME

Determining an expected outcome is an important component of the nursing process. It is equivalent to using a road map on a trip—it helps set the target. Expected outcomes are focused on the client and are written as a client outcome (e.g., the client will . . .), not as a nursing goal, (e.g., the nurse will . . .). The expected outcome relates to the human response. Usually, the response is reversed, modified, or corrected. For example, the client may demonstrate knowledge or have adequate gas exchange. Outcomes also list measurable criteria indicating that the outcome was attained.

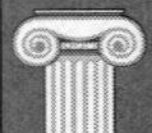

ETHICAL ISSUES IN NURSING

How Should Discrepancies Between Client Outcomes and Medical Management Outcomes Be Resolved?

Nursing care for clients is based upon several factors, including nursing diagnoses, nursing problem lists, and nursing care plans. Professional nurses can largely influence the course of their clients' progress by setting goals with their clients regarding client-related outcomes. These goals most often reflect the overall plan of care, which coincides with physician care plans. But what happens when the clients' outcomes do not jointly reflect medical management outcomes?

Setting priorities and evaluating plans of care may be a source of conflict between the nursing staff and the medical staff. Another source of conflict may be poor communication between the nursing staff and the medical staff. For example, the nursing staff may see certain discharge plans and client education as a priority for a particular client before discharge, but before such plans could be adequately implemented, the client is discharged. Perhaps if the nursing and medical staffs had been more open about each others' plans of care the discharge teaching could have been implemented sooner before the physicians discharged the client.

The nursing process is a very good way to provide quality client care. Nursing diagnoses and client outcomes focus on different areas of client management and are not a restatement of medical care. Therefore, communication between health care team members is important so that all activities might enhance overall client care.

Box 1–6. Guidelines for Writing Expected Outcomes

The expected outcome statement should

- Illustrate the absence or reduction of the human response or related factors identified in the nursing diagnosis
- Be realistic for the client to accomplish.
- Be realistic for the nurse's level of skill and expertise
- Be congruent with and supportive of other therapies
- Be valued by the client, family, and health care team
- Be written in observable and measurable terms
- Be written in terms of client outcomes, not nursing actions
- Be specific
- Include a time frame for achievement

Likewise, the criteria reverse, modify, or correct the original assessment of the signs and symptoms seen in the client. Outcomes also list the time frame for attainment. The time frame varies with the problem. The nurse needs to set realistic goals, and at times, the discernment of the time frame is difficult. Usually, working with a more experienced nurse provides some frame of reference in setting the outcome. Most acute care settings work with short-term outcomes; long-term outcomes are used in rehabilitation settings. Short-term outcomes may be met within hours, such as improvement in oxygenation, or in days, such as increase in comfort. Long-term outcomes may require months, such as learning to ambulate safely after a stroke. Other guidelines for writing expected outcomes are listed in Box 1–6.

The following is an example of a short-term outcome for the client with impaired gas exchange related to ineffective cough:

The client will have improved gas exchange in 2 days as evidenced by

Diminishing crackles in lungs,
Productive cough,
Afebrile,
Skin pink, warm, and dry,
Incentive spirometer to 750 ml, and
Being able to walk to the door without dyspnea.

In the above-mentioned example, the human response was impaired gas exchange. Each of the criteria are measurable and assist in determining to what degree the problem has been resolved. The criteria were developed by examining the clinical manifestations (signs and symptoms) present in the client originally that indicated that there was a problem with gas exchange.

Writing Outcomes for Collaborative Problems

Because the nurse cannot be directly responsible for the development and the treatment of a client's complications, the expected outcomes are expressed in a different format. The expected outcome for collaborative problems focuses on the nurse's recognition of the problem rather than the resolution of the problem. Therefore, the outcomes are written in the following format:

The nurse will monitor the client for clinical manifestations of hyperkalemia, as evidenced by (list the data to be assessed).

This format assists with differentiation of the monitoring function of nurses versus independent actions to resolve nursing diagnoses.

Planning Interventions

Once the outcome is determined, the process of planning care can begin. In the above-mentioned client's care, the nurse identifies interventions that assist the client in improving gas exchange. Some of these interventions are continued assessment of the patient's lung sounds, temperature, skin, and ability to use incentive spirometer. Other interventions focus on teaching the client how to cough and use of the incentive spirometer effectively. The nurse also encourages the client to ambulate and cough.

The interventions should be recorded for other nurses to follow and they must be clearly written. Examples of frequent errors in writing interventions are shown in Table 1-4.

Use of Standardized Care Plans

Standardized care plans are care plans written for clients with common problems. They serve as a memory guide for the nurse to provide care. They also help ensure that consistent care is given to all clients. These care plans are grouped by medical diagnosis and are an excellent resource for the novice nurse or when the nurse is unfamiliar with a client's condition.

Standardized care plans are not a substitute for individualized care. These care plans usually address physiologic and expected problems with various disease states. They cannot address how the client will respond as an individual to the health or illness. Therefore, they are an excellent supplement to a care plan, but they are not a substitute.

TABLE 1-4. Frequent Errors in Writing Interventions

Type of Error	Incorrectly Stated Intervention	Correctly Stated Intervention
Does not indicate quantity	Force fluids	Force fluids to 2500 ml/24 hours 1200 ml on days 1000 ml on evenings 300 ml on nights
Does not indicate frequency	Turn frequently	Turn q 2 hours: 8:00 supine 10:00 left side 12:00 right side 14:00 supine
Does not indicate exactly what is to be done	Wound care bid	Irrigate leg wound at 10:00 and 19:00 with ½ strength Betadine in NS. Repack wound with four opened 4 × 4's and cover with 5 × 9.

NURSING INTERVENTION

Nursing interventions are the actual implementation of the care plan. Nursing interventions are designed to promote, maintain, or restore the client's health. Nursing interventions have the following seven characteristics:

1. Be congruent with the overall plan of care,
2. Be based on scientific principles,
3. Be individualized to the client,
4. Be designed to provide a safe and therapeutic environment,
5. Consider the need for teaching and learning,
6. Use resources appropriately, and
7. Be clearly communicated.

Providing Safe Care

The nurse should identify what skills are required for providing the intervention. If necessary, the nurse may need to review a procedure prior to performing a skill, confer with another nurse before performing the skill, or at times (if it is safe for the client), delegate the skill to another member of the health care team. It is important to remember that when a skill is delegated to another health care team member, the registered nurse remains legally responsible for the client's outcome.

Another aspect of providing safe care is continuous monitoring for complications. There are many complications that can follow surgery, medication administration, and disease states. The nurse needs to be aware of potential complications and assess the patient continuously for their occurrence.

While the care is being given, the nurse continues to assess the client and evaluate his or her response to the care. The nurse also needs to consider which of the interventions could be modified if the client shows no progress toward the desired outcome.

Nursing Roles

Providing care falls into seven categories, according to Benner: helper role, teaching-coaching, diagnostic and patient monitoring, management of rapidly changing conditions, administering and monitoring therapeutic regimes, monitoring and ensuring quality of health care practices, and organizational and work role competencies.[3]

From this list, it is clear that nurses are involved in many areas of client care management. Some of these roles are very *independent*, such as the helper and teacher role. Other roles would be considered *dependent*, when a physician's order is required for the care to be given, such as the administration of medications. Still other roles are *interdependent*, such as monitoring or teaching the client with other health care providers, such as the physician, dietician, or physical therapist.

Rationale

At times, the scientific rationale for an intervention is required on a student care plan or listed within a standardized plan of care. It is important that the care given has its basis in scientific study, not in habit or old wives' tales. The use of rationale assists in identifying the professional nurse from other providers of health care. Advances in nursing research are continuing to provide more scientific basis for nursing care. This text lists rationale for each intervention within the care plans.

EVALUATION

The last step in the process is evaluation. Evaluation examines the degree of goal attainment and basically asks "Did the client achieve the goal he or she was supposed to?" and if not why not? Evaluation begins with collecting data about the client's health status, closely reexamining the outcome criteria. The degree of outcome attainment is determined, and a revised plan of care is established, if needed.

For example, in the above-mentioned outcome, the nurse would assess lung sounds and decide whether the degree of crackles was decreased and so on. If the criteria were met completely, the outcome was fully met.

If the outcome was not met, the nurse asks the following series of questions to illuminate the source of the problem:

Steps in Evaluation

WAS THE CORRECT DIAGNOSIS MADE?

At times, the human response was mislabeled or changed during the course of care. For example, a client was diagnosed with impaired swallowing, but after closer examination, the client's response was more correctly written as potential for aspiration related to impaired swallowing.

DOES THE PROBLEM STILL EXIST?

If the problem has been resolved, it can be deleted from the problem list or care plan. If it has become a lower priority, it should be left on the care plan but labeled as an inactive problem. For example, if a client expressed an interest in learning about a new medication but has since developed major complications, the problem of knowledge deficit must be placed as inactive until the client can focus on learning again.

WAS THE EXPECTED OUTCOME APPROPRIATE AND REALISTIC?

If the outcomes listed are inappropriate for the time frame given, the target date should be changed. When the target date is advanced, the interventions may also require some adjustment.

WERE THE INTERVENTIONS APPROPRIATE, COMPLETE?

Many times, the interventions are appropriate but just need to be continued for a longer period of time to achieve the expected outcomes.

Through these questions, the reasons for not meeting outcomes are identified, needed corrections are made, and the client proceeds through the nursing process again.

The process of evaluation can be seen in the following example:

The nurse is caring for a client with a fever due to an infection and the diagnosis of hyperthermia is made. A goal was set that the fever will be reduced to 37° C (98.6° F) in 4 hours. Interventions chosen included a tepid sponge bath and reducing bed linens.

After 4 hours, the client's temperature was still elevated and the nurse evaluated the goal. Was the correct diagnosis made?—yes the client did have fever. Does the problem still exist—yes, the client is still febrile. Was the goal appropriate and realistic—yes, it is possible (and desirable) to reduce fever within 4 hours. Were the interventions appropriate—yes, treating fever with a tepid bath is scientifically sound. Were all appropriate interventions used—no, the nurse could have given the client an antipyretic medication to assist with fever reduction at the hypothalamic level. So the client is treated again with acetaminophen, and the client's temperature decreases to near normal.

At times, even though the outcome was not met, nothing is wrong with the outcome or interventions except that more time is needed to meet the outcome. In this instance, the nurse can indicate that the plan needs to be continued as was originally designed and a later date should be planned for reevaluation.

The step of evaluation is critical in the process to be certain that goals are met. It is possible to learn a great deal from evaluating goals and interventions. Nurses should not expect that every goal set for every client will be met but instead should learn from the process.

Formal Evaluation Models

The previous discussion centered on the individual evaluation of a client's progress. This type of evaluation can be viewed as informal. There is also a formal method of evaluation through a system called quality assurance.

Quality assurance is the planned and systematic evaluation of care given to a group of clients. The organization most actively involved in formal quality assurance is the Joint Commission for Accreditation of Healthcare Organizations (JCAHO). The JCAHO evaluates the physical structure of health care agencies (e.g., hospitals) to ensure each has the appropriate space, equipment, safety regulations, policies, and procedures to give care safely. In addition, the JCAHO examines the outcomes a facility achieves with various groups of clients to ensure that acceptable results are being obtained. The groups of clients usually examined through quality assurance reviews are those who are seen in high volume, those who are at high risk of serious consequences if care is not provided correctly, and problem-prone clients.

FUTURE OF NURSING DIAGNOSIS

In the past, nurses worked from the medical diagnoses and served in a dependent role to the physician. Nurses were discouraged from making any type of diagnosis and instead charted items like "appears to be bleeding." The use of the nursing diagnosis has allowed nurses to diagnose and treat clients within the realm of nursing. This approach has been a significant change for the profession.

The future of nursing diagnoses also looks bright. The nursing diagnosis may be used to bill clients for nursing service rather than have nursing care as a portion of the room charge. In addition, collaborative research projects can begin to further refine the human response statement and identify interventions (see Nursing Research). Finally, if all nurses used the same language to identify client problems, students would have an easier transition to a staff nurse position.

NURSING RESEARCH

A group of nurse researchers listed 12 broad groups of interventions that were a portion of care of the integument. Through a Dephi-technique (a repeated survey), they asked other nurses to list actual activities that were performed within these groups to illuminate the breadth and depth of care given. The 12 groups of interventions were bathing, bed rest care, hair care, nail care, oral health maintenance, oral health promotion, oral health restoration, positioning, pressure management, skin care with topical treatments, skin surveillance, and wound care. For example, within the group of nurses providing bed rest care, these were some of the activities identified: monitor pulmonary status, place on therapeutic mattress, assist with activities of daily living, turn as indicated by skin condition, explain reasons for requiring bed rest, and keep bed linen clean, dry, and wrinkle free. All 12 groups as well as the interventions are listed in the article. Although the group was small, the work is significant in that it was beginning to build a pool of nursing interventions for the various nursing diagnoses.

▼▼▼

Titler, M., Pettit, D. et. al. (1991). Classification of nursing interventions for care of the integument. *Nursing Diagnosis 2* (2), 45–56.

ROLE OF NANDA

What is NANDA and what is its role? The organization was established in the early 1970s at St. Louis University by Christine Gebbie and Mary Ann Lavin, and was originally called the National Task Force for the Classification of Nursing Diagnosis, which was later shortened to the North American Nursing Diagnosis Association (NANDA). These nurses were concerned with accurately identifying a common terminology of client problems for use by ambulatory care nurses. For example, physicians everywhere know what a diagnosis such as hypertension means; yet, nurses were treating client problems as if each was different.

There was no system for classifying the problems that nurses treat, so there was no way to quantify nursing activities. This problem became very apparent when records were computerized and a coding system was needed to delineate what the nurses were doing.

The diagnostic labels are an attempt to specify just what it is that nurses are able to diagnose and treat. To make a diagnosis, as described earlier, specific cues had to be present. When nurses begin to use the same diagnosis, based on standard cues, data could be collected on the activities of nurses.

Nursing diagnoses have also fostered research, because nursing actions across the country can now be quantified and compared. Research is also continuing on the validation of the diagnoses and the cues that lead to any specific diagnosis.

NURSING RESEARCH AND THE NURSING PROCESS

The nursing process is also an excellent framework for nursing research. It is another standardized system used by nurses throughout the country, so comparisons can be made among apparently diverse groups. The use of nursing diagnosis and the nursing process also has improved nursing care standards that can be applied nationwide. A great deal of emphasis is placed on nursing care standards, because these provide a basis for what care is expected for a certain problem.

THEORETICAL OR CONCEPTUAL MODELS OF NURSING

What is a theoretical or conceptual model of nursing? Why do nurses need such a model? How do these models relate to the nursing process? You may have become familiar with a nursing model through your school of nursing. Many schools use either one of the established models or one that the faculty has decided best defines the practice of nursing for them.

Theories or conceptual models are a way to describe the phenomenon we call nursing. It should help to clarify the phenomenon of nursing so the critical elements can be identified and become the focus of practice. Models help us understand how nursing affects clients. It helps nurses define their beliefs about health and illness, and the way they can help clients move toward health or cope with their illness.

Nursing borrows theoretical knowledge from many professions such as sociology, psychology, medicine, and philosophy. There is, however, knowledge that is unique to nursing, and this knowledge is the basis of the models.

There are many theoretical or conceptual models of nursing practice. Whether these are conceptual models or theoretical models has been debated for years. This text is not the place to continue the debate. Whatever they are called, these models help nurses conceptualize their practice. The nursing process is the way we solve client care problems, whereas the conceptual models are the way we organize our practice as a whole. Nurses working in different clinical areas find certain models help them define their practice better than other models.

There are four basic concepts common to many nursing models: (1) the individual, (2) health, (3) nursing, and (4) environment. Many models also add the concept of adaptation, which is how the model defines these concepts and how these concepts relate to each other. Some theories are more interpersonal, identifying interaction between and among individuals. Some models are based on system theories that look at interactions between or among all factors in the system.

Florence Nightingale

The earliest model of nursing practice was defined by Florence Nightingale, the founder of nursing. Nightingale looked at both sick nursing, which is used with

TABLE 1–5. Nursing Models

Theorist	Components of Model	View of Nursing
Florence Nightingale	Environmental core concept of model; physical, psychological, and social environment, with patient condition and nature at center of model	Environmental theory of nursing. Sees manipulation of the environment as having an impact on patient's condition, as the function of nursing
Virginia Henderson	Human seen as having four components: biologic, psychological, sociological, and spiritual. Health and nursing other major concepts	Nursing focuses on the individual. The purpose is to assist the individual in maintaining health, recovering health, or achieving a peaceful death
Dorothea Orem	Systems model with three main systems: wholly compensatory, partly compensatory, and supportive-educative	Self-care theory. The function of nursing is to help the individual reach or return to a state of self-care
Myra Estrin Levine	Identifies four conservation principles: conservation of energy, conservation of structural integrity, conservation of personal integrity, and conservation of social integrity	Conservation principles model. Goal of nursing to maintain or restore individual to state of health by using principles of conservation
Martha E. Rogers	Uses general systems theory. Four major components: energy fields, openness, pattern, and four-dimensionality. Principles of homeodynamics: integrality, resonancy, and helicity	Principles of homeodynamics. Individuals seen as open system. Nursing is an art and science that is humanistic and humanitarian
Imogene M. King	Open systems model composed of personal systems, interpersonal systems, and social systems	Dynamic interactions system model. The goal of nursing is a transaction between nurse and client leading to attainment of client's goals
Betty Neuman	Health care systems model. Major components are stressors (extrapersonal, interpersonal, and intrapersonal) and reaction (includes levels of prevention)	Health care systems model. Individual at the core of model with flexible lines of resistance surrounding the person. The nurse manipulates the environment using primary, secondary, and tertiary prevention to help maintain the lines of resistance
Sister Callista Roy	Adaptation model with five elements: person, goal of nursing, nursing activities, health, and environment. Four adaptive modes also defined: physiologic function, self-concept, role function, and interdependence	The goal of nursing is to assess patient's adaptive behavior and stimuli that help promote adaptation. Adaptive responses are those that positively affect health
Jean Watson	Theory of human care. Concepts are person, health, environment, nursing, and human care	Nursing holds human caring as a moral ideal that guides transactions with patients leading to a transpersonal caring relationship

clients who are ill, and health nursing, for midwifery and, as she called it, practical health teaching. She defined the role of nursing as getting the person in the best condition possible for nature to act on. She saw nurses' major role as controlling and manipulating the environment to accomplish this goal.

Nightingale's model fits well into a nursing process format. She believed the environment was the focus of the assessment and interventions. This model seems very modern in spite of its age, because it is probably the first description of the nursing process.

Other theorists have proposed models of practice. Some of the more common ones are summarized on Table 1-5.

Sister Callista Roy

Sister Callista Roy has proposed a model that focuses on adaptive behaviors by the person and how these behaviors allow the person to cope (adapt) with stressors from the environment. The nurse's role is to assess the person's adaptive behavior and identify what is affecting this behavior, and then to manipulate the stimuli in such a way that the person is able to cope.

Roy's model differs in the use of the nursing process only in that her model offers first- and second-level assessments. First-level assessments are behavioral assessments, whereas second-level assessments consist of data about the focal, contextual, and residual stimuli impinging on the person. Analysis of this data yields a nursing diagnosis. Interventions are directed at manipulating the stimuli to achieve the client-centered goal.

Dorothea Orem

Dorothea Orem sees the role of the nurse very differently. Her model is based on maintaining or restoring the client to self-care. When the client is unable to maintain self-care, the nurse provides compensatory care to help the person until self-care can be restored. She believes that nursing should support and educate the clients so they can function as independently as possible.

Orem uses a three-step nursing process beginning with assessment that identifies why a person needs nursing care. This equates with the assessment and analysis phase of the standard nursing process. The second phase involves designing a nursing system and planning for the delivery of nursing care. This is similar to the planning phase of the standard nursing process. The next phase is the actual performance of nursing behaviors. This equates with the implementation and evaluation phases of the nursing process.

Betty Neuman

Betty Neuman is one of the theorists who uses systems theory in her model. This model views the person as an open system interacting with the environment. She sees nursing as helping to reduce the stress on individuals through primary, secondary, and tertiary preventions. The person is surrounded by flexible lines of defense, a normal line of defense, and then flexible lines of resistance.

Neuman's model begins with assessment of the stressors. Her actual process has three steps: (1) nursing diagnosis, (2) nursing goals, and (3) nursing outcomes. The levels of prevention are the interventions used in Neuman's model to stabilize and restore the lines of defense.

Myra Estrin Levine

Myra Estrin Levine views the role of the nurse as one of interaction with the client to promote the client's adjustment. Levine identifies four conservation principles that guide nursing interventions. The goal of nursing, according to Levine's model is to maintain or restore the client to a state of health through the conservation principles. Conservation means maintaining a proper balance within the client.

Levine's model is very similar to the nursing process. She sees the first step as observation of the client to decide on appropriate interventions, perform the interventions, and then evaluate their effectiveness in helping the client. The client is seen as dependent and in need of nursing care to adapt to the new state of health. The nurse decides how much the client is able to participate in the care or in decision making. This model is often used by critical care nurses because their clients are usually completely dependent and unable to do much for themselves.

Jean Watson

Jean Watson has developed a model of human care, with human caring as the moral ideal of nursing. This is considered a metaphysical theory because it goes beyond the phenomenologic approach commonly used in nursing. This model seems to approach nursing on a higher level, incorporating the concepts of soul and transcendence. This is a radical shift from usual nursing theories, moving beyond the scientific to a transcendent level.

Rather than the nursing process, Watson refers to the caring occasion that is the interaction between the nurse and the individual. She talks about transpersonal caring and caring transactions. These transactions are an exchange between the individual and the nurse leading to protection, enhancement, and preservation of the person's humanity, which in turn potentially leads to healing through restoration of dignity and inner harmony.

Application of Nursing Models

To better understand these models, we need to observe how each model would approach the same situation. We can use the case from the beginning of the chapter. John, a 19-year-old college freshman, injured his back while water skiing. He is hospitalized during August, on bed rest, in pelvic traction, and on medications to relax his muscles, and he may require surgery. His parents' insurance is paying for his hospital bills, but he has lost his summer job and may be unable to afford his college tuition and books this Fall. Also, if he has surgery, he will probably miss the first semester of school.

Roy would begin by assessing the stressors impinging on John. The first level assessments would look at John's behavior to see how that might be interfering with his ability to adapt. She might find that his anxiety about school and his future is causing increased tension, even muscle tension, stimulating his nervous (cognator) system to increase his pain and his back problem. The role function and interdependence functions are both affected.

After analysis the conclusion may be role failure related to physical immobility. The mutually established goal would be that the client should explore alternatives to returning to school next semester. Interventions would include helping him to develop other options so he can focus on his health. Evaluation would be based on whether or not his anxiety and tension have been decreased.

Orem would focus on the need for John to return to a state of self-care. She would begin by identifying why John needs nursing care, especially how his current problem is limiting his ability for self-care.

In John's case, his need for bed rest and traction to allow his back to heal are the factors that limit his self-care abilities. He will need assistance to help him until he can resume his self-care. The nurse would design a plan of care that would support him during this time of dependency. One part of the plan would be education on future care of his back to prevent recurrence of the problem. His ability to return to self-care would be the focus of evaluation.

Neuman would begin by looking at the stressors that have an impact on John's flexible lines of defense. The stressors John is experiencing are extrapersonal (feelings about missing school), interpersonal (role difficulties), and intrapersonal (anger over loss of funds and not going to school next semester).

At this point, primary prevention is not the focus, because the stressors have already had an impact on John's flexible lines of defense. Primary prevention is important in preventing stressors from developing related to John's immobility. Secondary prevention would begin immediately in dealing with his existing symptoms and, it is hoped, strengthen internal lines of resistance and return the flexible lines of defense to their normal position. One nursing diagnosis would probably be that John is in pain, and this pain is increasing his muscle spasms. Secondary methods of prevention would include treating the pain so no further problems occur and he can begin to heal.

Levine would assess John based on the principles of conservation. One principle that is important is the conservation of personal integrity, because John's sense of personal identity and self-worth may be challenged. This goal would require supportive interventions to prevent John from developing further problems. There might be some difficulties with John, because this model views the client as dependent and with a limited ability to participate in decision making. John might find this difficult because, at this time in his life, dependency is itself a problem.

Watson would look at this person as someone in need of human caring. The nurse would enter into a caring interaction with John to help him restore his dignity over the loss of his schooling. This model would look more at the distress this situation is causing John and how it is interfering with his life. The nurse would enter into a transpersonal (interpersonal) relationship with John leading to a higher level of knowledge and an opportunity for healing. If John were more at peace with himself and his situation, other options might become more apparent.

These models can help the nurse conceptualize nursing and plan client care. Nurses have to decide which of these models best fit their philosophies of nursing and of client care. More about these models and others may be found in a text devoted to conceptual models of nursing practice.

Summary

Nursing process is the problem-solving method used by nurses to provide nursing care. The process has five steps: (1) assessment, (2) diagnosis, (3) planning, (4) intervention, and (5) evaluation. Nursing diagnoses approved by NANDA and collaborative problems are the most common phrases used to describe client problems. Planning expected outcomes centers on the client's desired response to the health problem. Interventions are the actual nursing care performed for or with the client. The final step, evaluation, is the determination of whether or not expected outcomes were met by evaluating each of the outcomes.

Bibliography

1. Alfaro, R. (1990). *Applying nursing diagnosis and nursing process: A step by step guide* (2nd ed.) Philadelphia: J. B. Lippincott.
2. Aspinall, M. (1976). Nursing diagnosis—the weak link. *Nursing Outlook, 24,* 433–437.
3. Benner, P. (1984). *From novice to expert.* Menlo Park, CA: Addison-Wesley Publishers.
4. Carpenito, L. (1991). *Nursing diagnosis: Application to clinical practice.* Philadelphia: J. B. Lippincott.
5. Carpenito, L. & Duespohl, T. (1986). *A guide to effective clinical instruction.* Rockville, MD: Aspen Systems Co.
6. Cox, H., Hinz, M., et al. (1989). *Clinical applications of nursing diagnosis.* Baltimore: Williams and Wilkins.
7. Donahue, M. (1985). *Nursing: The finest art.* St. Louis: C. V. Mosby.
8. Fitzpatrick, J., & Whall, A. (1989). *Conceptual models of nursing: Analysis and application* (2nd ed.) Norwalk, CT: Appleton & Lange.
9. George, J. (Ed.) (1985). *Nursing theories: The base for professional nursing practice* (2nd ed.) Englewood Cliffs, NJ: Prentice-Hall, Inc.

10. Gordon, M. (1987). *Nursing diagnosis: Process and application* (2nd ed.) New York: McGraw-Hill.
11. Hall, L. (1955). Quality of Nursing Care. *Public Health News.*
12. Iyer, P., et al. (1991). *Nursing process and nursing diagnosis* (2nd ed.) Philadelphia: W. B. Saunders.
13. Kalish, R. (1983). *The psychology of human behavior* (5th ed.) Monterey, CA: Brooks/Cole.
14. King, I. M. (1981). *A theory for nursing.* New York: Wiley.
15. Levine, M. E. (1973). *Introduction to clinical nursing* (2nd ed.) Philadelphia: F. A. Davis.
16. Malinsky, V. (Ed.) (1986). *Explorations on Martha Rogers' science of unitary human beings.* Philadelphia: F. A. Davis.
17. Mundinger, M., & Jauron, G. (1975). Developing a nursing diagnosis. *Nursing Outlook, 23* (2), 94-98.
18. Neuman, B. (1982). *The Neuman systems model.* East Norwalk, CT: Appleton-Century-Crofts.
19. Nightingale, F. (1969). *Notes on nursing.* New York: Dover Publications, Inc.
20. Orem, D. E. (1985). *Nursing: Concepts of practice* (3rd ed.) New York: McGraw-Hill.
21. Riehl-Sisca, Joan. (1989). *Conceptual models for nursing practice* (3rd ed.) Norwalk, CT: Appleton & Lange.
22. Roy, C. (1975). The impact of nursing diagnosis. *AORN Journal, 21* (5), 1023-1030.
23. Roy, C. (1984). *Introduction to nursing: An adaptation model,* (2nd ed.) Englewood Cliffs, NJ: Prentice-Hall.
24. Sparks, S., & Taylor, C. (1991). *Nursing diagnosis reference manual.* Springhouse, PA: Springhouse.
25. Weber, G. (1991). Making nursing diagnosis work for you and your client. *Nursing & Health Care, 12* (8), 424-430.
26. Yura, H., & Walsh, M. (1967). *The nursing process: Assessing, planning, implementing, evaluation.* New York: Appleton-Century-Crofts.
27. Yura, H., & Walsh, M. (1983). *The nursing process: Assessing, planning, implementing, evaluation* (4th ed.). New York: Appleton-Century-Crofts.

Chapter 2

Nursing Practice

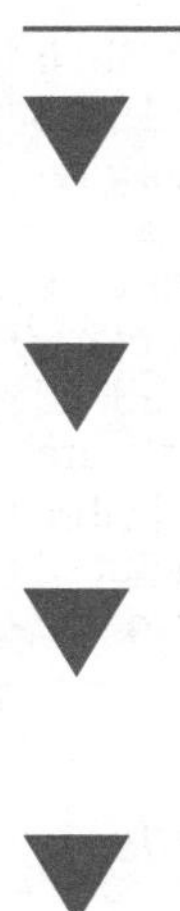

In the United States, nurses practice within a diverse and complex health care system. During the 1980s, the system experienced dramatic growth in scientific knowledge, coupled with an explosion of technology. This was also a period of increased competition and regulation. Finally, the financing of health care was revolutionized when prospective payment was introduced. These events have had a profound impact on the practice of nursing. Understanding who the major stakeholders are within the field of health care and understanding recent health care history are critical to the practice of professional nursing. The purpose of this chapter is to inform beginning practitioners of these changes and trends in order to prepare professional nurses for active roles in shaping the health care system of the 1990s and beyond.

The chapter is divided into four sections. The first presents an overview of those groups and institutions that are most concerned with the structure and function of the health care industry. In the second section, the various mechanisms for funding health care are defined and the industry's history over the past 70 years is reviewed. The third section highlights the richness and diversity of nursing practice, whereas the fourth section depicts some of the special client populations that nurses serve.

MAJOR STAKEHOLDERS IN THE UNITED STATES HEALTH CARE SYSTEM

Government

The role of government in the administration of health care cannot be overestimated. By the mid-1980s, over 40 per cent of health care dollars spent were funded by government programs, mostly (27 per cent) through Medicare (a federal program) and Medicaid (a joint federal-state initiative). Other important sources of federal government funding are the Department of Veterans Affairs (VA), which oversees the VA health care system, and the Department of Defense, which funds health care for the armed forces and their dependents. In addition, state and local governments support local indigent care through various mechanisms.[8]

As the major payor, the federal government has been active in regulating the health care industry. Approximately 40 per cent of hospital beds are occupied on any given day by Medicare recipients. Therefore, hospitals have great incentive to comply with regulations promulgated by the federal government because they can be fined or "de-certified" as a provider of care to Medicare clients if they fail to comply. This could result in the loss of millions of dollars of income for the hospital.

Government regulation is frequently opposed by the health care industry because it often affects the health care practitioner's autonomy. In 1991, for example, the Supreme Court upheld the right of the federal government to restrict health care providers in family planning clinics receiving federal funds from informing pregnant women about abortion options (Rust versus Sullivan). Since the Supreme Court ruling, health care workers in the clinics must alter their practice or be subject to penalty. Strong condemnation of this restriction was voiced by the American Nurse's Association (ANA) and the American Medical Association (AMA), among others. Congress has considered legislation to overturn the regulation.

The federal government is also the biggest source of funding for biomedical research and public health programs such as the Centers for Disease Control. By the late 1980s, more than $21 billion were spent on these programs annually.[8] This represents almost 5 per cent of every health care dollar spent. The growth of scientific knowledge related to health care is highly dependent on government funding. Nurse researchers are recipients of research grants through various government agencies, most notably the National Center for Nursing Research at the National Institutes of Health (NIH). Research funds are an important source of revenue for major medical centers and university affiliated hospitals.

Physicians

The role of physicians in the health care system in the United States is an important one. Physicians provide direct medical services to clients in a variety of settings, including offices, clinics, hospitals, and free-standing centers. In addition, physicians control 60 to 80 per cent of hospital costs through their decisions about the use of resources. As gatekeepers to inpatient care, physicians decide which clients to admit, where to admit clients, how long the client will stay, the quantity of ancillary services consumed, whether to perform surgery, when to initiate and when to discontinue treatment regimens, and which medications to prescribe.[19] Because physicians strongly influence health care use, health care agencies and consumers are often dependent on physicians. Agencies such as hospitals rely on their medical staffs to admit clients who generate income for the hospital. Therefore, physicians are customers of the hospital just as clients are. As a result, physicians and their lobby groups, such as the AMA, usually have strong political influence within hospital organizations, the health care system, legislatures, and government regulating agencies.

Many physicians have perceived a decline in their dominance and control of health care during the 1980s and early 1990s. This perceived and real loss has created anxiety and defensive tactics among some members of the profession toward a restructured health care system. The traditions that define medical practice, such as autonomy, professional control, solo medical practice, and fee-for-service entrepreneurialism, are being questioned and reformed. Some contend that physicians will enjoy less control in a restructured health care environment than they have enjoyed in the past.[11]

Hospital Administrators and Governing Boards

The chief executive and chief financial officers and the governing boards of hospitals strongly influence health care delivery in their institutions. In addition, a majority of hospitals are members of the American Hospital Association (AHA), which represents the industry's efforts to influence legislation, regulation, judicial decisions, and health policy. Recently, the AHA filed suit to stop the National Labor Relations Board from implementing new collective bargaining rules. The suit went to the Supreme Court, where the rules were upheld.[5] The AHA is also trying to block new regulations from the Health Care Financing Administration (HCFA), which will effectively decrease reimbursement for capital costs to hospitals from Medicare.[26]

Business and Industry

As health care costs rose in the past decade (about 8 per cent per year),[8] the influence of business and industry increased as well. Health insurance programs, such as Blue Cross/Blue Shield and commercial insurance, are purchased predominantly through employee benefit programs. As the cost of health care rises, insurance costs rise as well, forcing businesses to assume greater financial burdens to insure the health of their employees and their dependents. Nationally, health benefit costs amount to 26 per cent of corporate earnings; corporate medical care costs rose 21.6 per cent in 1990, and 20.4 per cent in 1989.[27] One major reason for the increase is the health care industry's practice of increasing charges to offset underpayment by Medicare, Medicaid, and other contracted payors. The result is that private sector, insured clients, and their employers pay more for care. During the past decade, business and industry leaders protested the increased costs and began to take collective action to drive costs down. Some of the strategies used have been increased deductibles, larger and more frequent copayments, reduced benefits and services, initiation of managed care programs, mandatory second opinions, precertification of admission, and increased contracting for care to health maintenance organizations (HMO) and preferred provider organizations (PPO). (See Box 2-1 for definition of these terms.)

In some areas of the country, industry leaders have formed coalition groups that lobby state government for laws to restrict health care spending and provide major reform for the health care system. Increasingly, large businesses have contracted for health care services directly with hospitals and physician groups demanding—and receiving—significant discounts for care. The influence of large employers is expected to remain strong within the health care industry.

The Public

The United States public has a stake in health care from several perspectives. First, the public are consumers of health care services. As consumers, they are concerned with quality, cost, and access to care. Many United States citizens believe health care is a right and should be universally available to all citizens regardless of cost. Paradoxically, however, most do not want to pay these costs in the form of increased taxes. The reality is, however, that those citizens who are uninsured (approximately 37 million) or underinsured do not have equal access to health care services that income and insurance provide.[12] Women and children are among those who suffer the most from this problem.[17] Because people have not reached a consensus as to the model for health care reform or the role government should play, a number of ideas are being explored by various interest groups.

The public also is composed of voters who can elect representatives to enact laws protecting their health care interests. Often, citizens band together in organized groups to influence the passage of health-related legislation that is favorable to their interests. In 1990, AIDS activist groups strongly lobbied Congress to ensure passage of the Ryan White bill (PL 101-381), which provided funds for AIDS education, service, and research. The American Association of Retired Persons (AARP) is another prominent group that actively supports health care legislation targeted for the elderly. Although there are many other consumer groups concerned with health care issues, AIDS activist groups and the AARP represent two of the larger and more vocal constituencies that are currently influencing the health care industry.

Overall, public values regarding health care are changing. Consumers are interested in receiving quality health care at a reasonable cost. In addition, the public has a more positive view of health promotion and illness prevention than in the past. The focus on a healthy lifestyle is in conflict with an illness-driven health care system, creating another impetus for change.[11]

Nurses

Nurses outnumber physicians, dentists, pharmacists, and every other single group of health care provider in the United States. As of March 1988, there were 2,033,032 licensed professional nurses in this country, of which 1.63 million were employed in nursing. Among those 1.63 million RNs, two thirds worked in hospitals, which is a distribution that has remained constant for more than a decade. Even as the supply of registered nurses has increased (45 per cent since 1977), the percentage employed in hospitals has been stable at 67 per cent. Most nurses are involved in direct patient care. Seventy-one per cent spend at least half their work time focused on patient care activities.[25]

The influence of such a large group of health care providers should be felt. The most frequently discussed impact of nursing within the industry, however, is the shortage of registered nurses. Despite their large numbers, demand for nurses continues to surpass supply. The epidemic of shortages since the late 1970s has generated the study and attention of various health care organizations, private foundations, and two federal Commissions on Nursing. These groups have attempted to identify the nature of the shortages, the characteristics of the supply, and long-term solutions to correct current and prevent future crises. Findings indicate that the current shortage is demand driven, and is not the result of a decreased supply of registered nurses. Chronic undercompensation of nurses has led to inappropriate use of professional nurses for non-registered nurse functions. The shortage is expected to continue. The consistent recommendation to correct the problem has been to increase compensation rates for registered nurses.

Nursing influence within health care is felt in other important ways as well. Nurses and other health care groups formed a coalition to successfully defeat a recent proposal from the AMA for a new health care worker, the Registered Care Technician (RCT). Under the leadership of organized nursing, the coalition represented more than one hundred professional and citizen groups opposed to the RCT.

In 1991, the American Nurses Association in collaboration with the National League for Nursing, the American Organization of Nurse Executives, the American Association of Colleges of Nursing, and other organized nursing groups, introduced *Nursing's Agenda for Health Care Reform.* The authors wrote "Nurses provide a unique perspective on the health care system. Our constant presence in a variety of settings places us in contact with individuals who reap the benefits of the system's most sophisticated services, as well as those individuals seriously compromised by the system's inefficiencies. . . . America's health care system is . . . very costly, its quality inconsistent, and its benefits unequally distributed. . . . In short, health care is neither fairly nor equitably delivered to all segments of the population."[2] Nursing's health care reform proposal attempts to address the cost-quality-access dilemmas facing the nation. This endeavor is a very proactive attempt by the nursing profession to significantly alter existing health policy.

VARIATIONS IN THE FINANCING OF HEALTH CARE SERVICES

Funding Mechanisms

Health care is paid for in various ways. The major funding programs are defined in Box 2-1.

The health care industry has evolved through significant phases over the past 70 years with regard to quality-cost-access. In order to understand current issues, it is useful for nurses to understand the past, which was characterized by two major periods—(1) the period of expansion and (2) the period of regulation and cost containment.

Period of Expansion in the Health Care Industry*

During the late 1920s, a Congressional committee studied various facets of health care organization and financing. Findings from that committee demonstrated that the cost of health care per illness had substantially increased with emergence of hospitalization as the appropriate method for treating illness.[16] These rising costs, coupled with the financial problems created by the economic depression of 1929, led to financial difficulties for community general hospitals. Consequently, the need to spread financial risk across the community was recognized. Prepayment plans for hospital care spread slowly during the 1930s and evolved into the Blue Cross system.[19]

There were two objectives of the Blue Cross plans: (1) to provide a stronger financial base for community hospitals, and (2) to move the risk of economic loss due to hospitalization away from single individuals to larger groups of people. These objectives were considered socially desirable, and as a result, Blue Cross and later Blue Shield organizations benefited from favorable legislation exempting them from some of the more stringent requirements for commercial insurance companies.[19]

Evolution of Blue Cross/Blue Shield plans and their availability to the average worker signaled the beginning of an era in which the actual cost of health care became separated from the person who consumed that care (the insurance effect). Such a separation causes the cost of health care to appear artificially low to the consumer, who, in turn, can afford to purchase more services.

Demand for health care services because of insurance grew very rapidly in the 1940s and 1950s. Owing to economic wage and price controls during and after World War II, salary increases to workers were very limited. Fringe benefits came into vogue as a means of attracting and retaining workers. Unions began bargaining for fringe benefits in lieu of unobtainable salary increases. As a consequence, health insurance became widely available to American workers and their families. Consumption of health care services, in turn, increased.

Another event of importance during the 1930s was the passage of the Social Security Act of 1935. This piece of legislation established as social policy the right of the aged to financial security. Although health care was not affected by this law at the time of its passage, the Social Security Act would later become the vehicle through which health care needs of the aged and the poor would be addressed.

After World War II, it was apparent that the nation's hospitals were obsolete and poorly distributed to meet the needs of the population. There had been great shifts in population from rural to urban areas during the war, and immediately after the war, the population began its "post-war baby boom." The private sector had difficulty in meeting the need for improvement.[3] Congress responded by passing the Hospital Survey and Construction Act of 1946, which is more generally known as the Hill-Burton Act.

The overt purpose of the Hill-Burton Act was to eliminate shortages of hospitals, especially in rural and economically depressed areas. Ratios of beds-to-population were used to measure shortage. Funds generated by the Hill-Burton Act were dispersed over a 28-year period (1946 to 1974). The act was amended over that time period to include not only construction of new facilities but modernization of existing facilities and, later, construction of emergency rooms and neighborhood health centers.[3]

Implicit within this legislation was the social policy of ensuring all people access to health care. The solution to the social problem of inadequate access was to construct more health care facilities. In order to ensure that individuals with limited ability to pay were actually served by the agencies receiving Hill-Burton Act money, the legislation stipulated a unique pay-back scheme. Each facility had to provide care to indigent clients, on an annual basis, which was equal in dollar value to the amount of money received by the hospital, prorated over a specified time period, usually 20 years. Much like a mortgage payment, the hospital provided free care each year equal to its annual repayment amount. These health services were provided, in lieu of payment, to those individuals with limited access due to poverty.

The Hill-Burton Act's approach to indigent care was a noble one but was not successful in providing access for all indigent clients. During the long pay-back period, the cost of health care increased dramatically due to increased technology and inflation. Many hospitals began meeting their obligations for free care in a few weeks' time each year. After those obligations were

---

* This sub-section and the one following were developed under Federal Contract (to the Division of Nursing in 1988 as part of a larger project). Grateful acknowledgment is made to the Division of Nursing for their funding support.

Box 2-1. Funding Programs

MEDICARE — a federally funded, federally administered national health insurance program for citizens aged 65 and older, and available for certain other clients, such as those with end-stage renal disease, regardless of age. Medicare began in 1966 and is paid for through payroll taxes of all workers (a portion of social security deductions) and through monthly premiums paid by recipients. The program covers both hospitalization and physician costs; however, deductibles and restrictions apply. The federal government instituted major changes in the way hospitals are reimbursed for Medicare clients in 1983. Previously, hospitals were reimbursed their costs plus an additional amount. Since 1983, hospitals have received compensation on a prospective basis. Under prospective payment, hospitals are paid one predetermined sum for a given diagnosis. Similar types of diagnoses and conditions are grouped together, weighted for severity or intensity of illness, and assigned a dollar value for compensation. These are called diagnostic related groups or DRGs. If the client's care for that diagnosis (acute myocardial infarction for example) costs the hospital *more* than Medicare's payment, the hospital *loses* money. If the costs are less than the reimbursement amount, the hospital can keep the profit. This system has caused dramatic changes in the process of care as hospitals struggle to survive financially.

MEDICAID — a joint federal-state program administered by the state governments. This insurance program provides limited funding for certain low income citizens' hospital costs and some medical care costs. Each state sets the income levels that determine eligibility for the Medicaid program. As a result, some states provide more services to more citizens than others can afford. The state must budget money from its own revenues for the program that the federal government matches using a ratio. The federal portion is always larger than the state portion.

BLUE CROSS and BLUE SHIELD — private not-for-profit health insurance companies set up through special legislation in the 1930s. The "Blues" are the largest single insurer outside of the federal government. Businesses and industry can purchase health care insurance for their employee groups from Blue Cross and Blue Shield. Both hospitalization and medical care insurance are available.

COMMERCIAL INSURANCE COMPANIES — such as AETNA, Traveler's, and Metropolitan Life that are for-profit businesses. These agencies usually sell a host of insurance packages, health insurance being just one. Businesses or individuals may opt to buy health insurance from a commercial carrier.

SELF-INSURANCE — increasing numbers of businesses now develop their own insurance programs for employees. The company sets aside monies (which can be millions of dollars) to cover the risk of their self-insurance program. Often, the company hires Blue Cross and Blue Shield or a commercial insurer to administer (receive, review, and pay out claims) their program for them.

HMO — a health maintenance organization is a system of bundled services. The client pays a monthly premium to the HMO, which entitles him or her to check-ups and preventive care, medical care, prescriptions, and hospitalization if needed. The HMO employs its own physicians, may own or manage its own hospitals, and employs other health care providers. Some HMOs charge the client a copayment for some services, such as prescriptions. The client is restricted in an HMO to using only HMO facilities and physicians. If clients choose to go outside the system, they must pay for some or all of their expenses. (There are specific exceptions for emergencies and for people who travel.)

PPO — a preferred provider organization is a group of physicians, usually at least one hospital, and sometimes ancillary providers as well that link together to form a system of care. This care system is marketed and sold, contractually, to employers. In this system of care, the physicians, hospital, and others remain independent agents who agree to treat certain clients (those who join the PPO) at discounted prices.

WORKMAN'S COMPENSATION — this is a federally mandated, state funded and administered insurance program available to workers injured on the job. Each employer is assessed a payroll tax, which funds this plan. Claims are filed through the employer in order to secure funds for treatment.

PRIVATE PAY — this term is used to describe clients who have no insurance and are responsible for payment of the entire health care bill themselves.

UNCOMPENSATED CARE — this is the health care delivered that cannot be or is not paid for by an insurance program or by clients themselves. Many private pay clients contribute to the amount of uncompensated care when they are unable to pay for the high costs of health care. Other sources of uncompensated care include the differences between what the care costs and what Medicare or Medicaid pays the provider. By law, providers cannot bill for the difference.

CAPITATION — a form of payment for health care services between the purchaser of care and the provider, which is often used when a large organization contracts for health services from a provider, such as a hospital or home health agency. The provider can get paid in one of two ways: either (1) a flat fee per incident of care (no care, no payment) or (2) the provider receives a flat fee per person enrolled in the health plan for a defined level of care, whether the enrollee seeks care or not. If few enrollees use the service, the provider does well financially. If not, the provider must care for every enrollee who seeks care regardless of whether the total money received covers the cost of all the care provided.

met, the hospital was not legally bound by the Hill-Burton Act to treat indigent clients. By the early 1970s, the bed shortage addressed by Hill-Burton legislation had reversed itself and an over-supply was thought to exist. In 1974, the act was allowed to expire.

The early 1950s included continued wage and price controls, growth of health insurance coverage among workers, and increased discussion of a national health insurance program. National health insurance was viewed as a means of insuring every United States citizen against economic loss due to the high cost of illness, regardless of employment status, age, or health status. This concern repeatedly asserted itself during Truman's administration. The medical and hospital lobby successfully fought such legislation as late as 1952.[17]

By the middle of the next decade, a new social problem was identified as the nation's priority: poverty. The War on Poverty during the Johnson administration (1963 to 1968) provided the impetus for passage of the first national health insurance plans, with the federal government as both the insurance carrier and the payor of a large portion of the premium. These insurance programs, known as Medicare and Medicaid, were passed as amendments to the Social Security Act in 1965. The social problem of poverty was translated more specifically into limited access to health care services by the elderly and the nonelderly poor as the result of inability of pay. The social policy expressed by both pieces of legislation implied that access to health care for all citizens was a right. Government had an obligation to ensure that right.

Funding for the Medicare hospitalization plan (Part A) is provided by a payroll tax collected from every worker who pays social security taxes. The medical payment component (Part B) for physician care is paid by the enrollee through monthly premiums. The Medicare program is administered by the federal government through the Department of Health and Human Services' Health Care Financing Administration.

Administration of Medicaid is delegated to the states, which must provide certain core services but are free to tailor other services to meet specific population needs. The states also determine eligibility requirements, and these vary considerably from state to state. Funding for Medicaid is provided by a matching formula specific for each state. The federal funds are always the greatest portion of each Medicaid dollar spent. States receive differing amounts of federal money (and, therefore, provide different ranges of care) because some states are able to match more federal dollars than others through larger state tax revenues.

Implementation of Medicare and Medicaid substantially increased the federal government's role (and to a lesser extent, the state governments' role) in the health care market. The federal government became the single largest purchaser of health care services. Subsequently, the government played a growing role in regulation of the health care industry relative to both cost and quality (see Bridge to Home Health Care).

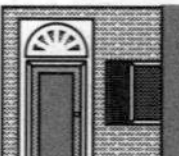

BRIDGE TO HOME HEALTH CARE

Federally Funded Home Health Services

Program	Eligibility	Requirements	Coverage
Medicare	65 years or older, plus some special other groups such as people with ESRD. Payment into Social Security or Railroad Retirement System	Homebound Needs intermittent skilled care Physician-prescribed treatment plan	Skilled nursing Physical therapy Speech therapy Occupational therapy Medical social work Home health aide Medical supplies and equipment
Medicaid	Meets income and categorical requirements that vary from state to state	Needs intermittent medically necessary care Physician-prescribed treatment plan Homebound	Nursing care Home health aide Medical supplies and equipment *At state's option:* Physical therapy Occupational therapy Speech therapy
Older Americans	Over 60 years of age Low income		Home-delivered meals (indirect) Transportation Home repair Information and referral Services may vary from state to state
Social Services Act*	Financial need (varies from state to state)		Homemaker/chore services
Veterans' Administration	Service-connected disability	Prior hospitalization at VA facility	Same as MEDICARE

*Not verified.

▼▼▼

Reprinted from *Home Health Care Nursing: Administrative and Clinical Perspectives* by S. Stuart-Siddal (ed.), p. 28, with permission of Aspen, Publishers Inc., © 1986.

Period of Regulation and Cost Containment

In 1974 Congress passed the National Health Planning and Resources Act (PL 93-641) requiring states to develop a statewide health plan for the use of resources. This act also required states to review providers' requests to initiate or expand health services.[3] This review process is known as Certificate of Need (CON) review and is still in force today. If the provider cannot demonstrate sufficient need for the service, the request is denied. This piece of legislation represents the first federal government effort to combine health planning and regulation in one program. It is also the first significant attempt to control health care costs through elimination of duplicate services and facilities. It was designed to curb the oversupply of facilities that arose during the period of expansion.

Results of the Certificate of Need regulation program demonstrated in research studies have been disappointing. Steinwald and Sloan reviewed eight empirical studies and concluded that "the current evidence . . . suggests that certificate-of-need controls, initiated by the states and mandated by PL 93-641, may be regarded as a classic example of regulatory failure."[22]

Some state governments undertook their own regulatory programs during the 1970s. Rate controls were in place in at least eight states by the end of the decade. According to Steinwald and Sloan, such programs "all respond to the evils of cost-based reimbursement—they seek to counteract the unrestrained nature of hospital reimbursement by superimposing constraints that the market cannot provide."[22]

The states with mandatory rate-setting programs represented the most stringent group of prospective reimbursement programs operating during the late 1970s. "Rates of increase in total hospital expenses in the eight mandatory states were 9.7 and 8.6 percent for the years of 1976-1977 and 1977-1978, respectively, versus 15.8 and 14.0 percent for the other states and the District of Columbia".[22] These data and other studies clearly indicated that prospective rate-setting was more effective in controlling health care costs than were the Certificate of Need controls. Reimbursement for Medicaid patients also had moved to a prospective system in many states, whether the state had mandatory rate setting or not.

The federal government, very much aware of the rising cost of health care and continuing as the nation's largest purchaser of care, began to look at methods of prospective reimbursement that could be used by the Medicare program. Research studies were under way at Yale and other centers to develop a system of prospective payment. These studies were closely followed and sometimes funded by the Department of Health and Human Services, previously called the Department of Health, Education, and Welfare.

The hospital industry adopted its own form of regulation in December 1977. Known as the Voluntary Effort (VE), it consisted of "joint activities at the state level by the American Hospital Association, the American Medical Association, and the Federation of American Hospitals (the for-profit hospitals' trade organization) to control the rate of growth of hospital costs."[22] The results of the VE were mixed. A study by the Congressional Budget Office indicated a small, nonsignificant negative effect on hospital expenditures. A second study did find a significant negative effect on cost per admission and cost per patient day. However, the study indicated that these cost savings were not passed on to the consumers because hospital profits increased during this same time period (1978 to 1980).[22]

The inability of various regulatory programs to control the rising cost of health care (from 9 per cent of the Gross National Product in 1978 to 13 per cent by 1992) became a priority issue with Congress. The nation was trying to recover from economic recession, and inflation in all sectors of the economy was of grave concern. In addition, the population was aging and the ratio of workers (who paid Medicare taxes for hospitalization insurance) to the aged (who consumed the dollars paid in by using hospital services) was shrinking. There were projections that the Medicare Trust Fund would be bankrupt by the mid 1980s.[1] (That did not occur; however, HCFA continues to take strong regulatory action to control spiralling Medicare costs.)

Not surprisingly, when Congress passed the Tax Equity and Fiscal Responsibility Act (TEFRA) in July 1982, it contained temporary caps on Medicare payments, and it directed the Secretary of Health and Human Services to develop a prospective payment system (PPS) for the Medicare program. The Secretary was instructed to report back to Congress by December 1982 on the status of such a system.

In December 1982, Secretary Richard Schweiker recommended to Congress that a PPS based on Diagnosis Related Groups (DRGs), developed by researchers at Yale, be used for all Medicare patients. In March 1983, Congress passed amendments to the Social Security Act authorizing such a system. This system was to replace the cost-based retrospective payment system used to determine Medicare payments to hospitals. All hospitals serving Medicare clients were to switch to PPS except for certain sole community providers, specialty hospitals, and some psychiatric units within general hospitals.

The program became operational on October 1, 1983. Hospitals were phased into the system over the next 11 months, whenever their fiscal year began. A formula was calculated for each hospital to determine its initial reimbursement rate under DRGs. Data were gathered from the hospital's own cost history (using a base year), and from a cost history by geographic region; additionally, there was a national rate. These rates were weighted and blended to determine the exact rate of reimbursement per DRG. There have been several adjustments in the blending since PPS was initiated. The goal is to move all hospitals toward one national rate; however, that has not yet occurred.

Government was not the only entity concerned with rising health care costs during the early 1980s. Business and industry also were very concerned because they paid the majority of health insurance premium costs for employees. Coalitions of local and regional business leaders were formed to discuss and to try to remedy the worsening situation. With the implementation of PPS for Medicare clients, these business coalitions were joined by Blue Cross Organizations and other commercial insurers. These new groups held a common fear: that hospitals would shift uncompensated costs generated by Medicare patients to patients who were still reimbursed retrospectively on a cost-plus basis. As a result of that fear, Blue Cross and other insurers have begun to restructure their payment systems to protect themselves from potential or actual cost shifting. These fears were warranted because cost shifting became and remains a reality.

There have been other results of PPS as well. Hospitals and other health care providers increasingly compete for non-Medicare clients who are more favorably reimbursed. Hospitals also compete for certain Medicare clients whose DRG rate has been profitable for the hospital. Much traditional inpatient care has been shifted to the outpatient system or to the client's home, where the cost of care is less. Insurers and providers have teamed up in creative arrangements designed to hold down costs and yet remain competitive. Such arrangements have caused alternative delivery systems to emerge, based on greater efficiency and decreased costs. Among those alternative systems are HMOs, PPOs, and independent practice associations (IPAs), among others. The number of outpatient surgical centers, free standing and hospital based, has increased rapidly, as have the numbers of free-standing emergency clinics.

Providers have turned increasingly to marketing in order to sell their system of health services to businesses and consumers. HMOs and PPOs, for example, seek to contract with employers to be the sole insurer or provider for employee groups. Capitation has emerged as a popular form of prospective payment used within these contractual arrangements. Medicare also is interested in capitation as a means for payment for its enrollees. In some regions of the country, Medicare enrollees already receive care through an HMO that receives capitation payments from the federal government. The American Hospital Association projected that the majority of Medicare clients would be covered by capitation by the early 1990s.[6]

Summary

The health care system in the United States has undergone rapid change since the early 1980s. The system is still in the midst of evolution, however, and the end product is difficult to foresee. Scarcity of and competition for human and financial resources are the dominant forces operating at present. This situation creates a dilemma with regard to social values of the past: health care as a right versus scarcity. Nurses must recognize and grapple with these forces and the dilemmas involved in order to play an active part in shaping the nation's future health care system.

What direction will the health care system in the United States take next? An interview with a nurse expert in health policy outlines priorities for this decade and beyond (Box 2-2).

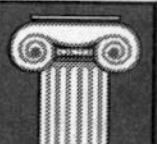

ETHICAL ISSUES IN NURSING

Can the Underinsured Client be Cared for Adequately?

A large percentage of the United States population is uninsured or underinsured for health care. The insurance situation in United States has thus created a two-tiered system of health care. One tier serves the more financially stable (private insurance, HMO/PPO plans, and the like), whereas the second tier serves the less financially stable (Medicare and Medicaid).

The dilemma with which health care workers are faced regarding this two-tiered system of health coverage has to do with the principle of justice. If health care services are to be just, or fair, then they must serve all persons equally, regardless of their ability to pay. Is the health care industry in United States just? Do all persons have equal access to health care?

Nurses work in a variety of settings. Settings include private hospitals, public hospitals, nursing homes, private offices, home health agencies, and homeless shelters. A client's economic background often determines at what type of health care facility she or he may be treated. Nurses in these various facilities must show respect for each client as a fundamental guiding principle in his or her treatment. Each nurse must consider the justice in her or his practice. Nursing may not always be involved in the medical treatment decisions dictated by financial considerations; however, nursing practice can always strive for justice within each context of care.

RICHNESS AND DIVERSITY OF NURSING PRACTICE

The discipline of nursing offers a wide variety of career opportunities across diverse settings. This section highlights the breadth of professional practice.

Hospital Practice

Eighty per cent of the total registered nurse population are employed in nursing. Of those 1.63 million nurses, the large majority (67 per cent) work in hospitals (over 1 million nurses). Between 1984 and 1988, the number of nurses working in hospitals increased by almost 100,000, although the percentage remained unchanged from previous years.[25]

Hospital practice offers a wide variety of options to nurses. The majority of hospital nurses work in staff nurse positions, giving direct, hands-on care to clients. Most staff nurses work with medical-surgical (adult and pediatric) clients. Other common areas of practice include critical care (cardiac, neonatal, pediatric, medical-surgical, perinatal), operating room, labor and delivery, recovery room, postpartum and newborn areas, emergency department, outpatient department, hospital-based home health care, and inpatient hospice.

The variety and intensity of experiences available to nurses in hospital practice have traditionally attracted new graduates. In addition, other employment settings often require nurses to have several years of hospital nursing practice before they can be hired. The familiarity with care requiring high technology systems and acutely ill clients has been viewed as an asset when practicing elsewhere, particularly in home health in which increased technology and skilled nursing care have allowed very sick clients to remain at home.

Among hospital nurses, over 14 per cent work in a leadership position. These positions include nurse executive, assistant administrator, supervisor, head nurse and nurse manager, and assistant nurse managers. These nurses are accountable for the day-to-day operation of the nursing department. They develop plans for and monitor resource use; they hire, train, and evaluate staff; and they monitor the quality of client care and take action to improve quality. Head nurses and their assistants typically manage the delivery of nursing care to clients on one or more nursing units or service areas. Nurses in higher leadership positions are responsible for increasingly larger systems of care such as all critical care areas, women and children's services, all medical-surgical units, or mental health services. Ultimately, the nurse executive is accountable for nursing practice throughout the institution. In addition, he or she is the link between professional practice within the hospital and the expectations, standards, and regulation of practice that originate from outside the hospital itself.

Nursing administration is an area of advanced practice within the discipline of nursing. Although the description in the preceding paragraph focuses on the role of hospital-based nurse administrators, the reader should be cognizant that nurses manage the practice of nursing and delivery of health care services within and across all settings.

Ambulatory Practice

The second most prevalent arena for nursing practice is ambulatory care. The number of nurses employed in this area increased by 29% between 1984 and 1988.[25] Ambulatory care nurses provide a diversity of services to clients. The largest number of ambulatory care nurses work in solo or group practice in physicians' offices.[25] Other areas of practice include free-standing emergency clinics, ambulatory surgery centers, occupational health positions, residential centers for senior citizens, dialysis centers, and rehabilitation centers. The term "ambulatory care" is applied to systems that serve "walk-in" clients, who return to their homes at the end of the visit.

Nurses in ambulatory practice offer a number of services to clients. Education, health counseling, health maintenance, and prevention and primary care are components of their role.[7] In some settings, nurses regularly administer hands-on, high technology care similar to that found in hospitals, for a limited period of time. This occurs most frequently within ambulatory surgery centers and emergency clinics, and in dialysis centers.

Occupational health nursing is a rapidly expanding area of ambulatory care. The focus of the occupational nurse's practice is a healthy worker who contributes to the productivity of the company. These nurses are also concerned with health maintenance, health promotion, and health education.[21]

Community Practice

Public health departments, visiting nurses' associations, and home health agencies are the prime settings for community practice (Bridge to Home Health Care). Public health nurses are employed by tax-supported

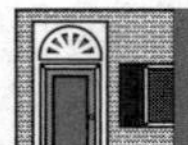

BRIDGE TO HOME HEALTH CARE

Health Care Personnel

The individuals who provide service to clients in their homes are human bridges to home health care. This is true whether the provider is a nurse, home health aide, physical therapist, occupational therapist, nutritionist, social worker, physician, or dentist. To maximize client outcomes of care, every member of the home health care team should follow some basic principles as they practice their specialty. These principles include the following:

1. You are a guest in someone's home. Your behavior needs to convey that you recognize that role.
2. Respect the client's cultural, religious, and ethnic heritage. Hesitate before contradicting that heritage because the client may not follow your advice anyway.
3. Almost every home health client has family members or significant others who will also offer advice and will serve as your advocate or foe. Try to develop them to be your advocates.
4. The client owns the health-related problem that initiated your home visits. That problem is just one portion of the client's past, present, and future life. Therefore, it is the client who experiences, learns to understand, and can ultimately solve that problem. It is your goal to help clients and their families become as independent as possible. Talk to your peers and supervisors when you sense you are losing that perspective.
5. Enjoy the unique autonomy and challenges of providing highly complex care in the home setting. Home health practice requires integration of high-technology skills, teaching, case management, and monitoring. Remember the necessity of communication with other members of the health care team. Because the home health nurse is usually responsible for judging whether or not the client can safely remain at home, other team members need to share this information through oral and written means.
6. Maintain your sense of humor.

Box 2–2. The Future of the Health Care System in the United States

The following is an interview with Virginia Trotter Betts, MSN, JD, RN, President, American Nurses' Association, and former Robert Wood Johnson Health Policy Fellow, 1987 to 1988. Questioner (Q) is Bonita Pilon, DSN, RN, CNAA, Assistant Professor, Vanderbilt University.

Q: When we review the history of our health care system over the past 70 years, we see it's been characterized by a period of expansion, and then a period of regulation and cost containment. Where is the nation heading next?

A: I think most people believe the next big era of health policy development is going to be in the area of quality and effectiveness, but I think to say that would imply that we have solved the problem of cost containment, which we have not. I believe, therefore, that the nation will continue to focus on cost, and only when effectiveness, initiatives, and quality measures also have an impact on cost will we truly move forward.

Q: So you believe that effectiveness is going to have to be tied up with cost; that we are going to be looking at these together?

A: I think that there was a belief for a while that the next big period in health policy, or trend in health care, would be to go from expansion to concerns about costs to concerns about quality. I believe that, in fact, we have never put to rest concerns about costs. People cannot think about quality in a pure way as yet.

Q: One issue that is raised repeatedly is that a patient's ability to purchase care does in fact determine what kind of care he or she receives, or certainly has a major impact on the patient's ability to have access to care. Many groups have called for major reform for our health care system with regard to access and reimbursement. Would you comment on what initiative the nursing profession has made with regard to health care reform, and on the initiatives other groups are making?

A: First of all, many, many organized groups have called for some kind of major reform in the health care system. The type of reform suggested varies from group to group. Some groups are really calling for rapid and radical reform. Nursing has long been concerned, as the hands-on provider, 24 hours a day in hospitals and nursing homes, about changing the type of care delivered, and how it's delivered, and to whom it's delivered, and when. The American Nurses' Association, in collaboration with the Tri-council for Nursing, went forward to the American people in May, 1991, with Nursing's Agenda for Health Reform. More than 65 specialty nursing organizations, representing more than 1,000,000 professional nurses, have signed on in support of this agenda. The reform paper, which is a statement of principles and a statement of directions, is being followed almost immediately by white papers to discuss the specifics. The Agenda identifies that problems in the American health care system are caused by access, cost, and quality issues and then describes what nursing wants to see happen to solve these problems.

Q: Where will this initiative go? Now that the ANA and other organized nursing groups have come forward with this very proactive stance on reforming our health care system, what are the next steps? How does this become action?

A: It becomes action at the federal, state, and local level. I think that it becomes action championed by nursing leaders. The president of the ANA and the president of the National League for Nursing (NLN), a member of the Tri-council and another organization that has been very interested in health policy, have been making the rounds in Washington with key Republican and Democratic leaders looking at proposals that they have on the legislative agenda, sharing the Nursing Agenda with them. The ANA evaluates every bill filed in Congress about health care to see how it fits with the overall direction of Nursing's Agenda. At the state and local level we are trying to make as many nurses as possible experts on the Agenda so they can talk with their state legislators and city officials.

Q: To your knowledge, has the nursing profession come forward with a proposal that is in direct opposition to any that have emerged from other organized groups? Specifically, I wonder about the American Medical Association (AMA), if indeed they have a proposal.

A: They do have a proposal. The last time I spoke publicly about Nursing's Agenda, I shared the podium with the president of a state medical association. At upcoming state nurses' association meetings, I and other officers of nursing organizations will be discussing our Agenda with the AMA as well as with the officers of the Health Insurance Association of America (HIAA), which also has a reform plan. Our proposals are all different. When you read them you will see that everyone is concerned about cost, quality, and access; however, when you analyze the solutions proposed by each group, differences emerge. There are two critical components to nursing's agenda. First, we have called for access—universal access—for all Americans. That universal access would be identified with a basic level of benefits. The nation has not indicated a willingness to provide open access to all health services without some control of cost, and some control of what basic benefits would entail. As you know, we currently ration health care by limiting access. Nursing believes that if we **must** ration, that rationing should focus on the package of health care benefits, not on eliminating certain people from necessary services. We further believe that a key component of health care has been overlooked in the past—access to primary care. Primary care is best delivered at convenient, familiar sites, or consumer-friendly sites such as the workplace, schools, and homes. This is much like the old public health model of 50 years ago, in which most had access to a primary provider who then made appropriate referrals when the scope of care

Box 2–2. The Future of the Health Care System in the United States (continued)

exceeded their practice. We moved away from that model during implementation of the entitlement and fee-for-service programs. We would like to go back to a program in which everyone has access to a health provider, there is a real focus on prevention and health promotion, and there is a focus on children. Our proposal calls for a major focus on children aged 0 to 18, with in-depth services for children, especially in schools. I think the country has been less than prudent in having put all of our health dollars into acute care. We are a society that in every area of life believes in a high-tech lifestyle. That's certainly true in health care. That's not to say that acute care, trauma care, and so forth aren't important. Nursing's position is that acute care should not and cannot take all of the resources out of the system.

Q: It's less than 10 years until the next century. Will health care reform be accomplished before then?

A: I believe the answer to that is yes. It's not just because I'm an optimist and want to see it happen. It's because of what makes policy. When does policy get made? That's when the benefits of doing something outweigh the costs. Some people say we can't reform health care, that we can't bring 37 million uninsured and 30 million under insured persons into the system, that we can't pay for any more health care. There are estimates that predict that the United States will spend almost $3 trillion on health care by the year 2000 if we change nothing about our system. This is an incredible cost of providing care; therefore, something has to happen. I believe whoever wins the presidential election in 1996, and the Congress that comes in with that president, will have to have put health care at the top of their domestic agenda. I expect dramatic reform after '96, and I think it will be caused by increasing lack of access to care. Consider the fact that most of us are just one step away from being uninsured because most people currently receive health insurance through their employer. As the employer makes efforts to cut costs, moving people to part-time, and as people lose jobs due to recession, there are more and more people among the ranks of the uninsured. I don't think the nation can tolerate it for much longer.

Q: You've talked about the era that will be coming; you've talked about how it might come about; you've discussed the forces that are moving agendas around in our country; and we've talked about a possible time frame for change. Is there anything else you'd like to add?

A: I would like to expand on how Nursing's Agenda for Health Care Reform is different from other plans. One of the differences is that people would get primary care and prevention. Another thing that we propose is that care should be given by the most qualified provider in the most appropriate setting. For nursing, with our tremendous growth in advanced practice nurses, we believe that there is a lot of room for other providers to come into the system, lowering costs and increasing access. This will make a big difference in our future health care system. I also think our proposal is the most definite about cost containment. We believe that there has to be, and we are committed to, both managed care and case management for continuity of care as well as a way of controlling the use of appropriate resources. Our Agenda also calls for controlled growth, for regional decisions about where certain procedures would be performed. We certainly believe that the current system has too much capacity for certain kinds of beds and not enough capacity for other kinds of services. We believe that there needs to be some direct governmental intervention regarding these issues. Those are risk-taking statements to make, considering 67 per cent of nurses work in hospitals. We believe, however, that there continue to be too many hospitals with too many vacant beds and there has to be a different way of distributing man-power and services. Our initial proposal is being followed by many white papers describing what the public health model of the future looks like; what care in the work place should look like; what's an appropriate package of mental health services; all of these are in process now. I'm pleased to say that with the ANA, many of the specialty nursing organizations are working together on our position papers. These people are the real experts in the content area. I believe that our agenda is a much richer proposal, coming from so many nurses, not from just one organization.

Q: One of the things that I hear you saying is that although nursing's agenda may, if it were totally adopted, change or limit the kinds of services found in acute care settings, nursing practice opportunities would be broadened far beyond hospital practice as we know it today. You have suggested that nurses would be an integral part of providing universal access to basic benefits when you speak of the public health model of the future.

A: I think that's what we in nursing know is happening already. Nursing practice is expanding well beyond the hospital into all sorts of settings. Nurses are seen as invaluable to the provision of hands-on service. What the profession believes is that one of the reasons that health care costs so much and has limited access, is because of both regulatory and legal barriers to practice. These barriers allowed some disciplines to offer services and other disciplines can only offer those services if the first discipline says it's ok. We believe that this should be a system where the consumer is allowed to choose. My favorite part of our plan is that it is clear that health care is the consumer's decision and that the consumer needs to take the responsibility for making healthy choices, living a healthy lifestyle. The consumer should seek out the most appropriate health provider, unbound by artificial barriers.

Q: It seems that the decade of the '90s will be fraught with much debate, and in the end, we believe, a radically different health care system will emerge, because it has to. Thank you, Dr. Betts, for sharing your expertise.

health departments. Because of the tax support, client services are provided free or for a very reduced fee. Nurses carry a case load of families that includes a range of ages and conditions across the health-illness continuum. These nurses are challenged to deliver health services in many settings: the home, school, and clinics (which often include providing care or advice on family planning, prenatal and new baby care, and sexually transmitted diseases). The nurse must draw from a broad knowledge base in nursing as well as in community resources. The goals of public health nursing are health maintenance and client independence.[12]

Home health care is a rapidly growing segment of the health care industry and is expected to continue its growth in the 1990s. Since 1972, the number of Medicare certified home health care agencies has grown from 2212 to 5800.[14] Factors such as an aging population and the rising costs of inpatient care have influenced the growth of this industry. The opportunity for nursing practice continues to expand as the number of agencies increases and more clients are cared for at home rather than in the hospital.

Home health clients require care of different intensity. Maintenance home care is used for clients who need assistance with personal care or homemaking and whose underlying medical condition is stable. Such care is not provided by registered nurses. Intermediate home care is used for clients with a relatively stable medical condition, but who require professional level care to promote rehabilitation or other improvement. Intensive-level home care is required by clients who have unstable, serious illnesses needing skilled nursing care. Such clients would likely be hospitalized if such care were not available. Registered nurses provide care in the home for clients in the last two categories.[10]

Community and public health nursing has also shown more growth in employment of nurses than hospitals in the last decade. The primary growth was among those nurses employed in nonhospital-based home health care agencies (other than visiting nurse associations).[25]

Nurses in community practice make independent assessments and decisions. The community setting promotes a highly autonomous practice.

Advanced Practice

Nurses in advanced practice are skilled specialists usually working with specific client populations both in the hospital and in the community. These specialists have acquired advanced education and experience in their area of practice.

Clinical nurse specialists (CNS) are the largest group of advanced practice nurses. Employed primarily in hospitals, these nurses have multifaceted roles that are performed differently in different settings, even within the same institution. The five components of the CNS role are educator, practitioner, researcher, consultant, and manager. Some CNSs work primarily in the practitioner role, often in collaboration with a group of physicians, providing highly skilled care to a specific group of clients (such as high-risk perinatal clients or heart transplant patients). The type of care provided by the CNS encompasses and surpasses that provided by the staff nurse.

Other CNSs focus more strongly on the educator role, teaching and role modeling expert skills to staff nurses, thus supporting client care more indirectly. All CNSs work in a consultant role at least part of the time. Nurses, physicians, and other health care providers frequently seek their input for solving complex care dilemmas for specific patients or groups of clients. CNSs are expected to be knowledgeable about the latest research developments within their area of practice and to add to the development of health care's knowledge base through research of their own.

The manager role of the CNS has traditionally been focused on the development of specific clinical programs within the hospital. For example, the CNS for cardiac surgery clients might be asked to develop a proposal for the care of pediatric open heart clients, whom the hospital anticipates admitting very soon. Such a proposal would specify the care needs and equipment support required based on the CNS's clinical expertise, as well as identify the education and training required for all staff involved in the care of these clients. The CNS would be expected to develop an educational program to prepare staff for these clients, implement the program, and evaluate the results.

A new type of advanced practitioner emerged in the late 1980s in response to changes within health care delivery. In order to improve the process of delivering inpatient care, many hospitals initiated a case management system of care. Nurse case managers work with specific client populations and the physicians treating those clients, as well as with the staff nurses managing the day-to-day client care. Their role is to improve the coordination of care for clients across nursing units, hospital departments, and into the community. Using pre-established collaborative case management plans and critical pathways for specific diagnoses, case managers work to keep the client moving toward a discharge within an acceptable time frame while maintaining or enhancing quality care.

Nurse case managers are found at different levels of the hospital organization. In some settings, CNSs function as case managers and, therefore, are not involved in direct client care activities on a specific unit. In other settings, most notably the New England Medical Center (Boston, MA), staff nurses function in a case management group practice across nursing units. Certain staff nurses in key units where specific types of clients reside during their hospitalization, form networks with each other and with the attending physicians. Nurses within these networks meet weekly to coordinate their case load of patients throughout the hospital stay and back to the community.

A third type of nurse case manager also emerged at the end of the 1980s. At Carondelet St. Mary's Hospital (Tucson, AZ), case managers are primarily based in the community, although they are employed by the hospital. These nurses follow a case load of frail elderly clients, multiple sclerosis clients, and others who are at risk for repeat admissions to the hospital due to both their medical and social situations. These nurse case managers strive to support the client toward independent living in the community and provide symptom management while monitoring them for signs of exacerbations of chronic illnesses. One of the goals of the program is to facilitate hospital admission early in the exacerbation period in order to avoid the most costly (and potentially the most devastating) portion of a hospital stay, such as emergency room and intensive care.

Nurse practitioners (NPs) are another type of nurse in advanced practice. These nurses have advanced education in the diagnosis and treatment of common, recurrent illnesses as well as in health maintenance and promotion. They are trained in advanced pharmacology and, in many states, have prescription-writing authority. Nurse practitioners work in community clinics, private practice, and in group practice with physicians. Licensure requirements vary from state to state, but NPs are required to be certified in their area of practice (e.g., family nurse practitioner, pediatric nurse practitioner, and geriatric nurse practitioner), and work under protocols established in collaboration with a precepting physician. The certification process is administered by the American Nurses Association and by some specialty organizations. Nurse anesthetists (CRNAs) and nurse midwives (CNMs) are two types of advanced practitioners who are certified through specialty organizations (i.e., Council on Certification of Nurse Anesthetists and the American College of Nurse Midwives).

Some advanced practice nurses establish an independent practice. Psychiatric–mental health specialists may open their own psychotherapy practice. Family nurse practitioners may choose to own and operate their own office practice. The laws governing the scope of practice and reimbursement vary across states. Some states have enacted legislation favorable to independent nursing practice, whereas others have not.

Advanced practice nurses, though practicing in a variety of settings, have a common foundation for their practice: advanced educational preparation. Most of the roles described in this section require a master's degree in nursing (MSN). These include the clinical nurse specialist and nurse practitioner. An MSN is also required for psychiatric nurses in independent practice who seek reimbursement from third-party payors. The nurse case manager role has not yet demanded master's preparation. However, institutions employing case managers set their own employment criteria; some agencies require the MSN, whereas others do not at this time.

VARIATIONS IN CLIENT POPULATIONS

Nurses work with clients who have diverse social, economic, and cultural backgrounds, all of which have an impact on the types of health care needs they may experience. In this section, some of the special populations that nurses serve are described.

Nursing Across the Lifespan

From before conception in a family planning clinic or infertility practice, to hospice care in the home, the presence of nurses is vital to the individual, the family, the community, and the nation. Nurses have special concerns for groups especially at risk for poor health outcomes. Nurses provide critical services to prenatal and perinatal clients, particularly those who are adolescent, living in poverty, single, and unemployed. Case finding, screening, referral, followup, and education are among the services that nurses provide to this at-risk group. These nursing services take place primarily in the community.

Among the neonatal-pediatric population, nurses again provide important services. Public health nurses follow at-risk neonates in the home after discharge from the hospital. They are most concerned with the stability of the family unit and its capacity to care for the preterm or otherwise compromised infant. Ongoing education and support are provided by the public health nurse.

Nurses in other ambulatory and community agencies monitor and support the growth and development of children. School nurses provide primary care and counseling to school-age children. These nurses are concerned with proper nutrition, prevention of substance abuse, and recognition of and intervention for child abuse at the first opportunity.

Nurses across various settings care for adult clients from the early 20s through old age. Most younger adults come in contact with nurses through occupational health programs or in acute care hospitals when accident or illness threatens the individual's health. Women in their childbearing years, a special segment of the adult population, are followed by nurses in community health practice as well as in hospital practice.

Middle-aged and older adults are cared for by nurses skilled in chronic care, acute-critical care, home care, and long-term care. The nurse plays a vital part in assisting this population with health promotion, disease prevention, symptom management, performance of activities of daily living, independent living to the fullest extent possible, and support for a dignified death. The number of frail elderly are increasing; nurses in geriatric practice provide multiple services to these clients at home, in the hospital, and in long-term facilities.

Geographic Variations in Practice

Nurses work with clients who live in a variety of settings, from the inner city to rural communities. The challenges, as well as the resources to meet those challenges, are often different in each area.

The rural nurse must be a skilled generalist who is able to assess and refer patients for secondary and tertiary care, which usually is many miles away. This nurse has limited resources to call on for consultation. There are relatively few clinical nurse specialists or other advanced practitioners working in rural areas.

Many rural communities have no hospital, and some do not have physicians. It is incumbent on the rural community health nurse to recognize abnormalities early in the course of illness, make timely referrals to far-away centers, and follow up clients to ensure they were treated. One of the greatest challenges for the rural population can be transportation to the city for care. Rural nurses work to facilitate the client and family's transition to the urban area and their return to the community.

Nurses practicing in inner city clinics and hospitals face other challenges. Public health clinics serve clients with limited ability to pay but who are in dire need of family planning services, prenatal care, pediatric services, and general health care. Nurses in both the clinic and the public hospital must be knowledgeable about the health practices and beliefs of many ethnic groups that have an impact on their client's ability to comply with the prescribed plan of care. Although nurses practicing in inner cities often have access to many health care experts for consultation, tax-supported hospitals and clinics are often underfunded, resulting in a chronic insufficiency of medical supplies, personnel, and beds. Nurses in these areas become expert at conserving and improvising to attain treatment goals.

Variations in Lifestyle

Nurses work with clients who live different lifestyles, often different from the lifestyle of the nurse. Homeless and substance abuse clients are two examples of such populations at risk that nurses serve.

Homeless clients are cared for in many ways across the country. The primary initiative among health care providers is to make health care accessible to these patients. In some cities, mobile health care vans travel from site to site offering primary care and referral. In other regions, walk-in clinics are open in the areas frequented by the homeless population. Homeless persons have special health care needs that range from diseases of the feet and legs due to walking, to mental health conditions. Nurses, particularly nurse practitioners and community health nurses, are critical to the provision of health care to these individuals and families.

People who abuse drugs, alcohol, or both also have special health care needs. In addition to their problems of addiction, the lifestyles they may lead in order to procure illegal substances and alcohol (e.g., prostitution, theft, violent crime) put them at considerable risk for illness, disease, and injury. They are also members of families and other communal groups and, therefore, are at risk of transmitting their addiction to unborn children, transmitting infectious diseases to others (such as hepatitis, AIDS, or other sexually transmitted diseases), or both. Nurses may encounter persons who are substance abusers in several ways. Nurses are active in the treatment of substance abuse at both inpatient and outpatient centers. They support and monitor the individual's acute detoxification and recovery period. Nurses in the community often confront clients who show signs of substance abuse in an attempt to gain client interest in referral for treatment. Among those persons who are not in recovery, nurses screen for and treat the undesirable health conditions that result from substance abuse. Community-based nurses also educate and counsel clients and their significant others about the dangers of addiction and ways to prevent the spread of infectious disease.

HIV Infection

One of the biggest challenges facing nursing and the health care community in general is the care of persons infected with human immunodeficiency virus (HIV, also known as AIDS). Nurses from across the country have risen to meet the challenge in clients' homes, in the community, and in acute care hospitals.

Nurse case managers work with AIDS patients in many large cities, coordinating and procuring necessary medical and social services. Clinic nurses in various sites across the United States give aerosol pentamidine treatments to prevent respiratory complications to outpatients. Nurse practitioners follow HIV clients from the onset of infection for their primary health care needs. Acute care nurses care for clients when they are hospitalized for exacerbations, and hospice nurses assist AIDS clients toward obtaining a dignified death at home. Nurses provide direct client care, emotional support, education, prevention counseling to friends and family, and support for self-care to AIDS clients. Wherever the need arises, nurses have come forth with compassion and concern to meet those needs.

Summary

The health care system in the United States is large and complex with many stakeholders (also see Box 2-3 for a comparison of health care in the United States and Canada). It is also a system under considerable pressure to change as a direct result of rising costs and lower accessibility to basic care for a growing number of citizens. This is the environment in which nursing practice takes place. This chapter has acquainted the reader with the political challenges facing the nation; it has also demonstrated that nurses are in the mainstream of service to both advantaged and disadvantaged client populations. Nurses play a critical role in delivering health care to the United States population. There are many who believe that nurses may be the key to revamping the health care system toward access to basic primary care for all citizens. The contribution of the nursing profession to the nation's health has never been so important as we move into the 21st century.

Box 2–3. Comparisons between the Canadian Health Care System and the United States Health Care System

As discussion and debate regarding health care reform intensify, there is increasing comparison of the United States health care system with the Canadian system. Some stakeholders suggest the Canadian model be adopted in the United States. Others are very much opposed to such a transformation. A brief overview of the Canadian system and selected comparisons to the system in the United States are described here.

The Canadian health care program is universal, comprehensive, publicly funded (with no financial access barriers for care), and privately delivered. All citizens are covered for all medically necessary services through a federal-provincial health insurance system. The United States system is not universal, comprehensive, or publicly funded except for Medicare and Medicaid enrollees (31 million and 19 million, respectively). These enrollees are subject to financial means tests (Medicaid) and copayment/deductible access barriers (Medicaid and Medicare). The majority of United States citizens (180 million) have private health insurance, largely financed through employers (82 per cent). Coverage varies widely, from minimal to comprehensive. Premium rates, copayments, and deductibles also vary by policy type.[18] An estimated 37 million Americans have no health insurance whatsoever.[24]

The Canadian system has evolved over more than 40 years, beginning at the provincial level. The federal-provincial funding arrangements vary across provinces, and administration and control of the program is unique within each province and the two territories. Provinces are single-source payers for both hospital and physician expenditures. There is a centralized locus of control, and the role of private insurance companies is limited by law. In the United States, private insurers are highly influential in the health care system, covering more than 77 per cent of the population.[23] The locus of control in the United States is dispersed over multiple-payer sources, making control of resources much more difficult.

Using a centralized control approach, each Canadian province (and territory) prospectively determines each hospital's global budget for the coming year. A global budget is the total or lump sum amount the hospital will receive for its services. Hospitals themselves determine the distribution of allocated funds within the institution. No deficit spending is permitted; hospitals must live within their budgets. Methods for adjusting the global budget vary by province. In Ontario (the most populated province), the Ministry of Health makes adjustments based on inflation, workload, approved new programs or expansion of existing programs, and increases in cost or volume related to certain services such as dialysis, oncology, neonatal intensive care, and cardiovascular surgery.[24] Within these constraints, hospitals must serve all patients who seek care.

Provincial governments also negotiate reimbursement rates with medical associations, and the fees are set prospectively. Aggregate physician expenditures are controlled in five provinces (which contain 80 per cent of the population) through a threshold approach. If physician expenditures within the province exceed what was budgeted due to increased volume of client services delivered, provinces can recoup their losses by adjusting future reimbursement rates downward or by paying current fees at a discount. This approach affects the total amount of money available to the medical profession for reimbursement and indirectly affects individual physician income.[18]

Like other provinces, Quebec negotiates expenditure targets for the total physician group; however, individual physician income targets are set as well. There are imposed ceilings on the quarterly gross billings of individual physicians, and if a physician exceeds the ceiling, he or she is reimbursed at only 25 per cent of the allowable rate for additional care delivered. The Ministry of Health also reimburses new physicians in rural areas at a higher rate than those opening practices in urban areas, thereby influencing the geographic distribution of care.[18]

Clearly, the Canadian government at the provincial level has much tighter control over health care expenditures than is found among the multiple payers in the United States. Other system-wide comparison data are displayed in the following table.

Selected Comparisons of United States and Canadian Health Care Systems

	Canada	United States
Health care as per cent of GNP	8.7 [1988]	11.2 [1987]
Per capita expenditures (U.S.$)	$1,556 [1989]	$1,973 [1987]
Length of stay (days)	8.1 [1988]	7.1 [1987]
Cost per hospital stay (U.S.$)	$2,014 [1988]	$3,532 [1987]
Cost per day (U.S.$)	$243 [1988]	$500 [1987]
Beds per 1000 population	7.1 [1986]	5.4 [1986]
Occupancy rate	83.8% [1988]	68.4% [1987]
Physicians per population ratio	486 [1985]	418 [1985]

GNP, Gross National Product.

Satisfaction surveys have indicated that 95 per cent of Canadians surveyed preferred their own health care system over a United States model whereas only 37 per cent of United States citizens surveyed preferred the United States system over the Canadian model.[4] Health status indicators for 1982 to 1984 reveal that Canada's infant mortality rate and age-standardized death rate for all causes were lower than those for the United States and that life expectancy at birth for males and females was slightly higher in Canada.[18] All expenditure and health status outcome data provide support for the apparent success of the Canadian model.

Can or should the United States replicate such a model? There is strong debate as to the feasibility of replicating the Canadian system in the United States. Canada has only one tenth the population (25 million versus 241 million) and only seven provincial and two territorial government structures in

Box continued on following page

Box 2–3. Comparisons between the Canadian Health Care System and the United States Health Care System (continued)

addition to the federal level. In contrast, there are 50 state governments with which the federal government would have to negotiate funding formulas. Moreover, the culture in the United States is substantially different with regard to government's role in the lives of citizens. Among Canadians, government is expected to design, implement, and support social programs.[18] In the United States there is much more emphasis on individual accountability and noninterference by government. The second critical factor that may prevent adoption of a Canadian-type model in the United States is the political environment. Congress and state legislatures are heavily influenced by special interest groups. A movement toward a centralized, single-payer system in the United States would likely produce intense opposition from hospital, physician, and health insurance lobbies, among others.

Finally, barriers to change may arise from among United States citizens who are adequately insured and enjoy health care "on demand." Shifting from the current open-ended system to a resource-controlled system would mandate care delivery on an "as needed" basis. Citizens would wait for elective services in some cases. Currently, only those uninsured (37 million) and underinsured United States citizens (19 million Medicaid plus unknown numbers of privately insured persons) are denied services or subject to delay. Under a single-payer, centralized control system, all citizens would be treated equitably within the health care system. Ability to pay would no longer separate the "haves" from the "have nots." Although many from both groups would welcome such a redistribution of health care resources, United States citizens would have to modify their expectations relating to health care services. As in Canada, there may be a gradual evolution to a single-payer system, and this evolution may begin at the state level. The decade of the 90s is the period in which the United States must resolve these issues.

Bibliography

1. Aiken, L. H., & Bays, K. D. (1984). The medicare debate—round one. *New England Journal of Medicine, 311,* 1196–1200.
2. American Nurses' Association (1991). *Agenda for health care reform.* Kansas City, Mo.: American Nurses' Association.
3. Bice, T. W. (1980). Health services planning and regulation. In S. J. Williams and P. R. Torrens (Eds.), *Introduction to health services* (pp. 267–321). New York: John Wiley.
4. Blendon, R. J. (1989). Three systems: A comparative survey. *Health Management Quarterly, 11,* 2–10.
5. Burda, D. (1991). Hospital industry regroups after Supreme Court upholds NRLB rule. *Modern Healthcare, 27* (17), 2–3.
6. Cherskov, M. (1987). Capitated payment will dominate by 1995: A study. *Hospitals, 61* (6), 83–84.
7. Daugherty, L. G., & Buchanan, G. J. (1985). Nursing role in ambulatory care. In L. L. Jarvis (Ed.), *Community health nursing: Keeping the public healthy* (pp. 263–275). Philadelphia: F. A. Davis.
8. Division of National Cost Estimates, Office of the Actuary, Health Care Financing Administration (1990). In P. Lee & C. Estes (Eds.), *The Nation's Health* (pp. 207–221). Boston: Jones & Bartlett.
9. Ethridge, P. (1991). A nursing HMO: Carondelet St. Mary's experience. *Nursing Management, 22* (7), 22–27.
10. Gallagher, B. M. (1985). Nursing role in home health care. In L. L. Jarvis (ed.), *Community health nursing: Keeping the public healthy* (pp. 337–350). Philadelphia: F. A. Davis.
11. Garner, J. S., et al. (1990). Strategic nursing management. Rockville, MD: Aspen.
12. Lewin, L. S. & Lewin, M. E. (1987). Financing charity care in an era of competition. *Health Affairs, 6* (1), 47–60.
13. Major, M. B. (1985). Nursing's role in public health. In L. L. Jarvis (Ed.), *Community health nursing: Keeping the public healthy* (pp. 311–325). Philadelphia: F. A. Davis.
14. National League for Nursing (1990). Improving the performance of nurse managers in home care. *A white paper.* New York: National League for Nursing.
15. Oberg, C. (1990). Medically uninsured children in the United States: A challenge to public policy. *Journal of School Health, 60* (10), 493–500.
16. Pilon, B. A., & Davis, S. (November, 1988). Health care delivery cost containment practices: History, current status, future directions. In N. Sanders (project director), *Cost management education for nurses.* Washington, D.C.: U. S. Department of Health and Human Services, Health Resources and Services Administration, Bureau of Health Professions, Division of Nursing (contract number 240-86-0064).
17. Poen, M. (1979). Politics, then health: The medicare compromise. In *Harry S. Truman versus the medical lobby* (pp. 174–209). Columbia, MO: University of Missouri Press.
18. Rakich, J. S. (1991). The Canadian and U.S. health care systems: Profiles and policies. *Journal of the American College of Healthcare Executives, 36*(1), 25–42.
19. Richardson, W. C. (1990). Financing health services. In S. J. Williams, & P. R. Torrens (Eds.), *Introduction to health services* (pp. 286–321). New York: John Wiley.
20. Rice, D. P. (1986). The medical care system: Past trends and future projections (1990). In P. Lee, & C. Estes (Eds.), *The Nation's Health* (pp. 72–93). Boston: Jones & Bartlett.
21. Silberstein, C. A. (1985). Nursing role in occupational health. In L. L. Jarvis (Ed.), *Community health nursing: Keeping the public healthy* (pp. 277–294). Philadelphia: F. A. Davis.
22. Steinwald, B., & Sloan, F. (1981). Regulatory approaches to hospital cost containment: A synthesis of the empirical evidence. In M. Olsen (Ed.), *A new approach to the economics of health care* (pp. 272–307). Washington, D.C.: American Enterprise Institute.
23. U.S. Department of Commerce, 1989. Statistical abstract of the United States, 1989. Washington, D.C.: Author.
24. U.S. Department of Health and Human Services, 1989. National medical expenditure survey: A profile of uninsured Americans, research findings 1. Publication No. PHS 89-3443. Washington, D.C.: Author.
25. U.S. Department of Health and Human Services, Public Health Service, Health Resources and Services Administration, Bureau of Health Professions, Division. (1990). *1988: The registered nurse population.* Washington, D.C.: Department of Health and Human Services.
26. White, J. (1991). Hospitals object to changes in capital payment policy. *Health Progress, 74* (4), 10–13.
27. Winslow, J. (January 29, 1991) Medical costs soar, defying firm's cures. *Wall Street Journal,* p. B1.

Unit

2

Holistic Aspects of Health Care

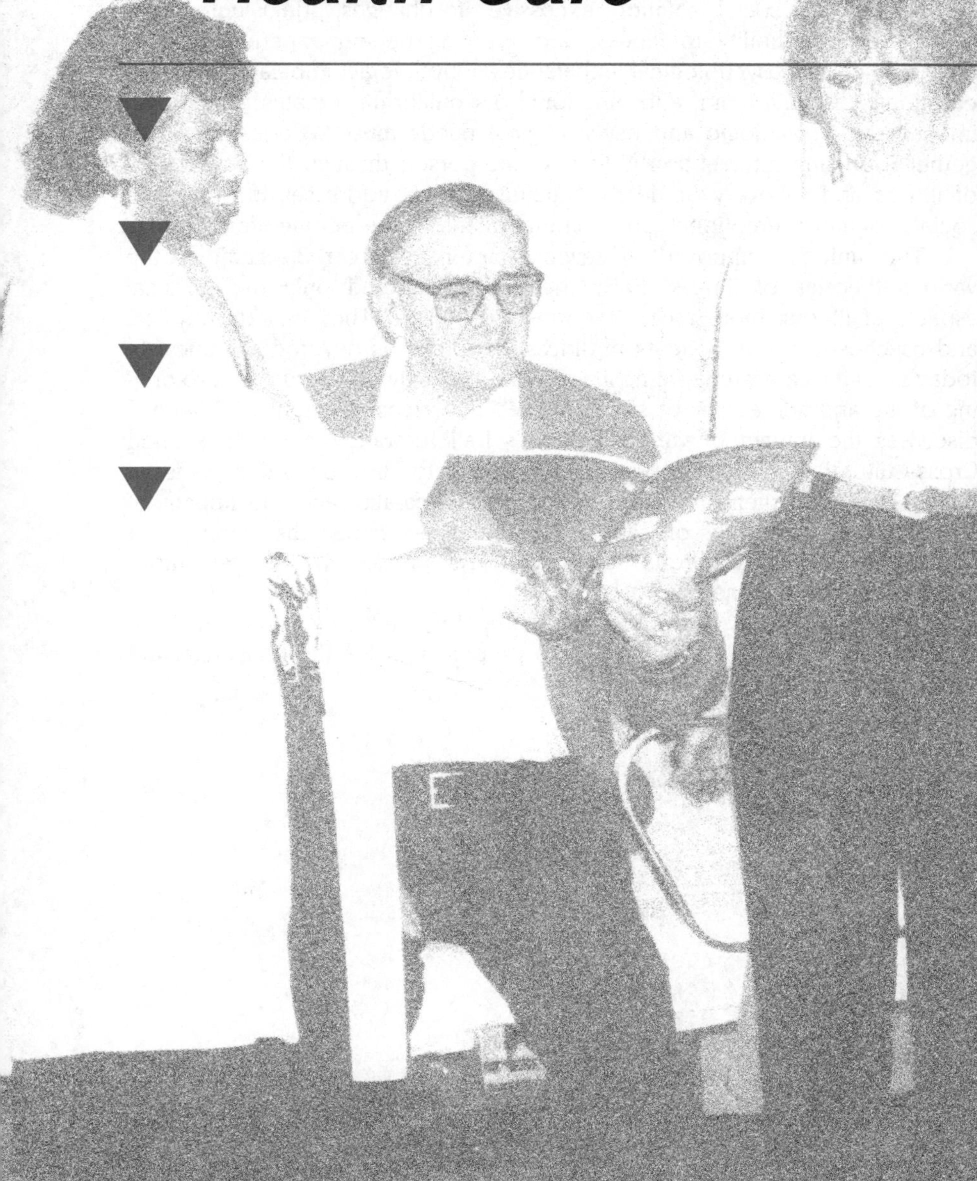

Chapter 1 considered the unique function of nursing and reviewed the nursing process. Nursing, we said, is the art of caring. Nurses use the five steps of the nursing process to care for others. Chapter 2 examined the nurse's role in health care of yesterday, today, and tomorrow.

In this unit, we consider how to care for the whole person. Although body and mind are susceptible to different types of stressors, we emphasize the interrelationship between body and mind and how physical problems create emotional problems and vice versa.

Stress (e.g., social isolation, excessive life changes, grief) increases a persons's susceptibility to illness, and every ill person experiences both physiologic and psychological imbalances. Physiologic imbalances create emotional disequilibrium, and emotional disequilibrium creates physiologic imbalances. Physiologic and psychological needs must be considered together if nursing intervention is to help the person through the experience of illness and recovery or death. Nursing process addresses the physical, social, cognitive, emotional, and spiritual needs of the people we care for.

This unit is composed of seven chapters. Chapter 3 examines the various theories of illness. Early theories considered only the physical aspects of illness; more recent theories are holistic. They include physical and psychosocial components of illness. Chapter 4 is devoted to ethics. In today's health care arena, almost everyone can stay alive, but the prolonging of life and sometimes of suffering presents ethical dilemmas. Chapter 5 discusses the impact of various people's beliefs about health. It is titled Cross-Cultural Nursing. Chapter 6 is devoted to the spiritual aspects of health care and clients. Chapter 7 addresses sexuality and the impact of illness on the sexuality of clients. Chapter 8 examines the family, and Chapter 9 describes chronic conditions. As people live longer, more chronic conditions emerge.

Nurses are firmly committed to caring for the whole client and the family of the client. This unit will help prepare you for the challenge and rewards of holistic nursing.

Chapter 3

Theories of Health and Illness

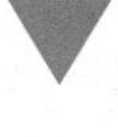

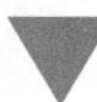

THEORIES OF CAUSATION OF ILLNESS

Who gets sick and why? It has been and is still a common question. Since early in human evolution there have been recordings of illness and its effect on the body and mind. Consider the stories from the Bible about Job and his multiple afflictions.

Ideas about the cause of illnesses have been influenced by the prevailing culture and scientific thought of the time. Early theories of disease causation regarded illness as a form of demonic possession. Healers of that age frequently used potions and chants to rid the body of the demon possessing it and causing the illness. Some people had holes cut into their skulls to enable evil spirits, which were believed to be causing disease, to leave the body (Fig. 3-1). Other cultures believed that illness was a punishment for sin. This concept is not uncommon in people living today and can cause significant stress for the client and family as they ponder over their past.

Historical Theories of the Causes of Disease

In the latter part of the 19th century, scientists began to unravel the basic causes of infectious disease. With the advent of Pasteur's germ theory, modern medicine was born. Pasteur proposed that a specific microorganism was capable of causing an infectious disease. Pasteur's theory was an important development in medical care and helped reduce the deaths from infection. The bubonic plague had killed about one fourth of the population of Europe in the sixth century. Smallpox infected three fourths of the population of Europe and killed or left people with severe scars or disfig-

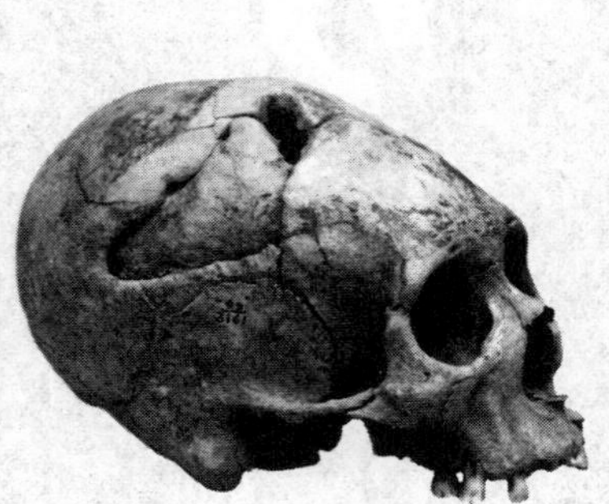
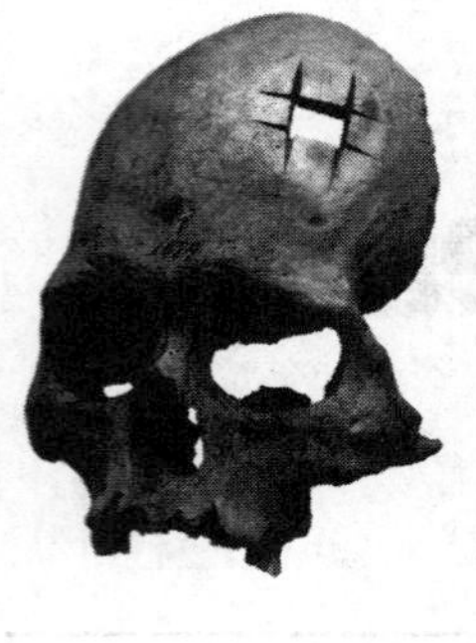
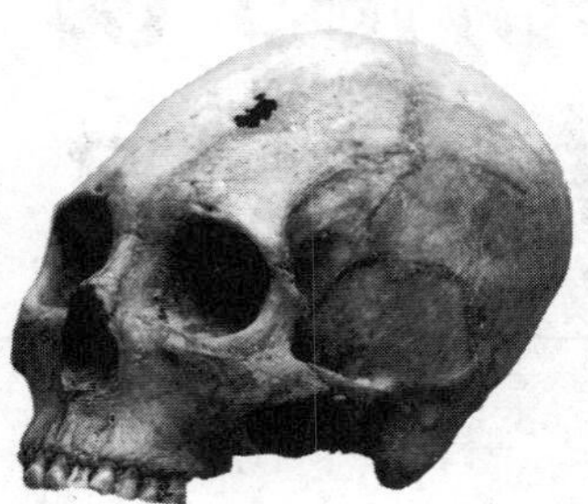

▲ *Figure 3–1*

Skull with trephine holes.

Holes were surgically made into the skulls in an attempt to treat disease. The purpose of the holes was to enable evil spirits, believed to cause disease, to leave the body. Ancient skulls show that people survived even though very large trephine holes were made. In fact, some skulls show multiple large holes that had healed. The practice still exists among primitive people in parts of Algeria and Melanesia, although it is fast becoming extinct. (Courtesy of American Museum of Natural History.)

urement. Even in recent times, infections can be a significant health problem. Poliomyelitis terrorized the United States in the 1940s and 1950s. Poliomyelitis killed many people and left many others paralyzed. Identification of the organism led to the development of the Salk and Sabin vaccines, which prevent poliomyelitis. In the mid-1970s, legionellosis, a previously unknown pneumonia-like infection, killed 29 people in Philadelphia. A causative organism was found, and this information led to treatment. In the early 1980s, some women who used superabsorbent tampons developed toxic shock syndrome. Again the organism was identified, and treatment methods were illuminated. The most recent infection to harm humans is acquired immune deficiency syndrome (AIDS). Again, the agent has been identified, and treatments are being developed.

Obviously, the germ theory cannot explain all diseases, and as science expanded, more complex theories were developed. The biomedical model explains disease as a result of malfunctioning organs or cells. Within this model, conditions can be classified as diseases if they have a recognized cause and if there is a consistently identifiable group of signs and symptoms. For example, diabetes mellitus is a disease caused by a malfunctioning pancreas. The signs and symptoms of early diabetes mellitus are polydypsia (increased thirst), polyuria (frequent urination), and polyphagia (increased hunger). The signs and symptoms of diabetes are directly related to an alteration in a physiologic process in the pancreas. The symptoms are due to an inability of the body to use sugar because there is no insulin to carry it into the cell.

The biomedical model focuses on the cause-and-effect relationships but tends to ignore the psychosocial components of diseases. For example, John is a 45-year-old businessman who develops diabetes mellitus. He is willing to change his lifestyle and give himself daily insulin injections, reduce his weight, and watch his diet more closely. His wife will do most of his cooking and will follow a diabetic plan. John can check his blood sugar at his office. In contrast, Jim is a 19-year-old college student with the same symptoms of diabetes and the same blood sugar levels as John. But the changes Jim needs to incorporate will not be as easy for him. He eats irregularly because of the scheduling of his classes, drinks on weekends with his friends, and cannot envision being able to monitor his blood sugar levels during the daytime hours. The biomedical model classifies both John and Jim as diabetics, yet the theory cannot explain the varying reactions to the disease due to age and personality and likelihood of compliance with the therapy.

Neither the germ theory nor the biomedical model can explain the widespread increase in noninfectious chronic diseases that affect modern civilizations. In the past, the high death rate from epidemics of infectious diseases meant that many people did not live long enough to develop chronic illnesses, especially those conditions that come about with aging. Even today, underdeveloped countries with high death rates from infectious diseases are less concerned with heart disease and cancer—ailments that plague industrialized nations.

The disorders that contribute to morbidity figures in developed nations today are ones in which a client's behavior, lifestyle and genetic background play an underlying role in the development of disease. For example, essential hypertension and coronary artery disease cannot be well explained through the biomedical model. The genetic background of the client, his lifestyle, his diet, and his stress response are aspects of the disease. It is becoming more common to probe the etiology of disease by examining the interrelationship of the client and the internal and external environment. Even infectious disease can be examined in a new light. Why does one person "catch a cold" when another person living in the same environment does not?

Newer theories of illness causation help to explain some of these issues. These new theories can be called a homeostatic or multicausal approach to illness because many factors within each client are examined.

Homeostatic Theories of the Causes of Disease

BERNARD AND CANNON

Claude Bernard, a 19th-century physiologist, laid the foundation for homeostatic theories. Bernard was the first scientist to describe the internal milieu or environment of the body. He hypothesized correctly that if an organism is to live, it must have the capacity to maintain its internal environment. Bernard described some of the mechanisms that regulate the balance of internal body processes. He also saw health and illness in a new and enlightening way. He defined health as the ability of the human organism to maintain its internal environment in a constant state despite the variations placed on it by the external environment. He postulated that illness was the result of an imbalance in the body's internal environment, or a disruption in the body's ability to communicate with the external environment. He also defined disease as an adaptive effort by the body to restore its balance. He saw these adaptive efforts as appropriate to the illness but incorrect in magnitude. For example, when the diabetic client cannot use sugar for energy, he or she uses fats and proteins. When fats are used for energy, an acid is produced that alters the body's acid-base balance. So using Bernard's theory, the diabetic client has attempted to adapt to the lack of sugar but has created a new problem—acidosis.

Walter Cannon, a 20th-century physician, developed the concept of feedback mechanisms to explain Bernard's theory of regulation of the internal environment. He recognized that the body's coordinated self-regulating, physiologic processes are needed to maintain a steady state. Cannon coined the term "homeostasis," which comes from the Greek word *homoios*, meaning like, and *stasis*, meaning standing. Cannon described homeostasis as a dynamic equilibrium, as opposed to a static equilibrium. A dynamic equilibrium is a flexible ongoing process to maintain certain factors within a given range. He cited the body's ability to maintain temperature, blood pressure, fluid and electrolyte balances, serum glucose levels, blood oxygen, and carbon dioxide levels in his theory.

Cannon also developed the concept of "fight or flight" to explain the body's reactions to emergencies. The fight-or-flight response prepares the body for muscular activity (e.g., running away) in response to a perceived or actual threat. The adrenal medulla is the pivotal organ for this response. It produces epinephrine (adrenalin) and norepinephrine, which increase the heart rate, respirations, blood pressure, and blood levels of glucose and shunts (moves) blood from the intestines into the muscles of the legs, heart, and lungs. All of these processes prepare the body to move quickly away from danger.

SELYE'S GENERAL ADAPTATION SYNDROME

Hans Selye further developed Bernard's work on the body's adaptation to dangers. Selye examined a framework to describe how people respond to stress, based on his own observations while caring for sick people. He observed that, regardless of the diagnosis, most clients had certain symptoms in common. They lost their appetite, lost weight, looked and felt ill, and had various muscle aches and pains. Selye called this response to illness a general adaptation syndrome (GAS) because it involved generalized changes, mediated by the sympathetic nervous system and adrenal cortices. Selye believed that the response to stress was measurable and described evidence of actual body changes. He noted that there was enlargement of the adrenal glands; shrinkage of the thymus, spleen, and lymph nodes; and the development of gastric and duodenal ulcers. Selye suggested that the entire body responds to stress in an attempt to maintain or adapt. But if the demand or the stressor continues, the adaptive capacity of the body may be exceeded and disease may result. These responses occur following any stressor, and they led Selye to describe stress as the nonspecific response of the body to any demand placed on it. Examples of stressors include extreme heat and cold, physical injury, intense physical exertion, infection, and anxiety. He also recognized that each person has a limited amount of energy to use when dealing with stress. Selye believed that a person must choose which stressors are worthy of response and which are not. He believed that controlling stress is necessary for survival.

In addition to the general adaptation syndrome, Selye described a local adaption syndrome (LAS). The LAS takes place in a single organ or specific section of the body. An example of LAS is inflammation, which is discussed in Chapter 18.

Selye suggested that both the GAS and LAS develop in three distinct stages: (1) the alarm reaction, (2) the stage of resistance, and (3) the stage of exhaustion. For example, the changes in the thymus, spleen, and lymph nodes and the development of gastric ulcers begins in Stage 1. Stage 2 occurs when the body starts to react and return to a homeostatic state. Stage 3 is the stage of exhaustion and occurs when the normal adaptational responses do not suffice to return the body to a steady state. Figure 3-2 describes the physical and psychological responses during the GAS.

Regulation of the GAS and LAS. The most important regulators of the GAS and LAS are the central and autonomic nervous systems and the pituitary and adrenal glands. The pituitary and adrenal glands release hormones that inhibit or stimulate the body's response to stress and defense mechanisms. Selye called the adrenal and pituitary hormones *adaptive hormones*. Adaptive hormones that inhibit excessive defense activities by the body include the glucocorticoids, which reduce inflammation. The other group of adaptive hor-

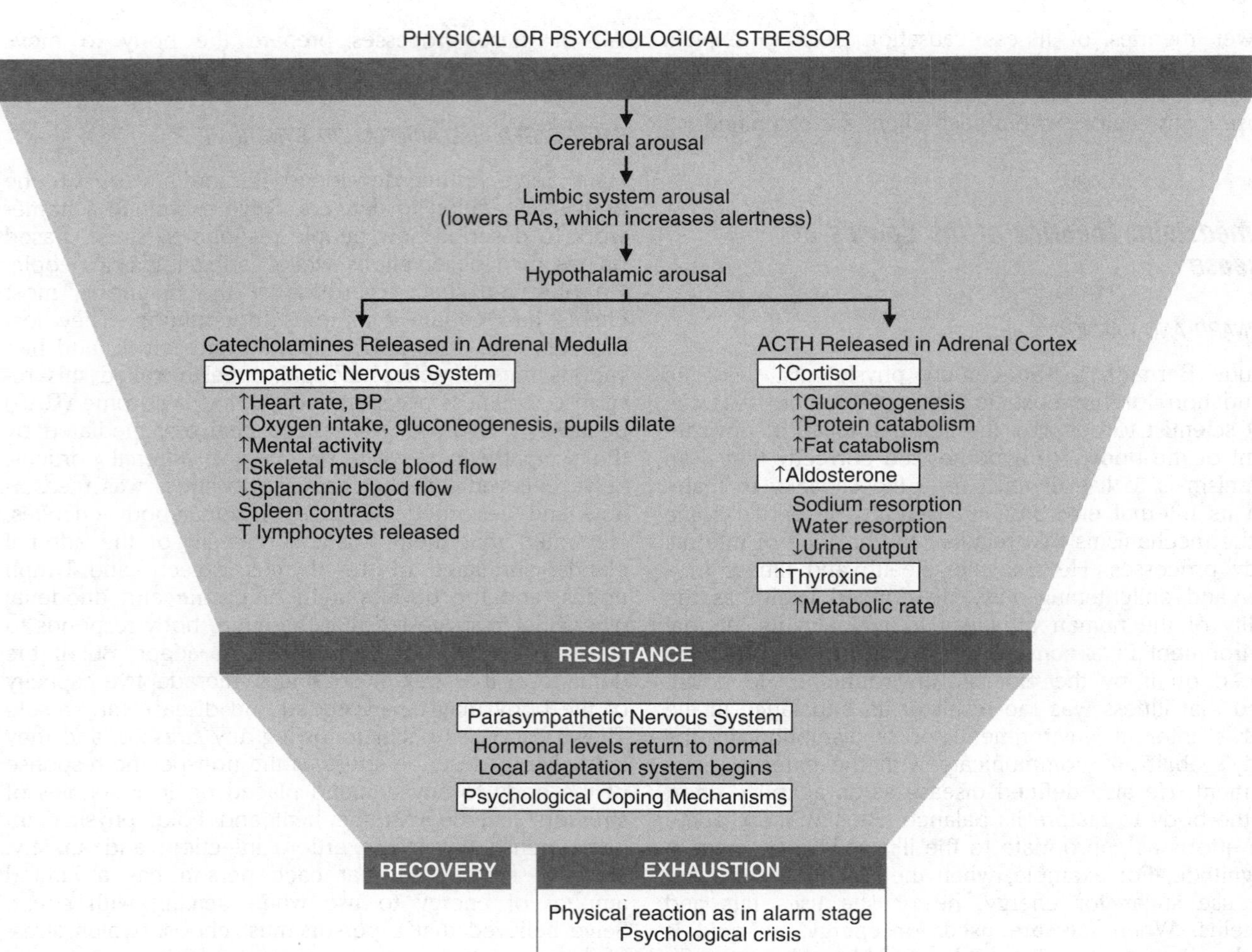

▲ *Figure 3–2*

The general adaptation syndrome.

mones are known as *proinflammatory corticoids* or *mineralocorticoids*. An example of a mineralocorticoid is aldosterone, which is secreted by the adrenal cortex and reduces the excretion of sodium for fluid balance.

The body's ability to resist stress and adapt to stressors depends on the proper balance of these hormones. In turn, the effect of these hormones on the body's resistance to stress depends on the individual's conditioning factors. Conditioning factors are circumstances that influence the GAS without being part of it. These factors can enhance or diminish the response to a stressor and include genetic predisposition, experience, mental attitude, diet, climate, lifestyle, and so forth. Because of the variability of the conditioning factors, different people respond differently to stressors. Conditioning factors help to strengthen the coping strategies through previous experiences with a stressor. Once a person has experienced a stressor, it is easier to develop an "I've been through this before and it will be OK" response.

Selye's theory that stress causes disease was based on the idea that excessive demands in a person's life produce high levels of hormones. These hormones lower the body's resistance to disease and cause organ damage. Such hormonal activity, when pronounced and prolonged, does seem to cause serious side effects, but a new question arises. Does the stress that a person experiences automatically cause distress when the person is repeatedly exposed to the same stressor?

MASON'S THEORY OF SPECIFICITY OF THE STRESS RESPONSE

John Mason reexamined Selye's concept of stress and proposed that there is a specific physiological response and a nonspecific psychological response. He also stated that the nonspecific response, as described by Selye, is actually a psychological reaction. Mason theorized that the stress response depended on psychological factors, such as the perception of the stressor rather than the stressor itself. He concluded that stress is primarily a psychological phenomenon rather than a physiologic one. The physiologic response, if one occurs, develops secondarily to the psychological response.

Mason also studied hormonal response to stressors. He found that 17-hydroxycorticosteroid (17-OHCS), epinephrine, and norepinephrine were released during specific stressors (e.g., heavy exercise and exposure to cold and heat) rather than in response to nonspecific stressors, as Selye had proposed. Mason found that 17-OHCS increases in response to an individual's first experiences with new stimuli, during the time an individual learns to avoid noxious stimuli, and when an individual receives punishment. Levels of 17-OHCS were found to increase during periods of sleep deprivation and in pilots during prolonged flights. There was a decrease in 17-OHCS during weekends. Mason also demonstrated that humans can *modify* the 17-OHCS response by coping effectively with a stressor. Research with parachute trainees over a 2-month period found that neuroendocrine responses to fear decreased only in those trainees who had mastered the technique of jumping. Thus, the stressor was no longer perceived as stressful because the person had dealt with it effectively.

Psychosocial Theories of Disease

Psychosocial theories of disease attempt to integrate physiologic, psychological, and social factors in order to explain disease.

LAZARUS'S CONCEPTS OF STRESS RESPONSE

Cognitive Appraisal. A newer understanding of why some people get sick when exposed to microorganisms whereas others remain healthy is revising popular concepts of what causes illness. Lazarus states that the degree of resistance to microbes depends largely on how well an individual is coping, which, in turn, depends on how one interprets problems—the "cognitive appraisal" of the stressor—and the chemical changes that occur in the brain and body. The brain appears to be the mediating physical structure between the body and the mind.

According to Lazarus, both stress and coping are processes, not events. Both change over time, partly as the result of interaction between the two processes. In the process of coping, the individual shapes as well as responds to a demand or stress. Coping may change the person's appraisal of the stressful experience and thereby influence what happens next.

Response to stress can have an impact on the client's resistance to diseases. Resistance to infectious disease, allergies, and possibly cancer depends upon a well-functioning immune system. People who cope poorly with stress have significantly impaired immune responses as seen by a diminished activity level in natural killer cells. These cells are a special type of leukocyte that destroys viruses and cancer cells without having previously encountered them.

Daily Uplifts and Hassles. Lazarus specifically looked at people's responses to daily hassles and daily uplifts. Daily hassles are the minor life events that everyone experiences. They are irritating, frustrating, and distressing demands met every day and include preparing routine meals, losing things, and getting delayed in traffic. Daily hassles also affect coping processes. The appraisal of the hassle will affect coping style. For instance, some people react philosophically to receiving a traffic ticket whereas others burn in anger. Still other people generate hassles by ineffective coping skills. People who do not manage their time effectively often feel pressured and out of control. They seldom find time for family or recreational activities. Self-generated hassles due to poor coping are more harmful to the person's health than hassles resulting from chance circumstances. This is because self-generated hassles tend to *recur* and are always *chronic in nature.* The student who always waits until the last minute to write a term paper will suffer much more from this self-generated hassle than the student who is occasionally late to class due to traffic congestion.

Lazarus also defined daily uplifts as buffers to the daily hassles. They provide relief from the daily hassles and come in three types. Daily uplifts act as breathers because they interrupt the intensity or frequency of the hassles. For example, reading an exciting novel or seeing a good movie provides a welcome escape from life's tiring demands. Other daily uplifts act as sustainers that provide people with the daily psychological nourishment needed to continue coping with life. An example of a sustainer is spending time with well-loved friends and family. Uplifts can also act as "restorers" that replenish the resources that have been depleted through harm or loss. Examples of "restorers" are prayer and meditation, resolving inner conflicts, and talking out problems with friends. Table 3-1 lists frequent hassles and uplifts as reported by a sample of 100 people. Lazarus' studies concluded that daily hassles are more significantly related to illness than are the major life events. The frequency of daily hassles also contributed more to the onset of illness than the intensity of the hassles.

THE CONCEPT OF HARDINESS

Hardiness has recently emerged as another variable that influences a client's response to stress. Hardiness is viewed as a personality component that moderates or buffers the response to stress. Clients who are hardy can remain healthy under stressful situations. They can also view the stressor as an opportunity to practice mastery and undergo personal growth.

Concepts of hardiness have been associated with health maintenance in the following three areas:

1. Control: the sense of mastery or self-confidence needed to appropriately appraise and interpret health stressors.

TABLE 3–1. Ten Most Frequent Hassles and Uplifts (N = 100) (items listed by frequency)

Hassles

1. Concerns about weight
2. Health of a family member
3. Rising prices of common goods
4. Home maintenance
5. Too many things to do
6. Misplacing or losing things
7. Yard work or outside home maintenance
8. Property, investment, or taxes
9. Crime
10. Physical appearance

Uplifts

1. Relating well with your spouse or lover
2. Relating well with friends
3. Completing a task
4. Feeling healthy
5. Getting enough sleep
6. Eating out
7. Meeting your responsibilities
8. Visiting, phoning, or writing someone
9. Spending time with family
10. Home (inside) pleasing you

Adapted from Kanner, A., et al. (1981). Comparison of two modes of stress measurement: Daily hassles and uplifts versus major life events. *Journal of Behavioral Medicine, 4, 14.*

2. Commitment: the presence of active involvement in efforts to maintain or improve health.
3. Challenge: the presence of flexibility and persistence in coping with health stressors.

Tools to measure or assess hardiness are being developed. Control is assessed by examining the client's sense that health and illness can be controlled (locus of control). Commitment is assessed by examining commitment to self and one's health. Challenge is assessed by examining the client's usual response to problems and illnesses.[13]

WOLFF'S THEORY OF STRESS, ORGAN MALADAPTATION, AND DISEASE

Harold Wolff was interested in how ineffective adaptation can lead to a breakdown in homeostasis and subsequently to disease. He studied people's responses to chronic stressors, such as a frustrating job or unhappy home life. Wolff believed that a person's "total life situation" with its accompanying joys, successes, and frustrations profoundly affects the person's susceptibility to disease. Like Bernard, Wolff hypothesized that disease often resulted from adaptive attempts to restore homeostasis, attempts that were appropriate in kind but incorrect in magnitude.

Wolff theorized that inappropriate attempts at adaptation occur in humans for several reasons. First, humans have highly developed nervous systems and can symbolize, recall the past, and project themselves into the future. Therefore, threats of possible danger and symbols of danger are just as important a cause of disease as are noxious chemicals, microbes, and mechanical forces. Second, humans are tribal creatures; people depend on other people for many of the satisfactions in life. Stressors are created by the need to be successful at work and in association with other people. In addition, modern life often forces people to associate with other people who are of different races, religions, outlooks, and cultural values. Finally, a person may respond inappropriately to other individuals because of unrealistic and distorted perceptions of human relationships. The basis for this distortion again lies in the human ability to symbolize and to consider both the past and future.

Wolff's research indicated that certain individuals consistently respond to frustrating situations through a response by a particular body system or organ, perhaps the stomach, muscles of the back, colon, or nasal mucous membranes. Mucous membranes (whether in the nose, stomach, rectum, bladder, or vagina) seem to be particularly susceptible to stress. This is probably because these membranes serve as a primary defense mechanism. Mucous membranes exhibit several stress reactions: edema, ischemia, increased friability, faulty absorption, ulceration, inflammation, and altered reactions to chemical substances. Such pathologic changes occur frequently in response to traumatic emotional situations. Pathologic changes that occur regularly and are combined with other chemical, biologic, or physical stressors can eventually lead to irreversible tissue damage, such as bleeding gastric ulcers.

LIFE CHANGE AND THE ONSET OF ILLNESS

Changes in life, such as the death of a spouse, create havoc in people's lives. Change is a form of stress to which people must learn to adapt, both psychologically and physically. Some life changes are universal and affect all people, e.g., the effects of aging, experiencing pain, changes in self-concept. Other life changes are personal and affect fewer people, e.g., the birth of a child, an accident, or a change in job responsibilities. Adaptation to the change requires energy. If the person is required to adapt to many significant changes over a short period of time, the person will become overextended, expend too much energy trying to adapt, and may become ill.

The belief that disease and life changes are strongly linked is very old. A psychiatrist in the 1930s began charting life events as a component of medical history. In the late 1960s the first attempt to quantify these changes was made by Holmes and Rahe.

Holmes and Rahe used a questionnaire to ask respondents to list major life changes based on the significance they held. The study was conducted in the United States and in other countries. Holmes and Rahe found that despite differences in lifestyles, education, cultures, and economic status, people tended to agree on the significance of the stress of various life events. A numerical weight was assigned to each of the events, the weights are called life change units. Once life events were weighted, they were ranked (Table 3–2). The death of a spouse ranks as the highest stressor.

Holmes and Rahe explored the relationship between the amount of change in a person's life and the subsequent illness. They discovered that the higher a person's life change score, the greater the likelihood that an illness would develop. The research appeared to indicate that people with a sufficiently high score of life change units suffer major illnesses within a relatively short period of time and that recent life events are precipitating factors that influence the timing of onset of illness but not the type of illness. Minor ailments, serious disease, depression, and suicide attempts typically follow a cluster of both positive and negative life change units.

There have been some problems with this approach to illness development. For the most part, studies have been performed on subjects who have a disease, such as myocardial infarction. Subjects have been asked to retrospectively review the number of life events that occurred in the time period preceding their illness. This approach may alter the validity of the data because of recall bias. Some people cope with illness by trying to find its cause. Therefore, they may have a bias in their recall of recent life events and life changes. In addition, more than one third of these events involve either marriage or work, and therefore, the instrument is focused toward younger, married, and working people. A study of men admitted to a Veteran's Administration hospital clearly revealed this bias. These men, for the most part, were unemployed, unmarried, and often homeless. They had major illness and major life stressors, but they scored low on the life change units scale. Finally, the scale does not take into consideration the stressfulness of non-events, "off-schedule" events, or chronic occurrences. For example, not getting a desired promotion (non-event) can be stressful. An unexpected "off-schedule" event, such as a pregnancy in a 45-year-old woman who believed that she had already raised her family, could not be marked on the scale. It should also be noted that the death of a child is not listed on the scale. Finally, anticipating an event could be as stressful as the event itself, and chronic occurrences of even minor life changes could create a great impact of stress. The impact of monotony on illness is also not covered in the Holmes and Rahe scale.

TABLE 3–2. Social Readjustment Rating Scale

Life Change Units	Major Life Events in Past 12 Months
100	Death of spouse
73	Divorce
65	Marital separation
63	Detention in jail institution
63	Death of close family member
53	Personal injury or illness
50	Marriage
47	Fired at work
45	Marital reconciliation
45	Retirement
44	Change in health behavior of family member
40	Pregnancy
39	Sexual difficulties
39	Gain of new family member
39	Business readjustment
38	Change in financial state
37	Death of close friend
36	Change to a different line of work
35	Change in number of arguments with spouse
31	Mortgage or loan over $10,000
30	Foreclosure of mortgage or loan
29	Change in responsibilities at work
29	Son or daughter leaving home
29	Trouble with in-laws
28	Outstanding personal achievement
26	Spouse began or ceased work
26	Began or ceased formal schooling
25	Change in living conditions
24	Revision of personal habits
23	Trouble with boss
20	Change in work hours or conditions
20	Change in residence
20	Change in schools
19	Change in recreation
19	Change in church activities
18	Change in social activities
17	Mortgage or loan less than $10,000
16	Change in sleeping habits
15	Change in number of family get-togethers
15	Change in eating habits
13	Vacation
11	Christmas
11	Minor violations of the law

From Holmes, T. H. & Rahe, R. H. (1967). The social readjustment rating scale. *Journal of Psychosomatic Research,* 2:214. Reprinted with permission of authors and Pergamon Press, Ltd.

DURATION OF STRESS

It is useful to distinguish four types of stressful events, based primarily on their duration: (1) acute, time-limited events (e.g., awaiting the results of a diagnostic test); (2) stress event sequences, in which a particular event initiates a series of stress events that occur over an extended period of time (e.g., bereavement); (3) chronic intermittent stressors, situations that occur and recur periodically (e.g., conflicts with family members); and (4) chronic stress situations (e.g., chronic disability). In stress event sequences and chronic stress conditions, stress reactions may occur over a long period of time. Further research is needed to determine the psychological and physiologic impact of these types of stressors. Most studies have been performed on acute stress response and measured autonomic nervous system and hormonal responses. Hormones such as cortisol rarely show chronic elevations, suggesting that the person may reach an equilibrium and constant coping efforts are not needed. We also do not know if different coping efforts are more effective with acute versus chronic stressors.

Mediators of the Stress Response

There is a growing consensus among stress researchers that in order to understand the relationship between stress and illness outcomes, the factors that modify or mediate the relationship must be clarified. Although stressors may produce temporary physiologic and psychological changes, most stressors are not followed by long-term illnesses. A stressor may produce an extreme reaction in one person and no reaction in another, or the same stressor may produce variable reactions in the same individual at different time periods. This suggests that there are factors that alter the responses to stressors. One factor that can alter a stress response is the environment, such as social supports, physical setting, and organizational factors. Social supports tend to buffer individuals from the potentially negative effects of stressors, and those people who have strong social supports may live longer and have a lower incidence of physical illness. Other factors are within the person, such as personality, personal resources, temperament, past history, and genetic variables. (Within the personal aspect of stress response is how the stressor is appraised and how the person copes with the stressors.) One coping style, the expression of emotion, especially anger, has been studied with interesting findings. One might think that the expression of anger would have a negative effect on illness outcome, but surprisingly the outcome after expressing negative emotions depends on the disease. Frequently expressing hostility and anger were shown to increase survival in persons with cancer. But in persons with lung disease, the expression of anger and other negative emotions increased their symptoms and they had negative physiologic changes (e.g., hypoxia).

BEHAVIOR PATTERNS

The relationship of behavior patterns, lifestyle, and stress to disease has been examined. An important study by Friedman and Rosenman described two behavior types: type A and type B. The original studies were performed to examine risk factors for coronary artery disease. Prior to these studies, it was believed that heart disease results from a diet that was too high in fat and cholesterol, lack of proper rest and exercise, excessive smoking, and a family history of heart disease. This theory focused on the hypothesis that heart disease can also evolve as a consequence of certain behavior types. Type A personality characterizes a person who is constantly mobilizing inner resources to combat real or imagined stresses. They are described as aggressive, often hostile, hard-driving, deadline-ridden people with a chronic sense of urgency. The type A person feels somewhat guilty when relaxing. Also, this person characteristically moves, walks, and eats rapidly and frequently does or thinks about two or more things at once. Job position does not appear to be a factor because type A behavior can be seen in all occupations.

In sharp contrast is the type B personality. This person characteristically takes life with all of its stresses in stride. Although this person often is intelligent and ambitious, the type B personality does not allow activity to become self-destructive. The person can relax without feeling guilty and work without a sense of time urgency. The basic attitude toward life is calm, optimistic, and self-confident.

It is possible to see a pure type A or type B person, but more frequently, people have some characteristics of both types. It is preferred to describe people as *predominately* type A or type B.

Friedman and Rosenman's research determined that the type A person between the ages of 35 and 60 was almost three times more likely to develop coronary artery disease than the type B person. In fact, the researchers concluded that the type B personality appeared to be almost immune to the onset of coronary artery disease. Although type A behavior patterns have a significant association with coronary heart disease, conclusions cannot be made that there is a direct relationship. In other words, a person with type A personality cannot be told that he will develop coronary artery disease nor can the person with type B personality be assured that he will not develop coronary heart disease. The exact relationship of type A to coronary artery disease is not clear. One possible explanation is that the continuous stress placed on the sympathetic nervous system results in increased fatty acid circulation. The fatty acids may begin to occlude arteries, which leads to coronary artery disease.

THE ROLE OF THE BRAIN IN ILLNESS

An expanded view of disease states that it is a *bio-psycho-social* process. This concept means that a person's body, mind and environment together determine whether illness develops. Illness occurs from increased vulnerability rather than from external agents that "cause" disease. The factors that affect the ability to cope include attitude, appraisal of stress, diet, and heredity. The bio-psycho-social risk factor concept of disease is a marked departure from the germ theory. Disease is not always seen as a pathologic change caused by a foreign force. Instead tissue damage is seen as more of the results of normal bodily processes gone awry or disrupted. These processes include the activity of neurotransmitters in the brain, the stress hormones of the adrenal glands and nervous system, and the helper and suppressor cells of the immune system. For example, excessive stress hormones (corticosteroids and catecholamines) can lead to artery damage or suppress the action of antibodies and natural killer cells, which protect the body from foreign invaders and tumor development. Deficient suppressor cells may permit overaction of the immune system to the point at which the body starts attacking itself, such as in rheumatoid arthritis.

The knowledge of how the brain profoundly affects the function of the neurotransmitters (chemical messengers) has greatly expanded current views about health and illness. In 1975, the endogenous analgesics, enkephalins and endorphins, were discovered. Since that time, other neurotransmitters have been discovered. And equally important to the development of illness is the knowledge that the function and balance of these transmitters can be influenced by drugs, viruses, bacteria, poor nutrition, defective genes, aging, or the perception of stress.

Another aspect of illness is the recognition that people are not either emotionally ill or physically ill. Illness is simply not an "either-or" matter. Ultimately, illness involves a combination of mind-body factors. These factors interact to produce symptoms experienced by the person. It is not uncommon to experience depression with physical illness or to have physical signs and symptoms of mental/emotional illness.

Historical Mind-Body Views. In general, early views of illness are difficult to reconstruct because only drawings, bony fragments, and surgical instruments remain. Apart from the treatment of wounds and broken bones, the folklore of medicine is the most ancient aspect of the art of healing because primitive physicians showed their wisdom by treating the whole person, soul as well as body. In early times, no division was made between physical illness and mental illness.

As humans progressed over time, various views on the body-mind relationship developed. At times, the mind and body were viewed as interrelated and, at other times, as divided and separate. Hippocrates, late in the fifth century, taught that both the mind and body were involved in illness. He said "It is more important to know what sort of person has a disease than to know what sort of disease a person has." This connection of the mind to the body was considered important until the Renaissance.

During the Renaissance, René Déscartes, the father of modern philosophy, developed a doctrine stating that there is a division of reality between the mind and the body. He believed that the mind contained the essence of thinking, consciousness, and the soul, whereas the body was just a machine. Therefore, the previous connections of the mind to the body were rejected. Religious and philosophical teachings were to focus on the mind and soul, whereas medicine concentrated on the physical body. This splitting of the mind from the body had significant impact on medical care. This dichotomous mind-body model of Déscartes, called *Cartesian dualism*, had tremendous impact on western thought. It was not until the work of Freud and others that described an unconscious element to human life that the Déscartes model was severely challenged. Freud's work developed an awareness of the significance of the emotions in mental and physical illness.

The task of reuniting the divided person in western culture has been difficult and is by no means complete. Various mind-body therapies have been developed in recent years. Biofeedback, autogenic training, and focused thought are some examples.

WOLF'S CONCEPT OF DISEASE AS A WAY OF LIFE

Stewart Wolf's theoretical approach focused on the role of the brain in regulating the body's process and in causing disease. The brain helps maintain an internal milieu and helps the body adapt to the external environment. The brain also provides the meaning and interpretation given to frustrations and problems of life. The response can markedly affect the body's functioning. The body needs high levels of epinephrine, blood glucose, and other hormones during times of physical threat when people must literally fight or flee. But when these responses occur inappropriately or chronically, the excess hormones can cause harm. The way the brain defines any situation can evoke inappropriate chemical and nervous system reactions. When people habitually act as if a frustration, disappointment, or loss is a matter of life and death, stating they "can't stand it," then the endocrine, musculoskeletal and autonomic nervous systems are called to respond. If people view life, as many coronary-prone individuals do, as requiring constant domination of things and people, such an attitude contributes to excessive outpouring of cholesterol, triglycerides, norepinephrine, adrenocorticotropic hormone (ACTH), and insulin. This attitude also contributes to deficient levels of pituitary growth hormone.

Data reveal that people who define their situation as hopeless may elicit an excessive conservation of oxygen, as if they were trying to hold their breath or "play dead" until hope returns. Breath holding can stimulate the vagus nerve and cause cardiac dysrhythmias. Disease, then, can arise from evoked reaction patterns that are meant to be protective when the person is physically threatened but are destructive when used inappropriately to fight symbolic battles. Wolf believed that disease cannot be separated from the total person, including the person's way of life and interpretation of what life means. He suggested that "disease is a way of life, the end result of a way that people react to life's problems."

SCHWARTZ'S MODEL OF THE BRAIN AS AN ADAPTIVE REGULATOR

Schwartz describes the role of the brain as an adaptive system that self-regulates the body. The brain is sensitive to the external and internal environment. It processes information, and through a "feedback" system with the peripheral organs, it maintains a stable internal environment. A common example of this process is the changes seen in the body when it is cold — shivering occurs and the skin becomes pale as blood is shunted away from the skin to prevent further loss of body heat.

Schwartz also describes a model of self-regulation and disregulation. According to the model, *attention* by the brain to external and internal environmental and psychophysiologic demands results in *connection* and *self-regulation.* The feedback loop stabilizes output and maintains homeostasis. Schwartz sees the correct functioning of the system as promoting ease or health. On the other hand, if the brain fails to pay attention to these demands (*disattention*), the result is *disconnection.* Disconnection results when the relationship between output and input or between the body and the brain becomes unbalanced and the feedback loop fails to stabilize output. The resulting disconnection of regulatory processes causes disregulation and disease. Thus, disattention is one condition that can lead to a disconnection between the brain and the body.

Consider the following example: Beth is a junior nursing student and has been under stress most of the semester trying to work and go to school. She has felt tired lately but has ignored the symptoms (disattention) and continued to work and attend class and clinical experiences (disconnection). Midterm arrives and the stress of studying for examinations causes Beth to become very ill (disregulation) and she cannot take an examination. Had Beth paid attention to the early warning signals from her body, made a connection between the growing fatigue and stressors, intervened to slow down her commitments and rest more frequently, she might have avoided becoming seriously ill and missing an examination.

Several implications about health and illness can be drawn from Schwartz's work. First, there is a degree of self-responsibility in maintaining health. This does not mean that people are necessarily responsible for becoming ill. Instead, individuals are responsible for detecting their body's feedback that indicates an imbalance is occurring. They also need to regulate themselves to correct the imbalance. And finally, people need to seek assistance to regain self-regulation.

The role of the brain in health and illness is fairly clear in Schwartz's work. The brain is central to any change in health because it is the mediator between the external and internal environments. Through the brain and its interpretations, a person can change the environment, leave it, engage in it, and decide to rest, to exercise, to diet, and so forth. The person has the power of the brain to move toward health or illness.

Genetic Aspects of Disease

In addition to research on the bio-psycho-social aspects of diseases, there has been much medical research in other areas of disease causation. Owing to elaborate technology, the field of genetics has been unlocked. Genetic aspects of diseases have been recognized for many years, but recent technology has allowed medical researchers to identify the actual gene containing the disorder. And in the past 5 years, therapy has been developed to treat the altered gene structure.

More than one fifth of the genes that exist in humans differ in form from one person to another. This remarkable degree of genetic variation among normal people is what accounts for the naturally occurring variations in people, such as height, hair color, intelligence, personality, and blood pressure. These genetic differences also have an impact on each person's ability to handle environmental challenges, including those that produce disease. There is some degree of genetic interaction with the environment in every disease. For example, most people get lung cancer from smoking cigarettes, yet some do not. Perhaps, it is the person's genetic make-up and tendency that allows him or her to kill early cancer cells. In certain diseases, however, the genetic component is so overwhelming that the disease occurs in a predictable manner. Such diseases are termed genetic disorders, and include diseases such as Huntington's chorea, which is a progressive neurologic disease. In 1990, medical researchers identified a single gene linked to lung cancer risk. New approaches to the treatment of genetic disease includes gene therapy. Gene therapy is the injection of DNA fragments into cells. The fragments find their way to the nucleus and repair enzymes so the cell can work normally again. In 1990, research was being conducted on the use of gene therapy in the treatment of Alzheimer's disease, muscular dystrophy, cystic fibrosis, and some forms of primary and secondary epilepsy.

THE EXPERIENCE OF ILLNESS

Obviously, it is important for the nurse to understand the various theories of illness causation, but perhaps, it is more important for the nurse to understand how a client may respond to being ill.

Illness usually refers to a group of symptoms or a condition underlying the symptoms. Illness behavior, on the other hand, describes the manner in which clients monitor their bodies, define and interpret their symptoms, take remedial action, and use the health care system. Clients perceive, evaluate, and respond to illness differently. The nurse may encounter clients who deny their symptoms, exaggerate their symptoms, or minimize their symptoms. Reactions to symptoms are influenced by the culture, the knowledge base of the client, the client's definition of health and previous interactions with the health care system. For example, if a client's definition of health was "not having cancer," then he or she is not as likely to comply with a treatment plan for diabetes, because he or she may not realize the seriousness of the disorder.

Various studies have been performed on illness behavior. For example, many studies of illness show that women report symptoms more frequently than men do and also that women use the services of physicians and psychiatrists more frequently than do men. Many explanations have been offered for these differences. Some researchers suggest that there may be an increased incidence of diseases in women, others suggest that women have a more sensitive perception of symptoms, and still others believe that women are more willing to acknowledge their symptoms and seek care. But before assuming that women are sicker than men, it is important to recognize that most medical research studies have been performed on men and, therefore, conclusions drawn recently about women using more medical services are based on a comparatively smaller sample. Cultural variations in response to illness are presented in Chapter 5.

The Sick Role

A client who becomes ill progresses through certain stages. These stages can be seen in clients who are acutely ill as well as in clients who have exacerbations of chronic illness. Even clients with "bad colds" may exhibit these behaviors.

STAGE 1: THE EXPERIENCE OF SYMPTOMS

During this stage, the client defines himself as sick, he recognizes that the symptoms are present, and he does not feel well. The most common symptom is pain, but other problems such as fever, cough, chills or malaise (generalized weakness) may be early signs. During this first stage, the client responds to illness in one of three ways. The client can (1) take action; (2) take no action; or (3) take counteraction.

Taking action is the use of self-diagnoses, self-treatment, or seeking help from a health care practitioner. Self-diagnosing can be through the use of previous knowledge and experience (e.g., "I have a cold") or through the use of medical self-help books. Self-diagnosing is common practice and usually is safe for minor ailments and illness. Self-diagnosing can become dangerous when the client makes the wrong diagnosis and, thereby, delays treatment. It is not uncommon for the neighbors and friends of nurses to ask for help and a diagnosis. The nurse should use caution in offering medical advice beyond her or his knowledge base. For example, if the nurse worked on an orthopedic floor in a hospital, she or he may not have the background to offer safe instructions for an eye problem. Even when the nurse knows about the illness, it is important to remember the potential legal ramifications of giving advice.

The second step in taking action is the practice of self-treatment. Again, with minor ailments or illness or for a chronic illness with which the client has had previous experience, self-treatment is usually safe. Billions of dollars are spent annually by Americans on over-the-counter medications to treat their own symptoms. The use of various agents can be greatly influenced by advertising and the client's friends and family members. Home remedies and folk medicine are other aspects of self-treatment. If the nurse is working in a community of clients who use folk remedies, such as herbs, the nurse should become familiar with these agents because they may interact with other treatments (see also Chap. 5, Cross-Cultural Nursing).

Not all forms of self-treatment have negative outcomes. Some degree of self-treatment is desirable because the client is managing his or her own health. And if every person saw a health care practitioner for every minor illness, the system would be overwhelmed. In addition, changes in diet, exercise, and rest and relaxation are positive forms of self-treatment.

If self-treatment does not relieve the symptoms, the client will probably seek the help of a health care practitioner. The type of practitioner selected depends on the client's economic and sociocultural background. Clients may choose to be examined by a physician or nurse practitioner, and others may see a herbalist, a chiropractor, or a spiritual healer. Some clients have forms of insurance that restrict them to the services of certain health care providers in order to control costs. Other clients have no insurance and often wait until their symptoms become unmanageable and then go to an emergency department in a local hospital. In the United States, it is illegal to refuse treatment to any client in the emergency department if he or she has a true emergency. Obviously, with increasing numbers of uninsured clients, emergency departments are overwhelmed with clients who might have been seen by other practitioners or at earlier stages of illness.

Taking no action is another possible response to the symptoms of illness. This response may be an "I'll wait and see" attitude on the part of the client or denial over the significance of the symptoms. For example, the client may say to himself "This chest pain is just indigestion. I'll take some antacids and wait to see if it will go away." Or perhaps the mere thought of having a heart attack is so frightening that the client simply denies the seriousness of the symptoms. "I've got four more reports to write yet this afternoon, I can't get sick now." Another group of clients may not know which physician to see or how to access the health care system in their community. For example, if a client is new to the community, he or she may be reluctant to look up the name of a physician in the telephone book or be unable to get an appointment without a long wait.

The client's lack of action may be rewarded if the symptoms disappear. However, if the symptoms persist or worsen, the client will be forced into action. Family members or friends may pressure the client to seek help, the client may be unable to work or rest comfortably, or the client may respond to the lack of symptom improvement and seek help voluntarily.

Taking counteraction is potentially the most harmful of all responses to illness. Taking counteraction is performing behaviors that attempt to disprove the seriousness or existence of the symptoms. An example would be the client who is not willing to accept a diagnosis of cancer and goes from one health practitioner to another until he finds one that tells him he does not have cancer. This form of response can actually threaten the client's life, because the client refuses to be labeled as ill. Because the client is not willing to seek appropriate help, the disease may worsen and he or she may die.

The client progresses into the next stage when he or she seeks treatment for the symptoms. The client seeks validation of the illness from others, gives up some normal activities, and assumes a sick role.

STAGE 2: THE DEPENDENT ROLE

The second stage of illness is accepting a dependent role and agreeing to follow a prescribed treatment plan. In a dependent role, a client requires assistance from others to meet basic human needs for daily living and needs emotional support, such as acceptance, approval, protection, and physical closeness. The client also must allow others to make decisions and carry out his or her usual tasks at work or home. It is during this stage that many clients enter the hospital. Parsons identified four aspects of the sick role. Although these aspects may not be seen in everyone, they are an important generalized description. Parsons stated that

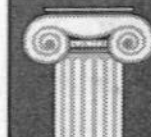

ETHICAL ISSUES IN NURSING

How Much Control Should We Have Over Our Health?

Our ideas regarding health and illness are shaped by many factors. How we deal with the stress of illness is greatly influenced by how we deal with life stressors of any kind. When a stressor is introduced into our lives, it interferes with whatever balance we have adjusted to. The most common response to such a stressor is to adapt our lives in order to keep the balance manageable. There is a feeling of safety as long as we feel we have control over the balance of our lives. Most day-to-day stressors are balanced successfully, because we have a large capacity to control the numerous variables that come our way. For example, the stress of a traffic jam may be reduced by taking an alternate route, or the stress of a final examination may be reduced by adequate preparation. A sense of control is very important to our sense of well being.

When illness strikes, our control over our health may be severely compromised. Disease may take over our cells without our knowledge until symptoms make the disease known to us. When symptoms of disease appear, we seek out help from health care providers. Clients go to see doctors and nurses for help in controlling their illness in order that the balance in their lives may be restored. Health care providers assess their clients and instruct them on recommended treatments. This model of health care is standard and it works very well, as long as clients comply with recommended treatments. A major dilemma arises, however, when clients fail to comply with the advice of their health care providers.

People have the right of autonomy, and in health care, autonomy may be exercised by compliance or by noncompliance with prescribed treatments. As health care providers, nurses must respect client autonomy and should try to avoid labeling clients as "problem clients" when they are noncompliant with care plans. It is difficult to understand why a client might not comply with a treatment that was beneficently prescribed; after all, the client came for advice on how to get better, so why doesn't he or she follow the advice?

Nurses may get caught in the middle with the noncompliant client. Insisting that the client comply is not the best approach to the problem. Nurses are in a great position to seek out why a client is not compliant. Perhaps the problem is that by noncompliance, the client feels more in control of the situation (even if the control does not benefit him or her). Perhaps there is a knowledge deficit that the nurse can rectify, or perhaps there is a resource problem inhibiting compliance (finances, transportation, family support), in which case the plan of care may need to be revised. There may be times, on the other hand, when the client makes a competent decision not to go along with treatment guidelines, and this is the end of the discussion. In that case, educational reinforcement may be the only resource the nurse can provide.

---

sick people are (1) exempt from usual social role responsibilities; (2) not morally responsible for being ill; (3) obligated to "want to get well"; and (4) obligated to seek competent help.

During this stage, most clients focus on their symptoms and abnormal body functions. Nurses can easily recognize clients in this stage, because the client is self-centered and introverted. The client often has no desire to hear about current events, talk about other people, or relate to concerns apart from himself. The client can become demanding and seemingly impatient.

STAGE 3: RECOVERY AND REHABILITATION

During this final stage of illness, the client begins the process of healing and recovery. This process may begin in the hospital and often concludes at home. Many insurance payment structures have reduced the number of allowable days for recovery in a hospital in order to control costs. In the future, nurses can expect that most clients will reach full recovery outside of an acute care hospital setting.

During this stage, the client is expected to return to an independent role and resume normal activities and responsibilities. Some clients become impatient with the length of recovery and lack of a quick recovery. Education may be required to reinforce the normal expectations for recovery for that client.

There is no usual timetable for the client to proceed through these stages. The nurse should assess the client's reaction to being ill and dependent. Some clients try too hard to become independent and may increase their risk of injury or delay healing. For example, some clients may refuse to have the nurse provide physical care and attempt to get up alone. Inappropriate independence may increase the risk of injury from orthostatic hypotension or other weakness. In contrast, some clients are reluctant or afraid to resume normal activities. They may fear pain, enjoy the dependent role, or be unclear about their role. For example, a client may refuse to get up to a bedside chair following surgery for fear of pain. The nurse should reinforce the need for and benefit of early ambulation (e.g., pain relief, lung expansion). At times, the nurse may need to be firm and almost demand that the client perform various activities. This is an awkward situation for both the nurse and the client. In general, the nurse needs to accept the client as an individual, examine the reasons for the behavior, continue to provide nursing care, and educate the client about the process of recovery.

Acute Illness in the Elderly

Older clients are more prone to injury, acute infections (especially respiratory), and other acute illnesses than are younger clients. This is due to the increased occurrence of chronic illness in the aged, combined with less reserve of energy and ability to respond to stress. It is common to see the aged client, who was mentally competent, frequently become confused during the stress of acute illness. Recovery from acute illness takes longer than in a younger client, and there is a risk that the previous level of functioning will not be regained. As early as possible in the recovery from acute illness the aged client should be ambulated, given range-of-motion exercises to keep joints in motion, have catheters discontinued to promote urinary continence, and

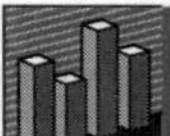

NURSING RESEARCH

This study describes the qualities of resilience that characterize elderly women who have adjusted successfully to major losses. A qualitative method was used to identify themes that describe the phenomenon of resilience. Analysis of data revealed five major themes that reflected the attitude of these women. These themes included a balanced perspective of life experiences (equanimity), persistence despite adversity and discouragement (perseverance), the belief in oneself and one's capabilities (self-reliance), realization that life has a purpose, valuing one's contribution to life and society (meaningfulness), and realizing that each person's life path is unique, some of which must be walked alone (existential aloneness).

Not all women can sustain a loss and survive. Some women withdraw, feeling helpless and vulnerable. Nurses are in a strategic position to promote resilience. Nurses can help clients through the initial reactions of shock and disbelief to a point of acceptance, with a commitment to live, not just survive. Interventions to assist the client include promoting a positive image of the client to herself, a belief in self, determination to go on, the use of humor, and spirituality.

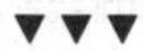

Waglid, G., & Young, H. (1990). Resilience among older women. *Image 22* (4), 252–255.

---

be engaged in social activities. Medications should be kept to a minimum to avoid overdosage or drug-drug interactions.

Common problems in the care of the aged client include management of dementia, depression, risk of falling, urinary incontinence, pressure ulcers, and contractures. Nurses should not presume that all elderly clients are weak and debilitated, though. Qualities such as resilience help many elderly clients through losses (see Nursing Research).

Deviant Sick Roles

In most societies, clients must do three things when they are sick: (1) accept that they are ill, (2) seek help, and (3) want to get well. Clients who do not follow these traditional roles are not common. Clients who are in a "deviant sick role" include those who (1) do not want to get well and do not comply with the prescribed treatments, (2) use their illness for secondary gains (e.g., money from an insurance or disability policy), (3) use their illness to avoid responsibilities, (4) do not care if they get well and act withdrawn, indifferent to care, and submissive, and (5) do not want to admit they are ill.

Another group of clients who do not demonstrate the normal reactions to illness are those clients who seek help more often than is apparently necessary. This group of clients includes people who have self-induced illness and those who have a heightened sense of their own bodily functions and quickly define themselves as ill.

The term hypochondriac is used to describe the group of clients who seek medical help frequently for minor problems. These clients are not helped by labeling them as hypochondriacs. They often are in need of care, and their symptoms often indicate a high level of anxiety. It is also important to remember that the person labeled a hypochondriac can develop a "true" illness and may be ignored because of the previous labeling.

There is another group of clients who experience illness but have no diagnosed physical cause for the problem. Clients with these problems often have recurrent headache and backache. Over the years, these clients were thought to be "acting ill" for secondary gain and their problems were treated through psychological methods. Commonly, little improvement is made in comfort or symptom management. As more is learned about health and illness, perhaps this type of illness will be better understood.

The term Munchausen's syndrome is sometimes used to describe clients who intentionally cause their own illness or pretend to be ill. These clients may enter the health care system with a variety of illnesses, such as nonhealing wounds or abdominal pain. When no physical cause of the illness can be found, the client can be approached about causing his own illness. Many times, the nursing staff feels angry about being tricked by the ability of the client to feign illness. Obviously, the client's illness is mental and requires the help of psychiatric professionals.

Crisis Intervention

Sometimes clients cannot cope with illness or hospitalization. In addition, family members may find that the client's illness or hospitalization is beyond their coping abilities. Not all stressors, such as illness or hospitalization, tax coping strategies, but at times the nurse may be faced with a client or family who are experiencing crisis.

Crisis is the emotional reaction to a stressful event. Recall that stress itself does not cause a crisis, but the cognitive appraisal of the event may lead to crisis. Crisis is not a disease state. Instead, it is a struggle to regain control of one's self and environment when the problem is perceived as insolvable. In general, the outcome of crisis depends on how the client deals with the crisis and what outside supports are available and used during the time of crisis.

INITIAL REACTION TO CRISIS

The client reacts to a stressful event using the typical coping mechanisms, also called relief behaviors. These coping mechanisms are used to lower or maintain anxiety. Coping mechanisms may be adaptive and include talking about the problem; or maladaptive, such as the use of alcohol or drugs. Regardless of the type of mechanism used, crisis exists when the coping mechanism does not allow the client to reach a lower level of anxiety.

TYPES OF CRISIS

There are two types of crisis situations (1) internal or developmental and (2) situational.

Internal or Developmental Crisis. Internal or developmental crisis occurs in response to stressors common to all or many persons during periods of transition or maturation. Stressors that occur in everyone include the process of maturing, which passes through predictable steps, as defined by Erikson. Each step has tasks that must be mastered before the person can move on to the higher level. When a person arrives at a new stage, the old coping styles are no longer effective and the new coping mechanisms have yet to be developed.

Consider the problem-solving methods that are learned through the process of maturing. A child may throw a tantrum when the child does not get what the child wants; an adult cannot act in such a way (and still be perceived as an adult). The adult has learned to explore other methods of problem solving. For a period of time during the transition to adulthood, the person is left without effective coping mechanisms and a maturational crisis occurs. The person in crisis is often filled with anxiety and has variations from normal behavior. Some common examples include the erratic behavior and mood swings seen during puberty and adolescence. Even adults have temporary maturational crises as they reach various stages in life. The empty-nest syndrome experienced by parents of children who grow up and leave home is an example. Erikson believes that how the crisis of one stage is solved affects the ability to move through the other stages. If a person lacks the support systems or role models to move through stages, resolution and finding another coping strategy may not occur. Unresolved problems and inadequate coping mechanisms can adversely affect what is learned in subsequent stages.

Stressors that are common to many people include the beginning of school, dating, marriage, divorce, hospitalization, illness, loss of a job, death of a family member, pregnancy, and change in financial status. The situations cited by Holmes are common examples of potential situational crises. Whether or not these situations result in crisis depends on the support available from caring friends and family members, and the person's general emotional status and ability to cope with the situation. The resolution of a situational crisis is centered around the resolution of the grief and anxiety that accompany it.

Situational Crisis. In sharp contrast to maturational crisis, a situational crisis arises from traumatic events. These stressors are not part of common everyday life; they are accidental. Examples of situational crises include natural disasters (fires, earthquake, flood), national disasters (wars), and crimes of violence (murder, abuse, rape).

Nurses may work with clients who are experiencing either type of crisis. Clients may require hospitalization following a situational crisis, such as a motor vehicle accident. Another client may have difficulty accepting a new diagnosis, or be hospitalized in an area of the country away from friends and family. Other clients may be hospitalized for medical or surgical illness during a period of maturational crisis. For example, a woman required surgery on the day before her youngest child was leaving home for college. Even though the surgery was necessary, she would be feeling torn that she was not present to be certain everything was in order for the child.

Box 3–1. Phases of Crisis

Phase 1: A person is confronted with a problem, stressor, or conflict that threatens the self-concept. He or she responds with anxiety. The increase in anxiety stimulates the use of usual problem-solving techniques and defense mechanisms in an effort to solve the problem and lower the anxiety.

Phase 2: If the usual defense mechanisms fail and the threat persists, anxiety continues to rise. This rise in anxiety produces extreme discomfort. The person's functioning becomes disorganized. He or she begins to make trial-and-error attempts at solving the problem and restoring a normal balance.

Phase 3: If the trial-and-error attempts fail, anxiety can escalate to severe and panic levels. These extreme levels of anxiety mobilize automatic relief behaviors such as withdrawal and flight. Some form of resolution may be made in this stage by either compromising needs or redefining the situation to make an acceptable solution.

Phase 4: If the problem is not solved, anxiety can overwhelm the person and lead to serious personality disorganization. This disorganization may be exhibited as yelling, confusion, running about aimlessly, immobilization with fear, violence against others, or suicidal behavior.

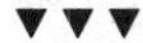

Adapted from Varcarolis, R. N. (1990), *Foundations of Psychiatric Mental Health Nursing.* Philadelphia, W. B. Saunders Company, p. 209; original data from Caplan (1964), Ewing (1978), Robinson (1973), and Hoff (1989).

Theories on Crisis and Crisis Intervention

Caplan described four distinct phases of crisis (Box 3–1). The first step begins with a conflict or a problem that threatens the self-concept. The client responds with increased feelings of anxiety and uses previous coping measures to reduce anxiety and solve the problem. One end to the situation is use of usual coping strategies and resolution of the crisis. This problem-solving process occurs quickly with most problems. When the usual coping mechanisms are ineffective, because the problem is new or the methods do not fit the problem, the client has to use a trial and error approach. If trial and error attempts to solve the problem fail, anxiety can escalate to severe or panic levels. This high level of anxiety may lead to the need for relief behaviors, such as withdrawal and flight, or redefining the problem. Redefining the problem may reveal areas or needs that can be compromised. If the problem is not solved, anxiety can overwhelm the client and crisis exists. At this stage, the client is not able to solve the problem and requires help.

RESEARCH ON CRISIS INTERVENTION

The study of crisis and crisis intervention began in the 1940s after a horrid fire in the Cocoanut Grove nightclub. Studies of the survivors of the fire revealed that acute grief was a normal reaction to a distressing situation. In addition, it was found that preventive interventions could eliminate or decrease some serious personality alterations and psychological consequences that follow severe anxiety. The outcome of these studies was a turning point for current crisis assessment and early intervention. The development of crisis services in hospitals and community clinics is a direct outcome from these studies. Common examples found in most communities include suicide prevention and crisis centers, and 24-hr hotlines for cocaine abuse, runaways, child abuse, rape victims, and battered women to provide emergency assessment and intervention.

Because the stress of being in crisis is so uncomfortable, crisis is self-limiting. Crisis usually lasts for a few days to a maximum of a few weeks (e.g., 6 weeks). The crisis will be resolved with or without intervention. However, the client who faces a crisis alone and without intervention is not likely to resolve the true problem and is more vulnerable to a repeat of the crisis. In contrast, the client who had some crisis intervention is more likely to find a positive method to solving the crisis and has a lesser chance of another problem.

Assessment. Crisis intervention is focused on the immediate problem causing the crisis. It begins with an assessment of the client's *perception of the event.* This initial assessment is critical because it allows the nurse to see the problem from the client's perspective. Some suggested questions to ask are

Has anything happened to you in the last few weeks or days that has been especially upsetting?
What was happening in your life before you started to feel the way you feel now?
What has brought you in for help at this time?
Describe how you are feeling right now.
How does this problem affect your life at the moment?
How do you see this problem affecting your life in the future?

The second step is to assess the client's *situational supports.* The support systems that the client has can provide an important source of energy, strength, financial assistance, services, and compassion. If the client has no support mechanism, the nurse may have to provide support to the client or request such support from within the agency. Some questions to ask to elicit the presence of supports are

With whom do you live?
To whom do you talk when you feel upset?
Who can you trust?
Who is available to you now?
Where do you go to church, school or other community-based activities?

The last portion of the assessment is to determine *coping strategies.* It is important to know what the client's usual coping strategies are so that some idea can be gleaned about why these strategies did not work with this event. In addition, previous coping strategies should be reused if appropriate. Finally, the level of anxiety should be determined, and if the client is in need, immediate intervention should be provided to prevent self-harm or harm to others. Some questions to ask in this portion of the assessment include

What has bothered you most about this illness?
How has it been a problem for you?
What have you done about the problem? Did it work?
What has been the most difficult thing in your life you have had to face until now? What did you do then?
Whom do you rely on the most? Whom do you expect will help you?
In general, how do things turn out for you?

The client's family is almost always affected by the crisis. Their reaction to the event needs to be assessed also. The nurse should assess the ability of the family members to help each other, to meet physical and emotional needs of the members, to communicate, to adapt to the situation, and to make decisions.

Nursing Diagnosis. The client in crisis often has high levels of anxiety. Once anxiety is at a moderate or severe level, the ability to problem solve is limited further. The immediate goal, therefore, is to reduce the anxiety by one level. For example, a client in a panic level could be assisted to a level of severe anxiety; severe to moderate anxiety; and moderate to mild anxiety. The client's family may also require intervention.

Once the anxiety level is decreased and the client can assist with problem solving, a realistic goal should be established. The client, not the nurse, must solve the problem. The nurse's role is to assist the client to gain new perspectives on the problem and thereby find constructive methods to solve the problem. If the nurse solves the problem for the client, the client does not learn to solve problems but instead learns to rely on the nurse. The nurse needs to be aware of his or her personal feelings and that the client's anxiety may be contagious. In addition, the nurse needs to be a caring person with excellent listening skills.

Summary

Disease has multiple causes. Many factors influence both health and illness. Some of these factors include stress and coping strategies. Understanding the many facets of health and illness helps the nurse provide more comprehensive care.

Bibliography

1. Aguilera, D. (1990). *Crisis intervention theory and methodology* (6th ed). St. Louis: C. V. Mosby.
2. Caplan, G. (1964). *Symptoms of preventive psychiatry.* New York: Basic Books.
3. Croushore, T. (1981). *Using crisis intervention wisely.* Philadelphia: Nursing Books, Intermed Communications.
4. Elliott, G. & Eisdorfer, C. (Eds.) (1982). *Stress and human health.* New York: Springer.
5. Ewing, C. (1978). *Crisis intervention as psychotherapy.* New York: Oxford University Press.
6. Friedman, M., & Rosenman, R. (1971). Type A behavior pattern: Its association with coronary heart disease. *Annals of Clinical Research 3,* 300-308.
7. Hoff, L. (1989). *People in crisis: Understanding and helping.* Menlo Park, CA: Addison-Wesley.
8. Holmes, T. & Romo, M. (1974). Subjects' recent life changes and the onset of myocardial infarction and coronary death. In E. Gunderson and R. Rahe (Eds.) *Life stress and illness.* Springfield, IL: Charles C Thomas, Publisher.
9. Holmes, T. & Rahe, R. (1967). The social readjustment rating scale. *Journal of Psychosomatic Research, 11,* 213-217.
10. Locke, S. & Heisel, J. (1977). The influence of stress and emotions on human immunity. *Biofeedback Self-regulation, 2,* 320.
11. Merz, B. (1990, Aug 17). Taking more steps toward gene therapy. *American Medical News, 3,* 16.
12. Parsons. T. (1951). *The social system.* New York: Free Press.
13. Pollock, S., & Duffy, M. (1990). The health-related hardiness scale: Development and psychometric analysis. *Nursing Research, 39*(4), 218-222.
14. Reed, D., et al. (1984). Psychosocial processes and general susceptibility to chronic disease. *American Journal of Epidemiology, 119*(3), 356-370.
15. Roberts, A. (1990). *Crisis intervention handbook.* Belmont, CA: Wadsworth Publishing Company.
16. Robinson, L. (1973). Psychiatric emergencies. *Nursing 73,* 7:43.
17. Temoshok, L., et al. (1983). *Emotions in Health and Illness.* New York: Grune and Stratton.

17a. Waglid, G., & Young, H. (1990). Resilence among older women. *Image, 22*(4), 252-255.

18. Wilson, H. & Kneisl, C. (1990). *Psychiatric nursing.* Menlo Park, CA: Addison-Wesley Publishers.
19. Wu, R. (1973). *Behavior and illness.* Englewood Cliffs, NJ: Prentice Hall.
20. Wyngaarden, J., Smith, L., Bennett, J. (1992). 19th ed. *Cecil textbook of medicine.* Philadelphia: W.B. Saunders.

Chapter 4

Ethics

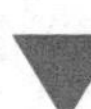

As a clinician, the contemporary nurse is frequently confronted with situations that require ethical decision making. Situations are often encountered in which the nurse can no longer refer to accepted standards, norms, or rules for guidance in ethical decision making. Frequent crisis situations force the nurse to make unprecedented choices that encompass ethical considerations. The prolongation of life, the institution of extraordinary means to sustain life, the dilemma of human experimentation, the need for informed consent, the promotion of beneficence and nonmaleficence, the promotion of autonomy and self-determination, and the consideration of justice as applied to the allocation of health care resources are only a few of the ethical dilemmas that confront the nurse in everyday practice.

The nurse needs to be aware of philosophic theories, concepts, and principles that underlie ethical decision making in clinical nursing practice. To enter into the ethical decision-making process, the nurse needs to have an awareness of ethics and a sense of certainty in analyzing ethical dilemmas. The nurse needs to be aware of the impact of beliefs, attitudes, values, rules, standards, past experience, and choices on the decision-making process. As a decision maker, the nurse should be familiar with a systematic process for reflective thinking and conscious choosing, and how this process interfaces with that of other decision makers. The nurse should be aware of ethical issues, and how these issues have an impact on contemporary nursing practice. Ethical decisions cannot and should not be made in isolation. As members of society, nurses have a responsibility to engage in shared decision making, particularly when the decisions are value laden, and when there frequently appears to be no "right" or "wrong" answer. Initially, a feeling of uneasiness may be sensed as the nurse begins to question those values that have been fostered over a lifetime, but the outcome of this experience may be a new sense of maturity. Situations that appeared to be clear in the past suddenly may become cloudy. The clarification of one's own values and the values of others assists the nurse in the development of a philosophy of nursing and client care. Once developed, this philosophy will assist in the implementation of care that is based on principles that serve to guide in decision making. Reflective thinking and conscious choosing will become automatic, and the burden of ethical decision making will be alleviated to some extent.

OVERVIEW

Ethics, or moral philosophy, is one branch of philosophy. The concern of ethics is the exploration and analysis of moral standards, judgements, choices, beliefs, and problems. As defined by McFadden[30] ethics is "that science which studies the morality of human acts through the medium of natural reason . . . directive of the moral acts of men's will according to basic rational principles . . . [It] teaches us how to judge accurately the moral goodness or badness of any human action" (p.1). McFadden reflects the critical elements of moral philosophy: the need for rationality and the need for guiding principles in the judgement of the moral rightness or wrongness, goodness or badness of human action. Also reflected in his writing are the realities that health care providers are being confronted with in clinical practice. The ushering in of life, the preservation of life, and the departing of life are very much a part of the nurse's practice. The search for guiding principles and the applicability of ethics to the client care situations are very real to the nurse who has confronted ethical dilemmas in nursing practice.

DEFINITIONS

A nurse needs to be aware of the nature of ethics as a systematic body of knowledge and as a directive and practical science that can be applied to daily living through reason and commitment.[30] Sahakian[35] differentiates between ethics and morals in noting that *ethics* pertains to the "study of morals or moral issues" whereas *morals* refers to the actual standards of conduct observed by individuals. Frankena[22] states that the term *ethical* may be used interchangeably with the word *moral*, and either the term *moral* or *ethical* may be considered as good or right. The nurse could consider *ethics* as the formal reasoning process for the exploration of the goodness or badness and rightness or wrongness of an action, and *morals* as those principles and standards the nurse refers to when determining the rightness or wrongness of an action.

Reflective thinking and conscious choosing are implied in the conduct of moral philosophy. Dewey,[18] referring to reflective morality (p. 3), proposes that reflective morality demands thinking, reasoning, and an appeal to an individual's conscience. He perceived reflection as being the process through which the moral decision maker seeks dependable principles when faced with an ethical dilemma that is difficult to decide in terms of the right decision or action. Nurses should also consider the personal, professional, and societal values and codes that guide them in their decisions and actions. Reflective thinking and confrontation of questions concerning actions, obligations, responsibilities, justifications, and principles enable the nurse to have a clearer perspective of ethical dilemmas and move the nurse toward freedom, autonomy, and accountability as a decision maker.[24]

The concept of *moral institution* is also important to the nurse. Moral institution is defined as a point of view for reasoning and judging that includes rules, ideals, virtues, principles, sanctions, codes, regulations, traditions, and moral beliefs that evolve from society and from an individual's personal experiences, history, and choices.[22, 24] The nurse should recognize that individuals have had their sense of morality fostered over a lifetime and from a variety of sources. One example of the early inculcation of morality is that of the development of the superego in early childhood. Awareness of right and wrong, and good and bad is frequently carried with an individual throughout childhood and into adulthood, and is reflected in an individual's conscience. Many individuals continue to refer to their basic beliefs, values, and ideals, which serve as their parameters for decision making. Personal experiences and choices also serve as the basis for everyday decision making, and rarely are these choices rationally examined in terms of their impact on decisions. Nurses, as social beings, strive to accommodate to the complex world around them. Their concern for other individuals further complicates the decision-making process.

Judgements and actions are frequently rationalized on the basis of rules and principles that guide the nurse in decision making. When exploring the meaning of ethics, it is evident that a continual process of valuing takes place in an individual during cognition and that these values are often expressed, for example, in the communication process. The importance of analyzing this valuing process becomes evident when considering nursing communication. Whether communicating with other nurses, families, or health care team members, nurses should be able to identify and express judgements and beliefs as rational, autonomous individuals.

When confronted with moral dilemmas, nurses need to engage in reflective thinking prior to and during the decision-making process. They need to consider personal, professional, and societal values and codes that guide them in their decisions and actions. Principles should be identified that can then serve as guidelines in the decision-making process.

PRINCIPLES

There are basic principles that serve as the foundation for ethical decision making. Beauchamp and Childress[9] identify the four basic principles: (1) justice, (2) respect for autonomy, (3) nonmaleficence, and (4) beneficence. The *American Nurses' Association's Code for Nurses with Interpretive Statements*[3] identifies one fundamental principle, the respect for persons, and seven basic principles: (1) beneficence (doing good); (2) nonmaleficence (avoiding harm); (3) autonomy (self-determination); (4) justice (treating people fairly); (5) fidelity (keeping promises); (6) veracity (truth telling); and (7) confidentiality (respecting privileged information). These principles can be used by nurses as the foundation for ethical decision making and to assist nurses in their determination of the right or the wrong choice that guides them in their direct and indirect actions.

Respect for the person is a broad, fundamental guiding principle. The *ANA Code for Nurses with Interpretive Statements*[3] identifies this principle as the supreme moral principle from which all other principles come. When these other principles are examined, it is easy to see how respect for the person is at the core of each.

Beneficence and Maleficence

The principles of *beneficence* and *maleficence* imply that the nurse should always do good and work to prevent harm. All health care providers should keep this principle in mind when making health care decisions. It is a basic principle that seems to be a major factor in the trust that develops between the health care consumer and the health care provider. The assumption is made by the consumer that this principle will not be violated, the goals and outcomes will be directed toward the good, and harm will not be intentional.

Autonomy

Another principle, *autonomy*, implies that the nurse will support freedom of choice, independence, and self-determination. Clients are given opportunities to make decisions, and informed consent is the basis for health care decisions. This principle seems to support the client's right to know, be informed, and be able to act on his or her own autonomous decision, and it excludes conditions of coercion and deception. It supports that clients should be able to determine the course of action that is consistent with their own beliefs, values, and choices, and that health care providers have no right to inflict on clients those decisions and actions that reflect their own beliefs, values, and choices, which may be inconsistent with the client's.

Justice

Another principle, *justice*, implies choosing the action that is most fair after reflecting on the claims or rights of the individuals involved in the decision-making process. Because we are social beings, we have certain obligations and commitments to other social beings. Part of this commitment is to distribute the 'good' in a way that most benefits other individuals and without discrimination or bias. This principle, when upheld, prevents unfair treatment of the sick, disabled, handicapped, indigent, or other classes of individuals. It addresses the allocation of scarce resources and development of an optimal level of care for all clients. The current health plan in Oregon is based on this principle—distribution of a basic level of care to all citizens of the state.

Fidelity and Veracity

The principles of *fidelity* and *veracity* are closely associated. These concepts imply that the nurse keeps any promises made to the client and does not make promises unless they can be kept. Also, the nurse always tells the client the truth. These issues can be problematic at times, because the nurse may not be the decision maker about when to give the client information as well as what information is to be given. For example, if a client has not been told the diagnosis but this client asks the nurse if that diagnosis is known, the nurse may be faced with a real dilemma. The principle of fidelity requires that promises be kept or that they not be made.

Confidentiality

The principle of confidentiality means that the nurse respects all privileged information about the client. A client must be able to assume that information given to a health care professional will be respected and not repeated. For example, consider a prominent client who is treated for a serious condition. This client could be personally ruined if the information was made public. The client must be able to trust that any such information will remain confidential or the client might not seek health care.

If the nurse is faithful to commitments, and these commitments reflect all the ethical principles, the nurse upholds these commitments. The nurse believes in doing good and avoiding harm. All clients are respected and clients are supported without discrimination or bias. The nurse respects the client's right to know, and informed choice always serves as the basis for decision making. Truthfulness and promise keeping are implicit, and clients actively and freely engage in decisions related to their personal care. Clients can trust that their confidences will be kept, no matter what circumstances prevail.

GUIDELINES FOR PROFESSIONAL PRACTICE

Parameters for nursing practice are also determined by the American Nurses' Association's *Standards of Nursing Practice*,[4] the American Nurses' Association's *Code for Nurses with Interpretive Statements*,[3] the American Hospital Association's *Patients' Bill of Rights*,[2] and state *Nurse Practice Acts. Nurse Practice Acts* and

Standards of Nursing Practice primarily address the nurse's use of the nursing process in the provision of care that is based on sound principles and substantive knowledge, which incorporates health teaching and counseling with a focus on health promotion, maintenance, and restoration. The *Standards*, in particular, indicate that nursing is client centered, and both documents reflect the need for nursing judgement that is ongoing and continuous in the nurse-client interaction. The *Code for Nurses* (Box 4-1) and the *Patients' Bill of Rights* (Box 4-2) also have many common elements that serve as guidelines for the nurse. The *Code for Nurses* addresses client dignity and uniqueness, privacy and confidentiality, client protection, nursing accountability and responsibility, maintenance of competence, informed judgement, participation in inquiry, the implementation and improvement of standards of care, enhancement of employment conditions to improve the quality of care, enhancement of nursing's integrity and image, and collaboration for the promotion of public health needs. The *Patients' Bill of Rights*, in addition, addresses the clients' rights to information, informed consent, timely responses to requests for services, information regarding human experimentation and the right to refuse treatment, continuity of care, explanations regarding treatment costs, and the need to explain hospital rules and regulations that influence the client's understanding of his role as a client.

These legal documents can serve as guidelines for decision making for the nurse who is confronted with situations that demand decision making because they entail ethical or legal problems. As the nurse becomes familiar with these documents, the commonalities begin to surface with respect to nursing obligations, judgements, and accountability. Box 4-3 summarizes some guidelines.

Box 4-1. American Nurses' Association's Code for Nurses

1. The nurse provides services with respect for human dignity and the uniqueness of the client unrestricted by considerations of social or economic status, personal attributes, or the nature of the health problems
2. The nurse safeguards the client's right to privacy by judiciously protecting information of a confidential nature
3. The nurse acts to safeguard the client and the public when health care and safety are affected by the incompetent, *unethical*, or illegal practice of any person
4. The nurse assumes responsibility and accountability for individual nursing judgements and actions
5. The nurse maintains competence in nursing
6. The nurse exercises informed judgement and uses individual competence and qualifications as criteria in seeking consultation, accepting responsibilities, and delegating nursing activities to others
7. The nurse participates in activities that contribute to the ongoing development of the profession's body of knowledge
8. The nurse participates in the profession's effort to implement and improve standards of nursing
9. The nurse participates in the profession's efforts to establish and maintain conditions of employment conducive to high-quality nursing care
10. The nurse participates in the profession's effort to protect the public from misinformation and misrepresentation and to maintain the integrity of nursing
11. The nurse collaborates with members of the health professions and other citizens in promoting community and national efforts to meet the needs of the public

▼▼▼

From American Nurses Association (1985). *American Nurses' Association: Code for nurses with interpretive statements*. Kansas City: American Nurses' Association.

Box 4-2. Patients' Bill of Rights

1. Considerate and respectful care
2. Current information regarding diagnosis, treatment, and prognosis
3. Informed consent
4. Right to refuse treatment and to be informed of consequences of that action
5. Privacy and discretion
6. Confidentiality
7. Reasonable response to request of patient for services
8. Information regarding relationships to other health care and educational institutions
9. Reasonable continuity of care
10. Advised as to use of human experimentation and right to refuse participation
11. Examination and reasonable explanation of bill, regardless of source of payment
12. Knowledge of hospital rules and regulations that apply to conduct as a patient

Adapted from American Hospital Association (1972). *Patients' bill of rights*. Chicago: American Hospital Association. Reprinted with permission of the American Hospital Association, copyright 1972.

Box 4-3. Selected Nursing Guidelines for Practice

- Nurses and clients should be informed
- Care should be systematically implemented
- Nursing knowledge and competence should be maintained
- Clients should be protected and safeguarded
- Professional integrity should be maintained
- Clients' rights should be upheld
- Clients should be treated with dignity
- Care should be individualized
- Care should be client centered
- Health teaching and counseling should be incorporated within plans of care
- Data should be accessible, communicated, and recorded
- Continuity of care should be maintained
- Goals of nursing should also extend to the broader public through collaborative efforts

ETHICAL THEORIES

In addition to basic ethical principles, codes, and professional guidelines for nursing practice, there are two basic ethical theories that offer substantive knowledge that the nurse can apply in practice. These theories are *deontology* and *teleology*. Using a deontological approach to ethics means that the person has a basic belief that moral judgements are based on factors other than the calculation of good over evil effects. This approach implies there is no right or wrong, or good or bad answer. The rules for ethical decision making using this theoretical approach are concerned with a right action, however. Some things are done simply because that is the right thing to do, regardless of the outcome. For example, if you believe in autonomy, then the person has the right to make a choice, regardless of the outcome.

Using a teleologic approach to ethics means that the primary consideration in determining the right action would be the ends or consequences of that action. The saying "the end justifies the means" comes from this theoretical approach. Approaching ethics from this perspective means there is a right or wrong outcome and that getting to the right or correct outcome is the important factor. This philosophy was in use, in the past, when prisoners were given medications or vaccines that might be harmful to them, that would speed the discovery of important medical treatments that would save many lives.

It is important for the nurse to be able to differentiate between the deontological and teleologic frames of reference for ethical decision making. If one health care provider is basically a deontologist, and another is a teleologist, a conflict can arise that may not be resolvable without mediation or negotiation. Deontologic and teleologic beliefs can be identified through application of the characteristics described in Tables 4-1 and 4-2. If the nurse can recognize some of these characteristics as personal beliefs, then the nurse can begin to comprehend how these beliefs influence decision making, and how values and beliefs are fostered in the nurse over a lifetime. Some people may find that they believe in both theories in part.

Because nurses are social beings, they have values and beliefs fostered in them from a variety of sources: home, friends, family, parents, teachers, society, education, literature, experience, and their choices throughout their lives. Because nurses are health care providers, they encounter many situations that cause conflict in their values and beliefs. For example, they witness a terminally ill client who has experienced a cardiac arrest. The nurse's first instinct is usually preserving life and, frequently, at any cost. The conflict arises when the nurse reflects on the situation, and considers all the facts. Perhaps the nurse believes in dignity, or the sanctity of life. On the other hand, the nurse also considers the cost to the family and to society. The nurse is faced with value conflicts and a dilemma that is not readily resolved. It is difficult to determine to whom or to what the nurse refers when confronted with these situations.

MODELS OF ETHICAL DECISION MAKING

Once familiar with the basic principles, codes, guidelines, and theories that can serve as substantive knowledge for ethical decision making in nursing, the nurse can use a systematic ethical decision-making model for

TABLE 4-1. Deontological Characteristics Compared with Nursing Beliefs

Deontological Characteristics	Nursing Beliefs
Never use a person as a means to an end	Do you believe that persons should not be sacrificed for the benefit of others?
The primary focus for decision making is not on the consequences of an action	Do you consider factors other than the outcomes or consequences of your decisions when making decisions?
Exceptionless rules	Do you believe that some rules should be upheld without exception?
High sense of duty	Do you recognize within yourself a high sense of duty?
Reference to reason and the will	Do you believe that you have a sense of reason and a will that assist you in determining right and wrong?
Universal principles	Do you recognize that some actions are always known to be right or wrong in similar situations?
Judeo-Christian ethic	Do you have some basic rules that have evolved from your religious beliefs that guide you in decision making?
Reference to covenant	Do you believe that there is a covenant for care that should not be violated?
Autonomy	Do you support the clients' need to make autonomous decisions?
Human dignity	Do you always respect the dignity of clients under all conditions?
Free choice	Do you believe that clients should be free to make choices related to their care?
Concern for the individual	Do you always plan your care on the basis of the individual client?
Uniqueness of humans	Do you always respect the client as a unique human being?
Actions are sometimes simply known to be right	Do you believe that some actions are simply known to be right, no matter what the circumstances?
Application of rules	Do you have basic rules that guide you in your decision making?

TABLE 4–2. Teleologic Characteristics Compared with Nursing Beliefs

Teleologic Characteristics	Nursing Beliefs
The moral status of an action is determined by the ends of that action	Do you believe that what matters in an action is the outcome or consequences of the action?
The primary question is "what is good?"	Do you ask yourself "what is good" when making decisions?
Calculation of good over evil effects	Do you try to balance the good over bad or evil effects when making decisions?
Rules are usually very general	Do you make decisions without reference to hardfast rules that are exceptionless?
The right action is that which produces benefit, advantage, pleasure, good, or happiness, or prevents mischief, pain, evil, or unhappiness	Do you believe that the right action can be calculated in terms of, for example, an increase in pleasure or a decrease in pain?
Outcomes are measurable and quantifiable	Do you sometimes make decisions on the basis of measurable or quantifiable outcomes in client care situations?
The right action produces the greatest amount of good in general or the greatest happiness for the greatest number	Do you believe that the right action is the one that promotes the greatest amount of good for everyone, or that the right action brings the greatest amount of happiness for the greatest number?
Distribution of goods	Do you believe that goods, such as health care resources, should be distributed evenly throughout society?
Justice	Do you recognize the need for justice and fairness in health care decision making?
Society	Do you frequently consider social consequences that may result from decisions?
Egalitarianism	Do you believe that all persons should be treated equally, for example, in relation to rights, privileges, and resources?
Proportional goodness	Do you believe that resources should be distributed proportionately among all members of society?

problem resolution when confronted with ethical dilemmas. There are a number of models that have been used by nurses to help them solve ethical dilemmas, including ones proposed by Murphy and Murphy,[31] Curtin,[16] and Levine-Ariff and Groh[27a] (Table 4–3). These models are very similar, offering the nurse a systematic way to look at ethical dilemmas. Table 4–4 compares the steps of the Murphy and Murphy model to the steps of the nursing process, showing the similarity between the two problem-solving methods.

Murphy and Murphy Model

We will use the Murphy and Murphy model as an example to discuss the process of ethical decision making. This model demands assessment, problem identification, data concerning the decision makers, establishment of alternatives, and an examination of the possible outcomes of each action based on principles, evaluation, and modifications arising from the evaluation.

ASSESSMENT

Initially, the nurse must be aware that a problem exists. For example, a terminally ill client has been admitted to the hospital and there are no clear policies related to the code/no code order for terminally ill clients.

IDENTIFICATION OF THE DILEMMA

The next step would be the identification of the existence of an ethical dilemma. The nurse may experience a feeling of uneasiness because of a value conflict or feel uncertain as to what the decision should be if the client experiences a cardiac arrest.

DECISION MAKERS

The nurse would then have to identify the persons who would be involved in making a decision related to the perceived dilemma. These individuals might be the client, family or significant others, physician, other team members, clergy, or even hospital administration and legal counsel. *Roles would have to be identified.* These roles could range from an autonomous client, to an advocate nurse or a guardian relative.

ALTERNATIVES

Those involved in making the decision would then have to explore the alternatives and the short-term and long-term consequences of each alternative. If an alternative were to write a no code order, there are

TABLE 4-3. Models for Ethical Decison Making

Steps in the Process	Murphy and Murphy	Curtin	Levine-Ariff and Groh
1	Identify the health problem	Get background information about the problem	Define the dilemma
2	Identify the ethical problem	Identify the ethical parts of the problem	Identify the medical facts
3	State who is involved in making the decision	Identify the ethical agents (people involved in making the decision)	Identify the nonmedical facts: A. Patient and family B. External factors
4	Identify the nurse's role	Identify all possible choices and the outcomes of those choices	Separate assumptions from facts
5	Consider as many alternatives as possible	Apply the relevant ethical theories, principles, and rules	Identify items needing clarification
6	Consider the long-range and short-range consequences of each alternative decision	Resolve the dilemma	Identify the decision makers
7	Reach a decision	Act on the decision	Review the underlying ethical principles
8	Consider how this decision fits into the nurse's general philosophy of patient care		Define alternatives
9	Follow this situation until the actual results of the decision are visible and use this information to help make future decisions		Follow up

Data from Murphy, M. A. & Murphy, J. (1976). Model for ethical decision making. *Nursing 76, 8,* 13–14; Curtin, L. L. (1978). A proposed model for critical ethical analysis. *Nursing Forum, 17,* 14; and Levine-Ariff, J., & Groh, D. H. (1990). *Nursing managers' bookshelf: Creating an ethical environment* (pp. 41–61). Baltimore: Williams & Wilkins.

TABLE 4-4. Comparison of Nursing Process and Murphy and Murphy's Ethical Decision-Making Model

Nursing Process	Murphy and Murphy Model
1. Assessment	1. Identify the health problem 2. Identify the ethical problem 3. State who is involved in making the decision
2. Analysis (diagnosis)	4. Identify your role
3. Planning	5. Consider as many alternatives as you can 6. Consider the long-range and short-range consequences of each alternative
4. Implementation	7. Reach your decision
5. Evaluation	8. Consider how this decision fits into your general philosophy of patient care 9. Follow this situation until you can see the actual results of your decision, and use this information to help you in making future decisions

many possible short-term consequences. It could cause the family grief, or it might disturb members of the health care team. On the other hand, it could support client autonomy and dignity, or it could be a relief for the family and health team members because the order might end a great deal of client suffering. The long-term consequences could be as varied as the short-term consequences, as could the consequences of a decision not to write the no code order.

MAKING A DECISION

Once the alternatives have been fully explored by the appropriate persons, a decision must be made.

Assuming the nurse is involved in the decision, the nurse should then reflect on whether or not the decision is consistent with the nurse's philosophy of client care ethics. If the nurse, for example, knows the client made a decision for a no code order and was fully informed, that freedom of choice was granted, and the nurse has a deontological philosophy, then the nurse will support the client's decision and feel comfortable with it. If, on the other hand, the client or family chose not to have a no code order written, the nurse with a teleologic philosophy would question the extreme cost to society. Rather than giving support to the client or family, the nurse would believe that the wrong decision was made.

EVALUATION

As a final step, the nurse needs to evaluate the outcome of the decision, so a baseline can be established for further decision making. If the outcomes are not consistent with the nurse's philosophy or beliefs, it could be that the nurse, when confronted with a similar situation, would choose alternatives before implementing action through ethical decision making. The use of an ethical decision-making model is a useful tool for any nurse who is often confronted with complex dilemmas. The nurse could use any of the models to reach similar solutions.

As one begins to analyze situations with ethical problems, basic principles begin to emerge. Sigman[37] has described the complexity of ethical choice in nursing and addresses the need for nurses to be responsible, accountable, and committed. She also notes that the nurse sometimes has to take a risk, and that choices may involve freedom, change, and justice. Nelson,[32] addressing the issue of authenticity, supports Sigman and notes that if the nurse is free to act in support of self-determination, the nurse also has to act in a way that will not violate the freedom or rights of others.

Given basic knowledge, principles, and guidelines for ethical decision making, the nurse can apply this knowledge in a way that will enhance decision making in clinical nursing practice. When confronted with conflicts, whether internal or external, the nurse can refer to guidelines and norms when engaging in problem resolution. Assessment, observation, and communication skills enhance the nurse's ability as an ethical decision maker. Reflective thinking and conscious choosing enable the nurse to make informed choices and act on choices as a rational decision maker.

RESEARCH IN ETHICS

In an International Council of Nurses' publication, Tate[39] reported on an ethics study that was based on data gathered from nurses and nursing students in 25 countries. Reflected within the study results were that common problems were perceived by nurses across many cultures and languages. Of particular notice was the nurses' feeling of being alone when confronted with ethical dilemmas. The fact that ethical problems are being encountered in daily nursing practice also was supported in studies by Chinn[14] and Sigman.[37]

In Scotland, Schrock[36] surveyed 131 nursing students and graduate nurses, exploring ethical issues that they were encountering or expected to encounter in their clinical nursing practice. Some of the issues identified as dilemmas were abortions, resuscitation, euthanasia, organ transplantation issues, and psychosurgery. Schrock noted the absence of everyday moral issues such as truth telling and confidentiality.

Applegate[5] explored ethical issues and decision-making patterns in 60 nurses employed in hospitals. Issues identified by the nurses were relationships, standards of care, terminal illness, congenital anomalies, setting priorities, and rights issues. Methods used by each nurse in making decisions were that he or she (1) communicates ethical opinions and judgements and/or seeks higher authority, (2) discriminates between right and wrong, (3) intervenes in spite of opposition, (4) intervenes without opposition, and (5) takes no intervention. One major conclusion was that these nurses were functioning beyond the ethical and legal parameters of nursing practice.

Mayberry[29] also explored methods of ethical decision making used by 167 hospital-based nurses. Kohlberg's[27] levels of moral reasoning were evaluated through administration of the Defining Issue Test to the nurses. The identified levels of moral reasoning were compared with the nurses' education, age, the amount of time in nursing practice, and the size of the employing hospital. Study results indicated that nurses are more apt to use an intuitive approach than critical inquiry or principled reasoning when solving ethical problems. Moral development, as well as principled decision making, was powerfully and consistently related to the nurse's level of education. The number of years in practice after formal schooling also affected the nurses' ability in principled reasoning. The fewer the years in practice, the greater was the nurse's ability in principled reasoning, which suggested to the researcher that formal education is significant in its contribution to principled reasoning.

The data also suggested that an individual's moral judgement may be strongly influenced by the work environment. Personal factors, such as obedience to authority within a hierarchy that represents a conventional level of reasoning, were frequently characteristics of head nurses. Increasing age and experience were considered by the researcher to be factors that contribute to the development of loyalty to peers and to the institution, as well as to a commitment to the organization's aims. The researcher recommended that nursing administrators have a responsibility to promote an environment in which nurses would have opportunities to engage in systematic ethical decision making, and selected strategies were suggested that would enhance nurses' ethical problem-solving skills.

The literature indicates that selected nursing studies have identified ethical issues confronting nurses in clinical practice. Ethical decision-making patterns used by nurses have been explored, as well as their patterns of moral reasoning. Research in nursing ethics is continuing to add to nursing's body of knowledge relating to ethics in nursing.

TOPICS OF ETHICAL CONCERN

The nurse is confronted with many ethical dilemmas on a daily basis. These dilemmas frequently cause conflict between the nurse and colleagues, clients, and families.

Conflicts also may arise from and be associated with specific situations, such as terminal illness, the allocation of scarce resources, or human experimentation. The complexity of ethical decision making is compounded by the variety of situations in clinical practice that confront the nurse with ethical dilemmas. The nurse is confronted with almost unlimited choices for which there are few clear guidelines to assist in ethical decision making.

Nonintervention

One action that has been reported by nurses in clinical practice situations is that of no intervention.[5] The *American Nurses' Association's Code for Nurses*[3] can provide the nurse with guidelines for this common dilemma. Nurses should remember that to not intervene is a conscious decision on the part of health care workers, and the outcome may be catastrophic for the client. For example, nurses have reported that clients have expired because of inappropriate nonintervention on the part of health care providers. An involuntary sterilization, which is intentionally performed on a mildly retarded client without the client's or guardian's consent while the client is having surgery, is an example of a client's rights being violated. The operating room staff allowed the procedure to be performed. The nurse, although feeling ambivalent, took no action to prevent the procedure from being performed. This is a violation of the tenets of the *American Nurses' Association's Code for Nurses.* The nurse had an ethical obligation to protect the client in any situation, and nurses should be aware that to not intervene is an unethical act. Nurses must become aware of the *Code for Nurses* and the implications of these responsibilities.

Violations of Legal and Ethical Standards in Health Care

The issues that confront nurses in clinical practice are often legal as well as ethical. In some states, reporting systems have evolved that encourage anonymous reporting of violations of the legal and ethical standards of health care practice. Once a violation is reported to the state regulatory agency, an initial investigation of the claim is conducted unknown to the person against whom the claim is made. If the regulatory agency finds cause for further investigation, a referral is made to the appropriate practice board for more extensive review. The health care practitioner may be unaware of the investigation of his or her practice until the claim is reviewed by two professional regulatory agencies. It is at this point that the practitioner is notified of the investigation.

Known as one form of "whistle blowing," these policies have caused some concern to health care providers. The discipline for the health care professions, as it is evolving historically, appears to be originating outside of the profession. One must question the accountability of health care professionals and how and why these reporting mechanisms have evolved. Support systems need to be developed within the professions to foster responsibility and accountability for the legal and ethical parameters of professional practice. Levine-Ariff and Groh in their book, *Creating an Ethical Environment,* discuss the need for nurses to work in an environment in which ethics are encouraged and supported.[27a] Their work discusses how to create such an environment.

ETHICAL CONCERNS FOR NURSES

Colleagues

The nurse may encounter problems related to colleague and peer competency. This competency could relate to a lack of skill, substance abuse, poor judgement, violation of standards, lack of emotional stability, lack of interpersonal skills, or a variety of other problems. The nurse may be confronted with situations such as being given wrong or contraindicated orders to carry out, or may be faced with the dilemma of procedural problems such as reporting the incompetence of a peer or colleague. When these dilemmas arise, support systems are often not available for the nurse. Communication channels may be blocked or unclear, and there may not be appropriate procedural policies within the institution. The nurse often feels alone when faced with this situation.

Clients and Families

The need for occasional separation of client and family often causes conflict and dilemmas for the nurse. If the nurse chooses to support client autonomy, dignity, and freedom of choice, it may mean that the nurse sometimes has to take on what appears to be an adversary position in relation to the family. Granting client privacy and confidentiality should be considered an implicit duty for the nurse. Problems arise in areas such as proxy consent, or who should speak for a client if the client is comatose, incompetent, a minor, or in a state of guardianship. Many states have begun to legalize the "Living Will" and "Durable Power of Attorney for Health Care." These documents provide a way for the client to arrive at health care decisions that must be made when the client is able to make informed decisions about himself or herself to be carried out when the client is unable to state these decisions. The states that recognize these forms as legal documents have a mechanism for the client's wishes to be followed. These documents are a perfect solution for the nurse who believes in client autonomy, because the client's wishes now have legal power. In December 1991, the federal government enacted a law mandating that every person admitted to a health care facility (including a nursing home) should have the Living Will and Durable Power of Attorney for Health Care explained to him or her and that the state laws governing these documents be explained. Booklets are available for use by these institutions to explain the implications of these documents to the client. It is hoped that this law will make more people aware of the options available to them for deciding their own care.

Not all states have these provisions, however, and not all clients have filled out these forms, so ethical choices still have to be made. Decisions must be made in relation to protecting the client and protecting the family as a unit. Situations arise in which the client and family, as well as other health team members, may differ as to their choices for action that will have an impact on the client's status. The nurse may experience a dilemma as the result of a difference in values based on the nurse's philosophic orientation. The nurse needs to develop an awareness of and an appreciation for the ethical decision-making process as a viable mechanism for problem resolution when he or she is confronted with difficult choices that entail ethical issues. In addition, the nurse needs to possess an awareness of the potential for ethical problems, particularly in relation to the client and his or her family. Basic knowledge and principles are needed if the nurse is to engage in ethical decision making, and many nurses are not prepared for the complex situations that arise in clinical practice.

Terminal Illness

Terminal illness often presents complex dilemmas for the nurse in clinical practice. Issues that may arise include, for example, the client's right to refuse treatment, the recognition and nonrecognition of the *Living Will* and *Durable Power of Attorney for Health Care*, questions of euthanasia, the institution and withdrawal of life support systems, the issue of resuscitate versus do not resuscitate orders, and basic ethical issues such as the quality of life versus the sanctity of life. It is a situation in which nurses should be prepared for ambivalence on the part of client, family, and health team members. Continuous support of the client as an autonomous, unique individual is required on the part of the nurse as the primary care giver. The nurse's level of maturity, philosophic orientation, and preparedness for ethical decision making have an impact on his or her ability to be supportive in the complex decisions related to terminal illness. The nurse may need a support system, and if this system is not readily accessible, he or she may once again feel alone when confronted with these situations. Some support systems include Ethics Committees and Nursing Ethics Rounds.

Allocation of Scarce Resources

Nurses are becoming more involved in issues related to the allocation of scarce resources. These resources may refer to personnel, space, equipment, finances, and other, more discrete entities, such as organ donation and transplantation. Resources in health care are not unlimited. In this highly technical society, it soon becomes apparent to the nurse that it may not be possible to meet all the demands of client requests for health service. The new health care system in Oregon addresses this issue specifically by providing a basic level of health care to all residents but limiting the extraordinary measures.

Specific unit services, such as nurses working in renal dialysis units, are often confronted with complex issues such as the unavailability of organs for transplant and the philosophic issue of the quality of life versus the quantity of life. Other complex issues such as organ procurement and transplantation confront the nurse. The introduction, maintenance, and withdrawal of life support systems become difficult issues that daily confront the nurse. Lack of availability of placement facilities for long-term care and lack of adequate resources for funding of health services may present dilemmas in clinical nursing practice. Because nurses are ethical decision makers, they must be aware of their philosophic orientation toward the allocation of scarce resources. Basic principles may be in conflict with each other, such as the commitment to the preservation of life versus the costs of treatment for the client, family, and society. The nurse should be aware of the health team's values on the allocation of scarce resources. Positions must be clarified and guidelines established to assist in decision making.

ETHICAL CONCERNS FOR CLIENTS

Many issues have been identified that have significant implications for clients as health care consumers and for nurses as health care providers. Those issues that have been clearly identified in the literature include clients' rights, informed consent, advocacy, confidentiality and privacy, and truth telling.

Clients' Rights

With advances in technology and the development of new treatment modalities, nurses are being confronted with issues such as the client's right to refuse treatment, therapeutic versus nontherapeutic experimentation, and clients' right to information and knowledge concerning their health status. Clients are becoming more involved in decisions related to their care. Clients' rights are being protected through the development of government regulations, state legislation, and professional guidelines. Documents such as the *Living Will*, *Durable Power of Attorney for Health Care*, and the *Patients' Bill of Rights* (see Box 4–2) provide clients with the ability to ensure that their wishes are carried out, if legally possible. Health care consumers, in general, are becoming more aware of their right to make care decisions. Nurses need to maintain an awareness of policies, procedures, guidelines, and regulations that affect clients' involvement in the decision-making process.

Informed Consent

Many factors violate the consent process in health care. If nurses truly believe that clients should be autonomous and self-determining, they will promote clients' rights to choose freely and to act on their choices without interference from others. Nurses will support clients' abilities to control their own decisions and actions with a sense of having power in the decision-making process. The nurse will promote respect for clients and support clients' rights.

Truth Telling

The nurse-client relationship includes an element of honesty as well as trust. If the nurse believes client autonomy and self-determination should be supported, the nurse will respond to the client with honesty, and the deceit of the client will not be supported. A nurse who believes that the end justifies the means may support client deceit based on a belief that the client is better off not knowing certain information. Nursing actions should be related to nursing concerns. Nurses need to maintain a constant awareness of the significance of the physician-client relationship and how this relationship also has an impact on the nurse, particularly in relation to giving information. The physician has the obligation to inform the client about medical issues, not the nurse. Clients, even when fully informed, may choose not to know the truth in a given situation, and all health care providers should be sensitive to the need to maintain significant care giver–client relationships.

APPROACHES TO RESOLVING PRACTICE PROBLEMS

When confronted with ethical issues in nursing practice, the nurse often experiences a sense of ambivalence in problem resolution. As nurses become better prepared to engage in ethical decision making, some of the feelings of ambivalence may be alleviated. Nurses need to maintain a constant awareness of current ethical issues confronting them in clinical practice. Some of the issues are readily apparent in the nurse's daily practice. Other sources of information should be sought through interaction with colleagues and peers, observance of the media, reading professional and lay literature, and participation in continuing education, both formal and informal (see Nursing Research).

Nurses should be assisted in the process of clarification of their beliefs, attitudes, and values, which serve as the basis for their ethical decision making. Opportunities should be afforded nurses to discuss ethical issues with other health care providers so they begin to recognize how their own personal and professional and others' beliefs, attitudes, and values have an impact on the decision-making process. Once they feel comfortable in this process, they should begin to identify those values that are most significant to them and begin to make choices on the basis of their values. The ultimate outcome of this experience will be the advancement of the nurse's ability to make reflective choices, and the nurse should be willing to support and defend those choices and actions based on a systematic decision-making process.

Policies and procedures should be developed that will assist nurses and other health care providers in their ethical decision making. These policies should be readily available to health care providers and developed with provider input. Appropriate channels of communication should be identified and made readily available to nurses who are confronted with ethical problems. For example, if a nurse confronts a situation in which a colleague has taken action that is not ethical, the nurse should know that there are clear lines of communication that should be followed for resolution of the problem.

Specific guidelines and protocols should be established for complex ethical situations that are frequently encountered in clinical practice. This is particularly rel-

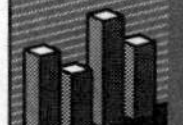

NURSING RESEARCH

Further research is needed in the area of ethics in nursing. Issues have been identified, ethical decision-making patterns and levels of moral reasoning have been explored, and recommendations for curriculum changes have been implemented in many nursing programs. Faculty in nursing are seeking advanced preparation to assist them in the integration of ethics throughout nursing curricula at all levels.

Many questions need to be explored in nursing practice and nursing education in order to add to the theoretical base for the discipline of nursing. Substantive knowledge, concepts, and principles must be identified if the knowledge is to be applied within nursing. A few examples of researchable problems follow:

- What type of support systems should be developed in the profession to foster responsibility and accountability for the ethical parameters of nursing practice?
- What criteria should be used for the institution and withdrawal of life support systems?
- What is the level of knowledge of clients in relation to their rights as clients within the health care system?
- How do nurses resolve their conflicts with other health care providers, clients, and family members?
- Can nurses identify the basic ethical principles that guide them in their ethical decision making?
- How do nurses resolve ethical conflicts in practice when system constraints impede intervention?
- Are nurses able to verbalize their attitudes, beliefs, and values that have an impact on their ethical decision making?
- How effective are ethical review boards in the resolution of ethical problems within health care institutions?
- What is the most effective method for preparing nursing students for ethical decision making in nursing practice?

evant in situations associated with terminal illness, which frequently involve both legal and ethical decision making. Protocols and guidelines have been developed for the implementation of documents such as the *Living Will* and *Durable Power of Attorney for Health Care* in states where these forms are recognized, and copies of the legislation should be available to health care providers for clarification. Nurses should be oriented to these documents and familiar with the hospital policies and procedures that are necessary to implement these documents. In states where these documents do not exist, nurses can initiate legislation for their acceptance.

Nurses also should become involved in the development and implementation of ethical review boards within their institutions. Criteria should be established for the selection of board members who represent health care providers, supporting professions, and the community at large. Policies and procedures should be established for referral of ethical situations to the ethical review board, and nurses should support and evaluate the outcomes of this process for its impact on nursing.

Criteria for the implementation and the withdrawal of life support systems for clients have been established in many health care settings and even in some state legislatures. Ethics committees exist in many institutions that help in the resolution of these complex issues. In institutions without these policies, nurses should be involved in the development of criteria prior to the implementation of policies and procedures within the institution. Protocols have been developed for documentation and recording of health care decisions, such as handling code versus no code orders, and criteria have been developed for the selection of all health care providers and personnel who will have input into these critical decisions. If an institution does not have these policies, the nurse must work for their development.

Nurses should become active on ethics committees within their institutions. In this way they can become involved in the development and implementation of appropriate consent forms and procedures that allow for individual differences in clients, such as level of cognition, reading levels, and language comprehension. Nurses should have a clear set of guidelines available that will assist them in implementing their appropriate role in the consent process. Channels of communication should be identified, such as how to involve the ethics committee, so nurses can seek appropriate guidance if confronted with a consent issue that requires nursing intervention.

Nurses, physicians, and other health care providers should have learning experiences such as ethical rounds, in which they can gain familiarity with systematic ethical decision-making procedures from a multidisciplinary perspective. Nurses should seek every opportunity to engage purposefully in the ethical decision-making process when appropriate, with the understanding that they are accountable for their decisions and actions in this situation in the same way that they are accountable for all of their decisions and actions.

Policies and procedures related to ethical problems should be revised on an ongoing basis as new issues are identified, analyzed, and evaluated. There should be a systematic plan developed for this process, and nurses should be held accountable. A professional commitment on the part of nursing personnel is required if a systematic process is to be implemented effectively.

Summary

The practice of professional nursing demands accountability for nursing actions and decisions. When confronted with issues in practice that demand ethical decision making, the nurse needs to be aware of his or her values, attitudes, and beliefs that influence the decision-making process. The nurse should be familiar with the standards that guide nursing practice and how these standards are applied within the clinical practice setting. The nurse should be willing to support clients' rights and recognize that health care providers also have rights. The assumption is made that rights are accompanied by obligations for clients as well as for health care providers. Within the clinical practice setting, support systems should be available for nurses, clients and families, and other health care providers who are confronted with ethical issues. Mechanisms should be made available for the resolution of problems, and these mechanisms should be developed with input from health care providers. Decision making should be collaborative and communication channels clearly delineated.

For the nurse, who often feels alone when confronted with ethical dilemmas, sometimes the most that can be done in a situation is to consciously engage in a rational, systematic decision-making process. There are few clear-cut, black or white decisions, and often the nurse is confronted with grays. Perhaps this is one unique ability of the professional nurse — the ability to gather data systematically, and to make judgements and decisions based on comprehensive valid information from a variety of sources. This ability, combined with authenticity, respect, and belief in individuals' rights to self-determination and autonomy, may be the key to ethical nursing practice, a practice that is guided by rights, obligations, and accountability.

Bibliography

1. Achetenberg, B., Sawyer, J., & Miller, C. (1983). *Code gray: Ethical dilemmas in nursing.* Boston: Boston Film/Video Foundation.
2. American Hospital Association. (1972). *Patients' bill of rights.* Chicago: Author.
3. American Nurses' Association. (1985). *Code for nurses with interpretive statements.* Kansas City: Author.
4. American Nurses' Association. (1973). *Standards of practice.* Kansas City: Author.
5. Applegate, M. I. (1981). *Moral decisions in selected clinical nursing practice situations.* Unpublished doctoral dissertation, Columbia University, New York.

6. Aroskar, M. A. (1977). Ethics in the nursing curriculum. *Nursing Outlook, 25*(4), 260-264.
7. Baier, K. Deontological theories. In W. T. Walsh (Ed.), *Encyclopedia of bioethics: Vol 1* (pp. 413-417). New York: Macmillan Publishing Co.
8. Baier, K. Teleological theories. In W. T. Walsh (Ed.), *Encyclopedia of bioethics: Vol 1* (pp. 417-421). New York: Macmillan Publishing Co.
9. Beauchamp, T. L., & Childress, J. F. (1989). *Principles of biomedical ethics* (3rd ed.). New York: Oxford University Press.
10. Benjamin, M., & Curtis, J. (1986). *Ethics in nursing* (2nd ed.). New York: Oxford University Press.
11. Bentham, J. (1907). *An introduction to the principles of morals and legislation.* Oxford: The Clarendon Press.
12. Bok, S. (1978). *Lying: Moral choice in public and private life.* New York: Pantheon Books.
13. Burnard, P., & Chapman, C. M. (1988). *Professional and ethical issues in nursing.* Chichester: John Wiley & Sons.
14. Chinn, P. L. (1979). Issues in lowering infant mortality: A call for ethical action. *Advances in Nursing Science, 4*(1), 63-78.
15. Curran, C. E. (1974). Paul Ramsey and traditional Roman Catholic natural law theory. In J. Johnson & D. Smith (Eds.), *Love and society: Essays in the ethics of Paul Ramsey* (pp. 47-65). Missoula, MT: American Academy of Religion and Scholars Press.
16. Curtin, L. L. (1978). A proposed model for critical ethical analysis. *Nursing Forum, 17,* 14.
17. Curtin, L. L. (1986). Autonomy, accountability, and nursing practice. In P. L. Chinn (Ed.), *Ethical issues in nursing* (pp. 11-20). Rockville, MD: Aspen Systems Corp.
18. Dewey, J. (1960). *Theory of the moral life.* New York: Holt, Rinehart, and Winston.
19. Evans, D. (1974). Paul Ramsey: Love and killing. In J. Johnson & D. Smith (Eds.), *Love and society: Essays in the ethics of Paul Ramsey* (pp. 19-46). Missoula, MT: American Academy of Religion and Scholars Press.
20. Fletcher, J. (1978). Situational ethics. In W. T. Walsh (Ed.), *Encyclopedia of bioethics: Vol 1* (pp. 421-424). New York: Macmillan Publishing Co.
21. Fowler, M. D. (1989). Ethical decision making in clinical practice. *Nursing Clinics of North America, 24*(4), 955-965.
22. Frankena, W. K. (1973). *Ethics* (2nd ed.). Englewood Cliffs, NJ: Prentice-Hall.
23. Fromer, M. I. (1986). Solving ethical dilemmas in nursing practice. In P. L. Chinn (Ed.), *Ethical issues in nursing* (pp. 81-87). Rockville, MD: Aspen Systems Corp.
24. Green, M. (1973). *Teacher as stranger.* Belmont, CA: Wadsworth Publishing Co.
25. Kant, J. (1969). *Foundations of the metaphysics of morals.* L. W. Beck (Trans.) and R. P. Wolff (Ed.). Indianapolis: The Bobs-Merrill Corp.
26. Kilpatrick, K. Y. (1986). Ethical issues and procedural dilemmas in measuring patient competence. In P. L. Chinn (Ed.), *Ethical issues in nursing* (pp. 111-122). Rockville, MD: Aspen Systems Corp.
27. Kohlberg, L. (1976). Moral stages and moralization. In T. Likona (Ed.), *Moral development and behavior* (pp. 31-53). New York: Holt, Rinehart, and Winston.
27a. Levine-Ariff, J., & Groh, D. H. (1990). Nursing manager's bookshelf: Creating an ethical environment (pp. 41-61). Baltimore: Williams & Wilkins.
28. Little, D. (1974). The structure of justification in the political ethics of Paul Ramsey. In J. Johnson & D. Smith (Eds.), *Love and society: Essays in the ethics of Paul Ramsey* (pp. 47-65). Missoula, MT: American Academy of Religion and Scholars Press.
29. Mayberry, M. A. (1986). Ethical decision making: A response of hospital nurses. *Nursing Administration Quarterly, 10*(3), 75-81.
30. McFadden, C. J. (1961). *Medical ethics* (2nd ed.) Philadelphia: F. A. Davis Co.
31. Murphy, M. A., & Murphy, J. (1976). Making ethical decisions systematically. *Nursing '76, 8*(5), 13-14.
32. Nelson, M. J. (1986). Authenticity: Fabric of ethical nursing practice. In P. L. Chinn (Ed.), *Ethical issues in nursing* (pp. 37-45). Rockville, MD: Aspen Systems Corp.
33. Pence, T. (1986). *Ethics in nursing: An annotated bibliography* (2nd ed.) New York: National League for Nursing.
34. Rhodes, A. M., & Miller, R. D. (1984). *Nursing and the law* (4th ed.) Rockville, MD: Aspen Systems Corp.
35. Sahakian, W. S. (1974). *Ethics: An introduction to theories and problems.* New York: Harper & Row.
36. Schrock, R. A. (1980). A question of honesty in nursing practice. *Journal of Advanced Nursing, 5*(2), 135-145.
37. Sigman, P. (1986). Ethical choice in nursing. In P. L. Chinn (Ed.), *Ethical issues in nursing* (pp. 21-36). Rockville, MD: Aspen Systems Corp.
38. Smith, D. H. (1974). Paul Ramsey: Love and killing. In J. Johnson & D. Smith (Eds.), *Love and society: Essays in the ethics of Paul Ramsey* (pp. 3-17). Missoula, MT: American Academy of Religion and Scholars Press.
39. Tate, B. L. (1977). *The nurses' dilemma: Ethical considerations in nursing practice.* Geneva: International Council of Nurses.

Chapter 5

Cross-Cultural Nursing

Over the past years, there has been a great influx of peoples into the United States (Fig. 5-1). As they undergo a necessary process of assimilation into the larger American population, people of all cultures bring with them a pride in their culture and a determination to preserve that culture. For us they offer rich cultural perspectives and traditions that encompass issues of health, happiness, and human existence.

All health professionals are finding themselves faced with an increasing number of clients from other cultures. There is a natural tendency to discount or belittle the attitudes, beliefs, and behaviors of others that appear alien or bewildering. However, with some effort at openness and understanding, the nurse can learn to appreciate each client and his or her differences. The nurse may also learn how to be responsive and work with the client and his or her beliefs and practices to maximize care. Likewise, the nurse might be able to better understand the client's misgivings about the conventional Western medical system, if the nurse understood the client's traditional medical system.

CROSS-CULTURAL CONCEPTS

Culture and Cultural Diversity

Culture can be defined as those things learned and transmitted from one generation to another that serve as a blueprint for living that guides the group's thoughts, actions, and sentiments. Culture can also be called socialization and is the process by which a person learns cultural meanings, beliefs, values, patterns of behavior, and methods of problem solving. Cultural variables affect not only a person's decisions and actions but also health care practices.

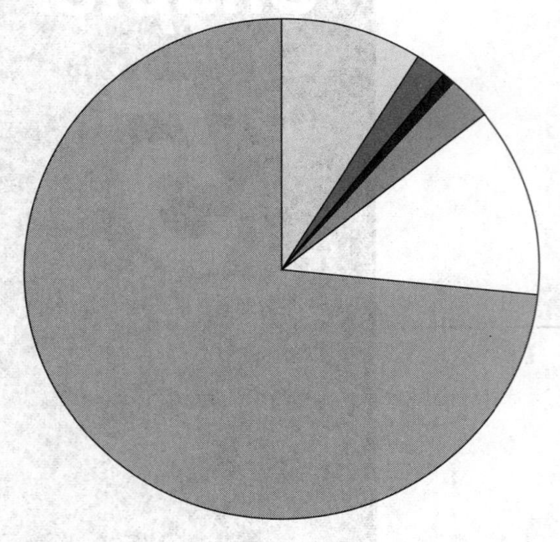

Selected Populations of the United States, 1990	
White	199,686,070
Per cent of total population	**73.3**
Black	29,986,060
Per cent of total population	**12.1**
American Indian, Eskimo, or Aleut	1,959,234
Per cent of total population	**0.8**
Asian or Pacific Islander	7,273,662
Per cent of total population	**2.9**
Other race	9,804,847
Per cent of total population	**1.9**
Hispanic origin (of any race)	22,354,059
Per cent of total population	**9.0**

▲ ***Figure 5–1***

Selected population percentages for the United States: 1990. (From the U.S. Department of Commerce, Bureau of the Census, 1990 Census.)

Cultural diversity is the overt and covert differences among people of different population groups with respect to their values, beliefs, language, physical characteristics, and general patterns of behavior. Cultural differences affect the client's choice of health care as well as his or her response to the health care team. The nurse must be aware of the client's cultural orientation without stereotyping the client. Treating all clients alike regardless of culture is unsafe. For example, some groups of clients express pain openly and others are stoic in pain. If the nurse derived conclusions about the degree of pain based on behaviors, one client could be overmedicated and the other undermedicated. Appreciation of another's culture begins with an understanding of one's own culture.

Uprooting

Uprooting is the movement or migration from one country to another. The United States has been described as a nation of immigrants, because only the Aleuts and Native Americans are indigenous to America. People cross geographic boundaries for many reasons. War may force some to be refugees. Religious differences may encourage people to seek others with similar beliefs. Some people choose to move on in an attempt to improve their financial status or to seek job opportunities. Finally, epidemics and disease may cause people to leave their homes in search of relief. The AIDS epidemic is a modern example of uprooting. Communities in developed and underdeveloped countries may reject a person with AIDS and force the individual into social isolation and uprooting.

The process of uprooting may cause a profound change in people. Many times the change is called "culture shock." Regardless of the reason for the move, the uprooted person has severed ties with the environment, people, relationships, family, and country. Uprooting has the potential to create positive change in a person, however, through self-development and personal growth.

On a smaller scale, hospitalization has been considered a situation of uprooting. With hospitalization, a client suddenly becomes dependent and is labeled as a "patient." In addition, communication patterns, words used, customs, and surroundings have changed.

Culture Shock

Culture shock is the reaction of people to an unfamiliar situation in which former patterns of behavior are no longer appropriate. Culture shock occurs when people are abruptly moved from one culture to another. Culture shock is also said to occur when clients are brought into the Western health care system.

Initially, the person tries to learn about the new culture and ask questions. Then the person begins to feel embarrassed or frustrated about mistakes made. The person may feel inadequate or alone. Eventually, the person develops new behaviors for the culture and is able to function effectively. There may be another type of culture shock if the person returns to the former culture after this time.

Taboos and Myths

All societies have taboos and myths. Taboos are proscribed acts that are thought to be harmful to self or others. Myths are stories that explain why people do what they do and why they believe what they believe. Interestingly, myths make sense to the people who believe them but are difficult to explain to outsiders.

In Western societies, many taboos exist. It is taboo to eat cats and dogs in Western societies, but beef is readily eaten. In India, the reverse is true. Likewise, other cultures have taboos. Some cultures forbid the discussion of certain topics, such as mentioning the name of a person recently deceased or exposing private parts.

An equal number of myths exist in Western health care. For example, Americans believe that eating worms, snakes, and lice would cause illness, yet in many other parts of the world, these foods are commonly eaten. The same food can be both a delicacy and taboo. There also may be taboos on the hospital ward, such as confronting a physician.

Cultural Imposition

Nurses must recognize that their own values, which are based on the Western health care system, are not superior and that they do not have the right to impose cultural practices on other people. Nurses must celebrate rather than condemn cultural diversity. It is hoped that as nurses are exposed to people from other cultures, they can appreciate and value the differences.

Sadly though, a true appreciation for difference seldom occurs. Instead, there is a tendency for the superior cultural group (by virtue of size, perceived status, or other factors) to impose its beliefs on a less dominant cultural group. This process is called cultural imposition. Cultural imposition is based on ethnocentrism, in which one group is totally convinced that it possesses the right ways and knowledge.

Ethnocentrism

Ethnocentrism is the belief and feeling that one's own way of life and way of viewing the world are desirable and actually superior to others. These feelings are fairly natural. In health care, ethnocentrism can be seen as a feeling that Western health care practices are superior to all other forms of health care. It is important to remember that all cultures in the world have some form of health care. In order to recognize cultural variations, the Western health care system is discussed first.

THEORIES OF HEALTH AND ILLNESS

Western Belief Systems

Anthropologists have developed a variety of frameworks to classify various theories of health and illness. Western societies believe in the germ theory. The germ theory began many years ago when infectious organisms were considered the main cause of illness. During that time, bacteria and their role in illness were discovered. At present, the theory relates a belief that illness has a known cause that is not supernatural, and if that cause can be identified, the disease can be treated or cured.

In Western societies, illness develops owing to problems with genetic transmission, exposure to toxic substances (e.g., tobacco, cocaine), excessive dietary intake of harmful substances (e.g., fat, alcohol), and infection with bacteria, fungi, and viruses. It is a Western belief that diseases are treatable and sometimes curable. Western medicine is also focused on risk reduction and prevention. The ill client may be seen in two ways: (1) as somewhat responsible for his or her own health conditions from risky behaviors or (2) a victim of the disease.

Western definitions of health used to be simply "the absence of illness." In recent years, health and wellness have been seen on a continuum and the theory recognizes that the client's perception of health is an important component of health.

Non-Western Belief Systems

In non-Western societies, there are two main theories of disease and health: (1) personalistic and (2) naturalistic medical systems. Personalistic medical systems contain the belief that illness is caused by a sensate agent, such as a deity, ghost, ancestor, evil spirit, witch, or sorcerer. The individual affected is a victim of aggression or is being punished for some reason. Illness is explained impersonally in the naturalistic system through the concept of equilibrium. All body elements, such as hot and cold humors, and yin and yang, are in harmony with the individual's natural and social environment. Illness occurs when equilibrium is disturbed. In the following paragraphs, a short description of various peoples' beliefs about health and illness is given. Data such as these are not meant to prejudice health care providers but to assist them to understand the possible beliefs of their clients.

Contained within the beliefs of naturalistic medicine are the concepts of humors and disease. Humoral pathology is a common belief in Latin America and India. There are four humors or fluids in the body—blood (hot and moist), phlegm (cold and moist), black bile (cold and dry), and yellow bile or choler (hot and dry). The major organs of the body (heart, brain, and liver) are thought to have certain quantities of dry, moist, hot, and cold fluids. Healthy people have adequate heat and moisture, and illness is attributed to excess hot or cold. Often, the terms hot and cold are used metaphorically and may not indicate a specific temperature. For example, pregnancy is considered to be a hot experience and so the woman must not eat foods classified as hot, such as pork. Only cold foods can restore equilibrium.

A similar system of belief exists in India. There are three humors, or dosha; they are phlegm, bile, and wind. Health is a manifestation of balance of the three humors. Illness occurs when an individual experiences an imbalance.

The traditional Navajo Indians believe that disease is disharmony caused by violating a taboo or attack by a witch. They also believe that following elaborate rituals can prevent illnesses. Health is demonstrated by harmony between the individual, earth, and the supernatural as well as the ability to survive difficult circumstances.

Likewise, traditional Hispanic cultures teach that illness is a punishment from God for wrongdoing as well as an imbalance between hot and cold properties. Health is a gift from God or good luck. Illness can be prevented by praying, being good, eating well, wearing medals, and working.

In traditional black cultures, disease is disharmony caused by spirits and demons. Health is harmony with nature. Illness can be prevented through a good diet, rest, and cleanliness. Some people use laxatives to "clean out the system" and wear copper and silver bracelets to prevent disease.

Traditional Chinese people believe that health is a balance between yin and yang factors and that health is a gift from one's parents and ancestors. Illness is caused by an imbalance of yin and yang, and may be due to overexertion or prolonged sitting. Illness can be prevented through better adaptation to nature. Illness is treated with foods, herbs, and curing methods that are thought to have hot or cold qualities. For example, acupuncture is considered a cold treatment for diseases due to excess yang. Moxibustion is a hot treatment for illness due to excess yin.

HEALTH CARE PROVIDERS

Western Practitioners

The most common Western health care provider is the physician. Other health care professionals provide care and can be sought out by the client. These people include nurse practitioners, physician assistants, doctors of osteopathy, and chiropractors.

Indigenous Healers

Various terms have been applied to healers practicing within personalistic and naturalistic systems. Titles such as "native healer," "traditional healer," "primitive healer," and "witch doctor" have been given to healers, but they have often been used in a negative sense, to mean "not as good" in comparison to Western practitioners. Therefore, the term "indigenous healer" should be used to refer to non-Western medical practitioners who are "of the culture."

A comprehensive definition of indigenous healers has been developed by the World Health Organization:

> . . . a person recognized by the community in which he lives as competent to provide health care by using vegetable, animal, and mineral substances and certain other substances based on the social, cultural, and religious background as well as on the knowledge, attitudes, and beliefs that are prevalent in the community regarding physical, mental and social well-being and the causation of disease and disability.[29]

CATEGORIES

Indigenous healers can be classified into four major categories:

- Those who have received an integrated training in modern and traditional systems of medicine, such as Hindu and Chinese medicine.
- Practitioners trained mainly in traditional medicine but who also have some knowledge of modern medicine, such as the village health worker.
- Indigenous practitioners without formal training but who have obtained diplomas in some particular system, such as that of India, after participating in correspondence courses.
- Those without institutional training who practice after a period of apprenticeship with an established indigenous healer.

The last category of indigenous healers can be further classified into herbalists, diviners, surgeons, bonesetters, and traditional birth attendants and spiritualists. All operate on various levels, with the simplest being the traditional birth attendants and herbalist and the more complex practitioner being the diviner and spiritualist.

CHARACTERISTICS

Characteristics of indigenous healers have been examined by Foster and Anderson,[9a] who have attempted to reverse commonly held myths of indigenous healers. First, most societies recognize distinct curing roles through the specialization of healers. A community may have a midwife, bonesetter, masseur, shaman (diviner), and herbalist. There is a hierarchy of status involved, and usually the greatest status is bestowed on the diviner.

Second, the decision to be a healer, especially a midwife or an herbalist, is often a personal one, although there are instances when the healer is "chosen." The term "shaman," which is Siberian in origin, often refers to healers who are elected by a spirit and who later maintain contact with that spirit during the curing process.

Third, there is usually a long period of training required of indigenous healers and they may be ritually certified by their teacher after completing training.

The fourth characteristic of an indigenous healer refers to the professional image upheld by the healer, which is not unlike that of the Western medical practitioner with his laboratory coat and stethoscope. Often, the indigenous healer dresses and behaves differently from other people in the community.

Fifth, indigenous healers receive payment in some form. The type of payment and the amount involved varies, but payment in some form is given to the healer.

Sixth, great prestige is usually given to the healers and their abilities are rarely questioned either by themselves or their clients. In fact, if a healer has been unsuccessful, blame is usually placed on the way the ritual was carried out, i.e., the person did not follow the directions exactly as they were given.

Finally, indigenous healers are often viewed with ambivalence by the community. Healers are expected to be all-knowing and highly skilled, and therefore, the people distrust and may even dislike the healer who holds so much power over them.

FUNCTIONS

The characteristics of indigenous healers should not be overshadowed by their function. The healer is not a simple curer who treats only symptoms. Instead, the healer is the individual who maintains harmony between the individual and his or her environment. Therapy provided by the healer consists of forgiveness and reestablishment of harmony with the supernatural. Also, the therapy is a mechanism to maintain social cohesion, because the person's family or neighbors may be involved in the cure.

Health care consumers throughout the world may seek the services of familiar indigenous healers. Nurses who are aware of the strengths and weaknesses of non-Western health care systems are more prepared to collaborate with indigenous healers, according to the client's desires (Nursing Research).

STRENGTHS AND WEAKNESSES

Positive features of indigenous healers recognized by health care consumers include the healers' acceptability and adaptability; the ability to perform psychological and sociological functions independent of the availability of biomedicine; possession of a large body of indigenous technical knowledge, ranging from group psychology to pharmacopoeia; the ability to treat a broad spectrum of disease; and often, the wisdom to refer clients to other healers or Western biomedical practitioners, as necessary.[26]

Weaknesses inherent within indigenous healing systems and their practitioners have been documented by Yoder, especially in regard to African healing systems.[30] First, knowledge of disease and the person's symptoms are subjective. That is, diagnosing illness depends on tactile and visual signs of dysfunction that may be difficult to verify. Second, indigenous healers may have only a limited number of diagnostic techniques available. Third, healers are educated on a broad continuum, from no formal training to being trained in established schools for healers. Therefore, the quality of care given by healers varies widely. Also, indigenous healers may be perceived as frauds by the public officials and be denounced by a country's formal health care system. Finally, indigenous healers and indigenous healing systems in general may be perceived as an embarrassing, shameful cultural legacy by those in society who have adopted a Western biomedical health care system. Also, clients who use indigenous healing systems may be reluctant to discuss their preferences with biomedical health care providers such as nurses.

Nurses can foster collaborative relationships with indigenous healers if they also acknowledge the strengths and weaknesses of their own biomedical Western health care system.

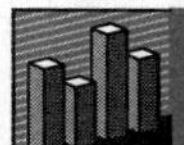

NURSING RESEARCH

On the Navajo Reservation in Arizona and New Mexico of the United States, certified nurse-midwives are incorporating indigenous beliefs with biomedical obstetric nursing care.[18] Families are encouraged to seek indigenous healers as they desire, and healers are welcomed in the hospital. Certified nurse-midwives wear necklaces made of juniper seeds, which are believed to promote a safe passage for the fetus from the uterus to the outside world. Birthing rooms in the hospital are equipped with traditional Navajo woven belts suspended from the ceiling. These belts are used during the second stage of labor as the client pushes. All client teaching, antepartum through postpartum, has been modified to include traditional Navajo beliefs and dietary preferences. Maternal hygiene and infant care teaching takes into consideration living arrangements that often consist of one-room hogans that do not have water or electricity. Clients have reacted favorably to the culturally sensitive care given by the certified nurse-midwives. They have been accepted into the community and participate in Navajo healing ceremonies as well.

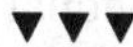

Goldstein, D. (1987). A traditional Navajo medicine woman . . . A modern nurse-midwife . . . Healing in harmony. *Frontier Nursing Service*, *62*(6): Winter.

Biomedical practitioners have access to a large fund of knowledge about disease through research and experience. Second, and perhaps most significant is biomedicine's access to powerful drugs in standardized doses. However, this strength may be undermined by unpredictable client compliance and insufficient stock, especially in developing countries. A third strength of biomedicine is surgical competence, which is widely recognized as positive by both the indigenous healer and the health care consumer.

In many parts of the world, however, the strengths of biomedicine have yet to be realized. This may be due to such negative factors as the inaccessibility and urban bias of biomedical practitioners, dependence on technology, and finally, the cost of biomedical Western health care.

Western Health Care Systems

The major problem in studying cultural differences is that the person is too close to his or her own culture to be objective. It is important, however, to examine one's own culture, because it is the view from which others see us.

The goal of any health care system is to mobilize the resources of the client, family, and society in resolving the client's problem. In addition, health care systems provide an explanation of illness, a rationale for treatment, and provide sanction for cultural norms.

VALUES

The American health care system has evolved to have the following values.

Optimal Health. Having optimal health is viewed as a right for all citizens. The eradication of illness and deformities, and the provision of many health services is now spoken of as both a human right and a civil right in our society. This emphasis on optimal health for all citizens is in sharp contrast to many cultures among the world. In many cultures, health is not a major concern and very little financial, social, or political support is given toward health promotion by these governments.

Democracy. With a democratic form of government, concerns about and programs to support health services and nationally sponsored health programs, such as Medicare, have come about. Again, this is in sharp contrast to other cultures in which the government is autocratic, with less direct concern for the citizens.

Individualism. The individual in American society has always been more important than the social group. Other cultures value the group, and the individual is subordinate and given much less respect and consideration.

Achieving and Doing. Americans are urged to work hard and be successful. Many Americans believe that they should be continually earning more money, getting a better job, and climbing the ladder of success. People in other cultures have learned to enjoy what they have and are not feverishly working toward some goal, material possession, or money.

Cleanliness. For Americans, cleanliness is next to godliness and to social success. Cleanliness is seen as related to having optimal health. Much time is spent on bathing, washing clothes, scrubbing floors, and so forth. Americans seem compulsive about cleanliness. There are very few cultures that emphasize cleanliness the way Americans do. Some people are comfortable with clutter and dirt around them and with having a weekly bath.

Time. Americans have a perpetual fixation about time and schedules. For Americans, time is extremely valuable and a lot of guilt ensues if time is lost or wasted. There are some cultures that do not have an instrument to keep time. There is also some evidence that the mental and physical health of these people is better than that of Westerners.

Automation. Automation and technology have a sharp impact on the American lifestyle. These machines are often able to do things instantly for us. Americans often expect instant health services, the finest in technology, and instant recovery from illness. Most other cultures have a willingness to accept illness, deformity, and even death as a natural part of life.

STEREOTYPES OF WESTERN MEDICINE

One of the biggest stereotypes of Western medicine is the misconception that it is omniscient and omnipotent. For the most part, Western medicine is based on scientific facts, and folk medicine is discounted as old wives' tales. Most health care providers are educated to believe that the science in Western medicine is the panacea to all of humankind's needs. Miracles bolstering this belief abound. Clients are brought back from the clutches of death. The heart, an organ that houses the soul in some cultures, is transplanted to save a life. Health care providers pound on chests, administer nearly lethal doses of medications, and usually succeed in curing the client.

Those people who do not want to participate or believe in our health care system are beyond our belief at times. But there are people who do not see Western medicine as a panacea. Sometimes, this disbelief is due to the method used to present the plan to the client. If the plan is presented with an attitude that the client's beliefs and treatments of health are incorrect, it is likely the client will not comply with the new plan.

TRANSCULTURAL NURSING

Leninger defined transcultural nursing as "a humanistic and scientific area of formal study and practice in nursing that is based on differences and similarities among cultures with respect to human care, health (or wellness), and illness originating from the person's cultural values, beliefs, and health practices and [the use of] this knowledge to provide cultural specific and culturally congruent nursing care to all people."[15] The concepts of transcultural nursing can be combined with the nursing process to provide care.

NURSING PROCESS IN CROSS-CULTURAL NURSING

Prerequisites to Cross-Cultural Care

DEVELOPING CULTURAL SENSITIVITY

Before beginning any form of assessment of a client from another culture, the nurse must be certain that the client can be approached in an objective method. Therefore, a prerequisite to assessment is to develop cultural sensitivity (Ethical Issues in Nursing).

Cultural sensitivity is defined as becoming aware and accepting of diversity among clients and peoples throughout the world. There are differences in the languages spoken, social behavior, belief systems, and manner of dress. All too often, people look for differences between themselves and not for similarities. These differences are usually seen as threatening. Prejudice and interpersonal tension decrease when people realize that they are more alike than they are different. A major difference between Americans and people of other cultures is variation in values and orientation.

Identifying commonalities among people of various cultures can serve as the first step in developing a greater sensitivity toward clients and families.

Cultural sensitivity also is defined as overcoming or recognizing ethnocentrism that occurs in everyone and trying to put those feelings aside. Nurses must convey respect for the client's values, beliefs, and customs. When the nurse treats the client with disdain or amusement, the client and family interpret this behavior as a lack of respect.

Assessment

Certain cultural components are present in all clients. Subtle as well as obvious differences exist. Some people may follow the cultural pattern exactly, and others may have chosen to deny it. It is important not to assume that any client has a prescribed cultural pattern. In order to determine the degree of cultural variation in clients an assessment should be performed.

Fong[9] and Orque, Bloch, and Monrroy[22a] have identified cultural assessment guidelines. Fong developed a model called the CONFHER model. The letters stand for *c*ommunication, *o*rientation, *n*utrition, *f*amily relationships, *h*ealth beliefs, *e*ducation, and *r*eligion. Bloch developed a list of questions to elicit information about the client. The two models are combined in Table 5-1.

HISTORY

Once a basic cultural assessment is performed on the client, the nurse can ask specific questions about the illness. The nurse should determine the client's beliefs about the cause of the illness. Does the client believe the disorder was caused by germs, lifestyle risks, spirits, punishment for past deeds, a curse, or an imbalance of nature's forces? From this discussion, the nurse can determine the sense of control the client feels he or she has over the illness. This sense of control, called locus of control, can be internal or external. A client with an external locus of control believes that disease just happens and there is nothing that can be done to prevent it from occurring. A client with an internal locus of control believes that there is a portion of disease that could be managed personally. For example, the client may believe that he or she can control the risk of heart disease by weight control and dietary management. The issue of locus of control has an impact when planning intervention. Specific questions that should be asked are

- What do you think caused your problem?
- Has the problem become better, worse, or stayed the same?
- What problems has your illness caused you?
- What are your fears concerning this problem?
- What have you been doing for this problem?
- What treatment do you think you need now?
- How should family members help in the treatment of the problem?

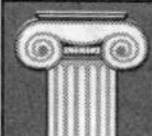

ETHICAL ISSUES IN NURSING

What Happens When the Nursing Care Plan Is in Conflict With a Specific Cultural Practice?

The term "cross-cultural" can mean several different things depending on the type of culture being described. For example, culture may mean a socioeconomic class or it may mean ethnic background. Cross-cultural nursing can mean nurses of different socioeconomic and ethnic backgrounds taking care of people from different socioeconomic and ethnic backgrounds.

Nurses who care for certain client populations need to become aware of the customs, beliefs, and ideals pertaining to the health care of those populations. There may be times when health care providers need to be sensitive to a specific cultural practice or practices that their clients may engage in (such as a spiritual ritual or a dietary request).

Problems arise in cross-cultural nursing when cultural differences are not understood or respected by those involved. Nurses who care for clients who are culturally different from themselves have an obligation to their clients to allow them the freedom to express their cultural diversities. These diversities may cause the nursing care plan to be altered in order to fit into the particular cultural habitat. There may be some cultural habits that are in total opposition to the health of a client (dietary restriction, for example). Once the nurse recognizes that a cultural change needs to occur, education may begin for the client and family in order that the change is not seen as a threat to the specific cultural lifestyle.

PHYSICAL ASSESSMENT

When performing a physical assessment, the nurse should be aware of cultural preferences for limiting bodily exposure, removing certain garments, and male-female relationships. At times, in order to obtain a complete examination, the client may need to accept a culturally forbidden practice. As often as possible, however, the nurse should work within the cultural parameters.

There are certain physical differences between people of various cultures, such as bone length, pelvic size, and number of vertebrae. These variations are discussed in the chapters in this text that focus on physical assessment of the various body systems.

HEALTH RISK APPRAISAL

Peoples of various cultures are at increased risk for various illnesses due to their cultural background. The nurse should be aware of these risks and examine the client's history and physical assessment findings for these risks. Chapter 11 discusses the risks of illness in the various cultures.

TABLE 5-1. Cross-Cultural Assessment

Communication Style

Is the interviewer in the correct proximity to the client (intimate or social zone)?

Are there nonverbal communication styles that need to be followed (e.g., bowing, speaking softly, touch restrictions)?

Which language does the client speak most frequently? Is an interpreter needed? Does the client speak English at all, have limited use of English, read and write in English?

Is there a need to vary the technique used to communicate with client (i.e., tempo of conversation, eye-body contact, topic restrictions, such as sexual matters, inclusion or exclusion of family members)?

Orientation

Does the client identify with a particular racial group (i.e., Asian, African, Native American)? or ethnic group (i.e., Chinese, Japanese, Mediterranean)?

Where was the client born? Where has the client lived recently?

How closely does the client adhere to traditional habits and values from his or her parents' cultural system?

What is the accepted behavior of the cultural group regarding the expression of emotions and feelings, religious concerns, and responses to illness and death?

Are there restrictions related to discussion of sexual matters, exposure of body parts, certain types of surgery (e.g., hysterectomy), discussion of dead relatives, and discussion of fears of the unknown? What does the client value or desire from the health care system?

Nutrition

Are there preferred ethnic foods?

Are there foods that are encouraged to be eaten or discouraged from eating while ill?

What is the usual style of food preparation?

What is the frequency of eating, time of eating, and utensils used?

What are the implications of the usual diet on the disease process?

Family Relationships

Who is in the family? What are their roles?

What is the family order (e.g., patriarchal, matriarchal)?

What is the position of women and children in the family structure? What is their role in decision making?

Are there key family members that need to be involved in health care decisions?

How is the family valued during illness (e.g., present all of the time, provides baths, brings food)?

Where does the family live? Will this environment be conducive to healing and recovery?

Health Habits

What cultural healing system does the client predominately follow (medicine men, herbalists, spiritualists, ministers)?

What religious system does the client follow (Christian Scientist, Seventh Day Adventist)?

How is illness explained (i.e., presence of evil spirits, imbalance of yin and yang, germ theory, inheritance)?

How does the client respond to pain and hospitalization?

Are there some disorders that the client is more prone to based on ethnic group (Sickle cell anemia, hypertension)?

Education

What is the highest level of education the client has attained? Do the level of education and ability to read allow comprehension of verbal and written materials on health care?

What is learning style (trial and error, didactic)?

Religion

Does the client's religion have a strong impact on how he or she relates to health and illness?

Do religious beliefs, sacred rites, and talismans play a role in the treatment of disease?

Are there religious restrictions that must be followed?

What is the role of significant religious persons during illness?

Modified from Fong, C. (1985). Ethnicity and nursing practice. *Topics in Clinical Nursing, 7*(3), 1-10; and Orque, M., et al. (1983). *Ethnic nursing care: A multicultural approach* (pp. 63-69). St. Louis: C. V. Mosby.

Nursing Diagnosis

There are many possible diagnoses for the client from other cultures. Most of these will focus on the physical nature of the illness. Specific diagnoses to support the client through the period of culture shock will be discussed here. A nursing diagnosis may be "Social isolation related to separation from cultural ties as evidenced by lack of family visits, little food consumption, and refusal of medical regimen."

Planning: Expected Outcomes

The client will experience less social isolation by feeling a reconnection to the culture as evidenced by finding an acceptable means to contact family, developing an extended family in the local area, consuming adequate amounts of food and fluids, establishing a method of communication, and discussing preferred treatment of the disorder.

Nursing Intervention

When planning interventions, the nurse must consider the client's cultural practices and how they compare or contrast with the Western health care system. For example, if the client is a dying Muslim, the family would stay with the client, wash the body before prayer time, turn the client to face Allah, and pray five times a day. These practices are certainly outside the normal routine for the hospital but should be allowed.

Frequently, clients from various countries will come for treatment of very serious illnesses. They have often saved money for years to allow a lifesaving surgery to be performed. Because of the cost, the client often comes alone or with just one other person. In these cases, there are few support systems for the client and significant other beyond themselves. The nurse should attempt to link the client and significant other to people in the area who are from the same culture or who are willing to work with such people.

Dietary practices vary greatly around the world. At times, the client's diet and the prescribed diet to facilitate healing are different. For example, Chinese clients often eat rice for every meal and pile all the food onto one plate. Because it is not possible to get rice for all three meals in the Western hospital, the nurse could work with the family to obtain the rice. However, if that amount of rice does not meet the needs for protein and fat, other food sources will have to be considered that are culturally acceptable. But it would be possible for the nurse to serve the Chinese client hot liquids, such as tea, rather than cold beverages.

If the client does not speak English, an interpreter can be used to facilitate conversation. The nurse should be certain that the client understands what is said, especially if a new medical treatment or surgery is planned. Nonverbal communication is commonly understood and can be used. If the client can read his or her own language, a list of terms in the primary language can be written alongside the terms in English. Then the client can point to the word and the nurse can immediately see its meaning. The nurse can also communicate with the client with the same tool. For example, the words drink, eat, sit in chair, pain, and the like can be on the list (Table 5–2).

Be certain to consider the role of communication within the culture. Do not assume that a lack of eye contact means disinterest in an Asian client. Be conscious of posture and nonverbal communication given by the client.

To meet the goal of compliance with the prescribed medical regimen, the nurse needs to determine the reasons for noncompliance. Perhaps the client has been treated by an indigenous healer. In this case, the nurse should seek information in a nonconfrontive manner about the healer's treatment.

Evaluation

The degree of goal attainment should be determined and adjustments in the interventions made accordingly.

INTERNATIONAL NURSING

International nursing focuses on developing national health policies, curriculum development in nursing education, the promotion of primary health care as directed by the World Health Organization, and international research efforts.

International nursing can be defined as any nursing care activity carried out by a nurse from a donor country in a host nation. The nurse providing the care was educated and has practiced nursing in the donor country. However, the nursing services are requested by and practiced in a host country. These services are contracted for a specific time period, and can range from a matter of days to many years.[8]

Terms such as multicultural, cross-cultural, transcultural, and transnational have been used as synonyms for international nursing.[2, 6, 17, 24] However, international nursing is a unique specialty, although it is related to transcultural nursing. As a specialty in nursing, international nursing reflects the different nursing needs in other countries. It requires the nurse to work within a system in which definitions of health may differ and unique skills are necessary for combining nursing knowledge and practice from both countries.

International nursing can be distinguished from transcultural nursing in a number of ways, although there is also some overlap. Two themes emerge from this international nursing focus. First, it becomes fully realized within the practice realm, although it may be based on transcultural nursing, anthropologic research, or both. Second, a national or *macro-perspective* is evident in international nursing.[12] This macro-perspective implies that nurses must be involved in policy making and health planning, because not only cultural forces but economic, political, educational, and historical forces affect health care. It is not enough to assess individuals. Sociopolitical and economic structures must also be evaluated.

Another dimension distinguishing international and transcultural nursing is the importance attached to primary health care in international nursing. Ministries of Health in many countries have committed their countries to primary health care, at least philosophically. Primary health care as an ideology for practice includes accessibility to health care services, involvement of individuals at the community level, health promotion, prevention and cure, appropriate technology, and integration of health with social and economic development.[26]

An individual working within an international nursing framework must be cognizant of the relationship and comprehensiveness of nursing and primary health care. This nurse may be actively collaborating with individuals involved in agriculture, natural resources, sanitation, nutrition, and textiles as well as members of the com-

TABLE 5-2. Phrases in Foreign Languages for Health Assessment and Examination

English	Spanish	Italian	French	German
General				
Good morning.	Buenos días.	Buon giorno.	Bonjour.	Guten Morgen.
What is your name?	¿Cómo se llama?	Come si chiama Lei?	Quel est votre nom?	Wie heissen Sie?
How old are you?	¿Cuántos años tiene?	Quanti anni ha?	Quel âge avez-vous?	Wie alt sind Sie?
Do you understand me?	¿Me entiende?	Mi capisce?	Me comprenez-vous?	Verstehen Sie mich?
Answer only . . .	Conteste solamente . . .	Risponda solamente . . .	Répondez seulement . . .	Antworten Sie nur . . .
Yes No	Sí No	Si No	Oui Non	Ja Nein
What do you say?	¿Qué dice?	Cosa dice?	Que dites-vous?	Was sagen Sie?
Speak slower.	Hable más despacio.	Parli più adaggio.	Parlez plus lentement.	Sprechen Sie langsamer.
Say it once again.	Repítalo, por favor.	Lo dica ancora una volta.	Répétez ça.	Wiederholen Sie das.
Show me . . .	Enséñeme . . .	Mi faccia vedere . . .	Montrez-moi . . .	Zeigen Sie mir . . .
Here There	Aquí Allí	Qui Qua	Ici Là	Hier Da
Which side?	¿En qué lado?	Quale lato?	Quel côté?	Auf welcher Seite?
Since when?	¿Desde cuándo?	Da quando?	Depuis quand?	Seit wann?
Right	Derecha	A destra	A droit	Rechts
Left	Izquierda	A sinistra	A gauche	Links
More or less	Más o menos	Più o meno	Plus ou moins	Mehr oder weniger
How long?	¿Cuánto tiempo?	Da quanto tempo?	Combien de temps?	Wie lange?
In a few days you may eat food.	Dentro de algunos días podrá comer.	Fra pochi giorni potrà mangiare.	Après quelques jours vous pouvez prendre de la nourriture.	In einigen Tagen dürfen Sie essen.
And remain on a diet.	Y estar a dieta.	E rimanga a dieta.	Et suivez un régime.	Und Diät halten.
You may eat . . .	Puede comer . . .	Potrà mangiare . . .	Vous pouvez manger . . .	Sie dürfen essen . . .
Two eggs	Dos huevos	Due d'uova	Deux oeufs	Zwei Eier
Toast	Pan tostado	Pane tostato	Du pain grillé	Geröstetes Brot
Bread	Pan	Pane	Du pain	Das Brot
Oysters	Ostras	Delle óstriche	Des huîtres	Die Austern
Chicken	Pollo	Pollo	Du poulet	Das Huhn
You may drink icewater.	Puede tomar agua con hielo.	Lei può bere acqua ghiacciata.	Vous pouvez boir de l'eau glacée.	Sie dürfen Eiswasser trinken.
Milk	Leche	Latte	Du lait	Die Milch
Tea	Té	Il té	Du thé	Der Tee
Coffee	Café	Il caffè	Du Café	Der Kaffee
Chocolate	Chocolate	La cioccolatta	Du chocolat	Die Schokolade
Beef bouillon	Caldo de carne	Brodo	Le bouillon	Die Bouillon
Bathe with hot water.	Báñese con agua caliente.	Faccia il bagno con acqua calda.	Bagnez-vous dans de l'eau chaude.	Baden Sie mit heissem Wasser.
Bathe with cold water.	Báñese con agua fría.	Si faccia il bagno con acqua fredda.	Baignez-vous dans de l'eau froide.	Baden Sie mit kaltem Wasser.
Bathe with alcohol.	Báñese con alcohol.	Si bagni con alcool.	Baignez-vous avec de l'alcool.	Reiben Sie sich alkoholab.
Apply bandage to . . .	Ponga un vendaje a . . .	Si metta una fasciatura . . .	Mettez un bandage à . . .	Verbinden Sie . . .
Apply ointment	Aplíquese ungüento.	Applichi un unguento.	Appliquez un onguent.	Verwenden Sie Salbe.
Keep very quiet.	Estése muy quieto.	Sia tranquillo.	Restez tranquille.	Verhalten Sie sich sehr ruhig.
You must not speak.	No debe hablar.	Non deve parlare.	Vous ne devez pas parler.	Sie dürfen nicht sprechen.
An operation will be necessary.	Tendrá que operarse.	Una operazione è necessaria.	Il faut que l'on fasse une operation.	Eine Operation ist notwendig.

TABLE 5-2. Phrases in Foreign Languages for Health Assessment and Examination Continued

English	Spanish	Italian	French	German
History Taking				
How do you feel?	¿Cómo se siente?	Come stà?	Comment vous sentez-vous?	Wie fühlen Sie sich?
Good	Bien	Bene	Bien	Gut
Bad	Mal	Male	Mal	Schlecht
Let me see . . .	Déjeme ver . . .	Mi lasci vedere . . .	Permettez-moi de voir . . .	Lassen Sie mich sehen . . .
Let me feel your pulse.	Déjeme tomarle el pulso.	Mi lasci sentire il polso.	Permettez-moi de vous tâter le pouls.	Lassen Sie mich Ihren Puls fühlen.
How does your head feel?	¿Cómo siente la cabeza?	Come si sente la testa?	Comment va votre tête?	Wie geht es Ihrem Kopf?
Your memory	Su memoria	La sua memoria	Votre mémoire	Ihr Gedächtnis
Is it good?	¿Es buena?	È buona?	Est-elle bonne?	Ist es gut?
Have you any pain in the head?	¿Le duele la cabeza?	Ha dolor di testa?	Avez-vous mal à la tête?	Haben Sie Kopfschmerzen?
Did you fall and how did you fall?	¿Se cayó, y cómo se cayó?	È caduto, e come è caduto?	Etes-vous tombé et comment êtes-vous tombé?	Sind Sie gefallen und wie sind Sie gefallen?
Did you faint?	¿Se desmayó?	È svenuto?	Vous êtes-vous évanoui?	Sind Sie ohnmächtig geworden?
Have you ever had fainting spells?	¿Ha tenido desmayos alguna vez?	È mai svenuto regolarmente?	Avez-vous jamais eu des évanouissements?	Habe Sie jemals Ohnmachtsanfälle gehabt?
Have you slept well?	¿Ha dormido bien?	Ha dormito bene?	Avez-vous bien dormi?	Haben Sie gut geschlafen?
Have you any difficulty in breathing?	¿Tiene dificultad al respirar?	Ha difficoltà di respirare?	C'est difficile à respirer?	Fällt Ihnen das Atemholen schwer?
Since when do you cough?	¿Desde cuándo tose Ud?	Da quando ha la tosse?	Depuis quand avez-vous la toux?	Seit wann husten Sie?
You cough a little?	¿Tose poco?	Tossisca pocco?	Toussez-vous un peu?	Hüsten Sie manchmal?
Do you expectorate much?	¿Escupe mucho?	Sputa molto?	Crachez-vous beaucoup?	Spucken Sie viel aus?
What is the color of your expectorations?	¿De qué color es el esputo?	Di che color lo sputo?	De quelle sont vos crachats?	Welche Farbe hat der Speichel?
The hearing	El oído	L'udito	L'ouïe	Das Gehör
Is it affected?	¿Está afectado?	È compromesso?	Est-elle changée?	Ist es angegriffen?
Do you have ringing in the ears?	¿Le pitan los oídos?	Le tentennano le orecchie?	Avez-vous des bourdonnements d'oreilles?	Haben Sie Ohrenbrausen?
Since when has your eyesight failed you?	¿Desde cuando ha disminuido su vista?	Da quanto tempo la sua vista È diminuita?	Depuis quand votre vue s'est-elle diminuée?	Seit wann hat Ihre Sehkraft nachgelassen?
Do you sometimes see things double?	¿Ve las cosas doble algunas veces?	Vede qualche volta le cose doppie?	Est-ce que la vue est double parfois?	Sehen Sie manchmal doppelt?
Tell me what number it is.	Dígame qué número es éste.	Mi dica che numero è.	Dites-moi quel est le numéro.	Sagen Sie mir welche Nummer es ist.
Tell me what letter it is.	Dígame qué letra es ésta.	Mi dica che lettera è.	Dites-moi quelle est la lettre.	Nennen Sir mir diesen Buchstaben.
Do you see things through a mist?	¿Ve las cosas a travès de una niebla?	Vede le cose come se fossero fra la nebbia?	Voyez-vous les choses à travers d'un brouillard?	Sehen Sie alles durch einen Nebel?
Can you see clearly?	¿Puede ver claramente?	Può vedere chiaro?	Pouvez-vous voir clairement?	Sehen Sie deutlich?

Table continued on following page

TABLE 5-2. Phrases in Foreign Languages for Health Assessment and Examination Continued

English	Spanish	Italian	French	German
History Taking *continued*				
Better at a distance?	¿Mejor a cierta distancia?	Meglio a distanza?	Mieux à distance?	Besser aus der Entfernung?
Nausea	Nausea	La nausea	La nausée	Die Ubelkeit
Does eating make you vomit?	¿El comer le hace vomitar?	Vomita dopo aver manginto?	Rendez-vous ce que vous mangez?	Erbrechen Sie nachdem Sie gegessen haben?
How are your stools?	¿Cómo son sus defecaciones?	Come va di corpo?	Comment allez-vous à la selle?	Wie ist der Stuhlgang?
Are they regular?	¿Son regulares?	Va regolarmente?	Allez-vous à la selle régulièrment?	Ist er regelmässig?
Have you noticed their color?	¿Se ha fijado en el color?	Si è accorto di che colore?	Avez-vous remarquè la couleur de vos selles?	Haben Sie auf die Farbe geachtet?
Are you constipated?	¿Está estreñido?	È stitico?	Etes-vous constipé?	Leiden Sie an Verstopfung?
Do you have diarrhea?	¿Tiene diarrea?	Ha diarrea?	Avez-vous la diarrhée?	Haben Sie Durchfall?
Have you any difficulty passing water?	¿Tiene dificultad en orinar?	Ha della difficoltà nell' urinare?	Avez-vous de la difficulté à uriner?	Haben Sie Schwierigkeiten beim Wasserlassen?
Do you pass water involuntarily?	¿Orina sin querer?	Urina involontariamente?	Urinez-vous involuntairement?	Lassen Sie den Harn ohne es zu wollen?
Are any of your limbs swollen?	¿Están hinchados alguno de sus miembros?	Si sente gonfio in qualche parte?	Avez-vous des membres gonflés?	Ist irgendeines Ihrer Glieder geschwollen?
How long have they been swollen like this?	¿Desde cuándo estan hinchados así?	Da quanto tempo che li ha così gonfi?	Depuis quand sont-ils gonflés comme ça?	Seit wann sind sie so angeschwollen?
Physical Assessment				
Look up.	Mire para arriba.	Guardi sù.	Regardez en haut.	Schauen Sie hinauf.
Look down.	Mire para abajo.	Guardi giu.	Regardez en bas.	Schauen Sie hinunter.
Look toward your nose.	Mire la nariz.	Si guardi il naso.	Regardez le nez.	Schauen sie auf Ihre Nase.
Look at me.	Míreme.	Mi guardi.	Regardez-moi.	Sehen Sie mich an.
Take a deep breath.	Respìre profundamente.	Prenda un gran respiro.	Respirez profondement.	Atmen Sie tief.
Cough.	Tosa.	Tossisca.	Toussez.	Husten Sie.
Cough again.	Tosa otra vez.	Tossisca ancora.	Toussez encore une fois.	Husten Sie noch einmal.
Open your mouth.	Abra la boca.	Apra la bocca.	Ouvrez la bouche.	Öffnen Sie den Mund.
Grasp my hand.	Apriete mi mano.	Mi stringa la mano.	Serrez-moi la main.	Drücken Sie mir die Hand.
Can you not do it better than that?	¿No puede hacerlo más fuerte?	Non può far meglio?	Vous ne pouvez-pas serrer plus fort que cela?	Können Sie nicht fester greifen?
Your arm feels paralyzed?	¿Parece que el brazo está paralizado?	Si sente il braccio paralizzato?	Est-ce que le bras vous paraît paralysé?	Ihr Arm erscheint Ihnen gelähmt?
Raise your arm.	Levante el brazo.	Alzi il braccio.	Levez le bras.	Heben Sie den Arm.
Raise it more.	Más alto.	Ancora di più.	Plus haut.	Höher.
Now the other.	Ahora el otro.	Adesso l'altro.	Maintenant l'autre.	Jetzt den andern.
Pain Assessment				
Have you any pain?	¿Tiene dolor?	Ha dolori?	Avez-vous mal quelque?	Haben Sie Schmerzen?

TABLE 5-2. Phrases in Foreign Languages for Health Assessment and Examination Continued

English	Spanish	Italian	French	German
Pain Assessment *continued*				
Where does it hurt?	¿Dónde le duele?	Dove le duele?	Où avez-vous mal?	Wo haben Sie Schmerzen?
Do you have pain here?	¿Le duele aquí?	Ha dolori qui?	Avez-vous mal par ici?	Haben Sie Schmerzen hier?
Do you have a pain in your side?	¿Le duele el costado?	Avete dolori al fianco?	Avez-vous mal au côté?	Haben Sie Seitenstechen?
Is it worse now?	¿Está peor ahora?	È peggio ora?	Est-ce que c'est encore pire maintenant?	Ist es jetzt schlimmer?
Does it still pain you?	¿Le duele todavía?	Fa male ancora?	Est-ce que ça vous fait mal toujours?	Schmerzt er noch?
Do you still have that heavy pain?	¿Le duele mucho todavia?	Ha ancora quel dolore pesante?	Avez-vous toujours la douleur pesante?	Habe Sie noch den drückenden Schmerz?
Does it pain you to breathe?	¿Le duele al respirar?	Le fa male respirare?	Votre respiration est-elle douloureuse?	Spüren Sie Schmerzen beim Atmen?
Shooting pains?	¿Dolores agudos?	Dei dolori acuti?	Des elancements?	Stechende Schmerzen?
As if one were pricking you with pins?	¿Como si estuvieran pinchándole con alfileres?	Come se fossero delle spille?	Comme si l'on vous piquâit avec des épingles?	Als ob man Sie mit Stecknadeln stäche?
Did you feel much pain at the time?	¿Sintió mucho dolor entonces?	Avete sentito molto dolore allora?	Est-ce que ça vous a fait beaucoup de mal alors?	Haben Sie gleich damals arge Schmerzen gespürt?
Show me where.	Enséñeme dónde.	Mi mostri dove.	Montrez-moi où.	Zeigen Sie mir wo.
In the abdomen?	¿En el vientre?	Nel ventre?	Dans le abdomen?	Im Leib?
The ankle	El tobillo	La caviglia	La cheville	Das Fussgelenk
The arm	El brazo	Il braccio	Le bras	Der Arm
The back	La espalda	Il dorso	Le dos	Der Rücken
The bones	Los huesos	La ossa	Le os	Die Knochen
The chest	El pecho	Il petto	La poitrine	Die Brust
The ears	Los oídos	Le orecchie	Les oreilles	Die Ohren
The elbow	El codo	Il gomito	Le coude	Der Ellenbogen
The eye	El ojo	L'occhio	L'oeil	Das Auge
The foot	El pie	Il piede	Le pied	Der Fuss
The gums	Las encías	Le gengive	Les gengives	Das Zahnfleisch
The hand	La mano	La mano	La main	Die Hand
The head	La cabeza	La testa	La tête	Der Kopf
The heart	El corazón	Il cuore	Le coeur	Das Herz
The leg	La pierna	La gamba	La jambe	Das Bein
The liver	El hígado	Il fegato	Le foie	Die Leber
The lungs	Los pulmones	I polmoni	Les poumons	Die Lungen
The mouth	La boca	La bocca	La bouche	Der Mund
The muscles	Los músculos	I muscoli	Les muscles	Die Muskeln
The neck	El cuello	Il collo	Le cou	Der Nacken
The nerves	Los nervios	I nervi	Les nerfs	Die Nerven
The nose	La nariz	Il naso	Le nez	Die Nase
The ribs	Las costillas	Le costole	Les côtes	Die Rippen
The shoulder blades	Las paletillas	Le scapole	Les omoplates	Die Schulterblätter
The side	El flanco	Il fianco	Le côté	Die Seite
The skin	La piel	La pelle	La peau	Die Haut

From: *Taber's cyclopedic medical dictionary* (16th Ed). Philadelphia: F.A. Davis.

munity in which health care services are being provided.

Although international and transcultural nursing are concerned with health beliefs and practices of different cultures,[8] collaboration is crucial within international nursing. Collaboration in international nursing exists at different levels. First, there is collaboration between the nurse from the donor country and the nurse from the host country. Second, there is national collaboration with Ministries of Health and their representatives. Finally, community collaboration exists as the international nurse secures the cooperation of the community for any health care project.

GLOBAL ORGANIZATIONS

The World Health Organization (WHO) is part of the United Nations. Created in 1948, WHO is concerned with international and public health problems.

A turning point for WHO occurred with the 1978 International Conference on Primary Health Care in Alma-Ata, USSR. During this conference, members were challenged to change health services with equity, through primary health care. The slogan from the conference became "Health for All by the Year 2000." Although it was viewed as an ambitious goal, WHO has made progress, and insight has been gained from programs that were not successful.[28]

Many countries have incorporated primary health care within their philosophies; however, access to health care is still limited in many countries, and success is sporadic. For example, from 1970 to 1980, immunization rates in some countries improved from 5 to 40 per cent. However, in less developed countries, immunization rates may still be less than 15 per cent.[27, 28]

In order to increase the impact of nurses working with WHO, global strategies were initiated. The Network of Collaborating Centers for Nursing Development was formally established in March, 1987, in Bangkok, Thailand. The goal is the creation of 30 centers throughout the world, with regional representation. Already, 14 centers have been established, which include the regions of Africa, the Americas, Europe, Southeast Asia, and the Western Pacific. These centers are creating a network of nursing leaders who are committed to implementing WHO's primary health care philosophy.[10]

The International Council of Nurses was initiated in 1900. According to its charter, member nurses make the following pledge:

> We, the nurses of all nations, sincerely believing that the best good of our profession will be advanced by greater unity of thought, sympathy and purpose, do hereby band ourselves in a confederation to further the efficient care of the sick and to secure the honour and interests of the Nursing Profession.[18]

Thus, the concept of a global nursing community was developed nearly a century ago through the International Council of Nurses. Every 4 years, an international conference is convened by the International Council of Nurses. Nurses worldwide gather to share new ideas and research, and networking is facilitated. Also, the International Council of Nurses has been committed to preparing nurses in primary health care since 1979. Between 1983 and 1985, the International Council of Nurses conducted seven regional workshops to prepare nursing leaders for primary health care[4] and their commitment continues through developing guidelines for implementing primary health care. In turn, these nursing leaders will educate other nurses, and so facilitate the growth of primary health care's philosophy from country to country.

Summary

The care of clients from other lands and cultures is becoming a common component of nursing practice. To enhance the quality of care given to the client, the nurse should understand and respect the differences in the client's health beliefs and practices.

Bibliography

1. Bergman, R. (1986). Nursing in a changing world. *International Nursing Review, 33,* 110.
2. Branch, M., & Paxton, P. (1976). *Providing safe nursing care for ethnic people of color.* Englewood Cliffs, NJ: Prentice-Hall.
3. Brink, P. (1984). Value orientations as an assessment tool in cultural diversity. *Nursing Research, 35,* 198.
4. Boyle, J., & Andrews, M. (1989). *Transcultural concepts in nursing care.* GlenView, IL: Scott Foresman.
5. Comos-Dias, L., & Griffith, E. (1988). *Clinical guidelines in cross-cultural mental health.* New York: Wiley.
6. Dawes, T. (1986). Multicultural nursing. *International Nursing Review, 33,* 148.
7. DeSantis, L. (1988). The relevance of transcultural nursing to international nursing. *International Nursing Review, 35,* 110.
8. Douglas, M., & Mobius, A. (1985). International nursing: Challenges and consequences. *Mobius 5,* 84.
9. Fong, C. (1985). Ethnicity and nursing practice. *Topics in Clinical Nursing, 7*(3), 1–10.

9a. Foster, G., & Anderson, B. (1978). *Medical anthropology.* New York: Alfred A. Knopf.

10. Glittenberg, J. (1990). Global network of World Health Organization collaborating centers for nursing. *Journal of Professional Nursing, 6*(3), 137.
11. Good, C. (1987). *Ethnomedical Systems in Africa.* New York: Guilford Publishers.
12. Ho, M. (1987). *Family therapy with ethnic minorities.* Beverly Hills, CA: Sage Publishers.
13. LaFargue, J. (1985). Mediating between two views of illness. *Topics in Clinical Nursing, 7*(3), 70–77.
14. Leninger, M. (1991). Transcultural nursing: The study and practice field. *Imprint, 38*(2), 55–66.
15. Leninger, M. (1988). Leninger's theory of nursing: Cultural care, diversity and universality. *Nursing Science Quarterly, 1*(4), 152–160.
16. Leninger, M. (1970). *Nursing and anthropology: Two worlds to blend.* New York: John Wiley & Sons.
17. Leninger, M. (1978). *Transcultural nursing: Concepts, theories and practices.* New York: John Wiley & Sons.
18. Levine, R., & Campbell, D. (1972). *Ethnocentrism: Theories of conflict, ethnic attitudes, and group behavior.* New York: John Wiley & Sons.
19. Lipson, J., & Melies, A. (1985). Culturally appropriate care: The case of immigrants. *Topics in Clinical Nursing, 7*(3), 48–56.

20. Louie, K. (1985). Transcending cultural bias: The literature speaks. *Topics in Clinical Nursing, 7*(3), 78-84.
21. Malone, R. (1990). The challenge of third world nursing. *American Journal of Nursing, 90*(7), 32-37.
22. Norbeck, E., & Lock, M. (1987). *Health, illness and medical care in Japan.* Honolulu: University of Hawaii Press.
22a. Orque, M., et al. (1983). *Ethnic nursing care: A multicultural approach.* St. Louis: C. V. Mosby.
23. Rothenburger, R. (1990). Transcultural nursing. *AORN Journal, 51*(5), 1349-1363.
24. Salmon, M. (1988). Health for all: A transnational model for nursing. *International Nursing Review, 35,* 107.
25. Tripp-Reimer, T. (1984). Cultural assessment: Content and process. *Nursing Outlook, 32*(2), 78.
26. Ulin, P. (1989). Global collaboration in primary health care. *Nursing Outlook, 37*(3), 134.
27. UNICEF (1987). *The state of the world's children.* New York: Oxford University Press.
28. World Health Organization (1987). *Evaluation of the strategy for health for all by the year 2000: Seventh report on the world health situation. (Vol 1): Global Review.* Geneva: World Health Organization.
29. World Health Organization (1976). *African traditional medicine.* Brazzaville: World Health Organization.
30. Yoder, P. (1982). Biomedical and ethnomedical practice in rural Zaire. *Social and Science Medicine, 16,* 1851.

ADDITIONAL READING ON SPECIFIC CULTURAL GROUPS

Ailinger, R. (1985). Beliefs about treatment of hypertension among Hispanic older persons. *Topics in Clinical Nursing, 7*(3), 26-31.

Boyle, J. (1991). Transcultural nursing care of Central American refugees. *Imprint, 38*(2), 73-77.

Boyle, J. (1989). Constructs of health and wellness in a Salvadoran population. *Public Health Nursing, 6,* 129-134.

Capers, C. (1985). Nursing and the Afro-American client. *Topics in Clinical Nursing, 7*(3), 11-17.

Egan, M. (1985). A family assessment challenge: Refugee youth and foster family adaptation. *Topics in Clinical Nursing, 7*(3), 64-69.

Foreman, J. (1985). Susto and the health needs of the Cuban refugee population. *Topics in Clinical Nursing, 7*(3), 40-47.

Giger, J., et al. (1991). Biologic variations in the Black patient. *Imprint, 38*(2), 95-105.

Hamilton, C. (1991). Nursing on the Navajo reservation. *Imprint, 38*(2), 121, 174.

Kelly, K. (1991). A nursing student's experience in Haiti. *Imprint, 38*(2), 69-72.

Louie, K. (1985). Providing health care to Chinese clients. *Topics in Clinical Nursing, 7*(3), 18-25.

Luna, L. (1989). Transcultural nursing care of Arab Muslims. *Journal of Transcultural Nursing, 1*(1), 22-26.

Orque, M., et al. (1983). *Ethnic nursing care: A multicultural approach.* St. Louis: C. V. Mosby.

Roberson, M. (1985). The influence of religious beliefs on health choices of Afro-Americans. *Topics in Clinical Nursing, 7*(3), 57-63.

Sobralske, M. (1985). Perceptions of health: Navajo Indians. *Topics in Clinical Nursing, 7*(3), 32-39.

Tripp-Reimer, T., et al. (1988). To be different from the world: Patterns of elder care among old order Amish. *Journal of Cultural Gerontology, 3,* 185-195.

Wenger, A. (1991). Culture-specific care and the older Amish. *Imprint, 38*(2), 80-93.

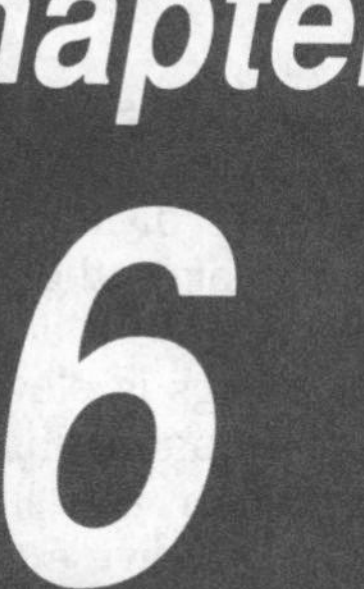

Spirituality

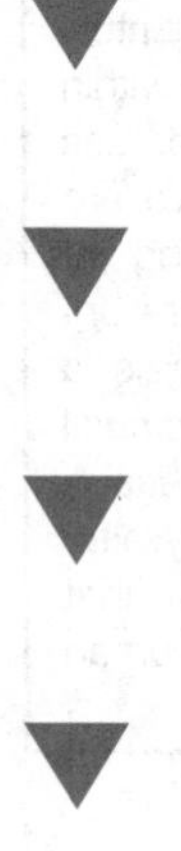

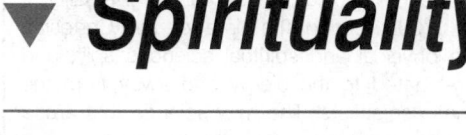

Who am I? Where did I come from? Why am I here? What is my place in the cosmos?

These and other questions like them constitute the spiritual search that engages each of us on our journey through life. The fact that a chapter on spirituality is included in a medical-surgical textbook represents an evolutionary step forward for the nursing profession. The spiritual domain represents a significant part of who we are. Any medical or surgical disorder of the body is reflected in an alteration of the mind and the spirit. Because of the holistic aspect of our being, each system has a direct or indirect effect on every other system.

CONCEPTS OF SPIRITUALITY

Spirituality is a broad concept encompassing values, meaning, and purpose. It is experienced when one turns inward to explore the human capacities of honesty, love, caring, wisdom, imagination, and compassion.[8] Spirituality can be described as a human need to search for the meaning and purpose of life.[29]

Spirituality comes from the term "spirit," which is derived from several ethnic and historical sources. In Latin, it meant "breath." The Greeks evolved the term from the root word "wind." Biblical sources describe spirit as the breath of God flowing through us. The definition of spirit found in Webster's Dictionary gives us the concept of spirit as the breath of life. Buddhists think of spirit in terms of inner light or truth. In contemporary times, we have come to think of spirit as divine animation, an inner guide, something greater than ourselves, something within ourselves, and in a variety of other conceptual ways.

Spirit can be seen as a multitude of animations, present at every level of existence from the simplest material to the divine. In pure matter, spirit is perhaps that which makes the electrons spin around their nucleus, affecting both animate and inanimate life.[14] Spirit in human beings is elevated to a higher plane, where it contains the animating principle seen in the lower forms of matter and life, but it also incorporates the principle of the divine that many call the soul.

FOSTERING SPIRITUALITY

The most important aspect of spirituality is recognizing that it is an essential need of human nature. There is something in each of us that seeks the spiritual. This yearning may vary in strength from person to person, but it is present all the same. It is the conscious seeking of the light, of the truth, or of the connection with the source that is the beginning point of those who quest to integrate spirituality into their nursing practice.

The exploration of one's spirituality is a process of unfoldment, a journey that may take a lifetime or a brief, poignant moment when the seeker suddenly discovers the light within. It is ongoing and continuous and is a part of every evolving nurse healer. One develops spirituality through a conscious decision to explore one's own inner self in relation to a larger cosmic consciousness. During the exploration process, there is an awareness, which may be gradual or abrupt, that there are new ways of viewing old situations. Once a person incorporates spirituality, he or she begins to shift and sort information for a fresh perspective as a transformational process is entered that incorporates a spiritual perspective in the delivery of health care (see Box 6-1).

There are a variety of skills and techniques used to assist people in developing their spirituality. These techniques are applicable for both the nurse and the client and are listed in Table 6-1. Questions such as these assist a person to delve more deeply into the conscious aspect of living. It is through an awakened consciousness that one grows spiritually.

Box 6-1. Spirituality: An Art or A Science?

There is wide debate about the placement of the spiritual sciences within the hierarchy of other sciences. Some scientists refute spirituality altogether because it is not precisely measurable or empirically verifiable. Historically, the word "science" meant logic, order, law, and universality. It was during the 1700s, during the time of the Cartesian dualism, that the physical and spiritual sciences split, and spirituality was relegated to the clergy and away from the emerging pragmatic scientists. The new science that arose was based solely on empiricism. (See also Chap. 3.)

At present, the pendulum is swinging back; the spiritual "arts" are rapidly being redefined and incorporated within the realm of science. After centuries of slow progress toward rational explanations of the physical world, we are entering a new level in the scientific understanding of mechanisms by which faith, belief, and imagination are unlocking the mysteries of healing.[2] At present, there is a whole new breed of scientists documenting that spiritual interventions and mystical openness are valid and measurable, and that spiritual interventions work to effectively alter the course of illness and disease. Some even postulate that the spiritual domain represents the apex of the human sciences.

RELEVANCE OF SPIRITUALITY TO NURSING PRACTICE

Emerging nursing models (i.e. Newman, Rogers, Travelbee and Watson) address spirituality directly in terms of human needs. Watson[31] states that the future of nursing belongs to caring more than curing, and that the entire profession is in process of redefinition. We are emerging from a traditional practice of objective, rational detachment into something far greater. Part of that greatness includes the renaissance of a holistic approach. As nursing redefines itself, it will reincorporate some of the forgotten aspects of our heritage—the role of spirit.

Watson[32] further states that "human caring theory allows the commitment and consciousness of the nurse to transcend (or at least attempt to transcend) the physical material surface and reach beyond to touch the human center of the person" (p. 176). When this occurs, we are less inclined to objectify persons and more inclined to see new caring and healing possibilities. The human caring process has an energy field of its own that exceeds the sum of each individual. We

TABLE 6-1. Techniques to Develop Spirituality

- Dream journeying
- Self-reflection
- Meditation
- Prayer
- Guided and/or individual retreats
- Psychological techniques
  - psychosynthesis
  - guided imagery
  - personal and group therapy sessions
- Travel
- Participating in transformational conferences
- Reflective contemplation of one's life with these questions
  - What is the meaning, purpose, and direction reflected in my life?
  - To what extent have I evolved on my life's journey?
  - How are my values operationalized in my day-to-day living?
  - What brings me pleasure; what causes me pain?
  - Am I doing what brings me pleasure and satisfaction in life? If not, why not, and how can I change the situation?
  - Am I achieving what I want to in my life?
  - Do I become still enough, often enough, to listen to the quiet, inner voice that directs my being?
  - How can I grow more fully?

Box 6–2. Spirituality Assessment Guide

Subjective Data—Does the client

Talk about spiritual needs or concerns?
Verbalize feelings about God, faith, prayer?
Feel that the illness affected his or her feelings about God?
Find any particular religious practices helpful?
Belong to any specific religious group or faith community?
Have someone or something to turn to for help and hope?
Feel lonely, depressed, abandoned?
Feel separated from spiritual connections?
Express bitterness, self-belittling thoughts? Project blame for illness?
Question the validity of faith? Verbalize inner conflicts about beliefs? Question the credibility of the religious system?
View illness as a form of punishment from God?
Have a form of belief that fosters or weakens faith and trust? Fosters or weakens self-esteem?
Express a preoccupation with thoughts of faith and illness?
Have access to spiritual resources?

Objective Data—Does the client

Pray before meals?
Read religious material?
Have religious materials nearby (e.g., rosary, medals)?
Express a reluctance to participate in spiritual or religious rituals?
Express anger or resentment toward religious or spiritual leaders?
Sleep listlessly, have disturbing dreams?

must remember that caring occurs in the metaphysical realm. We cannot see this realm, we can only experience it.

Meeting the spiritual needs of clients has become a recognized part of nursing care. Nursing care is not only to make clients well or prevent illness, "but to help those in health or illness to use the power within themselves as they evolve toward higher levels of consciousness."[25] Dennis conducted one of the first empirical studies of nurses' spirituality.[6] Data suggested that spiritual care is not a separate part of nursing, but that it is integral to nursing, as evidenced by the range of comments supporting spirituality in practice. (See Nursing Research.)

Nurses must be aware of their own spirituality in order to assist others in fulfilling their spiritual needs. People are not unidimensional in scope, but at least tridimensional; they are beings composed of body, mind, and spirit. When the physical domain of an individual is compromised, the mind and spirit are also involved. Guided by this understanding, the nurse can more easily facilitate the harmonious interconnections within and between persons. In addition, there is a stronger appreciation for the interpersonal and physical environments and for the Ultimate Other or God as understood by the individual.

SPIRITUALITY AND NURSING PROCESS

Those who suffer or those in spiritual crisis need nurses who allow and, on occasion, even encourage anger, tears, and the expression of sorrow. These people need sensitive caregivers who can say, "Yes, what happened to you is terrible and may make no sense from this perspective," rather than "Cheer up, it's not that bad." If this type of care is to be offered, nurses must be supported as they learn how to call forth the inner power and to empower their own personality.

NURSING RESEARCH

The purpose of this exploratory study was to discover and describe the components of spiritual care by nurses who provide such care. A qualitative approach was used with Watson's work on the spiritual aspect of human beings as a framework. Ten nurses who said they provided spiritual care from a nonreligious perspective were the sample. Data were analyzed by examining the interviews for incidents and facts and then grouping the data into Watson's categories.

The study found that spiritual care for these nurses was not a separate part of nursing but an integral portion of nursing care. The nurses believed that the human spirit is at the core of every client's existence and is the power that heals. Their goal was to bring forth the inner powers and nourish the subdued spirit.

Nurses who provide spiritual care need to be committed, fully prepared to use self as a healing tool, "able to stay within the moment," and willing to be seen as "different" from other nurses.

The process of providing such care includes the nurse honoring the client's uniqueness and setting up a safe environment for discussion, therapeutic touch, or quiet time. Significant others may or may not be helpful and may block spiritual care. Nurses noted that after such care was given, the clients express deep gratitude and the room was quieter. The hospital was generally not conducive or supportive to providing spiritual care. The nurses generally reported having encounters with clients that were an intimate exchange and like a soul-to-soul union that transcended the roles of nurse and client. For some nurses, this union occurred quickly, and for others, it only happened after many visits.

The study's implications are that if this type of care is to be offered, nurses need to be taught how to give such care. Nurses who work in hospital settings need empowerment if this type of care is to be given.

▼▼▼

Dennis, P. (1991). Components of spiritual nursing care from the nurse's perspective. *Journal of Holistic Nursing*, 9(1), 27–42.

Assessment

Spiritual calls for help seldom take the form of overt statements. Instead, they appear as subtle signs. Learning to recognize these signs will better prepare you to discuss and reinforce clients' religious beliefs. These signs may be statements such as, "Do you go to church? I have not been to church in a long time. What do the chaplains do in this hospital?" On the other hand, the questions may be profound and include philosophical inquiries about your perception of life after death or the meaning of life.

A second area of spiritual assessment involves the specific religious practices of a client. The nurse needs to question what these practices mean now during this time of stress and crisis. Some clients become more religious when they are in crisis and other coping mechanisms fail. Sometimes clients first explore their spiritual practice in the face of some new event (a serious illness, death of a loved one, or childbirth) that causes them to think about the hereafter. Many clients think of themselves as immortal until they are confronted with surgery or illness and come face to face with their own immortality. These events trigger the questions, such as "What is the meaning of life? Is there a heaven or hell? Why am I here?" In addition to collecting subjective data, the nurse may observe the environment for objective data (see Box 6–2).

Nursing Diagnosis

Spiritual distress (distress of the human spirit) has been accepted as a nursing diagnosis by the North American Nursing Diagnosis Association in 1989. The etiology of the condition may flow from various sources, including separation from religious or cultural ties, a change in beliefs or value systems, intense suffering during severe stress, or prolonged treatment. The defining characteristics (or symptoms) include anger against the deity or questions about the meaning of suffering being experienced. The client may joke in a macabre fashion, have nightmares, cry, act in a hostile or apathetic manner, express anger or resentment against religious figures, and cease participation in religious practices.

Planning: Expected Outcomes

The expected outcome for the client is decreased symptoms of spiritual distress with behaviors that may include the ability to experience forgiveness, connection to religious or cultural ties, a reaffirmation of faith or commitment to internal values, decreased feelings of guilt over past actions, or internal peace.

Nursing Intervention

Accepting others as they are, where they are—without the traditional concern for defining, controlling, and changing—permits the spirit to expand and express itself. So many people have lived a life of control, definition, and judgement that the spirit has been driven far below the surface.[27] Nurses who have awakened their own spirituality are inclined to encourage the expression of spirit in others.

Clients in spiritual distress need the nurse to offer support through active listening, to demonstrate concern and care, and to be available and sensitive to the expressed needs.

Other interventions include

- Clarifying the client's religious needs by (1) encouraging expression of thoughts and feelings, (2) talking about conflicts and their cause, and (3) seeking sources of strength and faith.
- Identifying supportive and helpful measures by communicating acceptance of and respect for the client's religious beliefs. The nurse should involve the client in the planning of spiritual care, including identification of objects, sacraments, and services that provide spiritual comfort.
- Making immediate changes necessary to accommodate the client's needs by providing privacy and time, contacting his or her denominational representative, and meeting special needs.
- Requesting clergy to help the client and family determine community resources for support.
- Direct participation with client when client expresses need.
- Encouraging the use of prayer and scripture.
- Other interventions specific to client.

When the nurse is asked personal questions about beliefs, she or he should attempt to give thoughtful answers and provide an environment for the client's self-exploration and self-expression. The nurse should not force her or his religious values onto the client. The nurse healer is like a tuning fork through which the client can begin to resonate with the consciousness of the universe.[17] Entering a client's room or walking through his or her front door, being open and vulnerable, without definitions and judgements, is sometimes just what is needed to assist another within the spiritual domain.

Many hospital environments do not provide spiritual care. However, despite the barriers, hospital nurses can transcend the situation while getting to the core of the person's experience, and can note positive environmental changes as a result of such care. As nurses become increasingly knowledgeable of methods of spiritual assessment and intervention, it is likely that there will be a more open environment for spiritual interventions.

Evaluation

Several approaches can be taken in evaluating the effectiveness of interventions for spiritual distress. These include (1) the relief of symptoms approach and (2) the values clarification approach.

RELIEF OF SYMPTOMS APPROACH

Is there a change in the client's verbalization, attitude, or both? Have the symptoms such as anger, guilt, depression, anxiety, and crying changed?

VALUES CLARIFICATION APPROACH

With use of values clarification tools, nurses can help clients identify their values. From these expressed values, short- and long-term goals consistent with the client's values and beliefs are formulated. From these written goals, then, the nurse and the client can determine if they were met and can reformulate new goals.

GRIEF

Grief is one of the most common human responses seen by nurses. It can be initiated by many things; death and illness are the most common. However, any loss, even the loss of a dream or life plan, can initiate a grief response. Consider the woman who has a miscarriage; not only has she lost the child but also the dreams she had stored, perhaps since her own childhood, for her child. Other losses of life plans may occur with forced or medically necessary retirement, institutionalization, divorce, or loss of a job.

Grief can be seen in clients, families, and even other health care providers in many clinical settings. Grief occurs in all ages and across all cultures. Whether it is offering support to a woman with a new diagnosis of breast cancer, caring for a client dying of AIDS, or helping a client after an amputation, nurses are frequently faced with the task of recognizing grief as well as providing appropriate interventions.

There are many emotional reactions to grief, and they are generally influenced by cultural background, socialization, and family structure. In 1969, Kubler-Ross[15] was one of the first to write about the process of dying and, thereby, the process of grief. She described five stages that all persons go through during the process of dying: (1) denial and isolation, (2) anger, (3) bargaining, (4) depression, and (5) acceptance. Other reactions may occur, however, such as fear, hostility, and retreat. Each of these responses should be recognized by the nurse as the client's attempt at coping and as part of the grief response.

A more contemporary concept of grief focuses on the fact that this process is not composed of a rigid set of stages with a predictable pattern of responses; the grief process is dynamic. Nurses cannot say "Well if Mr. Thompson is in denial today, by tomorrow he will be angry." The grief process is not that predictable. Some of the stages may be internal and may not be visible to the nurse. Other stages may never appear. Still other clients may clearly go back and forth between one stage and another.

A recent description of the grieving process recognizes some different aspects from Kubler-Ross. It is apparent that not only is grief dynamic but also individualized, pervasive, and normative. Every client does not have the same grief response when faced with the same medical condition. There are many factors that have an impact on grief, such as the nature of the loss, the relationship of the grieving person to the individual or object lost, and the presence of support systems.

Grief is also pervasive, affecting every aspect of the client's existence. Reported responses to grieving include physical (alterations in heart rate and blood pressure, crying, and gastrointestinal disturbances), social (withdrawal from social groups and difficulty forming new relationships), cognitive (preoccupation with thoughts of the lost object or person, thoughts of personal mortality, and inability to concentrate), affective (depression, sleeplessness), behavioral (inability to carry out daily activities), and spiritual (questioning religious beliefs or faith and questions about an afterlife).

Finally, grief has been described as normal. Despite the great variations in the grief response, grief is an expected response to loss. What constitutes a normal length of time for the grieving process is another question. Many years ago, a widow was expected to be in mourning for a year, wearing black during that time. There are limits to grief, beyond which time it becomes inappropriate or unacceptable. The boundaries of this period of time are dictated by culture and socialization. Grief that goes on after this acceptable period of time is called unresolved grief.

Stages of Grief

Four stages of the process of grief have been described: (1) shock and numbness, (2) searching and yearning, (3) disorientation and disorganization, and (4) resolution and reorganization.

Shock and numbness may leave one feeling as though time has stopped and engulfed in a fog or cloud. During this time, the griever may forget things, feel confused, or have a difficult time making decisions.

The stage of searching and yearning usually follows the initial period of shock. During this time, anger is usually present. The anger may be directed toward others or even the one who is lost. In many instances, guilt surfaces. The mourner can become convinced that if things had been done differently, the tragedy may have been averted. Feeling guilty is one way of grappling with the question of "why?" The search for the answers may help resolve the feelings of guilt.

Other feelings occurring during the second stage include difficulty in concentrating, physical symptoms, or feelings of emptiness and exhaustion. Sometimes, people even feel as though they are losing their minds because they cannot concentrate on anything. This stage may last for months and requires the sensitivity of a nurse who understands the grieving process.

The third stage involves disorientation and disorganization. This time is marked with more difficulties in concentration, or difficulty starting or continuing routine projects. Physical problems may appear as a result of sublimated emotions. During this period, grievers may not feel like preparing or eating food. If a loss of appetite occurs, this problem can contribute to increased depression. On the other hand, overeating can occur.

Sleeplessness is frequently another problem associated with grieving. If this problem occurs, the nurse might suggest exercise, warm baths, and listening to soothing music instead of watching television before bedtime.

In time, energy levels increase and the ability to make decisions returns. The body and mind prepare to move forward toward the fourth stage: resolution and reorganization. This period is easier if there are others to encourage and support the griever. This is why support groups are so valuable. When the griever joins a support group, he or she meets others who have gone through similar circumstances and have the strength to help newcomers.

What about nurses who care for dying clients? Do they experience grief over the loss? Nurses do experience grief. They often report feelings of helplessness, inadequacy, and question their beliefs, faith, and own health. Clinical areas that have large numbers of clients and families in grief states, such as oncology, critical care units, and burn units, often employ psychologists to assist with the staff's grief work.

SUFFERING

Suffering is submitting or being forced to submit to and endure a particular set of circumstances that is not under one's control. Suffering may be physical, psychological, spiritual, or social. It is in response to suffering that many, perhaps all of us, define ourselves, take on character and develop ethos (a guiding belief system). To the person suffering, though, suffering seems to be pointless.

To see the value of suffering we only have to ask "how would people behave if they did not have the capacity to suffer?" Such people could not bear grief, loss, or misfortune and, in effect, would give up much of the measure of their humanness. Our capacity to feel grief and to identify with the misfortune of others is the basis for our ability to recognize, empathize with, and care for our fellow human beings.

It is important to be careful about how we conceptualize suffering. It is seldom a means for character building but rather a test for character already built. Our reactions to suffering may reveal us as better or worse than we had thought ourselves to be. Suffering can just as easily destroy a person's ego structure as it can make us more resolute. In that respect it is useful to reflect on our reaction to someone suffering. Suffering has the potential to make another person a stranger. To the uninitiated, the first response may be to be repelled. Suffering makes people's otherness stand out in strong relief, but that otherness is exactly the condition necessary to force recognition of them and of ourselves. It is the obligation of those who care for the suffering to know how to minister to them in such a way as to include rather than exclude them from the human condition. One of our challenges as nurses is to bind the suffering and the nonsuffering into the same community. Our role is not to eliminate suffering and death but to sooth unnecessary suffering and untimely death.

A nurse may wonder why some lives seem so burdened with suffering whereas others seem untouched. When these situations occur, you may want to consider yourself or point out to your clients the analogy of a beautiful tapestry. Looked at from the right side, it is an intricately woven work of art, drawing together threads of different lengths and colors to make up a creative picture. However, when it is turned to the other side, you see a medley of many threads, some short, others

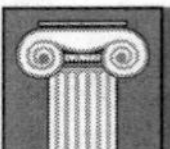

ETHICAL ISSUES IN NURSING

Should Spiritual Beliefs That Are in Opposition to Modern Medical Practices Be Respected?

A person's beliefs about his or her spiritual self is a very private and reflective matter. Some people follow spiritual guidelines accepted through organized religious institutions. Other people incorporate spiritual identities from sources including mysticism, new age phenomena, or naturalism. Personal beliefs, from whatever source, may have a great impact on a person's concept of health, illness, grief, and loss.

Spiritual healing through prayer, repentance, and positive thoughts is a practice demonstrated by certain religious groups. Christian Scientists, for example, believe that the healing of many of the bodies ills should come only through prayer. They also believe that certain illnesses that their children experience are caused by their own fears and errors of thought. The Christian Science church discourages parents from seeking medical treatment for their children (from medical practitioners other than their own Christian Science practitioners). There have been several cases in the recent past in which children of Christian Science parents have died from conditions that could very easily have been medically treated (bacterial meningitis, for example).

Freedom of religion is a right that should always be protected, but should spiritual beliefs that are in such opposition to common modern medical practices be respected in such an industrialized nation as the United States? Do parents have the right to impose their own spiritual guidelines on their minor children when such guidelines could cause physical impairment or possibly death?

Nurses are human beings, also, with human values and perhaps spiritual beliefs. During day-to-day nursing care, the spirituality of patients is not always assessed or considered as part of their care; however, spirituality can be a very important aspect of a client's treatment. It is important to be able to separate one's own beliefs from the beliefs of others so as not to impose one's own beliefs onto another. It is also important to be aware of one's own attitudes toward those who possess different spiritual ideas so that those attitudes do not interfere with the responsibilities as a health care professional.

long, some smooth and cut, others knotted and gnarled. Human life seen from the perspective of a tapestry may be viewed in a similar fashion. Moving away from the particular situation to the general scheme of things it is possible to view the individual situation from a spiritual perspective. Perhaps there is a large pattern into which all our lives fit. This pattern requires that some lives be twisted, knotted, or cut short, whereas others extend to impressive lengths and fine quality. This is not necessarily because one thread (person) is more deserving than another but simply because the pattern requires it. Looked at from the underneath, from our vantage point in this temporal life, the pattern of reward and punishment seems arbitrary and without design, but looked at from the outside, from a vantage point we cannot yet see, every twist and sorrow has its place in a great design that encompasses a creative work of art.

Grief and loss viewed from this perspective may help to alleviate individual suffering. Pointless suffering seen as a punishment for some unspecified sin or for some unknown reason is hard to bear. However, it is much more tolerable when viewed as a contribution to a great work of art, the tapestry of life, designed by a source far greater than ourselves.

RELIGION

Religion is an organized set of beliefs and practices expressing those beliefs. Religion is not a synonym for spirituality, although the words overlap in meaning.

It is common for clients who are ill, suffering, or dying to question their God and call on their religion for support. The religious practices of many clients offer support through periods of illness and at the time of death. Therefore, it is important for nurses to be aware of the impact of various religious beliefs and not interfere with the client's practice (see Ethical Issues in Nursing). Table 6-2 lists the various major religions and their beliefs and practices as it intertwines with health care.

TABLE 6-2. Religious Beliefs and Practices Affecting Health Care

Religious Group	Beliefs and Practices
WESTERN RELIGIONS *Judaism* Orthodox Jews and some Conservative Jewish groups	*Care of women:* A woman is considered to be in a ritual state of impurity whenever blood is coming from her uterus, such as during menstrual periods and after the birth of a child. During this time, her husband will not have physical contact with her. When this time is completed, she will bathe herself in a pool called a mikvah. Nurses need to be aware of this practice and be sensitive to the husband and wife because the husband will not touch his wife. He cannot assist her in moving in the bed, so the nurse will have to do this. An Orthodox Jewish man will not touch any women other than his wife, daughters, and mother. *Dietary rules:* (1) Kosher dietary laws include the following: No mixing of milk and meat at a meal; no consumption of food or any derivative thereof from animals not slaughtered in accordance with Jewish law; use of separate cooking utensils for milk and milk products; if a client requires milk and meat products for a meal, the dairy foods should be served first, followed later by the meat. (2) During Yom Kippur (Day of Atonement), a 24-hour fast is required, but exceptions are made for those who cannot fast because of medical reasons. (3) During Passover, no leavened products are eaten. (4) May say benediction of thanksgiving before meals and grace at the end of the meal. Time and a quiet environment should be provided for this. *Sabbath:* Observed from sunset Friday until sunset Saturday. Orthodox law prohibits riding in a car, smoking, turning lights on and off, handling money, and using television and telephone. Nurses need to be aware of this when caring for observant Jews at home and in the hospital. Medical or surgical treatments should be postponed if possible. *Death:* Judaism defines death as occurring when respiration and circulation are irreversibly stopped and no movement is apparent. (1) Euthanasia is strictly forbidden by Orthodox Jews, who advocate the strict use of life-support measures. (2) Prior to death, Jewish faith indicates that visiting of the person by family and friends is a religious duty. The Torah and Psalms may be read and prayers recited. A witness needs to be present when a person prays for health so that if death occurs God will protect the family and the spirit will be committed to God. Extraneous talking and conversation about death are not encouraged unless initiated by the client or visitors. In Judaism, the belief is that people should have someone with them when the soul leaves the body,

Table continued on following page

TABLE 6–2. Religious Beliefs and Practices Affecting Health Care Continued

Religious Group	Beliefs and Practices
	so family and/or friends should be allowed to stay with clients. After death, the body should be not be left alone until buried, usually within 24 hours. (3) When death occurs, the body should be untouched for 8 to 30 minutes. Medical personnel should not touch or wash the body but allow only an Orthodox person or the Jewish Burial Society to care for the body. Handling of a corpse on the Sabbath is forbidden to Jewish persons. If need be, the nursing staff may provide routine care of the body, wearing gloves. Water in the room should be emptied, and the family may request that mirrors be covered to symbolize that a death has occurred. (4) Orthodox Jews and some Conservative Jews do not approve of autopies. If an autopsy must be done, all body parts must remain with the body. (5) For Orthodox Jews, the body must be buried within 24 hours. No flowers are permitted. A fetus must be buried. (6) A 7-day mourning period is required by the immediate family. They must stay at home except for Sabbath worship. (7) Organs or other body parts such as amputated limbs must be made available for burial for Orthodox Jews, because they believe that all of the body must be returned to earth. *Birth control and abortion:* Artificial methods of birth control are not encouraged. Vasectomy is not allowed. Abortion may be performed only to save the mother's life. *Organ transplant:* Donor organ transplants generally are not permitted by Orthodox Jews but may be allowed with rabbinical consent. *Shaving:* The beard is regarded as a mark of piety among observant Jews. For the very Orthodox, shaving should not be done with a razor but with scissors or electric razor, because a blade should not contact the skin. *Head covering:* Orthodox men wear skull caps at all times, and women cover their hair after marriage. Some Orthodox women wear wigs as a mark of piety. Conservative Jews cover their heads only during acts of worship and prayer. *Prayer:* Praying directly to God, including a prayer of confession, is required for Orthodox Jews. Nurses should provide quiet time for prayer.
Reform Jews	*Care of women:* Reform Jews do not observe the rules against touching. *Dietary rules:* Reform Jews usually do not observe kosher dietary restrictions. *Sabbath:* Usually worship in temples on Friday evenings. No strict rules. *Death:* Advocate use of life support without heroic measures. Allow for cremation but suggest that ashes be buried in a Jewish cemetery. *Organ transplants:* Donation or transplantation of organs allowed with permission of a rabbi. *Head coverings:* Generally pray without wearing skull caps.
Christianity	
Roman Catholic	*Holy Eucharist:* For clients and health caregivers who are to receive communion, abstinence from solid food and alcohol is required for 15 minutes (if possible) prior to reception of the consecrated wafer. Medicine, water, and nonalcoholic drinks are permitted at any time. If a client is in danger of death, the fast is waived because the reception of the Eucharist at this time is very important. *Anointing of the sick:* The priest uses oil to anoint the forehead and hands and, if desired, the affected area. The rite may be performed on any who are ill and desire it. Clients receiving the sacrament seek complete healing, and strength to endure suffering. Prior to 1963, this sacrament was given only to clients at time of imminent death, so the nurse must be sensitive to the meaning this has for the client. If possible, the nurse calls a priest before the client is unconscious but may also call when there is sudden death, because the sacrament may also be given shortly after death. The nurse records on the care plan that this sacrament has been administered. *Dietary habits:* Obligatory fasting is excused during hospitalization. However, if there are no health restrictions, some Catholics may still observe the following guidelines: (1) Anyone 14 years or older must abstain from eating meat on

TABLE 6–2. Religious Beliefs and Practices Affecting Health Care Continued

Religious Group	Beliefs and Practices
	Ash Wednesday and all Fridays during Lent. Some older Catholics may still abstain from meat on all Fridays of the year. (2) In addition to abstinence from meat, persons 21 to 59 years of age must limit themselves to one full meal and two light meals on Ash Wednesday and Good Friday. (3) Eastern Rite Catholics are stricter about fasting and fast more frequently than Western Rite Catholics, so it is important for the nurse to know if a client is Eastern or Western. *Death:* Each Roman Catholic should participate in the anointing of the sick as well as the Eucharist and penance before death. The body should not be shrouded until after these sacraments are performed. All body parts that retain human quality must be appropriately buried or cremated. *Birth control:* Prohibited except for abstinence or natural family planning. Referral to a priest for questions about this can be of great help. Nurses can teach the techniques of natural family planning if they are familiar with them; otherwise, this should be referred to the physician or to a support group of the church that instructs couples in this method of birth control. Sterilization is prohibited unless there is an overriding medical reason. *Organ donation:* Donation and transplantation of organs are acceptable as long as the donor is not harmed and is not deprived of life. *Religious objects:* Rosary prayers are said using rosary beads. Medals bearing the images of saints, relics, statues, and scapulars are important objects that may be pinned to a hospital gown or pillow or be at the bedside. Extreme care should be taken not to lose these objects, because they have special meaning to the client.
Eastern Orthodox	*Holy Eucharist:* The priest is notified if the client desires this sacrament. *Anointing of the sick:* The priest conducts this in the hospital room. *Dietary habits:* Fasting from meat and dairy products is required on Wednesday and Friday during Lent and on other holy days. Hospital clients are exempt if fasting is detrimental to health. *Special days:* Christmas is celebrated on January 7 and New Year's Day on January 14. This is important to the care of a cleint who is hospitalized on these days. *Death:* Last rites are obligatory. This is handled by an ordained priest who is notified by the nurse while the client is conscious. The Russian Orthodox Church does not encourage autopsy or organ donation. Euthanasia, even for the terminally ill, is discouraged, as is cremation. *Birth control:* This as well as abortion is not permitted.
Protestant	*Holy Communion:* Notify clergy if the client desires.
Assemblies of God (Pentecostal)	*Anointing of the sick:* Members believe in divine healing through prayer and the laying on of hands. Clergy is notified if client or family desires this. *Dietary habits:* Abstinence from alcohol, tobacco, and all illegal drugs is strongly encouraged. *Death:* No special practices. *Other practices:* Faith in God and in the health care providers is encouraged. Members pray for divine intervention in health matters. Nurses should encourage and allow time for prayer. Members may speak in "tongues" during prayer.
Baptist (over 27 different groups in the United States)	*Holy Communion:* Clergy should be notified if the client desires. *Dietary habits:* Total abstinence from alcohol is expected. *Death:* No general service is provided, but the clergy does minister through counseling, prayer, and Scripture as requested by the client or family, and the client is encouraged to believe in Jesus Christ as Savior and Lord. *Other practices:* The Bible is held to be the word of God, so the nurse should either allow quiet time for Scripture reading or offer to read to the client.
Christian Church (Disciples of Christ)	*Holy Communion:* Open communion is celebrated each Sunday and is a central part of worship services. The nurse notifies the clergy if the client desires it, or the clergy may suggest it.

Table continued on following page

TABLE 6-2. Religious Beliefs and Practices Affecting Health Care Continued

Religious Group	Beliefs and Practices
	Death: No special practices. *Other practices:* Church elders as well as clergy may be notified to assist with meeting the client's spiritual needs.
Church of the Brethren	*Holy Communion:* Usually received within church, but clergy will give it in the hospital when requested. *Anointing of the sick:* Practiced for physical healing as well as spiritual uplift and held in high regard by the church. The clergy is notified if the client or family desire. *Death:* The clergy is notified for counsel and prayer.
Church of the Nazarene	*Holy Communion:* Pastor will administer if the client wishes. *Dietary habits:* The use of alcohol and tobacco is forbidden. *Death:* Cremation is permitted, and term stillborn infants are buried. *Other practices:* Believe in divine healing but not to the exclusion of medical treatment. Clients may desire quiet time for prayer.
Episcopal (Anglican)	*Holy Communion:* The priest is notified if the client wishes to receive this sacrament. *Anointing of the sick:* Priest may administer this rite when death is imminent, but it is not considered mandatory. *Dietary habits:* Some clients may abstain from meat on Fridays. Others may fast before receiving the Eucharist, but fasting is not mandatory. *Death:* No special practices. *Other practices:* Confession of sins to a priest is optional; if the client desires this, the clergy should be notified.
Lutheran (18 different branches)	*Holy Communion:* Notify the clergy if the client desires this sacrament. Clergy may also inquire about the client's desire. *Anointing of the sick:* The client may request an anointing and blessing from the minister when the prognosis is poor. *Death:* A service of Commendation of the Dying is used at the client's or family's request.
Mennonite (12 different groups)	*Holy Communion:* Served twice a year, with foot washing as part of ceremony. *Dietary habits:* Abstinence from alcohol is urged for all. *Death:* Prayer is important at time of crisis, so contacting a minister is important. *Other practices:* Women may wear head coverings during hospitalization. Anointing with oil is administered in harmony with James 5:14 when requested.
Methodist (over 20 different groups)	*Holy Communion:* Notify the clergy if a client requests it prior to surgery or another health crisis. *Anointing of the sick:* If requested, the clergy will come to pray and sprinkle the client with olive oil. *Death:* Scripture reading and prayer are important at this time. *Other practices:* Donation of one's body or part of the body at death is encouraged.
Presbyterian (10 different groups)	*Holy Communion:* Given when appropriate and convenient, at the hospitalized client's request. *Death:* Notify a local pastor or elder for prayer and Scripture reading if desired by the family or client.
Quaker (Friends)	*Holy Communion:* Because Friends have no creed, there is a diversity of personal beliefs, one of which is that outward sacraments are usually not necessary because there is the ministry of the Spirit inwardly in such areas as baptism and communion. *Death:* Believe that the present life is part of God's kingdom and generally have no ceremony as a rite of passage from this life to the next. Personal beliefs and wishes need to be ascertained, and the nurse can then act on the client's wishes.
Salvation Army	*Holy Communion:* No particular ceremony. *Death:* Notify the local officer in charge of the Army Corps for any soldier (member) who needs assistance. *Other practices:* The Bible is seen as the only rule for one's faith, so the Scriptures should be made available to a client. The Army has many of its

TABLE 6-2. Religious Beliefs and Practices Affecting Health Care Continued

Religious Group	Beliefs and Practices
	own social welfare centers, with hospitals and homes where unwed mothers are cared for and outpatient services provided. No medical or surgical procedures are opposed, except for abortion on demand.
Seventh-Day Adventist	*Holy Communion:* Although this is not required of hospitalized clients, the clergy are notified if the client desires. *Anointing of the sick:* The clergy are contacted for prayer and anointing with oil. *Dietary habits:* Because the body is viewed as the temple of the Holy Spirit, healthy living is essential. Therefore, the use of alcohol, tobacco, coffee, and tea and the promiscuous use of drugs are prohibited. Some are vegetarians, and most avoid pork. *Special days:* The Sabbath is observed on Saturday. *Death:* No special procedures. *Other related practices:* Use of hypnotism is opposed by some. Persons of homosexual or lesbian orientation are ministered to in the hope of correction of these practices, which are believed to be wrong. A Bible should always be available for Scripture reading.
United Church of Christ	*Holy Communion:* Clergy are notified if the client desires to receive this sacrament. *Death:* If the client desires counsel or prayer, notify the clergy.
Other	
Christian Science	*Dietary habits:* Because alcohol and tobacco are considered drugs, they are not used. Coffee and tea are often declined. *Death:* Autopsy is usually declined unless required by law. Donation of organs is unlikely, but is an individual decision. *Other practices:* Do not normally seek medical care, because they approach health care in a different, primarily spiritual, framework. They commonly utilize the services of a surgeon to set a bone but decline drugs and, in general, other medical or surgical procedures. Hypnotism and psychotherapy are also declined. Family planning is left to the family. They seek exemption from vaccinations but obey legal requirements (e.g., report infectious diseases and obey public health quarantines). Nonmedical care facilities are maintained for those needing nursing assistance in the course of a healing. *The Christian Science Journal* lists available Christian Science nurses. When a Christian Science believer is in the hospital, the nurse should allow and encourage time for prayer and study. Clients may request that a Christian Science practitioner be notified to come.
Jehovah's Witnesses	*Dietary habits:* Use of alcohol and tobacco is discouraged, because these harm the physical body. *Death:* Autopsy is a private matter to be decided by the persons involved. Burial and cremation are acceptable. *Birth control and abortion:* Use of birth control is a personal decision. Abortion is opposed based on Exodus 21:22–23. *Organ transplants:* Use of organ transplant is a private decision and if used must be cleansed with a nonblood solution. *Blood transfusions:* Blood transfusions violate God's laws and are therefore not allowed. Clients do respect physicians and will accept alternatives to blood transfusions. These might include use of nonblood plasma expanders, careful surgical techniques to decrease blood loss, use of autologous transfusions, and autotransfusion through use of a heart-lung machine. Nurses should check unconscious patients for medic alert cards that state that the person does not want a transfusion. Since Jehovah's Witnesses are prepared to die rather than break God's law, nurses need to be sensitive to the spiritual as well as the physical needs of the client.
The Church of Jesus Christ of Latter-Day Saints	*Holy Communion:* A hospitalized client may desire to have a member of the church priesthood administer this sacrament. *Anointing of the sick:* Mormons frequently are anointed and given a blessing before going to the hospital and after admission by laying on of hands. *Dietary habits:* Abstinence from the use of tobacco; beverages with caffeine such as cola, coffee, and tea; alcohol and other substances considered

Table continued on following page

TABLE 6-2. Religious Beliefs and Practices Affecting Health Care Continued

Religious Group	Beliefs and Practices
	injurious. Mormons eat meat but encourage the intake of fruits, grains, and herbs.
	Death: Prefer burial of the body. A church elder should be notified to assist the family. If need be, the elder will assist the funeral director in dressing the body in special clothes and will give other help as needed.
	Birth control and abortion: Abortion is opposed except when the life of the mother is in danger. Only natural means of birth control are recommended. Artificial means can be used when the health of the woman is at stake (including emotional health).
	Personal care: Cleanliness is very important to Mormons. A sacred undergarment may be worn at all times by Mormons and should only be removed in emergency situations.
	Other practices: Allowing quiet time for prayer and the reading of the sacred writings is important. The church maintains a welfare system to assist those in need. Families are of great importance, so visiting should be encouraged.
Unitarian Universalist Association	*Death:* Cremation is often preferred to burial.
	Other practices: Use of birth control is advocated as part of responsible parenting. Strong support for a woman's right to choice regarding abortion is maintained. Unitarian Universalists advocate donation of body parts for research and transplants.
Unification Church	*Baptism:* No baptism.
	Special days: Sunday mornings are used to honor Reverend and Mrs. Moon as the true parents, and members get up at 5:00 A.M., bow before a picture of the Moons three times, and vow to do what is needed to help the Reverend accomplish his mission on earth.
	Death: Believe that after death one's place of destiny will depend on his or her spirit's quality of life and goodness while on earth. In the afterlife, one will have the same aspirations and feelings as before death. Hell is not a concern, because it will not be a place as heaven grows in size. Persons who leave the Unification Church are warned that Satan may try to possess them.
	Other practices: All marriages must be solemnized by Reverend Moon in order to be part of the perfect family and have salvation. The church supplies its faithful members with life's necessities. Members may use occult practices to have spiritual and psychic experiences.
Islam	*Dietary habits:* No pork is allowed, nor alcoholic beverages. All halal (permissible) meat must be blessed and killed in a special way. This is called zabihah (correctly slaughtered).
	Death: Prior to death, family members ask to be present so that they can read the Koran and pray with the client. An Imam may come if requested by the client or family but is not required. Clients must face Mecca and confess their sins and beg forgiveness in the presence of their family. If the family is unavailable, any practicing Muslim can provide support to the client. After death, Muslims prefer that the family wash, prepare, and place the body in a position facing Mecca. If necessary, the health care providers may perform these procedures as long as they wear gloves. Burial is performed as soon as possible. Cremation is forbidden. Autopsy is also prohibited except for legal reasons, and then no body part is to be removed. Donation of body parts or organs is not allowed, because according to culturally developed law persons do not own their body.
	Abortion and birth control: Abortion is forbidden, and many conservative Muslims do not encourage the use of contraceptives because this interferes with God's purpose. Others feel that a woman should only have as many children as her husband can afford. Contraception is permitted by Islamic law.
	Personal devotions: At prayer time, washing is required, even by those who are sick. A client on bed rest may require assistance with this task before prayer. Provision of privacy is important during prayer.
	Religious objects: The Koran must not be touched by anyone ritually unclean, and nothing should be placed on top of it. Some Muslims wear taviz, a black

TABLE 6-2. Religious Beliefs and Practices Affecting Health Care Continued

Religious Group	Beliefs and Practices
	string on which words of the Koran are attached. These should not be removed and must remain dry. Certain items of jewelry such as bangles may have religious significance and should not be removed unnecessarily.
	Care of women: Because women are not allowed to sign consent forms or make a decision regarding family planning, the husband needs to be present. Women are very modest and frequently wear clothes that cover all of the body. During a medical examination, the woman's modesty should be respected as much as possible. Muslim women prefer female doctors. For 40 days after giving birth and also during menstruation, a woman is exempt from prayer because this is a time of cleansing for her.
American Muslim Mission	*Dietary habits:* In addition to refusing pork, many will not eat traditional black American foods such as corn bread and collard greens.
	Death: The family is contacted before any care of the deceased is performed. There are special procedures for washing and shrouding the body.
	Other practices: Quiet time is necessary to permit prayer. Members are encouraged to use black physicians for health care. Because these clients do not smoke their request for a nonsmoking roommate should be honored.
EASTERN RELIGIONS	
Hinduism	*Dietary Habits:* Some sects are vegetarian, believing meats and intoxicants to be too stimulating to the senses.
	Belief About Illness: View illnesses as a result of misuse of the body or a consequence of sins committed in a previous life. They do not oppose medical treatment, but view its effect as transitory. Believe that praying for health is the lowest form of prayer.
	Death: See death as a union with Brahman (God) achieved through prayers, ritual, purity, self-control, detachment, truth, nonviolence, charity, and compassion toward all creatures. Following death, one will be reborn (reincarnated) into a future life based on the behavior in this life. The record of behavior is called karma. Eventually, the process of rebirth stops which is called moksha. A priest may be called at the time of death, and may tie a thread around neck or waist as a blessing. The family washes the body, and it is cremated.
	Other practices: Offer daily worship at a shrine in the home. Daily offering to god, and morning and evening rites. Society is organized into castes, or strata. People are born into a caste, and the caste shapes one's entire life. Hindus practice a discipline of the mind and body, called yoga, to reach god. In the highest state, a meditating yogi does not see, hear, taste, feel or smell. Beyond good and evil, time and space, he is one with god.
Buddhism	*Death:* Believe that salvation depends on one's own right living. Believe in reincarnation. Can speed the process toward Nirvana, the goal of all humanity's striving, through acts of merit. Meditation, worship, and prayer are some of the acts of merit. Buddhists may drive themselves into more and more ritual or contemplation in the hope that their last moments of consciousness may be filled with thoughts worthy enough to elevate them to a higher existence. Last rights of chanting may be performed at bedside.
	Renunciation: The most important Buddhist feasts. Young boys are taught to despise the world's vanity and the boy spends a night in a nearby monastery.
Taoism/Confucianism	*General beliefs:* Founded on ethical principles of Confucius. God is not clearly defined as in other religions. Taoism is a mixture of magic and religion. Believe that humans and nature are inseparable, and that if heaven is upset, earth does not prosper. This relationship is described as yang and yin, which are two interplaying forces. When yang and yin are in balance, good occurs.
	Death: The dead are remembered in all festivals. The fate of the dead in the afterworld depends not only on the life they led but also on being properly honored after death. Otherwise they may become demons. Graves are mounds like those dedicated to the gifts of the soil. Graves and houses must be in harmony with the universe, otherwise evil will befall the occupants.

Modified from Carson, V. B. (1989). *Spiritual dimensions of nursing practice.* Philadelphia: W. B. Saunders.

Summary

There is a renaissance in recognizing and attending to clients' spiritual needs. Nurses are in a position to restore balance to the recently dominated technical-physical realm of nursing care. In the words of Plato: "As you ought not to attempt to cure the eyes without the head, or the head without the body, so neither ought you to attempt to cure the body without the soul . . . for the part can never be well unless the whole is well."

Bibliography

1. American Holistic Nurses' Association. (1986). *Standards for holistic nursing care.* Raleigh, North Carolina: American Holistic Nurses' Association.
2. Borysenko, J. (1987). *Minding the body, mending the mind.* New York: Bantam.
3. Carson, V. (1989). *Spiritual dimensions of nursing practice.* Philadelphia: W. B. Saunders.
4. Copp, L. (1990). The spectrum of suffering. *American Journal of Nursing, 90*(8), 35–39.
5. Cowles, K., & Rodgers, B. (1991). The concept of grief: A foundation for nursing research and practice. *Research in Nursing and Health, 14*(2), 119–127.
6. Dennis, P. (1991). Components of spiritual nursing care from the nurses' perspective. *Journal of Holistic Nursing, 9*(1), 27–42.
7. Dossey, B. (1991). Awaking the inner healer. *American Journal of Nursing, 91*(8), 31–33.
8. Dossey, B. (1989). Forward. *Journal of Holistic Nursing, 3*(3), vii.
9. Dossey, L. (1990). *Recovering the soul.* New York: Bantam.
10. Ferszt, G., & Taylor, P. (1988). When your patient needs spiritual comfort. *Nursing '88, 18*(4), 48–49.
11. Groer, M. (1991). Psychoneuroimmunology. *American Journal of Nursing, 91*(8), 33.
12. Harman, W. (1987). Further comments on . . . an extended science. *Noetic Sciences Review, 4,* 22–25.
13. Jowett, B. (1937). Charmides. In *The dialogue of Plato.* New York: Random House.
14. Keegan, G., & Keegan, L. (1987). Spirituality and the technological crisis. *Healing Currents, 11*(2).
15. Kennison, M. M. (1987). Faith: An untapped health resource. *Journal of Psychosocial Nursing, 25*(10), 28–33.
16. Kubler-Ross, E. (1969). *On death and dying.* New York: Macmillan Publishing Co., Inc.
17. Nagai-Jacobson, M., & Burkhardt, M. (1989). Spirituality: Cornerstone of holistic nursing practice. *Holistic Nursing Practice, 3*(3), 18–26.
18. Newman, M. (1989). The spirit of nursing. *Holistic Nursing Practice, 3*(3), 6.
19. North American Nursing Diagnosis Association. (1989). *Taxonomy I revised - 1989.* St. Louis: North American Nursing Diagnosis Association.
20. Peel, R. (1987). *Spiritual healing in a scientific age.* San Francisco: Harper & Row.
21. Peterson, E., & Nelson, K. (1987). How to meet your client's spiritual need. *Journal of Psychosocial Nursing, 25*(5), 34–39.
22. Peterson, E. A. (1985). The physical . . . the spiritual . . . can you meet all of your patient's needs? *Journal of Gerontological Nursing, 11*(10), 23–27.
23. Reed, P. G. (1986). Religiousness among terminally ill and healthy adults. *Research in Nursing and Health, 9,* 35–42.
24. Reed, P. G. (1987). Spirituality and well-being in terminally ill and hospitalized adults. *Research in Nursing and Health, 10,* 335–344.
25. Rogers, M. (1970). *An introduction to the theoretical basis of nursing.* Philadelphia: F. A. Davis.
26. Shaffer, J. (1991) Spiritual distress and critical illness. *Critical Care Nurse, 11*(1), 42–45.
27. Schunior, C. (1989). Nursing and the comic mask. *Holistic Nursing Practice, 3*(3), 16.
28. Shelly, J., & Fish, S. (1988). *Spiritual care* (3rd ed.). Downers Grove, IL: Intervarsity Press.
29. Sims, C. (1987). Spiritual care as a part of holistic nursing. *Imprint, 34*(6), 63–65.
30. Travelbee, J. (1971). *Interpersonal aspects of nursing.* Philadelphia: F. A. Davis.
31. Watson, J. (1985). *Nursing: The philosophy and science of caring.* Denver, CO: Association University Press.
32. Watson, M. J. (1988). New dimensions of human caring theory. *Nursing Science Quarterly, 1*(4), 175–181.

Chapter 7

Human Sexuality

Whether a client is male or female influences the nurse-client relationship. Although nurses are becoming more knowledgeable and comfortable with the topic of sexuality, it remains a topic that continually needs to be discussed in order to provide new information and to correct misinformation. This chapter provides an overview of human sexuality from a bio-psycho-sociocultural framework.

DEFINITION OF SEXUALITY

Because people were created as male and female, human sexuality is an intrinsic part of being human. Various definitions of sexuality exist. It has been described as the quality of being human,[9] the most intimate feelings of the human heart,[5] the totality of the human being,[10] and the ongoing process of recognizing, accepting and expressing oneself as a sexual being.[18] Therefore, the term sexuality represents a much broader concept than the word sex, which represents the physiologic act of sexual intercourse. Sexuality is a deep pervasive aspect of the total human personality and is present in some degree from birth to death.[8]

ELEMENTS OF SEXUALITY

In all biologic, psychological, sociologic and cultural arenas, sexuality involves both the self and other individuals. Sexuality is an ongoing process that changes with aging, acquisition of new roles in life, and interaction with other persons and the environment. Sexuality must be viewed within the context of one's whole life. It is important to view sexuality as multidimensional, because it embodies what we are and what we do.

Biologic Elements

EARLY DEVELOPMENT

Biologic differences between male and female are determined at conception. The female fetus has two X chromosomes, one from each parent. The male fetus has an X and Y chromosome, the X from the mother and the Y chromosome from the father. Initially, there is no outward difference in the appearance of the fetus. At about 7 weeks after conception, the male sexual organs begin to develop under the influence of the sex hormone, testosterone. At the same time, the female sexual organs develop due to a lack of testosterone, not due to the presence of estrogen.

Later during puberty, the hormones again assist to bring the female or male to full development. Females begin menstruation and develop secondary sex characteristics. Males begin to develop sperm and also secondary sexual characteristics.

ADULT SEXUAL RESPONSE

The adult has sexual intercourse for both pleasure and procreation. He or she has normally incorporated a firm gender identity and gender role. The structure and function of adult sexual organs are discussed in Chapter 73.

TABLE 7–1. Changes in Sexuality with Aging

	Men	Women
Middle-aged adult	Prolonged erection Decreased premature ejaculation Greater emphasis on touch Fertility intact Sexual arousal may diminish usually due to stress or illness Some men develop increased prostatic size	Cessation of menses, fertility varies Thinning of vaginal mucosa Sexual arousal peaks due to effects of androgens May be a fear of pregnancy
Older-aged adult	Decrease in size of penis and testes Increased refractory time after orgasm Decreased penile sensation Decreased force of ejaculation Slowed arousal Fertility varies Interferences due to the side effects of medications and illness	Loss of vaginal lubrication, decreased fat pad over the symphysis pubis, and friable mucosa due to loss of estrogen Infertile Interferences due to the side effects of medications and illness

MENOPAUSE

By definition, menopause is the last menstrual period and represents the end of the female reproductive ability. The term climacteric is the preferred term because it describes a process of decreasing production of estrogen by the ovaries, a change in the lining of the uterus, and a reduction in size of the vagina and clitoris.

AGING AND SEXUALITY

Sexuality is not related to age. In fact, just the opposite is true. People have a need for intimacy and touch throughout life. The ability to have sexual intercourse does not end at menopause. There are often some physical changes that occur with aging, and these changes may have an impact on sexual intercourse (Table 7–1).

Psychologic Elements

GENDER IDENTITY

Gender identity is the individual's sense of being male or female, and describes one's internal sense of masculinity or femininity. Gender role is a part of a person's identity.

Society has a substantial role in the development of gender identity. As soon as an infant is born, he or she is labeled as a boy or girl and given certain toys and certain colors of clothing. Likewise, adults respond to female and male children differently depending on their upbringing and personal parenting style. For example, it would be nontraditional for girls to be given trucks and cars to play with. Likewise it would be nontraditional for boys to have lace lining on their bluejeans.

As children grow, they encompass the information from society and their own knowledge of their bodies to develop their own sense of gender identity. By the age of 3 years, children know themselves as boys or girls. They also know that they cannot change their sex by changing their outward appearance with clothing or make-up.

GENDER ROLE

Gender role is the public expression of gender identity. Most social theorists believe that social influence (parents, peers, media) is the major developmental force in teaching or shaping gender roles. Gender roles are learned in school and at home. Formal learning typically includes specific information about the sexual organs, changes in the body with puberty, and the need to delay sexual intercourse until "one is old enough to be in love." The most influential learning comes from the sexual value system of the family and community. Children acquire these attitudes at an early age. Often, the pattern involves repression and avoidance of sexual topics and so sexuality may be perceived as a negative experience. Another influential source of learning includes the gestures, cues, and discussion that take place within the peer group.

All gender role behavior cannot be fully attributed to society, however, since there is a difference in the behavior of boys and girls even at an early age. It has been suggested that the sex hormones have an influence on the brain, which also influences behavior.[11] Gender role is one area of sexuality that overlaps to include psychological, biologic, and sociocultural components.

SEXUAL ORIENTATION

Sexual orientation is the preference for intimate relationships with a person of the opposite sex or the same sex. The vast majority of adults identify themselves as heterosexual, that is, having a clear, sustained, and erotic desire for a person of the opposite sex. About 10 per cent of adults define themselves as homosexual, that is, having similar desires for a person of the same sex. Men who desire intimate relationships with men are called homosexuals, or gay, and women who desire intimate relationships with women are called lesbians.

A very small number of people are bisexual, that is, they prefer intimate relationships with both sexes. Transsexual people (transvestites) are dissatisfied with their physical body because it does not match their feelings of gender identity. They often feel that they are really trapped in the wrong body.

Over the years, society has intermingled homosexuality and transvestism; however, they are not the same phenomenon. It is a common misconception that lesbians are women who want to be men, and gays are men who want to be women. Some gay men do have effeminate behaviors, and some lesbians have masculine behaviors. But most homosexual men and women are satisfied with their male or female gender.

Sociocultural Elements

Sociocultural components reflect the beliefs of a culture or society. These beliefs shape the development of a person as a sexual being. Social interaction is important to this process because role behaviors are modeled and social expectations learned. Religious and legal systems attempt to control or prescribe sexuality.[8] Sociocultural components also influence male and female sexuality and gender role behavior.

MALE AND FEMALE ROLES

Culture influences gender roles. Some cultures have clear distinctions of the appropriate roles for males and females. For example, the male role may be one of providing money to support the family (breadwinner) and the female role may be one of rearing children and caring for the household. Other cultures do not hold such sharp distinctions.

The Women's Liberation Movement of the 1970s has changed many gender role behaviors in North America. It is now more common for women to work outside the home, and it is becoming more acceptable for men to stay home to care for children. This role reversal is not without conflict, however. Many women and men have a difficult time switching roles. Women report feelings of overwork when trying to balance home, family, and work responsibilities. Likewise, some men appreciate having social approval to be more involved with child care; the others resent the extra demands.

Feminism is a belief pattern about the role of women that challenges the conventional ideas about gender. Feminism is not a new concept that began in the 1980s; the ideas of feminism have been thought and expressed for over 300 years.[17] Regardless of the time frame from which feminist thought was established, it has consistently turned the spotlight on a complex system of inequality for women in present society. Areas that have been explored include disadvantages in the workplace, including reduced pay for equal job responsibility; corporate ladder "glass ceilings," which have prevented women from being promoted to the top levels of management; exploitation as housewives and brutality as sexual objects; exclusion from political life; discrimination in areas such as religion, education, and athletics; and general silence in history about the accomplishments of women.[13, 17] Feminists have pushed society to obliterate sexism by legalizing changes to equalize economic disadvantages and produce equal political and educational opportunities.

SEXUAL PRACTICES

Social attitudes range from the nontraditional view of sex, which holds that each person must make an individual choice of appropriate behavior, to a traditional view, which holds that sex must occur only after marriage. The risk of acquiring a sexually transmitted disease or becoming pregnant, as well as religious beliefs, may also influence a person's decisions about sexual practices. When a person acts outside of the socially prescribed behaviors by having sex, acquiring sexually transmitted diseases, or becoming pregnant, there is often much guilt and internal conflict over the behavior. Nurses may frequently work with these clients and need to be able to put aside personal views and beliefs in order to assist the client. If the nurse has religious beliefs that prohibit involvement with certain clients, such as assisting in surgery during an abortion, the nurse should make these personal issues known to the nursing administrator.

Because gender identity, gender behavior, and sexuality norms differ from culture to culture and have changed over the years, it must be understood that the norms themselves are not what is important. It is more critical that the norms are understood and accepted by the persons in that culture or society. It is equally important that health care professionals work within the social norms and help clients without judging them against personal norms.

PSYCHOSOCIAL DEVELOPMENT OF MEN AND WOMEN

Erikson's Model of Male Development

Most studies of human development include Erik Erikson's childhood developmental stages. Erikson charted eight stages of life that were described as maturational crises of development.[7] The model is like a ladder, in which each step must be taken in order to ascend the ladder. If the stage is not passed through successfully, persistent problems develop. Likewise, even though a person passes through a stage, the stage is often revisited when new experiences (such as illness and hospitalization) uproot the progression. In 1978, Levinson also described male development and noted the presence of crisis periods, such as mid-life crisis.[14] During mid-life crisis, men consider their own mortality and begin to see how building on others, rather than standing alone, is a way to reach beyond the ability of the self and accomplish more in a lifetime. The combination of Erikson's and Levinson's models is shown in Figure 7–1.

Boyce's Model of Female Development

Female development is best explained through a separate model. Women are more concerned with emotions and feelings that occur in the course of activity.[4] Out of these feelings, women have come to realize that events are important to them only if there is a sense of attachment and affiliation with others. Many developmental psychologists describe the development of women as framed in a context of commitments made to others at various levels—to care for younger children, to manage the home, and to be responsible and dependable in relationships. A revised model to show the complexities of female development has been developed by Boyce (Fig. 7–2).

The model is framed by two arrows, which represent the context of commitment in which females develop. These commitments increase during the course of a woman's life. The longer arrows stemming from the bottom of the model represent generativity (a concern for future generations). Women sense a need for generativity from childhood on, and express these concerns through childrearing practices. In contrast, men sometimes do not see generativity as a concern until late in adulthood, when they ask what can they leave for the next generation. In contrast to the sharp steps of Erikson's model, the female model shows the developmental crises to be overlapping and circular. This structure shows that women can focus on more than one crisis at a time and become quite adept at juggling multiple issues. Overlapping circles represent periods of transition.

Women and men have a similar pattern of development in early childhood, which is based on developing a sense of trust and independence, represented by the three circles at the bottom of the model.

The first set of industry, identity, and intimacy circles represent the crisis about age 20, when the woman decides about a life choice of career, marriage, family or some combination of the three alternatives. These same issues reappear at age 30, when previous decisions are reexamined as the biologic clock is ticking away and shortening the time for childbearing.

The last circle is the crisis for integrity, and it occurs in middle adulthood. During this phase, issues about purpose and personal integration appear. Women deal with this issue sooner than men do, because typically

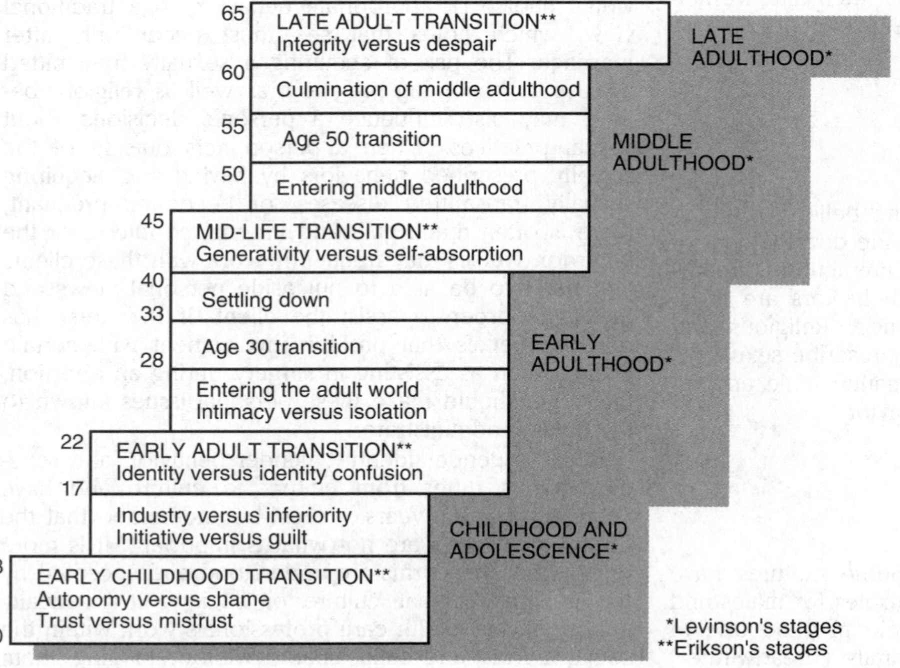

▲ *Figure 7–1*

Interrelationship of Erikson's and Levinson's models of male development. (From Boyce, M. [1985]. Female psychosocial development: A model and implications for counselors and educators. *Counseling and Human Development, 17*(6), 2. Reprinted by permission of Love Publishing Company, Denver, CO.)

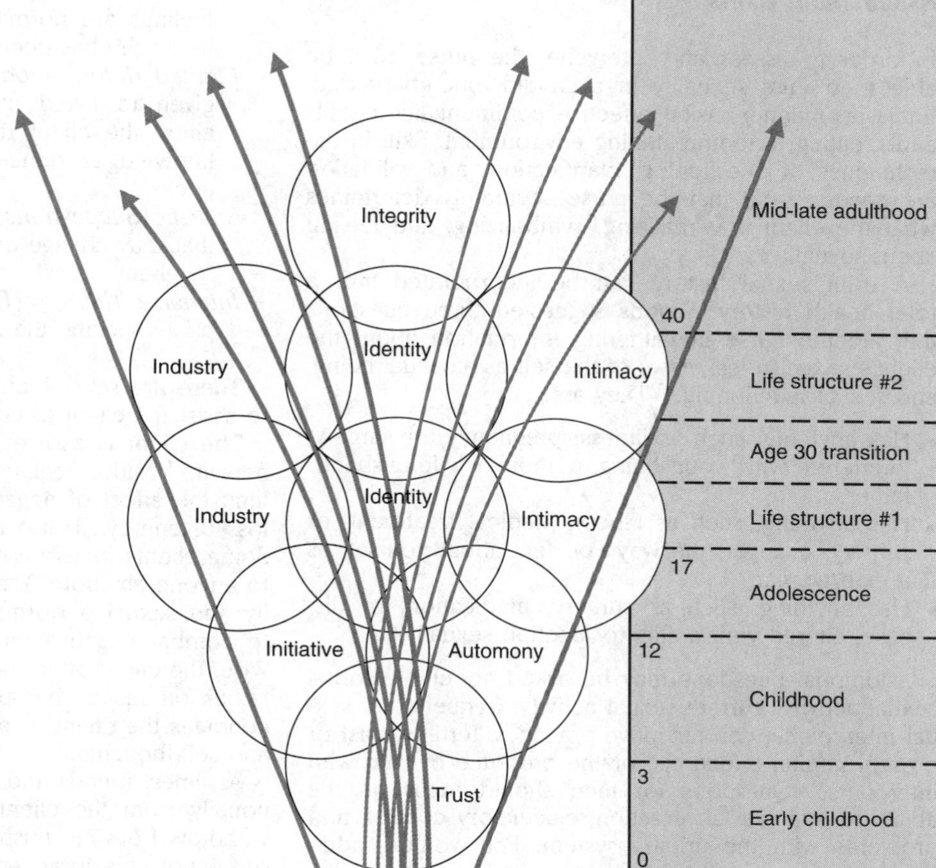

▲ *Figure 7–2*

A model of female psychosocial development. See text for discussion. (From Boyce, M. [1985]. Female psychosocial development: A model and implications for counselors and educators. *Counseling and Human Development, 17*(6), 10. Reprinted by permission of Love Publishing Company, Denver, CO.)

children leave home, the period for conception is ending, and perhaps a long-delayed career can begin.

THE NURSE'S ROLE IN PROMOTING SEXUAL HEALTH

The World Health Organization (WHO) developed the following definition of sexual health: "Sexual health is the integration of the somatic, emotional, intellectual, and social aspects of sexual beings in ways that are positively enriching and that enhance personality, communication, and love."[20] In other words, sexual health is the physical and emotional state of well-being that enables us to enjoy and act on sexual feelings.[3] These definitions provide a basis for delivery of nursing care.

Nurses care for the whole person as they assess and treat human responses to actual and potential health problems. Because sexuality is a quality of being human, the sexual aspects of clients should be addressed. Nurses knowledgeable about and comfortable with the topic of sexuality and comfortable with their own sexuality have the opportunity to promote sexual health. All nurses can integrate sexuality into client care by focusing on preventive, therapeutic, and educational interventions that help attain and maintain sexual health.

The nurse needs to be competent in four areas in order to promote sexual health. Those areas are (1) knowledge of subject matter related to sexuality; (2) skill in assessing and intervening with the client and family; (3) personal awareness of beliefs, attitudes, and values; and (4) awareness of how personal beliefs, attitudes, and values affect delivery of care to clients.[10]

Competency in these four areas involves three levels of learning. First, the nurse must overcome any sexual embarrassment which can be done by talking with other nurses, taking human sexuality courses, or through values clarification exercises.[8] Second, the nurse must be able to identify and understand sexuality problems. Third, the nurse is able to assist clients in dealing with sexual problems.

Knowledge Base

Because the subject of sexuality is complex, basic knowledge about human relationships, sexual development, reproduction, sexual expression, sexual dysfunction and disease, and sociocultural aspects of sex, marriage, and the family is needed.[10] Knowledge of moral, legal, and religious issues related to sexuality is also important.

Assessment Skills

In order to assess and intervene, the nurse must be able to discuss sexuality in a candid, unembarrassed, unbiased manner, using effective communication skills and creating a nonthreatening environment. Skill in the techniques of questioning, clarification, and validation are necessary so that the nurse accurately determines what the client is verbalizing, symbolizing, and feeling about sexuality.

A brief sexual history can be incorporated into a total health history. Woods suggested three questions that aid the nurse in gathering information about the client's sexual roles, views of the self as a sexual being, and sexual functioning.[19] They are:

- Has anything, such as illness, pregnancy, or surgery, interfered with your being a mother/wife/husband/father?
- Has anything, such as illness, medical treatment, or surgery, changed the way you feel about yourself as a man/woman?
- Has anything, such as surgery, medication, or disease, altered your ability to function sexually?

Additional questions may be asked about premarital sexual activity, current sexual activity, frequency of sexual intercourse, contraceptive practices, fertility, past or present genital infections, or the presence of pain with intercourse. Questions for men should focus on the ability to maintain an erection, ejaculatory control, and problems with the urinary system. For women, additional questions might relate to arousal and the ability to reach orgasm, menstrual history, obstetric history, or menopause if the client is beyond childbearing years. The nurse may conclude the interview by asking whether there are any questions or problems the client wishes to discuss with the nurse.

Intervention Skills

Once the problem is identified, the nurse must be able to offer the client help in an understanding, reassuring manner. The nurse creates an environment that supports sexual health by minimizing guilt and anxiety. Interventions may take the form of sex education, anticipatory guidance, or counseling. The intervention may involve initiating a referral for the client with a complex problem, offering suggestions for the problem, or simply listening to the client and offering reassurance. The nurse's goal is to facilitate the client's sexual adaptation to enhance or maintain health. Specific interventions that relate to specific disorders, such as mutilating surgery, cancer, and neurologic and musculoskeletal problems, are discussed in other chapters.

Annon developed the PLISSIT Model for Sexual Health Interventions.[2] The model is based on principles of learning theory and uses a behavioral approach to treatment of sexual problems. The model contains four levels: (1) *p*ermission, (2) *l*imited *i*nformation, (3) specific *s*uggestions, and (4) *i*ntensive *t*herapy. The model is clarified further in the following list:

Permission (P): Provides reassurance that sexual feelings are normal. Permission to continue what he or she has been feeling.

Limited Information (LI): Limited information is given to avoid overwhelming the client and to allow the client to ask questions. The nurse acknowledges concerns that are common experiences.

Specific Suggestions (SS): Suggestions are offered that may change or add to sexual approaches used by client.

Intensive Therapy (IT): Client is referred to appropriate specific therapy from trained professionals.

There are several other interventions the nurse uses to assist the client to cope with sexual concerns.

The client is assisted to feel good about himself or herself. Positive feelings and a positive image of self limit the effect of negative self-talk on self esteem and loss of energy. It also improves a sense of well being. Some clients focus on negative thoughts ("I'm no good to anyone anymore"), especially in the areas of sexuality and sexual performance. These clients are assisted to combat negative thoughts with positive ones. Likewise, the client often focuses on the loss of a body part rather on his or her positive features. The nurse encourages the client to develop a list of positive feelings and self-thoughts.

At times, friends and family members withdraw emotionally from the client. For example, a woman may withdraw from her husband following a stroke, because she is not able to accept his paralysis or aphasia. Actually, she often is expressing deeper feelings. Perhaps she is angry that she has to assume all of his responsibilities in the home, such as paying bills. Or his illness may remind her of the loss she would feel if he died, so she feels safer not gettting close. The husband realizes his wife's reactions; he, in turn, internalizes a negative self-image. The nurse encourages the client and spouse to discuss these feelings with the team of health care providers or with each other.

Coping with outward effects of treatment, such as alopecia (hair loss), weight loss, and loss of muscle mass during chemotherapy, requires some disguise. Wigs can cover hair loss, and wearing clothes that fit well will disguise weight loss. Infusion catheters can be hidden by clothing with high necks or long sleeves.

The nurse encourages the client to resume sexual activity slowly and not to feel rushed to perform. Many clients plan for sexual intercourse at certain times of the day, when their energy level is higher. For example, the client with lung disorders may have more energy in the late morning. If one client is weak or in pain, variations in the position for intercourse are suggested. Some clients cannot have physical intercourse, but experience pleasure from caressing.

The nurse advises the clients in the treatment of specific concerns. Women may need to use vaginal lubrication to reduce pain with intercourse. Condoms or spermicides can be used to reduce the risk of sexually transmitted disease. Men may have difficulty obtaining an erection or forceful orgasm. Various devices exist to facilitate erection. There are external pneumatic pumps which draw blood into the penile shaft for erection. Men can also have penile prosthesis implanted for erection. The feelings of weakened orgasm are common, for which there is no specific treatment.

Personal Awareness of Beliefs, Attitudes, and Values

A nurse's beliefs, attitudes, and values may affect the way a nurse delivers care. Certainly, the nurse is entitled to these beliefs, values, and attitudes, but the nurse must be aware of what they are and remain objective when providing care that involves any aspect of the client's sexuality.

Assessment of personal attitudes toward sexuality involves deciding whether the attitudes are positive or negative. Self-examination may be necessary to determine the root of negative attitudes and beliefs. If negative attitudes cannot be overcome or if a nurse is uncomfortable in discussing sexuality, other nurses should be asked to care for the client so that the negative attitudes are not communicated.

Some of the topics that should be considered when evaluating feelings, attitudes, beliefs, and values include reproduction, masturbation, dating, sexual activity such as petting and orgasm, sexual intercourse in marriage, sexual intercourse outside of marriage, childbearing, contraception, sterilization, abortion, venereal disease, homosexuality, bisexuality, transsexuality, and transvestism.[12] Not only should one identify the feelings but why they might have developed as they did. There are no right or wrong answers when it comes to these topics. However, it is important that the nurse be very familiar with personal values, beliefs, and attitudes so that their effect on practice can be determined.

Effects of Beliefs, Attitudes, and Values on Delivery of Care

Once beliefs and attitudes are assessed, it is important for the nurse to determine how they might affect his or her delivery of nursing care. For instance, do the attitudes and beliefs deny, inhibit, or allow for the sexuality of the client? Becoming open, nonjudgemental and accepting of others' sexuality and developing comfort in interviewing in the area of sexuality may be a difficult task for the nurse.[10] The nurse should not attempt to help another person with sexual problems until comfort with acceptance of others' sexuality and interviewing skills is accomplished.

MALE AND FEMALE COMMUNICATION STYLES

When discussing the issues concerning sexuality with men and women clients, the nurse may notice some differences in communication style between the sexes. Men often have difficulty quickly processing their thoughts into words. Men excel in relating logic and facts rather than feelings and relationships. Although this description does not fit all men, it may be helpful to know that there is nothing wrong with a man because he cannot express his feelings freely.

In comparison women, especially extroverted women, tend to process emotional information faster and express them without being cold and rational or wildly emotional. Women may be inclined to express feelings to a fault without regard to the listener's ability to receive and process the information.[11]

The nurse needs to consider these differences when setting up counseling sessions with men, women, or men and women together. If communication is a concern, explaining these biologic differences between men's and women's ability to communicate about feelings may decrease anxiety and facilitate communication.

ILLNESS AND SEXUALITY

Perhaps most clients and many health care professionals do not think about sexual activity occurring following surgery or illness. In fact, the mass media commonly portrays sex as an act between two healthy young adults. Sex is seldom portrayed in clients who have been injured or are debilitated. This social portrayal has influenced many health care providers not to think about sexuality as a component of the whole being. Sadly, it is often ignored in planning care.

If the client is wondering whether sexual activity would interfere with treatments or be permissible after surgery, the client should ask the physician. Sadly though, many clients are uncomfortable and do not ask. Likewise, many health care professionals do not view seriously ill clients as sexual people and fail to teach the client about sexual guidelines.

Sexuality and Chronic Conditions

The client with a chronic illness that interferes with oxygenation, such as pulmonary or cardiac disorders, may not have the physical stamina to have intercourse. These clients may find intercourse possible if they plan it around periods of increased energy, such as in the middle of the day. Medications such as nitroglycerin prior to intercourse may decrease the fear of angina. Following myocardial infarction, many clients have concerns about sexual intercourse. Fear of dying during sex is common. The nurse should facilitate discussion of concerns with the client, even if the nurse has to initiate the conversation.

Diabetes and other vascular disorders interfere with blood supply to the genitals, and reduces erection and orgasm. Clients with these conditions may benefit from surgery to restore the erectile tissues (see Chap. 75). If surgery is not feasible, the client may find satisfaction through touch and caressing.

Spinal cord injury results in the lack of sensation and inability to have an erection in men. Some clients can be taught methods to enjoy physical intercourse (see Chap. 32), and others are overwhelmed by the injury and psychologically do not feel whole enough to participate. These clients and their partners may benefit from counseling.

In clients with musculoskeletal disorders, such as arthritis, contracture may be too extensive or they may have too much pain to move into positions to facilitate intercourse. These clients can often be helped by experimenting with new positions.

Clients with cancer may feel alterations in their sexuality from alopecia, loss of body mass, loss of energy, nausea and vomiting, or pain. Young clients may not be able to have a child as a result of surgery, chemotherapy, or radiation therapy. These clients should be advised about the possibility of sperm or egg banking to preserve this function.

For most clients with cancer, sexual activity is not dangerous to health. In a few situations, however, sex can be hazardous. During recovery from surgery, sexual intercourse can strain the incision or cause bleeding. Intimate contact may also increase the risk of contracting infection, especially in clients who are being treated with radiation and chemotherapy. Radiation and chemotherapy suppress the immune system.

Sexuality and Surgery

Some surgical interventions may have a profound impact on the client's sexuality. Surgery to remove organs related to sexual intercourse or reproduction, such as the uterus, ovaries, external genitalia, penis, testes, or breasts, may leave the client feeling asexual. Also, extensive lower abdominal surgery and surgery on the pelvic floor decrease erectile function and ejaculation. Prostate surgery for cancer also decreases erectile function. Newer surgical techniques are being developed that spare nerves allowing partial or complete erection. These clients need assistance to build a new self-image that does not include these body parts. This process takes months to years to develop. Sometimes, reconstructive surgery can assist to restore form and function, such as breast reconstruction (see Chap. 72). Surgery that alters the physical appearance of other body parts not so clearly associated with reproduction can also have an impact on feelings of sexuality. Surgical removal of the bowel or bladder with the creation of a new external opening on the abdominal skin commonly has an impact on sexuality.

Sexuality and Hospitalization

Anyone who has ever been hospitalized can appreciate the sense of loss of control a person feels. Equal to this loss is often a loss of the sense of wholeness, of which sexuality is a part. Consider the 90-year-old woman, who has never married and now is hospitalized. When she was young, skirts were at the ankles. Perhaps she joined the ranks of promiscuous women who showed their lower legs and knees in public! She is asked to submit to a physical examination, a bath, being only partly dressed, and perhaps being catheterized. Nurses take these activities for granted, yet this woman has never revealed her body to anyone. Although this type of client is not common, her case best exemplifies the asexual treatment many clients receive. Nurses need to be aware of a client's need for privacy and control of their bodies.

On the contrary, some clients act out their sexual frustrations by using gestures, using obscene language or pinching or touching the staff. This behavior can occur for many reasons. Perhaps the client is confused, has lost a sense of control, feels asexual, feels a need for attention, or needs to test the limits set on him or her. The nurse needs to be firm with the client and tell the client that the behavior is not acceptable and limits should be set. Psychiatric treatment may be required.

Summary

Nurses have a primary role in promoting and maintaining the sexual health of individuals and groups. The nurse can assess clients' regular sexual concerns and sexuality, accurately identify problems, and intervene effectively. The extent of the nurse's role in promoting sexual health depends on client needs and the nurse's level of preparation.

Bibliography

1. American Nurses' Association. (1983). *Standards of maternal child health nursing practice.* Kansas City, MO: American Nurses' Association.
2. Annon, J. S. (1976). The PLISSIT model: A proposed conceptual scheme for the behavioral treatment of sexual problems. *Journal of Sex Education Therapy, 2,* 1–15.
3. Boston Women's Health Book Collective. (1985). *The new our bodies, ourselves.* New York: Simon & Schuster.
4. Boyce, M. (1985). Female psychosocial development: A model and implications for counselors and educators. *Counseling and Human Development 17*(6), 1–12.
5. Brower, L. (1967). Character education: A guideline for discussion of sexual behavior. *Journal of School Health, 39*(12), 715–722.
6. Chenitz, W. C., et al. (1991). *Clinical gerontological nursing.* Philadelphia: W. B. Saunders.
7. Erikson, E. (1968). *Identity: Youth and crisis.* New York: W. W. Norton.
8. Fogel, C., & Lauver, D. (1990). *Sexual health promotion.* Philadelphia: W. B. Saunders.
9. Fonesca, J. D. (1970). Sexuality—a quality of being human. *Nursing Outlook, 18*(11), 25.
10. Hogan, R. (1985). *Human sexuality* (2nd ed.). Norwalk, CT: Appleton-Century-Crofts.
11. Johnson, R. & Brock, D. (1988). Gender specific therapy. *Journal of Psychology and Christianity, 7*(4), 50–61.
12. Kempton, W. (1974). *A teacher's guide to sex education.* North Scituate, MA: Duxbury Press.
13. Lengermann, P. & Wallace, R. (1985). *Gender in America: Social control and social change.* Englewood Cliffs, NJ: Prentice-Hall.
14. Levinson, D. J. (1978). *The seasons of a man's life.* New York: Ballantine Books.

15. Mason, D. J., Backer, B. & Georges, C. A. (1991). Toward a feminist model for the political empowerment of nurses. *IMAGE: The Journal of Nursing Scholarship, 23*(2), 72–77.
16. Miller, J. B. (1976). *Toward a new psychology of women*. Boston: Beacon Press.
17. Sampselle, C. (1990). The influence of feminist philosophy on nursing practice. *IMAGE: The Journal of Nursing Scholarship, 22*(4), 243–247.
18. Shippee, R. (1979). *Touching and pleasuring behaviors in a well elderly population*. Master's thesis. Rochester, NY: University of Rochester.
19. Woods, N. F. (1984). *Human sexuality in health and illness* (3rd ed.). St. Louis: C. V. Mosby.
20. World Health Organization. (1975). *Education and treatment in human sexuality: The training of health professionals* (Report of a WHO meeting, Technical Report Series, No. 572).

Chapter 8

The Family

Nothing happens in isolation. System theory suggests that change in one part of a system may lead to change throughout the system. Application of this concept to the family system makes it apparent that whenever illness strikes one family member, all family members will be affected in some way. Depending on the circumstances, families may be required to make minor adaptations or completely reorganize their way of living.

The manner in which families respond to changes imposed by illness is related to the nature of the illness, the timing of the illness relative to individual or family developmental stages, and the functional level of the family. When families are successful in their adaptation to changes imposed by illness, there may be a buffering effect that diminishes the perceived severity of the disease and supports the ill member in coping with lifestyle changes and treatment restrictions. On the other hand, when families are unable to adapt, there may be role confusion, conflict, and feelings of isolation that significantly compromise supportive efforts.

THE FAMILY AS A CONCEPTUAL FRAMEWORK

The contemporary American family system should be viewed as a semi-closed system that is interactive and interdependent with changing social, economic, political, and cultural systems. Because of changes in systems outside the family, families are always facing significant threats to their survival as well as opportunities for growth. Analysis of the various changes influencing an individual family allows greater likelihood for understanding and supporting the unique strengths or weaknesses of a given family.

MAJOR CHANGES AFFECTING THE AMERICAN FAMILY

Change is evident today in the wide range of alternatives available to American families regarding lifestyle choices. In general, these changes can be inferred from statistical trends provided by the United States Census Bureau regarding life expectancy, changes in marriage, birth, and divorce rates, and changes in living arrangements.

Life Expectancy

The average life expectancy, which rose from 69.7 years in 1960 to 75.0 years in 1987, is projected to increase to 77.9 years in 2010. The proportion of the United States population over the age of 65 has increased, and this trend is predicted to continue. Between 1960 and 1987, the percentage of the population over the age of 65 increased from 9 to 12.2 per cent. Furthermore, by the year 2030, it is projected that the elderly will account for 22 per cent of the total population.

Marriage

The number of marriages has decreased from 11.1 (per 1000 population) in 1950 to 9.9 (per 1000 population) in 1986. The age of spouses at the time of first marriage has increased. For women, the median age at first marriage has increased from 20.6 years in 1970 to 23.3 years in 1986. During the same period, the increase for men has been from 22.5 years to 25.1 years.

Evidence of a change in traditional attitudes toward marriage also may be inferred from the increasing proportion of adults choosing to remain single. In 1970, 16.2 per cent of adults in the United States were single; in 1988, that percentage had increased to 21.9 per cent.

Divorce

Nearly half of all marriages eventually end in divorce; the median duration of a marriage is less than 7 years. The annual divorce rate almost doubled between 1950 (2.6 divorces per 1000 population) and 1988 (4.8 divorces per 1000 population). Consequently, the number of divorced people in the United States has increased from 4.3 million in 1970 to 13.9 million in 1988.

Birth

The birth rate (per 1000 women) in the United States has declined almost 55 per cent, from 118 in 1950 to 65.7 in 1987.

Living Arrangements

The proportion of American families composed of a legally married couple has declined from 75 per cent of the population in 1960 to 55 per cent in 1988. During the period between 1970 and 1988, the number of unmarried couples of the opposite sex sharing the same household increased 63 per cent.

Changes in the American family are seen also in the increasing proportion of single-parent families, most of which are headed by a female. In 1986, one of every five children in the United States lived in a single-parent home; this represents a twofold increase in the number of single-parent families since 1970.

In 1988, there were 10.8 million single-parent families headed by a female and 2.8 million headed by a male. The median family income of single-parent families headed by women was $15,346, whereas it was $26,827 in single-parent families headed by men.

PURPOSE OF THE FAMILY

Many authors have noted that as society changes, so do the structures and functions of the family. Although some see these changes as evidence of regression of the family system, others suggest that families have an incredible stability and flexibility that allows its basic purpose to persist. Friedman[10] states that the main purpose of the family is to mediate the needs of its individual members with that of society's needs. Satir[20] considers a family's purpose to be a "people-making factory" that nurtures its individual members and links them with society to promote the survival and growth of both. In order to fulfill this basic purpose, Duvall[7] delineates six basic tasks for all families (Box 8-1).

A DEFINITION OF THE FAMILY

The concept of family has been defined differently by a variety of theorists. The definition one chooses should depend on the context of the individual situation as well as one's personal perspectives. In order to avoid the tendency to incorrectly assume that all families

Box 8-1. Basic Tasks of the Family

Generating affection among family members
Meeting needs for continuity of companionship
Providing a sense of support and personal security
Providing a sense of satisfaction and purpose
Transmitting a sense of moral responsibility and social controls
Facilitating social placement and socialization of members

▼▼▼

Adapted from Duvall, E. M., & Miller, B. C. (1985). *Marriage and family development (6th ed).* New York: Harper & Row Publishers.

operate as one's childhood family, nurses should recognize the differences between their perspectives, values, and beliefs and those of their clients. In general, the family system is considered to involve people related in a traditional or nontraditional sense by marriage, blood, adoption, or friendship. In the most inclusive sense, family can be defined as a dynamic system of two or more people who are (1) emotionally involved with each other; and (2) live near one another. The term emotional involvement assumes reciprocal obligations and responsibilities within the context of a caring and committed relationship.[1] Two of the major theoretical frameworks underlying a definition of family include a structural-functional perspective and a developmental perspective.

THEORETICAL PERSPECTIVES

Structural-Functional Perspective

The structural-functional perspective arises from a social systems approach and focuses on analysis of the structure and functions of family units within a social context. Although this perspective is often criticized for seeming rigid or narrow in scope, it provides a firm and necessary foundation from which to build a more dynamic and comprehensive understanding of the family.

A family's structure refers to the general scheme of organization resulting in patterned interactions among its members (internal structure) as well as relationships with other family systems (external structure). Family functions refer to the tasks performed by the family system for maintenance of the family unit, for individual members, and for society.

STRUCTURE OF THE FAMILY

Owing to the pressures and demands created by complex, constantly changing internal and external environments, the structural patterns of families vary considerably among cultures and societal groups. Common family structures in America include (1) the nuclear family, (2) the family of origin, (3) the extended family, (4) the blended family, (5) single-parent families, (6) social contracts, and (7) communes.

The Family of Origin. The family of origin refers to the family into which an individual is born. This may also be called the family of orientation. The family of origin is highly significant for the transmission of culture and expectations regarding health and illness of its members. Nurses should be aware of potential role conflicts and confusion when there is a marked difference between a client's family of origin and present family structure.

The Nuclear Family. The nuclear family, also referred to as the family of marriage or the conjugal family, is composed of husband, wife, and their immediate children (natural or adopted). Historically, nuclear families have tended to have the highest income, to maintain relatively close generational ties, and to function according to traditional gender roles. Although this traditional idea of the American family was once the predominant family structure, it is no longer true today. Besides a declining number of nuclear families, there have also been significant changes within contemporary nuclear families relative to traditional gender roles and expectations.

The Extended Family. The extended family includes the nuclear family as well as other blood relatives who also may be members of the family of origin of the husband or wife. A typical extended family unit might include a nuclear family plus grandparents, uncles, aunts, or cousins who share household arrangements and responsibilities. Although the extended family has never been common in the United States, American families often maintain kin relationships through frequent contact, and exchange of information and resources.

The extended family has the potential to be very cohesive, effective, and supportive in times of crisis. Studies show that assistance during crises is most often sought from family members rather than outsiders. Obviously, this assistance can represent a significant strength for families as they cope with a member's illness.

On the other hand, the relationships between family generations also can be the source of strain in some situations. Research of three-generation families suggests that the middle generation is most likely to be the "giver" generation to both their parents as well as their children. Unfortunately, this can translate into an added stressor for the "sandwich generation" that may be undetected unless deliberate attempts are made to evaluate this possibility. Given the increase in life expectancy, it seems that the possible strain on this "sandwich generation" should receive greater attention in the future.

The Blended Family. The blended family, also called a reconstituted or step-family, refers to a family composed of an adult and at least one child from one marriage and an adult with or without children from a different marriage. The number of blended families is increasing dramatically to the extent that one of every three marriages in 1985 included at least one spouse who had been married before.

Blended families face complex and unique problems. Members do not share a common family history; thus, there may be different expectations for health maintenance and different strategies for coping with stress or illness. In addition, if one or both spouses perceived a sense of failure in their previous marriage, they may show greater than expected role strain and conflict in response to a family member's illness.

The Single-Parent Family. The single-parent family consists of one parent and one or more children.

These families occur when a single person adopts a child, when a child is born to an unmarried mother who chooses to raise the child alone, or when one spouse leaves the marriage relationship through divorce, separation, or death.

Often, single-parent families may confront social stigma in addition to role conflicts among members. When dealing with a family member's illness, single-parent families often face problems associated with inadequate financial or emotional resources for coping with the actual illness. For example, single-parent families typically have fewer funds available for preventive health care and less time available for visits to clinics or physicians' offices.

Interestingly, research has shown that the absence of a dual-parent household does not necessarily contribute to dysfunctional behavior for the individuals involved. Apparently, the manner in which the individuals cope with their situation is more important than the lack of one spouse within the same household.

Social Contract Families. Social contract families are also increasing; this family structure includes unmarried couples of the same or opposite sex who live together and may have children. These families exist because of an emotional commitment that is expressed in a social contract rather than a legal one. Because of social, financial, or external pressures, these relationships are sometimes temporary. According to the United States Census Bureau, the number of couples cohabitating (including gay and lesbian couples) doubled between 1970 and 1980. In 1985, social contract families represented 2.3 per cent of all couple households.

Communes. Communes may be one of two different types. First, there is the structure encompassing more than one monogamous couple with children; such households share facilities, resources, experiences, and child socialization responsibilities. A second type of commune may consist of a household of adults and children in which adults are "married" to each other and all are parents to the children. When illness strikes one member, there is the potential to have support of many members in responding to the crisis. Communes are declining in popularity in today's society.

FUNCTIONS OF THE FAMILY

In general, the particular structure of a family is less significant than a family's ability to perform functions considered necessary for growth of the family system and the individual members. Clements and Roberts[5] and Wright and Leahey[26] describe the family's functioning within the five broad areas of (1) management functions, (2) boundary functions, (3) communication functions, (4) educative and supportive functions, and (5) socialization functions.

Management Functions. Management functions refer to the decision making of adult members regarding resource allocation, use of power, establishment of rules, negotiation with other systems, providing financial support for members, and planning for the future. Within this function, the family may significantly influence the wellness of its members through expressed rules for health maintenance and health promotion practices. Management functions can be accomplished in different ways, but there should be general agreement among adult members on the manner chosen. More important, management functions should be the responsibility of adult members rather than of children. Nurses should be alerted to the need for further evaluation when someone other than an adult is primarily responsible for family management during an extended period.

Boundary Functions. The boundary function involves maintaining clear distinctions among the roles of individuals within a family, among generations, and with other systems. Studies demonstrate that when clear generational boundaries (the boundaries between children and their parents) are present, there is less likelihood of dysfunctional behavior than when these boundaries are not present.

In general, it is more difficult to maintain normal functioning in all areas when the family's boundaries are tightly closed or widely open. A family's boundaries should be permeable enough to permit others to enter for assistance in coping with illness changes. On the other hand, boundaries should be sufficiently defined to provide a sense of cohesion or connectedness among family members.

Communication Functions. Communication functions emphasize the patterns of interactions within families. Healthy communication patterns involve direct, clear communication styles that allow all members full and appropriate expression of either affection or conflict. On the other hand, dysfunctional communication styles may be rigid or of limited range. For example, one family may freely express conflict through frequent arguments but fail to demonstrate their affection openly. A different family may exhibit the opposite behaviors through open demonstration of affection but not conflict. If either of these patterns is observed, further evaluation may be warranted.

Emotional and Supportive Functions. Emotional and supportive functions involve the degree of genuine affection and support expressed in families. This may be likened to the concept of social support, which is defined as "information leading the subject to believe that he is loved and cared for."[6] Such support may have a mediating or buffering effect that facilitates regaining health or effectively coping with imposed changes. In healthy families, the degree of support is shared so that the needs of all family members are met the majority of the time instead of allowing one person to continually sacrifice for another.

Socialization Functions. The socialization function focuses on transmission of culture and role behavior in order to facilitate a member's functioning both in the family and in society. For example, parents socialize their children (and children socialize their parents) regarding societal expectations. In addition to societal expectations, there is also socialization regarding appropriate role behavior within the family. Each member has an identified position with accompanying role responsibilities and expectations.

Although there may be variation in role performance between families, the most common examples of family roles are those of spouse, parent, child, or sibling. The role expectations for such positions arise from multiple sources, including social norms, culture, other family members, and from within the individual holding the position. Healthy families are able to successfully negotiate role changes in order to cope with individual maturational or situational events surrounding individual family members.

LEVELS OF FAMILY FUNCTIONING

When the general family functioning is healthy, there is effective coping and adaptation to changes required by situational or developmental crises. However, there are several factors that are associated with a lower level of functioning that ultimately inhibits a family's ability to meet the needs of its members. Awareness of these factors allows nurses to plan for potential problems and develop appropriate intervention strategies.

One of the most useful frameworks for assessing a family's functional level has been developed by Tapia.[23] According to this perspective, families are viewed along a continuum of five levels ranging from a dysfunctional to a highly functional level. (See Figure 8-1.)

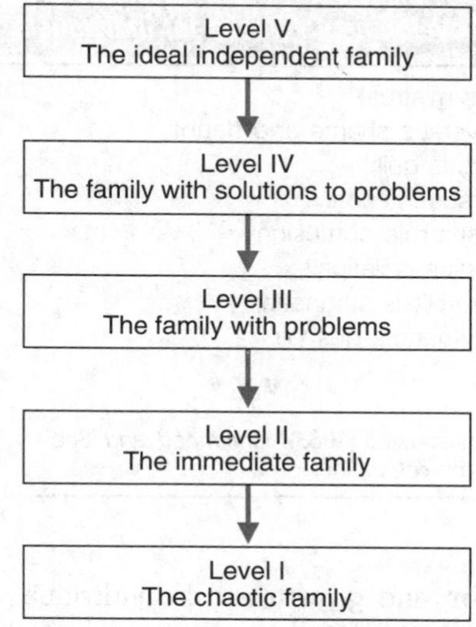

▲ *Figure 8-1*

Levels of family functioning. (Data from Tapia, J. [1972]. The nursing process in family health. *Nursing Outlook*, 20 [4], 267-270.)

The Chaotic Family. The chaotic family is highly disorganized and has difficulty in meeting the basic needs of its members. Frequently, adults are not able to meet their role expectations and responsibilities. As a result, children may assume adult roles and responsibilities. In addition, there may be abuse or neglect of individual members along with a pervasive sense of failure inside the family system. Interactions with outside systems are often marked by the chaotic family's distrust, hostility toward offers of assistance, and resistance to suggested changes. The chaotic family is at risk for ineffective coping and dysfunctional behaviors in response to illness of any member.

The Intermediate Family. Compared with the chaotic family, the intermediate family is less disorganized and better able to meet the members' basic needs. Although there is role confusion among members, the degree is not as pronounced. In addition, there is less community alienation and less abuse or neglect of family members. Although this family may sometimes be suspicious of outsiders, the intermediate family is generally more willing to accept offers of assistance than is the chaotic family.

The Family with Problems. The third level, the family with problems, might be considered "normal" despite the presence of problems. Although this family is generally able to meet basic needs, there is often role ambiguity and confusion between the parents owing to differences in their maturity levels. For example, when one parent is less mature than the other, it may lead to inappropriate role behaviors and conflicts that affect the entire family system. Compared with the intermediate family, this family is much less hostile and less suspicious of those outside the family system. With support and guidance, this family is able to recognize its problems and accept assistance or suggestions for necessary changes. Nurses working with this level of family should be aware that role changes due to illness may be more difficult than one might expect if no role confusion or ambiguity existed.

The Family with Solutions to Its Problems. The fourth level, the family with solutions to its problems, is able to meet basic needs and has clear role definitions for family members. Interventions planned with this family should be directed toward the changes imposed by illness rather than assessment and interventions related to dysfunctional family patterns.

The Ideal Independent Family. The fifth level, the ideal independent family, functions at a much higher level in fulfilling all members' physical, emotional, and social needs. These families communicate needs clearly, are highly receptive to health maintenance or health promotion strategies, and frequently are independent in identifying a problem area and seeking appropriate assistance. Generally, this family has been successful in coping with previous problems, thus demonstrating a significant strength that nurses should integrate into plans for care.

Developmental Perspectives

INDIVIDUAL DEVELOPMENT

An individual's developmental needs are described by Erikson (1963) as universal crises that are faced by all individuals. Successful achievement of these tasks leads

Box 8-2. Developmental Tasks for Individuals

Trust versus mistrust
Autonomy versus shame and doubt
Initiative versus guilt
Industry versus inferiority
Identity versus role confusion
Intimacy versus isolation
Generativity versus stagnation
Ego integrity versus despair

▼▼▼

Data from Erikson, E. (1963). *Childhood and Society*. New York: W. W. Norton & Co., Inc.

to satisfaction and growth for the individual as well as the family system (Box 8-2).

FAMILY LIFE CYCLE

In a similar manner, the family's life cycle can be seen as a series of inevitable tasks or crises that must be resolved in order for the family unit to achieve successful growth. As with individuals, the family's tasks are considered to apply universally to all family units as they seek to meet individual maturational needs as well as functional needs of society.

Within each stage of the family life cycle, there are certain tasks that must be achieved in order for the family to grow and survive. Awareness of these tasks, and the underlying key principles, can be used to facilitate a family's progress through the transition from one stage to the next. Since the transitional stage represents the time of greatest risk for development of dysfunctional behaviors, nurses should strive to pay special attention to families during this phase.

The developmental perspective of a family has evolved considerably since Duvall[7] conceptualized the family's life cycle as a series of eight stages, from initial formation through retirement. According to Duvall, a family's life cycle consists of the following eight stages: married couple, childbearing family, preschool-aged family, school-aged family, teen-aged family, launching center, middle-aged parents, and aging family members. Within each of these stages, achievement of certain tasks is necessary for successful growth and satisfaction.

As is apparent, the family life cycle stages are based on normative assumptions about families that are closely tied to the development of children. When these assumptions are not valid for an individual family, then the expected developmental tasks also lack validity. Obviously, contemporary dual-career or childless families do not meet the normative patterns originally assumed by Duvall. Partially in response to such concerns, many theorists have modified Duvall's original framework to make it more reflective of contemporary society. Box 8-3 displays a family life cycle, which incorporates more aspects to the family. Key principles and tasks are listed. Important potential health concerns are displayed within each stage. The nurse working with families can plan for usual health issues (e.g., family planning) as well as assess for other potential issues (e.g., drug abuse).[3, 11]

ALTERATIONS IN THE FAMILY LIFE CYCLE

Although most families go through the traditional stages of development described earlier, there are a significant number of families whose life cycle is altered in one way or another. Obviously, divorce and remarriage are major alterations to traditional family development because approximately 40 per cent of current marriages will end in divorce. Furthermore, approximately one half of all divorced couples will remarry within 3 years of the divorce.

Divorce. Whenever divorce occurs, there is disequilibrium in the entire life cycle of the family. In general, studies show that all divorcing families face additional stages in the divorce phase: (1) the decision to divorce, (2) planning the breakup of the family, (3) separation, and (4) finally, the divorce itself.[3] Many authorities agree that much of the mourning experienced during these stages is due to grieving for the loss of a relationship rather than the person. Obviously, this reaction can be magnified when illness or treatment restrictions represent additional losses.

Remarriage. Following divorce, there is reorganization of family structure and functioning so that significant relationships between parents and children, the extended family, and other systems must be renegotiated. If parents from the original nuclear family marry new spouses, then the remarried families must face the immediate task of restructuring roles, boundaries, and relationships. In essence, there is an "instant family" in which two families are forcibly blended together. Two of the most common problems seen in newly blended families are (1) development of adversarial relationships between step-parents and natural parents and (2) reversal of the hierarchy established in the single-parent family. As with other developmental transitions, this is a period of strain that is likely to lead to dysfunctional behaviors if it is not recognized.

WORKING WITH HIGH-RISK FAMILIES

Awareness of a family's developmental stage allows health professionals to anticipate the family's possible strengths or weaknesses for adapting to changes associated with illness. Although some families are successful in adapting to the changes imposed by illness, other families are unsuccessful. Research shows that families most likely to successfully adapt to illness are those in which there is harmony between the social environment and the developmental needs of the individual members.[18] On the other hand, families at the greatest risk for failing to adapt to a member's illness are those functioning at a low level for meeting basic needs (chaotic family), those families simultaneously experiencing a developmental transition and a member's

Box 8–3. Stages of Family Life Cycle and Related Health Concerns

Family Life Cycle Stage	*Key Principles*	*Stage-Related Family Tasks*	*Stage-Related Family Health Concerns*
Between families: the unattached young adult	Accepting parent-offspring separation	Differentiation of self in relation to family Development of intimate peer relationships Development of self in work	Adequate nutrition and exercise in light of single lifestyle Drug/alcohol abuse Management of sexual expression and functioning (birth control, abortion, sexually transmitted diseases) Management of work-related and interpersonal stress
The joining of families through marriage: the newly married couple	Commitment to new system	Formation of marital system Realignment of relationships with extended family to include spouse	Management of stress related to marital role adjustment Family planning Planning of pregnancy and birth
The family with young children (early childbearing, preschool-aged children, school children)	Accepting new generation of members into the system	Adjusting marital system to make space for a child or children Taking on parenting roles Realignment of relationships with extended family to include parenting and grandparenting roles Realignment and extension of relationships with community to include educational and child-care resources	Well-baby and child, including immunizations Management of acute and chronic child health problems Environmental safety Understanding of child's needs and abilities based on developmental level Management of role strain associated with expansion of family system
The family with adolescents	Increasing flexibility of family boundaries to include children's independence	Shifting of parent-child relationships to permit adolescents to move in and out of system Refocus on midlife marital and career issues Beginning shift toward concerns for older generation	Intensified interest of marital pair in health promotion and management of risk factors Management of tensions arising from adolescents' increasing pressure toward individualization and autonomy Heightened risk of adolescent substance abuse, automobile accidents, and other accidents
Launching children and moving on	Accepting a multitude of exits from and entries into the family system	Renegotiation of marital system as a dyad Development of adult-to-adult relationships between grown children and parents Realignment of relationships to include in-laws and grandchildren Dealing with disabilities and death of parents or grandparents	Management of stress arising from "reshaping" of family Dealing with children's separation from family Management of impact of aging grandparents, provision of assistance and care, coping with their death Dealing with emerging chronic health problems of marital pair

Box continued on following page

Box 8–3. Stages of Family Life Cycle and Related Health Concerns Continued

Family Life Cycle Stage	Key Principles	Stage-Related Family Tasks	Stage-Related Family Health Concerns
The family in later life (families of middle years, and families in retirement and old age)	Accepting the shifting of generational roles	Maintaining own or couple functioning and interests in face of physiologic decline; exploration of new familial and social role options Support for a more central role for the adult children Making room in the system for the wisdom and experience of the elderly; supporting the older generation without overfunctioning for them Dealling with loss of spouse, siblings, and other peers, and preparation for own death. Life review and integration	Promotion and maintenance of health Deterioration of physical or mental health or both, coping with loss of function, provision of assistance and care Management of stress generated by changing role relationships within marital dyad and among parents and children

▼▼▼

From Getty, C., & Humphreys, W. (1990). Family assessment: A base for nursing practice. In B. Bullough & V. Bullough (Eds.), *Nursing in the community* (pp. 242–271). St. Louis: C. V. Mosby.

chronic illness, and families in the middle generation. The occurrence of any of these situations deserves careful attention in order to identify a potential or actual problem in adapting to a member's illness (Box 8–4).

ASSESSMENT

Family assessment is the evaluation of interaction within a family system. The two major tools used in family assessment are the genogram and the ecosystems map. Family members should be encouraged to participate actively with the health professional during the development of these tools. Ideally, this procedure should be begun during admission and orientation to the health care agency.

Box 8–4. High-Risk Families

Chaotic, disorganized families
Middle-aged families with adolescent facing chronic illness
Families experiencing both a developmental transition and a major chronic illness

▼▼▼

From Rankin, S., & Weeks, D. (1989). Life-span development: A review of theory and practice for families with chronically ill members. *Scholarly Inquiry for Nursing Practice: An International Journal, 3*(1), 3–22. Used by permission of Springer Publishing Company, Inc., New York, NY, 10012; and Tapia, J. (1972). The nursing process in family health. *Nursing Outlook, 20*(4), 267–270.

The Genogram

The genogram is a schematic depiction of the intergenerational relationships of at least three family generations.[13] It is similar to a conventional genealogy chart or family tree. In this system, generations are placed on horizontal lines and children are denoted through vertical lines. The symbols used in genograms vary but generally, each person's name, age, date of birth, and any health problems should be noted. If a family member is deceased, both the cause and date of death should be indicated on the genogram (Figure 8–2).

The Ecosystems Map

The term ecosystems represents a synthesis of the concepts of ecology and general systems theory. Ecology is that branch of biology concerned with the interactive relationship of organisms with their environments. As with the genogram, the ecosystems map is intended to provide an easily understood schematic of the relationships of the family to the surrounding subsystems as well as the larger suprasystem. In developing an ecosystems map, the genogram should be placed in the center and labeled "family." Outer circles should be

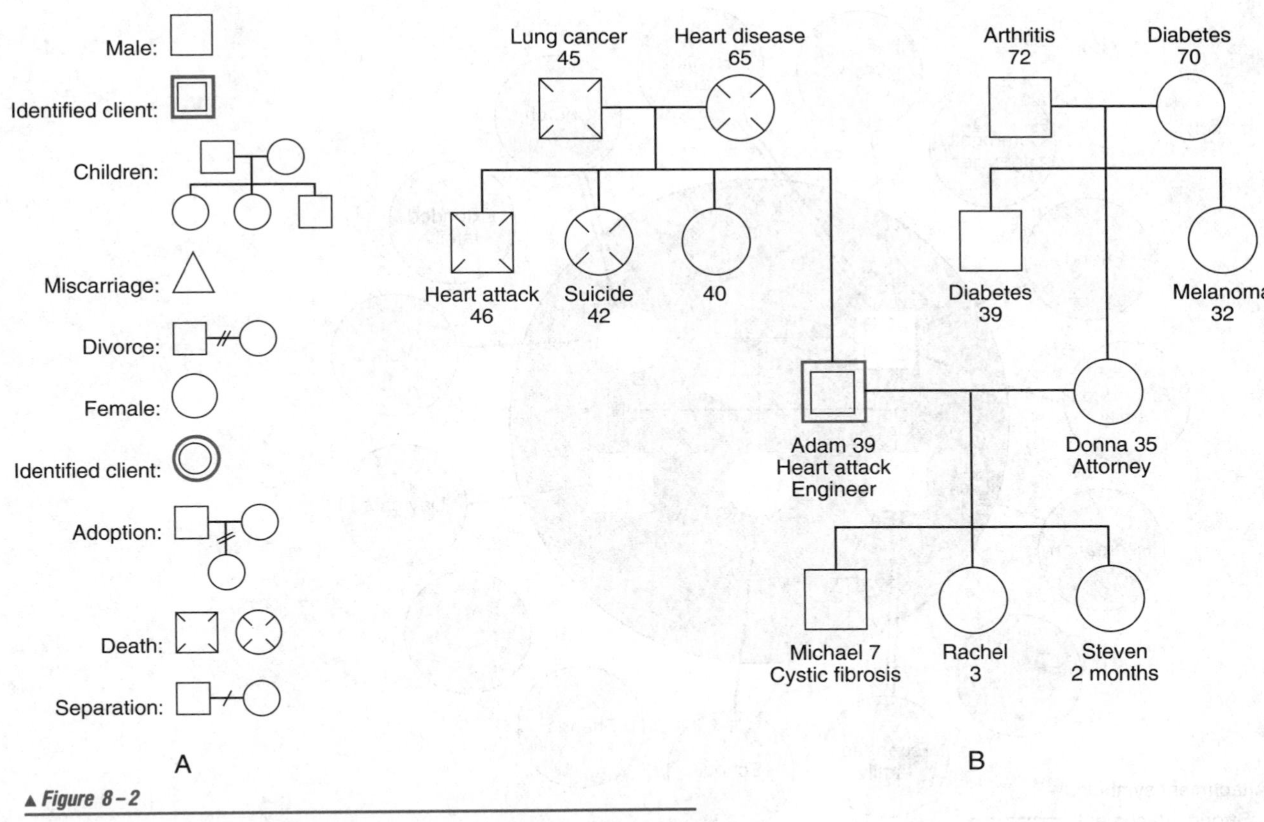

▲ *Figure 8–2*

A, Symbols to use in constructing a genogram. *B*, Example of a genogram.

drawn to indicate relevant suprasystems such as health agencies, educational institutions, and other family groups. Lines are drawn between the circles to indicate relationships. The strength of these relationships is indicated by the type of line drawn. Bold lines indicate strong relationships, dotted lines indicate weak relationships, and slashed lines indicate stressful relationships. The flow of energy can be indicated by arrows drawn adjacent to the circles (Fig. 8–3).

Comprehensive Summaries

After collection of data from a genogram, ecosystems map, and family interviews, the findings should be analyzed and integrated in a meaningful manner. An appropriate system should be developed for each health care agency or setting depending on philosophy, relevance, and practicality. Obviously, the system used in an emergency room is different from the system used in a long-term care facility.

Despite the actual style used, the nursing assessment of the family in medical-surgical nursing practice should be viewed as an ongoing process that is integral to professional nursing care. Initially, nurses in a medical-surgical setting should focus on a general macro-level assessment of the family relative to structure, function, and developmental status. If problems are detected, then micro-level assessment of that area may be warranted. Depending on the experience and philosophy of the nurse, the micro-level assessment may be conducted by the staff nurse during subsequent family sessions or the family may be referred to a nurse specialist in the appropriate area. For example, if a macro-level assessment indicates that a family is functioning at a low level (the chaotic family) and is likely to need further assistance following discharge, it may be appropriate to refer this family to a community health nurse for further evaluation. A family assessment tool is shown in Table 8–1.

NURSING DIAGNOSIS

A comprehensive family assessment leads to formulation of nursing diagnoses within two major areas: (1) those that focus on the family unit and (2) those that emphasize the individuals within the family.

Nursing Diagnoses Related to the Family System

Nursing diagnoses that focus on the family unit may involve altered family processes or ineffective family coping (disabling). The related factors of either diagnostic statement may be situational or developmental crisis, and the defining characteristics may vary considerably. The diagnostic statement of altered family pro-

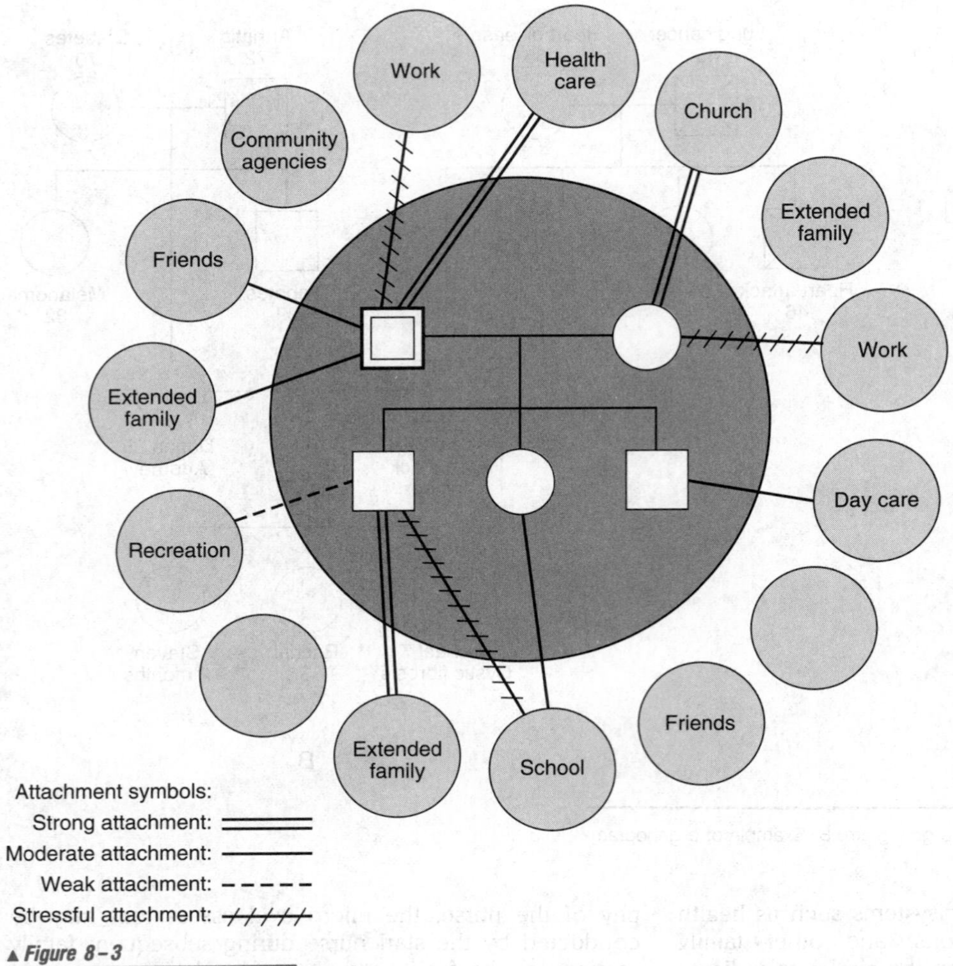

▲ *Figure 8–3*

Example of an ecosystems map.

cesses should be used for a normally healthy family unit that is challenged by the stress of acute or chronic illness. Some of the family behaviors that might indicate the appropriateness of this diagnostic statement include verbal outbursts, interference with necessary treatments, absence of family interaction, inappropriate communication patterns, and verbalization of fear, anxiety, or anger.

The nursing diagnostic statement of ineffective coping (disabling) should be used when the behavior of the family is considered to be destructive, not merely lacking in support. Some of the defining characteristics for this diagnosis include neglect or abuse of a family member (see Bridge to Home Health Care), depression, agitation, hostility, distortion of reality, and aggression.

Nursing Diagnoses Related to Individual Family Members

Nursing diagnoses that emphasize an individual family member's responses to the illness of a family member are generally related to fear, powerlessness, grieving, social isolation, and knowledge deficit. Even though the nursing diagnosis may focus on individual family members, they should also be viewed for their effect on the functions of the family unit and other family members.

Nursing Diagnoses Related to Special Client Populations

Although there is still a great deal of research needed on the role of the family in the illness experience of family members, there have been strides made within certain populations of patients. Two special populations of patients (critically ill patients and head-injured patients) have received special attention within adult medical-surgical nursing. Although there are commonalities between these groups relative to their needs, there are also significant differences that nurses should be cognizant of in order to provide a high level of nursing care. (see Nursing Research and Ethical Issues in Nursing).

TABLE 8–1. Family Assessment Guidelines

Family Demographics:
Demographic data: family name, address, telephone number
Family Structure: (The basis for assessing family structure may be a genogram or a chart that lists relevant data for each family member.)

Name	Age	Sex	Family Role	Occupation	Education
1.					
2.					
3.					
4.					

Family Functions:
Management:
How are decisions made? (give examples).
Who is responsible for providing economic income?
Has this changed because of a family member's illness?
How are the available family resources allocated?
Does one member require/receive more of the available resources than any other member?
How are home maintenance tasks divided?
Boundary (The ecosystems map may be used as a basis for discussion in this area.)
Who initiates and maintains relationships with the extended family, friends, and community agencies?
What, if any, are the problems in these relationships?
Communication
How frequently, and in what way, do members express anger?
How frequently, and in what way, do members express affection?
In general, is communication clear, open, and direct, or is it more likely to be evasive, covert, and circular?
Is there consistency between the verbal and nonverbal behavior of family members?
Emotional-Supportive
To what degree, and in what way, do family members provide support for one another?
In what ways does the family demonstrate cohesiveness and connectedness?
In what ways does the family encourage the individuality of its members?
Socialization
Who assumes responsibility for the education, care, and discipline of children?
Is this role/responsibility shared? How? Does this sharing create any problems?
Are each of the family members demonstrating appropriate role behavior and growth within and outside of the family? How is this growth exhibited?
Developmental Status
What is the family's stage in the life cycle?
What are the expected developmental tasks?
In what ways is the family meeting the stage-related tasks?
In what ways is the family having difficulty in this?
In what ways is the family meeting the stage-related health concerns?
In what ways is the family having difficulties with this?
What additional resources might be needed?
What are the individual developmental tasks for each member? (List each member separately.)
To what degree does the family foster or inhibit the individual members in meeting these tasks?
How has the illness situation influenced the development of individuals? of the family?
Summary
On the basis of assessment in all of the above-mentioned areas, list any identified problems and indicate the family's strengths and weaknesses for coping with the problem. In addition, indicate the type and availability of resources that will be needed to assist this family.

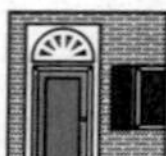

BRIDGE TO HOME HEALTH CARE

Elder Abuse Detection

Taking care of clients in the home setting cannot be done in a vacuum. When abuse of a patient is suspected, the patient, family, and caregivers must be incorporated into the total assessment and plan of care.

First, it is important to listen carefully to the patient and observe overt and covert behaviors. It may be difficult for the patient to admit that the caregiver is abusive. Also, the abusive caregiver usually does provide some positive support, whether it be financial, emotional, or assistance with activities of daily living, which allows the patient to continue to live in the community. The assessment also must confirm the caregiver's report of the client's condition. For example, if the caregiver attributes bruises to a fall, then it should be determined whether or not gait instability is consistent with the patient's physical condition.

Conversely, from a caregiver's perspective, there must be adequate instruction in areas such as nutrition, transfer, positioning, and ambulation to safely meet the patient's needs. The frustration of providing care may also contribute to abuse. The caregiver needs to be encouraged to have regular absences from the care.

It is helpful to use a multidisciplinary approach in the plan of care including the physician, social workers, homemakers, home health aides, and volunteers.

The home health care nurse must not be reluctant to confront suspicious situations in fear of jeopardizing rapport with the patient and family. Although maintaining a relationship is important, advocacy for the client should be the nurse's first priority.

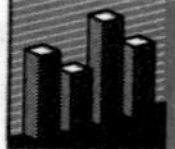

NURSING RESEARCH

According to Fife, the major needs of families of critically ill patients are for the relief of anxiety, the provision of information and support, proximity to the patient, a feeling of helpfulness to the patient, and various personal needs of family members. Consequently, nurses should be aware of the need to assist families of critically ill patients in their coping strategies as they seek to understand the illness as well as treatments, gain awareness of their feelings, and develop a realistically hopeful perspective.

When caring for families of head-injured patients, nurses should be aware that the major problem is often social isolation. The cause of a perceived or actual sense of social isolation may be due to a sense of embarrassment related to the ill family member's inappropriate behavior in public settings, the lack of time or finances to participate in social activities, and drastic changes in previous family and social relationships. In addition, the actual care required by some patients can be so physically and emotionally draining to family members that there is not enough energy left for negotiating social relationships and activities.

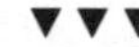

Fife, B. (1985). A model for predicting the adaptation of families to medical crisis: An analysis of role integration. *Image: The Journal of Nursing Scholarship, 18* (4), 108–112.

Rogers, P., & Kreutzer, J. (1984). Family crisis following head injury: A network intervention strategy. *Journal of Neurosurgical Nursing*, 16 (6), 343–346.

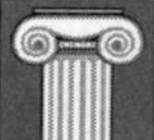

ETHICAL ISSUES IN NURSING

Should Organ Procurement and Donation Be Discussed with the Dying and Their Families?

For many clients, having a supportive family during times of illness is one of the most important aspects of their care. It is even possible for family roles to change during times of acute or chronic illness. Nursing assessments of clients should always, whenever possible, include assessments of family dynamics and interactions. Family assessments help the nursing staff better facilitate teaching, discharge planning, and follow-up care. Interactions between family members and nursing staff are usually pleasant encounters revolving around helping the client through his or her illness.

When a client's condition is such that death appears imminent, family members need the support of the health care team. It is at this most uncomfortable time that nurses have the opportunity to speak to clients and their families about organ donation. Ideally, this issue should be addressed prior to ill health or trauma, but the reality is that organ donation is not something many people plan prior to ill health or trauma.

How does a nurse approach an upset or grieving family about organ donation? Should they be approached about organ donation at all? Is there an ethical responsibility to discuss the procurement of organs with the dying and their family? Thousands of living persons are on waiting lists for organ transplants—should they have the opportunity to receive an organ from someone who no longer has need of it? Should we have to get consent to procure organs from the deceased? In some parts of the world, human organs are procured from the deceased automatically, without need of consent. In fact, consent is needed only in cases in which donation is not to occur.

Nurses need to be aware of their state laws and institution's policies regarding organ donation. It is not an easy task to discuss this matter with clients and their families, but nurses should assess their clients when the possibility for donation is present.

NURSING INTERVENTION

Once appropriate nursing diagnoses and goals have been formulated, interventions should be planned in recognition of the fact that there may be considerable variation between the needs of the family structure and the needs of individual members. For example, while the identified client is attempting to cope with terminal cancer, the spouse may be coping with an acute myocardial infarction, an adolescent daughter with an unwanted pregnancy, and a preschool-aged son with diabetes. There may also be competing needs based on differences in developmental transitions and tasks. Interventions for any family should always begin with understanding of therapeutic family communication techniques. Therapeutic communication with families facilitates effectiveness in using other strategies such as anticipatory guidance, networking, referral, and health teaching activities.

Therapeutic Family Communication

ENGAGEMENT

Therapeutic family communication consists of a four-step process that includes engagement, assessment, intervention, and termination.[26] The focus of the first stage, engagement, emphasizes the establishment and maintenance of a trusting relationship.

Jarvis[14] states that the ease with which trust is attained depends on the functional level of the family. When working with families that function at a low level, nurses should emphasize trust building by being consistent in their actions, setting clear limits, adhering to promises made, and developing patience when faced with negative behavior. As a trusting relationship is developed, nurses can be less directive and more collaborative in their communications.

During the engagement phase, nurses should attempt to remain essentially neutral and avoid confrontation. Each family member should be encouraged to express particular areas of concern or interest without fear of reprisal or argument.

ASSESSMENT

The second stage, assessment, focuses on greater exploration and identification of problem areas. During this stage, nurses should avoid the obvious extremes of reaching a conclusion prematurely or collecting irrelevant information. Communication patterns should be individualized to the functional level and maturity of the family members.

INTERVENTION

The third stage, intervention, is the working phase of therapeutic communication with families. During this phase, communication patterns may be directive or collaborative as needed to assist the family to make changes in their approaches to the identified problem.

TERMINATION

The final stage, termination, focuses on ending the relationship between the family and the nurse in a manner that will facilitate independent problem solving by the family in the future. Again, the degree to which this stage is possible is dependent on the level of family functioning and the illness situation.

Anticipatory Guidance

One of the most useful interventions available to all nurses working with families is that of anticipatory guidance or preparation for expected occurrences. Anticipatory guidance should be provided in relation to two types of changes: (1) those associated with illness and (2) those associated with developmental transitions. When the family knows what is expected, there is greater possibility that the response will be positive and adaptive rather than harmful and counterproductive.

For example, when working with the family of a middle-aged male before major surgery, nurses should provide anticipatory guidance for the family about possible behavioral changes likely to occur postoperatively. If a family is able to anticipate a short-lived depression following surgery, then there will be less energy spent on inappropriate strategies and anxiety. Consequently, more of the family's energy and resources will be available for meeting needs of other family members or the family system itself.

Networking

In addition to anticipatory guidance, networking sessions should also be part of the plan when working with families of medical or surgical clients. A network may be defined as a type of kinship bond occurring when people share an experience. The actual process of networking involves gathering the immediate and extended family along with friends and community ties in order to identify problems, generate possible solutions, and provide the necessary resources. Networking should be initiated with the client's entry into the health care system and continued into the community if necessary. Nurses should facilitate the development of networks that will continue following discharge without the intervention of health professionals.

An example of the network effect is frequently seen when families spontaneously discuss their members' illness in the hospital waiting areas adjacent to emergency rooms, intensive care units, or operating room suites. In effect, families who share their mutual concerns under such stressful conditions are providing support for each other as they attempt to understand and adapt to the various illness changes. Although the relationships that develop under these situations may provide valuable support initially, they are often temporary and do not provide the level of support needed to cope with long-term changes. However, nurses can plan networking strategies that will provide more lasting and substantive support for the family faced with long-term changes. An example of the effectiveness of networking strategies in coping with long-term changes has been demonstrated by Rogers and Kreutzer's

(1984) study of the families of head-injured patients. Frequently, it has been shown that planning for respite care allows the family to renew its energy and better support the ill member. Networking allows others to become aware of potential problems and provide support that otherwise might not be provided.

Referral

Part of the concept of networking involves referral to community agencies. Referral is indicated whenever it is likely that the client will continue to need assistance following discharge. It should be noted that the process of referral requires more than merely supplying names and addresses of agencies regarded by the nurse as appropriate for the family's needs. In order for the outcome of a referral to be productive, two additional factors need to be considered: (1) the meaning of the referral to the client and the family and (2) the receptivity of the responding agency. Obviously, referrals that a nurse considers appropriate may actually be resisted by a family if the community agency is seen as threatening or too inconvenient. Even when the family concurs on the necessity of a referral, the eventual outcome may be jeopardized if the receiving agency responds poorly. Therefore, a means for following up with families after a referral should be planned so that alternative strategies may be developed when necessary. As is apparent, collaboration between families and all members of the health team is essential for effective care.

Teaching

The advent of Diagnosis-Related Groups and subsequent early discharge from hospital settings makes the need for teaching more critical today than ever before. Nurses should be fully aware of a family's abilities to understand and provide care before family members are released from hospital care. Although many teaching activities planned with the families of medical-surgical clients necessarily focus on providing information regarding the illness and treatments encountered in the hospital, nurses should also focus on health promotion and health maintenance activities to be implemented following discharge.

Summary

Families can be viewed as contributing to illness or wellness, as professional care extenders, and as resources for ill family members. It is apparent that there is not a universally correct form for family structures or functions to assume. Family structures and functions, to a large degree, are shaped by the social milieu. Rather than attempting to impose an artificially contrived definition, it is more useful to focus on understanding a family's strengths and weaknesses, especially as they relate to health practices.

The future of professional nursing is likely to integrate the family more consistently into all phases of the nursing process. Therefore, it is critical that nurses thoroughly understand the structure, functions, and development of families. Once these concepts are assimilated, nurses will be prepared to assess families and develop strategies to support healthy functioning.

Bibliography

1. Bullough, B., & Bullough, V. (1990). *Nursing in the community.* St. Louis: C. V. Mosby Company.
2. Carpenito, L. (1991). *Nursing diagnoses: Application to clinical practice* (4th. ed.). St. Louis: J. B. Lippincott.
3. Carter, B., & McGoldrick, M. (1989). *The changing family life cycle: A framework for family therapy* (2nd ed.). Boston, MA: Allyn and Bacon.
4. Clemen-Stone, S., et al. (1991). *Comprehensive family and community health nursing* (3rd ed.). St. Louis: Mosby-Year Book, Inc.
5. Clements, I., & Roberts, F. (1983). *Family health: A theoretical approach to nursing care.* New York: John Wiley & Sons.
6. Cobb, S. (1976). Social support as a moderator of life stress. *Psychosomatic Medicine, 38,* 300-314.
7. Duvall, E., & Miller, B. (1985). *Marriage and family development* (6th ed.). New York: Harper & Row Publishers.
8. Erikson, E. (1963). *Childhood and society.* New York: W. W. Norton & Co., Inc.
9. Fife, B. (1985). A model for predicting the adaptation of families to medical crises: An analysis of role integration. *Image: The Journal of Nursing Scholarship, 18* (4), 108-112.
10. Friedman, M. (1986). *Family nursing: Theory and assessment* (2nd ed.). Norwalk, CT: Appleton-Century-Crofts.
11. Getty, C., & Humphreys, W. (1990). Family assessment: A base for nursing practice. In B. Bullough & V. Bullough (Eds.), *Nursing in the community* (pp. 242-271). St. Louis: C. V. Mosby
12. Gillis, C., et al. (1990). *Toward a science of family nursing.* Menlo Park, CA. Addison-Wesley.
13. Herth, K. (1989). The root of it all. *Journal of Gerontological Nursing, 15*(12), 32-37.
14. Jarvis, L. (1985). *Community health nursing: Keeping the public healthy* (2nd ed.). Philadelphia: F. A. Davis.
15. L'Abate, L., Ganahl, G., & Hansen, J. (1986). *Methods of family therapy.* Englewood Cliffs, NJ: Prentice-Hall.
16. Mechanic, D. (1977). Illness behavior, social adaptation, and the management of illness. *Journal of Nervous Mental Disorders, 165*(2), 79-87.
17. Minuchin, S. (1974). *Families and family therapy.* Cambridge, MA: Harvard University Press.
18. Rankin, S., & Weeks, D. (1989). Life-span development: A review of theory and practice for families with chronically ill members. *Scholarly Inquiry for Nursing Practice: An International Journal, 3*(1), 3-22.
19. Rogers, P., & Kreutzer, J. (1984). Family crises following head injury: A network intervention strategy. *Journal of Neurosurgical Nursing, 16*(6), 343-346.
20. Satir, V. (1972). *Peoplemaking.* Palo Alto, CA: Science and Behavior Books, Inc.
21. Spradley, B. (1990). *Community health nursing: Concepts and practice* (3rd ed.). Glenview, IL: Scott, Foresman/Little, Brown Higher Education.
22. Spradley, B. (1991). *Readings in community health nursing* (4th ed.). Philadelphia: JB Lippincott.
23. Tapia, J. (1972). The nursing process in family health. *Nursing Outlook, 20*(4), 267-270.
24. U.S. Bureau of the Census, Current Population Reports, Series P-25, No. 1018. (1989). *Projections of the population of the United States, by age, sex, and race: 1988-2080.* Washington, D.C.: U.S. Government Printing Office.
25. U.S. Bureau of the Census, Statistical abstract of the United States. (1990). *The national data book* (110th ed.). Washington, D.C.: U.S. Department of Commerce, Bureau of the Census.
26. Wright, L., & Leahy, M. (1984). *Nurses and families: A guide to family assessment and interventions.* Philadelphia: F. A. Davis.

Chapter 9

Chronic Conditions

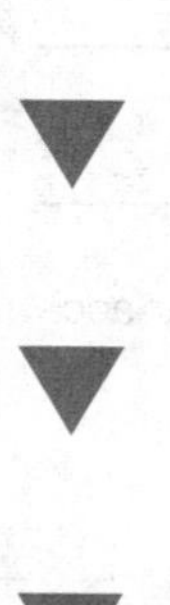

Chronic conditions constitute a major challenge to health care providers and health care delivery systems. There are more and more clients with chronic conditions due to an ever-growing number of elderly clients and increasing numbers of clients who survive major illnesses. Because chronic conditions cannot be cured, the client needs to learn to adapt to the condition. Helping a client adapt to a chronic illness challenges the health care system, health care providers, and society as a whole. Adaptation to chronic conditions is a complex and ongoing process that involves physiologic, sociologic, psychological, technologic, and time factors.

DEFINITION

Chronic conditions are long-term health problems due to an irreversible disorder, an accumulation of disorders, or a latent disease state.[13] Some chronic conditions cause irreversible change in the structure or function of one or more body systems. Other chronic conditions are chronic because no cure has been found. Developments in the fields of bacteriology, immunology, public health, and pharmacology have led to a rapid drop in mortality from previously fatal illnesses. Decreased mortality from acute illnesses has led to lengthened lifespans and a greater risk of accidents and illness that can develop into chronic conditions. Previously fatal diseases are becoming chronic conditions. Tuberculosis is an example of a previously chronic condition for which clients were isolated in sanitariums. Today tuberculosis is treatable and is preventable with vaccines.

The terms chronic illness, long-term illness, and chronic condition are used interchangeably. The term chronic condition is preferred because it is more consistent with a definition of health that includes components of wellness and illness.

The increased prevalence of chronic conditions in our society is due to many factors. Much knowledge about physiologic function has been generated during the past 40 years. Advances have been made in techniques and equipment for assessing and diagnosing alterations in physical function, supporting and sustaining life, combating infection, maintaining and restoring physical function, and compensating and substituting for lost physical function. More infants survive with congenital problems. More persons of all ages survive life-threatening episodes of acute illness and trauma with different degrees of residual deficits in physical or cognitive function. Chronic conditions that were once considered rare, such as dermatophytosis and amyotropic lateral sclerosis, are becoming more common because people are living longer. Illnesses previously viewed as acute, such as myocardial infarction, cerebral vascular accidents, and congestive heart failure, are now recognized to be acute episodes of chronic conditions. New illnesses such as acquired immunodeficiency syndrome (AIDS) and Lyme disease are being diagnosed. Implantable devices and transplants extend the chronic phase of chronic conditions.

Clients with chronic conditions are more visible. Beliefs about the rights of clients with chronic conditions and their role in society have changed. Having a chronic condition is no longer viewed as incompatible with maintaining social roles. Health was previously defined as the absence of illness. Health is now viewed as a continuum of wellness to death, with some degree of health being present until death. The revised definition of health recognizes the presence of abilities as well as deficits within illness and fits the client with a chronic condition well.

INCIDENCE

The incidence, visibility, and awareness of chronic conditions in our society and acute health care settings are greater than at any other time in history. Exact measurement of the incidence of chronic conditions is limited by variations in definitions of chronic illness found in the literature. According to the definition of chronic conditions used in the 1986 Department of Commerce census, approximately 50 per cent of the American population have one or more chronic conditions. It is estimated that more than 75 per cent of clients receiving care in acute care settings have one or more chronic conditions.

Chronic conditions can occur at any point in the lifespan. Some adults have chronic conditions that are present from birth or that are acquired during childhood or adolescence. Other clients acquire chronic conditions during adulthood. Common chronic conditions grouped according to age of onset and body system involved are listed in Table 9-1.

It is important to differentiate acute conditions from chronic conditions. An acute condition is caused by a disease that produces signs and symptoms soon after exposure to the cause, typically runs a short course, and usually ends with complete recovery or abrupt termination in death. Acute conditions may become chronic; for example, seasonal allergies may lead to lung conditions such as asthma.

A chronic condition is caused by a disease that produces signs and symptoms over a varying period of time, runs a long course, and only partially resolves. The symptoms of chronic conditions may subside with proper care. This period of time when the client is symptom free is called remission. The symptoms often return, a process called exacerbation.

TABLE 9-1. Common Chronic Medical Conditions

Body System	Onset Prior to Adulthood	Adult Onset
Neurologic	Epilepsy Cerebrovascular accident Tumors Blindness Deafness Head injury Spinal cord injury Aneurysm Cerebral palsy Spina bifida	Epilepsy Cerebrovascular accident Tumors Blindness Deafness Head injury Spinal cord injury Aneurysm Multiple sclerosis Migraine Dermatophytosis Amyotropic lateral sclerosis Huntington's chorea Myasthenia gravis
Cardiovascular	Congenital cardiac disease Sickle-cell Hemophilia	Hypertension Coronary artery disease Myocardial infarction Congestive heart failure Chronic anticoagulation Chronic lower extremity ischemia Angina Cardiomyopathies
Pulmonary	Asthma Hodgkin's disease Antitrypsin deficiency Cystic fibrosis	Asthma Hodgkin's disease Chronic obstructive pulmonary disease Leukemia Cancer
Digestive	Deficiencies Cystic fibrosis	Gastric ulcer Lactose deficiency Colitis Crohn's disease Cirrhosis Cancer

TABLE 9-1. Common Chronic Medical Conditions Continued

Body System	Onset Prior to Adulthood	Adult Onset
Renal and urinary	Neurogenic bladder Chronic renal failure	Neurogenic bladder Chronic renal failure Chronic urinary tract infection Cancer
Metabolic	Diabetes	Diabetes Hyperlipidemia
Musculoskeletal	Juvenile arthritis Paralysis or absence of limbs (congenital, traumatic, surgical)	Arthritis Paralysis or absence of limbs Low back pain Sarcoma Osteoporosis
Immune		Asthma Lupus erythematosus Scleroderma Arthritis Acquired immunodeficiency syndrome Tuberculosis
Other		Alcoholism

In the past, health care practice, education, and research have focused on acute illnesses. These conditions were life threatening and were the most common problems seen by health care providers. At present, most clients are hospitalized for exacerbations of chronic conditions rather than for acute illnesses. Because most clients with chronic illness are managed by themselves or by members of the family, it is common for the client and family to have more factual and experiential knowledge about the condition than the average health care provider. A comparison of chronic and acute illnesses is listed in Table 9-2.

Many nursing leaders have advocated the inclusion of more content on chronic illness and wellness into nursing education. Likewise, there is an increasing need for research to build nursing's knowledge base about chronic conditions.

THE PROCESS OF ADAPTATION

Physiologic Adaptation

Some changes in physiologic structure or function that are associated with chronic conditions are irreversible. Other physiologic changes are reversible. Treatment and lifestyle changes can slow the rate of some physiologic changes. Technology is available to compensate or substitute for some types of physical functioning. Adaptive tasks related to changes in physiologic structure or function are as follows:

- Changing lifestyle
- Controlling symptoms
- Learning about illness and treatment
- Managing the prescribed medical regimen
- Learning about techniques and devices that can substitute for lost function
- Acquiring skills in using these techniques and devices
- Monitoring body response to therapies
- Adjusting to changes in physical appearance and function during the course of the disease
- Capitalizing on physical and psychological strengths.

Psychological Adaptation

Psychological adaptation to a chronic condition is an ongoing process that overlaps other biologic and psychosocial processes associated with gains, losses, and challenges throughout the remainder of a client's lifespan. As with other ongoing processes, psychological

TABLE 9-2. Comparison of Chronic Illness and Acute Illness

	Chronic Illness	Acute Illness
Knowledge base of health providers	Broad, less commonly defined than acute illness	Focused, fairly well defined
Onset	Rapid or gradual	Rapid
Course	Ongoing process with transitions and changing demands Phases Diagnosis Chronic constant progressive remissions/exacerbations Terminal	Short, temporary
Outcome	Varying types and degrees of physical deficits Uncertain Different degrees of ongoing impact on personal, family, work, and recreational roles	Self-limiting (cure or death), no residual deficits Fairly predictable Temporary impact on personal, family, work, and recreational roles
Nursing/medical management	Long term; client/family co-managers	Short term

adaptation to a chronic condition is characterized by periods of changing demands and transitions. Predictable periods of changing psychological demands and transitions include onset and diagnosis, hospitalizations for treatment of the condition, exacerbation of illness, failure of treatments, and loss of self-care abilities. Some clients whose chronic condition has a terminal phase must also adapt to a shortened lifespan and the dying process.

Although chronic conditions are associated with disease-specific physiologic changes and outcomes, psychological adaptation of persons who have not experienced severe cognitive impairment has been found to be similar in clients with all conditions, and is not related to length of time since diagnosis. The psychological health of adults with different stages of chronic illnesses has been found to be similar to that of normal adults.

Clients adapt to the same diagnosis and phase of illness in very diverse ways. During the diagnostic phase, one client may appear overwhelmed and assume a lower level of physical, psychological, or social functioning than the physical condition warrants and another client may evidence minimal distress, maintain or regain a high level of physical, psychological, and social functioning and continue to adapt.

INITIAL ADAPTIVE TASKS

Psychological adaptive demands common to persons during the onset or diagnostic phase of a chronic condition are

- Coping with anxiety of not knowing, and fantasies and fears about what might be wrong;
- Coping with feelings of guilt;
- Tolerating the physical and emotional strain of tests and painful procedures;
- Balancing hopefulness and the possibility of a feared diagnosis; and
- Adapting to the health care system and different health care providers.

Although the onset or diagnostic period is a crisis period for the majority of clients, the adaptive behavior varies. Some clients may deny the diagnosis, or they accept the diagnosis but deny the feared implications. Other clients who have experienced symptoms over a period of time may experience a sense of relief that a diagnosis has been established because identification of the problem validates the existence of the problem and increases the potential for the alleviation of symptoms.

THREE PHASES OF PSYCHOLOGICAL ADAPTATION

A general pattern of psychological adaptation to personal change, loss, and threat of loss has been described by sociologists and psychologists.

Disbelief. The first phase of the pattern is commonly referred to as disbelief or resistance. Denial of the changes or the need for personal change is characteristic of this phase. This phase is similar to the stress "fight or flight" response and is believed to protect the client from being psychologically overwhelmed.

Developing Awareness. The second phase is developing awareness, which is characterized by withdrawal, preoccupation with the self, crying, depression, expression of anger toward others, or feelings of guilt, anger, being different, and being alone. In this phase, the client experiences acute awareness of what has been lost and grieves for what has been lost.

Integration. The third phase of integration is characterized by logical acceptance that change has occurred; keeping emotional distress within manageable limits; reestablishing a sense of self and meaning and purpose; revising life goals; learning to live with uncertainty; and achieving a new means to cope with one's environment.

Anniversary dates of onset, special events and birthdays, and subsequent losses in physical function may trigger sadness. Some persons have been described as experiencing ongoing chronic sorrow related to physical, social, and psychological losses.

GENERAL PSYCHOLOGICAL ADAPTIVE TASKS

A number of general psychological adaptive tasks are related to having and living with a chronic condition. These adaptive tasks include

- Coping with emotional responses of oneself and significant others to the illness experience;
- Coping with the uncertainty of diagnosis and treatment;
- Coming to terms with having a chronic condition;
- Restructuring one's life around the chronic condition;
- Restructuring schedules, priorities, and plans for the future;
- Negotiating new and altered relationships with oneself, family, friends, and the health care system;
- Developing attitudes, knowledge, and skills that enable oneself to actively participate in regimen management;
- Controlling symptoms;
- Preventing and handling acute health crises;
- Dealing with genetic concerns and issues in reproductive decision making; and
- Adapting to changes in physical abilities or appearance.

Personal resources that assist clients in accomplishing these adaptative tasks include life experiences, interests, memories, and the capacity to learn, change behavior, relate to others, solve problems, and express and change feelings. Literature related to psychological adaptation to chronic conditions focuses primarily on the distress component of psychological adaptation. The ways in which clients interpret physical, social, and psychological changes during the course of their illness and the methods they find effective in adapting to these ongoing changes are less well understood.

Different numbers and types of physiologic, psychological, and social events are appraised as distressful by

TABLE 9-3. Common Concerns, Fears, and Personal Changes Associated with Chronic Conditions

Concerns and Fears
Sense of self
Loss of control and predictability
Heightened sense of mortality
Loss of productivity
Loss of valued roles
Loss of relationships
Loss of opportunity or ability for sexual expression
Uncertainty about the future
Purpose and meaning in life
Fear of procedures
Fear of death
Personal Changes
Life plans and goals
Established roles and patterns of interacting within family and outside the home
Relationships with others
Daily routines
Loss of gratifying behaviors
Changes in health maintenance and management behaviors
Activity and sleep patterns
Financial resources
Appearance

clients having the same chronic condition for the same period of time. A number of concerns, fears, and personal change events are common to a variety of chronic conditions; these problems are identified in Table 9-3.

COPING BEHAVIORS

Clients with the same medical diagnosis and in the same phase of chronic illness use a variety of physical, cognitive, and verbal behaviors in managing distress. The type of behaviors used and the appraised effectiveness of the same type of behaviors are highly individual. Some coping behaviors are passive in nature, and others are active in nature. The behaviors are frequently categorized as emotion focused (affective) or problem focused. A number of behaviors fall into both categories.

Interestingly, some clients report that talking about their illness helps them cope, whereas others report that not talking about their illness helps them cope. Strategies reported as effective in managing distressful situations include avoiding, ignoring, accepting, thinking out, or changing the situation. Shopping, driving, going out to eat, and exercising are types of activities some find helpful in relieving stress. Other strategies found to be helpful include taking naps; seeking information and advice; changing values, attitudes, and goals; imagining the worst; hope; prayer; putting the problem in God's hands; humor; positive thinking; positive or negative self-talks; taking anger out on others; trying to maintain some control over the situation; trying to look at the problem objectively; drawing on past experiences; blaming someone else; and taking drugs, eating, smoking, or drinking alcohol.

Sociologic Adaptation

Health/illness roles of clients with chronic conditions overlap with social roles related to age, sex, family, work, and recreation. The degree of impact of health and illness roles on social roles ranges from minimal to severe, with health and illness roles being the dominant life roles. The degree to which clients adapt socially is influenced by changes in physical appearance, ability to communicate, ability to navigate the physical environment, and social resources (e.g., people, money, and community services). Society responds differently to clients with less visible and apparent chronic conditions than to those with more visible signs of illness. Social acceptance is influenced by cultural values and beliefs of oneself and others related to attractiveness, productivity, independence, self-reliance, normalcy, individual rights, and health and illness. These beliefs and values also influence availability of social resources, health services, and funding as well as job, recreational, and housing opportunities (see Bridge to Home Health Care).

Changing social beliefs about individual rights and normalcy have influenced state and federal legislation. This legislation has contributed to a decrease in attitudinal and architectural barriers to social integration as well as the increased availability of health care, housing, employment, and transportation for persons with chronic conditions. The 1990 passage of the Americans with Disabilities Act (PL 101-336) by Congress will further increase social options for persons with chronic conditions. Disability is defined as "physical or mental impairment that substantially limits one or more of an individual's major life activities." Passage of the act was motivated by economic as well as altruistic concerns. Equal access to society will increase social independence and provide opportunities for more disabled people to be employed taxpayers rather than dependent on tax-supported services. The Act addresses access to public accommodations and services, telecommunication relay services, and employment. Unlike previous legislation related to disability, this legislation holds the private sector accountable for the cost of compliance with the Act.

COMMUNICATION PATTERNS

Communication patterns between clients and families with chronic conditions and health care professionals have been described as changing over time and tending to move through three phases. Initially, clients and families have a naive trust in health care workers. A characteristic of this phase is the belief that health care professionals will provide a cure or do what is best for the client. This naive trust is followed by a phase of mistrust and anger. A major source of anger is lack of

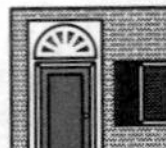

BRIDGE TO HOME HEALTH CARE

Chronic Illness Financial Issues and Support Services in the Community

Finding financial help and support services for the chronically ill client requires much patience and perseverance. A multidisciplinary approach and creative problem solving will enhance continuity of care when bridging this client from the hospital setting to the home environment.

Waiting periods for federal, state, county, and local services such as Medicare, Medicaid, Social Security Disability, and County assistance make early referral essential. Applications to these agencies can be initiated while the client is still hospitalized. A complete assessment should be made of the client's present and future needs. These assessments address not only physical but also financial, environmental, and emotional concerns. Evaluation should include information on the resources of the client, family, and community and their ability to provide these needs and what it takes to mobilize these resources. The home health care team should be sensitive to ethnic, cultural, privacy, and value issues of the client by affirmation of the client's choices and goals.

A tentative approach may provide temporary relief for the client's problem, but a more permanent or long-term solution is preferable and prevents the need to deal with the problem again. An example of this approach would be the client who has no money to purchase his or her medications. Finding a resource to help purchase several days' worth of medications may require only a phone call to a local philanthropic group. However, the long-term solution will require creative problem solving.

When you brainstorm for a solution, remember to include all members of the home health care team. Team members in addition to nursing personnel may be familiar with resources that are frequently used and with the staff members or volunteers who serve as the gatekeepers for those resources. Local churches, human service agencies, clubs, community action groups, and health service organizations can provide numerous resources for supportive care.

---

involvement in decision making. Over time, the second phase is replaced by guarded trust, with trust being placed in some health care professionals and not in others. Health care providers should be aware of these phases and work with the client, providing factual information without denying hope.

SOCIAL CHANGE EVENTS

Social change events commonly associated with having a chronic condition relate to roles and interaction patterns, mobility patterns, employment, living arrangements, recreation, finances, time and place for vacations, and health insurance coverage. Common adjustment tasks include preventing or adjusting to social isolation, normalizing, managing symptoms and treatments in social environments, maintaining physical mobility in the environment, changing present housing or locating new housing, dealing with rejection and discrimination, developing new social skills and social networks, teaching others about the chronic condition and how it interferes with a person's abilities, and learning about community resources.

FAMILY ADAPTATION

Because of the long-term nature of chronic conditions and the role of the family in health maintenance of its family members, a chronic condition is also a family condition. Families as well as the chronically ill client must cope with unusual ongoing adaptive tasks related to the presence of a chronic condition. Family adjustment tasks differ with different phases of the chronic condition. Adaptive tasks during the onset or diagnostic phase that are the same as those related to acute illness include pulling together, learning to cope with the acute care environment and treatment, and establishing relationships with care givers. Additional adaptive tasks during this phase that are specific to chronic conditions are identifying the meaning of the illness, assessing potential changes in the family, moving toward integration of temporary and permanent changes while maintaining a sense of continuity between past and present, and developing an attitude of flexibility toward future personal and family goals.

Additional adaptive tasks during the chronic phase include maintaining a sense of normalcy, adjusting to changing expectations of each family member, striving to balance family resources, and maintaining maximal autonomy of all family members despite the pull toward mutual dependency, care taking, or focus on the ill family member. If a terminal phase is associated with the chronic illness, families must also manage issues related to the death of the client, achieve resolution of mourning following the death of the client, and resume normal individual and family lives.

Some families are more effective than others in accomplishing adaptive tasks. The type of physical impairments, family resources, family perception, developmental stage of family members and family unit, behaviors of the client, and the health care environment are interrelated factors that have an impact on family adaptation. Some family units become stronger, whereas others disintegrate. (Assessment and interventions for the family are also discussed in Chap. 8.)

ETIOLOGY

There are a multitude of etiologies for chronic conditions; a few of the major ones are discussed.

Multifactorial Etiology

Multiple factors interact to cause a chronic condition. The interaction of the factors may be additive or synergistic; that is, they may combine to cause increased harm. For example, asbestos workers have an increased risk of lung cancer. If the asbestos worker smokes, the risk of lung cancer increases 30 times over those co-workers who do not smoke, and the risk increases 90 times over people who neither work with asbestos nor smoke.

Impact of Aging

The process of aging predisposes clients to chronic conditions. Young clients usually have short, intense, acute conditions from which they quickly recover. In contrast, elderly clients usually have long, drawn-out conditions with unpredictable degrees of recovery. It must be pointed out, though, that people in all age groups can develop a chronic illness. For example, an infant may be born with a heart condition, a child may develop diabetes, and a young adult may develop multiple sclerosis. In elderly clients, arthritis, diabetes, hypertension, and heart disease are the most common chronic illnesses.

Technology

Medical success has contributed to the unprecedented growth of chronic conditions. The treatment of infectious illness in children has allowed more people to live to older ages, when chronic illnesses are contracted. Likewise, the development of equipment to sustain life has changed the picture of medical care. For example, the use of dialysis for chronic renal failure has lengthened many lives. And as clients live by means of dialysis, health care providers learn more about the ongoing process of renal failure and living while attached to a lifesaving machine.

Race and Ethnic Background

Race or ethnic background predisposes clients to certain chronic conditions. Race-specific rates measure the association between disease occurrence and race. Data indicate that some conditions are more prevalent in certain races and, sadly, that nonwhite people (black, Native Americans, and Asians) also fail to receive necessary care for the illness. For example, nonwhites are three times more likely to die of hypertension than whites of the same age group. In a 1985 study, six causes of death were identified that together accounted for more than 80 per cent of excess mortality in nonwhite people.[21] The diseases and degree of excess mortality listed were

- Cancer — 16 per cent excess mortality among black males under age 70 and 10 per cent for black females
- Cardiovascular disease and stroke — 24 per cent of excess mortality among black males and 41 per cent among black females
- Chemical dependency, measured by deaths for cirrhosis of the liver, associated with excessive alcohol consumption — 13 per cent of excess mortality in Native American males and 22 per cent among Native American females
- Diabetes — 38 per cent of excess deaths among Mexican-born Hispanic females
- Homicides and accidents (unintentional injury) — 60 per cent of excess mortality among Hispanics under 65; 44 per cent of excess deaths due to unintentional injury in male Native Americans and 30 per cent in female Native Americans. Homicides and unintentional injuries account for 19 per cent of excess mortality among black males under 70 and 38 per cent for those under age 45. The figures for black females are 6 and 14 per cent, respectively. The study noted the association of these deaths with the use of drugs and alcohol.
- Infant mortality — 35 per cent of excess deaths in the first year of life among black females.

Cultural variations may also prevent illness. Mormons, who neither drink nor smoke, have lower cancer rates than the general population.

RISK FACTORS

Risk factors for chronic conditions are as varied as the number of conditions. Chronic illness can develop from an acute illness that is only partially resolved or as a sequela of other illnesses, such as long-standing diabetes.

Although no one is immune from aging, the early recognition of problems can lead to early treatment in some instances. Diagnoses are made earlier in clients with a scientific orientation to health (e.g., "I have to watch my cholesterol level"). These clients have routine check-ups to prevent illness and recognize early symptoms. Clients with a functional orientation to life ("I haven't felt well for months now") only seek medical care when they do not feel well or experience symptoms that interfere with the ability to carry out activities and demands of daily living.

In addition, some disorders have specific forms of medical management with fairly predictable outcomes. Cancer, diabetes, cardiovascular disease, and spinal cord injury have specific management regimens. These diseases can be successfully managed and leave a controllable level of residual defect. In contrast, treatment protocols are less clear cut for clients with multiple sclerosis, systemic lupus erythematosus, Alzheimer's disease, and severe brain injury. A clear understanding of the pathology of some diseases has not yet come about, which delays the development of an exact method of treatment and increases the chronic nature of the disorder.

PATHOPHYSIOLOGY

Chronic conditions interfere with the intake, transformation, and expenditure of physical energy for cellular metabolism, protein synthesis, and body system functioning or coordinated function of body systems. Nutrients and oxygen are primary sources of physical energy. If the intake of nutrients exceeds body energy requirements for basal metabolic processes and physical activity, the excess energy is stored as muscle and fat. The client experiences an increase in body weight. Factors contributing to weight gain in clients with chronic conditions are

- Polyphagia (excessive appetite) secondary to a central nervous system insult, corticosteroids, pickwickian syndrome, or certain endocrine disorders;
- Changes in taste;
- Anxiety;
- Depression; and
- Decreased mobility or sedentary lifestyle.

A number of factors associated with other chronic conditions contribute to energy deficits by interfering with the intake of nutrients, metabolism, or expenditure of energy. Social, psychological, and treatment factors as well as disease-related factors may limit intake of nutrients. The following list includes several of these factors:

- Inability to procure food secondary to physical, economic, transportation, or cognitive limitations;
- Lack of knowledge about adequate nutrition;
- Anorexia, nausea, and vomiting secondary to the disease process, medication or treatments, depressed mood, or anxiety;
- Changes in taste, smell, or vision;
- Inability to feed self;
- Decreased salivation;
- Impaired swallowing; and
- Changes in the structure of the mouth or esophagus.

The process by which nutrients are transformed into physical energy units may be altered by changes in the structure or function of the neurologic, musculoskeletal, circulatory, respiratory, endocrine, or digestive systems. Changes in these body systems may also interfere with the transport and use of energy. Additional energy may be required for physiologic functions and mobility. Body mechanisms can compensate for some changes in physical function; however, these mechanisms may become exhausted over time. When the physical energy demands of a chronic condition exceed the intake and processing of nutrients over time, the body uses reserves of fat and protein as physical energy sources. Use of fat reserves is characterized by a decrease in subcutaneous tissue. Use of protein is characterized by a decrease in visceral protein and muscle mass. The client's general resistance to physiologic stressors is impaired.

Neuroendocrine responses to psychological distress have been associated with the development of chronic conditions such as cardiovascular disease, peptic ulcers, asthma, ulcerative colitis, multiple sclerosis, cancer, and accidental trauma. Neuroendocrine response to distress has also been implicated as a factor in symptoms of anorexia, pain, fatigue, shortness of breath, and decreased immune response; progression of chronic conditions; exacerbations of chronic conditions; and delayed recovery from acute episodes of illness during the course of the chronic illness. Over time, adaptive energy from neuroendocrine sources is believed to become exhausted.

CLINICAL MANIFESTATIONS

As a general rule, the longer a client has a chronic condition, the greater the number of body systems involved. Some chronic conditions are characterized by an abrupt onset of symptoms, whereas others begin gradually over months or years.

Anorexia, fatigue, pain, shortness of breath, sleep disturbance, and impaired mobility are common clinical manifestations of many chronic conditions. Mobility and self-care abilities associated with the chronic phase of chronic conditions comprise a continuum ranging from complete independence, modified independence, and modified dependence to complete dependence. Many illness-related, treatment-related, and psychological factors contribute to immobility. Fatigue, pain, loss of sensation, muscle weakness, paralysis, spasticity, joint stiffness, braces or casts, and enforced chair or bed activity are common factors that contribute to immobility.

Complications

Adaptive responses to prolonged bed rest and decreased levels of mobility occur in the neurologic, cardiovascular, respiratory, digestive, renal, metabolic, integumentary, and immune systems as well as the musculoskeletal system. These adaptive responses, which are commonly referred to collectively as disuse syndrome, increase levels of disability. Common adaptive changes in body systems and nursing diagnoses related to the nursing diagnosis of High Risk for Disuse Syndrome are identified in Table 9-4.

Diagnostic Assessment

There are no specific diagnostic tests for chronic conditions as a whole. Because there are so many types of chronic conditions, specific assessments are used for each of the conditions.

MEDICAL MANAGEMENT

Because there are so many chronic conditions, medical management varies with the condition. A specific form of medical management that focuses on rehabilitation will be discussed here.

Patterns of health care delivery that have been expanded or implemented to address health care needs of persons with chronic conditions include rehabilitation centers, units, and programs; home health care; nurse-managed clinics; hospice care; and case management.

TABLE 9-4. Physiologic Changes Leading to Disease Syndrome

Body System	Physiologic Change
Neurologic	Decreased ability to concentrate
	Reduced stimulation of reticular activation system
	Brain stimulates self with visual and auditory hallucinations
	Sleep disturbance
Cardiovascular	Decreased stroke volume
	Increased heart rate
	Hypovolemia
	Postural hypotension
	Increased procoagulants
	Shortened thromboplastin time. Thromboembolism
	Compression of blood vessels of calves of leg
Pulmonary	Abdominal contents pushing against diaphragm
	Stress on inspiratory muscles
	Stasis of secretions
	Decreased lung volume
	Decreased intake of oxygen
Digestive	Diminished appetite
	Decreased metabolism
	Changes in insulin release pattern and effectiveness
	Decreased peristalsis
Integumentary	Larger surface area of skin bearing weight
	Evaporation of perspiration less efficient than when exposed to air
	Exposure to moist bed linens
	Pressure against bed impairs skin circulation
Renal	Stasis of urine in kidneys; urinary tract infection
	Increased excretion of calcium (formation of urinary calculi)
	Increased excretion of nitrogen
Musculoskeletal	Loss of muscle tone
	Loss of muscle mass
	Contractures
	Heterotrophic bone disease
	Osteoporosis
Immune	Decreased immunity

Rehabilitation

The first rehabilitation center was established approximately 40 years ago in New York by Dr. Rusk, who is known as the father of rehabilitation medicine. He was instrumental in establishing the medical specialty of physiatry, which focuses on physical medicine rehabilitation. Dr. Rusk's interest in rehabilitation evolved from practice experiences with soldiers during World War II. Dr. Rusk also had a personal experience in which he told the family of a woman who had a stroke that she would never walk or talk again. The family returned 1 year later with the woman, who was walking and talking.

Traditional goals of rehabilitation have been prevention of physical deformity, maintenance of physical function, restoration of function, client and family education, and reintegration of the client into his or her family and society. Strategies used to achieve these goals included using an interdisciplinary team approach, beginning discharge planning on admission, preventing deformity, maintaining skin integrity, and providing the family and the client with information and skills. Over the years, these strategies have also become integrated into acute care and are used to address the problems of chronic pain, cardiovascular disease, and chronic obstructive lung disease.

The original multidisciplinary team of physiatrist, nurses, physical therapists, occupational therapists, speech therapists, and psychologists has expanded to include dieticians, respiratory therapists, and practitioners from the newer disciplines of neuropsychology and recreational therapy. The team members apply their knowledge and skills in assisting clients in regaining functional abilities and acquiring knowledge and skills that maximize their ability to live with physical disability. Clients served are those with severe disability secondary to neurologic or musculoskeletal trauma (accidental and surgical) or illnesses. Many clients with chronic conditions such as arthritis, cancer, amytrophic lateral sclerosis, and multiple sclerosis would benefit from knowledge of assistive devices and techniques that compensate or substitute for lost physical function. Acquiring skills in using these devices and techniques would improve their functional levels. Unfortunately, many clients who could benefit from these services are not referred owing to health professionals' lack of knowledge about these services or third-party hesitancy to pay for these services.

The multidisciplinary approach and physical conditioning have been implemented in inpatient and outpatient rehabilitation programs for clients with cardiac diseases, chronic obstructive lung disease, and chronic pain. Exercise does not reverse pathophysiologic changes, but it is believed to condition muscles so that they work more efficiently and use less oxygen. Exercise also stimulates the production of endorphins that promote feelings of well being, increases production of high-density lipoproteins, assists in weight control, and increases exercise tolerance.

Illness Trajectory

A trajectory is the course of something indicating predictable direction and movement. In health care, the term trajectory is used to describe the process of any

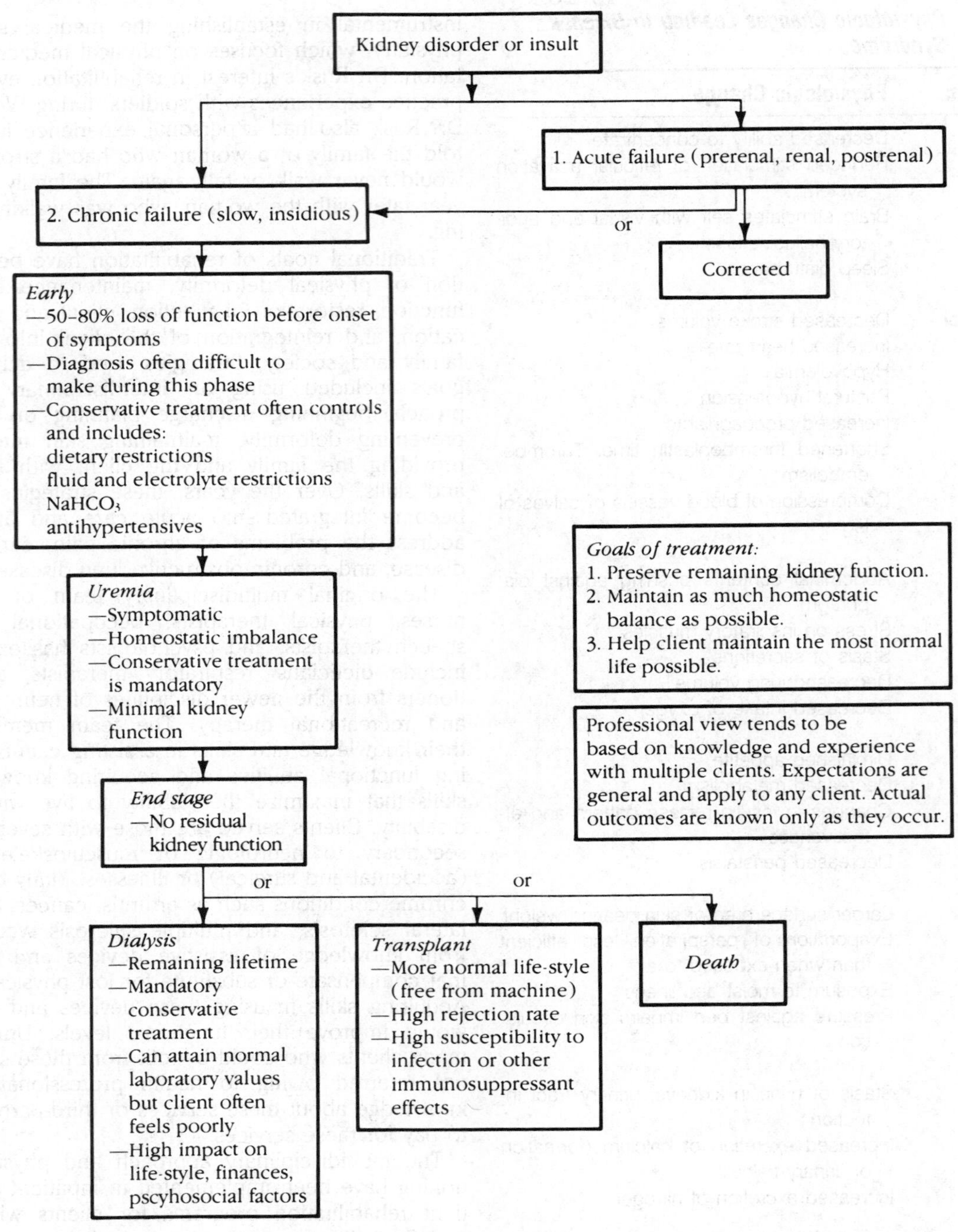

▲ **Figure 9–1**

Trajectory: Professional perception of renal failure. (From Lubkin, I. [1986]. *Chronic illness* [p. 27]. Boston: Jones and Bartlett © 1990, Boston: Jones and Bartlett Publishers. Reprinted by permission.)

disorder. A trajectory begins with a pathophysiologic event and ends with resolution of the problem or development of another problem (e.g., a complication). By taking into account a disorder's symptoms, phases, and treatment over time, it is possible to predict potential and probable outcomes. Physicians use the knowledge of disease trajectory to recognize probable outcomes and to plan treatments to correct, reverse, or slow a disease's progression. Nurses also use trajectories. Consider the extensive knowledge base nurses have on the postoperative recovery of clients. Nurses know that pain is managed with injections early in the course of disease and later with oral analgesia. Likewise, the client is assessed for possible complications along a trajectory (e.g., atelectasis, thrombus, and wound infection).

Illness trajectories seldom take into account the psychological aspects of a disease, because most of the time psychological adaptation is an individual variable in the disease. As more clients live, the quality of life must become an essential aspect of any disease trajectory.

Interesting twists to the development of illness trajectories have occurred. Consider the increasing number of infants who survive prematurity and clients saved through technologic advances. These clients would have never lived before, so a full trajectory of likely long-term complications is not known.

With the ongoing development and refinement of equipment and medications, the traditional disease trajectories have had to be redefined. An example of a redefined trajectory is in the client with end-stage renal disease. In the past, clients with end-stage renal disease would have died, but today these clients live through the use of dialysis and renal transplantation. Because dialysis keeps clients with end-stage renal disease alive but does not cure them, the client faces an ongoing battle of dialysis versus dying and transplant versus rejection.

Compounding the issue for the client are the medical opinions. Surgeons advocate transplants, arguing that they free the client from dialysis machines. Nephrologists advocate dialysis, pointing out the number of transplant rejections. Figure 9–1 is a trajectory of the physician's view of end-stage renal disease. Figure 9–2 represents the client's view of the same illness. The difference in concerns is obvious.

A trajectory can be used to plan and intervene to shape the course of the disease. With chronic illness, these tasks may go on at home or in the hospital. Once

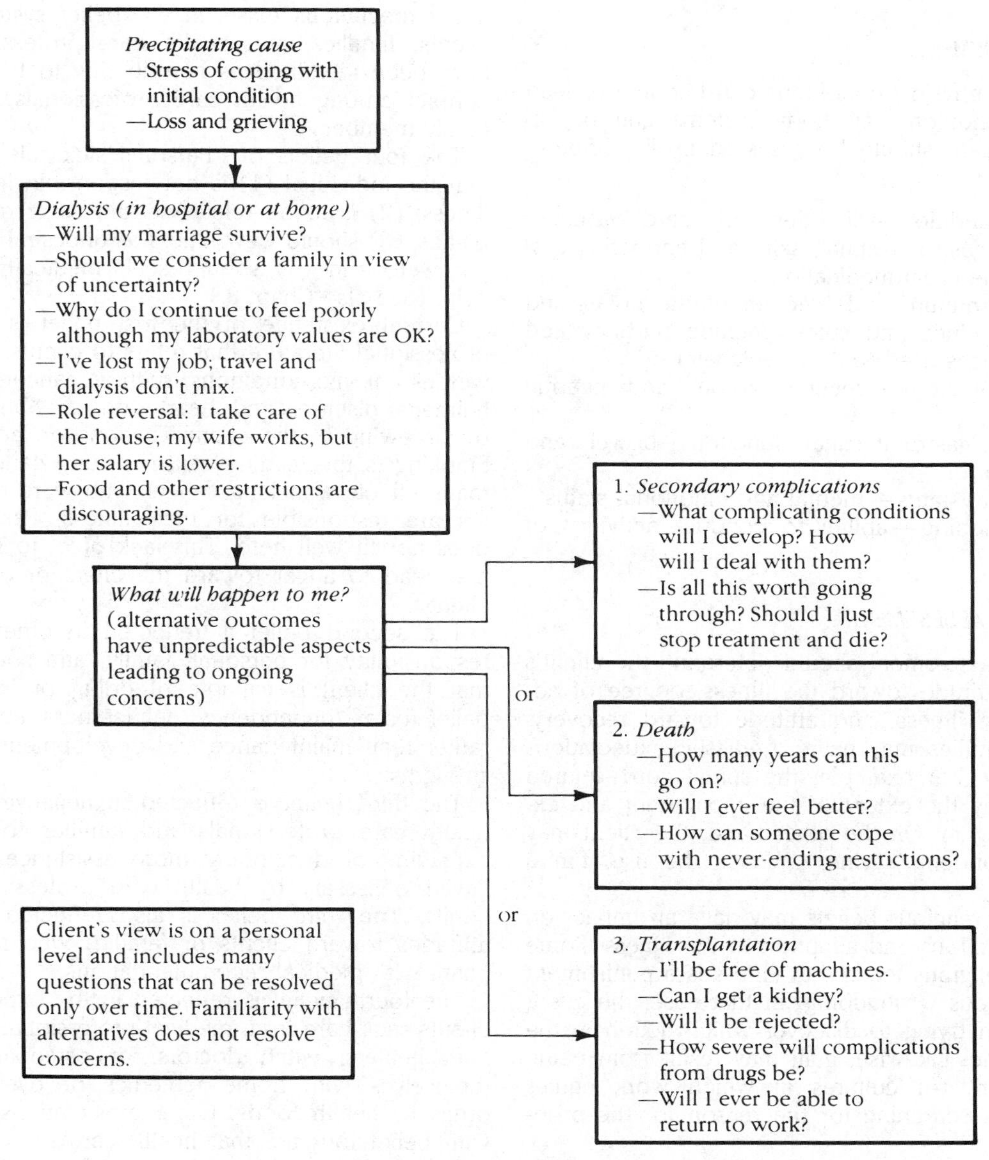

▲ **Figure 9–2**

Trajectory: A client's perception of renal failure. The client is a 30-year-old man who is married and has no children. Also, he is a salesman and is required to travel regularly. (From Lubkin, I. [1986]. *Chronic illness* [p. 28]. Boston: Jones and Bartlett © 1990, Boston: Jones and Bartlett Publishers. Reprinted by permission.)

a trajectory for a client is written out, it should be a part of the client's permanent record to provide continuity of care.

NURSING MANAGEMENT

Assessment

Because a chronic illness has a tremendous impact on the client and family, a complete assessment should be performed in the physical, psychological, and sociologic realms before developing a plan of care. Owing to the nature of chronic conditions, a cure is not expected. Therefore, facilitating the client's adaptation to the condition is the focus of assessment and the goal of care.

PHYSICAL ASSESSMENT

Because many physical conditions can become or lead to chronic conditions, all body systems can be involved. The client should be assessed in six different areas:

1. Physical condition—disorders of cardiovascular, pulmonary, gastrointestinal, skin, and endocrine systems. Include usual medications
2. Mobility—structure and function of the upper and lower extremities and spine. Include mobility and support devices used (e.g., wheelchair)
3. Sensory limitations—speech, vision, and hearing limitations
4. Renal and gastrointestinal function—bowel and bladder control
5. Psychological status—mental and emotional status
6. Basic functioning—ability to conduct activities of daily living

PSYCHOLOGICAL ASSESSMENT

Psychological assessment should determine the client's and family's attitude toward the illness, degree of adaptation to the illness, and attitude toward recovery. Clients and families may have unrealistic expectations about recovery. For example, the spinal cord-injured client may deny the extent of the impairment and expect to walk again. On the other hand, the client may become despondent, saying, "What's the use, I'm a cripple."

Cultural and religious beliefs may have an impact on the client's reactions and adaption to the illness. Some cultures and religions teach that illness is a punishment for some previous wrongdoing. In that case, the client may struggle in trying to discover which action in the past is to blame. Likewise, guilt may result from being unable to work (in cultures in which work equals worth) or from searching for the reason for the problem.

When performing a psychological assessment, the nurse must be open and nonjudgemental about the client's perception of the illness and process of recovery. If the nurse considers the client's reaction to illness wrong or silly, the client will not be open to discussing his or her true feelings.

SOCIOLOGIC ASSESSMENT

Sociologic assessment considers the degree of impact the condition has on health and illness roles.

Sick Role Expectations. Forty years ago, medical sociologist Talcott Parsons identified four beliefs and expectations about behaviors appropriate for ill persons that were dominant in our society and among health care professionals. These beliefs and behavioral expectations applied to persons with acute physical illness rather than to persons with psychiatric or chronic illness. Although beliefs and expectations about persons who are ill are changing, an element of these beliefs and expectations exists in the belief system of some clients, families, and health care professionals. They have been identified as contributing to frustration and conflict among health care professionals, clients, and family members.

The four beliefs of "Parson's sick role model" are that the individual (1) is not responsible for his or her illness, (2) is to be released from usual role responsibilities, (3) should view illness as undesirable and try to get well, and (4) should seek medically competent help. (See also Chap. 3.)

Current existence of the first belief is reflected in professional literature that refers to clients as victims of various chronic conditions, such as cancer, stroke, Alzheimer's disease, and heart attacks. Some disorders occur owing to the clients' actions or lack of action. Smoking is the leading cause of lung cancer. Because many clients with lung cancer who were or are smokers are responsible for their illness, Parson's model does not fit well here. This lack of fit to social norms may lead to anger toward the client or denial by the client.

The second belief is reflected in others' assuming responsibility for personal, family, and social activities that the client is capable of doing or learning. This belief fosters dependency, helplessness, and regression rather than maintenance and development of personal strengths.

The third belief is reflected in negative attitudes of health care professionals and families toward clients expecting or demanding more assistance than is believed necessary by health care professionals or the family. The third belief is also reflected in negative attitudes toward clients or families who are noncompliant with medical recommendations.

The fourth belief is reflected in the expectation that clients seek care from medical professionals rather than faith healers, witch doctors, or osteopaths or treat themselves with home remedies or over-the-counter drugs or health foods. Other expectations interrelated with belief four are that health care professionals will provide a cure and that following the medical regimen will result in a cure.

In addition to the response to illness and sick role, the nurse should consider the client's response to feel-

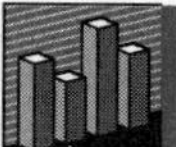

NURSING RESEARCH

Chronic illness in one parent of a family with children can cause disruption in many areas of the family's functioning. The ill adult must cope with changes in the family structure, changes in emotional and interpersonal relationships, loss or change in his or her ability to work, and physical changes from the illness. The purpose of this study was to explore the patterns of functioning in families with one chronically ill adult member.

The population studied contained 67 adults with conditions of cardiovascular disease, arthritis or collagen disorders, diabetes, and multiple sclerosis. A sickness impact profile was used to measure the perception of the severity of the chronic illness and a family environmental scale was used to measure social environmental characteristics.

The patterns of functioning were grouped into clusters. The highest cluster was that of cohesiveness. This cluster was characterized by cohesion, moral-religious values, and intellectual-cultural orientation. The second largest cluster were families in the moral-religious cluster. These families placed their highest emphasis on religion and moral values. These families placed less emphasis on the intellectual and cultural development issues.

It is hoped that these clusters that describe the patterns of family functioning can add to the understanding of how family dynamics can have an impact on client outcomes.

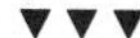

Stuifbergen, A. (1990). Patterns of functioning in families with a chronically ill parent: An exploratory study. *Research in Nursing & Health, 13*(1), 35–44.

ings of attractiveness, normalcy, productivity, self-reliance, and use of community services.

Demands of Illness. The demands of illness are the events or experiences that clients and families attribute to the illness that tax the family's personal and social resources and, thus, the family's well being.[8] Some demands result from the treatment of the condition, for example, changing work schedules to accommodate treatments or loss of strength due to side effects of the treatment. Likewise, the roles of the client may have to be assumed by other family members or friends. If the client is the breadwinner of the family, the tasks of earning a living will have to be assumed by another person. The demands of the illness are also affected by the perception of the client and family during the course of the illness. Initially, the illness may generate a lot of support from extended family members, because they can be freed from work for a few days. But as the disease process continues, the members may be difficult to call on because demands of work and family have drawn them back home. This puts all of the responsibilities on the immediate family and may create a temporary crisis until new support networks can be arranged (See Nursing Research Box).

ASSESSMENT TOOLS

Assessment tools found to yield reliable data about functional abilities of clients with chronic conditions are described in Table 9–5. The Barthel Index and the Rancho Los Amigos scale are commonly used in rehabilitation centers to quantify functional gains during the acute rehabilitation phase of recovery. The Functional Independence Measure (FIM) is a more recently devised instrument that is gaining acceptance.

These assessment tools can be used to quantify physical or cognitive abilities of clients in other settings. For example, the Rancho Los Amigos scale (Table 9–6) would be useful for quantifying changes in cognitive functioning evidenced by clients experiencing acute or chronic conditions that alter brain function. Levels of cognitive functioning in the scale are based on clinical observations of physical and cognitive behaviors evidenced by clients during recovery from severe head trauma. The scale contains indicators of changing abilities related to taking in, processing, and responding to information.

Nursing Diagnosis

PHYSIOLOGIC NURSING DIAGNOSES

A number of physiologic nursing diagnoses are commonly associated with a variety of chronic conditions and medications and treatments used in managing chronic conditions. Owing to the great number of chronic conditions, many related factors contribute to the diagnoses. These factors include age, type and degree of irreversible change in physiologic structure or function, type of treatment, and degree of physiologic adaptation. Nursing diagnoses of a physiologic nature common to several types of chronic conditions include

Activity Intolerance;
Disuse Syndrome, High Risk For;
Fatigue;
Fluid Volume, Deficit or Excess;
Health Maintenance, Altered;
Infection, High Risk For;
Injury, High Risk For;
Nutrition, Altered, Less than or More than Body Requirements;
Pain, Acute and Chronic;
Physical Mobility, Impaired;
Self-Care Deficit;
Thought Processes, Altered; and
Urinary Elimination, Altered.

PSYCHOLOGICAL NURSING DIAGNOSES

Potential nursing diagnoses of a psychological nature include

Anxiety;
Body Image Disturbance;
Decisional Conflict;
Diversional Activity Deficit;

TABLE 9–5. Assessment Tools

Physical Function	
Barthel Index	Nine categories: feeding, transfers, grooming, toileting, bathing, walking, climbing stairs, bowel and bladder control
PULSES	Six categories: *P*resence of medical conditions, *U*pper extremity (self-care), *L*ower extremity (walking), *S*ensory, *E*limination (bowel and bladder control), *S*ocialization
Index of Activities of Daily Living (ADL)	Six categories: bed activities, transfers, hygiene, dressing, feeding, and locomotion
Functional Independence Measure (FIM)	Eighteen categories: eating, grooming–upper body, dressing–lower body, toileting, bladder management, bowel management, transfers (bed, chair, wheelchair), transfers–toilet, transfers–tub or shower, locomotion, stairs, comprehension, expression, social interaction, problem solving, memory
Cognitive Function	
Rancho Los Amigos	Eight levels of responses: none, generalized, localized, confused-agitated, confused-inappropriate, confused-appropriate, automatic-appropriate, purposeful-appropriate
Pain	
McGill Pain Questionnaire	Comprehensive and modified versions. Modified—20 sets of sensory, affective, evaluative, and miscellaneous descriptors of pain. Includes pain intensity scale, and body location of pain
Visual Analog Scales	Numbers or faces for rating intensity of pain
Coping	
Ways of Coping Scale	Fifty cognitive and behavioral strategies used in managing distress
Jaloweic Coping Scale	Forty coping behaviors used to manage distress rated according to helpfulness

TABLE 9–6. Rancho Los Amigos Hospital: Scale of Cognitive Functioning

Level of Response	Behavior
I None	Unresponsive to auditory, visual, or tactile stimuli
II Generalized	Reacts inconsistently and nonpurposively to stimuli. Delayed and limited responses
III Localized	Reacts specifically but inconsistently to stimuli. Responses are related to type of stimuli presented, such as visually focusing on an object or responding to sounds
IV Confused-agitated	Extremely agitated and in a high state of confusion. Nonpurposeful and aggressive behavior. Unable to fully cooperate with treatments owing to short attention span. Requires maximal assistance with self-care
V Confused-inappropriate, nonagitated	Alert and can respond to simple commands on a more consistent basis. Highly distractible. Needs constant cueing to attend to an activity. Memory is impaired, with confusion regarding past and present. Can perform self-care activities with assistance. May wander, and needs to be watched carefully
VI Confused-appropriate	Shows goal-directed behavior, but still needs direction. Follows simple tasks consistently, and shows carry-over for relearned tasks. More aware of his or her deficits, and has increased awareness of self, family, and basic needs
VII Automatic-appropriate	Appears oriented in home and hospital, and goes through daily routine automatically. Shows carry-over for new learning, but still requires structure and supervision to ensure safety and good judgment. Able to initiate tasks in which he or she has an interest
VIII Purposeful-appropriate	Totally alert, oriented, and shows good recall of past and recent events. Independent in the home and community

Fear;
Grieving;
Growth and Development, Altered;
Hopelessness;
Knowledge Deficit;
Powerlessness;
Self-Esteem Disturbance; and
Spiritual Distress.

SOCIOLOGIC NURSING DIAGNOSES

Potential nursing diagnoses of a sociologic nature commonly associated with chronic conditions include

Communication, Impaired Verbal;
Decisional Conflict;
Diversional Activity Deficit;
Family Processes, Altered;
Parenting, Altered;
Powerlessness;
Role Performance, Altered;
Sexuality Patterns, Altered;
Social Interaction, Impaired; and
Social Isolation.

Planning: Expected Outcomes

The expected outcomes for the client with a chronic condition are directly related to the specific diagnosis. In general, a cure is not expected, and instead the client should be assisted to adapt to the condition. The client and family or care giver may need to be educated in order to control the condition and adapt to the change in roles. Long-term expected outcomes are usually written with months allowed for achievement.

Nursing Intervention

Interventions for the client with a chronic illness vary depending on the disorders the client is experiencing. Many times, interventions are collaborative among all health care providers. Regardless of the disorders the client has, there are some general tasks that the client must accomplish. Client education plans should center on these tasks. (See Client Education Guide.) In addition, the client needs to learn to adapt to the illness.

PROMOTING PHYSICAL ADAPTATION

The client's adaptation to chronic illness can be improved by changing medications, dosages or schedules, diet, and activity patterns. Identifying environmental or behavioral factors that exacerbate symptoms or reduce sleep can also increase feelings of wellness. Early detection of clinical manifestations of complications is also part of physical adaptation.

PROMOTING PSYCHOLOGICAL ADAPTATION

Interventions to enhance psychological adaptation during the onset or diagnostic phase include encouraging the client's active involvement in the diagnostic process and treatment decisions (see Ethical Issues in Nursing), facilitating expressions of feelings, and providing or helping clients seek appropriate information. Hospitalization during the chronic phase of a chronic condition may be perceived as a crisis episode by some clients. Other clients may view hospitalization during this phase as a reprieve from day-to-day hassles and concerns or as a period of hope. In the terminal phase of illness, one client may fear death and another client may view death as a preferred alternative to suffering and disability. Personal factors that are believed to contribute to the individual nature of psychological adaptation include hope, commitment, learned helplessness, appraisals of changes, and personal and social resources and coping strategies. Appraisals of change are based on an individual's given set of beliefs, commitments, knowledge and skills, previous losses, and threat of loss with this crisis. The ability to manage loss, the threat of loss, or challenge also differs among individuals.

PROMOTING SOCIOLOGIC ADAPTATION

Interventions that promote sociologic adaptation include referral to community resources or organizations for vocational rehabilitation and job skills training. Interventions that foster and support role changes include role playing of anticipated situations; imaginative role taking, in which the individual imagines how another person would respond to behaviors; and role modeling, in which the individual is introduced to another person who has the same chronic condition and has positively adapted to changes presented. With use of role modeling, the individual may gain practical tips about hunting for a job, finding accessible housing, and meeting new friends.

Role clarification is a strategy in which the individual is provided with information about behaviors necessary to accomplish a particular role. Reference group interaction is a strategy in which support groups with similar problems and concerns are found. These groups are helpful for exchanging ideas for solving problems.

Evaluation

The degree of goal attainment should be examined at regular intervals. The expected outcomes for clients with chronic conditions are obtained over the long term, and evaluation may be used as a formal process to examine outcome achievement and movement to another level of care within a rehabilitational center. For example, the client may no longer require complete care for activities of daily living and can be moved to a less skilled area of the hospital or center. Of course, the goal may not have been met. In these instances, the cause should be determined, keeping in

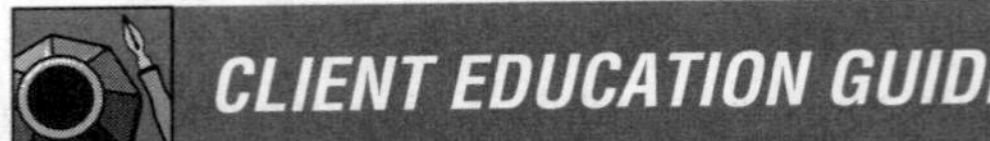

CLIENT EDUCATION GUIDE

Components of a Client Education Plan

Preventing and Managing a Medical Crisis

Most chronic illnesses exist in a balance of control and out of control, or crisis. The client needs to know the clinical indications that the disorder is becoming out of control, what to do to treat it, and when to notify the physician. For example, the diabetic needs to recognize hyperglycemia and hypoglycemia, begin treatment, and determine when to notify the physician. The client needs to learn to plan for these crises. The diabetic client should carry a blood glucose assessment device, sugar, and insulin at all times. Likewise, the asthmatic client should carry a bronchodilator, and the client with angina should carry nitroglycerin.

Managing Treatment Regimens

Most chronic illnesses require some degree of daily treatment. These treatments can range from taking one pill a day, to giving injections, to running a home dialysis unit. The ability of the client and family to follow the treatment should be assessed using the following guidelines:

1. Degree of difficulty in learning to follow the regimen. Are there several steps involved? Are there potential complications that may result from not using the equipment correctly? How much manual dexterity is required?
2. Amount of time required to implement the regimen. Does the activity require several hours or just a few minutes? How many times a day does the activity have to be performed?
3. Amount of discomfort and energy associated with the regimen. If the treatment is painful, will the client comply and will the family member be persuasive enough to have the client complete the treatment?
4. Visibility of the regimen to other people, and social acceptability of the disease regimen. If the equipment must be brought with the client (e.g., oxygen), social isolation may occur. If there has been a physical alteration, such as a tracheostomy or fistula, the client may be shunned by the public.
5. Effectiveness and speed of the regimen in treating the disorder or controlling symptoms. Some clients will follow a treatment regimen if progress can be seen, and others will stop the regimen once symptoms abate.

From these data, a teaching plan can be developed. The use of visiting nurses to monitor progress and assist with financial concerns should be considered.

Controlling Symptoms

Clients must learn to control symptoms so that they can participate in desired activities. Some clients can plan ahead so that needed items are available, such as buying adequate supplies before leaving on a trip. In addition, the client must carry needed supplies on an airplane rather than check them with the luggage, in the event that the luggage is lost. Likewise, some clients require special equipment to perform usual activities. The client with arthritis may benefit by using Velcro closures rather than zippers or buttons.

Reordering of Time

Some clients with chronic conditions have too much time or too little time. For example, clients forced into retirement because of a chronic condition may have too much time on their hands. In contrast, the client who spends hours each day conducting or undergoing the medical regimen may have very little time left to enjoy life. The client needs to be assisted to have the amount of free time desired to enjoy a high-quality life. Sometimes, a hobby or support group will help build supports and new interests. Examining the protocol used by the client in performing medical regimens may illuminate some areas in which time is wasted in the procedure, thereby freeing up time.

Adjusting to Changes in the Course of the Disorder

Some disorders have a stable course and others are very unpredictable. For example, chronic ulcerative colitis is usually quite stable, with predictable flare-ups, whereas multiple sclerosis is an erratic disorder. The client and family need to be taught the disease's trajectory and encouraged to be aware of probable changes. For example, depression is very common 4 to 6 months following stroke. The client and family need to be warned of the symptoms and taught management strategies.

Preventing Social Isolation

Because of the stigma of chronic disorders, the client and family may find it easier to withdraw from society than to face it. The nurse should prepare the client and family by easing adjustment back into society while in the hospital, especially when there is visible deformity, such as burn scars. The client should be encouraged to interact with society while in the hospital. Taking a trip to the gift shop or lobby will allow the client to experience some common reactions, such as staring. Then when the client returns, the feelings can be discussed with the nurse.

Attempting to Normalize Relations with Others

Clients should be encouraged not to become socially isolated but to normalize their lives and resume activities with others. Clients with visible deformity can often disguise the problem with scarves or makeup. Likewise, clients with dyspnea can disguise the fact that they are stopping to catch a breath while they look in a store window.

Some conditions cannot be disguised, and the client should be prepared for stares and comments by strangers. Eventually, the client becomes desensitized to these remarks and goes about his or her life.

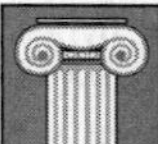

ETHICAL ISSUES IN NURSING

Who Should Make Decisions for Clients?

Caring for clients who have chronic illnesses can be very challenging for nurses. Nurses are called on to deliver many aspects of care to these clients, including helping ease the pain of their illness, listening to the client regarding feelings about his or her illness, assisting in the technological care of their disease process (e.g., dressing changes, tube feedings, IV infusions), and perhaps in helping patients work through their decisions about treatment options. Clients who are in the chronic stages of their illness may come to rely on nurses for care that may go beyond the realm of nursing practice. When decisions become overwhelming, clients might prefer that their health care providers make all the health care decisions for them. On the other hand, are health care decisions ever made for clients with chronic conditions without their input or consent simply because the client is thought to be unable to make the best choices for himself or herself?

There are three ethical principles involved here, the first being autonomy. All clients who are competent have the right to decide what medical treatments they want or do not want. Chronic illness may cause a client to become incompetent, but each client should be assessed carefully before deciding that they are truly not competent. Chronic illness is not always followed by incompetence.

The second and third principles, beneficence and paternalism, are closely related. Nurses act beneficently in many ways, that is, they perform activities that benefit the client, but these actions are not seen as taking away a client's autonomy. For example, crushing a pill for a client who has dysphagia and cannot crush his or her own medications is of benefit to the client but is hardly seen as a dilemma regarding autonomy. On the other hand, paternalism in its extreme form allows health care providers to make decisions for their clients, on their behalf, without their input.

It is sometimes the wish of a client that the nurse or doctor make decisions for them. Perhaps the client feels overwhelmed and simply does not know what to do, or perhaps the client feels that a nurse or doctor would make a better decision on their behalf. Is this any reason to act out of extreme paternalism? Clients with chronic illnesses are probably more vulnerable when it comes to making health care decisions. Nurses should be aware of this so that they do not exercise extreme paternalism when beneficence may be more appropriate. Clients should always be allowed to make their own informed decisions. Nurses may be able to help clients gain the knowledge they need in order to do so, which is a very important act of beneficence.

mind that the condition may have exacerbated and the expected outcomes and interventions may require revision.

ALTERNATIVE HEALTH CARE DELIVERY MODES

Home Health Care

Multidisciplinary home health care is not new. It is a pattern of care delivery that began in New York in the late 1950s due to the shortage of hospital beds. This pattern of care underwent a tremendous spurt of growth in the late 1970s, when the government instituted financial reimbursement for care based on diagnostic groupings (DRGs). (See Chap. 2.) Home health care agencies provide care to clients recovering from acute episodes of illness as well as to clients in the chronic and terminal phases of a chronic illness. Services provided include laboratory monitoring, intravenous therapy for antibiotics and chemotherapy, pump-driven feedings, respiratory support, peritoneal dialysis, physical therapy, parenteral nutrition, and a wide range of nursing services. Concern has been expressed about the quality of service provided by some of the home health agencies, and a movement has been started for the accreditation of home health agencies.

Hospice Care

The first hospice care program was implemented in this country in the late 1960s. Hospice care programs address health care needs of clients in the terminal phase of chronic illness. Some programs are acute-care based, some are based in long-term care agencies, and others are operated by community groups. Some are accredited by an outside agency, and others are not. Some are multidisciplinary, and others are not. Services provided are pain control, palliative and supportive care for clients, and supportive care and bereavement care for significant others. Care is provided in the home or in a hospice facility.

Nurse-Managed Clinics

Nurse-managed clinics are a revival of a concept of care that dates back to the early 1900s. The majority of these clinics focus on health maintenance. Some address physical and psychosocial needs of clients in the chronic phase of chronic illnesses with less defined treatments, such as multiple sclerosis, myasthenia gravis, and Parkinson's disease. Lack of reimbursement for these services has limited the growth of this type of care.

Case Management

Case management is a care delivery mode that was expanded in the late 1970s to incorporate concepts of continuity and efficiency in addressing long-term physical, psychological, and social needs of clients. The primary goals of case management are promotion of self-care, promotion of quality of life, and efficient use of resources. A health care professional, usually a nurse or social worker, assesses and monitors the availability of client needs and services. The type of monitoring may be intermittent or continuous. The case manager directly negotiates with the client, family, health care institutions, insurance companies, or businesses for health and social services needed by the client. The case manager is a consultant to clients and families, and empowers them in planning for and obtaining needed care.

Summary

The number of clients with chronic conditions is increasing and will continue to increase in our society. Nursing practice for these clients includes a complete understanding of the condition and its trajectory as well as the psychological adjustments and sociologic impact of the condition. The client and family must be assisted to adapt to the condition and recover some degree of normalcy in their lives.

Bibliography

1. Bronstein, K. S., et al. (1991). *Promoting Stroke Recovery.* St. Louis, Mosby.
2. Flavo, D., et al. (1982). Psychosocial aspects of invisible disability. *Rehabilitation Literature, 43*(1-2), 2-6.
3. Felton, B., & Revenson, T. (1987). Age differences in coping with chronic illness. *Psychology and Aging, 2*(2), 164-171.
4. Felton, B., et al. (1984). Stress and coping: An explanation of psychological adjustment among chronically ill adults. *Social Science Medicine, 18*(10), 889-898.
5. Folkman, S., & Lazarus, R. (1988). Coping as a mediator of emotions. *Journal of Personality and Social Psychology, 54*(3), 466-471.
6. Foxall, M., et al. (1985). Adjustment patterns of chronically ill middle-aged persons and spouses. *Western Journal of Nursing Research, 7*(4), 425-444.
7. Frank, R., et al. (1987). Differences in coping styles among persons with spinal cord injury: A cluster-analytic approach. *Journal of Consulting and Clinical Psychology, 55*(5), 727-731.
8. Fugate-Woods, N., et al. (1989). Supporting families during chronic illness. *IMAGE: The Journal of Nursing Scholarship, 21*(1), 46-50.
9. Gass, K. (1987). The health of conjugally bereaved older widows: The role of appraisal, coping and resources. *Research in Nursing and Health, 10*(1), 29-47.
10. Gurkles, J., & Menks, E. (1988). Identification of stressors and use of coping methods in chronic hemodialysis patients. *Nursing Research, 37*(4), 236-239.
11. Hickey, S. (1986). Enabling hope. *Cancer Nursing, 9*(3), 133-137.
12. Jalowiec, A., & Powers, M. (1981). Stress and coping in hypertensive and emergency room patients. *Nursing Research, 30*(1), 10-15.
13. Lambert, C., et al. (1989). Social support, hardiness and psychological well being in women with arthritis. *Image, 21*(3), 128-131.
14. Lancaster, L. (1988). Impact of chronic illness over the life span. *American Nephrology Nurses Association Journal, 15*(3), 164-168.
15. Leidy, N., et al. (1990). Psychophysiological processes of stress in chronic physical illness: A theoretical perspective. *Journal of Advanced Nursing, 13,* 478-486.

15a. Loomis, M., & Conco, D. (1991). Patients' perceptions of health, chronic illness, and nursing diagnoses. *Nursing Diagnoses 2*(4), 162-170.

16. Mailick, M. (1987). The impact of severe illness on the individual and family: An overview. *Social Work in Health Care, 5*(2), 117-128.
17. Make, B., & Paine, R. (1987). Pulmonary rehabilitation for COPD patients. *Hospital Practice, 22*(1A), 26-27, 31-34.
18. McNett, S. (1987). Social support, threat, and coping responses and effectiveness in the functionally disabled. *Nursing Research, 36*(2), 98-103.
19. Miller, Sr. P., et al. (1990). Stressors and stress management one month after myocardial infarction. *Rehabilitation Nursing, 15*(6), 306-310.
20. Miller, P., et al. (1985). Coping methods and societal adjustments of cardiovascular clients. *Health Values: Achieving High Level Wellness, 9*(4), 10-13.
21. National Center for Health Statistics. (1985). Vital statistics of the United States 1980, vol 11. Mortality, Part B, DHHS Pub No (PHS) 8501102. Washington, DC: US Government Printing Office.
22. Oppenbrier, D., et al. (1988). What patients want to know about home oxygen therapy. *American Journal of Nursing 88*(2), 198-201.
23. Parchert, M., & Simon, J. (1988). The role of exercise in cardiac rehabilitation: A nursing perspective. *Rehabilitation Nursing 13*(2), 198-201.
24. Pollock, S. (1986). Human responses to chronic illness: Physiologic and psychosocial adaptation. *Nursing Research, 35*(2), 90-95.
25. Reed, P. (1986). Religiousness among terminally ill and healthy adults. *Research in Nursing and Health, 9,* 35-41.
26. Reinhard, S. (1988). Case managing community services for hip fractured elders. *Orthopedic Nursing, 7*(5), 42-45.
27. Rolland, J. (1987). Chronic illness and the life cycle: A conceptual framework. *Family Process, 26,* 203-221.
28. Rubin, M. (1988). The physiology of bedrest. *American Journal of Nursing 88*(1), 50-55.
29. Segall, A. (1976). The sick role concept: Understanding illness behavior. *Journal of Health and Social Behavior, 17*(6), 163-170.
30. State University of New York Research Foundation (1990). *Functional Independence Measure.* Buffalo, NY: State University of New York.
31. Sutton, T., & Murphy, S. (1989). Stressors and patterns of coping in renal transplant patients. *Nursing Research, 38*(1), 46-49.
32. Turner, J., et al. (1987). Relationship of stress, appraisal and coping to chronic low back pain. *Behavioral Research Therapy, 25*(4), 281-288.
33. Turk, D., et al. (1980). A sequential criterion analysis for assessing coping with chronic illness. *Journal of Human Stress, 6*(2), 35-40.
34. Weinberger, M., et al. (1987). In support of hassles as a measure of stress in predicting health outcomes. *Journal of Behavioral Medicine, 10*(1), 19-31.

Unit 3

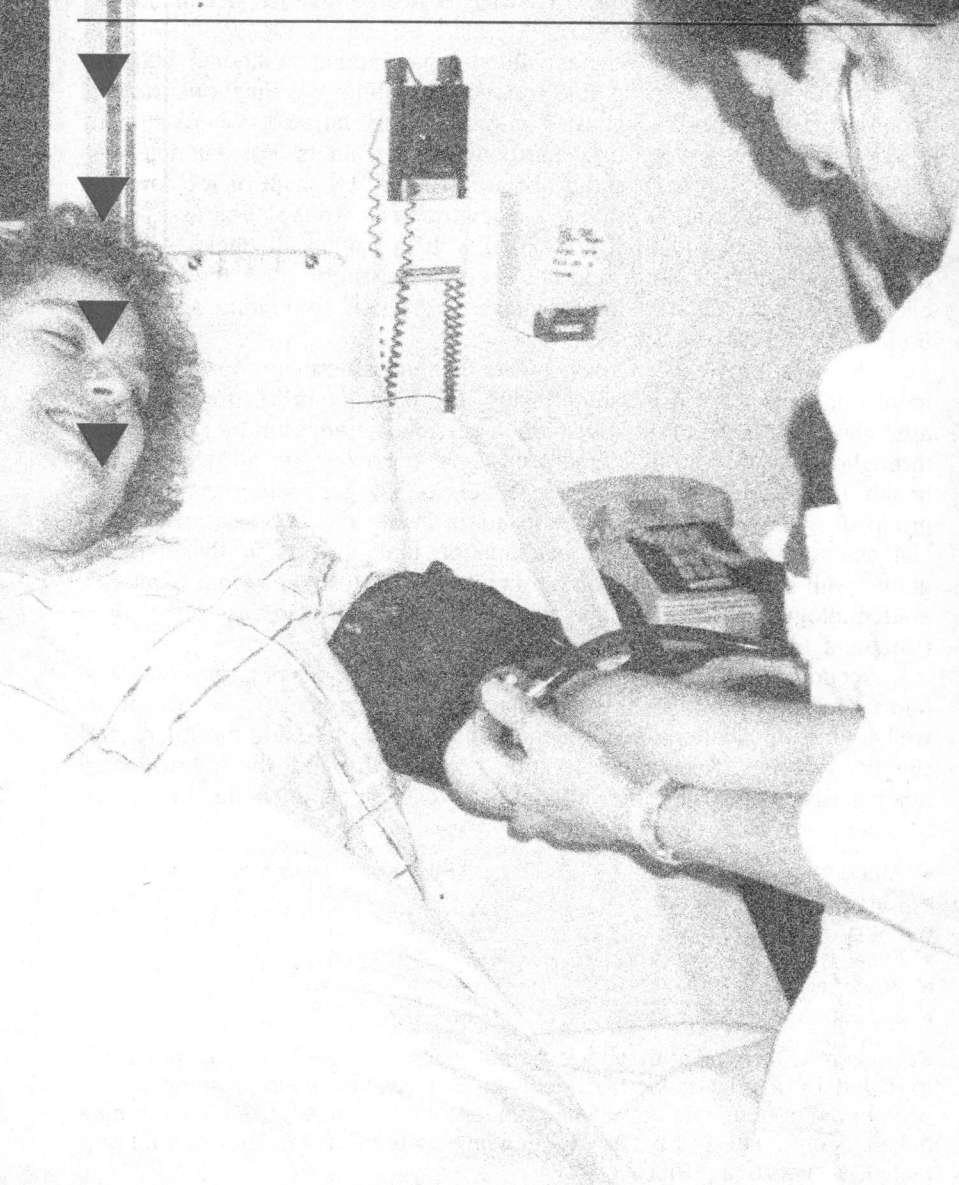

Health Promotion and Assessment

Nursing process is a planned, systematic method used to deliver skilled nursing care. It hinges on careful and thorough assessment of the client, which provides baseline data. Thorough nursing assessment enhances the nurse's ability to identify the client's specific needs, both physical and psychosocial.

The amount, depth, and level of skill used to assess a client will vary with the nurse's knowledge and expertise. Some assessment skills are basic, such as taking a temperature. Advanced assessment skills are learned and practiced so that the nurse may use them to provide direct interventions and to evaluate ill as well as healthy clients' health maintenance and preventive practices.

The nurse must be familiar with the parameters of human behavior and physiology before being able to recognize abnormal situations. Normal ranges for psychosocial behavior may be quite variable, whereas many physiologic manifestations have narrowly defined limits. For example, cell death occurs if body temperature becomes either too high or too low; the defined parameters are a matter of a few degrees. Thus skillful assessment requires careful observation, combined with the ability to decide whether that observation is or is not normal. The nurse also considers the individual client and the client's unique circumstances when comparing assessment findings to standardize norms.

This unit provides an overview of health assessment. Health assessment concepts, basic assessment skills, and parameters for normal ranges are given. Specific body system assessments are further delineated throughout the text to supplement this unit. For example, an occupational health nurse concerned with the incidence of gastroenteritis among a group of workers needs information about health risk appraisal, psychosocial assessment, and physical examination that appears in this unit, together with specific information about the gastrointestinal system (Unit 12), epidemiology (Chapter 25), and fluid-electrolyte and acid-base imbalances (Chapters 14–15).

Accurate nursing diagnosis is fundamental to nursing process. The nurse evaluates how the client reacts to the assessment process itself, as well as the implications assessment findings may have for the client and significant others. Keeping these considerations in mind, the following are nursing diagnosis categories common to clients experiencing health assessment procedures:

- Anxiety
- Knowledge deficit
- Pain
- Fear
- Powerlessness
- Situational low self-esteem

Consistent with nursing diagnosis format, each of these human responses is followed by a related factor identifying the specific cause leading to the problem. For example, a woman undergoing a breast examination may have anxiety related to never experiencing such an examination before and fear of a lump being found.

A client's specific nursing diagnoses are determined by individual needs and problems and not the medical diagnosis. Assessment skills are tools the nurse uses to facilitate the nursing process.

Assessment requires both skill and judgment. This unit provides basic information for the nurse to begin developing expertise in health assessment. Extensive practice is necessary for proficiency. The beginning nurse should also seek guidance from a skilled, competent practicing nurse. A broad knowledge base, repeated practice, and access to a mentor will assist the nurse in developing the ability to discriminate normal from abnormal.

Chapter 10

Health Promotion

Health promotion is about joyful living, actualizing our potentials, and being the best we can be. It is about cleaning up our air, our water, our cities, and ourselves. It is for the well-being of the individual and humanity; it is for and about creating a healthier internal and external environment for all living creatures on planet Earth. Health promotion has to do with the acquisition of mental, physical, and spiritual assets to protect and buffer us from disease as well as move us along the continuum toward high-level wellness.

DEFINITIONS

The term "health" has been defined in a variety of ways from a variety of sources. The most widely accepted definition is the classic 1947 World Health Organization description that states, health is "a state of complete physical, mental, and social well-being and not merely the absence of disease or infirmity" (p. 1).[40]

Likewise a variety of definitions for wellness have been proposed. A synthesized definition is that wellness is the quality or condition of being well, especially of being robust, healthy, and fit. Wellness is not simply the absence of symptoms but incorporates positive mental, physical, and spiritual well-being.

Health promotion is the process of fostering awareness, influencing attitudes and identifying alternatives so that individuals can make informed choices and change their behavior to achieve an optimal level of physical and mental health and improve their physical and social environment.

Health promotion programs are programs designed to improve the health and well-being of individuals and communities by providing people with the information, skill, services, and support they need to undertake and maintain positive lifestyle changes.

Self-responsibility means developing the awareness and ability to take action on behalf of oneself in order to achieve or maintain individual freedom, health, and well-being.

Risk factors are genetic, environmental, or lifestyle factors that increase the probability of developing an illness or disease.

A healthy lifestyle is a manner of day-to-day, positive, action-oriented living that works in a cumulative way to promote health and well-being.

Community is any group of people living together or having close interaction. It includes all people, service providers, support people, administrators, family, and friends who interact in any given setting.

HOLISM AND WELLNESS

Awakening to the importance of both individual and collective health-promoting behaviors is part of the paradigm shift of this age. Ferguson described the social transformation that is occurring concomitantly with the alteration in health behaviors.[12a] Because of the popularity of a holistic approach that began during the 1970s and continues to gain support today, people are focusing attention on a search for patterns of occurrence and causes for their symptoms. Figure 10-1 illustrates how every aspect of each individual being has an influence on every other aspect of oneself.

Because of our holistic makeup, each system has a direct or indirect effect on every other system. These patterns of action occur within the client and also between the client and the ever-changing environment. This permutation then provides an opportunity to constantly renew all areas of our being.

Halpert Dunn was the first person to define and describe the term wellness, a term and an ideal that was the precursor of the health promotion movement.[10] His now classic definition of what he termed "high-level wellness" is "an integrated method of functioning which is oriented toward maximizing the potential of which the individual is capable within the environment where he is functioning." Dunn stressed that wellness is an ongoing process directed toward higher potential, not a static goal, and that high-level wellness is a feeling of being "alive to the tips of the fingers, with energy to burn, tingling with vitality." He postulated that health professionals tend to focus on disease rather than wellness because their training is disease focused rather than wellness or prevention oriented. It is easier to fight against disease than to fight for a condition of greater wellness. Dunn's work may have

	BODY	MIND	SPIRIT
BODY	body body	mind body	spirit body
MIND	body mind	mind mind	spirit mind
SPIRIT	body spirit	mind spirit	spirit spirit

▲ *Figure 10-1*

Body-Mind-Spirit template. (From Keegan, L. & Dossey, B. [1987]. *Self-care: A program to improve your life* [p. 3]. Temple, TX: Bodymind Systems.)

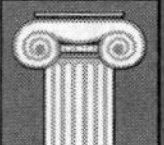

ETHICAL ISSUES IN NURSING

Do Persons Have an Obligation to Avoid Activities Known to Cause Illness that, in Turn, May Burden Society?

Every day there is something in the news about health maintenance or disease prevention. Research is constantly being cited telling us what foods, unsafe practices, or environmental substances cause cancer or disease. It can be a very confusing task to keep up with what one can do to prevent disease. Sometimes, persons can even become ill from something they are not aware of, such as through contaminated water or industrial waste. There are, however, many things people can do to stay healthy and perhaps prevent illness. We are faced with the following dilemma: Do persons have an obligation to avoid activities which are known to cause illness (i.e., smoking, alcohol abuse, high cholesterol diets, obesity and the like) that, in turn, may burden society? And, if they do not avoid such activities and illness occurs, does society have the obligation to care for them?

Modern research provides us with much information regarding the risk factors of disease. The public today are the most well-informed consumers ever. Even so, persons still choose to engage in activities that cause them to have ill health. Should persons be denied the freedom to choose activities, even if these activities cause them harm? Should the government impose sanctions on certain activities in order to prevent potential illness or disease, such as banning cigarette smoking (anywhere) or prosecuting pregnant women who drink alcohol? Should persons be held responsible for their own health-risking behaviors?

To hold persons responsible for their unhealthy behaviors is to hold them responsible for their illnesses that are directly related to such behaviors. Should society have to pay for health care resources used by persons whose illnesses were caused by their own irresponsible behaviors? Should health care workers have an obligation to care for such persons if they have to choose between treating such clients and treating a client, for example, with a congenital disease?

There are no easy answers to these questions. The best role nurses can adopt regarding these issues is that of educator. Education remains one of the best defenses health care providers can give to their clients.

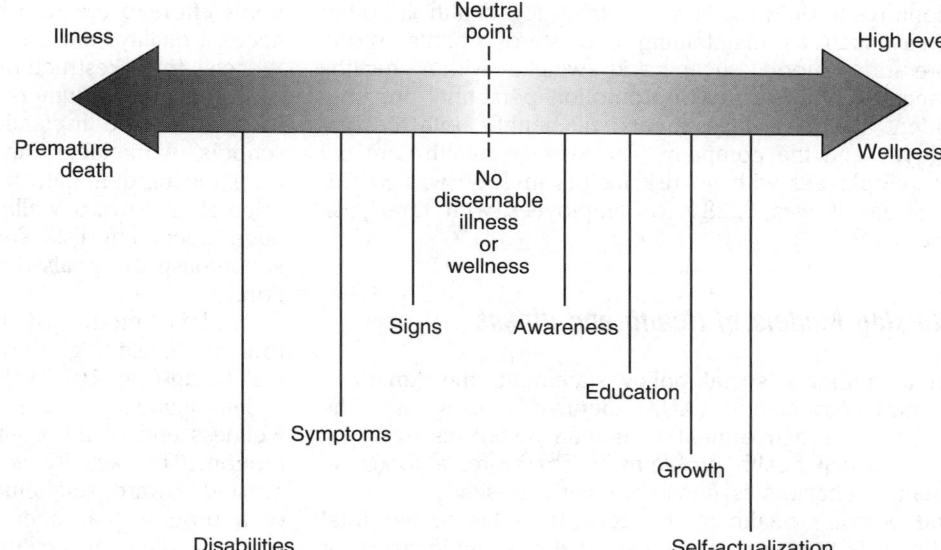

▲ *Figure 10–2*

Wellness model.

been stimulated by the work of medical historian Henry Sigerist.[33] He was the first person to describe the promotion of health as one of the four functions of medicine. The other three functions are prevention of illness, restoration of the sick, and rehabilitation. He believed health included a certain standard of living, good labor conditions, education, physical well being, and rest and recreation. This requires coordinated efforts of large groups, not only the individual.

Travis, a pioneer in the field of wellness, popularized the theoretical concept of wellness through developing and teaching the model illustrated in Figure 10–2.[6] The impact of this model resulted in the recognition that wellness requires attention; it does not happen automatically. The medical model represented on the left side of the figure brings the client back from illness or disease to a neutral point. The right side represents the potential for high-level health and wellness. It is this aspect the field of health promotion addresses. The objective of this model is to demonstrate how people can move from the point of illness or neutrality (no discernible illness or wellness) into the realm of high-level wellness, and to reduce the occurrence or recurrence of illness and disease.

HEALTH PROMOTION

Evolution of the Concept

The field of health promotion grew alongside the emerging ideology and practice of wellness that developed during the 1970s and 1980s. Initially, it found expression in Canada, with the publication of the Lalonde Report,[22] and in the United States, in the Surgeon General's Report "Healthy People."[37] Both of these documents discuss the significance of environmental factors in influencing health and do not limit themselves to a discussion of individual lifestyle or personal behavior issues, which hallmark the wellness movement. The Lalonde Report made recommendations in four equally weighted areas: (1) human biology, (2) environment, (3) lifestyle, and (4) health care organization. The Surgeon General's Report argued that "we are killing ourselves" not only by "our own careless habits" but also by polluting the environment and permitting harmful social conditions to exist. For the first time, attention was directed toward environmental concerns with issues such as toxic-agent control and occupational health and safety. This report was followed by the clearly articulated and measurable "Health Promotion/Disease Prevention: Objectives for the Nation."[38] This report listed specific activities for achieving each objective as proposed in "Healthy People." These publications also prompted agencies to focus on prevention and promotion through strategies of institutional change, legislation, and public policy and not merely in the realm of personal behavior change.[36] Labonte, a health educator, believes that the ultimate challenge is to create social and health conditions that allow all the world's citizens to achieve a state of good health.[20]

As data continue to grow in this field, evidence demonstrates that social class is one of the major risk factors for developing illness and disease.[18, 19, 23, 35] Social class and lifestyle behavior are so interrelated that they must be addressed together. Broad-based interventions that target all aspects of living, such as lifestyle behaviors and social, economic, political, and environmental factors are now under way (see Ethical Issues in Nursing).

Offering incentives in the workplace is the most recent innovation in health promotion. In 1991, 1053 United States companies were polled regarding monetary incentives for staying well. Nine per cent of the firms already offered financial rewards for healthy living, with numerous other firms ready to institute monetary reward programs. The concept started during the 1980s with the problem of smoking, when some insurance companies reduced premiums for nonsmokers. Now other companies are offering similar discounts contingent on promises to strive for health in other areas such as maintaining cholesterol counts, blood pressure, blood sugar, and weight within healthy ranges. Company health-promotion personnel are confident that these investments will benefit both the employee and the company. The average health care bill for employees with no risk factors in 1989 was $1273, whereas it was $2284 for employees with three risk factors.[42]

Nursing Models of Health and Illness

In a landmark social policy statement, the American Nurses' Association (ANA) defined nursing as, "the diagnosis and treatment of human responses to actual or potential health problems."[2] Therefore, a focus on health behaviors is consistent with nursing's focus on the person's health in the context of his or her total life.[1] It is the term "potential" that has significance for the area of health promotion.

The ANA's 1991 document "Nursing's Agenda for Health Care Reform" specifically addresses health promotion. The first paragraph of the executive summary states "America's nurses have long supported our nation's effort to create a health care system that assures access, quality, and services at affordable costs. . . . We call for a restructured health care system that will focus on the consumers and their health, with services to be delivered in familiar, convenient sites, such as schools, workplaces, and homes. We call for a shift from the predominate focus on illness and cure to an orientation toward wellness and care." The entire 22-page document lists specific goals and strategies to accomplish the goals directly related to health promotion.

Penders' model of health promotion is directed toward developing individual resources that enhance well-being (Fig. 10-3).[30]

Self-initiated activities with goals directed toward the wellness end of the continuum reflect true health promotion. This activity is one of always becoming, or moving toward self-actualization, and is characteristic of a process that occurs over an entire lifespan. An understanding of health promotion is necessary for client goal setting, outcomes, and the development of different patterns of health related behaviors.[9] Laffrey and associates agree that the focus on health promotion behavior "logically fits within the scope of nursing."[21]

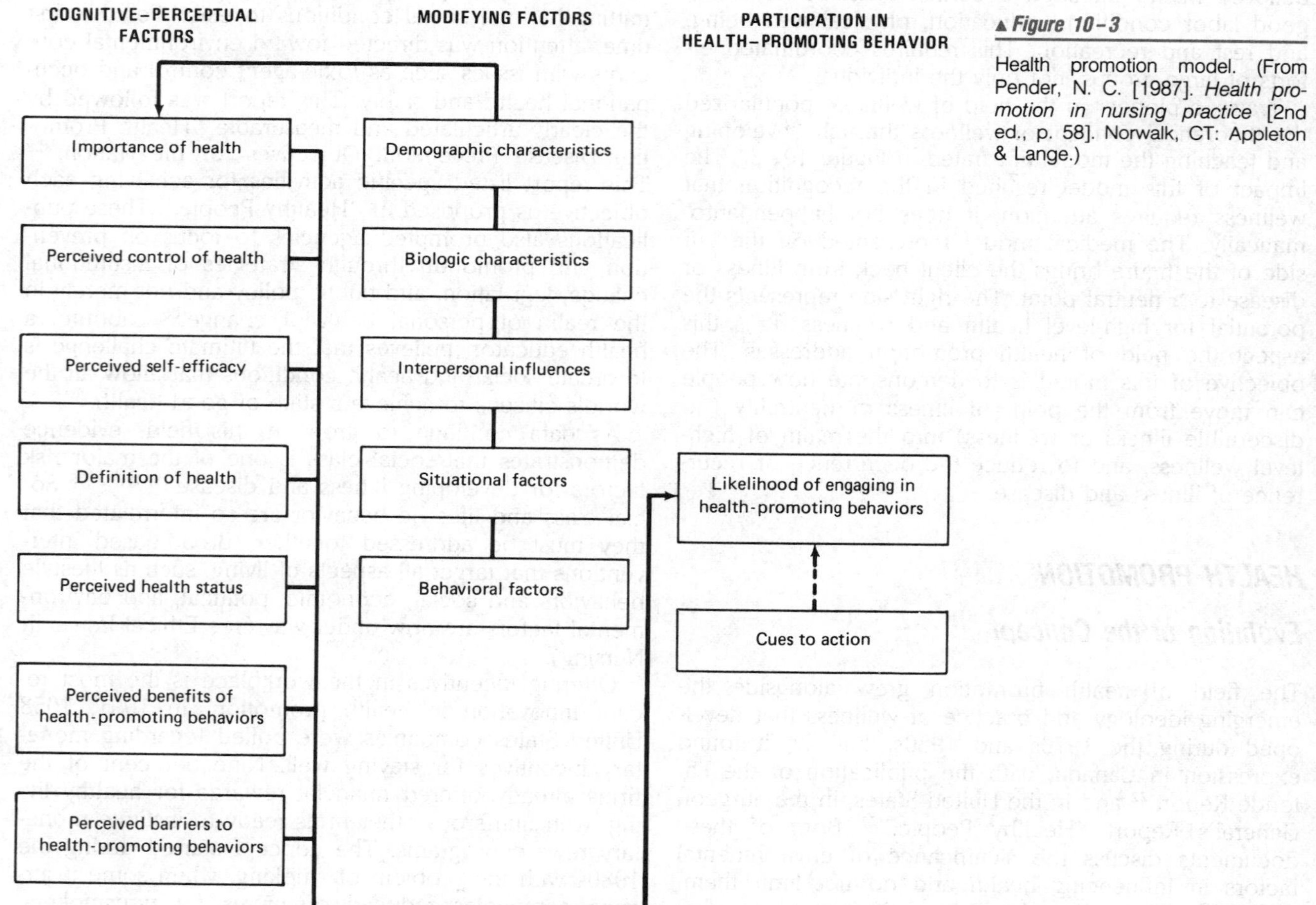

▲ *Figure 10-3*

Health promotion model. (From Pender, N. C. [1987]. *Health promotion in nursing practice* [2nd ed., p. 58]. Norwalk, CT: Appleton & Lange.)

Nurses must understand the complex social, political, and economic forces that shape clients' lives in order to promote health.[5] Nurses are charged with the responsibility of altering client attitudes toward health rather than altering the system itself. However, the nurse who is active in the social and political arena is in line with the ANA social policy statement that delineates involvement in social reform is within the realm of nursing practice. The policy states, among other concerns, the "provision for the public health through use of preventive and environmental measures and increased assumption of responsibility by individuals, families, and other groups."[2]

LEVELS OF PREVENTION

Preventive health care is more dynamic than health maintenance. This approach to health care has to do with health enhancement and promotion, whereas health maintenance is concerned with maintaining the status quo. When we think about the levels of prevention, there is a philosophical consideration that embraces a commitment to wellness and a conscious desire to prevent illness and disease. The levels of prevention are primary, secondary, and tertiary. Selected behaviors associated with these levels are identified in Table 10-1.

Primary Prevention

Primary prevention is concerned with prevention or delay of the actual occurrence of a specific illness or disease. A program of health enhancement activities can be developed to increase immunity and strengthen the body and mind. Everyday lifestyle behaviors can be examined by an individual himself or herself or by the nurse, who guides the client in primary prevention. The objective is to achieve maximum functioning in each health potential (Table 10-1).

Secondary Prevention

Secondary prevention refers to those health behaviors that promote the early detection and treatment of disease. When working with a client, the nurse first identifies the risk factors that cannot be modified but that leave the client vulnerable to disease. Using secondary prevention, the nurse analyzes assessment data for the purposes of deriving nursing diagnoses and identifying problems common to target populations who exhibit risk factors that are not modifiable. Emphasis is on the ranking of intervention priorities, nursing management approaches within the secondary prevention mode, and evaluation of outcomes. Data is obtained by interview, observation, and physical examination. The nurse then proceeds to work with the client to develop a means of early detection (Table 10-1).

TABLE 10-1. Behaviors Associated with Each Level of Prevention

Level of Prevention	Type of Behavior
Primary prevention	Stop smoking or do not start smoking
	Avoid overexposure to the sun
	Support antipollution legislation
	Practice safe sex, monogamy, or abstinence
	Obtain genetic counseling
	Design and follow a regular exercise plan
	Maintain ideal body weight
	Maintain low-cholesterol, low-fat, nutritious diet
	Wear seat belt and helmet
	Identify and eliminate stressors
	Limit alcohol intake, and never drink and drive
Secondary prevention	Obtain genetic counseling
	Screening for tuberculosis
	Obtain tonometry yearly after 40 for glaucoma screening
	Get yearly PAP smears
	Get biannual eye examinations
	Practice monthly self-breast and self-testicular examinations
	Get a physical examination yearly after age 40
Tertiary prevention	Have CBC drawn before chemotherapy
	Have speech therapy after a stroke
	Participate in cardiac rehabilitation
	Have breast reconstruction
	Participate in stroke/coma rehabilitation

IMMOBILITY: AN EXAMPLE OF SECONDARY PREVENTION

Immobility is a problem for a wide variety of clients. Using immobility as an example to examine secondary prevention, consider subconcepts that emerge if immobility is thought of as the prescribed or unavoidable restriction of movement in any area of the client's life. Types of immobility include physical, emotional or psychological, intellectual, and social. Causes of physical immobility may be (1) decreased energy from ischemia, hypoxia, malnutrition, and electrolyte imbalance; (2) lack of innervation as in central nervous system or peripheral nerve impairment; (3) decreased musculoskeletal strength as in endocrine diseases, disuse syndrome, and scar tissue formation; and (4) pain, which inhibits movement and the desire to move. Individual norms of mobility need to be considered when the nurse looks at problems of immobility. These complications may not be preventable, but signs of immobility can be detected early and, therefore, complications can be prevented.

Tertiary Prevention

Tertiary prevention is directed toward prevention of complications and rehabilitation after the disease or condition has already occurred (Table 10–1). In tertiary prevention, the nurse incorporates creative problem-solving approaches in the design, implementation, and evaluation of nursing intervention to support client's achievement of successful adaptation to known risks, optimal reconstitution and/or establishment of high-level wellness.

Continuing with the concept of immobility as the example, when a client remains immobile for any length of time, there is a risk of developing secondary disabilities such as muscle and joint degeneration, and metabolic and circulatory disturbances. The nurse who identifies immobility as a diagnosis will quickly develop a plan for prevention of disuse syndromes. The plan would implement (1) active exercise, (2) passive mobilization, and (3) frequent change of position. The nurse will develop outcome goals of optimal reconstitution within the parameters the client can achieve.

Risk Factors

Risk factors can generally be classified according to six categories (Fig. 10–4). The purpose of risk appraisal is to provide clients with a means of evaluation of health threats to which they may be vulnerable prior to the signs and symptoms of illness or disease.

Risk factors are a key to health promotion. Once identified, risk factors can be individually addressed and a primary prevention program initiated. There are numerous risk factors that, when left unattended or unacknowledged, can become life threatening. It is possible to uncover one or more of these risk factors during assessment. Some of the more common risk factors are

- Hypertension;
- Substance abuse;
- Smoking;
- Dietary indiscretion, deficiencies, and overindulgence (obesity);
- Sedentary lifestyle;
- Pollution, such as noise, air, and environment;
- Exposure to sexually transmitted diseases;
- Stress factors, such as chemical, environmental, and psychological;
- Genetic aberrations; and
- Fatigue and lack of sleep.

The approach to the assessment of risk factors for cardiovascular disease is detailed in Table 10–2. This is an example of risk factor analysis.

HEALTHY LIFESTYLES

Health promotion, like charity and other laudable virtues, should begin at home. Friedman believes that the family is the basic system in which health behavior is first learned.[14] Pratt finds that when families make commitments to improve and maintain their health through lifestyle modification, the health of all the individual members improves.[32]

The development of healthy lifestyle behaviors as early in life as possible usually results in higher levels of health and longevity for all family members. Benjamin Spock, author, political activist, and pediatrician, cites specific problems that have had a deleterious effect on the health of our young and, consequently, on the health of our nation as a whole (Table 10–3).[34]

Because of these social and economic problems, it becomes difficult to focus on health promotion behaviors. If we do not address these social situations, the result will be a continued deterioration of the nation's general health and well-being. We must emphasize the importance of the family unit in preparing children for a healthy future. Spock's recommendation is to teach children to develop an assertive sense, which, in turn, helps them to become intrinsically motivated. By the age of 19, out of every 200 children, only about one-quarter maintain the skills and talents (e.g., music, imagination, and interest in reading) they had at age 13. Spock found the difference in those who maintained their abilities and those who did not was whether or not they became intrinsically motivated. The family is the significant determinant, and this is the setting in which the initial teaching and learning process occurs. There are two characteristics the family needs to promote the development of intrinsic motivation and to foster a psychologically and physically healthy child. They are (1) the consistent offering of emotional support and (2) providing challenges and opportunities. Teens need to feel there is an emotionally secure environment to which they can return from the increasingly complex world outside the home. In addition, parents need to stimulate their children and offer them new opportunities for education and development.

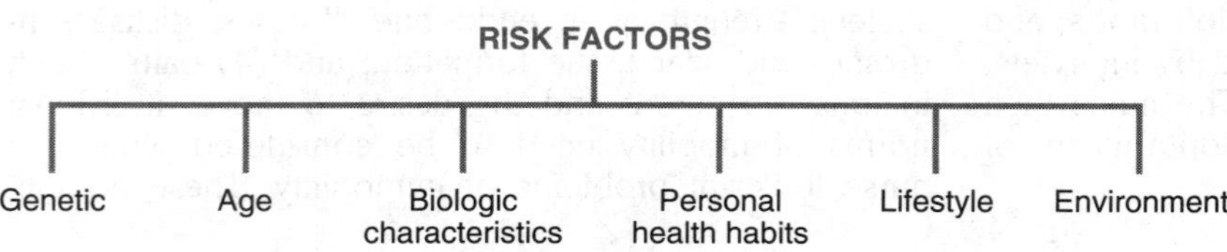

▲ **Figure 10–4**

Categories of risk factors. (From *Dietary Goals for the United States [1977]. U. S. Senate Select Committee on Nutrition and Human Needs* [Figure 6–8]. Washington, DC: Government Printing Office.)

TABLE 10-2. Risk Factor Appraisal for Cardiovascular Disease

Risk Factor	High Risk	Highest Risk
Sex/age	Women after menopause	Men over age 60
Family history of high blood pressure	Two blood relatives	Three of more blood relatives
Family history of heart attacks	One relative, before age 60	Two relatives, before age 60
Family history of diabetes	One or more relatives with NIDDM	One or more relatives with IDDM
Blood pressure† (degree of control somewhat modifiable)	Systolic: 160-200 Diastolic: 90-110	Systolic: > 200 Diastolic: > 110
Diabetes† (degree of control somewhat modifiable)	NIDDM uncontrolled or IDDM controlled	IDDM uncontrolled
Weight*	30 to 40 per cent overweight	50 per cent or more overweight
Cholesterol level†	240 to 280	Over 280
Serum triglycerides, fasting†	400 to 1000	Over 1000
Per cent of fat in diet†	30 to 50 per cent	Over 50 per cent
Frequency of recreational exercise*	Minimal	No activity
Frequency of occupational exercise*	Minimal	Sedentary occupation
Cigarette smoking*	20 to 40 a day	Over 40 a day
Stress at home*	High	Extremely high
Stress at work†	High	Extremely high
Behavior pattern (especially men)†	Type A	Type A
Use of oral contraceptives (women)†	Under 40 and use oral contraceptives	Over 40 and use oral contraceptives
Air pollution†	Moderate	High
Sleep patterns*	More than 8 hours sleep a night	4 to 6 hours sleep a night

* Modifiable risk factors
† Possibly modifiable risk factors
NIDDM, non-insulin-dependent diabetes mellitus; IDDM, insulin-dependent diabetes mellitus.

Developing Human Potential

It is within the domain of health promotion that we spend time in developing and maintaining our life potentials, or becoming the best and healthiest persons that we can be. The more time and energy we devote to developing our strengths, the less likely we are to develop problems. Two of the physical potentials, nutrition and exercise, will be discussed later in this chapter.

Figure 10-5 represents the circle of human potentials, each of which needs to be developed to maximize health. Each physical body is unique. Through our senses of sight, touch, taste, and smell, we gather experience of the world. When the body is nurtured, it increases in strength, vitality, energy, sexuality, and the capacity for language and connection with other potentials.

Our picture of the world is created uniquely from mental stimuli. It is through the logical process that one learns to fully understand, enjoy, and appreciate many of life's greatest pleasures. Growth is possible when one opens up to information, suggestions, and help.

Emotions are our feelings, the inner and outer responses to the events encountered in life. One of the greatest challenges we have is to acknowledge, own, express, and understand our emotions. Increasing attention to the development and balancing of this po-

TABLE 10-3. Social Problems That Affect Health and Well-Being

Demise of the extended family
The increasing disappearance of the small, tightly knit community
The numbers of mothers in the workplace. The National Center for Health Statistics (1990) reports that in 1988, 13.3 million children—60 per cent of all those age 5 or younger—were in a regular day care arrangement; this included half of all those children younger than age two. This statistic does not address the children cared for by friends, neighbors, and extended family members
Dissatisfaction with so many jobs. The primary gratification is the money, an extrinsic motivation, which adds to an increasing mercenary attitude
Divorce
Excessive competitiveness in all areas of American life
Jobs being more important than family
An increasing materialistic society

Data from Spock, B. "A Healthy Life," Lecture at Scott and White Clinic and Hospital, Temple, Texas, October 24, 1990.

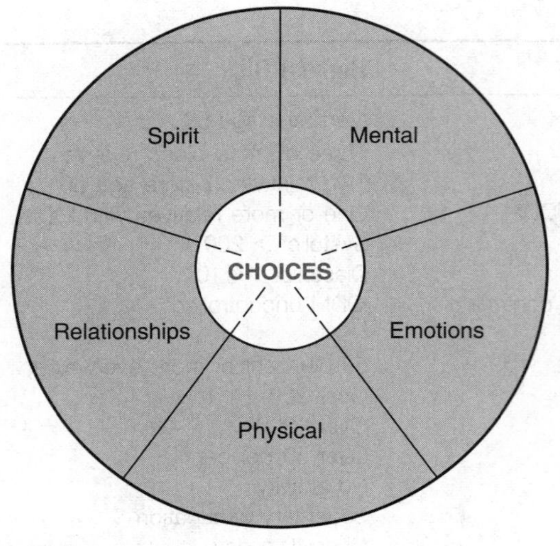

▲ *Figure 10-5*

The circle of human potentials.

tential allows our spontaneity and positive zest for living to emerge.

Spirit comes from our roots. It is related to the universal need to understand the human experience of life on Earth. Where did we come from? Where are we going? What is our purpose? Why do good and evil exist? What occurs after death? Who or what put this life form together? Development of the spiritual potential involves the development of our higher self, the transcendence of the experience of oneness, peace, harmony, and connection with the universe.

We cannot live purposeful lives without meaningful relationships. We may not share a house with anyone, but we all live in neighborhoods and are part of communities, cities, and states. We extend to our nation and even to the whole of planet Earth. The challenge in relationships is to extend ourselves and learn how to exchange our feelings of honesty, trust, intimacy, compassion, openness, and harmony. When we share our experiences, true interchange between individuals occurs. Something either positive or negative always occurs when people are together. It is through our attitude and orientation that we affect the outcome of all our encounters.

People have enormous capacity for making choices. These choices can be conscious or unconscious. Health and balance occur when the skill of effective choice making is used. Each of us is responsible for assessing our values and desires. No one else can make decisions for us.

Milio contends that the focus on choice is paramount in shaping the overall health for the person as well as the society as a whole.[24, 25] The range of choices is affected by personal resources, including awareness, knowledge, and beliefs in oneself and one's family. Time, money, support of family and friends, and the urgency of other priorities all influence what choices are made. Milio states that "most human beings, professional or nonprofessional, provider or consumer, make the easiest choices available to them most of the time." Nurses must be savvy to this when working with clients. Lifestyle behavior patterns are not isolated choices unrelated to social, personal, or economic circumstances.

Protecting the Environment

It is not enough to think solely in terms of ourselves or our immediate surroundings when we think of health promotion. At present, we are not just members of families, communities, states, or regions but we are intertwined with one another and linked as a global family. What affects one of us now has a ripple effect and affects us all. Because of the massive population explosion and congested urban living conditions, it is easy to affect another person's living environment. For example, it is possible to individually pollute the air by driving a car with a defective exhaust pipe, impinge on another person's auditory air space by playing loud music, or litter another person's visual space by discarding trash where it does not belong. In a larger, collective sense, we can cumulatively do much worse and pollute the environment to such a great degree that life itself is threatened.

Health promotion, because it addresses the whole self and the whole human family, must also address the protection of the environment. It is not within the scope of this chapter to delineate ways to do this but rather simply to awaken our awareness to the fact that each of us can play a role in cleaning, maintaining, and assisting to improve the conditions of the environment to the best of our ability.

Wellness experts Callander and Travis give us a number of areas to examine as we consider the health of our relationship to the planet.[6] They are recognizing/believing, conserving, water, consuming, eating, moving, and stepping forward.

RECOGNIZING/BELIEVING

We need a shift in consciousness. We must awaken to the fact that we are all interdependent and begin to think and act in an integrated and synergistic fashion rather than in the old way of fragmentation and competition.

CONSERVING

We routinely turn on lights and energy-consuming equipment without thinking of the environmental impact of our actions, such as more acid smoke billowing from coal-fired electric plants, additional spent nuclear fuel rods awaiting disposal, greater risk of coastlines damaged by oil spills, and more wild rivers being dammed up, diminishing wilderness habitat. We must practice energy conservation.

WATER

More than 10 million deaths worldwide result each year from waterborne diseases. Clean, safe drinking water, even in our industrialized nation, is rapidly becoming one of our scarcest commodities. The average American uses 60 gallons of water per day. Three-fourths of it is used in the bathroom, and as much as 40 per cent is wasted. Thirty to eighty per cent of residential water is used for lawn watering.

CONSUMING

Americans generate 160 million tons of garbage a year, which is 3½ pounds per person per day. The irony of this situation is that we have fewer places to put it. Since the early 1980s, two thirds of our landfills have been closed, and one third of those remaining will likely be filled to capacity and closed during the next 5 years. We keep toxic substances, such as furniture polishes, and toilet and oven cleaners, in our homes and dispose of them through the sewer systems, often contaminating domestic water supplies. Industry uses approximately 50 per cent of its paper, 8 per cent of its steel, 75 per cent of its glass, 40 per cent of its aluminum, and 30 per cent of its plastics for packaging. Every hour, Americans go through 2.5 million plastic beverage bottles, which may take years, or forever, to disintegrate.

EATING

Sixteen pounds of feed and 2500 gallons of water are required to produce 1 pound of meat, whereas only 25 gallons of water are needed to produce 1 pound of wheat. Insecticides and pesticides cause a danger to our health through indirect ingestion. The United States uses an estimated 2½ billion pounds of pesticides per year, at a cost of $6.6 billion. Up to 60 per cent of pesticides used on fruit and vegetables are used to improve the appearance of the produce.

MOVING

Our dependence on the automobile is at a great cost to the planet. Burning 1 gallon of fuel produces almost 20 pounds of carbon dioxide as well as nitrogen and sulfur oxides, hydrocarbons, and lead, causing air pollution, acid rain, and lead pollution.

STEPPING FORWARD

Global problems are complex and all pervasive. Nurses need to be knowledgeable and ready to speak out on behalf of the well-being of our world. It is the ideals, skills, and knowledge of each of us that, when recognized and applied, can make a positive difference in the health of the planet. We must act individually and collectively. Vote for your political candidates of choice, lobby for what you think is right, and garner legislative support for health promotion programs. By accepting the attitude that each of us can make our own little piece of the planet cleaner and healthier, Mother Earth will fare better and increase the likelihood of becoming healthier.

MOTIVATION

Nurses encounter clients during major health changes and, therefore, are in key positions to help them make decisions and adopt behaviors to significantly alter health.[39] If we are to effectively assist others with making healthy decisions and changes, we must function as role models as well as have an understanding of the concepts of motivation.

Both practice and research have demonstrated that giving information to clients does not, in itself, bring about healthy behaviors.[13] Nurses frequently give up trying to teach because of a lack of client motivation. When this occurs, clients are frequently labeled as noncompliant or difficult. Orem suggests that we alter our perspective and view this seeming lack of motivation in the light of self-care deficit theory of nursing.[29] In this theory, motivation is described as one of the power components that nurses can use to help people harness their energies. Through this approach, the nurse capitalizes on the client's strengths and empowers him or her to promote health. Pender also emphasizes the importance of the helping relationship in order to empower the client for self-determination.[30]

To motivate others to change health behaviors, several areas are involved. These areas include the following:

- The client must believe that the problem is solvable.[8]
- The client must see the solution as attractive.[3]
- The client must feel competent to carry out the behavior successfully.[4]
- The client must experience positive feedback and consequences.[15]

The role of the nurse then is to use multiple skills to enhance and empower clients to engage in healthy behaviors. Approaches include helping clients identify their values and explore feelings about themselves with emphasis on identifying strengths. Helping clients set their own goals (developing intrinsic motivation) will greatly enhance the likelihood of achieving the desired and articulated behavior changes. We need to assist our clients in differentiating between perceived and actual barriers, and promote behaviors to overcome the actual barriers. Whenever possible, nurses should model health and a joyful zest for living; in this way, we teach by providing a living example.

NUTRITION AND EXERCISE IN HEALTH PROMOTION

Nutrition and exercise are addressed together because they work synergistically to promote high-level wellness. The lack of good nutrition and sedentary living contribute to major risk factors, such as hypercholesterolemia, obesity, and muscular atrophy. When people begin to work on one of these two areas, often the other area receives attention at the same time.

Nutrition

Nutrition has moved into the forefront as a prominent component in health promotion and disease prevention. There is a correlation between what we eat and how we feel and the potential for development of diseases. Cardiovascular disease, cancer, and osteoporosis are three common afflictions that are directly related to nutrition to some degree. There are scores of other conditions related to poor nutrition that are perhaps less crippling but that clearly affect how we feel; dental caries, constipation, and acne are a few examples.

Nutritional Deficits

Deficits in nutritional intake can result in stunted growth, reduced metabolic function, and delayed or premature cessation of the reproductive system, and can put the body at risk for many less serious illnesses. Homeostatic mechanisms protect the body from temporary deficits, but chronic nutritional deprivation creates a susceptible host for the diseases of malnutrition. Two classic deficiency diseases are scurvy (vitamin C deficiency), and beriberi and pellagra (thiamine, niacin, and B complex deficiency). Malnutrition also increases susceptibility to infection and decreases the ability for wound healing.

Nutritional Excess

Overeating, or eating too many of the wrong foods, can also cause illness and disease. A large segment of our population, especially clients in the lower socioeconomic group, eat foods that are high in fats, sugar, protein, simple carbohydrates, caffeine, and alcohol. Over a period of time, diseases of overconsumption or malconsumption appear. Obesity, atherosclerosis, alcoholism, constipation, hypertension, and cardiorespiratory disorders and some cancers are all, to some extent, related to nutritional imbalance.

Balanced Nutrition

Healthy nutrition is the proper balance of nutrients, fiber, fluids, vitamins and, minerals. Whenever possible, foods should be free of chemicals, additives, preservatives, and toxins. Eat fresh foods, fruits, vegetables, legumes, and lean meats; avoid high-fat, overprocessed, and fried foods. The United States government recommends a decreased intake of fat and increased consumption of complex carbohydrates (Fig. 10–6). Clients who are beginning to assess their own food intake can use a food diary, as illustrated in Figure 10–7.

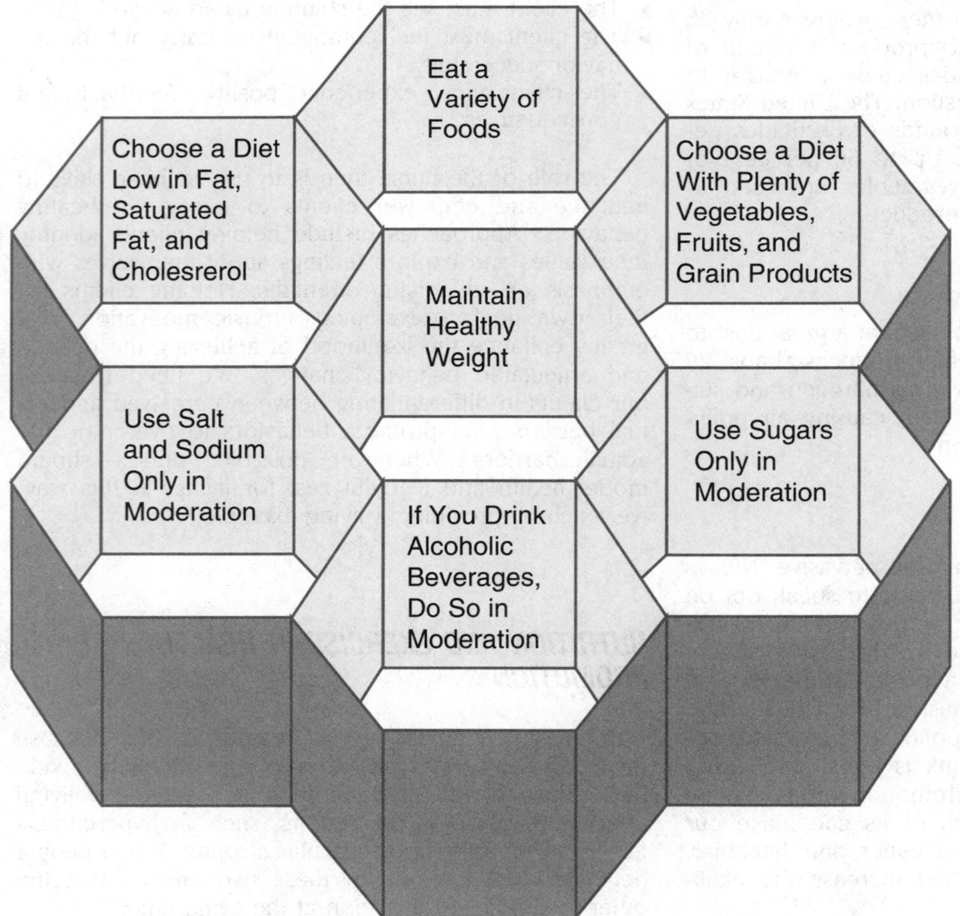
Eat a Variety of Foods
Choose a Diet Low in Fat, Saturated Fat, and Cholesrerol
Choose a Diet With Plenty of Vegetables, Fruits, and Grain Products
Maintain Healthy Weight
Use Salt and Sodium Only in Moderation
Use Sugars Only in Moderation
If You Drink Alcoholic Beverages, Do So in Moderation

▲ *Figure 10–6*

The seven guidelines for a healthful diet. (From the U. S. Department of Agriculture and the U. S. Department of Health and Human Services [1990]. *Dietary guidelines for Americans.* Washington, D. C.: U. S. Government Printing Office.)

Record *all* foods and drinks that you had during the day and during the night.

Day of the Week (Mon Tues Wed Thurs Fri Sat Sun)

Breakfast

Foods and Drinks — Amounts (cups, tbsps)

Lunch

Foods and Drinks — Amounts (cups, tbsps)

Dinner

Foods and Drinks — Amounts (cups, tbsps)

Snacks

Foods and Drinks — Amounts (cups, tbsps)

Do you take vitamin or mineral supplements? Yes______ No_______

Please list kind and how many per day.

▲ *Figure 10-7*

Food diary form. (From Dietary Goals for the United States. [1977]. *U. S. Senate Select Committee on Nutrition and Human Needs* [Figure 6-6]. Washington, D. C.: Government Printing Office.)

Exercise

Physical fitness is beginning to take on a whole new meaning. Until recently, fitness was directed primarily toward building muscle groups for the purpose of preparing for competition. A new way of thinking about fitness is depicted in Table 10-4.

Exercise, like nutrition, should be balanced and done on a regular basis. It cannot be effective if it is performed on a sporadic basis. The purpose of exercise is to tone and strengthen internal organs and the circulatory, respiratory, and musculoskeletal systems.

Exercise is more than calisthenics. The components of fitness are multiple, and all aspects should be part of the routine (Table 10-5).

A physical exercise program coupled with a wise nutritional diet is the most effective way to actualize physical health promotion. When eating and exercising wisely, one will develop improved strength and endurance, a more youthful appearance, increased vitality, good posture, and improved general physical stamina.

STRESS MANAGEMENT

All of us have experienced stress, but each of us has different perceptions and thoughts about it. What are your perceptions? Think of a recent stressful event at home or at work that involved you and someone else. How did you react? How did the other person react? Was there a different reaction to the same event? You realize that stress is an individual matter. No two people respond completely in the same manner. In any situation, one person may perceive it as a challenge,

TABLE 10–4. Old and New Fitness Paradigms

Old Fitness Paradigm	New Fitness Paradigm
Emphasis exclusively physical	An integration of the body and mind
Compared self with others	Noncomparative
Regulated calisthenics	Aerobic dancing to motivational music. Individually paced build up with machines that provide feedback. Motivation and subliminal tapes for individual challenge.
Competitive with others	Competition with self
Rigorous and punitive	Exhilarating and fun
Muscle building	Health building

Data from Keegan, L. (1988). Nutrition, exercise, and movement: Nourishing the bodymind. In B. Dossey, L. Keegan, C. Guzzetta, & L. Kolkmeier (Eds.), *Holistic nursing* (p. 163). Rockville, MD: Aspen Systems Corporation.

whereas the other perceives it as a serious stressor. The way in which you perceive it in each situation both directly and indirectly affects your health. Stress is discussed in detail in Chapter 3.

Coping Skills

There are many ways to cope with stress practically. Planning is one effective way to reduce adverse effects. For example, we prepare for predictable life changes such as marriage, job change, or retirement. We plan by establishing goals. Through planning, we develop a belief system that allows us to dictate our own life and our own experience. Setting goals facilitates this belief system because it serves as a reminder that we have the power to create new experiences in our own lives. Goals should include areas such as meaning and purpose, fun and play, exercise, nutrition, work, and relaxation.

The most widely practiced and possibly the most effective exercise for immediate stress reduction is to evoke the relaxation response. When first learning to do this, remove yourself from the source of stress, assume a relaxed posture, and begin taking deep breaths through your nose. Then consciously and progressively relax all your muscles. Begin thinking of your strengths and imagining a successful outcome. Realize that, in the great scheme of things, this event, whatever its nature, is only a minor event. Through these techniques, you can help to evoke the relaxation response, which includes a decrease in sympathetic nervous system activity and moving into an altered, quieted state of consciousness. As you begin to appreciate the effects of the simple progressive relaxation technique you may want to explore and develop more long-term stress management techniques such as biofeedback training, yoga, tai chi, meditation, and guided imagery.

Identifying Strengths

Everyone has both strengths and weaknesses. It is important to recognize this fact and take the necessary time to identify them. When using introspection for yourself or with a client, consider questions such as:

What do I like best about myself?
What are my personal strengths?

TABLE 10–5. The Components of Fitness

Flexibility: the ability to use a joint throughout its full range of motion and to maintain some degree of elasticity of major muscle groups

Importance:

- Provides increased resistance to muscle and joint injury
- Helps prevent mild muscle soreness if exercises are performed before and after vigorous activity

Muscle strength: the contracting power of a muscle

Importance:

- Daily activities become less strenuous as muscles become stronger.
- Strong abdominal and lower back muscles help prevent lower back problems.
- Appearance improves as muscles become firmer.

Cardiorespiratory endurance: the ability of the circulatory and respiratory systems to maintain blood and oxygen delivery to the exercising muscles

Importance:

- Increases resistance to cardiovascular diseases.
- Improves the ability to maintain actvity levels.
- Allows for a high energy return for daily activities.

Data from Spock, B. ''A Healthy Life,'' Lecture at Scott and White Clinic and Hospital, Temple, Texas, October 24, 1990.

Do I set goals for myself?
Am I able to complete goals I set for myself?
How do I perceive my personal strengths as a way of understanding these patterns?

The time taken to evaluate the source of strengths can help an individual build a belief system. Gaining knowledge of strengths and weaknesses can help us develop a sense of personal worth, which may be severely tested or even destroyed during periods of stress or crises. What people think affects their life patterns. When you work on acknowledging your strengths, you can call them to consciousness during periods of stress. Positive cognitive thoughts connect with all the human potentials so that the body behaves with positive responses. When you activate and act from your strengths, you are more likely to develop positive attitudes. With the development of positive attitudes, there will be a better chance of effectively coping with stress during the inevitable everyday life struggles that confront us all. Some of these interventions, such as recognizing strengths, provide active techniques that enable individuals to call up inner resources to combat stress on our journey toward becoming healthy people.

HEALTH PROMOTION AND THE OLDER ADULT

Since the turn of the century, the elderly population of the United States has multiplied approximately eight times. At present, there are approximately 25 million people over the age of 65; there is a distinct trend toward the graying of America. Life expectancy has risen from 47 years in 1900 to approximately 72 years at present, primarily as a result of effective control of smallpox, tuberculosis, diphtheria, and other infectious diseases. Consequently, an entire segment of the population has lived to an old age and is now ripe for participation in health promotion programs. For seniors, health promotion is not just for fun, cosmetic improvement, or to prevent some distant risk factor but is vital for enhancement and maintenance of current daily health.

Women are particularly vulnerable to problems of old age because they have a longer life expectancy than men. Women are more likely to become widowed, whereas men usually remain married up to the time of their death. Also, because there are more elderly women than men, women are less likely to remarry than widowers. Consequently, women have a lesser chance of retaining supportive relationships with spouses than do males.[27]

Health promotion programs for the elderly can be designed to address specific diseases or problems common to a particular population, or they can be more global in design. An example of a broad health promotion program is one that addresses maintenance of

Self-responsibility;
Nutritional intake;
Physical stamina, strength, and flexibility;
Control of own environment;
Intellectual capacities;
Financial self-reliance; and
Stress control.

Specific programs target particular problems such as hypertension, cancer screening, weight control, foot care, physical fitness, and other concerns. "Healthy People: The Surgeon General's Report on Health Promotion and Disease Prevention" recommends the use of health promotion programs to improve the overall health and quality of life for older adults and to reduce the average annual number of days of restricted activity due to acute and chronic conditions by 20 per cent, to fewer than 30 days per year for people aged 65 and older.

Wallingford Wellness Project (WWP)

One of the most widely known health promotion programs that focuses on the problems of older people is the Wallingford Wellness Project that operates in the suburbs of Seattle, Washington. Initially, this program was a federally funded project used to document and evaluate programs that focused on lifestyle changes. The program demonstrated that a comprehensive health promotion program for older people is effective, appropriate, and exciting. The outcome of the WWP program was a book by Fallcreek and Mettler entitled "A Healthy Old Age" that includes specific guidelines and detailed steps for setting community-based health promotion programs into operation. The other significant outcome of this program is the fact that after federal pilot funding ran out, the program continued operations and even grew in scope and design. Graduates from the WWP and other health promotion programs tend to move on to lead classes themselves in either the same program or to help develop new programs closer to home. Housing projects, high-rise apartment buildings, and neighborhood centers are prime sites for health promotion programs (see Bridge to Home Health Care).

Several features of the WWP are distinctive and may attribute to its long-term success. These factors should be considered when developing new programs. They include a participant-oriented focus, individual and community empowerment, an intergenerational focus, education, and communication skills and assertiveness training.

PARTICIPANT-ORIENTED FOCUS

Participants and potential participants should be involved in all phases of the project, from the development of the original plan to delivery and evaluation of the content.

INDIVIDUAL AND COMMUNITY EMPOWERMENT

The long-range goal of the training program is individual and community empowerment. Focus on helping

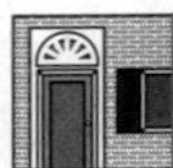

BRIDGE TO HOME HEALTH CARE

Health Fairs

A health fair offers an opportunity to combine health screenings and health education in a casual setting. There is enormous potential to attract a large number of individuals interested and concerned about their health. The desired outcome of the event should dictate the components included in the health fair. For example; if early detection of disease is a goal of the fair, a variety of health screenings ranging from blood pressure and vision screening to oral cancer, glaucoma screening, and pulmonary function can be included. If the desired goal is to raise awareness of individuals' health, health education displays provided by local non-profit organizations and hospitals are excellent opportunities to provide information on a wide variety of health topics. Most often, health fairs include a combination of both health screenings and education to the community.

Laboratory work is another component often included in health fairs. The method and results offered can vary from a total-cholesterol reading with instant results performed with a simple finger stick method to a fasting blood chemistry/coronary risk profile performed by venipuncture. Results should be mailed directly to the participant's residence to maintain confidentiality and to encourage self-responsibility for health. Generally, a fee is assessed if laboratory work is included, reflecting the cost of the profile. A health fair does not attempt to replace a physical examination by a physician but instead serves as a connecting link between the individual and their physician.

Several major cities across the United States host community-wide health fairs. These events are held in locations with ample parking and convenient access, including community centers, church halls, high school gymnasiums, social halls, shopping malls, and hospitals. Most communities are rich with human and financial resources to implement when planning a health fair. A network of non-profit agencies, hospitals, physician's offices, community groups and major corporations can play an important role in the successful health fair. Television and radio stations can also become involved in the health fair event by providing media support and advertisement.

Health fairs are a positive and upbeat way to blend existing resources to celebrate the health of any community.

---

participants develop maximum self-responsibility for their overall well-being.

INTERGENERATIONAL FOCUS

About one quarter of the participants in the WWP are under 60 years of age. The ages of the participants to date range from 13 to 84 years.

EDUCATION

The educational component emphasizes common sense health-related information and skills that are well within the grasp of most people. The need for extensive involvement of experts in the training program is minimized. This suggests that nurses are best used as guides, organizers, and resource people, but not as the key program instructors.

COMMUNICATION SKILLS AND ASSERTIVENESS TRAINING

Training in communication skills and assertiveness is a key program component. In the WWP, a course originally conceived as an environmental awareness and assertiveness course evolved to incorporate and emphasize a variety of communication skills. The development and application of these skills resulted in improved relationships with health care providers, friends and family members; working with others to secure desired products at local shopping places; and organizing to influence local legislation to enhance traffic safety provisions for older people.

ACTION STEPS

Nurses who want to work in the area of health promotion can seek positions with companies, schools and colleges, senior centers, municipalities, and health care agencies. Steps to develop programs should include

- Establishing goals and objectives.
- Performing needs assessment, and garnering participant involvement.
- Creating a participative learning climate.
- Facilitating interaction among participants.
- Developing teaching tools, such as handouts and audiovisuals.
- Developing independent teaching strategies, such as symposiums, panels, brainstorming sessions, readings, discussion sessions, demonstrations, case studies, interviews, role playing, problem solving, and field trips, for example.

Nurses working in the area of health promotion will be on the cutting edge of future health care roles. Wellness nursing made its impact in the 1980s; health promotion nurses will be the leaders into the next century.[7]

Summary

Health promotion is a key watch word for the 21st century. Nurses are encouraged to develop a consciousness that includes attention to the social, political, and economic aspects of the environment. Through reviewing health promotion, nurses will understand that human responses to health and illnesses, "are related to the structure of the social world, the economic, and political policies that govern that structure, and the human, social relationships that are produced by the structure and the politics." Once we recognize that establishing health promoting behaviors can alter the presence or absence of good health, then specific interventions must be delineated and diffused to the subsets of the population that can benefit. Portnoy believes that diffusion of programs generally lags behind their development.[31]

The process of diffusion can best be implemented and measured for effectiveness through research, practice, and evaluation. Nursing needs to strengthen its conceptual foundations to enable practitioners to better understand the parameters of and the means to promote health. If nurses are to enact changes at the social level, they need theoretical frameworks that are consistent with social, economic, and political forces.

RESOURCES

SAGE (Senior Actualization and Growth Exploration)
1713 Grove Street
Berkeley, CA 94709

SAGE began in 1974 and offers health promotion programs to older people, both in institutions and in the community. It makes use of a variety of approaches. The program offers books for purchase and a videotape for purchase or rental.

American Hospital Association
840 North Lake Shore Drive
Chicago, IL 60611

Publishes Coordinated activity program for the aged: A how-to-do-it manual.

Growing Younger
Healthwise, Inc.
P.O. Box 1989
Boise, ID 83702

This program works with neighborhood groups of older adults. Healthwise markets a training program and materials to assist other organizations to implement similar programs.

The Arthritis Self-Management Program
701 Welch Road, Suite 2208
Palo Alto, CA 94304

This program is located at Stanford University and has developed many materials specifically related to arthritis and self-care.

National Self-Help Clearinghouse
Graduate School and University Center/CUNY
33 West 42nd Street, Room 1227
New York, NY 10036

This organization provides information on various self-help programs across the country. It also publishes a highly informative bimonthly newsletter entitled "Self-Help Reporter" as well as other publications of interest.

National Clearinghouse on Aging
SCAN Social Gerontology Resource Center
P.O. Box 231
Silver Spring, MD 20907

The organization offers bibliographies on a variety of health promotion topics.

Bibliography

1. Allan, J. D., & Hall, B. A. (1988). Challenging the focus on technology: A critique of the medical model in a changing health care system. *Advances in Nursing Science, 3*(1), 22–34.
2. American Nurses' Association (1980). *A social policy statement.* Kansas City, MO: Author.
3. Briody, M. E. (1984). The role of the nurse in modification of cardiac risk factors. *Nursing Clinics of North America. 19,* 387–395.
4. Brown, S. J. (1989). Perceived self-efficacy and recovery from cardiac illness. *Research Review: Studies for Nursing Practice, 5*(4), 2.
5. Butterfield, P. (1990). Thinking upstream: Nurturing a conceptual understanding of the societal context of health behavior. *Advances in Nursing Science, 12*(2), 1–8.
6. Callander, M., & Travis, J. (1990). *Global wellness inventory.* Mill Valley, CA: Wellness Associates.
7. Clark, C. (1986). *Wellness nursing.* New York: Springer Publishing Co.
8. Ditto, P. H., et al. (1988). Appraising the threat of illness: A mental representational approach. *Health Psychology, 7*(2), 183–201.
9. Donnelly, E. (1990). Health promotion, families, and the diagnostic process. *Family Community Health, 12*(4), 12–20.
10. Dunn, H. (1961). *High-level wellness* (pp. 5–6). Arlington, VA: R. W. Beatty Co.
11. Dunn, H. (1980). *High level wellness.* Thorofare, NJ: Charles Slack.
12. Fallcreek, S., & Mettler, M. (1984). *A healthy old age.* New York: The Haworth Press.

12a. Ferguson, M. (1980). *The Aquarian conspiracy.* Los Angeles: J. P. Torcher.

13. Feuerstein, M., et al. (1986). *Health psychology: A psychobiological perspective.* New York: Plenum Press.
14. Friedman, M. M. (1962). *Family development.* Philadelphia: J. B. Lippincott.
15. Girdano, D. A., & Dusek, D. E. (1988). *Changing health behaviors.* Scottsdale, AZ: Gorsuch Scarisbrick Publishers.
16. Green, L. W., et al. (1980). *Health education planning: A diagnostic approach.* Palo Alto, CA: Mayfield Publishing Co.
17. Hann, M., et al. (1987). Poverty and health. *American Journal of Epidemiology, 125,* 989–998.
18. Holmes, T., & Rahe, R. (1967). Social readjustment rating scale. *Journal of Psychosomatic Research, 11,* 216.
19. Kitagawa, E. M., & Hauser, P. M. (1973). *Different mortality in the U.S.: A study in socio-economic epidemiology.* Cambridge, MA: Harvard University Press.
20. Labonte, R. (1986). Social inequality and healthy public policy. *Health Promotion, 1,* 314–351.
21. Laffrey, S. C., et al. (1986). Health behavior: Evolution of two paradigms. *Public Health Nursing, 3*(2), 92–100.
22. Lalonde, M. (1974). *A new perspective on the health of Canadians.* Ottawa: Government of Canada.
23. Marmoi, M. G. (1978). Employment grade and coronary heart disease in British civil servants. *Journal of Epidemiology and Community Health, 32,* 244–249.
24. Milio, N. (1976). A framework for prevention: Changing health damaging to health-generating life patterns. *American Journal of Public Health, 66,* 435–439.
25. Milio, N. (1981). *Promoting health through public policy.* Philadelphia: F. A. Davis.
26. Minkler, M. (1989). Health education, health promotion and the open society: A historical perspective. *Health Education Quarterly, 16*(1), 2–19.
27. Monk, A. (1979). Family supports in old age. *Social Work, 24*(6), 534.
28. O'Donnell, M. (1986). Definition of health promotion. *American Journal of Health Promotion, 1,* 4–5.
29. Orem, D. E. (Ed.) (1979). *Concept formalization in nursing: Process and product, (2nd ed.).* Boston: Little, Brown.
30. Pender, N. J. (1987). *Health promotion in nursing practice, (2nd ed.).* Norwalk, Conn.: Appleton & Lange.
31. Portnoy, B., et al. (1989). Application of diffusion theory to health promotion research. *Family Community Health, 12*(3), 63–71.
32. Pratt, L. (1976). *Family structure and effective health behavior.* Boston: Houghton Mifflin.
33. Sigerist, H. E. (1946). *The university at the crossroads: Addresses and essays.* New York: Henry Schuman.
34. Spock, B. (1990). *A healthy life.* Lecture at Scott and White Clinic, Temple, Texas, October 24.

35. Syme, S. L., & Berkman, L. (1976). Social class—Susceptibility and sickness. *American Journal of Epidemiology, 104*, 1–8.
36. Tones, B. K. (1986). Health education and the ideology of health promotion: A review of alternative approaches. *Health Education Research, 1*, 3–12.
37. U.S. Surgeon General. (1979). *Healthy people: The Surgeon General's report on health promotion and disease prevention.* Washington, D.C.: Department of Health, Education and Welfare.
38. U.S. Surgeon General. (1980). *Health promotion/disease prevention: Objectives for the nation.* Washington, D.C.: Department of Health and Human Services.
39. Utz, S. (1990). Motivating self-care: A nursing approach. *Holistic Nursing Practice, 4*(2), 13–21.
40. WHO (1986). World Health Organization report on concept and principles of health promotion. *Health Promotion, 1*(1), 73–76.
41. Who Cares for Kids Depends on Their Status. *The Wall Street Journal*, November 29, 1990.
42. Workplace: Paying workers for good health habits catches on as a way to cut medical costs. *Wall Street Journal*, Nov. 26, 1991.

Chapter

11

Health Assessment

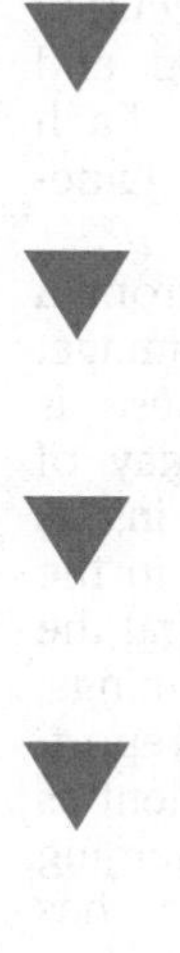

Health assessment focuses on the individual client. It is divided into two portions. The health history contains subjective information, whereas the physical examination is the objective information about a client's health status. The client is viewed as being a unique entity having complex spheres of interaction with physical and psychosocial environments. The nurse focuses on the client as an individual throughout the health assessment process. The health history interview is conducted free from bias or prejudice and without stereotyping the client. For example, an elderly client with several chronic health problems may or may not have actual health care needs requiring immediate intervention. Yet the potential for complex health problems exists for this particular client. Conversely, a young adult client in relatively sound physical health may appear "healthy" to the casual observer when, in fact, this client may have overwhelming psychosocial problems or needs affecting both his or her current and future health status. An individualized approach to health assessment provides a valid data base for further nursing care.

HEALTH HISTORY

Accuracy of Health History

The nurse assesses the accuracy and completeness of the information the client provides throughout the health history interview. Validation is important so that the data may be used to formulate accurate nursing diagnoses. It should be determined whether or not the client is an accurate historian, capable of and willing to provide the necessary information. The client may be unconscious or disoriented and, therefore, incapable of cooperating; willing to cooperate but hindered by circumstances, such as a client with a language barrier, or one who is overly anxious; or unwilling and mistrustful about cooperating with the nurse due to anger or depression. If the client cannot provide the necessary information, secondary sources of information should be sought, such as significant others or an interpreter for assistance. However, the nurse is aware that the content and accuracy of information may be influenced by the perceptions and biases of the secondary sources.

Computerization has affected the health history assessment process in some clinical settings, particularly ambulatory care. Computer programs for history taking result in accurate, reliable, and legible data displays. Data are recorded directly by either the client or nurse by means of interactive programs. Data also may be entered from a client-completed questionnaire, which is reviewed and validated by a nurse skilled in health assessment. Computerized health histories are complete because pertinent assessment areas are included in the programs and branching programs direct the nurse to collect additional data when the client responds with significant information.

Depth or Level of Health History

Many factors influence the depth or level of assessment. The setting for an interview may be less than ideal (e.g., the scene of a motor vehicle accident). The client's reason for seeking health care may preclude in-depth interviewing (e.g., a ruptured appendix). The client's attention span, energy, and comfort level may affect his or her ability to participate in an interview (e.g., pain). In an acute situation, the nurse collects data pertinent to the immediate problem and assesses the client's present health status. The nurse individualizes the health history interview to include the pertinent data while striving to be thorough. The data base is updated and enlarged as indicated and tolerated by the client's condition.

STEREOTYPING AND HEALTH ASSESSMENT

Stereotyping during the health history interview jeopardizes the nurse's ability to collect accurate data. False assumptions and generalizations about a client may lead the nurse to pursue avenues of questioning that alienate the client and interfere with development of client trust. The nontrusting client is reluctant to divulge sensitive information, perhaps fearing rejection or ridicule, resulting in inaccurate or missed nursing diagnoses.

Similarities among people result in their being grouped. For example, people may be of the same age, sex, or ethnic background, or they may share a common occupation, recreational activity, health risk behavior, or health problem. However, each person within a group is also an individual, possessing individual differences that make him or her unique. It is valid to identify reliable research findings concerning a group's characteristics or similarities and to apply those findings to an individual client who belongs to that group. However, as a rule, generalization is potentially harmful. This is especially true for generalizations grounded in assumptions or prejudice, or those based on the nurse's limited experience.

A client's physical appearance or presenting signs and symptoms may bias the nurse's perception of that client. Different etiologies may result in similar physical manifestations. For example, the nurse assumes that a client with an uneven, lurching gait and garbled speech is intoxicated or under the influence of a controlled substance. In fact, this particular client sustained a head injury in a motor vehicle accident and had a residual neurologic deficit. The nurse's initial inaccurate judgement may be costly both in wasted time and effort, and a strained nurse-client relationship. Each client is assessed as an individual. The following guidelines may reduce stereotyping.

The nurse does not manipulate information from a client to make it congruent with a stereotyped image. For example, a client with known alcohol abuse is being treated for a gastric ulcer. The second day of hospitalization, the client becomes agitated and insists that there are "bugs" coming out of the air vent in the room. The nurse does not see any bugs on entering the room and tells the client that he is imagining things; there are no bugs coming from the vent. In the report, the nurse tells the oncoming nurse that the client is having delirium tremens. Later, gnats are seen emerging from the air vent. But in the interim, the client has been labeled inappropriately.

The nurse does not assume that a client's reported symptoms all derive from the identified medical diagnosis. For example, a 24-year-old woman has low abdominal pain increasing in intensity with her menses. She is diagnosed as having endometriosis. Two years later, the woman begins to experience increased discomfort and her menses become more irregular, then cease. Her physician suspects that endometrial implants have caused pelvic adhesions, and the woman undergoes many tests, and surgery is planned. The woman is actually pregnant and has incurred some risk for the fetus because her symptoms were attributed to the previously mentioned diagnosis.

The nurse does not stereotype a client based on external appearance or behavior. False assumptions may result in the nurse omitting important parts of the assessment, resulting in an incomplete data base. For example, an elderly male client is admitted for hydronephrosis. He has a history of confusion. During the first night of hospitalization, the client becomes confused and combative. The staff assume that the client's increasing confusion and agitation are a result of being in an unfamiliar environment. But when blood work is drawn, the tests reveal that the client has a severe electrolyte imbalance that contributed to his confusion.

The nurse does not take a limited view and assess only a portion of the client. For example, a young male client is admitted to the emergency department following a motor vehicle accident. The client is unconscious and does not respond to questions. Assessment reveals that the right pupil is dilated and fixed, and the left pupil reacts to light. The emergency department staff prepare to insert an intracranial pressure monitoring probe, believing that cerebral edema is present. The client's wife arrives soon after and tells the staff that the client has had the dilated pupil ever since he was a teenager.

OBTAINING A HEALTH HISTORY

The health history interview process is affected by external (environmental and interpersonal) as well as internal (intrapersonal and physiologic) factors. The quality and quantity of data elicited are enhanced by the nurse's sensitivity to the client. The nurse's communication style is adapted to the specific circumstances.

When possible, the nurse assists the client to a comfortable position and setting. A quiet room with a door that closes decreases interruptions. Use of comfortable chairs that face each other, help establish rapport. Their distance apart is adjusted to the client's preference and sense of personal space. A moderate room temperature promotes comfort. Indirect lighting avoids glare and strong shadows that may distort the nurse's observation of the client's nonverbal cues.

The nurse speaks in a moderate tone of voice, calmly and patiently. The interview proceeds in a loosely structured manner and includes an introduction, a working phase, and a termination.

After introductions, the nurse explains to the client the nature and purpose of the health history interview. Nonprobing, client-centered questions and remarks help put the client at ease. The working phase is devoted to the health history interview. Until the nurse is comfortable with the interview format, a pocket-sized outline of the health history may be used as an aid. The nurse may keep *brief* notes during the interview; if so, the client is informed in advance so as not to disrupt the flow of the interview. Extensive note taking is discouraged because it conveys to the client that the nurse is not listening attentively. The nurse compiles the written history after the interview is completed. The nurse terminates the interview by summarizing highlights and providing the client with the opportunity to add or clarify information. The nurse also informs the client how the physical examination will proceed.

HEALTH HISTORY COMPONENTS

The health history includes the client's subjective data regarding (1) biographic and demographic information, (2) health risk appraisal, (3) psychosocial assessment, and (4) a review of the client's physical health history including the review of systems (ROS).

Sometimes a health history assessment is organized according to a nursing theory (e.g., Orem's theory of self-care) or by health behavior patterns (e.g., Gordon's functional health patterns). The format is a tool the nurse uses to collect comprehensive subjective data. In this chapter, the health history format integrates functional health patterns assessment and selected components of the medical history model that have been adapted to a nursing focus.

Biographic and Demographic Information

The extent and type of information recorded in the biographic and demographic data vary depending on the specific health care agency's protocol. Data include the client's full name, address and telephone number, a contact person, date and place of birth, sex, race, ethnic and cultural background, religious preference, marital status, occupation, Social Security number, type of health insurance coverage and policy number, name of primary health care provider, source of referral to the agency, source and reliability of the history information, and date of the health history interview.

The date of the health history interview is noted because the information is the client's baseline assessment. Should the client's health status change, the health history and physical examination will reflect the extent of the change over time.

Biographic and demographic data also provide clues about personal health risk. For example, the client's age and sex incur some health risk. Family history and the location of residence may also affect health risk (Fig. 11-1). Various health screening procedures are performed or recommended based on the client's age, sex, or other background data. Examples of recommended procedures include periodic pelvic examinations and monthly breast self-examinations for women and periodic prostate examinations and monthly testicular self-examinations for men.

Health Risk Appraisal

Health risk appraisal examines factors that affect a client's potential for developing a particular health problem. Risk factors are genetic or biologic (e.g., race, family history, personal history), behavioral (e.g., health habits such as smoking), or environmental (e.g., living in a locale with smog). Determining a client's health risk status identifies high-risk clients who may benefit from timely intervention. The nurse explains the difference between *being at high risk* of developing a potential health problem and the inevitability of *actually developing* a health problem. In health risk appraisal, the nurse assesses the client's willingness to modify or reduce his or her risk status. For example, a client who smokes is at higher risk of developing pulmonary diseases than a nonsmoker. The nurse may believe that the client *should* stop smoking. However, if the client has no desire to stop, teaching will be ineffective. This client may be labeled "noncompliant" by the health care team when the client is only adhering to a personal decision to keep smoking.

On the other hand, a female client who is at risk of developing osteoporosis tells the nurse that she is concerned and desires to reduce her risk. This client is receptive to teaching about increasing dietary calcium intake and engaging in regular weight-bearing activity.

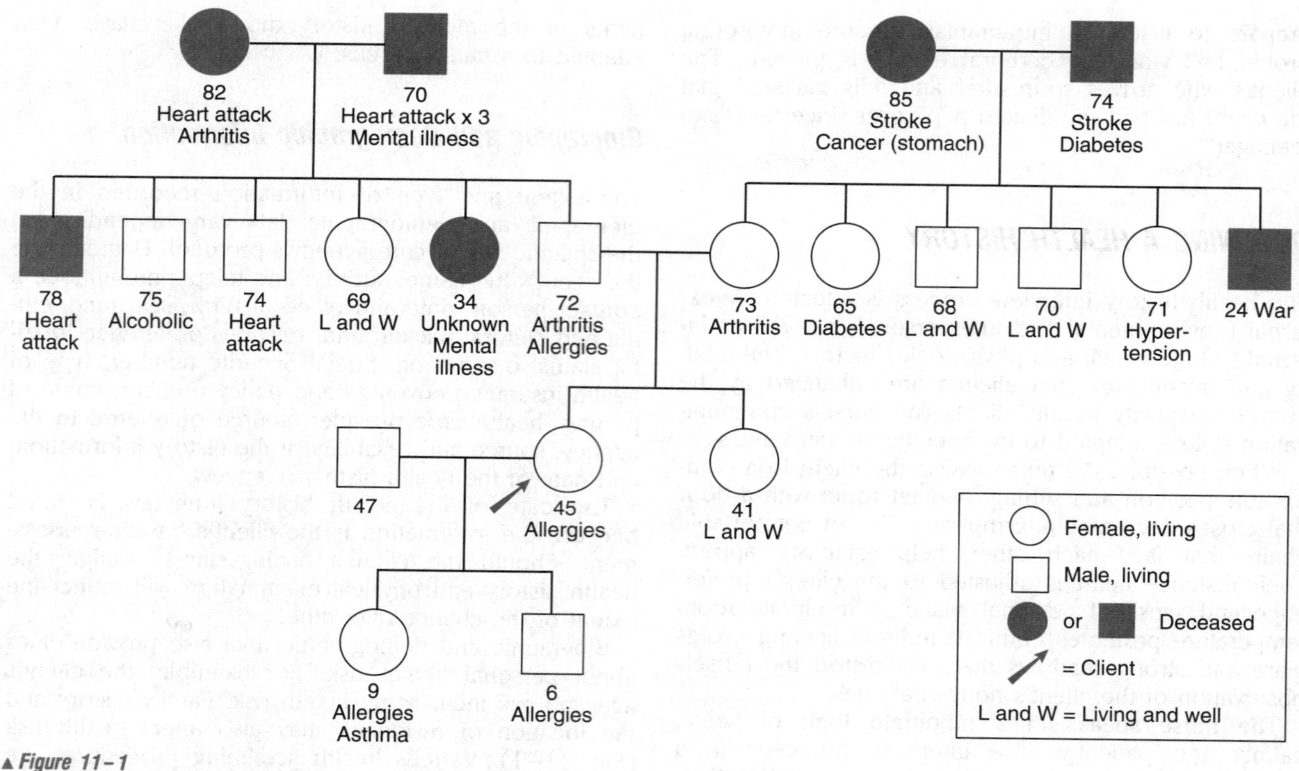

▲ *Figure 11–1*

Diagram of the family history for Mary C. Jones.

Health risk factors are categorized for assessment purposes. Some risk factors are potentially hazardous for many people (e.g., ground water pollution in a community dependent on wells for the water supply). Other risk factors may adversely affect a limited group of individuals (e.g., particle inhalation in workers who install insulation materials). And other risk factors are significant for a family group (e.g., genetic-linked diseases such as Huntington's chorea). Risk factor categories include race and genetic- or family-related, age-related, biologic, personal habits, lifestyle, environmental and occupational, and socioeconomic.

Table 11–1 summarizes examples of health risk factors, their commonly associated health problems, and suggested preventive client behaviors or screening procedures that may reduce a client's potential risk or facilitate early detection. Awareness of health risk factors may motivate a client to seek screening procedures and to practice preventive behaviors, particularly for health problems that are treatable or manageable through timely intervention. Knowledge of risk factors may assist a client to modify his or her personal risk profile by changing behaviors and habits. Environmental and occupational risk factors are more clearly linked with specific health problems and are usually more susceptible to change. Socioeconomic risk factors are less easily eliminated; however, their effects may be modified through skillful case finding and risk management.

The client's risk profile is assessed throughout the health history interview (see Box 11–1). A client with multiple risk factors linked to specific health problems is at greater risk for developing those problems than is the client with fewer or no risk factors. Hazardous occupations include firefighters, policemen, miners, heavy equipment operators, lumber and construction workers, factory and textile workers, musicians, and people who use chemicals or pesticides such as farmers, landscapers, gardeners, painters, and artists. A higher risk for accidental injury or trauma has been linked to multiple stressors, inadequate coping ability, mental and physical fatigue, decreased reaction time, and substance abuse. Stressors include strained interpersonal relationships, being a victim of physical or psychological abuse, inadequate financial resources, recent change in lifestyle, sensory stimulation overload, nutritional deficits, and hazardous environments, to name just a few examples. Lifestyle and personal habits affect one's health status significantly. Many risk factors in these categories are modifiable if the client chooses to do so.

Once the nurse has assessed a client's risk factor profile, the client's health risk status is evaluated. Each identified risk factor is examined with the client to determine whether or not its effects can be modified. Sharing the risk appraisal with the client in a nonjudgemental way provides the client opportunity to exercise autonomy regarding health care outcomes. The client must recognize that the risk factors have an effect on his or her quality of health. The client must also be willing to take initiative to change. If the client is interested in reducing health risks (e.g., stopping cigarette

Text continued on page 174

TABLE 11–1. Health Risk Appraisal, Screening, and Prevention

Risk Factor	Potential Health Problem	Screening and Preventive Measures: Self-Care	Screening and Preventive Measures: Professional Level
Race			
Black	Hypertension	Self-monitor BP Avoid salt in diet Maintain IBW See physician if systolic BP > 160 or diastolic BP > 90	Monitor if BP is elevated or client is taking antihypertensive medications
White (fair skin tones)	Skin cancer	Limit exposure to sun Wear protective clothing Use sunscreen with SPF 15 or above Perform monthly head-to-toe skin inspection See physician if change noted in any moles or birthmarks, or new growths or patches do not heal	Monitor skin lesions Skin biopsy or excision and follow-up treatment
Japanese	Stomach cancer	Know suspicious GI symptoms: pain, hematemesis, melena, weight loss, nausea, etc. See physician if symptoms develop	Follow up for laboratory tests and special diagnostic procedures
Hispanic	Diabetes mellitus	Regular exercise and weight control Consume balanced diet of no more than 30 per cent fats with complex carbohydrates Know symptoms of hyperglycemia: polydipsia, polyuria, polyphagia, and delayed wound healing See physician if symptoms occur	Diet counseling Follow up for laboratory tests, diagnostic procedures, and blood glucose monitoring and control
Native American	Alcohol abuse and related diseases	Abstinence Limit alcohol intake to 1 ounce per day or less if personal tendency (e.g., 1 to 2 mixed drinks or cans of beer) Know symptoms of alcoholism Join self-help support group such as Alcoholics Anonymous Seek professional help	Assessment of history and physical condition Referral to a detoxification program Counseling for client and family
Genetic or Family Related			
Overweight	Obesity-related disease	Monitor weight once per week Perform regular, sustained exercise Consume balanced diet (no more than 30 per cent fats, and calories should not exceed metabolic needs) Join self-help group such as Weight Watchers	Diet counseling Follow up by physician for moribund obesity (>100 per cent over IBW)
Diabetes	Diabetes or glucose intolerance	Regular exercise and weight control Consume balanced diet Know symptoms of hyperglycemia: polydipsia, polyuria, polyphagia, and delayed wound healing See physician if symptoms occur	Follow up for laboratory tests, special diagnostic procedures, and blood glucose monitoring and control
Hypertension	Cardiovascular disease	Regular, sustained exercise Consume balanced diet Avoid excess salt intake Maintain IBW Regular BP checks (self or professional)	Regular follow up by physician for diagnostic studies and laboratory work

Table continued on following page

TABLE 11-1. Health Risk Appraisal, Screening, and Prevention Continued

Risk Factor	Potential Health Problem	Screening and Preventive Measures: *Self-Care*	Screening and Preventive Measures: *Professional Level*
Genetic or Family Related			
Heart disease (onset before age 50)	Cardiovascular disease	See "Hypertension" Know symptoms of heart disease: chest pain, dyspnea, cyanosis Stop smoking Monitor resting pulse rate Low saturated fat diet Regular exercise	Annual physical examination, including ECG and laboratory tests Stop smoking clinics Diet counseling
Breast cancer (in mother or sister)	Breast cancer	Learn to perform BSE Perform BSE monthly	Regular professional breast examination as indicated for age and personal history Regular mammography as indicated for age (see Table 11-2)
Age Related			
Vision changes	Strabismus	Monitor for difficulty focusing, especially on near objects See ophthalmologist if symptoms occur Schedule regular eye examinations as indicated for age (see Table 11-2)	Follow up for complete eye examination and possible neurologic examination
	Visual acuity changes, cataracts, glaucoma, or macular degeneration	Monitor visual acuity See ophthalmologist if vision is "fuzzy," or seeing halos around lights Schedule regular eye examinations	Complete eye examination to screen for cataracts, glaucoma, and macular degeneration as indicated for age (see Table 11-2)
	Injury or trauma	Wear protective eye gear when engaging in activity likely to result in projectiles or blunt trauma, such as sports, woodworking, using high-speed machinery See ophthalmologist if injury should occur	Provide prompt diagnosis and treatment if injury occurs
Falls	Injury or trauma	Keep environment illuminated Remove loose scatter rugs Use a night-light Install handrails and grab bars Wipe up spills immediately	Provide prompt diagnosis and treatment if injury occurs
Self-medication errors	Over- or under-medicating	Request and use prepackaged unit dose medications Prepare medicines in a well-lit area Wear corrective lenses when preparing medicines	Careful assessment of medication history
Hearing problem	Presbycusis	Avoid exposure to loud noises Wear ear plugs when exposed to loud noise levels and limit length of exposure	Complete audiometric screening as appropriate for age and personal history
	Injury or trauma	Avoid putting sharp objects into ear canals Know symptoms of ear infections: pain, discharge from ear canal, vertigo, and fever See physician if symptoms occur	Follow up for prompt diagnosis and treatment if injury or infection occurs
Dental hygiene	Dental caries Periodontal disease Premature loss of teeth	Brush teeth regularly after meals and at bed time Floss teeth daily Have damaged teeth repaired or replaced promptly	Provide complete dental check-ups, and follow up annually Fluoride treatments as indicated for age and locale

TABLE 11-1. Health Risk Appraisal, Screening, and Prevention Continued

Risk Factor	Potential Health Problem	Screening and Preventive Measures: *Self-Care*	Screening and Preventive Measures: *Professional Level*
		Follow recommendations for fluoride treatments. Use fluoridated toothpaste Schedule regular dental check-ups	
Immune system integrity	Community-acquired infections	Keep immunizations current as recommended for age Elderly should receive vaccinations for influenza yearly and pneumococcus one time See physician if symptoms of infection occur	Provide prompt diagnosis and treatment if a contagious disease or infection is suspected
Impaired mobility	Falls	See self-care measures listed under falls related to vision changes Use mobility-assistance devices (e.g., cane or walker) Avoid hazardous surfaces such as wet floors and icy pavements	Provide prompt diagnosis and treatment if injury occurs
Biologic			
Hyperlipidemia, hypercholesteremia	Cardiovascular disease	Consume balanced diet low in saturated fats Exercise regularly Avoid or stop smoking Have blood lipid and cholesterol levels monitored periodically as recommended	Regular follow up for monitoring serum levels
Hyperglycemia	Diabetes mellitus	Consume diet low in fats and simple carbohydrates Include complex carbohydrates Exercise regularly Have blood glucose levels monitored periodically as recommended Self-monitor blood glucose levels if diabetic and following a prescribed medical regimen	Regular follow up for monitoring control of blood glucose levels Adjustment of medical treatment as indicated by laboratory results
Hypersensitivity reactions	Allergic reactions, including rhinitis, bronchospasm, asthma, eczema, and atopic dermatitis	Avoid known allergens Seek prompt medical treatment if self-care measures are ineffective Discuss with physician whether allergen sensitivity testing and treatment for desensitization is indicated	Provide prompt diagnosis and treatment if severe reactions or complications occur Initiation of desensitization therapy if indicated
Personal Habits			
Rest and sleep	Fatigue Lowered resistance to illness	Obtain sufficient sleep to feel rested on awakening (amount varies with individual need) Avoid sedatives See physician if chronic fatigue interferes with activities of daily living	Complete history and physical examination Evaluation in a sleep laboratory
Diet habits	Obesity, diabetes, hypertension, cardiovascular disease, irritability, depression, and hyper- or hypoactivity	Consume meals at regular times each day Eat three balanced meals per day Limit intake of salt, caffeine, refined sugar, and fats Perform regular exercise Monitor weight weekly	Regular follow up to monitor existing health problems Provide prompt diagnosis and treatment if a health problem arises

Table continued on following page

TABLE 11-1. Health Risk Appraisal, Screening, and Prevention Continued

Risk Factor	Potential Health Problem	Screening and Preventive Measures: *Self-Care*	Screening and Preventive Measures: *Professional Level*
Personal Habits			
		See self-care measures listed under obesity, diabetes, hypertension, and cardiovascular disease	
Calcium intake	Osteoporosis	Consume 800 mg of calcium per day in elemental form (men and menstruating women). In premenopausal women, 1000 mg per day. In postmenopausal women, 1500 mg per day Limit milk products as source of calcium; include other sources of dietary calcium, such as broccoli, carrots, green beans, spinach, collard greens, and rhubarb Engage in daily, weight-bearing activity such as walking	Follow up for periodic physical examination Possible estrogen hormone replacement therapy, when indicated Diet counseling
Fat intake	Colon cancer Possible breast cancer	Consume diet low in saturated fats, such as that found in beef. Substitute with fish, poultry, and beans Limit milk products and eggs Include fiber in diet such as from grains and cereals Know symptoms of colon cancer (blood in stool, change in bowel habits) and breast cancer (lump, discharge, pain) Have stool specimen tested for occult blood Perform BSE monthly See physician if symptoms develop	Follow up for laboratory tests and possible diagnostic procedures Diet counseling
Fiber intake	Colon cancer	Consume diet high in fiber, including cereals and grains, especially bran Know symptoms of colon cancer (see earlier) Have stool specimen tested for occult blood See physician if symptoms develop	Follow up for laboratory tests and diagnostic procedures Supplemental fiber to include in diet
Alcohol intake	Alcoholism Cancer of mouth, throat, esophagus, larynx, and liver Accidents, including those that result in death Cirrhosis Esophageal varices Pancreatitis Dementia	Abstinence, if high risk for alcoholism Limit alcohol intake to one ounce or less per day if no personal tendency (e.g., 1 to 2 mixed drinks or cans of beer) Know the symptoms of alcoholism Join self-help support group, such as Alcoholics Anonymous, if alcohol consumption interferes with performance of job or interpersonal relationships Seek professional help	Careful assessment of history and physical condition Referral to a detoxification program, if indicated Provide counseling Family counseling and support are often necessary (e.g., Al-Anon, Ala-Teen)
Drug abuse	Harmful side effects Drug interactions Allergic reactions Hepatitis	Use prescribed medications only as directed Discard outdated medications Limit use of over-the-counter drugs to only those necessary	Careful assessment of history and physical condition Referral to a detoxication program, if indicated Provide counseling

TABLE 11-1. Health Risk Appraisal, Screening, and Prevention Continued

Risk Factor	Potential Health Problem	Screening and Preventive Measures: *Self-Care*	Screening and Preventive Measures: *Professional Level*
	AIDS	Avoid recreational drug use Know symptoms of substance abuse Seek professional help If using intravenous drugs, do not share needles or syringes	Family counseling and support are often necessary Screening for AIDS or ARC
Tobacco use	Cancer of mouth or lung Cardiovascular disease Respiratory disease	Avoid tobacco use in any form Limit use, if unable to quit Know symptoms of tobacco-related health problems: persistent cough, oral sore that does not heal, hoarseness that persists, blood in sputum See physician if symptoms occur Have regular health check-ups Avoid exposing others to sidestream smoke Attend support group to help stop smoking, such as Smokers Anonymous	Follow up for laboratory tests and special diagnostic procedures Counseling for help to stop smoking Referral of family members (if indicated) for health assessment if exposed to sidestream smoke
Safety	Unintentional injury or death	Use safety equipment as indicated (seat belts, helmet, eye shield, life vest) Learn how to swim Never drink and drive. Appoint a designated driver Do not operate equipment or engage in hazardous activity if taking medication that causes drowsiness Develop safety awareness, e.g., learn to identify unsafe situations and avoid them or take corrective action	Thorough teaching about medications and their side effects Provide prompt diagnosis and treatment if an injury occurs
Sun exposure	Sunburn Skin cancer	See self-care measures listed under skin cancer related to race	See measures listed under skin cancer related to race
Lifestyle			
Lack of regular exercise	Obesity Cardiovascular disease	Engage in regular aerobic exercise (brisk walking, biking, jogging, swimming) at least three times per week for 30 to 40 minutes each Warm up prior to exercising to increase flexibility and reduce chance of injury Do not begin an exercise program until checked by physician for a baseline health assessment Follow professional advice regarding type of exercise program and intensity of training Wear appropriate gear for activity as protection Consume a balanced diet Know warning signals of when to stop exercising (e.g., dizziness, chest pain)	Baseline health assessment prior to beginning exercise program Provide prompt diagnosis and treatment if complications or injury occurs Periodic assessment of cardiovascular status and endurance
Stress and coping ability	Many health problems are related to high stress	Decrease level of stress whenever possible Develop a variety of coping skills	Provide counseling Refer to appropriate support system as indicated by the individual circum-

Table continued on following page

TABLE 11-1. Health Risk Appraisal, Screening, and Prevention Continued

Risk Factor	Potential Health Problem	Screening and Preventive Measures: Self-Care	Screening and Preventive Measures: Professional Level
Lifestyle			
	levels and inadequate coping	Practice relaxation techniques (e.g., biofeedback, imagery, meditation, self-hypnosis) Recognize effect stress has on self Develop a support network Modify lifestyle to reduce stress Seek professional help if needed	stances Teach regarding relaxation techniques Carefully assess and treat if psychosomatic health problems develop
Lack of self-care activities to promote health	Cancer of breast or testis	Monthly practice BSE or TSE Regular professional examination as indicated for age (see Table 11-2)	Periodic, regular examination by physician
	Cancer of the cervix	Obtain regular pelvic examination and Pap test as indicated for age and sexual activity status	Periodic, regular examination by physician, with follow up as necessary
	Vision and hearing problems	See self-care measures under age-related health problems	See measures listed under age-related health problems for vision and hearing
	Dental and gum disease	See self-care measures under age-related health problems	See measures listed under age-related health problems for dental hygiene
	Tetanus Influenza Pneumonia	Keep immunizations current See physician if complications of these diseases develop	Provide prompt diagnosis and treatment if an infectious disease occurs
	Cancer	Know the seven warning signs: change in bowel or bladder habits, a nonhealing sore, unusual bleeding or discharge, lump or thickening in breast or other area, difficulty swallowing or indigestion, change in mole or wart, and persistent cough or hoarseness See physician if these symptoms persist Know and follow current recommendations for prevention and early entry into the health care system	Follow up for laboratory tests and special diagnostic procedures Provide prompt diagnosis and treatment
High-risk sexual activity	Unplanned pregnancy	Use contraceptive method acceptable to self and partner Prenatal care	Provide counseling regarding options for contraceptives Provide counseling regarding pregnancy outcome options
	Cervical cancer	Abstain from early, frequent sexual activity Limit number of sexual partners Limit number of childbirths Schedule regular Pap test as recommended for age	Regular professional pelvic examinations and Pap tests as indicated by health behavior profile
	STDs, such as AIDS and herpes	Limit number of sexual partners Avoid anal intercourse Use condoms Avoid oral-genital intercourse Avoid oral contact with body fluids (semen, blood, feces, urine) See physician for regular, periodic assessment if engaging in high-risk sexual activity Know symptoms of STDs, e.g., sore on genitals or mucous membranes, dis-	Follow up for prompt diagnosis and treatment should STD be suspected Provide counseling regarding safe sex practices Refer to public health for contact and follow up of possible infected partners

TABLE 11-1. Health Risk Appraisal, Screening, and Prevention Continued

Risk Factor	Potential Health Problem	Screening and Preventive Measures: Self-Care	Screening and Preventive Measures: Professional Level
		charge from penis or vagina, abnormal bleeding, dyspareunia Refrain from sexual activity if symptoms of STDs develop	
Travel	Diseases endemic to locale	Obtain necessary vaccinations before departure Seek prompt treatment if illness develops while traveling or after return	Provide prompt diagnosis and treatment if illness occurs
Environmental and Occupational			
Sports	Fractures, sprains, and strains	Have a baseline health assessment prior to beginning a sport Wear protective gear to avoid injury (e.g., eye shield, helmet, padding) Follow recommendations for warm-up and cool-down exercises See physician if injury occurs Limit mobility of injured body part until rehabilitation begins	Provide prompt diagnosis and treatment of injuries Rehabilitation
Outdoor activity	Sunburn Skin cancer Frostbite Hypo- or hyperthermia	Wear protective gear appropriate for the weather Use sunscreen with an SPF of 15 or above Limit exposure to extremes of heat or cold Learn survival tactics relative to activity Know early signs of hypothermia (disorientation) and hyperthermia (dry, hot skin) Attempt to seek medical treatment as soon as possible if a problem arises	Provide prompt diagnosis and treatment if a problem occurs See measures listed under skin cancer related to race
Loud noise	Hearing loss	Limit exposure to loud music and machinery Wear protective ear plugs Have regular screening of hearing See physician if hearing loss is evident	Regular, complete audiometric screening, as appropriate
Chemical fumes, airborne particle exposure	Respiratory diseases Cancer	Provide adequate ventilation Wear protective gear (goggles, respirators) Limit exposure when possible (chemicals, dry cleaning fluid, film processing, mining, asbestos exposure, household cleaners) Reduce exposure by changing jobs, if necessary Know symptoms of possible disease, such as hoarseness, persistent cough, hemoptysis, chronic dyspnea See physician if symptoms of disease develop Avoid smoking	Prompt diagnosis and treatment if disease should occur
Stress-provoking activity	Cardiovascular disease Hypertension	Limit stress-provoking activity, when possible Learn stress management techniques (e.g., biofeedback, guided imagery)	Teach relaxation techniques Provide counseling regarding stress management Provide prompt diagnosis and treat-

Table continued on following page

TABLE 11–1. Health Risk Appraisal, Screening, and Prevention Continued

Risk Factor	Potential Health Problem	Screening and Preventive Measures: Self-Care	Screening and Preventive Measures: Professional Level
Environmental and Occupational			
		Practice stress management techniques regularly Know symptoms of cardiovascular disease See physician if symptoms develop	ment if a stress-related problem occurs
High-accident risk activity	Unintentional injury or death	Avoid high-accident risk activities Learn safety measures Practice safety measures so they become habitual Use safety equipment such as goggles, helmets Get sufficient rest Avoid alcohol, drugs, or medications known to cause drowsiness when engaging in high-risk activity Obtain treatment if injury occurs	Provide prompt diagnosis and treatment if an accidental injury occurs
Low-level electromagnetic radiation exposure	Cancer of brain or eye Leukemia Sarcoma Possible birth defects	Limit exposure Monitor immediate environment for radiation levels Promptly seek health assessment and treatment for possible problems	Provide prompt diagnosis and treatment if a health problem occurs
Socioeconomic			
Recent immigration	Diseases endemic to locale of origin or where traveled	Obtain necessary immunizations before departure See physician if symptoms of disease occur, especially during or after recent travel	Careful assessment of history and physical examination Provide prompt diagnosis and treatment if a health problem occurs
Lack of health insurance coverage	Delayed or postponed treatment of health problems Undetected health problems	Use free walk-in health care facilities	Refer client to social services or welfare agency for assistance with applying for available health care such as Medicaid or Medicare

AIDS, acquired immunodeficiency syndrome; ARC, AIDS-related complex; BP, blood pressure; BSE, breast self-examination; IBW, ideal body weight; SPF, sun protection factor; STDs, sexually transmitted diseases; TSE, testicular self-examination.

smoking or wearing seatbelts), the nurse intervenes either directly or indirectly. Approaches to behavior changes are discussed with the client. Direct interventions include teaching sessions to provide information and counseling, or to reinforce client behavior. Indirect interventions include referral to an appropriate community resource or other health care professional (e.g., nutritionist, smoking clinic, counselor, support group for substance abusers, diet support programs). The goals for the client are (1) to take responsibility for modifying those factors that can affect one's health and (2) to strive for optimal health. Box 11–1 illustrates how the nurse integrates health risk appraisal into the history interview.

HEALTH RISK APPRAISAL ACROSS THE LIFESPAN

Health risk appraisal related to a client's age and sex is consistent with assessment of the whole person. Certain health problems tend to occur more frequently depending on a client's age and sex. The risk profile changes with the age-related cohort. For example, after age 50, a client's risk of developing cancer of the bowel or breast increases compared with someone younger.

Specific screening procedures are performed during a complete health assessment in order to determine potential and actual health problems. For example, after the age of 40, glaucoma screening is recom-

Box 11–1. Health Risk Appraisal

Clinical Example: Health Risk Appraisal

Biographic and Demographic Data

S. W. is a white, 28-year-old, single, female self-employed fashion clothes designer. Self-insured. Admitted to surgical nursing unit for elective cosmetic surgery.

Health Management Activities

Annual examinations for teeth, vision, Pap smear. No breast self-examination.

Personal Habits

Denies smoking. Consumes one to two alcoholic drinks or glasses of wine most days. Uses own automobile frequently, wears seatbelts "when remembers to put them on." Uses tanning room at health spa twice a week for 30 minutes.

Diet

No restrictions, likes most foods. Prefers to limit sugar and salt intake. Typical 24-hour diet includes basic four food groups. Usually eats breakfast and dinner, lunch consumed "on the run." Dines out often with clients at restaurants.

Exercise

Jogs once per week for 2 to 3 miles and performs aerobics once per week at health spa.

Stress Management

Feels "moderate" pressure to succeed in business. Life becomes "hectic" when new fashion lines shown. Uses imagery for relaxation (usually effective). Denies current problems with stress management.

Sleep and Rest

Gets approximately 6 to 7 hours sleep per night and feels rested.

Sexuality

Sexually active since age 18. Admits to five or six partners in past 10 years, with one partner for past 2 years. Prescribed oral contraceptive for 6 years. Partner does not use condoms.

Past Medical History

No previous illness, injury, or surgery. No allergies.

Family History

Mother diagnosed with breast cancer at age 42; treated with surgery and is currently healthy. No other known family-linked health problems.

Health Risk Appraisal

S. W. is at risk for (1) breast cancer, (2) possible skin cancer, (3) automobile-related injury or death, and (4) possible sexually transmitted diseases, including acquired immune deficiency syndrome (AIDS). She also is at risk for health problems related to alcohol consumption, inadequate nutrition, inadequate exercise patterns, and a stress-producing lifestyle. There may be concerns about financial security that are explored with S. W. during further questioning.

mended every 2 years. For health maintenance and prevention, specific health management behaviors are recommended based on age. For example, routine childhood immunizations for contagious diseases are administered according to a schedule that correlates with the development of the immune system as well as to periods when exposure is most likely to occur. Adults may be deficient in routine immunizations or previous exposure to childhood contagious diseases. These clients are recommended to have screening titers and immunizations.

Recommendations for common screening procedures and health management behaviors across the lifespan are listed in Table 11–2. Recommendations change periodically as research and epidemiologic studies reveal new information about occurrence and newer, easily applied, sensitive screening methods are developed. The nurse is familiar with the most current recommendations.

Refer to Chapter 21 for a discussion of risk factors for developing the common types of cancer (Table 21–5), as well as primary risk factors and secondary type of cancer prevention (Table 21–6). Also see Table 21–8, the American Cancer Society Guidelines for early detection in asymptomatic populations.

Screening Tests or Procedures

When the nurse inquires if the client has had a *specific screening test or procedure*, such as an eye examination or mammograms, the client also is asked when the test was last performed and what the results were. The nurse uses this information to assess the client's health risk status and to recommend follow-up screening procedures.

Psychosocial Assessment

Psychosocial assessment is an important part of the health history. A complete psychosocial assessment, although lengthy, is essential to a client-centered approach.

TABLE 11-2. Health Risk Appraisal Across the Lifespan

Potential Health Problem	Recommended Preventive/ Screening Examination	Birth to 18 Months	2 to 6 Years	7 to 12 Years	13 to 18 Years	19 to 39 Years	40 to 64 Years	65 Years and over
Growth and Development Concerns	History—re: developmental disorders	Parent/family dysfunction. Physical, mental, emotional, and social growth. Behavioral and learning disorders				Relationships with significant others. Parenting behaviors. Job satisfaction.		Retirement planning; declining mental activity
			Discipline, school readiness		Sexual practices			
	Nutrition history	Breastfeeding, iron intake	Sweets, between-meal snacks, fats (saturated), cholesterol, sodium, iron, calcium			Fats (saturated), cholesterol, complex carbohydrates, fiber, sodium, calcium		
						Iron for women until menopause		
			Caloric balance and selection of exercise program					
	Complete physical examination	Birth and 2, 4, 6, 15, and 18 months	Every year until age 5	Every 2 years	Every 2 years	Every 5 years	Every 3 years	Every year
Vision Problems	Strabismus check, amblyopia	Every visit						
	Assessment of visual activity		Every year beginning at age 3	One time	One time	Every 2 to 5 years		Every 2 years
Hearing Problems	Audiometry	18 months	Every year				Every 3 years	Every year
Dental Problems	Assessment of teeth/cleaning	Every visit (baby bottle tooth decay)	Every 6 months beginning at age 3		Every year			
	Fluoride	+	+	+	+			
	Brushing and flossing		+	+	+	+	+	+
Infectious Diseases	Routine immunizations	DTP, OPV, MMR, Hib, HBV per protocol	DTP, OPV, MMR per protocol			MMR		
	Tine test	At age 1	One time	One time	One time	One time	One time	One time
	Tetanus-diphtheria booster				One time between 14 to 16 years	Every 10 years		
	Influenza vaccine					Every year if high risk under age 65		Every year
	Pneumococcal vaccine							One time

Accidents and Injuries	Automobile restraints	Car seats	Car seats until age 4; seat belts	+	+	+	+	+
	History—re: risk factors	Burns, falls, choking, poisoning	Poisoning, drowning, burns, bicycle accidents	Bicycle accidents burns, poisoning, firearms	Bicycle accidents, burns, firearms, drinking while driving, suicide	Drinking while driving, firearms, back injury, burns, suicide	Drinking while driving, burns, back injury, falls	Falls
Substance Abuse	History—re: use of tobacco, drug, alcohol			+	+	+	+	+
Birth Defects	Rubella titre				Unimmunized female			
	Amniocentesis					Over age 35		
Unplanned Pregnancy	Sex education			+	+	+	+	
	Contraceptive information				+	+	+	
Anemia	Hemoglobin and hematocrit	One time, early infancy	Age 3 and 5 years	Ages 8, 10, and 12	Ages 15 and 18	One time	Every 3 years	Every year
Bowel Cancer	Rectal Examination						Every year	
	Stool examination for occult blood						Every year beginning age 50	
	Sigmoidoscopy						Every 3 to 5 years after two negative tests taken 1 year apart, beginning age 50	
Breast Cancer	Breast self-examination					Every month		
	Professional examination					Every 3 years	Every year	
	Mammogram					One time between ages 35 and 39	Every 1 to 2 years until age 50; then every year until age 75	
Cervical Cancer/ Gynecologic Problems	Papanicolaou smear				Every 1 to 3 years if sexually active	Every year		
	Pelvic examination					Every year		

Table continued on following page

TABLE 11–2. Health Risk Appraisal Across the Lifespan Continued

Potential Health Problem	Recommended Preventive/ Screening Examination	Birth to 18 Months	2 to 6 Years	7 to 12 Years	13 to 18 Years	19 to 39 Years	40 to 64 Years	65 Years and over
Diabetes and Kidney Diseases	Urinalysis		One time at age 3	One time	One time	Every 1 to 3 years		Every year
Heart Disease	History—re: exercise program or physical activity			Every visit				
	Electrocardiogram (ECG)						One time	
Hypertension	Blood pressure		Every year beginning age 3	Every 1 to 2 years				Every year
Hyperlipidemia	Blood cholesterol level		Age 3 if family history			Every 1 to 3 years		Every year
Obesity	Height and weight	Every visit	+	+	+	+	+	+
Scoliosis	Back examination			Every year beginning age 8	Every visit			
Sexually transmitted Diseases (STDs)	VDRL/RPR				One time if sexually active	One time	One time	One time
	Chlamydial testing					+	+	+
	Gonorrhea culture					+	+	+
	HIV counseling and testing					+	+	+
Testicular/ Prostate Problems	Testicular self-examination					Every month	Every month	Every month
	Professional examination					Every 5 years	Every 2 to 3 years between 40 and 50/then every year	Every year

* Recommendations are subject to change, based on the most current information available. Recommendations in this table are based on guidelines from the American Academy of Ophthalmology, the American Academy of Pediatrics, the American Cancer Society, the American College of Obstetricians and Gynecologists, the National Heart, Lung, and Blood Institute, Centers for Disease Control, and the U.S. Preventive Services Task Force.

The list of preventive/screening services is not exhaustive nor are all services listed indicated for every client at every visit. Type and frequency of visits and services are determined by individual and family health history and personal habits.

DTP, Diphtheria and tetanus toxoids combined with pertussis vaccine; HBV, hepatitis B vaccine; Hib (or HbCV), *Haemophilus* b conjugate vaccine; MMR, measles, mumps, and rubella vaccine; OPV, oral polio vaccine; RPR, rapid plasma reagin test for syphilis; VDRL, Venereal Disease Research Laboratory test (a test designed to detect syphilis); +, ongoing preventive behavior (these items should be assessed during each contact with the client).

An individual's psychological status affects multiple areas of function that are vital to human development and behavior, such as intellectual development and capability, motivation, perception and insight, decision making, speech and communication, motor ability, sleep and rest patterns, and nutrition and elimination patterns, to name just a few. It is impossible to separate a human being into discrete components. Rather, the nurse considers the client as having multiple dimensions that include the psychological, sociologic, and physiologic. These dimensions interact and affect the individual's behavior and responses to the environment. Interrelationships among the psychological, sociologic, and physiologic dimensions are neither static nor always predictable. Human physiologic responses to health problems are usually more predictable and are objectively observed, whereas two individuals faced with identical problems rarely react the same way emotionally. For this reason, psychosocial assessment may be less reliable than objective assessment of physical findings. However, it is possible for the nurse to develop skill and expertise in psychosocial assessment.

Psychosocial assessment assists the nurse to understand a client's response to circumstances and events, which, in turn, influences the client's ability to function. This understanding enables the nurse to provide comprehensive care to clients and their significant others based on accurate nursing diagnoses. Barry[5] emphasizes that approximately two thirds of the disorders that nurses independently diagnose and treat are psychosocial. When applied to the medical-surgical client, accurate assessment of the client's responses to physical health problems is used to help the client return to an optimal level of function, both physiologic and psychological.

During the interview, the nurse focuses on developing a therapeutic relationship with the client. Because many of the topics in a psychosocial assessment are of a highly personal and sensitive nature, it is imperative that the nurse is tactful and nonjudgemental (see Ethical Issues in Nursing). Psychosocial assessment is integrated throughout the history interview, similar to health risk appraisal.

THE NATURE OF PSYCHOSOCIAL ASSESSMENT

Psychosocial assessment encompasses gathering information about a client's psychological patterns and social experiences. *Psychological patterns* are the individual, unique nonphysical components of a client, such as thoughts, feelings, motivations, mental status, personal strengths, and weaknesses. *Social experiences* are the parts of a client's life that are affected by or dependent on others. The term "*psychosocial*" denotes the melding of the two dimensions because it is impossible to separate the effects of psychological factors from those of social factors on an individual. Similarly, the psychosocial dimension intertwines with the physiologic dimension. All dimensions interact to produce a unique individual. Therefore, the client is viewed both as an individual and as a member of a unique and personal social network.

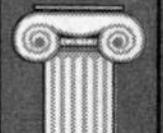

ETHICAL ISSUES IN NURSING

What Should Nurses Do with Confidential Information?

What should nurses do with confidential information? The information gained through client interviews and assessments is the basis by which a plan of care is initiated. In order for a person to feel comfortable in verbalizing all of their personal information, a sense of trust must be reached. This sense of trust may take a while to establish (over several office visits, days in the hospital, and home visits). Because of this, it is important that communication between health care providers and their clients be as open and nonthreatening as possible. The health care provider must be astute to verbal as well as nonverbal information. Client information, as a rule, should remain confidential, just as the medical record is confidential.

What happens when such confidential and perhaps sensitive information discloses situations that places confidentiality in an ethical dilemma? For example, a dilemma occurs when a client comes in for treatment of a sexually transmitted disease (STD) and does not want the spouse informed because he or she has engaged in an extramarital affair. On one hand, confidentiality should be protected. On the other hand, perhaps the spouse needs to be examined for possible STD infection as well. Another example centers around information gained from a client regarding illegal drug use. What obligation do health care providers have in keeping illegal activities confidential?

Issues of confidentiality can place the nurse in some very sensitive positions. When information on illegal practices or practices that may be harmful to others is revealed by a client, the nurse must decide what action should be taken. A client's right of confidentiality should always be respected, but when such confidentiality places a nurse in a legal dilemma, the nurse must inform the client that such a dilemma exists and that he or she must report such information. Clients do have a right to confidentiality, but they do not have the right to involve nurses in legal dilemmas. It is the nonlegal dilemmas, such as the STD example given above, that place nurses in uncomfortable positions. In these situations, the nurse may respect confidentiality by simply referring inquiries about the client back to the client and/or physician. The nurse may also help the client understand the possible consequences that his/her confidential information may have on themselves and/or others.

Psychosocial assessment requires sensitivity and interpersonal skills. The nurse's ability to establish a professional therapeutic relationship directly affects the quality and usefulness of the data collected. An atmosphere of trust between the client and nurse encourages the client to feel free to divulge sensitive psychosocial information. The nurse conveys interest to the client by listening attentively, making eye contact, and using skillful interview techniques. The nurse's personal value system may influence or bias his or her perception of a client's behavior and experiences. Self-awareness assists the nurse to be nonjudgemental. Unencumbered by bias, the nurse is likely to establish a trusting relationship with the client and to receive relevant information. The nurse's ability to make accurate observations and to share them with the client allows the client opportunity to validate the nurse's perceptions and inferences.

It is difficult to separate the dimensions of psychosocial assessment. Consideration of one or two dimensions while ignoring the others jeopardizes data completeness and accuracy. Significant information may be missed if the nurse does not consider all the dimensions and their relationships to each other. Likewise, because all dimensions are interrelated, both subjective and objective data are included in a psychosocial assessment. The nurse considers this when recording the data.

Table 11–3 gives examples of psychosocial information collected as part of the initial nursing history interview. Possible use and rationale are included.

PSYCHOSOCIAL RISK FACTORS

Eight factors have been identified to evaluate in clients adjusting to health problems. These include social history, level of stress experienced during the previous year, the client's usual coping pattern, neurovegetative changes, the client's understanding of the health problem, mental status, personality style, and the major psychosocial issues (reactions) to the health problem.

Social History. Social history includes information about the client's lifestyle, family members, and social network. The nurse asks whether or not others are available to provide emotional support to the client during stressful times. This includes nonhuman support systems such as pets.

Level of Stress Experienced During the Previous Year. The client's stress level is information the nurse assesses to determine the client's present situation including recent major stressors. Change and loss are two major influences that produce stress in individuals.

Usual Coping Pattern. The usual coping pattern refers to how the client copes with a serious problem or manages high levels of stress. The nurse asks the client to describe a particularly stressful situation and how it was managed. The nurse assesses whether the client's usual coping style is adequate for the current situation. Other coping strategies may be necessary.

Neurovegetative Changes. Neurovegetative changes include physical symptoms of neurophysiologic malfunctioning or changes in the client's usual physical patterns that indicate psychological stress. The stress response, regardless of its cause, results in altered neurotransmitter levels, such as norepinephrine and serotonin, which then affect the sympathetic and parasympathetic nervous systems. The client's usual body functions, such as sleep and rest patterns, appetite, energy level, sexual function, and elimination patterns, are affected.

Client's Level of Understanding About the Health Problem. The client's level of understanding is explored by the nurse. The client may not comprehend what has happened or could happen as a result of a health problem. The client's expectations of the health care team may be unrealistic. The nurse determines how threatening a particular health problem is and whether the client has been able to prepare psychologically for its effects.

Mental Status. Mental status refers to the current emotional, intellectual, and perceptual functioning of the client. If a dysfunction is noted, the nurse describes the problem. Areas assessed include general appearance, affect and mood, level of consciousness, orientation, memory, speech and communication, thought processes, ability to calculate, general fund of knowledge, abstract thinking ability, perception, judgement, and insight.

Personality Style. Personality style is the way a client usually interacts with others. Examples include dependent, independent, controlled, relaxed, dramatic, suspicious, accepting, self-sacrificing, superior, inferior, uninvolved, involved, mixed (a combination of two predominant styles), or no predominant style.

Major Psychosocial Issues. The development of major psychosocial issues (reactions) to health problems is highly individual and usually occurs as the client and significant others cope with the effects of illness. Reactions include disruption in the ability to trust, maintenance of self-esteem, retention of feeling in control, coping with loss and guilt, and maintenance of intimacy.

COMPONENTS OF PSYCHOLOGICAL ASSESSMENT

The psychological, sociologic, and physiologic dimensions include factors that the nurse assesses, such as behavior, mental status, personal strengths and motivation, values, beliefs, and lifestyle.

Behavior. Behavior is the client's activities that are observed by others. Although key to understanding the client, it is only a small portion of the client's complex nature. It is commonly accepted that all behavior has meaning but that the meaning is not always clearly understandable to others.

The nurse considers the client's behavior as being central to psychological assessment. Accurate assessment dictates that the nurse describe observed behavior rather than interpret it. "The client is crying" is an example of an observed behavior, whereas "The client is depressed" is a judgemental statement. Without further assessment, the nurse does not know why the client is crying. If the client tells the nurse, "I feel depressed," then the recorded statement reads, "States she feels depressed."

Behavior is verbal or nonverbal. *Verbal behavior* is what the client says. *Nonverbal behavior* is everything the client does that may be observed, such as posture, movement, facial expression, and voice tone. The nurse observes and records both verbal and nonverbal behavior while noting which data are subjective (verbal)

TABLE 11-3. Applying Psychosocial Assessment to the Nursing Process

Data	Guidelines/Techniques	Use and Rationale for Data
1. Name	a. The nurse introduces herself to the client by name, and includes her role and professional relationship to the client. How often and when the client may expect to talk to the nurse is explained	a. Stating one's name, role, and relationship can help decrease the client's initial anxiety
	b. The client is first addressed as "Mr. or Mrs. ____." The names of people who accompany the client are also requested and recorded	b. Being addressed by name and title is a sign of respect. It also helps the client feel welcomed. Determining and using the names of significant others helps reduce anxiety and conveys a message that the nurse knows who is included in the client's social support network
	c. The client and significant others are asked if they have a preference in how they like to be addressed, e.g., Ms., Mrs., by first name, or nickname. Using a client's first name is not done unless the client gives permission and the nurse reciprocates	c. The client may have a preference for or against using titles that designate marital status or sex. If addressed incorrectly, the client may resent the nurse's assumption
2. Sex	a. It is usually obvious that a client is either male or female except with infants or sometimes older children. It may be necessary to ask	a. Sex may be significant when the client is assigned to a bed or room in a health care facility
	b. The nurse does not assume or expect the client to have stereotypical roles or behavior based on sex	b. Human psychosocial responses to situations are more similar than different between sexes
3. Age	a. The exact number of chronologic years is asked. However, this information may be less important than the client's developmental stage, e.g., infant, toddler, preschool, school-age, adolescent, teenage, young adult, middle adult, older adult	a. Knowledge of human growth and development helps the nurse anticipate the client's needs. However, the nurse realizes that developmental theories depict the "average" client and are to be used only as a guideline because individual differences occur
4. Where the client has come from	a. The nurse asks the client where the usual residence is as well as where the client has just come from. This information is asked during informal conversation	a. The usual residence and where the client has last been may not be the same. The information is used to individualize care and reduce the client's anxiety
	b. The nurse asks how far and how long the client traveled to reach the health care facility, when the client was home last, whether the client must rely on others to get to and from the health care facility, whether the client has brought along personal care items such as a toothbrush or comb (if he or she is being admitted)	b. The client's response helps the nurse understand some of the psychosocial stressors (recent and possibly ongoing) that the client and significant others have had. The client's ability to relate this information (as well as information about the health problem) may be an indication of the client's mental status
5. Client's reason for seeking help	a. The nurse asks the client to state the reason for coming to the health care facility	a. The client's response may indicate *possible* concerns and anxieties of the client and significant others
	b. The nurse asks if this is a planned (elective) visit or unexpected emergency	b. An unanticipated visit or admission to a health care facility may cause increased stress or worry for the client and others. The client may have concerns about a job or obligations at work or home. Other people may need to be notified of the client's status
	c. The nurse asks whether the client is experiencing pain or discomfort and, if so, to describe it	c. Pain, discomfort, or anxiety may occupy the client's attention and energy, leaving little ability to cooperate with a history interview

Table continued on following page

TABLE 11–3. Applying Psychosocial Assessment to the Nursing Process Continued

Data	Guidelines/Technique	Use and Rationale for Data
	d. The nurse asks the client if the present health problem is acute and of recent onset or if it is part of a progressive, ongoing, or long-term problem	d. The client may understand more about a long-term health problem and possess insight into the nature of the current situation compared with that of an acute problem
6. Significant others	a. The nurse acknowledges others who accompany the client and asks if they have any questions	a. Regardless of their relationship to the client, these people are present at a stressful and possibly critical time. They also need attention to allay their concerns and anxiety, which may be conveyed to the client. The client may be able to relax if the significant others are also attended
	b. The nurse allows (if possible) a significant other to remain close by if the client requests this, regardless of familial relationship to the client (CAUTION: If an abuser/victim relationship is suspected, this request is denied)	b. This information provides insight about the client's social network and possible support systems (The client, if a victim of abuse, may be fearful or hesitant to have the abusing party present, especially if the reason for seeking health care is a result of an abusive episode)
	c. The nurse asks the client to identify which significant others are to be kept informed of the client's condition, especially in case of an emergency. The client may also request that certain people *not* be given information	c. Allowing the client to exercise autonomy promotes a feeling of being in control and reduces anxiety. The client may identify someone who is not family related. The client may also change these requests at a later time
7. Nonverbal communication	a. The nurse observes the client throughout the nurse-client interaction	a. Much may be learned from the client's nonverbal behavior. However, information communicated nonverbally is considered tentative until it is validated
	b. The client's body language is noted, such as posture, gestures, eye movements, eye contact, use of touch, reaction to being touched. The client may rely on gestures to help convey information	b. The client's actions guide the nurse's behavior and approach to how further assessment is conducted. For example, the client who distances him or herself from the nurse may need additional time and explanation to relax and be able to communicate important information
	c. The nurse notes the client's interactions with significant others	c. Information about the client's social network and support systems may be learned
8. Speech	a. The nurse listens carefully to the client for what is said and how it is expressed. Noted are the client's choice of words; the volume, tone, accent, and timing of speech; if there is any repetition; the use of silence; the energy and animation used to express words; and if there are any obvious speech disorders, such as slurring of words, stuttering, and inappropriate word use	a. Verbal communication may reveal the client's level of anxiety, such as rapid speech, repetition, and inappropriate laughter. Accentuation, word choice, or presence of a speech disorder reveals information about the client's comprehension, existence of a possible language barrier, or a possible neurologic problem

and which are objective (nonverbal). Observations, when validated by the client, assist the nurse in understanding the client's psychological status.

Mental Status. Mental status assessment consists of evaluating the client's behavior (verbal and nonverbal) and asking the client a series of questions to determine his or her level of consciousness. The following areas are included in a mental status examination: general appearance, motor behavior, affect, mood, speech and communication, thought processes and content, orientation, attention span, memory, general fund of knowledge, calculations, ability for abstract reasoning and thinking, perceptual distortion, judgement, and insight.

General Appearance. The nurse observes the client's posture, nonverbal behavior, facial expression, manner of dress with regard to the climate and occasion, grooming and hygiene, and attitude toward the assessment interview (e.g., cooperative, hostile, withdrawn).

Motor Behavior. The client's motor ability, gait, coordination, reaction time, unusual body movements (e.g., gestures, tics, tremors, foot tapping, hand wringing, grimacing, or other repetitive movements) are noted.

Affect. The nurse describes the observable, outward demeanor that depicts the client's current emotional state, such as fear, anger, resentment, depression, elation. In addition, the nurse notes whether or not the observed affect is congruent with the client's immediate circumstances. For example, "When informed that dismissal from the hospital was postponed because of an infection, the client first cried, then shouted at the nurse to leave the room."

Mood. Mood is the client's subjective description of a personal emotion that is pervasive and sustained. The nurse records whether or not the described mood is congruent with the client's present situation. For example, "The client stated she was 'happy and going to celebrate' when informed that the results of her tests were negative."

Speech and Communication (Language). The nurse evaluates the client's ability to understand and communicate by focusing on *how* the client talks, not the content of the client's speech. The nurse observes the client's tone of voice, pitch, rate of speech, spontaneity, coherence, articulation, length of responses, pauses, and pauses before replying to questions (latency).

Thought Processes and Content. The client's subjective responses and interpretations of daily living are reflected in his or her thought processes and content. The nurse assesses whether the client's speech progresses logically and whether the client's stream of thought is spontaneous, natural, organized, logical, relevant, coherent, and goal directed.

Orientation to Person, Place, Time, and Circumstances. The nurse asks the client to state his or her name and identify where he or she is. Ability to recall the date and time are also assessed. The nurse also asks the client to explain the reason for seeking health care.

Attention Span. The nurse assesses the client's ability to focus or concentrate on a task or activity over time. *Digit span* is a test of attention span in which the client repeats a series of 5 to 7 numbers forward and up to 5 numbers backward that have been identified by the nurse. The use of *Serial 7s and 3s* tests the client's attention span as well as calculation ability. The client is asked to subtract 7 (or 3) from 100 and continue to subtract by 7 (or 3) until unable to go any further.

Memory: Immediate, Recent, and Remote. The client is asked to recall information: within seconds (e.g., repeat a series of numbers); within several minutes to hours (e.g., recall specific words later during the interview); and within hours, months, or years (e.g., identify where the client grew up).

General Fund of Knowledge. The nurse asks the client to identify commonly known places, events, and people.

Calculations. The nurse asks the client to perform simple arithmetic calculations (addition, subtraction, multiplication, division) without the aid of pencil or paper.

Ability for Abstract Reasoning and Thinking. The client is asked to think beyond the concrete dimension by explaining a common proverb or by explaining similarities or differences between selected concepts. For example, "A bird in the hand is worth two in the bush." "What is the difference between a tree and a bush?"

Perceptual Distortion. The nurse asks the client to describe any illusions or hallucinations by asking specifically about each of the senses. For example, "Do you ever feel that you are hearing sounds that other people do not?"

Judgement. The client is asked to relate what he or she would do in a given situation such as when a prescribed medication has run out. Such questioning allows the nurse to assess the client's ability to make decisions.

Insight. The client is asked to explain in his or her own words what is the nature of the current health problem and what the expectations are for the health care team. The nurse evaluates whether the client demonstrates ability to perceive the self realistically and accurately.

When assessing mental status, the nurse individualizes questions to the client's circumstances. Variables affecting a client's ability to respond to specific questions include level of education, cultural background, degree of exposure to knowledge and information, familiarity with the nurse's language and vocabulary, and perceived acceptance of the client by the nurse. For example, it may be revealing to ask a teenager the name of a current popular singer but inappropriate to ask this same question of someone elderly. A client who has not progressed beyond a third-grade level of education may be incapable of performing complicated arithmetic calculations. A proverb widely known in one culture may have no meaning to someone from a different cultural background. Last, the nurse has access to correct answers for the questions asked, particularly those relating to the client's personal circumstances, such as the location of his or her home, date and place of birth, and family members.

Other Psychological Factors. The nurse assesses additional psychological factors such as motivation, personal strengths, values and beliefs, lifestyle, and formal psychological tests, while interacting with the client and significant others.

Motivation. Motivation is highly individual and is influenced by personal needs and desires, goals, hopes, and aspirations. The nurse attempts to determine the client's motivation for seeking health care and, if the client is ill, the motivation for returning to an optimal level of wellness.

Personal Strengths. The client's strengths are used by the nurse when planning care. Barry refers to *resources*, both internal and external, which are personal elements that determine an individual's capability to adapt to challenges and threatening stressors.[5] *Internal resources* are physiologic (e.g., immune system, nutritional state, physiologic defense systems, genetic predisposition to health, current state of each body system) and psychological (e.g., defense mechanisms, interpersonal style, usual conscious coping ability, current coping ability, and spiritual state such as the will to live). *External resources* include the social environment (e.g., usual coping style of the family, availability of social support, and the assessment skills of the health care givers) and the physical, economic, and cultural environments.

Values and Beliefs. The client's value system and beliefs determine whether or not the client views health care as worthwhile to pursue. The client's values and beliefs may be different from those of the nurse. However, the nurse accepts them as being valid for that particular client because they help provide insight to the client's behavior.

Lifestyle. Lifestyle data include information about the client's typical day and preferences for routines, habits, and activities of daily living.

Formal Psychological Tests. The nurse does not usually participate in formal psychological testing of clients. However, the nurse may use data from formal testing to supplement psychosocial data collected in nurse-client interactions and the health history. Nursing psychological assessment is concerned with the client as an individual and with the client's response to circumstances rather than with formal psychological diagnoses.

COMPONENTS OF SOCIOLOGIC ASSESSMENT

The *sociologic dimension* includes information about the client's social roles and functions. The nurse assesses the client's social network, socioeconomic status, lifestyle, sexuality, psychosocial development, and spirituality.

Social Network. All humans have need for being loved and feeling a sense of belonging. A social network is the group of people that surrounds, interacts, and sustains the client with intimacy, social integration, nurturing, reassurance, and assistance. The nurse becomes part of a client's social network when the client enters the health care system. However, the client continues to receive support from the established social network.

Social network data are collected by observing the client during interactions with family and visitors, asking questions about the client's interpersonal relationships, and determining whether there are certain individuals with whom the client prefers to maintain contact. The client may prefer to restrict access to specific visitors or telephone calls. The client may change these restrictions at any time. The nurse does not assume that only family members are the most significant people to the client. When planning care, the nurse includes the significant others who may be experiencing stress along with the client.

Socioeconomic Status. An individual's economic position within society is referred to as socioeconomic status. The nurse asks about factors that affect the client's financial and social well-being because they have implications for planning individualized health care. These include occupation, current employment status, work-related concerns, financial concerns, effect of the client's health status on the ability to work and finances, perceived effect that the client's socioeconomic status has on access to the health care system, educational background, and hopes and goals for the future.

Lifestyle. The client's usual daily patterns of living are referred to as lifestyle. Lifestyle is closely associated with socioeconomic status but also includes relationships with others. The nurse assesses the client's usual roles and functions, work and study habits, leisure and relaxation activities, type and location of residence, living arrangements, usual manner of transportation, proximity of close friends, importance and influence of cultural beliefs on diet and health-seeking behavior or treatment, health habits (e.g., use of alcohol, medications, nicotine, recreational drugs), stress level, methods used to relieve stress and their effectiveness, usual sleep pattern, and degree of satisfaction with current status.

Sexuality. Sexuality is the behavioral expression of one's sexual identity. It involves sexual relationships between people as well as the perception of one's maleness or femaleness. Many aspects of sexuality affect a client's health status and have significance in relation to nursing care and client outcomes. Aspects include physical health problems that affect sexual behavior (e.g., mastectomy, colostomy, skin lesions, venereal diseases, paralysis, physical deformities), concerns with sexual performance (e.g., impotence, premature ejaculation, inability to achieve orgasm, infertility), issues of sex role function (e.g., homosexuality, bisexuality, sexual ambiguity, transsexual surgery), and effects of environmental restrictions on sexual performance (e.g., residency in a long-term care facility) (see Chap. 7.)

Sexuality and sexual behavior remain sensitive topics for clients to discuss. The nurse does not allow personal beliefs and values to interfere with professional care but accepts and interacts with clients without judging them or their behavior.

Psychosocial Development. Psychosocial development is the client's level of growth and development. It includes the life developmental processes and phases of growth and maturation. Psychosocial development occurs across the lifespan and includes components that are physical, emotional, psychological, social, and cognitive. These components are not necessarily distinct from one another nor is the client's progress through life's stages and phases always predictable or inflexible. The nurse's understanding of human growth and development provides a foundation from which to assess the client.

Spirituality Assessment. Spiritual beliefs have implications for the client's well-being, such as sustaining hope or assisting with coping during periods of stress. The nurse includes spirituality assessment as part of the health history and explains to the client the purpose for asking about it (see Chap. 6). This portion of the history is usually addressed at the end of the interview after a trusting relationship is established. Because spirituality is very personal, the nurse respects a client's wish not to discuss this topic. However, the nurse asks whether there is someone special that the client prefers when spiritual support is needed.

GUIDE TO PSYCHOSOCIAL ASSESSMENT

The appendix to this chapter contains a psychosocial assessment format developed by Barry.[5] It is designed to assess the overall psychosocial functioning of the client and family. Questions are grouped according to Gordon's functional health patterns and are appropriate for general psychosocial assessment. When a specific area of distress or dysfunction is identified, a *focus assessment* is completed. A focus assessment narrows the general assessment and provides detailed information about the problem, enabling the nurse to identify the cause of the problem.

The nurse may collect psychosocial data that indicate a client has a psychiatric disorder. If this situation occurs, the nurse consults with other health care professionals such as a psychiatric clinical nurse specialist and the client's physician.

Physical Health History

REVIEW OF SYSTEMS

Physical health history is integrated with health risk assessment and the psychosocial history. In addition, the nurse conducts a head-to-toe review of systems (ROS). The ROS provides focus for the following physical examination. When the client reports a health problem, either past or current, the nurse proceeds with a *symptom analysis.*

Symptom Analysis. Symptom analysis is the client's description of the health problem's characteristics. Seven areas are included: location, quality, quantity, timing, precipitating factors, aggravating or relieving factors, and associated factors. In addition, the nurse asks the client to provide an opinion about the cause of the symptom or problem. Clients often have insight as to the nature and cause of their problems and sometimes express fears and concerns while discussing health problems with the nurse. These fears and concerns are explored in order to diagnose and treat clients' responses to health problems.

Location. The nurse asks the client to show where a symptom, such as pain, is located on the body while asking if the symptom moves or is stationary. For example, "Does the pain stay in one place or does it radiate to another part of your body?" Asking the client to point to the location of a symptom helps define its location.

Quality. The nurse assists the client to discriminate the quality of a symptom by using adjectives such as sharp, stabbing, dull, aching, continuous, intermittent, regular, irregular, searing, burning, numb, tingling, loose, solid, soft, hard, tight, crushing, etc.

Quantity. The nurse assists the client to describe the size, amount, number, or extent of the symptom or symptoms as well as the severity or intensity. Severity is quantified by asking the client to rate the symptom on a scale such as 1 to 5 or 1 to 10. The extent of a symptom's effect is assessed by asking the client to describe how the symptom has altered usual daily activities. For example, "Describe how the pain has interfered with what you usually do during the day. Does it keep you awake at night?"

Timing. Description of a symptom's timing includes onset, duration, and frequency. *Onset* refers to when a symptom first was noticed by the client (e.g., hours, days, months). *Duration* is how long the symptom lasts (e.g., minutes, hours, days, weeks). *Frequency* refers to how often a symptom occurs (e.g., every morning, once a week, every month).

Precipitating Factors. The nurse asks what the client was doing at the time the symptom was first noticed. Does the client have knowledge of what may have led to the symptom's occurrence?

Aggravating and Relieving Factors. The client is asked to recall whether there are any factors that alleviate the symptom or make it worse. For example, "Is there anything that makes the symptom go away or be less uncomfortable?" "Is there anything that makes the symptom get worse?"

Associated Factors. The nurse inquires specifically whether the client has noticed anything that happens in conjunction with the symptom. For example, "Does the symptom ever occur at other times or only when ________?"

When the client reports a symptom, the nurse assesses all the physiologic areas that are associated with the symptom or problem. For example, a client who reports epigastric pain will have an ROS for the gastrointestinal, endocrine, and psychological systems. The epigastric pain may be related to problems in any of these body systems.

ORGANIZING THE HEALTH HISTORY INTERVIEW

Data collected during the health history interview are organized by topical areas. The nurse uses a comprehensive, flexible format to collect data while allowing for in-depth focus assessment in areas of particular concern. The nurse develops an approach that includes a head-to-toe assessment of the client. Several guidelines assist the nurse to conduct a health history interview. Functional health patterns are presented as an example.

Functional Health Patterns

FHPs may be used by the nurse to collect health history data. This approach to assessment assists the nurse to identify the client's health patterns, deviations from these patterns, and actual or potential nursing diagnoses. Each of the 11 patterns has its own assessment criteria, which are listed in Table 11-4.

Health Perception and Health Management Pattern. The health perception and health management pattern describes the client's perception and understanding of the health status. This includes the client's lifestyle and behaviors to maintain and restore health and well-being.

Nutritional-Metabolic Pattern. The nutritional-metabolic pattern describes the client's food and fluid consumption in relationship to the body's metabolic needs. Adequacy of nutrient supply to local tissues is included in this pattern. Multiple factors influence the client's behavior in this pattern, such as physiologic (e.g., dehydration), pathophysiologic (e.g., peptic ulcer), psychosocial (e.g., the emotional significance of food), and socioeconomic (e.g., financial ability to purchase food).

Elimination Pattern. The elimination pattern focuses on the client's patterns of excretory function, including the bowel, bladder, and skin. Habits for excretory regularity and perceived difficulties in this pattern are assessed.

Activity-Exercise Pattern. The activity-exercise pattern describes the client's activities of daily living requiring energy expenditure. These include self-care measures, physical exercise, stamina, and leisure and recreational activities.

TABLE 11-4. Functional Health Pattern Assessment History Data

Functional Health Pattern	Health History Data
Health-perception–health management	Quality of usual and current health rated on a scale of 1 to 10
	Self-rating of the importance of health on a scale of 1 to 10
	Perceived ability to control and manage health
	Resources used in health management including primary care giver
	Self-care measures to maintain or prevent disruption of health status (e.g., risk management)
	Health habits (e.g., seatbelt use, diet, alcohol consumption, tobacco use)
	Complete description of present health problem (i.e., *chief complaint*)
	Expectations for outcome of current health problem
	Expectations for care givers
	Previous illnesses or hospitalizations, reaction to these events, and their outcomes
	Developmental history, including childhood illnesses and immunizations
	Ability to manage and comply with recommended treatment of health problems
	Current medications, including over-the-counter
	Allergies
	Environmental factors affecting health (e.g., occupation, home, leisure)
	Socioeconomic factors affecting health (e.g., financial concerns, health care insurance, living conditions)
	Knowledge and use of community resources to manage health
	Family history
Nutritional–metabolic	Recall of usual food and fluid intake for the past 24 hours
	Comparison of the 24-hour recall diet to typical pattern of diet intake

TABLE 11-4. Functional Health Pattern Assessment History Data Continued

Functional Health Pattern	Health History Data
	Quality of appetite Dietary restrictions (medical order) Food preferences and dislikes Use of food supplements (e.g., vitamins) Knowledge level of dietary recommendations (e.g., basic four food groups, recommended dietary allowances, special dietary guidelines) Past alterations in dietary habits (e.g., bulimia nervosa, anorexia nervosa) Usual weight Minimum and maximum weight range Recent weight gain or loss (how much? time span?) Social significance of food Who shops for food items? Who usually prepares meals? Religious or cultural beliefs affecting diet or meal preparation Ability to swallow and chew Are there any feeding problems?
Elimination	
Bowel	Usual bowel habits, including frequency, time of day, color, consistency, assistive devices used (e.g., laxatives, suppositories, enemas), constipation, diarrhea Change in bowel habits. Describe
Bladder	Usual frequency, amount, color of voiding Assistive devices used (e.g., self-catheterization) Problems with frequency, urgency, burning, retention, incontinence, dribbling, dysuria, polyuria, nocturia
Skin	Condition, color, temperature, turgor, lesions, edema, pruritus
Activity-exercise	Description of usual daily activities Weekend schedule, if different from daily Occupation-related activities Leisure activities including hobbies Description of exercise regimen Limitation in ambulation, bathing, dressing, toileting, and feeding Dyspnea with exertion Fatigue
Sleep-rest	Usual sleep habits including bedtime, hours of sleep obtained, wake-up time Problems falling asleep or staying asleep Sleep aids used, including medications, food, beverages, and sexual intercourse Rating of quality of sleep obtained (does client feel rested?) Periods of decreased wakefulness during the day Naps or rest periods
Cognitive-perceptual	Ability to understand Educational level obtained Self-rating of intelligence level Ability to communicate with others Ability to make decisions and the relative ease or difficulty experienced with decision making Ability to see, hear, feel, taste, smell Compensations made for sensory deficits and their effectiveness Problems with vertigo, heat or cold intolerance Pain (including a symptom analysis) Desire to learn
Self-perception–self-concept	Description of self, including strengths and weaknesses Major concerns

Table continued on following page

TABLE 11-4. Functional Health Pattern Assessment History Data Continued

Functional Health Pattern	Health History Data
	Health goals Body image and feelings about the self Level of satisfaction with current age Perceived developmental level Emotional status Effect of illness on self-perception Personal factors contributing to illness, recovery, health maintenance
Role relationship	Language, quality of speech and relevancy Ability to express self Family life, including family members and their relationships to client Roles client and family members fill Interpersonal relationships within family Support systems within family, including person client feels closest to Family-related problems or complaints, including living arrangements, parenting, marital problems, abuse Occupation and job-related role expectations Problems at work Societal relationships beyond family or work Most important person to client Type of neighborhood or community in which client lives Participation in social groups (e.g., church, clubs) Perceived contributions to society
Sexuality-reproductive	Level of satisfaction with role as male or female Anticipated changes related to health problem (e.g., fertility, libido, impotency, pregnancy, contraception, menstruation) Sexual activity, including how long client has been sexually active, number of partners, use of contraceptives Known exposure to venereal diseases including AIDS Level of satisfaction with intercourse Problems with intercourse (e.g., premature ejaculation, impotence, pain, bleeding)
Female	Menstrual history including age at menarche, description of typical cycle, last menstrual period, age at menopause or symptoms of menopause Obstetric history including number of pregnancies, number of births, problems during pregnancy or labor and delivery Practice of breast self-examination, knowledge of technique, compliance Last Pap test and results, frequency of pelvic examinations and Pap tests
Male	Circumcision Age at climacteric and description of symptoms experienced Date and results of last pelvic examination Practice of testicular self-examination, knowledge of technique, compliance
Coping-stress tolerance	Coping strategies used and their effectiveness Personal loss or major changes in past year Comfort and security needs Most stressful event in life and reaction to it Use of stress management techniques and their effectiveness (e.g., eating, sleeping, self-medication, counseling, exercise, biofeedback) Effect stress has on lifestyle and ability to function, including decision making
Value-belief	Most important value to client Sources of strength and hope Importance of religion, type, and frequency of worship Life goals Values influencing decision making and ability to resolve moral questions Recent changes in values or beliefs Conflict in values or beliefs with those of significant others Spirituality needs, particularly during time of illness or hospitalization

Sleep-Rest Pattern. The sleep-rest pattern refers to the client's usual habits for sleep, rest, relaxation, and energy level. Patterns are assessed for a 24-hour period to consider circadian rhythmicity.

Cognitive-Perceptual Pattern. The cognitive-perceptual pattern describes the client's ability to perceive, comprehend, and use information as well as the sensory functions.

Self-Perception and Self-Concept Pattern. The self-perception and self-concept pattern includes the client's view of self, including attitudes, identity, body image, sense of self-worth, and self-esteem.

Role Relationship Pattern. The role relationship pattern describes the client's roles in society and interpersonal relationships.

Sexuality-Reproductive Pattern. The sexuality-reproductive pattern refers to the client's satisfaction or dissatisfaction with sexuality and reproductive functions. These include sex role behavior and identification, physiologic and biologic functions, and sociocultural aspects of sexual behavior.

Coping–Stress Tolerance Pattern. The coping–stress tolerance pattern describes the client's general coping strategies and their effectiveness in managing stress. Included are the client's perception of stressors and their effect on the client.

Value-Belief Pattern. The value-belief pattern includes the values, beliefs (including spiritual), and goals that guide the client's choices and decisions, particularly in health care. Sources of strength and meaning for the client are identified.

Table 11–5 presents a health history interview guide organized according to functional health patterns including an ROS. The nurse notes areas already discussed and reduces repetitive questioning so as not to fatigue the client.

Text continued on page 204

TABLE 11–5. Health History Assessment Guide

Data	Example
Interview date	April 15, 1992
Biographic Data	
Full name	Mary C. Jones
Age	45
Sex	Female
Race	Caucasian
Nationality	United States citizen of central European background
Date and place of birth	December 1, 1946 in Springfield, MA
Significant others	Husband: John Jones Children: Jessica (age 8) and Jeremy (age 5)
Home address	123 Main Street Springfield MA
Phone number	888-8888 (Home)
Occupation	Housewife
Social Security Number	000-00-0000
Religion	Roman Catholic
Emergency contact	Husband—see above for home phone or work (888-0000)
Source of information and reliability	Client, reliable historian
Source of referral to agency	Insurance company
Health Insurance	Blue Cross/Blue Shield of MA
Health Perception–Health Management	
Reason for visit (also called "chief complaint" or "CC"). Recorded in the client's own words	"I need to have a complete history and physical examination for my insurance policy"
Current health status (also known as "history of present illness" or "HPI")	
A. *Usual health* Rating of usual and current health by the client	Rates quality of usual health as 8 out of 10 and current health as 6 out of 10 on a scale of 1 to 10, with 10 being the best possible
B. *Importance of health* Rating of health's importance to the client	Rates health importance as 9 out of 10, with 10 being the highest importance

Table continued on following page

TABLE 11-5. Health History Assessment Guide Continued

Data	Example
Health Perception–Health Management	
C. *Perceived control of health* Client's view of the extent health is influenced by self-care actions or by others	Has a certain amount of control and responsibility for health but realizes that some health problems cannot be avoided
D. *Resources used in health management* 1. Primary care giver	Gynecologist, Dr. Smith
2. Self-care measures to maintain health or prevent disruption of health a. Exercise b. Diet c. Safety measures d. Recreational drug use (how long used, type, amount, frequency) e. Tobacco (type, amount smoked per day and for how long, efforts to quit and success) f. Alcohol intake (type, amount and frequency, how long used) g. Self-monitoring procedures h. Regular screening procedures	Balanced diet including basic food groups. Tries to limit salt and saturated fat intake. No regular exercise regimen. Always uses seatbelts. Denies recreational drugs. Nonsmoker; although "tried a couple of times." One to two glasses of wine four to five times per week. No hard liquor. Wears safety goggles, work gloves, and closed shoes when gardening. Knows BSE and performs "every few months or so." Sees gynecologist every 1 to 2 years for routine pelvic examination and Pap smear. Mammograms every 2 years. Vision tested every 2 to 3 years when prescription change needed. Sees dentist once a year for routine cleaning and x-ray studies
E. *Description of each symptom or problem identified by client in the reason for visit* (i.e., symptom analysis) 1. Location 2. Quality 3. Quantity 4. Timing including onset, duration, and frequency 5. Precipitating factors 6. Aggravating or alleviating factors 7. Associated factors	Rates present health 6 out of 10 because of recent increased stress and back pain. "When I get tense, my lower back aches, especially if I sit too long." Also develops shoulder and neck stiffness and headache. Present lower back pain began 2 weeks ago after vacuuming. Aching sensation comes and goes. Uses heating pad to lower back at night and cervical pillow. Takes aspirin, 10 gr, alternating with acetaminophen, 10 gr, every 2 to 4 hours while awake, which takes edge off the ache. Denies straining back. States that income tax time is always stressful; also family is trying to place elderly parents in a long-term care facility. Takes care of parents' home as well as own household. Parents depend on client for shopping, cleaning, and transportation. Able to perform ADLs without limitation, although back pain is distracting and makes it hard to fall asleep at bedtime
F. *Review of biologic systems and functional health patterns related to the symptom or problem* See the ROS below for the type of information to elicit Record both significant positive and negative data	Include the ROS for musculoskeletal, neurologic, and psychiatric body systems. The functional health patterns of role relationships, coping and stress tolerance, sleep and rest, and activity and exercise should also be included for this client
G. *Client's perception of the symptom or problem* The client often has insight into the nature of the health problem. The client may also express fears and concerns that become apparent from comments or comparisons made to family, friends, or acquaintances	"I think I'm reacting to putting my parents in a nursing home. I just can't be responsible for two families and two households anymore. I'm not able to do the job I should for either family. My husband and kids resent all the time I spend with Grandma and Grandpa. I no longer have time for myself. I guess I am angry that I feel so caught in the middle"
H. *Client's expectations for outcome of the current health problem*	"I just want to pass this physical today. I know I've got other problems but somehow it'll work out"
I. *Client's expectations from care givers in the management of the current health problem*	"You can't solve my problems. But maybe you can tell me if there is anything wrong with my back or not"
Past health status (also known as "past medical history" or "PMH")	
A. *Developmental* The client is asked to identify known problems with growth and development, including prenatal or birth history, such as premature delivery, low birth weight	Full-term, vaginal delivery. No known problems with growth or development
B. *Immunizations*	Usual childhood immunizations. Last tetanus booster at 18

TABLE 11-5. Health History Assessment Guide Continued

Data	Example
C. *Past illnesses* 1. Childhood 2. Adulthood	Had measles (rubeola), chickenpox, mumps. Denies rubella, polio, whooping cough, scarlet fever, or rheumatic fever. Frequent bronchitis during childhood, but none as an adult. Denies asthma, tuberculosis, pneumonia, hypertension, heart problems, kidney problems, ulcers, diabetes, thyroid problems, stroke, seizures, migraine headaches, arthritis, anemia, cancer, or bleeding tendencies
D. *Allergies*	Hayfever and allergies to animal dander (itching, wheezing, eye irritation relieved by antihistamine such as diphenhydramine [Benadryl]). No known drug or food allergies
E. *Previous hospitalizations* Include client's reaction to these events and their outcomes	1959—Tonsillectomy & adenoidectomy 1964—Septoplasty 1969—Ganglion removal, right wrist 1974—Dilatation and curettage 1980—Dilatation and curettage 1983—Childbirth 1986—Childbirth All hospital stays were short term and uneventful. Satisfied with care and outcomes
F. *Previous surgery* Reasons procedures were performed, client's reaction to events and their outcomes	See "previous hospitalizations" 1967—Ganglion removal, right wrist 1973—Wisdom teeth extracted 1977—Sebaceous cyst removed, right thigh 1982—Mole excision, right scapula 1983—Mole reexcision, right scapula 1986—Tubal ligation All procedures without complications Satisfied with care and outcomes
G. *Serious injuries or accidents* Client's reaction and eventual outcomes	Suffered broken nose at some time during childhood, causing a deviated septum (corrected with surgery in 1964). No other major injuries
H. *Obstetric history* 1. Gravida (number of pregnancies and dates) 2. Para (number of births, infant weights, and health of babies) 3. Abortions 4. Miscarriages 5. Stillbirths 6. Complications	Gravida = 4, para = 2. Two full-term pregnancies resulting in live births of healthy infants. Two miscarriages, followed by dilatation and currettage, no abortions. No stillbirths. Pregnancies uncomplicated. Weight gain of approximately 20 lbs with each pregnancy 1983—Female infant, 8 lbs, 1 oz 1986—Male infant, 9 lbs, 3 oz
I. *Current medications* Include name, dose, frequency, route, reason for taking, desired effectiveness, side effects experienced. Include prescribed and over-the-counter drugs	Dyazide, one capsule, PO, prn prior to menses onset. For premenstrual fluid retention. No side effects. Reduces "bloating" and hand numbness Multiple vitamin with iron and calcium, one tablet, PO, qd. For diet supplement. No known side effects. Feels that she is getting minerals and vitamins needed to maintain health Acetaminophen, gr X, PO, q4h prn, alternating with ASA for headache, muscle aches, backache. Helps relieve discomfort Terfenadine (Seldane) 1 tablet twice daily. For relief of hay fever symptoms. Usually effective.
Psychosocial History A. *Environmental* 1. Job hazards	Not employed outside home. Unaware of problems with air or noise pollution. Some heavy lifting with housework. Fatigued from taking care of two households
2. Home hazards	Smoke detectors in home. Fire extinguisher kept in kitchen. Central heating and air conditioning. Several flights of stairs in home (carpeted). Home approximately 20 years old

Table continued on following page

TABLE 11–5. Health History Assessment Guide Continued

Data	Example
Health Perception–Health Management	
3. Neighborhood and community hazards	Lives in a middle-class white and blue collar neighborhood; most are single family homes. No industry in immediate area. City water supply. Relies on own car for transportation
B. *Socioeconomic factors*	
1. Financial concerns; can meet basic needs	"Money is tight" but has the necessities. Concerned whether family can afford placing parents in a long-term care facility
2. Health care insurance	Insured through husband's group policy. Seeking to increase coverage on life insurance policy
3. Knowledge of resources available to assist in health management. Use of services?	Uses gynecologist as primary care provider. Annual dental checks. Uses screening services through community health fairs. Rates knowledge of available services as "fair"
Family History. The purpose of the family history is to identify familial diseases that affect the client's health status and risk of potential health problems	
A. *Diagram* It is commonly displayed as a diagram of a family tree of blood relatives (parents, grandparents, siblings, children). Each person's health status is noted	See diagram of family history in Figure 11–1
1. Age (if alive), or age at time of death and cause of death	
2. Presence of significant illnesses or problems that client is presently experiencing	
3. A *key* to the diagram is included to aid interpretation	
B. *Summary statement*	
1. The client is asked specifically whether there is a family history or symptoms of certain health problems that exist in the family	Denies family history of kidney disease, anemia, hemophilia, epilepsy or seizures, migraines and headaches, hypertension, retardation, thyroid problems, tuberculosis, eating disorders (e.g., overeating, undereating, self-induced vomiting), obesity, or Huntington's chorea
2. A final opportunity is provided for the client to add information about the existence of any other type of health problem that tends to run in the family	Family history positive for heart disease, strokes, arthritis, mental illness, alcoholism, cancer (stomach), diabetes mellitus, allergies, and asthma
Nutritional-Metabolic	
Diet History. The purpose is to identify actual or potential nutritional deficits or metabolic demands that increase a client's risk of developing a nutritional problem	
A. *Usual diet* The client is asked to recall everything consumed during the past 24 hours, including quantities of portions. This diet is compared with the usual diet consumed. Food restrictions are noted, as well as the client's preferences and dislikes. The nurse asks specifically about intake of salt, sugar, calcium, fats, caffeine, fiber, and alcohol. Use of dietary supplements is noted	No medical dietary restrictions. Uses salt sparingly when cooking, and low saturated fat margarine. Does not prepare fried foods, although occasionally eats them if dining out. Eats breakfast and most dinners at home. Lunch usually at parents' home. Uses only 2 per cent fat milk. Drinks four to six cups regular coffee daily. Has one to two glasses (4 oz) wine with dinner four to five times a week. Puts milk in coffee; rarely drinks it by the glass. Eats hard cheese occasionally. Prefers fresh or frozen vegetables. No canned vegetables. No particular food dislikes. Uses sugar in baking. Takes vitamin and mineral supplement daily
	24-hour recall diet:
	Breakfast—Orange juice (8 oz); oatmeal, prepackaged, instant (1/2 cup); whole wheat toast (1 slice) with 1 tsp margarine; 2 cups coffee with 2 tbsp milk each
	Lunch—Canned chicken noodle soup (8 oz); whole wheat crackers (6); water (12 oz); chocolate chip cookies (four); two cups coffee with 2 tbsp milk each
	Dinner—Spaghetti (2 cups) with homemade tomato/meat sauce; Parmesan cheese (1 tbsp); tossed green salad (2

TABLE 11–5. Health History Assessment Guide Continued

Data	Example
	cups) with vinaigrette dressing; sourdough roll (1) with 2 tsp margarine; low-fat ice cream (1/2 cup)
B. *Appetite* The client is asked to describe appetite in relation to the foods consumed. Important to note is whether or not there has been a change in appetite. If so, is this change related to an identifiable event in the client's life?	No change in diet habits. Hearty appetite and could eat more but tries not to overeat. Treats self to candy bar about once a week. "There isn't much that disturbs my appetite. I feel worse if I miss or skip a meal, so I try not to"
C. *Knowledge level* The nurse asks the client to describe what system is used to guide diet planning to determine whether or not the client knows what is included in a balanced diet. If on a special or restricted diet, can the client recount the modifications to be followed?	"I use the basic four food groups to plan my family's meals. I don't get enough milk or milk products, which is why I started to take a vitamin pill. I do well with the fruit and vegetable and the grain and cereal groups. I'm not worried about my kids or husband, because they all drink more milk and eat more fruits than I do. We all probably eat too much meat but I try to use poultry, fish, and lean beef or pork. I never buy luncheon meats"
D. *Food preparation* The nurse asks who is responsible for food shopping as well as food preparation in the family. If it is someone other than the client, is this person knowledgeable about the client's special dietary needs? Are there religious or cultural beliefs that affect the client's diet or how meals are prepared?	"I do the food shopping for my family and for my parents. I also do the meal planning and cooking for all of us. I buy in quantity and cook up large batches that will feed all of us with leftovers. That way we get at least two meals out of it" "We all pretty much eat anything and everything except for individual dislikes. No one is on a special diet"
E. *Importance of food to the client* Is there any special significance of food (or lack of it) to the client?	"I love food and I like to experiment with new dishes. But I'd rather have something to eat instead of nothing"
F. *Weight* 1. What is the client's usual weight and the range that the weight varies (minimum-to-maximum)	Usual weight = 145 lbs Weight range = 136–154 lbs
2. Has there been a recent (within 6 months) weight gain or loss? If so, how much? A change in weight of 10 per cent or more increases the client's risk of developing related problems, such as malnutrition, protein deficiency, hypertension, diabetes, cardiovascular insufficiency	Denies recent weight change. Has been at usual weight for past 6 years, since last child was born
G. *Feeding problems* The client is asked to identify whether or not there has been difficulty with chewing or swallowing. Has there ever been treatment for such a problem in the past?	Denies problems with chewing or ability to swallow
Elimination	
Bowel	
A. The client is asked to describe usual bowel habits, including frequency of stools, time of day bowel movements occur, stool color and consistency. The nurse notes whether the client uses terms such as "constipation" or "diarrhea" to describe patterns	"I have a bowel movement every 1 to 3 days. It's usually formed, brown. It's not at any particular time of day, just whenever I feel the urge" Denies constipation, diarrhea
B. Does the client use assistive devices such as laxatives, enemas, or suppositories? If so, the nurse asks the client to identify the type used and the frequency that they are used. How long has the client required assistance to evacuate bowels?	Denies use of laxatives, enemas, or suppositories. If client feels constipated, tries to drink more liquids or includes more fruit in diet
C. The client is asked whether or not there has been a change in bowel habits (increase or decrease in frequency, amount, consistency, odor, color). If so, how long has the client noticed the change?	Denies change in bowel habits. Is rarely bothered with constipation or diarrhea

Table continued on following page

TABLE 11–5. Health History Assessment Guide Continued

Data	Example
Elimination	
Bladder	
A. The nurse asks the client to describe the usual urinary habits, including frequency of urination, amount, color, odor. Are there specific terms the client uses to describe patterns?	Urine usually medium yellow in color. Urinates upon arising and every 2 to 3 hours while awake, moderate amounts. Voids more often when has been drinking coffee, especially during the evening. Sometimes awakens to urinate once during the night
B. Does the client use assistive devices such as self-catheterization, running water, or applying pressure over the symphysis pubis? The client is asked to explain the purpose for using such devices and how long they have been used	Denies use of assistive devices for urination
C. The client is asked whether or not there has been a change in usual urinary habits such as an increase or decrease in frequency, urgency, burning, ability to empty bladder completely, dribbling, incontinence, pain with urination, nocturia	No recent change in urinary habits. Began having some problems with urgency and leaking of urine when laughing, coughing, sneezing, or straining, such as with lifting bags of groceries. This began after the birth of second child. Nocturia, as described earlier
Skin	
A. The client is asked to describe the overall condition of the skin (dry, oily), hair, and nails	Skin is dry. Applies moisturizing lotion after shower. Uses hand lotion frequently during the day. Denies dandruff or itching scalp. Nails are brittle
B. Have there been problems with itching or lesions? If so, how long has the problem existed?	No unusual lesions reported. Has had several "brown spots" removed in the past when mole was removed
Activity-Exercise	
A. *Usual daily activity* The nurse asks the client to describe a typical day's pattern for what activities are performed and the approximate times these occur. When are meals prepared and eaten? What time does the client leave home for school or work? Are rest breaks included in the day's schedule? Is the major activity of the day one that is sedentary, moderately active, or very active? What time does school or work end?	Gets up about 6:00 AM with husband. Likes to have time to wake up with breakfast and some reading before getting the kids up and ready for school. Both parents get breakfast ready. Kids leave for school at 8:00 AM. Client then does errands, grocery shopping, cleaning. Goes to parents' home around 10:30 AM. Helps them get cleaned up, does their housekeeping. Prepares their lunch and dinner to reheat later. Takes parents to doctor appointments, helps with their errands and shopping. Home by 4:30 PM to be with kids after school. Prepares family dinner. Evenings used to catch up on housekeeping, laundry, helping kids with school work
B. *Leisure and relaxation activities* The nurse specifically inquires about what the client does during leisure time. On days off from school or work, do the day's typical activities differ from the usual daily schedule? What hobbies does the client enjoy? Does the client believe there is sufficient time for hobbies or other interests?	Enjoys needlework and reading when has time, usually in evening after kids in bed. Doesn't have much time lately for hobbies. Spends weekends doing laundry, yard work, with family going to the library, zoo, or a movie. Kids are not involved in outdoor sports because of their allergies. Sister helps out with parents on weekends, which gives family a break. "I often wish I had more time for the things I like"
C. *Exercise regimen* The client is asked to describe the type of exercise regimen followed. How often does the client exercise (minutes or hours per day and number of days per week)? A combination of aerobic, stretching, and strengthening exercises is recommended for fitness	Denies any type of exercise program. States is usually tired by end of the day, and exercise is the last thing on her mind
D. *Problems in activity tolerance*	
1. Are there limitations in the client's ability to ambulate, bathe, dress, or with toileting? The client is asked to describe limitations and whether assistive devices are used, e.g., crutches, cane, walker, wheel chair, button hooks, reach extenders, splints	Denies limitations in ADLs. No assistive devices
2. Does the client tolerate ADLs without becoming short of breath?	Able to complete ADLs without dyspnea

TABLE 11–5. Health History Assessment Guide Continued

Data	Example
3. Does the client feel fatigued? The client is asked to describe fatigue in detail, for example, is the fatigue constant? Is it related to certain activities? What is the client's level of energy? Is the energy level sufficient to meet the demands of the daily schedule?	Admits to feeling tired lately. "I am trying to run two households and it is wearing me out." Usually has enough energy to do most tasks, but some days has difficulty getting everything done
Sleep-Rest	
A. *Usual sleep pattern* The client is asked to describe the usual sleep habits including customary bedtime, number of hours sleep per night, and typical wake-up time. Does the client have a regular or irregular pattern? Is wake-up time assisted by an alarm clock or does the client wake up unassisted?	Usually in bed by 11:00 PM and awakens at 6:00 AM when husband gets up to the alarm clock. Gets 7 hours sleep per night
B. *Sleep aids* The nurse asks the client whether or not assistive devices are used to induce sleep. These devices may include a particular food or beverage, medication, sexual intercourse, listening to music or a "white noise" audiotape, watching television, and reading. Are there bedtime rituals that the client performs to get ready for sleep, e.g., brushing teeth, warm bath, meditation?	No particular sleep aids used or rituals followed. "I'm usually tired by bedtime and just tumble in bed and fall asleep." Lately has been taking analgesia at bedtime to ease back pain and make it easier to relax and fall asleep
C. *Quality of sleep* The nurse asks the client whether enough sleep is obtained to feel rested upon awakening. Are there problems falling asleep or staying asleep? What does the client do to return to sleep? What is the client's reaction to sleep disruptions? Does the client experience periods of sleepiness during the day? Does the client take naps; if so, when? Do naps help refresh the client?	Feels rested upon awakening. No particular problems falling asleep except recently because of back pain. Wakes occasionally during night but usually returns to sleep without difficulty. Sometimes has problems with sleepiness after lunch and dozes off, especially if parents are napping. Naps help to get through rest of afternoon
Cognitive-Perceptual	
A. *Cognitive performance* 1. The client is asked if there are difficulties with understanding (comprehension) what others communicate. What was the highest level of formal education attained by the client? The client is asked to *rate* or quantify own intelligence level (e.g., average, above average, below average when compared with peers). Does the client remember things easily? Is the client able to communicate with others verbally? in writing? by other means?	Denies difficulty with understanding others. College graduate with degree in home economics. Rates intelligence as above average compared with others in immediate neighborhood. Usually no problem with remembering. Communicates verbally, writes
2. Decision-making ability is also assessed. Does the client have difficulty making decisions? Or is decision making performed readily? Is there a predominant style the client uses to make decisions such as slowly after lengthy deliberation or quickly?	Denies difficulty with decision making in most circumstances. Tries to consider all possible outcomes and consequences when making decisions. Admits to current indecision about placement of elderly parents in nursing home
B. *Perceptual abilities* 1. The nurse inquires about each sensory organ's function: Are there problems with vision, hearing, tasting, smelling, or feeling (vertigo, heat/cold intolerance)?	Wears eye glasses for myopia, astigmatism since age 10. Currently has corrective lenses for these problems plus presbyopia. Denies problems with hearing, tasting, smelling, or tactile sensation. No dizziness or heat or cold intolerance
2. Does the client use assistive devices to compensate for perceptual deficiences (e.g., eye glasses, hearing aid)? Are devices effective?	Eye glasses worn (see earlier). Are effective
3. Does the client verbalize concern that perceptual difficulties have affected lifestyle or self-image?	Denies problems with adjusting to visual changes. "My glasses are a part of me, I've worn them so long"

Table continued on following page

TABLE 11-5. Health History Assessment Guide Continued

Data	Example
Cognitive-Perceptual	
C. *Pain* Does the client have pain? A complete description is elicited (see the analysis of a symptom under the Health Perception and Health Management Pattern). What effect does the pain have on the client's ability to perform ADLs?	Reports intermittent back pain. See complete symptom analysis under FHP Health Perception and Health Management. No limitation of ADLs
Self-Perception and Self-Concept	
A. The client is asked to describe the self as others might perceive him or her. The nurse asks the client to include descriptions of the major strengths and areas that want or need strengthening	Describes self as honest, hard working, caring about family, tries to please others. Strengths include willingness to help when needed, keeping family healthy by preparing nutritious meals. Areas to improve include having more time for self, family, and hobbies
B. What are the client's primary concerns? What are the client's goals in seeking health care?	Major concern is to work out a plan for placement of parents. Does not want them to feel abandoned by her. Health care goal is to have a "normal" physical examination
C. Is the client satisfied with the age and stage of personal development attained? Does the client have strong feelings (positive or negative) about self?	Satisfied with age and developmental level. Enjoys parenting. Finds it hard to be part of the "sandwich generation," with responsibilities for children and elders. Likes and respects self
D. Has illness had an effect on the client's self-perception? What effect has illness had in the client's life?	Denies effects of illness on self-concept. Most health problems have been acute and short term with no lingering effects
E. The client is asked to describe the overall emotional status (worried, concerned, sad, upset, depressed) resulting from illness or other disruptions in health status. Does the client express a belief that there is control over what happens during illness and recovery?	Believes self to be cheerful, happy. No major problems with health status. Admits to being worried about back, but does not believe it is serious. Believes that there is a certain amount of control over health status and that some illnesses can be avoided by taking care of self. Believes that recovery is affected by one's attitude and willingness to improve
Role Relationship	
A. The client is asked to relate an opinion about the ability to express the self in words. The nurse notes the language used by the client and appropriateness to the topic under discussion	No difficulty expressing self in words and conveying ideas to others
B. *Family*	
1. The client is asked to identify family members and their relationship to the client	Immediate family of four: self, spouse, and two children, a daughter and son. One younger sister and parents
2. Ask the client to identify the roles that each family member fills (e.g., parent, spouse, sibling, child, breadwinner, homemaker, peacemaker, arbitrator)	Client is mother, wife, lover, homemaker, caretaker. Husband is main breadwinner and authority figure to children; is a loving spouse. Parents share in decision making for family. Children are school aged
3. Ask the client to describe family interpersonal relationships. Is there someone who the client feels especially close to for support?	Immediate family is close to one another. Main supports to client are husband and sister. Children have the "usual" sibling quarrels but generally get along well with each other
4. Are there problems within the family that have strained relationships, such as a change in living space, marital problems, abuse?	No major marital or family problems. Husband and children verbalize that client spends a lot of time with her parents and less time with them. Some resentment expressed that client is too tired to pay attention to them
C. *Job-related*	
1. What roles does the client fulfill related to occupation? employee? manager? negotiater? "boss"? friend? confidant?	Unemployed outside the home. Describes occupation as full-time homemaker and manager of two households. Confidant and friend to husband and sister. Caretaker to aging parents
2. What are the client's major responsibilities at work?	

TABLE 11–5. Health History Assessment Guide Continued

Data	Example
3. Are there work-related problems that concern the client?	
D. *Society*	
1. The client is asked to describe what social activities are engaged in that go beyond the level of the family. Who is the most important nonfamily individual to the client?	Has little time for outside social activities. Tries to attend church services weekly. Is unable to identify a significant support person outside family
2. In what type of neighborhood or community does the client reside? Is it open and friendly with neighbors who know one another? Or is it closed and distant?	Neighborhood is friendly; most people know one another's names. Little socialization among families because most people work outside the home. Children play with neighborhood friends. Prior to parents' caretaking, client used to socialize with one or two close friends who did not work outside the home. These people have since moved from community
3. Does the client participate in any organizations or social groups? If so, does the client fulfill particular roles within the group, such as elected office, active member?	No outside participation in social groups other than going to church. Used to be involved in Parent-Teacher's Association and was a classroom "mom" and teacher's aide
4. What does the client see as his or her most important contribution to society? This may include aspects of the client's occupation (e.g., being employed and taking care of dependents, providing an essential service) or family life (e.g., being an example or role model for children)	Most important contribution is to raise decent children who will become responsible adults
Sexuality-Reproductive	
Clients of Either Sex	
A. The client is asked to describe the level of satisfaction experienced with being either a male or female. Does the client ever desire to be of the opposite sex?	Satisfied with being female; has no desire to trade sex roles
B. Does the client have concerns that there will be changes in sexual functioning related to health problems, such as infertility, loss of libido, impotence?	Unconcerned with possibility of change in level of sexual functioning. Does not see this as applying to her at this time
C. How long has the client been sexually active? Can the client relate the number of sexual partners? Have contraceptive measures been used in these relationships? Is the client satisfied with the frequency and quality of sexual relationships?	Sexually active since age 19. One partner who is current spouse. Has used a variety of contraceptives including diaphragm, intrauterine devices, and birth control pills. Had tubal ligation following birth of second child. Satisfied with sexual relationship with husband
D. Has the client ever had or knowingly been exposed to venereal disease, including AIDS? What treatment was received, if so?	No known exposure to venereal disease. Periodic problems with vaginal infections, usually yeast. Treated with prescription from gynecologist
E. Are there problems with sexual intercourse, such as impotence, premature ejaculation, pain, bleeding? What effect have these problems had on the client and the ability to engage in sexual relationships?	Denies problems with sexual intercourse. Often feels too tired to engage in intercourse, and frequency is less than it could be. Admits that husband tries to understand her tiredness, but occasionally expresses resentment
Female Clients	
A. *Menstrual history* 1. Age at menarche 2. Description of typical cycle 3. LMP 4. Age at menopause or symptoms of menopause 5. Description of changes in menstrual cycle	Menarche at age 12. Cycle lasts approximately 23 to 28 days. Has had some cycles as often as 18 days. Duration of flow 5 days, first 2 days moderate to heavy then tapering. LMP = 4/2/92. Some cramping first day of flow but not unbearable
B. *Obstetric history* See Health Perception–Health Management	
C. *Health risk appraisal*	
1. Does the client know technique for breast self examination? How often does the client perform BSE?	Knows BSE technique. Performs 1 week after menses begins. States she knows BSE should be performed every month

Table continued on following page

TABLE 11–5. Health History Assessment Guide Continued

Data	Example
Sexuality-Reproductive	
When does the client perform BSE during the menstrual cycle (or when during the month if client is menopausal)?	but sometimes forgets and skips a month or so
2. Date of last pelvic examination? How frequently does the client have pelvic examinations performed? Date of last Pap test and results, if known? How frequently are Pap tests performed?	Last pelvic examination and Pap test 5/91; results were "normal." Examinations every 1 to 2 years
Male Clients	
A. The nurse asks the client if he is circumcised	
B. Client's age at climacteric and symptoms experienced, if any	
C. *Health risk appraisal*	
1. Date of last male pelvic examination and results, if known?	
2. Does the client know technique for TSE? How often does the client perform TSE?	
Coping–Stress Tolerance	
A. The nurse asks the client to describe typical coping strategies used when faced with a stress-provoking situation. How effective are these strategies? Does the client try to use a variety of strategies to adapt to new situations? Or does the client tend to rely on a limited number of techniques?	Strategy used to cope depends on the type of stressor. Minor annoyances usually cause client to get mad and yell, then can decide whether further reaction is worthwhile. Major stressors cause client to withdraw and try to think of ways to cope or resolve stress. During these times, the client can be impatient with her family
B. The client is asked to describe any losses or major changes that have occurred during the past year. What was the client's reaction to these events?	No major loss identified. Parents' deteriorating health and ability to care for themselves perceived as a major stressor. Initially, tried to take care of them at home but is no longer able to do so. Feels upset and unable to decide what to do
C. What does the client do to help meet own needs for comfort and security? Is there a specific behavior or individual who helps the client manage through stress-provoking incidents?	Talks to husband and sister when is unable to cope with parents. When children get on her nerves, tends to isolate herself and tells kids to leave her alone. "Time out" helps client regain equilibrium
D. The client is asked to describe an event that was the most stress-provoking and how the client reacted	Current situation with parents is most stressful event client can recall. Is having difficulty resolving situation. Feels torn and angry
E. The nurse asks the client to *rate* the current stress level on a scale of 1 to 10	Rates current stress level as 9 out of 10
F. Does the client practice a stress-management technique, such as eating a favorite "comfort" food, sleeping, taking medications, exercise, biofeedback, self-hypnosis? How effective are these techniques in assisting the client to cope with increased stress levels?	Most effective technique is to take time out for self when she reads or goes shopping. Usually feels refreshed and able to resume activity
G. What effect has stress had on the client? Have there been any changes in lifestyle because of stress, in the client's ability to function, or on the client's ability to make decisions?	"It's been hard. I have almost no time for myself anymore. There are days that are hard to get through because I feel I'm going in five different directions." Finds it more difficult to make decisions, even about simple matters
Value–Belief	
A. The nurse asks the client to identify the most important value that provides guidance in daily living	Identifies most important value in life as love and respect for others
B. Are there particular values that influence the client's style of decision making? Are there values that affect the client's ability to resolve problems in a moral conflict?	Tries to be honest and consider as many aspects as possible when faced with moral conflicts. Religion is important but will follow own conscience first

TABLE 11-5. Health History Assessment Guide Continued

Data	Example
C. Has there been a change in the client's values or beliefs? Has this change had an effect on the client's relationships with significant others?	Denies changes in values or beliefs that affect relationships with others
D. The client is asked to describe life goals. How does the client visualize the progress that has been made toward these goals? Is the client satisfied or dissatisfied with lifetime accomplishments thus far?	Goals are to raise healthy, happy children who will be responsible adults and to continue in marital relationship until "we both fade away into the woodwork." Satisfied with family but realizes that there is stress on the whole family because of placement issue with parents
E. Does the client have a preferred religion or religious practices that are important? How frequently does the client attend worship services? Does the client consider religion to be a major influence in life?	States a preference for being Roman Catholic because that is how she was raised. Observes major religious holidays (Easter, Christmas) but not the others and goes to church most weeks. Does not follow diet restrictions regularly. Religion is an influence on life but not the only one
F. Does the client follow particular health practices or restrictions that are based on religious beliefs or other personal convictions?	See earlier note re: diet. Tries to maintain healthy diet for self and family because it's easier to keep healthy than to be sick
G. Does the client express a need for spiritual support during times of illness? Is there a particular individual or practice that will assist the client to feel that spiritual needs are being met?	Unable to relate a need for religious support during illness because has never perceived a need. Closest support is from husband, children, and sister. Does use prayer during times of feeling overwhelmed
ROS	
The purpose of the ROS is to screen for health problems that the client may be unaware of or has not previously mentioned during the history interview. Each biologic system is reviewed, and each symptom or problem is thoroughly described by completing a symptom analysis (see Health Perception and Health Management)	
A. *General* The nurse asks the client whether or not the following symptoms occur: fever, chills, weight loss or gain, weakness, headaches, nausea, vomiting, fatigue, malaise, sweats or night sweats, mood changes	Denies fever, chills, recent weight loss or gain, weakness, nausea, vomiting, malaise, sweats, or night sweats. Occasional headaches from tension (see Current Health Status). Fatigue attributed to being responsible for two households (see Health Perception and Health Management). Denies mood changes but is short tempered with children and husband
B. *Skin* The client is asked about past skin problems, such as scars or birthmarks, and current skin problems, including changes in color, texture or surface temperature, sores that do not heal, bruising, skin eruptions, growths, rashes, moles, itching (pruritus), dryness, hair changes (loss, dryness, brittleness, use of dyes, dandruff), and nail changes (cracking, brittleness)	Denies problems with skin changes or pruritus. Hands dry from frequently being wet and the use of soaps. Uses hand lotion to soften. Previous moles on back surgically removed × 2 (see Past Health Status). No recurrence. Wears hat during summer when outdoors and uses sun screen. Denies problems with hair. Nails are brittle
C. *Hematopoietic* The nurse asks about anemia, abnormal bleeding or bruising (ecchymoses), easy bruising, fatigue, known exposure to radiation, leukemia, blood transfusions, presence of unusual antibodies (if known), and blood type (if known)	Denies problems with anemia, unusual fatigue, easy bruising or bleeding, leukemia, unusual antibodies. No known exposure to radiation except chest x-ray study on admission to college and for mammograms. No blood transfusions. Blood type is A+
D. *Endocrine* Have there been past problems with diabetes, goiter, thyroid, growth and development, treatment with hormones, heat or cold intolerance, neck surgery? Are there current problems with weakness, tremors, nervousness, dry skin or hair, heat and cold intolerance, excessive sweating, change in hair distribution or hirsutism, impotence, altered interest in sexual activity, increased urination, increased appetite or thirst?	Denies problems with diabetes, goiter, thyroid, growth and development, heat or cold intolerance, weakness, tremors, nervousness, excessively dry skin or nails, undue sweating, changes in hair distribution, hirsutism, increased hunger, thirst or urination. Often too tired to engage in sexual intercourse (see Sexuality)

Table continued on following page

TABLE 11-5. Health History Assessment Guide Continued

Data	Example
ROS	
E. *Head* The client is asked about past problems with head trauma. Are there current problems with headaches, fainting (syncope), dizziness (vertigo), seizures, recent head injury?	Denies fainting, syncope, dizziness, seizures, recent head injury. See Current Health Status, re: headaches
F. *Eyes* The nurse asks the client whether there have been past problems with glaucoma, cataracts, infection (e.g., "pink eye"), eye trauma, or if the client has an eye prosthesis. Present problems may include changes in vision, failing vision or blindness, blurred vision, double vision (diplopia), redness, pain, itching, discharge or drainage, glaucoma, cataracts, excessive tearing or dryness, light sensitivity (photophobia), or swelling. The client is asked when vision was last examined (date) and the results, if known. Does the client wear glasses or contact lenses? If so, when was the last change of prescription?	Denies problems with glaucoma, cataracts, trauma, failing vision, blurred vision, diplopia, excessive tearing or dryness, pain, photophobia, swelling, redness, itching, or drainage. Has had conjunctivitis several times in past when children have had it. Treated with Neobiotic eye drops, which were effective. Has photophobia sometimes with severe headaches; usually resolves when headache relieved. Wears eye glasses for myopia, astigmatism, and presbyopia. Last prescription change was at last examination in 1990
G. *Ears* The client is asked whether or not there have been past problems with hearing loss, ear infections, or earaches. Has the client had the ears pierced? Current problems may include difficulty hearing, deafness, ringing (tinnitus), dizziness (vertigo), pain, discharge, or sensitivity to noise. When was the client's hearing last tested? Does the client wear a hearing aid?	Denies problems with hearing loss, ear infections, earaches, deafness, tinnitus, vertigo, pain, discharge, or sensitivity to noise. Cannot remember when hearing was last tested, but it may have been while still in school
H. *Nose and Sinuses* The nurse asks the client about past problems with frequent colds, sinus infections, nasal stuffiness, or trauma. Are there current problems with nosebleeds (epistaxis), sinus infections, hay fever, allergies, postnasal drip, sneezing, discharge, pain, obstruction, or decreased sense of smell?	Denies problems with frequent colds, sinus infections, epistaxis, sneezing, postnasal drip, pain, obstruction, or decreased sense of smell. History of allergies and hay fever (see Past Health Status). Had suffered some sort of nasal trauma as a child, leading to deviated nasal septum; septoplasty in 1964. No problems now
I. *Mouth and Pharynx* Past problems include history of strep throat. Current problems include changes in taste, difficulty chewing, bleeding gums, increased saliva or dry mouth, mouth lesions, mouth pain, sore throat, hoarseness, or difficulty swallowing (dysphagia). Does the client use tobacco of any kind? If so, what type (cigarette, chewing tobacco, snuff), and how much and how often is tobacco used? When was the client's last dental examination and the results? The client is asked to describe dental hygiene habits that are practiced, including brushing and flossing	Denies problems with changes in taste, difficulty chewing or dysphagia, oral lesions, bleeding gums, missing or broken teeth, increased saliva or dry mouth, mouth pain, sore throat, or hoarseness. Denies use of tobacco. Last dental examination in 1991, no caries. X-ray studies taken. Usually brushes with a tartar control toothpaste twice a day (after breakfast and at bedtime). Flosses daily at bedtime
J. *Neck* Has the client had problems with goiter, neck injury, pain, or limited movement? Are there current problems with neck stiffness, pain, limited mobility, or lumps or swelling in the neck? Has the client ever had "swollen glands"?	Denies problems with neck pain and decreased mobility. Does have neck stiffness at times with headache, but none at present (see Health Perception and Health Management). Occasional swollen glands with sore throat resolve away when throat is better
K. *Breasts* Past problems include fibrocystic breast disease and cancer of the breast. Family history of breast cancer in mother or sisters increases client's risk status for cancer of the breast. Current problems include breast enlargement (gynecomastia), itching (pruritus), pain, ten-	Denies problems with fibrocystic breast disease, cancer of the breast, or family history of breast cancer. No gynecomastia, pruritus, pain or tenderness, skin or nipple changes, or nipple discharge. Practices BSE "occasionally," approximately every 2 to 3 months. Last mammograms were in 5/90, results were "normal." Took birth control pills approx-

TABLE 11–5. Health History Assessment Guide Continued

Data	Example
derness, skin changes (e.g., dimpling), nipple changes or discharge. Does the client practice BSE? If so, how often? Has the client ever had mammograms (if female)? If so, when was the last time x-ray studies were taken? What were the results of the mammograms? Does the client have a history of taking corticosteroids?	imately 5 years, with interruption for pregnancies. Stopped taking them after tubal ligation in 1986
L. *Lungs* Past problems include pneumonia, bronchitis, asthma, emphysema, wheezing, pleurisy, tuberculosis, and whooping cough. Present problems may include shortness of breath, difficulty breathing (dyspnea) either at rest or with exertion, wheezing, cough, blue-tinged nail beds or lips (cyanosis), pain with respiration, blood in sputum (hemoptysis), increased sputum production, or difficulty breathing without elevating the head (orthopnea). The nurse reviews the client's smoking history and when the last chest x-ray study was performed. When was the client's last tine test or PPD and what were the results? If the client is a smoker, does he or she have interest in quitting? What is the client's tolerance for exercise?	Denies problems with pneumonia, tuberculosis, asthma, wheezing, emphysema, bronchitis, pleurisy, or whooping cough. Had bronchitis as a child, but no longer a problem. No shortness of breath, dyspnea on exertion, dyspnea, cough, cyanosis, pain with respiration, hemoptysis, excess sputum, or orthopnea. Denies smoking history. Last chest x-ray study in 1964, results "normal." Last tine test in 1964, no reaction. Tolerates moderate exercise without dyspnea
M. *Heart* The nurse asks the client about past problems with rheumatic fever, congenital heart disease, heart murmur, high blood pressure, heart attack, sudden awakening at night with difficulty breathing (paroxysmal nocturnal dyspnea), coronary artery disease, hyperlipidemia, thyroid problems, palpitations, chest discomfort, or pain. Is there a family history of hypertension or heart attack before age 50? Has the client had cardiac surgery? Has the client had an electrocardiogram? If so, when, and does the client know the results? Has the client had other types of cardiac tests or examination? If so, when were they performed and what were the results? Does the client smoke? Are there current problems with fainting (syncope), palpitations, chest discomfort or pain, paroxysmal nocturnal dyspnea, weight gain, orthopnea, dyspnea on exertion, dizziness (vertigo), swelling of hands or feet (edema), heart racing or slowing?	Denies problems with rheumatic fever, congenital heart disease, heart murmur, high blood pressure, heart attack, paroxysmal nocturnal dyspnea, coronary artery disease, orthopnea, thyroid problems, palpitations, syncope, dizziness, chest pain. Never had an ECG or other heart tests. No recent weight gain or problems with edema. Nonsmoker. Family history positive for myocardial infarction on paternal side, and hypertension and stroke on maternal side
N. *Peripheral vascular* The client is asked whether there have been problems with varicose veins, diabetes, high blood pressure, pain in the legs or arms, edema, areas of discoloration or ulceration of the arms or legs, leg cramping, numbness, change in temperature of the extremities, nail changes, or hair loss on the extremities. Is there a family history of high blood pressure or stroke?	Denies problems with varicose veins, diabetes, leg or arm pain or cramps, discoloration of skin or nails, peripheral numbness, temperature changes in extremities, nail changes, high blood pressure or stroke. Family history positive for diabetes, stroke, and hypertension on maternal side
O. *Gastrointestinal* Has the client had past problems with ulcers, indigestion or heartburn, hernias, vomiting of blood (hematemesis), liver disease or hepatitis (type of hepatitis), gallbladder problems, pancreatic disease, appendicitis, or a history of alcoholism? Are there present problems with weight loss or gain, appetite change, food intolerances, belching, nausea or vomiting, diarrhea or constipation, changes in bowel habits, excess gas (flatulence), hemorrhoids, rectal fissure, rectal itching, abdominal pain or	Denies problems with indigestion or heartburn, hernia, hematemesis, hepatitis, gallbladder or pancreas problems, appendicitis, weight loss or gain, change in appetite, food intolerance, belching, nausea or vomiting, diarrhea, constipation, change in bowel habits, flatulence, hemorrhoids, fissures, rectal itch, abdominal pain or swelling, jaundice, clay-colored stool or melena, or incontinence. See Health Perception and Health Management for history of alcohol consumption. Denies use of laxatives, enemas, or suppositories. No history of undergoing diagnostic special x-ray

Table continued on following page

TABLE 11-5. Health History Assessment Guide Continued

Data	Example
ROS	
swelling, skin yellowing (jaundice), clay-colored stool, blood in stool or tarry stools, loss of bowel control (incontinence). Does the client admit to consuming alcoholic beverages, and if so, how much is consumed? Does the client use laxatives, enemas, or suppositories to assist bowel elimination? Has the client undergone x-ray studies of the abdomen or other special x-ray studies or examinations, such as a barium swallow, upper and lower gastrointestinal series, proctoscopy, liver scan, gallbladder x-ray studies? Is there a family history of alcoholism? Is there a family history of cancer of the stomach, liver, intestines, or colorectal area?	studies or procedures for the gastrointestinal system. Family history is positive for alcoholism on paternal side and for stomach cancer on maternal side. No other known family incidence of gastrointestinal cancer. See Elimination for description of bowel habits
P. *Urinary* The nurse asks the client about past problems with bladder infections, kidney problems, urinary tract stones, or STDs. Are there current problems producing a change in urinary habits, such as pain with urination (dysuria), frequency, urgency, difficulty starting urine stream (hesitancy), urine incontinence, getting up at night to urinate (nocturia), decreased amount of urine (oliguria) or increased amount (polyuria), dribbling, change in color of urine, low back pain or flank pain, or foaming of urine (albuminuria)? Does the client have a urethral discharge? Has the client undergone special test or x-ray studies of the urinary tract such as cystoscopy or intravenous pyelogram? Is there a family history of renal disease?	Denies problems with bladder infections, kidney problems, stones, or STDs. Reports no dysuria, nocturia, hesitancy, frequency changes, or change in urine characteristics. No change in urine stream. Has episodes of stress incontinence. See Elimination for description of urinary habits. Family history negative for urinary tract problems. Never has had special tests for the urinary system except for routine urinalysis with physical examinations
Q. *Genito-reproductive*	
1. *Female clients*	
a. Past problems include vaginal discharge, PID, STDs including herpes, endometriosis, infertility, gynecologic surgery, or abnormal Pap test	Denies past problems with vaginal discharge, PID, genital herpes, endometriosis, infertility, or abnormal Pap test. Intermittent vaginal yeast infections responsive to treatment. See Past Health Status for previous gynecologic surgeries
b. Menstrual history is recorded if not done previously. The nurse asks about menses onset (menarche), duration of menses, length of menstrual cycle, presence of bleeding between menses, last menstrual period, amount of bleeding, presence of premenstrual symptoms, dysmenorrhea, abnormal menstrual cycles, whether menopause has occurred (and if so, when), whether menopausal symptoms exist	See Sexuality and Reproductive Pattern for menstrual history
c. Obstetric history is also noted if not already recorded. The client is asked about the dates and number of pregnancies, live births, abortions, miscarriages, stillbirths, or complications. The birth weight and health of infants is noted	See Past Health Status for obstetric history
d. Current problems the client may experience include vaginal discharge, genital sores, STDs, itching, painful intercourse (dyspareunia), postmenstrual bleeding, postcoital bleeding, or sexual performance problems	Denies current problems with discharge, genital sores, STDs, pruritus, dyspareunia, spotting or bleeding between menses, or postcoital bleeding. No problems with sexual performance other than decreased frequency of intercourse from fatigue (see Sexuality-Reproductive Pattern)
e. The client is asked about use of contraceptives (type, length of use, problems)	No current use of contraceptives, has tubal ligation. See Sexuality-Reproductive Pattern for details
f. The date of last pelvic examination is noted and whether the client knows the result of the last Pap test	See Health Perception and Health Management Pattern and Sexuality-Reproductive Pattern

TABLE 11–5. Health History Assessment Guide Continued

Data	Example
g. Is there a family history of reproductive cancer such as of the uterus or ovaries?	Family history negative for reproductive problems
2. *Male clients*	
a. Past problems include hernia, prostate problems, STDs, infertility, or difficulty with sexual performance	
b. Current problems include testicular pain or mass, urethral discharge, genital sores, STDs, or problems with sexual performance	
c. Does the client perform TSE? If so, how often?	
d. Does the client use condoms during sexual intercourse?	
e. What is the date and results of the last male pelvic examination including prostate check?	
R. *Musculoskeletal* The nurse asks the client about past problems with fractures, strains, sprains, dislocations, arthritis, gout, backache, bursitis, osteomyelitis, scoliosis, or flat feet. Current problems may include joint or muscle pain or stiffness, joint swelling or tenderness, muscle weakness, muscle cramps or spasms, muscle atrophy, involuntary movements, uncoordinated movement, limited mobility, paralysis, or changes in gait. Has the client had x-ray studies of the skeletal system or special procedures such as electromyography? Is there a family history of musculoskeletal diseases such as arthritis or gout?	Denies past problems with sprains. Probable nose fracture as child, corrected with septoplasty in 1964. Intermittent backache usually after lifting and moving (see Current Health Status). Occasional stiff right wrist if overuses with repetitive motions. States "It's been like that ever since the ganglion was removed." No joint swelling, tenderness, or redness. Denies muscle cramps, weakness, or spasms. No involuntary movements, incoordination, weakness, paralysis, or limited range of motion. No history of scoliosis, bursitis, or arthritis. Family history positive for arthritis on paternal and maternal sides. No special procedures
S. *Nervous system* The nurse asks the client about past problems with loss of consciousness, fainting, seizures, paralysis, trauma to the nervous system, or stroke. Are there present problems with dizziness (vertigo), fainting (syncope), numbness (paresthesia), weakness (paresis), paralysis, headache, loss of balance, convulsions, uncoordinated or involuntary movements (e.g., tremors, tics, spasms, clumsiness), speech problems, or memory problems. Has the client had special procedures such as electroencephalography, lumbar puncture, or computerized tomography (CT scan)? Is there a family history of neurologic diseases such as CVA or stroke, seizures, or Huntington's chorea?	Denies problems with loss of consciousness, fainting, seizures, paralysis, paresis, parasthesia, loss of balance, incoordination, dizziness, speech or memory problems. Occasional headache (see Current Health Status). Hand numbness prior to menses relieved with triamterene (Dyazide). No special tests. Family history positive for CVA in maternal grandparents
T. *Psychiatric* The nurse asks the client about past problems with depression (especially if it had interfered with ADLs), anxiety attacks, memory problems, hallucinations, delusions, sleeping problems, or eating disorders, such as anorexia nervosa or bulimia nervosa. Current problems include mood swings, insomnia, nervousness, anxiety that interferes with ADLs, increased or decreased appetite, memory lapses. Are there problems with spouse, family or peers? Is there a family history of mental health problems?	Denies problems with depression, anxiety attacks, memory problems, hallucinations, delusions, insomnia, eating pattern or appetite changes, excessive nervousness, or mood swings. Feels family is under stress while she is spending more time with parents (see Role Relationship Pattern and Sexuality Pattern). Family history positive for "mental illness" on paternal side
Closure	
The nurse provides the client with the opportunity to give further information, clarify points, or ask questions by stating that the history interview is completed. It is appropriate	

Table continued on following page

TABLE 11-5. Health History Assessment Guide Continued

Data	Example
Closure	
to ask the client whether there are any questions he or she would like to ask of the nurse. The nurse then prepares the client for the physical examination	

This concludes the history portion of the health assessment of the client, Mary C. Jones. Based on these data, the nurse begins to formulate inferences about the health risk factors present in Ms. Jones and her tentative nursing diagnoses. The following example illustrates the health risk appraisal and tentative nursing diagnoses for Ms. Jones.

Health Risk Appraisal

1. Ms. Jones is at increased risk for problems with back strain because of the lifting done during housework and her stated level of fatigue
2. A tetanus booster is needed, because it has been more than 10 years since the last dose and Ms. Jones works outdoors in her garden and with tools
3. Reinforcement teaching is indicated for Ms. Jones to emphasize the reason for performing BSE on a regular monthly schedule
4. Ms. Jones is due for vision screening and mammograms because it has been approximately 2 years since these procedures have been performed
5. Further exploration of Ms. Jones' sources of calcium are indicated because her diet is deficient in calcium, increasing her risk for osteoporosis
6. Ms. Jones is at risk for situational crisis related to the need to resolve placement of her elderly parents in a nursing home. She (and her family) may need counseling to assist with the decision-making process

Tentative Nursing Diagnoses
(The following diagnoses are not listed in order of priority)

1. High Risk for Injury R/T fatigue, distraction, and frequency of physical activity associated with housekeeping chores
2. Decisional Conflict R/T disposition of elderly parents
3. Pain (intermittent backache) R/T frequency of lifting and moving, and possible use of improper body mechanics
4. Sexual Dysfunction R/T fatigue
5. High Risk for Altered Health Maintenance R/T sporadic practice of BSE, lack of screening mammography within past 2 years, lack of vision screening as recommended by health maintenance guidelines, and probable insufficient antitetanus titer
6. Stress Incontinence R/T childbirth and loss of muscle tone
7. Fatigue R/T prolonged excessive role demands and decisional conflict
8. Altered Family Processes R/T change in family roles
9. Diversional Activity Deficit R/T excessive long hours of stressful work and no time for leisure activities
10. High Risk for Altered Nutrition: Less than Body Requirements R/T possible insufficient calcium in diet

ADLs, activities of daily living; BSE, breast self-examination; CVA, cerebrovascular accident; LMP, last menstrual period; PID, pelvic inflammatory disease; PO, by mouth; PPD, purified protein derivative; ROS, review of systems; R/T, related to; STDs, sexually transmitted diseases; TSE, testicular self-examination.

RECORDING THE HEALTH HISTORY INTERVIEW

Interview data are recorded in the client's record according to specific agency protocol. The format is organized and may be a narrative, outline, or checklist with written supplementary comments. All pertinent data (both positive as well as negative findings) are recorded. Data are clear, concise, comprehensive, and consistent, with no gaps or areas of ambiguity. The nurse uses approved agency abbreviations and terminology whenever possible to promote communication among health care team members.

APPLYING THE NURSING PROCESS TO HEALTH ASSESSMENT

In health assessment, the nurse seeks to gather as much data about the client as possible, both subjective and objective. These data are analyzed to determine the client's needs and responses to potential and actual health problems. The nurse considers the client's preferences when formulating nursing diagnoses that are amenable to intervention. Establishing realistic goals and outcome criteria and planning interventions follow in logical order, as Box 11-2 illustrates.

Box 11-2. Applying Nursing Process to Health Assessment

Introduction

Mrs. L. is a 58-year-old, healthy-looking woman who visits a glaucoma screening booth at a health fair. The nurse integrates health assessment data and nursing process while talking to Mrs. L. and testing her visual acuity.

Biographic Data

Married. Has one married child who lives out of state. Works full time as a legal secretary.

Health Risk Appraisal

Mother had cataracts. Family history positive for hypertension. Nearsighted since age 10 and wears corrective lenses. Last eye examination 5 years ago. Has smoked one pack of cigarettes per day for 40 years.

Physical Health History

History negative for significant health problems. Postmenopausal. Reports seeing rings around lights and decreased side vision most noticeable when reading.

Physical Examination

Snellen chart results (with corrective lenses) are O.D. = 20/40, O.S. = 20/30, O.U. = 20/30. Visual fields to confrontation reveal superior fields less than those of the examiner. Pupils react sluggishly to accommodation. Further physical examination limited owing to setting.

Nursing Diagnosis

Altered health maintenance related to infrequent monitoring of vision by ophthalmologist.

Expected Outcomes

Long Term

Mrs. L. will maintain present visual acuity and prevent further loss of vision.

Short Term

1. Mrs. L. will verbalize understanding of the need for an immediate, complete ophthalmologic examination.
2. Mrs. L. will identify an ophthalmologist whom she will contact no later than tomorrow for an appointment.

Intervention

1. Discuss results of visual screening with Mrs. L. and their significance.
2. Explain risk factors for glaucoma and Mrs. L.'s risk profile.
3. Assist Mrs. L. to identify an ophthalmologist.
4. Provide Mrs. L. with pamphlets about glaucoma from the National Society to Prevent Blindness.
5. Give Mrs. L. a self-addressed, stamped postcard that is to be returned by the ophthalmologist after the first visit.

Evaluation

Long Term

Ask Mrs. L. to restate her understanding of the need to have regular visual check-ups by an ophthalmologist and to follow the recommended medical regimen for eye care.

Short Term

Ask Mrs. L. whom she plans to contact for an eye appointment and when she intends to do this.

Summary

The health history is the first component of health assessment. The history is the subjective data that guides the examiner to assess more fully specific concerns of the client or areas identified through health risk appraisal. The history can be recorded in many ways, such as through computerized data base assessments or on paper. Although a thorough history may seem to be time consuming, the data provided are very valuable in fully understanding the client and his or her special needs.

References

1. Alfaro, R. (1990). *Applying nursing diagnosis and nursing process: A step-by-step guide* (2nd ed.). Philadelphia: J. B. Lippincott.
2. Allen, P. T. (1986). Screening. In C. Edelman & C. L. Mandel (Eds.), *Health promotion throughout the lifespan* (pp. 142-158). St. Louis: C. V. Mosby.
3. American Academy of Pediatrics. (1988). *Guidelines for health supervision II* (2nd ed.). Elk Grove Village, IL: Author.
4. American Medical Association. (1983). Medical evaluations of healthy persons (Report of the Council on Scientific Affairs). *Journal of the American Medical Association, 249*, 1626-1633.
5. Barry, P. D. (1989). *Psychosocial nursing assessment and intervention: Care of the physically ill person* (2nd ed.). Philadelphia: J. B. Lippincott.
6. Braverman, B. G. (1990). Eliciting assessment data from the patient who is difficult to interview. *Nursing Clinics of North America, 25*, 743-750.
7. Brennan, P. F., & Romano, C. A. (1987). Computers and nursing diagnoses: Issues in implementation. *Nursing Clinics of North America, 22*, 935-941.
8. Cameron, C. T., & McNeil, E. L. (1976). The importance of history. *Journal of Emergency Nursing, 2*(3), 21-22.
9. Carpenito, L. J. (1989). *Nursing diagnosis: Application to clinical practice* (3rd ed.). Philadelphia: J. B. Lippincott.
10. Carson, V. B. (1989). *Spiritual dimensions of nursing practice.* Philadelphia: W. B. Saunders.

11. Clark, C. C. (1986). *Wellness nursing: Concepts, theory, research, and practice.* New York: Springer Publishing.
12. Cox, H. C., et al. (1989). *Clinical applications of nursing diagnosis: Adult health, child health, women's health, mental health, home health.* Baltimore: Williams & Wilkins.
13. Fuller, J., & Schaller-Ayers, J. (1990). *Health assessment: A nursing approach.* Philadelphia: J. B. Lippincott.
14. Gordon, M. (1987). *Nursing diagnosis: Process and application* (2nd ed.). New York: McGraw-Hill.
15. Halloran, E. J. (1988). Computerized nurse assessments. *Nursing and Health Care, 9,* 497-499.
16. Hart, C. R. (1975). *Screening in general practice.* New York: Longham Medical Group Limited.
17. Hill, L. H., & Smith, N. (1990). *Self-care nursing: Promotion of health* (2nd ed.). Norwalk, CT: Appleton & Lange.
18. Malasanos, L., et al. (1990). *Health assessment.* (4th ed.). St. Louis: C. V. Mosby.
19. Morton, P. G. (1989). *Health assessment in nursing.* Springhouse, PA: Springhouse.
20. North American Nursing Diagnosis Association (NANDA). (1990). *Ninth conference on the classification of nursing diagnosis.* St. Louis: Author.
21. Rahe, R. H. (1975). Life changes and near-future illness reports. In L. Levi (Ed.), *Emotions: Their parameters and measurement.* New York: Raven Press.
22. Saba, V. K. (1988). Taming the computer jungle of NISs. *Nursing and Health Care, 9,* 487-491.
23. Schneiderman, H. (1982, June). The review of systems, an important part of comprehensive examination. *Postgraduate Medicine, 71,* 151-158.
24. Sparks, S. M., & Taylor, C. M. (1991). *Nursing diagnosis reference manual.* Springhouse, PA: Springhouse.
25. Spradley, B. W. (1990). *Community health nursing: Concepts and practice.* Glenview, IL: Scott, Foresman and Company.
26. Tom, C. K. (1976). Nursing assessment of biological rhythms. *Nursing Clinics of North America, 11,* 621-630.
27. U.S. Preventive Services Task Force. (1989). *Guide to clinical preventive services: An assessment of the effectiveness of 169 interventions.* Baltimore: Williams & Wilkins.

Appendix 11-1

Barry Psychosocial Assessment Rating Scale

All questions in italics should be subjectively assessed by the nurse, rather than asked of the patient directly. Bold-faced statements advise the assessor on how to proceed.

Admitting Information

Name__________ Age_____ Date of admission__________
Date of assessment__________
Marital status S_____ M_____ W_____ D_____ How long?__________
Occupation__________
Years of education completed__________
Admitting diagnosis__________

HEALTH PERCEPTION–HEALTH MANAGEMENT

Patient's Perception of Illness

What was the original problem that caused you to come to the hospital?
On what date did you first become ill?
What caused this illness?
How do you feel about being in a hospital?
How can the physicians and nurses help you most?
How will this illness affect you when you are out of the hospital?
Do you think it will cause any changes in your life?
How will it affect your family?

Potential for noncompliance? Yes_____ No_____ Possible_____
Related to: _____ *Anxiety*
_____ *Negative side effects of prescribed treatment*
_____ *Unsatisfactory relationship with care-giving environment or care givers*
_____ *Other*
Explain
Potential for injury? Yes_____ No_____ Possible_____

NUTRITIONAL-METABOLIC

How does your current appetite compare with your normal appetite?
Same_____ Increased_____ Decreased_____
How long has it been different?_____
Has your weight fluctuated by more than 5 pounds in the last several weeks?
Yes_____ No_____
How many pounds?_____
What is your normal fluid intake per day? _____ml*
Your current intake? _____ml
Aspects of patient's illness or condition that could contribute to organic mental disorder?
No_____ Yes_____
Delirium type_____ Dementia type_____

---

*Nurse can substitute estimate of ml for patient's reported fluid intake.

Possible cause:

___***M***etabolic	___***A***rterial disease
Electrolytes	___***M***echanical disease
Other metabolic or endocrine condition	___***I***nfectious disease
___***E***lectrical disorder	___***N***utritional disease
___***N***eoplastic disease	___***D***rug toxicity
___***D***egenerative (chronic) brain disease	

ELIMINATION

What is your current pattern of bowel movements?
Constipated_____ Diarrhea_____ Incontinent_____
How does this compare with normal? Same_____ Different_____
Explain

What is your current pattern of urination?
How does this compare to normal? Same_____ Different_____
Explain

Possibility that emotional distress may be contributing to any change?
High_____ Moderate_____ Low_____

ACTIVITY-EXERCISE

What is your normal energy level? High_____ Moderate_____ Low_____
Has it changed in the past 6 months? Yes_____ No_____
To what do you attribute the cause?
How would you describe your normal activity level?
High_____ Moderate_____ Low_____
How may it change following this hospitalization?
What types of activities do you normally pursue outside the home?
What recreational activities do you enjoy?
Do you anticipate your ability to manage your home will be changed following your hospitalization?
Explain

Current self-care deficits?
Feeding_____ Bathing_____ Dressing_____ Toileting_____
Anticipated deficits following hospitalization?
Current impairment in mobility?
Anticipated immobility following hospitalization?
Alterations in the following?
Airway clearance_____ How?
Breathing patterns_____ How?
Cardiac output_____ How?
Respiratory function_____ How?
Potential for altered tissue perfusion, as manifested by altered cognitive-perceptual patterns?

SLEEP-REST

Normal Sleeping Pattern

How many hours do you normally sleep per night?_____
From what hour to what hour? _____ to _____

Changes in Normal Sleeping Pattern

Do you have difficulty falling asleep?
Do you awaken in the middle of night?
Do you awaken early in the morning?
Are you sleeping more _____ or fewer _____ hours than normal?
How many?_____

COGNITIVE-PERCEPTUAL

Are you feeling pain now?
  How severe?
  How often?
What relieves the pain?

What information does this client need to know to manage this illness/health state?
Ability to comprehend this information? Good_____ Moderate_____ Poor_____
  If poor, explain

Mental Status Examination

Level of awareness and orientation____________________
Appearance and behavior____________________
Speech and communication____________________
Affect (mood)____________________
Thinking process____________________
Related to: Inability to evaluate reality_____ Aging_____ Other_____
Explain

If there is a distortion of the thought process, a focus assessment (see note at the end of scale) is indicated.

Perception____________________
Abstract thinking____________________
Social judgement____________________
Memory____________________
  Impairment in short-term memory_____ Long-term_____
  Is there evidence of unilateral neglect? Yes_____ No_____
  Does not apply_____

SELF-PERCEPTION

Does the patient describe feelings of anxiety or uneasiness?_____
Is he or she able to identify a cause? Yes_____ No_____
Cause?

If he or she feels anxious but cannot identify a cause, assess for the major coping risks of physical illness below.

Is there anything you are frightened of during this hospitalization or illness?
  Yes_____ No_____ What is it?
How will this illness affect your future plans?
Normally, do you believe that you control what happens to you (internal locus of control) or do you believe that other people or events control what happens (external locus of control)?
  Internal locus of control_____ External locus of control_____
Will this illness affect the way you feel about yourself?
  How?
  About your body?

Psychosocial Risks of Illness

What are the major issues of this illness for this patient? For this family?

Use the following space to record patient and family comments illustrating how they are coping with these issues.

Trust *Patient____________________*
Family____________________
Self-esteem *Patient____________________*
Family____________________
Body Image *Patient____________________*
Family____________________
Control *Patient____________________*
Family____________________

Loss *Patient*______________________
*Family*______________________
Guilt *Patient*______________________
*Family*______________________
Intimacy *Patient*______________________
*Family*______________________

Could one or more of these issues be contributing to feelings of anxiety, hopelessness, powerlessness, or disturbance in self-concept?
*Yes*_____ *No*_____ *Possible*_____

If so, explain which ones and proceed with focus assessment.

ROLE-RELATIONSHIP

What is your occupation?
How many years have you been in this occupation?_____
Do you anticipate that this illness will have an affect on your ability to work?
Yes_____ No_____ How?
With whom do you live?
Are they supportive?
Who are the most important people in your life?
Do you ever feel socially isolated? Yes_____ No_____
Explain
Is there any indication in this history of social isolation or impaired social interaction?
*Yes*_____ *No*_____
Explain
*Ability to communicate. Within normal limits*_____ *Impaired*_____
Describe

Family History

Who are the members of your immediate family? What are their ages and how are they related to you? Please include deceased members and when they died.

Name of Family Member	Relationship to You	Age	Date of Death

What is your position in relation to your brothers and sisters? For example, are you the second oldest, the youngest. . .?

How often do you see your immediate family members?

What goes on in your family when something bad happens? What do most of the members do?
Have any of your relationships within your immediate and extended family changed recently?
Which ones?
How have they changed?
Is there any change in the way you parent your children? Yes_____ No_____
If so, to what do you attribute the cause?
_____New baby
_____Death of family member
_____Illness in other family member
_____Change in residence
Cause of change in residence
_____Other (describe)
What is your normal role within your family?
What role do the significant other people in your family play?
*Potential for disruption of these roles by this illness? High*_____ *Moderate*_____ *Low*_____
Explain
While the patient is describing the family, is there indication of uncontrolled anger or rage?

Yes_____ No_____

Related to a specific issue or person?

Explain

Open (trusting) or closed (untrusting) communication style in family? (Can be initially determined by statements and emotional expression of patient.)

Developmental stage of family

_____*Early married*

_____*Married with no children*

_____*Active childbearing*

_____*Pre-school or school-aged children*

_____*Adolescent children and children leaving home*

_____*Middle-aged children no longer at home*

_____*Elderly, well-functioning*

_____*Elderly, infirm*

Is there any other aspect of your family or the way your family normally operates that you think should be added here? What is it?

If any item discussed in this section appears to be a current stressor for this patient or family it can be assessed using a focus approach with the other items under Coping–Stress Tolerance pattern.

Interpersonal style

_____*Dependent*

_____*Controlled*

_____*Dramatizing*

_____*Suspicious*

_____*Self-sacrificing*

_____*Superior*

_____*Uninvolved*

_____*Mixed (usually two styles predominate)*

_____*No predominant personality style*

Write a brief sentence explaining your choice.

Response to you as the interviewer. Guarded?_____ Open?_____

Is the patient able to maintain good eye contact?

SEXUALITY-REPRODUCTIVE

Have you experienced any recent change in your sexual functioning? Yes_____ No_____

How?

For how long?

Do you associate your change in sexual functioning with some event in your life?

Do you think this illness could change your normal pattern of sexual functioning?

How?

Is this change in sexuality patterns related to

_____*Ineffective coping*

_____*Change or loss of body part*

_____*Prenatal or postpartum changes*

_____*Changes in neurovegetative functioning related to depression*

Explain

Use focus assessment if necessary.

COPING–STRESS TOLERANCE

Level of Stress During Year Before Admission

How long have you been out of work with this illness?

Have you experienced any recent change in your job?

Have you been under any unusual job stress during the past year?

What was the cause?

_____Retirement

_____Fired

_____Same job, but new boss or working relationship

_____Promotion or demotion

_____Other. Explain

Do you expect the stress will be present when you return to work?

The preceding questions should be adapted for students to a school situation.

Have there been changes in your family during the last 2 years? Which family members are involved? Include dates.

_____Death

Was this someone you were close to?

_____Divorce

_____Child leaving home

Cause?

_____Other

Has there been any other unusual stress during the last year that is still affecting you?

Describe

Any unusual stress in your family?

Describe

Normal Coping Ability

When you go through a very difficult time, how do you handle it?

_____Talk it out with someone
_____Ignore it
_____Withdraw from others
_____Get angry and yell
_____Get angry and clam up
_____Get angry and hit or throw something
_____Drink
_____Become anxious
_____Become depressed
_____Other (Explain)

How often do you experience feelings of depression?
In the past what is the longest period of time this feeling has lasted?
Have you felt depressed during the past few weeks? Yes_____ No_____
To what do you attribute the cause?

If rape trauma is the cause of this admission do not explore the psychological reaction with the patient until reading the report of the rape crisis counselor, who should have met with the patient within an hour of arrival at the emergency room. Either follow the recommendations on the report for ongoing assessment or proceed with gentle questioning about her current feelings.

What is the most serious trauma you have experienced?
What was the most difficult time you have experienced in your life?
How long did it take you to get over it?
What did you do to cope with it?

Potential for Self-Harm

This part of the assessment should be included if moderate to severe depression is present.

Have you ever thought of committing suicide? No_____ Yes_____

If yes, continue on.

What would you do to end your life? No plan_____ Plan_____
Describe
What would prevent you from committing suicide?

Substances That May Be Used as Stress Relievers

Smoking history
Do you smoke?_____ How long have you been smoking?_____ How many packs per day?_____
Alcohol use history
Do you drink?_____ How often?_____ How much?_____
Is there a history of alcoholism in your family?_____ Who?_____
Drug use
What prescribed medications are you currently using?

Name of Medication	***Dose or Schedule***	***Prescribing Physician***

Are you currently using any other drugs? Yes_____ No_____
What are they?
How long have you been using it (them)?
What is the usual amount?
How often?
Have you ever been treated for drug abuse?

Value-Belief

What is your religious affiliation?
Do you consider yourself active or inactive in practicing your religion? Active_____ Inactive_____
Is your pastor a supportive person? Yes_____ No_____
Explain
What does this illness mean to you?
Are you experiencing spiritual distress? Yes_____ No_____
Explain
What would you consider to be the primary cause of this spiritual distress (actual, possible, or potential)?
_____Inability to practice spiritual rituals
_____Conflict between religious, spiritual, or cultural beliefs and prescribed health regimen
_____Crisis of illness/suffering/death
_____Other (explain)
Do you expect there will be any disparity in your caregivers' approach that could present a problem for you? Any problems in the areas of
_____Spiritual rituals
_____Cause of illness
_____Perception of illness and sick role
_____Health maintenance
_____Communication
_____Problem solving
_____Nutrition
_____Family response
Explain
How has this illness affected your relationship with God or the supreme being of your religion?

Explain

The 11 functional health patterns were named by Marjorie Gordon in Nursing Diagnosis: Process and Application (New York, McGraw-Hill, 1987).

NOTE: This scale can be used in its entirety or to assist in developing psychosocial assessment criteria for individuals and families adapting to physical illness. When ineffective coping is occurring it can help the nurse to focus on the potential cause of the coping problem. The nurse's asking of specific questions about an issue is called a *focus assessment*. Effective nursing intervention and care planning can be enhanced by focusing on the cause of the problem.

From Barry, P.D. (1989). *Psychosocial nursing assessment and intervention: Care of the physically ill person* (2nd ed.). Philadelphia: J.B. Lippincott.

Chapter 12

Physical Examination

The physical examination follows the health history interview. Physical examination skills require use of the ears, eyes, and senses of touch and smell. Repeated practice is necessary to learn how to integrate these skills into the nursing repertoire. The nurse learns the techniques and correct use of the equipment as well as discriminates normal from abnormal findings.

Objective data are collected systematically during the physical examination to supplement and validate the client's subjective data. The nurse's ability to perceive the client in a holistic manner is enhanced when both subjective and objective data are evaluated together. It is not uncommon for the nurse to ask the client questions about abnormal physical findings. For example, if a mass is found during palpation, the nurse asks the client if the area is tender to touch. The client's reply is recorded in the physical examination portion of the data base (e.g., "nontender") even though it is subjective data. If the nurse is palpating a lump or mass that the client did not report initially during the history interview, the nurse asks if the client is aware of the mass's existence. If the client knows the mass is present or admits to related symptoms, the nurse proceeds with a complete symptom analysis. These subjective data are recorded as part of the health history.

Physical examination is a skill used by nurses in all types of settings. Health fairs, screening clinics, physician's offices, independent practice clinics, home health, and hospitals are just some of the areas where nurses use physical examination skills to assess clients' health. The extent and depth of the physical examination are determined by the client's needs.

For example, a home health nurse visits a client who has had total hip replacement surgery. During the first home visit, the nurse assesses the client to obtain baseline data. As recovery from the surgery continues, the client should be able to demonstrate increasing mobility and strength in the operative leg during subsequent home visits. Decreased mobility, guarding against leg movement, unequal leg length, and internal rotation of the operative hip are physical examination findings that indicate a hip prosthesis dislocation, a serious postoperative complication. Likewise, a coronary care unit nurse conducts periodic physical examinations of a client after a myocardial infarction to assess for changes that indicate a life-threatening complication has developed.

PURPOSE OF THE PHYSICAL EXAMINATION

The purpose of physical examination is to differentiate normal from abnormal physical findings. The nurse must have a thorough understanding of basic anatomy (structure) and physiology (function) as a foundation. From this foundation, skill and expertise develop, which enable the nurse to appreciate the wide range of findings that are considered "normal."

In addition to collecting baseline data, physical assessment skills are used to assist in making clinical judgements about a client's health status and evaluating the effectiveness of nursing and medical interventions. The examples of the home health and coronary care clients illustrate this point.

TYPES OF PHYSICAL EXAMINATION

Several types, or levels, of physical examination are performed, depending on the client's needs. A *screening physical examination* is an organized, superficial check of the major body systems for detecting abnormalities or possible problems. If the nurse detects a problem, the focus of the examination is directed to a *regional or branching examination*, which is an in-depth assessment of a specific body system. This chapter presents information that allows the nurse to perform a screening adult physical examination and regional examinations when indicated. A *complete physical examination* includes ancillary examinations and procedures such as x-ray studies and clinical laboratory tests and is beyond the scope of this text.

ACCURACY OF PHYSICAL EXAMINATION

The physical examination helps to validate data collected during the health history interview. As with the health history, the nurse strives to collect accurate, thorough physical data. If difficulty is encountered while a physical assessment technique is performed or the accuracy of a finding is questionable, the nurse consults with colleagues. A second opinion or evaluation of the client may be necessary for accurate data to be obtained.

PHYSICAL EXAMINATION AND NURSING PROCESS

An accurate data base is essential to the formulation of individualized nursing diagnoses. It may be misleading for the nurse to diagnose a problem on the basis of one assessment finding. Significant findings (i.e., data that are either abnormal or indicate a potential risk) cue the nurse to collect additional information. A complete assessment is necessary before data are grouped into patterns and the etiologic basis is determined. The initial physical assessment is the baseline for the client's functional ability. Physical assessment is also used as intervention (e.g., monitoring lung sounds) and to evaluate changes in the client's physical condition and determine whether expected outcomes have been achieved.

TECHNIQUES OF PHYSICAL EXAMINATION

There are four primary techniques used in physical assessment: inspection, palpation, percussion, and auscultation. These techniques enhance the data collected by the ears, eyes, and senses of touch and smell and are employed as indicated when each body region is examined (Fig. 12–1).

Inspection

Inspection is the systematic, deliberate visual examination of the entire client or a region. Inspection yields information about size, shape, color, texture, symmetry, position, and deformities. It is the first technique of examination and begins at the onset of the client-nurse interaction. For example, the nurse inspects the facial skin while collecting the history. Inspection is important and is completed before progressing to the "hands on" techniques of palpation, percussion, or auscultation.

Inspection is conducted in a well-lit setting. The body region or part being inspected is uncovered sufficiently to permit complete visualization while the rest of the client's body is draped to preserve modesty and comfort. During inspection, the nurse compares what is observed with the known parameters of normal findings in clients of similar age, sex, and racial background.

Inspection is enhanced by the use of special instruments such as a penlight, oto-ophthalmoscope, and various specula (e.g., nasal and vaginal) that permit visual access to body cavities and orifices (Fig. 12–2). Other equipment used during inspection includes tongue blades, marking pen, ruler, tape measure, skinfold calipers, goniometer, and eye charts.

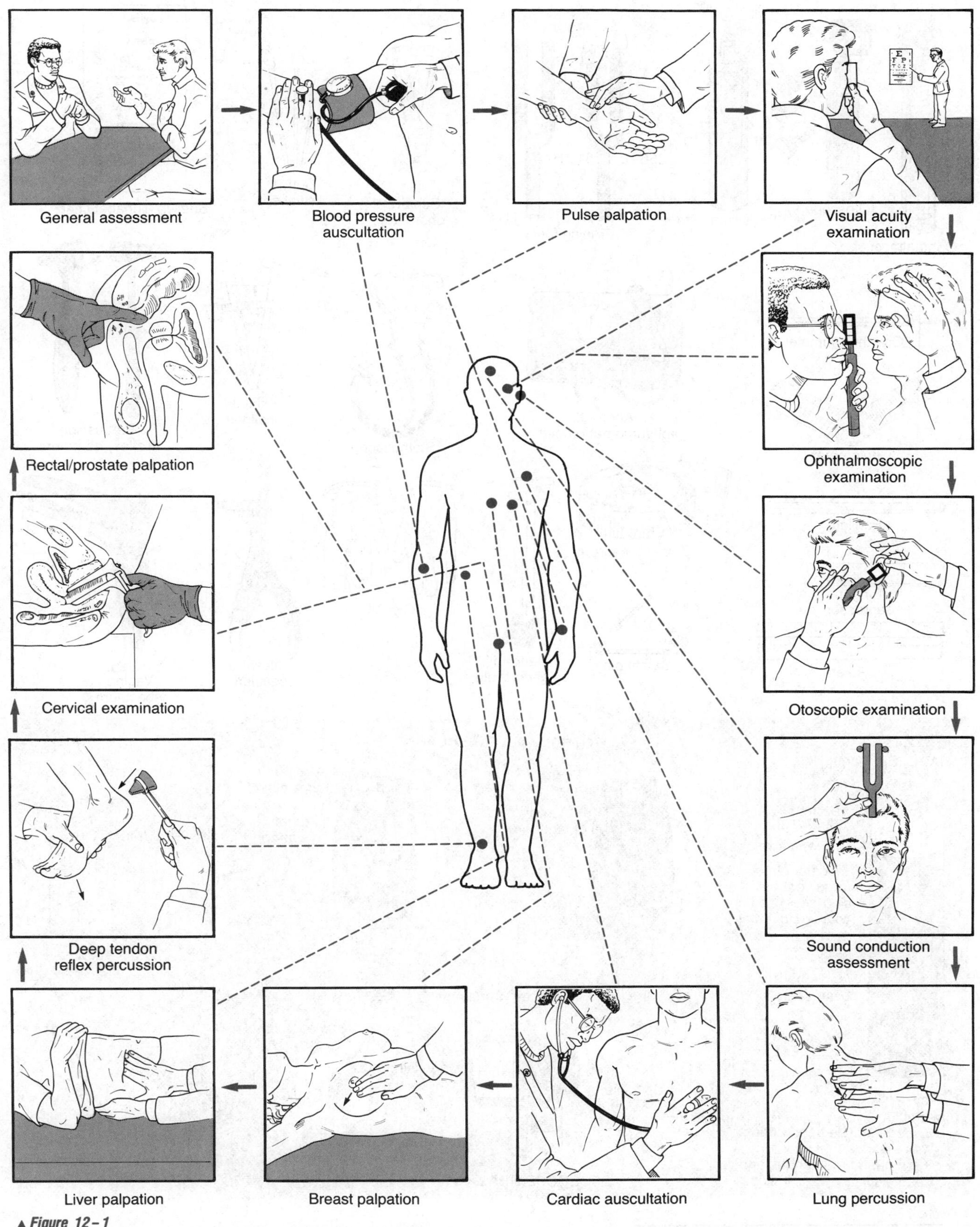

▲ **Figure 12-1**

Common head-to-toe screening physical assessments. Note that the examiner wears gloves for the pelvic, rectal, and prostate examinations.

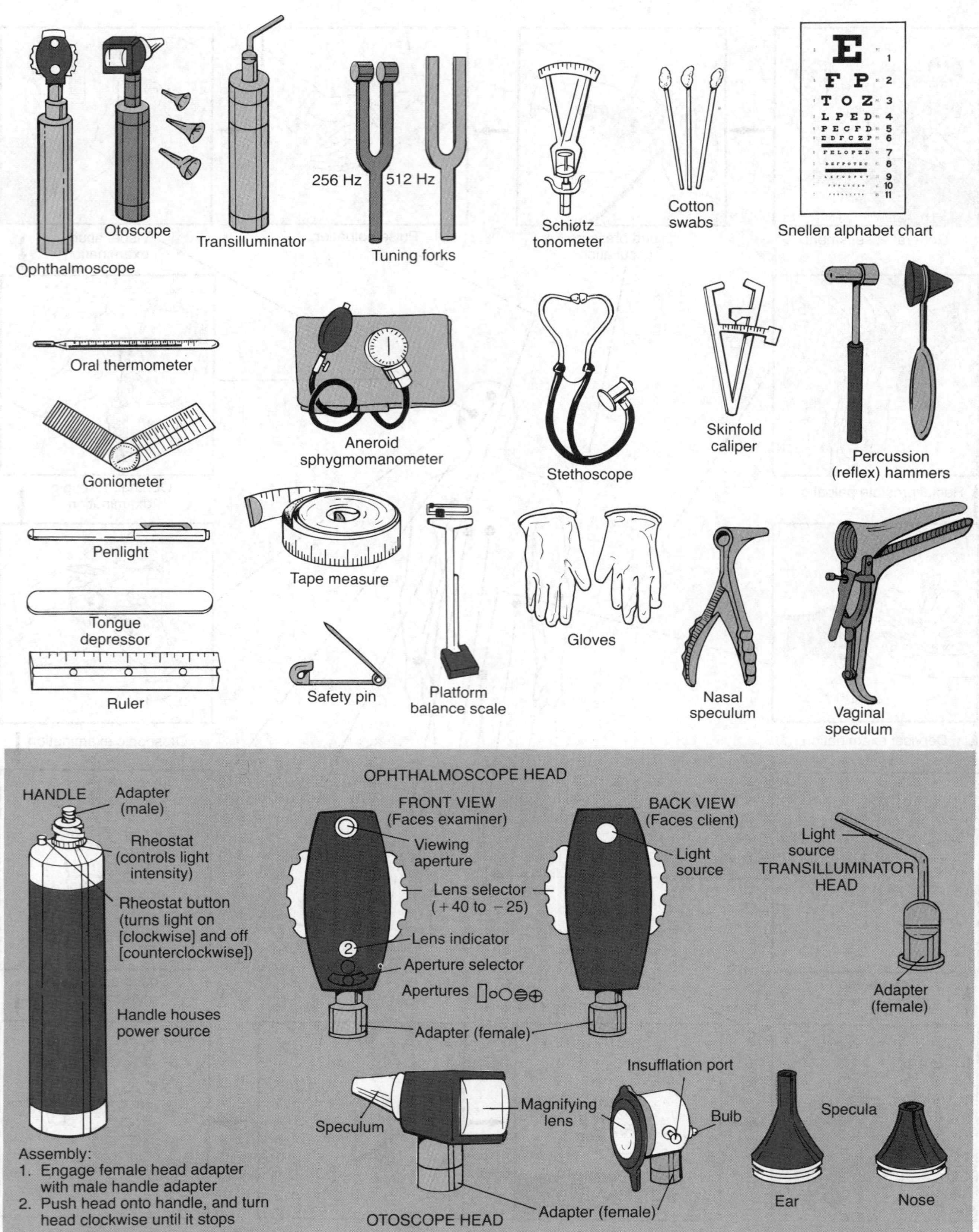
Ophthalmoscope
Otoscope
Transilluminator
256 Hz
512 Hz
Tuning forks
Schiøtz tonometer
Cotton swabs
Snellen alphabet chart
Oral thermometer
Goniometer
Aneroid sphygmomanometer
Stethoscope
Skinfold caliper
Percussion (reflex) hammers
Penlight
Tongue depressor
Ruler
Tape measure
Safety pin
Platform balance scale
Gloves
Nasal speculum
Vaginal speculum
OPHTHALMOSCOPE HEAD
HANDLE
Adapter (male)
Rheostat (controls light intensity)
Rheostat button (turns light on [clockwise] and off [counterclockwise])
Handle houses power source
FRONT VIEW (Faces examiner)
Viewing aperture
Lens selector (+40 to −25)
Lens indicator
Aperture selector
Apertures
Adapter (female)
BACK VIEW (Faces client)
Light source
Light source
TRANSILLUMINATOR HEAD
Adapter (female)
Assembly:
1. Engage female head adapter with male handle adapter
2. Push head onto handle, and turn head clockwise until it stops
Speculum
Magnifying lens
Insufflation port
Bulb
Adapter (female)
OTOSCOPE HEAD
Specula
Ear
Nose

▲ *Figure 12–2*

Equipment commonly used in physical assessment.

Palpation

Palpation, generally the second technique of physical assessment, is the use of touch. During palpation, varying amounts of pressure are exerted to determine information about masses, pulsation, organ size, tenderness or pain, swelling, tissue firmness and elasticity, vibration, crepitation, temperature, variation in texture, and moisture. In addition, palpation is used to assess masses for position, size, shape, consistency, and mobility.

The nurse uses the most sensitive parts of the hands and fingers to palpate specific characteristics. For example, the *fingertips or pads* are the most sensitive for fine touch and are used to palpate pulses, lymph nodes, and breast tissue. The *dorsum*, or back of the hand and fingers, is used to discriminate skin temperature. The *palmar surface* of the hand over the metacarpophalangeal joints and *ulnar aspect* are used to assess vibration of the lung with vocalization (tactile fremitus). Position, consistency, mobility, size, shape, and turgor are assessed by lightly grasping tissue between the *thumb and index finger.*

Palpation is facilitated when the client is relaxed and comfortably positioned. Muscle tension is minimized, which lessens the possibility of the nurse's mistaking such tension for muscle rigidity. Relaxation is promoted by having warm hands and short fingernails and using a gentle approach. Encouraging the client to take slow, deep breaths also assists relaxation. Tactile pressure is applied and increased gradually. Prolonged pressure results in decreased sensitivity in the nurse's palpating hand.

The client is asked to indicate tender areas before palpation. Tender areas are palpated last while the nurse observes the client for nonverbal signs of discomfort or pain. The nurse examines these areas, but this may result in the client's becoming uncomfortable and reluctant to endure further examination.

Palpation proceeds from light to deep (Fig. 12-3). In *light palpation*, the underlying tissue is depressed approximately 1 to 2 cm ($\frac{1}{2}$ to $\frac{3}{4}$ inch). After light palpation, the nurse uses deep palpation to determine the size and condition of underlying structures such as abdominal organs. For *deep palpation*, the nurse depresses the underlying tissue approximately 4 to 5 cm ($1\frac{1}{2}$ to 2 inches), proceeding cautiously because prolonged pressure can potentially injure internal organs. Deep palpation is accomplished with either one or both hands (i.e., bimanual). For *bimanual palpation*, the nurse places one hand lightly on the client's skin. This hand is the sensing hand. The other hand (active hand) is placed over the sensing hand and applies pressure. The sensing hand does not apply direct pressure and remains sensitive to underlying organ characteristics.

The nurse takes precautions when palpating. For example, an artery is palpated so that blood flow is not obstructed. The carotid arteries are not palpated simultaneously because of the possibility of restricting blood flow to the brain.

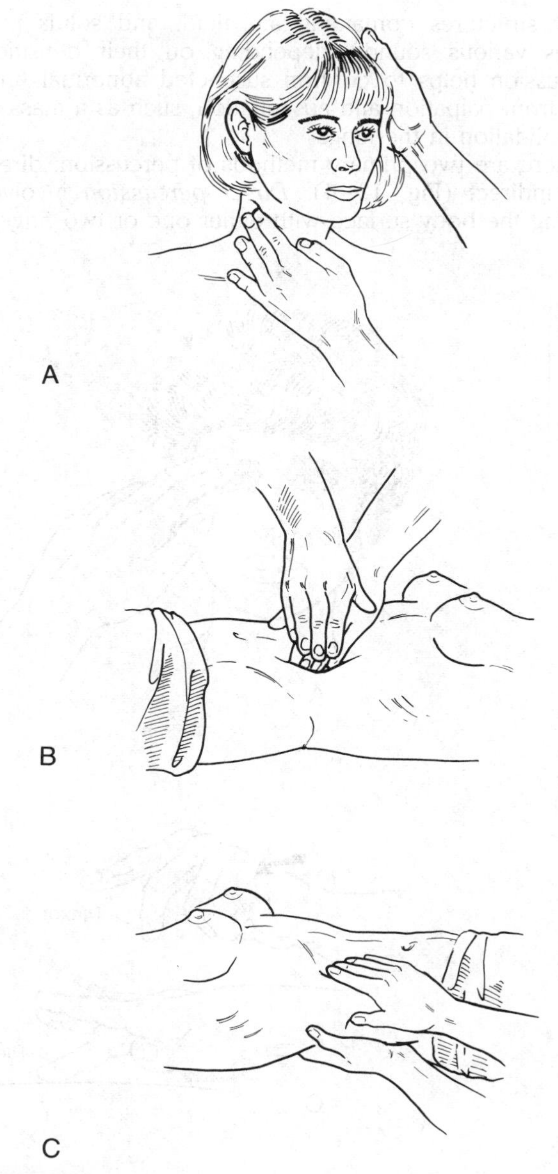

▲ *Figure 12-3*

Palpation techniques. *A*, Light palpation employs the lightest pressure possible to assess structures under the skin's surface, such as lymph nodes. *B*, Deep palpation is used to assess the condition of underlying organs such as in the abdomen using one or both hands. *C*, Bimanual palpation is used to trap and assess hard-to-palpate organs (e.g., kidney or spleen) or to stabilize an organ with one hand while the other hand palpates (e.g., liver).

Percussion

Percussion is a technique in which sound is produced by striking the client's skin in order to assess the underlying area. It is usually the third technique in physical assessment. Three to 5 cm of tissue depth can be examined by percussion. The sounds and tissue vibrations that result from percussion are evaluated in relation to the underlying body structures. Percussion of body structures containing air, fluid, and solids produces various sounds, depending on their densities. Percussion helps to confirm suspected abnormal findings from palpation and auscultation, such as a mass or consolidation in the lungs.

There are two primary methods of percussion, direct and indirect (Fig. 12–4). *Direct percussion* involves striking the body surface with either one or two fingers or the fist (i.e., blunt percussion). It is used primarily to assess the sinuses or over the thin chest wall of a child. *Blunt percussion* is performed to elicit tenderness from an underlying structure such as the liver or kidney and not to create a sound. Use of a reflex hammer is another example of blunt percussion.

Indirect percussion involves striking an intermediary finger or hand that is placed firmly on the body's sur-

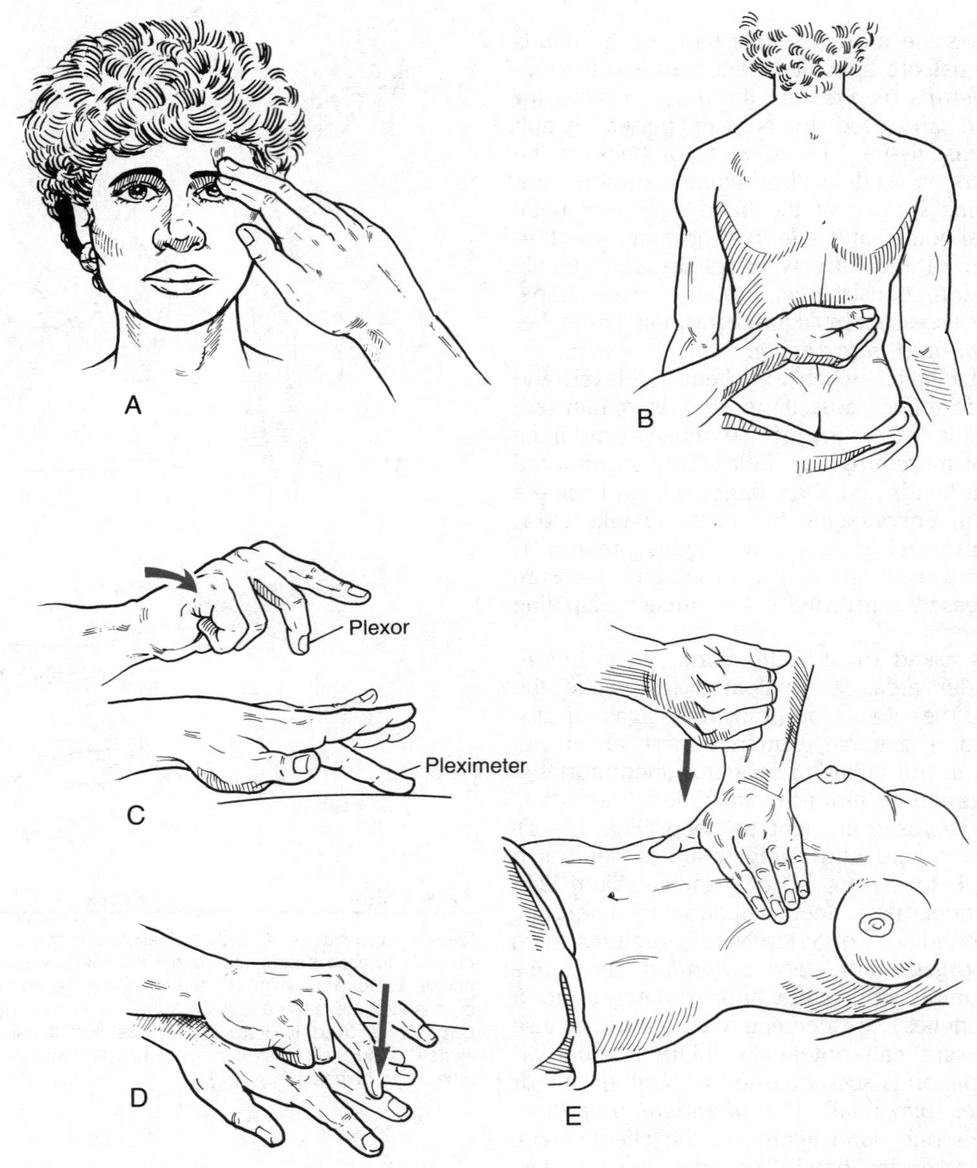

▲ **Figure 12–4**

Direct percussion. A, One or two fingers are used to percuss directly against the body's surface, such as an adult's sinuses to elicit tenderness or a child's thorax to assess sounds. *B*, The ulnar surface of the fist is used to gently strike the body's surface over an underlying organ such as at the costovertebral junction to assess for kidney tenderness. *Indirect percussion. C*, The pleximeter (distal phalanx of nondominant hand's middle finger) is placed firmly on the client's skin surface over soft tissue. The remaining fingers are hyperextended so that only the single joint is in contact with the skin. Failure to do this dampens (i.e., diminishes) the sound. The middle finger of the dominant hand is bent at its distal interphalangeal joint to create a hammer (i.e., plexor). *D*, The plexor moves in an arc to strike the pleximeter sharply and quickly at a perpendicular angle over the joint. The wrist remains relaxed and the forearm stationary to ensure a sharp blow. Resting the palm of the nondominant hand on the body surface, loose contact of the pleximeter with the skin surface, and delivering a weak blow with the plexor dampen the sound. The same amount of force is delivered with each blow for accurate comparison of sounds. A light, quick blow produces the clearest sound. The blows may be repeated rapidly three or four times to assess the sound. *E*, The palm of the left hand is placed over the area to be percussed, and the ulnar surface of the right fist is used to gently strike the left hand.

face. Indirect percussion requires dexterity and practice in order to become proficient. Refer to Figure 12-4 for discussion of the technique and common errors in technique.

Percussion results in five characteristic sounds.

Flatness. Flatness is a soft, high-pitched, short sound produced by very dense matter such as muscle. Percussion of the thigh will reproduce characteristic flat sound.

Dullness. Dullness is a soft to moderately loud sound of moderate pitch and duration. It is produced by less dense, mostly fluid-filled matter such as the liver and spleen and has a thudding quality.

Resonance. Resonance is a moderate to loud sound with low pitch and long duration. It results from the air-filled tissue of the normal lung and has a hollow quality.

Hyperresonance. Hyperresonance is a very loud, low-pitched sound of longer duration than resonance. It is produced by the overinflated, air-filled lungs of a client with pulmonary emphysema or a child's lung (because of a thin chest wall). Hyperresonance has a booming quality.

Tympany. Tympany is a loud, high-pitched, moderately long sound with a drumlike, musical quality. It results from enclosed, air-containing structures such as the stomach (gastric bubble) and bowel. It can be reproduced by percussing over a puffed cheek.

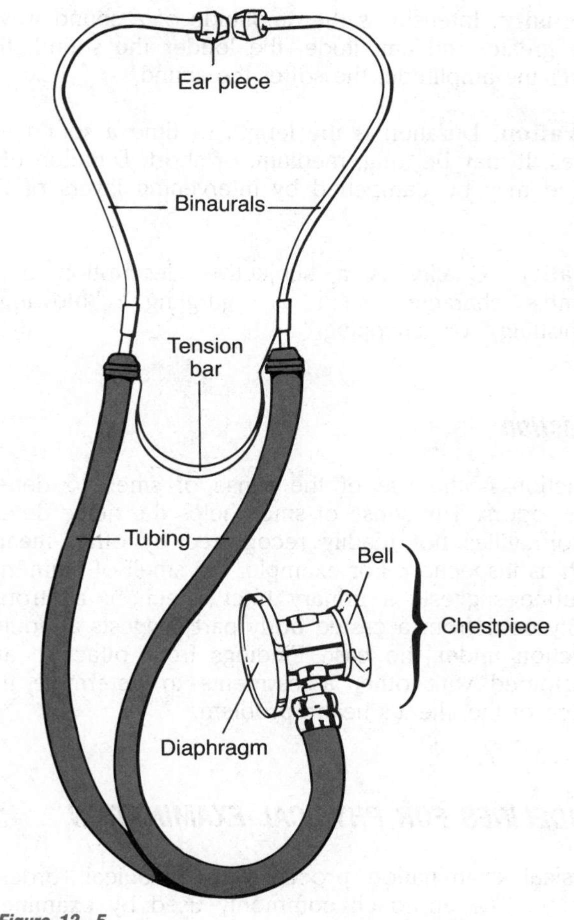

▲ ***Figure 12-5***

Stethoscope. The *bell* is used for low-pitched sounds such as bruits. The *diaphragm* is used to assess high-pitched sounds such as lung sounds and blood pressure. See text for further discussion.

Auscultation

Auscultation is listening to internal body sounds in order to assess normal sounds and detect abnormal sounds. It is the final step in examination. Auscultation is performed with use of a stethoscope to enhance sounds. The body sounds commonly assessed by auscultation include those produced by the heart, lungs, abdomen, and vascular system. The nurse becomes proficient at auscultation by knowing which sounds are produced by each body structure and the location at which they are most readily heard. Recognizing abnormal sounds is learned once the normal sounds have been mastered.

Acute hearing ability, a reliable stethoscope, and knowledge of how to use the stethoscope are essential to auscultation. Stethoscopes that amplify sounds are available for those who are hard of hearing. The basic stethoscope (Fig. 12-5) has a chestpiece with a bell and diaphragm and single or double tubing connected to double ear tubes (i.e., binaurals). A tension bar between the binaurals holds the earpieces firmly in place and reduces kinking of the tubing.

The *diaphragm* is held between the index and middle fingers firmly against the skin surface. It is used to hear high-pitched sounds such as lung sounds, heart sounds, and blood pressure. The *bell* is placed lightly in contact with the skin to hear low-pitched sounds such as murmurs and bruits. The *chestpiece* is placed on the skin so that it is between bones and not over them, because bone does not transmit sound readily. Snug-fitting *earpieces* occlude the external ear canal to enhance sound transmission from the chestpiece. The *tubing*, no longer than 12 to 15 inches for the best sound transmission, is kept free of contact with all surfaces to prevent extraneous noises.

A quiet environment is essential for accurate auscultation. The nurse concentrates on the body part being auscultated to determine what is causing the sounds that are heard. Once the nurse understands the source and characteristics of normal body sounds, recognition of abnormal sounds and their origin becomes easier.

There are four sound characteristics the nurse notes when auscultating.

Pitch. Pitch is the number or frequency of sound wave cycles per second. By varying the frequency, the pitch may be altered. For example, a high frequency results in a high-pitched sound, whereas a low frequency produces a low-pitched sound.

Intensity. Intensity is the amplitude of a sound wave. The greater the amplitude, the louder the sound; the lower the amplitude, the softer the sound.

Duration. Duration is the length of time a sound endures. It may be long, medium, or short. Duration of a sound may be dampened by intervening layers of tissue.

Quality. Quality is a subjective description of a sound's character, such as "gurgling," "blowing," "whistling," or "snapping."

Olfaction

Olfaction is the use of the sense of smell to detect body odors. The sense of smell helps the nurse detect abnormalities not readily recognized by other means such as inspection. For example, the smell of ammonia in urine suggests a urinary tract infection; a strong, musty odor from a casted body part suggests a wound infection under the cast. Findings from olfaction are considered with other assessments to determine the nature of the client's health problem.

GUIDELINES FOR PHYSICAL EXAMINATION

Physical examination proceeds in a logical, orderly fashion. The approach commonly used by examiners follows a head-to-toe system of organization so that findings are complete. This, however, is not an absolute rule, and the nurse who is beginning to use physical assessment skills practices and develops a system that is comfortable to use. Once a system is developed, the nurse uses it routinely to decrease inadvertent omission of portions of the examination. Successful physical assessment requires the nurse to be knowledgeable of both the techniques and the parameters of normal client findings. The following guidelines are provided for planning and conducting a physical examination.

Preparation of the Environment

1. The environment for physical examination is private, quiet, comfortable, and well lit.
2. An examination may be conducted in a special examination room in an office or clinic; in a client's bedroom in the home setting; or in the screened, enclosed area around a client's bed in a hospital room.
3. Extraneous noises are eliminated or controlled to allow the nurse to concentrate on the examination and to encourage the client to feel free to discuss problems or concerns.
4. The area is neither too warm nor too cool.

Preparation of Equipment

All necessary equipment is assembled and available before the examination is begun. Arranging equipment in order of use facilitates the examination. The nurse practices picking up equipment, holding it in the position of use, making adjustments, and assembling and disassembling. Equipment is also checked before use for adequate functioning. It is embarrassing as well as time-consuming to hunt for a replacement bulb for the oto-ophthalmoscope or to discover that the battery needs recharging in the middle of an examination.

Equipment commonly used in physical examination is described in Box 12-1 (refer also to Fig. 12-2). Additional equipment that may be used includes a goniometer, a Schiøtz tonometer, and substances to test taste and smell.

Preparation of the Client

The client is prepared physically and psychologically for the physical examination. Before beginning the examination, the nurse instructs the client to empty the bladder. If a urine specimen is needed for further testing, the client is instructed in the technique for collection at this time. An empty bladder facilitates examination of the abdomen, genitalia, and rectum.

Box 12-1. Equipment Commonly Used in Physical Examination

- cotton balls
- cotton-tipped applicators
- eye charts (Snellen, Stycar)
- examination gloves
- flashlight or floor lamp
- gauze sponges
- glass of water
- lubricant (water-soluble)
- ophthalmoscope
- otoscope (ear, nose specula)
- penlight
- reflex hammer
- ruler
- safety pin (sterile)
- skinfold calipers
- sphygmomanometer
- stethoscope (bell, diaphragm)
- supplies for tests (Pap, guaiac)
- tape measure
- thermometer
- tongue blades
- tuning forks
- vaginal speculum
- watch with second hand
- weight scale

DRAPING

Physical preparation also includes instructing the client to dress according to the type and extent of examination to be conducted. A hospital or paper gown and drapes provide privacy.

POSITIONING

During the examination, the client is assisted in assuming different positions to facilitate assessment. Figure 12-6 illustrates common positions for examination and the areas of the body that are assessed. The nurse considers limitations the client has that prevent optimal positioning, such as arthritis, back injury, joint deformities, or weakness. Alternative positions may have to be assumed for the examination to be completed. Several positions are uncomfortable and embarrassing. The client is kept in these positions only as long as required and is draped to prevent unnecessary exposure.

PSYCHOLOGICAL PREPARATION

The nurse approaches the client in a professional, calm manner. An organized, efficient approach coupled with a relaxed voice tone and facial expression puts the client at ease and promotes a relationship of trust. The client may feel anxious about the examination process and the possibility of the nurse's finding something abnormal. The nurse explains what will be done before proceeding so that the client knows what to expect and cooperates to the fullest extent possible.

The nurse first explains the physical examination in general terms and then provides a detailed explanation as each body system is examined. Simple terms are less confusing for clients to understand and are less threatening than complicated explanations. The nurse encourages the client to verbalize discomfort as the examination proceeds.

The nurse watches the client's facial expressions and body language throughout the examination. These nonverbal forms of communication may convey anxiety, fear, or concern. For example, the client may pull the drape closely around the body, or muscles may feel tight and tense. In extreme instances, the client may wish to stop the examination and the nurse complies. The client is never coerced to continue. The nurse does, however, attempt to explain the purpose of the examination and to clarify any client misconceptions.

Preparation of the Examiner

The nurse begins the physical examination on meeting the client by focusing on the client's appearance, movements, position, and reaction to the assessment process. A mental plan (assisted by a general outline or checklist) is helpful so that the major portions of the examination are included. The outline may include the general sequence of the examination and the methods, equipment, and techniques needed to examine each body system.

ORGANIZATION

Organization and efficiency provide a framework for a thorough physical assessment without wasting the time or energy of the nurse or the client. Position changes are kept to a minimum so that the client is not fatigued. The nurse uses a specific piece of equipment to examine an entire region or body system before returning it to the equipment tray. For example, the reflex hammer is used to test deep tendon reflexes in quick succession, proceeding from upper to lower extremities, while the client is either seated or supine.

SEQUENCE OF EXAMINATION

The importance of organizing the physical examination systematically has already been discussed. A suggested format for sequencing the adult general screening physical examination is presented in Table 12-1. This format integrates a head-to-toe approach incorporating regional assessments of the head and neck, upper extremities and spine, posterior and anterior thorax, abdomen, lower extremities and spine, and genitalia and rectum, as well as each body system. Each examiner develops an individual style and approach to physical assessment. The examination is sufficiently complete to obtain the data necessary to diagnose the client's responses to physical problems yet flexible enough to accommodate the client's individual needs.

KNOWLEDGE OF STRUCTURE AND FUNCTION

Anatomic landmarks are used as reference points both for locating areas to examine and in recording findings. Reference to an anatomy book is recommended for the nurse who is a beginning practitioner in physical examination. Table 12-2 presents common terms used to describe the location of findings in relationship to the anatomy. Additional descriptive terms and anatomic reference points are discussed further with the examination of the respective body systems.

THE ADULT GENERAL SCREENING PHYSICAL EXAMINATION

General Survey

The general survey begins the physical examination and includes observing the client's general appearance and behavior, taking vital signs, and measuring height and weight. Additional assessments include the anthropometric parameters of triceps skinfold thickness and midarm muscle circumference.

GENERAL APPEARANCE AND BEHAVIOR

The nurse evaluates observations regarding general appearance and behavior in relationship to the client's

Text continued on page 233

POSITION	AREAS EXAMINED	RATIONALE	CONTRAINDICATIONS
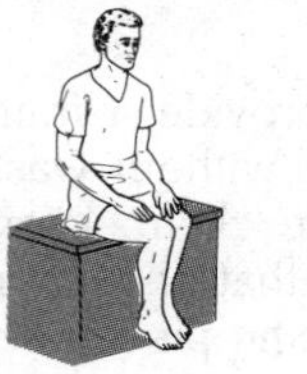 Sitting	Vital signs, head and neck, back, posterior and anterior thorax and lungs, breasts, axillae, heart, upper and lower extremities, reflexes	Sitting upright allows for full lung expansion and better visualization of upper body symmetry.	Elderly and weak clients may be unable to sit without support. Alternate position is supine with head of bed elevated.
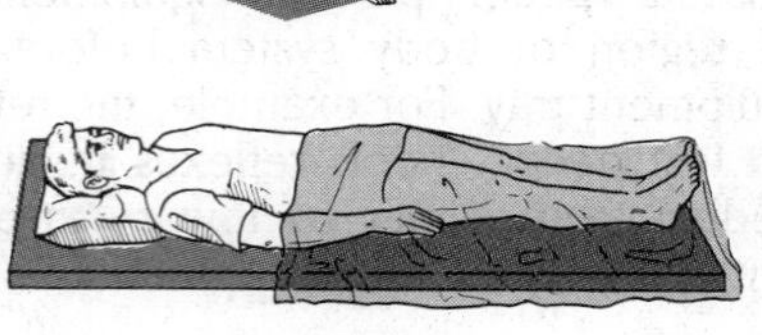 Supine	Vital signs, head and neck, anterior thorax and lungs, breasts, axillae, heart, abdomen, extremities, peripheral pulses	This is a relaxed position for most clients. It provides access to pulse sites and prevents contracture of abdominal muscles especially if a small pillow is placed under the knees.	Clients with cardiovascular and respiratory problems may be unable to lie flat without becoming short of breath. Alternate position is to raise head of bed. Clients with low back pain may be unable to lie flat without flexing the knees.
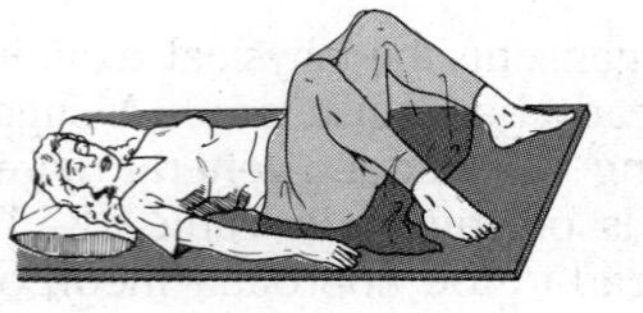 Dorsal recumbent	Vital signs, head and neck, anterior thorax and lungs, breasts, axillae, heart, abdomen, extremities, peripheral pulses, vagina	Flexed knees reduce tension on lower back and abdominal muscles and increase client comfort.	Same as for supine. Client should not raise arms over the head or clasp hands behind head as this increases contraction of abdominal muscles.
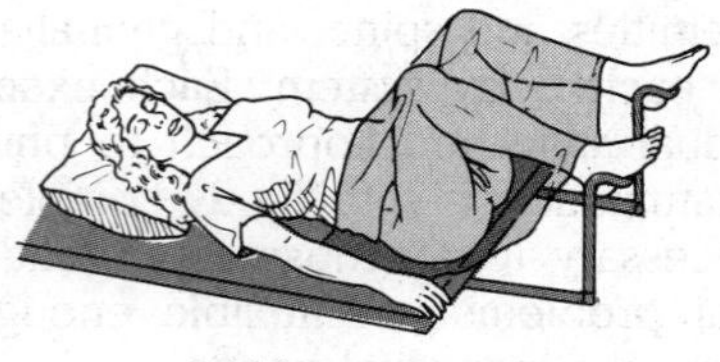 Lithotomy	Female genitalia, reproductive tract, and rectum	This position maximally exposes the genitalia and facilitates the insertion of vaginal speculum.	This position is assumed immediately before it is needed as it is embarrassing and uncomfortable. The client is kept draped. Clients with arthritis or joint deformity may be unable to assume this position. Alternate positions are dorsal recumbent or Sims.
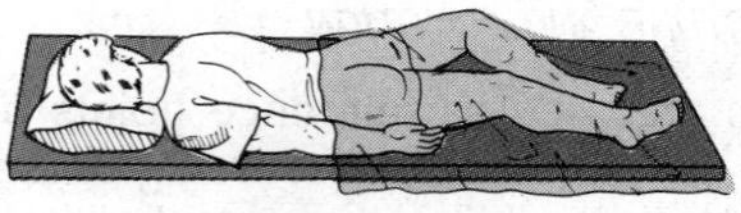 Sims (posterior view)	Rectum, vagina	Flexion of the upper hip and knee improves exposure of the rectal area.	Clients with deformities of the hip or knee may be unable to assume this position. Elderly and obese clients may be uncomfortable.
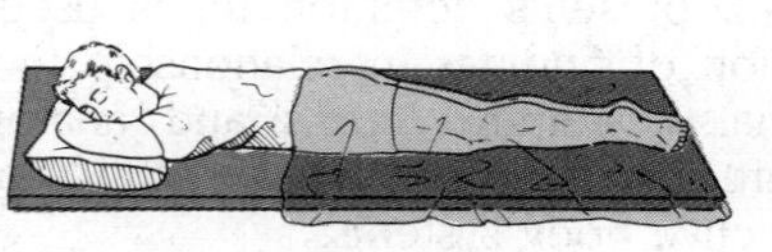 Prone	Posterior thorax, hip movement, popliteal pulses	This position is used to assess hip extension. Sometimes popliteal pulse palpation is facilitated in this position.	This position is not well tolerated by the elderly or clients with cardiovascular or respiratory problems.
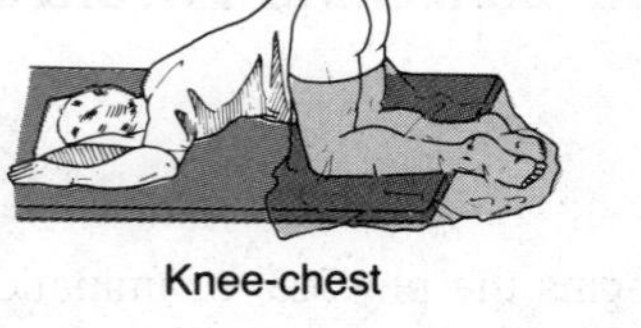 Knee-chest	Rectum, prostate	This position provides maximal exposure of the anal and rectal areas and facilitates insertion of instruments into the rectum.	Poorly tolerated by clients with cardiovascular or respiratory problems. Clients with difficulty flexing hips or knees may be unable to assume this position.
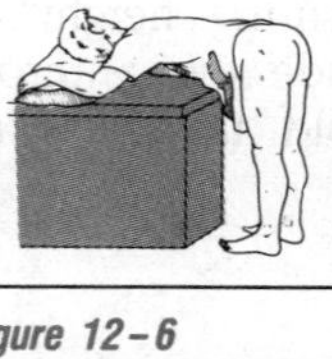 Standing, bent over examining table	Rectum, prostate	This is a more comfortable position than knee-chest and allows for palpation of the prostate gland.	This position is assumed immediately before it is needed as it is embarrassing. Clients with back problems may need assistance.

▲ **Figure 12-6**

Common physical examination positions and their application.

TABLE 12-1. Format for Integrated Head-to-Toe Screening Physical Examination

Assessment Area	Client Position or Activity*	Technique†	Equipment	What to Observe
1. General survey	► Standing and walking during entrance (a, c) ► Sitting during health history interview (a, c) ► Changing into examining gown (a, c, f) ► Walking to examining table (a, b, c, d, f) ► Sitting on edge of examining table (a, c, e, f)	► Inspection (a, b, c, d, e, f) ► Olfaction (a)		a. General appearance and behavior: apparent age; sex; race; general state of health; signs of distress; body build; posture; gait; obvious deformity; movements and gross ROM; skin color and texture of exposed areas; dress, hygiene, and grooming; body or breath odor; mental status (expression, affect, speech, memory, eye contact); level of consciousness; level of cooperation
			b. Balance scale with height measure	b. Height and weight measurements
				c. Balance, coordination (Romberg's test, arm drift)
			d. Snellen chart	d. Visual acuity (CN II)
			e. Thermometer; watch with second hand; sphygmomanometer; stethoscope	e. Vital signs: temperature; pulse; respirations; blood pressure including check for auscultatory gap
			f. Tape measure; skinfold calipers	f. Nutritional status: body frame (wrist circumference); MAC; TSF; MAMC; IBW
2. Head and neck	► Sitting on edge of examining table (a, b, c, d, e, f, g)	► Inspection (a, b, c, d, e, f, g) ► Palpation (a, b, c, d, e, f, g) ► Percussion (e) ► Auscultation (a, f, g) ► Olfaction (a, f)		a. *Head*
			(1) Tape measure	(1) Inspect and palpate skull size, shape, symmetry, contour, tenderness, lesions; measure circumference if abnormal size
				(2) Inspect hair and scalp: color, integrity; hair distribution and texture; presence of nits or lice; hygiene
			(3) Stethoscope	(3) Palpate temporal arteries: thickening, tenderness; auscultate for bruits if abnormality noted; rate amplitude
				b. *Face*
				(1) Inspect symmetry, skin color, hair distribution; facial movements (CN V and VII): clench jaws, puff cheeks, raise eyebrows, frown, eyelid strength
				(2) Palpate TMJ; temporal and masseter muscles (CN V); nodules
			(3) Cotton wisp; sterile safety pin	(3) Test facial sensation for light touch, pressure and pain (CN V) over forehead, cheeks, and jaw
				c. *Eyes*
			(1) Snellen chart; eye cover	(1) Visual acuity, if not performed earlier (CN II)
			(2) Eye cover; penlight or pen	(2) Visual fields (peripheral vision) by confrontation method (CN II)
			(3) Penlight or pen	(3) EOMs through six cardinal positions of gaze (CN III, IV, VI)
			(4) Penlight or pen	(4) Convergence and accommodation (CN III, IV, VI)
			(5) Eye cover	(5) Cover/uncover test (CN III, IV, VI) for movement
			(6) Penlight	(6) Corneal light reflex (CN III, IV, VI) for alignment (Hirschberg's test)

Table continued on following page

TABLE 12–1. *Format for Integrated Head-to-Toe Screening Physical Examination* Continued

Assessment Area	Client Position or Activity*	Technique†	Equipment	What to Observe
			(7) Penlight; cotton wisp; cotton applicator	(7) Inspect and palpate external eye structures: (a) Eyebrows' symmetry, alignment (b) Eyelashes' symmetry, hair distribution, direction of growth (c) Eyelids' position, skin characteristics, blinking (d) Lacrimal apparatus function (e) Eyeballs' symmetry, firmness (f) Conjunctivae and sclerae color, texture, lesions, foreign bodies (g) Corneas' texture, transparency; corneal reflex (CN V) (h) Anterior chambers' transparency, depth (i) Irises' and pupils' symmetry, color, size, reaction to light and accommodation (CN III, IV, VI)
			(8) Ophthalmoscope	(8) Inspect internal eye structures: red reflex, retina, retinal vessels, optic disc, macula and fovea
				d. *Ears*
			(1) Otoscope	(1) Inspect and palpate external ear structures: (a) Auricles' symmetry, placement, skin integrity, color, mobility, and tenderness over tragus (b) Ear canals' skin integrity, cerumen, obstruction, foreign body, discharge (c) Tympanic membranes' symmetry, color, light reflection, landmarks, scars, fluid
			(2) Tuning fork (512 Hz)	(2) Hearing acuity: response to normal conversation, whisper test, Weber's test for sound lateralization, Rinne's test for air and bone conduction of sound (CN VIII)
				e. *Nose and sinuses*
				(1) Inspect and palpate external nose alignment, symmetry, skin color, lesions, tenderness, discharge, nasal flaring, patency
			(2) Penlight	(2) Inspect vestibules' color, mucous membrane, septum alignment
			(3) Nasal speculum and penlight; or otoscope head with nasal speculum	(3) Inspect nares' mucosa for color, moisture; septum for alignment, masses, perforation; turbinates for color, exudate, inflammation
				(4) Palpate and percuss frontal and maxillary sinuses for swelling and tenderness
			(5) Penlight or transilluminator	(5) Transilluminate frontal and maxillary sinuses
			(6) Various substances to smell (coffee grounds, cinnamon, cloves, peppermint)	(6) Sense of smell (CN I) not usually tested, but if done, test with coffee grounds, cinnamon, cloves, peppermint
			f. Gloves; tongue blade; penlight	f. *Mouth and pharynx* (1) Inspect and palpate lips and oral mucosa for color, symmetry, texture, hydration, lesions, Stensen's ducts

TABLE 12–1. *Format for Integrated Head-to-Toe Screening Physical Examination* Continued

Assessment Area	Client Position or Activity*	Technique†	Equipment	What to Observe
				(2) Inspect teeth and gums and palpate gums for state of repair, hygiene, teeth alignment, missing teeth, gum bleeding, gum integrity
				(3) Inspect and palpate tongue and floor of mouth for symmetry, color, tongue position and size, texture, mobility, lesions, presence of papillae
				(4) Tongue mobility and strength (CN IX, XII)
				(5) Inspect Wharton's duct under tongue, floor of mouth, and base of tongue for lesions
				(6) Inspect roof of mouth, palates, and uvula for color, symmetry, texture, bone deformity
				(7) Test rise of uvula and soft palate with phonation (CN X)
				(8) Inspect tonsils and pillars for color, size, shape
				(9) Inspect pharynx for color, discharge on posterior wall
				(10) Test gag reflex (CN IX, X)
				(11) Note characteristics of voice, ability to swallow (CN IX, X)
				(12) Note presence of breath odor
			(13) Various substances to taste (sugar, salt, lemon juice, bitters)	(13) Test sense of taste (CN VII, IX) only if abnormality reported with sugar, salt, lemon juice, bitters
				g. *Neck*
				(1) Inspect neck muscles' symmetry, ROM, strength (CN XI); shrug shoulders
				(2) Palpate and inspect over parotid and submandibular salivary glands for swelling, tenderness
				(3) Palpate all cervical lymph nodes
				(4) Inspect and palpate trachea for symmetry and alignment
			(5) Stethoscope	(5) Inspect and palpate thyroid gland for symmetry, masses; auscultate for bruits if enlarged
			(6) Stethoscope	(6) Inspect and palpate carotid arteries; rate amplitude; auscultate for bruits
				(7) Inspect jugular venous distention
3. Upper extremities and spine	► Sitting on edge of examining table (a, b)	► Inspection (a, b) ► Palpation (a) ► Percussion (b)		a. *Upper extremities*
				(1) Inspect skin for lesions and palpate turgor
				(2) Inspect limbs for alignment and symmetry
				(3) Inspect fingernails and blanche to test capillary refill
				(4) Palpate peripheral pulses: brachial, radial, ulnar; rate amplitude
				(5) Palpate epitrochlear lymph nodes
			(6) Tape measure	(6) Inspect and palpate muscle groups for size, symmetry, tone; measure if appear unequal
				(7) Evaluate and rate muscle strength: upper arms, forearms, wrists, fingers
				(8) Inspect and palpate joints for swelling and tenderness, crepitus

Table continued on following page

TABLE 12–1. Format for Integrated Head-to-Toe Screening Physical Examination Continued

Assessment Area	Client Position or Activity*	Technique†	Equipment	What to Observe
			(9) Goniometer	(9) Assess ROM: shoulders, elbows, wrists, fingers; measure ROM if limitation noted
				b. *Spine*
			(1) Reflex hammer	(1) Test DTRs and rate response: biceps, triceps, brachioradialis; also test lower extremity DTRs: patellar, Achilles, and plantar cutaneous reflexes
				(2) Assess cerebellar functions: finger-to-toes; hand supination and pronation; finger-to-thumb opposition
4. Posterior thorax	► Sitting on edge of examining table; nurse goes around behind client (a, b, c)	► Inspection (a, b) ► Palpation (a, b) ► Percussion (a, b, c) ► Auscultation (b)		a. *Spine, ribs, muscles*
				(1) Inspect spine for alignment; palpate spine processes for tenderness; inspect skin integrity
				(2) Inspect rib cage for symmetry, shape, movement with respiration
				(3) Measure anteroposterior to lateral diameter
				(4) Inspect and lightly palpate paravertebral muscles for tenderness, spasm
				(5) Assess thoracic expansion (respiratory excursion)
				b. *Lungs*
				(1) Observe respiratory pattern
				(2) Palpate tactile fremitus and respiratory excursion
				(3) Percuss posterior and lateral thorax and diaphragmatic excursion
			(4) Ruler and pen	(4) Measure diaphragmatic excursion
			(5) Stethoscope	(5) Auscultate breath sounds, posterior and lateral thorax
			(6) Stethoscope	(6) Auscultate voice sounds if fremitus abnormal (bronchophony, egophony, whispered pectoriloquy)
				c. *Kidneys* Percuss over CVAs for kidney tenderness
5. Anterior thorax	► Sitting on edge of examining table; nurse goes around to right side of client (a, b, c, d, e) ► Sitting up and leaning forward (b, e) ► Sitting with arms at sides; with hands on hips; with arms raised over head (e) ► Supine, arm behind head (e) ► Supine, head elevated 30 degrees (f, g) ► Left lateral recumbent (f)	► Inspection (a, b, c, d, e, f, g) ► Palpation (a, b, e, f) ► Percussion (a) ► Auscultation (a, b, c, f)		a. *Lungs and thorax*
				(1) Inspect skin integrity
				(2) Observe respiratory pattern
				(3) Inspect rib cage for symmetry, movement with respiration, shape, use of accessory muscles
				(4) Palpate respiratory excursion
				(5) Palpate tactile fremitus
				(6) Percuss anterior thorax
			(7) Stethoscope	(7) Auscultate breath sounds and voice sounds (if fremitus abnormal)
				b. *Heart*
				(1) Inspect precordium for lifts, heaves, apical impulse
				(2) Inspect epigastrium for aortic pulsations
				(3) Palpate precordium for thrills, apical impulse, lift, heaves
			(4) Stethoscope	(4) Auscultate heart sounds with client sitting up, then leaning forward
			(5) Stethoscope	(5) Assess heart rate and rhythm
				c. *Carotid vessels*
			(1) Stethoscope	(1) Auscultate for bruits

TABLE 12-1. Format for Integrated Head-to-Toe Screening Physical Examination Continued

Assessment Area	Client Position or Activity*	Technique†	Equipment	What to Observe
				(2) Rate amplitude if not done during neck examination
				d. *Jugular veins* Inspect for distention
				e. *Breasts and axillae*
				(1) Inspect breasts in 3 positions for size, shape, symmetry, contour, skin characteristics, lesions
				(2) Inspect areolae and nipples for size, shape, color, contour, symmetry, lesions
				(3) Inspect axillae for rashes, masses, lesions, pigmentation
				(4) Palpate axillae for lymph nodes
				(5) Palpate breasts for lumps, masses, consistency
				► **Assist client to supine position**
				(6) Palpate breasts, areolae, and nipples with client supine and arm behind head
				f. *Heart*
				(1) Inspect precordium for lifts, heaves, apical impulse
				(2) Inspect epigastrium for aortic pulsations
				(3) Palpate precordium for thrills, lifts, heaves, apical impulse
			(4) Stethoscope	(4) Auscultate heart sounds with client supine, then in left lateral recumbent
				g. *Jugular veins*
				(1) Inspect for level of venous distention with client's head elevated 30 to 45 degrees; measure level of distention between angle of Louis and angle of jaw
				(2) Assess for hepatojugular reflux if right ventricular failure suspected
6. Abdomen	► Supine with arms relaxed at sides or crossed over chest; may have knees flexed slightly (a, b, c, d, e, f, i) ► Turned to right lateral recumbent (g, h)	► Inspection (a, i, j) ► Auscultation (a) ► Percussion (a, b, c, h, j) ► Palpation (a, b, d, e, f, g, h)		a. *Abdomen (general)*
				(1) Inspect skin integrity and characteristics: striae, venous pattern, hair distribution
			(2) Tape measure	(2) Inspect contour, symmetry, umbilicus, pulsations, peristalsis, rectus muscles with straining; measure girth if distention noted
			(3) Stethoscope	(3) Auscultate all quadrants for bowel sounds
			(4) Stethoscope	(4) Auscultate major vessels for bruits: abdominal aorta; renal, iliac, and femoral arteries
			(5) Stethoscope	(5) Auscultate over epigastrium for venous hum
			(6) Stethoscope	(6) Auscultate over liver and spleen for peritoneal friction rub
				(7) Percuss all quadrants for masses, tenderness, gastric bubble; over bladder and spleen
				(8) Lightly palpate all quadrants for masses, tenderness
				(9) Deep palpation for masses and tenderness, all quadrants

Table continued on following page

TABLE 12–1. *Format for Integrated Head-to-Toe Screening Physical Examination* Continued

Assessment Area	Client Position or Activity*	Technique†	Equipment	What to Observe
				(10) Assess rebound tenderness over RLQ and LLQ
				b. *Liver*
			(1) Pen	(1) Percuss liver size at RMCL and MSL and mark borders
			(2) Ruler	(2) Measure liver span at RMCL and MSL
				c. *Spleen*
				(1) Percuss spleen size
				(2) Percuss for splenic enlargement if indicated
				d. *Aorta* Palpate for area of pulsation in epigastrium
				e. *Inguinal areas*
				(1) Palpate femoral arteries and rate amplitude
				(2) Palpate inguinal lymph nodes, note characteristcs
				f. *Liver* Palpate for size, masses, nodules
				g. *Spleen* Palpate for size if enlargement suspected
				h. *Kidneys*
				(1) Palpate right and left kidneys for enlargement
				(2) Blunt percussion over CVAs (posterior thorax) for tenderness if not done earlier
			i. Tongue blade	i. *Abdominal reflexes* Assess each quadrant for presence of reflex
				j. Test for ascites if indicated
7. Lower extremities and spine	► Supine with arms relaxed (a, b) ► Prone if needed to assess popliteal lymph nodes (a)	► Inspection (a, b) ► Palpation (a) ► Percussion (b)		a. *Lower extremities*
				(1) Inspect skin for lesions, hair distribution
				(2) Inspect limbs for alignment and symmetry
				(3) Inspect toenails and blanche to test capillary refill
				(4) Palpate peripheral pulses: popliteal, posterior tibial, dorsalis pedis; rate amplitude
				(5) Palpate popliteal lymph nodes
				(6) Inspect for edema and palpate for pitting if present
			(7) Tape measure	(7) Palpate for phlebitis, varicosities; measure circumference of calves or thighs if phlebitis present
				(8) Assess for presence of Homan's sign
			(9) Tape measure	(9) Inspect and palpate muscle groups for size, symmetry, tone; measure if appear unequal
				(10) Evaluate and rate muscle strength: hips, hamstrings, quadriceps, ankles, toes, feet
				(11) Inspect and palpate joints for swelling, tenderness, crepitus
			(12) Goniometer	(12) Assess ROM: hips, knees, ankles, feet, toes; measure ROM if limitation noted

TABLE 12–1. Format for Integrated Head-to-Toe Screening Physical Examination Continued

Assessment Area	Client Position or Activity*	Technique†	Equipment	What to Observe
				b. *Spine* (1) Test DTRs if not done before at time of upper extremity evaluation; test patellar, Achilles, and plantar cutaneous reflex (2) Assess cerebellar functions; ability to slide heel down opposite shin; foot tapping
8. General neurologic and spine	► Supine with arms at sides, eyes closed (a) ► Walking heel to toe (b) ► Walking on toes, then heels (b) ► Hopping on each foot (b) ► Knee bends (b) ► Standing with arms relaxed at sides (c)	► Inspection (a, b, c)		a. *Sensory function*
			(1) Cotton wisp	(1) Test perception of light touch over symmetric dermatomes distally then proximally, trunk, face, neck
			(2) Sterile safety pin or needle	(2) Test perception of pain vs. pressure over symmetric dermatomes distally then proximally, trunk, face, neck
			(3) Tuning fork (128 Hz)	(3) Test perception of vibration distally on toes and fingers; progress proximally if abnormal
				(4) Test position sense, fingers and toes
			(5) Key, coins, safety pin, paper clip	(5) Test object identification, both hands (stereognosis)
			(6) Closed pen	(6) Test graphesthesia, both hands
			(7) Two sterile safety pins	(7) Test two-point discrimination, both index fingers
			(8) Test tubes filled with hot water and cold water	(8) Test temperature perception only if pain perception is impaired distally then proximally, trunk, face, neck
			(9) Finger touch	(9) Test point localization and tactile localization (double simultaneous stimulation) only if light touch perception is impaired
				► **Assist client to standing position**
				b. *Gross motor and balance* (1) Inspect gait and balance while client walks heel-to-toe, then on toes, then on heels (2) Observe balance while client stands on one foot, then the other (3) Observe balance and lower extremity strength while client hops on one foot, then the other (4) Observe balance and strength while client performs shallow knee bends
				c. *Spine* (1) Inspect spine from anterior, lateral, and posterior views for kyphosis, lordosis, or scoliosis (2) Assess spine ROM
9A. Genitalia (male)	► Standing facing nurse (a, b, c, d, e, f, g, h, i) ► Standing and performing Valsalva's maneuver (g, h, i)	► Inspection (a, b, d, f, g) ► Palpation (c, e, h, i)	A. Gloves worn throughout	A. *Male genitalia* a. Inspect pubic hair and skin, hair distribution, rashes, lesions, parasites
			b. Culture medium	b. Inspect penis: shaft, prepuce, glans, urethral meatus; culture discharge if present
				c. Palpate penile shaft for nodules, tenderness
				d. Inspect scrotum for size, symmetry, shape, swelling
				e. Palpate scrotum for presence of testes, epididymis, vas deferens
			f. Transilluminator or flashlight	f. Transilluminate scrotum if swelling or mass palpated

Table continued on following page

TABLE 12–1. Format for Integrated Head-to-Toe Screening Physical Examination Continued

Assessment Area	Client Position or Activity*	Technique†	Equipment	What to Observe
				g. Inspect inguinal areas for hernia, first with client standing quietly, then during Valsalva's maneuver h. Palpate for direct inguinal hernia with client at rest and performing Valsalva's maneuver i. Palpate for indirect inguinal hernia with client at rest and performing Valsalva's maneuver
9B. Anus and rectum (male)	▶ Standing and bending over examining table (a, c, f, g) ▶ Standing and bending over examining table, performing Valsalva's maneuver (b, d, e)	▶ Inspection (a, b, g) ▶ Palpation (c, d, e, f)	A. Gloves worn throughout	A. *Anus and rectum (male)* a. Inspect perianal skin integrity, color, excoriation, rash, lesions, fissures, ulcers, hemorrhoids b. Inspect anal area for rectal prolapse, fissures, fistulas, inflammation, hemorrhoids, polyps with client performing Valsalva's maneuver
			c. Lubricant	c. Palpate anus, anal canal, sphincter tone, anorectal junction, rectal walls, coccyx with client at rest d. Palpate anal sphincter tone during Valsalva's maneuver e. Palpate for a descending rectal mass with client performing Valsalva's maneuver f. Palpate prostate gland: median sulcus, two lateral lobes
			g. Hemoccult test; culture medium	g. Inspect gloved finger as it is withdrawn for stool and test stool for occult blood; obtain rectal culture if indicated ▶ **Female client is assisted to lithotomy position or dorsal recumbent**
10A. Genitalia (female)	▶ Lithotomy position if both external and internal genitalia examined (a, b, c, d, e, f, g, h, i, j, k, l, m, n) ▶ Dorsal recumbent if only external genitalia examined (a, b, c, d, e, f, g, h, i)	▶ Inspection (a, b, c, d, e, g, j, k) ▶ Palpation (f, h, i, l, m, n)	B. Gloves worn throughout	B. *Female genitalia* a. Inspect mons pubis; pubic hair distribution and texture; perineal skin for color, lesions, irritation, parasites b. Inspect labia majora edema, symmetry c. Inspect labia minora symmetry d. Inspect clitoris color, presence of lesions e. Inspect introitus and hymen f. Palpate Bartholin's glands if inflamed or enlarged for size, tenderness g. Inspect urethral meatus for discharge, inflammation, swelling
			h. Culture medium *change gloves if discharge present	h. Palpate Skene's glands for discharge and obtain specimen for culture if present i. Assess integrity of pelvic floor muscles: strength, presence of cystocele or rectocele, discharge of urine
			j. Vaginal speculum; light source; wooden spatula; cotton-tipped applicator; glass slides; fixative; culture medium	j. Insert vaginal speculum and inspect cervix; adjust light as needed; note shape, position, color, lesions, discharge; obtain cervical specimens if indicated: cervical scraping, endocervical swab, vaginal pool scraping k. Inspect vagina as speculum is removed: color, rugae, mucosa
			l. Lubricant	l. Palpate vagina and cervix for nodules, masses; cervix position, mobility, consistency, tenderness

TABLE 12-1. Format for Integrated Head-to-Toe Screening Physical Examination Continued

Assessment Area	Client Position or Activity*	Technique†	Equipment	What to Observe
				m. Bimanually palpate pelvic structures (1) Uterus (anterior wall and fundus) for masses, tenderness, position (2) Ovary and adnexa for ovary size, masses, tenderness
			n. Change gloves if vaginal examination performed; lubricant	n. Recto-vaginal palpation of uterus for masses, position, tenderness (Proceed with 10B, step c, and so on. Steps a and b will then be last.)
10B. Anus and rectum (female)	► Lithotomy position if done at same time as internal genitalia examination (a, b, c, d, e, g) ► Dorsal recumbent if done after external genitalia examination (a, b, c, d, e, f, g) ► Performing Valsalva's maneuver (b, d, e)	► Inspection (a, b, g) ► Palpation (c, d, e, f)	B. Gloves worn throughout	B. *Anus and rectum (female)* a. Inspect perianal skin integrity, color, excoriation, rash, lesions, fissures, ulcers, hemorrhoids b. Inspect anal area for rectal prolapse, fissures, fistulas, inflammation, hemorrhoids, polyps with client performing Valsalva's maneuver
			c. Lubricant	c. Palpate anus, anal canal, sphincter tone, anorectal junction, rectal walls, coccyx d. Palpate anal sphincter tone during Valsalva's maneuver e. Palpate for a descending rectal mass with client performing Valsalva's maneuver f. Palpate cervix through anterior rectal wall for shape, position, mobility, tenderness
			g. Hemoccult; culture medium	g. Inspect gloved finger as it is withdrawn for stool and test stool for occult blood; obtain rectal culture if indicated
11. Examination complete	► Sitting			After removal of fingers, assist client to clean perineum and to sit comfortably before leaving to allow client to dress

* Letters in parentheses after the client position or activity denote what the nurse observes.
† Letters in parentheses after technique denote when the nurse uses these skills to assist observations.
CN, cranial nerve; CVAs, costovertebral angles; DTRs, deep tendon reflexes; EOMs, extraocular movements; IBW, ideal body weight; LLQ, left lower quadrant; MAC, midarm circumference; MAMC, midarm muscle circumference; MSL, midsternal line; RLQ, right lower quadrant; RMCL, right midclavicular line; ROM, range of motion; TMJ, temporomandibular joint; TSF, triceps skinfold thickness.

background, that is, culture, educational level, socioeconomic status, and current health and illness status. Signs of problems or abnormalities direct the nurse to examine specific body areas thoroughly as the examination proceeds. For example, the client who is unkempt and has obvious body odor will need thorough examination of the hair, skin, and nails for assessment of hygiene. General appearance and behavior assessments include the following.

Apparent Age, Sex, and Race. The client's appearance may or may not be congruent with chronologic age, directing the nurse to assess each body system for potential problems related to the aging process. Other assessments are sex-specific and affect the type of procedures performed. Data are interpreted and recommendations are made for health teaching and further screening on the basis of the client's health risk profile (see Chap. 11).

Apparent State of Health. The nurse assesses whether the client looks "healthy," frail, or ill. Deformities or absent body parts are noted.

Signs of Distress or Discomfort. The client may display obvious signs of pain (wincing), anxiety (eyes darting around room), difficulty breathing (gasping), or other problems. The nurse adapts the examination to the client's needs by including only the necessary assessments. The ideal situation is that the client is comfortable and in no acute distress.

Body Build, Height, and Weight. The client's body build is assessed for proportionate distribution of

TABLE 12-2. Anatomic Terms Used to Describe Locations of Physical Findings

Term	Anatomic Location	Example
Anterior (ventral)	Toward or at front of body; situated in front of a reference structure	Trachea is anterior to esophagus
Contralateral	Pertaining to or on opposite side of body; opposite of ipsilateral	Right eye is contralateral to left eye
Deep	Below or away from surface of body	Aortic arch is deep to sternum
Distal	Farthest from the center or trunk of body or a reference structure; opposite of proximal	Hand is distal to elbow
Inferior (caudad)	Situated toward lower part of a reference structure, away from head	Umbilicus is inferior to xiphoid
Intermediate	Located between two extremes or body structures	Nose is intermediate to eyes
Ipsilateral (homolateral)	Pertaining to or on same side of body; opposite of contralateral	Left arm and leg are ipsilateral
Lateral	Located away from midline or medial plane of body or a reference structure; at or toward the side	Axillae are lateral to breasts
Medial	Located nearer midline or medial plane of body or a reference structure	Tibia is medial to fibula
Posterior (dorsal)	Toward or at back of body; situated behind a reference structure	Heart is posterior to sternum
Proximal	Nearest to point of attachment of an extremity to trunk of body or a reference structure; opposite of distal	Femur is proximal to tibia
Superficial	Located toward or on surface of body; opposite of deep	Pupil is superficial to lens
Superior (cephalad)	Situated toward head or upper part of a reference structure	Thorax is superior to abdomen

weight for height. Body build may be thin, obese, trim, or muscular and reflect the client's level of wellness, age, and lifestyle.

Posture. Posture reflects the client's mood or presence of a physical problem. The nurse observes the client's posture throughout the health assessment process. Normal findings are an erect posture while standing, with alignment of the shoulders and hips equally distributed over the knees and ankles. Sitting posture is with a straight back and slight rounding of the shoulders. Deviations from normal include stooping, slouching, or a curved posture.

Gait. Gait is observed as the client enters the examination room or ambulates. It is smooth and coordinated with arms swinging freely at the sides, opposite to leg movement. Head and face orient in the direction the client is moving. Shuffling steps and hesitancy are abnormal findings in a young or middle-aged adult. Devices to assist ambulation are noted.

Movements. The nurse observes the client's body movements as the examination proceeds. They are usually purposeful and controlled without tremors, tics, muscle fasciculations, signs of spasticity, or decreased muscle tone. Immobile body parts are noted.

Dress. The client's manner of dress is appropriate to the time of year, temperature, age, socioeconomic status, and current circumstances. The client who is sensitive to cold wears more layers or heavier clothing. A depressed client may wear clothing that is dull, unkempt, or mismatched.

Hygiene and Grooming. The nurse notes the client's cleanliness of hair, nails, skin, and clothes. Does the client present a pleasant image? The nurse considers what activity the client engaged in before the examination and if it affects the client's appearance.

Body and Breath Odor. These are noted in relationship to the client's activity level, such as strenuous exercise. Deficient hygiene may result in body and breath odors that are considered unpleasant or offensive. Odors include cigarette smoke, perfume, perspiration, alcohol, acetone, blood, decaying tissue, or odors associated with a disease process.

Mental Status. Mental status includes the client's level of consciousness, orientation, affect, speech, and thought processes. Refer to Chapter 11 for discussion of these assessments. If abnormalities are noted in these areas, the nurse proceeds with a full mental status assessment. Refer to Chapters 11 and 28 for discussion. The client is alert, responds to questions, and is not inattentive, drowsy, or comatose. The client's orientation to time, place, person, and situation is assessed as the health history interview progresses. Affect reflects the client's situation and is congruent with mood. Speech is clear, fluent, and appropriate to the topic of conversation. Voice tone is moderate. Thought processes are logical, coherent, and related to the subject being discussed.

Level of Cooperation. The nurse assesses the client's cooperation with the examination. Is the client interested, concerned, and willing to discuss information? Or is the client silent, withdrawn, hostile, angry, or

TABLE 12-3. Metropolitan Life's Table of Adult Weight Standards

Weights* for men (according to frame, ages 25-59) for greatest longevity†

Height‡ Feet	Height‡ Inches	Small Frame	Medium Frame	Large Frame
5	2	128-134	131-141	138-150
5	3	130-136	133-143	140-153
5	4	132-138	135-145	152-156
5	5	134-140	137-148	144-160
5	6	136-142	139-151	146-164
5	7	138-145	142-154	149-168
5	8	140-148	145-157	152-172
5	9	142-151	148-160	155-176
5	10	144-154	151-163	158-180
5	11	146-157	154-166	161-184
6	0	149-160	157-170	164-188
6	1	152-164	160-174	168-192
6	2	155-168	164-178	172-197
6	3	158-172	167-182	176-202
6	4	162-176	171-187	181-207

Weights* for women (according to frame, ages 25-59) for greatest longevity†

Height‡ Feet	Height‡ Inches	Small Frame	Medium Frame	Large Frame
4	10	102-111	109-121	118-131
4	11	103-113	111-123	120-134
5	0	104-115	113-126	122-137
5	1	106-118	115-129	125-140
5	2	108-121	118-132	128-143
5	3	111-124	121-135	131-147
5	4	114-127	124-138	134-151
5	5	117-130	127-141	137-155
5	6	120-133	130-144	140-159
5	7	123-136	133-147	143-163
5	8	126-139	136-150	146-167
5	9	129-142	139-153	149-170
5	10	132-145	142-156	152-173
5	11	135-148	145-159	155-176
6	0	138-151	148-162	158-179

Courtesy of Metropolitan Life Insurance Company, copyright 1983.
* Weight in pounds (in indoor clothing weighing 5 lb for men, 3 lb for women).
† Metropolitan no longer labels these weights "ideal" or "desirable," because these adjectives mean different things to different people.
‡ In shoes with 1-inch heels.

suspicious? Is the client relaxed and willing to engage in eye contact? Or is the client tense and avoiding eye contact?

HEIGHT AND WEIGHT

The nurse measures height and weight while the client is standing. This often is done immediately after the health history interview, before the client sits on the examination table. A balance scale (see Fig. 12-2) is preferable because of its greater accuracy. (Alternatives to the standing platform scale include bed and chair scales.) The standing scale has a telescoping ruler to measure height.

Height and weight are compared with tables such as that developed by Metropolitan Life Insurance Company (Table 12-3). Weight should fall within range for the client's sex, height, and body frame. (Determining body frame is discussed later.) Weight that is more than 20 per cent above or 10 per cent below the *ideal body weight (IBW)* indicates that the client is at increased risk for nutritional problems. To calculate IBW, the nurse uses a formula specific to the client's sex and body frame (Table 12-4).

BALANCE (ROMBERG'S TEST)

Balance is assessed after measurement of height and weight and before the client sits down. Romberg's test and the test for pronation assess cerebellar function. They may be done later during neurologic examination. The nurse instructs the client to stand quietly with

TABLE 12-4. Calculating Ideal Body Weight (IBW)

Adult Male*	Adult Female*
Take 106 lb for the first 5 ft of height; add 6 lb/inch for each additional inch over 5 ft	Take 100 lb for the first 5 ft of height; add 5 lb/inch for each additional inch over 5 ft

Small Frame Calculate 10 per cent of the amount for medium frame and subtract it from the first amount (i.e., IBW is 10 per cent *less* for individuals with small frames)

Large Frame Calculate 10 per cent of the amount for medium frame and add it to the first amount (i.e., IBW is 10 per cent *more* for individuals with large frames)

Example An adult male is 6′1″ tall with a large body frame. His IBW is calculated as follows:

6′1″ = 5 ft plus 13 in
First 5 ft of height = 106 lb
Additional height over 5 ft = (13) × (6) = 78 lb
Medium frame IBW = 106 + 78 = 184 lb
Allowance for large frame = (10%) × 184 = 18.4 lb
Large frame IBW = 184 + 18.4 = 202.4 lb

Data from The American Dietetic Association. (1981). *Handbook of Clinical Dietetics*. New Haven: Yale University Press.
* These formulas are for adults with a medium body frame. Adjust formulas for clients with small or large frames (adjustment is the same formula for both sexes).

hands at the sides and feet together. Once equilibrium is attained, the nurse instructs the client to close the eyes. The client should be able to stand upright with minimal swaying and no loss of balance. The nurse is close by and intervenes should the client begin to lose balance and fall. While standing, the client is instructed to raise and extend the arms in front to shoulder height, then close the eyes. The client is able to maintain the arms in extension with no downward drifting or pronation (pronation sign). (See other cerebellar assessments in Chap. 28.)

Once this portion of the examination is completed, the nurse may elect to test the client's visual acuity if the eye chart is located the correct distance from the examination table. Otherwise, visual acuity is tested when the eyes are examined.

The nurse instructs the client to sit on the edge of the examination table for assessment of vital signs and anthropometric measurements (refer to Table 12-1).

VITAL SIGNS

Once the client is comfortably seated, the nurse measures vital signs after a brief stabilization period. Body temperature and blood pressure are measured during the general survey. The nurse may measure specific vital signs during examination of the upper extremities or heart (peripheral pulse) and thorax (respirations). Refer to a nursing fundamentals textbook for discussion of the techniques of vital signs measurement, equipment selection, and interpretation of findings.

Temperature. Oral body temperature ranges from 96.8° to 99.5° F (36° to 37.5° C) with an average of 98.6° F (37° C). Temperatures above the normal range are *hyperthermic;* those below are *hypothermic.*

Pulse. Resting pulse rate ranges from 60 to 100 beats per minute (BPM). A rate above 100 BPM is *tachycardia;* below 60 BPM is *bradycardia.* The nurse notes general characteristics of the pulse, such as rhythm (regular or irregular), amplitude (weak or bounding), and pattern. Rhythm is regular with pulsations occurring at equal intervals and being of similar amplitude. Slight variation in rhythm occurs with respiration and is normal. *Pulse amplitude* is rated on a scale ranging from 0 to 3+ (Box 12-2).

Irregular patterns are described. Pulse amplitude that fades with inspiration and strengthens with expiration is *paradoxical* and is reported to the physician. If an irregular pulse is detected, the nurse auscultates the apical pulse while simultaneously palpating the radial pulse to assess for a *pulse deficit,* that is, the difference between the two pulse rates. This finding also is reported. Further discussion of pulse assessment is found in Chapter 41.

Respiration. Respirations range from 12 to 20 per minute; have a regular, smooth pattern; and are of consistent depth. They are quiet and effortless, without abnormal sounds such as wheezing. Respiratory depth reflects tidal volume (i.e., the amount of air taken in with each breath). The rise and fall of the client's chest is used to estimate whether respirations are shallow, moderate, or deep. The nurse notes the respiratory pattern and records its characteristics (Fig. 12-7). Further discussion of respiration assessment is found in Chapter 36.

Box 12-2. Rating and Recording Pulse Amplitude

The following scale is commonly used to rate and record pulse amplitude. Note that the rating 2+ is considered "normal." When the nurse records a pulse amplitude, it is expressed in relationship to the rating scale norm, for example, 3+/2+ (i.e., the pulse is rated 3+ on a rating scale in which 2+ is normal).

0 *Absent.* The pulse is indiscernible to palpation.
1+ *Weak, thready.* The pulse is difficult to palpate and easily obliterated by slight pressure.
2+ *Normal.* The pulse is easily palpable and can be obliterated only with strong pressure.
3+ *Bounding.* The pulse is easily palpable, forceful, and not easily obliterated by pressure.

Blood Pressure. Blood pressure varies greatly among individuals. Normal systolic pressure ranges from 100 to 140 mm Hg, and diastolic pressure ranges from 60 to 90 mm Hg. It is more accurate to evaluate consecutive blood pressure readings over time rather than make an isolated measurement for determining blood pressure abnormalities. *Hypotension* is a systolic pressure below 95 mm Hg or diastolic pressure below 60 mm Hg. *Hypertension* is a systolic pressure above 140 mm Hg or diastolic pressure above 90 mm Hg. The difference between the systolic and diastolic pressure readings (i.e., *pulse pressure*) is noted. A difference of more than 40 mm Hg is abnormal and is reported. A slightly elevated blood pressure may be considered a normal finding in the elderly.

The nurse assesses the client's blood pressure in both arms and compares the two readings. A pressure difference of 5 to 10 mm Hg between the two arms is normal. Larger differences are reported. The nurse assesses for an *auscultatory gap* the first time a client's blood pressure is measured. This phenomenon occurs as a period of silence between two levels of systolic pressures that may range as much as 40 mm Hg. Further discussion of blood pressure is found in Chapter 41.

BODY FRAME

The nurse assesses the client's body frame by measuring the wrist circumference and dividing it into the height. The resulting *r* value is compared with a chart to determine whether the client's body frame is small, medium, or large (Fig. 12-8). This information is necessary for calculating the IBW.

RESPIRATORY PATTERN	DESCRIPTION
A. Eupnea (Normal) 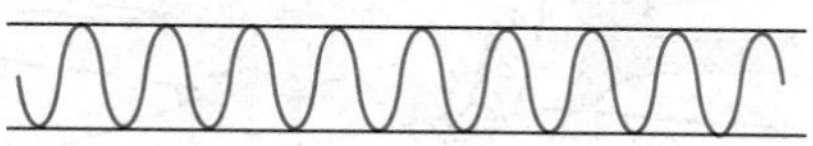	Rate = 12 to 20 breaths per minute Depth = Average tidal volume 350-500 ml (adults) Rhythm = Regular, occasional sigh breath deeper than baseline tidal volume I:E Ratio* = 1:2
B. Hyperventilation 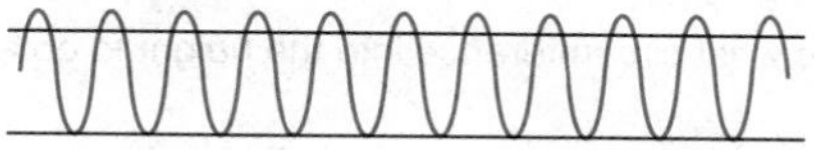	Rate = May increase Depth = Deep—large tidal volumes Rhythm = Usually regular I:E Ratio = Approaches 1:1 Comment = May be associated with CO_2 loss
C. Tachypnea 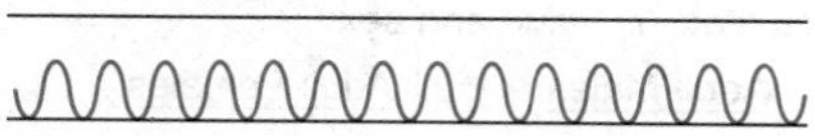	Rate = Rapid Depth = Shallow—small tidal volume with each breath Rhythm = Regular I:E Ratio = Approaches 1:1 Comment = May be associated with CO_2 retention
D. Bradypnea 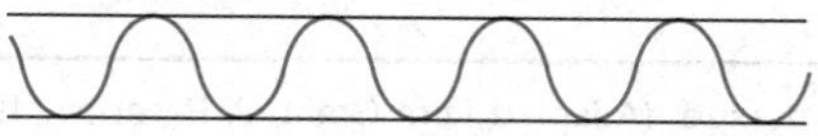	Rate = Slow Depth = Tidal volumes vary depending on the cause Rhythm = Regular I:E Ratio = 1:2
E. Apnea 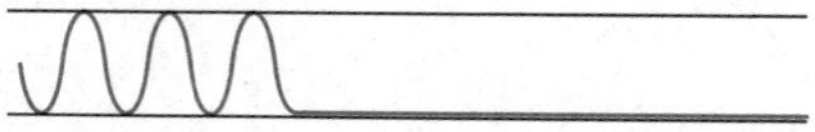	Complete absence of breathing Comment = May be of a temporary nature
F. Cheyne-Stokes 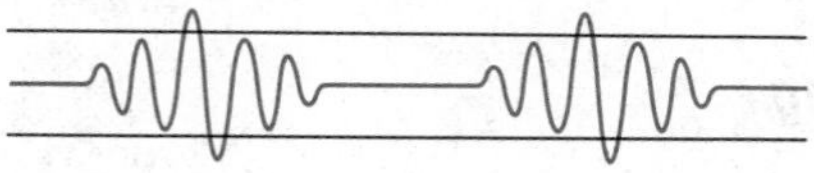	Rate = Variable Depth = Depth of each breath varies in a cyclical pattern: Shallow before and after apnea, deep with hyperventilation Rhythm = Apneic periods alternate with hyperventilation Comment = Regular-irregular—crescendo-decrescendo pattern
G. Biot's 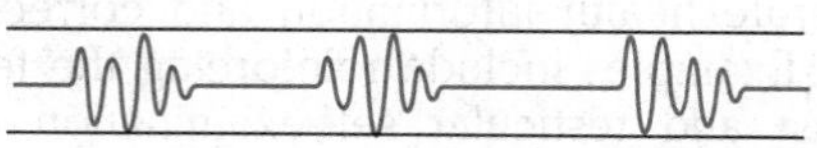	Rate = Variable Depth = Depth variable—predominantly shallow Rhythm = Unpredictable irregularity Comment = Long periods of apnea alternate with breathing periods
H. Kussmaul's 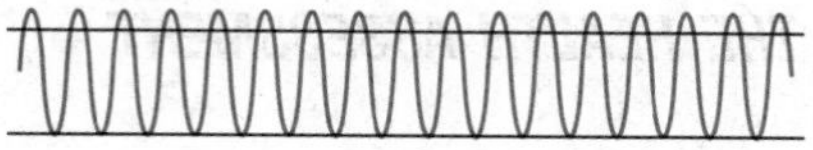	Rate = Rapid Depth = Deep without pauses Rhythm = Regular Comment = Associated with diabetic ketoacidosis
I. Apneustic 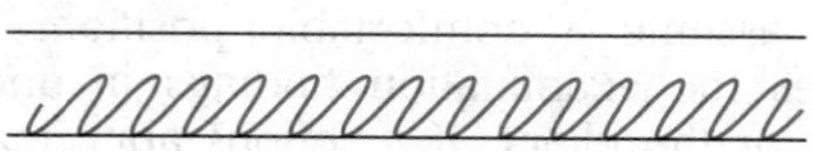	Rate = Rapid Depth = Shallow Comment = Prolonged inspiration followed by short, ineffective expiration

* Inspiration to Expiration (I:E) ratio

▲ **Figure 12-7**

Assessing respiratory patterns.

ADIPOSE TISSUE MEASUREMENT

The nurse measures the triceps skinfold thickness (TSF) and midarm circumference (MAC) to estimate the client's nutritional status. The TSF and MAC are used to calculate the midarm muscle circumference (MAMC), which is an indication of protein and calorie reserves. All measurements are compared with published norms for age and sex. The techniques for measuring TSF, MAC, and MAMC and their norms are shown in Figure 12–9.

SKIN COLOR

Overall skin color is assessed as the nurse interviews the client. A more thorough assessment is conducted as the nurse proceeds with the remainder of the physical examination. The nurse observes the client's face and visible skin surfaces for color tones that should be congruent with the client's stated race. Abnormal findings include pallor (paleness), flushing or a ruddy complexion, cyanosis (blue cast), jaundice (yellow cast), and areas of irregular pigmentation.

1. Measure the client's right wrist (in centimeters) at the point of smallest circumference, just distal to the styloid process of the radius and ulna.

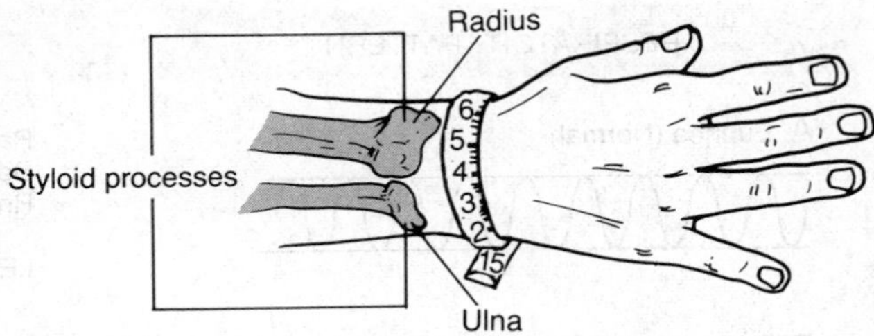

2. Obtain the client's height (in centimeters) without shoes.
3. Divide the client's wrist circumference into the height to obtain the "r" value:

$$r = \frac{\text{height (in cm)}}{\text{wrist circumference (in cm)}}$$

4. Use the chart shown to determine the client's body frame size based on the calculated "r" value and sex:

	Adult Males	Adult Females
Small frame	r > 10.4	r > 10.9
Medium frame	r = 9.6 – 10.4	r = 9.9 – 10.9
Large frame	r < 9.6	r < 9.9

▲ **Figure 12–8**

Calculating body frame size. (Adapted from Grant, J. P., et al. [1981]. Current techniques of nutritional assessment. *Surgical Clinics of North America*, 61, 437–463).

PROCESSING THE DATA

Comparison of Findings

The client is used as a "control" or self-standard for comparison during the physical examination. Findings from one side of the body are compared with those of the opposite side, or *bilaterally*. Even though both sides of the human body are not exactly identical (i.e., symmetric), similarities in structure and appearance are individualized and unique. Comparisons are useful and valid when the nurse assesses findings such as a joint deformity or extremity swelling.

Comparison to Known Standards

The nurse compares physical examination findings with known parameters of "normal" for the client's age, sex, and racial background. For example, decreased skin elasticity and loss of subcutaneous adipose tissue are normal findings for an elderly client but not for a thirty-year-old.

Suspected Problem Areas

The nurse examines known or suspected problem areas or regions carefully. Areas to include are those identified by the client during the health history interview as well as those the nurse predicts to be at risk on the basis of the client's history and reactions to the physical examination. For example, the client who reports difficulty swallowing receives a thorough assessment of mouth and neck structures. The nurse explains to the client why a particular portion of the examination is more thorough than is customary to allay anxiety.

Health Teaching

The physical examination process lends itself to health teaching; there are opportunities for providing the client with accurate health information and correcting misconceptions. Examples include reinforcing the techniques for breast and testicular self-examination and having the client perform a return demonstration.

TERMINATING THE HEALTH ASSESSMENT PROCESS

After completion of the physical examination, the nurse closes the gown or allows the client to dress (assisting if needed) and assume a comfortable position. The nurse summarizes the examination findings in understandable terms for the client. If a serious abnormality is found, the nurse consults with the client's physician or refers the client to a physician for further assessment after explaining the general nature of the abnormality found and the need for further examination.

Disposable, used equipment and supplies are discarded according to agency protocol. Nondisposable equipment is cleaned and restocked for future use.

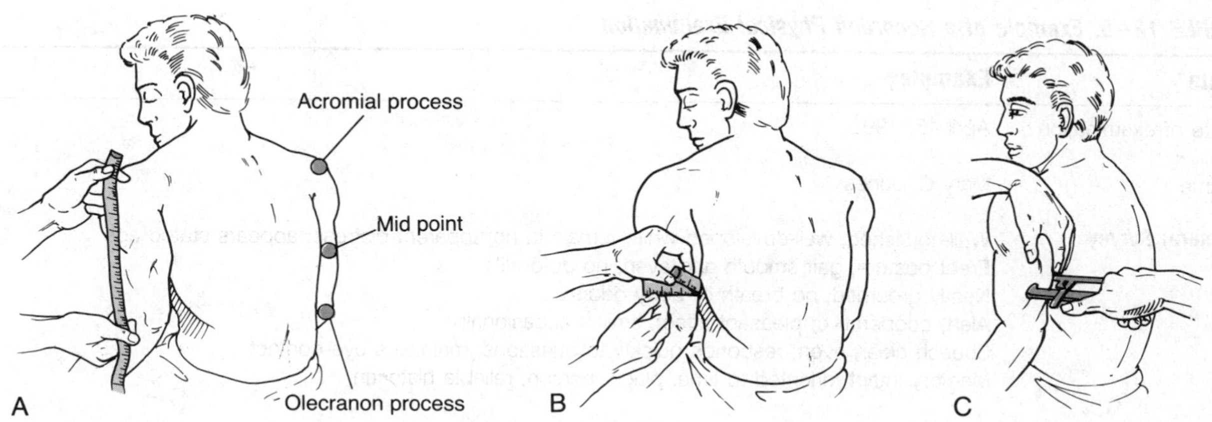

D Calculate the midarm muscle circumference (MAMC) using the following formula:
MAMC (in cm) = [MAC in cm] − [(0.314) × (TSF in mm)]

MEASUREMENT		STANDARD	90%	60%
Midarm circumference (MAC)	Men	29.3 cm	26.4 cm	17.6 cm
	Women	28.5 cm	25.7 cm	17.1 cm
Triceps skinfold (TSF)	Men	12.5 mm	11.3 mm	7.5 mm
	Women	16.5 mm	14.9 mm	9.9 mm
Midarm muscle circumference (MAMC)	Men	25.3 cm	22.8 cm	15.2 cm
	Women	23.2 cm	20.9 cm	13.9 cm

▲ *Figure 12–9*

Measuring adipose and skeletal muscle tissue to estimate the client's reserves of protein and calories. *A*, Locate the *midpoint* of the client's relaxed, nondominant upper arm by palpating the acromial and olecranon processes and measuring the distance between the two points with a tape measure. Mark the posterior aspect of the arm at the midpoint with a pen. *B*, Measure *midarm circumference (MAC)* at the midpoint, keeping the tape measure level. *C*, Just above the midpoint at the posterior aspect of the arm, grasp the client's skin and subcutaneous tissue between thumb and index finger, freeing it from the underlying muscle mass. Place the calipers at the midpoint just below the fold of grasped tissue. Squeeze the calipers until they are equilibrated at the "measure" markings for approximately 3 seconds. Read the measurement to the nearest mm. Repeat the readings two more times, allowing a rest period of 3 seconds between readings. Calculate the average of the three readings for the *triceps skinfold thickness (TSF)*. *D*, Compare the client's values for MAC, TSF, and MAMC to the following standards to determine nutritional risk status. *Undernutrition* is indicated by a measurement below 90 per cent of the standard. *Protein-calorie malnutrition* is indicated by a measurement of less than 60 per cent of the standard, especially for the MAMC. *Obesity* is indicated by a TSF measurement 120 per cent or more above the standard.

RECORDING PHYSICAL EXAMINATION FINDINGS

The nurse documents physical examination findings using accurate, descriptive terms. Vague, subjective terminology, such as "normal," "slight," "moderate," "healthy," or "poor," is avoided because it is easily misinterpreted by others. The nurse strives to be objective, concise, clear, and thorough in the recording. However, it is better to err on the side of verbosity than to describe a significant finding vaguely or inadequately.

During the examination, the nurse may briefly note abnormal assessment findings on a pad for later retrieval and detailed documentation. This avoids interrupting the flow of the examination to record detailed observations. After the examination, the nurse combines normal and abnormal findings in the final document. An example of a recorded screening physical examination for an adult client appears in Table 12–3.

HEALTH ASSESSMENT, NURSING DIAGNOSIS, AND NURSING PROCESS

After the collection of baseline data, which includes both the health history and the physical examination results, the nurse summarizes the client's health problems (Table 12–3). The client's areas of strength and health risk profile are assessed. Nursing diagnoses are formalized and prioritized. Tentative diagnoses formulated after the health history interview are reexamined and validated in light of the physical examination findings.

The nurse determines which health problems are nursing diagnoses and which are collaborative problems. Referrals are made when indicated so that the client receives continuity of care and either resolution or effective management of the health problems.

Summary

The physical examination is the second portion of physical assessment following the health history. The

TABLE 12-5. Example of a Recorded Physical Examination

Data*	Example†
Date of examination	April 15, 1992
Name	Mary C. Jones
General Survey	Well-nourished, well-developed white female in no apparent distress; appears stated age Erect posture, gait smooth and even, no deformity Neatly groomed; no breath or body odors Alert, cooperative; pleasant affect, smiles occasionally Speech clear, even; responds quickly to questions, maintains eye contact Memory intact, oriented to time, place, person; reliable historian
Vital Signs	T = 98.8° F; P = 84, regular; R = 16, even; BP = 116/72, left arm (sitting); BP = 114/74, right arm (sitting); no auscultatory gap
Nutritional Status	Height = 5′6″; weight = 143 lb; body frame = medium IBW = 130 lb; % IBW = 110% MAC = 28.4 cm (99.7% standard); TSF = 15.8 mm (95.7% standard); MAMC = 22.8 cm (98.3% standard) basically sedentary lifestyle with periods of moderate activity
Mental Status	Thought process clear, logical; active problem-solving behavior in resolving elderly parents' placement; wrinkles brow and looks down, sighs when discussing topic Articulate; no difficulty recalling recent or past events; serial sevens deferred
Integument	
Skin	Skin tones pink, even, darker on exposed extremities Warm, smooth, supple, well-lubricated; turgor immediate Fine tan or brown macules scattered over arms, legs, back, face Scars: under right scapula (2 cm), right wrist (3 cm), lateral right upper thigh (1 cm)
Hair	Light brown, thick hair; no dandruff or nits; no alopecia Fine light body hair, usual female distribution
Nails	Short, groomed, rounded with no cracking or peeling; cuticles intact; beds pink; immediate capillary refill upon blanching; no lesions; angle = 160°
Head	Normocephalic with no lesions or tenderness; face symmetric at rest and with movements; TMJ joint: no crepitus, full mobility; CN II–XII intact; CN I not tested; temporal artery 2+/2+ bilaterally, soft
Eyes	Acuity per Snellen chart with glasses: OD = 20/30, OS = 20/20, OU = 20/20 Full visual fields to confrontation; EOMs intact, no nystagmus; PERRLA, direct and consensual; cover/uncover test negative; corneal light reflections equal (Hirschberg's) Eyebrows symmetric, full, groomed; lashes full, outward curve Lids approximated when closed and rest at limbus borders when open; palpebral fissures equal; no lesions Lacrimal apparatus functioning Sclerae white, palpebral conjunctivae pink, bulbar conjunctivae clear; corneas and anterior chambers clear; globes firm; lenses clear Disc margins sharp with some nasal blurring; bilateral cup-to-disc ratio is 1:3, cups symmetric No A-V nicking; ratio is 2:3 Fovea not visualized
Ears	Auricles symmetric; no lesions or tenderness over tragus Canals with small amount of soft cerumen bilaterally; no tenderness or discharge TMs gray, cone of light at 4:00, right ear; at 7:00, left ear No retraction; landmarks visualized; no lateralization AC > BC, bilaterally; Whisper heard at 3 ft

TABLE 12–5. Example of a Recorded Physical Examination Continued

Data*	Example†
Nose and Sinuses	Nose straight; no nasal flaring, lesions, discharge, tenderness; bilaterally patent; septum midline; mucosa pink, moist Inferior, middle turbinates pale pink, edematous; clear discharge present; frontal and maxillary sinuses nontender, transilluminate
Mouth and Pharynx	Lips pink, symmetric, smooth, moist, without lesions or makeup Gingivae pink, intact; 28 teeth present, third molars absent, rest without caries; fillings in all second molars; no malocclusion Mucosa pink, smooth; no lesions; stensen's ducts visualized bilaterally Tongue midline with full mobility and strength, no lesions or fasciculation; papillae present, light white coating Saliva pool in floor of mouth Palates intact, smooth, symmetric, pink; palates and uvula rise in midline with phonation Pillars pink, tonsils absent Pharynx pink, clear mucus on posterior wall; gag reflex intact Voice clear, strong; swallows without difficulty; taste perception deferred
Neck	Symmetric; no masses or swelling; full ROM of cervical spine Trapezius muscle tender; no masses or stiffness Occipital, postauricular, postcervical, supraclavicular, superficial and deep cervical, preauricular, submental nodes nonpalpable Tonsillar and submandibular nodes felt bilaterally: 0.5 cm, soft, round, mobile, nontender Trachea midline, mobile, nontender; thyroid isthmus soft, rest of gland not palpable; no bruit JVD absent sitting upright, and in lower third of neck above sternal notch when supine; carotids 2+/3+ bilaterally, no bruit
Thorax and Lungs	A-P to lateral diameter is 1:2 Breathing quiet, unlabored without use of ancillary muscles or retractions; rate is 16, regular Thorax symmetric; no tenderness or masses; tactile fremitus within normal limits; resonant throughout; thoracic expansion equal; diaphragmatic excursion equal, 3 cm Breath sounds vesicular in periphery, no crackles or wheezes No CVA tenderness bilaterally
Heart	Precordium without lifts, heaves, or thrills Apical impulse at 5th ICS, 1 cm right of LMCL; diameter: 1.5 cm No pulsations in epigastrium Regular rhythm with apical rate of 82 S_1 and S_2 within normal limits; no splitting, gallops, murmurs, or rubs No changes in sounds with position changes
Peripheral Vascular	Brachial, radial, femoral, and posterior tibial pulses 2+/3+ bilaterally Ulnar, popliteal, and dorsalis pedis pulses 1+/2+ bilaterally Epitrochlear, vertical inguinal, and popliteal nodes nonpalpable Horizontal inguinal nodes palpable (2 in right groin, 1 in left groin), 1 cm, round, mobile, nontender; no edema Homan's sign negative bilaterally Calves nontender; varicosities absent
Breasts and Axillae	Breasts full, symmetric in all positions; skin smooth, even contour, no lesions Light, symmetric vascular pattern Areola and nipple symmetric bilaterally, no puckering or inversion Soft, no masses or discharge, nontender; axillae shaven No rashes, lesions, hyperpigmentation; nodes nonpalpable, nontender
Abdomen	Symmetric, flat with slight rounding over lower third Visible pulsations or peristalsis absent Umbilicus midline, inverted Rectus muscles intact at rest and with straining

Table continued on following page

TABLE 12–5. Example of a Recorded Physical Examination Continued

Data*	Example†
	Striae over lower quadrants Bowel sounds active all quadrants No vascular bruits, venous hum, or friction rubs Abdominal aortic pulsation in epigastrium palpable, thrusting, nonradiating Abdomen nontender, no guarding or rigidity; tympany throughout Liver span: 6 cm at RMCL and 4 cm at MSL; nonpalpable at RMCL Splenic dullness at LAAL, 6th ICS Kidneys nonpalpable; no rebound tenderness Inguinal areas, no bulging; see diagram for abdominal reflexes
Neurologic	Gross and fine motor coordination intact; Romberg's test negative, no arm drift or pronation; see Head for CN Performs rapid alternating movements and point-to-point maneuvers without difficulty Gait steady, maintains balance on toes and heels Sensation to light touch, pain, and vibration intact distally, over trunk, neck, and face Position sense of fingers and toes intact; stereognosis and graphesthesia present bilaterally Two-point discrimination: 2 mm on index fingers bilaterally; see diagram for DTRs and plantar reflex
Musculoskeletal	Muscle masses smooth, firm, nontender, and without fasciculations or lesions Strength equal at 5/5 bilaterally for all major muscle groups: neck, deltoids, triceps, wrists, fingers, grip strength, hips, hamstrings, quadriceps, ankles, and feet ROM is WNL for all joints Palpable crepitus in knees and shoulders; audible crepitus in right wrist Extremities symmetric, no deformity; spine straight; no kyphosis, lordosis, or scoliosis Paravertebral muscles nontender, soft; joints symmetric, nontender; no edema or nodules

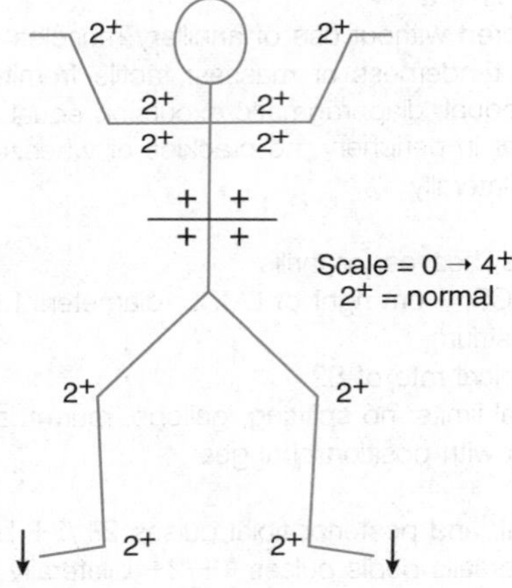

Data*	Example†
Genitalia	Mature, multiparous female external genitalia Pubic hair clean; skin: no lesions or parasites; no discharge or foul odor Labia majora and minora symmetric, slight gaping; clitoris midline, no lesions; introitus clean; Bartholin's glands nonpalpable; urethral meatus inside vaginal orifice, no discharge; pelvic floor relaxed, decreased tone Small cystocele palpated anteriorly with Valsalva's maneuver Cervix pink, round, orifice multiparous; no lesions; firm, mobile and nontender Vaginal mucosa intact, moist; no lesions; uterus midline, firm, nontender, no fibroids Adnexae nontender; no masses
Rectum	Perianal area: no rashes, lesions, or hemorrhoids at rest or with Valsalva's maneuver; sphincter intact No polyps, rectal tenderness, or masses; stool for occult blood negative
Summary	Generally healthy; myopia corrected with glasses; probable allergic rhinitis; cystocele

TABLE 12-5. Example of a Recorded Physical Examination Continued

Data*	Example†
Nursing Diagnoses	(The nursing diagnoses tentatively formulated after the health history interview are reviewed in light of the physical examination data. Diagnoses are validated, revised, added, or discarded after careful evaluation. The following diagnoses are not listed in order of priority. Refer to Chapter 11 for the list of tentative nursing diagnoses for Ms. Jones.) 1. Validated, no change. 2. Validated, no change. 3. Validated, no change. 4. Validated, no change. 5. Validated, no change. 6. Revised: Incontinence, Stress R/T childbirth, loss of muscle tone, and presence of cystocele. 7. Validated, no change. 8. Validated, no change. 9. Validated, no change. 10. Validated, no change. 11. Added: Altered Health Maintenence, High Risk for R/T exacerbation of allergic rhinitis.
Plan	(The nurse and client formulate a plan to address the nursing diagnoses after consulting together.) 1. Discuss with client referral to gynecologist for follow up on cystocele and stress incontinence. Teach about fluid intake, toileting, pelvic floor muscle strengthening exercises, perineal hygiene, and odor control. 2. Discuss with client current regimen for allergy self-care. If inadequate, seek referral to ENT or allergist. Teaching about regular schedule for prophylactic self-medication (OTC medications). 3. Review with client need for regular BSE and client's technique. Encourage her to make an appointment for mammography. 4. Review with client need for regular vision screening and glaucoma checks. Encourage her to make an appointment with her ophthalmologist. 5. Discuss with client need for tetanus toxoid booster. Can administer today with an order from clinic physician. 6. Discuss with client willingness to obtain counseling for self and family regarding placement issues for elderly parents. Obtain referral to Social Services to contact client regarding placement availability. 7. Encourage client to explore time management and to build in "personal time" and "family time." Discuss possibility of hiring a part-time homemaker for parents, or respite care for parents through a community organization or church. 8. Review with client principles of body mechanics and back safety (give pamphlet). 9. Review with client foods high in calcium that could be incorporated into diet. 10. Discuss with client benefits of including regular sessions of aerobic exercise into schedule. Explore possibilities of developing a schedule that builds gradually to include three to four sessions (minimum of 20 minutes each) per week.

* See text for data to collect.

† Client's history is in Chapter 11.

AC, air conduction; AP, anteroposterior; A-V, arterioventricular; BC, bone conduction; BSE, breast self-examination; CN, cranial nerve; CVA, costovertebral angle; DTRs, deep tendon reflexes; ENT, ear, nose, and throat; EOMs, extraocular muscles; IBW, ideal body weight; ICS, intercostal space; JVD, jugular venous distention; LAAL, left anterior axillary line; LMCL, left midclavicular line; MAC, midarm circumference; MAMC, midarm muscle circumference; MSL, midsternal line; OTC, over the counter; PERRLA, pupils equal, round, reactive to light and accommodation; RMCL, right midclavicular line; ROM, range of motion; R/T, related to; TMJ, temporomandibular joint; TMs, tympanic membranes; TSF, triceps skinfold thickness; WNL, within normal limits.

physical examination is the collection of objective data through inspection, palpation, percussion, and auscultation. Once all data are collected, the nurse compares the findings to known standards and makes appropriate referrals or provides health teaching.

Bibliography

1. American Dietetic Association. (1981). *Handbook of clinical dietetics.* New Haven: Yale University Press.
2. Bates, B. (1991). *A guide to physical examination* (5th ed.). Philadelphia: J. B. Lippincott.
3. Blackburn, G. L., et al. (1977). Nutritional and metabolic assessment of the hospitalized patient. *Journal of Parenteral and Enteral Nutrition, 1*(1), 11–22.
4. Braunwald, E. (1992). *Heart disease* (4th ed.). Philadelphia: W. B. Saunders.
5. Curtas, S., et al. (1989). Evaluation of nutritional status. *Nursing Clinics of North America, 24,* 301–313.
6. Grant, J. P., et al. (1981). Current techniques of nutritional assessment. *Surgical Clinics of North America, 61,* 437–463.
7. Jarvis, C. (1992). Physical examination and health assessment. Philadelphia: W. B. Saunders.
8. Kozier, B., et al. (1991). *Fundamentals of nursing* (4th ed.). Menlo Park, CA: Addison-Wesley.
9. Malasanos, L., et al. (1990). *Health assessment* (4th ed.). St. Louis: C. V. Mosby.
10. Morton, P. (1989). *Health assessment in nursing.* Springhouse, PA: Springhouse.
11. Potter, P., & Perry, A. (1989). *Fundamentals of nursing: Concepts, process, and practice* (2nd ed.). St. Louis: C. V. Mosby.
12. Solomon, E. P., et al. (1990). *Human anatomy and physiology* (2nd ed.). Philadelphia: W. B. Saunders.
13. Swartz, M. H. (1989). *Textbook of physical diagnosis.* Philadelphia: W. B. Saunders.
14. Thomas, C. L. (1989). *Taber's cyclopedic medical dictionary* (16th ed.). Philadelphia: F. A. Davis.

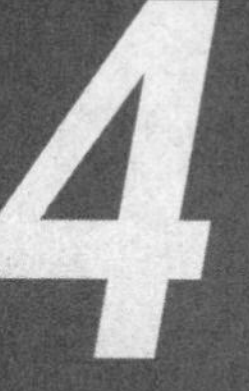

Unit 4

Common Health Disorders in Medical-Surgical Clients

This unit contains 10 chapters about common health disorders. These disorders are commonly seen in clients and commonly seen in the disorders presented throughout the rest of the text. The unit begins with a discussion of the cell. Through continued advances in medical science, disorders and their treatment are viewed from a cellular level. Fluid and electrolytes and acid-base balance are the first disorders addressed in this unit. These disorders reflect imbalances in cellular homeostasis. Certainly, when one thinks about common problems in clients, the problem of pain comes to light. Pain is a universal problem and the one that leads many people to seek health care. Sleep disorders can result from pain, anxiety, or physical alterations that interfere with ventilation. Because many clients require surgery, the nursing aspects of the perioperative experience are discussed in this unit. Surgery results in the creation of a wound and in bleeding; therefore, the concepts of wound healing and shock are found here. Finally, the concepts of neoplastic disorders (cancer) are discussed. Cancer of the various organs of the body is discussed again in each unit throughout the text; consequently, this unit gives you an overview of cancer and its treatments.

Chapter 13

▼ The Cell

Cells are the basic units or building blocks of all living organisms. Within the adult human body, there are approximately 60 trillion cells—each of them multiplying, reacting to stimuli, producing enzymes, and performing many other precise and highly specialized functions. It would take about 40,000 of your red blood cells to fill this letter "o." The healthy cell is a miniature chemistry laboratory, powerhouse, factory, and duplicating machine. However, aging, illness, or injury produces pathologic changes that alter normal cellular structures and function. These adverse changes in individual cells then produce adverse changes in the total organism.

Recent advances in the diagnosis and treatment of many disorders have made the knowledge of cellular structure and function an important component of client care. For many years, diseases were classified, studied, and treated as malfunctions of organs. A recent explosion in technology has allowed the study of the cell and its components. This knowledge have converted disease discussion and treatment into a cellular format. The cell and its components can be used to explain genetic disorders, aging, tumor biology, immune disorders, and neurologic diseases.

GENERAL STRUCTURE AND FUNCTION OF THE CELL

Structure

The cell is composed of a jelly-like material. Outside the nucleus, this material is called cytoplasm, and inside the nucleus, it is referred to as nucleoplasm. Scattered throughout the cytoplasm are tiny structures, called organelles ("little organs"), that perform various jobs within the cell, just as organs perform various jobs within the body (Figure 13-1). Most of the

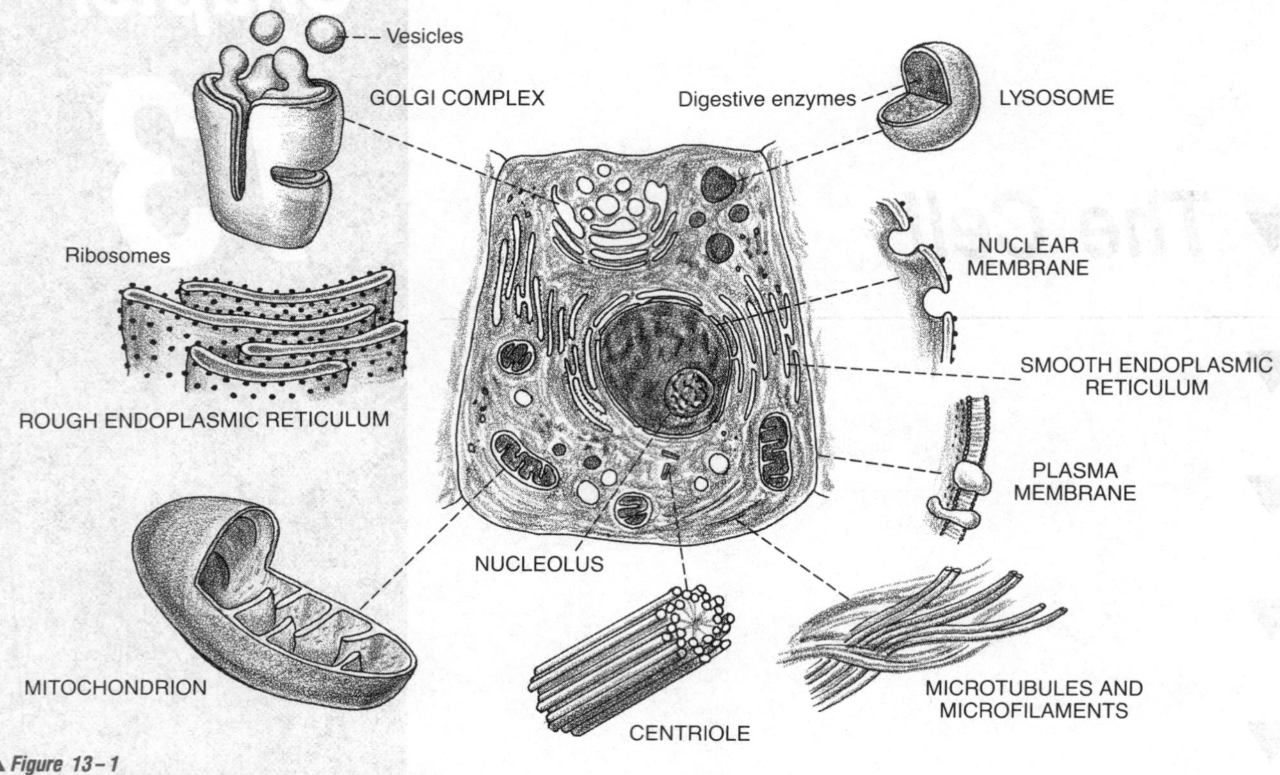

▲ *Figure 13-1*

Components of a cell as seen through the electron microscope.

organelles within the cell are enclosed by membranes. The membranes separate the organelles into different compartments. The separation allows chemical reactions to occur in one organelle without affecting the other portions of the cell.

Most of the cell (80 to 90 per cent) is water, containing amino acids, simple sugar, and other substances used to manufacture larger molecules. Water acts as a solvent for the chemicals within the cell and as a fluid vehicle in which chemical reactions can occur. Ten to twenty per cent of the cell is protein. Enzymes, which assist with various metabolic reactions, are also protein. Within each cell are electrolytes to assist with cellular activity and maintain a constant environment. The most common intracellular electrolytes are potassium, magnesium, phosphate, and bicarbonate.

Function

All human life begins as a single cell, with one half of the cell from the father and the other half from the mother. At conception, this fertilized egg is an *undifferentiated* cell. That is, their progeny cells have the ability to form an arm muscle, the heart's chamber, or the eye's iris. On about the seventh day after fertilization, the cells start to gradually become *committed* to develop a specific tissue with specific function. Once cells are fully differentiated they reproduce slowly, in an orderly manner, and have contact inhibition. Contact inhibition is a protective response that prevents the cells from dividing unless there is room and energy supplies to divide. Cancerous cells lose their contact inhibition. In addition, differentiated cells look different and have specific functions. A liver cell looks different and performs different functions than does a bone cell. Again, in cancer, the cells lose their differentiation and function. Their cycle of cellular reproduction is shown in Figure 13-2.

Although cells have their own unique special functions and attributes, they also share many characteristics. All cells reproduce, react to stimuli, and move either by ameboid motion or by means of cilia or flagella. Ameboid movement is defined as the "movement of the entire cell in relation to its surroundings such as the movement of white blood cells through tissues."[4] Cells also move by ciliary movement, which involves the wavelike movement of cilia on the cell surface. Cilia are short projections resembling hairs. They are filled with protein fibers called microtubules and are bounded by a plasma membrane. Movement of substances due to the simultaneous contraction of cilia occurs in the respiratory tract and in the fallopian tubes of the female reproductive tract. Flagella, which have the same basic structure as cilia except for a long tail, provide another form of cell movement. The tail of a sperm cell is the only example of a flagellum in the human.

The most important activities of cells are

Synthesis of protein molecules
Production of energy for cellular work

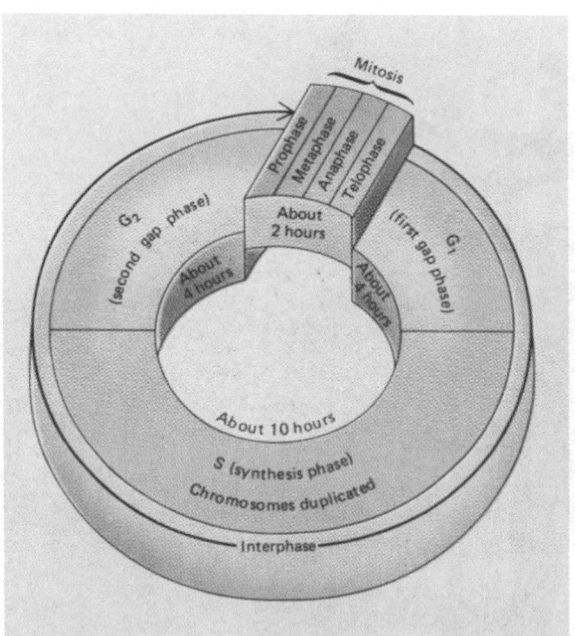

▲ **Figure 13-2**

Phases in the life cycle of a cell. Time relations are illustrative only: actual times vary with the cell type. (From Solomon, F. P., Schmidt, R., & Adragna P. [Eds.] [1990]. *Human Anatomy and Physiology*. Philadelphia: Saunders College Publishing.)

Maintenance of a homeostatic environment within the cell

Ingestion and assimilation by the cell of materials from the outside environment by means of active and passive transport, pinocytosis, and phagocytosis

Reproduction within unicellular organisms by means of simple division, and in higher organisms by means of mitotic division.

The cells of the skin and mucous membranes are replaced continually, at varying rates. The cells of the skin and mucous membranes, as well as the blood-forming, digestive, and reproductive system, are replaced at a higher rate than, for example, a liver cell. However, liver cell division rates increase with injury. Some cells such as smooth muscle cells have very limited replacement capabilities, reproducing once or twice in a lifetime. Striated muscle cells (heart and skeletal) and neurons are incapable of replacement and are considered permanent. This means that once a serious injury occurs, the damage is also permanent. For example, the person who is a paraplegic due to spinal cord injury will be permanently paralyzed because the spinal nerve cells (gray matter) cannot reproduce.

In essence, the body cells—like the body itself—must digest and assimilate substances, protect themselves by reacting to stimuli, reproduce, build products, and expend energy. Also, like the total organism, cells age, become sick and injured, lose their ability to function and to generate energy, die, and finally, decay.

STRUCTURE AND FUNCTION OF CELLULAR COMPONENTS

The cell has many parts: (1) the cell membrane, (2) the nucleus, and (3) the cytoplasm.

Cell Membrane

LIPIDS AND PROTEINS

The cell membrane, also called the plasma membrane, gives the cell its shape as well as providing many other functions. The cell membrane is composed of a lipid bilayer with a variety of proteins embedded in a mosaic pattern (Fig. 13-3). The lipids in the membrane present a barrier to the passage of materials. If the membrane were completely permeable, all material would pass freely in and out of the cell. The cell would then have the same content as the surrounding fluids and would quickly die. The lipid bilayer is almost totally impermeable to water and water-soluble substances, such as glucose, ions, and urea. On the other hand, oxygen, carbon dioxide, and alcohol, which are fat-soluble, are able to penetrate the lipid bilayer. The proteins in the membrane permit selective transport of water-soluble substances. Proteins that are water-soluble and are thought to be weakly bound to the surface are called peripheral proteins. Proteins that penetrate the lipid bilayer are called integral proteins. Some integral proteins form channels for small molecules to pass through.

The cell membrane also communicates with other cells and organs. It is equipped with certain proteins on its surface that permit other cells to recognize it. Based on this recognition, some cells bind together to form tissues.

The glycoproteins of the cell membrane play many diverse roles. They serve as the sites of ABO blood group antigens and histocompatibility antigens. Glycoproteins also act as receptors for hormones and enzymes. In addition, glycoproteins have a net negative charge, which causes adjacent cells to repel each other, thereby preventing cell adhesion and clumping. Finally, proteins such as fibronectin, a cell-surface glycoprotein, may act as a glue that causes cells to adhere to the connective tissue matrix. Fibronectin, which is continually shed from the cell surface, also helps regulate cell interactions and tissue organization. A schematic diagram of the cell membrane showing ways in which proteins associate with lipids is shown in Figure 13-3.

PASSIVE AND ACTIVE TRANSPORT

One function of the cell membrane is to control the exchange of substances into and out of the cell. The cellular membrane is selectively permeable, allowing only certain substances to enter and leave the internal environment of the cell. In some cases, the cell membrane allows molecules and ions to move passively into and out of the cell via diffusion or osmosis. Passive

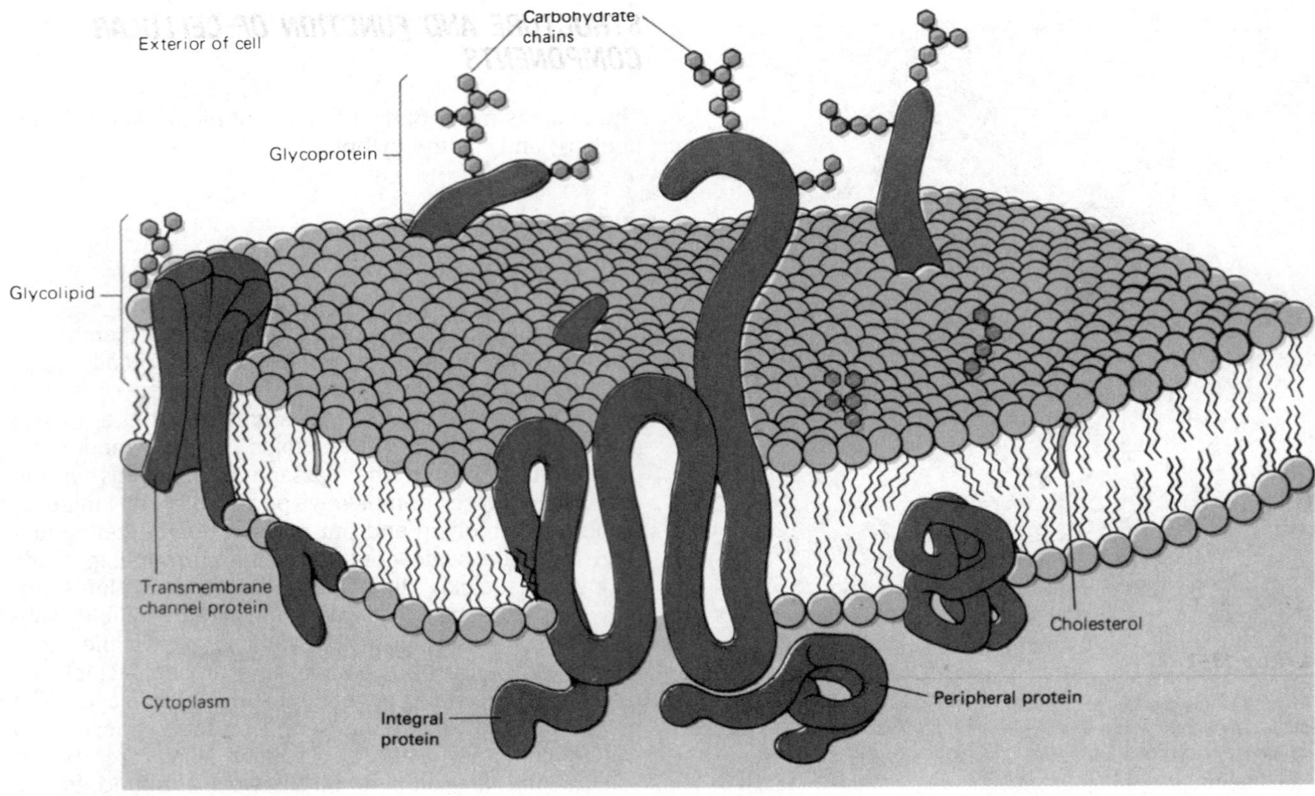

▲ *Figure 13-3*

The cell membrane is composed of a bimolecular layer of lipids, primarily phospholipid and cholesterol. Proteins can be attached or embedded in the membrane. Peripheral proteins are attached to the surface; integral proteins are embedded in the cell membrane. (From Solomon, Schmidt, & Adragna [Eds.] [1990]. *Human Anatomy and Physiology.* Philadelphia: Saunders College Publishing.)

movement requires no energy. However, other substances do require energy expenditure to cross the cellular membrane. Transport across a cellular membrane against a concentration, chemical, or electrical gradient is called active transport. An example of active transport is the sodium-potassium pump, which generates large amounts of sodium in the extracellular fluid and bloodstream and large quantities of potassium in the cell. Both sodium and potassium can diffuse (leak back) through the cell membrane, and an active mechanism using energy must operate to keep these ions in their respective compartments where they are needed.

PHAGOCYTOSIS AND PINOCYTOSIS

A second function of the cell membrane is to process information crossing the membrane. Information is exchanged via the interaction of neurotransmitters and cell membrane receptors. Cell membrane receptors bind with specific, extracellular molecules (e.g., a hormone), which triggers a series of events that result in changes in cell activities. For example, the binding of insulin to a cell membrane receptor triggers an increased uptake in glucose by the cell.

To take nutrients into the cell, such as proteins, the cell uses phagocytosis or pinocytosis. Pinocytosis (Greek, to drink) is the engulfment and ingestion of liquid droplets by the cell. Phagocytosis (Greek, to eat) is the engulfment and ingestion of large particles of matter such as bacteria and other cells.

Nucleus

The nucleus, an oval or spherical body, is the largest structure in the cell. All cells have nuclei except for mature red blood cells. The nucleus, which is the control center of the cell, governs (1) chemical reactions within the cell, (2) cell reproduction or mitosis, and (3) transmission of genetic information, which, in turn, determines the organism's hereditary characteristics.

MITOSIS

The nucleus contains deoxyribonucleic acid (DNA), the cell's genetic material. DNA provides the blueprint for all the body's structures and functions. DNA is contained in structures called chromosomes. Humans have 46 chromosomes, which are grouped into 23 pairs, one half of each pair originating from the father and the other half from the mother. The chromosomes themselves are composed of 50,000 to 100,000 genes, which are hereditary units. Many of the genes consist of encoded information that specifies the structure of proteins that constitute the enzymes and other components of the cell. Genes carry hereditary information concerning both the species and the individual characteristics of an organism. They transmit this vital information from generation to generation.

PROTEIN SYNTHESIS

In addition to chromosomes and genes, the nuclei of some cells contain one or more spherical bodies called nucleoli. These structures contain large amounts of ribonucleic acid (RNA). RNA carries the information concerning protein construction from the DNA of the nucleus to the ribosome, where proteins are produced.

RNA exists in three major forms, each of which is important to protein synthesis. Messenger RNA, produced by DNA, carries the genetic code from the nucleus to the cytoplasm. It dictates the sequence of amino acids to be synthesized in the protein. Transfer RNA carries activated amino acids to the ribosomes, the site of protein synthesis. Ribosomal RNA produces ribosomes, which are large genetic structures made up of RNA and proteins on which protein synthesis occurs.

DNA provides a template for the manufacturing of polypeptides (a chain of amino acids). DNA begins to make a protein by uncoiling the portion of the DNA double strand responsible for the specific protein. A complement to the template is made by messenger RNA (mRNA). mRNA leaves the nucleus and becomes associated with the ribosomes, in which the complete protein is made by rematching the sequence. Through this process, the genetic instructions in the DNA are safeguarded within the DNA for the life of the cell. Damage to the DNA can severely compromise cellular functions.

In such a complex operation as the transmission of heredity, mistakes are sometimes made in the process of copying the genetic information prior to cell division. Genes can be lost or they can change, or mutate. A mutation is a change and can be favorable, unfavorable, or neutral. Abnormal genes can cause structural and functional problems. Disease caused by alterations in genes include phenylketonuria (PKU) and sickle cell anemia.

GENETIC ENGINEERING

Biotechnologists are applying recent advances in genetic engineering to the prevention of diseases. Scientists have discovered restriction enzymes, which are proteins that can cut DNA at specific predictable sites, and DNA ligase, which is a genetic glue that can bind unrelated DNA fragments. By manipulating restriction enzymes and DNA ligase, scientists can now mix genes together or recombine them.

Also genes can be cut out of sections of human DNA molecules and joined to bacterial plasmids. Bacterial plasmids are small rings of nonessential DNA that (1) supply the coding for certain proteins and (2) have the capacity to easily incorporate human genes. Bacterial plasmids float freely in bacterial cells. The bacteria act as tiny factories, reproducing the protein encoded by the human genes, thereby creating new generations of a specific protein or product. Yeast also can be used to express recombinant human genes. Unlike bacteria, they can process or modify the protein in ways similar to the way human cells do. This makes the product more accessible to scientists, who must isolate the product or protein from the bacterial cell.

Currently, human insulin, interferon, and human growth hormone are being manufactured by bacteria and by yeast. Many enzymes are also genetically engineered in order to make them work more efficiently. In addition, researchers are attempting to manufacture human antibodies to specific tumors and viruses.

Cytoplasm

The cytoplasm is separated from the environment external to it by the cell membrane. Within the cytoplasm is the nucleus of the cell as well as other specialized organelles. Other organelles include the mitochondrion, endoplasmic reticulum, the Golgi apparatus, lysosomes, microtubules, microfilaments, and centrioles (see Fig. 13-1).

MITOCHONDRION

The mitochondrion is often referred to as the powerhouse of the cell, or as a tiny cell within a cell. Mitochondria are to the cell what an engine is to an automobile. They provide the cell with most of the energy it needs to perform its many activities.

The number of mitochondria per cell varies from a few hundred to a few thousand, depending on the energy requirements of the particular cell. Notably, the erythrocyte (red blood cell) is the only cell that does not contain mitochondria. Mitochondria replicate independently from the rest of the cell, and scientists postulate that they were at one time totally independent organisms much like bacteria.

The major functions of the mitochondria are (1) the oxidation of nutrients and (2) the changing of energy released by oxidation into adenosine triphosphate (ATP). ATP supplies most of the energy needed by the cell and is necessary for protein synthesis.

ENDOPLASMIC RETICULUM

The endoplasmic reticulum (ER) is a network of membranes shaped like tubules or channels that branch like miniature arteries throughout the cytoplasm. Proteins that are secreted by the cell or that are located on the cell surface are synthesized on the ER, which operates somewhat like a pipeline that transports materials throughout the cell as needed.

There are two types of ER, rough and smooth, each with its own functions. Rough ER is studded with ribosomes and plays a major role in synthesis of cell surface proteins such as hormone receptors, and secreted proteins, such as albumin, and peptide hormones, including as insulin and follicle-stimulating hormone. Other ribosomes are not attached to the ER surface and secrete their protein directly into the cytoplasm. Cell surface and secreted proteins are synthesized by the ER-bound ribosomes and extrude into the ER membrane. They can then be transferred to the Golgi apparatus by membrane vesicles and conjugated with carbohydrates on their way to the cell surface.

Smooth ER, on the other hand, has no ribosomes. It binds enzymes to its surface and is involved in the synthesis of certain nonprotein substances, such as steroids and lipids, including cholesterol and phospholipids. These substances are incorporated into the lipid bilayer of the ER itself, thereby causing the smooth ER to grow continually. Smooth endoplasmic reticulum in cells also (1) contributes to the detoxification and metabolism of drugs, toxins, and other foreign substances and (2) releases enzymes that control glycogen breakdown. In muscle cells, smooth ER sequesters and releases calcium ions, which are necessary for muscular contraction.

GOLGI APPARATUS

The Golgi apparatus, or complex, is a group of miniature sacs that process and modify proteins. Proteins are sorted and stored in vesicles until they are delivered to various destinations.

LYSOSOMES

The lysosome, a vesicle surrounded by membranes, is the cell's organ of digestion. Lysosomes arise from the Golgi apparatus by a process of budding. Lysosomes contain digestive enzymes that break down lipids, proteins, certain carbohydrates, DNA, and RNA into small molecules so that they can be oxidized for energy by the mitochondria. The hydrolytic enzymes split the organic substances that they contact into highly diffusible substances, such as amino acids and glucose. The membranes of the lysosome keep its potentially dangerous digestive enzymes separate from the rest of the cells. In the case of severe cell injury, the lysosomal enzymes are released and the entire cell is digested, a process called autolysis. Lysosomes are abundant in white blood cells whose principal activity is phagocytosis of foreign material (e.g., bacteria) in the body.

Lysosomes are also responsible for tissue regression, as in the uterus following pregnancy; in muscles during long periods of inactivity; and in mammary glands after lactation. This mechanism of lysosome release is unknown. In addition, lysosomes perform the function of removing injured cells or cell parts from damaged tissues so that new cells can replace the old ones in the process of repair.

MICROTUBULES AND MICROFILAMENTS

The microtubules and microfilaments are filamentous structures within the cytoplasm that play a role in cell support and cell mobility. Microtubules possibly maintain cell shape. Also, microtubules are involved (1) in streaming movements of the cytoplasm, (2) in the intracytoplasmic movements of organelles, (3) possibly in cell motility, and (4) in the lateral mobility of globular protein in the plasma membrane.

TISSUES AND ORGANS

Cells bond together according to their special functions to form definite units or structures called tissues. In turn, tissues unite to form individual organs. Four major specialized types of cells that unite into larger tissue units are

- Epithelial cells, which are arranged in sheets. They cover the outside of the body and form the absorptive covering that lines the inside of the body's cavities and tubular structures.
- Nerve cells, which form the highly specialized, irritable, and conductive nerve tissue. Injured or destroyed nerve cells cannot be replaced.
- Muscle cells, which allow mobility by contracting and relaxing.
- Connective tissue cells, which bind together and support other cells and tissues. They include blood cells and structural cells such as bones, tendons, and ligaments. Blood cells carry oxygen to the tissues and carry carbon dioxide and wastes from the tissues. Also, they defend the body against foreign substances. Structural cells build the bony scaffolding and form the critical intercellular proteins that bind together the cells of the body. Collagen is an important extracellular connective tissue protein.

Because groups of cells are specialized in function, the total organism suffers when any one group of cells breaks down. For example, the entire body depends on the ability of the heart muscle to contract and to propel blood throughout the body. If the cells of the heart muscle are damaged or destroyed, the entire organism suffers because of the resulting disruption in the circulation of oxygenated blood.

ALTERATIONS IN STRUCTURE AND FUNCTION OF THE CELL

The Aging Cell

Like the human beings they compose, cells age and die. In a young healthy client, cells are constantly and rapidly multiplying and dividing, and they function efficiently. In the elderly client, cells do not multiply or divide as rapidly. As cells age, they shrink in size, protein synthesis slows, the Golgi complexes begin to break apart, and the mitochondria may fragment. Ultimately, the aged cell dies and disappears. Its nucleus disintegrates and its cytoplasm liquefies. Different types of cells have different lifespans. For example, epithelial cells lining the intestinal tract live only about a day and a half, whereas red blood cells can live for 120 days.

At the opposite extreme are nerve cells, which have a potential life expectancy of 100 years. Immune cells appear to remain strong in numbers when people age but weaken in function. This characteristic results in increased incidences of autoimmune disease and tumors, and in susceptibility to infection. From the moment of fertilization, the human organism grows and develops. After maturity is reached, aging begins gradually. The processes that governs aging are always being researched as people try to slow down aging. Although theories on aging are numerous, little is known about the exact mechanism. The following discussion offers some thoughts on aging.

In the mature adult, some highly specialized cells such as nerve cells do not reproduce. Therefore, when these cells die, from injury or disease, they are not replaced and the remaining nerve cells must assume their functions. The additional work places stress on these cells and may hasten their death or aging. Eventually, the organ begins to lose some of its ability to function and the client may exhibit slowed functions. Other cells of the body retain their ability to reproduce and replace injured cells, such as the liver and pancreas. These organs age more slowly than do the brain and nerves. Another theory is that each person is born with a genetic clock that governs the person's lifespan. This theory is supported in part by the lifespans seen in various families.

Mechanisms of Cellular Injury

The extent of cellular injury depends on the nature and severity of the stressor, duration, vulnerability of the cells, blood supply to the cells, and differentiation of the cells. Because the liver metabolizes noxious chemicals and drugs, liver cells bear the brunt of toxic injury. Cardiac nerve cells are extremely vulnerable to hypoxia because they have a high rate of metabolism. Two clients may be exposed to the same injurious substance but may not sustain the same degree of injury. Modifying factors, such as nutritional status, can have a profound impact on the extent of injury. There is a point of no return with cellular injury at which cell death occurs. The exact mechanisms responsible for the transition from reversible to irreversible cellular damage are not clearly understood.

HYPOXIA

Hypoxia (inadequate tissue oxygenation) is a leading cause of cell injury and death. The hypoxic condition can arise secondary to (1) vascular disease, which impedes blood flow to tissues, and (2) anemia or monoxide poisoning, which results in the insufficient oxygenation of blood. Depending on the severity of the hypoxic state, cells may adapt, undergo injury, or die. For example, if the femoral artery is narrowed, the skeletal muscles of the legs may eventually atrophy. This is because the muscles' metabolic needs are compromised from the inadequate blood flow and oxygen. More severe hypoxia would result in cell injury or death. The most common cause of hypoxia is ischemia, or reduced blood supply. Ischemic injury is often caused by gradual narrowing of arteries (arteriosclerosis). This progressive hypoxia is better tolerated than sudden anoxia (total lack of oxygen) caused by a sudden obstruction in blood supply.

TEMPERATURE EXTREMES

Extreme heat damages cells by literally coagulating cytoplasmic protein. Even mild heat results in permanent cellular damage if it is applied over a prolonged period to clients with decreased circulation, such as peripheral vascular disease. Irreversible damage occurs in these cases because heat increases the metabolic needs of cells and tissues. This increase is dangerous because oxygen circulation to the cells is deficient and waste products from the increased metabolism cannot be carried away.

Cold injures cells by constricting the blood vessels, thereby decreasing the circulation of blood and oxygen to tissue cells. Freezing temperatures cause the intracellular water to crystalize, which destroys the cell's structure. Cold injury results in frostbite, which permanently injures involved tissues. Also, cold temperatures cause stasis of blood, which can lead to clot formation. The clots occlude arteries, resulting in ischemia and, ultimately, in cell death and necrosis.

IONIZING RADIATION

Radiation causes mutations, damages enzymes, and interrupts cell division. The fact that radiation can stop mitosis makes radiation therapy important in the treatment of cancer—a disease involving pathologic cell reproduction. Although radiation affects virtually all cells, certain cells are more susceptible than others. Reproductive cells, cells of the lymph nodes and gastrointestinal tract, and bone marrow cells, for example, are highly sensitive to radiation, whereas the cells of the cartilage, muscle, brain, and endocrine glands are relatively insensitive. Clients who work with radioactive materials or nuclear fission reactors, or who are receiving therapeutic radiation treatment are most susceptible to cellular trauma from radiation.

ELECTRICAL INJURY

Electrical energy generates heat when it passes through the body and may thus produce burns. It also interferes with neural conduction pathways and often causes death from cardiac arrhythmias. The extent of damage from electrical energy depends on its voltage and amperage, the tissue resistance, and the pathway of the current as it passes through the body. Electrical burns are discussed in Chapter 71.

CHEMICAL INJURY

Chemicals harm cells by destroying or injuring their structures and by disrupting their metabolism. The capacity of a chemical to produce cell injury depends on the strength and toxicity of the chemical. There are numerous chemicals that can cause cellular injury. Highly toxic substances are called poisons. Minute amounts of poisonous substances such as cyanide and arsenic cause death. Environmental chemicals, such as herbicides, pesticides, and air pollution, can cause cellular injury. The effect of lead ingestion has been studied. Lead-based paint, which tastes sweet, is often eaten by children. The lead destroys cells in the nervous system, affects blood cell production, and damages the kidneys. Carbon monoxide binds tightly to the hemoglobin molecule, preventing the normal exchange of oxygen and carbon dioxide. Therefore, cells cannot receive oxygen and become hypoxic.

BACTERIAL INJURY

Microorganisms such as bacteria injure cells mainly by means of the toxins they produce. Toxins are either endotoxins or exotoxins. An endotoxin is a substance produced by gram-negative bacteria. Endotoxins are released only when the microorganism dies. Endotoxins cause fever by acting on thermoregulators in the hypothalamus. Endotoxins are not easily neutralized by antitoxins. An exotoxin is excreted by a microorganism into a surrounding medium. Exotoxins are proteins and have very specific toxic effects. *Clostridium tetani,* the organism that causes tetanus, produces a neurotoxin that blocks inhibition in the spinal cord. The client has spasms of the airway and depression of the respiratory center. Exotoxins can be neutralized by antitoxins.

VIRAL INJURY

Viruses enter the cell and control the metabolism of the cell. Once in the cell, the virus uses the cell's energy and stable environment to survive and reproduce. Viruses do not produce endotoxin or exotoxins. Viruses have a strong membrane that allows them to resist breakdown by lysosomes after phagocytosis.

MECHANICAL INJURY

Cells can be damaged by physical impact or irritations. Examples of this type of injury include blisters from tight shoes, abrasions, lacerations, and contusions (bruises).

NUTRITIONAL IMBALANCE

If intake of carbohydrate, protein, fat, vitamins, or minerals is inadequate or if excess amounts of nutrients are consumed by the cell, the cell can be injured.

Inadequate protein intake decreases the function of the intestinal mucosa and pancreas, which decreases nutrient absorption. When plasma proteins (which hold fluid in blood vessels, especially albumin) are low, fluid moves into interstitial spaces, causing edema. In addition, the lack of proteins reduces production of immune system cells and increases the risk of infection.

Inadequate carbohydrate intake forces the body to use fats for energy, such as in conditions of starvation and diabetes due to lack of insulin.

In inadequate fat (lipid) intake, the body uses fatty acids stored in adipose tissue for energy. The metabolism of fat produces acid byproducts called ketones. Increased fat intake often causes deposits of fats in the heart, liver, and muscle.

Vitamins and minerals are not sources of energy but are used in metabolism and cell reproduction.

OTHER CAUSES OF CELLULAR INJURY

The cell can be injured in other ways as well. Light can damage cells of the cornea. Noise can damage the eardrum (tympanic membrane), the ossicles in the middle ear, and the organ of Corti in the inner ear. Prolonged contact with vibrating objects can alter the muscles and bone structure, as well as nerve conduction. Clients at risk for these injuries are those who work with machinery such as hand tools and air hammers.

Major Types of Cellular Alterations

The major cellular alterations are (1) genetic disturbances, (2) degenerations and infiltrations, and (3) disorders of cell growth, including malignant growth, atrophy, and hypertrophy.

GENETIC DISTURBANCES

If a cell carries a genetic abnormality, either newly acquired or hereditary, it may be exhibited in the cell as a disturbance of normal function. Cellular disorders of genetic causation are not apparent until the mutated gene is needed and is either nonfunctional or only partially functional.

INFILTRATIONS

Injured cells have observable changes in their cytoplasm and nucleus. Infiltration means that a substance that is external to the cell filters into the cell and damages its ability to function. For example, when large amounts of fat globules are deposited within the cell as the result of a metabolic systemic illness, the process is called fatty infiltration. Other infiltrates include water, glucogen, protein, and macopolysaccharides.

DISTURBANCES OF CELL GROWTH

Some major disturbances of cellular growth involve the problems of atrophy, hypertrophy, and precancerous changes (Fig. 13-4).

Atrophy

Atrophy is the wasting of a tissue or organ and a decrease in its size following the normal development of the structure. This condition is due to a decrease in either the number of cells or the actual size of the cells

Hyperplasia

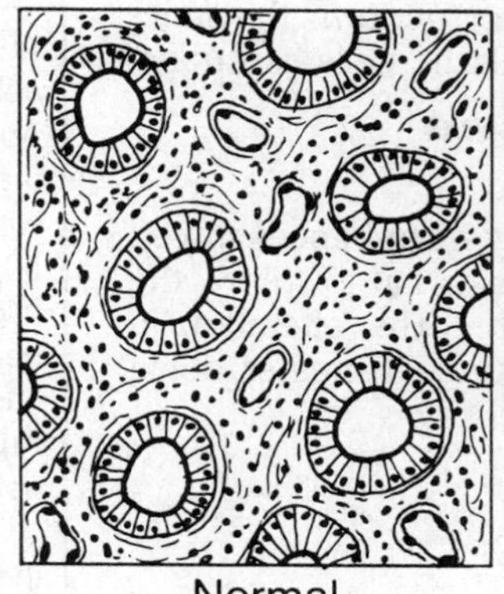

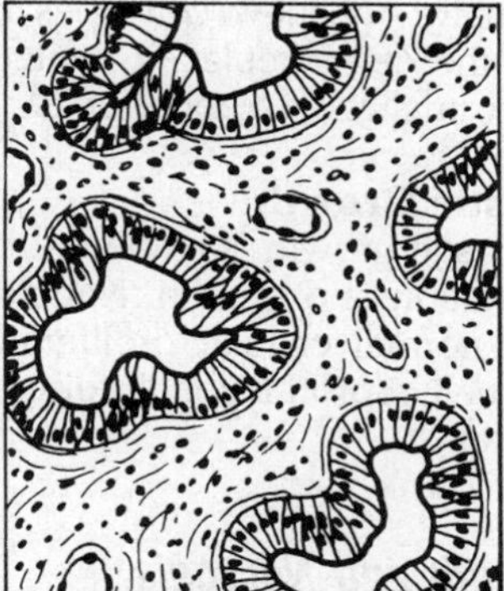

Metaplasia

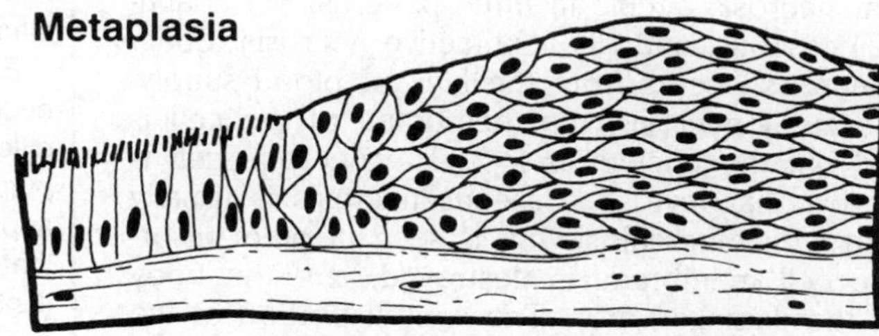

Dysplasia

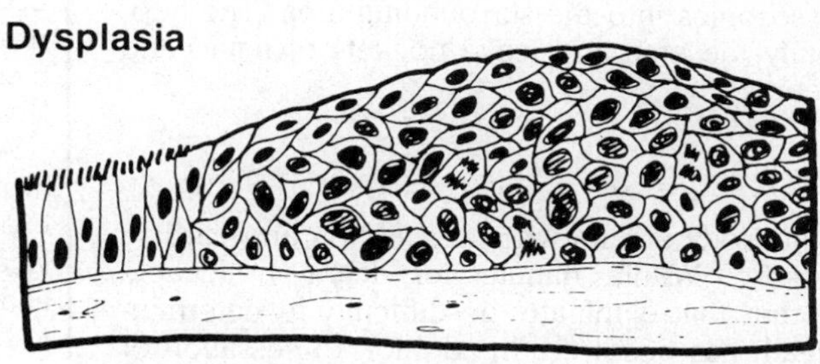

▲ *Figure 13-4*

Adaptive alterations in simple cuboidal epithelial cells. (From Kumar, V., et al. [1992] *Basic pathology* [5th ed.). Philadelphia, W. B. Saunders.)

composing a tissue or organ. Atrophy may follow disuse of an organ. For example, muscular atrophy may develop following denervation or prolonged immobilization. Because the adrenal glands normally secrete corticosteroids, atrophy of these glands can occur when large doses of corticosteroids are administered over a prolonged period. Finally, atrophy accompanies the normal physiologic aging process. Thus, the thymus gland atrophies when the child matures, and ovaries atrophy after menopause.

Hypertrophy

Hypertrophy is an increase in the size of an organ or tissue resulting from an increase in the size of the cells. Hypertrophy sometimes represents the response of an organ to a greater workload. For example, when the heart is subjected to great strain, the left ventricle of the heart enlarges, or hypertrophies, in order to handle the additional stress. A second example of hypertrophy is the increase in size of the biceps muscle in individuals engaged in regular, strenuous physical activity.

Dysplasia

Dysplasia is deranged cellular growth or a form of hyperplasia. It occurs from persistent severe injury or irritation. Hyperplasia is an increase in the number of cells. Hyperplasia can be an expected cellular response, such as increased cell regeneration and formation of calluses. Pathologic hyperplasia is usually a response to excessive hormone secretion. If the process continues, the cells can become cancerous. Metaplasia is the replacement of one mature cell type for another cell. Usually, the new cell does not perform the functions of the cell it replaced. Metaplastic cells can transform into malignant cancer cells.

Neoplastic Growth

Neoplastic growth is exhibited by disturbances in cell differentiation and growth. Neoplasms fail to follow the rules of normal cellular proliferation. This alteration in normal cell reproduction is discussed in greater detail in Chapter 20.

Cell Death and Necrosis

When cells die, the mitochondria swell, cell function stops, cell membranes rupture, and the lysosome releases enzymes to destroy the cell.

Cellular necrosis occurs in three patterns: (1) coagulative, (2) caseous, and (3) liquefactive necrosis. Coagulative necrosis occurs from the lack of blood supply. In this form of necrosis, the membrane of the cell is preserved but the nucleus is lost. The necrotic cell is removed by phagocytosis. Caseous necrosis is usually associated with tuberculosis but is seen in other disorders. The cell membrane is destroyed, and the body walls off the damaged area. The central portion of the walled off area looks cheesy and crumbly. Liquefactive necrosis is seen in brain tissues. Death of the neuron releases lysosomes into the surrounding area. The lysosomes liquify the area and leave pockets of liquid and cellular debris.

SOMATIC DEATH

Death of the body occurs when respiration and cardiac function cease. Within minutes of death, noticeable changes occur that eliminate the difficulty in determining that death has occurred. In addition to cessation of respiration and circulation, the skin becomes pale and yellow, body temperature falls until it reaches the temperature of the environment after 24 hours, blood pressure is absent, pupils become fixed and dilated, and limbs become rigid. The processes noted at death have been given specific names: algor mortis is loss of body temperature, livor mortis is a purple discoloration in dependent body tissues from blood stasis, rigor mortis is muscle stiffening. Rigor mortis affects the entire body within 12 to 24 hours and diminishes after 24 hours.

The legal and ethical issues surrounding death are difficult to think about. Clients who have suffered for a long time may ask that no extraordinary measures be used to prolong their life. Other times, the family of a patient who has sustained an irreversible traumatic injury may cling to any evidence of life in the patient. (The term "patient" as used here refers to a comatose client who cannot be an active participant in care.) The issue of promoting or facilitating death in the chronically ill is ongoing. The advances in medical care options, such as respirators and organ transplantation, have led to the development of specific criteria to document that brain death has occurred. These criteria are (1) coma with unresponsiveness, including the absence of brain stem reflexes (blinking, eye movement, pupil response to light and swallowing); (2) cessation of automatic breathing when patient is removed from respirator support; and (3) isoelectric electroencephalogram. Once the patient is declared dead, undamaged organs can be taken from the body and used in transplantation (see Chap. 24). Autopsy is performed if the

Box 13–1. The Value of Autopsy

Autopsy, or examination of the body after death, is invaluable for providing knowledge to clarify the cause of death. Autopsy can also serve as a monitor for clinical care and the quality of society's health. Despite the data gathered with autopsy, the rate has steadily declined—from nearly 50 per cent in the late 1940's to 15 per cent in 1984. One might think that as medical science has advanced, the need for autopsy has declined. But in fact, each generation has seen new diseases that are initially not recognized. Autopsy can assist with recognition and identification of new diseases.

The purpose of autopsy goes beyond providing data on the effectiveness of medical therapy. The family of the deceased may be reassured that everything necessary and possible was done for the patient. In addition, contagious illness and genetic illness can be identified and made known to the family. Autopsy also helps clarify the circumstances of violent and unexplained death.

Each state in the United States has its own laws on the need for permission for autopsy. Even though specific laws differ, there are some general similarities. Autopsy for the purpose of resolving medicolegal issues is ordered by an appropriate authority, such as a medical examiner. Death that is unexpected, occurring while in surgery, or in a patient who is not under physician's care falls into this category. When there is no medicolegal reason for ordering an autopsy, permission can be given only by next of kin. Usually, a patient cannot order his own autopsy before death. Once death has occurred, the body becomes the property of the next of kin, or if there is no next of kin, of a legal entity such as the coroner or sheriff.

An autopsy is performed in privacy and in a professional manner. An incision is made from the axilla to groin to expose internal organs. Organs are examined and weighed. In addition, microscopic study and chemical, toxicologic, and microbiologic analyses are performed. The ideal time to perform an autopsy is within 24 hours of death. Autopsy can be performed after embalming.

The family may be concerned about the final appearance of the patient at burial. Autopsy is customarily performed with great care so as not to disfigure the body. The family may meet with the pathologist and receive a copy of the findings. The cost of autopsy is usually built into the hospital costs; therefore, charges for autopsy do not appear on the bill.

cause of death is suspicious or if the family would benefit from knowing the cause of death (Box 13-1).

Summary

Cells are the basic units of life. Within the body, they serve many functions, from energy production to genetic transmission. In the past few years, the role of the cell in disease has become increasingly understood and, therefore, increasingly important in the care of clients. Many disorders are discussed as changes within the cell. This chapter reviewed the general structure and function of the cell, the cellular components, and tissues and organs. Mechanisms of cell injury and death were also reviewed.

Bibliography

1. Goldman, L. (1983). The value of autopsy in three medical eras. *New England Journal of Medicine, 308*(17), 1002-1006.
2. Guyton, A. C. (1988). *Basic human physiology: Normal function and mechanisms of disease* (7th ed.). Philadelphia: W. B. Saunders.
3. Hayflick, L. (1980, January). The cell biology of human aging. *Scientific American, 242,* 54.
4. McCance, K., & Huether, S. (1990). *Pathophysiology.* St. Louis: C. V. Mosby.
5. Robbins, S. (1984). *Pathologic basis of disease* (3rd ed.). Philadelphia: W. B. Saunders.
6. Solomon, E., et al. (1990). *Human anatomy and physiology.* Philadelphia: W. B. Saunders.
7. Weiss, L. M., et al. (1986, August 21). Clonal T-cell populations in lymphomatoid papulosis: Evidence of lymphoproliferative origin for a clinically benign disease. *New England Journal of Medicine, 315,* 475.
8. Wyngaarden, J. B., et al. (1992). *Cecil Textbook of Medicine* (19th ed.). Philadelphia: W. B. Saunders.

Chapter 14

Fluid and Electrolyte Balance

Physiologic homeostasis depends on normal fluid and electrolyte balance, and is important in both health promotion and treatment of disorders. Fluid and electrolyte imbalances commonly accompany illness. Severe imbalances may result in death. Such imbalances affect not only the acutely and chronically ill but also clients with faulty diets or those who take selected medications such as diuretics and glucocorticoid preparations. The nursing process is applicable to both the prevention and treatment of fluid and electrolyte imbalances. Every nurse must understand the process of fluid and electrolyte balance, identify clients at risk of imbalances, recognize early signs and symptoms of imbalances, intervene as appropriate, and evaluate the outcomes.

FLUIDS

Water and Fluid Balance

FLUID COMPARTMENTS

Water is the solvent responsible for the body's structure and function. Body water is located in two major fluid compartments—the intracellular fluid (ICF) compartment and extracellular fluid (ECF) compartment. The ECF is composed of interstitial (tissues) and intravascular fluid (plasma). Interstitial fluid lies outside the vascular fluid and cells and comprises 28 per cent of the total body water. It provides the cells with the external medium necessary for cellular metabolism. In the adult, approximately 60 per cent of body weight is water; two thirds of the water is intracellular, and one third of the water is extracellular fluid.

The ICF provides the cell with the internal aqueous medium necessary for its chemical functions. The ECF transports nutrients, electrolytes, and oxygen to cells and waste products for excretion; regulates heat; lubricates and cushions joints and membranes; and hydrolyzes food for digestive processes. Cerebrospinal fluid, lymphatic fluid, synovial fluid, and fluids in the eye are also part of the ECF.

FLUID PRESSURES

Body fluids shift between the interstitial space and the vascular space in the capillary as a result of differences in the hydrostatic pressure and the oncotic (colloid osmotic) pressure. Hydrostatic pressure is pressure due to water volume in the vessels. Oncotic pressure is the pressure exerted by plasma proteins. Filtration occurs at arterial ends of the capillaries because the hydrostatic pressure is greater than the oncotic pressure. Therefore, fluid is pushed out of the vessels into tissue space. At the venous end of the capillary, the oncotic pressure is greater than the hydrostatic pressure, and fluid is pulled back into the capillary from the interstitial space (Fig. 14-1).

There are some conditions in which this system does not work smoothly and fluid remains in the tissue spaces. When there is a low level of plasma/serum protein, oncotic pressure in the vascular fluid is decreased and less water is reabsorbed into the vascular space. Likewise, when the hydrostatic pressure is high because of fluid overload, the pressure gradient opposes fluid reabsorption into the venous end of the capillary. The functions of water are numerous, and without sufficient water, cells of the body deteriorate and life cannot be sustained.

REGULATORS OF FLUID BALANCE

Thirst, hormones, the lymphatic system, the nervous system, and the kidneys assist in the regulation of body fluids. These regulators may respond inappropriately to various stimuli and cause a fluid imbalance. Thirst is a primary factor in the maintenance of an intake of fluids. The kidneys are responsible for maintaining an adequate fluid output or retaining fluids (Fig. 14-2).

Thirst

The thirst center is located in the hypothalamus and is activated by an increase in ECF osmolality (concentration). Thirst may result from hypotension, polyuria, or fluid volume depletion.

Although thirst can be reported and is an important clinical manifestation of fluid imbalances, it is not a true indicator of fluid balance in all clients. The thirst mechanism may be depressed in the elderly and in clients with debilitating illnesses. Edematous clients, who have excess fluids, may be thirsty because the fluid is trapped in the interstitial spaces and is not contributing to cell osmolarity. Comatose and confused clients may have very high osmolarity but are unable to recognize the urge to drink. Finally, the client with hypo-osmolarity of the ECF will not experience thirst even though the fluid volumes are decreased. Hypo-osmolarity inhibits the thirst mechanism. It is also important to recognize the cultural variations in fluid consumption. In Western civilization, offering guests something to drink is common practice and may influence total fluid consumption.

Hormonal Influences

The antidiuretic hormone and aldosterone are the two major hormones influencing fluid balance.

Antidiuretic hormone (ADH), produced by the hypothalamus and stored in the neurohypophysis (posterior pituitary gland), is secreted when there is an increased plasma/serum osmolality (hyperosmolality), ECF volume depletion, pain, use of certain medications, or stress (emotional; physiologic, such as surgery, trauma, prolonged exercise). ADH promotes water reabsorption from the renal tubules. Stimulation of the thirst mechanism and ADH release usually occur concurrently in response to a body fluid deficit.

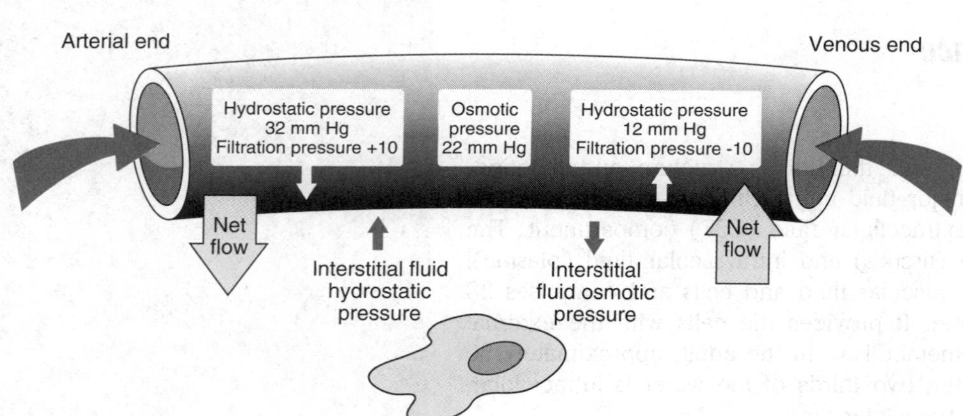

▲ **Figure 14-1**

Pressure differences within the capillary are responsible for the movement of fluids. Fluid moves out of the capillary at the arterial end due to hydrostatic pressure in the vessel exceeding the pressure in the tissues. Fluids return to the vessel at the venous end because the proteins (colloids) that remained in the vessel exert a pulling pressure on them. Under normal conditions, the movement of fluids is equal and neither dehydration nor edema results. These abnormal conditions occur when there is too much fluid, too few proteins, or changes in the capillary wall.

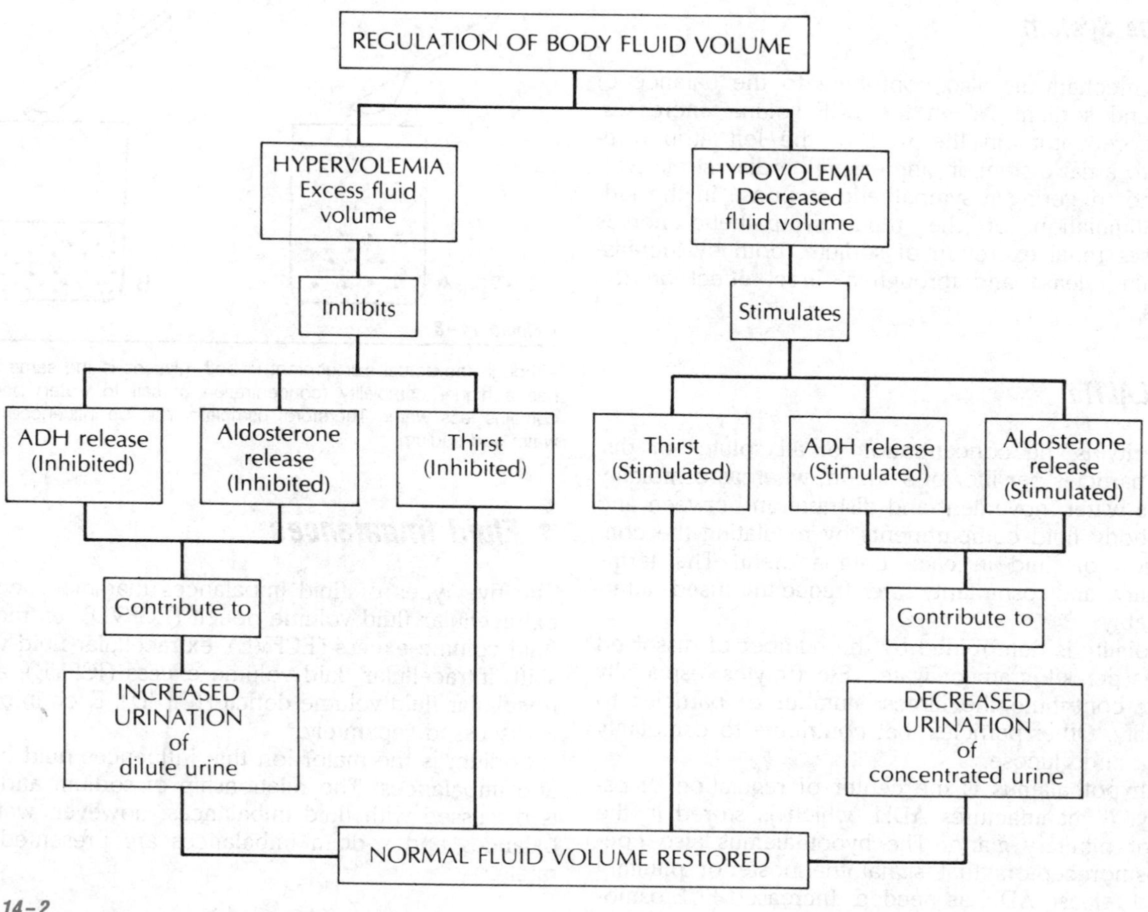

▲ **Figure 14–2**

Regulation of body fluid volume depends on ADH, aldosterone, and thirst. (From Sorensen, K. C., & Luckmann, J. [Eds.] [1986]. *Basic nursing: A psychophysiologic approach* [2nd ed.]. Philadelphia: W. B. Saunders.)

Factors suppressing ADH include hypo-osmolarity of the ECF, increased blood volume, exposure to cold, acute alcohol ingestion, carbon dioxide inhalation, and administration of some diuretics.

Aldosterone is secreted by the adrenal cortex and promotes sodium reabsorption and potassium excretion from the kidneys. Aldosterone secretion is stimulated primarily by the renin-angiotensin system. Renin, secreted by the juxtaglomerular apparatus of the kidney, converts angiotensinogen in the blood to angiotensin I. Angiotensin I is further converted to angiotensin II in the capillary beds. Aldosterone secretion can also be stimulated by an increase in potassium or decrease in sodium concentration in interstitial fluids and by adrenocorticotropic hormone (ACTH) release from the anterior pituitary.

Hypovolemia is a common clinical condition in which aldosterone is secreted to maintain homeostasis. When arterial blood pressure falls, renal blood pressure falls. Hypotension decreases the stretch in vascular smooth muscle in the afferent arteriole of the kidney, which increases renin release. Renin stimulates aldosterone, through multiple steps, which increases sodium retention and thereby fluid retention to raise blood pressure.

In addition to aldosterone, other circulating factors contribute to the regulation of sodium balance. Atrial natriuretic factors are peptides released from the atria in response to atrial distention. These factors increase the excretion of sodium and water. Renal prostaglandins and the renal renin-kinin system also increase sodium excretion.

Lymphatic System

Plasma protein and fluid escaping from the tissue spaces cannot be directly reabsorbed into the blood vessels. The lymphatic system plays an important role in returning any excess fluid and protein from the interstitial spaces to the blood.

Kidneys

The kidneys maintain fluid volume and the concentration of urine by filtrating the ECF through the glomeruli. Reabsorption and excretion of ECF occurs in the renal tubules.

Nervous System

Neural mechanisms also contribute to the balance of water and sodium. When the ECF volume increases, mechanoreceptors in the wall of the left atrium respond to atrial distention, increasing cardiac stroke volume and triggering a sympathetic response in the kidney. Stimulation of the renal sympathetic nerves decreases renal excretion of sodium, both by increasing renin release and through a direct effect on the kidneys.

OSMOLALITY

Osmolarity is the concentration of all solutes or dissolved particles per liter of solution, whereas osmolality controls water movement and distribution between and within body fluid compartments by regulating the concentration of fluid in each compartment. The terms osmolality and osmolarity are frequently used interchangeably.

Osmolality is determined by the number of dissolved particles per kilogram of water. Electrolytes, especially sodium, contribute the largest number of particles to osmolality. Other particles that contribute to osmolality are urea and glucose.

The hypothalamus is the center of regulation of osmolarity. It manufactures ADH, which is stored in the posterior pituitary gland. The hypothalamus also contains osmoreceptors that signal the posterior pituitary gland to release ADH as needed. Increased ECF osmolarity causes the osmoreceptors to stimulate ADH release. Conversely, when ECF osmolarity decreases, the osmoreceptors inhibit ADH secretion.

Osmolality is measured by calculating the concentration of solutes per kilogram of water. Sodium is the easiest solute to measure because it is abundant and readily accessible in the plasma and serum. Elevated serum sodium (hypernatremia) indicates a state of hyperosmolality, and decreased serum sodium (hyponatremia) indicates hypo-osmolality.

The serum sodium value does not signify the total amount of sodium in the extracellular fluid, but rather it indicates the relationship of the amount of water to dissolved sodium. To illustrate this point, consider two glasses of water, one full and the other half full (Fig. 14-3). To each, add 1 teaspoon of salt. The glass on the right would taste saltier, yet it contains the same amount of salt as the glass on the left. The solution in the glass on the right is more concentrated (hyperosmolality), or in other words, there is less water for the same amount of salt.

The range of serum osmolality (concentration of solutes in body fluid) is 275 to 295 mOsm/kg of water. When there are more milliosmols per kilogram (over 295 mOsm/kg of water), a hyperosmolar fluid results. Iso-osmolar fluid contains particles and water in equal proportion. Hypo-osmolar fluid has less particles than water. Calculating serum osmolality is shown in Box 14-1.

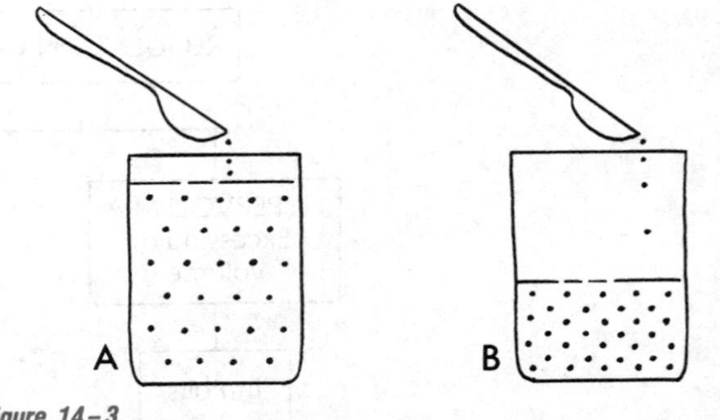

▲ Figure 14-3

Although the actual salt content in both glasses is the same, glass B has a higher osmolality (concentration of salt to water) because it contains less water. Therefore, osmolality can be influenced by both water and sodium.

▼ Fluid Imbalances

The five types of fluid imbalances that may occur are extracellular fluid volume deficit (ECFVD), extracellular fluid volume excess (ECFVE), extracellular fluid volume shift, intracellular fluid volume excess (ICFVE), and intracellular fluid volume deficit (ICFVD). Each imbalance is discussed separately.

Sodium is the major ion that influences fluid balance and imbalances. The relationship of sodium and water is discussed with fluid imbalances; however, water imbalances and sodium imbalances are presented separately.

EXTRACELLULAR FLUID VOLUME DEFICIT

Definition and Incidence

An ECFVD is a decrease in intravascular and interstitial fluids. ECFVD is a common and serious fluid imbalance that results in vascular fluid volume loss (hypovolemia). ECFVD can lead to cellular fluid loss owing to fluid shifting from the cells to the vascular fluid to restore fluid balance.

There are two major types of extracellular fluid volume deficits: (1) *hyperosmolar fluid volume deficit*, in

Box 14-1. How to Calculate Serum Osmolality

To calculate serum osmolality, the serum sodium (Na) level should be known. Additionally, the glucose and blood urea nitrogen (BUN) should be known. The first formula may be used as a rough estimate of the serum osmolality; the second formula gives a more exact serum osmolality value.

$$2 \times \text{serum Na} = \text{serum osmolality}$$

$$2 \times \text{serum Na} + \frac{\text{BUN}}{3} + \frac{\text{glucose}}{18} = \text{serum osmolality}$$

which the fluid loss is greater than the solute (sodium) loss, and (2) *iso-osmolar fluid volume deficit*, in which there is equal proportion of fluid and solute (sodium) loss.

Etiology and Risk Factors

ECFVD commonly occurs with severe vomiting or diarrhea, traumatic injuries with excessive blood loss, third space fluid shifts, and insufficient water or fluid intake.

Clients at risk for ECFVD include those who are elderly, confused, or debilitated; in diabetic ketoacidosis; losing large volumes of blood; having severe vomiting or diarrhea; having difficulty swallowing; unable to procure water because of physical restraint; or receiving an overabundance of intravenous glucose without saline or hypertonic tube feeding. The elderly are at risk because of their potential for depressed thirst mechanism. Prevention begins with adequate hydration. If fluids are being lost, fluid replacement should begin immediately by offering oral fluids or replacing fluid loss with intravenous solutions that contain saline as well as dextrose.

Pathophysiology

The pathophysiologic changes related to ECFVD are usually related to changes in sodium levels. Sodium has a major influence on water retention and water loss. Serum sodium concentration is increased with an ECFVD due to insufficient water intake or massive water loss. The increased serum sodium concentration causes ECFVD by shifting water from the cells to the vascular space to decrease the hyperosmolality that occurs with water loss. This shift causes cells to shrink and cellular dehydration to occur.

The pathophysiologic changes that relate to clinical manifestations of fluid volume deficit are explained in Table 14–1.

With a severe fluid volume deficit, vascular collapse

TABLE 14–1. Clinical Manifestations of Extracellular Fluid Volume Deficit and Their Pathophysiologic Basis

Clinical Manifestation	Pathophysiologic Basis
Thirst	Cells shrink, stimulating "thirst" osmoreceptors in the hypothalamus; with iso-osmolar fluid loss, thirst usually does not occur
Decreased skin turgor	Decreased interstitial fluid causes skin tissue to "stick together"
Dry mucous membranes; dry, cracked lips or tongue	Cells of mucous membranes and tongue "dry out"
Eyeballs soft and sunken (severe deficit)	Water tension in eyeballs decreased
Apprehension and restlessness; coma in severe deficit	Cerebral dehydration
Elevated temperature	Less fluid available for evaporation
Tachycardia	Pulse greater than 100 bpm may be due to circulatory compensation by the heart
Postural systolic blood pressure fall >15 mm Hg and diastolic fall >10 mm Hg	With iso-osmolar fluid loss, the plasma volume is inadequate owing to hypovolemia; systolic pressure begins to fall
Narrowed pulse pressure, decreased CVP and PCWP	Decreased venous return
Flattened neck veins in supine position	Decreased venous return
Weight loss	A lack of the water component of body weight
Oliguria (<30 ml per hour)	Due to the renal response to hypovolemia
Laboratory Findings	
Increased osmolality	Serum osmolality >295 mOsm/kg due to hypo-osmolar fluid loss (more fluid than solutes is lost)
Increased or normal serum sodium level	Hypo-osmolar fluid volume loss: serum sodium level >145 mEq/L; water is lost in greater amounts than sodium Iso-osmolar fluid volume loss: serum sodium level is within normal range
Increased BUN (>25 mg/dl)	The blood urea nitrogen (BUN) would be slightly elevated (25–35 mg/dl) because of hemoconcentration
Hyperglycemia (>120 mg/dl)	Sugar increases serum osmolality, thus causing diuresis and water loss; glucose levels may also be elevated owing to hemoconcentration
Elevated hematocrit (>55%)	With hypo-osmolar fluid loss, hematocrit will be increased owing to hemoconcentration; with iso-osmolar fluid loss (e.g., hemorrhage), hematocrit may be within normal range
Increased specific gravity	Increased solute to solvent ratio

and shock may occur. The major clinical manifestations are due to changes in the cerebral cells. If the ECFVD develops rapidly, the manifestations are more severe. Severe brain shrinkage during water deficit may cause vascular damage and intracerebral hemorrhage. When ECFVD occurs slowly, the brain cells adapt to the increased intracellular osmolality by producing extra intracellular particles (idiogenic osmoles), which prevent large amounts of water from leaving the cell.

Clinical Manifestations

With mild ECFVD, 1 to 2 L water and 2 per cent of the body weight is lost. Moderate ECFVD is evidenced by 3 to 5 L of water loss and a 5 per cent weight loss. In severe ECFVD, the water loss is increased to 5 to 10 L and the weight loss is increased to 8 per cent; the systolic blood pressure becomes alarmingly low as demonstrated by a reading of less than 70 mm Hg. Immediate medical management is necessary for severe ECFVD.

DIAGNOSTIC ASSESSMENT

An elevated serum osmolality (greater than 295 mOsm/kg) and a serum sodium level greater than 145 mEq/L could indicate a hyperosmolar fluid volume deficit. Other laboratory indicators of fluid volume deficit are increased blood urea nitrogen (BUN) and an elevated hematocrit. A low central venous pressure (CVP <2 mm H_2O) and a decreased pulmonary capillary wedge pressure (PCWP <6 mm Hg) are additional diagnostic indicators of fluid deficit.

Medical Management

Medical treatment of fluid volume deficit depends on the severity of the fluid deficit. If the fluid loss is mild, the fluid intake should be increased in accordance with the client's physical condition.

PHARMACOLOGIC MANAGEMENT

When a hyperosmolar fluid volume deficit is present, an intravenous solution of 5 per cent dextrose in water (D_5W) or 5 per cent dextrose in 0.2 per cent saline (D_5/0.2 per cent NaCl) may be prescribed. If the deficit has existed for more than 24 hours, it is dangerous to correct it too rapidly. Some authorities recommend that the maximal rate at which sodium solutions be infused is 2 mEq/L per hour. If fluid is given too rapidly, cerebral edema may result (see Ethical Issues in Nursing).

If hemorrhage is the cause of the ECFVD, blood replacement may be necessary when blood loss is greater than 1 L. In situations in which the blood losses are less than 1 L, normal saline and lactated Ringer's may be used to restore fluid volume.

The fluid needs of the client must be assessed within the context of the client's overall condition. A client with severe ECFVD and also severe heart or kidney disease will not be able to be given large volumes of fluid or sodium.

DIETARY MANAGEMENT

Clients experiencing fluid loss from diarrhea should avoid fatty or fried foods and milk products.

Nursing Management

ASSESSMENT

The client should be assessed for the typical clinical manifestations. In addition, the nurse should assess the client's ability to participate in the treatment plan. For example, can the client swallow? What site and what size intravenous line should be initiated?

NURSING INTERVENTION

Nursing Diagnosis: Fluid Volume Deficit R/T insufficient fluid intake, vomiting, diarrhea, hemorrhage, or third space fluid loss (ascites, burns).

Planning: Expected Outcomes. The client will have restored fluid balance, as evidenced by vital signs within normal range, return to baseline body weight, absence of the causative factor(s) of ECFVD, intake equals output, urine output of greater than 600 ml/day, skin turgor at or less than 2 seconds, and pink and moist mucous membranes.

Implementation. Vital signs should be assessed every 2 to 4 hours depending on the severity of the fluid loss, compared with baseline vital signs and marked differences reported. Positional blood pressure should be assessed to determine the degree of orthostasis. If the standing systolic blood pressure falls 10 to 15 mm Hg or more, the results should be reported and the client protected from injury while ambulating.

Urine output should be assessed hourly if ECFVD is severe; in mild cases, the urine output per shift and per day should be compared with intake for the same time frame. Absence of a urine output in 8 to 12 hours may indicate renal insufficiency due to decreased renal perfusion. Absence of adequate renal perfusion for several hours may result in permanent renal damage. Urine specific gravity measurements should also be noted every shift, because these data provide very objective measurements of osmolality.

Daily weight should be monitored. A loss of 2.2 pounds is equivalent to 1 L. An 8-pound weight loss equals approximately 3.5 L, which is indicative of a moderate fluid volume deficit.

The nurse should apply lotion to the skin to preserve skin integrity. The client's position should be changed every 2 hours, or more often if skin assessment dictates. Oral care should be given every 2 hours with a nonalcoholic base solution. Lips should be moistened frequently.

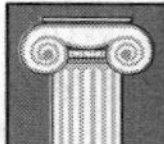

ETHICAL ISSUES IN NURSING

Should Hydration Measures Be Used on All Clients?

The electrolytes found in the body work together with amazing precision. Slight alterations in the electrolyte balance may cause physical symptoms as simple as muscle cramps or as grave as cardiac arrhythmias. Electrolyte imbalances may be caused by many different factors including dehydration, anorexia, severe dieting, medications, and illness. These imbalances may be corrected in many cases by the reintroduction, or the removal, of the electrolyte that is out of balance. This issue appears simple enough. However, what if a client refuses to have his or her electrolyte imbalance corrected, for instance, through hydration measures? Or, in the case of a client in a persistent vegetative state, what happens if the family wishes to cease hydration measures, which will ultimately assist in the client's demise?

The issue of hydration may be separated into two categories: life-sustaining and death-delaying. Life-sustaining measures of any kind mean to do just that—to sustain life. The ultimate goal may be to correct whatever is threatening life, which may be as simple as correcting an electrolyte imbalance. On the other hand, death-delaying measures are those that prolong the inevitable. Perhaps the disease process has matured beyond control, or a traumatic experience has rendered a person in a persistent vegetative state with no hope of recovery. In such cases, hydration may be considered a futile treatment, being used only to prolong the process of death.

Should hydration measures be used on all persons regardless of whether such measures are life-sustaining or death-delaying? Is hydration a basic measure of care that should never be denied to anyone for any reason? Do clients experience pain if they are not hydrated even if they are in a persistent vegetative state? Do nurses have the right to refuse to carry out orders not to hydrate clients if they believe this is a basic comfort never to be denied? By hydrating clients who no longer may benefit from its treatment effects, are we really just comforting ourselves as care givers?

It is not unlikely that nurses in all areas of health care will experience this type of dilemma sometime in their professional career. How a nurse reacts in a specific situation depends on many variables specific to that situation and his or her ethical feelings at the time. All cases concerning these issues should be evaluated case by case so as not to trivialize the end results of such actions taken.

Serum sodium, BUN, glucose, and hematocrit levels should be closely monitored in order to determine the serum osmolality.

Mild fluid volume loss can be corrected with oral fluid replacement, especially for the elderly and debilitated clients. If the fluid loss is moderate or severe, administration of intravenous fluids is indicated. Intravenous solutions need to be closely monitored. Overhydration may occur from excessive and rapidly infused intravenous fluids or in clients with preexisting renal or cardiac disorders. Clinical manifestations of fluid overload include dyspnea, crackles, and jugular vein engorgement.

EVALUATION

The degree of expected outcome attainment should be monitored after 8 and 24 hours for determining whether the ECFVD is being corrected. Revisions of the interventions may be required.

Modification of Plan of Care for the Elderly

The elderly client must be rehydrated slowly because of the frequent problems with renal and cardiac disease in that age group. Skin breakdown is also more common, and position changes will be needed more frequently. A frustrating problem is resistance on the part of the elderly client to eat or drink. The client may be fed with some success by members of the family. The nursing staff seldom has time to feed a client slowly, but that is one of the most effective interventions. Often, the client will forget that he or she has just drunk or eaten and in just a few minutes will eat or drink again.

Post-hospital Care

Follow-up care is based on the original problem. If the client was fluid deficient because of inadequate fluid intake, the client or responsible person will need to be taught how to be certain the client gets adequate fluids. For example, if the client is dehydrated owing to the use of too highly concentrated tube feedings, the use of additional water between feedings will be needed. If the client is fluid deficient as the result of a traumatic injury, the problem will most likely be resolved before dismissal.

EXTRACELLULAR FLUID VOLUME EXCESS

Definition

ECFVE is increased fluid retention in the intravascular and interstitial spaces. Sodium and water retention in the same proportion is referred to as iso-osmolar fluid volume excess. The serum sodium level may be within the normal range even though the actual sodium level is increased because of excess water retention.

Incidence

ECFVE frequently occurs in heart disease when there is pump failure. Excessive fluid volume and coronary insufficiency due to heart pump failure usually lead to congestive heart failure.

Etiology

ECFVE usually results from an increase in the total body sodium content. Causes of ECFVE include heart failure, renal disorders, cirrhosis of the liver, increased ingestion of foods containing high amounts of sodium such as packaged foods, excessive tap water enemas, and excessive amounts of intravenous fluids containing sodium.

Risk Factors

Clients with heart, kidney, or liver disorders are prone to the development of sodium and water retention. Likewise, clients with hyperaldosteronism, with Cushing's syndrome, and using glucocorticoids are at increased risk. Other risk factors include the use of hypotonic fluids to irrigate nasogastric tubes. Men who have undergone transurethral resection of the prostate and have a sodium-free irrigation during and after surgery are also at increased risk.

Preventive measures may be simple, such as decreasing salt intake or initiating medical treatment with digoxin and diuretics.

Pathophysiology

With a fluid volume excess (fluid overload), the fluid pressure is even greater than usual at the arterial end of the capillary. Fluid is pushed into the tissue spaces with greater force because venous pressure also exceeds oncotic pressure. Peripheral and pulmonary edema may result (Fig. 14–4*A*). As the fluid pressure increases in the tissues, it also increases in the left ventricle, which

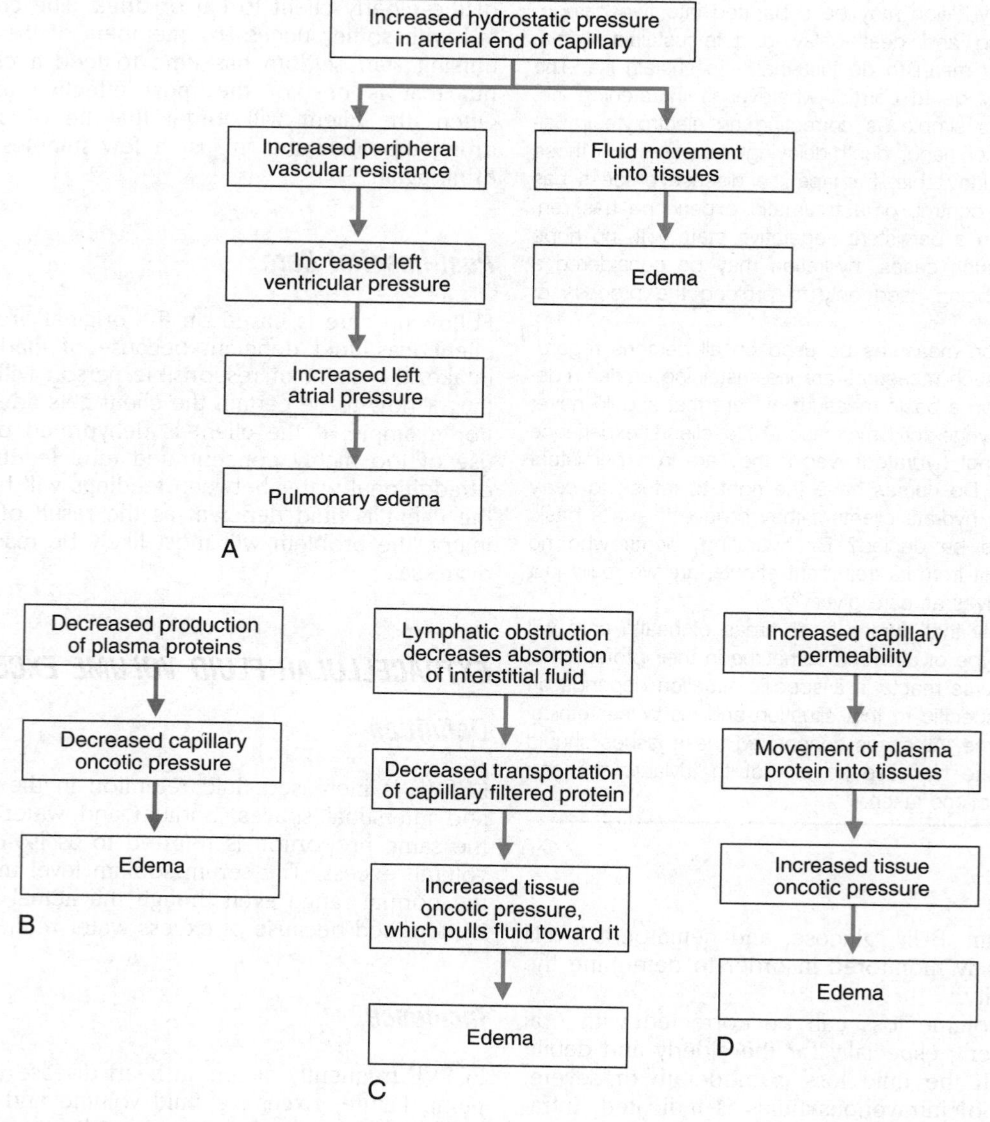

▲ **Figure 14–4**

Mechanisms of edema formation. *A*, Fluid overload. *B*, Decreased serum and albumin. *C*, Lymphatic obstruction. *D*, Tissue injury.

increases pressure in the left atrium. From the atrium, fluid will be forced backward across the alveolar-capillary membrane of the lungs, resulting in pulmonary edema. Pulmonary edema is commonly seen when the left side of the heart is distended and fails to pump adequately. If the right side of the heart fails, peripheral edema occurs through the same process. Left-sided heart failure leads to right-sided failure (and vice versa), so both pulmonary and peripheral edema may exist simultaneously.

When fluid overload results from renal disorders, there is a decrease in sodium and water excretion. Fluid volume rises, and the heart again must compensate for the increasing pressures; heart failure can result.

In clients with cirrhosis of the liver, the serum protein and albumin levels are decreased; therefore, the oncotic pressure is decreased in the vascular fluids, which results in less fluid reabsorption from the tissue spaces. Peripheral edema and ascites result (Fig. 14-4*B*).

When lymphatic channels are obstructed, tissue oncotic pressure rises and leads to edema (Fig. 14-4*C*). Edema due to increased capillary permeability is discussed in Chapters 18 and 71.

Congestive heart failure that is not corrected leads to kidney and liver failure that may be fatal. Multiple organ failures cause body water retention in massive amounts (anasarca), which is incompatible with life.

Clinical Manifestations

Some obvious indicators of severe fluid volume excess include dyspnea, engorged neck and hand veins, a bounding pulse, moist crackles in the lungs, and edema of the extremities. Table 14-2 lists the clinical manifestations with pathophysiologic bases of fluid volume excess.

DIAGNOSTIC ASSESSMENT

With fluid volume excess or fluid overload, concentration of solutes such as sodium is diluted. Reduced concentration of solutes lowers the serum osmolality

TABLE 14-2. Clinical Manifestations of Extracellular Fluid Volume Excess and Their Pathophysiologic Basis

Clinical Manifestation	Pathophysiologic Basis
Respiratory Manifestations	
Constant, irritating cough	Fluid accumulation in the alveolar sacs due to hypervolemia
Dyspnea	Due to fluid congestion in lungs
Crackles in lungs	Alveoli are congested with fluid owing to increased hydrostatic pressure
Cyanosis	A late symptom of pulmonary edema that results from impaired oxygen transport due to the capillaries being filled with fluid
Cardiovascular Manifestations	
Neck vein engorgement in semi-Fowler's position	Due to fluid overload and delayed right-sided heart emptying/filling
Hand vein engorgement	Due to peripheral vascular fluid overload
Bounding pulse, elevated blood pressure	Due to peripheral vascular fluid overload
S_3 gallop	Due to delayed ventricular filling and overdistention of ventricles from rapid filling during early diastole
Pitting edema of the lower extremities	Osmotic pressure in the venous end of the capillary exceeds interstitial pressure and fluid cannot return to the bloodstream
Sacral edema	Dependent edema in the supine client occurs in the sacral hollow rather than in the feet and legs, because the sacrum is the lowest place on the body
Weight gain	Due to fluid retention; for every 2.2 pounds gained, 1 L body fluid is retained
Neurologic Manifestations	
Change in level of consciousness	Malaise, confusion, headache, and lethargy are due to cerebral edema
Laboratory Findings	
Serum osmolality <275 mOsm/kg	Indicates a diluted body fluid in which there are fewer solutes in proportion to the water volume
Serum sodium <135 mEq/L–>145 mEq/L (low, normal, or high value)	Depending on the amount of sodium retention or water retention, the serum sodium level may be normal, decreased, or elevated
Decreased hematocrit	Due to hemodilution
Specific gravity below 1.010	Solvent in the urine exceeds solute

value to less than 275 mOsm/kg. Clients gain weight as a result of the excess fluid volume.

Medical Management

Diagnosis is determined by a clinical history of contributing and causative factors, drug history, signs and symptoms of fluid overload, and laboratory findings. The presence of pulmonary edema is a medical emergency requiring immediate interventions to prevent further respiratory distress.

PHARMACOLOGIC MANAGEMENT

Loop and potassium-wasting diuretics and a digitalis preparation are frequently prescribed for the treatment of ECFVE. These potent diuretics cause potassium to be excreted along with the sodium and water. To preserve potassium, a combination of potassium-wasting and potassium-sparing diuretics is frequently prescribed.

Digoxin, a digitalis preparation, is ordered to increase the force of myocardial contraction or to slow the heart rate if heart failure is the cause of ECFVE.

DIETARY MANAGEMENT

A low-sodium diet is prescribed in order to reduce fluid retention. Low-sodium diets are discussed later in this chapter.

Nursing Management

ASSESSMENT

Frequent assessments of breath sounds, palpation of the lower extremities for pitting edema, observation for hand and neck vein engorgement, and changes in vital signs are used to determine the presence of a fluid volume excess. When checking for neck vein engorgement, the nurse should note whether the jugular vein remains engorged when the client is in a semi-Fowler's position. Engorgement of neck veins in this position may indicate fluid overload. To check for hand vein engorgement, lower the hand until the peripheral veins are engorged. Then raise the hand above the level of the heart and observe the amount of time it takes for the veins to flatten. If the veins do not flatten within 3 to 5 seconds, fluid overload should be suspected.

Serum electrolyte values should be checked for abnormalities when the client is receiving diuretics. If the client is taking digoxin and a potassium-wasting diuretic, the client should be observed for signs and symptoms of digitalis toxicity and hypokalemia.

NURSING INTERVENTION

Nursing Diagnosis: Fluid Volume Excess R/T congestive heart failure, renal failure, or hypervolemia.

Planning: Expected Outcomes. The client's fluid balance will be improved, as evidenced by absence of dyspnea, clear chest sounds, absence of dependent edema, flat neck veins, peripheral vein emptying in 3 to 5 seconds, decreased body weight, and urine output exceeding intake.

Implementation. Vital signs should be monitored for bounding pulse or an elevated blood pressure every 4 to 8 hours. Auscultate breath sounds every 4 to 8 hours for crackles, noting changes and the location of adventitious sounds. Notify the physician if there is an increase in crackles. Assess for neck vein engorgement every 8 hours. Monitor daily weights. Edema does not usually occur unless there are 3 L or more of excess fluids. Intake and output should be evaluated every 4 to 8 hours in severe fluid excess, every shift in moderate levels of fluid excess. Assess for changes in level of consciousness. Palpate the lower extremities and sacrum for pitting edema each morning.

Monitor laboratory values for changes. Pertinent values include serum osmolarity, sodium level, hematocrit, potassium, and specific gravity of urine.

Fluid and sodium restrictions may be necessary. Instruct the client about the fluid restriction and the rationale for it. Be certain to include fluids on meal trays as part of the total fluids. The nurse should work with the dietician in planning for fluid restrictions. Oral medications should be scheduled at the time meals are eaten (as is possible); this will decrease the chance of extra fluids being used to swallow medications. Provide very cold fluids rather than warm or hot liquids, because this will decrease the sensation of thirst. Offer oral care frequently. When generalized edema is present, skin care is important for preventing pressure ulcers.

EVALUATION

The client's improvement should be assessed following every shift. Revisions in the plan of care may be required.

Modification of Plan of Care for the Elderly

The elderly client commonly develops ECFVE owing to the many other diseases that are present, such as congestive heart failure. In general, the interventions are the same except that the elderly client responds more slowly to them. The potential for drug-drug interaction should be assessed before any therapy is begun.

Post-hospital Care

DISCHARGE TEACHING

If the client is being dismissed on a low-sodium diet, the nurse should review the foods allowed on that diet. Canned foods should be avoided; fresh and frozen foods are permissible. The client (or person who does the cooking) should be taught to read the labels on food, if sodium level is not evident. The nurse should also ask if the client drinks softened water, which is high in sodium. The client may need to obtain water from another source.

EXTRACELLULAR FLUID VOLUME SHIFT: THIRD SPACE FLUID

Definition

A fluid volume shift is basically a change in the location of extracellular fluid between the intravascular and the interstitial spaces. There are two types of fluid shifts: (1) vascular fluid to interstitial space and (2) interstitial fluid to vascular fluid space. Fluid that shifts into the interstitial space and remains there is referred to as third space fluid. Third space fluid occurs in tissue injury from altered capillary permeability (e.g., inflammation, traumatic injury) and from increased vascular fluid volumes. Increased vascular fluid volume appears in the abdomen (ascites), pleural cavity, peritoneal cavity, and pericardial sac. Third space fluid is physiologically useless because it does *not* circulate to provide nutrients to cells.

Incidence

The incidence of third-space fluid shifts has not been recorded.

Etiology

Clinical causes of fluid shift from the vascular to the interstitial spaces may be a simple blister or sprain. Causes of massive fluid shifts from the vascular to interstitial spaces include crushing injuries, extensive burns, perforated peptic ulcer, intestinal obstruction, lymphatic obstruction, and large venous thrombosis. Pleural and pericardial fluid shifts are secondary to inflammatory responses to infectious, noninfectious, and autoimmune disorders.

Risk Factors

Clients at risk of third space fluids are those who have sustained major trauma (e.g., car accidents with major tissue injury) or had major surgery.

Pathophysiology

Tissue injury causes the release of histamine and bradykinin, which increases capillary permeability, allowing fluid, protein, and other solutes to shift into the interstitial spaces. There are two phases of fluid shift associated with tissue injury. The first phase is the fluid shift from vascular to interstitial spaces leading to a fluid volume deficit (hypovolemia) (Fig. 14–4*D*). The second phase is the shift from the interstitial to the vascular space leading to a fluid volume excess (hypervolemia). In the case of burns, the fluid shifts out of the vessels into the injured tissue spaces as well as normal (unburned) tissue. After 24 to 72 hours, the capillary permeability is restored, and fluid leaves the tissue spaces and returns to the vascular space. Adequate renal function is needed to excrete the excess fluid. Renal insufficiency may result in a fluid overload or hypervolemia. As the injured cell wall stabilizes, fluid is returned to the vascular spaces; a fluid overload may result without adequate kidney function. If renal function is normal in the second phase, the urine output may be as high as 3000 ml a day.

During the first phase of a fluid shift, severe hypovolemia may lead to vascular collapse and death. The fluid overload occurring during the second phase of a fluid shift may result in heart failure. If third spacing of fluids is due to major tissue damage, the cellular components (especially potassium) may also enter the vascular fluids and become toxic.

Clinical Manifestations

Clinical manifestations of a fluid shift from the vascular to the interstitial spaces are similar to the signs and symptoms of shock. Typical clinical manifestations include skin pallor, cold extremities, weak and rapid pulse, hypotension, oliguria, and decreased levels of consciousness. If the fluid is obstructing an organ, nerve, or vessel, other clinical manifestations may be noted. For example, bowel sounds may change character throughout the abdomen; extremities may become pale, cool, and pulseless.

When the fluid returns to the blood vessels, the clinical manifestations are similar to those of fluid overload. Signs may include a bounding pulse, crackles, engorgement of peripheral and jugular veins, and an increased blood pressure.

DIAGNOSTIC ASSESSMENT

Laboratory results may indicate an elevated hematocrit in relation to the hemoglobin and elevated BUN. Later, after fluids return to the bloodstream, laboratory results may indicate a decreased hematocrit and BUN. Other abnormal findings that may be seen depend on the area of the body affected.

Medical Management

Medical treatment begins with the determination of the cause of the fluid volume shift. When hypovolemia results from tissue injury such as burns or crush injury, a large volume of intravenous (iso-osmolar) fluid administration is required. The amount of fluid infusion may be three times greater than the urinary output. Generally, fluids are titrated for maintenance of an adequate blood pressure, PCWP, and urine output. If replacement is too overzealous, a fluid overload could occur. During the second phase, fluid administration and intake may need to be limited because of fluid influx from the tissue spaces to the vessels.

If the third spacing of fluid has occurred as a result of other processes, such as pericarditis and bowel obstruction, the fluid may have to be removed in order for the organ to retain its function (e.g., pericentesis).

Nursing Management

Shocklike symptoms are frequently present, so the client's vital signs should be assessed every hour to every 8 hours (depending on the condition of the client). If fluid loss is to the peritoneum (ascites) or extremities (peripheral edema), the fluid shift is slower, and changes in the vital signs are usually subtle.

Intravenous fluid replacement needs to be monitored. If fluids are administered too rapidly, hypervolemia (fluid overload) may occur. Frequent checks for chest crackles, difficulty in breathing, and neck vein engorgement are essential to prevent pulmonary edema with fluid volume excess. The abdominal girth of clients with ascites should be measured every 8 hours. If the extremities are involved, measure the circumference of the extremity and peripheral pulses every hour. The level of consciousness should be monitored and precautions taken for seizures. Frequent skin care to edematous areas during fluid shift is essential to prevent skin breakdown. As the fluid shifts back with the repair of tissue damage, intravenous fluid replacement is decreased.

Urine output should be monitored every hour to ensure at least 25 ml per hour. Urine output is usually reduced after tissue injury because of decreased renal circulation and the fluid shift into the injured tissue spaces. Three to five days after tissue injury, fluid returns to the circulation and excess fluid is excreted by the kidneys unless there is impaired renal function. The serum levels of BUN and ammonia should be monitored in clients with ascites.

A comparison of the fluids administered with the urine output and vital signs is a common practice in monitoring progress.

INTRACELLULAR FLUID VOLUME EXCESS: WATER INTOXICATION

Overview

Hypo-osmolar disorders result from either water excess or solute deficit and are mainly due to sodium loss. In water excess, the number of solutes is normal but diluted by excessive water. In solute deficit, the amount of water is normal, but there are too few particles per liter of water. In both cases, hypo-osmolality of vascular fluids exists and cellular swelling occurs.

Although intracellular fluid volume excess (ICFVE) is not as common a type of fluid imbalance as ECFVD and ECFVE, it presents a serious health problem if it is unrecognized and untreated. The most common cause of ICFVE is the administration of excessive amounts of hypo-osmolar intravenous fluids such as 0.45 per cent saline or 5 per cent dextrose in water. ICFVE may occur in clients who receive continuous D_5W intravenous fluids, those with brain injury or disease causing an increased antidiuretic hormone (ADH) production that increases water reabsorption from the renal tubules, or those who are elderly and consume excessive amounts of tap water without adequate nutrient intake. Increased ADH production may also follow the stress of surgery, pain, and narcotic use. Such reactions are described as secretion of inappropriate antidiuretic hormone (SIADH). Early administration of intravenous fluids containing some sodium chloride can prevent SIADH. Saline solutions increase the osmolality of vascular fluid and prevent hypo-osmolarity.

Hypo-osmolar fluids move by osmosis to maintain fluid equilibrium, forcing fluids to move from the lesser concentration (in the vessels) to the higher concentration (in the cells). Unfortunately, too much fluid accumulates in the cells, causing cellular edema. The cerebral cells are usually involved first, and a continued state of ICFVE may result in cerebral edema.

Common characteristics of ICFVE are headaches and behavioral changes (apprehension, irritability, disorientation, confusion), which are early signs of increased intracranial pressure. Pupillary changes and decreased motor and sensory function occur as pressure continues to build. Vital sign changes typify the late stages of increased intracranial pressure and include bradycardia, elevated blood pressure, widened pulse pressure, and increased respirations. The urine output may be normal or decreased with water intoxication. Table 14–3 lists the clinical manifestations of ICFVE and their pathophysiologic bases. The serum sodium level is decreased because of hemodilution.

Management

Treatment should begin when early signs of increased intracranial pressure are noted. ICFVE is treated by adding solutes to intravenous fluids. The use of D_5/0.45 per cent NaCl will help to correct ICFVE when the cause is water excess. Oral fluids such as juices or soft drinks should be given in addition to water and ice chips.

The nurse should have a high index of suspicion for clients who have received excessive amounts of D_5W or tap water or who have had a recent operation, pain, stress, and central nervous system (CNS) drug depressants. Notify the physician if the client's sensorium changes from baseline assessment.

Reflexes and pupillary response should be assessed. Intravenous therapy should be monitored every hour. Offer fluids containing solutes (juices, colas, broth) every hour if permitted. Monitor for changes in vital signs every hour to every 8 hours depending on client's condition. Monitor intake and output every hour to every 8 hours.

An increase in urine output is needed to decrease ICFVE; polyuria indicates that fluid has shifted to the vascular space from where it can be excreted. The

TABLE 14-3. Clinical Manifestations of Intracellular Fluid Volume Excess and Their Pathophysiologic Basis

Clinical Manifestation	Pathophysiologic Basis
Headaches, nausea, vomiting	CNS changes due to ICFVE cause increased intracranial pressure; cerebral cells absorb hypo-osmolar fluid more quickly than other cells do
Pupillary changes	Pressure on the third cranial nerve from increased cranial pressure
Behavioral changes: progressive apprehension, irritability, disorientation, confusion, drowsiness, decreased coordination	Swollen cerebral cells cause behavioral changes
Decreased muscle strength, unequal grasp, pronation drift	Cerebellar or basal ganglia swelling
Weight gain	Increased weight results from excess water retention
Severe CNS symptoms	Severe CNS changes occur when water excess progressively increases intracranial pressure and interferes with cell function
Vital signs: bradycardia with an increased systolic blood pressure (widened pulse pressure); increased respirations; neuroexcitability (muscle twitching); Babinski's response; flaccidity; projectile vomiting; papilledema; delirium; convulsions, coma	Vital signs changes are an ominous indicator of increased intracranial pressure and herniation of the brain stem
Laboratory Findings	
Serum sodium level <125 mEq/L	Low serum sodium level associated with hypo-osmolality
Decreased hematocrit	Hemodilution; ECF excess often accompanies ICF excess

client's weight should be checked daily to measure fluid gain or loss.

Administer prescribed antiemetics as needed to allow food and fluids to be ingested.

Safety measures are necessary when the client displays behavioral changes (confusion, disorientation). The bed should be kept in low position, and bedside rails should be raised. The client should be closely observed for protection from injury. An oral airway and suction equipment should be kept at the bedside in the event of seizures. The airway should be inserted only during the aura phase, never during the actual seizure. The seizuring client should be turned to the side, and the nurse should remain at the bedside. (See also Chapter 30 for care of the client during a seizure.)

INTRACELLULAR FLUID VOLUME DEFICIT

Hypernatremia and dehydration can become so severe that the cells become dehydrated. This condition is relatively rare, but if it does occur, the client develops symptoms of thirst, fever, oliguria and CNS changes (e.g., confusion, coma, and cerebral hemorrhage).

▼ ELECTROLYTES

Electrolytes are substances found in extracellular and intracellular fluid that dissociate into electrically charged particles known as ions. *Cations* are ions carrying a positive charge, and *anions* are ions carrying a negative charge. The positively charged electrolytes (cations) are sodium, potassium, calcium, and magnesium; the negatively charged electrolytes (anions) are chloride, phosphate, and bicarbonate. The electrolytes that are most plentiful in the cells are potassium, magnesium, phosphate, and proteinate. The most plentiful ions in the ECF are sodium, calcium, chloride, and bicarbonate. The principal cation in the ICF is potassium, and the principal cation in the ECF is sodium (Table 14-4).

TABLE 14-4. Distribution of Electrolytes in Body Compartment

Electrolyte	Extracellular Fluid (mEq/L)	Intracellular Fluid (mEq/L)
Cations		
Sodium	142	10
Potassium	5	156
Calcium	5	4
Magnesium	2	26
Total	154	196
Anions		
Bicarbonate	24	12
Chloride	104	4
Phosphate	2	40-95
Proteins	16	54
Other anions	8	31-86
Total	154	196*

From McCance, K., & Huether, S. (1990). *Pathophysiology. The basic biologic basis for disease in adults and children.* St. Louis. C. V. Mosby.

* This is the average value.

TABLE 14-5. Concentration of Electrolytes in Body Fluids

Fluid	Na^+ (mEq/L)	K^+ (mEq/L)	Cl^- (mEq/L)	HCO_3^- (mEq/L)
Saliva	33	20	34	0
Gastric juice*	60	9	84	0
Bile	149	5	101	45
Pancreatic juice	141	5	77	92
Ileal fluid	129	11	116	29
Cecal fluid	80	21	48	22
Cerebrospinal fluid	141	3	127	23
Sweat	45	5	58	0

From Smith, L. H., & Thier, S. O. (1981). *Pathophysiology: The biological principles of disease.* Philadelphia: W. B. Saunders. Adapted from Arieff, A. (1972). In M. H. Maxwell & C. R. Kleeman (Eds.), *Clinical disorders of fluid and electrolyte metabolism* (2nd ed.). New York: McGraw-Hill.

* The Cl concentration exceeds the Na^+, K^+ concentration by 15 mEq/L in gastric juice. This largely represents the secretion of H^+ by the parietal cells.

Electrolytes have major influences on (1) body water regulation, (2) acid-base regulation, (3) enzyme reactions, and (4) neuromuscular activity. Sodium concentration in the extracellular fluid assists in the maintenance of fluid balance. Sodium, potassium, chloride, bicarbonate, phosphate, and proteinate ions regulate acid-base balance within the body. The cations are necessary for the transmission of nerve impulses and stimulation of muscle activity. Concentration of electrolytes in various body fluids is shown in Table 14-5.

Because intracellular levels of electrolytes cannot be measured, all values for electrolytes are expressed as serum values. Serum values for electrolytes can be expressed as mEq/L or mg/dl. Both values are given in this text. Values reported as mEq/L can be converted to mg/dl by multiplying by 1.2.

▼ Sodium Homeostatic Mechanisms

Sodium balance is regulated by afferent and efferent mechanisms. Afferent sensing mechanisms in nerve endings recognize changes in sodium intake and extracellular fluid volume by sensing an increase or decrease in pressure. Afferent mechanisms are found in the atria, carotid sinus, liver, and kidneys. In addition, there are central nervous system receptors that respond to changes in the sodium concentration in the cerebrospinal fluid.

Efferent mechanisms include the glomerular filtration rate in the kidney. The renal glomerulus is a capillary system and, therefore, is subject to the effects of Starling forces. Blood enters the glomerulus and is driven by the systemic blood pressure. The pressure of the blood entering the glomeruli is high and favors filtration across the membrane. Blood proteins remaining in the vessel exert oncotic pressure to draw fluids back into the vessel. The glomerulus filters 1000 mEq of sodium every hour, and about 99 per cent of this is reabsorbed back by the renal tubules. Considering the enormous quantities of sodium that are normally handled by the kidney, any alteration in renal function can have an impact on sodium homeostasis.

Hormonal factors also control sodium homeostasis. These mechanisms include renin-angiotensin-aldosterone, prostaglandins, kallikrein, and natriuretic hormones. Renin is a hormone excreted in response to hypotension. Renin production results in increased angiotensin; angiotensin, in turn, increases aldosterone production for the adrenal cortex. Aldosterone stimulates net sodium reabsorption across the tubule.

Prostaglandins are secreted by the kidney and stimulate the production of renin. These hormones also maintain renal blood flow during periods of reduced blood volume. Kallikreins are high-molecular-weight proteins produced by the distal convoluted tubule and secrete kinin. Kinin is a potent renal vasodilator and increases renal excretion of sodium. The function of natriuretic hormone is not fully understood. It appears that this hormone plays a role in renal adaptation to uremia by decreasing sodium reabsorption.

▼ Sodium Imbalances

A sodium imbalance occurs when there is either a decrease in sodium or an increase in sodium concentration in the plasma. A sodium deficit is called *hyponatremia* and occurs when serum sodium levels are less than 135 mEq/L. Sodium excess is called *hypernatremia* and occurs when the serum sodium levels are greater than 145 mEq/L.

HYPONATREMIA

Definition

Hyponatremia is a serum sodium level below 135 mEq/L.

Incidence

Hyponatremia is said to be one of the most common electrolyte disorders, occurring in a wide variety of illnesses.

Etiology

The causes of hyponatremia usually are associated with the fluid volume status. Hyponatremia may occur when the total body water (TBW) is decreased. Four types of hyponatremia reactions that may occur are hypovolemic hyponatremia, euvolemic hyponatremia, hypervolemic hyponatremia, and redistributive hyponatremia. When sodium loss is greater than water loss, hypovolemic hyponatremia occurs. Euvolemic hyponatremia re-

TABLE 14-6. Pathophysiologic Factors in Hyponatremia (Serum Sodium < 135 mEq/L)

Etiology	Total Body Water	Body Sodium
Hypovolemic hyponatremia	↓	↓↓
Euvolemic hyponatremia	↑	Normal
Hypervolemic hyponatremia	↑↑	↑ or normal
Redistributive hyponatremia	Normal	Normal

sults when the TBW is moderately increased and the total body sodium remains at a normal level. Hypervolemic hyponatremia results when there is a greater increase in TBW than in total body sodium. In redistributive hyponatremia, there is no change in TBW or total body sodium; there is merely a water shift between the intracellular and extracellular compartments relative to the sodium concentration. Table 14-6 shows the relationship of total body water to body sodium with the various types of hyponatremia.

Hyponatremia may develop from SIADH. SIADH may follow many forms of drug therapy including chemotherapy, phenothiazines, morphine, and barbiturates.

Hyponatremia may also result from the kidney's inability to excrete sufficiently diluted urine. Normally, when hyponatremia and hypo-osmolality occur, diuresis (increased urine excretion) follows to promote sodium and water balance. Table 14-7 lists clinical conditions and disorders that may cause hyponatremia.

Risk Factors

Risk factors leading to hyponatremia are more prominent in the elderly, infants, and small children because of the variations in TBW. Clinical conditions such as vomiting and diarrhea or the diagnosis of cardiac and renal disorders increases the risk of hyponatremia. Clients with Addison's disease are at risk. Clients who are NPO, NPO and receiving intravenous solutions, and on potent diuretics without sodium replacement are also at risk. Early recognition of the high-risk clients may prevent a marked hyponatremic state.

Hyponatremia can also occur in healthy clients. Clients at risk include those who lose fluids through excessive perspiration and do not restore the lost sodium through fluid intake. Athletes and outdoor laborers are included in this category.

Pathophysiology

As the ECF concentration of sodium decreases, the sodium concentration gradient (difference) between the ECF and ICF also decreases. This hypo-osmolarity can lead to intracellular edema. The water in the ECF moves by osmosis into the cells. These changes also mean that there is less sodium to move across the excitable membrane, which usually results in delayed membrane depolarization. Excitable tissues vary in their response to decreased sodium; the most sensitive to changes are the CNS cells, leading to cerebral edema. Generally, the clinical manifestations reflect the decreased excitability or irritability of the membranes. The total body sodium and the ECF volume measures are used to categorize the hyponatremic state.

If the hyponatremic state and body fluid volume disorders are not corrected, potassium, calcium, chloride, and bicarbonate electrolyte imbalances may occur. Uncorrected hypovolemic hyponatremia may result in shock from continued ECF volume loss. This severe hyponatremic state leads to neurologic changes varying from confusion to convulsion and coma. A hypervolemic hyponatremic state, if not corrected, results in ECF volume excess and edema.

Clinical Manifestations

Clinical manifestations of hyponatremia vary with the cause and type of fluid volume imbalance present. A sodium deficit may occur in the presence of decreased, normal, or increased total body sodium and water. An assessment of the body fluid volume is helpful in the

TABLE 14-7. Causes of Hyponatremia

Etiology	Clinical Conditions and Disorders
Hypovolemic hyponatremia	Renal loss of sodium from diuretic use, diabetic glycosuria, aldosterone deficiency, intrinsic renal disease Extrarenal loss of sodium from vomiting, diarrhea, increased sweating, burns
Euvolemic hyponatremia	Sodium deficit resulting from syndrome of inappropriate secretion of antidiuretic hormone (SIADH) or the continuous secretion of ADH due to pain, emotion, medications
Hypervolemic hyponatremia	Edematous disorders resulting in sodium deficits: congestive heart failure, cirrhosis of the liver, nephrotic syndrome, acute and chronic renal failure
Redistributive hyponatremia	Pseudohyponatremia, hyperglycemia, hyperlipidemia

TABLE 14–8. Clinical Manifestations of Hyponatremia and Their Pathophysiologic Basis

Clinical Manifestation	Pathophysiologic Basis
Gastrointestinal Manifestations	
Nausea, vomiting, diarrhea, hyperactive bowel sounds, abdominal cramps	Sodium is abundant in the gastrointestinal tract Loss of gastrointestinal secretions causes a sodium loss
Cardiovascular Manifestations	
Decrease in diastolic blood pressure, tachycardia, profound orthostatic hypotension, weak pulse	Losses of sodium and water decrease the circulating fluid volume and may result in shocklike symptoms
Elevated blood pressure; full, rapid pulse	Dilutional hyponatremia with excessive fluid volume increases circulating fluids
Pulmonary Manifestations	
Changes in rate of respirations	Due to changes in CNS
Adventitious lung sounds	Fluid overload, congestive heart failure
Neurologic Manifestations	
Headache, apprehension, lethargy, confusion, slowed problem solving, flat affect, diminished muscle tone in the extremities, decreased deep tendon reflexes, weakness and tremor	Diluted body fluids move into the brain cells, affecting both cognition and reflexes; excitable membranes are less responsive to stimuli
Integumentary Manifestations	
Dry skin; pale, dry mucous membranes	Decreased interstitial fluids
Laboratory Findings	
Serum sodium <135 mEq/L	Serum sodium level of <135 mEq/L results in hyponatremia; symptoms become apparent when the serum sodium is <125 mEq/L
Urine sodium <40 mEq/L	Body sodium losses result in a compensatory decrease in urinary excretion of sodium
Serum osmolality <275 mOsm/kg	Sodium losses result in a decreased concentration of sodium in body fluids

determination of a sodium imbalance. With cardiac, renal, and liver disease, the total body sodium is usually high, although the serum sodium level may appear normal or low. In such instances, there is generally a greater increase in TBW than the sodium indicates.

A serum sodium level of less than 115 mEq/L will cause severe neurologic changes such as confusion or convulsions and may result in death due to excessive water shift to the intracellular compartment. When the serum sodium decreases slowly or is greater than 125 mEq/L, signs and symptoms may not be apparent.

With a loss of body fluids and sodium, the heart rate increases as a compensatory mechanism to overcome fluid and sodium losses. Cellular swelling causes neurologic and behavioral changes. Clinical manifestations and their pathologic basis are presented in Table 14–8.

DIAGNOSTIC ASSESSMENT

Diagnosis is based on the combination of clinical manifestations and serum laboratory values. Acute hyponatremia is a serum sodium concentration below 120 mEq/L with CNS manifestations.

Medical Management

Medical management begins by attempting to determine the cause of the hyponatremia and correcting it. The goal of treatment is to correct the body water osmolarity and therefore restore cell volume by raising the ratio of sodium to water in the ECF. The increased ECF osmolarity draws water from the cells and therefore decreases cellular edema. If the client has hyponatremia due to fluid volume excess, fluids will be restricted to allow the sodium to regain balance. If the serum sodium level declines below 125 mEq/L, sodium replacement is needed.

Rapid elevation of serum sodium concentrations to levels greater than 125 mEq/L is hazardous. Loss of fluids in and around the brain and shifting of electrolytes (such as potassium) are homeostatic mechanisms that prevent damage to the brain cells. The rapid correction of serum sodium levels may increase fluid volume levels and can result in damage to the CNS.

PHARMACOLOGIC MANAGEMENT

With moderate hyponatremia, 125 mEq/L, intravenous normal saline solution (0.9 per cent NaCl) or lactated Ringer's solution may be ordered. When the serum sodium level is 115 mEq/L or less, a concentrated saline solution such as 3 per cent NaCl is generally indicated. The administration of hypertonic solutions is irritating to peripheral veins. The client must be closely monitored for overhydration or hypernatremia when 3 per cent saline solution is administered. This is especially true for the client with a cardiac problem such as congestive heart failure or renal disease.

Many times, normal saline is administered in conjunction with furosemide. The diuretic increases urinary sodium loss and therefore reduces the risk of ECF volume expansion. Moreover, the diuresis induced by furosemide has much less sodium than does the ECF, which raises the serum sodium levels.

Drug therapy for hyponatremia from SIADH includes agents that antagonize ADH, such as demeclocycline and lithium.

DIETARY MANAGEMENT

A balanced diet is usually adequate therapy for mild hyponatremia (126 to 135 mEq/L). More severe hyponatremia may require sodium replacement. Foods high in sodium are listed in Box 14-2. If the client has hyponatremia due to excess fluids, a fluid-restricted diet may be prescribed. Fluids may be restricted to 800 to 1000 ml/day.

Nursing Management

ASSESSMENT

Nursing assessment focuses on data collection related to health problems and signs and symptoms manifested by the client with hyponatremia. The nurse should obtain a history of the cause of hyponatremia such as vomiting, diarrhea, and decreased intake of sodium. Likewise, a history of Addison's disease, steroid use, cerebrovascular accident, and renal, cardiac, or hepatic failure should be noted. Assessment should include checking serum sodium levels and estimating the serum osmolality. It is important to remember that in hyponatremic conditions such as hypervolemic hyponatremia, serum sodium levels may reveal normal to low readings. This misleading reading occurs in response to medical conditions that cause water to be retained in greater quantities than sodium.

The usual medications and over-the-counter medications should be noted. The elderly are especially prone to drug-drug interactions that may alter sodium balance. Urine output as well as recent fluctuations in body weight should be assessed. A diet history should be assessed to ascertain the amount of sodium consumed.

The client and family should be asked about behavioral changes, headaches, and increased sleepiness.

Physical assessment should include height and weight, with a calculation of ideal body weight for body frame. Turgor and peripheral vein filling time should be noted.

Box 14-2. Common Food Sources of Sodium

Sodium Amounts in Selected Foods

Foods High in Sodium (Approximately 250 Mg per Serving)

Pasta
- Cold cereal, 1 oz
- Corn chips, 14 chips
- Instant hot cereal, ½ cup
- Potato chips, 14 chips

Cheeses
- Natural cheese, 1 oz
- Processed cheese, 1 oz
- Creamed cheese, ½ cup

Meats
- Sausage, 1 oz
- Luncheon meats, 1 oz
- Frankfurters, 1 oz
- Cooked bacon, 2 slices
- Ham, 1 oz

Convenience foods
- Pizza, 2 to 3 slices
- Pot pies, 8 oz
- Ravioli, canned, 8 oz
- Soups (canned/dehydrated), 1 cup

Foods Low in Sodium (Less Than 50 Mg per Serving)

Fruits/vegetables
- Fresh, fruits or canned, ½ cup
- Fresh, frozen, ½ cup

Pasta
- Unsalted pastas, ½ cup
- Oatmeal, cooked, 1 cup
- Popcorn (unsalted), 1 oz
- Puffed rice, 1 cup
- Shredded wheat, 1 biscuit

Meats
- Fresh meat, 1 oz
- Fresh chicken, 1 oz
- Fresh fish, 1 oz

Beverages

▼▼▼

Data from: Laquarta, I., & Gerlach, M. (1990). *Nutrition in clinical nursing*. Albany, New York: Delmar Publishers; and Burtis, G., et al. (1988). *Applied nutrition and diet therapy*. Philadelphia; W. B. Saunders.

NURSING INTERVENTION

Collaborative Problem. Hyponatremia R/T vomiting, diarrhea, gastric suctioning, burns, SIADH, or surgery.

Planning: Expected Outcomes. The nurse will monitor the client for sodium levels to return to 135 mEq/L or above, the reduction of factors contributing to the hyponatremia, fluid and electrolyte losses and replacement, and symptoms of fluid and sodium imbalance.

Implementation. The nurse should have a high index of suspicion for hyponatremia in clients who have been NPO or NPO without sodium replacement in intravenous fluids; with nausea, vomiting, or abdominal cramps; and with neurologic changes or changes in mucous membranes or skin turgor.

Vital signs should be checked every 4 to 8 hours. Monitor serum sodium and osmolality levels. A serum sodium level of less than 125 mEq/L indicates the need for prompt medical care. Estimation of the serum osmolality can be accomplished by doubling the serum sodium level.

Monitor the type and amount of fluid intake. Fluid intake, whether oral or intravenous, should include sodium. If the client is receiving 3 per cent saline solution intravenously, the nurse observes for signs and symptoms of hypervolemia such as dyspnea, chest crackles, and neck vein engorgement. The intravenous flow rate should be regulated with the aid of an intravenous pump to decrease the risk of hypervolemia.

Irrigate nasogastric tubes and wound sites with normal saline solution to prevent further sodium losses. Distilled or sterile water irrigations will increase sodium loss. Promote the intake of fluids containing sodium such as broth and juices. Minimize the intake of ice chips. Ice chips can be made from saline to reduce the intake of tap water.

Intake and output should be closely monitored; hourly assessments should be performed if the client is acutely ill. Daily weights should be obtained to monitor fluid balance. Plan for fluid restriction if the hyponatremia is due to fluid volume excess. Be certain to coordinate fluid restriction with the dietician and schedule medications at the time of meals, as possible. Very cold fluids should be offered, rather than hot or warm liquids because very cold fluids satisfy thirst more.

If the client is confused or agitated, the nurse needs to provide mechanisms to reorient the client as well as provide safety measures. Extraneous noise may aggravate the client's mental status and should be eliminated as much as possible. Side rails should be elevated and the bed kept in low position when the nurse is not providing direct care. Seizures may develop. The client should be protected from injury during the seizure and the airway maintained. Oral airways and padded tongue blades can be inserted during an aura phase, but not during an active seizure. If the client experiences a seizure, the nurse should turn the client to the side, to keep the airway patent and reduce the risk of aspiration, and stay with the client, noting the events during the actual seizure.

EVALUATION

The client's serum sodium levels should return to normal. If the client remains hyponatremic, the interventions may require revision.

HYPERNATREMIA

Definition

Hypernatremia is a serum sodium level over 145 mEq/L.

Incidence

Hypernatremia occurs in approximately 1 per cent of hospitalized clients and carries a high mortality rate regardless of whether it has an acute or chronic onset.

Etiology

Hypernatremia is usually associated with water loss or sodium gain. It can occur with an increased, decreased, or normal total body sodium and water. The underlying cause of hypernatremia is a TBW deficit relative to the total body sodium content, which results in hyperosmolality. Common conditions leading to hypernatremia include impaired thirst, solute or osmotic diuresis, or excessive losses of water through the kidneys or other routes.

Body fluid loss causing hypernatremia may be due to renal or extrarenal (gastrointestinal, skin) problems. Hypernatremia can be classified into three types: (1) hypovolemic hypernatremia in which TBW is greatly decreased relative to sodium (loss of hypotonic fluid); (2) euvolemic hypernatremia in which TBW is decreased relative to the normal total body sodium (sodium gains in excess of water gains); and (3) hypervolemic hypernatremia in which TBW is normal or near-normal relative to the increased total body sodium (essentially a pure water loss). Hypervolemic hypernatremia is the least common type of hypernatremia. Table 14–9 gives disorders and conditions that may contribute to the development of hypernatremia.

Clients with untreated diabetes insipidus do not secrete ADH; however, they tend to be only mildly hypernatremic. The thirst mechanism is intact and stimulates the client to drink water and fluids, which helps to balance water losses and hypernatremia. (Diabetes insipidus is fully discussed in Chapter 30.)

Risk Factors

Populations at risk for developing hypernatremia are infants, the elderly, and debilitated persons. A common factor for the development of hypernatremia in each of these groups is inadequate water intake in conjunction with decreased thirst (hypodipsia). These clients are also at great risk of hypernatremia due to either an

TABLE 14-9. Causes of Hypernatremia

Etiology	Clinical Conditions and Disorders
Hypovolemic hypernatremia	Renal losses: osmotic diuresis, severe hyperglycemia Extrarenal losses: profuse diaphoresis, decreased thirst, diarrhea occurring with inadequate volume replacement or fluid replacement with hyperosmolar solutions
Euvolemic hypernatremia	Excess fluid losses from the skin and lungs Hypodipsia in the elderly and infants Diabetes insipidus
Hypervolemic hypernatremia	Administration of concentrated saline solutions; hypertonic feedings, excess mineralocorticoids Accidental or intentional salt ingestions; commercially prepared soups and canned vegetables

excessive water loss or insufficient fluid replacement associated with a febrile illness, vomiting, or diarrhea. The client with uncontrolled diabetes mellitus and renal disease is at high risk.

Maintaining hydration for the infant, the elderly, or a debilitated client by offering fluids and monitoring intake and output will help prevent sodium and water imbalances. Clients with congestive heart failure and renal disorders may need to have their sodium intake restricted.

Pathophysiology

Hyperosmolality of ECF resulting from hypernatremia promotes a shift of water from the cells to the ECF by the process of osmosis in an attempt to maintain fluid homeostasis. Loss of water from the cells causes cellular dehydration. The sodium gradient is higher between the ECF and the ICF. More sodium is available to move across the excitable membrane. This change results in earlier membrane depolarization even with a smaller stimulus. With mild hypernatremia, almost all excitable tissues are excited more easily and are called "irritable." The CNS is affected the most by hypernatremia, followed by skeletal, cardiac, and smooth muscles. If the hypernatremia occurred slowly or occurs chronically, the brain develops idiogenic osmoles to prevent fluid shifts in and out of the brain cells. The pathophysiologic changes that relate to clinical manifestations of hypernatremia are explained in Table 14-10.

The cardiac system is sensitive to the increasing sodium levels. Calcium must move into the channel for cardiac muscle contraction. The sodium competes with calcium in the calcium channels (slow channels of the heart), which depresses myocardial contractility. Myocardial depolarization, however, occurs more easily with the increased sodium levels.

Generally, the body responds to increased sodium levels by suppressing the effects of aldosterone and ADH. These two mechanisms normally increase the renal blood flow and cause excretion of sodium and water. Therefore, in the event of hypernatremia, there is a problem that cannot be normalized by homeostatic mechanisms.

There is a high mortality rate for untreated acute and chronic hypernatremia. Neurologic manifestations and death can result from cellular dehydration. If the vascular volume decreases, the pulse rate increases and eventually the blood pressure drops. As hypernatremia progresses, convulsions or coma or both occur.

Clinical Manifestations

Because two thirds of the body water is intracellular, primary water losses tend to cause only modest effects on circulating blood volume. Rather, the clinical manifestations are produced by the shrinkage of brain cells that results from increases in ECF osmolarity.

Mild hypernatremia is usually asymptomatic, and early nonspecific symptoms such as polyuria initially, then oliguria, nausea, and vomiting, may be overlooked. Orthostatic hypotension also may be present. As hypernatremia progresses (sodium level >155 mEq/L), neurologic symptoms occur as the consequence of cellular dehydration. Severe hypernatremia in children can result in permanent brain damage from brain contraction.

In hypernatremic conditions, the skin and mucous membranes tend to be dry, the tongue is rough and dry, and the skin is flushed. In moderate hypernatremic states, restlessness and weakness may occur followed by agitation, disorientation, and confusion. Cardiac symptoms include tachycardia and decreasing blood pressure.

DIAGNOSTIC ASSESSMENT

Hypernatremia is determined by the clinical manifestations and laboratory findings presented in Table 14-10. Because chloride is the major ECF ion to balance sodium, the serum chloride level is also higher.

Medical Management

To decrease total body sodium and replace fluid loss, either a hypo-osmolar electrolyte solution (0.2 per cent or 0.45 per cent NaCl) or 5 per cent dextrose in water is administered. These solutions will not cause a con-

TABLE 14–10. Clinical Manifestations of Hypernatremia and Their Pathophysiologic Basis

Clinical Manifestation	Pathophysiologic Basis
Gastrointestinal Manifestations	
Anorexia, nausea, and vomiting	Fluid retention in gastric cells
Integumentary Manifestations	
Skin dry and flushed; mucous membranes dry and sticky	Decrease of interstitial fluid in tissues
Thirst; tongue dry and rough; body temperature elevated	Less interstitial fluids to cool body by evaporation
Neurologic Manifestations	
Restlessness, agitation, irritability, lethargy, stupor, coma	Neurologic symptoms are the result of cerebral cellular dehydration
Muscle twitching, tremor, hyperreflexia, seizures; rigid paralysis in late stages	Neuromuscular irritability
Cardiovascular Manifestations	
Tachycardia, hypotension or hypertension	Blood pressure relative to the type of hypernatremia. If hypovolemic, pressure will be decreased. If hypervolemic, pressure will be increased
Erratic heart rate and blood pressure dependent on fluid status	Myocardial depression as sodium ions compete with calcium ions in slow channels of heart
Renal Manifestations	
Oliguria, dark and concentrated	Compensatory mechanism
Laboratory Findings	
Serum sodium >145 mEq/L	Hypernatremia is present when serum sodium level is >145 mEq/L
Serum osmolality >295 mOsm/kg	Sodium is the major solute of fluid concentration; hypernatremia increases serum osmolality

siderable dilution of body sodium; instead, the serum sodium level will be gradually decreased. D_5W, when administered continuously, is considered to be a hypo-osmolar solution because the dextrose is metabolized quickly and only water remains. When 5 per cent dextrose solutions are given, they must be given slowly to prevent osmotic diuresis, which aggravates the hypertonic state.

Sometimes normal saline is used for the volume-depleted client to provide fluid resuscitation. The saline is hypotonic in comparison with the serum and, therefore, allows the sodium level to decrease slowly. If the serum sodium level is lowered too rapidly, fluid will shift from the vascular fluid into the cerebral cells, causing cerebral edema. A general rule of thumb is that water replacement be administered to reduce serum sodium levels not more than 2 mEq/L/hr for the first 48 hours.

PHARMACOLOGIC MANAGEMENT

Hypernatremia due to sodium excess may be treated with D_5W and a diuretic such as furosemide (Lasix). When hypernatremia is due to diabetes insipidus, desmopressin acetate (DDAVP) nasal spray is commonly used to slow diuresis. In the past, vasopressin oil nasal spray had been used. Vasopressin has a 4- to 6-hour duration; however, DDAVP controls urine output for 20 hours.

DIETARY MANAGEMENT

Dietary restrictions of sodium are useful in preventing hypernatremia in high-risk clients. Dietary restriction will not bring a high sodium level down to normal, however. Clients with renal disease may need sodium restricted to 500 to 2000 mg/day. Often fluids must also be restricted. Compliance with this degree of restriction is often difficult.

Clients with diabetes insipidus who are receiving antidiuretic medications must be taught to avoid excessive water intake.

Nursing Management

ASSESSMENT

The client should be assessed for usual clinical manifestations. Again the nurse should have a high index of suspicion for those high-risk clients (e.g., head-injured clients). A medication history should be used to assess for drugs that contain sodium, such as cough medicine and corticosteroids. Likewise, the diet history should be assessed for sodium consumption. Serum sodium levels should be checked, and the serum osmolality needs to be estimated.

The nurse should monitor the condition of the client's oral mucous membranes. Oral membrane assessment scores are very effective means of assessment (see Chapter 52).

NURSING INTERVENTION

Collaborative Problem. Hypernatremia R/T decreased thirst or excessive administration of salt solutions or impaired secretion of sodium and water.

Planning: Expected Outcomes. The nurse will monitor the client for response to intravenous fluid replacement of hypo-osmolar electrolyte solutions, absence of signs and symptoms of hypernatremia, and return of normal sodium levels.

Implementation. Water and fluids should be offered frequently to the elderly and clients with debilitating diseases in order to prevent body fluid loss and hypernatremia. However, increasing fluid intake in clients with congestive heart failure or severe renal disease is usually contraindicated. Encourage clients to drink decaffeinated fluids and to avoid alcohol. Caffeinated fluids and alcohol increase fluid loss, which can result in an increase in the serum sodium level.

Depending on the client's condition, vital signs should be assessed every 4 to 8 hours, and skin care should be given every 2 to 4 hours. Intake and output should be assessed every 8 hours, and body weight should be assessed daily.

Monitor changes in the serum sodium, serum osmolality, and symptoms of hypernatremia. Detection of the early symptoms of altered mental status (agitation, irritability, confusion) can prevent the progression of hypernatremia. Seizure precautions should be initiated.

Fluid replacement with or without sodium should be closely monitored by the nurse. The nurse should check for symptoms of osmotic diuresis when D_5W is continuously used. Signs and symptoms of cerebral edema may be apparent.

Nursing Diagnosis: Oral Mucous Membranes, Altered R/T inadequate volume of oral secretions.

Planning: Expected Outcomes. The client will have improved condition of oral mucous membranes, as evidenced by oral mucous membranes pink, moist, and intact; increased oral mucous membrane score on assessment tool; reporting no oral discomfort; and being able to consume fluids without pain.

Implementation. The client should be given or offered oral care every 2 hours with a nonalcoholic mouthwash. Lemon-glycerin swabs should also be avoided because they dry the membranes and may cause pain. If only lemon-glycerin swabs are available, they should be diluted with water before use. A soft toothbrush should be used to prevent injury to the mucosa. Lips should be moistened with a petrolatum-based lubricant. Cool, nonacidic fluids such as apple juice are generally tolerated best.

EVALUATION

The nurse evaluates whether or not the goals of preventing and correcting fluid imbalance and hypernatremia have been met. If abnormal laboratory findings and symptoms remain, this information should be conveyed to the appropriate health professional.

The client's oral mucous membranes should be evaluated every shift to detect a lack of improvement.

Post-hospital Care

DISCHARGE TEACHING

The client may require dietary education to reinforce need for fluid and sodium restriction. The client should also be taught to avoid over-the-counter medications high in sodium as well as to recognize clinical manifestations of hypo- and hypernatremia.

▼ Potassium Imbalances

Approximately 96 per cent of potassium is in intracellular fluid and 4 per cent is in the intravascular fluid. Potassium is also plentiful in the gastrointestinal tract. Intracellular potassium (K) has a value of 150 mEq. However, body potassium levels can be obtained only through the measurement of plasma. Therefore, the range of serum potassium is very narrow (3.5 to 5.0 mEq/L). It is vitally important that the potassium level be maintained within this narrow range in order to avoid potassium imbalance. Alterations in potassium are extremely serious problems; if the serum potassium level is less than 2.5 mEq/L or greater than 7.0 mEq/L, cardiac arrest could result.

Potassium Homeostatic Mechanisms

Potassium has many functions within the body. It assists in the regulation of intracellular osmolality. Potassium also promotes the transmission and conduction of nerve impulses and the contraction of skeletal, cardiac, and smooth muscles. It promotes enzyme action for cellular metabolism, promotes glycogen storage in the liver, and assists with the maintenance of acid-base balance. A potassium deficit is associated with alkalosis; a potassium excess is associated with acidosis.

Normal daily potassium requirements are 40 to 60 mEq/L. Potassium is poorly stored in the body, so daily potassium intake is necessary. A standard diet contains 50 to 100 mEq/day. Foods rich in potassium include vegetables, fruits, dry fruits, nuts, and meats. An increased sodium intake promotes potassium loss. Eighty to 90 per cent of potassium is excreted through the kidneys, and the remainder is excreted in feces. Renal excretion of potassium is influenced by plasma potassium concentration, blood flow into the kidney, acid-base status, and various hormones.

ACID-BASE ALTERATION

The potassium level is affected by acid-base imbalances. Alkalosis can cause hypokalemia. In an alkalotic state, hydrogen moves out of the cells to correct the alkalosis, and potassium shifts into the cells, thus lowering the serum potassium level. In acidosis, the reverse is true; potassium levels rise.

HORMONAL INFLUENCE

Insulin promotes potassium uptake by the cells. Insulin-deficient clients frequently develop hyperkalemia. The mechanism whereby insulin promotes potassium uptake is controversial. Data suggest that insulin directly stimulates the sodium-potassium pump.

Glucagon increases plasma levels of potassium. Again, the mechanism is not fully understood; it appears that glucagon stimulates potassium release from the liver and may promote potassium movement in muscle cells.

Adrenocortical hormones such as cortisol and aldosterone promote potassium excretion and sodium retention via the kidneys. During stress, cortisol and aldosterone levels are increased; thus, potassium excretion is promoted. Catecholamines also affect potassium concentration. Beta-adrenergic agonists promote cellular uptake of potassium. Adrenergic mechanisms may also stimulate a sensor in the CNS for potassium homeostasis.

In contrast with beta-adrenergic stimulation, alpha-adrenergic agonists increase plasma potassium concentration. Hepatic stores of potassium are released, and muscle storage is altered.

Epinephrine, which has both alpha- and beta-adrenergic properties, causes an initial, transient rise in potassium. The beta-adrenergic properties subsequently become dominant, and the major effect is a lowering of plasma potassium levels.

HYPOKALEMIA

Definition, Incidence, and Etiology

Hypokalemia is a serum potassium level of less than 3.5 mEq/L; it is a common electrolyte disorder. The many causes of hypokalemia are listed in Table 14–11.

Risk Factors

The elderly and the young are at a higher risk for development of hypokalemia. The body does not preserve potassium; thus, potassium deficit frequently occurs in relation to an inadequate nutrient intake. Clients taking potassium-wasting diuretics or those who have a severe tissue injury are prone to develop hypokalemia.

Prevention of hypokalemia can be accomplished by eating foods rich in potassium or taking potassium supplements. The serum potassium level should be closely monitored when a client has a renal disorder and is taking potassium supplements.

Pathophysiology

When the serum potassium levels decrease, there is an increased potassium gradient between the cell and the plasma. The increased gradient causes the resting membrane potential to increase, thus reducing excitability. Therefore, cell membranes are less responsive to stimuli. The respiratory system is profoundly affected

TABLE 14–11. Causes of Hypokalemia

Etiology	Clinical Conditions and Disorders
Gastrointestinal losses	Vomiting, diarrhea, nasogastric suctioning, intestinal fistula, laxative abuse, excessive tap water enemas
Dietary changes	Malnutrition, starvation, potassium-free diet, some weight reduction diets, potassium-free intravenous solutions when there is no dietary intake
Medications	Potassium-wasting diuretics (thiazide, loop of Henle, and osmotic), steroids (cortisone preparations), ingestion of large amounts of licorice (aldosterone-like effect), gentamicin, amphotericin B, digitalis preparations, and beta-adrenergics promote potassium loss
Redistribution of potassium	Insulin moves glucose and potassium back into cells; potassium loss from osmotic diuresis; in diabetic acidosis, alkalosis causes potassium to shift into cells in exchange for the hydrogen ion
Disorders	Cushing's syndrome, diuretic phase of acute renal failure, alcoholism, hyperaldosteronism

TABLE 14-12. Clinical Manifestations of Hypokalemia and Their Pathophysiologic Basis

Clinical Manifestation	Pathophysiologic Basis
Gastrointestinal Manifestations	
Anorexia, vomiting, diarrhea, ileus, distention	Smooth muscle contraction slowed
Musculoskeletal Manifestations	
Muscle weakness, paralysis, leg cramps, muscle flabbiness	Slowed smooth and skeletal muscle contraction
Cardovascular Manifestations	
Dysrhythmias, vertigo, postural hypotension, flattened T wave, prominent U wave, slow weak pulse	Increase in cell excitability; prolongation of myocardial repolarization Dysrhythmias are more pronounced when the client is taking a digitalis preparation
Respiratory Manifestations	
Shallow respirations, shortness of breath	Weakness of the respiratory muscles due to a decrease in muscle contractions
Neurologic Manifestations	
Fatigue, lethargy, decreased tendon reflexes, confusion, depression	Decreased transmission and conduction of nerve impulses
Renal Manifestations	
Polyuria, decreased serum osmolality, nocturia	Inhibition of the kidney's ability to concentrate urine
Laboratory Findings	
Serum potassium <3.5 mEq/L	Hypokalemia is present when serum potassium level is <3.5 mEq/L
Serum osmolality <275 mOsm/kg	Polyuria, which leads to a loss of body potassium and other solutes

through depression of nervous and muscle synapses. Contraction of muscle groups is slowed, and respiratory movement and ventilation are slowed. Cardiac function is also affected. The pulse is thready and often slow. Electrocardiogram (ECG) changes are common and include a depressed ST segment, a flat T wave, and a U wave. Skeletal muscle contraction is slowed. The client may have transient irritability to profound confusion. Hypokalemia suppresses gastrointestinal function, which leads to paralytic ileus.

Clinical Manifestations (Table 14-12)

The clinical manifestations of hypokalemia include a decreased serum potassium level, abnormal electrocardiography, and signs and symptoms related to gastrointestinal, cardiac, renal, and neurologic disturbances. The serum potassium level and the ECG provide clues to the severity of potassium deficit. With severe hypokalemia, the ECG findings may indicate a depressed, prolonged ST segment, a depressed or inverted T wave, and a U wave. Observable signs and symptoms may not be apparent with mild hypokalemia (3.3 to 3.4 mEq/L), especially if the decrease is gradual. In such instances, the potassium imbalance may go undetected until the serum potassium level continues to fall (Fig. 14-5). With severe hypokalemia, cardiac arrest may occur.

DIAGNOSTIC ASSESSMENT

Hypokalemia is determined by clinical manifestations and laboratory findings consistent with low potassium levels.

Medical Management

Medical management is focused on determining and correcting the cause of the imbalance. Medical care is also directed by the level of the potassium and clinical manifestations. Extreme hypokalemia requires cardiac monitoring.

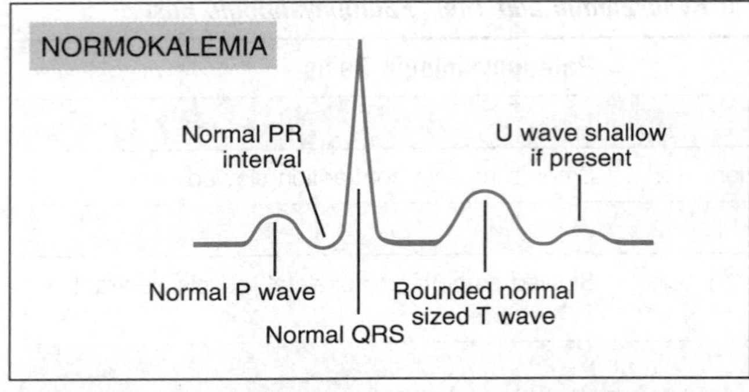

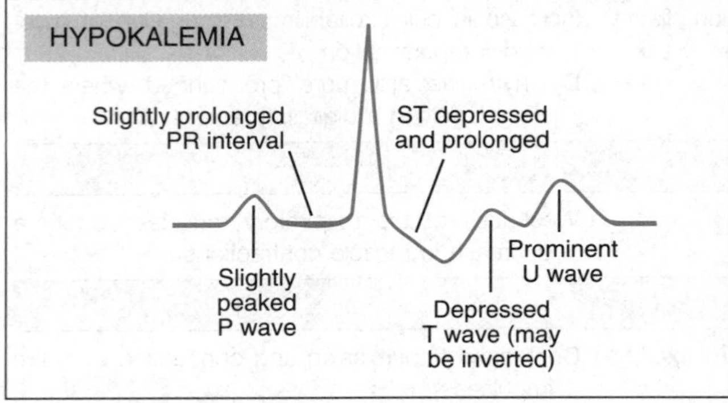

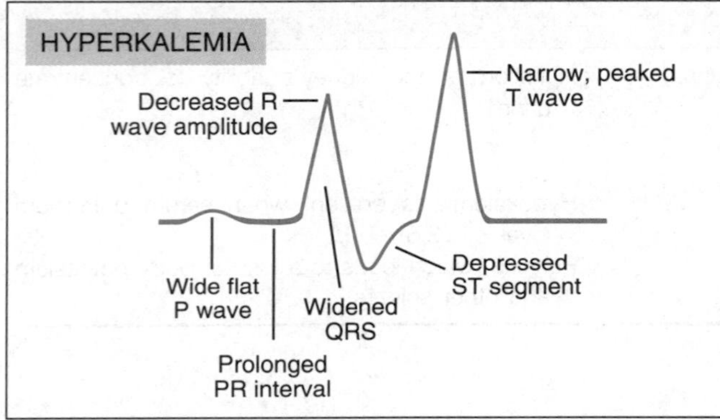

▲ ***Figure 14–5***

ECG changes with potassium imbalance. (From McCance, K. L., & Huether, S. E. [1990]. *Pathophysiology: The basic biologic basis for disease in adults and children*. St. Louis: C. V. Mosby.)

PHARMACOLOGIC MANAGEMENT

Oral potassium replacement therapy is usually prescribed for mild hypokalemia (serum potassium 3.3 to 3.5 mEq/L) or for preventive purposes. Oral potassium chloride or potassium gluconate is available in liquid or tablet form. Potassium is extremely irritating to the gastric mucosa; therefore, the drug must be taken with one-half to one glass of water or juice or during meals.

Potassium chloride can be administered intravenously for moderate or severe hypokalemia. Potassium is *NOT* given intramuscularly and *NEVER* given as a bolus (intravenous push) injection. Potassium given intravenously *MUST ALWAYS BE DILUTED IN INTRAVENOUS FLUIDS.* Giving potassium by intravenous push may result in cardiac arrest. Potassium can be given in 10 to 20 mEq/h diluted in intravenous fluids if the client is on a heart monitor.

Clients with serum potassium levels between 3.0 and 3.4 mEq/L need approximately 100 to 200 mEq of intravenous potassium for the serum potassium level to be raised 1 mEq/L. If the client's serum potassium level is less than 3.0 mEq/L, it takes approximately 200 to 400 mEq of intravenous potassium to raise the serum potassium level 1 mEq/L. Potassium is irritating to the blood vessels, so it has been recommended that 20 to 40 mEq of potassium be mixed in a liter of intravenous fluids for clients with mild and moderate hypokalemia. Clients with severe hypokalemia need 40 to 80 mEq in a liter of fluid. High concentrations of potassium are extremely irritating to the heart muscle. Thus, correcting a potassium deficit may take several days.

For clients who are NPO, usually after surgery or with intestinal problems that prevent eating, a maintenance dosage of potassium is required. A common dose is 40 mEq/day in the intravenous solution.

DIETARY MANAGEMENT

Administering foods high in potassium will help correct the problem as well as prevent further potassium losses. The adult recommended allowance of potassium is 1875 to 5625 mg. Common sources of foods containing potassium are listed in Box 14–3.

Nursing Management

ASSESSMENT

Nursing assessments focus on data collection related to the health problem and the clinical manifestations and laboratory findings associated with hypokalemia. The nurse should obtain a history to ascertain the cause of hypokalemia. Specific questions related to inadequate dietary intake of potassium and potassium losses due to vomiting, diarrhea, and drugs (diuretics, cortisone) are necessary. Assessment should include checking the serum potassium level and assessing for cardiac, gastrointestinal, and neuromuscular changes.

The nurse should maintain a high index of suspicion for clients who have prolonged nasogastric suctioning, are NPO without intravenous potassium supplements, or have renal disease.

NURSING INTERVENTION

Collaborative Problem. Hypokalemia R/T vomiting, diarrhea, Cushing's disease, cortisone therapy, or decreased intake.

Planning: Expected Outcomes. The nurse will monitor the client for serum potassium level returning to normal range, absence of complications related to intravenous administration of potassium chloride, and absence of signs and symptoms of cardiac and neuromuscular changes associated with hypokalemia.

Box 14–3. Common Food Sources of Potassium

Potassium Amounts in Selected Foods

High in Potassium (Average 7 mEq Per Serving)

- Vegetables (½ cup cooked or 1 cup raw)
  - Artichokes
  - Broccoli
  - Brussels sprouts
  - Cabbage
  - Carrots
  - Celery
  - Collards
  - Cucumber
  - Mushrooms
  - Spinach
  - Tomatoes
- Fruits
  - Apricots, fresh, 4 medium
  - Apricots, canned, 4 halves
  - Apricots, dried, 7 halves
  - Banana, 7 inches
  - Cantaloupe, ¼ small
  - Guava, 1 medium
  - Honeydew melon, ⅛ medium
  - Nectarine, ½
  - Orange, 1 small
  - Prunes, 3 medium
  - Strawberries, 1¼ cup
  - Tangerine, 2 medium
  - Watermelon, 1¼ cup
- Beverages
  - Brewed coffee
  - Tomato juice
  - Vegetable juice cocktail, unsalted

Low in Potassium (Average 3 mEq Per Serving)

- Vegetables
  - Corn, ⅓ cup
  - Sweet potato, yams, ¼ cup
  - Lima beans, ⅓ cup
  - French fried potatoes, 10
- Fruit
  - Apple, 1 small
  - Apple juice, ½ cup
  - Applesauce, ½ cup
  - Blueberries, ¾ cup
  - Cranberries, 1¼ cup
- Beverages
  - Coffee, instant
  - Cola
  - Cranberry juice cocktail, ⅓ cup
  - Ginger ale
  - Noncarbonated soft drinks
  - Root beer
  - Lemon-lime soda

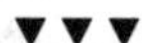

Data from Mahan, K. L. & Arlin, M. (1992). *Food, nutrition & diet therapy* (8th ed.). Philadelphia: W. B. Saunders.

Implementation. Intravenous potassium chloride is usually given for correcting potassium deficit and for maintaining potassium balance. Intravenous potassium chloride *MUST BE DILUTED IN INTRAVENOUS FLUIDS; IT CANNOT BE GIVEN AS AN INTRAVENOUS PUSH.* A large loading dose of potassium can cause cardiac arrest; thus, intravenous solution bags should always be agitated before hanging. The usual dose of intravenous potassium is 20 to 40 mEq in a liter of intravenous solution. Intravenous potassium is irritating to veins and can cause phlebitis; thus, the rate of flow must be carefully monitored. Intravenous fluids with potassium chloride are usually delivered by a controlled infusion pump to assist with maintaining the correct intravenous flow rate.

Serum potassium levels should be closely monitored by the nurse. If the serum potassium level is less than 3.0 mEq/L, the potassium deficit will take longer to correct and requires a larger dose of potassium. Care should also be taken that continuous correction does not cause hyperkalemia. The nurse should continue to assess for signs and symptoms of potassium deficit. Neuromuscular changes are more pronounced with moderate and severe hypokalemia. Renal function should also be assessed. Monitor bowel function because constipation may be a problem. Clients on digitalis derivatives are at risk for digitalis toxicity if hypokalemic; assess apical pulses for dysrhythmia.

Nursing Diagnosis: Injury, High Risk for R/T muscle weakness and hypotension.

Planning: Expected Outcomes. The client will remain free of injury, as evidenced by no falls or near falls.

Implementation. The nurse must employ safety measures to reduce the risk of injury. The bed must be kept in low position with side rails up. Before the client ambulates, the path should be cleared of obstacles and the client should wear shoes to prevent slipping. An ambulation belt should be worn by the client and used by the nurse. Restraints should be used as needed to prevent inadvertent harm.

Nursing Diagnosis: Nutrition, Altered: Less than Body Requirements R/T insufficient intake of foods rich in potassium.

Planning: Expected Outcomes. Client will increase dietary potassium intake to correct hypokalemia, as evidenced by selecting a diet consisting of potassium-rich foods such as bananas, cantaloupe, and nuts, consuming 1875 to 5625 mg of potassium each day, consuming oral potassium supplements as prescribed to decrease or prevent potassium deficit, and an absence of signs and symptoms of hypokalemia.

Implementation. Instruct the client to choose and consume foods rich in potassium, such as fruits, fruit juices, dry fruits, vegetables including potatoes (potato skins are very rich in potassium), and nuts such as peanuts. Some fruits have more potassium than do others; bananas, cantaloupe, and honeydew melons have twice as much potassium as oranges do. Meats and milk have a moderate amount of potassium. If the client is taking a liquid or tablet potassium supplement, the client should be instructed to take the potassium in or with at least one-half glass or more of water or juice.

EVALUATION

The nurse evaluates whether the expected outcomes have been met: the serum potassium level is within normal range; the client is free of signs and symptoms of hypokalemia; and the client did not suffer from any preventable adverse effects of potassium therapy. A revision of the plan of care may be required if outcomes are not met.

Modification of Plan of Care for the Elderly

The elderly have frequent problems with hypokalemia, mostly owing to the use of diuretics. Dietary intake may also be low because of fatigue. Foods may need to be pureed or finely chopped to facilitate eating. In addition, small frequent meals or fluids in between meals may be complied with more easily. Colas seem to be effective in decreasing nausea. In addition, colas are fairly high in potassium.

Post-hospital Care

DISCHARGE TEACHING

The client or whoever cooks in the home needs to be taught which foods are high in potassium. In addition, prolonged cooking of vegetables may result in potassium and vitamin loss. These foods should be steamed or cooked quickly.

HYPERKALEMIA

Definition

Hyperkalemia is an elevated potassium level over 5.0 mEq/L. Hyperkalemia is rare in clients with normal kidney function but may develop in clients with renal insufficiency or renal failure.

Incidence

Because 80 to 90 per cent of potassium is excreted in the urine, clients with severe traumatic injuries—when potassium has left intracellular spaces owing to direct cellular injury (e.g., burns)—develop hyperkalemia. The presence of shock in these clients compounds the problem because of low circulating vascular fluids and diminished kidney function.

Etiology

The three major causes of hyperkalemia are (1) retention of potassium within the body caused by decreased or inadequate urine output; (2) excessive release of potassium from the cells due to traumatic injury, burns, or acidosis; and (3) excessive intravenous infusions containing potassium. All three potential causes of hyperkalemia limit the ability of the kidneys to excrete the excess potassium. Because the kidney is responsible for the majority of potassium excretion, the underlying cause of hyperkalemia is related to decreased kidney function. Disorders that decrease or inhibit secretion of aldosterone may also cause hyperkalemia. Hyperkalemia does not usually occur from increasing dietary potassium intake, unless the potassium is administered in large doses, either orally or intravenously. Table 14–13 lists the causes of hyperkalemia.

Risk Factors

Clients at risk for hyperkalemia are those with insufficient renal function and decreased urinary output. Hyperkalemia may occur with excessive or rapid infusion of intravenous fluids with potassium even though there is adequate urine output.

Prevention of hyperkalemia is essential because a rapid elevation of serum potassium could cause cardiac arrest. Intravenous infusion of fluids with potassium chloride for clients with limited renal function and low urine output should be carefully monitored and given very slowly or not at all. Solutions containing potassium should be infused by intravenous pumps. Urinary output should be assessed hourly when the client is receiving a potassium supplement.

Pathophysiology

Hyperkalemia decreases the cell membrane's threshold, causing the cell to become more excitable. This results in increased nerve and muscle irritability. As hyperkalemia becomes more severe, muscles become weak and paralyzed. Weakness and paralysis of the respiratory muscles may result.

Cardiac effects due to hyperkalemia usually do not occur until the serum potassium level is greater than 7.0 mEq/L. Hyperkalemia causes a disturbance in the cardiac conduction, which can be noted on the ECG strip. Changes include a peaked, narrow T wave; a prolonged PR interval; a depressed ST segment; and a widened QRS complex (see Fig. 14–5). As a result, ventricular contraction of the heart muscle is slowed and cardiac output decreases. Cardiac arrest may result.

Pathophysiologic changes as they relate to clinical manifestations of hyperkalemia are described in Table 14–14.

TABLE 14–13. Causes of Hyperkalemia

Etiology	Clinical Conditions and Disorders
Retention of potassium	Renal insufficiency, renal failure, decreased urine output after surgery, adrenal insufficiency, Addison's disease, hypoaldosteronism, potassium-sparing diuretics, blood for transfusion that is 2 weeks old or more (as blood ages, hemolysis of the red blood cell occurs, which releases the intracellular potassium into the surrounding fluids)
Excessive release of cellular potassium	Severe traumatic injuries, crushing injuries, severe burns, severe infection, metabolic acidosis; after open-heart surgery or surgery that requires a perfusion pump
Excessive intravenous infusions or oral administration of potassium	Excessive and rapid intravenous administration of potassium; excessive administration of large doses of oral potassium

Clinical Manifestations

Clinical manifestations are related to the serum potassium level. The client may develop clinical manifestations in many body systems, including gastrointestinal, cardiac, renal, and neurologic systems. Mild to moderate hyperkalemia causes muscle irritability, whereas severe hyperkalemia causes muscle weakness. When a serum potassium level reaches 6.0 mEq/L, paresthesia (numbness, tingling), tachycardia, and intestinal colic

TABLE 14–14. Clinical Manifestations of Hyperkalemia and Their Pathophysiologic Basis

Clinical Manifestation	Pathophysiologic Basis
Cardiovascular Manifestations	
First tachycardia, and then bradycardia ECG changes: peaked, narrow T waves; wide QRS complex; depressed ST segment; widened PR interval	Disturbances in cardiac conduction, especially through the Purkinje fibers and atrioventricular node, which may lead to ectopic beats; prolonged diastole
Ectopic beats Hypotension	Increase in pacemaker and ectopic foci excitability
Weaker cardiac contraction	Cardiac arrest results with severe potassium elevation
Gastrointestinal Manifestations	
Nausea, explosive diarrhea, intestinal colic, hyperactive bowel sounds (especially over splenic flexure)	Increased smooth muscle contraction, increased peristalsis
Neuromuscular Manifestations	
Paresthesia (tingling sensation), muscle weakness and later flaccid muscle paralysis, muscle cramps	Increased neuromuscular irritability of the skeletal muscles; elevated serum potassium levels cause the muscle to become weak owing to a depolarization block in the muscle
Renal Manifestations	
Oliguria and later anuria	Usually due to preexisting renal dysfunction; limits potassium excretion in the urine
Laboratory Findings	
Serum potassium >5.0 mEq/L	Hyperkalemia is present when serum potassium level >5.0 mEq/L
Serum osmolality >295 mOsm/kg	Oliguria or anuria causes an accumulation of potassium and other solutes, thus increasing the osmolality of body fluids
Serum creatinine >1.5 mg/dl BUN >25 mg/dl	Oliguria or anuria causes an elevation of creatinine and urea nitrogen in the intravascular fluids

may be apparent. As the serum potassium approaches 7.0 mEq/L and above, there are serious cardiac and neuromuscular changes. Evidence of cardiac changes can be seen in ECG strips. The T wave of the ECG becomes more peaked as the serum potassium level rises, and the QRS complex and PR intervals widen.

DIAGNOSTIC ASSESSMENT

Hyperkalemia is determined by clinical manifestations and laboratory findings as presented in Table 14–14. Low urinary output and renal function determined by BUN and serum creatinine levels are important indicators of risk of hyperkalemia because renal failure decreases potassium excretion.

Medical Management

Potassium elevation must be corrected before levels become severe. When the serum potassium level is 5.0 to 5.5 mEq/L, restriction of dietary potassium intake may be all that is needed. However, if the potassium excess is due to metabolic acidosis, correcting the acidosis with sodium bicarbonate promotes potassium uptake into the cells. Improving urine output usually decreases the elevated serum potassium level. Potassium-wasting diuretics might be used.

When hyperkalemia is severe, immediate actions are needed to avoid severe cardiac disturbances. These measures may include (1) intravenous calcium gluconate infusions to decrease the antagonistic effect of potassium excess on the myocardium and (2) infusion of insulin and glucose or sodium bicarbonate to promote potassium uptake into the cells. These methods for decreasing potassium excess usually provide temporary relief, and repeating these methods may not help.

As hyperkalemia persists or increases, a cation exchange resin such as polystyrene sulfonate (Kayexalate) may be given orally or rectally. This treatment stimulates the exchange of a potassium ion for a sodium ion in the intestinal tract; the potassium ion is then excreted in the stool. Because Kayexalate can be constipating, sorbitol may be combined with Kayexalate to prevent constipation and induce diarrhea. For rectal administration, it is given as a retention enema. In marked renal failure, peritoneal dialysis or hemodialysis may be needed.

Nursing Management

ASSESSMENT

Nursing assessment focuses on the clinical manifestations of and laboratory findings associated with hyperkalemia. The nurse should assess the urinary output especially when the client is to receive oral or intravenous potassium preparations. A decrease in urine output should be reported.

The serum potassium level must be closely monitored with high-risk clients and clients who are receiving potassium supplements. A serum potassium level greater than 7.0 mEq/L results in cardiac disturbances. If this is not corrected or the level increases, cardiac arrest can result. The ECG strips need to be assessed for narrowed, peaked T waves, depressed ST segment, and widening of the QRS complex and PR interval.

The flow rate of intravenous fluids with potassium should be closely monitored. A rapidly infused intravenous fluid with potassium may cause hyperkalemia. The potassium in the intravenous fluid is irritating to the vein and subcutaneous tissue. Assess for phlebitis and infiltration into the subcutaneous tissues, which can cause sloughing and tissue necrosis.

NURSING INTERVENTION

Collaborative Problem. Hyperkalemia R/T renal dysfunction, shock from traumatic injuries, or burns.

Planning: Expected Outcomes. The nurse will monitor the client for return of serum potassium level to normal levels, presence of adequate (30 ml/hr) urinary output, absence of signs and symptoms of neuromuscular changes, and apical pulse rate within normal range and without dysrhythmia.

Implementation. The nurse should have a high index of suspicion for those disorders that may cause hyperkalemia. Continued assessment of signs and symptoms of hyperkalemia must be ongoing, and changes need to be reported immediately. Numbness and tingling of the extremities are early signs of hyperkalemia. Muscle weakness and flaccid muscle paralysis are symptoms of more severe hyperkalemia.

The urine output should be closely monitored every hour to every 8 hours, depending on the client's condition. Changes such as a urine output of less than 25 ml/hr or less than 600 ml/day should be reported immediately. Most of the body's excess potassium is excreted in urine.

If the client is to receive a blood transfusion and is at risk of hyperkalemia, the nurse must notify the blood bank so that "old" blood (i.e., blood more than 2 weeks old) is not given to the client.

Methods prescribed for the correction of hyperkalemia should be closely monitored by the nurse. If the client is taking a digitalis preparation and the potassium correction is too rapid, hypokalemia may result. A hypokalemic state could enhance the action of digitalis and cause digitalis toxicity. Serum potassium levels and signs and symptoms of hyperkalemia and hypokalemia need to be continually assessed.

Collaborative Problem. Potential for dysrhythmias R/T hyperkalemia.

Planning: Expected Outcomes. The nurse will monitor for dysrhythmias, assess ECG recording every hour, and intervene according to protocols or notify the physician.

Implementation. The nurse should monitor ECG recordings and report ECG changes that are related to hyperkalemia (see Assessment). Cardiopulmonary resuscitation may be required but is seldom successful with severe hyperkalemia because the heart muscle will not respond. Insulin and glucose may be given to reduce potassium levels temporarily. The client should be assessed for decreased cardiac output as a result of bradycardia. The chest should be auscultated for crackles, the urine monitored for a decreased output, and the extremities assessed for peripheral edema. The nurse needs to report abnormal findings.

EVALUATION

The client's status should be evaluated every hour if the client has severe hyperkalemia. Revisions in the plan of care may be required.

Post-hospital Care

DISCHARGE TEACHING

The client will need to closely adhere to a diet low in potassium if the hyperkalemia is a chronic problem, such as with renal failure. Knowledge of food preparation is important because cooking styles can affect potassium levels.

▼ Calcium Imbalances

Calcium (Ca), an extracellular and intracellular cation, has a normal serum range of 4.5 to 5.5 mEq/L or 9 to 11 mg/dl. Approximately 99 per cent of the body's calcium is in bone and teeth. The other 1 per cent is in tissue and intravascular fluid, of which half is bound to protein, mostly albumin, and the remaining half is free, ionized calcium. The total serum calcium level does not indicate the exact amount of free, active calcium in the body. When albumin is low, it may give a false normal serum calcium level. Instead, levels of serum ionized calcium (iCa) can be used to determine calcium deficit or excess in critically ill clients.

CALCIUM AND PHOSPHORUS HOMEOSTATIC MECHANISMS

Calcium has many functions in the body. It acts as a catalyst in the transmission and conduction of nerve impulses and stimulates the contraction of skeletal, smooth, and cardiac muscles. Calcium maintains normal cellular permeability. Increased serum calcium levels decrease cellular permeability, and decreased serum calcium levels increase cellular permeability. It promotes coagulation of blood in all phases but mostly the prothrombin to thrombin phase. Calcium promotes absorption and utilization of vitamin B_{12}. Finally, calcium promotes strong and durable bones and teeth. Calcium is excreted in the urine and feces.

Vitamin D promotes calcium absorption from the gastrointestinal tract, whereas phosphorus (phosphate) inhibits its absorption. Therefore, calcium and phosphorus counterbalance each other.

Normal levels of serum calcium are also maintained by parathyroid hormone (PTH) in conjunction with the bones. The bones act very effectively to remove excess calcium from the blood. However, when the bones have become saturated with calcium salts, the resulting rise in calcium levels in the interstitial fluid affects the parathyroid gland. There is a decrease in PTH secretion and an increase in urinary calcium excretion. Phosphorus and calcitonin from the thyroid gland act quickly to inhibit removal of calcium from the bone, thus decreasing the serum calcium level (Fig. 14-6).

Conversely, when the level of serum calcium falls even slightly, PTH secretion increases (Fig. 14-6). Within minutes, calcium is reabsorbed through the kidneys; bone resorption occurs within hours, and increased absorption from the gastrointestinal tract occurs within days.

Like calcium, most phosphorus in the body resides in the skeleton. Sources of phosphorus are numerous in poultry and meat. Phosphorus is an integral part of the energy systems in the body (ADP and ATP). Deficiency is extremely rare. Phosphorus depletion can occur as a result of prolonged and excessive intake of antacids. Symptoms of phosphorus deficiency are weakness, anorexia, malaise, and bone pain. Excessive phosphorus levels can occur with renal failure, hyperthyroidism, phosphate poisoning, and severe hemolytic anemia.

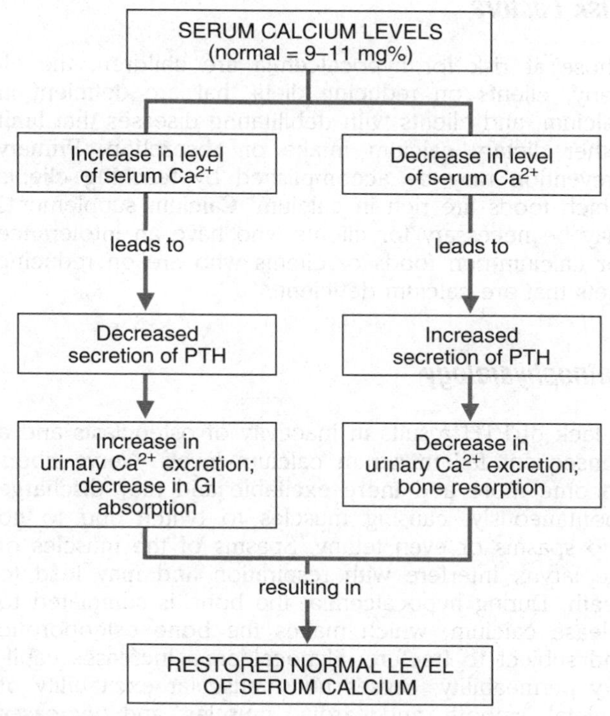

▲ *Figure 14-6*

PTH regulation of serum calcium level.

TABLE 14-15. Causes of Hypocalcemia

Etiology	Clinical Conditions and Disorders
Dietary changes	Inadequate dietary calcium intake, vitamin D deficiency, or both; excess intake of phosphorus combines with calcium, so neither electrolyte is absorbed
Gastrointestinal changes	Malabsorption of fat in the intestine
Calcium binding	Metabolic alkalosis (because there is less ionized calcium), multiple transfusion of stored blood (which is combined with citrate for storage)
Disorders	Renal failure with hyperphosphatemia, acute pancreatitis (which causes release of lipases into soft tissue spaces, so that free fatty acids that are formed bind with calcium), burns, Cushing's disease), hypoparathyroidism, liver disease, inadvertent removal of the parathyroid gland with thyroidectomy
Medications	Magnesium sulfate, colchicine, neomycin inhibit PTH secretion; aspirin, anticonvulsants, estrogen alter vitamin D metabolism; phosphate preparations decrease serum calcium level; steroids decrease calcium mobilization; loop diuretics reduce calcium absorption from the renal tubules; antacids and laxatives decrease calcium absorption

HYPOCALCEMIA

Definition, Incidence, and Etiology

Hypocalcemia is a serum calcium level below 4.5 mEq/L or 8.5 mg/dl. Hypocalcemia is a common and potentially serious electrolyte disorder that occurs more frequently in children and the elderly. Overcorrection of acidosis may also lead to hypocalcemia, because too much calcium is bound to protein. There are many causes of hypocalcemia; they are listed in Table 14-15.

Risk Factors

Those at risk for hypocalcemia are children, the elderly, clients on reducing diets that are deficient in calcium, and clients with debilitating diseases that limit either dietary calcium intake or absorption. Primary prevention may be accomplished by teaching clients which foods are rich in calcium. Calcium supplements may be necessary for clients who have an intolerance for calcium-rich foods or clients who are on reducing diets that are calcium deficient.

Pathophysiology

A lack of PTH results in inactivity of osteoclasts and a consequent fall in serum calcium levels. Nerve fibers become more and more excitable and may discharge spontaneously, causing muscles to twitch and to go into spasms or even tetany. Spasms of the muscles of the larynx interfere with respiration and may lead to death. During hypocalcemia, the bone is stimulated to release calcium, which makes the bone osteoporotic and subject to fracture. Hypocalcemia increases capillary permeability; causes neuromuscular excitability of skeletal, smooth, and cardiac muscles; and decreases blood coagulation, which results in bleeding. Severe hypocalcemia causes neuromuscular excitability that results in tetany. If it is untreated, convulsions and death can occur. An acute hypocalcemia may cause cardiac insufficiency and cardiac dysrhythmias. Pathophysiologic changes as they relate to clinical manifestations of hypocalcemia are explained in Table 14-16.

Clinical Manifestations

Most of the clinical manifestations of hypocalcemia can be attributed to increased neuromuscular excitability. Numbness and tingling of the hands, toes and lips, irritability, anxiety, dysrhythmias (prolonged QT interval), carpopedal spasm, seizures, laryngeal stridor, and prolonged bleeding time are common.

With prolonged hypocalcemia, cataracts may develop because of increased uptake of sodium and water by the lens. In addition, pathologic fractures and trophic changes, such as dry, sparse hair and rough skin, may be seen.

DIAGNOSTIC ASSESSMENT

Hypocalcemia is suspected in clients with a history that indicates risk; clinical manifestations and laboratory findings are presented in Table 14-16.

Medical Management

Medical management is focused on determining and correcting the cause of the hypocalcemia. Other medical management is dictated by the level of the serum calcium.

PHARMACOLOGIC MANAGEMENT

Asymptomatic hypocalcemia is usually corrected with oral calcium gluconate, calcium lactate, or calcium chloride. It is best to give the calcium supplement 30 minutes before meals for better absorption and with a glass of milk because vitamin D is necessary in the absorption of calcium from the intestine. Acute hypocalcemia with tetany needs immediate correction. In-

TABLE 14–16. Clinical Manifestations of Hypocalcemia and Their Pathophysiologic Basis

Clinical Manifestation	Pathophysiologic Basis
Neuromuscular Manifestations	
Tetany symptoms: twitching around mouth, tingling and numbness of fingers, carpopedal spasms, facial spasm, laryngospasm, and later convulsions	Hypocalcemia causes increased neuromuscular excitability/irritability, producing hyperactivity of the motor and sensory nerves
Presence of Trousseau's and Chvostek's signs	
Respiratory Manifestations	
Dyspnea, laryngeal spasm	Increased nerve conduction leading to tetany
Gastrointestinal Manifestations	
Increased peristalsis, diarrhea	Calcium absorption from the intestine is decreased; decreased calcium increases smooth muscle contraction
Cardiovascular Manifestations	
Dysrhythmias, palpitations	Increase in cell excitability
Musculoskeletal Manifestations	
Pathologic fractures	Calcium loss from bone due to osteoporosis causes bone to be brittle
Hematologic Manifestations	
Prolonged bleeding time	Intrinsic pathway for blood coagulation is inhibited
Laboratory Findings	
Serum calcium <4.5 mEq/L (<9 mg/dl) iCa <2.2 mEq/L (<4.4 mg/dl)	Hypocalcemia is present when serum level is <4.5 mEq/L (9 mg/dl)

travenous calcium chloride or calcium gluconate (10 per cent) is given slowly to avoid hypotension, bradycardia, and other arrhythmias. Usually intravenous calcium is diluted in a liter of D_5W. Saline solutions are not used because sodium tends to promote calcium loss.

DIETARY MANAGEMENT

Chronic or mild hypocalcemia can be treated in part by having the client consume a diet high in calcium. Foods high in calcium are listed in Box 14–4. If hypocalcemia is secondary to parathyroid deficiency, the client must avoid high-phosphate foods (e.g., milk products, carbonated beverages). Maintenance needs are met through calcium and vitamin D supplements.

Nursing Management

ASSESSMENT

The nurse should have a high index of suspicion for those clients at risk for hypocalcemia and present with clinical manifestations. If neuromuscular and cardiac symptoms are present, the hypocalcemic state is usually severe. Assessing the medications and diet the client is taking is important. If the client is taking a digitalis preparation, administration of calcium will enhance the action of digitalis and may cause digitalis toxicity. Clinical manifestations of digitalis toxicity include bradycardia (pulse rate <60), nausea, vomiting, and blurred vision. The client's diet may also give clues to hypocalcemia due to malnutrition or lack of calcium intake.

The nurse needs to assess the client's cardiac status by noting changes in the ECG and heart rate. Changes would include a weak pulse, and the ECG recording may show a prolonged QT interval.

Two tests used to check for increased neuromuscular excitability and tetany are the Trousseau's and Chvostek's signs. The Trousseau's sign is carpopedal spasm (contraction of the fingers and hand). It is best elicited by inflating a blood pressure cuff on the upper arm for 1 to 5 minutes, constricting circulation. A positive test result is carpopedal spasm. The Chvostek's sign is spasm of the muscles innervated by the facial nerve. It is best determined by tapping the client's face lightly (over the facial nerve) below the temple. Spasm of the face, lip, or nose would indicate a positive test for tetany (Fig. 14–7).

Box 14-4. Common Food Sources of Calcium

Calcium Content of Selected Foods

Foods High in Calcium (Over 100 Mg per Serving)

- Dairy Products
  - Cheese, all types
  - Ice cream, 1 cup
  - Milk, 1 cup
  - Yogurt, low-fat with fruit, 1 cup
- Other Foods
  - Oatmeal, instant, $\frac{3}{4}$ cup
  - Rhubarb, cooked, 1 cup
  - Spinach, frozen, $\frac{1}{2}$ cup
  - Tofu, regular $\frac{1}{2}$ cup

Foods Low in Calcium (Below 25 Mg per Serving)

- Apple, 1 medium
- Banana, 1 medium
- Chicken breast, baked, 3 oz
- Ground beef, lean, 3 oz
- Oatmeal, cooked, 1 cup
- Pasta, cooked, 1 cup
- Vegetable juices

Data from Laquarta, I., & Gerlach, M. (1990). *Nutrition in clinical nursing*. Albany, New York: Delmar Publishers; and Burtis, G., et al. (1988). *Applied nutrition and diet therapy*. Philadelphia: W. B. Saunders.

NURSING INTERVENTION

Collaborative Problem. Hypocalcemia R/T diarrhea, pancreatitis, renal failure, or decreased intake.

Planning: Expected Outcomes. The nurse will monitor the client for resolution of hypocalcemia: serum calcium level, dysrhythmias, absence of tetany symptoms, and adequate peripheral perfusion.

Implementation. The nurse monitors peripheral pulses and vital signs, especially the heart rate and ECG recordings, every hour to every 4 hours depending on the client's condition. The nurse should check the arterial blood gases for the presence of acid-base imbalances. As the acidotic state is being corrected, the nurse needs to monitor for tetany.

If the client is receiving intravenous calcium, the nurse needs to monitor the intravenous site for infiltration or phlebitis every hour. Calcium chloride is extremely irritating to the subcutaneous tissue; if infiltration occurs, sloughing of the tissue can result.

Symptomatic hypocalcemia should be assessed by testing of the Chvostek's and Trousseau's signs. The serum calcium level should be closely monitored and changes reported.

Nursing Diagnosis: Injury, High Risk for R/T increased neuromuscular irritability resulting from hypocalcemia.

Planning: Expected Outcomes. The client will be free of injury associated with calcium deficit, as evi-

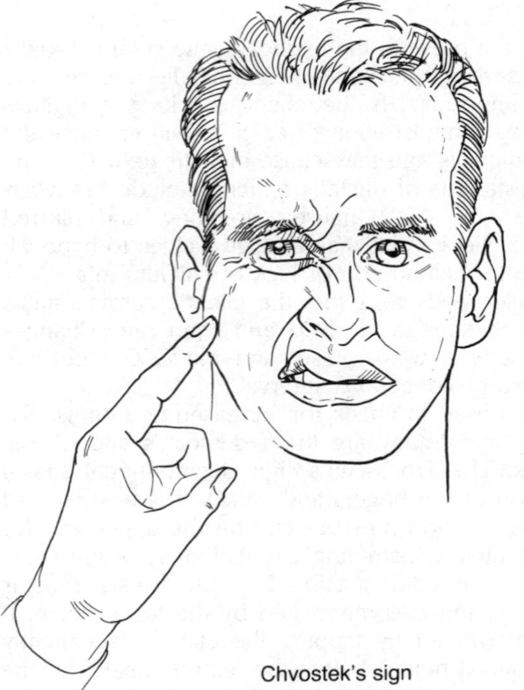

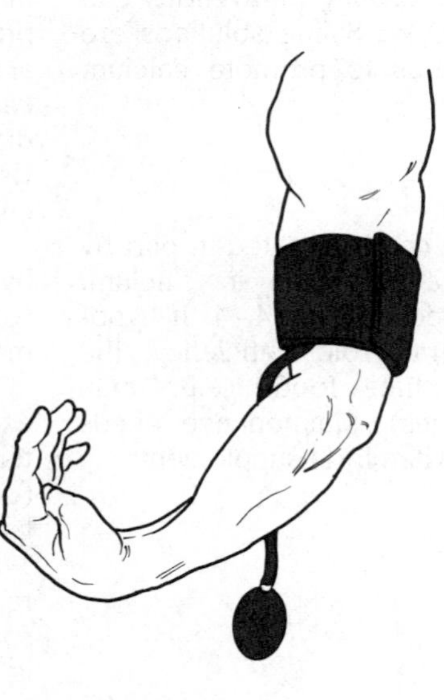

▲ **Figure 14-7**

Chvostek's and Trousseau's sign.

denced by no falls or near falls and no pathologic fractures.

Interventions. Use caution in turning or moving the client to prevent inadvertent pathologic fractures. Walk the client with an ambulation belt and use precautions (e.g., extra personnel) to lift or move the client in and from bed.

Nursing Diagnosis: Health Maintenance, Altered R/T knowledge deficit regarding foods high in calcium.

Planning: Expected Outcomes. The client will have an improved knowledge base regarding dietary correction of hypocalcemia, as evidenced by selecting a diet to replace calcium loss and using oral calcium supplements or providing intravenous calcium replacement.

Implementation. The client should be instructed about foods that are rich in calcium, such as milk, cheese, yogurt, and vegetables. Oral calcium supplements should be taken before meals and with milk that contains vitamin D for better absorption. Instruct the client who is on a reducing diet to check with the physician for diet approval. Use caution if hypocalcemia is due to hypoparathyroidism. For these clients, phosphorus intake should be decreased by omitting milk and milk products. Instead, calcium and vitamin D supplements should be used.

EVALUATION

The degree of attainment of expected outcomes should be reviewed and modifications made in the plan of care as needed.

Modification of Plan of Care for the Elderly

Elderly clients may have difficulty incorporating large amounts of food and fluids containing calcium into the diet. Part of the difficulty is in adjusting long-established eating habits. Many elderly clients drink very little milk because it used to be a high-priced food item that adults gave up in favor of children drinking milk. The nurse can help the client find other sources of milk that are palatable and obtainable.

HYPERCALCEMIA

Definition

Hypercalcemia is a serum level over 5.5 mEq/L or 11 mg/dl.

Incidence

Hypercalcemia can occur in any age group. It is a common electrolyte disorder that can create serious physical complications.

Etiology

The three most common causes of hypercalcemia are metastatic malignancy, hyperparathyroidism, and thiazide diuretic therapy. Severely high levels of calcium are usually due to a malignancy. The most common of malignancies that may cause hypercalcemia include lung, breast, ovarian, prostatic, bladder, multiple myeloma, leukemia, lymphoma, kidney, and head and neck cancers. These cancers can cause bone destruction from metastasis or increase secretion of ectopic PTH.

Other causes of hypercalcemia include prolonged immobilization, excessive intake of calcium supplements and vitamin D, calcium-containing antacids, and hypophosphatemia. With hypophosphatemia, the serum calcium level is increased and the kidneys are unable to excrete the excess calcium. Metabolic acidosis can also decrease calcium elimination, thus increasing the serum calcium levels. Severe hypercalcemia may result in hypercalcemic crisis, which carries a 30 to 50 per cent mortality rate.

Risk Factors

Calcium loss from the bone, increasing the serum calcium level, can occur with many malignancies. Severe hypercalcemia may be fatal; thus, the serum calcium levels must be monitored. Early treatment may prevent a hypercalcemic crisis. Mobilization is an important factor in the prevention of calcium loss from the bone. Bones maintain calcium because of the pressure exerted on them by carrying body weight; therefore, during bed rest the bone can lose calcium.

Pathophysiology

Because calcium levels are increased, there is a lesser gradient between the cell and the serum. There is also an increased amount of calcium in the cell. Therefore, the threshold becomes more difficult to achieve, and the cell membrane becomes refractory to depolarization. As a result, cardiac and smooth muscle activity is decreased. Calcium in the bloodstream impairs renal function, and it precipitates as a salt, forming renal stones. Some cancer tumors destroy the bone, whereas others, such as lung and breast cancers, cause an ectopic PTH production. Hypophosphatemia is a complication of excessive PTH production that promotes calcium retention. A shortened QT segment and depressed T waves may be seen on ECG. Pathophysiologic changes as they relate to clinical manifestations of hypercalcemia are explained in Table 14–17.

Hypercalcemic Crisis

A hypercalcemic crisis occurs when calcium levels reach 15 mg/dl. This level of serum calcium can cause cardiac dysrhythmias (widened T wave, and shortened QT interval). Hypokalemia may occur as the body

TABLE 14–17. Clinical Manifestations of Hypercalcemia and Their Pathophysiologic Basis

Clinical Manifestation	Pathophysiologic Basis
Gastrointestinal Manifestations	
Anorexia, nausea, vomiting, constipation, decreased peristalsis, distention	Slowed gastrointestinal transit time Increased calcium enhances hydrochloric acid, gastrin, and pancreatic enzyme release
Neuromuscular Manifestations	
Mild to moderate hypercalcemic state: weakness, fatigue, depression, difficulty in concentrating Severe hypercalcemic state: extreme lethargy, depressed sensorium, confusion, and coma	Neurologic depression
Cardiovascular Manifestations	
Dysrhythmias, heart block ECG changes: shortened ST segment and lengthened QT interval Digitalis toxicity Critical: cardiac arrest	Delayed transmission due to prolonged repolarization
Renal Manifestations	
Polyuria, kidney stones, renal failure	Decreases the glomerular filtration rate; causes osmotic diuresis and volume depletion; reduces the kidney's ability to concentrate urine and results in polyuria
Musculoskeletal Manifestations	
Bone pain, fracture	Metastatic cancer to the bone causes bone pain, which can be severe; decalcification of bones may cause osteoporosis and spontaneous fractures
Laboratory Findings	
Serum calcium >5.5 mEq/L (>11.5 mg/dl)	Hypercalcemia is present when serum calcium level is >5.5 mEq/L (11.5 mg/dl)
ABGs pH <7.45 HCO_3^- >26 mEq/L	Acidotic state inhibits calcium excretion from the kidneys

wastes potassium rather than calcium. Usual treatment includes hydration with 6 to 10 L normal saline in 24 hours and etidronate disodium (Didronel) therapy. These actions are designed to lower the calcium level in 36 to 48 hours.

Clinical Manifestations

The clinical manifestations of hypercalcemia are determined by the serum calcium level but in general are nonspecific. Mild hypercalcemia (near 11.5 mg/dl or 5.5 mEq/L) is usually asymptomatic. In mild cases, the serum calcium level may increase momentarily when the client consumes calcium-containing antacids or a large dose of an oral calcium supplement and the kidneys are initially unable to eliminate the excess. In moderate hypercalcemia (serum calcium level of 13 mg/dl or 6.2 mEq/L), symptoms usually include anorexia, nausea, vomiting, polyuria, fatigue, lethargy, and dehydration. As the hypercalcemic state progresses to severe levels, the client becomes more lethargic and confused, and coma may result. In some instances, clients may complain of deep bone pain.

DIAGNOSTIC ASSESSMENT

Hypercalcemia is determined by clinical manifestations and laboratory findings presented in Table 14–17.

Medical Management

Treatment consists of correcting the underlying cause. In addition, the clinical manifestations may require some additional forms of treatment.

PHARMACOLOGIC MANAGEMENT

Immediate correction of moderate and severe hypercalcemia is essential. Intravenous normal saline (0.9 per cent NaCl), given rapidly with furosemide to prevent fluid overload, promotes urinary calcium excretion. Antitumor antibiotics such as plicamycin (mithramycin) inhibit the action of PTH on osteoclasts in bone tissue and result in a reduction of decalcification and a decrease in the serum calcium level. Calcitonin decreases the serum calcium level by inhibiting the effects of PTH on the osteoclasts and increasing urinary calcium excretion. Corticosteroid drugs decrease calcium levels by competing with vitamin D, thus resulting in decreased intestinal absorption of calcium. Intravenous phosphate decreases the serum calcium level; however, it should be used cautiously because it may result in severe calcification of various tissues. Sometimes thiazide diuretics are changed to furosemide or some other diuretic that does not retain calcium. If the cause is excessive use of calcium or vitamin D supplements or calcium-containing antacids, these agents should be either avoided or used in a reduced dosage. A newer form of therapy is the use of etidronate disodium. This drug reduces serum calcium by reducing normal and abnormal bone reabsorption of calcium and secondarily by reducing bone formation. The client needs to be hydrated with normal saline before administration and given loop diuretics to enhance urine output and calcium excretion following administration of the drug.

DIETARY MANAGEMENT

Forcing fluids will assist in adequately hydrating the client and flushing excess calcium through the kidney.

Surgical Management

Surgery may be used to remove ectopic PTH-secreting tumor.

Nursing Management

ASSESSMENT

The nurse should have a high index of suspicion for those clients at risk for hypercalcemia or with early symptoms of this disorder. When the nurse notes an elevated serum calcium level, the nurse should assess the client for signs and symptoms of neuromuscular and cardiac changes associated with hypercalcemia. An accurate nursing history may identify factors such as excessive use of calcium supplements or calcium-containing antacids that could cause a mild to moderate hypercalcemia. A drug history is important for determining whether the medications the client is taking could be affected by the hypercalcemic state. For example, an increased calcium level enhances the action of digoxin; thus, digitalis toxicity may result.

The client's hydration status should be assessed for fluid volume depletion caused by hypercalcemia. ECG changes and the state of the client's sensorium should be reported.

NURSING INTERVENTION

Collaborative Problem. Hypercalcemia R/T metastatic lesions, hyperparathyroidism, thiazide therapy or increased intake of calcium.

Planning: Expected Outcomes. The nurse will monitor the client for resolution of hypercalcemia: serum calcium levels returning toward normal, adequate urine output, no cardiac dysrhythmias, neurologic changes, no pathologic fractures, and no severe weakness.

Implementation. Vital signs, including ECG, should be assessed every 4 to 8 hours. The presence of dysrhythmias or changes in sensorium should be reported. Bowel sounds should be assessed every 8 hours. Calcium levels should be closely monitored. Fluid intake should be increased, unless contraindicated (congestive heart failure), to dilute the calcium level. Acid-ash foods and fluids that contain acid should be encouraged, such as cranberry and prune juices. Urine should be strained to capture renal calculi (stones). Caution should be used with mobilization to reduce the risk of fractures.

Nursing Diagnosis: Health Maintenance, Altered R/T excessive ingestion of calcium supplements and/or calcium-containing antacids.

Planning: Expected Outcomes. The client's knowledge of the complications of calcium-containing drugs will be improved, as evidenced by decrease in or elimination of supplemental dosage of calcium, substitution of calcium-free antacids or decrease in the use of calcium-containing antacids, and return of serum calcium level to normal range.

Implementation. Instruct the client to avoid use of calcium supplements. Sodium intake is increased, unless contraindicated (sodium promotes calcium loss through the kidney). High-fiber foods may be suggested to prevent constipation associated with hypercalcemia.

Nursing Diagnosis: Injury, High Risk for R/T potential pathologic fractures, mental confusion, and immobility.

Planning: Expected Outcomes. The client will sustain no injury as evidenced by no falls or near falls and no reports of bone pain or extremity swelling, loss of motion, or ecchymosis.

Implementation. Safety precautions are necessary when the client is displaying symptoms of confusion or is extremely lethargic or comatose. The client should be turned and moved with extreme caution and adequate assistance given for prevention of injury. Back braces, tripod canes, and walkers may be used to facilitate safer ambulation. The bed should be in low position with side rails elevated. Clinical manifestations of fractures (bone pain, ecchymosis) should be reported immediately.

EVALUATION

The nurse evaluates whether the expected outcomes have been achieved and the client's serum calcium level is normal. Revisions in the plan of care may be required.

DISCHARGE TEACHING

The client and family should be taught to continue an acid-ash diet, force fluids, and avoid calcium-containing medications. The client should also be taught to report clinical manifestations of renal calculi (flank pain, hematuria) or cardiac dysrhythmias (irregular pulse, palpitations).

▼ Magnesium Imbalances

Magnesium (Mg) is the second most abundant intracellular cation. Magnesium's actions in the body and the clinical manifestations of imbalances are similar to those of potassium. Magnesium is absorbed from the small intestine and excreted in the urine. Fifty per cent of the body's magnesium is stored in bone, 49 per cent is in intracellular fluid, and 1 per cent is in the extracellular fluid. In the plasma/serum, 30 per cent of the magnesium is bound to protein, 15 per cent is combined with anions, and 55 per cent is in a free, ionized form. Magnesium is absorbed from the small intestine in the same site where calcium is absorbed; therefore, malabsorption problems will affect both electrolytes. Magnesium is excreted in the urine and in small amounts in feces.

The functions of magnesium include the transmission and conduction of nerve impulses and the contraction of skeletal, smooth, and cardiac muscles. It is responsible for the transportation of sodium and potassium across the cell membrane, through the sodium-potassium pump. It influences utilization of potassium, sodium, and protein and activates enzymes that are necessary for the metabolism of carbohydrates and protein. Finally, magnesium promotes vasodilation of peripheral arteries and arterioles.

An increased calcium or phosphorus intake can decrease magnesium absorption from the intestines. Conversely, a low calcium level increases magnesium absorption from the intestines. Magnesium inhibits PTH, which results in a decrease in the amount of calcium released from the bone, thus promoting a calcium deficit.

Magnesium has been used for the treatment of acute myocardial infarction. It acts to decrease dysrhythmias, especially the digoxin-induced ventricular dysrhythmias. It is frequently selected when other treatment modalities have failed, especially when the client has hypokalemia.

Box 14–5. Common Food Sources of Magnesium

Magnesium Content of Selected Foods

Foods High in Magnesium (Above 75 Mg per Serving)

- Cashews, roasted, 1 cup
- Chili, with beans, 1 cup
- Halibut, baked, 3 oz
- Swiss chard, cooked, ½ cup
- Tofu, ½ cup
- Wheat germ, ¼ cup, toasted

Foods Low in Magnesium (Below 25 Mg per Serving)

- Chicken breast, 3 oz
- Fruits
- Egg, 1
- Green peas, frozen, ½ cup
- Ground beef, 3 oz
- White bread, 1 slice

▼▼▼

Data from Mahan, K. L., & Arlin, M. (1992). *Food, nutrition & diet therapy* (8th ed.). Philadelphia: W. B. Saunders.

HYPOMAGNESEMIA

Overview

Hypomagnesemia is a serum magnesium level below 1.5 mEq/L or below 1.8 mg/dl. Magnesium deficits are rare among healthy individuals because magnesium is abundant in foods and water. Magnesium deficits are seen in critically ill clients and alcoholic clients. Administering magnesium-free parenteral fluid solutions may increase the hypomagnesemic state.

Hypomagnesemia may be present but overlooked because tests for serum magnesium levels are not routinely ordered until there is a severe deficit. Magnesium deficits often accompany a potassium or calcium deficit. Cellular magnesium deficits can occur in the presence of normal serum values.

Major health problems causing hypomagnesemia are inadequate intake of magnesium or intestinal malabsorption and gastrointestinal or renal losses.

Clients who are prone to an inadequate intake of magnesium include those with severe or chronic malnutrition, alcoholism, and prolonged intravenous or hyperalimentation therapy without magnesium replacement.

Hypomagnesemia can lead to increased transmission of action potentials owing to an increased release of acetylcholine. Greater releases of acetylcholine increase transmission from nerve to nerve and nerve to muscle. Therefore, magnesium deficiencies can cause cardiac dysrhythmias as a result of myocardial irritability and neuromuscular changes such as tetany. The client can also develop psychological disorders such as depression, psychosis, and confusion. Gastrointestinal changes include decreased contractility leading to anorexia, nausea, and abdominal distention.

Alcoholism, when accompanied by liver disease, decreases intestinal absorption as the enzymes necessary for absorption are decreased. In addition, excessive amounts of phosphorus in the intestine (usually from antacids) will inhibit the uptake of magnesium from the intestinal villi. Clients with prolonged losses of fluids from the gastrointestinal tract (diarrhea, draining intestinal fistulas, laxative abuse), hyperparathyroidism, prolonged diuretic therapy, and in the diuresis phase of acute renal failure are prone to excessive loss of magnesium. There are also medications that interfere with renal handling of magnesium as either a primary action or side effect. The primary drugs are diuretics and antibiotics. Furosemide, osmotic and thiazide diuretics, aminoglycoside antibiotics (gentamicin, tobramycin), amphotericin B, corticosteroids, and digitalis are the usual offenders.

Severe hypomagnesemia causes neuromuscular symptoms such as presence of Chvostek's and Trousseau's signs, tetany, and convulsions. Cardiac dysrhythmias include premature ventricular contractions; atrial or ventricular fibrillation; and ECG changes including prolonged QT intervals, widened QRS complex, flat or inverted T waves, and ST segment depression. Clients having a magnesium deficit and who are taking digoxin could develop toxic effects of digitalis.

A magnesium deficit affects the potassium-sodium pump, causing hypokalemia. Hypomagnesemia also inhibits PTH, so the serum calcium levels may also be low.

Management

Treatment of hypomagnesemia includes oral magnesium replacement in the form of magnesium-containing antacids or parenteral magnesium sulfate. Increasing dietary intake of magnesium will also help prevent further loss.

Nursing diagnoses for magnesium imbalances are similar to the other nursing diagnoses for electrolyte imbalances: injury, high risk for; nutrition, altered; decreased cardiac output. The majority of nursing intervention falls within the collaborative problem of hypomagnesemia.

Vital signs and ECG recordings should be monitored every 4 to 8 hours depending on the client's condition. Tachycardia and cardiac dysrhythmias may indicate hypomagnesemia. Serum magnesium, potassium, and calcium levels should be monitored. Clients who are extremely confused will need protection from harm with restraints or constant monitoring.

The administration of magnesium replacements needs to be closely monitored. Slowly administer magnesium diluted in intravenous solution. Rapid infusion of magnesium sulfate can cause a hot or flushed feeling.

Clients should be taught which foods are rich in magnesium to prevent magnesium deficiency or to correct a mild deficit. These foods are listed in Box 14-5.

HYPERMAGNESEMIA

Overview

Hypermagnesemia is a serum magnesium level over 2.5 mEq/L (3.0 mg/dl). It is a rare disorder. Hypermagnesemia may occur with renal insufficiency, excessive use of magnesium-containing antacids or laxatives, severe dehydration from ketoacidosis, disorders that decrease the synthesis of aldosterone (e.g., Addison's disease or adrenalectomy), or overuse of intravenous magnesium sulfate for controlling premature labor or pregnancy-induced hypertension. Extreme hypermagnesemia has a sedative effect on the neuromuscular system, which causes muscle weakness. It blocks the release of acetylcholine from the myoneural junction, thus decreasing muscle cell activity. The respiratory muscles are affected, and respiratory paralysis may result.

With mild hypermagnesemia, peripheral vessels dilate, causing hypotension. Severe hypermagnesemia causes a delayed conduction of the myocardium that could cause premature ventricular contractions and lead to heart block.

Lethargy, drowsiness, loss of deep tendon reflexes, muscle weakness, respiratory paralysis, and loss of consciousness are the clinical manifestations in the CNS. Cardiac clinical manifestations include hypotension and ECG changes. Mild hypermagnesemia prolongs PR and QT intervals. High levels widen QRS complexes, elevate the T wave, and lead to heart block.

Management

Treatment for hypermagnesemia is decreasing the use of intravenous magnesium sulfate administration and speeding up its elimination. A saline infusion with a diuretic increases renal elimination of magnesium; however, the side effect of the treatment is a loss of calcium. Hypocalcemia may intensify the hypermagnesemic state. Calcium antagonizes magnesium; thus, intravenous calcium salts in solution have been used for extreme hypermagnesemia. Clients with respiratory distress due to severe magnesium excess may need ventilatory assistance. If renal failure is present, hemodialysis may be necessary.

Vital signs, respiratory function, ECG recordings, urinary output, and the state of sensorium should be assessed every hour to every 4 hours depending on the condition of the client. The bed should be in low position, side rails should be raised, and restraints should be used if the client is confused. Clients should be taught to avoid constant use of laxatives and antacids containing magnesium, especially if urinary output is decreased. Encourage the client to eat foods containing fiber and drink adequate fluids to promote fecal elimination. Intravenous calcium salts should be available for emergency use for reversing the effects of severe hypermagnesemia.

Summary

Fluid and electrolyte disorders are fairly common problems. The nurse needs to maintain a high index of suspicion for the disorders because the clinical manifestations can be vague. Interventions are focused on correcting the underlying etiology and preventing injury during acute phases.

Bibliography

1. Bidani, A. (1986). Electrolyte and acid-base disorders. *Medical Clinics of North America, 70*(5), 1013.
2. Bullock, B., & Rosendahl, P. (1988). *Pathophysiology* (2nd ed.). Boston: Scott, Foresman and Co.
2a. Burtis, G., et al. (1988). *Applied nutrition and diet therapy*. Philadelphia, W. B. Saunders.
3. Cannon, P. (1989). Sodium retention in heart failure. *Cardiology Clinics, 7*(1), 49-59.
4. Carroll, H., & Oh, M. (1989). *Water, electrolyte and acid-base metabolism* (2nd ed.). Philadelphia: J. B. Lippincott Co.
5. Chernow, B., et al. (1989). Hypomagnesemia in patients in postoperative care. *Chest, 95*(2), 391-396.
6. Davis, K., & Attie, M. (1991). Management of severe hypercalcemia. *Critical Care Clinics, 7*(1), 175-189.
7. German, K. (1987). Fluid and electrolyte problems associated with diabetes insipidus and syndrome of inappropriate antidiuretic hormone. *Nursing Clinics of North America, 22*(4), 785.
8. Gershan, J., et al. (1990). Fluid volume deficit: Validating the indicators. *Heart and Lung, 19*(2), 152-156.
9. Giesecke, A., Grande, C., & Whitten, C. (1990). Fluid therapy and the resuscitation of traumatic shock. *Critical Care Clinics, 6*(1), 61-71.
10. Heitkemper, M., & Bond, E. (1988). Fluid and electrolytes: Assessment and interventions. *Journal of Enterostomal Therapy 15*(1), 18.
11. Kamel, K. S., et al. (1990). Urine electrolytes and osmolality: When and how to use them. *American Journal of Nephrology, 10*(2), 89-102.
12. Karb, V. (1989). Electrolyte abnormalities and drugs which commonly cause them. *Journal of Neuroscience Nursing, 21*(2), 125-128.
13. Kee, J. (1986). *Fluids and electrolytes with clinical applications* (4th ed.). New York: John Wiley and Sons.
14. Kee, J. (1991). *Laboratory and diagnostic tests with nursing implications* (3rd ed.). Norwalk, CT: Appleton and Lange.
15. Kokko, J., & Tannen, R. (1986). *Fluids and electrolytes*. Philadelphia: W. B. Saunders.
15a. Laquarta, I., & Gerlach, M. (1990). *Nutrition in clinical nursing*. Albany, New York: Delmar Publishers.
15b. Mahan, K. L., & Arlin, M. (1992). *Food, nutrition & diet therapy* (8th ed.). Philadelphia: W. B. Saunders.
16. McCance, K., & Huether, S. (1990). *Pathophysiology: The basic biologic basis for disease in adults and children*. St. Louis: C.V. Mosby.
17. Olinger, M. (1989). Disorders of calcium and magnesium metabolism. *Emergency Medical Clinics of North America, 7*(4), 795-819.
18. Salem, M., et al. (1991). Hypomagnesemia in critical illness. *Critical Care Clinics, 7*(1), 225-247.
19. Stein, J. H. (1988). Hypokalemia, common and uncommon causes. *Hospital Practice, 23*(3A), 55-70.
20. Sterns, R. (1991). The management of hyponatremic emergencies. *Critical Care Clinics, 7*(1), 127-141.
21. Van Hook, J. (1991). Hypermagnesemia. *Critical Care Clinics, 7*(1), 215-223.
22. Votey, S., et al. (1989). Disorders of water metabolism: Hyponatremia and hypernatremia. *Emergency Medical Clinics of North America, 7*(4), 749-765.
23. Watson, J. (1987). Fluid and electrolyte disorders in cardiovascular patients. *Nursing Clinics of North America, 22*(4), 805.
24. Williams, M. (1991). Hyperkalemia. *Critical Care Clinics, 7*(1), 155-173.
25. Zaloga, G. (1991). Hypocalcemic crisis. *Critical Care Clinics, 7*(1), 191-199.
26. Zull, D. (1989). Disorders of potassium metabolism. *Emergency Medical Clinics of North America, 7*(4), 771-793.

Chapter 15

Acid-Base Imbalances

Normal function of body cells depends on regulation of hydrogen ion concentration (H^+) within very narrow limits. Acid-base imbalances occur when these limits are exceeded and are recognized clinically as abnormalities of serum pH. Because acid-base imbalances may result from disease of virtually any body system, their incidence in clinical settings is very high. The nurse is responsible, along with other health professionals, for the prevention, detection, and intervention in acid-base disorders.

REGULATION OF ACID-BASE BALANCE

The symbol pH stands for the negative log of the hydrogen ion. It is used to express the degree of acidity or alkalinity of a solution. A pH of 7.0 is neutral, having an equal number of acids and bases. An acidic solution has a pH below 7.0; an alkaline solution has a pH above 7.0. Because pH is the *negative* log, a rise in pH reflects a fall in H^+ and vice versa.

Normal serum pH is 7.35 to 7.45. Cell function is seriously impaired when pH falls to 7.2 or lower or rises to 7.55 or higher. Rapid *rates* of change in pH are especially detrimental. Serum pH below 6.8 or above 7.8 may be incompatible with life.

Three physiologic systems act interdependently to maintain normal serum pH: excretion of acid by the *lungs,* excretion of acid or reclamation of base by the *kidneys,* and buffering of excess acid or base by the *blood buffer systems.*

Regulation of Volatile Acid by the Lungs

Volatile acids are acids that can be converted to gases. The lungs are the major organs of acid elimination, excreting approximately 13,000 mEq/day of acid in comparison to 40 to 80 mEg/day excreted by the kidneys. The lungs excrete carbonic acid (H_2CO_3) in its gaseous form, carbon dioxide (CO_2).

CO_2, produced by body cells as an end product of aerobic carbohydrate metabolism, diffuses into the blood, where it reacts with water to form carbonic acid. Carbonic acid may then dissociate, releasing free H^+ into the blood to decrease pH. This reversible *hydrolysis reaction* is shown.

$$H_2O + CO_2 \rightleftarrows H_2CO_3 \rightleftarrows HCO_3^- + H^+$$

It is apparent from this equation that CO_2 and H_2CO_3 are directly related. As CO_2 rises, acid rises (pH falls), and vice versa. As carbonic acid reaches the lungs via venous blood, CO_2 is exhaled. The lungs are able to respond relatively quickly to pH changes, acting within a matter of hours to restore normal or near-normal acid-base proportions. The rate of CO_2 excretion by the lungs depends on the rate of alveolar ventilation. As ventilation increases (i.e., as tidal volume or respiratory rate increases), CO_2 excretion increases and pH rises. Conversely, when ventilation is decreased, less acid is excreted, and pH falls.

The hydrolysis equation also demonstrates that some of the CO_2 entering the blood ultimately forms the base bicarbonate (HCO_3^-). A small amount of HCO_3^- is formed in the plasma, but most is formed in erythrocytes. CO_2 diffuses into erythrocytes, in which the hydrolysis reaction occurs rapidly owing to the presence of *carbonic anhydrase,* a catalytic enzyme. The bicarbonate anion then diffuses out of the erythrocyte into the plasma while the chloride anion moves in. This *chloride shift* is necessary to maintain electroneutrality inside the red blood cell. HCO_3^- formed in this way accounts for the major portion (80 per cent) of CO_2 transported in the blood. Small amounts are transported in dissolved form (8 per cent) or in combination with hemoglobin or other proteins (12 per cent). The actual amount of carbonic acid in the blood is negligible (0.0006 per cent).

Regulation of Fixed Acids and Bicarbonate by the Kidneys

Acids that cannot be converted to a gaseous form must be eliminated in the urine. These include sulfuric and phosphoric acid produced by protein metabolism, ketoacids produced by incomplete lipid metabolism (as in diabetic ketoacidosis), and lactic acid produced by anaerobic carbohydrate metabolism (as in shock or hypoxemia). Regulation of acid-base balance by the kidneys is slower than that of the lungs; it takes several days for significant changes in urine pH to be clinically apparent.

Renal tubular cells are able to secrete H^+ into the urine until the pH of the urine falls to about 4.5. Presence of *urinary buffer systems* allows the tubular fluid to accept large quantities of H^+ while the degree to which urinary pH falls is limited.

BUFFER SYSTEMS

Buffer systems consist of a weak acid (one that does not readily release free H^+) with a salt of its conjugate base. The pH of buffered solutions tends to be fairly stable in spite of the addition of strong acid or base because the buffer system combines with the added acid or base to convert it to a weaker form. Buffer systems do *not* eliminate acid or base from the body; rather, they minimize pH changes by forming acids or bases that do not readily dissociate into free ions. Because only the free H^+ contributes to pH, changes in pH are minimized.

The three principal buffers in renal tubular fluid are bicarbonate, ammonia, and phosphate. All three systems start within the renal tubular cell, in which the hydrolysis reaction occurs at rapid rates because of the presence of carbonic anhydrase.

In the *bicarbonate system,* the conjugate pair consists of carbonic acid and sodium bicarbonate ($NaHCO_3$). H^+ ions from the hydrolysis reaction are secreted into the urinary filtrate in exchange for sodium from the dissociated salt (Fig. 15–1*A*). The sodium is then actively transported to the extracellular fluid, accompanied by HCO_3^-, which was also formed in the tubular cell from the hydrolysis reaction. It is important to note that for each H^+ secreted, a bicarbonate ion is returned to the blood. Meanwhile, in the tubule, the H^+ ions combine with HCO_3^- from the dissociated salt, forming carbonic acid, which in turn forms CO_2 and H_2O in a reversal of hydrolysis. CO_2 is reabsorbed into the blood for excretion by the lungs; the H_2O is eliminated in the urine.

Ammonia (NH_3) is generated in renal tubular cells from amino acids such as glutamine. NH_3 gas diffuses into the tubular fluid, in which it can combine with H^+ to form ammonium (NH_4^+), which cannot be reabsorbed into the tubular cell (Fig. 15–1*B*). NH_4^+, "trapped" in the tubule, combines with Cl^- (from NaCl) and is excreted in the urine. Na^+ is reabsorbed along with HCO_3^- from the tubular cell.

The *phosphate* buffer operates similarly (Fig. 15–1*C*). $Na_2^{2+}HPO_4^{2-}$, present in the filtrate, exchanges hydrogen for sodium. $H_2PO_4^-$ is then excreted in the urine; Na^+ and HCO_3^- enter the blood.

THE ROLE OF OTHER ELECTROLYTES

The role of the kidneys in regulating serum bicarbonate and hydrogen ion concentrations is greatly influenced by the concentrations of other electrolytes. When potassium (K^+) is present in excessive amounts in tubular cells (hyperkalemia), K^+ is secreted in place of H^+. In hypokalemia, increased amounts of H^+ are secreted. When H^+ is low, selective K^+ loss occurs. In acidosis at the tissue level, extracellular H^+ tends to shift intracel-

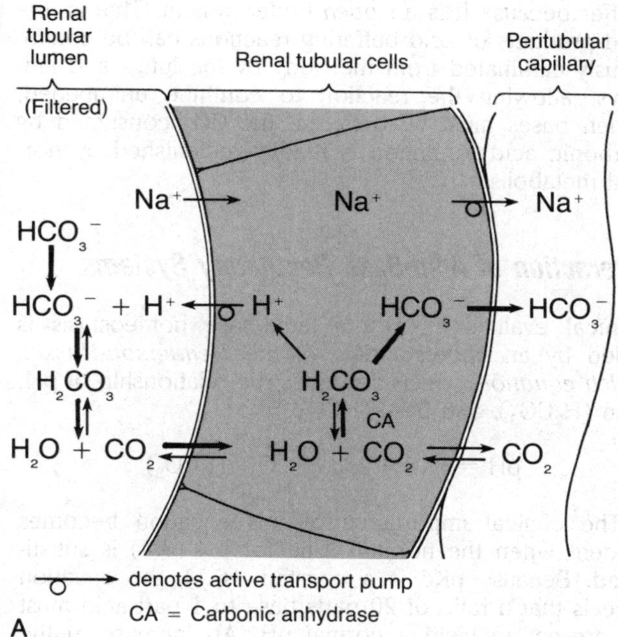

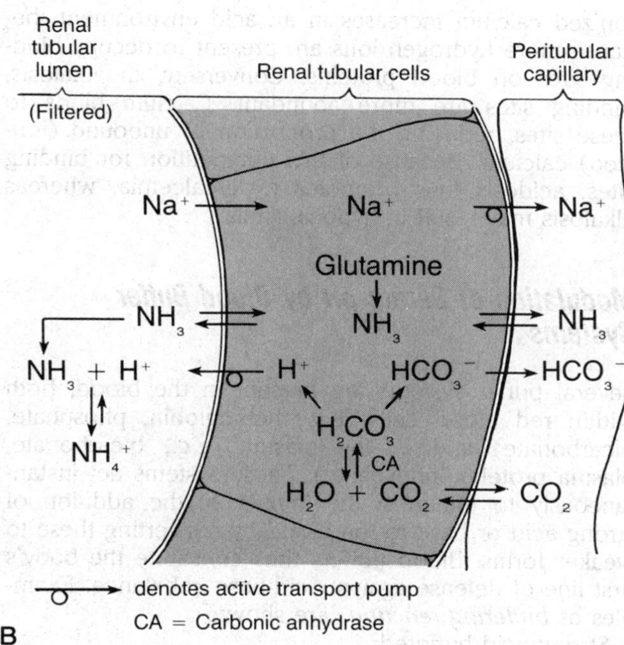

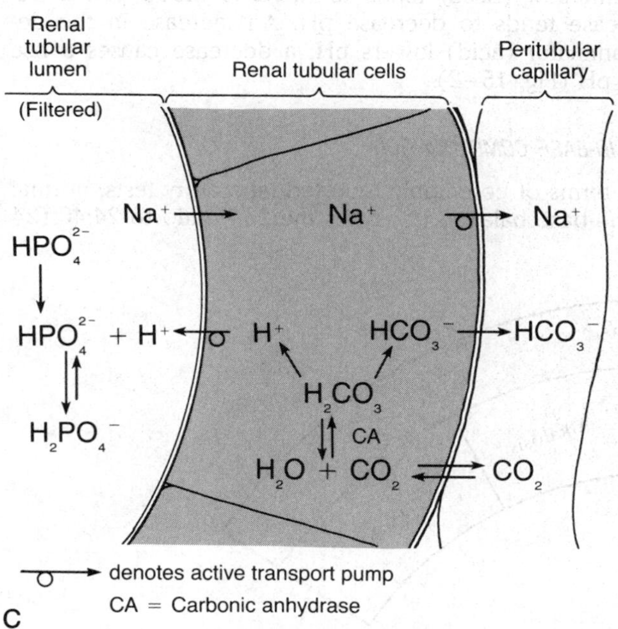

▲ ***Figure 15–1***

Urinary buffer systems. *A*, Bicarbonate buffer; *B*, ammonia buffer; *C*, phosphate buffer. (Data from Rose, B. D. [1984]. *Clinical physiology of acid-base and electrolyte disorders* (2nd ed.). New York: McGraw-Hill Book Co.)

lularly while K^+ moves into the blood. Early in acidosis, K^+ excess occurs in the extracellular fluid because of this exchange. True hyperkalemia develops more gradually, as the kidney secretes H^+ instead of K^+. This concept has clinical implications in that if acidosis is corrected too rapidly (as with rapid infusion of sodium bicarbonate), an undetected hypokalemia may result as K^+ moves back into cells. (Twenty-five per cent of deaths due to diabetic ketoacidosis result from this mechanism.)

Bicarbonate reabsorption is also influenced by sodium regulation, which is in turn dependent on blood volume. As a consequence of hypovolemia, the renin-angiotensin-aldosterone system is activated, and the adrenocortical hormone aldosterone stimulates $NaHCO_3$ reabsorption in the distal tubule of the nephron.

Because of the chloride shift in the red blood cells, chloride levels in the blood vary inversely with bicarbonate. When a chloride deficit exists (as is often the case with hyponatremia), bicarbonate is reabsorbed in increased amounts by the kidney. Chloride levels may, therefore, be elevated in acidosis caused by loss of bicarbonate in the urine, as in renal tubular acidosis, or by intestinal losses through enteric drainage or diarrhea.

Serum calcium (Ca^{2+}) exists in both ionized and nonionized forms in the plasma; however, only the ionized form is electrochemically active. The proportion of ionized calcium increases in an acid environment, because more hydrogen ions are present to occupy binding sites on blood proteins. Conversely, in alkalosis, binding sites are more abundant. Calcium binds to these sites, reducing the proportion of unbound (ionized) calcium. Because of this competition for binding sites, acidosis thus promotes hypercalcemia, whereas alkalosis may result in hypocalcemia.

Modulation of Serum pH by Blood Buffer Systems

Several buffer systems are present in the blood, both within red blood cells (e.g., hemoglobin, phosphate, bicarbonate) and in the plasma (e.g., bicarbonate, plasma proteins, phosphate). These systems act instantaneously to minimize the impact of the addition of strong acid or base to the blood by converting these to weaker forms. Blood buffers thus constitute the body's first line of defense against acid-base imbalance. Examples of *buffering reactions* are shown.

Strong acid buffered:

$$HCl + (H_2CO_3/NaHCO_3) \rightarrow NaCl + H_2CO_3$$

Strong base buffered:

$$NaOH + H_2CO_3 \rightarrow NaHCO_3 + H_2O$$

Whereas hemoglobin is present in the greatest concentration, *plasma bicarbonate* is the most effective buffer because it is an *open* buffer system. That is, the end products of acid buffering reactions can be continuously eliminated from the body by the lungs and kidneys, allowing the reaction to continue unimpeded. When bases must be buffered, the CO_2 consumed by carbonic acid formation is readily replenished by normal metabolism.

Interaction of Acid-Base Regulatory Systems

Clinical evaluation of total acid-base homeostasis is aided by an understanding of the *Henderson-Hasselbalch equation*, which describes the relationship of pH, acid (H_2CO_3), and base (HCO_3^-).

$$pH = pKc + \log (HCO_3^-/H_2CO_3)$$

The clinical importance of this equation becomes evident when the normal value for pH (7.4) is substituted. Because pKc is a constant (6.1), the equation reveals that a ratio of 20 parts base to 1 part acid must be present to yield a normal pH. An increase in the numerator (base) tends to increase blood pH; a decrease tends to decrease pH. An increase in the denominator (acid) lowers pH; a decrease causes a rise in pH (Fig. 15-2).

ACID-BASE COMPENSATION

In terms of commonly reported laboratory tests, normal acid-base balance translates the 20:1 ratio to 24:40 (24

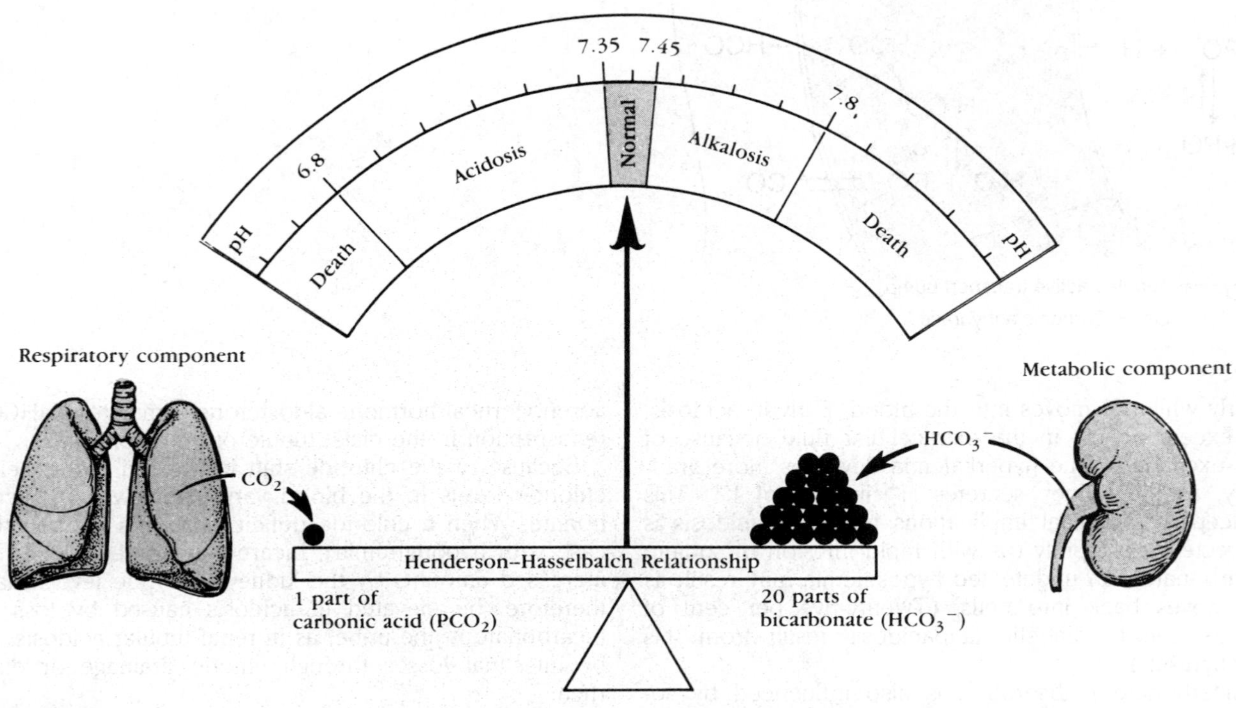

▲ Figure 15-2

Regulation of acid-base balance. (From Bullock, B. & Rosendahl, P. [1992]. *Pathophysiology: Adaptations and alterations in function* (3rd ed.). Glenview, IL: Scott, Foresman and Company. Used with permission.)

mEq/L HCO_3^- to 40 mm Hg $PaCO_2$) (Fig. 15-3). $PaCO_2$ is the partial pressure of carbon dioxide in arterial blood. When primary disease processes alter either the acid or base component of the ratio, the lungs or the kidneys (whichever is unaffected by pathologic change) act to restore the 20:1 ratio and normalize pH. This process is known as acid-base *compensation.* When kidney disease impairs excretion of fixed acids, for example, the respiratory system can increase ventilation to "blow off" excess acid as CO_2. The kidneys can compensate for retention of acid (CO_2) in respiratory failure by retaining more HCO_3^-.

The blood buffers act to modulate pH changes but do not eliminate acid or base from the body. The lungs or kidneys alter actual amounts of acid and base, but regulation by these systems is not instantaneous. The lungs respond within minutes, but maximal compensation takes up to 24 hours. The kidneys may require up to 72 hours to achieve optimal compensation. Compensation does not usually result in complete return of pH to the normal range. More typically, compensation brings pH to within 50 to 75 per cent of normal.

ACID-BASE CORRECTION

Although compensatory responses for primary acid-base disorders may nearly restore the 20:1 ratio of base to acid, the actual amounts of acid and base remain abnormal. Thus, compensation must be differentiated from *correction,* in which not only is the ratio restored, but absolute quantities of $PaCO_2$ and HCO_3^- are returned to the normal range. Correction occurs only with resolution of the underlying disorder.

DISORDERS OF ACID-BASE BALANCE

Definition

The four general classes of acid-base imbalance are respiratory acidosis, respiratory alkalosis, metabolic acidosis, and metabolic alkalosis. *Acidosis* refers to any pathologic process causing a relative excess of acid (volatile or fixed) in the body. *Acidemia* is excess acid in the blood. The presence of acidemia does not necessarily confirm an underlying pathologic process; technically it is merely a laboratory finding. The same distinction may be made between the terms *alkalosis* and *alkalemia*; alkalosis indicates a primary condition resulting in excess base in the body. Although efforts have been made to standardize acid-base terminology, the terms are often used interchangeably in clinical practice.

Incidence

The incidence of acid-base imbalances in clinical settings is high. A recent study of 110 consecutive admissions to a general hospital revealed an overall incidence of acid-base imbalances of 56 per cent. The most common disorder was respiratory alkalosis (26

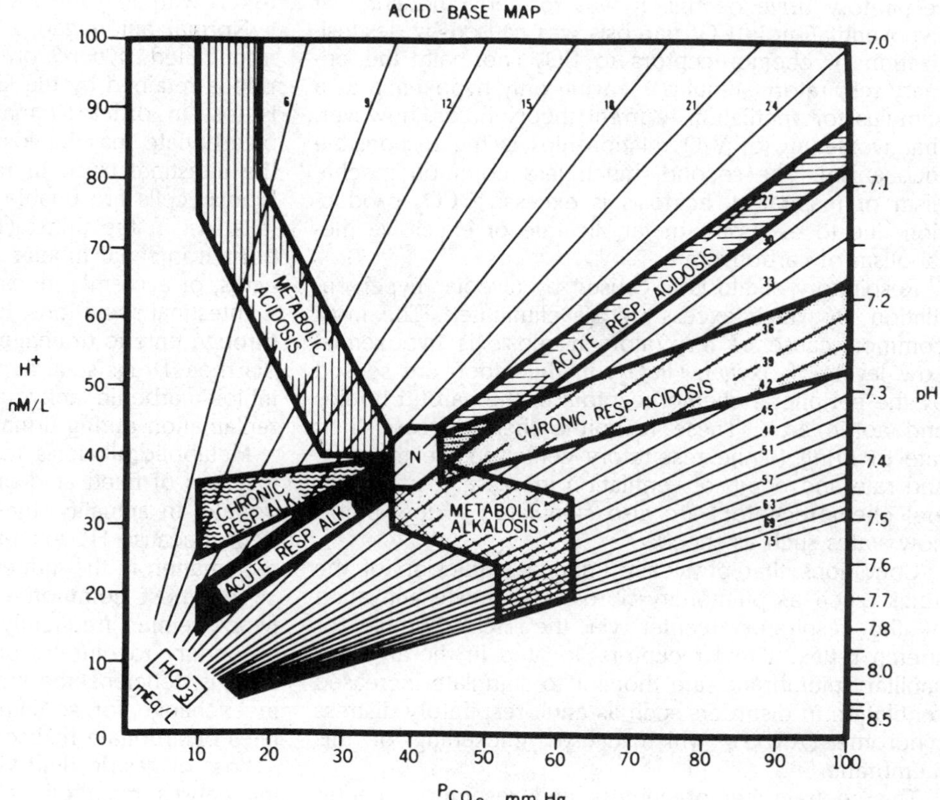

▲ **Figure 15-3**

Acid-base map. To use the acid-base map, the pH is plotted on the vertical axis and the $PaCO_2$ is plotted on the horizontal axis. The point at which the values intersect is noted. If it falls outside the normal (N) area or the 95 per cent confidence bands for the major primary disorders, it most likely represents a mixed acid-base imbalance. A point falling within one of the bands does not rule out mixed disorder, however. (From Halstad, C., & Halstad, J. [1981]. *The Laboratory in Clinical Medicine.* Philadelphia: W. B. Saunders Company. Used with permission.)

cases), followed in order by respiratory acidosis (16), metabolic alkalosis (10), and metabolic acidosis (6). Eleven persons had more than one acid-base imbalance concurrently.[13]

Overview of Acid-Base Disorders

Table 15-1 summarizes pathophysiologic mechanisms, common etiologic factors, clinical manifestations, and medical management of the four imbalances.

RESPIRATORY ACIDOSIS/ALKALOSIS

Respiratory acidosis is nearly always due to hypoventilation. Chronic respiratory acidosis is most commonly caused by chronic obstructive pulmonary disease (COPD). In end-stage disease, pathologic changes lead to airway collapse, air trapping, and disturbance of ventilation-perfusion (V/Q) relationships. Acute respiratory acidosis also occurs in these clients when superimposed respiratory infection or concurrent cardiac disease increases the work of breathing. Hypoventilation with resultant respiratory acidosis is also seen in diseases of the neuromuscular junction in which diaphragmatic movement is impaired (such as Guillain-Barré syndrome) and in depression of the medullary respiratory center by drugs or lesions of the central nervous system (CNS).

Respiratory acidosis may be caused iatrogenically by inadequate mechanical ventilation or by excessive oxygen administration to clients with COPD. In the latter case, CO_2 narcosis results when blunting of the central respiratory drive occurs. It was formerly thought that hypoventilation in CO_2 narcosis was caused by desensitization of chemoreceptors to CO_2 (normally the primary respiratory stimulus), leaving only hypoxemia as a stimulus for ventilation. Current theory holds, however, that worsening of V/Q relationships is the responsible mechanism. The second, much less common mechanism of respiratory acidosis is excessive CO_2 production due to excessive metabolic rate or excessive metabolism of carbohydrate.

Respiratory alkalosis is caused by alveolar hyperventilation, in which excess CO_2 is eliminated. The most common cause of respiratory alkalosis is hypoxemia. Low levels of oxygen (PaO_2) in the blood are sensed by the peripheral chemoreceptors in the carotid bodies and aortic arch. These receptors then increase their rate of firing to the respiratory center in the medulla, and rate and depth of ventilation increase. The peripheral chemoreceptors are also stimulated in low blood flow states such as shock.

Conditions that physically impede expansion of the lungs (such as pulmonary fibrosis) stimulate activation of the respiratory center via the Hering-Breuer or stretch reflex. The J receptors, located in the alveolar-capillary membrane, are thought to stimulate increased ventilation in disorders such as adult respiratory distress syndrome (ARDS), which causes thickening of this membrane.

The central chemoreceptors and respiratory center may be stimulated excessively by chemicals or toxins. In the case of salicylate (aspirin) overdose, it is interesting that adults usually exhibit respiratory alkalosis, whereas children more often have metabolic acidosis due to the acid ingestion. The reason for this is unknown. Other conditions that may overstimulate the respiratory center include CNS lesions or trauma, fever, exercise, extreme emotional stress, or severe pain.

METABOLIC ACIDOSIS/ALKALOSIS

Metabolic acidosis may be caused by two different mechanisms: accumulation of fixed acid or loss of base. These mechanisms may be differentiated clinically by the presence or absence of a high *anion gap* (A^-). Normally, the anion gap is 12 to 14 mEq/L. A^- is calculated by subtracting the sum of the major anions, bicarbonate and chloride, from the sodium concentration. The principle of electroneutrality forms the basis for this calculation. When acidosis is the result of addition of fixed acid (as in lactic acidosis), bicarbonate is consumed in buffering, and the anion gap increases. When acidosis is due to loss of bicarbonate, however, chloride levels increase to maintain electroneutrality, and the anion gap does not change.

Common causes of high anion gap acidosis include azotemic renal failure, in which acid end products of protein metabolism cannot be effectively excreted because of impaired glomerular filtration; diabetic ketoacidosis, in which ketoacids accumulate owing to accelerated lipid metabolism in the absence of insulin; and lactic acidosis, a consequence of anaerobic carbohydrate metabolism. Less commonly, ingestion of toxins with acid metabolites is the cause.

Normal anion gap acidosis, due to loss of base, is also called *hyperchloremic metabolic acidosis*. Chloride is retained by the kidney when excess bicarbonate is lost in order to maintain electroneutrality. Excess bicarbonate may be lost through either the kidneys or the intestinal tract. In renal tubular acidosis, the renal tubular cells are unable to reabsorb bicarbonate; thus, it is lost in the urine. (Because glomerular filtration is normal in renal tubular acidosis, accumulation of fixed acids, or azotemia, does not occur.)

Intestinal secretions, high in bicarbonate, may be lost through enteric drainage tubes (e.g., ileostomy) or with diarrhea. Drugs such as acetazolamide (Diamox), which inhibit carbonic anhydrase, interfere with bicarbonate reclamation during urinary buffering.

Metabolic alkalosis may be caused by either abnormal loss of fixed acid or excess accumulation of bicarbonate. In actuality, these mechanisms are interdependent, because H^+ excretion is accompanied by HCO_3^- reclamation in the kidney and in gastric cells.

The most common cause of metabolic alkalosis is hypokalemia, frequently seen in hospitalized clients secondary to diuretic or steroid therapy. When potassium is deficient, the kidneys secrete H^+ into the urine in exchange for sodium. This process, in turn, stimulates bicarbonate reabsorption.

Loss of gastric fluid via nasogastric suction or vomiting causes metabolic alkalosis due to loss of hydro-

TABLE 15-1. Overview of Acid-Base Imbalances

Mechanism	Etiology	Clinical Manifestations	Treatment
Respiratory Acidosis			
Hypoventilation	COPD Neuromuscular disease Guillain-Barré Myasthenia gravis Respiratory center depression Drugs Barbiturates Sedatives Narcotics Anesthetics CNS lesions Tumor Stroke Iatrogenic disorders Inadequate mechanical ventilation CO_2 narcosis	Dyspnea Disorientation or coma Dysrhythmias pH below 7.35 $PaCO_2$ above 45 mmHg Hyperkalemia Hypoxemia	Treat underlying cause Support ventilation Correct electrolyte imbalance Intravenous $NaHCO_3$*
Excess CO_2 production	Hypermetabolism Sepsis Burns Excess carbohydrate intake Total parenteral nutrition Enteral feeding		
Respiratory Alkalosis			
Hyperventilation	Hypoxemia Emphysema Pneumonia ARDS Impaired lung expansion Pulmonary fibrosis Ascites Scoliosis Pregnancy† Thickened alveolar-capillary membrane Congestive heart failure ARDS Pneumonia Pulmonary embolism Chemical stimulation of respiratory center Bacterial toxins (sepsis) Ammonia (hepatic failure) Salicylates (aspirin overdose) Traumatic stimulation of respiratory center CNS trauma CNS tumor Increased intracranial pressure Excessive exercise Extreme stress Severe pain	Tachypnea Hyperpnea‡ Giddiness, dizziness, syncope, convulsions, or coma Weakness, paresthesias, tetany pH above 7.45 $PaCO_2$ below 35 mmHg Hypokalemia Hypocalcemia	Treat underlying cause Increase CO_2 retention Mechanical hypoventilation CO_2 rebreathing§ Sedation

Table continued on following page

TABLE 15–1. Overview of Acid-Base Imbalances Continued

Mechanism	Etiology	Clinical Manifestations	Treatment
Metabolic Acidosis			
Fixed acid excess	Renal failure Diabetic ketoacidosis Lactic acidosis Injested toxins Aspirin Antifreeze	Hyperventilation (compensatory) Drowsiness, confusion, or coma Headache pH below 7.35 HCO_3^- less than 22 mmHg Anion gap greater than 16 if excess acid Hyperchloremia if base deficit $PaCO_2$ normal or slightly decreased	Treat underlying cause Correct electrolyte imbalance Intravenous $NaHCO_3$*
Base deficit	Renal tubular acidosis Carbonic anhydrase inhibitors Acetazolamide (Diamox) Mafenide acetate (Sulfamylon Acetate Cream)		
Metabolic Alkalosis			
Fixed acid loss (with resultant base excess)	Hypokalemia Diuresis Steroids Gastric fluid loss Vomiting Nasogastric aspiration	Hypoventilation (compensatory) Dysrhythmias pH above 7.45 Hypokalemia Hypocalcemia $PaCO_2$ normal or slightly increased	Treat underlying cause Administer KCl Intravenous acidifying salts* (e.g., NH_4Cl) in extreme cases
Excessive HCO_3^- intake	Milk-alkali syndrome Overcorrection of acidosis with $NaHCO_3$ Massive transfusion of whole blood		
Excessive HCO_3^- reabsorption	Hyperaldosteronism Licorice intoxication		

* Use of therapeutic compensation, e.g., intravenous acid or base administration, is controversial. (See text.)
† In the third trimester of pregnancy, the hormone progesterone also stimulates respiration.
‡ Restrictive lung disorders may preclude increased tidal volume.
§ Specific measures include breathing into a paper bag or increasing tubing dead space with mechanical ventilation.

chloric acid (HCl). When HCl is lost, new HCl must be produced by gastric cells via the hydrolysis reaction. H^+ is secreted into the stomach with Cl^-; the HCO_3^- produced in the reaction is reabsorbed into the blood in exchange for chloride.

Hyperaldosteronism leads to metabolic alkalosis via increased renal tubular reabsorption of sodium and subsequent loss of potassium. Rarely, excessive licorice ingestion (e.g., 20 to 40 g) causes metabolic alkalosis owing to its structural similarity to aldosterone. Overcorrection of acidosis with $NaHCO_3$ administration may cause alkalosis, as can massive transfusion of whole blood. The citrate anticoagulant used for storage of blood is metabolized to bicarbonate. Packed red blood cells contain much less citrate; thus, their use in multiple transfusion is preferred.

MIXED ACID-BASE DISORDERS

Mixed acid-base disorders, in which two primary acid-base imbalances coexist, are frequently seen in clinical situations. In cardiac arrest, for example, lactic acid quickly accumulates as a result of anaerobic metabolism; carbonic acid is elevated because of respiratory arrest. In COPD, underlying respiratory acidosis may be complicated by metabolic alkalosis secondary to diuretic or steroid therapy.

Prevention

The nurse must maintain a high index of suspicion in *clients at risk* for acid-base imbalance. These include (1) clients with known disease of the pulmonary, cardiovascular, or renal systems; (2) clients who manifest hypermetabolic states, as in fever, sepsis, or burns; (3) clients receiving total parenteral nutrition or enteral tube feedings high in carbohydrate; (4) mechanically ventilated clients; (5) insulin-dependent diabetics; (6) clients with vomiting, diarrhea, or enteric drainage; and (7) the elderly, whose age-related decreases in respiratory and renal function may limit their ability to compensate for acid-base disturbances.

The *normal aging process* results in decreased ventilatory capacity as well as loss of alveolar surface area for gas exchange; thus, the elderly are prone to respiratory acidosis due to hypoventilation and to respiratory alkalosis due to hypoxemia. Elderly persons are frequently taking multiple medications for hypertension or cardiovascular disease; these drugs may contribute to hypokalemia and metabolic alkalosis. Respiratory compensation in this condition is compromised owing to the structural and functional changes mentioned. Decreased cardiac output in the aging person diminishes renal perfusion and glomerular filtration. Aldosterone is less effective in the elderly, as is ammonia buffering. These changes limit renal compensation for respiratory imbalances and place the individual at higher risk for metabolic imbalance.

Clinical Manifestations

Ventilatory disturbance is present in all imbalances, either as a contributing cause in respiratory imbalances or as a compensatory response in metabolic imbalances. Acidosis depresses the central nervous system; alkalosis stimulates it. Ultimately, severe, untreated acidosis and alkalosis both lead to coma.

DIAGNOSTIC ASSESSMENT

Electrolyte imbalance nearly always coexists with acid-base imbalance owing to the mechanisms previously discussed. Symptoms resulting from abnormal levels of specific ions are seen. Abnormalities of serum pH, $PaCO_2$, or HCO_3^- typical of the specific disturbance are seen on arterial blood gas (ABG) reports. (See later discussion of ABG analysis.)

Medical Management

Treatment in acid-base imbalances is directed toward removing the underlying cause, if possible. Respiratory infections contributing to ventilatory failure are managed with appropriate antibiotic therapy. Use of pharmaceutical agents that depress the respiratory control center is curtailed. Enteral feedings that supply more than 50 per cent of calories in the form of carbohydrate are replaced if metabolic CO_2 production is excessive. Dialysis may be indicated in renal failure or overdose of toxins. Support of ventilation may be required, in the form of pharmacologic intervention, hydration, pulmonary hygiene, oxygen therapy, and possibly continuous mechanical ventilation. Correction of any coexisting electrolyte imbalance is also indicated.

Therapeutic compensation for severe pH derangement is controversial. In acidosis, for example, intravenous administration of sodium bicarbonate may have an immediate beneficial effect on pH. Eventually, however, blood levels of CO_2 rise because HCO_3^- fuels the hydrolysis reaction in reverse. In severe alkalosis, intravenous administration of HCl or an acidifying salt such as ammonium chloride or arginine hydrochloride might be employed. These agents are highly toxic to the liver and kidneys, however, and cause red blood cell hemolysis if they are administered too rapidly.

Nursing Management

ASSESSMENT

Findings of comprehensive *physical assessment* of ventilatory status, cardiovascular function, and fluid balance must be documented with careful analysis of trends. Laboratory values that should be noted include electrolytes, blood urea nitrogen, creatinine, serum lactate, and *arterial blood gases (ABGs).*

The nurse's knowledgeable interpretation of ABGs is critical for timely, appropriate intervention in acid-base disturbances. Often, ABG results are first reported to the nurse, who is the communication link between respiratory therapists and physicians regarding potential changes in client status or treatment. Whereas ABG interpretation is essential to diagnosis and treatment of acid-base imbalance, it must be emphasized that ABG findings are of value only when they are considered in the context of the total clinical picture. The recommended procedure for evaluation of ABGs is detailed in Box 15-1. The data from ABGs can also be interpreted by using the acid-base map (Fig. 15-3).

Nursing Diagnosis: Several *nursing diagnoses* may apply to the management of underlying causes and clinical manifestations of acid-base disturbances. Examples of these diagnoses, along with priority nursing interventions, are shown in the Care Plan for the Client with Acid-Base Imbalance. Acid-base imbalances per se are perhaps best conceptualized as *collaborative problems,* however, in that the interventions of several health care professionals including nurses, respiratory therapists, and physicians are required for effective treatment.

NURSING INTERVENTION

Planning: Expected Outcomes. The expected outcomes for the client with acid-base imbalances when collaborative problems are used entail monitoring for clinical manifestations of the imbalances. Likewise, the nurse monitors clinical manifestations of the imbalances following treatment. Expected outcomes for nursing diagnoses are shown in the Care Plan for the Client with Acid-Base Imbalance.

Implementation. *Protection of the client* from injury during diagnostic procedures is a priority nursing responsibility. Before radial puncture for obtaining an arterial specimen for ABGs, the Allen test should be performed to ascertain adequate ulnar circulation (see Chap. 36). The Allen test is done by first having the

Box 15–1. Analysis of Arterial Blood Gases

Step 1: Classify the pH

Normal: 7.35–7.45
Acidemia: below 7.35
Alkalemia: above 7.45

Step 2: Assess $PaCO_2$

Normal: 35–45 mm Hg
Respiratory acidosis: above 45 mm Hg
Respiratory alkalosis: below 35 mm Hg

Step 3: Assess HCO_3^-*

Normal: 22–26 mEq/L
Metabolic acidosis: below 22 mEq/L
Metabolic alkalosis: above 26 mEq/L

Step 4: Determine presence of compensation

Compensation present: $PaCO_2$ *and* HCO_3^- are abnormal (or nearly so) in *opposite* directions, e.g., one is acidotic and the other alkalotic.†

Compensation absent: One component ($PaCO_2$ or HCO_3^-) is abnormal, the other normal.

Step 5: Identify primary disorder, if possible

If pH is clearly abnormal: Acid-base component most consistent with pH is primary disorder.

If pH is normal or near-normal: The more deviant component is probably primary.‡ To verify, note whether pH is on acidotic or alkalotic side of 7.4. The more deviant value should be consistent with this pH.

Step 6: Classify degree of compensation, if present

Partial compensation: Evidence of compensation, but pH is still abnormal.

Complete compensation: Evidence of compensation, pH is normal.

* Base excess (BE) is also reported with ABGs and is a second index of metabolic status. Normal BE is −2 to +2. Because fluctuation in BE exactly parallels that of bicarbonate, it is not necessary to classify both.

† It is possible, but less likely, that two opposing primary imbalances (e.g., a mixed disorder) are present, which results in the *appearance* of compensation. The detection of mixed disorders is facilitated by the use of acid-base maps or nomograms (Fig. 15–3), but a mixed disorder cannot always be differentiated from compensation.

‡ It is unlikely that the more deviant value represents compensation, because the body does not overcompensate for imbalance. When pH approaches the normal range, compensatory mechanisms are no longer triggered.

client tightly close the hand into a fist. The nurse then occludes both the radial and ulnar arteries by applying pressure over the pulse points. The client's hand is then opened; it will have a blanched appearance due to lack of blood. The nurse then releases the ulnar pressure. If ulnar circulation is adequate, color will return to the hand within 10 to 15 seconds. The test should then be repeated with release of the radial artery. Failure to assess collateral circulation could result in severe ischemic injury to the hand if damage to the radial artery occurs with arterial puncture.

Critically ill clients commonly have femoral or radial arterial catheter systems from which blood specimens are drawn. Frequent sampling can result in significant blood loss if an open system is used. Nursing research has demonstrated that a minimum discard specimen of 2 ml is sufficient to clear the arterial line of heparinized solution before aspiration of blood for ABG testing (see Nursing Research). Recently introduced closed systems (e.g., the VAMP system) allow reinstillation of initially aspirated heparinized solution and blood. Nursing responsibilities for clients with arterial lines are discussed in Chapter 43.

The nurse is also responsible for minimizing errors in ABG analysis due to faulty specimen collection and handling. Potential sampling errors, their consequences, and nursing implications are summarized in Table 15–2.

Despite quality control procedures, erroneous blood gas data are sometimes reported. The nurse should suspect sampling error or transcription error when the reported values lack internal consistency or external congruity. Internal consistency means that the values make sense when considered as a whole. An alkalotic pH, for example, is inconsistent with excess $PaCO_2$ *and* a deficit of HCO_3^-. External congruity means that the ABG findings are consistent with other laboratory data as well as with clinical assessment findings. The client with a pH of 7.10 should appear profoundly ill.

SUPPORTIVE CARE

Supportive care involves preserving an *acceptable* (not necessarily normal) pH and preventing life-threatening

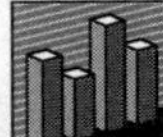

NURSING RESEARCH

Using an in vitro model (time-expired human red cells from banked blood), the researchers tested 319 arterial blood gas (ABG) specimens drawn from an arterial line system that had a typical dead space of 1 ml. The discard sample was intentionally varied from 0 to 5 ml in 0.5 ml increments in random order. A 1 ml ABG sample was drawn after each discard. Statistically significant differences in ABG values were found between the samples drawn after 0 to 1.5 ml discard and the samples drawn after 2 ml or greater discards. Small discard samples were associated with lowered PCO_2 and HCO_3^-. The authors concluded that a minimum 2 ml discard sample is required to ensure accuracy of ABG specimens drawn from arterial lines.

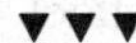

Preusser, B., Lash, J., Stone, K., et al. (1989). Quantifying the minimum discard sample required for accurate arterial blood gases. *Nursing Research, 38*(5), 276–279.

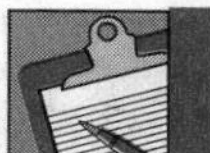

CARE PLAN

The Client with Acid-Base Imbalance

Nursing Diagnosis/ Collaborative Problem	Planning: Expected Outcomes	Implementation: Nursing Interventions	Rationales
Ineffective Breathing Pattern and Impaired Gas Exchange	Client will have improved breathing patterns and gas exchange as evidenced by: • respiratory rate WNL • no dyspnea • clear breath sounds • ABGs WNL • SaO_2 above 95%	Monitor respiratory status: rate, volume, patterns, breath sounds, ABGs, SaO_2	There are clinical manifestations of respiratory impairments.
		Position for optimal ventilation; reposition frequently	Ventilatory problems exist in all acid-base disorders. Repositioning allows ventilation of all lung fields.
		Offer fluids if allowed.	Fluids help thin secretions facilitating expectoration.
		Intervene in pain, fever, or anxiety if present.	Pain, fever, and anxiety increase respiratory rate.
		Teach and encourage coughing and deep-breathing. Suction prn.	Coughing, deep breathing, and suctioning help maintain airway patency and ventilation.
Sensory-Perceptual Alteration	Client will have decreased sensory perceptual alterations as evidenced by: • orientation in all spheres	Observe and attend as necessary to ensure safety. Restrain prn.	Physical restraints are one method to ensure safety.
		Assess level of consciousness and orientation.	Decreasing levels of consciousness and disorientation may indicate cerebral hypoxia.
		Reorient as necessary.	Reorientation assists the client to understand and participate in care.
Altered Peripheral Tissue Perfusion	Client will have adequate peripheral tissue perfusion as evidenced by: • full pulses in extremities • immediate capillary refill • skin warm and dry	Assess skin color, temperature, peripheral pulses, capillary refill.	Decreased peripheral tissue perfusion causes pallor, cool skin, decrease pulse quality, and slowed capillary refill.
		Maintain comfortable room temperature and provide warm blankets if needed.	External warmth will improve peripheral tissue perfusion.
		Assess pressure points for skin breakdown.	Decreased perfusion to the skin increases risk of pressure ulcers.
Anxiety	Client will have decreased anxiety as evidenced by: • decreased statements about anxiety • decreased nonverbal signs (eyes darting, fidgeting)	Assess verbal and nonverbal behavior for cues to anxiety.	Anxiety is seen in conditions leading to cerebral hypoxia. Clients often report anxiety prior to other objective symptoms.

Care Plan continued on following page

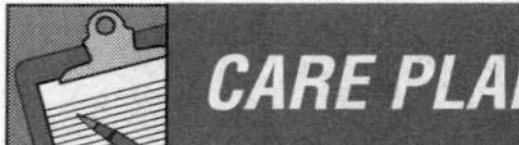

CARE PLAN

The Client with Acid-Base Imbalance Continued

Nursing Diagnosis/ Collaborative Problem	Planning: Expected Outcomes	Implementation: Nursing Interventions	Rationales
		Assess client and family coping.	Ineffective coping increases anxiety and anxiety is contagious.
		Reduce environmental stress if possible	Stressors in the environment may increase anxiety and oxygen consumption.
		Establish therapeutic relationship: acknowledge client's anxiety, listen to client's concerns, provide factual information, reinforce positive coping.	The nurse's calm manner and therapeutic communication can decrease anxiety.
Risk for Injury	Client will sustain no injury as evidenced by: • maintaining adequate (or previous quality) of pulses and perfusion of extremities • developing no clinical manifestations of complications from mechanical ventilation or oxygen therapy	Perform Allen test prior to arterial puncture.	Determines patency of ulnar and radial arteries.
		Monitor infusion rates of fluids, $NaHCO_3$, or HCl if ordered. Observe carefully for response.	These drugs are tissue irritants.
		Use quality control measures to maximize ABG accuracy.	Prevents unnecessary re-drawing ABGs.
		Monitor mechanical ventilation parameters carefully; assess for deteriorating status.	Impairment of lung tissue may result from mechanical ventilation which would further impair oxygen.
		Monitor response to oxygen therapy. Assess for possible CO_2 narcosis if indicated.	The client's response to oxygen should be monitored before oxygen levels are increased.
		Monitor electrolyte levels; assess for symptoms specific to imbalance associated with identified acid-base abnormality.	Early detection of abnormalities improves treatment.
Fatigue	Client will have improved energy level as evidenced by: • being able to perform more of own ADLs • fewer statements of fatigue • ambulating to chair or walking with less assistance • remaining up for longer periods of time	Assess client's energy level.	Ongoing assessments provide data to monitor fatigue.
		Assist client with ADLs as indicated.	Client should be encouraged to perform ADLs within energy limits to prevent further muscle wasting.
		Provide a quiet environment.	Decreases oxygen consumption.
		Organize nursing care to provide periods of uninterrupted rest.	Stress and illness increase need for rest.
		Promote optimal nutrition.	Fatigue may be due to inadequate nutrition.

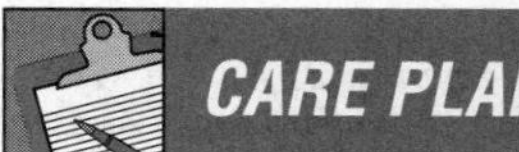

CARE PLAN

The Client with Acid-Base Imbalance Continued

Nursing Diagnosis/ Collaborative Problem	Planning: Expected Outcomes	Implementation: Nursing Interventions	Rationales
Fluid Volume Deficit and Decreased Cardiac Output	Client will have adequate fluid volume and cardiac output as evidenced by: • blood pressure WNL • urine output > 30 cc per hour • skin turgor responsive < 2 seconds • immediate capillary refill • no abnormal heart sounds (S_3 and S_4) • stable body weight intake = output	Monitor for signs related to contributing cause, e.g., shock, dehydration, diabetic ketoacidosis.	There are multiple etiologies of acid-base imbalances.
		Monitor for signs of azotemia.	Evaluation of BUN and creatinine may increase risk of metabolic acidosis.
		Assess vital signs, skin turgor, capillary refill, heart sounds.	Signs of dehydration and cardiac disorders which may increase risk of acid-base balance.
		Promote rest to decrease metabolic demand.	Decreases oxygen demand.
		Monitor weight and fluid balance.	Weight change is the most accurate measure of fluid balance. Fluid imbalance may lead to acid-base imbalance.

deviations in pH. The nurse optimizes respiratory and renal function through positioning, pulmonary hygiene, and hydration. The nurse intervenes in helping clients cope with the anxiety that often accompanies—and may contribute to—acid-base imbalance. The nurse collaborates in the administration of drug therapy, oxygen therapy, and mechanical ventilation when indicated. In extreme circumstances in which therapeutic compensation (intravenous administration of acid or base) is required, the nurse is knowledgeable about potential risks of this therapy and carefully monitors administration rates and therapeutic response.

TABLE 15-2. Sources of Error in Sampling of Arterial Blood Gases

Sampling Error	Effect	Nursing Implications
Air bubbles in syringe	↑PaO_2 ↓$PaCO_2$ ↑pH	Expel all air bubbles immediately Do not agitate syringe Do not use any sample that appears frothy
Inadvertent venous sample or venous contamination of arterial sample	↓PaO_2 ↑$PaCO_2$ ↓pH	Avoid use of femoral artery Use short-beveled needle Do not overshoot artery and then withdraw to "catch" it Watch for autofilling of syringe with arterial puncture Verify questionable results with new sample
Anticoagulant effects: alteration of pH	↓pH	Use lithium heparin, if possible Use 1:1000 units/ml concentration Use minimum 2-ml discard sample with arterial line aspiration
Anticoagulant effects: dilution of sample	↑pH ↓in all other values	Use syringe with minimal dead space Use dried heparin if available
Effects of metabolism of white blood cells in sample	↓PaO_2 ↑$PaCO_2$ ↓pH	Place sample in ice water immediately Have sample analyzed within 20 minutes Have sample analyzed immediately if client has leukocytosis

Data from Malley, W. J. (1990). *Clinical blood gases: Application and noninvasive alternatives.* Philadelphia: W. B. Saunders Co.

Corrective interventions address the underlying causes of *primary* acid-base imbalances and are the mainstay of treatment in such disorders. Compensatory imbalances are not treated but instead resolve spontaneously as the primary disorder is reversed. Chapters on the specific diseases responsible for acid-base imbalances should be consulted for detailed discussion of appropriate nursing intervention.

EVALUATION

The client's status should be evaluated frequently, because many acid-base imbalances are life threatening. Revisions in the plan of care may be required.

Summary

Normal function of all body cells depends on the regulation of acid-base balance. The kidneys, lungs, and blood buffers can usually balance acids and bases. Disorders of the lungs, kidneys, and metabolism can impair the balance, leading to respiratory or metabolic acidosis or alkalosis. Nurses play an instrumental role in early detection of high-risk clients.

Bibliography

1. Anderson, S. (1990). ABGs: Six easy steps to interpreting blood gases. *American Journal of Nursing, 90*(8), 42–45.
2. Brenner, M., & Welliver, J. (1990). Pulmonary and acid-base assessment. *Nursing Clinics of North America, 25*(4), 761–770.
3. Bullock, B., & Rosendahl, P. (1988). *Pathophysiology: Adaptations and alterations in function* (2nd ed.). Glenview, IL: Scott, Foresman and Co.
4. Carpenito, L. (1991). *Nursing care plans and documentation: Nursing diagnoses and collaborative problems.* New York: J. B. Lippincott Co.
5. Feeney-Stewart, F. (1990). The sodium bicarbonate controversy. *Dimensions of Critical Care Nursing, 9*(1), 22–28.
6. Holloway, N. (1988). *Nursing the critically ill adult* (3rd ed.). Menlo Park, CA: Addison-Wesley Publishing Co.
7. Malley, W. (1990). *Clinical blood gases: Application and noninvasive alternatives.* Philadelphia: W. B. Saunders Co.
8. Mathewson, M., & Mathewson, R. (1987). Establishing acid-base balance. *Critical Care Nurse, 7*(5), 77–80, 82–85.
9. Maxwell, M., et al. (1987). *Clinical disorders of fluid and electrolyte metabolism* (4th ed.). New York: McGraw-Hill Book Co.
10. Metheny, N. (1987). *Fluid and electrolyte balance: Nursing considerations.* Philadelphia: J. B. Lippincott Co.
11. Middaugh, R., et al. (1988). Current considerations in respiratory and acid-base management during cardiopulmonary resuscitation. *Critical Care Nursing Quarterly, 10*(4), 25–33.
12. Mountain, R., et al. (1990). Acid-base disturbances in acute asthma. *Chest, 98*(3), 651–655.
13. Palange, P., et al. (1990). Incidence of acid-base and electrolyte disturbances in a general hospital: a study of 110 consecutive admissions. *Recenti Progressi in Medicina (Roma), 81*(12), 788–791.
14. Preusser, B., et al. (1989). Quantifying the minimum discard sample required for accurate blood gases. *Nursing Research, 38*(5), 276–279.
15. Rice, V. (1987). Acid-base derangements in the patient with cardiac arrest. *Focus on Critical Care, 14*(6), 53–61.
16. Shapiro, B., & Walton, J. (1988). *Clinical application of blood gases* (4th ed.). Chicago: Year Book Medical Publishers.
17. Taylor, L., & Stephens, D. (1990). Arterial blood gases: clinical application. *Journal of Post-Anesthesia Nursing, 5*(4), 264–272.

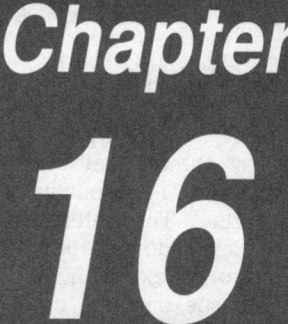

Pain Assessment and Intervention

Pain prompts people to seek health care more often than any other symptom.

How would you define pain? Does your definition include ideas, such as a feeling of agony, distress, or suffering? Or did you define it in a structural or physiologic manner and say that pain results from stimulation of nerve endings? Your definition probably includes some personal words reflecting your own painful experiences. The pain you have experienced is the only pain you know.

We all know that others experience pain. Ultimately, however, pain is defined by each of us from our own personal experiences. Perhaps pain is simply whatever a person says "hurts."

In this chapter, a variety of definitions of pain are discussed, along with many ways in which pain can be treated. Nurses are in an excellent position to work with the client in pain and to help that client overcome the pain. This is an important but not an easy task. This chapter makes that care easier.

DEFINITIONS OF PAIN

Pain is a multidimensional phenomenon; therefore, it is difficult to define. It is a personal and subjective experience with few or no objective measurements. Pain has been defined in many different ways by health care practitioners. Some of the definitions enhance the nurse's ability to assess the client who is in pain by helping the nurse to focus on specific aspects of the pain experience. The nurse may find pain control a difficult problem faced in providing total care for individual clients. It is, however, one of the most important areas of care, because people cannot function fully when they are in pain. Pain is best viewed as an experience, not merely as a symptom.

Medical Definition

Mountcastle[79] defined pain as "that sensory experience evoked by stimuli that injure or threaten to destroy tissue, defined introspectively by every man as that which hurts." The International Association for the Study of Pain[50] defines pain as "an unpleasant sensory and emotional experience associated with actual or potential tissue damage, or described in terms of such damage." This is the accepted medical definition of pain. Although this definition is useful, it defines pain in terms of tissue damage rather than what the client is experiencing. Tissue damage is not associated with all types of pain, such as a headache. Other definitions may prove more useful for the practicing nurse.

Psychological Definition

Sternbach[93] defines pain as "an abstract concept which refers to (1) a personal, private sensation of hurt; (2) a harmful stimulus that signals current or impending tissue damage; and (3) a pattern of responses to protect the organism from harm." This definition contributes to the nurse's understanding of the client's pain. It focuses on pain as something that belongs to the client, because pain is both personal and private. Sternbach's definition also reminds the nurse that pain can and does often have a protective function.

Nursing Definition

McCaffery,[66] a nurse, defined pain as "whatever the experiencing person says it is and existing whenever the person says it does." This definition makes the client the expert about his or her own pain. Because clinical pain is subjective in nature and no objective measures of it exist, the only people who can accurately define their own pain are the people experiencing that pain.

In spite of its subjective nature, the nurse is charged with accurately assessing and helping to relieve the client's pain. McCaffery's definition helps nurses achieve this goal.

THE PROCESS OF PAIN

Pain is a complex phenomenon. It is elicited by threatened or actual tissue damage that stimulates nociceptive (pain-sensitive) neural receptors. Pain also may be caused by damage to the pain transmission system itself. However, these stark statements do not actually help nurses understand a client's actual pain experience. It is like describing the experience of a sunset as the physical stimulation of the retina! We do need to know about pain receptors and their pathways to the brain, but nurses need a broader understanding of what may happen when pain is perceived, reacted to, and acted on. One way to gain this understanding is to conceptualize pain as a process made up of the *transduction, transmission,* and *modulation* of pain; *perception* of pain; and *reaction* to pain. Examining each of the parts of the process helps the nurse better understand the pain experience and better treat the client in pain.

Transduction, Transmission, and Modulation of Pain

Pain transduction, transmission, and modulation are physiologic processes dependent on an intact peripheral and central nervous system.

PAIN TRANSDUCTION

The train of events that leads to pain begins when pain fibers are excited by multiple types of stimuli. The stimuli consist of mechanical events (such as stretching of organs or pressure), heat or cold, and chemical changes (such as ischemia). Specific fibers react to any of these stimuli. The fibers are classified as mechanical, thermal, or chemical nociceptors. Fast pain is usually elicited by the mechanical and thermal type receptors (A-delta fibers), whereas slow pain can be elicited by all receptors (C fibers).

Fast pain is the pain that occurs in about 0.1 second when painful stimuli are applied. It is often referred to as sharp, pricking, acute, or electric pain. It is transmitted through type A-delta pain fibers. It is the pain felt when the skin is cut or an electric shock is felt. Fast pain is due to a more superficial stimulus, so it is rare in deep tissues.

Slow pain is pain that begins 1 or more seconds after stimulation and increases slowly over seconds or minutes. This pain is also known as burning, aching, throbbing, or chronic pain. It is often associated with tissue destruction and is felt in both superficial or deep tissues. It is transmitted through the more primitive type C fibers.

A wide variety of chemical substances, including bradykinin, serotonin, histamine, substance P, and acetylcholine and others, are especially significant in stimulating the slow pain that often follows tissue injury. These substances are released when tissue is damaged by injury, disease, or inflammation. These substances enhance nociceptive input and, therefore, increase pain.

Nerve receptors for pain (nociceptors) differ from the complex receptors for vision and other senses. Nociceptors are simply free nerve endings occurring in almost all types of tissue. Nociceptors react only to changes very close to them, and they require a relatively high level of stimulation to be activated. The chemical mediators, mentioned previously, increase the pain input into the nociceptors. However, once the threshold of the nociceptors is exceeded, they actively continue to communicate the presence of painful stimulus (slow adaptation). Nociceptors also can become sensitized so they continue to discharge long after the stimulus is removed. Most is known about pain originating from receptors in the skin. It is assumed that pain receptors in deeper tissues are similar, but they may operate differently.

PAIN TRANSMISSION

Once nociceptors are stimulated, the impulse they discharge travels as electric activity to the spinal cord and on to the brain. This electric activity becomes the experience of pain when it reaches the brain. There are no pain impulses as such, that is, impulses from nociception are not actually "pain" because pain is a complex phenomenon. However, if the neural pathway for these impulses is blocked, pain is also blocked because the impulses do not reach the brain. Pain pathways can be blocked by (1) surgically cutting them, (2) medications that inhibit the activity of the pathway's fibers, (3) natural (endogenous) methods of blocking portions of the pain pathway, and (4) other procedures.

Nerve fibers that carry somatosensory information from the body periphery to the spinal cord include A-beta, A-delta, and C fibers. A-type fibers have a myelin sheath that speeds up information transmission. A-delta fibers transmit pain. A-beta fibers are larger and carry other sensory information such as touch. C fibers transmit pain more slowly because they have no myelin sheath.

Pain sensation following stimulation of A-delta fibers differs from that following C fiber stimulation. A-delta activity is felt as a sharp, easily localized pain. C fiber activity is felt more slowly after painful stimulation. It is persistent, dull, and aching and is difficult to localize. Recall when you hit your elbow. A sharp, well-localized sensation occurred first (A-delta activation), followed by a persistent, dull, aching sensation (C fiber activation).

These afferent fibers enter the dorsal root of the spinal cord, which transmits the pain impulses. The fibers separate as they enter the cord and then reform in the dorsal horn. This area receives, transmits, and processes sensory impulses. The afferent nociceptors end at the level of the first and second laminae. The substantia gelatinosa (SG) is found in the second and third laminae, hypothesized to be the gating mechanisms described in the gate-control theory.

Different transmission pathways in the spinal cord contribute to the experience of various qualities of pain, such as slow pain versus fast pain. The major spinal tract carrying information to the brain is the spinothalamic tract. These ascending tracts transmit impulses through the spinal cord. Some fibers in this tract lead directly to the thalamus. From there, they pass to the somatosensory cortex, which is involved in discriminating the quality and localization of the pain.

Other fibers branch diffusely out to the many areas of the brain associated with emotion and motivation. The direct path of pain from the spinal cord to the thalamus to the somatosensory cortex is called the neospinothalamic tract, a tract that occupies the more lateral portion of the cord. This pathway contains few synapses, allowing for more rapid conduction of impulses. It projects into the posterior nucleus of the thalamus and is important in providing discriminative functions, such as the location, intensity, and duration of the painful stimulus.

The diffuse path of pain leads to more diverse brain centers, such as the reticular formation, medulla, hypothalamus, and limbic structures of the brain. It is called the paleospinothalamic tract and is more medial within the cord. This multisynaptic tract provides for slower conduction. It is associated with the unpleasant emotional component of pain and with the autonomic responses to pain.

Other ascending pathways include the spinoreticular tract, the spinomesencephalic tract, and the spinocervical tract.

PAIN MODULATION

There is a great deal of variation in the way clients perceive similarly painful stimuli. The pain modulation system is one reason this variance occurs. There is a variety of mechanisms that contribute to this modulation (Fig. 16-1).

Modulation via the Dorsal Horn. The dorsal horn was once considered a simple relay for impulses but is now known to contain extremely complex circuitry and multiple biochemical agents that both transmit and modulate nociceptive input. The dorsal horn is now thought to modulate the nociceptive impulses rather than simply receive and transmit these impulses. A high degree of sensory processing of the sensory impulses occurs at this level.

Modulation via Descending Pathways. The descending serotoninergic inhibitory fibers originate in the periaqueductal gray matter (PAG) of the midbrain and descend downward into the nucleus raphe magnus (NMR). Neurons from the PAG project downward into the dorsal horn at the first and fifth lamina levels. The neurotransmitters serotonin and substance P are released into these areas, contributing to the modulation of pain.

Modulation via Endogenous Chemicals. Some chemical compounds released by injury or inflammation stimulate nociceptors, for example, histamine, bradykinin, serotonin, substance P, and prostaglandin E. Pain may be reduced by drugs that block these agents, such as steroids, aspirin, and other nonsteroidal anti-inflammatory drugs (NSAIDs) that reduce inflammation and block prostaglandins. There is also a naturally occurring system within the nervous system called the analgesia system.

This analgesia system, described in Guyton,[47] has three major parts: "1) the *periaqueductal gray area* of the mesencephalon and upper pons surrounding the aqueduct of Sylvius. Neurons from this area send their signals to 2) the *raphe magnus nucleus,* a thin midline nucleus located in the lower pons and upper medulla. From here the signals are sent down the dorsolateral columns in the spinal cord to 3) a *pain inhibitory complex located in the dorsal horns of the spinal cord.*" At this point in the system, pain can be blocked.

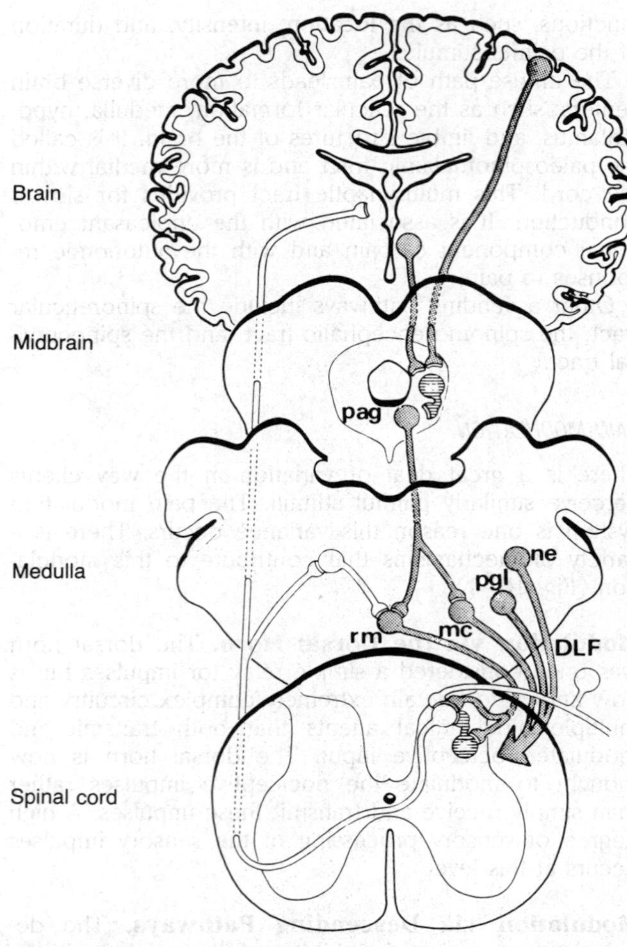

▲ *Figure 16-1*

Pain-modulating network. Diagram of critical structures that contribute to control of pain-transmission neurons. The network includes connections from midbrain periaqueductal grey *(pag)* to medullary nucleus raphe magnus *(rm)*/recticularis magnocellularis *(mc)* and, via the dorsolateral funiculus *(DLF)*, to the spinal cord dorsal horn. Additional bulbospinal pathways potentially relevant to analgesia arise from the nucleus paragigantocellularis *(pgl)*, which also receives input from pag and the noradrenergic medullary cell groups *(ne)* lateral to pgl.

In addition to this brain stem to spinal cord network, connections from neocortex and hypothalamus to the PAG have been documented. Hypothalamic stimulation produces analgesia. The role of the cortex in pain modulation is unknown.

At the spinal level, descending pathways inhibit nociceptive projection neurons through direct connections as well as through interneurons in superficial layers of the dorsal horn.

There is evidence that endorphin-containing interneurons *(cross hatched)* in PAG and dorsal horn play an active role in pain modulation.

(From Fields, H., & Basbaum, A. (1984). Endogenous pain control mechanisms. In P. Wall & R. Melzack [Eds.], *Textbook of pain.* New York: Churchill Livingstone.)

Other compounds are associated with pain transmission. Their action occurs at various points in the pain pathways described earlier. Substance P, a neuropeptide, appears to be a pain-specific neurotransmitter that is present in the spinal cord's horn (at the gate in the gate-control model), among other places. Other neuropeptides undoubtedly facilitate pain transmission.

Other peptides are associated with inhibiting pain. A group of naturally occurring (endogenous) peptides have properties similar to those of morphine and other narcotic analgesics. The central nervous system has specific neuroreceptors that bind morphine. The body also manufactures opium-like compounds called endogenous opioids, or endorphins, that bind to these sites and have analgesic properties. The term endorphins actually refers to a group of peptides with similar properties, two of which are β-endorphin and enkephalin. Electric and other stimulation of brain stem centers provide a profound analgesic effect, which can block pain in the analgesia system and appears related to endorphin release.

Other neurotransmitters are involved in the downward inhibition of pain. Serotonin, which facilitates pain in nociceptors, also acts as one of the transmitters in the descending pain inhibition system. The background level of many of these neurotransmitters varies throughout the day. Pain sensitivity is higher (lower pain threshold) in the afternoon than in the morning. Also, an individual's analgesic requirement may differ at different times of the day. There is increasing evidence that people who experience chronic pain may be deficient in some neurotransmitter.

Remember, nociceptors and the various areas of the brain activated by pain dictate a complex response to painful stimuli. Painful stimulation provides (1) information about the character, intensity, and location of the stimuli and (2) motivation to behave, for example, to act to reduce the pain, to avoid the cause of pain, to guard the injured area, and to remember the circumstances that caused the pain to avoid it in the future.

Perception of Pain

Pain perception or interpretation is the second phase of the pain process. Once pain has been received and transmitted, it must be perceived or interpreted. Because every individual perceives or interprets based on his or her individual experience, this is one point at which pain becomes different for each person.

Pain perception does not depend solely on the degree of physical damage. It is generally agreed that psychosocial factors influence a person's experience of pain. Although there is little consensus about the specific effects of these factors, it is known that anxiety, experience, attention, expectation, and the meaning of the situation in which injury occurs affect pain perception. Brain activities, such as distraction or anxiety, may also affect the severity and quality of the pain experience.

In the past, pain was viewed as a primary sensation, and motivational and cognitive processes were believed to influence only our reaction to pain. However, it now seems apparent there are mechanisms within the body that can modify pain-related neural impulses even before they are transmitted to the brain. Thus, pain is likely to be determined by a relative balance between the sensory peripheral input and mechanisms of central control (brain) input to gating mechanisms in the spinal cord.

Sensory mechanisms by themselves do not completely explain why nerve lesions do not always produce pain. Also, they do not explain why, when these lesions do produce pain, the pain is usually not continuous. The gate-control theory (see section on gate-control theory) proposes that the presence or absence of pain is determined by the balance between the sensory and central inputs to the gate-control system. In addition to the sensory influences on the gate-control system, there is an input to the system from higher levels of the central nervous system, opening the gate. For example, central nervous system (CNS) lesions associated with hyperalgesia and spontaneous pain could have this effect. On the other hand, any CNS condition or activity that increases the flow of descending impulses tends to close the gate.

The first point the nurse needs to consider, therefore, is the client's pain threshold. This is defined as the lowest perceivable intensity of stimuli that is transmitted as pain. The pain threshold may vary based on physiologic factors such as inflammation or injury near pain receptors, but essentially it is similar for all people if the central and peripheral nervous systems are intact.

The second part of pain perception is the individual's tolerance for pain. Tolerance is different for each person who experiences pain. This may vary within each person based on many subjective factors, such as the meaning of the pain and the setting. It really refers to the amount of pain the client is willing to endure. Some individuals have a high tolerance, that is, they can tolerate a lot of pain without distress, whereas others have a very low tolerance. Only the individual, not the health care team, can tell what the client's tolerance level is. The nurse must remember this and remember that pain tolerance can vary from situation to situation.

Another aspect that will alter a person's perception of pain is his or her experience with pain. This may be the reason that people assume infants do not have pain. When the infant feels pain, it is simply that the infant has no experience with pain and, therefore, is unable to interpret it, and cannot communicate what is being felt. The reverse is also true. When a person has a bad experience with pain, the anticipation that future pain may be as bad can make any pain worse.

Response to Pain

The client's reaction to pain adds even more variation to the pain process. There are many variables in this part of the process, including situation, culture, age, sex, cause of pain, tolerance, value and meaning of pain, and various psychological factors such as fear, anxiety, and depression. Each of these factors is discussed so the nurse will be better able to understand the client's experience.

SITUATIONAL FACTORS

The situation associated with the pain will influence the client's response to it. If a person experiences severe pain but is in a formal or crowded situation, the person's response may be very different from that if he or she were alone or in a hospital. Another example might be the woman who has an exploratory laparotomy for ovarian cancer. Although she may feel pain, it seems better if the diagnosis proved to be benign. The nurse must decide whether or not the client's expression of pain is being influenced by the setting.

SOCIOCULTURAL FACTORS

Race, culture, and ethnicity are critical factors in an individual's response to pain. These factors influence our responses and, especially, our responses to pain. We learn much about how to respond to pain and other experiences from our family and our ethnic peer group.

Zborowski's[109, 110] studies on cultural and ethnic influences on pain are considered the classic studies conducted in this area. He identified four major groups, Old American, Italian, Irish, and Jewish and looked at how each responded to pain (Table 16–1).

Racial groups also differ in the way they react to pain. Blacks may react differently from whites. Black society is considered to be a matriarchal society, which may influence the reaction to pain. Davitz and Davitz[26] report that Southern blacks are more vocal in their reports of pain than Northern blacks. Blacks are more likely to stop treatment as soon as any symptoms abate. Problems also may arise because of the view these clients have of health care team members. They often have difficulty communicating what they are feeling to white doctors and nurses.[26, 48]

Hispanics often view health as the absence of illness. Stoicism is valued in this culture. They believe that difficulties and illness should be borne with dignity. There may be many folk beliefs associated with illness in this group, so any treatment has to fit into their patterns of belief. If the client is not convinced that the pain is related to an illness, he or she might refuse treatment for it.[72]

There are characteristics of many other groups, such as stoicism among Asians. One of the most important things the nurse can remember is that clients of any culture may deal with pain in a wide variety of ways. The problem arises when the nurse does not recognize the client's way of dealing with pain or does not accept it. More study on the cultural influences of pain is needed. Davitz and Davitz[26] have looked at the effect of the nurse's culture on assessment of pain in relationship to the client's culture. Again, they recommend that more research is needed to clarify the effect that culture has on both pain assessment and pain expression.

TABLE 16–1. Cultural Responses to Pain

Culture	Response to Painful Stimuli
Old American (English)	Stoic reaction to pain Often display "stiff upper lip philosophy" Find pride in ability to tolerate high levels of pain without showing distress, so often refuse interventions to relieve pain Want to know cause of pain on an intellectual level
Irish	Denial of pain common, so expression of pain limited and minimized Equate pain with illness and death, so they are unwilling to admit to the presence of pain Unwilling to accept interventions to relieve pain, because doing this would be admitting to the pain Do not want to know about pain Exhibit some degree of martyrdom
Italian	Suffer loudly and want everyone to know about the pain they are experiencing Often seen to react out of proportion to the painful stimuli Enjoy the sympathy and secondary gains associated with their verbal reports of pain Have no desire to know about their pain; however, they do want it relieved May exhibit some degree of martyrdom
Jewish	Suffer their pain loudly, and family often closely involved with the suffering Reaction to painful stimuli often seen as being out of proportion to stimuli Do want to know exact cause of pain in great detail, want pain relieved immediately, and may even seek a second opinion Most concerned with the meaning of the pain

Data from Zborowski, M. (1969). *People in pain.* San Francisco: Jossey-Bass.

AGE

Age may release a client from culturally imposed norms in relation to pain expression. A young girl in a stoic culture may be allowed to cry because of pain. Children are usually given greater freedom of action, but boys may have more restrictions on their behavior.

There is controversy associated with information about pain in the elderly. There is no reason to assume that pain reception is altered in the elderly unless some damage has occurred in the CNS. The transmission and perception might be slowed with aging, but this does not diminish the pain that is felt. Physical factors such as paralysis or aphasia may change response to pain, but it does not mean that pain is not occurring, only that the older client might be having difficulty responding. This is a very important point for the nurse to remember; lack of response does not mean lack of pain in older adults. Even confused clients need to be closely assessed because their expression of pain may be altered. It is vital that the nurse remembers that altered expression does not mean there is no pain.

Older adults may assign different meanings to their pain. Pain is often thought of by the elderly as a natural part of aging. This is interpreted in two ways. First, they may think it is natural and, therefore, something to be simply endured as a normal part of the aging process. Second, it may be seen as a part of aging and, therefore, should be denied because it means they are getting old. Many older adults are hesitant to express pain for fear of being labeled as a complaining elder. Again, careful assessment of the older person's pain is important for the nurse.

SEX

Sex may be more of an influence than many other factors. In most cultures in the United States, little boys are expected to show less expression of pain than little girls. As they grow older, men are also expected to express pain less than women. This does not mean that men feel pain less, only that they are assumed to show it less. In most cultures, men will be less expressive in their reports of pain. As men age, they may be allowed more freedom to express their pain.

MEANING OF PAIN

The meaning of a person's pain is a factor that influences his or her response to pain. Again, pain caused by childbirth may be responded to differently from pain caused by a surgery. If the cause of pain is known, it may help the client respond to it. If the cause is unknown, more negative psychological factors such as fear and anxiety come into play and the pain can be misinterpreted, resulting in an inappropriate response.

Pain that is associated with a threat to body image may be much worse than pain that is not. Think of the client who has a devastating alteration in body image such as a radical neck dissection, or a client with an amputation. If the client's psychological response to the pain is not considered, the nurse may not completely understand the client's suffering.

ANXIETY

The degree of anxiety the client is experiencing also may influence the client's response to pain. It is not possible to separate the mind from the body, so pain always has both physiologic components and psychological components. When anxiety is high, pain is felt as greater. Anxiety is often related to the meaning of the pain. If the cause is unknown, anxiety is likely to be higher and the pain is worse.

OTHER FACTORS

Other factors that also may alter pain reaction are (1) fatigue and insomnia, (2) stress, (3) experience with pain, and (4) depression and the associated isolation.

Therapeutic Implications of the Pain Process

Therapeutic implications of current knowledge of pain include the following:

- Pain control might be achieved by selectively influencing the large, rapidly conducting fibers (C fibers). Decreasing small fiber input (A-delta fibers) and enhancing large fiber input may close the gate. Also, any procedure that reduces sensory input lessens the opportunity for summation and pain.
- A better understanding of the physiology and pharmacology of the (SG) and other central control mechanisms may lead to new ways of controlling pain with medications that excite or inhibit activity.
- Experience, attention, emotion, and other psychological factors influence pain perception and pain response by acting on the spinal cord's pain transmission system. Pain management includes motivational and cognitive aspects of an individual's pain experience.
- Stimulation or blocking the production of various endogenous CNS chemicals may prove very useful in controlling transmission of pain in the CNS and blocking its transmission to the central cortex.

THEORIES OF PAIN

Specificity Theory

The specificity theory was described by Descartes in the 17th century. This theory is based on a belief that specialized pathways for pain transmission exist. It was thought that free nerve endings existed in the periphery that acted as pain receptors. These nerves were believed to be capable of receiving painful stimuli and transmitting the impulses on highly specific nerve fibers. The sensation would then be transmitted through the dorsal horns and SG to the thalamus and finally to the higher cortical areas. Pain would be interpreted in these higher areas, and a response would occur.

This theory did not address the multidimensional characteristics of pain, viewing it simply as a sense like all the other senses. It is mainly a biologic explanation of a highly complex process.

Gate-Control Theory

The physiology of pain transmission and perception is less well understood than the underlying physical structure (anatomy). There are various theoretical models that attempt to explain how neural units interact during the experience of pain. One such model is the gate-control theory, described more than 25 years ago and revised periodically. It explains many aspects of pain and how pain may be controlled by thoughts, emotions, and action.

In 1965, Melzack and Wall[75] presented the first version of the gate-control theory. They suggested the existence of a gate that could either facilitate or inhibit the transmission of pain signals. The gate is controlled by the dynamic function of certain cells in the spinal cord's dorsal horn. The fibers bringing information about pain from tissue synapse for the first time in laminae of the dorsal horns. Laminae II is known as the SG. The SG is visually distinct from other laminae when the spinal cord is inspected in cross section. Melzack and Wall proposed that the SG is the anatomic location of the gate. Both A-delta, small-diameter fibers that carry information about pain, and C fibers, large-diameter fibers that carry information such as touch, converge in the SG. Also, fibers sending their pain-inhibitory information down from the brain act here. They come from areas such as the PAG, hypothalamus, NMR, and locus ceruleus.

Melzack and Wall[75] proposed that a spinal cord transmission cell (T cell) exists in the SG. Depending on its input from other cells, the T cell either facilitates pain transmission (opens the gate) or inhibits pain transmission (closes the gate). The gate can be influenced (opened or closed) by information from various sources. Activity from large-diameter fibers (carrying information, such as touch) can inhibit pain transmission (close the gate); for example, one rubs one's elbow after banging it to ease the pain, thereby closing the gate.

Whether the gate is open or closed, it can be influenced by fibers carrying information from many different brain centers down to the T cells. According to this theory, information from non-pain fibers or information from the brain can reduce or totally block pain information before it is experienced. When the gate is open, pain information influences multiple centers in the brain. When working together, these centers produce the complex but integrated responses that occur in a client experiencing pain. The model suggests, however, that the brain also can influence whether or not the gate is open. Thus, factors such as attention, memory, thinking, and emotion may either inhibit or enhance the transmission of pain signals.

A recent version of the gate-control theory (called Mark II by Melzack and Wall[76]) is presented in Figure 16-2. The newer model emphasizes the probability that there is an inhibitory system within the brain stem that also acts as a gate inhibiting pain transmission. This brain stem inhibitory circuit has been described in detail by Basbaum and Fields[9] who believe that the system involves structures in the midbrain, medulla, and the spinal cord. Activation of cells in the midbrain's PAG (by electric stimulation, opiate analgesic drugs, or possible psychological factors), in turn, stimulates structures in the medulla. These medullary structures then project to and inhibit spinal pain transmission fibers. Pain itself might activate this system. Under some circumstances, it acts as a natural control mech-

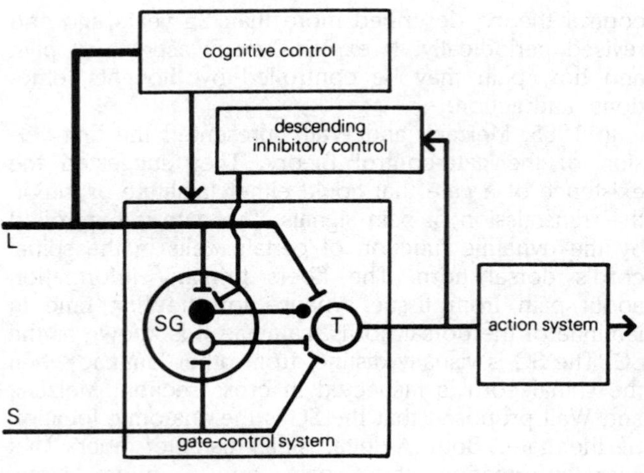

▲ Figure 16-2

The gate-control theory: Mark II. The new model includes excitatory *(white circle)* and inhibitory *(black circle)* links from the substantia gelatinosa *(SG)* to the transmission *(T)* cells as well as descending inhibitory control from brain stem systems. The round knob at the end of the inhibitory link implies that its action may be presynaptic, postsynaptic, or both. All connections are excitatory, except the inhibitory link from SG to T cell. (From *The challenge of pain* by Ronald Melzack and Patrick D. Wall. [Penguin Books, 2nd edition, 1988], copyright © Ronald Melzack and Patrick D. Wall, 1982, 1988.)

anism that limits the severity of the pain experience, such as in the soldier severely injured in battle who is unaware of pain.

TYPES OF PAIN

It is important for nurses to realize that there are many different types of pain, to participate knowledgeably in nursing clients experiencing pain. There are various ways of discussing types of pain including

- Onset or time of occurrence, such as postoperative pain (see Chap. 19);
- Duration, such as chronic or acute pain;
- Severity or intensity, such as severe or mild, or 0 to 10 on a scale;
- Mode of transmission, such as normal pain pathways or referred pain;
- Location or source, such as superficial, deep, or central pain;
- Causation, such as pain due to receptor stimulation or nerve damage, or psychophysiologic pain;
- Causative forces or agent, such as spontaneous, self-inflicted, or other pain.

Acute Pain

Acute pain is usually of short duration (less than 6 months) and has an identifiable, immediate onset, such as fast pain. It is also seen as having a limited and often predictable duration, such as postoperative pain, which usually disappears as the wound heals. It has the characteristics of fast pain and is often described in the same sensory terms, such as sharp, stabbing, and shooting.

Acute pain is seen as a useful and limiting pain in that it indicates injury and motivates the individual to get relief by treatment of the pain and usually the cause. Acute pain is usually reversible or controllable with adequate treatment.

Figure 16-3 illustrates that as pain increases, so does a person's anxiety, until a certain point is reached. The individual then does something to get relief before the pain becomes even more severe.

Clients suffering from acute pain can often come to terms with that pain because of the meaning or the limited nature of the pain, such as with the pain of childbirth. When the pain is relieved, the client again appears perfectly normal.

The physiologic response to acute pain is due to stimulation of the sympathetic nervous system. The client will probably exhibit the following symptoms: (1) increased or decreased blood pressure, (2) tachycardia, (3) diaphoresis, (4) tachypnea, (5) focusing on the pain, and (6) guarding the painful part.

Chronic Pain

Chronic pain is usually considered pain that lasts more than 6 months (or 1 month beyond the normal end of the condition causing the pain) and has no foreseeable end except very slow healing, such as burns, or death. It is continual or persistent and recurrent. There is some disagreement as to whether or not acute recurrent pain, such as migraines or sickle cell crisis, should be classified as chronic pain, but they usually are. The acute nature of this pain means that the nurse should be very careful when treating these clients as simple chronic pain clients.

Other characteristics of chronic pain include that it often has an identifiable cause (although the cause may

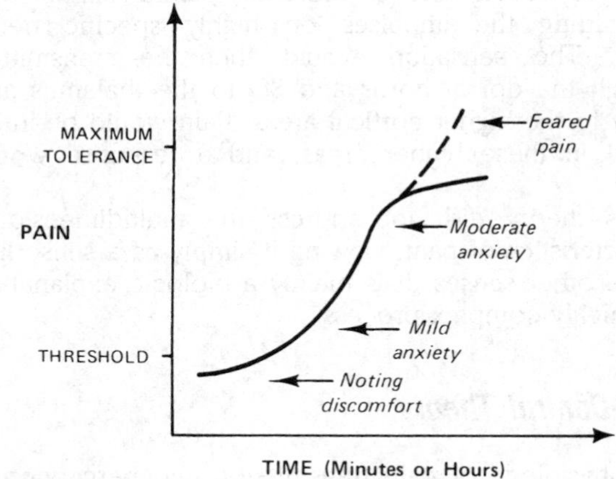

▲ Figure 16-3

Sequence of reactions to acute pain. (From Sternbach, R. A. [1974]. *Pain patients—traits and treatment* [p. 6]. New York: Academic Press.)

be difficult to determine); is often described using affective terms, such as hateful or sickening; has the qualities of slow pain; and is often much more difficult to treat than acute pain. It is considered a useless pain because it is not usually a sign of impending damage. For example, a client immobilized with severe rheumatoid arthritis pain may be further crippled by that immobility. Chronic pain is often called either chronic malignant (cancer) or chronic nonmalignant pain.

Chronic pain is often frustrating and difficult for a person to live with. It gives no clues about how to lessen it. Health care providers may feel frustrated and incompetent when their attempts to relieve chronic pain are ineffective. However, if nurses understand the anatomy, physiology, and psychosocial aspects of chronic pain, they can be very helpful to the client. Professionals can intervene before extreme suffering occurs.

Clients experiencing continuous or continually recurring chronic pain often become increasingly engrossed by their illness. They may seem fearful, tense, fatigued, and depressed. Many individuals with an unending chronic pain become withdrawn and isolated. Their pain often exhausts them both physically and mentally.

An individual's mental response to pain depends on the duration and possibly the intensity of the pain. Pain that is constant, continuous, and moderate is often described by clients as far more difficult to bear than pain that is paroxysmal and intense.

Figure 16-4 depicts the course of chronic pain—it includes months and years of pain, not minutes or hours. Chronic pain is associated with withdrawal and despair. Anxiety gives way to depression.

The sympathetic arousal associated with acute pain diminishes over weeks or months as severe pain itself persists. Sympathetic adaptation occurs over time. The nurse must remember, however, that absence of the expected expression of severe pain does not mean that the pain is gone. The nurse must depend on the client's report of pain, not symptoms one expects to see. An example of severe chronic pain is causalgia. With causalgia, the nerve trunk itself is damaged, and prolonged, intense pain is experienced. Causalgia is often a cause of many types of chronic pain.

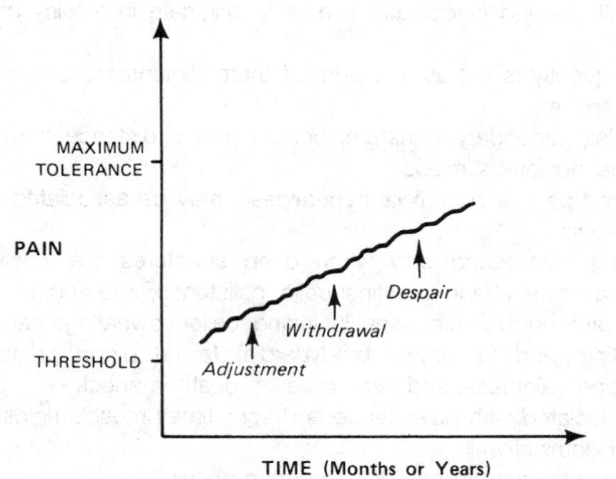

▲ *Figure 16-4*

Sequence of reactions to chronic pain. (From Sternbach, R. A. [1974]. *Pain patients—traits and treatment* [p. 8]. New York: Academic Press.)

Intractable, chronic pain states, producing prolonged and intense bombardment of the central nervous system, are very difficult to bear. The client may become suicidal or at least take no steps to prolong life. Two days before her death, Alice James (sister of Henry James) wrote in her journal, "I am being ground slowly on the grim grindstone of physical pain, and on two nights I had almost asked for K's lethal dose; but one steps hesitantly along such unaccustomed ways, and endures from second to second."

Most clients have major affective and behavioral changes when experiencing pain for prolonged periods. Such changes may be compounded, and chronic pain syndrome can develop. Characteristics of clients experiencing chronic pain syndrome include

- Depressed mood;
- Increased or decreased appetite and weight;
- Drastically restricted activity level, leading to reduced work capacity, poor physical tone, and increased depression;
- Social withdrawal;
- Preoccupation with physical symptoms; and
- Poor sleep and chronic fatigue, which may result from inactivity, analgesics, and depression, as well as pain.

Some clients with chronic pain may not exhibit any of the above-mentioned symptoms, or they may exhibit only a few. However, once these changes take place, they may become more significant to treatment than the pain's original physical source.

Unfortunately, psychosocial implications about pain sometimes reinforce the idea that clients may "make too much fuss" over their pain. Clients with significant pain are rightfully resentful and angry if told this (either verbally or nonverbally), such as "your pain is all in your head." Such statements are not helpful and are based on (1) inadequate knowledge of the physical basis of pain, (2) behavioral consequences of having to endure persistent pain, (3) inadequate understanding of various therapies, and (4) the subjective nature of the pain experience (it is felt by the client, and if the client feels it, it is real).

Some psychosocial theories of pain attempt to explain variations in pain from one client to another, such as why some clients experience pain with little tissue damage. Examples of such theories include the following:

- Pain results from hostility, either following the repression of hostility or as an expression of guilt for overt hostility.
- Pain arises in individuals of pain-prone personality. They use pain as communication and emotional expression.
- Pain arises from a threat to the integrity of the body. Pain is termed psychogenic when the threat is not apparent to the outside observer.

Current knowledge does not support any of the previously mentioned theories. More often, chronic pain syndrome results from poor assessment and treatment during the initial acute pain episode or its transition to chronic pain. To date, there is no universally accepted psychological theory of pain.

Cutaneous or Superficial Pain

Two types of cutaneous pain are (1) pain with an abrupt onset and a sharp or sting quality, and (2) pain with a slower onset and a burning quality. Cutaneous pain may be delineated by having the client point to the painful area. It may occur along each segment representing a portion of the body surface innervated by one dorsal root. A dermatome or skin segment is an area of skin supplied by one dorsal root. Each spinal nerve has a dorsal or sensory root. The boundaries of dermatomes may appear to be distinct in anatomic drawings, but nerve distribution actually overlaps. Irritation of one posterior root produces pain in the adjacent dermatomes. A spinal nerve attaches to the spinal cord with two roots—anterior and posterior. The anterior root contains efferent nerve fibers that carry impulses from the central nervous system to the periphery of the body. The posterior root contains afferent nerve fibers that carry impulses from the body's periphery toward the CNS.

Cutaneous pain is relatively uncomplicated because it is directly perceived and readily localized, that is, the client can indicate exactly where it hurts.

Deep Somatic Pain

Pain in the somatic structures is a complicated phenomenon. Somatic structures are those of the body wall, such as muscles and bone.

Table 16–2 compares deep pain with cutaneous pain. The main difference between cutaneous and deep sensibility (i.e., the capacity to receive stimuli and respond to them) is the different nature of the pain evoked by harmful (noxious) stimuli. For example, unlike cutaneous pain, deep pain (1) is poorly localized, (2) may produce nausea, and (3) is frequently associated with sweating and blood pressure changes.

Deep somatic pain is generally diffuse, less localizable than cutaneous pain. This is because the area supplied by one posterior nerve root (sclerotome) is less well defined than a dermatome and does not correspond with a dermal segment. Also, pain from deep structures frequently radiates (spreads) from the primary site (e.g., pain from a lumbar disc is felt along the sciatic nerve).

Somatic structures vary in their sensitivity to pain. Highly sensitive structures include tendons, deep fascia, ligaments, joints, bone periosteum, blood vessels, and nerves. Skeletal muscle is sensitive only to stretching and ischemia. Bone and cartilage respond to extreme

TABLE 16–2. Comparison of Cutaneous and Deep Pain

Characteristic	Cutaneous Pain	Deep Pain
Quality	Sharp, bright sensation or burning; felt superficially	Primarily dull and aching May be described as boring, crushing, throbbing, or cramping, or (if less intense) as a soreness or hurting
Duration	Typically short	Often fairly long
Localization	Tends to be precise Pain is often experienced as a point, surface, or line	Often diffuse and inaccurate; seems to originate in a fairly broad area Pain frequently is felt as if it were of three dimensions and occupied space
Hyperalgesia	May occur; of a primary nature	May exist; secondary in nature; occurring at a distance from the original noxious stimulus In referred pain, a superficial hyperalgesia may be associated with deep pain
Nausea	Never occurs	Sickening pain found only when deep structures are involved, such as in renal and intestinal colic, gallstones, and angina
Associated symptoms	May be hyperalgesia, paresthesia, tickling, burning, or itching Also associated with brisk movements, a quick pulse, and a sense of invigoration	Due to autonomic responses including pallor, sweating, nausea, vomiting, and (at times) bradycardia, fall in blood pressure, syncope, faintness, and perhaps even death in shock Also associated with quiescence and sometimes muscle rigidity of the abdominal wall Muscle contraction and tenderness often occur Segmental spread of pain frequently noted Pain may not remain confined to original spinal segment but may spread into one or more adjacent segments

pressure and chemical stimulation (e.g., rheumatoid arthritis, osteomyelitis).

Visceral Pain

Usually, the term viscera refers to abdominal viscera. Actually, however, a viscus (plural, viscera) is any of the large interior body organs occupying any body cavity, such as the cranial, thoracic, abdominal, or pelvic cavities. The word splanchnic pertains to the viscera. Thus, visceral pain also may be called splanchnic pain.

Visceral pain tends to be diffuse, poorly localized, vague, dull pain. Nerve fibers innervating body organs follow the sympathetic nerves to the spinal cord. This may be the reason why autonomic symptoms (e.g., diarrhea, cramps, sweating, hypertension) frequently accompany visceral pain. Typical visceral pains include acute appendicitis, cholecystitis, inflammations of the biliary and pancreatic tract, gastroduodenal disease, cardiovascular disease, pleurisy, and renal and ureteral colic.

Most viscera are not sensitive to stimuli that cause pain in somatic structures (such as cutting, burning, or pressure). This is understandable. Because viscera are not normally exposed to such traumas, the body does not 'need' a response system. Although these types of stimuli do not produce pain in most viscera, other stimuli may cause severe pain, for example, violent or abnormal contractions of hollow viscera such as the ureters and alimentary tract.

Visceral pain differs from cutaneous pain in that highly localized damage to the viscera rarely causes severe pain, whereas such damage to the body surface would cause pain. An example would be a surgical cut, such as in the gut, does not cause pain, whereas such a cut on the skin would cause severe pain. If the stimulus to the viscera causes diffuse stimulation of nerve endings, then the resulting pain is severe, as in ischemia of the gut.

Visceral pain is transmitted through the sympathetic and parasympathetic fibers of the autonomic nervous system, with the pain being referred to the body surface, often in sites at a far distance. Parietal pain is transmitted directly into the spinal nerves, with the pain being felt directly over the painful area. Referred pain due to visceral disease follows dermatome patterns that somatic referred pain does not.

Visceral pain also may be sent through the nerve fibers in the parietal pleura, pericardium, or peritoneum and is called parietal pain. Parietal tissue is well supplied with spinal nerves instead of sympathetic nerves. Pain starting in the parietal tissue is often very sharp in nature.

Referred Pain

Deep pain may arise from disease of the viscera or from a lesion of a deep somatic structure (e.g., vertebra, muscle, interspinous ligament). However, both visceral and somatic pain are usually referred to a segment of skin because visceral fibers synapse at the level of spinal cord close to fibers innervating some subcutaneous tissues.

Referred pain is peculiar because it is sometimes intense although there is little or no pain at the point of noxious stimuli. For example, myocardial ischemia is not felt as pain in the heart; rather, it is felt as left arm, shoulder, or jaw pain. The fibers innervating these areas are close to those innervating the myocardium, resulting in the referred pain.

Identification of the segment of the spinal cord that is involved in transmitting referred pain is diagnostically helpful. Pain arising from a deep structure, whether a viscus or a deep somatic structure, has a referred segmental distribution, or a pattern of pain, determined according to the spinal cord segment supplying the structure.

Referred pain is often baffling and requires careful assessment. Examples of common patterns include pleural pain from the diaphragm referred to the shoulder, and the pain of cholecystitis referred to the back and in the angle of the scapula. Figure 16–5 illustrates common sites of referred pain.

PATHOLOGIC PAIN SYNDROMES

Deafferentation or Neuropathic Pain

The types of pain discussed so far involve the stimulation of nociceptors by chemical, mechanical, or thermal (heat or cold) stimuli. Because they involve nociceptors, they are sometimes referred to as nociceptive pain. Severe pain also can be caused by nervous system damage, when the flow of afferent nerve impulses has been partially or completely interrupted. This type of pain is called neuropathic pain or deafferentation. (Other names include hyperpathia or spontaneous pain). Most neuropathic pain syndromes have similar features including the following:

- Pain is often present in the absence of stimulation or an obvious pathologic process to account for the pain, such as nonvascular peripheral neuropathies.
- Pain is present in the absence of stimulation, with damage to small caliber nerves that may be found on diagnostic studies, such as burning feet in a diabetic client.
- When nonpainful stimulation is applied to the area where pain is felt, the pain sensation often increases, such as sensitivity of postherpetic neuralgia.
- Although change in other somatosensory sensations, such as touch or position sense, may occur, the common finding is a change in pain sensation due to damage to the normal pathways for pain transmissions, such as thalamic pain.
- Pain may appear to arise from a body part that has its pain pathway to the brain destroyed. This seeming paradox (pain in the absence of a pathway) has given rise to such terms as phantom or phantom-like pain.

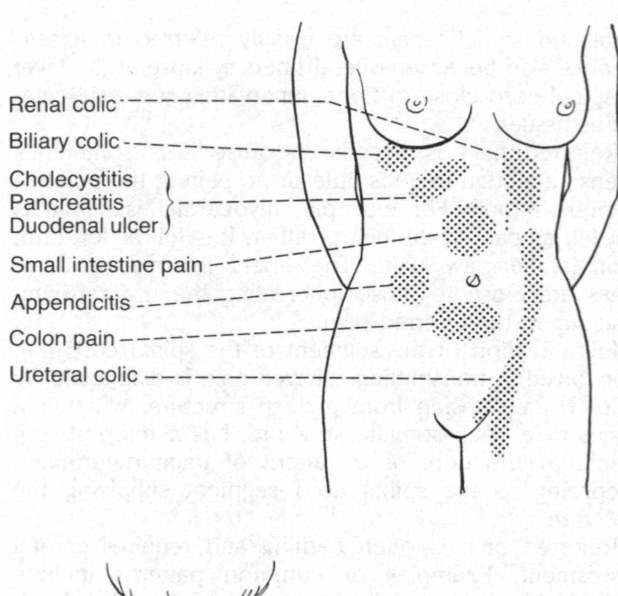

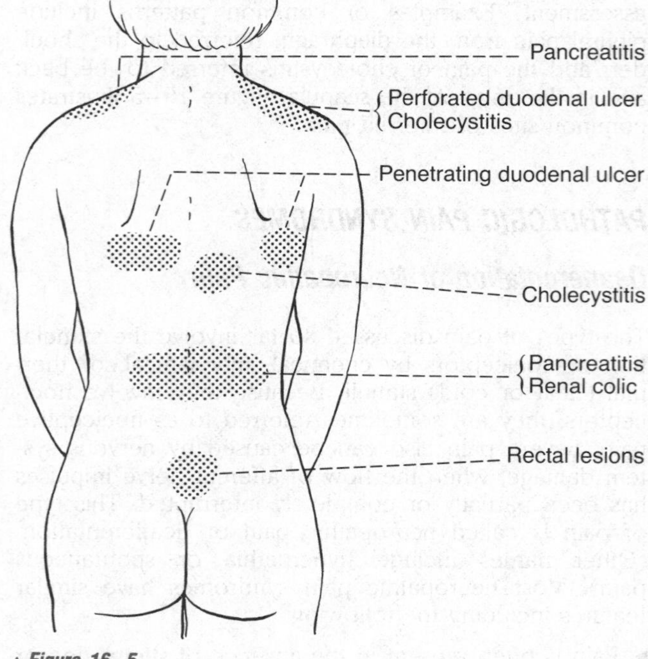

▲ **Figure 16-5**
Areas of referred pain.

The lesions that cause neuropathic pain can occur at any location in the pain pathway. There may be damage to peripheral nerves as well as lesions of the spinal cord, brain stem, and thalamus and other subcortical and even cortical areas.

Pain of Muscular and Bony Origin

Ligaments, joint capsules, fascia, tendons, and muscle all vary in the density of their innervation. The periosteum is most sensitive. Spontaneous pain may occur from spasm, rupture, ischemia, inflammation, or other disturbances of the ligaments, tendons, muscles, and periosteum of bones and joints. The muscular ischemia of intermittent claudication and occlusive vascular disease induces pain in the extremities. Also, it is the basis of the pain of coronary occlusion. Although chemical irritants injected into muscles may give rise to considerable pain, muscular pain usually occurs in association with stretching, ischemia, or forceful or sustained contractile activity.

The sustained clenching of muscles or their continued overuse may produce muscular pain. The primary cause of muscle pain does not appear to be muscle tension but rather the compression or constriction of blood vessels within the muscle or traction on periosteum.

When muscle pain causes a sustained reflex contraction of the muscle, a vicious circle may occur. The contraction successively increases muscular pain, and the pain gradually radiates into adjacent areas. A large proportion of headaches, especially those accompanied by stiffness or tenderness in the neck and occipital region, originate from the sustained contraction of underlying neck and scalp muscles (see the section on headache).

Vascular Pain

The precise mechanism of vascular pain is not understood but is believed to originate from some pathologic condition of the vessels or perivascular tissues. Some pain-producing chemical substances also seem significant.

The blood vessels are often involved in various pain syndromes. Blood vessels are believed to be associated with pain induced by cold. Also, distortion of the cranial vessels by pulling, displacement, or distention is the source of a large proportion of headaches. These include migraine headaches and headaches associated with arterial hypertension, brain tumors, and variations in the hydrodynamics of the cerebrospinal fluid (e.g., increased intracranial pressure).

Pain Due to Inflammation

Inflammation is one of the most common pathologic conditions influencing pain sensitivity. Inflammation can be caused by numerous harmful agents, such as bacterial or chemical agents, or stressors, such as heat, cold, or trauma. Gross assessment findings associated with the inflammatory process are redness, swelling, heat, and pain. Inflammatory pain is secondary to the distention of stretch-sensitive tissue (i.e., periosteum, pleura) and the direct effect of released neuroregulators on afferent nerve endings. Principal chemical causes (mediators) of the inflammatory response are histamine, substance P, bradykinin, prostaglandins, and leukokinins. All of these mediators are highly acidic. Increased acidity at the site of the injured tissue seems to heighten sensitivity in pain fibers. This allows less stimulation to cause a sensation of pain and makes pain more intense (e.g., if one has a paper cut then the mildest touch, usually nonpainful, can cause pain).

These acidic mediators are also capable of provoking pain directly.

In the chest, the parietal pleura is richly supplied with pain endings through the intercostal nerves and through the phrenic nerve, on the surface of the diaphragm.

The visceral pleura in the chest, however, is insensitive to pain. The bronchi, on the other hand, are sensitive to pain. Elsewhere and throughout their serous surfaces, the visceral pericardia is insensitive to pain, with the exception that the lower portion of the fibrous pericardium appears to have pain fibers from the phrenic nerve.

Pain in the gastrointestinal (GI) tract is common. It appears to arise mainly from the tract's muscular and serous coats. GI pain seems to occur when intestinal mucosa is inflamed, ulcerated, or otherwise abnormal, or when the visceral muscles contract strongly or pass into spasm. Thus, while the wall of the intestine is not sensitive to cutting, burning, or crushing, it does produce pain under other conditions, such as widespread ischemia.

Abdominal pain may also occur when body organs perforate and their contents drain into the peritoneal cavity. Intraperitoneal fluids that may accumulate are listed next, from the most irritating to the least irritating:

- Pancreatic enzyme fluid
- Gastric or duodenal fluid
- Fecal fluid from the colon, appendix, or small bowel
- Bile
- Urine
- Blood
- Lymph

The parietal peritoneum, the mesentery, and many blood vessels are sensitive to injuries such as cutting, stretching, and handling. Also, the mucosal lining of the urethra, bladder, ureters, and kidney pelvis is sensitive to nociceptive pain and stretching.

Central Pain

Pathologic pain due to CNS injury (central pain) often results from infarction, tumor, or other localized damage to the spinal cord, the brain stem, or areas of the brain itself.

Central pain is often severe, constant, and difficult to treat. It can occur with any type of disorder that causes CNS damage, including cancer, diabetes, stroke, multiple sclerosis, or trauma.

THALAMIC PAIN

Thalamic pain is one of the most common types of central pain. Thalamic pain is the perception of pain in one half of the body, occurring after thalamic injury. It usually is constant and subject to spontaneous aggravation (increases in pain without serious injury). The intensity of thalamic pain may also be increased by specific stimuli, such as sudden temperature changes, anxiety, and emotional stress. Overreaction to stimuli may occur, so that stimuli that normally are not painful may be painful. Also, there may be an unusually prolonged time lag between the initiation of a painful stimulus and the feeling of pain. The feeling of pain may then long outlast the stimulus. Frequently, signs of autonomic dysfunction (such as increased perspiration, cyanosis, and lowered skin temperature) may accompany the pain. People with central pain often find it difficult to describe the quality of their sensations. Others describe pain as boring, cold, burning, aching, or gnawing.

Vascular lesions of the thalamus, which involve the lateral nucleus of the thalamus, are the most common thalamic source of central pain. However, tumor, trauma, or inflammation of this area may also produce thalamic central pain. When thalamic infarct or thrombosis occurs, the pain usually does not begin for several weeks.

Thalamic pain may range in intensity from paresthesias (sensations of numbness, tingling, or prickling) to agonizing, boring, burning pains that are often associated with a feeling that the hand or foot is being twisted. Following a thalamic infarct (cerebrovascular accident [CVA], i.e., stroke), these often excruciating thalamic pains may involve an entire half of the body.

Thalamic pain may be intensified by emotional disturbances. Increased emotional lability (e.g., unmotivated crying or laughing) is often associated with this syndrome.

The thalamic syndrome is produced by thalamic lesions. Typically, it consists of the following four *assessment findings* on the side opposite the lesion: (1) transient hemiparesis or hemiplegia; (2) loss of deep sensation and impairment of superficial sensation; (3) tremor, ataxia, and choreoathetoid movements; and (4) spontaneous, excruciating pain, hyperalgesia, and excessive reaction to stimulation of involved bodily areas. Hyperpathic pain (pain of greater intensity than normally expected) may be present in the entire contralateral half of the head and body, or smaller contiguous areas may be affected.

Clients experiencing thalamic syndrome overrespond to stimuli such as pinprick, stroking, and deep pressure on the involved area of the skin. Bright light, sudden noises, temperature changes (cold especially), fatigue, debilitation, and apprehension all intensify the pain. Such clients may laugh or cry without apparent motivation, since extreme emotional lability is a part of their illness.

The *mechanism* by which central pain occurs is not precisely known. It is speculated that "irritation" at the lesion site or "reduction of central inhibition" are important factors. Also, since psychological stress obviously aggravates central pain, it is believed that regardless of what the specific pain mechanism is, pain production is somehow connected to those neurologic circuits that relate to emotions.

Careful neurologic assessment is essential before a person with "thalamic pain" can be treated, so that a possible surgical lesion is not overlooked.

PAIN FROM LESIONS OF THE CEREBRAL CORTEX

These lesions (e.g., brain tumors and other mass lesions), as well as cortical ischemic lesions resulting from cerebrovascular occlusive disease, may involve the cerebral cortex and not the thalamus. They may produce central pain in the opposite (i.e., contralateral) side of the body.

Peripheral Pathologic Pain

POSTHERPETIC NEURALGIA

One type of pathologic pain presenting histologic changes in nerve structure is postherpetic neuralgia. After the extremely painful vesicles of herpes zoster have subsided and disappeared, some people experience persistent, severe, intractable pain in the area of the original skin eruption. This is postherpetic neuralgia or postherpetic pain. This syndrome is very annoying and tormenting. Its unrelenting pain may cause sleepless nights and unbearable days. Some individuals are willing to undergo anything in hope of relief. However, the results of therapy may be poor and the postherpetic pain may continue. Neurologic pain is often treated with anticonvulsants or tricyclic antidepressants, such as phenytoin or amitriptyline.

The cause of postherpetic neuralgia is not fully understood. However, scarring and degenerative changes involving the spinal cord, ganglia, nerve trunks, and skin may be important factors.

CAUSALGIA

The pain syndrome of causalgia typically follows peripheral nerve injury. The brachial plexus and the median and sciatic nerves are involved most frequently. Although peripheral nerve damage is the usual cause, other conditions may rarely precipitate the problem. Examples of these are sprains, bruises, fractures, amputations, and arterial and venous occlusions.

Assessment findings with causalgia include burning pain that is often severe, persistent, diffuse, spontaneous, and aggravated by motion, touch, or emotional stimuli. A client with causalgia may appear apathetic and haggard. The pain may cause emotional disturbance if it is prolonged. If the suffering increases in intensity and the area of involvement spreads, intractable pain may lead to severe depression and even suicide.

As with many types of deafferentation pain, virtually any stimulus may set off paroxysms of excruciating pain (e.g., drafts of air, eating, temperature changes, contact with clothing). Consequently, a client may try to prevent pain by keeping the affected joints rigid or by wrapping the part in a moist cloth. Because of a realistic fear of severe pain, a client experiencing causalgia may adopt elaborate precautions to prevent the paroxysms of pain from being triggered. Those who do not understand a client's suffering or the reasons for these actions may view the actions as absurd and unreasonable. Such judgements only further hurt the client and cause additional suffering.

Generally, causalgia is associated with dystrophic and vasomotor changes, that is, reflex sympathetic dystrophy. This disorder of the sympathetic nervous system may follow not only injuries to nerves but also those to blood vessels, or it may follow fractures or sprains. Assessment findings of reflex sympathetic dystrophy include rubor or pallor, sweating or dryness, edema, pain, or skin atrophy.

TRIGEMINAL NEURALGIA (TIC DOULOUREUX)

This severe lancinating pain occurs along the sensory area of the fifth or ninth cranial nerves. The paroxysmal attacks of pain may be triggered by minimal stimuli, such as drafts of cold air, temperature changes, clothing against the area, eating, or talking, or even without any stimulus. This pain occurs as a result of a mild mechanoreceptive stimulus rather than a painful stimulus. The pain is described as feeling like a sudden electric shock. The severity of the attacks may lead the client to try to avoid all triggering by not talking or even eating, and the client becomes weak and often depressed.

Often, this condition can be treated with simple drug therapy. Carbamazepine (Tegretol), used to treat epilepsy, is usually effective in the treatment of this painful condition. Surgery, with the severing of the sensory portion of the fifth cranial nerve also relieves the pain. This procedure leaves the motor function intact but causes anesthesia of the affected side of the face.

PHANTOM PAIN

Following amputation of a body part (e.g., limb, breast), a client may feel phantom sensations in the area of the amputation, as if that part were still present. These abnormal sensations (paresthesias) commonly include feelings of itching, pressure sensations, tingling feelings, or "pins and needles."

Although phantom sensations are relatively common, phantom pain is less common. Most phantom paresthesias are tolerable, but some types of phantom pain are severe. A formerly painless phantom area may gradually become painful. More typically, however, phantom areas that pose severe problems tend to be painful immediately after amputation.

When phantom pain does occur, throbbing, burning, stabbing, boring, or vicelike sensations are experienced in the amputated area. Pain quality varies widely. Phantom pain also may be experienced as cramped, twisted, and abnormal posturing of a phantom limb.

With abnormal posturing sensations, the phantom limb feels as if it were being held immovably rigid in spite of the client's desire to change its position. The fist of an amputated hand may feel clenched so tightly that the nails are tearing into the palm. Clients with amputated legs or feet may experience their missing toes as cramped and curled. This type of pain does not occur in clients who maintain the feeling they can move the phantom limb voluntarily.

Exacerbations of the conditions may be precipitated by fatigue, excitement, sickness, weather changes, emotional stress, and other stimuli.

Stump pain (pain in the tissues adjacent to the amputation) is often associated with phantom pain. However, it is not necessarily related to it. Clients who have phantom pain usually experience some stump discomfort with their phantom pain, but some clients have phantom pain without stump pain.

HEADACHE

Headache is probably the most common pain felt by most people. There are many causes of headaches, with both intracranial and extracranial structures being involved. The brain itself is almost insensitive to pain, although the venous sinuses, tentorium, dura, some of the cranial nerves, and associated vasculature all are pain sensitive. One of the most sensitive areas in the brain is the middle meningeal artery. Changes in the intracranial pressure, either increases or decreases, may lead to headaches because the pressure changes cause the pain-sensitive structures in the head to shift. For example, when the client undergoes a lumbar puncture, the loss of cerebrospinal fluid leads to a decreased cushioning of the brain and a downward displacement of the pain-sensitive structures.

Many extracranial structures are sensitive to nociceptive stimuli. These structures include the skin, subcutaneous tissues, muscles, arteries, and periosteum of the skull. Problems in the eyes, sinuses, ears, teeth, nose, and jaws also may lead to headaches.

There are many types of headaches of intracranial origin. Vascular headaches are a common type of intracranial headache. These headaches can be caused by a variety of problems, such as hypertension, sepsis, hypoxia, and various drugs. Other causes of intracranial headaches include infection, hemorrhage, and as mentioned, changes in intracranial pressure.

Probably the most well-known headache of intracranial origin is the migraine. Although the exact cause of migraines is unknown, it seems to involve some abnormality of the vasculature. Clients suffering from migraines often experience prodromal symptoms, ranging from nausea to visual and auditory changes. One theory is that something triggers extreme vasospasm in some of the arteries in the cranium, leading to ischemia, which would explain the prodromal symptoms. The combination of vasospasm and ischemia leads to a decrease in vascular tone, causing vasodilation for 24 to 48 hours, with intense pulsating of these vessels. This process may cause stretching of intracranial and extracranial arteries, including the temporal artery, causing the migraine pain. Shifting of pain-sensitive structures in the head also may lead to pain.

Headaches of extracranial origin also are common and have many causes. The mechanisms of these headaches are similar to those causing headaches of intracranial origin. Stimuli such as traction, distention, dilation and spasms of vessels, irritation of nerves, and inflammation of various structures can cause them. The common types of extracranial headaches are muscle tension, temporomandibular joint syndrome, ocular, sinus, dental, and otic.

Headaches of both intracranial and extracranial origin are best treated by first identifying the cause and, if possible, treating it. Medications such as aspirin, muscle relaxants, ergotamine, and dexamethasone are used to treat a variety of headaches. The nurse should carefully assess the client to identify the cause so correct treatment can be started.

Malignant Pain

Cancer pain is a common pain syndrome because one in three people in the United States develops cancer. Cancer pain is uncommon in some cancers such as leukemia. However, pain occurs in 60 to 80 per cent of clients with solid tumors.

This pain syndrome has multiple causes. Some pain is caused by pressure on or displacement of nerves. Pain also may result from interference with blood supply or blockage within hollow organs. A common cause of cancer pain is metastasis of cancer to the bone. This type of pain can occur as a result of pathologic fracture with resultant muscle spasms, or as the spine is involved and nerves are affected. Another cause of the pain is iatrogenic causes such as surgery, radiation therapy, and chemotherapy. Immobility and inflammation also can lead to pain.

Treatment of this pain syndrome is also difficult because it has a variety of causes. Bone pain usually responds to a combination of radiation therapy and NSAIDs, whereas other pain may require narcotic analgesics such as morphine. The client and the nurse must know and believe that cancer pain is controllable if adequate and correct medications are used in adequate amounts.

Pain of Psychological Origin

PRETENDED PAIN

Very rarely, a nurse may meet a client who says that pain is being experienced and who is seeking treatment for pain but who actually has no pain. This is referred to as malingering. Such clients are aware that they are not experiencing pain. They may make this pretense to

- Avoid a task;
- Obtain possible economic gain, e.g., money to compensate for an injury;
- Obtain narcotic analgesics or other psychoactive drugs to which they have become physically or psychologically dependent; and
- Obtain attention or sympathy from others (such clients usually lack more effective social coping techniques).

Never assume that pain is pretended. An accurate diagnosis of pretended pain is difficult to make and is rarely made correctly. Much suffering has resulted when clients actually experiencing pain were treated as if they were just pretending.

PSYCHOGENIC PAIN

The term psychogenic pain is often used but is difficult to define. Psychogenic pain refers to pain believed to be due primarily to emotional factors rather than to physiologic dysfunction. Clients experiencing psychogenic pain have a real pain experience.

Psychogenic pain is different from pretended pain. Although psychogenic pain starts without a physical basis, repeated severe stress probably alters the complex physiology of pain transmission, modulation, and perception. The pain the client feels is real to that client, and the tension or stress the client is feeling may lead to pronounced physiologic changes. Unfortunately, this diagnosis is often assigned prematurely to a client's pain, when careful assessment would uncover a treatable physiologic dysfunction (such as either the cause of the pain or a result of the stress). Obtaining pain relief from a placebo does not mean the client is not experiencing pain (see section on placebo). Psychogenic pain requires that the cause be found and treated.

When the psychogenic effect of stress, anxiety, fear, and anger produce painful alterations in physiology, this can be called psychophysiologic pain. For example, stress can produce chronic excessive muscle contraction, as if the client were continually prepared to meet danger. In turn, this chronic muscle contraction can produce pain. Most often, this occurs in the scalp muscles (muscle contraction or tension headache, see section on headache) and postural muscles. Stress also can produce visceral changes that can result in painful structural damage over a long period.

ASSESSMENT

Because pain is a subjective experience, one of the priorities for adequate treatment of pain is an accurate assessment. Assessment, however, is highly influenced by the client's ability to delineate aspects of the pain experience accurately. If the client cannot communicate clearly (i.e., child, unconscious, aphasic), then this aspect of the pain assessment is altered. Without the subjective information, it is very difficult to intervene correctly, except by trial and error.

Blocks to Accurate Pain Assessment

MYTHS AND MISCONCEPTIONS ABOUT PAIN

Many myths and misconceptions exist about pain (Table 16-3). These may influence the nurse's assessment of the client's pain. If nurses continue to believe these myths, then adequate pain assessment and relief are hampered.

Just because pain is a subjective phenomenon, that does not mean it is not real. All pain is real to the individual who is experiencing it. This does not mean that a physical cause can always be found. Sometimes, the cause is obscure, such as with many nerve pains, and it is difficult to determine an accurate diagnosis. The inability to identify a specific diagnostic cause does not negate the pain.

Pain of psychological origin is also very real. Think of the last time you had a tension headache. The cause is purely psychological—tension. Knowing that fact does not make the pain any less; in fact, a tension headache is usually very painful and very difficult to treat. Psychological stimuli lead to physiologic responses, and one such response can be pain. The nurse must remember that pain is always a combination of physiologic and psychological stimuli.

There are both physiologic and psychological responses to acute pain. These responses, however, vary over time as adaptation occurs. Initial physiologic responses are due to sympathetic stimulation that causes increased blood pressure, and pulse and respiratory rate; dilated pupils; and diaphoresis. The initial psychological responses are usually a focusing on the pain, with a report of pain, crying or moaning, increased muscle tension, and guarding of the painful part. With time, the client with even extremely severe pain develops an adaptive response. The adaptive physiologic response is a return to normal vital signs and other physiologic parameters. The adaptive psychological responses include a shifting away from the pain, reporting pain only if directly asked, sleepiness, decreased physical activity, and often a blank facial expression.

Although some of the responses to pain are predictable, how much pain any given stimulus causes in an individual is not. It is impossible to predict how much pain something will cause. When the members of the health care team make this sort of assumption, they are usually wrong. You may hear comments like, "A 3rd-day post op hysterectomy client should not be having that much pain." No one except the client can tell how much pain is occurring.

The only way the nurse can overcome these myths, misconceptions, and prejudices is through education. By knowing the facts about pain, pain assessment, and pain treatment, the nurse can provide more complete care for the client.

Client Misinformation About Pain

Often, one of the major blocks to accurate assessment of the client's pain is the client. If the health care team members still have myths and misconceptions about pain, then it is likely the client also has been misinformed about pain and pain control. Clients pick up on the expectations of the health care team about their own pain. Clients have learned quickly that they are often expected to tolerate certain levels of pain and not to complain excessively. They have also learned to be afraid of pain medications, especially narcotics.

A major nursing responsibility, therefore, is to educate the client about pain and pain control. The nurse needs to help clients see that it is clients who are the experts on their pain, not the health care team. The

TABLE 16-3. Common Pain Myths, Misconceptions, and Facts

Myth/Misconception	Fact
Pain that is real has an identifiable cause	There is always a cause for pain, but it may be very obscure and must be assessed carefully. Also pain that has a psychological origin is just as real as pain of physiologic origin
There are predictable signs that a client in pain will exhibit	Pain is unpredictable in the physiologic changes that are produced. Even severe pain may not produce the typical pain symptoms. Lack of pain expression does not mean lack of pain
Very young or very old clients do not experience as much pain	All clients with an intact CNS experience pain. Age is not a determinant of pain, although it may influence expression
Pain is predictable. Certain stimuli produce predictable amounts of pain for all clients	Pain is individualized. There is no standard pain produced by a particular stimulus. An identical surgical incision in different people produces different amounts of pain
The health care team is the expert about the client's pain. They know how much pain the client should be feeling and how it should be treated	The person experiencing the pain is the only expert on that pain. The client is the only one who knows whether any given treatment works
Nurses can best assess pain using their own definitions of pain and cultural beliefs and values about pain	Using your own values and beliefs to assess another's pain is a mistake. Everyone defines pain for themselves, in terms of their own values and beliefs. The only way to understand the client's pain is to have the client tell you about it
A person can learn to increase tolerance to pain and that is good. With prolonged pain, a person's tolerance increases	High pain tolerance has no value in and of itself. There is no reason for a client to suffer unnecessarily. Prolonged pain actually lowers the client's tolerance of pain
If people can sleep then they are not in pain	Pain is exhausting. People will sleep, however poorly, in spite of pain. People with severe or prolonged pain often sleep because of exhaustion. Sleep may also be how the client escapes from pain
Clients with chronic pain often have psychological problems	Clients with any unrelieved pain may experience depression or anxiety. If pain continues, then these other symptoms may increase, but they are caused by the pain, not the reverse
If distraction or other noninvasive pain relief methods work for the client, then the pain is not real	Noninvasive pain relief methods can be very effective in relieving both acute and chronic pain. You must believe the client's pain and the method of relief he or she chooses, as long as it does not hurt anyone

Data from McCaffery, M., & Beebe, A. (1989). *Pain: Clinical manual for nursing practice.* St. Louis: C. V. Mosby.

nurse is also responsible for helping the client provide an accurate pain history and assessment.

When discussing or documenting pain, avoid saying that a client complains of pain. This term tends to invalidate or minimize the client's experience, as if the client is fussing unnecessarily. It is more accurate and helpful simply to use the word states or reports.

When discussing pain (e.g., with those experiencing it) or when documenting pain, avoid using the word attack. Feeling that one is under attack may produce a greater feeling of powerlessness, such as feeling like a victim. Victim is another word best avoided in these situations, for similar reasons. Use the term episode rather than attack to promote self-control and a sense of being able to do something to manage the episode.

Basic Principles

Ongoing assessment of pain is vital. This ongoing assessment should include subjective and objective assessment, that is, the individual's verbal descriptions of the pain and observations of a person's behavior.

Each person has a basic human need to be free of

pain and discomfort. Human beings are motivated to avoid pain. Pain can occur as a result of inadequate satisfaction of other basic human needs. For example, if the need to eliminate urine is not met because urinary stones block the bladder outlet, pain occurs. Similarly, if a person does not experience affection and caring from someone else (i.e., to satisfy the need for love and belonging), some form of psychogenic pain may occur. Part of nursing assessment is to identify any unmet needs that may contribute to a person's pain.

Pain assessment is difficult because there are no objective tests for pain. Also, psychic and somatic factors interact indivisibly. Each person experiences and expresses pain uniquely, and attaches personal meanings or explanations to pain experiences.

The personal meanings nurses attach to pain may interfere with their assessments. For example, nurses may interpret a person's pain according to their own personal experiences rather than from the person's point of view. The frequent exposure nurses have to others experiencing pain may lead them to underestimate the significance of this pain.

Personal meanings attached to pain result from personal pain experiences throughout life and may arise from a person's (1) individual experiences and (2) sociocultural experiences. The cultural and familial role modeling a person is exposed to as a child teaches the person such things as

- What pains are appropriate or inappropriate to talk about
- Behavior that is appropriate or inappropriate when one experiences pain
- Circumstances likely to produce pain, which should therefore be avoided
- Various methods to avoid or relieve pain
- "Reasons" why one may experience pain, such as punishment, testing by supernatural or divine powers, or because of bad thoughts
- Possible consequences of pain, such as attention or lack of attention from others, imminent death.

A pain experience is also affected by personal factors:

- Pain expectancy (the anticipation of pain)
- Pain acceptance (willingness to experience pain)
- Pain apprehension (generalized desire to avoid pain)
- Pain anxiety (the anxiety pain provokes because of its associated mystery, loneliness, helplessness, threat)

Pain evokes emotional responses that may have behavioral expressions. Observations of behavior provide a nurse with some understanding of a person's feelings and of what pain means to a particular person. By accepting behaviors and trying to understand their origins, nurses can help individuals experiencing pain. To do this well, nurses must (1) accurately observe clients' behavior, (2) listen to all that clients say, and (3) never judge clients or jump to conclusions.

Perception of pain is influenced by such factors as

- Integrity of a client's nervous system,
- State of consciousness,
- Age,
- Physical state (fatigue, debility, lack of sleep, and prolonged suffering all reduce a client's ability to tolerate pain) (Fig. 16-6), and
- Emotional state (worry, fear, and anxiety reduce a client's ability to tolerate pain).

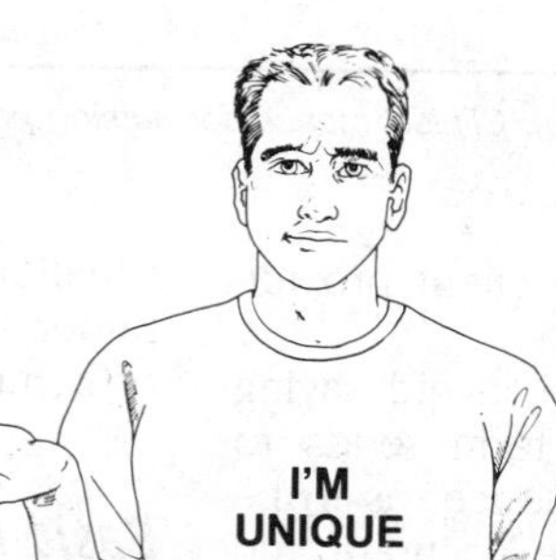
PSYCHOSOCIAL INFLUENCES
Family and occupational roles—Past experiences—Spiritual belief system
Meaning of pain—Cultural/societal influences—Sexual identity and stereotypes
Communication skills—Level of growth and development—Motivations
Personality—Presence of fear—Level of excitement or distraction at time of injury
Attitude toward pain—Level of anxiety—Fatigue
PAIN THRESHOLD
GENERAL STATE OF HEALTH
PAIN INTENSITY
PAIN FREQUENCY
INTEGRITY OF NERVOUS SYSTEM PATHWAYS
AGE
PHYSICAL INFLUENCES
(SLEEP, STRESS)
PAIN TOLERANCE
UNDERLYING CAUSE OF PAIN
PAIN QUALITY
PAIN LOCATION
PAIN DURATION
TYPE OF PAIN
PRIOR EXPERIENCE WITH PAIN
I'M
UNIQUE
!

▲ **Figure 16-6**

Factors influencing responses to pain.

History

An accurate history is essential to assess a client's pain experience. A detailed symptom analysis (see also Chap. 11) is performed using the following guidelines.

LOCATION

To determine the location of the client's pain, ask the following questions:

- Where in the body is the pain? (Use a figure of a person and have the client point to or mark painful areas.)
- Is the pain inside (internal) or on the surface (external)?
- Is the pain always in these areas?
- If the pain is in more than one spot, are the pains equal, or does one trigger the others?
- Is the pain on both sides of your body; if so, is it the same on each side?

EXTENSION OR RADIATION

To determine the extension and radiation of the client's pain, ask the following questions:

- Does the pain extend from where it started? Does it cover a wide area, or can you point to where it is?
- Is there a pattern in which the pain spreads?
- Is the pain on the surface or deep inside?

ONSET AND PATTERN

To determine the onset and pattern of the client's pain, ask the following questions:

- When did the pain begin? Is it a regular pain, or does it vary? Does it occur in cycles, such as at the same time every day, every month, or every spring?
- What triggers the pain? Are there specific things that always trigger it? Can you identify any particular patterns?
- Does the pain begin suddenly or gradually over time? Is it continuous, or does it vary? Are there separate episodes of pain? If so, does the pain go away completely between episodes, or does it just get better?
- Has the pain pattern changed at all since it began?
- Has your lifestyle changed since the pain began?

DURATION

To determine the duration of the client's pain, ask the following questions:

- How long does the pain last? Are you free of pain between attacks?
- Is the pain constant, intermittent, rhythmic, pulsating, or throbbing?

CHARACTER OR QUALITY

To determine the character or quality of the client's pain, ask the client to describe it.

- Is the pain dull, sharp, throbbing, burning, "electric," or shooting? (If the client cannot describe the pain, offer terms like those on the McGill-Melzack Pain Questionnaire[75] [Fig. 16–7]. When recording the history, record the client's exact terms.)

PRECIPITATING, AGGRAVATING, AND ALLEVIATING FACTORS

To determine the factors that precipitate, aggravate, and alleviate the client's pain, ask the following questions:

- What seems to trigger the pain? Can you identify a specific cause or event that always or sometimes precedes the pain?
- Does anything alter the pain? Does anything make it worse, such as smoking, drinking alcohol, eating, heat, or tension? Is there anything that makes the pain better?
- What helps relieve the pain, such as rest, activity, heat or cold, or medications?

INTENSITY

To determine the intensity of the client's pain:

- Ask: On a scale of 0 to 10, with 0 being no pain and 10 being the worst pain you can imagine, how would you rate your pain now? How would you rate it at its worst? How would you rate it at its best? (When treatment starts, always have the client rate the pain before and after treatment.)
- Note what nonverbal signs of pain the client exhibits, such as grimacing, crying, moaning, sleeping, appearing exhausted, or remaining immobile.

ASSOCIATED SYMPTOMS

To determine whether there are any symptoms associated with the client's pain ask:

- Are there any other problems caused by your pain? Do you have any nausea, restlessness, insomnia, excessive sleeping, or loss of appetite?

EFFECT ON ACTIVITIES OF DAILY LIVING

To determine how the client's pain affects activities of daily living, ask:

- Does the pain interfere with work, sleep, driving, eating, schoolwork, sexual relations, housework, social activity, or other activity (Box 16–1)?
- Has the pain caused any changes in your lifestyle?
- When did you last have a good night's sleep?

METHODS OF PAIN RELIEF

To determine how the client obtains pain relief, ask:

- What do you do to relieve the pain? (Ask about both invasive and noninvasive pain relief methods.)
- What has *not* worked to relieve your pain?

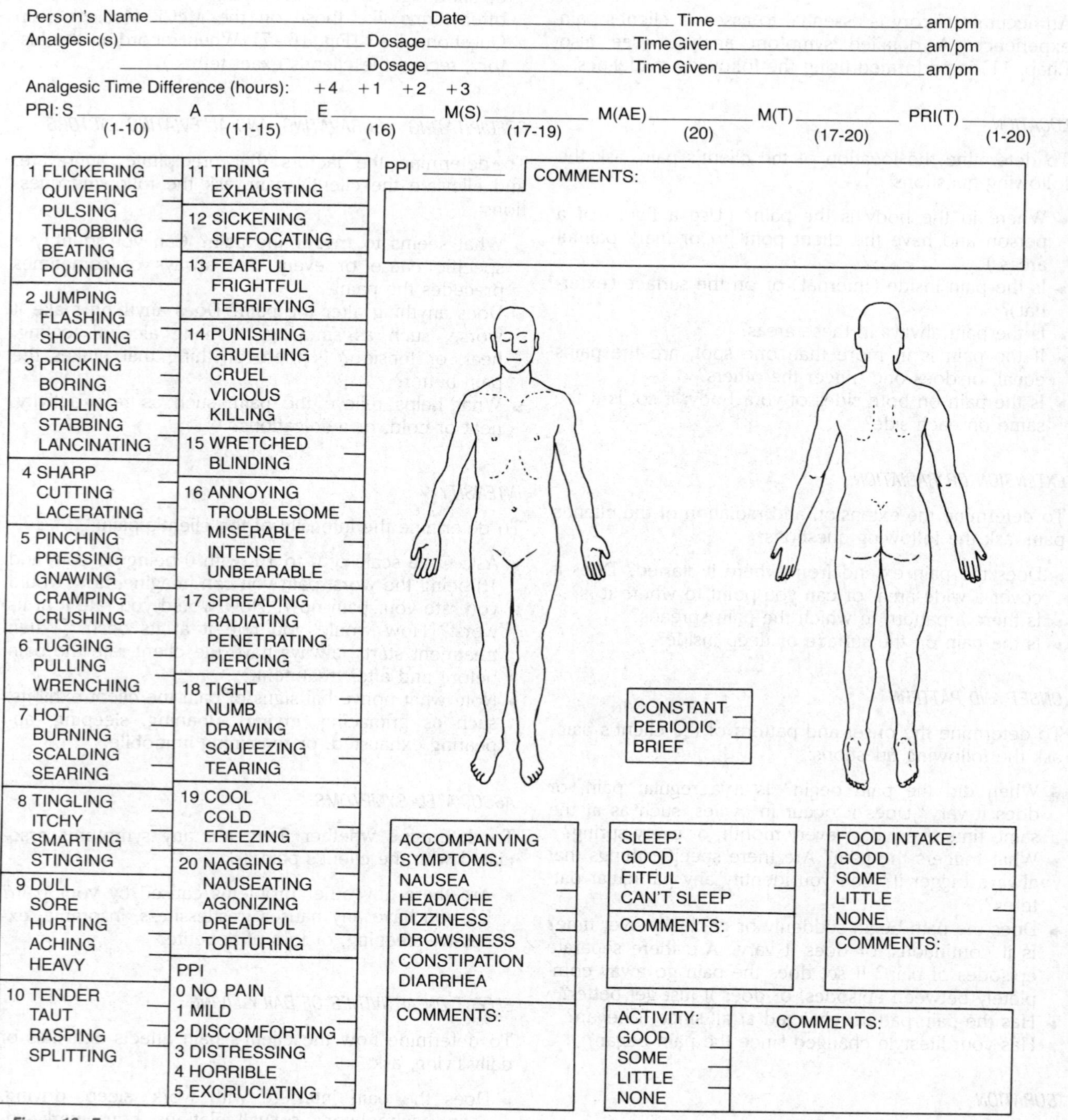

McGill - Melzack Pain Questionnaire

Person's Name ________ Date ________ Time ________ am/pm

Analgesic(s) ________ Dosage ________ Time Given ________ am/pm

________ Dosage ________ Time Given ________ am/pm

Analgesic Time Difference (hours): +4 +1 +2 +3

PRI: S ____ (1-10) A ____ (11-15) E ____ (16) M(S) ____ (17-19) M(AE) ____ (20) M(T) ____ (17-20) PRI(T) ____ (1-20)

1 FLICKERING, QUIVERING, PULSING, THROBBING, BEATING, POUNDING

2 JUMPING, FLASHING, SHOOTING

3 PRICKING, BORING, DRILLING, STABBING, LANCINATING

4 SHARP, CUTTING, LACERATING

5 PINCHING, PRESSING, GNAWING, CRAMPING, CRUSHING

6 TUGGING, PULLING, WRENCHING

7 HOT, BURNING, SCALDING, SEARING

8 TINGLING, ITCHY, SMARTING, STINGING

9 DULL, SORE, HURTING, ACHING, HEAVY

10 TENDER, TAUT, RASPING, SPLITTING

11 TIRING, EXHAUSTING

12 SICKENING, SUFFOCATING

13 FEARFUL, FRIGHTFUL, TERRIFYING

14 PUNISHING, GRUELLING, CRUEL, VICIOUS, KILLING

15 WRETCHED, BLINDING

16 ANNOYING, TROUBLESOME, MISERABLE, INTENSE, UNBEARABLE

17 SPREADING, RADIATING, PENETRATING, PIERCING

18 TIGHT, NUMB, DRAWING, SQUEEZING, TEARING

19 COOL, COLD, FREEZING

20 NAGGING, NAUSEATING, AGONIZING, DREADFUL, TORTURING

PPI: 0 NO PAIN, 1 MILD, 2 DISCOMFORTING, 3 DISTRESSING, 4 HORRIBLE, 5 EXCRUCIATING

PPI ____ COMMENTS:

CONSTANT, PERIODIC, BRIEF

ACCOMPANYING SYMPTOMS: NAUSEA, HEADACHE, DIZZINESS, DROWSINESS, CONSTIPATION, DIARRHEA. COMMENTS:

SLEEP: GOOD, FITFUL, CAN'T SLEEP. COMMENTS:

FOOD INTAKE: GOOD, SOME, LITTLE, NONE. COMMENTS:

ACTIVITY: GOOD, SOME, LITTLE, NONE. COMMENTS:

▲ *Figure 16–7*

The McGill-Melzack Pain Questionnaire, adapted for the study of narcotic drugs. The descriptors listed at left comprise four groups: 1 to 10, sensory; 11 to 15, affective; 16, evaluative; 17 to 20, miscellaneous. The rank value for each descriptor is based on its position in the word set. Total rank values comprise the pain-rating index (PRI). The present pain intensity (PPI) is based on a scale from 0 to 5. The drawings are used to designate the site of pain. (From Bonica, J. J. [1980]. *Pain* [p. 145]. New York: Raven Press.)

Physical Examination

Begin the examination by having the client show where the pain is and describe how it feels. Remember that the client is the expert on the pain and is the one who can best describe and pinpoint it.

Objective signs of pain can be divided into three categories: sympathetic responses, parasympathetic responses, and behavioral responses. These responses are not diagnostic of pain, but they may give clues about its cause.

Box 16-1. Effects of Pain on Daily Living Scale

Instructions

On a scale of 0 (no pain) to 5 (maximum pain), the client should indicate the areas of life currently affected and the severity of the interference. If the client's current level of pain is less than that usually felt, the client also should be asked to rate the most pain (effects) ever experienced in these areas.

Sleep
Appetite
Concentration
Work and School
Interpersonal Relationships
Marital Relations and Sex
Home Activities
Driving and Walking
Leisure Activities
Emotional Status (mood, irritability, depression, anxiety)

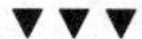

From E. Matassarin-Jacobs, unpublished presentation, *Pain Assessment*, Chicago, Illinois, May 1981. Reprinted with permission.

SYMPATHETIC RESPONSES

Sympathetic responses are often associated with low to moderate pain intensity or superficial pain. They signify that body defenses are mobilized and that the fight or flight response has begun. Objective signs include pallor, increased blood pressure, increased pulse, increased respirations, skeletal muscle tension, dilated pupils, and diaphoresis.

PARASYMPATHETIC RESPONSES

Parasympathetic responses are often associated with pain of severe intensity, or with deep pain. In parasympathetic responses, body defenses may collapse in an attempt to lessen the effects of an external threat. Signs and symptoms of a parasympathetic response include decreased blood pressure, decreased pulse, nausea and vomiting, weakness, prostration, pallor, and possible loss of consciousness.

BEHAVIORAL RESPONSES

The client may

- Assume a posture that minimizes pain, such as lying rigidly, guarding, drawing up the legs, or assuming the fetal position;
- Moan, sigh, grimace, clench the jaws or fist, become quiet, or withdraw from others;
- Blink rapidly;
- Cry, appear frightened, exhibit restlessness;
- Have a drawn facial expression;
- Have twitching muscles;
- Withdraw when touched; and
- Hold or protect the painful area, or remain motionless.

VISUAL DESCRIPTOR SCALE

No pain | Slight pain | Moderate pain | Severe pain | Worst pain

VISUAL ANALOG SCALE

No pain | Worst pain

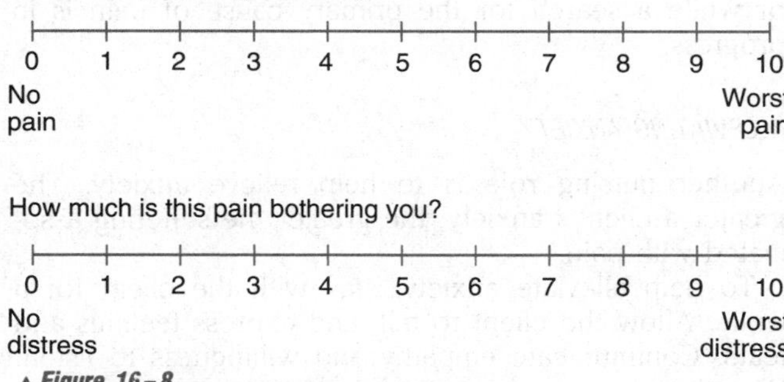

▲ *Figure 16-8*

Visual analog and visual descriptor scales.

Tools Used to Assess Pain

The simplest pain assessment tools to use for both nurse and client are the visual analog or visual descriptor scales. These scales can be combined with numbers and verbal anchors (Fig. 16-8). These tools are easy to use and provide the client and nurse a way to quantify pain. Another common assessment tool used to assess pain is the McGill-Melzack Pain Questionnaire (see Fig. 16-7). Although this tool is complex and more difficult than others to use, it can be very useful.

NURSING INTERVENTION

Basic Principles

When caring for a client in pain, identify and remove the cause whenever possible. Work with the client in seeking ways to reduce or remove pain. Listen to what the client thinks will help, and decide with the client and other health care team members what should be done. Allow the client a sense of control over the pain experience, rather than promote a feeling that the client is helpless in the grip of an episode of pain.

Also, it is important to make frequent reassessments and evaluations and adjust nursing interventions accordingly. Realize that an intervention that is helpful at one time for one client is not necessarily helpful at another time for another client—or even for the same client.

Also remember that the quality of your relationship with the client in pain may be as important as the pain-relieving skills that you use. Create a relationship characterized by genuineness, warmth, empathy, and respect.

The client's basic human needs, such as those for food and elimination, should also be met. If they are, pain or discomfort (physical and psychological) may be reduced or even eliminated.

Although specific therapy is, whenever possible, directed at removing the cause of the client's pain, you must also intervene for other problems that aggravate pain. Such problems include coughing, anorexia, diarrhea, and constipation. Management of these ancillary problems may also be used for palliation when the primary cause of pain cannot be treated or removed, or while a search for the primary cause of pain is in progress.

ALLEVIATING ANXIETY

Another nursing role is to help relieve anxiety. The greater a client's anxiety, the greater the suffering associated with pain.

To help alleviate anxiety, stay with the client for a while. Allow the client to talk and express feelings and fears. Communicate empathy and willingness to listen. Give the client some sense of control by encouraging input into the nursing care plan and by encouraging the client to practice self-directed pain-prevention or pain-reduction techniques, such as use of meditation. Use therapeutic touch or other measures, such as giving a back rub and applying a cool cloth to relieve physical tension, promote comfort, and help the client relax. Do what you can to relieve the pain, and be sure that the client understands that everything possible is being done. Always seek help if the client's pain is not being controlled and anxiety is increasing. Finally, inform the client whenever a procedure is likely to be painful, and encourage the client to express the pain.

DISTRACTION OR DIVERSION

Another nursing measure used for clients in pain is distraction, or diversion. Generally, the intensity of a client's suffering depends on the extent to which pain dominates consciousness. Pain perception, therefore, can be reduced by reducing the client's conscious awareness of pain. Distraction, which reduces this conscious awareness of pain, usually works better with mild pain than with severe pain, especially if used alone, without medication as an adjunct.

Distraction may take many forms. Occupational therapy, conversation, reading, watching television, listening to the radio, meditation, self-hypnosis, biofeedback, and autosuggestion are a few forms of distraction that may be helpful. It is important to remember, however, to check with the client to determine what works best for him or her. To some clients, for example, small talk, idle chatter, and excessive noise are tiring rather than helpful. Likewise, some clients find that low background noise such as a radio playing very softly is relaxing, whereas others find this same stimulus irritating and tension producing.

When seeking to use distraction to relieve pain, encourage clients to use any methods that they have found helpful in the past to relieve pain, provided that these methods are not harmful or bothersome to others.

Another means of distraction is to involve the client in self-care, such as deep breathing, turning, and moving the legs. Be sure to give specific, clear instructions such as "concentrate on slow, deep breathing, in through the nose and out through the mouth for about 10 breaths" or "hold onto the side rail of the bed and turn to your right side."

Distraction is also useful during painful procedures. However, you must be careful to maintain a delicate balance between keeping the client informed and focusing his or her attention on other things. Be sure to use appropriate timing and a sincere manner, or the client may feel that you are discounting his or her pain.

COMBATTING ANTICIPATORY FEARS

Anticipatory fears are those fears that occur prior to an experience of pain-producing stimuli. Help prepare clients to meet pain realistically by talking with them about the pain they fear.

Before painful procedures, talk with the client about what he or she can expect. This method may encourage relaxation and reduce muscle resistance that, in itself, could produce pain. Discuss the kind of pain or discomfort that the client may expect. For example, "You will feel a sharp prick." "You will probably feel some pressure, which may be uncomfortable but should not be painful." Clients who are given information about the sensation they can expect have less anticipatory distress and are more relaxed throughout the procedure than are those who are not prepared in this way.

Also before painful procedures, help clients assume body alignment and positions that will help them tolerate painful procedures more comfortably. For example, place a pillow between the client's legs if a side-lying position is required.

For preoperative clients, assure the client that he or she will be given adequate medication to control postoperative pain. If a postoperative client's analgesics are prescribed on a prn basis, give the medication at the prescribed intervals for the first 24 to 72 hours after surgery. Analgesics given around the clock provide better pain control and less sedation than analgesics provided on a more intermittent basis. Make sure that the client knows that if the medication is not offered, he or she should ask for it at regular intervals.

If a client who receives prescribed, scheduled analgesics is worried about pain, review with the client the times when the medication may be given. The routine of giving analgesics on a scheduled basis should be used to treat chronic pain, especially malignant pain.

Reassure clients who will require pain-relieving medications that you will promptly supply them as necessary. Clients who know this in advance are less likely to request medication unnecessarily or too early in anticipation of pain.

In addition to the measures outlined earlier for reducing anticipatory fear, teach the client techniques for reducing stress (see Chap. 3) and help the client to communicate pain to other health care providers, such as the physician.

PROVIDING PHYSICAL CARE

Effective physical nursing care for clients experiencing pain is directed at reducing mechanical, chemical, and thermal stressors that lower pain tolerance (Bridge to Home Health Care). This includes protecting clients from local irritations or inflammations such as infection or thrombosis, muscle spasm or muscle strain, interference with local blood supply and venous and lymphatic drainage, distention of hollow visceral organs such as the bowel and bladder, and further damage to traumatized tissue.

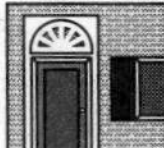

BRIDGE TO HOME HEALTH CARE

Pain Management

When evaluating pain management in the home health care client, a complete assessment is very important. In assessing pain, it is necessary to evaluate physical, social, emotional, and spiritual pain because each of these adds to the total pain experience. A plan of care can then be decided on that may include intervention in each of these areas, and may well include a multidisciplinary approach.

When medical intervention includes medication, instructing the client and family is very important. Explanation of the action and scheduling of the medication increases compliance. Teaching about side effects, and assessing and treating side effects, is also vital in promoting compliance. Untreated side effects often result in a client's decreasing use of the medication to avoid those effects. Recognizing the difference between chronic and acute pain is also necessary because the treatment may differ. Scheduling may well be the single most important instruction in the use of analgesics for chronic pain. Use of adjuvant therapy for pain control should also be considered because this often increases the effectiveness of the analgesic.

Fear of addiction is often a major problem. Explaining that medication taken correctly for pain will not cause addiction is essential. The client should be assured that pain can and will be relieved.

When dealing with intractable pain, it is important to consider various methods of analgesia such as continuous, patient-controlled analgesia pumps, time-released skin patches, sustained released oral medications, and suppositories.

Individualizing care is essential, and the various options available should be recognized. Providing the medical team with an assessment of the client's condition and home situation will help the team arrive at the safest, most effective pain management possible.

There are several important principles of physical nursing care. Identify the source of pain, and eliminate or reduce the pain. Handle sensitive or injured tissue carefully. Always perform painful procedures when pain-relieving medications are producing their maximal effect. Check drainage tubes frequently to ensure that they are not caught, stretched, pulled, kinked, or looped, and that they are positioned correctly.

Additional important principles of physical care include protecting the client from fatigue and helping the client get a good night's sleep, because overtiredness decreases pain tolerance.

It is also important to be alert to inflammation and ischemia caused by immobilization. If pain is caused by swollen body parts, elevating these parts may help. Likewise, a position of semiflexion may reduce the pain of joint disorders. Consult with the physical therapy department about mobilization, positioning, and supportive devices that might be used to relieve pain.

If the client is experiencing pain from muscle spasms, a position change may help. Frequent muscle changes with good body alignment may also prevent painful muscle contractures. Know exactly what you are going to do before moving clients who are experiencing pain. Listen to the client's advice about the move. Whenever possible, allow them to control the movement.

Additional physical care measures include gentle massage and applications of heat and cold. Gentle massage may help relieve muscle pain and prevent clot formation. However, never vigorously massage the client's calf, and teach the client never to do this. Blood clots may form in that area, and massage could dislodge the clots and possibly cause a fatal embolism! Application of heat and cold may block pain, as explained by the gate-control theory.

ADMINISTRATION OF PAIN-RELIEVING MEDICATION

Too often nurses view the administration of pain-relieving medications as all they need to do for pain management. The nurse must remember that medication can be more effective when combined with other pain relief techniques. When the nurse administers medication plus repositioning, a back rub, or simple interaction with the client, the effectiveness of the treatment may increase. Simply giving an injection or a pill does not replace thoughtful, comprehensive pain management.

Therapeutic interaction with someone experiencing pain may include (1) facilitating the client's expression of feelings, which gives the client a feeling of being cared for; (2) providing support, assurance, and understanding that may relieve present pain or prevent future pain; and (3) teaching the client self-management of pain.

Numerous medications are used in pain relief. They are administered in a variety of ways—by mouth, rectum, topical application, inhalation, or injection. Medications may be injected by subcutaneous, intramuscular, and intravenous routes. Also, certain medications are sometimes injected spinally, paravertebrally, or into selected nerves to produce nerve blocks. The latter types of injections are performed by physicians, and nurses often assist with the procedures.

MANAGING CHRONIC INTRACTABLE PAIN

Chronic intractable pain (pain that cannot be satisfactorily relieved) causes additional difficulties for people experiencing it. Clients experiencing chronic intractable pain may be helped by applying the psychological and physical nursing interventions discussed earlier. Nursing and medical therapeutic regimens must be coordinated and consistent, to ensure a unified approach.

MANAGING PROGRESSIVE PAIN

Clients experiencing progressive pain may be helped by the methods described in this chapter (Fig. 16-9). One important difference is that these individuals may require pain-relieving medications routinely as a preventive measure (in the same way that vasodilators are routinely taken by clients with ischemic heart disease). Some clients hesitate to take pain-relieving medications routinely for fear of addiction. However, clients experiencing pain because of widespread cancer have a disorder that requires pain-relieving medications. Thus, they are no more addicted to narcotics than clients with heart disease are addicted to vasodilators. Help clients and their significant others understand this important point.

Noninvasive Interventions

BEHAVIORAL TECHNIQUES

It was not until the end of the 19th century that scientific attention was given to physiologic phenomena that accompany various yogic disciplines, hypnotism, and spiritual practices. It is now well known that activities such as meditation, relaxation, and hypnosis cause various physiologic changes. For example, peripheral blood vessels may dilate, blood sugar levels may change, and muscle tension is reduced. Thus, techniques such as these can be used to manage pain and promote healthy living.

A variety of behavioral techniques can reduce pain in many clients. These noninvasive techniques are more desirable than invasive methods and should be used whenever possible. It is important for the nurse to remember, however, that most of these techniques require a great deal of client participation. Some clients may be emotionally or developmentally unable to participate in these activities. Assess the client carefully before encouraging these methods.

It may be possible to teach clients a combination of these techniques to maximize their opportunities for self-control over symptoms. When a client is able to use these techniques successfully to control pain, this in no way indicates that the pain is primarily psychological in origin. Such techniques may close the gate in the spinal cord or activate the descending analgesic system.

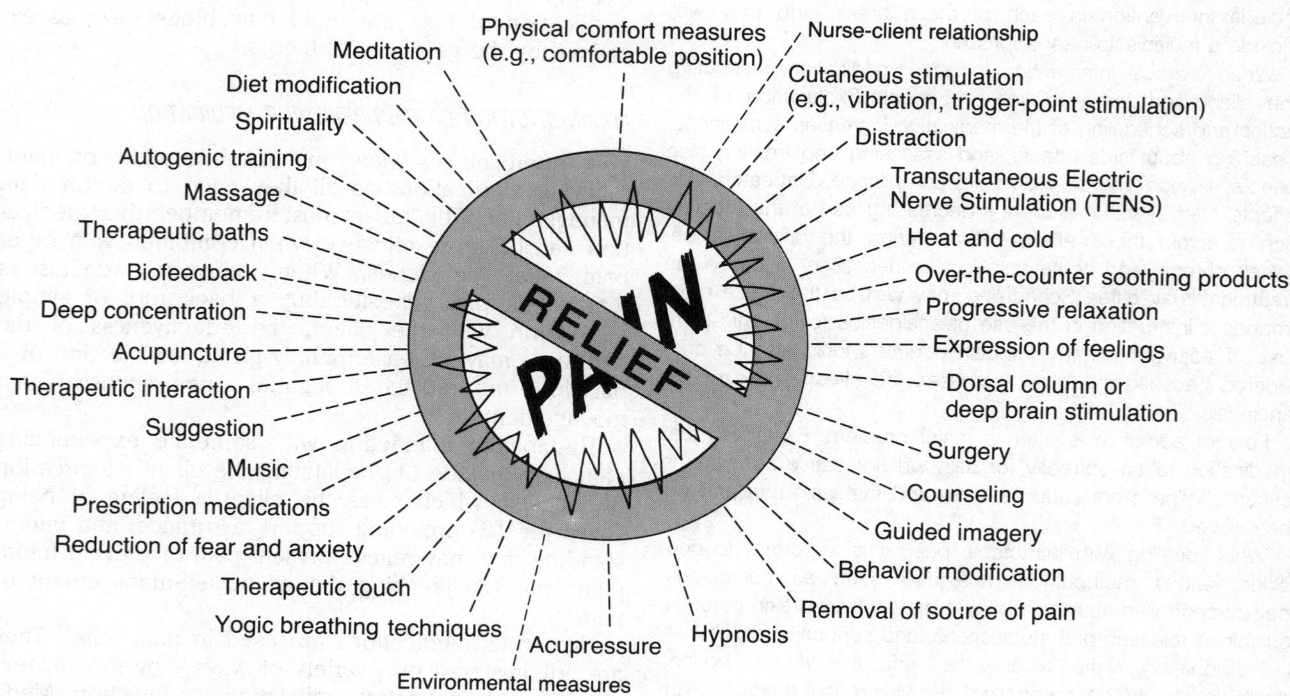

▲ Figure 16-9

Pain relief measures.

Many of the noninvasive techniques require the cooperation and even active participation of the client. It is difficult, however, to teach people who are already in severe pain. We must teach clients before a painful procedure or a painful period occurs, if possible. Clients with chronic pain may require longer times for the teaching so they do not become overstressed with this new information.

Learning plays an important role in chronic pain. Unfortunately, health care providers often react to an indication of pain in ways that promote and strengthen pain behaviors. For example, many health care professionals are accustomed to working with clients experiencing acute pain and to responding to their reports of pain. However, when using behavior control methods, health professionals attend to a client when the client is not reporting pain or demonstrating pain behavior. Increases in pain severity and related functional impairment may occur without worsening the underlying disease when pain behaviors are reinforced. For example, when a client's pain behavior is reinforced, that client may inhibit his or her range of motion or activities of daily living.

Clients experiencing chronic pain over long periods often learn to (or become conditioned to) display a complex set of pain behaviors. Then, by using these pain behaviors, they actually reinforce their feelings of pain. For example, grimacing, guarding, and vocalizations can have a reinforcing effect by making other people respond to the client's pain.

When clients have learned pain behaviors, modification of these behaviors can be helpful. There are several behavioral modification techniques in which the person controls what is happening, including meditation, hypnosis (see section on hypnosis), operant conditioning, biofeedback, autogenic training, and progressive relaxation training.

Meditation. Meditation focuses the attention of people experiencing pain away from their pain. It also provides energy and peace to the meditator. Meditation involves simply sitting comfortably and quietly with oneself and focusing attention. Focuses vary. Examples include flow of the breath, a mantra, and a picture or mental image of a great spiritual being or peaceful place. Sometimes the meditator communicates with a great spiritual being. There are many meditation techniques, some with a spiritual base, such as Siddha meditation. Meditation is easily practiced anywhere and involves no special equipment. The positive experiences available through meditation are available to anyone, including individuals experiencing pain.

Autogenic Training. The purpose of autogenic training is to help individuals be self-motivated. The technique teaches relaxation and physiologic control by a system of self-suggestion in which people repeat phrases to themselves suggesting changes toward relaxation and self-control. This may help clients who resist more directive forms of hypnosis.

Progressive Relaxation Training. Progressive relaxation training (PRT) is used to treat various physical and psychosocial problems, including pain. The client is taught to gradually tighten, then deeply relax, various muscle groups, proceeding systematically from one area of the body to the next. The deep relaxation produced by this method can decrease anxiety and excessive muscle contraction, and promote the onset of sleep. Audiotape cassettes are available to guide clients through PRT.

Guided Imagery. Imagery is a way to relieve pain through several mechanisms. First, using imagery is a way to help clients distract themselves from their pain, which may increase their pain tolerance. Second, imagery may produce a relaxation response that helps produce muscle relaxation and relieve pain. Last, the image can be a healing one, designed not only to relieve the pain, but possibly to diminish the source of the pain.[91] Imagery is often combined with relaxation and biofeedback to produce a multifocal pain relief technique.

The image the client uses in this technique could be a complex scene that requires the client to think of each detail. This image would increase distraction. The image might be a relaxing scene such as a beach or meadow, which would help with the relaxation response, or the image could be one that visualizes the pain being worn away, until it is so small it can be blown away. This is an example of a more healing image.

Rhythmic Breathing. Rhythmic breathing is a method of both relaxation and distraction. This method can be combined with rhythms such as music, a ticking clock, or a metronome. The technique does not require a lot of concentration because once the client begins the process, it takes on an automatic quality. This method focuses the client's attention away from the pain and on the breathing and the rhythm.

Operant Conditioning. An operant conditioning program does not cure pain. However, it can help reduce associated functional impairment. Operant conditioning is a program designed for clients whose high levels of pain behavior interfere with their ability to function. It is not used for clients whose pain is caused by progressive, rather than stable, organic disease.

A successful operant conditioning program fully informs the client and significant others of every element before proceeding. The purposes of an operant conditioning program are (1) to reduce pain behaviors by withdrawing positive reinforcement for such behavior, (2) to increase the client's well behaviors by programming positive reinforcement when the client increases well behaviors, (3) to teach significant others to reinforce well behaviors and not to reinforce the pain behaviors, and (4) to refer clients having pain to other health professionals who can help with other functional impairments once the limitation of pain is successfully removed. An example of (1) is not attending to a client's verbal or nonverbal demonstrations of pain, such as saying that washing dishes is too painful. An example of (2) is attending a client when the person is not demonstrating pain behavior: for example, by praising the client for performing a task that previously was not done because of pain.

Biofeedback. Biofeedback refers to a wide variety of techniques that provide a client with information about changes in bodily functions of which the client is usually unaware, such as blood pressure. Biofeedback equipment provides a client with immediate, continuous information. Some clients learn to use this information to control previously involuntary functions. The purpose of biofeedback in pain management is to teach the client self-control over physiologic variables that relate to the pain, such as muscle contraction, blood flow.

Information used to reduce muscle contraction is obtained by an electromyogram (EMG) recorded from body surface electrodes. (Needle EMG electrodes are not used.) Changes in blood flow are produced by monitoring skin temperature, which increases with increased blood flow. Depending on the equipment used, individuals can self-monitor their changes through (1) auditory displays (decreases in muscle contractions are heard as decreases in the pitch of a tone) or (2) visual displays (increases in skin temperature are seen as increases on a dial). A client using biofeedback tries to change the display of information in the desired direction, such as to reduce muscle contraction (relax muscle tension) and to reduce blood flow. The continuous, precise information received shows the effectiveness of the effort and often helps a client learn physiologic control of these functions.

Biofeedback can be performed at home with purchased or rented biofeedback equipment under the guidance of a suitably prepared health care worker. Alternatively, it may be performed in an office or clinic setting with a biofeedback therapist or other specialist, such as a nurse prepared for this role. The cost for this equipment is fairly high.

ESTABLISHING A THERAPEUTIC RELATIONSHIP

The client must be able to establish a therapeutic relationship with the nurse or someone else on the health care team. Pain is a very lonely state of being. Clients suffering from pain often find their world shrinking until sometimes the pain becomes the only focus. When the health care team cannot relieve the client's pain, the impulse is to stay away, thereby increasing the client's sense of isolation and loneliness. When the nurse is unable to help in any other way, the nurse can stay with the client. By setting up a therapeutic relationship with the client, the nurse can decrease the client's sense of isolation and the nurse can actually be a distraction for the client.

THERAPEUTIC TOUCH

Therapeutic touch is a type of holistic pain management. It is a derivative of the laying on of hands. If the human body is thought of as having energy fields, therapeutic touch is a way to realign these fields. Unlike some of the behavioral techniques, this technique requires learning and practice on the part of the nurse.

Therapeutic touch involves three steps. First, the nurse must be centered, or focused in a meditative state. This helps the nurse become aware of the vibrations in the surrounding energy fields. In the second step, the nurse assesses the field. The hands are passed over the client's body at a distance of 2 to 6 inches to pick up on changes of the client's energy field. The last step is treatment. During this step, the nurse helps to clean up the client's energy field and return it to normal.

CUTANEOUS STIMULATION

Cutaneous stimulation refers to the stimulation of the skin to relieve pain. This technique draws its rationale from the gate-control theory of pain transmission. Cutaneous stimulation activates the large diameter fibers, which, in turn, close the gate to painful stimuli. The stimulus can consist of a wide variety of stimuli such as cold, heat, massage, vibration, menthol application, and transcutaneous nerve stimulation (TENS). The nurse should remember that a back rub is one of the best methods of providing cutaneous stimulation. It is particularly relaxing at bedtime and may block pain so the client can sleep easier.

Cutaneous stimulation can decrease the intensity of pain the client feels and, in some instances, eliminate it. It also can help change the sensations in a painful or noxious area to a more pleasant sensation, such as warmth. This process may also be seen as a form of distraction, because the client usually focuses on the sensation being created rather than the pain.

Cutaneous stimulation can be applied to the unaffected side and still elicit positive benefits. This is because the fibers cross within the spinal cord. This method is particularly useful when an area is too painful to be directly stimulated, such as with burns.

This method of pain relief also may produce prolonged pain relief. It has been theorized that cutaneous stimulation may cause the body to secrete the natural pain killers—endorphins.

HYPNOSIS

An individual's reaction to pain can be significantly altered by hypnosis. Hypnosis is based on suggestion and the process of focusing attention.

Various procedures may be used to relieve pain following induction of a trance state including (1) suggestion to alter the character of the pain or the individual's attitude toward it, (2) body disorientation and dissociations, and (3) anesthesia and analgesia for superficial and deep sensation.

In situations of chronic pain, posthypnotic suggestion may be used in combination with autohypnosis (self-hypnosis) to provide prolonged relief. Many hypnotic subjects successfully learn to use deliberate spontaneous trance induction or autohypnosis.

Hypnosis cannot change organic lesions that are producing pain. However, it can often reduce discomfort. It is not without hazards. However, the procedure itself is fairly simple and innocuous compared with the administration of many anesthetic and analgesic drugs.

Hypnosis may be used as an adjunct to other pain-relieving therapies. Alteration of pain by hypnosis should be performed by those who are aware of the possible diagnostic implications of pain in the medical management of a person's disease. A hypnotherapist must be skilled and informed, and the client selected to avoid untoward effects.

MUSIC

Music is another way to relieve pain. It works in several ways. Music can be the background to relaxation tapes that help the client relax. The use of music can be more specific, such as having the client sing. It can be used as a specific distraction. Some clients find the use of a radio and headphones a quiet way to listen to distracting music without bothering others with the noise. These radios also allow the client to turn the music up or play it softly. When using this method, make sure to let clients pick the kind of music most suited for them.

There are also other types of tapes available to promote relaxation. These include nature sounds, such as birds, water, and rainstorms. These tapes also can help the client form images to use to decrease the pain.

ACUPRESSURE

Acupressure is a noninvasive pain relief method based on the principles of acupuncture. In this case, pressure, massage, or other cutaneous stimulations are applied over acupuncture points. Charts are available that pinpoint each of the pressure points. Stimulation is accomplished in a variety of ways such as a circular massage, pressure with the thumbs, or cold applied to the pressure point.

Invasive Interventions

An analgesic is a pharmacologic substance that diminishes or eliminates pain without producing unconsciousness. An anesthetic is a pharmacologic substance that, in addition to abolishing pain, generally causes loss of feeling and sensation. Many analgesics, depending on mode of action and route of administration, act as anesthetics when given in larger doses. There are many different types of anesthesia. General anesthesia is usually accompanied by loss of consciousness and amnesia. Local anesthetics produce anesthesia in a restricted area of the body without loss of consciousness. (Anesthetics are also discussed in Chap. 19.)

A technique frequently used in minor surgery and other procedures is infiltration of a local anesthetic into the skin and subcutaneous tissue to produce loss of sensation or local anesthesia. The same agent injected near a sensory nerve causes anesthesia in the distribution of the nerve, that is, regional anesthesia. Often, nerves are mixed in function; that is, they carry both sensory and motor fibers. Hence, a nerve block may cause motor weakness or paralysis, in addition to loss of sensation, in the appropriate area. A nerve block is the application of a pharmacologic substance that inhibits nerve conduction (e.g., to numb the mouth).

Local anesthetic agents may be applied topically (e.g., spinal anesthetic for surgery), infiltrated locally, used for specific nerve blocks, or administered intravenously, depending on the reason for their use. An example of a local anesthetic given intravenously is one below a tourniquet for extremity surgery, such as Bier block. However they are applied, local anesthetic agents act by temporarily blocking nerve impulses between the peripheral structures and higher centers. Such blocks are reversible because the nerves regain their function over a period of minutes to hours.

Prolonged nerve blocks are produced by neurolytic agents, such as phenol and alcohol, which destroy the nerves. Neurolytic blocks may not be truly permanent because nerve fibers regrow after several months. However, the growth is often disorganized. Hence, the sensation from these nerve fibers is often abnormal or painful. Consequently, neurolytic blocks are generally used only in terminally ill persons with a short life expectancy, such as those with cancer-related pain.

LOCAL ANESTHESIA

Local anesthetics are chemically divided into two classes, the esters and the amides. The esters, of which procaine (Novocain) is an example, are metabolized in the plasma, are less heat stable than the amides, and account for most of the rarely occurring allergic reactions to local anesthetics. The amides lidocaine (Xylocaine) and bupivacaine (Marcaine, Sensorcaine) are metabolized in the liver.

Procaine produces analgesia in 3 to 10 minutes, usually lasting less than 1 hour. It is one of the least toxic of the local anesthetics. Procaine is not effective for topical use.

Lidocaine is one of the most commonly used local anesthetics. It has a wide range of applications, including topical and intravascular block. A Bier block (see section on nerve blocks) is an example of an intravascular block.

Bupivacaine is long acting (4 to 8 hours) but has a slow onset. It is four times more potent than lidocaine and four to six times more toxic. Therefore, a lower concentration is used. Bupivacaine appears to block sensory nerves in preference to motor nerves when used in low concentration. Thus, good analgesia may result without accompanying motor weakness.

Local anesthetics are usually vasodilators, increasing blood flow into the area in which they are injected. Thus, they shorten the duration of their own action by enhancing their own vascular absorption. Adding epinephrine, a vasoconstrictor, to local anesthetic solutions prolongs the anesthetic effect by decreasing the vascular uptake of the anesthetic, allowing it to stay in contact with the nerve tissue for a longer period.

Caution. Epinephrine-containing solutions are not used for nerve blocks of the penis, fingers, or toes where vasoconstriction could cause inadequate blood flow and necrosis of the distal extremity.

In addition to prolonging anesthesia, epinephrine-containing local anesthetic solutions offer other advantages. The supplementary use of a vasoconstrictor reduces the possibility of the anesthetic's reaching a toxic blood level. The toxicity of local analgesic drugs depends on their concentration in the blood. This, in turn, depends on the speed of absorption. Vasoconstricting medications delay absorption of a local analgesic solution and thus prevent a suddenly high blood concentration. This gives the body more time to metabolize and detoxify the medication. Vasoconstrictors also inhibit bleeding in the area of the injection.

TOPICAL LOCAL ANESTHESIA

Dilute solutions of local anesthetics may be applied topically in the form of pastes, sprays, or other preparations. They may reduce the severe pain of burns, abrasions, and necrosis of the mucous membranes and skin. Remember, once an area is anesthetized, it does not transmit painful sensation, so the area is at greater risk for injury.

Caution. Cocaine, a highly toxic agent, is sometimes used for topical anesthesia (perhaps in an atomizer for topical spray). However, cocaine should never be used for infiltration anesthesia (i.e., injected) because it is highly toxic.

Toxic reactions to overdoses of topical medications can easily occur. Therefore, use dilute solutions of these medications and take care not to exceed the recommended total dose.

If topical anesthetic agents are applied to burned or abraded skin or mucous membranes, absorption of the medication is almost as rapid as that following intravenous administration!

ANALGESIA

Various factors are considered in selecting the most effective analgesic for a specific client. These include the etiology, quality, intensity, duration, and distribution of the client's pain. The World Health Organization[108] has formulated a tool called an analgesic ladder, which is used to aid in the decision of what pain medications to use for cancer pain. The first step is to use non-opioids (such as aspirin) with or without adjuvants (such as hydroxyzine). If the pain persists or increases, step 2 uses weak opioids (such as codeine) plus non-opioids with or without adjuvants. If the pain persists or increases, step 3 uses strong opioids (such as morphine) with or without non-opioids with or without adjuvants.

Systemic analgesic drugs are the most prevalent and most frequently used means of pain control. Analgesics are the most commonly prescribed drugs and, therefore, are the most widely used of all medications. They are also purchased extensively over the counter. This is not unexpected, because pain is usually the first symptom of injury, and most diseases begin with or include pain at some time during their course.

Mechanisms of Analgesia. Analgesics do not all act in the same way. For example, acetylsalicylic acid and other NSAIDs act peripherally and do not seem to alter CNS processing. They also decrease the inflammation and, therefore, the source of pain. On the other hand, opiates and alcohol control the reaction to pain as well as raising the pain perception threshold.

Generally, opiate (narcotic) analgesics modify the central reception of pain within the central nervous system by (1) blocking the facilitating reflexes and thus raising the pain threshold; (2) interrupting the pathways that transmit pain impulses in the brain and thus modifying central perception, interpretation, and reaction to the painful stimulus; and (3) depressing reflex activity and thus modifying the central perception of pain and reducing psychogenic pain.

Opiate analgesics, including local anesthetics, can raise or obliterate the pain threshold. The pain threshold is the stimulus intensity at which a person perceives pain (Table 16–4).

Some analgesics, such as morphine and alcohol, besides affecting the perception of pain, also affect the response to pain. Thus, clients receiving these medications may report some pain is still felt but the pain no longer bothers them. It is important to remember that these drugs do nothing to decrease the source of pain, only the response to it.

Opioid analgesics have long been thought to produce their effects in the brain. In addition to their activity in the brain, special narcotic receptors have now been identified. Multiple receptor sites exist within and outside the central nervous system. The three major opioid receptors are the mu, kappa, and sigma (Table 16–4). The mu receptors mediate analgesia, respiratory depression, and euphoria. Kappa receptors also mediate analgesia and respiratory depression, and in addition, mediate sedation and miosis (pupil constriction). Sigma receptors cause psychotropic reactions (e.g., hallucinations, euphoria).

NSAIDs act in several ways. As mentioned earlier, they are anti-inflammatory in action, and because the swelling associated with inflammation is a cause of the pain, these drugs help relieve this pain. NSAIDs are also prostaglandin inhibitors. Remember that prostaglandins sensitize pain receptors to mechanical and chemical stimulation. By blocking prostaglandin synthesis, NSAIDs prevent stimulation of nociceptors. These

TABLE 16-4. Drug Actions at Specific Receptor Sites*

Drug Classification	Specific Drugs	Type of Opioid Receptor: Mu	Kappa	Sigma
Pure opioid agonists	Morphine, codeine, and all other opioids	Agonist	Agonist	No action
Pure opioid antagonist	Naloxone (Narcan) or naltrexone (Trexan)	Antagonist	Antagonist	Partial antagonist
Mixed, agonist-antagonists opioid	Pentazocine (Fortral or Talwin)	Antagonist	Agonist	Agonist
	or nalbuphine (Nubain)	Antagonist	Partial agonist	Agonist
	Buprenorphine (Buprenex)	No action	Agonist	Agonist
	or butorphanol (Stadol)	Partial agonist	Unknown action	No action

* Agonist means it enhances the action of that receptor. Partial agonist means it acts as a weak stimulant of the receptor when given alone, but can block the action of a pure agonist. Antagonist means it blocks the action of that receptor.

Adapted from Lehne, R. A., et al. (1990). *Pharmacology for nursing care.* Philadelphia: W. B. Saunders Co.

drugs work peripherally, not centrally, although some types may have some as yet undefined central action.

Because analgesics work on a variety of sites by differing mechanisms, a combination of analgesics is sometimes prescribed. Giving an NSAID plus an opioid can relieve severe visceral pain while also relieving the peripheral muscle aches and pains.

Types of Analgesics. Analgesics are usually divided into two classes on the basis of their clinical effectiveness: (1) strong opiates (agonists) and agonist-antagonist analgesics, and (2) weak non-opiate, antipyretic analgesics and NSAIDs (Box 16-2).

Each class is distinguished by what type of pain it relieves and where in the nervous system it seems to work, rather than on its analgesic potency. Generally, opiate analgesics are given to relieve severe central pain; non-opiate analgesics are given for peripheral pains, such as muscle aches, headaches, and pains of inflammatory origin.

Box 16-2. Some Types of Analgesic Medications

Antipyretic-analgesic agents

Para-aminophenol derivatives
Nonsteroidal anti-inflammatory drugs (NSAIDs)

Narcotic agonists

Morphine and its congeners
Morphinians
Phenylpiperidines
Phenylheptylamines

Narcotic antagonists

Pure antagonists
Mixed agonist-antagonists
Partial agonists

Weak Non-Opiate Analgesics

Nonsteroidal Anti-Inflammatory Drugs. NSAIDs were originally developed to treat arthritis. They are effective, however, in treating a number of mild to moderate pains of nonarthritic origin. NSAIDs act to decrease inflammation, but it is their ability to block prostaglandin synthesis that is thought to be responsible for most of their pain-relieving properties. As described earlier, prostaglandins are mediators of painful stimuli. Aspirin is one of the oldest NSAID pain relievers and one of the most widely used. Many others, however, exist today, and if one is ineffective for the client, another can be tried. A comparison of the analgesic quality of NSAIDs and aspirin is given in Table 16-5.

The most common problem associated with NSAIDs is GI upset and possible bleeding. These agents also inhibit platelet aggregation, increasing the risk of hemorrhage. Clients taking NSAIDs must be monitored closely for the development of peptic ulcers. In clients who are taking high doses of NSAIDs for long periods of time, mainly those clients with arthritis, histamine H_2-receptor antagonists such as ranitidine may be used.

Nonanalgesic Pain Relievers. A number of other drugs not typically associated with analgesics may be effective for certain types of pain. Tricyclic antidepressants such as amitriptyline (Elavil) are very effective when used for neuropathic pain. They can be given daily at bedtime so the drowsiness associated with them helps the client sleep. Other drugs that are effective in treating neuropathic pain are phenytoin (Dilantin) and carbamazepine (Tegretol). Nerve compression and bone pain may respond to dexamethasone (Decadron). Hydroxyzine (Vistaril) and diphenhydramine (Benadryl) are effective against a variety of pains.

Muscle relaxants, such as baclofen (Lioresal) and

TABLE 16–5. Weak Analgesic Equianalgesic Chart

Medication	PO Dosage (mg)	Comments
Aspirin (ASA)	650	*ASPIRIN 650 MG PO IS THE ANALGESIC DOSE WITH WHICH ALL OTHER DRUGS IN THIS TABLE ARE COMPARED* Aspirin is best NSAID if client tolerates; much less expensive Major side effect is GI irritation and bleeding Contraindicated in clients with history of ulcers or with active bleeding or on anticoagulants; also in children with a viral illness Available in enteric coated form
Acetaminophen	650	Acetaminophen has less anti-inflammatory effect; however, still effective weak analgesic with fewer side effects May be given in combination with NSAIDs Use with care in clients with renal or hepatic disease
Sodium salicylate	1000	Same as aspirin, but fewer GI side effects and less bleeding tendencies
Ibuprofen (Motrin)	200	Available in 200 mg doses as nonprescription forms; 400 mg is prescription dose Effective, with similar but fewer side effects than aspirin Rapid onset, but shorter duration than aspirin
Naproxen (Naprosyn)	250	Relatively long action (8 to 12 hours) Side effects similar to aspirin
Indomethacin (Indocin)	25	Very effective NSAID, but with high incidence of GI side effects Cannot be given to clients with aspirin sensitivity
Codeine	32	Weak narcotic Often combined with Tylenol as Tylenol #3 (30 mg codeine + 325 mg acetaminophen) or aspirin as Empirin #3 (30 mg codeine + 325 mg aspirin) Can cause severe constipation in high or prolonged doses Effectiveness increased by giving Tylenol #3 with two more acetaminophen
Meperidine (Demerol)	50	Narcotic with usual side effects (see Table 16–9)
Oxycodone	5	Available in combination with aspirin or acetaminophen and as a suppository Good analgesic potential, especially during first two hours after administration Side effects similar to other narcotics
Hydrocodone	5	Available in combination with 500 mg of acetaminophen as Vicodin Similar to oxycodone
Pentazocine (Talwin)	30	Available in 50-mg scored tablets High incidence of psychomimetic effects
Propoxyphene hydrochloride (Darvon)	65	Used for mild to moderate pain May cause GI symptoms Considered mild narcotic
Propoxyphene napsylate (Darvon-N)	100	Similar to Darvon

GI, gastrointestinal; NSAID, nonsteroidal anti-inflammatory agent.

diazepam (Valium), are used to treat muscle spasm associated with pain.

Phenothiazines are not appropriate for pain relief. They are good antiemetics; however, when given for pain, they simply increase sedation, hypotension, and respiratory depression. A phenothiazine, promethazine (Phenergan), should never be used for pain relief. Promethazine actually increases the perception of pain, even in doses as low as 12 mg.[70]

Strong Opiate (Narcotic) Analgesics. Opiates are generally used when other methods of pain relief are not feasible, have failed, or the pain is moderate to severe. Although physical dependence and tolerance can occur when potent analgesics are given, this does not mean that these medications should be withheld. Tolerance and physical dependence are very unlikely to occur in short-term pain therapy.

Examples of opiate analgesics are morphine and various morphine-like agents, such as opiate agonists. Agonists are opiates that stimulate the activities of selected pain receptor sites (see Table 16-4). Antagonists are drugs that counteract both the CNS and analgesic effects of opiates. Some drugs are combinations of agonists and antagonists, such as butorphanol (Stadol) and pentazocine (Talwin). The morphine-like drugs differ from morphine only in individual characteristics such as rate of onset, duration of action, route of administration, adverse side effects, and chemical configuration.

Narcotic Agonists. The pharmacologic action of all opiate agonists is similar to those of their parent compound, morphine. They all share certain desirable and undesirable characteristics (Box 16-3).

Narcotic Antagonists. A pure antagonist, naloxone, reverses the effects of narcotics, both side effects and analgesia. It has no agonist effects, that is, it produces no analgesia or CNS depression. This drug would be used only to counteract against an overdose of a narcotic.

Narcotic Agonist-Antagonists. The combined agonist-antagonist drugs act in two ways. When they are given following long-term use of narcotics, they will reverse the narcotic and can precipitate acute withdrawal. When the combination agents are given alone, they produce analgesia and the positive effects of opioids without as many side effects. They are less likely to produce respiratory depression, although many of them are more likely to produce psychomimetic effects.

Methadone. Methadone is a potent, long-acting narcotic analgesic that gained popularity in the management of cancer pain before the development of the newer long acting forms of morphine. Unlike most morphine preparations, methadone has a long plasma half-life. This long plasma half-life, when repeated doses are given, may account for methadone's longer duration of analgesic action. The long plasma half-life of methadone also poses certain problems. Elderly clients and individuals with compromised hepatic and renal function should be monitored closely for signs of overdosage. The long plasma half-life also necessitates close monitoring of any client receiving repeated doses of this medication because cumulative effects develop. If the client becomes oversedated, the dosage should be reduced or the intervals between administration lengthened.

Box 16-3. Effects of Morphine and Opiate Agonists as an Analgesic

Desirable Effects

Effective analgesia
Relief of anxiety
Euphoria*
Sedation*

Undesirable Effects

Psychologic dependence
Tolerance
Physical dependence
Mental clouding
Dysphoria
Nausea, vomiting
Spasmogenic effects
Euphoria*
Sedation*
Constipation*
Respiratory depression*
Suppression of cough reflex*

▼▼▼

Data from Houde, R. W. (1974). The use and misuse of narcotics in the treatment of chronic pain. *Advances in Neurology, 4*, 527.

* May be either desirable or undesirable depending on circumstances.

Complications of Opiate Analgesics. *Respiratory depression,* one complication of narcotic analgesic therapy, is caused by diminished sensitivity of the respiratory center to carbon dioxide. All narcotics can potentially produce respiratory depression, but this does not have to be a life-threatening problem, because this effect can be rapidly reversed with a narcotic antagonist. This potential problem should not interfere in any way with the proper use of narcotics to relieve pain in clients of all ages. The development of respiratory depression is not necessarily dose related because even lesser amounts of a narcotic may produce respiratory depression. The problem is related more to individual differences and the type of pain being experienced rather than the medication used. Narcotic agonist-antagonists cause respiratory depression to a lesser degree than do narcotics. Narcotic antagonists, such as butorphanol and nalbuphine, also cause respiratory depression, although the extent of respiratory depression is limited. Rather than limit the use of narcotic analgesics, the nurse must carefully assess each client after giving the pain medication for the occurrence of any side effects.

Deaths that occur secondary to narcotic poisoning are usually due to respiratory depression. With morphine, maximal respiratory depression usually occurs within 7 minutes of intravenous administration, within 30 minutes of intramuscular administration, and within 90 minutes of subcutaneous administration.[95] It is very important to remember these time ranges when assessing the client's respiratory status following administration of narcotics. For poisoning to occur, however, doses well above the therapeutic level would have to be given.

Treatments for respiratory depression include arousing the client, establishing a patent airway, administering an opiate antagonist such as naloxone, and providing artificial ventilation as necessary.

Circulatory depression is a second complication of opiate analgesics. In a supine client, therapeutic dosages of morphine or synthetic opioids have very little effect on blood pressure and cardiac rate or rhythm. However, some clients experience orthostatic hypotension when moving from a supine position to a head-up or standing position. This hypotension is secondary to a direct dilating action on the peripheral blood vessels caused by the opiates, which reduces the capacity of the cardiovascular system to respond to gravitational shifts. Avoid abrupt body position changes in clients who have received opiates. For this reason, opiates are used very cautiously in clients with decreased blood volume.

Opiates may precipitate *nausea and vomiting* owing to their action on the brain stem centers. Morphine-like drugs also affect the vestibular system, which also can produce these symptoms. Changing the type of opiate used may stop the side effect, or the addition of an antiemetic agent may help.

Constipation, another complication of morphine and other opiates, results from increased smooth muscle tone and decreased motility of the gastrointestinal tract. Opiates diminish the propulsive peristaltic contractions in the small and large intestine and delay the passage of gastric contents through the duodenum. Tolerance does not develop to constipation as it does to the other side effects of opiates. Clients taking opiate analgesics need to follow some type of bowel regimen to prevent constipation. A diet high in roughage with plenty of fluids and stool-softening medications (such as Colace or Pericolace) is common prophylactic treatment. It is better to prevent constipation than to begin treatment after it develops.

Paresthesias may complicate the use of intramuscular opiate analgesics. The intramuscular injection of analgesic agents is generally not irritating to the local tissues. However, two exceptions are meperidine and methadone. Subcutaneous methadone may cause local tissue irritation. Both subcutaneous and intramuscular meperidine cause local tissue irritation and induration, and frequent administration can lead to severe fibrosis of muscle tissue.

If any analgesic is deposited in the region of a nerve when it is injected intramuscularly, paresthesia and paresis may result along the course of the nerve. Proper injection techniques prevent nerve injury.

Physical dependence, another complication of opiate analgesics, is defined as the altered physiologic state produced by repeated administration of a drug. When the drug is stopped abruptly, physiologic symptoms of withdrawal occur. Continued administration of the drug is necessary to prevent withdrawal syndrome. Physical dependence on opioids can develop as well as dependence on other substances such as alcohol, barbiturates, and nicotine.

Physical dependence is not an addiction, but it is an involuntary physiologic response that is an expected effect of the drug when it is taken for a time and then stopped. The nurse must observe the client for these physiologic symptoms. Gradual withdrawal of the medication can usually prevent this response.

Clients who receive a therapeutic dose of morphine several times a day develop some physical dependency in approximately 2 weeks. This means that if morphine were suddenly discontinued, a withdrawal syndrome would occur. Assessment findings that indicate a withdrawal syndrome include diarrhea, lacrimation, sweating, dilated pupils, restlessness, tremor, and anorexia. Most symptoms, if untreated, subside in 5 to 10 days. Withdrawal symptoms can be avoided by gradually (over 1 to 2 weeks) reducing and, finally, by discontinuing a client's opiate intake as the pain decreases.

Tolerance to opioid analgesics, another of their complications, is characterized by a shortened duration of pain relief, a decrease in peak analgesic effect, and an increase in the amount of opiate needed to relieve pain. An example of tolerance is when pain has been adequately controlled by a particular dosage of opiate, but it begins to be less effective for the same length of time. A higher dose is needed to obtain the desired effects. The usual treatment for tolerance when pain relief is necessary is to increase the analgesic dose or decrease the interval between doses.

Addiction, another complication of opioid analgesics, is a behavioral pattern of drug use characterized by (1) overwhelming involvement with the use of a drug (compulsive use) and securing a supply of it, and (2) a high tendency to relapse after withdrawal from the drug, that is, to begin taking it again. The vast majority of clients who take opiate analgesic medication for pain do not become addicted.

Factors Influencing the Effectiveness of Analgesics

Relative Analgesic Potency. Relative analgesic potency refers to the ratio of the doses of two analgesics required to produce the same effect. Estimates of relative analgesic potency provide a basis for prescribing the dose when changing from one analgesic to another, or from one route of administration to another. The equianalgesic table (Table 16-6) gives examples of the common analgesics and their relative analgesic potential compared with morphine. The nurse will find this information useful when assessing analgesic effectiveness.

TABLE 16-6. Narcotic Equianalgesic Chart

Drug	IM Route (mg)	PO Route (mg)	Peak (Hr)	Duration (Hr)	Comments
Morphine	10	20 to 60	1/2 to 1 IM 1/2 to 2 PO	4 to 5 IM 4 to 5 PO	*MORPHINE 10 MG IM IS THE ANALGESIC DOSE WITH WHICH ALL OTHER DRUGS IN THIS TABLE ARE COMPARED* PO dose varies from three to six times the IM dose, depending on form used Also comes in rectal suppositories, timed release, and for spinal injection
Buprenorphine (Buprenex)	0.3–0.4	N/A	1/2 to 1 IM	5 to 6 IM	Agonist-antagonist Can produce withdrawal from narcotics More likely to produce nausea and vomiting Respiratory depression rare but severe and not easily reversed by naloxone
Butorphanol (Stadol)	2	N/A	1/2 to 1 IM	4 to 5 IM	Agonist–antagonist Can produce withdrawal from narcotics May produce psychomimetic effects, but less than pentazocine Contraindicated in people with cardiac abnormalities
Codeine	130	200	1/2 to 1 IM 2 PO	4 to 5 IM 3 to 4 PO	More toxic in higher doses than morphine Causes more nausea and vomiting and is extremely constipating Adding 650 mg of acetaminophen or aspirin will significantly increase analgesic effect
Fentanyl (Sublimaze)	0.05	N/A	1/4 IM	1 1/2 IM	Commonly used for anesthetic, IV Substituted for high dose morphine in terminally ill clients May be used in PCA or epidural
Hydromorphone (Dilaudid)	1.5	7.5	1/2 to 1 IM 1/2 to 2 PO	3 IM 3 to 4 PO	Shorter acting than morphine Also available as rectal suppository or high potency injection 10 mg/ml
Levorphanol (Levo-Dromoran)	2	4	1/2 to 1 IM 1/2 to 2 PO	4 to 5 IM 4 to 5 PO	Longer acting than morphine when given in repeated, regular doses Good alternative to methadone Drug accumulates, so analgesic effect may increase with repeated doses Subcutaneous route better than IM
Meperidine (Demerol)	75	300	1/2 to 1 IM 1/2 to 2 PO	2 to 4 IM 2 to 4 PO	Shorter acting than morphine Biotransformed to normeperidine, a toxic metabolite that stimulates the CNS *Oral dose of 300 mg not recommended*

Table continued on following page

TABLE 16-6. Narcotic Equianalgesic Chart Continued

Drug	IM Route (mg)	PO Route (mg)	Peak (Hr)	Duration (Hr)	Comments
					Effects of normeperidine not reversed by naloxone Normeperidine has a long half-life so it is even more dangerous with repeated doses
Methadone (Dolophine)	10	20	1/2 to 1 IM 1/2 to 1 PO	up to 12 IM up to 12 PO	Long plasma half-life, so regular doses lead to accumulation of drug and increased analgesia Dosage must be carefully titrated over time
Nalbuphine (Nubain)	10	N/A	1/2 to 1 IM	4 to 5 IM	Agonist-antagonist Similar to butorphanol Longer acting and less likely to cause hypotension than morphine Less respiratory depression
Oxycodone	N/A	30	1 IM	3 to 4 IM	Faster onset and higher peak effect than most oral narcotics Available in United States as fixed dose of 5 mg in drugs such as Percodan and Percocet; therefore, less effective
Oxymorphone (Numorphan)	1-1.5	N/A	1/2 to 1 IM	4 to 5 IM	Also available as rectal suppository 10 mg by suppository equivalent to 10 mg IM morphine
Pentazocine (Talwin)	60	180	1/2 to 1 IM 1/2 to 2 PO	4 to 5 IM 4 to 5 PO	Agonist-antagonist Similar to butorphanol but much higher incidence of psychomimetic effects
Propoxyphene (Darvon)	N/A	500	1/2 to 2 PO	4 to 5 PO	May be used for mild to moderate pain *Never given in 500 mg dose* Doses of 65 to 130 mg usual

CNS, central nervous system; IM, intramuscular; IV, intravenous; N/A, not available; PCA, patient controlled anesthesia.
Data from McCaffery, M., & Beebe, A. (1989). *Pain: Clinical manual for nursing practice.* St. Louis: C. V. Mosby.

Time Action. The time action of an analgesic agent results from factors such as pain intensity, size of dose, and the person's ability to absorb, biotransform, and eliminate the medication. The duration of action for each analgesic listed in Table 16-6 is based on a dose that produces a peak effect equivalent to that of morphine. The time of peak effect and the duration of action of a particular narcotic can vary with the route of administration. For instance, the peak analgesic effect of intramuscular morphine occurs between 30 minutes and 1 hour after administration. The peak analgesic effect of orally administered morphine occurs from 1 1/2 to 2 hours after administration. The duration of analgesic action of orally administered narcotics is usually somewhat longer than those given intramuscularly.

The nurse should be aware of information about peak and duration of analgesics so painful activities can be planned to coincide with these periods.

Several new forms of morphine have been developed. An oral liquid can be given for more rapid but short-acting effects. A controlled-release form also exists. With the long-acting morphine, the onset is somewhat slower, but the duration ranges from 8 to 12 hours.

Oral Potency. Narcotics differ in the degree to which they are active as they are absorbed from the intestine and pass through the liver and into the systemic circulation. This difference in absorption accounts for the different oral doses listed on Table 16-6 for oral morphine. The older tablets had a low bioavailability and, therefore, required higher doses. The newer forms of morphine, such as Roxanol, are much more bioavailable and, therefore, the dosages of these are lower than the older oral form.

Failure of health care providers to recognize differences in the oral and intramuscular potencies of narcotics can lead to undertreatment of a client's pain.

Principles and Methods of Analgesic Administration

Preadministration Assessment. The goal of analgesic administration is to provide pain relief while maintaining the ability of the client to be in control of the environment and participate in care. Assessment of a client before and after administering an analgesic is necessary to ensure safe and adequate pain relief. Factors to be assessed prior to analgesic administration include

- Drug allergies or sensitivities;
- Other medications the client is taking;
- Body weight;
- Individual pain experience;
- Other individual characteristics, such as age, general state of health, mental status, probable duration of pain, and probable life expectancy;
- Cardiac, respiratory, renal, and nervous system status; and
- Previous response to analgesics.

Drug Allergies or Sensitivities. Before administering an analgesic such as morphine, ensure that the client does not have a history of untoward reactions to the medication. When possible, ask the client or significant others, and review the chart or other documentation for such information.

Other Medications Being Taken. Clients on monoamine oxidase (MAO) antidepressants should not receive meperidine (Demerol).

Body Weight. Ten mg of morphine per 70 kg of body weight is considered standard. This produces satisfactory analgesia in about 70 per cent of clients with moderate-to-severe postoperative pain. Some clients require higher or lower doses. The analgesic effect is dose related. Review documentation concerning the client's body weight, or ask the client or significant others as necessary.

Individual Pain Experience. As we have seen, variation exists in pain experiences. There is no way to tell for certain how much, if any, pain an individual is experiencing from a particular health problem or intervention (e.g., surgery). Likewise, one cannot know what dosage of analgesics is needed to control a client's pain. One method of treating postoperative pain is to administer a standard medication and dosage following a particular surgical procedure, and then to increase or decrease the potency of subsequent doses on the basis of an evaluation of the response to the initial dose. This is referred to as titrating the amount and kind of analgesic needed in accordance with client's statements about pain and pain relief (Ethical Issues in Nursing).

Other Individual Characteristics. A client's age determines, to a great extent, the length of time an analgesic will be effective. Clients older than 70 years of age respond to a standard dose of morphine as though they had received three to four times the dosage given to clients aged 18 to 49 years. In other words, three hours after the medication is administered, about 20 per cent of 70-year-old people are no longer receiving pain relief from a standard dose of morphine. However, 50 per cent of clients aged 18 to 49 years are no longer receiving pain relief under the same circumstances.

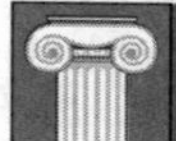

ETHICAL ISSUES IN NURSING

Pain: Who Is the Expert?

Pain is a very relative term. People experience pain in many different ways. What might be considered painful to one person may not be considered so by another. Even so, health care providers tend to conceptualize what type and intensity of pain a certain person should experience for a certain type of illness, trauma, medical-surgical procedure, and postoperative course. If persons do not conform to such ideas concerning the type of pain response they are experiencing, such as in the case of a person with a low pain threshold, then he or she may be labeled as a 'weakling' or as having a 'dependent' personality (perhaps if they frequently ask for pain medications).

It is useful for health care providers to anticipate the type and degree of pain a client may experience for a given condition in order to better care for him or her. What would happen, however, if a certain client did not fit into the anticipated pain experience and pain medication schedule? Perhaps pain medication of a certain type was ordered every 4 hours, but the client began to complain of severe pain 2 hours after administration. Should the nurse assess the client's complaint of pain? Certainly, there are physical signs that should be assessed in these clients, such as blood pressure, heart rate, wound appearance, and the inspection of the area in which the pain is located. After having assessed the client's complaint, what should the nurse do? Should the nurse tell the client no matter what, he or she must wait 2 more hours until the next dose of medication is due? (after all, a client should not have that much pain after a simple procedure such as XXXXXXXXX). Should the nurse try diversional activities to help the client forget his or her pain? Should the nurse call the doctor and report the client's complaint and physical assessment?

It is apparent that in some cases, clients may, indeed, be dependent on certain pain medications, which would cause them to ask for frequent doses. However, it is wrong to assume that all clients have such dependencies, or may develop such dependencies if given pain medications frequently. Nurses must not pre-judge a client's pain by whatever personal standards they may have. The obligation exists to assess clients' complaints of pain and address such complaints on an individual basis without preconceived notions about what type of pain they 'should' or 'should not' be experiencing.

An older client tends to receive pain relief from a narcotic for a longer time than a younger client. This difference in duration of action may relate to the speed with which a narcotic is cleared from the body. A younger client clears a narcotic (opiate) faster than an elderly client. Also, people with debilitating diseases, whether old or young, have a heightened sensitivity to the effects of narcotics.

Also, assess a client's general mental status, the probable duration of the pain, and the client's probable life expectancy in planning drug therapy for pain relief. A mentally anxious client may benefit from a mild tranquilizer or antihistamine in addition to an analgesic. A client whose life expectancy is relatively short may be given narcotics more readily than a client with a chronic pain problem that will probably continue for a long period of time. When it appears that a client will require prolonged therapy for relief of chronic pain, the side effects of analgesics must be considered.

Body System Assessment. Because all analgesics have the potential to produce mild-to-severe side effects, it is important to assess a client's cardiac, respiratory, renal, and nervous system status before administering analgesics. Hepatic function is also assessed since the role of the liver in detoxifying analgesics is important. The presence of increased intracranial pressure is cause for concern.

Potent narcotic analgesics are contraindicated in the presence of increased intracranial pressure. This is because narcotics further increase cerebrospinal fluid (CSF) pressure. This increase is secondary to carbon dioxide retention (increased arterial carbon dioxide tension), which always follows narcotic-induced respiratory depression (see the section on complications of opiate analgesics). Clients who are being artificially ventilated do not experience respiratory depression and carbon dioxide retention after receiving morphine. Hence, they can receive narcotics in spite of an elevated CSF pressure.

As a general rule, morphine is not given to clients who have internal abdominal injuries, respiratory distress, or head injuries. In all three of these conditions morphine may cause vomiting, with serious effects.

With head injuries (in addition to the danger of increasing CSF pressure, discussed earlier), internal cerebral hemorrhage may be present. Cerebral hemorrhage depresses the respiratory center, and morphine could worsen the condition. Also, the fact that morphine affects pupil size[52] makes assessments of pupil size inaccurate and misleading. These assessments are important following head injuries.

Previous Response to Analgesics. A number of instruments have been developed to assess and document pain location, pain severity, pain character, and the client's response to analgesic medications. Any of the instruments may be used as long as they help the nurse accurately assess the client's response to the analgesic.

Methods of Administration

Nurse-Administered (Demand) Analgesia. The traditional method of treating pain is by nurse-administered pain medication on a schedule, or on an as-needed basis. This system has advantages. For example, it allows the nurse to assess the pain, helps the nurse detect or avoid untoward reactions or side effects due to the analgesic, and permits dose adjustment as necessary. It is also the best for clients who are unable to control their own pain for a variety of physical or psychological reasons. However, in spite of these advantages, it is unfortunate that with this system pain is often significantly undertreated.[69] Undertreatment may occur because (1) it is difficult to assess the severity of another person's pain (unless the client is asked directly), (2) overconcern about possible narcotic side effects and fear of inducing narcotic addiction are often present in both the client (and significant others) and health care providers, (3) too low a dose of medication is ordered,[64] and (4) the interval between doses is too long. Also, with this system, the client experiencing the pain becomes dependent on others for pain relief. The client's pain may be worsened by anxiety about whether the nurse will give the next dose in time to prevent the return of severe pain.

Intermittent dosing causes wide swings in blood levels of the analgesic, resulting in sedation following one dose and unacceptable pain levels preceding the next dose. This problem could be lessened if the nurse administers prn medications on a regular basis for clients with acute pain. If the medication is administered regularly rather than intermittently, the peaks and valleys of pain management are avoided.

Patient-Controlled Analgesia. One way to avoid some of the problems concerning nurse-administered pain medication is to use patient-controlled analgesia instead. This method entails using an intravenous infusion pump, which contains the analgesic and is controlled by the client. The client can self-administer a dose of analgesic by pressing a button that then releases a preset dose of analgesic. The pumps are programmed to deliver preset demand doses of analgesic until a maximum dose is reached. There is then a minimal interval when no further analgesic can be administered. With this system, the clients control the administration of their own pain medication, within the limits set by the program.

There are many advantages to this system. First, the client usually reports that pain control is much better. This system also seems to relieve the client's anxiety about waiting for the nurse to administer the drug, thereby lowering the dose needed to relieve pain. This system also increases the client's independence. Another benefit is improved pulmonary function and fewer postoperative complications, probably because of the decreased sedation produced by this form of administration.[44]

Studies have shown that clients using these devices adjust their analgesic doses to a near-constant blood concentration. This method provides the best analgesia with minimal side effects. As the pain lessens, clients adjust themselves to lower doses, and finally stop taking the analgesic. Clients using patient-controlled analgesia report superior analgesia with a lower incidence of side effects compared with the traditional nurse-administered method.

There are some potential problems associated with patient-controlled analgesia. The success of this method depends on the nurse's understanding of the system and on how well the client is taught to use this system. If the client is taught properly, this method is usually successful. Failures can often be traced to a poor understanding on the part of either the client or the nurse.

Intraspinal Analgesia. A new advance in the treatment of severe pain, such as postoperative pain, or of chronic malignant pain is a method of injecting narcotics intrathecally or epidurally (Fig. 16-10). The epidural space is outside the dura mater of the spinal cord and brain. The intrathecal space is inside the dura mater and contains the spinal fluid. The dorsal horns of the spinal cord contain receptors for endogenous opioid substances. These receptors also bind narcotics and provide excellent pain relief of long duration (8 to 24 hours) without also causing sympathetic and motor nerve blockade. Relatively small doses provide high concentrations of the narcotic in the spinal fluid that bathes the dorsal columns of the spinal cord. These concentrations are far higher than those that occur in the spinal fluid following similar doses given by standard parenteral routes.

Repeated bolus doses, patient-controlled administration, or a constant infusion of the narcotic may be given through a small catheter placed in the epidural or intrathecal space. These catheters have been left in place for days to months without adverse effects. All the precautions observed for epidural and intrathecal nerve blocks (see the section on nerve blocks) also apply to the placement of intraspinal catheters. Possible side effects of administering narcotics by this route include pruritus, urinary retention, and delayed respiratory depression occurring 6 to 12 hours after a dose of medication. Low doses of naloxone may reverse these side effects without reducing analgesia.

Caution: Before giving a dose of narcotics through an epidural catheter, carefully aspirate the catheter to ensure that there is no return of CSF. If CSF is aspirated, it is assumed that the catheter has migrated from the epidural space to the intrathecal space. Because an intrathecal dose of narcotics is about one-tenth that of an epidural dose, marked and potentially severe side effects (e.g., respiratory depression) occur rapidly.

Daily or every other day inspect the catheter insertion site for indications of infection (e.g., redness or swelling) and change the dressings. If they become moist or otherwise soiled, change the dressings.

Clients may experience exceptional analgesia from

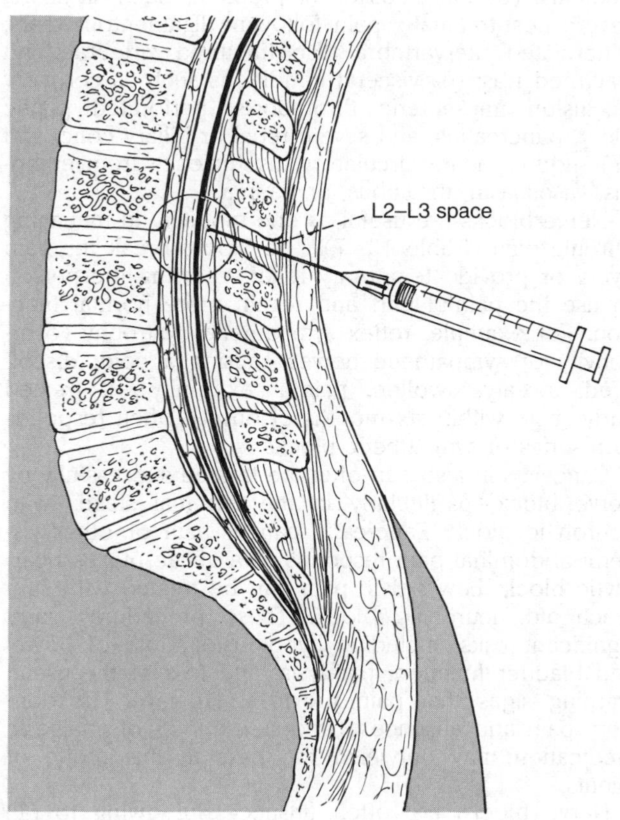

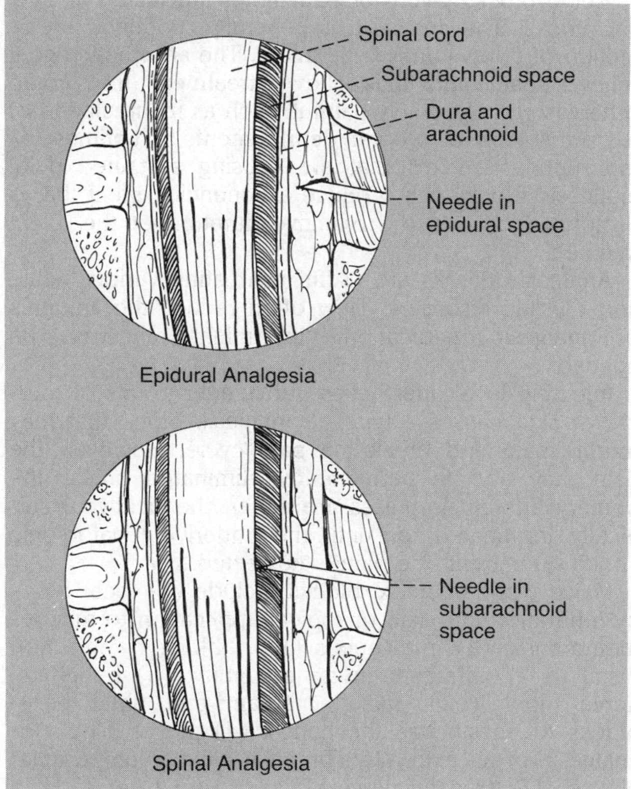

▲ **Figure 16-10**

Epidural and spinal analgesia. *Top circle,* A small amount of analgesic medication, such as preservative-free morphine sulfate, is injected into the L2-L3 space just outside the dura mater, that is, into the epidural space. *Bottom circle,* Analgesic medication is injected intrathecally into the subarachnoid space, which contains the cerebrospinal fluid.

epidural or intrathecal narcotics. It may then be possible to reduce or stop the previous regimen of parenteral or oral narcotics.

Nerve Blocks. Nerve blocks are commonly used for operative procedures as well as in pain clinics.

Essentially, nerve blocks are performed by injecting various substances (e.g., local anesthetics) close to nerves, thereby blocking their conductivity. They may be used to produce a complete, reversible interruption of nervous pathways for the following purposes:

- To eliminate a local focus of pain-producing stimulation or nervous irritation
- To interrupt the perception of pain, either at the source of the pain or anywhere along the peripheral afferent neurons
- To interrupt reflex mechanisms that are maintaining abnormal activity in blood vessels, glands, or skeletal or smooth muscle
- To eliminate reflex responses to pain (e.g., tachycardia, hypertension) by directly infiltrating skeletal muscle and other involved structures

Some irreversible nerve-blocking procedures are also possible. These procedures are often used in managing pain associated with cancer. The nerves may regenerate to some extent, with an associated return of sensory and motor functions (see the section on intraspinal narcotics).

Nerve blocks given for pain relief are called analgesic blocks. The analgesia is generally produced by injection of a local anesthetic agent. The anesthetic agent relieves pain and thus allows treatment that could otherwise be extremely painful, such as manipulation of a painful joint or wound débridement. Sometimes, by interrupting reflexes that are causing sustained pain, analgesic blocks can produce a beneficial effect that is prolonged beyond the effective duration of the agent injected.

Analgesic blocks are useful in treating various acute and chronic disorders. They often reduce the amounts of analgesic medication that might otherwise be needed.

Injecting local anesthetics into tender points of muscle or skin causes a type of analgesic block that may modify pain and break the pain cycle. However, the pain may not be permanently eliminated unless the primary afferent impulses are either chemically or surgically terminated, or until the underlying pathologic condition causing the pain is corrected.

Major types of nerve blocks include (1) local block by infiltration into skin or topical application to mucous membranes; (2) intravenous (Bier) block by injection distal to a tourniquet in an extremity; (3) peripheral nerve block (e.g., radial, median, and ulnar nerve blocks to anesthetize the hand); (4) plexus block for analgesia of an extremity (brachial plexus, lumbosacral plexus); (5) somatic nerve block of spinal nerves by a paravertebral or intercostal approach; (6) prevertebral sympathetic (autonomic) block (Fig. 16-11); (7) epidural block (caudal and segmental spinal epidural block); (8) subarachnoid spinal block; and (9) blocks of the cranial nerves.

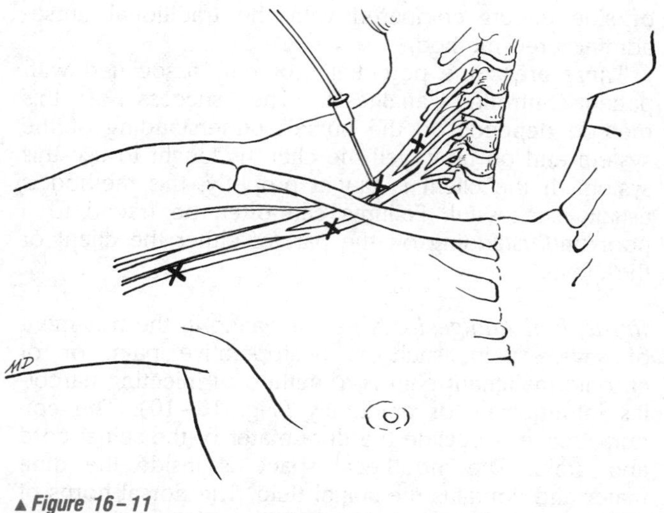

▲ **Figure 16-11**

Nerve block of the brachial plexus may be performed at one of several levels. The "X" marks indicate (from distal to proximal) the axillary, infraclavicular, supraclavicular, and interscalene approaches.

Examples of some acute painful situations that may be relieved with nerve blocks include (1) childbirth; (2) herpes zoster; (3) some neuralgias; (4) thrombophlebitis; (5) musculoskeletal problems such as acute, severe post-traumatic pain following ligamentous tears, a herniated intervertebral disc, fractured vertebrae, and fractured ribs; (6) visceral conditions such as coronary occlusion, mesenteric thrombosis, perforated peptic ulcer, pancreatitis, and severe renal or biliary colic; and (7) sudden, acute circulatory insufficiency from embolus, vasospasm, thrombus, or trauma.

Nerve blocks are useful as one modality in managing chronic pain (Table 16-7). The blocks break the pain cycle or provide temporary relief, allowing the person to use the painful part and regain more normal function. For example, reflex sympathetic dystrophy (overactivity of sympathetic nerves causing a cold, discolored, sweaty, swollen, painful extremity), if treated early (e.g., within six months of onset), often responds to a series of sympathetic blocks.

Cancer pain also can often be treated successfully by nerve block, particularly in the terminal stages with neurolytic block. Pancreatic cancer pain or other visceral abdominal pain responds to a celiac plexus neurolytic block. Low pelvic pain can be treated with subarachnoid neurolytic block. These procedures carry significant risks, including hypotension, loss of bowel and bladder function, paralysis, and loss of the useful warning signs that pain provides. However, freedom from pain and absence of the side effects of analgesic medication may outweigh the risks in this group of clients.

Nerve blocks are often unsuccessful owing to (1) difficulties in identifying the pain pathways or in locating the correct nerve for injection and (2) the complexity of pain psychophysiopathology. Some additional

TABLE 16-7. Indications for Therapeutic Nerve Blocks for Chronic Pain

Indications	Types of Nerve Block
Causalgia and other reflex sympathetic dystrophies Acute herpes zoster and postherpetic syndrome	Blockade of appropriate sympathetic pathways Occasionally, epidural or subarachnoid injection of neurolytic agents (phenol or alcohol) to interrupt preganglionic pathways
Chronic pancreatitis Upper abdominal cancer	Blockade of celiac plexus (injection of neurolytic agents)
Chronic myofascial pain dysfunction syndromes	Infiltration of trigger areas with anesthetic agents
Chronic back pain with nerve root irritation (no myelographic evidence of acute herniated intervertebral disc)	Injection of steroids and a local anesthetic into subarachnoid or epidural space Continuous epidural techniques (to provide profound muscle relaxation as an adjunct to bed rest and traction)
Post-traumatic and postinfectious neuralgia	Intercostal nerve blocks
Terminal stage of metastatic cancer in people with clearly unilateral and well-circumscribed pain	Subarachnoid block with neurolytic agents
Painful spasticity	Fanwise injections of 45 per cent alcohol into clonic and stretched muscle belly (to decrease muscle tone and clonus)

From Ghia, J. N., et al. (1979). Therapeutic nerve blocks for chronic pain. *American Family Physician, 20,* 74.

problems occur because only small amounts of solution can be injected at one time.

Nerve blocks are contraindicated in people who (1) are receiving anticoagulant medication, (2) have an infection at the site of injection, or (3) are in shock, especially if extensive vasomotor paralysis will be produced or if large amounts of local anesthetic are required. They should be used cautiously for people who are psychoneurotic, psychotic, or cachectic.

Caution. Because of potential complications, have resuscitative equipment and necessary drugs readily available to combat untoward reactions when nerve block procedures are performed.

Complications of nerve blocks include systemic toxic reactions related to peak blood concentrations of local anesthetics. These reactions are likely to involve the heart and central nervous system. Early assessment findings indicating the onset of these complications include lightheadedness, numbness of the tongue and lips, nausea, tinnitus, and hypertension or hypotension. The complications may culminate in loss of consciousness, seizures, and cardiac arrest. These complications may be prevented or minimized by (1) individualizing the dose to the person, (2) using a test dose, (3) administering appropriate premedication, and (4) having readily available resuscitative medications and equipment (including oxygen, suction, adequate intravenous access, and appropriate monitoring). If a systemic toxic reaction occurs, treatment should immediately be directed to establishing a clear airway, providing oxygen and adequate ventilation, and ensuring a good pulse and blood pressure. Convulsions are effectively treated with diazepam. Complications such as pneumothorax, inadvertent subarachnoid (spinal) block, postinjection neuropathy, respiratory dysfunction and paralysis, and hematoma relate to needle misplacement. Other complications relate to vasoconstrictor overdose or to idiosyncratic or allergic drug reaction.

Following a nerve block procedure, make the following assessments, and document the findings:

1. Indications of complications or untoward effects.
2. The client's descriptions of symptoms and pain relief or continued presence of pain.
3. The apparent amount, type, and duration of pain relief.
4. Instructions to client about reporting changes in pain.
5. Analgesics administered.

Such assessment may continue for several weeks to help evaluate the effectiveness of the nerve block. If alcohol is used for the block, the maximal effects do not occur for several days.

NEUROSURGERY FOR PAIN RELIEF

For a client suffering from long-standing pain, the problem can become totally absorbing, completely dominating the client's life. The lives of significant others are also affected by the client's prolonged pain and the client's responses to it. When such pain is alleviated by surgical interruption of pain pathways and pain perception is abolished, the problem is not entirely solved. Because of the complicated nature of chronically painful conditions, such clients frequently require long-term counseling and rehabilitative measures after surgery. Once pain relief is obtained by surgery, function must be restored and new goals found. Occupational therapy may be necessary. The client's significant others should be included in the therapeutic approaches used.

When a client is experiencing persistent, intractable pain of high intensity, and less invasive modalities of treatment fail, neurosurgical procedures may be considered. Such procedures attempt to relieve pain by interrupting parts of nervous system tracts that relay sensations to the brain from their point of origin.

The goal of neurosurgical procedures for pain relief is to provide pain relief without causing the loss of other sensations, such as the loss of all feeling in an area or loss of movement following some procedures. Many procedures are used only in terminally ill clients because relief may be short-lived. In some clients, the same pain returns, and in others, the pain becomes even worse. Neurosurgical approaches should be used cautiously in clients with chronic pain.

These operations may be performed peripherally or centrally (on the spinal cord or brain). In addition, surgery on the autonomic nervous system (sympathectomy) may be performed alone or in combination with other procedures for the pain of causalgia or vascular disease.

Summarized next are some of the neurosurgical procedures performed for pain management (Fig. 16–12).

Neurectomy interrupts cranial or peripheral nerves by an incision. This procedure is used when pain is localized to a small part of the body. Neurectomies are performed infrequently because it is difficult to isolate sensory and motor fibers. Also, regeneration of the cut peripheral nerve fibers may occur, causing pain to return. There has been some success in treating localized pain, such as trigeminal neuralgia and tic douloureux. When a cranial neurectomy is performed, a craniotomy is necessary.

Rhizotomy is the interruption of the anterior or posterior nerve root area close to the spinal cord. Either a surgical procedure takes place or a radiofrequency electrode needle is used. Rhizotomy is performed when pain is more widely distributed than that occurring in a small area of the body. This technique is not generally useful for diffuse cancer pain because the extent of denervation and laminectomy is too extensive. Unpleasant dysesthesias may result from this procedure, such as "pins and needles" or crawling skin sensations.

Chordotomy or spinothalamic tractotomy is the surgical interruption of pain-conducting pathways within the spinal cord. An incision a few millimeters in length is made in the anterolateral pathway opposite the side on which pain is located. When pain is midline in nature, a bilateral chordotomy must be performed. A laminectomy is necessary for this surgery.

Percutaneous cervical chordotomy is a preferred procedure for the relief of intractable pain in persons who are poor surgical risks or who have terminal cancer. It is used for lateral pain below T4. The operation is relatively simple, it is well tolerated, and there is a short convalescence period and a low morbidity rate. However, individuals with pre-existing respiratory disease are at a greater risk. By means of this procedure, a surgical incision is avoided and stereotaxic destruction of the anterolateral spinothalamic tracts is possible. Percutaneous chordotomy is a simplified form of surgical chordotomy that interrupts or destroys the conduction of pain in the pain pathways of the spinal cord. The procedure is performed under local anesthesia by inserting a radio frequency electrode needle into the neck, below and behind the mastoid process. X-ray control is used to guide the needle into the spinal cord. There, a thermal lesion is produced by passing radiofrequency current through the needle and heating the tip. This process coagulates a small area of nerve tissue at the tip of the needle. Some physicians believe that percutaneous chordotomy is simpler, more accurate, and safer than surgical chordotomy. A lateral cervical approach and an anterior approach have been used.

Tractotomy is the surgical division of the anterolateral pathway in the brain stem. Morbidity and mortality rates are high and limit the usefulness of this procedure in pain management. A craniotomy is necessary to accomplish this procedure.

Gyrectomy involves removal of the postcentral gyrus (part of the sensory cortex of the brain) corresponding to the painful part. This procedure is performed in an attempt to remove the registration of pain within the cortex of the brain.

Hypophysectomy is accomplished by destroying the pituitary gland, usually by injecting it with absolute alcohol. This technique may bring relief of pain associated with advanced cancer.

Prefrontal leukotomy, medial frontal leukotomy, cingulotomy, and frontal lobectomy are all procedures that interrupt the connections of the frontal lobe to the rest of the brain. To varying degrees, these procedures permanently change the client's personality. Hence, these interventions are reserved for only those clients most seriously affected by intractable pain and whose pain has not responded to other therapies.

Remember: When sensory nerves are cut, the tissues that no longer receive sensory innervation become highly susceptible to injury. With sensory innervation gone, feelings of pain, pressure, and temperature are no longer present. Therefore, injury can occur without the client's even being aware that it has happened. Because the interruption of sensory nerve pathways deprives body tissues of these protective mechanisms, this procedure is usually not carried out unless other less radical treatment measures have failed.

Once such procedures are performed, the individual (and significant others as appropriate) must be taught how to protect the affected area from damage. Frequent inspection of the area for indications of tissue damage is essential because the individual cannot feel when tissue damage has occurred.

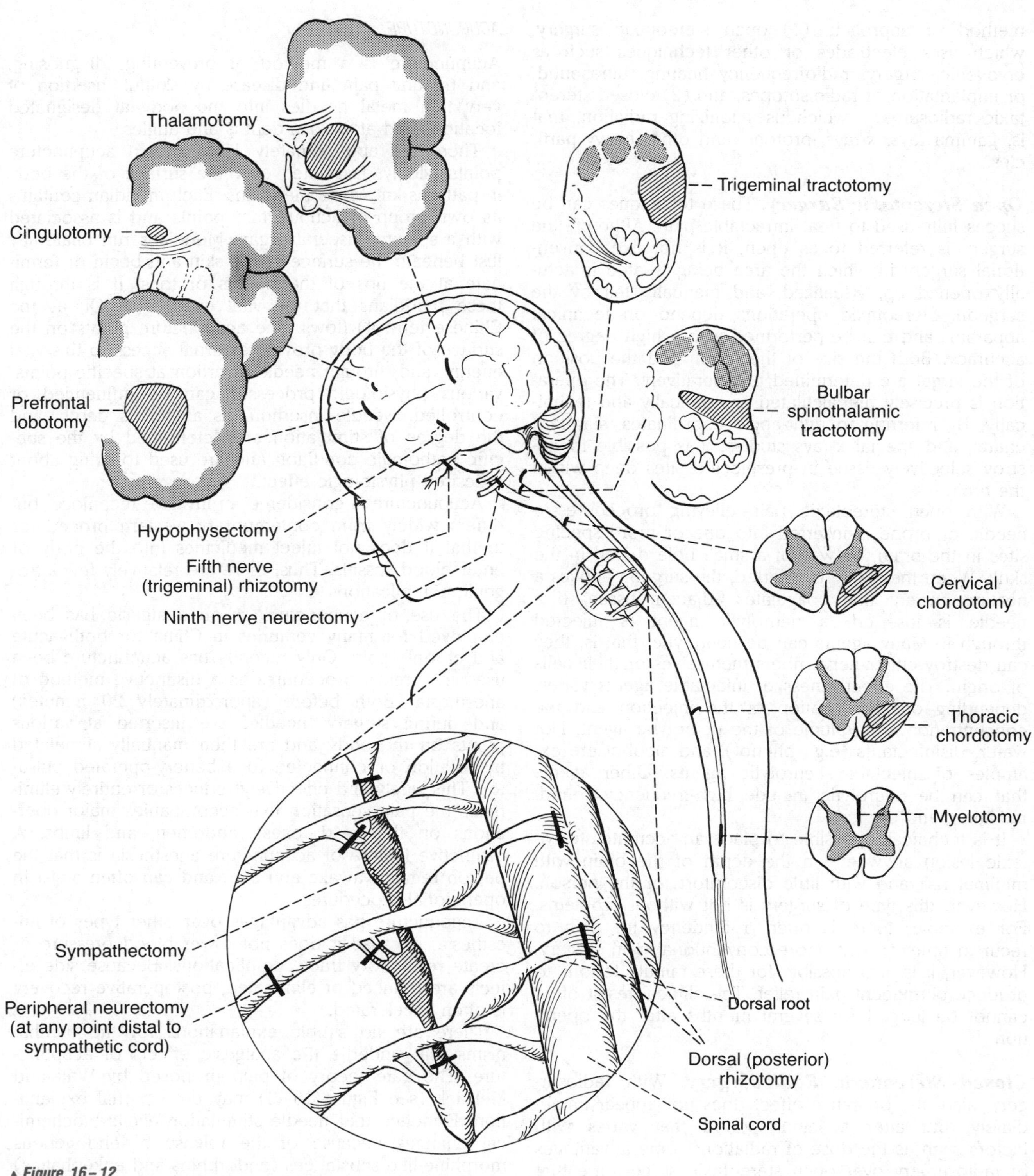

▲ *Figure 16-12*

Diagram of various surgical procedures designed to alleviate pain.

Stereotaxic Pain Surgery. The techniques of stereotaxic surgery can be used to treat some types of pain by sectioning deep fiber tracts in the brain. The word stereotaxic refers to precise positioning in space. In relation to surgery, it refers to precisely locating operative sites deep within the body—frequently within the cranium—by instrumentation from outside the body.

Stereotaxic brain surgery, aimed at modifying cerebral function by sectioning tracts and destroying nuclei, can be divided into two categories according to method of approach: (1) open stereotaxic surgery, which uses electrodes or other techniques such as cryogenic surgery, radiofrequency heating, ultrasound, or implantation of radioisotopes; and (2) closed stereotaxic radiosurgery, which uses ionizing radiation, that is, gamma rays, x-rays, protons, and other heavy particles.

Open Stereotaxic Surgery. These techniques can be successfully used to treat intractable pain. Although the surgery is referred to as open, it is not like conventional surgery in which the area being treated is actually opened up, visualized, and manually felt by the surgeon. Stereotaxic operations depend on technical apparatus and can be performed with a high degree of accuracy. Both the size of the lesion and the position of the target are determined preoperatively. The operation is precisely precalculated anatomically and technically. By referring to right-angle coordinates, standard charts, and special x-rays studies, it is possible to destroy selectively tissue in preselected sites deep within the brain.

With open stereotaxic pain-relieving procedures a needle or probe is inserted into one or more specific sites in the brain, by way of a small hole drilled in the skull. When the probe is inserted, the surgeon applies a heating current that coagulates adjacent tissue. If a needle is inserted, a neurolytic agent is injected through it. Many agents can be neurolytic, that is, they can destroy either nerve fibers themselves or their cells of origin. The effectiveness of injectable agents varies, depending on the location of the injection and the concentration and volume of the neurolytic agent. Hot water, disinfectants (e.g., phenol), and alcohol are examples of injectable neurolytic agents. Other agents that can be neurolytic include high-frequency sound, radiation, and dry ice.

It is technically possible to place an accurate stereotaxic lesion anywhere in the depth of the brain with minimal risk and with little discomfort for the person. However, this type of surgery is not without problems. For example, there is often a tendency for pain to recur in time, as with more conventional pain surgery. However, it is also possible for these minute lesions to produce permanent pain relief. The clinical result often cannot be judged for several months after the operation.

Closed Stereotaxic Radiosurgery. With radiosurgery, also, the operative effect does not appear immediately, but after a latent period that varies with factors such as the dose of radiation. Some advantages of radiosurgery over open stereotaxic surgery are that (1) there is no operative shock and practically no mortality risk, (2) the risks of infection and bleeding are eliminated, and (3) the person can leave the hospital the day after the procedure. A lesion produced by radiosurgery continues to enlarge for several months. Thus, care must be taken to ensure that the ultimate size of the lesion does not produce undesirable side effects.

ACUPUNCTURE

Acupuncture is a method of preventing, diagnosing, and treating pain and disease by skillful insertion of very thin metal needles into the body at designated locations and at various depths and angles.

There are approximately 1000 known acupuncture points widely distributed over the surface of the body in patterns known as meridians. Each meridian contains its own group of acupuncture points and is associated with a specific visceral organ. Meridians run bilaterally just beneath the surface of the skin and begin or terminate at the tips of the fingers or toes. It is through these meridians that the vital energy (or Qi, as the Chinese term it) flows. The acupuncture points on the surface of the body provide external access to this vital energy, and through needle insertion at specific points, various physiologic processes can be influenced or controlled. Needle insertion, its angle, its depth, and the degree of stimulation are determined by the specific pathologic condition and are used to bring about a desired physiologic effect.

Acupuncture is considered an invasive technique, but differs widely from contemporary western procedures in that it does not inject medicines into the body or enter blood vessels. Thus, there are relatively few iatrogenic complications.

The use of acupuncture as an analgesic has been employed for many centuries in China for both acute and chronic pain. Only recently has acupuncture been used in surgical procedures as a distinctive method of anesthesia. Both before (approximately 20 minutes) and during surgery, needles are inserted at various points on the body and are then manually stimulated by rotation or connected to a battery-operated pulsator. This safely and effectively reduces or entirely eliminates the pain sensation that accompanies major operations on the head, chest, abdomen, and limbs. A distinctive feature of acupuncture anesthesia is that the person remains awake and alert and can often assist in operational procedures.

Acupuncture has advantages over other types of anesthesia, because it does not lower blood pressure or create respiratory tract complications. Because side effects are reduced or eliminated, postoperative recovery is often accelerated.

There are no simple explanations for the mechanisms that underlie the analgesic effects of acupuncture. The gate theory of pain proposed by Wall and Melzack (see Figure 16–2) may be a partial explanation. Evidence that needle stimulation elicits biochemical changes because of the release of endogenous morphine-like substances (endorphins and enkephalins) is another possible theory.

STIMULATION THERAPY

The relief of chronic pain by electric stimulation became a new clinical management technique after Melzack and Wall proposed the gate-control theory of pain transmission. The gate-control theory describes a spinal cord-modulating mechanism in which one type of sensation, such as vibration or light touch, can impede the transmission of another sensation, such as pain. The former sensations are transmitted by larger, more rapidly conducting fibers in the peripheral nerves. These sensations reach the spinal cord sooner than sensations traveling in the small fibers that conduct painful impulses. Because sensations such as vibration or light touch reach the spinal cord before the painful impulses, they can activate a pool of modulating neurons and block the incoming pain signal. Another explanation is that the electric stimulation causes release of the body's own pain-relieving substances—endorphins. Electric nerve stimulators can activate the large fibers and produce a tingling or vibratory sensation that blocks painful stimuli.

It is known that the dorsal columns carry most light touch and vibratory sensations to higher centers. The idea developed that stimulating the dorsal columns directly could achieve a wider area of stimulation and pain relief. Other techniques involve the thalamus, including implanting electrodes and the use of continuous stimulation for pain relief.

Transcutaneous Electric Nerve Stimulation. Transcutaneous electric nerve stimulation (TENS) developed from the need to screen clients prior to dorsal column stimulator implants (see later). The screening apparatus was then found to relieve pain effectively in many clients. Success with TENS depends on the client's understanding of, interest in, and motivation to use the apparatus, as well as the skillfulness of application of the device by the clinician (Table 16-8). Thoroughly familiarize the client with the TENS equipment, such as how to operate the machine and adjust electric settings. Involve significant others as appropriate in learning and teaching sessions, as shown in the Client Education Guide. The client may need their help in applying the machine to areas that are difficult to reach, such as below the shoulder blades.

Usually, a superficial nerve close to the pain is selected for stimulation. Electrode placement depends on the site of the pain. Positive and negative poles are usually placed within several inches of each other. Voltage and pulsation are controlled by the client wearing the device. Before application, the electrodes are moistened with electrode jelly to ensure proper conduction. Both the skin and the electrodes are cleaned every 8 hours, and fresh jelly is applied. When stimulation is not effective, the entire painful area is explored for subsequent electrode placement.

The overall efficiency of TENS in individuals with chronic pain is about 25 per cent. TENS has been reported to be less effective for pain due to cancer than for other types of pain.

Percutaneous Epidural Dorsal Column Stimulation. A single (unipolar) electrode or two (bipolar) insulated-wire electrodes are placed through the skin (i.e., percutaneously) into the spinal epidural space. The dorsal column may then be temporarily stimulated to evaluate the mechanism's effectiveness in obtaining pain relief before permanent implantation of a stimulator. It is a necessary part of the assessment of a client to evaluate whether or not a permanent stimulator would be beneficial.

Local anesthesia is injected into the tissue overlying the interspinous space. A curved needle is inserted and the wire electrode is gently passed through the needle into the epidural space. After the electrode has been manipulated into proper position under fluoroscopy, the needle is withdrawn and the electrode left in place. This procedure is then repeated at the same place or at a different interspace to place the second electrode. The electrodes are then attached to an external power source, by which the person can control the amount of dorsal column stimulation received.

Dorsal Column Spinal Cord Stimulation. Success with this type of pain therapy requires careful assessment and selection of the client experiencing pain. The pain must have a definitively diagnosed organic cause. Individuals selected should previously have tried many other types of pain management techniques and therapies in attempts to relieve their pain. Initial screening is performed with a percutaneous epidural dorsal column stimulator (see earlier). If the person experiences pain relief from this temporary technique, a dorsal column stimulation implant is surgically placed.

The implant stimulation device is a transistorized receiver that is surgically implanted. Electrode wires run into the epidural space and to an external transmitter. In a surgical procedure, a subcutaneous pocket is formed for the receiver. This pocket is usually in the infraclavicular region of the abdomen. Electrodes are passed subcutaneously from the receiver to a laminectomy incision. Electrode leads are threaded into the epidural space. Usually, the laminectomy is performed in the thoracic or lumbar region.

Relief of chronic pain from the dorsal column stimulator may diminish with time, and results have not been as encouraging as was hoped. Implantation of peripheral nerve stimulators is safer and easier than implanting dorsal column stimulators.

Intracranial Stimulation. Use of this device is becoming more common. It is considered for individuals whose pain is diffuse in nature and unresponsive to other treatments. This therapy is an alternative to destructive intracranial procedures. Under local anesthesia, a stimulating electrode is inserted into the posterior end of the third ventricle. The proximal end of the electrode is connected to a battery-driven stimulator, which is operated by the person. There is some evidence that the enkephalin levels in the cerebrospinal fluid may be increased by this technique.[9]

RADIATION THERAPY

Because it may cause multiple complications, radiation therapy is not usually used to treat benign pain states if the condition can be managed by more conservative

TABLE 16-8. Troubleshooting TENS Units

Following are some common problems of TENS use and some simple solutions. But remember, *always* turn the TENS unit off before checking it.

Problem	Solution
No stimulation	Change batteries
	Make sure batteries are inserted correctly
	Check that lead wires are plugged in securely at both ends
	Make sure electrodes are in total contact with the skin
	Look for corrosion on battery contacts
	Replace electrodes
	Check for defective wires
Cuts in and out	Check that both ends of the lead wire are plugged in securely
	Replace defective leads
	Check that batteries are securely in place
	Make sure electrodes are in total contact with the skin
	Check that amplitude is turned up enough
Skin irritation	Remove preoperative skin antiseptic
	Discontinue use temporarily if necessary
	Treat rash (leave open to air; use skin cream)
	Reposition electrodes so they are not on irritated area
	Replace electrodes if necessary
	Change type of electrode if desired
	Make sure electrodes are in total contact with the skin
	Try a protective film (such as Skin-Prep), cream (such as Uniderm), or nonprescription cortisone cream
	Try a different adhesive tape
	Wash electrode (if made of reusable carbon rubber)
	Discontinue using TENS if problem does not resolve
Unpleasant sensation (itching, burning, pricking—without rash)	Use a different type of electrode
	Lower pulse-width dial
	Increase distance between electrodes
	Check electrode adhesion
	Try another brand of TENS
Unpleasant sensation (too intense, feels obnoxious, too distracting)	Turn down amplitude dial
	Turn down pulse-width dial
	Adjust rate
	Try another style of electrode
	Turn unit on less frequently
	Change electrode location
	Try another brand of TENS
Nausea	Reposition electrodes
	Vary rate, pulse width, amplitude
	Try another brand of TENS
	Discontinue using TENS if problem does not resolve
Headache	Turn down pulse-width dial
	Turn down amplitude dial
	Use shorter stimulation period (turn off more often)
	Use fewer electrodes and place them farther apart
	Reposition electrodes
	Vary the rate
	Try different brand of TENS
	Discontinue using TENS if problem does not resolve

From Meyer, T. H. (1982). TENS: Relieving pain through electricity. *Nursing 82, 12*, 57. Reprinted with permission from Nursing 82, Copyright 1982, Springhouse Corporation, 1111 Bethlehem Pike, Springhouse, PA 19477-0908. All rights reserved.

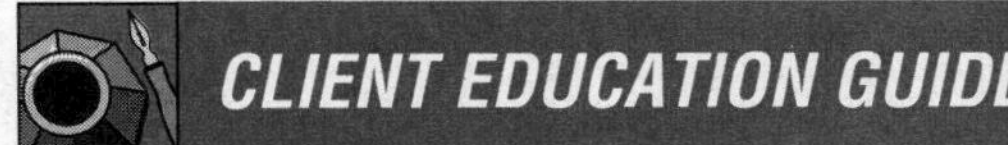

TENS Units

Teaching and learning activities are very important for a client using a TENS unit. Teaching for clients using a TENS unit includes the following items:

- A shock will not occur, and electrocution need not be feared.
- Wash the electrode sites and apply skin cream.
- Apply electrodes properly; if they are not lying flat and making full surface contact, a burn may occur.
- You may conceal the unit's wires so that they are not visible to others.
- Use the TENS unit for as long as directed. (Regimens for the use of TENS units are highly individualized.)

measures. Radiation therapy, however, is extensively used in treating pain due to malignant conditions, such as bone pain. It is also very useful in reducing the size of tumors pressing on nerves and other organs.

PLACEBOS

A placebo is thought of as a harmless, but useless, treatment designed to make the client better. It has been defined as any treatment that produces an effect in the client because of its intent, not because of anything specific in the nature or therapeutic properties of the treatment.[68] If the client responds to a placebo, the client is said to be placebo positive.

Unfortunately, placebos given instead of pain medications are not harmless. If nothing else, they usually require the nurse to lie to the client about what is being given. When the client discovers what has been done, all faith and trust in the health team is lost. The nurse must question why the placebo is being ordered. If the client is placebo positive, this only proves that the client is one of the one third of the population who respond positively to placebos. The problem arises when the client's response is considered to mean that the client's pain is not real.

There are many myths associated with response to placebos. These seem to have as a basis, a disbelief of the client's report of pain. Any client who reports pain must be believed, because that pain is real for the client. The nurse should always closely question the use of placebos in the place of adequate pain medication. It is unethical to lie to a client, and placebos are a lie.

Modification of Plan of Care for the Elderly

It is important for the nurse to be aware of problems associated with pain assessment and treatment in the elderly. There are many myths associated with both pain and treatment in this age group (Table 16-9). Some of these points were discussed previously in the section on response to pain.

TABLE 16-9. Misconceptions and Facts About Pain in the Elderly

Misconceptions	Facts
Pain is a natural part of the aging process	Pain does not accompany aging unless there is some specific disease process present. Older clients are more likely to suffer from chronic diseases such as arthritis, but without disease, there should not be pain
Pain perception decreases with aging	If the CNS is intact, then there is no alteration in pain perception. Pain response may be affected by a variety of factors, such as aphasia or paralysis. Lack of pain response, however, does not mean lack of pain
Narcotics should never be used in the elderly. They are too dangerous	Narcotics are appropriate to treat severe pain in the elderly as long as the changes in sensitivity are accounted for. The elderly may have more problems biotransforming and excreting these medications, so lower doses and longer intervals between doses are safer
If the older person is confused, pain medications should not be given because they will increase the client's confusion	Pain itself can cause confusion in the elderly. It may interfere with sleep and rest, leading to confusion. Confusion often resolves once the client has been adequately treated for pain
If the elderly client is showing signs of depression and chronic pain, the pain is caused by the depression. If the depression is treated, the pain will disappear	Depression is a normal response to, not a cause of, pain. Depression may influence the client's ability to cope with the pain, but is not the cause of it. When the pain is relieved, the depression will probably disappear

When administering analgesics to the elderly, the nurse should be aware of the physiologic changes in these clients. The distribution of drugs are altered by aging. There is usually a higher percentage of body fat in the elderly which could increase the accumulation of fat-soluble drugs, such as the lower muscle mass, resulting in the need for a lower dosage. Serum proteins are also lower, which will affect the dosage needed of any drug that is bound to plasma proteins. This is important because NSAIDs are such drugs and are commonly used to treat some chronic pains, such as arthritis.

The liver is the major site of drug biotransformation. Aging alters the liver, and therefore, the biotransformation of drugs may change in an unpredictable way. Drugs such as acetaminophen are biotransformed more slowly, but other drugs may not be affected. The interval between doses may have to be lengthened to avoid this problem.

Excretion of drugs is also affected due to changes in renal mass, blood flow, glomerular filtration rate, and tubular secretion. Again, the length of time drugs remain in the body is longer, so lower doses and longer intervals are needed. The clearance of morphine from the plasma is also decreased. This means that morphine remains in the body longer at higher concentrations. Giving lower doses at longer intervals will compensate for this problem.

There are other factors that may alter drug therapy in the elderly. Intramuscular injections may be poorly absorbed because of the decrease in muscle mass. The possible alterations in circulation also may affect distribution of injected drugs.

To treat pain adequately in the elderly, the nurse must rely on careful observation of the effectiveness of the treatment. If oversedation or other problems occur, the dose of the drug should be decreased. Problems associated with pain medication and the elderly, however, should never mean that they are not being adequately treated for their pain.

Summary

Pain is a complex phenomenon, and it is one of the most common problems nurses face. Pain is an almost universal experience (except for the few clients who feel no pain), but, at the same time, it is a unique experience for each client. The nurse is in a good position to help the client with pain. The nurse can help the client communicate with the physician when pain relief is not sufficient. The nurse can establish a relationship with the client to help the client learn new ways of controlling pain.

The subject of pain control is changing constantly. New information about the physiology of pain transmission and control serves to broaden the options available to help the client in pain. Nurses are becoming even more knowledgeable about pain and its control. Nurses have an ever-expanding role to play in the treatment of clients' pain.

Bibliography

1. Abram, S. E. (Ed.) (1990). *The pain clinic manual.* Philadelphia: J. B. Lippincott.
2. Adler, R. (1981). The differentiation of organic and psychogenic pain. *Pain, 10,* 249.
3. Akil, H., et al. (1984). Endogenous opioids: Biology and function. *Annual Review of Neuroscience, 7,* 223.
4. Ament, P. (1982). Concepts in the use of hypnosis for pain relief. *Journal of Medicine, 13,* 233.
5. Angarola, R. T. (1986). Narcotic analgesics: Fear and responsibilities. *Journal of Pain and Symptom Management, 1,* 77.
6. Arnoff, G. M., et al. (1983). A review of follow-up studies of multidisciplinary pain units. *Pain, 16,* 1.
7. Bailey, L. M. (1986). Music therapy in pain management. *Journal of Pain and Symptom Management, 1,* 25.
8. Barnett, D. C., & Hair, B. (1981). Use and effectiveness of transcutaneous electrical nerve stimulation in pain management. *Journal of Neurosurgical Nursing, 13,* 323.
9. Basbaum, A. I., & Fields, H. L. (1978). Endogenous pain control mechanisms: Review and hypothesis. *Annals of Neurology, 4,* 451.
10. Basbaum, A. I., Fields, H. L. (1984). Endogenous pain control systems: Brainstem spinal pathways and endorphin circuitry. *Annual Review of Neuroscience, 7,* 309.
11. Boguslowski, M. (1980). Therapeutic touch: A facilitator of pain relief. *Topics in Clinical Nursing, 2,* 27.
12. Bonica, J. J. (1959). *Clinical applications of diagnostic and therapeutic nerve blocks.* Springfield, IL: Charles C Thomas.
13. Bonica, J. J., et al. (Eds.) (1990). *The management of pain (vols I and II, 2nd ed.).* Philadelphia: Lea & Febiger.
14. Chapman, C. E. (1991). Can the use of physical modalities for pain control be rationalized by the research evidence? *Canadian Journal of Physiological Pharmacology,* (5)*69,* 704–712.
15. Chapman, D., et al. (1985). Pain measurement: An overview. *Pain, 22,* 1–31.
16. Chapman, C. R., & Turner, J. A. (1986). Psychologic control of acute pain in medical settings. *Journal of Pain and Symptom Management, 1,* 9.
17. Choiniere, M., et al. The pain of burns: Characteristics and correlates. *Journal of Trauma, 29*(11), 1531–1539.
18. Choiniere, M., et al. (1990). Comparison between patients' and nurses' assessments of pain and medication efficacy in severe burn injuries. *Pain, 40*(2), 143–152.
19. Cleeland, C. S. (1984). Assessing pain in cancer: The patient's role. In: *The Management of Cancer Pain.* Nutley, NJ: Roche Laboratories, 1984.
20. Cleeland, C. S. (1984). Impact of pain on the patient with cancer. Proceedings of National Conference on Cancer Therapy. *Cancer, 54* (Suppl), 2635.
21. Cleeland, C. S. (1986). Behavioral control of symptoms, introduction. *Journal of Pain and Symptom Management, 1,* 36.
22. Cohen, F. (1980). Postsurgical pain relief: Patient's status and nurses' medication choices. *Pain, 9,* 265–274.
23. Concilus, R., et al. (1989). Continuous intravenous infusion of methadone for control of burn pain. *Journal of Burn Care and Rehabilitation, 5*(10), 406–409.
24. Cousins, M. J., Mather, L. E. (1984). Intrathecal and epidural administration of opioids. *Anesthesiology, 61,* 276.
25. Crawford, M. E., et al. (1983). Pain treatment on outpatient basis utilizing extradural opiates. A Danish multicentre study comprising 105 patients. *Pain, 16,* 41.
26. Davitz, L. L., & Davitz, J. R. (1980). *Nurses response to patients' suffering.* New York: Springer Publishing.
27. Digregorio, G. J., & Kozin, S. H. (1986). Adjuvant drug therapy for pain. *American Family Physician, 33,* 227.
28. Donovan, M., et al. (1987). Incidence and characteristics of pain in a sample of medical-surgical inpatients. *Pain, 30,* 69–78.
29. Donovan, M. I.: Relaxation with guided imagery: A useful technique. *Cancer Nursing, 3,* 27.
30. Dowman, R. (1991). Spinal and supraspinal correlates of nociception in man. *Pain, 45*(3), 269–281.
31. Drain, C. B., & Cain, R. S.: The nursing implications of postoperative pain. *Military Medicine, 146,* 127.

32. Dubner, R., & Bennett, G. J.: Spinal and trigeminal mechanisms of nociception. *Annual Review of Neuroscience, 6,* 381.
33. Duncan, D. J., & Driscoll, D. M. (1991). Burn management. *Critical Care Nursing Clinics of North America, 2*(3), 165–267.
34. Falk, D. (1982). Antidepressants for pain. *Aches and Pains, 3,* 8.
35. Ferrer-Brechner, T. (Ed.) (1990). *Common problems in pain management.* Chicago: Year Book Medical Publishers.
36. Fields, H. L. (Ed.) (1990). *Pain syndromes in neurology.* Boston: Butterworths.
37. Fields, H. L., et al. (1991). Neurotransmitters in nociceptive modulatory circuits. *Annual Review of Neuroscience, 14,* 219–245.
38. Fishman, B., et al. (1988). The Memorial pain assessment card: Reliability and validity for cancer pain. *Journal of Pain and Symptom Management, 3*(3), S23.
39. Foley, K. M. (1982). The practical use of narcotic analgesics. *Medical Clinics of North America, 66,* 1091.
40. Foley, K. M. (1985). Adjuvant analgesic drugs in cancer pain management. In G. M. Arnoff (Ed.), *Evaluation and treatment of chronic pain.* Baltimore: Urban & Schwarzenberg.
41. Foley, K. M., & Rogers, A. (1981). The management of cancer pain (Vol. 2) *The rational use of analgesics in the management of cancer pain.* Nutley, NJ: Hoffman-LaRoche, Inc.
42. Friedman, F. B. (1983). PRN analgesics: Controlling the pain or controlling the patient? *RN, 46,* 67.
43. Gaukroger, P. B. (1991). Paediatric analgesia: Which drug? Which dose? *Drugs, 1*(41), 52–59.
44. Graves, D. A., et al. (1983). Patient-controlled analgesia. *Annals of Internal Medicine, 99,* 360.
45. Griffin, M. (1986). In the mind's eye. *American Journal of Nursing, 86,* 805.
46. Grinde, J. W., et al. (1984). Pain management by epidural analgesia: The challenge for nursing. *Heart and Lung, 13,* 105.
47. Guyton, A. C. (1991). *Textbook of medical physiology* (5th ed.). Philadelphia: W. B. Saunders.
48. Harwood, A. (Ed.) (1981). *Ethnicity and Medical Care.* Cambridge, MA: Harvard University Press.
49. Heidrich, G., et al. (1985). Efficiency and quality of ibuprofen and acetaminophen plus codeine analgesia. *Pain, 22,* 385.
50. International Association for the Study of Pain (1986). Pain terms: A current list with definitions and notes on usage. *Pain, 3*:S216–S221.
51. Inturrisi, C. E. (1984). Pharmacology of narcotic analgesics. In: *The management of cancer pain.* Nutley, NJ: Roche Laboratories.
52. Jaffe, J. H., & Martin, W. R. (1980). Opioid analgesics and antagonists. In A. G. Gilman, et al. (Eds.), *The pharmacological basis of therapeutics* (6th ed.). New York: Macmillan.
53. Johnson, A., et al. (1991). Inhibition of burn pain by intravenous lignocaine. *Lancet, 2*(338), 151–152.
54. Jong, A. (1985). Ethical issues in pain management. In G. M. Arnoff (Ed.), *Evaluation and treatment of chronic pain.* Baltimore: Urban & Schwarzenberg.
55. Kantor, T. G. (1984). Nonsteroidal anti-inflammatory analgesic agents in management of cancer pain. In *The management of cancer pain.* Nutley, NJ: Roche Laboratories.
56. Karoly, P. (1985). The assessment of pain: Concepts and procedures. In P. Karoly (Ed.), *Measurement strategies in health psychology.* New York: Wiley Interscience.
57. Klinman, A. (1985). Control of pain associated with advanced malignancy. In G. M. Arnoff (Ed.), *Evaluation and treatment of chronic pain.* Baltimore: Urban & Schwarzenberg.
58. Kopala, B., & Matassarin-Jacobs, E. (1984). Sensory-perceptual-pain assessment. In J. Bellack & P. Bamford (Eds.), *Nursing assessment: A multidimensional approach* (pp. 310–357). Monterey, CA: Wadsworth.
59. Kutz, I., et al. (1983). The role of relaxation in behavioral therapies for chronic pain. *International Anesthesiology Clinics, 21,* 193.
60. Lloyd, J. W., et al. (1981). Selective hypophysectomy for metastatic pain. *British Journal of Anaesthesiology, 53,* 1129.
61. Lund, P. C. (1982). The role of analgesic blocking in the management of cancer pain: Current trends. A review article. *Journal of Medicine, 13,* 161.
62. Lytle, S. A., et al. (1991). Postoperative analgesia with epidural fentanyl. *Journal of the American Osteopathic Association, 91*(6), 547–550.
63. Mackersie, R. C., & Karagianes, T. G. (1990). Pain management following trauma and burns. *Critical Care Clinics, 6*(2), 433–449.
64. Marks, R. M., & Sachar, E. J. (1973). Undertreatment of medical inpatients with narcotic analgesics. *Annals of Internal Medicine, 78,* 173–181.
65. McCaffery, M. (1979). *Nursing management of the patient in pain* (p. 11). Philadelphia: J. B. Lippincott.
66. McCaffery, M. (1981). *Nursing management of the patient with pain* (2nd ed.). Philadelphia: J. B. Lippincott.
67. McCaffery, M. (1984). Improving interactions between the patient with cancer pain, the health team, and the family. In *The management of cancer pain.* Nutley, NJ: Roche Laboratories, 1984.
68. McCaffery, M., & Beebe, A. (1989). *Pain: Clinical manual for nursing practice.* St. Louis: C. V. Mosby.
69. McCaffery, M., & Hart, L. L. (1976). Undertreatment of acute pain with narcotics. *Nursing 76, 10,* 1586–1591.
70. McGee, J. L., & Alexander, M. R. (1979). Phenothiazine analgesia: Fact or fantasy. *American Journal of Hospital Pharmacy, 36,* 633–640.
71. McGuire, D. B. (1984). The measurement of clinical pain. *Nursing Research, 3*(33), 152–156.
72. Meinhart, N. T., & McCaffery, M. (1983). *Pain: A nursing approach to assessment and analysis.* Norwalk, CT: Appleton-Century-Crofts.
73. Melzack, R. (1987). The short form McGill pain questionnaire. *Pain, 30,* 191–197.
74. Melzack, R., et al. (1987). Pain on a surgical ward: A survey of the duration and intensity of pain and the effectiveness of medication. *Pain, 29,* 67–72.
75. Melzack, R., & Wall, P. (1982). *The puzzle of pain.* New York: Basic Books.
76. Melzack, R., & Wall, P. (1983). *The challenge of pain.* New York: Basic Books.
77. Moore, D. E., & Blacker, A. M. (1983). How effective is TENS for chronic pain? *American Journal of Nursing, 83,* 1175.
78. Moret, V., et al. (1991). Mechanisms of analgesia-induced hypnosis and acupuncture: Is there a difference? *Pain, 45*(2), 135–140.
79. Mountcastle, V. B. (1980). *Medical physiology* (p. 391). St. Louis: C. V. Mosby.
80. Oden, R. V. (Ed.) (1989). Management of postoperative pain. *Anesthesiology Clinics of North America, 1*(7), 111–362.
81. Ohnhaus, E. E., & Adler, R. (1975). Methodological problems in the measurement of pain: A comparison between the verbal rating scale and the visual analog scale. *Pain, 1,* 379–384.
82. Paris, P. M. (1986). Hypnosis. *Emergency Medicine, 18,* 63.
83. Paris, P. M. (1986). Narcotics. *Emergency Medicine, 18,* 66.
84. Paris, P. M. (1986). Pain in perspective. *Emergency Medicine, 18,* 28.
85. Paris, P. M. (1986). Transcutaneous nerve stimulation. *Emergency Medicine, 18,* 57.
86. Perez, S. (1984). Reducing injection pain. *American Journal of Nursing, 84,* 645.
87. Perry, S., & Heidrich, G. H.: Placebo response: Myth and matter. *American Journal of Nursing, 81,* 720.
88. Porter, J., & Jick, H.: Addiction rare in patients treated with narcotics. *New England Journal of Medicine, 302,* 123.
89. Schroeder, M. E. (1986). Neurolytic nerve block for cancer pain. *Journal of Pain and Symptom Management, 1,* 91.
90. Selbst, S. M. & Clark, M. (1990). Analgesic use in the emergency department. *Annals of Emergency Medicine, 19*(9), 1010–1013.
91. Simonton, O. C., et al. (1978). *Getting well again.* New York: Bantam Books.
92. Sorkin, L. S. (1991). Nociceptive transmission within the spinal cord. *Mt. Sinai Journal of Medicine, 58*(3), 208–216.
93. Sternbach, R. (1968). *Pain: A psychophysiological analysis* (p. 12). New York: Academic.
94. Stewart, R. (1986). Nitrous oxide. *Emergency Medicine, 18,* 49.

95. Stimmel, B. (1983). *Pain, analgesics, addiction: The pharmacologic treatment*. New York: Raven Press.
96. Taylor, A. G., et al. (1984). Duration of pain condition and physical pathology as determinants of nurses' assessments of patients in pain. *Nursing Research, 1* (33), 4-8.
97. Teske, K., et al. (1983). Relationships between nurses' observations and patients' self-reports of pain. *Pain, 16*, 289.
98. Todd, E. M. (1985). Pain: Historical perspectives. In G. M. Arnoff (Ed.), *Evaluation and treatment of chronic pain*. Baltimore: Urban & Schwarzenberg.
99. Tollison, C. D. (Ed.) (1989). *Handbook of chronic pain management*. Baltimore: Williams & Wilkins.
100. Toomey, T. C., et al. (1988). Relationship between perceived self-control of pain, pain description, and functioning. *Pain, 45*(2), 129-133.
101. Twycross, R. G., & Lack, S. A. (1983). *Symptom control in far advanced cancer: Pain relief*. London: Pitman Books, 1983.
102. Wall, P. D., & Melzack, R. (Eds.) (1989). *Textbook of pain*. Edinburgh: Churchill Livingstone.
103. Warfield, C. A. (Ed.) (1991). *Manual of pain management*. Philadelphia: J. B. Lippincott.
104. Whitt, J. R. (1984). Relieving chronic pain. *Nurse Practitioner, 9*, 36.
105. Wild, L. (1990). Pain management. *Critical Care Nursing Clinics of North America, 2*(4), 537-547.
106. Willis, W. D. (1985). The pain system. Basel, Switzerland: Karger.
107. Woodforde, J. M., & Merskey, H. (1972). Some relationships between subjective measures of pain. *Journal of Psychosomatic Research, 16*, 173-178.
108. World Health Organization. (1986). *Cancer pain relief*. Geneva, Switzerland: World Health Organization.
109. Zborowski, M. (1952). Cultural components in responses to pain. *Journal of Sociological Issues, 8*, 16-30.
110. Zborowski, M. (1969). *People in pain*. San Francisco: Jossey-Bass.

Chapter 17

Sleep and Sensory Disorders

A 21-year-old has spent about 7½ years of life sleeping. Just what is sleep, and why do people spend so much time sleeping?

DEFINITION

Sleep can be defined as a state of unconsciousness during which the cerebrum rests and from which a person can be aroused by external stimuli.

Sleep pattern disturbance is a nursing diagnosis that is defined as a disruption of sleep time that causes discomfort or interferes with a desired lifestyle.[7] The sleep pattern disturbance may relate to one of over 60 sleep disorders identified in the International Classification of Sleep Disorders, presented in Box 17-1.

Physiology of Sleep and Arousal

The sleep-wake cycle is one of the circadian rhythms of the body. It follows an approximate 24-hour cycle linked to light and dark. The timing of the sleep-wake cycle and other circadian rhythms, such as body temperature, is controlled, at least in part, by the superchiasmatic nucleus in the anterior hypothalamus. Located above the optic chiasm, this area receives input from the retina, which provides information about darkness and light. The superchiasmatic nucleus controls the production of melatonin, which is believed to be a potent sleep inducer.[41, 42]

Sleep is a naturally occurring, readily reversible altered state of arousal, characterized by a decreased responsiveness to the environment.

Box 17–1. International Classification of Sleep Disorders*

I. Dyssomnias
  A. Intrinsic Sleep Disorders
    1. Psychophysiological Insomnia
    2. Narcolepsy
    3. Obstructive Sleep Apnea Syndrome
    4. Central Sleep Apnea Syndrome
    5. Periodic Limb Movement Disorder
    6. Restless Legs Syndrome
  B. Extrinsic Sleep Disorders
    1. Inadequate Sleep Hygiene
    2. Environmental Sleep Disorder
  C. Circadian Rhythm Sleep Disorders
II. Parasomnias
  A. Arousal Disorders
    1. Sleepwalking
    2. Sleep Terrors
  B. Sleep-Wake Transition Disorders
  C. Parasomnias Usually Associated with REM Sleep
    1. Nightmares
    2. Sleep paralysis
  D. Other Parasomnias
    1. Sleep Bruxism
    2. Sleep Enuresis
    3. Primary Snoring
III. Sleep Disorders Associated with Medical/Psychiatric Disorders
  A. Associated with Mental Disorders
  B. Associated with Neurologic Disorders
  C. Associated with Other Medical Disorders
IV. Proposed Sleep Disorders

* The table includes a partial listing of common sleep disorders. Used with permission from the Diagnostic Classification Steering Committee, Thorpy MJ, Chairman (1990). *International classification of sleep disorders: Diagnostic and coding manual.* Rochester, MN: American Sleep Disorders Association.

The mediator of arousal and of sensory stimulation is the reticular activating system (RAS). The RAS is located in the brain stem and contains projections between to the thalamus and cortex. The diffuse network of neurons in the RAS is in a strategic position to monitor ascending and descending stimuli through feedback loops.[32]

Although the RAS provides the anatomic framework for arousal, it is the neurotransmitters that serve as the chemical messengers.[32] The onset of sleep and each subsequent sleep stage is an active process involving delicate shifts in the balance of several of these neurotransmitters.

The transition from the awake state to non-rapid eye movement (NREM) sleep is marked by decreases in the concentration of serotonin (5-HT), norepinephrine, and acetylcholine. The later transition to rapid eye movement (REM) sleep is marked by a dramatic increase in acetylcholine and further drops in serotonin and norepinephrine.[17, 42] As REM sleep continues, the concentrations of serotonin and norepinephrine build up, eventually stopping REM sleep. Cholinergic activation with the release of acetylcholine seems to reestablish REM sleep.[17, 42] The continuous interaction of these two systems is thought to produce the normal alterations between NREM and REM sleep.[14] Other neurotransmitters, such as GABA and dopamine, are also believed to have a part in the reciprocal processes involved in the shift in sleep state.

All of these neurotransmitters are actively involved in waking processes as well. For example, neurons that produce serotonin and norepinephrine play a role in the modulation of sensory input, mood, energy, and information processing, including attention, learning, and memory.[17] Thus, it can be seen that imbalances in these neurotransmitters induced through sleep pattern disturbances, medications, or diseases may reciprocally affect not only sleep but aspects of sensory processing, mood, and cognition.

SLEEP STAGES

Sleep can be defined behaviorally, functionally, and electrophysiologically. By using the electroencephalogram (EEG), sleep can be divided into REM and NREM sleep. NREM can be further divided into stages 1 through 4. The stages vary in depth but are characterized by lack of eye movement, low, fragmented cognitive activity, maintenance of moderate muscle tone, and slower but generally rhythmic respirations and pulse rate. As individuals progress from stage 1 to stage 4 sleep, the waveforms recorded by EEG become more synchronized, slower, and of greater amplitude (Fig. 17–1).[43]

Stage 1 is very light sleep. Respirations begin to slow, and muscles relax. At sleep onset, there may be some erratic breathing as well as sudden myoclonic jerks (sleep starts) as the body shifts from the awake to asleep state. Stage 1 is such a light stage of sleep that persons wakened from it will often claim that they were not asleep at all.

Stage 2 is still light sleep. The brain waves are mixed frequently and low voltage in pattern, with bursts of activity called sleep spindles and large amplitude waves called K complexes.[14, 42] More than 50 per cent of sleep is in stage 2.

Stages 3 and 4 are known as slow wave sleep (SWS), named for the characteristic high-voltage, low-frequency delta waves. Respirations become slow and even. The pulse and blood pressure fall. Oxygen consumption by muscle tissues and urine formation are decreased.

Dreams that occur during these NREM stages of sleep are generally thoughtlike ruminations of recent events and current concerns, with little story line.[17]

REM sleep is characterized by low-voltage, random fast waves, as in stage 1. Clients in REM sleep have the characteristic rapid eye movements, erratic respirations and changes in heart rate, and very low muscle tone (see Figure 17–1). During REM sleep, ventilation primarily depends on the movement of the diaphragm

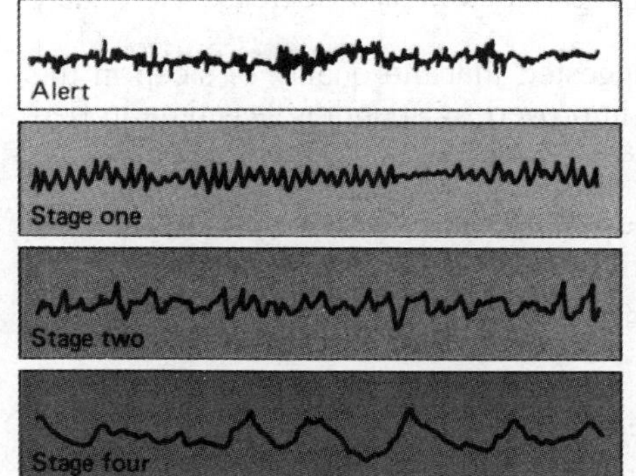

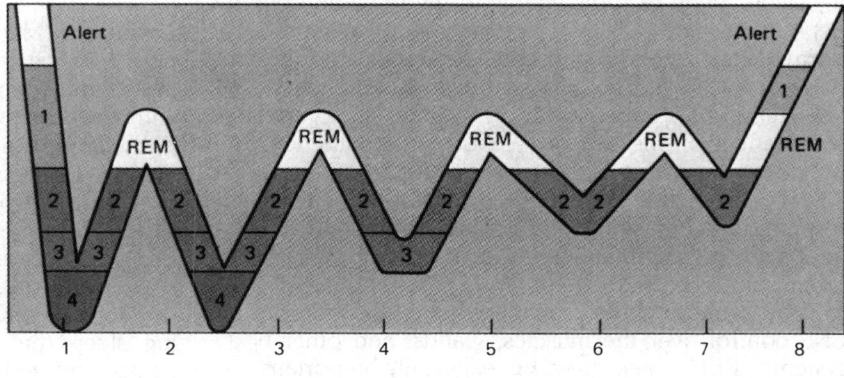

▲ *Figure 17–1*

A, The electrical activity of the brain during various stages of sleep can be shown on EEGs. *B*, During the night, a person goes through three to five cycles. Each cycle includes a sequence of sleep stages. (From Solomon, E. P., Schmidt, R. R., & Adranga, P. J. [1990]. Human anatomy and physiology [2nd ed.]. Philadelphia: Saunders College Publishing.)

because intercostal and accessory muscle tone is markedly diminished, and all postural and nonrespiratory muscles are essentially paralyzed.[39] The ventilatory response to hypoxia and hypercapnia is decreased. Thermoregulation is significantly reduced. Dreams in REM sleep are vivid, story-like, emotional, and bizarre.

Most persons move through an orderly progression of sleep stages from 1 to 4 and back through 3 to 2 before initiating a period of REM (see Fig. 17–2). Although this is the typical progression, it is not essential or always seen. Atypical progressions are characteristic of some of the sleep disorders, such as narcolepsy, in which REM is entered almost immediately after sleep onset.

In adults, each sleep cycle through the various stages lasts about 90 minutes. During the first few cycles, more time is spent in SWS, whereas later in the sleep period, the percentage of REM sleep increases.[43]

Wide variations exist among individuals in relation to sleep patterns.[43] By explaining the range of these variations, the nurse can help clients to seek a pattern that leaves them feeling reasonably refreshed and alert. Eight hours of undisturbed sleep at night with no daytime naps has become the assumed ideal pattern in North American society. However, some adults do well on 6 hours or less; other healthy adults require 10 hours or more of nighttime sleep. Even young adults often waken once or twice a night, and with aging, such wakenings are more frequent. New evidence suggests that humans may tend to have a biphasic sleep pattern similar to that followed in warmer climates, where the siesta is a normal part of the day's schedule.[10]

CHANGES IN SLEEP PATTERNS IN THE ELDERLY

The elderly spend more time in bed, take longer to fall asleep, have increased nocturnal wakefulness, and experience more sleepiness during the day than do younger adults.

With aging, the percentage of stage 4 decreases considerably and REM sleep decreases somewhat, with more time spent in stage 1. REM sleep is more evenly distributed through the night. Sleep latency, the time it takes to get to sleep, increases, as does the average length of time it takes to get back to sleep after arousal.[43] Elevated levels of norepinephrine and age-related respiratory dysfunction may be responsible for sleep fragmentation. Other problems, such as pain and nocturnal dyspnea, may also decrease effective sleep. About one third of the elderly experience sleep apnea, and this condition is exacerbated by the use of sleep medications.

Hospitalization affects the quality of sleep of both nocturnal and other sleep time for the elderly. There is often a lack of light and dark cues in the hospital and a lack of activity or exercise to cause fatigue. In addition, there are unfamiliar sights and sounds, and frequent awakenings for vital signs and other interventions that disturb sleep. Finally, the elderly client often is in a poorer state of health and has more worry, anxiety, tension, and fatigue than does an older adult who is not hospitalized. These factors also decrease the quality of sleep.

It has been suggested that the quality of sleep in the elderly might be improved by spending less time in bed during the day and avoiding sleep medications. Daytime sleepiness is often associated with nighttime wakefulness. This process starts with a cycle of daytime naps to compensate for inadequate nighttime sleep, followed by nighttime wakefulness due to daytime sleep.

THE NEED FOR SLEEP

A lot of information is known about the architecture of the sleep cycle, but much less is known about the need for sleep. Sleep restores energy to the brain and central nervous system (CNS). Sleep seems to restore both normal sensitivities of and balance among the different parts of the CNS. This process might be likened to the "resetting" of a baseline on a machine. Sleep also has some effect on the rest of the body. Sympathetic activity decreases, whereas parasympathetic activity occasionally increases. Arterial blood pressure, pulse, and respiration decrease; skin vessels dilate; the gastrointestinal system sometimes increases its activity; and skeletal muscle relaxes.

SWS is important for building protein and restoring CNS control over the muscles, glands, and other body systems. REM sleep may be especially important for maintaining mental activities, such as learning, reasoning, and emotional adjustment.

INCIDENCE

Almost one third of the general population has some problems with sleep during any given year. Among hospitalized clients, the incidence of sleep pattern disturbance has been found to range from 27 to 76.5 per cent.

ETIOLOGY

Sleep and sensory disturbances are frequently associated with illness and hospitalization. These disturbances may be secondary to situational and environmental stressors, or they may be associated with the illness itself or with pre-existing disorders. Often, the relationship is reciprocal, in that the disorder decreases sleep and the decreased sleep affects the disorder. The specific etiologies of various sleep disorders are covered in the discussion of each problem.

RISK FACTORS

Risk factors that reduce or prevent adequate sleep include drugs, such as caffeine and alcohol; sedatives and barbiturates, which alter the structure of sleep; stress; changes in the environment; and various disorders that have an impact on respiration during sleep.

CLINICAL MANIFESTATIONS AND MEDICAL MANAGEMENT

Dyssomnias

The dyssomnias are sleep disorders in which there is difficulty initiating or maintaining sleep (insomnias), or excessive sleepiness. These disorders may arise predominantly from within the body (intrinsic), from external sources (extrinsic), or from disruptions of circadian rhythm.[9] The intrinsic sleep disorders are discussed first.

INTRINSIC SLEEP DISORDERS

Insomnia. Many persons experience transitory periods during which they have difficulty initiating or maintaining sleep. The onset or exacerbation of illness with or without hospitalization may precipitate such difficulty. These sleep pattern disturbances are most often associated with disrupted or inconsistent sleep habits (*inadequate sleep hygiene*) or environmental disruptions. These disorders do not constitute insomnia, but they do predispose individuals to insomnia.

A much smaller proportion of the population have developed persistent difficulty in initiating or maintaining sleep that does not respond to improved sleep habits and removal of precipitating factors.[9] An estimated 4 to 5 per cent of the population define themselves as insomniacs.[48]

Psychophysiologic insomnia is characterized by learned sleep-preventing associations and heightened physiologic responses to stress.[9] The perceived difficulty sleeping can be confirmed by polysomnographic recording, which usually shows the same pattern of long sleep latency or fragmentation that the patient describes. The total sleep time is often within normal range but is felt to be inadequate, becoming a focal point of concern for the client. These persons often find that they can fall asleep unintentionally in low-stimulus situations such as watching television but feel increased arousal when they go to bed. They also may find it easier to get to sleep in places other than their usual bedroom, having become conditioned to their bedroom as a place of sleepless nights.

Management of insomnia is complex. Clients often feel that they have already tried the usual interventions to promote sleep. Sleep habits may be erratic out of a tendency to take advantage of whatever sleep they can get. Sleep should be consolidated or restricted by curtailing time in bed to the minimum believed necessary with a consistent rising time.[15] Relaxation exercises can be helpful but should initially be practiced at times other than bedtime so that by the time they are introduced at bedtime they are effective. Referral to a sleep specialist or psychologist who can work with the client over a period of time should be considered.

Narcolepsy. Narcolepsy is one of the disorders characterized by excessive sleepiness. The client experiences repeated episodes of drowsiness followed by brief naps, especially when engaged in monotonous activities. Most narcoleptic clients also experience *cataplexy*, a sudden loss of muscle tone at times of unexpected emotion (e.g., fright). Several other sleep-related abnormalities are commonly experienced by clients with narcolepsy. On initial wakening, they may experience *sleep paralysis* for 1 to several minutes, during which time they cannot move. This condition, like the other manifestations of narcolepsy, is thought to be linked to a malfunctioning of the mechanism controlling REM sleep, but the REM that is expressed is normal. It just occurs at the wrong time. Another REM-like manifestation is *hypnagogic hallucinations*, hallucinatory experiences that occur at sleep onset or awakening.[1] Some persons experience sleep paralysis or one of the other associated manifestations without narcolepsy, but when seen together with excessive sleepiness, they comprise the narcolepsy tetrad.[9]

On polysomnography, the most characteristic finding is sleep-onset REM periods. An multiple sleep latency test showing sleep latency of less than 5 minutes and REM periods occuring at sleep onset at least twice during the five test periods is used to confirm the diagnosis.[1, 22]

Susceptibility to narcolepsy is a genetically heterogeneous condition with autosomal dominance in some cases. The prevalence is about 0.3 to 1.6/1000 in the United States. The incidence is higher in Japan and lower in Israel.[1, 22]

The effects of the disease on lifestyle are significant, with 60 to 80 per cent of clients reporting episodes of having fallen asleep at work, driving, or both.[1] The associated disruption of social and occupational roles and self-esteem is a major contributing factor to the depression and personality disorders frequently seen in clients who have narcolepsy.[12] Impaired release of neurotransmitters such as dopamine may be a factor in both the narcolepsy and associated depression.[1]

Medical management for narcolepsy usually consists of low doses of stimulants to improve alertness and tricyclic antidepressants to control cataplexy.[1, 41]

Good sleep hygiene should be emphasized in counseling clients experiencing narcolepsy. It is important that they maintain a regular schedule with adequate nocturnal sleep. Regular naps at times that they are prone to increased sleepiness can be recommended. Safety is a major issue. Clients may need assistance in coping with the disruptive potential of their condition on family, work, and social roles.

Sleep Apnea Syndrome. Sleep apnea is characterized by recurrent periods of cessation of breathing for 10 seconds or longer occurring at least five times per hour. Sleep apnea can be differentiated as obstructive and central nervous system apnea.

Obstructive Sleep Apnea. In obstructive sleep apnea (OSA), respiratory efforts are apparent but ineffective against a collapsed or obstructed upper airway. As hypoxia ensues, the client eventually awakens to breathe. The frequent awakenings impair the normal sleep cycle. With sleep, the muscles of the upper airway relax and may occlude an airway that is already narrowed by enlarged soft tissue structures, jaw structure, or obesity. Repeated microarousals lead to excessive daytime sleepiness in most patients. A few, particularly the elderly, may present with insomnia.

OSA affects over 1 per cent of the adult male population.[25] A much smaller percentage progresses to the classic Pickwickian syndrome, characterized by obesity, severe sleep apnea, daytime hypercapnia, and cor pulmonale.[21]

Referral to a sleep disorders center should be considered for clients observed to have repeated periods of apnea (one a minute or more than 15 to 20 periods an hour) lasting longer than 10 seconds, whether or not these periods are associated with snoring. Because OSA is particularly common among males who are obese with short, thick necks and who are heavy snorers, these clients should be observed during sleep for apneic periods. Question clients regarding the degree of daytime sleepiness, with particular concern for safety in relation to driving and occupational activities.

Milder cases of OSA, in which excessive daytime sleepiness is not yet a concern, may respond to weight reduction and measures to facilitate sleeping in positions other than on the back. However, once the apneas are observed to occur most nights and in all body positions, more definitive treatment is usually required.

Many such clients regularly use continuous positive airway pressure (CPAP) and may bring a CPAP unit with them to the hospital. As at home, the CPAP mask should be applied securely over the nose, held in place by the headband, and turned on whenever the client is ready to go to sleep. Clients with OSA need to be closely monitored when recovering from anesthetic and receiving narcotics. A note should be made on the health record at the time of admission that the client has OSA. It is imperative that the anesthetist and recovery room staff are alerted. It may be requested that the CPAP unit accompany the client to the recovery room.

Question any order for benzodiazepines or other hypnotic drugs for clients with OSA, chronic obstructive pulmonary disease (COPD), or loud snoring.[12, 33] Teach clients with such conditions that alcohol also may worsen their symptoms because of its selective effect in relaxing the muscles of the upper airway and depression of arousal.

Uvulopalatopharyngoplasty is the most common surgical procedure for OSA. By resecting the uvula, posterior portion of the soft palate, tonsils, and any excessive pharyngeal tissue, the propensity to obstruction and snoring can be reduced in some patients.[44] Tracheostomy also may be required.

Central Sleep Apnea Syndrome. Central sleep apnea is characterized by apneic periods during which there is no apparent respiratory effort. It may be seen with CNS lesions, such as in stroke or brain stem involvement, but is most commonly mixed with obstructive sleep apnea. Cheyne-Stokes respirations are common. CPAP is the usual treatment. As with OSA, sedative and hypnotic drugs should be avoided. In severe cases with CNS involvement, use of diaphragmatic pacemakers or mechanical ventilation may be required.

Periodic Limb Movement Disorder. Another disorder that may contribute to daytime sleepiness and frequent nocturnal wakenings is periodic limb movement disorder. Originally described as nocturnal myoclonus, it is characterized by periodic episodes of repetitive, stereotypic leg movements that occur during sleep, causing partial arousals.[9, 23] The diagnosis can be confirmed during polysomnography with surface EMG of the anterior tibial muscles. Periodic limb movement disorder is common in the elderly. Clonazepam, a benzodiazepine, or baclofen, a skeletal muscle relaxant, may be ordered to diminish the magnitude of the movement and arousals. The anti-parkinsonian drug carbidopa-levodopa (Sinemet) and the tricyclic antidepressant, imipramine, seem to act more directly and almost eliminate the movements. However, most of the other tricyclic antidepressants aggravate the condition. For some clients, the use of transcutaneous electric nerve stimulation (TENS) before sleep has been found to be helpful.[23]

Restless Legs Syndrome. Restless legs syndrome involves annoying crawling sensations of the legs while at rest, which cause an almost irresistible urge to move.[9, 23] The syndrome is often most severe prior to sleep onset. Clients with restless legs syndrome almost always have periodic limb movements during sleep. Treatment is similar to that used for period limb movements.

EXTRINSIC SLEEP DISORDERS

All of the preceding dyssomnias are classified as intrinsic. The extrinsic sleep disorders encompass a range of factors from environmentally to chemically induced. Some factors temporarily present in hospitalized clients are discussed in the section on Hospital-Acquired Sleep Disturbances.

In the general population, the most frequently seen extrinsic sleep disorders are the circadian rhythm sleep disorders: *time zone change syndrome* and *shift work sleep disorder*. In taking a nursing history, be alert to a history of long-time shift work.

Elderly and chronically ill clients who live alone may be vulnerable to *irregular sleep-wake pattern*. In this disorder, the prolonged ignoring or absence of external cues to time, such as regular mealtimes, work periods, and daylight, leads to erratic periods of sleeping and wakefulness. Internal circadian cues may also be dampened as a result of aging or diffuse brain disease.[9, 14]

Management strategies for circadian rhythm disorders include maintenance of a regular schedule (e.g., persons who regularly work night shift are encouraged to maintain their same sleep schedule on nights off), and exposure to natural sunlight. Phototherapy is now being used in some situations to facilitate adjustments in circadian rhythms as well as in the treatment of seasonal affective disorder.[8, 24]

Parasomnias

The parasomnias are disorders that occur during sleep but that usually do not produce insomnia or excessive sleepiness.[9] The underlying pathologic mechanism may involve partial arousal or abnormalities in sleep-wake transition. As many as 5 per cent of Americans may suffer from some form of parasomnia.[14]

AROUSAL DISORDERS

Partial arousals typically occur during SWS.[9] *Sleep walking*, also known as somnambulism, may include semipurposeful behavior, such as dressing, but may be lacking in coordination and appropriateness, such as voiding in the closet. The occurrence of sleep walking in adults is often associated with anxiety.[14] *Sleep terrors* are sudden arousals from SWS accompanied by screaming, tachycardia, tachypnea, diaphoresis, and other manifestations of intense fear.[9] If awakened, the person is often disoriented and has little recall of the nature of the dream image. Sleep terrors typically occur in young children but may develop in adults.

SLEEP-WAKE TRANSITION DISORDERS

Sleep-wake transition disorders are common in the general population, rarely causing enough disruption to be legitimately called disorders. As mentioned earlier, *sleep starts* is the technical name for the sudden jerking movement of the legs that often occurs just as a person is falling asleep. The frequency and intensity may be greater with high caffeine intake, stress, or intense physical activity prior to going to bed. *Sleep talking* may also be more frequent during times of stress.

PARASOMNIAS ASSOCIATED WITH REM SLEEP

As with the other parasomnias, those associated with REM sleep may be distressing but are seldom serious. *Nightmares* are frightening dreams arising in REM sleep for which the person often has vivid and detailed recall on wakening. These dreams are in contrast to night terrors, which occur in SWS and for which there is little recall. *Sleep paralysis* is one of the classic signs of narcolepsy but can occur in isolation. At sleep onset or wakening, persons experience episodes of one to several minutes during which they are unable to move. This may be an extension of the normal state of low muscle tone during REM sleep.

OTHER PARASOMNIAS

These parasomnias are not specifically associated with a particular sleep stage. *Sleep bruxism* refers to grinding of the teeth during sleep and may lead to dental damage. *Sleep enuresis*, or bed-wetting, may occur in adults in association with other disorders such as OSA.[9] *Primary snoring* is distinguished from OSA by its rhythmic nature without episodes of apnea or hypoventilation.

Sleep Disorders Associated with Medical and Psychiatric Disorders

These secondary sleep disorders are of particular relevance in considering problems common to medical-surgical clients. Whereas some clients have a pre-existing sleep disorder of the dyssomnia or parasomnia type, other clients develop a sleep disorder as a secondary result of disease or its manifestations. By thinking of the physiology of normal sleep, the nurse can be alert to medical-surgical clients who are at particular risk for sleep pattern disturbance.

NEUROTRANSMITTER IMBALANCES

Neurotransmitter imbalances predispose persons to sleep pattern disturbances.[40] These imbalances may be disease related or drug induced.

Parkinson's disease is an example of a condition in which neurotransmitter imbalances may be related to sleep disorders. Over 70 per cent of persons being treated for Parkinson's disease, which results from a deficiency of the neurotransmitter dopamine, report sleep pattern disturbances.[9] Insomnia is the most frequent initial concern, followed by sleep fragmentation, disturbances in the sleep-wake schedule, and visual hallucinations. The factors that may contribute to sleep disturbance associated with Parkinson's disease are shown in Table 17–1.

Depression is accompanied by sleep disturbance in at least 90 per cent of persons.[9] Milder forms of depression and those occurring in young persons are often associated with sleep-onset insomnia; more major depressions are characterized by broken sleep and early morning wakening. There appears to be some relationship between the pathogenesis of depression and REM sleep mechanisms, in that depressed persons deprived of REM sleep often show improved mood.[33] The action of tricyclic antidepressants in suppressing REM sleep has been proposed as the primary mechanism underlying their effectiveness in treating depression.[40]

Neurotransmitter imbalances may also contribute to the sleep disturbances frequently seen in persons with *Alzheimer's disease* and other dementias. The most typical pattern with dementias is frequent wakenings, with agitation progressing to a loss of sleep-wake consolidation.[40] Assessment of sleep patterns, minimization of care giver–initiated wakenings (e.g., for toileting), and ensuring a regular bedtime may help to reduce nocturnal and daytime agitation.[6, 19] Because the incidence of sleep apnea is higher in individuals with Alzheimer's disease, possibly as a result of associated neuronal degeneration in the brain stem, the nocturnal respiratory patterns of these persons should be carefully assessed, with referral to a sleep disorders center if apnea is suspected.[18] The sleep-wake cycle may be completely reversed in the client with Alzheimer's disease. The client may nap during the daytime and be awake all night, restless, agitated, and wandering.

HEAD INJURY

Head injury of all degrees of severity affects sleep patterns. The appearance of differentiated sleep stages on EEG in comatose patients* with severe head injuries is a favorable prognostic indicator. Sleep stages indicate that connections between the brain stem, diencephalon, and telencephalon are intact and allowing shifts between NREM and REM sleep to occur.[2, 33] However,

* The term "patient" as used here refers to a comatose client who cannot be an active participant in care.

TABLE 17–1. Factors That May Contribute to Sleep Disturbance in Parkinson's Disease

Pathogenesis	Intermediary Factor	Sleep Disturbance
Primary		
Dopamine deficiency and associated neurotransmitter imbalance	Altered sleep-wake regulation	Sleep fragmentation. Reduced REM and slow wave sleep
Secondary		
Bradykinesia and rigidity	Reduced number of body shifts	Discomfort Wakenings to change position
Tremor and periodic leg movements.	Arousals	Daytime somnolence
Abnormal upper airway and chest wall motor activity (particularly when autonomic abnormalities are present)	Decreased depth and rate of breathing.	Wakenings. Daytime somnolence
Dementia (seen in some clients with Parkinson's disease)	Further breakdown of sleep-wake cycle	Wakenings. Daytime somnolence Increased confusion at night
Prolonged treatment with levodopa and bromocriptine	Medication-induced sleep disruption, with or without toxicity	Vivid dreaming, sleep terrors, myoclonus, and vocalizations

even in mild head injury, some degree of sleep disturbance may persist for several months after the injury.[35] Teaching clients and their families that this unsettled sleep is a typical part of *postconcussion syndrome* can allay anxiety and hasten functional recovery. For those clients in the confused-agitated stage of recovery resulting from more severe head injury, use of environmental cues such as light and darkness, regularity of daily schedule, and appropriate daytime exercise and activity can help to restore the sleep-wake cycle. Haloperidol (Haldol), which is often given to confused, agitated patients, blocks the activity of dopamine. This disruption in the delicate neurotransmitter balance may lead to insomnia. Thus, the health care team must balance the option of controlling agitated behavior with its associated high consumption of energy, with the undesirable side effect of increasing sleep fragmentation through medication (Table 17–2).[38]

HORMONAL IMBALANCES

Hormonal imbalances also contribute to sleep pattern disturbance. *Hyperthyroid* clients tend to have fragmented, short sleep periods with an excess of SWS.[14] *Hypothyroidism* is characterized by excessive sleepiness, and polysomnographic recordings show a reduction in the proportion of slow wave sleep.

Clients with *diabetes mellitus*, particularly type I, may experience hypoglycemic attacks during the night. Besides the usual symptoms of sweating, palpitations, hunger, and anxiety that the client may recognize as a hypoglycemic reaction, the nurse should be alert to complaints of nightmares and early morning headaches.[31] If these symptoms are present, blood sugar levels should be checked at regular intervals during the night. Insulin dosage or timing may need to be changed. Diabetic clients who have developed autonomic neuropathy have a higher prevalence of breathing abnormalities during sleep because of the associated dysfunction of autonomic control of respiration, and thus, nocturnal breathing patterns should be assessed in those with symptoms.[30]

Sleep patterns normally vary across the menstrual cycle in response to estrogen and progesterone levels. During the latter part of the cycle, when progesterone levels are higher, the first REM sleep period occurs earlier and some studies have shown sleep disturbances to be more frequent.[26, 49] Women with *premenstrual syndrome* tend to have less SWS throughout the menstrual cycle than their asymptomatic peers. *Postmenopausal* women are at higher risk for snoring and OSA.

RESPIRATORY DISORDERS

Nocturnal *asthmatic* attacks are common in cases of poorly managed asthma, contributing to frequent wakenings in up to 70 per cent of persons with asthma.[9, 49] Bronchial resistance increases during the early morning hours, even in healthy persons, as does sensitivity to histamine.

Chronic airway limitations (CAL), such as asthma and emphysema, contribute to difficulty initiating sleep, frequent arousals with shortness of breath or cough, and chronic fatigue. Oxygen saturation may fall, particularly during REM sleep, when ventilation depends on the diaphragm, which, in advanced CAL, is often flattened and inefficient.[20, 34] In addition, ventilation and perfusion are altered. Arrhythmias are common during sleep in clients with advanced respiratory disease, especially when oxygen saturation falls below 60 per cent.[9] Pulmonary artery pressure increases secondary to the pulmonary vascular constriction induced by the low oxygen desaturation and the destructive processes of the underlying disease.

Ventilatory responses to hypoxia and hypercapnia are decreased during sleep even in normal persons.[3] Clients with advanced respiratory disease are even more vulnerable, and therefore, hypnotics and other central nervous system depressants that depress arousal should be given with greater caution.

Some of the medications used in the treatment of CAL, such as the theophylline preparations, may contribute to insomnia. Anxiety and depression associated with effects of the disease may further exacerbate the tendency toward fragmented sleep. The nurse aims to provide a calm, secure, and relaxed environment for these clients. Stimulants such as caffeine may need to be avoided.

The recumbent posture for sleeping is problematic for many persons with respiratory disorders. They can be encouraged to use several pillows or have the head of the bed elevated; during acute episodes, they may find it more comfortable to sleep in a reclining chair.

CARDIOVASCULAR DISORDERS

Up to 25 per cent of *hypertensive* persons have been found to have OSA.[49] An association between snoring and hypertension has also been documented. Thus, it is important that nurses assess hospitalized clients who have hypertension or who snore while having repeated apneic periods during sleep.

In clients with severe *congestive heart failure*, periodic breathing of the Cheyne-Stokes type occurs, particularly during sleep stages 1 and 2, resulting in significant hypoxemia, frequent arousals, increased stage 1 sleep, and reduced total sleep time.[13]

The variability of heart and respiratory rates during REM sleep may be a factor in *nocturnal angina*.[49] Clients recovering from *myocardial infarction* are often deprived of sleep during their stay in a critical care unit and then may experience REM rebound on transfer to a step-down or standard unit. The greater cardiac demands during REM sleep may put some additional strain on the recovering heart, making continued nursing surveillance during this period particularly important.[27]

GASTROINTESTINAL DISORDERS

Gastric acid secretion normally decreases during sleep, but persons with *duodenal ulcers* have higher than average levels of secretion.[49] Recurrent wakenings with epigastric pain are common, especially in the first 4 hours after sleep onset,[9] and antacids or histamine antagonists may need to be administered.

Gastroesophageal reflux (heartburn) can be more

serious when it occurs during sleep because the longer exposure of the esophagus to gastric acid can lead to esophagitis.[33] Hypnotics should be used cautiously with these clients because the suppression of arousal makes them more vulnerable to esophagitis and pulmonary aspiration. In addition, the nurse may suggest that these clients avoid eating within 3 hours of bedtime, consider use of antacids or histamine antagonists, and in severe cases, raise the head of bed on blocks to decrease the likelihood of reflux and subsequent aspiration. Some forms of antacids cause slight regurgitation by effervescing (e.g., Gaviscon). These drugs can be extremely soothing to the lower esophagus.

OTHER DISORDERS

Numerous other disorders seem to have some impact on or association with sleep. Any condition that results in *pain* or *impaired mobility* has the potential to disrupt sleep. Various skin conditions such as atopic *eczema* are associated with decreased REM sleep.[49] Unrefreshing sleep and chronic fatigue along with diffuse musculoskeletal pain are among the diagnostic criteria for *fibrositis*. On EEG, persons with this condition often show a unique pattern of alpha waves intruding into SWS, producing what is called "alpha-delta activity."[9] Because the symptoms tend to be vague, clients

TABLE 17-2. Selected Drugs That Influence Sleep

Category Example	Action	Nursing Implications
Benzodiazepines	Sedative/hypnotic; thought to act at the level of limbic system and reticular formation; inhibit GABA	Consider half-life and duration of sedative effect Teach client to avoid alcohol and other CNS depressants Metabolized more slowly in the elderly, resulting in longer duration, lower dose
Triazolam (Halcion)	rapid acting (half-life 2 to 3 hours)	Effective for sleep-onset insomnia. Rebound insomnia may occur on discontinuation
Oxazepam (Serax)	half-life 10 to 25 hours	Given for its antianxiety effect; also enhances sleep maintenance
Diazepam (Valium)	half-life 20 to 100 hours	Observe for daytime drowsiness
Antihistamines Diphenhydramine (Benadryl)	Sedative effect as well as antihistamine	May decrease sleep latency
Narcotics Morphine	CNS depressant	REM rebound on discontinuation may lead to bizarre dreams
Antidepressants Amitriptyline (Elavil)	Most tricyclics have some sedative effect as well	Suppress REM May aggravate periodic limb movements
Fluoxetine (Prozac)	mild stimulant	May aggravate insomnia with initial use
Alcohol	CNS depressant	Decreases sleep latency but contributes to frequent wakenings Decreases REM and deep sleep Regular use leads to sleep disturbance that may persist long after withdrawal
Caffeine	CNS stimulant	Contributes to increased sleep latency and more frequent wakenings
Propranolol (Inderal)	Beta-adrenoceptor blocker that readily crosses the blood-brain barrier	May contribute to frequent wakenings
Antihypertensives Clonidine (Catapres)	Centrally acting sympatholytic	Suppresses REM May contribute to insomnia

CNS, central nervous system; GABA, gamma-aminobutyric acid; REM, rapid eye movement.

are often discouraged with the inability of health care professionals to diagnose and treat this condition. The nurse may be in a position to encourage referral of these persons to a sleep disorders center.

The effect of sleep or sleep deprivation on some disorders can be useful for diagnostic purposes. For example, the typical occurrence of erections in healthy males during REM sleep is being used as a diagnostic measure in differentiating sources of *impotence*.[33] These REM-associated erections are also the reason why the nurse needs to be careful when securing an in-dwelling catheter on any male client, allowing sufficient amount of loop to accommodate an erection.

Sleep deprivation and erratic sleep patterns reduce the seizure threshold, which is an important point for the nurse to consider in assessment and teaching of clients with *epilepsy*. Seizure activity may also be a cause of sleep disturbance. Partial and focal seizures can arise in all phases of sleep, including REM; generalized tonic-clonic seizures are more likely to occur during SWS than REM.[11] The tendency of sleep deprivation to trigger seizure activity is used diagnostically, in that clients may be required to stay awake all night prior to a sleep-deprived EEG. Some treatment regimens for clients susceptible to nocturnal seizures involve selective suppression by medication of those sleep stages in which the client's seizures most frequently occur.

Hospital-Acquired Sleep Disturbances

Persons may report difficulty getting to sleep, wakening frequently with difficulty getting back to sleep, or early morning wakening. The etiology and interventions are somewhat different.

Sleep-onset difficulty is a common problem in hospitals because of the strange environment and anxieties associated with illness and hospitalization. A sleep latency time of 20 to 30 minutes is within the normal range for most adults. Environmental control and conservative relaxation measures such as a back rub should be tried before resorting to a hypnotic. The short-acting hypnotics such as the benzodiazepine triazolam (Halcion) are most effective with this type of insomnia.

If a hypnotic is given, monitor the client's safety in getting up at night. Most hypnotics cause some degree of anterograde amnesia, meaning that otherwise cognitively intact clients may become somewhat disoriented, forgetting where they are. The longer acting hypnotics also result in some hangover effect. An increased risk of hip fractures from falls has been documented in persons who are taking long-acting benzodiazepines.[37]

Sleep maintenance disturbance may be associated with sustained use of or withdrawal from a variety of medications and related substances. Alcohol hastens sleep onset but leads to wakening later in the night. In acute intoxication, REM sleep is suppressed. Abrupt withdrawal, as occurs with hospitalization, may trigger massive REM rebound. In chronic alcoholics, sleep architecture remains disturbed even several years after abstinence. Sustained use of or withdrawal from antidepressants, monamine oxidase inhibitors, propranolol, and phenytoin can also contribute to insomnia.[42]

Other factors that contribute to sleep fragmentation include a variety of stimuli that tend to waken persons in the middle of the night. Internal stimuli, such as pain, discomfort, and the urge to void, are frequent disturbers of sleep. Sleep disorders, such as sleep apnea and periodic limb movement, are more frequently exhibited as excessive somnolence, but they do trigger wakenings from which some persons have difficulty getting back to sleep. Hospitalization provides an opportunity for nursing surveillance, which may be instrumental in detecting these disorders as distinct from those disturbances triggered by natural or transitory stimuli.

External stimuli include environmental factors, such as noise, light, and temperature, as well as disruptions from other persons. The nurse can reduce nocturnal stimuli by darkening the client's room. This can be accomplished by turning lights off (except for a small

NURSING RESEARCH

Sleep deprivation has been identified as a research priority by critical care nurses. It is thought to be a major factor in the development of intensive care unit psychosis, a state of delirium observed in 10 to 20 per cent of clients who have had open heart surgery. In this descriptive study, the investigators obtained polysomnographic recordings of the sleep patterns of 10 subjects during one or more of their first 3 nights in a critical care unit and compared them with 12 age- and sex-matched healthy subjects who slept in a sleep laboratory. The results indicated a wide variability among the critical care unit subjects but no significant differences among the 3 nights. The critical care subjects had significantly less total nocturnal sleep time, spent significantly more time awake and in stage 1 sleep, and had a significantly greater number of sleep stage shifts than did the healthy subjects. The sample size for this study was small, but the results are comparable to those of similar studies.

The authors suggest implications for critical care nurses based on the study results and their personal observations during data collection regarding noise and light control, postponement of routine laboratory work and nursing care until clients waken, and spacing of monitoring to allow sustained periods of uninterrupted sleep.

Their findings have implications for medical-surgical nurses as well. Clients transferred from critical care units can anticipate experiencing some degree of sleep deprivation. Besides planning interventions to promote sleep for these clients, nurses working with all types of hospitalized clients should monitor care-giver wakenings, and noise and light levels in client sleeping areas.

▼▼▼

Richards, K. C., & Bairnsfather, L. (1988). A description of night sleep patterns in the critical care unit. *Heart & Lung*, *17*(1), 35–42.

night light for safety purposes) and closing curtains. To reduce nocturnal stimuli the nurse may also reduce as many sources of noise as possible, such as avoiding unnecessary conversation, minimizing equipment noise, and closing the client's door, if possible. Also, the nurse may adjust the temperature by providing bed coverings according to client preference, and by modifying room temperature directly by adjusting the thermostat or air conditioner when possible, or indirectly through closing curtains and adjusting ventilation. The nurse may also remove disturbing objects to create a pleasant, tidy environment. An example is removing equipment associated with painful procedures. Other means of reducing nocturnal stimuli include spacing necessary care-giving activities (e.g., turning, taking vital signs) to allow periods of 90 minutes or more of undisturbed sleep and, where possible, synchronizing these activities with periods when the client is already awake. Finally, the nurse may coordinate the nature and timing of interruptions by other care givers (e.g., for laboratory testing or chest physiotherapy) to preserve periods of undisturbed sleep.

Early-morning wakening is frequently seen among the elderly. Sensitivity to environmental disturbances increases toward morning for all age groups but even more so for the elderly. Clients who are disturbed by early morning wakening should be screened for indications of depression.

Sleep deprivation is of particular concern for clients in critical care units. The noise level, 24-hour lighting, and frequency of care-giver interruptions create a situation of sensory overload and sleep deprivation, which is thought to be a major contributing factor to postoperative psychosis (see Nursing Research).[43]

Clients who have had *surgery* are also at risk for sleep pattern disturbance. The etiology is unclear but may be related to the length and type of anesthetic, postoperative analgesia, or mechanisms associated with the procedure itself.[4, 33, 49] REM and SWS are suppressed. Whereas recovery to presurgical patterns is fairly rapid following more minor surgery such as herniorrhaphy, it may take 4 to 6 weeks for the client's sleep patterns to return to normal after open heart surgery with cardiopulmonary bypass. Specific assessment of sleep quality and quantity should be incorporated into the care of all surgical patients.

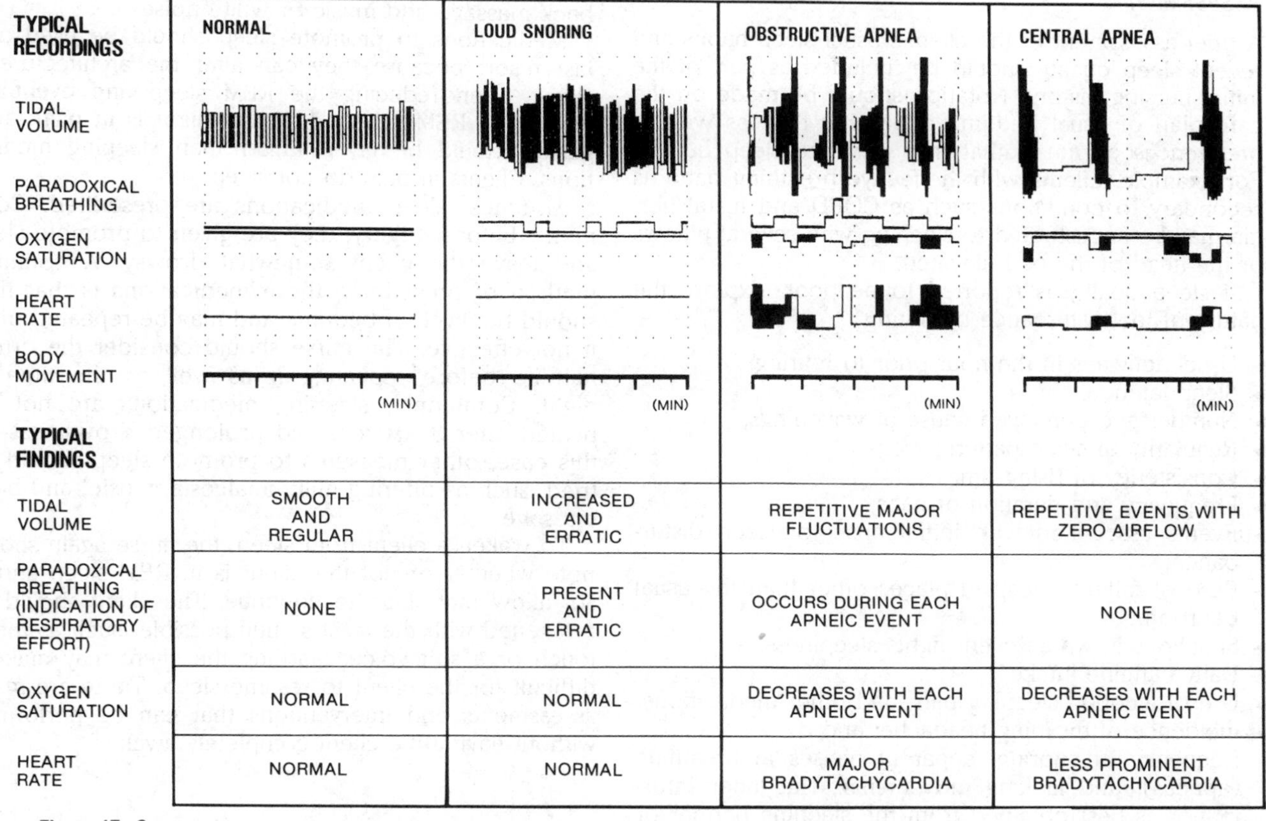

TYPICAL RECORDINGS
NORMAL
LOUD SNORING
OBSTRUCTIVE APNEA
CENTRAL APNEA
TIDAL VOLUME
PARADOXICAL BREATHING
OXYGEN SATURATION
HEART RATE
BODY MOVEMENT
(MIN)
(MIN)
(MIN)
(MIN)
TYPICAL FINDINGS
TIDAL VOLUME
SMOOTH AND REGULAR
INCREASED AND ERRATIC
REPETITIVE MAJOR FLUCTUATIONS
REPETITIVE EVENTS WITH ZERO AIRFLOW
PARADOXICAL BREATHING (INDICATION OF RESPIRATORY EFFORT)
NONE
PRESENT AND ERRATIC
OCCURS DURING EACH APNEIC EVENT
NONE
OXYGEN SATURATION
NORMAL
NORMAL
DECREASES WITH EACH APNEIC EVENT
DECREASES WITH EACH APNEIC EVENT
HEART RATE
NORMAL
NORMAL
MAJOR BRADYTACHYCARDIA
LESS PROMINENT BRADYTACHYCARDIA

▲ **Figure 17–2**

Polysomnography used to determine the presence of sleep disorders. These examples are taken from a screening system that may be used in a person's home (as opposed to a laboratory), where sleep patterns are more typical. Screening studies can differentiate between obstructive (i.e., peripheral) sleep apnea and central sleep apnea, as well as loud snoring and normal sleep patterns. When a sleep disorder is identified, further assessment is needed, including EEG and ECG readings to further define the cause of the problem. (Courtesy of Vitalog, Mountain View, CA.)

Diagnostic Assessment

The primary diagnostic test for sleep disorders is polysomnography (Figure 17–2). Clients may be referred to a sleep disorders center for an over-night recording of EEG, electrooculograph (EOG), and submental electromyograph (EMG) from surface electrodes. Depending on the purpose of the investigation, other types of monitoring may include continuous recording of arterial oxygen saturation by ear or finger oximeter, airflow as detected by monitoring expired CO_2, respiratory movements by means of transducers placed around the chest and abdomen, and electrocardiograph (ECG) and heart rate from standard limb leads.

A multiple sleep latency test may also be performed to assess impairment of daytime alertness. The multiple sleep latency text is performed following a standard overnight polysomnogram. The time required for clients to fall asleep when in a relaxed state is evaluated at 2-hour intervals, with each nap limited to 10 minutes. The type of sleep is also assessed, making the test particularly useful in diagnosing narcolepsy, a condition in which clients typically have sleep-onset REM periods.[47]

Nursing Management

ASSESSMENT

A brief assessment of the client's usual sleep habits and recent sleep quality should be included as part of the initial nursing history. Notation should be made on the care plan of usual bedtime and rising time as well as preferences or rituals that may enhance sleep quality. For example, clients with ineffective breathing patterns secondary to conditions such as COPD and hiatal hernia may be accustomed to sleeping with several pillows or the head of the bed elevated.

If sleep quality is reported to be poor, explore the nature of the disturbance by noting

- Usual activities in the hour prior to retiring;
- Sleep latency;
- Number and perceived cause of wakenings;
- Regularity of sleep pattern;
- Consistency of rising time;
- Frequency and duration of naps;
- Events associated with initial onset of sleep disturbance;
- Ease of falling asleep in places other than the usual bedroom;
- Situations in which client fights sleepiness;
- Daily caffeine intake;
- Use of alcohol, sleeping pills, and other medications;
- incidence of morning headache; and
- frequency of snoring, apparent pauses in breathing (apneas), and kicking movements. The latter information is best obtained from the sleeping partner or observed by a nurse while the client is in the hospital.

Objective data may include visible signs of fatigue and lack of sleep, such as induration of the eyes, lack of coordination, drowsiness, and irritability.

NURSING INTERVENTION

Nursing Diagnosis: Sleep Pattern Disturbance R/T hospitalization.

Planning: Expected Outcomes. The client will have improved sleep patterns within 48 hours as evidenced by sleeping for 6 to 8 hours at one time, stated feeling of less fatigue, and, decreased irritability.

Implementation. The client's usual bedtime routine should be followed as closely as possible. For example, if the client watches television before sleeping, attempt to make this possible. Nursing assessments and interventions should be scheduled into blocks of time to allow 90 to 120 minutes of uninterrupted sleep. If the client is noted to be in REM sleep (by seeing the eyes move about), the nurse should not wake the client but wait until that sleep cycle is over. The environment should mimic nighttime, with lights dimmed and quiet maintained. External warmth with extra blankets should be offered. Milk has tryptophan, which promotes sleep, and should be offered if the client's condition allows its use. Other techniques used to promote sleep include back massage and music or white noise.

Medications to promote sleep should be used as a last resort because they can alter the architecture of sleep, often reducing the REM sleep and eventually leading to REM rebound. If the client is in pain, analgesics should be given rather than sleeping medications. Clients in pain do not sleep.

At times, sleep medications are prescribed. Commonly before surgery, they are given to promote sleep and leave the client somewhat drowsy. A common method of prescribing these medications is that they should be given at bedtime and may be repeated once if not effective. The nurse should consider the drug's half-life before repeating it as well as the time of night. Commonly, sleeping medications are not repeated after 3 AM to avoid prolonged drowsiness. In this case, other measures to promote sleep should be tried, such as offering milk, analgesia, music, and back massage.

To waken a client from sleep, the nurse again should note whether or not the client is in REM sleep and, if so, allow that stage to continue. The client should be awakened with the least stimuli possible, such as a soft touch or a soft voice. Startling the client may make it difficult for the client to resume sleep. There are many assessments and interventions that can be performed without having the client completely awake.

EVALUATION

The degree of expected outcome attainment should be determined and revisions made in the intervention or outcomes. Many sleep disturbances are due to the effects of aging and cannot be corrected at all; others are temporary and due to the stress of hospitalization. These temporary stress problems may be corrected only after the client returns home.

Follow-Up Care

Clients with sleep disturbances may need follow-up care with repeated studies to determine whether or not the problem was corrected. The elderly client should be taught about the effects of aging on sleep and how to make the most of the new sleep patterns. Clients with long-term sleep disorders need ongoing care to determine the effectiveness of the treatments.

HOSPITAL-ACQUIRED SENSORY DISTURBANCES

Each person has an optimal level of sensory input that facilitates a sense of well-being and optimal cognitive and motor performance.[29] Sensory input comes from environmental and internal sources. Sensory input is received through peripheral receptors, transmitted via afferent neurons up the spinal cord, and channeled through the hypothalamus to the cortex, where it is interpreted in relation to previous patterns of experience.

Persons at risk for sensory overload or deprivation include those who are experiencing

A new or unfamiliar environment,
Altered sensory input, and
Altered cognitive processing.

Classification

SENSORY OVERLOAD

Sensory overload is a state in which the degree and nature of sensory input exceeds the tolerance level of the individual, resulting in feelings of distress and hyperarousal with impaired thinking and problem-solving ability.

SENSORY DEPRIVATION

Sensory deprivation is a state in which the overall sensory input is decreased. With the overall reduction in stimuli, persons become more sensitive to the stimuli that are present in the environment and often supplement it with increasing internal stimuli, such as by daydreaming or reminiscing.[46]

Prevention

The nurse can minimize the risk of sensory disturbances by explaining not only procedures but also the sights and sounds in the client's environment (e.g., the intercom).

Clients who have had limited prior experience with hospitalization or with aspects of the related technology are at risk for sensory overload because they lack memories and knowledge to make sense out of much of their new environment.

Likewise, clients whose sensory input is restricted or distorted are at risk for sensory deprivation in the sense that the stimuli are inappropriate to their needs. For example, a client with a spinal cord injury may be kept in a supine position for several weeks during which time the field of vision is limited to the ceiling and the portions of the room that can be seen from each side.

Another major high-risk group of clients are those experiencing alterations in thought processes such as occur with stroke, head injury, or Alzheimer's disease. Explanations for these clients should be kept simple and concrete. The environment should be structured and simplified, with the incorporation of normalizing cues (e.g., drapes open to sunlight, and familiar pictures and objects).

Associated factors that can increase the risk of sensory overload include confinement, lack of ability to control the environment, and pressures relating to time, decision making, and complex task performance.[29]

Consider the risks for an elderly, slightly deaf woman recovering from a fractured hip. She is confined to bed for much of the day except for her physiotherapy session and short walks with the nurses. Learning to use the walker is a complex task. The faces surrounding her are strange. It is difficult to hear what the nurses are saying, so she just nods. She does hear a hissing, gurgling sound coming from above her head. She does not know that the sound comes from oxygen bubbling through water for humidification. She also hears a name that sounds like hers come booming out of the wall occasionally. She does not understand about intercom systems. The nights are the worst because then everything looks strange and unfamiliar.

This inability to integrate incoming stimuli may be exhibited as confusion.[36] Sensory overload from an excess of poorly understood environmental stimuli may be superimposed on disturbed cerebral metabolism from electrolyte disturbance, drugs, organic brain disease, and cardiopulmonary problems.[36, 45] The nurse should monitor the client for abnormal laboratory values and possible drug toxicity or interactions, with particular attention to implications of slower metabolic processes in elderly persons.[33] For more information on assessing the confused patient, see Chapter 29.

Summary

The adequacy of sleep and rest, and the appropriateness of the quality and degree of sensory stimulation are important factors to consider in caring for clients with acute or chronic illness. In this chapter, disorders of sleep and sensory stimulation have been discussed with consideration of the reciprocity between these processes, illness, and hospitalization. The nurse can play a pivotal role in environmental modification and client teaching to minimize the impact of sleep and sensory disturbances.

Bibliography

1. Aldrich, M. S. (1990). Narcolepsy. *The New England Journal of Medicine, 323*(6), 389-394.
2. Alexandre, A., Colombo, F., Nertempi, P., & Benedetti, A. (1983). Cognitive outcome and early indices of severity of head injury. *Journal of Neurosurgery, 59*, 751-761.
3. Anthonisen, N. R., & Kryger, M. (1986). Sleep and breathing in patients with lung disease. In N. Edelman & T. Santiago (Eds.), *Breathing disorders of sleep* (pp. 205-224). New York: Churchill-Livingstone.
4. Aurell, J., & Elmquist, D. (1985). Sleep in the surgical intensive care unit: Continuous polygraphic recording of sleep in nine patients receiving postoperative care. *British Medical Journal, 290*, 1029-1032.
5. Closs, J. (1988). Patients' sleep-wake rhythms in hospital: Part 2. *Nursing Times, 84*(2), 54-55.
6. Cohen-Mansfield, J., & Marx, M. S. (1990). The relationship between sleep disturbances and agitation in a nursing home. *Journal of Aging Health, 2*(1), 42-57.
7. Cox, H. C., Hinz, M. D., Lubno, M. A., Newfield, S. A., Ridenour, N. A., & Sridaromont, K. L. (1989). *Clinical applications of nursing diagnosis*. Baltimore: Williams & Wilkins.
8. Czeisler, C. A., & Allan, J. S. (1988). Pathologies of the sleep-wake cycle. In R. L. Williams, I. Karacan, & C. A. Moore (Eds.), *Sleep disorders: Diagnosis and treatment* (2nd ed., pp. 109-129). New York: John Wiley & Sons.
9. Diagnostic Classification Steering Committee, Thorpy MJ, Chairman (1990). *International classification of sleep disorders: Diagnostic and coding manual*. Rochester, MN: American Sleep Disorders Association.
10. Dinges, D. F., & Broughton, R. J. (1989). *Sleep and alertness: Chronobiological, behavioral and medical aspects of napping*. New York: Raven Press.
11. Feldman, R. (1983). Management of underlying causes and precipitating factors in epilepsy. In T. Browne, & R. Feldman (Eds.), *Epilepsy: Diagnosis and management* (pp. 129-138). Toronto: Little Brown & Co.
12. Fredrickson, P. A., Richardson, J. W., Esther, M. S., & Lin, S. (1990). Sleep disorders in psychiatric practice. *Mayo Clinic Proceedings, 65*, 861-868.
13. Hanly, P. J., Willar, T. W., Steljes, D. G., Baert, R., Frais, M. A., & Kryger, M. H. (1989). Respiration and abnormal sleep in patients with congestive heart failure. *Chest, 96*(3), 480-488.
14. Hauri, P. J. (1982). *The sleep disorders: Current concepts*. Kalamazoo, MI: Upjohn.
15. Hauri, P. J., & Exther, M. S. (1990). Insomnia. *Mayo Clinic Proceedings, 65*, 869-882.
16. Hickey, J. (1986). *Neurological and neurosurgical nursing* (2nd ed.). Philadelphia: J. B. Lippincott.
17. Hobson, J. A. (1988). Homeostasis and heteroplasticity: Functional significance of behavioral state sequences. In R. Lydic & J. F. Biebuyck (Eds.), *Clinical physiology of sleep* (pp. 199-220). Bethesda, Maryland: American Physiological Society.
18. Hoch, C. C., Reynolds III, C. F., & Houck, P. R. (1987). Sleep apnea in Alzheimer's patients and the healthy elderly. *Scholarly Inquiry for Nursing Practice, 1*(3), 221-235.
19. Hoch, C. C., Reynolds III, C. F., & Houck, P. R. (1988). Sleep patterns in Alzheimer, depressed and healthy elderly. *Western Journal of Nursing Research, 10*(3), 239-256.
20. Johnson, M. W., & Jemmers, J. E. (1984). Accessory muscle activity during sleep in chronic obstructive pulmonary disease. *Journal of Applied Physiology, 57*(4), 1011-1017.
21. Kaplan, J., & Staats, B. A. (1990). Obstructive sleep apnea syndrome. *Mayo Clinic Proceedings, 65*, 1087-1094.
22. Karacan, I., & Howell, J. W. (1988). Narcolepsy. In R. L. Williams, I. Karacan, C. A. Moore (Eds.), *Sleep disorders: Diagnosis and treatment* (pp. 85-105). New York: John Wiley & Sons.
23. Krueger, B. R. (1990). Restless legs syndrome and periodic movements of sleep. *Mayo Clinic Proceedings, 65*, 999-1006.
24. Lahaie, U. (1991). Shift-workers and seasonal affective disorder. *Canadian Nurse, 87*(5), 33-34.
25. Lavie, P. (1983). Incidence of sleep apnea in a presumably healthy working population: A significant relationship with excessive daytime sleepiness. *Sleep, 6*(4), 312-318.
26. Lee, K. A., Shaver, J. F. A., Giblin, E. C., & Woods, N. F. (1990). Sleep patterns related to menstrual cycle phase and premenstrual affective symptoms. *Sleep, 13*(5), 403-409.
27. Littrell, K. D., & Schumann, L. L. (1989). Promoting sleep for the patient with a myocardial infarction. *Critical Care Nurse, 9*(3), 44, 46-49.
28. Lipowski, Z. J. (1983). Transient cognitive disorders (delirium, acute confusional states) in the elderly. *American Journal of Psychiatry, 140*(11), 1426-1436.
29. Lipowski, Z. J. (1975). Sensory and information inputs overload: Behavioral effects. *Comprehensive Psychiatry, 16*(3), 199-221.
30. Lugaresi, E., Cirignotta, F., Mondini, S., Montagna, P., & Zucconi, M. (1988). Sleep in clinical neurology. In R. L. Williams, I. Karacan, C. A. Moore, (Eds.), *Sleep disorders: Diagnosis and treatment* (2nd ed., pp. 245-263). New York: John Wiley & Sons.
31. McCance, K. L., & Huether, S. E. (1990). *Pathophysiology: The biologic basis for disease in adults and children*. St. Louis: C. V. Mosby.
32. Mitchell, P. H. (1988). Consciousness: An overview. In P. H. Mitchell, L. C. Hodges, M. Muwaswes, & C. A. Walleck (Eds.), *AANN's neuroscience nursing* (pp. 57-66). Norwalk, CT: Appleton & Lange.
33. Orr, W. C. (1985). Sleep pathophysiology in medicine and surgery. In T. Riley (Ed.), *Clinical aspects of sleep and sleep disturbance* (pp. 159-180). Toronto: Butterworth Publishers.
34. Parkosewich, J. A. Sleep-disordered breathing: A common problem in chronic obstructive pulmonary disease. *Critical Care Nurse 6*(6), 60-64.
35. Parsons, L. C., & Ver Beek, D. (1982). Sleep-awake patterns following cerebral concussion. *Nursing Research 31*(5), 260-264.
36. Rasin, J. H. (1990). Confusion. *Nursing Clinics of North America, 25*(4), 909-918.
37. Ray, W., Griffen, M., & Downey, W. (1989). Benzodiazepines of long and short elimination half-life and the risk of hip fracture. *JAMA, 262*(23), 3303-3307.
38. Reimer, M. (1989). Sleep pattern disturbances related to neurological dysfunction. *Axon, 10*(3), 65-68.
39. Remmers, J. E. (1990). Sleeping and breathing. *Chest 97*, 77S-80S.
40. Reynolds III, C. F., & Kuppfer, D. J. (1987). Sleep research in affective illness: State of the art circa 1987. *Sleep 10*(3), 199-215.
41. Richardson, J. W., Fredrickson, P. A., Siong-Chi, L. (1990). Narcolepsy update. *Mayo Clinic Proceedings*, 65, 991-998.
42. Robinson, C. (1986). Impaired sleep. In V. K. Carrieri, A. M. Lindsey, & C. M. West (Eds.), *Pathophysiological phenomena in nursing* (pp. 390-417). Philadelphia: W. B. Saunders.
43. Shaver, J. L., & Giblin, E. C. (1989). Sleep. *Annual Review of Nursing Research, 7*, 71-93d.
44. Shepard, J. W., & Olsen, K. D. (1990). Uvulopalatopharyngoplasty for treatment of obstructive sleep apnea. *Mayo Clinic Proceedings, 65*, 1260-1267.
45. Sloane, P. D., & Mathew, L. J. (1990). The therapeutic environment screening scale. *The American Journal of Alzheimer's Care and Related Disorders & Research*, 22-26.
46. Suedfeld, P. (1985). Stressful levels of environmental stimulation. *Issues in Mental Health Nursing, 7*, 83-104.
47. Thorpy, M. (1988). Diagnosis, evaluation, and classification of sleep disorders. In R. L. Williams, I. Karacan, & C. A. Moor (Eds.), *Sleep disorders: Diagnosis and treatment* (2nd ed.; pp. 9-25). New York: John Wiley & Sons.
48. Welstein, L., Dement, W. C., Redington, D., Guilleminault, C., & Mitler, M. M. (1983). Insomnia in the San Francisco Bay Area: A telephone survey. In C. Guilleminault & E. Lugaresi, (Eds.), *Sleep/wake disorders: Natural history, epidemiology, and long-term evaluation* (pp. 73-85). New York: Raven Press, 1983.
49. Williams, R. L. (1988). Sleep disturbances in various medical and surgical conditions. In R. L Williams, I. Karacan, & C. A. Moore, Sleep disorders: Diagnosis and treatment (2nd ed.). New York: John Wiley & Sons.

Wound Healing

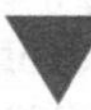

This chapter focuses on tissue injury and repair. Injury is common and is seen in clients who sustain trauma and those who have undergone surgery. Another group of clients with tissue injury are those with pressure ulcers. In the latter part of this chapter, pressure ulcers are closely studied.

Tissue injury is common, and the body is well equipped with mechanisms of defense. These defense mechanisms include intact skin and mucous membranes, phagocytes within the blood, and the immune and inflammatory responses.

STRUCTURE AND FUNCTION OF THE DEFENSE MECHANISMS

FIRST-LINE DEFENSE MECHANISMS

The first line of defense includes the skin and other organs and secretions to reduce the risk of injury. When these systems function normally, little tissue injury occurs (Table 18-1). Of course, many agents are able to overcome the structural, chemical, or biologic defenses. When invasion or trauma occurs, the second line of defenses is set into action.

SECOND-LINE DEFENSE MECHANISMS

The white blood cells (WBCs) provide the major second line of defense. These defense mechanisms are called general or nonspecific responses because they occur in response to any form of injury. In addition to the WBCs, the immune system provides antibodies. The second-line defenses are examined first by their structure (cell type) and then by their function (cell processes).

TABLE 18-1. Nonspecific First-Line Defense Mechanisms

Type of Defense	Defense Mechanism
Organ-Based	
Skin and mucous membrane	Surface cells provide a waterproof shield; membranes emit a secretion that traps foreign material and microorganisms
Lymph nodes	Filter and devour foreign materials; house lymphocytes and monocytes
Spleen	Contains masses of lymphocytes (called nodules); filters blood slowly to allow lymphocytes a greater chance of coming into contact with microorganisms
Liver	Houses macrophages, called Kupffer cells; filters and purifies portal system blood
Bone Marrow	Produces blood cells
Mechanical	
Flushing action of body fluids	Sweeps bacteria from the body
Chemical	
Perspiration	Contains acetic acid and salt, which kill pathogens
Gastrointestinal fluids	Highly acidic secretions kill pathogens
Vaginal secretions	Acids produced by harmless bacteria to control growth of other pathogens
Enzymes	Lysozyme, an enzyme present in tears, saliva, mucus and skin secretions as well as many cells and internal fluids, works in tandem with blood cells to combat pathogens
Biological	
Flora	Inhibit the growth of pathogens

Structure

LEUKOCYTES

The term leukocyte means white blood cell, and it is a general name for many types of WBCs. Leukocytes are a powerful mobile defense system. These cells originate from stem cells in the bone marrow. There are two major types of mature leukocytes: granular and agranular. Some leukocytes mature in the bone marrow and others mature at various body sites. Leukocytes are released into the circulation at the time of injury and migrate to the sites of injury.

Granular Leukocytes. Granular leukocytes are formed in the bone marrow. There are three types of granular leukocytes: (1) neutrophils, (2) eosinophils, and (3) basophils. The names given to these cells are derived from their appearance after staining. Neutrophils stain a neutral color, eosinophils stain red, and basophils stain blue. The granules (sacs of fluid) in granular leukocytes contain potent enzymes that destroy ingested bacteria, stimulate tissue response to allergens, and mediate inflammation.

Neutrophils. Neutrophils are sometimes called polymorphonuclear leukocytes (PMNs or polys) because of their irregularly shaped nuclei. Neutrophils compose about 60 per cent of the circulating WBCs. They are a vital defense mechanism because they are both the first and most numerous cell type to arrive at any area of disease or injury. Their role, along with tissue macrophages, is to phagocytize injurious agents.

Eosinophils. Eosinophils are granulocytes that have a large number of lysosomes containing (1) biochemical mediators to inactivate serotonin and histamine and (2) a caustic protein capable of dissolving the surface membrane of parasites. Eosinophils play a major role in allergic reactions by releasing enzymes to inactivate histamine. Eosinophil levels increase in clients with allergic responses and those with parasitic infections, such as malaria.

Basophils. The third type of granulocyte is the basophil. Basophils represent less than 1 per cent of the circulating WBCs. Despite their small number, they are important defense mechanisms. Basophils increase in number during inflammation and with allergy. Basophils are similar to mast cells. Both cells release leukotrienes and prostaglandins, histamine, bradykinin, and serotonin into the circulation. These vasoactive substances mediate inflammation.

Agranular Leukocytes. Agranular leukocytes are the second major group of leukocytes and include lymphocytes and monocytes.

Lymphocytes. The lymphocytes are formed in the lymphoid tissues of the tonsils, intestines, and bone marrow, and they mature in the lymph nodes, thymus, and spleen. Lymphocytes are fairly numerous small cells, forming about 25 to 33 per cent of the total WBC count. Lymphocytes are controlled by the adrenocortical hormones. Therefore, clients on steroid therapy have decreased numbers of lymphocytes as well as atrophy of lymphoid tissues. This change places the steroid-dependent client at increased risk of infection.

There are two types of lymphocytes: *bursal-equivalent lymphocytes* or B cells and *thymus-derived lymphocytes* or T cells. T and B cells provide specific immune responses. T cells provide cell-mediated immunity and B cells provide antibody-mediated immunity. Both types of cells are produced in and are released from the bone marrow. On their way to the lymphatic tissues, future T cells stop in the thymus for processing. There are three types of T cells. The first type are cytotoxic T cells, sometimes called killer T cells. These cells recognize cells with foreign antigens on their surface and destroy them, without the assistance of complement. The second type are helper T cells, which assist other T cells. The third type are suppressor T cells, which inhibit the activity of the helper and cytotoxic T cells. B cells mature in a lymphatic organ in animals, called the bursa of Fabricus, but an equivalent organ has not been found in humans. However, in humans, B cells are processed as they form. B cells provide immunity by producing antibodies through plasma cells. Plasma cells are the cells that produce antibodies and release them into the circulation. B lymphocytes also generate antibodies that neutralize toxins and, in conjunction with complement, can lead to bacterial destruction.

The immunoglobulins provide a specific form of immunity rather than producing a general response such as that provided by the leukocytes. The immunoglobulins are capable of remembering past contact with pathogens (in this case called antigens). They produce antibodies with specific memory for certain antigens. This form of defense is seen most often in transplant rejection, and hypersensitivity reactions (see Chap. 24).

Monocytes. Monocytes are leukocytes that have a similar function to the neutrophils. They migrate to areas of injury, but they arrive slowly and do so in smaller numbers, but their lifespan is 3 to 4 times longer than that of the neutrophil. A large portion of monocytes enter the tissues and become macrophages. In the tissue, these cells continue to phagocytize large numbers of bacteria. If the need arises, these cells can reenter the circulation and become mobile macrophages.

TISSUE MACROPHAGE SYSTEM

The tissue macrophage system consists of mobile macrophages and fixed tissue macrophages. Collectively, this system has been called the reticuloendothelial system. These cells are like sentries and are located strategically throughout the body, waiting to act. Fixed macrophages are found in the lymph nodes, spleen, liver, lungs, blood vessels, and bone marrow. The tissue macrophages have differing names depending on their location (Fig. 18-1). The mobile macrophages are called monocytes (see earlier). Like the other phagocytes, macrophages ingest, neutralize, and destroy foreign substances and organisms. For example, macrophages entrap old red blood cells and prepare the hemoglobin for reprocessing. In addition to phagocytosis, the macrophage secretes angiogenesis factor. This substance stimulates the formation of new blood vessels from the ends and sides of severed vessels. Macrophages are inactivated by tissue hypoxia. Most important, the macrophage forms antibodies to combat infections.

PLATELETS

Platelets, also called thrombocytes, are not complete cells. They are tiny fragments of membrane-enclosed cytoplasm that are pinched off from megakaryocytes, which are giant cells in the bone marrow. Each megakaryocyte can yield several thousand platelets. Platelets have no nucleus so their lifespan is brief, typically less than 10 days.

CELLULAR PRODUCTS

There are three cellular products that also assist the body in its fight against invaders: (1) interferon, (2) interleukins, and (3) lymphokines.

Interferon. Interferon produces an antiviral protein. It does not kill viruses but prevents them from infecting healthy cells. When they are invaded by viruses or other organisms (such as bacteria, fungi and protozoa), some cells secrete interferon. Once a cell has been exposed to interferon, the new viruses that are produced in it are less able to infect other cells. Interferon has no effect on cells already infected with a virus. Interferons also stimulate natural killer (NK) cells. NK cells recognize body cells that have been altered by viruses and quickly destroy them before they can multiply. Interferon has been used in the treatment of viral infection and cancer. Recombinant DNA techniques have been used to produce interferon, and it is being used to treat some forms of viral infections and cancer.

Interleukins. Interleukins are chemical substances that serve as messengers between leukocytes. Interleukins enhance the response of the leukocytes to foreign cells.

Lymphokines. Lymphokines are produced by the T cells in the immune system, but they assist with inflammation. Lymphokines assist the macrophages to be more effective in the site of local injury through a number of processes.

Function

At the time of injury, many actions occur simultaneously. For purposes of discussion, they will be separated into vascular response, phagocytosis, chemical mediators, plasma protein mediators, the "walling off" effect, and the immune response. Figure 18-2 depicts the entire time line of wound healing.

VASCULAR RESPONSE

Within seconds after an injury, regardless of the source, blood vessels constrict to stop bleeding and reduce exposure to bacteria. Vessels with large diameters undergo contraction of their smooth muscle walls to

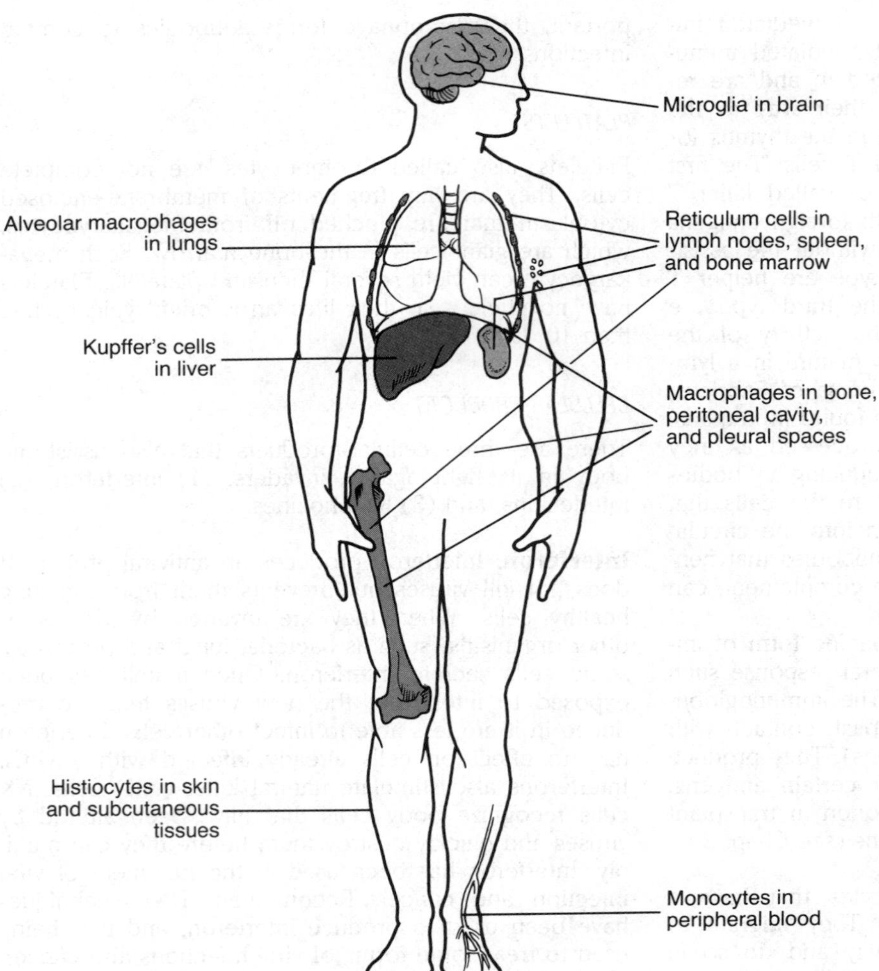

▲ **Figure 18-1**

The monocytes are mobile macrophages that are capable of wandering through the tissues. A large portion of monocytes enter tissue, become macrophages, and remain in the tissues for months. In the tissues, they serve as a first line of defense and phagocytize large quantities of bacteria, viruses, necrotic tissue, and other foreign particles.

cause constriction. Platelets, activated by the injury, aggregate to form a clot and stop bleeding. At the same time, the plasma protein system begins to form a fibrinous meshwork. When the platelets come in contact with the fibrin meshwork across the open vessel wall they become sticky and adhere (aggregate) to the fibers forming a plug. This meshwork of clotted blood and serum covers the wound while it heals and keeps the microorganisms near the site of greatest phagocytic activity. Platelets also release chemicals that promote clotting such as adenosine diphosphate (ADP) to attract other platelets and a type of prostaglandin to activate other platelets.

Capillaries dilate 10 to 30 minutes after injury and remain dilated for some time because of serotonin released by the platelets. The capillary dilation causes the classic signs of warmth and redness seen with inflammation. When the vessels dilate, the flow of blood slows and extra blood and oxygen are brought into the injured area.

PHAGOCYTOSIS

The process of phagocytosis, the engulfment and destruction of microorganisms, dead cells, and foreign material, involves four steps. The first step is the recognition of the target cell by the phagocyte and adherence to the phagocyte. This step is facilitated by the opsonization process in the complement system. The second step is the engulfment or ingestion of the material. The phagocyte surrounds the target cell with pseudopods (false feet). The pseudopods are lined with a membrane-bound vesicle to prevent harmful effects to the phagocyte. The third step is fusion of the lysosomes within the phagocyte with the organism. The final step is destruction of the target cell. This process requires oxygen and, usually, the phagocyte kills its target cell with hydrogen peroxide. When the phagocyte dies at the site of inflammation, its cellular contents are released, including the contents of its lysosomes. The destructive chemicals in the lysosome can digest surrounding tissues and stimulate the other components of inflammation. The liver secretes a plasma protein, α-1-antitrypsin, that inhibits destruction by many of the lysosome's contents.

The amount of oxygen in the wound influences the effectiveness of phagocytic cells. Both macrophages and neutrophils can function in an anaerobic environment, but their ability to effectively digest bacteria is slowed. Macrophages are inactivated when tissue levels of oxygen are below 30 mm Hg.

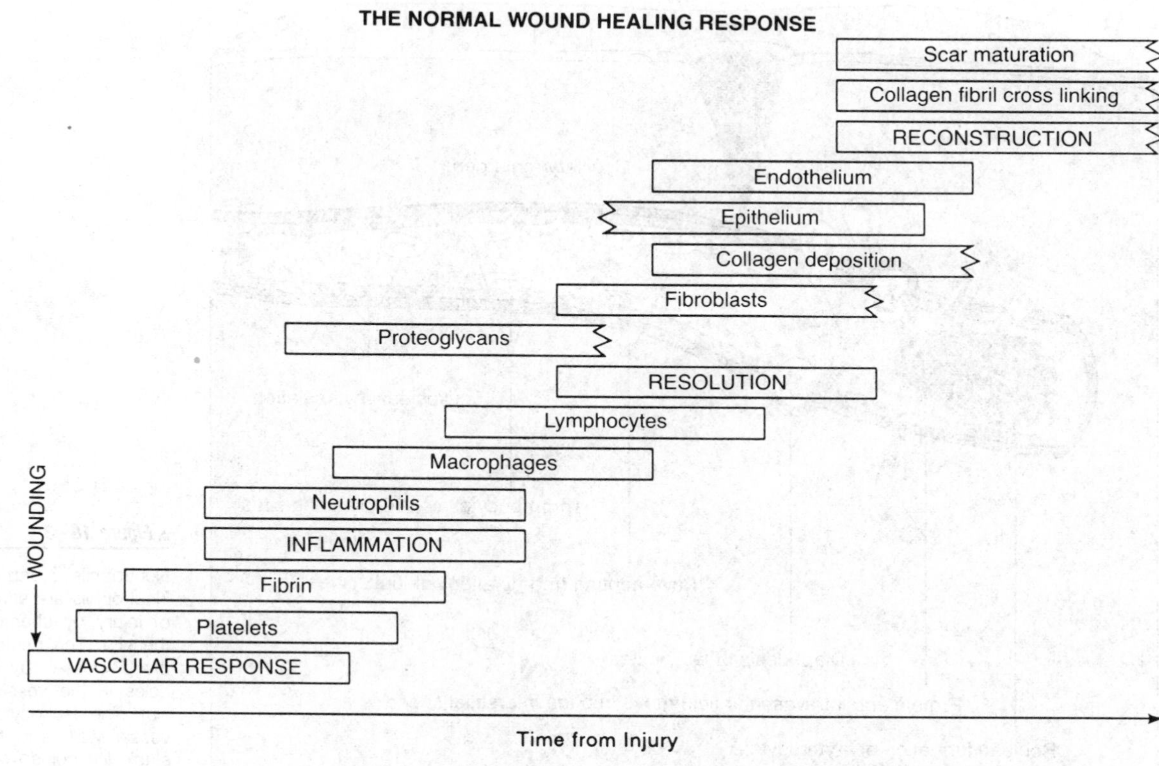

▲ *Figure 18–2*

The normal wound healing response. Wound healing proceeds through three phases: (1) the vascular response, (2) resolution of the wound, and (3) reconstruction of the wound. There are many components of each step. (From Cohen, I., et al. [1992]. *Wound Healing.* Philadelphia: W.B. Saunders.)

Neutrophils are the first phagocytic cells to arrive at the injured site, appearing within 6 to 12 hours of injury. They are attracted to the injury site by chemotaxis. The slowed flow of blood allows the neutrophil to leave the center of the bloodstream and line the walls of the capillaries, a process called pavementing (also called marginating) because they line up like bricks on a sidewalk. Histamine stimulates the cells lining the capillary to constrict, creating spaces in the wall. Neutrophils, which are normally too large to squeeze through the lining, can pass through the capillary wall and enter the site of tissue injury to begin phagocytosis, through a process called diapedesis (Fig. 18–3). Neutrophils phagocytize bacteria, dead cells, and cellular debris. They subsequently die and are removed in the form of pus through the epithelium or the lymphatic system. These cells are short lived, with a half-life of 6 hours, but they are effective in clearing a wound of debris if bacteria are not excessive in number (greater than 100,000 per gram of tissue).

Monocytes are the next phagocyte on the scene, stimulated by neutrophils and lymphokines. The monocyte develops into a macrophage at the site of injury. These cells perform the same function (phagocytosis) but for a longer time. Macrophages have a greater role in chronic inflammation, and the process is discussed later. In addition, the macrophage is a critical cell in wound healing because it secretes angiogenesis factor (AGF). AGF stimulates the formation of new blood vessels at the end of injured vessels.

Eosinophils and basophils may also migrate to the injured area. Eosinophils will help control the inflammatory response by secreting antihistamine. Eosinophils also produce a caustic protein, which dissolves the surface membranes of parasites. Basophils serve the same role as mast cells.

CHEMICAL MEDIATORS

Mast cells are found in the tissue and are similar to basophils found in the blood. Mast cells are filled with histamine and neutrophil chemotaxic factor, substances called vasoactive amines. Histamine and serotonin cause capillary dilation. The mast cell is stimulated by many factors, such as physical injury (wounds, burns, x-ray exposure), chemical injury (toxins, snake and bee venom), or immunologic means (the trigger of hypersensitivity reactions seen in allergy).

Mast cells synthesize leukotrienes and prostaglandins. These two chemicals cause the same responses as histamine, except that the response they generate lasts longer. Prostaglandins also cause pain. They tend to appear in later stages of inflammation. Leukotrienes and prostaglandins are produced from arachidonic acid released from the mast cell membrane. Aspirin and other nonsteroidal anti-inflammatory agents block the production of prostaglandins and can assist in reducing inflammation and pain. Leukotrienes and prostaglandins increase vascular permeability, and enhance the action of neutrophils. The increase in blood flow brings in

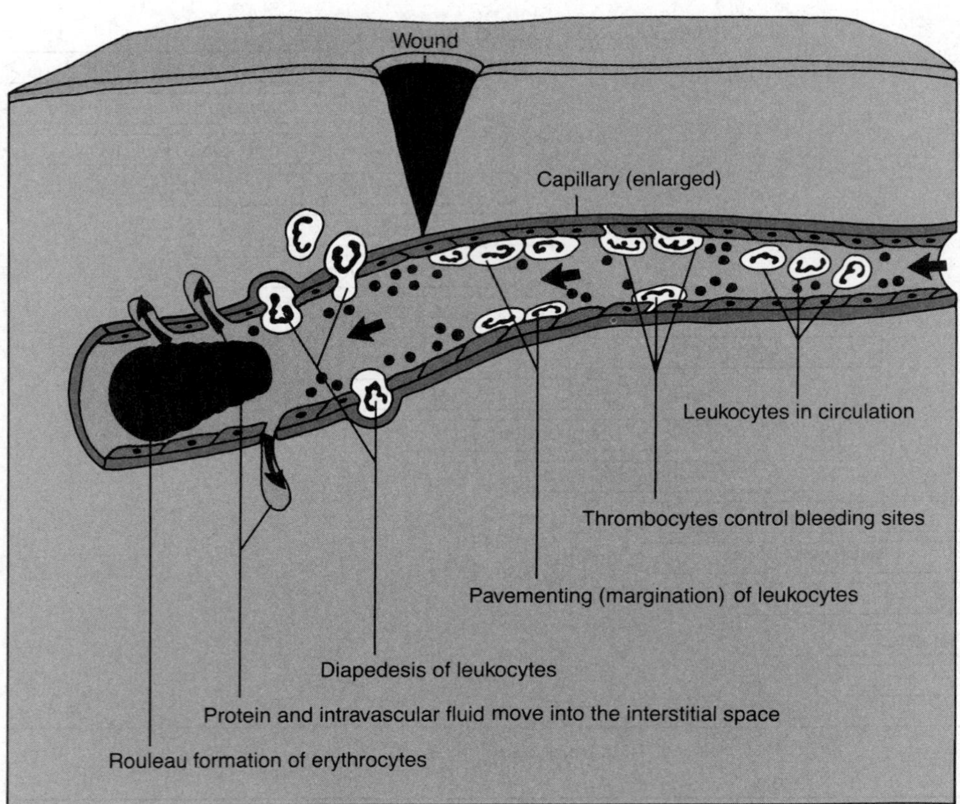

▲ *Figure 18–3*

Neutrophils and phagocytosis. Neutrophils are attracted to the site of injury by chemotaxic factors at the site. The neutrophil leaves the blood vessel by sliding through holes in the vessel wall (diapedesis). The leukocytes also line the vessel wall, and the erythrocytes stack like coins (rouleau formation) in order to slow blood flow.

more nutrients and WBCs. Bradykinin also causes vasodilation, induces pain, and facilitates the action of the leukocyte.

PLASMA PROTEIN MEDIATORS

There are three important plasma proteins that assist to mediate the inflammatory response: (1) the complement system, (2) the kinins, and (3) the clotting system.

Complement System. The complement system is composed of a group of plasma proteins that normally lie dormant in the blood, interstitial fluid, and mucosal surfaces. The complement system is activated by microorganisms (or antigen-antibody complexes). Complement causes three events to occur that promote inflammation. The first event is vasodilation of the capillaries, which increases blood flow to the area. The vessel walls open up, which allows the movement of plasma into the area. Plasma dilutes toxins secreted by the organisms, brings nutrients necessary for tissue repair, and carries phagocytes into the area. This fluid shift brings about the classic sign of edema in an inflamed area. The second aspect of complement activation is promotion of the movement of leukocytes into the area. This process is called *chemotaxis*. The final aspect of complement activation is the coating of microbes with opsonin to make them vulnerable to phagocytosis (opsonization). Many bacteria have an outer capsule that resists phagocytosis without opsonin.

Kinin. Kinin is a plasma protein involved in inflammation. Early in injury, kinins increase vascular permeability (open up blood vessel walls) and allow the leukocytes to enter the tissue through diapedesis. Later in the inflammatory process, kinin acts with prostaglandin to cause pain and smooth muscle contraction, and to increase leukocyte chemotaxis. Kinin increases vascular permeability, fluid in the wound, and the number of leukocytes available to assist with phagocytosis. The primary kinin is bradykinin.

Clotting System. Plasma proteins form a portion of the clotting system (blood coagulation). When bleeding occurs, fibrin forms a meshwork at bleeding sites. In addition to forming a clot to stop bleeding, this meshwork traps exudate, microorganisms, and foreign bodies. The meshwork keeps organisms contained in an area where there are the greatest number of phagocytes. This prevents the spread of infection to other sites and begins the process of healing and tissue repair.

"WALLING OFF" EFFECT

The "walling off" effect occurs in the damaged area to prevent the spread of injurious agents to other body tissues. The lymphatics and spaces in the tissues are blocked by fibrinogen clots so that fluid barely flows through the area.

The process of "walling off" the area is partly dependent on the invading agent. For example, staphylococci invade and destroy nearby tissues quickly and, therefore, the process of "walling off" also develops quickly to control the spread. In contrast, streptococci do not cause an intense reaction in the tissues and can digest the walls. This allows the streptococci to multiply and spread. As a result, streptococcal infections have a much greater tendency to invade other organs (such as the heart valves) and are associated with a higher mortality rate.

THE IMMUNE RESPONSE

Nonspecific defense mechanisms destroy pathogens and prevent the spread of infection while specific defense mechanisms are being mobilized. Specific defenses are a later form of defense but are directed at a known pathogen. Several days are usually required to activate specific immune responses, but once they are activated, these processes are extremely effective. There are two types of specific immunity: (1) cell-mediated immunity and (2) antibody-mediated immunity. These types of immune responses are discussed in Chapter 23. The number of lymphocytes does not increase with acute inflammation but does rise in chronic inflammation. Therefore, they do not appear to be a major portion of second-line defenses.

▼ TISSUE INJURY AND REPAIR

Regardless of the wound's etiology, wound healing follows a predictable course. Events can be described in three phases: (1) the inflammation, (2) wound healing with resolution and reconstruction, and (3) maturation of scar.

INFLAMMATION

Overview

Inflammation is a series of physiologic responses to tissue injury induced by trauma or an immune response to a foreign object. It is nonspecific and it occurs in the same way regardless of the type of injury and occurs even on second exposure to the same injury. The inflammatory response is essential for the repair and restoration of the structure and function of damaged tissues.

The inflammatory response occurs whenever injury has occurred. Cellular injury can occur from trauma, oxygen or nutrient deprivation, chemical agents, microorganism invasion, temperature extremes, or ionizing radiation. Inflammation also occurs when dead cells are present.

Many of the cells previously discussed have a role in the inflammatory process. The nurse must recognize inflammation as an expected response to tissue injury and not necessarily a pathophysiologic process. Although inflammation can cause additional tissue injury, it is an adaptation to injury. The purpose of inflammation is to limit the effects of harmful bacteria or injury by destroying or neutralizing the organism, and by limiting its spread throughout the body. The inflammatory response thereby sets up proper conditions to promote tissue repair. Unlike the immune response which is slow and deliberate, using a system of specific antibodies, the effects of inflammation are immediate.

Chronic Inflammation

Chronic inflammation is differentiated from acute inflammation by its duration, because chronic inflammation lasts for more than 2 weeks. Chronic inflammation can arise from incomplete resolution of an acute process of inflammation. The chronically inflamed wound has purulent drainage (suppuration) and does not heal completely. A common example of chronic inflammation is seen when foreign objects are not removed from the tissues (e.g., splinter, glass, dirt). Chronic inflammation can also occur when certain forms of bacteria cannot be killed by phagocytes. For example, the organisms that cause tuberculosis, syphilis, and leprosy have cell walls with a very high lipid and wax content, which makes them impermeable to the phagocyte.

The lymphocyte and tissue macrophage are the major phagocytes in chronic inflammation. When the body is unable to kill the invading organisms during the acute stage of inflammation, it attempts to protect surrounding tissues from further invasion by building a wall, around the infected site. The wall is called a granuloma. Some forms of infection, such as fungi, parasites, and perhaps, antibody-antigen reactions (autoimmune disease), result in granuloma formation. Tuberculosis is a good example of granuloma formation. When the client develops tuberculosis, a thick wall forms around the mycobacterium. The bacteria continue to live in the walled-off area, and it is soon filled with dead tissue. As the tissue dies, the cellular enzymes are released and the fluid leaves the granuloma. The empty sac remains for the life of the client, and is called a Ghon complex.

Clinical Manifestations

The clinical manifestations of inflammation have been recorded for thousands of years and include redness (rubor), swelling (tumor), heat (calor), pain (dolor), and loss of function (functio laesa). With the development of the microscope, the cellular activity that occurs with inflammation was discovered. There are both local and systemic responses to inflammation.

LOCAL MANIFESTATIONS

Because the response to inflammation is the same regardless of the cause, the symptoms of inflammation are relatively consistent. Tissues are red, warm, painful, and swollen and have limited mobility. In addition, an inflammatory exudate is formed. The exudate dilutes the toxins released by bacteria, brings certain nutrients to the wound, and carries phagocytes for defense.

TABLE 18–2. Inflammatory Exudates

Type	Appearance	Significance
Hemorrhagic, sanguinous	Bright red or bloody	Small amounts expected after surgery or trauma. Large amounts may indicate hemorrhage. Sudden large amounts of dark red blood may indicate a draining hematoma
Serosanguinous	Blood-tinged yellow or pink	Expected for 48 to 72 hours after injury or trauma. A sudden increase may precede wound dehiscence
Serous	Thin clear yellow	Expected for up to 1 week after trauma or surgery. A sudden increase may indicate a draining seroma
Purulent	Thin, cloudy, foul smelling. May be thick if filled with dead cells and necrotic tissues	Usually indicates infection. May drain suddenly from an abscess (boil)
Catarrhal	Thin, clear mucus	Seen with upper respiratory infection
Fibrinous	Thin, usually clear, may be yellow or pink, tinged or cloudy	Occurs with severe inflammation

There are various types of exudate depending on the stage of inflammation and its cause. Serous exudate is seen in early inflammation and is composed of water with a small amount of colloids, ions, and phagocytic cells. A blister would be a common example of serous exudate. Purulent exudate is filled with more leukocytes (pus) and is common in chronic inflammation from "walled-off" lesions. The drainage from an abscess would typify this exudate. Other forms of exudate are fibrinous, seen in forms of pneumonia, and *hemorrhagic* or *sanguinous,* which occurs when the exudate is composed of blood. Initially, a wound has sanguinous drainage, which then progresses to serosanguinous and finally to serous drainage (Table 18–2).

SYSTEMIC MANIFESTATIONS

There are three systemic reactions to inflammation: (1) fever, (2) leukocytosis (a rise in the number of white blood cells), and (3) an increase in the number of plasma proteins. Fever is caused by a pyrogen (fever-causing chemical) released from leukocytes, macrophages, and tumor necrosis factor (TNF). Prostaglandins act on the hypothalamus in the brain to reset the internal thermostat. Fever is usually adaptive because some of the bacteria are sensitive to even slight increases in temperature. However, fever can be detrimental if it is extreme or prolonged. Therefore, the temperature is monitored closely to avoid harm to the client. The client may also experience malaise, nausea, and anorexia, weight loss, and tachypnea and tachycardia.

DIAGNOSTIC ASSESSMENT

Leukocytosis is due to the increase in the number of leukocytes in circulation to combat infection. Sometimes, in an effort to combat infection the bone marrow releases immature leukocytes, called banded neutrophils or "bands." When the number of immature neutrophils is high, the client is said to have a "left shift." At times, the release of immature cells means that the body is having difficulty combating the infection with mature cells. (Interpretation of the WBC differential is shown in Table 18–3.)

The sedimentation rate also rises with inflammation. The sedimentation rate (or "sed rate") is the rate at which cells settle to the bottom of a glass test tube. Increased levels of fibrinogen cause the red blood cell to stack (like coins) and, therefore, settle more quickly. Additionally, the plasma proteins rise during inflammation (e.g., fibrinogen, C-reactive protein). Most are released by the liver, and they are collectively called acute-phase reactants. They provide components of coagulation, transportation, and complement production.

Management

Since the inflammatory response is a desired response to promote wound healing, sometimes the client only requires supportive care. The degree of inflammation is monitored to determine whether or not it is leading to healing. The area of inflammation is often elevated or wrapped to reduce edema. Analgesics may be required for pain control. Temperature is monitored and treated with antipyretics when it reaches levels that are detrimental to the client (e.g, over 38.3° C [101° F]).

If the inflammation is in response to a probable invasion by organisms, antibiotics may be prescribed. If the edema is causing a detrimental alteration in tissue perfusion, anti-inflammatory agents may be required.

The diet of the client with inflammation should be high in (1) vitamin C, to aid in the synthesis of collagen; (2) protein, to aid in the formation of blood cells and tissue; and (3) fluids, to remove metabolic waste

TABLE 18–3. Interpretation of the Differential Counts within a CBC

Cell Type	Function	Normal Value	Significance of Change
Segmented neutrophils (segs)*	Mature neutrophils act as phagocytes	50 to 60 per cent	Elevated with infection A "left shift" means that many bands (immature) cells are present as the body fights infection. A "right shift" is the presence of more mature cells, seen with liver disease and pernicious anemia
Band neutrophils	Immature neutrophils	3 to 8 per cent	Elevated in acute stages of infection
Lymphocytes	Produced by lymphoid tissue, participate in humoral response	25 to 40 per cent	Elevated in infectious mononucleosis, cytomegalovirus infection, infectious hepatitis. Decreased in AIDS, Cushing's syndrome, chronic uremia, and following trauma (e.g., burn injury)
Monocytes	A second line of defense, increasing in chronic infections	2 to 8 per cent	Elevated in chronic bacterial infection, viral disease, Hodgkin's disease, multiple myeloma, and some forms of leukemia
Eosinophils	Phagocytic, destroy antigen-antibody complexes before they can harm the body	1 to 4 percent	Elevated in allergic disorders, and parasitic infections. Decreased in infectious mononucleosis, congestive heart failure, pernicious anemia, and during the use of steroids, epinephrine, and thyroxin

*To calculate the absolute neutrophil count:

$$\text{Absolute neutrophil count} = \frac{\text{Total per cent of neutrophils (segs + bands)} \times \text{WBC count}}{100}$$

When the absolute neutrophil count falls below 1000/mm^3, the client is said to be "neutropenic" and precautions must be taken to prevent infection.

and rehydrate the client, especially if the client has been febrile.

In certain areas of the body, such as the brain and extremities, the edema that accompanies inflammation can be detrimental to tissue perfusion. These clients may require surgery to release pressure in the area and restore blood flow. Burr Holes and fasciotomy are examples of these operations, and are discussed in Chapters 30 and 71, respectively.

Clients with visible injury causing inflammation should be assessed for the resolution of bleeding in the area, adequate blood flow, and nerve conduction distal to the area. The frequent assessment (every 2 hours) of the circumference of the area will provide data to indicate whether or not the area is becoming markedly edematous. In order to measure the same site, the area on the client should be marked with a pen. In addition to assessing the circumference, the nurse should assess for pulses, capillary refill, sensation, and movement in areas distal to the inflammation. The edema from the inflammatory response may restrict blood vessels and entrap nerves in the area. Dressings or casts over the affected area can also form a constriction. The nurse should monitor the level of WBCs, differential counts, and temperature as indicators of infection.

Objects that may become entrapped in edematous tissues, such as rings, should be removed. The inflamed area should be elevated. Application of cold compresses will cause vasoconstriction and decrease the amount of edema. However, prolonged use of cold compresses may lead to rebound vasodilation and increase the risk of tissue injury. Vasoconstriction can also decrease the inflow of new blood and, thereby, slow the removal of toxins and waste from the site of injury.

There is controversy about the use of heat and cold in the management of injury. Some researchers advocate the use of heat to bring in more blood and phagocytes to clean up the wound. In clinical practice, the use of ice seems to be preferred to control the extent of inflammation and pain. Some physicians order ice for 24 to 72 hours to control inflammation, and then heat to remove the accumulated waste products.

Fluids should be forced, if they are not contraindicated. The diet should be high in protein and vitamin C. Antibiotics and anti-inflammatory agents should be given as prescribed.

WOUND HEALING

Definition

Wound healing is the process of tissue regeneration that completely restores structure and function to an injured area. Wound healing is most apparent on the skin but occurs in all areas of the body. Bones, tendons, organs, and tissues can regenerate cells and restore function. The most favorable outcome of healing is the complete return to normal structure and function. This outcome is possible if tissue damage is minor, no complications occur, and the destroyed tissues are capable of regeneration. Body tissues have varying capabilities for regeneration. For example, the gastrointestinal lining of mucous membrane is completely regenerated. Deep skin injury regenerates with scar, which restores only a barrier. The central nervous system (CNS) cannot regenerate damaged cells. Therefore, damaged tissues in the CNS may be repaired with scar tissue, but they cannot be regenerated to regain their original function.

The process of wound repair begins with inflammation. Sometimes the inflammatory phase is called the reaction phase of wound healing. The inflammatory process cleans the wound and provides the fundamental steps for wound healing.

Incidence

The incidence of tissue injury and repair is impossible to measure. There have been statistics recorded on specific injuries, such as burns (see Chap. 71). Surgical incisions and traumatic lacerations are perhaps the most common causes of tissue injury.

Etiology

WOUND HEALING INTENTION

Primary Intention. The repair of a wound centers on processes that fill the wound with new tissue, cover or seal the wound, and contract the wound. These three aspects of wound healing vary depending upon the type of wound and its healing. A surgical incision is usually clean and heals through the process of collagen synthesis. An incision has had minimal tissue loss and its edges are usually approximated (brought together) with sutures, staples or tape. Therefore, very little sealing or contracture is needed for healing. This process of healing is called *primary intention* (Fig. 18-4). The eventual scar is usually thin and flat.

Secondary Intention. Other wounds do not heal as easily or as neatly. Consider open wounds like pressure sores or abrasions. These wounds require the regeneration of much more tissue than does an incision. The processes of the reconstructive phase take much longer, increase the risk of infection, and lead to healing by contraction and the formation of scar tissue. Healing by this mechanism is *secondary intention*.

Wounds healing by secondary intention have a prolonged phase of inflammation with the macrophage and lymphocyte as the predominant cells. There is more time required for phagocytosis of necrotic tissue, growth of granulation tissue, and epithelization. The extent of cell migration for epithelization is limited, and the process may not heal the wound. If the wound cannot heal by epithelization, it becomes covered with eschar (dried protein and dead cells). Although the eschar covers the wound, it is also tissue that is prone to infection and must be removed for complete healing. Sometimes, the healing of these wounds is hastened by the application of skin grafts or musculocutaneous flaps (see Chap. 72).

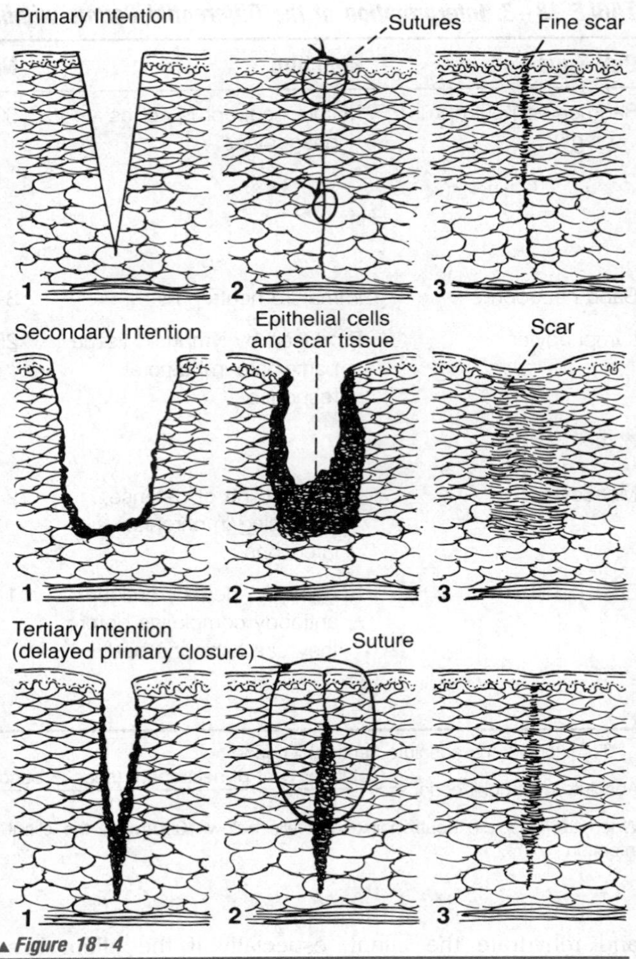

▲ **Figure 18-4**

Primary, secondary, and tertiary intention (delayed primary closure) wound healing.

Tertiary Intention. Certain wounds may be contaminated and, although they could be closed by primary intention (e.g., sutured closed), they are not. Because of the increased risk of infection, these wounds are closed later when they are free of debris. This type of wound closure is called healing by *tertiary intention*, or *delayed primary closure*.

Risk Factors

Even though the incidence of surgical incisions cannot be reduced, there are many precautions taken during surgery to increase healing and are a form of primary risk reduction. For example, bleeding is controlled, sterility is maintained, and the wound edges are brought together (approximated). Secondary risk reduction occurs through the management of disorders that delay wound healing. Disorders that decrease oxygenation or nutrition, decrease the inflammatory reaction, or increase bacterial growth must be controlled in order to facilitate healing. Secondary risk management can occur by providing the client with a diet that is high in protein and vitamins (especially vitamin C), and oxygen via inhalation or through hyperbaric oxygen. Stress on the wound should be avoided, especially 5 to 10 days after the injury when tensile strength is at its lowest level. Clients who are steroid dependent will have delayed wound healing, because these medications reduce the inflammatory response, thereby slowing wound healing. Tertiary risk reduction is the assessment of complications of wound healing, which is discussed at the end of the chapter.

Pathophysiology

NORMAL WOUND HEALING

In order to discuss the problems of wound healing, the normal processes of wound healing are reviewed first (Fig. 18–5). Normal wound healing occurs in three phases. During inflammation, phagocytosis of foreign material and exudate débrides (cleans) the wound. The actual process has been described earlier as a form of secondary defense mechanism.

The second phase of wound healing is the reconstruction phase. This phase contains the processes of collagen deposition, angiogenesis, granulation tissue development, and wound contraction. Initially, the fibrin clot must be dissolved.

Collagen Deposition. Fibroblasts, normally found in the connective tissues, are brought into the wound by various cellular mediators. They are the most important cells in the reconstructive phase of healing, because they synthesize and secrete collagen, elastin, and proteoglycans. These substances reconstruct the connective tissue. Initially, collagen is gel-like, but within several months, it reforms along lines of mechanical stress, which adds strength to the wound.

Angiogenesis. The development of new blood vessels in the wound bed can be identified through clinical assessment. Initially, the skin edges of a wound are

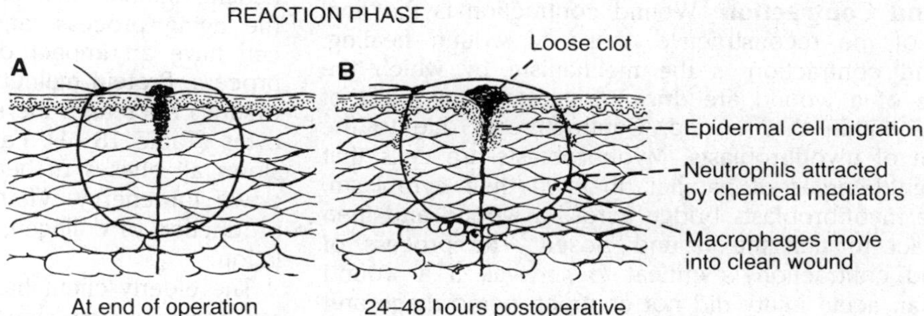

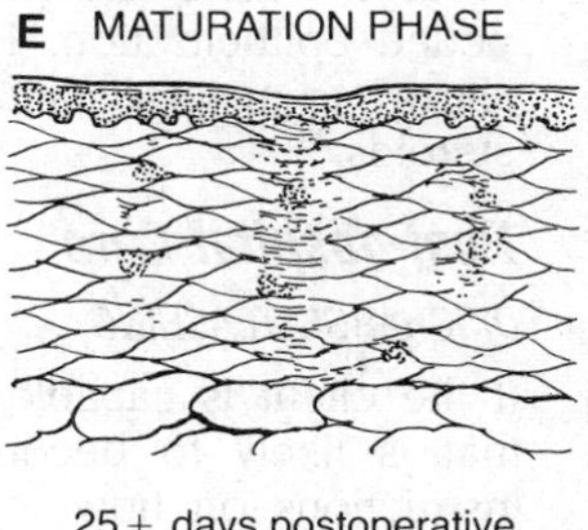

▲ *Figure 18–5*

The healing of an incised, sutured skin wound.

bright red and bleed easily. Microscopically, angiogenesis begins within hours of injury. The endothelial cells in preexisting vessels begin to produce enzymes that break down the basement membrane. The membrane opens, and new endothelial cells build a new vessel. New lymphatics grow through the same process. There are many factors that promote or retard angiogenesis. Perhaps one of the most important factors is adequate oxygenation.

Granulation Tissue. This new tissue grows onto the wound from the surrounding edges. Granulation tissue is filled with new capillary buds, which gives it a red, granular appearance. It is also surrounded by fibroblasts and macrophages. The fibroblasts secrete collagen. The macrophages continue to débride the wound and stimulate the fibroblasts and the process of angiogenesis. As granulation tissue is being formed, the process of epithelization begins. This is the process by which epithelial cells grow onto a wound from surrounding edges and the lining of hair follicles. The follicle is lined with epidermal cells but exists in the dermis. Eventually, the migrating cells contact similar cells from the other edges and stop migrating. At this point, they begin to differentiate into the various layers of epidermis. Epithelization can be hastened if a wound is kept moist.

Wound Contraction. Wound contraction is the final step of the reconstructive phase of wound healing. Wound contraction is the mechanism by which the edges of a wound are drawn together as a result of forces within that wound. Contracture is due to the action of myofibroblasts. Myofibroblasts are cells that contain bundles of parallel fibers in their cytoplasm. These myofibroblasts bridge across a wound and then contract to pull the wound closed. The process of wound contraction is critical to survival. If a wound from an acute injury did not contract, hemorrhage and infection would be lethal complications in all acute injuries. On the other hand, the contracture of scar can produce profound deformities. The contracture of scar can pull the chin onto the chest or contract a joint. Contracture also occurs in internal organs, such as the intestine, breast and liver.

FACTORS THAT DELAY WOUND HEALING

Wound healing is a process with several phases. The nonhealing wound results from the impairment of one or more of those processes. Factors that lead to delayed healing may be intrinsic (within the wound) or extrinsic (elsewhere within the client).

Intrinsic Factors. In wound infection, the inflammatory response is prolonged and healing is delayed. Wounds will not heal while infection is present. Infection can develop when the defense mechanisms are weakened, thus allowing a normal bacterial load to become overwhelming. Alternatively, the bacterial load can be greater than the body's defenses can handle. In healthy clients, the critical number is 100,000 bacteria per gram of tissue. Above that number, the body loses control over bacterial proliferation and invasion and infection is present. (This threshold number for bacteria holds true for all kinds of bacteria except for group B streptococcus, which can cause infection in lesser quantities.) The diagnosis of infection is through quantitative wound biopsy cultures. This test requires 24 to 48 hours to process, so most of the time the client is given a broad-spectrum antibiotic while awaiting results. Sometimes, foreign bodies within the wound provide a source for infection. Examples include soil, hematomas (accumulations of blood), and bone fragments.

An adequate blood supply is essential for all aspects of wound healing. The blood supply can be restricted through disorders of the heart, vessels, or the lungs. Hypoxia impairs the delivery of oxygen and nutrients to the wound, and the action of the various defensive cells. Neutrophils require oxygen to generate hydrogen peroxide to kill the pathogens. Likewise, fibroblast and collagen proliferation are slowed. The only aspect of wound healing that can proceed in hypoxic states is angiogenesis.

Smoking causes vasoconstriction and hypoxia because of the carbon monoxide in the smoke. In addition to limiting oxygen supply, smoking increases atherosclerosis and platelet aggregation. These conditions further restrict the amount of oxygen in the wound.

Extrinsic Factors. Extrinsic factors that delay wound healing include malnutrition, changes associated with the aging process, and other disorders. Malnutrition can have an impact on several areas of the healing process. Protein malnutrition (especially the amino acid cystine) decreases the synthesis of collagen and leukocytes (Table 18–4). Fat and carbohydrate malnutrition slows all phases of healing because protein is broken down for energy. Vitamin deficiency leads to slowed production of collagen, immune responses, and coagulation.

The elderly client has decreased initial inflammatory responses, which slows the process of healing. The aged client may have decreased circulation, which delays WBC migration to the site and phagocytosis. In addition, the client may be malnourished and have concurrent disorders that retard healing.

Diabetes is a disorder that predisposes many clients to difficulty in wound healing because of impaired collagen synthesis, angiogenesis, and phagocytosis. Atherosclerosis, especially of small vessels, is also common in diabetes and impairs tissue oxygen delivery. Diabetic neuropathy further impairs healing by interrupting the neurologic control of healing (e.g., reducing vasodilation and the protective sensation of pain).

The use of steroids slows healing by inhibiting collagen synthesis. Clients who are taking steroids have decreased wound strength, inhibited contraction, and impeded epithelization. Fortunately, vitamin A has been shown to reverse the healing impairments caused by steroids.[28]

Post-hospital Care

DISCHARGE TEACHING

If the client is capable of caring for a wound or area that is likely to become inflamed, he or she needs instructions on how to elevate the extremity, how to

TABLE 18-4. Nutrients and Wound Healing

Nutrient	RDA for Healthy Adults	Clinical Manifestations of Deficiency	Implementation
Water	2,000 ml	Dry mucous membranes Oliguria, thirst	Provide adequate water through fluids and food, monitor weight and intake and output
Protein	46 to 53 g/day depending on sex and weight (or 0.8 g/Kg)	Delayed wound healing Impaired immune response, inflammation	Need to increase protein intake through various sources up to 1.5 g/Kg/day
Calories	1500 to 3500/day depending on level of activity	Delayed wound healing Muscle wasting complex	May need a fivefold increase with major wounds (e.g., burns). Carbohydrates should provide 50 to 60 per cent of calories
Vitamin A	800-1,000 μg	Slowed epithelialization and collagen synthesis, decreased resistance to infection because there is a decreased number of macrophages produced	Increase intake to 25,000 units in major wounds. Vitamin A may reverse the effects of glucocorticoids on wound healing
Vitamin B_6	1.6-20 μg	Decreased protein synthesis, perhaps decreased collagen strength Slowed hemoglobin and antibody production	Must be increased as protein intake is increased
Folate	200 μg	Slowed protein synthesis	Increase intake, especially when wound infection is present
Iron	10 to 12mg/day (males) 10 to 15mg/day (females)	Slowed healing due to lack of oxygen transportation	Monitor hemoglobin, encourage foods with iron or administer $FeSO_4$
Zinc	12 to 15 mg	Decreased immunity and slowed collagen synthesis	Increase intake when wounds are present

use heat or ice, the medication regimen, and clinical manifestations of edema and infection that must be reported.

MATURATION OF SCARS

The final phase of wound healing is called the maturation phase. Collagen deposition, tissue regeneration, and wound contraction all began in the reconstructive phase. The initial scar is bright red, thick, and blanches with pressure. This phase ends about 2 weeks after injury, but the processes of healing are not complete and continue for 1 to 2 years. During the maturation phase, the scar is remodeled, capillaries disappear, and the scar tissue regains about two thirds of its original strength. The scar becomes mature, and appears thin and white instead of red and raised.

WOUND HEALING BY PRIMARY INTENTION

Medical Management

Medical management centers on getting the client in the best condition for the processes of healing to work. Disorders that delay wound healing should be stabilized.

Wound drainage tubes can be placed into the dead space created during surgery. Drainage of a wound is indicated when actual or potential fluid accumulation threatens the healing process. The drain facilitates removal of blood and bacteria from the wound. Drains are also placed when a dead (vacant) space has been created. Dead space is created during surgical procedures that involve large wound dissections or removal of a tumor or body organ.

Nursing Management

The client's wound should be assessed twice daily. The incision normally appears somewhat pink and swollen, but the erythema should not extend outside the edges. Drainage is initially sanguinous, proceeding to serosanguinous, and then to serous. If a drain is in place, the volume and type of fluid should be assessed hourly immediately after surgery. If a reservoir is attached to the drain, the volume of drainage can be measured by markings on the reservoir. If the drainage is emptied from the reservoir, universal precautions must be followed for its disposal. In addition, if the drainage is caustic (e.g., bile) the skin around the site must be protected with agents such as skin preps or stoma adhesives.

The wound that is healing by primary intention should be protected from further trauma, kept free of pulling forces that stretch the sutured skin, kept clean but not washed (water carries microorganisms into the wound along the sutures), protected from the external environment with dressings, and kept free from pressure.

Dressings should be applied using a sterile technique, but sterile gloves are usually not required. The side of the dressing that will not touch the client's incision can be held by the nurse's clean gloved hands and taped in place. The type of dressing used will change as the wound responds to treatment. The nurse should use dressings that best suit the wound. Gauze dressings are the most common dressing used on a wound healing by primary intention.

Post-hospital Care

DISCHARGE TEACHING

The client should be taught how to care for the incision, the indications of wound infection, and when to return for suture removal. Sutures in areas where scarring must be controlled (e.g., the face) are removed in 4 to 7 days; in other areas, sutures are usually removed in 7 to 10 days. Sutures in the hand and foot are removed in 1 to 2 weeks or more.

WOUND HEALING BY SECONDARY INTENTION

Medical Management

The goal of management is the same as with wound healing by primary intention. Clients with wounds healing through the process of granulation often have other problems, such as venous insufficiency and diabetes. These disorders decrease blood flow (and thereby oxygen) into the wound and delay healing. Medical management may include the use of oxygen and vasodilators to restore arterial flow, elevation to promote venous drainage, and antibiotics to reduce infection. The client's diet should be high in carbohydrates, fat, protein, iron, and vitamins because all of these components are required for wound healing.

It is imperative to avoid applying solutions on and in the wound that impair wound healing. For example, iodine, hydrogen peroxide, and Dakin's solution were once commonly used for wound care. It is now known that these solutions damage the wound and further delay healing.

DÉBRIDEMENT

Surgical Débridement. Before beginning wound treatment, all necrotic tissue must be removed. Débridement of necrotic tissue can be accomplished by using a variety of therapies. Surgical débridement is the most effective and permits immediate treatment to the wound bed after the eschar is removed. The wound size, depth of the wound, contamination, and client status influence whether or not the client is in satisfactory condition to tolerate a surgical intervention that may require general anesthesia or sedation.

Surgical débridement is carried out under sterile conditions and usually occurs in the operating room or outpatient surgical setting. Risks associated with general anesthesia, blood loss, and infection are of major concern. This procedure is used for a larger wound or a wound that involves a thick eschar that could not be permeated by any topical agent.

Mechanical Débridement. Mechanical débridement provides another treatment option for the high-risk client. The effectiveness of irrigation is a result of the hydraulic force created by water pressure. High-pressure irrigations, above 8 psi, remove debris, bacteria, and necrotic tissue. Low-pressure irrigations, less than 8 psi, are more useful in removing foreign bodies and exudate (Fig. 18–6). The greater the fluid volume used, the more rapidly the contaminants will be eliminated. Irrigation with continuous pressure and flow from a pulsating jet device is more effective than irrigation with a bulb syringe.[44]

Barrier precautions need to be taken with masks or goggles, gowns, and gloves because it is common for the nurse to be sprayed with contaminated solutions. The client may also need protection. Irrigation with pulsating devices is contraindicated in clients with wounds of the neck, eyes, or dura and in those with exposed blood vessels. To prevent further contamination of adjacent tissues, pressure should not be increased beyond the prescribed level.

Mechanical débridement can also be accomplished by using wet-to-dry dressings. The moist dressing is placed in the wound, allowed to dry, and then removed. The drying dressing causes debris, necrotic tissue, exudate, and drainage to adhere to it. The wound is débrided as the dressing is gently removed. The wet dressing is obtained by saturating an all-gauze dressing with the prescribed solution and wringing the dressing out until it is just moist. The moist dressing should be placed in the wound and left long enough to begin to dry (4 to 6 hours). The packing must be removed while the dressing is slightly damp to avoid disrupting the granular bed. Bleeding should not occur when the dressing is removed. If the dressing is too dry to pull

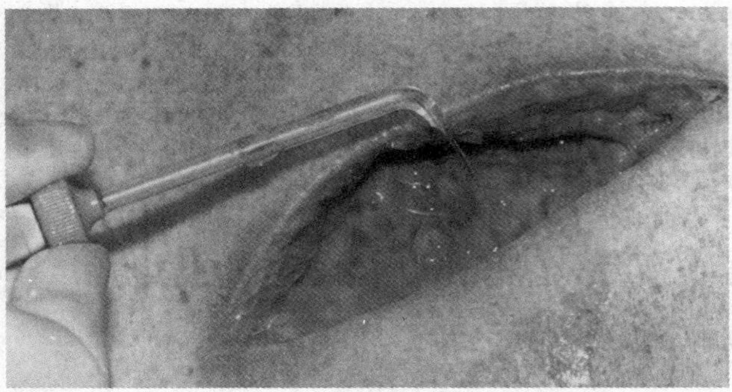

▲ Figure 18–6

Incision and drainage of thoracolumbar abscess with débridement by the Water Pik. (From Trelstad, A., & Osmundson, D. [1989]. Water Piks: Wound cleansing alternative. *Plastic Surgical Nursing, 9* [3], 117.)

off, moisten it with sterile normal saline before attempting to remove it. This treatment, however, is nonselective and can remove new granulation tissues as well as necrotic tissue, creating an environment that retards healing.

To avoid the risk of damaging new tissue growth often experienced with wet-to-dry dressings, chemical agents, such as enzymes and autolytic, vapor-permeable dressings, offer nonsurgical options when surgery is not indicated or places the client at risk. Enzymatic chemicals are expensive and require diligent care. When enzymatic preparations, such as fibrolysin (Elase) or sutilains (Travase), are used, the eschar must first be scored and then the enzymatic ointment applied. A moist saline dressing is placed over the ointment. The ointment is used until the eschar separates from the wound surface. These agents require frequent dressing changes and must be used only on the necrotic tissue.

The vapor-permeable dressings also offer another therapy alternative for removing necrotic tissue. The occlusion created by the dressing hastens the separation of the necrotic tissue by keeping wound fluids in intimate contact with the wound surface and trapping macrophages and leukocytes. These wound fluids contain enzymes that lyse dead tissue. This process is called autolytic débridement and uses the client's wound healing capabilities and the wound healing process to destroy necrotic tissues. This wound therapy facilitates granular tissue formation, speeds cell migration and epithelialization, and prevents further necrosis.[17]

CLOSURE

Once the wound is clean, surgery may be used to speed healing and decrease the risk of infection and contracture. Skin grafts are commonly used to replace the epidermis. The partial-thickness burn wound is the best example of a wound that could heal by secondary intention but is often grafted to speed healing and reduce infection and scarring. Cutaneous or musculocutaneous flaps can also be used to close a large wound (see Chap. 72).

Box 18-1. Assessing a Wound

When assessing a wound, be certain to obtain the following points of information:

1. What is the size of the wound? Use objective measures to indicate length and width (such as cm or mm). Avoid terms such as "size of a grape." Use a sterile gloved finger or cotton swab to measure depth. Consider using photographs to provide a baseline and serial evaluations.
2. Where is the wound located anatomically?
3. What is the color of the wound? A red wound is a new wound or one that is not infected. It is healing properly and is filled with red granulation tissue and fragile capillaries. A yellow wound is covered with yellow or ivory eschar. It may contain pus, debris and exudate. A black wound is completely or partially covered with black or brown necrotic eschar.
4. Is there granulation tissue or epithelial tissue? Granulation tissue is red, shiny, and bumpy; epithelial tissue looks like pale skin.
5. Are there sinus tracts or are the edges undermined? Use a gloved hand or swab to measure the extent. Indicate the location.
6. Are there signs of infection in the wound? Look for erythema extending beyond the edges of the wound, as well as warmth, edema, and odor, and purulent exudate. (Consider systemic signs also.)
7. Is there any drainage? Note the color, odor, approximate amount by the number of dressings saturated, and consistency.
8. What is condition of the surrounding skin? Is it intact, red, indurated, or macerated?

Modified from Faller, N., & Lawrence, K. (1991). Nursing to promote healing. *Ostomy/Wound Management, 32* (1), 43–46, 48; and Cuzzel, J. (1988). The new RYB color code. AJN, 88 (10), 1342–1346.

Nursing Management

ASSESSMENT

The history of the present illness should include the client's beliefs about the causes and contributing factors of the wound, previous methods used in treatment, and degree of success.

The nursing history should include information about the client's medical history, previous surgery, current and past medications used (especially steroids), nutritional state (what type of diet has the client been eating? any supplements?), degree of immobility, level of continence, circulatory status, and presence of infection.

Psychosocial assessment should include the client's age, occupation, living situation, financial status, health care benefits, roles and responsibilities, cultural and spiritual beliefs, body image and self-esteem and probable ability of client to learn self-care and comply with the treatment plan.

Physical assessment of the client should include height and weight; degree of range of motion; muscle wasting and level of activity; assessment of circulatory, status such as peripheral pulses, color, and temperature of extremities; and lung sounds. The wound requires complete assessment (see Box 18-1). Data about the wound should be documented clearly to allow for objective evaluation at a later date.

The nurse should also examine the laboratory values for hemoglobin, hematocrit, oxygen saturation, arterial oxygen pressure, albumin, WBCs and lymphocytes. These values indicate the degree of oxygenation and nutritional impairment that may be contributing to the wound's lack of healing. Generally, the lower the serum albumin level, the higher the risk of delayed healing.

NURSING INTERVENTION

Nursing Diagnosis: Skin Integrity, Impaired R/T delayed wound healing secondary to impaired circulation.

Planning: Expected Outcomes. The client will have improvement in skin integrity, as evidenced by a smaller wound within 1 week and no signs of infection in the wound.

Implementation. The treatment of a wound includes the removal of its cause(s), the correction of underlying problems that are delaying healing, and the initiation of topical (or systemic) treatments to facilitate healing. The wound's appearance should be used as a guide in planning interventions.

Protection for Red Wounds. Wounds that are red require protection.[12] Red wounds are filled with granulation tissue and are beginning to heal. These wounds should not be treated with lotions, ointments, or soaps because they may irritate or infect the area. Topical vasodilators can be used to stimulate capillary flow to the wound but require a physician's order. If the wound is shallow, a thin layer of antibiotic ointment and a nonadhering dressing (or synthetic dressing) should be used to cover it. If the wound is deep, saline-moistened gauze can be used to pack the wound, but the dressing should not dry out before changing it. A dried dressing removes the granulation tissue and new epithelium.[12] If a wound is healing, the wound should be kept moist to facilitate healing (Fig. 18–7).

Cleaning of Yellow Wounds. Wounds that are yellow require cleaning.[12] Yellow wounds are covered with soft necrotic eschar. These wounds need to have the eschar removed so that healing can begin. The wound needs débridement, and this usually can be accomplished with whirlpool baths to soften and lift the eschar, in combination with wet-to-dry dressings. Gauze dressings are applied wet and removed when dry. The necrotic tissue sticks to the gauze and is removed with each dressing change. The wound can also be irrigated with a syringe or by having the client hold the wound under a faucet or shower. There are some dressings that assist with débridement. Film dressings can be used. They are left on the wound for approximately 3 days (or changed sooner if they leak). Hydrocolloidal wafers and gels can also be used but are left on longer. These dressings work by promoting autolysis. Because there is a risk of infection, the area around the dressing must be assessed carefully for signs of infection.

Débridement of Black Wounds. Wounds that are black need débridement.[12] The risk of infection rises in proportion to the amount of necrotic tissue present. Infection is a serious risk for the client with immunosuppression. Clients with neutropenia do not have enough macrophages to combat the pathogens in the wound. Therefore, even small wounds increase the risk of sepsis in the client. Decreased tissue oxygenation from impaired blood flow compounds the problem because the macrophages require oxygen for phagocytosis.

Systemic antibiotics seldom stop infection because they cannot penetrate through the avascular tissues. Topical antibiotics do not penetrate the avascular es-

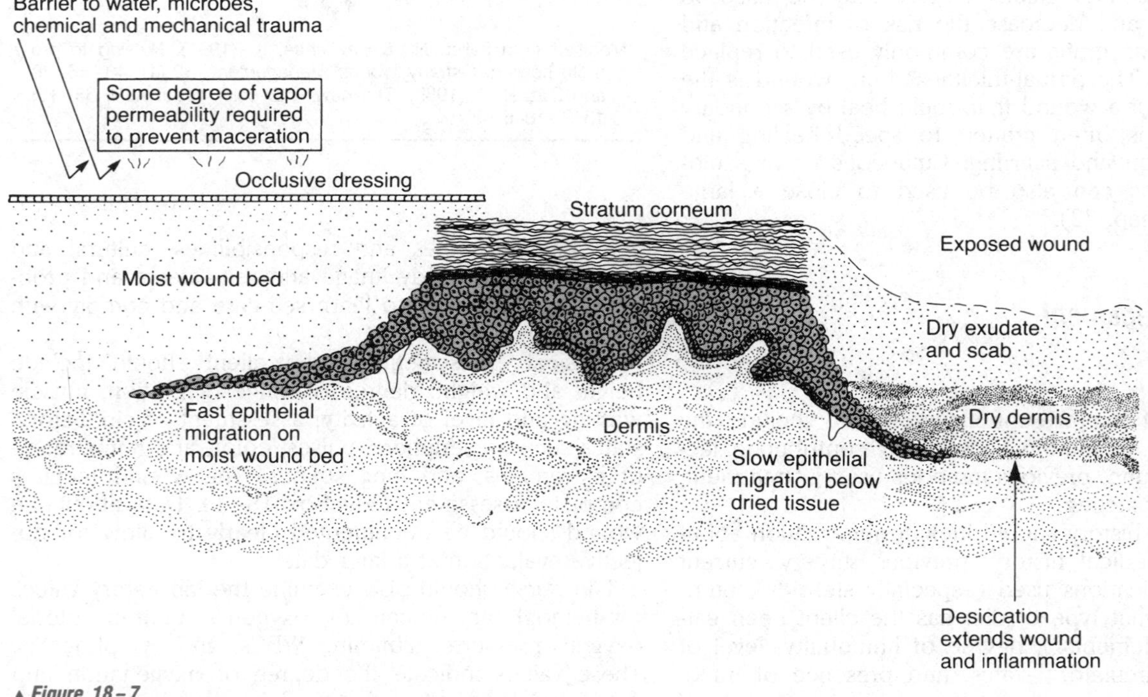

▲ *Figure 18–7*

Wound healing under an occlusive dressing. (Adapted from Winter, G. D., & Scales, J. T. [1963]. Effect of air drying and dressings on the surface of a wound. *Nature, 197,* 91–92. Copyright 1963 Macmillan Magazines Limited.)

char either. Timely débridement is a must to remove the eschar and reduce the risk of infection and the physical obstacle to granulation.

Sometimes, the eschar can be removed to the level of red, bleeding tissues. The wound then requires protection to begin healing. At other times, the top layer of eschar is removed by débridement by a chemical agent or natural sloughing, leaving a yellow eschar. This yellow wound requires aggressive cleaning.

Other Interventions. In addition to local wound care, the client must be provided with a diet that is high in protein, fat, carbohydrates, vitamins, and minerals to facilitate healing. Regardless of the client's actual body weight (e.g., obese), this is not the time to begin a weight loss diet. The wound must be healed first. If the client cannot or will not eat, the use of tube feeding and/or hyperalimentation should be considered.

If the client is immobile or incontinent, adequate prevention must be given to reduce the incidence of new areas of skin breakdown. If the wound is due to lack of venous return, the leg will require elevation. If it is due to lack of arterial flow, it should be positioned flat. Disorders such as diabetes mellitus and cardiovascular disease should be controlled as well as possible.

Dressings. Gauze dressings still remain the most cost-effective dressing. Gauze is used as a dry cover for surgical wounds or wounds that will heal by primary intention (Table 18-5). Wet-to-dry gauze dressings can be used for nonselective débridement of wounds. More absorbent dressings should be used with exudating wounds. Only woven gauze dressings (e.g., Kerlix, Nu-Gauze, Surgipad) should be used in a wound. The non-woven gauze (Sof-Kling) is meant as a secondary dressing for outer wrapping.

If the wound edges are friable or if the wound will be disrupted when the dressing is removed, a nonadhering dressing (Adaptic, Telfa) can be used. The nonadherant dressing can be impregnated or nonimpregnated. The intent of this dressing choice is that when this dressing is removed, the disruption of the wound bed will be minimal.

Wound healing is optimized in a moist environment. When the environment is moist, collagen synthesis and granulation tissue formation are enhanced, cell migration and epithelial resurfacing occurs more rapidly, and scab, crust, and eschar cannot form. This moist environment, however, does create a medium conducive to infection. It is essential to differentiate between normal wound inflammation in the presence of colonizing microorganisms and the environment that results from invading microorganisms.

Transparent films, hydrocolloids, gels, and hydrogels are not only moisture retentive but are also useful for autolytic débridement of the wound. If the wound produces exudate, several absorption dressing products can be used. Absorption dressings, calcium alginates, and hypertonic saline dressings can be used. Foams can also be used for absorption and autolytic débridement. Table 18-5 describes the actions, indications and nursing implications for various categories of wound dressings.

The selection of the dressing type will change as the wound responds to treatment. Careful assessment and reassessment will indicate progress, or lack of progress,

TABLE 18-5. Indications and Implications of Wound Dressings

Type of Dressing	Examples	Indications for Use	Nursing Implications
Non-adhering		Shallow open wounds	Require a second dressing or tape because they are nonadhesive
Non-impregnated	Telfa		
Impregnated	Adaptic Vaseline Gauze		Nonabsorbent, occlusive, not traumatic to remove
Gauze	4 × 4 gauze dressing	Wet-to-dry débridement, wound packing	Moderately absorbent; can be used as wound packing for shallow wounds; use long strips of gauze to pack deep wounds
Transparent films	Bio-occlusive, Omniderm, Op-Site, Tegaderm	Coverage of shallow wounds (skin tears) or intravenous sites	Adhesive; therefore, no secondary dressing is needed. Retain moisture, semipermeable, water resistant
Hydrocolloids and hydrogels	Duoderm, Intrasite, Restore, 3M Tegasorb Biolex Wound Gel, Clearsite, Vigilon	Shallow ulcers, as will provide autolytic débridement Hydrogels have cooling effect	Retain moisture, occlusive or semipermeable, water resistant, adhesive; require replacement because the dressing melts
Exudate absorbers	Bard Absorption Dressing, Envisan	Deep wounds with eschar	Retain moisture, absorbent, promote autolytic débridement

Data from Krasner, D. (1991). Resolving the dressing dilemma: Selecting wound dressings by category. *Ostomy/Wound Management, 35* (4), 62, 64-70.

in wound healing. As the wound changes, variations in the dressing materials are made so that healing is maximized. There is no single dressing that will provide the optimum atmosphere required during all healing stages of the wound.

EVALUATION

The ongoing healing in the wound should be assessed frequently (every 24 hours), especially if the risk of infection remains high. Revisions in the plan of care may be required if healing is not progressing.

Post-hospital Care

DISCHARGE TEACHING

The client with alterations in skin integrity will require long-term care. Appropriate referral to the home health agency should be made. Financial status, home environment, and support systems must be evaluated. Third-party reimbursement may cover supplies, equipment, and nursing care.

The client or family should demonstrate dressing removal, wound cleansing, and dressing application before discharge. The client may need to incorporate lifestyle changes into the activities of daily living in an effort to promote healing. Detailed instructions should be provided to the client, family, and home health care nurse for home use.

Planning for discharge should begin several days before dismissal so that the home situation can be appraised and necessary supplies and equipment obtained. The client should be alerted to signs of complications, such as infection, and given directions on when and how to contact the physician in the case of an emergency.

At home, a balanced diet with frequent high-protein snacks should continue. Vitamin and mineral supplements should be taken as directed by the physician. Proper use of dressing materials and supplies is emphasized in order to minimize waste and help decrease the overall cost of treatment. Physician follow-up is needed to monitor the progress of wound healing and evaluate response to treatment.

CHRONIC NONHEALING WOUNDS

Chronic nonhealing wounds are a challenge. They may be unhealed wounds that should have healed by any of the three intentions, but generally they are nonhealed wounds of secondary intention. The factors that lead to nonhealing are the extrinsic and intrinsic factors discussed earlier in this chapter. Not all of these factors can be eliminated, however. Problems such as infection can usually be controlled with dressings and antibiotics. Clients cannot be made younger, and some clients will refuse to stop smoking, even though their leg wound is due to inadequate circulation. At times, bypass surgery may be required to bring in adequate blood flow. The use of cultured epithelial grafts and hyperbaric oxygen are relatively new treatments in the care of nonhealing wounds (Fig. 18-8). Wound healing accelerators are being studied.

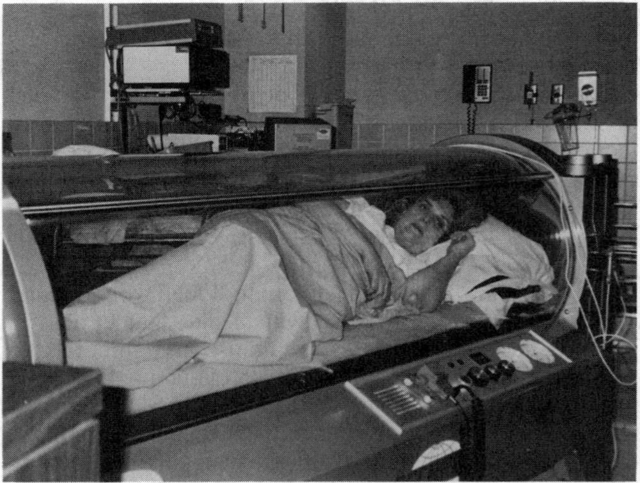

▲ Figure 18-8

Client receiving hyperbaric oxygen (HBO) treatments. HBO is the administration of oxygen at greater than atmospheric pressure. Oxygen is greatly increased in the tissues, and neovascularization, fibroblast activity, collagen synthesis, and phagocytosis are increased to speed wound healing.

▼ COMPLICATIONS OF WOUND HEALING

IMPAIRED COLLAGEN SYNTHESIS

In the wound sutured in surgery, the nurse is able to determine the presence of newly synthesized collagen by what is known as a "healing ridge" just under an intact suture line. When this ridge is not present 5 to 7 days after suturing, the nurse should suspect slowed collagen synthesis and treat the wound with special care.

WOUND INFECTION

Clinical manifestations of wound infection include increased drainage, erythema around the entire wound (not just the edges), development of purulent drainage, fever, leukocytosis, and general malaise. The infected wound is slow to heal and may become disrupted.

Medical Management

Wound infection is a serious consequence and delays wound healing. Topical antimicrobials can be used as the primary treatment. Ideal antimicrobials would be broad spectrum and preserve the regenerating tissues.

But all of the antimicrobials compromise wound healing to some degree by being low in effectiveness against a particular organism or by interfering with healing.

A variety of topical agents can be used to either cleanse or disinfect the wound. Table 18-6 describes enzymatic, cleansing, antiseptic, and antibacterial agents that may be used. A word of caution must be given for the use of disinfectants. They can retard healing and destroy tissue growth.

Hydrogen peroxide breaks down into water and oxygen. When it is used in a wound, it must be rinsed thoroughly with normal saline to remove any trapped oxygen before it can be absorbed by the tissues. Providone-iodine, acetic acid, and sodium hypochlorite are used only in debris-contaminated, infected, and malodorous wounds. These agents are cytotoxic and inhibit granular tissue growth and damage endothelial cells and fibroblasts.[38]

Nurses should be able to assess the WBC differential to assist with the diagnosis of infection. When a client has infection that is not being controlled by mature neutrophils, immature ones are released into the blood. These immature leukocytes are called "bands" or "stabs" as a result of their appearance under the microscope.

The WBC counts and percentages are commonly monitored data. These studies are called differential counts and assist in diagnosing the type of infection. For example, a client with a bacterial infection would have an elevated neutrophil count, whereas a client with allergy would have an elevated eosinophil count. Differential counts are delineated in Table 18-3.

WOUND DISRUPTION

Dehiscence, the interruption of a previously intact suture line (see Fig. 19-11, Chap. 19) is frequently preceded by the client experiencing a sharp pain in the suture line, or a cough and increased serosanguinous drainage from the wound. Evisceration, the opening of a wound with exposure of internal organs, is obviously more serious than dehiscence. If a client experiences evisceration, the nurse should cover the exposed organs with sterile wet dressings, notify the physician, and prepare the client for surgery.

SCARRING

Scarring is a normal part of wound healing. Some scars will become barely visible and others will remain very visible throughout the client's lifetime. Factors that affect scarring are discussed in Chapter 72.

Hypertrophic scars are scars that are raised above the suture line. They may be painful and itch. In general, hypertrophic scars tend to regress over time. Keloids are scars that extend well beyond the suture line (Fig. 18-9). These scars tend to occur in black and Mediterranean clients. They can be excised from a wound but unfortunately tend to recur.

TABLE 18-6. Topical Agents Used in Treatment of Open Wounds

Agent	Indications	Impact on Wound Healing
Antiseptic Solutions		
Normal Saline	Moisten dry eschar; keep a clean wound healing by secondary intention	Speeds healing as solution is iso-osmolar, and it keeps the wound bed moist
Hydrogen peroxide	Used to dissolve clotted blood in a wound	Retards healing, do not use as a dressing on an open wound
Providone-iodine (Betadine)	Use for preparation of intact skin. May be used to clean very contaminated wounds	Retards healing, does not penetrate eschar
Dakin's solution	Used 1/4 to 1/2 strength to clean contaminated wounds	Retards wound healing
Acetic acid	Used to treat wounds contaminated with *Pseudomonas*	
Antibiotic Solutions and Ointments		
Neomycin, bacitracin and polymyxin B combination	Used to clean wounds contaminated with gram-negative and gram-positive bacteria	Increase epidermal healing but may sensitize tissues
Polysporin	Treatment of gram-negative organisms	Unknown
Silver sulfadiazine	Wounds with eschar (e.g., burns). Effective against gram-negative and gram-positive organisms	Enhances epidermal healing
Gentamycin	Most effective against gram-negative organisms, but its use may promote resistance in hospital flora	Unknown
Bacitracin	Effective against gram-positive organisms	May enhance epidermal healing

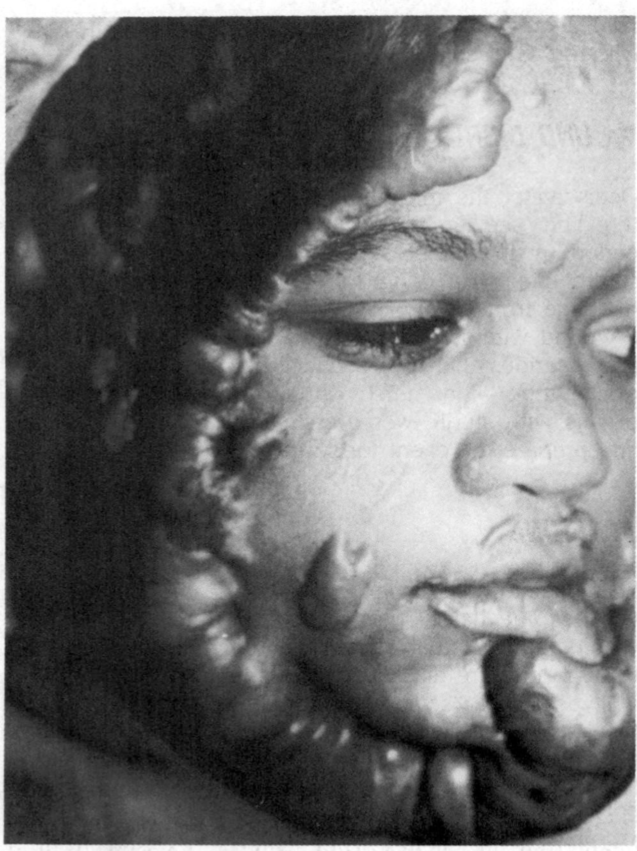

▲ Figure 18–9

Keloid formation. Keloids are overgrowth of scar tissue above and beyond the normal boundaries of the scar. They are fairly resistant to treatment. (From Moncada, G. A. [1984] Trouble-shooting the problem wound. *Plastic Surgical Nursing, 4* [1], 23.

PRESSURE ULCERS

Definition

A pressure ulcer is an alteration in the skin integrity. Pressure ulcers occur commonly in areas subject to high pressure from body weight on bony prominences. Pressure ulcers have also been called bed sores and decubitus ulcers. The word decubitus comes from the Latin word decumbere, which means to lay down. The ulcers were so named because they are common in bedridden clients.

Incidence

The incidence of pressure ulcers is variable because there are certain groups of clients at risk. About 24 to 27 per cent of elderly clients have pressure ulcers and about 25 to 40 per cent of spinal cord-injured clients have pressure ulcers at any given time. Because of the mix of clients in acute care hospitals, the prevalence is near 3 per cent.[38]

Etiology

Pressure ulcers develop when soft tissue (skin, subcutaneous tissue and muscle) are compressed between a bony prominence and a firm surface for a prolonged period of time. The period of time before breakdown varies between clients; very debilitated clients can have permanent tissue damage in less than 2 hours.

Risk Factors

The risk factors leading to pressure ulcers are intrinsic and extrinsic. In addition, incontinence, immobility, and skin shearing can also lead to breakdown.

PREVENTION

Prevention of pressure ulcers begins with identifying the client at risk. Risk factors for alteration in skin integrity can be determined by assessing sensory perception, moisture, activity, mobility, nutrition, and friction and sheer. The Braden Scale (Fig. 18–10) is an assessment tool that evaluates both sensation and physiologic risk.

The high-risk client will need frequent position changes. A trapeze bar, turning sheet, or transfer board can be used to prevent shearing injury to the skin. Frequent shifting of body weight prevents ischemia by redistributing the weight and allowing blood to recirculate.

Pressure-reducing devices may also be helpful. These are either static or dynamic. Static pressure reduction comes from air, flotation of gel or water, and foam mattresses. Dynamic pressure reduction devices are the alternating air flow pressure mattresses and specialty beds, which include air-fluidized beds, the low-air-loss bed, and the three-layer air cushions. These devices do not prohibit capillary blood flow to the skin.

Besides reducing the pressure on the skin, fluid and nutrition intake must be evaluated. Nutritional status must be adequate enough to promote healing and prevent deterioration. The dietician should be consulted to evaluate nitrogen balance and suggest dietary modifications.

The incontinent client must be kept as dry as possible. Stool or urine can contaminate an existing wound or create an environment that will result in a loss of skin integrity. Stool or urine becomes an irritant and places the client at risk for skin breakdown.

Pathophysiology

Continuous pressure on soft tissues between bony prominences and hard surfaces compresses capillaries and occludes the blood flow. If the pressure is relieved, a brief period of rebound capillary dilation (called reactive hyperemia) occurs and no tissue damage occurs. If pressure is not relieved, the microthrombi form in the capillary and completely occlude blood

RISK PREDICTORS FOR SKIN BREAKDOWN

Patient's Name__________ Evaluator's Name__________

					Date of Assessment			
SENSORY PERCEPTION ability to respond to discomfort	1. **Completely limited:** Unresponsive to painful stimuli, either because of state of unconsciousness or severe sensory impairment, which limits ability to feel pain over most of body surface	2. **Very limited:** Responds only to painful stimuli (but not verbal commands) by opening eyes or flexing extremities. Cannot communicate discomfort verbally, OR has a sensory impairment which limits the ability to feel pain or discomfort over one half of body surface	3. **Slightly limited:** Responds to verbal commands by opening eyes and obeying some commands, but cannot always communicate discomfort or need to be turned, OR has some sensory impairment which limits ability to feel pain or discomfort in one or two extremities.	4. **No impairment:** Responds to verbal commands by obeying. Can communicate needs accurately. Has no sensory deficit which would limit ability to feel pain or discomfort				
MOISTURE degree to which skin is exposed to moisture	1. **Very Moist:** Skin is kept moist almost constantly by perspiration and urine. Dampness is detected every time patient is moved or turned. Linen must be changed more than one time each shift	2. **Occasionally Moist:** Skin is frequently, but not always kept moist, linen must be changed two to three times every 24 hours	3. **Rarely Moist:** Skin is rarely moist more than three to four times a week, but linen does require changing at that time	4. **Never Moist:** Perspiration and incontinence is never a problem, linen changed at routine intervals only				
ACTIVITY degree of physical activity	1. **Bedfast:** Confined to bed	2. **Chairfast:** Ability to walk severely impaired or nonexistant and must be assisted into chair or wheelchair. Is confined to chair or wheelchair when not in bed	3. **Walks occasionally:** Walks occasionally during day, but for very short distances, with or without assistance. Spends majority of each shift in bed or chair	4. **Walks frequently:** Walks a moderate distance at least once every 1 to 2 hours during waking hours				
MOBILITY ability to change and control body position	1. **Completely Immobile:** Unable to make even slight changes in position without assistance	2. **Very limited:** Makes occasional slight changes in position without help but unable to make frequent or significant changes in position independently	3. **Slightly limited:** Makes frequent though slight changes in position without assistance but unable to make or maintain major changes in position independently	4. **No limitations:** Makes major and frequent changes in position without assistance				
NUTRITION usual food intake pattern	1. **Very Poor:** Never eats a complete meal. Rarely eats more than 1/3 of any food offered. Intake of protein is negligible. Takes even fluids poorly. Does not take a liquid dietary supplement, OR is NPO and/or maintained on clear liquids or IV for more than 5 days	2. **Probably Inadequate:** Rarely eats a complete meal and generally eats only about one half of any food offered. Protein intake is poor. Occasionally will take a liquid dietary supplement, OR receiving less than optimum amount of liquid diet or tube feeding	3. **Adequate:** Eats over half of most meals. Eats moderate amount of protein source one to two times daily. Occasionally will refuse a meal. Will usually take a dietary supplement if offered, OR is on a tube feeding or TPN regimen which probably meets most of nutritional needs	4. **Excellent:** Eats most of every meal. Never refuses a meal. Frequently eats between meals. Does not require a dietary supplementation				
FRICTION AND SHEAR	1. **Problem:** Requires moderate to maximum assistance in moving. Complete lifting without sliding against sheets is impossible. Frequently slides down in bed or chair, requiring frequent repositioning with maximum assistance. Either spasticity, contractures or agitation leads to almost constant friction	2. **Potential Problem:** Moves feebly Independently or requires minimum assistance. Skin probably slides against bedsheets or chair to some extent when movement occurs. Maintains relatively good position in chair or bed most of time but occasionally slides down	3. **No Apparent Problem:** Moves in bed and in chair independently and has sufficient muscle strength to lift up completely during move. Maintains good position in bed or chair at all times					
				Total Score				

Key: 16, minimum risk; 13–14, moderate risk; 12 or less, high risk;
NPO, nothing by mouth; IV, intravenously; TPN, total parenteral nutrition.

▲ ***Figure 18–10***

Braden scale. (Courtesy of Barbara Braden.)

flow. A blister may form initially and if there has been damage to only the superficial tissues. Damage to underlying tissues creates a necrotic area of tissue. The necrotic tissue undergoes the process of inflammation as the body tries to clear it and ready the tissue for healing.

Clinical Manifestations

The clinical manifestations of pressure ulcers have been described in four stages (Fig. 18-11). Ulcers most commonly occur on the greater trochanter, heel, sacrum, and ischial tuberosities (Fig. 18-12).

Medical Management

The medical and surgical management of pressure ulcers begins with the management of the client with a wound healing by secondary intention (see earlier discussion). In addition, the client may be placed on low-pressurized beds to reduce the risk of further ulcers (Fig. 18-13).

Surgical Management

Surgical repair is frequently performed on Stage III and IV ulcers, on ulcers over 2 cm in diameter and in clients who can tolerate surgery. In stage III ulcers, undamaged tissue near the wound is rotated to cover the ulcer. In stage IV ulcers, musculocutaneous flaps are often used (see Chap. 72).

Nursing Management

ASSESSMENT

The assessment of the client at high risk for the development of pressure ulcers should include the risk factors. Braden's tool (see Fig. 18-10) has been developed to assist the nurse in predicting which clients are at greatest risk. In addition, laboratory data on hemoglobin, hematocrit, albumin, total protein, and lymphocytes should be assessed. It is important to realize that risk prediction must be an ongoing assessment. Objective data about the pressure ulcer should be noted (see Box 18-1).

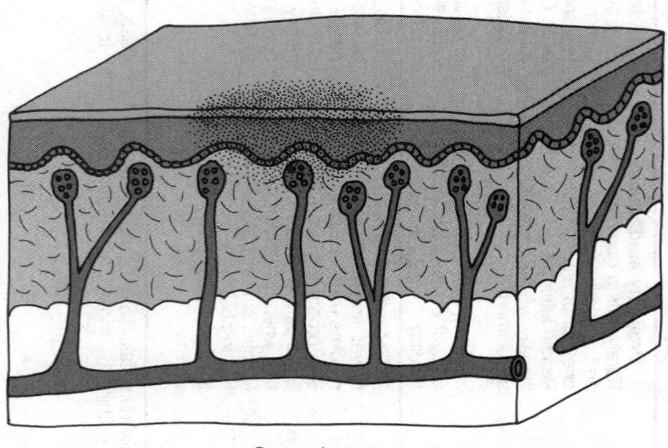

Stage I

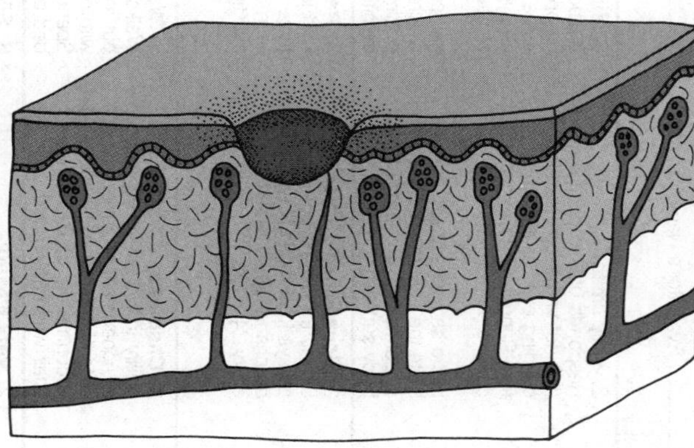

Stage II

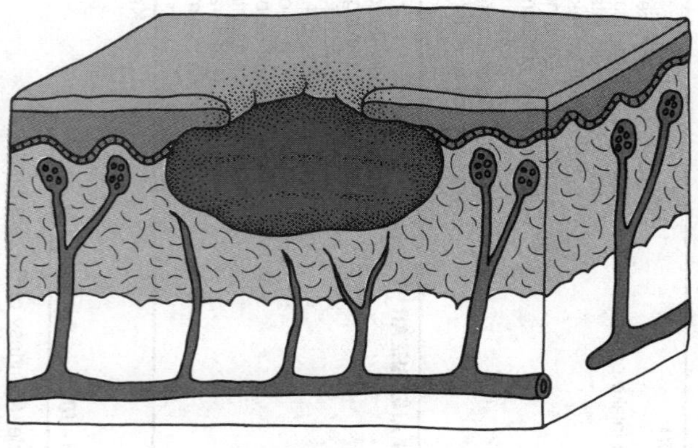

Stage III

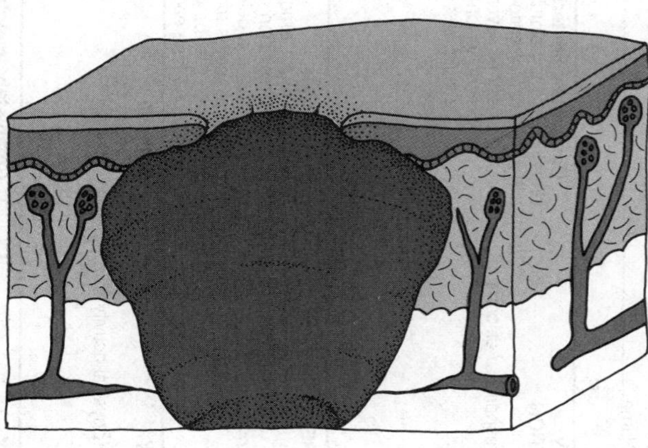

Stage IV

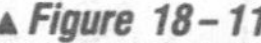

▲ **Figure 18-11**

Stages in the development of pressure sores.

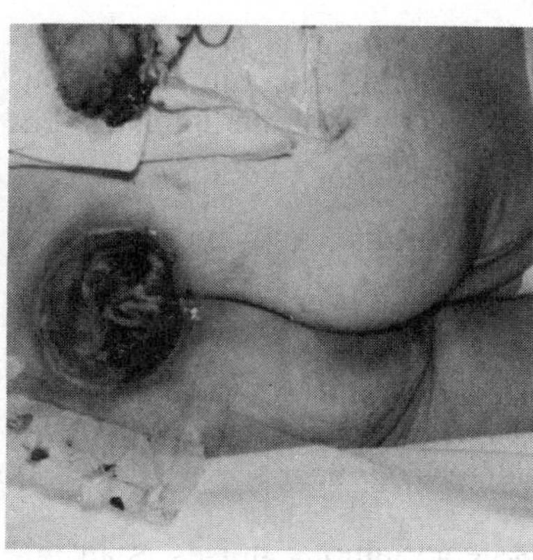

▲ Figure 18-12

Pressure sore.

NURSING INTERVENTION

Nursing Diagnosis: Skin Integrity, Impaired, High Risk for R/T pressure over bony prominences.

Planning: Expected Outcomes. The client will reduce the risk of impairment in skin integrity, as evidenced by no actual tissue breakdown and no persistent reddened areas.

Implementation. Preventive measures to reduce the risk of pressure ulcers cannot be overemphasized. In 1992, the United States Department of Health and Human Services developed guidelines for prediction and prevention of pressure ulcers in adults.[36] These guidelines are summarized here:

1. All clients at risk should have a systematic skin inspection at least once a day, paying particular attention to the bony prominences. Results of skin inspection should be documented.
2. Skin should be cleansed at the time of soiling and at routine intervals. The frequency of skin cleansing should be individualized according to need and/or client preference. Avoid hot water, and use a mild cleansing agent that minimizes irritation and dryness of the skin. During the cleansing process, care should be used to minimize the force and friction applied to the skin.
3. Minimize environmental factors leading to skin drying, such as low humidity (less than 40 percent) and exposure to cold. Dry skin should be treated with moisturizers.
4. Avoid massage over bony prominences. Current evidence suggests that massage over bony prominences may be harmful.
5. Minimize skin exposure to moisture due to incontinence, perspiration, or wound drainage. When these sources of moisture cannot be controlled, underpads or briefs can be used that are made of materials that absorb moisture and present a quick-drying surface to the skin. For information about assessing and managing urinary incontinence, refer to *Urinary Incontinence in Adults: Clinical Practice Guideline* (available from AHCPR). Topical agents that act as barriers to moisture can also be used.
6. Skin injury due to friction and shear forces should be minimized through proper positioning, transferring, and turning techniques. In addition, friction injuries may be reduced by the use of lubricants (such as corn starch and creams), protective films (such as transparent film dressings and skin sealants), protective dressings (such as hydrocolloids), and protective padding.
7. When apparently well-nourished clients develop an inadequate dietary intake of protein or calories, caregivers should first attempt to discover the factors compromising intake and offer support with eating. Other nutritional supplements or support may be needed. If dietary intake remains inadequate and if consistent with overall goals of therapy, more aggressive nutritional intervention such as enteral or parenteral feedings should be considered.

For nutritionally compromised individuals, a plan of nutritional support and/or supplementation

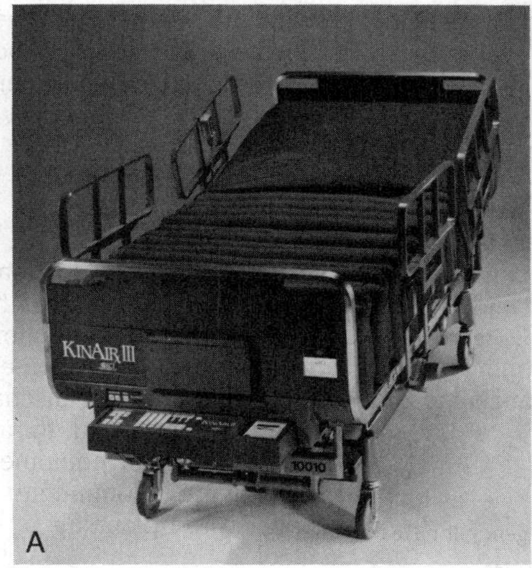

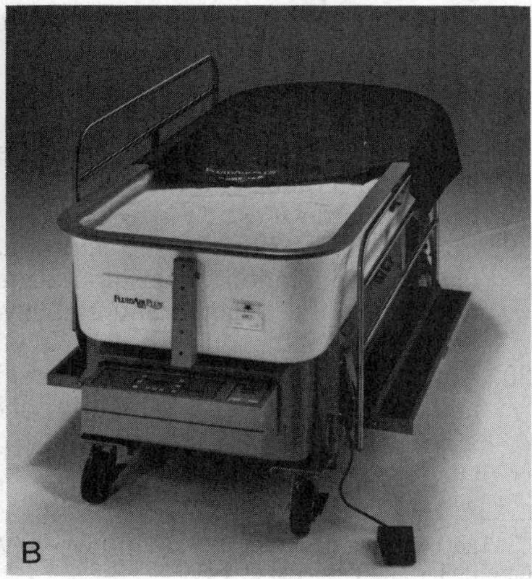

▲ Figure 18-13

A, An air-flotation, low air-loss support surface that provides pressure relief. Used in care of clients who are at high risk for skin breakdown. *B*, A fluid air bed. These beds feel like waterbeds but are composed of air-fluidized silicone beads. Used in care of clients who cannot tolerate turning or have only one turning surface. (Photos courtesy of KCI Medical Therapeutic Services, San Antonio, TX.)

should be implemented that meets individual needs and is consistent with the overall goals of therapy.

8. If the potential exists for improving the individual's mobility and activity status, rehabilitation efforts should be instituted if consistent with the overall goals of therapy. Maintaining current activity level, mobility, and range of motion is an appropriate goal for most individuals.
9. Interventions and outcomes should be monitored and documented.
10. Any individual in bed who is assessed to be at risk for developing pressure ulcers should be repositioned at least every 2 hours if consistent with overall patient goals. A written schedule for systematically turning and repositioning the individual should be used.
11. For individuals in bed, positioning devices such as pillows or foam wedges should be used to keep bony prominences (such as knees or ankles) from direct contact with one another, according to a written plan.
12. Individuals in bed who are completely immobile should have a care plan that includes the use of devices that totally relieve pressure on the heels, most commonly by raising the heels off the bed. Do not use donut-type devices.
13. When the side-lying position is used in bed, avoid positioning directly on the trochanter.
14. Maintain the head of the bed at the lowest degree of elevation consistent with medical conditions and other restrictions. Limit the amount of time the head of the bed is elevated.
15. Use lifting devices such as a trapeze or bed linen to move (rather than drag) individuals in bed who cannot assist during transfers and position changes.
16. Any individual assessed to be at risk for developing pressure ulcers should be placed when lying in bed on a pressure-reducing device, such as foam, static air, alternating air, gel, or water mattresses.
17. Any person at risk for developing a pressure ulcer should avoid uninterrupted sitting in any chair or wheelchair. The individual should be repositioned, shifting the points under pressure at least every hour or be put back to bed if consistent with overall patient management goals. Individuals who are able should be taught to shift weight every 15 minutes.
18. For chair-bound individuals, the use of a pressure-reducing device such as those made of foam, gel, air, or a combination is indicated. Do not use donut-type devices.
19. Positioning of chair-bound individuals should include consideration of postural alignment, distribution of weight, balance and stability, and pressure relief.
20. A written plan for the use of positioning devices and schedules may be helpful for chair-bound individuals.*

* The complete pamphlet is available from the Agency for Health Care Policy and Research at 1-800-358-9295.

There are many devices that may be used to relieve pressure on the skin. In general, they are not substitutes for nursing care but lengthen the intervals between back care and repositioning.

Nursing Diagnosis: Skin Integrity, Impaired (pressure ulcer), High Risk for R/T to lack of awareness of the need to reposition.

Planning: Expected Outcomes. The client will have healing of the ulcer, as evidenced by development of granulation tissue and decreasing ulcer size.

Implementation. Consistency among nurses is an important aspect in achieving wound healing. It is important to develop and use scientific protocols in ulcer care and use them. It is also important to give one protocol time to work before changing to another one.

The ulcer must be cleaned in order to heal. The approach that differentiates treatment of wounds according to color (red-yellow-black) will work for pressure ulcers. In addition, all of the intrinsic and extrinsic factors that lead to the ulcer's formation must be addressed.

EVALUATION

The degree of goal attainment should be measured on every shift, because pressure ulcers can develop quickly. As the wound heals, the degree of goal attainment should be assessed every 3 to 4 days.

Post-hospital Care

DISCHARGE TEACHING

Clients at high risk for pressure ulcers should be referred to home health agencies before discharge so that devices to reduce pressure can be obtained for home use. The family and client need to understand the importance of frequent turning. If the client is wheelchair bound and has arm function, the client should be taught to lift the body with the arms off of the chair twice every hour for repositioning. Clients who are incontinent need to wear protective pads to absorb the urine or stool and be assessed often. The United States Department of Health and Human Services has developed a patient guide for preventing pressure ulcers.[36]

FOLLOW-UP CARE

If the client is going home with an unhealed ulcer, the client and family must be taught wound care, wound assessment, and sometimes, the administration of intravenous antibiotics. These interventions should be taught prior to the day of discharge, so that return demonstrations can be used to ascertain learning. In addition, procurement of equipment is often necessary, and this takes time. Community nurses need to be involved early in the planning of discharge of the client with an ulcer.

Summary

Wound healing is a complex process but often goes on with little effort on the part of the client. It is only when the wound does not heal or pressure ulcers develop, that the many steps in wound healing are evident. Pressure ulcers are a significant problem especially in the elderly and the paralyzed client. Nurses need to be diligent in their care of these special clients to prevent pressure ulcers.

Bibliography

1. Alterescu, V. (1989). The financial cost of inpatient pressure ulcers to an acute care facility. *Decubitus, 2* (3), 14-23.
2. Bergstrom, N., et al. (1987). The Braden scale for predicting pressure sore risk. *Nursing Research, 36* (4), 205-210.
3. Black, J. (1991). Reconstructive surgery in the elderly. *Plastic Surgical Nursing, 11* (4), 151-162.
4. Black, J., & Black, S. (1987). Surgical management of pressure ulcers. *Nursing Clinics of North America, 22* (2), 429-438.
5. Braden, B., & Bergstrom, N. (1989). Clinical utility of the Braden scale for predicting pressure sore risk. *Decubitus, 2* (3), 44-51.
6. Braden, B., & Bryant, R. (1990). Innovations to prevent and treat pressure ulcers. *Geriatric Nursing, (4),* 182-186.
7. Brown, S. (1990). Behind the numbers of the CBC. *RN, 53* (2), 46-51.
8. Cohen, I., et al. (Eds.) (1992). *Wound healing.* Philadelphia: W.B. Saunders.
9. Cohburn, L. (1990). Preventing pressure ulcers: How to recognize and care for patients at risk. *Nursing 90, 20* (12), 60-63.
10. Copper, D. (1990). Optimizing wound healing. *Nursing Clinics of North America, 25* (1), 165-180.
11. Curtis, A., et al. (1990). Hyperbaric oxygen therapy—An overview. *Plastic Surgical Nursing, 10* (2), 63-68.
12. Cuzzell, J. (1988). The new RYB color code. *AJN, 88* (10), 1342-1346.
13. Cuzzell, J., & Stotts, N. (1990). Trial and error yields to knowledge. *AJN, 90* (10), 53-61.
14. Cuzzell, J., & Wiley, T. (1987). Pressure relief perennials. *AJN, 87* (9), 1157-1161.
15. Dealey, C. (1991). The size of the pressure-sore problem in a teaching hospital. *Journal of Advanced Nursing, 16,* 663-670.
16. Deloach, E.D., et al. (1992). Osteomyelitis underlying severe pressure sores. *Contemporary Surgery, 40* (5), 25-32.
17. Faller, N., & Lawrence, K. (1991). Nursing to promote healing. *Ostomy/Wound Management, 32* (1), 43-46, 48.
18. Frantz, R. (1989). Pressure ulcer costs in long-term care. *Decubitus, 2* (3), 56-57.
19. French, E., & Sifner, K. (1991). A method for consistent documentation of pressure sores. *Rehabilitation Nursing, 16* (4), 204-207.
20. Goodman, T., et al. (1990). Skin ulcers. *AORN Journal, 52* (1), 24-37.
21. Goss, R. (1992). Regeneration versus repair. In I. Cohen et al. (Eds.), *Wound healing.* Philadelphia: W.B. Saunders.
22. Green, E., & Katz, J. (1991). Practice guidelines for management of pressure ulcers. *Decubitus, 4* (1), 36-42.
23. Holmes, R., et al. (1987). Combatting pressure sores—nutritionally. *AJN, 87* (10), 1301-1303.
24. Hotter, A. (1990). Wound healing and immunocompromise. *Nursing Clinics of North America, 25* (1), 193-203.
25. Jones, P., & Milliman, A. (1990). Wound healing and the aged patient. *Nursing Clinics of North America, 25* (1), 263-277.
26. Kaminski, M., & Devin, G. (1989). Nutritional management of decubitus ulcers in the elderly. *Decubitus, 2* (4), 20-30.
27. Krasner, D. (1991). Resolving the dressing dilemma: Selecting wound dressings by category. *Ostomy/Wound Management, 35* (4), 62, 64-70.
28. Lawrence, W. (1992). Clinical management of nonhealing wounds. In I. Cohen, et al. (Eds.), *Wound healing.* Philadelphia: W.B. Saunders.
29. Maklebust, J. (1991). Pressure sore update. *RN, 54* (12), 56-62.
30. McCance, K., & Huether, S. (1990). *Pathophysiology.* St. Louis: C. V. Mosby.
31. Meehan, M. (1990). Multisite pressure ulcer prevalence study. *Decubitus, 3* (4), 14-17.
32. Messer, M. (1989). Wound care. *Critical Care Nursing Quarterly, 11* (4), 17-27.
33. Munro, B., et al. (1989). Pressure ulcers: One bed or another? *Geriatric Nursing, 10* (4), 190-192.
34. Neuberger, G. (1987). Wound care. *Nursing 87, 17* (2), 34-37.
35. Olson, B. (1989). Effects of massage for prevention of pressure ulcers. *Decubitus, 2* (4), 32-37.
36. Panel of the Prediction and Prevention of Pressure Ulcers in Adults (1992). *Pressure ulcers in adults: prediction and prevention: clinical practice guidelines.* A CPR Publication No. 92-0050. Rockville, MD: Agency for Health Care Policy and Research, Public Health Service, U.S. Department of Health and Human Services.
37. Sater, B., et al. (1991). A protocol for the management of patients at high risk for pressure sores. In W. Chenitz, et al. (Eds.), *Clinical Gerontological Nursing.* Philadelphia: W.B. Saunders.
38. Sayler, J. (1988). Wound management in the home: Part II. *Home Healthcare Nurse, 6* (3), 29-34.
39. Shannon, M., & Skorga, P. (1989). Pressure ulcer prevalence in two general hospitals. *Decubitus, 2* (4), 38-43.
40. Smith, A., & Malone, J. (1990). Preventing pressure ulcers in institutionalized elders: Assessing the effects of small unscheduled shifts in body position. *Decubitus, 3* (4), 20-24.
41. Smith, T. (1989). Management of difficult or chronic wounds. *Topics in Emergency Medicine, 11* (1), 45-55.
42. Sparks, S. (1992). Nurse validation of pressure ulcer risk factors for a nursing diagnosis. *Decubitus, 5* (1), 26-35.
43. Stone, J. (1991). Pressure sores. In W. Chenitz, et al. (Eds.), *Clinical Gerontological Nursing.* Philadelphia: W.B. Saunders.
44. Trelstad, A., & Osmundson, D. (1989). Water Piks: Wound Cleansing Alternative. *Plastic Surgical Nursing, 9* (3), 117-119.
45. Wiseman, D., et al. (1992). Wound dressings: Design and Use. In I. Cohen, et al. (Eds.), *Wound healing.* Philadelphia: W.B. Saunders.

Chapter 19

Perioperative Nursing

Caring for perioperative clients is a challenging and gratifying specialty. Over the last 20 years, dedicated researchers and practitioners have made tremendous advances in surgical intervention and postoperative care. Operations that were once considered last-resort measures are now termed routine. Clients no longer spend weeks in bed following surgery, which was a common practice in the past. Advances in anesthesia and surgical techniques allow clients to recover quickly from surgery and return home to productive lives.

A major change in the past decade is the emergence of outpatient surgery centers and ambulatory surgery. Estimates vary, but market analysts predict that during the 1990s, more than 60 per cent of all surgical care will be provided on an ambulatory basis.[22] This development will change the focus of nursing care because of the brief time the client spends in the hospital or clinic. Knowledge of nursing process, technical skills, and responsibility for all phases of the client's perioperative experience becomes essential to the nursing care of the surgical client.

What is perioperative nursing, and what special skills does it require? The perioperative nurse prepares clients and their families or significant others physically and emotionally for surgery. Surgery is traumatic. Any surgical procedure, however minor, carries some degree of risk. The nurse also helps prepare clients and families or significant others cognitively, emotionally, and spiritually following psychosocial assessment. The client being prepared for surgery is awaiting the unknown and is often in a state of anxiety.

Experienced perioperative nurses are alert to the emotional turmoil many clients and their significant others experience preoperatively. These nurses recognize that surgery inevitably involves expense, discomfort, emotional and physiologic stress, and disruption of the client's life. Nursing assessment and interventions are planned accordingly.

The scope of perioperative nursing practice consists of three phases: preoperative, intraoperative, and postoperative.

Preoperative Phase. The scope of perioperative practice commences with the preoperative phase. This phase begins when the decision for surgical intervention is made and ends with transfer of the client to the operating room bed. Nursing activities range from a baseline assessment of the client during the preoperative interview at the clinic or at home and continues with assessment in the preoperative area or surgical suite on the day of surgery.

Intraoperative Phase. The scope of perioperative nursing practice continues into the intraoperative phase of the surgical experience. This phase begins when the client is transferred to the operating room bed and ends when the client is admitted to the postanesthesia recovery area (PAR). In this phase, nursing interventions range from recognizing improper positioning and the potential for injury, to implementing corrective measures, and evaluating cardiopulmonary assessment data.

Postoperative Phase. The scope of perioperative nursing practice ends with the postoperative phase of the surgical experience. The client's postoperative period begins with admission to the postanesthesia recovery area and ends with the resolution of the surgical sequelae. Nursing activities range from communicating pertinent information about the client's surgery to postanesthesia nursing staff to a postoperative evaluation in the clinic or client's home.

The nursing process is applied throughout the entire perioperative period to ensure that the client's physical and emotional needs are met. Meeting these needs enhances the client's ability to withstand the trauma of surgery and return quickly to preoperative condition.

BASIC CONCEPTS

The word *perioperative* refers to events during the entire surgical period, from preparation for surgery to recovery from the temporary effects of surgery and anesthesia. This period is divided into the preoperative, intraoperative, and postoperative phases.

Overview

Historically, *surgeons* bored holes in the patient's skull to provide a means 'for disease to escape.' Modern technology and advances in surgical technique and anesthesia have made procedures such as transplants and open heart surgery commonplace.

For many types of surgery the client is admitted, surgery is performed, and the client is discharged the same day. To decrease the cost of care, infection rate, and client recovery, many types of surgery are performed in ambulatory care settings (also known as surgicenters, same-day surgery centers, or outpatient surgery centers).

DEFINITIONS AND SURGICAL PROCEDURES

Common prefixes and suffixes can explain the type of procedure the client will undergo. Table 19-1 outlines some common surgical terminology.

Surgical procedures are categorized by purpose, extent, and urgency of the procedure. Knowledge of these categories may aid nurses in planning care for all phases of the client's surgery. Table 19-2 outlines the main categories of surgical procedures.

STRESS AND THE PERIOPERATIVE CLIENT

Stress must be considered in the care of the perioperative client. Surgery increases stress on all body systems, and stress can be exhibited psychologically or physically. Stress is a collective term used to describe the many psychological and physiologic factors that cause neurochemical changes within the body.

TABLE 19-1. Common Surgical Terminology

Term	Definition
Prefixes	
supra-	Above; beyond
artho-	Joint
chole-	Bile or gall
cysto-	Bladder
encephalo-	Brain
entero-	Intestine
hystero-	Uterus
mast-	Breast
meningo-	Membrane
myo-	Muscle
nephro-	Kidney
neuro-	Nerve
oophor-	Ovary
pneumo-	Lung
pyelo-	Pelvis; kidney pelvis
salpingo-	Fallopian tubes
thoraco-	Chest
viscer-	Organ; especially abdominal
Suffixes	
-oma	Tumor; swelling
-ectomy	Removal of organ or gland
-rrhaphy	The suturing or stitching of a part or an organ
-scopy	Looking into
-ostomy	Making an opening or stoma
-otomy	Cutting into
-plasty	To repair or restore
-cele	Tumor, hernia, swelling
-itis	Inflammation of

TABLE 19-2. Categories of Surgical Procedures

Procedure	Definition
Purpose	
Diagnostic	To confirm a diagnosis
Exploratory	To estimate the extent of disease and/or to confirm a diagnosis
Curative	To remove or repair damaged or diseased tissue or organs
Ablative	Involves removal of diseased organ
Reconstructive	Partial or complete restoration of a damaged organ or tissue to its original appearance and function
Constructive	Repair of a congenitally defective organ by improving its function or appearance
Palliative	Relieves symptoms but does not cure underlying disease
Extent	
Major	Extensive; involves significant, serious risk; may involve significant loss of blood, serious complications
Minor	Minimal, few serious complications; involves minimal loss of blood
Urgency	
Emergency	Must be performed immediately to (1) maintain life; (2) maintain organ or limb function; (3) remove a damaged organ; or (4) stop hemorrhage
Imperative	Requires surgical intervention within 24–48 hours.
Planned or required	Surgical intervention is important, but it can be scheduled several weeks or months in advance
Elective	Performed for the person's well-being but is not absolutely necessary
Optional	Surgery performed simply for individual's preference. It is not needed

Stressors in the perioperative client include pain, tissue damage, blood loss, anesthesia, fever, and immobilization. The stressful stimuli imposed by surgery promote the stress response by combining both psychological (anxiety, fear of unknown) and physiologic (blood loss, anesthesia, pain, immobility) factors.

In response to the stress of surgery, the body mobilizes its defenses to maintain homeostasis. The systemic responses to surgical stress are outlined in Table 19–3. The success of the stress response in maintaining homeostatic balance is determined by a person's age, physical condition, and the duration of stress. The ability to withstand the stress of surgery and anesthesia is decreased significantly in aged or debilitated persons. In the perioperative period, the nurse must be able to assess stress in the client and intervene to prevent and reduce complications.

The Practice of Perioperative Nursing

Technologic advances and a change in the surgical setting have contributed to the expanded practice of perioperative nursing. The safety and welfare of the client is the primary goal during all phases of the perioperative experience.

Nurses have different roles and have varied responsibilities for the care of the surgical client. All contribute to the safe recovery of the operative client. The *staff nurse* is responsible for the care of the client in the preoperative and postoperative period. The nurse's role includes teaching, the physical preparation, assessment, and discharge of the client. The *operating room nurse* is responsible for the safe care of the client during surgery. The operating room nurse's role may include visiting clients preoperatively to assess their needs and prepare them for surgery. *Nurse anesthetists* are responsible for the safe delivery of anesthesia during surgery. *Post-anesthesia care unit nurses* care for clients in the immediate post-anesthesia and postoperative period. After a client is stable and ready to be transferred, the client is cared for by a *staff nurse* on a general surgery floor or in an intensive care or specialized unit, or he or she may go home. Because so many types of surgery are now performed on an outpatient basis, some staff nurses in ambulatory care units or outpatient centers care for clients throughout the entire perioperative period.

The Association of Operating Room Nurses (AORN) has developed standards of nursing care and provides a basic model by which the quality of nursing practice can be measured for the operative client. The American Nurses Association (ANA) has developed standards of medical-surgical practice that outline standards for the nursing care of the preoperative and postoperative client. The American Association of Nurse Anesthetists (AANA) has developed standards of practice for the nurse anesthetist. The American Society for Post Anesthesia Nursing (ASPAN) has also developed perioperative standards.

Surgery is a unique experience for the individual. Nursing is challenged to provide excellent care in all phases of the operative experience. Perioperative nursing has become highly sophisticated and specialized, but the client always remains the focus of the process. In the following units, the nurses' role in each phase of the operative experience is discussed.

PREOPERATIVE NURSING

Careful preparation of individuals undergoing surgery during the preoperative period decreases operative risk and promotes postoperative recovery. In the case of emergency surgery, time may not permit complete preoperative assessment, care planning, and teaching. Nevertheless, essential preparation must be thorough.

Generally, preoperative preparation can take place in any of four places: (1) in the physician's office before admission to the health care facility, (2) on admission

TABLE 19–3. Responses to Surgical Stress

Response to Surgical Stress	Adaptive Response	Maladaptive Responses
Vasoconstriction peripherally with increased coagulability	Blood increased to vital organs, away from periphery; increased clotting to decrease blood loss	Decrease in renal profusion possible; clotting and thrombus formation increase
Tachycardia with increased cardiac output, blood pressure, and coronary artery dilation	Increased perfusion of myocardium; increased oxygen perfusion to vital organs	Increased demand on heart possibly leading to heart failure; hypertension
Sodium and water retention secondary to increased ADH and aldosterone secretion	Increased volume to prevent hypovolemia, maintenance of blood pressure and cardiac output	Hypervolemia, circulatory overload, hypertension, and heart failure
Increased gastric acidity and decreased peristalsis	Blood shifted from large intestine to more vital areas	Paralytic ileus and stress ulcers
Bronchial dilation	Increased oxygen exchange, improved ventilation	No maladaptive change
Protein catabolism	Increased amino acids for wound healing	Negative nitrogen balance, eventual lack of tissue repair unless reversed
Proliferation of granulation and connective tissue	Increased wound healing	Development of excessive scar tissue and adhesions
Increased blood sugar and mobilization of fat stores	Increased energy available	Increased blood sugar detrimental to diabetics
Increased cortisol with increased anti-inflammatory response	Increases blood sugar	Possible infection if antiinflammatory effect is prolonged
Increased metabolic rate	Increases energy available for adaptation	Increased heat loss may lead to hypothermia and shivering, with increasing oxygen demand

ADH, Antidiuretic hormone.

and during the days before the operation, (3) the night before surgery if the client is in the hospital, and (4) the morning of surgery on admission.

The preoperative period begins once the client is scheduled for surgery and ends at the time of transfer to the surgical suite. During this phase, the nurse begins a complete assessment and establishes a plan of care based on individual physical and psychosocial needs. Preoperative care focuses on preoperative teaching of the client and family to reduce anxiety and decrease postoperative complications.

General Preoperative Preparation

NURSING ASSESSMENT OF THE CLIENT UNDERGOING SURGERY

Each client responds differently to surgery. Many variables influence a person's physiologic and psychological responses to the surgical experience. These include the (1) physical and mental status, (2) extent of the disease, (3) magnitude of the surgery, (4) social and financial resources, and (5) psychological and physiologic preparation for surgery. When considered collectively, these variables reveal the degree of risk for a client undergoing surgery. Therefore, nursing assessment includes all these factors.

PHYSIOLOGIC NURSING ASSESSMENT OF THE CLIENT UNDERGOING SURGERY

Physiologic nursing assessment before surgery includes information about (1) age, (2) presence of pain, (3) nutritional status, (4) fluid and electrolyte balance, (5) presence of infection, (6) cardiovascular function, (7) pulmonary function, (8) renal function, (9) gastrointestinal function, (10) liver function, (11) endocrine function, (12) neurologic function, (13) hematologic function, (14) medication history, (15) presence of trauma, (16) health habits, and (17) social history.

Age. Infants, young children, and older adults have the lowest tolerance to the stressful effects of surgery. Consequently, their perioperative needs differ from those of older children, adolescents, and adults.

Infants. Immature organ development makes the infant less resistant to surgical stress. Monitor the infant's vital signs closely. Also, the fluid and electrolyte balance of infants and young children is easily disrupted. It is important, therefore, to measure fluid intake, urine volume, and body weight accurately before and after surgery. Infants have decreased resistance to infection; therefore, assess postoperative wound status every 4 hours.

Older Adults. Like extreme youth, old age produces physiologic changes that increase surgical risk. Physiologic changes and presence of disease in the older adult's cardiovascular, pulmonary, musculoskeletal, gastrointestinal, hepatic, and renal systems may affect surgical outcomes. Chronic conditions also increase risk for older adults undergoing surgery.

Some of the conditions that increase the risk include malnutrition, anemia, dehydration, atherosclerosis, chronic obstructive pulmonary disease (COPD), diabetes mellitus, and many others. These are examples of common problems in older adults that should be corrected or controlled before surgery, if possible. A nutritious diet and adequate fluids help to counteract these problems, thus reducing the client's operative risk (Table 19-4).

Presence of Pain. Pain (see Chap. 16) is an important physiologic indicator that must be carefully monitored. During the preoperative nursing assessment, ask the client to describe the pain and how it began. Learn if the pain developed rapidly, gradually, or in one explosive burst. Determine the regularity of the pain—whether it is constant or intermittent—and if anything has helped relieve it.

Judging the client's reaction to pain is as important as assessing the nature of the pain. Reactions vary from panic to apparent indifference; making it difficult to observe exactly what an individual is experiencing.

Nutritional Status. Nutritional status directly correlates with intraoperative success and postoperative recovery. The client who is well nourished preoperatively is better prepared to handle surgical stress and to return to optimal health after surgery.

Two major problems are nutritional deficiencies and excess. Nutritional deficiencies primarily affect clients with chronic illnesses, cancer, gastrointestinal conditions (e.g., ulcerative colitis, pyloric stenosis, bulemia), and advanced age. Nursing intervention for clients who are malnourished preoperatively includes encouraging a high intake of carbohydrates (for energy), protein (for wound healing), and vitamins (for healing), especially vitamin K (for proper blood coagulation). Total parenteral (TPN) or enteral nutrition may be administered for several days to a week before surgery.

TPN plus lipids consists of total nutritional replacement with vitamin and mineral supplements. Enteral nutrition involves feeding directly through a tube placed into the stomach or small intestine. Enteral nutrition is also called tube feeding. Both methods help improve a client's nutritional status before surgery and are often continued postoperatively until satisfactory gastrointestinal function returns.

TABLE 19-4. Interventions for Physical Changes in Older Adults Undergoing Surgery

Physical Change	Nursing Interventions
Cardiovascular	
Decreased cardiac output Moderate increase in blood pressure Decreased peripheral circulation Arrhythmias	Know what anesthesia is used Monitor vital signs carefully Encourage early ambulation and leg exercises Assess for hypo or hypertension or hypothermia Baseline EKG, note any changes
Respiratory	
Decreased vital capacity Reduced oxygenation of blood	Assess for pulmonary aspiration Monitor respirations carefully Vigorous pulmonary hygiene Postoperatively—auscultate lung sounds Oxygen saturation monitor
Renal	
Decreased renal blood flow and glomerular filtration rate Decreased ability to excrete waste products	Monitor urine output q 1 to 2 hours during immediate postoperative period Evaluate intake and output Monitor fluid and electrolyte status
Musculoskeletal	
Decrease in lean body mass Increase in spinal compression Increased incidence of osteoporosis and arthritis	Assess level of mobility Position on operating table with padding to reduce trauma to bones and joints Spine, limbs, and pressure points may be padded to prevent fractures Early ambulation or exercises to individual's ability Provide adequate nutrition Provide effective pain management
Sensorimotor	
Decreased reaction time Decreased visual acuity Decreased auditory acuity	Orient client to environment Plan individual teaching, allow time to reinforce teaching Provide a safe environment

EKG, electrocardiogram

If possible, obesity should be corrected before elective surgery. A severely obese client faces a greater surgical risk than a client of normal weight because of the following problems:

- Obese clients frequently suffer from hypertension, congestive heart failure, and metabolic problems such as diabetes mellitus. These complicate the operative and postoperative course.
- Adipose tissue increases the technical difficulty of surgery. Incisions are usually larger than normal, and the tissue is weaker. This increases the risk of postoperative infection, incisional hernias, and wound dehiscence and evisceration.
- An obese client is more susceptible to postoperative pulmonary complications. Obesity decreases the efficiency of coughing and deep breathing. The pressure of the abdominal contents on the diaphragm and lungs decrease expansion, leading to hypotension.

Treating obesity before surgery requires a reducing diet; mild exercise, if possible; and assessing and controlling conditions such as hypertension and diabetes mellitus, often with medications.

Fluid and Electrolyte Balance. Dehydration and hypovolemia (fluid volume deficit) predisposes a client to complications during and after surgery. Dehydration results from prolonged vomiting, diarrhea, and bleeding, coupled with inadequate fluid intake. To correct dehydration, fluids are usually administered intravenously during the preoperative period.

Electrolyte imbalances also increase operative risk. It is particularly important to correct sodium, potassium, calcium, and magnesium deficiencies as well as acid-base disturbances before surgery through diet and intravenous infusions. Assessment and management of fluid and electrolyte imbalances is discussed in detail in Chapter 14.

Infection. Any infection, even a minor cold, can adversely affect surgical outcome. When the surgical site is near the lymphatic glands draining an infection, the likelihood of postoperative wound infection increases. During preoperative assessment, document such symptoms as sneezing, coughing, sore throat, elevated temperature, and the presence of skin lesions, boils, or rashes. Also, note an elevated white blood count (WBC). Communicate these findings to the surgeon or anesthesiologist, because all these factors increase surgical risk. It may be necessary to reschedule surgery.

A low WBC also can be dangerous for a client. A low WBC may mean that the client is more susceptible to infection. A client who is immunosuppressed is a great risk of postoperative infections. Clients who test positive to human immunodeficient virus (HIV) are at increased risk for postoperative infections, also.

Cardiovascular Function. Cardiac conditions that increase operative risk include angina pectoris, a myocardial infarction within the last 6 months, uncontrolled hypertension, congestive heart failure, and peripheral vascular disease. All cardiac conditions could lead to decreased tissue perfusion, and peripheral vascular disease could impair wound healing in an extremity.

Assess all clients for elevated blood pressure; slow, rapid, or irregular pulse; edema; cold, cyanotic extremities; weakness; and shortness of breath. Laboratory and diagnostic studies, which are often ordered before surgery to determine cardiovascular function, include electrocardiogram, hemoglobin, hematocrit, and serum electrolytes.

Preoperative treatment of clients with cardiovascular disease includes rest, a low-sodium or low-cholesterol diet, heart medications such as digoxin, and the judicious administration of fluids. An attempt is made to get the client's cardiovascular system in the best condition possible before surgery.

Pulmonary Function. Pulmonary conditions such as COPD, emphysema, asthma, and bronchitis increase operative risk because they impair CO_2 and O_2 diffusion in the alveolus and predispose the client to pulmonary infection.

To evaluate pulmonary conditions, assess the client for shortness of breath, wheezing, clubbed fingers, chest pain, and coughing with expectoration of copious or purulent mucus. Question the client carefully about smoking habits. Obtain a history of any respiratory allergies and infections. A chest x-ray study is ordered for diagnostic purposes on all clients.

Often a baseline arterial blood gas study is obtained to evaluate pulmonary function in a client with known respiratory disease, as are pulmonary function studies (see Chaps. 35 and 36). Clients with severe respiratory disease are usually treated preoperatively with aerosol therapy, postural drainage, and antibiotics. Clients who still smoke are strongly encouraged to stop before surgery. To help prevent postoperative respiratory complications, these clients need careful preoperative instruction and practice in deep breathing and coughing exercises.

Renal Function. The surgical client needs adequate renal function to eliminate protein wastes, preserve fluid and electrolyte balance, and clear anesthetic agents. Emergency surgery must be performed, however, whatever the client's renal function. Conditions that increase operative risk by affecting urine elimination include advanced renal insufficiency, acute nephritis, and benign prostatic hypertrophy. In older men, benign prostatic hypertrophy may obstruct the normal flow of urine and predispose them to urinary tract infection.

To assess renal status, observe for symptoms of frequency, dysuria, and anuria. Also observe the appearance of the urine. Document and report urine that is cloudy or bloody rather than clear amber.

The most commonly ordered preoperative tests to assess renal function are urinalysis, blood urea nitrogen (BUN), and creatinine.

Urinalysis, performed on either a clean voided specimen or a catheterized specimen, checks urine for the presence of

- Red or white blood cells, which may indicate an infection or tumor;

- Casts, which may indicate renal disease;
- Protein, which may indicate renal disease;
- Glucose, which usually indicates diabetes; and
- Specific gravity (if below 1.010, the kidney may be unable to concentrate urine; if elevated over 1.025, the client may be dehydrated).

BUN and creatinine are serum studies that test the ability of the kidney to excrete urea and protein wastes. Elevated levels may simply reflect dehydration, although they may mean more serious problems exist. Serious renal disease and urinary infections must be treated, if possible, before surgery.

Gastrointestinal Function. The clients gastrointestinal system should be functioning well before surgery to prevent more postoperative problems. Impaired nutrition may be related to an altered gastrointestinal function. The client should be questioned about normal bowel functioning, so postoperative expectations for return of function are appropriate. Clients with a long history of constipation may have more difficulty postoperatively than those with regular bowel function.

Liver Function. Liver disease, such as cirrhosis, increases risk because an impaired liver is unable to detoxify medications and anesthetic agents or to metabolize carbohydrates, fats, and amino acids. In addition, inadequate liver function is associated with poor wound healing and a higher rate of infection. Clients with a history of alcoholism or ascites require a careful examination of liver function before surgery. Because these clients are usually malnourished and debilitated, the surgeon generally orders a high-calorie diet, intravenous solutions, and vitamins during the preoperative period.

Endocrine Function. Endocrine function, particularly that of the thyroid, must be monitored carefully preoperatively to minimize operative risk. Hyperthyroidism can lead to thyroid storm or thyroid crisis, with symptoms of hypertension, tachycardia, and hyperthermia and, therefore, should be treated medically preoperatively (see Chap. 62). Likewise, hypothyroidism increases the risk of hypotension and cardiac arrest during the administration of anesthesia, and it should be recognized and treated before surgery.

Diabetes mellitus predisposes a client to infection and to poor tissue healing and swings of blood sugar more profound than usual. Cardiovascular and renal complications also increase surgical risk for a client with diabetes. The client with well-controlled diabetes is more likely to respond well to surgery. Chapter 61 discusses in detail the care of clients with diabetes mellitus.

Neurologic Function. The nurse should conduct a thorough neurologic physical assessment before surgery to determine the client's baseline function. Testing generally includes assessing cranial nerves, reflex response of the upper and lower extremities, sensory reflexes, and cerebellar response (see Chap. 28).

Serious neurologic conditions, such as uncontrolled epilepsy or severe Parkinson's disease, increase surgical risk. Important neurologic preoperative findings include severe headache, frequent dizziness, lightheadedness, ringing in the ears, unsteady gait, unequal pupils, and a history of convulsions.

Hematologic Function. Clients with blood coagulation disorders are at risk of hemorrhage and hypovolemic shock during and following surgery. Five factors pointing to abnormal hematologic factors are

- A history of bleeding tendencies;
- Symptoms such as easy bruising, excessive bleeding following dental extractions and shaving, and severe nosebleeds;
- The presence of hepatic or renal disease;
- Use of anticoagulants; and
- Abnormal bleeding time, prothrombin time, or platelet counts (see Chaps. 45 and 46).

Blood transfusions are used less frequently than in past years because of the fear of AIDS and hepatitis B transmission. If possible, clients are encouraged to donate their own blood before surgery (autologous blood transfusion) for use during or after. Blood transfusions are discussed in Chapter 46.

Use of Medications. Many clients take prescribed and nonprescribed medications that may increase operative risk by (1) increasing coagulation time or (2) interacting unfavorably with the anesthetic. Some of the medications that may result in complications include

- Anticoagulants including aspirin, which cause clotting abnormalities;
- Antibiotics, which combine with some muscle relaxants to increase postoperative respiratory depression;
- Tranquilizers, which decrease blood pressure and, thus, increase the risk of shock; they also potentiate the effects of narcotics and barbiturates;
- Thiazide diuretics, which can create potassium depletion;
- Steroids, which cause hypofunction of the adrenal cortex and, thus, impair physiologic response to the stress of anesthesia and surgery; their anti-inflammatory effects also delay wound healing and increase the risk of infection. Steroid replacement also needs to be increased before, during, and after surgery;
- Monoamine (MAO) inhibitors, which can cause hypertensive crisis when combined with anesthetic agents;
- Anti-parkinsonian drugs, which cause hypotension or hypertension when combined with anesthetics;
- Street drugs and alcohol abuse, which increase the tolerance to narcotics; and
- Hypoglycemics, which require dosage alteration and close monitoring of the blood sugar.

When performing a nursing preoperative assessment, document whether the client has any drug allergies or reactions or is currently taking any prescribed or over-the-counter medications. Surgical risk is increased (1) if the client is allergic to the anesthetic or (2) if medications the client is taking interact adversely with the anesthesia. Clients often forget to list some medications they are taking. They also sometimes fail to recognize that nonprescription medications may pose a threat and, consequently, do not mention them. Therefore, question clients very carefully and obtain as complete a list of medications as possible. The physician's decision to discontinue, reduce, or continue preoperative medications is based on the client's surgical risk (Table 19–5).

Presence of Trauma. When surgery must be performed following a traumatic incident (e.g., gunshot wound, stab wound, serious accident, severe fall), document details of the event as precisely as possible. If the client was shot or stabbed, try to find out the nature of the weapon, its size and shape, and the client's position when the incident occurred. If the client was injured in a fall or accident, ask questions such as "what was the client's position when the accident occurred?" and "was consciousness lost?" The answers may help to determine whether or not there is an underlying, undetected condition that may increase surgical risk (e.g., epilepsy, coronary artery disease, uncontrolled diabetes mellitus). Be especially alert to signs of severe trauma warranting surgery in children. Young children are often unable to talk about what happened to them. Some children are victims of child abuse, and the trauma may have been inflicted on them by an adult in their environment. If abuse is suspected, report the findings to the surgical team and proper authorities. Also, remember that adults can be abused, often by a spouse.

Health Habits. The client undergoing surgery who smokes or abuses drugs has an increased surgical risk. The client who smokes has reduced hemoglobin levels and, therefore, less oxygen available for tissue repair. Smokers are more susceptible to thrombus formation because of the hypercoaguability of their blood and their increased rate of arteriosclerosis. Smokers are also more likely to have damage to their lung tissue, including COPD, and chronic bronchitis. Smokers

TABLE 19–5. Examples of Medications and Possible Effects on the Operative Client

Medications	Possible Effects
Antibiotics	
Gentamicin (Garamycin) Penicillin	Produces mild respiratory depression, may mask infection, and affects metabolism of muscle relaxants
Antiarrhythmics	
Propranolol hydrochloride (Inderal)	Affects client's tolerance of anesthesia. Interacts with epinephrine used in local anesthesia
Quinidine gluconate (Quinate)	Depresses cardiac function
Procainamide hydrochloride (Pronestyl)	Potentiates anesthetics that are neuromuscular blockers
Antihypertensives	
Methyldopa (Aldomet) Captopril (Capoten)	May alter response to muscle relaxants and narcotics. May cause intraoperative or postoperative hypotensive crisis
Corticosteroids	
Dexamethasone (Decadron) Hydrocortisone sodium (Solu-Cortef) Prednisone (Deltasone)	Delays wound healing; masks infection; increases risk of hemorrhage; increases serum glucose; decreases stress response (needs replacement during surgery)
Anticoagulants	
Heparin sodium Warfarin sodium (Coumadin) Aspirin	Increases risk of hemorrhage intraoperatively and postoperatively
Glaucoma medications	
Pilocarpine hydrochloride	May cause respiratory or cardiovascular collapse during surgery
Antidiabetic Agents	
Chlorpropamide Glipizide Glyburide Insulin	Insulin needs decrease when client is to receive nothing by mouth. Insulin levels may fluctuate during healing because of dietary and activity restrictions

should stop smoking at least a week before elective surgery.

Clients undergoing surgery who use alcohol or drugs may experience withdrawal symptoms during hospitalization. Their surgical course may be complicated by poor nutrition, as well as unpredictable reactions to the anesthetic agents. Remember, even two drinks a day can lead to withdrawal symptoms and the need for increased analgesia and anesthesia.

Clients who lead a sedentary lifestyle may have a complicated postoperative course because of poor muscle tone, limited cardiac and respiratory reserve, and decreased stress response to the physical demands of surgery.

Clients who are HIV positive have several areas of increased surgical risk. If their immune systems are affected, they are at a much higher risk of developing a postoperative infection and of being unable to fight that infection. If they have developed *Pneumocystis carinii* pneumonia, they are at increased risk of anesthetic and postoperative pulmonary complications.

Social History. The client's marital status, significant others, and support systems should be thoroughly explored. The client's occupation should also be identified because it may be a source of difficulty after surgery if the client is unable to return to work. It is also important to determine whether the client has insurance or whether this surgery will cause severe financial hardship.

Because all of these factors could increase the client's stress and interfere with healing, the nurse should be aware of these potential risks that may jeopardize a successful surgical intervention.

Psychosocial Aspects of Preoperative Preparation

Everyone is somewhat fearful of surgery. The extent to which a client fears surgery depends on his or her personality, general responses to stress, mental health, and preconceptions about surgery and anesthesia.

Fear of the unknown is one of the most important causes of preoperative anxiety. During the preoperative phase, clients also may fear postoperative pain, the discovery of cancer, the loss of an organ or limb, anesthesia, vulnerability while unconscious, threat of loss of job or financial security, loss of social and familial roles, disruption of lifestyle, separation from significant others, and even death.

Clients respond differently to fear. Some respond by becoming silent and withdrawn, childish, belligerent, evasive, tearful, or clinging. Most clients feel helpless when admitted to a health care facility. We need to remember that although surgery may become common place to the health care professional, it is a frightening experience to the client.

Based on the nursing assessment, a number of interventions may be appropriate for the preoperative client. First, provide explanations and printed information about the health care facility routines, visiting hours, mealtimes, the location of the chapel and waiting room, and so forth. Explain the procedures involved in the planned surgery to allay the client's anxiety. The client should have a complete idea of what the preoperative, intraoperative, and postoperative course entails. Consult with the physician before speaking to the client about specific or technical details. Explain all nursing care and any possible discomfort that may result as a consequence of nursing interventions. Also, tell the client what you will do to minimize any discomfort. If the client is scheduled to go to the intensive care unit after surgery, ask what the client already knows or has heard about intensive care. At this point, take time to clarify any misconceptions or incorrect information.

Allow the client to take the lead in asking questions concerning surgery and the postoperative period. Provide the client with essential information, such as nothing-by-mouth (NPO) status and preoperative procedures, but then provide only as much additional information as the client wishes to know. If the client is very withdrawn, depressed, or apprehensive, use your communication skills to encourage expression of fears and concerns. For example, tell the client that preoperative fear is normal and that it is not unusual to experience anxiety. Invite the client to share concerns. Find out if the client knows someone who had similar surgery and what the outcome was. Often a client's fears may be rooted in the stories of unpleasant experiences that happened to others.

Whenever possible, introduce the client or family to others who have successfully undergone similar surgery. If this is not possible preoperatively, it may be done after surgery. You may want to contact support groups such as the local laryngectomy or colostomy organization, for instance, and ask for a volunteer to visit the client.

Identify discharge needs of the client based on their planned surgical procedures and current health status. Referrals for assistance could include

- Local visiting nurse or home health care services;
- Local chapters of the Cancer Society, Heart Association, and Diabetes Association, for example;
- Local mastectomy, laryngectomy, colostomy support groups;
- Medic Alert Foundation;
- Malignant hyperthermia hotline;
- Local senior citizens' assistance program;
- Substance abuse treatment programs or groups;
- Emergency social services;
- Local sexual assault center (American law requires that suspected sexual abuse of minors be reported);
- Child protection services; and
- Emergency legal assistance

Find out the client's religious preference and arrange for a visit from clergy, if the client so desires. Finally, include the client's significant others in preoperative discussions whenever possible. Provide them with information they can use to assist in reducing the client's preoperative anxiety.

Handling fears in these ways can smooth the preoperative experience. Studies show that clients who are calm and emotionally prepared for surgery withstand anesthesia better and experience fewer postoperative complications.

Preoperative Assessment

HISTORY

Data gathered during a purposeful history help detect problems that may arise preoperatively or postoperatively. The manner is which the history is conducted plays a large part in determining the degree of preoperative and postoperative anxiety the client experiences.

The history allows clients to explain their understanding of impending surgery. This information can be used to determine clients' learning needs. The preoperative history also allows the nurse to

- Establish rapport with the client and significant others.
- Begin a psychosocial assessment of the client. This information is valuable in developing the preoperative and postoperative teaching care plan. For example, a client who is apprehensive preoperatively may need more frequent or repetitive instruction and more reinforcement than a less anxious client.
- Reassure the client and significant others, and answer general questions about the surgery, the health care facility, and so forth.

Specific information to obtain during the preoperative history concerns

- Previous surgery and experience with anesthesia;
- Responses of family members to previous surgery and anesthesia;
- Whether the client has had any serious illnesses;
- Previous and current medications (prescription or over-the-counter);
- Allergies and reactions, any dietary restrictions;
- Alcohol, nicotine, or recreational drug use;
- Current symptoms or discomforts;
- Occupation;
- Religious affiliation;
- Significant others (Is the client single or married? How many dependents does the client have?);
- Whether the client has any questions about the surgery; and
- Chronic illnesses, such as arthritis, migraines, back pain.

In addition to helping the nurse establish valuable preoperative baseline data, this information uncovers the need for supportive services. If a client will need assistance after returning home, the nurse can initiate discharge plans.

PHYSICAL EXAMINATION

A physical examination is performed on all clients undergoing surgery to determine baseline data and identify conditions that may interfere with the administration of anesthesia or produce problems postoperatively.

A complete physical examination should be performed, paying special attention to cardiac and respiratory systems. Baseline vital signs are obtained as one determination of the client's risk for postoperative complications. Any abnormal vital sign is significant and may cause a postponement of surgery until the problem is treated. Abnormal breath sounds may indicate the need for respiratory therapy both before and after surgery, or the need for bronchodilators. Clients with abnormal cardiac findings will need further evaluation to determine whether or not they can withstand the stress of surgery and anesthesia. Physical examination also should reveal any problems with joint mobility or deformities that may interfere with operative positioning as well as their postoperative course. Special consideration of the elderly should include cardiac, respiratory, renal, and musculoskeletal assessment.

PREOPERATIVE DIAGNOSTIC TESTS

Routine diagnostic tests are ordered less often than in past years. Now clients have specific tests ordered based on their health status to identify potential problems that would interfere with the surgery. Table 19-6 identifies commonly requested preoperative laboratory tests.

INFORMED CONSENT

Anyone undergoing any invasive procedure must sign a permit. This legal document signifies that the client is giving informed consent for the procedure. The permit guards the client against unwanted invasive procedures. It also protects the health care facility and health care professionals.

A signed consent is necessary for each invasive procedure. The client must receive a full explanation of the operation before signing the permit. Pictures and diagrams may be necessary for complete understanding of the surgical procedure. Moreover, the client must be told about potential risks, complications and disfigurement that may result from the surgery, anesthesia, who will perform the surgery, and whether or not organs or body parts may be removed. The client should be informed about alternative treatments. The surgeon should explain the procedure in terms the client readily understands. Ensure that the client receives an honest, accurate, and fair statement of what to expect during and after surgery, and understands the consent form before signing.

The procedure for obtaining a signed consent varies from state to state and according to the policy of the health care facility. Generally, the surgeon explains the surgical procedure, possible risks and complications, and alternatives. The nurse, however, may obtain and witness the client's signature on the operative permit (dependent on health care facility policy).

Adults sign their own operative permit unless they are unconscious or mentally incompetent. In such cases, a relative or guardian is responsible for consent (see Ethical Issues in Nursing). If the relative or guard-

TABLE 19-6. Preoperative Diagnostic Tests

Test	Normal Ranges (may vary with different labs)	Purpose
Serum potassium	3.5 to 5.0 mEq/L	To identify hyperkalemia or hypokalemia
Serum sodium	136 to 145 mEq/L	To identify hypernatremia, hyponatremia, dehydration, or overhydration
Serum chloride	96 to 106 mEq/L	To identify hyperchloremia, hypochloremia, or metabolic alkalosis
Glucose	60 to 100 mg/dl	To identify hypoglycemia or hyperglycemia
Creatinine	0.7 to 1.4 mg/dl	To identify acute or chronic renal disease
Blood urea nitrogen (BUN)	10 to 20 mg/dl	To identify impaired liver or kidney function or excessive protein or tissue catabolism
Hemoglobin (Hgb)	Female: 12.0 to 15.0 g/dl Male: 13.0 to 17.0 g/dl	To identify the presence and extent of anemia
Hematocrit (Hct)	Female: 36 to 45 per cent Male: 39 to 51 per cent	To identify the presence and extent of anemia
Prothrombin time (PT)	11 to 18 seconds	To identify dysfunction of blood clotting (prothrombin level)
Partial thromboplastin time (PTT)	35 to 45 seconds	To identify deficiencies of coagulation factors
Chest x-ray study	No abnormal heart or lung lesions	To determine size and contour of heart, lungs, and major vessels
Electrocardiogram (EKG)	Normal rate and rhythm	To determine the electrical activity of the heart.

ian is out of state, the physician can secure consent over the telephone in the presence of one or two witnesses on the same line. If no relative or guardian can be found, the court can appoint one.

Children under the legal age must be signed for by the child's parent or legal guardian. If the child's family cannot be present to sign the permit, consent can be obtained from a parent by telephone, wire, or letter. When a minor's relatives cannot be located, a court order may be needed to permit surgery, depending on state laws.

Once the operative permit is signed, it becomes a permanent part of the client's record. Make sure it accompanies the record to the operating room.

The client may choose to obtain a second opinion regarding their need for surgery. One resource is the Second Surgical Opinion Hotline, available Monday through Friday from 8 am to 12 midnight Eastern time at 800-638-6833 (nationwide) or 800-492-6603 (in Maryland). This hotline provides the names of surgeons in the client's area who will give a second opinion in nonemergency situations. These surgeons do not treat persons who consult them and, thus, have no financial interest in the outcome of the surgery. Most insurance carriers, Medicare, and Medicaid encourage second opinions and will pay for them.

SPECIAL CONSIDERATIONS

Medications. In preparing the client for surgery it is important to assess what routine medications they are taking so their care can be planned safely. Table 19-5 outlines some major medications and possible untoward side effects that may be anticipated.

Clients must be interviewed carefully about what medications they are taking, and nurses need to assess the individual's medication history. Nurses, in consultation with the physician, must intervene to stop medications, reduce dosage, or anticipate possible medication side effects.

The Older Adult. Another consideration in the care of the operative client is the care of the older surgical client. Normal physiologic changes place the older client at increased risk when surgical intervention is needed. Table 19-4 outlines major physiologic changes that occur as a result of surgery and appropriate nursing interventions.

Preoperative Teaching

Preoperative teaching is an important component in the client's operative experience. Numerous research stud-

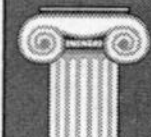

ETHICAL ISSUES IN NURSING

Should Clients Who Have a "Do Not Resuscitate" Order Undergo Surgery?

Surgical procedures are performed to enhance the lives of those receiving them. Such procedures may be elective (such as a cosmetic procedure), scheduled, but not emergent (such as a thyroidectomy), or emergent (such as emergency trauma procedures). In most instances, the clients undergoing surgery hope to have whatever problem they are experiencing corrected so they might go on living a normal life. There are times, however, when problems cannot be surgically corrected and such surgical procedures result in a poor outcome or possibly death.

No surgery is without risk, even for the most healthy of clients. There are cases when very unhealthy patients might require surgical procedures. The risks of surgery are, of course, far greater for these clients than for more healthy patients. If any of these clients need resuscitative measures during surgery, there should be no question that the operating room staff would administer such measures. There is really no dilemma present for such cases. On the other hand, what should be done in the operating room for clients who have a "do not resuscitate" (DNR) order but experience cardiac or respiratory arrest on the operating table? Should the surgical staff honor the DNR order? Is a DNR order valid in the operating room? Should a client with a DNR order undergo a surgical procedure in the first place?

In most hospitals and surgicenters, DNR orders are not honored in the operating room. The client may have a 'DNR' preoperatively and postoperatively, but during surgery, if there is a need for resuscitative measures, such measures should be administered. Nurses in operating room settings should be aware of what their institution's policies are regarding DNR orders in the operating room. No matter what a nurse's personal belief may be regarding this issue, he or she must comply with whatever laws or policies are in place at the institution where he or she practices. However, the question remains as to whether or not clients who have a DNR order should undergo surgical procedures.

---

ies have supported the value of preoperative instruction in both decreasing the postoperative complications and decreasing the length of stay. Client's teaching needs, anxieties, and fears about the surgery must be assessed individually.

The timing of preoperative teaching is highly individualized. Ideally, there will be enough time for the client to be given instructions and time to answer questions. If teaching is done several days in advance, the client may forget. On the other hand, clients who are taught immediately before the surgery may be too anxious to comprehend what is being taught. In many cases, the client is admitted the same day of the surgery. Hopefully, they will have received written or verbal instructions prior to this time and the nurse will be able to reinforce instructions and answer questions. A phone interview is conducted in many ambulatory surgery units.

Preoperative teaching decreases anxiety and encourages clients to participate actively in their own care. The basic areas that must be covered in preoperative teaching are

- Deep breathing and coughing exercises,
- Turning and extremity exercises,
- Pain control methods that will be offered, and
- Postoperative equipment.

DEEP BREATHING EXERCISES

Breathing and coughing exercises help expand collapsed lungs and prevent postoperative pneumonia and atelectasis. Demonstrate correct deep breathing by inhaling slowly through the nose, distending the abdomen, and exhaling slowly through pursed lips. After you have demonstrated the method, ask the client to perform it (Figure 19–1). Have the client

- Sit on the edge of the bed or lie supine, with knees flexed to relax the abdominal musculature (the client may lie on either side if lying on the back is impossible);
- Place hands on the abdomen;
- Inhale through the nose until the abdomen balloons outward; and
- Exhale through pursed lips while contracting the abdominal muscles.

Instruct the client to use this breathing method as often as possible, preferably five to ten times every hour during the postoperative, immobilized period.

COUGHING EXERCISES

For this exercise, the client may be in a sitting or lying position. Show the client how to splint an incision. Splinting minimizes pressure and helps to control pain when the person is coughing. Instruct the client to lace the fingers and hold them tightly across the incision before coughing. A small pillow or folded towel held over the incision also facilitates splinting. Have the client take a deep breath, exhaling through the mouth, before coughing from deep in the lungs. Encourage the client to perform deep breathing exercises *before* coughing, to stimulate the cough reflex.

Incentive spirometers are used to promote lung expansion. They promote alveolar inflation and strengthen respiratory muscles. Their use also helps prevent atelectasis in the postoperative client. They should be used about 10 times an hour after surgery.

TURNING EXERCISES

The client also needs to practice turning from side to side, using the side rails to assist movements. Turning prevents venous stasis and respiratory problems. Teach the client to turn every 1 to 2 hours during the postoperative period.

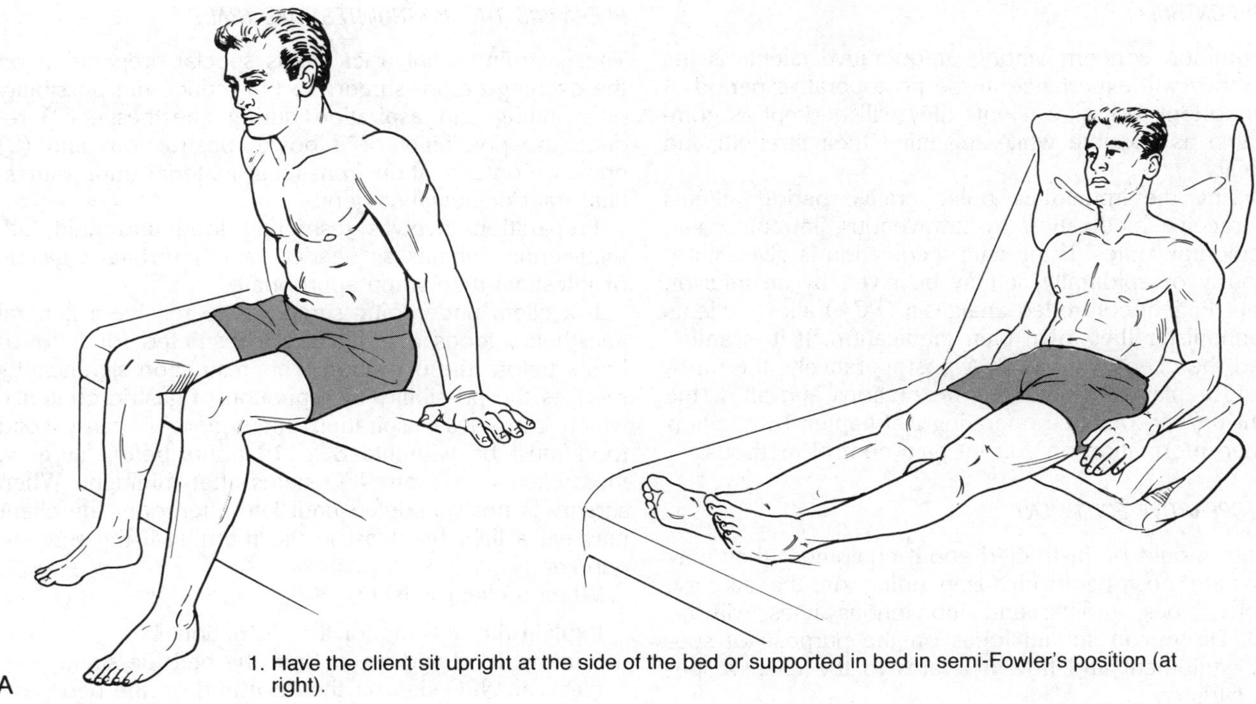

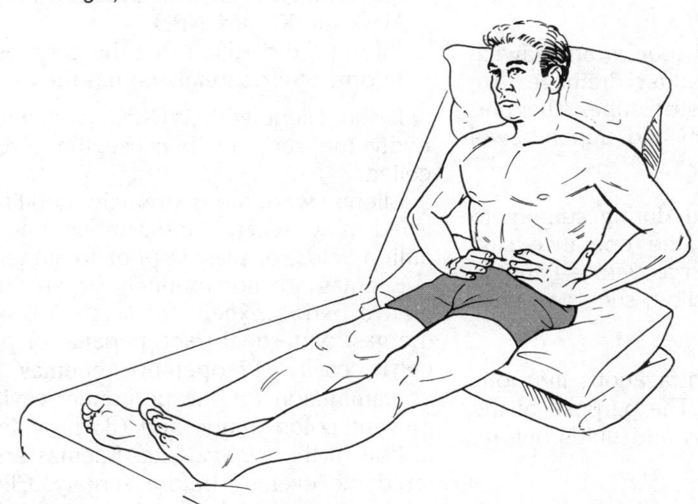

2. Instruct the client to place his or her hands on the abdomen to feel whether the chest rises to indicate that the lungs are expanding.
3. Have the client inhale through the nose until the abdomen distends.
4. Instruct the client to exhale through pursed lips while contracting the abdominal muscles.
B
5. Have the client repeat this exercise every hour during the first postoperative day.

▲ **Figure 19-1**

Deep (diaphragmatic) breathing after surgery.

EXTREMITY EXERCISES

Finally, the client should practice extremity exercises. Ask the client to flex and extend each joint, particularly the hip, knee, and ankle joints, keeping the lower back flat as the leg is lowered and straightened. Have the client move each foot in a circular motion. These exercises help prevent circulatory problems, such as thrombophlebitis, by facilitating venous return to the heart.

Antiembolism stockings are used on the lower extremities preoperatively, intraoperatively, and postoperatively combined with turning and leg exercises help to prevent thrombophlebitis or thromboemboli formation. Newer sequential compression stockings to massage legs rhythmically are being used for even more effective prevention of clots.

Encourage ambulation after the surgery when appropriate. Ambulation helps prevent postoperative complications. Include a projected schedule for postoperative ambulation in your preoperative teaching program.

PAIN CONTROL

A common concern among preoperative clients is the pain they will experience in the postoperative period. It is important to assure clients they will be kept as comfortable as possible while regaining their strength and mobility.

During the immediate postoperative period, clients will receive medication by intravenous, intramuscular, or epidural routes. If the pain medication is given intravenously or epidurally, it may be given by an infusion pump. Patient-controlled analgesia (PCA) allows clients to administer their own pain medication. If it is anticipated the client will use PCA postoperatively, the nurse should explain the operating instructions and allow the client time to practice operating it. Chapter 16 contains further information on current pain control methods.

POSTOPERATIVE EQUIPMENT

Clients should be instructed about equipment they may anticipate postoperatively. Depending on the surgery, various tubes, drains, and intravenous lines will be used. Discussion should focus on the purpose of specific equipment and how it relates to the client's specific surgery.

Tubes. The most common type of tube is an indwelling catheter for the purpose of bladder drainage. Another common tube is the nasogastric tube. The purpose is to decompress the stomach and upper bowel and to drain stomach contents.

Drains. Drains are usually inserted during surgery to promote evacuation of fluid from the operative site. They act by either wick action, such as with a Penrose drain, or with a mild amount of suction, such as with a Hemovac or Davol drain.

Intravenous Infusion Devices. Intravenous infusions are usually started prior to surgery. The purpose of the infusion is to administer medications and fluids before, during, and after surgery.

Physical Preparation

PREPARING THE SKIN

Usually the operative area is cleansed the night prior to surgery with an antiseptic such as povidone-iodine (Betadine) to decrease the number of microorganisms on the skin.

Opinions differ as to preoperative skin preparation. Recent research studies show that not removing hair at all, clipping hair, or using electric razors are associated with a lower rate of infection than traditional shaving.[1] The Centers for Disease Control recommends that if shaving is necessary, it can be performed in the operating room prior to surgery. The nurse responsible for skin preparation should conduct a preoperative assessment for any skin abrasions, lacerations, or signs of infection at the operative area.

PREPARING THE GASTROINTESTINAL TRACT

The gastrointestinal tract needs special preparation on the evening before surgery to (1) reduce the possibility of vomiting and aspiration during anesthesia, (2) reduce the possibility of a bowel obstruction, and (3) prevent contamination from fecal material during intestinal tract or bowel surgery.

Preparation involves restricting food and fluid, administering enemas as needed, and inserting a gastric or intestinal tube when appropriate.

If a client undergoing surgery is to receive a general anesthetic, foods and fluids are restricted for 8 to 10 hours before the operation. This restriction significantly reduces the possibility of aspiration of gastric contents, which can cause aspiration pneumonia. Because solid food must be withheld 8 to 10 hours before surgery, most clients have an NPO status after midnight. When surgery is not scheduled until late afternoon, the client may eat a light breakfast in the morning if the surgeon permits.

When a client is NPO,

Explain the reasons for the restriction
Remove food and water from the bedside stand
Place an NPO sign on the door and on the bed
Mark the Kardex NPO
Inform the dietitian that the client is awaiting surgery
Inform other caretakers that the client is NPO

If the client who is NPO consumes food or fluids, notify the surgeon, because the surgery may be cancelled.

Clients who are extremely debilitated or malnourished may receive intravenous infusions of glucose, amino acids, or plasma prior to surgery.

Enemas are not routinely ordered during the preoperative period except for surgical procedures involving the gastrointestinal tract, perianal or perineal areas, and pelvic cavity. Preoperative enemas help (1) prevent contamination for the peritoneal cavity with feces, (2) prevent colon injury, and (3) provide adequate visualization of the surgical site. Enemas are usually administered the evening before surgery. Clients who are admitted the same day as the surgery may be instructed to take one or more enemas at home the night before surgery. This will require excellent teaching to ensure the client knows how to administer the enemas correctly and what results are expected. Some clients may require further bowel cleansing on the morning of surgery after admission to the facility.

Gastrointestinal tubes are usually inserted during surgery, if they are to be used at all. This procedure is usually performed for clients undergoing major abdominal or intestinal tract surgery.

Many types of surgery require special preparations. The specific protocol for each surgical procedure is usually available at the health care facility.

PREPARING FOR ANESTHESIA

The anesthesiologist or nurse anesthetist visits the client before surgery to perform a complete respiratory, cardiovascular, and neurologic examination. Generally, the topics discussed with the client during the examination include the type of anesthesia planned and the sensations the client will experience when undergoing anesthesia. Fears the client has concerning anesthesia also are addressed.

PROMOTING REST AND SLEEP

The preoperative client will rest more completely on the night before surgery if he or she is physically comfortable, mentally at ease, and adequately sedated. Measures to reduce preoperative sleeplessness and restlessness include a well-ventilated room, a comfortable clean bed, a backrub, and a warm beverage (if fluids are not contraindicated). With same-day surgery admissions, the client may be at home the night before surgery and must get up very early to get to the hospital for surgery. They still need to be encouraged to get as much sleep as possible before surgery. Encourage apprehensive clients to take ordered sleep medication the night before surgery to help them to sleep.

Always remember to talk in a positive manner with the client as you give preoperative care, and listen to any doubts or fears the client may have concerning surgery.

Preparing the Client on the Day of Surgery

EARLY MORNING CARE

Immediate preoperative preparation begins at least 1 to 2 hours before surgery for clients in the hospital and as soon as same day admission clients come into the hospital. At this time, the nurse asks whether the client has any questions or concerns. Continue to assess for signs of anxiety. Communicate any surgical delays to the client and significant others.

The following preoperative interventions help promote safety during surgery:

- Take and record the vital signs. Some increase in blood pressure or pulse are common because of anxiety. However, if marked differences from baseline information appear, report them to the surgeon. They might signify, for example, a respiratory infection and may require delay of surgery.
- Check the identification band to make sure it is legible, accurate, and securely fastened to the client.
- If a skin preparation has been ordered, check that it has been completed accurately and thoroughly.
- Check for and carry out any special orders such as administering enemas or starting an intravenous line.
- Verify that the client has not eaten for the last 8 hours. Check that fluids have been restricted, although sometimes the physician will order clients to take their usual oral medications with a small sip of water (often medications such as digoxin).
- Ask the client to void; measure and record the amount of urine (if indicated).
- Assist the client with oral hygiene, if necessary.
- Remove dentures or bridgework that could obstruct the airway if left in place. Store these and other valuable items according to health care facility policy or give them to family members.
- Have the client remove jewelry. Many facilities allow the client to keep wedding bands on as long as they are taped securely. If jewelry is removed, store them according to policy or give them to the family. Assist the client with the removal of hairpins, wigs, or prosthesis.
- If the client is wearing a hearing aid, notify the operating room nurse. Leave it in place so operating room personnel know it is there and can communicate with the client.
- Assist the client in donning a hospital gown, protective head cap, Ace wraps, or antiembolic hose, if these items have been ordered.
- Remove colored nail polish from at least one nail for the pulse oximeter (although the device can accurately read oxygen saturation levels through light-colored polish). Remove make-up so skin color can be observed.

To prevent omissions in preoperative nursing interventions, most facilities supply nurses with a preoperative checklist. As each intervention on the list is completed, the nurse initials it.

PREOPERATIVE MEDICATIONS

Prior to administering preoperative medications, check to be sure that the operative permit and transfusion permit (if required) are correctly signed and attached to the client record. These must be signed and witnessed before the client receives any medication that will alter his or her consciousness (such as a narcotic or tranquilizer).

The purposes of various preoperative medications are to allay anxiety, decrease pharyngeal secretions, reduce side effects of anesthetic agents, and create amnesia.

The pharmacologic preparation of the client for anesthesia is based on many variables, including a client's age and physical and psychological condition, the type of surgery, and the specific anesthesia to be administered.

Table 19–7 presents an overview of common preoperative medications. Specific drug choices are based on the individual client variables, the goals for sedation, and the potential for undesirable side effects. Preoperative medications may be given in the preoperative area or on the nursing unit prior to the client leaving for surgery. If the preoperative medication is given on the unit, the nurse is responsible for raising the bed side rails. Lower the window shades, and turn off bright lights. *Instruct the client not to get up without assistance, because medications may cause drowsiness or dizziness.* Once the client is calm and drowsy, disturb the client only when necessary and then briefly and quietly. Observe the client for side effects from medication such as hypotension or respiratory depression.

TABLE 19-7. Commonly Used Preoperative Medications

Generic Name	Trade Name	Desired Effects	Undesired Effects
Tranquilizers			
Diazepam	Valium	Decrease anxiety	May cause dizziness, clumsiness, or confusion
Droperidol	Inapsine	Decrease anxiety Produce an antiemetic effect	Anxiety Hypotension during and after surgery
Sedatives			
Midazolam hydrochloride	Versed	To induce desired sleepiness and reduce anxiety	Hypotension, undesired respiratory depression
Promethazine	Phenergan	Same as for droperidol	Hypotension during and after surgery
Secobarbital sodium	Seconal sodium	Decrease anxiety Promote sedation	Disorientation, especially in elderly patients
Pentobarbital sodium	Nembutal sodium	Same as for secobarbital sodium	Same as for secobarbital sodium
Analgesics			
Morphine sulfate	—	Relieve pain Decrease anxiety Sedation	Respiratory depression Hypotension Circulatory depression Decreased gastric motility causing potential for vomiting
Meperidine hydrochloride	Demerol	Same as for morphine sulfate	Same as for morphine sulfate
Anticholinergics			
Atropine sulfate	—	Control secretions	Excessive dryness of mouth, tachycardia
Glycopyrrolate	Robinul	Same as for atropine sulfate	Same as for atropine sulfate
Histamine-H_2 Receptor Antagonists			
Cimetidine (See Table 54-2 for other H_2 antagonists)	Tagamet	Inhibit gastric acid production	Some mild dizziness, diarrhea, somnolence, and rash

TRANSPORTING THE CLIENT TO SURGERY

When surgical personnel call for the client, gently transfer the client to a stretcher (making sure you have enough help to transfer the client safely). Cover the client with blankets for protection from drafts, and then secure with a restraining belt. Make sure the client record accompanies the client to the operating room. Make the trip to surgery as smooth as possible so the sedated client does not develop nausea and dizziness. Avoid rapid walking and swinging the cart around corners.

The nursing unit should prepare the client's room for postoperative care as follows:

- Arrange furniture so the stretcher can easily be brought to the bedside.
- Make a surgical bed.
- Set out an emesis basin.
- Bring in additional equipment, such as the blood pressure cuff, intravenous standard, suction, and oxygen equipment as anticipated.
- Ensure that all equipment is in working order.

Caring for Significant Others

During surgery, the significant others usually wait in a designated surgical lounge. If they must leave the facility for any reason, ask them for a phone number where they can be reached. Provide the phone number of the client's unit.

When discussing surgery with significant others, be aware of information previously given by the surgeon regarding the immediate surgical outcome and eventual prognosis. You can then answer questions confident the information you give agrees with previous statements.

Prepare significant others for nasogastric tubes, chest

tubes, suction equipment, respiratory equipment, intravenous infusions, dressings, or monitoring equipment the client might require. Inform significant others when the surgery is completed (this may be done by waiting room personnel). Make certain the surgeon knows who is waiting for information on the client.

Reassure significant others that the length of time the client is gone may not reflect the actual length of surgery. There are often unpredictable delays that might cause the client to wait before surgery. Reassure the family if this has happened to the client so they will not worry.

INTRAOPERATIVE NURSING

The intraoperative phase of the perioperative experience begins as the client is placed on the surgical bed and ends with admission to the post-anesthesia care unit. The nursing care during this phase focuses on the client's emotional well-being as well as physical factors such as safety, positioning, maintaining asepsis, and controlling the surgical environment. Clients are highly dependent on the nurse for their needs during this phase.

In the preoperative area, the nurse is responsible for reviewing the record for completeness, ensuring proper identification of the client, client safety, and providing emotional support. It is important to deal with the fears and concerns of a frightened or agitated client. A relaxed client undergoes anesthetic induction easier than one who is anxious. If the client still seems anxious despite sedation and reassurance, notify the surgeon or anesthesia personnel.

Procedures vary among institutions, but after admission to the operating room, the client is moved to the operating room bed. At this time, the client is identified by the surgeon, anesthetized, positioned, has the skin prepared, and is draped for surgery.

Members of the Surgical Team

The surgical team is a group of highly trained individuals who must work together as a coordinated team for the welfare and safety of the client undergoing surgery. The team is composed of surgeon, anesthesiologist or nurse anesthetist, circulating nurse, scrub nurse or technician, and assistants.

The surgeon heads the surgical team and makes the major decisions concerning the course of surgery, such as whether to remove an organ, amputate a limb, or make radical or extensive repairs. The surgeon must be alert at all times to the changing physiologic needs of the client undergoing the stress of surgery.

The anesthesiologist (a physician) or nurse anesthetist (a registered nurse (RN) with special additional education) alleviates pain and promotes relaxation with medications. These specialists must (1) maintain the client's airway; (2) ensure that the client has an adequate oxygen and carbon dioxide exchange; (3) infuse blood, fluids, and medications to maintain hemodynamic stability; (4) monitor the client's circulation and respiration; and (5) alert the surgeon immediately about any complications.

The circulating nurse is an RN who acts as the manager of the operating suite. During an operation, the circulating nurse (1) checks that all equipment is working properly before the surgery; (2) ensures sterility of the instruments for surgery; (3) assists with positioning the client; (4) performs a skin preparation on the client, if ordered; (5) alerts team members of any break in sterile technique; (6) assists the anesthesiologist or anesthetist with monitoring vital functions, such as urine output and blood loss; (7) labels specimens, and (8) coordinates activities with other departments such as x-ray and pathology. The circulating nurse ensures that staff conversation and traffic are kept to a minimum. The sedated surgical client may confuse or misinterpret conversation overheard.

The circulating nurse promotes smooth and safe function of the operating suite by bringing needed supplies and medications to the operating table; assisting with the sponge, sharps, and instrument counts; and removing unneeded items or specimens. The Joint Commission on Accreditation of Healthcare Organizations recommends that only registered nurses perform this role.

The scrub person, who may be a registered nurse or a surgical technologist, assists the surgeon during the procedure by handing instruments, sutures, and other supplies. During the surgery, the scrub person maintains an accurate count of sponges, sharps, and instruments in the sterile field.

The direct assistants to the surgeon are usually other surgeons or surgical residents who plan a career as surgeons. Registered nurses and certain experienced paraprofessionals may act under the surgeon's direction as surgeon's assistants too.

The surgical team may include other members of the health care team when surgical procedures so dictate. For example, a pathologist may be requested to identify a pathologic process if it is discovered. An x-ray technician may be needed to perform various radiologic procedures while the client is on the operating table. A cardiopulmonary perfusionist may be required to assist during cardiothoracic surgery.

Anesthesia in Surgery

Anesthesia means the absence of pain ('an' meaning without, and 'esthesia' meaning awareness or feeling). Anesthesia is an artificially induced state of partial or total loss of sensation, occurring with or without loss of consciousness. The purpose of anesthesia is to produce muscle relaxation, block transmission of nerve impulses, suppress reflexes, and cause loss of consciousness.

Clients are generally anxious about receiving anesthesia. Some are concerned about the adequacy of analgesic effects. Others are concerned about being "put to sleep" with a drug. Some clients wonder if they will talk during anesthesia or experience nausea and vomiting after surgery. Reviewing the client's preoperative nursing assessment reveals some of these fears and concerns and allows the surgical nursing staff to offer continued support. A smile, a cordial introduction, and a warm touch help allay clients' fears in a threatening and strange environment.

The decision as to the type of anesthesia to be used is made largely by the anesthesiologist in consultation with the surgeon and client. The anesthetic agents chosen for a client's surgical procedure depend on many variables. These include (1) age and physical condition of the client; (2) type, location, and duration of the surgery; (3) degree of technical intricacy of the surgery; (4) previous anesthetic history; and (5) personal preference, expertise, and judgement of the anesthesiologist or nurse anesthetist. Also, the client undergoing surgery may prefer one type of anesthesia over another (e.g., spinal anesthesia rather than general anesthesia). A client's preference should be considered as part of the total profile when the type of anesthesia is selected.

There are two major classifications of anesthesia: (1) general and (2) regional. General anesthetics block pain stimulus at the cerebral cortex. General anesthesia is a drug-induced depression of the central nervous system that is reversed either by metabolic elimination in the body or by pharmacologic means. General anesthetic agents produce analgesia, amnesia, and unconsciousness, characterized by the loss of reflexes and muscle tone.

Regional anesthetics block the pain stimulus (1) at its origin, (2) along afferent neurons, or (3) along the spinal cord. Unlike general anesthesia, regional anesthesia produces a loss of painful sensation in only one region of the body and does not result in unconsciousness. The client also may receive sedative agents that produce drowsiness. The client might receive epidural narcotics, which have a systemic effect and produce some drowsiness. Table 19–8 illustrates the goal, method of administration, and assessment of these two major types of anesthesia.

GENERAL ANESTHESIA

Effects of General Anesthesia. The body systems affected by general anesthetics are the neurologic, respiratory, and cardiovascular systems. General anesthesia is best suited for surgery of the head, neck, and upper torso; prolonged surgical procedures; or for clients who are unable to lie quietly for a prolonged period of time. General anesthetic agents affect all tissues in the body to some degree.

The anesthesiologist or nurse anesthetist continually monitors body systems and tissues during induction of anesthesia, maintenance of the anesthetized state, and emergence of the client from anesthesia. These specialists understand when body systems are functioning adequately, and they recognize and intervene when systems are unstable. The depth of anesthesia is monitored by observing changes in respirations, oxygen saturation and tidal CO_2, heart rate, urine output, and blood pressure.

Stages of General Anesthesia. The four stages of anesthesia are described in Table 19–9. Although not apparent with all anesthetics, all stages may be seen if the drug is given slowly. Clients emerge through all three stages after the anesthetic agents are discontinued.

Administration of General Anesthesia. General anesthesia can be administered by inhalation, intravenous, rectal, or oral routes. Inhalation and intravenous meth-

TABLE 19–8. Types of Anesthesia

Type	Goal	Administration	Assessment
General			
	Total loss of consciousness and sensation; produces amnesia by blocking awareness centers in brain	Intravenous Inhalation Rectal	Loss of reflexes and muscle tone
Regional			
	Reduce all painful sensations in one region of the body without inducing unconsciousness:		
	▶ Block transmission of nerve impulses at their origin	Topical Local infiltration	Produces analgesia over specific tissue area
	▶ Block transmission of nerve impulses along afferent neurons	Field block Nerve block Intravenous regional	Produces analgesia over specific area of body
	▶ Block transmission of nerve impulses along spinal cord	Spinal Epidural block	Produces analgesia over specific region of body

TABLE 19-9. The Four Stages of Anesthesia

Stage	From	To	Assessment	Nursing Interventions
I: Onset	Anesthetic administration	Loss of consciousness	Client may be drowsy or dizzy May experience auditory or visual hallucinations	Close operating room doors. Keep room quiet. Stand by client to assist, if necessary
II: Excitement	Loss of consciousness	Loss of eyelid reflexes	Increase in autonomic activity Irregular breathing Client may struggle	Remain quietly at client's side. Assist anesthetist, if needed
III: Surgical anesthesia	Loss of eyelid reflexes	Loss of most reflexes Depression of vital functions	Client is unconscious Muscles are relaxed No blink or gag reflex	Begin preparation (if indicated) only when anesthetist indicates stage III has been reached and client is under good control
IV: Danger (death)	Vital functions too depressed	Respiratory and circulatory failure	Client is not breathing May or may not have a heartbeat	If arrest occurs, respond immediately to assist in establishing airway. Provide cardiac arrest tray, drugs, syringes, long needles. Assist surgeon with closed or open cardiac massage

ods are the most common routes of administration. Table 19-10 describes the most common general anesthetic agents in use and their implications for nursing.

Balanced Anesthesia. Balanced anesthesia is the practice of selecting drug combinations based on the individual client's need with consideration of the type of surgery. Balanced anesthesia is typically achieved with a combination of inhalation agent, narcotic, and muscle relaxants.

TYPES OF GENERAL ANESTHESIA

Intravenous Anesthesia. When general anesthesia is administered intravenously, the client experiences an extremely rapid induction. Unconsciousness generally occurs about 30 seconds after the initial intravenous administration. Intravenous anesthesia is most commonly used as an induction agent before inhalation anesthetics are given. However, intravenous anesthesia is sufficiently potent to be used alone in such minor procedures as dental extractions or pelvic examinations. Examples of intravenous anesthetics include thiopental sodium and ketamine.

Inhalation Anesthesia. Inhalation anesthesia is a mixture of volatile liquids or gas and oxygen. The mixture is given through a mask or through an endotracheal tube inserted directly into the trachea (Fig. 19-2). These anesthetics are advantageous because of their ease of administration and elimination through the respiratory system.

When inhalation anesthesia is administered by mask, the gases generally flow into the mask via a finely

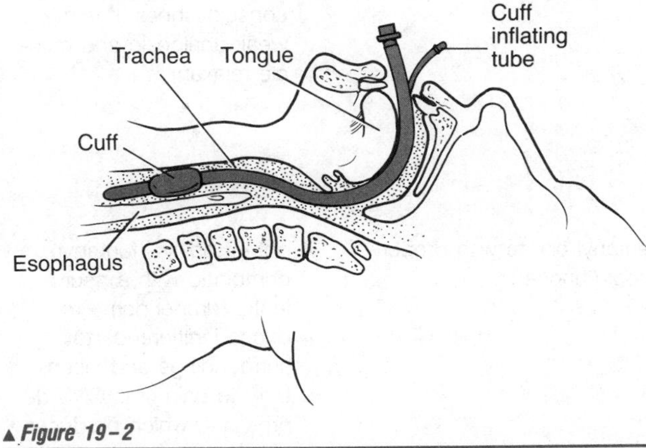

▲ *Figure 19-2*

Correct placement of endotracheal tube for anesthesia administration.

TABLE 19-10. General Anesthetic Agents

Drug	Action	Side Effects	Nursing Implications
Inhalation Agents			
Nitrous oxide	Gas with very low anesthetic potency, so it must be used with other agents. Highest analgesic effect of all agents; little or no effect on BP or P, no muscle relaxant properties	Minimal side effects; little or no hypotension or respiratory depression. Low incidence of malignant hypothermia	Monitor vital signs, especially BP and P; monitor effects of CNS depressants for 24 hours after administration
Halothane (Fluothane)	Volatile liquid with high anesthetic potency, so it could be used alone. Has weak analgesic effect; causes a moderate decrease in BP and a large decrease in respirations, and is only a mild muscle relaxant	Hypotension, depression of myocardium with decreased cardiac output, bradycardia, respiratory depression, sensitizes heart to catecholamines, malignant hyperthermia, hepatitis, postoperative mild nausea and vomiting, and decreased urine output	Monitor all vital signs closely; monitor temperature for signs of malignant hyperthermia; keep client warm during recovery, and watch for severe shivering; avoid use of catecholamines (epinephrine or norepinephrine); monitor liver function after surgery; monitor urine output closely
Enflurane (Ethrane)	Volatile liquid with fairly high anesthetic potential. Has weak analgesic effect, causes moderate decrease in BP, a large decrease in respirations, and is moderate muscle relaxant	Hypotension, respiratory depression, blocks labor, minimal sensitization of heart to catecholamines, and seizures with high doses	Do not give to clients with history of seizures; monitor vital signs, especially BP, P, and respirations; and is not for use during labor
Isoflurane (Forane)	Volatile liquid with high anesthetic potential. Has weak analgesic effect, causes moderate decrease in BP, a large decrease in respirations, and is a moderate muscle relaxant. Produces profound vasodilation	Hypotension related to vasodilatory effect; respiratory depression; and suppresses uterine contractions	Does not sensitize heart to catecholamines, so it can be used with epinephrine and norepinephrine; monitor vital signs; and avoid rapid position changes, because it may lead to hypotension due to vasodilation
Intravenous Drugs			
Thiopental sodium (Pentothal)	Short-acting barbiturate that produces rapid unconsciousness. It is a weak analgesic and muscle relaxant	Respiratory depression with momentary apnea after injection, retrograde amnesia, myocardial depression, hypotension, headache, and shivering	Monitor for allergic reactions; monitor respiratory function closely, especially during induction; monitor vital signs; can not be mixed with solutions containing atropine, diturbocurare, or succinylcholine; and avoid extravasation
Fentanyl citrate with droperidol (Innovar)	A potent opioid (fentanyl) combined with a neuroleptic (droperidol). Produces indifference to surroundings and insensitivity to pain. It is CNS depressant, which produces calming, analgesia, and reduced motor activity	Emergence delirium with hallucinations, hypotension, vasodilation, nausea and vomiting, laryngospasm, respiratory depression, shivering, and apnea	Use with caution in clients with head injuries, increased intracranial pressure, COPD, hepatic or renal dysfunction, bradyarrhythmias, or with elderly; monitor vital signs; maintain patient airway; decrease narcotic doses

TABLE 19-10. General Anesthetic Agents Continued

Drug	Action	Side Effects	Nursing Implications
Intravenous Drugs			
			to $\frac{1}{4}$ or $\frac{1}{3}$ for the first 24 hours postoperatively; when Innovar is used for induction, fentanyl (Sublimaze) alone is used for maintenance of anesthesia
Ketamine hydrochloride (Ketamine)	Produces state of dissociative anesthesia. Causes sedation, immobility, analgesia, amnesia, and unresponsiveness to pain	Delirium, hallucinations, disturbing dreams, tonic and clonic movements, respiratory depression, hypotension or hypertension, decreased or increased pulse, nystagmus, increased salivation, laryngospasms, and mild nausea and vomiting	Contraindicated in clients with history of CVA and severe hypertension; use with caution in clients with alcoholism, or elevated CSF; maintain airway; do not give in same syringe as barbiturates; keep all stimulation to a minimum as client emerges from anesthesia; use diazepam if hallucinations occur or delusions are severe; excellent for anesthesia in young and elderly

calibrated vaporizer controlled by a machine. When an endotracheal tube is used to give anesthetic, the gases flow directly into the client's tracheobronchial tree.

Many different liquids and gases are used in inhalation anesthesia. Two commonly employed volatile liquid anesthetics are halothane and isoflurane. A commonly used gas anesthetic is nitrous oxide.

As mentioned earlier, an intravenous anesthetic is often administered before the use of inhalation anesthetic. This process promotes a rapid transition from the conscious stage to the surgical anesthesia stage (from stage 1 to stage 3). In this case, the early stages of anesthesia typically are not seen.

Although ether rarely is used today, it is important historically as one of the oldest known anesthetics. It produces a deep and prolonged anesthesia that rarely results in cardiovascular complications, the leading medical cause of perioperative mortality in adults. Consequently, ether is sometimes used for high-risk individuals, but its highly explosive properties make it a dangerous and less desirable choice.

Rectal Anesthesia. Rectal anesthesia is administered via a rectal tube. This form rarely is used today, although it is useful when anesthetizing a child or when facial surgery makes it difficult to maintain an airway. Intravenous or liquid inhalation agents are instilled into the rectum. Methohexital sodium is one anesthetic agent that may be administered rectally. It is absorbed by the rectal mucosa and delivered to the central nervous system (CNS) via the circulatory system. Because rectal anesthesia is used only during induction, it must always be supplemented with other types of anesthetic agents.

MUSCLE RELAXANTS

Muscle relaxants are administered intravenously and are given mainly to facilitate intubation, relax the muscles within the surgical field, ease laryngospasms, and relax muscles for controlled ventilation. When given with muscle relaxants, potent general anesthetics can be administered in smaller, and thus safer, doses.

Muscle relaxants are classified as depolarizing and nondepolarizing agents that block the transmission of nervous impulses to the muscle fibers (Table 19-11). This block produces temporary paralysis of voluntary muscles, including the muscles that control respiration. Hence, respiration must be supported mechanically when muscle relaxants are employed. Respirations in clients who have received muscle relaxants must be closely monitored for at least 1 hour after the relaxants appear to have worn off because paralysis may recur.

Examples of the common muscle relaxant agents include succinylcholine (Anectine), D-tubocurarine (DTC), pancuronium (Pavulon), and vecuronium (Norcuron).

LOCAL ANESTHESIA

Local anesthetics are useful in many clinical situations. Local anesthetics can be used for local effects and also can be administered to function as central, peripheral, intravenous, regional, retrobulbar, or transbronchial nerve blocks. These anesthetic agents block the con-

TABLE 19-11. Muscle Relaxants

Drug	Action	Side Effects	Nursing Implications
Pancuronium bromide (Pavulon)	Nondepolarizing agent; prevents acetylcholine from binding to receptors on muscle end plate, blocking depolarization	Tachycardia, hypertension, prolonged dose-related apnea, allergic reaction, and excessive sweating and salivation	Use carefully in older or debilitated clients or clients with or in clients with renal, hepatic, or pulmonary disease, myasthenia gravis, or thyroid disease; measure intake and output carefully; have resuscitation equipment available; do not mix in syringe or solution with barbiturates; and neostigmine reverses effect
Vencuronium bromide (Norcuron)	Nondepolarizing agent; prevents acetylcholine from binding to receptors on muscle end plate, blocking depolarization	Transient tachycardia; prolonged dose-related apnea, redness, itching, and induration	Has no effect on cardiovascular system. Use with caution in clients with hepatic disease, obesity, or neuromuscular disease; tolerated well in renal disease; reversed with anticholinesterase and neostigmine. Have emergency resuscitation equipment available
Succinylcholine chloride (Anectine)	Depolarizing agent that prolongs depolarization of muscle end plate	Increased or decreased pulse rate and blood pressure, dysrhythmias, increased intraocular pressure, prolonged respiratory depression, malignant hyperthermia, postoperative muscle pain, excessive salivation, and hypersensitivity	Monitor vital signs; maintain patent airway; postoperative stiffness is normal; drug of choice for short procedures; keep emergency resuscitation equipment on hand; repeat infusions can prolong apnea; and is reversible with neostigmine

duction of impulses in nerve fibers without depolarizing the cell membrane (Table 19-12).

Sometimes, epinephrine is added to the local anesthetic agent to provide a more prolonged effect. Epinephrine causes local blood vessels to constrict, thus delaying absorption of the anesthetic agent. Epinephrine should be used with caution in elderly clients with cardiovascular or liver disease.

Types of Local Anesthesia. There are several anesthetic techniques using local anesthesia: (1) topical, (2) local infiltration, (3) field block, (4) peripheral nerve block, (5) spinal, (6) epidural, (7) caudal, and (8) intravenous regional block.

Topical Anesthesia. Topical anesthesia may be directly applied onto an area to be desensitized. The anesthetic may be a solution, ointment, gel, cream, or powder. This short-acting form of anesthesia can block peripheral nerve endings in the mucous membranes of the vagina, rectum, nasopharynx, and mouth. Topical anesthesia is used in minor procedures such as a rectal examination when painful hemorrhoids are present, or before a bronchoscopic examination to desensitize the bronchi.

One drug commonly used for topical anesthesia is cocaine, in a 4 to 10 per cent solution. This agent is for topical use only, and it is primarily used to anesthetize the eye and the mucous membranes of the nose, mouth, and urethra. Cocaine is highly toxic. If accidentally injected, it may cause severe excitement and seizures, followed by shock, respiratory failure, and cardiac arrest. Emergency resuscitation equipment must be available.

Other agents used for topical anesthesia include tetracaine, procaine, mepivacaine, bupivacaine, and lidocaine. To avoid an anaphylactic reaction from previous sensitization to anesthetic agents, check the client's drug allergies before topical anesthesia is applied. (see Table 19-12)

Infiltration Anesthesia. Local anesthesia involves the injection of an anesthetic agent, such as lidocaine (Xylocaine), into the skin and subcutaneous tissue of the

TABLE 19-12. Local and Topical Anesthetic Agents

Drug	Action	Side Effects	Nursing Implications
Local Agents			
Bupivacaine (Marcaine)	Amide type local anesthetic that blocks depolarization, preventing generation and conduction of nerve impulses. When combined with epinephrine, it has prolonged action	Edema, anaphylaxsis. Rarely, anxiety, convulsions, respiratory arrest, cardiac arrest, blurred vision, and shivering	Contraindicated for children under 12, for spinal or paracervical block or topical anesthesia; use with caution in older clients, or clients with hepatic disease or allergies; onset 4 to 15 minutes, duration 3 to 6 hours; and keep resuscitative eqiupment available
Chloroprocaine hydrochloride (Nesacaine)	Ester type local anesthetic that blocks depolarization, preventing generation and conduction of nerve impulses	Anaphylaxis, edema. Rarely, anxiety, convulsions, respiratory arrest, cardiac arrest, blurred vision, and shivering	Contraindicated for clients with allergies to "caines," CNS disease; use cautiously with older adults; check solution for particles or discoloration; keep resuscitative equipment available; and do not use solution with preservative for caudal or epidural blocks
Lidocaine hydrochloride (Xylocaine)	Amide type local anesthetic that blocks depolarization, preventing generation and conduction of nerve impulses. When combined with epinephrine, it has prolonged action	Edema, anaphylaxis, arrhythmias, or rarely, anxiety, respiratory arrest, cardiac arrest, and tinnitus	Contraindicated in clients with hypersensitivity, severe hypertension, septicemia, spinal deformities, or neurologic disorders; use cautiously with older clients and clients with heart block, general drug allergies, or in severe shock; use solutions with epinephrine only in body areas with good blood supply; and use preservative free solution for spinal, epidural, and caudal blocks
Topical Agents			
Benzocaine (Americaine)	Blocks conduction of impulses at sensory nerve endings	Sensitization rash, possible tolerance	Contraindicated in clients with history of hypersensitivity to "caines"; discontinue if rash develops; avoid contact with eyes; avoid inhalation when using spray; has short duration of action; do not use over infected area; and if used rectally, clean area well first
Ethyl chloride (Ethyl Chloride Spray)	Produces local anesthesia by producing sensation of cold	Frostbite, tissue necrosis from prolonged use, muscle spasms, and increased pain	Do not apply over broken skin; protect adjacent skin; avoid contact with eyes; avoid inhalation; highly flammable, do not

Table continued on following page

TABLE 19–12. Local and Topical Anesthetic Agents Continued

Drug	Action	Side Effects	Nursing Implications
Topical Agents			
			use near open flame; and very short duration
Tetracaine hydrochloride (Pontocaine)	Blocks conduction of impulses at sensory nerve endings	Local sensitization and rash	Do not use in hypersensitive clients; cleanse rectal area well before applying; and do not use if rash develops
Cocaine	Ester type topical anesthetic, block uptake of norepinephrine by adrenergic neurons	CNS stimulation, euphoria, decreased fatigue, tachycardia, vasoconstriction, and hypertension	For topical use only; produces psychological dependence with prolonged or repeated use, schedule II narcotic; use cautiously with clients with history of severe hypertension or heart disease; when combined with epinephrine, it can lead to cardiovascular toxicity; and monitor vital signs closely

BP, Blood pressure; CNS, central nervous system; COPD, chronic obstructive pulmonary disease; CSF, cerebrospinal fluid; CVA, cerebrovascular accident; P, pulse.

area to be incised. Local anesthesia blocks only the peripheral nerves around the area of the incision.

When a local anesthetic is administered, the physician must not allow the needle to slip into one of the veins. If a local anesthetic agent is given intravenously by accident, cardiovascular collapse or convulsions may result. For this reason, the physician must always aspirate before injection to ensure the needle is not in a vein.

Field Block Anesthesia. In a field block, the area proximal to the incision is injected and infiltrated with local anesthetics, thereby forming a barrier between the incision and the nervous system. This procedure contrasts with local anesthesia, in which only the area of the incision is injected. Thus, a field block actually walls in the area around the incision and thereby prevents transmission of sensory impulses to the brain from that area. Precautions to avoid intravenous administration must be taken in performing field blocks.

Peripheral Nerve Block Anesthesia. A nerve block anesthetizes individual nerves or nerve plexuses rather than all the local nerves anesthetized by a field block. Nerve blocks may be used to anesthetize, for example, a finger (digital nerve block), the entire upper arm (brachial plexus nerve block), or the chest or abdominal wall (intercostal nerve block). Nerves most commonly blocked are those within the brachial plexus and the intercostal, sciatic, and femoral nerves. Drugs commonly used as nerve blocks are lidocaine, bupivacaine, and mepivacaine. The anesthetist attempts to inject the anesthetic along the nerve, rather than into the nerve, to decrease the risk of nerve damage. Once the drug has been injected, it takes several minutes to anesthetize the area.

Nerve blocks, like local infiltration blocks, can produce severe systemic responses if the drug is accidentally injected into a blood vessel. Because epinephrine causes vasoconstriction, particularly of the extremities, surgery performed below the wrist or ankle typically uses anesthetics that do not contain epinephrine.

Spinal Anesthesia. Spinal anesthesia is achieved by injecting certain local anesthetics into the subarachnoid space (Fig. 19–3). Autonomic nerve fibers are the first to be affected by spinal anesthesia and the last to recover. Following autonomic blockage, spinal anesthesia blocks the following fibers in this order: touch, pain, motor, pressure, and proprioceptive fibers. Recovery is in reverse order.

Spinal anesthesia can be used for almost any type of major procedure performed below the level of the diaphragm, such as hysterectomy and appendectomy. Figure 19–4 illustrates the proper positioning for spinal anesthesia.

Within minutes after induction of spinal anesthesia, the client experiences a loss of sensation and paralysis of first the toes, then the feet and legs, and finally, the abdomen.

Spinal anesthesia offers many advantages for clients undergoing surgical procedures involving the lower half of the body. Major benefits are that it

- Is a relatively safe method of anesthesia,
- Provides excellent muscle relaxation,

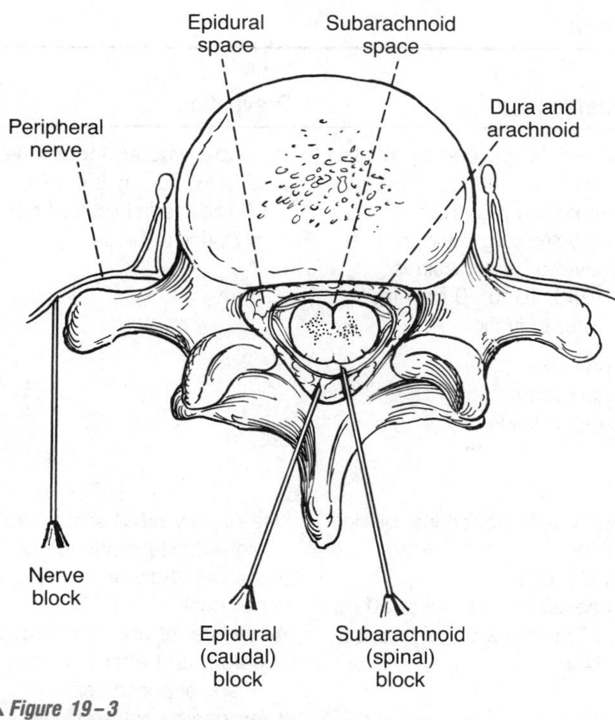

▲ **Figure 19-3**

Cross section of the spinal cord, showing injection sites for anesthesia.

- Does not cloud the client's consciousness or alertness (anxious clients, however, can be given a small dose of barbiturates to enable them to rest or even sleep throughout the operation),
- Can be used for clients with a full stomach, because they will be awake to maintain their airway if they vomit.

Complications of spinal anesthesia are listed in Table 19-13 with their causes, prevention, and intervention. Remember that a client who has undergone spinal anesthesia is a candidate for serious neurologic, respiratory, or cardiovascular problems.

As the anesthetic agent wears off, monitor the client carefully. Return of motion to the extremities is checked by asking clients to move their toes. However, clients who can wiggle their toes have not necessarily recovered completely from the spinal anesthetic. An ability to move the toes simply means that the motor blockade is wearing off, although autonomic blockade may still be present. Clients who are still experiencing autonomic blockade are prone to hypotension despite having the ability to move toes and extremities. Continue to monitor vital signs and for return of sensation.

Epidural Anesthesia. Epidural block is achieved by introducing an anesthetic agent into the epidural space (see Fig. 19-3). The epidural space is generally entered by a needle at the thoracic, lumbar, sacral, or caudal interspaces. The needle is carefully positioned in the epidural space, without penetrating the dura and entering the subarachnoid space. When the needle is properly positioned, the cerebrospinal fluid (CSF) cannot be aspirated.

Epidural block, like spinal anesthesia, produces autonomic blockade. Hypotension can result. Respiratory depression or paralysis also may occur if the level of the block is too high and affects respiratory muscles.

Caudal Anesthesia. This type of anesthesia is produced by injecting the local anesthetic into the caudal or sacral canal. Caudal anesthesia is a variation of epidural anesthesia. This method of regional anesthesia is commonly used in obstetric clients.

Intravenous Regional (Extremity) Block Anesthesia (Bier Block). Regional anesthesia of a limb can be achieved through an agent such as lidocaine, which is injected into a vein of the limb to be anesthetized. A pneumatic tourniquet applied to the anesthetized area prevents the lidocaine from circulating beyond the area undergoing the procedure. This type of anesthesia is used most commonly for short procedures on the extremities.

OTHER TYPES OF ANESTHESIA

Acupuncture. Acupuncture is an age-old Chinese pain-killing technique that works by the insertion of long, thin needles into specific acupuncture points located along channels called *meridians* that run throughout

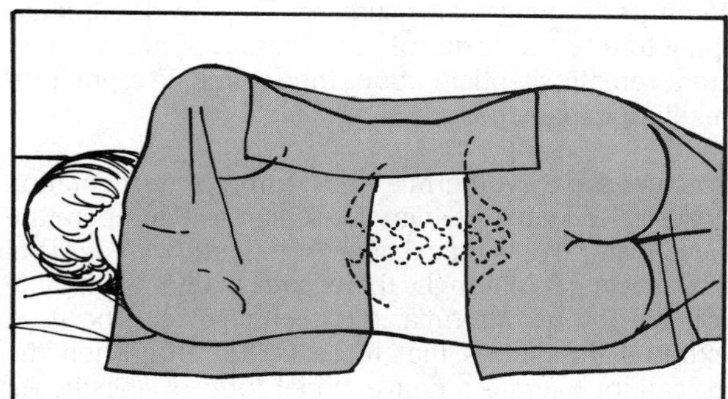

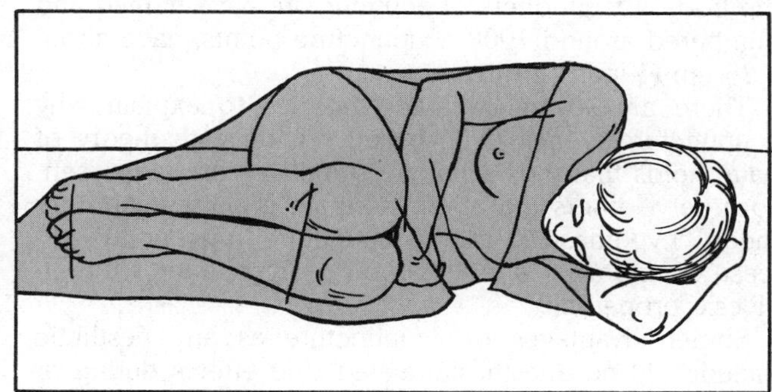

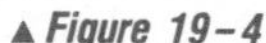

▲ **Figure 19-4**

Proper positioning for spinal anesthesia administration.

TABLE 19-13. Complications and Discomforts of Spinal Anesthesia

Complications and Discomforts	Causes	Intervention	Prevention
Hypotension	Paralysis of vasomotor nerves; usually occurs shortly after induction of anesthesia	Administer oxygen by inhalation Vasoactive drugs Trendelenburg position if level of anesthesia is fixed, 10 to 20 minutes after induction	In people who are not prone to CHF, 500 to 800 ml of IV fluids, administered rapidly prior to block
Nausea and vomiting	Occurs mainly during abdominal surgery, owing to traction placed on various structures within abdomen or hypotension	Ephedrine Antiemetics Oxygen fluids	
Headache (can be extremely painful and may last a week)	Cerebrospinal fluid (which cushions the brain) is lost through dural hole; leakage of fluid and loss of cushioning effect increased by 1. use of a large spinal needle 2. poor hydration	Apply tight abdominal binder Fluids Analgesics In severe cases, inject 10 ml of person's blood to plug hole	Use of very small spinal needle reduces incidence of spinal headache to 0.9 per cent Administer IV and oral fluids before and after induction of spinal anesthesia Keep person flat and quiet 6-8 hours postoperatively
Respiratory paralysis	Occurs if drug reaches upper thoracic and cervical cord in large amounts or in heavy concentrations	Artificial respiration	Avoid extreme Trendelenburg position before level of spinal anesthesia set, i.e., 10 to 20 minutes following induction
Neurologic complications (e.g., paraplegia, severe muscle weakness in legs)	Paralysis postoperatively may be due to 1. unsterile needles, syringes, and anesthetic medications 2. preexisting diseases of CNA (e.g., multiple sclerosis and spinal cord tumors), which cause paralysis, rather than spinal anesthesia itself	See Unit VI	Strict sterile technique Heat-sterilized medications and instruments Careful preoperative neurologic examination to ascertain presence of neurologic disease

CNS, Central nervous system.

the body. Practitioners of acupuncture have named and numbered around 1000 acupuncture points, each about 0.25 cm ($\frac{1}{8}$-inch) in diameter.

There are several western theories to explain why acupuncture works. One, based on the gate theory of pain, holds that the technique stimulates the larger sensory nerve fibers that carry nonpain impulses. Another theory hypothesizes that acupuncture triggers the release of endorphins, endogenous polypeptides with analgesic properties.

Some advantages of acupuncture as an anesthetic include (1) no anesthesia-related side effects during or after surgery, (2) less blood loss during surgery, and (3) reduced need for postoperative analgesia, because acupuncture's pain-killing effects persist for several hours.

When performing major surgery, Chinese doctors use acupuncture as a form of anesthesia. Some western doctors remain skeptical about the technique's practical pain-killing capabilities.

Cryothermia. Cryothermia is a form of refrigeration anesthesia. Because a very low surface temperature reduces pain, the surgical site is treated with ice before operating. Although there are many acceptable alternatives to cryothermia, this technique can be used in extreme conditions that threaten life and when the client cannot tolerate a conventional form of anesthesia.

Hypnoanesthesia. Hypnosis is an altered state of consciousness in which the person experiences a heightened state of concentration. As an anesthetic, hypnosis alleviates pain through relaxation, suggestion, and intense concentration on a particular object or sound to the exclusion of other distractions, including pain. Exactly how hypnosis relieves pain is unknown.

Some therapeutic hypnoanesthesia techniques currently used include

- Symptom suppression in which the client blocks awareness of the pain through concentration;
- Symptom substitution in which the client substitutes warmth, pressure, or tingling for the sensation of pain; and
- Time distortion in which the therapist suggests to the client that the period of pain is very brief when in reality it may last for hours

Hypnoanesthesia has been used successfully in obstetrics and in certain dental procedures, but not every person is susceptible to hypnotic suggestion. Moreover, it must be carried out by a carefully and specially trained practitioner. Like cryothermia, there are better alternatives to anesthesia, especially for major surgery.

Nursing Care During Surgery

PROVIDING EMOTIONAL CARE

The client's emotional well-being is paramount during the operative phase. Before anesthesia, the nurse is responsible for ensuring that the client feels secure and that anxieties have been addressed.

If the client is awake during the procedure, the nurse should explain the procedure and support and reassure the client. When the client is recovering from the anesthesia, explanations and reinforcement of teaching should be given.

ASSISTING WITH CLIENT POSITIONING

The operating room nurse understands the various operative positions as well as the physiologic changes that occur when a client is placed in a specific position. Essential factors to consider when positioning a client on the operating room bed include (1) site of operation, (2) age and size of client, (3) type of anesthetic used, and (4) pain normally experienced by the client on movement, such as from arthritis. The position must not hinder respiration, circulation, apply excessive pressure to the skin surfaces, or limit surgical exposure. The following surgical positions are shown in Figure 19–5:

- The *dorsal recumbent* position, commonly used for hernia repair, mastectomy, or bowel resection.
- The *Trendelenburg* position permits displacement of the intestines into the upper abdomen and is often used during surgery of the lower abdomen or pelvis.

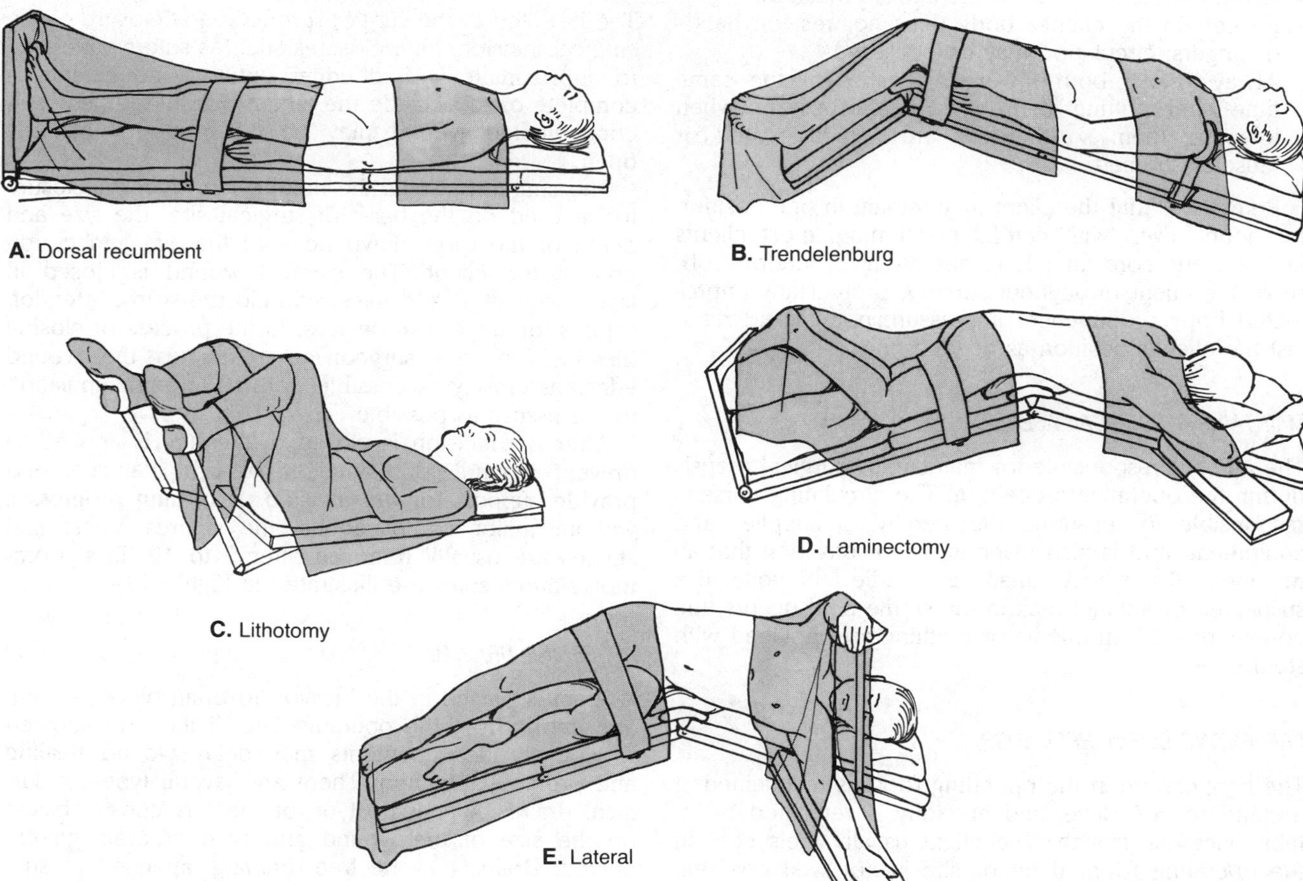

▲ **Figure 19–5**

Five surgical positions.

- The *lithotomy* position exposes the perineal and rectal areas, and is ideal for vaginal repairs, dilatation and curettage, and most rectal surgeries.
- The *laminectomy* position is used during surgical procedures involving the spine.
- The *lateral* position is used for clients undergoing kidney, chest, or hip surgery.

Whatever the client's position on the operating room bed, there are certain general considerations and rules of safety to observe:

- Explain to the client in simple, understandable terms, why the positions and restraints are necessary.
- Preserve the client's dignity and avoid undue exposure.
- Secure the client to the table with well-padded straps, usually placed above the knees. Nerves, muscles, and bony prominence are padded to prevent nerve and tissue damage.
- Maintain adequate respiratory exchange and vascular circulation to permit the exchange of gases. Avoid pressure on the chest and on body parts, because pressure can impair or slow circulation, resulting in the pooling of blood. Slow blood flow predisposes a client to thrombus formation.
- Do not allow the client's extremities to dangle over the sides of the table, because this may impair circulation or cause nerve and muscle damage.
- Avoid excessive strain on the client's muscles.
- Be certain the client's body does not rest on hands or fingers; circulation may be occluded.
- Always move both lower extremities at the same time when putting them up in the stirrups and when lowering them so the hips are not dislocated or muscles strained.

Remember that the client may remain in one position for hours. Even with careful positioning, most clients feel stiff and sore after long operations. Therefore, observe the client throughout surgery, protect any unprotected bony prominence or pressure points, and readjust the client's position as needed.

MAINTAINING SURGICAL ASEPSIS

The nurse is responsible for maintaining surgical asepsis during the operative procedure. The circulating nurse is responsible for ensuring the sterility of supplies and equipment, and is also responsible for ensuring that all members of the health team use sterile technique. If a suspected or actual break in the sterile field occurs, the contaminated instruments or clothing are replaced with sterile ones.

PREVENTING CLIENT HEAT LOSS

The temperature in the operating room is maintained at a standard cool level and humidity is regulated to inhibit bacterial growth. The client usually feels cold in the operating room if he or she is not well covered. The client loses heat from the skin and from the area open for surgery. When tissues that are not covered with skin are exposed to the air, the heat loss is greater. The client should be kept as warm as possible to minimize heat loss without causing vasodilation that could cause more bleeding.

MONITORING FOR MALIGNANT HYPERTHERMIA

Malignant hyperthermia is a genetic disorder characterized by uncontrolled skeletal muscle contraction, leading to potentially fatal hyperthermia. It occurs in clients carrying this genetic disorder who receive a combination of succinylcholine, inhalation agents (especially halothanes), and other factors (such as stress, infection, and trauma). This condition can occur within 30 minutes of anesthesia induction or may occur several hours after the surgery. The initial sign is usually skeletal muscle rigidity, followed by cardiac arrhythmias and a hypermetabolic state. The client's fever can rise as high as 104° F (43° C). Unless the triggering event is stopped and attempts are made to cool the body, death can result. Dantrolene, a muscle relaxant, can be used to decrease the skeletal muscle rigidity. There is no screening test for this disorder; however, if there is a family history of this problem, general anesthesia should be used only if absolutely necessary (and then the client monitored very closely).

ASSISTING WITH SURGICAL WOUND CLOSURE

The last step in the surgical procedure is closure of the surgical incision. Skin closures such as sutures are used to approximate wound edges until wound healing is complete or to occlude the lumen or a blood vessel. A contaminated wound may be left open or partially open.

The surgeon selects the method and type of closure to be used on the basis of surgical site, the size and depth of the surgical wound, and the age and condition of the client. The surgical wound is closed in layers with sutures, staples, skin closure strips, retention sutures, or zipper-like devices. In the process of closing the incision, the surgeon approximates the wound edges as closely as possible, with as little manipulation to the tissues as possible.

After the incision is closed, a dressing is applied to prevent wound contamination, absorb drainage, and provide support for the incision. If healing progresses without major complications, the sutures, clips, and staples are usually removed after 7 to 10 days. Common skin closures are illustrated in Figure 19–6.

ASSESSING DRAINAGE

A drain is placed in the incision to drain blood, serum, and debris from the operative site. If they are allowed to collect, these contents may delay wound healing and promote infection. There are several types of surgical drains. A specific type of drain is chosen based on the size of the wound and type of drainage expected. Drains may be free draining, attached to suction, or a self-contained drainage with suction.

The nurse is responsible for assessing that the drain-

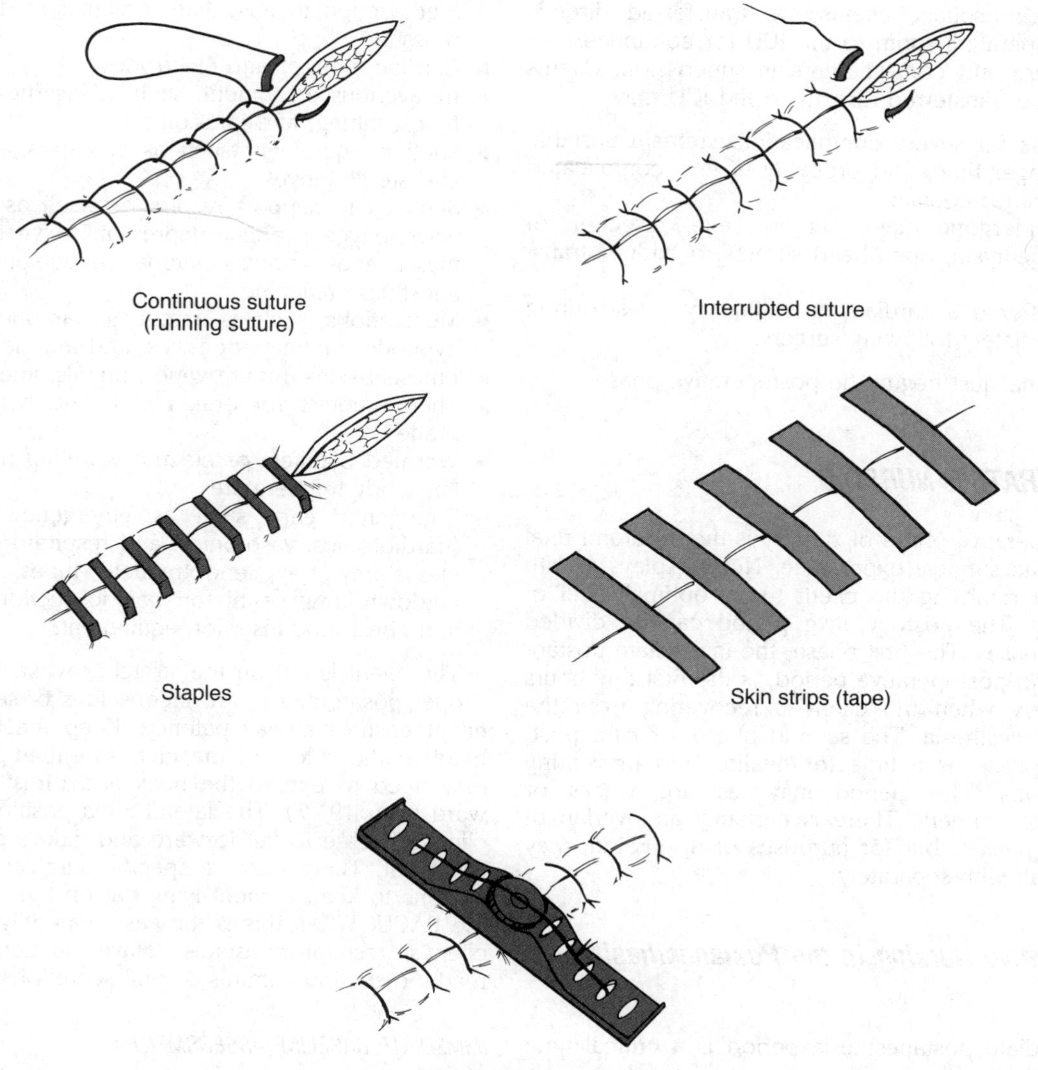

▲ *Figure 19–6*

Skin closures.

age is flowing freely through the system. Drains are usually removed when the drainage is reduced to an insignificant amount.

TRANSPORTING THE CLIENT TO THE POSTANESTHESIA OR INTENSIVE CARE UNIT

Following the operation, a member of the surgical team generally dresses the client in a clean gown, then assists with the transfer of the client to a stretcher. During this transfer, the operating room personnel avoid exposure, which may be embarrassing and predisposes the client to heat loss, respiratory infections, and shock. Also, avoid rough handling, which may strain the client's sutures and conveys lack of concern for the client's comfort and feelings. Finally, avoid hurried movements and rapid changes in position that predispose the client to hypotension. In particular, the client must be moved gradually from the lithotomy to the horizontal position and from the prone to the supine position, and he or she must be moved carefully after receiving spinal or epidural anesthesia. When moving or transferring a client after surgery, always have adequate help to prevent injuries to staff or the postoperative client. Very large clients and clients going to intensive care unit (ICU) are often placed directly into their beds.

After moving to the stretcher, the client should be covered with warm blankets and secured with safety belts. The side rails of the stretcher must be up to ensure the client's safety in case the client becomes agitated during transport from the operating room. The anesthesiologist or the nurse anesthetist, as well as another member of the operating room professional staff and sometimes the surgeon or assistant, accompany the client to the postanesthesia care unit (PACU).

In some hospitals, clients are transferred directly from the operating room to the ICU for continued specialized care and constant nursing supervision. Clients who may be transferred directly to the ICU may

- Be at risk for severe complications, remain unstable for a longer time, and probably have a complicated postoperative course;
- Have undergone major surgery (e.g., resection of aortic aneurysm, open heart surgery, or kidney transplant); or
- Have suffered a cardiac or respiratory arrest during or immediately following surgery.

The client has just begun the postoperative phase.

POSTOPERATIVE NURSING

The postoperative phase of surgery is the third and final phase of the surgical experience. Nursing plays a critical role in returning the client to an optimal level of functioning. The postoperative period can be divided into two phases. The first phase, the immediate postanesthesia and postoperative period, is the first few hours after surgery when the client is recovering from the effects of anesthesia. The second phase, or later postoperative phase, is a time for healing and preventing complications. This period may last for weeks or months after surgery. There is certainly an overlap of these two phases, but for purposes of discussion, they will be dealt with separately.

Postoperative Nursing in the Postanesthesia Care Unit

The immediate postanesthesia period is a critical time for the client. Close observation is important. The client's vital psychological functions must be supported until the effects of the anesthesia abate. Until then, the client is dependent, drowsy, and may be unable to call for assistance. In PACU, nurses assess the client during recovery from the immediate effects of surgery and intervene as appropriate.

ASPAN has described the goal of the postanesthesia nurse as "to assist the client in returning to a safe physiological level after an anesthetic by providing safe, knowledgeable, individualized nursing care to clients and their families in the immediate postanesthesia phase."[3]

ADMISSION TO THE POSTANESTHESIA CARE UNIT

The PACU nurse has special education in the care of clients recovering from surgery. Before the arrival of each client from the operating room, the nurse checks that the following equipment is functioning and ready for use:

- Sphygmomanometer or automatic blood pressure monitor
- Stethoscope to auscultate breath sounds and blood pressure
- Cardiac monitor and electrodes
- Intravenous equipment, such as insertion equipment, fluids, tubing, and infusion pumps
- Suction equipment such as catheters, sterile saline, and sterile gloves
- Supplies to support respiration such as artificial airways, oxygen, tongue depressors, oxygen tubing with masks and cannulas, intubation equipment, and an anesthesia machine
- Medications, such as narcotics, narcotic antagonists, hypnotics, antihypertensives, and muscle relaxants
- Emesis basins, mouth wipes, urinals, and bedpans
- Thermometers for oral, rectal, and tympanic membrane
- Warmed blankets or electric warming units to maintain body temperature
- Emergency cart, such as emergency medications (cardiotonics, vasotonics, and respiratory drugs), tracheostomy tray, endotracheal tubes, defibrillator, cutdown tray, ventilator, gastric suction equipment, and chest tube insertion equipment.

The client is left on the stretcher while in the PACU. Proper positioning of an unconscious or semiconscious client ensures airway patency. Keep the adult client's head to the side and the chin extended forward; you may need to extend the neck and thrust the jaw forward (Fig. 19-7). The lateral Sims position allows the client's tongue to fall forward and mucus or vomitus to drain out. There may be specific surgical or anatomic reasons to keep a client lying flat on the back while in the PACU. When this is the case, carefully monitor the client's respiratory status. Have suction equipment ready to suction vomitus or oral secretions.

IMMEDIATE BASELINE ASSESSMENT

On admission, the PACU nurse

- Assesses airway patency and support as needed. Assesses for the presence of hoarseness, croup, stridor, wheezes, or decreased breath sounds:
- Applies humidified oxygen via nasal cannula or face mask;
- Records vital signs (blood pressure, heart rate, strength, and regularity, respiratory rate and depth, oxygen saturation, skin color, and temperature);
- Assesses the client's level of consciousness, muscle strength, and ability to follow commands.
- Observes the client's intravenous infusions, dressings, drains, and special equipment.
- Remains at the client's bedside, continuing close observation of the client's condition.

After the client has been positioned safely and the baseline vital signs status has been ascertained, the nurse receives a verbal report from the members of the operating room team and a detailed report of events from the anesthesia personnel.

The following questions should be answered during the report:

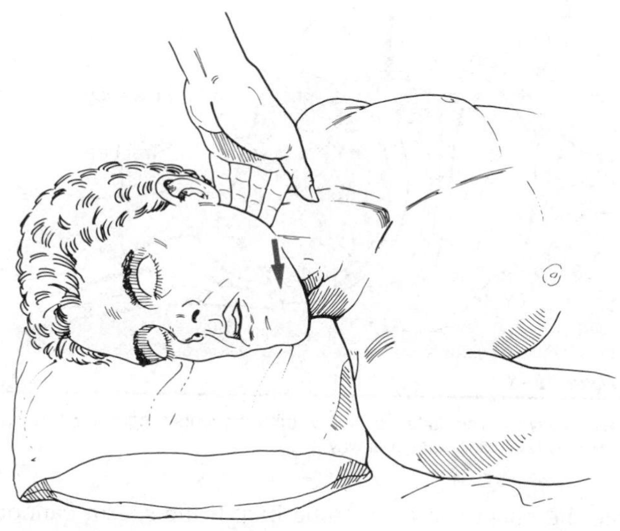

▲ *Figure 19-7*

Position of hand to move jaw forward after anesthesia. Fingers are placed behind angle of jaw. As jaw is moved, tongue comes forward, opening the airway.

- What operative procedure was performed?
- What were the client's vital signs in the operating room?
- What were the client's blood loss, fluids or blood infused, and urine output?
- What is the client's general condition?
- What are the client's medical diagnosis, pertinent medical history, and daily medications?
- What anesthetic agents, narcotics, muscle relaxants, antibiotics, and steroids has the client received?
- Did the client suffer any complications during surgery? What interventions were instituted? What were the outcomes?
- What pathologic disorders were encountered during surgery? Was cancer or some other unexpected problem discovered? When will the client be told that the cancer (or other problems) is present?
- Are there any specific symptoms or complications to observe? What symptoms should be reported immediately?
- Are there physician orders to be carried out immediately?

With the anesthesiologist present, the PACU nurse then reviews the client's record, noting specifically (1) the anesthesia record for intravenous medications and blood received during surgery, and (2) the length of time the client was in surgery. Ideally, a preoperative nursing assessment and nursing history are available in the record for comparison with the postoperative assessment.

Following the baseline nursing assessments, review of the client's record, and postoperative verbal report, the PACU nurse assesses and documents routine observations. Observations to document include

- Time of admission of the client to the PACU.
- The absence of reflexes, such as the pharyngeal reflex. Clients admitted to the PACU without pharyngeal reflex are positioned on their side. **The nurse stays at the bedside until the client's gag reflex returns.**
- Level of consciousness. What is the response to stimuli such as light or touch? Does saying the client's name or giving simple commands bring a response? Is the client moving voluntarily or making audible or intelligible sounds?
- Temperature and vital signs. Monitor the vital signs every 15 minutes until they are stable or more often as necessary. In some hospitals this assessment continues until the client leaves the PACU. Monitor the temperature on admission and at intervals until the client is discharged as established by PACU policy. Usually, clients must achieve a minimum temperature of greater than 36° C (96.8° F) before they are discharged from the PACU.
- Skin color and dryness. Dusky, pale, cold, wet skin is one important sign of shock and should be considered with blood pressure. Also, observe the lips and nail beds for pallor and cyanosis. Consider this information in relationship to oxygen saturation and hemoglobin.
- Condition of the dressing, (whether it is dry or soiled, or intact)? If soiled, note the color, type, and amount of drainage.
- Drainage tubes, such as T-tube, gastric tube, urinary catheter, or wound drains. Is the T-tube unclamped and attached to a gravity drainage system? Are gastric, chest, and intestinal tubes attached to suction as ordered? Ensure that tubes drain freely, that there are no kinks in the tubes, and that the client is not lying on them. Note the volume of drainage and color. Note any abnormalities in the appearance of the urine.
- Intravenous infusion. Note the type of intravenous solutions that are running. Also, check the amount of intravenous solution left in the bottle and the rate of infusion. Redness, soreness, and swelling at the insertion site may indicate that the solution has infiltrated. Note medications added to the intravenous solution or orders.
- Infusion of blood products or colloid infusion, or if one is ordered. Check the rate of drip, and watch carefully for signs of a reaction.
- Maintenance of the client's comfort and safety. Side rails always must be up. Maintain proper body alignment, and turn the client from side to side if he or she is still unconscious. Offer psychological support.
- Pain. Observe and interview client about pain. Initiate analgesia in consultation with anesthesia personnel or PACU policy.

After completing the assessment, the nurse performs an assessment that relates to the specific surgical procedure. In most health care facilities, the nurse and other PACU staff record their observations on a post-anesthesia recovery assessment form. Finally, the nurse carefully reviews the physician's order sheet for further instructions and medication orders.

ASSESSMENT AND INTERVENTIONS FOR IMMEDIATE POSTOPERATIVE COMPLICATIONS

Nursing intervention during the immediate postoperative period centers on performing interventions to prevent or treat complications. The most common immediate postoperative complications that occur are those related to spinal anesthesia and those affecting respiratory, cardiovascular, and renal systems and those affecting fluid and electrolyte balance.

Complications of Spinal Anesthesia. An important nursing intervention for the client who has received spinal anesthesia is to check the blood pressure, heart rate, and depth of breathing every 10 to 15 minutes during the recovery period. If the blood pressure begins to fall rapidly or if breathing becomes labored, notify the surgeon or anesthesiologist at once so interventions can be started promptly.

Transient hypotension may occur as blood pools in the lower extremities. Elevating the client's feet can quickly reverse this problem. Clients who have undergone spinal anesthesia and who are discharged from the PACU still require monitoring. Watch them for sudden drops in blood pressure and other signs of shock.

Respiratory Complications. Respiratory complications that occur in the PACU are usually due to airway obstruction or hypoventilation. Airway obstruction is caused by mucus or vomitus collecting in the back of the throat, the tongue relaxing to obstruct the airway passage, aspiration, or pre-existing problems such as chronic obstructive pulmonary disease (COPD) or pulmonary edema.

The primary intervention to prevent respiratory complications is ensuring that the airway is patent. All clients receive oxygen. In the immediate postoperative period, the minimally responsive client's head may be turned to the side and the chin extended forward to prevent respiratory obstruction. An oral or nasal airway may be placed to help maintain airway patency and tongue control. It is a hollow rubber or plastic tube, through the nose or mouth, that passes over the base of the tongue and keeps the tongue from falling back and obstructing the anatomic airway (Fig. 19–8). Airways should not be taped in place. As clients awaken and the gag reflex returns, they may spit it out. When the gag reflex has returned, the PACU nurse may remove the airway for the responsive client who is unable to remove it him or herself. Its continued presence could irritate or stimulate vomiting or laryngospasm. The client who is unable to clear mucus or vomitus from the throat requires suctioning immediately.

Some clients are intubated and ventilated. They require close monitoring and suctioning as needed. When the client is extubated, observe for the development of laryngospasms. If the client develops crowing respirations after extubation and is not moving air, he or she is probably experiencing a laryngospasm. If this problem develops, the client could progress to respiratory arrest. The nurse should immediately attempt to ventilate the client using an Ambu bag. If the spasm cannot be broken, the client may require a tracheostomy.

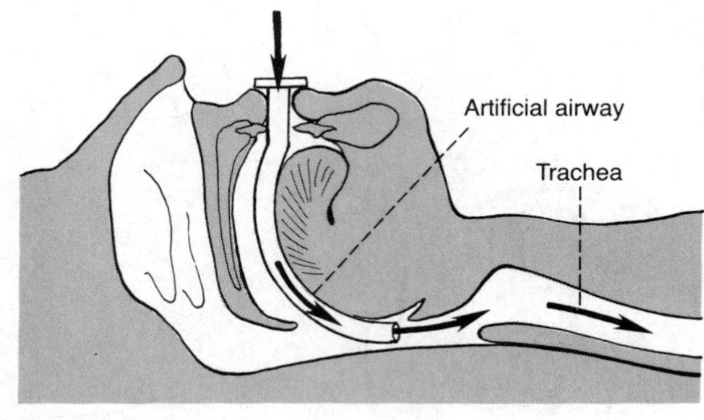

▲ **Figure 19–8**

Artificial airway. The flattened, hollow tube prevents tongue from falling back and occluding natural airway.

Other major respiratory problems include respiratory distress or depression, wheezing, and aspiration. Interventions may include the continued administration of oxygen, positive pressure airway support, or narcotic antagonists. Reversal agents such as naloxone hydrochloride (Narcan), are administered to reverse the narcotic effect or neostigmine with glycopyrrolate (Robinul) to reverse muscle relaxants.

Cardiovascular Complications. Common cardiovascular complications include cardiac arrhythmias, hypertension, and hypotension resulting in shock. When assessing a client for postoperative cardiovascular complications, remember that a slight increase in a client's heart rate after surgery may be normal. However, a significant increase or decrease in the preoperative heart rate or the development of new dysrhythmias requires observation. ASPAN Standards recommend that clients in the PACU should be connected to a cardiac monitor. In this way, diagnosis and treatment can be started immediately.

Causes of postoperative cardiac dysrhythmias include hypovolemia, pain, electrolyte imbalances, hypoxemia, and acidosis. When dysrhythmias develop, the PACU nurse monitors the client's blood pressure, oxygen saturation, and ventilation. When ventilatory status is inadequate, the nurse institutes airway management. The nurse also consults with the surgeon and anesthetist, and intervenes with prescribed medications.

Postoperative hypotension can have numerous causes, including inadequate ventilation, effects of anesthetic agents or preoperative medications, rapid position change, pain, fluid or blood loss, and peripheral pooling of blood after regional anesthesia. A drop in blood pressure slightly below a client's preoperative baseline range is common after surgery. However, a significant drop in blood pressure, accompanied by an increase or decrease in heart rate, may indicate hemorrhage, circulatory failure, or fluid shifts. In addition to hypotension, symptoms of shock include a weakened, thready pulse; cold, moist, pale, or cyanotic skin; and increased restlessness and apprehension.

When a client appears to be going into shock, the PACU nurse (1) applies oxygen or increases the rate of delivery; (2) places the client in Trendelenburg position, if the position is not contraindicated by the surgical procedure, or raises the client's legs above the level of the heart; (3) increases the rate of the intravenous fluids; (4) notifies the anesthesiologist and surgeon; (5) administers medication or additional fluid volume as ordered; and (6) continues assessment on a one-to-one basis.

Clients in PACU also may develop hypertension. Older clients with a history of hypertension may exhibit hypertensive episodes after the stress of surgery. If the blood pressure rises above the baseline, the PACU nurse should consult with the anesthesiologist or surgeon and administer antihypertensive medications as ordered.

Complications Involving Renal Function and Fluid and Electrolyte Balance. Changes in renal function and fluid and electrolyte balances also may develop soon after surgery. Surgery and anesthesia stimulate the secretion of antidiuretic hormone (ADH) and aldosterone, which cause fluid retention. Urine volume decreases regardless of the fluid intake. Fluid and electrolyte maintenance following surgery requires astute nursing assessment and intervention. Avoid fluid overload while maintaining blood pressure, cardiac output, and adequate urinary output. Nursing interventions must include assessment of intake and output, blood pressure, pulse, and serum electrolytes. Any significant changes should be reported to the anesthesiologist or surgeon.

Temperature Alterations. Malignant hyperthermia, as stated, can develop in the operating room or in the PACU. The PACU nurse must assess for the severe muscle contractions and increased temperature (see the section on Malignant Hyperthermia).

Hypothermia is another potential problem in the PACU. The heat loss from operating room can continue in the PACU if the client is not warmed sufficiently. Warming is a delicate balance between maintaining the client's temperature without overwarming and causing excessive vasodilation (which could cause fluid shifts and a decrease in BP). Warm blankets are applied to maintain the client's body temperature.

Pain. Clients must be assessed carefully in PACU for postoperative pain. If the client becomes restless and states they are in pain, they should be medicated. The nurse consults with the anesthesiologist to determine the appropriate medication and dosage for this client. After the client receives a pain medication, many PACUs have a policy requiring them to be closely monitored for another hour or until stable.

Other Complications. Diabetic clients require extra monitoring and care in PACU. The stress of surgery can cause fluctuations in the client's blood sugar. Blood glucose monitoring is conducted in the PACU and, based on the results, intravenous regular insulin may be ordered (see Chap. 61).

Clients who are on steroids also require special care in the PACU. The client should be assessed for the development of addisonian crisis. If the blood pressure drops, the pulse increases, and the client appears to be in shock, a low level of cortisol may be the problem. Intervention is immediate replacement with intravenous hydrocortisone (see Chap. 63).

DISCHARGE FROM THE PACU

Common criteria to evaluate the client's readiness for discharge from the PACU are

- The client has recovered (a criterion score of 10 on the PACU assessment form) from the effects of anesthesia. This requires a stay of about 1 to 2 hours in the PACU.
- The vital signs are stable at the preoperative level.
- There is only moderate or light drainage from any site.
- The physiologic effects of narcotic medication have stabilized. This requires about ½ hour from the time of administration.
- The client has regained a satisfactory level of consciousness and can maintain a patent airway.
- Essential postoperative care has been completed by the PACU personnel.
- Urine output is adequate, at least 30 ml/hour for an adult. The amount must be monitored and recorded.
- Staff on the clinical unit to which the client is to be transferred have been alerted, a report has been given on the client's condition, and the unit is prepared to receive the client.
- Thorough documentation of the client's progress in the PACU is included in the client's permanent medical record.

A client who has undergone ambulatory surgery, in an in-patient or outpatient facility, requires the same level of monitoring and support if general or regional anesthesia was used. After surgery, the client remains in the PACU until fully awake, possibly until the client voids and tolerates oral fluids, and then may be transported to a special area to prepare for discharge.

To prepare for discharge following ambulatory surgery, the client (1) receives complete postoperative written and verbal instructions, (2) knows when and how to seek help for any problems that may arise, and (3) has transportation home with assistance by a competent individual. The next day there will be a follow-up phone call by the staff.

TRANSFER TO THE CLINICAL UNIT

After meeting the PACU discharge criteria, the client can be returned to the appropriate clinical unit to complete recovery. Clients who have experienced complications in the PACU generally may be transferred to the intensive care unit for continued close observation.

Postoperative Nursing on the Clinical Unit

To carry out postoperative care, certain preparations need to be made on the clinical unit. These preparations include the following:

- A clear passageway to the client's bed to ensure easy transfer.
- Clean bed linen, with pads if excessive drainage is anticipated. Keep additional blankets available.
- Necessary equipment that is contingent on the type of surgery, such as an emesis basin, intravenous pole, tissues, suction apparatus, and oxygen administration equipment.

The PACU nurse calls the clinical unit to notify the staff that the client is ready for transfer. The client is transferred to the unit, accompanied by a PACU nurse. The nursing staff helps move the client into bed, ensuring the client's body is in correct alignment and a comfortable position. All tubes and equipment are identified and adjusted appropriately. The PACU nurse gives a verbal report that includes client's history, condition, the operative and PACU course, and any special orders that were initiated or need to be initiated.

The family and significant others should be notified of the client's status. The surgeon usually discusses the surgical procedure and outcome with the client, family, and significant others. Thus, the nurse needs to be aware of the client's condition and of the information given to the client, family, and significant others by the surgeon.

ASSESSMENT ON THE CLINICAL UNIT

The nurse on the unit makes an initial assessment of the client after the transfer. The assessment should include the status of respiratory, cardiovascular, and neurologic systems, and assessment of the surgical wound, intravenous lines, tubes, client position, and level of pain.

Respiratory Status. Assess for a patent airway. Listen for breath sounds and assess their character. Check the quality, depth, and rate of respirations. Remember that skin color and temperature also indicate the degree of oxygen exchange. Pale or dusky skin may signal poor oxygen exchange and the possible recurrence of narcotic effects. Cyanosis is a very late sign of hypoxia.

Cardiovascular Status. Assess vital signs, skin color, temperature, and degree of moistness. Assess for any abnormal pulses.

Neurologic Status. Assess the client's level of consciousness or ability to move extremities, and assess the lingering effects of regional anesthesia.

Surgical Wound. Assess the dressing and any drainage present. The nurse should measure and record the area of drainage to compare later assessments for changes.

Intravenous Lines. The nurse assesses the intravenous line for patency, type of fluid infusing, and rate.

Tubes. The nurse assesses any drainage tubes (e.g., nasogastric tube or chest tube) as to whether to attach it to suction or to use gravity drainage. Note and record the amount of drainage.

Position. Assess the client for proper positioning to promote ventilation and decrease pain.

Pain. The nurse assesses the client for pain. Comfort measures are initiated. The need for pain control through the use of narcotic analgesics is assessed. It is vital that pain be managed if the client is to comply with instructions for coughing, deep breathing, and ambulation.

ESTABLISHMENT OF POSTOPERATIVE GOALS

The client has now entered the next phase of the postoperative course. At this point, a postoperative care plan is developed. This plan should include an assessment of the client's needs and goals as well as nursing interventions. Nursing diagnoses will be used to specify and define postoperative problems and guide the plan of nursing care.

Goal 1: Restore Homeostasis and Prevent Complications. Surgery upsets the body's homeostatic balance, disrupting fluid and electrolyte balance, vital signs, and body temperature. Therefore, nursing care is directed toward restoring the client's normal balance, which, in turn, helps prevent complications.

One of the nurse's primary goals in caring for the postoperative client is to prevent complications after surgery. No matter how seemingly minor the surgery, the danger of postoperative complications is present. Complications have caused death following relatively simple surgeries such as tonsillectomies and hernia repairs.

Postoperative complications can develop (1) directly in the wound, (2) in organs bordering on the operative site or far removed from it, (3) in body cavities, or (4) as a result of the client's medical condition. Complications may arise immediately after surgery or may develop later. Some authorities arbitrarily define a postoperative complication as any untoward event arising within 30 days after surgery. Complications may result directly from the surgical procedure, or may be a consequence of the condition being treated. For example, abdominal surgery may lead to an abdominal-peritoneal abscess, which, in turn, causes intra-abdominal infection. In this instance, the surgery itself resulted in a postoperative complication.

Complications are particularly common after a devastating illness or difficult surgery. These include disorders such as stress ulcer, renal failure, and hepatic failure. Most cardiovascular complications (e.g., cerebrovascular accident, myocardial infarction, pulmonary embolism) and virtually all life-threatening infections (e.g., peritonitis) follow some critical event such as postoperative shock or hemorrhage, or preoperative rupture of an organ.

Preventing postoperative complications promotes rapid convalescence and saves time, expense, worry, pain, and even life itself. Know the symptoms of postoperative complications, and be able to recognize them quickly. Once postoperative problems develop, they are difficult to treat. One complication often leads to others, thereby prolonging morbidity and dependence. For example, the client who develops pneumonia following surgery has limited mobility that may possibly lead to thrombophlebitis, constipation, and further respiratory stasis. With pneumonia, appetite decreases and the client may develop a negative nitrogen balance that, in turn, slows wound healing. Fever and diaphoresis can result in fluid and electrolyte imbalances. Intravenous fluids probably will be ordered, but then this intervention causes additional discomfort, triggers a possible infection, and prolongs immobility. Additionally, these problems cause psychological reactions in the client and significant others.

One of the most common complications following surgery is postoperative shock. Causes include bleeding and hemorrhage (hypovolemic shock), sepsis (septic shock), cardiac arrest and myocardial infarction (cardiogenic shock), drug sensitivity (anaphylactic shock), transfusion reactions, pulmonary embolism, and adrenal failure.

Table 19–14 discusses, in brief, each type of shock, its causes, assessments, and interventions. See Chapter 20 for further information on shock.

Goal 2: Maintain and Promote Adequate Airway and Respiratory Function. Respiratory complications are among the more common complications that may occur in the postoperative period. Early assessment of respiratory problems can lead to immediate treatment.

Symptoms of pulmonary complications include increased temperature, restlessness, dyspnea, tachycar-

TABLE 19–14. Types of Shock

Cause	Assessment	Intervention
Bleeding (hypovolemic shock)	Check wounds, drain sites, open wounds; central venous pressure low; bleeding usually in peritoneal or pleural cavities or retroperitoneal areas	Blood administration and immediate ligation of bleeding vessel by surgeon; measure arterial blood gases
Sepsis (septic shock)	Culture of blood or suspicion of gram-negative bacterial source of septicemia; tachycardia, hypotension, oliguria, fluid retention, respiratory failure	Massive intravenous antibiotics, fluids, corticosteroids may be ordered
Cardiac arrest, myocardial infarction or arrhythmias (cardiogenic shock)	Check for pulse irregularities, electrocardiogram; absence of pulse and cyanosis suggest cardiac arrest; AST aids diagnosis of infarction; central venous pressure is high	Dependent on specific cause; general measures: oxygen; sedation; and cardiopulmonary resuscitation, if needed
Drug sensitivity (anaphylactic shock)	Obscure clinical picture; history of drug sensitivities is vitally important; urticaria and edema may aid diagnosis	Epinephrine, antihistamines, corticosteroids may be ordered; maintain airway, O_2 by mask or prongs, intravenous line, cardiac monitor, reassurance, arrange for ICU bed
Transfusion reaction (contaminated or incompatible blood)	Smears of blood show gram-negative orgaisms; shock rapidly follows blood administration	Discontinue blood; corticosteroids, massive doses of antibiotics intravenously may be ordered
Pulmonary embolism	No specific signs; chest pain, hemoptysis suggest diagnosis; angiography can make diagnosis; obesity, previous cardiac difficulties, cancer, pelvic operations, immobility, and increased age are associated factors	Embolectomy, fibrinolytic agents to dissolve clots are promising and may be ordered. O_2 by mask or prongs, arterial blood gases, ECG, cardiac monitor, pain relief, chest film
Adrenal failure	Must be diagnosed by suspicion or history of steroid therapy, lack of other causes	Intravenous corticosteroids (hydrocortisone) may be ordered

Adapted by permission from Liechty, R. D. 1985 Postoperative care. In R. D. Liechty & R. T. Soper (Eds.), *Synopsis of Surgery*. (5th ed.). St. Louis: C. V. Mosby Co.

ECG, Electrocardiogram.

dia, hemoptysis, pulmonary edema, altered breath sounds, and thick viscous sputum (with chest pain, if the client has pneumonia).

Pulmonary problems typically develop in the first 48 hours after surgery. Postoperative respiratory complications may be caused by one or several of the following factors:

- Pre-existing respiratory infections (colds, flu, and sore throats) that were not resolved during the preoperative period.
- Respiratory infection following surgery.
- Use of anesthetics, endotracheal tubes, and oxygen—all of which irritate the tracheobronchial tree and cause increased mucous secretions.
- Aspiration of vomitus.
- Prolonged immobility of the client on the operating table during lengthy surgery.
- A history of smoking.
- Respiratory disease prior to surgery (e.g., asthma, chronic bronchitis, COPD).
- Depressive effects of many narcotics (especially codeine) on the cough reflex.
- Collapse of the lung during surgery or inadequate reexpansion of lung tissue following surgery.
- Severe postoperative pain, which makes the client reluctant or unable to turn, cough, or breathe deeply.
- Surgery with a high abdominal or chest incision, which causes the client to neglect deep breathing exercises because of pain.
- Extreme debilitation and old age, which lower the client's resistance to pulmonary infections.
- Prolonged postoperative immobility, which leads to decreased chest expansion, pooling of mucus in the bronchi, and hypostatic pneumonia.

The most common postoperative respiratory problems are atelectasis, pneumonia, and pulmonary emboli.

Atelectasis is the most common of these problems. Atelectasis is defined as collapse of the alveoli in sections of a lung. Assessment includes increased pulse, increased temperature, and decreased breath sounds on auscultation. The chest x-ray study verifies areas of consolidation.

Pneumonia is an acute infection causing inflammation of lung tissue. Typical assessment findings include an elevated temperature, tachycardia, tachypnea, productive cough, dyspnea, crackles, and a dullness over area of consolidation.

Pulmonary emboli, either a blood clot or a fat emboli, can occur after any major surgery, especially those involving the abdomen or long bones. It is a potentially fatal complication. It occurs when there is a passage of thrombi into the pulmonary vasculature. Assessment includes severe dyspnea, intense pleural pain, apprehension, fever, and hemoptysis.

Although the etiology of each respiratory complication is different, some basic nursing interventions may prevent these and other pulmonary complications. Rigorous attention to these interventions is essential to prevent respiratory complications. First, provide preoperative instruction regarding moving, coughing, and deep breathing exercises. After surgery, coach the client during the performance of these exercises. Encourage the client to breathe deeply every one to two hours in the manner described earlier. Encourage the client to cough every 1 to 2 hours. Splint the client's incision so coughing will be less painful and less likely to cause the incision to rupture. Check the color and consistency of mucus expectorated following coughing. If a respiratory infection is present, the mucus may be thick, colored, and emit an odor. Adequately hydrate the client. Fluids thin mucous secretions. If the client is receiving intravenous infusions, make certain the infusions drip properly and are administered on time. If the client can tolerate oral fluids, encourage fluid intake.

Assist the client to ambulate as early as possible. Assess the client for respiratory depression and suppression of cough, especially if the client is receiving narcotics (e.g., morphine) for pain. If respirations are depressed, notify the surgeon so a different narcotic can be prescribed. Assess and report symptoms of respiratory infection. If pneumonia develops, nasotracheal suctioning may be necessary to stimulate a cough. Also, antibiotics and antipyretics may be prescribed.

Encourage the client to stop smoking prior to surgery and postoperatively. Encourage the use of an incentive spirometer every 1 to 2 hours after surgery. This device provides physiologically correct exercise that encourages deep, prolonged, voluntary inspiration. It also promotes maximal alveolar inflation, helps restore and maintain lung capacity, and strengthens respiratory muscles (Fig. 19-9). Finally, perform respiratory assessment and chest auscultation as part of routine postoperative care.

Goal 3: Maintain Adequate Cardiac Function and Promote Tissue Perfusion. Any surgical client is at risk of developing cardiac or perfusion problems, but clients at most risk are the elderly and clients with a history of cardiac or peripheral vascular disease. Two common problems that may occur in the postoperative client are thrombophlebitis (and possibly embolism) and myocardial infarction.

Thrombophlebitis usually involves a thrombus of the peripheral veins, usually the calf veins. It develops because of direct pressure on the walls of veins during surgery or from venous stasis.

Postoperative thrombophlebitis generally occurs 7 to 14 days after surgery. Dehydration and inadequate circulation resulting from hemorrhage can result in circulatory stasis and increased blood coagulability, both of which can cause thrombophlebitis. The great danger of thrombophlebitis is that a clot will break loose from the vein wall and travel as an embolus to the client's lungs, heart, or brain.

Symptoms of phlebitis include redness, swelling, and tenderness of the extremity, and the presence of a Homans' sign. Preventive measures for thrombophlebitis include postoperative leg exercises, early ambulation, antiembolic support stockings, adequate hydration, and low-dose heparin.

Myocardial infarction occurs during the first 72 hours after surgery. The nurse must assess high-risk clients—

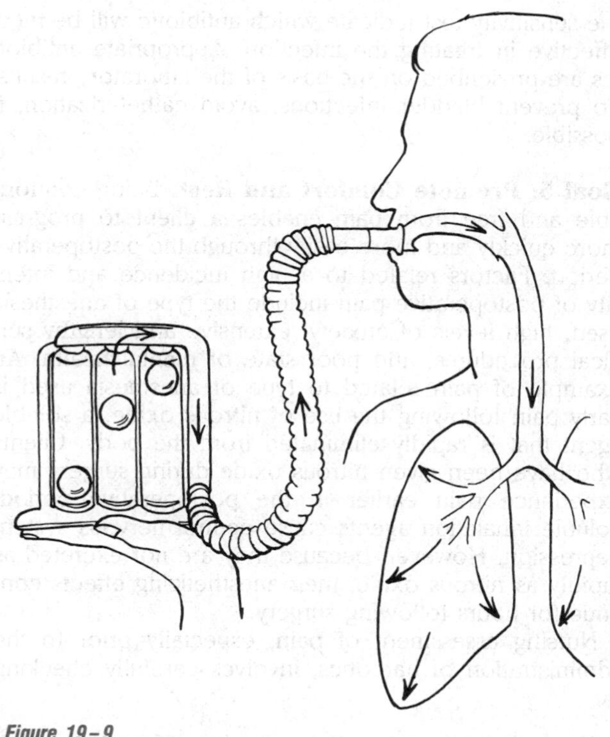

▲ Figure 19-9

Using incentive deep-breathing exerciser to promote alveolar inflation, restore and maintain lung capacity, and strengthen respiratory muscles.

those with a history of dysrhythmias or heart disease, or any client over 70 years of age. Because anesthesia might mask chest pain, the nurse should observe the client for dyspnea, tachycardia, cyanosis, or dysrhythmias. Interventions and nursing care for the client with a myocardial infarct are discussed in depth in Chapter 42.

Another postoperative condition that can occur related to tissue perfusion is blood loss. In the postoperative client, this can be the result of a pre-existing condition, blood loss during the surgery, or a postoperative complication.

Clients who are at high risk of experiencing blood loss postoperatively are those with pre-existing medical conditions, a history of aspirin use, a history of anemia or clotting disorders, and the elderly.

Signs and symptoms of blood loss in the postoperative client include postural hypotension, tachycardia, tachypnea, decreased urine output, cool clammy skin, and decreased level of consciousness. Laboratory data should include hemoglobin, hematocrit, and clotting studies (PT, PTT, and platelet count).

Treatment of blood loss is accomplished with plasma expanders, albumin, large volumes of fluid, salvage of blood with the cell saver, and possibly, transfusion therapy. Whole blood may be used, but packed red blood cells are administered more commonly. Fresh frozen plasma or coagulation factors are used if the client has a coagulation problem. Blood transfusions are covered in detail in Chapter 46. The importance of intelligent nursing care for the client needing transfusion therapy is critical to success in maintaining adequate tissue perfusion.

Goal 4: Maintain Adequate Fluid and Electrolyte Balance and Adequate Renal Function. After surgery, it is crucial to promote adequate fluid and electrolyte intake and output. Postoperative imbalances can lead to retention of metabolic wastes, neurologic and cardiac problems, and problems of overhydration or underhydration.

The goals of postoperative fluid and electrolyte therapy are twofold: (1) to give sufficient fluids to maintain extracellular fluid and blood volume (proper fluid volume ensures adequate blood pressure, cardiac output, and urinary flow); and (2) to prevent fluid overload with resultant congestive heart failure and pulmonary edema.

Normal fluid and electrolyte adjustments during the first 3 to 4 days following surgery include

- Renal retention of water and sodium
- Expansion of extracellular fluid (ECF) in excess of sodium (Na^+) and chloride (Cl^-),
- A transient decrease in ECF Na^+ and Cl^-,
- An increase in potassium (K^+) excretion, and
- A decrease in hematocrit as a result of expansion of ECF.

Normal fluid and electrolyte adjustments during the fifth through seventh days following surgery include

- Diuresis,
- Return of ECF volume to normal,
- Serum Na^+ returns to normal, and
- Reduction of K^+ concentration in urine.

Further information on fluid and electrolyte alterations can be found in Chapter 14.

Principal causes of postoperative dehydration and electrolyte deficits are (1) failure to replace deficits existing before surgery, (2) inadequate replacement of normal postoperative losses, and (3) excessive postoperative losses as a result of sweating, hyperventilation, wound drainage, gastrointestinal tract drainage, diarrhea, diuresis, or vomiting.

Principal causes of fluid overload are the administration of excessive amounts of intravenous fluids and inadequate renal function with low urine output.

Principal causes of respiratory acidosis (many of which cause hypoventilation), are

- Narcotics, some of which reduce respiratory efficiency, especially in the elderly;
- Postoperative pain and bulky, uncomfortable dressings that make clients reluctant to cough and deep breathe;
- Abdominal distention, a common postoperative problem, that crowds the diaphragm and makes breathing deeply difficult;
- Surgery with a high incision involving the diaphragm that reduces ventilation, such as hiatal hernia repair and gallbladder surgery;

- Postoperative complications, such as atelectasis, pneumonia, and bronchitis that cause respiratory obstruction and poor ventilation.

Nursing interventions that prevent fluid and electrolyte imbalances include

- Record intake and output accurately;
- Assess serum electrolyte values and report abnormal findings to the surgeon immediately;
- Obtain an order for an antiemetic (e.g., Compazine) if the client develops nausea and vomiting;
- Irrigate nasogastric suction tubes properly (see Chap. 54);
- Instruct the client to cough and deep breathe deeply to prevent respiratory acidosis;
- Give oral fluids to the client as soon as active peristalsis is present and they can be tolerated.

To help promote and maintain renal function following surgery, encourage fluids when the client is able to tolerate them. Before administering oral or parenteral fluids, check the fluid limits set by the physician. Remember to administer fluids cautiously during the early postoperative period while ADH is being released. 'Forcing' fluids too soon can result in dangerous overhydration.

Adequately record intake and output in the intake and output record for at least 48 hours after surgery. A client with a fluid restriction, or anyone whose intake is being closely monitored, may need close observation for a week or more. Check the physician's order, consult with the physician and nursing staff, and use your own judgement to decide when documentation of fluid intake and output can be discontinued.

The well-hydrated client generally is able to void 6 to 8 hours after surgery. An inability to void after surgery may be caused by anesthesia (especially spinal or epidural), pain, fear, unfamiliar surroundings, or the client's position.

Signs of bladder distention are fullness above the symphysis pubis that can palpated (usually indicating more than 250 ml in the bladder) and voiding 30 to 60 ml of urine every 20 to 30 minutes (indicating retention with overflow).

Possible nursing interventions include

- Running tap water so the client hears it,
- Pouring warm water over the female perineum,
- Assisting the male to sit or stand at the bedside (if not contraindicated),
- Administering prescribed pain medication, and
- Inserting a straight or indwelling catheter, as ordered.

Catheterization is the most common cause of postoperative urinary tract infection. Symptoms of urinary tract infection generally occur between the third to fifth day after catheterization and include dysuria, frequency, and fever.

Intervention for urinary tract infections involves first sending a specimen of the urine to the laboratory for culture and sensitivity testing. The culture results indicate the organism causing the infection. The results of the sensitivity test indicate which antibiotic will be most effective in treating the infection. Appropriate antibiotics are prescribed on the basis of the laboratory results. To prevent bladder infections, avoid catheterization, if possible.

Goal 5: Promote Comfort and Rest. Being comfortable and free from pain enables a client to progress more quickly and more easily through the postoperative period. Factors related to a high incidence and intensity of postoperative pain include the type of anesthesia used, high levels of anxiety, extensive and lengthy surgical procedures, and poor state of mental health. An example of pain related to type of anesthesia used is early pain following the use of nitrous oxide, a soluble agent that is rapidly eliminated from the body. Clients who have been given nitrous oxide during surgery may experience pain earlier in the postoperative period. Soluble inhalation agents cause central nervous system depression. However, because they are not excreted as rapidly as nitrous oxide, their anesthetizing effects continue for hours following surgery.

Nursing assessment of pain, especially prior to the administration of narcotics, involves carefully checking for

- Hypotension or hypertension, although pain can either cause an increase or decrease in blood pressure.
- Pressure points beneath a cast or splint. Relieving pressure by splitting the cast or cutting a window (usually done by a physician) may decrease pain.
- Distended bladder. Obtain an order for catheterization if the client is unable to void.
- Abdominal distention and flatulence. A rectal suppository may decrease gas pain. Flatus is a common postoperative problem, that is often alleviated by ambulation.

Nursing measures that help alleviate pain include

- Comfort measures, such as changing the client's position, straightening bed linen, giving a back rub with lotion, and applying a cool cloth to the hands and face.
- Administration of narcotics, such as morphine, meperidine, and codeine. Narcotics are used primarily during the first 24 to 72 hours after surgery to relieve pain.

A newer option is the use of PCA, which allows the client to self-administer postoperative analgesia (often morphine, meperidine, or fentanyl). Note in Figure 19–10 that the PCA system is basically a pump that can be programmed to deliver a precise dose of analgesic when the client pushes the control button. A system also can be set up that delivers a continuous dose with the client able to trigger an increase in the dosage as needed. An indwelling intravenous line carries the analgesic into the client's circulatory system.

The PCA system has the following advantages:

- Clients, who are the experts on their own pain, can monitor and meet their own analgesia needs.

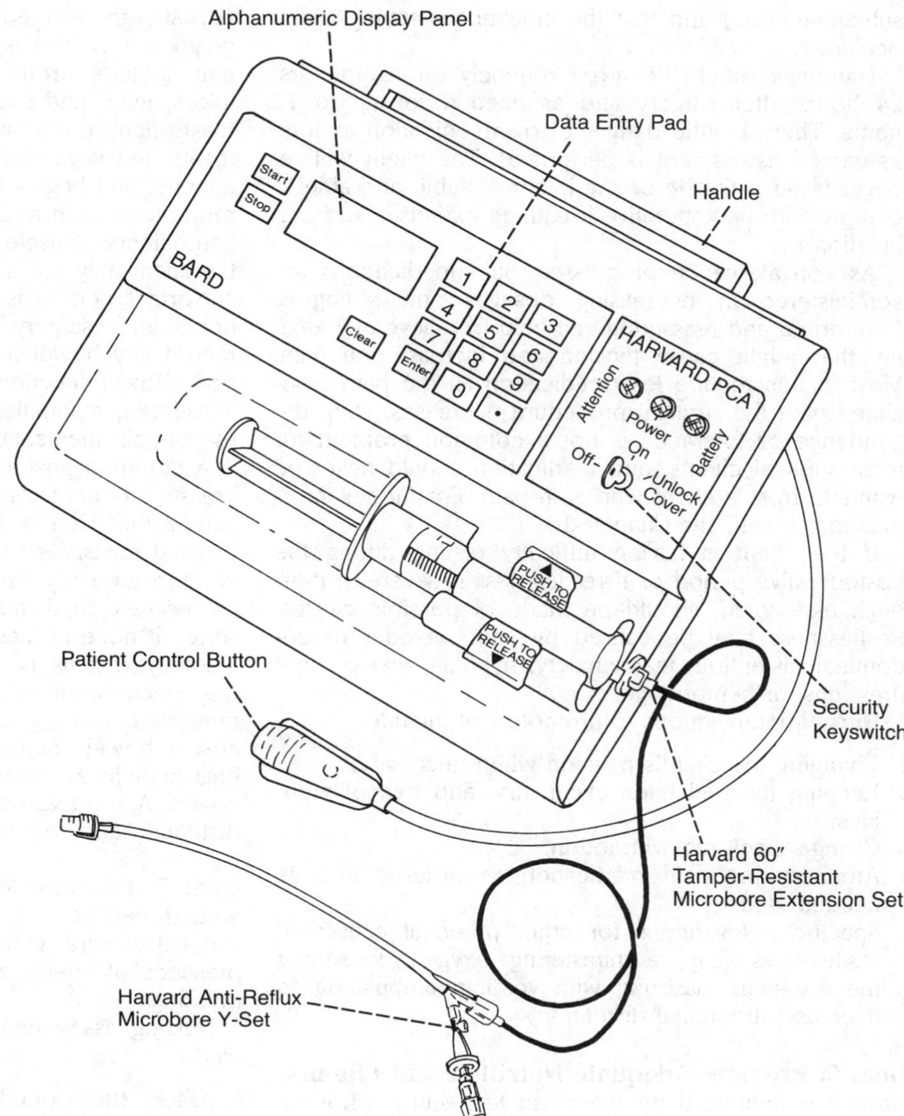

▲ **Figure 19–10**

A PCA device allows individuals to control their own pain relief postoperatively. (Courtesy of Bard Electro Medical Systems, Inc., Englewood, CO.)

- PCA allows a constant blood level of analgesic, in contrast to an intramuscular injection, which delivers a bolus of pain medication that tapers off over hours.
- Clients can self-administer small amounts of analgesia, sparing them the difficult cycles of escalating pain and heavy sedation.

The pump is provided with safety features to prevent overdosing. An average setting for a PCA device is 1 mg morphine administered not more often than every 6 minutes; however, the setting for each client is based on the client's pain, body size, surgery, and physician choice. With one set-up, the client must push the button to receive medication; there is no automatic administration. With another set-up, the client receives a steady dosage that the client can augment as needed. After receiving a dose of medication, there is a pre-set time (e.g., 6 minutes), during which the machine will not deliver more medication. Contrary to what some health care providers expect, postoperative clients do not overmedicate themselves. Most clients balance between pain relief and sedation. Studies have shown that clients using PCA (1) use less medication, (2) are able to ambulate earlier, and (3) recover pulmonary function sooner, as a result of increased activity levels.

On most PCA devices, the following settings can be programmed: (1) flow rate (dosage), (2) flow type (continuous or intermittent), (3) number of milligrams per dose, and (4) time required between injections. In addition, the device records (1) the number of injection attempts, (2) the number of injections actually given, (3) a low battery, (4) an error in the system set-up, (5) little or no remaining infusion, (6) an unauthorized entry to the system, and (7) an occlusion or excessive pressure in the line.

Assessing intravenous catheter patency during PCA is the nurse's responsibility. Ensure that the intravenous line remains patent (so the analgesic is not deposited subcutaneously) and that the intravenous tubing is not occluded.

Narcotics should be given routinely during the first 24 hours after surgery and as needed for up to 72 hours. There is little danger of overmedication as long as careful assessment is performed. The client will recover faster if the he or she is comfortable and able to comply with postoperative breathing exercises and ambulation.

As convalescence progresses, pain medications are administered in decreasing dosages and strengths. Comforting and reassuring can help to relieve any anxiety that might cause tension and increase the pain. Most clients require less medication as the pain associated with the surgical procedure decreases. Drug dependence or tolerance is not a common problem for most surgical clients, and medication should never be withheld from a client who is in pain. For further information on pain, see Chapter 16.

If the client is having difficulty resting during the postoperative period or if restlessness is severe, a thorough assessment should be made of possible causes. Restlessness may be caused by pain, bladder or abdominal distention, fear, anxiety, hypoxia, wet or tight dressings, or hemorrhage.

Nursing interventions to promote rest include

- Changing the client's position when necessary;
- Keeping the bed linen clean, dry, and free of wrinkles;
- Giving a back rub with lotion;
- Administering pain medication as ordered and as needed; and
- Specific interventions for other potential causes of restlessness (e.g., administering oxygen, loosening the dressings, assisting with voiding, ambulating to decrease abdominal distention).

Goal 6: Promote Adequate Nutrition and Elimination. It is beneficial for the client to resume a normal diet as soon as possible after surgery. A normal diet promotes an early return of gastrointestinal function, aids in wound healing, and is psychologically healthy for the client.

Nursing assessments to be made prior to feeding a client postoperatively are the presence of positive bowel sounds and that the abdomen is soft and palpable.

Certain surgical procedures (e.g., abdominal exploration and cholecystectomy) may require that the client abstain from oral fluids and food until the bowel sounds return, usually within about 24 to 48 hours after surgery. Clients who are unable to eat for longer periods (after gastric or bowel resection) may have a nasogastric tube in place, which, because of its decompressive properties, removes flatus and stomach secretions. Clients who are allowed nothing by mouth for a prolonged period after surgery usually receive nutritional support with hyperalimentation.

For the first 24 to 36 hours following surgery, many clients are nauseated and have episodes of vomiting. Antiemetics may be ordered for the nausea. If nausea persists, the surgeon should be notified. The initial postoperative diet is usually clear liquids. These liquids may include broth, tea with lemon and sugar, fruit juices, jello, and soups. Early solid foods may include toast, light cornstarch puddings, and easily digested meats and vegetables. As the client regains his or her appetite and begins to eat well, a full diet is ordered to promote vitamin and mineral balance and proper nitrogen balance. Muscle substance and strength return, and the client may regain weight slightly.

Normal peristalsis returns during the first 48 to 72 hours after surgery. It is important for the nurse to record any bowel movements in the postoperative period. Bowel function can be impaired by immobility, anesthesia, manipulation of abdominal organs, and the use of pain medications.

A common postoperative discomfort related to a decrease in peristalsis is abdominal distention. This causes the client a feeling of fullness and discomfort. Nursing measures to prevent and treat abdominal discomfort are early ambulation, adequate fluid intake and an increase in dietary fiber. A rectal tube may be inserted if none of these interventions work.

Paralytic ileus is a postoperative complication that may occur when a portion of the bowel stops normal peristalsis. Nursing assessment includes diminished or absent bowel sounds, abdominal distention, and feelings of fullness. X-ray studies often reveal a distended bowel. A nasogastric tube may be inserted to prevent distention and vomiting until bowel function resumes.

Goal 7: Promote Wound Healing. Factors affecting wound healing are location of the incision, type of surgical closure, nutritional status, presence of disease, presence of infection, and the presence of drains and dressings.

Nursing assessments to promote wound healing include

- Assess the wound for signs of infection, such as redness, drainage, odor, pain, and induration;
- Observe the wound for edema, bleeding, and color;
- Observe the wound for approximation of the suture line; and
- Monitor drains, and assess the color, consistency, and amount of drainage.

Maintaining strict asepsis during surgery and the postoperative period is the single most important factor in promoting wound healing.

Wound infections are often evident within 36 to 48 hours postoperatively, although most symptoms appear about 5 to 7 days after surgery. Important factors that predispose a client to develop wound infections are

- *Obesity.* Adipose tissue is difficult for the surgeon to approximate and suture, and it does not heal readily.
- *Debilitation.* Clients debilitated by cancer, malnutrition, or ulcerative colitis have a lowered resistance to infections.
- *Advanced age.* Elderly clients, particularly those with arteriosclerosis and poor circulation, have lowered defenses against infection.

- *Lengthy, complicated operations.* Complex operations are stressful and lower resistance. The longer the client is in surgery, the longer the tissues are exposed, making them more susceptible to infection.
- *Therapy with steroids, irradiation, and anticancer medications.* Certain medications and treatments affect the immune system and reduce the body's leukocyte counts dramatically.
- *The presence of other diseases.* Hypogammaglobinemia, diabetes mellitus, obstructive jaundice, ulcerative colitis, uremia, leukemia, aplastic anemia, and malignant neoplasms, in particular, lowers resistance to wound infection.
- *Failure to maintain asepsis* in the operating room or during wound dressing changes
- *Preoperative organ rupture or sepsis,* such as occurs with a ruptured appendix, perforated ulcer, or abscess drainage. When the organ is also infected prior to surgery, the wound is usually considered contaminated and infected.

Studies show that the general attitude of the staff toward controlling infection is an important factor in maintaining infection control. Health care personnel are sometimes careless in aseptic technique because they fail to recognize the importance of asepsis. Inservice education that concentrates on the principles of asepsis is one important way to prevent wound infections.

The organism most commonly responsible for wound infections is methicillin-resistant *Staphylococcus aureus* (MRSA), a gram-positive, nonmotile organism. Staphylococci produce a golden-yellow pus. These organisms can be transmitted to the surgical wound from contaminated wound-dressing equipment or from staff who harbor the organism in their noses and throats as resident flora.

Clients with infected surgical wounds must be isolated from clients with clean wounds in order to stem the transmission of infections. Other organisms frequently responsible for wound infections are *Escherichia coli, Proteus vulgaris, Aerobacter aerogenes,* and *Pseudomonas aeruginosa.* Infectious diseases are covered in more detail in Chapter 25.

Wound dehiscence and evisceration are possible complications of improper wound healing. Wound dehiscence is an opening of the wound edges (Fig. 19–11). Wound evisceration is the protrusion of internal organs (such as loops of bowel) through the incision (Fig. 19–11). Malnourished, chronically ill, or obese clients are most prone to wound dehiscence and evisceration. Related causal factors are wound infection, faulty closure of the wound in surgery, and severe stretching of the abdominal wall as a result of coughing and vomiting.

Although wound dehiscence or evisceration can occur at any time, they generally develop on the sixth to seventh day after surgery. At this time, the client's incision is weakest because the sutures may have been removed, wound infection is likely to be present, and pulmonary complications may cause excessive pressure when the client coughs. Preventing wound dehiscence and evisceration includes splinting the wound during vigorous coughing or movement, preventing wound infection, and providing adequate nutrition and hydration. Obese or debilitated clients can wear a binder to increase the support to the suture line. Any wound can rupture. However, midline abdominal incisions are the most prone to dehiscence and evisceration.

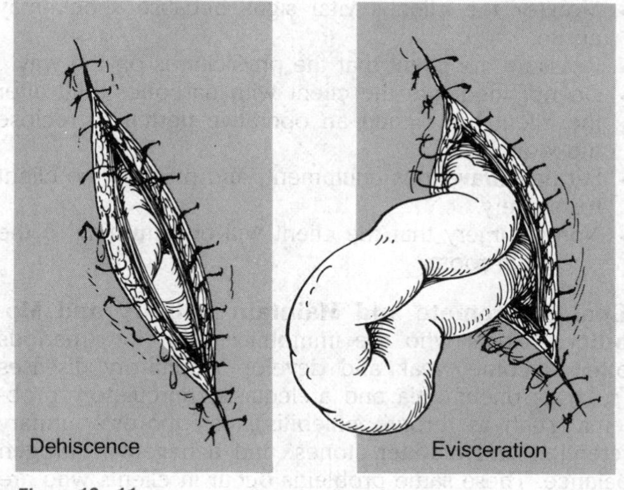

▲ **Figure 19–11**

Wound dehiscence and evisceration require immediate attention. Have someone notify the surgeon. Using sterile technique, cover the wound site with gauze or a sterile towel moistened in sterile saline. Take measures to prevent shock (see text). Do not leave the person's side.

When an abdominal wound ruptures suddenly, evisceration may occur because coils of intestine protrude from the incision. When the wound edges part slowly, a gush of pinkish serous drainage is usually the major sign of dehiscence. The client feels something give way. In any postoperative client, sudden, profuse, pink, serous drainage from the wound is an ominous sign and must be investigated immediately!

Intervention for wound dehiscence and evisceration involves immediate closure of the wound under general or local anesthesia. The nurse's role in the event of wound dehiscence and evisceration includes the following:

- Remain calm.
- Place the client in bed in semi-Fowler's position with the knees slightly gatched. If the wound has not completely opened or has not eviscerated, this position may prevent further tear.
- Ring the emergency bell, pull on the call light, or use the phone to tell the hospital operator to notify the nurse's station on your floor to send help immediately.
- Have another nurse notify the surgeon while you remain with the client.
- Cover any protruding coils of intestine with sterile dressings moistened with sterile normal saline; if sterile supplies are not available, use clean towels or dressings.
- Moisten the towels and dressings frequently with sterile normal saline.

- Monitor the client's vital signs because shock may ensue.
- Reassure the client that the physician is on the way.
- Do not medicate the client with narcotics until after the client has signed an operative permit to reclose the wound.
- Set up intravenous equipment, and prepare the client for surgery.
- Notify surgery that the client will be returning to the operating room.

Goal 8: Promote and Maintain Activity and Mobility. Clients who are immobilized for long periods often become weak and develop respiratory diseases (such as pneumonia and atelectasis), circulatory problems (such as thrombophlebitis), osteoporosis, urinary retention and bladder stones, and a negative nitrogen balance. These same problems occur in clients who are immobilized after surgery.

After surgery, complications from immobility may be prevented by encouraging the client to (1) move around in bed, (2) cough and deep breathe, and (3) flex the ankles and legs. Allow the client to assume personal care as soon as possible to promote early movement. Encourage and assist with ambulation, if it is not contraindicated by the physician. Remember that clients vary. Some clients are ready to move or walk about more quickly than others. Allowing the client to return to physical activity as soon as possible after surgery can hasten recovery, shorten his or her hospital stay, and decrease the client's expenses.

Goal 9: Provide Adequate Emotional Support and Foster Positive Body Image. Surgery has different meanings and implications for each client. Recognize these differences and individualize your psychological approach to each client and significant others as they progress through the surgical experience. The degree of psychological support the client needs depends on the client's social support as well as the type of surgery performed. A client whose postoperative course is complicated needs much more psychological support than the client who recovers quickly.

Maladaptive coping behavior may occur in response to a loss or change associated with surgery. Surgical incisions can alter a client's body image. Some surgeries that are at high risk to cause a change in a client's body image are surgeries of the face, head, neck, breast, or gynecologic or genitourinary system. The onset of problems with coping with these changes may occur in the immediate or extended postoperative stage.

Assessment may reveal passivity, depression, reduced involvement in self-care, sleep disturbances, increased pain and use of analgesics, and hyperactivity. The client also may experience the onset of stress-related symptoms, such as gastrointestinal dysfunction and cardiovascular problems.

Nursing intervention primarily involves providing psychological support. Draw the client and significant others into discussions of anticipated changes and about how they feel these postoperative changes will affect their lives. Encourage the expression of feelings. Provide empathetic listening. Reassure these clients that the grieving process they are going through is normal and that it will pass with time. Arrange support groups and community referrals for the client and significant others.

Goal 10: Plan for Discharge. Discharge planning and teaching should begin at the time of the client's admission to the hospital. Most clients are discharged within 5 to 7 days after major surgery and sometimes even sooner. Early discharge planning is a necessity.

Specific instructions that the client needs to receive prior to discharge should include

Wound care (signs of infection),
Activity restrictions,
Dietary instructions,
Postoperative medication instruction,
Personal hygiene,
Follow-up appointment with surgeon or clinic.

Because of the anxiety associated with discharge, written instructions should be given to the client and family or significant others for reference.

The type of planning and instruction required varies with each individual and type of surgery. Discharge teaching instructions need to be clear, and they must reinforce the material the client learned during the preoperative period and recovery. Teaching plans and the client's understanding need to be included in their care plan and documented in their chart.

Finally, know the quality of the client's support systems, because you may need to involve community resources for follow-up care. Contacting community resources such as mental health facilities and home health agencies helps to ensure continuity of care.

Summary

The nurse plays a critical role in the postoperative care of the client. Today, surgery ranges from outpatient procedures to complex inpatient procedures. No matter what type of surgery is performed, however, the client needs a great deal of expert nursing care. The quality of that nursing care can determine whether or not the client has a successful perioperative experience.

Bibliography

1. Alexander, J. W. (1983). The influence of hair-removal methods on wound infection. *Archives of Surgery, 118,* 347.
2. Alverson, E. (1987). The preoperative interview: Its effect on perioperative nursing empathy. *AORN Journal, 45,* 1150–1159, 1162–1164.
3. American Society of Postanesthesia Nurses (1986). *Standards of nursing practice.* Richmond, VA: Author.
4. Andrews, D. R., & Taylor, C. (1985). Documenting postanesthesia recovery. *American Journal of Nursing, 85,* 290–291.
5. Applegeet, C. J. (1987). Nursing aspects of outpatient surgery. *Urologic Clinics of North America, 14*(1), 21.
6. Ashby, D. M. (1987). Balancing fluids and electrolytes in the PACU. *Journal of Post Anesthesia Nursing, 2,* 114–116.

7. Association of Operating Room Nurses (1988). *Standards of Nursing Practice*. Denver: Author.
8. Atkinson, L. J., & Kohn, M. L. *Berry and Kohn's introduction to operating room techniques*. New York: McGraw-Hill.
9. Baida, M. R. (1978). Nursing care in use of local anesthesia. *AORN Journal, 28,* 855-858.
10. Bailes, B. K. (1989). Perioperative nursing research, part IV: Intraoperative phase. *AORN Journal, 49,* 1397-1409.
11. Barrett, J. E. (1985). Helping your postoperative patient breathe easier with incentive spirometry. *Nursing '85, 15*(10), 64.
12. Birdsall, C., et al. (1988). How is autotransfusion done? *American Journal of Nursing, 88,* 108-111.
13. Blackwood, S. (1986). Back to basics: The preop exam. *American Journal of Nursing, 86,* 39-44.
14. Boucher, B. A. (1986). The postoperative adverse effects of inhalation anesthetics. *Heart and Lung, 15,* 590-608.
15. Bray, C. A. (1986). Postop pain: Altering the patients experience through education. *AORN Journal, 43,* 672, 674-675, 677.
16. Brent, N. (November/December, 1987). How informed are you about consents? *Nursing Life, 6,* 37-39.
17. Burden, N., & Iyer, J. (1987). Local anesthesia: Not always benign. *Journal of Post Anesthesia Nursing, 2,* 45-50.
18. Burge, S. (1986). How painful are postop incisions? *American Journal of Nursing, 86,* 1263A, 1266D, 1266H.
19. Chitwood, L. B. (1987). Unveiling the mysteries of anesthesia. *Nursing '87, 17*(2), 52-55.
20. Cramer, C., & Ring, V. (1987). Preoperative care unit: An alternative to the holding room. *AORN Journal, 46,* 464-472.
21. Crawford, F. J. (1985). Ambulatory surgery: The elderly patient. *AORN Journal, 41,* 3566-3569.
22. Curtin, L. (1984). Ambulatory surgery: Organization, finance, and regulation. *Nursing Management, 15,* 22-24.
23. Cuzzell, J. Z. (1988). The new RYB color code. *American Journal of Nursing, 88,* 1342-1346.
24. Davis, N. B. (1987). Suturing techniques and material. In Rothrock, J. C. (Ed.). *The RN first assistant*. Philadelphia: J. B. Lippincott.
25. Devine, E. C., & Cook, T. D. (1986). Clinical and cost-saving effects of psychoeducational interventions with surgical patients: A meta-analysis. *Research in Nursing and Health, 9*(2), 89-96.
26. Drain, C. B., & Christoph, S. S. (1987). *The recovery room: A critical care approach to post anesthesia nursing (2nd ed.)*. Philadelphia: W. B. Saunders.
27. Dripps, R. D., et al. (1988). *Introduction to anesthesia (7th ed.)*. Philadelphia: W. B. Saunders.
28. Erbostoesser, M. (1989). Care of the patient with malignant hyperthermia. *Journal of Post Anesthesia Nursing, 3,* 71-74.
29. Faherty, B. S., & Grier, M. R. (1982). Analgesic medication for elderly people post surgery. *Nursing Research, 33,* 369-372.
30. Fay, M. F. (1987). Drainage systems: Their role in wound healing. *AORN Journal, 46,* 442-455.
31. Feldman, M. E. (1988). Inadvertent hypothermia: A threat to homeostasis in the postanesthetic patient. *Journal of Post Anesthesia Nursing, 3,* 82-87.
32. Felver, L., & Pendarvis, J. H. (1989). Electrolyte imbalances: Intraoperative risk factors. *AORN Journal, 49,* 992-1008.
33. Foster, C. G. (1979). Effects of surgical positioning. *AORN Journal, 30,* 219-232.
34. Fraulini, K. E., & Borchardt, A. C. (1988). Guide to solving postanesthesia problems. *Nursing '88, 18*(5), 66-86.
35. Fraulini, K. E., & Gorski, D. N. (1983). Don't let perioperative medications put you in a spin. *Nursing '83, 13,* 26-30.
36. Frost, E. A. M. (1985). *Recovery room practice*. Boston: Blackwell Scientific.
37. Gibson, J. R., et al. (1985). Geriatric anesthesia: Minimizing the risk. *Geriatric Clinics of North America, 1,* 313-320.
38. Girard, N. J., et al. (1988). Autologous salvage of blood: Perioperative nursing considerations. *AORN Journal, 47,* 492-502.
39. Goulart, D. (1987). Preoperative teaching for surgical patients. *Perioperative Nursing Quarterly, 3*(2), 8-13.
40. Groah, L. K. (1983). *Operating room nursing: The perioperative role*. Reston, VA: Reston Publishing.
41. Gruendenemann, B. J., & Meeker, M. H. (1987). *Alexander's care of the patient in surgery*. St. Louis: C. V. Mosby Co.
42. Hardy, E. B., et al. (1988). Rewarming patients in the PACU: Can we make a difference? *Journal of Post Anesthesia Nursing, 3,* 313-316.
43. Hardy, J. D. (1988). *Hardy's textbook of surgery (2nd ed.)*. Philadelphia: J. B. Lippincott.
44. Hill, G. J. (1988). *Outpatient surgery (3rd ed.)*. Philadelphia: W. B. Saunders.
45. Hogan, P., & Bells, S. (1986). How to handle postanesthetic hypertension. *Nursing '86, 16*(5), 58-63.
46. In style: Staples, clips, zippers. (1983). *Nursing Life, 3*(12), 4.
47. Iscenheur, M. L. (1988). Quality of interpersonal care: A study of ambulatory surgery patient's perspective. *AORN Journal, 47,* 1414-1419.
48. Isreal, S. J., & De Kornfeld, T. J. (1987). *Recovery room care (2nd ed.)*. Chicago: Year Book Medical Publishers.
49. Ivey, D. F. (1987). Local anesthesia: Implications for the perioperative nurse. *AORN Journal, 45,* 682-689.
50. Jackson, M. F. (1989). High risk surgical patients. *Journal of Gerontological Nursing, 14,* 8-15.
51. Kempe, A. R. (1987). Patient education for the ambulatory surgical patient. *AORN Journal, 45,* 500-507.
52. Kneedler, J. A., & Dodge, G. H. (1987). *Perioperative patient care (2nd ed.)*. Boston: Blackwell Scientific Publications.
53. Kneedler, J. A., & Purcell, S. K. (1989). Perioperative nursing research, part II: Intraoperative chemical and physical hazards to personnel. *AORN Journal, 49,* 829-854.
54. Kneedler, J. A., & Purcell, S. K. (1989). Perioperative nursing research, part III: Potential intraoperative biological hazards to personnel. *AORN Journal, 49,* 1066-1079.
55. Kuhn, M. (1990). *Pharmacotherapeutics: A nursing process approach*. Philadelphia: F. A. Davis.
56. Latz, P. A., & Wyble, S. J. (1987). Elderly patients: Perioperative nursing implications. *AORN Journal, 46,* 238-253.
57. Leyder, B. L., & Piper, B. (1986). Identifying discharge concerns: A study. *AORN Journal, 43,* 1298-1302.
58. Lindeman, C. A. (1988). Patient education. *Annual Review of Nursing Research, 6,* 29-60.
59. Litwak, K., & Parnass, S. (1988). Practical points in the management of postoperative nausea and vomiting. *Journal of Post Anesthesia Nursing, 3,* 275-277.
60. Mattison, M., & McConnell, E. A. (1988). *Gerontologic nursing: Concepts and practice*. Philadelphia: W. B. Saunders.
61. McCaffery, M. (1985). Narcotic analgesia for the elderly. *American Journal of Nursing, 85,* 296-298.
62. McConnell, E. A. (1987). *Clinical considerations in perioperative nursing*. Philadelphia: J. B. Lippincott.
63. Montanari, J. (1986). Action STAT! Wound dehiscence. *Nursing '86, 16*(2), 33.
64. Mortensen, M., & McMullen, C. (1986). Discharge score for surgical outpatient. *American Journal of Nursing, 86,* 1347-1349.
65. Matassarin-Jacobs, E. (Ed.) (1990). *Saunders review for NCLEX-RN*. Philadelphia: W. B. Saunders.
66. Neuberger, G. B. (1987). Wound care: What's clear, what's not. *Nursing '87, 17*(2), 34-37.
67. Norheim, C. (1986). Spinal anesthesia: As bad as it sounds? *Nursing '86, 16*(4), 42-44.
68. Nyamathi, A., & Kashiwabara, A. (1988). Preoperative anxiety: Its effects on cognitive thinking. *AORN Journal, 47,* 164-170.
69. Pierce, S. F., & Campbell, M. (1988). Return of bladder function: A research study. *AORN Journal, 47,* 702-703, 706-712.
70. Poland, V. (1985). Ambulatory surgery: Freestanding centers look beyond the early years. *AORN Journal, 42,* 105-108.
71. Rothrock, J. C. (1989). Perioperative nursing research. Part I. Preoperative psychoeducational interventions. *AORN Journal, 49,* 597-614.
72. Sabiston, D. C., Jr. (1991). *Textbook of surgery: The biological basis of modern surgical practice*. Philadelphia: W. B. Saunders.
73. Schwartz, S. I. (1984). *Principles of surgery (4th ed.)*. New York: McGraw-Hill.
74. Silo, H. M. S. (1989). Perioperative nursing research, part V: Intraoperative recommended practices. *AORN Journal, 49,* 1627-1635.
75. Spearing, C., & Cornell, D. J. (1988). Incentive spirometry: Inspiring your patients to breathe deeply. *Nursing '88, 17*(9), 50-51.
76. Stroud, M. D. (1986). Assessing the elderly PACU patient. *Journal of Post Anesthesia Nursing, 1,* 107-111.

77. Sullivan, D. (1985). Complications from intraoperative positioning. *Orthopaedic Nursing, 4*(4), 56–59.
78. Taylor, D. L. (1988). The healing process: From the inside out. *Nursing '88, 18*(6), 36–67.
79. Taylor, T. H., & Major, E. (Eds.). (1987). *Hazards and complications of anaesthesia.* New York: Churchill-Livingstone.
80. Walker, M. L. (1986). Growing old: Increased surgical risks in the elderly. *AORN Journal, 43,* 887–890.
81. Wetchler, B. V. (1985). Postanesthesia scoring system: Discharging ambulatory surgery patients. *AORN Journal, 41,* 382–384.
82. Williams, B., & Baer, C. (1990). *Essentials of clinical pharmacology.* Springhouse, PA: Springhouse Corporation.
83. Wolcott, M. W. (1988). *Ambulatory surgery and the basics of surgical care (2nd ed.).* Philadelphia: J. B. Lippincott.
84. Worley, B. (1986). Pre-admission testing and teaching: More satisfaction. *Nurse Manager, 17*(2), 32–33.
85. Young, M. E. (1987). Fever in the postoperative patient. *Focus on Critical Care, 14*(2), 13–18.
86. Young, M. E. (1988). Malnutrition and wound healing. *Heart and Lung, 17*(1), 60–65.

Shock

Shock is a complex clinical problem occurring all around us in homes and health care facilities and on streets. Unfortunately, shock sometimes occurs when it could and should have been prevented.

Shock is an emergency often requiring team action by many health care providers, including nurses, physicians, laboratory technicians, pharmacists, and respiratory therapists. It is a life-threatening condition associated with generalized circulatory inadequacy.

Shock causes thousands of deaths and unknown numbers of permanent injuries each year. Because shock is potentially lethal, it is essential that nurses be able to identify clients at risk for developing shock, recognize the early assessment findings indicating shock, and initiate prescribed therapy before shock ensues.

Identifying accurate, individualized interventions is paramount to the nursing process and to appropriate care of the client in shock. Nursing diagnoses that are common for the client in shock include Tissue Perfusion, High Risk and Fluid Volume Deficit.

This chapter discusses three major classifications of shock: hypovolemic, cardiogenic, and distributive. Various etiologic factors related to each classification are also addressed. Included in the discussion are the pathophysiologic mechanism of shock, its complications, and its medical and nursing management.

DEFINITION

Much confusion exists about definitions and classifications of shock. Shock is defined as inadequate tissue perfusion. Inadequate tissue perfusion can be caused by various disorders that result in decreased oxygenation at the cellular level. This inadequate oxygenation leads to an abnormal physiologic state in which there is inadequate cellular metabolism and accumulated waste products in cells. If the condition is untreated, cell and organ death occurs.

INCIDENCE

The incidence of occurrence among the various forms of shock differs widely. Hypovolemic shock occurs most commonly and develops when the intravascular volume decreases to the point that compensatory mechanisms are unable to maintain adequate tissue perfusion and normal cellular function.

Cardiogenic shock occurs in 15 to 20 per cent of all clients following myocardial infarction (MI) (heart attack) and has at least an 80 per cent mortality rate. Cardiogenic shock occurring after an MI usually happens when 40 per cent or more of the myocardium has been damaged.

Some amount of neurogenic shock is seen with all spinal cord injuries. The more dramatic cases of neurogenic shock are seen with cervical spine injuries. The duration of neurogenic shock is usually 1 to 6 weeks, provided there has been no irreparable cord injury.

The incidence of occurrence for both septic and anaphylactic shock is variable. Clients who are at risk for either type of shock should be monitored closely.

ETIOLOGY

Shock is commonly discussed in three major categories: hypovolemic, cardiogenic, and distributive. The major causes of each type are listed here and discussed in the following sections.

- **Hypovolemic shock** is due to inadequate circulating blood volume resulting from hemorrhage with actual blood loss, burns with a loss of plasma proteins and fluid shift, or dehydration with a loss of fluid volume.
- **Cardiogenic shock** is due to inadequate pumping action of the heart because of primary cardiac muscle dysfunction or mechanical obstruction of blood flow caused by myocardial infarction, valvular insufficiency due to disease or trauma, cardiac dysrhythmias, or an obstructive condition, such as pericardial tamponade or pulmonary embolus.
- **Distributive shock** is due to changes in blood vessel tone that increase the size of the vascular space without an increase in the circulating blood volume. This results in a relative hypovolemia (total fluid volume remains the same but is redistributed). Distributive shock is further divided into three types: anaphylactic shock, a severe hypersensitivity reaction resulting in massive systemic vasodilation; neurogenic shock, interference with nervous system control of the blood vessels, such as with spinal cord injury, spinal anesthesia, or severe vasovagal reactions due to pain or psychic trauma; and septic shock, due to a release of vasoactive substances.

Hypovolemic Shock

The primary event precipitating hypovolemic shock is a decrease in the circulating blood volume so large that the body's metabolic needs cannot be met. Hypovolemic shock may be due to loss of plasma within the blood or blood itself. Conditions that may cause a reduction in the circulating volume include hemorrhage, burns, and dehydration.

HEMORRHAGE

Hemorrhage is the loss of blood. Hypovolemic shock develops when there is a significant decrease in a client's intravascular blood volume. Assessment findings indicative of hypovolemic shock may begin to appear with a blood volume deficit of 15 to 25 per cent, or about 500 to 1500 ml in an adult with a normal circulating volume. Shock fully develops if a previously healthy client loses about one third of the normal circulating blood volume.

The loss of smaller amounts of blood may cause shock in clients less able to compensate rapidly (e.g., the elderly with decreased vascular tone and impaired cardiac function). The extent to which a client develops shock after blood loss also depends on the length of time over which the blood loss occurs. Clients with slow blood loss over a period of days or weeks tolerate their blood loss better than do those whose blood loss occurs rapidly over minutes or hours. Hypovolemic shock due to trauma is typically due to hemorrhage. The classes of hemorrhage and the associated assessment findings are listed in Table 20-1.

BURNS

Hypovolemic shock due to burns occurs most often in clients with large partial-thickness or full-thickness burns. It is caused primarily by a shift of plasma from the vascular space into the interstitial space or loss through the surface of the burn wound. Also, after a burn injury, there is a shift in the fluid components of the intravascular, interstitial, and intracellular spaces. In addition to these fluid losses or shifts, burned clients may have cardiac dysfunction due to the presence of *myocardial depressant factor (MDF)*. MDF affects the contractility of cardiac muscle by depressing myocardial muscle function. The result is impaired cardiac output, even in the presence of a normal circulating volume. Shock related to burns is discussed in Chapter 71.

Other conditions that may produce fluid shifts similar to those in burns include nephrotic syndrome, severe crush injuries, starvation, and conditions causing plasma fluids to accumulate in the abdominal cavity (e.g., cirrhosis of the liver, pancreatitis, and bowel obstruction).

DEHYDRATION

Shock may also occur from either decreased oral fluid intake or significant losses of fluid. Examples of situa-

TABLE 20–1. Assessment Findings and Classifications of Acute Hemorrhage

Assessment Finding	Class I	Class II	Class III	Class IV
Blood loss (%)	15	15–30	30–40	>40
Blood loss (ml)	<750	1000–1250	1500–1800	2000–2500
Pulse rate/min	<100	>100	>120	>140
Respiratory rate/min	Normal (14–20)	20–30	30–40	>35
Blood pressure	Normal	Normal or slightly increased	Decreased	Not obtained
Pulse pressure	Normal	Narrowed	Narrowed	Narrowed
Capillary refill	Normal	Prolonged	Prolonged	Prolonged
Skin circulation	Pale, pink, cool	Slightly pale, cool	Pale, cold, moist	Cyanotic, cold, clammy
Level of consciousness	Slightly anxious	Mildly anxious	Anxious/confused	Confused, lethargic, or obtunded
Urine output (ml/hr)*	30 or more	25–30	5–15	Negligible
Intravenous fluid replacement	Crystalloid at 3 ml/1 ml of blood loss	Crystalloid at 3 ml/1 ml of blood loss	Crystalloid plus blood	Crystalloid plus blood

Data from American College of Surgeons Committee on Trauma guidelines.
* Assumes a normal 70-kg male.

tions in which inadequate oral fluid intake may occur are (1) rigorous exercise causing fluid loss due to both sweating and insensible fluid loss through the respiratory tract and (2) hot environments. Loss of fluid, leading to dehydration-induced hypovolemic shock, may occur in clients with excessive urine output or prolonged vomiting or diarrhea. With a prolonged fluid deficit, all compartments—intravascular, interstitial, and intracellular—are depleted.

Cardiogenic Shock

Clients with hypovolemic shock may develop cardiogenic shock. This happens because the rapid heart rate initiated to compensate for decreased volume and to increase the cardiac output does not allow time for the coronary arteries to fill with blood. Because these arteries supply blood to the myocardium, myocardial oxygen supply is impaired. Also, the increased heart rate increases the myocardium's need for oxygen. In addition, the decreased venous return associated with hypovolemia results in decreased coronary artery perfusion and inadequate oxygenation of the myocardium. Finally, shock results in the release of MDF and lactic acid, which decreases myocardial function.

Cardiogenic shock results primarily from an inability of heart muscle to function adequately or mechanical obstructions of blood flow to or from the heart.

MYOCARDIAL INFARCTION

Impaired heart muscle action is most often caused by myocardial infarction (see Chapter 43). With myocardial infarction, coronary artery obstruction occurs. Then the area of myocardium that normally received blood through that artery fails to receive its blood supply. The area is then inadequately perfused with blood and oxygen, and ischemia and necrosis of that tissue occur. This area of dead or dying tissue impairs contractility of the myocardium, and the cardiac output decreases.

Impaired myocardial contractility also occurs with traumatic cardiac contusion, cardiomyopathy, and congestive heart failure.

Clients with cardiogenic shock may also develop some degree of hypovolemic shock. This is most often due to therapeutic use of diuretics or edema in interstitial spaces in the extremities or other dependent areas (due to inadequate cardiac pumping activity and venous congestion).

VALVULAR INSUFFICIENCY AND CARDIAC DYSRHYTHMIAS

Other causes of cardiogenic shock include valvular cardiac insufficiency from trauma or disease; myocardial aneurysms (usually due to previous myocardial infarction or congenital abnormalities); rupture of a valvular papillary muscle; rupture of a ventricle; aortic stenosis; mitral regurgitation; cardiac tamponade; or cardiac dysrhythmias. Inadequate myocardial function causes an accumulation of blood in the left atrium and ventricle and in the pulmonary venous circulation, with resultant marked pulmonary congestion.

OBSTRUCTIVE CONDITIONS

Mechanical obstructions to blood flow causing cardiogenic shock include a large pulmonary embolism, pericardial tamponade, and tension pneumothorax. An embolus is usually the result of a blood clot that breaks loose in a client with deep vein thrombosis. This embolus travels through the venous system to the right side of the heart and out into the pulmonary artery. The size of the embolus determines at what point it lodges in the pulmonary artery. A large embolus can inhibit perfusion of a major portion of the lung field, resulting in an increased workload for the heart. Pericardial tamponade is an accumulation of blood or fluid in the pericardial space that compresses the myocardium and interferes with the myocardium's ability to contract adequately. Tension pneumothorax is a significant amount of air in the pleural space compressing the heart and great vessels and thus interfering with venous return to the heart.

Distributive Shock

Distributive shock (also sometimes called vasogenic shock) results from inadequate vascular tone. With distributive shock, the blood volume remains normal. However, the size of the vascular space increases dramatically because of massive vasodilation. Thus, there is a disproportion between the amount of blood available and the size of the capillary space.

After extensive vasodilation, blood pressure, return of venous blood to the heart, and cardiac output are decreased. As with other forms of shock, tissue anoxia and cell destruction result.

The massive vasodilation present with distributive shock can be due to several major causes.

ANAPHYLACTIC SHOCK

Distributive shock induced by vasoactive substances released during an allergic reaction is called anaphylactic shock.

NEUROGENIC SHOCK

When shock occurs as the result of loss of innervation to the vessels, as from spinal cord injury or spinal anesthesia, it is called neurogenic shock or spinal shock.

SEPTIC SHOCK

Distributive shock resulting from massive sepsis and the release of toxins or vasoactive substances leads to septic or toxic shock.

Each of the three basic types of shock—hypovolemic, cardiogenic, and distributive—has a different primary cause. However, sometimes shock is due to combinations of problems that do not fit into a single category.

The initial clinical course and initial intervention for the various primary events causing shock differ, depending on the etiologic factor. However, whereas factors that may initiate shock vary, the underlying problem is always inadequate tissue perfusion.

RISK FACTORS

Risk factors for the various forms of shock are numerous and varied. However, for a few shock states, the risk factors are identifiable.

Any client experiencing major trauma may be at risk for hypovolemic or neurogenic shock. A client with a history of previous myocardial damage is at risk for cardiogenic shock when conditions that stress the heart occur.

The client receiving immunosuppressive therapy, or the client with a disease process that impairs the immune system, is at risk for developing septic shock.

Anaphylactic shock would be anticipated in a client exposed to an allergen that previously caused a significant allergy reaction.

Primary prevention is not usually an option for shock, although clients with marked sensitivity to allergens can be desensitized to reduce the risk of an allergic response. Early recognition is important in any of the shock states. Early recognition allows earlier treatment, which will decrease the risk of complications and death.

PATHOPHYSIOLOGY

Blood Circulation and Tissue Perfusion

ADEQUATE BLOOD CIRCULATION

The circulatory system consists of three major components: the heart, large blood vessels, and microcirculation. The microcirculation is also called peripheral circulation, capillary circulation, and terminal vascular bed. Each component of the circulatory system is designed for and concerned with separate and distinct intrinsic activities. However, all the component parts function interdependently. An alteration in one part affects the other parts.

Activities of the heart and large blood vessels are regulated by the brain's vasomotor center, autonomic nervous pathways, and monitoring devices (baroreceptors and chemoreceptors) in the walls of the heart and large blood vessels. Baroreceptors are sensory nerve terminals stimulated by pressure changes. Chemoreceptors are receptors stimulated by chemical substances, such as carbon dioxide and lactic acid.

Once blood flow passes the arteriolar sphincters and enters the tissues, it becomes the microcirculation and is regulated by a completely different set of devices, primarily chemical in nature. The microcirculation is governed locally by vasoactive substances (i.e., affecting blood vessels) released into the area by the actions of various different types of cells. This local regulation is a sensitive mechanism that can adjust blood flow from moment to moment according to tissue needs.

For adequate blood circulation to occur, three factors must function effectively together:

- circulating blood volume, or the total amount of blood in the body;
- vascular tone, or the resistance of the blood vessels (amount of vasoconstriction or vasodilation); and
- cardiac pump, or the pumping action of the heart.

When these three components of the circulatory system are functioning properly, mean arterial pressure (MAP) is maintained at normal levels (70 to 105 mm Hg). MAP is the average effective pressure that drives blood through the systemic organs.[24] If MAP is not maintained at normal or near-normal levels, tissues are inadequately perfused.

INADEQUATE BLOOD CIRCULATION

Compensatory Mechanisms. If one of the three factors of adequate blood circulation fails, other parts of the system initiate compensatory mechanisms. For example, vascular tone may increase (causing vasoconstriction and reduced vascular capacity), and cardiac pump action or blood volume may increase. Thus, as long as two of these basic factors can maintain a satisfactory compensatory action, adequate blood circulation can be maintained even though the third factor is not functioning normally. However, if compensatory mechanisms fail or if more than one of the three factors necessary for adequate circulation malfunction, circulatory failure results, and shock develops.

Stages of Shock

Shock is a clinical syndrome that is usually in a constant state of flux. A client in shock may progress through various stages of the condition. These stages are termed compensated, decompensated, and progressive.

COMPENSATED STAGE

During the initial or compensated stage of shock, cardiac output is slightly decreased. The body will, however, attempt to compensate for the decreased cardiac output. During this stage, the body's compensatory mechanisms are able to maintain blood pressure (BP) within a normal to low-normal range and are able to maintain tissue perfusion to the vital organs.

The microcirculation has the potential capacity to hold a tremendous volume of blood. Nonetheless, the capillaries normally are relatively ischemic, containing only about 6 to 7 per cent of the body's volume of blood. Typically, blood flow through the capillary bed is influenced by the varying needs of the cells located near the vessel. The capillaries open in rotation on demand of the cells adjacent to them. The size of the body's larger blood vessels is regulated by the autonomic nervous system. However, this is not so for the microcirculation. Arteriole and capillary sphincters are separate mechanisms governed by different controls.

The microcirculation is amazingly autonomous as a functional entity. Its patterns of behavior (in both normal and abnormal situations) are highly independent of those vasomotor influences affecting the systemic circulation lying next to it. The systemic circulatory bed and the microcirculatory bed apparently do not have sensing devices that would allow a unified, coordinated response throughout the entire circulation. Thus, events occurring within one bed do not influence events in the other. As shall be seen next, the relative autonomy of the microcirculation and the lack of coordination between it and the systemic circulation are important in determining the course of events in shock.

During the compensatory phase, the systemic circulation and microcirculation work together. Both undergo a major readjustment in which their activities are coordinated to preserve the entire system.

Compensation occurs because decreased cardiac output causes decreased blood flow through the capillaries, which results in decreased hydrostatic pressure within the capillaries. As the hydrostatic pressure decreases to a level below that of the surrounding tissues, fluid moves from the higher pressure tissues into the lower pressure vascular system, thereby increasing circulating volume. The decreased cardiac output also stimulates the sympathetic nervous system. The vasoconstriction caused by this stimulation and the accompanying tachycardia further maintain blood pressure.

DECOMPENSATED STAGE

If shock and the compensatory vasoconstriction persist, the body begins to decompensate and the systemic circulation and microcirculation no longer work in unison. As vasoconstriction continues, the microcirculation dilates. This dilation causes decreased venous return and decreased circulation of reoxygenated blood.

Lactic acidosis occurs as a result of anaerobic metabolism from the decreased oxygen delivery, which causes increased capillary permeability and relaxation of the capillary sphincters. Relaxation of the sphincters allows increased blood in the capillaries and increased capillary pressure. This increased pressure, along with the increased capillary permeability, allows fluid to move back into the tissues. In doing so, the microcirculation has reversed its pattern and is trying to secure for itself (and the tissue it supplies) more of the limited supply of available blood. Thus, the blood supply is progressively retained in the capillary bed. In other words, blood "pools" in the microcirculation. Because the cells demand greater perfusion time, many or most of the capillaries remain open at any one time. This increases the vascular space in the microcirculation.

Increased vascular capacity, decreased blood volume, or decreased heart action reduces the mean arterial blood pressure.

$$\text{Mean arterial blood pressure} = \frac{\text{systolic} + 2 \times \text{diastolic}}{3}$$

In turn, the pressure gradient for the venous return of blood decreases. This also contributes to venous "pooling" of blood, decreased venous return to the heart, and decreased cardiac output.

Because there are no feedback systems within the body to change this pattern, the events become progressively more severe. Eventually, the circulation is totally disrupted. Once the vascular space enlarges (owing to vasodilation of the microcirculation), even a normal blood volume cannot fill all these small vessels and the larger ones as well. The result is a low central venous pressure and inadequate venous return to the right side of the heart, with a further decrease in cardiac output.

This resultant decrease in circulating volume and capillary flow does not allow adequate perfusion and oxygenation of the vital organs. With the prolonged decrease in capillary blood flow, the tissues become hypoxic. This process is described in Figure 20–1.

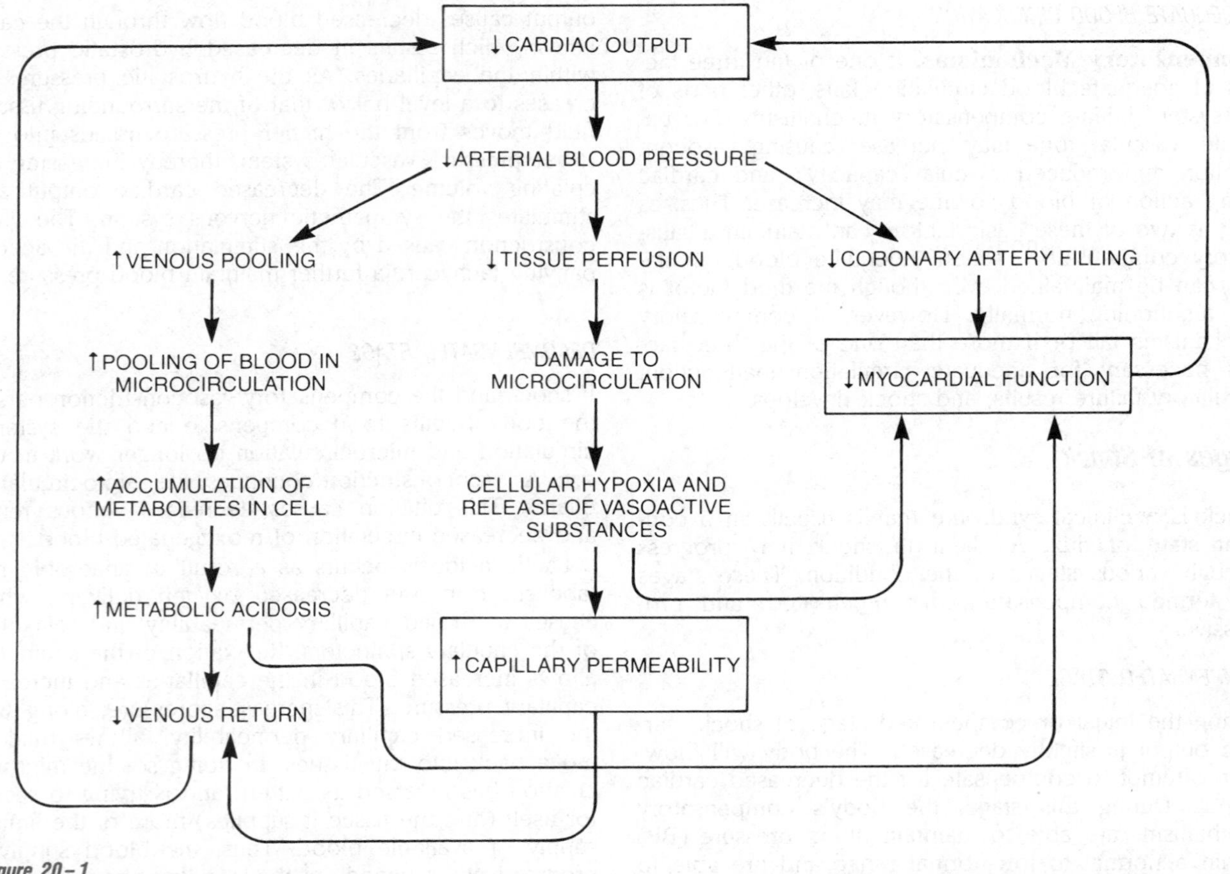

▲ **Figure 20-1**

Vicious circle of events occurring in shock. The shock syndrome can be initiated anywhere in the circle, depending on the precipitating cause, e.g., impaired myocardial function due to myocardial infarction, blood loss due to trauma, or the release of vasoactive toxins due to sepsis. Hypovolemic shock resulting from blood loss, for example, results in decreased arterial blood pressure, setting in motion a cascade of events that worsen the shock state.

PROGRESSIVE STAGE

The progressive stage of shock occurs if the cycle of inadequate tissue perfusion is not interrupted. The shock state becomes progressively more severe, even though the initial cause of the shock is not itself becoming more severe. Cellular ischemia and necrosis lead to organ failure and death of the client.

Systemic Effects of Shock

Shock is a condition that affects every system within the body. The following is a discussion of the systemic effects of shock.

RESPIRATORY SYSTEM

Despite many advances in shock prevention, early recognition, and management, respiratory failure continues to be a major cause of death with shock. The magnitude of this problem surfaced during the Vietnam War when soldiers sustaining massive injuries and profound blood loss were successfully resuscitated only to die several days later from adult respiratory distress syndrome (ARDS). (ARDS is discussed in detail in Chap. 39.)

Respiratory Alkalosis/Acidosis. As previously emphasized, shock produces prolonged circulatory insufficiency. This leads to variable and inadequate perfusion of certain organs and tissues, particularly at the microcirculation level. Such circulatory deprivation results in tissue hypoxia and anoxia.

In response to the change in oxygenation, the rate and depth of respirations are increased. This results in respiratory alkalosis. However, the cellular hypoxia is not due to impaired gas exchange but to inadequate tissue perfusion. Therefore, the increased respiratory effort does little to correct the problem.

Hypoxia and anoxia can be tolerated for a short time. However, as the time lengthens, the chances for recovery diminish. A lack of oxygen appears to stimulate the development of the progressive stage of shock. The greater the difference between the amount of oxygen available and the amount needed, the more rapidly progressive shock develops. If sufficient oxygen is available to the cells to meet the body's needs, progressive shock is less likely to occur.

Metabolic Acidosis. To function properly, cells depend on adequate circulation to receive nutrients, electrolytes, and oxygen and to remove waste products. Oxygen and nutrients are essential to life because they make possible complex chemical transformations resulting in the synthesis of adenosine triphosphate (ATP). ATP is the ultimate source of energy for life processes.

When oxygen is not present, ATP is produced through a different set of reactions called anaerobic metabolism. Production of ATP in this manner is a useful emergency measure. However, it is inefficient, compared with the normal process of aerobic (oxidative) metabolism. Anaerobic metabolism produces anaerobic metabolites, such as lactic acid (which causes intracellular acidity with consequent cellular damage) and substrates of the adenylic acid system (which depress the heart) (Fig. 20-2).

Because lactic acid is not exhaled, it accumulates in tissue fluids. This causes them to become increasingly acidic. Eventually, metabolic acidosis is produced. During metabolic acidosis, blood pH, PCO_2, and bicarbonate fall. Pyruvate, lactate, phosphate, and sulfate rise. Unless circulation is restored, the acidotic reaction resulting from metabolic acidosis ultimately kills the cells. The buildup of lactic acid causes such a severe local acidosis that cellular enzymes are inactivated. As a result, the cells soon die.

Respiratory alkalosis or respiratory acidosis (induced by pulmonary ventilatory or diffusion changes) may be superimposed on the metabolic acidosis. As perfusion and oxygen delivery to the tissues decrease, cellular energy production decreases. To compensate, cells increase anaerobic metabolism, which results in the buildup of lactic acid in the cell. As the pH of the cells decreases, lysosomes within the cell explode, releasing

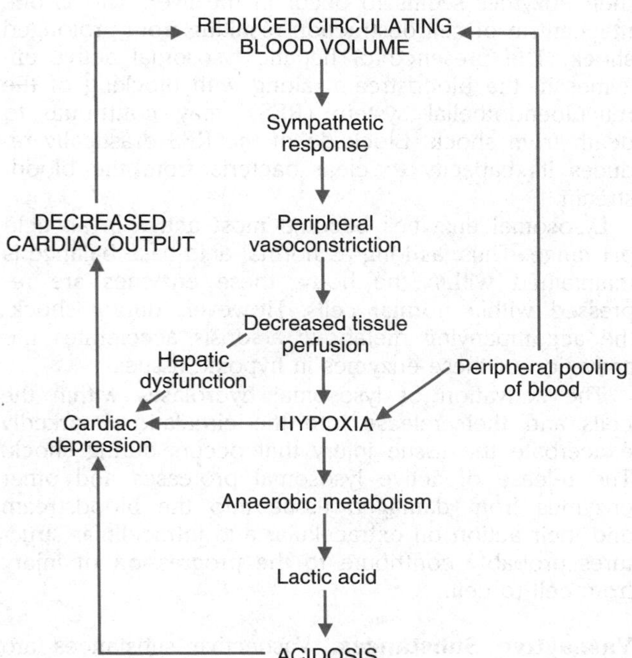

▲ *Figure 20-2*

Shock leads to tissue hypoxia, with blockage of normal aerobic metabolism. Lactic acid accumulates, resulting in tissue acidosis. (Modified from Condon, R. E., & Nyhus, L. M. [1978]. Manual of surgical therapeutics. © by Robert E. Condon and Lloyd M. Nyhus.)

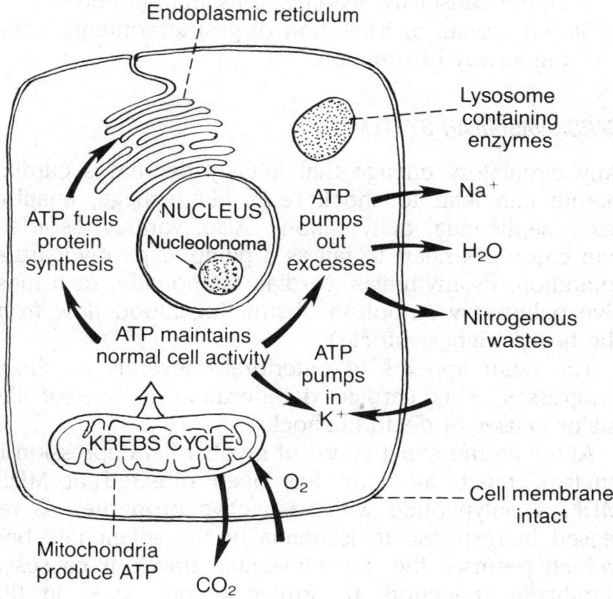

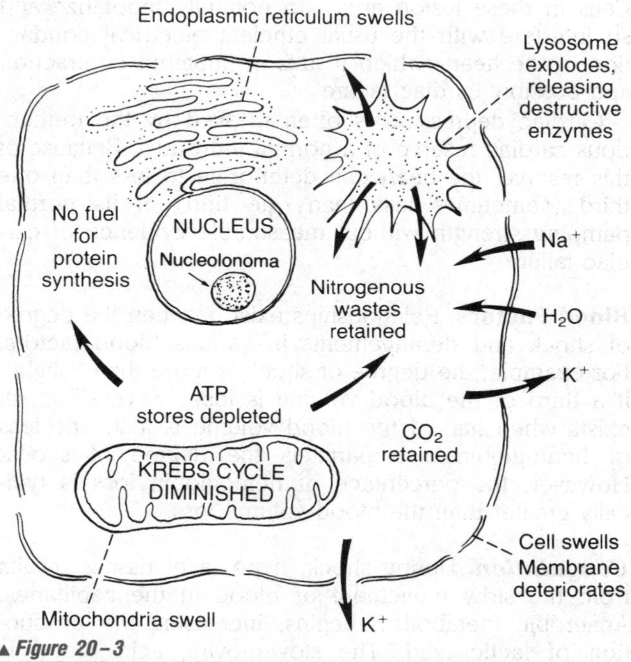

▲ *Figure 20-3*

A, Normal cell. *B*, Alterations in cell function during late shock.

powerful, destructive enzymes. These enzymes destroy the cellular membrane and digest the cell contents. Once this process begins, the cellular changes are irreversible. The end result is cellular death (Fig. 20-3).

Some causes of respiratory failure during shock in addition to those discussed earlier are

- Respiratory overload due to fever, infection, or metabolic acidosis;
- Cerebral arterial insufficiency, which obtunds the gag

and cough reflexes as well as the respiratory center sensitivity, leading to aspiration; and

Stupor, coma, or aspiration of gastric contents, causing airway obstruction.

CARDIOVASCULAR SYSTEM

Any circulatory change that initially decreases cardiac output can lead to shock (e.g., hemorrhage, anaphylaxis, septicemia, dehydration). Also, various disorders can cause the heart to fail as a pump (e.g., myocardial infarction, dysrhythmias, cardiac tamponade, or a massive pulmonary embolism obstructing blood flow from the heart's right ventricle).

The heart appears to deteriorate severely as shock progresses. This cardiac deterioration is one of the major causes of death in shock.

Although the exact cause of myocardial depression is unclear, much attention has been directed at MDF. MDF, a polypeptide with vasoactive properties, is released in response to ischemia of the splanchnic bed (which perfuses the gastrointestinal tract). It causes a significant reduction in cardiac output, even in the presence of a normal circulating volume of blood. Another factor may be myocardial zonal lesions, which appear in the myocardium after ischemia or infarction. Cells in these lesion areas do not fully repolarize and so interfere with the usual efficient electrical conduction in the heart, which results in impaired contraction and possibly cardiac failure.

Cardiac depression is often masked by the tremendous cardiac reserve of a normal individual. Because of this reserve, the heart can deteriorate to less than one third (sometimes less than one fifth) of its normal pumping strength without measurable evidence of cardiac failure.

Blood Factors. Relationships exist between the degree of shock and derangements in various blood factors. For example, the degree of shock is more than "slight" if a third of the blood volume is lost. "Severe" shock exists when half of the blood volume is lost. The loss of hemoglobin also parallels the degree of shock. However, the percentage of hemoglobin loss is typically greater than the blood volume loss.

Coagulation. During shock, hypoxia of tissues results from the slow movement of blood in the capillaries. Anaerobic metabolism begins, increasing the production of lactic acid. The slow-moving acid blood is hypercoagulable; however, it will not actually coagulate unless some clot-initiating factor is present. Such factors include bacterial toxins and thromboplastin of red blood cells (liberated by hemolysis). Hemolysis (destruction of red blood cells with the liberation of hemoglobin) accompanies trauma, especially when massive crushing injury occurs. When any of these factors is present, along with the stagnant, acidic blood of shock, widespread intravascular clotting may occur in the vessels. This disorder is called disseminated intravascular coagulation (DIC) (see Chap. 46).

DIC is associated with multiple thrombi or emboli that are deposited in the microvascular circulation, with resultant organ obstruction and increased tissue ischemia. As blood attempts to flow through partially obstructed vessels, widespread hemolysis may occur. When red blood cells are destroyed, hemoglobin is liberated. Anemia occurs because the liberated hemoglobin is excreted by the kidneys.

As DIC progresses, clotting factors are depleted, causing an inability for normal clot formation in the presence of hemorrhage. Treatment of the precipitating cause and anticoagulant therapy need to be started as soon as possible for maximal effectiveness. DIC is a serious complication of shock and can be fatal.

Carbon Dioxide. Sluggish circulation also results in decreased removal of carbon dioxide (CO_2) from the tissues. Increased CO_2 dilates arterioles located in active tissues and constricts those in nonactive tissues. Because of the heart's increased activity, excessive CO_2 is produced in the myocardium. This directly dilates the coronary arteries leading to the myocardium, which allows the myocardium to receive more arterial blood (with its oxygen and nutrients). CO_2 is also a powerful stimulant of the vasoconstrictor center in the sympathetic nervous system. With vasoconstriction of nonactive tissues, blood is shunted to the more active tissues, which have a greater immediate need of it.

Enzymes. Lysosomal enzymes are released in dead cells undergoing autolysis. They are also released just before cell death due to cellular anoxia or some other form of injury. For example, these enzymes may be liberated as a result of trauma and endotoxins. During shock, the disruption of lysosomes and the release of their enzymes seems to occur in the liver. This is one mechanism of cell destruction resulting from prolonged shock. The presence of hepatic lysosomal active enzymes in the bloodstream, along with blocking of the reticuloendothelial system (RES), may contribute to death from shock. Blockade of the RES drastically reduces its capacity to clear bacteria from the bloodstream.

Lysosomal enzymes become most active in an acid pH range. Thus, as long as normal acid-base balance is maintained within the body, these enzymes are repressed within normal cells. However, during shock, the accompanying metabolic acidosis accelerates the activation of these enzymes in hypoxic tissues.

The activation of lysosomal hydrolases within the cells and their release into the circulation markedly exacerbate the tissue injury that occurs during shock. The release of active lysosomal proteases and other enzymes from damaged tissue into the bloodstream and their action on extracellular and intracellular structures probably contribute to the progression of injury from cell to cell.

Vasoactive Substances. Vasoactive substances are highly variable in promoting vasoconstriction or vasodilation in a client experiencing shock. The influence they exert may be altered by factors such as pH, specific tissue (e.g., heart, lung), presence of drugs or other substances, serum electrolyte levels, and sensitivity of the end organ.

Catecholamines. Catecholamines, such as epinephrine and norepinephrine, are present early in shock. Their general effects are to increase blood flow to the brain, heart, and striated (skeletal) muscle and to decrease blood flow to the skin, kidneys, and splanchnic bed. Although the initial effect of vasoconstriction in the skin, kidneys, and splanchnic bed serves to increase the intravascular volume, sustained vasoconstriction contributes to stagnant hypoxia and cellular death.

Histamine. Histamine causes vasodilation, increased capillary permeability, bronchoconstriction, coronary vasodilation, and cutaneous reactions (flares, wheals). The effects of histamine are especially obvious in anaphylactic and septic shock.

Vasoactive Polypeptides. Bradykinin, angiotensin, and MDF are among the more important vasoactive polypeptides that appear to play significant roles in shock.

- Bradykinin (a kinin peptide) is known to produce vasodilation, increased capillary permeability, smooth muscle relaxation, pain, and infiltration of an area with leukocytes. Kinins appear to be most active in late shock. They may be a factor in the development of pulmonary insufficiency associated with shock.
- Angiotensin results from the action of renal renin on angiotensinogen. This potent substance causes vasoconstriction and increased vascular resistance. Although similar to norepinephrine in effect, angiotensin may have fewer negative effects. The role of angiotensin in sodium and water retention (through the stimulation of aldosterone secretion) is discussed under the sympathoadrenal response.
- MDF is a vasoactive polypeptide that contributes to cardiac failure in clients in shock by depressing cardiac muscle contraction.

NEUROENDOCRINE SYSTEM

Neuroendocrine responses during shock are defensive reactions that occur during the body's stage of resistance in the general adaptation syndrome (GAS), discussed in Chapter 3. Remember, the length of the stage of resistance varies among clients and is determined by a body's ability to compensate for its deficiencies. Hence, one client may be able to combat shock longer than another may. For example, a previously healthy client may have a longer stage of resistance against shock than will a client who is debilitated before shock develops.

Adrenal Response. Some basic features of the neuroendocrine responses are (1) the release of epinephrine and norepinephrine from the adrenal medulla, which results in increased respiratory and heart rates, increased BP, increased blood flow to organs, and decreased blood flow to peripheral tissues; and (2) the release of mineralocorticoids (which control fluid and electrolyte balance) and glucocorticoids (which affect energy and tissue resistance) from the adrenal cortex.

Increased production of adrenocortical mineralocorticoid hormones occurs. The main mineralocorticoids, aldosterone and desoxycorticosterone, help to increase intravascular fluid volume by stimulating the kidneys to retain sodium and hence water. The renal tubular conservation of sodium occurs with any type of fluid loss or blood volume depletion. Aldosterone is essential in this conservation of sodium. Because water is retained in the body along with sodium, urine excretion is diminished during shock. This fluid is retained in the bloodstream in an effort to increase the blood volume. Increasing the volume of blood in this way is aimed at increasing venous return, cardiac output, and blood pressure.

Pituitary Response. Of major importance in regulating water and sodium balance are aldosterone and the antidiuretic hormone (ADH), also called vasopressin. ADH is produced by the posterior pituitary gland. The blood's osmolality (osmotic concentration) increases with dehydration. This stimulates osmoreceptors in the hypothalamus to release ADH from the posterior pituitary gland. Via the blood, the ADH is carried to the kidneys. There it causes the body to retain water.

Various components of the sympathoadrenal (sympathetic part of the autonomic nervous system and adrenal medulla) response to a major stressor are shown in Figure 20–4.

Metabolic Response. Generally, the hormonal response to stress rapidly provides fuel for the body's various tissues, organs, and systems. These fuels (e.g., amino acids, fatty acids, glucose, sodium, and water) are produced by the breakdown of food into sugars, fatty acids, and amino acids. Then these are chemically converted into energy, resulting in the formation of ATP. ATP is the main source of energy produced and used inside the body's cells.

The glucocorticoids, particularly hydrocortisone, mobilize energy stores. During the initial phase of shock, the body's small stores of available carbohydrate are rapidly depleted. Then it becomes necessary to mobilize protein and fat stores to meet the body's energy requirements. Protein catabolism and negative nitrogen balance occur as part of the metabolic response, because of gluconeogenesis (resulting from glucocorticoid action) and starvation.

Neurologic Response. With shock, cerebral blood flow and, thereby, cerebral metabolism may become insufficient to maintain normal mental functioning and level of consciousness. Brain cells are highly sensitive to a shortage of oxygen and glucose. When the brain becomes hypoxic, the cerebral vessels dilate to restore blood flow. Likewise, blood is diverted to the brain from the other less-vital organs.

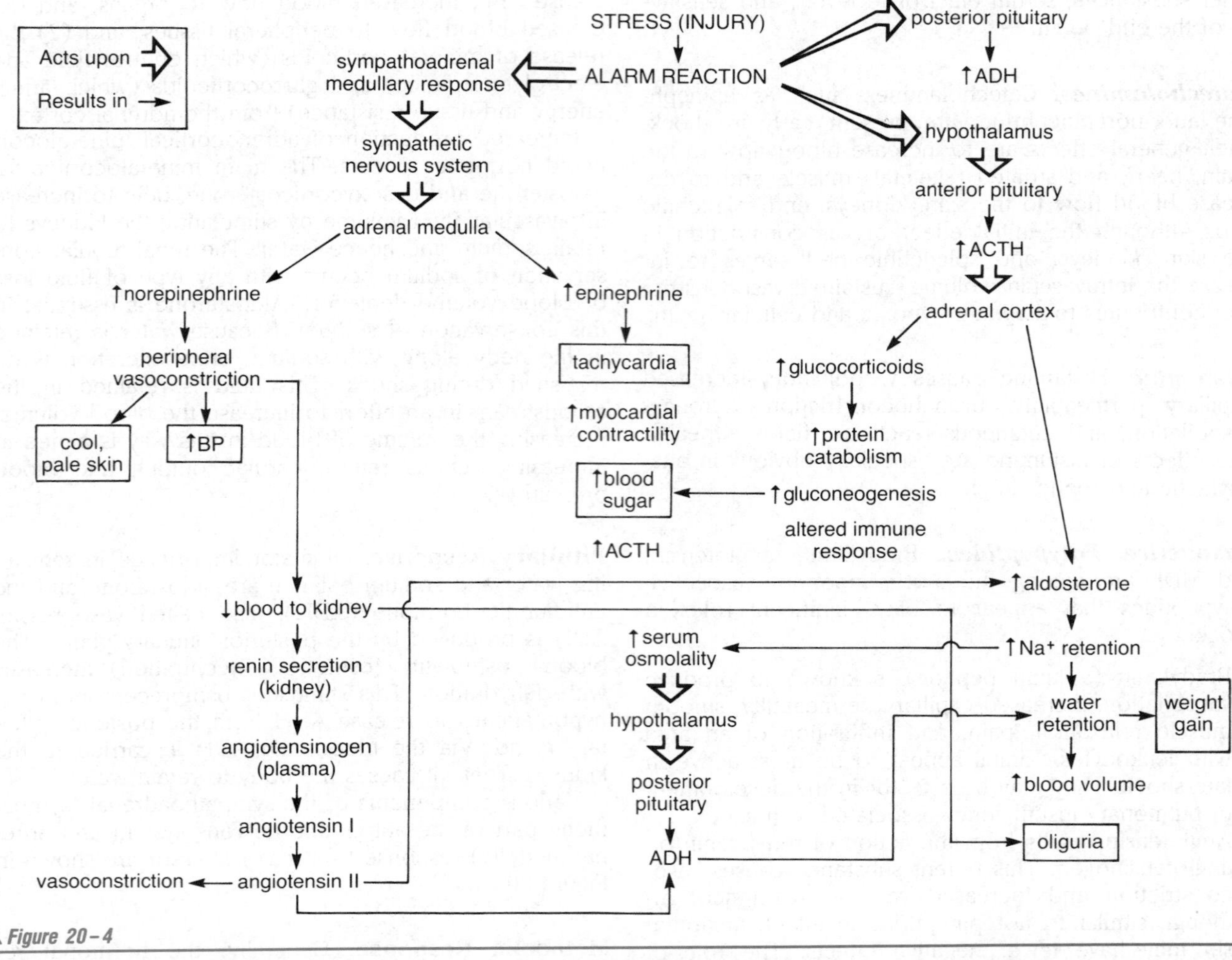

▲ *Figure 20–4*

Components of the sympathoadrenal response to major stressor. Readily observed clinical signs as well as laboratory values are indicated by boxes.

IMMUNE SYSTEM

All forms of shock severely depress the reticuloendothelial system (RES) and antibacterial defense mechanisms. The capacity of the RES to remove bacteria and the constantly formed endotoxins from the bloodstream is greatly reduced. Alterations occur in immunologic factors circulating in the bloodstream.

Alterations in the blood itself are partially due to tissue hypoxia and impairment of monitoring activities of the RES. Indeed, the stasis, sludging, tendency to venular thrombosis, impaired capillary permeability, and subnormal vascular reactivity that occur during shock can all be traced to RES dysfunction.

Toxic Agents. The impaired ability of the RES to ward off toxic agents is critical. Reduced blood flow through the intestines during shock impairs the vitality of intestinal tissue so extensively that bacterial products from the intestines gain access to the bloodstream. Further compounding the problem is the fact that the client in a state of shock is more susceptible than normal to bacterial products, particularly bacterial endotoxins, because interference with the RES reduces the ability to withstand stress.

GASTROINTESTINAL SYSTEM

Because various tissues have differing oxygen requirements, some organs are irreversibly damaged before other tissues reach a stage of destruction. For example, the musculoskeletal system is not damaged, yet the liver and small intestine suffer damage. Microcirculatory failure appears greater in abdominal visceral tissues. Yet, even there the changes are not uniform.

Biliary (Liver) Function. Shock causes serious changes in functions of the liver and the intestines. Because parts of these changes are interrelated, these structures are discussed together.

The visceral (splanchnic area) blood vessels are those most strongly constricted by reflex sympathetic nervous system activity and by vasopressor agents. Thus, visceral circulation is highly susceptible to the dangerous effects of prolonged vasoconstriction during shock. The liver and intestines both suffer from this impaired circulation and appear to be sources of toxic materials.

The liver has an important role in metabolizing carbohydrate, protein, and fat. It is also a major detoxifying organ. Normally, the liver protectively traps and disposes of toxic materials (released from the bowel contents) that are products of bacterial enzyme actions. During shock, the anoxic liver develops metabolic deficiencies and, probably, an impaired ability to detoxify. In addition, enhanced bacterial invasion of the liver from the intestine apparently occurs. Also, the anoxic liver may itself release vasotoxic substances.

The liver plays a key role in visceral circulation. During shock, pooling of blood occurs in the visceral area. Pooling of blood in the liver and portal bed may occur from masses of agglutinated (clotted) blood plugging numerous small hepatic vessels, sinusoids, and intrahepatic radicles of the portal vein and hepatic artery. A prolonged, extreme resistance to portal blood flow may lead to stagnation of blood in the portal system. This presumably results in the backing up of blood into the vessels of the intestines, adding to mucosal congestion and pooling of blood within intestinal capillaries.

The depressed protective action of the reticuloendothelial system (previously discussed) permits the release of bacterial endotoxins (e.g., *Escherichia coli, Brucella melitensis*). These agents seem to destroy the integrity of the microcirculation.

Gastrointestinal Function. Gastrointestinal changes now appear to have a more vital role in the progression of shock than was previously thought. The submucosa of the intestine becomes ischemic early in shock. If the period of congestion and subsequent stagnant anoxia is prolonged, actual tissue necrosis and loss of integrity of intestinal mucosa occur. The intestinal arterioles and venules seem highly susceptible to the extensive vasoconstriction that occurs during shock. The massive amount of tissue destruction within the intestines that results from vasoconstriction and tissue anoxia is sufficient to cause death even if bacteria are not present. Bacteria and their toxins contribute to shock by escaping into the systemic circulation because of destruction of the intestinal mucosa barrier.

RENAL SYSTEM

Urinary Production and Circulation. The rate of urine production reflects visceral blood flow and body fluid balance. Thus, urinary output indicates the status of circulation through the vital organs. Adequate urine output indicates adequate circulation even if the arterial blood pressure is below normal.

During shock, urine output should be measured and compared with normal urine production. The normal rate of urine excretion from the kidneys is 1 ml/min, or 60 ml/hr. A client who becomes acutely hypovolemic or is experiencing a redistribution of circulating volume cannot maintain an hourly output of 40 to 60 ml of urine. Decreased urine output (oliguria) typically occurs in shock. Often during shock, the urine output may stop completely (anuria). When this occurs, the client is said to be in renal shutdown or renal failure.

Capillary Blood Pressure and Glomerular Filtration. Glomerular filtration within the kidneys depends on the pressure at which the blood is circulating through the glomerular capillaries. Usually, the average capillary pressure of blood is much higher in the kidneys' glomeruli than in other capillaries. Interestingly, under usual circumstances, the kidneys can maintain this heightened capillary pressure in the glomeruli in spite of changes in systemic blood pressure. Afferent arterioles supplying the glomeruli dilate as the blood pressure falls and constrict as it rises. However, eventually this adaptive mechanism cannot protect the kidneys against damage from a falling systemic blood pressure.

During shock, when the blood volume and blood pressure decline steadily, glomerular filtrate is progressively reduced. Because it cannot be excreted by the kidneys, sodium, along with the water, leaves the body through the sweat glands. Damaged kidneys lose their crucial ability to regulate electrolyte and acid-base balance.

Inadequate perfusion of renal capillaries is believed to be the cause of early renal failure in shock. The afferent and efferent arterioles constrict, shunting blood away from the glomeruli. Later, if shock persists, actual renal shutdown occurs from focal tubular necrosis. Unfortunately, vasoconstriction in the kidneys may continue for a long time after the systemic blood pressure is restored to normal levels.

Renal Ischemia. The kidneys may suffer from renal ischemia during shock because microcirculatory failure has a predilection for abdominal visceral tissues. Because the kidneys have a high rate of metabolism, they are highly susceptible to injury of the tubule cells when the blood supply is deficient. When injury to the kidneys is extensive and renal failure ensues, tubular necrosis occurs. With appropriate intervention, including careful fluid administration, the kidneys can repair this condition. Normal kidney function returns after 10 to 14 days.

Oliguria does not contraindicate the administration of large volumes of fluid in the treatment of shock. In fact, restoring renal capillary perfusion along with that of other vital capillaries restores urine volume production as long as tubular necrosis is not already present. Indeed, fluid administration may prevent renal tubular necrosis.

A large amount of tissue damage (e.g., crush injuries) may cause a release of myoglobin from muscle tissue. Because the myoglobin molecule is large, a type of mechanical renal failure may result from attempts to excrete large amounts of the myoglobin.

CLINICAL MANIFESTATIONS

General Signs and Symptoms of Shock

Because the body is made up of many cells, which may function or malfunction at different stages of metabolic impairment, shock causes many diverse signs and symptoms. Subjective complaints are usually nonspecific and may not be particularly helpful to the clinician who is attempting diagnosis and treatment. The individual may report feeling sick, weak, cold, hot, nauseated, dizzy, confused, afraid, thirsty, and short of breath. Observable and measurable signs and symptoms are often conflicting in nature. BP, cardiac output, and urinary output are usually—but not always—decreased. Respiratory rate is usually increased. Variable indicators of shock include alterations of heart rate, core body temperature, skin temperature, systemic vascular resistance, and skin color. Dyspnea, diaphoresis, and altered sensorium may be present.

Early recognition of shock is vitally important. Treatment may become very difficult if shock is not suspected or recognized until the development of overt hypotension, cyanosis, and a clammy, cold skin. The classic clinical manifestations associated with hypovolemic shock are illustrated in Figure 20-5. Assessment findings due to other types of shock are similar to these; however, specific symptoms of other forms of shock are also discussed.

Assessment findings common to all types of shock are discussed in the following paragraphs. Defining characteristics peculiar to any one type of shock are discussed afterward in relation to the specific shock types.

RESPIRATORY

Rapid respirations (tachypnea) typically occur during shock owing to decreased tissue perfusion. The respiratory rate increases as the blood's oxygen-carrying capacity decreases. Also, the respiratory rate increases because the accumulation of excessive amounts of CO_2 stimulates the respiratory center. As discussed earlier, tachypnea results in respiratory alkalosis.

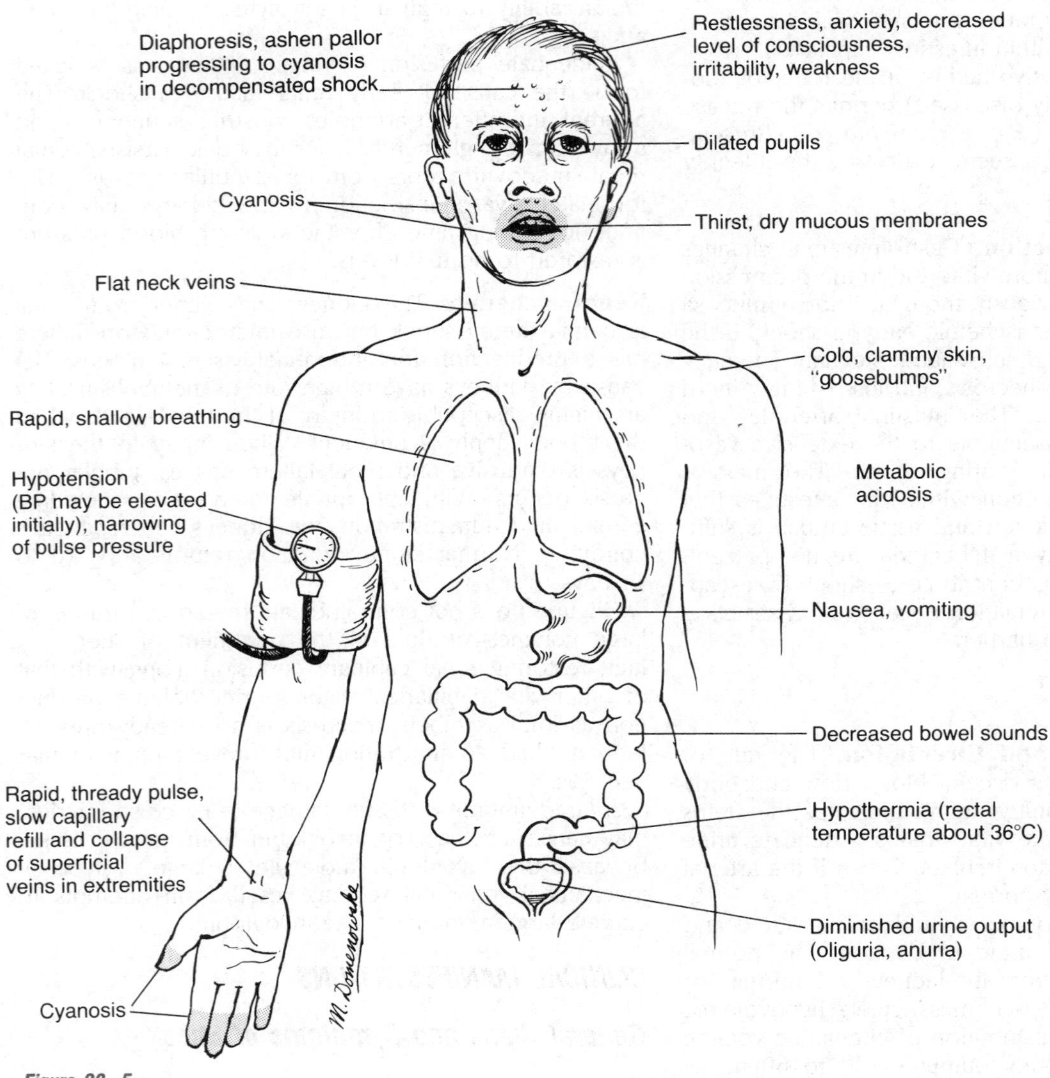

▲ *Figure 20-5*

Subjective and objective assessment findings for a person with hypovolemic shock. (See text for details.)

CARDIOVASCULAR

Pulse. Generally, the pulse rate increases (tachycardia) in shock from increased sympathetic stimulation. This occurs in an attempt to maintain adequate cardiac output when the blood's circulating volume is declining.

In addition to being increased, the pulse is typically weak and thready. At the onset of shock, the pulse rate does not relate as directly to the severity of the shock as does the BP. This is because in the early stage of shock, worry, excitement, and fear may influence the heart rate out of proportion to the underlying conditions. However, when emotional factors are no longer significant, serial observations of the pulse rate over a period of time are highly useful to (1) assess the client's condition and the direction of the shock state and (2) evaluate the effectiveness of intervention. Elderly clients (with and without various degrees of heart block) are an exception to this. Their heart rates may show little change in spite of the presence of conditions causing circulatory failure (e.g., hemorrhage). The pulse rate may become extremely slow in the terminal stages of shock and is usually slow in neurogenic shock.

Blood Pressure. The BP relates inversely to the heart rate. Thus, a decreased BP is accompanied by an increased heart rate. The systolic BP indicates the integrity of the cardiac mechanism, the arteries, and the arterioles. The diastolic BP indicates the resistance of blood vessels. The amount of peripheral resistance (or vasoconstriction) is indicated by the level of the diastolic BP.

For example, an increasing diastolic BP indicates increasing peripheral blood vessel resistance. Conversely, a declining diastolic BP indicates decreasing peripheral resistance. When the diastolic BP falls significantly, vasoconstriction is being lost as a compensatory mechanism. When vasoconstriction is replaced by marked vasodilation, there is no resistance to the blood flow, and adequate BP is difficult to maintain.

Usually, the BP begins to fall when the total blood volume is decreased by about 15 to 20 per cent. However, some people lose as much as 25 per cent of their total blood volume without having a fall in BP. This is especially true in young adults; therefore, in young adults, falling BP is a *very* late sign of shock.

Typically, as shock progresses, the systolic and diastolic BPs drop—the systolic pressure dropping more than the diastolic. The pulse pressure also falls, because it is equal to the difference between the systolic and diastolic blood pressures.

During shock, the pulse pressure is actually more significant than is the BP, because it tends to parallel the cardiac stroke volume. The pulse pressure is affected by stroke volume (amount of blood ejected by the left ventricle during contraction) and peripheral resistance. If the stroke volume is decreased from a decreased circulating blood volume, the pulse pressure decreases. In shock, the pulse pressure may decrease even in the presence of an acceptable systolic BP. This may provide a clue to worsening of the shock. In shock, the pulse pressure is often less than 20 mm Hg.

In order to supply the myocardium with blood (i.e., to maintain coronary circulation), a minimal systolic BP of 60 to 70 mm Hg is necessary. In interpreting BP readings, the nurse needs to know what the client's BP was previously. A systolic BP of 100 mm Hg or less is significant for clients whose systolic BP usually ranges from 110 to 140 mm Hg. When a client is in a supine position, a decline in BP may be a late finding. It is important to note that hypotension by itself (without other abnormal assessment findings) is not shock. Healthy clients often have BP readings lower than textbook normals.

Additional problems need to be considered in assessing BP and make it (particularly the systolic BP) an unreliable criterion for assessing the presence and severity of shock.

In the early, compensated stages of shock, BP changes are generally unreliable because the arterial pressure may actually be normal or slightly elevated even though shock is present. In fact, blood volume deficits of a liter or more may occur even though arterial and venous pressures are normal or elevated.

When severe vasoconstriction is present, the BP may be normal even though the circulation is actually highly inadequate. Also, conversely, the blood flow may be adequate even though the BP is decreased (e.g., because of mechanisms such as vasodilation).

Valuable information about the level of arterial pressure in vasoconstricted clients can be gained by assessing the strength of the femoral pulses. It may also be appropriate to use a Doppler instrument (Chapter 44) to obtain an accurate peripheral blood pressure.

Level of Consciousness. Early in shock, hyperactivity of the sympathetic nervous system with increased secretion of epinephrine usually causes the client to feel anxious, nervous, and irritable. Anxiety and worry are seen in the client's facial expressions.

Assessment findings associated with lack of blood to the brain are determined by the suddenness with which the shock develops and by its severity. With sudden, severe shock, the body may not have time to initiate its compensatory adjustment mechanisms. Consequently, the brain is deprived of its blood supply. The client may feel dizzy and faint on sitting up from a horizontal position. Fainting and unconsciousness may occur. If shock develops gradually over a period of hours, early assessment findings may include apathy and confusion, or the opposite, restlessness and unusual alertness.

The systolic BP is important in maintaining blood flow to the brain. A cerebral perfusion pressure (CPP) of at least 50 mm Hg is required to deliver blood to the brain (CPP = MAP − ICP [intracranial pressure]). Usually, a decrease in systolic BP is accompanied by a reduced flow of blood to the brain. However, the brain's vessels, like those of the heart, are not constricted by the vasoconstrictor center in the medulla oblongata. Thus, blood from the peripheral vessels can be shifted to the brain as an emergency compensatory measure.

A client's level of consciousness decreases as circulation to brain tissue becomes increasingly impaired.

Confusion, agitation, and restlessness may occur. In trauma situations, restlessness can be mistaken for pain. When this happens, if narcotics are given, the client's situation may be worsened.

In decompensated shock, apathy may ensue. Drowsiness and stupor are more likely to occur in shock related to severe infection than in shock caused by trauma and hemorrhage. Ultimately, a comatose condition may be reached.

RENAL

A decreased urine volume often is the earliest sign of developing shock. It may occur even while the arterial BP and pulse remain stable. Urine output is one of the most sensitive indices in shock. However, it should be kept in mind that any form of shock that develops very rapidly (e.g., due to trauma) shows other symptoms before decreased urine output is noticed.

Urine output should be kept above 0.5 ml/kg/hr (approximately 35 ml in an average adult 70-kg male). If the hourly output diminishes significantly, treatment must be instituted to prevent renal failure. Urine flow of less than 20 ml/hr can cause acute tubular necrosis from inadequate renal circulation.

Signs and Symptoms of Specific Types of Shock

All forms of shock have altered cardiac output and altered tissue perfusion. The mechanism by which these occur may be different, however. The assessment findings of shock in general have been discussed. The following is a discussion of some clinical manifestations for each type of shock.

HYPOVOLEMIC

Sympathetic nervous stimulation results in decreased tissue perfusion to the skin, causing the skin to feel cool and clammy and to appear pale. In later stages, diaphoresis occurs because of reduced aldosterone secretion. When aldosterone secretion is decreased, sodium can no longer be retained in the body. Consequently, water cannot be retained, and it leaves the body via the sweat glands.

Cyanosis may indicate either decreased tissue perfusion or decreased oxygenation or both. Cyanosis is a late sign of decreased oxygenation and should not be the principal defining characteristic for diagnosis of decreased oxygenation in any form of shock.

Initially, urine osmolality and specific gravity increase because of sodium and water reabsorption, which attempts to support circulating volume. As altered tissue perfusion and the hypovolemic shock progress, urine osmolality and specific gravity decrease owing to the kidneys' inability to reabsorb sodium and water.

CARDIOGENIC

As in hypovolemic shock, there is stimulation of the sympathetic nervous system due to decreased cardiac output and decreased blood pressure. The sympathetic nervous system causes decreased tissue perfusion to the skin and all of its resultant clinical manifestations.

Because of the impaired muscle action or mechanical obstruction that caused the cardiogenic shock, blood is inadequately pumped through the heart. This results in a "back-up" of blood. When the shock is due to right-sided heart failure, this "back-up" will be evidenced as jugular venous distention. (See Chaps. 42 and 39 for discussions of cardiac tamponade and tension pneumothorax.)

DISTRIBUTIVE

Anaphylactic. Initially, the client may complain of a vague feeling of uneasiness or a feeling of impending doom. The massive vasodilation that occurs with anaphylaxis may cause complaints of headache as well. This may be followed by severe anxiety, dizziness, disorientation, and loss of consciousness.

Respiratory involvement may be manifested through a variety of symptoms. The initial complaint may be of feeling as though there were a lump in the throat. This is due to laryngeal edema and is followed by hoarseness, coughing, dyspnea, and stridor. Diffuse wheezes and prolonged expiratory phase are heard on auscultation.

Additional complaints may include pruritus and urticaria. Direct observation may also demonstrate edema of the eyelids, lips, or tongue (angioedema).

Neurogenic. In neurogenic shock, interruption or loss of sympathetic innervation is experienced. The result is abnormal distribution of fluid volume. Clinical manifestations of neurogenic shock are basically the same as those for shock in general. Some exceptions are related to heart rate, BP, skin temperature, and skin moisture. Because of loss of sympathetic control, the client experiences bradycardia and hypotension (which cannot be corrected because of loss of the ability to vasoconstrict). Below the level of injury, skin temperature takes on the same temperature as the room (poikilothermia). There is also an inability to sweat, so skin feels dry to the touch.

Septic. In the early stages of septic shock, the body experiences massive vasodilation. Warm, dry, flushed skin is apparent during this stage of septic shock. It is the increased perfusion of the skin that gives this stage the name "warm shock."

During later stages, the release of MDF and decreased venous return result in decreased perfusion and "cold shock." At this point, skin becomes pale, cold, clammy, and mottled. Body temperature drops to subnormal levels. Auscultation of the lungs reveals crackles and wheezes, which develop secondary to pulmonary congestion. In addition to the clinical manifestations seen with shock in general, level of consciousness changes seen may include drowsiness and stupor progressing to coma.

Diagnostic Assessment

Assessment of respiratory status can be accomplished to some degree by noninvasive procedures. Spirometry measures tidal volume and minute volume. A pulse oximeter assesses arterial oxygen saturation. A fiberoptic probe is placed on the client's skin (either on the pinna of the ear or on a finger), and oxygen saturation of the arterial blood is determined by the amount of light transmitted through the skin. Corneal oxygen sensors may also be used to assess arterial oxygen saturation. The pulse oximeter does not replace arterial blood gas (ABG) analysis, which provides information about PaO_2, $PaCO_2$, and pH. However, it may be valuable in determining when ABGs are needed.

The $PaCO_2$ is measured by arterial blood gas analysis for determining whether the metabolic acidosis that occurs with shock is being effectively combated by hyperventilation. A low $PaCO_2$ along with low pH and bicarbonate levels (metabolic acidosis) indicates that hyperventilation is trying to compensate. However, a rising $PaCO_2$ in the presence of a persistently low pH indicates that respiratory assistance is needed. It will also be important to monitor PaO_2 levels to determine whether the client is being adequately oxygenated. (See Chap. 37 for discussion of therapeutic respiratory interventions.)

Central venous pressure (CVP) measurement is one of the first invasive assessments made in the presence of shock. CVP is an important means of estimating fluid loss.

Other noninvasive assessment and monitoring tools are the cardiac monitor and the 12-lead electrocardiogram (ECG). Laboratory studies include a complete blood count and chemistries. Other specific studies, such as blood alcohol levels, may be indicated for certain clients.

MEDICAL MANAGEMENT

It is difficult to know when shock actually exists and when therapy should begin. Treatment should generally be instituted for shock whenever at least two of the following three conditions occur: (1) systolic BP of 80 mm Hg or less; (2) pulse pressure of 20 mm Hg or less, and (3) pulse rate of 120 or more.

Methods for treating inadequate tissue perfusion vary according to the specific cause of a client's shock state. Thus, assessment and an accurate differential medical diagnosis, which established the specific cause of the shock state, form the basis for treatment. The differential medical diagnosis is usually readily made unless the shock is in an advanced stage, in which several specific forms of shock may exist at the same time. Some forms of shock usually easily recognized are hypovolemic shock due to extensive burns and cardiogenic shock with severe chest pain and electrocardiographic readings indicating acute myocardial infarction. Septic shock is probably the most difficult shock diagnosis to make because of its insidious onset and confusing symptoms.

Management of the client in shock largely depends on the stage of shock, cause of the shock, and resources (e.g., personnel, equipment, supplies) available for care. Detailed discussion of interventions appropriate for each type of shock is beyond the scope of this book. The emphasis here is on treatment of hypovolemic shock, with occasional reference to other forms of shock. However, remember that the overall goal in treating all forms of shock is to achieve optimal tissue perfusion and oxygenation. Therefore, many aspects of care are similar for all types of shock.

The primary aim in treating shock is to increase tissue perfusion. Unless this is accomplished early, subsequent therapeutic measures are of no avail, and death can be anticipated. Identifying and managing the cause of shock is part of the process in achieving a satisfactory outcome.

The therapeutic management of shock has changed markedly over recent years. Lowering the head, raising the feet, and administering potent vasoconstrictor drugs were once the foundation of treatment for a client in shock. Now, emphasis is placed on adequate fluid resuscitation, positions that do not interfere with pulmonary ventilation, and the use of medications having both vasoconstrictor and vasodilator effects.

As with many other areas of clinical care, clear-cut and final answers concerning the treatment of shock cannot be presented. Shock intervention as discussed in this chapter is in the process of change. The informed nurse must keep up to date with changes. As with any care, recognize that intervention for shock is individualized and follow specific physician prescriptions or agency guidelines. The management of the client in shock is presented as collaborative management in this section. Nursing management is discussed later in the chapter.

Of central importance in current shock intervention is establishing and maintaining an adequate circulating blood volume. In addition, other treatment adjuncts are necessary. The adjuncts facilitate the distribution of blood to the body and enhance the perfusion and oxygenation of the tissues with the circulating blood.

During shock intervention, all of the basic pathophysiologic changes associated with the development of shock must be corrected. Some problems that must often be treated are the vascular problem of vasoconstriction, with the diminished tissue perfusion it causes; the intravascular problem of coagulation and sludging of blood cells; and the extravascular problem of extravasation of fluid into the extravascular space.

Characteristically, impaired tissue perfusion is correctable during early shock. However, it may be fatal if treatment is not received or is inadequate. In the later stages of shock, impaired tissue perfusion apparently becomes "irreversible," leading to death in spite of treatment. However, treatment for "irreversible" shock is never abandoned while the client remains alive. Before a client's shock state is viewed as probably irreversible, the following therapies must have been attempted:

Restoration of circulating volume
Identification and treatment of occult bleeding
Identification and treatment of any factors interfering with cardiopulmonary functioning
Identification and treatment of overwhelming infection

Treating the Shock

Treatment modalities discussed in the following pages can be divided into two major categories: (1) those used to treat the shock state itself and (2) those used to prevent or treat complications of shock through early symptom intervention. Interventions discussed in the following sections include respiratory support, positioning, circulatory assist devices, intravenous fluid therapy, vasoactive and other medications, renal support, and gastrointestinal tract support.

RESPIRATORY SUPPORT

A client in shock must be assessed immediately for ascertaining that the airway is open and functioning. If necessary, ensure ventilation by resuscitation. Circulatory improvement depends on adequate respiratory function. By increasing the rate of pulmonary ventilation (through spontaneous or mechanical hyperventilation), it is possible to compensate for minor degrees of metabolic acidosis. This increased "blowing off" of carbon dioxide with hyperventilation restores acid-base balance.

Endotracheal intubation or tracheostomy may be performed to rest an exhausted client during severe or prolonged shock and to correct respiratory failure. Remember that these interventions interfere with the client's ability to speak.

In all types of shock, regardless of cause, supplemental oxygen is administered to protect against hypoxemia. Oxygen can be delivered via nasal cannula, mask, high-flow non-rebreathing mask, endotracheal tube, or tracheostomy tube. If the client is being mechanically ventilated, be certain oxygen is connected to the bag-valve device in case the equipment fails and manual ventilation is required.

For the prevention or treatment of hypoxia, positive end-expiratory pressure (PEEP) may be added when the client is being mechanically ventilated. This assists in preventing atelectasis and provides a higher PaO_2 for the client at a lower oxygen concentration setting.

In addition to the respiratory support measures mentioned, nursing care also includes vigorous pulmonary hygiene and chest physical therapy, including vibration, percussion, and postural drainage.

Sometimes the interventions discussed cannot establish optimal tissue oxygenation. In these instances, hyperbaric oxygenation or extracorporeal membrane oxygenation may be used.

Hyperbaric oxygenation involves the administration of 100 per cent oxygen under 2 to 3 atmospheres of pressure. This raises tissue oxygen tension to normal or above-normal levels. Hyperbaric oxygenation requires the use of special chambers, which usually are available only in highly specialized institutions (see Chap. 18).

Extracorporeal membrane oxygenation is most commonly used in adults as a temporary intervention for refractory ARDS. Arterial and venous catheters are inserted, and some of the client's blood is diverted through them into a machine that artificially oxygenates the blood. This is a relatively expensive form of therapy and is usually done only in large medical centers.

CIRCULATORY ASSIST DEVICES

Mechanical devices that assist circulation or decrease the heart's workload are commonly used as temporary measures in managing clients in shock. Examples of these include the military or medical antishock trouser (MAST suit), intra-aortic balloon pump, and external counterpulsation device. (See Chap. 42 for more information.)

MAST Suit. A MAST suit (Fig. 20–6) encases the body in a one-piece, three-chambered (two leg chambers and one abdominal chamber) suit from the lower costal margin to the ankles. The perineal area is accessible for urinary catheter insertion. The leg and abdominal chambers connect to a foot pump and gauges. All or some of the chambers are inflated until the pressure pop-off valve is activated or until the BP improves. When all valves are closed, a MAST suit can sustain an internal air pressure of up to 104 pounds per square inch.

Usually, suit inflation dramatically improves the client's blood pressure in 1 or 2 minutes. The external pressure provided by the MAST suit causes increased vascular resistance and decreases the diameter of the blood vessels in the abdomen and legs. This results in impedance of blood flow and decreases leakage into the tissues. Cardiac output increases, and arterial BP improves.

MAST suits are most often used in trauma situations occurring outside the hospital setting for management of massive blood loss with no obtainable BP, fluid loss other than hemorrhage, and cardiac arrest due to severe fluid or blood loss. Also, they help further decrease bleeding in areas being compressed, immobilize fractures of the femur and pelvis, and facilitate insertion of the intravenous line by increasing upper extremity cardiac output and vein filling.

In trauma situations, a MAST suit is usually not deflated until the client is in the operating room and the surgical team is completely ready to treat bleeding areas. X-ray studies can be performed with the suit on without difficulty.

Massive shock or cardiac arrest can occur if the suit is quickly deflated or removed rather than deflated gradually along with restoration of blood volume with intravenous fluids. Before removing a MAST suit, gradually deflate it over a period of several minutes, 5 mm Hg at a time. During this period, closely monitor the client's BP. Intravenous fluids are administered to raise the BP to the level it was before deflation began. Deflating the suit too fast causes the client to rapidly go

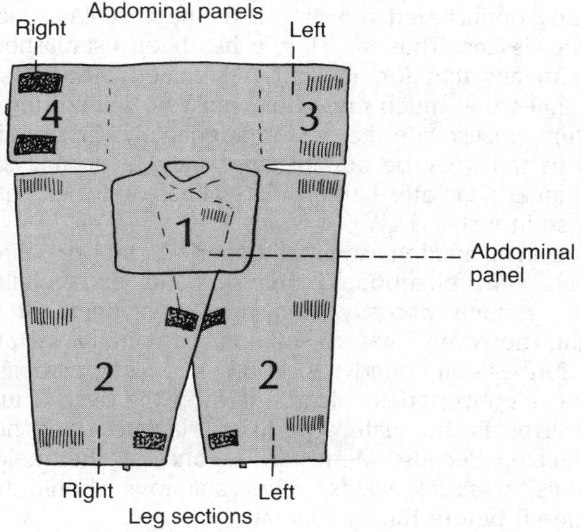

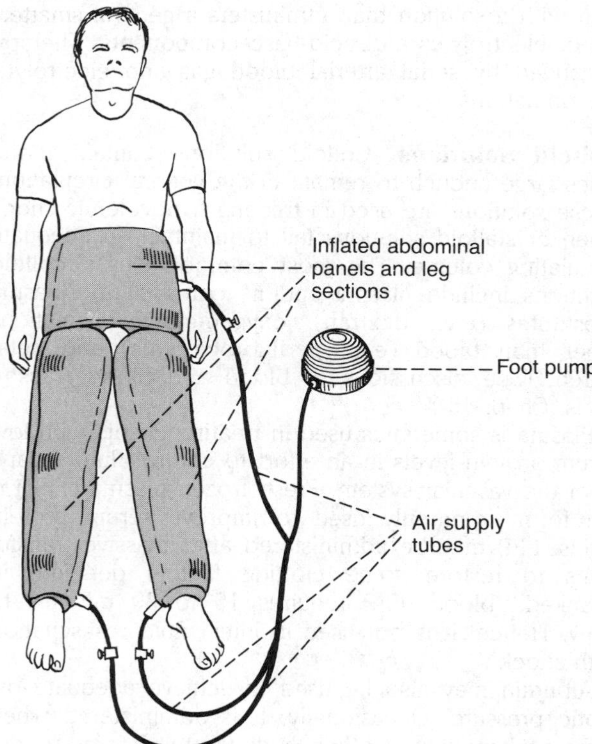

▲ *Figure 20–6*

MAST suit or pneumatic antishock garment. *A*, The suit is composed of two leg compartments and an abdominal compartment. *B*, The MAST suit in place. Abdominal and leg compartments are attached to air tubes and a foot pump for inflation. (See text for further discussion.)

back into shock, because the circulating blood volume has not been adequately restored.

A potential problem that should be remembered is that a MAST suit causes lactic acid to build up in tissues compressed by the suit because circulation to those tissues is decreased. When the suit is deflated and circulation returns to those areas, the lactic acid is sent into circulation, leading to increased acidosis.

Intra-aortic Balloon Pump (IABP). An IABP is used primarily for individuals with cardiogenic shock and after open heart surgery. The heart's ability to pump blood adequately is augmented by a balloon-tipped catheter placed in the descending thoracic aorta. The catheter is attached to a gas-driven unit that inflates during diastole and deflates just before systole. This counterpulsation displaces blood back into the aorta and improves coronary artery circulation. Details of the IABP are found in Chapter 42.

External Counterpulsation Device. This device uses the same general principles as an IABP but is applied externally to the legs. The legs are encased in air- or water-filled tubular bags connected to a pumping unit. Pressure is applied to the legs during diastole and is released in systole.

POSITIONING

A client in shock is usually positioned in a modified shock position with the lower extremities elevated about 45 degrees, knees straight, trunk horizontal or very slightly raised, and neck comfortably positioned with the head level with the chest or slightly higher (Fig. 20–7). This position promotes increased venous return from the lower extremities without compressing the abdominal organs against the diaphragm.

Elevating the legs mobilizes blood that has pooled in the lower extremities. As a result of gravity, the additional circulating blood increases venous return to the heart, thus improving cardiac output. The position is of temporary value in moderate hypovolemia. However, it does not help severe hypovolemia, because the extremities have very little blood in them in such a state. Generally, the modified shock position is not used with cardiogenic shock, when there is already circulatory overload.

The Trendelenburg position (head down, with legs elevated at least 30 cm above the head) was once the classic shock position but in this form is no longer

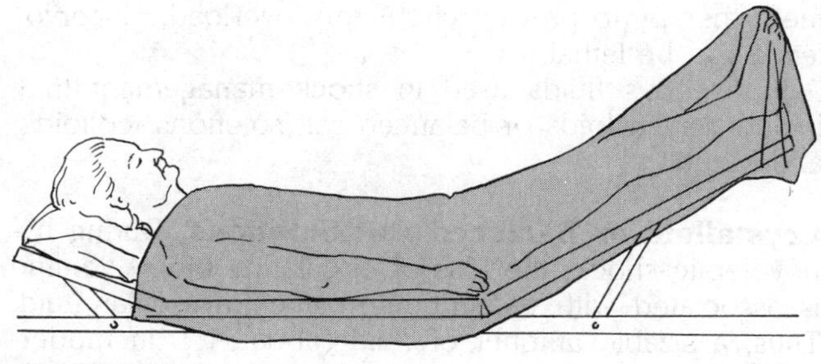

▲ *Figure 20–7*

Positioning of the person in shock. This position is a modification of the Trendelenburg position and includes elevating the legs, leaving the trunk flat, and elevating the head and shoulders slightly.

used for shock management. This position compresses the client's abdominal contents against the diaphragm, thus interfering with pulmonary excursion. Also, it promotes a congestion of blood in the brain, possibly contributing to cerebral edema. Because the Trendelenburg position was used for such a long time, possibly some of your colleagues incorrectly use its name for the modified shock position described. Thus, it is important to determine exactly what the standard shock position is in settings in which you practice.

FLUID THERAPY

All forms of shock involve a decreased effective circulating blood volume. In most forms of shock, this is due to the external or internal loss of whole blood, plasma, or relatively protein-free plasma water, or a combination of these.

The mainstay of hypovolemic shock therapy is expansion of circulating blood volume by intravenous administration of blood or other appropriate fluids. Fluid replacement should be administered through large-bore peripheral lines, central venous lines, or both.

Various fluids are given to correct specific problems, such as electrolyte or protein deficiencies or other defects of the blood, including acidosis and hyponatremia. However, in treating hypovolemic shock, the immediate results of therapy seem to depend less on the type of fluid administered for fluid replacement than on the amount of fluid administered. Generally, enough fluid is given to exceed the normal blood volume. In part, this "extra" fluid is required because the vascular space is expanded owing to dilation of the microcirculation. Additional fluid is also administered to replace intracellular fluid that was mobilized into the circulation as an early response to the hypovolemia.

In replacing fluids, enough volume must be administered to fill the client's capillaries and run through into the veins. Such fluid replacement maintains the central venous pressure and provides an adequate venous return to the heart. This promotes additional cardiac output. In addition, adequate fluid replacement decreases the blood catecholamine level and thus produces a vasodilation that promotes capillary flow. Adequate flow of fluids in the capillaries in turn perfuses tissues and prevents sludging and coagulation of blood within the vessels. Carefully monitor intravenous fluid replacement therapy to prevent circulatory overload. Hypervolemia can be lethal.

Intravenous fluids used in shock management may include crystalloids or balanced salt solutions, colloids, and blood.

Crystalloid or Balanced Salt Solutions. During hypovolemic shock, the loss of circulating blood volume is associated with redistribution of extravascular fluid. Thus, a sizable amount of fluid (about 4 L in moderately severe shock) leaves the interstitial space. This is in addition to fluid lost from the circulating volume. Thus, fluid replacement therapy must replace both blood lost from the circulation and fluid lost from the interstitial space. About two thirds of the crystalloid solution administered moves out of the vascular space into the tissues. Thus, a 3:1 rule has been established, which means that for a client's estimated blood loss, three times that much crystalloid must be administered to volume-resuscitate the person adequately. Crystalloid solutions that may be administered include normal saline, Ringer's lactate, half-normal saline, or 5 per cent dextrose in water (D_5W).

Electrolyte solutions such as Ringer's lactate or saline buffered with bicarbonate help expand extracellular volume, reduce viscosity, and prevent sludging. It is thought, however, that a solution containing lactate might further compound the problem of lactic acidosis. Lactate is converted to bicarbonate by the liver. Thus, if the liver is adequately perfused, lactate does not accumulate. Because perfusion is one of the major problems in shock states, other solutions should be considered before Ringer's lactate.

Abnormalities of electrolyte and acid-base balance are corrected with the specific substance needed rather than with a solution that administers a general smattering of electrolytes and acid-base components. Therapy is gauged by serial arterial blood gas and electrolyte determinations.

Colloid Solutions. Colloid solutions contain molecules large enough to remain in the general circulation. These solutions are used in treating hypovolemic shock when crystalloid solutions fail to maintain an adequate circulating volume. The most commonly used colloid solutions include plasma and its components, plasma substitutes (e.g., dextran), oxygen-carrying solutions other than blood (e.g., perfluorocarbons) and hetastarch. (See discussions of blood and blood transfusions, Chap. 46.)

Plasma is sometimes used in treating clients with low serum protein levels in an effort to control fluid escape from the vascular system. Fresh frozen plasma (FFP) is the form commonly used to improve serum protein levels. FFP may be administered after massive transfusions to restore some clotting factors deficient in "banked" blood. FFP requires 15 to 30 minutes to thaw. Hence, it is not used in initial fluid resuscitation with shock.

Albumin may also be used to achieve adequate osmotic pressure. Occasionally, it is administered when sufficient amounts of other fluids fail to restore an adequate circulating volume. Use of albumin is controversial because it may move into the pulmonary interstitial space, drawing water along with it. Thus, albumin may contribute to the development of ARDS.

Dextran may be used in both high- and low-molecular-weight forms. By initiating therapy with low-molecular-weight dextran and then progressing to high-molecular-weight forms, the incidence of hypersensitivity reactions to dextran can be decreased. The advantage in using dextran is that it contains large size molecules that should effectively and rapidly expand the intravascular volume.

Dextran can interfere with blood type and crossmatch procedures and with clotting factors. It should, therefore, be used only after type and crossmatch have been done and until blood is available for transfusion.

Although the administration of crystalloids, albumin, and blood has been the standard treatment of hypovolemic shock for many years, several new substances have recently been introduced for shock management. Perfluorocarbons such as Fluosol-DA are nonblood, oxygen-carrying solutions that remain in the circulation for about 12 to 24 hours. Major problems associated with use of perfluorocarbons relate to limited immediate availability (the product must be stored frozen) and accumulation of the chemicals in the body. A significant advantage is that Fluosol-DA is acceptable to clients whose religious beliefs prohibit the use of blood products. Fluorocarbons are largely experimental at this time. Hetastarch is another solution with limited use as a volume expander in shock situations.

Blood. When hemorrhage is the primary cause of shock, the rapid administration of large volumes of packed cells may be necessary. Type-specific, crossmatched blood is the most desirable form of blood replacement. However, if the client is hemorrhaging, it may be necessary to administer type-specific, uncrossmatched blood; O-negative blood; or O-positive, low–antibody titer blood.

When shock resulting from hemorrhage is treated, crystalloid is usually given as an initial emergency treatment to sustain blood pressure. Later, the acute anemia resulting from the hemorrhage must be corrected by administration of packed cells for prevention of hypoxemia.

During fluid replacement, a normal red blood cell mass should be maintained. Fluids given in excess of normal volume should be fluids other than blood so that they can be easily removed from the circulation by the kidneys once the shock is corrected. If the normal red blood cell mass is exceeded, it is difficult for the body to get rid of the excess red blood cells after the vascular volume contracts to normal (after adequate perfusion of tissues with blood is achieved). Also, because dangers are involved in blood transfusions, blood should not be used as long as another fluid can satisfactorily maintain an adequate oxygen-carrying capacity and can sufficiently increase blood volume.

Autotransfusion. Autotransfusion involves collecting and retransfusing blood into the same client. Autotransfusion is commonly used in the prevention or treatment of existing hypovolemic shock due to hemorrhage.

As mentioned earlier, the volume of fluid given generally exceeds estimates of blood or fluid loss or volume deficit. Sometimes up to 8 to 12 L fluid may be administered in only a few hours.

Often, fluid replacement is the only treatment required for shock. However, it is difficult to evaluate whether fluid replacement is adequate.

Internal losses of circulating fluid volume, including whole blood, into areas of traumatized tissue, infection, and so forth are difficult to estimate. If a vasoconstrictor drug has been administered or if prolonged vasoconstriction occurs, an additional considerable loss of circulating volume may also occur owing to vasoconstriction. Large volumes of intravenous fluid may be administered either until systemic blood pressure, urine volume, and lactate levels become relatively normal or until central venous or pulmonary artery pressures, or both, elevate.

Infusion of blood or other fluids usually continues only as long as the CVP is low, that is, below 10 cm H_2O or 2 mm Hg. When the CVP is higher than normal (e.g., above 15 cm H_2O or 7 mm Hg), benefit cannot be expected from the continued infusion of fluids or blood beyond maintenance amounts. When the CVP is low and the lungs are clear, with no indications of congestive heart failure, fluids are administered to improve the return of blood to the heart. However, some clients have a normal or low CVP in spite of faulty left ventricular function. They readily develop congestive failure or pulmonary edema. Thus, a low or normal CVP does not always mean that fluid administration is advisable.

Intravenous fluid administration should be stopped before extremely high elevations of pulmonary artery pressure occur if there is an adequate systemic response. Adequate volume of circulating fluid causes an adequate venous return to the right side of the heart and increases the right-sided output. Pulmonary artery hypertension may develop if continued pulmonary obstruction is present because of coagulation in the microcirculation and to vasoconstriction. This appears as increased pulmonary artery pressure. In the presence of right-sided heart failure, this increased pressure may back up through the right heart, causing an abnormal elevation in the CVP. Vasodilators may help open this partially blocked pulmonary microcirculation.

PHARMACOLOGIC MANAGEMENT

Unfortunately, the management of shock easily lapses into treating the client's BP rather than promoting tissue perfusion. Because shock is a complex syndrome with differing causes, various medications may be used. This discussion is divided into vasoactive and other medications.

Vasoactive Medications. As their name implies, vasoactive medications affect blood vessels. Included in this discussion of vasoactive medications are vasoconstrictors, vasodilators, and combination vasoconstrictor-vasodilator medications (Table 20–2).

Opinion differs about the use of vasoconstrictors and vasodilators in treating shock. In general, vasoconstrictors increase peripheral resistance, whereas vasodilators decrease peripheral resistance, allowing greater blood flow in tissues.

Vasoconstrictors. Vasoconstrictors elevate the systemic blood pressure. However, the excessive vasoconstriction they cause may actually impede rather than enhance tissue perfusion.

Whereas the use of vasoconstrictors during shock is being critically evaluated, they do favorably increase blood flow to the brain and heart. This may particularly benefit elderly clients who cannot tolerate prolonged, severe hypotension because of arteriosclerotic narrowing of their coronary or cerebral arteries. Reduced tis-

TABLE 20-2. Vasoactive Medications Used in Shock Management

Medication	Action
High-dosage dopamine (Intropin); norepinephrine (Levophed); phenylephrine (Neo-Synephrine)	Systemic vasoconstriction, especially in the gastrointestinal tract, skin, and kidney
Amrinone (Inocor); epinephrine (Adrenalin); dobutamine (Dobutrex); isoproterenol (Isuprel)	Increased heart rate, increased contractility
Amrinone; dobutamine; epinephrine; isoproterenol; nitroprusside (Nipride)	Vasodilation of blood vessels in heart and skeletal muscle
Low-dosage dopamine	Vasodilation of renal and mesenteric blood vessels
Amrinone; nitroglycerin (Tridil); nitroprusside; phentolamine (Regitine)	Relaxation of vascular smooth muscle

sue perfusion when arterial pressures are below 60 to 70 mm Hg may precipitate myocardial infarction or a cerebrovascular accident.

Vasoconstrictor agents may be used briefly in shock if compensatory vasoconstriction is unable to maintain blood flow to vital organs. They may also be used to correct hypotension secondary to vasoconstrictor nerve paralysis, as in spinal anesthesia or conditions associated with massive vasodilation. However, vasoconstricting agents should not be used exclusively but should be given concomitantly with intravenous fluids in an attempt to restore adequate circulation and perfusion.

Perfusion of vital organs with blood is impossible when systolic BP is below 50 mm Hg. Usually, the goal of using vasoconstrictors is to achieve and maintain a mean BP of 70 to 80 mm Hg. This maintains a BP level sufficient to perfuse tissues. Generally, attempts to increase the BP beyond this level are not advisable because vasoconstrictors increase the heart's oxygen demand and may cause fatal dysrhythmias.

Major adverse effects of vasoconstrictors include

- Increased myocardial oxygen consumption
- Ventricular dysrhythmias. Continuous electrocardiographic monitoring is essential during administration of vasoconstrictors. Prompt administration of antidysrhythmic medications may be necessary.
- Decreased blood flow to kidneys and splanchnic area
- Excessive or sudden rise in arterial BP, which may precipitate heart failure
- Overloading of the vascular system, because vasoconstricting medications must be diluted before administration
- Pulmonary edema or left ventricular decompensation. Vasoconstrictors elevate blood pressure by constricting peripheral vessels. This can dangerously overload the pulmonary circulation. If indications of these problems appear, immediately slow the intravenous flow to a minimum, notify the physician, and elevate the head of the bed to reduce respiratory distress.
- Gangrene of the fingers and toes may result from prolonged vasoconstriction.

Carefully monitor arterial blood pressure during vasoconstrictor administration. Watch for undesirable BP elevations. Carefully adjust intravenous flow to establish and maintain the desired blood pressure. Inspect intravenous sites frequently for evidence of infiltration.

Vasodilators. Agents that induce vasodilation or inhibit vasoconstriction may promote recovery from shock. These include adrenergic blocking agents, ganglionic blocking agents, and direct-acting peripheral vasodilators.

Adrenergic blockade prevents the following harmful effects of prolonged vasoconstriction in shock: prolonged vasoconstriction increases pressure in capillaries, hence promoting fluid loss from the vascular to the interstitial compartment; and prolonged vasoconstriction alters blood flow, especially in the splanchnic area. As a result, considerably more blood passes through channels that do not permit an exchange of metabolites with tissue cells. Cellular nutrition is thus impaired, and waste products accumulate. Not only does adrenergic blockade prevent these changes in circulation, it may also induce opposite beneficial changes.

Vasodilators may be helpful during shock when vasoconstriction is severe and persists even though fluids have been infused in what should be adequate amounts for fluid replacement. As discussed, during shock, peripheral blood vessels are fully constricted owing to the large output of norepinephrine (a compensatory action by the body). Vasodilators may be administered to try to inhibit vasoconstriction so the blood can be redistributed. That is, blood trapped peripherally would become available to enhance tissue perfusion, and the vascular volume increases.

Vasodilation, after an adequate circulating blood volume is restored, may improve capillary flow, tissue perfusion, and cellular metabolism, increasing the client's chances of survival. When shock is caused by hypovolemia, rapid and adequate fluid replacement is essential before vasodilators are used. Vasodilators are dangerous because they lower arterial blood pressure if they are given while circulating blood volume is deficient. This is because while the circulating blood volume is inadequate, the body depends on vasoconstriction to try to maintain arterial pressure. However, when the vascular space is full and cardiac venous return is adequate, vasodilation should open arterioles in the lungs and elsewhere. This lets blood circulate, increasing cardiac output and capillary perfusion without lowering systemic blood pressure. In fact, a vasodilator may produce a dramatic, sustained rise in the systemic arterial pressure. Remember that clients with cardiogenic shock after myocardial infarction may be volume depleted. If a client's volume status is unclear, a fluid challenge may be performed before vasodilators are given.

Continually monitor blood pressure and CVP when vasodilator drugs are being used. Usually, a mean blood pressure of 70 mm Hg is acceptable. However, if abrupt severe hypotension occurs, administration of the vasodilator is generally stopped and fluid administration increased.

CVP drops substantially if peripheral resistance markedly decreases. Blood volume needs to be expanded as the vascular space enlarges, and CVP measurements are used to determine the amount of fluid needed to fill the enlarging vascular space. The rate of fluid replacement is adjusted to maintain the desired CVP. It is serious if the CVP continues to fall in spite of fluid replacement. This means that the rate and volume of fluid replacement are not sufficient to meet the client's physiologic needs.

Keep clients receiving vasodilators lying relatively flat. Elevation of the head could produce dangerous orthostatic hypotension. Older clients may have sclerotic blood vessels and may not tolerate the hypotension that may accompany administration of vasodilators. In this situation, a cardiogenic drug (such as dobutamine) may be given with the vasodilator to increase cardiac output. This helps maintain or raise the blood pressure.

Vasoconstrictor medications are sometimes given in combination with vasodilator medications. This may be done to offset the profound effects that may occur with some vasoconstrictors. This may also be done to provide the benefits both types of drugs have to offer.

Other Medications. Included in this section are antibiotics, heparin, steroids, calcium, histamine H_2-receptor antagonists, naloxone, diphenhydramine hydrochloride (Benadryl), narcotics, and cardiotonic medications.

Antibiotics. Antibiotics are essential when shock is due to infection. If septic shock is suspected, a blood specimen for culture and sensitivity is taken at once, and broad-spectrum antibiotics are started even though the specific infectious organism has not yet been identified. When the blood sample is drawn, samples of urine, sputum, and fluid from draining wounds, sinuses, and so forth are also taken for culture. The antibiotic selected depends on the cause of the infection treatment and should not be initiated until after all cultures have been taken.

Antibiotics may be administered along with appropriate surgical management to clients with open or potentially contaminated wounds who are experiencing hypovolemic shock.

Heparin. The anticoagulant effect of heparin may help prevent or treat some complications of shock. The dosage is usually adjusted according to clotting studies. Heparin may be used in treating myocardial infarction because of the tendency for small thrombi to form on or near large areas of infarction. These can move and cause systemic emboli. Heparin is also used because of the prolonged immobility often associated with shock. Immobility predisposes individuals to venous thrombosis and pulmonary emboli. The treatment of DIC may include heparin administration to minimize consumption of clotting factors. Also, heparin may be appropriate for people with ARDS if the primary cause of the respiratory insufficiency is believed to be from DIC or massive microembolism.

Steroids. Steroids may be given during shock intervention. Examples of synthetic glucocorticoids are prednisone, prednisolone, methylprednisolone, triamcinolone, and dexamethasone. Glucocorticoids (e.g., cortisone, hydrocortisone) have an established place in treating some types of shock. However, the therapeutic use of the mineralocorticoids (e.g., aldosterone and desoxycorticosterone) is not satisfactorily established.

The precise action of steroids is unknown. However, some possible actions include

- Antitoxic effect. In treating shock, steroids may counteract the detrimental effects of gram-negative endotoxins. Steroids may help mobilize the inactive pools of venous blood that reduce cardiac output in toxic shock. If administered early, steroids may improve the survival rate of clients with septic shock
- Antiplatelet aggregating effect; may help minimize pulmonary damage associated with shock
- Stabilizing lysosomal membrane and preventing intracellular release of enzymes
- Increasing blood volume by increasing sodium retention
- Cardiotonic (e.g., increased cardiac output) as well as vascular effects. Glucocorticoids may counteract the reduced cardiac output and the increased total resistance to blood flow that are the basic hemodynamic problems with shock. Thus, they may be administered for shock to increase blood flow and decrease blood resistance, augmenting the beneficial effects of vasoconstricting medications. In large doses, glucocorticoids may promote a more adequate blood pressure level as a result of improved systemic blood flow. When they are used, it is recommended that glucocorticoids be given early rather than as a last resort.

Some physicians give steroids in combination with vasoconstricting medications to treat shock. Steroids may help clients with protracted hypotension associated with severe allergic (hypersensitivity) reactions.

Complications may accompany steroid therapy in the high dosage ranges used in treating shock. These include acute gastrointestinal bleeding; aggravation of diabetes; and inhibition of the antibody response. The lack of antibody response makes the client susceptible to uncontrollable infection.

Calcium. Calcium is needed for normal functioning of the nervous and cardiovascular systems and for blood clotting. The value and dosages of calcium in treating shock are not clear. However, calcium may be administered if impaired cardiac function is evident.

Calcium may precipitate toxic effects in a person who has received digitalis. It is given only with extreme caution to such a person. Monitor for evidence of digitalis toxicity (e.g., bradyarrhythmias or tachyarrhythmias, ST-segment depression).

Calcium chloride should be given intravenously only. Calcium gluconate may be given intramuscularly but is very irritating to tissues. Whereas calcium chloride and calcium gluconate are both available as 10 per cent solutions, they are not identical in concentration. Do not substitute one for the other.

Indications of hypocalcemia may be subtle. Careful assessment is essential. (See discussions of calcium in Chap. 14.)

Histamine H_2-Receptor Antagonists. Cimetidine, famotidine, and ranitidine are histamine H_2-receptor antagonists, which inhibit gastric acid secretion. Any of them may be administered to a client experiencing shock for preventing stress ulcers, which are often lethal complications of severe illness or injury. They are commonly given intravenously to the client in shock and may be prescribed in combination with oral antacids.

Naloxone (Narcan). This opiate antagonist is commonly used to treat narcotic and synthetic narcotic overdosages. During stress, opiate-like substances known as enkephalins and endorphins are released from the brain. Although the mechanisms of action are not clear, endorphins may play a role in capillary bed vasodilation found in all forms of shock. Studies indicate that when naloxone is administered to animals not in shock, no significant cardiovascular effects are noted. However, when administered during shock, naloxone reverses the hypotension and decreases cardiac contractility. It is believed that naloxone blocks the effects of endorphins and enkephalins.

Diphenhydramine Hydrochloride (Benadryl). Anaphylaxis or less severe allergic reactions are treated with this antihistamine. This medication acts primarily to relieve symptoms associated with anaphylaxis rather than to stop the release of histamine. Therefore, epinephrine is always administered first in treating anaphylaxis.

Narcotics. The need for pain relief may be obvious in clients experiencing different types of shock. However, the use of narcotics for pain management may unfortunately be dangerous for them. Narcotics interfere with vasoconstriction, and vasoconstriction may be the only way the client's blood pressure is being maintained.

Morphine sulfate, however, causes pooling of blood in the extremities and contributes toward the decrease of anxiety. These effects may prove useful for the client in cardiogenic shock.

Do not administer narcotics to a client suffering from acute, multiple trauma without first knowing that the blood volume is adequate. Narcotic administration causes vasodilation, which results in severe hypotension or shock. Also, if a narcotic is administered intramuscularly to a client in shock, it may not be completely absorbed because of the vasoconstriction that is present. Then, because the client experiences little or no pain relief, a second injection may be given. Once fluid resuscitation is complete and the circulating volume is restored, the client may absorb both doses of the narcotic and go back into shock. Therefore, no one in shock should be given intramuscular medications.

When narcotics are appropriate for a client in shock, they are most effective if administered intravenously in small doses. When caring for trauma victims, especially those with massive injury, remember that the extent of the injury does not necessarily coincide with the amount of pain being experienced. Careful assessment is necessary once narcotic administration seems safe (in terms of the client's hemodynamic status). Assess the client's blood pressure more closely after the intravenous administration of narcotics to watch for hypotension.

When caring for clients experiencing shock, carefully make nursing diagnoses concerning pain and impaired gas exchange. Restlessness is an assessment finding common to both and can thus be easily misinterpreted. Too often, clients who are restless, especially trauma victims, are given narcotics because their behavior is incorrectly interpreted as resulting from pain. However, the restlessness frequently is actually due to hypoxia, and narcotics worsen the problem. The decision to administer narcotics is often a nursing decision. It is important to assess the need for these medications carefully. Attention to positioning, splinting of injured areas, breathing techniques, and comfort measures may provide safer and more effective pain relief than narcotics will. (Pain is discussed in detail in Chap. 16.)

Cardiotonic Medications. Medications that improve myocardial contraction are basic in treating those forms of shock that decrease cardiac output (e.g., hypovolemic shock and cardiogenic shock.

- Digitalis. Digitalis is often used if there is evidence of cardiac failure. By strengthening and slowing the heart beat, digitalis supports a weakened heart and may reduce the heart rate to a more normal level. It is not given to clients who are already digitalized.
- Lidocaine, bretyllium, quinidine, and procainamide may treat dysrhythmias that tend to reduce cardiac efficiency. However, these medications do reduce myocardial contractility.
- Atropine may treat bradycardias, which predispose clients to cardiogenic shock.

RENAL SUPPORT

Impaired kidney function and acute renal tubular necrosis may result from inadequate renal tissue perfusion as discussed earlier. In an attempt to prevent acute renal damage, the urine output is monitored with an indwelling catheter, and diuretics (e.g., furosemide) may be given. Correcting metabolic acidosis (see Chap. 15) and using other measures to increase blood volume and improve cardiac output also benefit the kidney as well as other tissues. If tubular necrosis is present, peritoneal dialysis or hemodialysis may be needed until regeneration of functioning renal tubular epithelium occurs. (Chap. 49 discusses management of renal disorders in detail.)

THERMOREGULATION

Even though a person in shock may feel cold and may be hypothermic, do not apply heat to the skin. Heat application dilates peripheral blood vessels and draws blood away from the vital organs (where it is life-sustaining) into the vessels of the skin. This interferes with the body's initial compensatory mechanism of peripheral vasoconstriction. Also, heat increases the body's metabolism. In turn, this increases the need for oxygen and puts an added strain on the heart.

This does not mean that the person is kept in a cold environment. The environment is kept warm because it is important that the person not become chilled. Chilling and shivering require energy expenditure needed to maintain vital functions. Also, chilling contributes to sludging of blood in the microcirculation. Hypothermia slows the heart, increases the likelihood of ventricular fibrillation, and inhibits the body's reparative processes.

NASOGASTRIC SUCTION

Recall that an early physiologic response to shock is a decrease in splanchnic circulation. This reduces blood supply to the stomach and bowel, causing inadequate gastrointestinal tissue perfusion and delayed gastric emptying; thus, vomiting with aspiration of gastric contents into the lung may develop. For this reason and for diagnostic purposes, nasogastric suction is often used during treatment for shock. A double-lumen, 16-French nasogastric tube (Salem sump tube) is usually used for adults. The tube is connected to continuous suction rather than to intermittent suction.

Assess gastric aspirate periodically for blood. Guaiac solution or Hemoccult tablets and reagent check for blood; litmus paper checks the pH to determine the acidity of the stomach. Promptly report new findings of blood or increases in the amount of blood. Antacids are commonly instilled through the tube when the pH is acidic in an attempt to minimize the formation of stress ulcers.

When shock is caused by gastrointestinal bleeding, other nasogastric tubes may be used. For example, if the suspected cause of bleeding is a gastric ulcer, a 36-French Ewald tube may be used. This tube's many large holes facilitate saline lavage and removal of blood clots. If esophageal varices are suspected or present, a Sengstaken-Blakemore tube is often used. This triple-lumen tube exerts pressure on the lower portion of the esophagus and the upper portion of the stomach, where varices are most prominent. Pressure is created by esophageal and gastric balloons inflated with air. Gentle traction is applied to keep the balloons in proper position (see Chap. 53).

It is a nursing responsibility to maintain proper nasogastric suction and to irrigate the tube as prescribed. Remember that aspiration of gastric contents into the lungs may occur even though a nasogastric system is operating properly. Periodic assessment of the client's pulmonary system is essential.

The medical management of shock has been discussed in general. Tables 20-3 to 20-5 identify some of the specific interventions for hypovolemic, cardiogenic, and distributive shock.

TABLE 20-3. Summary of the Management of Hypovolemic Shock

Etiology	Clinical Situation	Intervention*
Blood loss	Massive trauma Gastrointestinal bleeding Ruptured aortic aneurysm Surgery Erosion of vessel due to lesion, tubes, or other devices DIC	Stop external bleeding with direct pressure, pressure dressing, tourniquet (as last resort) Decrease intra-abdominal or retroperitoneal bleeding by applying MAST suit Administer crystalloids Transfuse with fresh whole blood, packed cells, fresh frozen plasma, or platelets if significant improvement does not occur with crystalloid administration; administer crystalloids as well Use nonblood plasma expanders (albumin, hetastarch, dextran) until blood is available Autotransfusion if appropriate
Plasma loss	Burns Accumulation of intra-abdominal fluid Malnutrition Severe dermatitis DIC	Administer albumin, fresh frozen plasma, hetastarch, or dextran along with crystalloids
Crystalloid loss	Dehydration (e.g., diabetic ketoacidosis, heat exhaustion) Protracted vomiting, diarrhea Nasogastric suction	Isotonic or hypotonic saline with electrolytes as needed to maintain normal circulating volume and electrolyte balance

* Assumes that airway management and cardiac monitoring are ongoing.

TABLE 20-4. Summary of Management of Cardiogenic Shock

Etiology	Clinical Situation	Intervention*
Myocardial disease/injury	Acute myocardial infarction Myocardial contusion Cardiomyopathies	Fluid challenge with up to 300 ml of normal saline solution or Ringer's lactate to rule out hypovolemia, unless congestive failure or pulmonary edema is present Insert CVP or pulmonary artery catheter; monitor cardiac output, pulmonary artery pressure, and pulmonary capillary wedge pressure; administer intravenous fluids to maintain left ventricular filling pressure of 15–20 mm Hg Administer dopamine or dobutamine Vasodilators (e.g., sodium nitroprusside) Diuretics (e.g., mannitol or furosemide) Cardiotonics (e.g., digitalis) Glucocorticosteroids† Rotating tourniquets if pulmonary edema present (rarely done) Intra-aortic balloon pump or external counterpulsation device if unresponsive to other therapies
Valvular disease or injury	Ruptured aortic cusp Ruptured papillary muscle Ball thrombus	Same as above: if rapid response does not occur, provide for prompt cardiac surgery
External pressure on the heart interferes with heart filling or emptying	Pericardial tamponade due to trauma, aneurysm, cardiac surgery, pericarditis	Relieve tamponade with ECG-assisted pericardiocentesis; repair surgically if it recurs
	Massive pulmonary embolus	Thrombolytic (streptokinase) or anticoagulant (heparin) therapy
	Tension pneumothorax	Relieve air accumulation with needle thoracostomy or chest tube insertion
Cardiac dysrhythmias	Tachyarrhythmias Bradyarrhythmias Electromechanical dissociation	Treat dysrhythmias; be prepared to initiate CPR, cardiac pacing

* Assumes that airway management and cardiac monitoring are ongoing.
† Controversial.

SURGICAL MANAGEMENT

Surgical interventions that can help in shock states are limited; however, they may be very useful in trauma situations. In hypovolemic shock due to trauma, surgery can be performed in an attempt to control sources of bleeding. Once bleeding has been controlled, interventions aimed at restoring adequate fluid volume will be more effective.

NURSING MANAGEMENT

Assessment

Because a client's condition can change rapidly in shock, frequent nursing assessment is essential. Documentation of progress and response to intervention needs to be concise yet convey the client's status minute by minute.

Initiate a flow sheet containing all pertinent data in an easily read format. This flow sheet must accompany the client at all times. At the bedside, immediate laboratory assessments are essential in treating shock. Blood chemistries, blood gases, oxygen saturations, and electrolytes need to be determined frequently and reported promptly so therapy can be adjusted to the client's rapidly changing physiologic status.

NONINVASIVE AND INVASIVE TECHNIQUES

Various invasive and noninvasive techniques are used to assess a person's status during shock and to evaluate the effectiveness of interventions.

Noninvasive Techniques. Because nurses often provide health care in settings other than hospitals, it helps to know about assessment and monitoring techniques that do not require sophisticated machinery or invade body tissues or cavities. These noninvasive techniques can be performed rapidly and relatively easily, and they require little equipment and are readily observable.

The first step in assessing a person in shock is a general overview, giving attention as necessary to the ABCs—airway, breathing, and circulation. Once the airway is patent, air exchange is adequate, a pulse is present, and the cervical spine is immobilized (if it is a trauma situation), perform a rapid, cursory initial head-to-toe physical assessment. The initial assessment goal is to identify major problems and gross abnormalities. Give further, detailed attention to specific injuries or problems after shock is stabilized.

With the use of physical assessment skills, the following observations should be made:

- Airway patent; presence of noisy respirations, obstructions
- Breathing; respiratory rate and effort
- Circulation; pulse present; skin color and temperature
- Level of consciousness; orientation ×3 (i.e., person, place, time); ability to move extremities, sensation in all extremities; hand-grasps; response to verbal and painful stimuli; pupil size and reaction to light; presence of abnormal posturing; and so on to evaluate neurologic function
- State of hydration and perfusion of the skin (e.g., capillary refill time <3 seconds); condition of mucous membranes, sclera, and conjunctiva; presence of pallor or cyanosis

TABLE 20–5. Summary of Management of Distributive Shock

Etiology	Clinical Setting	Intervention*
Anaphylactic shock	Allergy to food, medicines, dyes, insect bites, or stings	Prepare for surgical management of the airway Decrease further absorption of antigen (e.g., stop intravenous fluid, place tourniquet between injection/sting site and heart if feasible) Epinephrine (1:1,000) 0.3–0.5 ml given intramuscularly, sublingually, or by inhalation, or 0.01 mg/kg *or* Epinephrine (1:10,000) 0.5–10 ml given intravenously slowly over 5–10 minutes Intravenous fluid resuscitation with isotonic solution MAST suit may be useful Diphenhydramine hydrochloride 50–100 mg intramuscularly Aminophylline intravenous drip for bronchospasm Steroids Vasopressors (e.g., norepinephrine, metaraminol bitartrate, high-dosage dopamine) Gastric lavage for ingested antigen Ice pack to injection or sting site Meat tenderizer paste to sting site
Septic shock	Often gram-negative septicemia but also caused by other organisms in debilitated, immunodeficient, or chronically ill clients	Identify origin of sepsis Apply MAST suit Vigorous intravenous fluid resuscitation with normal saline, D_5W, or colloids Antibiotic therapy: in initial phase, until sensitivities are reported, broad-spectrum coverage may include a combination of penicillin, aminoglycoside, and clindamycin or chloramphenicol Dopamine or dobutamine, norepinephrine, metaraminol bitartrate, isoproterenol, digitalis, calcium Naloxone Diphenhydramine hydrochloride Steroids (dexamethasone, methylprednisolone) Temperature control (both hypothermia and hyperthermia are noted) Heparin if DIC develops
Neurogenic (spinal) shock	Spinal anesthesia Spinal cord injury	Treat bradycardia with atropine Vasopressors (e.g., norepinephrine, metaraminol bitartrate, high-dosage dopamine, and phenylephrine may be given
Vaso-vagal reaction	Severe pain Severe emotional stress	Place person in a head-down or recumbent position Give atropine if bradycardia and profound hypotension; eliminate pain

* Assumes airway management and cardiac monitoring are ongoing.

- Fullness of neck veins, which may suggest cardiogenic shock
- Position of trachea; tracheal deviation may indicate tension pneumothorax
- Respiratory pattern; chest wall expansion; chest wall bulges or defects
- Heart sounds
- Presence and location of pain
- Abdominal sounds, distention, rigidity
- Circumference of abdomen or extremities
- Peripheral pulses
- Presence of lacerations, contusions, ecchymosis, petechiae, purpura (also check for bruising over flank area)
- Bone deformities
- Presence of medical alert tags or bracelets

After potentially life-threatening problems are treated, take complete vital signs. It is important to take postural vital signs if it is safe to do so. Do not take postural vital signs if the client has multiple traumatic injuries; if there is evidence of vertebral, pelvic, or femoral fracture; or if hypotension already exists. Clients with postural hypotension should not be sent to the x-ray department for upright films until they are adequately volume resuscitated. If the x-ray films must be taken, clients require constant attendance by a nurse who monitors vital signs, administers intravenous fluids if necessary, and provides guidance to x-ray department personnel regarding movement, positioning, and timing of studies.

Measurement of postural vital signs is indicated under the following circumstances:

History or presence of significant blood loss
Unexplained tachycardia
History of fluid loss (e.g., diarrhea, vomiting, diuretic therapy, or third space loss)
Unexplained syncope
Blunt chest or abdominal trauma
Abdominal pain
Unexplained hypotension

Alternative Methods of Obtaining Blood Pressure. Often when a client is in shock it is difficult to hear the BP with a standard stethoscope. Two commonly used techniques to obtain BP measurements are palpation of radial or brachial pulse during deflation of the BP cuff and use of a Doppler instrument (see Chap. 46). When palpation is used, the first palpable pulse noted during deflation of the cuff is the systolic BP. Document the BP as such (e.g., 90/palp). A Doppler amplifies arterial and venous pulsations by ultrasonography. Various Doppler probes are available and are used instead of a stethoscope to measure the BP. The systolic BP is easily heard by placing the probe over the brachial artery after applying transmission gel. The diastolic BP is not readily obtainable when the Doppler is used.

For clarity and accuracy, document the method by which BP readings are taken (in addition to the readings themselves) and if palpation or a Doppler monitor is used. This is important because these readings may be higher or lower than those obtained in the standard way with a cuff and stethoscope. Likewise, document whether readings are obtained by automatic BP machines even though readings from these machines may not differ from those taken in the standard way.

Direct measurement of arterial BP by use of an arterial line often is done during shock. Discussion of arterial lines is found in Chapter 42.

An accurate core temperature measurement is important in assessing a person in shock. Sometimes an indwelling flexible rectal probe connected to a continuous display monitor is more accurate and less traumatic than are intermittent rectal temperature measurements with a standard thermometer. Core temperature can also be obtained if the client has a thermodilution (Swan-Ganz) catheter in place.

Oral temperature measurement is not accurate or safe. During shock, the buccal mucosa is poorly perfused, and the client should be receiving oxygen by mask or nasal prongs. (Because clients in shock are hypoxemic, the procedure of removing the oxygen long enough to obtain an oral temperature is not routinely recommended.)

For assessment and evaluation purposes, electrical activity of the heart needs to be continuously monitored in all clients in shock, regardless of age. Nurses caring for clients experiencing shock need to be able to initiate cardiac monitoring, recognize cardiac dysrhythmias, and initiate treatment for any potentially lethal dysrhythmias that occur (see Chap. 43).

During the initial resuscitation period, it may be more appropriate to place the ECG monitor electrodes on the client's shoulders rather than on the chest. This placement does not interfere with chest film findings. Also, it allows better access to the chest for thoracic procedures such as insertion of chest tubes, pericardiocentesis, and CVP line placement. Once the client is stabilized, the monitor electrodes may be moved to the chest.

Invasive Techniques

Hemodynamic Monitoring. Measurement of the central venous pressure (CVP) is one hemodynamic technique that may be used in initial shock management, especially with hypovolemic shock. However, because the CVP is of limited value, peripheral intra-arterial lines or a pulmonary artery catheter is inserted as soon as possible. Peripheral arterial catheters are commonly used in shock to measure arterial BP and mean arterial pressure and to obtain blood samples for chemical and blood gas analysis. These catheters are usually placed in the radial and brachial arteries. Pulmonary artery and pulmonary capillary wedge pressure measurements are monitored to assess left-sided heart function and to guide fluid administration. These pressures are measured through a Swan-Ganz catheter. The pulmonary capillary wedge pressure corresponds to the left ventricular end-diastolic pressure. This is the pressure in the heart's left ventricle just before contraction. A rise in this pressure in a client with cardiogenic shock may indicate left-sided heart failure. A low value in a client with hypovolemic shock may indicate that volume replacement is needed. In a client with septic shock, lower values would be expected during the warm phase and higher values during the cold phase.

Depending on the type of Swan-Ganz catheter used, additional measurements may be obtained. Some catheters have a fiberoptic tip that allows measurement of the saturation of hemoglobin with oxygen in the venous blood. This venous saturation measurement is abbreviated SvO_2. The SvO_2 is measured in the pulmonary artery, just before the blood's reoxygenation in the lungs. This reading gives an average of the tissue's uptake or use of oxygen in the body. The normal range for SvO_2 is 60 to 80 per cent. When the SvO_2 falls below 60 per cent, it may indicate either decreased arterial oxygenation or increased tissue oxygen demand. If the SvO_2 is greater than 80 per cent, the indication, in relation to shock, is that the oxygen is unable to reach the tissues or to be extracted by the tissues even if the oxygen can reach them.

Most Swan-Ganz catheters also have a thermistor bead just proximal to the balloon. This may be used to determine cardiac output by a thermodilution technique. A fourth lumen opens at the level of the right atrium, and CVP measurements can be obtained through this lumen.

Cardiac Output Monitoring. Cardiac output, measured in liters per minute, is the amount of blood pumped by the left ventricle into the aorta each minute. During shock, cardiac output may be decreased because of myocardial damage resulting from a myocardial infarction or, in hypovolemic shock, from inadequate volume replacement.

Because of the widespread use of Swan-Ganz catheters and the ease of performing measurements, cardiac outputs are used in managing all types of shock. These measurements assess overall cardiac function and function of the heart's left ventricle. Factors that may alter cardiac output include heart rate, peripheral resistance, age, body size, exercise, and (in persons with cardiac problems) decreased filling or emptying of the left ventricle.

Cardiac index is the cardiac output divided by the body surface area. Cardiac output as a separate reading does not take into account the amount of tissue that needs to be perfused. By figuring body size into the calculation, a more accurate assessment is obtained.

Urine Output Monitoring. An indwelling urinary catheter is a simple means of monitoring a client during shock. Continuously measuring urine flow provides important information about peripheral blood flow and kidney function. Because the amount of urine excreted during shock is often very small, it is important to have an accurate, calibrated urine collector. In some settings, the catheter may be attached to a urimeter collector or to a more complex electric urimeter.

Urine volume changes can be highly important as an index of the success or failure of therapy. Minimal or absent urine output indicates treatment is not successful. Increasing urine output is a favorable sign. Assess the client's urine output routinely and record it at least every hour.

Nursing Intervention

NURSING DIAGNOSIS

Some potential nursing diagnoses for the client in shock are listed in Table 20-6.

Planning: Expected Outcomes. Nursing care of the client with shock is complex. Frequent reassessment of the client and nursing activities is essential because the client's status often changes rapidly. Specific nursing and medical interventions vary according to individual needs and the setting in which care is delivered (e.g., emergency room versus intensive care unit). However, four major outcomes of care are desired:

tissue perfusion and cellular function return to normal,
metabolic demands are met,
further injury is prevented, and
coping of the individual and significant others is effective.

TABLE 20-6. Potential Nursing Diagnoses for Client in Shock

Airway Clearance, Ineffective
Breathing Pattern, Ineffective
Gas Exchange, Impaired
Tissue Perfusion, Altered: cerebral, cardiopulmonary, renal, gastrointestinal, peripheral
Decreased Cardiac Output
Fluid Volume Deficit
Nutrition, Altered: Less than Body Requirements
Constipation
Activity Intolerance
Physical Mobility, Impaired
Injury, High Risk for
Sensory/Perceptual Alterations: visual, auditory, kinesthetic, gustatory, tactile
Sleep Pattern Disturbance
Skin Integrity, Impaired
Skin Integrity, High Risk for Impaired
Self-Care Deficit: feeding, bathing/hygiene, dressing/grooming, toileting
Body Image Disturbance
Self-Esteen Disturbance
Role Performance, Altered
Personal Identity Disturbance
Anxiety
Fear
Pain
Communication, Impaired Verbal
Spiritual Distress (Distress of the Human Spirit)
Thought Processes, Altered
Family Coping, Compromised, Ineffective
Family Processes, Altered
Grieving, Anticipatory

Implementation. Other nursing considerations in caring for clients in shock include

- Continuous assessment of the client. Cardiovascular and respiratory changes can occur rapidly, and intervention must be promptly adjusted accordingly. Document observations clearly and concisely.
- Help the client (and family) to feel physically and emotionally comfortable. For the client in shock, this helps reduce the physical need for oxygen and nutrients and promotes rest.
- Facilitate the expression of concerns and questions by the person and family. For example, try to reduce the client's fears and anxieties about what is happening and about the equipment being used.
- Keep equipment and supplies (e.g., suction, emergency drugs) available and in working order.
- Implement appropriate, planned nursing interventions to prevent complications that can develop from enforced immobilization.
- Provide adequate pain relief, because pain intensifies shock. Base this intervention on careful assessment.

A client in shock is extremely ill and may die. In addition, the stress of the situation is compounded by emergency medical treatment with all the people, equipment, and movement this entails. During shock management, nurses have numerous delegated medical care activities to attend to. However, there must be sufficient nursing resources to provide psychosocial care (e.g., reassurance, emotional support) to the client and family. All of these people involved may be frightened, anxious, perhaps confused, and certainly very dependent.

Keep the client's family informed of what is happening. They need information on which to base decisions. Because of their anxiety, the nurse may need to calmly repeat information several times. Remember that the client and significant others may be experiencing "psychological shock." Often they need (and greatly appreciate) opportunities to discuss with care providers their important concerns.

Do not keep loved ones away from the client unnecessarily. There may be times when, because of limited space, they have to wait in another room for a while. However, they should not be kept away long. They should not be asked to leave their loved one without being given a reasonable explanation of why it is necessary.

A client experiencing shock requires emotional support. When caught up in the sudden drama of an emergency or critical care, health professionals sometimes forget that the experience and setting are often new and very frightening for the client. Unfortunately, "dehumanization" of the client may occasionally occur during the rush of emergency treatment. Whether a client appears to be conscious or not, always explain what is happening. Keep the atmosphere as quiet and orderly as possible. Eliminate unnecessary chatter. Commonly, recovered clients remember hearing what was said and were aware of what happened to them even though they seemed unconscious.

Among nurses' greatest responsibilities are those of providing support, comfort, and advocacy to clients receiving care and to their significant others. In nursing clients who are critically ill and experiencing shock, this is very important.

Evaluation

The expected outcomes should be evaluated frequently; revisions in the plan of care may be required hourly to maintain tissue perfusion.

POST-HOSPITAL CARE

Shock must be fully resolved before a client is transferred or discharged (unless the client is being transported for the treatment of shock). Clients who have survived shock find that recovery of the precipitating problem is delayed. They may also experience some feelings of confusion, depression, or grief when they realize that they lived through a very critical illness.

Summary

This chapter has discussed shock under three major classifications: hypovolemic, cardiogenic, and distributive. The pathophysiology, complications, and medical and nursing management have been presented. Shock is a critical condition with a potentially high mortality rate. Early diagnosis and intervention are necessary for the best possible outcomes.

Bibliography

1. Aguilar, M. M., & Hartley-Winkler, M. (1990). CAVHD during extracorporeal membrane oxygenation. *Dialysis and Transplantation, 19*(8), 436–439.
2. Barone, J. E., & Snyder, A. B. (1991). Treatment strategies in shock: Use of oxygen transport measurements. *Heart and Lung, 20*(1), 81–85.
3. Bell, T. N. (1990). Disseminated intravascular coagulation and shock: Multisystem crisis in the critically ill. *Critical Care Nursing Clinics of North America, 2*(2), 255–268.
4. Blansfield, J. (1990). Emergency autotransfusion in hypovolemia. *Critical Care Nursing Clinics of North America, 2*(2), 195–199.
5. Burns, K. M. (1990). Vasoactive drug therapy in shock. *Critical Care Nursing Clinics of North America, 2*(2), 167–178.
6. Charette, A. L. (1989). Bridging the gap between hemodynamics and monitoring. *Critical Care Nursing Clinics of North America, 1*(3), 539–546.
7. Collins, A. S. (1990). Gastrointestinal complication in shock. *Critical Care Nursing Clinics of North America, 2*(2), 269–277.
8. Daily, E. K. (1989). Use of hemodynamics to differentiate pathophysiologic causes of cardiogenic shock. *Critical Care Nursing Clinics of North America, 1*(3), 589–602.
9. Gardner, P. E. (1989). Cardiac output: Theory, technique, troubleshooting. *Critical Care Nursing Clinics of North America, 1*(3), 577–587.
10. Gawlinski, A. (1989). Saving the cardiogenic shock patient. *Nursing, 19*(12), 34–41.

11. Goran, S. F. (1989). Vascular complication of the patient undergoing intra-aortic balloon pumping. *Critical Care Nursing Clinics of North America, 1*(3), 459-467.
12. Houston, M. C. (1990). Pathophysiology of shock. *Critical Care Nursing Clinics of North America, 2*(2), 143-149.
13. Hoyt, N. J. (1990). Preventing septic shock: Infection control in the intensive care unit. *Critical Care Nursing Clinics of North America, 2*(2), 287-297.
14. Jillings, C. R. (1990). Shock: Psychosocial needs of the patients and family. *Critical Care Nursing Clinics of North America, 2*(2), 325-330.
15. Karch, A. M., & Boyd, E. H. (1989). *Handbook of drugs and the nursing process.* Philadelphia: J. B. Lippincott.
16. Lancaster, L. E., & Rice, V. (1990). Nurse care planning: Overview and application to the patient in shock. *Critical Care Nursing Clinics of North America, 2*(2), 279-286.
17. Lancaster, L. E. (1990). Renal response to shock. *Critical Care Nursing Clinics of North America, 2*(2), 221-233.
18. Lekander, B. J., & Cerra, F. B. (1990). The syndrome of multiple organ failure. *Critical Care Nursing Clinics of North America, 2*(2), 331-342.
19. Ley, S. J. (1988). Fluid therapy following intracardiac operation. *Critical Care Nurse, 8*(1), 26-36.
20. Lorenz, A. (1989). Lactic acidosis: A nursing challenge. *Critical Care Nurse, 9*(4), 64-73.
21. Martin, E., Harris, A., Johnson, N., et al.: (1989). Autotransfusion systems. *Critical Care Nurse, 9*(7), 65-73.
22. McCormac, M. (1990). Managing hemorrhagic shock. *American Journal of Nursing, 90*(8), 22-27.
23. Mims, B. C. (1989). Physiologic rationale of SvO_2 monitoring. *Critical Care Nursing Clinics of North America, 1*(3), 619-628.
24. Mohrman, D. E., & Heller, L. J. (1991). *Cardiovascular physiology.* New York: McGraw-Hill.
25. Perkins, S. B., & Kennally, K. M. (1989). The hidden danger of internal hemorrhage. *Nursing, 19*(7), 34-41.
26. Phoenix, J. (1990). Low blood pressure: how to investigate this ominous sign. *Nursing, 20*(11), 34-39.
27. Rice, V. (1991). Shock, a clinical syndrome: An update. Part 1. *Critical Care Nurse, 11*(4), 20-27.
28. Rice, V. (1991). Shock, a clinical syndrome: An update. Part 2. The stages of shock. *Critical Care Nurse, 11*(5), 74-82.
29. Rice, V. (1991). Shock, a clinical syndrome: An update. Part 3. Therapeutic management. *Critical Care Nurse, 11*(6), 34-39.
30. Rice, V. (1991). Shock, a clinical syndrome: An update. Part 4. Nursing care of the shock patient. *Critical Care Nurse, 11*(7), 28-40.
31. Roach, A. C. (1990). Antibiotic therapy in septic shock. *Critical Care Nursing Clinics of North America, 2*(2), 179-186.
32. Robins, E. V. (1990). Burn shock. *Critical Care Nursing Clinics of North America, 2*(2), 299-307.
33. Scherer, P. (1989). Shock trauma. *American Journal of Nursing, 89*(11), 1440-1445.
34. Schott, K. E. (1990). Intra-aortic balloon counterpulsation as a therapy for shock. *Critical Care Nursing Clinics of North America, 2*(2), 187-193.
35. Schumann, L. L., & Remington, M. A. (1990). The use of naloxone in treating endotoxic shock. *Critical Care Nurse, 10*(2), 63-71.
36. Siskind, J. (1990). Handling hemorrhage wisely. *Nursing, 20*(3), 137-143.
37. Stroud, M., et al. (1990). Cellular and humoral mediators of sepsis syndrome. *Critical Care Nursing Clinics of North America, 2*(2), 151-160.
38. Summers, G. (1990). The clinical and hemodynamic presentation of the shock patient. *Critical Care Nursing Clinics of North America, 2*(2), 161-166.
39. Teplitz, L. (1989). Clinical close-up on atropine. *Nursing, 19*(11), 44-47.
40. Teplitz, L. (1989). Clinical close-up on dopamine. *Nursing, 19*(12), 50-53.
41. Teplitz, L. (1989). Clinical close-up on epinephrine. *Nursing, 19*(10), 50-53.
42. Vaughan, P., & Brooks, C. (1990). Adult respiratory distress syndrome: A complication of shock. *Critical Care Nursing Clinics of North America, 2*(2), 235-253.
43. Young, L. M. (1990). DIC: The insidious killer. *Critical Care Nurse, 10*(10), 26-33.

Chapter 21

Basic Concepts of Neoplastic Disorders

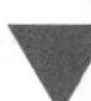

BASIC PRINCIPLES

Caring for clients with cancer is one of the most significant tasks facing health care professionals today. Currently, cancer is the second leading cause of death in the United States, exceeded only by cardiovascular disease. Cancer claims nearly 500,000 lives per year and disrupts many thousands more. It will strike at least one in four people in this country and about one in three will survive the encounter. Within the United States and throughout the world, cancer has a tremendous economic and sociologic impact. It influences people in every realm of their lives: physical, emotional, spiritual, cognitive, social, and economic.

In the past decade, cancer research has made significant strides toward solving the mysteries of cancer causation and the many problems of cancer treatment. The National Cancer Institute has set a target for the year 2000 to reduce the nation's cancer mortality to 50 per cent or less.

Nurses in all areas of practice are likely to come into contact with people who are ill with cancer, and, therefore, must be familiar with its diagnosis and treatment. More important, the nurse is often the professional in closest contact with clients and is in a unique position to teach prevention and to practice early detection.

The first task in understanding the complex disease of cancer is being able to define some commonly used terms associated with the disease. It is vital that both the client and the health care provider have a mutual understanding of the terms associated with cancer so the disease and its treatment can be discussed without confusion.

The word cancer, abbreviated Ca, is a term that frightens most people. Cancer is synonymous with the term malignant neoplasm. Other terms that suggest malignant neoplasm include tumor, malignancy, carcinoma, and aberrant cell growth. Strictly speaking, these words are not interchangeable.

The term cancer is a collective term describing a large group of diseases characterized by uncontrolled growth and spread of abnormal cells. This group of diseases (1) arises from different tissues and organs, (2) differs greatly from one another in appearance and growth, (3) may follow very different courses of development in their hosts, and (4) responds differently to the variety of therapies applied to them.

The word neoplasm is derived from the Greek word *neos*, which means new, and *plasia*, which means growth of new tissue. Therefore, a neoplasm is defined as an abnormal new growth of tissue that serves no useful purpose and may harm the host organism.

A neoplasm can be either benign or malignant. Benign is defined as a usually harmless growth that does not spread or invade other tissue. Malignant is defined as a harmful tumor, capable of spread and invasion of other tissues far removed from the site of origin. Other important terms can be found in Table 21 – 1.

Cancer is a disease of the cell in which the normal mechanisms of control of growth and proliferation are disturbed.

TABLE 21 – 1. Cancer Terminology

Terms	Definitions
Anaplastic	Tumor cells that are completely undifferentiated and bear no resemblance to cells of tissues of their origin
Hyperplasia	An increase in the number of normal cells in a normal arrangement in a tissue or organ. Usually leads to an increase in the size or part and an increase in functional activity
Metaplasia	The replacement of one type of fully differentiated cell by another fully differentiated cell in another part of the body where the second cell type does not normally occur
Dysplasia	An alteration in the size, shape, and organization of differentiated cells. Cells lose their regularity and show variability in size and shape, usually in response to an irritant. It reverts to normal when the irritant is removed but may transform to a neoplasia
Metastasis	The ability of neoplastic cells to spread from the original site of the tumor to distant organs, spreading as the same cell type as the original neoplastic tissue
Carcinoma	A form of cancer that is composed of epithelial cells that tend to infiltrate surrounding tissues and may eventually spread to distant sites
Oncogene	Cancer genes that are altered versions of normal genes.
Proto-oncogenes	Repressed oncogenes existing in normal cells which can be activated by many different factors and cause the host cell to become malignant
Tumor	Usually synonymous with neoplasm

The Challenge of Cancer Nursing

For too many people, the word cancer means death. As recently as 20 years ago, cancer was usually incurable. Today, because of advances in early diagnosis and treatment, more and more people are living after the diagnosis has been made. In fact, more than 5 million Americans with a history of cancer are alive today. It is estimated that more than 1 million Americans will be diagnosed with cancer during 1991, and during the same year more than 500,000 Americans will die from their disease. The figures are large and many are affected by the experience of cancer and its sequelae.

Nurses are involved in all phases of the cancer experience: prevention, detection, diagnosis, treatment, rehabilitation, survivorship, and palliative and terminal care. Cancer nursing skills are vital in all health care settings because clients are seen in the home, office, clinic, acute care setting, rehabilitation setting, and hospice.

Perhaps the greatest role any nurse can play is by assisting individuals in the prevention and early detection of cancer. Nurses meet a variety of people daily (family, friends, coworkers), and there is always an opportunity to teach and encourage good health habits. Nurses can and must take advantage of time spent with the general public to engage in health promotion teaching and encourage individuals to follow cancer prevention guidelines.

The nurse, whether a generalist or a specialist, assists in caring for clients in all phases of the cancer experience. Through teaching, using clinical expertise, research, and supporting the client, the nurse delivers the highest quality of care possible to a group of clients requiring intensive nursing services.

Cancer occurs in all strata of our society. It strikes people of all ages, socioeconomic and cultural backgrounds, and both sexes. It is the second leading cause of death in the United States, affecting one in three to four persons. Nurses are in the unique position to influence and care for clients in all phases of the cancer experience. Rather than being seen as a uniformly terminal illness, cancer is now seen as more of a chronic illness, or at least one with a long trajectory.

Epidemiology

Epidemiology is the study of the distribution and determinants of diseases and health problems in human populations. The goal of an epidemiologic study is the control or prevention of the health problem. An epidemiologic approach to cancer evaluates patterns of the disease, identifies possible causes, and infers relationships between patterns of disease and determining factors. Although the etiologic factors (causes) of many cancers remain unknown, some epidemiologic studies have helped to identify those factors that underlie theories of causation. The knowledge gained from epidemiologic findings gives the nurse greater insight into the magnitude of cancer risk or complications.

The National Cancer Institute (NCI) established the Surveillance, Epidemiology, and End Results (SEER) Program in 1973 as a way to report population-based data in site-specific incidences of cancer, mortality, and survival rates. This report is based on a sample of 12 per cent of the population in this country and includes six large cities around the country (San Francisco, Oakland, Detroit, New Orleans, Atlanta, and Seattle). It also contains data from six states (New Jersey, Utah, Connecticut, New Mexico, Hawaii, and Iowa) and the Commonwealth of Puerto Rico. This is an ongoing project from NCI and provides a great deal of information about different geographic areas and ethnic groups.

Incidence

The *incidence rate* for cancer reflects the number of new cases occurring in a given population at risk during a specified time. The incidence gives a perspective on the current magnitude of the problem and provides a source for establishing future priorities in cancer control programs (Fig. 21-1). Factors that influence cancer incidence and deaths include sex, age, geographic location, socioeconomic status, ethnic background, personal habits (including diet), occupation, and personal and family histories of cancer or precancerous conditions.

The incidence of reported cases of cancer has been increasing steadily since 1900. There are at least three reasons for this apparent increase. First, all diagnostic methods are more precise today than in the past. Thus, people who would have died from what were believed to be unknown causes or pulmonary hemorrhage in the past are now correctly diagnosed with cancer. Second, the gathering, analysis, and publication of cancer statistics have become more sophisticated over the years. Formerly, many cases of cancer were not included in the yearly reports on cancer morbidity and mortality. Finally, people are living longer than even a few decades ago. Older adults are at greater risk for many cancers; therefore, the incidence of cancer is higher now than when people died younger. Therefore, the apparent rise in the incidence of cancer is somewhat misleading. It may simply reflect more precise diagnostic and statistical methods combined with the trend toward a longer lifespan.

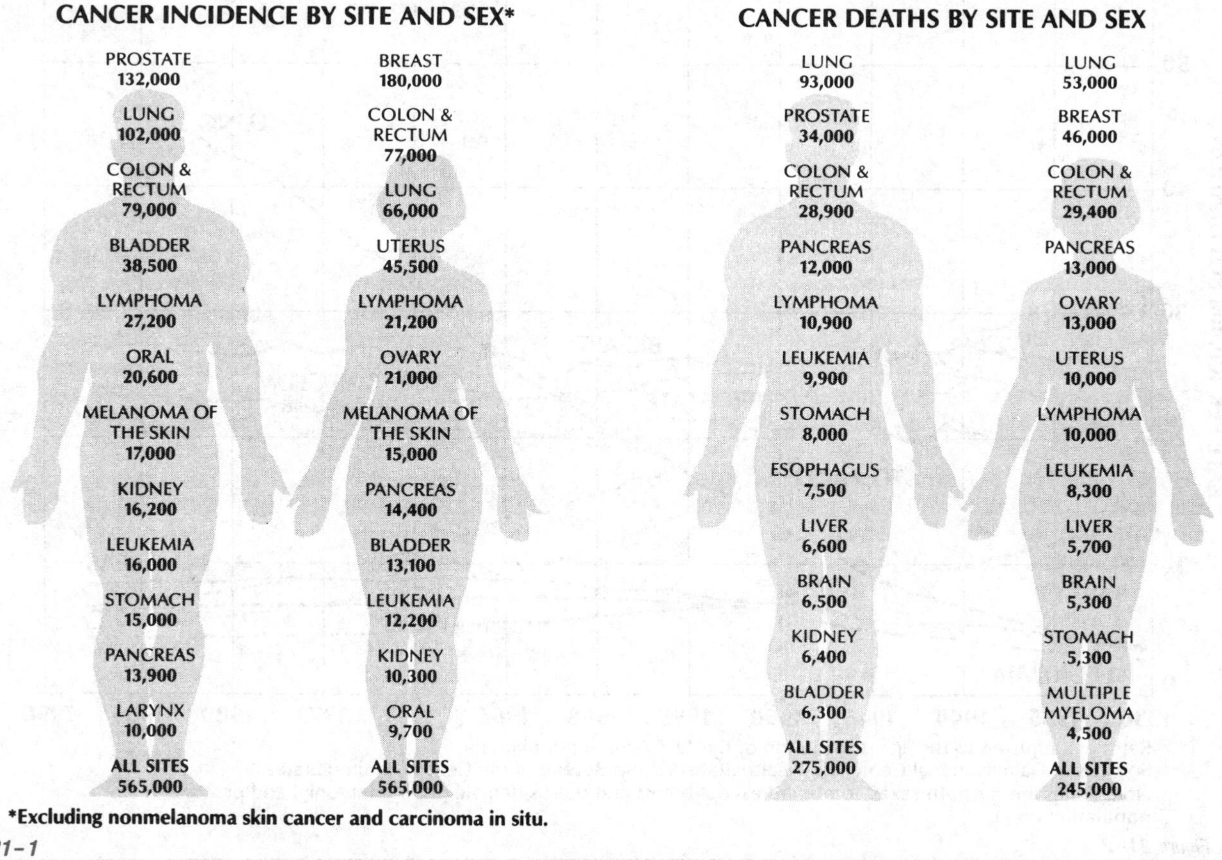

CANCER INCIDENCE BY SITE AND SEX*

PROSTATE 132,000	BREAST 180,000
LUNG 102,000	COLON & RECTUM 77,000
COLON & RECTUM 79,000	LUNG 66,000
BLADDER 38,500	UTERUS 45,500
LYMPHOMA 27,200	LYMPHOMA 21,200
ORAL 20,600	OVARY 21,000
MELANOMA OF THE SKIN 17,000	MELANOMA OF THE SKIN 15,000
KIDNEY 16,200	PANCREAS 14,400
LEUKEMIA 16,000	BLADDER 13,100
STOMACH 15,000	LEUKEMIA 12,200
PANCREAS 13,900	KIDNEY 10,300
LARYNX 10,000	ORAL 9,700
ALL SITES 565,000	**ALL SITES 565,000**

***Excluding nonmelanoma skin cancer and carcinoma in situ.**

CANCER DEATHS BY SITE AND SEX

LUNG 93,000	LUNG 53,000
PROSTATE 34,000	BREAST 46,000
COLON & RECTUM 28,900	COLON & RECTUM 29,400
PANCREAS 12,000	PANCREAS 13,000
LYMPHOMA 10,900	OVARY 13,000
LEUKEMIA 9,900	UTERUS 10,000
STOMACH 8,000	LYMPHOMA 10,000
ESOPHAGUS 7,500	LEUKEMIA 8,300
LIVER 6,600	LIVER 5,700
BRAIN 6,500	BRAIN 5,300
KIDNEY 6,400	STOMACH 5,300
BLADDER 6,300	MULTIPLE MYELOMA 4,500
ALL SITES 275,000	**ALL SITES 245,000**

▲ *Figure 21-1*

Cancer incidence and deaths by site and sex—1992 estimates. (From American Cancer Society [1992]. *Cancer facts and figures—1992.* Atlanta, GA: American Cancer Society.)

Mortality

The *mortality rate* is the number of deaths that occur in the population at risk in a specific period (Fig. 21–2). The data used to determine mortality rates are from death certificates. Although there is a chance some of that information is inaccurate or incomplete, it is a solid beginning in helping describe and determine the number of deaths attributed to cancer.

Survival

Generally, clinicians consider the client who is alive and without evidence of the disease for at least 5 years after diagnosis of cancer as cured. Although the 5-year determination is arbitrary, in many cancers, this waiting period decreases the probability that the condition will recur or spread.

Survival data for the most common cancer sites are displayed in Figure 21–3. A 5-year relative survival rate of 50 per cent is expected in many of the cancers listed. The lower survival in blacks for most cancer classifications is striking. This difference may be due to a variety of factors, including limited access to health care, no or little insurance, no primary health care provider, homelessness, poverty, lack of knowledge regarding early diagnosis and treatment, attitude toward primary and secondary prevention, and greater exposure to carcinogens.

Survival analysis is used to evaluate the effectiveness of cancer therapies, determine whether or not the interval between disease onset and treatment initiation could be modified to reduce cancer morbidity or mortality, and develop hypotheses regarding cancer risk factors.

Trends

The change in 5-year relative survival rates can be seen in Table 21–2. Although the 5-year survival rate has increased from 36 to 45 per cent from 1960 to 1986 when races are combined, not all cancers have seen this 9 per cent survival increase. In fact, cancer of the oral cavity and pharynx, liver, pancreas, esophagus,

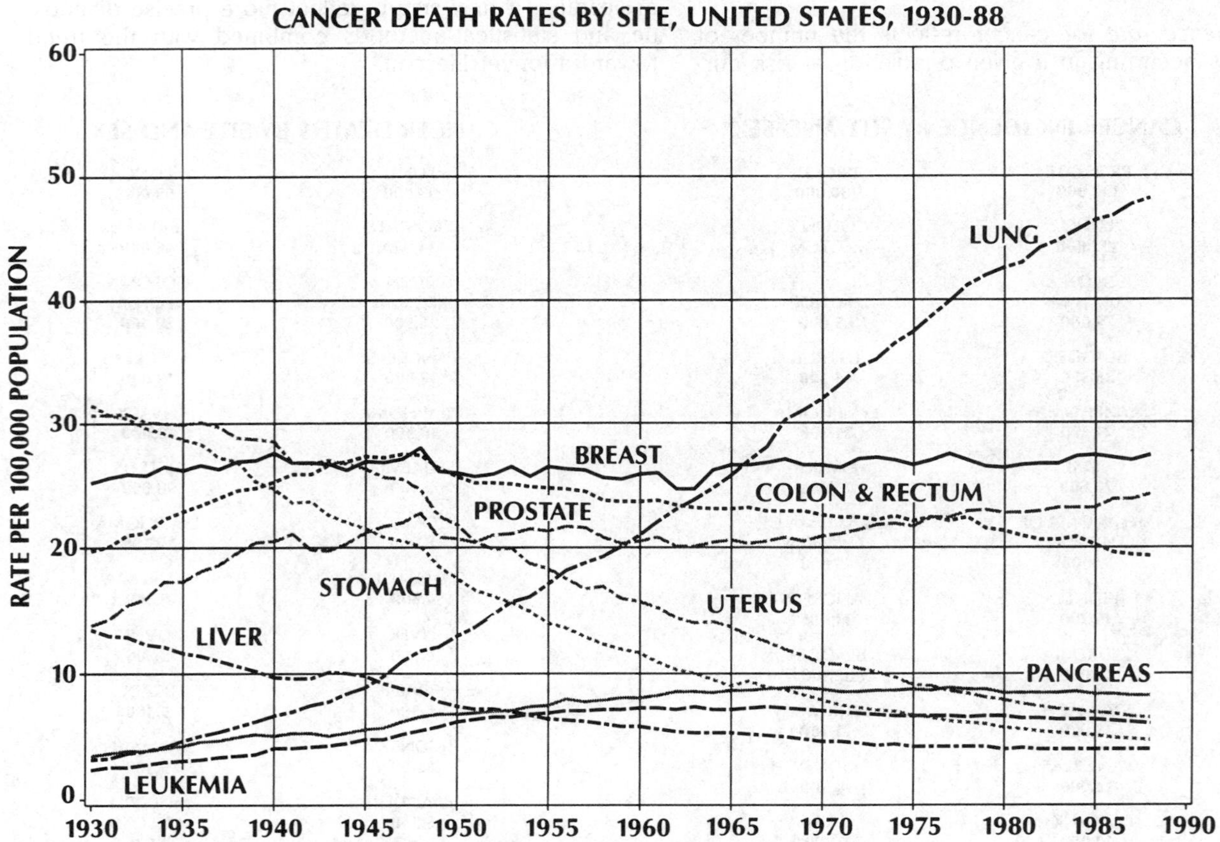

▲ *Figure 21–2*

Cancer death rates by site, United States, 1930 to 1988. (From American Cancer Society [1992]. *Cancer facts and figures—1992.* Atlanta, GA: American Cancer Society.)

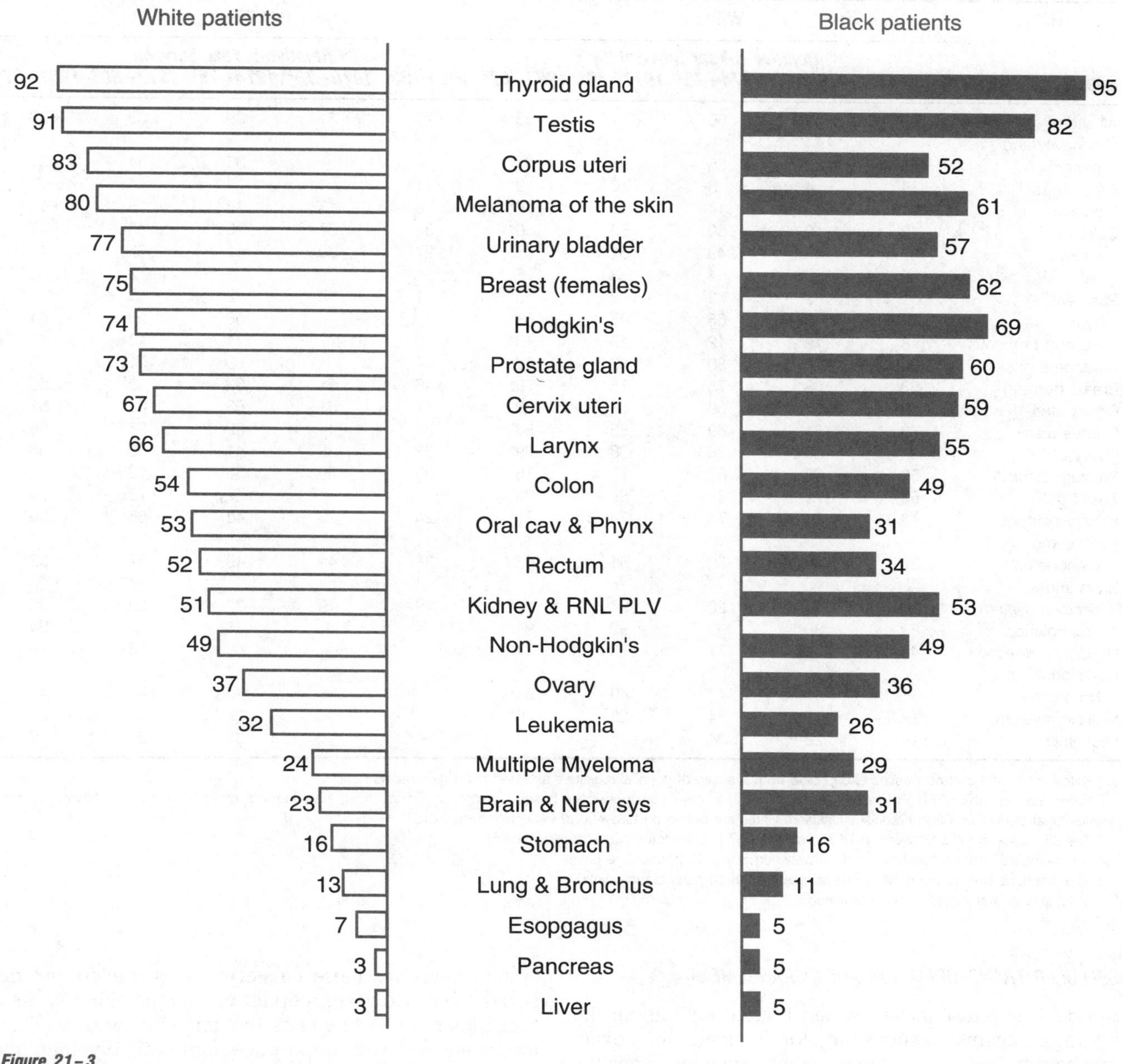

▲ *Figure 21-3*

Five-year relative survival rates. (From Greenwald, P., & Sandik, E. J. [Eds.] [1986]. Surveillance in cancer control objectives for the nation: 1985–2000. NCI Monograph no. 2. Washington, DC: United States Government Printing Office.)

and colon have decreased or increased less than 5 per cent. At the same time, the survival rate for Hodgkin's disease and prostate, testicular, and bladder cancers has increased by at least 25 per cent.

Despite significant advances in detection, diagnosis, and treatment, cancer continues to be a significant health problem. It is believed that 75 per cent of all cancers could be prevented if primary prevention (such as stopping smoking) was initiated against known causative factors by the government, industry, and the public.[44] Prevention and early detection of cancer must be a high priority to further decrease cancer morbidity and mortality rates.

Pathogenesis

The exact causes and methods of the development of cancer are unknown. The following two theories are common explanations for the development of cancer.

TABLE 21-2. Trends in Survival by Site of Cancer, by Race: Cases Diagnosed in 1960-63, 1970-73, 1974-76, 1977-80, 1981-87

	White					Black				
	Relative 5-Year Survival					Relative 5-Year Survival				
Site	1960-63[1]	1970-73[1]	1974-76[2]	1977-80[2]	1981-87[2]	1960-63[1]	1970-73[1]	1974-76[2]	1977-80[2]	1981-87[2]
All sites	39	43	50	51	53*	27	31	39	39	38
Oral cavity and pharynx	45	43	55	54	54	–	–	35	34	31
Esophagus	4	4	5	6	9*	1	4	4	4	6*
Stomach	11	13	14	16	16*	8	13	16	16	17
Colon	43	49	50	53	58*	34	37	46	48	47
Rectum	38	45	49	51	55*	27	30	41	37	44
Liver	2	3	4	3	5	–	–	1	3	5
Pancreas	1	2	3	2	3*	1	2	2	5	4
Larynx	53	62	66	67	68	–	–	59	58	54
Lung and bronchus	8	10	12	13	13*	5	7	11	12	11
Melanoma of skin	60	68	80	82	82*	–	–	69†	51‡	70
Breast (female)	63	68	75	75	78*	46	51	63	63	63
Cervix uteri	58	64	69	68	68	47	61	63	62	57
Corpus uteri	73	81	89	86	84*	31	44	62	56	56
Ovary	32	36	36	38	39*	32	32	41	40	36
Prostate gland	50	63	67	72	76*	35	55	58	62	63*
Testis	63	72	79	88	93*	–	–	77†	73‡	94
Urinary bladder	53	61	74	76	79*	24	36	48	55	59*
Kidney and renal pelvis	37	46	52	51	53	38	44	49	57	52
Brain and nervous system	18	20	22	24	24*	19	19	27	28	33
Thyroid gland	83	86	92	92	94	–	–	87	92	94
Hodgkin's disease	40	67	71	73	77*	–	–	68	73	74
Non-Hodgkin's lymphoma	31	41	47	49	51*	–	–	48	49	45
Multiple myeloma	12	19	24	25	26*	–	–	27	32	28
Leukemia	14	22	34	36	36*	–	–	31	30	29

[1] Rates are based on End Results Group data from a series of hospital registries and one population-based registry.

[2] Rates are from the SEER Program. They are based on data from population-based registries in Connecticut, New Mexico, Utah, Iowa, Hawaii, Atlanta, Detroit, Seattle-Puget Sound, and San Francisco-Oakland. Rates are based on follow-up of patients through 1988.

* The difference in rates between 1974-76 and 1981-87 is statistically significant ($p < 0.05$).

† The standard error of the survival rate is between 5 and 10 percentage points.

‡ The standard error of the survival rate is greater than 10 percentage points.

– Valid survival rate could not be calculated.

CELLULAR TRANSFORMATION AND DERANGEMENT

Although scientists have learned a great deal about the etiologic agents responsible for cancer, the exact mechanism by which these agents transform healthy cells into neoplastic cells remains obscure. One accepted premise is that cancer develops as a result of genetic alteration caused by one or more etiologic agents, resulting in uncontrolled cellular reproduction and growth. When a defective cell divides, the new cells contain the defective genetic code within the DNA. Over time, defective cells divide and multiply, and the malignancy grows.

IMMUNE RESPONSE FAILURE

Researchers are actively pursuing the role of immunity in preventing, controlling, and treating cancer. According to the immune theory of cancer control, cancer cells continually form within the body. The immune system perceives these cancer cells as foreign and destroys them. However, certain conditions either cause a breakdown or overwhelm the immune system. Thus, the malignant cells reproduce more rapidly than the immune system can destroy them.

Supporting this theory is the data from postoperative heart and kidney transplant clients. These clients are intentionally immunosuppressed to prevent the rejection of their transplanted organs. The risk of developing cancer is at least 80 times greater among clients who have undergone transplantation surgery than among the population as a whole. Further support for this theory comes from data on clients with AIDS. These clients have a much higher incidence of a number of cancers such as non-Hodgkin's lymphoma and Kaposi's sarcoma. The immunodeficiency of acquired immune deficiency syndrome (AIDS) makes these clients more susceptible to cancers.

Investigators are trying to determine whether the immune system controls the spontaneous regression of tumors, a mysterious phenomenon. Spontaneous regression of cancers occurs in about one out of every 100,000 cases. The role of the immune system in bringing about this seemingly miraculous change remains a provocative and unanswered question.

Etiology

There are approximately 150 types of cancers found in humans, and there are probably at least 500 different cancer-causing agents. Researchers suspect that cancer results from multiple agents working together.

VIRUSES

The study of viruses as carcinogens is one of the most rapidly advancing areas in cancer research today. Researchers now have proof that viruses cause cancer in animals.

The study of viruses in tumors has led researchers to discover oncogenes. Oncogenes are small segments of genetic DNA that have the ability to transform normal cells into malignant cells, independently or incorporated with a virus.

Viruses probably do not, as single agents, cause cancer. However, viruses may be one of multiple agents acting to initiate carcinogenesis. Viruses have been associated with hepatocellular carcinoma, T-cell lymphoma, T-cell leukemia, Burkitt's lymphoma, nasopharyngeal carcinoma, and cervical cancer.

CHEMICAL AGENTS

Some of the most common chemical carcinogens include tar, soot, asphalt, aniline dyes, hydrocarbons, crude paraffin oil, fuel oils, nickel, and arsenicals. Most of these agents cause cancer only after close and prolonged contact, and persons affected are usually workers in industries where these chemicals are used or occur as byproducts such as tanning, die making, refineries, and battery-making factories.

Because organisms have different metabolic systems, potential carcinogens are metabolized one way in some organisms and in other ways in other organisms. It may be that some organisms, humans included, are more sensitive than others to certain carcinogens because of their metabolic differences.

PHYSICAL AGENTS

Physical carcinogens cause cellular damage just as chemical carcinogens do, except their action is physical in nature. Radiation and asbestos are both physical carcinogens.

Two forms of radiation can lead to cancer: ultraviolet radiation and ionizing radiation. Ultraviolet radiation from the sun can cause changes in DNA structure that can lead to malignant transformation if it is not repaired. Both basal and squamous cell carcinomas of the skin as well as melanoma are linked to ultraviolet exposure.

Ionizing radiation can cause permanent DNA mutation when exposure is excessive. This mutation may transform into a malignant growth if the DNA repair is incomplete. The vast majority of radiation exposure is from natural sources (radon, cosmic, terrestrial, and internal radiation). Preventive measures are usually focused on minimizing exposure to manufactured sources of radiation such as x-rays and isotopes, which are used in medical diagnosis and treatment.

In the United States, asbestos, a carcinogenic fiber, contributes significantly to the occurrence of bronchogenic cancer and mesothelioma. There is a strong synergistic relation between tobacco smoke and asbestos. The mechanism of action of asbestos is unknown, but it is thought to be a promoter rather than an initiator of the cancer.

DRUGS AND HORMONES

Scientists have demonstrated that a relationship exists between hormonal secretion, action, tumor development, and growth. Exactly what the relationship is remains obscure. Do hormones actually cause normal cells to change into cancer cells? Do hormones act only to promote the growth of tumors caused by other factors? The answers to these questions lie in future research.

One of the most controversial topics in carcinogenesis is the role of estrogen. Animal studies have shown that estrogen is involved in the development of breast cancer. Human studies indicate that estrogen is related to human breast cancer but in a poorly defined manner.

Cancer chemotherapeutic agents are carcinogenic, and cancer clients are at risk for future development of leukemia and other cancers (see Chap. 22 for further discussion on this topic).

Predisposing Factors

In addition to the carcinogens described, there are also predisposing factors that influence the host's susceptibility to various etiologic agents.

AGE

Cancer affects people of all ages. However, older people develop cancer more readily than do younger individuals. Many cancers, such as prostate, colon, and some chronic leukemias, have increased incidence in older clients. Older people may be more susceptible to cancer simply because they have been exposed to carcinogens longer than younger people. Also, as individuals age, their immune system ages and becomes less active. The immune response failure theory suggests that this problem alone could make the clients more susceptible to cancers.

Also, there are cancers that occur within very narrow age ranges. Testicular cancer is found in men from about 20 to 40 years of age. Ovarian cancer is more common in women over 55 years of age. There are a number of cancers that occur mainly in childhood, such as Ewing's sarcoma, certain acute leukemias, Wilms' tumor, and retinoblastoma.

SEX

Women are more susceptible to certain types of cancer than men are, and vice versa. Since 1949, more men than women have died from all types of cancer. The increased incidence of cancer deaths among men apparently relates to the higher incidence and mortality of lung cancer, which is currently almost twice that in women. More women, however, are smoking, leading to an increase in the rate in women. Lung cancer is now the leading killer of both men and women. Oral cancer death rates are almost twice as high for men as for women.

GEOGRAPHIC LOCATION

The incidence of different types of cancer varies on a geographic basis. For example, the incidence of stomach cancer is higher in Japan than in the United States. On the other hand, breast cancer is rare in Japan but has a high incidence in the United States, Europe, and Israel. These differences may reflect the influence of environmental factors (diet, customs, pollutants in the environment) rather than genetic differences between races and nationalism. This explanation seems likely because when Japanese women live in the United States, their rate of breast cancer is the same as that of other women in the United States.

Differences exist among parts of this country also. In highly urbanized areas, colon cancer is more prevalent than in rural areas. The industrialized areas have higher amounts of polluted air, so rates of lung cancer are higher. In rural areas, particularly among farmers, skin cancer is more common. Colon cancer is more common in the industrialized northeast and Great Lakes region. The greater susceptibility in certain geographic areas is probably related to exposure to different carcinogens, especially environmental ones.

OCCUPATION

People in certain jobs are more susceptible to certain cancers because of their greater contact with specific carcinogens. For example, workers in asbestos factories have a higher incidence of lung cancer due to their chronic exposure to asbestos. People who work around hydrocarbons, especially benzene, have a higher rate of bladder cancer. Radium miners and the people who paint the iridescent dials on watches have a higher incidence of leukemia from the exposure to radioactivity. Radiologists also have a high rate of leukemia.

HEREDITY

There are a number of cancers that provide evidence of a heritable predisposition to cancer. Fanconi's anemia, ataxia-telangiectasia, and xeroderma pigmentosum are examples of autosomal recessive conditions that predispose persons to a variety of malignancies. Familial polyposis coli, retinoblastoma, Wilms' tumor, and neurofibromatosis are examples of autosomal dominant disorders that follow classic Mendelian patterns of inheritance.[35] Breast, ovarian, and colon cancers also show a familial pattern.

DIET

The role of diet in the causation of cancer, for the most part, is unclear. What is known is that intake of cured, pickled, smoked, salted, preserved, and unrefrigerated food has been linked to stomach cancer. The high amount of fat in the average diet of people in this country and the incidence of breast and colon cancer show a striking correlation. There is a similar correlation between excessive meat consumption in this country and colon cancer.[45] Although the potential for substantial reduction in cancer incidence by dietary modification alone appears remote, a diet rich in fruits and fiber and low in animal fats is desirable for many health reasons.

It is important to note that a multitude of fad anticancer diets and drugs prey on the ignorance and fear of many clients. Before a specific diet is condoned as helpful in the fight against cancer, it is vital to evaluate its overall nutritional content and to be aware of any harmful effects it may generate.

STRESS

Recent research suggests a strong link between stress and cancer. In brief, stress may increase the risk of cancer. Chronic physical or emotional stress preys on the hypothalamus, the portion of the pituitary gland that regulates hormone and immune systems. Increased stress causes hormonal or immunologic changes, or both, which, in turn, spur the growth and proliferation of cancer cells.

PRECANCEROUS LESIONS

Precancerous lesions and some benign tumors may undergo transformation later into cancerous lesions and tumors. Common precancerous lesions include pigmented moles, burn scars, senile keratosis, leukoplakia, and benign adenomas or polyps of the colon or stomach. All of these lesions need to be periodically assessed for malignant changes.

Impact of Cancer

PHYSICAL

Physical changes can occur in the client throughout the cancer experience. The malignant tumor itself may cause obvious disfigurement or internal organ changes even prior to diagnosis. For example, some skin cancers are potentially disfiguring and colon cancer can cause a great deal of internal change, including obstruction, before diagnosis.

Treatment for a malignant tumor also may cause the client to experience physical changes. Surgery may be mutilative, as in the amputation of a breast or an arm. Radiation therapy may cause changes in body functions and skin integrity. Chemotherapy may lead to hair loss, weight gain or loss, and skin pigmentation changes.

It is important for the health care provider to recognize the fact that even though the body has been changed by treatment to increase survival, it has still been changed. Clients, along with their families, need to adjust to the changes that treatment may produce.

Clients, therefore, live not only with the physical indicators of the disease, but with the sequelae of its treatment as well.[25] Although some of the physical changes of cancer are a result of its treatment, the changes impact on a client's self-concept, self-esteem, and general feelings of worth and acceptance (see Chap. 22 for further discussion).

PSYCHOSOCIAL

Historically, studies of individuals with cancer were used to identify unique psychosocial responses to cancer, describe types of coping behaviors, and guide health care professionals in assisting the client with cancer adjust to the diagnosis, the demands of treatment, and the requirements of living with cancer. The variability of psychosocial responses is increased by the fact that clients bring their own sets of values, beliefs, attitudes, resources, and coping mechanisms to the cancer experience.

Anxiety, along with depression, has been described as the most common psychosocial reaction among clients with cancer.[16] It is vital to realize that each client diagnosed with cancer reacts to the diagnosis differently and has unique concerns and problems regarding the diagnosis and treatment. Each client copes with the cancer experience in his or her own way.

Health professionals can guide and facilitate open communication between the client, family, and health care provider to reduce anxiety and depression and increase feelings of hopefulness. The nurse can help the client in many ways. First, the nurse can help the client recognize the manifestations of anxiety. Often, simply helping the client identify these behaviors can help the client cope more effectively. If the client is suffering from severe depression, the nurse should spend time with the client and possibly suggest counseling. It is also helpful for the client to know that these are normal feelings associated with the diagnosis and treatment of cancer. There are many support groups (such as I Can Cope, Make Today Count, New Voice Club) available for these clients to help them establish effective support systems.

FINANCIAL

Impact on Client and Family. The diagnosis and treatment of cancer are expensive. Medical intervention is technical and lengthy. Not surprisingly, the financial consequences of the illness are a major concern to the cancer client. Sometimes, even if the client has health insurance, the amount the client is required to pay can be astronomical. The client without private insurance may be unable to afford needed care. Medicaid, in some states, will not pay for expensive treatments such as bone marrow transplants (BMT). A BMT can cost from $100,000 to $1,000,000, more than most individuals can afford. Moving cancer care to outpatient, ambulatory care centers or the home helps decrease the cost. Unfortunately, not all procedures can be administered outside the hospital. Primary and secondary prevention methods also can help lower the cost either by preventing the cancer or by treating it sooner.

Depending on the type and stage of cancer, a client may find it necessary to work fewer hours, to find a different line of work, or in extreme cases, to stop working altogether. If the client is the main source of income and insurance benefits, a change, decrease, or loss of work may have catastrophic consequences. It has been reported that up to 80 per cent of clients with cancer return to work after diagnosis and treatment of cancer.[18]

Because a social stigma is still associated with the diagnosis of cancer, clients may be denied their former jobs or job benefits (insurance included) when their cancer becomes known to those in the workplace. It is, however, illegal to terminate someone based on the diagnosis of cancer. The Federal Rehabilitation Act of 1973 prohibits discrimination against an employee based on a real or perceived handicap. Many states also protect cancer clients against job discrimination. Unfortunately, there is no federal protection against the loss of insurance that occurs. It has been estimated that 25 to 30 per cent of individuals with cancer face some form of insurance discrimination.[19] The COBRA federal law requires employers with 20 employees or more to offer a continuation of group medical coverage to those individuals whose circumstances warrant reducing or changing work hours or to those who must leave a job.[17]

To help the client and family deal with the overall cancer experience, it is necessary to discuss personal financial obligations and responsibilities and the changes diagnosis and treatment may bring.

Impact on the Economy. Cost may be direct or indirect. Direct costs involve cancer prevention, diagnosis, and treatment. It also includes payment for chronic and acute care facilities, nursing and medical services, research, and professional education. Indirect costs include loss of national productivity due to the absence of clients with cancer from the work force.

Cancer also affects the economy of the society. In this time of limited access to health care, questions are being raised about the cost of cancer care. Cancer care cost an estimated $104 billion in 1990. As technology advances and medical costs increase, the cost of cancer care will become even greater in the future. It is unlikely that this nation can afford the ever-increasing cost of health care.

Research

Both physicians and nurses contribute to cancer research. Medical research focuses on the natural history of the disease, new treatment approaches, and singular versus multimodal approaches to medical treatment. Nursing research focuses on the client with cancer and the client's family rather than on the cancer and may include biologic, psychological, and social aspects.[27] The Oncology Nursing Society (ONS) has fostered a great deal of nursing research. The *ONS Standards of Nursing Practice* include a statement about the importance of research and the need for the oncology nurse to be actively involved.

CLINICAL TRIALS

The National Cancer Institute (NCI) has developed a method of testing new cancer treatments, especially chemotherapy. There are several stages to this method, commonly known as Phase I, II, III, and IV Clinical Trials. Information is available on these trials from the Physician's Data Query (NDQ), a computer program accessible by modem, through a medical library, or by calling 1-800-4-Cancer. Each phase has well-defined guidelines. Phase I studies determine the maximum tolerated dose of a new agent and assess its toxicity. Phase II trials determine the efficacy of the agent in different types of cancer. Phase III trials compare the new agent to the standard treatment, and in Phase IV trials, the agent is given to large numbers of clients with the same tumor type to confirm its efficacy. If an agent successfully meets the criteria of the clinical trials, Food and Drug Association (FDA) approval is granted and the agent is approved to treat specific cancers.

ETHICAL ISSUES

Ethical issues related to cancer research include informed consent, which encompasses client competence; disclosure and understanding of information; voluntariness; and confidentiality. Although in any given institution it may be the physician's responsibility to obtain informed consent prior to the client's inclusion in a research protocol, it is always the nurse's responsibility to ascertain a client's competence, understanding of the given information, and voluntariness prior to the initiation of any treatment or therapy.

CHARACTERISTICS OF NORMAL CELLS

Chapter 13 explores general characteristics of normal cells. Specific characteristics of normal cells that help us understand changes that occur in neoplastic cells are (1) the cell cycle, (2) differentiation, and (3) contact inhibition.

The Cell Cycle. The concept of the cell cycle has increased researchers' understanding of how both normal and neoplastic cells replicate (Fig. 21–4). The cell's replication cycle is divided into the following intervals, or steps, with the letter G standing for "gap" — the interval separating mitosis (M) and synthesis (S).

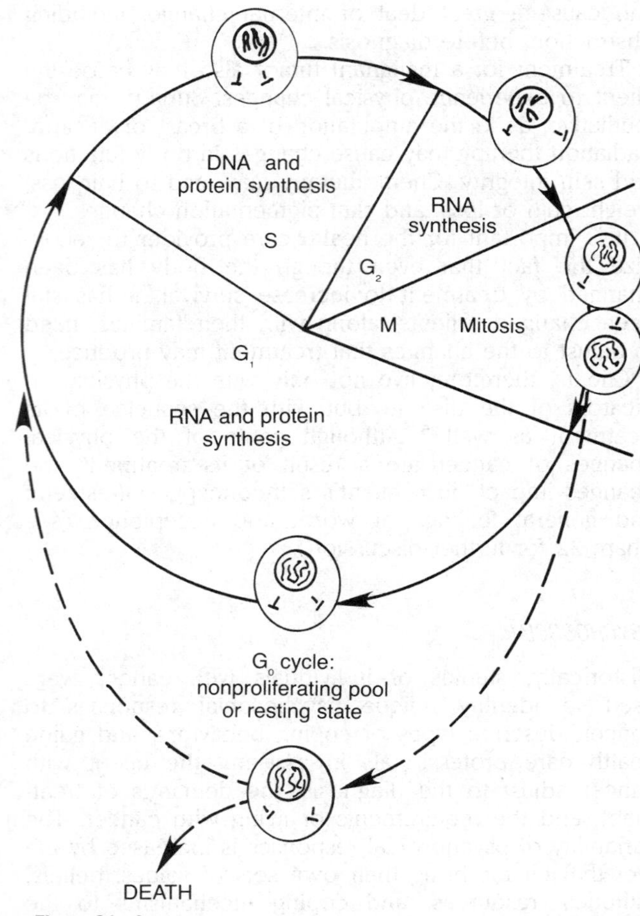

▲ Figure 21–4

The cell cycle. Periods of DNA synthesis (S) and mitosis (M) are divided by gaps (G) in which the cell is in a resting state (G_0), producing substances in preparation for DNA synthesis (G_1), or producing proteins and some RNA in preparation for mitosis (G_2).

Step 1a: G_0. The interval in which the cell is at rest (until a trigger in the immediate environment signals the beginning of the G_1 interval). Some cells do not replicate, or they replicate so infrequently that they are always said to be in G_0 state.

Step 1b: G_1. The interval in which RNA and protein are synthesized. The period of time the cell is in G_1 varies, depending on the type of cell and the proliferative activity of the tissue. With high activity, G_1 interval is short. The interval lengthens when activity is low. The acquisition of the ability to begin DNA synthesis marks the termination of G_1.

Step 2: S. Synthesis of both the DNA and proteins of new chromosomes occurs. The interval of time is probably 6 to 8 hours. It varies in certain cell populations and under different circumstances.

Step 3: G_2. Biochemical processes, including synthesis of some RNA, occur in preparation for mitosis. Little is known about this phase, which may last only a few hours.

Step 4: M. Actual division of the cell—mitosis—occurs, producing two daughter cells. The duration of this phase usually ranges from less than an hour to a few hours.

In the normal mature organ, cell cycling is carefully controlled so that the organ maintains its function. Cells that die are replaced, but no extra cells are produced. Researchers are investigating the mechanisms of this control, which is not fully understood at this time.

Differentiation. In the embryo, genetically identical cells assume various structures and functions. One muscle cell looks like all the other muscle cells but not much like a kidney or liver cell. This process is called differentiation.

Contact Inhibition. When normal cells are grown outside the body on culture plates, they exhibit an interesting characteristic called contact inhibition. Normal cells spread freely about the culture medium until they contact another cell. Then they adhere to each other and align themselves in parallel fashion. The cells grow until they reach the edges of the container, covering the surface in a single layer. At this point active growth stops.

PREVENTION AND ASSESSMENT

Cancer Cell Growth

Tumor growth is related to increased numbers of cells. Cells may increase in number by (1) shortening the length of the cell cycle, (2) increasing the fraction of cells going through the cell cycle, or (3) decreasing cell loss. At one time, researchers believed that neoplastic cells divided much more rapidly than other cells in the body. This rapid division was thought to account for the mass of cells that developed. Later, investigators discovered that some normal cells proceed through the cell cycle faster than neoplastic cells. The current belief is that the fraction of proliferating cells in a tumor is higher, thus accounting for the tumor mass. There is also a decrease in cell death, with the ratio of cell death to cell birth being altered.

The concept of doubling time is central to the study of tumor growth. Theoretically, cancer could start as a single abnormal cell that divides to form two cells, then four cells, and so on. Provided that the amount of time for the cell cycle remains constant, the tumor mass would double each time the cell cycle went from mitosis to mitosis (Fig. 21-5).

Although some tumors steadily enlarge, this factor does not entirely account for their growth. There is some indication that tumors may cycle faster early in their growth. Also, cycling times vary with the type of tumor. Cell losses are considerable in all tumors, and may counterbalance new cell output in some. Approximately 20 doublings will occur before a 1-mm^3 tumor is produced. This is the smallest mass that could be detected clinically. At 30 doublings, the mass would be about 1 cm^3, weighing 1 g, still a small lesion by any standards. Ten more doublings bring the mass to 1 kg, but only five more doublings bring the mass to 32 kg, or half of body weight! Another five doublings and the tumor would weigh about 1000 kg.

Clearly, the cell cycle of a tumor is of great clinical significance. First, the slower the cell cycle of the tumor, the longer it is before the tumor can be identified. Second, Figure 21-5 shows that the preclinical period of growth is approximately two thirds of the total growth period. This fact helps us to understand how metastasis or spread of a tumor occurs, even when the original tumor is small. It also explains why the physician requires a long period of time following removal of the tumor before being assured that the client is cancer free.

Neoplastic Cell Division and Differentiation

Despite research advances, investigators still have unanswered questions about cancer. What is a cancer cell? How does it differ from a normal cell, and what are the factors that cause cancer cells to develop? To better define abnormal cells and explain why they develop, researchers are learning more about normal cells and their regulation at the genetic level.

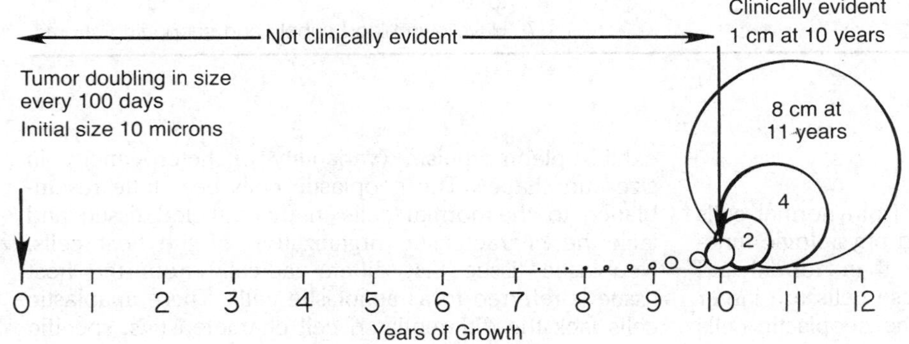

▲ *Figure 21-5*

Tumor growth. Doubling time related to tumor size.

TABLE 21–3. Normal Cells Versus Malignant Cells

Characteristic	Normal Cells	Malignant Cells
Mitotic cell division	Mitotic division leads to two daughter cells	Mitosis leads to multiple daughter cells that may or may not resemble the parent. Multiple miotic spindles
Appearance	1. Cells of same type homogeneous in size, shape, and growth 2. Cells cohesive, form regular pattern of expansion 3. Uniform size to nucleus 4. Have characteristic pattern of organization 5. Mixture of stem cells (precursors) and well-differentiated cells	1. Cells larger and grow more rapidly than normal. Pleomorphic, i.e., heterogeneous in size and shape 2. Cells not as cohesive, irregular patterns of expansion 3. Larger, more prominent nucleus 4. Lack characteristic pattern of organization of host cell 5. Anaplastic, lack of differentiated cell characteristics, specific functions
Growth pattern	1. Do not invade adjacent tissue 2. Proliferate in response to specific stimuli 3. Grow in ideal conditions (e.g., nutrients, oxygen, space, correct biochemical environment) 4. Exhibit contact inhibition 5. Cell birth equals or is less than cell death 6. Stable cell membrane 7. Constant or predictable growth rate 8. Cannot grow outside specific environment (e.g., breast cells grow only in breast)	1. Invade adjacent tissues 2. Proliferation in response to abnormal stimuli 3. Grow in adverse conditions such as lack of nutrients 4. Do not exhibit contact inhibition 5. Cell birth exceeds cell death 6. Loss of cell control a result of cell membrane changes 7. Growth rate erratic 8. Able to break off cells that migrate through bloodstream or lymphatics, or seed to distant sites and grow in other sites
Function	1. Have specific, designated purpose 2. Contribute to the overall well-being of the host 3. Cells function in specific predetermined manners, such as cells in the thyroid secrete thyroid hormone	1. Serve no useful purpose 2. Do not contribute to the well-being of the host, parasitic, actually feed off host without contributing anything 3. If cells function at all, they do not function normally, or they may actually function to cause damage, such as malignant lung cancer cells that secrete ACTH and cause excessive stimulation of the adrenal cortex
Other	1. Develop specific antigens, characteristic of the particular cell formed 2. Chromosomes remain constant throughout cell division 3. Complex metabolic and enzyme pattern 4. Cannot invade, erode, or spread 5. Cannot grow in presence of necrosis or inflammation	1. Develop antigens completely different from a normal cell 2. Chromosomal aberrations occur as cell matures 3. Have more primitive and simplified metabolic and enzyme pattern 4. Invade, erode, and spread 5. Grow in presence of necrosis and inflammatory cells such as lymphocytes and macrophages 6. Exhibit periods of latency that vary from tumor to tumor 7. Have own blood supply and supporting stroma

ACTH, adrenocorticotropic hormone.

CHARACTERISTICS OF NEOPLASTIC CELLS

Appearance. Neoplastic cells differ from normal cells in appearance, pattern of growth, and physiologic function. The cells themselves are larger than normal and grow more rapidly. The nuclei of these cells are larger and more prominent than normal. The neoplastic cells exhibit pleomorphism (variability or heterogeneity in size and shape). The neoplastic cells bear little resemblance to the normal cells in the afflicted tissue and lack the characteristic organization of the host cells. Neoplastic tissue that differs radically from the host tissue is referred to as anaplastic cells. These anaplastic cells lack the differentiated cell characteristics, specific functions, and organization of normal cells (Table 21-3). Differentiated cells are functionally and structurally specialized, and are often nondividing.

Growth. The growth patterns of neoplastic cells also differ from those of normal cells. These cells flourish in antagonistic physical, chemical, hormonal, and viral environments. Neoplastic cells invade adjacent tissue. Malignant cells grow and proliferate in response to abnormal stimuli. Neoplastic cells grow well under adverse conditions that would keep other cells from growing. The growth rate is also very erratic.

There is a loss of cellular control in neoplastic cells, as a consequence of changes in the cell membrane. They exhibit increased mitosis, with multiple miotic spindles, leading to the development of more than the normal two daughter cells at the end of mitosis. The normal limits of replication do not exist in neoplastic cells, which leads to uncontrolled replication. Also, neoplastic cells do not exhibit contact inhibition, and cell birth exceeds cell death.

Neoplastic cells also exhibit other growth characteristics that normal cells do not. Neoplastic cells are able to break off proliferative cells that enter the circulation and migrate away from their tissue of origin. These cells form emboli that lodge in distant areas, where they are able to extravasate (leak out) from the vessels and begin new proliferation in foreign tissues. Neoplastic cells are also able to invade lymphatic channels and move with the lymph to other nodes. They also can seed throughout body cavities, such as the peritoneal cavity.

Function. Malignant cells, unlike normal cells, serve no useful purpose. The result of neoplastic growth is an abnormal tissue mass that does not contribute in any way to the well-being of the host. If the malignant cells function at all, they do not function normally and may even act in a way that causes damage to the host. For example, a functional tumor of the thyroid gland produces excess amounts of thyroid hormone, leading to a hypermetabolic state.

Other Differences. Malignant cells exhibit other differences that normal cells do not. First, they develop antigens that are completely different from those associated with normal cells. Chromosomal aberrations also occur as the malignant cell matures. There is a return to a more primitive and simplified metabolic and enzyme pattern, and these cells can invade, erode, and spread.

Malignant cells can be seen as actually parasitic, that is, they feed off the host without contributing anything. They occupy space, draw nutrition and sustenance from the host, and provide nothing useful in return. Neoplastic cells grow in adverse conditions, such as in the presence of necrosis and inflammatory cells, lymphocytes, and macrophages. Malignant cells also exhibit varying periods of latency. When the cells group to form tumors, they develop their own blood supply and supporting stroma (structure).

Growth of Neoplastic Tumors

Neoplastic cells mass together to form neoplastic tissue growths or tumors. What accounts for the growth and spread of these tumors?

Some neoplastic cells have the ability to spread from the original site of the tumor to distant organs of the body. This characteristic is called metastasis. The word is derived from the Greek words *meta*, meaning beyond, and *stasis*, meaning standing. The capacity of a neoplastic tumor to metastasize to other sites is a major characteristic of malignancy, and it distinguishes malignant from benign growths.

Researchers do not fully understand the mechanisms of tumor spread at this time. Studies have revealed that the walls of tumor cells are different from those of their normal counterparts. Furthermore, the "contact inhibition" noted in normal cells is extremely variable in tumor cells.

For the purposes of study, the metastatic process may be divided into three stages (Fig. 21-6).

Stage 1 involves invasion of neoplastic cells from the primary tumor into surrounding tissue, and penetration

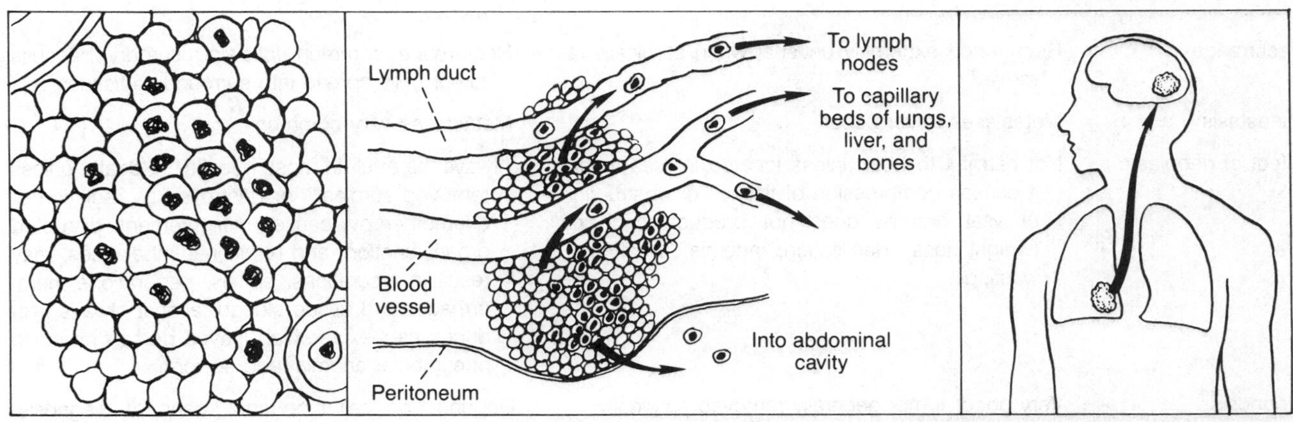

▲ *Figure 21-6*

Three stages of the metastatic process.

of blood and/or lymph vessels. Tumor invasion may be caused by any of the following:

- Increasing tumor size, leading to tissue pressure and mechanical expansion.
- Loss of tumor cell cohesiveness, with increasing motility.
- Destruction of the host stroma (the supporting tissues of an organ).
- Factors in the host response to tumor cell invasion.

Stage 2 involves spread of tumor cells via the lymph or blood circulation or by direct expansion. The lymphatic system provides the most common pathway for initial spread of cancer cells. The spread may be to the lymph nodes draining the region of the primary site. Distant lymph nodes may be affected later in the disease or if the regional lymph nodes are obstructed by inflammation or other processes. Lymph node involvement is seen in about one half of all fatal cancers. The blood vessels (including both veins and arteries) carry cancer cells from the primary tumor to the capillary beds of the lungs, liver, and bones. Metastatic spread to distant organs and tissues is almost always the result of cells moving through the bloodstream. Direct expansion of tumors in body cavities occurs as cells travel throughout the cavity to develop new growth on other serosal surfaces. Cancers of the ovary are often said to seed the entire peritoneal cavity. Primary tumors of the central nervous system appear to spread by direct extension, or via gravity, in the cerebral fluid. Direct extension of tumors to directly adjacent tissues also occurs. For example, some breast cancers spread directly to the chest wall.

Stage 3 involves establishment and growth of tumor cells at the secondary site. The tumor develops its own vascularization in the new site and has the ability to infiltrate adjacent tissue. Researchers have observed that certain tumor cells for unknown reasons have an affinity for certain sites.

TABLE 21-4. A Comparison of the Characteristics of Benign and Malignant Neoplasms

Characteristic	Benign Neoplasm	Malignant Neoplasm
Speed of growth	Grows slowly, usually continues to grow throughout life unless surgically removed; may have periods of remission	Usually grows rapidly, tends to grow relentlessly throughout life; rarely, neoplasm may regress spontaneously
Mode of growth	Grows by enlarging and expanding; always remains localized; never infiltrates surrounding tissues	Grows by infiltrating surrounding tissues; may remain localized (in situ) but usually infiltrates other tissues
Capsule	Almost always contained within a fibrous capsule; capsule does not prevent expansion of neoplasm but does prevent growth by infiltration; capsule advantageous because encapsulated tumor can be removed surgically	Never contained within a capsule; absence of capsule allows neoplastic cells to invade surrounding tissues; surgical removal of tumor difficult
Cell characteristics	Usually well differentiated; mitotic figures absent or scanty; mature cells; anaplastic cells absent; cells function poorly in comparison with normal cells from which they arise; if neoplasm arises in glandular tissue, cells may secrete hormones	Usually poorly differentiated; large numbers of normal and abnormal mitotic figures present; cells tend to be anaplastic, i.e., young, embryonic type; cells too abnormal to perform any physiologic functions; occasionally a malignant tumor arising in glandular tissue secretes hormones
Recurrence	Recurrence extremely unusual when surgically removed	Recurrence common following surgery because tumor cells spread into surrounding tissues
Metastasis	Metastases never occur	Metastases very common
Effect of neoplasm	Not harmful to host unless located in area where it causes compression of tissues or obstruction of vital organs; does not produce cachexia (weight loss, debilitation, anemia, weakness, wasting)	Always harmful to host; results in death unless removed surgically or destroyed by radiation or chemotherapy; causes disfigurement, disrupted organ function, and nutritional imbalances; may result in ulcerations, sepsis, perforations, hemorrhage, and tissue slough; almost always produces cachexia, which leaves person prone to pneumonia, anemia, and so forth
Prognosis	Very good; tumor generally removed surgically	Depends on cell type and speed of diagnosis; poor prognosis indicated if cells are poorly differentiated and evidence exists of metastatic spread; good prognosis indicated if cells still resemble normal and there is no evidence of metastasis

TABLE 21-5. Classification of Neoplasms by Tissue of Origin

Tissue of Origin	Benign	Malignant
Connective tissue		Sarcoma
Embryonic fibrous tissue	Myxoma	Myxosarcoma
Fibrous tissue	Fibroma	Fibrosarcoma
Adipose tissue	Lipoma	Liposarcoma
Cartilage	Chondroma	Chondrosarcoma
Bone	Osteoma	Osteogenic sarcoma
Epithelium		Carcinoma
Skin and mucous membrane	Papilloma	Squamous cell carcinoma
Glands	Polyp	Basal cell carcinoma
		Transitional cell carcinoma
	Adenoma	Adenocarcinoma
	Cystadenoma	
Pigmented cells (melanoblasts)	Nevus	Malignant melanoma
Endothelium		Endothelioma
Blood vessels	Hemangioma	Hemangioendothelioma
		Hemangiosarcoma
Lymph vessels	Lymphangioma	Lymphangiosarcoma
		Lymphangioendothelioma
Bone marrow		Multiple myeloma
		Ewing's sarcoma
		Leukemia
Lymphoid tissue		Malignant lymphoma
		Lymphosarcoma
		Reticulum cell sarcoma
		Lymphatic leukemia
Muscle tissue		
Smooth muscle	Leiomyoma	Leiomyosarcoma
Striated muscle	Rhabdomyoma	Rhabdomyosarcoma
Nerve tissue		
Nerve fibers and sheaths	Neuroma	Neurogenic sarcoma
	Neurinoma (Neurilemoma)	
	Neurofibroma	(Neurofibrosarcoma)
Ganglion cells	Ganglioneuroma	Neuroblastoma
Glial cells	Glioma	Glioblastoma
		Spongioblastoma
Meninges	Meningioma	Malignant meningioma
Gonads	Dermoid cyst	Embryonal carcinoma
		Embryonal sarcoma
		Teratocarcinoma

As previously mentioned, the cell cycle time and host factors determine the length of time necessary to detect metastatic growth. If the cells replicate quickly, a tumor may attain a size of 1 cm within months. If the cells proliferate slowly, it may be many years before the metastatic lesion is large enough to be detected.

The growth of metastatic tumors puts severe stress on the person both physiologically and psychologically. As the tumor burden (the amount of tumor in the body) increases, fewer metabolic resources are available for normal cells.

Common Metastatic Sites. Although there is no clear explanation about the exact mechanism of metastasis, the metastatic sites of many tumors are fairly predictable. The predilection of certain tumors for particular sites may be due to the ability of the tumor to live within only certain tissues, or it may be due to some other unknown factor. The five most common sites of metastasis are the lymph nodes, liver, lung, bone, and brain.

Factors Influencing Metastasis. The spread of cancer, although not fully understood, appears to be dependent on a variety of factors. These include the host factors such as the immune system, age, and hormonal environment. Many other factors such as pregnancy, stress, and trauma to the malignant tumor seem to increase spread. Other factors such as steroids, aspirin, the immune system, and radiation and chemotherapy appear to both increase and decrease the spread, but these factors are not predictable. Anticoagulants, conversely, seem to decrease the spread of malignant cells.

Classification of Neoplasms

BENIGN VERSUS MALIGNANT

Neoplastic tumors are classified as either benign or malignant. Deciding whether a tumor is benign or malignant is probably the most important decision a physician must make when treating a person with a neoplastic growth.

The word benign comes from the Latin *bene*, meaning good, and *genus*, which means sort. Thus, a benign tumor is a "good sort of tumor," a tumor of limited growth. A benign tumor, however, does occupy space. Consequently, if it is located near a vital tube or organ, it could be fatal. As a rule, though, the person with a benign tumor has a good prognosis because the tumor can be readily excised.

Malignant tumors, on the other hand, represent a serious threat to the life and well-being of the host. Table 21-4 compares the characteristics of these two major types of neoplasms.

TISSUE OF ORIGIN

Neoplasms are classified not only as benign or malignant but also according to the tissue from which they arise. Almost all names for tumors end in the suffix *oma*, meaning tumor (Table 21-5). This suffix is usually attached to a term for the parent tissue of the tumor. Thus, adenoma comes from the Greek *aden*, or gland, plus *oma*. When more than one parent tissue enters into the formation of a neoplasm, the names of the tumors are even more descriptive. For example, an adenomyoma is a benign neoplasm that contains both glandular and muscle cells.

Because epithelial tissues vary greatly, benign tumors of epithelial origin are classified according to either their microscopic appearance (e.g., adenoma) or their macroscopic appearance (e.g., polyp, from the Greek *polys* [many] + *pous* [foot]).

Three of the most common benign tumors listed in Table 21-5 are the fibroma, lipoma, and leiomyoma.

The fibroma may grow anywhere in the body, but it very frequently makes its home in the uterus. Fibromas are generally small, but occasionally they grow to great size. These encapsulated, relatively harmless tumors do not cause symptoms unless, because of their location, they press on a bone or nerve. Fibromas are easily removed surgically.

The lipoma, a very common benign tumor, arises in adipose tissue. Lipomas rarely cause symptoms, but they are poorly encapsulated and may put pressure on surrounding tissues as they expand.

The leiomyoma, a benign neoplasm of smooth muscle origin, is the most common benign tumor in women. Leiomyomas may develop anywhere in the body, but they most commonly grow in the uterus. Rarely (in approximately 1 per cent of cases), these tumors become malignant.

Let us now consider the classification of malignant tumors. A malignant tumor that arises from epithelial tissue is called a carcinoma, whereas a malignant neoplasm that arises from mesenchymal origins (i.e., blood vessels, lymphatics, nerve tissue) is called a sarcoma (Greek *sarc* means flesh).

Three representative examples of malignant neoplasms are carcinoma in situ, fibrosarcoma, and bronchogenic carcinoma.

Carcinoma in situ is a neoplasm of epithelial tissue that remains confined to the site of origin. In situ carcinoma typically affects the cervix, and it may occur in squamous epithelium in other parts of the body. This form of cancer is, by definition, localized, and thus can be removed surgically. However, it is well to remember that in situ carcinoma can become invasive, eroding into surrounding tissues.

The malignant fibrosarcomas are similar to benign fibromas. Fibrosarcomas tend to grow in the same sites and may originate as benign fibromas, later becoming malignant. These bulky, well-differentiated tumor masses are usually responsive to surgery. Fortunately, fibrosarcomas rarely metastasize.

Bronchogenic carcinoma accounts for 90 per cent of all cases of lung cancer. Bronchogenic carcinoma usually develops in the lower trachea and lower bronchi. Surgical excision of the tumor is the intervention of choice. However, this type of cancer readily gives rise to metastases, and if this occurs, surgery is contraindicated.

Prevention

RISK ANALYSIS AND MODIFICATION

Although cancer is the second most common cause of death in this country, many forms of cancer have identifiable risk factors and are preventable (Table 21-6). Some cancers can be prevented through primary prevention. However, some cancers cannot be prevented from occurring. For these cancers, there is secondary prevention, or early detection. Dietary modifications are among the important ways to reduce the occurrence of cancer in general (Fig. 21-7).

The nurse needs to know the risk factors for each client and the common factors for each type of cancer. Tables 21-7 and 21-8 identify specifics of primary and secondary preventions with which the nurse should be familiar.

SCREENING

Primary prevention is the ideal method of cancer control. Not all cancers can be prevented, however, so early detection is also a major tool in the fight against cancer. Nurses must emphasize to the public the importance of finding the cancer and eradicating it early, before the cancer begins to metastasize from the primary site. The public needs to realize that manifesta-

TABLE 21-6. Risk Factors and Prevention Levels for Common Cancers

Type of Cancer	Risk Factors and Level of Prevention
Lung	Smoking, all types (P); high levels of indoor radon (P); occupational and environmental industrial pollutants (P); air pollution (P); family history of lung cancer (S); secondary cigarette smoke (P)
Breast	Family history of breast cancer, especially on maternal side and occurring before menopause (S); history of previous breast or other gynecologic cancer (S); Jewish (S); single (P,S); nulliparity (P,S); early menarche, late menopause (S); birth of first child after 30 (P,S); ? history of benign breast disease (S); diet high in fat (S); high alcohol intake (S); higher socioeconomic groups (S); increasing age (S); whites (S)
Colon/rectal	Low-fiber, high-fat diet (P); history of ulcerative colitis, colon cancer, breast or female genital cancer, or bladder cancer (S); increasing age (S); obesity (P); sedentary lifestyle (P); family predisposition (S); history of colorectal adenomas (S)
Bladder	Smoking (P); men (S); whites (S); high alcohol consumption (P); aniline dye, print, coal, tar, and pitch workers, apparel, textile, and leather industry, and painters (S); ? saccharin use (P); schistosomiasis (S); treatment with cyclophosphamide (S); exposure to asbestos (P,S)
Cervical	Black women (S); early frequent intercourse with multiple sex partners (P,S); multiparity (S); intercourse with uncircumcised males (P,S); chronic cervicitis (S); history of genital herpes or HPV (P,S)
Skin	Exposure to ultraviolet light (P); history of excessive sunbathing and/or sunburn before age 20 (P); fair skinned, fair hair (S); increasing age (S); history of dysplasic nevi, burns, topical ulcers, scars from squamous or basal cell carcinoma (S); family history of melanoma (S); PUVA treatment for psoriasis (S); outdoor workers (P,S); organ transplant recipients (S)
Prostate	Increasing age (S); black men (S); industrial exposure to cadmium (P,S); ? diet high in fats and sugar (P); ? history of venereal disease (P,S); ? sexual activity (P,S)
Ovarian	History of breast cancer (S); nulliparity or first pregnancy after 30 (S); white, upper income groups (S); history of pelvic radiation (S)
Uterine/endometrial	Obesity (P); history of hypertension, diabetes mellitus, or menstrual disorders (P,S); higher socioeconomic groups (S); nulliparity (P,S); infertility related to anovulation (S); long-term use of conjugated estrogens (P,S); Stein-Leventhal syndrome (S)
Testicular	Whites (S); cryptorchidism (S); age, 20 to 40 years old (S); family history (S); DES exposure in utero (S); atrophic testicles (S)
Oral	Smoking (P); smokeless tobacco or snuff (P); heavy alcohol use (P); vitamin B complex and iron deficiencies (P); poor oral hygiene, poor dental care, or ill-fitting dentures (P); pipe smoking or long-term exposure to sun (lip) (P,S)
Gastric	Family history (S); blood group A (S); atrophic gastric mucosa (S); gastric ulcers (P,S); pernicious anemia (S); history of gastric resection (S); stomach polyps (S); lower socioeconomic groups (S); intake of nitrates and nitrosamines (P); nonwhites (S); eating smoked foods, especially fish and mutton (P); eating pickled foods (P); eating rice treated with talc (P)
Leukemia	Age, childhood for acute and old age for chronic (S); exposure to benzene (P,S); poultry farmers (S); exposure to radiation (P,S); explosive and rubber cement workers, radiologists, distillers, dye users and painters, radium miners and chemists, and radium dial painters (P,S); Down's or Klinefelter's syndrome (S); men (S); an identical twin with leukemia (S); viruses (S); immunologic factors (S); genetic factors (S); intake of drugs such as melphalan, cyclophosphamide (Cytoxan), or chloramphenicol (P,S)

?, possible risk factor, not yet proved; P, primary prevention; S, secondary prevention; DES, diethylstilbestrol; HPV, human papilloma virus; PUVA, ultraviolet light.

Data from Groenwald, S., et al. (1990). *Cancer nursing: Principles and practice* (2nd ed.). Boston: Jones and Bartlett.

tions of a malignant disease can mimic those of other less serious disease processes. Currently, two of three people diagnosed with cancer die from it. Early detection could raise the survival rate to 50 per cent.

The individual's age, personal health history, and family history may indicate risk factors and are vital to the early detection of cancer. Nurses can help in this educational process by emphasizing the need for an *annual physical examination*, by stressing the importance of a *yearly Papanicolaou (Pap) test* for women, and by teaching women the technique for *breast self-examination (BSE)* and teaching men the technique for *testicular self-examination (TSE)*. Chapters 74, 75, and 78 describe these examinations in detail.

DIETARY DEFENSES AGAINST CANCER

INCREASED INTAKE OF:	REDUCED INTAKE OF:
High-fiber foods such as raw fruits and vegetables and whole-grain cereals	Salt-cured, smoked, and nitrite-cured foods
Dark green and deep yellow fruits and vegetables rich in vitamins A and C	Fats and oils, especially from animal sources
Cabbage, broccoli, cauliflower, brussels sprouts, and kohlrabi	Alcoholic beverages
	Excess calories leading to obesity

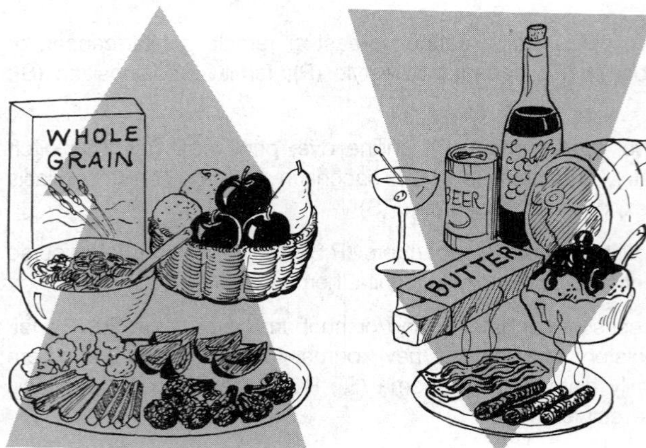

▲ *Figure 21-7*

Dietary changes to reduce cancer risks.

Increasing public awareness of cancer's warning signals is the role of every nurse (Box 21-1). Table 21-9 summarizes the American Cancer Society's (ACS) most recent guidelines for screening asymptomatic populations.

The nurse should remember that it is a normal human response to procrastinate in scheduling an examination when cancer is suspected. People are frightened by the thought of cancer. They do not always realize that cancer is curable when found early. Early detection always improves survival. Part of the process of screening clients is educating them as well.

The ACS strongly supports public education programs for cancer prevention and early detection. The nurse needs to support these measures to help reduce the risk of cancer (see Ethical Issues in Nursing).

Diagnosis

What specifically is involved in cancer detection? The primary health care provider employs both general and special techniques in a complete cancer diagnostic examination. General techniques include obtaining the client's history, including familial and environmental histories (see Chap. 11), performing a thorough physical examination, and ordering and evaluating laboratory examinations of the client's blood, tissue, sputum, urine, and other specimens.

PSYCHOSOCIAL ISSUES DURING DIAGNOSIS

When people undergo the diagnostic process associated with suspicious lumps or other cancer symptoms, they are usually somewhat afraid and anxious. They are experiencing unfamiliar and possibly painful tests.

In the past, if the diagnosis was cancer, there was often a debate about whether or not to tell the client the diagnosis. Today, nurses and physicians respect the client's right to know the diagnosis and all options for treatment. Consequently, health care professionals must face the difficulty of telling a client what is usually seen as bad news. One problem, however, is that health professionals have as many feelings and fears about this diagnosis as the client. They do not want to be the bearers of bad tidings, fearing that this diagnosis may destroy a client's will to live, which could result in the client giving up or committing suicide. Most clients exhibit much more strength than expected, and giving up or suicide is a rare response. Therefore, these are not valid reasons or valid excuses for avoiding our responsibility to the individual. If support is to be provided through a difficult period, nurses must be able to discuss the diagnosis, treatment, care, and expected outcomes with the client and significant others.

When working with clients undergoing diagnosis, the nurse should consider the following points. First, it usually is helpful to give the client the information over time. If the client knows the alternatives that are being ruled out during the diagnostic process, the confirmation of one alternative, even if unpleasant, will not be as much of a shock. Having time to prepare for an event is part of successful coping. Second, the nurse should gear explanations to the client's level of understanding. Listen to the clients and the terms they are choosing. Sometimes they avoid the word cancer and use tumor or growth instead. If the diagnosis of cancer is made, make sure that the client understands the terms the physician is using. Third, clients will need to hear information several times and often from several people they trust. Often, clients repeat the same questions several times. Sometimes, clients are reluctant to take up the time of the busy nurse or physician with their repeated questions. Clients need to feel that the nurse is willing to take the time to talk with them. The nurse should communicate the client's need to other members of the health care team as well. Finally, at the time the diagnosis is confirmed, the client needs to know what alternatives are available. There should be time for the client to assimilate the information before being asked to make choices about interventions. The nurse needs to be informed about the diagnosis and plan of care, about the disease and interventions in general, and about what the client actually knows.

If the diagnosis of cancer is made, expect a wide variety of reactions to the diagnosis. This will be a period of crisis for the client. This time is marked by fear, denial, withdrawal, anger, and other reactions to a crisis situation. A few clients will say that they do not want to hear anything about the disease or treatment.

TABLE 21-7. Avoid Those Factors That Might Lead to the Development of Cancer (Primary Prevention)

Smoking	Cigarette smoking is responsible for 90 per cent of lung cancer cases among men and 79 per cent among women—about 87 per cent overall. Smoking accounts for about 30 per cent of all cancer deaths. Those who smoke two or more packs of cigarettes a day have lung cancer mortality rates 15 to 25 times greater than nonsmokers
Sunlight	Almost all of the more than 600,000 cases of basal and squamous cell skin cancer diagnosed each year in the United States are considered to be sun related. Epidemiologic evidence shows that sun exposure is a major factor in the development of melanoma and that the incidence increases for those living near the equator
Ionizing radiation	Excessive exposure to ionizing radiation can increase cancer risk. Most medical and dental x-rays are adjusted to deliver the lowest dose possible without sacrificing image quality. Excessive radon exposure in homes may increase risk of lung cancer, especially in cigarette smokers. If levels are found to be too high, remedial actions should be taken
Nutrition and diet	Risk for colon, breast, and uterine cancers increases in obese people. High-fat diets may contribute to the development of cancers of the breast, colon, and prostate. High-fiber foods might help reduce risk of colon cancer. A varied diet containing plenty of vegetables and fruits rich in vitamins A and C may reduce risk for a wide range of cancers. Salt-cured, smoked, and nitrite-cured foods have been linked to esophagus and stomach cancer
Alcohol	Oral cancer and cancers of the larynx, throat, esophagus, and liver occur more frequently among heavy drinkers of alcohol especially when accompanied by cigarette smoking or chewing tobacco
Smokeless tobacco	Use of chewing tobacco or snuff increases risk of cancer of the mouth, larynx, throat, and esophagus and is a highly addictive habit
Estrogen	Estrogen treatment to control menopausal symptoms increases risk of endometrial cancer. However, including progesterone in estrogen replacement therapy helps to minimize the risk. Consultation with a physician will help each woman to assess personal risks and benefits
Occupational hazards	Exposure to several different industrial agents (nickel, chromate, asbestos, vinyl chloride, etc.) increases risk of various cancers. Risk from asbestos is greatly increased when combined with cigarette smoking

From American Cancer Society (1992). *Cancer facts and figures—1992.* New York: American Cancer Society.

TABLE 21-8. Actions to Diagnose a Cancer or Precursor as Early as Possible (Secondary Prevention/Early Detection)

Breast cancer detection	The American Cancer Society recommends that screening mammography begin by age 40. Women age 40 to 49 should have mammography every 1 to 2 years, depending on physical and mammographic findings. Women age 50 and older should have mammograms yearly. The ACS recommends the monthly practice of breast self-examination (BSE) by women 20 years and older as a routine good health habit. Clinical examination of the breast should be done every 3 years from ages 20 to 40 and then every year
Colorectal	The American Cancer Society recommends three tests for the early detection of colon and rectum cancer in people without symptoms. A digital rectal examination by a physician during an office visit should be performed every year after the age of 40; the stool blood test is recommended every year after 50; and the proctosigmoidoscopy examination should be carried out every 3 to 5 years, based on the advice of a physician
Pap test	For cervical cancer, women who are or have been sexually active, or have reached age 18, should have an annual Pap test and pelvic examination. After a woman has had three or more consecutive satisfactory normal annual examinations, the Pap test may be performed less frequently at the discretion of her physician

From American Cancer Society (1992). *Cancer facts and figures—1992.* New York: American Cancer Society.

Box 21–1. Cancer's Seven Warning Signals

Change in bowel or bladder habits
A sore that does not heal
Unusual bleeding or discharge
Thickening or lump in breast or elsewhere
Indigestion or difficulty in swallowing
Obvious change in wart or mole
Nagging cough or hoarseness

If YOU have a warning signal, see your doctor!

They cope by saying, "Don't tell me anything. Just do what you have to do." Because this is probably a temporary coping strategy, remain sensitive to clients' requests for no information now, knowing that later they will probably want to know more.

The goal of care, during this time, is to help the client cope with the diagnosis, recommended treatment, and prognosis. People cope in different ways during a crisis situation. Nevertheless, the nurse can help the client explore new and more effective coping strategies. The foundation for successful coping is receiving accurate information about the situation and possible solutions.

It is also important for the client to be both physiologically and psychologically intact enough to under-

TABLE 21–9. American Cancer Society Guidelines (1991) for Early Detection of Cancer in Asymptomatic Populations

Test	Age	Sex	Frequency
Chest x-ray study			No longer recommended for smokers to screen for lung cancer
Sputum cytology			No longer recommended for smokers to screen for lung cancer
Physical examination	40+	M,F	Yearly for all people over 40, including examination of skin, lymph nodes, mouth, thyroid, breast, testes, rectum, and prostate
Health teaching	20	M,F	Teach proper diet, exercise, health habits, breast and testicular self-examination, avoidance of sunlight, and stop smoking
Breast self-examination (BSE)	20+	F	Every month after menses before menopause. After menopause, monthly, on any specified day such as the first or last of the month
Mammography	35 to 40	F	Baseline mammogram between 35 and 40. Between 40 and 49, a mammogram should be done every 1 to 2 years and yearly after 50. High-risk women should check with their physician
Pap smear	18+	F	Sexually active women should have Pap smears regardless of age. Should be performed yearly until there are three negative examinations in a row. At this point, they can be performed yearly or as physician advises
Pelvic examination	20 to 40, 40+	F	Every 3 years, earlier if sexually active. Yearly after 40
Endometrial tissue sample	at menopause	F	High-risk women (obese, abnormal uterine bleeding, estrogen therapy, history of infertility, diabetes, hypertension, and failure to ovulate) should have this test performed at menopause
Testicular self-examination (TSE)	20 to 40	M	Monthly, on a set date such as the first of the month, following a shower
Digital rectal examination	40+	M,F	Annually for rectal cancer in men and women and prostate in men
Fecal occult blood	20 to 40, 40 to 49, 50+	M,F	Done per physician's recommendation, women at higher risk. Done per physician's recommendation. Yearly
Proctoscopy, flexible sigmoidoscopy	50+	M,F	Examination annually for 2 years and, if negative, then every 3 to 5 years
Oral examination	20+	M,F	Annually
Breast physical examination	20 to 40, 40+	F	Every 3 years. Annually

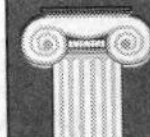

ETHICAL ISSUES IN NURSING

Who Should Be Screened for Cancer and What Tests Should Be Used?

There are several ethical dilemmas associated with the screening tests for cancer. First, not all screening tests are as effective as others. Screening tests can be very expensive. Who should be screened is another important point. Should everyone be screened, or should only those at highest risk be screened routinely (for example, age and race are specific risks for many cancers)?

To be most effective tests should be (1) specific for one type of cancer in one anatomic site, (2) reliable, (3) acceptable to the client, and (4) economical in terms of the cost-benefit ratio. The question then becomes, should only those tests that meet these standards be used?

There are no correct answers; however, those at highest risk for a disease are a priority for screening.

stand and use the information. The client should not be physically suffering, and he or she must have a sense of control over the situation. The nurse must be especially aware of the client's feelings. Hospitalization makes most people feel helpless and out of control, all of which interferes with coping.

If the nurse can help the client cope successfully during the period of diagnosis and beginning of treatment, the client may cope better during the entire course of the disease. People with cancer and their significant others often demonstrate great strength as they learn to deal with their fears and with the difficulties of being treated for cancer.

HISTORY AND PHYSICAL ASSESSMENT

The first step in the diagnostic process is obtaining a complete history and physical examination of the client. Some cancers are linked with certain genetic and environmental factors. Nurses must, therefore, learn about the health of the client's family members, the work history of the client, and the environment in which the client lives. (Review Chaps. 11 and 12) for the health history and physical assessment.) There is a great deal of information that can be obtained from the history and physical assessment.

When a malignant tumor is in its early stages, there are often few symptoms. Clinical manifestations usually appear once the tumor has grown to a sufficiently large size to cause one or more of the following problems:

- Pressure on surrounding organs or nerves;
- Distortion of surrounding tissues;
- Obstruction of lumen of tubes;
- Interference with the blood supply of surrounding tissues;
- Interference with organ function;
- Disturbance of body metabolism;
- Parasitic use of the body's nutritional supplies; and
- Mobilization of the body's defensive responses, resulting in inflammatory changes.

Common clinical manifestations that may arise secondary to cancer include weight loss, weakness or fatigue, central nervous system (CNS) alterations, pain, and hematologic and metabolic alterations. Close assessment of such symptoms may reveal that they are directly or indirectly related to the tumor growth.

Anorexia, weight loss, weakness, and fatigue are related to the body's inability to consume and use nutrients appropriately. Mechanical interference by tumors, malabsorption, paraneoplastic endocrine secretions (such as excessive secretion of thyroid hormones), and tumor use of nutrients may all contribute to a cycle that must be interrupted or that results in general physical debilitation.

The client who has difficulty with vision, speech, coordination, or memory may be experiencing primary or metastatic CNS disease. Increased intracranial pressure caused by tumor growth may cause headache, lethargy, nausea, or vomiting.

Although pain is not a common early symptom of cancer, it may occur as a result of obstruction or destruction of a vital organ, pressure on sensitive tissues or bone, or involvement of nerves. If it occurs and is not adequately treated, it may become constant and progressively severe. Bone cancer is particularly painful because the rigidity of bone allows for little or no expansion as the tumor cells proliferate. It also becomes more painful because pathologic fractures produce instability and muscle spasms.

Unexplained anemia often indicates a malignancy. Hematologic changes also include leukopenia, leukocytosis, and bleeding disorders, which, in some diseases, may occur before local symptoms. Metabolic manifestations such as Cushing's syndrome, hypercalcemia, inappropriate antidiuretic hormone (ADH) secretion, and carcinoid syndrome also signify the possibility of malignant disease.

A localized tumor usually produces symptoms related to increased pressure or obstruction in a single region. Metastatic disease and extensive tumors of major organs may display a variety of local and systemic symptoms.

CANCER-SPECIFIC DIAGNOSTIC EXAMINATIONS

The ideal diagnostic test would find cancer at the beginning, when it is composed of only a few cells. It would be specific for one type of cancer, and a positive test would provide a definitive diagnosis. It should also be inexpensive, easy to perform, and noninvasive. Unfortunately, no such text exists. Some laboratory tests can detect cancer when there are 10^4 cells, whereas the more routine laboratory and x-ray examinations detect cancer when 10^7 cells are present. A general physical assessment does not detect most tumors until there are 10^8 cells, and cancer is symptomatic at about 10^{10} cells.

RADIOGRAPHIC PROCEDURES

Basic X-ray Studies. X-ray studies are particularly useful in diagnosing obstructive tumors of the gastrointestinal, respiratory, and renal tracts. They are also valuable in identifying bone malignancies and, aided by computers, help pinpoint the location of brain tumors and the degree to which the tumors are compressing surrounding tissues.

Radioisotope Studies (Scans). Isotopes are capable of entering into the same chemical reactions and the same metabolic processes in the body as stable elements. When a radioactive isotope enters a person's body, the fate of the element can be followed, or traced, by scanning machines. Abnormal tissue appears different on the scan because the isotope is metabolized differently by this tissue. Thyroid, bone, brain, liver, lung, and spleen are areas of the body most frequently scanned for diagnostic purposes.

When diagnostically employed, radioisotopes are used as tracers. A tracer is a material that can be administered to the client, either orally or by injection. The isotope is then identified, located, and traced by a radiosensitive apparatus as the radioactive material circulates through the body and concentrates in particular organs and tissues.

The scintillation scanner is a device for locating and pinpointing malignant growths by measuring the uptake of a radioisotope. This scanner is passed back and forth over the area of the body that is being studied.

Radioisotopes are useful in the diagnosis of cancer and other diseases for several reasons. First, radioisotopes can be administered in extremely small doses, e.g., one billionth of a gram of a radioisotope can be used for administration as a tracer dose. With such small doses, the body absorbs a minimal amount of radiation, and consequently, the cells suffer no damage. Thus, radioisotopes can be employed diagnostically without the danger of cellular destruction.

Second, radioisotopes can be used to study the functions of specific organs and tissues. A classic example of this type of study is the ^{131}I uptake test that is used to evaluate thyroid function. If the examiner suspects the presence of thyroid disease, the client receives a tracer dose of radioactive iodine (^{131}I). The radioactive iodine circulates to the thyroid gland and there converts into thyroxine in precisely the same manner as regular (nonradioactive) iodine. The scintillation counter or scanner can then trace, locate, and measure tagged atoms to determine the presence of disease.

Radioisotopes are also employed to measure blood volume, blood circulation rate, red blood cell turnover, cardiac output, and lung blood flow, using the same types of procedures.

Finally, radioisotopes are used to locate tumors and lesions within the brain, kidneys, liver, lungs, pericardium, and bones. Certain radioisotopes have an affinity for particular organs or tissues; for example, ^{131}I has an affinity for thyroid tissue, ^{198}Au has an affinity for the liver, and so forth. In some cases, if the organ harbors a malignant tumor, the tagged atoms will tend to concentrate in the area of tumor growth. Consequently, a scan of the organ will reveal a high uptake of the radioisotope at the site of the tumor. For example, ^{131}I is used to locate cancerous tissues that have metastasized from the thyroid gland to other parts of the body. An area in which the concentration of a radioisotope is unusually high is called a hot spot. In other cases, the tagged atoms tend to concentrate less densely in the diseased portion of the organ than in the normal portion. The area of less concentration of a radioactive isotope is called a cold spot.

An organ scan is a simple and completely painless procedure. There are three steps involved.

1. *Administration of the radioisotope.* The client receives a tracer dose of the appropriate radioisotope either orally or by injection.
2. *Waiting period.* Before the scanning procedure can be performed, the radioisotope must be assimilated by the organ under study. The length of time required for assimilation varies. A brain scan should be performed 1 1/2 hours after an injection of radioactive mercury, and 18 to 48 hours after an injection of radioiodinated human serum albumin (RIHSA).
3. *The scanning procedure.* The client is asked to lie still and breathe normally while the scintillation scanner measures the radioactive atoms concentrated in the organ under study and records its findings. Sedation before this procedure may help the restless, agitated, or anxious client.

Computed Tomography (CT or CAT) Scan. The computed axial tomogram is an x-ray technique that produces sequential cross-sectional body images at progressive depths. CT scans can help differentiate malignant and nonmalignant masses, and accurately identify their size and location. Occasionally, an oral or intravenous contrast agent is administered to increase the sensitivity of the CT scan. Always check for an allergy to the dye.

Depending on the area to be scanned, the client may be placed on a restricted diet. Clients should be taught that they will lie on a table and the x-ray machine will move around them. This is a painless test unless an intravenous contrast dye, which may cause a burning sensation on injection, is given. The dye also may cause nausea, vomiting, flushing, itching, and a bitter taste. The x-ray machine is very noisy and could frighten the client if he or she is not warned.

Mammogram. A mammogram is a radiologic examination using a minimal and safe amount of radiation to allow visualization of breast masses, differentiating tumors from fibrocysts. The breast is compressed between two plates. The use of compression decreases the amount of radiation that must be used to visualize the tumors. Some women, particularly those with multiple fibrocysts in the breast, will find the compression uncomfortable; otherwise, the examination is painless. Two views are taken of the breast, a craniocaudal and a lateral view.

Angiogram. Angiography is used infrequently to check the resectability of tumors. This examination involves the injection of a radiopaque dye that circulates to the tumor, and then a radiographic study is performed.

This procedure clearly outlines the blood supply of the tumor and surrounding structures.

Depending on the site of the angiography, the client may be placed on a restricted diet. Clients may be sedated before the examination to help them relax and lay still during the test. The skin over the injection site is cleaned, shaved if necessary, and anesthetized. The radiopaque dye injected may cause some feelings of nausea, vomiting, flushing, itching, or a bitter or salty taste. Check whether or not the client has an allergy to the dye before it is administered.

After the test, a pressure bandage is applied to the site of the cannulization. This site is then immobilized for up to 24 hours. If a cutdown (an incision to locate the vein) is used, then the site is sutured and wound care should be done.

Lymphangiogram. The lymphangiogram is a very useful diagnostic test because it examines the lymphatic system, the primary site of metastasis for tumors with good lymphatic drainage. Although the test cannot rule out metastasis, it is an excellent marker when there is known disease because it can show tumor growth or remission.

The lymphangiogram cannot be performed for 48 hours after another contrast study. There is no preparation before this examination except client teaching. The nurse should explain to the client that the test is fairly long and uncomfortable. The test is performed by injecting blue dye into the interdigital webs of the feet. This dye is picked up by the lymphatic system so it can be cannulized. The skin on each foot over the lymphatics is anesthetized and cutdown performed so cannulas can be inserted to infuse the dye. The dye may take several hours to infuse into the lymphatics of the abdomen. X-ray studies are then obtained.

After the test, the client should drink plenty of fluids. The dye may continue to discolor the urine for several days. The feet also will remain tinted blue for a long time after the test. The client must return the following day for follow-up x-ray studies.

BLOOD STUDIES

A variety of blood tests can be performed to help diagnose cancer (Table 21-10). Some of the more routine tests, such as the complete blood count (CBC) and differential, do not test for specific types of cancer but indicate the presence of any number of problems. Other blood tests, such as tumor markers and biochemical tests, including the acid phosphatase, identify the extent of a particular type of cancer. These specific tests, however, are not used to make the diagnosis of cancer but only to check its progression.

CYTOLOGIC EXAMINATION

Papanicolaou Test (Pap Smear). This valuable diagnostic test was developed by George N. Papanicolaou in 1943. Its original purpose was to discover cancer of the cervix during the early, noninvasive, asymptomatic stage. Today, the test is also used to detect early cancers of the digestive, respiratory, and renal tracts and, occasionally, those of the breast. The Pap smear is employed to evaluate responses to chemotherapy and radiation therapy as well as to detect malignant disease when it recurs postoperatively.

Materials that can be examined by Pap smears include (1) cervical scrapings, (2) bronchial secretions and washings obtained by bronchoscopy, (3) urine sediment, (4) coughed-up sputum, (5) aspirated gastric secretions, and (6) mammary gland discharge fluid.

The method for obtaining a Pap smear is fairly simple. First, the examiner either scrapes cells from a tissue (e.g., the cervix) or obtains cells by aspirating fluid or sediment from an organ (e.g., the stomach or bronchi). Next, the examiner fixes the smear by immersing it in a chemical solution of equal parts of ether and 95 per cent ethyl alcohol. Finally, the fixed slide is allowed to dry. It is then stained and evaluated.

The laboratory technique used to analyze the Pap smear is called exfoliative cytology, which means the examination of desquamated or sloughed-off cells. Under the microscope, the cells may have either a normal or an anaplastic appearance. Cells are graded on the following five-point scale:

Class I: normal
Class II: inflammation
Class III: mild to moderate dysplasia
Class IV: possibly malignant
Class V: probably malignant

If the Pap smear indicates a Class II finding, the smear is simply repeated in 3 months. If the test reveals a Class III finding, the Pap smear will be repeated in 6 weeks to 3 months, and if it is still Class III, a biopsy is performed. If the Pap smear is Class IV or V, a biopsy is performed immediately.

BIOPSY

A biopsy is the surgical excision of a small piece of tissue for microscopic examination. Physicians most commonly use this method to either rule out or confirm a diagnosis of malignancy.

The client is usually scheduled for minor surgery. If the site for biopsy is easily accessible (e.g., cervix, breast), drape the person appropriately and assist with the administration of a local anesthetic. Then, the surgeon removes a piece of the suspicious tissue. Additional procedures (e.g., bronchoscopy, cystoscopy, and sigmoidoscopy) are necessary for an internal tumor.

There are two types of biopsy procedures. The type used depends on the size of the tumor and the purpose of the biopsy. If the suspicious tumor is small, the entire tumor is excised for examination. This is called a total or excisional type of biopsy. If the tumor is large, only a part of the neoplasm is excised. This procedure is termed a subtotal or incisional type of biopsy. There is some question as to the safety of the subtotal biopsy. Some surgeons believe that this procedure opens vascular channels and releases tumor cells that may then metastasize to other sites during the time when the excised tissue is being examined. However, there are no studies to date that definitely confirm this fear.

Following the excision, the pathologist prepares a

TABLE 21–10. Laboratory Blood Tests for Cancer

Test	Reference Values	Conditions in Which Levels Are Altered
Hematologic Tests (CBC)		
Hemoglobin	M: 14 to 18 g/dl F: 12 to 16 g/dl	↓ in anemia, nonspecific, may indicate malignancy
Hematocrit	M: 40 to 54 ml/dl F: 37 to 47 ml/dl	↓ in anemia, nonspecific, may indicate malignancy
Leukocytes (WBC)	4500 to 11,000 mm^3	↑ in leukemia and lymphomas ↓ in leukemia and metastatic disease to bone marrow
Per cent neutrophils	54 to 62 per cent	↑ in AML, CML, and lymphoma ↓ in leukemia, carcinoma, myeloma, sarcoma, and bone marrow depression
Per cent lymphocytes	25 to 33 per cent	↑ in ALL and CLL, multiple myeloma, lymphoma, and carcinoma ↓ in Hodgkin's disease, nonlymphocytic leukemias, lymphosarcoma, and bone marrow depression
Per cent monocytes	3 to 7 per cent	↑ in Hodgkin's disease, lymphoma, monocytic leukemia, CML, and multiple myeloma ↓ in hairy cell leukemia
Per cent eosinophils	1 to 3 per cent	↑ in CML ↓ in Hodgkin's disease and bone marrow depression
Per cent basophils	0 to 1 per cent	↑ in CML and Hodgkin's disease
Platelets	150,000 to 300,000 mm^3	↑ in myeloproliferative disorders, CML, and Hodgkin's disease ↓ in ALL, AML, multiple myeloma, and bone marrow depression
Blood/Serum Tests		
Acid phosphatase	0.11 to 0.60 milliunits/ml	↑ in metastatic prostate cancer
ACTH	10 to 80 pg/ml (in AM)	↑ in lung cancer
Alkaline phosphatase	20 to 90 milliunits/ml	↑ in cancer of bone or bone metastasis, liver cancer, lymphoma, and leukemia
Calcitonin	Undetectable	↑ in medullary thyroid cancer > 100 pg/ml
Calcium	9.0 to 11.0 mg/dl	↑ in bone metastasis, breast cancer, leukemia, lymphoma, multiple myeloma, lung, kidney, bladder, liver, and parathyroid cancers
Gastrin	<200 pg/ml	↑ in gastric and pancreatic cancer
IgG	500 to 1900 mg/dl	↑ in IgG myeloma
IgA	60 to 333 mg/dl	↑ in IgA myeloma
IgM	45 to 145 mg/dl	↑ in IgM Waldenstrom's macroglobulinemia
IgD	0.5 to 3.0 mg/dl	↑ in IgD myeloma
IgE	500 ng/ml	↑ in IgE myeloma
LDH	100 to 190 milliunits/dl	↑ in liver cancer and liver metastasis, lymphoma, acute leukemia
Lysozyme	4 to 13 mg/L	↑ in AML and CML
Parathyroid hormone	430 to 1860 ng/L	↑ in squamous cell lung, kidney, pancreatic, and ovarian cancers
Serotonin	50 to 200 ng/ml	↑ in carcinoid syndrome
SGPT	5 to 35 milliunits/ml	↑ in metastatic liver cancer

TABLE 21–10. Laboratory Blood Tests for Cancer Continued

Test	Reference Values	Conditions in Which Levels Are Altered
Blood/Serum Tests *Continued*		
SGOT	7 to 40 milliunits/ml	↑ in metastatic liver cancer
Testosterone	M: 275 to 875 ng/dl F: 23 to 75 ng/dl	↑ in adrenal and ovarian cancers
Uric acid	M: 2.5 to 8.0 mg/dl F: 1.4 to 7.0 mg/dl	↑ in leukemia and multiple myeloma ↓ in Hodgkin's disease, multiple myeloma, and lung cancer
Tests for Tumor Markers		
AFP	<10 ng/ml	↑ in lung, nonseminomatous testicular, pancreatic, colon, and stomach cancers, and choriocarcinoma
CA-125	<35 units	↑ in ovarian cancer
Calcitonin	<100 pg/ml	↑ in medullary thyroid, small cell lung, and breast cancers, and carcinoid
CEA	0 to 2.5 ng/ml nonsmokers <3.0 ng/ml smokers	↑ in colorectal, breast, lung, stomach, pancreatic, and prostate cancers
Estrogen receptors	Positive > 10 femtomoles/mg	↑ in breast cancer
HCG	0 to 5 IU/L	↑ in choriocarcinoma, germ cell testicular, lung, liver, stomach, pancreatic, endometrial, and liver cancers
Progesterone receptor assay	Positive > 10 femtomoles/mg	↑ in breast cancer
Prostatic acid phosphatase	0.26 to 0.83 u/L	↑ in metastatic prostate cancer
PSA	0 to 4 ng/ml	↑ in prostate cancer
CA-19-9		↑ in pancreatic and colon cancer
CA-15-3		↑ in breast cancer

ACTH, adrenocorticotropic hormone; AFP, alpha-fetoprotein; ALL, acute lymphocytic leukemia; AML, acute myelogenous leukemia; CBC, complete blood count; CEA, carcinoembryonic antigen; CLL, chronic lymphocytic leukemia; CML, chronic myelogenous leukemia; HCG, human chorionic gonadotropin; PSA, prostate-specific antigen; SGOT, serum aspartate aminotransferase; SPGT, serum alanine aminotransferase.

frozen section and/or a permanent paraffin section in order to examine the specimen. To prepare a frozen (or rapid) section, the tissue is immediately frozen. Then the pathologist cuts the tissue into thin sections and examines the tissue slices under the microscope. The main advantage of the frozen section is the speed with which the section can be prepared and the diagnosis made. Only minutes are required. In contrast, the slower, more classic method of embedding the tissue in paraffin takes about 24 hours. However, the paraffin section provides the pathologist with clearer detail than does the frozen section.

Needle or aspiration biopsy is used mainly to obtain tissue samples for identification from the liver, kidney, spleen, lung, or breast. The physician aspirates a core of tissue from a suspicious nodule or mass rather than excising it.

ULTRASOUND PROCEDURES

The ultrasound uses high-frequency sound waves to visualize the interfaces around organs and within pathologic masses. Special equipment is used to detect and map echoes of varying densities from various organs and tumors. This technique is used to detect lesions in the female pelvis, abdominal lymph nodes, prostate through a transrectal approach, and other areas of the body. One advantage of this procedure is that it is a noninvasive way to demonstrate and follow the growth of neoplasms without radiation exposure.

Preparation for the test includes cleansing the bowel with enemas if the abdominal area is to be tested and having the client drink 6 to 8 glasses of water without voiding before the test. The water distends the bladder, used as a landmark for a pelvic ultrasound, and the client is not allowed to void until after the test. The test is painless, with only a slight pressure being felt. A lubricant gel is applied, but is easily wiped off after the test. The client is allowed to void after the test is completed.

DIRECT VISUALIZATION

An endoscopy involves direct visualization of the gastrointestinal tract, a bronchoscopy of the lungs, a laryngoscopy of the larynx, a colposcopy of the cervix and vagina, a cystoscopy of the bladder, a laparoscopy of the pelvic or abdominal cavities, and so on. These tests use a rigid or flexible scope, which allows the physician to view the internal anatomy directly, without major surgery. During these tests, suspicious areas can be examined, tissue samples and aspirates taken for biopsies, the extent of the disease staged, and pathologic processes excised. These tests are discussed in detail in later chapters.

MAGNETIC RESONANCE IMAGING

Magnetic resonance imaging (MRI) identifies abnormalities by creating sectional images of the body, without the use of contrast dyes or radiation. MRI provides clear images of internal structures in response to the magnetic field created by harmless low-energy radio waves. MRI can be used to detect, localize, and stage malignancies of the central nervous system, spine, head and neck, and musculoskeletal system.

All materials that might be affected by a magnet should be removed before the test. This test cannot be performed if any material affected by a magnet cannot be removed such as a pacemaker or surgical clips. The test is painless, although some clients may feel somewhat claustrophobic because of the narrow tunnel in the machine where they must lie. Inform clients that the machine makes a loud hammering sound during the test, so they will not be frightened. If an intravenous contrast dye is used to enhance the image, the client may experience some nausea, vomiting, and itching. There is no specific nursing care required after the test. As with all diagnostic tests, the client must be supported while awaiting the results.

ANTIGEN SKIN TESTING

Recall that the immune system apparently plays a vital role in preventing tumor growth and in destroying those tumors that do develop. The immune response can be repressed by (1) immunosuppressive medications, (2) physical or emotional stress (which stimulates the release of plasma cortisol), (3) smoking, (4) alcohol, and (5) blocking agents released by the tumor. A repressed immune response usually indicates a poor prognosis. The dinitrochlorobenzene (DNCB) skin test is one method currently used to assess whether or not the person has a properly functioning immune system. Approximately 90 to 95 per cent of healthy clients can be sensitized to the chemical DNCB when it is placed on a small area of the skin. The healthy individual develops a positive response (redness, itching, perhaps blistering) within 24 to 48 hours. When given a second

TABLE 21–11. The TNM Staging System

Tumor	
T0	No evidence of primary tumor
TIS	Carcinoma in situ
T1 T2 T3 T4	Progressive increase in tumor size and involvement
TX	Tumor cannot be assessed
Nodes	
N0	Regional lymph nodes not demonstrably abnormal
N1 N2 N3	Increasing degrees of demonstrable abnormality of regional lymph nodes. (For many primary sites, the subscript a, e.g., $N1_a$, may be used to indicate that metastasis to the node is not suspected; and the subscript b, e.g., $N1_b$, may be used to indicate that metastasis to the node is suspected or proved.)
NX	Regional lymph nodes cannot be assessed clinically
Metastasis	
M0	No evidence of distant metastasis
M1 M2 M3	Ascending degrees of distant metastasis, including metastasis to distant lymph nodes

TABLE 21–12. Comparison of Staging and the TNM System

Stage	TNM Classification	Criteria
Stage I	**T1, N0, M0**	Clinical examination reveals a mass limited to the organ of origin. The lesion is operable and resectable with only local involvement, and there is no nodal and vascular spread. This stage affords the best chance for survival (from 70 to 90 per cent).
Stage II	**T2, N1, M0**	Clinical examination shows evidence of local spread into surrounding tissue and first-station lymph nodes. The lesion is operable and resectable, but because of the greater local extent, there is uncertainty as to completeness of removal. The specimen shows evidence of microinvasion into capsule and lymphatics. This stage affords a good chance of survival (50 per cent ± 5 per cent)
Stage III	**T3, N2, M0**	Clinical examination reveals an extensive primary tumor with fixation to a deeper structure, bone invasion, and lymph nodes of a similar nature. The lesion is operable but not resectable, and gross disease is left behind. This stage affords some chance of survival (20 per cent ± 5 per cent)
Stage IV	**T4, N3, M+**	There is evidence of distant metastasis beyond the site of origin. The lesion is inoperable. There is little chance of survival (<5 per cent)

From Rubin, P (Ed.) (1983). *Clinical oncology for medical students and physicians: A multidisciplinary approach* (6th ed.). New York: American Cancer Society.

(challenge) dose of DNCB 14 days later, the individual then develops a delayed cutaneous hypersensitivity response (a raised red site) on the skin.

The DNCB skin test is useful in several ways. First, it acts as a diagnostic aid. For example, clients who have a negative reaction or who cannot be sensitized to DNCB are said to be anergic (i.e., have diminished ability to react to specific antigens). This signals inadequacy of the immune response. Second, DNCB can assess the client's immunocompetence before and during radiotherapy and chemotherapy. Remember that both of these modalities can suppress the immune system. A candidate for immunotherapy (see Chap. 22) is tested prior to therapy to determine his or her immune function. Clients in immunotherapy programs are monitored throughout their therapeutic regimen to determine their response to therapy.

Staging and Grading

When a neoplastic growth is definitely diagnosed, it must be further defined in terms of its extent. This diagnostic process, called *staging*, involves a systematic search for (1) the characteristics of the primary tumor (using clinical examination and pathologic examination), (2) involvement of the lymph nodes (using clinical examination, lymphangiography, and perhaps needle biopsy), and (3) evidence of metastasis, based on knowledge of the natural history of the disease.

The TNM system is the accepted system for staging today. In this system, T stands for tumor, and T1-T4 defines the increasing tumor size. N refers to the regional lymph nodes, and N1-N3 indicates advancing nodal disease. M refers to metastasis, with M0 meaning no evidence of metastasis and M+ referring to the presence of metastasis. Table 21-11 summarizes the TNM staging system.

The older system of staging was the simple Stage 0 to V method. Table 21-12 compares the two systems. Several types of tumors are still staged using older systems, such as Clark's classification for malignant melanomas and Duke's classification for colorectal cancer. Clark's classification considers the level of invasion of melanomas, and Duke's system refers to the depth of invasion of colorectal cancer. Hodgkin's disease uses the Ann Arbor classification that refers to both the distribution of the tumor and the associated symptoms.

The *tumor grade* is an evaluation of the extent to which tumor cells differ from their normal precursors. Low numeric grades, Grade I or II, mean the cells are well differentiated and deviate minimally from the normal cells. High grades, Grade III or IV, refer to cells that are poorly differentiated and the most aberrant compared with the normal cells.

The histologic grade is determined by a pathologist. Tumor grading involves a histologic and anatomic description of the malignant neoplasm. Staging and grading information guides the physician in the choice of intervention and in estimating the client's prognosis.

Assessment of the Client's Physical Performance

There are scales that help assess the client's ability to continue activity. A common scale is the Karnofsky Performance Status Scale (Table 21-13). This scale can help the nurse assess the effect of the cancer on the client's physical activity and guide interventions to assist with deficits.

TABLE 21-13. Karnofsky Performance Status Scale

Condition	Percentage	Comments
Able to carry on normal activity and to work. No special care is needed	100	Normal; no complaints; no evidence of disease
	90	Able to carry on normal activity; minor signs or symptoms of disease
	80	Normal activity with effort; some signs or symptoms of disease
Unable to work. Able to live at home, care for most of personal needs. A varying degree of assistance is needed	70	Cares for self; unable to carry on normal activity or to do active work
	60	Requires occasional assistance but is able to care for most needs
	50	Requires considerable assistance and frequent medical care
Unable to care for self. Requires equivalent of institutional or hospital care. Disease may be progressing rapidly	40	Disabled; requires special care and assistance
	30	Severely disabled; hospitalization is indicated, although death is not imminent
	20	Hospitalization is necessary; very sick; active supportive treatment necessary
	10	Moribund; fatal processes progressing rapidly
	1	Unconscious
	0	Dead

From Baird, S.B., et al. (1991). *Cancer nursing: A comprehensive textbook.* Philadelphia: W.B. Saunders.

Summary

Cancer is a disease that strikes one in three to four people in the United States. It is a condition most nurses will work with at some point during their careers. An understanding of the basic principles concerning its development, prevention, and early detection is essential for every nurse.

Bibliography

1. Achterberg, J., et al. (1976). *Stress, psychological factors and cancer.* Fort Worth, TX: Medicine Press.
2. American Cancer Society (1990). *Cancer facts and figures.* New York: American Cancer Society.

2a. American Cancer Society (1992). *Cancer facts and figures.* New York: American Cancer Society.

3. American Cancer Society (1984). *Nutrition and cancer: Cause and prevention.* New York: American Cancer Society.
4. American Nurses' Association & Oncology Nursing Society (1987). *Standards of oncology nursing practice.* Kansas City, MO: American Nurses' Association.
5. Baird, S. B., et al. (1991). *Cancer nursing: A comprehensive textbook.* Philadelphia: W. B. Saunders.
6. Barber, H. (1986). Ovarian cancer. *Ca: A Cancer Journal for Clinicians, 36,* 149-183.
7. Bassett, M., & Krieger, N. (1986). Social class and black-white differences in breast cancer survival. *American Journal of Public Health, 76,* 1400-1403.
8. Beahrs, O. H., et al. (1988). *American Joint Committee on Cancer: Manual for staging of cancer* (3rd ed.). Philadelphia: J. B. Lippincott.
9. Benedict, W. (1987). Hereditary factors: Human cancer susceptibility genes. *Proceedings of the second national conference on cancer prevention and detection.* New York: American Cancer Society.
10. Benner, P., & Wrubel, J. (1989). *The primacy of caring.* Menlo Park, CA: Addison-Wesley.
11. Blesch, K. (1986). Health beliefs about testicular cancer and self-examination among professional men. *Oncology Nursing Forum, 143,* 29-33.
12. Breslow, L., & Cumberland, W. G. (1988). Progress and objectives in cancer control. *Journal of the American Medical Association, 259,* 1690-1694.
13. Briton, L. A., & Fraumeni, J. F. (1986). Epidemiology in uterine and cervical cancer. *Journal of Chronic Diseases, 39,* 1051-1065.
14. Cannon-Albright, L. A., Skolnick, M. H., Bishop, T., Lee, R. G., & Burt, R. W. (1988). Common inheritance of susceptibility to colonic adenomatous polyps and associated colorectal cancers. *New England Journal of Medicine, 319,* 533-537.
15. Centers for Disease Control (1985). Behavioral risk factors surveillance in selected states. *Journal of the American Medical Association, 256,* 697-698.
16. Clark, J. (1990). Psychosocial dimensions: The patient. In S. L. Groenwald, et al. (Eds.), *Cancer nursing: Principles and practice* (2nd ed., pp. 346-364). Boston: Jones and Bartlett.
17. Consolidated Omnibus Budget Reconciliation Act (COBRA) (1986). 42 U.S.C. 300 bb *et seq.*
18. Crothers, H. M. (1986). Employment problems of cancer survivors: Local problems and local solutions. In American Cancer Society, *Proceedings of the workshop on employment, insurance, and the patient with cancer* (pp. 51-57). New Orleans: American Cancer Society.
19. Crothers, H. M. (1987). Health insurance: Problems and solutions for people with cancer histories. In American Cancer Society, *Proceedings of the 5th national conference on human values and cancer* (pp. 100-109). San Francisco: American Cancer Society.
20. Eddy, D. A. (1985). Screening for cancer in adults. *CIBA Foundation Symposium, 110,* 88-109.
21. Eddy, D. M. (1986). Secondary prevention in cancer: An overview. *Bulletin of the World Health Organization, 64,* 421-429.
22. Frank-Stromborg, M. (1986). The role of the nurse in early detection of cancer: Population 66 years of age and older. *Oncology Nursing Forum, 13,* 107-115.
23. Frank-Stromborg, M. (1988). Nursing's role in cancer prevention and early detection: Vital contributions to attainment of the Planning, goals/expected outcomes year 2000 goals, *Cancer, 62,* 1833-1838.
24. Frank-Stromborg, M. (1989). Reaction to the diagnosis of cancer questionnaire (RDCQ): Development and psychometric evaluation. *Nursing Research, 38,* 364-369.
25. Frank-Stromborg, M., & Wright, P. (1984). Ambulatory cancer patients' perception of the physical and psychosocial changes in their lives since the diagnosis of cancer. *Cancer Nursing, 7,* 117-130.
26. Frost, P., & Fidler, I. J. (1986). Biology of metastasis. *Cancer, 58,* 550-553.
27. Grant, M. M., & Padilla, G. V. (1990). Cancer nursing research. In S. L. Groenwald, et al. (Eds.), *Cancer nursing: Principles and practice* (2nd ed., pp. 1270-1279). Boston: Jones and Bartlett.
28. Greenwald, P., & Sondik, E. (Eds.) (1986). Cancer control objectives for the nation. *National Cancer Institute Monograph, 1985-2000.* (NIH Publication No. 86-2880). Washington, DC: United States Government Printing Office.
29. Gritz, E. R. (1988). Cigarette smoking: The need for action by health professionals. *Ca: A Cancer Journal for Clinicians, 38,* 194-212.
30. Groenwald, S., et al. (1990). *Cancer nursing: Principles and practice.* Boston: Jones and Bartlett.
31. Hakama, M. (1986). Scientific basis of screening in early detection. *Cancer Detection and Prevention, 9,* 139-143.
32. Karnofsky, D. A., & Burchenal, J. H. (1949). The clinical evaluation of chemotherapeutic agents in cancer. In C. M. MacLeod (Ed.), *Evaluation of chemotherapeutic agents.* New York: Columbia University Press.
33. Larson, P. J. (1986). Cancer nurses' perception of caring. *Cancer Nursing, 9,* 86-91.
34. Lewandowski, W., & Jones, S. L. (1988). The family with cancer. *Cancer Nursing, 11,* 313-321.
35. Levine, E. G., et al. (1989). The role of heredity in cancer. *Journal of Clinical Oncology, 7,* 527-540.
36. Miller, A. B. (1986). Screening for cancer: Issues and future direction. *Journal of Chronic Diseases, 39,* 1067-1077.
37. Page, H., & Asire, A. (1985). *Cancer rates and risks* (3rd ed.). (NIH Publication no. 85-691). Washington, DC: United States Government Printing Office.
38. Palmer, S. (1986). Dietary considerations for risk reduction. *Cancer, 58,* 1949-1953.
39. Polit, D., & Hungler, B. (1977). *Nursing research: Principles and methods.* Philadelphia: J. B. Lippincott.
40. Rubin, P. (Ed.) (1983). *Clinical oncology for medical students and physicians: A multidisciplinary approach* (6th ed.). New York: American Cancer Society.
41. Simonton, C. O., et al. (1978). *Getting well again.* New York: Bantam Books.
42. Stoll, B. A. (1985). *Screening and monitoring of cancer.* New York: John Wiley & Sons.
43. Stromborg, M., et al. (1986). Carcinogens: Are some risks acceptable? *American Journal of Nursing, 86,* 814-817.
44. Stromborg, M. F., & Bourque-Nord, S. (1979). A cancer detection clinic: Patient motivation and satisfaction. *Nurse Practitioner, 4*(10), 10-11, 51-52.
45. Willet, W. (1989). The search for the causes of breast and colon cancer. *Nature, 338,* 389-394.
46. Wynder, E., et al. (1986). Diet and breast cancer in causation and therapy. *Cancer, 58,* 1804-1813.
47. Yasko, J. M., & Greene, P. (1987). Coping with problems related to cancer and cancer treatment. *Ca: A Cancer Journal for Clinicians, 37*(2), 106-125.

Chapter 22

Treatment Modalities for Neoplastic Disorders

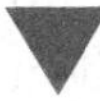

PSYCHOSOCIAL ASPECTS OF CANCER

Cancer is a feared and dreaded disease for several reasons. It may present in an advanced stage with no symptoms. Compliance with vigorous and sometimes disfiguring treatment does not guarantee a cure. In addition, cancer may recur after many years of remission. A healthy lifestyle does not ensure that a person will escape from the disease.[43]

Great variability exists in the distress, changes, and effects of cancer on the lives of the clients and their families. Responses to cancer depend on the (1) client and the client's psychological make-up, (2) family and social community of the client, and (3) disease, disabilities, and disfigurements it may cause.

Cancer can affect the client at all levels of functioning. Intellectual function can be clouded by physical distress or medication. The client's self-concept is affected by the physical changes and changes in role or function. The client who was the caretaker of the family may become dependent on others and the consumer of family savings and resources. The young adult, striving for independence, may need to revert to an earlier level of dependency. Changes in body image occur in most clients. Weight loss, alopecia, and skin changes can result from treatment. Radical surgical procedures can produce devastating and permanent changes in appearance and function. Procedures such as laryngectomy, glossectomy, quadrant resection, hemicorpectomy, or pelvic exenteration produce changes that may be humiliating and overwhelming to the client.

The diagnosis of cancer has an impact on the entire family. The daily life of the family is changed. If the client is the caretaker, other family members will need to assume this role. If the family functions poorly before the illness, then the additional stress may increase the dysfunction.

Imposed on the intrinsic complexity of individuals, families, and cultures is the variability of cancer as a disease. Some cancers are relatively easy to treat and have a reliable potential for cure, whereas others require extensive, rigorous treatment without a guarantee of cure. Symptoms vary among clients as well. Some may have considerable physical distress whereas others have none.

Although each cancer experience is unique to any individual, clients with cancer have some common problems during particular time points in the illness continuum. All clients undergo a period of diagnosis and initial treatment. If the cancer is considered curable and the client completes definitive treatment for the cancer, a period of survivorship ensues. This is characterized by watchful waiting for disease recurrence.[47] Those clients who have metastatic disease at the time of treatment or who have a cancer recurrence must deal with the chronicity of the disease.

Specific psychosocial problems, assessment, and intervention strategies are addressed for each of the distinct phases of the cancer continuum: (1) diagnosis and treatment, (2) survivorship, (3) recurrent disease and palliation, and (4) terminal illness.

DIAGNOSIS AND TREATMENT

Cancer clients reach the point of diagnosis in many ways. Clients may have had vague symptoms, that is, weight loss and fatigue, that have been ignored or the cause of some anxiety for weeks or months. They may have symptoms such as pain or abdominal bloating that evaded diagnosis. Many times, cancer is found inadvertently during routine examinations. Often, the client suspects cancer, but many clients are shocked when the diagnosis is made. The diagnostic period may be lengthy and extremely distressful. This period is filled with anxiety over each test result, especially when staging procedures are done. Over 70 per cent of clients consider the time of diagnosis and treatment as the most distressful in the cancer experience.[67]

Most clients fear death during the first few months of the cancer experience. Weisman called this stage the existential plight. Whether clients can express their fears or not, it is an underlying cause of distress.[67] During diagnosis, the magnitude of the problems becomes apparent. Is the disease curable or not? Will the disabilities be temporary or permanent? What types of physical impairment will occur? What will be the side effects of treatment? Will the symptoms be relieved? Will the client be able to return to work? What adjustments have to be made in family life or work? Will finances be adequate? What plans need to be abandoned? Which changes in lifestyle will be temporary and which permanent?

Clients must not only deal with specific problems but also the emotional distress experienced throughout this time. They may feel angry and frustrated because their lives have been changed; they may feel isolated or may worry about being abandoned by family and friends. They may be shocked and unbelieving that they are the ones with cancer.

It must be stressed that there is great variability in client's reactions. Some have minimal distress, whereas others may be overwhelmed and devastated. The magnitude and intensity of emotions and problems depend on the clients psychological make-up, social support, resources, and the disease itself.

Coping is the dynamic process by which a client responds to a problem to bring about relief or equilibrium. Weisman's studies of cancer clients and their coping identified coping styles used by many cancer clients (Box 22-1). Denial that is a part of coping allows a client to "repudiate what cannot be avoided, by substituting a more favorable or agreeable idea."[47] Denial can be useful to the newly diagnosed client when the sheer number of problems may be overwhelming. Denial is harmful when it prevents the client from seeking appropriate treatment. Awareness and denial can exist at the same time.

Clients who are good problem solvers or who cope well confront reality, avoid excessive denial, remain flexible, accept support, and remain hopeful and optimistic. Clients who cope poorly use avoidance and excessive denial; they are pessimistic and feel hopeless.[47] Factors that enable or hinder coping are listed in Box 22-2.[32]

To assess the psychosocial needs of the client, the nurse must be knowledgeable of the general types of emotions and problems of clients with cancer and sen-

Box 22-1. General Coping Strategies

- Seek more information (rational inquiry)
- Share concern and talk with others (mutuality)
- Laugh it off; make light of situation (affect reversal)
- Try to forget; put it out of your mind (suppression)
- Do other things for distraction (displacement/redirection)
- Take firm action based on present understanding (confront)
- Accept but find something favorable (redefine/revise)
- Submit to the inevitable; fatalism (passive acceptance)
- Do something, anything, however reckless or impractical (impulsivity)
- Consider or negotiate feasible alternative (if x, then y)
- Reduce tension with excessive drink, drugs, danger (life threats)
- Withdraw into isolation; get away (disengagement)
- Blame someone or something (externalize/project)
- Seek direction; do what you're told (cooperative compliance)
- Blame yourself; sacrifice or atone (moral masochism)

From Weisman, A. (1979). *Coping with cancer* (p. 23). New York: McGraw-Hill.

Box 22-2. Enabling and Hindering Factors in Coping with Cancer

Enabling Factors

Social support systems
Perception of control
Hardiness
Humor
Positive appraisal
Hopefulness
Positive comparisons
Religiosity
Self-esteem
Information seeking
Open communication
Social skills
Problem-solving ability

Hindering Factors

Denial
Avoidance
Helplessness
Powerlessness
Hopelessness or despair
Depression
Guilt
Erosion of autonomy
Isolation or withdrawal
Wishful thinking
Anger or hostility
Blaming others
Noncompliance

From Jalowiec, A., & Dudas, S., (1991). Alterations in patient coping. In S. Baird, R. McCorkle, & M. Grant (Eds.), *Cancer nursing: A comprehensive text* (pp. 806–820). Philadelphia: W. B. Saunders.

sitive to their expression by the client. Asking tactful questions will determine the accuracy of the nurse's perception. The complexity and uniqueness of each client requires validation of that client's individual problems.

Families also should be assessed for their coping ability. Use of a specific family assessment tool often is not possible, but high-risk families can be readily identified. Families who use excessive denial, exhibit strong anger and guilt, or are particularly demanding may be at increased risk of dysfunction. When the client is the pivotal family person or when the family has had a previous experience of cancer, family needs may be increased.[42]

Coping strategies of the clients must be identified. Once defined, interventions to (1) help clients deal with their emotions and (2) solve specific problems can be used.

Expressing emotions may be difficult for many clients. Nurses can help clients by listening actively to clients and maintaining a noncritical relationship with the client that allows expression of negative feelings. Referrals to counseling or more formal methods of emotional expression such as music or art therapy may be appropriate, if available. Providing social support and improving the client's sense of control helps reduce anxiety. Stress reduction or relaxation techniques can be taught. Many clients are encouraged by speaking with former clients. Programs such as Reach to Recovery and Cansurmount (American Cancer Society) provide this opportunity.

Informational needs predominate during the diagnostic and treatment periods. Tests, procedures, and treatments, which are often very technical and complicated, need to be taught to the client. During this time of anxiety and stress, the simplest explanation is usually the most appropriate and all that the client can assimilate. Misconceptions need to be identified and corrected.

The specific problems of clients can be addressed by helping the client to identify the problem, providing information when necessary and referring the client to appropriate resources.

The diagnostic period is one of great distress. Clients are vulnerable and fragile. They need compassion and caring, sensitivity and understanding. A relationship of trust and confidence helps carry the client through this time of uncertainty and threat.

SURVIVORSHIP

Clients who have completed curative treatment enter an indeterminate period of survivorship. As increasing numbers of clients are being cured of cancer, more attention is being focused on the physiologic and psychological needs of this group. Clients have organized into advocate groups to provide mutual support and to lobby for legislation to address some of their specific needs in employment and insurance coverage.

The time of survivorship has been divided into a time of extended survival followed by a period of permanent survival.[47] The transition between these periods is not precise but evolves as the time passes and cancer does not recur.

The period of extended survival maybe one of physical fatigue and limitation, depending on the extent of treatment (see Bridge to Home Health Care). Physical rehabilitation to improve functioning may dominate the client's energy in this early period. Efforts must focus on returning the client to the previous level of functioning. The long-term physical effects of cancer treatment are now becoming apparent as data accumulate, especially from pediatric cancer clients. The physical effects may range from minimal restriction to life-threatening complications. Effects can be organ specific, such as cardiomyopathy or pulmonary fibrosis, or general, such as fatigue. The potential for developing a second malignancy as a result of primary treatment exists, although it rarely occurs. Routine follow-up and long-term health care need to be established with the client at this time.[40]

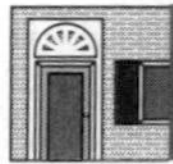

BRIDGE TO HOME HEALTH CARE

Supporting the Client with Cancer

The home health care nurse functions as a vital link that ensures continuity of care as the cancer client goes home following surgery, chemotherapy, and/or radiation therapy. Still stunned by the reality of the disease, the cancer client requires considerable emotional support to aid in the management of symptoms. It is hoped that symptom management will result in a renewed sense of well-being and determination to continue to participate in life despite the illness. Emotional support means simply showing you care through touch and active listening. When all else is forgotten, that touch and that kind word will provide comfort.

Teaching quickly becomes the focus of the home health nurse's visit as the cancer client begins to relax again in his own home and really hears other information that will help him or her feel better. Be familiar with the rationale for your suggestions and present them when appropriate. Start with simple basic information about nutrition and fluid intake. Teaching should include information such as eating a sizeable breakfast because the appetite wanes with the day, eating small frequent meals, eating foods at room temperature, avoiding fatty or fried foods, avoiding spicy foods, using a supplement such as a powdered instant breakfast between meals to boost caloric intake and give energy, and taking nausea medication regularly so eating is possible. Drink lots of water to support blood pressure, flush the bladder, and replace fluids that might be lost through vomiting and diarrhea. Pay attention to mouth care, watch for the development of mouth sores and report them immediately, use a soft tooth brush, keep lips moist, and rinse the mouth before and after meals. Elimination is always a major concern of clients. If diarrhea is the problem, increase fluids; use nutmeg, apples, or bananas to slow peristalsis; use vitamins A & D ointment on the rectum after washing; and use prescribed medication. If constipation is the problem, increase fluids, fiber, and activity. A concoction of prune juice, milk of magnesia, and sodium biphosphate (Phospho-Soda) is just one remedy.

Fatigue remains a troublesome and universal symptom. Clients must be reminded that it is okay to take the time needed for recovery, and that a longer recovery period is likely with each succeeding treatment. Clients in treatment are likely to be affected by low blood counts. Stress the necessity of avoiding sick people, have the client take his or her temperature twice a day, teach good handwashing, suggest avoiding bumping or cutting the skin, and have the client use an electric shaver. Pain, actual or potential, frightens all cancer clients. Two simple suggestions go a long way to promote comfort. They are (1) take medication on a scheduled rather than an as-needed basis, and (2) reorder medication 1 week before the supply is depleted.

Psychologically, the period of extended survival is one in which clients must resocialize into previous roles or adjust and reorganize their lives. The possibility of recurrence may dominate their lives. Plans may be suspended. Decisions concerning changing jobs, buying a house, starting a family, or retirement may be difficult in the face of the uncertainty of recurrence. Referral to support groups of survivors may be helpful.

Employment discrimination has been a problem for cancer survivors. Although clients with a cancer history have proved themselves to be dependable and productive, studies show that as many as 84 per cent of blue collar workers and 38 per cent of white collar workers experience some type of discrimination in employment.[54] Over the years, these issues have been rectified by state laws protecting the rights of the disabled.

Like employment, obtaining insurance coverage for a client with a cancer history has been difficult, exorbitantly expensive, and sometimes impossible. Legislative efforts over the past decade have rectified some of these problems. Insurance discrimination can be legally appealed. Federal programs such as Cobra (Consolidated Omnibus Budget Reconciliation Act) protect the insurance coverage of an employee for 18 months following employment termination. Many states have passed comprehensive health insurance plans to provide coverage for clients who are unable to obtain commercial insurance. Clients who have difficulty with insurance coverage should be directed to the American Cancer Society, their state Department of Human Rights, or Insurance Department. The booklet *Facing Forward* from the National Institute of Health provides detailed informational resources.

With time, problems abate and clients become permanent survivors. The experience of cancer is indelibly printed on their life. They are forever changed. Amazingly, most clients cope very well and courageously face the difficulties in their life. For many, the experience has caused a reappraisal of goals and values, making life richer and more meaningful.

RECURRENT DISEASE AND PALLIATION

The recurrence of cancer provides the basis for a chronic phase of the cancer experience. Most clients with cancer live with the threat or reality of recurrent disease. Recurrence, at the very least, signifies that the disease is in control and that the individual is not. Weisman[67] describes the impact that this phase has on the client as "the hope for a cure" becomes the "struggle for existence."

With recurrent disease, therapy may once again be used to eradicate or stabilize the disease process. Yet, although subsequent recurrent disease may occur, it is usually the first recurrence that involves surprise, shock, and disbelief. Thus, it is important for the nurse to assess the client's coping skills and provide assistance in helping to mobilize resources and support. Many cancers have a propensity for recurrence, including adult acute leukemias, non-Hodgkin's lymphoma, breast, and lung cancers.

Physical impairment may be increased and quality of life may be limited owing to disease or treatment. The client who previously verbalized an optimistic outlook may now express a more guarded attitude. It is vital for the nurse to maintain open communication and to be sensitive to the informational and support needs of the client and family with cancer.

Palliative care and palliative treatment are two distinct options for the client with cancer. Palliative treatment (surgery, radiation therapy or chemotherapy) may be used to alleviate complications caused by persistent tumor growth. For example, surgery may be used to manage a malignant obstruction or radiation therapy to reduce or prevent paralysis from spinal cord compression.

Palliative care is the provision of symptom management and psychosocial support provided by a multidisciplinary health care team. It is important that the nurse communicates that symptoms can be managed successfully and that resources are available to assist in providing supplies and support. Palliative care is effective in decreasing the stress related to advanced cancer and provides the client and family with options to assist them as the disease enters the terminal phase of illness.

THE TERMINALLY ILL

More than 50 per cent of clients with cancer die from their disease. The time from diagnosis to death ranges from weeks to years. Not all clients with cancer become terminally ill. Some clients die during the initial treatment, whereas others die from treatment complications. Many clients, however, reach an endpoint at which time their cancer no longer responds to treatment and disease progression cannot be controlled. Now the goals of treatment are directed toward supportive care of the client and family until death occurs.

During the past 25 years, hospice care has become the standard of care for terminally ill cancer clients in the United States. This philosophy of care emphasizes symptom control and pain management, providing comfort and dignity for the client during the dying process.

Hospices date back to medieval times and were way stations for weary and sick travellers during the Crusades. Mostly, they were run by Christian religious orders. The Irish Sisters of Charity opened the first hospice specifically for the dying in the mid-19th century in London. However, it was not until 1967 when Dr. Cicely Saunders opened the St. Christopher's hospice in London and pioneered techniques for adequate pain control that the modern concept of hospice care emerged.[41]

The first hospice in the United States was opened in 1974 in New Haven, Connecticut. Since that time, more than 1600 hospices have been opened in the United States. The hospice can be connected with a hospital, community, home care agency, or skilled nursing facility. The basic characteristics of a hospice program include:

- Control of client symptoms and pain relief;
- Treatment of client and family as a unit;
- Provision of care by a physician-directed interdisciplinary team;
- 24-hour, 7-day coverage;
- An autonomous hospice administration providing coordinated home care with back-up inpatient services;
- Use of trained volunteers to augment staff services;
- Structured systems of staff support;
- Bereavement follow-up; and
- Services given based on need and not ability to pay.

To qualify for hospice services, clients must have a life expectancy of less than 6 months and be on only supportive treatment.[41]

When cancer clients reach the point at which treatment is no longer effective, they are considered terminally ill (Ethical Issues in Nursing). Some clients can accept or resign themselves to the approaching end of their life; others cannot and will continue to seek treatment beyond reasonable limits.

Cancer clients approach death in as many ways as they approach life. Some try to remain active despite tremendous physical limitations. Others may withdraw into depression. This period is a time of suffering for

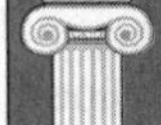

ETHICAL ISSUES IN NURSING

Who Should Decide the Continuation or Cessation of Cancer Treatment?

Great strides have been made in these modern times in the treatment of neoplastic disorders. No longer is the word *cancer* always equated with death. There is much hope in the treatment of certain cancerous conditions. Oncology nursing has become a very specialized area of practice. Even though this is true, and even though much has been learned, disease processes that cannot be cured remain, and patients with these diseases must rely on care.

Are there times when a client should accept from the health care provider that nothing more can be done—that treatment options are futile? Are physicians obligated to treat clients with therapies that are hopeless even if the client might want such therapies? On the other hand, are there times when a client can say they wish no more treatment—no more chemotherapy, radiation therapy, or even surgery—even if there is a chance that such treatments might be helpful? Perhaps they believe the end stages of their life would be better lived without the side effects of such treatments.

Nursing care for clients with cancer presents many challenges. The nurse must be sensitive to the emotional aspect of their client's illness, be skilled with the technical aspects of care (such as in chemotherapy), be available to teach both client and significant others about the disease process and treatments, and be a health care advocate for the client. If a client decides that he or she no longer wants treatment, the nurse must put all of his or her skills to work to help meet the client's current and anticipated needs. If treatment is no longer an option for a client, the nurse is there to provide care for the client and perhaps significant others.

To cure should not always be seen as success and not to cure as failure. Caring can be just as successful as curing when curing is not an option. Nurses have an important role in the caring process of a client's illness, especially when such care is exercised during the final stages of life.

both client and family as the physical loss of function and the psychological pain of anticipated and real losses in relationships and roles are intensified.

Nursing care of the terminally ill addresses pain and symptom management while maintaining the dignity of the client and promoting the maximum quality of life. As family members become caretakers, they must be taught simple nursing skills and pain management. Open communication and continued revalidation of the concerns and needs of client and family need to be maintained.

Family members need constant reassurance that they are providing good care. Although it is often a new and unfamiliar experience, most families are able to focus their energies and strengthen their family bonds through the experience of caring for a dying family member. When death occurs, families are usually physically exhausted but psychologically strengthened.

Clients without families or friends to function as primary caretakers have few options for their care. A few free-standing hospices exist to provide them with care. Many nursing homes have hospice programs. Clients without insurance or financial means are less fortunate.

Masterful use of ordinary nursing skills, combined with creative symptom management and compassion for the client and family suffering, is the essence of hospice nursing care. When all else has failed, nursing care remains to ameliorate the suffering of the dying. In return, the nurse is witness to the essence of human life and the courage of the human spirit.

Nurses are encouraged to plan, implement, and evaluate the care of the client with cancer using the high incidence problem areas in oncology identified in Box 22–3. If these areas are thoroughly assessed and evaluated for each client during each phase of the cancer experience, the physical and emotional distress of cancer may be minimized.

> Beyond what machines and medicines and procedures can do for the patient, the act of caring remains a powerful weapon in the fight against disease. It is the one thing that medical technology can never replace. When everything is done that can be done, compassion is the only thing that brings beauty and meaning to our lives. It is the irreplaceable gift.[61]

MEDICAL TREATMENT AND NURSING CARE FOR CLIENTS WITH CANCER

Goals of Intervention

The major objective of cancer therapy is to treat the client effectively with the appropriate therapy for a sufficient duration so a cure results with minimal functional and structural impairment.[7] If a cure is not possible, important alternate goals are to (1) prevent further metastasis, (2) relieve symptoms, and (3) maintain a high quality of life for as long as possible. Decisions made at the time of first diagnosis are crucial, because early aggressive intervention usually offers the best hope of cure.

Box 22–3. High Incidence Problem Areas in Oncology

Prevention and early detection
Coping
Nutrition
Mobility
Sexuality
Circulation
Information
Comfort
Protective mechanisms
Elimination
Ventilation

From American Nurses' Association & Oncology Nursing Society (1987). *Standards of oncology nursing practice.* Kansas City, MO: American Nurses' Association.

Methods for treating clients with cancer include chemotherapy, surgery, radiation therapy, biotherapy, and bone marrow transplantation. The choice of method depends on the tumor type, extent of disease, and the client's physical status. Often, a client is treated with a combination of methods rather than a single therapy. This approach is called combined modality therapy. Combined modality therapy is used when appropriate to the tumor, because it produces greater tumor cell kill.

Surgery

Surgery plays a major role in the diagnosis, staging, and treatment of cancer. It is also an integral part of rehabilitation and palliation of clients with cancer. It is used with less frequency as a method of cancer prevention.

DIAGNOSTIC SURGERY

The diagnosis of cancer is established by microscopic identification of malignant cells from tumor tissue. There are a variety of methods used to obtain tissue for diagnostic purposes. The biology of the tumor, size, location, and proposed method of treatment determine which method of biopsy should be used.

Cytology Specimens. Cytology specimens can be obtained from tumors that tend to shed cells from their surface. Tumor cells can often be obtained from cytologic examination of fluids aspirated from effusions, ascitic fluid, or endoscopic brushings.

Needle Biopsy. Needle biopsy is a simple method of obtaining tissue samples. In a fine-needle aspiration, tumor cells are withdrawn from the tumor by a needle and syringe. A core-needle biopsy is essentially the same procedure; however, the needle is larger and a core of tissue is obtained. This allows the pathologist to examine the cells with their spatial relationships intact, whereas aspiration biopsy provides individual cells or clumps of cells for review. Needle biopsies are useful in obtaining samples from tumors in subcutaneous tissue, muscle, breast, pancreas, liver, and lung.

Cytology and needle biopsies are relatively simple procedures. Care must be taken to obtain needle biopsies from areas that will be surgically removed if the tumor is malignant, because malignant cells can be deposited in the needle tract. A negative biopsy does not prove the absence of cancer but rather may be an indication of inadequate or misplaced tissue sampling. Negative biopsies must be pursued with additional biopsies.

Incisional Biopsy. An incisional biopsy surgically removes a small sample of tissue for examination. It is performed during endoscopic examinations of the bronchus, stomach, bladder, and colon and in removal of samples of large tumor masses in which a diagnosis must be made before definitive surgical treatment. Surgical techniques are used to prevent seeding of tumor cells in the biopsy site. As with the needle biopsy, cancer can be proved with a positive result but not ruled out with a negative one. When negative results are obtained, additional biopsies may be attempted.

Excisional Biopsy. An excisional biopsy removes all of the tumor mass and provides the pathologist with an entire sample. It is used for small tumors (2 to 3 cm. in size) in which the biopsy also may serve as the treatment if the tissue margins contain no tumor cells. If tumor cells remain, a wider excision is required. Excisional biopsies are useful in skin cancers, melanomas, and in breast cancer.

STAGING

Cancer staging is the process of determining the extent of disease as the basis for treatment decisions. Clinical staging, such as x-ray studies or scans are sufficient for most types of cancer. Staging information is also obtained during surgery for cancer treatment. For example, the true stage of colon cancer is usually determined after surgery, when the regional lymph nodes are examined for the presence of tumor cells.

In Hodgkin's disease, although radiation therapy and chemotherapy are the primary treatment modalities, a surgical laparotomy may be required to obtain tissue samples of lymph nodes to ascertain the precise extent of the disease. Laparotomies are often required for the accurate staging of ovarian cancer as well.

CURATIVE SURGERY

Primary Lesions. Surgery is performed in the treatment of 55 per cent of clients with cancer. Forty per cent of clients are treated with surgery alone. Cancers that are localized to the organ of origin and the regional lymph nodes are potentially curable by surgery.

Historically, the generally accepted concept of tumor growth was as an orderly sequence of growth from the organ of origin to the adjacent tissue, regional lymph nodes, and eventually, systemically to distant sites. The logical surgical approach for this type of growth was the widest excision possible of the tumor, surrounding tissue, and regional lymph nodes. Thus, radical surgery became the standard for cancer treatment. Analysis of treatment results, however, demonstrated that despite radical excisions, tumors recurred.[64a] Current concepts in tumor biology hold that tumors probably begin shedding cells into the systemic circulation throughout their growth and, therefore, combinations of local therapies, surgery, and radiation must be combined with systemic therapies, chemotherapy, and biotherapy to improve client survival.

When surgery is performed with curative intent, the extent of the excision is determined by the type of tumor. For slow-growing tumors, such as those of the skin, a wide local excision may be sufficient. Tumors of the colon and breast that spread to the regional lymph nodes are removed with an en bloc excision of the tumor and the regional lymph nodes. Large tumors, such as sarcomas, which tend to spread locally without metastasizing are removed with radical excisions, such as amputations. In all surgical procedures, various operative techniques, such as glove changing, instrument cleaning, and wound irrigation with cytotoxic agents, are used to prevent dissemination of tumor cells into the operative field.

Recurrent Lesions. Cancer that recurs locally can be resected, resulting in occasional cure, remission, or both. Local recurrences of sarcomas, colon, breast, and skin cancers have been successfully excised, resulting in cures.

Metastatic Lesions. Solitary metastatic lesions that appear in the lungs, liver, or brain can be removed to effect a surgical cure. Excision of metastatic lesions is considered if no other evidence of disease exists and the metastatic lesion appeared after a relatively long disease-free interval. The metastatic lesion must exhibit some degree of stability and be refractory to chemotherapy and radiotherapy. Metastatic renal cell carcinomas, sarcomas, melanomas, and colon carcinomas have been removed in selected clients, resulting in cures or prolonged survival times.

PALLIATIVE SURGERY

Because surgical procedures carry an inherent potential for morbidity, use of surgery in palliative care is carefully considered and used only if the risk/benefit ratio is favorable. Examples of palliative surgery that can benefit the client with cancer and improve quality of life include procedures that (1) reduce pain, (2) relieve airway obstructions, (3) relieve obstructions in the gastrointestinal and urinary tracts, (4) relieve pressure on the brain or spinal cord, (5) prevent hemorrhage, (6) remove infected and ulcerating tumors, and (7) drain abscesses.

RECONSTRUCTIVE SURGERY

Advances in reconstructive surgery offer a different perspective of rehabilitation to the client who has experienced curative surgery. Restoration of form and function is possible in varying degrees, depending on the site and extent of surgery. Reconstructive surgery may be performed concurrently with the radical procedure or delayed for optimal outcome. The major goal of reconstructive surgery is to improve the client's quality of life by restoring maximal function and appearance.

PREVENTIVE SURGERY

The client at unusually high risk for cancer may elect to have preventive surgical intervention. Certain conditions or diseases increase the risk of cancer occurrence so significantly that removal of the target organ is justified to prevent cancer development. Clients with familial polyposis have a 50 per cent risk of developing colon cancer by the age of 40. By the age of 70, all clients with this inherited trait have developed colon cancer. Clients with ulcerative colitis also have an increased risk for colon cancer. Prophylactic subtotal colectomies are indicated for this group of clients.[55] Clients with multiple high-risk factors (see Chap. 20) may consider prophylactic surgery. Prophylactic mastectomy, although infrequently indicated, is a form of preventive therapy.

NURSING MANAGEMENT

Although many aspects of surgical care for the client with cancer are similar to all surgical clients (see Chap. 19 and those chapters that address surgery of a specific body system), some differences exist.

Preoperatively, clients with cancer may be nutritionally compromised and require hospitalization before surgery. Those who have had adjuvant or palliative chemotherapy or radiotherapy may have low blood counts, which need correction before surgery. Clients undergoing a palliative surgical procedure must have their pain assessed from the perspective of normal postoperative pain in addition to pain secondary to tumor invasion.

Unfortunately, the current insurance-driven practices of shortened hospital stays leave little time for preoperative assessment of the client's psychological equilibrium. It is critical, however, that nurses preoperatively evaluate the client's understanding of the proposed surgery and the changes it involves. Some clients anticipate surgery with relief because it represents a physical removal of the tumor and the endpoint of what may have been a protracted diagnostic interval. On the other hand, the client may suffer from great anxiety if the extent of the tumor is unknown preoperatively and the procedure will determine the curability or noncurability of the disease.

Radiation Therapy

One half of all clients with cancer receive radiation therapy (RT) at some point during their disease course. RT may be used as a primary, adjuvant, or palliative treatment modality. As a primary treatment modality, RT is the only treatment used and provides local cure of the cancer (e.g., early stage Hodgkin's disease). In the adjuvant setting, RT can be used either preoperatively or postoperatively to aid in the destruction of cancer cells. In addition, it can be used in conjunction with chemotherapy to treat disease in sites not readily accessible to systemic chemotherapy, such as the brain. Chemotherapy also can be combined with RT and is administered before the RT dose in an attempt to potentiate the effects of RT. RT also can be used as a palliative treatment modality to relieve pain due to obstruction, pathologic fractures, spinal cord compression, and metastasis.

HOW RADIATION THERAPY WORKS (RADIOBIOLOGY)

RT is the use of high-energy ionizing rays to treat a variety of cancers. Ionizing radiation destroys the cell's ability to reproduce by damaging the cell's DNA. Rapidly dividing cells, such as some cancer cells, are more vulnerable to radiation than are slower dividing cells. Furthermore, normal cells have a greater ability than cancer cells to repair the DNA damage from radiation.

Radiosensitivity, the relative susceptibility of tissues to radiation, depends on the individual cells and the characteristics of the tissue itself. A highly radiosensitive tumor is greatly affected by radiation because it divides rapidly, is well vascularized, and has a high oxygen content.

TYPES OF RADIATION THERAPY

RT can be administered from a variety of sources. Sources can be divided into those used outside the body (external RT) and those used inside the body (internal RT).

External Radiation Therapy. External RT is usually administered by high-energy x-ray machines (e.g., the betatron and linear accelerator) or machines containing a radioisotope (cobalt 60 [^{60}Co]).

The major advantage of the high-energy x-ray machines is their skin-sparing effect. This means that the maximum effect of radiation occurs within the tumor deep in the body and not on the skin surface.

Neutron beam therapy delivered from a cyclotron particle accelerator is currently used to treat many types of cancers, including salivary gland tumors, sarcomas, and tumors of the prostate and lung.

Internal Radiation Therapy. Internal RT involves the placement of specially prepared radioisotopes directly into or near the tumor itself or into the systemic circulation. The two major types of internal RT are the sealed source, in which the radioactive material is enclosed in a sealed container and the unsealed source, in which the radioactive material is administered systemically, such as by injection or orally.

Sealed-Source Radiation Therapy (Brachytherapy). Sealed-source RT includes intracavity and interstitial therapy. In intracavity therapy, the radioisotope, usually 137 cesium (^{137}Cs) or 226 radium (^{226}Ra), is placed into an applicator, then placed into the body cavity for a carefully calculated time, usually 24 to 72 hours. Intracavity radiation therapy is used to treat cancers of the uterus and cervix.

In interstitial therapy the radioisotope of choice (e.g., iridium 192 [^{192}Ir], iodine 125 [^{125}I], ^{137}Cs, gold 198 [^{198}Au], or radon 222 [^{222}Rn]) is placed into needles, beads, seeds, ribbons, or catheters and then implanted directly into the tumor. For example, clients with prostate cancer may receive implanted seeds as therapy. Implants may be left in the tumor either temporarily (e.g., when ribbons, needles, or catheters are used) or permanently (prostatic seeds), depending on the half-life of the radiation source being used.

Unsealed-Source Radiation Therapy. Unsealed sources are used in systemic therapy. Radioisotopes may be administered intravenously or orally. For example, sodium phosphate (^{32}P) is administered intravenously to treat polycythemia vera. 131 Iodine (^{131}I) is given orally in very low doses to treat Graves' disease (see Chap. 62) or in high doses to treat thyroid cancer.

FACTORS THAT DETERMINE SIDE EFFECTS OF RADIATION THERAPY

Several factors determine the side effects of RT. The size of the treatment field is important. If a small area is treated, the client will tolerate a higher dose of radiation than if a larger area is treated. Different areas of the body are affected differently by radiation. In general, only the area in the treatment field is affected by the radiation. For example, hair loss occurs only in the area being treated with radiation. The total dose of radiation is also related to the side effects a client may experience. A client receiving 5000 centigrays (cGy) for cure probably will experience more side effects than someone receiving 2000 cGy for palliation.

In general, skin toxicities, fatigue, and anorexia may occur with RT to any site, whereas other side effects occur only when specific areas are involved in the treatment field. Strohl provides a comprehensive review of symptom management of acute and chronic RT reactions.[60]

The goal of RT is to destroy the malignant tumor without harming the surrounding tissues. Several factors help achieve this goal. Fractionation refers to dividing the total radiation dose into small, frequent doses. A common dosage schedule for external radiation therapy is 150 to 200 cGy, 5 days per week for a total of 4 to 5 weeks. Fractionation increases the probability that tumor cells will be in a vulnerable phase of the cell cycle when treated. Fractionation also allows normal cells time to repair themselves.

Another way in which normal cells are spared is to alternate the sites of entry (ports) of radiation. For example, radiation for cervical cancer can be directed at the cervix through the front, back, and sides of the body. The maximum effect of the radiation beam is on the cervix, with the normal tissues receiving only a portion of the total dose. Additionally, customized shielding "blocks" may be created to protect normal tissues from ionizing rays.

ROLE OF RADIATION IN CANCER RESEARCH

Radiation is a vital area in medical research. Radioactive isotopes are being attached to monoclonal and polyclonal antibodies to treat certain tumors on an investigational basis.[5, 12] Intraoperative radiation is being used in several centers in the United States in an attempt to deliver a high dose of radiation directly to the tumor, with little damage to normal structures in the beam pathway.[37]

Another area of research involves the use of hyperthermia with RT. Hyperthermia and radiation therapy work together in three ways: (1) hypoxic tumor cells are radioresistant but heat sensitive, (2) tumor cells in the S phase of replication tend to be radioresistant but heat sensitive, and (3) heat directly impairs the repair process of irradiated cells.

Hyperthermia can be provided locally, regionally, or to the entire body. Local hyperthermia is usually generated with electromagnetic coupling or ultrasound. Regional hyperthermia may involve perfusion with heated solutions. Whole-body hyperthermia can be accomplished by placing the client in a heated enclosure, such as a heated water tank or a water-heated space suit. Studies involving hyperthermia continue and may prove to significantly potentiate the efficacy of radiation therapy.[64]

In addition, the use of radiosensitizers and radioprotectors is being explored. Radiosensitizers and radioprotectors are chemical compounds that may be used to change the effect of radiation on cells and tissues.[65] Because hypoxic cells are resistant to radiation, research is being directed toward increasing the oxygen supply to the tumor. Radiosensitizers are chemical agents that take the place of oxygen in hypoxic cells and, thus, promote radiation effectiveness. Agents under current investigation include metronidazole, misonidazole, and desmethylmisonidazole. Radioprotectors are compounds that are selective for normal healthy tissues and also enhance tumor radiosensitivity.

RADIATION SAFETY

Three key principles to follow to protect nurses and others from excessive radiation exposure are distance, time, and shielding.

Distance. The greater the distance maintained from the radiation source, the less the exposure to ionizing rays. Distance and radiation exposure are inversely related. Thus, as the square of the distance from the source increases, the intensity of radiation decreases. For example, if a person stands 4 feet away from a source of radiation, the person is exposed to approximately one fourth the amount of radiation the person would receive at 2 feet (Fig. 22–1).

Time. The less time that is spent close to the radiation source, the less the amount of radiation exposure. Min-

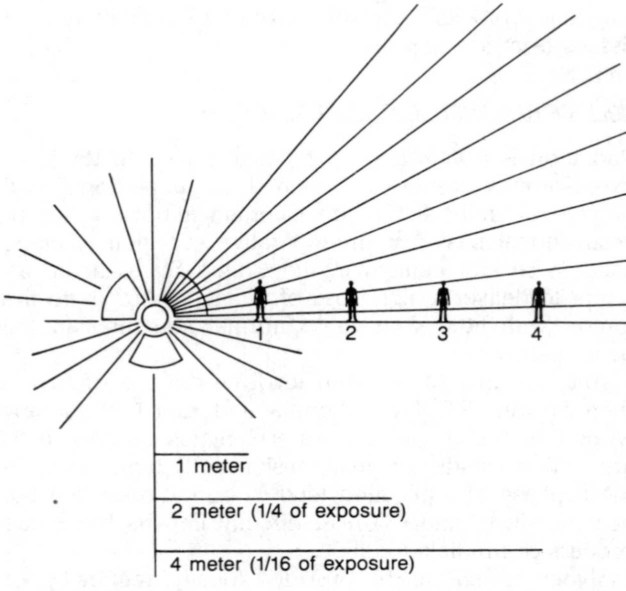

▲ Figure 22-1

Radiation safety. (From Sedhom, L. N., & Yann, M. I. Y. [1985]. Radiation therapy and nurses' fears of radiation exposure. *Cancer Nursing,* 8, 129–134.)

imal exposure time should be promoted, although client care needs must still be met. A nurse's exposure time is generally limited to 30 minutes of direct care per 8-hour shift.[26]

Shielding. The choice of whether or not to use shielding devices to decrease exposure depends on the source of radiation. X-rays and gamma rays are blocked as the thickness of the lead shield increases. Individuals routinely working with x-rays or gamma rays wear lead gloves or aprons in situations that present the risk of exposure.

Radiation Safety Standards. The United States Nuclear Regulatory Commission requires that radiation exposure be kept as low as reasonably achievable.[63] All institutions using radioactive materials must have written policies concerning radiation protection. In addition, a radiation safety officer who is licensed by the United States Atomic Energy Commission to work with radioactive materials must be available at all institutions using radioactive materials.

Monitoring devices such as a film badge are required by law and provide a record of an individual's exposure.[27] Film badges should not be shared. The film badge provides a measure of whole-body exposure.

NURSING MANAGEMENT

The general precautions listed earlier apply to all forms of internal RT, both sealed and unsealed sources. However, because sealed and unsealed sources differ from each other in certain respects, each type requires additional precautionary measures for safe use.

Sealed Sources. Sealed sources of internal radiation differ from unsealed sources in that the radioisotope is completely enclosed by nonradioactive material. Thus, the radioisotope cannot circulate through the client's body, nor can it contaminate urine, sweat, blood, or vomitus. Consequently, the client's excretions are not radioactive. However, radiation exposure can result from direct contact with the sealed radioisotope, such as touching the container with bare hands or from lengthy exposure. After-loading devices have been developed in which an empty applicator (the product that holds the radiation source) is placed during the operative procedure, and the radioactive source is not loaded until the client returns to the hospital room. The radioactive source can then be automatically removed each time entry by health care personnel is necessary. Thus, the use of after-loading devices has helped to decrease exposure. *Clients with radioactive implants require a private room and bath.* Client rooms at the ends of halls or stairwells may be designated for use because their location provides a decreased chance of exposure to others. Institutions with a high volume of radiation implants may have specially designed rooms with lead-shielded walls.

A lead container and a pair of long-handled forceps always should be present in the client's room. If the source becomes dislodged from the client, forceps should be used to pick up the source, which should then be placed immediately in the lead container. Generally, the radiation therapist and the radiation safety officer are notified immediately of the situation.[6, 25]

Unsealed Sources. Unsealed sources used for internal radiation therapy are colloid suspensions and come into direct contact with body tissues. Unsealed sources are given intravenously, orally, or by instillation directly into a body cavity. Because the source is not encased in a protective container, a potential contamination hazard exists. The isotope may be excreted in any body fluid. Clients are instructed to flush the toilet several times after each use for several days, depending on the radiation source used.[73]

Table 22-1 summarizes radiation safety precautions. Nurses use these guidelines for their own protection as well as for the protection of other staff and visitors. Clients receiving internal radiation therapy should be taught about the precautions that must be followed and why they are necessary.

Chemotherapy

DRUG DEVELOPMENT AND CLINICAL TRIALS

The era of modern chemotherapy can be considered to have begun in 1948 with the introduction of nitrogen mustard.[59] Since that time, scientists have continued to search for medications to treat neoplasms.

The National Cancer Institute methodically screens 50,000 compounds each year, of which only a few become commercially available. First, pharmacologic studies are carried out in the laboratory. If these experiments demonstrate antitumor activity and the absence of prohibitive toxicity, the drug advances to supervised clinical trials in humans.

Phase I trials determine the maximum tolerated dose with acceptable toxicity, define drug side effects, and provide information on bioavailability and pharmacologic data. During this phase, an investigational drug is given to a small number of human subjects for the first time. Although the drug has been tested in the laboratory and in animals, it is not known how humans will respond. No direct benefit in terms of disease remission can be guaranteed. Because these trials may involve significant risks for the client and only minimal, if any benefit, they are offered only to those whose cancer has spread and would not be helped by other known treatments. Safety, comfort, and ethical considerations are primary nursing concerns during this phase of clinical trials.

The information obtained in phase I trials is then used to conduct phase II trials that determine the effect of the drug on various types of cancer. After tumor specificity has been determined in phase II, a phase III trial then compares the investigational therapy against an established form of treatment for a particular type of cancer. This phase often involves randomization (random selection of who is treated with the usual therapy and who will receive the new treatment).

Nursing responsibilities associated with caring for a client participating in a clinical trial include documentation of treatment benefits and side effects, anticipation of adverse reactions and early recognition of toxicity, management of side effects, preparation for diagnostic procedures, and client education.[21] Important questions a client should ask when considering participation in a clinical trial are described in a client education pamphlet prepared by the National Cancer Institute, *What Are Clinical Trials All About?*[48]

TABLE 22-1. Radiation Safety Precautions and Rationales for Internal Implants

Safety Precaution	Rationale
Place the client in a private room	Prevents undue exposure to other clients and to nurses caring for these clients
Plan care well so minimal time is spent in direct contact with client with implant	The nurse should not spend more than 1/2 hour per shift with the client to limit amount of radiation exposure. Plan care well in advance, change linens less frequently, prepare meal trays outside the room, and work as quickly as possible. If client can get up, have him or her sit as far as possible from bed while nurse changes linen. The nurse can spend more time with the client at a distance of 20 feet, where exposure will be minimal
Provide care for client standing at client's shoulder (for cervical implants) or at foot of bed (for head and neck implants), avoiding any close contact with unshielded areas	The client's body will provide increased shielding for the nurse
If prolonged contact or care of unshielded area, use lead aprons or lead shield	Lead will decrease radiation exposure to the nurse
Never care for more than one client with a radiation implant at the same time	Caring for more than one client with an implant could expose the nurse to unnecessarily high amounts of radiation
All health care personnel should wear appropriate monitoring devices	Records must be kept to monitor the exact amount of radiation exposure for each person in contact with the client. If any single employee is receiving too high an amount, this person should not be assigned to care for radiation clients for a while
The room should be marked with appropriate signs stating the presence of radiation. The kardex should also be appropriately marked, and a sign should also be posted in the room	All personnel (and visitors) should be adequately warned of the presence of radiation so that undue exposure does not occur
Carefully check all linens or other materials removed from the bed for the presence of foreign bodies	If the client has excessive drainage requiring frequent linen changes, the linen may be examined with a Geiger counter to be certain no portion of the implant is lost. Careless discarding of the linens could lead to unnecessary exposure of personnel to radiation
Keep long-handled forceps and a lead-lined container available on the nursing unit or in the client's room while the implant is in place	In case of accidental dislodgement of implant, use long-handled forceps to pick up implant and place it in the lead-lined container. Notify radiation therapy department immediately

OBJECTIVES OF CHEMOTHERAPY

The objective of cancer chemotherapy is to destroy all malignant tumor cells without excessive destruction of normal cells. Chemotherapy is a systemic intervention and is appropriate when disease is widespread or when the risk of undetectable disease is high.

Chemotherapy leads to a cure for many clients with cancer. Guidelines for treating curable cancers stress early aggressive therapy. Another important use of chemotherapy is to control tumor growth when a cure is not possible. Chemotherapy may also be given for palliation (alleviation of symptoms such as pain or obstructions) without curing the underlying disease. Many clients with cancer have benefitted from an extended lifespan and an improved quality of life as a result of chemotherapy.

In recent years, chemotherapeutic agents have come into use as adjuvant therapy. This means that after initial treatment with either surgery or radiotherapy, medications are used to eliminate any remaining cancer cells. The client at high risk for recurrence but with no evidence of current disease may be a candidate for adjuvant therapy. Adjuvant therapy is now well established in the treatment of breast cancer. Neoadjuvant chemotherapy refers to the initial use of chemotherapy to reduce the bulk and lower the stage of a tumor, making it amenable to cure with subsequent local therapy.[38,39]

Significant advances in the field of chemotherapy have been made in the last 30 years. Twelve types of cancer are now considered curable with chemotherapy, even in advanced stages.[38] Unfortunately, these 12 tumors account for only about 10 percent of all cancers. The most common types have not yet shown a significant response to systemic therapy, and in the intermediate and less favorable groups of cancer, the responses to chemotherapy are mainly temporary.[38, 39] The chemosensitivity of specific neoplasms is summarized in Box 22–4.

Box 22–4. Chemoresponsiveness of Selected Tumors

Cures in Advanced Cancers

Gestational trophoblastic tumors
Acute lymphoblastic leukemia (children)
Acute lymphoblastic leukemia (adults)
Acute myeloblastic leukemia
Non-Hodgkin's lymphoma (children)
Diffuse large cell lymphoma
Hodgkin's disease
Burkitt's lymphoma
Testicular tumors

Cures with Adjuvant Chemotherapy

Wilms' tumor
Osteogenic sarcoma
Rhabdomyosarcoma

Minor Responses with Chemotherapy/Adjuvant Chemotherapy, No Demonstrable Prolongation of Life

Non–small cell lung cancer
Head and neck cancer
Large bowel cancer
Cancer of the adrenal cortex
Soft tissue sarcoma
Stomach cancer
Pancreatic cancer
Liver cancer
Cervical cancer
Melanoma

Complete and Partial Remissions with Uncertain Prolongation of Survival with Chemotherapy/Adjuvant Chemotherapy

Multiple myeloma
Ovarian cancer
Endometrial cancer
Neuroblastoma

Complete Remissions with Increased Survival with Chemotherapy/Adjuvant Chemotherapy

Small cell carcinoma of the lung
Acute myeloblastic leukemia
Non-Hodgkin's lymphoma, indolent
Chronic granulocytic leukemia
Breast cancer
Prostate cancer
Hairy cell leukemia

From Krakoff, I. H. (1991). Cancer chemotherapeutic and biologic agents. *Ca-A Journal for Clinicians, 41,* 265–266.

BASIS OF ACTION OF CHEMOTHERAPY

The phases of mitosis are common to all cells. Normally, cells respond to the body's need for growth, repair, or regeneration in an orderly manner and cease production by entering a resting phase or slowing growth when the need is met. At any given time, normal cells may be found in all phases of growth. Cancer cells reproduce in the same manner as normal cells. However, growth occurs in an uncontrolled manner. In general, cells that are actively dividing are the most sensitive to chemotherapy.

Chemotherapy directly or indirectly disrupts reproduction of cells by altering essential biochemical processes. The desired outcome is control or eradication of all malignant cells.

Experiments and clinical experience suggest that most types of chemotherapy do not kill all cancer cells during one exposure.[59] According to the cell kill hypothesis, only a percentage of cancer cells will be killed with each course of chemotherapy. Repeated doses of chemotherapy, therefore, must be used.

The use of medications in combination, known as combination chemotherapy, has been consistently far superior to single-agent therapy.[38, 39] When combined, medications destroy malignant cells more effectively and produce fewer side effects. Combination chemotherapy is now the standard, and the regimens are complex and cyclic. An example of a chemotherapy regimen for Hodgkin's disease is shown in Table 22–2.

TABLE 22-2. MOPP Regimen

M = Nitrogen Mustard	6.0 mg/m² IV	Day 1 and 8
O = Oncovin	1.4 mg/m² IV	Day 1 and 8
P = Procarbazine	100.0 mg/m² PO	Day 1 to 14
P = Prednisone	40.0 mg/m² PO	Day 1 to 14

Repeat cycle every 28 days for a minimum of 6 cycles

CLASSIFICATION OF CHEMOTHERAPY

Chemotherapeutic agents generally are classified according to their pharmacologic action and effect on the cell generation cycle. However, the method by which cancer cells are inhibited or destroyed is not always known. Common chemotherapeutic drugs are classified in Box 22-5.

Box 22-5. Classification of Chemotherapy

Alkylating Agents

Busulfan (Myleran)
Chlorambucil (Leukeran)
Cyclophosphamide (Cytoxan)
Cisplatin (Platinol)
Carboplatin (Paraplatin)
Ifosfamide (IFEX)
Mecholethamine (Mustargen)
Melphalan (L-PAM, Alkeran)
Thiotepa

Antimetabolites

Cytarabine (Ara-C, Cytosar)
Methotrexate
5-Azacytidine
5-Fluorouracil (5-FU)
Floxuridine (FUDR)
6-Mercaptopurine (6-MP)
6-Thioguanine (6-TG)
Hydroxyurea (Hydrea)

Antitumor Antibiotics

Bleomycin (Bleoxane)
Dactinomycin (Actinomycin-D)
Daunorubicin (Daunomycin)
Doxorubicin (Adriamycin)
Mitomycin C (Mutamycin)
Mitoxantrone (Novantrone)
Plicamycin (Mithramycin)

Nitrosureas

Carmustine (BCNU)
Lomustine (CCNU)
Semustine (Methyl-CCNU)
Streptozocin (Zanosar)

Vinca (Plant) Alkaloids

Vinblastine (Velban)
Vincristine (Oncovin)
VP-16 (Etoposide, VePesid)
VM-26 (Teniposide)
Vindesine (Eldisine)

Steroids and Hormones

Androgen

Testosterone propionate
Fluoxymesterone (Halotestin)
Testolactone (Teslac)
Methyltestosterone

Estrogen

Diethylstilbestrol (DES)
Ethinyl estradiol (Estinyl)

Antiestrogens

Tamoxifen (Nolvadex)
Leuprolide (Lupron)

Progestins

Delalutin
Megestrol (Megace)
Medroxyprogesterone (Depo-Provera, Provera)

Adrenal Cortical Compounds

Cortisone acetate
Prednisone
Dexamethasone (Decadron)
Methylprednisolone sodium succinate (Solu-Medrol)
Hydrocortisone sodium succinate (Solu-Cortef)

Antiadrenal

Aminoglutethimide

Miscellaneous Agents

DTIC (Dacarbazine)
mAMSA
Hexamethylmelamine (HXM)
L-Asparaginase (Elspar)
Procarbazine hydrochloride (Matulane)

Data from Chabner, B. A., & Myers, C. E. (1989). Clinical pharmacology of cancer chemotherapy. In V. T. DeVita, S. Hellman, S. A. Rosenberg (Eds.): *Cancer: Principles & practice of oncology* (3rd ed.). Philadelphia: J. B. Lippincott; Krakoff, I. H. (1991). Cancer chemotherapeutic and biologic agents. *Ca-A Journal for Clinicians,* 41, 270-276.

ADMINISTRATION OF CHEMOTHERAPY

Depending on the clinical setting, chemotherapy may be administered by the physician, staff nurse, or specialized team member, such as the oncology clinical nurse specialist or intravenous therapist. Only adequately prepared registered professional nurses who are skilled in administering chemotherapy should assume responsibility for its administration to ensure quality of client care and maintain the highest standards of client and personnel safety.[51] Recommendations for course content, clinical practicum, and nursing practice can be found in the Oncology Nursing Society *Cancer Chemotherapy Guidelines*.[51]

Safe Preparation, Handling, and Disposal. The safe administration and disposal of chemotherapeutic agents is controversial. Although evidence suggests that these agents may be carcinogenic, no valid and reliable studies have verified the risks of exposure to the health care provider.

Undue exposure to antineoplastic drugs can occur from three major routes: (1) inhalation of aerosols, (2) absorption through the skin, and (3) ingestion of contaminated materials.[22] Several organizations including the Occupational Safety and Health Administration, the National Study Commission on Cytotoxic Exposure, and the Oncology Nursing Society have prepared guidelines for the safe preparation, handling, and disposal of antineoplastics.[49-51] The use of gloves and gowns during preparation and administration and the use of a Biologic Safety Cabinet for drug preparation is included in these guidelines.

Antineoplastic agents and their metabolites are found in the excreta and body fluids of clients undergoing chemotherapy. For this reason, it is recommended that gloves and disposable gowns be worn when handling body secretions such as blood, vomitus, or excreta from clients who have received chemotherapy within the previous 48 hours.[51]

CHEMOTHERAPY ADMINISTRATION ROUTES

Appropriate routes of medication administration are determined by the properties of the medication and the purpose of the therapy. Some agents may be safely administered by a variety of routes. Therapy may be systemic or local.

Intravenous Routes

Peripheral Access. Large veins in the forearm are the preferred peripheral access sites. Avoid areas of impaired lymphatic drainage, phlebitis, invading neoplasm, hematoma, inflamed or sclerosing areas, areas of impaired venous circulation, the lower extremities, and sites distal to a recent venipuncture site.

Vascular Access. In the past, vascular access devices (VADs) were placed as a last resort in clients with poor venous access. Today, because chemotherapy regimens are complex and supportive care is extensive, they are being used during the initial treatment of clients with leukemia and in those requiring continuous chemotherapy, total parenteral nutrition, multiple access, parenteral fluids and antibiotics, and frequent blood draws. Client selection criteria for VAD placement are listed in Table 22–3.

These catheters are usually inserted into one of the major veins of the upper chest. The brachial or cephalic vein in the forearm is used for nontunneled peripheral access devices. The distal catheter tip is advanced to the level of the superior vena cava at or above the junction of the right atrium. Proper catheter tip placement is confirmed by fluoroscopy or radiography.

A variety of VADs are currently available, including (1) tunneled catheters that are subcutaneously tunneled for several inches from the catheter exit site to the venous insertion site, (2) nontunneled catheters that enter the vein 1 inch from the exit site, and (3) totally implanted venous access ports that lie completely beneath the skin. Examples of various types are shown in Figure 22–2*A* to *D*. There are advantages and disadvantages to each type of device, including factors such as maintenance requirements, ease of use, cost, ease of insertion, longevity, and affect on body image.

The most frequently reported complications are infection and catheter occlusion. The prevention of VAD infections centers on catheter care, daily assessment for signs and symptoms of infection, and client education. Intraluminal occlusion may occur secondary to a blood clot or precipitate. Prevention strategies include proper flushing, vigilance for drug incompatibilities, and adherence to proper drug dilutions. Procedures for the care and maintenance of vascular access devices vary with each clinical setting. Nursing management strategies for VADs are extensively described elsewhere.[52, 70]

Extravasation Management. Careful assessment of the intravenous site is required during and after the infusion of antineoplastic agents because some agents have the potential to cause tissue damage if extravasated (infiltrated). Nonvesicant agents have no significant soft tissue toxicities. Vesicant chemotherapeutic agents are capable of causing or forming a blister, causing tissue destruction, or both. Irritant drugs are capable of producing venous pain at the site and along the vein, with or without an inflammatory reaction. Criteria to determine whether or not an extravasation is present include pain, erythema, swelling, and lack of a blood return.

Procedures for management of extravasation are controversial and unique to each clinical setting. Institutionally approved guidelines for the management of extravasation should be readily available. Guidelines for the management of extravasation are included in the Oncology Nursing Society *Cancer Chemotherapy Guidelines*.[51]

Less Common Administration Routes. Regional chemotherapy allows high concentrations of chemotherapy to be directed to localized tumors. Methods of regional administration include topical, intrathecal, intracavitary, and intra-arterial chemotherapy. Although intra-arterial infusions involve some risk, major organs or tumor sites do receive maximal exposure with limited serum levels of medications. As a result, systemic side effects are minimal.

TABLE 22-3. Client Selection Criteria for a Vascular Access Device

Criterion	Low Priority	High Priority
Frequency of venous access	Infrequent	Frequent
Longevity of treatment	Short term	Long term, indefinite
Mode of administration	Intermittent single injections	Continuous infusions Home infusion
Venous integrity	Administration of nonvesicant/nonirritant drugs No previous intravenous therapy Both extremities available Venous access with two or fewer venipunctures	Administration of vesicant/irritating drugs Venous thrombosis/sclerosis due to previous intravenous therapy Venous access limited to one extremity Prior tissue damage due to drug infiltration Multiple (>2) venipunctures to secure venous access
Client preference	Client does not prefer a vascular access device	Client prefers a vascular access device

Reprinted from the *Oncology Nursing Forum*, with permission from the Oncology Nursing Press. Goodman, M. S., & Wickham, R. (1984). Venous access devices: An overview. *Oncology Nursing Forum, 11* (5), 16-23.

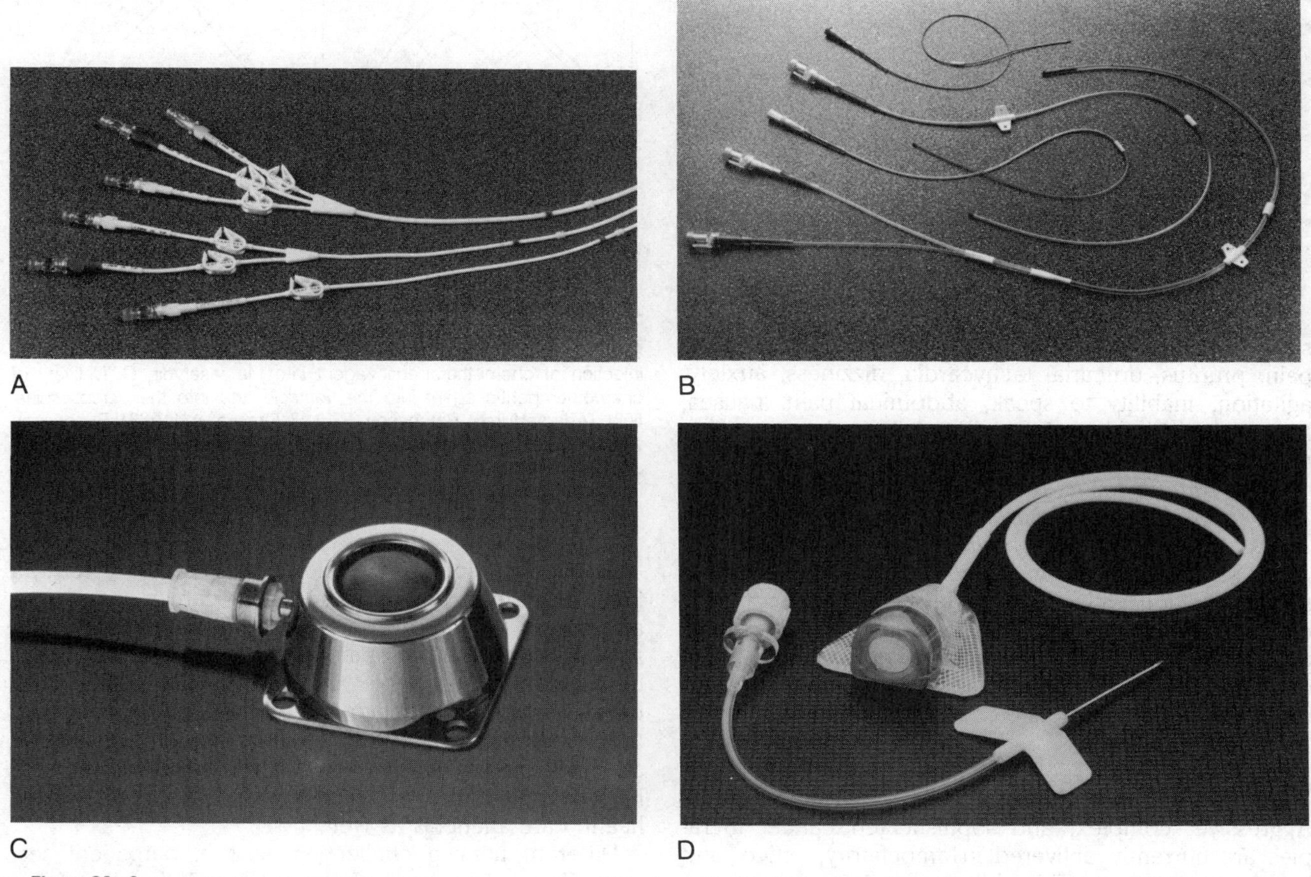

▲ ***Figure 22-2***

Venous access devices. *A,* Single-lumen, double-lumen, and triple-lumen Hickman catheters (C. R. Bard, Inc.) with VitaCuff (Vitaphore Corporation, courtesy of Davol Inc.); *B,* single-lumen and double-lumen Groshong catheters (C. R. Bard, Inc., courtesy of Davol Inc.); *C,* Port-A-Cath Access System (courtesy of Pharmacia Deltec Inc., St. Paul, MN); and *D,* Norport-SP, a side-entrance port (courtesy of Norfolk Medical Products, Inc., Skokie, IL). (From Baird, S. B., et al. [Eds.] [1991]. *Cancer nursing: A comprehensive textbook.* Philadelphia: W. B. Saunders.)

Most medications given systemically are not effective against central nervous system (CNS) tumors because they cannot cross the blood-brain barrier. The physician may instill chemotherapeutic agents into the CNS through a reservoir placed in the ventricle (Fig. 22-3) or via a lumbar puncture.

Intracavitary therapy instills the medication directly into areas such as the abdomen, bladder, or pleural space. Intraperitoneal chemotherapy is an innovative intervention option for cancer involving the intra-abdominal area, such as ovarian cancer. With this method, a high concentration of a chemotherapeutic agent is delivered to the actual tumor site with minimal exposure of healthy tissues, thereby decreasing toxic side effects.

HYPERSENSITIVITY REACTIONS TO CHEMOTHERAPY

Hypersensitivity reactions to chemotherapy, although rare, can be serious and life threatening. The antineoplastic agents most commonly implicated in the development of immediate hypersensitivity reactions are L-asparaginase, cisplatin, and bleomycin.[11]

When administering a drug with anaphylactic potential, take precautions to ensure client safety, such as the following:

- Obtain an allergy history from the client
- Administer a test dose when ordered by the physician
- Stay with the client the entire time the drug is being administered
- Have emergency equipment and drugs readily available
- Obtain baseline vital signs
- Establish a free-flowing intravenous line for the administration of fluids and emergency drugs should the need arise

The signs and symptoms of an immediate hypersensitivity reaction include dyspnea, chest tightness or pain, pruritus, urticaria, tachycardia, dizziness, anxiety, agitation, inability to speak, abdominal pain, nausea, hypotension, decreased sensorium, flushed appearance, and cyanosis.

If an anaphylactic reaction is suspected, immediately stop drug administration, maintain intravenous access with 0.9 per cent saline, and notify the physician. Maintain the airway, and place the client in a supine position with the feet elevated unless contraindicated. Monitor the client's vital signs every 2 minutes until he or she is stable. Administer epinephrine, aminophylline, diphenhydramine, and corticosteroids based on the physician's orders.

OUTPATIENT CHEMOTHERAPY ADMINISTRATION

Aggressive, complex, and sophisticated cancer therapies are currently delivered in ambulatory, office, and home care settings. This shift in the provision of services from the traditional hospital setting is a result of cost-containment efforts, consumerism, advanced technology, competition, and nursing competence.[76]

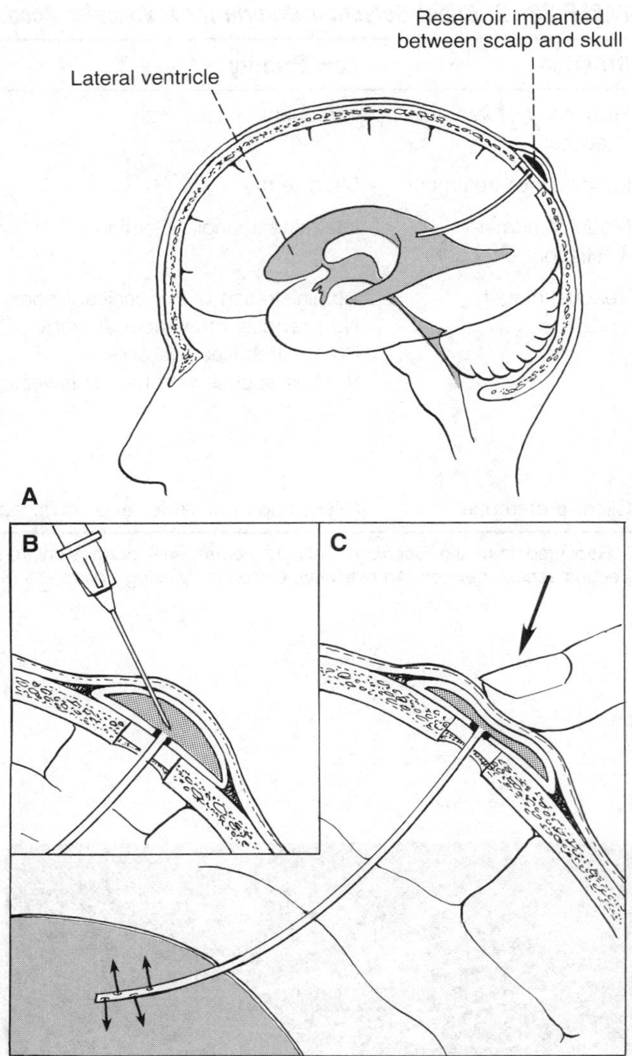

▲ **Figure 22-3**

Omaya reservoir. *A*, Placement of Omaya reservoir in ventricle. *B*, Injection of chemotherapeutic agent into the reservoir. *C*, Delivery of chemotherapeutic agent into the ventricle and into the cerebrospinal fluid. (Adapted from Ratcheson, R. A. & Omaya, A. [1968]. Experience with the subcutaneous cerebrospinal fluid reservoir. *New England Journal of Medicine,* 279, 1026. Reprinted by permission of The New England Journal of Medicine.)

Cost containment is a major consideration in today's health care environment. Outpatient care is less costly and allows for the maintenance of a more normal lifestyle. Technical developments such as venous access devices and implantable and external infusion pumps make it possible to deliver chemotherapy, hyperalimentation, antibiotics, blood components, and parenteral and epidural analgesics outside the hospital. Increasingly sophisticated support is available from home health care agencies as well.

Different nursing challenges exist in outpatient settings. First, a high level of commitment is required from the client and care givers. Both require education regarding complex treatment regimens; identification, prevention, and treatment of symptoms experienced at home; the operation of medical equipment; and the care of a variety of vascular access devices. Second, a mechanism for immediate access to health care personnel is required. Finally, when chemotherapy is administered in the home setting, provisions must be made for the safe handling and disposal of cytotoxics to minimize client, family, and nurse exposure.

When the chemotherapeutic medication is obtained from the health care facility, it should be labeled as cytotoxic, carefully capped and securely sealed, and packed in an impervious material for transportation. The family or nurse can obtain the medication.

When preparing the medication in the home for administration, the nurse should be sure to work in an area away from food and anywhere the family, particularly children, congregate. The area should be cleaned and covered with a plastic backed pad. The nurse can then assemble all needed materials for the chemotherapy administration on this absorbent surface. The nurse should use the same precautions for administering the chemotherapy used in the hospital setting.[4]

The waste materials can be disposed of in biohazard containers obtained from medical supply companies, or empty coffee cans with reinforced lids can be used for sharp instruments. All empty containers and tubing should be placed in sealable plastic bags with appropriate labels. These items are then returned to the health care facility for proper disposal.[50]

If spills occur in the home, the nurse should wear a protective gown, gloves, and goggles to clean it up. The area should be wiped completely with disposable absorbent towels and then washed three times with detergent and rinsed. All materials used should be placed in sealable plastic bags and disposed of as hazardous waste.

The client may excrete the chemotherapeutic agents for 48 hours after administration. Blood, emesis, and excreta may be considered contaminated during this time. The client should not share a bathroom with children or pregnant women during this time. Any contaminated linens or clothing should be washed separately, and then can be washed a second time with the rest of the laundry. All contaminated disposable items should be sealed in plastic bags and disposed of as hazardous waste.[50]

TOXIC EFFECTS OF CHEMOTHERAPY

Antineoplastic medications are capable of damaging and destroying not only malignant cells but also certain normal cells. Normal cells most vulnerable to antineoplastic medications are those that divide and proliferate rapidly, specifically cells of the bone marrow, hair, and mucosa. Damage to these cells can result in myelosuppression, alopecia, oral mucositis, and diarrhea. In addition to these effects on proliferative cells, drugs may exert organ specific toxicities resulting in cardiac, renal, pulmonary, hepatic, reproductive, and neurologic dysfunction. A summary of the multiple potential side effects and toxicities of antineoplastic agents is found in Box 22–6.

Side effects are evaluated or graded according to the degree of severity. Mild to moderate side effects generally do not warrant discontinuing the drug or decreasing the dose. More severe or unexpected toxicities require careful evaluation and dose reduction. Risk factors for the development of toxicities are listed in Box 22–7.

The onset of side effects of chemotherapy may be acute or delayed. Acute toxicities tend to occur in tissues composed of rapidly dividing cells, are frequently intermittent in nature, and generally resolve with complete recovery; in contrast, late effects tend to occur in different tissues and may produce lifelong problems.[56] The client and all health care providers must be aware of, monitor for, and report side effects. A discussion of the more common acute side effects of chemotherapy follows.

Myelosuppressive Effects. Myelosuppression is one of the most common side effects of chemotherapeutic drugs. It is also one of the most lethal. Infection and bleeding as a result of diminished white cell and platelet production are two common causes of death in cancer clients. For this reason, complete blood counts must be checked before administration of myelosuppressive drugs and must be monitored periodically after drug administration.

The time after chemotherapy administration when the white cell or platelet count is at the lowest point is referred to as the *nadir*. For the majority of myelosuppressive agents, the nadir occurs within 7 to 14 days after drug administration. Knowledge of blood count nadirs assists the nurse in predicting when the client is at greatest risk for infection and bleeding.

Granulocytopenia, also known as neutropenia, predisposes the client to infection, especially by opportunistic endogenous organisms. Neutrophils are the first and most numerous type of cell to arrive at any area of disease or tissue injury. When the number of neutrophils is substantially reduced, one of the body's prime defenses against infection is impaired.

The absolute neutrophil count (ANC) is calculated by multiplying the white blood cell count (WBC) by the per cent of granulocytes in the differential: ANC = WBC × % granulocytes. Neutropenia has commonly been defined as an ANC less than 1000 cells/mm^3.[53] The frequency of infection increases as the ANC decreases below 500/mm^3, and the longer the client remains neutropenic.[53]

It is essential that clients are taught measures to protect against infection:

- Maintain adequate nutrition and fluid intake
- Avoid crowds, people with infections, and clients who have been recently vaccinated with live or attenuated vaccines
- Avoid contact with animal excrement, such as bird, cat, and dog feces
- Immediately report any signs and symptoms of infection, such as fever over 38°C (100°F), cough, sore throat, chills or sweating, or frequent or painful urination
- Maintain personal hygiene, especially handwashing

Box 22–6. Systemic Chemotherapeutic Effects

Gastrointestinal

Nausea and vomiting
Constipation
Anorexia
Stomatitis
Esophagitis
Taste alterations
Diarrhea
Weight loss
Pharyngitis

Integumentary

Dermatitis
Alopecia
Perianal ulcers
Vulvular ulcers
Hyperpigmentation
Photosensitivity
Nail changes

Hematopoietic

Anemia
Thrombocytopenia
Neutropenia

Genitourinary

Nephrotoxicity
Urine color change
Hemorrhagic cystitis
Hyperuricemic nephropathy

Hepatic

Hepatotoxicity
Cirrhosis
Hepatic fibrosis
Portal hypertension

Reproductive

Amenorrhea
Sterility
Loss of libido
Impotence
Azoospermia
Gonadal dysfunction
Menopausal symptoms
Irregular menses
Gynecomastia
Oligospermia

Cardiac

EKG changes
Arrhythmias
Cardiomyopathy, chronic heart failure
Tachycardia

Pulmonary

Pneumonitis
Pulmonary fibrosis

Metabolic

Tumor lysis syndrome

Neurologic/Sensory-Perceptual

Ototoxicity
Subacute meningeal irritation
Peripheral neuropathy
Cranial nerve neuropathy
Autonomic neuropathy
Cerebellar toxicity

Data from Hydzik, C. A. (1990). Late effects of chemotherapy: Implications for patient management and rehabilitation. *Nursing Clinics of North America, 25,* 423; Ruccione, K., & Weinberg, K.: (1989). Late effects in multiple body systems. *Seminars in Oncology Nursing, 5,* 4.

- Get adequate rest and exercise
- Avoid indiscriminate use of antipyretics because they can mask fever.

Because infections are associated with increased morbidity and mortality, infection must be treated promptly and aggressively in the neutropenic client. The typical signs and symptoms of infection are often absent because these clients are not able to produce an adequate inflammatory response to infection. Fever is the single most important and often the only sign of infection in the neutropenic client.[53] The development of fever in a neutropenic client should be treated as a medical emergency and mandates prompt assessment, diagnosis, and initiation of antibiotic therapy. Manage-

Box 22–7. Risk Factors for Chemotherapy Toxicity

- Drug dose, route, method of administration
- Extent of cancer and overall physical condition
- Prior chemotherapy and/or radiation therapy
- Concomitant organ dysfunction or illness
- Age
- Nutritional status
- Self-care behavior
- Combination vs. single agent therapy

Adapted from Goodman, M. S. (1989). Managing the side effects of chemotherapy. *Seminars in Oncology Nursing, 5* (2)(Suppl 1), 29.

ment includes culturing all suspected infection sites, use of protective isolation, and the administration of broad-spectrum antibiotics.

Thrombocytopenia increases the client's risk for bleeding. A high risk of hemorrhage exists when the platelet count is less than 20,000/mm^3. Fatal CNS hemorrhage or massive gastrointestinal hemorrhage can occur when the platelet count is less than 10,000/mm^3. Clients should be instructed to report

- Bleeding gums;
- Increased bruising, petechiae, or purpura, especially on lower extremities;
- Hypermenorrhea;
- Tarry colored stools, blood in urine, coffee-ground emesis;
- Hemoptysis; and
- Epistaxis.

Controversy exists as to whether or not clients should receive prophylactic transfusions when platelet counts reach a certain level, or emergent transfusions when bleeding is noted.[17] Platelet products include multiple or random donor, single donor, and HLA matched.

Anemia may cause fatigue, headache, dizziness, fainting, pallor, dyspnea, palpitations, and tachycardia. Packed red blood cell transfusions may be required to relieve symptomatic anemia.

Additional precautions are necessary when administering blood components to selected groups of oncology clients. Cytomegalovirus-negative products are required for cytomegalovirus-negative clients undergoing bone marrow transplant. Irradiated products are transfused to severely immunocompromised clients to prevent graft-versus-host disease from occurring secondary to the transfusion of immune-competent lymphocytes present in donor platelet and packed cell products. Leukocyte-poor products are indicated for clients with a history of repeated nonhemolytic febrile transfusion reactions. They are also used as a prophylactic measure to prevent alloimmunization to leukocytes. A comprehensive discussion of transfusion practices in the oncology setting can be found in the study written by McGuire and Braine.[44]

Gastrointestinal Effects. Gastrointestinal effects of chemotherapy include nausea and vomiting, anorexia, taste alteration, weight loss, oral mucositis, diarrhea, and constipation.

Nausea and vomiting are two of the most dreaded side effects of chemotherapy. However, contrary to client fears, nausea and vomiting are not universal. The emetic potential of a particular chemotherapeutic regimen depends on the drugs given, the dose and route of administration, and the client's susceptibility to emesis.[9]

Adequate control is an essential aspect of client compliance with chemotherapy. Uncontrolled nausea and vomiting can result in anorexia, malnutrition, dehydration, metabolic imbalances, psychological depression, and treatment noncompliance.[45]

Management of nausea and vomiting has greatly improved during the last decade because of heightened interest and research. Successful management depends on an understanding of the pathophysiology of the symptoms, recognition of patterns of nausea and vomiting, and an appreciation of pharmacologic and nonpharmacologic interventions.[28]

Recent research indicates that the vomiting center, located in the medulla oblongata, is responsible for coordinating the act of vomiting.[20] It is postulated that stimulation of the vomiting center occurs via a variety of pathways and is mediated by a variety of neurotransmitters.[45] Pharmacologic blockade of these potential neurotransmitters is the hypothesized mechanism of action of drugs used as antiemetics.

Three common patterns of nausea and vomiting have been described. Anticipatory nausea and vomiting occur before the administration of therapy. Acute, post-therapy nausea and vomiting occur within the first 24 hours following therapy. Delayed nausea and vomiting refers to symptoms that persist or develop 24 hours after chemotherapy.

Antiemetics are usually prescribed 6 to 12 hours prior to the administration of chemotherapy and are continued every 4 to 6 hours for at least 12 to 24 hours, or as long as the symptoms persist.[75] Specific drug combinations, doses, and schedules are described elsewhere.[28, 45] Ongoing evaluation is essential to find the most effective dose, schedule, and combination of drugs for each client.

Nonpharmacologic interventions include adjusting oral and fluid intake, relaxation, exercise, hypnosis, biofeedback, guided imagery, and systemic desensitization.[20, 28]

Anorexia and weight loss occur as a result of the disease process as well as the treatment. The client with cancer is at risk for protein-calorie malnutrition. Many variables may alter the client's ability to ingest food via the oral route. Common problems that may interfere with oral intake include anorexia, nausea and vomiting, early satiety, taste alterations, dry mouth, stomatitis, esophagitis, viscous saliva, lactose intolerance, pain, diarrhea, and constipation.

Assessment of nutritional status includes

- Current and normal weight and height,
- Caloric intake,
- Anthropometric measurements,
- Laboratory values (albumin, transferrin, creatinine, lymphocyte count, nitrogen balance),
- Diet history (previous and current), and
- Physiologic factors (difficulty in swallowing, malabsorption, taste alterations).

When medically appropriate, enhance oral nutrition by relaxing any dietary restrictions and emphasizing the need for a high-protein, high-calorie diet with fortification from either natural food sources or commercial supplements. Monitor the client's nutritional status by daily calorie counts and assessment. If the nutritional requirements cannot be met orally, another method must be considered. Enteral or intravenous feedings are two possibilities (see Chaps. 53 and 54 for a detailed discussion of these alternate methods).

Stomatitis or oral mucositis is the term used to describe inflammation and ulceration of the mucosal lining of the mouth. Consequences of stomatitis include pain, decreased nutritional and fluid intake, and oral infections.

An oral hygiene program should start before therapy and continue throughout treatment. A plan for oral care includes a dental examination prior to and during therapy, thorough and gentle cleansing to avoid further trauma, moisturization if saliva is decreased or absent, avoidance of alcohol and smoking, culture and appropriate coverage for infections, and topical anesthetics and analgesics for pain or discomfort.[13] Dietary modifications during periods of stomatitis include avoiding extremely hot or cold foods, spices, and citrus juices; eating soft foods; and taking nutritional supplements.

Diarrhea is most often the result of antimetabolite drugs. A low-residue or liquid diet is usually advised. Electrolytes and intake and output should be carefully monitored. Scrupulous perineal hygiene is encouraged, especially in the neutropenic client. Antidiarrheals may be prescribed.

Constipation is frequently the result of vinca alkaloid effects on bowel peristalsis. Other causes of constipation include narcotics, immobility, decreased fluid and bulk intake, tumor invasion of the gastrointestinal tract, and depression. Preventive measures include increasing fluid and bulk intake, administering stool softeners prophylactically, increasing activity, and administering laxatives when necessary.

Cutaneous Effects. Alopecia is a common side effect of many antineoplastic agents. The degree of hair loss depends on the specific drug, dosage, and method of administration. Alopecia is temporary, with regrowth often occurring before chemotherapy ends, although the hair color and texture may change. Approaches to lessen or prevent chemotherapy-induced alopecia remain controversial and subject to further research. One such method is the use of scalp hypothermia to decrease the blood flow to the hair follicle and, thereby, reduce contact between the drug and epithelial cells.

A variety of skin reactions may occur in the client receiving chemotherapy, such as the following:

- Red patches (erythema) or hives (urticaria) at the drug injection site or on other body parts. These reactions generally disappear within several hours.
- Darkening of the skin (hyperpigmentation) in the nail beds, mouth, on the gums or teeth, or along the veins used for chemotherapy or the condition may be generalized. Hyperpigmentation usually occurs 2 to 3 weeks after the administration of chemotherapy and continues for 10 to 12 weeks after therapy completion.
- Sensitivity to sunlight (photosensitivity). This may result in an acute sunburn after just a short exposure to the sun. The sensitivity disappears once treatment stops.
- Radiation recall. This skin reaction may occur in clients who received radiation therapy prior to the administration of chemotherapy. When chemotherapy is given several weeks or months later, a recall reaction occurs in the previously irradiated skin area. Skin effects range from redness, shedding or peeling, to blisters and oozing. After the skin heals, it is permanently darkened.[76]

Reproductive Effects. The effects of chemotherapy on gonadal function and reproductive capacity may be temporary or permanent. Azoospermia, oligospermia, and sterility have been documented in males. Amenorrhea, menopausal symptoms, and sterility have been noted in females.

However, not all clients experience these effects to the same degree. Preliminary studies suggest that the effects of chemotherapy on gonadal function vary with respect to the client's age at time of therapy, drugs administered, and total drug dosage.[2] Surgery and radiation therapy may likewise produce temporary or permanent sterility. Therefore, in clients who have received combined modality therapy, the effect of any one modality on reproductive function is less defined.

Administration of antineoplastic agents during the first trimester of pregnancy generally increases the risk of spontaneous abortion and fetal malformations.[36] Second and third trimester chemotherapy exposure may result in low birth weight or prematurity, although successful pregnancy outcomes have been reported.[36] For these reasons, many physicians advise the use of birth control during cancer treatment and for up to two years following the completion of treatment.

Pregnancies conceived after cytotoxic chemotherapy have about the same chance for successful outcomes as do normal pregnancies.[2] However, the genetic effects of chemotherapy may not be evident for several generations of offspring. Therefore, the unpredictability of the occurrence, degree, or duration of genetic damage should be discussed with the client and spouse or significant other.

Pretreatment sperm banking offers the possibility of retaining reproductive capacity for some clients. More in-depth discussions of fertility considerations, procreative alternatives, and sexuality with respect to the cancer client are found in the studies conducted by Kaempfer and colleagues[36] and Yarbro.[74]

NURSING MANAGEMENT

Assessment. A thorough client evaluation is necessary before cytotoxic drugs can be administered. By reviewing the client's medical history, the nurse can identify potential risk factors for chemotherapy toxicity, such as a history of impaired cardiac, pulmonary, or renal function. The severity and duration of side effects experienced since the previous course of therapy must be carefully assessed as well.

Abnormal laboratory values may indicate the development of organ specific toxicities. Drug doses may be modified or delayed based on these results.

The client's chart should have either a copy of the formal drug protocol or a written summary of the planned chemotherapy regimen. Chemotherapy doses are usually based on body surface area (m^2), which is determined by the client's height and weight. Clear and complete chemotherapy prescriptions include the name of the drug, dosage/m^2 and total dose, administration route, administration rate for intravenous infusions, and frequency of administration. Plans for antiemetic coverage, hydration, diuresis, and electrolyte supplementation are frequently included as well.

Before administering antineoplastic agents, consult with the pharmacist and review chemotherapy drug handbooks and investigational drug protocols for detailed information regarding drug actions, dosages, administration guidelines, and potential side effects.

Client and Family Education. Client and family education about chemotherapy and the identification, prevention, and management of side effects are primarily nursing functions. Behavioral objectives for chemotherapy client education are identified in Box 22-8.

Bone Marrow Transplantation

Early efforts to cure leukemia with supralethal radiation and bone marrow transplantation (BMT) began in the 1950s.[34] Current advances in cell typing, prevention and treatment of graft-versus-host disease, antimicrobial therapy, and management of marrow aplasia have broadened the application for BMT to a variety of cancers as well as aplastic anemia and immune deficiency diseases.[16, 72] BMT is a unique treatment modality with the singular goal of cure. It is a complex therapy with a high potential for complications.

Box 22-8. Behavioral Objectives for Chemotherapy Knowledge Deficit

Client demonstrates knowledge related to rationale for treatment with chemotherapy

- Verbalizes the need for chemotherapy
- States understanding of the use of chemotherapy in conjunction with other treatment modalities, if applicable
- States expected response to treatment

Client demonstrates knowledge of treatment plan and schedule

- Identifies drugs to be given and frequency and duration of administration
- Identifies studies and procedures that will be performed prior to administration of chemotherapy
- Identifies follow-up studies and procedures to be performed

Client demonstrates knowledge of potential side effects of drugs

- Identifies side effects that may occur
- States self-management strategies to control side effects
- States signs and symptoms to report to health care persons
- Identifies procedures for reporting signs and symptoms

Adapted from Somerville, E. T. (1991). Knowledge deficit related to chemotherapy. In J. C. McNally, et al. (Eds.), *Guidelines for cancer nursing practice* (2nd ed., pp. 36-39). Philadelphia: W. B. Saunders.

BMT allows the client to receive lethal and potentially more effective doses of chemotherapy and radiation therapy without regard to hematopoietic toxicity. The damaged bone marrow is replaced by healthy donor marrow.

There are three types of donor bone marrow: allogeneic, syngeneic, and autologous. An autologous BMT is the most common type of transplant performed and is often referred to as a rescue. The marrow donor is also the recipient. The bone marrow is generally harvested during disease remission, may or may not be chemically treated, and is stored (frozen) to be reinfused later. Autologous BMTs (ABMT) are now common for solid tumor diseases that are chemotherapy sensitive, radiosensitive, or both.[68] These tumors include breast, ovarian, testicular, neuroblastoma, and lung (small cell and non-small cell) cancers. In addition, ABMTs are being performed for hematologic malignancies such as Hodgkin's and non-Hodgkin's lymphoma, myeloma, and acute and chronic leukemias when a human leukocyte antigen (HLA) match is unavailable. In these cases, once the bone marrow is harvested, the marrow may be purged (treated) with the use of a biophysical, pharmacologic, or immunologic agent to kill any cancer cells present while sparing the normal cells.[57]

In an allogeneic BMT, the marrow donor is usually a sibling or parent with a similar HLA tissue type. In rare instances, an unrelated donor, found through the National Bone Marrow Registry or through a local tissue typing drive may be the donor.[66] A syngeneic BMT uses bone marrow from an identical twin (see also Chap. 24).

Another type of BMT is the peripheral blood stem cell harvest (PBSC). Clients who do not have an HLA-matched donor or who are unable to withstand general anesthesia for the ABMT harvest procedure may be candidates for PBSC. A PBSC transplant is when the client's peripheral blood stem cells are harvested by leukopheresis, processed, and stored. The client then receives lethal doses of chemotherapy, RT, or both and then the PBSC are reinfused.

The transplant process consists of several phases: conditioning, harvest, marrow infusion, pre-engraftment, and engraftment. The time of the bone marrow harvest depends on the type of transplant being performed. In ABMT and PBSC transplants, the harvest is obtained before the initiation of the conditioning regimen. Clients undergoing a bone marrow harvest procedure need to be instructed on the procedure and requirements after the procedure.[29] Conditioning refers to the immunosuppression treatment regimen (chemotherapy, RT, or both) used to eradicate all malignant cells, provide a state of immunosuppression, and create space in the bone marrow for the engraftment of the new marrow.

Marrow is usually infused 48 to 72 hours after the last dose of chemotherapy or RT. Potential side effects include fluid overload, development of micropulmonary emboli, and hypersensitivity reactions to the white cells present in the marrow.[68]

Once the marrow has been infused, the client starts an arduous upward battle. Potential complications include infection; bleeding; renal insufficiency; gastrointestinal effects, veno-occlusive disease (VOD), a condition in which the small veins of the liver become obstructed; and graft-versus-host disease. Management of these transplant complications is beyond the scope of this chapter.[14, 69]

Biologic Response Modifiers

The search to understand and manipulate the human immune system has fascinated scientists for decades. Evidence exists that under the proper circumstances, malignant tumors are susceptible to immune surveillance and subsequent destruction. Thus, the quest to isolate and identify effective biologic agents continues.

In the last decade, four major technologic advances have assisted scientists in their search. These advances include an increased understanding of the complex cellular nature of the immune system; advances in genetic engineering, making it feasible to produce recombinant biologic agents; advances in molecular biology; and refined and advanced laboratory equipment and computer systems.[30, 33]

Biologic response modifiers are defined as those agents that are capable of modifying the relationship between the tumor and the host by strengthening the host's immune function. Clark and Longo identified three major categories of biologic response modifiers according to their mechanism of action: (1) agents that restore, augment, or modulate the host's normal immune function; (2) agents that have direct antitumor effects; and (3) agents that demonstrate other biologic effects, such as interference with a tumor cell's ability to metastasize, promotion of cell differentiation, or tumor cell transformation.[10]

Biologic response modifier agents currently in use in the clinical setting include a variety of interleukins (IL), including IL-1, IL-2, IL-3, IL-4; alpha interferon (IFN); monoclonal antibodies (MoAbs); tumor necrosis factor (TNF); and colony-stimulating factors (CSF), granulocyte-macrophage (GM-CSF), granulocyte (G-CSF), and erythropoietin (EPO). Several of these agents, such as G-CSF, GM-CSF, and EPO, have received Food and Drug Administration (FDA) approval and are available on the market.

Interleukins are substances produced by lymphocytes and function to promote normal hematopoiesis. IL-2 is responsible for the growth of T cells and augments various other T-cell activities and enhances natural killer cell function. Clients with tumors previously unresponsive to standard therapy, such as renal cell carcinoma, melanoma, and non-Hodgkin's lymphoma, have responded to therapy with IL-2. Phase I and II clinical trials continue in an attempt to document the efficacy and therapeutic use of IL-2.

Major toxicities reported with IL-2 therapy include an increased capillary permeability that may produce hypotension, ascites, pulmonary edema, and generalized weight gain.[35] Additionally, integumentary changes occur and may include generalized redness, rash, pruritus, and occasionally, skin desquamation. Toxicities with IL-2 vary greatly with the dose of drug administered. Higher doses produce greater toxicities and require astute clinical management.

IFNs are small proteins that have cellular activity in three areas: antiviral, immunomodulatory, and antiproliferative. IFN received FDA approval for use in hairy cell leukemia in 1986, and in 1989, the drug's clinical indications were broadened to include AIDS-associated Kaposi's sarcoma. Currently, clinical trials are being conducted to investigate its use in other hematologic (particularly chronic leukemias) and solid tumors.

Toxicities appear to be dose related, with lower doses of IFN exhibiting few side effects, whereas high doses may require therapy to be interrupted or stopped.[24] A flulike syndrome is a common side effect of IFN therapy and may include the following symptoms: fever, chills, tachycardia, muscle aches, malaise, fatigue, and headaches. Continued use of IFN produces a tachyphylactic response such that these symptoms decrease in intensity over time. Premedication with acetaminophen and diphenhydramine assists in providing client comfort.

MoAbs have the potential of providing the specificity now lacking in other types of treatment modalities. They can be used either diagnostically or therapeutically. Diagnostic use may include the early detection of cancer by identification of surface markers of tumor cells, or as a delivery agent of radioisotopes to the tumor site to aid in tumor visualization. Therapeutically, MoAbs may be used to deliver immunotoxins, such as ricin, chemotherapeutic agents, and radioactive isotopes directly to the tumor site.[12] To date, MoAbs have demonstrated limited success as a therapeutic option, and clinical trials continue for a variety of cancers.

CSFs are naturally occurring growth factors that mediate hematopoiesis.[23] Generally, CSFs have been named for the major cell lineage they mediate: GM-CSF affects both the granulocyte and macrophage lineage; G-CSF affects only granulocytes; IL-3, or multi-CSF, targets the early cell lineage; and erythropoietin affects erythrocyte production. Erythropoietin was FDA approved in 1989 for use in clients with anemia secondary to end-stage renal failure. Two additional CSFs were FDA approved in February of 1991—G-CSF and GM-CSF for cancer-related neutropenia.

G-CSF is administered by subcutaneous injection, intravenous short infusion, or intravenous continuous infusion daily, starting at least 24 hours after chemotherapy is completed. The recommended dose of G-CSF is 5 mcg/kg/day. It is important to note that G-CSF (Neupogen) is not compatible with saline. The drug is continued for 10 to 14 days, or until the client's absolute neutrophil count is greater than or equal to 10,000 cells/mm^3. When G-CSF is discontinued, a 50 per cent decrease in circulating neutrophils will occur within 1 to 2 days, and a return to pretreatment values occurs within 1 to 7 days. Thus, it is essential that the drug be continued beyond the expected nadir period for optimal benefit. G-CSF is well tolerated, with minimal toxicities reported. The most commonly reported side effect is bone pain, and the problem appears to occur more frequently in high doses administered intravenously. It is hypothesized that the bone pain is the result of the marrow expansion that occurs from the rapid increase in the neutrophil pool. Clients report pain in bone areas that have large marrow reserves such as the pelvis, sternum, and long bones.

GM-CSF can be administered by continuous intravenous infusion (over 2 hours) or by subcutaneous injection daily. The recommended dose of GM-CSF is 250 mcg/m^2/day for 21 days starting 2 to 4 hours after reinfusion of autologous bone marrow and at least 24 hours after chemotherapy and at least 12 hours after radiotherapy is completed.

GM-CSF (Leukine and Prokine) is not compatible with dextrose. GM-CSF should be discontinued if the absolute neutrophil count exceeds 20,000 cells/mm^3. For clients receiving either G-CSF or GM-CSF, monitoring of the complete blood count with a differential is recommended twice weekly during therapy to avoid potential complications of excessive leukocytosis. Currently, the use of erythropoietin in clients with cancer is under clinical investigation.

Because most biologic agents are still investigational, it is important for the nurse to understand the potential side effects of the agent to be administered and to be prepared for and continually assess and document the client's response to therapy. Client and family teaching is of the utmost importance because many clients will seek investigational therapy when standard therapy fails to achieve a tumor response.

SECOND MALIGNANCIES

The term second malignancy refers to the occurrence of new, unrelated neoplasms following initial cancer therapy. The risk of carcinogenesis associated with RT and chemotherapy is under intense investigation. Determination of treatment-related risks is complicated by the interaction of additional risk factors such as the natural history of the disease, genetic predisposition, age, immune status, and environmental factors.[31]

An increased risk of leukemia and solid tumors has been noted following treatment of childhood malignancies, Hodgkin's disease, multiple myeloma, non-Hodgkin's lymphomas, gastrointestinal cancers, lung cancer, and ovarian cancer.[15] Acute nonlymphocytic leukemia following treatment with alkylating agents and solid tumors following RT account for the majority of second cancers.

Most treatment-related leukemias occur within the first 10 years following treatment. Acute nonlymphocytic leukemia that occurs following cancer therapy is exceedingly refractory to therapy and almost uniformly fatal within 6 months of diagnosis.

In contrast to leukemia, most radiation-related cancers appear after 10 years. The majority of these cancers occur either within the direct field of radiation or in the organs surrounding it. The relationship of chemotherapy alone to subsequent solid tumor development is not as clear.

When instructing clients and families about treatment-related risks, it is important to remember that the risk of second malignancy is small and must be balanced against the benefits of therapy for a life-threatening disease. Once therapy is completed, the nurse should emphasize the importance of life-long surveillance.

CANCER RESOURCES

Many resources (patient and/or professional emphasis) are available on request. The following list identifies a few key resources for the nurse caring for the client and family with cancer to contact for further information.

Oncology Nursing Society (ONS)
501 Holiday Drive
Pittsburgh, PA 15229-2749
(412) 921-7373

Office of Cancer Communications
National Cancer Institute
Building 31, Room 10A24
Bethesda, MD 20892
1-800-4-CANCER

American Cancer Society (ACS)
1599 Clifton Road NE
Atlanta, GA 30329
(404) 320-3333

National Coalition for Cancer Survivorship
323 Eighth Street SW
Albuquerque, NM 87102
(505) 764-9956

Bibliography

1. American Nurses' Association & Oncology Nursing Society (1987). *Standards of oncology nursing practice.* Kansas City, MO: American Nurses' Association.
2. Averette, H. D., et al. (1990). Effects of cancer chemotherapy on gonadal and reproductive capacity. *Ca-A Cancer Journal for Clinicians, 40,* 199–209.
3. Baird, S., et al. *Cancer nursing: A comprehensive text.* Philadelphia: W. B. Saunders.
4. Barry, L. K., & Booher, R. N. (1985). Promoting the responsible handling of antineoplastic agents in the community. *Oncology Nursing Forum, 12*(5), 41–46.
5. Bucholtz, J. (1987a). Radiolabeled antibody therapy. *Seminars in Oncology Nursing, 3*(1), 67–83.
6. Bucholtz, J. (1987b). Radiation therapy. In C. Ziegfeld (Ed.), *Core curriculum for oncology nursing* (pp. 207–224). Philadelphia: W. B. Saunders.
7. Carbone, P. P. (1990). Progress in the systemic treatment of cancer: Concepts, trials, drugs, and biologics. *Cancer, 65,* 625–633.
8. Chabner, B. A., & Myers, C. E. (1989). Clinical pharmacology of cancer chemotherapy. In V. T. DeVita, S. Hellman, & S. A. Rosenberg (Eds.), *Cancer: Principles & practice of oncology* (3rd ed., pp. 349–395). Philadelphia: J. B. Lippincott.
9. Clark, R. A., et al. (1989). Antiemetic therapy: Management of chemotherapy-induced nausea and vomiting. *Seminars in Oncology Nursing, 5*(2, Suppl. 1), 53–57.
10. Clark, J. W., & Longo, D. L. (1986). Biological response modifiers. *Mediguide Oncology, 6,* 1–10.
11. Craig, J. B., & Capizzi, R. L. (1985). The prevention and treatment of immediate hypersensitivity reactions from cancer chemotherapy. *Seminars in Oncology Nursing, 1*(4), 285–291.
12. Dillman, J. B. (1988). Toxicity of monoclonal antibodies in the treatment of cancer. *Seminars in Oncology Nursing, 4,* 107–116.
13. Eilers, J. G. (1988). Oral cavity problems experienced in cancer treatment. In *Nursing management of common problems* (pp. 9–16) (A.C.S. NO. 3480.06-PE). New York: American Cancer Society.

14. Ford, R. & Ballard, B. (1988). Acute complications after bone marrow transplantation. *Seminars in Oncology Nursing, 4*(1), 15-24.
15. Fraser, M. C., & Tucker, M. A. (1989). Second malignancies following cancer therapy. *Seminars in Oncology Nursing, 5*(1), 43-55.
16. Freedman, S. E. (1988). An overview of bone marrow transplantation. *Seminars in Oncology Nursing, 4*(1), 3-8.
17. Fuller, A. K. (1990). Platelet transfusion therapy for thrombocytopenia. *Seminars in Oncology Nursing, 6*(2), 123-128.
18. Goodman, M. (1989). Managing the side effects of chemotherapy. *Seminars in Oncology Nursing, 5*(2, Suppl 1), 29-52.
19. Goodman, M. S., & Wickham, R. (1984). Venous access devices: An overview. *Oncology Nursing Forum, 11,* 16-23.
20. Grant, M. (1988). Nausea and vomiting. In *Nursing management of common problems* (pp. 16-24) (A.C.S. NO. 3480.06-PE). New York: American Cancer Society.
21. Gross, J. (1986). Clinical research in cancer chemotherapy. *Oncology Nursing Forum, 13,* 59-65.
22. Gullo, S. M. (1988). Safe handling of antineoplastic drugs: Translating the recommendations into practice. *Oncology Nursing Forum, 15,* 595-601.
23. Haeuber, D., & DiJulio, J. E. (1989). Hemopoietic colony stimulating factors: An overview. *Oncology Nursing Forum, 16*(2), 247-255.
24. Hahn, M. B. & Jassak, P. F. (1988). Nursing management of patients receiving interferon. *Seminars in Oncology Nursing, 4*(2), 95-101.
25. Hassey, K. (1985). Demystifying care of patients with radioactive implants. *American Journal of Nursing 85,* 788-792.
26. Hassey, K. (1987). Principles of radiation safety and protection. *Seminars in Oncology Nursing, 3*(1), 23-29.
27. Hilderley, L. J., & Hassey Dow, K. (1990). Radiation oncology. In S. B. Baird, R. McCorkle, & M. Grant (Eds.), *Cancer nursing: A comprehensive textbook* (pp. 246-265). Philadelphia: W. B. Saunders.
28. Hogan, C. M. (1990). Advances in the management of nausea and vomiting. *Nursing Clinics of North America, 25,* 475-497.
29. Holcombe, A. (1987). Bone marrow harvest. *Oncology Nursing Forum, 14*(2), 63-65.
30. Hood, L. A., & Abernathy, E. (1991). Biologic response modifiers. In S. Baird, R. McCorkle, & M. Grant (Eds.), *Cancer nursing: A comprehensive text* (pp. 321-343). Philadelphia: W. B. Saunders.
31. Hydzik, C. A. (1990). Late effects of chemotherapy: Implications for patient management and rehabilitation. *Nursing Clinics of North America, 25,* 423-446.
32. Jalowiec, A., & Dudas, S. (1991). Alterations in patient coping, In S. Baird, R. McCorkle, & M. Grant (Eds.), *Cancer nursing: A comprehensive text* (pp. 806-820). Philadelphia: W. B. Saunders.
33. Jassak, P. F. (1990). Biotherapy. In S. Groenwald, M. Frogge, M. Goodman, & C., Yarbro (Eds.), *Cancer nursing principles and practice* (pp. 284-306). Boston: Jones and Bartlett.
34. Jassak, P. F., & Porter, N. A. (1990). Bone marrow transplantation. In K. M. Sigardson-Poor & L. M. Haggerty (Eds.), *Nursing care of the transplant recipient* (pp. 280-306). Philadelphia: W. B. Saunders.
35. Jassak, P. F., & Sticklin, L. A. (1986). Interleukin-2: An overview. *Oncology Nursing Forum, 13*(6), 17-22.
36. Kaempfer, S. H., et al. (1985). Fertility considerations and procreative alternatives in cancer care. *Seminars in Oncology Nursing, 1*(1), 25-34.
37. Kinsella, T. J., & Sindelar, W. F. (1985). Newer methods of cancer treatment: Intraoperative radiotherapy. In V. T. DeVita, S. Hellman, & S. Rosenberg (Eds.), *Cancer: Principles and practice of oncology* (2nd ed., pp. 2293-2304). Philadelphia: J. B. Lippincott.
38. Krakoff, I. H. (1987). Cancer chemotherapeutic agents. *Ca-A Cancer Journal for Clinicians, 37,* 93-105.
39. Krakoff, I. H. (1991). Cancer chemotherapeutic and biologic agents. *Ca-A Cancer Journal for Clinicians, 41,* 264-277.
40. Loescher, L. J., et al. (1989). Surviving adult cancers, Part I: Physiologic effects. *Annals of Internal Medicine, 111*(5), 411-432.
41. McCabe, S. V. (1982). An overview of hospice care. *Cancer Nursing,* 103-108.
42. McCaffery, D. (1989). Family issues in cancer care: current dilemmas and future directions. *Journal of Psychosocial Oncology, 6* (1/2), 199-211.
43. McGee, R. F. (1990). Overview of psychosocial dimensions. In S. L. Groenwald, M. Frogge, M. Goodman, and C. Yarbro (Eds.), *Cancer nursing: Principles and practice* (2nd ed., pp. 342-345). Boston: Jones and Bartlett.
44. McGuire, D. B., & Braine, H. G. (Guest Eds.) (1990). Blood component therapy. *Seminars in Oncology Nursing, 6*(2), 89-177.
45. Morrow, G. R. (1989). Chemotherapy-related nausea and vomiting: Etiology and management. *Ca-A Cancer Journal for Clinicians, 39,* 89-104.
46. Morton, D. L., et al. (1989). Principles of surgery. In S. I. Schwartz (Ed.). *Principles of surgery* (pp. 331-381). New York: McGraw-Hill.
47. Mullan, F. (1985). Seasons of survival: Reflections of a physician with cancer. *New England Journal of Medicine, 313,* 270-273.
48. National Cancer Institute. (1986). *What are clinical trials all about?* (NIH Publication No. 86-2706). Washington, D.C.: U.S. Government Printing Office.
49. National Study Commission on Cytotoxic Exposure (1984). *Recommendations for handling cytotoxic agents.* Providence, RI: Rhode Island Hospital.
50. Occupational Safety and Health Administration (Jan. 29, 1986). *Work practice guidelines for personnel dealing with cytotoxic (antineoplastic) drugs.* (OSHA Instruction Publication No. 8-11). Washington, D.C.: Office of Occupational Medicine.
51. Oncology Nursing Society (1988). *Cancer chemotherapy guidelines: Module I, II, III, IV, V.* Pittsburgh, PA: Author.
52. Oncology Nursing Society (1989). *Access device guidelines: Recommendations for nursing education and practice, Module I, II, III.* Pittsburgh, PA: Author.
53. Oniboni, A. C. (1990). Infection in the neutropenic patient. *Seminars in Oncology Nursing, 6*(1), 50-60.
54. Quigley, K. M. (1989). The adult cancer survivor: Psychosocial consequences of cure. *Seminars in Oncology Nursing, 5*(1), 63-69.
54a. Relman, D.A., et al. (1992). Identification of the uncultured bacillus of Whipple's disease. *The New England Journal of Medicine, 327*(5), 293-301.
55. Rosenberg, S. A. (1989). Principles of surgical oncology. In J. T. DeVita, S. Hellman, and S. A. Rosenberg (Eds.), *Cancer: Principles and practice of oncology* (3rd ed., pp. 236-246). Philadelphia: J. B. Lippincott.
56. Ruccione, K., & Weinberg, K. (1989). Late effects in multiple body systems. *Seminars in Oncology Nursing, 5*(1), 4-13.
57. Schryber, S., et al. (1987). Autologous bone marrow transplantation. *Oncology Nursing Forum, 14*(4), 74-80.
58. Somerville, E. T. (1991). Knowledge deficit related to chemotherapy. In J. C. McNally, J. Campbell Stair, and E. T. Somerville (Eds.), *Guidelines for cancer nursing practice* (2nd ed., pp. 36-39). Philadelphia: W. B. Saunders.
59. Spiegel, R. J., & Muggia, F. M. (1983). Cancer chemotherapy. In S. B. Kahn, R. R. Love, C. Sherman, & R. Chakrovorty (Eds.), *Concepts in cancer medicine* (pp. 337-366). Orlando, FL: Grune & Stratton.
60. Strohl, R. (1988). The nursing role in radiation oncology: Symptom management of acute and chronic reactions. *Oncology Nursing Forum, 15*(4), 429-434.
61. Theisen, A. (1991). The irreplaceable gift. *Journal of the American Medical Association, 266*(9), 1283.
62. U.S. Department of Health and Human Services. (1990). *Facing Forward: A Guide for Cancer Survivors* (NIH PUBL NO 90-2424). Washington, D.C.: National Cancer Institute.
63. United States Nuclear Regulatory Commission. (1981). *Instruction concerning risks from occupational radiation exposure.* Regulatory Guide 8:29, Washington, DC.: Office of Nuclear Regulatory Research.
64. Valdagni, R., et al. (1988). Important prognostic factors influencing outcome of combined radiation and hyperthermia. *International Journal of Radiation Oncology, Biology, Physics, 15,* 959-972.

64a. Veronisi, U. (1987). Rationale and indications for limited surgery in breast cancer. *World Journal of Surgery, 11,* 493–498.
65. Wasserman, T. H., & Kligerman, M. (1987). Chemical modifiers of radiation effect. In C. A. Perez, & L. W. Brady (Eds.), *Principles and practice of radiation oncology* (pp. 360–376). Philadelphia: J. B. Lippincott.
66. Weinberg, P. A. (1991). The human leukocyte antigen (HLA) system, the search for a matching donor, national marrow donor program development, and marrow donor issues. In M. Whedon, (Ed.), *Bone marrow transplantation: Principles, practice, and nursing insights* (pp. 3–19). Boston: Jones and Bartlett.
67. Weisman, A. (1979). *Coping with cancer.* New York: McGraw-Hill.
68. Whedon, M. (1991a). Autologous bone marrow transplantation: Clinical indications, transplant process and outcomes. In M. Whedon (Ed.), *Bone marrow transplantation: Principles, practice, and nursing insights* (pp. 49–69). Boston: Jones and Bartlett.
69. Whedon, M. (Ed.) (1991b). *Bone marrow transplantation: Principles, practice, and nursing insights.* Boston: Jones and Bartlett.
70. Wickham, R. S. (1990). Advances in venous access devices and nursing management strategies. *Nursing Clinics of North America, 25,* 345–364.
71. Wickham, R. (1988). Techniques for long-term venous access. In *Nursing management of the patient receiving chemotherapy* (pp. 9–20) (ACS No. 3480.03-PE). American Cancer Society.
72. Wingard, J. R. (1991). Historical perspective and future directions. In M. Whedon (Ed.), *Bone marrow transplantation: Principles, practice, and nursing insights* (pp. 3–19). Boston: Jones and Bartlett.
73. Wood, H. (1985). Radiation therapy implants. In B. L. Johnson & J. Gross (Eds.), *Handbook of oncology nursing* (pp. 567–589). New York: John Wiley & Sons.
74. Yarbro, C. H. (Ed.) (1985). Sexuality and cancer. *Seminars in Oncology Nursing, 1*(1).
75. Yasko, J. M., & Greene, P. (1987). Coping with problems related to cancer and cancer treatment. *Ca-A Cancer Journal for Clinicians, 37*(2), 106–125.
76. Yasko, J. M., & Rust, D. (1989). Trends in chemotherapy administration. *Seminars in Oncology Nursing, 5*(2, Suppl 1), 3–7.

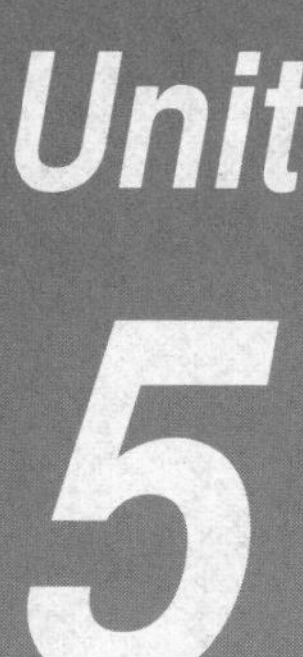

Immunologic Disorders

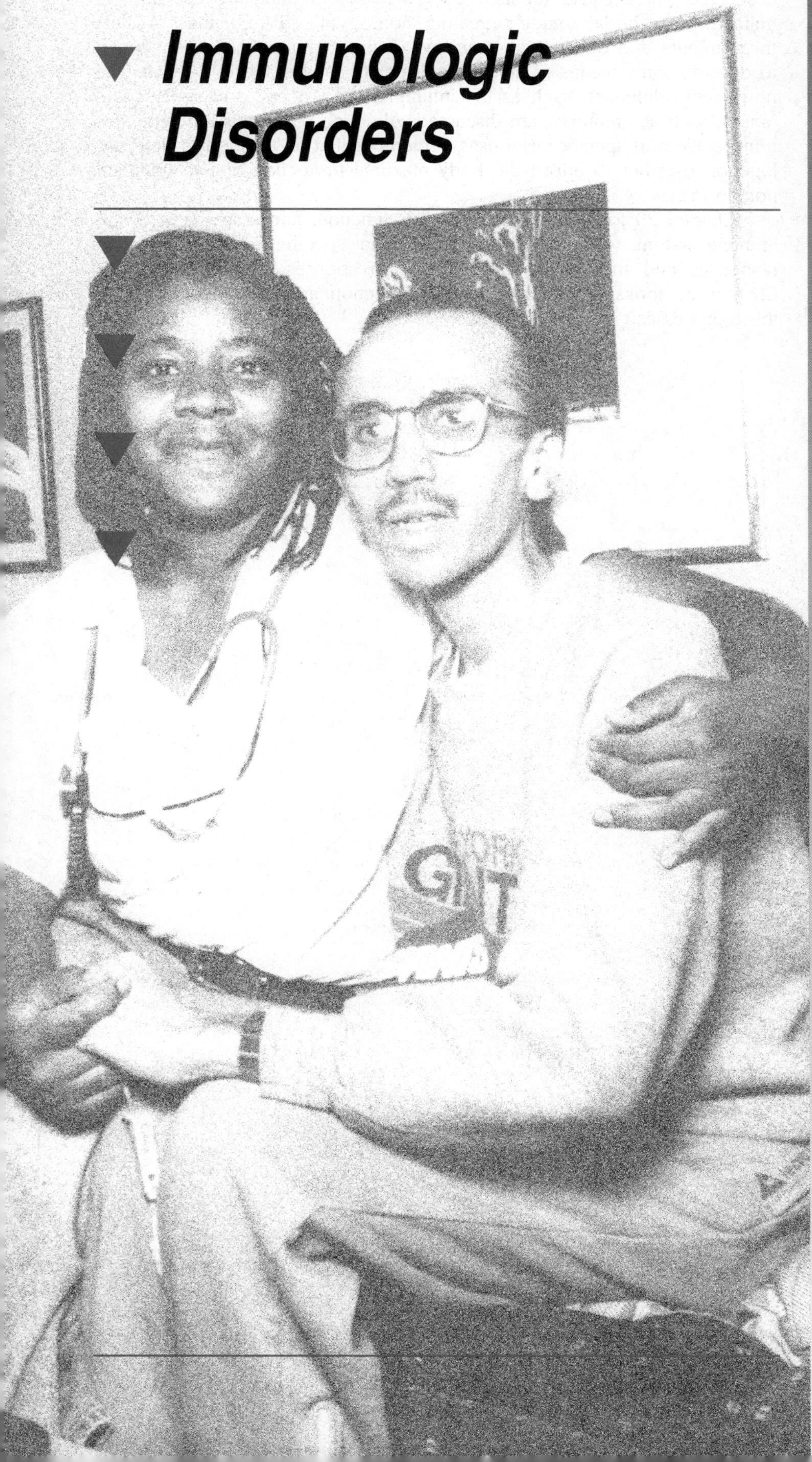

Bacteria and viruses have always plagued humans and animals. These tiny, unseen enemies cause damage by entering and attacking the internal milieu of the body, thereby creating homeostatic disturbances. Against these minute and dangerous organisms, living creatures have been forced to develop some means of defense in order to survive and reproduce. The nonspecific defenses, such as the inflammatory process, and specific defenses, such as immunity, are discussed. Although the discussion separates nonspecific and specific responses, remember that all the body's defenses function together to afford the body maximal protection and to maintain homeostasis.

Chapter 23 focuses on the structure, function, and assessment of the immune system, whereas Chapter 24 looks at specific immune protective responses and the implications of these responses for transplantation. Chapter 25 looks at the processes of infection and the implications of these processes.

Unit photo courtesy of Marilu Halamandaris, *Caring Magazine,* National Association for Home Care.

Chapter 23

Structure, Function, and Assessment of the Immune System

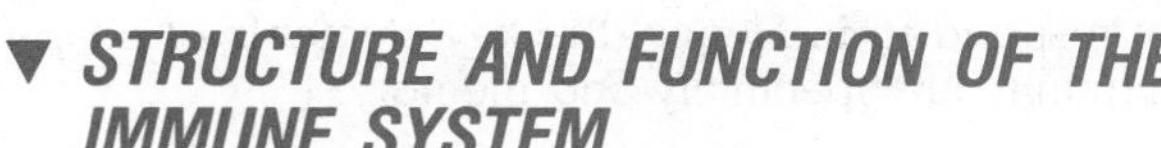

STRUCTURE AND FUNCTION OF THE IMMUNE SYSTEM

The immune system is an intricate network of specialized cells, tissues, and organs designed to allow us to exist in an environment that often includes hostile microorganisms. The system has evolved to protect and defend the body against invasion by bacteria, viruses, fungi, and parasites. It also seeks out and destroys malignantly transformed cells. The significance of a healthy immune system is apparent in states or diseases characterized by immunodeficiency, such as occurs in HIV infection or in patients on immunosuppressive medication. Without an effective immune system, an individual is at risk for the development of overwhelming infection, malignant disease, or both. On the other hand, excessive or inappropriate activity of the immune system can result in autoimmune disease, hypersensitivity states, or immune complex disease.

SELF AND NONSELF

The basis of immunity depends on the immune cells' ability to distinguish self from nonself. All cells of the body contain specific cell surface markers or molecules that are as unique to that person as one's fingerprints. The immune system recognizes these cell markers and tolerates them as self, in other words producing self-tolerance. These cell markers are present on the surface of all body cells and are known as the major histocompatibility complex (MHC) proteins. Because they were initially discovered on leukocytes, in humans they are commonly called human leukocytic antigens (HLA). A cluster of genes, called the MHC genes, are located on chromosome 6, and they encode for the HLA proteins. An individual inherits one maternal and one paternal chromosome 6. Since each of these genes has as many as 25 varieties, there are innumerable different HLA combinations. Thus the HLA pattern varies widely from person to person but is the same in identical twins and similar in siblings. The rejection of foreign or transplanted tissue occurs because the recipient's immune system recognizes that the surface HLA proteins of the donor's tissue are different than that of the recipient's.

The MHC self-markers are classified as either class I or class II. Class I markers are present on all body cells, whereas Class II markers are restricted to the surfaces of macrophages and B lymphocytes. Besides labeling our body cells as self, these cell surface markers play a significant role in the immunologic recognition between the different types of lymphoid cells and between lymphocytes and antigen-presenting cells (APC).

It is now known that having certain HLA proteins increases an individual's susceptibility to some diseases. Such diseases encompass many that affect the joints, endocrine glands, and skin including rheumatoid arthritis, Graves' disease, psoriasis, and many others. This association between specific HLA patterns and disease is of a statistical nature. This means that not all individuals with a certain HLA pattern will develop the disease, but they have a greater probability for its development than the general population. Furthermore, this association may be strong for some diseases and weak for others. Although several theories exist as to how the MHC genes might be involved in disease susceptibility, none yet has been proved.

Any foreign substance in the body that does not have the characteristic cell surface markers of that individual and is capable of eliciting an immune response is referred to as an antigen. Bacteria, viruses, parasites, foreign tissue cells, and even large protein molecules are antigenic. Smaller molecules, called haptens, can also become antigenic or elicit an immune response by combining with larger molecular weight substances. On encountering an antigen, the immune system recognizes it as nonself, and the appropriate immune response is mounted against the antigen. A single bacterium contains hundreds of antigenic sites and, therefore, has multiple sites capable of stimulating an immune response.

The antigenic determinants or subunits of an antigen that elicit an immune response are called epitopes. Epitopes are molecules that protrude from the surface of an antigen and actually combine with an antibody (Fig. 23–1). Each antigen may display hundreds of epitopes. The more epitopes there are, the greater the antigenicity of a substance and the greater the immune response. Antibodies are produced in response to an antigen and are protein molecules structured so that they interact only with the antigen that induced their synthesis, much like a key is made to fit a lock.

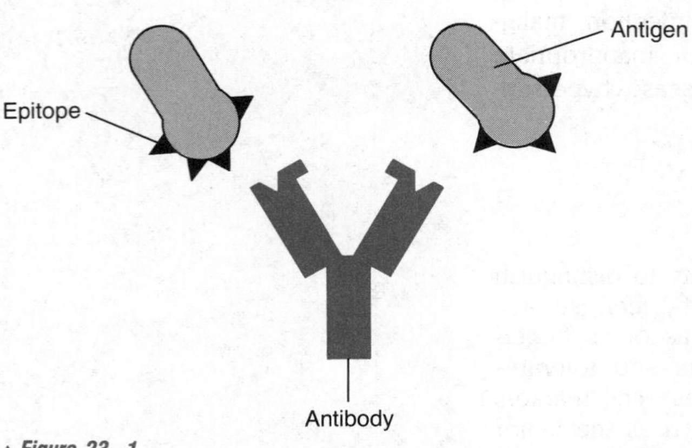

▲ **Figure 23–1**

Epitopes protrude from the surface of an antigen and combine with the appropriate receptor of an antibody, much like a key fits a lock.

TYPES OF IMMUNITY

Two types of immunity are recognized; (1) innate and (2) adaptive immunity. Innate immunity is nonspecific and acts as the body's first line of defense, guarding against potential pathogens and preventing them from becoming established as an overt infection. Adaptive immunity is stimulated when a pathogen gains entry to the body, and it produces a specific response to the invader. Furthermore, adaptive immunity has memory, so when the invader is encountered again, it can more rapidly respond to it. Hence, the key elements of adaptive immunity are specificity and memory.

Innate Immunity

The defenses of the innate immune system consist of a variety of physical barriers, biochemicals, and cellular defense mechanisms designed to prevent the establishment of potential pathogens within the body. Most organisms enter the body by penetrating the epithelial surfaces of the respiratory, gastrointestinal, and genitourinary tracts. However, these portals of entry are protected by many physical and biochemical defenses, including the skin barrier, acid secretions, which produce an unfavorable pH, and lysozymes that destroy cell walls of bacteria. Phagocytic cells that engulf and destroy foreign particles, including microorganisms, are also part of innate immunity. So, too, are the natural killer (NK) cells, which indiscriminately attack and destroy virus-infected cells and tumor cells. In addition, a number of proteins, produced nonspecifically in response to potential pathogens, are also part of the innate immune system. These include proteins of the complement system, acute phase proteins, and interferons. The complement system is a series of proteins that, when activated, enhance phagocytosis, inflammation, and lysis of microorganisms. Acute phase proteins are produced by the liver in response to an infection. One such protein, called C-reactive protein, promotes binding of complement to microorganisms, which enhances their phagocytosis. Interferons are a family of related proteins that are produced by either virally infected body cells or activated T lymphocytes. When released, they confer a state of antiviral resistance in uninfected body cells.

Adaptive Immunity

The recognition of a foreign antigen and the formation of memory cells against an antigen are the hallmarks of specific adaptive immunity. It is mediated by the actions of B and T lymphocytes and can be acquired actively or passively. Active acquired immunity refers to protection acquired by introduction of an antigen into a responsive host. The antigen can be introduced deliberately, as in vaccinations, or naturally from exposure in the environment. For example, contact with the virus causing chicken pox stimulates an immune response against this virus and will confer resistance or immunity upon reexposure to this pathogen. Vaccinations refer to immunization with antigens administered to protect against infectious disease. Whole or parts of weakened or killed microorganisms or their toxic products are injected into or ingested by a responsive host. This process will not produce the disease but will stimulate an immune response and provide resistance to this organism when it is naturally encountered in the environment. More recently, the use of recombinant technology allows vaccination by the injection of synthetic antigen and avoids the use of human or animal serum, which can stimulate allergic reactions. The hepatitis B surface antigen (HBsAg) used to produce the hepatitis B vaccine, for instance, is obtained from recombinant yeast cells that have been genetically altered to produce large quantities of HBsAg.

Active acquired immunity is possible because of immunologic memory. This refers to the ability of immune cells to recall prior exposure to an antigen and respond in an accelerated and augmented fashion. How effective this immunity is and how long it lasts depends on the type of antigen, its amount, and how it enters the body. For example, certain vaccines, such as tetanus toxoid, must be readministered at certain intervals to maintain immunity; whereas, one-time exposure to other disease-causing organisms or vaccines can produce immunity for an indefinite period. Other variables, such as heredity, also affect the strength and effectiveness of a person's immune response and, hence, the degree and duration of active acquired immunity.

Passive acquired immunity is obtained when antibodies, antisera (serum that contains antibodies), or sensitized lymphocytes produced by one person are transferred to another. The transplacental transfer of antibody (IgG) from mother to fetus, the transfer of antibody (IgA) to an infant through breast milk, or the receipt of immune serum globulin (gamma globulin) are examples of passive acquired immunity. Passive immunotherapy for cancer occurs when a cancer patient's lymphocytes are sensitized against tumor antigens in vitro (outside the body) and reinfused to combat the same tumor cells in vivo (inside the body). Passive acquired immunity produces immediate protection but does not result in the formation of memory cells and consequently is short lived. It lasts only until the antibodies are degraded which may be a few weeks or months. Any injection of immune serum has the potential to produce an allergic reaction called serum sickness in the recipient.

CELLS OF THE IMMUNE SYSTEM

The immune system contains an immense arsenal of cells aimed at protecting the body against foreign invasion. The total number of circulating leukocytes or white blood cells (WBC) is 4000 to 10,000 cells per cubic millimeter of blood. This count does not include those leukocytes that have marginated along the vascular endothelial surface or entered tissue spaces or lymphatics. Infection stimulates WBC production from hematopoietic tissue and leads to an increase in the circulating number of WBCs (leukocytosis). Leukopenia, a decrease in the total number of circulating WBCs, occurs in conditions marked by bone marrow suppression or increased peripheral destruction of WBCs, which might occur with splenomegaly.

Five classes of leukocytes are recognized: (1) neutrophil, (2) eosinophil, (3) basophil, (4) monocyte, and (5) lymphocyte. Each of these cell types has a specific function in the immune response (Table 23-1). Measurement of the subcategories of leukocytes, or a differ-

TABLE 23-1. Types of White Blood Cells

Type	% of Total WBC	Function
Neutrophils Bands (immature) Segmented (mature)	40 to 75	Phagocytosis
Eosinophils	2 to 5	Phagocytosis Allergy Suppresses inflammation Decreases granulocyte migration
Basophils	0.2 to 0.5	Inflammatory mediator release
Monocytes (macrophages)	2 to 6	Phagocytosis Monokine production
Lymphocytes	20 to 35	Adaptive immunity Cell-mediated immunity Humoral immunity

WBC, white blood cells.

ential count, provides important diagnostic information concerning the etiology of disease, be it due to inflammation, allergy, infection, or leukemia.

Granulocytes: Neutrophils, Eosinophils, and Basophils

Because of the granular appearance of their cytoplasm, the neutrophils, eosinophils, and basophils are collectively referred to as granulocytes. The granulocytes are short lived (2 to 3 days) compared with monocytes and macrophages which may live for months or years.

The neutrophils are phagocytic cells and account for about 40 to 75 per cent of blood leukocytes. Neutrophils leave the vascular compartment and enter tissue spaces searching out bacteria or cell debris, which they can phagocytize and destroy. Neutrophils are attracted to and migrate toward various chemicals called chemoattractants. An example of a chemoattractant is C5a, a protein of the complement system (see the section on Complement). In response to a chemoattractant, neutrophils will marginate or adhere to the endothelial surface of blood vessels and move through the capillary wall (i.e., diapedisis) (Fig. 23-2). In the process of phagocytosis, which literally means cell eating, the bacteria or debris are engulfed and taken up into the phagocytic cell and contained within a cytoplasmic vacuole. The granules of neutrophils contain enzymes that are released into the vacuoles and assist in digesting the organisms or debris. Neutrophils cannot replicate and die following phagocytosis. The accumulation of dead neutrophils contributes to the formation of pus.

The process of phagocytosis results in an excess or burst of oxygen consumption called a respiratory burst. It produces toxic oxygen radicals such as superoxide and hydrogen peroxide. Oxygen radicals are used within the phagocytic vacuole to degrade the ingested organism or debris but can be released extracellularly. In excess, oxygen radicals can cause damage to normal body tissue in the area of neutrophil activation. Such damage has been implicated in a variety of immune-based diseases. For example, oxygen radicals have been linked to the damage that occurs in inflamed arthritic joints and in the pulmonary vascular endothelial injury seen in the adult respiratory distress syndrome that often complicates septic shock.

During infection, the bone marrow produces and releases an increased number of neutrophils in various stages of development. Immature neutrophils have horseshoe-shaped nuclei and are called bands, whereas the nuclei of mature neutrophils are segmented or divided into lobes. An increase in circulating neutrophils is called neutrophilia, and when the condition is characterized by an excess number of immature neutrophils, it is called a left shift. Conversely, a right shift describes neutrophilia that is marked by an increased percentage of mature neutrophils. (This nomenclature reflects the traditional practice of illustrating neutrophil maturation by depicting the most immature cells on the left side of the page and the more mature on the right side.) An increased ratio of immature to mature neutrophils places an individual at greater risk for infection because immature neutrophils have less phagocytic activity than mature cells. Neutropenia, or a decreased number of circulating neutrophils, is primarily seen in hematologic malignancies, cytotoxic therapy, or aplastic anemia.

Eosinophils account for 2 to 5 per cent of leukocytes, and although they are phagocytic, they are not as effective as neutrophils. They contain many cytoplasmic granules filled with enzymes, which can be released on appropriate stimulation. Eosinophils are thought to protect humans against helminth (parasitic worm) infections, such as intestinal pinworms and tapeworms. Eosinophils deactivate inflammatory mediators by releasing histaminase, which deactivates histamine, and aryl sulphatase, which deactivates the slow reactive substance of anaphylaxis (SRS-A). Generally, eosinophils dampen down the inflammatory response and decrease granulocyte migration into the inflammatory site. Eosinophilia is often seen with allergic reactions.

Basophils comprise less than 0.2 per cent of leuko-

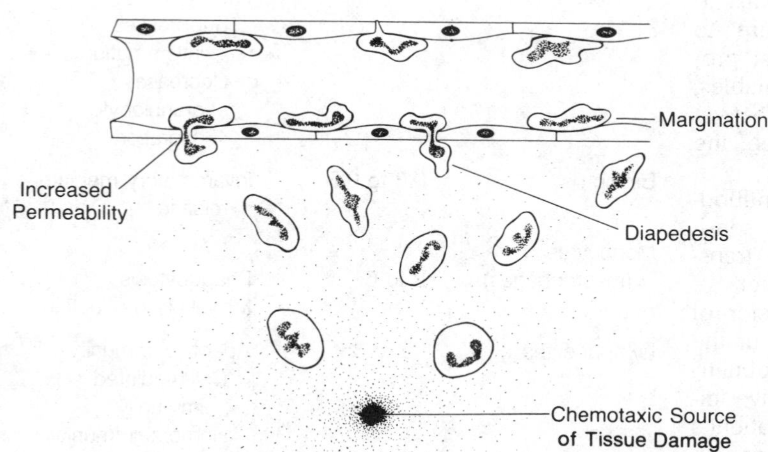

▲ **Figure 23-2**

Movement of white blood cells by the process of chemotaxis toward an area of tissue damage. (From Miller, M. J. [1983]. Pathophysiology [p. 149]. Philadelphia, W. B. Saunders.)

cytes and are similar to mast cells. They contain granules made up of heparin, SRS-A, and eosinophil chemotactic factor of anaphylaxis. These chemicals are released on appropriate stimulation, such as by allergens.

Monocytes/Macrophages

Of the nongranulocytes, the monocytes are the largest in size and they account for 2 to 6 per cent of the total WBC count. Monocytes circulate in the blood, but when they migrate to tissues, they mature into macrophages. For instance, the lung contains alveolar macrophages, whereas macrophages lining the blood sinusoids of the liver are called Kupffer's cells. Macrophage literally means big eaters. They are responsible for removing particulate antigens, such as damaged or aged cells and cellular debris, by phagocytosis (Fig. 23-3).

Macrophages also serve as APCs because they present antigen to specific lymphocytes in the following manner. On encountering antigen, that is, nonself, the macrophage will phagocytize and process it so that the foreign antigenic determinants are expressed on its surface membrane. In this form, the antigen is then presented to specific lymphocytes and lymphocyte activation occurs. Macrophages also participate in the defense against tumor cells and secrete numerous molecules called monokines that assist in the immune and inflammatory response. Some macrophage secretory

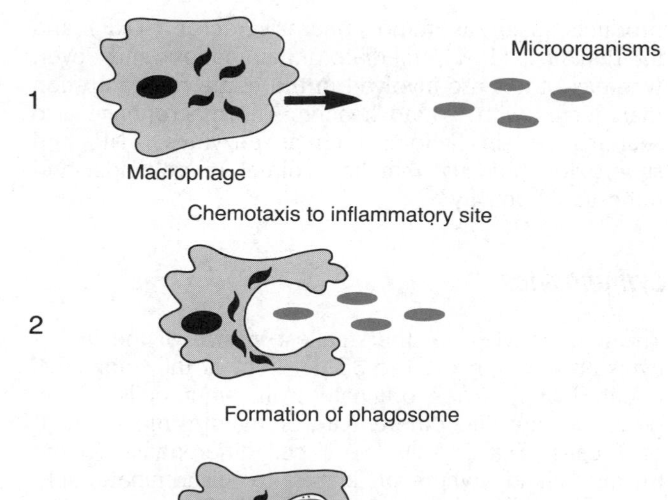

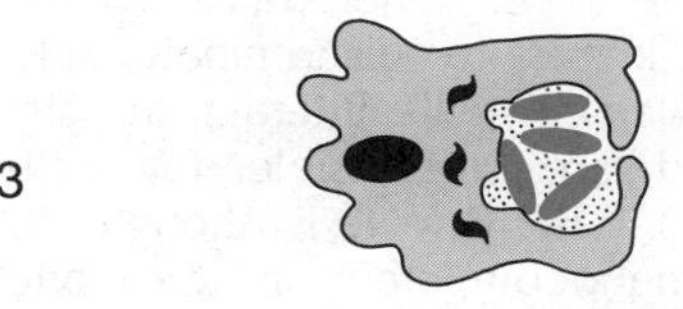

▲ *Figure 23-3*

(1) Macrophages migrate to an inflammatory site by chemotaxis. (2) Macrophages engulf the microorganisms by extending pseudopodia around them. A phagosome or phagocytic vacuole forms around the microorganisms. (3) Lysosomes attach to the phagosome and release their enzymes, which destroy the microorganisms.

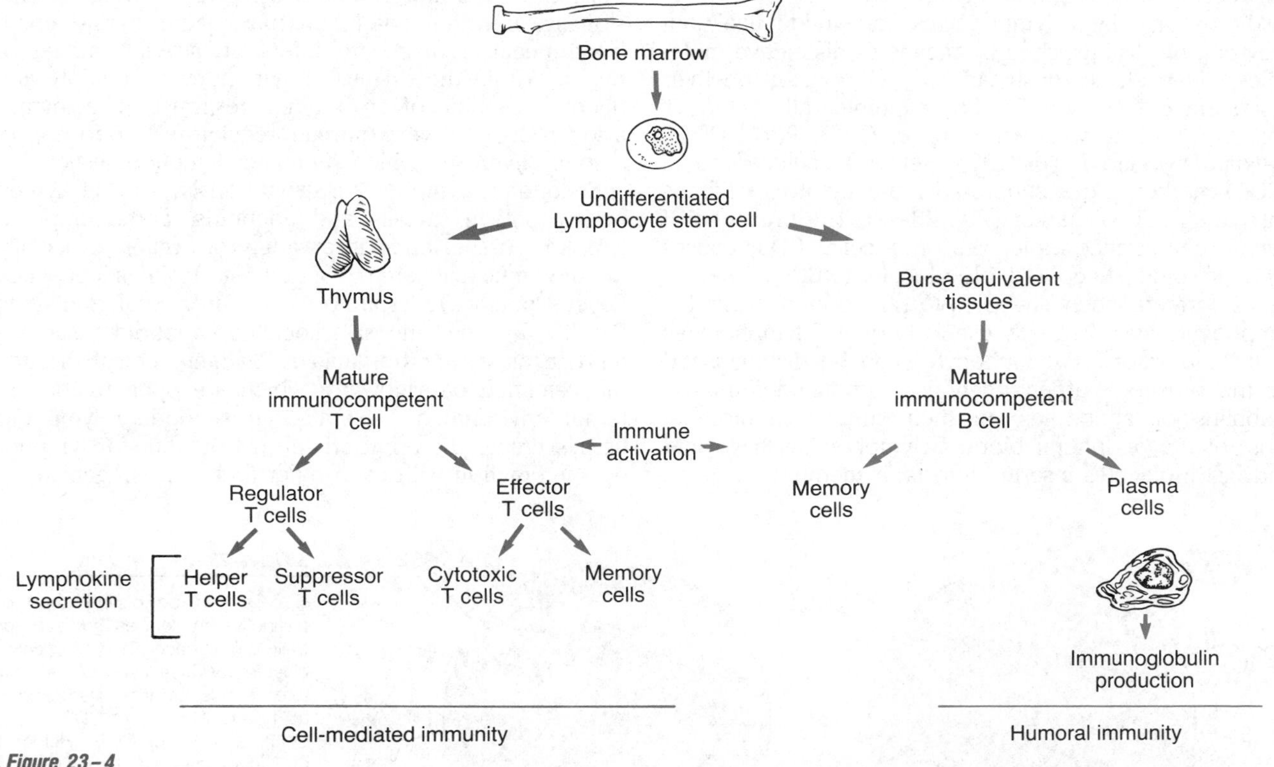

▲ *Figure 23-4*

The pathway of lymphocyte maturation. Undifferentiated lymphocyte stem cells are derived from the bone marrow. Those stem cells that are processed in the thymus differentiate into mature immunocompetent T cells, whereas those that are "processed" in bursa equivalent tissues (most likely the bone marrow) become mature immunocompetent B cells. Activation of either T or B cells by antigens leads to proliferation of immune cells that mediate either cell-mediated immunity or humoral immunity.

products, such as tumor necrosis factor (TNF) and interleukin-1 (IL-1), mediate inflammation and fever, whereas others are involved in the tissue reorganization that occurs with wound healing. The macrophage also secretes certain factors, such as enzymes, TNF, and superoxide radicals, that have direct microbicidal and tumoricidal activity.

Lymphocytes

The lymphocytes are the smallest in size of the leukocytes and comprise 20 to 35 per cent of the total WBC count. Lymphocytes originate from stem cells in the bone marrow and differentiate or mature into either B or T cells (Fig. 23–4). The T cell differentiates in the thymus gland, where it learns to discriminate self-antigen from nonself-antigen. T cells interact directly with cellular targets and are responsible for cell-mediated immunity (CMI). The B cell is thought to mature and become immunocompetent in the bone marrow. (The differentiation of B cells was first discovered in the bursa of Fabricius, which is lymphoid tissue located in the hindgut of birds. Hence, the site of B cell differentiation in mammals is often referred to as bursa equivalent tissue.) When stimulated by an antigen, B cells further differentiate into plasma cells, which secrete soluble molecules called antibodies into the body's fluids. Antibodies mediate humoral immunity. Both T and B lymphocytes continually recirculate between blood, lymph, and lymph nodes.

Microscopically T lymphocytes appear identical, but they can be distinguished by means of distinctive molecules called cluster designations (CD) located on their cell surface (Fig. 23–5). For example, all mature T cells carry markers known as T_2 (or CD2), T_3 (or CD3), T_5 (or CD5), and T_7 (or CD7). Helper T cells carry a T_4 (CD4) marker and a suppressor, and cytotoxic T cells carry a T_8 (CD8) marker (Fig. 23–5). The presence of certain cell surface molecules on T cells (CD2) causes them to bind sheep red blood cells (RBCs). The rosettes formed when sheep RBCs are bound around a lymphocyte was originally used to count T lymphocytes in the laboratory. B lymphocytes can be distinguished by the presence of endogenously produced immunoglobulins or antibodies on their surface membrane. Most of the peripheral blood B lymphocytes have IgM and IgG molecules inserted into their membranes.

Another group of large lymphocytes lack conventional surface antigen receptors. Functionally, they are identified by their ability to kill certain tumor cells and virus-infected cells without prior sensitization or activation. Hence, they are called NK cells. NK cells can also attack certain targets coated with IgG antibody, and this process is referred to as antibody-dependent cellular cytotoxity (ADCC).

THE LYMPHOID SYSTEM

Throughout the body, there are multiple portals of entry for disease-causing microbes to penetrate. Because the purpose of the immune system is to rapidly encounter and respond to any foreign invader, it is not surprising that the cells, tissues, and organs comprising the lymphoid system are widely distributed throughout the body. Furthermore, the mobility of immune cells allows them to circulate and move in and out of tissues so that they can survey the body for pathogens, cellular debris, virus-infected cells, and tumor cells (i.e., immune surveillance).

The bone marrow and the thymus are the primary lymphoid organs (Fig. 23–6). The bone marrow is the soft tissue inside the hollow of long bones and is a major site for proliferation and maturation of immune cells from undifferentiated stem cells. The thymus is a multilobed gland located in the mediastinum anterior to and above the heart. The thymus is large in the newborn and child and gradually involutes with age. Occasionally, transient involution may occur during childhood because of severe infection, stress, trauma, or burns. Within the thymus, T lymphocytes multiply and become capable of an immune response. The thymus also produces several immunoregulatory hormones, including thymosin, which stimulates lymphopoiesis.

Secondary lymphoid organs consist of the lymph nodes, spleen, tonsils and adenoids, and clumps of lymphoid tissue found in a variety of organs, especially in the mucosal areas of the gastrointestinal (i.e., Peyer's patches), respiratory, and urogenital tract (see Fig. 23–7). The mucosa-associated lymphoid tissue defend against microorganisms gaining entry through mucosa-lined passageways, which are open to the external environment. Overall, the secondary lymphoid tissues create the appropriate environment for lymphocyte interaction with each other and with antigens.

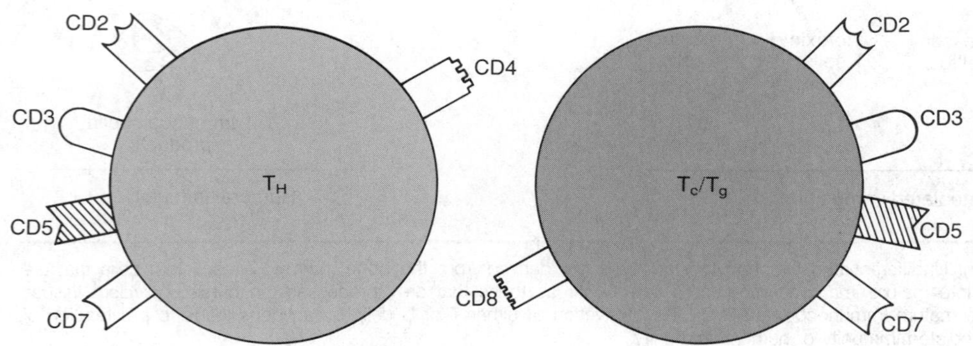

▲ Figure 23–5

T cells can be distinguished by distinctive molecules located on their cell surface. They are called cluster designations (CD). All mature T cells carry markers known as T_2 (or CD2), T_3 (or CD3), T_5 (or CD5), and T_7 (or CD7). Helper T (T_H) cells carry a T_4 (CD4) and suppressor (T_s) and cytotoxic T cells (T_c) and cytotoxic T cells carry a T_8 (CD8) marker.

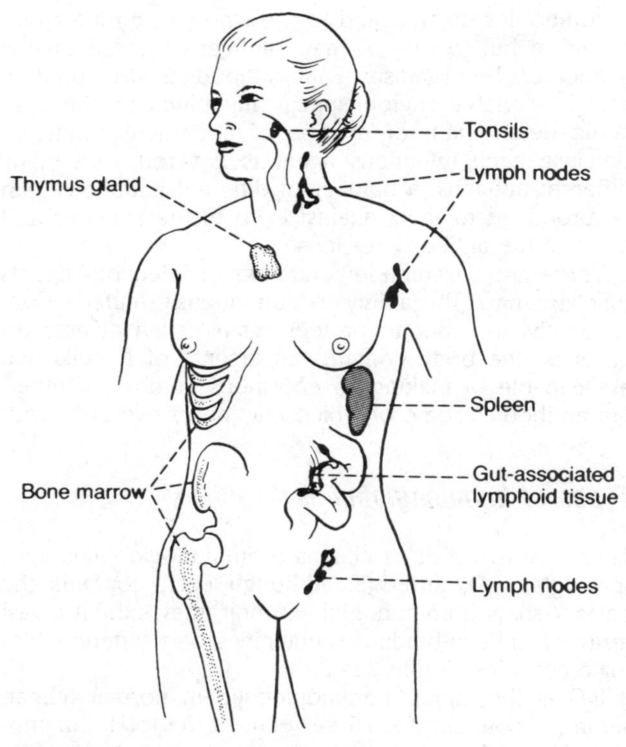

▲ *Figure 23-6*

Organs of the immune system. The bone marrow, spleen, lymph nodes, tonsils, and gut-associated lymphoid tissue function in both specific and nonspecific immunity, whereas the thymus functions primarily in specific immunity.

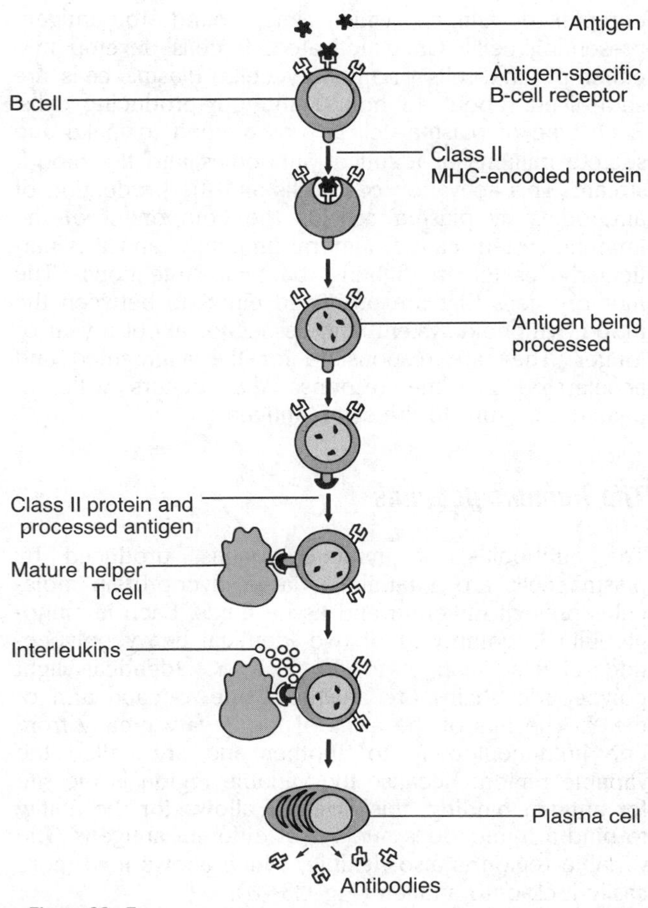

▲ *Figure 23-7*

Activation of B cells to make antibody. The B cell uses its receptor to bind matching antigen, which it engulfs and processes. The B cell then presents a piece of antigen, bound to class II protein, on its surface. The complex binds to the mature helper T cell, which releases interleukins that transform the B cell into an antibody-secreting plasma cell. (Redrawn from Schindler, L. W. [1990]. *Understanding the immune system.* Washington, D.C.: National Institutes of Health.)

There is a continuous recirculation of lymphocytes between the blood vessels and the lymphatic vessels, which parallel the venous system. While recirculating, lymphocytes percolate through the lymph nodes and some may temporarily take up residence there. The lymphocytes eventually return to the circulation through the thoracic duct or right lymphatic duct.

The lymph nodes are dispersed along the lymphatic vessels and form clusters in the neck, axillae, abdomen, and groin. They are small, encapsulated, round or kidney-shaped structures and have an indentation, or hilus, where blood vessels enter and leave the node. The nodes have separate areas housing aggregates of B and T lymphocytes.

Fluid from the interstitial space of the tissues is drained by the lymphatic vessels. This fluid then filters through the lymph nodes, where any foreign antigen can be enmeshed and presented to lymphocytes. The lymphocytes then proliferate, and the node enlarges and becomes palpable. Enlarged nodes are a useful diagnostic sign of infection or malignant disease. Scavenger phagocytic cells are also strategically placed along the blood sinuses of the lymph nodes and remove particulate antigens filtering through the node.

The spleen is located in the upper abdomen and contains two types of tissue: (1) the red pulp and (2) the white pulp. The red pulp contains phagocytic cells that dispose of damaged or aged red blood cells, and the white pulp contains lymphoid tissue. This tissue is organized with separate compartments for either B or T cells, which can be stimulated when antigen filters through the spleen. Although the spleen is not essential for life, individuals whose spleens have been damaged by trauma or disease, such as sickle cell anemia, are much more susceptible to infection.

B LYMPHOCYTES AND THE ANTIBODY RESPONSE

The surface of B lymphocytes are coated with immunoglobulin or antibody. When the appropriately matched antigen is detected by a B cell, the surface immunoglobulin will latch onto it or bind it. This binding of antigen will signal the B cell to proliferate and differentiate (Fig. 23-7). Unlike T cells, B cells do not need to recognize antigen in association with MHC molecules but can be stimulated by free antigen or complexed antigen which has bound to antigen-presenting cells. Once activated, B cells develop into either plasma cells or memory cells. Plasma cells are short-lived (about 48 hours) antibody-producing cells. Each type of plasma cell is programmed to make and secrete millions of identical antibodies into the bloodstream. This activation of B cells and the production of antibodies by plasma cells is the component of the immune system called humoral immunity, and it is particularly useful in fighting bacterial infections. The memory cells that are produced circulate between the blood, lymphoid system, and tissues for about a year or longer. They are responsible for the augmented and accelerated immune response that occurs with repeated exposure to the same antigen.

Antibodies do not bind to the whole of an infectious organism but to one of many antigens located on the surface of the organism. Each antibody is structured so that its variable region specifically binds to the antigenic determinant or epitope of a particular antigen. Because each infectious agent is covered with many different antigens, a number of different antibodies can be produced to react against each of the antigens and escalate the antibody response.

There are a tremendous number of infectious agents that also have the ability to continuously mutate. Consequently, in order to protect against such diverse organisms, the body contains an arsenal of B cells that are capable of making an enormous number of different antibodies some of which may never even be used.

The Immunoglobulins

The antibodies, or immunoglobulins, produced by plasma cells are a family of large glycoprotein molecules present in serum and tissue fluids. Each immunoglobulin is composed of two identical heavy polypeptide chains shaped to form a Y. Identical light polypeptide chains are attached, one to each arm of the Y. The tips of the arms of the Y vary greatly from one immunoglobulin to another and are called the variable region. Because the variable region is the site for antigen binding, this diversity allows for the ability to bind a tremendous number of different antigens. The variable region is also flexible, which allows it to more easily lock onto antigen (Fig. 23-8).

The stem of the Y is identical in all antibodies of the same class and is referred to as the constant region (Fc). The Fc region inserts itself into the surface membrane of B lymphocytes and other cells that carry an Fc receptor, such as macrophages and neutrophils. B lymphocytes carry membrane-bound immunoglobulin of the same binding specificity as that produced by the terminally differentiated plasma cell.

Types of Immunoglobulins

There are five distinct classes of immunoglobulins: IgG, IgA, IgM, IgD, and IgE. Although each contains the basic Y-shaped immunoglobulin unit, they exhibit a vast array of antigen-binding specificities and different biologic activities (Table 23-2).

IgG is the major immunoglobulin in normal human serum, accounting for 75 per cent of the total immunoglobulins. It is monomeric, meaning it is composed of one Y-shaped immunoglobulin unit. IgG can leave the vascular compartment and enter tissue spaces to seek out infectious organisms. By opsonizing or coating microorganisms, it speeds their uptake by phagocytic cells. IgG can activate the complement cascade, which, in turn, amplifies the immune response. It is the only immunoglobulin that can cross the placenta and offer some protection to the newborn during the first few months of life.

IgA comprises approximately 15 per cent of the immunoglobulin pool. It is present in the circulation but also in seromucous secretions, such as saliva, tears, colostrum, breast milk, and secretions of the respira-

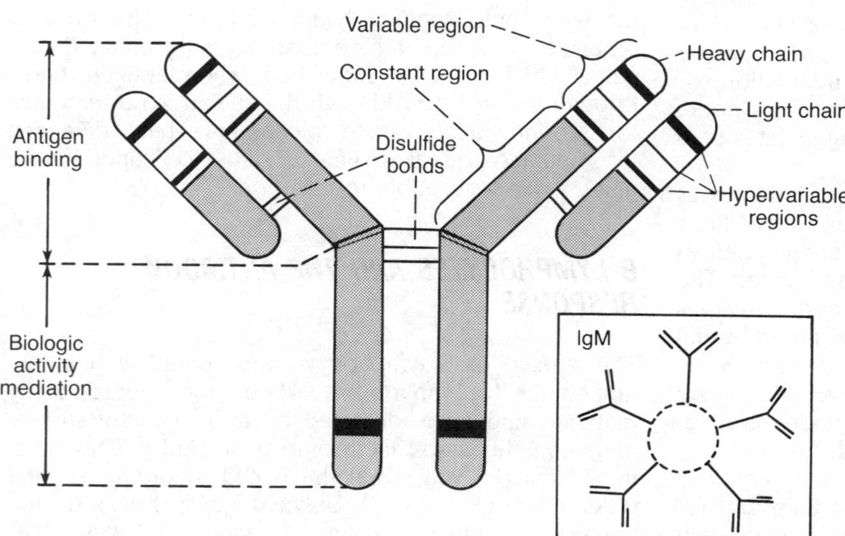

▲ *Figure 23-8*

The immunoglobulin molecule (IgG) consists of two heavy chains joined by disulfide bonds to two light chains. Both chains have regions of constant and of variable amino acid sequences. All five major immunoglobulin classes are composed of variations of this structure; combinations form pentamers of the IgM molecule for example (see inset). The antigen-binding portion of the Y is responsible for immunologic specificity of the IgG molecule; the biologic activity mediation portion is responsible for facilitating complement, phagocytosis, phagocytic cell specificity, and IgG transport across the placenta.

TABLE 23–2. Classes and Characteristics of Immunoglobulins

Class	% of Total	Characteristics
IgG	75	Present in the circulation and tissue spaces Opsonizes antigen Activates complement Transferred transplacentally First Ig synthesized in secondary immune response
IgA	15	Present in the circulation and seromucous secretions Prevents adherence of microorganisms to mucosal surface
IgM	10	Present primarily in the circulation Powerful agglutinating antibody First Ig of the primary immune response Activates complement
IgE	<1.0	Mediates hypersensitivity reactions Binds to mast cells and triggers mediator release
IgD	<1.0	Lymphocyte differentiation Full function unknown

tory, gastrointestinal, and reproductive tracts. Secretory IgA is often called antiseptic paint because it prevents the adherence of microorganisms to the mucosal surface and provides the primary defense against local infections. Unlike monomeric IgA, which is confined to the circulation, secretory IgA is a dimer containing two Y subunits linked together by a peptide chain called a J chain. When it is secreted, it links up with a secretory piece or molecule released from the epithelial cells of whatever organ it is being secreted from. The secretory piece is believed to increase its resistance to proteolytic enzyme digestion, especially in the gastrointestinal tract.

IgM represents about 10 per cent of the total plasma immunoglobulin. It has a pentameric structure containing five Y-subunits linked together to form star-shaped clusters. As a result of its large size, it tends to remain in the blood, where it is effective against gram-negative bacteria. It is a powerful agglutinating agent, producing large clumps of antigen that can be more readily phagocytized. IgM is the major early antibody seen in the primary immune response and the most efficient activator of the complement cascade.

IgE is normally present in trace amounts within the blood. It binds to the surface of mast cells, where it triggers the release of chemical mediators, such as histamine, which produce the symptoms of allergy.

IgD comprises less than 1 per cent of the total circulating immunoglobulins. However, it is present in large numbers on the cell membrane of circulating B lymphocytes. Its precise role is unknown, but it may be involved in antigen-triggered lymphocyte differentiation.

Actions of Antibodies

Antibodies carry out a number of roles in the immune response. Generally, they neutralize the invader or make it more vulnerable to attack from macrophages and neutrophils. They can opsonize antigen and precipitate soluble antigen, all of which make it more susceptible to phagocytosis by macrophages. Antibodies can directly bind to bacterial toxins and neutralize them. IgG and IgM can activate the complement cascade, liberating molecules that amplify the immune response. By binding to macrophages with their Fc region, they arm macrophages and assist them in their cytotoxic role. Antibodies can also coat foreign cells or tumor cells and make them vulnerable to attack by leukocytes. This is called antibody-dependent cell-mediated cytotoxicity.

Monoclonal Antibodies

Monoclonal antibodies are immunoglobulin molecules that are synthesized from a single family or clone of B lymphocytes. Because cells from a specific clone of B lymphocytes have the same genetic composition, they produce the same type of antibody. Monoclonal antibodies can be produced in large quantity in laboratory cell cultures by a hybrid cell or hybridoma. A hybridoma is a hybrid cell created by fusing a B lymphocyte with a long-lived neoplastic cell. It secretes a single specific antibody, or monoclonal antibody. The importance of monoclonal antibodies is that they are homogeneous and capable of binding to a specific target and mediating its neutralization or destruction. For example, human monoclonal antibodies have been produced against the toxic portion of gram-negative bacterial endotoxin, which is the mediator of septic shock. The clinical use of monoclonal antibodies provides a specific immunotherapy for clients with gram-negative sepsis.

Primary and Secondary Immune Response

After exposure to an antigen, there is a delay or latent period in which little or no antibody can be measured in the serum (Fig. 23–9). It is during this latent period that the B cell recognizes antigen and differentiates into a plasma cell. By 4 to 10 days after the initial exposure, serum antibody levels rise with IgM appearing first and then IgG. This is the primary immune response, and usually, the peak levels of antibody rapidly decrease; however, memory cells are produced, which are able to recall this antigen. Memory cells recirculate for several years through body tissues and lymphoid organs, seeking reexposure to the specific antigen they are programmed to target.

On reexposure to the same antigen, the antibody is produced within 1 to 2 days, and the level is often 50 times greater than that of the primary response. The levels also remain elevated for a longer period of time

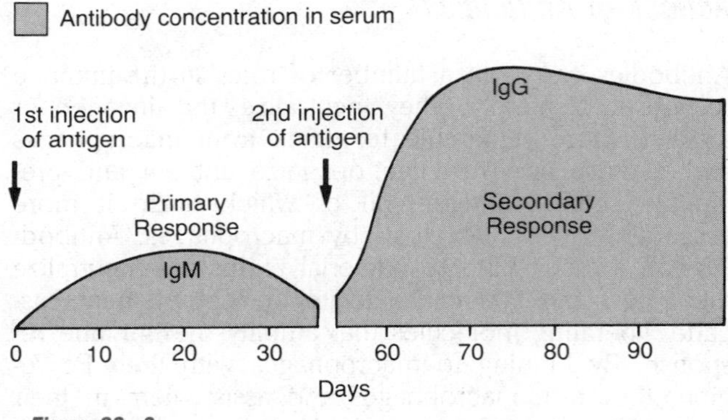

▲ *Figure 23-9*

Primary and secondary antibody response. The second exposure of an antigen to the host causes a more rapid, stronger, and longer-acting response than the first exposure, owing to the presence of memory cells. IgM is most often produced in the primary response, whereas IgG is more likely to be produced predominantly in the secondary response.

and fall off slowly over the course of months. Thus, the secondary immune response occurs faster, is more intense, and has a longer duration of peak antibody titer, all due to the presence of memory cells. With subsequent exposure, the antibody response can be boosted to even higher levels.

Complement

The complement system consists of a group of proteins that circulate in the blood in an inactive form, but when activated, the system provides a potent mechanism for initiating and amplifying inflammation. When triggered, a domino-like effect is set into motion, whereby each activated complement component will, in turn, act on the next in an exact sequence of precisely regulated steps, producing what is termed the complement cascade (Fig. 23-10). Activation of the complement cascade is referred to as complement fixation. The physiologic consequences of complement activation are (1) opsonization of microorganisms and immune complexes, which facilitates their phagocytosis; (2) chemotaxis and activation of phagocytes, including macrophages and neutrophils; and (3) lysis of target cells.

The complement cascade can be triggered by antigen-antibody complexes, which activate the classical pathway, or by the polysaccharide component of the microorganism's cell membrane, which activates the alternate pathway. It is thought that the classic pathway probably represents a recently evolved adaptive mechanism, while the alternate pathway provides nonspecific or innate immunity.

As the cascade progresses, various protein fragments are activated, some of which have specific effects. For example, protein fragments called anaphylatoxins, which have powerful vasoconstrictive effects as well as actions that increase vascular permeability, are produced. C5a is the most powerful anaphylatoxin. Another protein, C3b, opsonizes microorganisms and immune complexes, enhancing their uptake by phagocytes, which contain a receptor for C3b. The final phase of the complement cascade produces a protein called the membrane attack complex (MAC). The MAC inserts itself into the surface membrane of target cells, allowing water to enter the cell and causing the cell to swell and lyse.

T LYMPHOCYTES AND CELL-MEDIATED IMMUNITY

CMI includes any immune response in which antibodies play a subordinate role. CMI is vital in protecting the body against invasion by viruses, slow-growing bacteria, and fungal infections. It is responsible for immune surveillance, searching for abnormal clones of cells, which may be malignant. Such cells can be destroyed by so-called cytotoxic or killer cells, preventing them from becoming established tumors. However, malignantly transformed cells can often evade detection by the immune system, which is called immunologic escape.

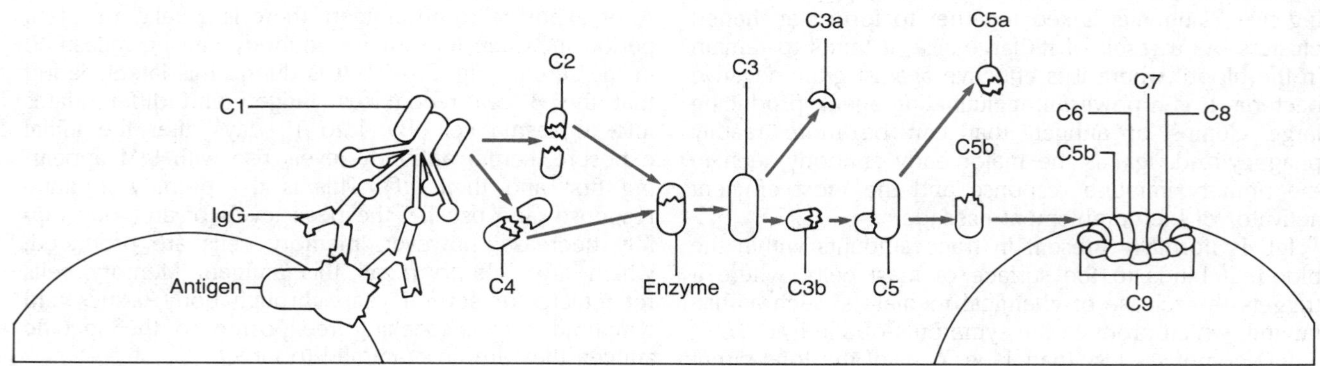

▲ *Figure 23-10*

The classic complement pathway becomes activated when the first complement molecule, C1, recognizes an antigen-antibody complex. Each of the remaining complement proteins, in turn, performs its specialized job, cleaving or binding the complement molecule next in line. The end product is the cylindric membrane attack complex. (Redrawn from Schindler, L. W. [1990]. *Understanding the immune system.* Washington, D.C.: National Institutes of Health.)

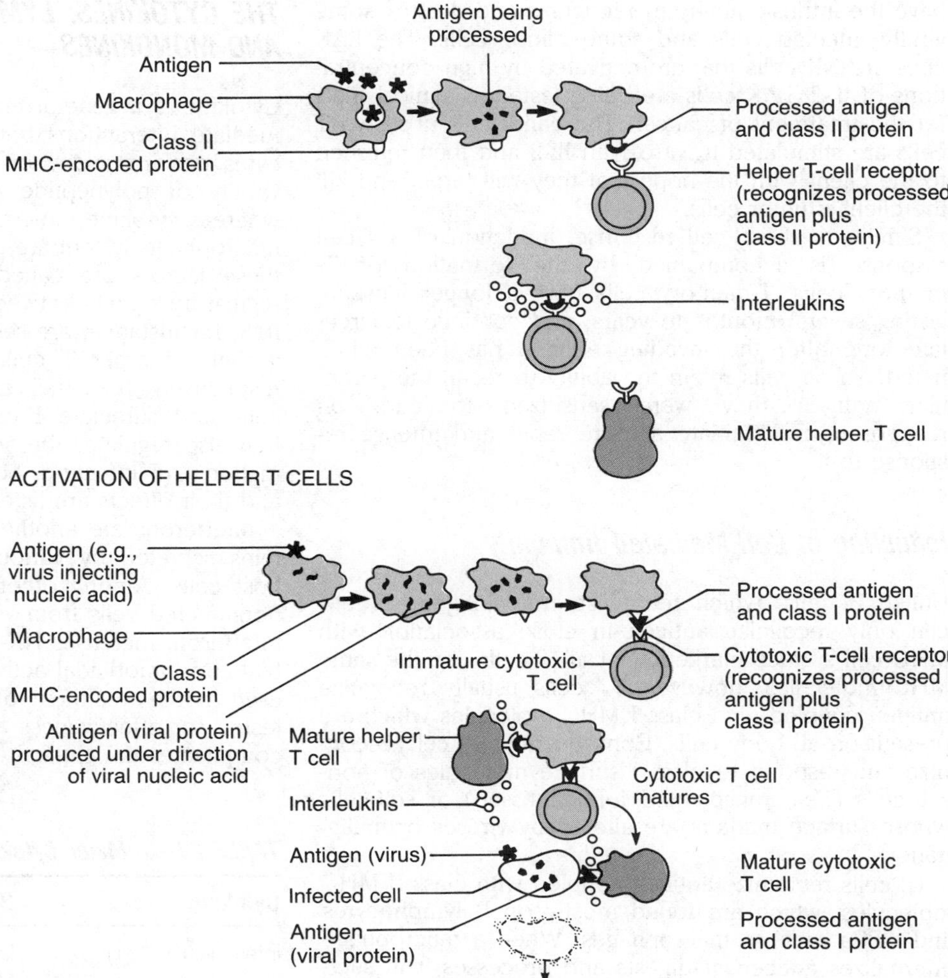

▲ ***Figure 23-11***

Activation of cytotoxic T cells. After the macrophage internalizes and processes antigen, it presents antigen fragments on its surface. Antigen combined with class II protein attracts the helper T cell; interleukins help the T cell mature. Antigen plus the class I protein binds to the cytotoxic T cell; aided by the helper T cell, the cytotoxic T cell matures. (Redrawn from Schindler, L. W. [1990]. *Understanding the immune system.* Washington, D.C.: National Institutes of Health.)

This component of the immune system also recognizes and reacts to foreign tissue cells. Consequently, it is the component of the immune response that is largely responsible for the rejection of transplanted tissue. Delayed hypersensitivity reactions, such as contact dermatitis or the tissue damage accompanying transplant rejection and some autoimmune disease, are also mediated by CMI. Many of the actions of T lymphocytes occur by the cells themselves or through the secretion of factors called lymphokines. Although humoral and cell-mediated responses are often discussed separately, it is important to realize that these two arms of the immune system work together and any failure in one can alter the effectiveness of the other.

The T lymphocytes play a predominant role in CMI. There are a variety of T cell subsets. Some are called regulatory T cells and include the T-helper (T_H) cells and the T-suppressor (T_S) cells. These cells are essential in controlling and modulating both CMI and the humoral immune response. For example, T_H cells assist B cells to mature and produce antibody by secreting interleukins originally called B-cell growth factor and B-cell differentiation factor. They also modulate the growth and function of a variety of T cells. The T_H cell is the primary target of the human immunodeficiency virus (HIV). The invasion and eventual destruction of the T_H cells by HIV is the basis for the immune deficiency and subsequent development of opportunistic infection and malignancy in the acquired immune deficiency syndrome (AIDS) patient.

The function of the T_S cell is to suppress or turn off both B- and T-cell responses. It may be involved in some forms of immunologic tolerance, prevention of autoimmune diseases, and regulation of the IgE response.

Other types of T cells include the cytotoxic T (T_C) cell, which can directly attack target cells and destroy them. The primary function of T_C cells is to recognize and eliminate virus-infected cells. When a virus invades a cell, its antigens are expressed on the invaded cell's surface. The T_C cells recognize these antigens in association with the host cell's class I MHC molecules. The T_C cell then releases various enzymes into the vicinity of the virus-infected target cell membrane, which, together with various lymphokines, causes cytotoxic damage and death of the target cell (Fig. 23-11).

Other cytotoxic cells include the NK cell and the lymphocyte-activated killer (LAK) cell. The NK cells have the intrinsic ability to recognize and destroy some virally infected cells and some tumor cells. The LAK cells are NK cells that are activated by high concentrations of IL-2. LAK cells are being tested in clinical trials for the treatment of cancer. The cancer client's own T cells are stimulated in vitro with IL-2 and then returned to the client with the hope that they will target and kill the client's tumor cells.

Similar to the B-cell response, induction of a T-cell response is accompanied by the formation of T-memory cells. T-memory cells have a longer lifespan, lasting several months to years, and continue to circulate long after the invading antigen has been eliminated. These cells retain the ability to recall the particular antigen they were sensitized to and, on reexposure, will initiate a more rapid and intense response to it.

Induction of Cell-Mediated Immunity

Unlike B cells, which recognize free antigen, T cells can only recognize antigen in close association with MHC cell surface markers. Not all T cells use the same MHC molecules, however. T_C cells usually recognize antigen coupled with class I MHC molecules which are present on all body cells. Consequently, T_C cells recognize and respond to class I surface molecules of non-self-cells (i.e., transplanted foreign tissue) or self-cells whose surface markers are altered by viruses or malignancy.

T_H cells recognize antigen coupled with class II MHC molecules, which are found mostly on B lymphocytes and APCs such as macrophages. When a macrophage internalizes antigen, it digests and processes it in such a way that the antigenic determinants of the invader are expressed on its own cell surface in close association with its MHC class II molecules. The T_H cell then binds to this complex, and the macrophage secretes IL-1, which stimulates the T_H cell to proliferate, mature, and carry out its functions.

Clonal Selection and Expansion

As a whole, the immune system can recognize and respond to millions of antigens; however, the lymphocytes capable of responding to one particular antigen are a very small part of the total number. Yet, they are capable of mounting a large-scale attack on the invading antigen because of what is termed clonal selection and expansion. When the small number of appropriately matched lymphocytes encounter their antigen, they are stimulated to proliferate and mature into effector cells. As a result, enough cells are available to effectively respond to the antigen. In other words, the antigen stimulates the appropriately matched clone or family of lymphocytes to proliferate and differentiate into effector cells or memory cells. Clonal selection and expansion occurs for antibody-producing B cells and also for T cells responsible for cell-mediated immunity.

THE CYTOKINES: LYMPHOKINES AND MONOKINES

Cytokine is a general term for cell-derived factors that mediate interactions between cells. T and B lymphocytes perform many of their functions by secreting a variety of polypeptide cytokines called lymphokines, whereas cytokine molecules secreted by the monocyte/macrophage system are called monokines. A number of these factors are called interleukins, which serve as regulatory signals between various leukocytes. IL-2 and IL-3, for instance, are secreted by T cells and stimulate growth of other T cells and colonies of stem cells, respectively. IL-4, IL-5, and IL-6 are also secreted by T cells and stimulate B-cell growth and differentiation. IL-6 also regulates the acute phase response of inflammation and infection. Some of the principal cytokines and their effects are listed in Table 23–3.

Interferons are another group of heterogeneous proteins secreted by various leukocytes and by infected host cells. Among other functions, interferons protect noninfected cells from viral invasion. One type, gamma interferon, increases NK-cell activity and the antimicrobial and tumoricidal activity of macrophages. It is being used in the treatment of cancer patients and is being tested for effectiveness against infection that too often complicates the clinical course of trauma victims.

TABLE 23–3. Major Cytokines

Cytokine	Principal Effects
Interleukin-1 (IL-1)	Lymphocyte activation Macrophage and neutrophil stimulation Stimulation of acute phase proteins Fever and sleep Pituitary hormone regulation
Interleukin-2 (IL-2)	Enhances T-cell growth and function
Interleukin-3 (IL-3)	Stimulates differentiation of hematopoietic cells (colony-stimulating factor)
Interleukin-4 (IL-4)	B-cell growth factor
Interleukin-5 (IL-5)	B-cell growth and differentiation
Interleukin-6 (IL-6)	B-cell growth and differentiation Stimulates the acute phase response
Tumor necrosis factor (TNF)	Activates macrophages, granulocytes, and cytotoxic cells Cachexia Mediates septic shock Increases leukocyte adhesion Enhances antigen presentation
Colony-stimulating factor (CSF)	Stimulates division and differentiation of bone marrow stem cells
Interferon	Antiviral factor

When activated by either lymphocytes, tumor cells, or bacterial cell products, such as endotoxin, monocytes and macrophages synthesize and secrete a number of regulatory mediators called monokines. Two of these monokines that have been studied in more detail include IL-1 and TNF.

IL-1 is responsible for a variety of effects that accompany infection. IL-1, originally called endogenous pyrogen, produces the febrile response by acting on the temperature-regulating center in the hypothalamus. It also produces the sleepiness that occurs with infection. IL-1 can activate T cells, B cells, and other tissue cells, such as osteoclasts, chrondrocytes, and fibroblasts.

Initially, TNF was found to produce necrosis of tumor cells and weight loss or cachexia in laboratory animals. Based on the latter observation, TNF has also been called cachectin. TNF is now known to have numerous actions, and many of these occur in synergy with other cytokines, especially IL-1. Some of the effects of TNF are of obvious benefit, but under certain conditions, TNF can produce harmful effects.

One of the protective effects of TNF is its tumoricidal action. It produces necrosis of tumors predominantly by choking off the blood supply feeding these growths. Clinical trials testing the effectiveness of TNF as a form of cancer treatment have had variable success. Recently, lymphocytes obtained from a patient's tumor have been given the genes for TNF and then infused back into the patient to test their ability to more effectively target and attack the patient's tumor. TNF also provides protection against various infecting organisms by activating eosinophils, neutrophils, and macrophages and cytotoxic cells such as NK and K cells.

TNF has a number of effects that can be harmful especially in a septic patient. In response to overwhelming bacterial invasion, TNF initiates a series of reactions, including endothelial cell, macrophage, and neutrophil activation. Various mediators are released, leading to platelet aggregation and fibrin deposition, which eventually cause intravascular coagulation and tissue damage. As a result of these effects, TNF is thought to be the major mediator responsible for the circulatory collapse and widespread tissue damage that characterize septic shock. Antibodies, which have been directed against TNF, are now being examined for their potential usefulness in combating the eventual organ failure and rate of high mortality that accompanies septic shock.

FACTORS AFFECTING IMMUNITY

Genetics

Immune function is greatly influenced by a number of factors. An individual's genetic make-up is just one factor that provides the foundation for one's immune system and, subsequently, one's susceptibility/resistance pattern to immunologically related disease. In the most extreme case, various immunodeficiency diseases can be congenitally acquired as a consequence of an embryologic insult or an enzyme defect, such as adenosine deaminase (ADA) deficiency. With ADA deficiency an individual has little, if any, immunocompetence and is highly susceptible to any pathogen. Currently, the administration of genetically engineered cells containing the genetic code for ADA is being tested as a potential therapeutic approach for ADA deficiency. Genetic predisposition also influences the expression of allergy and autoimmune disease, such as rheumatoid arthritis and myasthenia gravis. Genetic differences in one's immune surveillance may also account for the familial tendency associated with the development of certain forms of cancer.

Age

The very young and the elderly are more susceptible to infection. As a result of immaturity, components of both the innate, humoral, and cell-mediated immune responses are underdeveloped in the newborn. Maternal transfer of IgG to the fetus equips the newborn with IgG for the first few months of life. By this time, the infant begins to synthesize his or her own immunoglobulins, although at a very minimal level. Initially, the infant's immunoglobulin response is primarily IgM. The immunity of the breastfed infant also is bolstered by receiving secretory IgA and immune cells from breast milk. Immunization of an infant typically does not begin until approximately 3 months of age, because prior to this time, the infant is incapable of producing antibody and memory cells in response to the antigen in the vaccination. By about 1 year of age, the infant produces 60 per cent of the adult level of IgG, 75 per cent of the adult level of IgM, and 20 per cent of the adult level of IgA.

In the elderly, the thymus has atrophied and there is a decrease in thymic hormones. T-lymphocyte activity is depressed, especially delayed hypersensitivity reactions. However, there is an increase in activity of T_S cells, which may mediate suppression of various components of the immune system. The titers of natural and induced antibodies are lower in the elderly because of the depression of B-lymphocyte function. Furthermore, the elderly exhibit an increase in the frequency of autoantibodies directed against cell nuclei and thyroid cells and also an increase in rheumatoid factor. These changes may account for the increased frequency of autoimmune disease in the aged population. Overall, these changes in immune function undoubtedly increase the susceptibility of the elderly to infection and may also account for the increase in malignancies observed with advanced age.

The decline in immune function with age may be related to the presence of chronic illness in the elderly. Certain diseases, such as diabetes mellitus, chronic renal failure, and liver disease are characterized by impaired immune function. The elderly also have impaired physical barriers to infectious agents, such as breakdown of skin and mucous membranes and decreased muscle mass. The immune system interacts with the endocrine system and changes in hormone levels that occur with aging may further contribute to impaired immunity. Finally, poor nutrition, which is common in this age group, may also impair immune function.

Nutrition

Adequate nutrition is vital to promote optimum immune function. Protein deficiency impairs humoral and cell-mediated immune responses because proteins are required for the proliferation of leukocytes, the synthesis of immunoglobulins, and the proteins of the complement cascade. On the other hand, diets high in calories, especially fats, appear to be involved in the development of autoimmunity.

Trace elements, such as copper and zinc, and vitamins are important in maintaining a healthy immune system. For example, zinc deficiency leads to thymus involution and a decrease in T-cell number and function. Low levels of zinc can also depress NK-cell activity. Vitamin A deficiency increases an individual's susceptibility to infection because it is required for a normal humoral immune response.

Despite these factors, the immune system is very robust. It requires extreme changes in nutrition or frank malnutrition before it is affected. A normal diet is usually adequate in proteins, vitamins, and minerals, but significant nutritional deficiencies can occur in the critically ill patient with impaired gastrointestinal function, renal failure, and in catabolic states, such as burns and sepsis, as well as in chronic illness marked by cachexia as seen with cancer.

Medications

A large number of medications can depress the immune system. Some medications may be taken specifically for their anti-inflammatory or immunosuppressive properties, whereas others taken for unrelated indications have side effects that suppress immunity. Bone marrow depression refers to the decreased ability of the bone marrow to produce peripheral blood cells from the precursor stem cells. Many drugs also produce bone marrow depression as a side effect. For example, antibiotics, such as the cephalosporins and penicillin, and antipsychotic drugs, such as the phenothiazines, can depress the bone marrow. Glucocorticoids are commonly given for a large number of conditions and produce many anti-inflammatory and immunosuppressive effects, including a decrease in phagocytic cell activity and the production of immunoregulatory cytokines. The administration of high doses of glucocorticoids is associated with the increased susceptibility to infection and delayed wound healing.

Stress

For decades, stress has been linked to immunosuppression. Acute physical stressors, such as trauma and burns, are accompanied by depressed immune cell function, and if the affected individual survives the initial insult, he or she will be at risk for infection. Emotional stress, such as grieving the loss of a loved one, is also marked by immunosuppression. The mechanisms connecting stress and immunity have only more recently been discovered. Stress, both emotional and physical, triggers activation of the autonomic nervous system and the endocrine system. Both of these systems can, in turn, affect the immune response. For example, a number of organs and tissues of the immune system, such as the thymus gland, bone marrow, spleen, and lymph nodes, are directly innervated by the autonomic nervous system. Typically, stress-triggered norepinephrine secretion produces immunosuppression. Some nerve cells that are activated by stress can even produce and secrete various lymphokines of the immune system and, hence, can regulate immune activity.

A number of so-called stress hormones secreted by glands of the endocrine system also modulate immune activity. The best known stress hormone is cortisol, secreted by the adrenal cortex, which has multiple anti-inflammatory and immunosuppressive effects. However, other hormones released during stress, such as pituitary endorphins, growth hormone, prolactin, thyroid hormones, and reproductive hormones, also influence immune cell function. Furthermore, the link between the immune and endocrine systems appears to be a "two-way street" because secretory products from the immune system, such as interleukin-1, can also affect endocrine gland secretion. The relationship between the immune, endocrine, and nervous systems and the client's psychological make-up has evolved into the science of psycho-neuro-immuno-endocrinology.

▼ ASSESSMENT OF THE IMMUNE SYSTEM

Allergies always follow sensitization to an allergen, so one of the primary diagnostic tools is a complete history to determine possible allergies, including food, medication, insect, or pollen sensitivities. The history is followed by a complete physical examination.

HISTORY

The health history focuses on the chief complaint and present allergies, the past medical history for allergies, family history, psychosocial history including lifestyle and stress management, and review of systems (ROS). The client ideally is the source for the history, although significant others such as parents or spouse or other family members may be valuable sources of information.

Chief Complaint

The client may report allergy symptoms such as rhinitis, sneezing, nasal stuffiness, postnasal drip, sore throat, voice changes, hoarseness, wheezing, persistent cough, dyspnea, malaise, fatigue, rashes, pruritus, vomiting, diarrhea, intestinal colic, excessive tearing, or altered hearing acuity. Symptoms vary depending on the nature of the allergen and the client's individual sensitivity pattern. The nurse completes a symptom analysis (see Chap. 11) for each reported symptom to assist in the identification of the allergen. The major types of allergens include inhalants (e.g., pollens, molds, spores, dust, mites, and animal dander); contact agents (e.g., dyes in clothing, fibers, cosmetics, metals in jewelry, plant oils and secretions, topical drugs, and numerous chemicals); ingested agents (e.g., foods, food additives, drugs); and injectable agents (e.g., drugs, vaccines, and insect venom).

Past Medical History

The nurse asks the client about past episodes of allergic reactions. The client is asked to relate whether or not there is a seasonal pattern associated with these episodes, the symptoms that developed, and the treatment for these allergies and their effectiveness. Specifically, inquire about drug allergies and food allergies or sensitivities. Has the client ever suffered an anaphylactic reaction? Or has the client ever been hospitalized for an allergic reaction? Has the client had previous series of treatment for desensitization with allergy shots? If so, were the treatments effective?

Family History

The client is asked to identify allergies and sensitivities in family members, particularly atopic reactions. The nurse attempts to determine the specific problem, the accompanying symptoms, and course of treatment.

Psychosocial History and Lifestyle

Information about the client's physical environment and psychosocial patterns is important in obtaining a complete allergy history. The nurse asks about both the home and work (or school) environments. Are there pets in the home? Are houseplants or fresh-cut flowers part of the home? What type of vegetation is in the immediate vicinity of the home or workplace? Ask the client to describe the type of heating and cooling systems both in the home and at work. If food-related allergies are suspected, the client is asked to keep a food diary, including descriptions of any reactions to ingested foods. The nurse encourages the client to discuss his or her level of stress and whether there is a relationship to the appearance of allergic symptoms. Also ask how the client reacts to outbreaks of allergic symptoms. For example, some clients break out in hives when they are under psychological or emotional stress. Their appearance triggers more emotional stress, which, in turn, leads to further outbreaks of hives. A cycle develops that is difficult to interrupt.

Review of Systems

Prior to the physical examination, the nurse asks the client about the following problems.

- General: Fatigue, malaise, unusual reactions to insect bites or medications, including over-the-counter drugs.
- Integumentary: Rashes, urticaria, itching, scratching, dryness, scaling.
- Eyes: Dark circles around the eyes, excessive tearing, rubbing or blinking, conjunctivitis, styes.
- Ears: Altered hearing acuity, feeling of fullness in the ears, ruptured tympanic membranes.
- Nose: Sneezing, sniffling, rhinitis, nasal polyps, nasal voice quality, nose twitching or rubbing, nasal stuffiness, recurrent epistaxis, postnasal drip.
- Throat: Swollen lips or tongue, frequent clearing of the throat, sore throat, itching of the throat or neck, hoarseness.
- Respiratory: Wheezing, dyspnea, frequent cough, ineffective cough.
- Gastrointestinal: Diarrhea, vomiting, cramping, food intolerances.

PHYSICAL EXAMINATION

The client with allergies should receive a head-to-toe physical examination. The nurse focuses on the area that is target for the allergen for in-depth assessment.

▼ Assessment of the Lymphatic System

Disorders of the lymphatic system may result from inflammation (lymphangitis), an increased amount of lymph (lymphedema), or enlargement of the lymph nodes (lymphadenopathy). A complete history and physical examination help determine the cause of the problem and direct the eventual treatment. Included in the assessment of the lymphatic system are the peripheral lymph nodes, liver, and spleen. Assessment of the liver and spleen is discussed in Chapter 57.

HISTORY

The history for the lymphatic system focuses on the client's chief complaint, history of present illness, past medical history, psychosocial history and lifestyle, and ROS.

Chief Complaint

The client may report localized swelling over an underlying lymph node (or nodes) or generalized swelling and edema of an extremity. Other symptoms include pruritus, increased redness or streaks (indicating cellulitis), pain, tenderness, fever, malaise, anorexia, headache, and irritability. The nurse conducts a symptom analysis (see Chap. 11) to determine the location, onset, and duration of the problem, and accompanying symptoms such as drainage and increased warmth over the area.

History of Present Illness

The nurse asks the client about infections, both systemic and local. These infections may be associated with breaks in the skin, ingrown nails, fungal infections, or puncture wounds. Lymphedema can result from congenital deformity of the lymph vessels or as a result of altered structure and function. Therefore, the nurse asks the client about surgery or trauma to extremities, radiation therapy, and presence of a malignancy or neoplasm, which may have interrupted lymphatic flow and drainage from an area. Ask whether elevation relieves swelling of an affected extremity and whether or not a dependent position leads to increased swelling.

Past Medical History

Inquire about previous problems with swelling, injury, or trauma to extremities including surgery. Has the client had a systemic infection, immunologic reaction, or neoplastic disorder? If so, ask the client to describe the specific disorder and its treatment. For example, a client who has had axillary node dissection accompanying a mastectomy often has upper extremity edema of the ipsilateral side. The nurse also asks about disorders affecting the vascular system such as congestive heart failure, renal disease, and peripheral vascular problems because these disorders are often accompanied by edema of the extremities. Specifically ask about allergies to iodine or seafoods such as shellfish. Diagnostic studies of the lymphatic system use an iodine-based contrast medium.

Psychosocial History and Lifestyle

The nurse inquires about the effect the problem has had on the client's emotional status and coping abilities. Disorders involving the lymphatic system may result in a variety of psychological and emotional reactions ranging from disregard to obvious distress. The client may be disturbed by an altered body image, particularly if the deformity is evident. Edema can interfere with function and coordination of extremities, resulting in clumsiness or awkward movements and difficulty with performing activities of daily living (ADL). If symptoms are related to a neoplastic disorder, the client may express fear or anxiety, especially if it is a recurrent problem. The nurse remains sensitive to the client's expressed and unexpressed emotions during the history and physical examination.

Review of Systems

The client is asked to describe problems in the following areas:

- General: Malaise, fatigue, fever, lassitude, chills, sweating, pruritus.
- Head and neck: Localized swelling, pain or tenderness; swollen nodes; headache; irritability.
- Cardiovascular: Hypertension; congestive heart failure; peripheral vascular disorders such as varicose veins; edema of the hands, feet, or legs.
- Gastrointestinal: Anorexia; hepatomegaly, splenomegaly.
- Renal: Kidney disease including renal failure.
- Immunologic: Recent infections such as influenza, measles, mononucleosis, viral infections; neoplasms including lymphoma; injury or trauma resulting in break in the skin barrier; date of last tetanus toxoid injection.

PHYSICAL EXAMINATION

The portions of the lymphatic system accessible to physical examination are the superficial lymph nodes, liver, and spleen. Examination of the liver and spleen is discussed in Chapter 57. The techniques used to examine superficial lymph nodes are inspection and palpation. The nurse uses a methodical approach when examining lymph nodes in order not to overlook single nodes or chains of nodes. The nodes of the head and neck, supraclavicular areas, axillae, and epitrochlear areas are most easily palpated while the client is sitting. Inguinal and popliteal nodes are more accessible when the client is lying.

Inspection

The nurse inspects the surface overlying nodes for masses or scars, looking for bilateral symmetry. If masses are seen, the nurse palpates the area and compares it with the contralateral side.

Palpation

Palpation is used to assess lymph nodes for size, shape, consistency, discreteness, mobility, and tenderness. The nurse uses the finger pads of the middle three fingers in a gentle, circular motion to palpate over the nodes. The finger tips stay in contact with the skin and slide the skin's surface over the underlying nodes. Excessive pressure is avoided because it obliterates small, palpable nodes. Lymph nodes are not normally palpable, yet it is common to find small (1 cm or less diameter), round, soft, single, mobile, nontender nodes particularly in the cervical and inguinal areas. Nodes that are large (greater than 1 cm diameter), hard, feel matted together, fixed to underlying structures, or tender are abnormal findings, and their characteristics are described thoroughly.

Specific guidelines for palpating the *head and neck lymph nodes* are given in Table 23–4. The location of these nodes is shown in Figure 12–3. The nurse uses a methodical approach when examining head and neck nodes in order to be thorough. These nodes normally

TABLE 23-4. Sequence and Palpation Technique for Lymph Nodes in the Head and Neck

Nodes	Location	Palpation Technique
Occipital	Posterior at base of skull and lateral to cervical spine	Flex client's neck forward slightly to relax trapezius. Palpate right and left node centers simultaneously
Posterior auricular (mastoid)	Behind auricle of ear, over outer surface of mastoid process	Palpate over both mastoid processes simultaneously
Posterior cervical chain	Along anterior edge of trapezius, in the posterior triangle	Flex client's neck to relax trapezius muscles. Palpate slowly against the trapezius muscles, progressing from the mastoid processes toward the clavicles
Supraclavicular (scalene)	Above the clavicle, in the angle formed by the clavicle and the sternocleidomastoid	Flex client's neck sharply with one hand and encourage the client to relax the shoulders so that clavicles drop. Palpate one side at a time with fingers over client's right clavicle lateral to sternocleidomastoid. Ask the client to inhale deeply while pressing in and behind clavicle. Repeat using right hand to palpate client's left node centers.
Superficial (anterior) cervical chain	Along and over (anterior to) the sternocleidomastoid, in the anterior triangle	Flex client's neck forward to relax sternocleidomastoid. Palpate one side at a time. Palpate slowly against the sternocleidomastoid, progressing from the clavicle toward the jaw
Deep cervical chain	Under the sternocleidomastoid	Flex client's neck laterally toward the side being examined to relax muscles and soft tissue. Palpate one side at a time. Hook thumb (on one side) and fingers (on the other side) around the sternocleidomastoid muscle to feel deep to the muscle. Progress from the jaw toward the sternum
	Along anterior edge of sternocleidomastoid, in the anterior triangle	With client's neck still flexed laterally, palpate along anterior edge of sternocleidomastoid from the sternum to the jaw angle. Repeat on opposite side of neck
Tonsillar	Near angle of jaw at the jaw margin	Flex client's neck slightly in midline. Palpate behind both jaw angles simultaneously
Submandibular (submaxillary)	Along medial border of mandible, between the angle of the jaw and the chin	Palpate along medial borders of mandible from angle of jaw toward the chin. Palpate right and left node centers simultaneously
Submental	At the midline, posterior to the tip of the mandibles under the chin	Palpate with one hand under client's chin just behind tip of mandible. Steady client's head with free hand if necessary
Anterior auricular	In front of tragus of ear	Palpate right and left sides simultaneously, anterior to tragus and posterior to the temporomandibular joint

are nonpalpable. However, small, mobile, nontender nodes are common because they enlarge with repeated local and systemic infections. The lymph nodes accessible to examination in the arms are the *epitrochlear chains*. These nodes are located in the groove between the biceps and triceps muscles, proximal to the medial epicondyle of the humerus. They are usually nonpalpable. *Axillary nodes* are usually examined during assessment of the anterior thorax, as part of the breast examination. See Chapter 78 for discussion of axillary lymph node palpation. The superior (horizontal) and inferior (vertical) chains of the *inguinal lymph nodes* are nonpalpable although small, soft, mobile, nontender nodes are common. The inguinal area is normally free of bulges or masses. The lymph nodes examined in the lower extremities are the *popliteal nodes*. The popliteal nodes are located in the popliteal fossae on the lateral aspects and are normally nonpalpable.

If an extremity appears edematous, the nurse measures its circumference and compares it to the contralateral extremity. Differences of less than 1 cm (about $\frac{1}{2}$ in) are considered within normal limits.

DIAGNOSTIC TESTS

HIV Testing

ENZYME-LINKED IMMUNOSORBENT ASSAY (ELISA)

This test is the first one performed when HIV infection is suspected. Although this is a relatively inexpensive, quick, and easy test, there tends to be a high rate of false-positive results; in other words, the ELISA is a highly sensitive test but not necessarily very specific for HIV.

WESTERN BLOT

The Western Blot is a more specific test for the presence of the HIV antibody. It is also more expensive and labor intensive compared with the ELISA.

The usual course of events when a client requests testing for HIV includes the following steps: (1) Pretest counseling is provided, and the informed consent is signed; (2) Serum is drawn and tested by ELISA for the presence of the HIV antibody, and if this test is negative, the tests stop here; (3) If the test is positive twice by ELISA, then a Western Blot is performed, and if this is also positive, the client is considered HIV positive and, therefore, infected with HIV; (4) If the Western Blot is negative, a confirmatory test is often run, and if this is still negative, the client is considered HIV negative. Most laboratories will confirm positive results by running the Western Blot a second time.

Allergic Skin Testing

In addition to blood tests, skin testing confirms sensitivity to a specific allergen. These tests involve placing a known antigen on or directly below the skin (intradermal) to check for the presence of antibodies. The antigen can be applied in one of three methods: (1) scratch test, (2) patch test, or (3) intradermal test. In the first test (also known as a tine or prick test), the allergen is applied to a superficial scratch that cuts the outer layer of skin. For a patch test, the antigen is applied directly to the skin, and then covered with a gauze dressing. Intradermal testing involves injecting a small amount of the antigen into the intradermal layer of the skin. Intradermal testing is the most accurate method, but carries a higher risk of severe allergic reactions.

Often, nurses administer skin tests and interpret test results. To interpret results, observe for the following reactions. An immediate reaction (i.e., appearing within 10 to 20 minutes after the injection) marked by erythema and wheal formation denotes a positive reaction. Positive reactions indicate an antibody response to previous exposure to this antigen, and suggest the client is allergic to the particular substance causing the reaction (see Chap. 24, Fig. 24-1). Negative reactions may be inconclusive, indicating the need for further assessment. Negative results may indicate that (1) antibodies have not formed to this antigen, (2) the antigen was deposited too deeply into the skin (e.g., subcutaneously), or (3) the client is immunosuppressed as a result of disease or therapies (e.g., chemotherapy, steroids, and radiation therapy).

Problems arising from skin testing range from minor itching to anaphylaxis. Itching and discomfort at the injection site, for example, are common and can be relieved by the application of cool compresses and topical steroids. Ulceration of the injection site is best treated by keeping the area clean and dry. Anaphylactic shock is a rare but potentially lethal complication of skin testing. A client with a history of an anaphylactic reaction to a substance should never be skin tested for an allergy to that substance. This is especially true of allergens such as penicillin, which can produce lethal anaphylaxis in susceptible clients. Anaphylaxis is treated with emergency oxygen administration, epinephrine subcutaneously, intravenous aminophylline, and intravenous antihistamines, as necessary.

Food Allergy Testing

Food allergies can be tested by skin testing or by either food challenges or an elimination diet. In the challenge test, suspected foods are given to the client in progressively larger doses until a reaction is evoked. Symptoms of a reaction range from the typical erythema, itching, and rash to vomiting or diarrhea. Symptoms such as fatigue, depression, or restlessness are not conclusive of an allergy.

In the elimination diet, foods are eliminated from the diet one by one until the symptoms are relieved. This may indicate allergies to food additives or foods themselves.

Bone Marrow Assessment

Chapter 45 discusses bone marrow aspiration.

Lymphatic Assessment

Diagnostic assessment of the lymphatic system can be found in Chapters 45, 46, 57, and 78.

Lymphangiogram

A lymphangiogram is a test that allows visualization of the lymphatic system to assess the presence of malignancy (lymphoma) or metastatic disease (testicular cancer) in tumors involving the lymphatic system or with typical lymphatic spread. The test involves the injection of an oil-based dye into the lymphatic system. The tops of the feet are first deadened using local anesthesia, and a blue dye is injected into the top of the feet that is picked up by the lymphatics. A cut down is done with a catheter inserted into the lymphatic channel and an oil-based dye injected. The feet are elevated to aid in distribution of the dye throughout the lymphatic system. X-ray studies are taken to visualize the lymphatic system.

The test takes several hours on the first day, and follow-up x-ray studies are performed the next day. The dye itself is excreted very slowly, taking months to more than a year for it to be completely excreted. The dye is excreted through both the urine and respiratory system.

Possible adverse reactions associated with the test include fever, allergic reaction to the dye, infection at the incision site, and possible pulmonary oil embolism. The client should monitor the site of the incision closely for infection. The client should be told that the urine will have a bluish discoloration for a while after the test and the tops of the feet may remain blue for months. The client also should be told to report any fever, signs of redness or swelling at the incision, or respiratory distress to the physician.

Summary

The immune system is an extremely complex system. Understanding the structure, function, and assessment of the immune system helps the nurse provide more consistent and appropriate care for the client with inflammatory, infectious, or immune disorders.

Bibliography

1. Cohen, J. (1988). The self, the world, and autoimmunity. *Scientific American, 258,* 52-60.
2. Galant, S. P. (1980). Development of host resistance in the fetus and newborn. *Perinatology-Neonatology 4,* 16-19.
3. Golde, D. W. (1991). The stem cell. *Scientific American, 261,* 86-93.
4. Grady, C. (1988). Host defense mechanisms: An overview. *Seminars in Oncology Nursing, 4,* 86-94.
5. Griffen, J. (1986). Nursing care of the immunosuppressed patient in an intensive care unit. *Heart and Lung, 15,* 179-188.
6. Gurevich, I. (1985). The competent internal immune system. *Nursing Clinics North America, 20,* 151-161.
7. Hokyt, N. J. (1989). Host defense mechanisms and compromises in the trauma patient. *Critical Care Clinics of North America, 1,* 753-765.
8. Klein, J. (1990). *Immunology.* Boston: Blackwell Scientific.
9. Klein, D. M., & Witek-Janusek, L. (1992). Advances in immunotherapy for sepsis. *Dimensions in Critical Care Nursing, 11,* 75-89.
10. McConnell, E. (1986). Leukocyte counts: What the counts tell you. *Nursing '86,* 16: 42-43.
11. McDevitt, H. O. (1985). The HLA system and its relation to disease. *Hospital Practice, 20,* 57-72.
12. Nossal, G. J. V. (1987). Current concepts—immunology: The basic components of the immune system. *New England Journal of Medicine, 316,* 1320-1325.
13. Old, L. J. (1988). Tumor necrosis factor. *Scientific American, 258,* 59-76.
14. Reckling, J. (1987). Understanding immune system dysfunction. *Nursing '87, 87,* 34-42.
15. Rennie, J. (1990). The body against itself. *Scientific American, 260,* 106-115.
16. Roit, I. M., Brostoff, J., & Male, D. K. (1989). *Immunology.* Philadelphia: Lippincott.
17. Rosenthal, C. H. (1989). Immunosuppression in pediatric critical care patients. *Critical Care Nursing Clinics of North America, 1,* 775-785.
18. Schwab, R. (1989). Host defense mechanisms and aging. *Seminars in Oncology, 16,* 20-27.
19. Sheehan, C. (1990). *Clinical Immunology.* Philadelphia: Lippincott.
20. Stites, D. P., Stobo, J. D., & Wells, J. V. (Eds.) (1987). *Basic and Clinical Immunology,* Norwalk: Appleton & Lange.
21. Tafuro, B. (1985). The extremes of age: The newborn and the elderly at increased risk for development of infection. *Nursing Clinics of North America, 20,* 181-190.
22. Tribett, D. (1989). Immune system function. Implications for critical care nursing practice. *Critical Care Nursing Clinics of America, 1,* 725-740.
23. Virella, G., Goust, J. M., & Fudenberg, H. H. (Eds.) (1990). *Medical Immunology.* New York: Marcel Dekker.
24. Weigle, W. (1989). Effects of aging on the immune system. *Hospital Practice, 24,* 112-119.
25. Young, J. D. & Cohn, Z. A. (1988). How killer cells kill. *Scientific American, 258,* 38-44.

Chapter 24

Nursing Care of Clients with Altered Immune Systems

The immune system controls the body's response to invading foreign substances. A functioning immune system can help protect the body from a wide variety of pathogens. On the other hand, an immune system that is malfunctioning predisposes the client to the development of a wide variety of disorders ranging from severe infection to autoimmune disease. Chapter 23 describes the normally functioning immune system; this chapter looks at alterations in the immune system and how these changes affect the client.

HUMAN IMMUNODEFICIENCY VIRUS

Definition

In 1981, astute observation by several physicians in San Francisco and New York witnessed the onset of a new spectrum of diseases known as acquired immunodeficiency syndrome (AIDS). Homosexual men in the United States presented with opportunistic infections, most commonly *Pneumocystis carinii* pneumonia, and rare malignancies, such as Kaposi's sarcoma. Because of the prevalence of AIDS in the homosexual community, it was suspected that the causative agent was sexually transmitted, similar to that of hepatitis B. By 1982, AIDS was identified in other populations, including injection drug users, recipients of blood or blood products, heterosexual partners of clients with AIDS, and children. The causative agent, human immunodeficiency virus (HIV), was isolated from clients with AIDS in 1983. Shortly after this discovery, screening tests for the detection of HIV antibody were developed. Since March 1985, all blood products have been routinely screened for the presence of HIV antibody. Anonymous testing sites have been established to facilitate voluntary screening of those who participate in high-risk behaviors.

The development of AIDS represents an advanced stage of disease along a continuum that ranges from asymptomatic HIV infection to the development of this most serious and debilitating condition. Historically, the diagnosis of AIDS was made once the development of one or more clinical diseases took place that indicated an underlying cellular immunodeficiency (Box 24-1). A revised classification system has been proposed, which emphasizes the importance of the CD4+ lymphocyte count, the laboratory parameter that defines those clients with AIDS. The client must either test positive for HIV or have no other reason for the immunodeficiency. AIDS strikes during the prime of life; it affects most clients between the ages of 20 and 49 years.

Since the onset of the epidemic in the early 1980s, there has been significant confusion about several important issues, including nomenclature and disease progression. Much of the confusion has stemmed from the controversial nature of the populations initially infected as well as the changing face of scientific knowledge and medical treatment.

The nomenclature of HIV infection/HIV disease has taken on several forms over the past decade. In 1982, the Centers for Disease Control (CDC) developed the case definition for AIDS and AIDS-related complex (ARC). This definition has been revised several times (see Box 24-2) until it reached the proposed form in 1991 (Box 24-3). The usefulness of the earlier definitions was limited to epidemiology and surveillance rather than to the clinical area. The 1991 definition was proposed in order to simplify the process of reporting and classifying cases of AIDS and to create some consistency with which to record the number of clients with severe HIV-related immunosuppression.

Box 24-1. Case Definition for AIDS

For national reporting, a case of AIDS is defined as an illness characterized by one or more of the following "indicator" diseases:

One or more of the following diseases *must be present* in order for a client to have AIDS. Numbers 1 through 12 require that the client have no other cause of immunodeficiency; numbers 13 through 22 indicate a diagnosis of AIDS regardless of the presence of other causes of immunodeficiency provided that there is laboratory evidence for HIV infection.

1. Candidiasis of the esophagus, trachea, bronchi, or lungs.
2. Cryptococcosis, extrapulmonary.
3. Cryptosporidiosis with diarrhea persisting more than 1 month.
4. Cytomegalovirus disease of an organ other than liver, spleen, or lymph nodes in a client more than 1 month of age.
5. Herpes simplex virus infection causing a mucocutaneous ulcer that persists longer than 1 month; or bronchitis, pneumonitis, or esophagitis for any duration affecting a client more than 1 month of age.
6. Kaposi's sarcoma affecting a client less than 60 years of age.
7. Lymphoma of the brain (primary) affecting a client less than 60 years of age.
8. Lymphoid interstitial pneumonia and/or pulmonary lymphoid hyperplasia (LIP/PLH complex) affecting a child less than 13 years of age.
9. *Mycobacterium avium* complex or *M. kansasii* disease, disseminated (at a site other than or in addition to lungs, skin, or cervical or hilar lymph nodes).
10. *Pneumocystis carinii* pneumonia.
11. Progressive multifocal leukoencephalopathy.
12. Toxoplasmosis of the brain affecting a client more than 1 month of age.
13. Bacterial infections, multiple or recurrent (any combination of at least two within a 2-year period), of the following types affecting a child less than 13 years of age: septicemia, pneumonia, meningitis, bone or joint infection, or abscess of an internal organ or body cavity (excluding otitis media or superficial skin or mucosal abscesses) caused by *Haemophilus, Streptococcus* (including pneumococcus), or other pyogenic bacteria.
14. Coccidioidomycosis, disseminated (at a site other than or in addition to lungs or cervical or hilar lymph nodes).
15. HIV encephalopathy (also called HIV dementia, AIDS dementia, or subacute encephalitis due to HIV).
16. Histoplasmosis, disseminated (at a site other than or in addition to lungs or cervical or hilar lymph nodes).
17. Isosporiasis with diarrhea persisting more than 1 month.
18. Lymphoma of the brain (primary) at any age.
19. Other non-Hodgkin's lymphoma of B-cell or unknown immunologic phenotype and the following histologic types: noncleaved lymphoma, immunoblastic sarcoma.
20. Disease caused by *M. tuberculosis,* extrapulmonary (involving at least one site outside the lungs, regardless of whether there is concurrent pulmonary involvement.
21. *Salmonella* (nontyphoid) septicemia, recurrent.
22. HIV wasting syndrome: findings of profound involuntary weight loss more than 10 per cent of baseline body weight *plus* either chronic diarrhea (at least two loose stools per day for more than 30 days) or chronic weakness and documented fever (for more than 30 days intermittent or constant) in the absence of a concurrent illness or condition other than HIV infection that could explain the findings.

Adapted from the Centers for Disease Control (1987). Revision of the CDC surveillance case definition for acquired immunodeficiency syndrome. *Morbidity and Mortality Weekly Report, 31*(Suppl. 1), 3-15.

Box 24–2. 1993 Revised HIV Classification System for Adolescents and Adults

The revised CDC classification system for HIV-infected adolescents and adults emphasizes the importance of CD4+ lymphocyte testing in the clinical management of HIV-infected clients. The classification system is divided into laboratory and clinical categories as follows.

Laboratory Categories

Category 1: Greater than or equal to 500 CD4+ cells
Category 2: 200 to 499 CD4+ cells
Category 3: Less than 200 CD4+ cells

Clinical Categories

Category A: One or more of the following conditions occurring in an adolescent or adult with documented HIV infection. Conditions listed in categories B and C must not have occurred.

- Asymptomatic HIV infection
- Persistent generalized lymphadenopathy (PGL)
- Acute (primary) HIV infection with accompanying illness or history of acute HIV infection

Category B: Symptomatic conditions occurring in an HIV-infected adolescent or adult that are not included among conditions listed in clinical category C and that meet at least one of the following criteria:

1. The conditions are attributed to HIV infection and/or are indicative of a defect in cell-mediated immunity.
2. The conditions are considered by physicians to have a clinical course or management that is complicated by HIV infection.

Examples of conditions in clinical category B include but are not limited to

- Bacterial endocarditis, meningitis, pneumonia, or sepsis
- Candidiasis, vulvovaginal; persistent for more than 1 month, or poorly responsive to therapy
- Candidiasis, oropharyngeal (thrush)
- Cervical dysplasia, severe; or carcinoma
- Constitutional symptoms, such as fever (>38.5° C) or diarrhea lasting more than 1 month
- Hairy leukoplakia, oral
- Herpes zoster (shingles), involving at least two distinct episodes or more than one dermatome
- Idiopathic thrombocytopenic purpura
- Listeriosis
- *Mycobacterium tuberculosis* infection, pulmonary
- Nocardiosis
- Pelvic inflammatory disease
- Peripheral neuropathy

Category C: Any condition listed in the 1987 surveillance case definition for AIDS and affecting an adolescent or an adult.

- The conditions in clinical category C are strongly associated with severe immunodeficiency, occur frequently in HIV-infected clients, and cause serious morbidity or mortality.
- According to the proposed classification system, HIV-infected clients would be classified on the basis of both.

1. The lowest accurate (not necessarily the most recent) CD4+ lymphocyte determination; and
2. The most severe clinical condition diagnosed regardless of the client's current clinical condition.

Adapted from the U.S. Department of Health and Human Services, Public Health Service, CDC (1993). Revised classification system for HIV infection for adolescents and adults. November 15, 1993.

Incidence

HIV disease represents one of the most devastating conditions to appear in modern times. Current research suggests that HIV is probably a new disease that has occurred as a result of mutation of a closely related virus, called the simian immunodeficiency virus. Retrospective studies have shown that HIV was present in Africa, Europe, and the United States over the past 30 years. The disease has grown to epidemic proportions since 1981; by mid-1991, 174,893 cases of AIDS (in the United States) had been reported to the CDC. Because only AIDS is reportable to the CDC, statistical information is somewhat limited concerning those with the earlier form of infection or disease. It is estimated that worldwide over 10 million people are HIV-positive; by the year 2000, it is projected that 15 to 20 million people will be HIV-positive, with 1 million in the United States alone. According to World Health Organization statistics, the major incidence of AIDS remains in the United States; however, the disease has been reported worldwide. Other countries with a relatively high incidence include Brazil, France, Uganda, Tanzania, Germany, Canada, Haiti, and the United Kingdom.

Etiology

The CDC first used the name AIDS in the fall of 1982. The etiologic agent was initially named lymphadenopathy-associated virus (LAV) by the French and human T-cell lymphotropic virus, variant III (HTLV-III) by scientists in the United States. In 1986, the virus was renamed HIV. This term is now commonly accepted throughout the world.

Besides the logarithmic increase in incidence, AIDS has an extremely high mortality rate; over 90 per cent of clients who develop the most severe form of the disease will die within 4 years of an AIDS diagnosis.

In the United States, the incidence of HIV disease is not evenly distributed. Cases of HIV infection tend to occur in areas with high concentrations of participants in high-risk behaviors. According to the CDC, states with the highest occurrence are New York, California, Florida, Texas, and New Jersey.

Since 1989, there has been a decrease in the incidence of AIDS in white gay men but an increase in intravenous drug users. Black and Hispanic communities are disproportionately represented in the number of AIDS cases in the United States. The incidence of infection is especially increasing in women. Minority women are even more dramatically affected by AIDS. According to the CDC, 52 per cent of women with AIDS are black and 19 per cent are Hispanic. In the United States, AIDS has become the fifth leading killer of women of childbearing age. Although the percentage of AIDS in children has not increased dramatically, it is expected that the incidence will rise as the number of HIV-infected women continues to increase.

Risk Factors

Transmission of HIV occurs through horizontal transmission (from either sexual contact or parenteral exposure to blood and blood products) or through vertical transmission (from HIV-infected mother to infant). Several cases of HIV transmission through breast milk have been reported. No other routes of transmission have been shown to exist. HIV is not transmitted by casual contact. Transmission always involves exposure to some body fluid from an infected client. The greatest concentrations of virus have been found in blood, semen, cerebrospinal fluid, and cervical/vaginal secretions. HIV has been found in low concentrations in tears, saliva, and urine, but no cases have been transmitted by these routes. It is believed that the amount or concentration of the virus, the length of exposure, and the route of transmission all play important roles in transmission of the virus.

Sexual activity remains the number one route of transmission in the United States. Sexual activity between men and between men and women can result in transmission of HIV. At the time of this writing, sexual activity between women has resulted in only two reported cases of HIV infection; therefore, lesbian women maintain one of the lowest risks for acquiring HIV infection. Although the majority of cases of AIDS in the United States (60 to 70 per cent) and Europe have occurred as a result of male homosexual activity, the incidence of heterosexual transmission is on the rise. Some factors that increase the risk of sexual transmission include multiple sexual partners, receptive anal intercourse, the presence of open lesions in the genital area, and sexual exposure without some form of barrier such as a condom.

Parenteral transmission occurs when there is direct blood to blood contact with a client infected with HIV. This can occur through sharing of contaminated needles and drug paraphernalia (works), through transfusion of blood or blood products, by accidental needlestick injury to a health care worker, or from blood exposure to nonintact skin or to mucous membranes. The rate of transmission to a health care worker from a needlestick involving a known HIV-positive client is 0.47 per cent.

There is recent evidence that the use of crack cocaine (which is smoked, not injected) results in an alarmingly high rate of HIV infection. Some investigators have speculated that this may occur because of the frequent practice of exchanging this drug for sexual favors, which therefore increases the number of sexual partners. The fact that crack costs significantly less than other drugs has led to its use in younger populations; therefore, there is concern that this will lead to an increased incidence of HIV in adolescents.

Although the mechanism is not completely clear, it is believed that perinatal transmission of HIV can occur at various stages of gestation. The likelihood of an infant's acquiring HIV infection from the mother ranges from 20 to 50 per cent. In other words, 50 to 80 per cent of babies born to infected mothers will not be infected with HIV. The incidence of AIDS in infants directly correlates with the geographic distribution of intravenous drug use in the United States. The method of delivery, whether vaginal or cesarean, does not appear to alter the transmission rate. HIV transmission has been attributed to breastfeeding; therefore, the CDC recommends that HIV-positive women should not breastfeed.

There is general consensus that the spread of HIV, similar to any communicable disease, is preventable through education that focuses on knowledge about transmission and risk reduction strategies. Interventions aimed at reducing a client's risk of acquiring HIV infection needs to be based on a thorough assessment of the client's sexual practices and past or present use of drugs. Clients need to be counseled on safer sexual practices, avoidance of sharing needles, or methods of cleaning drug paraphernalia. Assisting the injection drug user to gain access to drug treatment facilities is an essential aspect of nursing care aimed at reducing the risk of HIV transmission both for the individual and the client's family.

Women considering pregnancy who participate in high-risk behaviors, or have sexual partners who do, should be offered HIV testing and counseling. Information regarding the risk to the infant and the mother needs to be discussed, as well as methods of reducing risks during pregnancy. Currently, the National Academy of Sciences recommends that all pregnant women be offered the option of being tested for the presence of HIV.

Health care workers need to employ universal precautions (Box 24–3) when handling all body fluids or when they engage in procedures that may possibly place them at risk (i.e., phlebotomy, handling of specimens).

Pathophysiology

HIV-1 is a member of the lentivirus subfamily of human retroviruses. Diseases caused by lentiviruses are characterized by an insidious onset with progressive involvement of the central nervous system and may result in disorders of the immune system. A retrovirus belongs to the family Retroviridae and is characterized by the presence of reverse transcriptase. HIV infects T-helper

Box 24–3. Universal Precautions

Universal precautions are intended to prevent parenteral, mucous membrane, and nonintact skin exposures of health care workers to blood-borne pathogens. Universal precautions apply to blood and to other body fluids containing visible blood, semen, vaginal secretions, cerebrospinal fluid, synovial fluid, pleural fluid, peritoneal fluid, pericardial fluid, and amniotic fluid. Universal precautions do not apply to feces, nasal secretions, sputum, sweat, tears, urine, and vomitus unless they contain visible blood.

Barrier Guidelines

1. Disposable gloves (vinyl, latex) should be worn when in contact or when there is potential for contact with blood, body fluids, or other fluids that may contain human immunodeficiency virus (HIV). Gloves should be removed after each client contact. Rubber gloves can be used for equipment cleaning.
2. Hands should be washed between clients, after any exposure, and after removal of gloves.
3. Protective eyewear, face shields, and/or masks should be worn during procedures that may aerosolize blood.
4. Impervious gowns should be worn when there is potential for exposure to large quantities of blood, such as in the labor and delivery area or emergency room.

Needle Precautions

1. Needles should never be recapped after use; keep in mind that most needlesticks are the result of missed needle recapping.
2. Do not cut, break, or bend needles after use; this may release aerosolized blood from the needle shaft.
3. Do not leave used needles lying around.
4. Do not dispose of needles in ordinary receptacles; instead, use appropriately labeled, impermeable needle containers.

Adapted from the Centers for Disease Control (1988). Update: Universal precautions for prevention of transmission of human immunodeficiency virus, hepatitis B virus, and other bloodborne pathogens in health-care setting. *Morbidity and Mortality Weekly Report, 37*(3), 377–388.

cells (T4 lymphocytes), macrophages, B cells, and certain cells in the brain and central nervous system. T-helper cells are infected more readily than are other cells, and their subsequent depletion is responsible for the devastating symptoms and opportunistic infections associated with HIV disease. This depletion of the T-helper cell occurs in the following steps:

1. Once inside the host, HIV attaches to the target cell membrane by way of its receptor molecule, CD4+.
2. The virus is uncoated, and the RNA enters the cell.
3. The enzyme known as reverse transcriptase is released; thereby, the viral RNA is transcribed into DNA.
4. This newly created DNA moves into the nucleus and the DNA of the cell.
5. A provirus is created when the viral DNA integrates itself into the cellular DNA or genome of the cell.
6. The cell becomes confused once the provirus is in place, and its genetic material is no longer pure cell but part virus.
7. The cell may function abnormally.
8. The host cell dies, and viral budding occurs; the new virus proceeds to infect other cells.

Once the initial HIV infection takes place, the virus may remain latent inside the cell for an undetermined length of time. Some form of activation must occur for viral replication to begin. The exact mechanism that causes activation is still being investigated. Some of the theories being explored include the possibility that other infectious agents (such as cytomegalovirus, Epstein-Barr virus, and parasitic infection), environmental antigens, drugs, toxic substances, and genetic factors play a role in cell activation.

HIV-2 is distinctly different from HIV-1 but has many similarities. HIV-2 was first described in West Africa in 1986. The majority of clients with HIV-2 infection in Africa experience a syndrome similar to AIDS; others have ARC type symptoms, whereas others remain asymptomatic. HIV-2 is most commonly spread through sexual intercourse. To date, cases of HIV-2 are rare in the United States, but the CDC and the Food and Drug Administration initiated a surveillance program for HIV-2 in 1987 anticipating that occasional cases of infection with this virus will occur.

The main target of HIV infection is the T4 or CD4+ cell. Once these cells are infected, either they are changed and rendered nonfunctional or their actual number is depleted. The normal number of T4 cells for clients with an intact immune system is between 700 and 1300 T4 cells/mm^3. The T4 (helper cells) to T8 (suppressor cells) ratio is also measured. The normal ratio of T4 to T8 cells is approximately 2 : 1. In clients with HIV infection, this ratio is typically reversed so that there are more suppressor cells, compared with helper cells. Opportunistic infections most commonly occur when the T4 cell count drops below 200. HIV-related malignancies and neurologic disease can occur at higher T4 cell counts. Remaining T4 cells may become dysfunctional and exhibit (1) decreased ability to release lymphokines, (2) decreased cytotoxicity, (3) decreased help to the B cells for immunoglobulin synthesis, (4) decreased ability to proliferate in mixed lymphocyte cultures, and (5) unresponsiveness to specific antigens.

Infection by HIV can also result in leukopenia, which frequently results in a white blood cell count less that 3500 cells/mm^3. Immune thrombocytopenia is also seen along the entire spectrum of HIV infection. Platelet counts may drop to a level that requires frequent intervention to prevent hemorrhage. Zidovudine, intravenous immune globulin, and steroids have been shown to be effective in treating HIV-related thrombocytopenia. In rare cases, splenectomy may be indicated when thrombocytopenia is unresponsive to conventional therapy.

The CDC also developed a classification system in 1987 in an attempt to outline the stages of illness (Table 24-1). This system viewed HIV disease in stages rather than as a continuum of disease states. The proposed HIV classification system revision (see Box 24-2) is consistent with the revised AIDS surveillance case definition, which views HIV disease as a process along a continuum.

Clinical Manifestations

The first stage is often one of acute infection (CDC category A), or the process of being exposed to HIV and becoming antibody-positive (also known as seroconversion). Some clients experience a mononucleosis-like illness consisting of fever, malaise, lymphadenopathy, rash, and, at times, aseptic meningitis; others remain asymptomatic throughout the seroconversion phase.

Once a client is HIV positive, the continuum begins with a period of remaining asymptomatic. Although the length of the asymptomatic state varies for each client, it commonly ranges from 7 to 10 years. These clients usually feel well and are able to carry on their usual activities. They are faced, however, with risks of transmission and anxiety over planning for the future. Persistent generalized lymphadenopathy (PGL), defined as lymph node enlargement persisting for longer than 3 months, with greater than 1 cm enlargement at more than one extrainguinal site and with no other explanation for the lymphadenopathy, is frequently found in the earlier phase of HIV infection. Early HIV infection is classified by the CDC as category A (see Box 24-2).

HIV disease begins to develop as the immune system becomes depleted or ineffective as a result of the virus's effect on the T-helper cell. During this phase, symptoms develop, either alone or in combination, that reflect the damage done to the body's defenses. Some of these symptoms include skin rashes, fevers, fatigue, drenching night sweats, persistent diarrhea, weight loss, PGL, oral thrush, oral hairy leukoplakia, and vaginal yeast infections. The CDC classification system describes these clients as belonging to clinical category B.

The most severe form of HIV disease (CDC category C) involves the development of clinical disease indicative of severe immunosuppression (any condition listed in the 1987 surveillance case definition for AIDS; see Box 24-1). Although clients with constitutional signs may have debilitating symptoms (i.e., severe diarrhea and weight loss), clients with clinical category C disease, in general, have more severe immune suppression. The AIDS-associated malignancies and neurologic disease may occur at higher T-helper cell counts, whereas opportunistic infections more commonly occur when the T-helper count drops below 200.

These clients are usually very ill and frequently require hospitalization during their acute infection. It is not unusual, however, for these clients (especially when first diagnosed) to return to a high level of functioning once the infection is treated and maintenance therapy is begun.

TABLE 24-1. Centers for Disease Control Classification System for HIV Infection

Group I	Acute Infection
Group II	Asymptomatic infection
Group III	Persistent generalized lymphadenopathy with nodes 1 cm or more at two or more extrainguinal sites for more than 3 months
Group IV	Other disease
Subgroup A	Constitutional symptoms
Subgroup B	Neurologic disease
Subgroup C	Secondary infectious diseases
Category C-1	Specified secondary infectious diseases listed in the CDC surveillance definitions for AIDS
Category C-2	Other specified secondary infectious diseases
Subgroup D	Secondary cancers
Subgroup E	Other conditions

Adapted from the Centers for Disease Control (1986). Classification system for human T-lymphotropic virus III/lymphadenopathy-associated virus infection. *Morbidity and Mortality Weekly Report*, *35*, 334-339.

Another phase of HIV disease, not truly captured by the CDC case definition or classification system, is advanced or terminal AIDS. Within this phase, clients often have experienced multiple opportunistic infections or malignancies, have some form of neurologic disease, developed toxic reactions such as bone marrow suppression or intolerance to known therapies, and have little in the way of energy or nutritional stores to combat the persistent devastation of HIV infection on an already depleted immune system. In addition to the more common constitutional symptoms, clients with advanced AIDS often experience some form of pain. Pain may be related to physical symptoms such as peripheral neuropathies, myalgias, or malignancies; but psychogenic pain may be experienced by these clients as well.

DIAGNOSTIC ASSESSMENT

Many clients infected with HIV will develop the antibody in about 6 to 12 weeks. Testing for the presence of the antibody is done in two stages: first with the enzyme-linked immunosorbent assay, and then for confirmation with the Western blot. It is important the clients receive posttest counseling, whether they test positive or negative. HIV-positive clients will have many questions and concerns about insurance, medical care, and access to support services. Clients who test HIV-negative need to be counseled about any high-risk behaviors as well as the need for retesting if it has been 12 weeks or less since a possible exposure. There have been only rare instances when it took more than 12 months to detect the HIV antibody, and these reports remain controversial. Several other HIV detection tests are available, including p24 antigen detection, viral culture, and the polymerase chain reaction technique. Because these assays are expensive and still investigational, they continue to be reserved mainly for pediatric and research purposes.

OPPORTUNISTIC INFECTIONS

Because nurses frequently care for clients with opportunistic infections, it is important that these unusual infections be demystified by acquiring an understanding of the type of infection, the target organs, and the methods of treatment and prevention.

***Pneumocystis carinii* Pneumonia.** *Pneumocystis carinii* pneumonia (PCP) is the number one killer of clients with AIDS. PCP is caused by the protozoal pneumocyst; until 1981, it was seen only sporadically in clients with certain malignancies or in those receiving immunosuppressive therapy. Its incidence has increased dramatically since the onset of the AIDS epidemic. The target organ is the lung, although extrapulmonary pneumocystosis has occurred in clients with AIDS. Those clients who develop PCP almost always have clear evidence of immunosuppression, such as a low T-helper cell count (often less than 200). PCP commonly has an insidious onset. Clients with the HIV infection often have nonspecific symptoms such as fever, fatigue, and weight loss for weeks to months before the onset of respiratory symptoms. Nonproductive cough and dyspnea are the most common presenting symptoms. Clients may be mildly or very symptomatic. The respiratory rate is generally increased. Lung sounds are usually clear, and a chest radiograph may reveal bilateral diffuse interstitial infiltrates or be normal. Pulse oximetry typically reveals a low oxygen level at rest; but even more suggestive of PCP is a decrease in the oxygen level with trending (called desaturation).

Definitive diagnosis requires seeing *Pneumocystis* organisms in bronchial secretions or in lung tissue. This can be accomplished by bronchoscopy, transbronchial lung biopsy, or sputum induction. Treatment options include a 3-week course of trimethoprim-sulfamethoxazole (Bactrim or Septra), parenteral pentamidine, or dapsone-trimethoprim. It is important to note that in clients with AIDS, there is a high frequency of adverse reactions (especially rash and fever) to trimethoprim-sulfamethoxazole. Because PCP ultimately occurs in 80 to 90 per cent of clients with AIDS, it is important to prevent either the first episode or recurrences of this opportunistic infection. PCP prophylaxis is indicated for any HIV-infected client with fewer than 200 T4 lymphocytes. Currently there are several regimens used for PCP prophylaxis, including (1) oral trimethoprim-sulfamethoxazole, (2) oral dapsone, (3) aerosolized pentamidine, and, rarely, (4) parenteral pentamidine. Which regimen is most efficacious and the appropriate dosage are still under debate and investigation.

Cytomegalovirus. Infection with cytomegalovirus (CMV), a member of the herpesvirus family, is extremely common in clients with AIDS. Depending on the socioeconomic conditions of the population, anywhere from 40 to 100 per cent of adults have been infected with CMV and have formed an antibody to it; yet, in immunocompetent hosts, it remains latent and does not cause clinical disease. In clients with AIDS, infection with CMV can cause various clinical illnesses, including chorioretinitis, pneumonitis, esophagitis, colitis, encephalitis, adrenalitis, and hepatitis.

CMV chorioretinitis is the most common of these manifestations; early symptoms include mild visual impairment and deficits of peripheral vision. On funduscopic examination, areas of hemorrhage, exudate, or necrosis are seen. Lesions may sometimes lead to blindness, depending on the location and extent of involvement. Treatment modalities include intravenous gancyclovir or foscarnet. Both of these regimens require lifelong therapy and the placement of a permanent indwelling intravenous catheter.

CMV colitis is manifested by watery diarrhea and weight loss. Diffuse pulmonary infiltrates on the chest film and symptoms of dyspnea, increased respiratory rate, and hypoxemia are suggestive of CMV in the lungs. CMV may also be disseminated in clients with AIDS and result in fevers, malaise, weight loss, and pancytopenia.

Diagnosis of CMV disease is made by biopsy and the search for intranuclear or intracytoplasmic inclusion bodies. Autopsy reports and clinical studies have indicated that almost 90 per cent of AIDS clients develop invasive CMV during the course of their illness.

Herpes Simplex. Herpes simplex virus (HSV) can cause disease in both normal and immunocompromised hosts. Ulcerative HSV infection that lasts longer than 1 month in a client with the HIV infection is diagnostic of AIDS. Reactivation of HSV is common in clients with AIDS and includes extensive disease of the mouth, esophagus, and genital and perirectal areas. In severe cases, HSV may result in encephalitis. In the normal host, HSV lesions typically heal over 7 to 10 days; but in clients with HIV disease, these lesions may take 4 weeks or longer to heal and may result in deep ulcerations and scarring. Tingling and burning at the site of the vesicle and later blister formation are the first symptoms. Severe pain at the location of the lesions is not unusual. In the case of esophageal HSV, pain and difficulty swallowing are the presenting symptoms. Diagnosis is made by clinical evidence, viral culture, or biopsy. Acyclovir is the agent of choice for all HSV infections. Acyclovir is available in oral, topical, and intravenous preparations; the best route of administration is based on the location and severity of the infection. Foscarnet has also been used to treat severe HSV infections when acyclovir resistance was suspected.

Toxoplasmosis. Toxoplasmosis, or infection with *Toxoplasma gondii,* a protozoan, causes focal neurologic symptoms in clients with AIDS and is recognized as the major opportunistic infection of the central nervous system. Infection with *T. gondii* is the result of reactivation of a latent infection that causes headache, seizures, hemiparesis, lethargy, and focal encephalitis. Some clients may experience a subtle change in personality or cognitive ability. A computed tomographic scan of the head with contrast will usually show multiple ring-enhancing mass lesions. Brain biopsy is the only definitive diagnostic method but is rarely used because of the risks associated with this procedure. Standard medical management includes the combination of pyrimethamine and sulfadiazine.

Cryptosporidium. *Cryptosporidium* is also a protozoan parasite that results in intestinal infection manifested by watery diarrhea, malaise, nausea, and abdominal cramps. Diarrhea and abdominal pain usually occur after food ingestion. Clients with AIDS have been known to lose 10 to 15 liters of stool per day, which results in severe dehydration. The diagnosis of cryptosporidiosis is made by stool culture. There is still no known effective therapy, but the addition of zidovudine has shown some benefit in those not previously taking this antiretroviral medication. Clinical trials are under way using various medications to control the symptoms. Management focuses on alleviation of symptoms associated with dehydration, fluid and electrolyte imbalance, and weight loss.

Isospora belli. *Isospora belli* is a protozoan also responsible for intestinal infection that causes symptoms similar to those of cryptosporidiosis. Diagnosis is based on the identification of the parasite in stained fecal smears. The main difference between isosporiasis and cryptosporidiosis is that isosporiasis responds readily to therapy. Oral trimethoprim-sulfamethoxazole is the treatment of choice. Both of these intestinal parasites have a high frequency of recurrence in clients with AIDS; therefore, chronic suppressive therapy is often indicated.

***Mycobacterium avium* Complex.** *Mycobacterium avium* complex (MAC) is an environmental bacterium, present in soil and water, that causes gastrointestinal, respiratory, or disseminated disease in immunocompromised hosts. In clients with AIDS, it is usually found when severe immunosuppression is present and after multiple opportunistic infections have occurred. Symptoms of infection include fever, weight loss, anemia, and neutropenia; it may cause chronic diarrhea, malabsorption, and extrabiliary obstruction. Special blood culture techniques and biopsy of target organs, such as the bone marrow, lymph nodes, liver, and spleen, can demonstrate MAC infection. Disseminated disease can be revealed through bronchial washings or sputum induction. MAC is resistant to standard antituberculous drugs. Multiple-drug regimens have been used in MAC infection, including amikacin, ethambutol, clofazimine, ciprofloxacin, and rifampin. The profound side effects of these drugs and the variable response to treatment have prompted much controversy about whether to attempt to treat this infection at all. Drug trials are under way to examine various drug regimens for treatment of MAC infection.

The incidence of *Mycobacterium tuberculosis* (MTB) infection is increasing in clients with HIV infection. Tuberculosis is a more rapidly progressing disease in these clients and may occur at any time throughout the spectrum of HIV infection. Fever, weight loss, night sweats, fatigue, and lymphadenitis are the most common presenting symptoms. HIV-associated MTB infection is often extrapulmonary and disseminated to other organs, particularly the kidneys, liver, spleen, lymph nodes, blood, skin, gastrointestinal tract, and bone marrow. Diagnosis is made by culture or by chest radiography if the lungs are involved. A tuberculin skin test should be done with use of a control such as *Candida;* because anergy is frequently found in clients with HIV infection, false-negatives may result. Two- or three-drug regimens are used to treat MTB infection; most commonly, ethambutol, isoniazid, rifampin, and pyrazinamide are among the choices. All clients with HIV infection should be screened for tuberculosis by having a Mantoux skin test with a control done every 6 months. Clients with advancing HIV disease may need periodic chest radiographs because they are likely to be anergic.

Candida albicans. *Candida albicans* is a fungus that causes infection of the mouth, esophagus, and vagina of clients with HIV infection. Oral and vaginal candidiasis may be present in HIV-infected clients at any time along the continuum. Candidiasis appears as a white, thick, cottage cheese–like exudate on the affected mucosa. An atrophic form can also be seen as a smooth red patch usually on the hard or soft palate, buccal mucosa, or dorsal surface of the tongue. Angular cheilitis, or cracks and fissures at the corners of the mouth, frequently accompanies thrush. Difficulty or pain with swallowing or retrosternal burning may signal candidiasis of the esophagus. The diagnosis of *Candida* esophagitis is made by examination and culture of lesions. When esophagitis is considered, endoscopy may be necessary. Topical therapy, such as clotrimazole or nystatin, is useful in oral candidiasis; miconazole is used in vaginal candidiasis. Systemic antifungal therapy is indicated for severe disease and includes ketoconazole and fluconazole. Chronic suppressive therapy is sometimes required.

Cryptococcus neoformans. *Cryptococcus neoformans* is a fungus that can cause meningitis or disseminated disease. In clients with AIDS, there is often an insidious onset. Presenting symptoms include headache and subtle mental status changes that may progress to fever, focal neurologic signs, seizures, and coma. Diagnosis is made by lumbar puncture looking for a measurable cryptococcal antigen titer. Treatment consists of intravenous amphotericin B followed by chronic suppressive therapy, which may include periodic infusions of amphotericin B or oral administration of fluconazole.

Histoplasmosis. Histoplasmosis is a fungal infection that results from reactivation of a latent infection. In clients with AIDS, the clinical manifestations are more severe than in other immunocompromised clients. Symptoms include persistent fever and weight loss. Histoplasmosis may initially present on the skin. Diagnosis is made by bone marrow culture or biopsy. The treatment is amphotericin B followed by chronic suppressive therapy with amphotericin B, ketoconazole, or itraconazole (*investigational*).

Coccidioidomycosis. Coccidioidomycosis, caused by the fungus *Coccidioides immitis*, is associated with respiratory symptoms and disseminated disease in immunosuppressed clients. This disease usually occurs only in clients with a history of travel in endemic areas such as Mexico, Central and South America, Nevada, Utah, New Mexico, and western Texas. Although still a rare disease, it is associated with a high mortality rate. Nonspecific symptoms such as malaise, fever, weight loss, cough, and fatigue are often present. Chest radiography reveals unilateral or bilateral reticulonodular or nodular infiltrates. Diagnosis is made by sputum examination after bronchoscopy. Cultures of bone marrow, blood, urine, lymph nodes, and liver are frequently positive. Amphotericin B is the treatment of choice. Relapses are extremely common.

HIV-ASSOCIATED MALIGNANCIES

HIV-associated malignancies include Kaposi's sarcoma (KS) and AIDS-associated lymphoma. KS, a neoplasm of the vascular endothelium, is the most common neoplasm affecting clients with AIDS. AIDS-associated KS is often aggressive and disfiguring. KS is more common in homosexual and bisexual men, compared with other high-risk groups. It typically presents as a purplish-red lesion that is not painful or pruritic. The lesion can be flat or indurated and will frequently progress to a nodule over time. Lesions may appear anywhere on the skin and may include the lymph nodes, mucous membranes, and viscera. Treatment for KS centers on balancing the risk of treatment with the risk of opportunistic infection. Radiation therapy, chemotherapy, and interferon-alpha are all used, depending on the location and extent of involvement. Symptomatic therapy is also used for palliation of disfigurement, lymphedema, skin breakdown, and pain.

Non-Hodgkin's lymphoma, Burkitt's-like lymphomas, and malignant lymphomas of the central nervous system can be classified as AIDS-associated malignancies. Prognosis tends to be poor because of an inadequate response to chemotherapy and lack of adequate bone marrow reserve for completion of needed therapy. Although these neoplasms occur less often than KS does, survival is significantly shorter when they are present.

HIV NEUROLOGIC DISEASE

HIV neurologic disease can involve the central and peripheral nervous systems. AIDS dementia complex is characterized by cognitive, motor, and behavioral dysfunction. Early symptoms involve difficulty with concentration and memory. Complaints of slowness in thought process or having difficulty in conversations are common. Personality changes, irritability, apathy, depression, and withdrawal usually occur as the dementia progresses. Motor dysfunction sometimes accompanies cognitive changes and may result in poor balance and coordination. Falls may become frequent, and a slow deliberate gait may ensue.

Neuropsychiatric testing may be performed at various intervals to monitor symptoms. Cerebral atrophy on neurodiagnostic imaging is a nearly universal finding in AIDS dementia complex. The use of zidovudine (Retrovir, ZDV, and formerly known as AZT) has been used successfully in treating AIDS dementia. Symptomatic therapy is aimed at treating the depression or mania; ensuring safety is essential. Prognosis is poor, and end-stage dementia leaves the client lying in bed with a vacant stare, unable to ambulate and often incontinent.

Peripheral nerve disease, although not an AIDS-defining condition, is a common complication of the HIV infection. The most common of these neuropathies presents as a burning or tingling sensation of the feet, legs, or hands. Neuropathies may be further complicated by the addition of certain antiviral medications (ddI, ddC) that are discussed later. Treatment involves symptomatic therapy. Amitriptyline has been reported to have some benefit in treating these neuropathies.

HIV WASTING SYNDROME

HIV wasting syndrome is characterized by progressive weight loss (greater than 10 per cent of body weight), cachexia, persistent fevers, and diarrhea. These clients usually appear quite ill and debilitated. Evaluation in order to rule out other causes for the presenting complaints must take place before this complex group of symptoms is named wasting syndrome. Nutritional support, symptomatic treatment, and antiretroviral therapy are used with varying degrees of success.

Medical Management

PHARMACOLOGIC MANAGEMENT

The medical management of HIV infection is aimed at controlling the replication of the virus and thereby delaying further destruction of the immune system. Zidovudine (also known as Retrovir, ZDV, and formerly AZT) is an antiretroviral agent that has been shown to prolong survival and reduce mortality in clients with HIV infection. The use of zidovudine is indicated for anyone with HIV infection with a T4 helper cell count less than 500. The most worrisome side effects associated with zidovudine include anemia and neutropenia. Complete blood counts are monitored at frequent intervals throughout the course of therapy. Serious side effects are easily managed by blood transfusion, temporarily withholding the medication, or reducing the dosage. Some additional adverse experiences that have been reported include nausea, headaches, muscle pain and weakness, and fatigue. The dose of zidovudine has been modified to include the current standard of 100 mg every 4 hours five times per day. Various doses and schedules are being investigated, including 300 mg/day and a schedule of 200 mg every 8 hours.

Dideoxyinosine (ddI) is a nucleoside analog approved for use in clients with HIV infection who have demonstrated intolerance to zidovudine or who have had significant disease progression despite treatment with this drug. Dideoxycytidine (ddC) is still under investigation; it is available through clinical trial participation and the expanded access program. Both ddI and ddC are antiretroviral agents that inhibit replication of the virus. The main side effects include peripheral neuropathy, diarrhea, and pancreatitis. Both drugs are in clinical trials comparing their efficacy with zidovudine. Studies are also looking at the combination of zidovudine and these agents.

Vaccines both to prevent HIV transmission and to treat those already infected are being developed. Scientists predict that the availability of such vaccines will take another 5 to 10 years before general distribution is possible.

Emphasis on prevention (prophylaxis) of opportunistic infections has sparked new fields of study in the management of HIV. As mentioned earlier, the standard of care is to initiate prophylaxis against PCP once a client's T4 cell count drops below 200. There continues to be much controversy over the use of "200" as the time for initiation; many clinicians argue that a T4 cell count below 300 should be the starting point for prophylaxis, especially when thrush or oral hairy leukoplakia has occurred. Studies are under way to examine methods of preventing other opportunistic infections, such as CMV, MAC, and systemic fungal infections.

DIETARY MANAGEMENT

The immune system needs protein, carbohydrates, fat, vitamins, and minerals in sufficient quantity to maintain optimal functioning. Therefore, nutrition is an essential component of the management of clients with the HIV infection. Eating well not only enhances the immune system but can serve to maintain a normal lifestyle and appearance.

A complete nutritional assessment is key to any educational strategy aimed at improving general nutrition. Because weight loss is frequently seen as HIV disease progresses, it is important to evaluate other factors (mechanical or infectious) that may be responsible. Disorders that occur in the upper gastrointestinal tract include oral ulcerations/lesions, mucositis, periodontitis, dysphagia, odynophagia, nausea, and vomiting. All of these may result in an alteration in nutritional status. Many of these symptoms are due to infection and therefore are amenable to medical and nursing management. Routine dental care is essential for clients with HIV infection. Progressive disease to the gingivae and teeth can occur as a result of HIV infection and thereby affect the desire (taste changes) and ability to eat a well-balanced diet.

The lower gastrointestinal tract disorders include diarrhea and malabsorption, although often these can be attributed to an identifiable infectious agent. Treatment results in resolution of or improvement in symptoms and subsequent weight gain. HIV infection itself can lead to disorders of the digestive tract, and unfortunately these symptoms respond poorly to treatment. Constipation is frequently a problem for clients on methadone or for those requiring narcotic analgesics for pain management. A diet that includes increasing amounts of fiber, six to eight glasses of water per day, and some form of regular exercise is recommended.

HIV wasting syndrome or the profound involuntary weight loss that occurs in some clients with advanced HIV disease is characterized by a weight loss of greater than 10 per cent of baseline body weight, either chronic diarrhea for more than 30 days or chronic weakness, and fever that is present constantly without any other explanation. This syndrome places extraordinary demands on available nutrients. Oral and enteral nutritional supplements are frequently used to combat the rapid weight loss and debilitation.

A well-balanced diet is generally recommended for all clients with the HIV infection. Dietary guidelines need to include foods that take into account the cultural and economic background of the client. Many experts also suggest that the addition of a multiple vitamin with B complex is desirable for ensuring adequate intake of essential vitamins and minerals.

Because of the increased energy requirements during times of infection, the body often demands more than is able to be consumed. For these clients, nutritional supplements are used. These supplements provide vitamins and minerals besides extra protein and calories. Products such as Ensure Plus, Sustacal H C, and Carnation Instant Breakfast are frequently added two to three times per day to the daily diet.

HOLISTIC THERAPIES

Many clients with HIV turn to holistic or complementary therapies in addition to traditional Western health care practices. Some of these therapies include acupuncture, meditation, guided imagery, massage, and spiritual healing. The goal of such interventions is to empower clients to take an active part in the healing process. Psychoneuroimmunology is an exciting new field of research that is exploring the connection between the mind and the central nervous system and their relationship to the immune system. Although some of these therapies are met by skepticism, especially by Western medicine, it appears that these therapies frequently offer clients control over their altered health state by allowing active participation in the healing process.

Surgical Management

The surgical management of clients with HIV is limited to the placement of a venous access device, surgical intervention for treatment of malignancies, or biopsy.

Venous access devices, such as a Groshung catheter, are used to facilitate frequent blood drawing, administration of intravenous medications (gancyclovir), hyperalimentation, and transfusions.

Nursing Management

ASSESSMENT

Understanding the real risk of HIV transmission is the first step in providing comprehensive nursing care. HIV is a fragile virus that demands a set of conditions in order to cause infection. For health care workers, there must be mucous membrane contact or a break in the skin in order for the virus to invade the bloodstream. Even an inoculation of infected blood from an accidental needlestick accounts for less than five seroconversions in a thousand (0.47 per cent). Compared with all other infectious diseases (i.e., hepatitis), HIV infection is the most difficult to contract in the health care setting, but its potential devastation warrants careful adherence to universal precautions (see Box 24-3).

The institution of universal precautions was recommended by the CDC in 1987. This method was adopted in an attempt to protect health care workers from blood or other body fluids that may contain HIV or hepatitis B virus. Because the majority of clients infected with these viruses will not be known or apparent, this system works under the premise that all clients need to be considered capable of transmitting the viruses.

Most of the infections that afflict clients with HIV infection cannot be transmitted. Opportunistic infections, such as with *Pneumocystis carinii, Toxoplasma gondii, Mycobacterium avium-intracellulare,* and *candida,* are not transmissible. Viruses such as herpes and bacteria such as *Mycobacterium tuberculosis* can be transmitted to the immunocompetent host. Careful adherence to good hygiene and universal precautions is essential. Hepatitis B infection tends to be very common in clients with the HIV infection; therefore, immunization is recommended for health care workers who have regular contact with these clients.

The major responsibility of the professional nurse in the care of clients with HIV infection involves support of immunocompetence. This is accomplished through assessment of those factors, both physical and psychosocial, that affect the immune system and the development of intervention strategies aimed at minimizing further deterioration of the body's defenses.

The skin is the body's first line of defense and is frequently affected by HIV infection. Cutaneous hypersensitivity reactions to medications and environmental antigens is seen often, and skin breakdown due to various viruses (HSV, varicella zoster) and fungi (tinea) can lead to further invasion and systemic disease. Open wounds may take slightly longer to heal and frequently cause scarring. Clients with a history of psoriasis or eczema may have severe exacerbations of these conditions. Nail changes are frequent and occur as a result of fungal infection or medications. Zidovudine has been shown to cause hyperpigmented changes in nails, especially in black and Hispanic clients. Hair changes are also seen; thinning of the hair is the most common. The nursing assessment includes a complete history of any skin conditions and allergies. Examining for rashes, ulcerations, vesicles, lesions, pruritus, dryness, scaling, bruising, color changes, and violaceous lesions is essential. Intervention is aimed at defining the cause and eliminating it, if possible (medication or environmental allergen), or treating the infection or dermatologic condition. Prevention of further sequelae involves teaching clients the basics of routine skin care and observation. Skin care should include daily bathing (showers are preferred if a client has fungus involving the feet or groin), the use of lotions or creams to prevent dry skin and cracking, and observation of any rashes or lesions. Hair care includes washing with gentle shampoos and avoidance of excessive washing, brushing, and chemicals such as dyes. Nails need to be kept clean and cut to reduce fungal and bacterial infections.

The mucous membranes are vulnerable to attack by various antigens, especially when there is evidence of cellular immunodeficiency and an interruption or break in the membranes occurs. The oral, vaginal, and rectal mucosa are particularly susceptible to the effects of HIV. The history should include information about prior history of oral, vaginal, or rectal lesions (i.e., HSV); oral hygiene and dental practices; history of vaginal infections; and the presence of pain or bleeding in any of these locations. Assessment includes examination for oral ulcerations or lesions (violaceous lesions in the mouth may be suggestive of KS); thick, white, curdlike exudate, suggestive of oral thrush; linear white striations on the lateral aspect of the tongue, or white plaques, suggestive of oral hairy leukoplakia; bleeding or hypertrophy of the gums; and the condition of existing teeth or dentures. The presence of a white, thick vaginal discharge is suggestive of vaginal candidiasis. The presence of vesicular lesions, ulcerations, and condylomata (warts) in the vaginal and rectal areas needs to be ascertained. The nasal mucosa is susceptible to herpetic lesions and may contain perforations when clients use inhaled cocaine. Intervention is based on defining the cause and initiating appropriate treatment. Teaching proper oral, vaginal, and rectal hygiene is extremely important. Oral care needs to include brushing after meals with a soft toothbrush, daily flossing (interventions need to be modified if bleeding is a concern), scheduling regular dental visits, and using oral rinses such as saline or quarter-strength hydrogen peroxide to enhance bactericidal effect. Rectal and vaginal care includes avoidance of enemas, douches, or other chemicals that interrupt the normal flora; routine skin care; avoidance of sexual activities that may result in breaks in the mucosa; and observation for the presence of any interruption in the integrity of the mucous membranes.

Appetite and weight changes are frequent occurrences associated with HIV infection and disease. Whether these changes lead to obesity or cachexia, both can adversely affect immune system functioning.

Profound weight loss is readily associated with HIV infection; however, some clients, especially early in the course of disease, actually have a weight gain. Sometimes this is a result of appetite changes due to medication, stress, or drug detoxification. Most clients experience weight loss at some time during the course of HIV infection. This can be due to an increase in metabolism, active infection, HIV itself, depression, medication side effects, or active substance abuse. Nursing care needs to focus on identification of the underlying cause, monitoring weight and dietary intake, and evaluating the effect that the weight change has on the client's self-image. In addition to education regarding the components of a balanced diet, advice regarding beginning an exercise (as tolerated) program may enhance the client's sense of general well-being and should be included in the plan of care.

Substance abuse, whether of alcohol or drugs such as heroin or cocaine, has potential deleterious effects on the immune system. The actual abuse of the chemical substance is not the only problem; the behaviors that frequently surround substance abuse can have a negative impact on the client's health. The abuse of alcohol and illicit drugs often involves "binging," which places the focus on acquisition and use of the substance of choice. Whether the binge lasts for days or months, it frequently results in omission of prescribed medications, poor dietary intake, inadequate rest, and missed follow-up appointments. Nursing care focuses on assessment of the potential/actual substance abuse and includes defining the substance of choice, the frequency of use, financial considerations, and how these affect family, job, and interpersonal relationships. Nurses need to evaluate the client's desire to change this behavior and to refer the client to appropriate services. It is important to call attention to the substance abuse and offer assistance even if it is refused. Many experts in the field of substance abuse agree that most clients are approached numerous times before they finally obtain help.

Many studies have proposed a connection between stress/coping and the immune system. Throughout the spectrum of events that follow the initial HIV-positive diagnosis, there are periods of overwhelming stress. Some of these stressful times include (1) initially finding out that one is HIV-positive; (2) concern about who to tell, job, and insurance security; (3) notification of past, present, or future sexual partners; (4) the death of friends, lovers, or family members from AIDS; (5) development of HIV-related signs and symptoms; (6) receiving the AIDS diagnosis; and (7) dealing with terminal illness. Nurses need to assess the current stressor and coping patterns. If substance abuse has been a past coping mechanism, it is important to identify this by discussing the potential for relapse with the client. Using stress reduction techniques and referral to counseling or support groups may also be helpful.

Besides supporting immunocompetence, nurses play an important role in evaluating the client's level of functioning. Because intervention strategies need to be tailored to the client's ability to carry out such an intervention, it is essential to obtain an adequate data base. This data base should include assessment of the client's energy level, sleep patterns, comfort level, mobility, spirituality, sexual functioning, and relationships. All of these areas can be affected by both the HIV disease itself and the process of coping with the many complex issues surrounding this disease. Nurses need to be cognizant of these factors when developing individual plans of care in order that realistic goals are established.

Because many clients with HIV disease experience multiple losses, it is important for nurses to assist these clients in maintaining a realistic sense of hope in the face of multiple changes. Some of the changes and losses experienced include loss of function (decreased strength, mental acuity), change in social roles, loss of self-esteem, loss of social support, housing changes, changes in sexuality and childbearing options, loss of financial security or job, and finally loss of control over one's own life decisions. Understanding the losses is the first step in helping clients with HIV infection cope and maintain hope in the face of adversity.

NURSING INTERVENTION

There are many nursing diagnoses appropriate for the client with AIDS (Box 24–4). The five highest priority diagnoses are discussed in detail. Nursing care for clients with symptomatic AIDS centers on management of the symptoms, support of immunocompetence, and psychosocial support and counseling.

Nursing care for clients with AIDS focuses on the response to the opportunistic infections or malignancy, issues of death and dying, support for the family or significant others, and restoration to an optimal level of functioning.

In caring for the client with AIDS, remember use of universal precautions to protect the nurse. Handling of any needle or sharp instrument needs to be done with extreme care (see Box 24–3). If a needlestick or mucous membrane splash does occur, immediately report this event to the appropriate department. Some early studies have suggested that using zidovudine (AZT) after occupational exposure may interfere with transmission; however, prophylaxis must be started within 24 hours after exposure.

Nursing Diagnosis: Breathing Pattern, Ineffective R/T congestion and weakness secondary to PCP, CMV, pulmonary KS, MAC, tuberculosis, pneumonitis, pneumothorax, and anxiety.

Planning: Expected Outcomes. The client will breathe with minimal difficulty, as evidenced by a decrease in dyspnea and less effort with breathing.

Implementation. Infection of the lung is very common in clients with AIDS and PCP, and it continues to be the most frequent AIDS-defining diagnosis; therefore, ineffective breathing pattern is a major problem of clients with HIV infection.

Nurses need to assess the client's respiratory status for rate, rhythm, regularity of respirations, use of acces-

Box 24–4. Common Nursing Diagnoses for Clients with HIV Infection Diseases

- Infection (any body organ), High Risk for R/T cellular immunodeficiency
- Breathing Pattern, Ineffective R/T PCP, CMV infection, pulmonary KS, MAC infection, tuberculosis, pneumonitis, pneumothorax
- Nutrition, Altered: Less than Body Requirements R/T persistent diarrhea, malabsorption, increased metabolic rate, anorexia, stomatitis, infection
- Skin Integrity, Impaired R/T malnutrition, KS, immobility, infection (HSV, histoplasmosis, CMV, varicella zoster, candidiasis)
- Social Isolation R/T stigma, fear, cultural and religious mores, risk for HIV transmission
- Diarrhea R/T infection, diet, medications
- Sleep Pattern Disturbance R/T anxiety, depression, withdrawal from drugs (heroin, cocaine, methadone), pain, night sweats, side effect of medications
- Pain R/T side effects of medications, infections, immobility, lymphadenopathy, lymphedema secondary to KS, lymphoma, headaches due to central nervous system infection, peripheral neuropathy, severe myalgias, psychogenic pain related to anxiety and fear of death
- Activity Intolerance R/T fatigue, weakness, arthralgia, myalgia, side effects of medications, dyspnea, fever, malnutrition
- Thought Processes, Altered R/T central nervous system disease (toxoplasmosis, cryptococcosis), CMV infection, KS, lymphoma, HIV infection
- Body Image Disturbance R/T diagnosis, KS lesions, alopecia from chemotherapy or HIV infection, weight loss, depression, social stigma, change in sexuality
- Grieving, Anticipatory R/T multiple losses, including health, independence, friends, social activities, job, housing, life, and loss of control
- Anxiety R/T HIV diagnosis, fear of death, fear of disclosure
- Knowledge Deficit R/T disease progression, treatment options, transmission, and methods of preventing transmission
- Sexual Patterns, Altered R/T safer sex practices, abstinence, fear of transmission, impotency secondary to medications
- Injury, High Risk for R/T weakness, HIV encephalopathy and cognitive changes, neuromuscular changes
- Sensory/Perceptual Alterations: Auditory/Visual R/T hearing loss secondary to medications and visual loss related to infection (CMV)
- Role Performance, Altered R/T parenting, childbearing, supporting
- Individual Coping, Ineffective R/T the diagnosis of HIV disease

sory muscles, presence of adventitious breath sounds, cough, skin color, general appearance, and level of consciousness. A patent airway must be maintained at all times. Administer medications and oxygen as ordered and monitor for side effects. The head of the bed should be elevated and the client monitored frequently to lessen anxiety during times of dyspnea. Monitor the results of arterial blood gas analyses, pulmonary function tests, and other pertinent laboratory studies. Provide teaching before any procedures including bronchoscopy, lung biopsy, or radiographic imaging. Encourage the client to report any changes such as increased dyspnea or cough. Help the client with activities of daily living (ADLs) and support the client and significant others.

Nursing Diagnosis: Activity Intolerance R/T fatigue, weakness, anemia, arthralgia, myalgia, dyspnea, fever, malnutrition, or motor dysfunction secondary to neurologic disease.

Planning: Expected Outcomes. The client will maintain a level of activity compatible with the stage of disease, avoiding immobility as long as possible, as evidenced by a balance of rest and activity and absence of complications associated with immobility.

Implementation. A change in activity tolerance becomes a common finding as AIDS progresses. AIDS itself can cause severe fatigue, and the many medications and opportunistic infections are capable of decreasing a client's activity level, thereby affecting the client's ability to perform daily activities such as working and caring for self or family. Nurses need to assess the pre-illness activity tolerance in order to establish the client's usual energy level.

Second, the current degree of activity needs to be determined. Assess the client's need for sleep and rest. Assist the client with ADLs. Encourage the client to engage in regular exercise and rest as tolerated. Teach the client energy conservation measures and evaluate response to instructions. Establish a time with the client and family or significant others for rest while the client is hospitalized and educate other staff about this protected time. Encourage the client to eat and maintain an adequate dietary intake during periods of activity intolerance. Administer ordered treatment for underlying infections, pain, anxiety, sleeplessness, or malnutrition.

Nursing Diagnosis: Pain R/T lymphadenopathy, peripheral neuropathy, lymphedema secondary to KS, lymphoma, severe myalgia, headache secondary to central nervous system infection, and psychogenic pain related to fear and anxiety over death.

Planning: Expected Outcomes. The client will have pain controlled or relieved, as evidenced by client's statements and increased activity for the client.

Implementation. The pain experienced by clients with AIDS needs to be carefully assessed. Nurses and clients alike expect to have pain with cancer, whereas clients with AIDS are expected to waste away without significant painful experiences. Nurses need to perform a pain assessment that includes assessing for location, onset, duration, time of day of occurrence, precipitating or alleviating factors, characteristics, and frequency of the pain. The client would quantify the pain by describing its intensity on a scale of 0 to 10 (0 being no pain). In collaboration with the physician, appropriate pain relief in the form of anti-inflammatory, antianxiety, or analgesic agents may be used. See Chapter 16 for more information on pain control.

Clients with a history of injectable drug abuse are particularly concerned about the potential of being inadequately medicated because of either past illicit drug use or a high tolerance for narcotics. The use of established schedules or client-controlled analgesia works well in these situations. Provide alternative measures for pain relief such as massage, visualization, and touch. Assess the effectiveness of any therapy that is administered and monitor for side effects. Support is essential at this phase, because clients with AIDS frequently associate the need for chronic pain medication with death and dying and therefore delay requesting pain relief.

Nursing Diagnosis: Knowledge Deficit R/T transmission of the disease and the need for proper nutrition, adequate rest and exercise, and good health practices.

Planning: Expected Outcomes. The client will understand disease transmission and the need for proper nutrition, adequate rest and exercise, and good health practices, as evidenced by client's statements and absence of transmission to others, maintenance of body weight, adequate activity level, and good health practices.

Implementation. Nursing care of asymptomatic AIDS clients includes education strategies aimed at reducing the risk of transmission. This includes safe sex counseling, avoidance of sharing of needles or instructions on cleaning the works (paraphernalia used in the injection of drugs) or both, care of household items, and proper disposal of items soiled with body fluids.

Health maintenance also is important at this stage. This includes instruction on maintaining adequate nutrition, weight management, exercise, smoking cessation, and stress reduction. Early disease detection methods need to be included in care planning, including screening mammography, Pap smears, breast self-examination, testicular self-examination, and Mantoux testing. Counseling and support around the issue of social stigma, potential losses to body image and childbearing potential, changes in sexuality, and premature loss of life need to be included in the nursing care planning.

Nursing Diagnosis: Spiritual Distress, High Risk for R/T terminal illness.

Planning: Expected Outcomes. The client will come to terms with terminal nature of disease, as evidenced by client's statements and acceptance of approaching death.

Implementation. Nursing care in the late stages focuses on palliative care, symptom management, and emotional support for the client, family, and significant others. The ethical dilemmas of advanced life support, ability to care for surviving children, and use of experimental treatments are major concerns.

EVALUATION

The nurse must evaluate client outcomes on the basis of the established plan of care. If these goals have not been achieved, the plan and interventions must be revised to meet the client's needs.

Modification of Plan of Care for the Elderly

To date, there is little information regarding HIV infections in the elderly, because this tends to be a disease that affects a younger population (ages 20 to 49 years). Limited experience has suggested that clients with HIV who are older (more than 45 years of age) may have a more rapid rate of disease progression than do their younger counterparts.

Post-hospital Care

Discharge planning for clients with AIDS involves evaluation of the client's home health care needs (see Bridge to Home Health Care). It is essential to identify, early in the hospitalization, the person who will care for the client upon discharge. The second step is to evaluate the home itself (if there is one). The availability of laundry, toilet, and cooking facilities is important. The safety of the client in the home needs to take precedence. The availability of reimbursement sources is often neglected by nurses in the plan of care, but this often dictates the amount of care a client can receive and can greatly affect a decision to go home versus a hospice approach. Confidentiality is a very important concern for home health care. The client may wish that only certain individuals know about the HIV diagnosis. These wishes must be honored for both legal and ethical reasons.

DISCHARGE TEACHING

Discharge teaching needs to include information on any medications, access to follow-up care, location of local support networks, knowledge about transmission of HIV or any coexisting infections (i.e., tuberculosis), and care of any central or peripheral intravenous lines, when appropriate.

HOME HEALTH CARE NEEDS

Once a complete discharge package is put together, the work of the home health care agency begins. A "case management" approach is frequently used to coordinate needed services for clients at home. Often there are several case managers from different agencies who work together to provide comprehensive home health care services. For clients with HIV infection, the

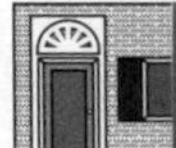

BRIDGE TO HOME HEALTH CARE

Home Health Care Guidelines for Care Givers and Clients with HIV

Maintain personal hygiene; wash hands frequently. Care givers should wear gloves for actual or potential contact with body fluids or if the care giver's hands are chapped or have open sores. Kitchen and bathroom facilities may be shared provided normal sanitary practices are observed.

- Wash dishes and silverware in hot, soapy water, or use dishwasher.
- Clean kitchen counters with sponges and scouring pads to remove food particles. Do not use the same sponge to clean bathroom spills.
- Clean refrigerator frequently to control molds.
- Clean up spills of body fluids or waste immediately with a solution of 1 part bleach to 10 parts water. A bleach solution should be used to disinfect kitchen and bathroom floors, showers, sinks, and toilet bowls.
- Towels and washcloths should not be shared without laundering.
- Toothbrushes, razors, enema equipment, and sexual toys should not be shared.
- Clothes and linens can be washed in the usual manner unless soiled with body fluids; bleach should then be used.
- Sanitary napkins, tampons, and any bloody dressings should be wrapped in a plastic bag, then placed in a plastic-lined trash collector.
- Needles or sharp instruments should be handled carefully. Needles should not be recapped; dispose of them in an impenetrable sealed container, for example, a coffee can with a plastic lid or a plastic milk jug.

Clients with AIDS do not have to remove pets from the household if certain precautions are taken:

- Do not allow outdoor cats to use an indoor litter box. Have someone else change litter boxes and birdcages, when possible; if this is not feasible, use gloves.
- Do not handle animals with diarrhea or those that appear ill.
- Wash hands after handling animals.

care typically involves a multidisciplinary team including nurses, social workers, nutritionists, physical therapists, and clergy. Many locations also have volunteer groups that provide additional support to clients with HIV infection. These individuals are frequently referred to as "buddies." HIV buddies come from all walks of life and usually have a common interest in helping those with HIV infection. These individuals will often help with ADLs, transportation, cooking, shopping, and pleasure activities. The HIV buddy program has served to enhance the lives of many clients with HIV infection, especially those who have been disenfranchized from their family and community.

The nurse providing home health care needs to assess the home situation for safety. Frequent mental status and functional assessments are important for establishing whether home care is the most suitable setting. Issues of child care for women with HIV infection are just coming to the forefront. To date, there is little support for childcare in the home during terminal illness. Many care givers are concerned about transmission of HIV in the household. Education must be done with respect to the correct methods of disposal and disinfection of contaminated items, care of pets in the home, and care of personal care items such as razors and toothbrushes (see Bridge to Home Health Care). The nurse needs to facilitate access to follow-up appointments through either arranging transportation or providing written reminders for clients with a memory impairment.

Hospice care is an option once a client with HIV disease has reached the end of the HIV continuum. Hospice usually involves a less than 6-month prognosis and the willingness of the client to waive aggressive treatment and instead search out palliative, comforting care at the end of life. Hospice care is provided either in the home or in a separate facility. Home hospice is designed for clients with a primary care giver. The care giver assumes 24-hour accountability for care and in return is assisted and supported in this care by a hospice team. A hospice facility is preferred when there is no primary care giver in the home or when the safety or nursing care needs surpass that which the average person could provide, even with significant support in the home. Both forms of hospice are beneficial to clients with terminal illness because they provide specialized services in symptom management and care of the dying.

HYPERSENSITIVITY DISORDERS

Although the immune system protects the body from harmful invaders, an overactive or overzealous response is detrimental. Overreaction to a substance, or hypersensitivity, is often referred to as an allergic response. Although "allergy" is widely used, the word "hypersensitivity" is more appropriate; this term designates an increased immune response to the presence of an antigen (in this case referred to as an allergen) that results in tissue destruction.

Predisposing Factors

The occurrence and intensity of hypersensitivity responses depend on several factors: host defenses, the nature of the allergen, the concentration of the allergen, the route of allergen entrance into the body, and the exposure to the allergen.

HOST DEFENSES

Some clients are more prone to allergies than others are for reasons that are unclear. About one in four Americans have serious allergies. The term "atopy" is used to distinguish clients who seem to have familial tendencies for allergies. Atopic clients produce IgE antibodies to allergens rather than IgG or IgM antibodies.

NATURE OF THE ALLERGEN

Like all antigens, allergens are usually high-molecular-weight proteins. However, some haptens (e.g., penicillin) are highly allergic. A hapten is a low-molecular-weight substance that binds with an antigenic substance to elicit an allergic response.

CONCENTRATION OF THE ALLERGEN

Higher concentrations usually result in hypersensitivity responses of greater intensity.

ROUTE OF ALLERGEN ENTRANCE INTO THE BODY

Routes include inhalation, injection, ingestion, or direct contact. Most allergens are inhaled.

EXPOSURE TO THE ALLERGEN

Hypersensitivity responses occur after initial exposure. The first contact with the substance causes a primary immune response, slower and less severe than the secondary immune response, which occurs with subsequent exposure to the allergen. Also, if much time elapses between each contact with the allergen (e.g., several years), the immune response diminishes.

Types of Hypersensitivity Reactions

There are two general categories of hypersensitivity reaction: immediate and delayed. These designations are based on the rapidity of the immune response. Recent research, however, suggests there is a biochemical and a cellular component in both types of reaction. Immunoglobulins mediate immediate reactions, whereas T cells govern delayed hypersensitivity responses. Humoral responses occur more rapidly than cell-mediated responses do.

In addition to the delayed and immediate categories, hypersensitivity reactions are divided into four main types (Table 24–2): (1) immediate/anaphylactic, (2) cytolytic/cytotoxic, (3) immune complex, and (4) cell-mediated delayed.

TYPE I ANAPHYLACTIC HYPERSENSITIVITY

This response is a rapidly occurring reaction mediated by IgE antibodies. The allergen stimulates IgE production, which in turn causes mast cell degranulation. Mast cells release histamine and leukotrienes (formerly slow-reacting substances of anaphylaxis [SRS-A]). Mast cells cause vasodilation and increased capillary permeability, which promotes fluid loss into the interstitial space. Leukotrienes cause spasm of the bronchial smooth muscles, which elicits an asthmalike response. Table 24–3 outlines other chemical mediators of these reactions.

Anaphylactic shock represents the most severe form of type I hypersensitivity. Initial manifestations of anaphylaxis may include localized itching, edema, and sneezing. These seemingly innocuous problems are followed in minutes by wheezing, dyspnea, cyanosis, and circulatory shock.

Anaphylaxis requires immediate emergency treatment. Common causes of anaphylaxis are listed in Table 24–4. See Chapter 80 for a discussion of emergency care of clients with anaphylaxis.

Prevention is the key in anaphylaxis. A careful nursing history reveals individual susceptibility to such reactions. Always mark known allergies clearly on the per-

TABLE 24–2. Types of Hypersensitivity Reactions

	Type	Causative Component	Pathologic Process	Reaction
I	Immediate/anaphylactic	IgE	Mast cell degranulation ↓ Histamine and leukotriene release	Anaphylaxis Atopic diseases Skin reactions
II	Cytolytic/cytotoxic	IgG IgM Complement	Complement fixation ↓ Cell lysis	ABO incompatibility Drug-induced hemolytic anemia
III	Immune complex	Antigen-antibody complexes	Deposition in vessels and tissue walls ↓ Inflammation	Arthus reaction Serum sickness Systemic lupus erythematosus Acute glomerulonephritis
IV	Cell-mediated delayed	Sensitized T cells	Lymphokine release	Tuberculosis Contact dermatitis Transplant rejection

TABLE 24-3. Chemical Mediators of the Allergic Reaction

Mediator	Function
Histamine	Increased vascular permeability → erythema Increased respiratory airway resistance → increased cAMP
Leukotrienes (formerly SRS-A)	Increased vascular permeability Increased smooth muscle contraction
Eosinophil chemotactic factor of anaphylaxis (ECF-A)	Increased eosinophils to site
Neutrophil chemotactic factor	Increased neutrophils to site
Heparin	Anticomplement action Anticoagulation
Bradykinin	Slow smooth muscle contraction Increased vascular permeability Increased mucous secretions Stimulation of pain fibers
Platelet-activating factor	Secretion and aggregation of platelets

TABLE 24-4. Common Agents Causing Anaphylaxis

Drugs	
Penicillins (most common)	Vancomycin
Cephalosporins	Amphotericin B
Tetracyclines	Polymyxin
Streptomycin	Bacitracin
Kanamycin	Aspirin, other anti-inflammatory agents
Neomycin	Colchicine
Heparin	Tranquilizers
Protamine	
Foods	
Seafoods	Citrus fruits
Eggs	Strawberries
Nuts	Legumes
Insect Venoms	
Hymenoptera (honeybees, wasps, yellow jacket, hornets, fire ants)	
Biologicals	
Heterologous antisera (especially equine)	
Enzymes	
Hormones	
Vaccines (especially egg-cultured types)	
Blood Products	
Plasma	
Cryoprecipitate	
Whole blood	
Gamma globulin	
Allergen Extracts	
Skin-testing agents	
Desensitization	
Diagnostic Agents	
Bromsulphalein dye	
Iodinated contrast media	

manent health record, nursing Kardexes, and nursing care plans.

Special identification bracelets worn by the client at all times or signs placed on the client's bed also help. If the physician suspects a client might be allergic to a certain medication or substance, the physician will order an intradermal skin test. A localized reaction to such a test may be an indication that a more severe reaction will occur if the full dose is given.

Atopic allergies are less severe forms of type I response. These reactions commonly occur; 15 to 25 per cent of people in developed countries suffer from atopic allergies. Atopic allergies include hay fever (allergic rhinitis), some types of bronchial asthma, atopic dermatitis, some food and drug allergies, and urticaria. Urticaria is an area of localized edema and itching resulting from exposure to an allergen, most commonly a food or drug. Table 24-5 lists some clinical manifestations of allergic reactions to selected medications.

TYPE II CYTOLYTIC OR CYTOTOXIC HYPERSENSITIVITY

These reactions are complement-dependent and thus involve IgG or IgM antibodies. The antigen-antibody complex and complement attach to a cell, usually a circulating blood cell, with resultant cell lysis. During blood transfusion, blood group incompatibility causes cell lysis, which results in a transfusion reaction. The antigen responsible for initiating the reaction is a part of the donor red blood cell membrane.

Manifestations of a transfusion reaction result from intravascular hemolysis of red blood cells. They include

- headache and back pain (flank)
- chest pain similar to angina
- nausea and vomiting
- tachycardia and hypotension
- hematuria
- urticaria

Transfusions of more than 100 ml of incompatible blood can result in severe, permanent renal damage, circulatory shock, and death. Therefore, stop the transfusion immediately, maintain an open intravenous line, check the client's vital signs, and notify the physician immediately when these problems develop. For de-

TABLE 24-5. Clinical Manifestations of Allergic Reactions to Selected Medications

Drug	Systemic Manifestations	Cutaneous Manifestations
Penicillin	Anaphylaxis Serum sickness syndrome Pulmonary alterations (e.g., bronchial asthma) Vasculitis	Contact dermatitis Urticaria Rash Pruritus
Sulfonamides	Hepatic alterations Vasculitis Polyarteritis Renal disturbances Hematologic alterations	Rash Pruritus Exfoliative dermatitis Erythema multiforme Purpuric eruptions Photosensitivity
Salicylates	Bronchial asthma	Angioneurotic edema Urticaria Pruritus
Para-amino-salicylic acid	Fever Löffler's syndrome (pulmonary infiltrate with eosinophilia) Hepatic alterations Hematologic alterations	—
Phenytoin sodium (Dilantin)	Eosinophilia Lymphadenopathy Hepatic alterations	Erythema multiforme
Barbiturates	—	Rash Exfoliative dermatitis Fixed eruptions

tailed nursing interventions related to transfusion reactions, see Chapter 46.

TYPE III IMMUNE COMPLEX HYPERSENSITIVITY

Immune complex disease results from the formation or deposition of antigen-antibody complexes in tissues. The molecular size of the antigen-antibody complexes is an important feature in eliciting immune complex disease. Larger complexes are rapidly cleared by phagocytic cells. The smaller complexes formed in antigen excess persist longer in the circulation because they are not as easily captured by phagocytic cells in the spleen and liver. Inflammation results and leads to acute or chronic disease of the organ system in which the immune complexes were deposited.

Immune complex-mediated inflammation is produced by IgG or IgM antibodies, antigen, and complement. The mediators of inflammatory injury include the complement cleavage peptides, which can degranulate mast cells and basophils. Also, release of lysosomal granules from white blood cells and macrophages causes further tissue injury.

The antigen may be tissue fixed or released locally, as in Goodpasture's disease, in which circulating antibodies react with autologous antigens in the glomerular basement membranes of the kidneys and result in inflammation of the glomerulus. Alternatively, antigen-antibody complexes may form in the joint space, with resultant synovitis, as in rheumatoid arthritis. The antigen may also be circulating, as in serum sickness. Antigen-antibody complexes are formed in the bloodstream and get trapped in capillaries or deposited in vessel walls, causing urticaria, arthritis, arteritis, or glomerulonephritis. The Arthus reaction is a localized area of tissue necrosis that results from immune complex hypersensitivity.

Serum sickness is another type III hypersensitivity response, which develops 6 to 14 days after injection with foreign serum. Deposition of complexes on vessel walls causes complement activation with resultant edema, fever, inflammation of blood vessels and joints, and urticaria. Today, classic serum sickness is rare because large doses of heterologous sera (e.g., horse antisera to human lymphocytes) are seldom used.

However, the serum sickness-like reaction may occur after administration of such medications as penicillin, sulfonamides, streptomycin, thiouracils, and hydantoin compounds. Rather than being dominated by cutaneous vasculitis, these reactions more often manifest with fever, arthralgias, lymphadenopathy, and urticaria. This illness is usually benign and self-limiting. It resolves after the offending medication is discontinued.

Nursing care of the client with serum sickness depends on the severity of the reaction. For a mild reaction, care includes control of fever and pain with aspirin and antihistamines. A severe reaction may require steroids for control of the problem.

Serum sickness can be prevented by avoiding allergen exposure. Nursing assessment includes obtaining an allergic history and information about previous reactions to drugs or vaccines. Document findings in the client's chart, care plan, Kardex, and medication record so that risk of subsequent exposure is minimized.

TYPE IV CELL-MEDIATED OR DELAYED HYPERSENSITIVITY

In cell-mediated hypersensitivity, sensitized T cells respond to antigens by releasing lymphokines, which direct phagocytic cell activity. This reaction occurs 24 to 72 hours after exposure to an allergen. Delayed hypersensitivity is induced by chronic infection (e.g., tuberculosis) or by contact sensitivities, as in contact dermatitis.

Type IV reactions occur after the intradermal injection of tuberculosis antigen or purified protein derivative. If the client has been sensitized to tuberculosis, sensitized T cells react with the antigen at the injection site. The reaction leads to edema and fibrin deposits, which result in the induration characteristic of a positive tuberculosis reaction.

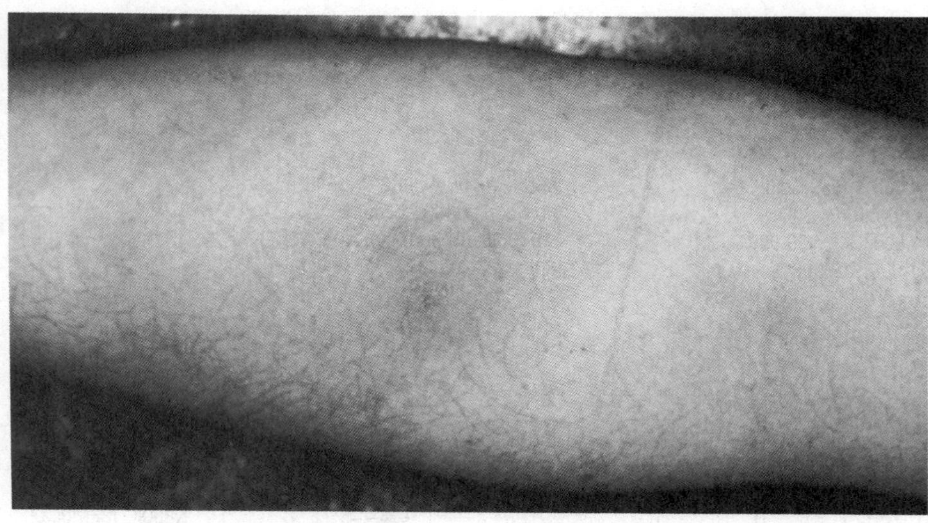

▲ *Figure 24-1*

Delayed hypersensitivity reaction. This positive reaction to intradermal challenge with tuberculin supplies a convenient window through which to observe the cell-mediated inflammatory processes at work. (From Dwyer, J. M. [1983]. The cell-mediated immune system. In Dwyer, J. M., et al., *Management of the immune-compromised patient.* Berkeley, CA: Pharmaceutical Division of Miles Laboratories, Inc.)

Graft-versus-host disease (GVHD) and transplant rejection are also type IV reactions. In GVHD, immunocompetent donor bone marrow cells (the graft) react against various antigens in the bone marrow recipient (the host), which results in a variety of clinical manifestations including skin, gastrointestinal, and hepatic lesions. Further details of transplant rejection and GVHD are discussed later.

Contact dermatitis is another type IV reaction that occurs after sensitization to an allergen, commonly a cosmetic, adhesive, topical medication, drug additive (such as lanolin added to lotions), or plant toxin (such as poison ivy). With the first exposure, no reaction occurs; however, antigens are formed. On subsequent exposures, hypersensitivity reactions are triggered, which leads to itching, erythema, and vesicular lesions.

Diagnostic Assessment

Laboratory tests also provide valuable data, especially when they are evaluated with consideration of a history of allergic responses. Common tests include assays of IgE levels: radioallergosorbent test, radioimmunosorbent test, and paper radioimmunosorbent test. These tests reveal elevated levels of IgE, but a normal or even decreased level may occur in IgE-mediated sensitivities. The last two tests are more sensitive. Elevated serum eosinophil levels also suggest hypersensitivities.

Pulmonary function studies may also be done to evaluate the status of the respiratory system from asthma attacks. Ventilatory capacity and lung volume are both abnormal in asthma. This test can also indicate the presence of complications such as pneumothorax.

In addition to blood tests, skin testing confirms sensitivity to a specific allergen. These tests involve placing a known antigen on or directly below the skin (intradermal) to check for the presence of antibodies. The antigen can be applied in one of three methods: scratch test, patch test, or intradermal test. In the first (also known as a tine or prick test), the allergen is applied to a superficial scratch that cuts the outer layer of skin. For a patch test, the antigen is directly applied to the skin and then covered with a gauze dressing. Intradermal testing involves injecting a small amount of the antigen into the intradermal layer of the skin. Intradermal testing is the most accurate method but carries a higher risk of severe allergic reactions.

Nurses often administer skin tests and interpret test results. To interpret results, observe for the following reactions. An immediate reaction (i.e., appearing within 10 to 20 minutes after the injection) marked by erythema and wheal formation denotes a positive reaction. Positive reactions indicate antibody response to previous exposure to this antigen and suggest the client is allergic to the particular substance causing the reaction (Fig. 24-1). Negative reactions may be inconclusive, indicating the need for further assessment. Negative results may indicate that (1) antibodies have not formed to this antigen, (2) the antigen was deposited too deeply into the skin (e.g., subcutaneously), or (3) the client is immunosuppressed from disease or therapies (e.g., chemotherapy, steroids, radiation therapy).

Problems arising from skin testing range from minor itching to anaphylaxis. Itching and discomfort at the injection site, for example, are common and can be relieved by the application of cool compresses and topical steroids. Ulceration of the injection site is best treated by keeping the area clean and dry.

Anaphylactic shock is a rare but potentially lethal complication of skin testing. A client with a history of an anaphylactic reaction to a substance should never be skin tested for an allergy to that substance. This is especially true of allergens such as penicillin that can produce lethal anaphylaxis in susceptible clients. Anaphylaxis is treated with emergency oxygen administration, epinephrine subcutaneously, intravenous aminophylline, and antihistamines intravenously as necessary.

Food allergies can be tested by skin testing or by either food challenges or an elimination diet. In the challenge test, suspected foods are given to the client in progressively larger doses until a reaction is evoked. Symptoms of a reaction range from the typical ery-

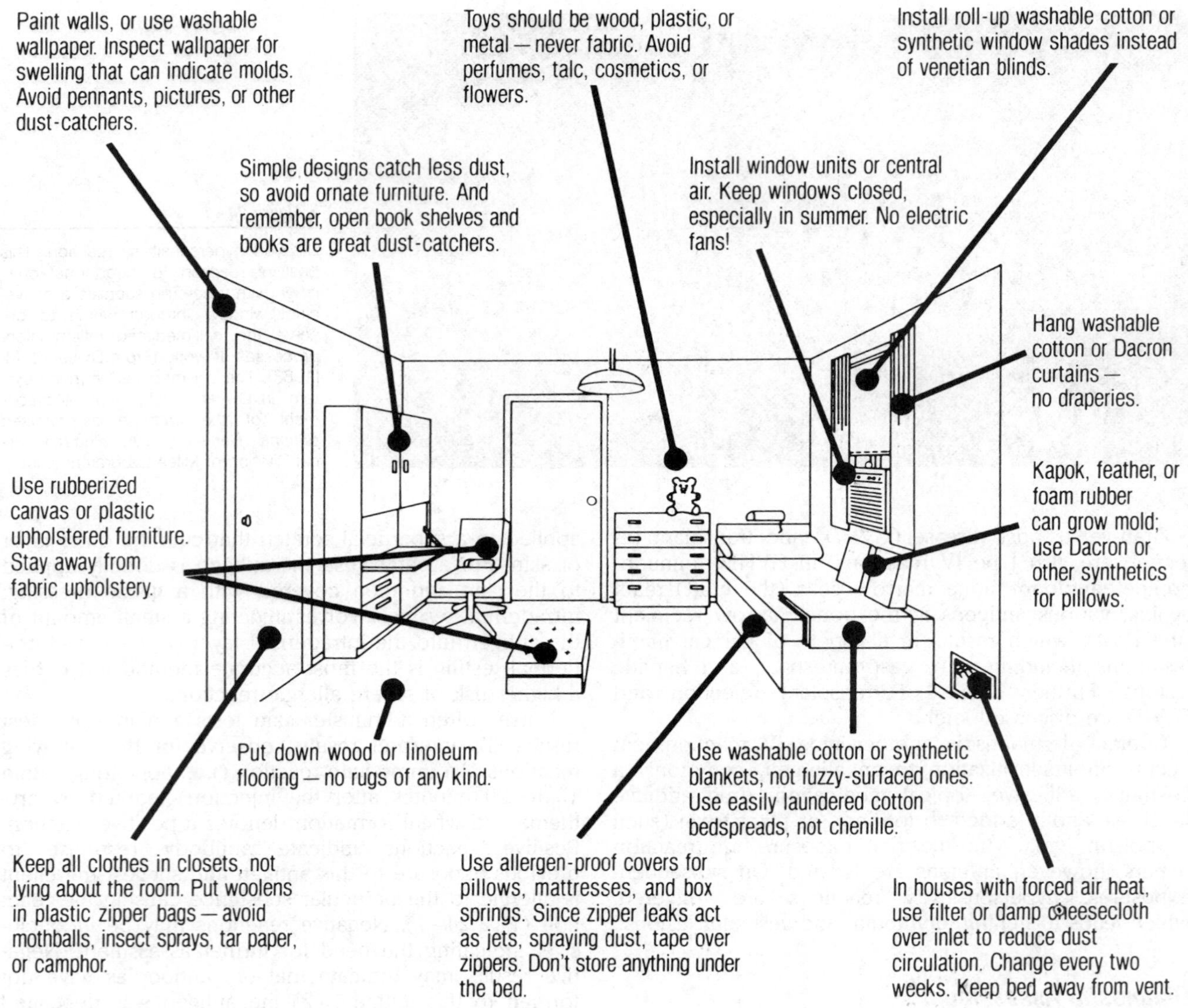

Paint walls, or use washable wallpaper. Inspect wallpaper for swelling that can indicate molds. Avoid pennants, pictures, or other dust-catchers.
Toys should be wood, plastic, or metal — never fabric. Avoid perfumes, talc, cosmetics, or flowers.
Install roll-up washable cotton or synthetic window shades instead of venetian blinds.
Simple designs catch less dust, so avoid ornate furniture. And remember, open book shelves and books are great dust-catchers.
Install window units or central air. Keep windows closed, especially in summer. No electric fans!
Hang washable cotton or Dacron curtains — no draperies.
Use rubberized canvas or plastic upholstered furniture. Stay away from fabric upholstery.
Kapok, feather, or foam rubber can grow mold; use Dacron or other synthetics for pillows.
Put down wood or linoleum flooring — no rugs of any kind.
Use washable cotton or synthetic blankets, not fuzzy-surfaced ones. Use easily laundered cotton bedspreads, not chenille.
Keep all clothes in closets, not lying about the room. Put woolens in plastic zipper bags — avoid mothballs, insect sprays, tar paper, or camphor.
Use allergen-proof covers for pillows, mattresses, and box springs. Since zipper leaks act as jets, spraying dust, tape over zippers. Don't store anything under the bed.
In houses with forced air heat, use filter or damp cheesecloth over inlet to reduce dust circulation. Change every two weeks. Keep bed away from vent.

▲ **Figure 24–2**

Controlling the environment of a room. (Courtesy of A. H. Robins Company, Richmond, VA.)

thema, itching, and rash to vomiting or diarrhea. Symptoms such as fatigue, depression, or restlessness are not conclusive of an allergy.

In the elimination diet, foods are eliminated from the diet one by one until the symptoms are relieved. This may indicate allergies to food additives or foods themselves.

Medical Management

Allergies are chronic problems that require prolonged and often multiple treatments. The client often requires a combination of treatments ranging from avoidance of known allergens to environmental control and immunotherapy.

Avoidance of the allergen is often the easiest, cheapest, and safest way of dealing with allergies. However, identification of the specific allergen is sometimes difficult, especially if the client refuses or cannot afford or locate allergen-testing services. Sometimes, even if the allergen can be identified, complete avoidance may not be possible, such as with pollens, dust, and some food additives.

Environmental control sometimes helps eliminate airborne allergens. Figure 24–2 illustrates ways to desensitize a room. These environmental controls, combined with air filters that remove small particles from the air, can help eliminate many allergens for the client.

PHARMACOLOGIC MANAGEMENT

Clients with atopic allergies can have their symptoms alleviated or controlled by many prescription and over-the-counter medications. Usually, clients will self-administer these agents, although in some settings the nurse or family members administer them. Instructing clients about these medications, however, is always an important nursing responsibility.

Antihistamines are the major group of prescription and over-the-counter drugs used to alleviate symptoms. These medications decrease sneezing, rhinorrhea, itching, and other symptoms of allergic rhinitis. Newer agents (such as terfenadine, Seldane) do not cause the drowsiness that limited the use of older medications.

Decongestants (oral sympathomimetics) help relieve the nasal congestion. These drugs can be combined with antihistamines to treat multiple symptoms of the allergy. The nasal sprays of these agents can be used for several days to treat the nasal congestion; however, overuse of these agents can lead to rebound congestion and exacerbation of the nasal symptoms secondary to chemical rhinitis.

Corticosteroids, anti-inflammatory agents, and immunosuppressant agents can be used to treat a variety of symptoms associated with allergies. Topical steroids can be used to treat dermatitis and other skin manifestations (i.e., urticaria). Beclomethasone dipropionate (Beconase) is a steroidal aerosol useful in treating allergic rhinitis. It has fewer side effects than dexamethasone does. This drug is also available via inhalation for asthma.

Cromolyn sodium is another topical or aerosol medication used to treat allergic rhinitis and asthma. It helps prevent the release of chemical mediators, such as histamine and leukotrienes from mast cells.

Immunotherapy (sometimes called desensitization therapy) is designed for type I, IgE-mediated hypersensitivity reactions. Precise doses of allergens are injected at intervals over a prolonged period. The doses are increased gradually over time. Immunotherapy increases IgG antibody levels and may increase suppressor T-cell function. It also decreases IgE binding to allergens. The decrease in IgE binding occurs because allergens bind more readily to IgG. Therefore, immunotherapy mitigates the hypersensitivity response. Although there is some controversy regarding the efficacy of this treatment, it is widely used. The greatest success has been achieved with allergic rhinitis (hay fever) and Hymenoptera sensitivity (bee, yellow jacket, wasp, and hornet stings).

Nurses often administer these injections and assess and treat side effects. Clients are asked to wait at least 20 minutes after receiving the injections so immediate reactions can be treated. Side effects are similar to those seen in skin testing. Sometimes, clients are taught to administer the desensitization injections to themselves. In this case, the nurse will teach clients proper injection technique and signs of any untoward reactions to the medication.

ORGAN TRANSPLANTATION

Histocompatibility

With recent advances in technology and immunology, organ and tissue transplantation is becoming commonplace. Thus, nurses need to (1) gain a clear understanding of the immunology on which this intervention is based and (2) learn how to assess and provide intervention for clients with their transplants. See the specific chapters (such as Chap. 50 for renal transplants) for specific information on each type of transplant.

There are several different types of transplant. *Syngeneic* transplants are between genetically identical members of the same species (identical twins); they are also called *isograft. Allogeneic* transplants are between individuals of the same species (e.g., human to human). *Autologous* transplants are grafts within the same species (e.g., skin graft from leg to hand, on the same client). *Xenogeneic* transplants are between individuals of different species.

In all cases of graft rejection, the cause is incompatibility of cell-surface antigens. As expected, there is a better chance of graft acceptance with autologous or syngeneic transplants, because the cell-surface antigens are identical.

A major role of the immune system is to distinguish between self and nonself. This fact is the major problem facing the candidate for transplantation: the immunologic response of the client to the donor's tissues. This ability to distinguish between self and nonself is central to proper immune function.

The identification process causes problems, however, when a tissue or organ from one client or animal (donor) is transplanted to another client or animal (recipient). In the immunocompetent recipient, the client's immune system recognizes the transplanted tissue or organ as "foreign" (nonself) and produces antibodies and sensitized lymphocytes against it. The cell-mediated delayed hypersensitivity response causes damage or destruction to the donated tissue. Graft rejection is the term describing the immune responses leading to graft destruction by the recipient's immune system.

The closer the match between the donor's and recipient's antigens, the less chance rejection will occur. Although many hundreds of antigens may differ between donor and recipient, certain antigens are critical for a successful transplant. These are (1) ABO and Rh antigens present on red blood cells and (2) histocompatibility antigens. Most important in this latter group is the human leukocyte antigen (HLA). To increase compatibility and decrease the chance of graft rejection, physicians and scientists attempt to match donors and recipients who have similar immune characteristics, especially those involving the ABO, Rh, and HLA antigens.

Genes in the area known as the major histocompatibility complex (MHC) on the sixth chromosome contain the human histocompatibility antigens. All people inherit one MHC zone from each parent. Histocompatibility antigens reside on the surface of most body cells. There are five specific HLAs within the MHC: HLA-A, HLA-B, HLA-C, HLA-D, and HLA-DR. HLA-A, HLA-B, and HLA-C are referred to as class I antigens and the others as class II antigens. Class I antigens are those recognized by the host during the rejection process. Class II antigens are found mainly on B cells, activated T cells, and macrophages. These antigens act to stimulate the proliferation of helper T cells, activating killer T cells, and antibody-producing B cells.

The process of finding compatible donors and recipients is called tissue typing. After tissue typing of the donor and recipient, the laboratory performs a matching procedure called the mixed lymphocyte culture. Various lymphocyte antibodies form after blood transfusions, pregnancy, (prior) exposure to foreign bodies, or infections. In the mixed lymphocyte culture, lymphocytes from the donor are mixed with serum from the recipient and then observed for immune responses. This test can determine whether antibodies incompatible with the donor have been formed by the recipient (a positive crossmatch). If the crossmatch is positive, the transplant will fail; therefore, a negative test is necessary for a successful transplant.

Graft Rejection

Rejection is actually the body's normal immune response to the invasion of foreign tissue (the transplanted tissue or organ). Although this response is normal, it is not the desired response after a transplant. The physiologic mechanisms in rejection (the normal immune response) involve B lymphocytes forming antibodies and T lymphocytes producing cell-mediated immunity. Acute rejection is caused by the T-lymphocyte activity and chronic rejection by that of B lymphocytes.

There are three basic kinds of rejection: hyperacute, acute, and chronic.

HYPERACUTE REJECTION

Allografts transplanted into presensitized recipients may be rejected very quickly. This rejection may occur from the time of the transplant up to 48 hours after the transplant. These recipients have preformed cytotoxic antibodies to donor antigens as well as sensitized lymphocytes, which reject the graft immediately. Rejection occurs before vascularization takes place.

The symptoms of hyperacute rejection include general malaise and high fever. In renal transplants, the kidney becomes infiltrated with leukocytes, which results in thrombosis of arterioles and glomerular capillaries. In cardiac transplants, the heart becomes hard and a mottled purple.

Hyperacute rejection is not treatable; removal of the rejected tissue or organ is the only way to stop the reaction. The client must then be maintained until another transplant can be arranged.

ACUTE REJECTION

This occurs usually within 3 months but may occur as late as 2 years after the transplant. The graft becomes vascularized in 2 to 3 days. In acute rejection, the response is primarily a cell-mediated one. The reaction begins when the recipient becomes sensitized to the donor antigens. Memory cells are formed that can trigger rapid rejection of a subsequent transplant of the same histocompatibility type.

In 6 to 10 days, the first signs of rejection may be observed. Sensitized lymphocytes and macrophages appear at the graft site. Later, the vascular bed itself begins to deteriorate, and the graft becomes necrotic.

Acute rejection is treatable with immunosuppressant medications including corticosteroids, azathioprine, cyclophosphamide, antithymocyte globulin (ATG), cyclosporin A, and OKT_3 (Table 24–6). Intravenous methylprednisolone sodium succinate (Solu-Medrol) is usually given first with good response (i.e., rejection reversed). Repeated episodes of acute rejection can lead to permanent damage of the organ.

CHRONIC REJECTION

Months or even years after the transplant, function of the transplanted tissue or organ may deteriorate gradually. The problem is a recurring, continuing problem. Antibodies and complement play a role in this type of rejection, causing arteriolar narrowing due to deposition of fibrin, platelets, and complement along vessel walls. The body tries to repair the endothelial damage that leads to intimal proliferation, necrosis, and collagen deposits, which further blocks circulation.

The symptoms of chronic rejection are related to deterioration of the organ function. In renal transplants, there is a gradual increase in serum creatinine and blood urea nitrogen, electrolyte imbalance, weight gain, hypertension, decreasing urine output, and peripheral edema. In cardiac transplants, there is myocardial fibrosis and increasing blockage of the coronary arteries, which leads to myocardial ischemia and infarction. In liver transplants, there is progressive thickening of the hepatic arteries and narrowing of the bile ducts, which leads to progressive liver failure. In pancreatic rejections, the vessels begin to thicken, which leads to fibrosis and a decrease in insulin secretion and hyperglycemia.

Clients with chronic rejection may be asymptomatic. Others will demonstrate symptoms directly related to failure of the transplanted organ.

Treatment is not usually successful for chronic rejection. It is a gradual, progressive deterioration. Antirejection medications may slow the process, so it is years before the organ fails completely and retransplantation is required.

Graft-Versus-Host Disease

A different type of rejection occurs when the transplanted material is an allogeneic bone marrow transplant. GVHD is a variation of the traditional graft rejection but involves the same immunologic principles. GVHD occurs with bone marrow transplantation in which immunocompetent donor cells are infused into an immunosuppressed recipient. Thus, if rejection occurs, it is the immunocompetent T lymphocytes from the graft (i.e., the donated marrow) rather than the host cells that cause the problem.

TABLE 24–6. Medications Used in Transplants

Medication	Action	Side Effects	Nursing Implications
Azathioprine (Imuran)	Inhibits DNA and RNA, blocks antibody production	Leukopenia, bone marrow depression, pancreatitis, liver dysfunction, immunosuppression	Monitor for signs of liver dysfunction; monitor CBC; warn client to avoid people with known infections; teach client signs of even mild infection to report; avoid IM injections if client is thrombocytopenic
Cyclosporine (Sandimmune)	Inhibits action of T lymphocytes and cell-mediated immunity	Hypertension, tremor, infection, gum hyperplasia, hirsutism, nephrotoxicity, hepatotoxicity, flushing	Monitor BUN and creatinine, liver function studies; always given in conjunction with corticosteroids; monitor levels of drug because oral absorption is erratic; give dose daily, at same time of day; give with meal to decrease nausea; comes suspended in olive oil, so administer in juice or milk, in glass so container does not absorb drug; stress to client importance of never varying or stopping medication without physician's approval
Antithymocyte globulin (ATG)	Either alters T-cell function or eliminates antigen-reactive T cells to inhibit cell-mediated immunity	Leukopenia, hemolysis, hypotension, chest pain, dyspnea, laryngospasms, nausea, vomiting, serum sickness (horse serum), anaphylaxis	Client should be skin-tested before first dose; do not use in clients allergic to horse serum; solution very heat-sensitive, keep refrigerated; monitor client for signs of infection; use filter when administering drug
Muromonab-CD3 (OKT_3)	IgG antibody, reacts in T-lymphocyte membrane to block T-cell function and proliferation; may reverse rejection, but carcinogenic and used with caution	Chest pain, fever, nausea, vomiting, severe pulmonary edema, dyspnea, increased incidence of malignant lymphomas	Used only in cases of acute rejection not responding to other agents; monitor cardiopulmonary system closely during administration; assess for signs of fluid overload; administer antipyretic before drug to decrease chills and fever
Methylprednisolone sodium succinate (Solu-Medrol)	Anti-inflammatory, prevents leukocyte infiltration during rejection, decreases antibody production and inhibits antigen-antibody reaction	Infection, delayed wound healing, peptic ulcers, hypertension, congestive heart failure, hypokalemia, weight gain, hyperglycemia; withdrawal symptoms if stopped suddenly	Monitor client for infection; teach client to prevent infection; tell client not to decrease or stop dose suddenly because of possibly life-threatening reaction; treat side effects symptomatically; give with food or antacids to prevent ulcers.
Cyclophosphamide (Cytoxan)	Action similar to azathioprine, used mainly when cyclosporine or azathioprine not tolerated	Bone marrow depression, leukopenia, nausea, vomiting, hemorrhagic cystitis, alopecia	Monitor for infection; teach client to avoid infections and notify physician at first sign of infection; increase fluid intake and encourage client to void every 2 hours; monitor CBC regularly

BUN, blood urea nitrogen; CBC, complete blood count; IM, intramuscular.

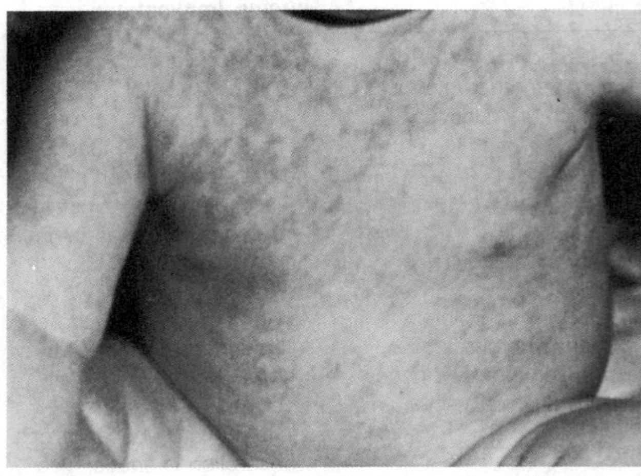

▲ Figure 24–3

Erythroderma of trunk and extremities in child with graft-versus-host disease.

GVHD has acute and chronic forms. Acute GVHD manifests itself as early as 1 to 100 days after transplant, with a peak time of onset in 30 to 50 days. Chronic GVHD usually occurs or persists later than 100 days. The major organs affected by GVHD are the skin, liver, and gastrointestinal tract. Skin involvement often begins with an erythematous rash, which may progress to a severe, sloughing stage. Figure 24–3 shows erythroderma of the trunk and extremities.

Abnormalities in liver function tests (as evidenced by increased liver enzymes and bilirubin), right upper quadrant pain, hepatomegaly, and jaundice signal liver involvement. Gastrointestinal tract manifestations of GVHD include nausea and vomiting, mild to severe diarrhea, malabsorption, ileus, and sloughing of intestinal mucosa.

Chronic GVHD resembles autoimmune collagen vascular disease, such as lupus erythematosus. Skin changes resemble scleroderma-like fibrosis. The same organs are affected in chronic and acute forms; however, in chronic GVHD, the changes are less than in the acute form.

Prevention of GVHD is similar to that of transplant rejection and involves immunosuppression of the recipient. For further information on bone marrow transplants, see Chapters 22 and 46.

Criteria for Transplantation

The basic criteria for transplantation include the following:

- The presence of end-stage disease in a transplantable organ.
- Failure of conventional therapy to treat the condition successfully.
- Progression of problems associated with the organ failure that in themselves may be fatal.
- The absence of untreatable malignancy or irreversible infection.
- The absence of disease that would attack the transplanted tissue.
- The client is able to survive the surgical procedure.

The first, fourth, fifth, and sixth criteria apply to all transplants, whereas the second is mainly for liver and heart, and the third for pancreas and kidney. Different institutions apply other criteria, such as age limits and the absence of drug or alcohol abuse.

For kidney transplants, the most common organ transplant procedure, the candidates have end-stage renal disease without systemic infection or major uncontrollable complication. For heart transplants, candidates have irreversible end-stage cardiac disease. Cardiomyopathy and left ventricular disease are the most common causes. The client should not have severe renal, pulmonary, or liver complications. Heart-lung transplant candidates have terminal cardiopulmonary disease or end-stage cardiac disease associated with severe pulmonary disease. The client should not have severe pulmonary hypertension or other serious organ failure.

Candidates for liver transplants suffer from end-stage liver disease, congenital biliary abnormalities, inborn errors of metabolism, chronic active hepatitis, sclerosing cholangitis, vascular disorders, fulminant disease such as hepatitis B, and cirrhosis. Clients with continuing alcoholism are evaluated carefully before transplant. If the clients are willing to enter substance abuse recovery programs, they are considered for transplant. Candidates for pancreatic transplants are usually diabetics who have progressive disease of other organs (kidney, heart) and are often also scheduled for kidney transplant.

Corneal transplants are done on clients with corneal opacity or ulceration. Skin transplants are typically done on clients with severe burns, which make autografts impossible. Bone marrow transplants are done for clients with leukemia, aplastic anemia, genetic hematopoietic disorder, or experimentally on others with late-stage malignant disease (however, these are usually autologous transplants). Criteria for selection of bone marrow transplant candidates are mainly based on the stage of disease and the potential for improvement.

Donor Procurement and Preparation

Organ procurement is a subject that makes many health care professionals uncomfortable. They hesitate to approach a family of a potential donor when the family is suffering the potential loss of their loved one. There is, however, a federal requirement that request protocols for donation exist in the hospital, or the hospital risks losing Medicare and Medicaid reimbursement. Most states now have laws requiring that families be given the opportunity for organ donation.

Families often have been very receptive to possible donation as a living memorial to their loved one. The approach must be sensitive, sincere, and stated in the most positive way possible. Many institutions have set up organ procurement nurses or teams that handle this process. The request for organ donation occurs only after the family has been completely informed about the hopelessness of the situation. The discussion can be initiated by asking the family if their loved one ever thought about organ donation and how they feel about this option.

Organ donors typically have been either living relatives or cadavers. More recently, however, living unrelated donors have been used for bone marrow transplants (see Chaps. 22 and 46). The most ideal living donor is an identical twin, who will have the same genetic make-up. Close relatives with similar genetic make-up are the most common living donors.

Cadaver donors are usually people who have died suddenly, often in accidents that spare the vital organs, who have signed organ donor cards or whose family gives permission for the donation. The organs are removed from cadaver donors when they are declared brain dead. The organs must remain viable until they can be used for transplant. The primary concern, at this point, is adequate perfusion of the organs. Once the family has agreed to the transplant, all costs are assumed by the organ procurement organization. There are many ethical considerations associated with donor procurement (see Ethical Issues in Nursing).

The potential donor, living or cadaver, must undergo thorough assessment for eligibility for donation to be determined. The donor must be free of communicable diseases, especially hepatitis B and HIV infection. The involved organ cannot be diseased; therefore, diabetics are often unable to donate most organs. The presence of a malignancy is also usually a contraindication, except the cornea and skin if they are not involved. Of course, the donor must be histocompatible with potential recipients.

Not all organs from a cadaver donor may be suitable for transplant. Heart donors should be less than 40 years old without cardiac disease or chest trauma. The heart has the shortest hypothermic preservation time (about 4 hours). Heart-lung donors are even harder to find because size is an additional criterion. The donor must also have good pulmonary function without history of any pulmonary disorder.

Kidney donors may be 1 to 65 years old, with normal renal function. Size is a problem only with children.

Liver donors can be living or cadaver. Live donors have been used for adult to child donations in the last few years. Liver donors must have well-perfused organs; therefore, only those on a ventilator with adequate perfusion are eligible. The donor should be less than 50 years old. MHC compatibility is not a concern for liver transplants because this does not seem to affect rejection. Size is important because the liver bed limits available space for transplantation.

Pancreas donors can be living or cadaver; therefore, the islet cells or distal pancreas can be taken from living relatives. Total pancreas transplants must come from cadaver donors. The donor must be younger than 55 years of age.

Bone marrow is transplanted only from living donors. For autologous transplants, the marrow is donated by the client, frozen, and then returned to the client after treatment.

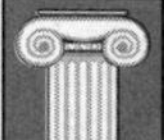

ETHICAL ISSUES IN NURSING

Do Transplant Clients Have an Obligation to Comply with Their Post-Transplant Self-Care?

The transplantation of human organs from one client into another is a major miracle of modern medicine. These transplants give life to clients who would surely die without such procedures. Although certain organ transplant operations are common these days, the postoperative course that transplant clients go through may be very complicated. Organ transplant clients must take medications for help in preventing rejection of the "foreign" part. These medications alter one's immune system, causing one to be immunosuppressed. The postoperative transplant regimen can be quite rigorous, and clients must be counseled regarding this before surgery.

All transplant clients feel a sense of gratitude for being given a second chance at life. Most usually follow their postoperative course of treatment rigidly. There will be times, however, that organ rejection will take place, even though everything was done by the clients as ordered. The dilemma faced by the health care providers of transplant clients has to do with clients who do *not* follow their postoperative treatment regimens or who abuse their bodies in such ways that may cause organ rejection. Examples of this include the liver transplant client who continues to drink alcohol or any transplant client who does not follow dietary and medication protocols. With limited availability of organs for transplant, should clients be strictly screened and those showing potential lack of postoperative treatment compliance be placed on a longer waiting list than those who show more promise in compliance with treatment orders? Do transplant clients, by accepting organs, have an obligation to take care of themselves as prescribed by their physicians in order not to "waste" their transplanted organs?

Nurses who care for posttransplant clients have a duty to reinforce their clients' treatment protocols. Those clients who choose not to comply with such protocols pose many challenges to the nurses caring for them. When clients do not comply with their treatments, nurses need to seek out reasons in order to identify problems. Perhaps a client's reason for noncompliance might be misunderstanding of the treatment, or perhaps there is a financial constraint that might need social work intervention. Nurses must be aware of potential problems due to possible lack of compliance in their clients in order that maximal benefit might come to such transplant clients.

All living donors must be in good health without severe disease. Kidney donors must have normally functioning kidneys. Kidney disease is often genetic, so with living donors, assessment must be made for the presence of the same genetic disorder. The donor's ability to withstand the transplant must be a prime consideration.

The nurse is responsible for continuing care of the potential cadaver donor so that the organs are maintained in prime condition. Continued evaluation will require that specimens be collected and that vital signs be assessed continually. A great deal of physical care is required for ensuring that the organs are adequately perfused, which includes managing parenteral fluids to maintain adequate blood pressure, medications, and ventilatory support. These potential donors are usually in critical care areas where they can receive continuous monitoring and care.

Many donors have suffered head injuries and require strict control of fluids for control of cerebral edema. The restriction of fluids often leads to a decreased perfusion of the kidneys and other organs. Once brain death has been established, the donor is rehydrated to improve perfusion. Antibiotics may also be initiated.

Living donors and the families of cadaver donors must be given a great deal of psychological support. The living donor often seems to be forgotten in the joy of a successful transplant. This client has undergone major surgery and requires expert physical and psychosocial nursing care. The families of cadaver donors often find the usefulness of their loved one's organs of help in their grief. These families should not be forgotten in the rush to transplant the organs successfully.

The organ to be transplanted is removed under sterile conditions for both living and cadaver donors. With living donors, the organ is transplanted immediately. With cadaver donors, once the organs are removed, they must be transplanted immediately or preserved at 4° C in a special electrolyte solution. The organs are then transported to the recipient's hospital as soon as possible for transplantation. The kidney can last about 48 hours with hypothermic preservation; the liver lasts 18 to 24 hours; the pancreas about 18 hours; and the heart-lung about 4 hours. Corneas and skin can be preserved for longer periods.

Nursing Management

PRETRANSPLANTATION

Before the transplant, the priority nursing intervention is to maintain the health of the recipient. The client's disease as well as any other problems that develop during the pretransplant period must continue to be vigorously treated. The client must be monitored closely for the development of any new problems and must be protected as much as possible from developing an infection or other problem that might delay the transplant. Clients should have careful dental screening and receive any needed treatment before the transplant. Also, any chronic condition, such as ulcers or gastritis, should be adequately treated before the stress of a transplant. Any condition that can be resolved before the transplant should be done because the immunosuppressed client will be at much greater risk from any disease after the transplant. The client should be in the best health possible for the transplant.

Immunosuppressants may begin before the transplant in some cases. In the case of clients undergoing bone marrow transplant, the recipient's marrow must be destroyed before the transplant (see Chaps. 22 and 46 for further information).

The psychosocial care of the transplant recipient is very important for the nurse. These clients are often very ill and may have some unrealistic expectations about the outcome. The nurse must listen closely to what the client is saying and what the client's expectations are. Many transplant programs include psychological evaluation and follow-up, but expert nursing care is of vital importance. All concerns are usually addressed in multidisciplinary conferences. The family or significant others should also be assessed for their coping abilities and strategies.

Once the decision is made to undergo transplant, the client is placed on a transplant list with others awaiting the availability of the same organ. This wait can be unbearable for the client and significant others. The client, however, must continue treatment of the underlying disease and maintain a high level of wellness.

One issue that is often discussed before the transplant is the client's ability to comply with therapy after the transplant. Often, it is the client's failure to comply with therapy that has led to the organ failure and the need for transplant. The question is raised whether this client is capable of compliance and, therefore, whether the client is an acceptable candidate. Organs are rare, and there are many needy candidates. An ethical question arises whether clients "responsible" for their own illness are appropriate transplant candidates. There is no one answer to this question. Clients are screened, and the reasons for past noncompliance are explored. If there is strong evidence that clients will not be able to comply with the complex posttransplant regimen, they will probably not be placed on the transplant list.

Nutrition is important before the transplant. Many clients may be malnourished and need extra vitamins and protein before the procedure. Liver transplant clients need to have the ascites reduced and may need total parenteral nutrition to reach a better physical condition for the transplant.

There is a great deal of teaching that must be done before the transplant. The client must be instructed in pulmonary exercises for preventing postoperative respiratory problems. Teaching about the posttransplant medication and treatment regimen is also begun preoperatively. The client should also be thoroughly taught about what to expect throughout the transplant, from the uncertainty of the waiting period to the intensive care required postoperatively. Some of the appropriate nursing diagnoses for transplant clients are in Box 24–5. Specific care for each type of transplant can be found in the appropriate chapter.

The financial impact of the transplant on the family and on society must also be considered. The transplant surgery is extremely expensive. Many clients are not employed at the time of the transplant, having left their jobs as their diseases progressed. Posttransplant medications alone may cost between $5000 and $10,000 a year. Many of these clients have only Medicare, and perhaps Medicaid, to provide insurance coverage. Those with coverage often find they have reached their policy limit.

Box 24–5. Common Nursing Diagnoses and Collaborative Problems for the Client Undergoing a Transplant

- ▶ Knowledge Deficit R/T transplant procedure, postoperative course, posttransplant self-care requirements, and medication regimen
- ▶ Anxiety R/T end-stage organ disease and pending transplant
- ▶ Breathing Pattern, Ineffective, High Risk for R/T surgical procedure and need for ventilator
- ▶ Fluid Volume Excess, High Risk for R/T postoperative fluid management
- ▶ Pain R/T surgical procedure
- ▶ Infection, High Risk for R/T immunosuppressant medications
- ▶ Individual and Family Coping, Ineffective, High Risk for R/T possible rejection phenomena
- ▶ Tissue Perfusion, Altered, High Risk for R/T leakage or thrombosis at graft anastomosis sites
- ▶ Injury, High Risk for R/T side effects of immunosuppressant medications
- ▶ Activity Intolerance R/T posttransplant weakness and fatigue
- ▶ Home Maintenance Management, Altered, High Risk for R/T posttransplant activity intolerance

In the United States, without national health insurance, many clients simply cannot afford transplants. Financial costs also affect the nation. In this time of increasingly scarce health care resources, the cost of a transplant and client maintenance must be considered. Many policy makers argue that the cost of transplantation is simply not worth the quality of life posttransplant recipients face. It is not an easy question, and there are no easy answers. Nursing research is being conducted in areas of quality of life after transplants to address some of these issues.

POSTTRANSPLANTATION

In many ways, care after a transplant is the same as the care after any major abdominal or cardiothoracic surgery (see Chap. 19). Infection control, however, is even more important for these clients because of the immunosuppression required by the transplant. Nosocomial (hospital-associated) infections can be fatal in these clients, so the nurse must be meticulous about preventing them. Strict aseptic technique must be used in working with these clients, especially with indwelling urinary catheters and intravenous lines.

A variety of complications, other than organ rejection, are possible after transplant (Table 24–7). These must be anticipated and, if possible, prevented. Postoperative nursing care of clients receiving specific transplants is discussed in the appropriate chapters.

Fluid and electrolyte balance is vital postoperatively. The client's intake and output must be measured carefully so signs of fluid imbalance can be diagnosed early and treated before complications occur. Fluid balance is monitored hourly in most clients and determined by subtracting output plus 500 ml for insensible fluid loss from intake for a 24-hour period. Wound care and care of all tubes are also vitally important. Tubes in transplant clients range from nasogastric to chest and other drainage tubes.

TABLE 24–7. Potential Posttransplant Complications

Organ	Potential Complications
Kidney	Rejection, fluid and electrolyte imbalances, acute tubular necrosis, posttransplant diabetes, problems related to immunosuppression (e.g., infections), renal artery thrombosis or leakage at anastomosis sites, decreased renal function, hypertension, renal abscess
Liver	Rejection, fluid and electrolyte imbalance, clotting disorders, posttransplant diabetes, problems related to immunosuppression (e.g., infections), hepatic artery or vein thrombosis or leakage at anastomosis sites, liver failure, subphrenic abscess, atelectasis and pneumonia secondary to ascites, peritonitis.
Heart (lung)	Rejection, posttransplant diabetes, problems related to immunosuppression (e.g., infections), thrombosis or leakage at anastomosis sites, heart (lung) failure, pulmonary hypertension, mental status changes, effusion
Pancreas	Rejection, problems related to immunosuppression (e.g., infections), thrombosis or leakage at anastomosis sites for total replacement, decreased pancreatic function, peritonitis, pancreatic abscess
Bone marrow	Graft-versus-host disease, clotting disorders, problems related to immunosuppression (e.g., infections), agranulocytosis, failure of engraftment

Client teaching about these potential problems is an important nursing function. The educational program for a transplant client is complex and often must be taught and mastered in a short time under less than ideal conditions. The nurse must do everything possible to facilitate client learning.

The focus of nursing care after transplant, in addition to the prevention of infection, is on the prevention of rejection. Early recognition of rejection leads to early treatment, which improves the chances that rejection can be reversed. The pathophysiology of rejection has been covered earlier in this chapter. The actual symptoms of rejection vary with the affected organ (see appropriate chapters for each specific organ).

All clients receive immunosuppressant therapy, but when rejection actually occurs, the doses of the immunosuppressants must be increased. The nurse must then watch the client closely for the side effects and potentially toxic effects of these medications.

Each medication administered has its own particular side effects (see Table 24–6). These drugs produce immunosuppression and, therefore, possible infection. Clients and significant others must understand their medications, the side effects, and adverse effects. Often clients with transplants are also taught to keep track of their own laboratory values as well as to understand them.

Clients on cyclosporine must be closely monitored for signs of nephrotoxicity. In renal transplant clients, this must be carefully differentiated from rejection. If the cyclosporine level is not elevated, then rejection is the possible cause of fever and graft tenderness.

When the immunosuppressant ATG is begun, the nurse must closely assess the client for anaphylaxis. Skin testing is usually done first to assess for possible allergy. The nurse should have diphenhydramine hydrochloride (Benadryl) and epinephrine on hand in case of an adverse reaction.

Psychosocial care is also extremely important at this point. The client often plummets from the joy of survival to the dark depression of possible rejection. The client needs a great deal of emotional support at this point and needs to focus on the reality of the situation. Clients often assume the worst once rejection begins, even if the rejection is minor and expected. If the rejection is serious, the client still needs to understand the reality of the situation and to receive help to understand it. Significant amounts of research have been done in this area.

Long-Term Follow-up Care

The posttransplant client requires follow-up care for a prolonged period. The client will continue immunosuppressant therapy, which can usually be gradually decreased over time.

Infection is one of the most serious prolonged problems after transplant. The client must be continually vigilant to avoid obvious potential sources of infection. This includes precautions such as avoiding crowds, wearing a mask when out in public, and immediately seeking treatment for even a minor infection. Prevention of infection, however, remains the priority.

Immunosuppressant medications have major side effects, and much of the posttransplant client's long-term care needs revolve around controlling these side effects. Clients must learn what to do to control these problems. The common side effects are given in Table 24–6. It is important to help the client understand that although the side effects from these medications can be severe and even fatal, these medications are necessary to maintain the viability of the transplant. The client must decide between the often distressing side effects of the immunosuppressants and survival of the transplant. Although this is discussed thoroughly before the transplant, clients often seem dismayed when reality sets in.

Future Considerations

The future for organ transplantation continues to grow. The use of living donors who share their liver, kidney, pancreas, or bone marrow with the recipient exemplifies this. As improvements in antirejection medications continue, transplants are increasingly successful with prolonged survival.

Renal grafts have a success rate of 85 per cent for the first year and about 60 per cent thereafter. Heart transplant survival has similar rates, with about 80 per cent success in the first year and 60 per cent after. Pancreatic transplants successfully produce insulin, which eliminates diabetes. Bone marrow transplants are very successful in good matches. Remember that GVHD and recurrence of the cancer in bone marrow transplants are the problems, rather than rejection. At present, there have not been enough heart-lung transplants to assess long-term survival and benefits accurately.

Liver transplants have previously not had good success in many clients because of the severity of illness before the transplant is performed. As these transplants have become more frequent, clients can be transplanted sooner before their health deteriorates completely. This has helped increase the survival rate in these clients.

The nurse has a major role to play in the future of transplantation. Nurses are becoming increasingly involved in procurement. Nurses also provide care to the potential donors in intensive care units. The nurse must provide increasingly complex care to keep the organs viable and then provide the complex care required by the recipient.

Organ transplantation will continue to grow in this country, and the nurse's involvement should grow with it. The role of the nurse in helping this client learn self-care is vital.

Summary

The immune system is a complex, interrelated system that affects the whole body. The nurse must understand this system in order to provide clients with complete and individualized care. This chapter covers a wide variety of disorders ranging from AIDS, to allergies, to transplantation. The care of these clients requires complex interventions for meeting the wide variety of problems they exhibit. The nurse must be able to plan and implement complex care to meet the needs of these clients.

Bibliography

1. American Hospital Association, American Medical Association, United Network for Organ Sharing (UNOS). (1988). *Required request legislation: A guide for hospitals on organ and tissue donation*. Richmond, VA: UNOS.
2. Anderson, J. A., & Adkinson, N. F., Jr. (1987). Allergic reaction to drugs and biologic agents. *Journal of the American Medical Association, 258,* 2834–2840.

3. Austen, K. F. (1987). Diseases of immune-mediated injury. In E. Braunwalk, et al. (Eds.), *Harrison's principles of internal medicine* (11th ed., pp. 1407-1414). New York: McGraw-Hill.
4. Barrett, J. T. (1988). *Textbook of immunology* (5th ed.). St. Louis: C. V. Mosby.
5. Bellanti, J. A. (1985). *Immunology III.* Philadelphia: W. B. Saunders.
6. Centers for Disease Control. (1987). Recommendation for prevention of HIV transmission in health care settings. *Morbidity and Mortality Weekly Report, 36*(Suppl. 2), 1-3.
7. Centers for Disease Control. (1987). Revision of the CDC surveillance case definition for acquired immunodeficiency syndrome. *Morbidity and Mortality Weekly Report, 36*(Suppl. 1), 3-15.
8. Centers for Disease Control. (1988). Update: AIDS worldwide. *Morbidity and Mortality Weekly Report, 37,* 286-295.
9. Centers for Disease Control. (1991). Women and AIDS: the growing crisis. *HIV/AIDS Prevention Newsletter, 2*(1), 1-19.
10. Cerilli, J. G. (Ed.). (1988). *Organ transplantation and replacement.* Philadelphia: J. B. Lippincott.
11. Chmielewski, C. (1987). Early recognition of infection after renal transplantation. *ANNA Journal, 14,* 389-391.
12. Claman, H. N. (1987). The biology of the immune response. *Journal of the American Medical Association, 258,* 3011-3031.
13. Colonna, J. O., et al. (1988). The quality of survival after liver transplantation. *Transplantation Proceedings, 20*(Suppl. 1), 594-597.
14. Condemi, J. J. (1987). The autoimmune diseases. *Journal of the American Medical Association, 258,* 2920-2929.
15. Costa, A. J. (1988). Anaphylactic shock: guidelines for immediate diagnosis and treatment. *Postgraduate Medicine, 83*(4), 368-373.
16. Creticos, P. S., & Norman, P.S. (1987). Immunotherapy with allergies. *Journal of the American Medical Association, 258,* 2874-2880.
17. Dault, L. A., et al. (1989). Reversing cardiac transplant rejection with orthoclone OKT_3. *American Journal of Nursing, 89,* 953-955.
18. Delafuente, J. C. (1985). Immunosenescence: clinical and pharmacologic considerations. *Medical Clinics of North America, 69*(3), 475-483.
19. Dickerson, M. (1988). Anaphylaxis and anaphylactic shock. *Critical Care Nursing Quarterly, 11,* 68-74.
20. Dindzans, V., et al. (1988). Medical problems before and after transplantation. *Gastrointestinal Clinics of North America, 17,* 19-31.
21. Farrell, M. L. (1987). Orthoclone OKT_3: a treatment for acute renal allograft rejection. *ANNA Journal, 14*(6), 373-376.
22. Flaskerud, J. H. (1989). *AIDS/HIV infection: A reference guide for nursing professionals.* Philadelphia: W. B. Saunders.
23. Flye, M. W. (Ed.). (1989). *Principles of organ transplantation.* Philadelphia: W. B. Saunders.
24. Fowler, M. B., & Schroeder, J. S. (1986). Current status of cardiac transplantation. *Modern Concepts of Cardiovascular Disease, 55*(8), 37-41.
25. Freedman, S. (1988). An overview of bone marrow transplantation. *Seminars in Oncology Nursing, 4*(1), 3-8.
26. Fuller, B. F. (1985). Organ graft rejection: the biological process. *AORN Journal, 14*(4), 738-745.
27. Gallo, R. C. (1988). HIV—the cause of AIDS: an overview on its biology, mechanisms of disease induction, and our attempts to control it. *Journal of AIDS, 1,* 521-535.
28. Gee, G., & Moran, T. (1988). *AIDS: Concepts in nursing practice.* Baltimore: Williams and Wilkins.
29. Grady, C. (1988). Host defense mechanisms: an overview. *Seminars in Oncology Nursing, 4*(2), 86-94.
30. Graziano, F. M., & Bell, C. L. (1985). The normal immune response and what can go wrong. *Medical Clinics of North America, 69*(3), 439-452.
31. Graziano, F. M., & Lemanske, R., Jr. (1989). *Clinical immunology.* Baltimore: Williams and Wilkins.
32. Griffin, J. (1986). *Hematology and immunology: Concepts for nursing.* Norwalk, CT: Appleton-Century-Crofts.
33. Gunderson, L. (1985). Teaching the transplant recipient. *The Journal of Heart Transplantation, 4*(2), 226-227.
34. Hathaway, D. K., et al. (1987). Psychosocial assessment of renal transplant recipients. *Dialysis and Transplantation, 16,* 442-444.
35. Hess, N. J., et al. (1985). Complete isolation: is it necessary? *The Journal of Heart Transplantation, 4*(4), 458-459.
36. Hofflin, J., et al. (1987). Infectious complications in heart transplant recipients receiving cyclosporine and corticosteroids. *Annals of Internal Medicine, 106,* 20-126.
37. Hoth, D. F., & Myers, M. W. (1991). Current status of HIV therapy: antiretroviral agents. *Hospital Practice, 1,* 94-117.
38. Katz, P. (1985). Clinical and laboratory evaluation of the immune system. *Medical Clinics of North America, 69*(3), 453-464.
39. Keown, P. A., et al. (1987). Cyclosporine: a double-edged sword. *Hospital Practice, 22*(5), 207-220.
40. Kusne, S., et al. (1988). Infections after liver transplantation: an analysis of 101 consecutive cases. *Medicine, 67,* 132-143.
41. Lichtenstein, L. M. (1988). Anaphylaxis. In J. B. Wyngaarden & L. H. Smith, Jr. (Eds.), *Cecil's textbook of medicine* (18th ed., pp. 1956-1958). Philadelphia: W. B. Saunders.
42. Lichtenstein, L., & Fauci, A. (1985). *Current therapy in allergy, immunology, and rheumatology.* St. Louis: C. V. Mosby.
43. Lockey, R. F., & Bukantz, S. C. (1987). *Principles of immunology and allergy.* Philadelphia: W. B. Saunders.
44. Maddeux, M. S. (1989). The pharmacology and complications of immunosuppressive therapy. *Problems of General Surgery, 6*(2), 85-96.
45. McGuire, T., & Almgren, J. (1987). Complications associated with bone marrow transplantation. *Highlights on Antineoplastic Drugs 3,* 16-20.
46. Meisenhelder, J. B., & La Charite, C. L. (1989). *Comfort in caring: Nursing the person with HIV infection.* Illinois: Scott, Foresman & Co.
47. Meister, N. D., et al. (1986). Returning to work after heart transplant. *Journal of Heart Transplantation, 5*(2), 154-160.
48. Migliori, R. J. & Simmons, R. L. (1988). Infection prophylaxis after organ transplantation. *Transplantation Proceedings, 20*(3), 395-399.
49. Mills, G., et al. (1985). An evaluation of an inpatient cardiac patient/family education program. *Heart and Lung, 14*(4), 400-406.
50. Montagnier, L. (1988). Origin and evolution of HIV's and their role in AIDS pathogenesis. *Journal of AIDS, 1,* 517-520.
51. Morris, P. J. (Ed.). (1988). *Kidney transplantation principles and practice* (3rd ed.). Philadelphia: W. B. Saunders.
52. Murdock, D. K., et al. (1987). Rejection of the transplanted heart. *Heart and Lung, 16*(3), 237-245.
53. Ota, B. (1983). Administration of cyclosporine. *Transplantation Proceedings, 15*(4), 3111-3123.
54. Randall, B. J. (1986). Reacting to anaphylaxis. *Nursing '86, 16*(3), 34-39.
55. Rao, K. V., & Anderson, R. (1988). Long-term results and complications in renal transplant recipients. *Transplantation, 45,* 45-52.
56. Richard, C. J. (Ed.). (1986). *Comprehensive nephrology nursing.* Boston: Little-Brown.
57. Rollins, B. J. (1986). Hepatic veno-occlusive disease. *American Journal of Medicine, 81,* 297-306.
58. Ruggiero, M. (1988). The donor in bone marrow transplantation. *Seminars in Oncology, 4*(1), 9-14.
59. Sande, M. A., & Volberding, R. A. (1990). *The medical management of AIDS* (2nd ed.). Philadelphia: W. B. Saunders.
60. Santangelo, J., & Schnack, J. (1991). Primary care intervention and management for adults with early HIV infection. *Nurse Practitioner, 16*(6), 9-15.
61. Schade, R. R. (1987). The changing indicators for liver transplantation. *Transplantation Proceedings, 19*(Suppl. 3), 2-6.
62. Sebesin, S. M., et al. (1987). Status of liver transplantation. *Annals of Surgery, 200,* 524-534.
63. Sechrest, L., & Pitz, D. (1987). Commentary: measuring the effectiveness of heart transplant programmes. *Journal of Chronic Disease, 40*(Suppl. 1), 155S-158S.
64. Selwyn, P. A. (1989). Issues in the clinical management of intravenous drug users with HIV. *AIDS, 3*(Suppl. 1), 201-206.
65. Simmons, R. G., et al. (1988). Quality of life after kidney transplantation. *Transplantation, 45,* 415-421.
66. Sinclair, B. P. (1991). Epidemiology and transmission of infection by human immunodeficiency virus. *NAACOG's Clinical Issues in Perinatal Women's Health Nursing, 1*(1), 1-9.

67. Smith, S. L. (1986). Immunosuppressive drugs used in clinical practice. *Critical Care Nursing Quarterly, 9*(1), 19–24.
68. Steinhiser, S. A., et al. (1987). OKT_3 for the treatment of patients with acute renal allograft rejection. *ANNA Journal, 14*(2), 127–129.
69. Stites, D. P. (1989). *Basic and clinical immunology* (6th ed.). Norwalk, CT: Appleton and Lange.
70. Tutschka, P. J. (1987). Complications of bone marrow transplantation. *American Journal of Medical Science, 294*(2), 86–90.
71. Widman, F. K. (1989). *An introduction to clinical immunology*. Philadelphia: F. A. Davis.
72. Williams, B. A. H., et al. (1991). *Organ transplantation: A manual for nurses*. New York: Springer.
73. Wyngaarden, J. B., & Smith, L. H. (1988). *Cecil's textbook of medicine* (18th ed.). Philadelphia: W. B. Saunders.
74. Unanue, E., & Benacerraf, B. (Eds.). (1984). *Textbook of immunology* (2nd ed.). Baltimore: Williams and Wilkins.

Chapter 25

Nursing Care of Clients with Infectious Diseases

For one brief moment in human history (circa 1950–1980), management of infectious disease did not dominate health care practice. During those years, morbidity and death from infectious diseases had plummeted as a result of multifaceted efforts in social, public health, and medical control. Environmental sanitation had curbed such killers as yellow fever, cholera, typhus, malaria, typhoid fever, and plague. International immunization programs had eradicated smallpox. Organized efforts to immunize all children lowered the occurrence of vaccine-preventable diseases, particularly measles, mumps, rubella, diphtheria, tetanus, and polio. Improved living conditions and personal hygiene had altered the occurrence of debilitating parasites and severe gastrointestinal infections. The widespread availability of sulfa and antibiotics quelled the fear of deadly tuberculosis, syphilis, gonorrhea, bacterial meningitis, scarlet fever, and rheumatic fever. Nosocomial (hospital-acquired) infections, which had earlier succumbed to medical asepsis, responded to further control with antibiotics; and medical technology continued to produce anti-infective agents to match the newly developing antibiotic-resistant organisms. Life for many was no longer determined by fear of infectious disease; thus, health professionals were allowed to turn their attention to preventing and managing chronic disease.

This brief moment in history did not last. The 1980s brought new infectious agents, such as *Legionella* and the human immunodeficiency virus (HIV), further reminders of human vulnerability to infectious disease. Hepatitis, tuberculosis, sexually transmitted diseases, and the vaccine-preventable diseases persist, spread, and continue to kill. Antibiotic-resistant organisms flourish, particularly in the hospital; and organisms that are normally nonpathogenic create devastating disease in the immunocompromised. In addition, many of the major killers of the past, such as cholera and yellow fever, continue to cause death and destruction in many parts of the world, thus reminding us of the need for vigilance everywhere.

All persons, particularly health care professionals, must maintain a vigilant attitude (see Ethical Issues in Nursing). Such an attitude centers on preventing infectious disease rather than relying on treating it. Prevention requires understanding of the infection process, the transmission chain, and the control measures that break the chain. This chapter describes the process of infection, the chain of transmission, and selected aspects of control. This chapter also presents tables on the chain of transmission of selected infectious diseases. These tables summarize major information highlighted in this chapter for each disease. The reader is referred to other chapters for information on nursing care of clients with specific infectious diseases.

THE PROCESS OF INFECTION

Infection is a process by which an organism establishes a parasitic relationship with its host. The process begins with transmission of an infectious organism (sometimes called an agent, pathogen, or pathogenic agent). Infection may end in infectious disease, a condition that depends on the response of the host to the invader. The entire process and its outcome hinges on a complex interaction of the pathogen, an environment conducive to transmission of the organism, and a susceptible human host. This agent, host, and environment interaction is a prerequisite to infectious disease occurrence, and all infectious diseases must be viewed in their unique multicausal context.

Even after successful transmission of a pathogen, the host may experience more than one possible outcome. The pathogen may merely contaminate the body surface. The process ends there if the host's first-line defenses, such as intact skin or mucous membranes, block the pathogen from further invasion. Successful invasion and replication of the pathogen is called colonization. The period of time when the pathogen is replicating but before it can be shed from the host is called the latent period. During latency, host inflammatory and immune responses may ward off the organism or its products, thus preventing tissue damage; or the pathogen or its products may begin destroying undefended or poorly defended tissue, producing infectious disease. Disease symptoms herald the end of the incubation period. By definition, infectious disease is the pathophysiologic response of a host to the destructive action of the pathogen, to its toxic products, or to the host immune responses to fight the pathogen. This pathophysiologic response is generally symptomatic. An asymptomatic pathologic response is called subclinical infection.

An important point to note is that an asymptomatic host can still transmit a pathogen. The host may harbor

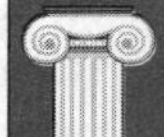

ETHICAL ISSUES IN NURSING

Do Health Care Workers Have the Right to Refuse Care to HIV-Infected Clients?

Infectious diseases have been around as long as human beings have been on earth. Most such diseases are no longer a threat to societies, thanks to years of research and modern medical technology. It was not until the discovery of the human immunodeficiency virus (HIV) in the early 1980s that such intense interest was restored to the study of infectious diseases, namely, the diseases that HIV caused—acquired immunodeficiency syndrome (AIDS) and AIDS-related conditions. The most frightening aspects of this virus continue to be that no one is immune to its destructive nature and, more important, that although medical research has discovered how HIV can be transmitted and has begun to provide treatment protocols, no effective treatment for the cure of AIDS or AIDS-related conditions has evolved. At present, the acquisition of HIV is ultimately fatal. The transmission of the virus poses potential risk to health care workers who provide care for clients infected with HIV. This risk, of course, depends on the *kind* of care provided, particularly if there is potential for the exchange of blood and body fluids.

The ethical question that must be addressed is whether health care workers have a right not to provide care to HIV-infected clients. This question is important for several reasons. One is the severity of the disease. Clients infected with HIV become very ill and are in great need of health care. Another reason is the fatal nature of the virus. In caring for an infected client, there may be a chance that this fatal disease could be transmitted to the health care worker. A third consideration is the availability of care—do all clients, no matter what the circumstances, have a right to health care? Also, do health care workers have a blind obligation to care for all clients, even if it places their own health at risk? On the other hand, do clients have the right to know the HIV status of their health care workers? Should HIV-infected health care workers be allowed to work, even if their work involves little or no risk of transmission of the disease to their clients?

The Centers for Disease Control (CDC) have set up guidelines for the care of all clients regarding precautions for the transmission of disease. These universal precautions should be used on all clients regardless of their disease status. If such precautions are used, the transmission of any disease by blood or body fluids is extremely limited. Nurses care for clients from all walks of life. Some clients may have the HIV virus and not know it. Some might have other diseases, such as hepatitis, which are similarly transmitted. It is of the utmost importance that nurses and all other health care providers exercise universal precautions with all clients.

Nurses do need to examine their own feelings about caring for clients who may have infectious diseases. There are no easy answers to the dilemmas that have surrounded HIV. Nurses and other health care workers do have an obligation to keep up with research regarding infectious diseases and should be responsible for taking appropriate precautions in caring for all clients. Such precautions are in the best interest of both the health care workers and the clients.

a pathogen in sufficient quantities to be shed at any time after latency and toward the end of the incubation period. This time period when an organism can be shed is called the period of communicability. It usually precedes symptoms and coincides with part or all of clinical disease, sometimes extending to convalescence. The communicable period, like the incubation period, varies with different pathogens and different diseases. The chain of transmission tables, which are presented later in this chapter, describe specifics on these time periods for each disease.

THE CHAIN OF TRANSMISSION

Infection begins with transmission of a pathogen to a new host. Determinants of successful transmission include a pathogenic agent, a reservoir, a portal of exit from the reservoir, a mode (mechanism) of transmission through the environment, a portal of entry into a new host, and a susceptible host. This sequence of events is called the chain of transmission. Each of the links in the chain is described.

Pathogen

Humans coexist with many microorganisms in complex, mutually beneficial relationships. Nonetheless, many organisms are parasitic, maintaining themselves at the expense of their host. Some parasites arouse a pathologic response in the host and are called pathogens or pathogenic agents. In one sense, pathogens are very ineffective parasites because they stimulate a disease response, which may harm the host and eventually kill the pathogen.

The ability of pathogens to elicit disease in the host explains why they are sometimes called etiologic agents of infectious disease. One must remember, however, that pathogens can produce disease only when the host is susceptible. Also, nonpathogens, that is, normal flora organisms, can also produce disease when the host is immunocompromised and defenseless. So, the etiology of infectious disease is always multicausal even though the term "etiologic agent" may be used to describe a pathogen. See the chain of transmission tables for the etiologic agents for each of the diseases summarized.

All microorganisms can be distinguished by certain intrinsic properties. These include shape, size, structure, chemical composition, antigenic make-up, growth requirements, viability under adverse environmental conditions, and ability to produce toxins. These properties provide the basis for identification and classification of organisms like bacteria, viruses, mycoplasmas, rickettsiae, chlamydiae, fungi, protozoa, and helminths. Knowledge of the properties permits diagnosis of a specific pathogen in specimens of body fluids, secretions, or exudates. The property of viability is important because it determines the pathogen's ability to survive in a free state outside its host. Viability is a function of how well an organism can withstand environmental conditions such as drying, sunlight, or heat. It is important in considering ways of interfering with the mechanisms of indirect transmission.

Pathogens also vary in how they interact with their human host. Means of interaction encompass the pathogen's mode of action, infectivity, pathogenicity, virulence, toxigenicity, and antigenicity. These are discussed next.

The mode of action of a pathogen refers to how the organism produces a pathologic process. There is great variation here. Some intracellular pathogens, like viruses, invade cells and interfere with cellular metabolism, growth, and replication, whereas others invade and cause hyperplasia, necrosis, and cell death. Some pathogens, such as tetanus bacillus, produce a toxin that interferes with intercellular responses. Others, such as group A beta-hemolytic streptococcus, stimulate a pathologic immune response in the host. Larger parasites, such as roundworms, interfere with the function of the whole gastrointestinal system. Some viruses, like cytomegalovirus, herpes, and varicella zoster, create a persistent latent infection. The deadly HIV virus causes immune suppression by destroying T-helper lymphocytes.

Infectivity refers to the pathogen's ability to invade and replicate in the host. The invasiveness of some pathogens is facilitated by enzymes produced by the organism. These enzymes dissolve host connective tissue or protect the pathogen from host defenses. Infectivity is high in measles because it takes very few viruses to establish infection. Infectivity is low in tuberculosis.

Pathogenicity is the ability of the organism to always induce disease. This depends on the organism's speed of reproduction in the host, the extent of tissue damage, and the strength of any toxin that is released. The rabies virus is highly pathogenic; infection with it always results in disease. Poliomyelitis virus and *Mycobacterium tuberculosis* have low pathogenicity.

Virulence refers to the potency of the pathogen in producing severe disease and is measured by case-fatality rate (the proportion of cases that die). Some pathogens, such as the rabies virus or HIV, are highly virulent. In contrast, herpes simplex and herpes zoster are much less virulent. Some pathogens have changed their virulence over time. Syphilis, for example, was frequently a fatal disease in medieval periods.

Toxigenicity, the amount and destructive potential of released toxin, is closely related to virulence. Some bacteria secrete water-soluble antigenic exotoxins that are quickly disseminated in the blood, causing potentially severe systemic and neurologic manifestations. Diphtheria and tetanus are examples of such a pathologic process. Endotoxins comprise the cell lining of some pathogens and cause local inflammation and destruction of the cells in which the pathogen invades. This is the case with *Shigella* and its action in the intestinal tract.

Antigenicity, the ability of a pathogen to stimulate an immune response in the host, varies greatly between organisms and with the site of their invasion and dissemination in the body. Generally, organisms that invade and localize in tissue initially stimulate a cellular (T-cell) response. Organisms that disseminate quickly stimulate a humoral or antibody response. Some organisms, such as the influenza virus, have the potential to alter their antigenic characteristics.

One additional characteristic of pathogens and their interaction with their host is worth noting. Many parasites have the ability to adapt to new hosts over time. An example is the plague bacillus, *Pasteurella pestis*. Before 1900, this organism resided in domestic rats and fleas. With environmental control of domestic rats, the bacillus has taken up residence in wild rodents and their parasites, thus maintaining its viability in nature.

Reservoir

A reservoir is an environment in which an organism can live and multiply. This can be a person, animal, arthropod, plant, soil, food, or other organic substance or combination of substances. The reservoir provides the essentials for survival of the organism at specific stages in its life cycle. Some parasites have more than one reservoir but require only one. An example is the yellow fever virus, which can maintain life in either humans or mosquitoes. A few parasites require more than one reservoir. Such is the case with *Schistosoma,* which is parasitic in snails and humans at different growth stages. Other parasites, such as most sexually transmitted organisms, require only a human reservoir.

Both human and animal reservoirs may be diseased and, therefore, also be hosts. If diseased, the host may be a symptomatic or asymptomatic case or be a carrier of the pathogen. A carrier maintains an environment that promotes growth, multiplication, and shedding of the parasite without exhibiting signs of disease.

Portal of Exit

The portal of exit is the place (and body secretions, excretions, or exudates) from which the parasite escapes the reservoir. Generally, this is the site of growth of the organism and corresponds to the system of entry into the next host. For example, the portal of exit for gastrointestinal parasites is generally the feces, and the portal of entry into a new host is the mouth. As is the case with other links in the transmission chain, there is variability here. Hookworm eggs, for example, are shed in the feces, but hookworm larvae enter through the skin of a person walking barefoot in soil containing hatched eggs. Common portals of exit include secretions and fluids (respiratory secretions, blood, tears, vaginal secretions, semen), excretions such as urine and feces, open lesions, and exudates. Some organisms, such as HIV, have more than one portal of exit. Knowledge of the portal of exit is essential for preventing transmission of a pathogen.

Mode of Transmission

Organisms can have one or more than one route of transmission from the reservoir to a new host. Two main routes are direct and indirect transmission. Direct refers to immediate transfer from one person to another as in sexual contact, biting, touching, kissing, or direct projection of respiratory mucous droplets. Indirect transmission implies a vehicle of transmission: a living vector, a common vehicle, or a fomite (inanimate object). Living vectors can carry the pathogen internally as a biologic vector or externally by mechanical means. Common vehicles include water, soil, food, milk, biologic products, and air. Airborne transmission requires that the pathogen survive in dried form in the air until it is inhaled. Fomites include inanimate objects like needles, eating utensils, and urinary catheters.

Portal of Entry

A pathogen may enter a new host by ingestion, by inhalation, through contact with mucous membranes, percutaneously, or transplacentally. There is variation with each infectious disease as to the number of organisms and the duration of the exposure required to start the infectious process in a new host.

Susceptible Host

When it comes to infectious diseases, not all humans are created equal; some are more susceptible than others. A susceptible host has personal characteristics and behaviors that increase the probability of an infectious disease developing. Biologic and personal characteristics such as age, gender, ethnicity, and heredity influence this probability. General health and nutritional status, hormonal balance, and the presence of concurrent disease also play a role. Likewise, living conditions and personal behaviors such as drug use, eating, hygiene, and sexual practices all influence the risk of exposure to pathogens and resistance once exposed. Susceptibility is also influenced by the presence of anatomic and physiologic defenses, sometimes called lines of defense.

The first-line defenses are external and act to bar invasion of pathogens. These defenses are nonspecific in that they act against any invading pathogen. First-line defenses include physical and chemical barriers and the body's own natural flora of organisms. Physical barriers include intact skin and mucous membranes; oil and perspiration on skin; cilia in respiratory passages; gag and cough reflexes; peristalsis in the gastrointestinal tract; and the flushing action of tears, saliva, and mucus. All act to remove organisms before they have an opportunity to invade. The chemical composition of body secretions such as tears and sweat together with the pH of saliva, vaginal secretions, urine, and digestive juices further prevents or inhibits growth of organisms. Compromise in any of these natural defenses increases host susceptibility to pathogen invasion.

Another important first-line defense is the normal flora of microorganisms that inhabits the skin and mucous membranes in the oral cavity, gastrointestinal tract, and vagina. These parasites are indigenous to specific tissue. They generally coexist with their host in a mutually beneficial relationship as long as they do not wander from the specific tissue. Through a mechanism called microbial antagonism they control the replication of potential pathogens. The importance of this mechanism is evident when it is disturbed. An example of disturbance is the overgrowth of *Candida albicans* (thrush) that results from extensive antibiotic therapy that destroys normal flora in the oral or vaginal cavity.

Some normal flora can become pathogenic under specific conditions, such as immunosuppression or displacement of the pathogen to another area of the body. The opportunistic infections experienced by clients with symptomatic HIV infection are an example of the former condition. The latter is seen when *Escherichia coli,* ordinarily normal flora in the gastrointestinal tract, becomes pathogenic when it invades the urinary tract. Displacement of normal flora is a common cause of nosocomial (hospital-acquired) infections. Invasive procedures increase the risk of displacing these organisms.

The second line of defense, the inflammatory process, and the third line, the immune response, share several physiologic components. These include the lymphatic system, leukocytes, and a multitude of chemicals, proteins, and enzymes that facilitate the internal defenses. For discussion of inflammation and wound healing, refer to Chapter 18. See Chapter 23 for description of the structure and function of the immune system.

CONTROL OF TRANSMISSION

Transmission of infectious disease can be controlled by breaking the transmission chain at only one link. The link most amenable to control varies with characteristics of the organism, its reservoirs, the type of pathologic response it produces, and available technology for control. In general, the aim is to break the chain at the most cost-effective point or points. That is the point at which the greatest number of people can be protected with available technology with use of the least amount of resources.

Some pathogens can be controlled by interventions directed at inactivating them through disinfection, sterilization, or use of anti-infective drugs. Such is the case with *Staphylococcus aureus*. Other pathogens can be controlled best by eradicating their nonhuman reservoirs. This is accomplished through environmental sanitation, particularly water treatment; food and milk safety programs; and control of animals, vectors, rodents, sewage, and solid wastes.

Transmission from the portal of exit can often be prevented by detecting and treating clients shedding a pathogen, such as gonococcus. Other prevention methods include proper handling and disposal of secretions, excretions, and exudates; isolation of infected clients; and quarantine of contacts. Specific isolation precautions, based on knowledge of the transmission chain for individual infections, have been recommended by the Centers for Disease Control (CDC). The precautions were designed to prevent transmission of pathogens among hospitalized patients, health care personnel, and visitors (see Box 25-1). The category-specific recommendations from the CDC (1983) together with the 1991 recommended universal precautions are given in Box 25-2 and Chapter 24. Specific recommendations for each disease are also highlighted in Tables 25-1 through 25-4.

Transmission to a new portal of entry can be prevented by environmental disinfection; use of barrier precautions (gloves, masks, condoms); proper handling of food, milk, and water; protection from vectors; personal hygiene and avoidance of high-risk behaviors (unsafe sexual practices, intravenous drug use, recapping needles); and effective *handwashing.*

Host susceptibility can be decreased through active and passive immunization, positive health practices, avoiding risky behaviors, and maintaining the first-line defenses. The last is an important consideration for the nurse caring for clients whose health status has already been compromised by disease or diagnostic and treatment procedures. Specifically, the nurse can strengthen

Text continued on page 590

Box 25-1. Methicillin-Resistant *Staphylococcus aureus*

Methicillin-resistant *Staphylococcus aureus* (MRSA) is a strain of staphylococcus that is resistant (cannot be killed) to antibiotics, including the aminoglycosides, penicillins, cephalosporins, and others. Over the past 10 years, MRSA and other resistant strains of *S. aureus* have become the most common causes of hospital- and community-acquired infections. MRSA is virulent and because of its resistance to antibiotics is a feared organism. MRSA usually develops when multiple antibiotics are used in the treatment of infection and in clients who are elderly, debilitated, having surgery or multiple invasive procedures, or being treated in critical care units. Unfortunately, inanimate objects can also serve as reservoirs for the bacterium. Items such as the telephone, sphygmomanometer, side rails, and tray tables have been infected.

Not only are clients at risk, but also health care providers can become "colonized" by the bacterium. The term "colonized" means that a healthy person carries the organism and potentially can infect others with it, although she or he does not feel ill.

MRSA is difficult to eradicate once it has been introduced into a hospital or nursing home by a client. A client infected with it is usually treated with intravenous vancomycin. Colonized carriers can be treated with a variety of medications including topical antibiotics for colonized nasal passages and shampoos with disinfectants for skin and hair colonization. Some health care providers have lost their jobs because of chronic colonization with MRSA.

It is perhaps more important to prevent MRSA, because it is not easily treated. Some suggested precautions include thorough handwashing with a mild iodine-containing soap and establishing community-wide infection control policies on the placement of clients who are infected with MRSA. Sometimes potentially infected clients are isolated when they are transferred to other agencies until all culture reports are returned. Honest reporting of infected clients would reduce unnecessary costs.

Box 25–2. Category-Specific Isolation Precautions

Strict Isolation

Strict isolation is an isolation category designed to prevent transmission of highly contagious or virulent infections that may be spread by both air and contact.

Specifications for Strict Isolation

1. Private room is indicated; door should be kept closed. In general, clients infected with the same organism may share a room.
2. Masks are indicated for everyone entering the room.
3. Gowns are indicated for everyone entering the room.
4. Gloves are indicated for everyone entering the room.
5. Hands must be washed after touching the client or potentially contaminated articles and before taking care of another client.
6. Articles contaminated with infective material should be discarded or bagged and labeled before being sent for decontamination and reprocessing.

Diseases Requiring Strict Isolation

Diphtheria, pharyngeal
Lassa fever and other viral hemorrhagic fevers, such as Marburg virus disease*
Plague, pneumonia
Smallpox*
Varicella (chickenpox)
Zoster, localized in immunocompromised client or disseminated

Contact Isolation

Contact isolation is designed to prevent transmission of highly transmissible or epidemiologically important infections (or colonization) that do not warrant strict isolation.

All diseases or conditions included in this category are spread primarily by close or direct contact. Thus, masks, gowns, and gloves are recommended for anyone in close or direct contact with any client who has an infection (or colonization) that is included in this category. For individual diseases or conditions, however, one or more of these three barriers may not be indicated. For example, masks and gowns are not generally indicated for care of infants and young children with acute viral respiratory infections; gowns are not generally indicated for gonococcal conjunctivitis in newborns; and masks are not generally indicated for clients infected with multiply resistant microorganisms, except those with pneumonia. Therefore, some degree of "overisolation" may occur in this category.

Specifications for Contact Isolation

1. Private room is indicated. In general, clients infected with the same organism may share a room. During outbreaks, infants and young children with the same respiratory clinical syndrome may share a room.
2. Masks are indicated for those who come close to the client.
3. Gowns are indicated if soiling is likely.
4. Gloves are indicated for touching infective material.
5. Hands must be washed after touching the client or potentially contaminated articles and before taking care of another client.
6. Articles contaminated with infective material should be discarded or bagged and labeled before being sent for decontamination and reprocessing.

Diseases or Conditions Requiring Contact Isolation

Acute respiratory infections in infants and young children including croup, colds, bronchitis, and bronchiolitis caused by respiratory syncytial virus, adenovirus, coronavirus, influenza viruses, parainfluenza viruses, and rhinovirus
Conjunctivitis, gonococcal in newborns
Diphtheria, cutaneous
Endometritis, group A streptococcus
Furunculosis, staphylococcal in newborns
Herpes simplex, disseminated, severe primary or neonatal
Impetigo
Influenza, in infants and young children
Multiply resistant bacteria, infection, or colonization (any site) with any of the following:

1. Gram-negative bacilli resistant to all aminoglycosides that are tested. (In general, such organisms should be resistant to gentamicin, tobramycin, and amikacin for these special precautions to be indicated.)
2. *Staphylococcus aureus* resistant to methicillin (or nafcillin or oxacillin if they are used instead of methicillin for testing).
3. *Pneumococcus* resistant to penicillin.
4. *Haemophilus influenzae* resistant to ampicillin (beta-lactamase-positive) and chloramphenicol.
5. Other resistant bacteria may be included if they are judged by the infection control team to be of special clinical and epidemiologic significance.

Pediculosis
Pharyngitis, infectious, in infants and young children
Pneumonia, viral, in infants and young children
Pneumonia, *Staphylococcus aureus* or group A streptococcus
Rabies
Rubella, congenital and other
Scabies
Scalded skin syndrome, staphylococcal (Ritter's disease)
Skin wound or burn infection, major (draining and not covered by dressing or dressing does not adequately contain the purulent material) including those infected with *Staphylococcus aureus* or group A streptococcus
Vaccinia (generalized and progressive eczema vaccinatum)

Respiratory Isolation

Respiratory isolation is designed to prevent transmission of infectious diseases primarily over short distances through the

*A private room with special ventilation is indicated.

Box 25–2. Category-Specific Isolation Precautions Continued

air (droplet transmission). Direct and indirect contact transmission occurs with some infections in this isolation category but is infrequent.

Specifications for Respiratory Isolation

1. Private room is indicated. In general, clients infected with the same organism may share a room.
2. Masks are indicated for those who come close to the client.
3. Gowns are not indicated.
4. Gloves are not indicated.
5. Hands must be washed after touching the client or potentially contaminated articles and before taking care of another client.
6. Articles contaminated with infective material should be discarded or bagged and labeled before being sent for decontamination and reprocessing.

Diseases Requiring Respiratory Isolation

Epiglottitis, *Haemophilus influenzae*
Erythema infectiosum
Measles
Meningitis
  Haemophilus influenzae, known or suspected
  Meningococcal, known or suspected
Meningococcal pneumonia
Meningococcemia
Mumps
Pertussis (whooping cough)
Pneumonia, *Haemophilus influenzae,* in children (any age)

Tuberculosis Isolation (AFB Isolation)

Tuberculosis isolation (AFB isolation) is an isolation category for clients with pulmonary tuberculosis who have a positive sputum smear or a chest film that strongly suggests current (active) tuberculosis. Laryngeal tuberculosis is also included in this isolation category. In general, infants and young children with pulmonary tuberculosis do not require isolation precautions because they rarely cough, and their bronchial secretions contain few AFB, compared with adults with pulmonary tuberculosis. On the instruction card, this category is called AFB (for acid-fast bacilli) isolation to protect the client's privacy.

Specifications for Tuberculosis Isolation (AFB Isolation)

1. Private room with special ventilation is indicated; door should be kept closed. In general, clients infected with the same organism may share a room.
2. Masks are indicated only if the client is coughing and does not reliably cover mouth.
3. Gowns are indicated only if needed to prevent gross contamination of clothing.
4. Gloves are not indicated.
5. Hands must be washed after touching the client or potentially contaminated articles and before taking care of another client.
6. Articles are rarely involved in transmission of tuberculosis. However, articles should be thoroughly cleaned and disinfected or discarded.

Enteric Precautions

Enteric precautions are designed to prevent infections that are transmitted by direct or indirect contact with feces. Hepatitis A is included in this category because it is spread through feces, although the disease is much less likely to be transmitted after the onset of jaundice. Most infections in this category primarily cause gastrointestinal symptoms, but some do not. For example, feces from clients infected with "poliovirus" and coxsackieviruses are infective, but those infections do not usually cause prominent gastrointestinal symptoms.

Specifications for Enteric Precautions

1. Private room is indicated if client's hygiene is poor. A client with poor hygiene does not wash hands after touching infective material, contaminates the environment with infective material, or shares contaminated articles with other clients. In general, clients infected with the same organism may share a room.
2. Masks are not indicated.
3. Gowns are indicated if soiling is likely.
4. Gloves are indicated for touching infective material.
5. Hands must be washed after touching the client or potentially contaminated articles and before taking care of another client.
6. Articles contaminated with infective material should be discarded or bagged and labeled before being sent for decontamination or reprocessing.

Diseases Requiring Enteric Precautions

Amebic dysentery
Cholera
Coxsackievirus disease
Diarrhea, acute illness with suspected infectious etiology
Echovirus disease
Encephalitis (unless known not to be caused by enteroviruses)
Enterocolitis caused by *Clostridium difficile* or *Staphylococcus aureus*
Enteroviral infection
Gastroenteritis caused by
  Campylobacter species
  Cryptosporidium species
  Dientamoeba fragilis
  Escherichia coli (enterotoxic, enteropathogenic, or enteroinvasive)
  Giardia lamblia
  Salmonella species
  Shigella species
  Vibrio parahaemolyticus
  Viruses—including Norwalk agent and rotavirus

Box continued on following page

Box 25–2. Category-Specific Isolation Precautions Continued

Yersinia enterocolitica
Unknown etiology but presumed to be an infectious agent
Hand, foot, mouth disease
Hepatitis, viral, type A
Herpangina
Meningitis, viral (unless known not to be caused by enteroviruses)
Necrotizing enterocolitis
Pleurodynia
Poliomyelitis
Typhoid fever *(Salmonella typhi)*
Viral pericarditis, myocarditis, or meningitis (unless known not to be caused by enteroviruses)

Drainage/Secretion Precautions

Drainage/secretion precautions are designed to prevent infections that are transmitted by direct or indirect contact with purulent material or drainage from an infected body site. This newly created isolation category includes many infections formerly included in wound and skin precautions, discharge (lesion), and secretion (oral) precautions, which have been discontinued. Infectious diseases included in this category are those that result in the production of infective purulent material, drainage, or secretions, unless the disease is included in another isolation category that requires more rigorous precautions. For example, minor limited skin, wound, or burn infections are included in this category, but major skin, wound, or burn infections are included in contact isolation.

Specifications for Drainage/Secretion Precautions

1. Private room is not indicated.
2. Masks are not indicated.
3. Gowns are indicated if soiling is likely.
4. Gloves are indicated for touching infective material.
5. Hands must be washed after touching the client or potentially contaminated articles and before taking care of another client.
6. Articles contaminated with infective material should be discarded or bagged and labeled before being sent for decontamination and reprocessing.

Diseases Requiring Drainage/Secretion Precautions

The following infections are examples of those included in this category provided they are not (1) caused by multiply resistant microorganisms; (2) major draining (and not covered by a dressing or dressing does not adequately contain the drainage) skin, wound, or burn infections, including those caused by *Staphylococcus aureus* or group A streptococcus; or (3) gonococcal eye infections in newborns. See contact isolation if the infection is one of these three.

Abscess, minor limited
Burn infection, minor limited
Conjunctivitis
Decubitus ulcer, infected, minor or limited
Skin infection, minor or limited
Wound infection, minor or limited

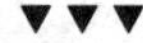

Centers for Disease Control (1983). *CDC guidelines for isolation precautions in hospitals.* HHS publication number CDC 83-8314. Atlanta: The Center.

TABLE 25–1. Chain of Transmission for Acute Bacterial and Viral Gastroenteritis

	Campylobacter Enteritis (Traveler's Diarrhea)	*E. coli* Diarrhea (Traveler's Diarrhea)	Shigellosis (Bacillary Dysentery)	Epidemic Viral Gastroenteritis	Rotavirus Gastroenteritis
Pathogen	*Campylobacter jejuni* and *C. coli*	Enterotoxigenic, invasive, or enteropathogenic strains of *E. coli*	Four different groups of *Shigella* bacteria, with many strains	Many viruses; Norwalk virus most common	Many types of rotaviruses
Reservoir	Domestic and wild animals and birds	Humans, who are often asymptomatic; cattle	Humans	Humans	Humans; pathogenicity of animal viruses undetermined
Transmission	Ingestion of water, food, or raw milk contaminated with organism from feces; contact with infected animals or infants; fecal-oral	Fecal contamination of food, water, baby formula, or fomites; transmitted to infant during delivery; fecal-oral, by hand	Direct or indirect fecal-oral transmission from infected person or carrier, usually by hand	Fecal-oral route; food-borne and water-borne transmission	Fecal-oral; possibly fecal-respiratory

TABLE 25-1. Chain of Transmission for Acute Bacterial and Viral Gastroenteritis Continued

	***Campylobacter* Enteritis (Traveler's Diarrhea)**	***E. coli* Diarrhea (Traveler's Diarrhea)**	**Shigellosis (Bacillary Dysentery)**	**Epidemic Viral Gastroenteritis**	**Rotavirus Gastroenteritis**
Host susceptibility	Persons of all ages	Infants very susceptible; travelers to developing countries; persons living in unsanitary conditions also susceptible; duration of acquired immunity unknown	Highest in children under 10 years old; outbreaks common in crowded living conditions, day care; more severe in children and elderly and debilitated persons; strain-specific antibodies develop	Infants and adults; short-term (14 weeks) immunity may follow infection with specific serotypes	Infants and young children; by age 3 years, most persons have acquired antibodies against most serotypes
Incubation period	3-5 days; range: 1-10 days	10-72 hours	12-96 hours	Usually 24-48 hours; range: 10-50 hours	24-72 hours
Period of communicability	Several days to weeks throughout course of infection; usually 2-7 weeks; carriers are rare	Duration of fecal excretion of organism, possibly weeks	During acute infection to 4 weeks after illness; carrier state may persist for months	During acute stage and up to 48 hours after diarrhea stops	During acute stage and as long as virus is shed (up to 30 days)
Isolation precautions	Enteric precautions for duration of illness		Enteric precautions until 3 fecal cultures are negative for *Shigella*	Enteric precautions for duration of illness	

Adapted from Grimes, D. (1991). *Infectious diseases*. St Louis: Mosby-Year Book.

TABLE 25-2. Chain of Transmission for Food-borne Diseases

	Staphylococcal Food Poisoning	**Botulism**	***Clostridium perfringens***	***Vibrio parahaemolyticus***	***Bacillus cereus***
Pathogen	Several enterotoxins of staphylococci; stable at boiling temperature	Toxins produced by *Clostridium botulinum* in anaerobic conditions; destroyed by boiling	Type A strains of *C. perfringens* (*C. welchii*)	*V. parahaemolyticus* (many types)	*B. cereus*, an aerobic spore-former that produces two enterotoxins—one heat-stable, causing vomiting, and one heat-labile, causing diarrhea
Reservoir	Humans; cows with infected udders; dogs and fowl	Soil, water, and intestinal tract of animals and fish	Soil and gastrointestinal tract of humans and animals	Marine silt, coastal waters, fish, and shellfish	Soil; commonly found in raw, dried, and processed foods
Transmission	Ingestion of food containing staphylococcal toxin, which formed while food was held at room temperature	Ingestion of food in which toxin has formed; generally home-canned vegetables, fruits, and meats; also onions and potatoes cooked and held at room temperature	Ingestion of food, especially meat, contaminated by soil or feces; spores survive normal cooking temperatures, germinate, and multiply during cooking and reheating	Ingestion of raw or undercooked contaminated seafood; food contaminated with seawater	Ingestion of food that has been kept at ambient temperatures after cooking, permitting multiplication of the organism

Table continued on following page

TABLE 25-2. Chain of Transmission for Food-borne Diseases Continued

	Staphylococcal Food Poisoning	Botulism	*Clostridium perfringens*	*Vibrio parahaemolyticus*	*Bacillus cereus*
Host susceptibility	All clients whose cooking practices favor growth of organisms in food; no immunity develops from exposure				
Incubation period	30 minutes–7 hours, usually 2–4 hours	12–36 hours	6–24 hours; usually 10–12 hours	4–96 hours; usually 12–24 hours	1–6 hours for disease causing vomiting; 6–20 hours for disease causing diarrhea
Period of communicability	Noncommunicable	Noncommunicable	Noncommunicable	Noncommunicable	Noncommunicable
Isolation precautions	None	None	None	None	None

Adapted from Grimes, D. (1991). *Infectious diseases.* St Louis: Mosby-Year Book.

TABLE 25-3. Chain of Transmission for Meningitis and Encephalitis

	Meningococcal Meningitis	Pneumococcal Meningitis	*Haemophilus* Meningitis	Viral Meningitis (Aseptic)	Viral Encephalitis
Pathogen	*Neisseria meningitidis*, with many subgroups	*Streptococcus pneumoniae*, many serotypes	*Haemophilus influenzae,* six serotypes; type B responsible for 90% of *Haemophilus* meningitis	Most viruses (e.g., mumps, herpes, and polio) produce the syndrome	A variety of viruses, commonly the *herpes virus*
Reservoir	Humans	Humans; many carriers	Humans	Humans	Humans
Transmission	Direct contact with droplets from respiratory passages of infected clients and carriers	Direct and indirect contact with discharges from respiratory passages	Direct contact with droplets from respiratory passages	Not transmitted at this stage	Direct contact with droplets from respiratory passages or other excretions harboring the virus
Host susceptibility	Children under 5 years and clients in crowded living conditions; susceptibility to clinical disease is low; many carriers; group-specific immunity of unknown duration follows infection	Infants and elderly most susceptible; follows pneumococcal pneumonia; immunity for specific type persists for years	Children 2 months to 3 years most susceptible; otitis media may be a precursor; immunity of unknown duration follows infection	Children, elderly, and immunocompromised clients and those unimmunized against vaccine-preventable viral diseases	Depends on viral disease
Incubation period	2–10 days; usually 3–4 days	1–3 days for pneumonia	2–4 days	Depends on virus and associated viral disease	Depends on viral disease
Period of communicability	Until organism is not present in discharges: within 24 hours of treatment with sulfonamides	Until organism is not present in respiratory discharges: 24–48 hours after antibiotic treatment	Prolonged; until organism is not present in nasal discharge		Depends on viral disease
Isolation precautions	Respiratory isolation for 24 hours after initiation of antibiotic therapy			Respiratory isolation for duration of hospitalization	

Adapted from Grimes, D. (1991). *Infectious diseases.* St Louis: Mosby-Year Book.

TABLE 25-4. Chain of Transmission for Streptococcal Throat, Scarlet Fever, and Rheumatic Fever

	Streptococcal Throat	Scarlet Fever	Rheumatic Fever
Pathogen	*Streptococcus pyogenes* (group A streptococcus of approximately 70 serologically distinct types)	Three erythrogenic toxins	Group A beta-hemolytic streptococcus
Reservoir	Humans	Humans	Humans
Transmission	Direct or intimate contact with person or carrier; may follow ingestion of contaminated food	Contact with respiratory secretions containing *Streptococcus*	Contact with respiratory secretions containing *Streptococcus*
Host susceptibility	Children age 3-15 years most susceptible	Permanent acquired immunity from active disease with type of toxin; second attacks due to different toxin	Persons who have suffered one attack are predisposed to a recurrent episode after group A streptococcal upper respiratory infections
Incubation period	1-3 days	2-4 days (range: 1-7 days)	3-35 days after clinical strep throat (average: 19 days)
Period of communicability	Untreated, uncomplicated cases: 10-21 days; complicated: weeks to months; antibiotic-treated: 24-48 hours	Not communicable	Not communicable
Isolation precautions	Respiratory isolation for 24 hours after onset of antibiotic therapy	None	None

Adapted from Grimes, D. (1991). *Infectious diseases.* St Louis: Mosby-Year Book.

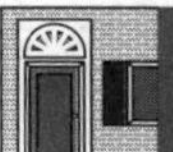

BRIDGE TO HOME HEALTH CARE

Infection Control

Preventing spread of the infectious disease to the family, the home health nurse, and perhaps the community, is the primary goal when preparing for the client to return to his or her home. The home environment of the client needs to be evaluated. The home health care nurse needs to consider what area of the home can best meet the client's total medical needs as well as what may be required to contain the infection. The nurse will need to work with the family in deciding these matters. In addition, evaluating the home will provide the nurse with an opportunity to teach the family about practical matters involved in caring for the family member with an infectious disease.

How the disease is transmitted from person to person is the basis for client and family education. For example, a feces-borne illness such as hepatitis A requires a good sewer system, easy access to toileting, and means to wash the hands.

The home health nurse who will be caring for the client on a regular basis needs to consider not only the safety of the client and his family but the nurse's safety as well. Some questions that should be asked are:

- How should needles and syringes be disposed of safely?
- How should soiled dressings and gloves be disposed of?
- How is equipment kept clean?
- How should hands be washed?

A list of helpful hints for home health care follows:

1. Handwashing is the best protection against transmission of infectious diseases, and it is essential after the nurse provides direct care and when gloves are removed.
2. Staff should leave extraneous clothing and equipment outside the client's area and take in only items that are needed.
3. Equipment needed on a regular basis such as the blood pressure cuff and stethoscope should be in the room at the beginning of home health care. When it is no longer needed, equipment should be bagged or covered and taken to the appropriate area for decontamination and reprocessing. Disposable equipment should be contained, labeled, and discarded.
4. The nursing case should be adequately supplied with gloves, masks, gowns, and disposable plastic aprons. Some plastic bags of different sizes should be carried for the nurse's own use as well as to demonstrate to the client's family how to handle soiled linens and trash.
5. Paper towels are useful when working in the client's area. The nurse can use them as a clean surface during care and to wipe the hands.
6. Before going into the client's area, the nurse should plan what will she be doing and gather the items needed.

Bridge to Home Health Care continued on following page

7. It is important to remember that isolation or precautions can have a negative effect on the family, resulting in depression. Help the family to feel comfortable with the techniques needed for isolation. Encourage them to visit with the client and not just to be with him or her during care.
8. Should the client have a feces-borne infectious disease such as hepatitis A or salmonellosis, it is important to show the family how to bag and launder soiled linens. It is equally important to demonstrate how to bag and dispose of soiled paper products such as linen savers that cannot be flushed down the toilet. Remind the family to wash their hands afterwards.
9. If the client has hepatitis A or salmonellosis, the family as well as the client should be reminded that he or she is not to handle raw food, such as lettuce or tomatoes, until the physician believes the client is past the infectious stage.
10. In treating clients with blood-borne illnesses, the family should be taught what to do if the client accidentally cuts himself or herself; for example, to clean the blood off the bathroom counter with household bleach and water. Sharing razors or toothbrushes should be discouraged.
11. Last, the nurse should protect herself at all times. Good handwashing practices and safe handling of needles are a must.

---

defenses of clients by providing preprocedure instruction and postprocedure assistance to encourage deep breathing, coughing, ambulation, bladder emptying, and asepsis of invasive sites. Turning and providing skin care to an immobilized client also protect the defenses. Maintaining hydration and electrolyte balance and ensuring adequate fluid and nutrition intake strengthen resistance. Administering anti-infectives as ordered and instructing clients and care givers on proper use of anti-infectives are important, not only in treatment but also in preventing drug resistance. In addition, using asepsis with all invasive procedures and avoiding all unnecessary invasive procedures are essential for preventing transmission of infection (see Bridge to Home Health Care).

Health professionals should be concerned about improving their own resistance and decreasing their own susceptibility to infectious diseases. One important approach is to maintain one's immunization status. This means being adequately immunized for hepatitis B, measles, mumps, rubella, polio, tetanus, and diphtheria. The 1991 CDC recommendations for immunization of health care workers are given in Table 25-5.

No infectious disease control program can be effectively implemented or evaluated without a mechanism for monitoring the occurrence of infectious diseases. That is why reporting infectious disease is so very important. According to government regulations, certain diseases must be reported to the local health authority. Some states require that additional diseases endemic to their area be reported. State laws vary regarding who is responsible for reporting. In general, the responsibility falls to physicians, laboratories, and others who are aware that a reportable disease has not been reported (nurses!).

Summary

Infectious diseases have been killers of humans throughout recorded history. For most of this time, except for a respite from circa 1950 to 1980, conquering infection has been the focus of health care.

The nurse's role in preventing, detecting, and treating infectious disease is a vital one. The nurse must be aware of the entire chain of infectious disease occur-

TABLE 25-5. 1991 CDC Recommendations for Immunization of Health Care Workers

Disease	Recommendation
Hepatitis B	Three-dose series of HB vaccine for pre-exposure protection
Polio	Primary series of oral poliovirus vaccine in childhood is sufficient
Tetanus/diphtheria	Booster dose of Td every 10 years after primary series of diphtheria and tetanus toxoids; tetanus toxoid may be repeated in 5 years if a dirty wound is sustained
Measles	College entrants and health care workers who do not have evidence of immunity to measles (physician-diagnosed measles or laboratory evidence of immunity) should have documentation of two doses of measles vaccine received on or after their first birthday; vaccine can be given as MMR*
Mumps	A single dose of live mumps vaccine received on or after the first birthday is sufficient; vaccine can be given as MMR*
Rubella	A single dose of live attenuated rubella vaccine received on or after the first birthday is sufficient; vaccine can be given as MMR*

*There is no evidence suggesting an increased risk from live measles, mumps, or rubella (MMR) vaccination to persons already immune to these diseases as a result of previous vaccination or natural disease.

From Centers for Disease Control (1991). Update on adult immunization: recommendations of the Immunization Practices Advisory Committee (ACIP). *Morbidity and Mortality Weekly Report, 40* (RR-12).

rence, especially transmission, so that steps can be taken to prevent accidental transmission. The nurse plays an important role in infection control, both in directly limiting the spread of disease and in teaching others how to avoid transmission. Clients are often discharged from health care facilities earlier than in the past, and it is important that the client and significant others understand infection control. The nurse must provide this information.

Bibliography

1. Benenson, A. (Ed.) (1990). *Control of communicable diseases in man* (15th ed.). Washington, DC: The American Public Health Association.
2. Centers for Disease Control (1983). *CDC guidelines for isolation precautions in hospitals*. HHS publication number CDC 83-8314. Atlanta: The Center.
3. Centers for Disease Control (1987). Recommendations for prevention of HIV transmission in health-care settings. *Morbidity and Mortality Weekly Report, 36*(2S), 3-17.
4. Centers for Disease Control (1989). 1989 sexually transmitted disease treatment guidelines. *Morbidity and Mortality Weekly Report, 38*(S-8), 1-43.
5. Centers for Disease Control (1991). Update on adult immunization: recommendations of the Immunization Practices Advisory Committee (ACIP). *Morbidity and Mortality Weekly Report, 40*(RR-12), 1-19.
6. Fox, J., et al. (1970). *Epidemiology, man and disease*. New York: Macmillan.
7. Fuerst, R. (1983). *Frobisher & Fuersts microbiology* (15th ed.). Philadelphia: W.B. Saunders.
8. Grimes, D. (1989). Potential for infection. In J. Thompson, et al. (Eds.), *Mosby's manual of clinical nursing* (2nd ed., pp. 1616-1618). St. Louis: C.V. Mosby.
9. Grimes, D. (1991). *Infectious diseases*. St. Louis: Mosby-Year Book.
10. Holmes, D., & Mardh, R. (Eds.) (1983). *International perspectives on neglected sexually transmitted diseases*. New York: McGraw-Hill.
11. Jawetz, E., et al. (1984). *Review of medical microbiology* (16th ed.). California: Lange Medical.
12. Shovein, J., & Young, M. S. (1992). MRSA: Pandora's box for hospitals. *American Journal of Nursing, 92*(2), 49-52.
13. Wehrle, P. F., & Top, F. W. Sr. (1981). *Communicable and infectious diseases* (9th ed.). St. Louis: C.V. Mosby.

Chapter 26

Nursing Care of Clients with Connective Tissue Disorders

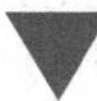

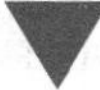

OVERVIEW

Connective tissue disorders (collagen diseases) include diseases such as rheumatoid arthritis, systemic lupus erythematosus (SLE), polyarteritis nodosa, polymyositis, dermatomyositis, and scleroderma. Genetic factors appear to be significant in the development of these conditions. They are also classified as autoimmune disorders.

Collagen diseases (1) produce widespread changes in collagenous connective tissue, (2) cause problems involving almost every organ, (3) may be autoimmune in nature, (4) are difficult to diagnose, (5) have no cure, and (6) are not preventable. Treatment for autoimmune conditions (mainly to control the symptoms) includes corticosteroids, ionizing radiation, and salicylates.

These conditions have features in common, and differentiation between them is often difficult. Common features include myocarditis, endocarditis, pericarditis, pleuritis, peritonitis, vasculitis, myositis, and sometimes, nephritis.

Laboratory tests may reveal Coombs-positive hemolytic anemia, thrombocytopenia, leukopenia, immunoglobulin excesses or deficiencies, antinuclear antibodies, antibodies to DNA and RNA, rheumatoid factors, false-positive serologic tests for syphilis, elevated muscle enzymes, and changes in acute phase-reactive proteins. Some of these laboratory findings also may occur in asymptomatic clients, suggesting the possibility of the presence or future development of a connective tissue disease.

Often anatomic, immunologic, and histologic findings overlap from one disease to another. Although serologic tests may help establish a differential diagnosis, they are not specific. The various conditions do tend to differ in their prognosis, clinical patterns, and response to treatment.

The term *autoimmunity* describes an inappropriate reaction by the immune system in which antibodies form against self-antigens, which are mistaken as foreign. Autoimmune responses are not as rare as once thought, and not all are harmful. For instance, autoantibodies may arise following tissue injury and may develop against cardiac muscle after myocardial infarction. Such antibodies help the body rid itself of damaged or necrotic self-components.

The term autoimmune disease implies that autoantibodies are important in the etiology or pathogenesis of the disorder. These diseases have been classified as systemic or organ specific (Table 26-1). Clients, particularly older ones, are often afflicted with one or more autoimmune diseases.

Etiology

The etiology of autoimmunity remains obscure, but five factors are thought to contribute to this state: (1) altered antigens, (2) cross-reactive antibodies, (3) viral factors, (4) hormonal factors, and (5) genetic factors. None of these elements are a complete explanation for autoimmune disease, but they do offer clues to the direction of future research in this area.

ALTERED ANTIGENS

Tissues may break down naturally, or in response to some stimulus, so autoantibody production may occur. Tissue injury may cause cells that do not normally circulate to be released into the bloodstream and to be recognized as foreign. For example, testicular cells, which do not normally circulate in the bloodstream, may be released after a vasectomy. They may elicit an autoantibody response because the immune cells do not recognize them as self, a normally circulating cell.

CROSS-REACTIVE ANTIBODIES

The body may elicit an immune response to a foreign antigen that is very similar structurally to a self-antigen. For example, the streptococcal antigen that causes rheumatic fever is very similar to heart tissue antigen. The antibodies produced to the streptococcal antigen may cross-react with heart tissue and damage the heart.

VIRAL FACTORS

Viruses may damage cells, allowing the release of antigens that do not normally circulate (i.e., causing altered antigens). Viruses also may damage the regulatory T cells, promoting faulty regulation of the immune response. The occurrence of multiple autoimmune disorders in the same client suggests a breakdown in suppressor T-cell activity.

HORMONAL FACTORS

Autoimmune diseases have a much higher incidence in women than in men. In SLE, for example, the female-to-male ratio is 10:1. This suggests hormonal influence on the immune response.

GENETIC FACTORS

Identical twins have a higher incidence of the same autoimmune disease than do nonidentical twins. Thus, it may not be simply environmental factors that lead to autoimmunity. Autoimmune disease increases with age, which may indicate that genetic errors accumulate in cells as one ages. It is known that regulatory T-cell function decreases with age, so there may be a link between the loss of this suppressor regulation and the development of autoimmunity.

Pathophysiology

There are three ways in which the autoimmune response causes disease: (1) the action of autoantibodies on cell surfaces, (2) the circulation and deposition of small immune complexes, and (3) the activation of sensitized T lymphocytes.

THE ACTION OF AUTOANTIBODIES ON CELL SURFACES

Destruction of cells or tissues occurs by direct antibody-mediated cellular cytotoxicity (e.g., autoimmune hemolytic anemia and thrombocytopenia), interference with receptors (e.g., myasthenia gravis and Graves' disease), or complement activation (e.g., basement membrane disease).

THE CIRCULATION AND DEPOSITION OF SMALL IMMUNE COMPLEXES

Soluble antigen-antibody complexes (made up of one antibody and one or more antigens) are small enough to invade and deposit in the capillaries (butterfly rash of SLE), the synovium of joints (rheumatoid arthritis), and the basement membrane of cells (as occurs with renal damage in SLE and Goodpasture's syndrome). These complexes cause tissue damage via activation of the complement system.

THE ACTIVATION OF SENSITIZED T LYMPHOCYTES

Sensitized T cells cause tissue destruction by the release of lymphokines (e.g., polymyositis).

RHEUMATOID ARTHRITIS

Definition

Arthritis is defined as joint inflammation. Rheumatoid arthritis (RA) is a chronic, systemic, progressive, inflammatory connective tissue disorder affecting mainly

TABLE 26-1. Autoimmune Diseases and Associated Antibodies

Automimmune Disease	Antibody
Organ-Specific Diseases	
Myasthenia gravis	Antibody to acetylcholine
Graves' disease	Thyroid-stimulating antibody
Hashimoto's thyroiditis	Antibodies to thyroglobulin and microsomal antigens
Insulin-resistant diabetes mellitus	Antibodies to insulin receptor
Insulin-dependent diabetes mellitus	Antibodies to islet cells
Pernicious anemia	Antibodies to gastric parietal cells and to vitamin B_{12}-binding sites of intrinsic factor
Addison's disease	Antibodies to adrenal cells
Idiopathic hypoparathyroidism	Antibodies to antigens of parathyroid cells
Spontaneous infertility	Antibodies to sperm
Premature ovarian failure	Antibodies to interstitial cells and corpus luteum cells
Pemphigus	Antibodies to intercellular substance of skin and mucosa
Bullous pemphigoid	Antibodies to basement membrane zone of skin and mucosa
Primary biliary cirrhosis	Antibodies to mitochondrial antigens
Autoimmune hemolytic anemia	Antibodies to red blood cells
Idiopathic thrombocytopenic purpura	Antibodies to platelets
Idiopathic neutropenia	Antibodies to neutrophils
Systemic Diseases	
Goodpasture's syndrome	Antibodies to basement membrane
Rheumatoid arthritis	Antibodies to gamma globulin and antinuclear antibodies
Sjögren's syndrome	Antinuclear antibodies, and autoantibodies against salivary duct antigens
Progressive systemic sclerosis (scleroderma)	Antinuclear antibodies, antibodies against the ribonuclease-sensitive component of ENA
Polymyositis	Antinuclear antibodies
Systemic lupus erythematosus	Antibodies to nuclear antigens, double-stranded and single-stranded DNA, ribonucleoprotein, ENA, RBCs, platelets, neuronal cells, and gamma globulin

ENA, anti-extractable nuclear antigen. Adapted from Stites, D.P., et al. (1984). *Basic and clinical immunology* (5th ed.). Los Altos, CA: Lange Medical Publications.

the small, peripheral joints in a pattern of symmetric distribution (Fig. 26-1).

Incidence

Women are affected with rheumatoid arthritis 2 to 3 times more often than are men; however, women who are taking or have taken oral contraceptives are less likely to develop RA. Although it may occur at any age, rheumatoid arthritis is most common in people between the ages of 20 and 40. The incidence of RA is about 1 to 3 per 100. It is characterized by unexplained periods of exacerbation and remission.

RA effects primarily synovial joints but also may involve the cervical spine and temporomandibular, sternoclavicular, manubriosternal, shoulder, elbow, hip, and ankle joints and the cricoarytenoid cartilages of the

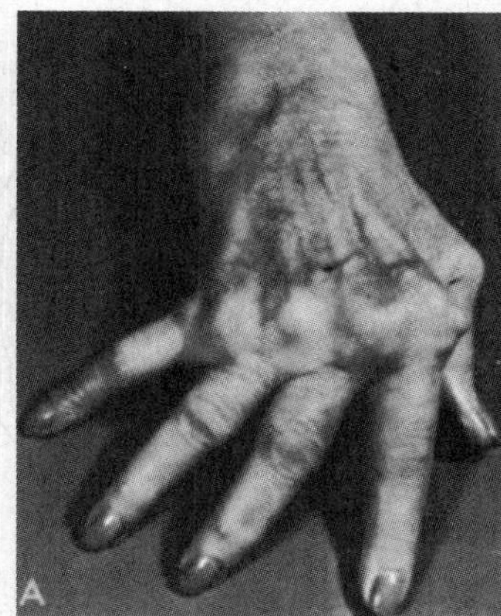

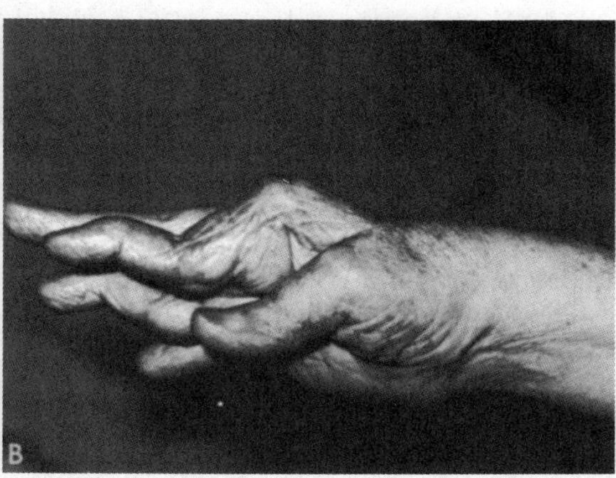

▲ *Figure 26-1*

Hand deformities characteristic of chronic rheumatoid arthritis. *A*, Subluxation of metacarpophalangeal joints with ulnar deviation (ulnar drift) of digits. *B*, Hyperextension ("swan neck") deformities of proximal interphalangeal joints. (From Wyngaarden, J. B., & Smith, L. H. Jr. [1982]. *Cecil Textbook of Medicine* [16th ed.] Philadelphia: W. B. Saunders Co.)

larynx. Articular and periarticular structures are progressively destroyed by chronic proliferative synovium, which replaces involved structures with granulation tissue.

Etiology

The etiology of RA is unknown, although there are many and varied theories about its cause. Some speculate that the disease is caused by (1) an unidentified virus or some other microorganism, (2) metabolic aberrations, or (3) immunologic mechanisms. A genetic basis may exist, and RA may be caused by a combination of factors.

The immunologic theory is currently the most prevalent. Rheumatoid factor, unusual antibodies of the IgM or IgG type or both, develops against the IgG antigens. These complexes lodge in the synovium and other connective tissues. The result is local and systemic inflammation.

Risk Factors

There are no specific risk factors for the development of RA. There are risk factors, however, for exacerbation of the disease, including the presence of physical and emotional stress. Controlling stress can help the client keep the disease in remission.

Pathophysiology

The pathologic process involved in RA are type III (immune complex) and type IV (cell-mediated) reactions. If unarrested, pathologic changes in RA pass through four stages (Fig. 26-2): (1) synovitis, (2) pannus formation, (3) fibrous ankylosis, and (4) bony ankylosis.

In stage 1, involved joint(s) become inflamed with a proliferative type of inflammation, initially localized in the joint capsule, primarily in the synovial membrane (synovitis). Tissue thickens with edema and congestion.

In stage 2, pannus gradually develops. This layer of inflammatory granulation tissue is derived from synovial membrane extending over the articular surface into the joint interior. It appears reddish and rough and adheres tightly to underlying cartilage by invasion and lysis, interfering with cartilage nutrition. Additional destruction may occur as pannus granulation develops on contiguous areas and in subchondral bone, progressively damaging the joint capsule and subchondral bone.

In stage 3, fibrous ankylosis, with subluxation and distortion of the affected joint, occurs as granulation tissue becomes invaded with tough fibrous tissue and is converted to scar tissue that inhibits or prevents joint movement.

In stage 4, bony ankylosis (firm bony union) may then develop as the fibrous tissue calcifies and changes into osseous tissue.

Although joint involvement is the most obvious manifestation of RA, other body tissues also are affected by this inflammatory process. RA is a systemic disease, attacking all connective tissue. Nonarticular connective tissue may be diffusely involved, such as, the collagen in lungs, heart, muscles, blood vessels, pleura, or tendons. Collagen is a scleroprotein present in connective tissue. Vasculitis may occur in the eyes, nervous system, and skin, producing thrombosis and ischemia.

As the disease destroys the joints, the client experiences pain, stiffness, and swelling. If the disease can be diagnosed early and treated successfully, permanent joint deterioration may not occur. About 25 per cent of clients with RA have a remission possibly lasting up to 25 years. Some clients experience spontaneous remissions without any treatment. It is difficult to predict the expected rate of disease progress. Many clients lead active, productive lives. With early, intensive treatment, only slight lifestyle modification may be needed. Some clients, however, seem to progress rapidly to deformity and limitation of joint movement in spite of aggressive therapy.

Clinical Manifestations

Figure 26-3 shows the common manifestation of RA. Even in well-established, chronic arthritis, the client typically has periods of increased and severe symptoms

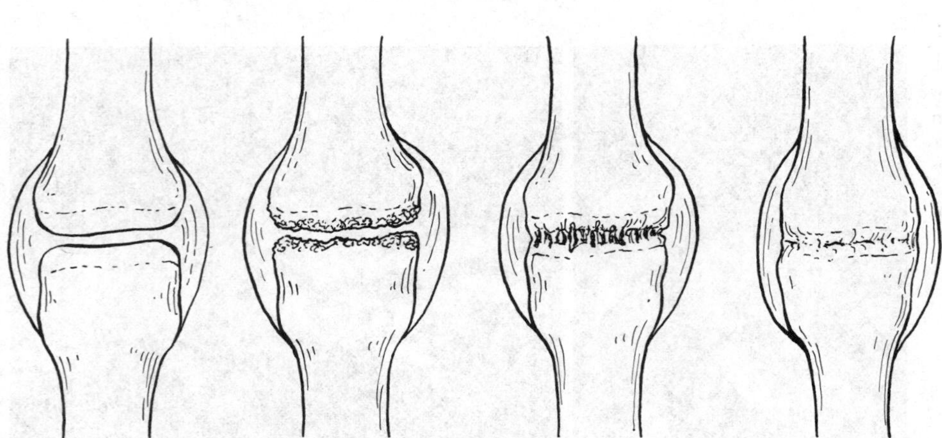

▲ *Figure 26-2*

Pathologic changes of the joint in rheumatoid arthritis. *A*, Joint capsule synovial inflammation with synovitis. *B*, Inflammation progression to pannus formation. *C*, Fibrous ankylosis. Inflammation subsided. *D*, Bony ankylosis. (See text.)

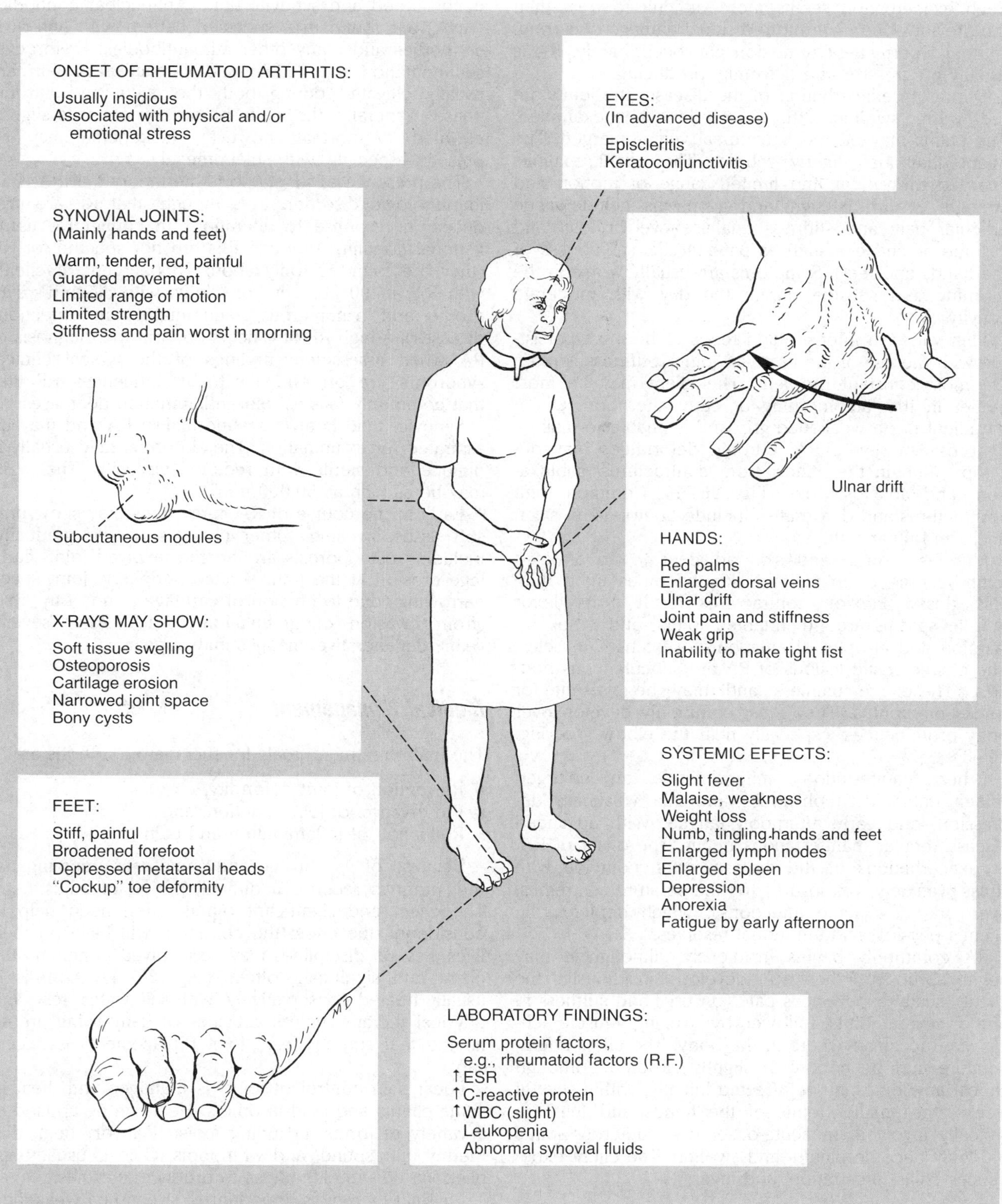
ONSET OF RHEUMATOID ARTHRITIS:
Usually insidious
Associated with physical and/or emotional stress
EYES:
(In advanced disease)
Episcleritis
Keratoconjunctivitis
SYNOVIAL JOINTS:
(Mainly hands and feet)
Warm, tender, red, painful
Guarded movement
Limited range of motion
Limited strength
Stiffness and pain worst in morning
Ulnar drift
Subcutaneous nodules
HANDS:
Red palms
Enlarged dorsal veins
Ulnar drift
Joint pain and stiffness
Weak grip
Inability to make tight fist
X-RAYS MAY SHOW:
Soft tissue swelling
Osteoporosis
Cartilage erosion
Narrowed joint space
Bony cysts
SYSTEMIC EFFECTS:
Slight fever
Malaise, weakness
Weight loss
Numb, tingling hands and feet
Enlarged lymph nodes
Enlarged spleen
Depression
Anorexia
Fatigue by early afternoon
FEET:
Stiff, painful
Broadened forefoot
Depressed metatarsal heads
"Cockup" toe deformity
LABORATORY FINDINGS:
Serum protein factors,
e.g., rheumatoid factors (R.F.)
↑ESR
↑C-reactive protein
↑WBC (slight)
Leukopenia
Abnormal synovial fluids

▲ Figure 26–3

Common assessment findings in rheumatoid arthritis.

and times of relative comfort and remission. Remissions occur most often, however, early in the disease. Each exacerbation seems more difficult to treat than the previous one, with more residual damage occurring. Although permanent remission can occur rarely, RA is usually progressive and deformity producing.

During an exacerbation of the disease, the joints are red, warm, swollen, stiff, and tender when examined. The palms may be red and dorsal veins enlarged. The client may be slightly febrile. The client exhibits guarded movement and limited range of motion and strength. Prodromal signs and symptoms include vague articular pain and stiffness, malaise, weight loss, and vasomotor changes such as paresthesias (numbness of the hands and feet). Symptoms are usually worse in the morning and subside during the day with moderate activity.

Pain varies in intensity and tends to be most persistent with the use of the involved joints. Stiffness is often the most constant problem. The client may be most limber in the late morning or early afternoon. Often, the client has a weakened grip and is unable to make a tight fist. In severe RA, chronic deformities may develop, often in the hands, from contractures, subluxation, and ankylosis (see Fig. 26–1). Common joint contractures and deformities include boutonnière, swan neck, and ulnar drift.

Muscles, bones, and skin adjacent to an affected joint become atrophic, and skin becomes tight, thin, and glossy. Flexion contractures result from flexor muscle spasms around inflamed joints, and reflex relaxation and atrophy of antagonistic extensor muscles. The characteristic lesions of RA are subcutaneous nodules. These are painless and may be present for weeks or months. They most commonly develop over bony prominences, especially near the elbow (see Fig. 26–3).

Other manifestations may include an enlarged spleen, enlarged lymph nodes, anorexia, weakness, depression, and early afternoon fatigue. With advanced disease, ocular manifestations occur. The onset of RA, or exacerbations of the disease, often coincide with stress (anxiety, exposure to temperature extremes, overwork, and acute infections), which depletes the client's physical and emotional reserves.

RA commonly begins insidiously, although it may begin abruptly. When RA develops insidiously, the client usually experiences pain (on use) and stiffness in one or several joints, followed by swelling. Muscle aching may occur anywhere in the body. The client's temperature may be normal or slightly elevated. Although almost any joint may be affected initially, within several weeks, the smaller joints of the hands and feet are typically involved. In acute-onset RA, numerous joints suddenly become painful and swollen. The client experiences chills, prostration, and fever.

DIAGNOSTIC ASSESSMENT

Laboratory findings help establish a diagnosis of RA. Serum protein abnormalities are often present, such as rheumatoid factors (RFs) (large protein molecules). Specifically, 7S and 19S IgM and 7S IgG RF are found in the blood and synovial fluid. Antinuclear antibodies (ANA) are found in a speckled pattern with anti-DNA antibodies and many other autoantibodies. Erythrocyte sedimentation rate (ESR) and C-reactive protein are usually elevated during both the acute and chronic phase. Generally, the white blood cell count is slightly elevated or normal; however, leukopenia may be present, especially with splenomegaly.

The presence of RF supports the theory that RA is an immunologic disorder. It is thought that RF are produced in response to alterations in connective tissue gamma globulin. Although RFs are not specific for RA (they are found in only about 75 per cent of clients with RA, in 90 per cent of clients with Sjögren's syndrome, and in numerous granulomatous and infectious diseases), a high RF titre helps confirm the diagnosis of RA when assessment findings of the typical clinical syndrome are present. Treatment influences RF titer that commonly falls as joint inflammation decreases.

Synovial fluid is always abnormal in RA and may be aspirated for examination. The abnormal fluid usually is opaque and sterile with reduced viscosity. The WBC may be as high as 50,000/mm^3.

Early in the course of RA, x-ray films may show only soft tissue swelling. Other changes appear gradually, including osteoporosis around the involved joint, cartilage erosion at the joint surface periphery, joint space narrowing (due to erosion of cartilage), and bony cysts (from invasion of granulation tissue). After several years, degenerative changes may appear.

Medical Management

The main treatment goals for rheumatoid arthritis are

- ▸ Prevention of joint deformity,
- ▸ Preservation of joint function, and
- ▸ Reduction of inflammation and pain.

Because of its chronic and sometimes crippling nature, arthritis requires a difficult period of adjustment. The client and significant others often need help in considering the effect the condition will have on their lives. Several disciplines may be involved in helping the client and significant others (Fig. 26–4). Arthritis is usually treated conservatively, with salicylates, rest, and physical therapy, unless activities of daily living are so limited that surgery (e.g., joint replacement) is necessary.

Local pain control of joints is managed with heat in some clients and cold in others. Heat can be applied in a variety of forms, including moist heat, dry heat, diathermy, ultrasound, and whirlpools. Cold is usually applied via crushed ice packs to produce anesthesia.

Physical therapy is important to strengthen weakened muscles and improve function. Deformities can be minimized and corrected by an active positioning and exercise program. Pain can be controlled by teaching clients how to regulate activities in ways that will not

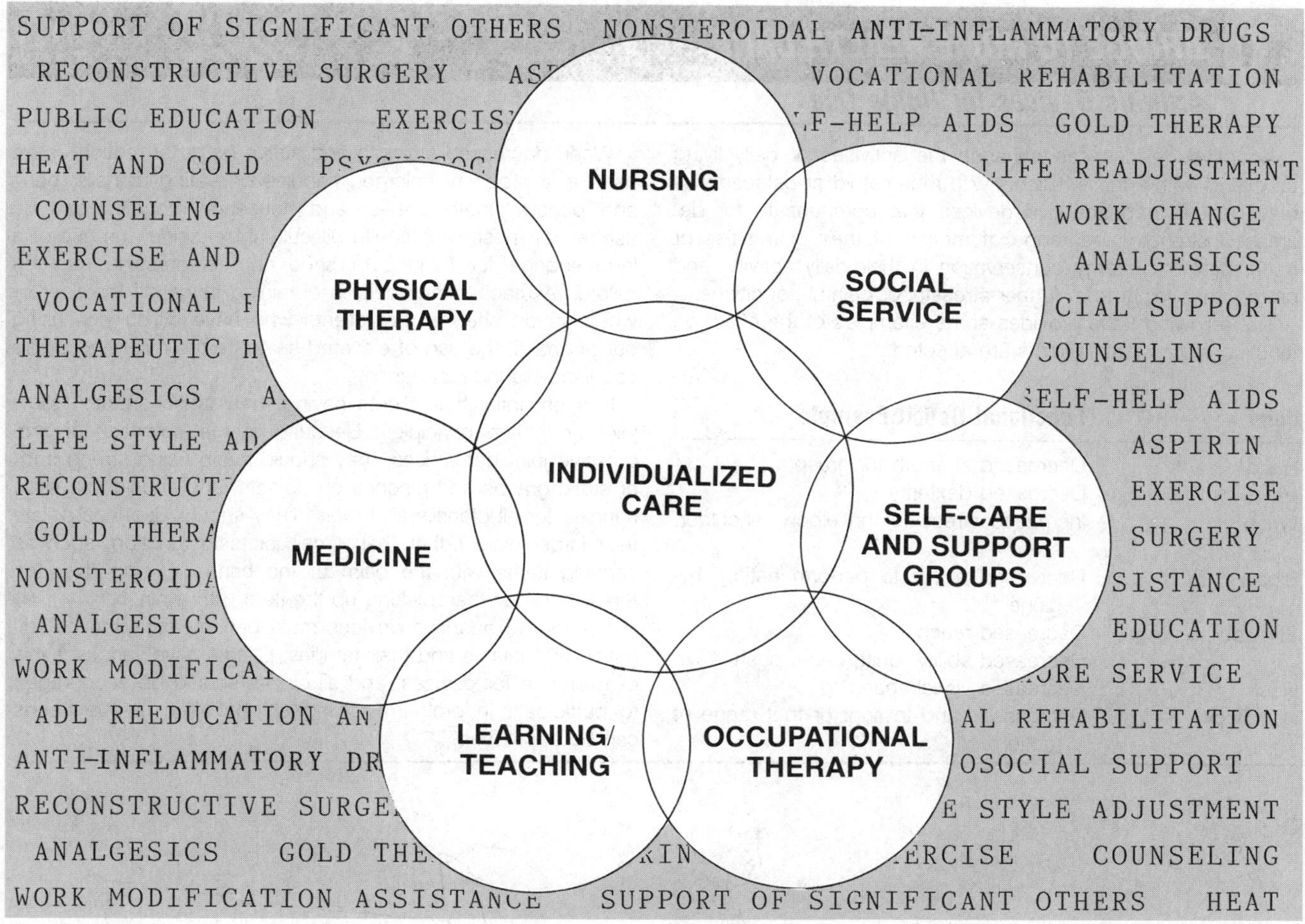

▲ *Figure 26–4*

Circles of care for a person with rheumatic diseases.

increase pain. Clients can be taught isometric exercises and progressive resistance methods of isotonic strengthening exercises.

Most clients with arthritis do not need assistive devices to help with activities of daily living, but these may be used occasionally if severe loss of range of motion occurs. Many such aids are available, including devices that assist a client to grab, hold, and carry objects or to cut food (see Bridge to Home Health Care). A client with limited shoulder, elbow, wrist, or hand movement may find dressing difficult. Careful selection of clothing is important, especially the choice of closing and fastening mechanisms. In general, zippers are easier to manage than snaps or buttons. Clothing is now available with Velcro fasteners, which are ideal for clients with arthritis. Grooming aids are available to help with combing hair, brushing teeth, shaving, and clipping nails.

Continuous immobility can increase pain. Exercise of all joints can actually relieve pain (Fig. 26–5). Because clients often hesitate to move as a result of fear that pain will increase (and it does hurt more at the start of exercise), emphasize to the client and significant other the importance of exercise. It may be helpful to take aspirin 1/2 hour before exercising, providing the client does not overexercise, because aspirin raises the pain threshold. Isometric exercises are important in maintaining muscle function even when splints are applied. When there is only slight joint involvement, isotonic exercises are best. Exercises are the most important single part of the physical therapy program for a client with rheumatoid arthritis.

When correctly performed, massage may help relieve pain and muscle aching. *Never massage acutely inflamed joints* because it may aggravate inflammation. Instruct clients because they may have a tendency to rub inflamed, aching joints. The client should massage over surrounding muscles, not over joints.

Occupational therapy also should be involved in the care of the client with RA. Occupational therapy can provide the client assistance with activities of daily living. They also can provide splints and other assistive devices to help the client function as normally as possible.

PHARMACOLOGIC MANAGEMENT

Medication may be prescribed to decrease inflammation and reduce pain.

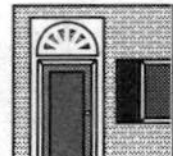

BRIDGE TO HOME HEALTH CARE

Arthritis Devices for Home Use

Adaptive devices can enhance the activities of daily living for clients with arthritis. Clients with rheumatoid or osteoarthritis may benefit from adaptive devices that compensate for decreased strength and range of motion of their extremities or trunk, promote energy conservation in their daily activity, and protect their joints from further stressful or painful conditions.

The following table provides some examples of the effect on function when specific joints are affected:

Joint	Functional Deficit Example
Hand	Decreased strength for grasp Decreased dexterity
Wrist	Increased stress to the elbow, shoulder, spine
Elbow	Decreased ability to perform eating, hygiene
Shoulder	Decreased reach Decreased ability to lift, carry, push
Neck	Decreased visual scanning
Hip, Back	Decreased hand to floor or foot range of motion

When decreased strength and active range of motion of the hand is a problem, enlarged handles on eating utensils, pens and pencils, toothbrushes, and household handles can be useful. For those clients with difficulty in reaching, the use of a long sponge for bathing or shoe horn in dressing may be helpful. A reacher may help in obtaining items off the floor or when up on shelves. For clients who have difficulty in rising out of chairs, the use of elevated seats on the toilet and chairs can increase independence.

It is essential that clients having rheumatoid arthritis follow joint protection principles. Because of the potential for progressive joint deformities, they should avoid using strong and/or static grasps and pinches on objects, and should use large handles for all utensils and tools. They should also incorporate their large joints rather than small joints in function, such as carrying items with the palm of the hand or hung over the forearm, rather than picking up the item with a pinch.

The use of adaptive devices must be determined in coordination with clients and their families. Clients have various levels of tolerance for devices, and all clients should be encouraged to participate in problem solving so that their unique needs can be addressed.

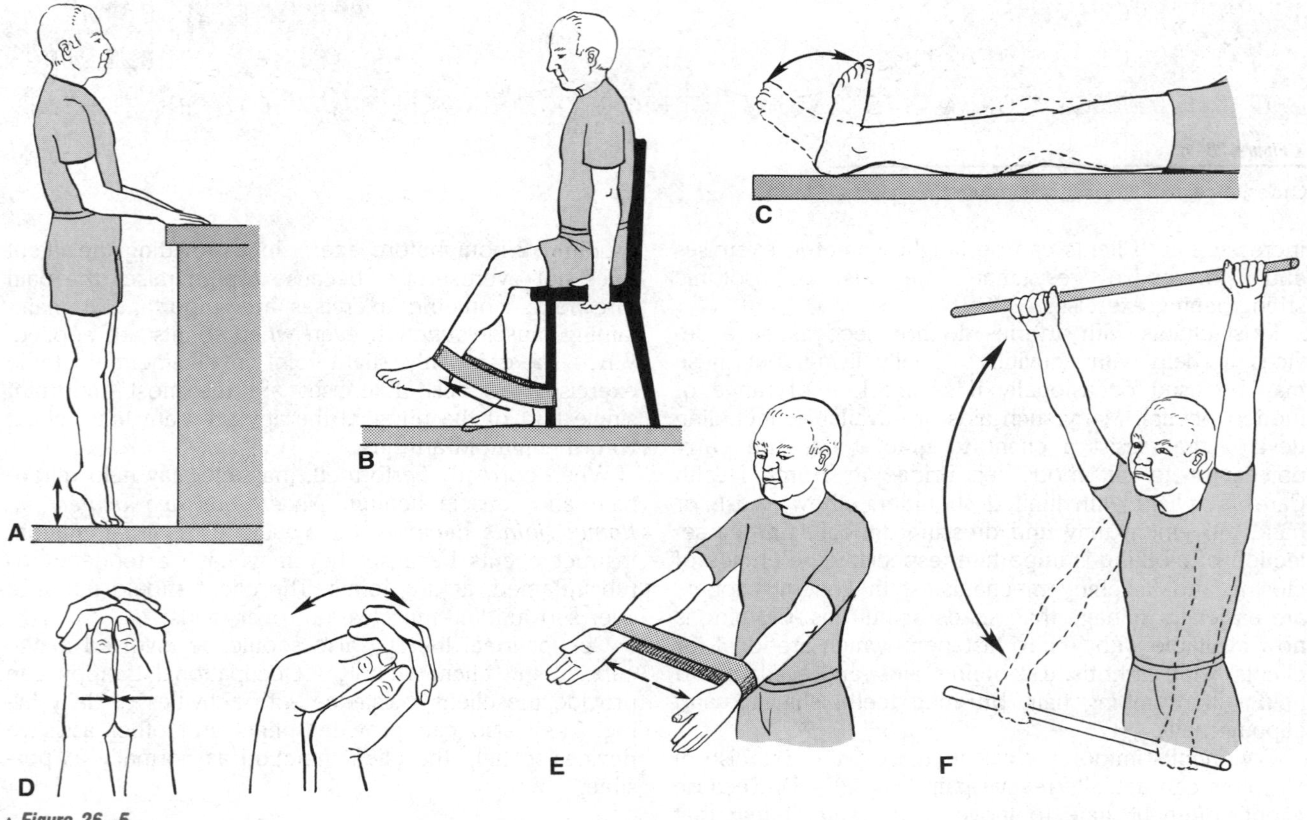

▲ *Figure 26–5*

Exercises helpful for arthritic people to increase flexibility, improve circulation and muscle tone, and prevent further movement restriction. *A*, Stand alternately on tiptoes and flat of foot. *B*, Knee scissor. Loop a cloth ring (e.g., bandage) around chair leg. Move leg from normal position to extend cloth ring. *C*, Quadriceps setting. *D*, Palm presses. Press palms together. Bend wrists as shown. *E*, Side pull. Loop cloth ring over wrists. Pull arms against resistance of cloth ring. *F*, Wand exercise. Holding a short pole, move arms from thigh level to above head.

Aspirin or Sodium Salicylate. Salicylates are the mainstay of pharmacologic treatment for arthritis. They are analgesic, anti-inflammatory, relatively safe, and inexpensive. Analgesia is achieved with small doses, and large doses are needed to reduce inflammation. Frequent doses (three to four times a day) are required, even when pain is not present, to keep blood salicylate levels high. Aspirin is usually prescribed in doses sufficient to produce mild symptoms of drug toxicity, e.g., tinnitus. Once such symptoms are produced, the dose is reduced slightly. Aspirin is available in various forms: plain or soluble tablet, enteric-coated, with buffers added, and as a suppository.

Other Nonsteroidal Anti-Inflammatory Drugs. If aspirin is ineffective or not tolerated, nonsteroidal anti-inflammatory drugs (NSAIDs) may be used. Compliance may be better with these agents because they have a simpler dosage schedule. Like aspirin, they are anti-inflammatory, analgesic, and antipyretic. Phenylbutazone (Butazolidin) is not used frequently because of the danger of developing agranulocytosis. Indomethacin (Indocin) is another drug that is usually not well tolerated by clients and may produce gastrointestinal bleeding. There are a number of commonly prescribed NSAIDs including ibuprofen (Motrin), naproxen (Naprosyn), tolmetin (Tolectin), sulindac (Clinoril), and ketoprofen (Orudis). The effects of these drugs vary among individuals. Several NSAIDs may have to be tried until the most effective one is found. These drugs also cause some gastrointestinal side effects, but when taken with food and a histamine receptor antagonist such as ranitidine (Zantac), they seem to be tolerated better than aspirin.

Corticosteroids. Adrenocorticosteroids are often used in treating RA, but these drugs are not without potentially serious side effects. Side effects of corticosteroids can worsen some features of the disease. Prolonged use can create severe side effects that are more serious and difficult to treat than the arthritis itself. Severe adrenal insufficiency may follow withdrawal of the medication. Corticosteroids are prescribed in the smallest dose permitting functional improvement, and the dose is reduced as soon as possible. The dosage must be increased during major stressful situations such as illness or surgery if the client is steroid dependent.

Intra-Articular Injections of Corticosteroids. These injections may be helpful to suppress inflammation temporarily in specific joints and are most effective with acute inflammation in smaller joints. Fluid is removed from the joint before injecting the medication. If there is any possibility of infection, corticosteroids are *never* injected.

Antimalarials, Gold Salts, and D-Penicillamine. These are remissive agents used to treat RA, sometimes with NSAIDs or steroids, if these medications alone are not sufficient to control the disease. Although they are not immunosuppressants, these drugs seem to halt progression of RA. The onset of action is slow (1 to 8 weeks) so prolonged administration is necessary. Gold salts and D-penicillamine may lead to leukopenia, thrombocytopenia, proteinuria, and skin rashes.

Immunosuppressive (Cytotoxic) Agents. The most common cytotoxic agent used to treat RA is methotrexate. This drug acts as an immunosuppressant, blocking the inflammatory process of RA. The dosage used to treat RA is much lower than the dose used to treat cancer. The side effects are also fewer than those associated with doses to treat cancer.

DIETARY MANAGEMENT

There is no particular dietary modification required in the management of RA. The client is encouraged to eat a nutritious diet. If clients are overweight, they are taught to lose weight to relieve stress on the affected joints.

Surgical Management

Surgical procedures may be helpful for clients with arthritis. Surgery may be used to relieve symptoms such as pain, improve function, and correct deformities. Previously, surgery was only considered late in the course of arthritis, often after severe joint destruction or deformity had developed. Preventive surgery (to prevent deformities) is now used during early phases of the disease. Surgery may be performed when there is active arthritis.

TENDON TRANSFERS AND OSTEOTOMY

Among the numerous types of surgical procedures used in the treatment of RA are tendon transfers and osteotomy. Tendon transfers can prevent progressive deformity caused by muscle spasm. Nodules or bony tumors (exostoses) may be surgically removed, and flexion contractures may be surgically relieved. Osteotomy (excising or cutting through bone) may improve the function of deformed joints or limbs. For example, a femoral head osteotomy may give symptomatic relief by changing the position of the head of the femur when it is being subjected to impact stress against the acetabulum.

SYNOVECTOMY

Synovectomy (removal of synovia), such as of the elbows, wrists, fingers, or knees, may be used in treating RA to help maintain joint function. Early synovectomy helps prevent recurrent inflammation. With RA, joint destruction begins in the synovial tissue and then proceeds to involve bone, cartilage, and other structures.

JOINT REPLACEMENT

Implants composed of Vitallium, stainless steel, and polyethylene (for cups, such as those used to replace the acetabulum) have been developed for reconstructive joint surgery. These are used to replace joints as small as those of the fingers or great toe up to joints as large as the shoulder or hip.

Recently, techniques for joint replacement have changed considerably. In the past, the cement used to hold the replacement prostheses in place created problems. The cement, methyl methacrylate, held the implant for a limited time and could cause problems during insertion by causing nerve damage from heat and hypotension.

Newer implants are made with a porous metal coating and are inserted with a tight fit, known as a press fit. The implant is placed very snugly against the bone, and within about 6 weeks, new bone tissue grows between the pores and grafts to the new prosthesis. The bony growth serves as the fixation mechanism that holds the device in place. The implant appears to hold for an indefinite time.

Prostheses and procedures for joint replacement are currently changing and developing. Each prosthesis and procedure has its own advantages and potential complications. It is essential that nurses know the exact procedure and prosthesis to be used for each client so specific preoperative preparation and postoperative care can be planned. These procedures include the arthroplasty, hemiarthroplasty, and total hip replacement.

Hip Arthroplasty. Severely involved arthritic hips can be very disabling. Severe hip pain can interfere with sleep, prevent walking, and impair or prevent sexual enjoyment. Arthrodesis of the hip is contraindicated in RA because (1) the disease is generalized, and (2) the other hip often becomes involved. Arthroplasty may be performed for RA to relieve pain and restore joint motion.

Two types of hip arthroplasty may be performed: (1) hemiarthroplasty, in which either the femoral head or the acetabulum is replaced, and (2) total hip replacement, in which the femoral head and acetabulum are both replaced.

Hemiarthroplasty. Either the head of the femur or the acetabulum may be replaced. Hemiarthroplasty is used not only to treat arthritic joints but also in the early stages of necrosis of the head of the femur or in the presence of post-traumatic pseudoarthrosis of the femoral neck. The acetabulum would not be replaced in the latter two examples. Permitting the operated leg to move into adduction before adequate healing has occurred can ruin an arthroplasty.

Total Hip Replacement (Fig. 26–6). Total hip replacement is performed if arthritis involves both acetabulum and femoral head. A total hip replacement also may be performed for complications of femoral neck fractures, failure of previous reconstructive surgery (such as osteotomy and femoral head replacement), complications of congenital hip disease, and pathologic fractures from metastatic cancer.

If both hips are involved, surgery is usually performed on the most severely affected hip and then the other one several weeks later, when the client has recovered from the first operation. If the client is in excellent condition otherwise, both hips can be operated on together. Total hip replacements are not performed if an infection is present. With total hip replacement, the femoral head and acetabulum are both replaced by prostheses.

Total Knee Replacement (Fig. 26–6). This procedure is performed to relieve pain and increase stability and function in a knee severely affected by osteoarthritis or RA. The tibial, femoral, and patellar joint surfaces are replaced. The choice of implant depends on the degree of joint destruction.

Preoperative care is the same as for total hip replacement. Possible postoperative complications include infection, thrombophlebitis, pulmonary embolism, fat embolism, peroneal nerve palsy, skin breakdown, technical failure, synovial herniation, loosening of the prosthesis, and stress fracture.

Postoperative care is similar to that for total hip replacement, although there is more emphasis on active exercises because dislocation is not a problem due to the anatomy of the knee.

A compression dressing immobilizes the knee in maximum extension immediately after surgery. The dressing is removed on third postoperative day, and a posterior plaster shell or knee immobilizer is used as a resting splint and during ambulation. A resting splint is used to keep the knee in extension for about a month.

Isometric quadriceps-setting exercises begin on the first postoperative day. Teaching may be conducted preoperatively in the physician's office. As pain decreases and voluntary muscle control improves, increase exercising to active straight leg raising. Exercise both ankles actively to prevent thrombophlebitis.

After the compression dressing is removed, start gentle, active assistive range-of-motion exercises and continue a progressive exercise program to increase muscle strength and range of motion in the operated knee.

Once the client has 90-degree knee flexion and good voluntary quadriceps muscle control (can actively raise a straight leg and initiate active knee extension against gravity), start ambulation. Partial weight-bearing usually begins about 1 week after surgery or sooner. At about 2 weeks or less, weight bearing is permitted to the point of pain.

A posterior splint or immobilizer may be used during early gait training, such as when the client uses parallel bars and is on crutches.

The client is discharged with detailed instructions for a home exercise program. Stationary bicycle exercise can be helpful for at least 1 year after surgery.

Flexion contractures can develop after total knee replacement. To prevent this complication, keep the operated knee extended whenever the client is in bed. Use a trochanter roll beside the affected leg in bed to prevent external rotation.

Swelling also can be a problem. Keep the leg elevated with a pillow under the leg (including the ankle). This position also promotes full extension with the aid of gravity. Whirlpool baths may help the person obtain knee flexion and full extension.

Other Total Joint Replacements. Replacement surgery is possible for elbow, shoulder, finger, and ankle joints, although they are not as common as hip and knee replacements (Fig. 26-7). Finger joint replacement is performed for clients with loss of finger joint function due to RA. The metacarpophalangeal and proximal interphalangeal joints are most commonly replaced.

Infection and dislocation are the two most common postoperative complications following any joint replacement. Methods of preventing these problems are discussed later.

Nursing Management

ASSESSMENT

The assessment of the client with rheumatoid arthritis varies slightly depending on whether this is a new condition or an ongoing one.

In clients who are just being diagnosed with the disease, assessment should center around symptoms, the way the client has been treating them, how the disease has affected their lives, and their knowledge of the disease and treatment. Their coping abilities are also important to assess at this point, since they are now faced with a progressively, debilitating chronic illness.

Clients who have had the disease should be assessed for changes in functional ability, deformities, and tolerance of treatment. It is important with these clients to continue to assess both their compliance with therapy and their continued ability to cope with this disease and all its changes.

Physical assessment includes inspecting all joints for signs of inflammation, deformity, or limitation of normal movement. Assessment of the whole client is required, not just the joints, because arthritis is a systemic disease. Organs possibly affected include the heart, blood vessels, eyes, and peripheral nerves.

As mentioned earlier, all clients with rheumatoid disease require a thorough psychosocial assessment. The disease affects the client's whole life. The impact of the disease and how client is coping with it are vital areas for the nurse to assess. Chronic disease such as RA requires the client to cope and adapt to an entire new lifestyle. Chapter 3 discusses theories of health and illness and the effects of chronic disease on clients.

NURSING INTERVENTION

For the client with rheumatoid arthritis, the following plan of care would be appropriate.

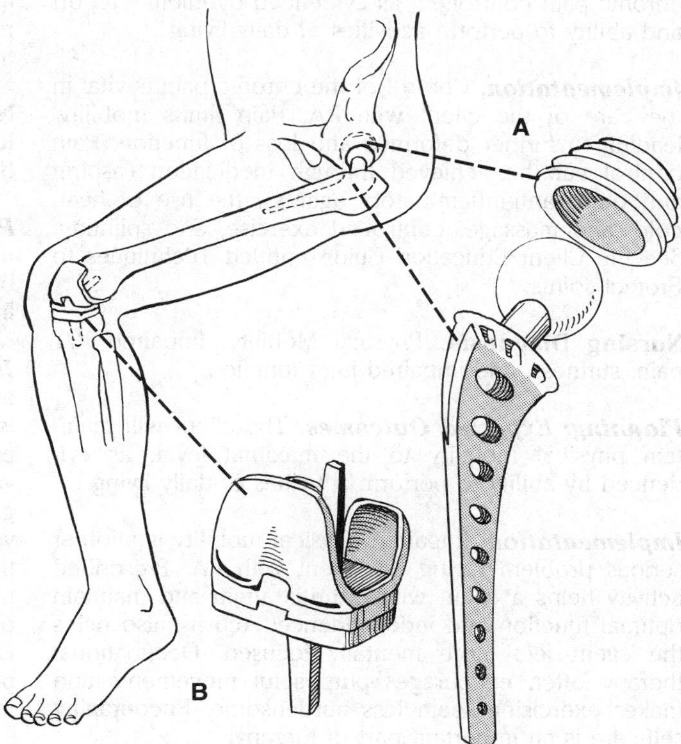

▲ *Figure 26-6*

A, Total hip joint replacement. A cementless prosthesis allows porous ingrowth of bone. *B*, Total knee joint replacement using a tibial metal retainer and a femoral component. The femoral component is chosen individually for each person according to the amount of healthy bone present.

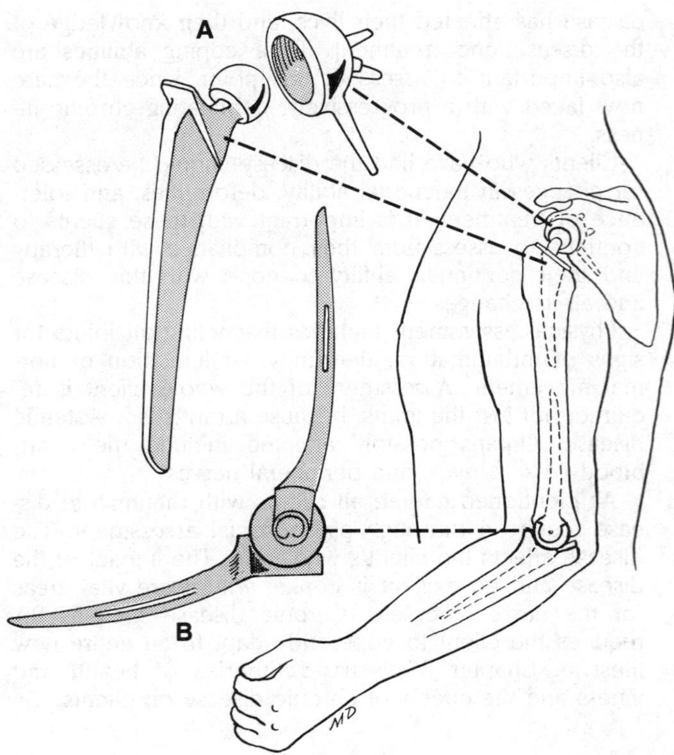

▲ *Figure 26-7*

A, Total shoulder replacement using two components. *B*, Total elbow joint replacement using one prosthesis.

Nursing Diagnosis: Chronic Pain R/T inflammation, joint deformity, and joint destruction.

Planning: Expected Outcomes. The client will have chronic pain controlled, as evidenced by client's report and ability to perform activities of daily living.

Implementation. Control of the chronic pain is vital in the care of the client with RA. Pain limits mobility, leading to further deformity and loss of function. Pain control can be achieved through medication (aspirin and other anti-inflammatory agents), the use of heat, cold, and massage, controlled exercise, and splinting. See the Client Education Guide entitled Techniques to Protect Joints.

Nursing Diagnosis: Physical Mobility, Impaired R/T pain, stiffness, and impaired joint function.

Planning: Expected Outcomes. The client will maintain physical mobility to the maximal level, as evidenced by ability to perform activities of daily living.

Implementation. Impaired physical mobility is another serious problem facing the client with RA. Prescribed activity helps a client with arthritis attain and maintain optimal function and independence. Activity also helps the client feel more mentally focused. Occupational therapy often encourages purposeful movements and makes exercising seem less burdensome. Encouraging self-care is an important part of therapy.

During exercise, a client may experience pain for a short time. If pain lasts for several hours after exercise, the program may be excessive and need modification. Rest and activity must be balanced. Fatigue is common, and overactivity can increase inflammation. Exercise must be performed within the limits of the client's pain tolerance.

Nursing Diagnosis: Fatigue and Activity Intolerance R/T systemic inflammation, anemia, and impaired mobility.

Planning: Expected Outcomes. The client will have minimal fatigue and tolerate activity, as evidenced by a balance of rest and activity and ability to maintain usual lifestyle.

Implementation. The fatigue and activity intolerance are common problems associated with RA. Because RA is a systemic disease, both physical and emotional rest are important. The amount of systemic rest needed varies, depending on the severity of the disease at any given time. With extensive systemic and articular involvement, complete bed rest is indicated for a limited time for its anti-inflammatory effect. Generally, the more acute the disease and/or the greater the number of joints involved, the greater the benefit of bed rest. Bed rest, however, should not be maintained for long periods because it may lead to other problems of immobility that can make the disease worse.

For bed rest to be effective, the bed must be firm

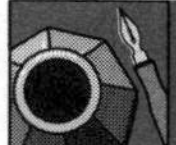

CLIENT EDUCATION GUIDE

Techniques to Protect Joints

The following techniques reduce stress to joints, tendons, ligaments, and capsules.

- Respond to pain. If pain lasts more than an hour or two after activity, stop doing that particular activity for a while.
- Use your biggest muscles. For example, women should carry a shoulder bag rather than a handbag; push doors open with your arms rather than with your hands or fingers.
- Alternate between light and heavy tasks. Do not do all your heavy tasks at once. Take frequent breaks and rest between tasks.
- Minimize joint stress that may lead to deformity, for example, use a large, wide pen rather than a thin one; use lightweight equipment and devices; maintain a good, comfortable posture; change position frequently.
- Plan for rest, for example, take a walk where you can sit down if you need to.
- Conserve energy. Make activities that are really important to you a priority. Eliminate unnecessary tasks.
- Assess your joints. If they are warm or swollen, use them as little as possible. Put them through range-of-motion exercises only once a day.
- Assess the tasks you must do, such as your work. What is the least painful way to accomplish these tasks? Be sure you do the tasks in this way.
- What are your horizontal and vertical reaching areas? Move items into these ranges.
- Avoid prolonged or unnecessary bending, stretching, reaching, stair climbing, or prolonged grip.
- Use simultaneous motion with smooth, continuous movements, such as dusting or putting dishes away with both hands.
- Sit to work as much as possible because standing places more stress on hip and knee joints and uses more energy. Do remember to get up and move around at intervals.

and the client positioned to prevent deformities (footdrop, fixation of the joints in extension, flexion contractures). Use devices such as footboards, splints, and sandbags to maintain proper body alignment. The client should lie flat on the back, with affected joints in positions of extension for long periods (periodically up to 10 hours a day while on bed rest). Extension is important to combat flexion contractures. Place a small pillow or folded towel only under the head. A small pillow may be placed under the ankles to straighten the knees. Position arms with palms upward by placing small pillows or folded towels under elbows or wrists to maintain extension. Use sandbags and trochanter rolls as needed to maintain proper body alignment. Many clients do not find this a comfortable position and need help to appreciate the reasons for maintaining it.

Resting joints involved with RA helps reduce articular inflammation. Weight-bearing joints may be rested by complete bed rest. Splints may be used to rest inflamed joints. Splints are removed periodically and the joints exercised to prevent fibrous ankylosis. Intervention is needed to prevent complications of immobility during periods of limited activity, such as during bed rest or while in a wheelchair (see Chaps. 65 and 66).

During periods when the client is not on bed rest, the client must learn to balance rest and activity. Rest periods should be planned between all activities causing fatigue. The client needs to learn to do the most important activities first while his or her energy is at the highest. Activities that can be eliminated should be in order to save the client's strength.

Nursing Diagnosis: Self-Care Deficit, High Risk for Possibly Total, R/T joint deformity, pain, fatigue, and immobility

Planning: Expected Outcomes. The client will be able to perform self-care activities with minimal pain, as evidenced by client's maintaining activities of daily living.

Implementation. Proper posture and body alignment are important for clients with RA. Teach clients to look at their posture in a mirror and consciously attempt to sit and stand erect.

When a client begins ambulation, take care to avoid aggravating flexion deformities by weight bearing. Until these contractures are corrected, supports may be required (crutches, braces) during ambulation. Properly fitting shoes are important to support feet and make ambulation safer.

When hips, knees or both are involved, it may be most comfortable for the client to sit on a straight-backed armchair elevated 3 to 4 inches higher than ordinary chairs. The added height prevents excessive hip and knee flexion and makes it easier for the client to get in and out of the chair. Similarly, elevation of toilet seats also helps. Grab bars on or beside the toilet are helpful. It also may help to have the client's bed raised between 10 and 30 degrees.

Often, the knees of a client with arthritis become stiff after sitting for a while. Teach the client to flex and extend the knees several times before standing up. Limbering up helps the client stand up more easily and feel steadier. Similarly, periodic flexion and extension of the knees while seated may make sitting more comfortable.

Self-care is important for the client. Occupational therapy is often involved in this intervention. The occupational therapist can help with assistive devices to make self-care possible, even with joints that have become deformed. They also can provide splints for the client so further joint deformity can be limited.

Nursing Diagnosis: Individual Coping, Ineffective, High Risk for R/T pain, self-care deficits, chronic illness, role changes, and impaired mobility.

Planning: Expected Outcomes. The client will cope with chronic debilitating nature of disease, as evidenced by client's statements and compliance with therapy.

Implementation. As stated, the nurse must assess the client's coping with this life-altering, chronic disease. The client must learn to cope with this chronic condition so his or her life can continue as normally as possible.

If the client is having difficulty adjusting to the changes this disease is producing, the nurse should plan to spend time with the client discussing ways that the client might handle the alterations. Some clients may require further counseling and help with stress management to handle the changes. Sometimes, a counselor (a nurse clinical specialist, psychologist, or psychiatrist) may be necessary to help the client learn methods of adjustment.

Nursing Diagnosis: Health Maintenance, Altered R/T knowledge deficit regarding the disease, physical therapy, medication, and alterations in lifestyle.

Planning: Expected Outcomes. The client will understand the disease, physical therapy, medication, and alterations in lifestyle, as evidenced by client's statements and compliance with treatment regimen.

Implementation. When providing the client with medications to control the symptoms of RA, use this opportunity to teach the client about them. Teach the client to take aspirin with food to reduce gastric irritation. It also may help to take aspirin with antacids. There is increasing concern, however, about the aluminum content of antacids. Advise the client to watch for signs of bleeding, such as dark stools, bruising.

When the client is taking NSAIDs, advise the client to take the medication with food to minimize possible gastric irritating effects. Some clients also may be given histamine receptor antagonists such as ranitidine (Zantac) to prevent any gastrointestinal irritation or ulcer formation. In older clients, piroxicam (Feldene) appears to increase the risk of peptic ulcer disease, so it should be used with caution in this age group. Also, warn the client that the effects of these medications may not be apparent for several weeks.

Clients who take corticosteroids should always carry identification stating they are receiving steroid therapy. Such identification advises health professionals of the client's condition if emergency treatment is required.

For the client who has a total joint replacement, an appropriate plan of care would include the following items.

Nursing Diagnosis: Knowledge Deficit R/T surgery, postoperative restrictions, and rehabilitation.

Planning: Expected Outcomes. The client will understand the proposed surgery, postoperative restrictions, and rehabilitation, as evidenced by client's statements and compliance with postoperative regimen.

Implementation. The care of the client who will have joint replacement is another focus of the plan of care. Preoperative preparation is similar to that for any client undergoing major surgery (see Chap. 19). Besides the usual preparation, the client requires specialized teaching about the postoperative course.

Total hip and total knee replacement will be used as the prototypes of total joint replacement experienced by these clients. Clients requiring total hip replacement may be admitted to the hospital 1 day before surgery to allow thorough assessment and to begin preoperative teaching.

Teach the client and significant others about the procedure and what the client can expect after surgery. Discuss the procedure and goals of treatment with the client and significant others. Assess ambulation and identify areas in which the client may need extra help postoperatively. Teach the client how to use crutches, a walker, or both. Encourage the client to practice using crutches or a walker. Assist the client to practice moving from bed to a chair or a wheelchair without flexing the hip more than 90 degrees to prevent dislocation of the prosthesis.

With nursing assistance, physical therapists assess the client preoperatively and teach postoperative exercise. If the exercises are not understood preoperatively, the client may not be able to do them effectively after surgery, when pain and anxiety may be present. Exercises include quadriceps setting, gluteal setting, isometric hip extension and abduction exercises, as well as upper extremity strengthening exercises to prepare for crutch walking or use of a walker. Encourage the client to practice the exercises regularly.

Nursing Diagnosis: Injury, High Risk for R/T postoperative complications such as dislocation of the prosthesis, thrombophlebitis.

Planning: Expected Outcomes. The client will not suffer injury related to postoperative complications and will heal normally, as evidenced by absence of dislocation of the prosthesis and no thrombophlebitis.

Implementation. General postoperative nursing interventions are discussed in Chapter 19. Postoperative interventions for clients following hip surgery are discussed in Chapter 67. Here, it is necessary to emphasize only those points that are particularly relevant for clients after total hip replacement.

Postoperatively, keep the affected leg in an abducted position and in straight alignment while the client is recumbent. The surgeon may order support hose to prevent deep vein thrombosis. An abduction splint or four pillows are used postoperatively. Most splints can be adjusted for the desired amount of abduction.

Encourage and supervise prescribed exercises such as quadriceps setting. Muscle strengthening of the gluteal muscles helps prevent dislocation, because muscular control replaces the function of the hip capsule. Dislocation of the prosthesis and infection are possible early postoperative complications. Document and report indications of complications immediately. Following hip replacement, prevent hip flexion greater than 90 degrees and leg adduction. Both can cause dislocation.

With some surgical procedures, the greater trochanter (with attachment of the abductor muscles) is transferred to the distal position on the femur to increase the efficiency of the abductor mechanism. When such a transfer is made, the greater trochanter is usually held in its new position by wires. The transfer must be protected until it heals in place (4 to 6 weeks). In this situation, progressive abduction exercises must be limited. Excessive exercise may cause nonunion or fracture of the osteotomy site. Follow the surgeon's orders concerning movement and positioning.

The client is usually mobilized at the bedside on the first or second postoperative day. This may mean standing at the bedside briefly or being assisted to a chair. Be careful not to flex the hip joint greater than 90 degrees, and maintain abduction of the legs to prevent dislocation.

While the client is supine, turn the client to the unaffected side and give back care every 2 hours. The client is turned with the splint in place so abduction is maintained. The client should be medicated well before this procedure to prevent any pain caused by the turning. The client's position must be changed frequently to help prevent complications of immobility.

Assess nerve function and circulation in the affected leg every 1 or 2 hours (or as directed by the physician) for the first day or so, then as often as the client's condition warrants. This includes assessment of bilateral pulses and quality, skin color and temperature, capillary refill in the toes, and movement of joints distal to the surgery.

Pink-tinged sputum may appear postoperatively and is believed to result from some of the cement leaking into circulation and being excreted through pulmonary alveoli. It is important, therefore, to know the type of replacement procedure that has been performed. This complication is not dangerous, but it should be documented and must be distinguished from pulmonary emboli.

Assess the client's position frequently while the client is in bed. Prevent external rotation or abduction of the affected leg and flexion of the hip of more than 90 degrees. Progressive ambulation follows, such as use of parallel bars, crutches or walker, and finally, a cane.

Physical therapy may be started as early as the fourth or fifth postoperative day. In addition to helping the client ambulate, physical therapy may include gentle, active assisted range-of-motion exercises in sling suspension (within the pain-free range). Until discharge, the client continues exercises that increase range of motion and strengthen hip muscles.

On the third to fifth postoperative day, the physician may allow the client to lie prone twice a day for 20 to 30 minutes to prevent hip flexion contractures. The client may be required to continue this practice at home after discharge.

The nurse must be aware of the risk of adrenocortical insufficiency or addisonian crisis occurring in clients who are taking steroids to treat their arthritis. When subjected to the stress of surgery, steroid-dependent clients may exhibit signs of adrenocortical insufficiency. These symptoms would include tachycardia, hypotension, diaphoresis, and a decreasing level of consciousness. This condition resembles hypovolemic shock, although in this case there is no bleeding and the client is not hypotensive. If there is abrupt cessation of adrenalcorticoids, hypotension and diuresis can occur.

Treatment for adrenocortical insufficiency or addisonian crisis is intravenous cortisone administration, often in the form of Solu-Cortef. Once the client's level of steroids is increased, the symptoms resolve very rapidly. The nurse should be aware of the possibility of this complication developing and be sure that the client receives ordered increased doses of steroids to prevent the crisis situation.

The client is also at risk for thrombophlebitis after total hip replacement. The surgery itself, positioning during surgery, and impaired mobility all contribute to the development of thrombophlebitis. To prevent the development of phlebitis, support stockings are applied to the client preoperatively and are maintained postoperatively. Another preventive measure used by some physicians is low-dose heparin. Heparin can be given subcutaneously in doses of 5000 units every 12 hours. This helps to prevent thrombophlebitis without significantly increasing the risk of hemorrhage. Exercising the unaffected leg also helps prevent clot formation.

The usual period of hospitalization for total hip replacement varies from 5 to 10 days. If clients still require extensive rehabilitation, they are sent to rehabilitation centers or extended care facilities until they are able to function independently or with limited assistance. Total hip replacement often produces dramatic results. Clients often find their pain relieved and movement increased markedly and rapidly.

Before discharge, the client and significant others should be given a list of written instructions for home health care. The most important instruction is that the client not flex the hip greater than 90 degrees to prevent the hip from dislocating and to avoid extremes of internal rotation, adduction, and flexion of the hip. Exercises to be performed also should be included in the instructions (Fig. 26-8). These restrictions continue for 6 months to 1 year after surgery.

Nursing Diagnosis: Infection, High Risk for R/T implanted prosthesis and possible immunosuppression related to drug therapy.

Planning: Expected Outcomes. The client will not develop an infection in implanted prosthesis, as evidenced by a normal white blood cell count, temperature, absence of purulent drainage, and no sign of inflammation.

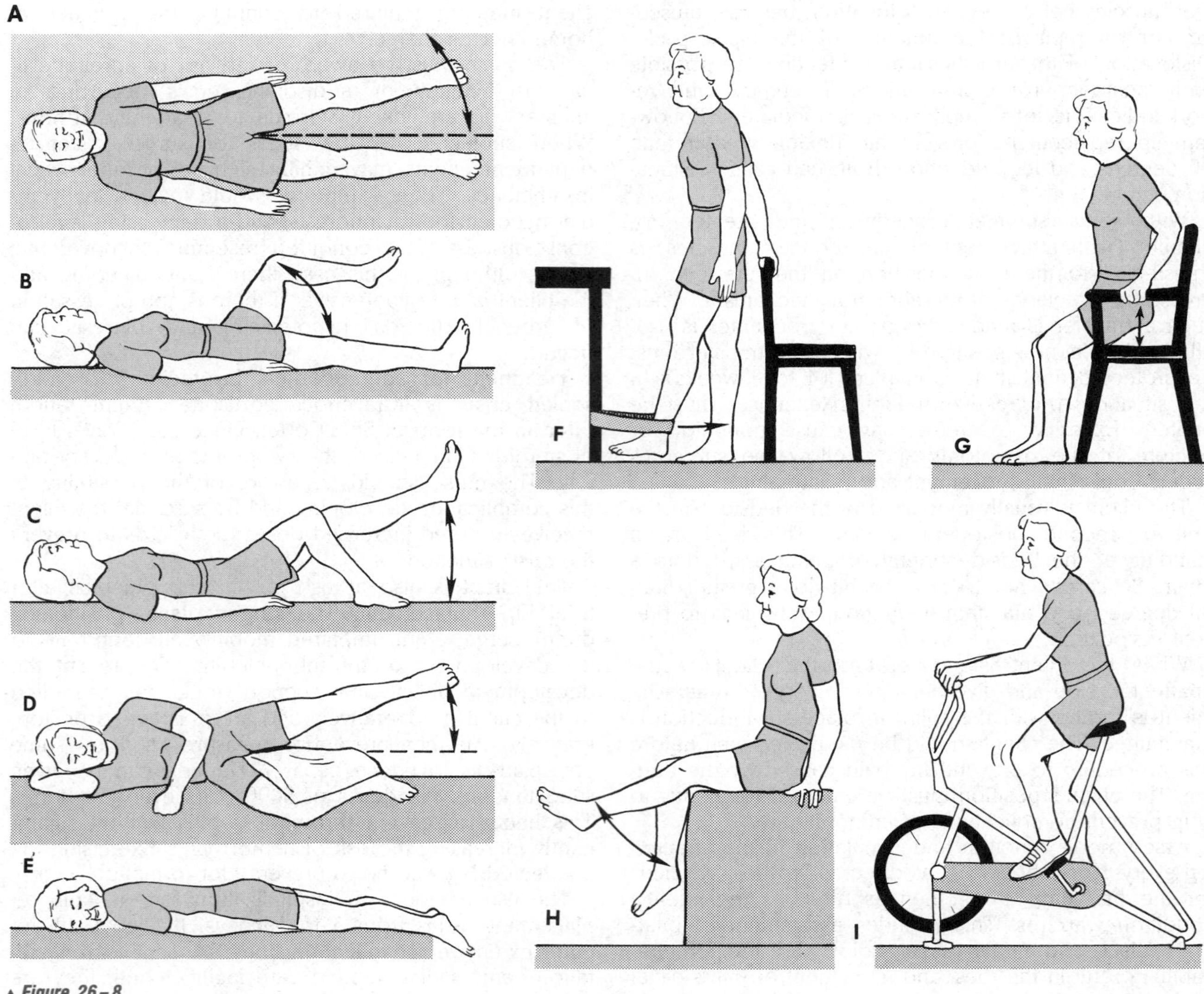

▲ *Figure 26–8*

Rehabilitative exercises after total hip replacement. *A*, Lie on back and gently swing leg away from body and return to midline. *B*, While supine, raise hip and knee as shown to increase ROM and strengthen hip flexors. *C*, While supine, straight leg raise to strengthen quadriceps muscle. *D*, Lie on unoperated side and raise operated leg straight up toward ceiling to strengthen hip abductors and adductors. *E*, Lying prone stretches flexor muscles of the hip and prevents flexion contractures. *F*, Using a resistive material (rubber tubing), put tubing on ankle and secure to sturdy object. Try to pull operated leg back to midline to increase power of quadriceps. *G*, Raise self gently out of a chair to increase strength of upper extremities. Good preparation for crutch walking. *H*, Raise leg from a sitting position to increase ROM and strengthen quadriceps tone. *I*, Stationary bicycling is one of the last exercises to be added to a post-total hip replacement exercise program. This increases ROM, provides warm-up before and after exercises, and increases cardiovascular capacity.

Implementation. Prevention of infection is another priority in the client after hip replacement. These clients are at high risk for infection for several reasons. First, a foreign body has been implanted in the client. Although the material used produces little inflammation, it is a potential source of infection because of the trauma of surgery. The client also may have been receiving anti-inflammatory agents, especially steroids or cytotoxics, which increase the risk of infection. This places the total joint replacement client at a greater risk of infection.

Usually the client is started on prophylactic broad-spectrum antibiotics during surgery, and this therapy is continued for several days after surgery, even if there is no sign of infection. If the client begins to exhibit any sign of infection in the operative site such as redness, fever, purulent drainage, or increasing incisional pain, any drainage is cultured and aggressive antibiotic therapy is begun.

Other preventive measures range from the use of staples for wound closure because they are associated with a lower infection rate and the use of strict aseptic technique when handling dressings or wound drains. Drainage from the wound drains is usually less than 600 ml/24 hours or 200 ml/8 hours unless the client has been heavily hydrated with plasma expanders such as dextran. In this case, the amount of output from these drains can easily triple. Therefore, intake and output totals should be carefully calculated to assess fluid balance.

The dressing applied immediately after surgery is usually heavy and bulky, and is left in place (but carefully assessed) until the surgeon removes it 2 to 3 days postoperatively. The wound is either then recovered with a light dressing or sometimes left open to the air. The wound is usually cleansed each shift according to the surgeon's orders.

EVALUATION

The nurse must assess whether the goals have been met for the client with rheumatoid arthritis who has had surgery. If these goals have not been met, the nurse must revise the plan and interventions to better meet the client's needs.

Modification of Plan of Care for the Elderly

Although the age of onset for RA is between 20 and 40 years of age, the client who is treated for the disease is often an older adult. The care is essentially the same; however, immobility, deformity, and joint destruction can be more severe in this age group. Elderly clients are more susceptible to the side effects their decreased mobility may cause including more rapid loss of function.

Older clients may have adapted to the RA very well but often find any further deterioration more difficult to handle. Elderly clients also may have more trouble recovering following an acute exacerbation of the disease. They also may be slower in their recovery from total joint replacement. They may require prolonged hospitalization in an extended care facility until they regain adequate mobility to function independently or with some assistance and safely.

Post-Hospital Care

DISCHARGE TEACHING

The discharge instructions that the client and significant others must receive are given in the Client Education Guide entitled Discharge Instructions for the Client After a Total Hip Replacement and Figure 26–8. It is important for the client to know which activities are allowed and which may cause problems. Clients should be reminded that this surgery does not cure their arthritis and that they will need to continue therapy for their disease.

HOME HEALTH CARE NEEDS

There are some alterations that need to be made to the home for the client with severe arthritis and for the client after total hip surgery. These alterations include devices such as ramps, good lighting, and modifications in floor plans that help the client maintain independence longer.

The client who has a total hip replacement needs assistive devices added to the home such as a riser on the toilet seat, a good chair for sitting, and grab bars in the bathroom. These devices should be installed before the client returns from the hospital.

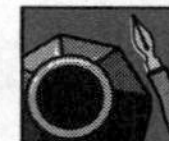

CLIENT EDUCATION GUIDE

Discharge Instructions for the Client After a Total Hip Replacement

- Do not cross one leg over the other—keep the knees apart.
- Do not flex the hip when putting on shoes and stockings. Use assistive devices such as long-handled shoe horns and extenders with clothespins, or have someone help you put them on.
- Do not sit continuously for longer than 1 hour. Stand, stretch, and take a few steps periodically to prevent hip flexion contractures.
- Do not sit in low, reclining, or rocking chairs. Low, soft seats require more than 90 degrees of hip flexion to stand up. Sit in a firm, high chair with arms. Use a raised toilet seat. Place a very secure bar beside the toilet to help you stand up. Use of tub baths are not allowed.
- Do lie prone twice a day for 30 minutes.
- Do place a pillow between the knees when lying down to prevent hip adduction and maintain abduction.
- Follow detailed exercise prescriptions, including quadriceps setting, range-of-motion exercises, and activity limitations. The most important exercises to rebuild hip muscles are abduction exercises (spreading legs apart) and extension exercises (pushing the knee backward into the bed). Stationary bicycle exercises may help when an adequate range of hip flexion is achieved (see Fig. 26–8*I*).
- Avoid actions that place a strain on the hip joint, such as excessive bending, heavy lifting, jogging, and jumping.
- Use crutches or a walker for as long as prescribed by the physician. (Full weight bearing without crutches may be allowed as early as 4 weeks after surgery or later if the physician requires). Then use a cane in the hand opposite the operated leg. See Chapter 66 for proper use of assistive devices.
- Climb stairs carefully after discharge from the health care facility (see Chapter 66 for proper ways to climb stairs with crutches).
- Wear support stockings on the unaffected leg and an ace wrap on the affected leg until there is no swelling in the legs or feet and full activities are resumed.
- Do not drive a car for 6 weeks after surgery unless authorized by the physician.
- Take prophylactic antibiotics if undergoing procedures that may cause bacteremia, such as tooth extraction.

FOLLOW-UP CARE

The client may require outpatient physical therapy or even a visiting therapist to maintain optimal function and to complete rehabilitation after total joint replacement surgery.

SYSTEMIC LUPUS ERYTHEMATOSUS

Definition

SLE is a chronic, inflammatory, autoimmune disease. Lupus comes from the Latin word for wolf, referring to a belief in the 1800s that the rash of this disease was caused by a wolf bite. The characteristic rash of lupus is red, leading to the term erythematosus.

Incidence

SLE occurs most commonly in younger women between the ages of 15 and 40. It is almost 10 times more common in women than in men. It is more common in black women, with a rate of about 1 per 250, with the rate for white women about 1 per 700.[29] SLE has a familial tendency, and when one twin has the disease, the other twin has a 60 to 70 per cent chance of developing it.

SLE may be drug induced. Four features separate this condition from spontaneous SLE. In the drug-induced syndrome, (1) men and women are affected equally, (2) nephritis and central nervous system features do not usually occur, (3) depressed serum complement and antibodies to DNA are present, and (4) symptoms revert to normal when the offending drug is withdrawn, although serologic abnormalities may persist for months or years.

Etiology

SLE is an autoimmune disease involving diffuse inflammatory changes of the vascular and connective tissue. There is some evidence of a genetic predisposition to the disease because of the incidence in families and twins. There is a theory that the genetic predisposition for the disease is present in some clients and a virus or some other agent triggers it and the disease occurs. This theory is as yet unsupported.

Although the exact etiology of SLE is unknown, causes of disease exacerbation have been identified. These include sunlight and other forms of ultraviolet light, physical and emotional stress, and pregnancy.

There is a form of drug-induced SLE associated with adverse reactions to some drugs, including procainamide (Pronestyl) and hydralazine (Apresoline). Some drugs, phenytoin (Dilantin) and phenobarbital, are known to produce a SLE-like syndrome. The drug-induced problems resolve when the drugs are discontinued. Sometimes, a short course of steroids are needed to completely eradicate the symptoms.

Risk Factors

This is not a preventable disease; however, the exacerbations might be prevented. Control of stress, avoidance of sunlight and ultraviolet light, and prevention of pregnancy can help delay exacerbations of SLE.

Pathophysiology

SLE is a chronic, progressive, systemic, inflammatory connective tissue disease. It produces inflammatory, biochemical, and structural changes in the vascular and connective tissue as well as in the viscera, joints, fascia, tendons, and bursae. SLE is characterized by remissions and exacerbations and often has an insidious onset.

Several abnormal serum protein factors and ANA may be found with SLE that suggest an autoimmune mechanism is occurring. These ANA mainly affect the DNA within the cell nuclei, leading to the formation of immune complexes in serum and organ tissues. The complexes can cause vasculitis, or inflammation of the vessels, leading to a decrease of oxygen in the organs and tissues. They may also directly invade the organs, causing inflammation and damage.

Characteristic histologic findings are lupus erythematosus (LE) cells and extracellular masses called hematoxylin bodies. However, LE cells may be found in many diseases and may or may not be demonstrated with SLE. Most clients with SLE have a mild to moderate, normochromic anemia. The ESR is usually elevated, a mild leukopenia is often present, and serum globulins may be increased.

The leading cause of death in clients with SLE is renal failure from the kidney involvement. There is some degree of kidney involvement causing progressive changes within the glomeruli in most clients with SLE. With progression of SLE nephritis, the glomeruli become increasingly abnormal and accumulate immune complex deposits. Once 50 per cent of the glomeruli have been affected, the client will show signs of renal failure.

The heart is the other major organ involved with SLE, and cardiac involvement is the second leading cause of death in these clients. The immune complexes deposit in the coronary vessels, myocardium, and pericardium. CNS involvement, usually leading to cerebral infarction, is the third leading cause of death.

In general, the clinical pattern and prognosis of SLE are variable. The illness may develop rapidly and have an acute fulminant course. More commonly, it develops insidiously and becomes chronic with remissions and exacerbations. The survival rate has improved dramatically in recent years, although the disease is still potentially fatal. More than 95 per cent of clients are alive 5 years after diagnosis. Improvements in treatments mean that clients can now live for many years.

Clinical Manifestations

Assessment findings in acute disease may include fever, musculoskeletal aches and pains, butterfly rash on the face, pleural effusion, basilar pneumonia, generalized lymphadenopathy, pericarditis, tachycardia, gallop rhythm, hepatosplenomegaly, nephritis prostration, delirium, convulsions, psychosis, and coma.

Clients with SLE often present with nonspecific symptoms, such as weight loss, fever, malaise, and lethargy. In some clients, the symptoms are very insidious and resemble other conditions such as arthritis because of the joint involvement. Many of the clinical hallmarks of SLE are due to the deposition of immune complexes in the tissues.

Assessment findings in chronic SLE are variable depending on the organs involved but may include fever, malaise, weight loss, cutaneous discoid LE lesions, erythema of exposed skin, generalized lymphadenopathy, severe hemolytic anemia, thrombocytopenic purpura, hypersplenism, pericarditis, tachycardia, gallop rhythm, peripheral vascular syndromes (e.g., Raynaud's phenomena, gangrene), ulcerative mucous membrane lesions, abdominal pains, nausea, vomiting, anorexia, bloody stools, hepatic dysfunction, hepatomegaly, focal glomerulitis progressing to glomerulonephritis, myalgia, arthralgia, neuritis, hemiplegia, psychosis, convulsions, and coma.

An SLE-like syndrome is seen in 20 per cent of children receiving anticonvulsant medications. Drug-induced SLE can be distinguished from acute or chronic SLE by the following characteristics: a low frequency of renal and central nervous system involvement, absence of antibody to native DNA, usually normal serum complement levels, and prompt resolution of the symptoms after discontinuation of the medication.

DIAGNOSTIC ASSESSMENT

In addition to the physical findings of SLE, laboratory tests reveal

- Presence of LE cells (autoantibodies); the severity of SLE usually correlates with the degree of LE cell formation;
- Decreased complement levels;
- Presence of immune complexes in the serum;
- Presence of immune antibodies to DNA and antinuclear antibodies;
- Decreased levels of red blood cells, white blood cells, and platelets;
- Increased gamma globulin fraction due to increased antibody production; and
- An elevated ESR.

Other abnormal findings are those given previously for any autoimmune disease. At some point, abnormalities in the kidneys show up on an intravenous pyelogram (IVP); a barium enema would reveal colonic ulceration; a magnetic resonance imaging (MRI) study might reveal central nervous system involvement; and an electrocardiogram or echocardiogram might show cardiac changes.

Medical Management

Treatment of SLE is based on the organ systems involved in the disease. The treatments are essentially pharmacologic in nature. Dialysis may be used to treat the renal failure if it develops.

PHARMACOLOGIC MANAGEMENT

Treatment of SLE is similar to the treatment of RA and other autoimmune, connective tissue disorders. These treatments include the following:

- Nonsteroidal anti-inflammatory agents such as aspirin and ibuprofen.
- Antimalarial drugs, although the action of these medications in SLE is unclear. These agents are helpful, especially in clients with predominantly cutaneous and joint involvement.
- Corticosteroids, agents that ameliorate the systemic inflammatory manifestations of the disease.
- Cytotoxic agents, the use of which is controversial because of the serious side effects. However, they are used in severe, refractory cases of SLE including alkylating agents (cyclophosphamide) and antifolates (methotrexate).
- Plasmapheresis, which is used to remove circulating autoantibodies and immune complexes from the blood before organ and tissue damage occurs. The efficacy and safety of this therapy is also controversial.

Note the order of these therapies. The agents associated with the least serious side effects are tried first. Success of pharmacologic intervention is often difficult to evaluate because spontaneous remissions may occur.

DIETARY MANAGEMENT

Dietary factors are thought to influence the development of autoimmune diseases. Therefore, some clinicians recommend dietary alterations. Restriction of L-canavanine (a nonprotein amino acid found in alfalfa sprouts) is sometimes suggested because this substance is thought to be an inducer of autoimmune diseases. Other studies suggest that diets high in calories may enhance autoimmunity. If this is true, a reduction in calories may decrease the formation of antibodies to DNA. However, dietary modifications are still in the experimental stages.

Nursing Management

The goals of care for the client with SLE focus on:

Maintenance of skin integrity,
Promotion of a healthy lifestyle and reduction of stress,
Maintenance of proper nutrition,
Relief of discomfort,
An increase in the client's independence, and
Maintenance of emotional well-being.

Intervention for clients with SLE depends on how they respond to the condition and on the severity and specific types of clinical manifestations. In a newly diagnosed client, the nurse can expect knowledge deficits with respect to the diagnosis itself, prescribed drug therapies, and the prognosis. Provide the client and significant others with teaching to help relieve anxiety and avoid misunderstandings. This is particularly important in terms of the prescribed medications. Advise the client and significant others of the actions, side effects, and potential interactions of prescribed medications.

During exacerbations, provide physiologic support to prevent skin breakdown, maintain nutritional and metabolic status, and minimize the risk of opportunistic infection. Also, provide emotional support to the client facing a chronic, potentially fatal disease.

Affected clients may experience a grieflike reaction following diagnosis, with exacerbations, or both. It is important to allow for verbalization of these feelings. In such situations, be supportive and understanding, and when necessary, refer the client or significant others for counseling.

The client will be followed closely for the development of organ failure associated with SLE. Information concerning care of the client with renal failure can be found in Chapter 50. For care of clients with the other problems associated, see the appropriate sections.

PROGRESSIVE SYSTEMIC SCLEROSIS (SCLERODERMA)

Progressive systemic sclerosis (PSS) is commonly known as scleroderma, although the skin is not the only organ system affected by the progressive sclerosis. Actually, this is a connective tissue disease characterized by fibrosis and degenerative changes of the skin, synovium, digital arteries, and parenchymal and small arteries of the internal organs.

PSS is less common than SLE but has a higher mortality rate. It is two to three times more common in women as men, occurs between the ages of 30 to 50, and is not more common in any race.

The cause of PSS is unknown, although abnormal serologic features suggest an altered immune status.

There are two forms of PSS: (1) CREST syndrome and (2) progressively fatal PSS.

CREST syndrome is a group of symptoms involving *c*alcinosis (calcium deposits), *R*aynaud's phenomenon (vasospasms of small peripheral arteries or arterioles), *e*sophageal dysfunction (impaired motility), *s*clerodactyly (scleroderma of the digits), and *t*elangiectasia (spider-like hemangiomas). This condition can progress rapidly but is still characterized by periods of exacerbation and spontaneous remission.

Progressively fatal PSS is associated with a generalized skin thickening and invasion into internal organs.

Common clinical manifestations include subcutaneous edema, fever, and malaise. The skin becomes thickened and hidelike and loses normal skin folds. Ulcerations around the fingertips and subcutaneous calcification occur. Polyarthritis and polyarthralgias are also present. Dysphagia due to esophageal dysfunction, from abnormalities in motility and later from fibrosis, occurs in about 90 per cent of clients. Fibrosis and atrophy of the gastrointestinal tract cause hypermotility and malabsorption.

Diffuse pulmonary fibrosis and pulmonary vascular disease are reflected by low oxygen-diffusing capacity and decreased lung compliance. Hypertensive uremic syndrome, resulting from obstruction in small renal vessels, is serious.

Mild anemia is often present. An elevated ESR and hypergammaglobulinemia are also common. RF may be present in a small number of clients.

PSS typically progresses slowly. When death occurs, it is usually from infection, or renal or cardiac failure. Treatment for the disease is supportive and symptomatic. The primary goal of medical treatment is to trigger a remission of the disease. Steroids and immunosuppressants are used to treat the disease, often in high doses.

Nursing interventions are directed at control of symptoms. One of the major areas of concern is skin care to prevent breakdown and ulceration. The skin should be carefully inspected daily so any injury or breakdown is noted and treatment begun immediately. The client should be taught to use gentle soaps and nonalcohol astringent lotions to maintain skin integrity.

Helping the client control acute pain, which is sometimes associated with Raynaud's phenomenon, polyarthralgia, and polyarthritis, is another important nursing function. The client must learn to avoid activities that might trigger pain. This includes actions such as joint protective behaviors, avoiding extreme cold, wearing gloves when hands are exposed to cold (even when removing food from the freezer), eliminating smoking, and resting the painful part when pain is acute.

If the client is experiencing esophageal dysfunction, modification of the diet may be necessary. Clients usually tolerate small, frequent, bland feedings better than three regular meals a day. The client also should learn to sit up for at least 1 hour after meals to help the food move into the stomach. Histamine receptor antagonists and antacids may be prescribed to help the acidity some clients feel.

The client will need continued follow-up care and monitoring. As with SLE, the client also will need psychosocial support to cope with this chronic debilitating disease. Encourage the client to continue to receive psychological support as needed after hospitalization.

SJÖGREN'S SYNDROME

Sjögren's syndrome is a chronic inflammatory disorder associated with a decrease in lacrimation and salivation due to immune complexes obstructing these secretory ducts. The client exhibits dry eyes (keraconjunctivitis sicca), a dry mouth (xerostomia), and a dry vagina in women. The client also may exhibit swelling of the parotid gland and lacrimal ducts.

This condition affects mainly women, and almost half of the clients with Sjögren's syndrome also exhibit another connective tissue disorder, especially RA.

Diagnostic tests reveal hypergammaglobulinemia and

the presence of RF, ANA, and anti-extractable nuclear antigen (anti-ENA). Autoantibodies against salivary duct antigens are also found.

If the client also has RA, the treatment is directed at the arthritis. Artificial tears are used to keep the eyes moist and prevent corneal abrasions. Artificial saliva can be used for the xerostomia. If untreated, the client can develop visual problems, oral ulcerations, dental caries, and dysphagia.

POLYMYOSITIS AND DERMATOMYOSITIS

Polymyositis is an acute or chronic inflammatory disorder of the striated muscles causing symmetric weakness. When there is a rash associated with polymyositis, it is referred to as dermatomyositis. As with other connective tissue diseases, they are characterized by periods of remission and exacerbation, and are chronically progressive.

This disorder is twice as common in women as in men and occurs equally among all races. Clients between the ages of 30 and 60 are most likely to get the disease. Polymyositis may be associated with a malignancy.

Diagnostic tests reveal positive ANA and focal deposition of complement, IgG, and IgM in vessels of the involved muscles.

Clinical manifestations of the disease beside the symmetric muscle weakness and rash include polyarthralgia, polyarthritis, and Raynaud's phenomena. Clients with dermatomyositis have characteristic heliotrope B (lilac) rash and periorbital edema. The muscle weakness can lead to problems with speaking and swallowing.

These disorders are treated with high-dose corticosteroids and immunosuppressants. Nursing care is mainly supportive. The client's ability to swallow should be monitored closely so that aspiration does not occur.

VASCULITIS

This is actually a group of disorders including polyarteritis nodosa, systemic necrotizing vasculitis, and allergic agranulomatosis angiitis, all of which result in necrotizing inflammation of the blood vessels. With these disorders, the circulating immune complexes are deposited in the blood vessels.

With these disorders, there is inflammation and damage to large and small vessels, resulting in end-stage organ damage. The specific symptoms vary depending on the organs affected. Steroids are the treatment of choice for these disorders.

SPONDYLOARTHROPATHY

This group of diseases includes ankylosing spondylitis (also known as Marie-Strümpell disease, or rheumatoid spondylitis), Reiter's syndrome, and psoriatic arthritis. The first two disorders are more common in men, and the latter disorder is more common in women. The disease is associated with the HLA-B27 antigen. RF is absent in the serum.

The major characteristic of these disorders are progressive joint fibrosis (especially of the vertebral column with ankylosing spondylitis), synovitis, and inflammation of skin, mucous membranes, and at the site of ligament insertion into the bone.

The specific manifestations associated with ankylosing spondylitis include iritis, arthritis or arthralgia, weight loss, and malaise. Compression of the chest wall from the vertebral ankylosing may lead to respiratory dysfunction. It is most commonly found in Caucasian men under age 40 years.

The specific characteristics of Reiter's syndrome are that it is most common in young Caucasian men and follows venereal disease or dysentery. The disorder is characterized by arthritis, conjunctivitis, and urethritis. Other symptoms may include a ringlike inflammation of the glans penis (circinate balanitis) and skin lesions.

All the disorders are treated with steroid therapy and aggressive physical therapy. Nonsteroidal anti-inflammatory agents may be used to treat the joint pain.

POLYMYALGIA RHEUMATICA AND CRANIAL (GIANT CELL) ARTERITIS

Polymyalgia rheumatica is a clinical syndrome occurring more commonly in women than in men. It is a disease of aging, rarely occurring before the age of 60 years. It is characterized by pain and stiffness in the neck, shoulder, back, and pelvic girdle especially in the morning. Headaches or painful areas on the head may be present. The client also may have a low grade fever or temporal arteritis.

Laboratory findings include an elevated ESR, mild anemia, and possible elevation of immune globulins. Steroids usually produce symptomatic relief within days.

Giant cell arteritis is also known as temporal or cranial arteritis. This is also a disease of older clients. The client often has symptoms of polymyalgia rheumatica for months, then suddenly develops the severe headaches associated with temporal arteritis.

The onset of this disorder is usually sudden, with severe pain often appearing in the temporal area. The pain also may be felt in the occipital area, face, jaw, or side of the neck. It is usually associated with hyperesthesia, which makes any touch exquisitely painful. The client may experience visual changes including sudden onset of blindness in one or both eyes.

It is very important to diagnose and treat this disorder before blindness occurs. Because older women are often affected, their complaints of decreased vision and headaches are sometimes ignored as normal aging. Treatment is with corticosteroids, which are highly effective in controlling this disorder.

SECONDARY ARTHRITIS

Whipple's Disease

Whipple's disease is a secondary arthritis associated with a gastrointestinal disorder. The disease was first described in the early 1900s as a condition characterized by arthralgias, diarrhea, abdominal pain, and weight loss. Other manifestations include fever, lymphadenopathy, and increased skin pigmentation. The disease can affect almost every organ system in the body.

Whipple's disease occurs most commonly in middle-aged white men. Although an organism was described as the cause, it was not isolated until 1992 when *Tropheryma whipelii* was isolated and cultured.[27a]

Treatment of Whipple's disease consists of antimicrobials (usually broad spectrum) and corticosteroids for the arthralgias. The disease may go into remission with these agents.

Other Diseases

Other conditions that may produce arthritis include Crohn's disease, ulcerative colitis, tuberculosis, hyperthyroidism, hyperparathyroidism, sickle cell anemia crisis, and psoriasis. Treatment for the primary condition usually leads to a decrease in the severity of the arthritis.

Summary

The immune system is a highly complex system. Diseases involving this system are also complex in nature. Autoimmune diseases are also complex in nature; an immune system attacking the self. The nurse must help clients with autoimmune diseases adjust to a wide variety of life changes. These clients will require a great deal of teaching, an important function of the nurse. The care of the client is also complex and difficult, because most of these diseases have no cure. The nurse plays a vital role in the care of these clients.

Bibliography

1. Balow, J. E. (1988). Lupus as a renal disease. *Hospital Practice, 23,* 129–135, 139–140, 142–144.
2. Benson, C. H. (1988). Arthritis and sexuality. *Journal of Urological Nursing, 7,* 370–372.
3. Blaha, J. D., & Pickett, J. C., (Eds.). (1985). Controversy on total knee arthroplasty. *Clinical Orthopedics, 192S,* 2–112.
4. Blake, S. A. (1985). Non-cemented femoral prostheses: Intraoperative focus. *Orthopaedic Nursing, 4*(1), 42–44.
5. Brassel, M. P. (1988). Pharmacologic management of rheumatic diseases. *Orthopaedic Nursing, 7*(2), 43–51.
6. Burlinghame, M. B., & Delafuente, J. C. (1988). Treatment of systemic lupus erythematosus. *Drug Intelligence and Clinical Pharmacology, 22,* 283–288.
7. Doheny, M. O. (1985). Porous coated femoral prosthesis: Concepts and care considerations. *Orthopaedic Nursing, 4*(1), 43–45.
8. Farrell, J. (1986). *Illustrated guide to orthopedic nursing* (3rd ed.). Philadelphia: J. B. Lippincott.
9. Fessel, W. J. (1988). Epidemiology of systemic lupus erythematosus. *Rheumatic Disease Clinics of North America, 14,* 15–23.
10. Fritzler, M. J. (1985). Antinuclear antibodies in the investigation of rheumatic diseases. *Bulletin on the Rheumatic Diseases, 35*(6), 1–10.
11. Hess, E. V. (1988). Rheumatoid arthritis complicated by vasculitis. *Hospital Practice, 23,* 50–54, 57, 61–64.
12. Ignatavicius, D. D. (1987). Meeting the psychosocial needs of patients with rheumatoid arthritis. *Orthopaedic Nursing, 6*(3), 16–20.
13. Joseph, N. (1989). Arthritis medications from A to Z. *Caring, 8*(1), 14–16.
14. Kaplan, H. (1985). Who should get gold and when? *Rheumatology in Practice, 3,* 53–57.
15. Klipple, J. H. (1990). Systemic lupus erythematosus, treatment-related complications, superimposed on chronic disease. *JAMA, 263*(13), 1812–1815.
16. Lambert, V. A. (1987). Coping with rheumatoid arthritis. *Nursing Clinics of North America, 22,* 551–558.
17. Levy, R. N., et al. (1985). Progress in arthritis surgery: With special reference to current status of total joint arthroplasty. *Clinical Orthopedics, 200,* 299–321.
18. Lieberman, J. D., & Schatten, S. (1988). Treatment: Disease-modifying therapies. *Rheumatic Disease Clinics of North America, 14,* 223–239.
19. Lorish, C., et al. (1989). Missed medication doses in rheumatic arthritis patients: Intentional and unintentional reasons. *Arthritis Care Research, 2*(1), 3–9.
20. McCarthy, D. J. (Ed.) (1989). *Arthritis and allied conditions: A textbook of rheumatology* (11th ed.). Philadelphia: Lea & Febiger.
21. Morrey, B. F., & Kavanagh, B. F. (1987). Cementless joint replacement: Current status and future. *Bulletin on the Rheumatic Diseases, 37*(4), 1–7.
22. Mourad, L., & Droste, M. (1988). *The nursing process in the care of adults with orthopedic conditions* (2nd ed.). New York: John Wiley & Sons.
23. Partridge, A. J. (1984). Determination of Social Security disability in rheumatic disease. *Clinical Rheumatology in Practice, 2,* 275–280.
24. Perricone, N. (1984). Overview of joint anatomy and physiology: A basis for understanding and assessing rheumatic conditions. *Occupational Health Nursing, 32*(7), 352–355.
25. Pfeiffer, C. A., & Wetstone, S. L. (1988). Health locus of control and well-being in systemic lupus erythematosus. *Arthritis Care Research, 1*(3), 131–138.
26. Phillips, K. F. (1983). The use of gold therapy with rheumatoid arthritis. *Orthopaedic Nursing, 2*(4), 31–34.
27. Pigg, J., et al. (1985). *Rheumatology nursing: A problem-oriented approach.* New York: John Wiley & Sons.

27a. Relman, D. A., et al. (1992). Identification of the uncultured bacillus of Whipple's disease. *The New England Journal of Medicine, 327*(5), 293–301.

28. Rothfield, N. F. (1989). The diagnostic pictures of systemic lupus erythematosus. *Hospital Practice, 24,* 37–46.
29. Schumacher, H. R., Jr. (Ed.) (1988). *Primer of rheumatic disease.* Atlanta: The Arthritis Foundation.
30. Schlegel, S. I., & Paulus, H. E. (1986). Update on NSAID use in rheumatic diseases. *Bulletin on the Rheumatic Diseases, 36*(6), 1–8.
31. Smeltzer, K. J. (1987). Fibromyalgia: The frustration of diagnosis and treatment. *Orthopaedic Nursing, 6*(3), 28–31.
32. Spindler, C. E. (1984). Audiovisual preoperative teaching for the total hip patient. *Orthopaedic Nursing, 3*(1), 30–40.
33. Steinberg, A. D., & Klinman, D. M. (1988). Pathogenesis of systemic lupus erythematosus. *Rheumatic Disease Clinics of North America, 14,* 25–41.
34. Stites, D. P., et al. (1984). *Basic and clinical immunology* (5th ed.). Los Altos, CA: Lange Medical Publications.
35. Strang, E. L., & Johns, J. L. Nursing care of the patient treated with continuous passive motion following total knee arthroplasty. *Orthopaedic Nursing, 3*(6), 27–32.
36. Townes, A. S. (1987). The "mask" of lupus. *Hospital Practice, 22,* 93–97, 101–103, 107–108.
37. Walsh, C. R., & Wirth, C. R. (1985). Total knee arthroplasty: Biomedical and nursing considerations. *Orthopaedic Nursing, 4*(1), 29–34.
38. Ziminski, C. M. (1985). Treating joint inflammation in the elderly: An update. *Geriatrics, 40,* 73–76, 79–81, 85, 88.

Neurologic Disorders

Unit

6

The nervous system is the body's most organized and complex structural and functional system. It profoundly affects both psychological and physiologic function. This unit discusses the importance of the nervous system to human function and the major consequences of neurologic disorders. The onset of neurologic problems may be sudden (e.g., traumatic spinal cord severance or ruptured aneurysm) or insidious (e.g., Parkinson's disease or multiple sclerosis). Providing nursing care for clients experiencing neurologic disorders is challenging, demanding extensive knowledge of neurologic structure and function and neurologic disease processes.

Neurologic problems can be frightening and even devastating to the client and significant others involved, especially if the process is irreversible. Many such problems produce varying degrees of physical or psychosocial dependency or both. Physical disabilities may limit self-care. Memory loss and confusion may occur. Subtle or gross changes in consciousness may occur, and the client may not be responsible for his or her behavior for a time. A grief reaction is common and appropriate for both the client and significant others when permanent or even temporary changes occur. A client's entire way of life may be altered.

This unit provides the information necessary to plan appropriate nursing care for clients experiencing neurologic problems in both acute and rehabilitative stages. Chapter 27 is an overview of neurologic structure and function. Chapter 28 describes the overall assessment of clients with neurologic problems. Among the disorders chapters, Chapter 29 discusses the care of clients with a loss of protective function; the nursing care of clients with cerebral disorders is explored in Chapter 30; Chapter 31 focuses on nursing care of clients with degenerative neurologic disorders; and disorders of the spinal cord, cranial nerves, and peripheral nerves, and accompanying nursing care are discussed in Chapter 32.

Chapter 27

Structure and Function of the Nervous System

The intent of this chapter is to present the anatomy and physiology of the nervous system that is necessary to understand alterations in neurologic function and the disorders of the nervous system. The central nervous system is discussed first, followed by a description of the protective and nutritional structures. Next, the peripheral nervous system and the autonomic nervous system are described. The cells of the central nervous system — neurons and neuroglia — and their functions including nerve impulse transmission are described. Finally, nervous system regeneration and normal aging are presented.

STRUCTURAL DIVISIONS OF THE NERVOUS SYSTEM

Central Nervous System

The brain and spinal cord are referred to as the central nervous system. These structures are protected by a rigid bony encasement, three layers of membranes, a fluid cushion, and a blood-brain barrier.

BRAIN

Cerebral Cortex. The brain tissues have a gelatin-like consistency. This semisolid, pinkish-gray organ weighs about 1400 g (3 lb) in the adult. The brain (encephalon) has five major divisions: (1) telencephalon, (2) diencephalon, (3) midbrain, (4) pons and cerebellum, and (5) medulla oblongata. The telencephalon, diencephalon, and upper midbrain are referred to as the cerebrum. The cerebrum is divided vertically into two sections called cerebral hemispheres. Each hemisphere is composed of a cortex, white matter tracts (myelinated and unmyelinated axons), the basal ganglion, and a portion of the corpus callosum. The corpus callosum is a bundle of nerve fibers that connects one cerebral cortex with the other (Fig. 27-1).

The outermost layer of the cerebral hemisphere (the cerebral cortex) is composed of gray matter (predominantly nerve cell bodies and dendrites) formed into raised projections or gyri. The grooves between the gyri are called sulci. The pattern of the gyri and sulci is not the same in each hemisphere. Each cerebral cortex is divided by major sulci into six lobes: the frontal, parietal, occipital, temporal, central (insula), and limbic lobes (Fig. 27-2).

Both the left and right cortex interpret sensory data, store memories, learn, and form concepts. However, the left cortex is better able to carry out sequential analysis involving an orderly, logical, systematic assessment of the parts. The left cortex deals well with language, mathematics, abstraction, and reasoning. The right cortex is best at using the entire sensory experience at one time. The right cortex deals well with visual-spatial information and activities such as dancing, gymnastics, and art appreciation.

In the frontal lobes, the precentral gyrus (the motor cortex) controls voluntary motor activity. The area anterior to the precentral gyrus (the premotor area) is also associated with voluntary motor activities. The prefrontal areas control attention over time (concentration). Motivation, ability to formulate or select goals, ability to plan, ability to initiate/maintain/terminate actions, ability to self-monitor, and ability to use feedback (called executive functions) are also carried out by the prefrontal areas. These same areas may well contribute to reasoning and problem-solving activities. The prefrontal areas additionally inhibit the limbic and vegetative areas of the cerebrum. Clients with frontal lobe injuries are often unable to concentrate, appear unmotivated and apathetic, and are unable to plan and problem solve.

Each parietal lobe, located posterior to the central sulcus of Rolando, contains a primary somatic (tactile) receptive area and the somatic (tactile) association areas. The postcentral gyrus and the posterior portion of the paracentral lobule (see Fig. 27-2) are the primary receptive areas for tactile sensations. The association areas occupy the remainder of the parietal lobe. Concept formation and abstraction are carried out by the parietal association areas. The right parietal areas deal with spatial orientation and body awareness. The left parietal areas deal with written language (reading), right-left orientation, and mathematics.

Each occipital lobe contains a primary visual receptive area and visual association areas. The primary visual cortex is on either side of the calcarine sulcus (see Fig. 27-2). The other areas of the occipital cortices are visual association areas. Visual memories are stored in these visual association areas, which contribute to a client's ability to visually recognize and understand his or her environment.

Each temporal lobe is located under (caudal to) the lateral sulcus. The temporal lobe contains a primary auditory receptive area and secondary auditory association areas. Spoken language memories are stored in

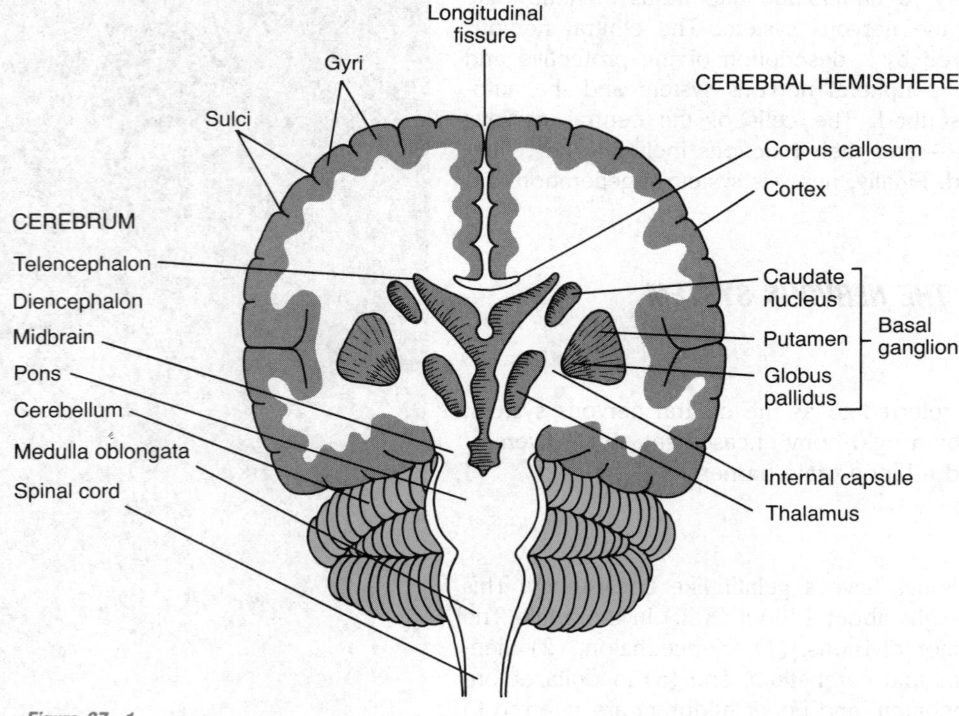

▲ *Figure 27-1*

Brain structures (coronal section).

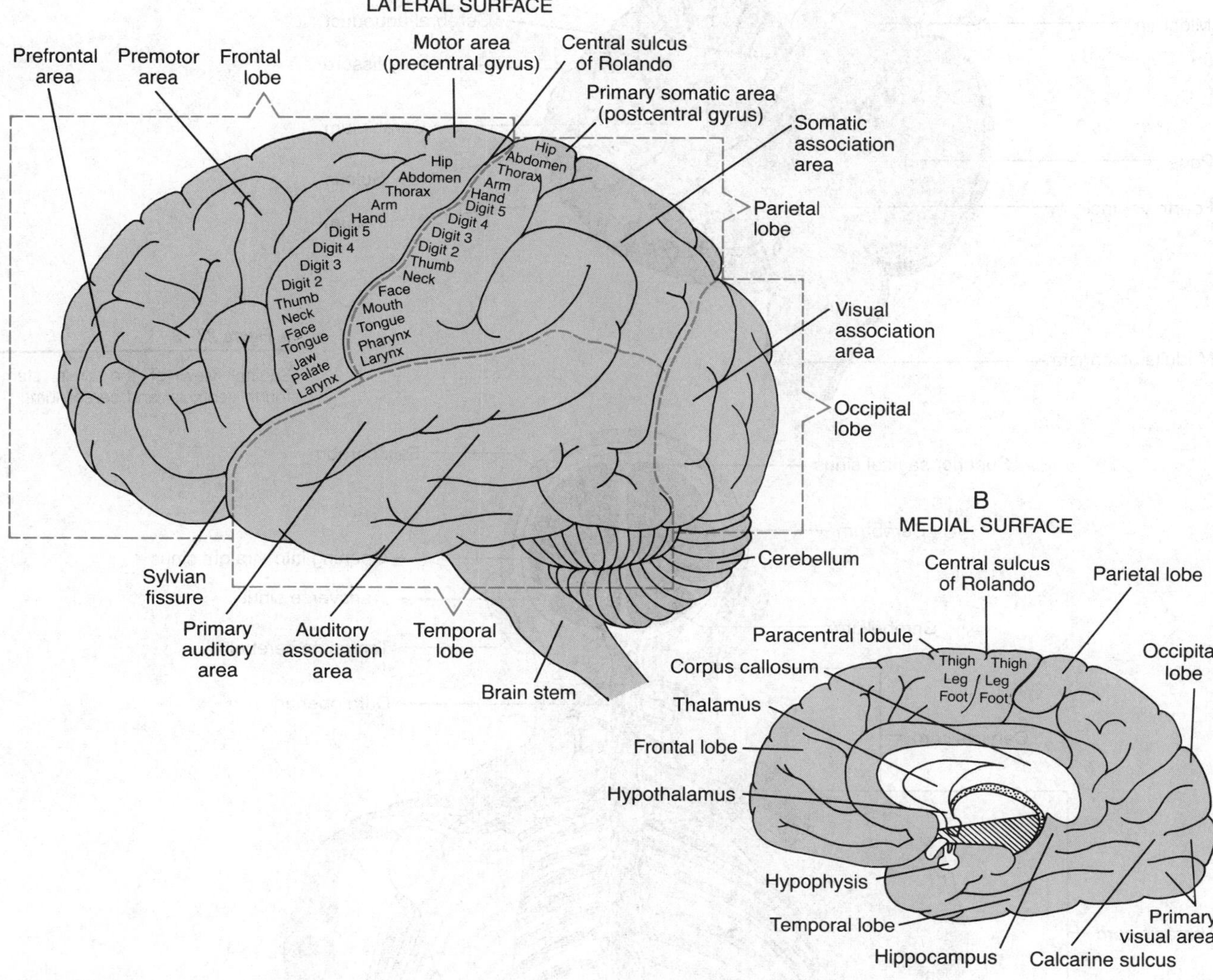

▲ *Figure 27–2*

Lateral and medial surfaces of the cerebrum.

the left temporal auditory association areas. All other sound memories that are not language—such as music, various animal sounds, and other noises—are stored in the right temporal auditory areas. Damage to these temporal lobe areas leaves the client unable to understand spoken language or unable to recognize music or other environmental sounds.

The limbic lobe is located at the core of the cerebrum and mediates affect. Some limbic structures control the transfer of short-term memory stores, called recent memory, into permanent memory stores, which are then held in the association areas of the parietal, temporal, and occipital association areas. Injury to this memory transfer system causes amnesia.

Basal Ganglia. The basal ganglion is a group of subcortical gray matter buried deep in each of the cerebral hemispheres. The basal ganglia serve as processing stations linking the cerebral cortices to certain thalamic nuclei (see Fig. 27–1). The basal ganglia are thought to integrate activities involved in the initiation and direction of voluntary movement and motor responses. The basal ganglia play a significant role in the regulation of stereotyped movement such as walking.

Internal Capsule. The internal capsule, shaped like an open fan, is composed of white matter pathways ascending to and descending from the cerebral cortex (see Fig. 27–1).

Brain Stem. The brain stem is composed of the diencephalon, midbrain, pons, and medulla oblongata (see Fig. 27–1; Fig. 27–3). Some authorities do not include the diencephalon as part of the brain stem.

The diencephalon, within the cerebrum, is continuous with the midbrain. The thalamus, the largest component of the diencephalon, is a processing center that coordinates and regulates the activity of the cerebral

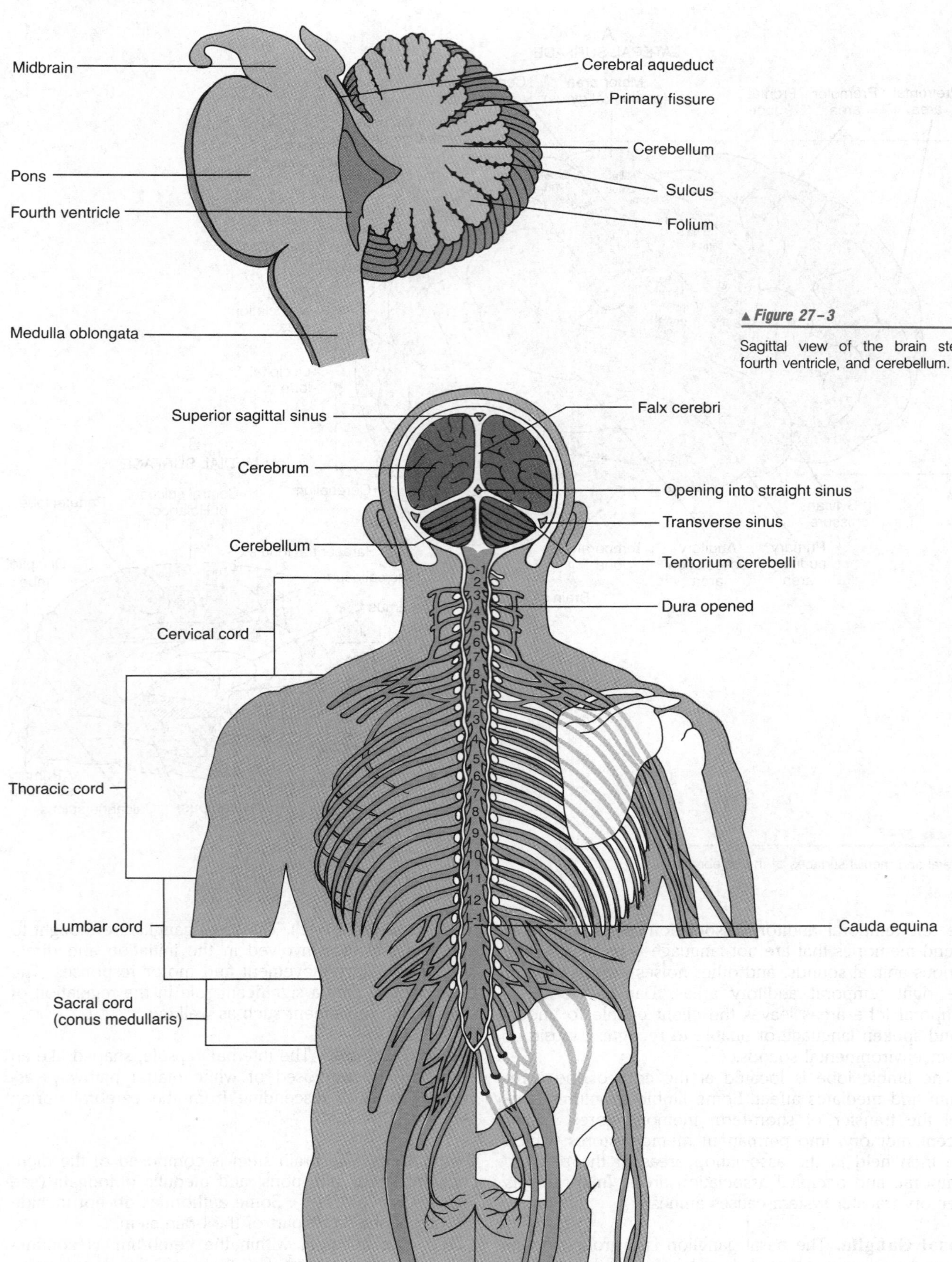

▲ *Figure 27-3*

Sagittal view of the brain stem, fourth ventricle, and cerebellum.

▲ *Figure 27-4*

The cranial vault, vertebral column, and peripheral nerves.

TABLE 27-1. Brain Stem Structures and Their Functions

Structures	Function
Midbrain	
Superior colliculi	Involved with optic system
Inferior colliculi	Involved with auditory system
Cerebral aqueduct	
Origin of CN III and IV	
Ascending sensory pathways	
Red nuclei	Involved with motor control
Paired crura cerebri	Afferent and efferent cerebellar pathways
Substantia nigra	Involved with basal ganglia function
Descending motor pathways	
Pons	
Fourth ventricle	
Nuclei of inferior colliculus	Major processing station in auditory pathway
Nuclei of CN V, VI, and VII and other pontine nuclei	
Ascending sensory pathways	
Medial lemniscus, auditory pathway	Proprioceptive pathways
Descending motor pathways	
Medial longitudinal fasciculi	Efferent pathway to spinal cord
Pyramids (corticospinal and corticobulbar tracts; corticopontine fibers)	Voluntary motor function Descending efferent pathways
Reticular formation	
Pontine nuclei and its pontocerebellar fibers	
Medulla Oblongata	
Fourth ventricle	
Central canal	
Ascending sensory pathways	
Medial lemniscal pathways	Proprioceptive pathways
Spinothalamic tracts	Pain pathways
Trigeminothalamic tracts	Tactile, temperature pathways
Lateral lemnisci	Audition pathways
Nuclei of CN X, XI, and XIII	
Olive and vestibular-cerebellar systems	
Descending motor pathways	
Pyramids	Voluntary motor function

cortex. It integrates information going to the cortex, projects motor signals, serves an energizing function, and contributes to affectual expression. The thalamus is connected with the cerebral cortex and subcortical nuclei on the same side (ipsilaterally).

The hypothalamus forms the base of the diencephalon. Hypothalamic functions fall into two major domains—the maintenance of a relatively constant internal body environment (homeostasis) and behavioral patterns. Within the hypothalamus are centers initiating sympathetic and parasympathetic nervous system activities, regulating body temperature, controlling endocrine gland secretions, and regulating emotional expression. Signals to the hypothalamus come from the midbrain, thalamus, neocortex, limbic lobe, olfactory system, and vascular system. Commands from the hypothalamus are complex and carried out by both nervous system pathways and the endocrine system.

The midbrain, pons, and medulla oblongata are continuous segments composed of ascending pathways, the reticular formation, cranial nerves and their nuclei, and descending autonomic and motor pathways (Fig. 27-4 and Table 27-1). The reticular formation is composed of reticular nuclei, ascending reticular pathways, and descending reticular pathways. One component of the reticular formation, the reticular activating system, controls the sleep-wake cycle and consciousness. Dysfunction in this system may produce unconsciousness (coma).

Cerebellum. The cerebellum is composed of gray and white matter. The cortex of the cerebellum is a thin layer of gray matter arranged in parallel long and deep gyri, called folia, and separated by cerebellar sulci (see Fig. 27-4). Deeper fissures divide the cerebellum into lobes. Underlying the cortex is a white matter core of fibers traveling to and from the cerebellar cortex. Within the white matter are deep cerebellar nuclei, the axons of which travel to other portions of the brain.

Pathways traveling to the cerebellum originate in the

brain stem and spinal cord nuclei and pass outward to the cerebellar cortex. They carry impulses to the cerebellar cortex; for example, information from the motor cortex is sent to the cerebellar cortex.

The output from the cerebellum is produced by the deep nuclei. The axons from these neurons travel to brain stem nuclei. The influence of the cerebellum on motor activity is carried out indirectly through many different pathways.

The cerebellum plays a background role for all movement (simple and complex). The cerebellum functions to coordinate the activity of groups of muscles by regulating muscle tension. This prevents tremor during movement and thereby maintains stability in movement (balance). Thus, the cerebellum controls and coordinates motor movements. The client with cerebellar damage exhibits weakness, intention tremor, and incoordination.

SPINAL CORD

The spinal cord, that portion of the central nervous system surrounded and protected by the vertebral column, is continuous with the medulla and lies within the upper two thirds of the vertebral canal (the cavity within the vertebral column). The lower spinal cord terminates caudally in a cone-shaped structure known as the conus medullaris at the level of the first (L1) and second (L2) lumbar vertebrae. The spinal cord is subdivided into four areas: (1) the cervical cord, (2) the thoracic cord, (3) the lumbar cord, and (4) the sacral cord (the conus medullaris) (see Fig. 27-4).

Within the spinal cord, butterfly-shaped gray matter (cell bodies and unmyelinated and some lightly myelinated fibers) is surrounded by lightly myelinated and heavily myelinated fibers (white matter) arranged in tracts that extend up and down the spinal cord (Fig. 27-5). The cell bodies are grouped into clusters of nuclei and laminae (a defined group or column of cells). The tracts are arranged into three paired columns: the posterior columns, lateral columns, and ventral columns.

Ascending Pathways. Information from peripheral receptors is transmitted through the nervous system by ascending pathways. In the major ascending pathways, the first neuron in the pathway (first-order neuron) has its cell body in a ganglion located outside of the central nervous system. The second neuron (second-order neuron) has its cell body within the central nervous system. The third-order neuron has its cell body in the thalamus. Throughout the spinal cord and brain stem, neurons with short axons interact with these neurons. The ascending pathways eventually terminate in the cerebral and cerebellar cortex. The ascending pathways belong to one of three groups: the anterolateral system, the posterior column system, and the spinocerebellar system; the functions of the ascending systems are presented in Table 27-2.

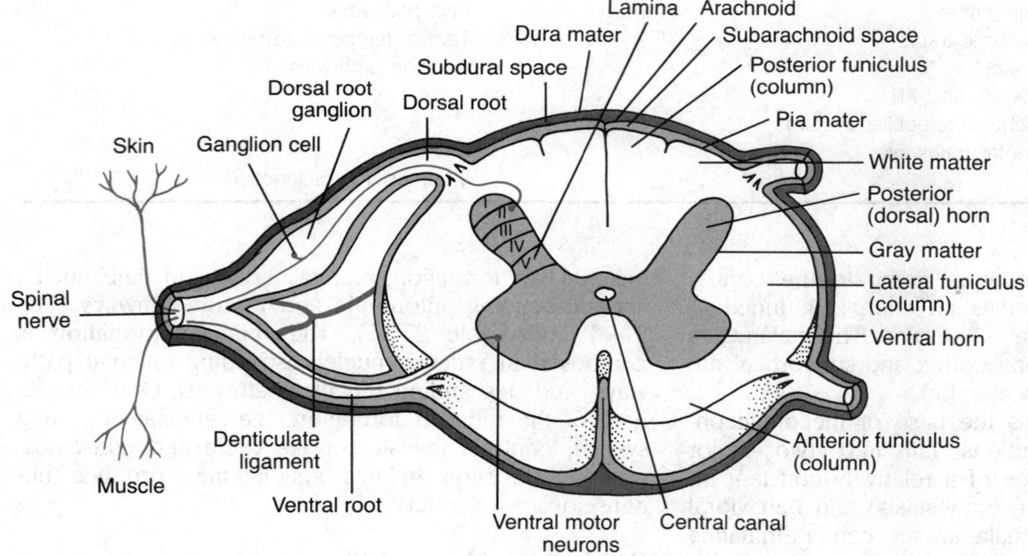

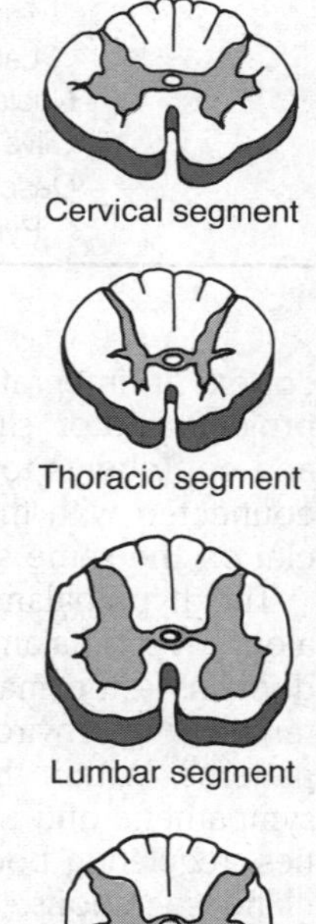

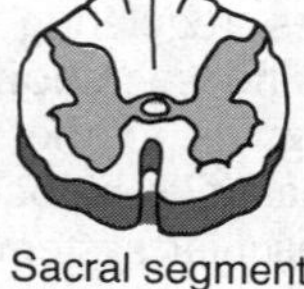

▲ *Figure 27-5*

Spinal cord and surrounding meninges.

TABLE 27-2. Ascending Systems Within the Central Nervous System

System	Tracts Within System	Function of Tract
Anterolateral system (tracts ascend through the anterolateral part of the spinal cord)	Lateral (direct) spinothalamic tract (neospinothalamic pathway, lateral pain system)	Thermal and pain pathway
	Anterior spinothalamic tract	Light (crude) touch
	Indirect spinoreticulothalamic tract (paleospinothalamic pathway, medial pain pathway)	Pain pathway
	Spinotectal tract	Unknown
Posterior column system	Posterior column (fasciculi gracilis and cuneatus)	Touch-pressure Sense of position and movement of joints (kinesthetic sense) Vibratory sense
	Spinocervicothalamic pathway	? Role in tactile and kinesthetic sensation
Spinocerebellar system	Anterior spinocerebellar tracts Posterior spinocerebellar tracts Cuneocerebellar tracts Rostral spinocerebellar tracts	Proprioceptive information from muscles, tendons, and joints

Intrinsic Neural Circuits. Chains of neurons (intrinsic neural circuits) that once activated follow a specific set of motor responses create the basic muscle tone necessary for motor movement and protect the muscle unit from overstretching. The descending motor pathways influence these intrinsic neural circuits in the spinal cord.

Some intrinsic reflex circuits create stereotyped patterns of movement (flexion and extension) that are the basis for posture and forward progression. Other reflex circuits are the basis for spinal cord reflexes, which include the myotatic (deep tendon, stretch) reflex, the flexor withdrawal reflex, the crossed extension reflex, and the extensor thrust reflex. Viscerosomatic reflexes can also excite or inhibit the motor neurons, producing changes in muscle tone and even movement.

Neuromuscular spindles monitor muscle length. As a muscle contracts, the neuromuscular spindle within the muscle becomes shorter, which reduces the rate of spindle firing to the motor neuron in the ventral horn, making continued contraction of the muscle impossible. Tone, residual tautness of the muscle, exists because some muscle fibers in a muscle are always contracted. This is primarily a function of the muscle spindle.

The Golgi tendon organs are tension detectors responding to increased tension within a tendon. As the tension within the tendon increases, these endings increase their rate of firing, which increases the inhibitory stimulation to the motor neurons. The Golgi tendon organs protect against excessive stretch of tendons and muscles.

Descending Pathways. The descending motor pathways from the cerebrum to the spinal cord (and brain stem) are composed of motor neurons (commonly referred to as upper motor neurons). These pathways cross (decussate) to travel downward on the opposite side in the medulla oblongata. Thus, motor control comes from the opposite (contralateral) motor cortex. Upper motor neurons provide voluntary control over motor movements and generally decrease the spinal reflex activity. Loss of these descending pathways results in loss of voluntary movement (paralysis) and increased (hyperactive) reflexes and increased muscle tone (spasticity).

Within the reticular formation of the lower brain stem are the descending neurons of the autonomic nervous system. These neurons receive signals from the hypothalamus, other brain levels, and cranial nerves. Signals from these neurons are carried via the reticulospinal fibers to neurons within the spinal gray matter, which in turn synapse with preganglionic neurons of the sympathetic and parasympathetic nervous systems.

PROTECTIVE AND NUTRITIONAL STRUCTURES

Cranium and Vertebral Column. Eight bones that fuse early in childhood compose the cranium. The fused junctions are called sutures. The cranium predominantly encloses the brain structures and serves as a source of protection (see Fig. 27-4).

The floor or basilar plate of the cranial vault has three depressions, called fossae. The frontal lobes lie in the anterior fossa. The anterior temporal lobes and the base of the diencephalon lie in the middle fossa. The cerebellum rests in the posterior fossa. The floor contains many openings (foramina) from which cranial nerves, blood vessels, and the spinal cord exit the cranial vault. The floor of the cranial vault supports the undersurface of the brain and can be fractured in some head injuries.

The vertebral column, a flexible series of vertebrae,

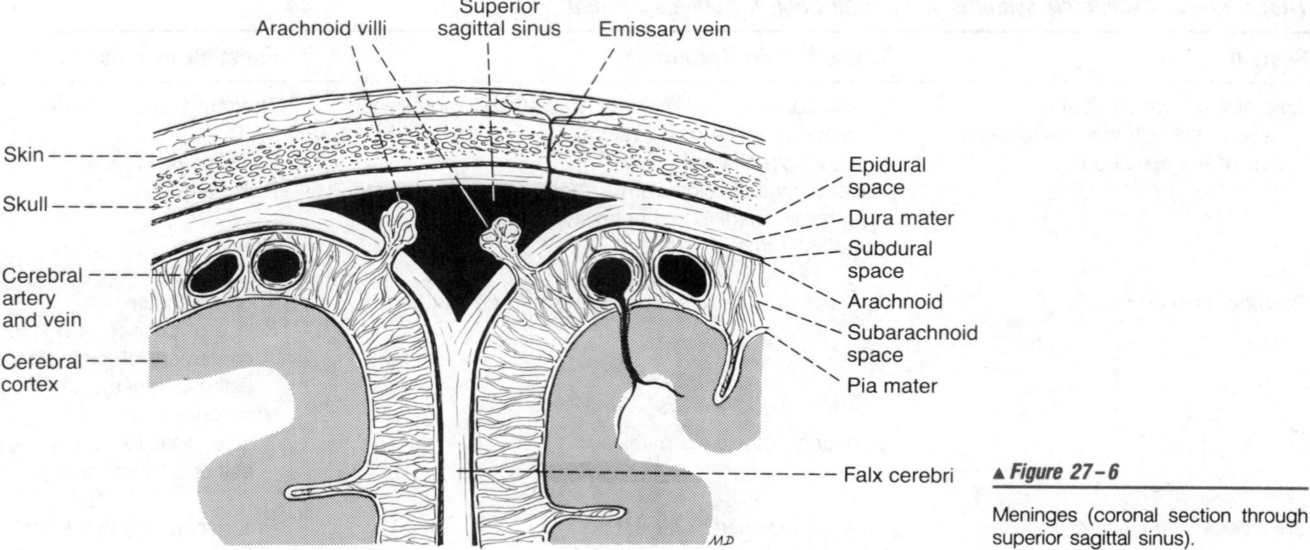

▲ *Figure 27-6*

Meninges (coronal section through superior sagittal sinus).

surrounds and protects the spinal cord. The vertebral column consists of 7 cervical vertebrae, 12 thoracic vertebrae, 5 lumbar vertebrae, 5 sacral vertebrae fused into a sacrum, and a coccyx. Ligaments hold the vertebrae together, and discs between the vertebrae prevent the bones from rubbing together. In the adult, the vertebral column is much longer than the spinal cord; the spinal cord ends at L1-L2.

Meninges. The meninges, three layers of connective tissue surrounding the brain and spinal cord, are predominantly for protection (see Figs. 27-4 and 27-5; Fig. 27-6). Each layer—pia mater, arachnoid, and dura mater—is a separate but continuous membrane.

The pia mater is a vascular layer of connective tissue and is so closely connected to the brain and spinal cord that it follows every sulci and fissure. This layer serves as a supporting structure for blood vessels passing through to the tissues of the brain and spinal cord. The pia mater and astrocytes (support cells of the central nervous system) together form a membrane that prevents harmful products from entering the central nervous system. This membrane is part of the blood-brain barrier.

The arachnoid mater is a thin layer of connective tissue; it extends from the top of each gyrus to the top of the adjacent gyrus. It does not extend into the sulci and fissures. This layer and the pia mater form the subarachnoid space, which contains cerebrospinal fluid. Meningitis, an inflammation of the meninges, is an infection of the pia and arachnoid mater.

The cranial dura mater is a tough, nonstretchable membrane with two layers. The outer dura mater is actually the membrane (periosteum) of the cranial bones. The inner dura mater forms the plates that separate the two cerebral hemispheres (falx cerebri) (see Fig. 27-4), the cerebrum and the lower brain stem/cerebellum (tentorium cerebelli) (see Fig. 27-4), and the roof of the pituitary fossa (diaphragma sellae). Venous sinuses, which collect venous blood for return to the heart, are located between the dural layers (see Fig. 27-6).

There is a potential space called the subdural space between the inner dura and arachnoid that can fill with blood and fluid, especially after head trauma. An epidural space exists between the dura mater and the periosteum, which likewise can fill with blood and fluid after head injury.

The meninges anchor the spinal cord. The pia mater, which closely surrounds the spinal cord, continues from the tip of the conus as a threadlike structure, called the filum terminale, to the end of the vertebral column where it is anchored into the ligament on the posterior side of the coccyx. The denticulate ligaments, paired strips of epidural tissue, extend laterally from the pia mater to the dura mater to suspend the spinal cord from the dura (see Fig. 27-5). The subarachnoid space extends below the level of the spinal cord to the second sacral (S2) vertebral level. The subarachnoid space is the area of needle placement during a lumbar puncture.

Cerebrospinal Fluid and Ventricular System. Cerebrospinal fluid (CSF) is a clear, colorless fluid composed of the substances listed in Table 27-3. Approximately 135 ml of CSF circulates through the ventricles and within the subarachnoid space (80 ml in the ventricles and 55 ml in the subarachnoid space). The pressure of the fluid when a client is lying on his or her side is 180 mm of water. The flow of CSF is due to the pressure difference between the arterial system and the subarachnoid system.

Most CSF is made in the choroid plexus of the lateral, third, and fourth ventricles. The choroid plexus is a network of blood vessels within the pia mater that is in direct contact with the lining of the ventricle. The choroid plexuses together make approximately 300 ml of CSF per day.

The ventricular system is a series of cavities within the brain. CSF flows from each of the lateral ventricles

TABLE 27-3. Composition of Cerebrospinal Fluid

Constituent	Normal Value
Na^+	148 mmol/L
K^+	2.9 mmol/L
Cl^-	125 mmol/L
HCO_3^-	22.9 mmol/L
Glucose (fasting)	50-75 mg/100 ml
pH	7.3
Protein	15-45 mg/100 ml
Albumin	80%
Gamma globulin	6-10%
Cells	
White (lymphocytes)	0-4/mm
Red	0/mm

via a foramen (foramen of Monro) into the third ventricle (Fig. 27-7). CSF drains from the third ventricle through the cerebral aqueduct into the fourth ventricle. From the fourth ventricle, CSF passes via one of three foramina (two foramina of Luschka and one foramen of Magendie) into the cisterna magna and from there throughout the subarachnoid space. Eventually, the CSF circulates upward into the region of the superior sagittal sinus (see Fig. 27-6) where it is absorbed across the arachnoid granulations because of a pressure difference into the venous system. The arachnoid granulations are extensive tufts of pia-arachnoid that along with the inner dura extend into the superior sagittal sinus and permit one-way flow of CSF into the sinus (see Fig. 27-6). If a blockage occurs within the ventricular system or in the arachnoid granulations, CSF accumulates, a condition known as hydrocephalus.

The brain and spinal cord float in the CSF, which absorbs shocks, thus cushioning the central nervous system. CSF also prevents the brain from tugging on meninges, nerve roots, and blood vessels.

Blood-Brain Barrier. Three barriers exist: a blood-brain barrier; a blood-CSF barrier; and a brain-CSF barrier. The primary role of these brain barriers is to regulate and maintain an optimal and stable chemical environment for neurons. Brain barriers are either physical barriers or physiologic processes (specifically transport systems) that slow movement of certain substances from one central nervous system compartment to another by regulating ion movement between the compartments. Tight junctions of the endothelial cells lining the capillaries, pores of the capillaries of the choroid plexuses, the basement membrane next to the choroid plexuses, and the pial-glial membrane serve as the physical barriers. An intact blood-brain barrier may prevent some drugs from crossing into the brain. This must be taken into consideration when medications are prescribed for nervous system disorders.

Blood Supply. The brain requires one third of the cardiac output and uses 20 per cent of the body's oxygen. It makes energy almost exclusively from glucose. The gray matter has higher metabolic needs than white matter does. The brain receives 800 ml of blood flow per minute. This blood flow can be regulated by metabolic end products (e.g., the ability of carbon dioxide to alter the vascular tone of cerebral vessels). By this means, the brain ensures that its blood flow is adequate.

The vertebral arteries and the internal carotid arteries (Fig. 27-8) provide the arterial supply to the brain. The vertebral arteries branch from the subclavian arteries, travel through the transverse foramina in the cervical vertebrae, and enter the cranial vault through the foramen magnum. The vertebral arteries are located on the anterolateral surface of the medulla. At the junction of the medulla and pons, the vertebral arteries join to form the basilar artery. The basilar artery bifurcates at the midbrain level to form two posterior cerebral arteries. The vertebral artery system supplies the brain stem, cerebellum, lower portion of the diencephalon, and medial and inferior regions of the temporal and occipital lobes.

The internal carotid arteries branch from the common carotid arteries and enter the cranial vault at the base of the skull. The internal carotid arteries pass through the cavernous sinus and bifurcate into the an-

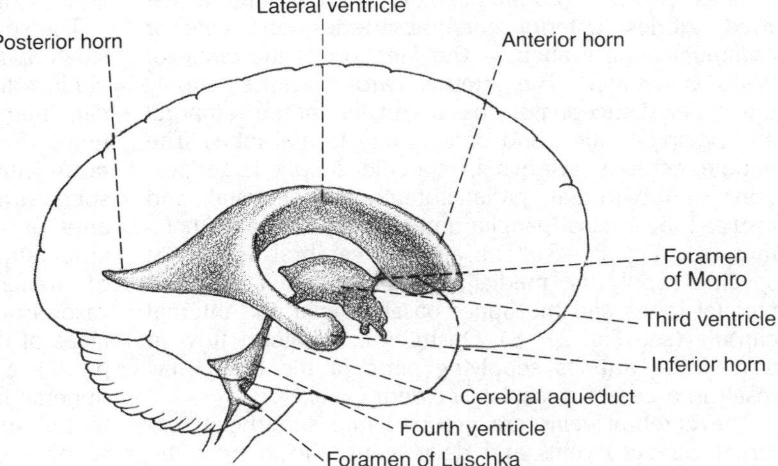

▲ *Figure 27-7*

The ventricular system, lateral view.

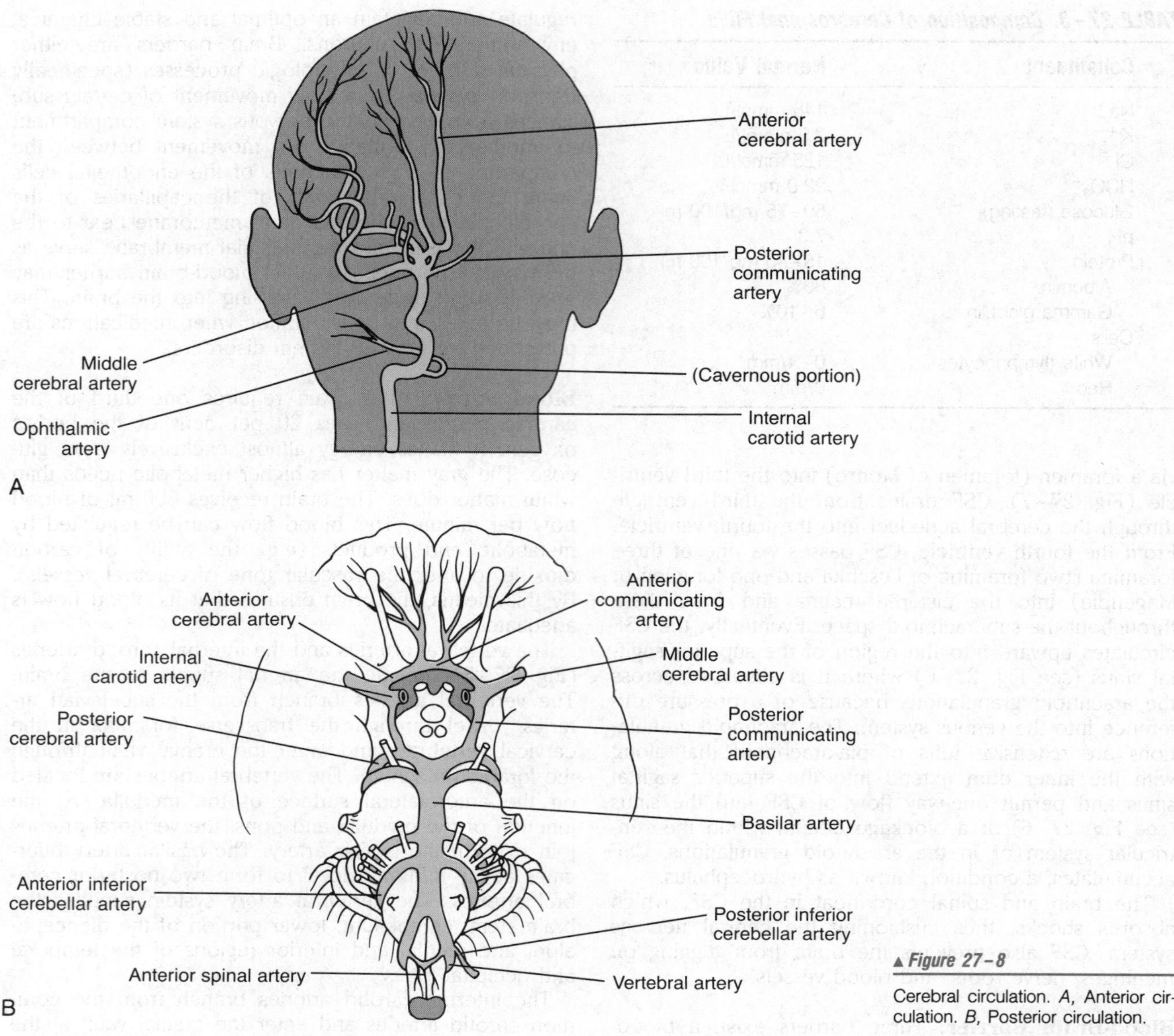

▲ *Figure 27–8*

Cerebral circulation. *A,* Anterior circulation. *B,* Posterior circulation.

terior and middle cerebral arteries. Near this bifurcation, the circle of Willis, a ring of blood vessels at the base of the brain, is formed by the posterior cerebral arteries, posterior communicating arteries, internal carotid arteries, anterior cerebral arteries, and anterior communicating branches. The function of the circle of Willis is debated. The internal carotid arteries supply the upper diencephalon, basal ganglia, lateral temporal and occipital lobes, and parietal and frontal lobes. The middle cerebral arteries in specific supply large portions of the frontal, parietal, temporal, occipital, and insular lobes; basal ganglia; internal capsule; and thalamus (see Fig. 27–8). The anterior cerebral arteries in specific supply the medial portions of the frontal and parietal lobes and the upper basal ganglia and internal capsule (see Fig. 27–8). Obstruction of blood flow in any of the arteries supplying parts of the brain may result in a cerebrovascular accident (stroke).

The cerebral veins are grouped into superficial (external, surface) veins and deep veins. Blood from the upper lateral and medial cortices drains into the superior sagittal sinus flowing occipitally through other sinuses until it reaches the right jugular vein. The deep veins drain into the internal cerebral vein through venous sinuses and into the left internal jugular vein.

The spinal cord derives its arterial blood supply from small spinal arteries that branch off larger arteries, including the vertebrals, ascending cervical, deep cervical, intercostal, lumbar, and sacral arteries. These arteries form the three main arteries of the spinal cord—the anterior spinal artery and a pair of posterior spinal arteries that extend the length of the cord. The anterior and posterior spinal arteries arise from the intracranial portion of the vertebral arteries. A network of branches from this arterial system, called arterial vasocorona, is located on the anterior and lateral surfaces of the spinal cord. Subcommissural branches supply the anterior two thirds of the cord except the peripheral anterior and lateral funiculi, which are supplied by the arterial vasocorona. The posterior spinal arteries supply the remainder of the cord.

The venous distribution is similar to the arterial distribution of the spinal cord. The venous system drains into the venous sinuses located between the dura mater and the periosteum of the vertebral column.

Peripheral Nervous System

The cranial and spinal nerves with their branches and their ganglia make up the peripheral nervous system. Each cranial and spinal nerve is composed of an axon, neurilemma cells with their neurilemma sheaths, and the connective tissue coverings to offer structural support and provide a network of blood vessels and the interstitial spaces essential for nerve impulse conduction.

SPINAL NERVES

The spinal nerves develop from a series of nerve rootlets that collect laterally as spinal roots. The dorsal root emerges from the posterolateral cord (see Fig. 27–5). The ventral root emerges from the anterolateral spinal cord (see Fig. 27–5). Thirty-one pairs of spinal nerves are formed (see Fig. 27–4). The specific area of inner-

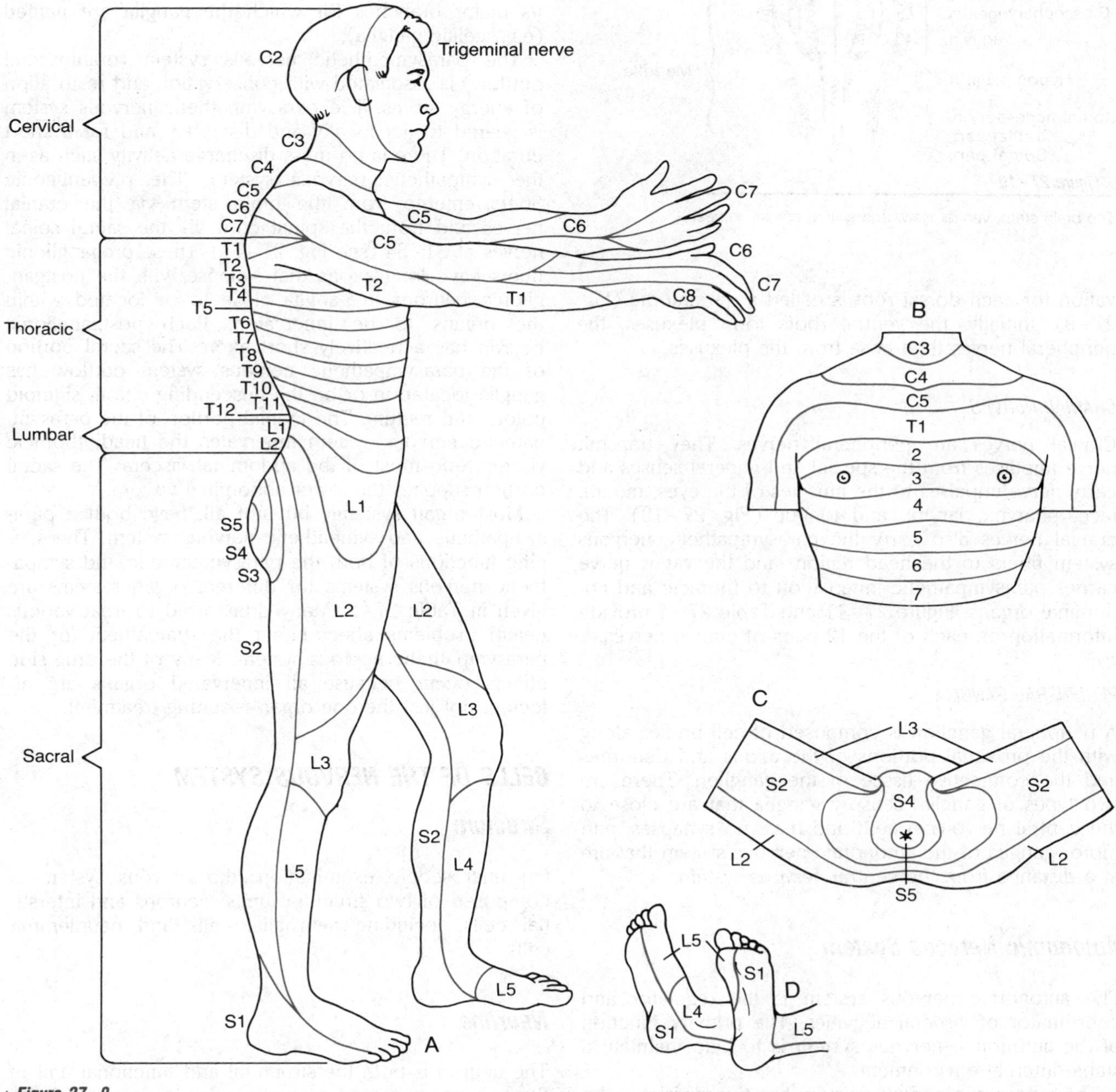

▲ Figure 27–9

Dermatomes indicate distribution of spinal nerves. Solid lines divide spinal cord regions (i.e., cervical, thoracic, lumbar, sacral). Dotted lines indicate spinal cord segments, or dermatomes. *A*, Torso and limbs. *B*, Anterior chest. *C*, Perineum. *D*, Feet. Dermatomes are used during assessment to identify specific areas of sensory impairment (e.g., touch, pain, temperature).

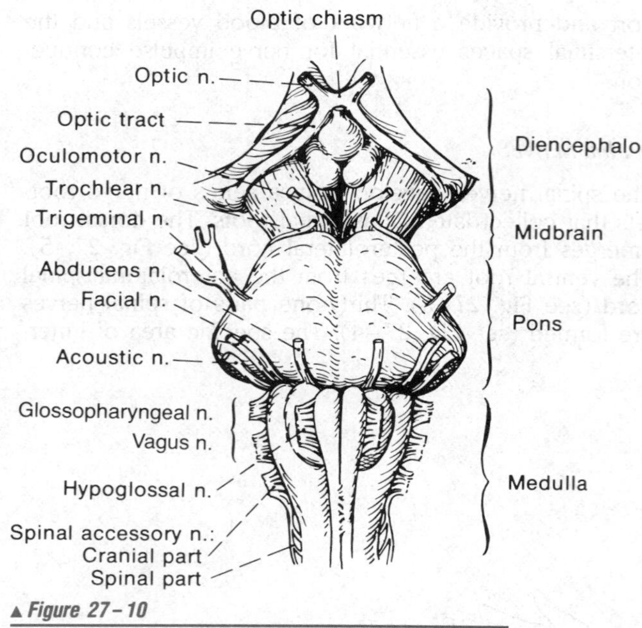

▲ *Figure 27–10*

The brain stem, ventral view, and exiting cranial nerves.

vation for each dorsal root is called a dermatome (Fig. 27–9). Initially, the ventral roots form plexuses; the peripheral nerves then arise from the plexuses.

CRANIAL NERVES

Cranial nerves are peripheral nerves. They transmit nerve impulses from the special and general senses and carry nerve impulses to the muscles of the eyes, mouth, face, pharynx, larynx, and tongue (Fig. 27–10). The cranial nerves also carry the parasympathetic nervous system fibers to the head region, and the vagus nerve carries parasympathetic innervation to thoracic and abdominal organs. Figure 27–11 and Table 27–4 provide information on each of the 12 pairs of cranial nerves.

PERIPHERAL GANGLIA

A peripheral ganglion is composed of cell bodies along with the proximal portions of the axons and dendrites and the connective tissue of the ganglion. There are two types of ganglia: sensory ganglia that are close to the central nervous system and have no synapses; and motor ganglia of the autonomic nervous system that are at a distance from the central nervous system.

Autonomic Nervous System

The autonomic nervous system is the regulator and coordinator of visceral activities. The primary function of the autonomic nervous system is to help maintain a stable internal environment.

The autonomic nervous system has two divisions, the sympathetic and parasympathetic nervous systems. These two systems are highly integrated and act together. The sympathetic system (thoracolumbar outflow) coordinates activities that are used to handle stress. The sympathetic nervous system is geared for action as a whole for sustained periods. All the preganglionic neurons of the sympathetic nervous system emerge from the spinal cord via the motor (ventral) roots of the thoracic and upper two lumbar spinal nerves (T1 to L2) (see Fig. 27–11). The preganglionic neurons terminate and synapse with postganglionic neurons located in the paravertebral ganglia or in the prevertebral ganglia. The paravertebral ganglia form a chain (a series of ganglia) located on and along the entire length of the vertebral column. The prevertebral ganglia are located in close proximity to the aorta and its major branches for which the ganglia are named (e.g., celiac ganglia).

The parasympathetic nervous system (craniosacral outflow) is associated with conservation and restoration of energy stores. The parasympathetic nervous system is geared to act locally and discretely and for a short duration. There is no mass discharge activity such as in the sympathetic nervous system. The preganglionic fibers emerge from the brain stem via the cranial nerves and from the spinal cord via the sacral spinal nerves at S1–S4 (see Fig. 27–11). These preganglionic fibers have long axons that synapse with the postganglionic neurons in ganglia close to or located within the organs to be innervated. Each postganglionic neuron has a relatively short axon. The sacral portion of the parasympathetic nervous system outflow has ganglia located in or on the descending colon, sigmoid colon, and rectum. The cranial portion of the parasympathetic nervous system innervates the head, thoracic viscera, and most of the abdominal viscera. The sacral portion supplies the lower abdominal viscera.

Most organ systems, but not all, have both a parasympathetic and sympathetic nervous system. The specific functions of both the parasympathetic and sympathetic nervous systems for different organ systems are given in Table 27–5. Many drugs used to treat various health problems affect either the sympathetic or the parasympathetic nervous system. Many of the drug side effects occur because all innervated organs are affected, not just the one organ requiring treatment.

CELLS OF THE NERVOUS SYSTEM

Structure

On microscopic examination, the nervous system is composed of two structural units: neurons and interstitial cells, including neuroglial cells and neurilemma cells.

Neurons

The neuron is both the structural and functional unit of the nervous system. A typical neuron is composed of a cell body (nerve cell) and threadlike processes that include one axon and several dendrites (Fig. 27–12).

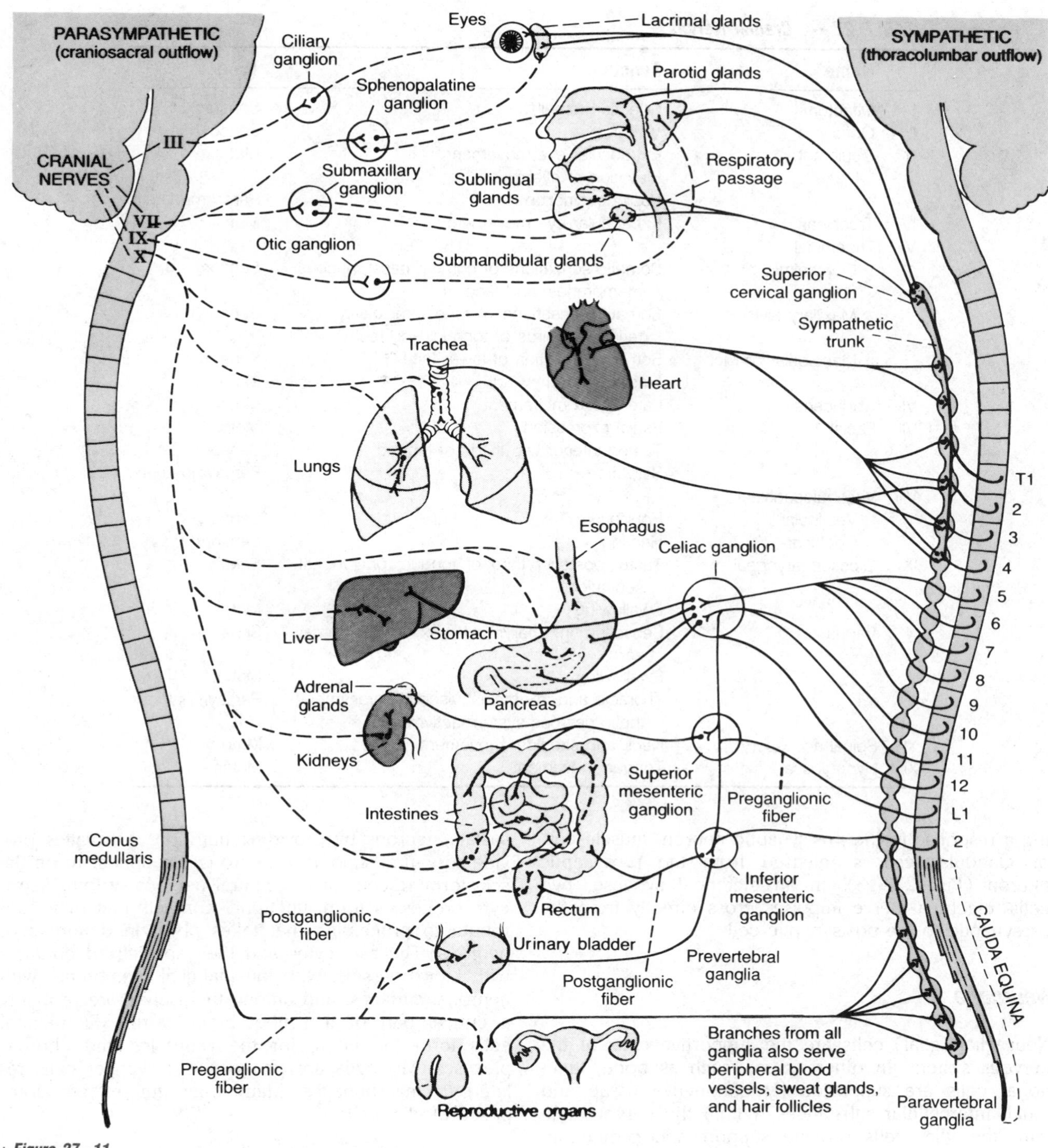

▲ *Figure 27-11*

Diagrammatic representation of autonomic nervous system.

Many neurons have their axons covered by myelin. Such axons are called myelinated nerve fibers. The sheaths of myelin are not continuous but broken into sections called nodes of Ranvier. Both the myelin and the gaps in myelin increase the speed of nerve impulse transmission.

The nerve cell contains structures typical of all cells. The neuron also contains some structures specific to neurons, including microtubules and neurofilaments.

Microtubules and neurofilaments are threadlike structures. The straight, long, unbranched neurofilaments are rigid structures that may provide strength and rigidity to the long slender dendrites and axons. Microtubules are finer filaments that provide a transport system within the cell.

Synapses are areas of specialized contact between neurons, or neurons and effector organs. In a chemical synapse, a chemical neurotransmitter capable of evok-

TABLE 27-4. Cranial Nerves

	Name	Function	Type
I	Olfactory	Olfaction (smell)	Sensory
II	Optic	Vision	Sensory
III	Oculomotor	Extraocular eye movement	Motor
		Elevation of eyelid	
		Pupil constriction	Parasympathetic
IV	Trochlear	Extraocular eye movement	Motor
V	Trigeminal		
	Ophthalmic division	Somatic sensations of cornea, nasal mucous membranes, and face	Sensory
	Maxillary division	Somatic sensations of face, oral cavity, anterior two thirds of tongue, and teeth	Sensory
	Mandibular division	Somatic sensation of lower face	Sensory
		Mastication (chewing)	Motor
VI	Abducens	Lateral eye movement	Motor
VII	Facial	Facial expression	Motor
		Taste, anterior two thirds of tongue	Sensory
		Salivation	Parasympathetic
VIII	Vestibulocochlear		
	Vestibular	Equilibrium	Sensory
	Cochlear	Hearing	Sensory
IX	Glossopharyngeal	Taste, posterior third of tongue; pharyngeal sensation	Sensory
		Swallowing	Motor
X	Vagus	Sensation in pharynx, larynx, and external ear	Sensory
		Swallowing	Motor
		Thoracic and abdominal visceral parasympathetic nervous system activities	Parasympathetic
XI	Spinal accessory	Neck and shoulder movement	Motor
XII	Hypoglossal	Tongue movement	Motor

ing a response in the postsynaptic neuron, muscle cell, or glandular cell is released from the presynaptic neuron (Fig. 27-13). In an electrical synapse, two cells' electrical nerve impulses cross directly from the presynaptic to the postsynaptic cell.

Neuroglia

Neuroglial (glial) cells are the supportive cells of the nervous system. In other tissues, such as bone, functional cells are supported by connective tissue and tough intercellular substances. Within the nervous system, the glial cells provide support and protection. Neuroglia compose approximately half of the total brain and spinal cord and are 5 to 10 times more numerous than neurons. Neuroglia function to assist the neurons to carry out their function. Glial cells control the ion concentrations within the extracellular space; provide high-energy compounds to neurons; form and maintain myelin sheaths; and may contribute to the transport of nutrients, gases, and waste products between neurons and the vascular system and CSF.

Four types of neuroglial cells exist (Fig. 27-14). Oligodendrocytes form sheaths around neurons and sustain myelin in the central nervous system. They also sustain neurons by providing nutrition. Astrocytes provide structural support to neurons and appear to be the scar-forming cells of the central nervous system. Astrocyte processes form junctional contacts that may contribute to processing that takes place in dendrites of neurons. The astrocytes and their specialized contacts with blood vessels, with the pial-glial membrane, with neuronal surfaces, and among themselves are probably a critical part of the blood-brain barrier. Ependymal cells form the lining for the ventricles and choroid plexuses. Microglia are phagocytic scavenger cells related to macrophages. Many brain tumors are composed of glial cells.

Function and Impulse Conduction

RESTING POTENTIAL

A neuron not conducting a nerve impulse is called a resting cell. A resting cell is a charged cell, however, because there is a difference in electrical potential between the interstitial fluid outside of the neuron and the intracellular fluid within the neuron (Fig. 27-15). The inside of the nerve cell is electrically negative, compared with the interstitial fluid. A resting potential

TABLE 27–5. Functions of the Autonomic Nervous System

Organ System	Results of Parasympathetic Stimulation	Results of Sympathetic Stimulation
Eye and lacrimal gland	Constriction (miosis) of pupil Accommodation of lens to near vision Secretion of tears by lacrimal glands	Dilation (mydriasis) of pupil Slight elevation of upper eyelid Possibly some accommodation to far vision
Glands of nose and mouth	Vasodilation in glands Secretion of profuse watery secretion	Vasoconstriction and diminished blood flow Sparse, thick, viscous mucous secretion
Heart	Slower heart rate Decreased stroke volume Probable constriction of coronary arteries	Increased heart rate Increased stroke volume Dilation of coronary arteries
Lungs	Constriction of bronchi and bronchioles Increased secretion of the glandular cells of the tubes	Dilation of bronchi and bronchioles
Digestive system	Increase in contractility, motility, and tone Relaxation of muscle sphincters Increase in secretion of digestive glands	Decrease in contractility, motility, and tone Constriction of muscle sphincters Inhibition of secretion Increased glucose in the bloodstream
Genital system	Engorgement of erectile tissues Active secretion of accessory glands of reproductive system	Ejaculation
Urinary system	Increased motility and tone of ureters Increased urination as a result of detrusor contraction	Relaxation of detrusor muscle
Blood vessels	Dilation of blood vessels to digestive system, glands of head and face, kidney, and ureters	Dilation of coronary arteries and arteries to voluntary muscles Constriction of blood vessels to digestive system and the skin
Sweat glands and pilomotor (hair) muscles of the skin		Secretion by sweat glands Contraction of pilomotor muscles
Adrenal glands		Release of epinephrine and norepinephrine

measured in millivolts results from this difference in electrical potential between the two compartments. The resting membrane potential is −70 to −100 mV.

Interstitial fluid has a much higher concentration of sodium and chloride ions. Intracellular fluids have a much higher concentration of potassium and organic protein ions. The differential concentrations of sodium, potassium, and chloride are produced and maintained across the semipermeable cell membrane by active transport systems (biologic pumps).

Calcium ions act as a "cement" and play a role in membrane excitability. When calcium is low, sodium leaks into the neuron and resting potential is lowered, which makes the cell more excitable and results in the cell's firing spontaneously. This happens when a client is experiencing tetany. When calcium is high, sodium is less able to enter the neuron. The neuron is less excitable and harder to fire.

NERVE IMPULSE

A nerve impulse is an electrochemical phenomenon involving a sequence of ion exchanges (see Fig. 27–15). If the axon's membrane potential is lowered to a critical point, called threshold value, an action potential (nerve impulse) is generated. This action potential passes along the axon to all parts of the neuron. The axon responds with an all-or-none response, that is, the stimulus either generates an action potential or it does not. A strong stimulus will produce the same action potential as a weaker one.

The generation of an action potential has two phases

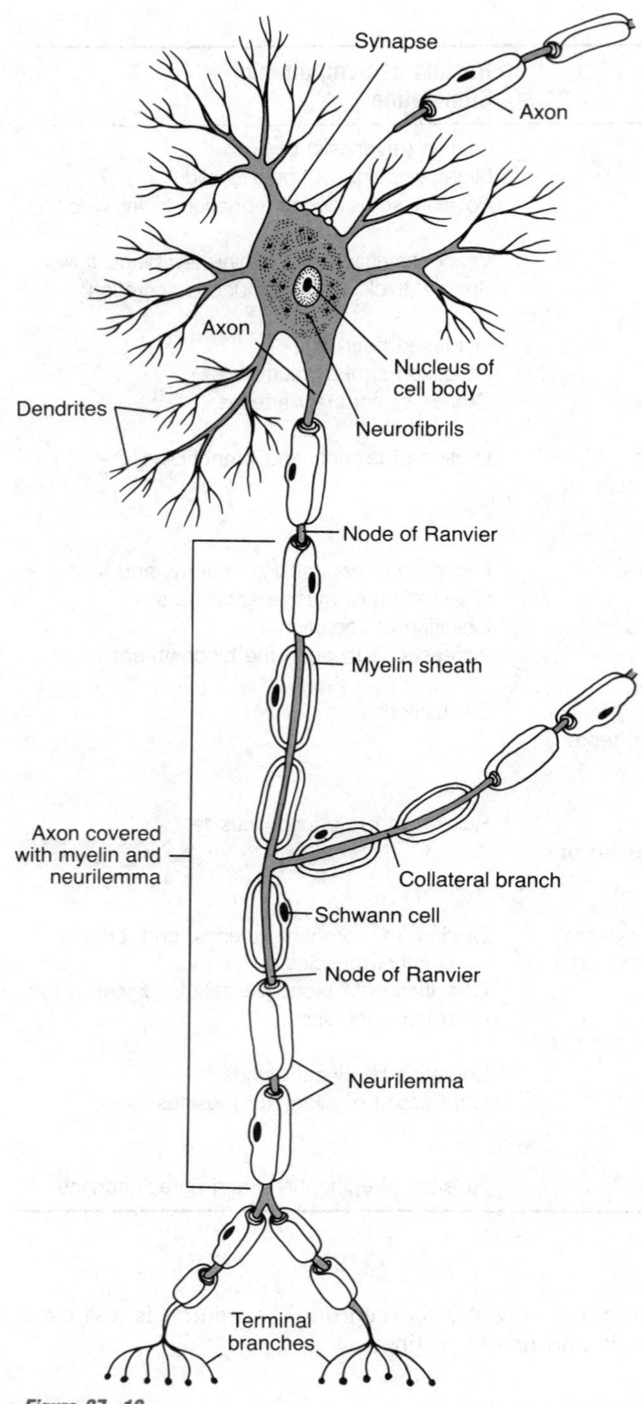

▲ *Figure 27-12*

A neuron, the basic element of the nervous system.

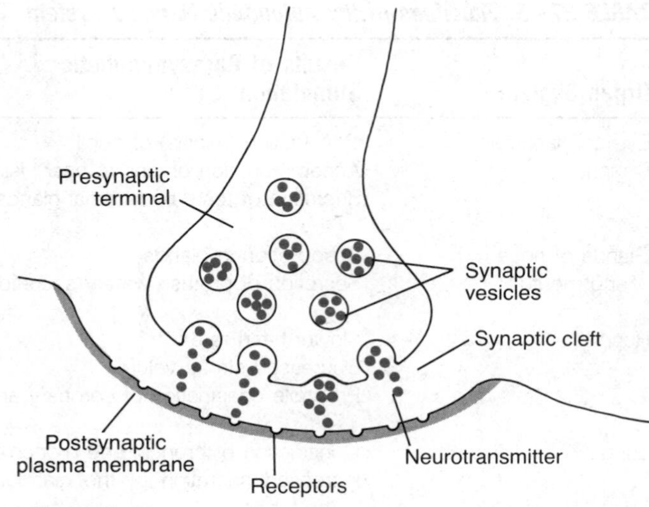

▲ *Figure 27-13*

The chemical synapse.

related to permeability of the cell membrane. The first phase involves an influx of sodium, a positively charged ion, into the cell; electronegativity changes from −70 to −90 mV to +30 to +50 mV. This change is called depolarization (see Fig. 27-15). Depolarization passes down the nerve. The nerve fiber gains sodium and loses potassium during the passage of an action potential (nerve impulse).

The sodium influx is immediately followed by the second phase, an increased permeability of the plasma membrane to potassium. Loss of potassium ions from within the cell continues until the resting potential of the membrane is reestablished (see Fig. 27-14). This process occurs within a millisecond or so after the action potential. Later, the sodium is actively pumped out of the cell.

In an unmyelinated nerve fiber, there is a smooth progressive movement of the action potential. In a myelinated nerve, the action potential spreads by a discontinuous conduction (saltatory conduction) from one node of Ranvier to the next node of Ranvier.

SALTATORY CONDUCTION

Saltatory conduction allows a faster speed of conduction. Each node of Ranvier is a site of self-regeneration of the nerve impulse because ion exchange readily occurs between the intracellular compartment and the interstitial compartment. Additionally, the myelin sheath prevents ion flow away from the nerve fiber. In demyelinating diseases like multiple sclerosis, the myelin sheath is damaged, and nerve impulse conduction is impaired; dysfunction such as weakness, incoordination, and tremor is produced.

REFRACTORY PERIOD

After an action potential is generated, each segment of the nerve fiber is not able to conduct another action potential for a millisecond. This is called the absolute refractory period. During this time interval, sodium is not able to enter the nerve cell. After the absolute refractory period, there is a period called the relative refractory period when only a stimulus stronger than ordinary will produce an action potential.

CHEMICAL SYNAPSE

The synapse acts as a one-way valve, allowing transmission of an action potential in only one direction

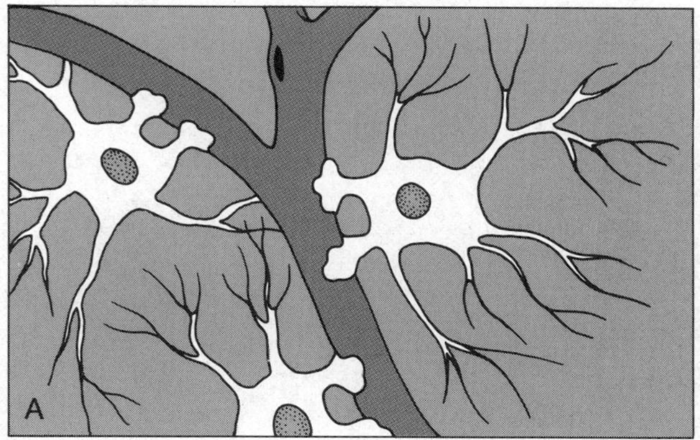

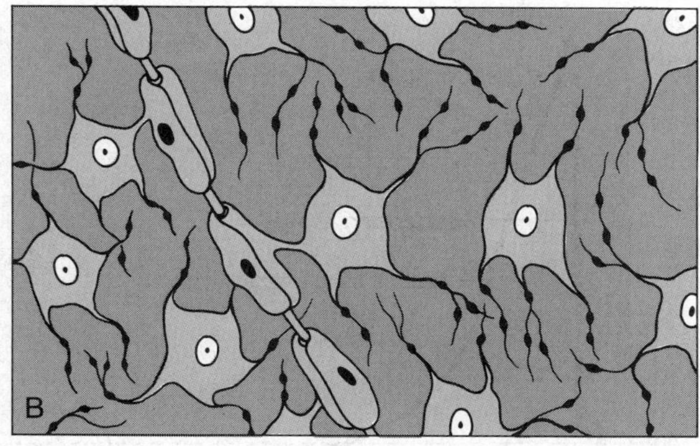

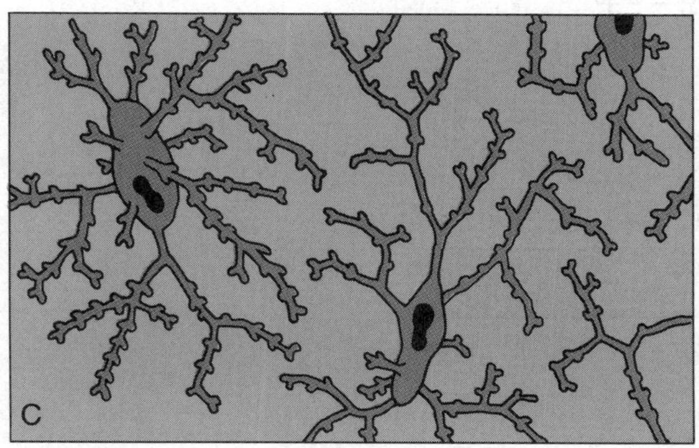

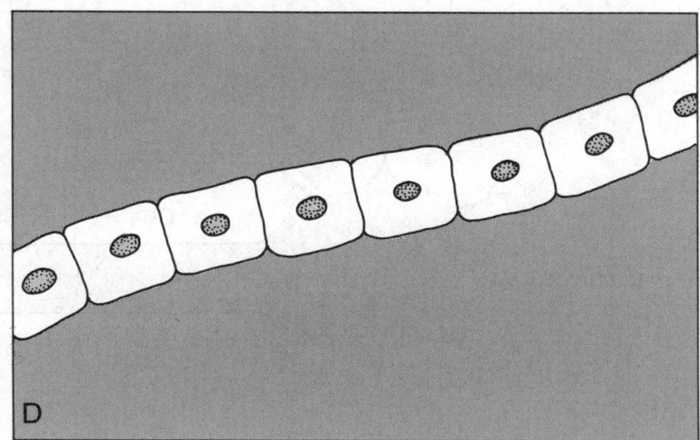

▲ *Figure 27-14*

Neuroglial cells. *A*, Astrocytes. *B*, Oligodendrocytes. *C*, Microglia. *D*, Ependymal cells.

from the presynaptic neuron to the postsynaptic neuron. When the action potential reaches the presynaptic terminal of the axon, neurotransmitters are released. Each neurotransmitter influences specific receptor sites on the postsynaptic membranes of neurons, muscles, and glands (see Fig. 27-15). A list of some of the common neurotransmitters is presented in Box 27-1. Two types of responses may be elicited. An excitatory response is manifested by depolarization. An inhibitory response is manifested by hyperpolarization. Many nervous system diseases are caused by alterations in neurotransmitters. For example, Parkinson's disease is due to decreased dopamine. Likewise, many drugs alter the amounts of neurotransmitters throughout the nervous system, with resultant undesired side effects such as abnormal movements or emotions.

Each neuron synapses with many other neurons. This potential for the neuron to excite or inhibit numerous other neurons because of its branching is called the principle of divergence. Each neuron of the central nervous system also has the potential to be excited and inhibited by many other neurons. This converging of the activity of many neurons onto one neuron is called the principle of convergence.

RECEPTORS

Three types of peripheral receptors exist: (1) fibers actually ending at the body surface, (2) naked or encapsulated nerve endings in the tissues, and (3) endings that synapse on specialized cells. Receptors are biologic transducers, using the stimulus of one form of energy to initiate the "electrical" energy of the nerve impulse—mechanical energy, chemical energy, light energy, and thermal energy. Although sensory receptors may be stimulated by more than one form of energy, each receptor is especially sensitive to a particular form of energy.

Receptors exhibit a phenomenon known as adaptation, a decreased receptor sensitivity in response to steady continuous stimuli. Slowly adapting receptors are able to maintain the lower rate of discharge for minutes to even hours. Fast-adapting receptors' bursts of impulses terminate in less than a second after initiation of the stimulus. The mechanism of adaptation is not known.

Receptors respond more effectively to change than to steady continuous stimulation.

REGENERATION

Nerve cell bodies are not able to regenerate. Regeneration is possible, however, if just the axon is injured. Initially, there is breakdown of the myelin sheath and axon. The axon swells and fragments while the myelin sheath disintegrates distal to the injury. The cell body takes up water. Macrophages phagocytize the breakdown products.

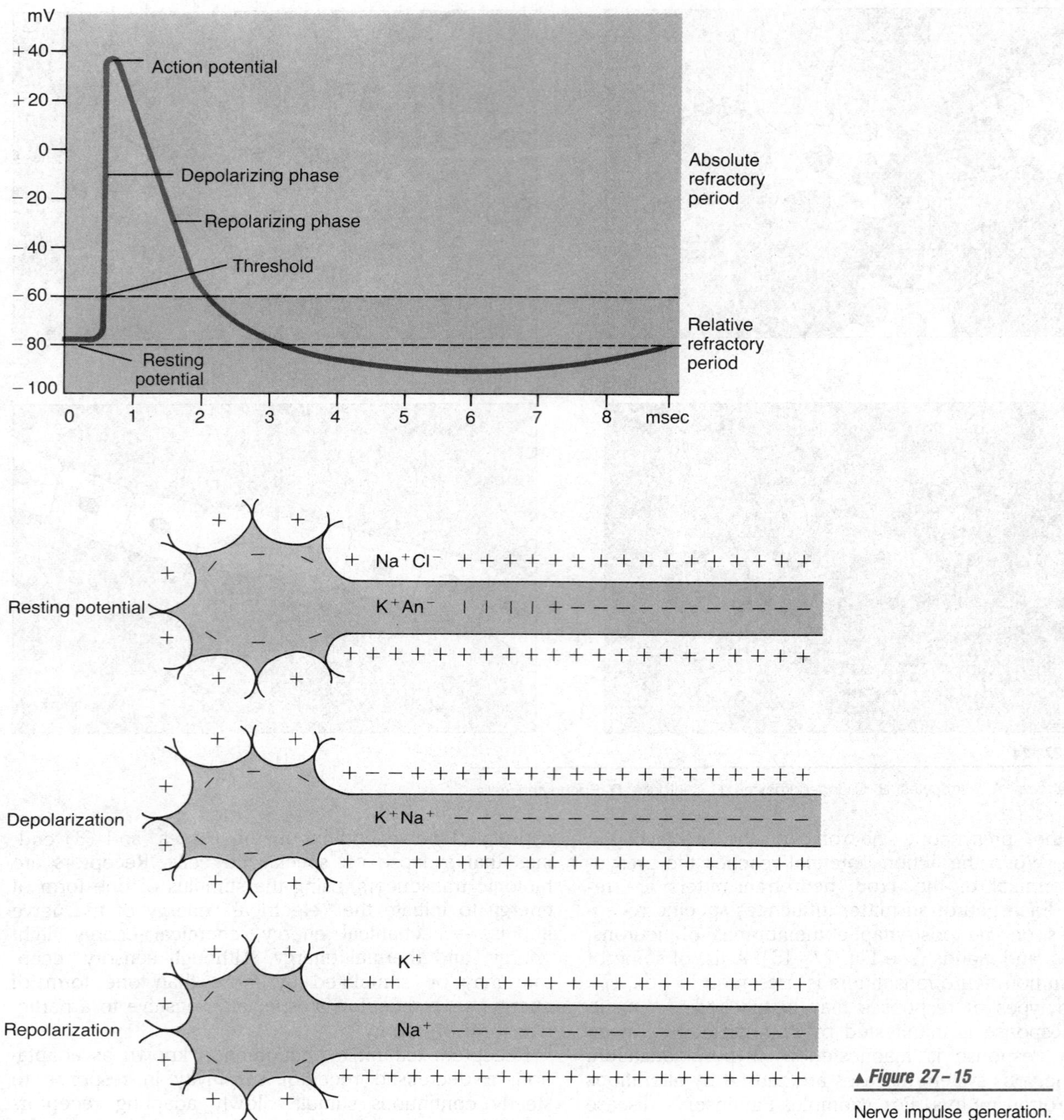

▲ **Figure 27-15**

Nerve impulse generation.

Neurilemma cells near the injury and in the entire segment distal to the injury undergo cell multiplication. These neurilemma cells form continuous cords (tubes) of cells that maintain the nerve fiber pattern. Neurilemma cells migrate into the emerging space.

The injured axon tip forms a new plasma membrane. Within a few days after injury, sprouts emerge from the tip. Peripheral nerve sprouts enter the distal stump and often come in contact with a neurilemma cord, which serves as a guide. The regenerating axon grows along the cord at a rate of 4 mm/day. Later, the neurilemma cells encapsulate the regenerating nerve fibers. With time, the axon and myelin sheath both thicken. Axons within the central nervous system sprout and form growing tips but appear unable to sustain the metabolic responses necessary for extensive regeneration. It is thought that the axon tip is not able to penetrate the glial scar formed at the injury site, such as after spinal cord injury.

An uninjured axon may sprout a collateral branch at a node of Ranvier that may enter into an adjacent denervated neurilemma cord. Collateral nerve regeneration occurs in both the peripheral and central nervous systems, for example, after peripheral nerve trauma or

Box 27–1. Common Neurotransmitters

Acetylcholine
Dopamine } Catecholamines
Norepinephrine } Catecholamines
Epinephrine } Catecholamines
5-Hydroxytryptamine (serotonin)
Gamma-aminobutyric acid (GABA)
Glycine
Enkephalin

inflammation of a peripheral nerve such as in Bell's palsy.

EFFECTS OF NORMAL AGING ON THE NEUROLOGIC SYSTEM

Neurons undergo senescence. Intracellular, cellular, and biochemical changes occur. Lipofuscin accumulates in the cell. Neurofibrillary tangles and senile plaques develop. The neurons decrease in number after 30 years of age; the neuroglial cells increase in size and number. The number of dendrites decreases. The axons' diameters thin, and the receptors decrease in number.

There is a decrease in the amount of available neurotransmitters by the age of 65 or 70 years. Oxygen consumption is decreased. Neuronal activity decreases, which is evidenced by a decrease in the frequency and amplitude of brain waves on an electroencephalogram. Conduction velocity (speed of transmission) decreases by about 10 per cent, thereby increasing response time.

Summary

The central nervous system is composed of the brain and spinal cord. These structures are protected by the skull and vertebrae, protective membranes, cerebrospinal fluid, a blood-brain barrier, and various cells.

The neuron is the structural and functional unit of the nervous system. The typical neuron is composed of a cell body, one axon, and several dendrites. The impulses along the nerve are carried through the action of several electrolytes and neurotransmitters. Unfortunately, only the axon (which is covered with myelin) is able to regenerate. Therefore, injury or disease and changes with aging create permanent losses of function within the central and peripheral nervous systems.

Bibliography

1. Boss, B. J., & Stowe, A. C. (1986). Neuroanatomy. *Journal of Neuroscience Nursing, 18*(4), 214–230.
2. Brown, D. R. (1980). *Neurosciences for allied health therapies.* St. Louis: C.V. Mosby.
3. deGroot, J., & Chusid, J. G. (1988). *Correlative neuroanatomy and functional neurology.* East Norwalk, CT: Lange.
4. Conway-Rutkowski, B. L. (1982). *Carini and Owens' neurological and neurosurgical nursing.* St. Louis: C.V. Mosby.
5. Guyton, A. (1992). *Basic neuroscience* (2nd ed.). Philadelphia: W. B. Saunders.
6. Kandel, E. R., & Schwartz, J. H. (1985). *Principles of neural science.* New York: Elsevier.
7. Kandel, E. R., & Schwartz, J. H. (1979). *Neuroanatomy and neurophysiology.* Gainesville, FL: Department of Neurosciences, University of Florida.
8. Noback, C. R., & Demarst, R. J. (1985). *The human nervous system. Basic principles of neurobiology.* New York: McGraw-Hill.
9. Solomon, E., et al. (1990). *Human anatomy and physiology.* Philadelphia: Saunders College Publishing.

Chapter 28

Assessment of Clients with Neurologic Disorders

The assessment of a client experiencing a neurologic disorder is a nursing challenge. Neurologic disorders can range from simple to complex with widespread involvement of the central nervous system (CNS). Some neurologic disorders have profound consequences on activities of daily living and even on survival. Neurologic assessment is used by physicians and nurses to establish a baseline of client data. This baseline is used to compare ongoing assessments, diagnose actual and potential health problems, plan the management of client care, and evaluate the client's outcomes. Some of these functions are physician-oriented assessments, and others are assessments shared by nurses and physicians. Because of the complexity of the nervous system, the neurologic assessment is both multifaceted and lengthy. There are three main components to a neurologic assessment: (1) a comprehensive history, which includes symptom analysis; (2) a neurologic physical examination; and (3) general and specific neurodiagnostic studies.

The physician's assessment of the client with neurologic disorders is usually focused on the organic basis of the disorder. Physicians assess the client's clinical manifestations to pinpoint the anatomic location of the disorder, for example, the brain versus the spinal cord. The cause of the signs and symptoms is identified, for example, a tumor versus trauma. These data are combined with all other data and allow a medical diagnosis to be made, from which a treatment plan is determined.

The focus of the nurse's assessment is both anatomic and functional. The nurse makes continuous observations of the client and compares them with baseline data. Astute observations are essential because most neurologic changes occur subtly. Nurses also collect data on the ability of the client to function physically (e.g., self-care deficit) and mentally (e.g., confusion and altered problem solving). Finally, because many neurologic disorders are very serious, the nurse provides skillful, crisis-oriented support for the client and significant others.

This chapter presents basic neurologic assessment procedures. Additional assessment techniques are discussed throughout this unit for other specific neurologic disorders.

HISTORY

The purpose of the history is to determine past and present health status and to obtain a description of the onset of the current illness. It includes biographic data, the chief complaint and history of present illness, past medical history, family history, psychosocial history, and review of systems.

Biographic Data

Biographic data include demographic, administrative, and insurance data. Often included is (1) personal profile, or brief description of the client, (2) source of the history (e.g., client or significant other), and (3) the client's mental status (indicating the reliability of the data). Neurologic problems often affect mental status, sometimes making it difficult to get an accurate history directly from the client.

Chief Complaint

The nurse obtains a detailed description of the events leading the client to seek care. The sequence of signs and symptoms development is explored, including onset, precipitating factors, and duration. The nurse avoids suggesting symptoms to the client and uses open-ended questions. For example, ask the client to describe what a headache feels like rather than asking whether it feels throbbing or dull.

The onset of symptoms and their progress are important to determine. Neurologic disease processes should be described with great accuracy, to facilitate the diagnostic process. Data regarding symptom characteristics and their progression are elicited using a symptom analysis (see Chap. 11).

The health history guides the nurse in the following physical examination. For example, a complaint of dizziness cues the nurse to focus on examination of the eyes, ears (vestibular), and cerebellar function instead of motor and sensory functions. A detailed neurologic examination is indicated in situations in which the client reports behavioral changes, altered level of consciousness, growth and development problems, pain, changes in motor or sensory function, infection, or trauma. The nurse is alert to assess for neurologic problems that may be related to other problems such as alcohol and recreational drug use, metabolic imbalances, or metastatic lesions.

Past Medical History

The past medical history encompasses previous illnesses, hospitalizations, childhood and infectious diseases, medications, perinatal period, growth and development, family history, and psychosocial history and lifestyle. Neurologic illnesses often subtly affect a client's ability to function in an integrated fashion. The nurse asks about changes in consciousness, vision, speech, motor or sensory functions, headaches, seizures, dizziness, vertigo, gait, and body posture.

CHILDHOOD AND INFECTIOUS DISEASES

Data are collected regarding common childhood diseases and immunizations. Diseases associated with neurologic sequelae include rubeola (measles), influenza, and meningitis. Ask whether or not the client has been immunized for polio, tetanus, and measles.

MAJOR ILLNESSES AND HOSPITALIZATIONS

There are a number of major illnesses associated with neurologic changes such as diabetes mellitus, pernicious anemia, cancer, infections, and hypertension. Advanced liver disease and renal disease result in metabolic disturbances such as fluid and electroyte imbalances and acid-base changes that affect mental function. Inquire about hospitalization, injury, or surgery for problems related to the neurologic system such as head trauma, seizures, stroke, or crushing tissue injury. Has the client had any neurologic diagnostic studies performed, such as an electroencephalography (EEG), electromyography (EMG), or computed tomography (CT) scan? Results of such diagnostic studies provide valuable data for future comparison.

MEDICATIONS

The medication history includes all medications that the client is taking or has taken, both prescription and over-the-counter medications. Specifically, ask about aspirin, anticonvulsants, CNS stimulants and depressants, sedatives, anticoagulants, narcotics, tranquilizers, and antihypertensive medications. Many preparations for allergies and colds contain ingredients that cause drowsiness. Inquire about the current use of recreational drugs or past use, type of drug, and duration of use.

GROWTH AND DEVELOPMENT

The client's history of growth and development may help determine whether or not neurologic dysfunction was present at an early age. The perinatal history may include data about in utero exposure to viruses (rubella), maternal consumption of alcohol and tobacco or other drugs, and radiation. Ask the client whether gestation was full term or premature, because premature birth increases risk of neurologic damage from inadequate oxygenation and intracranial bleeding if ventilator support was used. A difficult or prolonged labor and delivery can result in hypoxia or use of forceps for delivery, with consequent central and peripheral neurologic damage.

The nurse asks the client when major developmental tasks such as walking and talking occurred. Was the client able to participate in games, sports, and other childhood activities with peers? Were there any problems with coordination, balance, or agility?

FAMILY HISTORY

The nurse asks the client about the family history of neurologic disorders to determine whether genetic risk factors are present. Inquire about the familial occurrence of epilepsy, Huntington's disease, amyotrophic lateral sclerosis, muscular dystrophy, hypertension, stroke, mental retardation, and psychiatric disorders.

PSYCHOSOCIAL HISTORY AND LIFESTYLE

An understanding of personal psychosocial factors (e.g., educational background, level of performance, and personality changes) enhances accurate assessment. The nurse specifically inquires about changes that have occurred in the client's daily routines. Ask about changes in sleep patterns, exercise routines, hobbies and recreation, occupation, perceived stressors, and sexual interest and performance. Is the client at risk from exposure to neurotoxic fumes or chemicals, such as pesticides, paints, or bonding agents (glue), or is he or she in an inadequately ventilated living or work space?

REVIEW OF SYSTEMS

The client is asked to describe symptoms associated with the neurologic system such as behavior changes, mood swings, loss of consciousness, seizures, memory deficits, motor function problems (e.g., unstable balance, tics, tremors), and sensory function problems (e.g., pain, paresthesia or tingling, paralysis). Significant data related to the neurologic assessment include those given in Box 28-1. Detailed questions for the review of systems are found in Chapter 11, Table 11-5.

The client with a neurologic problem may be unaware of its presence. The nurse attempts to supplement and corroborate the client's history and review of systems with a family member or significant other who knows the client well. Ask specifically about mental or physical changes that have been noticed.

PHYSICAL EXAMINATION

The neurologic physical examination is intended to detect abnormalities in neurologic functioning. Variations in the client's age, physical condition, and level of

Box 28-1. Significant Data Related to the Neurologic Assessment

Eye

Visual loss
Diplopia

ENT

Infections
Hearing loss
Tinnitus
Dizziness
Vertigo
Voice change
Dysphagia
Changes in taste or smell
Experiences of unusual smells

Cardiovascular

Syncope
Palpitations
Hypotension
Hypertension
Vertigo
Transient ischemic attacks
Stroke

Neurologic

Weakness
Numbness
Paresthesias
Headache
Pain
Altered memory or thinking
Speech difficulty
Vomiting
Vertigo
Ataxia
Fainting
Seizures
Any loss of consciousness
Distortions of reality
Use of consciousness-altering drugs
Disorientation
Altered sleep patterns
Changes in ability to speak, read, or understand language
Changes in memory for recent or remote events
Changes in ability to concentrate

Skin

Hair and nail changes

Musculoskeletal

Tremor
Weakness
Altered coordination
Staggering
Difficulty climbing stairs

consciousness determine how detailed the examination can be. The components of a comprehensive neurologic examination are described here. Adaptations to the examination in response to various situations are presented.

The comprehensive neurologic examination consists of mental status, language and communication, cranial nerve assessment, motor response, sensory response, reflexes, and vital signs. A suggested sequence of physical examination is as follows:

1. Vital signs
2. Pupils
3. Mental status including language and communication
4. Head, neck, and back
5. Motor system
6. Sensory function
7. Reflexes
8. Cranial nerves

Vital Signs

Neurologic disorders can cause life-threatening changes in a client's vital signs. An example is the classic triad of hypotension, bradycardia, and hypothermia seen in spinal cord injuries. Inadequate perfusion of vital organs may result from hypotension if the blood pressure is not supported.

Another example of a neurologically mediated change in vital signs is the rise in pulse pressure that accompanies a rise in intracranial pressure. The body attempts to provide adequate supplies of oxygen and glucose to the brain by increasing the blood flow to the brain to compensate for increased intracranial pressure. Changes in vital signs can indicate neurologic changes in clients in whom the neurologic examination has limited usefulness, such as in unresponsive clients or those who are pharmacologically paralyzed.

Pupils

Evaluation of the eyes provides information about cranial nerve function, intracranial pressure, and the client's ability to follow commands. The reactivity of the pupils to light is assessed first. As in all aspects of the neurologic examination, symmetry in speed and degree of response is assessed. Approximately 20 per cent of the population has anisocoria (unequal pupils). The reaction of both pupils to direct light is assessed first, and then the consensual response is assessed. Consensus involves shining a light into one eye and watching the other pupil for constriction. If the constriction is not seen, then consensus is negative for that eye, which is an abnormal finding. Assessment of direct and consensual pupillary reactions provides information about the functioning of the third cranial nerve (oculomotor) and intracranial pressure. As intracranial pressure increases, the oculomotor nerve is compressed. Depending on the cause, the compression may be unilateral, as in a right-sided subdural hematoma, or bilateral, as seen with generalized edema secondary to head injury. The first indication of increasing intracranial pressure is hippus, a rapid constriction and dilation of the pupils. If the pressure is not relieved, the pupils become larger in size and less reactive until they are fixed and dilated (blown pupil). A fixed and dilated pupil indicates increased intracranial pressure of such severity that the oculomotor nerve is unable to function. This is a poor prognostic sign, because herniation of the brain and death may be imminent.

Assessment of extraocular movements and accommodation provides information on the functioning of cranial nerves III, IV, and VI and the client's ability to understand and obey commands. Extraocular movements are assessed by asking the client to follow the examiner's finger with the eyes. The examiner then moves the finger in different directions and observes for an inability to move one or both eyes in a particular direction (gaze palsy). Accommodation involves the examiner holding a finger approximately 12 inches in front of the client's nose. The client is asked to watch the finger as it is brought toward the nose. The eyes should deviate toward the nose and the pupils constrict. Both accommodation and extraocular movement assessment require an alert client who is able to follow verbal or visual cues. The extraocular movements of blind clients can be assessed by asking them to look in different directions. Direct and consensual responses also can be assessed in uncooperative or unconscious patients. The term "patient" is used in this chapter to describe the client who is unconscious and who cannot be an active participant in care. The family is considered the client in these situations.

Nystagmus is the rapid back-and-forth movement of the eyes. The movement may be horizontal or vertical. Although some individuals are born with nystagmus, the condition usually indicates brain stem dysfunction or dilantin toxicity.

Mental Status

Document general data about the client's mental status (e.g., level of consciousness, orientation, memory, mood and affect, intellectual performance, judgement and insight, speech, and thought content). Mental status examination is discussed in Chapter 11.

The *level of consciousness* (LOC) is the most sensitive indicator of changes in the neurologic status of a client. Consciousness is maintained by function of the cerebral hemispheres and the reticular activating system. LOC is tested using stimuli to determine arousability. Stimuli include verbal, visual, tactile, and noxious agents or painful pressure.

When assessing LOC, stimuli are provided and observations are made regarding the response. Start with visual cues, such as walking in front of the client, and note the response. If a response is not elicited, provide stimulation by use of the voice. Touch and painful (noxious) stimuli are used only if the client does not respond to the milder forms of stimulation. If the nurse must use painful stimuli to elicit a response, it should be a central stimulus, such as a sternal rub, and not fingernail pressure, which is local. Noxious stimuli are also discussed in Chapter 29.

The Glasgow Coma Scale is an assessment tool designed to note trends in a client's response to stimuli (see Chap. 29). Terms used to describe LOC include alert, lethargic, stuporous, semicomatose, and comatose.

Establish orientation to time, place, person, and event (or situation). (What is your name? What day is this? What kind of place is this? Where are you? What brought you to the hospital today?) Identify gross deficits in long- and short-term memory by using simple tests. For example, long-term memory is tested during history taking when the client is asked to give a past medical history. (Of course, there must be another source to validate such data.) Test short-term memory by giving the client three words to remember (e.g., red, Broadway, three), and asking the client to immediately repeat the words and repeat the same words in a few minutes.

Assess mood and affect both by the way the client appears (e.g., euphoric, depressed) and the reports of significant others. Is the client's affect appropriate to the situation?

Intellectual performance includes the fund of knowledge and calculation ability. Ask the client to identify commonly known people, places, events, and the like. Assess calculation ability by asking the client to subtract 7 from 100, then 7 from the remainder and so on. Judgement and insight include reasoning, abstract thinking, and problem solving, as well as the client's perception of the situation. Assess reasoning, abstract thinking, and problem solving for indications of major thought content problems. Listen to the way the client answers questions. Are the answers logical? Do they relate to the question? Clients can be asked to explain a proverb such as "a rolling stone gathers no moss." Assess problem solving by describing a problem situation and asking the client to give a solution. For example, "If a lion killed a leopard, which one would be alive?" or "Is my aunt's uncle a man or a women?" Be careful to ask such questions in a way that does not appear to judge the client's intelligence. Assess insight by asking the client to give an opinion of what may be the cause of the chief complaint.

Language and communication are used to assess the client's speech as well as thought processes, comprehension, and intellectual abilities. Assess speech for articulation problems (usually motor disorders) or problems in language understanding or expression (aphasic disorders). Assess the client's ability to communicate and understand verbally, in writing, mathematically, and nonverbally. During the initial interview, note the client's speech characteristics (e.g., fluency, words used, composition of sentences, questions asked). Does the client spontaneously initiate speech? Does the client repeat the examiner's words? Are the words appropriate? (Note the client's nonverbal behavior.) Does the client understand the questions that are asked? Can the client follow commands? (Ask the client to identify the right and left thumbs.) This tests the client's ability to comprehend the spoken word. Ask the client to read from a newspaper or magazine and ask what is the meaning of the words. Have the client copy several words or sentences on a piece of paper while noting the client's ability to form letters as well as copy. Ask the client to perform simple addition, subtraction, multiplication, and division without aid of pencil and paper. Ask the client to verbally identify several common objects, such as a pen, a key, and a coin.

If the client is expressively aphasic, mental status can still be assessed. Ask questions that can be answered with a yes or no response, or a head nod. Asking the same question using different phrasing will help identify whether or not the client is actually oriented. In the clinical setting, the nurse could go on from here and include assessment of speech patterns (i.e., fluent dysphasia, nonfluent dysphasia, global aphasia, dysarthria, and other disturbances).

Head, Neck, and Back

Head, neck, and spine are examined by inspection, palpation, auscultation, and percussion. The head is inspected for size, shape, contour, and symmetry. The nurse notes any ecchymosis or bruising around the eyes or behind the ears. "Raccoon eyes" are indicative of a anterior basilar skull fracture and appear as bruising around the eyelids with a triangular shape underneath the eyes; the sclerae are white, and there is an increased spread between medial canthi. Also note any drainage from the nares, bruising behind the ears over the mastoid (Battle's sign), and presence or absence of drainage from the ears.

The skull is palpated lightly for nodules or masses and to supplement abnormal inspection findings. If there are open or draining areas, the nurse wears gloves. The skull normally feels smooth and firm. Areas of bogginess or depressions are abnormal. Palpation of neck muscles may identify masses or areas of tenderness.

The spine is inspected and palpated for alignment, noting any deviation from the normal curvatures. Gentle percussion over the spinous processes may produce pain or tenderness. The paravertebral muscles are palpated for masses, tenderness, and spasm. Auscultation of major neck vessels and other vessels may reveal bruits or other abnormal sounds indicative of pathology. Tumors, vascular disorders, traumatic disorders, and problems involving the vertebrae and surrounding muscles may be detected through examination.

Motor System

Assessing the motor system thoroughly involves numerous procedures. The following discussion focuses on the screening examinations and common abnormalities.

Included in the motor examination are muscle size, muscle strength, tone, coordination, gait, station, and movement disorders.

MUSCLE SIZE

Inspect major muscle groups bilaterally for symmetry. Inspect the trunk, and intercostal and abdominal muscles.

MUSCLE STRENGTH

Assess muscle power. Ask the client first to walk on the heels, then on the toes. Ask the client to stand and hold the arms straight out in front with palms up, and then to maintain this posture with eyes closed. A "drift" is said to be present if one arm moves upward or if one hand begins to pronate and fall lower than the other arm. Also, assess major muscle groups against resistance (see Chap. 65). Muscle strength is assessed and rated on a five-point scale in all four extremities, comparing one side to the other as follows:

5/5 = Normal full strength. Muscle is able to move actively through full range of motion against the effects of gravity and applied resistance
4/5 = Muscle is able to move actively through full range of motion against the effect of gravity with weakness to applied resistance
3/5 = Muscle is able to move actively against the effect of gravity alone
2/5 = Muscle is able to move with support against the effect of gravity
1/5 = Muscle contraction is palpable and visible; trace or flicker movement occurs
0/5 = Muscle contraction or movement is undetectable

Assessment of specific muscle groups can be completed to assess deficits in certain areas, such as spinal cord disorders. Disorders of muscle strength may be exhibited by weakness on one side of the body, in both lower extremities, or in both upper and lower extremities.

If an asymmetry is detected, the client and/or family are asked if this is a long-standing or new finding. The age and physical condition of the client should be considered when interpreting the results of muscle strength testing. One would not expect the same strength from a physically fit young client as from an elderly or debilitated client.

If abnormalities are found in muscle power, more detailed assessment may be conducted with procedures such as EMG, discussed later in this chapter.

MUSCLE TONE

Muscle tone is assessed while moving each extremity through passive range of motion. When tone is decreased (hypotonic), the muscles are soft, flabby, or flaccid. Increased muscle tone exists if the muscles are resistant to movement, rigid, or spastic. Note the presence of abnormal flexion or extension posture.

MUSCLE COORDINATION

Muscle coordination assessment includes testing rapid alternating movements, point-to-point maneuvers, and maintenance of truncal balance and head position. To test rapid alternating movements, ask the client to touch (approximate) each finger to the thumb quickly in succession. Alternatively, ask the client to pat the thighs first with palms, then with the back of the hands. In point-to-point testing, the examiner holds up an index finger approximately 18 inches away from the client. The client is asked to first touch his or her nose with a finger, then the examiner's index finger. This is repeated several times while the examiner moves the index finger to different points. The test is performed bilaterally for both the client's right and left hands. Lower extremity coordination is tested by asking the client to place the heel of the foot below the opposite knee and then to slide the heel down the shin toward the great toe. Repeat for the opposite leg.

Disorders related to coordination are indicative of cerebellar or posterior column lesions. The defining characteristics of cerebellar dysfunction include ataxia, intention tremor, nystagmus, ocular dysmetria (inability to gaze on an object), and dysdiadochokinesia (arresting one motor impulse and substituting an opposite one).

GAIT AND STATION

Assess gait and station by having the client stand still, walk, and walk in tandem (i.e., one foot in front of the other in a straight line). Walking involves the functions of motor power, sensation, and coordination. The ability to stand quietly with feet together requires coordination and intact proprioception. If the client has difficulty standing, further assessment is needed to determine whether the client is weak or unsteady. If the client is weak, the nurse needs to protect the client from falling. Terms used to describe gait disorders include

- *Ataxic.* Staggering and unsteady
- *Double step.* Alternate steps differ in length or rate
- *Dystonic.* Irregular and nondirective
- *Dystrophic or broad-based.* Legs far apart, and weight shifting from side to side (waddling)
- *Equine.* High stepping
- *Festinating.* Walking on toes at an accelerating pace
- *Helicopod.* Feet (or foot) makes a half circle with each step
- *Hemiplegic.* Paralyzed on one side, paralyzed limb swings outward, foot drags, arm on affected side does not swing freely.
- *Parkinsonian.* Short, accelerating steps; shuffling; posture forward-leaning; head, hips, and knees flexed; difficult to start and stop
- *Scissors.* Legs cross while walking with short, slow steps
- *Spastic.* Stiff, short steps; toes catch and drag; legs held together; and hips and knees flexed
- *Steppage.* Foot and toes lifted high, heel comes down heavily
- *Tabetic.* High steps, foot slaps down

Examine the muscles for fine and gross abnormal movements. Examples of fine movements are fasciculations (involuntary ripples or twitches occurring while relaxed), which may indicate lower motor neuron disease. Examples of more grossly abnormal movements, often representing extrapyramidal disease, include

- *Akinesia.* Reduced body movement in the absence of weakness or paralysis. Habitual movements (e.g., swinging arms) are limited or absent.
- *Athetosis.* Gross, writhing, wormlike movements of body, face, or extremities.
- *Ballismus.* A form of chorea. Involuntary dramatic movements of arms and legs. Hemiballismus involves only one side.
- *Bradykinesia.* Slow movement.
- *Chorea.* Discrete, jerky, purposeless movements in distal extremities and face.
- *Dystonia.* Prolonged twisting movements.
- *Myoclonus.* Sudden muscle contractions of varying intensity, which may involve a small part of one extremity or the entire body; may violently fling a client to the floor.
- *Tic.* Involuntary movement of groups of muscles in stereotypical patterns. May be physical or psychogenic in origin. Pathologic causes of tics include Tourette's syndrome and tic douloureux.
- *Tremors.* Involuntary trembling or quivering. May vary in direction, amplitude, rhythmicity, parts involved, speed, and timing in relation to rest or activity. Types include parkinsonian, familial, and senile.

Move all joints through a full range of passive motions. Abnormal findings include pain, contractures, and muscle resistance.

Test for apraxia (inability to carry out a learned movement on command in the absence of weakness or paralysis). Ask the client to perform common activities, such as tying shoes or combing hair. True apraxia is present only if a client can do the activity spontaneously but cannot do it on request.

Sensory Function

The sensory function examination incorporates assessment of responses to superficial and mechanical sensations as well as cortical discrimination. Sensory assessment involves testing for touch, pain, vibration, position (proprioception), and discrimination. Assessing hearing, vision, smell, and taste is also sensory assessment. Sensory assessment may identify dermatomes (skin area innervated by various nerves) having absent, reduced, exaggerated, or delayed sensation. Dermatomes are shown in Figure 27–9, and are discussed in Chapter 27.

An unresponsive patient can only be tested for response to painful stimuli (e.g., reflex withdrawal of limbs, wincing, grimacing). A complete sensory examination is only possible on a conscious client because it requires cooperation. Always test sensation with the client's eyes closed. Help the client become as relaxed as possible.

Conduct sensory assessment systematically. Test a particular area of the body, and then test the corresponding area on the opposite side. Proceed in a systematic fashion until all dermatomes are tested. Test the extremities first, then the trunk. Document any asymmetric findings, that is, those varying from one side to the other. If the client has a sensory loss, document the area of loss and where normal sensation begins. Sensation assessment may be documented on a body chart of dermatomes.

SUPERFICIAL SENSATION

Superficial sensations are tested by stimulating the skin in symmetric areas on each side of the body according to the dermatome distribution. Superficial pain is tested by alternating the sharp and dull ends of a sterile safety pin.

Touch and Pain. Ask the client to close the eyes and say that there will be a sharp and a dull stimulus. Demonstrate how sharp and dull feel. Touch the client with the dull end of the safety pin. Then apply a painful stimulus by using the pin's sharp end. Moving from the fingers to the shoulders, alternate the two stimuli inconsistently (so the client cannot predict which is being used) and ask the client to distinguish between which is sharp and which is dull. Then test the toes to the thigh. Finally, test the anterior and posterior trunk and buttock. Keep in mind the dermatomal pattern while testing. Where there is a loss of the sense of pain, test for temperature awareness. Otherwise, it is not necessary to test for temperature, because pain and temperature travel on related pathways.

In an unconscious client, deep pain is used to elicit a sensory response when superficial pain does not produce such a response. The minimal amount of stimulus is used. Means of producing noxious stimuli include rubbing the sternum, applying pressure to the orbital rim, squeezing the sternocleidomastoid muscle, or squeezing the clavicle. The client's response to noxious stimuli is noted. The following responses are those most commonly seen when painful stimuli are applied:

Localization—the client pushes the stimulus away.

Flexion withdrawal—the client pulls away from the stimulus.

Decorticate posturing (abnormal flexion)—the client pulls the fists up toward the chest and extends the legs. This indicates damage to the cortex of the brain.

Decerebrate posturing (abnormal extension)—the client extends and outwardly rotates the arms and extends the legs. This indicates damage to the cerebellum.

No response—there is no visible movement to painful stimulus.

Other Modalities. Other modalities for testing superficial sensation in the conscious client include using a cotton wisp to assess light touch. Follow the same guidelines as for testing superficial pain sensation, stimulating symmetric areas of the dermatomes.

Temperature sensation is not assessed routinely, and the test is performed only when pain and light touch

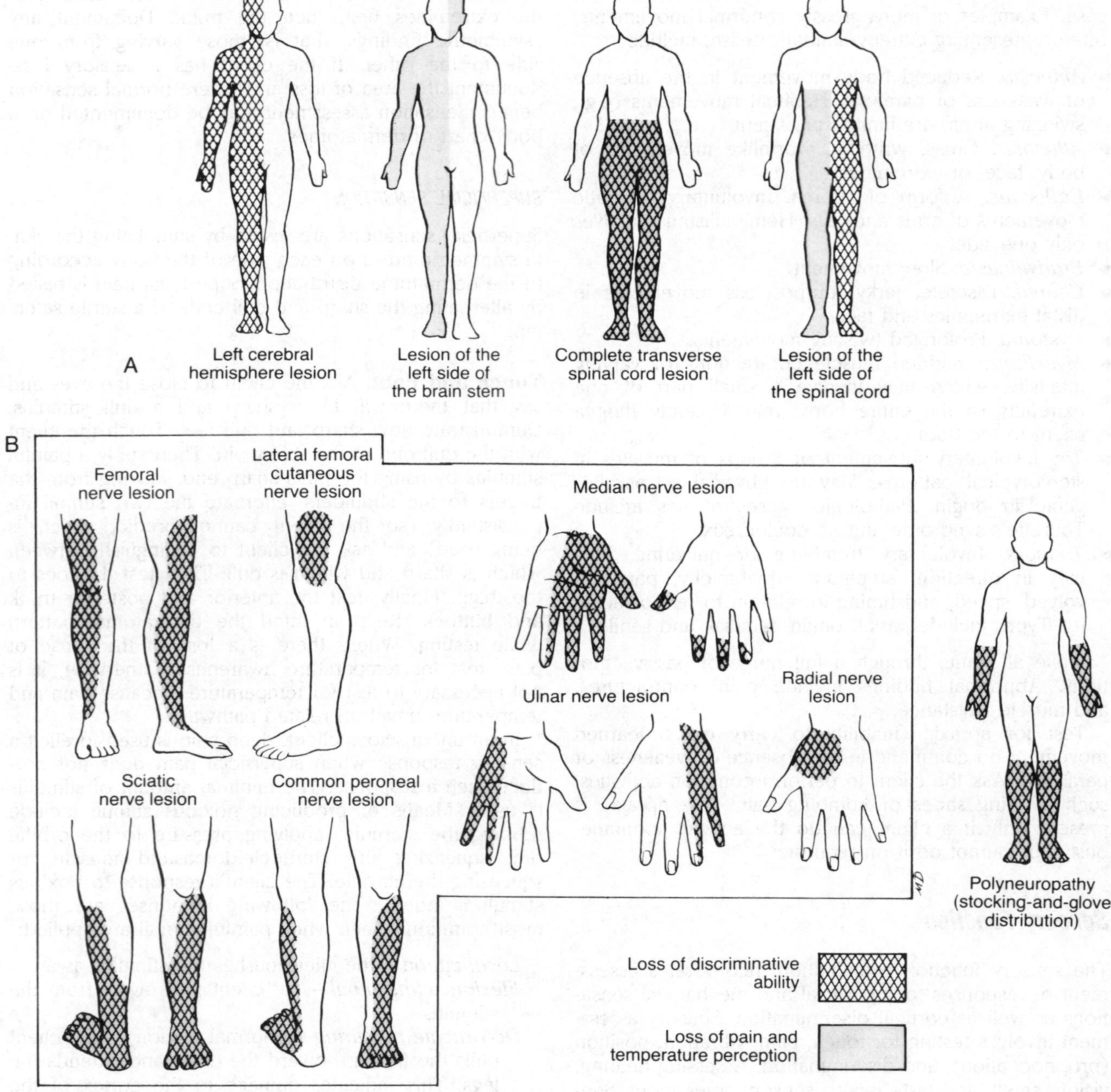

▲ *Figure 28–1*

Patterns of sensory loss with (*A*) brain and spinal cord disorders and (*B*) peripheral nerve lesions.

responses are abnormal. If performed, use test tubes, one filled with warm water and one with cold water (test first to ensure that the hot tube is not too hot). Assess each major dermatome symmetrically.

MECHANICAL SENSATION

Mechanical sensations are assessed by vibration and proprioception.

Vibration. Use a tuning fork to test for vibration. Place the end of a vibrating tuning fork on a distal bony prominence such as a finger or great toe joint. Ask the client to indicate when and where vibration (not touch) is felt. If vibration is not felt, move proximally to the wrist or elbow or foot or ankle.

Proprioception. Test sense of body position by holding the side of the client's finger tips, then the great toes, between thumb and index finger. As each of the client's fingers and toes are gently flexed and extended, ask the client to state when movement is felt and in what direction. If impairment is detected, test more proximal joints.

DISCRIMINATION

Cortical discrimination depends on the ability to discriminate superficial and deep sensations. Discrimination tests the integrative functions of sensation and memory in the brain's parietal lobe. Included are tests for stereognosis, graphesthesia, extinction phenomenon, and two-point stimulation.

To test stereognosis (i.e., discernment of the form and configuration of objects felt, or three-dimensional discrimination), place three small, familiar objects one at a time in the client's hands, such as coins, keys, or a paper clip, and ask the client to identify each.

To test graphesthesia (recognition of the form and configuration of written symbols), trace different separate letters and numbers on the client's palm with the blunt end of a pen, asking the client to identify each.

To test for the extinction phenomenon (simultaneous stimulation), simultaneously prick the client's skin at the same place on both sides of the body, and ask the client to say whether one or two pricks are felt.

To perform two-point stimulation, simultaneously prick the client's skin with two pins at varying distances apart to identify the smallest distance in which the client can perceive two pricks. Normal distances for loss of two-point stimulation discrimination: upper arms, 75 mm; thighs, 75 mm; back, 40 to 70 mm; chest, 40 mm; forearms, 40 mm; palms, 8 to 12 mm; toes, 3 to 8 mm; fingertips, 2.8 mm; tongue, 1 mm.

Sensation abnormalities may include

dysesthesias (well-localized irritating sensations, warmth, cold, itching, tickling, crawling, prickling, and tingling)
paresthesias (distortions of sensory stimuli, e.g., light touch may be experienced as burning or painful sensation)
anesthesia (absent sense of touch)
hypesthesia (reduced sense of touch)
hyperesthesia (pathologic overperception of touch)
hypalgesia (reduced sensation to pain)
hyperalgesia (increased sensation to pain)
analgesia (absence of pain sensation)
astereognosis (loss of sense of three-dimensional discrimination)

Figure 28-1 summarizes patterns of sensory loss. Sensory changes are part of the normal aging process. Careful assessment of such changes is the basis of nursing intervention for elderly clients. Table 28-1 is an assessment guide.

Reflex Activity

Muscles normally contract and relax promptly. This response can be elicited by striking a muscle with a reflex hammer. Reflex activity assessment, always a part of neurologic assessment, provides information about the nature, location, and progression of neurologic disorders.

NORMAL REFLEXES

Two types of reflexes are normally present: (1) superficial, or cutaneous, reflexes and (2) deep tendon, or muscle-stretch, reflexes.

Superficial (Cutaneous) Reflexes. Superficial (cutaneous) reflexes are elicited by cutaneous or mucous membrane stimulation. The stimulus is produced by stroking a sensory zone with an object that will not cause damage. Examples of superficial reflexes are the abdominal reflex, plantar reflex, corneal reflex, pharyngeal ("gag") reflex, cremasteric reflex, and anal reflex.

Abdominal Reflex. Scratching the skin on an abdominal quadrant normally contracts the abdominal muscle in that quadrant, and the umbilicus moves toward the stimulated side.

Plantar Reflex. Scratching the foot's outer aspect of the plantar surface (outer sole) from the heel toward

TABLE 28-1. Assessment of Neurologic Sensory Changes in the Elderly

Sensory Function	Assessment Technique	Observation
Hearing	Ask client questions using normal voice tone and volume. Vary position in relationship to client, such as face-to-face or facing away from client	Note client's response to direct questions when asked by examiner from the varying positions. Does client respond or not respond when face to face with examiner? When examiner's back is toward client?
	Rub thumb and index finger together lightly next to client's ear. Test each ear separately	Note client's ability to hear the sound in each ear, as well as discern the distance between examiner's fingers and client's ear
Vision	*Acuity*	
(instruct client to wear corrective lenses, if usually worn)	Ask client to read from a newspaper, first with one eye then the other eye (instruct client to cover one eye then the other eye with hand), and second with both eyes together	Note client's ability to see regular size print versus the headlines and fine print. Note distance at which client holds printed material from eyes

Table continued on following page

TABLE 28–1. Assessment of Neurologic Sensory Changes in the Elderly Continued

Sensory Function	Assessment Technique	Observation
	Color	
	Ask client to identify colors from a color wheel containing red, orange, yellow, green, blue, and purple	Note client's ability to identify primary colors (red, yellow, blue) as well as inability to identify any color
	Peripheral Vision	
	Instruct client to look straight ahead while examiner holds one finger on each side of client's head at eye level, just outside client's shoulder line	Note whether client can see both fingers. If one or no fingers is seen, visual deficit is present
	Depth Perception	
	Ask client to identify which one of two objects is nearer (select two objects in the room)	Note client's ability to identify which object is nearer. Also note whether client is able to estimate the distance between the two objects accurately within 1 inch
Position sense (instruct client to keep eyes closed)	Instruct client to identify when various body parts are flexed or extended passively by the examiner. Test each arm (at shoulder), thumbs and index fingers (grasp at the sides), and legs (at hip). Ask client to identify whether body part is being flexed or extended	Note client's ability to identify whether a body part is being moved or not. Also note whether client can identify whether joint is being flexed or extended
Vibration (instruct client to keep eyes closed)	Ask client to identify when vibration is felt. Use a tuning fork, set it into vibration, and place on bony prominences. Begin at distal carpal and phalangeal joints and progress proximally to wrists and ankles, elbows/knees, and iliac crests and acromion processes. Alternate vibration with nonvibrating tuning fork	Note client's ability to identify vibration versus lack of vibration, as well as whether sensation is diminished or absent at distal joints. If vibration is felt at distal joints, more proximal joints are usually not tested
Temperature (instruct client to keep eyes closed)	Ask client to identify whether an object feels hot or cold when placed against the skin. Use two test tubes, one filled with hot water, the other with cold water. Place tubes in an alternating pattern against the hands then arms, as well as the feet then legs	Note client's ability to discriminate hot from cold. Also note whether client is able to identify both hot and cold distally as well as proximally, that is, below the elbow and knee versus above elbow and knee
Smell (instruct client to keep eyes closed)	Ask client to identify various aromas. Test each nare separately by instructing client to occlude one nare at a time with index finger. Use familiar smells such as instant coffee or chocolate	Note client's ability to identify various aromas accurately
Taste (instruct client to keep eyes closed)	Ask client to differentiate between two flavors of familiar foods with similar textures, such as two flavors of hard candy or a cracker and a firm cookie	Note client's ability to discriminate between two flavors as well as ability to identify the different flavors
Light touch (instruct client to keep eyes closed)	Brush client's skin lightly with cotton wisp over scattered areas including face, hands, arms, trunk, feet, and legs	Note client's ability to discriminate sensation of being touched, comparing one side to the other. Does client feel cotton on both sides, one side, or not at all?
Deep pressure	Gently squeeze client's Achilles tendons, calf muscles, and forearm muscles	Note whether client verbalizes discomfort and/or withdraws extremity

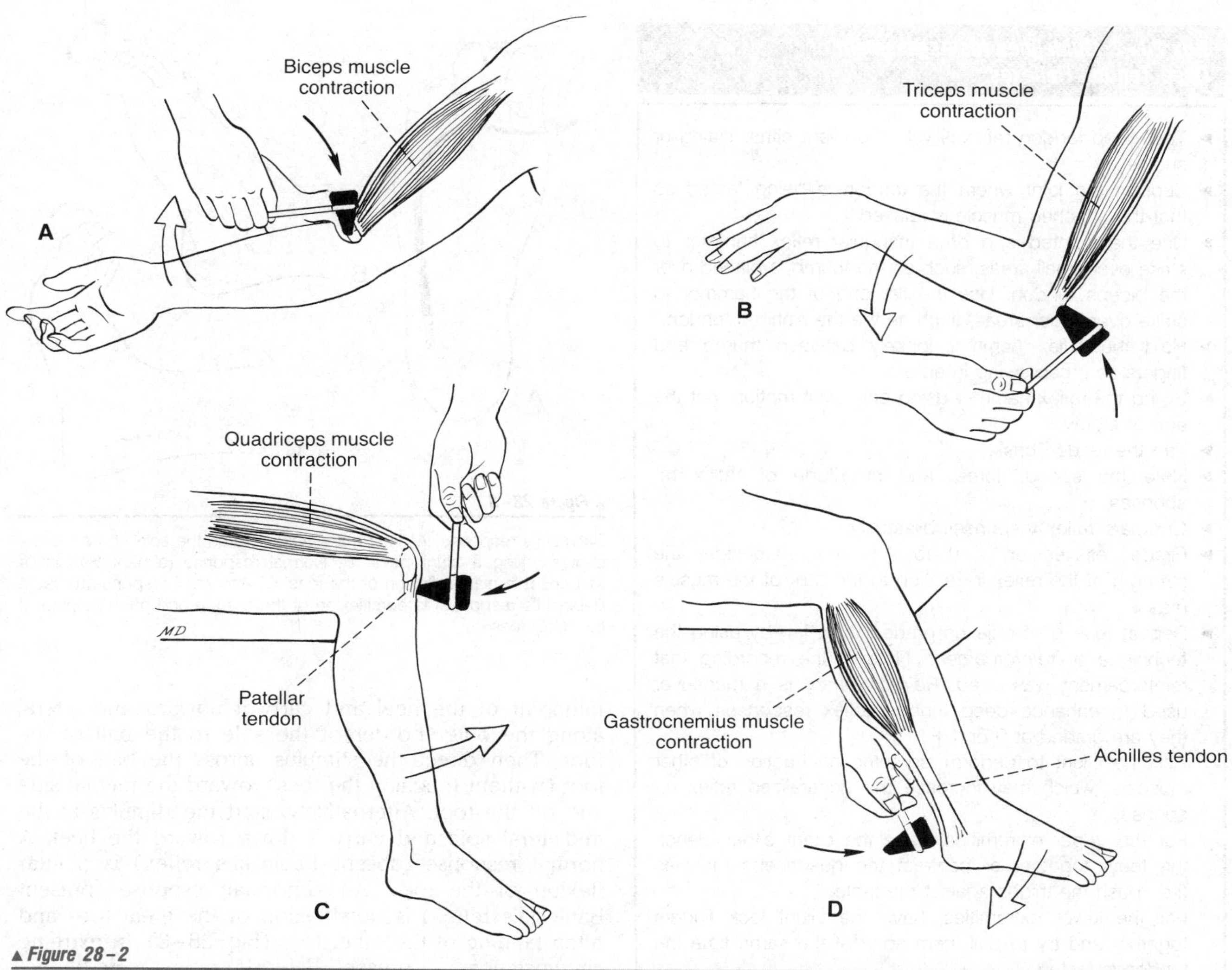

▲ *Figure 28–2*

Deep tendon (muscle stretch) reflexes. *A*, Biceps jerk (C5–C6); *B*, triceps jerk (C7–C8); *C*, patellar reflexes (C5–C6); *D*, ankle jerk (L3–L4).

the toes normally contracts or flexes the toes and sometimes the foot.

Corneal Reflex. Gently touching the cornea with a wisp of cotton causes reflex blinking. (For example, to test the left eye, have the client look up and to the right and bring the cotton wisp in from the side so the client cannot see the hand. Then very gently touch the outer edge of the cornea.) In an unconscious client, the corneal reflex can be tested by holding the eyelids open and placing a drop of sterile saline on the cornea. This technique prevents inadvertent corneal abrasions.

Pharyngeal ("Gag") Reflex. Gentle stimulation with a tongue blade at the back of the throat and pharynx normally produces gagging. The corneal and pharyngeal reflexes are usually assessed with the cranial nerves, discussed later in this chapter.

Cremasteric Reflex. Stroking the inner thigh of a male normally elevates the ipsilateral testicle. There is no counterpart reflex in a female.

Anal Reflex. Stimulate the perianal skin or gently insert a gloved finger into the rectum. Normal response is contraction of the rectal sphincter.

Deep Tendon (Muscle Stretch) Reflexes. Deep tendon reflexes are also called muscle stretch, or myotatic, reflexes because reflex muscle contraction normally results from rapidly stretching the muscle. This is produced by striking a muscle's tendon of insertion sharply with a sudden, brief blow using a reflex hammer (Fig. 28–2 and Box 28–2).

Reflex sites commonly assessed include the Achilles tendon, patella, biceps, and triceps.

- An *ankle jerk* (plantar flexion of the foot) is produced by tapping the Achilles tendon.
- A *knee jerk*, *quadriceps jerk*, or *patellar reflex* (leg extension) is produced by tapping the quadriceps femoris tendon just below the patella.
- A *biceps jerk* (forearm flexion) is produced by tapping the biceps brachii tendon.
- A *triceps jerk* (forearm extension) is produced by tapping the triceps brachii tendon at the elbow.

Box 28–2. Guidelines for Assessment of Deep Tendon Reflexes

- Test deep tendon reflexes with the client either sitting or supine.
- Support the joint where the tendon is being tested so that the attached muscle is relaxed.
- Use the pointed end of a triangular reflex hammer to strike over small areas, such as the thumb is placed over the biceps tendon. Use the flat end of the hammer to strike over larger areas, such as the the Achilles tendon.
- Hold the reflex hammer loosely between thumb and fingers so it can swing in an arc.
- Swing the reflex hammer using only wrist motion, not the arm or elbow.
- Tap the tendon briskly.
- Note the speed, force, and amplitude of reflex responses.
- Compare reflex responses bilaterally.
- Grade reflexes on a 0 to 4+ scale. Consider the strength of the reflex in relation to the bulk of the muscle mass.
- Repeat testing of reflexes graded 0 or 1+ by using the technique of *reinforcement.* Note in the recording that reinforcement was used. *Reinforcement* is a maneuver used to enhance deep tendon reflex responses when they are graded at 0 or 1+.

  Ask the client to perform isometric contraction of other muscles, which may increase the generalized reflex response.

  For the upper extremities, have the client either clench the teeth together or contract the quadriceps muscles (i.e., push the thighs against the table).

  For the lower extremities, have the client lock fingers together and try to pull them apart at the same time the tendon is tested.

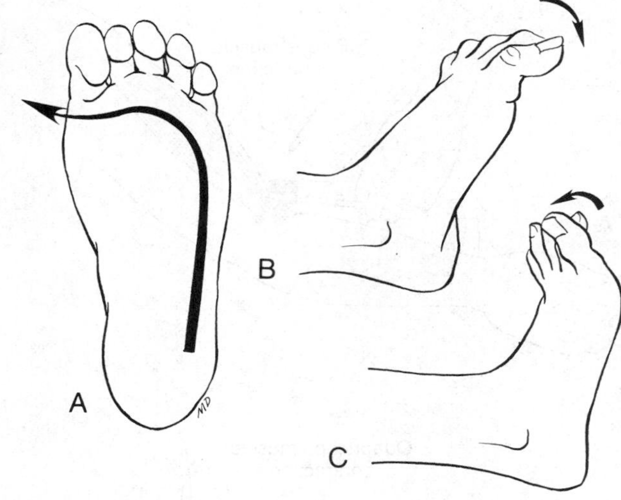

▲ *Figure 28–3*

Babinski's response. *A*, Test maneuver: Scratch the sole of the foot as shown, using a blunt point. *B*, Normal response (absent Babinski's response) is plantar flexion of the toes. *C*, Abnormal response (present Babinski's response) is dorsiflexion of the big toe and often fanning of the other toes.

Other Normal Reflexes. Some other normal reflexes involve structures other than skeletal muscles. For example, reflex mechanisms help maintain respiration and keep blood pressure within normal limits. Reflex salivation may follow taste (or smell) of food. Flashing a light in an eye causes pupils of both eyes to constrict (*light reflex,* or *pupillary reflex;* see also the section on pupil assessment).

ABNORMAL REFLEXES

Pathologic (abnormal) reflexes are reflexes that do not normally occur. Their presence indicates neurologic disorders, often related to the spinal cord or higher centers.

These responses include Babinski's, jaw, palm-chin (palmomental), clonus, snout, rooting, sucking, glabella, grasp, and chewing reflexes.

Babinski's Reflex. Babinski's reflex is tested by gently scraping the sole of the foot with a blunt point. To elicit the Babinski's reflex, start the stimulus at the midpoint of the heel and carry it upward and lateral along the outer border of the sole to the ball of the foot. Then direct the stimulus across the ball of the foot (without touching the toes) toward the medial side and off the foot. Alternatively, start the stimulus at the midlateral sole and carry it down toward the heel. A normal response (absent Babinski's reflex) is plantar flexion of the toes. An abnormal response (present Babinski's reflex) is dorsiflexion of the great toes and often fanning of the other toes (Fig. 28–3). In extreme circumstances, a present Babinski reflex may be ac-

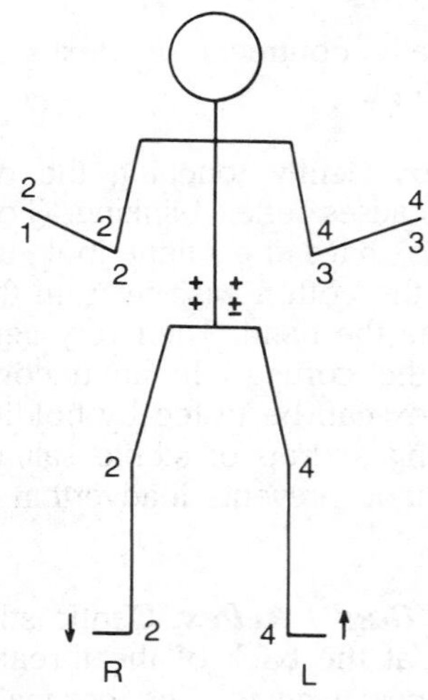

▲ *Figure 28–4*

Documentation of muscle stretch and superficial reflexes in left hemiparesis. Muscle stretch reflex grades: grade 0, absent; grade 1, diminished; grade 2, normal; grade 3, brisker than normal; grade 4, hyperactive (clonus). Superficial reflex grades: grade 0, absent; grade ±, equivocal or barely present; grade +, normally active.

companied by dorsiflexion of the foot at the ankle and flexion at the knee and hip.

When exaggerated deep reflexes are present, superficial reflexes are usually diminished or absent, and pathologic reflexes (e.g., Babinski's reflex) also exist.

Jaw Reflex. Jaw reflex (jaw contracts and closes the mouth as a result of downward tapping on the lower jaw, when the mouth is relaxed and passively hanging partially open) occurs rarely in healthy individuals, but is noticeably present in some disorders, e.g., sclerosis of the lateral columns of the spinal cord. Jaw reflex is also called mandibular reflex or jaw jerk.

Palm-Chin (Palmomental) Reflex. Palm-chin (palmomental) reflex produced by vigorous, rapid irritation on the mound of the palm at the thumb's base with a blunt instrument causing the chin muscles to pull up on the same side.

Clonus. Clonus is rapidly alternating joint flexions and extensions, resulting from continuous rhythmic contractions of a stretched muscle. This is not like a normal stretch reflex, which typically produces one reflex action. With clonus, the action continues.

Snout Reflex. A brisk midline tap above or below the mouth results in pursing of the lips.

Rooting Reflex. Stroking the side of the face causes the mouth to open and the head to turn to the stimulated side.

Sucking Reflex. Touching the lips with a blunt object results in movement of the tongue, lips, and jaws.

Glabella Reflex. Tapping the forehead between the eyebrows results in sustained closure of the eyelids.

Grasp Reflex. Placing an object in the palm of the hand causes the fingers to curl around the object.

Chewing Reflex. A tongue blade placed between the teeth results in the jaws closing tightly.

GRADING REFLEX ACTIVITY

Superficial reflexes are graded 0 (absent), ± (slightly present), and + (normally active). Deep reflexes are graded from 0 through 4 +; 2 + is normal. Although 1 + or 3 + responses are not considered normal, they may not be significant findings (Fig. 28-4). Asymmetric responses are much more significant. Abnormal reflexes may be present in both neurologic and metabolic disorders. Table 28-2 summarizes important reflexes.

TABLE 28-2. Important Reflexes

Reflex	Method	Effect	Localization
Tendon Reflexes			
Biceps reflex	A blow on the examiner's thumb placed over the biceps tendon	Flexion of elbow	C5 and C6
Brachioradialis reflex (supinator)	Styloid process of radius is tapped while forearm is in semiflexion and semipronation	Flexion of elbow, fingers, and hand with supination of forearm	C5 and C6
Triceps reflex	Strike on triceps tendon just above the olecranon	Extension of elbow	C6 to C8 (C7 primarily)
Patellar reflex (knee jerk)	Tap on patellar tendon	Leg extends	L2 to L4
Achilles reflex (ankle jerk)	Tap on Achilles tendon	Plantar flexion of foot	S1 and S2
Superficial Reflexes			
Corneal reflex	Light touch at the corneoscleral junction	Closure of eyelids	CN V and CN VII
Palatal and pharyngeal reflexes	Light touch to soft palate and pharynx	Elevation of palate; gagging	CN IX and CN X
Abdominal reflexes	Stroke skin of upper, middle, and lower abdomen toward umbilicus	Contraction of abdominal wall toward stimulus	Upper—T7 to T9 Middle—T9 to T11 Lower—T11 to T12
Cremasteric reflex	Stroke medial surface of upper thigh	Elevation of scrotum and testicle	T12 to L2
Anal reflex	Stroke perianal region	Contraction of external anal sphincter	S3 to S5
Plantar reflex (normal)	Stroke sole of foot	Flexion of toes	L4 to S2
Plantar reflex (pathologic; Babinski's sign)	Stroke sole of foot	Dorsiflexion of great toe and fanning of other toes	L4 to S2

Adapted from Mitchell, P.A., et al. (1988). *AANN's neuroscience nursing: Phenomena and practice.* Norwalk, CT: Appleton and Lange.

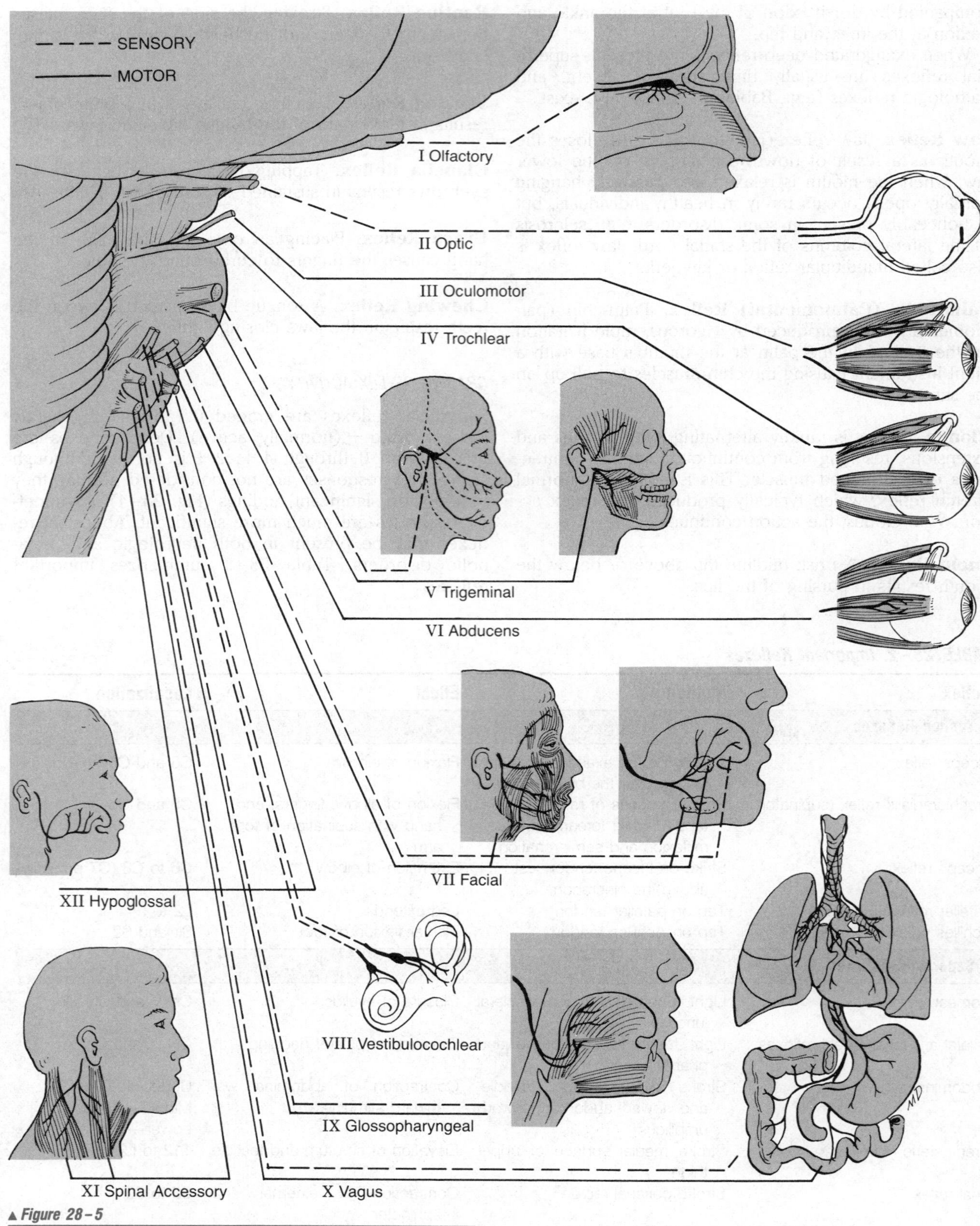

▲ *Figure 28–5*

Distribution of cranial nerves. Study this figure along with Table 28–3.

Cranial Nerves

The cranial nerves (CN) are referred to by specific name or number. Cranial nerve examination is important for three reasons.

First, half of all the cranial nerves innervate eye function. Therefore, careful examination of eye function provides considerable information about the cranial nerves.

Second, cranial nerves III through XII arise in the brain stem. Thus, testing their functions gives information about the brain stem.

Finally, normal cranial nerve function requires an appropriately received input stimulus that produces an appropriate response (output). When testing cranial nerves, failure to get a normal response may mean (1) failure to receive stimuli (input failure), (2) failure to respond appropriately (output failure), or (3) a combination of input and output failure. Determining which problems exist is often a challenge. For example, vision is a function of CN II, and pupillary light response is a function of both CN II and CN III. However, pupillary light response cannot be tested in a blind person because testing this reflex requires intact CN II and III (Fig. 28-5 and Table 28-3). The structure and function of the cranial nerves are discussed in Chapter 27.

TABLE 28-3. Neurologic Assessment Guidelines

Functional Category	Specific Category	Area of Nervous System Involved	Assessment Technique	Examples of Dysfunction
1. Consciousness (awareness of self and environment)	Arousal response to verbal, tactile, and visual stimuli	Reticular activating system (mesencephalon, diencephalon) Both hemispheres	Is client alert, what is attention span? Is there normal response to visual and auditory stimuli? Reaction to loud noises, shaking, deep pressure over eye orbits or sternum? Are vital signs, pupils, and reflexes normal?	Elevation: Insomnia, agitation, mania, delirium Depression: Somnolence, lethargy, semicoma, coma
2. Mentation	Thinking	Cerebral hemispheres plus specific regional functions	Is client oriented (time, place, person)?	Disorientation
	Insight, judgement, planning	Frontal lobe, with association fibers to other areas of cerebrum	Does client recognize implications of illness? Are goals congruent with abilities? How would client respond to given situation (e.g., house on fire)?	Lack of judgement, inattention to grooming, appearance, and personal habits
	Fund of information	Basic biologic intellect (frontal lobe) integrated into other areas	Calculation ability, knowledge of current events consistent with educational level. Who is U.S. President?	Impairment-functioning not congruent with level of education
	Memory	Temporal lobe and association to most other areas of cortex		
	Recent:		Recent memory: What was eaten for breakfast? What happened one day ago?	Recent memory: organic brain disease
	Past:		Past memory: Recall past events during taking of history	Lapses of memory for past events may coincide with past CNS problems (i.e., trauma, infection, psychic trauma)

Table continued on following page

TABLE 28–3. Neurologic Assessment Guidelines Continued

Functional Category	Specific Category	Area of Nervous System Involved	Assessment Technique	Examples of Dysfunction
	Feeling (affect) (congruence of response to stimulus)	General and bifrontal (Usually involves both hemispheres)	Compare observed with expected reactions. Are emotions labile? Appropriate?	Blunted affect. Hysteria, schizophrenia, bilateral frontal lobe lesions
	Perceptual distortions (illusions, hallucinations)	General and specific cortical areas in hallucinations	Observations for behavior indicating perceptual problems Ask client	Irritative lesions of cortex may → hallucinations. (Occipital cortex → visual, postcentral gyrus → somatic sensation uncus → smell)
3. Language and speech	*Dysarthria* (defects in articulation, enunciation, and rhythm in speech)	Impairment of muscles of tongue, palate, pharynx, or lips. (May be due to ↓ impulses or incoordination) Brain stem, cerebellum, or extraneural causes CN: V, VII, IX, X, XII	Have client repeat a difficult phrase (i.e., "Susie sells seashells by the seashore")	Slurring, slowness, indistinctness, nasality, break in normal speech rhythm (i.e., speech of a drunk, amyotrophic lateral sclerosis, pseudobulbar palsy, myasthenia gravis)
	Dysphonia (abnormal production of sounds from larynx)	Many extraneural causes Recurrent laryngeal nerve problems (part of vagus) CN: X	Is client hoarse? Whispered voice is intact Use indirect laryngoscopy findings	Compression of recurrent laryngeal nerve by bronchogenic CA of left main stem bronchus Left atrial hypertrophy
		Medulla (area of nucleus of vagus nerve)		Brain stem tumors, occlusion of posterior inferior cerebellar or vertebral artery
	Aphasia (inability to use and understand written and spoken words)	Fluent (receptive) left temporal and parietal lobes	Observe: vocal expression, written expression, comprehension of spoken, written language, and gesture communication	Cerebrovascular disease of middle cerebral artery Trauma, tumor, abscess, etc., in left temporal and parietal lobe areas
		Nonfluent (expressive) Broca's area (lateral) inferior portion of frontal lobe of dominant side Global (combined)		
	Agnosia (inability to recognize objects or symbols by means of senses)	Primarily in parietal temporal and occipital areas	Sense organs intact? Can the client recognize objects by sight, touch, hearing, etc?	Cerebrovascular disease
4. Motor function	Expression (facial)	CN: VII	Symmetry of smile, frown, raising eyebrows	Central facial weakness (upper motor neuron dysfunction); weakness of lower half of face Causes: Cerebral vascular accident, corticobulbar tract

TABLE 28–3. Neurologic Assessment Guidelines Continued

Functional Category	Specific Category	Area of Nervous System Involved	Assessment Technique	Examples of Dysfunction
				Peripheral facial weakness (lower motor dysfunction); weakness of entire half of face Causes: Bell's palsy, brain stem tumor, fracture of temporal bone
	Eating (chewing, swallowing)	CN: V, VII, IX, X, XII	Strength of masticator muscles, gag reflexes, ability to swallow	Tetanus, peripheral spasm of muscle. Amyotrophic lateral sclerosis, medullary tumor. Pseudobulbar palsy may be associated with dysarthria
	Eye movements	CN: III, IV, VI	Extraocular movement, pupil size, reactivity, pupils equally react to accommodation, diplopia, nystagmus	Cerebral peduncle pressure → CN: III dysfunction, cavernous sinus thrombus → CN: III, IV, VI, problem Muscular problems (i.e., myasthenia gravis, hyperthyroid), Horner's syndrome (ptosis, constricted pupil), anisocoria
	Moving	Motor precentral gyrus (pyramidal) and cerebellar systems, basal ganglia, CN: XI, spinal cord, upper motor neuron, (brain → anterior horn cell via corticospinal tract)	Gait, heel-to-toe walking, presence or absence of involuntary movements, coordination, muscle tone, mass, strength, Romberg reflex, ability to shrug shoulders and to rise from chair	*Upper motor neuron* Brain and cord-sparing anterior horn cell Tone ↑ ↑ (spastic) Bulk ↓ due to atrophy of disuse Reflexes ↑ ↑ due to loss of central inhibition No fasciculations Frequent clonus
		Lower motor neuron (motor cells of cranial nerves and anterior horn cells → peripheral muscles) Involves brain, midbrain, cerebellum, and spinal cord		*Lower motor neuron* Segment anterior horn cell peripheral nerve Tone ↓ ↓ (flaccid) Bulk ↓ due to tone loss Reflexes ↓ or absent due to loss of anterior horn cell

Table continued on following page

TABLE 28-3. Neurologic Assessment Guidelines Continued

Functional Category	Specific Category	Area of Nervous System Involved	Assessment Technique	Examples of Dysfunction
				Fasciculations No clonus *Cerebellar problem* → Loss of coordination and balance
5. Sensory function	Seeing	CN: II Optic, occipital lobe	Acuity, visual fields, fundoscopy	Field test: loss in retina or optic nerve → loss in eye involved, optic chiasm → bitemporal hemianopsia. Optic tract → homonymous hemianopsia, parietal lobe → quadrant problems (inferior), temporal lobe → superior quadrant problems ↑ ICP → papilledema (raised disc → hemorrhage)
	Smelling	CN: I Temporal lobe (uncus)	Ability to detect familiar odors	Usually ↓ smell due to extraneural causes (i.e., upper respiratory infection, allergy, smoking), olfactory groove Meningioma, olfactory hallucinations
	Hearing	CN: VIII Cochlear division, temporal lobe	Acuity of hearing, presence or absence of unusual sounds, Weber and Rinne tests.	May have conductive (nerve ok) or neural hearing loss. Ménière's syndrome (tinnitus, hearing loss, vertigo, and nystagmus), basilar skull fracture → otorrhea Brain stem vascular dysfunction or tumors → ↓ hearing
	Taste	CN: VII, IX	Ability to differentiate sweet, salt, sour, and bitter	Brain stem lesions → ↓ taste Extraneural causes, smoking, poor oral hygiene
	Feeling (sensory)	Peripheral nerves → Dermatomes → Spinal cord → Tracts (leading to) Pain-temperature tactile, anterolateral system, proprioception, stereognosis, dorsal roots thalamus (leading to) somasthetic area (postcentral gyrus)	Pain: pinprick Touch: cotton touched to skin Proprioception: check where digit is in space Vibration: place vibrating tuning fork on bony prominence Temperature: test tubes of cold and warm	Polyneuropathy, (i.e., diabetes, anemia) Spinal cord lesions → Dermatome alterations Upper pons → thalamus, contralateral loss Thalamus → contralateral loss + paresthesia

TABLE 28–3. Neurologic Assessment Guidelines Continued

Functional Category	Specific Category	Area of Nervous System Involved	Assessment Technique	Examples of Dysfunction
		(parietal lobe)	water laid against skin; person identifies whether hot or cold	Thalamus → cortex → cortical sensory loss
6. Bowel and bladder function	Bowel function	Afferent Spinal nerve S3-S5 External sphincter (voluntary control)	Check for fecal impaction or incontinence	Fecal incontinence with lesions of S3, 4, 5
		Internal sphincter Spinal nerve S3-S5 Autonomic nervous system	Check muscle tone	Anal anesthesia–conus medularis and tabes dorsalis May be extraneural causes
	Bladder function	Autonomic nervous system Afferent Spinal nerve T9-L2 & S2-S4 Pudendal nerve	Feel when bladder is full, complete emptying. Does client have urgency, frequently?	Urinary incontinence Flaccid bladder
		Efferent Spinal nerve T11-L2 External sphincter (voluntary) Spinal nerve S2-S4		Spastic bladder May be extraneural causes

OLFACTORY (CRANIAL NERVE I): SMELL

Ask the client to smell and then identify an aromatic, nonirritating odor (e.g., coffee, isopropyl alcohol, toothpaste) with each nostril with the eyes closed. Test with several different odors. If the client can perceive any one smell, consider the nerve functional. Although inability to smell (called anosmia) may develop in elderly people, problems such as basal skull fracture or olfactory groove tumor also may be present. Other possible causes of anosmia include cribriform plate fracture and an olfactory bulb or a tract tumor.

OPTIC (CRANIAL NERVE II): VISION

Assessing the optic nerve involves (1) inspecting the globe for foreign bodies, cataracts, inflammation, or other obvious abnormalities, (2) testing visual acuity, (3) testing visual fields, and (4) examining eye fundus with an ophthalmoscope. (Details of eye assessment are in Chap. 33.) Test visual acuity generally by having the client read from a newspaper, a sign (from a distance), or a Snellen chart while wearing glasses (if usually worn). Refraction errors are not significant in neurologic assessment. Test visual fields to determine whether vision is absent in one or more directions or a portion of the visual field, such as half of the visual fields, the middle portion, or both sides. Such losses may indicate various problems and may correlate with the area of the brain involved. Gross inspection of the eyes and examination of the fundus can provide information about neurologic disease. Possible causes of abnormal findings include trauma to orbit or eyeball; fracture of optic foramen; diabetic retinopathy; laceration or blood clot in the brain's temporal, parietal, or occipital lobes; and increased intracranial pressure (ICP) (e.g., papilledema).

OCULOMOTOR (CRANIAL NERVE III), TROCHLEAR (CRANIAL NERVE IV), AND ABDUCENS (CRANIAL NERVE VI): EYES AND EYE MOVEMENT

CN III controls pupil constriction and elevation of the upper lid. Pupils should be equal in size and round. Note pupil size prior to shining a light into the client's eyes. Document each pupil's size and shape. Approach the pupil from the temporal side while the client looks straight ahead. Test each pupil for both direct and consensual responses (pupillary constriction) to a light. A direct response occurs in the eye being tested. A consensual response occurs in the other eye at a slightly slower rate. Test accommodation (eyes able to focus on both near and far objects) by having the client look across the room (away from the light source) and then look at the examiner's fingers, held about 6 inches from the client's nose. Normally, the lens shape changes and the pupils constrict. The notation "PERRLA" indicates these functions are normal (i.e., *p*upils *e*qual, *r*ound, *r*eactive to *l*ight, and *a*ccommodation). Destruction of part of CN III can cause ptosis (drooping) of the eyelid. Disorders or pressure on a specific side of CN III can cause the ipsilateral pupil to dilate, the eyelid to droop, and the eye to deviate outward.

CN III, IV, and VI coordinate to control eye movements in all six cardinal directions of gaze (see Chap. 33). The function of these nerves is tested in various ways. Ask the client to move the eyes in the six directions. Alternatively, move an object in the six cardinal directions, and ask the client to follow it with the eyes. If a client has diplopia (double vision) but no muscle weakness can be demonstrated, shine a light so it reflects on both eyes. The area of reflection is normally symmetric, meaning that the client has a conjugate gaze. In dysconjugate gaze, the light's reflection is asymmetric (i.e., not the same in both eyes). If extraocular movements are intact, document as "EOMs intact." Also observe for nystagmus (involuntary eye movements) (see the section on pupils). Possible causes of abnormal findings include pressure on oculomotor, trochlear, or abducens nerves at the brain stem due to fractured orbit, increased ICP, tumor at or trauma to base of the brain. An inability to look down or to walk down steps because of a visual disturbance could be related to CN IV dysfunction. Failure of an eye to move laterally in an outward direction is associated with compression of or damage to CN VI.

TRIGEMINAL (CRANIAL NERVE V)

CN V has a motor and a sensory division. The motor division innervates the muscles of mastication. Test CN V function by asking the client to clamp the jaws, open the mouth against resistance, open the mouth widely, move the jaws from side to side, and make chewing movements. A normal CN V allows all these activities. Document any asymmetry in the temporal muscles. The sensory division mediates all sensations for the entire face, scalp, cornea, and nasal and oral cavities. With the client's eyes closed, test sensations such as pain (e.g., pinprick), touch (e.g., wisp of cotton), and temperatures (e.g., hot and cold test tubes of water) on both sides of the face from the top of the head (vertex) to the chin. Test the corneal reflexes by gently touching the cornea with a sterile wisp of cotton or gently stroke the eyelash. The normal response is brisk eyelid blinking. The corneal reflex involves CN V and CN VII. CN V is the afferent (sensory) arc while CN VII controls closure of the eye (motor). Possible causes of abnormal findings include tumor at or trauma to base of brain, fractured orbit, and trigeminal neuralgia.

FACIAL (CRANIAL NERVE VII)

CN VII has a motor and sensory division. The motor division innervates muscles controlling facial expression. Observe the face for symmetry and the ability to use facial muscles. Ask the client to smile, frown, raise the forehead and eyebrows, tightly close the eyes and resist attempts to open them, whistle, show the teeth, and puff out the cheeks. Test the anterior part of tongue for taste by asking the client to close the eyes and protrude the tongue. Then place a taste substance on one side of the anterior tongue. Have the client keep the tongue protruded while identifying the taste. Ask the client to rinse the mouth or drink a small amount of water before testing the other side. Test taste on each side with sweet, salty, acidic or sour (e.g., vinegar or lemon), and bitter (e.g., coffee). Common abnormalities noted include loss of the nasolabial fold, inability to close the eye and blink reflexively, facial asymmetry, drooling, difficulty swallowing secretions, loss of tearing, and loss of taste on anterior two thirds of the tongue. Possible causes of abnormal findings include Bell's palsy, temporal bone fracture, and peripheral laceration or contusion to the parotid region.

VESTIBULOCOCHLEAR OR ACOUSTIC (CRANIAL NERVE VIII)

CN VIII is a sensory nerve with two divisions, cochlear and vestibular. The cochlear nerve permits hearing. Test auditory acuity by having the client listen to and report on a whispered voice, rustling fingers, or a tuning fork at various distances from the ear. Test bone and air conduction with a tuning fork. Audiometry may be used for a precise assessment. The vestibular nerve helps maintain equilibrium by coordinating the muscles of the eye, neck, trunk, and extremities. Equilibrium tests include the Romberg and caloric tests (oculovestibular reflex) and electronystagmography. (For details on hearing and equilibrium assessment see Chap. 34.) Possible causes of abnormal findings include Ménière's syndrome and acoustic neuroma.

GLOSSOPHARYNGEAL (CRANIAL NERVE IX) AND VAGUS (CRANIAL NERVE X)

Because of the overlapping innervation of the pharynx, assess CNs IX and X together. Ask the client to open the mouth widely and say "Ah." Observe the position and movement of the uvula and palate. Do they rise midline? Test the gag reflex by gently touching the pharynx on each side with a tongue depressor. This normally elicits a brisk gag response. Assess the client's ability to swallow with a small amount of water. Test the posterior third of the tongue for taste, as with the seventh cranial nerve (may be performed when testing CN VII). Dysfunction of CN IX includes loss of taste and sensation of glossopharyngeal pain. Ask the client to cough and to speak to test CN X. Damage to CN X causes an ineffectual cough and a weak, hoarse voice. To differentiate areas of weakness, ask the client to vocalize different sounds: "kuh kuh" (soft palate), "mi mi" (lips), "la la" (tongue). Possible causes of abnormal findings include brain stem trauma, neck trauma, brain stem tumors, and stroke.

SPINAL ACCESSORY (CRANIAL NERVE XI)

CN XI innervates the sternocleidomastoid muscle and the upper portion of the trapezius muscle. To test, ask the client to (1) elevate the shoulders (with and without resistance), (2) turn (not tilt) the head to one side (and then the other), (3) resist attempts to pull the chin back toward midline, and (4) push the head forward against resistance. Disorders may produce drooping of a shoulder, muscle atrophy, weak shoulder shrug, or turn of the head. Possible causes of abnormal findings include neck trauma, radical neck surgery, and torticollis.

HYPOGLOSSAL (CRANIAL NERVE XII)

CN XII innervates the tongue. Ask the client to open the mouth widely, stick out the tongue, and rapidly move the tongue from side to side and in and out. Document any deviation of the tongue to the side. Assess tongue strength by having the client push the tongue strongly against the inside of the cheek while pressure is applied to the area externally. Possible causes of abnormal findings include neck trauma associated with major blood vessel damage.

Autonomic Nervous System

Clinical manifestations of disorders of the autonomic nervous system occur in many body systems. This unit focuses on neurologic disorders (e.g., heatstroke, autonomic dysreflexia). Disorders of other portions of the autonomic system can be seen in cardiac, urinary, digestive, reproductive, and endocrine sections of the text.

Clinical manifestations of autonomic disorders include (1) altered perspiration patterns; (2) faulty body temperature regulation (hypothermia and hyperthermia); (3) abnormal pulse rate and pilomotor responses; (4) skin, vasomotor, and pupillary changes; and (5) digestive changes.

When assessing for autonomic disturbances, ask about polyuria and abnormal motility of the gastrointestinal tract. Examine the abdomen for evidence of bowel and urinary bladder distention. Changes in thirst, energy, potency, libido, weight, and appetite may also be significant.

Examine the client's skin, mucous membranes, hair, and nails for trophic changes. Such changes occur in various diseases causing loss of innervation, including the autonomic nerve supply. Trophic changes may be indicated by (1) changes in the affected area's sweating, temperature, and color (e.g., pallor, cyanosis, and erythema); (2) nails that may become curved, brittle, broken, and thickened; (3) skin that may be painlessly ulcerated, thickened, atrophied, pigmented, oily, scaly, and rough or tight, shiny, and dry; (4) oily, brittle, and dry hair with hair loss or abnormal hair growth; and (5) pressure sores in denervated regions of the skin, beginning in areas subjected to prolonged pressure. Palpitation (i.e., a rapid heart rate felt by the client) may also indicate autonomic dysfunction.

Table 28-3 is an overall neurologic assessment guide.

FUNCTIONAL ASSESSMENT

A client with a neurologic disorder is usually experiencing problems that disrupt basic function either permanently or temporarily. The client's ability to cope effectively with activities of daily living (ability to meet basic needs) is often altered. For example, a client may have problems seeing, hearing, breathing, walking, talking, or eating. Remember that a client with a neurologic disorder may be frustrated just trying to do the things most people take for granted.

There are many tools for functional neurologic nursing assessment. They are based on the principle that the main purpose of nursing is to help clients cope effectively with changes (actual or potential) in daily living and self-care. The tools provide a systematic method of using daily observations that may become the basis for nursing intervention.

CLINICAL APPLICATIONS

The initial assessment for diagnosis and triage of the clients with a possible neurologic deficit includes a history, brief physical examination, and a neurologic examination. The initial neurologic examination usually consists of assessment of the level of consciousness using the Glasgow coma scale, pupillary response, focal motor and sensory abnormalities in all four extremities, and brain stem function via assessment of corneal response (Box 28-3).

The initial assessment provides the baseline for comparison when serial assessments are completed. When recorded on a time-oriented flow sheet, changes in the client's status can be quickly identified. The frequency of serial assessment is determined by the client's diagnosis and may be as frequent as every 15 minutes. The nurse has an important responsibility to monitor the client's progress and report any unexpected deviations.

Thorough assessment and reporting of changes in a client serve a major role in determining the plan of care. Often, the client's current condition, for example, a decreased level of responsiveness and a change in pupillary reaction, is compared with initial data.

Because nurses are with clients continuously, it becomes the nurse's responsibility to develop sound assessment skills and recognize trends in the client's condition that warrant further care. In no other area of practice are subtle changes as important to detect and act on than in the care of the client with neurologic disorders.

DIAGNOSTIC TESTS

The complexity of the CNS combined with the relative inaccessibility of the brain requires indirect techniques to study it. Early techniques such as lumbar puncture, plain x-ray study, pneumoencephalography, and EEG have provided the foundation for new techniques that allow direct visualization of the brain structure, blood supply, and metabolism. Air contrast studies, such as pneumoencephalogram and ventriculogram, were performed for client assessment prior to the development of CT and magnetic resonance imaging (MRI). The nurse may find the results of these tests recorded in the history of a client who has had neurologic disorders for

Box 28–3. The Initial Neurologic Examination

The sequence in which the neurologic examination is performed and the amount of time devoted to each section is dictated by the client's situation. For example, assessment of the head-injured client in the emergency room requires evaluation of vital signs, pupil reactivity, level of consciousness, and motor response. These clients may not be stable or cooperative enough to complete the cranial nerve and sensory response assessment. Spinal cord–injured clients, however, are usually coherent and able to participate in the sensory examination. This information is essential for documenting changes in the status of spinal cord–injured clients.

As clients become more stable and cooperative, the examination can be performed in more depth and with less frequency. It should be remembered that neurologically impaired clients frequently experience fluctuations in status. This requires the nurse to alter the assessment schedule and technique to detect and report these fluctuations.

The following are suggested modifications in the screening neurologic examination based on the client's initial presentation.

- Initial examination for diagnosis and triage:
  - Client history based on chief complaint
  - Physical examination including vital signs
  - LOC
  - Pupil response
  - Brain stem function (corneal reflex)
  - Motor and sensory function in all four extremities
- If the client is conscious and stable:
  - Complete baseline neurologic examination
  - Focused examination at prescribed levels
- If the client is conscious and unstable:
  - Quick baseline physical assessment
  - Frequent focused examinations until stable
  - Vital signs
  - LOC
  - Pupil response
  - Brain stem function
  - Motor and sensory function in extremities
  - Spinal cord function
- If the client is unconscious yet stable:
  - Vital signs
  - LOC and arousal
  - Cranial nerve function
  - Motor and sensory function
  - Pathologic reflexes
- If the client is unconscious and unstable:
  - Vital signs
  - LOC
  - Cranial nerve function
  - Motor and sensory function relative to the ability to test for these
  - Pathologic reflexes
  - Frequent focused examination on ongoing basis (hourly or more often)
- If the client is suspected to have spinal cord involvement:
  - Motor function in detail with testing of specific muscle groups
  - Sensory function
  - Reflexes
  - Bowel and bladder function
  - Vital signs

many years. These tests use air to provide contrast so that various portions of the brain can be viewed by x-ray study. The tests were painful and had potentially serious side effects. Today's neurodiagnostic studies are much safer for the client. The tests begin with the least invasive and move to the most invasive forms.

The focus of nursing care for the client having diagnostic assessment is centered on physical and psychological preparation for the study. The nurse also plans for the specific assessments that will need to be made after the study is completed, such as continued neurologic assessment. Prior to the study, the nurse should provide education to the client and family about the purpose of the study, the preparation needed, and the client's role during the test. The nurse may also have to assist the client to reduce anxiety about the test, and can usually reduce anxiety by providing information and answering questions. Serial scans may be necessary when the client has an evolving disease (e.g., cerebral bleeding) that reveals more pathology in 2 or 3 days than within the first 24 hours.

After the diagnostic procedures have been performed, the nurse assesses the client for possible side effects and neurologic changes and assists the client to understand the results of the studies as needed.

Noninvasive Tests

SKULL AND SPINAL X-RAY STUDIES

Skull x-ray studies reveal the size and shape of the skull bones, suture separation in infants, fractures or bony defects, erosion, calcification, sella turcica erosion, and pineal gland shift (after age 12). Spinal x-ray studies show fractures, dislocation, compressions, curvature, erosion, narrowed spinal cord, and degenerative processes.

Nursing Intervention. Some clients with neurologic disorders require nursing support throughout an x-ray study, especially clients who are confused, combative, or ventilator dependent. Whenever a client is unable to act as a self-advocate, a nurse is required. If the client has a suspected spinal fracture, the neck is immobilized prior to moving the client to make the x-ray films. A lateral view of the cervical spine is taken first because the x-ray study can usually be taken with minimal movement to determine whether fractures have occurred. Metal items should be removed from body parts undergoing the x-ray procedure, for example, barrettes. Nurses should document thick or heavy hair, because hair may affect interpretation of the x-ray film.

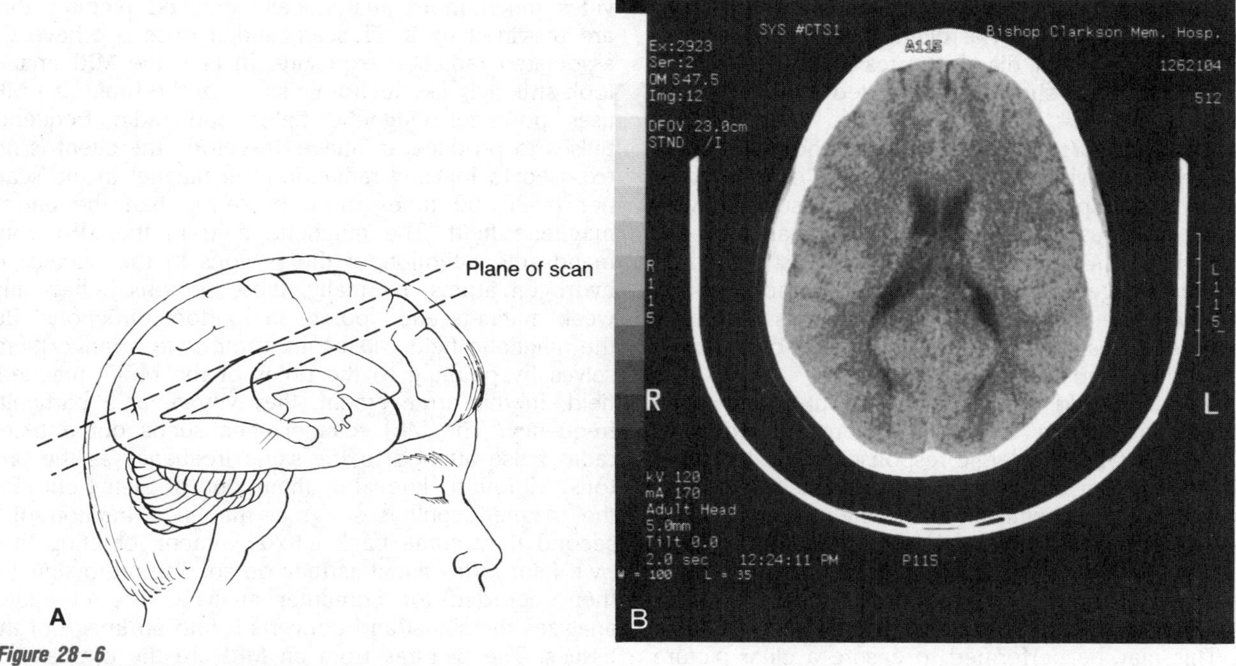

▲ **Figure 28–6**

CT scan. *A*, CT scans are taken at various cross sections of the brain. This figure illustrates the cross section used for the scan shown in *B*.

COMPUTED TOMOGRAPHY AND MAGNETIC RESONANCE IMAGING

Computed Tomography. The CT scan is a highly informative diagnostic test based on the principle of tissue density using the computer to analyze data. The primary purpose of CT scans is to detect intracranial bleeding, space-occupying lesions, cerebral edema, and shifts of brain structures. Infarctions, hydrocephalus, and cerebral atrophy can also be identified. Aneurysms and arteriovenous malformations (AVMs) are best detected by angiogram. The basilar cisterns and posterior fossa are not as well visualized on the CT scan. These areas have a large density contrast between the bone and air-filled sinuses.

CT scans are completed by having x-ray beams pass through the brain in many slices to provide cross-sectional pictures (Fig. 28–6). The computer amplifies tissue density differences to visualize structures, such as bone, blood vessels, and tissues. As the beam passes through the head, some of the radiation energy is absorbed by the structures of the brain and skull, with the remainder passing through onto a sensitive electronic detector. The amount of radiation absorbed depends on the density of the tissue it passes through, with bone absorbing the most and air the least. On the CT scan, bone appears white and air appears black. Once the data are in the computer, various slices can be created. For example, coronal slices may best visualize a pituitary tumor, but sagittal slices would assist with diagnosis of facial bone fractures. The CT scan can be performed quickly—within about 20 minutes—not including data analysis. The radiation exposure from CT scans has been reduced to a level similar to that of a chest x-ray study. The results of the CT scan are usually recorded on x-ray film for a permanent record.

Nursing Intervention. Providing information about the CT scan is the major focus of nursing intervention. Prior to the test, ascertain that informed consent has been obtained, and answer any questions the client and family have about the CT scan and explain the following items.

Fasting usually is not required for CT of the head, but ask whether or not the client tends to become nauseated easily and adjust the intake of food and fluids accordingly. For example, some clients prefer a light breakfast to reduce nausea and others prefer to have an empty stomach.

Explain that a contrast agent often is given. Because the agent (also called dye) is iodine based, ask whether the client has known allergies to iodine, contrast dyes, or shellfish. (See the section on the use of contrast.)

Remove any objects from the hair before the examination, including wigs, barrettes, earrings, and hair pins. The client's hair should be combed smoothly.

The client's role in the scan should be explained. The client will be positioned supine and the head placed into the donut-shaped ring of the scanner. The table is moved by the technologist from a control room during the scan to direct the study toward different levels of the head. The client should expect to hear mechanical noises coming from the scanner as it scans. Some clients will feel claustrophobic during the test but should be assured that it is possible to communicate with the technologist during the scan. Finally, the client will be asked to remain still during the scan. If the client is unable to comply, sedation, or even general anesthesia, may be required.

Following the test, the client should be assessed for reactions to contrast media as well as other specific assessments, such as presence of hematoma at the injection site and the quality of pulses in the extremity used to inject the dye. The client can resume normal activities, unless other diagnostic tests are planned. Diuresis from the dye should be expected.

Use of Contrast Agents. Certain pathologic conditions are better visualized with the use of a contrast agent. For example, tumors are better visualized with contrast, whereas bleeding and edema can be seen better without it. The use of the contrast agents is potentially dangerous. They may irritate blood vessels. Clients who are sensitive to contrast agents may have allergic reactions, and if untreated, these clients may develop anaphylactic shock.

The nurse should ask the client about a known allergy to contrast dye or possible allergy to iodine or shellfish. The type of allergic response should be noted on the record; for example, "client states she develops hives from eating shellfish." Some clients report allergies, but when asked to explain the reaction, they state that they "feel warm" when given the dye. This is a normal reaction, not an allergic one. Some clients will be given contrast dye even though they report allergy to it. This may be performed to ensure a clear picture and assist with diagnoses. To reduce the severity of the reaction, these clients are pretreated with an antihistamine or corticosteroids. Therefore, the nurse should not assure the client with a reported allergy to dye that contrast dye will not be given. Even if the client states that he or she has no history of allergy, the client should be observed for symptoms of an allergic reaction following the injection of contrast dye. Some anaphylactic reactions have occurred with the first dose of dye.

The nurse should instruct the client that it is common to feel a hot, flushed sensation and a metallic taste in the mouth when the dye is injected. The client should report any difficulty breathing or pruritus (itching) to the personnel in the radiology department. After the procedure has been completed, the client can usually resume normal activities. Diuresis will occur shortly after the use of contrast agents. Replacement fluids may be needed, and the client should be assessed for fluid balance. The fluid balance in clients with renal or cardiac disease should be assessed carefully after a series of tests requiring intravenous contrast agents.

Complications rarely occur but may include local and systemic allergic reactions, spasm or occlusion of the vessels by a clot, and bleeding at the injection site. The nurse should assess the affected extremity for color, warmth, pulses distal to the injection site, bleeding/hematoma formation, and ability to move the site.

In addition, the nurse should assess the client for clinical manifestations of an allergic reaction, which include restlessness, tachypnea, respiratory distress, facial flushing, urticaria, nausea, and vomiting. The client should be assessed for these reactions after the dye is injected, because clients have had respiratory and cardiac arrests while undergoing x-ray study. Emergency equipment always should be available.

Magnetic Resonance Imaging. MRI is a diagnostic tool similar to CT. The advantages are that MRI provides much more anatomically detailed pictures than are provided by a CT scan, and it does not have the associated radiation exposure. In fact, the MRI images look strikingly like anatomic slices of the brain. An MRI uses powerful magnetic fields and radio frequency pulses to produce an image; therefore, the client is not exposed to ionizing radiation. The magnet in the scanner is 30,000 times more powerful than the earth's magnetic field. The magnetic field in the MRI commands the attention of the protons in the nucleus of hydrogen atoms. Normally, these protons behave like weak magnets and "point" in random directions. But the magnetic field causes the protons to arrange themselves by pointing to the poles of the MRI's magnetic field. In this arrangement, they vibrate at a particular frequency. The MRI scanner then sends out a timed radio pulse attuned to the same frequency as the protons' vibration, knocking them out of alignment. But the magnetic pull is so great that in a fraction of a second they come back into alignment, emitting their own faint radio signal as they do so. The radio signal is then recorded for computer analysis. The computer analyzes the signal and converts it into an image of the tissues. The pictures from an MRI are the opposite of the CT. Bone appears black on MRI and is white on CT scan. A contrast agent is often used to augment the images (Fig. 28-7).

Advantages of MRI are that it

- Does not expose the client to radiation
- Is able to provide results fairly rapidly
- Is safe even when contrast dye is used
- Is cost effective when compared with other diagnostic invasive procedures, such as surgery
- Is able to visualize the optic chiasm, posterior fossa, brain stem, and spinal cord
- Is able to detect disorders that cause loss of myelin from the nerves, such as multiple sclerosis, which was previously undetectable
- Is able to detect disorders of blood flow, such as an aneurysm
- Is able to visualize soft tissues.

Disadvantages are that it

- Is an expensive diagnostic test
- Is not available in all areas
- Is not able to provide detail of bones because they appear black
- Is not able to be used during pregnancy
- Requires the client to tolerate close surroundings
- Requires the client to lie still
- Is not able to be used on clients with pacemakers, ear or eye implants, cardiac valve replacements, joint replacements, or old aneurysm clips (modern clips are compatible with MRI), metal fragments in the body (e.g., the eye), and on some types of ventilators. The powerful magnet in the MRI can interfere with the functioning and position of these metal devices.

Nursing Intervention. The client and family should be taught about the purpose of the test, the sensations that the client will hear and feel during the examination, and the client's role during the test.

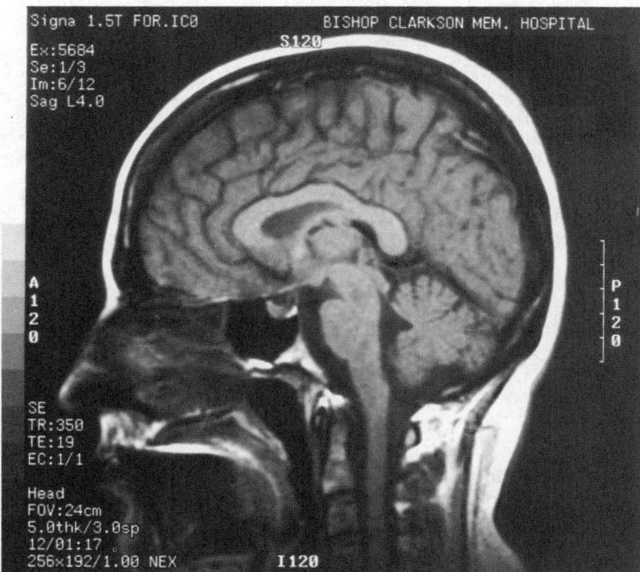

▲ *Figure 28–7*

Normal MRI. Sagittal section showing cerebrum, ventricles, cerebellum, and medulla of the brain.

Prior to the test, the client should remove all metal-containing objects, such as the bra, jewelry, and watches. Such objects may be drawn into the magnetic field by the powerful magnet and become harmful projectiles. Any internal metal objects should be noted for the physician, such as prostheses and pacemakers. Intravenous fluid pumps need to be removed from the client during the test. Special precautions are needed for clients with pulse oximeters. The cord from the sensor to the finger cannot be coiled around the body or any body part because it may cause a burn.

Normally, the client can eat and take any prescribed medication prior to the examination. If the use of a contrast agent is planned, the nurse should ask whether the client tends to become nauseated easily and should adjust the intake of food and fluids accordingly. For example, some clients prefer a light breakfast to reduce nausea and others prefer to have an empty stomach.

The client will lie supine on a padded table and move through the imager. The client may be asked to lie still while the test is in progress. There will be tapping noises from the scanner while the images are being taken. Some clients will feel claustrophobic during the test, but should be assured that it is possible to communicate with the technologist during the scan. The examination will take about an hour. Following the test, the client can resume previous activities. Expect diuresis if a contrast agent was used.

Clinical Aspects of Computed Tomography and Magnetic Resonance Imaging. The ability to clearly visualize the brain with the use of the CT scan and MRI has been a significant step in the care of the client with neurologic disorders. The specific location of tumors and areas of bleeding has allowed neurosurgeons greater precision with surgical procedures. Other disorders such as multiple sclerosis can be diagnosed with the aid of the CT and MRI scans. MRI uses magnetic fields to excite hydrogen in the body. Future imaging might use phosphorus or sodium ions to give additional physiologic information, such as early warning signals of impending myocardial infarction or stroke.

POSITRON-EMISSION TOMOGRAPHY

Positron-emission tomography (PET) allows the visualization of physiologic function in body areas. Often, the function of diseased tissue is different from normal tissues. The client is given doses of strong radioactive tracers, and the high concentration of tracers creates signals that are picked up by a scanner. The tracers, although potent, have a very short half-life, which makes their use safe. The tracers release positive electrons, which emit a signal when they come in contact with electrons. PET has three primary uses: (1) to determine the amount of blood flow to specific body tissues, (2) to reveal how adequately tissues use blood or nutrients, such as oxygen, and (3) to map specific receptors, such as medications or neurotransmittors. PET can be used to measure cerebral blood flow, cerebral glucose metabolism, and oxygen extraction. PET is used in the diagnosis of stroke, brain tumors, and epilepsy, and to chart the progress of Alzheimer's disease, Parkinson's disease, head injury, schizophrenia, and manic-depressive illness.

One major disadvantage is that PET is expensive. PET requires its own positron to manufacture high-energy radioactive tracers; a PET system can cost 5 million dollars initially. As a result of the cost of PET, a modification of the test has been developed. It is called a single photon emission computed tomography (SPECT). This test uses less precise but more stable and more readily available isotopes to measure cerebral blood flow rather than metabolic activity, as is measured with the PET. The test appears to be an effective diagnostic tool.

Nursing Intervention. The client and family should be taught about the purpose of the test, the sensations that the client will hear and feel during the examination, and the client's role during the test. In contrast to CT and MRI, the PET scanner is absolutely quiet. Clients need to fast for 4 hours prior to the scan. If the client is diabetic, it is preferred that the blood sugar be below 150 g/dl. Clients who are agitated may require sedation prior to the scan.

ELECTROENCEPHALOGRAM

An EEG is a measurement of the electrical activity of the superficial layers of the cerebral cortex. It demonstrates the electrical potentials from neuron activity within the brain in the form of wave patterns. The intensity and pattern of electrical activity is influenced by the reticular activating system. The characteristics of the wave depend on the degree of cortical activity. Several distinct wave patterns are found in recordings of clients without brain disorders. Wave patterns are called delta, theta, alpha, or beta depending on their appearance (amplitude and frequency). EEG waves are

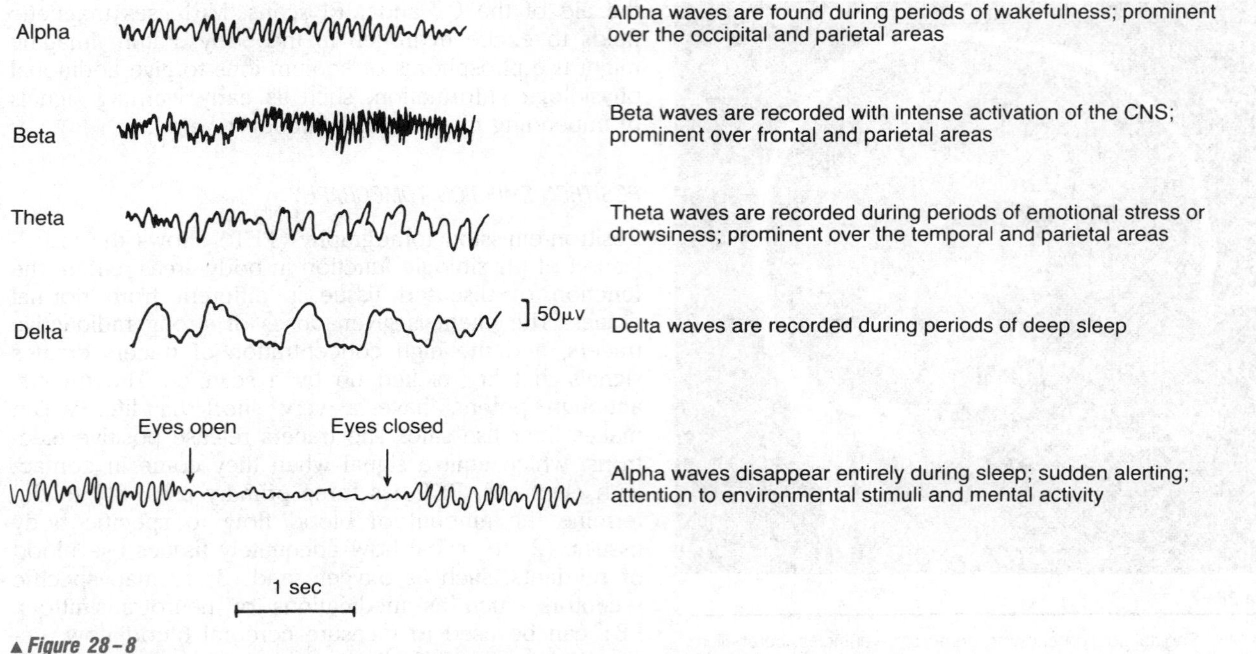
Alpha
Alpha waves are found during periods of wakefulness; prominent over the occipital and parietal areas
Beta
Beta waves are recorded with intense activation of the CNS; prominent over frontal and parietal areas
Theta
Theta waves are recorded during periods of emotional stress or drowsiness; prominent over the temporal and parietal areas
Delta
50µv
Delta waves are recorded during periods of deep sleep
Eyes open
Eyes closed
Alpha waves disappear entirely during sleep; sudden alerting; attention to environmental stimuli and mental activity
1 sec

▲ *Figure 28-8*

EEG waves. (Modified from Guyton, A. C. [Ed.] [1991]. *Textbook of medical physiology* [8th ed]. Philadelphia: W. B. Saunders.)

shown in Figure 28-8. The pattern of EEG waves changes with aging and disease; for example, beta activity increases with age.

Electrodes are attached to the client's scalp (Fig. 28-9). The waveforms are amplified and recorded on a moving paper strip, similar to an EKG. EEGs are interpreted according to brain wave characteristics, frequency, and amplitude.

Brain activity as recorded on an EEG correlates with the cerebral blood flow. A constant supply of oxygen, blood, and glucose is needed to meet the metabolic demands of the brain. Decreased cerebral blood flow causes cerebral hypoxia and causes changes in mentation and decreased electrical activity on the EEG. EEG can detect hypoxia in the brain prior to permanent damage to cerebral tissues.

If the client is comatose or unable to be moved, EEG can be performed at the bedside. For routine diagnostic examination, the client is taken to an EEG laboratory for a more controlled environment. The client's scalp is cleaned, and electrodes are applied to the scalp and earlobe (for reference) with collodion. Leads can also be placed in the nasopharynx to assess disorders in the temporal lobe. The first portion of the test is performed with the client as relaxed as possible to obtain a baseline recording. Further readings are taken while the client is hyperventilating, sleeping, or viewing flickering lights. Hyperventilation alters acid-base balance (respiratory alkalosis) and decreases cerebral blood flow. Flickering lights may trigger seizures. Sleep may evoke abnormal EEG patterns not present while the client is awake. The client may be kept awake the night preceding the test or sedated to induce sleep.

An EEG is useful in assessing clients with any type of seizure disorder. An EEG is diffusely abnormal in various metabolic disturbances, toxic conditions (e.g., drug overdose), coma, organic brain syndrome, and infections such as meningitis and encephalitis. The EEG may be used in the operating room to monitor cerebral activity during surgery on the blood vessels in the head or neck. Sleep patterns in depressed clients may also be assessed with EEGs. Some clients are assessed for temporal lobe epilepsy by using a 24-hour EEG recording. An EEG is also used to assist in diagnosing narcolepsy and impotence.

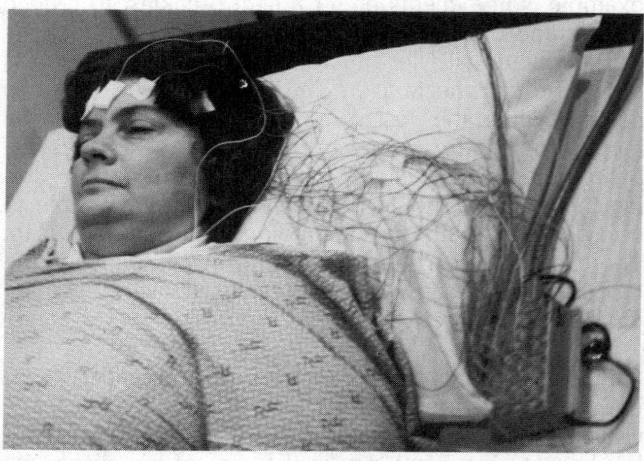

▲ *Figure 28-9*

Client undergoing an electroencephalogram (EEG).

Absence of EEG waves (flat lines) on EEG may be one of the criteria for defining brain death. Studies on comatose patients show that findings of the EEG have a high correlation with the survival or death of the client in a coma.

Nursing Intervention. The purpose of the test and the procedure should be explained to the client and family. The client and family may need to be reassured that electricity does not enter the brain (shock is not given) and the machine is not able to read the mind. Before the EEG is performed, the client's hair must be shampooed. Stimulants, (e.g., coffee, alcohol, tea, cola, and cigarettes), antidepressants, tranquilizers, and anticonvulsants should be avoided for 24 to 48 hours prior to the test. Sometimes sleep is withheld for many hours. Normal meals should be consumed because a lowered serum glucose will alter the test results. If the client will be asked to sleep for a portion of the test, sleep should be minimized the night before the test. The client will be asked to relax during the test, because anxiety can block alpha rhythms and produce artifacts from increased muscle tone in the head and neck. The nurse should be sure to send adequate supplies (i.e., intravenous fluids or oxygen) to the laboratory.

If the EEG is being performed to evaluate the possibility of brain death, it is important to keep artifacts to a minimum. Artifacts can be caused by the manipulation of electrodes, electrical interference, cycling of respirators, and even walking in the room. Institutional guidelines should be followed for the avoidance of artifacts when EEG is performed at the client's bedside.

Following the EEG, the client can resume previous activity, medications, and diet. If seizure activity is possible, seizure precautions need to be followed. The hair can be washed and acetone may be required to remove the collodion from the scalp and hair.

EVOKED POTENTIAL STUDIES

Evoked potential (EP) studies are a form of EEG in which the client's brain waves are monitored as the client is given various stimuli. The test is used to assess the function of the cerebral hemispheres and the brain stem. A variety of types of stimuli are used, such as auditory, somatosensory, and visual. Typical stimuli include flashing lights, buzzing tones, and peripheral nerve stimulation. EP can be used to assess blindness, deafness, and brain stem injury. Specific brain signals can be accentuated and others filtered out, allowing assessment of brain waves from other areas. EP studies are carried out in the same fashion as EEGs. EP studies can detect abnormalities even if the client is sedated or paralyzed with neuromuscular blocking agents. Some clinicians believe that EP studies are more reliable than clinical assessments in predicting neurologic recovery in comatose, head-injured clients.

Nursing interventions are the same as for the client having an EEG, except in the explanation of the variations between the tests.

TESTS FOR VASCULAR ABNORMALITIES

Noninvasive tests are useful in assessing cerebral vascular disease.

Ophthalmodynamometry. Ophthalmodynamometry compares the retinal artery pressures in both eyes. It may help diagnose extracranial vascular disease. While the retina is observed through an ophthalmoscope, pressure (or suction) is applied to the eyeball by a dynamometer, and readings are obtained.

Doppler Ultrasonography. Doppler ultrasonography may be used to measure blood flow (including direction and velocity) in the supraorbital region. In occlusion or stenosis of the internal carotid artery, the direction of blood flow is altered (reversed) in the supraorbital artery, which may be detected by ultrasonography.

Doppler Scanning. This is a test combining Doppler ultrasonography with pulse echo. Visual representation of moving blood is obtained. Mobile artery and vein imaging system is commonly used.

Quantitative Spectral Phonoangiography. This is a noninvasive method of assessing the extent of carotid stenosis by spectral analysis of bruits arising from the carotid bifurcation.

Invasive Tests

LUMBAR PUNCTURE

A lumbar puncture (LP, or spinal tap) is the insertion of a needle into the subarachnoid space in the lumbar region of the spine below the level of the spinal cord. Cerebral spinal fluid can be withdrawn or substances can be injected into this space.

LP is performed for assessment and therapeutic purposes. LP enables assessment of cerebrospinal fluid (CSF) pressure and collection of CSF for evaluation. When meningitis or subarachnoid hemorrhage is suspected, the CSF is examined for white blood cells and blood. *Myelogram* is an x-ray study in which a contrast agent is injected into the subarachnoid space after CSF is removed in order to examine the spinal canal.

Therapeutically, LP is used to administer spinal medications and anesthetics and, on occasion, to reduce dangerously high intracranial pressure by removing CSF. The CSF pressure drops 5 to 10 mm of water pressure for each millimeter of CSF removed. Usually, only 5 to 10 ml are removed, but this procedure can reduce intracranial pressure by 50 to 100 mm.

Even though LP is generally a safe procedure, it does have some potential hazards. The procedure can be uncomfortable for the client. The client will feel pressure in the lower back and may experience pain if a nerve root is touched with the needle during insertion. The potential complications of LP are CSF leakage (see spinal headache), infection, intervertebral disc damage, and herniation of the brain due to increased intracranial pressure. A space-occupying lesion within the cranium, such as a tumor or bleeding, increases intracranial pressure. Therefore, LP is not performed in clients with papilledema (a sign of increased intracranial pressure), suspected intracranial lesions, or increased intracranial pressure or infection of the skin at the puncture site. CT scans are used in these clients to rule out masses before a LP is performed. If an LP were performed in clients with increased intracranial pressure, there would be a rapid decrease in pressure within the CSF around the spinal cord. This change in pressure might allow the structures within the brain to drop (herniate) into the spinal canal. The process of herniation creates pressure on the vital centers in the medulla (cardiac and respiratory centers) and could cause sudden death.

Nursing Intervention

Prior to Procedure. The client and the family need to be taught about the purpose of lumbar puncture, the sensations that the client will feel during the examination, and the client's role during the examination. An informed consent form must be signed by the client prior to the test. The bladder and bowels should be emptied, if possible. The client will need to lie on one side with the legs pulled onto the abdomen and head tucked into the chest in order to open the spaces between the vertebrae. It will be important for the client to lie still during the test.

The necessary equipment should be assembled in the client's room. Spinal tap trays are available, which contain all needed equipment. In addition, the nurse should have laboratory request forms and a marking pencil to label the bottles of spinal fluid.

During the Procedure. LP to remove a sample of CSF is described here. The same general principles apply to any LP procedure, however.

Position the client on the side (lateral recumbent) with the back close to the edge of the bed. Place a pillow under the flank so that the spinous processes are horizontal. Use additional pillows between the client's knees and under the head to keep the spine horizontal. Ask the client to draw the knees up to the abdomen and chin onto the chest (Fig. 28-10). Help the client maintain this curved position to separate and increase spaces between the vertebrae so that the needle can be inserted more easily. Stand in front of the client and place one hand behind the client's knees and the other

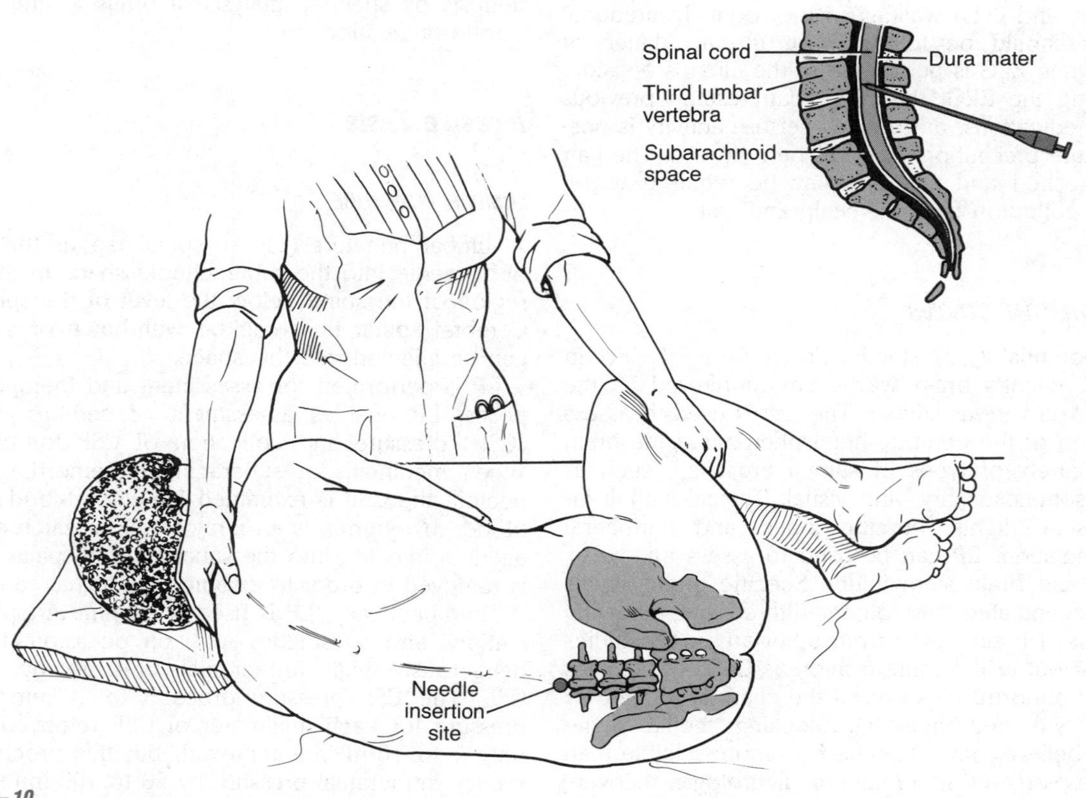

▲ Figure 28–10

Lumbar puncture (LP). Position the client as shown (i.e., laterally, with knees drawn up to abdomen and chin brought down to chest). This position curves the spine, thus increasing space between the vertebrae. The sterile LP needle is inserted as shown between the third and fourth (or fourth and fifth) vertebrae, and enters the subarachnoid space.

around the neck. Keep the client's upper shoulder from falling forward, thus preventing rotation of the spine. (An alternative position is with the person sitting up with head and chest bent toward the knees.)

After a local anesthetic is given, a small needle will be placed into the space between the vertebrae in the lower back. The needle is inserted well below the end of the spinal cord, so there is no danger of paralysis.

The needle bevel is usually held parallel to the longitudinal fibers of the dura. This position limits the size of the dural tear and reduces the risk of CSF leak. A little local pain may occur as the needle passes the dura mater. Ask the client to mention additional discomfort because it may indicate misplacement of the needle. In adults, the needle is inserted about level with the top of the iliac crests (hip bones) or at the next lower vertebral level (usually between the third and fourth or fourth and fifth lumbar vertebrae). In adults, the spinal cord normally ends at the lower border of the first lumbar vertebra. Thus, the puncture site is low enough to avoid spinal cord injury.

When the needle has entered the subarachnoid space, the physician removes the stylus and attaches a stopcock and manometer. A manometer measures CSF pressure. The first stabilized CSF pressure reading is the opening pressure. Normal opening CSF pressure with the person in a horizontal position is 6 to 13 mm Hg or 80 to 180 mm of H_2O. Pressures over 200 mm of H_2O are abnormal. Normally, CSF oscillates (fluctuates) in the manometer, readily responding to coughing, straining, and changes in the person's breathing. If there is a blockage in the spinal canal, the CSF pressure may not oscillate.

CSF specimens are collected in a series of small sterile test tubes, numbered in sequence of collection (e.g., No. 1, No. 2). Two to three ml of CSF are collected in each tube; 8 to 10 ml may be removed. The needle is withdrawn, and a dry sterile dressing is placed over the puncture site.

In adults, CSF is assessed for cells, chloride, glucose, protein, pressure, and lactate dehydrogenase (LDH). Table 28-4 lists common abnormalities of CSF. When sending CSF, the first vial obtained is not assessed for blood because it may contain blood from the puncture.

Following the Procedure. Vital signs should be recorded after an LP. Sometimes, lying flat for 3 hours is prescribed. The client can eat and drink, as was done prior to the test. Forcing fluids will help restore CSF volume. If the CSF measurement indicated a high intracranial pressure, the client should be assessed for decreasing levels of consciousness, indicating increasing intracranial pressure.

Postlumbar puncture headache (spinal puncture headache, spinal headache) is typically throbbing, bifrontal, and suboccipital, developing a few hours to several days after an LP. The headache is probably due to continuing CSF leakage through the opening in the dura made by the needle. As a result of the leak, the CSF circulating around the cranium is depleted. The fluid loss allows abnormal movement of the brain in the skull. When the brain moves, tension is placed on the meninges and venous sinuses, which causes pain. The headache is usually relieved when the client lies down and is made worse by sitting up or a sudden jolt of the head. Such headaches usually disappear within 24 hours but may last for several days.

To reduce the risk of postlumbar puncture headache, have the client remain in bed following the examination. Although physician's orders may differ on the length of time, an average time in bed is 3 hours. Fluids should be encouraged to replace the CSF withdrawn during the test. Once a headache begins, treatments may include bed rest in a dark, quiet room, and the administration of analgesics and fluids. If the headache continues, an epidural blood patch may be required. Blood is withdrawn from the client and injected into the epidural space, usually at the LP site. The blood acts as a fibrin patch to seal the hole in the dura and prevent further CSF leakage. Blood patches cannot be performed when the client has bleeding tendencies or infection at the puncture site.

MYELOGRAPHY

Myelography is an x-ray examination of the spinal cord and vertebral canal following introduction of contrast media into the spinal subarachnoid space (Figure 28-11). It is used to study the spinal canal and subarach-

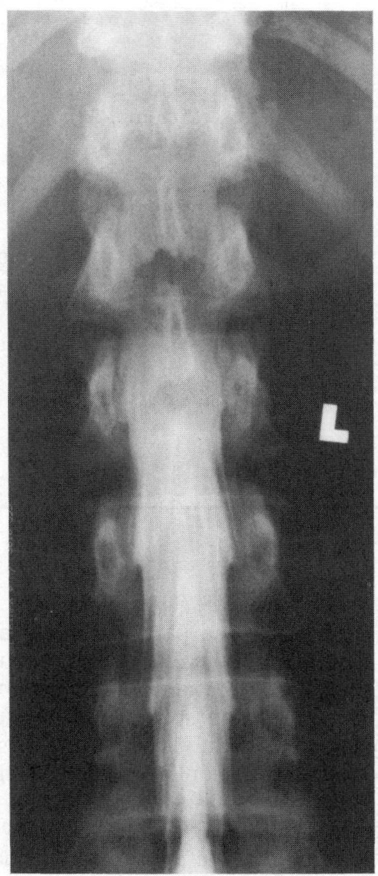

▲ **Figure 28-11**

Myelogram of lumbar spine shows contrast flowing throughout subarachnoid space without obstruction.

TABLE 28-4. Normal CSF Values and Significance of Abnormal Values

Substance	Normal Value (Conventional Units)	Significance of Abnormal Values
Blood	None; CSF should be clear	Gross blood is seen in CNS hemorrhage. Rarely, there are some blood cells in the first tube of CSF collected, because of trauma during the tap. The collection of specimens in sequence should be marked, so that it is possible to determine whether the blood in the first tube is more than the last tube. If the CSF is grossly bloody, other tests may not be able to be performed
Cells	0 to 5 mononuclear	Increased neutrophils may be seen in bacterial infections such as bacterial meningitis. Lymphocytes may be increased in tuberculosis and some viral disorders
Enzymes (LDH)	10 per cent of serum level	Elevated with inflammations and bacterial meningitis
Glucose	50 to 75 mg/dl, should be 20 mg less than serum glucose level	Glucose level is lowered in bacterial infections, because bacteria use sugar. Some types of tumors also lower CSF glucose. Be certain to compare CSF glucose with serum glucose. Ideally, a serum specimen should be drawn 30 minutes before an LP, because it takes glucose about 30 to 60 minutes to diffuse into the CSF
Protein Albumin	15 to 45 mg/dl 29.5 mg/dl (80%)	Increased proteins may be seen in degenerative disorders and brain tumors. Lesions that interrupt the blood-brain barrier also increase proteins because there is an increased diffusion from the blood into the brain tissues
IgG Oligoclonal Bands	<14% of total protein Absent	IgG and oligoclonal bands (an abnormal type of protein band seen on immunoelectrophoresis) is often present in multiple sclerosis and neurosyphilis
Pressure	70 to 180 mm H_2O	Elevated in bacterial meningitis, cerebral bleeding, and tumors. Decreased in conditions that obstruct CSF flow, such as tumors of the spinal canal

noid space. This study is a particularly valuable assessment tool when the spinal cord is thought to be compressed (e.g., by herniated intervertebral disc or tumor encroaching on the spinal subarachnoid space). Myelography is also useful in diagnosing such spinal cord pathology as intramedullary tumors, syringomyelia, and AVMs.

Preparation for a myelogram includes hydration for at least 12 hours before the procedure. In the radiology department, a lumbar puncture is performed, a small amount of CSF is withdrawn, and the contrast material is injected. With the needle in place, the person is turned on the abdomen and secured to the table by foot and shoulder supports. While the radiologist follows carefully with fluoroscopy, the table is slowly tilted. This procedure causes the column of dye to move up or down within the subarachnoid space, permitting visualization of the desired areas. Standard films are taken of these areas. The contrast material used is water soluble and is not removed from the spinal column.

Nursing Intervention. Following the myelogram, the client may have to remain flat in bed or with the head of the bed elevated 15 to 30 degrees, depending on the type of dye used. Usually, the client remains in bed 6 to 8 hours and then resumes normal activity. Encourage the person to take extra fluids. Assess neurologic status frequently. Back pain (ranging from mild discomfort to severe pain) in the area of the needle insertion may develop and may last a few days. Also, the person may experience a stiff neck and headache for a few days, particularly if the contrast medium was allowed to rise to high cervical levels. This discomfort is usually relieved by lying flat and the administration of fluids and analgesics. (See also nursing intervention for LP.)

CISTERNAL PUNCTURE

On rare occasions, access to the CSF cannot be made by LP and cisternal puncture may be used. Cisternal puncture is puncture of the cisterna magna (a small reservoir of CSF between the cerebellum and medulla). A physician introduces a short-beveled needle below the occipital bone, between the first cervical lamina and the rim of the foramen magnum. Cisternal puncture is performed either to drain CSF or to obtain a CSF specimen when there is a block in the spinal subarachnoid space or if LP is contraindicated. If the client has a lesion on the spinal cord, the top edge of the lesion can be determined by contrast injected via the cisternal puncture.

Position the client at the edge of a treatment table or bed, lying on the side with a sandbag under the head to keep the cervical spine and head straight with the thoracic spine. Flex the client's head forward and hold it firmly in position. Following skin preparation, local anesthetic may or may not be injected. A cisternal needle with stylet in place is inserted to a depth of about 5 cm.

Subsequent assessments and interventions are essentially the same as with LP.

CEREBRAL ANGIOGRAPHY

A cerebral angiogram is the injection of contrast into an artery to visualize intracranial circulation (Fig. 28-12). Angiography is the procedure used most often to visualize aneurysms, AVMs, major vessel displacement, vascular occlusion, and thrombi. Not only is cerebral angiography an invasive procedure, but it is a test in

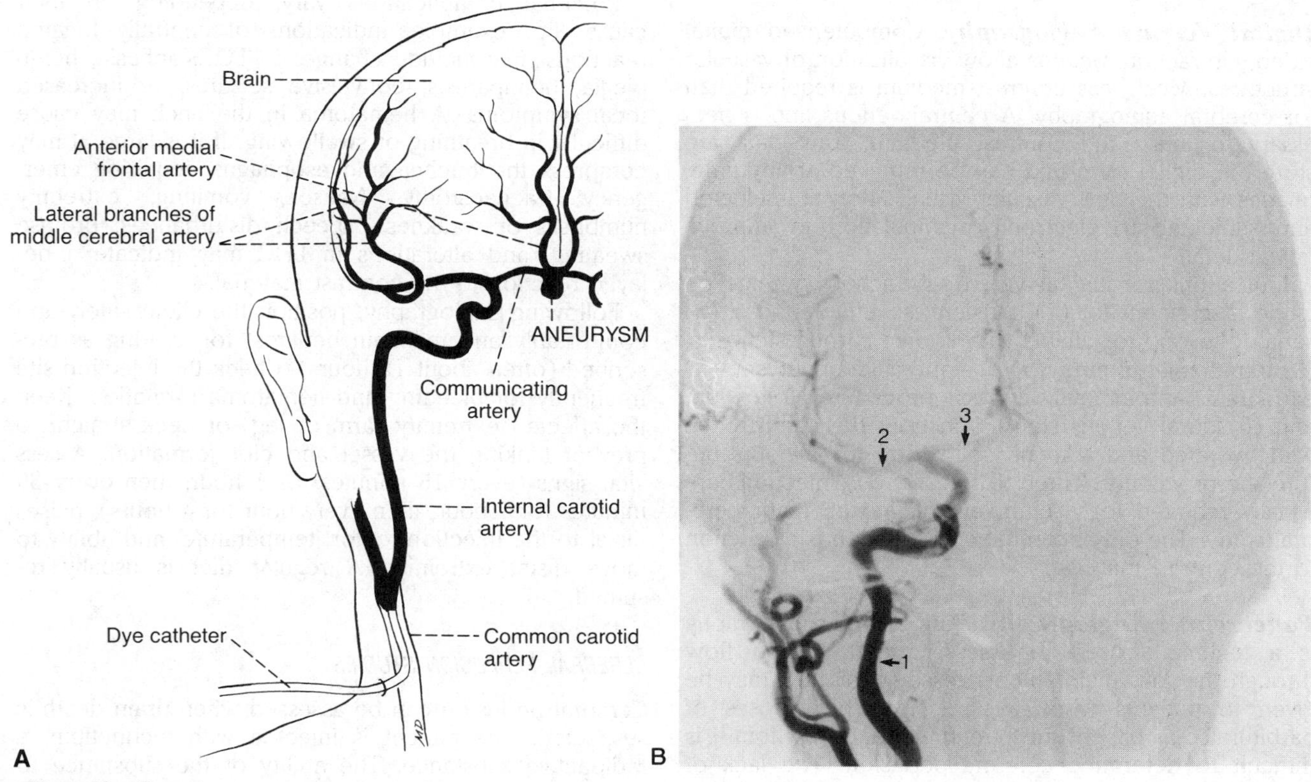

▲ *Figure 28-12*

Cerebral angiography allows x-ray visualization of the brain's vascular system when a contrast dye is injected arterially. *A*, Illustrates insertion of dye through a catheter in the common carotid artery, subsequently outlining vessels of the brain. *B*, Angiogram using subtraction technique. (1) Internal carotid, (2) middle cerebral, and (3) middle meningeal arteries.

which small errors can result in permanent disability or death. Meticulous attention must be given to the client before, during, and following angiography.

The procedure is performed by inserting a catheter (a soft needle) into the femoral artery and then guiding the catheter through the use of a fluoroscope into the carotid-vertebral arteries. This approach has replaced previous approaches in which the carotid, vertebral, or brachial vessels were punctured directly. The use of the femoral artery is less traumatic, and local complications, such as infection or bleeding in the puncture site, occur away from the neck. Once the vessels are reached, the contrast agent is injected and a series of x-ray studies are taken from lateral, anteroposterior, and oblique approaches. Sequential views of the vessels show the movement of the dye in the vessels. After the catheter is removed, a sterile dressing is placed over the puncture site and firm pressure is applied to the site for 10 minutes to prevent hematoma formation. Sandbags and a pressure dressing may be used to provide firm pressure. Ice bags may also be used to provide pressure and relieve tenderness. The injection site may be tender.

Interventional Angiography. Interventional angiography is a recent advance in client care. This technique uses a polymer glue or Gelfoam (a material that stops bleeding) to occlude feeding vessels in tumors or AVMs.

Digital Venous Angiography. Computerized digital video subtraction systems allow visualization of vascular structures. Much less contrast medium is required than for cerebral angiography. A central venous line is necessary to inject the contrast medium. Raw data are stored in digital form and can be retrieved at any time. Images with the best vascular visualization are selected and subjected to electronic manipulation to improve image detail.

Indications for digital video subtraction systems include assessment for (1) transient ischemic attacks, (2) serial follow-up for clients with known carotid stenoses, (3) intracranial tumors, (4) postoperative aneurysm, (5) extracranial-intracranial bypass procedure follow-up, and (6) dural venous sinuses. Instruct the client to be well hydrated and take no solid food for 2 hours before the procedure. Three to four venous injections are usually required for a complete diagnostic craniocerebral study. The only potential complication is a reaction to the contrast material.

Pancerebral Angiography. Pancerebral angiography is a technique used to assess cerebral blood flow through the four major blood vessels. This test may be given to patients who have received high doses of barbiturates as part of their treatment and in whom it is difficult to determine cerebral perfusion. The lack of intracranial blood flow through the four major vessels is an absolute indication of brain death.

Nursing Intervention. The client and the family should be taught about the purpose of the test, the sensations that the client will experience during the test, and the client's role during the procedure. Prior to the test, the client may not take anything by mouth for 4 to 6 hours but should be well hydrated prior to that time. Intravenous fluids may be prescribed. The nurse should document the neurologic status of the client to serve as a baseline after the examination. The client should remove any metal items from the hair, such as barrettes, and earrings. Allergies to iodine should be reported. During the test, the client will be given an injection of local anesthetic prior to the placement of the catheter. There will also be a warm flushed feeling when the dye is injected. (See also the section entitled "The Use of Contrast Dye.") While the angiogram is being conducted, the client is continually assessed for neurologic deterioration.

Following the test, the nurse must assess the client closely for complications. Complications are rare but include (1) local and systemic allergic reactions to the contrast dye, (2) spasm or occlusion of the vessel by a clot, (3) hemorrhage, and (4) obstructive clot formation above a femoral injection site. Assess for reactions to the contrast dye. Spasm or occlusion of the target vessel(s) causes symptoms similar to those of a stroke. (Stroke, or cerebral vascular accident, is discussed in Chap. 30.) Clot formation at the injection site also causes ischemic reactions in the affected area. These adverse reactions are usually reversible, but rarely cause permanent damage.

Potential complications vary, depending on their cause. For example, indications of centrally located reactions may include changes in LOC, aphasia, hemiplegia, hemiparesis, convulsive seizures, or increased focal symptoms. A hematoma in the neck may cause difficulty in breathing or swallowing. If it is large, it may compress the trachea and esophagus, requiring emergency tracheostomy. Nausea, vomiting, extremity numbness or weakness, speech disturbances, profuse sweating, and alterations in LOC may indicate a delayed reaction to the contrast material.

Following angiography, position the client safely and comfortably and maintain bed rest for as long as prescribed (often about 12 hours). Check the injection site frequently for bleeding and hematoma formation. Keep the affected extremity (arm or leg) or neck straight to prevent kinking the vessel and clot formation. Assess vital signs (every 15 minutes for 1 hour, then every 30 minutes for 1 hour, then every hour for 4 hours), pulses distal to the injection, color, temperature, and ability to move distal extremity. A regular diet is usually resumed.

CEREBRAL PERFUSION STUDIES

Cerebral perfusion can be assessed when brain death is suspected. The patient is injected with technetium, a radioactive substance. The ability of the substance to perfuse from blood vessels into brain tissue is assessed with a scanner. In patients who are clinically brain dead, there is no uptake of the substance by the cerebrum or cerebellum. The substance is injected at the bedside, and the scanner can be brought to the bedside to evaluate perfusion. This test allows appropriate medical care to continue when brain death cannot be determined, and conversely, medical care can stop for those patients who are brain dead. The nurse's role in this test is informing the patient's family about the significance of the test and its findings. Once the patient is declared brain dead, it is the end of meaningful life. The family may need help accepting the results of this very final test.

CALORIC TESTING

The oculovestibular reflex, or caloric test, is a diagnostic examination providing information about the function of the vestibular portion of the eighth cranial nerve. It aids in the differential diagnois of cerebellum and brain stem lesions (see also Chap. 29).

The test is performed by introducing either cold or hot water into the external auditory canal. A current then flows through the endolymphatic fluid. Typically, when the vestibular eighth cranial nerve is normal, stimulation of the auditory canal with hot water produces a rotary nystagmus away from the side of the irrigated ear. When cold water is used, the normal response is rotary nystagmus toward the irrigated ear. (Nystagmus is involuntary, rapid eyeball movement.)

If pathology exists, nystagmus does not occur. Sometimes unpleasant symptoms, such as vertigo, dizziness, nausea, and vomiting occur. Warn the client of the possibility of these symptoms and give supportive nursing intervention if they occur. Caloric tests are contraindicated in clients with perforated ear drums or with acute labyrinthine disease.

As with pupil signs, abnormalities in eye movements help to localize the area of a disorder. They also help differentiate between structural and metabolic causes of coma.

Bithermal caloric tests assess vestibular function. Alternate ear irrigations of hot and cold water are performed. Similar, although more specific, findings are obtained. Nystagmus is measured by electronystagmography.

ELECTROMYOGRAPHY

EMG uses an electromyograph to measure and document electrical currents produced by skeletal muscles, called muscle action potentials. Small needle electrodes are inserted into muscles. The electrical potentials of each muscle are amplified, transmitted to an oscilloscope, and displayed on a screen. The recording can be made audible and documented on paper (Fig. 28-13).

EMG can provide objective information that is helpful in diagnosing various neuromuscular diseases. EMG can differentiate between primary muscle disease and disease secondary to denervation. It helps identify specific primary muscle diseases. It may indicate a defect in transmission at the neuromuscular junction, such as myasthenia gravis. It can help to differentiate diseases of the anterior horn cells from those primarily of peripheral nerves. Peripheral nerve degeneration and regeneration can often be monitored with EMG before any clinical changes appear.

A nerve conduction velocity study is often performed in conjunction with EMG, which studies the excitability and conduction velocities of motor and sensory nerves. It is helpful in diagnosing diseases of peripheral nerves. A stimulating electrode and a recording electrode are placed to test specific nerves (usually on a limb). The time required for the passage of a nerve impulse from the point of stimulation to the point of recording is measured precisely. Conduction velocity is calculated. Both motor and sensory modalities are altered in peripheral nervous system disorders (e.g., carpal tunnel syndrome), whereas only motor fibers are affected in

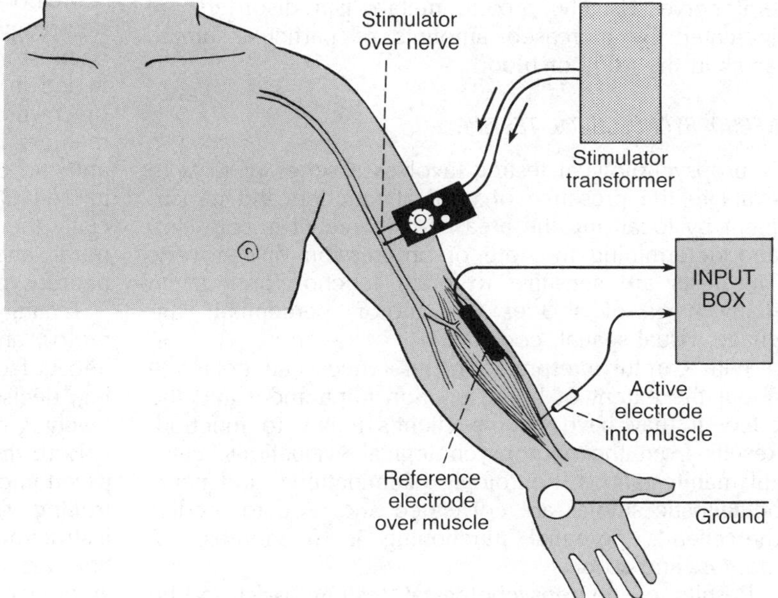

▲ **Figure 28-13**

Electromyography measures and documents electrical currents produced by skeletal muscles. A stimulator is placed over the peripheral nerve being tested. A small pin is inserted into the muscle being assessed for nerve innervation, and a ground is placed on the client's skin.

chronic diseases of the anterior horn cell or motor nerve roots.

Nursing Intervention. Explain the procedure to the client and significant others. They are often concerned about the outcome of the test. They may be very anxious and stressed. The person should avoid all stimulants, depressants, or sedatives for 24 hours before the test. There may be some discomfort when the electrodes are inserted. If many muscles are tested, there may be some residual discomfort. The client may experience a mild electrical shock during the procedure. The client lies flat and may be asked to move various muscles at specific times during the test.

MUSCLE BIOPSY

Muscle biopsy is used in diagnosing neuropathies and myopathies. It is useful in distinguishing between neurogenic and myopathic processes. However, muscle histologic findings are nonspecific for any neurogenic atrophy. An electromyogram is helpful in locating those muscle areas that are most abnormal. It is important that areas that have been traumatized by needle electrodes be avoided when tissue is taken for biopsy.

CELLULAR ASSESSMENT

Chromosome analysis is used to (1) assist diagnosis of some abnormal neurologic conditions and (2) provide the basis for genetic counseling in families with evidence of congenital neurologic malformations. Chromosomes can be prepared for microscopic examination from tissue culture of cells obtained from peripheral blood, bone marrow, or skin.

Mental retardation and convulsive seizures may result from neurologic dysfunction associated with inborn errors of metabolism. Diagnosis of disorders of carbohydrate and lipid metabolism may require measurements of specific enzyme concentration in blood cells or tissue biopsied from brain, muscle, liver, or peripheral nerve. Usually, protein metabolism disorders are indicated by increased amounts of particular amino acids in the urine or blood.

NEUROPSYCHOLOGICAL TESTING

Neuropsychological testing involves a series of tests to evaluate the presence of cortical function and impairment by localizing the area and degree of impairment, and determining the rate of progression or recovery. The tests are sensitive to brain function and gauge many types of abilities (i.e. motor, perceptual, language, visual-spatial, cognitive).

With careful interpretation, inferences can be made about the extent of brain function impairment and the effect it may have on the client's ability to function. Results from the neuropsychological evaluations, clinical manifestations, neurologic examinations, and neurodiagnostic studies are correlated and used to predict the client's potential functioning in 6 months, 12 months, and so on.

Results of neuropsychological testing assist in the diagnosis of specific cognitive dysfunction and the development of an individualized rehabilitation program. Serial testing is valuable to monitor rehabilitative progress and recovery in clients with problems such as head injury and epilepsy.

There is poor correlation between the degree of brain damage as revealed, for example, by CT scan and neuropsychological testing. A small lesion can create a large functional deficit, and in contrast, a large lesion may only cause small changes. There are even instances in which testing clearly demonstrates brain dysfunction in the absence of a demonstrable lesion on CT scan.

A client may be referred for neuropsychological assessment in the acute phase or months after an injury. For example, after a head injury in which the physical neuro-assessment is normal and the EEG reveals only mild generalized abnormalities, the client may complain of being unable to work because of persistent headaches. Recommendations from testing may be made about treatment, including educational and vocational rehabilitation.

Neuropsychological tests measure deficits in coping skills by assessing the skills directly. They may be helpful when deficits in adaptive abilities are suspected. An individual test may be performed in the case of a disorder with only one specific symptom, or a complete series of tests with extended evaluation may require several hours or days of testing. The client's level of performance is compared with scores that represent normal levels of performance. General measures of intelligence (e.g. Wechsler Adult Intelligence Scale) as well as tests for emotional and personal adjustment, such as the Minnesota Multiphasic Personality Inventory are used.

Testing may be nonspecific in implicating the presence of brain damage or very narrow in scope with sensitivity to certain areas of the brain. Results may indicate that something is wrong but not be able to identify the problem specifically.

Memory loss is common following head injury and in neurologic disorders. Skills such as reading, which have been stored in the brain over the years, may be retained in contrast to new learning or short-term memory, which may be impaired. The client's impaired memory may interfere with the nurse's ability to teach and the client's ability to learn. Knowing that a brain-injured client has damage to the limbic system, especially the hippocampus, amygdala, or areas of the temporal and prefrontal lobe, is a good indicator for neuropsychological testing to determine memory loss.

Testing will identify problems in cognitive, psychomotor, and affective domains. Left hemisphere lesions impair factual information functions like problem solving, decision making, and judgement. Client and family teaching must be modified to address these deficits.

Both the right and left hemispheres are involved with psychomotor learning, with the right hemisphere controlling visual and spatial abilities and the left verbal instructions and sequencing of activities. Repetition and time are needed for the individual to perform activities automatically.

Memory loss diagnosed from damage to the right or left hemisphere causing affective learning deficits can be improved with role modeling, one-to-one, and group therapy.

The nurse's documentation of client behavior and functional abilities assists the neuropsychologist in following the individual's progress and recovery.

Summary

The neurologic assessment of a client begins like all assessments do, with the history of the disorder and then proceeds to the physical examination. The physical examination of the client can be lengthy because of the complexity of the CNS. The neurologic examination includes the assessment of cognition, sensation, motor function, and reflexes. The complexity and length of time required to complete the assessment may tend to make the examiner want to omit sections to speed up the process. Before omitting any sections, it is important to realize that these assessments often provide the baseline for further evaluation and at times legal proof of a client's status.

Common diagnostic tests include LP, CT and MRI scans, and angiography. The nurse needs to understand how the test is performed so that the client can be adequately prepared and appropriate follow-up assessments can be conducted.

Bibliography

1. Barker, E., & Moore, K. (1992). Neurological assessment. *RN, 55* (4), 28-35.
2. Carnavali, D. L., & Enloe, C. (1986). Assessment in the elderly. In D. Carnavali & M. Patrick (Eds.), *Nursing management for the elderly* (2nd ed., pp. 26-49). Philadelphia: J. B. Lippincott.
3. el-Mallakh, R. (1987). CSF evaluation in neurologic disease. *American Family Physician, 35* (6), 112-118.
4. Fuller, J., & Schaller-Ayers, J. (1990). *Health assessment: A nursing approach.* Philadelphia: J. B. Lippincott.
5. Henneman, E. (1989). Clinical assessment and neurodiagnostics. *Critical Care Nursing Clinics of North America, 1* (1), 131-142.
6. Jarvis, C. (1992). *Physical examination and health assessment.* Philadelphia: W. B. Saunders.
7. Lauren, N., et al. (1989). Cerebral perfusion imaging with technetium-99m HM-PAO in brain death and severe central nervous system injury. *Journal of Nuclear Medicine, 30* (10), 1627-1635.
8. Lower, J. (1992). Rapid neuroassessment. *American Journal of Nursing, 92* (6), 38-48.
9. Lundgren, J. (1990). Computerized EEG: Applications and interventions. *Journal of Neuroscience Nursing, 22* (2), 108-112.
10. Malasanos, L., et al. (1990). *Health assessment* (4th ed.). St. Louis: C. V. Mosby.
11. Marshall, S., et al. (1990). *Neuroscience critical care.* Philadelphia: W. B. Saunders.
12. McDonagh, A. (1991). Getting your patient ready for a nuclear medicine scan. *Nursing 91, 21* (2), 53-57.
13. McGruder, J., et al. (1988). Headache after lumbar puncture: Review of the epidural blood patch. *Southern Medical Journal, 81* (10), 1249-1252.
14. Mitchell, P. A., et al. (1988). *AANN's neuroscience nursing: Phenomena and practice.* Norwalk, CT: Appleton and Lange.
15. Morton, P. (1989). *Health assessment in nursing.* Springhouse, PA: Springhouse.
16. Norris, M., et al. (1989). Needle bevel direction and headache after inadvertent dural puncture. *Anesthesiology, 70* (5), 729-731.
17. Potter, P., & Perry, A. (1989). *Fundamentals of nursing: Concepts, process, and practice* (2nd ed.). St. Louis: C. V. Mosby.
18. Reid, R., et al. (1989). Clinical use of technetium-99m HM-PAO for determination of brain death. *Journal of Nuclear Medicine, 30* (10), 1621-1626.
19. Rogers, A., & Dykstra, C. (1989). EEGs: A closer look at a familiar diagnostic test. *Journal of Neuroscience Nursing, 21* (4), 227-233.
20. Sand, T. (1989). Which factors affect reported headache incidence after lumbar myelography? A statistical analysis of publications in the literature. *Neuroradiology, 31* (1), 55-59.
21. Solomon, E. P., et al. (1990). *Human anatomy & physiology* (2nd ed.). Philadelphia: W. B. Saunders.
22. Swartz, M. H. (1989). *Textbook of physical diagnosis.* Philadelphia: W. B. Saunders.
23. Thomas, C. L. (1989). *Taber's cyclopedic medical dictionary* (16th ed.). Philadelphia: F. A. Davis.

Chapter 29

Nursing Care of Clients with a Loss of Protective Function

The brain serves many functions in the body. Unlike other body systems that monitor and regulate a group of functions, such as the gastrointestinal tract regulates digestion, the nervous system monitors and regulates all other body systems. Some of these functions are self-protective and include the ability to think, be awake, respond appropriately to the environment, and move about. Other functions are automatic and include the regulation of body temperature and protective reflex responses. When these protective functions are lost, the symptoms reflect the complexity of the nervous system. Clients with a loss of protective function may have mild symptoms, such as the inability to blink; or more serious symptoms, such as the inability to move; or life-threatening symptoms, such as irreversible coma. The term "patient" is used in this chapter to describe the client who is comatose. It is assumed that such a client cannot be an active participant in care, and the family serves as the client in these circumstances.

DISORDERS OF CONSCIOUSNESS

Definition

Consciousness is a state of being that has two important aspects: wakefulness and awareness of self, others, and time. Awareness of time includes the past, present, and future events. Therefore, a client can be awake but confused about the time of day or year. The nurse should never assume that a client who is awake and looking about is aware of self, others, surroundings, and time without fully assessing the client (see Ethical Issues in Nursing).

Unconsciousness can be sustained, lasting for a few hours or longer, or brief, lasting for a few seconds to an hour or so. To produce unconsciousness, a disorder must (1) disrupt the ascending reticular activating system that is found in the center of the brain stem and thalamus; (2) significantly disrupt the function of both cerebral hemispheres; or (3) metabolically depress the cerebrum or reticular activating system, such as drug overdose. Coma is a state of sustained unconsciousness in which the patient does not respond to verbal stimuli, may have varying responses to painful stimuli, may not move voluntarily, may have altered respiratory patterns, may have altered pupil responses to light, and does not blink. In general, the longer the state of unconsciousness lasts, the more likely it is due to a permanent disorder in the structure of the brain (and irreversible) rather than a temporary alteration in the function (and reversible).

Incidence

The incidence of disorders of consciousness would be difficult to measure. There are a great number of patients who temporarily lose consciousness when they faint. There are also a lesser number of patients who have been in a coma for years.

Etiology

Three kinds of disorders produce sustained unconsciousness (Fig. 29-1). They are: (1) structural lesions in the brain that place pressure on the brain stem or in the posterior fossa, which destroy the reticular formation; (2) metabolic disorders, which impair the cerebrum and the arousal functions by decreasing the supply of oxygen or allowing waste products to accumulate; and (3) psychogenic causes, in which the patient looks comatose but self-awareness is usually intact, such as is seen in catatonia. Refer to a psychiatric nursing text for discussion of psychogenic coma.

Structural causes of unconsciousness include brain tumors, concussion and head trauma, and cerebral hemorrhage. The etiology of primary brain tumors is unknown. The brain can be a site of metastatic tumors from many organs. Automobile and motorcycle accidents, assault with guns and knives, and falls are common etiologic factors for head injury. Trauma physically damages the brain, and the brain is further damaged as a result of the edema and hemorrhage that follow.

There are many metabolic causes of coma. The term "metabolic" is used to describe problems that did not begin in the brain but began in another system and eventually caused a disorder in the nervous system. Hypoxia is a common cause of metabolic brain disorders. Blood loss, high altitudes, or carbon monoxide poisoning may deprive the brain of oxygen. Ischemia, the loss of blood to the brain, may occur with cardiac

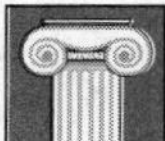

ETHICAL ISSUES IN NURSING

How Can Nurses Serve as Advocates to Confused Clients?

States of consciousness can be altered by many different factors, including disease, emotional stress, fatigue, poor nutrition, alcohol abuse, age-related pathologic changes, and sedation by medication. Such altered states may be temporary, as when one is under the influence of alcohol or sedative medications, or more permanent, like the result of Alzheimer's disease or any other disease process affecting cerebral activity. When a client experiences a change in consciousness, he or she may or may not be able to make rational decisions, particularly decisions about health care.

There is little question regarding the decision-making capabilities of someone who is in a more permanent altered state of mind, or is conscious. A client who is in a coma or has severe senile dementia would never be deemed competent to make personal health-related decisions. A surrogate would always need to be consulted to make health-related decisions for these clients (i.e., on their behalf, in their best interest). It is the client who is experiencing a transient altered state of mind who may erroneously be deemed competent to make health care decisions on his or her own behalf. The following is a true case presentation that illustrates the dilemma regarding this issue.

A 23-year-old gang member presented to the emergency room of a local hospital with a puncture wound to the left eye and surrounding facial tissue. He was alone and was not combative. The smell of alcohol was heavy on his breath, and the stat alcohol level confirmed that he was legally intoxicated. The ophthalmology surgeon examined him and decided that he must have surgery as soon as possible for preventing possible loss of vision. The surgeon had the client sign a consent for surgery form; however, she would have to wait to operate until a second alcohol level could be drawn, approximately 2 hours later, because the client could not go to surgery with an elevated blood alcohol level. The nurse caring for the young man noticed that the consent form was signed while his blood alcohol level was high. She approached the surgeon and explained that such an "informed" consent was not valid, because the client was temporarily incompetent to sign such a document, and that another consent must be obtained before surgery when the client's blood alcohol level was within normal limits. The surgeon did not think that this was necessary but did obtain a second consent when the client was no longer incompetent because of alcohol intoxication.

This case is an excellent example of the nursing role as client advocate. However tragic the loss of vision might have been for this client, he had a right to informed consent. Informed consent can never be obtained from a client who is not capable, for whatever reason, of understanding what he or she is consenting to. Nurses have an obligation to speak out when they believe, on the basis of their knowledge of the client, that their client's competence to make health care decisions is in doubt.

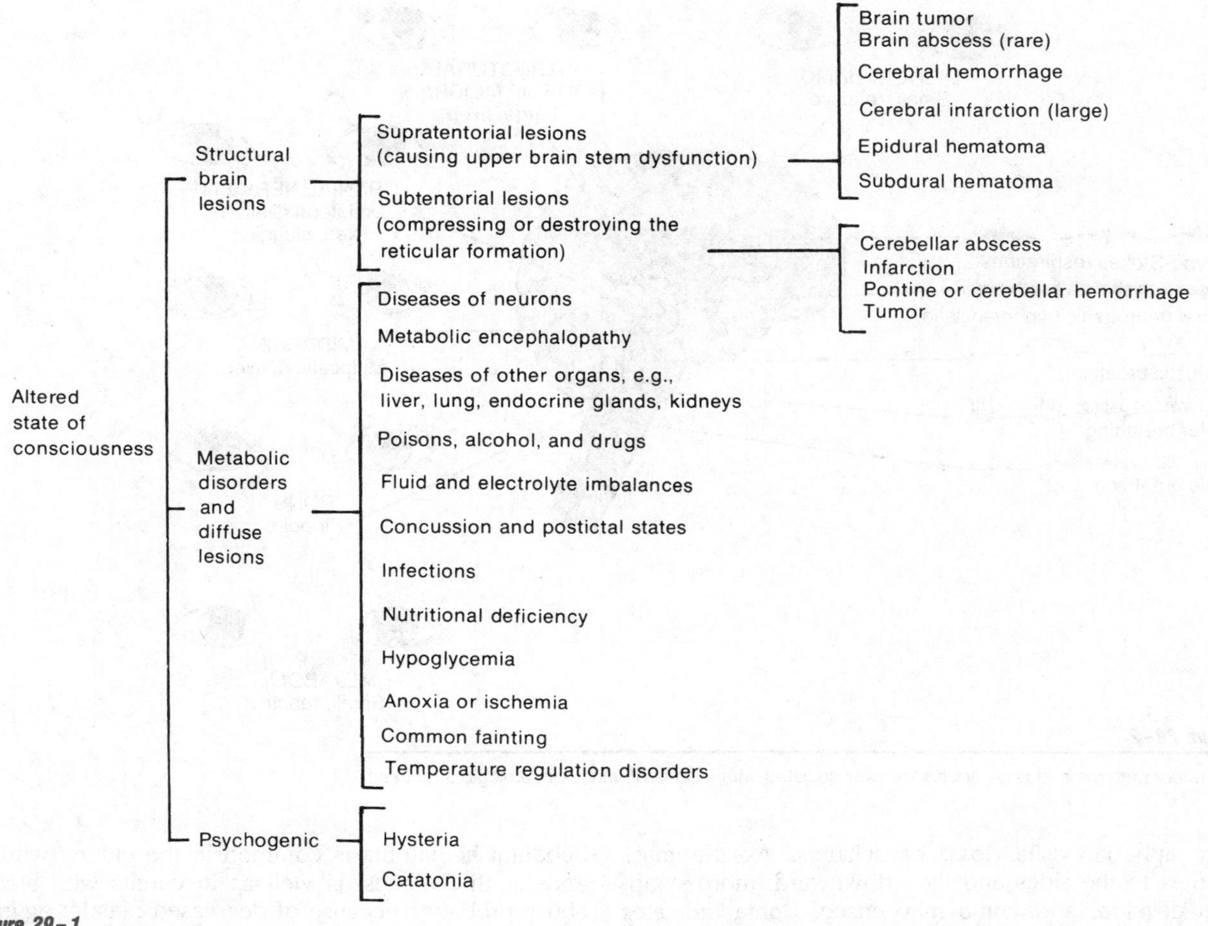

▲ *Figure 29-1*

Some causes of altered states of consciousness. (Note: *Supratentorial* lesions are located *above* the dura roofing in the cerebellum, which separates the cerebellum from the cerebrum. *Subtentorial* lesions lie *beneath* the dura roofing in the cerebellum.)

disorders in which the cardiac output is decreased, such as cardiac arrest or even fainting. Disorders of the liver, lungs, and kidney may produce coma because of the accumulation of metabolic waste products. Finally, there are many agents that have impact on the metabolism of neurons: poisons; hypoglycemia; fever; infection, such as encephalitis; and fluid, electrolyte, or acid-base imbalance.

Risk Factors

Risk factors for sustained unconsciousness are discussed with the various disorders later in this chapter.

Pathophysiology

Decreased levels of consciousness are most often due to disorders in the reticular activating system of the brain stem and thalamus. Conditions such as confusion and decreased attention span can be due to disorders of one of the cerebral hemispheres, such as stroke. Coma itself is due to extensive damage to both cerebral hemispheres or the reticular activating system.

Masses within the brain alter the functioning of the brain in many ways; a common symptom is a decreasing level of consciousness. Masses or lesions, whether they are growing tumors, edema, or bleeding, place pressure on the brain. Because the brain is encased in the cranium, there is no space within the skull for the expanding brain. The pressure is exerted down toward the spinal canal. This pressure slows blood and cerebrospinal fluid (CSF) flow in and out of the brain and reduces cerebral function. The level of consciousness and ability to move purposefully are affected. When pressure reaches the midbrain or diencephalon, vital functions such as heart rhythm and respiration are affected. The client's outcome is based on the location of the mass, the size and rate of enlargement, and the amount of edema and necrosis in brain tissues (see also Increased Intracranial Pressure).

Masses can be located in the supratentorial area (above the dura roofing the cerebellum) of the brain and cause a fairly predictable set of symptoms. Supratentorial lesions can involve the entire cortical or subcortical level of the brain tissue, such as with hemorrhage. The disorder may also be located in one hemisphere, such as with stroke. These masses first produce symptoms such as headache, sensorimotor de-

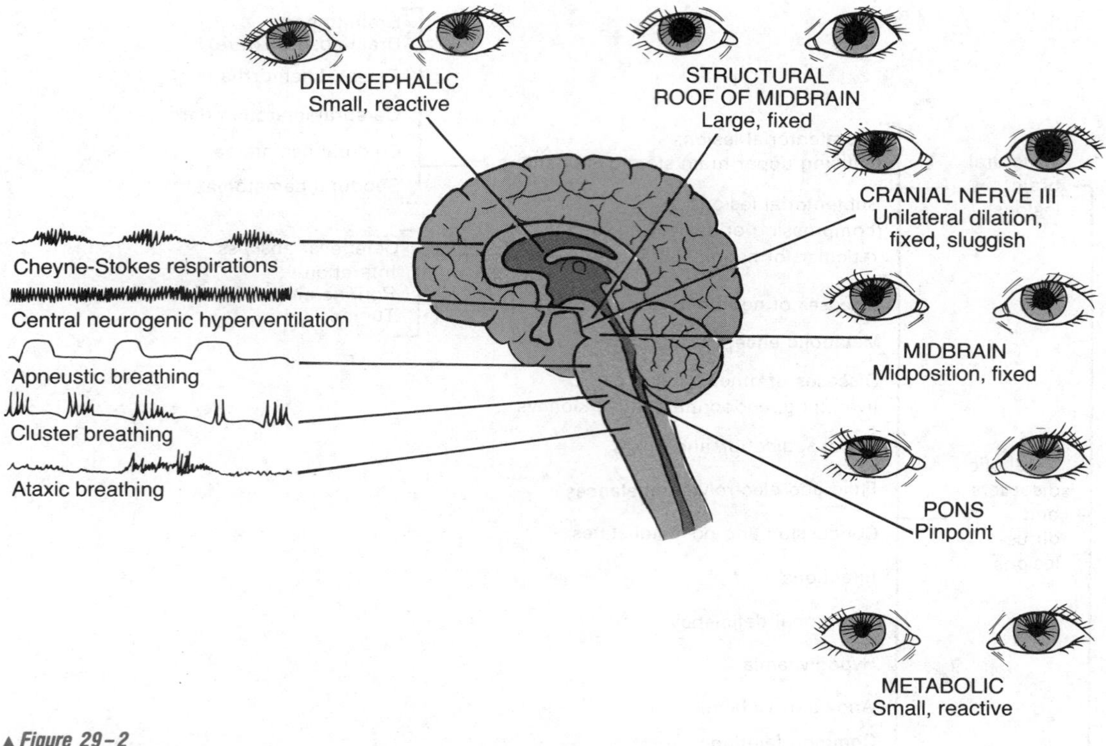

▲ *Figure 29-2*

Respiratory patterns and pupil appearances associated with lesions of various neurologic structures.

fects, aphasia, visual loss, or seizures. As the mass enlarges to the sides and then downward, more symptoms develop, and coma may ensue. Coma indicates that the mass has grown and compressed structures deep in the brain.

Infratentorial disorders (beneath the dura roofing the cerebellum) cause the client to lose consciousness in two ways: (1) by directly affecting the reticular activating system or its pathways or (2) by invading the brain stem or decreasing its blood supply. Lesions in this area also produce unusual respiratory patterns. The cerebrum houses the center for rhythmic breathing. This center's function is lost as consciousness decreases, and the lower brain stem regulates breathing by responding to changes in the carbon dioxide levels. The result is a very irregular breathing pattern and depth (Fig. 29-2). The cranial nerves are commonly trapped by the mass or edema in the brain, and various cranial nerve palsies can be seen. Specific patterns of pupil sizes and amount of reaction to light occur when pressure is exerted at various locations.

A blow to the head is a common cause of decreased consciousness and coma. At the time of impact, the brain can be lacerated, bruised, or contused as it is jarred within the cranium. In addition, the brain can suffer diffuse injury as tissues are torn and sheared. A common problem after head injury is the accumulation of blood between the skull and dura (epidural hematoma) or beneath the dura (subdural hematoma). Epidural hematomas are common when an unprotected head is injured, such as in assault victims, bicyclists and motorcyclists without helmets, and baseball players. Subdural hematoma is common in the elderly who fall and hit their heads as well as in clients with alcohol abuse problems because of decreased platelet aggregation. In addition to the direct injury to the brain tissue and the pressure caused by accumulating blood, clients with head injury may also have injury to their chests or airways, which increases the risk of hypoxia.

Metabolic disorders producing coma do so through various mechanisms. Infection of the brain, such as encephalitis, causes inflammation of the meninges and brain tissues. Hyperglycemia and hypoglycemia starve the cells of needed glucose for metabolism. Overdoses of sedative drugs suppress the central nervous system, especially the centers for breathing. Failure of the liver, kidney, and lungs allows metabolic waste to accumulate, which poisons the neurons.

There is a marked increase in the metabolic needs of the patient in a coma. When these nutritional needs are not met, malnutrition increases the patient's morbidity and mortality. Malnutrition and negative nitrogen balance will also retard healing. Immunodeficiency, which follows protein malnutrition, increases the risk of infection and sepsis. Malnutrition can also lead to pressure ulcers, stress ulcers, weight loss, skeletal muscle wasting, and lung tissue catabolism. The loss of lung tissues can lead to diaphragm weakness and reduction in respiratory function. Finally, starvation can lead to death.

Some patients in coma slowly awaken and begin to respond normally. They often require physical and speech therapy for restoration of previous levels of function. Irreversible coma, also called cerebral death, is due to damage to the cerebral hemispheres so that the patient is unable to respond to the environment. The brain stem and cerebellum remain intact and functional so that vital functions, such as heart, lung, and gastrointestinal function, continue. Patients can remain in irreversible coma for years. It is these patients, and the maintenance of their feeding and fluids, that have inspired great ethical and legal debates.

Brain death is irreversible damage to cerebrum, cerebellum, and brain stem. The damage is so severe that there is no hope for recovery and the patient's life must be maintained with a respirator and vasoactive drugs. General agreement is that brain death has occurred when there is no discernible evidence of cerebral activity or brain stem activity.

The clinical criteria for brain death are

- Completion of all appropriate and therapeutic procedures
- Unresponsive coma with absence of motor and reflex response
- No spontaneous respiration (apnea)
- No oculocephalic response or oculovestibular response with fixed and dilated pupils
- Isoelectric (flat) electroencephalogram (EEG)
- Persistence of the above signs for 30 minutes to 1 hour and for 6 hours after the onset of coma and apnea
- Confirming tests indicating the absence of cerebral circulation (optional)[16]

Clinical Manifestations

Data seen in the client with a structural lesion on the supratentorial areas of the brain point to the area of the mass. For example, if the client has a mass in the temporal lobe, early symptoms may include headaches or focal (located in one area, such as the hand) seizures. As the mass expands, symptoms change. The mass places pressure on nearby areas as well as the diencephalon. The client may develop a unilateral sensorimotor deficit (cannot raise the right leg or has numbness in the right leg), aphasia, and a deficit in the visual field (blind in the left visual field). These clients usually have intact pupillary reflexes and oculovestibular reflexes. If the mass is not detected or cannot be treated and progresses, the client will eventually develop coma.

Infratentorial lesions produce different symptoms. Infarct or bleeding in the midbrain or pons produces coma from the start. These clients may have a history of brain stem dysfunction or a sudden onset of coma. Oculovestibular abnormalities are present. Abnormal respiratory patterns also develop as the cranial nerves are trapped by the mass or edema.

An important difference in coma caused by a metabolic disorder is the presence of bilateral or symmetric symptoms, because the disorder affects the entire brain rather than just one section. The client usually develops confusion and stupor before any physical signs are noticed. Physical signs include tremor, asterixis (flapping tremors of the hands), myoclonus (a single, sudden jerking movement), and seizures. Pupillary response is normal. Depending on the underlying cause, acid-base imbalances may be noted. For example, metabolic acidosis would be present in a patient in a diabetic coma.

Clients with unresponsiveness from a psychiatric disorder, rather than a true coma, do not have the same manifestations. These clients have intact eyelid muscles and their eyelids close tightly; the pupils are small but react normally; oculocephalic responses are unpredictable; and oculovestibular stimulation produces the normal nystagmus. Motor tone is inconsistent, no pathophysiologic reflexes are present, and the EEG is normal.

The clinical manifestations of structurally induced and metabolic coma are presented in Table 29-1.

Level of Consciousness. The level of consciousness is the most critical clinical piece of data assessed in the comatose patient and clients with decreasing levels of consciousness. There are many components of level of

TABLE 29-1. Clinical Manifestations of Metabolically Induced and Structurally Induced Coma

Manifestation	Metabolically Induced Coma	Structurally Induced Coma
History	Behavioral changes	Frontal headache Local seizures
Typical problem	Hepatic coma Diabetic ketoacidosis	Tumor or bleeding in one area
Pupillary reaction (CN II)	Preserved	Unequal reaction
Pupillary size	May be midposition and fixed from anticholinergics Fixed and dilated from anoxia Pinpoint from opiates	May be unequal Midposition from injury to the midbrain Pinpoint from injury to the pons Large from herniation
Corneal reflex	Present and equal	Unequal, may be absent
Extraocular movement (CN III, IV, VI)	Eyes rove, calorics intact, doll's eyes absent	May have gaze paresis from a trapped CN III
Extremity movement	Moves both sides equally	Weakness or absent movement on one side
Abnormal posturing	Absent	Present (decerebrate, decorticate)
Reflexes	Deep tendon reflexes present and equal Plantar flexion	Deep tendon reflexes unequal Babinski's response
Response to pain	Equal	Unequal

Data from McCance, K., & Huether, S. (1990). *Pathophysiology,* St Louis: C. V. Mosby; and Wyngaarden, J.B., et al. (1992). *Cecil Textbook of Medicine* (19th ed.). Philadelphia: W. B. Saunders.

consciousness assessments, such as degree of orientation, level of alertness, and ability to problem solve or follow directions. A client who is awake, alert, and fully oriented to self, others, place, and time is considered to be fully conscious. As changes in the level of consciousness occur, the client can be improving or deteriorating. From the normal alert state, consciousness deteriorates in stages, each having its own definition.

- *Confusion:* the loss of the ability to think rapidly and clearly; an impairment in judgement and decision making.
- *Disorientation:* beginning loss of consciousness. Disorientation to time is followed by disorientation to place and the inability to recognize others. The last step of disorientation is the inability to know self. Sometimes referred to as "disoriented times 3" meaning time, place, and person.
- *Lethargy:* a lack of spontaneous movement or speech. The client is easily aroused with speech or touch but is not oriented to person, place, or time.
- *Obtundation:* reduced ability to be aroused and limited response to the environment. The client sleeps unless stimulated with speech or touch. Verbal response to questions is minimal, perhaps a grunt or nod.
- *Stupor:* a condition of deep sleep or unresponsiveness from which a patient may be aroused only with vigorous, sometimes painful, stimulation. Patients respond by withdrawing from or grabbing at the source of pain.
- *Coma:* no motor or verbal response to the environment or any stimuli, even deep pain or suctioning.[12]

In the clinical setting, these terms can be confusing, and their true meaning is debatable. The nurse should document the behavior to validate the terminology chosen.

Pattern of Breathing. Respiration is a complex process controlled by the cerebrum, pons, and brain stem. Disorders causing coma and decreased levels of consciousness also commonly cause respiratory abnormalities. Changes in respiratory rate and rhythm occur from many different processes. Compression of the medulla causes respiratory failure, and rapidly expanding lesions in the cerebellum may lead to respiratory arrest. Common abnormal respiratory patterns are shown in Figure 29-2.

Airway obstruction and aspiration are common complications in unconscious patients. An obstructed airway leads to inadequate gas exchange, which in turn causes (1) carbon dioxide retention, contributing to vasodilation, and cerebral edema, increasing intracranial pressure, or (2) decreased arterial oxygen levels, resulting in decreased oxygen delivery to the brain. Respiratory failure will occur if a patient has insufficient lung ventilation and inadequate gas exchange. Respiratory failure may be prevented by oxygen administration and assisted ventilation.

Eye Movement. The cranial nerves exit through the brain stem; when the cranial nerves are compressed, eye movement is impaired. Eye movements in the comatose patient are uncoordinated, and pupillary response is abnormal. The eyes of an awake and alert client at rest normally gaze straight ahead. Eyes normally track together to look at something. When the eyes move in such a way, gaze is said to be *conjugate.* Dysconjugate gaze or conjugate deviation of the eyes at rest indicates a disorder of one or more of the ocular muscles due to weak muscles or to damage to the cranial nerves supplying the eye muscles (CN III, IV, and VI). There are no involuntary eye movements. Several types of abnormal involuntary eye movements may occur, however: ocular bobbing, that is, the eyes appear to be slowly jumping up and down; or roving eye movements, that is, the eyes slowly wander or move around.

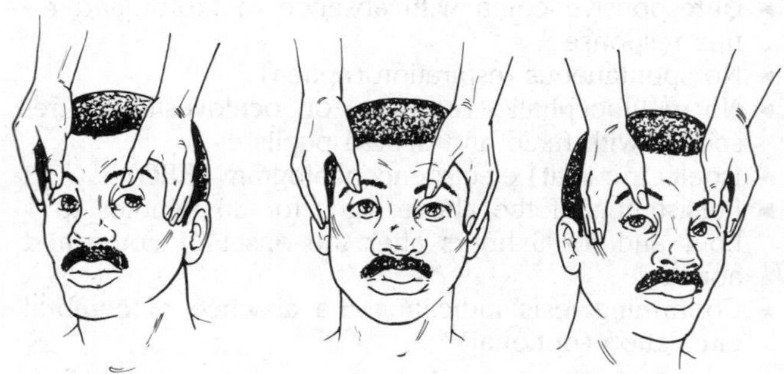

A. NORMAL REACTION:
Eyes move from side to side when head is turned

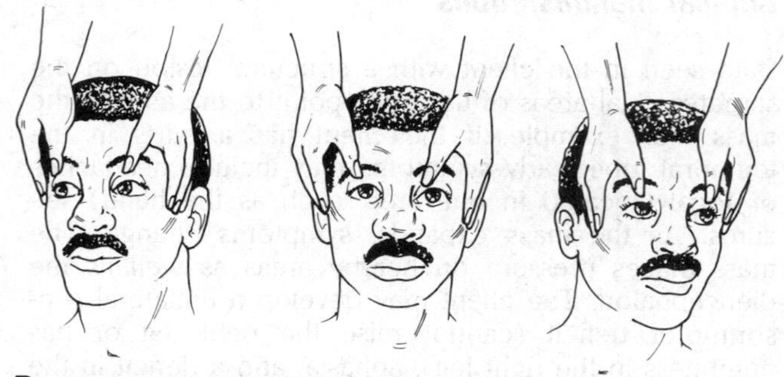

B. ABNORMAL REACTION:
Eyes remain in fixed position in skull when head is turned

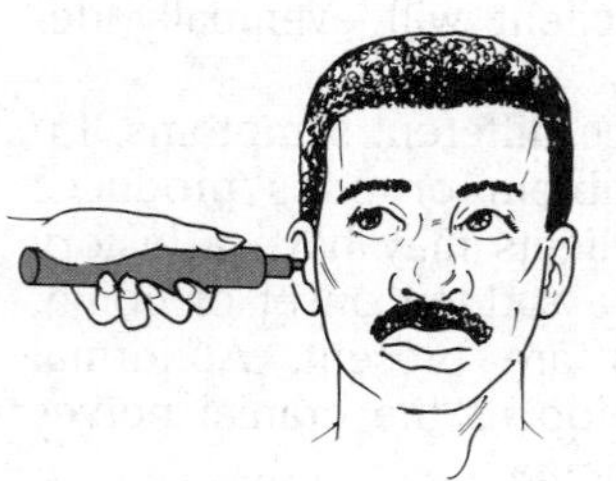

C. NORMAL CALORIC:
Eyes deviate to side of ice water application

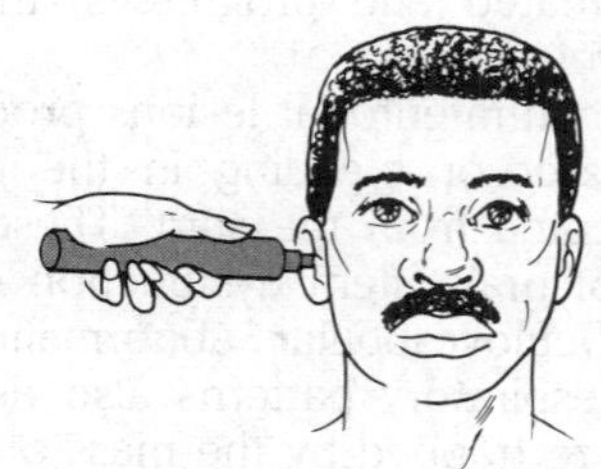

D. ABNORMAL CALORIC:
Eyes do not deviate

▲ **Figure 29-3**

A and *B*, Normal and abnormal doll's eye test (oculocephalic response). *C*, and *D*, Normal and abnormal caloric test (oculovestibular response).

Doll's eyes (oculoreflexic response) are abnormal reflexic eye movement when the head is suddenly turned. Doll's eyes are present if, when the head is rotated to the left, the eyes move to the right and vice versa. The presence or absence of doll's eyes can also be assessed. See the section on diagnostic assessment later in this section (Fig. 29-3).

Pupillary Changes. The reticular activating system within the brain stem is adjacent to the area that controls the pupil's size and reaction to light. Therefore, pupillary changes are used in the assessment of brain stem function. Severe cerebral hypoxia and ischemia cause pupils to become fixed and dilated. Hypothermia may also fix the pupils. There are also several medications that affect pupil size and reaction to light. These medications include large doses of atropine and scopolamine, which fix and fully dilate the pupil; miotics, which constrict the pupil; midriatics, which dilate the pupil; narcotics (especially morphine), which cause the pupils to become pinpoint in size; and barbiturates, which produce fixed pupils (see Fig. 29-2).

Motor Response. Motor response is the most powerful predictor of outcome in patients with severe neurologic impairment.[13] The client may respond to commands such as "raise your right arm" within a reasonable time. Other clients may not respond to verbal requests but are noted to have purposeful movement, that is, to withdraw from a painful stimulus. For example, the patient may push away a suction catheter. As consciousness decreases further, the patient may only draw up the knees and arms without directing any response toward the stimuli.

The patient may also exhibit some abnormal motor movements and postures. Posturing is the presence of abnormal flexion and extension (decorticate and decerebrate posturing) due to hyperreflexia because the brain has lost the ability to inhibit muscle contraction. Both postures occur in patients with severe brain dysfunction (e.g., herniation of the brain stem), lesions pushing on the midbrain and pons from the posterior fossa, and advanced metabolic coma. Both types of posturing usually appear in response to painful stimulation in patients with profound coma. The postures may also appear without stimulation. The postures may be so intense that the bed shakes as spasms of rigidity pass through the body. At times, shivering, hyperpnea, and teeth clenching may accompany the posturing.

Decorticate posturing is abnormal flexion of the arms, wrists, and fingers with the arms abducted. The legs are fully extended and internally rotated, with the feet in plantar flexion. Decerebrate posturing is abnormal extension of the legs in a position similar to decorticate posture. The arms are stiffly extended and abducted and the hands hyperpronated. Decorticate and decerebrate postures are shown in Figure 29-4.

Other motor signs in a patient with cerebral hemisphere damage may include (1) primitive sucking or snout reflexes, (2) strong reflexic hand grasp, (3) restlessness, (4) resistance to passive movement, (5) hemiplegia, (6) hemiparesis, and (7) seizures.

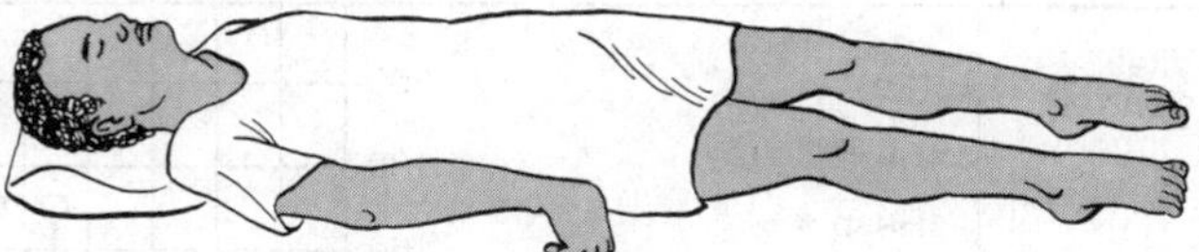

A. Extension posturing (decerebrate rigidity)

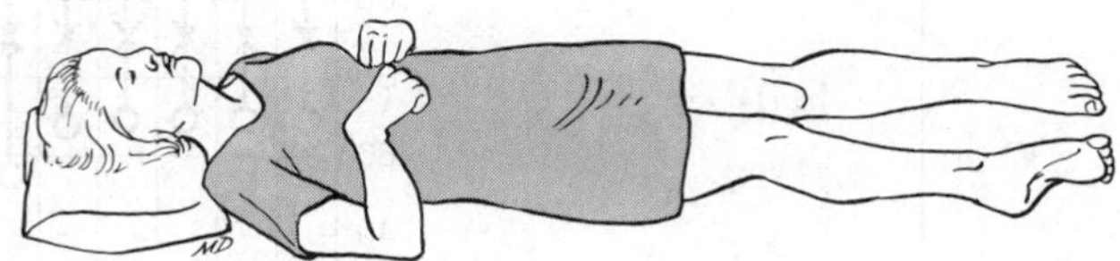

B. Abnormal flexion (decorticate rigidity)

▲ ***Figure 29-4***

Pathologic posturing occurring in clients with severe brain injury.

The most severe impairment of motor function is bilateral flaccidity. True flaccidity, the absence of any movement or tone in response to deep painful stimuli, is one of the criteria for measuring brain death. Therefore, great caution is used in determining whether flaccidity is present. Disorders such as stroke and spinal cord injury also may produce flaccidity.

Vital Signs. Wide variations in vital signs may occur in patients with various levels of consciousness. Some changes relate directly to the cause of the unconsciousness. Others relate to complications of the initial disorder, treatment, or immobility, such as shock, cardiac dysrhythmias, fluid and electrolyte imbalances, and hypertension. Some conditions causing coma produce autonomic nervous system instability because of impairment of the hypothalamus. These disorders may cause a wide variation in blood pressure, pulse, and body temperature.

Cushing's Changes. Cushing's changes may develop with increased intracranial pressure (ICP). These changes include decreased pulse and increased systolic blood pressure with diastolic pressure remaining the same (or rising slightly) to create a widened pulse pressure. These physiologic responses are an attempt to restore adequate blood flow through compressed cerebral vessels. Cushing's changes are not a reliable warning of increasing ICP because they do not always occur, and when they do occur, they are often late in the course of rising pressure. They are sometimes difficult to differentiate from other causes of hypertension or slowing pulse rate (Fig. 29-5).

PROGNOSIS

In the past, little information was available on which to base a prediction about the outcome of a patient in coma. Most of the time, a "wait and see attitude" was used. It is important for the family and the health care team to have some idea of the probable eventual outcome for the patient. It is discouraging and inappropri-

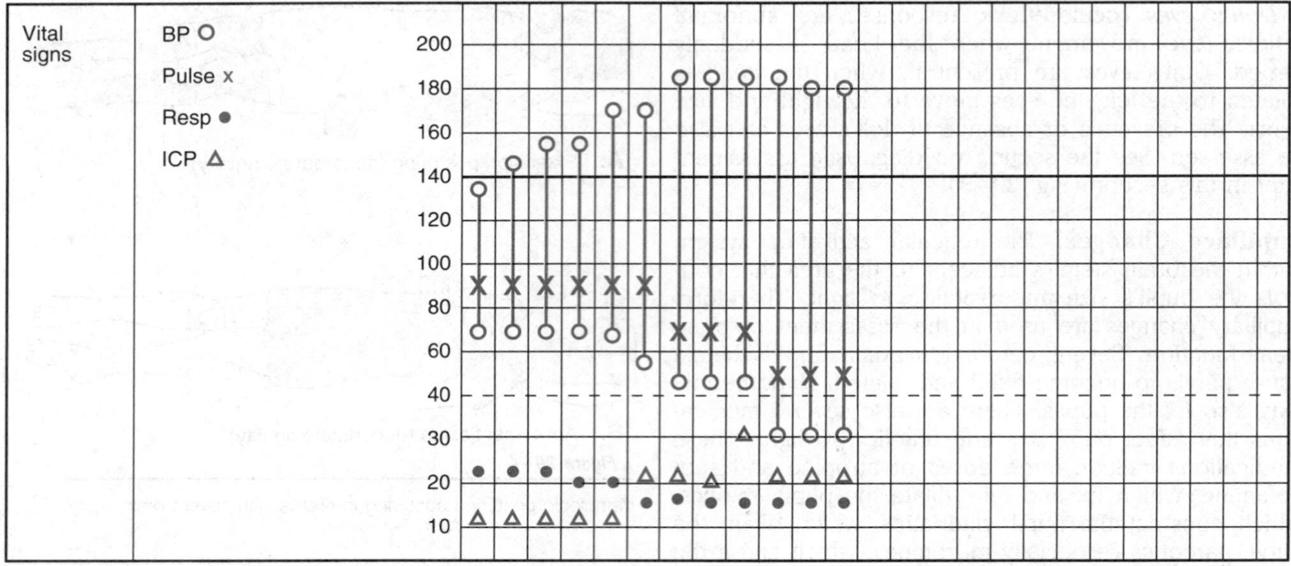

▲ *Figure 29–5*

Cushing's response (Cushing's triad) includes bradycardia, systolic hypertension, and bradypnea that occur from pressure on the medulla. These signs often occur with intracranial hypertension or herniation syndrome.

ate to vigorously treat a patient with no chance of recovery, but it is even more inappropriate to deny treatment to a patient with a reasonable chance of recovery.

It has been demonstrated that the absence of pupillary, corneal, or oculovestibular responses during early stages of coma is highly predictive of mortality or significant morbidity (e.g., vegetative state). The recovery of these responses and a return to purposeful movement correlate with a better prognosis. Patients who lapse into coma from metabolic disorders have an extremely poor prognosis if the coma lasts for more than 1 week.

DIAGNOSTIC ASSESSMENT

A computed tomographic (CT) scan or magnetic resonance imaging (MRI) usually provides data that indicate whether the cause of the coma is structural. Tumors or areas of bleeding will be evident on the scan. Sometimes the patient will require emergency surgery to remove the mass or drain the fluid and thereby release pressure.

A lumbar puncture can be done in patients when it is known from data provided by the CT or MRI scans that there is no expanding intracranial mass. Lumbar puncture can assist with the diagnosis of infection or bleeding as a cause of coma. CSF may be cloudy or bloody when the client has an infection or bleeding into the ventricles or the subarachnoid space.

An EEG can be used to determine whether the patient is comatose because of continuous seizures. EEG results are abnormal in many patients in metabolic coma and do not serve as a clear diagnostic tool.

In some comatose clients, doll's eyes can be noted without specially testing for the response. Doll's eyes can also be tested, and this is a rapid method for detecting potential abnormalities of the brain stem. This test can be done only on unconscious patients because this is an abnormal response and does not occur in awake clients or clients without brain stem problems. While the eyes are held open, the patient's head is rapidly turned from side to side. Doll's eyes are present if, when the head is rotated to the left, the eyes move to the right and vice versa (see Fig. 29–3). Do not perform the doll's eye test on comatose patients with suspected or known cervical spine injury. The head movement could produce permanent spinal cord damage.

Patients in metabolic coma, except barbiturate and phenytoin (Dilantin) poisoning, retain ocular reflexes. The presence of brisk doll's eyes movement indicates a decrease in the level of consciousness with an intact brain stem. The absence of doll's eyes movement in a comatose patient does not always mean that the brain stem is not functioning. Other agents and disorders can block the eye's response. Neuromuscular drugs, such as succinylcholine, and Meniere's disease, which destroys the labyrinth in the ear, cause absent oculocephalic response.

If oculocephalic responses are absent, oculovestibular (caloric) tests can be performed to test the third, sixth, and eighth cranial nerves (see Chap. 27). A normal response occurs when the eyes have conjugate movement and nystagmus. Nystagmus is the involuntary oscillation of the eyeballs and may be horizontal, vertical, oblique, rotary, or mixed with various rates of movement. The occurrence of roving eye movements and the failure to produce nystagmus with the instillation of warm or cold water into the ear canal indicates a decrease in consciousness with an intact brain stem. Absent cold caloric responses do not always indicate brain stem disorder. The use of ototoxic drugs, barbiturates, sedatives, phenytoin, or tricyclic antidepressants or the presence of Meniere's disease may produce a false caloric test. Use caution when assessing the oculovestibular response in clients with head trauma because they may have sustained a ruptured tympanum (eardrum).

Medical Management

The goal of medical management of the patient in coma is to remove or correct the cause. Frequently, time is required to perform all the tests to find the specific cause. In the interim, the patient's brain must be protected from further injury.

The patient's airway and circulation must be maintained. A nasal or oral airway may be inserted for a short time. If the patient is completely unresponsive, an endotracheal tube is carefully inserted, avoiding injury to the cervical spine. The head-injured patient may be hyperventilated while on a ventilator for reducing $PaCO_2$ to between 27 and 30 mm Hg. Hyperventilation is an effective way to reduce cerebral blood flow when coma is due to bleeding. Caution is used, however, to avoid decreasing blood supply to areas of the brain where blood flow is already reduced because of effects of the injury. Circulation is maintained by monitoring blood pressure and using vasoactive agents to keep mean systolic blood pressure above 80 mm Hg. If the patient is breathing without assistance, the airway and respirations need to be closely monitored because the airway may become obstructed and aspiration may occur as consciousness decreases.

Initial assessments of the comatose patient include

- depth of consciousness by observing responses to stimuli and presence of localizing neurologic symptoms indicating focal intracranial disease
- pupil sizes and reactivity to light for indications of increased ICP or other causes of coma
- deep and superficial reflexes (e.g., are they overactive, underactive, absent, unequal on the body's two sides, or unaltered?) (see Chap. 28). Reflex assessment is particularly valuable in comatose patients because it provides objective information about the condition without requiring conscious participation. Corneal reflex is assessed.
- response to painful stimuli. Other aspects of sensory assessment are not possible or are unreliable in patients with reduced consciousness.
- evidence of trauma. Trauma may be the result of coma rather than the cause of it (e.g., bitten tongue may result from a seizure). Examine ears for ruptured eardrums.
- determination of serum glucose level if symptoms suggest a metabolic disorder.
- history from significant others (or observers of what has happened) when possible.

Immediate interventions include treatment of common causes of coma while assessment of neurologic status continues.

Glucose is given after blood is drawn to reverse potential insulin reactions. Thiamine is commonly given because many comatose patients are malnourished and subject to Wernicke's encephalopathy, especially if they are given glucose.

If the patient is having repetitive seizures, coma and brain damage can follow; the patient is given intravenous diazepam to stop the seizures. If the patient is not intubated, the airway needs to be closely monitored because of the effects of the diazepam.

Many metabolic causes of coma lead to acid-base and fluid imbalances. The patient's acid-base balance should be restored quickly. Fluid imbalances should be restored slowly for preventing rebound fluid shifts into the brain. Fluids may be given if the patient is dehydrated or withheld if the patient is fluid overloaded. Normal saline and hypertonic saline are the fluids of choice because these fluids will not passively move into the brain and increase edema.

Cultures are taken of the blood, nose, throat, and wounds (if present). Once the cultures are taken, antibiotics are given to combat any infection. Body temperature should be brought to within 3 degrees of normal.

At one time, barbiturates were the most common cause of overdose, but there are many more choices of drugs today. Most emergency departments have lists of antidotes to reverse specific agents. Many times, however, the specific drug ingested is not known. Narcotic overdose is common and reversed with naloxone (Narcan). The nurse needs to be aware that the duration of action of naloxone is 2 to 3 hours shorter than that of most narcotics, and the drug may need repeating. Cocaine overdose can be treated with diazepam. Patients with cocaine overdose often have cardiac arrhythmias and irregular respirations also. Gastric lavage may be used to remove ingested agents.

Once the emergency care is given, medical management centers on trying to diagnose and treat the cause of the coma. Body functions are maintained, and complications that may slow recovery or cause residual problems are prevented. If the coma is prolonged, the patient is begun on nasogastric tube feeding for promotion of nutrition and prevention of muscle wasting. The complications from immobility, such as pneumonia and pressure ulcers, are continually assessed and treated.

Surgical Management

Most cases of coma cannot be cured by surgery alone, but if the cause of the coma is bleeding or tumor within the brain, the patient will require emergency surgery. ICP monitors may also be placed (see later).

Nursing Management

ASSESSMENT

Frequent, systematic, and objective nursing assessment including neurologic status and mental status is essential. Serial observations are important for comparison.

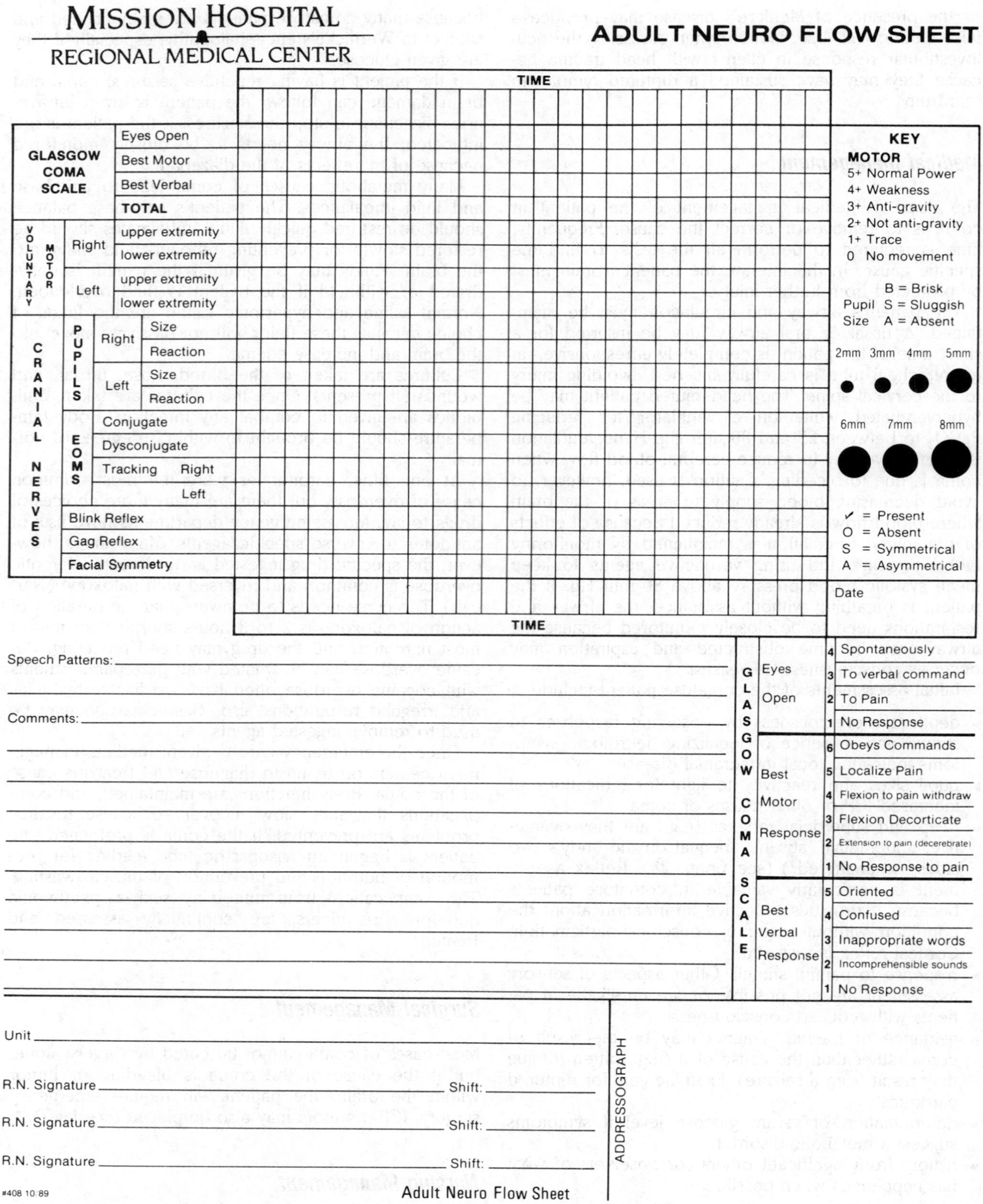

MISSION HOSPITAL
REGIONAL MEDICAL CENTER

ADULT NEURO FLOW SHEET

			TIME
GLASGOW COMA SCALE	Eyes Open		
	Best Motor		
	Best Verbal		
	TOTAL		
VOLUNTARY MOTOR	Right	upper extremity	
		lower extremity	
	Left	upper extremity	
		lower extremity	
CRANIAL NERVES — PUPILS	Right	Size	
		Reaction	
	Left	Size	
		Reaction	
CRANIAL NERVES — EOMS	Conjugate		
	Dysconjugate		
	Tracking	Right	
		Left	
CRANIAL NERVES	Blink Reflex		
	Gag Reflex		
	Facial Symmetry		

KEY

MOTOR
5+ Normal Power
4+ Weakness
3+ Anti-gravity
2+ Not anti-gravity
1+ Trace
0 No movement

Pupil Size
B = Brisk
S = Sluggish
A = Absent

2mm 3mm 4mm 5mm

6mm 7mm 8mm

✓ = Present
O = Absent
S = Symmetrical
A = Asymmetrical

Date

TIME

GLASGOW COMA SCALE			
Eyes Open	4	Spontaneously	
	3	To verbal command	
	2	To Pain	
	1	No Response	
Best Motor Response	6	Obeys Commands	
	5	Localize Pain	
	4	Flexion to pain withdraw	
	3	Flexion Decorticate	
	2	Extension to pain (decerebrate)	
	1	No Response to pain	
Best Verbal Response	5	Oriented	
	4	Confused	
	3	Inappropriate words	
	2	Incomprehensible sounds	
	1	No Response	

Speech Patterns: ______

Comments: ______

Unit ______

R.N. Signature ______ Shift: ______

R.N. Signature ______ Shift: ______

R.N. Signature ______ Shift: ______

ADDRESSOGRAPH

#408 10.89

Adult Neuro Flow Sheet

▲ **Figure 29–6**

Neurologic observation chart. (Courtesy of Mission Hospital Regional Medical Center, Mission Viejo, CA.)

NEUROLOGIC FLOW SHEET

1. Glasgow Coma Scale (GCS). Three areas are assessed: Best eye opeing, Best motor response, and Best verbal response. Assign the appropriate numerical score for each category (1st box—best eye, 2nd box—best motor, and 3rd box—best verbal). Place the total score in the fourth box (total score 3-15).

2. Voluntary Motor is evaluated by assessing each extremity on both the right and left side. Note **symmetry vs. asymmetry.** In the cooperative patient, voluntary motor strength is assessed by asking the patient to close their eyes and hold their arms straight ahead with palms up for about 30 seconds. The leg strength is evaluated by asking the patient to push downward against the examiner's hands.

Scoring: Normal power (5+) is the score given if the patient's arms stay in the same position and/or if the legs have equal strong power.

Weakness (4+) is the score given if one of the pt.'s arm drifts downward (hands may pronate) or if the leg strength is diminished. Some resistance to force is noted.

Anti-gravity (3+) is the score given if the patient is able to move an extremity above the plane of gravity (ie flexing & extending a hand up/down against gravity).

Not anti-gravity (2+) is the score given to a patient who can move the extremity back and forth on the bed but not against the forces of gravity.

Trace movement (1+) is the score given to a patient who can move an extremity slightly.

No movement (0) is the score given if a patient cannot move the extremity.

3. **Cranial Nerve Exam:**

Pupillary response: Each pupil is assessed individually. Note the size of the pupil prior to shining the light into the eye. Place your hand at the bridge of the nose to block light to the opposite eye. Using the penlight, shine the light from outside the right eye to midpoint across the eye to assess the direct light reflex. Note the pupillary constriction (Brisk, sluggish, or non-reactive) in the right eye. Also, observe for constriction in the left pupil (consensual light reflex). Repeat the above steps for the left eye observing the direct light reflex in the left eye and the consensual reflex in the right eye. Document the pupil size (prior to light in the eye) and the reaction on the flow sheet.

Extra-ocular movements (EOMS's) are tested on patients who are awake enough to follow instructions. Ask the patient to follow your fingers with his eyes without moving the head. Move your fingers in a figure H and observe both eyes as they move across/up/down. **Conjugate eye movements** occur when both eyes move in parallel motion. **Dysconjugate eye movements** occur when the eyes do not move in a lateral direction together (one eye may move laterally while the other is fixed or moves in another direction). **Tracking** occurs when the patient is consciously following someone's or something's movement around the room. Place a check for present or a 0 for absent.

The Blink reflex is elicited by lightly stroking the patient's eyelashes. When the eyelids are closed, the eyelids will flutter slightly if the reflex is present. In the conscious alert patient, observe for blinking. Place a check for present or a 0 for absent.

The Gag reflex is evaluated by asking the alert, cooperative patient to cough or swallow. If the patient is unable to do so or is unconscious, take a long cotton tipped swab and stroke the back of the patient's throat. Note if the reflex is present (place a check) or absent (place a 0).

Muscles of the face: Note the muscle symmetry of the facial muscles. Note the ability of the eyelids to open spontaneously and equally. Ask the patient to close their eyes as tightly as possible. Note asymmetry. Ask the patient to smile—note the corners of the mouth to identify symmetrical patterns. Ask the patient to frown/wrinkle his forehead—note the symmetry of the muscles. Place a S for symmetrical and an A for asymmetrical.

Speech patterns: Note if speech is clear, slurred, rambling, or aphasic.

Comments: Utilize this section to elaborate on any abnormal findings or document other pertinent data.

Sign your name and document shift worked. Complete the date/unit and addressograph. The Neurological flow sheet is for a 24 hour period. Each day at 7 am, obtain a new flow sheet. Document your findings in the appropriate time box.

▲ ***Figure 29-6*** Continued

Even if assessment findings seem insignificant for long periods, documentation provides an objective pattern and an important baseline for future observations.

Take "neuro checks" as often as every 15 minutes during the first few hours of unconsciousness. They are often continued hourly for several days.

Periodically assess the entire body, observing for lacerations, bruises, ulcerations, fractures, dislocations, and contractures. Also note skin color, texture, and temperature. Inspect dressings frequently for purulent or bloody drainage and head dressings for CSF leakage.

The following questions may guide nursing assessment of an unconscious patient.

- What is the patient's level of consciousness?
- Is the airway patent? Is the patient hemodynamically stable? Are circulation and respiration adequate? Is skin, nail bed, and mucous membrane color appropriate?
- Is heart rate slowing and diastolic and systolic blood pressure widening? If so, these indicate increased ICP. Document and report immediately.
- Are pupil responses normal, that is, equal size and reactive to light? Are corneal responses present? Are eye movements abnormal?
- Are any normal reflexes absent (e.g., corneal, blink, gag reflexes)? Are any abnormal reflexes present (e.g., Babinski's reflex)? Absence of the corneal reflex usually indicates problems in the first division of the fifth cranial nerve (see Chap 28).
- In what position are the head, limbs, and trunk? Does the patient change these positions? Is the neck rigid or stiff? Are there other indications of meningeal irritation? Are there changes in muscle tone? Is paralysis evident? Is the patient making any voluntary movements?
- Are any focal or generalized seizures occurring? Carfully document their onset and progression.
- Is the patient incontinent? Is the abdomen distended?
- Are there any indications of fluid-electrolyte imbalances?
- If the patient has sustained head injuries or had cranial surgery, is there any periorbital or facial edema?
- Does the patient respond to painful stimuli? Is the patient resistive to care? Is spontaneous behavior occurring?

Glasgow Coma Scale. The most commonly used neurologic assessment tool in clinical care is the Glasgow Coma Scale (GCS). This scale provides objective measurement of three essential components of the neurologic examination. The level of consciousness, pupil reaction, and motor activity are scored. Vital signs are also recorded. The total of the three scores can range from 3 to 15. The patient who is unresponsive to painful stimuli, does not open the eyes, and is flaccid has a score of 3. The client who is oriented, opens the eyes spontaneously, and follows commands scores 15. Because the scoring of the GCS is based on the client's ability to respond and communicate, the nurse should always note whether the client (1) is intubated and cannot speak; (2) has eyes that are swollen closed; (3) is unable to communicate in English; (4) has a hearing loss; or (5) is blind.

The first GCS score recorded on the patient becomes the baseline coma score. Subsequent scores allow assessment of trends or changes in neurologic status. The scale can also be used to recognize disorders as well as predict outcomes. It is imperative that the nurse use consistent criteria for patient assessment. Specific behaviors indicating a given score should be used. If there are variations in scoring criteria, the value of the scale is lost and serious changes in the client's condition can be overlooked or treated unnecessarily (Fig. 29-6).

Level of Consciousness. The most important part of neurologic examination is the assessment of the level of consciousness to determine the state of alertness and the level of arousability. For patients with decreased levels of consciousness, serial and detailed assessments are required until the patient is fully awake and oriented.

Consciousness is often expressed on a continuum ranging from "fully alert" to "deep coma" with levels in between. For eliminating confusion over terms such as lethargy, obtundation, and the like, the GCS is useful for scoring behavioral responses. Use of the GCS will verify subtle changes in the patient.

Eye Opening. Observe the eye opening without speaking to the client. Does the client open the eyes and look around? If the eyes are closed, call the client's name. If there is no response, raise your voice or shout. If there is still no response, a painful stimulus should be used to see if a response can be elicited (Fig. 29-7). Avoid supraorbital pressure if the face is traumatized. Use nail bed compression for an older client with thin skin.

Verbal Response. Verbal responses assess orientation of the client to self, environment, and time. The nurse should ask appropriate questions, such as, What is your name? Where are you? What is the date today? and so on. The conversation should include information that can be verified by family, such as address or employer. Many times slight degrees of confusion will not be noticeable until the nurse spends some time with a client. The nurse may find the apparently oriented client asking the same question a few hours after it was originally answered. Likewise, the client may have "learned" the answers to common questions such as "What is your name?" and "What hospital are you in?" Therefore, it is helpful to reassess a client after a few hours to check memory, or challenge the client with varying questions.

Motor Response. Motor responses are assessed by asking the client to follow specific commands, such as "raise your right arm" or "wiggle your toes." The client should not be asked to squeeze the nurse's hand because grasp is a reflexic response that occurs in clients

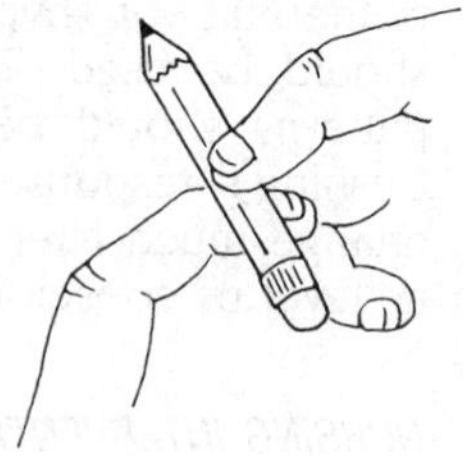

Placing a pencil or pen across the fingernail bed and applying firm pressure produces a constant noxious stimulus and a minimum amount of tissue trauma.

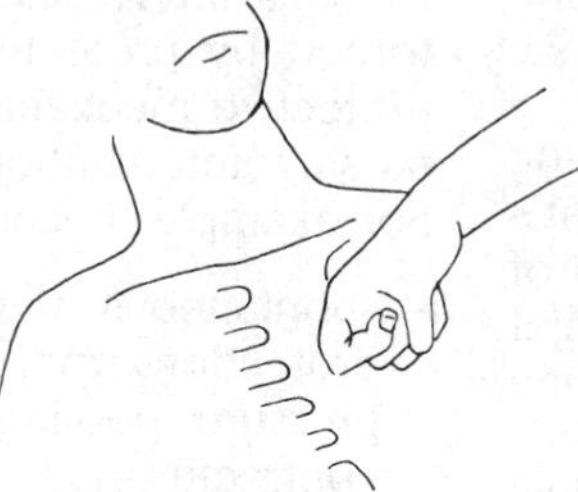

Sternal rub or compression is a common form of noxious stimulus but may, over time, cause severe tissue trauma. In the elderly, in whom bones may be very brittle, it can also cause fractured ribs and/or accompanying pulmonary complications.

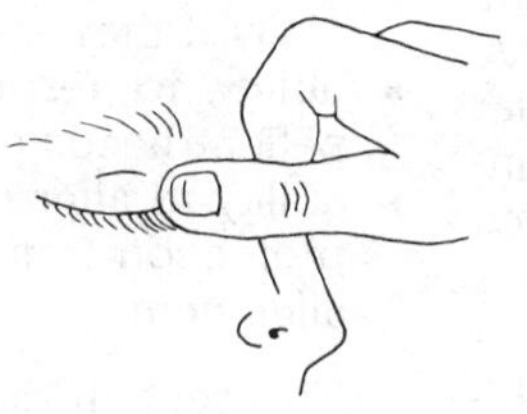

Supraorbital pressure is not recommended as a noxious stimulus when testing for eye opening response. The grimacing associated with supraorbital pressure may actually cause eye closure.

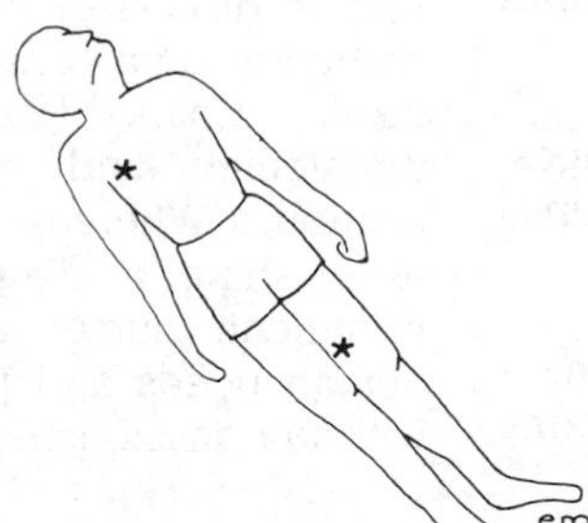

Pinching various parts of the extremity or trunk is the most appropriate stimulus when a response in each extremity is desired. Examples of where to apply stimulus are shown.

▲ Figure 29–7

Painful or noxious stimuli may need to be used to elicit a response from a patient in a coma or with decreased levels of consciousness. (From Marshall, S., et al. [1990]. *Neuroscience critical care: Pathophysiology and patient management.* Philadelphia: W.B. Saunders.)

with head injury. If agency protocol lists grasp as a neurologic assessment, the nurse can ask the client to "let go" after grasping, to measure the cognitive ability to control movement. Clients who are unable to follow commands are given a painful stimulus, and their response is assessed. The patient may respond by localizing (trying to remove the stimulus), withdrawing, or posturing; or no response may be elicited, with the patient remaining motionless and flaccid. Compare the right and left sides and upper and lower extremities. Record the best response while noting any abnormality as all four limbs are scored.

These three components are scored on the GCS. In addition to documentation on the GCS with a number, at times the nurse will document the neurologic status on the chart. Avoid using phrases such as "disoriented times 3" or "stuporous." Instead, record the specific data, such as "states it is 1968 and that Taft is president." In addition, describe the most obvious findings, such as aphasia and inability to move a specific limb. If the GCS score decreases, perform a detailed neurologic assessment and notify the physician immediately. A significant change in the level of consciousness, including a decrease of one point of the GCS, indicates cerebral dysfunction.

Pupillary Response. A pupil check includes assessing pupil appearance and physiologic response. Remember that the affected pupil is usually on the same side (ipsilateral) as the brain lesion, whereas the motor and sensory deficits are usually on the opposite side (contralateral). Be sure to determine whether the patient has an artificial eye before doing a pupil assessment. This mistake has occurred, and the pupil in the prosthetic eye has been reported as "fixed."

Pupil Equality. Document pupil equality with a labeled drawing of the relative size of each pupil, for example, R • L ●.

Pupil Size. Estimate the size of each pupil in millimeters.

Pupil Position. For example, note whether it is at midline or deviated from midline.

Pupil Reaction to Light. To assess pupil reaction, bring the light toward the eye from the side of the patient's head and shine it directly into the pupil. Constriction of the pupil should occur. Assess whether the other pupil responds to the light (consensual response). Determine how quickly the pupils react (e.g., briskly, sluggishly). This examination tests the fact that the light stimulus, once it travels along the optic nerve, stimulates the brain stem bilaterally.

Pupil Shape. If the shape is not round, describe the shape (e.g., oval) and document with a drawing. Assess whether each pupil has regular borders. Irregular borders may mean midbrain damage. Anisocoria, unequal pupils, occurs in about 17 per cent of the population, with one pupil about 1 mm larger.

Pupil Accommodation. Normally, the size of the pupil adjusts to accommodate varying focal lengths. It is usually tested by having the client focus on a distant object and then quickly focus on something close. Pupils should change size depending on focal length.

Eye Movement. Document eye movement changes. Observe the position of the eyes when checking pupils and involuntary movements.

Motor Activity. Motor activity assessment is the measure of strength on voluntary movement of the arms and legs.

If a client cannot cooperate with testing, paralysis may be difficult to detect. Observe the client carefully. If a client is restless, paralysis may become obvious because the paralyzed part will not move as other body parts move. Additional information may be obtained by (1) comparing the tone of one side of the body with the other, (2) lifting the arms or legs on both sides and watching them return to the bed, and (3) observing the position of the limbs at rest.

If a client can cooperate, assessing "drift" may show subtle tone alterations. To do this, have the client hold both arms up in front of the body with palms upward and eyes closed. Muscles are weak if one arm "drifts" (i.e., moves downward) or the hand pronates.

Vital Signs. Vital signs should be assessed every 15 minutes until the client regains full consciousness. Body temperature should be monitored every 2 hours. If hypothermia or hyperthermia occurs, a rectal probe should be used. Trends in vital signs and respiratory patterns should be analyzed. Vital signs change in a Cushing's response when ICP increases, but vital signs change much later than do other neurologic signs such as level of consciousness.

NURSING INTERVENTION FOR COMATOSE PATIENTS

Unconscious patients are completely dependent on others because their protective reflexes are impaired. Nursing intervention provides the safety normally afforded by protective reflexes. Recall what the normal protective mechanisms are and identify critical areas of nursing intervention required for unconscious clients. For example, because

- spontaneous movement is lost, the patient needs protection from skin breakdown due to prolonged pressure, pooling of secretions in the lungs, and joint contractures.
- ability to swallow or cough is lost, the patient needs protection from choking and alternative ways of maintaining nutrition and fluid-electrolyte balance.
- blink reflex is lost, the eyes need protection (especially if they are open).
- ability to respond to the environment is lost, the patient needs protection from environmental hazards.
- ability to alter body position is lost, the patient needs protection from injury by being positioned in correct alignment.

This section discusses intervention appropriate for all unconscious patients regardless of the cause of the coma. Intervention specific to particular etiologic factors is discussed in other sections of the book (e.g., diabetic coma, Chap. 61; unconsciousness from anesthesia, Chap. 19). Unconsciousness is often life-threatening and requires aggressive medical intervention. Whereas physicians are concerned with establishing a diagnosis and prescribing appropriate treatment, nurses are responsible for meeting basic human needs and preventing complications associated with unconsciousness.

Collaborative Problem. High risk for airway obstruction R/T loss of swallowing, gag, and coughing reflexes.

Planning: Expected Outcomes. The nurse will monitor the patient for signs of airway obstruction, as evidenced by abnormal lung sounds, unequal lung expansion, stridor, cyanosis or pallor, abnormal arterial blood gas values, and increasing ICP.

Implementation. Airway obstruction is the most common source of harm to patients with decreased consciousness. Initial care of an unconscious patient includes clearing the airway immediately and loosening all tight clothing, especially around the neck. Never move a recently injured or unconscious patient without using a collar to protect the neck if there is any possibility of spinal injury. Maintain a patent airway by the jaw-thrust method (i.e., place fingers at the angle of the jaws and pull the jaw forward). Remove and store any dentures or bridge work. These could cause airway obstruction or could be swallowed and broken.

Noisy respirations or obvious efforts to breathe indicate partial airway obstruction. When possible, remove the cause of obstruction. Place the patient in a lateral of semiprone position to facilitate drainage of pulmonary secretions and to prevent the tongue from falling into the posterior pharynx and occluding the airway. Do not position the patient on the back, unless intubated, because this position can compromise respirations. In addition to the tongue's occluding the airway, secretions may pool in the pharynx and be aspirated.

For initial airway management, an oral airway can be inserted in an unconscious patient. Endotracheal intubation may be required to maintain airway patency or improve ventilation with use of a ventilator.

For extended airway management, a tracheostomy may be required to (1) allow long-term continuous mechanical ventilation, (2) facilitate the removal of tracheobronchial secretions, and (3) seal off the esophagus from the trachea to prevent aspiration (see Chap. 37).

Nursing Diagnosis: Aspiration, High Risk for R/T ineffective airway clearance and absent gag reflex.

Planning: Expected Outcomes. The patient will exhibit no signs of aspiration, as evidenced by clear lung sounds, no stridor, afebrile, minimal amounts of clear mucus upon suctioning, and PaO_2, $PaCO_2$, and pH within normal limits.

Implementation. Aspiration is a common cause of death in unconscious patients. Keep suctioning equipment available. Often, an open route for tracheal suction is lifesaving for a comatose patient. Assess breath sounds every hour or two in acutely ill patients. Monitor the results of arterial blood gas analysis and pulse oximetry to determine the degree of oxygenation provided by ventilators or oxygen. Perform frequent tracheobronchial suctioning to prevent or decrease the accumulation of secretions from immobility, the lack of a cough and sigh reflex, or pneumonia. Even though suctioning increases ICP, the damage from hypoxia and hypercapnia requires that the removal of secretions be ongoing. While suctioning, the nurse should monitor the electrocardiogram for dysrhythmias (e.g., premature ventricular contractions) due to hypoxia.

A comatose patient may lack pharyngeal reflexes and is therefore unable to swallow. Never give a comatose patient fluids to swallow. Secretions accumulate in the posterior pharynx and may be aspirated. Turn the patient from side to side every 2 hours to facilitate drainage of secretions and prevent pneumonia. Suction the posterior pharynx and upper trachea frequently.

While performing mouth care, place a comatose patient well over onto the side to prevent aspiration. If facial paralysis is present, keep the affected side uppermost. Keep the mouth open by placing a padded tongue blade or soft roll between the teeth. At times, a second nurse assisting will facilitate oral care by holding the mouth open and suctioning. Pay close attention to the roof of the mouth in patients who mouthbreathe for long periods. Crusts may form, break off, and be aspirated.

Never suction the nasal passages in patients who have had brain surgery or head injuries. The suction catheter can cause further trauma and increase the risk of CSF leak.

Nursing Diagnosis: Tissue Perfusion, Altered Cerebral, High Risk for R/T increased ICP.

Planning: Expected Outcomes. The patient will maintain normal cerebral perfusion, as evidenced by maintaining or improving level of consciousness; maintaining or improving GCS score; ICP is less than or equal to 15 mm Hg, having no restlessness, irritability, or headache; and having no pupillary changes, no seizures, no widening pulse pressure, no respiratory irregularity, and no hypertension or bradycardia.

Implementation. Place the patient supine with the head of the bed elevated 30 degrees. The patient's head should be maintained in a neutral position to facilitate venous drainage from the brain. Extreme rotation and flexion of the neck are avoided because these positions compress the jugular veins and increase ICP. Extreme hip flexion is also avoided because this position increases intra-abdominal and intrathoracic pressure, which increases ICP. As coma lightens, the patient may become disoriented and combative, making it challenging to keep them positioned in an ideal position. The nurse will have to assess each patient to determine whether the use of restraints is necessary or if their use will cause further agitation. Agitation will further increase ICP. The patient will probably be treated with osmotic or loop diuretics or corticosteroids to reduce cerebral edema. The nurse needs to monitor the response to these medications. Because the signs of increasing ICP may develop slowly, the continued assessment of the patient is critical. Cerebral edema usually peaks within 72 hours after trauma and gradually subsides over the next few weeks. Additional interventions for clients with increased ICP are discussed later in this chapter. Some patients have ICP monitors inserted for close monitoring of increasing pressure. The monitors are described in the Bridge to Critical Care.

Nursing Diagnosis: Oral and Nasal Mucous Membranes, Altered, High Risk for R/T NPO status, inability to swallow, mouth breathing, and unconsciousness.

Planning: Expected Outcomes. The patient will maintain intact oral and nasal mucous membranes, as evidenced by having oral and nasal mucous membranes pink, moist, and without lesions, crusts, or bloody drainage.

Implementation. Inspect the patient's mouth daily, using a flashlight and tongue depressor. Keep the lips coated with a water-soluble lubricant to prevent encrustation, drying, and cracking. Carefully inspect a paralyzed cheek for crusts or other conditions requiring care.

Provide oral hygiene to prevent (1) excessive drying of oral mucous membranes and (2) complications such as parotitis, aspiration, and respiratory tract infections.

Brush the patient's teeth with a small toothbrush at least twice a day. Clean the oral mucous membranes (especially the roof of the mouth), tongue, and gums with toothettes. Avoid agents containing lemon or alcohol (or dilute them) because these agents dry the membranes. Then, rinse the mouth. Gauze wrapped around a tongue depressor or toothbrush (and saturated with dilute mouthwash) may help with aspects of oral care.

While performing mouth care for an unconscious patient, suction excess secretions to prevent aspiration. It is easier if two nurses perform mouth care together. One nurse does the cleaning while the other suctions as necessary.

Nasal passages may become occluded because an unconscious patient is unable to sniff, blow, sneeze, or clear the nose. To clear the nasal passages of mucus and crust formations, gently swab the nose with an applicator moistened with water or normal saline. Then, apply a thin coat of water-soluble lubricant with a cotton-tipped applicator.

Do *not* clean the nasal passages or ears of patients who have had brain surgery or head injuries. If bleeding occurs from the ears or nose, or if CSF (a watery discharge) appears to be draining from these areas, notify the physician.

Nursing Diagnosis: Skin Integrity, Impaired, High Risk for R/T immobility and loss of protective reflexes.

Planning: Expected Outcomes. The patient will have intact skin, as evidenced by no reddened areas over bone prominences, no areas or signs of skin irritation or dryness, and no signs of corneal irritation.

Implementation. Provide nursing intervention for all "self-care" needs, including bathing, hair care, and skin and nail care. Patients often scratch themselves as the depth of unconsciousness lessens; therefore, keep nails trimmed. Patients who are comatose for long periods may be lifted occasionally into a bathtub half filled with warm water. It may be helpful to apply superfatted solutions (e.g., castile, baby oil, or cold cream) instead of a bath every fourth or fifth day to prevent loss of cutaneous oils and skin irritation and dryness. If vaginal discharge or odor occurs, cleansing douches may be prescribed. Unconscious women need perineal care, especially during menstruation.

Keep the cornea moist by instilling methyl cellulose (0.5 to 1 per cent) solution. Apply protective eye shields or close the eyelids with adhesive strips if the corneal reflex is absent, if the eyes are open, or if they appear irritated. These measures prevent corneal abrasion and irritation.

When the patient cannot respond to local tissue hypoxia from being in one position for an extended period of time, the risk of pressure ulcers increases. Patients in a coma should be placed on special mattresses or beds (Fig. 29–8). However, the use of these special beds does not eliminate the need to assess the skin and rub the skin every 4 hours. In addition, the nutritional needs of the patient must be met in order to reduce the risk of pressure ulcers.

Collaborative Problem. High risk for contractures, R/T immobility.

Planning: Expected Outcomes. The patient will have no signs of contractures, as evidenced by full range of motion in all joints; no evidence of flexion contractures in wrists, elbows, and knees; and no signs of footdrop.

Implementation. Maintain extremities in functional positions by providing proper support. Hand rolls prevent flexion contracture of the fingers. Cock-up arm splints prevent wristdrop. Splints, casts, or high-topped tennis shoes help properly support feet. Remove support devices every 4 hours for skin care and passive exercises.

Nursing Diagnosis: Nutrition, Altered: Less than Body Requirements R/T inability to eat secondary to unconsciousness.

Planning: Expected Outcomes. The patient will demonstrate signs of adequate nutrition, as evidenced by weight remaining stable; consuming adequate calories for age, height, and weight; intake equaling output; incisions/wounds healing within 12 to 14 days; hemoglobin, blood urea nitrogen, total lymphocyte count, and albumin levels within normal limits for age and sex.

Implementation. Intravenous fluids are begun on admission for comatose patients. Initially the intravenous site provides access to the circulatory system for the administration of medications. Because fluid intake is restricted and glucose is avoided to control cerebral edema, an intravenous infusion cannot be considered nutritional support.

Just because a patient is comatose, the nurse should never assume that hunger is not present and calorie intake is decreased. In fact, the opposite is true; caloric needs are increased in patients with head injury. Nutritional and fluid needs of comatose patients are usually met through nasogastric feedings. If the patient does not have paralytic ileus or delayed gastric emptying and if bowel sounds are audible and gastric residual volumes are less than 100 ml/hr, nasogastric feedings are started. An unconscious patient cannot swallow fluids normally. To prevent aspiration, do not give food or liquids by mouth.

The nutritional requirements that follow brain injury are complex; a complete nutritional assessment with anthropometric tests, laboratory tests, and clinical examination is essential. There is a marked increase in metabolic needs with severe brain injury. Malnutrition increases the morbidity and mortality of neurologically

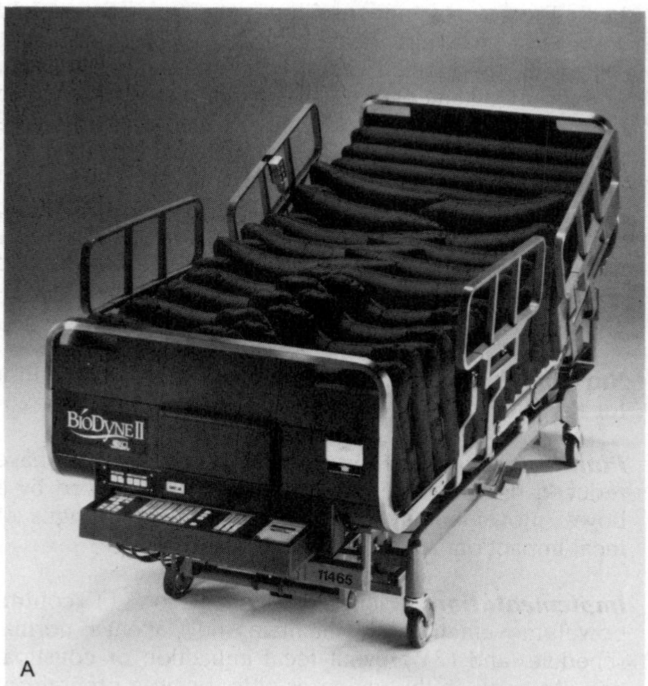

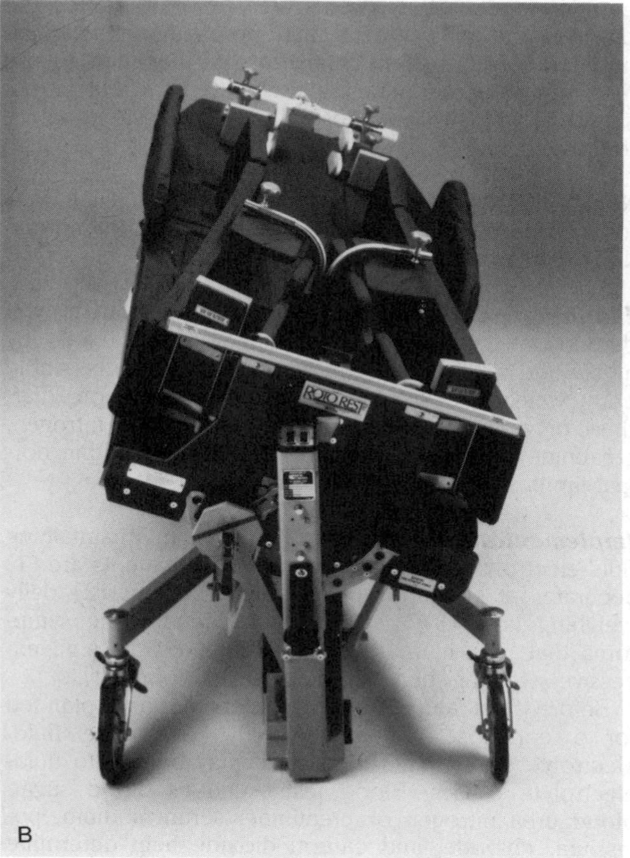

▲ **Figure 29–8**

A, BIODYNE, an oscillating air support surface. *B*, ROTO REST, an oscillating bed. Both devices are used to treat hypoxemia and to reduce the incidence of nosocomial pneumonia. ROTO REST is also used for clients with spinal cord injury and skeletal traction.

ill patients and may cause diarrhea and delayed gastric emptying from malabsorption. Healing will not take place in the presence of a negative nitrogen state. Immunodeficiency with increased risk for infection, sepsis, stress ulcers, weight loss, skeletal muscle protein wasting, and lung tissue catabolism leading to diaphragm weakness with respiratory reduction occur from prolonged calorie and protein deprivation. Starvation can lead to death.

Nursing responsibilities in tube feeding unconscious patients are critical because they (1) cannot communicate and (2) may have lost protective cough and gag reflexes. The possible complications from nasogastric feeding include

- vomiting and aspiration if the stomach is overfilled
- tube dislocation into trachea or lungs, causing aspiration. Unconscious patients are often restless. Watch that they do not pull out the tube. Aspiration may occur if a feeding tube is pulled out during a feeding session or whenever it is unclamped. During feeding sessions, cloth wristlets or wrist restraints may be needed. When tube feeding a person, elevate the head of the bed at least 30 degrees to minimize possible aspiration if the tube is displaced. Always check tube placement with a stethoscope, residual volume, and gastric distention before feeding. Gastrointestinal distention can increase ICP. Never tube feed a patient in the supine position unless all other positions are impossible.
- ulcerated, crusted nares
- tracheoesophageal fistula, that is, breakdown of the anterior esophageal wall from prolonged contact between the nasogastric tube and a tracheostomy tube. Indicated by gastric contents in tracheal excretions, this requires immediate treatment.
- gastric mucosa trauma if the tube's distal end hardens, as may happen over time

As consciousness returns and the client begins to respond to verbal stimuli and has a gag reflex, test the client's ability to suck and swallow liquid. Before the test, position the client sitting up and have suction equipment nearby in case it is needed. Use a thick juice, nectar, or ice chips rather than water. A thicker consistency is easiest to swallow. Place about 1 teaspoonful of liquid into the back of the mouth. Observe for swallowing. Suction as needed to prevent aspiration. If a client cannot suck through a straw or drink from a glass owing to facial paralysis, place fluids into the unaffected side of the mouth with an Asepto syringe. Watch for difficulty in swallowing. Suction as needed.

Swallowing can be stimulated by having the client lean the head forward and, after taking fluid, quickly tipping the head backward. Stroking the anterior neck may also promote swallowing.

Once a client can safely swallow, begin small oral liquid feedings, progressing to a soft diet. Discontinue tube feedings only when the client can take adequate nutrition orally. Many clients are fed orally during the daytime and tube fed at night to maintain adequate nutrition. When a client begins to eat independently, be reassuring and encouraging. Remind the client to eat slowly and to swallow. Position the client sitting up as tolerated.

Nursing Diagnosis: Fluid Volume Deficit, High Risk for R/T inability to drink fluids and respond to normal thirst mechanisms.

Planning: Expected Outcomes. The patient will demonstrate signs of fluid balance, as evidenced by intake and output equal for 24, 48, and 72 hours; stable body weight; no signs of excessive perspiration, diarrhea, or vomiting; serum glucose, blood urea nitrogen, creatinine, sodium, potassium, and chloride within normal limits.

Implementation. Important aspects in maintaining fluid-electrolyte balance in unconscious patients are (1) accurate intake and output documentation; (2) daily weighing; and (3) assessing and documenting symptoms that may increase fluid volume deficit (e.g., excessive sweating, polyuria, diarrhea, or vomiting).

Before fluid and electrolyte intervention is planned for a comatose patient, carefully assess the fluid-electrolyte status. The coma itself may be due to fluid-electrolyte causes. Blood tests such as blood sugar, blood urea nitrogen or creatinine, serum sodium, potassium, chloride, and carbon dioxide help determine fluid-electrolyte status (see Chaps. 14 and 15). Dehydration and water intoxication (true hyponatremia) are common causes of electrolyte imbalance associated with coma.

Overhydration and intravenous fluids with glucose are always avoided because cerebral edema may follow. Diuretics may be prescribed to correct fluid overload and reduce edema. The nurse should monitor the response to these medications. For evaluating the response to any diuretic, the indwelling catheter should be emptied before the diuretic is administered. When evaluating the response, the nurse should consider the diuretic given, the dose, and renal status.

Nursing Diagnosis: Injury, High Risk for R/T unconsciousness and immobility.

Planning: Expected Outcomes. The patient will sustain no injury, as evidenced by no abrasions or bruises and no falls from bed.

Implementation. Keep side rails up on the bed and bed in lowest position whenever the patient is not receiving direct care or is unattended. Observe seizure precautions for anyone with a history of seizure and for patients who could have a seizure for the first time.

Give adequate support to limbs and head when moving or turning an unconscious patient. Limbs without tone may dislocate if they are allowed to fall unsupported. Always turn an unconscious patient toward you or someone else, to stop the patient's rolling off the bed. Protect an unconscious patient from external sources of heat (e.g., heating pads, radiators).

Protect the patient from injury during seizures or periods of agitation (e.g., use padded side rails, keep the patient's nails short and clean). Medication may be prescribed to control seizures or hyperexcitability.

Avoid oversedation because it impedes assessment of level of consciousness and impairs respiration. Do not restrain the patient unless it is absolutely necessary because restraint is likely to increase confused and combative behavior. Do not leave unstable patients unattended.

Nursing Diagnosis: Incontinence, Bowel, High Risk for R/T unconsciousness.

Planning: Expected Outcomes. The patient will have reduced risk of bowel incontinence, as evidenced by a bowel movement every 2 to 3 days and no signs of fecal impaction.

Implementation. Plan intervention to (1) control bowel movements, (2) maintain the patient's normal schedule, and (3) prevent fecal impaction or constipation. As soon as the patient is able, begin a program of bowel retraining. Maintain a regular schedule of stool softeners, suppositories, and digital removal at approximately the same time each day. Frequently examine the abdomen for distention. Constipation and fecal impaction may occur. Small, frequent liquid stools may indicate impaction.

Nursing Diagnosis: Family Processes, Altered, R/T family member in a coma.

Planning: Expected Outcomes. The family members will exhibit positive coping behaviors, as evidenced by showing an ability to problem solve, not neglecting needs of other family members, and asking questions about the patient indicating that previous teaching has been understood.

Implementation. The significant others of a comatose patient are often very stressed. It is difficult for the family not to be able to communicate with the patient and at times not know whether the patient will recover. The nurse should include them in the patient's care as much as they can be involved and wish to be involved. It is important that the family see the patient receiving quality, professional, caring nursing care. A very caring behavior for the comatose patient and family is for the nurse to talk to the patient as if he or she could understand. Initially, this behavior will seem awkward for the nurse, but in time it will feel appropriate. Tell the patient that he or she will be turned to the side, bathed, and so on. Because the sense of hearing is the first sense to return as consciousness returns, the patient may hear the nurse speaking. Comatose patients have awakened and reported that they remember hearing specific voices.

The family is often in a state of shock, needing someone to recognize their need and help them through this difficult situation. They may experience various conflicting, perhaps irrational emotions, for example, guilt and anger. The nurse should reinforce information provided by the physician to the significant others, for example, what happened to the patient and the treatment being planned or given. The explanation may not be understood initially and will need to be repeated. Be sure to explain the function of all the "tubes" that can be seen by the family. The family can be overwhelmed by the presence of many tubes (i.e., intravenous line, catheter, ventilator) and perceive the patient to be in critical condition, when this may not be the case. When the patient is not expected to survive, the family should be told of the prognosis and be given the opportunity to be as involved as is possible with the decisions about care.

Allow the significant others to stay with the patient, when and where this is possible. At times, the members of the family may become vigilant in attending and stay at the patient's bedside continuously. Encourage the family members to care for themselves also by encouraging adequate meals and sleep. Have them consider using external support systems (e.g., neighbors and church groups). Tell them that they will be called if any significant changes occur, and ask them to leave a phone number where they can be reached. Encourage family members to call the nurses if they have questions or concerns.

Some hospitals, especially tertiary care centers, have "family homes" that provide the family members who travel a long distance to the hospital a place to stay and be close to the hospital and patient.

EVALUATION

The patient may remain comatose for a few hours or even months. Therefore, some expected outcomes have brief time frames (e.g., airway obstruction) and others are prolonged, requiring frequent reevaluation (e.g., family coping).

Modification of Plan of Care for the Elderly

The aged patient in a coma requires no different care, except that the nurse should be vigilant in assessing for the complications of immobility. The aged patient is at higher risk of all complications of immobility, especially pressure ulcers and pneumonia. For male patients, urinary retention is common because of prostatic enlargement. Finally, the common disorders of aging that might be the cause of the coma should be assessed for fully (e.g., diabetic coma).

Post-hospital Care

The site for discharge from an acute care setting is totally dependent on the condition of the patient and the cause of the coma. If the patient is still in a coma and recovery is expected, placement in a rehabilitation center may be planned. If the patient is in a coma and is not expected to awaken but may live for a time with nutritional support, placement in a skilled nursing center is common. Some comatose patients awaken and make a complete recovery while in the hospital, for example, those patients with diabetic coma. If the comatose patient is determined to be brain dead, the family may be approached for organ donation. Funeral arrangements can begin from the hospital for these patients.

DISCHARGE TEACHING

The nurse's role in discharge of the comatose patient centers on communication with the receiving nurses and family. If the patient is ventilator-dependent or combative, special consideration will be required for transport to the new facility. A complete plan of care should be provided also.

CONFUSIONAL STATES

Definition

Confusion is a mental state marked by alterations in thought and attention deficit followed by problems in comprehension. Confusion is accompanied by a loss of short-term memory and often irritability alternating with drowsiness.

Incidence

The true incidence of confusion has not been measured, but the condition is common. Confusion is a common symptom of many neurologic and metabolic disorders. In addition, the remarkable rise in longevity due to medical and environmental progress has extended life and dramatically increased the incidence of degenerative neurologic disorders.

Etiology

There are many causes of confusion. Common causes of acute confusion are alcohol withdrawal and drug ingestion. Confusion can also follow fever, heart failure, head injury, or anesthetics. Other causes of confusion are hypoxia, hypoglycemia, severe fluid and electrolyte disorders, sepsis, liver and renal failure, poisons, and drug overdose. Dementia is a chronic form of severe confusion affecting memory, judgement, and abstract thought resulting in the loss of personal and social independence in a previously competent individual. Alzheimer's disease is the most common cause of dementia. The remaining portion of dementia is caused by stroke, other neurologic diseases, and other treatable disorders. This section discusses the care of clients who have varying degrees of cognitive changes. The specific care required by the client with Alzheimer's disease and other disorders is discussed in Chapter 30.

Risk Factors

Risk factors leading to confusion vary with the specific etiologic factors. In general, the proper management of various diseases, such as diabetes mellitus, would reduce the incidence of confusion. Disorders such as Alzheimer's disease have no known prevention at this time.

Pathophysiology

Three mechanisms account for the development of acute confusion: (1) damage to the brain with swelling or loss of oxygen, blood, or both (functional disorder); (2) impairment of the action of the nervous system by chemicals or other substances (metabolic disorder); and (3) the rebound overactivity of a previously depressed center in the brain. Injury to the brain results in increased ICP (see later). Chemicals that cross the blood-brain barrier, such as alcohol, impair the metabolism of the neuronal cells. When the drug action wears off or the client is withdrawn from the drug, the lower centers in the brain are overactive. This overactivity accounts for the development of acute confusion, combativeness, and other abnormal behaviors.

Chronic confusional states are due to disorders that cause brain tissue destruction, biochemical imbalances, or compression of the brain. For example, clients with Alzheimer's disease have a lack of acetylcholine, a neurotransmitter that is necessary for short-term memory. Other disorders causing chronic confusion may be inherited, be due to viruses (e.g., Creutzfeldt-Jakob disease), or follow diseases (e.g., encephalitis).

Clinical Manifestations

The earliest sign of a metabolic brain disorder is a disorder of attention. The client may report the loss of concentration or appear preoccupied. At the same time, restlessness, emotional lability, insomnia or drowsiness, and vivid nightmares may begin. Clients may appear anxious and fear that they are "going crazy." As the disorder progresses, stupor and coma develop. Data seen in the client are reflective not of personality but of the cause of the disorder. For example, barbiturate/alcohol abuse and withdrawal and liver disorders cause agitated delirium. In contrast, anoxia and kidney and lung disorders cause a more quiet response. Disorders that develop rapidly are more likely to cause an agitated response than are those that develop slowly.

Fluctuations in cognition (the ability to think and reason) are common in clients with metabolic brain disorders. Clients may be totally out of context one moment and lucid the next. Some of the fluctuations are due to the environment, and delirious clients become more disoriented at night, in unfamiliar surroundings, and in situations in which restraints are used, unfamiliar noises are heard, or unfamiliar people are seen. The lack of a window in the room has caused many clients to become disoriented.

The client will commonly have difficulty with immediate recall and ability to abstract. Loss of memory for recent events is a hallmark of metabolic brain disorders (sometimes called organic brain disease). Clients who are delirious quickly lose orientation to time. Normal subjects can readily recall six or seven digits forward and five or six backward and identify the commonalities between an orange and an apple or a tree and a bush. Delirious clients cannot do this. However, the client's general intelligence level can have an impact on the data seen. If possible, the level of education should be known before assessment.

Perceptual errors (e.g., mistaking the nurse for a daughter) as well as hallucinations, illusions, and delusions are common accompaniments of delirium.

Hallucinations are sensations occurring in the absence of external stimuli. A client may hear, see, feel, smell, or taste something that is not present. The client may or may not realize that the experience is "unreal."

Illusions differ from hallucinations in that illusions are the misinterpretation of something in the environment. For example, if a client sees a shadow on the drape and mistakes it for a real person, the client is experiencing an illusion.

Delusions are thoughts or beliefs that have no basis in fact. For example, a client may think that he has been robbed or poisoned, when there is no basis for this thought.

DIAGNOSTIC ASSESSMENT

There are no specific diagnostic tests for confusion. The client would have a CT or MRI scan for determining whether there is a structural cause of the confusion, such as a tumor. In addition, a series of laboratory studies would be performed to determine whether there is a metabolic cause. Common studies include a complete blood count, electrolyte determinations, vitamin B_{12} and folate levels, thyroid and liver function studies, drug toxicity screening tests, and an electroencephalogram. A lumbar puncture may be performed for the analysis of CSF.

Medical Management

The medical management of the confused client begins by determining the cause of the confusion and correcting it if possible. When no specific cause is found, the medical management focuses on controlling symptoms. At times, haloperidol can be given to calm agitation. Nutritional needs must also be monitored.

Surgical Management

There are no operations for confusion, unless the confusion is due to a structural disorder such as a tumor or hematoma. For those clients, craniotomy may be performed to remove the growth or accumulation of blood.

Nursing Management

ASSESSMENT

The confused client needs a thorough history. The history should include the onset of the confusion, past medical illness, work and occupation history, and past injuries. Past medical illness, such as diabetes or liver failure, may be out of control and the cause of the confusion. The client may have been exposed to heavy metals or toxic waste during employment. Past injuries, especially head injury, are important to record. Depending on the level of confusion, the client may not be able to answer each question, and the nurse may need to rely on the family or others who have been with the client. Specific questions to determine how well the client was able to handle routine financial transactions or home safety such as with cooking, dressing, and driving will help determine whether the client will be safe to return home or need placement in a nursing home at discharge. At times the family may report a change in personality, such as apathy, social isolation, disinterest in current events, and irritability. These data should be recorded because they may be symptoms of Alzheimer's disease.

The confused client needs ongoing assessment with use of the Glasgow Coma Scale (see Fig. 29–6) or the mini–mental state form. The nurse should analyze the data collected to determine whether the confusion is improving, worsening, or remaining the same.

The confused client is often combative and argumentative. The nurse should assess whether the client is able to refrain from self-injury or injury to others. If not bedfast, the client may wander about and get lost or injured if harmful items are not recognized (e.g., knives).

NURSING INTERVENTION

Nursing Diagnosis: Thought Processes, Altered R/T memory loss and lack of self-protective behavior.

Planning: Expected Outcomes. The client will have improved thought processes, as evidenced by improving score on mini–mental state form and reported less hallucinations, illusions, and delusions.

Implementation. The confused client will benefit from having consistency in the environment and routine. Objects should be kept in the same place, such as the tray table and bedside chair. If possible, the same staff should care for the client. When the routine is changed, the client should be given short explanations as the events occur, such as "You need an x-ray" and "Please sit in the wheelchair." Telling the client that "in 2 hours an x-ray tech will be coming to take you for a CAT scan" will be neither remembered nor understood.

The nurse should reorient the client as often as necessary. The nurse should speak quietly and slowly and repeat as necessary. Clients with chronic untreatable confusion do not benefit from reorientation and may become more agitated when the nurse attempts to reorient them. For these select clients, the nurse can avoid reorienting and "go along" with the confusion. Of course, when the client has a risk of injury, safety precautions must be foremost. Clocks and calendars in the room will also help with reorientation. The use of familiar objects is helpful because remote memory is intact. For example, the use of a quilt from home on the bed may help the confused client recognize the bed as his or her own.

Unfamiliar noise should be reduced because it adds to the confusion. The client's room should be quiet and softly lit without producing shadows.

Nursing Diagnosis: Injury, High Risk for R/T unpredictable behavior.

Planning: Expected Outcomes. The client will sustain no injury and not injure others.

Implementation. The client must be protected from self-injury. The client should be in a room near the nursing station so that frequent assessments can be performed. In addition, the bed should be in low position and the side rails should be up at all times when the client is not attended. The use of side rails and the low bed position do not guarantee that the client will not fall but remind the client of the location and slow the client down as he or she attempts to get out of bed. Therefore, the nurse must continue frequent assessments. Physical restraints should be used cautiously. Some clients become more agitated as they resist the restraint. When restraints are used, the nurse must be certain to remove the restraint every 4 hours to assess the skin beneath it and allow or provide range-of-motion exercises. Chemical restraint (e.g., tranquilizers) should also be used cautiously, and the nurse should assess for the side effects of the drugs, including increased confusion and tremors (extrapyramidal symptoms). The nurse must remember that the client is not in control of his or her behavior. It is unpredictable, irrational, and impulsive. The client may be frightened and suspicious. Comments made by the client should not be taken as personal insults by the nurse. The client should never be "punished" for inappropriate behavior or comments.

Nursing Diagnosis: Sleep Pattern Disturbance R/T daytime napping and nighttime hallucinations.

Planning: Expected Outcomes. The client will have improved sleep patterns, as evidenced by sleeping 4 to 6 hours continuously at night and not sleeping as often during the day hours.

Implementation. Nighttime interventions should be planned to allow 4 to 6 hours of uninterrupted sleep. (Recall that a sleep cycle requires 2 to 3 hours and the loss of REM sleep can increase confusion.) When the nurse enters the room at night, the client should be assessed for rapid eye movement (REM). When REM is present, the client should be allowed to complete the

REM portion of the sleep cycle and the nurse should return later to care for the client.

The client should be kept active during the day hours so that there is some fatigue by nighttime. Daytime sleeping is a difficult pattern to break, and the client may have to be "kept awake" in order for the pattern to be reversed. For the elderly client, the normal changes in sleep with aging need to be considered, such as the increased use of short naps and less sleep during the night. Sleeping medications are seldom given to confused clients because they often alter sleep cycles and deplete the client of REM sleep.

Nursing Diagnosis: Family Coping, Ineffective R/T unfamiliar behavior of the client or stress of providing continual care for the client at home.

Planning: Expected Outcomes. The client's family will demonstrate improved coping strategies, as evidenced by improved use of support systems and appropriate analysis of the client's condition.

Implementation. When confusion is a new problem for the client, the family will be distressed by the behavior. The nurse should explain to the family that the client is not able to control behavior or speech at this time. The nurse should assess whether the client becomes calm or agitated when the family is present and advise visitation accordingly. If possible, the need for and use of restraints should be explained to the family, before they see the client. The family may be very surprised to see a member of the family "tied to the bed." Advance explanations can avert some of this reaction. There have also been instances in which the client suffered an injury because the family did not understand the purpose for the restraints and untied them.

If the client's confusion is due to a chronic disease, such as Alzheimer's disease, the family may need to find support systems to provide continual supervision of the client in the home. The nurse should also advise the family to have legal counsel determine the client's competency and determine the need for guardianship or durable power of attorney.

EVALUATION

The degree of goal attainment should be assessed at regular intervals. If expected outcomes have not been met, the plan of care may need revision or, more commonly, the degree of confusion will require more time to abate and the expected outcome will need a new time frame.

Modification of Plan of Care for the Elderly

The confused aged client is a common problem; therefore, most interventions discussed in the preceding are directed at that population. It is also common, but incorrect, to think that elderly clients have a marked deterioration in mental function. In general, most elderly clients have difficulty recalling new information, but the remote memory is intact. In addition, the incidence of depression occurs in 20 to 30 per cent of the elderly. Depression may follow the loss of friends, spouse, health, and independence and may lead to symptoms such as memory loss and confusion.

If the client is restrained, the nurse must continually assess the skin under the restraint as well as on bone prominences because the client is confined to one position.

Post-hospital Care

The discharge of a confused client from the hospital varies with the cause of confusion. If the confusion is acute and full recovery is expected, sometimes the client can go home under the care of family members. If the confusion is chronic, the client will need either care or supervision at home or placement in a nursing home. See also the care of the client with Alzheimer's disease at home in Chapter 31.

INCREASED INTRACRANIAL PRESSURE

Definition

Intracranial pressure (ICP) is the pressure exerted in the cranium by its contents: the brain, blood, and cerebrospinal fluid (CSF). The pressure is measured via the CSF. The normal pressure of CSF is 5 to 15 mm Hg or 60 to 180 mm H_2O. Pressures over 250 mm H_2O are called increased ICP and are a symptom of a serious underlying disorder. The pressure of CSF at the lumbar area, such as that recorded during a lumbar puncture, may not reflect the ICP. If the CSF flow is obstructed between the brain and the spinal cord, the lumbar pressure could be normal and the ICP very high.

Incidence

Increased ICP occurs commonly in clients with brain tumors, head injury, meningitis, encephalitis, subarachnoid hemorrhage, and disorders that alter the flow of CSF, such as stenosis of the aqueducts and hydrocephalus.

Etiology

Increased ICP is most often associated with a rapidly expanding lesion (e.g., bleeding), an obstruction to the outflow of CSF (e.g., tumor), or increased CSF formation (e.g., cerebral edema).

Risk Factors

Clients at the highest risk of developing increased ICP are those who have expanding masses in the brain.

Common clients are those who have had an injury to the head, surgery on the brain, hydrocephalus, brain tumors, and bleeding (e.g., subarachnoid hemorrhage).

Increased ICP can be reduced by proper positioning of the high-risk client, use of diuretics, and intracranial monitoring for early detection of rising pressures. The use of seat belts decreases the incidence of serious head injury and therefore would reduce problems from increased ICP.

Pathophysiology

The skull is a hard bony container filled with the brain tissue, blood, and CSF. The pressure within the cranium is maintained by the amount of brain tissue and the pressure of the blood and CSF. The Monro-Kellie hypothesis, a theory for understanding ICP, states that since the bony skull cannot expand, when one of the three compartments expands, the other two must compensate by decreasing in volume in order for the total brain volume and pressure to remain constant.

As a mass enlarges, initial compensation in the skull is through displacement of CSF into the spinal canal or back into venous blood through the arachnoid mater. The ability of the brain to adapt to increasing pressure without increasing ICP is called compliance. The movement of CSF is the first and the major compensatory mechanism, but it can accommodate increasing intracranial volume only to a point. When the ability of the brain to be compliant is exceeded, the ICP rises, the client develops symptoms, and other compensation efforts to reduce pressure begin.

The second form of compensation is by reducing blood volume in the brain. When blood flow is reduced by 40 per cent, cerebral tissue becomes acidotic. When 60 per cent of blood flow is lost, the EEG begins to change. This stage of compensation alters cerebral metabolism and eventually produces brain tissue hypoxia and areas of brain tissue necrosis.

The last stage of compensation and the most lethal is displacement of brain tissue across the tentorium, under the falx cerebri or through the foramen magnum into the spinal canal. This process is called herniation and often results in death.

It is important to remember that the brain is supported within various intracranial compartments. The supratentorial compartment contains all the brain tissue from the midbrain upward. This section is divided into two right and left chambers by the tough inelastic fibers of the falx cerebri. The supratentorial compartment is separated from the infratentorial compartment (containing brain stem and cerebellum) by the tentorium cerebelli (Fig. 29-9). It is also important to remember that the brain is capable of some movement within these compartments. When pressure rises in one compartment, pressure is placed on surrounding areas of lower pressure.

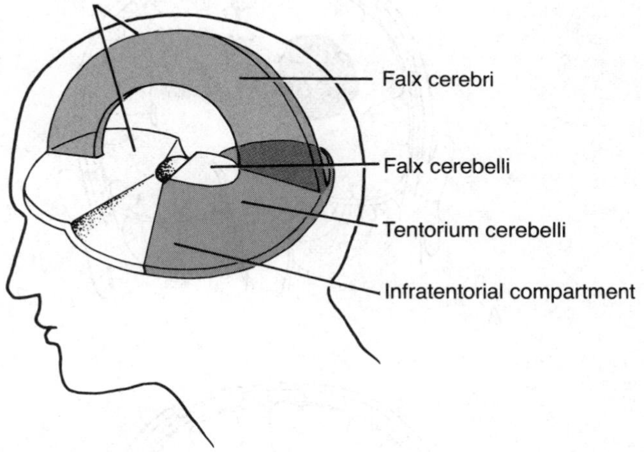

▲ *Figure 29-9*

The intracranial compartments. The supratentorial compartment contains all the brain tissue from the midbrain upward. This compartment is divided into two chambers—right and left—by the falx cerebri. The supratentorial compartment is separated from the infratentorial compartment (containing the brain stem and cerebellum) by the tentorium cerebelli.

HERNIATION SYNDROMES

There are four types of herniation syndrome. These conditions occur late in the course of increased ICP and represent the body's last attempt to restore normal brain volume and pressures (Fig. 29-10).

Central Transtentorial Herniation. Central transtentorial herniation is the end result of downward displacement of one or both of the cerebral hemispheres. As the cerebrum is compressed, it displaces the diencephalon and midbrain through the tentorial notch. An early indication of central transtentorial herniation is a change in the level of consciousness.

The following stages occur during the progression of central transtentorial herniation syndrome and reflect the compromised areas of brain.

Diencephalon Impairment. Diencephalon impairment causes early changes in level of consciousness. The client may have a headache and other symptoms such as nausea and vomiting. Subtle behavior changes such as agitation or apathy, or both, occur. If tissue displacement continues, the level of consciousness becomes lethargy, gradually progressing to stupor and coma. Pauses, sighs, or yawns may interrupt respirations. Cheyne-Stokes respirations gradually develop. The pupils are small but react to light, although the reaction may not be apparent without close scrutiny. Ocular movements may be roving. They may also be conjugate, with doll's eyes phenomenon and characteristic caloric test findings. Motor signs include increased tone and bilateral positive Babinski's response (Chapter 27). Gradually the grasp reflex may emerge, and finally flexion (decorticate) posturing (see Fig. 29-4) to painful stimuli appears on one side.

Midbrain-Upper Pons Stage Deterioration. The midbrain-upper pons stage of deterioration is characterized by progressive signs of brain stem failure. Cheyne-Stokes respirations change to central neuro-

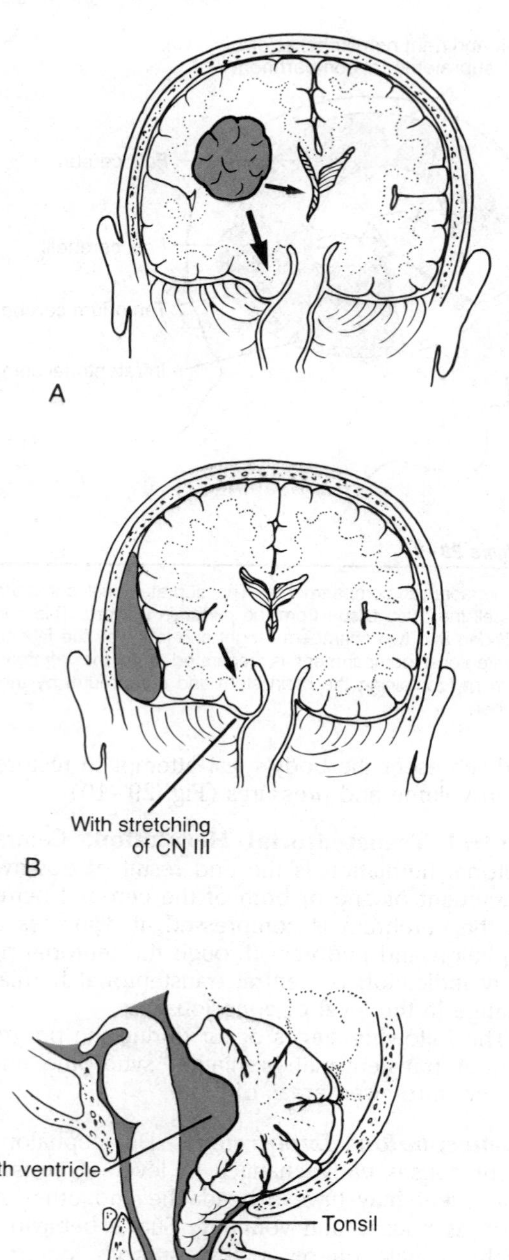

▲ *Figure 29-10*

Types of herniation syndromes. *A*, Central transtentorial herniation syndrome. Lesion centrally placed or superior in cranium may compress central and midbrain structures. Assessment findings include confusion and loss of consciousness. This may be followed by a dilated pupil and other signs of herniation. *B*, Lateral or uncal herniation syndrome. Lateral lesion within cranium causes pressure on midbrain. Assessment findings include headache, some confusion, and often a dilated pupil on same side of lesion. Client may lapse into coma. *C*, Tonsillar herniation syndrome occurs when the cerebellar tonsils are driven between the posterior arch of the atlas and the medulla and compressed.

genic hyperventilation, and the pupils dilate and fix at midposition. Eye movement responses to oculovestibular or oculocephalic testing become more difficult to elicit. When a response appears, although both eyes move, they are frequently dysconjugate (do not move together). Flexion (decorticate) posturing changes to bilateral extension (decerebrate) rigidity in response to painful stimulation. The client may develop extension rigidity spontaneously. During this stage, signs of pituitary and hypothalamus disruption may appear, including the onset of diabetes insipidus and wide swings in body temperature and other vital signs.

Lower Pontine–Upper Medullary Stage Deterioration. The patient appears calmer. The prognosis is very poor. Breathing patterns change and appear normal, except that the rate is faster and the depth shallow. Pupils do not change, but eye movements are not stimulated by the caloric test. The client is flaccid.

Medullary Stage Deterioration. The medullary stage is terminal. Respirations become slower and irregular, the pulse may be either slow or fast, and blood pressure drops. Finally breathing stops, pupils dilate widely, and death occurs.

Lateral Transtentorial Herniation. Lateral transtentorial herniation occurs from masses in or along the temporal lobe. As the temporal lobe is compressed, the uncus and hippocampal gyrus will herniate through the incisura, compressing the third cranial nerve, the midbrain, and the posterior cerebral artery. Symptoms include loss of oculomotor and pupil function from third cranial nerve compression, dilation of the ipsilateral pupil, and decerebrate posturing. At times, a respiratory dysfunction called central neurogenic hyperventilation will be noted also.

The following stages occur as lateral herniation syndrome progresses.

Early Third Nerve Stage. The early third nerve stage, with characteristic dilation of the ipsilateral pupil, is the first stage. Light reaction in the dilated pupil is usually present but sluggish. This may last for several hours and is usually the only early observable sign. Other "neuro sign" changes occur later. Notify physician immediately.

Lateral (uncal) herniation usually progresses very rapidly once the client begins to show signs of deterioration.

Late Third Nerve Stage. The late third nerve stage progresses rapidly. The client becomes stuporous, then comatose. The affected pupil fully dilates. Extraocular movements are at first abnormal, then disappear. Contralateral hemiplegia appears, followed by extension posturing (decerebration). The need for treatment is urgent.

Midbrain–Upper Pons Stage. If treatment fails, the client progresses to the midbrain–upper pons stage. The other (nondilated) pupil dilates and becomes fixed. Neurogenic hyperventilation and bilateral extension (decerebrate) posturing occur. Eye movements are impaired or absent. It is then not possible to differentiate further deteriorations from those of central tentorial herniation syndrome.

Tonsillar Herniation. Herniation of the cerebellar tonsils through the foramen magnum, compressing the medulla and the upper portion of the spinal cord, is called tonsillar herniation. Symptoms include quadriparesis and erratic changes in blood pressure, pulse rate, and breathing. The pupils become small, and there are disturbances in conjugate gaze. This syndrome occurs most often in clients with cerebellar bleeding and occurs rapidly over just a few minutes.

Cingulate Herniation. When the frontal lobes of the cerebrum are compressed, the cingulate gyrus is pressed under the falx cerebri; this process is called cingulate herniation. Symptoms include signs of severe increased ICP as the ipsilateral anterior cerebral artery is compressed, causing ischemia, congestion, and edema.

BRAIN SWELLING AND BRAIN EDEMA

The terms "cerebral edema," "brain swelling," and "increased ICP" are sometimes used interchangeably, but they are not the same. Cerebral edema and brain swelling are causes of increased ICP. An increase in brain bulk due to an increase in cerebral blood volume is called brain swelling. Brain edema, in contrast to brain swelling, is an increase in the water content surrounding the tissues of brain, such as the extracellular spaces or the white matter, or within the cells themselves. The distinction between these two conditions is important because the interventions differ.

After head injury, edema develops as a result of a disruption of the blood-brain barrier. This type of edema is similar to other forms of edema, such as that seen in a sprained ankle. The fluid contains electrolytes, proteins, and even blood. Edema reaches its maximum within 48 to 72 hours after brain surgery or injury. The fluid returns to the systemic circulation via the CSF or the venous systems. This form of edema is treated with corticosteroids to stabilize the cell walls and reduce fluid shifts.

Brain swelling occurs when blood vessels within the brain dilate. Brain swelling appears to be the major mechanism responsible for increasing ICP and decreasing the size of the ventricles when compensation occurs. This form of swelling is usually treated with hyperventilation, which causes the cerebral vessels to constrict.

Clinical Manifestations

Symptoms of increased ICP are due to the pull on the cerebral blood vessels by swelling tissues and pressure on the pain-sensitive dura mater and various structures within the brain and back of the eye. Increased ICP is actually several entities occurring at the same time, rather than one process. No single set of clinical manifestations occurs in all clients. Indications of increased ICP relate to the location and the cause of the raised pressure and the speed and extent of its development.

The symptoms of increased ICP are subtle, and the nurse must be diligent in observing for changes in the client's condition. Symptoms include any alteration in level of consciousness, restlessness, irritability, confusion, and a decrease in the GCS score. In addition, the client may have changes in speech, pupillary reactions, motor or sensory changes, or cardiac rate and rhythm changes. Headache, nausea, vomiting, or blurred or double vision (diplopia) may be reported. Remember that the optic nerve is an extension of the brain, and increased tension within the skull is transmitted to the optic nerve, where it can be directly observed. Papilledema has no symptoms, and often the client is surprised to hear about the seriousness of the disorder on the basis of an eye examination. Cushing's triad of increased systolic pressure, widened pulse pressure, and irregular respirations is a late response to increased ICP and often indicates that herniation is occurring.

The variety of symptoms and the vagueness of those indicating increased ICP have led to the development of more reliable forms of determining ICP, such as ICP monitors. Early detection and treatment of increased ICP can greatly improve client outcome because increased ICP precedes clinical signs and symptoms.

DIAGNOSTIC ASSESSMENT

Clients with symptoms of increased ICP have various studies performed to locate the lesion or other cause. Common diagnostic studies include the CT and MRI scans. Usually a lumbar puncture is not performed because of the risk of herniation of the brain stem when the pressure of CSF in the cord is lower than in the cranium. Continuous ICP monitoring is commonly used in clients with increased ICP. The equipment monitors the level of ICP and sometimes can drain extra CSF to lower pressure.

Medical Management

INTRACRANIAL PRESSURE MONITORING

Continuous ICP monitoring is used for clients experiencing conditions associated with potentially elevated ICP (e.g., head trauma, pre- and postoperative aneurysms, tumors, posterior fossa lesions). However, ICP monitoring supplements rather than replaces serial clinical observations of the client's condition.

There are several methods of ICP monitoring. The most common types measure CSF pressure in the ventricles or subarachnoid space. Each type works differently and has advantages and disadvantages (see Bridge to Critical Care on various monitoring methods). Most health care facilities have a standard procedure for setting up and maintaining the monitors.

Advantages of ICP monitoring are the following.

- Pressure increase may be recognized and treated before the onset of signs and symptoms.
- Some systems allow ventricular fluid drainage above a set pressure. The system becomes part of treatment as well as assessment.
- Delays in bringing the client to definitive treatment (e.g., surgery) can sometimes be avoided.

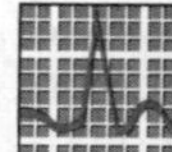

BRIDGE TO CRITICAL CARE

Intracranial Pressure (ICP) Monitoring

Guidelines for Management of ICP

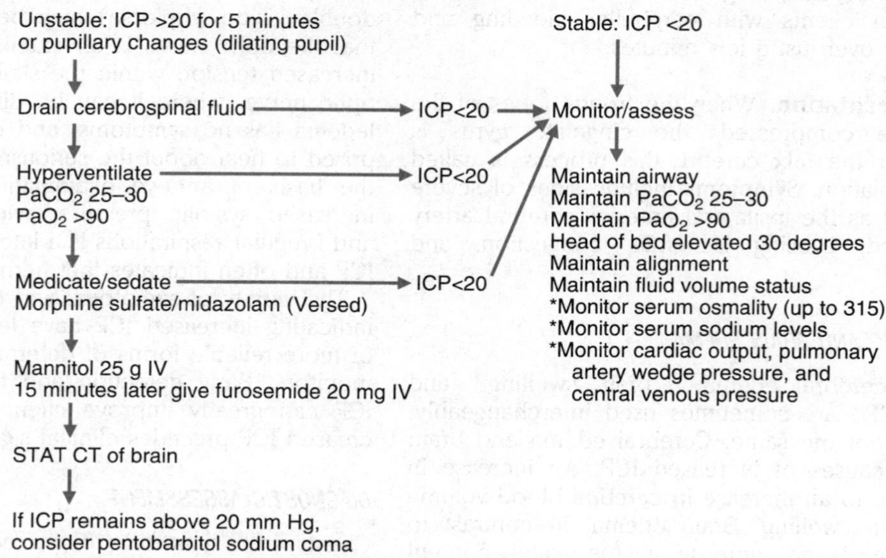

Intracranial Pressure Waveforms

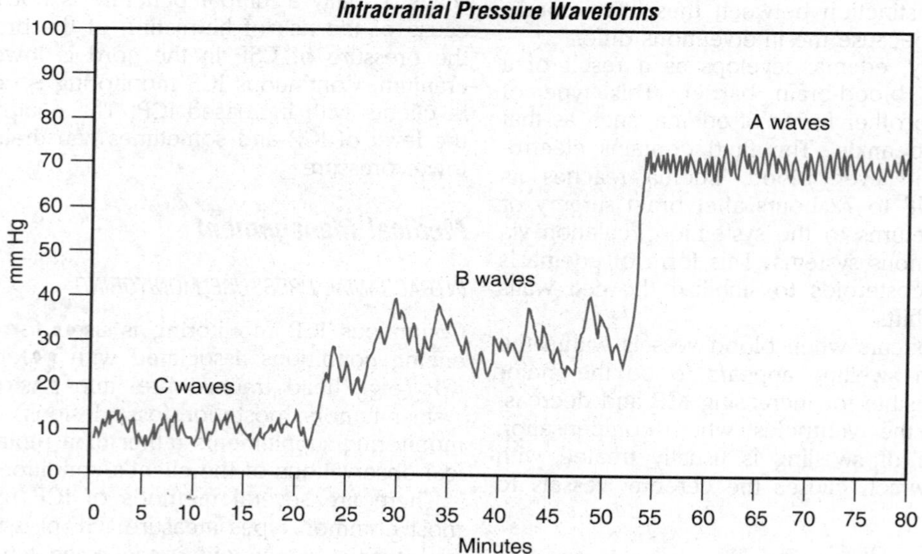

The shape of the waves is influenced by cardiac pulsations and respirations as well as by ICP. The waves have been named A, B, and C waves.

C waves occur four to eight times per minute and reflect fluctuations in arterial pressure. C waves are not considered significant.

B waves occur at intervals of 30 seconds to 2 minutes and represent increases in ICP to 50 mm Hg.

A waves are most pronounced when the cranial contents are increased. These waves, also called plateau waves, also called plateau waves, represent recurrent ICP elevations to 100 mm Hg. A waves may be caused by coughing or straining but, if recurrent or sustained, may indicate a reduced ability of the brain to compensate. The client may also show other signs of increasing intracranial pressure.

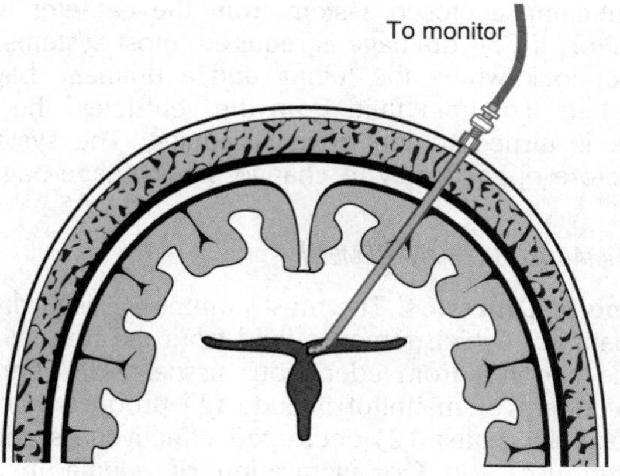

Ventricular Catheter (Ventriculostomy)

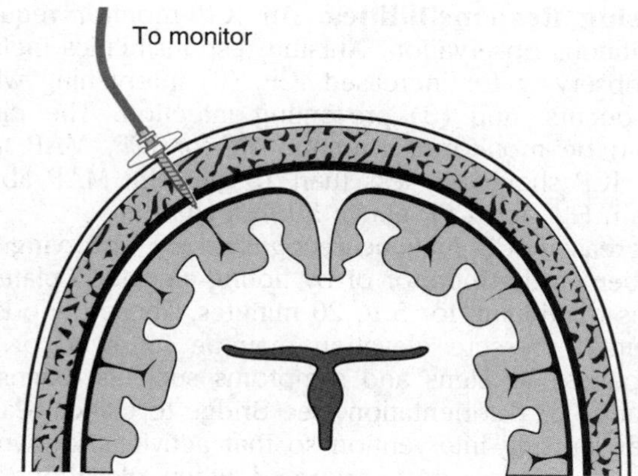

Subarachnoid Screw (bolt)

General Interventions for Intracranial Pressure Monitoring

- Ensure that the tubing is long enough to allow the client to be moved in bed but not longer than 14 feet. Tubing longer than 14 feet may cause inaccurate readings.
- Be careful to prevent kinks in the tubing.
- Place the transducer and screw (or catheter) at the preset level of the transducer to take a reading.
- Use sterile technique when working with the device.
- Monitor for signs of infection.
- Flush the catheter if the readings dampen.
- Check for the following if inaccurate readings occur:
  Leaks in the system
  Differences in the height of the transducer and the device
  Kinks in the tubing
  Client performing the Valsalva maneuver
  Obstruction in the system

- ▸ The effectiveness of other types of treatment can be monitored.
- ▸ Sustained pressure waves (plateau waves) can be detected.
- ▸ Intracranial compliance can be measured.
- ▸ Level of ICP elevation can provide prognostic information.
- ▸ Cerebral perfusion can be calculated.
- ▸ ICP monitoring is of particular value for clients who require paralyzing drugs (e.g., curare for mechanical ventilation) or are being treated with barbiturate-induced coma or induced hypothermia, because key changes in the "neuro signs" of these clients are not easily assessed.
- ▸ The effect of nursing intervention on ICP can be monitored. The timing of procedures known to raise ICP (e.g., suctioning) can be altered to coincide with periods of "lower" pressure.

Measuring Compliance and Cerebral Perfusion. Monitoring ICP also allows another method of determining intracranial compliance. Compliance is a measure of how much "slack" is present, that is, how much intracranial contents can expand within the nondistensible skull before the fit becomes "tight" and intracranial contents are compromised. A very compliant system is one in which "slack" exists. A noncompliant system is tight or has little "slack." Measuring compliance identifies low compliance, that is, when a small increase in volume would produce a large increase in ICP.

Compliance is tested by introducing a known volume of fluid into the ventricle and measuring its effect on ICP. Detecting a change in the critical relationship between volume and pressure allows early treatment before the onset of signs and symptoms or sustained elevated ICP.

Measurements of cerebral perfusion pressure (CPP) can be made with ICP monitors. CPP is the amount of blood flow from the systemic circulation required to provide adequate oxygen and glucose for brain metabolism. A normal brain can survive with a CPP of 30 mm Hg, but an injured brain requires a CPP of 50 mm Hg. Because ICP is normally 0 to 15 mm Hg, the mean arterial pressure (MAP) needs to be at least 60 mm Hg to produce an adequate CPP. In cases of profound increased ICP, the MAP and ICP become the same, and brain perfusion ceases.

$$CPP = MAP - ICP$$

Nursing Responsibilities. An ICP monitor requires continuous observation. Nursing responsibilities include (1) observing for increased ICP, (2) intervening when this occurs, and (3) preventing infection. The client should be monitored continuously for ICP, MAP, and CPP. ICP should be less than 15 mm Hg, MAP above 70 mm Hg, and CPP above 50 mm Hg.

Increased ICP may be recognized by observing the number on the monitor or by noting elevated (plateau) waves continuing for 5 to 20 minutes. These periods of sustained pressure elevation may be followed or accompanied by signs and symptoms such as extension posturing or disorientation (see Bridge to Critical Care).

Plan nursing intervention so that activities known to increase ICP are not performed when elevations are present (e.g., suctioning, excessive hip flexion, turning the client). Administration of endotracheal lidocaine has been helpful in limiting the effect of suctioning on ICP. Space out interventions so that a stair-step rise in ICP does not occur. Other problems that may contribute to increased ICP are (1) excess water in the respirator tubing, (2) excess secretion production causing a rise in PCO_2, (3) an endotracheal tube taped tightly over the jugular veins, retarding venous circulation from the head, and (4) discussing the client's condition at the bedside (see Nursing Research).

Avoid ICP catheter infections by (1) keeping the area around the catheter site clean and dry, (2) documenting and reporting leakage from the catheter, and (3) maintaining a closed system from the catheter to the monitor. If CSF drainage is required, most systems have a stopcock where the tubing and a drainage bag are attached. To drain fluid from the ventricles, the stopcock is turned to the drainage tubing. The system is therefore opened only to change the drainage bag.

NURSING RESEARCH

There are many nursing interventions that have been shown to have an effect on intracranial pressure (ICP), such as positioning, head rotation, and suctioning. This study examined the effect of emotionally referenced conversation that reflected an actual nursing report on the client's condition and a conversation that was composed of predetermined dialogue unrelated to the client's condition. The ICP measurements at baseline were compared with those recorded during the two types of conversation. Clients served as their own controls. T-test was used to analyze mean scores of the minimum, maximum, and average ICP measurements before, during, and after both conversations. The data collected revealed a wide variation in client responses, and it is concluded that the effect of conversation on ICP is related to the client's level of consciousness, not specially to conversation. Clients with a rating of less than 5 on the Glasgow Coma Scale may not interpret verbal language and therefore conversation of any nature may not have an effect on patients with ICP. Other clients were influenced by conversation.

Future studies should be done by comparing the response to conversation at various levels of consciousness as measured by points on the Glasgow Coma Scale, the effect of family conversation, and gentle tactile stimulation.

▼▼▼

Johnson, S., et al. (1989). Effects of conversation on intracranial pressure in comatose patients. *Heart and Lung, 18*(1), 56–63.

PHARMACOLOGIC MANAGEMENT

Osmotic Diuretics. The most commonly used diuretic is mannitol, which removes fluid from the normal brain tissue and not from edematous tissue. Side effects of large doses of mannitol include (1) production of hyperosmolar states, (2) decreased effectiveness with repeated use, and (3) aggravation of edema in some clients.

Loop Diuretics. Treatment with a nonosmotic diuretic like furosemide (Lasix) inhibits reabsorption of sodium and chloride at the proximal portion of the ascending loop of Henle. This drug is often given in varying doses ranging from 10 to 40 mg, alone or in combination with hyperosmolar agents to control cerebral edema. For older clients at risk for congestive heart failure, furosemide may improve the cardiovascular status. Watch for electrolyte disturbances, ototoxic effects, nausea, and vomiting. Monitor vital signs carefully.

Steroids. Steroids, such as dexamethasone (Decadron), may be used. The exact mechanism by which steroids work is unknown, but some physicians believe they are useful in controlling edema, especially brain tumor edema. Their use is controversial. Antacids or H_2-blockers may also be prescribed to control gastrointestinal irritation and hemorrhage.

Antihypertensives. Sustained arterial hypertension over 160 mm Hg is treated. Caution is used to avoid agents that cause peripheral vasodilation along with cerebral vasodilation. Beta blockers have been used in conjunction with other antihypertensives to block effects on cerebral vessels.

Anticonvulsants. Treatment of seizures after head injury requires anticonvulsants. Seizures increase metabolic requirements, cerebral blood flow, cerebral blood volume, and ICP even in paralyzed patients. Phenytoin (Dilantin) and phenobarbital are the usual agents. Seizures are discussed in Chapter 30.

Barbiturate Therapy for Uncontrolled ICP. Some clients require large doses of barbiturates for treatment of uncontrolled ICP. The use of this treatment requires sophisticated monitoring capacity and trained personnel, but its use has shown increased survival.

The client must be placed on a ventilator and have a Swan-Ganz catheter inserted. Pentobarbital is the drug of choice, and the client is given a loading dose of 5 to 10 mg/kg by slow intravenous injection. While the drug is infused, the client's blood pressure (MAP) is closely monitored because pentobarbital is a cardiac depressant. If the loading dose is sufficient to reduce ICP, a maintenance dose of 100 to 200 mg/hr is administered until pressure is under control. Pentobarbital is tapered slowly. It is important to monitor the serum level of the drug daily; the dose should be reduced if the serum levels exceed 5 mg/100 ml.

Assessment of the pupils should continue while the client is being treated. Even though the client is in a deep coma, the pupils will dilate if the brain stem becomes compressed. If pupils become dilated, the physician should be notified. Arterial pressure must be monitored closely, and systemic arterial pressure should not be allowed to fall below 70 mm Hg. Temperature should also be monitored because barbiturates reduce metabolism and have a concurrent cooling effect on the body. If temperature falls below 91.4° F (33° C), the patient should be warmed.

MECHANICAL VENTILATION

Hyperventilation, induced by a ventilator or by manual ventilation, is an important adjunct to management. It induces hypocapnia, which reduces cerebral blood volume and ICP. This intervention may be lifesaving while a client is being prepared for other treatments. Manual hyperventilation is sometimes done during ICP elevations or when sudden clinical signs of deterioration appear.

Surgical Management

Various surgical techniques are used to treat clients with increased ICP. Optimally, the cause is located and removed. Other techniques include (1) surgical placement of a shunt to allow drainage if CSF is blocked and (2) decompressive surgery. The latter is done by removing some brain tissue (e.g., part of the temporal lobe) to give the remaining structures room to expand. If compliance is low at surgery, the bone flap removed to gain access to the brain is not replaced or the dura may not be closed. Subsequent surgery is then required to repair the defect.

Nursing Management

Whether or not hyperventilation is used, pay meticulous attention to maintaining respiratory function. Assess an intubated client often. Frequent arterial blood gas samples are drawn. Acid-base imbalances are corrected to ensure adequate oxygenation.

Maintain a patent airway by suctioning to prevent buildup of carbon dioxide and elevation of ICP. Adequately oxygenate intubated clients before each passage of a suction catheter. Because hyperinflation as well as the addition of positive end-expiratory pressure raises ICP, keep the passage of a suction catheter as brief as possible. Never exceed 15 seconds. The use of lidocaine via the endotracheal tube may reduce elevations in ICP. Do not suction via the nose because drainage may indicate CSF leak and it is important to be able to observe it. (See discussion of suctioning in Chap. 37.)

It is also important to prevent venous obstruction. Raise the head of the bed 30 degrees. Avoid turning the client's head sharply to either side, and keep the head in alignment with the rest of the body. Maintain a regular bowel program because excessive strain can cause a Valsalva maneuver, which can result in venous back-up and increased ICP.

Fluid administration for clients with increased ICP is controversial. Administer fluid exactly as prescribed. Currently the tendency is to use a slightly hypertonic solution (e.g., 5 per cent dextrose in half-normal saline). Such fluid remains in the vascular space and therefore contributes less to cerebral edema. Balanced salt solutions are generally used, but other solutions may be required if complications occur that render the client hemodynamically unstable.

It is important to avoid the use of fluid (e.g., dextrose 5 per cent in water) that moves rapidly into the brain to cause edema. Remember to document the fluid administered with medications and in keeping monitoring devices open (e.g., indwelling arterial catheter lines). A large amount of fluid can be administered by these routes. The types and amounts of such fluids must be taken into account.

The actual amount of fluid infused per hour is determined by various factors. Never infuse more than the prescribed amount. If fluid therapy falls behind, consult the physician. This is especially important for a client with low intracranial compliance. Also remember that mechanical ventilation causes a client to retain fluid.

Increased temperature in clients with increased ICP raises the metabolic rate and aggravates ICP further. Therefore, hyperthermia requires vigorous treatment with cooling measures and prescribed medication.

▼ ALTERATIONS IN BODY TEMPERATURE

For maintenance of a normal body temperature, heat gain must equal heat loss. Heat is produced by metabolism or acquired from the environment. The regulation of body temperature is primarily through blood flow to the skin. Cutaneous blood flow is regulated by the hypothalamus. When the blood flow to the skin increases, the skin becomes red and warm. Heat is lost through the skin by conduction, radiation, or convection. When these mechanisms are not effective in reducing temperature, sweating begins, and evaporation is used to lose heat. If the body is too cold, cutaneous vessels control temperature by vasoconstriction. The skin becomes pale and cool as blood is shunted toward warm internal organs. If it is necessary to increase temperature, metabolic heat production increases, and shivering occurs.

There is a small range of normal temperature in the body. In a resting client, oral temperature is normally 96.8° to 100.4° F (36° to 38° C). Central nervous system function is impaired when the body temperature varies 4 degrees from this range. Seizures commonly occur when the temperature exceeds 106° F (41° C).

Irreversible changes in the brain occur with a temperature of 111° to 113° F (44° to 45° C).

The term *hyperthermia* is often used to describe a client who has an elevation in body temperature. There are many etiologic agents of hyperthermia, including malfunction of the thermoregulatory center in the hypothalamus, prolonged exposure to heat, loss of water, infection, cocaine toxicity, alcohol withdrawal, and salicylate overdose. This section focuses only on hyperthermia from hypothalamic disorders and heat exhaustion.

DISORDERS IN THE HYPOTHALAMIC CENTERS

The body's thermoregulatory centers in the hypothalamus may malfunction as a result of cerebral edema, after a cerebrovascular accident (stroke), after head injury, as a result of brain tumors, or in association with herniation syndrome. Hyperthermia exceeding 106° F (41.4° C) is most common in clients with central nervous system hemorrhage.

Fever is best understood from the hypothalamus level, and the best example is the thermostat used to regulate the home. The anterior hypothalamus regulates body temperature by balancing the heat gain and loss. During fever, the "thermostat" in the hypothalamus increases, and the common symptoms of fever occur. Heat is produced from shivering muscles and heat conservation (feeling cold) until the blood reaching the hypothalamus matches the thermostat setting. When the temperature of the blood exceeds the hypothalamic thermostat, sweating and vasodilation occur until the body cools to the thermostat setting. In clients with injury to the brain, the action of the hypothalamus can be impaired, and the client can develop hyperthermia. Hyperthermia also increases the demand for oxygen, cardiac output, and pulse rate. These changes can increase ICP and decrease cerebral perfusion. When untreated, hyperthermia can lead to acidosis, hypovolemia, cardiac dysrhythmias, and electrolyte imbalance.

Comatose patients may develop central nervous system hyperthermia (hyperpyrexia) because of damage to the hypothalamus. These fevers are difficult to control. Symptoms of hyperthermia include prolonged temperatures over 106° F (41.4° C), warm skin over the trunk, and cool extremities. The fever is not preceded by chilling. The client does not perspire, and cutaneous blood vessels do not dilate, so body temperature continues to rise. Hyperventilation and seizures may occur. Before hyperthermia from central nervous system disorders is diagnosed, other causes of fever, such as infection, must be considered.

Interventions for hyperthermia are aimed at reduction of body temperature. When body temperature is 101° F (38.4° C), the nurse should keep the room temperature at 70° F (21° C) and remove excess blankets and clothing. Keep the client from being improperly exposed. Cooling blankets may be used if temperature continues to rise. When the cooling blanket is used, be certain to provide frequent skin care. Inspect the skin every hour or two and cover the cooling blanket with a sheet or bath blanket. Monitor the client's temperature continuously with a rectal probe. Rapid cooling may induce serious dysrhythmias and hypothermia. These physical methods of reducing temperature are combined with the use of antipyretics for improved therapeutic effects.

Administer antipyretics as prescribed. These drugs inhibit prostaglandin synthesis and reduce the set point (thermostat) in the hypothalamus. If physical methods to reduce temperature are used when the thermostat in the hypothalamus is set higher, shivering and vasoconstriction will occur in an effort to raise core temperature to match the thermostat. The ideal treatment of fever is the combination of antipyretics and physical methods to promote heat dissipation.

HEATSTROKE

Heatstroke is an emergency and requires immediate treatment for survival. There are two forms of heatstroke: classic heatstroke and exertional heatstroke.

Classic heatstroke is seen most commonly in the poor, the elderly, the chronically ill, patients with heart disease, the obese, and alcoholics. Hot humid weather lasting 3 days or more increases the risk of heatstroke in these clients. The stress of the heat increases the demand on the heart. In addition, certain medications increase the risk of heatstroke. Some medications decrease the ability to sweat: antihistamines, beta-blockers, anticholinergics, and phenothiazines. Other medications increase heat production: amphetamines and neuroleptics.

Exertional heatstroke is more common in laborers, farmers, military recruits, athletes (especially football players and long-distance runners), and clients who work in boiler rooms or foundries. Symptoms of this form of heatstroke are similar to classic heatstroke except that these clients sweat. They tend to develop lactic acidosis and have more severe bleeding problems.

HEAT EXHAUSTION

Heat exhaustion is a common disorder that occurs after sustained exposure to heat for more than 3 days. It is caused by a lack of water or salt or both.

Heat exhaustion from loss of water occurs most often in the elderly, the infirm, or unconscious patients because they are unable to verbalize their thirst. It is also seen in clients who supplement their diet with salt tablets but inadequate water. Heat exhaustion from a loss of water is dangerous because it increases the risk of heatstroke. Symptoms of heat exhaustion include intense thirst with dehydration, fatigue, muscle incoordination, agitation, and impaired judgement.

Symptoms of central nervous system disorders are present with heat exhaustion and may include coma and bizarre behavior. In addition, the body temperature exceeds 104° F (40.6° C); the skin is hot, dry, and flushed; and the client is hypotensive as a result of shunting of blood into the peripheral circulation for cooling. Once cooling begins, the client may develop seizures, muscle rigidity, and tremors. Other symptoms may include respiratory alkalosis, hemorrhage, liver and renal problems, and dysrhythmias.

Heat exhaustion from lack of salt occurs mainly in clients who have moved to hot climates and not yet acclimated to the weather. These clients fail to replace their fluid and salt loss through perspiration with lightly salted fluids. The symptoms include weakness, fatigue, severe headache, and muscle cramps. Dehydration, thirst, and weight loss do not commonly occur.

Management

Prevention is key to treatment of this disorder. The rooms of elderly clients in nursing homes should be well supplied with fresh water during hot summer months. Ample water should be included in tube feedings when there is risk that water is being lost through evaporation, perspiration, or respiration. Further treatment includes replacement of water and salt loss, rest, and removal of the client from the source of the heat. If the client requires rehydration by intravenous therapy, hypertonic fluids are usually given at 2 mEq of sodium per hour. Acclimatization, the process of cardiovascular, endocrine, and exocrine adaptation to warm environments, requires about 2 weeks. During this time, the client should increase oral intake even though thirst is not felt.

HYPOTHERMIA

Hypothermia can occur accidentally through exposure to environmental cold, as a response to illness, or can be induced as a form of treatment. Hypothermia can also occur with central nervous system disorders, congestive heart failure, uremia, diabetes mellitus, drug overdose, and acute respiratory failure.

Hypothermia is induced during some surgical procedures to reduce blood flow to the area and blood loss. Some clients with near-drowning and during treatment for Reye's syndrome have been treated with hypothermia. Hypothermia decreases tissue metabolism by reducing demands for oxygen and glucose. It also reduces blood pressure, pulse, and cerebral function. Cerebral blood flow is reduced about 6 per cent for every centigrade degree the body temperature is reduced below normal.

Hypotension and somnolence often accompany hypothermia. When body core temperature drops to 30° C (86° F), ventricular dysrhythmias occur. At temperatures below 26.7° C (80° F), unconsciousness develops, and below 24° C (75° F), apnea and asystole occur. Rewarming of the client (in induced hypothermia) occurs slowly by either turning off the cooling blanket or warming the client through the blanket. The client may develop acidosis from the return of acidotic blood and waste from the peripheral tissues that were not completely perfused during the hypothermic state.

Cooling blankets are a common technique for induction of hypothermia. The client may be placed in barbiturate coma before hypothermia to control physiologic response to the rapid cooling, such as shivering.

Interventions for the client during hypothermia include continuous assessment. Hemodynamic lines will be placed to monitor cardiac and pulmonary function. Internal temperature probes will be required to monitor temperature. The remainder of the care is the same as for any patient in coma.

Summary

The loss of protective function can range from temporary states of confusion to coma and death from increased ICP. The early detection of neurologic problems is critical for improving the chances of full recovery.

Bibliography

1. Changaris, D., et al. (1987). Correlation of cerebral perfusion pressure and Glasgow Coma Scale to outcome. *Journal of Trauma, 27*(9), 1007–1013.
2. Crutchfield, J., et al. (1990). Evaluation of a fiberoptic intracranial pressure monitor. *Journal of Neurosurgery, 72*(3), 482–487.
3. Cutchins, C. (1991). Blueprint for restraint free care. *American Journal of Nursing, 91*(7), 36–44.
4. Folstein, M., et al. (1985). The meaning of cognitive impairment in the elderly. *Journal of the American Geriatric Society, 33*(4), 228–235.
5. Foreman, M. (1990). Complexities of acute confusion. *Geriatric Nursing, 11*(3), 136–139.
6. Foreman, M. (1986). Acute confusional states in the hospitalized elderly: A research dilemma. *Nursing Research, 35*(1), 35.
7. Franges, E., & Beideman, M. (1988). Infections related to intracranial pressure monitoring. *Journal of Neuroscience Nursing, 20*(2), 94–103.
8. German, K. (1988). Interpretation of ICP pulse waves to determine intracerebral compliance. *Journal of Neuroscience Nursing, 20*(6), 344–348.
9. Hollingsworth-Fridlund, P. et al. (1988). Use of the fiber-optic transducer. *Heart and Lung, 17*(2), 111–117.
10. House, M. (1990). Cocaine. *American Journal of Nursing, 90*(4), 40–45.
11. Laurin, N., et al. (1989). Cerebral perfusion imaging with technetium-99m HM-PAO in brain death and severe central nervous system injury. *Journal of Nuclear Medicine, 30*(10), 1627–1635.
12. McCance, K., & Huether, S. (1990). *Pathophysiology*. St. Louis: C.V. Mosby.
13. Marshall, S., et al. (1990). *Neuroscience critical care*. Philadelphia: W.B. Saunders.
14. Newbern, V. (1991). Is it really Alzheimer's? *American Journal of Nursing, 91*(2), 50–54.
15. Palmer, M., & Wyness, A. (1988). Positioning and handling: important considerations in the care of the severely head-injured patient. *Journal of Neuroscience Nursing, 20*(1), 42–46.
16. Plum, F., & Posner, J. (1980). *The diagnosis of stupor and coma*. Philadelphia: F. A. Davis.
17. Raimond, J., & Taylor, J. (1986). *Neurological emergencies: Effective nursing care*. Rockville, MD: Aspen Publishers.
18. Sherman, D. (1990). Managing acute head injury. *Nursing 91, 20*(4), 46–51.
19. Wallack, C. (1987). Intracranial hypertension: interventions and outcomes. *Critical Care Quarterly, 10*(1), 45–57.
20. Youmans, J. (1990) *Neurological surgery (3rd ed.)*. Philadelphia: W.B. Saunders.
21. Zegeer, L. (1989). Oculocephalic and vestibulo-ocular responses: significance for nursing care. *Journal of Neuroscience Nursing, 21*(1), 46–55.

Chapter 30

Nursing Care of Clients with Cerebral Disorders

CEREBROVASCULAR DISORDERS

Cerebrovascular disorders are those problems that result from inadequate blood supply to the brain. Stroke is probably the first disorder that comes to mind in considering cerebrovascular disorders. Although stroke is the most common problem, cerebrovascular disorders encompass other disorders of blood supply to the brain. This section addresses vascular lesions of the brain including aneurysms and arteriovenous malformations (AVMs).

CEREBROVASCULAR ACCIDENT

Definition

A cerebrovascular accident (CVA) or stroke is infarction (death) of a specific portion of the brain due to insufficient blood supply. Stroke can occur from an occlusion (blockage) of one of the major vessels feeding the brain, a partial or complete obstruction of a major intracranial vessel, or hemorrhage within the brain. The blood vessel affected determines the area and extent of infarction.

Incidence

Cerebrovascular disorders are the third most common cause of death in the United States (preceded by heart disease and cancer). The incidence rate of stroke is approximately 0.5 to 1.0 per 1000 people.[3] Fortunately, the incidence of stroke has been declining for the past 30 years, in part as a result of the improved control of hypertension, increased diet conscious-

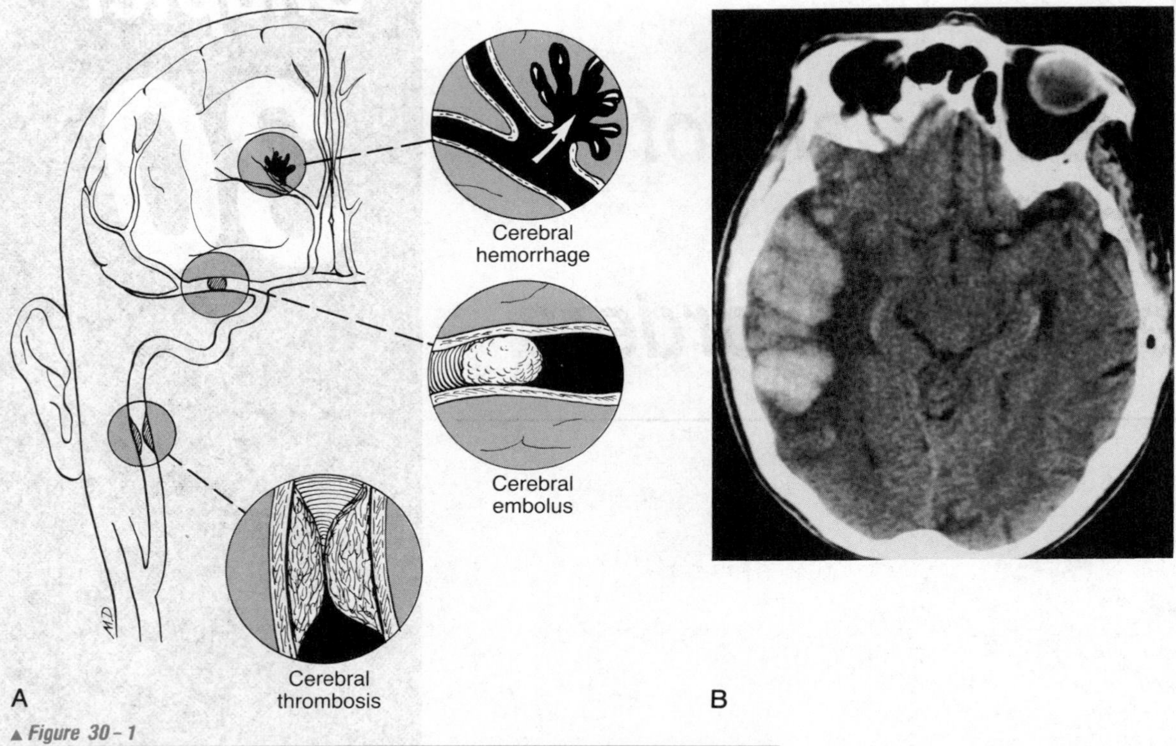

▲ Figure 30-1

A, Events causing stroke. *B*, An MRI showing hemorrhagic stroke in the left cerebrum.

ness, and a reduction in smoking in some segments of the population.

Several other important facts about stroke are noteworthy. There is a higher incidence and death rate for stroke in blacks than in whites in the United States. Stroke is found equally in men and women, with a greatly increased incidence after age 75.[21]

Etiology

Narrowing or complete closure of one of the vessels supplying the brain is the most common cause of CVA. The most common causes of CVA are thrombosis, embolism, and hemorrhage. Stroke is less common from vascular compression or arterial spasm (Fig. 30-1).

THROMBOSIS

Thrombosis is the most common cause of stroke and is usually due to atherosclerosis. Rarely, occlusion is secondary to inflammatory reactions in vessel walls. Thrombosis may occur anywhere along a carotid artery or its branches. A common site is at the bifurcation of the common carotid into the internal and external carotid arteries.

EMBOLISM

Cerebral embolism is the occlusion of a cerebral vessel by emboli (i.e., fragments of clotted blood, tumor, fat, bacteria, or air). Typically, cerebral embolism is associated with heart disease in which fragments of clotted blood or bacterial vegetations are released from the heart's walls or valves and lodge in the cerebral arterial system. The embolus most often lodges at the bifurcation of the middle cerebral artery. The incidence of cerebral embolism increases after the age of 40 years.

INTRACEREBRAL HEMORRHAGE

Intracerebral hemorrhage results from rupture of a cerebral vessel that causes bleeding into brain tissue. Intracerebral hemorrhage, due to arteriosclerosis and hypertension, is most common after age 50 years. These hemorrhages usually produce extensive residual function loss and have the slowest recovery of all types of stroke. Large hemorrhages usually come from arteries. Small ones may come from the veins and capillaries. Bleeding may also occur from subarachnoid hemorrhage or vascular malformations. The effects of intracerebral hemorrhages depend on the site and extent of the hemorrhage. Brain herniation causes death in more than 50 per cent of clients within the first 3 days after intracerebral hemorrhage.

SPASM

Cerebral arterial spasm, due to some irritation of the outer part of the arterial wall, reduces blood flow to the area of brain supplied by the constricted vessel.

Box 30–1. Risk Factors Related to Stroke

Prior ischemic episodes
Cardiac disease: myocardial infarction (emboli of the heart, especially with arrhythmias), coronary artery disease, left ventricular hypertrophy, congestive heart failure
Diabetes mellitus
Atherosclerotic disease of intracranial and extracranial vessels
Hypertension
Polycythemia
Hypercholesterolemia
Smoking
Oral contraceptive use
Emotional stress
Obesity
Family history of stroke
Age (incidence increases with age)
Note: With some of these risk factors, the client has a choice (e.g., whether to smoke, overeat, or use oral contraceptives). Also, some strokes may be prevented or minimized by activities such as stress reduction and by a proper balance of diet, rest, and exercise.

Spasm of short duration does not necessarily cause permanent brain damage.

COMPRESSION

Compression of cerebral vessels may result from a tumor, large blood clot, swollen brain tissue, or other disorders.

Risk Factors

Box 30–1 lists risk factors related to stroke. Primary prevention focuses on education of the public. Maintenance of appropriate body weight and of cholesterol levels within normal limits lessens the likelihood of stroke, as does avoidance of smoking and oral contraceptives.

Although clients cannot change their age or family health history, there are other factors amenable to secondary prevention. Medical management and control of diabetes, hypertension, and cardiac disease decrease the stroke risk factors these diseases present. Clients need education regarding the interaction of various disease processes and how these diseases can increase the severity of each other.

Tertiary prevention addresses those individuals who have already experienced CVA. In this situation, the goal is to prevent complications related to the present stroke and future infarctions. Immobility carries significant complication risks. Injury related to paralysis and aspiration are other potential complications. Prevention of future CVAs involves minimizing all identifiable risk factors. This may represent a major change in lifestyle for the client who smokes and eats a high-fat diet. Aspirin, antiplatelet drugs, and antihypertensives may be prescribed.

Pathophysiology

To understand the pathophysiology of cerebrovascular diseases, it is important to review (1) how the brain receives its blood supply, (2) what areas of the brain are supplied by various major vessels (Fig. 30–2), and (3) the physiology of cerebral circulation (see Chap. 27).

Cerebral infarction is deprivation of blood supply to a localized area of the brain. The extent of infarction depends on factors such as the location and size of an occluded vessel and the adequacy of collateral circulation to the area supplied by the occluded vessel.

Blood supply to the brain may be altered (slowly or rapidly) by local disorders (e.g., thrombi, emboli, hemorrhage, or vascular spasms) or by generalized disorders (e.g., hypoxia from lung and heart disorders). Atherosclerotic disease often affects arteries leading to the brain but affects vessels within the brain much less often. Thrombi may form on atherosclerotic plaques, or blood may clot in an area of stenosis in which the bloodstream is slowed or turbulence occurs. Thrombi that break loose from a blood vessel wall become emboli carried in the bloodstream.

Thrombosis produces (1) ischemia in the brain tissue supplied by the affected vessel and (2) edema and congestion in the surrounding areas. The area of edema may cause greater dysfunction than the infarct itself. The edema may subside in a few hours or sometimes after several days. As the edema subsides, the client begins to improve and may regain some functions that were impaired by the edema. CVA from thrombosis is usually not fatal, unless the infarct is massive.[10]

Occlusion of cerebral vessels by an embolus causes necrosis and edema similar to that following thrombosis unless the embolus contains bacteria. If it is septic and the infection extends beyond the walls of the vessel, an abscess forms or encephalitis develops (see Encephalitis). If the infection remains contained within the occluded vessel, an aneurysmal dilation of the vessel (mycotic aneurysm) may develop. This is dangerous because cerebral hemorrhage may occur if the aneurysm ruptures.

Most hemorrhages into the brain are caused by the rupture of arteriosclerotic and hypertensive vessels. Most intracerebral hemorrhages are very large; therefore, it is not surprising that hemorrhage into the brain causes the most fatalities of all cerebrovascular diseases. Although recovery is possible after intracerebral hemorrhage, it is less likely and less complete than is recovery from stroke caused by thrombosis or embolus.

If cerebral circulation is interrupted extensively, cerebral anoxia develops, that is, lack of oxygen to the brain. In an adult, the changes caused by cerebral anoxia may be reversible for up to 4 to 6 minutes. Changes are always irreversible if cerebral anoxia lasts longer than 10 minutes. Cerebral anoxia may be caused by various disorders, the main one being cardiac arrest.

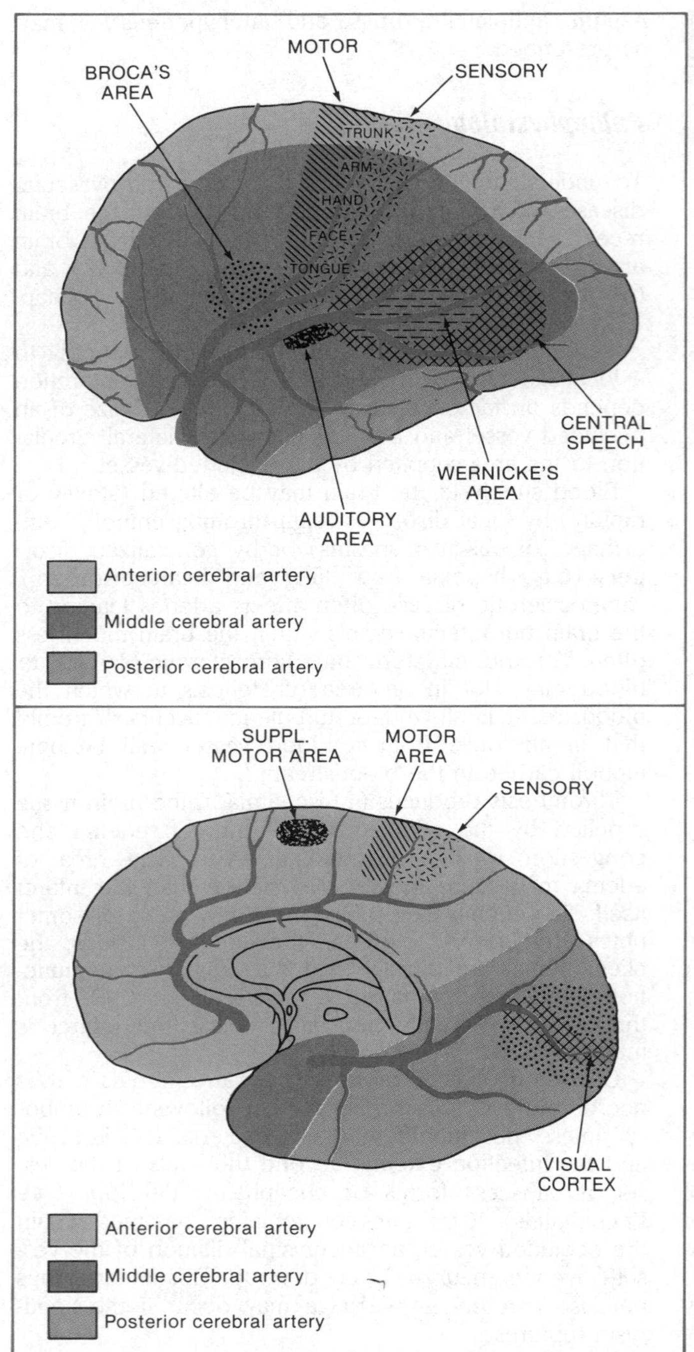

▲ *Figure 30–2*

Areas of the brain supplied with blood from the branches of the cerebral artery. (From Wyngaarden, J., & Smith, L. [1988]. *Cecil textbook of medicine*. [18th ed.]. Philadelphia: W. B. Saunders.)

Clinical Manifestations

Although they are not often recognized, focal warning signs may occur in clients with stenosis of the great vessels in the neck. Such warning signs may precede severe paralysis by a few hours or days. They include hemiplegia, transient loss of speech, and paresthesias involving half of the body. These manifestations are called transient ischemic attacks (TIAs) and should not be ignored (see later).

Five events that may precede cerebral hemorrhage in hypertensive clients are

1. severe occipital (back of head) or nuchal (nape of neck) headaches
2. vertigo (dizziness) or syncope (fainting)
3. motor or sensory disturbances (e.g., tingling, paresthesias, transient paralysis)
4. nosebleeds (epistaxis)
5. retinal hemorrhages

TABLE 30-1. Clinical Manifestations of the Various Causes of CVA

Cause	Clinical Manifestations
Thrombosis	Tends to develop during sleep or within 1 hour of arising Ischemia is produced gradually; therefore, the clinical manifestations develop more slowly than those caused by hemorrhage or emboli Relative preservation of consciousness Hypertension
Embolism	No discernible time pattern, unrelated to activity Clinical manifestations occur rapidly, within 10-30 seconds and often without warning; no headache May have rapid improvement Relative preservation of consciousness Normotension
Hemorrhage	Typically occurs during active, waking hours Severe headache occurs (if client is able to report symptoms) Rapid onset of complete hemiplegia, occurs over minutes to 1 hour; most likely form to be fatal Usually results in extensive, permanent loss of function with slower, less complete recovery Rapid progression into coma Nuchal rigidity

Other findings associated with strokes include headache, vomiting, seizures, coma, nuchal rigidity, fever, hypertension, electrocardiographic abnormalities (e.g., prolonged ST segment), sclerosis of peripheral and retinal vessels, confusion, disorientation, memory impairment, and other mental changes. Depending on the hemorrhage or infarct site, focal neurologic findings may be present (e.g., weakness or paralysis, sensory loss, language disorder, and reflex changes).

Table 30-1 correlates clinical manifestations of CVA with the cause. Table 30-2 correlates clinical manifestations with the area of brain affected.

SPECIFIC DEFICITS AFTER CVA

There are many deficits that occur with CVA. They depend on the area of the brain damaged as well as the side of the brain (e.g., dominant). The client may have more than one of the following deficits or have very little impairment after CVA.

Hemiplegia. Hemiplegia is paralysis of one side of the body. Complete hemiplegia involves one half of the face and tongue as well as the arm and leg of the same side. Hemiplegia results from damage to the (1) motor area of the cortex or (2) pyramidal tract fibers. Hemorrhage or clot in the brain's right side causes left-sided hemiplegia, and vice versa. This is because nerve fibers cross over in the pyramidal tract as they pass from the brain to the spinal cord. Other cortical areas may be affected, producing localized symptoms (e.g., hemianesthesia, hemianopia, apraxia, agnosia, aphasia).

Muscles of the thorax and abdomen are usually not paralyzed because they are innervated from both cerebral hemispheres. Sudden hemiplegia usually results from cerebral thrombosis, that is, occlusion of an artery supplying part of one side of the brain, which leads to impairment of function originating in that area.

When voluntary muscle control is destroyed, strong flexor muscles overbalance the extensors. This can cause serious deformities. For example, a hemiplegic client's affected arm tends to rotate internally and adduct, because adductor muscles are stronger than the abductors. Also, the elbow, wrist, and fingers tend to flex. The affected leg tends to rotate externally at the hip joint, flex at the knee, and plantar flex and supinate at the ankle joint (Fig. 30-3).

Aphasia. Aphasia, a defect in using and interpreting the symbols of language, is caused by a cerebral cortex disorder. Aphasia may involve any or all aspects of language use, such as speaking, reading, writing, and the understanding of spoken language. Aphasia may be (1) sensory (receptive aphasia), affecting speech comprehension, or (2) motor (expressive aphasia or executive aphasia), affecting speech production.

Sensory aphasias involve loss of the ability to comprehend written, printed, or spoken words. For example, with auditory or acoustic aphasia ("word deafness"), clients have difficulty understanding what is being said. They are not deaf. They hear sound but cannot make sense out of it because they cannot understand the symbolic communication associated with the sound. Visual aphasia ("word blindness") is similar. Affected clients cannot read words but can see them. They cannot understand the symbolic content of printed or written symbols.

Motor aphasias include aphasias in which the ability to write, make signs, or speak is lost. For example, with motor aphasia, words may be recalled, but the client cannot combine speech sounds into words and syllables. Pure motor or pure sensory aphasias are rare. Most aphasias are mixed (expressive-receptive), affecting both expressive and receptive elements.

Most aphasias are partial rather than complete. The severity of aphasia varies with the area and the extent of cerebral damage. Severe damage may deprive the client of any meaningful relationship with the environment. Global aphasia (total aphasia) is so extensive that neither expressive nor receptive language abilities are retained.

Aphasia is caused by pathologic lesions affecting specific locations in the cortex (Table 30-3). The most common cause of aphasia is vascular disease of the brain, especially involving the middle cerebral artery. Aphasia may occur if blood supply to a client's speech center is cut off. Aphasia is associated with hemiplegia

TABLE 30–2. Clinical Manifestations of CVAs Associated with Area of Brain Affected

Location	Middle Cerebral Artery	Anterior Cerebral Artery	Posterior Cerebral Artery	Internal Carotid Artery	Vertebral-Basilar System	Anteroinferior Cerebellar (Lateral Pontine)	Posteroinferior Cerebellar
Motor changes	Contralateral hemiparesis or hemiplegia	Contralateral hemiparesis, foot and leg deficits greater than arm, footdrop gait disturbances	Mild contralateral hemiparesis (with thalamic or subthalamic involvement) Intention tremor	Contralateral hemiparesis with facial asymmetry	Alternating motor weaknesses Ataxic gait, dysmetria (uncoordinated actions)	Ipsilateral ataxia Facial paralysis	Ataxia Paralysis of larynx and soft palate
Sensory changes	Contralateral hemisensory alterations Neglect of involved extremities	Contralateral hemisensory alterations	Diffuse sensory loss (thalamic)	Contralateral sensory alterations	Numbness of the tongue	Ipsilateral loss of sensation in face, sensation changes on trunk and limbs	Ipsilateral loss of sensation on face, contralateral on body
Visual or ocular changes	Homonymous hemianopia Inability to turn eyes toward affected side	Deviation of eyes toward affected side	Pupillary dysfunction (brain stem) Loss of conjugate gaze, nystagmus Loss of depth perception Cortical blindness Homonymous hemianopia	Heminanopia Ipsilateral periods of blindness (amaurosis fugax)	Double vision Homonymous hemianopia Nystagmus, conjugate gaze paralysis	Nystagmus	Nystagmus
Speech changes	Dyslexia, dysgraphia, aphasia	Expressive aphasia	Perseveration Dyslexia	Dysphagia	Dysarthria, dysphagia		Dysarthria, dysphagia, dysphonia
Mental changes		Confusion, amnesia Flat affect, apathy Shortened attention span Loss of mental acuity	Memory deficits		Memory loss Disorientation		
Other changes	Vomiting may occur	Apraxia (inability to carry out purposeful movements in nonaffected areas)	Visual hallucinations	Mild Horner's syndrome Carotid bruits	Drop attacks Tinnitus, hearing loss	Horner's syndrome Tinnitus, hearing loss	Horner's syndrome Hiccoughs and coughing

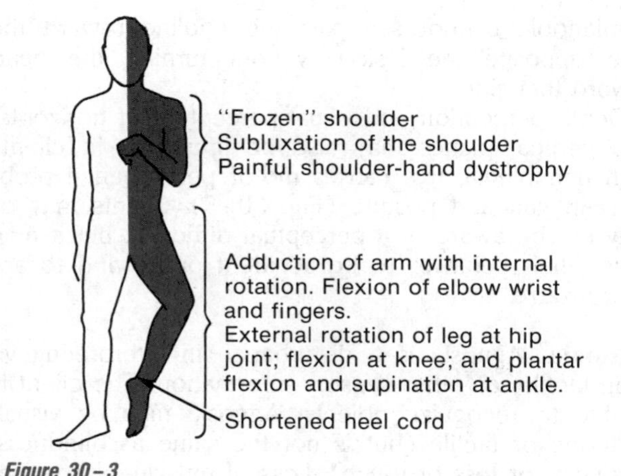

▲ *Figure 30–3*

Hemiplegic deformities to be prevented. Note that the elbow is bent, the wrist is flexed, and the fingers are curled into palmar flexion; the knee is bent and the heel cord shortened. (Illustration by K. C. Sorensen.)

involving the dominant hemisphere. The speech center for a right-handed client is located in the left cerebral hemisphere. The speech center for a left-handed client may be in the brain's right side. Thus, a right-handed client with a right-sided hemiplegia may have aphasia, because the speech center is in the damaged left hemisphere.

Apraxia. Apraxia is a condition in which a client can move the affected part but cannot use it for specific purposeful actions (e.g., walking, speaking, or dressing). The part is not paralyzed or uncoordinated. An apraxic client can conceive or conceptualize the content of messages to send to muscles (e.g., "stand"). However, it is impossible to reconstruct the motor patterns or schema necessary to convey the impulse message. Thus, accurate "instructions" do not reach the limb from the brain, and the desired action or movement does not happen.

Apraxia ranges from relatively simple to highly com-

TABLE 30–3. Types of Aphasia

Type of Aphasia	Clinical Manifestations	Affected Brain Area
Global aphasia	Spontaneous speech absent or limited to a few stereotyped words Comprehension reduced to client's name or few words	Posterior and anterior cortical areas
Nonfluent aphasia	Telegraphic speech, conjunctions and pronouns not used Repetition and reading aloud impaired Naming may show paraphasias Auditory and reading comprehension intact Frustration, agitation, depression	Anterior speech area Right-sided hemiplegia
Fluent aphasia	Severe disturbance in auditory comprehension Speech is well articulated but lacks meaningful content, is unrelated to questions, has paraphasias Client seems unaware he or she does not make sense; reading and writing are impaired	Posterior language area
Conduction aphasia	Fluent, halting speech; word finding pauses; paraphasias Comprehension good, naming disturbed, reading unimpaired; writing shows errors in spelling, word choice, syntax	Supramarginal gyrus and arcuate fasciculus between anterior and posterior areas
Anomic aphasia	Word finding difficulty, inability to name objects on confrontation Repetition good May have alexia (inability to read) and/or agraphia (inability to write)	Can be caused by lesions in many parts of dominant hemisphere
Articulation disturbances (dysarthrias)	Buccofacial apraxia (inability to control muscles needed for speech) Dysfluency (stuttering or stammering)	Lesions between supramarginal gyrus and frontal lobe Etiology not known

From Chenitz, W., et al. (1991). *Clinical gerontological nursing.* Philadelphia: W. B. Saunders; adapted from Strub, R., & Black, F. W. (Eds.)(1985). *The mental status examination in neurology.* Philadelphia: F. A. Davis.

plex disorders. It may occur in any or all modalities and may vary from one modality to another; for example, a client may have less difficulty writing than speaking, or vice versa.

In hemiplegic clients, apraxic and agnosic states generally occur along with other symptoms. Such clients are at great risk of injury and have a poor prognosis for functional recovery.

Visual Changes. Lesions in the parietal and temporal lobes may interrupt visual fibers of the optic tract (en route to the occipital cortex) and produce visual defects. A lesion on one side of the brain produces a defect in the opposite half of the visual field. Such defects occur in the same visual field of each eye.

Visual deficiency problems are often associated with hemiplegia and may prevent the client from seeing recognizable cues. Visual disorders may interfere with a client's ability to relearn motor skills and increase the risk of accidents.

Homonymous Hemianopia. Homonymous hemianopia (Fig. 30-4) is defective vision or visual loss in the same half of the visual field of each eye, so the client sees only one half of normal vision. For example, the client may see clearly on one side of the midline, but nothing on the other side. Clients with homonymous hemianopia cannot see past the midline toward the side opposite the lesion without turning the head toward that side.

Depth perception and visual perception of horizontal and vertical planes may also be impaired. In clients with hemiplegia, this causes motor performance problems in gait and posture (Fig. 30-5). Clients may or may not be aware of a perceptual difficulty, but it may cause their behavior to be accident prone and to appear bizarre.

Agnosia. Agnosia is a disturbance in interpreting visual, tactile, or other sensory information. The client is unable to recognize objects. Agnosia may be visual, auditory, or tactile (but is not the same as blindness, deafness, or loss of touch). Loss of muscle-joint sensation may be accompanied by inaccurate beliefs about the position of a limb in space or its existence or ownership. For example, a man with agnosia may not feel his arm is part of his body, he may be unaware of his arm's position, or he may deny that a limb is paralyzed when it is.

Another type of agnosia affects only one half of external space. Objects on one side are correctly interpreted, whereas those on the other side are not; for example, a client may be able to tell time only if it is between 12 and 6 o'clock and not between 6 and 12

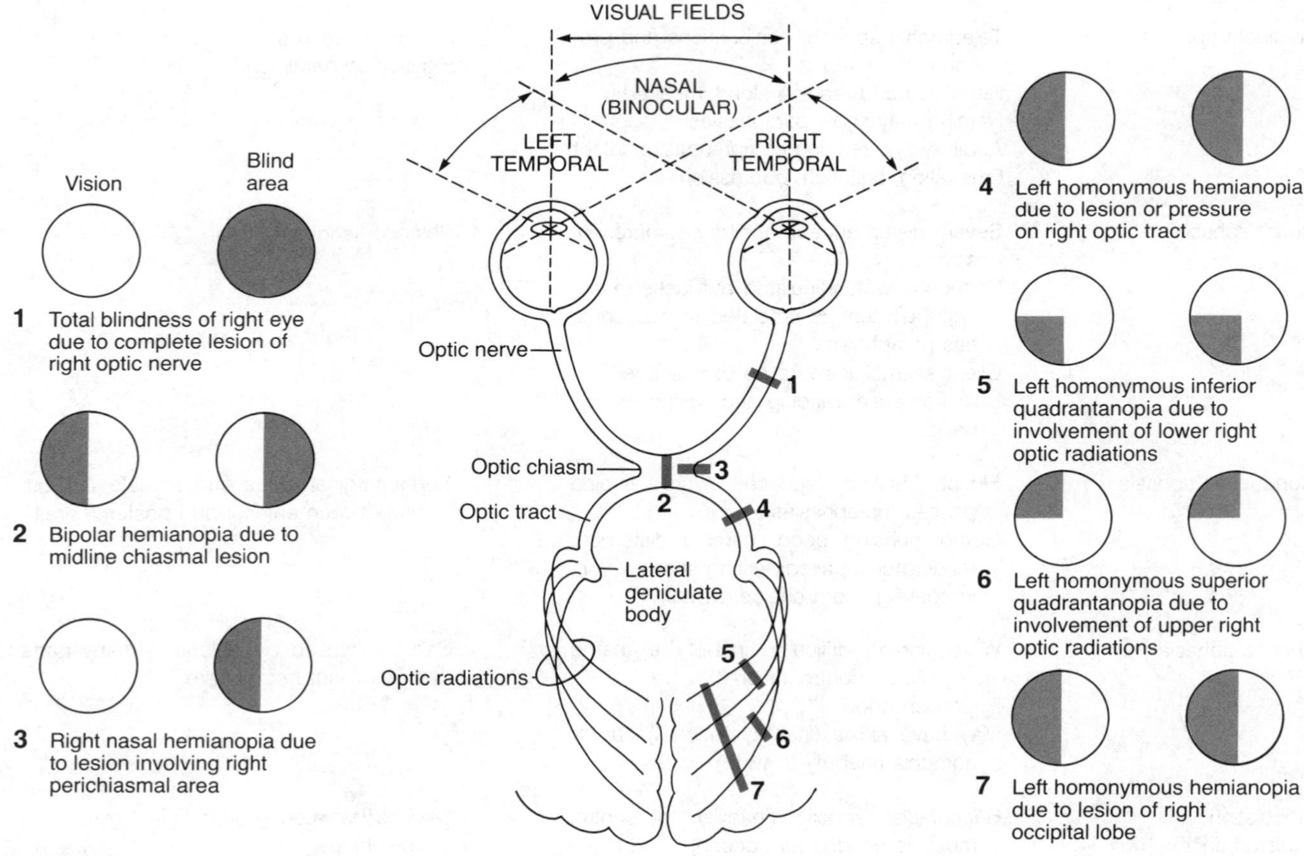

▲ ***Figure 30-4***

Visual field defects associated with optic nerve lesions.

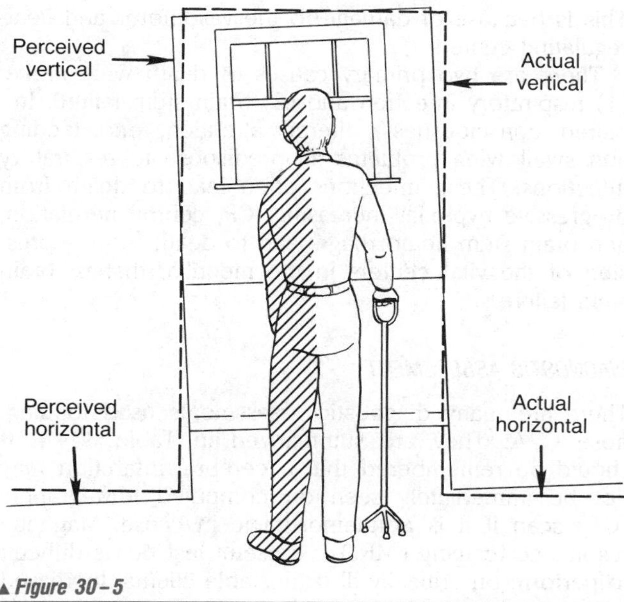

▲ Figure 30–5

Perceptual disturbance in hemiplegia. Such disturbances can be unpleasant and unsafe to experience.

o'clock. A client with this condition (neglecting the left half of space) usually has a right brain injury causing left hemiplegia and tends to avert the head and eyes to the right.

A client with visual agnosia sees objects but is unable to recognize or attach meaning to them. Disorientation occurs because of inability to recognize environmental cues, familiar faces, or symbols. Such a client may examine objects curiously but be unable to know their function. This can cause considerable self-care deficit when common, necessary objects such as silverware, clothing, or toilet articles are unfamiliar.

Visual agnosia greatly increases risk of injury because the client cannot recognize danger or symbols warning of danger. Extensive visual agnosia can produce such extreme behavioral effects that the client may be inaccurately diagnosed as having diffuse dementia.

Dysarthria. Dysarthria (anarthria) is imperfect articulation that causes difficulty in speaking. It is important to differentiate between dysarthric and aphasic speech. With dysarthria, the client understands language but has difficulty pronouncing words and may slur them, enunciating poorly. There is no disturbance in grammar or in phrase or sentence construction. A dysarthric client can understand verbal speech and can read and write (unless the dominant hand is paralyzed, absent, or injured).

Dysarthria is due to cranial nerve dysfunction. It may result from weakness or paralysis of the muscles of lips, tongue, and larynx or from a loss of sensation. In addition to speaking problems, clients with dysarthria often have difficulty chewing and swallowing food because of poor muscle control. Dysarthria is a problem for clients with bulbar disorders.

Kinesthesia. Kinesthesias are alterations in sensation. They occur on the affected side of the body and include (1) hemianesthesia (loss of sensation), (2) paresthesia (feelings of heaviness, numbness, tingling, prickling, heightened sensitivity), and (3) loss of muscle-joint sense. Hemianesthesia is generally incomplete and may not be noticed by the client. Paresthesia occasionally manifests in a hemiplegic client as persistent, boring pain, that is, thalamic pain (see Chap. 16). Proprioception and postural sense disturbance may occur with loss of muscle-joint sense. This may interfere seriously with the ability to ambulate because of lack of balance control and inappropriate movements. The risk of falling is high because of the tendency to misplace the feet when walking.

Incontinence. Bowel and bladder incontinence do not result from all types of stroke. There is no physiologic reason for a client with a unilateral hemisphere lesion to be incontinent. Incontinence in hemiplegic clients occurs because of (1) inattention, (2) memory lapses, (3) emotional factors, or (4) inability to communicate.

Shoulder Pain. Many clients have severe pain in the affected shoulder after CVA. This pain can be so severe that it restricts mobility and self-care because of the lack of balance and loss of range of motion (ROM). The problem can be aggravated by overstretching from turns and transfers. Some clients have experienced subluxation (partial dislocation) of the shoulder both from having the shoulder pulled on and from the weight of the arm pulling it. Chronic subluxation results in shoulder-hand syndrome (characterized by a painful or frozen shoulder and hand edema).

Horner's Syndrome. Horner's syndrome is the paralysis of sympathetic nerves to the eye, causing sinking of the eyeball, ptosis of the upper eyelid, slight elevation of the lower lid, constriction of the pupil, and lack of tearing in the eye.

Unilateral Neglect. Unilateral neglect is described as a deficit of looking, listening, touching, and searching as opposed to a deficit of seeing, hearing, feeling, or moving. Clients with neglect often have intact vision but will not look at or search for specific areas of the environment. Clients with injury to the temporoparietal lobe, inferior parietal lobe, lateral frontal lobe, cingulate gyrus, thalamus, and striatum most commonly develop neglect. Because of the dominance of the right hemisphere in directing attention, neglect is most commonly seen in clients with right hemisphere damage. Clinical manifestations of neglect appear on the contralateral side to the lesion and include failure to attend to one side of the body, failure to report or respond to stimuli on one side of the body, failure to use one extremity, and failure to orient the head and eyes to the one side.[12]

Other Deficits. The client may also have difficulty in localizing objects within the environment and estimating their size or distance. The client may have difficulty finding routes or following directions to new places. This is due in part to problems with memory, spatial perception, and loss of direction.

Some clients will lose their ability to recognize numbers; this will prohibit them from using a phone or telling time. The client may also have an inability to discriminate right from left.

There are various portions of the brain that assist with behavioral control and coping. The cerebral cortex interprets various stimuli. The temporal and limbic areas modulate emotional responses to stimuli. The hypothalamus and pituitary coordinate the motor cortex and language areas. The brain can be seen as an inhibitor of emotions, and when the brain is not fully functional, emotional reactions and responses lack this inhibition.

After CVA, clients are often emotionally labile, confused, forgetful, and frustrated. They tend to burst into tears or (less commonly) laughter without provocation. Clients may also use profanity, which is often termed automatic language. Also, they may appear highly distressed but not feel distress. This condition is not the same as an affective depressed state.

Other emotional or behavioral reactions may occur, including

- severe mood swings
- social withdrawal (especially in aphasic and dysphasic clients)
- inappropriate sexual behavior
- outbursts of frustration and anger
- regression to earlier behavior, perhaps childlike

Complications

Complications of stroke depend primarily on the location of the lesion or infarcted tissue. If the brain stem is affected, blood pressure fluctuations, altered respiratory patterns, and cardiac dysrhythmias are all possible. Aspiration, immobility, and injury related to the client's not realizing his or her physical limitations are other potential complications.

Coma can follow stroke from various causes. The blood supply to the brain stem or reticular activating system may have been directly occluded. Likewise, the deep structures of the thalamus that relay information to the cerebral cortex may be involved. Vascular occlusion of the internal carotid artery or one of its major branches may also decrease the level of consciousness. Sometimes, the cerebral edema that follows stroke may produce midline shifts resulting in coma.

Strokes due to occlusal disease (thrombus, embolus) rarely cause sudden death. When sudden death does occur, it is usually due to heart failure. However, if an intracerebral hemorrhage ruptures into the ventricles, symptoms of increased intracranial pressure (ICP) develop, and the outcome is fatal. When stroke is fatal, death may occur within 3 to 12 hours but is more usual between 1 and 14 days after the original episode. Typically, with any type of fatal stroke, a rise in temperature, heart rate, and respiratory rate occurs along with deepening coma several hours or days before death. This is because of damage to the vasomotor and heat-regulating centers.

There are two primary causes of death with stroke: (1) respiratory infection and (2) brain stem failure. Impaired consciousness, altered attention, and feeding and swallowing problems all predispose to respiratory infections. These infections often lead to death from progressive hypoxia. Increasing ICP, central herniation, and brain stem hemorrhage lead to death from depression of the vital centers in the medulla, that is, brain stem failure.

DIAGNOSTIC ASSESSMENT

There are many diagnostic assessments used to diagnose CVA. They are summarized in Table 30–4. It should be remembered that a cerebral infarction may not be immediately seen on computed tomographic (CT) scan if it is nonhemorrhagic in cause. Magnetic resonance imaging (MRI) is a useful test but is difficult to perform on critically ill or unstable clients. Increased ICP must be ruled out before a lumbar puncture is performed in order to minimize the risk of herniation.

Medical Management

Medical management of the client after CVA is directed toward (1) preserving life, (2) minimizing residual deformity, (3) reducing ICP, and (4) preventing extension or recurrence. Specific treatment goals and interventions are used in the treatment of the various causes of CVA.

The client is placed at bed rest with the head elevated to 30 degrees to reduce ICP and facilitate venous drainage. Sometimes, external ventriculostomy drainage is used for a few days to reduce pressure from cerebrospinal fluid (CSF) accumulation. Blood pressure and level of consciousness (LOC) are closely monitored. The goal is to maintain blood pressure enough to prevent another stroke or hemorrhage but not to the point at which cerebral perfusion is decreased. Because many clients with hemorrhagic stroke have a history of hypertension, it is common to maintain their systolic blood pressure at 150 to 160 mm Hg. Fluids are administered carefully for avoidance of fluid volume excess and further cerebral ischemia. The client may require continuous mechanical ventilation and may develop coma.

Rehabilitation begins during this acute period after the CVA. Interventions directed at preserving ROM and muscle tone are beneficial. In addition, the family is taught about the condition of stroke and what they can do to promote the client's independence.

OCCLUSIVE STROKE

The sudden occlusion of a major artery or blood supply to a large portion of the brain is usually poorly tolerated, especially in the elderly. If the dominant hemisphere is involved, aggressive medical management may not be considered if there is slim rehabilita-

TABLE 30–4. Diagnostic Assessment Findings in Cerebrovascular Disorders

	Intracerebral Hemorrhage	Cerebral Thrombosis	Cerebral Embolism	Subarachnoid Hemorrhage	Vascular Malformation and Intracranial Bleeding
History and related disorders	Suspect diagnosis, especially if other hemorrhagic manifestations are present, and in acute leukemia, aplastic anemia, thrombocytopenic purpura, and cirrhosis of the liver	Evidence of arteriosclerosis, especially coronary, peripheral vessels, aorta; associated disorders: diabetes mellitus, xanthomatosis	Evidence of recent emboli: (1) other organs (spleen, kidneys, lungs), extremities, intestines; (2) several regions of brain in different cerebrovascular areas	History of recurrent stiff neck, headaches, subarachnoid bleeding	History of repeated subarachnoid hemorrhages, epilepsy
Special findings	Hypertensive retinopathy, cardiac hypertrophy, and other evidence of hypertensive cerebrovascular disease may be present	Evidence of arteriosclerotic cardiovascular disease frequently present	Cardiac dysrhythmias or infarction (source of emboli usually in the heart)	Subhyaloid (preretinal) hemorrhages Focal neurologic signs frequently absent; nuchal rigidity, positive finding of Kernig's and Brudzinski's signs	Subhyaloid (preretinal) hemorrhages and retinal angioma Focal neurologic signs; cranial bruit
CSF	Grossly bloody	Clear	Clear	Grossly bloody	Grossly bloody
Skull radiography	Shift of pineal to opposite side	Calcification of internal carotid artery siphon visible; shift of pineal to opposite side may occur	Pineal apt to show little if any displacement	Partial calcification of walls of aneurysm sometimes noted	Characteristic calcifications in skull films may be present
Cerebral angiography	Hemorrhagic area seen as vascular zone surrounded by stretched and displaced arteries and veins	Arterial obstruction or narrowing of circle of Willis (internal carotid, etc.)	Arterial obstruction of circle of Willis branches (internal carotid, etc.)	Typical aneurysmal pattern in circle of Willis arteries (internal carotid, middle cerebral, anterior cerebral, etc.)	Characteristic pattern showing cerebral arteriovenous malformation
Brain scan	May show increased uptake in affected cerebral area; most marked in 2–3 weeks, with diminution or clearing thereafter			Apt to be normal	Increased uptake may be seen in area of arteriovenous malformation
Echoencephalography	May show shift of midline toward opposite side in clients with a cerebral lesion acting as a mass				
Computed tomography (CT) and magnetic resonance imaging (MRI)	May show area of hematoma, infarct, or the like with distortion or shift of ventricles				

From Chusid, J. G. (1985). *Correlative neuroanatomy and functional neurology* (19th ed.). Los Altos, CA: Lange Medical Publications.

tive potential. The choices of whether to pursue aggressive treatment focus on a number of factors. How old is the client? What other disorders are present, and how stable are these problems? How large is the area of infarction? What is the potential for rehabilitation? At present, the treatment for the majority of clients with large areas of infarction is supportive care. It is hoped that future research can improve the treatment outcomes for these clients.

EMBOLIC STROKE

The usual cause of embolism is cardiac disorders. Atrial fibrillation, cardiac valve disorders, valve prostheses, and bacterial endocarditis are common disorders that result in thrombus formation. The thrombi break loose (embolize) and travel to the brain. Treatment is directed at resolution of the underlying problem for preventing further emboli.

HEMORRHAGIC STROKE

Treatment of hemorrhagic stroke depends in part on the condition of the client when first seen. A client who is seen with a severe headache but who is fully conscious will probably survive no matter what the therapy. The client who is in a coma is likely to do poorly despite intensive medical or surgical intervention.[16]

Hypoxia often occurs in these clients because of inadequate ventilatory effort. Intubation and continuous mechanical ventilation may be required to prevent injury to the brain from hypoxia.

Often intracranial hemorrhage is accompanied by hyperthermia. This condition increases oxygen use by the brain at a time when the oxygen supply is compromised. Antipyretics may be prescribed. In addition, a hypothermia blanket or ice packs may be required to reduce body temperature. Causing the client to shiver should be avoided, however, because shivering increases oxygen consumption and ICP.

STROKE IN EVOLUTION

In clients in whom the cerebral infarction is still evolving, the eventual area of defect is controllable. Treatment centers on improving cerebral blood flow by avoiding fluid volume deficits and hypotension. In addition, hypoxia is also controlled by administration of oxygen and maintenance of a patent airway. The use of tissue plasminogen activator (tPA) and other medications to dissolve the clot has been met with mixed results.

PHARMACOLOGIC MANAGEMENT

Steroids or osmotic diuretics may be used to reduce ICP. Hypertension is commonly controlled with antihypertensives and diuretics.

Anticoagulants are commonly used initially through intravenous routes and then orally. Monitoring of clotting times is important for preventing overanticoagulation, which increases the risk of bleeding.

Headache and neck stiffness can usually be treated with mild analgesics, such as codeine and acetaminophen. Stronger narcotics are usually avoided; these agents sedate the client and can make neurologic assessment inaccurate.

If the client develops seizures, phenytoin (Dilantin) or phenobarbital may be used. Barbiturates and other sedative agents are avoided. If the client develops fever, antipyretics may be prescribed.

DIETARY MANAGEMENT

Because of the high risk for aspiration, choking, excessive coughing, and vomiting, oral food and fluids are generally withheld for 24 to 48 hours. If the client cannot eat or drink after 48 hours, alternative feeding routes are used, such as tube feeding or hyperalimentation. When the swallowing mechanism has returned, the client can be fed orally.

Surgical Management

Several criteria are used to determine candidates for rapid evacuation of the hematoma in clients with hemorrhagic stroke or bleeding on the dominant side. Clients who usually survive surgery are those who are under the age of 70, or who open their eyes and follow commands on the unaffected side. Another guide commonly used in the determination of the need for surgery is ICP. Pressures below 20 mm Hg are usually managed without surgery; pressures above 30 mm Hg often require surgery. Clients who have large areas of blood removed have been shown to recover a substantial portion of speech. Clients with relatively large areas of superficial cerebral bleeding or shifts may also require surgery. Likewise, clients who suddenly deteriorate from lethargy to unconsciousness may benefit from surgery. Surgery is usually not performed on clients with bleeding in the basal ganglia or thalamus.

Surgery is also performed on some intracranial aneurysms and on the carotid arteries (carotid endarterectomy) to reduce the risk of CVA. These operations are discussed later in this chapter.

Nursing Management

ASSESSMENT

The initial assessment of the client with CVA is very important. The assessment must be complete and accurate to provide a baseline for ongoing assessments. The client who is awake and alert should be taught about the pathologic process and instructed to inform the nurse about any changes in sensation, movement, or function regardless of how minor they may seem. Increasing neurologic deficit indicates either progression of the infarct or ischemia of the area from cerebral edema or bleeding. Changes in neurologic assessments must be reported promptly to the physician. Neurologic assessment and the Glasgow Coma Scale are discussed in Chapters 28 and 29.

A complete history of the presenting problem as well as past medical and social history will provide data about the problem source of the CVA. For example, a history of hypertension or cardiac valvular disorders is commonly associated with CVA.

Ongoing assessments of the neurologic status and vital signs are imperative. These assessments may be required as often as hourly for unstable clients. Assessment data must be analyzed, and if the client is deteriorating (decreasing LOC, changes in motor or sensory function, pupillary changes, respiratory difficulty, development of visual or perceptual defects or aphasia), the physician should be notified. Assessment of hemiplegia includes the repeated assessment of motor function (spontaneous movement), sensation, and reflex activity.

Nursing Diagnosis: Tissue Perfusion, Altered Cerebral, High Risk for R/T increased ICP.

Planning: Expected Outcomes. The client will experience no increase in ICP, as evidenced by type A waves, no reports of headache, no decreases in LOC, and stable or improving Glasgow Coma Scale score.

Implementation. The client's ICP should be monitored hourly. The physician should be notified of sustained rises in pressure. Ongoing neurologic assessments must be performed frequently and comparisons made with previous data.

Delirium and restlessness should be controlled, with sedatives if necessary. The nurse should be certain, however, that preventable causes of restlessness, such as a full bladder, bowel impaction, or pain, are not the cause. Restraints should be avoided, because they often increase agitation.

Fever should be treated with antipyretics. Sometimes a hypothermia blanket or ice packs may be required to bring down a high temperature rapidly. Shivering should be avoided. Sometimes keeping the client's feet warm will prevent shivering. For other clients, the use of phenothiazines may be required.

Straining with stool or with excessive coughing, vomiting, lifting, or use of the arms to change position should be avoided. Mild laxatives and stool softeners are often prescribed.

Nursing Diagnosis: Physical Mobility, Impaired R/T paralysis.

Planning: Expected Outcomes. The client will have maximal physical mobility, as evidenced by absence of tendon contractures, joint ankylosis, and muscle shortening and effective use of adaptive devices.

Implementation. Proper positioning, turning, and exercising of a hemiplegic client can prevent many deformities and complications.

Positioning. Change a hemiplegic client's position every 2 hours. Position the client mainly on the unaffected side, with brief periods on the affected side or supine to relieve pressure. When positioning on the affected side, make sure that body weight does not harm paralyzed limbs. Allow the client to sit upright for short periods only, because this position can contribute to hip flexion deformity. Do not place a pillow under the affected knee when the client is supine. This encourages flexion deformity and impedes circulation. If there is a tendency to develop hyperextension of the knee, however, place a folded towel under the knee for short periods while the client is lying supine. When the client is on one side, do not flex the upper thigh acutely (also to avoid hip flexion deformity). Position the client prone for 15 to 30 minutes several times a day, with a small pillow under the pelvis (from the umbilicus to the upper third of the thigh) to hyperextend the hip joints.

Prevent footdrop by avoiding pressure, performing frequent passive ROM exercises, and having the client sit in a chair as soon as possible with the feet flat on the floor. A footboard prevents the weight of bedclothes from causing footdrop and heel cord shortening and plantar flexion. High-top tennis shoes can also be worn in bed to keep the foot at 90 degrees of flexion.

A trochanter roll, extending from the crest of the ilium to midthigh, prevents external hip rotation by wedging under the projection of the greater trochanter and stopping the femur from rolling.

Support the affected leg when turning and positioning a hemiplegic client. Complete hip dislocation can occur if the flaccid leg falls forward and downward when the client is turned onto the unaffected side. Place a pillow between the client's legs to provide support. At night, apply a padded posterior splint to the affected leg to maintain correct positioning and prevent leg flexion.

When the client is in bed, prevent adduction of the affected shoulder by placing a pillow in the axilla, between the upper arm and chest wall, to keep the arm abducted about 60 degrees. Keep the arm slightly flexed in a neutral position. Place the forearm on another pillow in a modified "Statue of Liberty" position, with the elbow above the shoulder and the wrist above the elbow. This position stretches the shoulder's internal rotators. Elevating the arm also helps prevent edema and resultant fibrosis.

Place the affected hand in a position of function, that is, slight supination with fingers slightly flexed and thumb in opposition. Use a hand roll or splint to prevent finger flexion and thumb adduction. Frequent passive ROM exercises are important. If the wrist and fingers are spastic, use a splint (Fig. 30-6) to prevent flexion contracture. Some physicians believe the common practice of giving a client a ball of yarn or a rubber ball to squeeze is harmful because it promotes flexion when extension is desirable.

Exercises in Bed. Encouraging clients with hemiplegia to exercise while they are still in bed not only prepares

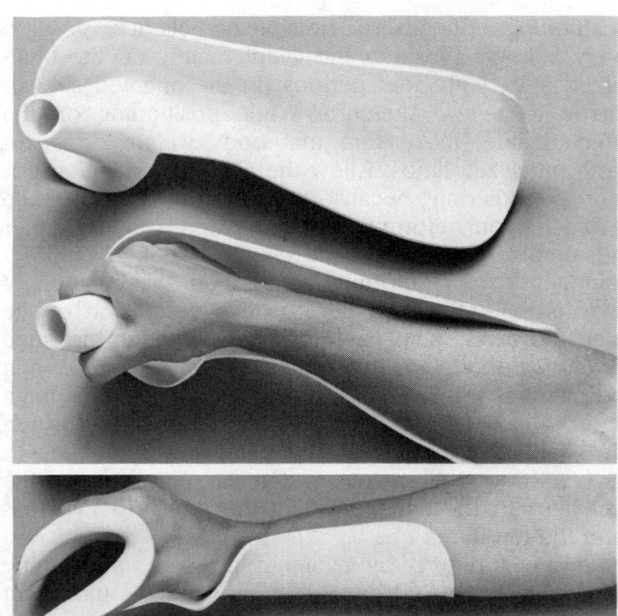

▲ Figure 30–6

Hand splints. (Courtesy of Rolyan Medical Products, Menomonee Falls, WI.)

for later activities but also offers hope and a sense of optimism about recovery. A hemiplegic client can learn to move the paralyzed leg by sliding the unaffected leg under it to lift and move the paralyzed leg. Hourly gluteal muscle setting and quadriceps muscle setting exercises during the day help prepare for later ambulation. Begin with 5 repetitions and increase gradually to 20 repetitions each time. Instruct the client as follows.

- Gluteal setting: "Pinch" or contract the buttocks together and count to five. Then relax and count to five. Repeat.
- Quadriceps setting: Contract the quadriceps muscles, on the anterior portion of the thigh, while raising the heel and trying to push the popliteal space down against the mattress. While keeping the muscle contracted, count to five; then relax and count to five. Repeat. Perform on each extremity if possible. Start quadriceps setting exercise as soon as the client is conscious. The quadriceps muscle is the most important in giving knee joint stability in walking.

Range-of-Motion Exercises. Perform passive ROM exercises four times daily after the first 24 hours following a stroke unless otherwise prescribed. Motor impulses usually begin to return between 2 and 14 days afterward. The affected part (initially flaccid) becomes spastic as the spinal cord motor systems establish their autonomy. Potential for contractures increases. Passive exercises are more difficult to perform once affected muscles begin to tighten. Do not force extremities beyond the point of initiating pain or continuous spasm.

Frequent passive ROM exercises prevent joint immobility, tendon contractures, and muscle atrophy and weakness. They also stimulate circulation and help reestablish neuromuscular pathways.

Once some voluntary movement returns, encourage the client with assisted movements. Support paralyzed arms during such movements with sling-suspensions. As movement strength increases, resisted movements may strengthen weakened muscles and help restore muscle bulk.

The weight of an immobile arm may cause (1) pain and movement limitation ("frozen shoulder") due to shoulder joint fibrositis or (2) subluxation, that is, incomplete dislocation of the shoulder joint. Prevent these by supporting a completely flaccid arm in a sling when the client is walking and on a pillow when the client is in bed or seated in a chair. Teach the client to use the unaffected hand to lift the paralyzed arm from the sling periodically and put it through ROM exercises. Exercise each finger separately. Also teach the client, while in bed, to (1) exercise the affected arm by grasping it at the wrist with the unaffected hand and raising it above the head and (2) stretch and rub the fingers of the affected hand several times each day.

Sitting Up. Help the client out of bed as soon as it is medically permitted. Remember, however, that hemiplegia severely affects the client's balance. Assistance is needed to provide security and safety. Raise the client's head slowly in bed to reduce the risk of injury from orthostatic hypotension.

When the client first sits up, support the paralyzed side, especially the back and head. Gradually the client learns to sit alone with the head of the bed elevated, and then to sit on the edge of the bed, with feet on a firm surface. Help the client maintain balance by extending the affected arm and placing its palm flat on the bed. Be patient and encouraging as the client regains balance.

Eventually the client learns to raise the paralyzed leg with the unaffected leg and swing both legs laterally over the side of the bed onto the floor. It is safest to have the client pivot on the unaffected leg. Therefore, position the chair at a right angle to the unaffected side.

Wheelchair. A hemiplegic client needs to learn safe transfers from bed to chair, commode, or wheelchair. One method is shown in the Client Education Guide. The client with unilateral paralysis can propel a wheelchair with the unaffected arm and leg; also, one-arm-drive wheelchairs are available. Once in a wheelchair, a client's level of independence increases greatly.

Using a wheelchair is helpful, but walking is best. A tilt table may be used to assume a standing position if there is difficulty with balance. Begin standing practice as soon as the quadriceps muscles on the unaffected side have normal strength. Have the client seated on the edge of the bed. Encourage the client to rise, using the muscle power of the unaffected leg. The client may tend to swing around toward the affected side. Gradually, the client learns to take increasing amounts of weight onto the weaker side. In spite of weakness in the affected limb, a hemiplegic client often develops an

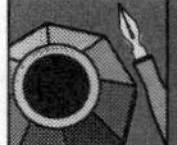

CLIENT EDUCATION GUIDE

Transfer to Wheelchair

Transfer from bed to wheelchair by a hemiplegic client. (Shading on right side of client indicates the affected side.) Lock the wheelchair for safety and keep it placed beside the bed on your nonaffected side. Use your nonaffected arm and leg (*A* and *B*) to move your affected arm and leg. As your legs drop over the edge of the bed, swing your torso up to a sitting position (*C*). Push yourself up to a standing position (*D*) by using your nonaffected arm and leg. Reach across the wheelchair (*E*) to grasp the far arm of the chair, and turn to seat yourself.

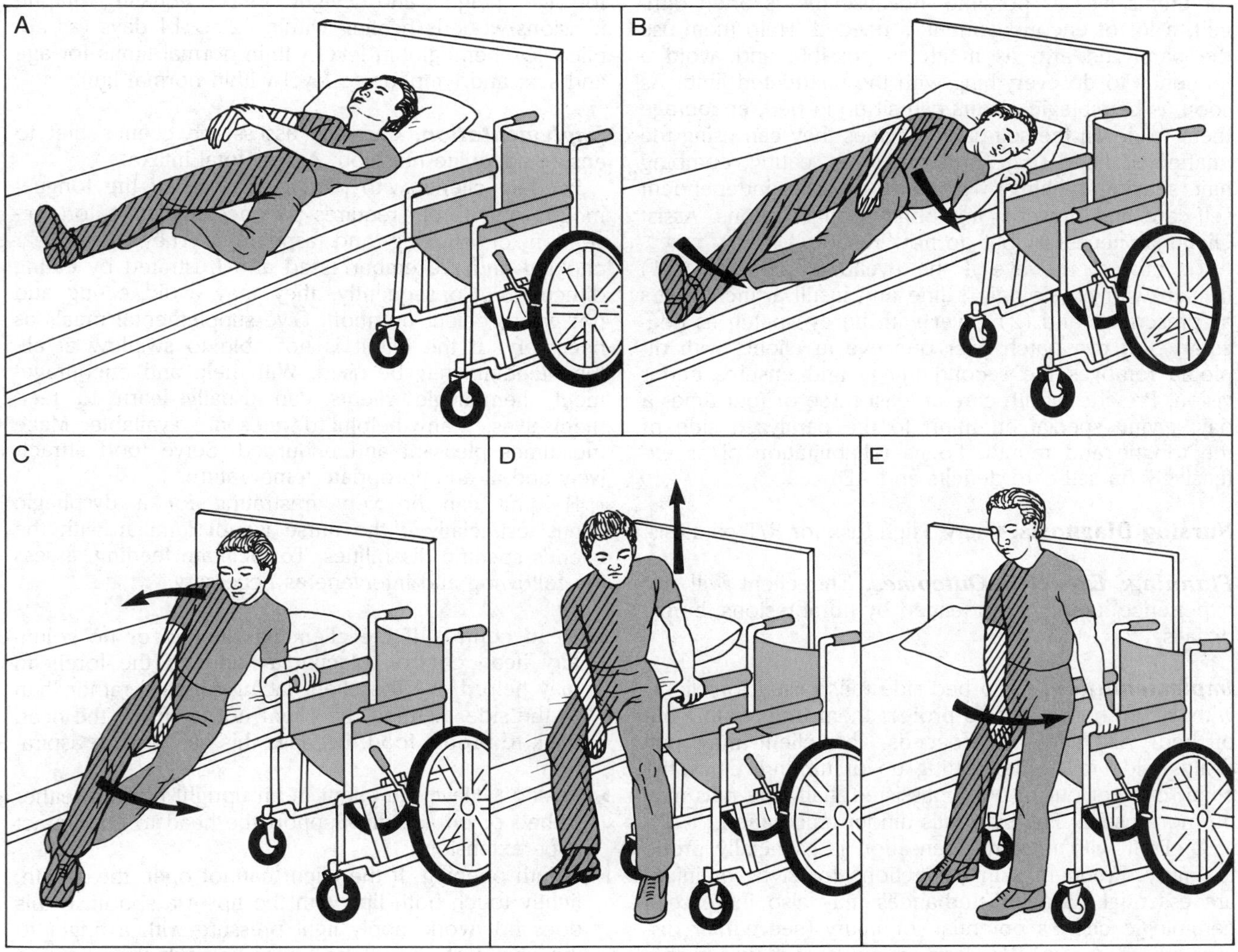

extensor reflex (reflex patterns of extension), which facilitates standing.

Most hemiplegic clients can be taught to walk. Remind them to keep body weight forward over the feet. Practice is important for learning to walk correctly. Incorrect habits, once developed, may be difficult to overcome later. Supervise clients carefully until they can safely walk alone without fear of falling. When walking, the client should not show circumduction, toe scraping, or any other characteristics of hemiplegic gait. Heel-toe walking with a reciprocal gait pattern is the goal of ambulation.

Bracing. Decisions regarding leg bracing are usually made after practice at standing and walking has started. Hemiplegic clients often do not need leg braces. However, if needed, the most commonly used short leg brace for hemiplegic clients is a double-bar 90-degree ankle stop with a posterior metal calf band. An orthopedic-type oxford shoe, properly fitted, is the support for the brace. Teach the client and family how to (1) apply and remove the brace, (2) observe skin for breakdown and give proper skin care, and (3) care for the brace itself.

Nursing Diagnosis: Self-Care Deficit R/T paralysis.

Planning: Expected Outcomes. The client will perform as many activities of daily living (ADLs) as possible, as evidenced by use of adaptive devices and techniques and recognition of limitations.

Implementation. At first, a client experiencing a stroke may need considerable help with all self-care activities (e.g., washing, eating, grooming).

It is important for hemiplegic clients to do as much for themselves as possible. Because this is often difficult, a lot of encouragement is needed. Help them use the paralyzed arm as much as possible and avoid a tendency to do everything with the unaffected limb. As soon as hemiplegic clients can sit up in bed, encourage them to do all the self-care activities they can using the unaffected hand (e.g., brushing teeth, eating, combing hair, shaving, bathing). This helps preserve independent self-care and prevents immobility complications. Assist clients as necessary but do not "rush in."

To protect the eye if the eyelid is paralyzed, (1) irrigate with physiologic saline and instill artificial tears as prescribed and (2) cover with an eye patch as necessary. An eye patch over one eye in clients with diplopia removes the second image and ensures better vision. Provide mouth care at least three or four times a day, giving special attention to the paralyzed side of the tongue and mouth. Focus rehabilitation plans extensively on self-care deficits and ADLs.

Nursing Diagnosis: Injury, High Risk for R/T paralysis.

Planning: Expected Outcomes. The client will not experience injury, as evidenced by no abrasions, burns, or falls.

Implementation. Keep bed side rails raised for clients with recent hemiplegia to protect them from rolling out of bed. As recovery proceeds, the client may pull against side rails when sitting up or turning. Once the client can get out of bed unassisted, half side rails may be more useful. Full side rails hinder ambulation.

A client with impaired sensation is especially prone to injury. Frequent skin inspections for signs of injury are essential. Visual disturbances may also increase a hemiplegic client's potential for injury (see earlier discussion of agnosia). Paralysis on one side makes clients prone to falls. Remind them to walk slowly, rest adequately between intervals of walking, use effective lighting, and look where they are going.

Nursing Diagnosis: Aspiration, High Risk for R/T loss of swallowing reflex.

Planning: Expected Outcomes. The client will develop no clinical manifestations of aspiration, as evidenced by no choking while eating, no coughing while eating, no fever, and no rales or rhonchi.

Implementation. Assess the client for clinical manifestations of aspiration, such as fever, dyspnea, crackles and rhonchi, confusion, and decreased PaO_2 in arterial blood gases. Use caution in feeding the client, either orally or by tube (see later).

Nursing Diagnosis: Nutrition, Altered: Less than Body Requirements R/T inability to swallow secondary to paralysis.

Planning: Expected Outcomes. The client will demonstrate signs of adequate nutrition, as evidenced by weight remaining stable; consuming adequate calories for age, height, and weight; intake equaling output; incisions/wounds healing within 12 to 14 days (as applicable); hemoglobin level within normal limits for age and sex; and lymphocyte level within normal limits.

Implementation. Carefully assess the client's diet to ensure adequate nutrition. Assess total intake.

Feeding clients with partial paralysis of the tongue, mouth, and throat requires patience and care for prevention of choking and aspiration. They often fear choking and are embarrassed and frustrated by eating difficulties. Consequently, they may avoid eating and not get sufficient nutrition. Give supplemental meals as necessary. If the client is not able to swallow at all, tube feeding may be used. With help and encouragement, hemiplegic clients can usually learn to feed themselves. Many helpful devices are available. Make mealtimes pleasant and unhurried. Serve food attractively and at an appropriate temperature.

Feeding can be very frustrating for a dysphagic client, especially if the nurse is not familiar with the client's specific disabilities. To facilitate feeding, assess the following and intervene as necessary.

- Head control. If the client has limited or no voluntary head control, placing a hand on the forehead may help. Have the client facing forward rather than to the side. Remind the client not to throw the head back to propel food, because this can lead to aspiration.
- Position. Have the client in an upright position either in bed or on a chair. Support the head to counteract hyperextension.
- Mouth opening. If the client cannot open the mouth, lightly touch both lips with the tip of a spoon. If this does not work, apply light pressure with a finger to the chin just below the lower lip. Ask the client to open at the same time. Stroking the muscle under the chin (digastric muscle), without crossing the midline, also stimulates mouth opening.
- Mouth closing. If a client cannot close the lips, swallowing is more difficult. Stimulate lip closure by (1) stroking the lips with a finger or ice or (2) applying gentle pressure just above the upper lip with your thumb or forefinger.
- Sucking. If a client cannot remove food from a spoon, the sucking reflex needs strengthening. Place a small disc at the end of a short straw and have the client drink through it. Gradually lengthen the straw and use thicker liquids as sucking strengthens.
- Tongue movement. Tongue movement can be im-

proved by (1) lightly touching various parts of the cheek with a tongue blade to encourage the tongue to move to that place, (2) icing weak tongue muscles, (3) applying pressure to soft tissue under the mandible to correct tongue protrusion, and (4) walking a tongue blade from the tip of the tongue to the back (this inhibits tongue thrust and stifles the gag reflex).

- Saliva secretion. Ice (plain or a popsicle) stimulates saliva secretion.
- Swallowing. A dysphagic client must concentrate on swallowing. A quiet environment, free from distractions, is helpful. Feed the client slowly and offer small amounts. Alternate liquids with solids whenever possible to prevent food from being left in the mouth. Place food in the unaffected side of the mouth. After clients have swallowed, teach them to check for food on the paralyzed side by turning the head to the unaffected side and checking with the tongue (see Bridge to Home Health Care).

Nursing Diagnosis: Communication, Impaired Verbal R/T aphasia secondary to CVA.

Planning: Expected Outcomes. The client will be able to effectively communicate, as evidenced by the client's needs being understood and met, and the client indicating understanding of the communication of others.

Implementation. Communication involves the dual processes of sending and receiving language. Although either can be affected, after initial recovery, the expressive defect commonly is greater than the receptive. Such clients may understand more than they can respond to.

Most aphasic clients regain some speech through speech therapy or spontaneously recover. Because this does not always occur, speech therapy should be started early. If speech therapy was not initiated early, clients may be helped by speech therapy 2 years or more after the time of origin of the speech disorder. Occasionally, residual brain function is not adequate for an aphasic client to relearn the complicated processes of communication.

Nurses often continue and reinforce lessons a speech therapist has initiated. Remember, the client may have a short attention span. Use every encounter to encourage and support communication, yet be careful not to cause fatigue. The following guidelines may help in communicating with aphasic clients.

- When a client cannot understand spoken words, repeat simple directions until they are understood (e.g., "Drink this juice"). Do not shout. The client can hear. Speak slowly and clearly. Talk without pressing for a response. Also use nonverbal methods of communication.
- When a client cannot identify objects by name, give practice in receiving word images. For example, point to an object and clearly state its name (e.g., "hand," "glass").
- When a client has difficulty with verbal expression, give practice in repeating words after you. Begin with simple words and then progress (e.g., "Yes," "No," "Here is breakfast").
- When working with an aphasic client, practice expanded speech (a slower rate) and self-pacing (give the client time to respond).
- Help the aphasic client's family to communicate with her or him. Act as a model for such communication. Be calm, patient, and gentle. Explain how damaging it can be to the client's self-image if others appear embarrassed or amused by his or her attempts to communicate. Likewise, the family should not do all the speaking for the client.
- Listen and watch carefully when an aphasic client attempts to communicate. Try hard to understand. This reduces the client's frustration.
- Anticipate an aphasic client's needs, to reduce feelings of communication helplessness.
- When talking to a client with receptive difficulty, stand within 6 feet and face the client directly. Grad-

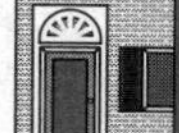

BRIDGE TO HOME HEALTH CARE

The Client with Swallowing Difficulties

Swallowing problems can be short- or long-term problems associated with cerebrovascular accident, radiation therapy, and esophageal problems. Bridging care to the home for these clients may require consultation with rehabilitation specialists with nursing and occupational therapy backgrounds.

Positioning is of primary importance when feeding. Ninety degrees flexion at the hips and 45 degrees flexion of the neck puts the client in the position that best facilitates swallowing. With the client in a chair or wheelchair, pillows can be placed behind the lower back to ensure the 90-degree angle at the hips. Prevent leaning to one side by using cushions on the weak side. The upright position is maintained for 30 to 45 minutes after the meal.

Oral care is necessary after all meals, because pocketing may occur as a result of a late or absent swallow reflex or secondary to reduced strength of pharyngeal muscles. Aspiration can occur long after the meal if pockets of food are not removed.

If impaired attention or memory is a problem, reducing distractions in the environment, giving clear and simple directions, and allowing clients adequate time to chew and swallow may be effective. If drooling is a problem, the client should eat in front of a mirror and chew on the strong side of the mouth.

If a delayed swallow reflex is noted, a puréed diet with encouragement of a dry swallow between bites and cuing the client to tuck his chin toward his chest while swallowing may be effective.

A pamphlet is available for professionals working in rural areas through the University of Montana at Missoula's Research and Training Center on Rural Rehabilitation Services, (406) 243-5481.

ually shift topics of conversation and say when you are going to change the topic.

- If the client has word deafness, give simple directions and repeat these until understood.
- If the client has naming aphasia, practice naming frequently used objects to give practice in recalling word images.
- If the client has motor aphasia, encourage practice in trying to repeat words and sounds after you.

Always try to put aphasic clients at ease. Reduce the feelings of panic that may occur when they first realize that they cannot communicate as before. The fact that others understand the problem helps. Offer calm reassurance. Demonstrate the call bell and allow practice. When they appear ready, introduce picture or word cards or picture books to facilitate communication temporarily.

Aphasic clients often express their emotional state by irritability and "moodiness." These frustrated clients are often anxious, bewildered, and depressed. Emotional lability may also be present. Accept such behavior in a matter-of-fact but kind manner without embarrassment.

Assessment of dysarthria usually includes examination of the peripheral speech mechanism, tests for specific speech skills, otolaryngologic consultation, and assessment of the client's functional ability based on the clarity of speech in conversation. Speech therapy is beneficial for many dysarthric clients.

Nursing Diagnosis: Thought Processes, Altered R/T impaired cerebral blood flow, altered sensations, and faulty interpretation of environmental stimuli.

Planning: Expected Outcomes. The client will have reduced confusion, as evidenced by recall of information, improved Glasgow Coma Scale scores, decreased agitation, and cooperation with interventions.

Implementation. Prevent intellectual regression and disorientation. Reorient the client as consciousness returns. Continually reorient a confused and aphasic client. Position a calender and a clock where the client can see them. Cerebrovascular diseases contribute to many behavioral deviations including confusion, memory loss, language disorders, and lability. Additional changes in behavior may be due to alterations such as in body image, sensation, vision, mobility, and perception. Cerebral edema may also increase confusion. Imagine what it would be like to regain consciousness after a stroke and find the right half of your body numb and paralyzed and that you cannot talk. Perhaps you cannot even understand what is said to you. This is the plight of many hemiplegic, aphasic clients. Empathetic understanding is necessary as the client regains consciousness after a stroke.

Nursing Diagnosis: Sensory/Perceptual Alterations, Visual R/T physiologic changes associated with CVA.

Planning: Expected Outcomes. The client will successfully compensate for altered sensory perceptions, as evidenced by safely performing ADLs and safely moving through the environment.

Implementation. Approach the client from the side that is not visually impaired. Position the call light and phone on that side. If possible, position the bed so that the side that is not visually impaired is toward the center of the room. Teach clients to position the head to increase the visual field. Warn hemiplegic clients to be very careful when crossing streets because they may not see traffic approaching from the affected side.

A client with perceptual defects benefits from simplicity. A busy or noisy environment is difficult to interpret and may increase confusion.

Reduce decision making and complexity. For example, (1) obtain clothing that is simply designed and easy to put on; (2) give brief, simple directions; and (3) prepare food trays with a minimum number of utensils, dishes, and foods.

Nursing Diagnosis: Unilateral Neglect R/T damage to portions of the right hemisphere.

Planning: Expected Outcomes. The client will be free of unilateral neglect, as evidenced by being free from injury, demonstrating an awareness of the neglected body side, and developing an ability to compensate for neglect.

Implementation. Initially, the nurse adapts the environment to the deficit by focusing on the client's unaffected side. Personal care items and bedside chair and commode are kept on the unaffected side. Extremities are positioned in correct alignment. Gradually, focus the client's attention to the affected side. Move personal items, bedside chair, and commode to the affected side. Assist client from affected side. Have the client groom the affected side first. Cue the client to scan the entire environment.[12]

Nursing Diagnosis: Individual Coping, Ineffective R/T physiologic changes and frustration associated with CVA.

Planning: Expected Outcomes. The client will develop effective coping strategies, as evidenced by appropriate lifestyle modifications, utilization of the assistance of others, and appropriate social interactions.

Implementation. The term "coping" refers to the use of all forms of coping strategies: emotional, cognitive, support systems, and risk appraisal. After CVA, the client may experience grief over lost motion, inability to speak, alterations in sensation and vision, and loss of roles within society (see Ethical Issues in Nursing). These reactions can be understood when the extent of the change and dysfunction in a client's life is appreciated. Be understanding and kind. Supportive statements are often helpful, such as "I am sure it's hard for you not to be able to dress alone."

Care for clients with hemiplegia so that their dependency is minimized. Praise all successes, however small. When necessary, point out disruptive or inappropriate behavior kindly and ask them to stop. Arrange the environment and anticipate needs to reduce frustration. Significant others often need help to understand these behaviors. It is often difficult for them to see their loved one behave in these ways. They may feel at a loss about what to do and need the nurse's support as much as the client does.

Psychosocial Nursing Diagnoses: Various psychosocial nursing diagnoses may be appropriate for clients experiencing stroke, depending on the client and the circumstances. These include Family Processes, Altered; Diversional Activity Deficit; Anxiety; Fear; Powerlessness; Self-Esteem Disturbance; and Social Isolation. Include significant others in the plan of care. Let them help care for the client if they want to. Provide them with the information they need to understand the client's condition. Many clients with strokes are in intensive care units (ICUs) during their acute phase. The complexity of equipment and activity within an ICU may be frightening to the client and significant others. Provide opportunities for questions and discussion; explain carefully what is happening. Give frequent reassurance and support.

INTERVENTION AFTER THE ACUTE PHASE OF STROKE

During the convalescent stage, residual defects from a stroke are treated, and intervention is directed toward helping the client function at the maximum capacity. Clients with stroke and their families face difficult adjustments as the acute stages pass and residual disabilities become obvious. A multidisciplinary rehabilitative team may help to assist and support clients during this time. Assessing the functional abilities of the client and setting realistic goals are part of this approach. Tasks the client and significant others face include

- learning to use intact strengths and abilities to compensate for impaired functions
- learning to become independent in ADLs, such as bathing, dressing, and eating
- developing behavior patterns that are likely to prevent symptom recurrence. Medications should be taken as prescribed. Diet may require modification. Advise the client to stop smoking and to engage in stress-reducing activities. Encourage following a prescribed exercise program to promote better physical health and mental well being.

EVALUATION

The degree of outcome attainment should be evaluated on an ongoing basis. After CVA, some outcomes are achieved early (e.g., cerebral perfusion); others may require rehabilitation (e.g., self-care deficit). It is important to monitor progress toward outcomes, working with both the client and the family.

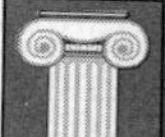

ETHICAL ISSUES IN NURSING

Who Should Judge Quality of Life?

The quality of life is important to most clients, in sickness or in health. "Quality" is a very relative term and is best described by each client at a given stage of his or her life. What clients consider quality in health might be significantly altered when illness strikes or anytime there is a change in lifestyle (i.e., employment, financial situation, family, and the like). Clients assess and reassess the quality of their lives day by day. We may not always consciously state what the quality of life is today, but nevertheless, how we feel about our life at a given moment is an important part of who we are. The best judge of the quality of life is each individual client, not someone else. However, health care workers are constantly being placed in positions of judging the quality of their clients' lives.

Cerebrovascular disorders can significantly change a client's life. Clients who have had a stroke may experience such life changes, which in turn alter the way they view the quality of life. Perhaps they can no longer speak clearly or perform many of the tasks that they used to. Perhaps their stroke was so severe they can no longer care for themselves. In severe cases, perhaps the stroke has left them dependent on machines and unaware of their existence.

When possible, nurses should be aware of how their clients feel their illness has affected the quality of their lives. This may help health care providers better understand how illness has emotionally affected their clients. In cases in which clients are unable to make their quality of life judgements known, it is easy for health care providers to make quality of life judgements for them. It is not uncommon to hear a nurse say, "I don't understand why we are continuing to treat Mr. X. I would not want to live that way." This statement may be true for the nurse, but it may not be true for the client being described.

Quality of life judgements are best made by each client about himself or herself, with the situation of life at the present time taken into account. Nurses who care for clients who can no longer judge their own quality of life must be sensitive not to judge the client's quality of life from their own personal perspective.

Modification of Plan of Care for the Elderly

Because CVA strikes the elderly population more than any other, the nursing care discussed here does not have to be significantly altered for the elderly client. It must be remembered that elderly clients often have multiple medical problems that must be monitored and treated simultaneously.

Post-hospital Care

DISCHARGE PLANNING

Clients who have experienced CVA often are transferred to a rehabilitation unit after they are medically stable. If this transfer moves the client a long distance from home, it may be stressful for the client and family, particularly an elderly spouse. During acute hospitalization, the spouse's and family's ability to care for the client should be assessed. If both partners are elderly or in poor health, placement in a nursing home may be the only option. This can create feelings of guilt and abandonment. Emotional support must be provided to both the client and family members. Education in how to choose a nursing home and how to monitor care can be helpful.

If the client is to be discharged home, the family needs clear understanding of the residual deficits. The family and client need to have realistic expectations about the client's abilities; yet, encourage independence when and where the client is able.

TRANSIENT ISCHEMIC ATTACKS

Definition

TIAs are brief, reversible episodes of neurologic dysfunction caused by temporary, focal cerebral ischemia. A TIA is analogous to angina pectoris. TIAs are also called intermittent cerebrovascular insufficiency or "mini stroke."

Incidence

Because of the variable presentation and duration, it is difficult to determine the incidence of TIAs. It is estimated that 25 to 50 per cent of all clients who experience CVA had a previous TIA.

Etiology

During a TIA, a transient decrease occurs in blood supply to a focal area of the cerebrum or brain stem. Many factors can cause this ischemia. Occlusive disease of the extracranial cerebral vessels is the most common cause of TIAs. The most frequent site of occlusion is the origin of the internal carotid artery. In addition to the carotid artery system, occlusions may occur in the vertebrobasilar system. Emboli can also cause TIAs. Common sources of emboli include the heart valves and breakdown of plaque.

Risk Factors

The risk factors and preventive measures of TIAs are essentially the same as those of CVAs. The pathophysiology is also similar; the major differences are the duration and permanency of symptoms.

Clinical Manifestations

Clinical manifestations vary with TIAs, depending on which area of brain is affected. Transient symptoms by TIAs include (1) visual, auditory, or vestibular disturbances; (2) motor and sensory disturbances; (3) headache; (4) slowed mental processes; and (5) seizures.

Generally, TIAs last only minutes (often 2 to 15 minutes) to an hour. Sometimes they last only a few seconds; other times, for as long as 24 hours. Although TIAs are often recurrent, some clients have only one or two episodes. TIAs may occur for as long as 2 years before cerebral infarction, or clusters of TIAs may first appear only a few hours or days before a cerebral infarction. Between episodes, neurologic assessment findings are usually normal.

Clients experiencing TIAs are often afraid that they are having a CVA. They need emotional support and education during this stressful time. The diagnostic work-up as well as the symptoms themselves can produce anxiety. Thorough, simple explanations of upcoming events can help.

DIAGNOSTIC ASSESSMENT

TIAs are diagnosed by the client's reported symptoms. The causes of the TIA and potential risk of CVA are diagnosed by (1) auscultation and palpation of a carotid bruit, (2) Doppler studies of the carotid, (3) CT to rule out CVA, and (4) echocardiogram to rule out mural thrombosis. If the Doppler reveals 70 per cent narrowing of the carotid, the results are considered significant of cerebrovascular disease. Angiograms are used to illuminate niches in the carotid plaque, which may have broken free (Fig. 30–7).

Medical Management

Preventing the progression of a TIA to a CVA is the goal of medical management. Antihypertensives, antiplatelet drugs, or aspirin may be prescribed. In some instances, warfarin (Coumadin) may be administered to prevent clot development. Every effort is made to determine the cause of the TIAs.

Surgical Management

If vascular insufficiency is detected in the distribution of the middle cerebral artery, an extracranial-intracranial bypass may be performed. This procedure surgically anastomoses the superficial temporal artery to the middle cerebral artery, thereby increasing blood flow to the brain.

A more frequently performed procedure is carotid endarterectomy. Surgery is usually performed only on stenotic arteries, not those that are totally occluded. A client may require bilateral extracranial-intracranial bypass and endarterectomy. Duration between surgeries is determined by the client's tolerance of the procedure

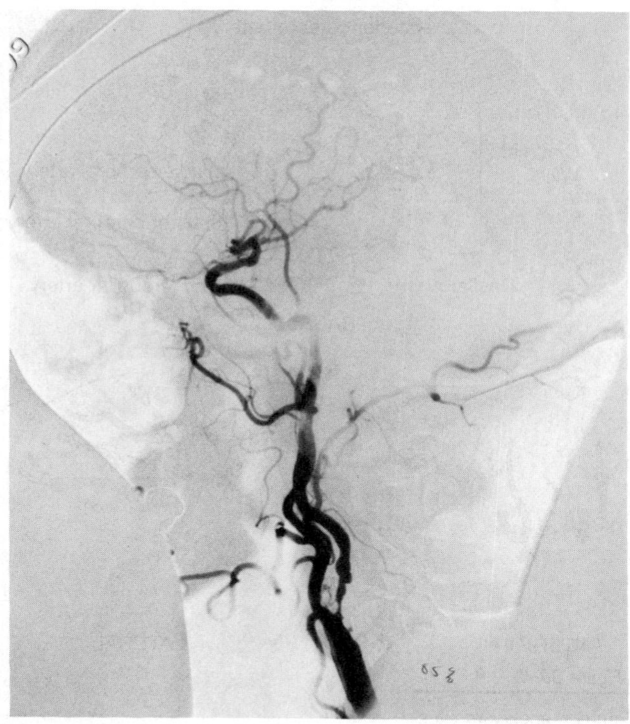

▲ Figure 30–7

Subtraction angiogram taken before an endarterectomy reveals an 85 per cent occlusion of internal carotid artery.

and the likelihood of symptom progression from the remaining stenotic vessel.

Carotid endarterectomy is performed through an incision on the anterior border of the sternocleidomastoid muscle (Fig. 30–8). The vessel is clamped, and the plaque (sometimes called atheroma) is dissected. The client is at increased risk of decreased cerebral perfusion during the operation. For some clients, a temporary blood supply is created by shunting blood through other vessels to the brain. Clients often treated with shunts include those with contralateral stenosis of the carotids, neurologic deficits, known decreases in cerebral blood flow, a history of CVA, and a stroke in evolution. Once the plaque is resected, the incision is closed with a drain in place. A pressure dressing is applied to reduce the risk of hematoma formation.

Serious neurologic complications include (1) embolization during surgery, causing cerebral occlusion and ischemia; (2) clotting (thrombosis) of the artery at the endarterectomy site, causing cerebral ischemia; (3) increased ICP due to intracranial hemorrhage; and (4) inadequate cerebral perfusion from intolerance of the temporary artery clamping during surgery.

Nursing Management

The care of clients undergoing an extracranial-intracranial bypass is the same as that of clients having other types of cranial surgery. Careful assessment of vital signs and neurologic function is essential. Changes in status must be reported immediately. In addition, the surgical anastomosis creates a pulse that should be palpated during vital sign assessments. This pulse is located just below the curve of the incision. If the pulse changes in character, the surgeon should be notified immediately.

Postoperative care after carotid endarterectomy is most important during the first 24 hours. Keep the head in a straight position to help maintain airway patency and to minimize stress on the operative site. Elevate

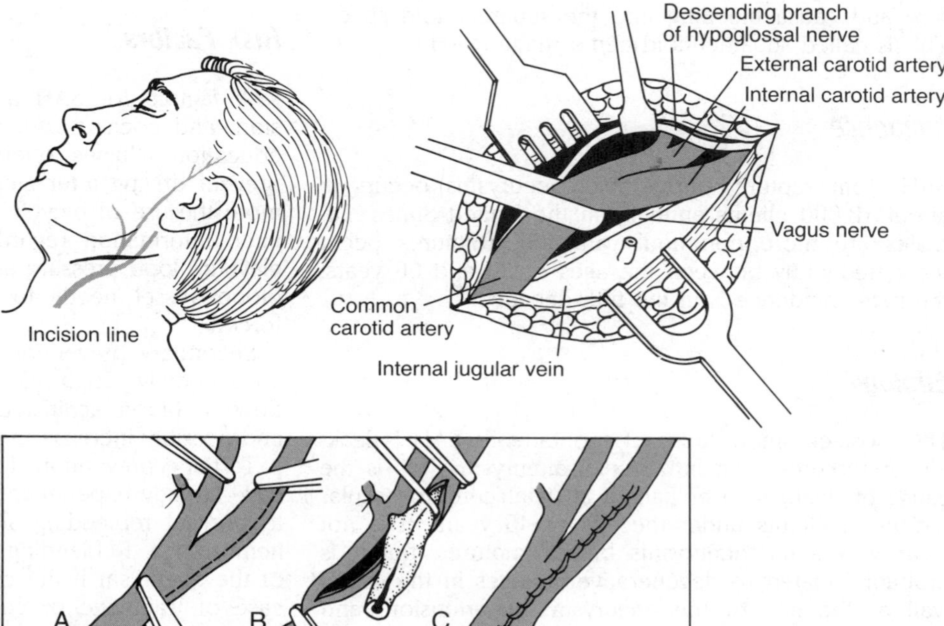

▲ Figure 30–8

Carotid endarterectomy. An incision is made along the carotid bifurcation, and plaque is removed. Sometimes portions of the artery are removed also and reconstructed with vein grafts or Dacron.

the head of the bed when vital signs are stable. Frequently assess the client's breathing pattern, pulse, and blood pressure. Blood pressure must be maintained between 120 and 170 systolic to ensure cerebral perfusion. Labile blood pressure is a common problem after surgery. Baroreceptors located in the lining of the carotid sinus are one of the primary mechanisms of maintaining normotension. Manipulation of the baroreceptors during surgery causes a short-term disruption in regulation. Observe the operative site. Airway obstruction can occur from excessive swelling of the neck or hematoma formation there. Also perform a neurologic assessment of the client's pupillary reactions, LOC, and motor and sensory function. Immediately report indications of deterioration of neurologic impairment. Local applications of cold to the operative site may be prescribed.

Assess the function of the following cranial nerves: facial (VII), vagus (X), spinal accessory (XI), and hypoglossal (XII) (see Chap. 28). Cranial nerve damage is usually temporary but may last for months. The most common cranial nerve damage causes vocal cord paralysis or difficulty managing saliva and tongue deviation. Horner's syndrome may result from damaged sympathetic nerve fibers. This is usually temporary.

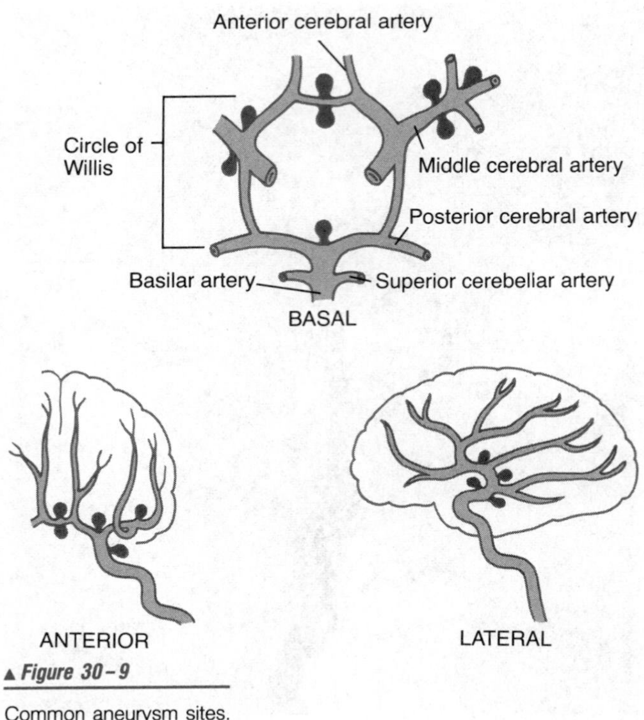

▲ *Figure 30–9*

Common aneurysm sites.

INTRACRANIAL ANEURYSM AND SUBARACHNOID HEMORRHAGE

Definition

Intracranial aneurysms are congenital, traumatic, arteriosclerotic, or septic weakenings or outpouchings in vessel walls. Ninety per cent of aneurysms are congenital. Eighty per cent occur on the circle of Willis (Fig. 30–9).[23] Sometimes these aneurysms weaken, leak, or rupture and cause bleeding into the subarachnoid space. This is called subarachnoid hemorrhage (SAH).

Incidence

SAH from ruptured intracranial aneurysms occurs in about 18,000 clients annually in the United States. Females are more commonly affected. Ruptures occur most frequently between the ages of 30 and 60 years; the peak incidence is in the fifth decade.[16]

Etiology

The most common cause of spontaneous SAH is leaking or rupture of an intracranial aneurysm. This is the cause of death in over half of all fatal cerebrovascular lesions in clients under the age of 45 years. It is not clear why some aneurysms bleed (rupture), but it is probably related to degenerative changes in the vessel wall at the site of the aneurysm, hypertension, and constant stress caused by the force of blood flow, particularly at a bifurcation. Meningeal vessel rupture from head trauma is another cause of subarachnoid bleeding. Spontaneous hemorrhage that is not associated with trauma may be caused by blood dyscrasias, primary or metastatic intracranial tumors, vascular anomalies (e.g., angiomas or AVMs), central nervous system (CNS) infections, or intracerebral hemorrhages spreading to the subarachnoid space.

Risk Factors

Risk factors for SAH include head trauma, hypertension, and cocaine use. Primary prevention focuses on education. Nurses often participate in campaigns to prevent driving after alcohol consumption and to promote the use of bicycle and motorcycle helmets. Similarly, information regarding the ability of cocaine to elevate blood pressure and possibly trigger rupture of a blood vessel needs to be made available and reinforced.

Secondary prevention involves treating hypertension appropriately. High blood pressure can increase the flow of blood against a weakened blood vessel wall and possibly increase the chance of aneurysm rupture.

Tertiary prevention focuses on those clients who have already experienced SAH. The goal in this case is to prevent rebleeding and complications of the initial hemorrhage. Rebleeding is prevented by early clipping of the aneurysm if the client's condition allows. In the case of traumatic or cocaine-induced SAH, hypertension is controlled as closely as possible. The nurse can minimize or prevent the complications associated with immobility, aspiration, or injury related to paralysis.

Pathophysiology

Fusiform and saccular aneurysms are the two most common types of cerebral aneurysm (Fig. 30–10). Both are caused by a congenital weakness in artery walls. Saccular (berry) aneurysms are the most common. More than one aneurysm may be present. Saccular aneurysms usually have a "neck" or narrowed portion attached to the vessel. Most develop around the anterior portion of the circle of Willis at the junction of the posterior communicating and the internal carotid arteries. Fusiform aneurysms most often occur on the larger basilar and carotid arteries. Usually, these aneurysms do not rupture. They develop from atherosclerotic changes that impair vascular elasticity. Almost one third of clients who have a ruptured aneurysm die from the initial hemorrhage.[10] Dissecting aneurysm occurs when the intima of the vessel wall is torn. Blood escapes the lumen of the vessel through the tear. Eventually, the expanding mass occludes the vessel.

The blood within the CSF causes irritation of the meninges. It also clots in the subarachnoid space and obstructs CSF flow, leading to hydrocephalus and increased ICP. After an aneurysm ruptures, a clot forms at the site of the hemorrhage. This reduces the risk of rebleeding for a few days. As the clot begins to dissolve, the possibility of rebleeding increases. The greatest risk is about 1 week after the initial hemorrhage.

There are several complications of SAH that may affect intervention.

REBLEEDING

Rebleeding is a major complication that may occur at any time in an untreated SAH. Rebleeding commonly occurs within the first few days after hemorrhage, but may occur anytime over the first few months. Mortality is high following rebleeding. Definitive management of rebleeding is clipping of the aneurysm. Antifibrinolytic agents may be used in situations in which surgery is not an option. These agents prevent dissolving of the clot. A disadvantage is that the agents cause vasospasm.[13]

VASOSPASM

Vasospasm is a narrowing of a vessel lumen. Vasospasm is a major concern because of its location. Aneurysms commonly occur in the circle of Willis; therefore, when vasospasm occurs in the major vessels, the major cerebral vessels are affected. Spasm usually occurs in the vessel adjacent to a ruptured aneurysm and may spread throughout all the major vessels at the base of the brain. Vasospasm produces symptoms of ischemia and, if extensive and prolonged, results in infarction and permanent neurologic deficit.

It is theorized that the breakdown of blood after SAH is the etiologic factor behind vasospasm. Research has identified several breakdown products that affect the contractility of vessel walls.

HYDROCEPHALUS

Hydrocephalus is caused by blood in the subarachnoid space that prevents adequate CSF circulation. It often occurs in the acute stage that follows SAH and contributes to increased ICP. Hydrocephalus often resolves spontaneously but may be treated by short-term external ventriculostomy to help decrease ICP. Hydrocephalus may develop again after several weeks, this time more slowly, producing dementia and ataxia. Chronic hydrocephalus is usually treated with a ventriculoperitoneal or a ventriculoatrial shunt.

Clinical Manifestations

An aneurysm is usually asymptomatic until it ruptures. Occasionally, there are mild premonitory indications such as mild headache, confusion, fainting, or vertigo. However, the onset of the hemorrhage is usually sudden. The client experiences a sudden, severe headache, typically in the occipital area and often accompanied by vomiting. Often the client says, "This is the worst headache I have ever had." The client may lose consciousness immediately, may become confused and lethargic and gradually comatose within hours, or may remain conscious and coherent. Generalized seizures may occur. There are often signs of meningeal irritation (e.g., stiff neck and leg and back pain) due to blood in the subarachnoid space. Focal neurologic deficits include cranial nerve involvement (usually the third and sixth cranial nerves) and motor weakness (usually monoparesis or hemiparesis).

Clinical manifestations of SAH have been divided into five grades for classification of severity of the neurologic deficits associated with the blood (see Box 30–2). Clients over age 50 years are classified one grade higher than their signs indicate. Prognosis varies from good to grave as the client progresses from grade I to grade V.

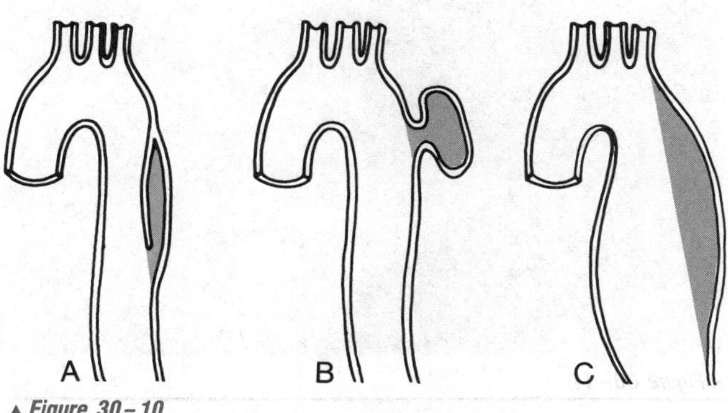

▲ Figure 30–10

Aneurysm types. *A*, Dissecting. *B*, Saccular. *C*, Fusiform.

Box 30–2. Grading the Severity of Subarachnoid Bleeding

Grade I	Minimal bleeding, alert, no neurologic deficit, no symptoms, slight nuchal rigidity
Grade II	Mild bleeding, alert, headache, minimal neurologic deficit (e.g., third nerve palsy, stiff neck)
Grade III	Moderate bleeding, drowsy or confused, headache, stiff neck, with or without neurologic deficit
Grade IV	Moderate to severe bleeding, semicoma, moderate to severe hemiparesis, early decerebrate posturing
Grade V	Severe bleeding, coma, decerebrate or decorticate posturing, moribund appearance

DIAGNOSTIC ASSESSMENT

Diagnosis of SAH is usually based on history and physical examination. CT scan may identify blood in the subarachnoid space, intracerebral clots, and large clots surrounding an aneurysm. Lumbar puncture usually confirms the presence of blood in the subarachnoid space. Variations occur in the pressure, color, and cell content of CSF, depending on the timing of the lumbar puncture in relation to the hemorrhage.

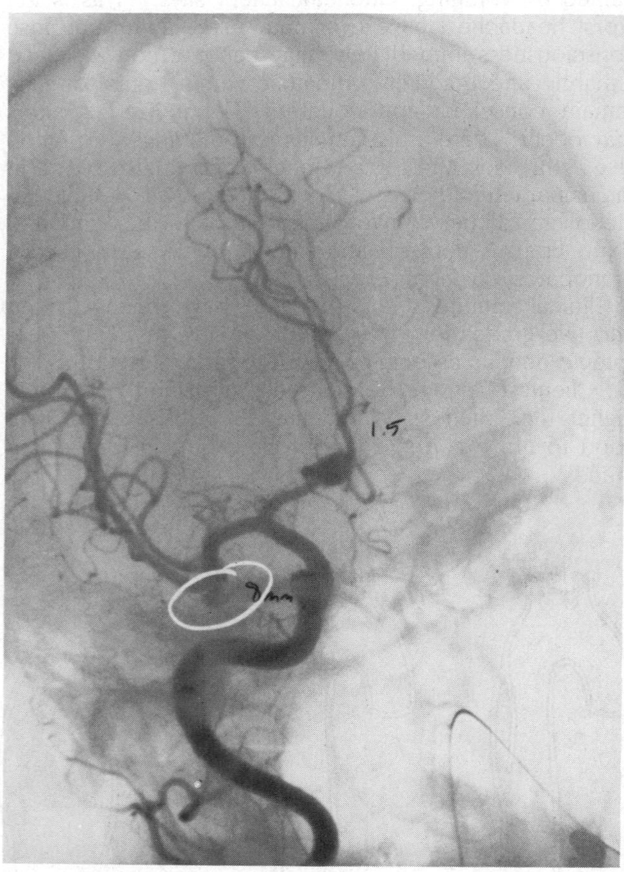

▲ **Figure 30–11**

Angiogram revealing aneurysm of the right middle cerebral artery and right anterior communicating artery.

Angiography is the definitive diagnostic test. A 4-vessel study provides adequate visualization of the carotid and vertebral-basilar circulation. An angiogram usually demonstrates (1) the aneurysm's structure and location, (2) the vessels supplying the aneurysm, and (3) the presence or absence of an intracerebral clot or vasospasm of any vessels surrounding the aneurysm or distal to it (Fig. 30–11). Depending on the client's condition and the physician's philosophy, the angiogram may be done immediately or when the client stabilizes. (See Chap. 28 regarding cerebral angiography.)

Medical Management

Medical intervention focuses on management of the systemic effects of SAH and vasospasm. Systemic effects include neurogenic pulmonary edema, cardiac arrhythmias, and stress ulcers. Although no definitive prevention or cure exists for cerebral vasospasm, there are treatment modalities. Hypertensive, hypervolemic hemodilution can minimize the impact of vasospasm. Systolic blood pressure is maintained between 100 and 150 mm Hg. The increase in volume and pressure forces blood through spastic vessels. Untreated vasospasm leads to ischemic stroke. Another theory of etiology for vasospasm is the influx of calcium into the muscular layer of the blood vessel wall. Nimodipine, which is a calcium channel blocker, has been administered in an effort to inhibit this influx. Research is ongoing in the use of this and other drugs in the treatment of vasospasm. This is usually accomplished by infusion of serum albumin. This colloid helps maintain the high intravascular volume by osmosis. Albumin also results in hemodilution. Low hematocrit reflects decreased blood viscosity. The less viscous the blood is, the easier it flows through narrowed vessels. If the hypervolemia does not adequately elevate blood pressure, the vasopressors may be instituted.

Nonsurgical measures to decrease ICP often include (1) restricting fluids, (2) administering dexamethasone (Decadron) and osmotic agents, (3) elevating the head of the bed 20 to 30 degrees, and (4) maintaining a patent airway to prevent increased PCO_2.

Surgical Management

Surgical obliteration of the aneurysm with a metal clip or suture eliminates the risk of rebleeding. Clipping is performed through a craniotomy to expose the aneurysm. The aneurysm is isolated, and a clip is placed over the neck of the aneurysm. Many neurosurgeons advocate surgery as soon as possible after rupture. Early surgery is not recommended for all clients, however. Clients with grades IV and V SAH are not operated on because early surgery may contribute to morbidity or mortality. Also, if vasospasm is present, most surgeons will delay surgery. Operating while vessels are in spasm has been shown to increase the morbidity and mortality. Unfortunately, medical instability, delay in transfer from one hospital to another, or client or family reluctance to consent to surgery may delay prompt surgery. Studies have shown that clients who enter the hospital in relatively good condition after the rupture of an aneurysm have only a 50 per cent chance of leaving the hospital in good condition when surgery is delayed.[23]

Nursing Management

Nursing care of the client with SAH is a complex task taking place in an ICU. The condition of the client may range from alert and oriented to comatose and ventilator-dependent. This is a disorder of sudden onset, often striking young people in the prime of their lives. Helping the family to understand what has happened and what is being done can be time-consuming. Explanations may need to be repeated frequently. Nurses can help family members to develop realistic expectations.

ASSESSMENT

Assessing arterial blood pressure is especially important after SAH. Elevated arterial pressure may contribute to further bleeding from the ruptured aneurysm. At the same time, pressure sufficient to maintain cerebral perfusion pressure must be maintained. Administer vasoactive agents as prescribed and evaluate the effects carefully. Ask the physician for an ideal blood pressure range. If the blood pressure goes above or below that range, contact the physician. Assess and document vital signs frequently, especially blood pressure. Observe carefully for changes in the client's status, particularly a decrease in LOC or progression of motor weakness, and notify the physician of significant changes.

NURSING INTERVENTION

Attempt to provide a quiet, calm environment for clients with SAH. This may be difficult to do in a busy ICU. Evaluate the client's response to visitors and adjust visiting schedules as needed (see Nursing Research). Keeping a restless client quiet and in bed for an extended period of time is difficult, especially if visual problems or attention deficits preclude reading or watching television as diversion. Avoid sedation whenever possible.

Individualized aneurysm precautions are followed during the acute stages of SAH in an attempt to prevent rupture of the vascular abnormality. They may also be used after surgery and in clients with AVMs. Typical aneurysm precautions include the following.

Elevation of the Head. Elevate the head of the bed 15 to 30 degrees, as prescribed. Advise the client to avoid straining. Place necessary items such as the call bell within easy reach. Assist with position changes and turning. During these activities, encourage the client to relax and not to tighten muscles. Advise the client to minimize turning the head and not to rotate or flex the neck. Isometric or active exercises are not permitted. Passive ROM exercises are acceptable.

Avoidance of Valsalva's Maneuvers. Avoid creating a vagal effect, and limit the duration and frequency of Valsalva's maneuvers. Valsalva's maneuvers occur with activities such as passing urine, sneezing, coughing, straining at stool, bending, and vomiting and during suctioning. Avoid rectal stimulation or straining at stool. Enemas are contraindicated, because a vagal effect may result from distention of the lower colon. Do not use rectal thermometers; they may precipitate Valsalva's maneuver. Manage bowel elimination with prescribed stool softeners and mild laxatives. A client whose condition allows (grades I and II) may be permitted by the physician to use a commode. Constipation, bedpan use, and the effort of expelling even a soft stool with weakened abdominal muscles increase Valsalva's effort. Taking a deep breath when it is necessary to perform Valsalva's maneuver reduces the strain. Teach this activity to the conscious client.

Administration of Analgesics and Sedatives. Administer prescribed medications such as analgesics for comfort and sedatives to promote rest. Avoid oversedation, because the client must be easily aroused as

NURSING RESEARCH

Correlation between presence of family members and changes in intracranial pressure (ICP) is the concept investigated by this study. The research was designed to use the ICP readings routinely obtained every 15 minutes. In addition, ICP readings were obtained every 5 minutes during family visits. Twenty-four patients who required ICP monitoring and were 14 years of age or older made up the study population.

In addition to recording ICP measurements, the investigator recorded the incidence of cerebrospinal fluid drainage and occurrence of client care procedures. Medications that affected ICP were also recorded.

The author reported 7 cases of significant decrease in ICP during family visits, 11 cases of nonsignificant decrease in ICP, and 6 cases of nonsignificant increase in ICP.

An important point of this study is the realization that not every client responds in the same way to family visits. It is up to the nurse to carefully assess each client's response and then individualize the visiting schedule on the basis of that response. Also, as the client's level of consciousness improves, he or she may be less able to tolerate the stimulation of family visits.

▼▼▼

Hendrickson, S. L. (1987). Intracranial pressure changes and family presence. *Journal of Neuroscience Nursing, 19*(1), 14.

necessary for neurologic assessment. Phenobarbital may be prescribed for sedation and because it also helps prevent seizures.

Careful monitoring of neurologic status, hemodynamic parameters, and systemic functioning is required. See care of the client after craniotomy later in this chapter. Prompt identification of changes, notification of the physician, and intervention are the keys to improving client outcome.

ARTERIOVENOUS MALFORMATION

These congenital malformations consist of tangles of thin-walled blood vessels without intervening capillaries. Arterial and venous blood shunt together. Hence, perfusion of brain tissue cannot occur through them. The vessels may "leak" small amounts of blood or they may rupture, causing hemorrhage into the subarachnoid space or brain, depending on the location of the bleeding AVM. Whereas some AVMs are huge, others are microscopic. Most commonly, they occur in the posterior portions of the cerebral hemispheres. Over time, they may change in size. Large AVMs may decrease somewhat, whereas small ones may enlarge. Bleeding into brain tissues usually produces focal neurologic clinical manifestations. However, cerebral infarction or ischemia may occur without rupture. A ruptured AVM produces clinical manifestations and laboratory results similar to those of SAH. The smaller AVMs are most prone to rupture.

Aneurysm precautions (see SAH) may be prescribed. About half of AVMs can be completely removed surgically. Laser intervention may be used preoperatively to decrease the size of the AVM, or neuroradiologic procedures may be performed to reduce the AVM's blood supply. (These procedures may also be used on inoperable AVMs.) Other techniques that may be used to reduce the size of AVMs include (1) use of radiation energy from a proton beam, (2) detachable balloon procedures, (3) artificially embolizing (clotting) the AVM, or (4) ligating the AVM's feeding arteries. These interventions are not without such hazards as initiating hemorrhage or infarction or enlarging the area of ischemia.

VASCULAR LESIONS OF CEREBRAL VEINS AND SINUSES

Lesions do not often occur in the small cerebral veins. However, these vessels may be affected by extension of infectious or thrombotic processes from the large dural sinuses. Focal neurologic symptoms occur from occlusion of the cortical and subcortical veins. The large dural sinuses may become thrombosed from infection within or from the epidural or subdural spaces. In adults, the dural sinuses may be occluded by trauma, tumor masses, or conditions such as the formation of clots in polycythemia.

The superior sagittal, lateral, and cavernous dural sinuses are most often thrombosed. The superior sagittal sinus is less commonly affected by infective thrombosis than is the lateral or cavernous sinus. Thrombosis of the lateral sinus is usually secondary to otitis media and mastoiditis. It is rare because of effective antibiotic treatment of these conditions.

Cavernous sinus thrombosis is typically secondary to suppurative processes in the orbit, nasal sinuses, or upper half of the face. The infection commonly first involves one sinus and then rapidly spreads to the opposite side. The client is acutely ill and has a septic febrile reaction and pain in the eye. Visual acuity may or may not be affected, and pupillary reactions may or may not be preserved. The pupils may be small or dilated, the cornea may be cloudy, and corneal ulcers may develop. Formerly fatal, cavernous sinus thrombosis can now be treated with antibiotics and possibly anticoagulants.

Carotid-cavernous sinus fistula may develop after head trauma or occur spontaneously. In this condition, there is an abnormal communication between the carotid artery and the cavernous sinus. This abnormality allows rapid blood flow into vessels not accustomed to such rapid flow. Carotid-cavernous sinus fistula results in several characteristic symptoms that are discussed later.

Exophthalmos is protrusion of the eyeball and is caused by blood flowing in a retrograde fashion into the ophthalmic veins from the cavernous sinus. These veins dilate and can displace the eyeball laterally and inferiorly. The displacement may be severe enough to prevent the eyelids from closing. Rapid flow through veins surrounding the orbit may result in palpable ocular pulsations.

Dilation and arterial blood flow through the small veins of the sclera and conjunctiva cause chemosis. This edema surrounding the cornea may herniate beyond the eyelids. These symptoms require vigilant eye care for preventing irreversible damage to the affected eye. The eye must be kept lubricated and protected from trauma. Traditional eye patches have limited usefulness in exophthalmos because pressure from the patch may actually cause tissue damage. Plastic bubbles, which allow protrusion of the eye and assist in maintaining a moist environment, are available.

Visual impairments and extraocular palsies can result from changes in blood vessels and cranial nerves. Changes in blood flow also cause headaches and bruits. The bruit may be the first symptom the client actually complains of. Sleeping may be difficult because the bruit tends to become louder when the client is lying down and the surrounding noise is less.

The treatment goal in carotid-cavernous sinus fistula is to eliminate the fistula while patency of the carotid artery is maintained. This may be accomplished by embolization of the fistula. Embolization is accomplished by introduction of a catheter via the femoral artery. When the catheter is properly positioned, the fistula is occluded. In most cases, this is accomplished by inflating a balloon and detaching it from the catheter. Other materials have also been used for embolization.

Obliteration of the fistula usually results in reversal of the symptoms. If the carotid artery is sacrificed or occluded, the client may develop symptoms of ischemia. If collateral circulation is inadequate, the client may experience CVA. A baseline neurologic assessment should be obtained before the procedure and then repeated frequently after the procedure. Any change from baseline should be reported to the physician immediately.

▼ TUMORS

INTRACRANIAL TUMORS

Definition

Intracranial tumors can be defined in several different ways. Primary tumors develop from CNS tissue. Secondary tumors have metastasized from other locations in the body. Intra-axial tumors originate from glial cells within the cerebrum, cerebellum, or brain stem. These tumors infiltrate and invade brain tissue. Extra-axial tumors have their origin in the skull, meninges, cranial nerves, or pituitary gland. These tumors have a compressive effect on the brain.

Incidence

Intracranial tumors are second only to cerebrovascular disease as the most common endogenous neurologic problem; 14,000 new cases of primary brain tumor develop yearly in the United States. Tumors of this type occur equally in males and females of all age groups. Heredity is not a significant risk factor in brain tumors, except for tumors of neurofibromatosis and tuberous sclerosis (Table 30–5). Metastatic brain tumors are even more frequent than primary tumors.[29]

Etiology

The etiology of secondary tumors can be traced to the primary site from which they metastasized. This site is often the lung or breast. No clear etiologic factor has been established for any of the primary intracranial tumors. Although the type of cell that gave rise to the tumor can often be identified, the mechanism causing the cells to act abnormally remains unknown. Primary intracranial tumors do not metastasize to other sites in the body.

Risk Factors

Because the etiologic mechanism of primary intracranial tumors is uncertain, there are no specific risk factors or primary and secondary preventive measures identified. Aggressive treatment of the primary site may prevent the development of metastatic tumors. Unfortunately, such treatment is not always successful, and not all clients can tolerate aggressive treatment. These clients may develop metastatic tumors.

Tertiary prevention addresses those clients who have an intracranial tumor. Depending on the location of the lesion and type and extensiveness of medical intervention, the client may exhibit various neurologic deficits. Tertiary prevention focuses on preventing complications associated with these deficits.

Pathophysiology

Both benign and malignant intracranial tumors are potentially fatal. The outcome depends on the tumor location, size, and type. Benign tumors (e.g., neurinomas, meningiomas) may be cured with early diagnosis and surgery. However, gliomas and metastatic intracranial tumors are often fatal. These tumors are the subject of extensive ongoing research.

Intracranial tumors cause death by infiltration and compression of brain tissue. Not only are the tumors space-occupying lesions, but they often produce considerable cerebral edema. The skull is rigid and has little room for expansion of the contents. Brain tumors progressively increase ICP, which causes brain stem herniation and death.

Cranial nerves may be compressed or invaded by benign or malignant tumors, or they may be the primary site of tumors. Papilledema (edema and hyperemia of the optic disc) from optic nerve head swelling, retinal vein enlargement, and eventually hemorrhages into the nerve and adjacent retina occur. The underlying pathophysiologic mechanism of papilledema is not clearly understood, but the cause may be increased pressure in the central retinal vein due to obstructed venous return from the eye.

Clinical Manifestations

As with other cranial disorders, the symptoms associated with an intracranial tumor correlate with the area of the brain involved.

Localized clinical manifestations are caused by destruction, irritation, or compression of the part of the brain in or near the tumor. Blood supply to the affected area is also impaired. Localized manifestations include (1) focal weaknesses (e.g., hemiparesis), (2) sensory disturbances (e.g., anesthesia or paresthesia), (3) language disturbances, (4) coordination disturbances (e.g., staggering gait), and (5) visual disturbances (e.g., diplopia [double vision] or visual field deficit [hemianopia]). As an intracranial tumor enlarges, it shifts intracranial structures and may produce brain stem herniation.

General signs and symptoms are caused by generalized cerebral function disturbance resulting from edema and increased ICP. They include the following.

HEADACHES

Headaches (localized or generalized) are often most severe in the frontal or occipital region. They are usually intermittent, are of increasing duration, and may be

TABLE 30–5. Types of Intracranial Tumors in Adults

Type of Tumor	Frequency of Occurrence	Characteristics
Glioma (malignant)	50% of all intracranial tumors	Rapid growth and infiltration
Astrocytoma	38% of all gliomas 6–10% start as benign but may become malignant	Can infiltrate large areas of brain, making complete excision impossible
Glioblastoma multiforme	50% of all primary brain tumors	Very invasive, vascular tumor Often causes cerebral edema Originates from various cell types
Oligodendroglioma	Less than 5% of all gliomas	Client may present with a long history of seizures
Metastases	20% of all intracranial tumors	It may be the increased ICP that causes death rather than the primary tumor
Pituitary adenomas (benign)	7–10% of all intracranial tumors	May cause visual disturbances, Cushing's syndrome, hypertension, acromegaly, and dysfunction of the reproductive system
Acoustic neuroma (benign)	5% of all intracranial tumors	Arises from Schwann cells in the vestibular portion of CN VII Slow-growing, encapsulated tumor Often symptoms of unilateral nerve compression are seen
Granuloma (benign)	Unknown	Composed of granulation tissue May develop after sarcoidosis, fungal infection, tuberculosis, syphilis infection, or intestinal parasite infections
Cholesteatoma (benign)	Unknown	Slow-growing epidermal tumor Extensive spread may make complete excision impossible
Chordoma (malignant)	Unknown	Locally invasive, slow-growing Usually originates at the base of the cranium Complete removal is often impossible
Meningioma (benign)	Unknown	Frequently recur if partial excision is done
Primary brain lymphoma	Increasing in frequency in AIDS and non-AIDS populations	Involves the brain diffusely, producing infiltrating, multicentric tumors that lie deep within the brain, unresectable; responds temporarily to radiation

intensified by a change in posture or straining. Recurrent, severe headaches in a client previously free of them or recurrent headaches in the morning, increasing in frequency and severity, suggest intracranial tumor and need assessment.

NAUSEA AND VOMITING

Nausea and vomiting may occur late in tumor progression. Vomiting may not be related to meals. Nausea may be marked.

PAPILLEDEMA

Papilledema ("choked disc") is common in clients with intracranial tumors and may be the first sign. Early papilledema does not cause visual acuity changes. Prolonged papilledema causes optic atrophy and severely diminished visual acuity.

SEIZURES

Seizures, focal or generalized, are common in clients with intracranial tumors, especially cerebral hemisphere tumors. Seizures are often the first indication of intracranial tumors, especially in clients without an obvious seizure cause (e.g., head injury).

DIZZINESS AND VERTIGO

Dizziness and vertigo may develop from intracranial circulatory impairment.

MENTAL STATUS CHANGES

Mental status changes may accompany intracranial tumor (e.g., lethargy and drowsiness, confusion, disorientation, and personality changes).

The clinical course of a client with an intracranial tumor varies with the specific type of tumor present. For example, a client with a low-grade glioma who has undergone partial surgical excision of the tumor followed by radiation may survive 5 to 15 years. In contrast, a glioblastoma multiforme grows rapidly and may cause death within 6 months to a year, even with radiation.

DIAGNOSTIC ASSESSMENT

A complete history from the client or family, followed by a thorough physical examination, is especially important. If intracranial tumor is suspected, the following diagnostic studies may be performed: (1) CT scan or MRI scan; (2) plain skull and chest radiographs (to rule out metastatic carcinoma); and (3) electroencephalogram (EEG) and radionuclide scans. An angiogram is used when an intracranial tumor is strongly suspected but a CT scan does not provide sufficient information. Angiograms are very helpful in making a differential diagnosis of masses and for planning surgery. A lumbar puncture is performed provided increased ICP does not exist (Figs. 30-12 and 30-13).

Medical Management

Intervention depends on the type and location of an intracranial tumor and the client's condition. Sometimes chemotherapy is used (e.g., methotrexate, CCNU, and BiCNU). Intrathecal (placed within the CSF) methotrexate is currently used. Nitrosourea (carmustine, BiCNU), and lomustine (CCNU), are lipid-soluble compounds that easily cross the blood-brain barrier. Carmustine can be administered directly into the tumor with biodegradable, timed-release wafers.

Surgical Management

STEREOTACTIC RADIATION THERAPY

A stereotactic needle biopsy may confirm the diagnosis of a brain tumor and help in planning chemotherapy and radiation therapy. Radiation therapy is often used to slow tumor growth and improve the quality of life. Radiation may be administered in the conventional manner or via several innovative systems. The Gamma Knife uses multiple lower-dosage radiation sources. These sources are arranged around the client's head in a helmet device to focus on the tumor. In radiosurgery, a linear accelerator is used to deliver the radiation. The single radiation source is moved in arcs around the client's head, again focusing on the tumor. The benefit of these systems is that the area being irradiated can be clearly identified. This minimizes the effect on healthy brain tissue. These techniques can also be used on tumors or AVMs that are surgically inaccessible. In brachytherapy, radioactive seeds are inserted, through catheters, into the tumor. These seeds are left in place for approximately 2 days and then removed to minimize radiation to healthy brain tissue. This technique can be used after traditional radiation treatments.

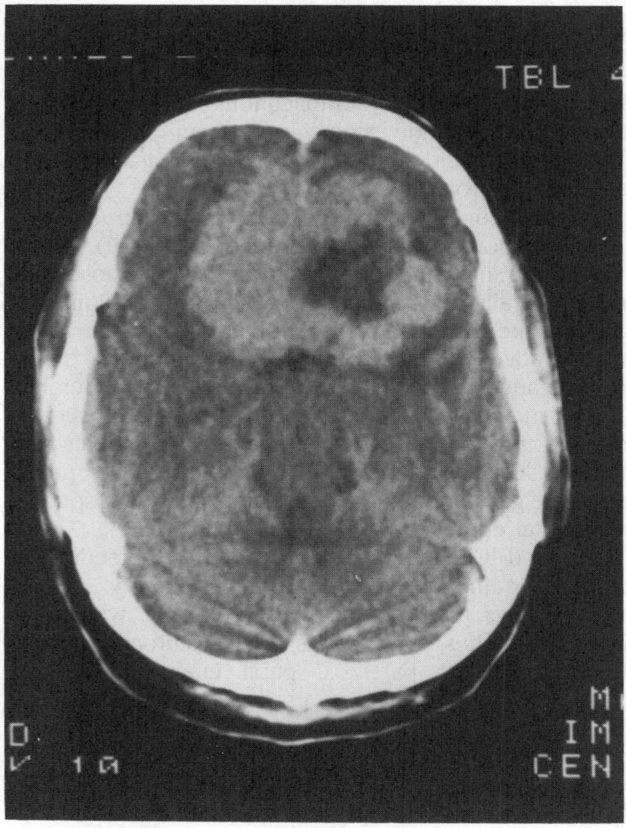

▲ **Figure 30-12**

MRI revealing a midline frontal meningioma.

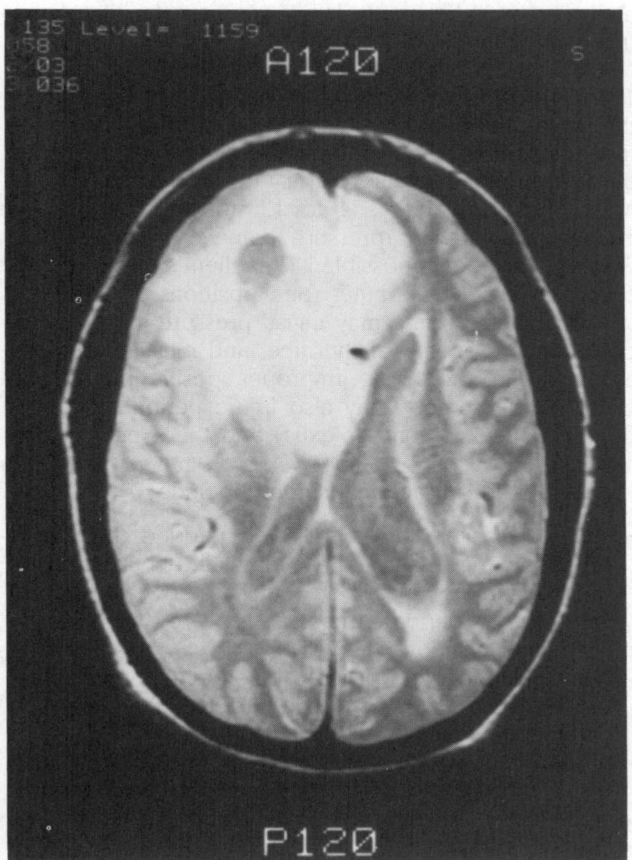

▲ **Figure 30-13**

MRI showing a mixed glioma in the right frontal lobe with ventricular compression.

CRANIOTOMY

A craniotomy is a surgical opening into the skull made in various ways:

- Osteoplastic bone flap: The bone flap remains attached and hinged to muscles and other structures (Fig. 30–14).
- Free-form flap: A section of cranium is cut away from its attachments and temporarily removed.
- Enlarging burr hole: Bone is gradually removed by a rongeur until enough brain is exposed for the procedure.

A craniectomy (in which a portion of cranium is permanently removed) is sometimes performed for decompression, that is, to relieve pressure on brain structures by providing space for expansion. After some craniectomies (e.g., if large), a protective prosthesis made of methyl methacrylate is later surgically inserted.

Intraoperative Care. Local or general anesthetics may be used for intracranial surgery. Local anesthesia is used when the client's response to manipulation of the brain must be assessed during surgery. Potential problems associated with local anesthesia include discomfort, inability to control the airway, nausea, vomiting, straining, and coughing. Some of these activities may detrimentally increase ICP. All general anesthetics alter cerebral dynamics. However, they facilitate control of the client's vital functions.

Positioning. The client must be carefully positioned during intracranial surgery for prevention of postoperative positioning complications. Pressure sores may form because intracranial surgery may be prolonged (e.g., 12 hours; typical length is 4 to 12 hours), and position changes (to prevent pressure damage to nerves and tissues) may be impossible. The client's head is supported in a special frame. (See positions listed in the following.) The frame may cause pressure sores on the client's head, edema of the face, and muscle soreness, especially in the neck. Improper positioning of the client during surgery may also injure peripheral nerves (e.g., peroneal, brachial plexus) and the eyes and eyelids.

Positions for intracranial surgery include

- supine. Pressure areas are well padded, but tissue breakdown (pressure sores) may still occur with prolonged surgery unless preventive care can be provided (e.g., periodic massage toward the pressure site, slight position changes).
- lateral. Support and protect the shoulders and pelvis. Avoid excessive head flexion to facilitate oral and pulmonary drainage.
- prone. This position may interfere with cardiac and respiratory function. It increases risk of postoperative atelectasis and pressure sores. Support and protect the iliac crests, knees, and chest.
- sitting. This position may be used for posterior fossa or cervical surgery. Potential complications include venous air embolism and cardiac or pulmonary distress.

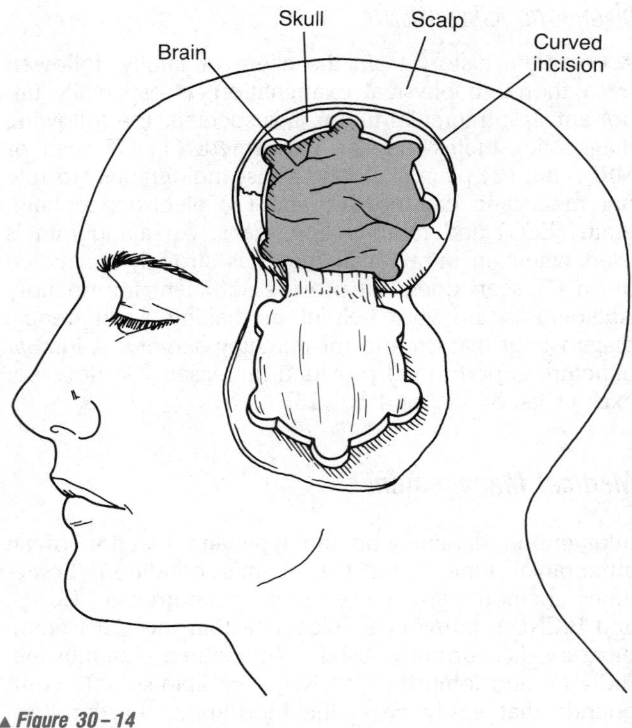

▲ ***Figure 30–14***
Craniotomy with osteoplastic bone flap.

Complications of Intracranial Surgery

General postoperative complications after intracranial surgery may include atelectasis, pneumonia, cardiac irregularities, fluid and electrolyte imbalances, and renal and gastrointestinal disorders.

Potential complications with any major surgery may be very serious, possibly fatal (see Chap. 19). Those from intracranial surgery may be fatal or psychosocially and physically devastating because of the significant functions performed by the structures involved. Some postoperative complications gradually improve; others are permanent. Potential complications with intracranial surgery may vary, depending on the area of surgery and the procedure being performed. Examples are memory loss, paralysis, loss of or impaired special senses (e.g., blindness), loss of or impaired speech, and mental confusion.

Increased ICP (due to cerebral edema or bleeding) is the major complication of intracranial surgery. Assessment findings may include decreased LOC with associated headaches, visual and speech disturbances, muscle weakness or paralysis, pupil changes, seizures, vomiting, and respiratory changes (see Chap. 29 also).

Conventional management of increased ICP includes osmotic diuretic therapy, intubation with hyperventilation to reduce ICP and prevent hypoxia, steroid administration, and elevation of the client's head (see Chap. 29). Further surgical intervention may be necessary, depending on the suspected cause of the increased

ICP. The surgeon may place a catheter in the brain to drain excess fluid or blood from a ventricle or another fluid-filled space. A Jackson-Pratt suction drain (Fig. 30-15) may be surgically inserted if a large cavity remains after removal of a tumor or large hematoma. During brain surgery, the brain may become quite edematous and expand so that the surgeon cannot close the dura. Sometimes a craniectomy is performed to permit expansion of such an edematous brain. Rarely, a client with an expanding brain tumor has a small craniectomy performed to provide for expansion when the tumor grows.

CSF leak may be indicated postoperatively by saturation of the surgical head dressing or drainage from the ear (otorrhea) or nose (rhinorrhea) of clear, thin fluid that dries in concentric circles. CSF leaks are managed with antibiotics. If they do not spontaneously close, a dural patch may be used to repair the site.

Management. Nursing intervention includes observing the client carefully for serous (or blood) drainage from the ears or nose. CSF drainage from the nose (CSF rhinorrhea) is usually preceded by bleeding from the nose and may not be recognized until bleeding stops.

Drainage from the nose or ears may be clear, serosanguineous, or frankly bloody. Distinguish between blood that is draining from local trauma (fractured nose) and blood containing CSF from a meningeal tear. Also, a clear wet "halo" or watery pale ring encircles a bloody spot on sterile gauze when CSF is in the drainage. Clear fluid draining from the nose may be either CSF or normal watery mucus. Keto-Diastix helps distinguish these fluids (i.e., a positive sugar reaction is often present with CSF; a negative sugar reaction may occur with mucus).

Gently place a sterile pad near the outer opening of the client's ear or nose for absorbency, or place a loosely slung external bandage (e.g., sterile pad) over the external ear to absorb the discharge. Replace these dressings as soon as they become moist. Do not pack cotton or gauze in the nose or ear. This obstructs the free flow of fluid and acts as a reservoir for infection.

Assess and document color, consistency, and approximate amount of drainage. Position the client as prescribed so that free drainage of the CSF is possible. A position with the client's head elevated about 20 degrees is often prescribed. Do not allow the client to remain for long in a position that allows stasis of the CSF drainage. Teach the client to observe the drainage and to be aware of signs of infection.

Never attempt to clean or suction the ears or nose of any head-injured client until the physician allows. These activities can introduce infection into the CNS. Instruct a head-injured client not to cough, sneeze, or blow the nose. These activities increase the likelihood of meningitis and may allow air to enter the cranial cavity (forming a pneumocele that may further increase ICP).

Body temperature regulation may be erratic after intracranial surgery. Hypothermia can result from excessive body dehydration due to the client's condition before surgery. Hyperthermia may be secondary to blood in the cranium or underlying infection. Postoperative respiratory complications are the most common cause of hyperthermia. When the hypothalamus has been operated on or manipulated, wide variations in temperature regulation may occur if nerves governing temperature regulation have been disturbed.

Seizures may occur in clients with intracranial surgical lesions (see Seizure Disorders later in chapter). There may be only one seizure or many, possibly progressing to status epilepticus. Because seizures increase metabolic activity, which increases ICP, they are suppressed by anticonvulsants (usually phenytoin). These are often prescribed prophylactically, preoperatively or during surgery, if the surgeon manipulates the cerebral cortex. Typically, seizure activity greatly increases the brain's metabolic needs and may cause further brain damage.

Meningitis (see later in chapter), when it develops, typically appears 2 to 3 days after surgery. Usually it is caused by irritation of the meninges due to infection or blood in the subarachnoid space. Meningitis may also develop with prolonged use of intracranial monitoring

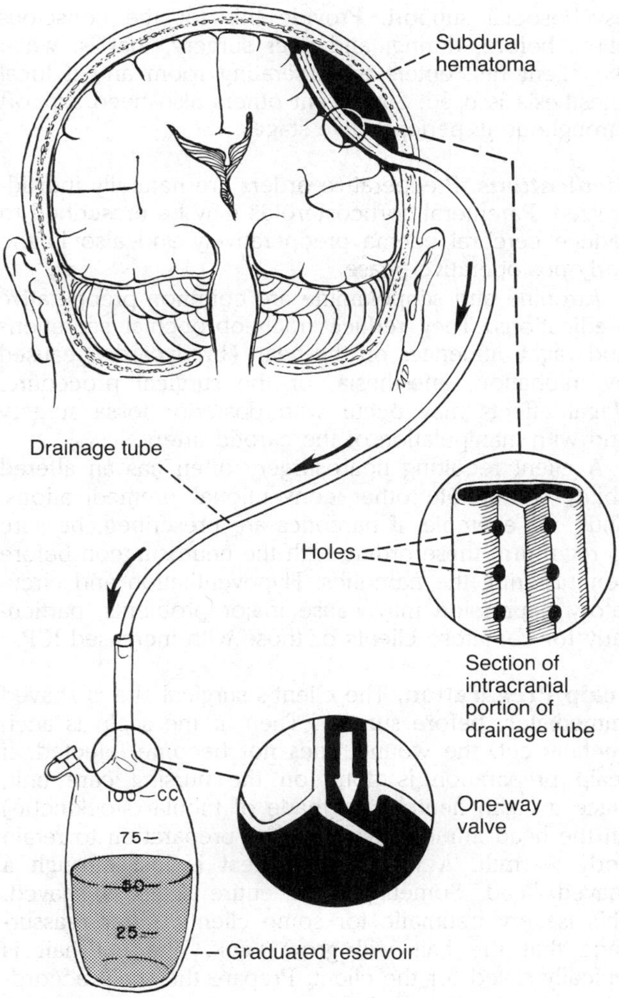

▲ **Figure 30-15**

Jackson-Pratt suction drain. (See text for discussion.)

devices. Assessment findings indicating meningitis may include chills, fever, nuchal rigidity, headache, irritability, decreased LOC, and increased sensitivity to light. It is essential for all care providers to practice infection prevention measures (e.g., handwashing) meticulously when caring for clients after intracranial surgery (e.g., when doing dressing changes, working with monitoring devices).

Ecchymosis and periorbital edema are commonly present after intracranial surgery but are usually transient. Nursing intervention to promote comfort may include use of cool moist packs of normal saline over the eyes and insertion of prescribed lubrication (artificial tears or ointment) into the eyes.

Stress ulcer is a frequent complication if the acute postoperative course is prolonged and requires complex management in an ICU setting. Hyperacidity of gastric secretions and decreased production of gastric mucus can cause gastritis with ulceration and frank hemorrhage. The development of stress ulcer is probably secondary to insult to one or several major organ systems. Steroid administration and mechanical ventilation are also predisposing factors. Intervention includes administering prescribed antacids or histamine-blocking agents and monitoring gastric contents to keep the pH above 4.5.

Clients who have had surgery in the posterior fossa have the risk of additional postoperative complications because the surgical site is close to vital brain stem structures. Cardiac arrhythmias and air embolism may relate to the positioning of the client during surgery. Other complications relate to eighth, ninth, tenth, eleventh, and twelfth cranial nerve dysfunction (e.g., hearing loss, inability to swallow, aspiration, and impaired airway protection).

Nursing Management

PREOPERATIVE ASSESSMENT

Assess and document the following about the client.

- Vital signs; LOC; orientation to person, place, time; ability to follow instructions; pupil size, equality, and reaction to light (Glasgow Coma Scale score); skin color and palpable skin temperature (cool, warm).
- Limb movements; limited or exaggerated movements; strength in extremities (grip); any paresis or paralysis; sensory abnormalities; edema; indications of skin pressure, burns, irritations, abrasions, bruises, or hematomas.
- Manifestations of increasing ICP or pulmonary congestion. Report these findings immediately.
- Any other abnormal findings (e.g., indications of dehydration, seizures, aphasia, visual or auditory problems).

These assessment findings provide preoperative baseline data for comparison with postoperative assessment findings. It is thus possible to determine if a client's condition is improved, is worsened, or remains unchanged in the various assessed parameters as a result of the neurosurgery.

Clients with suspected or known brain tumors are frightened and apprehensive. They and their significant others require the nurse's kindness, patience, and understanding. Often clients have questions about the nature of brain tumors and about brain surgery. Find out whether the client has been told about the malignancy and what else has been discussed concerning diagnosis and treatment. Answer questions as appropriate.

PREOPERATIVE NURSING INTERVENTION

Preoperative preparation for intracranial surgery generally differs little from that for general surgery. This is particularly true for nonemergency surgery when the client's general condition is stable. Preparation for intracranial surgery includes the following.

Psychosocial Preparation. Having one's skull opened and brain structures operated on is major surgery and obviously a frightening experience. This is true both for the client undergoing the surgery and for the significant others. All these individuals require sensitive, skilled psychosocial support. Provide this for the conscious client before, during, and after surgery, that is, when the client first enters the operating room and if local anesthesia is used. Significant others also need support throughout all perioperative stages.

Medications. Preoperative orders are naturally individualized. Parenteral corticosteroids may be prescribed to reduce cerebral edema preoperatively and also in the early postoperative phase.

Atropine and scopolamine are common preoperative medications. They reduce tracheobronchial secretions and vagal influences on the heart (bradycardia) caused by intubation, anesthesia, or the surgical procedure. Vagal effects may occur with posterior fossa surgery and with manipulation of the carotid artery.

A client requiring neurosurgery often has an altered ability to tolerate other conventional premedications. Thus, for example, if narcotics are prescribed, be sure to reconfirm these orders with the neurosurgeon before administering the narcotics. Hypoventilation and circulatory depression may cause major problems, particularly for comatose clients or those with increased ICP.

Scalp Preparation. The client's surgical site is shaved immediately before surgery. Then, if the scalp is accidentally cut, the wound does not become infected. If scalp preparation is done on the nursing care unit, place a clean neuro cap (made of tubular stockinette) on the head immediately after the preparation to retain body warmth. A lot of body heat is lost through a shaved head. Sometimes the entire scalp is shaved. This is very traumatic for some clients. Offer reassurance that the hair will grow back. The cut hair is typically saved for the client. Prepare the scalp according to the situation and the preoperative instructions. A shampoo may be ordered before the head is shaved. If so, during the shampoo, examine the scalp closely for unusual conditions (e.g., lesions, dermatitis, infection).

Antiembolism stockings and sequential compression devices are typically applied before the client goes to the operating room.

POSTOPERATIVE ASSESSMENT

The frequent and thorough neurologic assessment of the client after neurologic surgery is essential. These clients can deteriorate quickly. Vital signs and neurologic signs are usually assessed every hour until the client is stable and then every 2 hours. LOC, ability to move extremities, and speech are assessed. The dressing is inspected for drainage. Intake and output must be carefully documented each hour. Monitor electrolytes, especially serum glucose, sodium potassium, osmolarity, and hematocrit. Take appropriate measures to keep electrolytes within normal range while avoiding extremes of hydration. The response of the client and significant others to the surgery should be evaluated. This is a very stressful experience, particularly if the tumor was malignant or the client experiences neurologic deficits after surgery.

Observe the client carefully for focal or generalized seizure activity. Such activity requires prompt, aggressive nursing and medical intervention. The client must be protected from harm and seizures stopped as quickly as possible, because continuous seizure damages the brain. Immediately report a seizure to the physician. Do not restrict the client's movement during the seizure, but provide physical protection. Administer medication promptly, if ordered.

Frequently assess the condition of the head dressing. Inspect it and the underlying sheet for evidence of bleeding or CSF leak. Immediately report and document such evidence (see Head Trauma). Assess (character, estimated amount) and document prolonged oozing bleeding or oozing wound drainage. Sometimes a small amount of bloody drainage occurs on the dressing if a catheter or drain is in place. Immediately call this to the attention of the neurosurgeon, who may elect to place a stitch at the insertion site to stop this localized bleeding and to anchor the catheter or drain.

Assess whether the dressing is comfortable. It should not be constrictive around the client's head or ears or over the eyes. Sometimes the dressing fits tightly and is down over the eyes; it should remain above the eyes. Does the dressing appear to be too tight? Neurosurgeons usually prefer to perform the first head dressing change personally after intracranial surgery. The nurse may reinforce the initial dressing if it becomes contaminated before the first dressing change (e.g., from serosanguineous drainage). Nurses usually perform subsequent dressing changes.

Examples of residual neurologic deficits are provided in the following, stated in terms of nursing diagnoses. Others have been previously mentioned. Nursing assessment may be the first assessment process to identify some postoperative residual neurologic deficits.

Appropriate referrals to rehabilitation specialists (e.g., speech therapists or physical therapists or for vocational rehabilitation) facilitate recovery. They may help the client and significant others to experience hope, personal growth, and recovery and to build effective coping skills.

Postoperative Intervention

Nursing Diagnosis: Tissue Perfusion, Altered Cerebral, High Risk for R/T increased ICP.

Planning: Expected Outcomes. The client will maintain normopressure cerebral perfusion, as evidenced by maintaining or improving level of consciousness; maintaining or improving Glasgow Coma Scale score; no restlessness, irritability, or headache; no pupillary changes; no seizures; and no widening pulse pressure, respiratory irregularity, hypertension, or bradycardia.

Implementation. The nurse continuously assesses the client's neurologic status, comparing postoperative findings to preoperative status. The parameters within the Glasgow Coma Scale are common indicators.

During the acute phase of care after intracranial surgery, correct postoperative positioning of the client is extremely important to prevent pressure on the brain's operative site, prevent or minimize ICP increases, facilitate tissue perfusion (circulation), and prevent pressure sores or promote their healing.

Positions allowed vary with the type of surgery performed and specific postoperative orders. If in doubt, always double-check orders before placing the client in a questionable position. Incorrect positioning of a client after intracranial surgery may have serious, possibly fatal consequences. Make certain to know whether the client's head is to be elevated or kept flat. The client may not be positioned on the operative side if there is no bone flap. To help ensure proper positioning, post a sign clearly stating safe and unsafe positions for the client. Some guidelines for typical positions after intracranial surgery are presented.

Supratentorial Surgery. After surgery above the brain's tentorium, the client's head is usually elevated 30 degrees to promote venous outflow through the jugular veins. If central lines are present for hemodynamic monitoring purposes, assess and document pulmonary artery or central venous pressure readings at least every 4 hours. If the client is to remain in this head-elevated position, be certain to take these readings consistently while the client is in this position and document the position.

Do not lower the client's head (or the head of the bed) in the acute phase of care after supratentorial surgery for any procedure without a written order from the neurosurgeon.

The neurosurgeon may order the client's head to remain flat after supratentorial surgery to remove a chronic subdural hematoma. Clients with this problem are usually older and their brains are less expandable.

When the hematoma is removed, a large space may remain between the dura and brain. To allow the brain to reexpand, the client lies flat. There may also be a Jackson-Pratt drain to remove fluid buildup in the space. Increased ICP rarely occurs with chronic subdural hematomas.

Infratentorial Surgery. After surgery below the brain's tentorium, the client may be kept flat, without head elevation, to prevent pressure on brain stem structures. The client is turned every 2 hours but never onto the back. This would cause very serious, possibly life-threatening pressure on vital brain stem structures.

Do not elevate the client's head (or the head of the bed) in the acute phase of care after infratentorial surgery for any procedure without written permission from the neurosurgeon.

Posterior Fossa Surgery. The client is typically positioned on the sides, with a pillow under the head for support, and not on the back. This protects the operative site from pressure and minimizes tension on the suture line (very important if wound closure was difficult).

If a bone flap was surgically removed for decompression (to allow further expansion of an already edematous brain), place the client only on the unoperated side or back. This facilitates brain expansion. The client should be turned from the back to the unoperated side, but not to the operated side if a bone flap is not present.

Other interventions to reduce ICP are discussed in Chapter 29 and include diuretics and CSF drainage techniques.

Also, if a client is neurologically unstable (loses consciousness, is sleepy, or is weak) and the ICP elevation is within a critical range (more than 20 mm Hg), avoid procedures that require a flat position (e.g., daily weight-taking). Such a position dangerously elevates ICP.

When a client who must remain head-elevated is positioned on the side (for a position change), support the head. For example, prop the head on a small pillow or folded blanket or apply a soft cervical collar to prevent the head from turning and thus decreasing venous outflow (reduced venous outflow from the head elevates ICP). When the client is in the side-lying position, place a pillow between the legs to maintain good body alignment, to make the client comfortable, and to protect the knees from pressure sores. However, avoid sharp hip flexion, which increases ICP. Increased intra-abdominal pressure in turn increases intrathoracic pressure, and this decreases venous outflow.

Nursing Diagnosis: Infection (Wound and Meningitis), High Risk for R/T loss of primary defenses (incision).

Planning: Expected Outcomes. The client will exhibit no signs or symptoms of infection, as evidenced by no fever, timely wound healing, no induration or abnormal drainage amounts or color from wound, and no clinical manifestations of meningitis.

Implementation. For preventing wound infection and possible meningitis, use sterile technique during dressing changes. Place a Telfa dressing over the incision site or around a drain or catheter insertion site to keep this area clean, dry, and free from abrasion by the overlying bulky dressings. During dressing changes, inspect the operative site and sites around drains or catheters for edema and signs of infection. Document and report these assessment findings.

As postoperative edema subsides and the client's wound heals and improves, replace bulky dressings with modified dressings to suit individual needs. For example, sutures are usually kept covered with Telfa pads, and a stockinette cap is placed over the client's head. To remove dried flaky skin and residue, soften the scalp with baby oil or glycerin and then gently wash the head with soap and water. Do not cause any tension on the suture line. While giving wound care, assess the suture line and wound healing. Document and report any sutures inadvertently left in place, openings in the suture line, or other complications of wound healing.

Nursing Diagnosis: Nutrition, Altered: Less than Body Requirements R/T inability to eat secondary to unconsciousness.

Planning: Expected Outcomes. The client will demonstrate signs of adequate nutrition, as evidenced by weight remaining stable; consuming adequate calories for age, height, and weight; intake equaling output; incisions/wounds healing within 12 to 14 days; hemoglobin level within normal limits for age and sex; and lymphocyte level within normal limits.

Implementation. A client with an uncomplicated postoperative course after intracranial surgery usually requires minimal intravenous maintenance and electrolyte therapy. As the level of wakefulness improves and the swallowing and gag reflexes return, the client usually begins a clear liquid diet and progresses to diet as tolerated. Total food and fluid intake may be curtailed to minimize overhydration and cerebral edema.

If complications delay recovery and nutritional needs are not being met, or if the client's nutritional status is impaired by ill health, nasogastric feedings may be prescribed once the swallowing reflex and peristalsis are present. To minimize the subsequent development of diarrhea (which commonly accompanies tube feedings), keep feedings cold with a piggyback ice bag, infuse the feedings at a continuous rate with an infusion pump, and avoid using elixir-based medications.

Collaborative Problem. Airway obstruction, high risk for R/T cerebral edema, decreased level of consciousness, or neck edema.

Planning: Expected Outcomes. The client will show no signs of airway obstruction, as evidenced by clear lung sounds; full, equal lung expansion; and quiet respirations.

Implementation. Assess respiratory parameters frequently to avoid hypercapnia and to ensure maximal oxygenation of the brain (cerebral oxygenation). Arterial lines or pulse oximetry may be used. Maintain airway patency. However, do not suction through the nose. CSF is protected by the nasal membrane. If the nasal membrane is torn during suctioning, CSF will leak and infection may result. If ICP is markedly increased, do not suction longer than 15 seconds at one time. Prolonged suctioning increases thoracic pressure. This, in turn, increases ICP because of decreased venous return. Hyperventilate between each pass of the catheter.

Monitor arterial blood gases after intracranial surgery to ensure adequate oxygenation. If cerebral edema is a problem, the client may require hyperventilation for prevention of hypercapnia.

Nursing Diagnosis: Incontinence, Bowel, High Risk for R/T unconsciousness.

Planning: Expected Outcomes. The client will have reduced risk of bowel incontinence, as evidenced by formed stool every 2 to 3 days and no incontinence.

Implementation. If diarrhea becomes uncontrollable, reduce tube feedings in concentration and rate until it subsides. Typically, the intravenous fluid infusion rate is increased to replace fluid loss from diarrhea and to maintain adequate hydration. If it is still not possible to maintain adequate nutrition and there is only minimal lessening of the diarrhea (or if there is evidence of neurologic deterioration), total parenteral nutrition (TPN) may be ordered. The main advantage of TPN is its high-calorie, high-protein content. This maximizes the client's nutritional state rapidly, which promotes the possible return of normal gastrointestinal function. Consult a fundamentals of nursing text for nursing interventions for clients receiving intravenous therapy, tube feedings, and TPN.

Nursing Diagnosis: Communication, Impaired Verbal R/T aphasia or dysarthria.

Planning: Expected Outcomes. The client will be able to effectively communicate, as evidenced by the client's needs being understood and met, and the client indicating understanding of the communication of others.

Implementation. After intracranial surgery, speech disorders may occur as a result of decreased circulation to the brain during surgery or surgical trauma to the areas of the brain governing speech. Interventions for aphasia are discussed earlier.

Nursing Diagnosis: Contractures, High Risk for R/T immobility.

Planning: Expected Outcomes. The client will have no signs of contractures, as evidenced by full ROM in all joints; no evidence of flexion contractures in wrists, elbows, and knees; and no signs of footdrop.

Implementation. After intracranial surgery, the client remains on bed rest for at least 24 hours. Nursing care to prevent complications of immobility is imperative. After 24 hours, passive ROM exercises are usually begun. Increased ICP or physiologic instability may delay these activities beyond 24 hours.

Frequent position changes (to other safe positions) are important. Prepare the client (and other nurses) for the move. Explain what each nurse should or should not do during the move. Remember that even though a client appears to be unconscious, hearing may be intact. Turn the client very carefully using a turning sheet, and always have adequate help to prevent injury to the client and nursing staff. Do not make the client strain to assist with changing positions because straining may dangerously elevate ICP. For use during turning, position a turning sheet on the bed so that it extends well above the client's head. Protect and support the head and any weak extremities to prevent injury and to maintain a safe position.

When the client's condition is stabilized, movement to the bedside chair is ordered. In the ICU setting, the client is most easily lifted on a drawsheet by several care givers from the bed directly onto a reclining chair. Once the client is secured in the chair, the head of the chair is slowly elevated. This is done in gradual increments until the full upright position is tolerated. If a chair is not available, help the client to dangle his or her legs over the side of the bed. Remain present for safety and support in both situations. Closely assess for dizziness or faintness. Before and after the transfer, auscultate and document the blood pressure to assess for postural hypotension. As improvement continues, self-care and other activities are gradually resumed.

Nursing Diagnosis: Self-Care Deficit, High Risk for R/T weakness, cognitive impairments.

Planning: Expected Outcomes. The client will perform as many ADLs as possible, as evidenced by the use of adaptive devices and techniques and recognition of limitations.

Implementation. Extensive self-care deficits may be present after intracranial surgery. They may be due to factors such as neuromuscular impairment, perceptual or cognitive impairment, pain, severe anxiety, or weakness. Self-care deficits may include those related to bathing/hygiene, feeding, toileting, or dressing/grooming. Careful nursing assessment is required to meet the client's needs in these areas and to promote a return to maximal possible self-care. The client should be encouraged to perform ADLs as he or she is able.

Nursing Diagnosis: Self-Esteem Disturbance R/T operative or postoperative complications.

Planning: Expected Outcomes. The client will develop effective coping strategies, as evidenced by appropriate lifestyle modifications, use of the assistance of others, and appropriate social interactions.

Implementation. Postoperative complications of devastating proportions may occur after intracranial surgery. They can profoundly disturb the client's self-esteem, role performance, and personal identity. Also, there may be body image changes that are difficult for the client to accept. Nurses can assist the client and significant others to deal with these threatening issues.

If a defect remains in the skull after surgery, it may be helpful for the surgeon to discuss possible cranioplasty before the client sees the defect. Cranioplasty is the surgical repair of the defect with a custom-made implant. Naturally, it may be depressing for the client to experience a disturbance in self-esteem due to such a body image change, and the client may fear additional surgery. However, cranioplasty not only can improve the client's appearance but also protects the area of the skull defect.

Nursing Diagnosis: Thought Processes, Altered R/T surgical resection, cerebral edema, sleep deprivation.

Planning: Expected Outcomes. The client will recognize limitations and attempt to minimize them, as evidenced by participation in prescribed therapies, consideration of physical capabilities during activities, and verbalization of limitations and adaptations.

Implementation. Alteration in thought processes may be temporary (e.g., due to sleep deprivation, cerebral swelling) or permanent (e.g., due to surgical trauma) after intracranial surgery. If thought process disturbances continue to persist, the nurse may make suggestions for living with this problem. For any brain function change (verbal thought, memory), neuropsychological testing helps establish parameters of dysfunction.

Nursing Diagnosis: Pain R/T scalp incision.

Planning: Expected Outcomes. The client will experience adequate pain relief, as evidenced by verbalization of improvement in comfort level without excessive drowsiness or lethargy, the ability to rest without interruption by pain, and the ability to participate in therapies without hindrance by pain.

Implementation. Do not jar the client's bed or otherwise cause sudden movements that worsen the pain. Keep the environment quiet, calm, and dimly lit. Administer prescribed medications as indicated for pain relief. Acetaminophen or codeine may be prescribed for pain relief. Evaluate the effectiveness of pain-relieving medications. Check for allergies to medications. If the client vomits from inability to tolerate medication, ICP may be seriously elevated.

Nursing Diagnosis: Family Processes, Altered R/T irreversible changes in client after surgery.

Planning: Expected Outcomes. The family members will exhibit positive behaviors, as evidenced by the ability to problem solve; care for all members of the family as needed; and ask questions about showing concern toward the client as appropriate, showing that they have understood previous conversations.

Implementation. Family members are also affected by the client's postoperative changes. Some are able and willing to help the client and themselves grow and meet postoperative challenges. Others are unable to adapt effectively in this way, finding it difficult to accept changes in the client.

Facilitating the expression of concerns, providing support and understanding, careful listening, and an unhurried empathetic manner may all help the client and significant others if postoperative problems occur (e.g., paralysis, infection, speech disorders, skull defects) or if the surgery seems unsuccessful. The client and family may also experience spiritual distress, powerlessness, or anticipatory grieving if the surgery was not successful and the client is unimproved, has postoperative complications, or is dying.

EVALUATION

The degree of expected outcome attainment should be evaluated on a regular basis. Some expected outcomes, such as ICP and cerebral perfusion, will need to be met before discharge from the ICU. Other expected outcomes, such as improved cognition and speech, may require months to obtain. Setting appropriate and achievable outcomes with the client and family is important.

Post-hospital Care

DISCHARGE TEACHING

Many clients can be discharged home and return to a gratifying life after brain surgery. Others will require short-term or ongoing rehabilitation to achieve complete recovery. Still others will never regain complete competence because of the amount of brain tissue damaged from the disorder and surgery. For these clients, the greater burden rests on the family to provide ongoing care either at home or in a nursing home.

Family support groups are available through many hospitals to families with brain-damaged members. These groups help the significant others to know they are not alone. Clinical nurse specialists in neuroscience are often the facilitators for these groups. Participation by both client and significant others should be encouraged. Care should be taken to include everyone who is important to the client, not just those who are legal relatives.

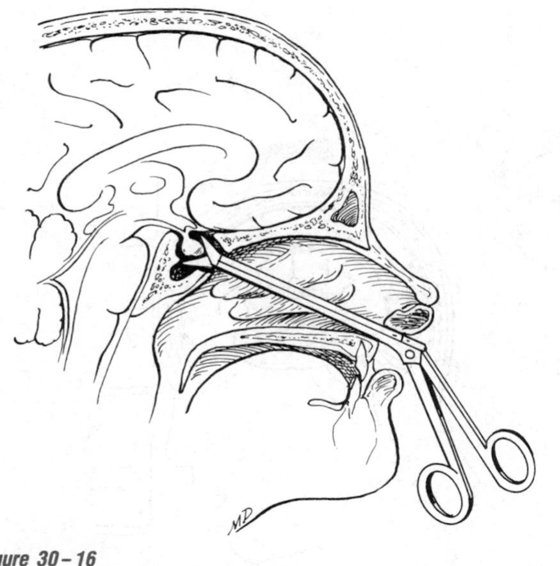

▲ Figure 30-16

Transsphenoidal hypophysectomy for the excision of pituitary tumors.

PITUITARY TUMORS

Pituitary tumors cause the client to develop visual field defects, irregular or absent menstrual cycles, infertility, decreased libido, impotence, decreased body hair, and decreased production of other stimulating hormones. Most of these tumors occur in the anterior lobe and are benign, small, and encapsulated. They can usually be removed successfully with surgery. The procedure is called transsphenoidal hypophysectomy. The operation is performed through the nose to avoid entering the cranium (Fig. 30-16).

After surgery, the client is positioned with head elevated. The nose is packed to control bleeding. Postoperative care is similar to that of other clients after craniotomy.

A fairly common effect from pituitary edema is the development of transient diabetes insipidus due to a lack of secretion of antidiuretic hormone (ADH). Clients with diabetes insipidus have large volumes (2 to 15 L/day) of dilute urine. Aside from the inconvenience of polyuria, the client often will suffer no serious side effects from diabetes insipidus, unless the client is deprived of water. When this happens, circulatory collapse (hypovolemic shock) and hypertonic encephalopathy will occur as a result of fluid shifts in the brain.

Usual treatment is with intravenous or inhalation vasopressin (Pitressin) or desmopressin (DDAVP). Long-acting forms of these agents can be used for chronic diabetes insipidus. After pituitary surgery, the client will also require hormones for replacement of those lost with tissue resection.

Nursing intervention for diabetes insipidus or syndrome of inappropriate antidiuretic hormone (SIADH) involves

- accurate intake and output documentation
- assessing urine specific gravity every 2 hours
- assessing for indications of fluid and electrolyte imbalances
- documenting and reporting changes in the client's status or therapy
- explaining the condition to the client and significant others, emphasizing the need for fluid balance (i.e., avoiding overhydration or dehydration)
- explaining the reasons for medication, when and how to take it, and any side effects to the client and significant others

▼ HEAD TRAUMA

INJURIES TO THE SCALP, SKULL, OR BRAIN

Definition

Head trauma may be defined as any injury to the scalp, skull, or brain.

Incidence

In the United States, a head injury is experienced approximately every 16 seconds. Head injury is often classified as minor or mild, moderate, and severe. Minor head injuries occur in over half a million Americans every year. Of these, more than 290,000 are hospitalized, and 150,000 experience disability lasting 1 month or more.

Moderate injuries, resulting in disability for 3 months or more, occur to approximately 60,000 to 75,000 clients per year. Fatal head injuries occur over 140,000 times per year. Head trauma results in more deaths than all other causes combined for Americans under the age of 34 years.

Etiology

Motor vehicle accidents are the foremost cause of head injuries. Other causes are assaults, falls, and accidents.

MECHANISMS OF INJURY

Head injuries are caused by a sudden force to the head (Fig. 30-17). The results are complex. Three mechanisms contribute to head trauma: (1) acceleration, (2) deceleration, and (3) deformation. An acceleration injury occurs when the immobile head is struck by a moving object. If the head is moving and hits an immobile object, a deceleration injury occurs. This can be seen in an auto accident when the head hits the steering wheel. In an acceleration/deceleration injury, a moving object hits the immobile head, and then the head hits an immobile object. Deformation refers to injuries in which the force results in deformation and disruption of the integrity of the impacted body part (e.g., skull fracture).

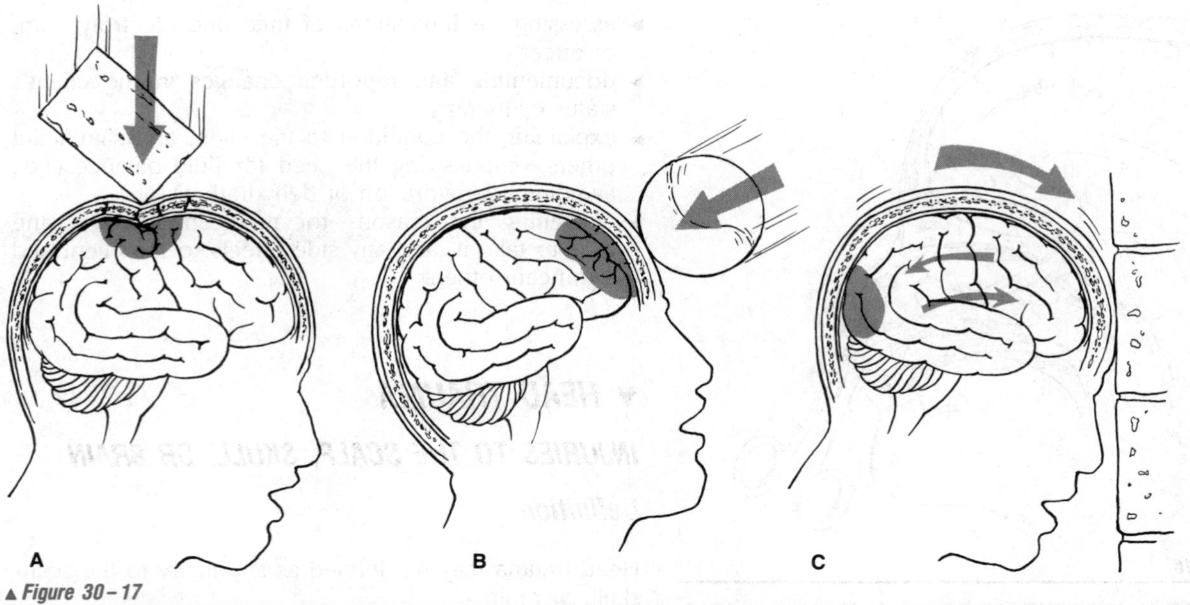

▲ *Figure 30–17*

Some mechanisms of head injury. Head injury results from penetration or impact. *A*, A direct injury (blow to skull) may fracture the skull. Contusion and laceration of the brain may result from fractures. Depressed portions of the skull may compress or penetrate brain tissue. *B*, In the absence of skull fracture, a blow to the skull may cause the brain to move enough to tear some of the veins going from the cortical surface to the dura. Subsequently, subdural hematoma may develop. Note areas of cerebral contusion *(shaded)*. *C*, Rebound of the cranial contents may result in an area of injury opposite the point of impact. Such an injury is called a contrecoup injury. In addition to the three injuries depicted, secondary phenomena may result from the injury and cause additional brain dysfunction or damage. For example, ischemia, especially cerebral edema, may occur, elevating intracranial pressure.

Head trauma is also categorized by describing the injury (e.g., blunt or penetrating trauma or a coup or contrecoup injury). Acceleration/deceleration injuries often result in blunt trauma. These are complex injuries involving several cranial structures, including brain parenchyma and vessels. Because the brain is able to move within the skull, movement of the brain can result in injuries at different locations. The brain is partially tethered down (at its base) and is also suspended in CSF. Therefore, a blow to the skull can cause the hemispheres to twist on the fixed brain stem. As the brain moves, it scrapes over the skull's irregular inner prominences, bruising and lacerating brain tissue. Disruption of the brain's small surface blood vessels may occur. Changes in vascular integrity may lead to fluid shifts and petechial hemorrhages. Cranial nerves, nerve tracts, larger blood vessels, and other tissues may be stretched, twisted, or rotated and their functions disrupted.

Penetrating injuries include those made by foreign bodies (e.g., knives or bullets) or those made by bone fragments from a skull fracture. The damage caused by a penetrating injury often relates to the velocity with which a penetrating object pierces the skull and brain. Bone fragments from a skull fracture may cause local brain injury by lacerating brain tissue and damaging other structures (e.g., nerves and blood vessels). If a major blood vessel is severed or ruptured, a large clot (hematoma) may form, with damage to adjacent or even remote structures (e.g., brain compression from one of the herniation syndromes). Thus, a secondary event, a hematoma, can also cause extensive brain tissue damage.

High-velocity objects (e.g., bullets) produce shock waves in the skull and brain. The shock waves may significantly damage brain structures beyond those in the object's path. "Explosion" of brain substance may occur, although lacerations and tissue maceration are more common. Frequently, low- and high-velocity penetrating wounds create an open communication between the external environment and the cranial cavity. Thus, infection is a possible complication. These penetrating wounds are commonly treated surgically with debridement and wound closure.

A coup injury occurs immediately at the point of impact. Because of movement within the skull, the same blow may cause injury on the opposite side of the brain, that is, a contrecoup injury. (Contrecoup is derived from a French word meaning reverse-blow.) In addition there are often multiple areas of injury along the line of the blow's force. Tissues around major injured areas often swell, which increases damage to the brain (Fig. 30–18).

Injuries may also be classified according to the structure damaged (e.g., brain stem) and whether they are primary or secondary. Primary head injury refers to impact damage, the severity of which is estimated by initial signs and symptoms. Secondary or delayed events that follow head injury include edema, hemorrhage, or infection. These processes can significantly impede recovery or even cause death from what initially appeared to be a mild injury.

Risk Factors

The major factor contributing to the occurrence of head injury is alcohol consumption. Alcohol slows reflexes and alters cognitive processes and perception. These physiologic changes increase the chances of being involved in an accident or altercation.

Primary prevention centers on the education of clients of all ages. Children should be taught the importance of safety restraints in cars and of bicycle helmets. The use of motorcycle helmets and the dangers of driving after drug or alcohol ingestion are necessary information for older children and adults. Secondary prevention is not an issue in head trauma because other health conditions do not increase the incidence of head trauma. Pre-existing conditions may have an impact on recovery from head injury.

Tertiary prevention focuses on preventing or minimizing the complications of head trauma. At-the-scene care by trained professionals, stabilization, and transportation to tertiary care centers improve outcomes. At the time of an accident, many clients suffer primary, irreversible brain injury, which ultimately causes death. The most common causes of such deaths are brain stem hemorrhage and diffuse axonal injury throughout the brain due to the impact.

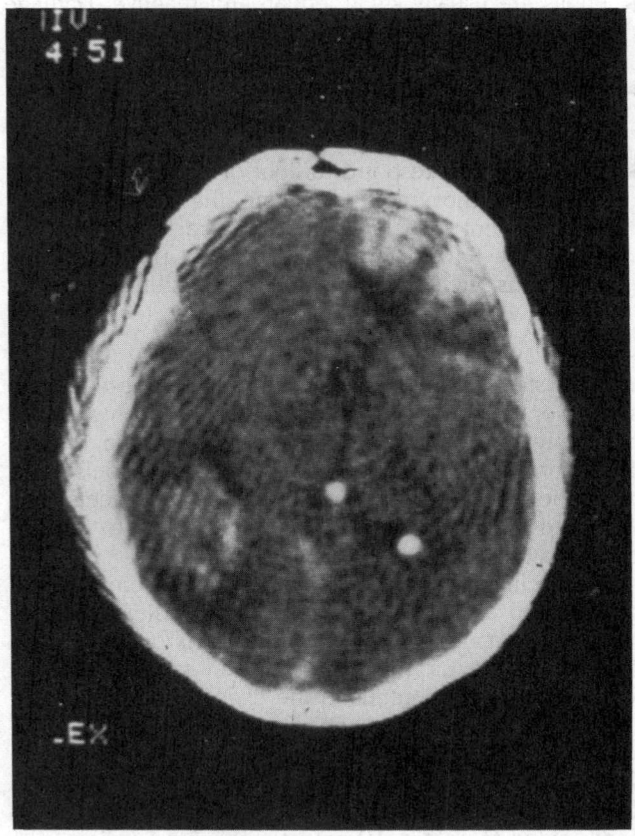

▲ Figure 30–18

MRI showing coup-contrecoup injury after head injury.

Pathophysiology

Primary head injuries include injuries to the scalp, skull, or brain or all of these. The injuries result from the original impact.

SCALP INJURIES

Scalp injuries can cause lacerations, hematomas, and contusions or abrasions to the skin. These injuries may be unsightly and bleed profusely. Clients with minor scalp injuries not accompanied by damage to other areas do not require hospitalization.

SKULL INJURIES

Skull fractures are often caused by a force sufficient to cause both fracture and brain injury. The fractures in themselves do not mean brain injury is also present. However, skull fractures often cause serious brain damage. Depressed skull fractures injure the brain by bruising it (abrasion) or by driving bone fragments into it (lacerations). The site of a fracture and the extent of brain injury may not correlate.

There are three types of skull fracture.

Linear Skull Fractures. Linear skull fractures appear as thin lines radiographically and do not require treatment. They are important only if there is significant underlying brain damage.

Depressed Skull Fractures. Depressed skull fractures may be palpated and are seen radiographically. Surgery may be required within the first 24 hours after injury if the depression is as deep as the skull thickness. Depressed fractures may be associated with bone fragments penetrating into brain tissue. When this occurs, the area is usually surgically explored and debrided.

Basilar Skull Fractures. Basilar skull fractures occur in bones over the base of the frontal and temporal lobes. They are rarely seen radiographically.

Basilar skull fractures, depressed fractures, and other open (compound) fractures all allow communication between the exterior environment and the brain. Infection is therefore a possible complication. (See later discussion of brain abscess and meningitis.)

BRAIN INJURIES

There is a wide variety of brain injuries (see Mechanisms of Injury). A single classification of brain injuries does not exist. However, the terms open, closed, contusion, and concussion are often applied to brain injuries. Open head injuries are those that penetrate the skull. Closed injuries are from blunt trauma.

Concussions. A concussion is head trauma that may result in loss of consciousness for 5 minutes or less and retrograde amnesia. There is no break in the skull or dura, and no visible damage on the CT or MRI is seen. The client usually presents with headache and dizziness and may complain of nausea and vomiting. The duration of amnesia may directly correlate with severity of the concussion.

Contusions. Contusions cause more extensive damage than do concussions. Contusions damage the brain substance itself, causing multiple areas of petechial and punctate hemorrhage and bruised areas. Diffuse axonal injury resulting in anatomic disruption of the white matter may result from serious contusions. Microscopic nerve fiber lesions also occur. Abnormalities may be mainly in one area of the brain, but other areas may also be injured. This is particularly true of brain stem contusions, which are a very serious type of lesion.

Nuchal rigidity (involuntary stiffness of neck muscles) may indicate cervical spine (C-spine) injuries, meningeal irritation, or subarachnoid bleeding after head injury.

Clinical Manifestations

SKULL FRACTURES

Other than a history of head injury, clients with skull fractures may not have clear symptoms of their injury. They may develop other clinical signs including (1) CSF or other drainage from the ear or nose, (2) various cranial nerve injuries, (3) blood behind the eardrum, (4) periorbital ecchymosis (bruise around the eyes), and (5) later, a bruise over the mastoid (Battle's sign).

Indications of cranial nerve damage may occur at the time of the initial injury or may develop later. They include

- vision loss (e.g., blindness, blurred vision) from optic nerve damage
- hearing loss with postural vertigo and nystagmus from auditory nerve damage
- loss of the sense of smell (bilaterally or unilaterally) from olfactory nerve damage
- squint or fixed dilated pupil and loss of some of the eye movements from oculomotor nerve damage
- facial paresis/paralysis (unilateral) from facial nerve damage.

CONTUSIONS

There are various clinical manifestations in clients with contusions. This is partly because of the numerous areas of damage. Contusions are often associated with other serious injuries, including cervical fractures. Secondary effects (e.g., brain swelling and edema) accompany serious contusions. Increased ICP and herniation syndromes may result.

Contusions may be divided into cerebral contusions and brain stem contusions.

Cerebral Contusions. These contusions can be diagnosed only if the client is alert, although they may be present in comatose patients. Assessment findings vary, depending on which areas of the cerebral hemispheres are damaged. An agitated, confused head-injured client who remains alert may have a temporal lobe contusion. Hemiparesis in an alert head-injured client may indicate a frontal contusion. An aphasic head-injured client may have a frontal-temporal contusion. Other findings indicate contusions in other areas. Remember that although these findings correlate with cerebral contusion, they do not rule out other abnormalities such as a developing mass or lesion. Adverse changes in the client's condition require immediate medical attention. They may indicate treatable complications.

Brain Stem Contusions. Brain stem contusions render a client immediately unresponsive or partially comatose because of significant brain stem disruption. Typically, an altered LOC continues for at least several hours and usually days or weeks. The client may regain partial consciousness within hours or remain in a coma.

Damage to the reticular activating system may render the client permanently comatose. Other neurologic abnormalities are present and are usually symmetric (i.e., on both sides of the body). Some may be lateralized (asymmetric, on one side of the body only), indicating development of a secondary event such as a hematoma.

In addition to the altered LOC that is always present with brain stem contusion, respiratory, pupillary, eye movement, and motor abnormalities may occur.

- Respirations may be normal, ataxic, periodic, or very rapid.
- Pupils are usually small, equal, and reactive. Damage to the upper brain stem (third cranial nerve) may cause pupillary abnormalities.
- Loss of normal eye movements may occur because pathways controlling eye movements traverse the midbrain and pons.
- The client may respond to light or noxious stimuli by purposeful movements, pushing the stimulus away. Or the client may have no response to stimuli, that is, may be flaccid. In the presence of profound LOC alterations, flexion and extension posturing may be elicited with or without noxious stimuli (see Chapter 28).

Brain stem contusions do not usually injure the brain stem alone. Swelling or direct injury to the hypothalamus may produce autonomic nervous system effects. The client has a high temperature, has rapid pulse and respiration, and perspires profusely. These effects may wax and wane but, if sustained, can lead to serious complications.

These clinical manifestations often vary from one observation to another (whereas findings indicating a developing hematoma are more consistent). Careful documentation of assessment findings is important to identify patterns or trends in the client's condition.

DIAGNOSTIC ASSESSMENT

There is a high association of cervical fracture with head injury; therefore, lateral cervical spine radiographs are obtained before the client's head is moved. CT scans and radiographs are also obtained to assess for

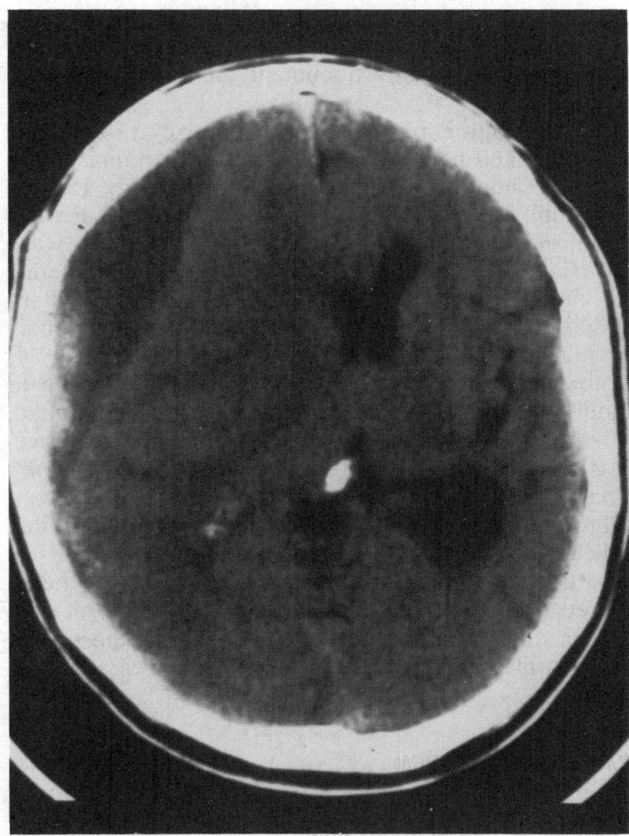

▲ Figure 30-19

MRI showing chronic subdural hematoma with an area of acute bleeding causing a severe midline shift.

fractures and areas of bleeding or brain shift (Figure 30-19). Lumbar puncture can also be used to assess for bleeding within the subarachnoid space.

Medical Management

A complete history is taken of the mechanism of injury. These data allow the physician to determine the probable extent of injury. Diagnostic findings are reviewed.

Open head wounds should be covered and pressure applied to control bleeding unless there appears to be underlying depressed or compound skull fracture. Do not attempt to remove foreign objects or any penetrating objects from the wound. Uncomplicated scalp wounds (that do not lie over depressed or compound skull fractures) are anesthetized locally, cleansed, and sutured.

Simple skull depressions are electively treated by surgically elevating the depressed bone fragment and repairing the dura if it is lacerated. All bone fragments are removed. Compound depressed skull fractures are immediately treated surgically. The scalp, skull, and devitalized brain are débrided, and the wound is cleansed thoroughly. Unless all foreign material is removed, a brain abscess develops. Débridement of a penetrating wound or depressed skull fracture frequently leaves a cranial defect that is cosmetically unsightly. The defect is surgically corrected by cranioplasty.

SEVERE HEAD INJURY

Major goals in the care of severely head-injured clients are (1) the prompt recognition and treatment of hypoxia and acid-base disturbances that can contribute to cerebral edema increasing ICP resulting from factors such as cerebral edema or expanding hematoma and (2) stabilization of other conditions.

Few clients die instantly from head injury. However, many head-injured clients die within the first few minutes after injury from shock or impaired respiration. Early death may also result from brain stem damage. Rigorous intervention is started immediately because severe brain trauma is associated with high morbidity and mortality rates.

Some clients survive initial head trauma only to develop intracranial mass lesions such as expanding hematomas (e.g., epidural and subdural hemorrhages), which may be fatal unless promptly diagnosed and treated. Severe cerebral swelling often follows brain injury. It is probably the most common cause of death in clients who survive the initial injury and who do not develop intracranial mass lesions.

Clients with traumatic head injuries often have other major injuries. These include facial fractures, lung and heart injuries, cervical fractures, abdominal injuries, and musculoskeletal injuries. Facial fractures and lung injuries may contribute to respiratory insufficiency. Airway obstruction and decreased ability to breathe (e.g., from pulmonary contusion, flail chest, pneumothorax) contribute to respiratory insufficiency and poor oxygenation of the brain and other tissues. Brain death may result.

Hemorrhagic shock in clients with multiple trauma is rarely caused by head injury alone. Frequently it relates to (1) ruptured abdominal organs or (2) musculoskeletal injuries (e.g., fractured femur and pelvis). Circulation may be further compromised by cardiac contusion and associated arrhythmias. Head injuries can also cause arrhythmias and further complicate the client's recovery.

The medical management of severely head-injured clients focuses on supporting all organ systems while recovery from the injuries takes place. This involves ventilatory support, management of nutrition and gastrointestinal function, and management of fluid balance and elimination. Head trauma has impact on all systems of the body, and managing these effects requires a holistic perspective. Clinical manifestations must be evaluated as stemming from the head injury or arising from a complicating process.

Fluids are usually managed carefully for avoidance of either over- or underadministration. Parameters such as central venous pressure and urinary output are used to guide fluid intake. Because severely head-injured clients are given nothing by mouth, potassium is commonly given through the intravenous line.

PHARMACOLOGIC MANAGEMENT

Antiseizure medications, such as phenytoin, are begun on admission. Even though seizures early in the course of head injury are uncommon, if they occur, brain injury can intensify because of alterations in oxygenation from impaired ventilation and increased ICP. Corticosteroids have not been shown to be of benefit after head injury and may cause further problems, so they are usually not prescribed. Histamine antagonists, such as cimetidine, are given to reduce the risk of stress ulcers. Mild analgesics may be prescribed, such as acetaminophen or codeine. Antibiotics may also be prescribed. Osmotic diuretics may be required to reduce ICP.

DIETARY MANAGEMENT

Initially the client is given nothing by mouth until peristalsis returns, commonly after 5 days. Feeding is begun via nasogastric tube because metabolic needs increase after head injury. The risk of aspiration with nasogastric feeding must be prevented by feeding the client with head elevated and monitoring pulmonary changes. Hyperalimentation can also be used, but some clients develop hyperglycemia from the solution. Hyperglycemia can further cerebral anoxia, and blood glucose levels should be monitored carefully.

Nursing Management

ASSESSMENT

A history of how a client was injured is helpful in understanding the nature of a head injury. When accident witnesses accompany a newly head-injured client to the care facility, obtain as much information as possible about the accident and the client's neurologic responses at the scene of the accident. Especially try to find out if the client lost consciousness.

As soon as possible after head injury, assess and document the client's vital signs and neurologic status. This initial assessment establishes a baseline for later observations. Carefully document all assessment findings.

In the health care facility, the frequency of assessing vital signs and neurologic status varies according to the client's condition. However, it is usually every 15 minutes until the client is stable and within limits for age and previous conditions. It may be necessary to wake up a head-injured client hourly for assessment during the first 24 to 48 hours after injury. Parameters assessed include (1) LOC and responsiveness, (2) pupillary diameters and responses to light, (3) vital signs, (4) motor strength, (5) speech, (6) vision, (7) reaction to auditory and painful stimuli, (8) response to command, (9) spontaneous activity, and (10) general responsiveness to stimulation. The Glasgow Coma Scale is commonly used.

Promptly report to the physician any findings that indicate the possible development of complications. It is particularly difficult to assess the condition of a head-injured client who has ingested large amounts of alcohol or other drugs before injury because these substances may obscure significant clinical assessment findings.

NURSING INTERVENTION

Nursing of the head-injured client is found in the care plan for the head-injured client.

EVALUATION

The degree of attainment of expected outcomes should be assessed often in the early phases of care. Later in rehabilitation, expected outcomes may require weeks for full attainment. Because the care of the head-injured client goes on in many areas of a health care setting (i.e., ICU, a general nursing unit, a rehabilitation unit), complete communication about the client, family, and goals should always be a part of any care plan.

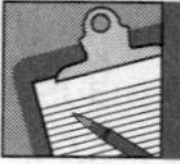

CARE PLAN

The Head-Injured Client

Nursing Diagnosis/ Collaborative Problem	Planning: Expected Outcomes	Implementation: Nursing Interventions	Rationales
Paralysis, High Risk for R/T undiagnosed cervical fractures	The nurse will monitor for development of progressive motor/sensory deficit; increased neck pain, stiffness, bruising; bilateral paralysis	Immobilize head and neck until cervical injury ruled out by examination/x-ray study (cervical collar, sandbags, spine board)	The cervical spine needs to be immobilized until it is certain no fracture exists
		Avoid flexion, hyperextension, rotation of neck	
		If respiratory resuscitation needed, use jaw thrust maneuver	Hyperextension of the neck increases risk of injury
		Assess/document leg, hand, arm, and shoulder move-	Cervical fracture may cause weakness or paresthesias

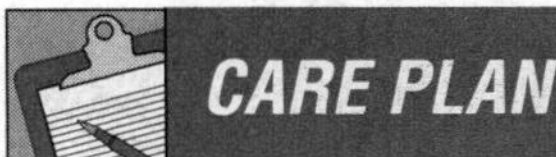

CARE PLAN

The Head-Injured Client Continued

Nursing Diagnosis/ Collaborative Problem	*Planning: Expected Outcomes*	*Implementation: Nursing Interventions*	*Rationales*
		ment and strength hourly and prn	in the extremities
		Assess sensory deficits	
		Assess for neck pain, stiffness, bruising	Bleeding in the subarachnoid space causes tissue irritation
Airway Clearance, Ineffective R/T coma or bleeding into airway	Client will have effective airway clearance, as evidenced	Maintain a patent airway	The airway may be occluded from blood, vomitus, or secretions
		Clear mouth/oropharynx of foreign bodies (e.g., teeth)	
	By upper airway free of secretions	Suction oropharynx and trachea q 1–2 hr and prn (suction nasopharynx after basilar fracture ruled out)	
	Regular respiratory rate (16–22), rhythm, amplitude		
	Breath sounds present both lung bases	Assess respiratory rate, rhythm, amplitude q 1–2 hr or prn	Respiratory rate may be altered if brain stem is injured
	Symmetric chest movement		
	Trachea midline	Check breath sounds and chest excursions q 1–2 hr	Breath sounds indicate air movement
	Absence of dyspnea, agitation, confusion, yawning	Monitor ABGs (initially, daily, and prn)	Indicate arterial oxygen, carbon dioxide, and pH
	Absence of aspiration		
	ABGs normal with PaO_2 greater than 90 mm Hg and PCO_2 between 30 and 35 mm Hg	Position semiprone, lateral position	Facilitates drainage of secretions and prevents aspiration *after* cervical spine stabilized
	Chest film clear	Administer humidified oxygen as indicated	Oxygen is used to prevent cerebral hypoxia
		Assist/maintain endotracheal intubation, tracheostomy, and mechanical ventilation as needed	Mechanical ventilation may be required to supplement ventilatory efforts
Tissue Perfusion, Altered Cerebral R/T hypotension, intracranial hemorrhage, hematoma, or other injuries	Client will have adequate cerebral tissue perfusion, as evidenced by	Assess LOC/responsiveness hourly or prn, including alertness, orientation	Alterations in LOC are first indications of increasing ICP
	Stable, improving LOC	Assess pupillary size, position, response to direct and consensual responses q 1–4 hr	Pupillary changes commonly accompany head injury
	GCS of 9 or above		
	Temperature less than 38.5° C		
	Equal and reactive pupils (PERLA)		
	Intact consensual light reflex		
	Intact extraocular movements	Assess EOM q 1–4 hr	Increasing ICP often traps CN III affecting eye movement
	Stable/improving motor response (hand, arm, and leg movements)	Cognitive function may be impaired by edema and inadequate blood flow	Voluntary movement requires functional brain areas (cerebrum, cerebellum, and parietal lobes)
	Stable/improving response to painful stimulation	Note verbalization and response to verbal command by checking hand grip and release, leg movement, dorsiflexion, and plantar flexion q 1–4 hr	
	ICP remains less than 15 mm Hg		
	Mean arterial pressure at about 100 mm Hg		
	Systolic pressure greater than 90 mm Hg	In unconscious client, note spontaneous movement,	Denotes level of coma

Care Plan continued on following page

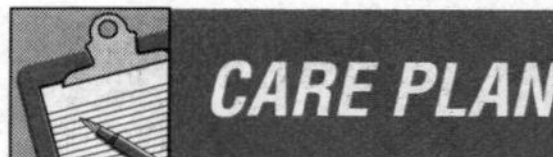

CARE PLAN

The Head-Injured Client Continued

Nursing Diagnosis/ Collaborative Problem	Planning: Expected Outcomes	Implementation: Nursing Interventions	Rationales
	Stable vital signs Normal sinus rhythm Urine output of at least 30 ml/hr Absence of hemorrhage Hgb/Hct WNL CVP WNL	withdrawal to pain q 1–4 hr	
		Report/record/assess more frequently if any deterioration	Early recognition of neurologic changes is imperative
		Monitor temperature q 2 hr; report temperature greater than 38.5° C and maintain normothermia with antipyretic agents or hypothermia blanket	Hyperthermia commonly accompanies head injury; blood is an irritant to the meninges; temperature is reduced as it increases cerebral metabolism
		Monitor cardiovascular and pulmonary status	Maximizes oxygenation and perfusion of brain tissue
		Vital signs q 1–4 hr	Changes may indicate increasing ICP
		Maintain head of bed elevation at least 30 degrees or as prescribed; keep head in neutral position (use sandbags)	Facilitates venous and CSF drainage
		Monitor I&O q 1–4 hr	Fluid overload and dehydration can impair cerebral circulation
		Avoid extreme hip flexion	Increases intrathoracic pressure and thereby intracranial pressure
		Monitor ECG pattern continuously	Dysrhythmias reduce cardiac output
		Monitor Hgb and Hct	Continued loss of blood decreases cerebral perfusion
		Assess for signs of bleeding: abdomen, chest, pelvis, long bones, extremities	Other injuries may be undetected
		Check for hematuria	Indication of renal or urinary trauma
		Control active bleeding from scalp by compression	Compression is effective in reducing blood loss
		Administer blood/blood products	Restore blood volume
Physical Mobility, Impaired R/T motor, sensory, or proprioceptive deficits, depressed consciousness level	Client will maintain physical mobility, as evidenced by not developing contractures and maintaining baseline ROM in all uninvolved joints	Early ROM exercises	Maintains joint mobility and muscle tone
		Footboard and/or foot supports	Maintains functional strength and alignment of extremities
		Prevent contractures: splints to maintain functional position of hands, arms, legs, and feet	
		Physical therapy as needed	
Skin Integrity, High Risk for Impaired R/T immobility and lack of awareness to turn	Client will have intact skin, as evidenced by Absence of skin redness, abrasions, breakdown	Check signs of skin redness, especially over ears, shoulders, elbows, sacrum, hips, heels, and toes q 4–8 hr	Bone prominences are the first body areas to develop skin impairment

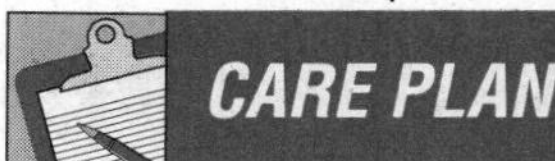

The Head-Injured Client Continued

Nursing Diagnosis/ Collaborative Problem	Planning: Expected Outcomes	Implementation: Nursing Interventions	Rationales
		Massage q 2–4 hr; avoid bony prominences if red	Massage stimulates blood supply, rubbing bony prominences may increase tissue shear
		Turn q 2 hr	Permits tissue perfusion
Tissue Integrity, High Risk for Impaired R/T lack of reflexic movement	Client will have intact tissues, as evidenced by Eyes free of irritation, inflammation Mucous membranes moist, absence of infection	Check corneal reflex, eye care q 4 hr: apply artificial tears and tape eye(s) closed prn	Blinking or use of artificial tears resupplies the cornea with fluid
		Mouth care q 4 hr; check for infection (thrush)	Stomatitis can occur in clients who are NPO; thrush may also develop, a side effect from antibiotics
Nutrition, Altered: Less than Body Requirements	Client will maintain usual weight, as evidenced by Caloric intake range of 2000–3000 (NG) daily Protein intake 50–60 g daily (adults) not to exceed 1 g/kg Minimal residual nasogastric (NG) feeding	Monitor daily weights Assess I&O q 8 hr Monitor daily caloric and protein intake (note: for every gram protein, 50 ml of water is required for excretion) Monitor NG residuals Hold next feeding per orders	Weight is an accurate indicator of nutrition Intake should equal output to avoid fluid overload or dehydration A catabolic state will delay wound healing Residuals indicate delayed gastric emptying
Fluid Volume Deficit, High Risk for R/T tube feeding and lack of ability to respond to thirst	Client will have fluid balance, as evidenced by I&O nearly equal every 24 hr Urine specific gravity WNL Skin turgor at 3 seconds Tongue moist and pink Normal serum electrolyte, BUN, creatinine, and Hct	Assess for signs of dehydration, electrolyte imbalance, and uremia by monitoring skin turgor, electrolytes, BUN, creatinine, Hct, urine specific gravity, I&O	Skin turgor will increase with dehydration because of loss of interstitial fluids Electrolytes and specific gravity will rise with dehydration
		Give additional free water with tube feeding to meet daily requirements	Free water will replace water lost to perspiration and respiration that is not replaced by drinking
Injury, High Risk for R/T restlessness and confusion	Client will remain free of injury, as evidenced by Oriented to time, place, person Absence of neurologic changes Absence of pain or other sources of discomfort ABGs WNL	Orientate prn Assess client for pain or other sources of discomfort	Assists client in understanding what has happened Pain and pain response increase ICP
		Decreases stressors: noxious stimuli, visceral discomfort (pain, chills, fever) Provide appropriate sedation as ordered, e.g., Haldol, Sublimaze Restrain if only alternative	Noxious stimuli increase ICP Facilitates management and ventilation Restraints may increase agitation

Care Plan continued on following page

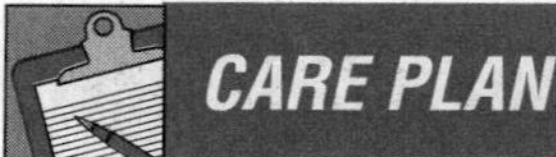

CARE PLAN

The Head-Injured Client Continued

Nursing Diagnosis/ Collaborative Problem	Planning: Expected Outcomes	Implementation: Nursing Interventions	Rationales
		Give emotional support	Emotional support may decrease anxiety
Sleep Pattern Disturbance R/T frequent assessments and loss of REM sleep	Client will obtain sleep, as evidenced by two 90-minute periods of uninterrupted sleep	Plan interventions together unless ICP rises during assessments or activity	Allows periods of no interruptions
		Allow visiting only to the extent client can tolerate it	Family may stimulate client and prohibit sleep
		Keep environmental stimuli to a minimum	Promotes a quiet environment for rest
Urinary Elimination, Altered R/T lack of awareness of bladder distention, unconsciousness	Client will have adequate urinary elimination, as evidenced by Urine output 30–50 ml/hr Absence of bladder distention Absence of urinary infection	Assess I&O q 8 hr (when stable)	Data to assess urine output
		Assess client for urinary retention, overflow, incontinence	Symptoms of urinary disorders
		Intermittent catheterization preferred to indwelling urinary catheter	Decreases risk of infection
		Bladder training program as soon as possible	Promotes self-care
		Monitor daily for signs of UTI	Catheterization increases risk of UTI
Constipation, High Risk for R/T loss of muscle tone, reflexes, and inactivity	Client will regain usual bowel habits, as evidenced by Normal bowel sounds Absence of paralytic ileus, distention, impaction Regular bowel evacuation	Auscultate for bowel sounds every shift	Bowel sounds indicate peristalsis
		Check for impaction daily	Unconscious patients will not have an urge to move their bowels
		Administer stool softeners, laxatives, suppositories, or enemas as needed	Treatments for constipation cause bowel evacuation
		Add water to diet	Replaces water loss with colonic reabsorption
		Use tube feedings	Increase the bulk in stool with fiber
Thought Processes, Altered R/T memory deficit, impaired reasoning ability, altered LOC, confusion, speech impairment, sensory deprivation	Client will have intact thought processes, as evidenced by Minimal/absent memory impairment Appropriate verbalizations Appropriate behavior patterns Establishes method of communication Participates in retraining and rehabilitation activities	Orientate to person, time, and place daily and prn	Reorientation to assist clients' memory
		Explain all nursing activities before initiating	Decreases agitation
		Avoid sensory overload	Decreases agitation
		Devise alternative methods of communication as needed	Provides a mechanism to communicate with client
		Side rails up, bed low	Decreases risk of injury
		Consult with rehabilitation therapists	Develops continuity of plans
		Involve client and significant others in care planning and goal setting	Family members and client need to have mutual goals

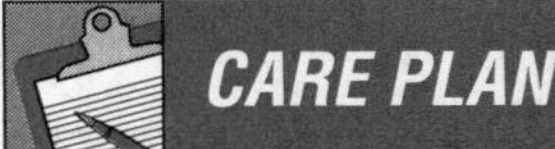

The Head-Injured Client Continued

Nursing Diagnosis/ Collaborative Problem	Planning: Expected Outcomes	Implementation: Nursing Interventions	Rationales
Seizures, High Risk for R/T brain injury, hypoxia, electrolyte imbalance, hyperthermia, fluid volume alterations	The nurse will monitor for seizure development, protect from injury, and maintain airway during seizure	Prevent/protect from injury	Client is unable to protect self
	Patent airway	Check adequate airway; do not force a tongue blade into mouth	Clients do not "swallow their tongues" during seizures
		Observe onset, progression, duration of seizures	Assists with diagnosis of location of epileptogenic focus
		Position client on side postictally; suction prn; monitor vital signs, duration postictal phase, onset status epilepticus	Maintains patent airway
		Administer antiepileptic drugs as prescribed	Head injury increases risk of seizure
Altered Health Maintenance R/T knowledge deficit on seizure management	Client will be able to manage seizure risk, as evidenced by verbalizing of understanding of seizures, medications, precipitating factors, community resources, safety measures by client and family members	Initiate client education opportunities to include medication instruction, precipitating factors, safety measures, community resources	Epilepsy is a chronic disorder, education is a critical aspect of nursing management
At Risk for CSF leak, meningitis, and diabetes insipidus	The nurse will monitor for complications of head injury: CSF leak, meningitis, diabetes insipidus	Observe for otorrhea or rhinorrhea	CSF may leak through nose or ears
		Test clear watery fluid for glucose	CSF rhinorrhea is clear
		Observe blood-tinged fluid for "halo sign"	CSF contains glucose and dries in concentric rings
		Apply a drip pad, change when wet	Wet dressings facilitate movement of organisms
		Do not suction nasally if anterior fossa fracture is present or if basilar fractures have not been ruled out	Suction catheter may pierce dura
		Instruct not to blow nose or cough or inhibit sneeze; sneeze through open mouth	Withholding a sneeze forces bacteria backward
		Aseptic technique when working with Richmond screws, incisions, drains	Prevent CNS infection
		Give antibiotics as prescribed	Reduces risk of infection
		Monitor I&O q 1–8 hr	Diabetes insipidus causes polyuria
		Assess skin turgor daily Daily weights if indicated Report urine output over 200 ml/hr for 2 consecutive hr	Clients can become dehydrated if fluid not replaced
		Monitor electrolytes and serum/urine osmolality and urine specific gravity	Sodium and osmolality can become altered because of fluid imbalance

Care Plan continued on following page

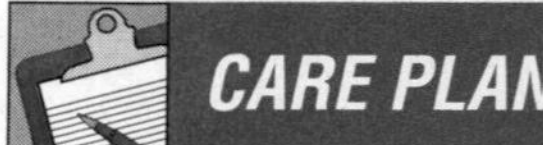

CARE PLAN

The Head-Injured Client Continued

Nursing Diagnosis/ Collaborative Problem	Planning: Expected Outcomes	Implementation: Nursing Interventions	Rationales
Posttraumatic Syndrome: High Risk for headache, dizziness, irritability, fatigue, insomnia, emotional lability, psychogenic symptoms	Client will reduce risk of posttraumatic syndrome as evidenced by Verbalizing of anxieties Verbalizing of understanding of posttraumatic syndrome symptoms	Encourage client and significant others to talk about anxieties, fear/symptoms Reassure of temporary nature of symptoms Assist with a graded plan of rest, activity	Facilitate understanding and participation

ABGs, arterial blood gases; ADH, antidiuretic hormone; BUN, blood urea nitrogen; CNS, central nervous system; CSF, cerebrospinal fluid; CVP, central venous pressure; ECG, electrocardiogram; EOM, extraocular eye movements; GCS, Glasgow Coma Scale; Hct, hematocrit; Hgb, hemoglobin; I&O, intake and output; ICP, intracranial pressure; LOC, level of consciousness; REM, rapid eye movement; ROM, range of motion; UTI, urinary tract infection; WBC, white blood cells; WNL, within normal limits.

Modification of Plan of Care for the Elderly

Although most head injuries do not occur in the elderly population, these clients experience more complications. An elderly client may be less able to tolerate respiratory problems or cardiac dysrhythmias. The presence of chronic obstructive pulmonary disease or congestive heart failure can make managing ventilation and fluid balance more difficult. If any type of mental impairment was present before the injury, recovery to full independence is less likely. Rehabilitation may be impeded by poor stamina and medical complications.

Post-hospital Care

DISCHARGE TEACHING

Clients with possible head injury or mild head injury are usually hospitalized for observation for a minimum of 6 hours (ideally for 48 hours) because of the risk of extradural hemorrhage (see later). This observation period is essential for clients who lose consciousness after the head injury, even if the period of unconsciousness lasts only minutes or seconds. If the client is sent home, clear instructions are required to assess for complications (see Client Education Guide).

REHABILITATION

Almost any client who is hospitalized for more than 48 hours because of a head injury will require some rehabilitation. This treatment may take place in an inpatient or outpatient setting, depending on the client's condition. Rehabilitation, which can include physical, occupational, speech, and cognitive therapy, is essential in returning the client to maximal function. Nurses play a major role in the rehabilitation of a head-injured client and significant others. Even if physical disabilities are not present, cognitive rehabilitation can greatly improve the likelihood of the client's leading a productive life. The rehabilitation of clients with brain injuries is challenging. Often, community reintegration is unsuccessful. Some problems have found improved success with interdisciplinary techniques that include development of cognitive skills, comprehensive techniques, social skills, emotional adjustment, leisure skills, physical fitness, and health maintenance. Most clients require 6 months in such a program.[25]

COMPLICATIONS AFTER HEAD TRAUMA

Overview

Secondary events after head injury (problems occurring soon after the primary injury) often cause rapid deterioration in the injured client's condition. Among these secondary events are (1) hemorrhage, with hematoma formation (epidural, subdural, and intracerebral); (2) infections, including meningitis and brain abscess; (3) secondary brain swelling and edema; and (4) carotid artery occlusion. All may turn a relatively "benign" head injury into a disastrous event (Fig. 30-20).

EARLY COMPLICATIONS

Epidural Hematoma (Extradural Hematoma). An epidural hematoma forms between the skull and the dura (i.e., outer meninges). It occurs in about 1 to 2 per cent of all head injuries and is usually associated with skull fracture. An epidural hematoma occurs from injury to the extracerebral blood vessels, most often the middle meningeal artery and vein.

Assessment findings usually reveal acute clinical manifestations because the bleeding is often arterial. Bleeding is almost always continuous, and a large clot forms, separating the dura from the skull. Bleeding ceases only with medical interventions or death. Occasionally, an epidural clot develops slowly, and the

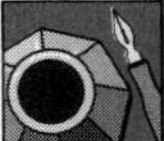

CLIENT EDUCATION GUIDE

Assessment for Complications After Head Injury

Any client who has sustained a head injury should be observed for 24 hours. The client should be taken to the hospital immediately if any of the following things occur.

- Increased drowsiness or confusion
- Inability to be awakened
- Vomiting
- Convulsions
- Bleeding or drainage from the nose or ears
- Weakness in either arm or either leg
- Loss of feeling in either arm or either leg
- Blurring of vision
- Slurred speech
- Enlargement or shrinkage of one pupil

client remains asymptomatic for a week or even a month before neurologic changes become evident.

With a "classic" epidural hematoma, the client (1) is unconscious immediately after head trauma, (2) then awakens and is quite lucid, and (3) later lapses into coma. Focal signs usually appear first (e.g., rapid deterioration in LOC, pupil dilation and eye movement paralysis on the same side as the hematoma). Hemiparesis on the opposite side or seizures may also occur. The client may deteriorate rapidly, showing signs of increasing ICP and tentorial herniation until death occurs from respiratory arrest.

There may be no indications of extradural hemorrhage immediately after the initial trauma. Within several hours, the hematoma may grow to a critical level, and the client deteriorates rapidly and may die. For this reason, head-injured clients are usually hospitalized for observation even after apparently minor injuries.

Skull radiography, CT scan, and arteriography may confirm the diagnosis. Rapid diagnosis and prompt intervention are essential with epidural hematoma. Careful, ongoing assessment of neurologic status is also necessary. Notify the physician immediately of significant changes.

Management. Intervention includes lowering the ICP with hyperventilation by mechanical ventilation or by manually ventilating the client with an Ambu bag. An epidural clot may be surgically evacuated through burr holes (Fig. 30-21), twist drills, or a craniotomy. Reasons for surgery include (1) removing the hematoma and (2) draining and ligating bleeding vessels.

Subdural Hematoma. Subdural hematoma (SDH) is a collection of blood in the subdural space (i.e., between the dura [other meninges] and arachnoid [middle meninges]). Blood escaping into the subdural space is not absorbed but becomes organized or encapsulated by the dura. As a blood clot forms, blood cells within the clot's membrane lyse, forming a fluid of high osmotic character. This draws water from the surrounding subarachnoid space into the clot, which produces a gradually increasing intracranial mass. Large clots may produce such high ICP that cerebral herniation occurs, and death may result.

SDH may be classified as acute, subacute, or chronic, depending on how rapidly signs and symptoms develop. Another classification recognizes only acute and chronic, combining the acute and subacute categories.

Acute SDH is symptomatic within 24 hours of injury.

Subacute SDH is symptomatic several weeks after injury.

Acute and Subacute SDH. Acute SDH usually results from brain laceration, with a tear in the arachnoid allowing blood (from the small pial veins bridging the subdural space) and CSF to collect in the subdural space. In addition to brain damage, severe brain swelling is usually present. Occasionally, acute SDH results from a ruptured saccular aneurysm or an intracerebral hemorrhage if tearing of the arachnoid over the source of the hemorrhage occurs. Acute SDH is seen in approximately 24 per cent of clients with severe head injuries.

Acute subdural hematomas are a serious complica-

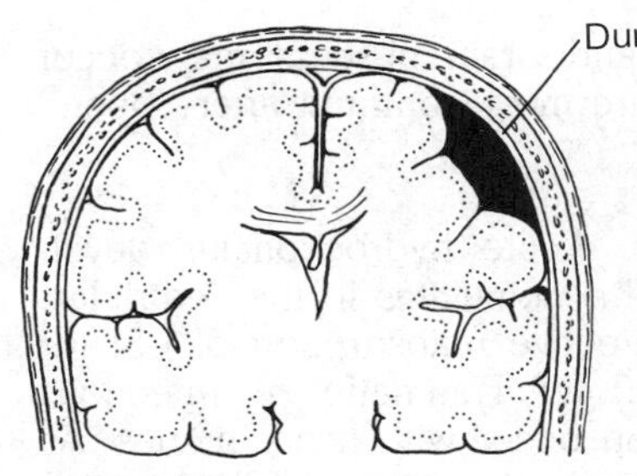

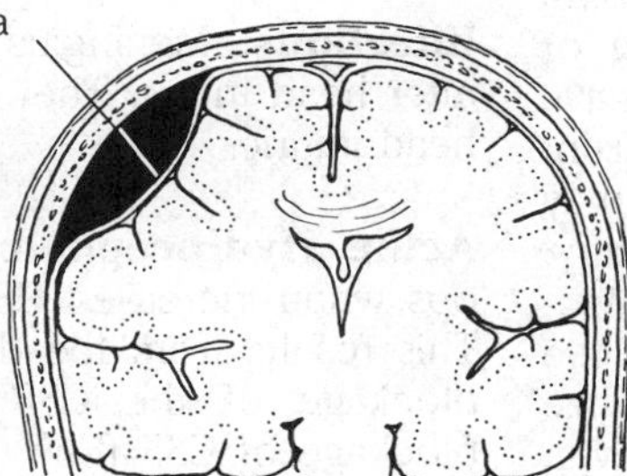

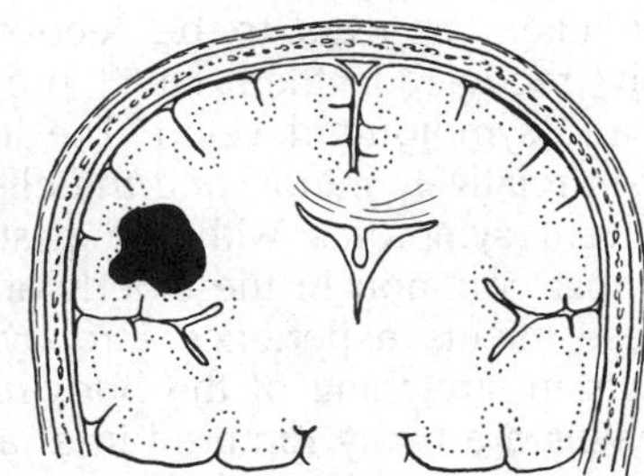

▲ **Figure 30-20**

The formation of hematoma after head injury.

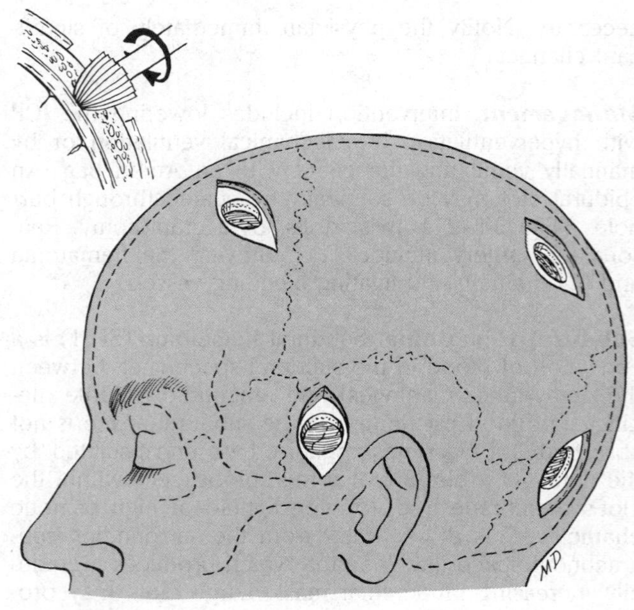

▲ **Figure 30-21**

Placement of burr holes in skull.

tion requiring prompt treatment because they compress and distort an already damaged, edematous brain.

The assessment findings with an acute SDH are similar to those with acute epidural hematoma. The onset and development of the clinical manifestations may be somewhat slower because the bleeding is more often venous (rather than arterial, as in most epidural hematomas). Symptom recognition may be difficult because SDH is often associated with moderate or severe brain injury. Subtle changes in LOC and development of lateralizing (on one side) changes (e.g., hemiparesis, pupillary dilation, extraocular eye movement paralysis) are important findings.

A client developing an acute SDH may remain unconscious after injury or may have a variable LOC (depending on the extent of injury). A conscious client usually has a headache. The client may become irritable and confused and lapse into coma or show fluctuating LOC. Symptoms of increasing ICP occur.

Chronic SDH. Chronic SDH often develops weeks or months after the initial head injury. Gradually the blood clot causes pressure on the brain. There is an interval during which the client appears to be recovering or seems completely recovered; then later, progressive neurologic signs and symptoms develop. The initial injury may have been relatively minor, and the client may not associate current symptoms with the past injury. Chronic SDH is most common in the elderly and alcoholic clients. These clients experience atrophy of the brain, which results in stretching of the bridging veins. These stretched veins are easily ruptured in a fall, even if it does not result in other injuries. Elderly or alcoholic clients may not even recall the mechanism of injury.

The client may become drowsy, inattentive, and incoherent and display personality changes. Headaches are another prominent symptom. These indications of chronic SDH may be overlooked until focal or lateralizing signs appear (e.g., hemiparesis, pupil signs). Changes in LOC continue and may fluctuate widely. An injured client and significant others need to be aware of indications of this possible complication so that they can seek medical help early if necessary.

Clinical assessment of subdural hematomas is similar to that for epidural hematomas. CT scan is definitive, but if it is unavailable, arteriography may be used. Surgical intervention usually consists of placing several burr holes or performing craniotomy to remove the hematoma. Treatment results depend on the client's condition before surgery.

A client who has had evacuation of a chronic SDH usually has a drain placed in the cavity to prevent reaccumulation of the fluid and blood. These clients are typically kept flat during the immediate postoperative period. This allows the brain to reexpand and fill the cavity, without the effects of gravity hindering the reexpansion.

Intracerebral Hematoma. Intracerebral hematomas occur less often than epidural or subdural hematomas do and are caused by bleeding directly into brain tissue. They may occur at the area of injury or some distance away. These hematomas are often hypertensive in nature and may occur deep within the brain. Surgical resection may cause as much damage as the clot itself and is usually not performed unless the clot is easily accessible.

Assessment findings are similar to those occurring with epidural or subdural hematomas, although hemiplegia is more common than hemiparesis. Many assessment findings relate to the lesion's "mass effect," for example, increased ICP. Various other clinical manifestations may also be present, depending on the location of the intracerebral hematoma. A diagnosis is established as with other types of hematomas.

Brain Swelling and Edema. Serious head injuries are almost always associated with brain swelling and edema. The skull is a closed box with little room to accommodate these changes. A "mass effect" occurs once the space is filled and ICP increases. Clinical manifestations of compromised brain function develop.

Infections. Meningitis and brain abscess may occur after head injury. They are most common after "open" head injuries.

Acute Hydrocephalus. Acute hydrocephalus develops when increased CSF accumulates in the ventricles. This results from the defective reabsorption of CSF or blockage of the CSF flow. Traumatic or infectious blockage of CSF flow can occur with head injuries. As the CSF pressure rises, signs of increased ICP develop. Intervention includes surgical shunting or the placement of a ventriculostomy.

Arteriovenous Aneurysms. Arteriovenous aneurysms are often caused by traumatic laceration of the internal carotid artery (as it passes through the cavernous sinus). Typical injuries are penetration by missiles or sphenoid bone fracture. Assessment findings include exophthalmos, distended orbital and periorbital veins, and cranial nerve paralysis. These result from increased tension in the cavernous sinus due to accumulated arterial blood. Surgery may be necessary to ligate the internal carotid artery in the neck and the internal carotid and ophthalmic arteries intracranially.

Carotid Artery Occlusion. Trauma either directly to the carotid artery or to the head may rapidly occlude the carotid artery partially or completely. Trauma to the rest of the body may also result in occlusion of the carotid or other arteries. Assessment findings with carotid artery occlusion are similar to those of a stroke (see earlier). Indications of carotid artery occlusion are difficult to diagnose in a client with an already altered neurologic state, but they illustrate the importance of the careful nursing observation of all changes.

Adult Respiratory Distress Syndrome (ARDS). Some clients with head injuries and other trauma develop ARDS that may not respond well to conventional therapy. ARDS is characterized by altered pulmonary capillary permeability leading to leakage of fluid into interstitial and intra-alveolar spaces. This produces hypoxemia (often profound and unresponsive to high levels of inspired oxygen), pulmonary congestion, atelectasis, and ventricular failure. The cause of ARDS is unknown. In the head-injured client, perhaps damage to the hypothalamus leads to massive sympathetic outflow. Conventional intervention with intubation, mechanical ventilation, and oxygen is generally used. Positive end-expiratory pressure may be necessary to treat extreme, unresponsive hypoxemia (see also Chapter 39).

Traumatic Delirium, Automatic Behavior. On regaining consciousness after several days of unconsciousness that follow head injury, a client's behavior may be noisy, generally disturbed, and confused. Such a client is usually experiencing traumatic delirium resulting from cerebral irritation. It is important to remember that a client experiencing traumatic delirium is not deliberately being difficult. During this temporary phase, the client needs protection, reassurance, and care such as during other delirious states. This partially confused state may remain even after the client can speak clearly and is able to cooperate in some activities. The family needs complete explanations and reassurance. They are often upset with the client's behavior.

After this phase comes a time in which the client appears to have fully regained mental faculties. The client may be up and about, may recognize others, and may cooperate, yet memory of these events is impaired. This is a state of automatic behavior during which the client has no memory of day-to-day events and yet is able to carry on activities in a seemingly normal manner.

Posttraumatic Syndrome (Postconcussional Syndrome). This is a set of complications emerging in the recovery phase after head injury that may continue for months or years. Posttraumatic syndrome generally occurs in clients who have sustained a "minor" head injury. Assessment findings include headache, poor concentration (especially in reading), dizziness, unsteadiness related to sudden head movements, irritability, sensitivity to noise, insomnia, restlessness, hyperhidrosis, depression, personality changes, nervousness, impaired memory, anxiety, alcohol intolerance, and easy fatigability. Although as many as half of head-injured clients may experience these symptoms in mild form for a short time, the symptoms are not appropriately referred to as posttraumatic unless they persist for weeks or even years and impair the client's employability.

Posttraumatic syndrome is seen in clients (1) whose condition progressively worsens, (2) whose extent of injury does not correlate with the severity of the syndrome, and (3) who tend to have complex overlapping neurologic and psychogenic symptoms. Whether the symptoms arise from brain damage or are psychogenic in origin is not known and is the subject of much controversy. Sometimes an organic cause cannot be found by physical examination, but careful neuropsychological testing demonstrates abnormalities compatible with brain damage.

Management. Intervention for posttraumatic syndrome is usually supportive. The client and family may be relieved to know that this syndrome does sometimes occur after head injury. Explain that the problems usually diminish and eventually clear. Supporting the client and family usually alleviates the anxiety. If not, professional counseling may be helpful. Cognitive rehabilitation may be useful to help the client compensate for memory impairment and attention deficits.

LATE COMPLICATIONS

Unfortunately, a head-injured client is prone to various complications and sequelae. These include not only problems related to the head injury itself but also the complications of any serious illness that requires immobilization for a period of time. See discussion of Complications of Intracranial Surgery earlier in chapter for a complete discussion.

▼ SEIZURE DISORDERS

EPILEPSY

Definition

Epilepsy, derived from the Greek word *epilepsia,* means to take hold of or to seize. In early times, epilepsy was viewed as being of divine origin and was called "the sacred disease" because it was thought that someone with epilepsy was "seized" or "struck down" by the gods. Today, it is known that epilepsies are paroxysmal neurologic disorders causing recurrent episodes of (1) loss of consciousness, (2) convulsive movements or other motor activity, (3) sensory phenomena, or (4) behavioral abnormalities.

Epilepsy is always recurrent. An isolated, single seizure does not mean a client has epilepsy. Epilepsy is not a single disorder. There are many types of recurrent seizures. Acute cerebral disturbance, producing seizures, can usually be demonstrated on an EEG.

The following are important definitions.

- Seizure: a paroxysmal, uncontrolled, abnormal discharge of electrical activity in the brain's gray matter; causes events that interfere with normal function; a symptom rather than a disease.
- Prodromal phase: precedes some seizures and may last minutes or hours; a vague change occurs in emotional reactivity or affective responses (e.g., depression or anxiety).
- Aura: generally, a brief sensory experience (e.g., a feeling of weakness, dizziness, strange sensations in an arm or leg, numbness, an odor) that occurs at the onset of some seizures. An aura may localize the area of the brain from which the seizure originates. For instance, a seizure arising from a focus in the motor strip could produce twitching in the client's thumb. A focus in the temporal lobe could cause a client to experience an unpleasant odor. Usually, an aura precedes other manifestations of the seizure by only a few seconds. Occasionally, an aura gives the client enough time to lie down before seizure activity occurs or may not be followed by a complete seizure.
- "Epileptic cry": a cry, occurring in some seizures, caused by a thoracic and abdominal spasm, which expels air through the narrowed spastic glottis.
- Ictus, post-ictal: ictus is synonymous with seizure; post-ictal refers to that time immediately after a seizure during which the client usually experiences some change in consciousness, behavior, or activity.

Also, occasionally, simulated convulsive episodes occur in clients with psychiatric disorders. Clients experiencing this type of seizure seldom have epilepsy. These are not "true" seizures.

Incidence

Approximately 0.5 to 1.0 per cent of people in the United States have epileptic seizures.[1]

Etiology

The etiology of seizures varies remarkably in adults, brain tumors being the most common. When a seizure disorder begins after the age of 20 years in the absence of head trauma, the client has a 10 per cent chance of having a brain tumor. Seizures are often the first symptom of an intracranial mass. Head trauma is another common cause of seizures in young adults. With severe closed head injuries, seizures occur in a small percentage of clients. However, with open head injuries in which skull and dura are penetrated, the incidence of seizures rises markedly. Posttraumatic seizures most often occur within the first year after head injury. Hence, many neurosurgeons prescribe prophylactic anticonvulsants for clients with head injuries for a year after injury.

Risk Factors

Arteriosclerotic cerebrovascular disease is the most common cause of seizures in clients over age 50 years. These episodes usually accompany a stroke due to infarct or intracerebral hemorrhage. In other vascular lesions (e.g., AVMs), seizures may be the first symptom.

CNS infections frequently produce seizures, either in their acute phase or chronically thereafter. Virus infections, which cause brain destruction, and postinfectious encephalitis can cause persistent seizures. Likewise, meningitis, especially in children, and brain abscesses are often accompanied by seizures.

Toxic substances that interfere with brain metabolism or with the supply of oxygen or glucose to the brain can cause seizures. Lead intoxication, usually in children, can result in lead encephalopathy and persistent seizures. Alcohol is one of the most frequently ingested toxins and can cause seizures either during ingestion or during withdrawal. Chronic substance abuse, especially of barbiturates, can lead to seizures when the drug is withdrawn (see Chap. 79).

The causes of symptomatic epilepsy (due to organic or other known factors) are multiple, including hyperpyrexia, CNS infections, cerebral hypoxia, toxic agents or poisons, metabolic intoxications and disturbances, convulsive agents, cerebral trauma, brain defects, electrical stimulation, expanding brain lesions, anaphylaxis, and degenerative brain disorders. Seizures resulting from these factors may be transient symptoms and may not recur after treatment of the primary disorder. However, if a permanent lesion or scar remains in the CNS, seizures may persist.

Genetic factors are associated with epilepsy beginning in childhood but decrease in importance with age. A tendency to cerebral dysrhythmia is inherited, not the actual seizure disorder itself. These seizures are usually labeled idiopathic epilepsy, because no specific causes can be found. A genetic predisposition to epilepsy exists in monozygotic twins.

The causes of seizures relate somewhat to the age of onset. Idiopathic epilepsy most often begins before age 20 years and rarely after age 30 years. Seizures beginning in newborns and infants are often due to congenital brain defects, birth injuries, or metabolic problems such as anoxia, hypoglycemia, or hypocalcemia. Although the underlying cause may be perinatal, seizures may not begin for many years, often during puberty. After age 20 years, generalized seizures usually have an identifiable cause.

Pathophysiology

Seizures occur from a malfunction of hypersensitive neurons in the cerebral cortex and the limbic centers in the hippocampus. These cells are called the epileptogenic focus. The membrane of the cell is more permeable, which makes the cell more likely to become activated by hyperthermia, hypoxia, hypoglycemia, hyponatremia, sensory overload, and certain phases of sleep. These cells begin by firing in increasing frequency and amplitude. When the intensity of the discharges reaches a threshold, it spreads to adjacent normal neurons and spreads over the entire cerebral cortex, the basal ganglia, thalamus, and brain stem. Discharges in the brain stem cause muscle contraction and loss of consciousness. The excitation of the cells can further spread to the spinal cord.

Eventually, inhibitory neurons in the cortex, anterior thalamus, and basal ganglia slow the neuronal firing. This inhibition interrupts the seizure and produces an intermittent contraction-relaxation phase. As the epileptogenic neurons are exhausted and inhibitory processes build, the seizure stops. These later events depress CNS action and impair consciousness. This period of impaired consciousness after a seizure can be seen as sleep, confusion, or fatigue. It is called a post-ictal state.

Seizure activity increases the need for adenosine triphosphate by 250 per cent and cerebral oxygen consumption by 60 per cent. To meet these demands, the cerebral blood flow increases by 250 per cent during a seizure, but supplies of oxygen and glucose are readily consumed. If the seizure is ongoing (such as in status epilepticus), severe hypoxia and lactic acidosis may occur. These conditions may result in brain tissue destruction.

Clinical Manifestations

There are various types and classifications of seizures. Table 30-6 presents one classification. Seizures can be divided into two major groups: (1) generalized seizures, which begin bilaterally without local onset and show diffuse EEG abnormalities; and (2) partial seizures (focal epilepsy), which begin in one localized area of the brain's cortex and produce abnormalities in one area of the EEG.

TABLE 30-6. Classification of Seizures

Generalized
Tonic-clonic seizures (grand mal) Absence (petit mal) Minor motor seizures (akinetic, myoclonic, atonic)
Partial (focal)
Partial seizures with motor components Partial seizures with sensory components Partial seizures with complex symptoms Partial seizures that secondarily generalize

GENERALIZED SEIZURES

About one third of seizures are generalized. The most common types of generalized seizures are (1) grand mal (generalized tonic-clonic), (2) petit mal (absence), and (3) "minor motor" seizures (e.g., akinetic, myoclonic, and atonic).

Generalized (Tonic-Clonic) Seizures. Although these are the type of seizures most associated with epilepsy, they actually make up only about 10 per cent of all seizures. A grand mal seizure typically proceeds as follows.

- Sudden loss of consciousness.
- Tonic phase, in which the entire body stiffens in rigid tonic contraction (Fig. 30-22*A*). If standing or sitting, the client falls stiffly to the floor. A cry may be uttered. Respirations are interrupted temporarily, and the client may become cyanotic. Jaws are fixed and the hands clenched. Eyes may be opened widely; the pupils are dilated and fixed. This tonic phase lasts 30 to 60 seconds.
- Clonic phase begins next with rhythmic, jerky contraction and relaxation of all body muscles, especially the extremities (Fig. 30-22*B*). The client is usually incontinent of urine or feces and may bite the lips, tongue, and inside of the mouth. Excessive saliva is blown from the mouth, which creates a froth at the lips.

An entire grand mal seizure may last from 2 to 5 minutes, after which the client relaxes and remains totally unresponsive for a time. The client may rouse briefly and then go into a post-ictal sleep lasting 30 minutes to several hours. This may be followed by general fatigue, depression, confusion, or headache, all

A

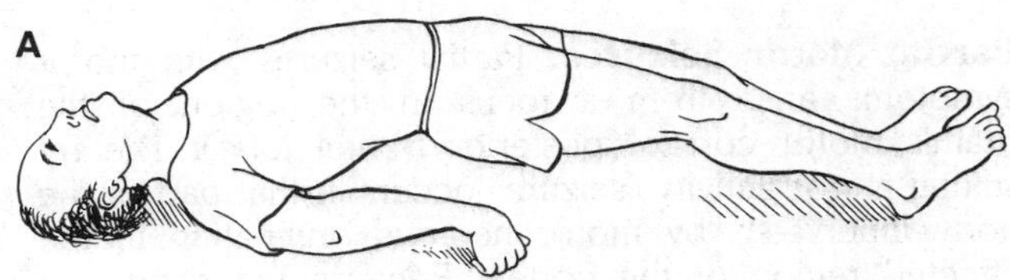

Grand mal, tonic

B

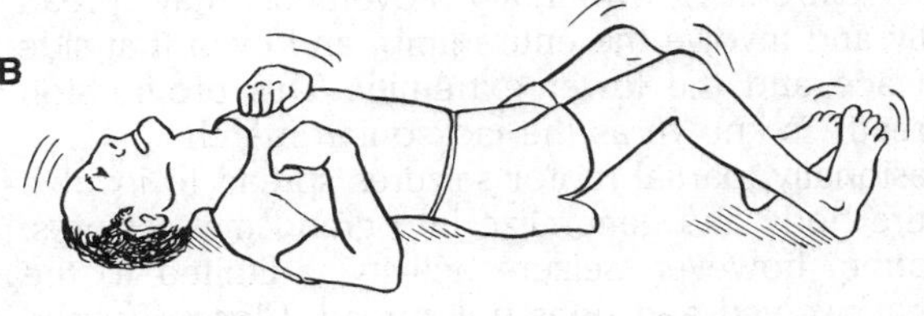

Grand mal, clonic

▲ **Figure 30-22**

Tonic and clonic phases of grand mal seizures.

of which gradually clear. The client has complete amnesia for the seizure episode and may feel nauseated, stiff, and sore. Falling during the seizure may cause injury. Grand mal seizures vary in frequency from many times daily to once or twice a year.

Petit Mal (Absence) Seizures. These "little," or minor, seizures usually begin during childhood and are primarily limited to childhood and early adolescence. Petit mal seizures consist of brief periods of altered consciousness (periods of "absence") lasting 5 to 30 seconds. They may diminish or disappear after puberty. Grand mal or partial seizures may develop at any time in clients who have had petit mal seizures. Petit mal seizures may be idiopathic (undetermined etiology) or may be secondary to identifiable disorders such as birth injuries or acute febrile childhood infections.

Minor Motor Seizures. Three other types of generalized seizures, referred to as minor motor seizures, are (1) myoclonic, (2) akinetic, and (3) atonic. Minor motor seizures are often difficult to treat. Myoclonic seizures are characterized by involuntary jerking contractions of major muscles. The contractures are often so intense that the client is thrown to the floor. Akinetic seizures are characterized by momentary loss of muscle movement. Atonic seizures cause a total loss of muscle tone, and the client falls to the floor. Occasionally, a client may have atonic along with myoclonic seizures. Often, the client needs to stay in bed with side rails up or must wear a protective helmet to prevent head injuries from frequent violent falls.

PARTIAL (FOCAL) SEIZURES

Partial seizures are the most common type of epilepsy. Various symptoms occur, depending on the part of the cerebral cortex involved; (1) partial motor seizures, (2) partial sensory seizures, and (3) partial seizures with complex symptoms (partial complex seizures, psychomotor seizures) are discussed.

Partial Motor Seizures. Partial seizures with motor symptoms arise from a focus in the region of the brain's motor cortex (posterior frontal lobe). The resulting motor activity (seizure) occurs in that part of the body innervated by motor neurons originating in the affected region of the cortex. Because the hand and fingers have the largest cortical representation, most focal motor seizures begin with convulsive twitching in an upper extremity. Involuntary movements may spread centrally and involve the entire limb, and even that side of the face and the lower extremity. This progression or "spread" is known as the jacksonian march.

Occasionally, partial motor seizures spread to involve the entire body and generalize into grand mal seizures. More often, however, seizure activity is limited to the first area involved and does not spread. Close observation of the area of origin and of any progression of movements is important in identifying the precise area of cerebral cortex involved.

Partial Sensory Seizures. Partial seizures with sensory symptoms may be transient. If such a seizure arises from a focus in the parietal area, the client experiences sensory phenomena such as numbness and tingling in the affected area. If the focus is in the occipital region, the client may experience bright, flashing lights in the field of vision opposite the side of the focus. Involvement in the posterior temporal area of the dominant hemisphere (usually the left) causes difficulty with speaking or total speech arrest.

Partial Seizures with Complex Symptoms. These seizures usually arise in the anterior temporal lobe. They are also called psychomotor seizures and partial complex seizures. These seizures frequently begin with an aura, or recognizable sensation, that helps localize the focus. Often the aura consists of a sense of "rising" or "welling up" in the epigastric region or the experiencing of an unpleasant odor. Visual distortions and feelings such as "déjà vu" are common.

The most characteristic parts of a psychomotor seizure are the automatisms during the seizure (i.e., purposeless, repetitive activities such as lip-smacking, chewing, patting a part of the body, or picking at clothes) while the client is in a dreamy state. Inappropriate or asocial behavior may also automatically occur during the seizure. This unusual behavior may cause the client to be viewed as psychotic or otherwise mentally disturbed. However, some abnormalities are very subtle and may not be detected by an untrained observer.

Temporal lobe seizures usually last 2 to 3 minutes but may last up to 15 minutes. The client is usually unaware of any activity during the seizure and may be confused or drowsy post-ictally. Attempts to restrain the client during a seizure may cause combative and uncooperative behavior.

Partial Seizures that Secondarily Generalize. Such a seizure starts from a particular focus, and then the electrical discharges spread throughout the brain. Clinically, the client first shows focal signs; one side of the face moves, and then the whole body becomes involved. Consciousness is lost if the discharges spread through the brain.

Complications

STATUS EPILEPTICUS

Status epilepticus is a state in which a client has continuous seizures or seizures in rapid succession lasting at least 30 minutes. A client experiencing status epilepticus may remain comatose and have repetitive seizures for hours. This state is exhausting and dangerous to the client. There are many kinds of status epilepticus. Status epilepticus may be precipitated by the sudden withdrawal of anticonvulsant medication.

Status epilepticus is a medical emergency. During a seizure, the brain's metabolic needs increase dramatically. If these heightened requirements continue without opportunity for the body to recover, the supply of glucose and oxygen to the brain becomes inadequate, and permanent brain damage may occur.

Treatment of status epilepticus is best carried out in a setting with emergency equipment and skilled personnel. Intervention for status epilepticus includes

- maintaining a clear airway. Prevent aspiration by positioning and suctioning, and provide adequate oxygenation. Pulmonary edema may occur. Intubation may be necessary.
- assessing the client constantly. Even when seizures are controlled, the client may be unconscious for a while. If a client does not awaken within 2 hours, careful reassessment is needed. Document and report recurrent seizures immediately.
- protecting the person from injury (e.g., padded side rails)
- administering prescribed emergency anticonvulsant therapy to terminate seizures and prevent exhaustion. Intravenous infusion is begun immediately and maintained during treatment. The medication of choice is intravenous lorazepam (Ativan) given slowly until the seizures stop. Other possible medications include diazepam (Valium), phenobarbital, or phenytoin (Dilantin). Because all of these medications may depress respirations, emergency ventilation equipment should be readily available. Phenobarbital may depress consciousness for a prolonged period. Intravenous phenytoin may cause cardiac arrhythmias, so it is given slowly while the heart rate is monitored.

If status epilepticus is not controlled by medication, general anesthesia may be used. If the client is placed on general anesthesia or neuromuscular blockade agents such as vecuronium bromide (Norcuron), there must be continuous EEG monitoring. Absence of signs of seizure does not mean the seizure has stopped.

Clients in status epilepticus are especially difficult for significant others to watch. They need ongoing support. Always explain to them the treatment that is being used. After the seizures have been controlled, maintenance anticonvulsants are prescribed.

DIAGNOSTIC ASSESSMENT

Assessment of a client experiencing seizures includes

- history: prenatal, birth, and developmental history; family history; age of seizure onset; history of all illness and trauma; complete description of seizures including precipitating factors and post-ictal symptoms
- psychosocial assessment including mental status examination
- complete physical examination, including a detailed neurologic examination
- skull radiographs
- EEG, which helps to (1) locate the focus of abnormal electrical discharges if present, (2) establish a diagnosis of epilepsy, and (3) identify specific types of seizures. However, a normal EEG does not always exclude a diagnosis of epilepsy, and EEG abnormalities do not always confirm the diagnosis. During a seizure, EEG abnormalities involve all portions of the cortex. Between seizures, clients with epilepsy may show EEG abnormalities not characteristic of seizure disorders.
- CT scan to detect congenital abnormalities or any masses (e.g., tumors)

Occasionally, diagnostic tests such as lumbar puncture, cerebral angiography, MRI, positron emission tomography (PET), and single photon-emission computed tomography (SPECT) may be helpful.

Medical Management

Intervention for epilepsy includes (1) eliminating factors that may cause or precipitate seizures, (2) improving the client's physical and mental health, (3) specific medical treatment, and (4) possible surgical treatment. The main focus in intervention for epilepsy is preventing seizures from occurring.

PHARMACOLOGIC MANAGEMENT

The most effective method of controlling seizures that have no treatable cause (tumors, infections, metabolic disturbances) or no identifiable cause is the use of anticonvulsant drugs, also called antiepileptic drugs. There are many such drugs. Large doses of a single anticonvulsant are often more helpful than are smaller doses of several drugs. Ideally, initial treatment begins with a single drug (primary anticonvulsant) until either seizure control is attained or unacceptable side effects appear. If side effects become intolerable before seizures are controlled, other drugs are used. Combining medications does not appear to be effective because drug-drug interactions decrease effectiveness.[1] Promising new medications are being investigated, including lamotrigine, felbamate, and vigabatrin. Current antiepileptic agents are shown in Table 30-7.

Medical intervention focuses on prescribing anticonvulsants that will arrest or prevent a client's seizures. Developing such a program requires weeks of medication trial and error and adjustment. During this time, the client and significant others must closely observe the effects of the medication and carefully document any seizure activity. The client must take the medication regularly as prescribed to maintain a blood level of the medication. Antiepileptic agents require time to take effect. Taking this medication after a seizure or when a seizure feels imminent is not effective. A certain antiepileptic level in the blood must be continually maintained. If a client feels a need to change the medication regimen, medical consultation is essential before acting.

Surgical Intervention

For approximately 75 per cent of people with seizures, medical management with antiepileptic agents and fol-

TABLE 30–7. Antiepileptic Agents

Classification of Seizure	Medication	Side Effects
Focal and generalized	Primary	
	Phenytoin (Dilantin)	Mental dullness, ataxia, diplopia, hypertrophy of gums
	Carbamazepine (Tegretol)	Nystagmus, ataxia, rash, blood dyscrasias
	Phenobarbital	Mental changes, withdrawal seizures if drug is stopped abruptly
	Primidone (Mysoline)	Emotional and mental changes including depression, irritability, impotence; withdrawal seizures if drug is not discontinued slowly
	Valproate (Depakene)	Transient nausea, potential bleeding problems, liver damage
	Secondary	
	Succinimides	
	Phensuximide (Milontin)	Drowsiness, headache
	Methsuximide (Celontin)	Drowsiness, headache
	Benzodiazepines	
	Diazepam (Valium)	Respiratory depression, lethargy, ataxia
	Clonazepam (Clonopin)	Drowsiness, exacerbation of childhood hyperactivity, withdrawal seizures, and status epilepticus if drug is removed too quickly
	Ancillary	
	Acetazolamide (Diamox)	Anorexia, numbness of extremities
Petit mal seizures	Primary	
	Ethosuximide (Zarontin)	Gastric distress, nausea, dizziness, drowsiness
	Valproate (Depakene)	See above
	Clonazepam (Clonopin)	See above
	Secondary	
	Trimethadione (Tridione)	Hemeralopia ("glare effect"), blood immune disorders
Other minor motor seizures		
Akinetic-atonic seizures	Same drugs as for focal and major generalized seizures	See above
Myoclonic seizures	Phenytoin (Dilantin)	See above
	Valproate (Depakene)	See above
	Clonazepam (Clonopin)	See above

low-up suffice. The remaining people continue to have seizures. For about 5 per cent of people with epilepsy, surgery is a last resort to control the disease. When seizures do not respond to medication, surgical therapy may be considered. The safest and most effective surgical treatment is cortical resection of the anterior temporal lobe for complex partial seizures.[7,10] Criteria for resection include (1) failure of the medical approach and (2) localization and identification of a focus of abnormal discharge that is easily accessible surgically and is located in dispensable cortex. Cortical resection is a lengthy surgery. The client must be awake during most of it. It is important that the client be highly motivated and psychologically well prepared.

Thorough assessment is necessary before cortical resection, including (1) several EEGs and/or PET studies to locate the epileptogenic site, (2) neuropsychological testing, (3) CT scan, and (4) cerebral angiogram with Wada's procedure to determine hemisphere dominance and location of the speech center. The functional supremacy of one cerebral hemisphere is critical to language function. Wada's test is a method of determining which side of the brain is dominant. An injection of sodium amytal is introduced into the left internal carotid artery. If the left hemisphere is dominant, speech is arrested for 1 or 2 minutes, followed by misnaming and misreading for 8 to 9 minutes altogether. After 30 minutes, the process is repeated in the right internal carotid artery.

Other surgical interventions may be considered. Epileptic foci are not identified by standard scalp EEGs in some clients. Electrodes may then be surgically implanted into the brain's deeper structures to help localize the focus. Some neurosurgeons advocate stereotactic procedures in an effort to (1) destroy foci, (2) interrupt pathways of electrical activity, or (3) alter the activity of cortical neurons. These procedures have not been very successful. Occasionally, more drastic surgical procedures, such as division of the corpus callosum and anterior commissure or hemispherectomy, are used.

Some seizures are caused by brain lesions that can be surgically removed (e.g., operable brain tumors, cysts, or abscesses). (See previous discussion.)

Nursing Management

Epilepsy is not usually treated by hospitalization. However, a client may initially be hospitalized for assessment, diagnosis, and education and again later if seizures become uncontrolled or if status epilepticus develops.

Nurses have a role in supporting and educating clients with epilepsy and their significant others. Provide information about (1) how anticonvulsants prevent seizures, (2) the importance of taking prescribed medication regularly, and (3) care during seizures. Plan with the client ways to make taking medication part of daily activities (e.g., keeping medication by the toothbrush). Also, help the client identify factors that precipitate seizures and ways of avoiding these factors. Such factors include increased stress, lack of sleep, emotional upset, and alcohol use.

It is important for a client with epilepsy to live as normal a life as possible. The client and family must learn to accept the condition and not exaggerate it or overprotect the client. Whereas certain dangerous activities should be avoided or performed with special safeguards (e.g., swimming or horseback riding), a wide range of activities can still be enjoyed. Driving motor vehicles depends on local laws and the client's medical control of seizures.

A regular pattern of adequate diet, fluid intake, sleep, and moderate recreation and exercise is helpful. Alcoholic beverages are contraindicated.

Clients with epilepsy should always wear or carry identification stating that they have epilepsy and providing the name of their physician.

Clients with epilepsy often have a poor self-image, feelings of inferiority, self-consciousness, guilt, anger, depression, and other emotional problems. These can be overcome by education and the support and understanding of significant others and care providers.

The client may be frightened and anxious about future seizures (e.g., Where will I be when it happens? What will I be doing? Who will be with me?). Social attitudes about epilepsy have improved greatly over recent years, yet more public education is required to reduce fears and misinformation about epilepsy and to teach appropriate actions if a seizure is witnessed. Some adults with epilepsy have difficulty finding or keeping employment and may benefit from vocational rehabilitation or counseling.

Various organizations are working at public education, introduction of appropriate legislation, and assisting people with epilepsy. In the United States, these include the National Epilepsy League, Inc., at 130 North Wells St., Chicago, IL 60606; and the National Association to Control Epilepsy, Inc., at 22 East 67th St., New York, NY 10021. Similar organizations exist in other countries.

NURSING MANAGEMENT DURING A SEIZURE

The client who is seizuring usually requires only protection from the environment. For example, objects should be moved out of the way and the client placed in bed so he or she does not strike the floor. Some clients will require airway management, and this usually can be done by turning the client over onto one side.

Observers' comments about a client's seizures can be very helpful in making a diagnosis, especially if they can describe minute detail, including the sequence in which phenomena occurred.

Assessment during the seizure involves

Duration of the seizure
Where the seizure began
Did eyes deviate?
Were the respirations labored or frothy?
Was client incontinent?

When the client continues to seizure without periods of rest or no seizure activity, the client is in *status epilepticus*. This is an emergency condition and, if not treated swiftly, will result in irreversible brain damage or death. When a client is in status epilepticus, the airway must be managed and endotracheal intubation may be required. The underlying cause of the seizure is initially assessed through laboratory studies for blood chemistry, liver function tests, and toxicology (for cocaine and heroin). Status epilepticus is treated with diphenylhydantoin to a total dose of 15 to 18 mg/kg by slow intravenous push (no more than 50 mg/min). The client must also be assessed for bradycardia and heart block while the medication is given. If this agent is not effective, diazepam or lorazepam can be used. If the diazepam or lorazepam is not effective, phenobarbital (15 to 20 mg/kg) can be used to bring on a barbiturate coma and suppress brain activity. This step is used only after all others have been tried and did not work. The client in barbiturate coma is ventilator-dependent and requires care in an intensive care unit.

Post-hospital Care

DISCHARGE TEACHING

The client and family should be taught that epilepsy is a chronic disorder and it requires long-term management. Even though the client does not actively seizure, it is important to take daily medication. Phenytoin, a common antiepileptic medication, leads to excessive gum tissue (gingival) growth. Brushing 2 to 3 times daily helps retard its growth. Some clients have excess gingival tissues excised every 6 to 12 months. Medications may also cause diplopia and ataxia.

If the client is able to recognize that certain activities trigger the seizure, the activities can be avoided or the client can be desensitized in some cases. For example, flickering lights can trigger seizures. Fluorescent lights and flickering shadows from trees on the road while driving during the late afternoon are common culprits. If the client has an aura, precautions should be taken immediately to prevent self-injury from the impending seizure; for example, lie down on the ground.

For some clients, the psychosocial impact of epilepsy is overwhelming. Because most seizures occur without warning, many clients spend their lives anticipating inappropriate behavior, embarrassment, and self-injury. In many states, clients with epilepsy may be prohibited from driving a car until they are seizure-free for 1 year. Some epileptics cannot find work if they admit to having seizures. These factors contribute to a higher incidence of depression among clients with epilepsy.

When discussing the long-term impact of epilepsy with the client, the nurse needs to be empathetic as well as realistic. It is hoped the client can accept the limitations of the disorder on lifestyle and not be overwhelmed by it.

Family Education. The client's family needs to know what to do for the client in the event of a seizure. The client should be protected from self-injury. Clothing should be loosened, the client's head protected from impact, and sharp objects in the environment removed. The client should not be forcibly restrained during a seizure but protected from self-injury. Hard objects or fingers should not be inserted into the mouth; clients do not swallow their tongues. When the seizure is over, the client should be positioned on the side to allow oral secretions to drain from the airway. Someone should stay with the client until full consciousness has returned. An ambulance should be called if the client's seizure lasts for over 10 minutes; another seizure occurs before consciousness returns; or there is respiratory difficulty, there is evidence of injury, or the client is pregnant.

▼ INFECTIONS

NEUROLOGIC INFECTIONS

Almost any pathogenic microorganism may invade the nervous system and related structures (e.g., neurologic parenchyma, coverings, and blood vessels). Neurologic infectious syndromes may be categorized according to the main area of involvement (e.g., meningeal subdural and epidural infections) or by causative mechanism. This section discusses (1) bacterial or pyogenic infections, (2) viral infections, (3) fungal infections, and (4) parasitic infections.

Bacterial or Pyogenic Neurologic Infections

In bacterial infections, the invading organisms reach the CNS by (1) the vascular system after systemic or bloodstream infection or (2) direct extension from adjacent cranial structures (e.g., infection entering through cranial fracture or fracture through mastoid or nasal sinuses). Infection may also be accidentally introduced into the CNS during invasive procedures.

BACTERIAL MENINGITIS

Overview. Bacterial meningitis is an inflammation of the arachnoid, pia and intervening cerebrospinal fluid. The infection spreads throughout the subarachnoid space about the brain and spinal cord and usually involves the ventricles. Approximately 20,000 to 25,000 cases of meningitis occur yearly in the United States.[27] Factors predisposing to bacterial meningitis include (1) head trauma, (2) systemic infection, (3) postsurgical infection, (4) meningeal infection, (5) anatomic defects, and (6) other systemic illness. When pathogenic organisms enter the subarachnoid space, an inflammatory reaction occurs, with resultant (1) CSF clouding, (2) exudate formation, (3) changes in subarachnoid arteries (e.g., engorgement with blood, rupture, thrombosis), and (4) congestion of adjacent tissues. The pia-arachnoid becomes thickened, and adhesions form, especially in the area of the basal cisterns. Little change occurs in brain structure in the early stages of meningitis.

Almost any bacteria entering the body can cause meningitis. The most common are meningococcus *(Neisseria meningitidis),* pneumococcus *(Streptococcus pneumoniae),* and *Haemophilus influenzae.* These organisms are often present in the nasopharynx. It is not known how they enter the bloodstream and the subarachnoid space. *S. pneumoniae* and *N. meningitidis* occur most often in adults.

Clinical manifestations initially include headache, prostration, chills, fever, nausea, vomiting, back pain, stiff neck, and generalized seizures. The client may be irritable at first, but as the infection progresses, the sensorium often becomes clouded, and coma may develop. Clients experiencing meningitis appear acutely ill and confused, stuporous, or semicomatose. A petechial or hemorrhagic rash may develop. Temperature is moderately elevated, and pulse and respiratory rate are increased. Blood pressure is usually normal. The client usually shows signs of meningeal irritation. Signs of meningeal irritation include (1) nuchal rigidity (rigidity of the neck), (2) positive finding of Brudzinski's sign, and (3) positive finding of Kernig's sign. Brudzinski's and Kernig's signs are elicited as follows.

Brudzinski's Sign. With the client supine, lift the head rapidly up from the bed. If meningeal irritation is present, forward neck flexion produces flexion of both thighs at the hips and flexure movements of the ankles and knees (Fig. 30–23*B*).

Kernig's Sign. Begin with the client recumbent and the thigh flexed at a right angle to the abdomen, with the knee flexed at a 90-degree angle to the thigh. Then extend the lower leg. In meningeal irritation, extending the leg upward causes pain, spasm of the hamstring muscles, and resistance to further leg extension at the knee (Fig. 30–23*A*).

Medical diagnosis is made by assessment of signs and symptoms and is confirmed by isolating the causative organism from CSF. Gram's stain is performed on the CSF and reveals the organisms in 70 to 80 per cent

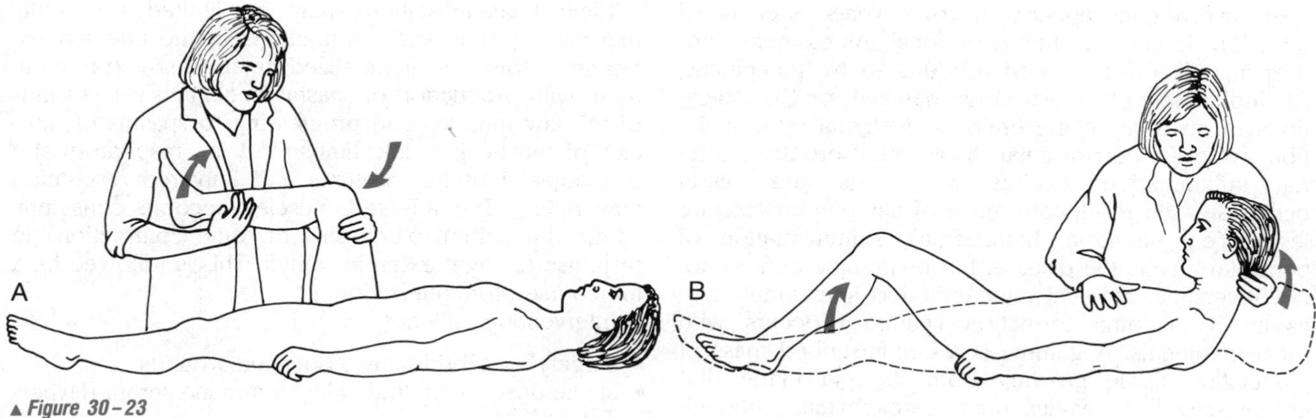

▲ Figure 30-23

Assessments of meningeal irritation. *A*, Kernig's sign. *B*, Brudzinski's sign. (See text for discussion.)

of cases.[27] In cases in which the organism cannot be identified, bacterial antigens can be determined. Cases of *H. influenzae* are frequently diagnosed with this technique. Clients with bacterial pneumomeningitis show (1) moderately elevated CSF pressures, (2) elevated CSF protein (over 100 mg/dl), (3) decreased CSF glucose (40 mg/dl), and, usually, (4) increased cell count (100-10,000/cm) with predominantly polymorphonuclear leukocytes.

Management. Bacterial meningitis is a medical emergency. If untreated, it can be fatal within hours to days. Intervention for bacterial meningitis depends on the causative microorganism and the source of the infection. Large doses of the appropriate antibiotic are usually prescribed four to six times daily for 10 days. With the exception of chloramphenicol, the common antibiotics do not readily penetrate the normal blood-brain barrier. Fortunately, meningeal inflammation improves passage. High doses of penicillins and third-generation cephalosporins are preferred agents. Antibiotics are given intravenously; their dosage is not reduced as the client improves because the blood-brain barrier recovers as inflammation subsides and high doses are required in order to reach the CSF. Adequate fluid and electrolyte balance are maintained. Assess neurologic status frequently (possibly as often as hourly) to detect early signs of increasing ICP and seizures. Anticonvulsants may be prescribed for seizures. If the primary focus of infection is located (e.g., in parasinuses or mastoid, cranial osteomyelitis), surgery may be indicated when the acute phases of meningitis have subsided.

The use of antibiotics has reduced the mortality rate of all types of bacterial meningitis. Prognosis varies according to the causative organism. Mortality is less than 5 per cent.[27] Deaths most often occur in newborn infants and elderly clients. Complications are rare but may include septic shock, vasomotor collapse, seizures, and increased ICP due to hydrocephalus, brain swelling, and fluid overload. Residual neurologic deficits are rare.

NEUROSYPHILIS

Neurosyphilis (i.e., syphilis affecting the nervous system) is due to CNS invasion by *Treponema pallidum* (spirochete causing syphilis) (see also Chap. 77). Neurosyphilis does not always develop in clients with syphilis. The organism invades the CNS after the original infection. Inflammatory changes in the CSF occur 13 to 18 months after infection.

There is a resurgence of primary and secondary syphilis (now estimated at 14.7 cases per 100,000). If these cases are not treated, about 7 per cent will develop some form of neurosyphilis.[34]

Assessment findings with neurosyphilis vary depending on involvement of the meninges, blood vessels, and brain parenchyma. Neurosyphilis is asymptomatic for the first few years after infection. The only indications of the condition during this time are CSF abnormalities (e.g., increased white blood cells with or without increased protein and positive serologic reaction). Unless lumbar puncture is done and these CSF abnormalities are found, the condition remains undetected at this stage.

CLINICAL MANIFESTATIONS

The clinical mainifestations of neurosyphilis are conventionally divided into acute syphilitic meningitis, cerebrovascular syphilis, tabes dorsalis and syphilitic dementia. These syndromes can occur alone or in combination.

Acute Syphilitic Meningitis. Symptomatic meningeal syphilis occurs during the first months to a year or two after the primary infection. Clients usually have headache, asymmetric cranial nerve abnormalities, no fever, and meningeal signs. Without treatment this form progresses to the other types.

Cerebrovascular Syphilis. Cerebrovascular neurosyphilis may develop any time after the primary infection but usually within the first year. Generally, meningeal involvement appears 6 to 7 years after initial infection. It may be diffuse or focal. Assessment findings include (1) increased ICP due to hydrocephalus, (2) indications of cranial nerve damage, or (3) indications of invasion of the brain parenchyma by granulation tissue. Cerebrovascular involvement produces arterial inflammation leading to fibrosis and vessel occlusion. The results are those of any cerebrovascular lesion (e.g., aphasia, hemiplegia). Administration of penicillin arrests the disease, but neurologic deficits are not reversible. Surgical intervention is sometimes necessary. Granuloma formation (gumma) occurs with focal meningitis. A gumma is a circumscribed mass of granulation tissue growing from the pia mater that compresses and invades brain parenchyma. Although the symptoms of diffuse syphilitic meningitis respond to penicillin, intracranial gummas do not, and surgical removal is necessary.

Tabes Dorsalis. Tabes dorsalis results from degenerative changes in the dorsal root entry zones or ganglia. It is also called progressive locomotor ataxia because ambulation is affected. The posterior spinal cord columns shrink, and fibrosis develops. Assessment findings include (1) sudden episodes of shooting pain usually in the legs; (2) ataxia due to sensory defects; (3) a peculiar "slapping" gait; (4) urinary overflow incontinence; (5) Arygll Robertson pupils, which are defined as pupils that do not have a light reflex but do constrict during accommodation; they may occur in disorders other than neurosyphilis such as multiple sclerosis, epidemic encephalitis, diabetes mellitus, midbrain and pineal tumors, and chronic alcoholism; (6) absent deep tendon reflexes; (7) loss of proprioception; and (8) various scattered paresthesias, e.g., zones of hyperesthesia (diminished sensitivity) and hypalgesia (excessive pain sensitivity). Charcot joints develop (i.e., painless arthropathies characterized by joint enlargement, hypermobility, and deformity). Painful tabetic crises may involve the epigastrium, bladder, and rectum. Penicillin arrests the condition and provides minimal symptomatic improvement.

Syphilitic Dementia. Syphilitic dementia is chronic meningoencephalitis, which destroys cerebral cortex. It is characterized by progressive physical and mental deterioration. Penicillin may arrest the disease, but the deficits remain. Without treatment, death occurs within months to a few years.

DISORDERS DUE TO BACTERIAL TOXINS

Toxins produced by several pathogenic bacteria have a special affinity for the nervous system, causing, for example, tetanus, diphtheria, and botulism.

Tetanus. Tetanus is caused by the anaerobic spore-forming rod *Clostridium tetani.* The spores produce a toxin when introduced into a wound. The toxin suppresses spinal and brain stem inhibitory neurons and may act directly on skeletal muscle at the point of entry.

Clinical manifestations may be limited to painful muscular spasms and contractions in the affected extremity. However, generalized tetanus is more common, with production of spasms beginning with trismus of the jaw muscles and progressing to spasms of muscles of the neck, trunk, limbs, and the respiratory and pharyngeal muscles. Seizures and impaired respiration may occur. The affected muscles become constantly rigid, with painful paroxysms of tonic contractions in response to slight external stimuli. This is followed by a full course of immunization.

Intervention includes

- surgery to débride any associated wounds
- single dose of antitoxin (hyperimmune serum [Hyper-Tet])
- ten-day course of penicillin G. (Tetracycline, erythromycin, and chloramphenicol are alternate agents.)
- respiratory support, including possible mechanical ventilation
- Chlorpromazine, meprobamate, or diazepam to control muscle spasms
- nasogastric feeding if client has dysphagia
- prophylactic anticoagulation to prevent thrombus

The overall mortality rate for tetanus is 25 to 50 per cent, even in modern facilities with extensive resources. Tetanus is best prevented by immunization and regular booster doses of toxoid.

BRAIN ABSCESS

Overview. A brain abscess is a collection of either encapsulated or free pus within brain tissue arising from a primary focus elsewhere (e.g., ear, mastoid sinuses, nasal sinuses, lungs, or primary bacteremia). Brain abscess occasionally follows penetrating head trauma or intracranial surgery. Staphylococcus is the most common organism in trauma-related cases. *Toxoplasma* is the usual agent found in clients with HIV infection. Brain abscesses vary in size. A large abscess may involve most of one cerebral hemisphere. Other abscesses are microscopic. Brain abscesses are relatively rare. They may occur at any age but more commonly occur in clients under age 30 years.

In its early stages, the abscess produces inflammation, necrotic tissue, and surrounding edema. Within several days, the center of the abscess is purulent, and a wall of granulation tissue forms, encapsulating the abscess. Infection may spread through thin places in the capsule, and other abscesses may develop.

Clinical manifestations of a brain abscess are essentially the same as with any space-occupying brain lesion. Headache and lethargy are the most common symptoms. Clinical indications of infection (e.g., fever, chills) are present about half the time. Other early findings include (1) drowsiness and confusion, (2) transient focal neurologic disorders (e.g., weakness on one side, loss of speech), and (3) depressed mental status. Early signs and symptoms may improve or subside, and within a few days or weeks, indications of increasing ICP may develop (e.g., recurrent headaches, changes in LOC, and focal or generalized seizures).

Medical diagnosis of brain abscess is made through CT and MRI.

Management. Pyrogenic brain abscess may be treated with antibiotic therapy alone or antibiotics combined with surgical aspiration or excision. Needle aspiration may be performed stereotactically guided by CT imaging while the client is under local anesthesia. Antibiotics commonly include penicillin. Corticosteroids may also be given to reduce cerebral edema. When antibiotics are used to treat the abscess, follow-up CT scans are used to monitor progress.

The current mortality rate is 5 to 15 per cent, depending on the location of the abscess and the client's pre-existing problems. Age, cause, number of abscesses, or use of corticosteroids does not affect outcome.[24]

Viral Infections

Neurologic viral infections are usually associated with systemic viral infections and can be devastating. Viruses may enter the body (1) via the respiratory system, mouth, or genitalia or (2) from an insect or animal bite. The organism invades the CNS via the cerebral capillaries and choroid plexus or along peripheral nerves. Viruses multiply in the body and cause viremia. Some viruses appear to have an affinity for specific cell types within the CNS.

There is no adequate treatment for most CNS viral infections. Immunizations are available for a few viral conditions (e.g., poliomyelitis and rabies). They are not available for most viral encephalitides, however. Currently, mass immunization is practical only for acute anterior poliomyelitis. The best control of other viral disorders is probably to identify and eliminate vectors responsible for their transmission.

VIRAL MENINGITIS

Acute viral meningitis ("aseptic" meningitis) is most often due to mumps virus or one of the picornaviruses. Aseptic meningitis infecting the subarachnoid space usually resolves within 2 weeks.

Clinical manifestations include mild symptoms. The client may be drowsy and photophobic, may have a headache and pain when moving the eyes, and may experience neck and spine stiffness on flexion. Other generalized symptoms include weakness, rash, and painful extremities. Fever and signs of meningeal irritation may be present. Physical examination reveals presence of Brudzinski's and Kernig's signs. Acute and convalescent serologic testing and appropriate viral cultures may identify the specific virus involved.

Intervention for clients with aseptic meningitis is symptomatic. Keep the client at bed rest during the acute phase. Plan intervention to relieve headache, control fever, and increase comfort. If seizures occur, anticonvulsants are prescribed.

VIRAL ENCEPHALITIS

Encephalitis is inflammation of the brain parenchyma. Many viruses can cause encephalitis. The two most common are arthropod-borne (arbo)virus encephalitis and herpes simplex type I virus encephalitis. Also, the viruses that cause viral meningitis (see preceding) may cause severe viral encephalitis. They become very destructive when they invade brain parenchyma. The course of the illness is unpredictable. Death occurs in about 10 per cent of affected clients. Herpes simplex encephalitis has a much higher mortality rate (10 to 40 per cent). Of the clients who recover, about 20 per cent have some disability (e.g., mental deterioration, personality changes, hemiparesis). (Residual disability is even higher in eastern equine encephalitis.)

Viral encephalitis is an acute febrile illness. Clinical manifestations include (1) meningeal irritation, (2) seizures, (3) confusion and delirium, (4) stupor or coma, (5) aphasia, (6) motor involvement (e.g., hemiparesis and asymmetric reflexes), and (7) involuntary movements.

Arbovirus Encephalitis. Arboviruses multiply in a blood-sucking vector (e.g., mosquito or tick) and are transmitted to humans by the insect's bite. The incidence of diseases caused by arboviruses is characteristically seasonal and geographic. Become familiar with those in your location. In the United States, they occur in late summer and early fall. The most common types are St. Louis and eastern and western equine encephalitis.

The infection sites are usually microscopic and scattered throughout the cerebral gray and white matter except for eastern equine encephalitis, which may destroy major parts of a lobe or hemisphere. Two thirds of clients who develop eastern equine encephalitis either die or develop severe residual disabilities (e.g., mental retardation, seizures, blindness, deafness, speech disorders, hemiplegia).

Clinical manifestations with all arbovirus encephalitides are similar. The onset is gradual in adults and older children, with headache, nausea, vomiting, listlessness, and fever. After a few days, seizures, stiff neck, stupor, and coma develop. Photophobia, hemiparesis, and asymmetric reflexes may be present. Fever and neurologic signs subside within 2 weeks if the client does not develop irreversible CNS changes or die.

Herpes Simplex Virus Encephalitis. This form of encephalitis occurs any time of year and throughout the world, particularly in middle-aged adults. The gradually evolving initial clinical manifestations are similar to those with other acute encephalitides. However, because this virus has an affinity for the inferomedial portions of the frontal and temporal lobes, the client soon becomes acutely ill with headache, fever, vomiting, and, often, seizures. Signs of a localized lesion develop, including visual field deficits. If not aggressively treated, temporal lobe swelling leads to transtentorial herniation, coma, and brain death.

The prognosis is grave but not hopeless. The mortality rate is above 30 per cent, and the client may die within 2 weeks. Of those who survive, many are left with severe neurologic and mental disabilities (e.g., global dementia, seizures, aphasia).

Intervention for herpes simplex encephalitis is a 10-day course of intravenous acyclovir, an antiviral agent. To be effective, it must be given early in the course of the disease. A biopsy may be done in an attempt to identify the herpes virus. Although biopsy is definitive for the disease, there are risks. MRI has been shown to be an effective diagnostic tool. Intervention for herpes simplex encephalitis is intravenous acyclovir. Despite treatment, the course of the disease may continue.

Nursing intervention is a challenge. An acutely ill client is often restless and combative and exhibits bizarre behavior. Such clients need careful protection from injury, and the family requires sensitive support. If residual behavior changes and mental deterioration develop, help the family adjust to changes in the client.

ACUTE ANTERIOR POLIOMYELITIS

Acute anterior poliomyelitis ("polio," infantile paralysis) is characterized by (1) destruction of motor cells (particularly anterior horn cells in the spinal cord and brain stem, especially the medulla) and (2) flaccid paralysis of muscles innervated by affected neurons. Poliomyelitis is caused by one of three types of poliovirus and spreads from the gastrointestinal tract to the nervous system.

Associated paralysis may or may not occur. If present, paralysis may be spinal or bulbar. Spinal paralysis, restricted to spinal segments, is flaccid, asymmetric, and scattered in distribution. It tends to be more severe in one extremity (most often a leg). Involvement of the diaphragm and intercostal muscles or damage to the respiratory center in the medulla oblongata may produce respiratory paralysis. Occasionally, transient bladder paralysis occurs. Bulbar paralysis involves the muscles supplied by the cranial nerves because bulbar nuclei are affected. These muscles may be paralyzed alone or in combination with spinal musculature. Bulbar paralysis is often unilateral. Respiratory paralysis results from reticular formation lesions. Protein levels in the CSF are elevated. It is difficult to distinguish polio from Guillain-Barré syndrome (see Chapter 31). However, for practical purposes, no other acute disorder produces headaches, stiff neck, fever, and asymmetric flaccid paralysis without sensory loss coupled with an increase in white blood cells in the CSF.

Clients with respiratory muscle paralysis need intensive care. Mechanical ventilation at the first sign of respiratory embarrassment greatly increases the client's chances of recovery.

Since the 1950s, mass immunization programs have significantly reduced the incidence of acute anterior poliomyelitis worldwide. The best time for this immunization is in infancy. Trivalent oral poliomyelitis vaccine has almost completely replaced both the inactivated (Salk) and monovalent (Sabin) vaccines because it is so easy to administer and supervise. A few infections secondary to other enteroviruses in unvaccinated clients occasionally occur.

Post-polio Syndrome. Post-polio syndrome is a recently recognized disorder affecting survivors of polio. This syndrome is characterized by new onset of progressive muscle weakness, fatigue, decreased endurance, pain in the joints and muscles, and respiratory problems beginning 30 or more years after the original attack. Clients may experience any or all of these symptoms. The etiology and pathophysiology of this syndrome are not well understood, particularly because the interval between the original illness and the post-polio syndrome is so long.

Post-polio syndrome can be very discouraging to clients who have successfully adapted to a certain level of disability. Further restriction of physical capabilities is difficult for the client and significant others to accept. Emotional support is as vital as teaching the client to balance rest and activity and to utilize new adaptive techniques. Development of respiratory difficulty may be particularly frightening to those clients who required ventilatory support with an iron lung (a respirator that encompassed all of the body except the head) during their initial illness.

Fungal Infections

Fungi may cause meningitis, meningoencephalitis, intracranial thrombophlebitis, or brain abscess. CNS fungal infections are rare. When they do occur, these infections are usually complications from another condition (e.g., leukemia, organ transplant, diabetes, collagen vascular disease) that interferes with the body's normal flora or suppresses immune response.

- Coccidioidomycosis mainly involves the lungs; it occasionally spreads to the meninges.
- Cryptococcosis is the most frequent CNS fungal infection. The cryptococcus, a common soil fungus, can cause granulomatous meningitis (i.e., small granulomas and cysts within the cortex, and large granulomas and cystic nodules deep within the brain). This organism is an opportunist, and the incidence of cryptococcosis has risen since the onset of the AIDS epidemic. Assessment findings vary, and diagnosis is confirmed by finding *Cryptococcus neoformans* in the CSF. If untreated, this infection is fatal within a few weeks.
- Mucormycosis, a malignant infection of cerebral vessels, is a rare complication of diabetic acidosis. It begins in the nose and paranasal sinuses and spreads to the brain. It may be associated with fungal meningitis.

CNS fungal infections produce clinical manifestations similar to those of bacterial infections. The main interventions for these infections are intravenous amphotericin B combined with flucytosine for 4 to 6 weeks. With this treatment, recovery is almost certain, except for clients with advanced infections or other overwhelming, fatal diseases. Cryptococcal meningitis in clients with AIDS is highly refractory and has a 50 to 60 per cent relapse rate.

Parasitic Infections

The parasite most commonly affecting the CNS is *Cysticercus*. The tapeworm, in larval form, causes a systemic infection. Pork may contain tapeworms. If it is eaten in a raw or undercooked state, the tapeworm is passed into the human gastrointestinal tract, where it grows. It enters the bloodstream and establishes a cyst within an organ. The cyst, which may be 3 to 15 mm in diameter, contains the larva of the tapeworm. These larvae die approximately 18 months after infection. Calcification of the cyst and inflammation follow. Clients may have more than one cyst.

CT scan or MRI identifies the cysts. Cysticercosis titers may be identified in blood and CSF; however, surgical biopsy is often performed to confirm the diagnosis. Praziquantel is the drug used to treat cysticercosis. The mechanism of action is to eliminate the tapeworm from the gastrointestinal system. If pharmacologic treatment is ineffective, surgical excision of the cyst may be recommended.

▼ BULBAR DISORDERS, SYNCOPE, AND HEAD PAIN

BULBAR DISORDERS

Some neurologic disorders involve the lower brain stem, altering bulbar function (e.g., difficulties in respiration, talking, swallowing, and coughing). Such conditions include tetanus, myasthenia gravis, and bulbar poliomyelitis.

Bulbar involvement is evidenced by hoarseness, dysarthria, pooling of food and saliva in the pharynx, increased oropharynx secretions, inability or difficulty swallowing (dysphagia), hypoxia, and laryngeal stridor. Airway obstruction, pulmonary aspiration, and asphyxia may occur. Mortality is high with bulbar disorders.

When caring for clients with bulbar dysfunction, watch for early indications of hypoxia (e.g., anxiety, restlessness, apprehension, sleeplessness, increasing respiratory effort, increasing pulse rate). Early indications of hypoxia may be very subtle (e.g., apparently insignificant requests by the client).

Quickly assess for possible causes of airway obstruction if hypoxia is possible. A tracheostomy and possibly mechanical ventilation may be needed. Many clients with bulbar problems are conscious but immobile and have difficulty speaking. Their progressive loss of respiratory function is terrifying. Thorough, ongoing assessment and supportive communication help reduce distress. Technical skills also reassure the client that respiration will be maintained.

Nursing intervention for clients with bulbar involvement is similar to that described for clients with altered states of consciousness. This is especially true for assessing vital signs, preventing deformities, and maintaining patent airway and fluid balance.

To test clients' ability to swallow, have them sit up with head slightly flexed. Do not tilt the head backward because this opens the airway. Offer a small amount of nectar (e.g., thick, fruity juice such as apricot nectar) or firm gelatin. (The consistency of these foods is easier to swallow than water.) Watch to see if they are able to swallow. If aspiration occurs, suction the fluid quickly from the back of the mouth and throat.

Before feeding, give mouth care to keep the mouth clean and induce salivation. Soft foods are easiest for dysphagic clients to swallow. Avoid milk products. Offer liquids in a small glass or cup. The client may not be able to suck or swallow when using a straw. Clients with progressive dysphagia may need tube feeding or gastrostomy to maintain adequate nutrition. Make sure they obtain enough calories.

The extent of bulbar paralysis and return of muscle function varies. A client with persisting partial bulbar paralysis is particularly disabled and may need a permanent tracheostomy tube. When suction equipment is needed in the client's home, someone must be taught to use it efficiently. Eating, drinking, and common colds are all potentially hazardous for clients with bulbar problems.

SYNCOPE (FAINTING)

Syncope (fainting) is a transient loss of consciousness lasting from a few seconds to 1 to 2 minutes. Syncope most often occurs when a client is standing. Prodromal symptoms, experienced for a few seconds before consciousness is lost, include dizziness, sweating, epigastric discomfort, and lightheadedness. While unconscious, the client (1) is pale or ashen color, (2) perspires heavily, (3) feels cold to touch, and (4) has a weak pulse and dilated pupils. On recovering consciousness, the client is usually mentally alert immediately but may feel weak.

Syncope most often results from a sudden decrease in brain circulation. The most common type is vasovagal syncope with a sudden loss of resistance in the peripheral blood vessels. Blood then pools in the dilated peripheral vessels and circulation to the brain becomes inadequate, which causes cerebral ischemia. Vasovagal syncope is often associated with gastrointestinal disturbances, anxiety, and tension states and may be precipitated by emotional or environmental stress. At the onset of symptoms, the client should either lie down or sit with the head lowered between the knees.

The second most common cause of syncope is orthostatic hypotension. Cerebral ischemia occurs when a client with impaired cardiovascular reflexes suddenly assumes an erect posture and an excessive drop in blood pressure occurs. Usually, orthostatic hypotension occurs without obvious organic illness other than advancing age. However, it may also relate to various central or peripheral nervous system conditions (e.g., Parkinson's disease, after sympathectomy, diabetic neuritis). Orthostatic hypotension can usually be controlled if the client exercises the legs before sitting up, exercises them again while sitting on the edge of the bed, and then stands up very slowly. This gradual change from lying down to standing up often prevents fainting. Some clients require abdominal support and leg bandages. Recurrent syncopal episodes require further assessment.

HEADACHES

Headaches, the most common of pains, may occur either in the absence of organic disease or as a manifestation of serious disease. Most headaches are transient and of only moderate or slight severity. However, a few are chronic, intense, and recurrent over a period of months or years.

Headache is a symptom of an underlying disorder, rather than a disease itself. The cause of headache must be identified so that appropriate treatment can be given.

Clients often self-treat headaches with over-the-counter medications available without prescription. Most headaches do not indicate serious disease. However, encourage clients with persistent or recurrent headaches to seek neurologic assessment. Serious disorders that typically produce headache include intracranial tumors and infections; bacterial or viral meningitis; acute systemic infections; head injuries; cerebral hypoxia; severe hypertension; and acute or chronic diseases of the eye, ear, nose, or throat.

There are many types of headaches. The most common are (1) migraine; (2) cluster headaches; (3) tension headaches (muscle contraction headaches); and (4) head pain related to the eyes, ears, teeth, and paranasal structures (Fig. 30–24). Some clients experience several types of headaches (e.g., migraine and tension headaches are often associated).

Assessment with headaches includes detailed history, psychosocial assessment, and physical examination. Neurologic assessment is particularly important. Possible neurologic diagnostic tests include skull radiographs, CT scan, EEG, and lumbar puncture with CSF examination.

History includes asking about (1) pain localization, intensity, and paths of radiation; (2) character of the headache (sharp, dull, throbbing); (3) mode of headache onset, duration, and frequency; (4) way in which headaches stop; (5) presence of localized tenderness; (6) associated phenomena or precipitating factors; and (7) familial incidence.

Migraine Headaches

OVERVIEW

Migraine headaches are paroxysmal disorders characterized by recurrent throbbing headaches. Headache episodes begin during puberty or ages 20 to 40 years. Generally, they decrease in frequency and severity with advancing years. Migraines affect about 5 to 10 per cent of the population. Women are more susceptible than men are. Migraine headaches usually occur at irregular intervals. Their frequency varies from several times a week to only several times a year.

The pathophysiology of migraine is complex. The vascular theory is currently accepted, which states that early neurologic symptoms are due to constriction of intracranial vessels. The later intense, throbbing headache is due to dilation of extracranial and intracranial branches of the external carotid artery. The underlying mechanism causing this periodic spasm and dilation of vessels is not known.

Psychosocial factors also influence migraine headaches. They tend to occur in clients who have "perfectionist" tendencies. Migraine episodes may be precipitated by various, often repetitive conditions such as fatigue, excess sleep, hunger, refractive errors, bright light, surprises, mental and emotional excitement, excessive smoking, high altitudes, or drinking alcoholic beverages. Certain foods seem to precipitate migraine episodes (see Client Education Guide). There appears to be a familial character to these headaches. Oral contraceptives may exacerbate migraines or induce their onset in women previously free from significant headaches. Headaches often occur during menstruation and are rare during pregnancy.

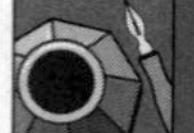

CLIENT EDUCATION GUIDE

Preventing Migraine Headaches

There are many things that can trigger a migraine headache. It is important for the client to find out what triggers the headache and avoid the trigger, if possible; if avoidance of the trigger is not possible, adjust the dose of medication.

Adjusting Medications During Menstrual Cycles. Menstruation and ovulation may trigger migraines. If medications are taken for migraines, a larger dose may be required during these times.

Recognizing Dietary Triggers. Alcohol increases the size of blood vessels (vasodilation) and may increase headache. Some foods contain beta-phenylethylamine and should be considered possible triggers. These items include chocolate, cheese, citrus fruits, coffee, pork products, and dairy products. The lack of eating may lower blood sugar and also lead to headache. In this case, small frequent meals may avert headaches.

Identifying the Role of Stress. Stress may trigger migraines. If stressors cannot be reduced, then medications may need to be increased. Heat intolerance (such as vacationing in warm climates) may increase headaches. Other factors related to stress that may trigger headaches include fatigue, excess sleep, and bright sunlight causing a glare from water, roads, or car hoods.

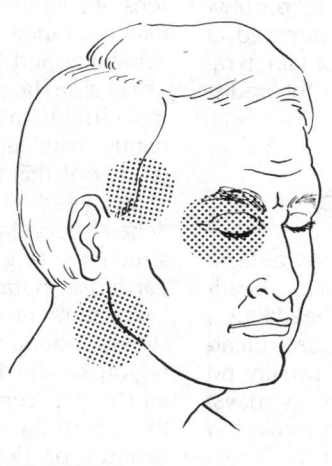

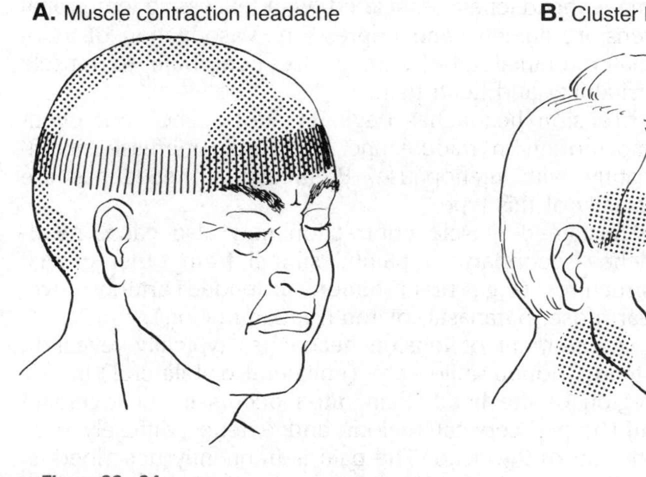

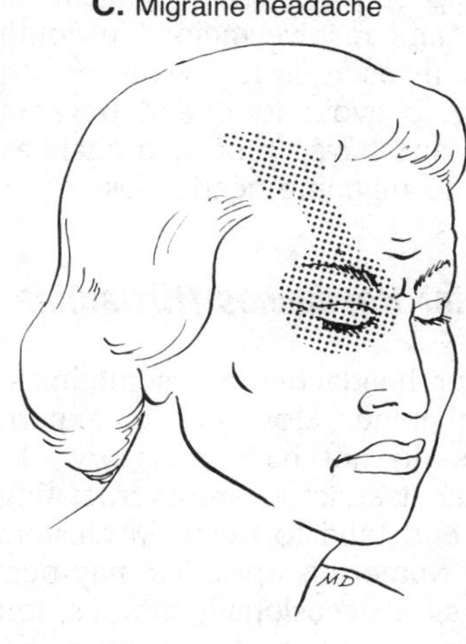

▲ Figure 30-24

Types of headache. Shaded areas show regions of greatest pain.

There are numerous variants of the migraine syndrome and many variations among clients.

Classic or Typical Migraine. The headache may be preceded by an aura or prodromal phase in which the client may feel depressed, irritable, restless, and perhaps anorexic. The client may also experience transient neurologic disturbances, including visual phenomena (flashes of lights, bright spots, distorted vision, diplopia, transitory impaired vision), vertigo, nausea, diarrhea, abdominal pain, paresthesias (numbness or tingling of lips, face, or extremities), or transient hemiparesis. Prodromal symptoms may last a few minutes or several hours.

A migraine headache has a "crescendo" quality. It gradually increases in severity until the pain becomes intense and all-encompassing. Pain varies in intensity from mild discomfort to a prostrating, throbbing pain that forces the client to seek seclusion and lie in bed in a darkened room. The pain may be described as viselike, dull and boring, pressing, throbbing, or hammering. Initially throbbing in nature, the pain may later become a steady ache. The pain is usually unilateral and may be localized to the front, back, or side of the head. It may begin at any part of the head, often the temple and the eye areas. Prodromal symptoms and head pain rarely occur in the same location in every episode.

During an acute migraine episode (often 4 to 6 hours), the client is acutely ill and may be extremely irritable. Various somatic signs and symptoms accompany severe episodes (e.g., photophobia, nausea, vomiting, vertigo, tremor, diarrhea, and excessive sweating or chilliness). The common symptoms of nausea and vomiting explain why many clients call migraine headaches "sick headaches." There is usually a general hypersensitivity of all the sensory organs, and the client withdraws from light and sound. Arteries of the head may become prominent, and the amplitude of their pulsations increases. The client's scalp may be very tender. Swelling, redness, and excessive tearing of the eyes and swelling of the nasal mucosa (sometimes accompanied by epistaxis) may occur.

Atypical or Common Migraine. This headache begins suddenly, with or without prodromal symptoms; may be generalized or unilateral; and may or may not be accompanied by nausea and vomiting.

MANAGEMENT

Treatment of migraine headaches involves prevention of episodes and treating the two phases of migraine, that is, vasoconstriction and vasodilation. Treatment of an acute migraine episode varies with symptom intensity. The transient neurologic symptoms are not treated. Analgesics such as acetaminophen or acetylsalicylic acid may relieve a mild headache. More severe headaches respond to ergot preparations, but only if they are taken 30 to 60 minutes after headache onset. Ergot must be taken before the vessels become rigid from edema in their walls. Ergot may be prescribed orally, intravenously, or rectally. Once a migraine headache becomes intense, ergot is of little value, and a stronger analgesic such as codeine sulfate, diphenhydramine hydrochloride (Benadryl), or meperidine may be more effective.

Some sources recommend reducing the pain of migraine by applying pressure on the common carotid artery and the affected superficial artery. Lying in a dark, quiet room with ice on the back of the neck is often helpful during an acute episode.

Between migraine attacks, the client is usually in a normal state of health. If migraine episodes occur as often as once a week or more, preventive treatment may be possible. Beta-adrenergic blockers (propranolol [Inderal]), the medication most often used, may reduce the frequency of episodes or abolish them completely. Some clients with migraine benefit from relaxation techniques, biofeedback, or counseling directed at preventing episodes by helping the client understand tensions and resolve major life conflicts. Another prophylactic measure is following a restrictive diet directed at trying to avoid food and beverages that contain tyramine and have vasoactive qualities that seem to predispose to migraine headaches.

Cluster Headaches (Histamine Headache)

Cluster headaches are sometimes classified as a form of migraine. Most clients experiencing cluster headaches do not have a history of migraine headaches. Cluster headaches are excruciatingly painful, are unilateral, and tend to occur in clusters. There is usually no aura. Numerous episodes may occur within a few days, weeks, or occasionally months, followed by a remission with no symptoms for months or years. Then the headaches again recur in clusters. Men are affected five times more often than are women. Episodes usually begin in middle life and are often worsened by alcohol consumption. Recurrent episodes are dreaded by the client because of the intense suffering they cause.

A cluster of episodes subsides as suddenly and inexplicably as it began. Cluster headache may recur at irregular intervals for many years, often related to times of stress, anxiety, or emotional upset. The mechanism underlying cluster headaches is not well understood but is believed to be vascular in origin. These headaches were formerly believed to be caused by sensitivity to histamine.

Individual cluster headaches begin suddenly and may last only a few minutes or as long as 2 to 3 hours. Often they begin at night at approximately the same time. During an episode, the client experiences excruciating, throbbing, or steady pain arising high in the nostril and spreading to one side of the forehead, around and behind the eye on the affected side. The nose and affected eye water, and the skin reddens on the affected side. Nasal congestion and conjunctival infection are common.

Intervention for cluster headaches is ineffective because of the shortness of episodes. The client is acutely ill during the attack and desires to be alone and quiet. Applying cold relieves some clients. Indomethacin (Indocin) is the medication of choice. Tricyclic antidepressants can also be used in treatment. Supportive care is important, because clients with cluster headaches often become depressed over their condition and fearful of recurrent episodes. Some feel they cannot survive another episode.

Tension Headaches (Muscle Contraction Headaches)

Tension headaches result from the long-sustained contraction of skeletal muscles around the scalp, face, neck, and upper back. The muscles become tender, and as a result, the client then tenses more. This prolonged muscle contraction is the primary source of many headaches associated with excessive emotional tension, anxiety, and depression. Vasodilation of associated cranial arteries may also contribute to muscle irritability and head pain.

Tension headaches begin in adolescence but occur most often in middle age. They may increase significantly with menopause. Premenstrual headaches are usually of this type.

Sustained muscle contraction may also cause headaches secondary to painful stimuli from other cranial structures (e.g., brain tumor; distended arteries; eye, ear, nose, paranasal, or tooth inflammation).

Assessment of tension headaches typically reveals a steady, nonpulsatile ache (unilateral or bilateral) in any region of the head. Pain often occurs in the occipital and upper cervical regions and extends diffusely over the top of the head. The pain is frequently described as feelings of tightness, fullness, drawing sensations, or pressure. The pain of tension headache may be localized, or frequent changes may occur in location and intensity. Sometimes these headaches are fleeting but recurrent.

The onset of tension headaches is more gradual than with migraine headache. Nausea and vomiting may accompany tension headache but occur as a late reaction to pain. Also, the headache may be accompanied by dizziness, tinnitus, or lacrimation, or these symptoms may be elicited by pressing on the tender muscles. Palpation may demonstrate contracted muscles with localized painful areas or nodules. Pain may be precipitated or aggravated by combing the hair, by wearing a hat, or by exposure to cold. Tension headaches may be unrelieved for weeks, months, or years.

Tension headaches are treated when possible by removing the primary source of stimulation (e.g., treating diseased teeth). Clients with prolonged or recurrent muscle tension headaches of psychological origin may be helped by psychotherapy. Symptomatic treatment for the headaches themselves includes massaging affected muscles, applying local heat, rest, and various relaxation techniques. Sometimes, local injections of procaine are helpful. Tension headaches respond best to a medication that combines a non-narcotic analgesic with an anxiety-relieving drug. Occasionally, a stronger analgesic is needed (e.g., codeine sulfate).

Head Pain Related to Other Structures

Headaches may result from errors of refraction, glaucoma (with increased intraocular pressure), inflammation, and ocular muscle equilibrium disturbances (see Chap. 33).

Pain associated with sinus infection is usually due to irritation and inflammation of sinus openings. (Sinus walls are less sensitive.) The pain of a sinus headache may be relieved or eliminated by decongestants and analgesics. Sometimes antibiotics are needed. Surgery to drain the sinuses may also be required (see Chap. 38).

Summary

Cerebral disorders can range in severity from life-threatening disorders such as head injury and stroke to mere nuisance problems such as headache. Because of the complexity of brain disorders and the emotional reactions the client and family have to these problems, neurologic nursing is one of the most challenging areas of practice. Common nursing problems center on cerebral perfusion and cognition as well as assisting the client to a maximal level of functional rehabilitation.

Bibliography

1. Adams, B. A., Clancey, J. K., & Eddy, M. S. (1991). Malignant glioma: Current treatment and perspectives. *Journal of Neuroscience Nursing, 23*(1), 15-20.
2. Andrus, C. (1991). Intracranial pressure: dynamics and nursing management. *Journal of Neuroscience Nursing, 23*(2), 85.
3. Cammermeyer, M., & Evans, J. E. (1988). A brief neurobehavioral exam useful for early detection of postoperative complications in neurosurgical patients. *Journal of Neuroscience Nursing, 20*(5), 3.
4. Dean, E. (1991). Clinical decision making in the management of the late sequelae of poliomyelitis. *Physical Therapy, 71*(10), 752-761.
5. Dring, R. (1989). The informal caregiver responsible for home care of the individual with cognitive dysfunction following brain injury. *Journal of Neuroscience Nursing, 21*(1), 42.
6. Fontaine, D. K. (1989). Measurement of nocturnal sleep patterns in trauma patients. *Heart and Lung, 18*(4), 402.
7. Gilman, S. (1992). Advances in neurology. Part 2. *New England Journal of Medicine, 326*(25), 1671-1676.
8. Godbole, K. B., et al. (1991). A head injured patient: caloric needs, clinical progress and nursing care priorities. *Journal of Neuroscience Nursing, 23*(5), 290.
9. Goldberg, S. (1986). *Clinical neuroanatomy made ridiculously simple.* Miami: Medmaster.
10. Hauser, W. A. & Hesdorffer, D. C. (Eds.) (1990). *Epilepsy: Frequency, causes and consequences.* New York: Demos Press.
11. Hodges, K. & Root, L. M. (1991). Surgical management of intractable seizure disorders. *Journal of Neuroscience Nursing 23*(2), 93-98.
12. Kalbach, L. R. (1991). Unilateral neglect: Mechanisms and nursing care. *Journal of Neuroscience Nursing, 23*(2), 125-129.
13. Kassell, N. F., Haley, E. C., & Torner, J. C. (1986). Antifibrinolytic therapy in the treatment of aneurysmal subarachnoid hemorrhage. *Clinics of Neurosurgery, 33,* 137-141.
14. Keller, C., et al. (1989). Psychological responses in aphasia: theoretical considerations and nursing implications. *Journal of Neuroscience Nursing, 21*(5), 290.
15. Krause, E. A., et al. (1991). Radiosurgery: A nursing perspective. *Journal of Neuroscience Nursing, 23*(1), 24-28.
16. Marshall, S. B., et al. (1990). *Neuroscience critical care: Pathophysiology and patient management.* Philadelphia: W. B. Saunders.

16a. Mattson, A. J., & Levin, H. S. (1990). Frontal lobe dysfunction following closed head injury. *The Journal of Nervous and Mental Disease, 178*(5), 282.

17. Mitchell, M. (1989). *Neuroscience nursing: A nursing diagnosis approach.* Baltimore: Williams & Wilkins.
18. Origitano, T. C., et al. (1990). Sustained increased cerebral blood flow with prophylactic hypertensive hypovolemic hemodilution ("triple-H" therapy) after subarachnoid hemorrhage. *Neurosurgery, 27*(5), 729.
19. Palmer, M., & Wyness, M. A. (1988). Positioning and handling: important considerations in the care of the severely head-injured patient. *Journal of Neuroscience Nursing, 20*(1), 42.
20. Plylar, P. A. (1989). Management of the agitated and aggressive head injury patient in an acute hospital setting. *Journal of Neuroscience Nursing, 21*(6), 353.
21. Pulsinelli, W. & Levy, D. (1992). Cerebrovascular diseases—principles. In J. Wyngaarden, L. Smith, & J. Bennett. (Eds.), *Cecil textbook of medicine.* Philadelphia: W. B. Saunders.
22. Rivara, F. P., et al. (1988). The public cost of motorcycle trauma. *Journal of the American Medical Association, 260*(2), 221.
23. Sabiston, D. (1991). *Textbook of surgery* (14th ed.). Philadelphia: W. B. Saunders.
24. Simon, R. (1992). Parameningeal infections. In J. Wyngaarden, L. Smith, & J. Bennett (Eds.), *Cecil textbook of medicine.* Philadelphia, W. B. Saunders.
25. Smigielski, J., et al. (1992). Mayo Medical Center brain injury outpatient program: Treatment procedures and early outcome data. *Mayo Clinic Proceedings, 67*(8), 767-774.
26. Stewart-Amidei, C. (1989). Hypervolemic hemodilution: A new approach to subarachnoid hemorrhage. *Heart and Lung, 18*(6), 590.
27. Swartz, M. N. (1992). Bacterial meningitis. In J. Wyngaarden, L. Smith, & J. Bennett (Eds.), *Cecil textbook of medicine.* Philadelphia, W. B. Saunders.
28. Tosch, P. (1988). Patients' recollections of their posttraumatic coma. *Journal of Neuroscience Nursing, 20*(4), 223-228.
29. Vick, N. A. (1992). Intracranial tumors: General considerations. In J. Wyngaarden, L. Smith, & J. Bennett, (Eds.), *Cecil textbook of medicine.* Philadelphia: W. B. Saunders.
30. Whitney, C. M., & Daroff, R. B. (1988). An approach to migraine. *Journal of Neuroscience Nursing, 20*(5), 284.
31. Willis, D. (1991). Intracranial astrocytoma: pathology. Diagnosis and clinical presentation. *Journal of Neuroscience Nursing, 23*(1), 7.
32. Willis, D., & Harbit, M. D. (1989). A fatal attraction: cocaine related subarachnoid hemorrhage. *Journal of Neuroscience Nursing, 21*(3), 171.
33. Wilson, S. F., et al. (1988). Determining interrater reliability of nurses' assessments of pupillary size and reaction. *Journal of Neuroscience Nursing, 20*(3), 189.
34. Wyngaarden, J., Smith, L., & Bennett, J. (1992). *Cecil textbook of medicine.* Philadelphia: W. B. Saunders.
35. Youmans, J. R. (Ed.) (1990). *Neurological surgery: A comprehensive reference guide to the diagnosis and management of neurosurgical problems.* Philadelphia: W. B. Saunders.

Chapter 31

Nursing Care of Clients with Degenerative Neurologic Disorders

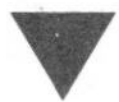

ALZHEIMER'S DISEASE

Definition

Alzheimer's disease is a form of dementia. Dementia involves progressive decline in two or more areas of cognition, usually memory and one or more of the following: language, calculation, visual-spatial perception, constructional praxis, judgement, abstraction, and personality change. Dementia of the Alzheimer's type (DAT) comprises at least half of all dementias (see Chap. 29 for a general discussion of dementia).

Prevalence

Recent studies have shown that the prevalence of DAT is higher than previously expected.[6,23] DAT occurs in 10 to 15 per cent of people over age 65, 19 per cent of people over age 75, and 47 per cent of people over age 85. The incidence of DAT increases greatly with increasing age.

Etiology/Risk Factors

The cause of DAT has not been found, although several risk factors have been identified. As can be seen by the statistics listed earlier, increasing age is a risk factor. DAT can be a genetic disorder. A defect associated with chromosome 21 has been found in some families with early-onset DAT, and a defect associated with chromosome 19 has been found in some families with late-onset DAT. However, the lack of 100 per cent concordance in studies of identical twins implies that environmental, metabolic, and other factors also may play a role. Head trauma, lack of education, and myocardial infarction have been shown to be risk factors,[14] although the reasons for their being risk factors are not fully understood. Some have postulated that aluminum intoxication, disordered immune function, and viral infection are causes of DAT; however these factors have not yet been proved.[3]

Pathophysiology

Alios Alzheimer first described presenile dementia in 1907. He used a new staining technique of human brain tissue to demonstrate the pathology. The changes he noted are now termed *neurofibrillary tangles* and *neuritic plaques* (Figure 31-1). These are abnormal proteins that accumulate in the brain. The neuritic plaque is a cluster of degenerating nerve terminals, both dendritic and axonal, that contains amyloid protein. The precursor of this protein, amyloid precursor protein, is coded by a gene on chromosome 21 and an adjacent "housekeeping" gene that regulates the daily functioning of cells. A hypothesis, based on studies of clients with Down syndrome (who develop the characteristic pathologic features of DAT), proposes that accumulation of amyloid protein leads to DAT.[14] Neurofibrillary tangles are abnormal neurons in which the cytoplasm is filled with bundles of abnormal protein called *paired helical filaments*. Neuritic plaques and neurofibrillary tangles are located in areas of cell loss in the brain of the person with DAT. These areas are the association areas of the neocortex and the hippocampus, which account for the cognitive decline. The term "association" is used to describe all the intellectual activities of the cerebral cortex. These functions include learning and reasoning, memory storage and recall, language abilities, and even consciousness.

In addition to structural changes, there are neurotransmitter changes in the brains of clients with DAT. A decline in cholinergic neurons in the basal nucleus leads to loss of choline acetyltransferase in the neocortex and hippocampus. Also affected are neuronal systems that project to the neocortex: the noradrenergic locus ceruleus and the serotonergic dorsal raphe nucleus in the brain stem. These two areas also contain neurofibrillary tangles. Involved neurons in the neocortex include those using corticotropin-releasing factor, somatostatin, and glutamate.[14]

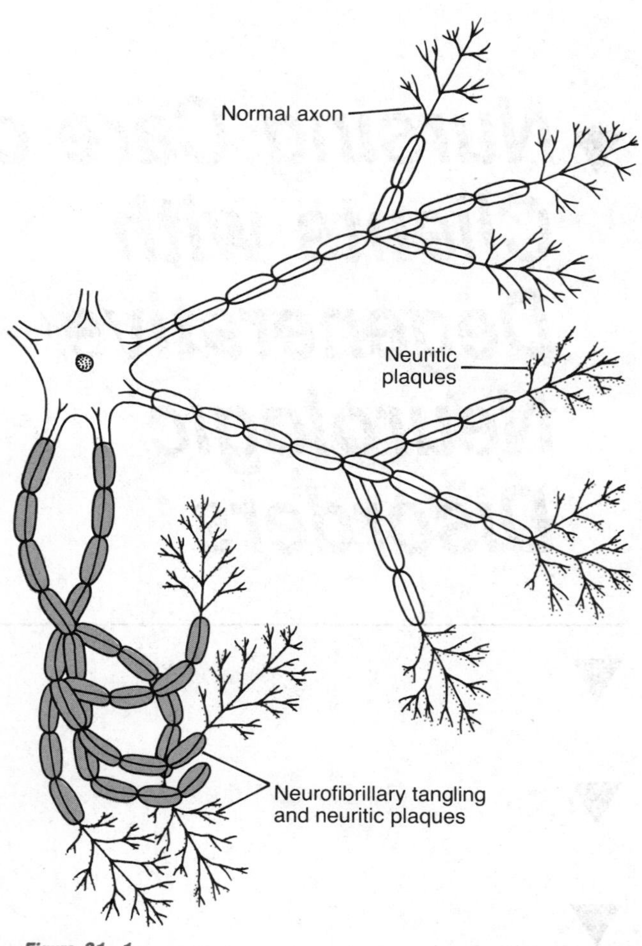

▲ *Figure 31-1*

Neurofibrillary tangles. Neurofibrillary tangles replace the normal neuronal cytoplasm in Alzheimer's disease and some other neurologic disorders. The tangles are often seen with senile plaques and appear throughout the cortex, hippocampus, and amygdala. The number of plaques and tangles correlates roughly with the severity of the dementia. *A*, Normal axon. *B*, Senile plaques on ends of axon. *C*, Neurofibrillary tangles and senile plaques replacing normal axon.

Clinical Manifestations

Clinically, Alzheimer's disease is characterized by a relentless impairment of decision making that generally begins insidiously and can progress for a decade or so. The onset of DAT typically occurs in late middle age (age 65 and older), although some familial cases occur in the fifth and sixth decades. The clinical progression of symptoms is usually divided into three stages (Table 31-1). The sequence of loss of higher cognitive functions is a helpful clue for establishing the clinical diagnosis. Memory disturbance is usually the first feature of the disease. Family members or co-workers often notice the memory loss before the individual does. The individual may demonstrate poor judgement and problem-solving skills and become careless in work habits and household chores. He or she may do well in familiar surroundings and be able to follow well-established routines but lack the ability to adapt to new challenges. The person may become irritable, suspicious, or indifferent.

TABLE 31-1. Common Clinical Manifestations in Each Stage of Dementia of the Alzheimer's Type

Stage I (duration of disease 1 to 3 years)

Memory—new learning defective, remote recall mildly impaired
Visuospatial skills—topographic disorientation, poor complex constructions
Language—poor wordlist generation, anomia
Personality—indifference, occasional irritability
Psychiatric features—sadness or delusions in some
Motor system—normal
EEG—normal
CT/MRI—normal
PET/SPECT—bilateral posterior parietal hypometabolism/hyperfusion

Stage II (duration of disease 2 to 10 years)

Memory—recent and remote recall more severely impaired
Visuospatial skills—poor constructions, spatial disorientation
Language—fluent aphasia
Calculation—acalculia
Praxis—ideomotor apraxia
Personality—indifference or irritability
Psychiatric features—delusions in some
Motor system—restlessness, pacing
EEG—slowing of background rhythm
CT/MRI—normal or ventricular dilatation and sulcal enlargement
PET/SPECT—bilateral parietal and frontal hypometabolism/hypoperfusion

Stage III (duration of disease 8 to 12 years)

Intellectual functions—severely deteriorated
Motor—limb rigidity and flexion posture
Sphincter control—urinary and fecal incontinence
EEG—diffusely slow
CT/MRI—ventricular dilatation and sulcal enlargement
PET/SPECT—bilateral parietal and frontal hypometabolism/hypoperfusion

EEG, electroencephalogram; CT, computerized tomography; MRI, magnetic resonance imaging; PET, positron emission tomography; SPECT, single photon emission computed tomography.

From Cummings, J. L., & Benson, D. F. (1992). *Dementia: A clinical approach.* Boston: Butterworth-Heinemann.

In the second stage of illness, the client may demonstrate language disturbance, characterized by impaired word finding and circumlocution (talking around a subject rather than directly about it). Later, spontaneous speech becomes increasingly empty and paraphasias (words used in the wrong context) are used. The person may repeat words and phrases used by him- or herself (palilalia) or others (echolalia). Motor disturbance (apraxia) is characterized by difficulty in using everyday objects like a toothbrush, comb, razor, and utensils. Apraxia combined with forgetfulness can create serious safety problems. The individual may leave a burner on in the kitchen or forget to extinguish a cigarette. Indifference worsens and restlessness with frequent pacing appears. Hyperorality (the desire to take everything into the mouth to suck, chew, or taste) may develop. Swallowing may become difficult. Depression and irritability may worsen, and delusions and psychosis may appear. The person fears personal harm, theft of property, or infidelity of the spouse. He or she may see bugs crawling in the bed or throughout the house. Wandering at night is common. Occasional incontinence may occur.

In the final stage, virtually all mental abilities are lost, including speech. Voluntary movement is minimal, and the limbs become rigid with flexor posturing. Urinary and fecal incontinence is frequent. The person has lost all ability for self-care.

DIAGNOSTIC ASSESSMENT

Because there is no definitive test for DAT, the diagnosis is made by exclusion of known causes of dementia (e.g., toxic/metabolic alterations, drug side effects, cerebrovascular disease, neoplasm, and infection). Diagnosis of DAT requires the presence of dementia involving two or more areas of cognition, insidious onset, steady progression, and normal alertness.[17] When these criteria are applied, 9 of 10 individuals given this diagnosis have DAT confirmed at autopsy. Postmortem examination of the brain is the only way DAT can be definitively diagnosed. The brain is viewed under the microscope for the presence of neuritic plaques and neurofibrillary tangles.

Diagnostic assessments such as the electroencephalogram (EEG), computerized tomography (CT), and magnetic resonance imaging (MRI) are sometimes used in the diagnosis of DAT. In general, these studies rule out other causes of dementia, such as seizures and cerebral bleeding, but do not diagnose DAT. Changes on EEG, CT, and MRI do not appear until the later stages of DAT. Finally, laboratory studies are currently being performed to assist in the diagnosis of DAT looking at beta-amyloid protein.

Medical Management

There is no cure for DAT. Results of studies in which acetylcholine precursors (choline, lecithin, and deanol) and anticholinesterase agents (physostigmine and tetrahydroaminoacridine) are used to enhance memory and cognitive function have been disappointing. Pharmacologic therapy is primarily aimed at treating behavior problems, although behavioral and environmental manipulations are often more effective (see later). Low-dose antipsychotic agents, like haloperidol, can be effective for agitation and confusion. The lowest effective dose should be used and should be given just before bedtime. Sometimes, twice-a-day dosing is required. Adverse side effects such as akathisia (motor restlessness), parkinsonian symptoms, tardive dyskinesias, orthostatic hypotension, anticholinergic symptoms (urinary retention and confusion), and sedation should be monitored. Antidepressants (e.g., nortriptyline and desipramine) that have few anticholinergic side effects, fluoxetine, and trazadone are helpful for depression.[14] Table 31-2 lists drugs that can be used to treat behavioral problems in DAT.

TABLE 31-2. Pharmacologic Treatment of Behavioral Problems in Dementia of the Alzheimer's Type

Problem	Treatment
Suspiciousness, paranoia, sundowning:	1. Behavioral 2. Environmental 3. Correct sensory impairment 4. Low-dose antipsychotics a) Haloperidol 0.25-1 mg/day b) High-potency phenothiazine 1-4 mg/day c) Watch for akathisias, parkinsonism, sedation, falls
Anxiety:	1. Treat underlying physical problems (pain, dyspnea, urinary urgency, sensory impairment) 2. Acute, short-lived—reassurance 3. Related to confusion—antipsychotics 4. Diffuse, chronic—long-acting benzodiazepine (low dose)* 5. Avoid: non-benzodiazepine sedative-hypnotics, esp. barbiturates 6. Role of buspirone unclear
Acute catastrophic reactions:	1. Haloperidol 2-5 mg IM 2. lorazepam 1 mg IM
Insomnia:	1. Environmental/behavioral 2. If associated confusion, low-dose antipsychotic 3. If associated depression, antidepressant a) Nortriptyline b) Trazadone 4. Intermediate-acting benzodiazepine (e.g., temazepam, lorazepam, oxazepam)* 5. Antihistamine (diphenhydramine) a) Particularly useful if restlessness with antipsychotic rx (?treating akathisia or parkinsonian symptoms) 6. Chloral hydrate
Angry or violent outbursts:	1. Very difficult to control 2. Behavior log key 3. ?Relationship to pain or other physiologic stimuli a) Arthritis b) GU problems c) Constipation 4. Low-dose antipsychotic 5. Trazadone 6. Carbamazepine 7. Propranolol (?) 8. Lithium (dubious)

IM, intramuscularly; GU, genitourinary.

* May cause disinhibition or increased confusion. Rebound anxiety at the end of a dosing interval may be a problem with chronic use.

Reprinted with permission of the American Geriatrics Society, Alzheimer disease: Basic and Clinical Advances, by Katzman R., & Jackson, J., *Journal of the American Geriatrics Society,* 39, 517-525, 1991.

Nursing Management

ASSESSMENT

When DAT is suspected, a complete history should be taken to assess for other causes of dementia. Data should be obtained from the client, family, and coworkers (if possible). Secondary sources are used because the client is often unaware of a problem with thought processing and minimizes it. The nurse should ask specific questions about difficulties with activities of daily living, increasing forgetfulness, and changes in personality. Past medical history should be assessed for previous head injury or surgery, recent falls, headache, and family history of DAT. A mini-mental state examination may provide objective data for ongoing evaluation of the client (see Chap. 29).

DAT has a profound impact on psychosocial behaviors. The nurse should ask about the client's reactions to changes in routine or in the environment. It is not uncommon for a client with DAT to become very agitated over small changes. Likewise, apathy, social isolation, and irritability may be noted. As the brain continues to atrophy and the limbic system becomes dysfunctional, the client displays paranoia, uses abusive language, and becomes suspicious of others.

DAT also has a profound impact on the family. The nurse needs to assess the family for strengths and weaknesses, the ability to provide care for the client, and financial concerns. In large centers, the assessment of the client and family is performed through a team approach.

NURSING INTERVENTION

Nursing Diagnosis: Communication, Impaired Verbal R/T neuronal degeneration.

Planning: Expected Outcomes. The client's needs will be communicated effectively, as evidenced by making his or her needs known and interacting meaningfully with others.

Implementation. In the initial stage of DAT, the client's receptive and expressive language skills are relatively intact. The nurse must be prepared to adapt to the communication level of the client. If the client speaks only single words or short phrases, the nurse should do likewise. It is best to speak slowly and simply, with firm volume and low pitch. The tone of voice should always be calm and reassuring and project control of the situation. However, when language becomes impaired in the second stage of the illness, the nurse must be prepared to apply new techniques for communicating with the client.

Bartol[2] wrote in 1979 a very useful guide for nurses that is still appropriate today. Nonverbal behavior can provide the nurse with clues. Clients with DAT often avert their eyes, look down, back away, and increase hand gesturing when they do not understand. If they are frustrated, angry, or hostile, they may increase motor activity by pacing, rattling door knobs, waving their arms or shaking their fists, frowning, raising their voice volume and pitch, or tightening their face muscles. These behaviors should signal staff to increase their alertness, search for the cause of the distress, and prepare to intervene. Interventions can include (1) decreasing environmental stimuli, (2) approaching the client calmly and with assurance, (3) taking care not to place any more demands on the client, (4) distracting the client, (5) making sure that all verbal and nonverbal communication cues are concordant, and (6) using multiple sensory modalities (visual, auditory, and tactile) to send the message. The client's memory loss can be an advantage in distracting him or her from the stressful situation. If removed from the situation and provided a calm, nonthreatening environment, the client may forget why he was upset. Bartol suggested that nurses can elicit listening behavior from DAT clients by reaching out and touching, holding a hand, putting an arm around the waist, or in some way maintaining physical contact with the client. Dementia sufferers can perceive nonverbal behavior from others and can become agitated or upset if they sense negative nonverbal behavior from others.

The identification of pain or discomfort in clients with advanced DAT is also difficult. Hurley[12] has developed a tool to facilitate assessment. Behavioral indicators of discomfort include noisy breathing, negative vocalization (constant muttering, making noise with a negative quality), sad or frightened facial expression, frown, tense body language, and fidgeting.

Nursing Diagnosis: Thought Processes, Altered R/T neuronal degeneration.

Planning: Expected Outcomes. The client will have improved thought processing, as evidenced by exhibiting retention of information to maximal capacity, maintaining orientation to maximal capacity, and sharing meaningful life experiences.

Implementation. Because memory deficit occurs in all stages of DAT, the nurse must continually apply interventions to enhance memory. The nurse should reorient the client as necessary by placing a calendar and clock in obvious places. Because DAT clients' long-term memory is retained longer than their short-term memory, the nurse should allow clients to reminisce. The nurse should be aware of a client's past so experiences can be shared meaningfully. Repetition is useful for ensuring maximal retention of information by the client.

Nursing Diagnosis: Injury, High Risk for R/T impaired judgement and forgetfulness.

Planning: Expected Outcomes. The client's physical and environmental safety will be maintained, as evidenced by the absence of physical injury and the existence of a safe living environment.

Implementation. Impaired judgement, forgetfulness, and motor impairment can make any environment unsafe for the client with DAT. In the home, electrical devices, toxic substances, loose rugs, hot tap water, inadequate lighting, and unlocked doors can be sources of injury. Family members should be educated on how to eliminate these safety hazards. In the inpatient setting, nurses should ensure that clients cannot leave the premises without being noticed, that they wear an identification badge in case they become lost, and that doors and windows be secured. Dangerous objects should be kept out of reach, and potentially dangerous activities, like cooking, should be supervised.

Nursing Diagnosis: Self-Care Deficit R/T loss of memory and motor praxis.

Expected Outcomes. The client will have activities of daily living (ADLs) completed, as evidenced by completing the tasks he or she is capable of performing and receiving assistance with ADLs he or she is incapable of performing.

Implementation. The client with DAT should be encouraged to do as much as possible, as long as it is safe and appropriate. The nurse must carefully balance helping the client with maintaining his or her autonomy. This will boost the client's confidence and self-respect, which can be very fragile during the early and middle stages of the disease. The client should be given plenty of time to complete a task. Constant encouragement, urging, and reminding the client in a step-by-step approach is necessary.

Nursing Diagnosis: Incontinence, Urge R/T neuronal degeneration and forgetfulness.

Planning: Expected Outcomes. The client will have optimal continence of bladder and bowel, as evidenced by having clean, dry clothing and bedding as much as possible; having intact skin; and voiding appropriately in the bathroom.

Implementation. DAT clients develop urge incontinence as cortical neurons degenerate and no longer provide inhibition of the micturition and defecation responses. Anticipation of elimination needs and scheduled voiding and defecation times can help in the initial stages. The client may show nonverbal signs of needing to void or defecate, like restlessness, grasping the genital area, or picking at clothing. Sometimes, the client may forget where the bathroom is located. Having clear, bright signs indicating where the bathroom is and frequently taking the client there may help control incontinence. Fluid intake after the dinner meal can be restricted to help maintain continence during the night. A bowel program can be arranged to coincide with the client's usual pattern. In the later stages of DAT, clients may need to wear incontinence pads during the day and external urinary drainage devices at night. Indwelling catheters should be avoided because of the risk of infection and injury.

Nursing Diagnosis: Care Giver Role Strain R/T grieving the loss of a family member to DAT, change in social role, and intense demands for time commitment and provision of care.

Planning: Expected Outcomes. The family will demonstrate decreased role strain, as evidenced by voicing their emotional concerns, seeking appropriate assistance, and providing adequate care for the client.

Implementation. Family members and especially care givers (usually a spouse or adult child) of clients with DAT face a great deal of emotional and physical burden. Family members grieve the loss of the person they used to know. Each decline in cognitive function becomes another source of grief. Jones and Martinson[13] describe two stages of grief in the family. The process of grief begins during the care giving stage and continues after the client's death. Normal family routines are lost, and the relationship between the family member and the dementia sufferer changes. Morris et al.[19] summarized studies of the factors that affect the emotional well being of care givers of dementia sufferers. The behavior problems most likely to be reported by care givers are incontinence, overdemanding behavior, and the need for constant supervision. Wives tend to experience a higher degree of emotional burden as care givers than do husbands. Paradoxically, the closer the emotional bond between care giver and dementia sufferer, the less the strain for the care giver. Conversely, a low past level of intimacy is associated with an increased level of both perceived strain and depression in the spouse care giver. Care givers are most likely to be depressed if they feel a loss of control over their spouse's behavior, if they feel unable to cope with the impact of care giving, and if they perceive the situation to be stable and to affect everything. Studies have not determined that formal support of the care giver (home visits by special practitioners, chore workers, and day care) relieves the care giver's burden more than informal support (family member visits and support groups). The Alzheimer's Disease and Related Disorders Association has local chapters that offer support groups in many major cities in the United States. The toll free number is 1-800-272-3900 for information on nearby local chapters.

A variety of options are available to care givers. Chore service workers can help with household chores and relieve the care giver of these duties. Other paid help can provide in-home respite care by observing the dementia sufferer while the care giver tends to business outside the home, seeks social interaction, or meets recreational needs. Adult day care provides time away from home for the dementia sufferer. Day care usually offers a lunchtime meal as well as several hours of scheduled activities that are tailored to the client's abilities. These activities may include games, crafts, music, and exercise. Respite care involves admission to an extended care facility for a few days to a few weeks to allow the care giver time to recover from the demands of providing 24-hour care. Nursing home care is usually the final, and most difficult and trying, option for a care giver. This decision creates guilt, self-doubt, and anxiety. However, it is often the only option when the care giver suffers burnout and becomes unable to provide adequate care. Table 31–3 lists helpful nursing guidelines for meeting family needs.

When the person with DAT reaches the terminal stage of illness, questions about end-of-life treatments arise. Should a feeding tube be used to provide nourishment? Should antibiotics be used to treat pneumonias or other infections? Should cardiopulmonary resuscitation be used? Ideally, decisions about these questions are raised and discussed with the client, before he or she loses decisional capacity, and with family members. Two forms of advance directives (means of expressing one's wishes about life-sustaining treatment after losing mental capacity to make informed decisions) are available. One is the living will, a written document, signed by the individual (while he or she is still mentally capable of making informed decisions) in the presence of a witness, that lists conditions under which the person wishes life-sustaining treatments to be withheld or withdrawn. The other is a durable power of attorney for health care. This is a legal document in which the individual (while still mentally capable) assigns a person to act on his or her behalf in matters of health care decisions if the individual loses decisional capacity (e.g., becomes demented).

EVALUATION

The nurse continually evaluates the degree of expected outcome attainment. In the case of the client with DAT, this includes evaluation of outcomes focused on improving verbal communication; facilitating memory; preventing injury; enhancing self-care; maintaining continence; and, perhaps most important, bolstering care giver and family coping strategies. Most of the nursing care of persons with DAT is provided in an outpatient setting or in a nursing home.

Post-hospital Care

DISCHARGE TEACHING

Family members should be interviewed to determine their understanding of the diagnosis and prognosis of DAT and to allow them to discuss their concerns about caring for the client. Do they know about community resources? Do they have someone to call when they can no longer cope with care giving? The home environment should be evaluated before the client is sent home from the hospital to ascertain safety issues (see Bridge to Home Health Care). Is the home on a busy street? Can doors be secured so that the client cannot get out without supervision? Are potentially dangerous appliances out of reach?

MULTIPLE SCLEROSIS

Definition

Multiple sclerosis (MS) is a progressive degenerative disease that affects the myelin sheath of neurons in the

TABLE 31-3. Nursing Guidelines for Meeting the Needs of the Family of the Client with Dementia of the Alzheimer's Type

Goals	Selected Interventions
Physical	
Monitor chronic health problems or physical limitations of family caregiver.	Obtain health history of family care giver to identify past and new health problems.
Identify development of new health problems.	Support family in following through with routine health examinations.
	Refer family member(s) to physician when health problems are observed.
	Assess family's understanding of medical management of own health problems.
	Teach family members to preserve own health in order to continue caring for patient with Alzheimer's disease.
Identify cues for stress.	Emphasize family's need for adequate nutrition, hydration, exercise, and rest.
Examine somatic health problems.	Help family members to be alert to signs of care giver stress.
Psychosocial	
Assist family to cope positively with stress.	Intruct family to get respite regularly for rest and relaxation.
	Teach stress management techniques (i.e., relaxation, supportive relationships, goal setting, time management, diversion).
Identify destructive methods of coping (i.e., alcohol, drugs, tobacco, over- or under-eating, physical abuse of patient).	Refer family to physician, therapist when stress remains unmanageable even with social or psychological resources.
	Refer signs of physical abuse to adult protective services.
Assess family dynamics.	Recognize the family's role, discuss capacity to provide care, and give reinforcement for care provided.
Assist family members to deal with role change and conflict.	Counsel family in dealing with role conflicts, unmet expectations, or interpersonal conflicts.
	Teach family the need to maintain roles and social activities outside care-giving experience.
	Administer burden interview.
	Reinforce family's attempt to cope.
	Acknowledge family fears of being unable to continue with care giving.
If need for support identified, direct family members to sources.	Refer family to a support group to share with others in similar situations.
	Refer family to nearest office on aging or Alzheimer's Disease and Related Disorders Association, Inc. (ADRDA) to identify benefits in community available to AD patients.
Identify family's mixed emotions (i.e., depression, anger, resentment, pity, embarrassment, guilt).	Listen to family and facilitate sharing of emotions and feelings in supportive, empathetic environment.
Identify alternative plans for care if family members or social support systems become unable to provide care or are ineffective.	Counsel and support family if patient placed in care of other (i.e., day care, respite service, home care, nursing home); allay feelings of guilt.
	Facilitate family meeting to identify time for socialization.
Identify financial limitations.	Encourage family to be specific about financial limitations.
	Offer family referrals (legal, financial, or social service) for information on eligibility for private, county, state or federal financial support for home services, and advice and counsel regarding power of attorney or guardianship, trust or estate planning.
Assess family's ability to make funeral plans.	Help family anticipate and cope with grief process.
	Assist family in making prefuneral arrangements.
	Address family's fear regarding the possible role of heredity in development of AD and assist in making decision regarding autopsy.
Environmental	
Identify compatibility of environment with family and patient.	Conduct a family meeting to discuss relationship of family, patient, and environment.
Assess learning needs regarding patient care tasks.	Teach management of concurrent physical health problems of the AD patient.
	Include family in development of patient care plan.

Table continued on following page

TABLE 31–3. Nursing Guidelines for Meeting the Needs of the Family of the Client with Dementia of the Alzheimer's Type Continued

Goals	Selected Interventions
Environmental	
	Teach family to encourage AD patient to continue daily habits to extent possible.
	Complete behavior problems checklist.
	Anticipate likely problems and teach how to manage them.
	Teach environmental modification (consistent, simple, calm routines) to maximize family endurance and enhance safety.
	Teach family to relate to patient with creative connectiveness (touch, humor, flexibility, reminiscence, music, planned activities).
Assess family need and desire for information about AD and how it affects patient's behavior.	Assist family to understand symptoms related to memory loss, nature of the illness, symptoms, stages of disease progression, and behavior manifestations.
	Provide written material to reinforce education and understanding (i.e., *The 36 Hour Day, Coping and Caring: Living with Alzheimer's Disease*; literature from local, state, or national ADRDA chapters).
	Supply ADRDA 24-hour hotline number: 1-800-621-0379.

Adapted from Stevenson, J. P. (1990). Family stress to home care of Alzheimer's disease patients and implications for support. *Journal of Neuroscience Nursing, 22*(3), 185.

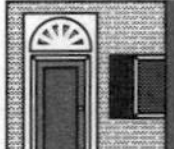

BRIDGE TO HOME HEALTH CARE

The Client with Alzheimer's Disease

Bridging hospital care to home health care of the client with Alzheimer's disease requires creativity and good communication patterns with the client's physician and care givers as well as the client. Nocturnal wandering is a significant problem in providing home health care for this client. Wandering presents numerous safety problems and is a constant challenge to providers. The use of sedatives and restraints has been found to be counterproductive, leading to confusion, physical injuries, and increased physical care needs such as toileting and positioning.

Sleep assessments are often not performed in the hospital environment. Care givers may not receive information related to the client's activities during the night while hospitalized. Bridging to home health care requires thorough assessment of the client's sleeping habits, activity during the day, number of and reasons for arousal during the night, amount of daytime sleeping, sleep aids used, and side effects of any medication. This information will assist in problem solving.

White noise from a fan, air conditioner, or a sound generator has been effective in stimulating sleep. Use of a "Wanderguard" to elicit an alarm if the client leaves the house or enters a potentially dangerous room, such as the kitchen, can enable the care giver to rest at night. Other safety interventions involve removal of knobs from the stove, keeping the living areas free from clutter and scatter rugs, and keeping the environment well lighted. A quiet and structured environment also serves to minimize confusion.

central nervous system (CNS). The myelin sheath is essential for normal conduction of nerve impulses to and from the brain and spinal cord. Patches of myelin deteriorate at irregular intervals along the nerve axon, causing slowing of nerve conduction.

Incidence

The onset of MS usually occurs between ages 20 and 40, and it affects women twice as often as men. Whites are affected more often than Hispanics, blacks, or Asians. The disease is most prevalent in the colder climates of North America and Europe. If someone is born in an area of high risk for MS and moves to an area of low risk after age 15, he or she carries the risk of the country of origin.

Etiology

The exact cause of MS is unknown. Most theories suggest that MS is an immunogenetic–viral disease: that is, an immune-mediated demyelination triggered by viral infection. A genetic susceptibility apparently alters the body's immune response to viral infection. MS is 15 to 20 times more common in first-degree relatives of affected persons.[20] The interaction between the CNS and the immune system is very complex. Several hypotheses have been put forth:[24] (1) MS is an immune reaction directed against myelin antigens by way of T cell entry into the CNS through endothelial cells, (2) myelin is an "innocent bystander" that is destroyed as a consequence of an immune reaction occurring within the CNS, and (3) MS is due to immune-mediated destruction of virus-infected oligodendrocytes.

Risk Factors

A variety of precipitating factors can precede the onset or an exacerbation of MS. They include infection, physical injury, emotional stress, pregnancy, and fatigue. Most pregnancy-related exacerbations occur 3 months postpartum and may relate more to the stress of labor and fatigue during the puerperium than to the pregnancy itself.

Pathophysiology

Myelin is a highly conductive fatty material that surrounds the axon and speeds conduction of nerve impulses along the axon. In MS, plaques form along the myelin sheath, causing inflammation, edema, and eventually, scarring and destruction (Figure 31–2). Plaques are characterized by primary demyelination and death of oligodendrocytes in the center of the lesion. Initially, perivascular inflammatory cells invade the myelin-covered axons in the CNS. This is followed by extensive gliosis or scarring by astrocytes and aberrant attempts at remyelination, with oligodendrocytes proliferating at the edges of the plaque. When edema and inflammation subside, some remyelination occurs but is often incomplete. Although plaques may occur anywhere in the white matter of the CNS, the areas most commonly involved are the optic nerves, cerebrum, and cervical spinal cord.

MS has two major courses: exacerbating remitting and chronic progressive. In the former case, the client has episodes of neurologic dysfunction (exacerbations) from which he or she recovers and is able to function normally (remission). In some cases, the recovery from each exacerbation is not complete, causing a stepwise decline in function with each exacerbation. In the second major course of MS, the client experiences a steady decline in neurologic function that can occur over several years. In acute, fulminant cases, the decline may occur rapidly within a year or two. Life expectancy is about 85 per cent of the general population. The usual cause of death is bacterial infection of the lungs, bladder, or pressure ulcers.

Clinical Manifestations

The random distribution of MS plaques leads to a variety of clinical manifestations: weakness or tingling sensations (paresthesias) of one or more extremities due to involvement of the cerebrum or spinal cord, vision loss from optic neuritis, incoordination due to cerebellar involvement, and bowel and bladder dysfunction as a result of spinal cord involvement. Seizures may develop in some clients.

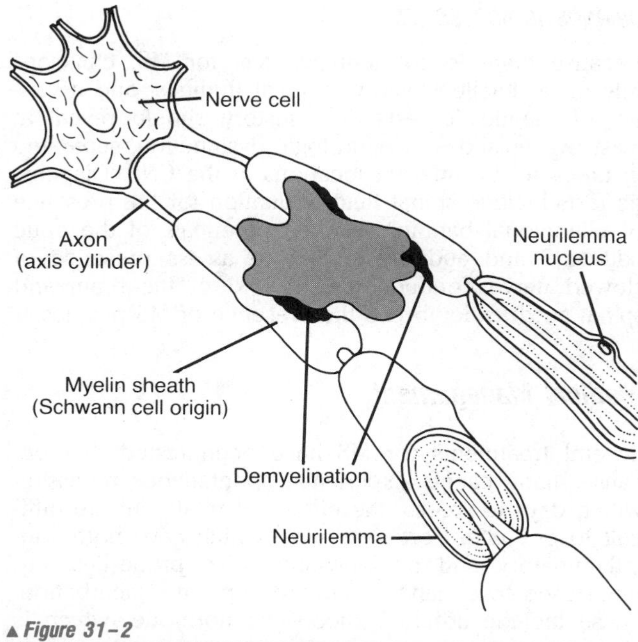

▲ *Figure 31–2*

Changes in the nerve sheath with multiple sclerosis. Myelin is made by the oligodendrocyte and coats peripheral nerves, facilitating nervous impulse. In multiple sclerosis, the myelin degenerates in patches, making nerve transmission erratic.

Bladder dysfunction can have several forms, depending on which neural pathways are affected. Dysfunction may involve hesitancy, frequency, loss of sensation, incontinence, and retention. There may be increased or decreased detrusor, bladder neck, or external sphincter tone or a combination of these problems. The ultimate bladder dysfunction, however, is usually a hyperreflexic bladder in association with sphincter dyssynergia (sphincter contraction during detrusor contraction).[5] Proper diagnosis of the type of bladder dysfunction requires a good history, laboratory assessment of kidney function, and a search for and identification of infection. If bladder emptying is defective, further investigation using urography, cystoscopy, and urodynamic studies should be performed.

Stool incontinence and constipation are commonly experienced by clients with MS. Dysfunction can result from one or more of the following factors: spinal cord lesion, immobility, dehydration, medications, and nutritional deficiencies.

Fatigue is a common symptom in MS. It usually worsens as the day progresses. Spasticity can reduce energy; inhibit motor control; and interfere with self-care, sexuality, vocational responsibilities, and recreation.

Because MS strikes young adults during their years of establishing a family and an occupation, the impact of the disease can be devastating. Depression often occurs in MS clients, but it is not clear whether depression is a reaction to disability or a function of the disease itself.[1]

DIAGNOSTIC ASSESSMENT

Because there is no definitive test for MS, clinicians rely on a detailed history, clinical findings, and a variety of diagnostic tests. The history should reveal at least two episodes of neurologic dysfunction, separated in time and in different locations in the CNS. Diagnostic tests include spinal fluid evaluation for the presence of oligoclonal banding, evoked potentials of the optic pathways and auditory system to assess presence of slowed nerve conduction, and MRI of the brain and spinal cord to determine the presence of MS plaques.

Medical Management

Several treatments for MS have been tested, but because many clients experience spontaneous remission within days to weeks, the effects of treatment are difficult to evaluate. Corticosteroids, which have both anti-inflammatory and immunosuppressive properties, are often used to enhance recovery from an exacerbation. These include adrenocorticotropic hormone, which is given intravenously, and prednisone, which is given orally. Despite the popularity of these therapies, clear evidence of their efficacy does not exist.[7] Likewise, there is no convincing evidence that either cyclophosphamide (Cytoxan), an alkylating agent with broad immunosuppressive properties, or plasma exchange is an effective treatment for chronic progressive MS.[7]

Several strategies are available for the variety of complications that occur with MS.[5] Interventions for bladder and bowel dysfunction, fatigue, weakness, spasticity, and ataxia are described later under the nursing diagnoses. Areas of numbness should be inspected regularly to prevent injury and development of pressure ulcers. Skin should be kept dry and free of urine and feces. A pressure-distributing seat cushion should be used for wheelchair-bound clients with insensate buttock skin. Some clients may experience painful dysesthesias or pain syndromes like trigeminal neuralgia. Drugs like carbamazepine (Tegretol), phenytoin (Dilantin), and amitriptyline (Elavil) are often helpful. Transcutaneous electrical stimulation is also helpful. Blindness or severely impaired vision may occur and will require referral to Services for the Blind for rehabilitation. Cognitive and perceptual impairment necessitates psychometric and functional testing for accurate assessment and rehabilitation services.

Nursing Management

ASSESSMENT

If the client is being assessed for possible MS, the nurse should assess the client for clinical manifestations of the disorder. Ocular symptoms are very common. Likewise, as a result of the fluctuations of clinical manifestations, the client may report a past history of similar findings that went away.

If the client is being hospitalized for an exacerbation of MS, the nurse should focus on the client's ability to perform ADLs as well as other areas that require fine motor movements. Gross motor activities such as walking may also be impaired and lead to problems with bowel and bladder continence (see the Nursing Research Box).

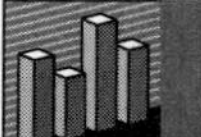

NURSING RESEARCH

This study examined self-assessments of health patterns over a 5-year period in clients with multiple sclerosis (MS). Health patterns are composites of interrelationships between the client and the environment that have occurred in the past. Health patterns include way of life, functions, abilities, and social relationships and are influenced by heredity, culture, and values.

Four areas were studied: (1) fine and gross motor movement, (2) socializing and recreation, (3) sensory and communication, and (4) intimacy. Symptoms occurred in all clients in all four areas and validated that clients with MS must learn to cope with a wide array of clinical manifestations. Fine and gross motor movement and intimacy declined in all groups. There was little change in socializing, perhaps because the disease had already affected social interactions.

It is important that nurses have a full understanding of the clinical manifestations of MS and the impact it has on many body functions so that health teaching with the client and family can focus on anticipation of needs. The client will benefit from knowing the various symptoms that are part of MS and what resources are available, such as a motorized wheel chair.

▼▼▼

Gulick, E., & Bugg, A. (1992). Holistic health patterning in multiple sclerosis. *Research in Nursing and Health, 15*(3), 175–186.

Nursing Diagnosis: Urinary Elimination, Altered R/T bladder dysfunction.

Planning: Expected Outcomes. The client will maintain urinary continence and normal bladder filling, as evidenced by residual volumes of less than 100 ml, application of appropriate bladder elimination procedures, and verbalization of personal satisfaction with urinary elimination status.

Implementation. The following interventions are for neurogenic bladder, the most common type of bladder dysfunction in MS. Fluid intake should be maintained at 2000 ml/24 h. Ideally, 400 to 500 ml with each meal and 200 ml at midmorning, midafternoon, and late afternoon. Avoidance of fluid intake after the evening meal reduces the need for bladder emptying during the night. Voiding should be attempted every 3 hours during waking hours. If voiding is not successful, a catheter should be inserted into the bladder and then removed once emptying is complete. This is called *intermittent catheterization*. If the volume of catheterized urine exceeds 500 ml, the catheterization schedule may need to be more frequent. The client should be instructed on how to do self-catheterization if he or she is capable. A clean red rubber catheter can be reused for up to 1 week, as long as it is washed thoroughly with soap and water and placed in a clean, tightly sealed plastic bag after every catheterization. Sterile equipment is not required for ongoing self-catheterization.

Nursing Diagnosis: Constipation R/T immobility and demyelination.

Planning: Expected Outcomes. The client will have bowel movements of normal consistency and frequency.

Implementation. A high-fiber diet, bulk formers, and stool softeners are useful for maintaining stool consistency. Adequate fluid intake also assists bowel elimination; 2000 ml should be taken. Laxatives and enemas should be avoided. A bowel program should be performed every other day, approximately 45 minutes after the largest meal, to take advantage of the gastrocolic reflex. Rectal evacuation may be augmented by the use of glycerin or bisacodyl (Dulcolax) suppositories or digital stimulation.

Nursing Diagnosis: Activity Intolerance R/T fatigue.

Planning: Expected Outcomes. The client will demonstrate improved activity tolerance, as evidenced by maintaining a balance among work, rest, and exercise/recreation; performing ADLs without excessive fatigue; using energy-saving devices and techniques; avoiding elevations in environmental and body temperatures; and consuming a diet adequate in calories and protein for body size, frame and age.

Implementation. Because fatigue can be precipitated by warm temperatures, the environment should be kept cool. If air conditioning is unavailable, cool baths and ice packs may help lower body temperature.

The nurse should assist the client to plan activities at his or her peak energy level, which is usually in the morning. This schedule promotes optimal synchrony between circadian rhythms and the client's physical demands. The client should plan for periods of rest throughout the day. Collaboration with the physical and occupational therapist can reveal methods to reduce energy consumption with repeated tasks and apply adaptive devices for ambulation and toileting. The drug amantadine (Symmetrel) may alleviate fatigue in some clients.

Nursing Diagnosis: Physical Mobility, Impaired R/T spasticity, ataxia, weakness, and contractures.

Planning: Expected Outcomes. The client will achieve optimal physical mobility, as evidenced by improved or maintained range of motion in all joints, optimal control of spasticity, and effective use of adaptive aids.

Implementation. Although some clients are bothered by painful muscle spasms, others may rely on spasticity to stabilize weak limbs during transfers and ambulation. Spastic muscles must be stretched at least twice daily through their full range of motion. The drug baclofen (Lioresal) provides synaptic inhibition of spinal reflexes, which can reduce spasticity, although it can increase weakness and fatigue in some clients. Diazepam (Valium) and dantrolene (Dantrium) are other antispasmotic drugs. Surgical intervention or nerve blocks may be necessary if contractures develop.

Strengthening exercises for muscle weakness (paresis) must be done with caution because they can aggravate paresis by causing muscle fatigue. However, selective strengthening of nonaffected or less affected muscles can enhance physical function and well being. Range-of-motion exercises should be performed at least twice daily. Active movement is preferable to passive movement. Correct body alignment should be maintained to reduce the risk of contractures. Splints may help maintain position and provide support for weak hands and ankles. Ataxia and tremor of the extremities can be lessened by the use of small weights applied to the distal extremities or the use of weighted utensils. Weakness and fatigue can aggravate ataxia. Ambulation aids such as a cane or a walker may be necessary.

Nursing Diagnosis: Self-Esteem Disturbance R/T loss of independence and fear of disability.

Planning: Expected Outcomes. The client will achieve improved self-concept, as evidenced by verbalizing awareness that personal goals and body image will need to be adjusted, willingness to maintain appropriate independence, and positive self-thoughts and statements about self.

Implementation. Regardless of the cause of disturbance in self-concept, the nurse should carefully assess the individual and family history for presence and type of depressive episodes and the clinical manifestations. Previous treatment for depression should be identified, including psychotherapy and drug therapy. By assessing the client's problem-solving strategies, the nurse can identify coping behavior strengths and defense mechanisms such as denial, avoidance, or intellectualization that the client may use to mask depression. The client's social support system should also be evaluated because this contributes to his or her sense of well being. Grieving the loss of function in MS can lead to a reactive depression and require provision of support group therapy for both the client and family. Some clients may not benefit from this kind of therapy, however, because they may see people whose condition is much worse than their own and may fear developing that level of disability.

EVALUATION

The degree of expected outcome attainment should be evaluated on an ongoing basis. Most outcomes are long term and may require weeks to months to attain.

Post-hospital Care

The client with MS needs to have a clear understanding about the unpredictableness of this disorder. The client may be symptom free for many weeks to months, even years, and then develop further symptoms. If the client can identify stressors that exacerbate the symptoms, sometimes these stressors can then be avoided.

HOME HEALTH CARE

Clients experiencing a decline in self care abilities may require aids to perform ADLs and ambulate, such as wheelchairs or canes. The performance of ADLs may be enhanced if the counters and/or table tops are adjusted to a comfortable working height. The nurse works in combination with the physical therapist, occupational therapist, social worker, and home health nurse to identify, purchase, and teach the client how to use ADL aids.

PARKINSON'S DISEASE

Overview

Parkinson's disease (PD) is an idiopathic syndrome characterized by disability from tremor and rigidity. There are various other forms of parkinsonism that cause similar symptoms but have known causes. They include postencephalitic parkinsonism, which occurred after the large epidemic of encephalitis in 1919; athereosclerotic parkinsonism, which results from ischemia in the basal ganglia; drug-induced parkinsonism, which occurs after long-term use of phenothiazines; toxin-induced parkinsonism, which can result from carbon monoxide, mercury, or manganese exposure; and trauma-induced parkinsonism, resulting from injury to the midbrain.

PD is the focus of this section because it is the most common form of parkinsonism. PD involves degeneration of dopamine-producing cells in the substantia nigra, which leads to degeneration of neurons in the basal ganglia. Once cell loss in the substantia nigra reaches 80 per cent, symptoms appear. The cause of nigral cell degeneration is not known.

PD most often develops in people in their 60s. It occurs worldwide. About 1 per cent of people over age 50 have PD. PD has three cardinal features: tremor, rigidity, and bradykinesia. Early in the disease, the client may notice a slight slowing in the ability to perform ADLs. This is called *bradykinesia*. A general feeling of stiffness (rigidity) may be noticed, along with mild diffuse muscular pain. Tremor is a common early sign that usually occurs in one of the upper limbs. It occurs at rest and involves a coarse "pill-rolling" movement of the thumb against the fingers, which can vary in intensity and distribution. Voluntary movement stops or reduces the tremor in some people; however, others have tremor during voluntary movement (intention tremor).

Bradykinesia makes voluntary movements difficult to execute. When symptoms are severe, total lack of movement (akinesia) may occur and the client is literally frozen in one spot. Bradykinesia also affects the gait. Initially there may be a slight stiffness of one leg while walking, and the corresponding arm may be held flexed at the elbow and abducted at the shoulder. The person may catch or drag one foot. Later, when both sides of the body are involved, the typical shuffling gait with short steps may develop. There is lack of associated swinging of the arms while walking. In advanced PD, the client stands with head, shoulders, and spine flexed forward, giving the appearance of a stooped posture (Figure 31-3).

The face of someone with advanced PD appears stiff, masklike, and without expression. The speech is low in volume, monotonous in tone, and slow. Words are poorly articulated (dysarthria). Saliva may flow involuntarily from the mouth because of the lack of spontaneous swallowing.

Rare complications of PD are (1) oculogyric crisis, in which the eyes fix upward and to one side or downward, and (2) blepharospasm, which causes almost total closure of the eyelid. Various autonomic effects may accompany PD, including decreased lacrimation (tearing) and sexual capacity, constipation, incontinence, excessive perspiration, and heat intolerance.

PD does not usually affect intellectual ability; however, 15 to 20 per cent of PD sufferers do develop a dementia similar to Alzheimer's disease. Mood disturbance can occur, and emotional stress may intensify signs and symptoms.

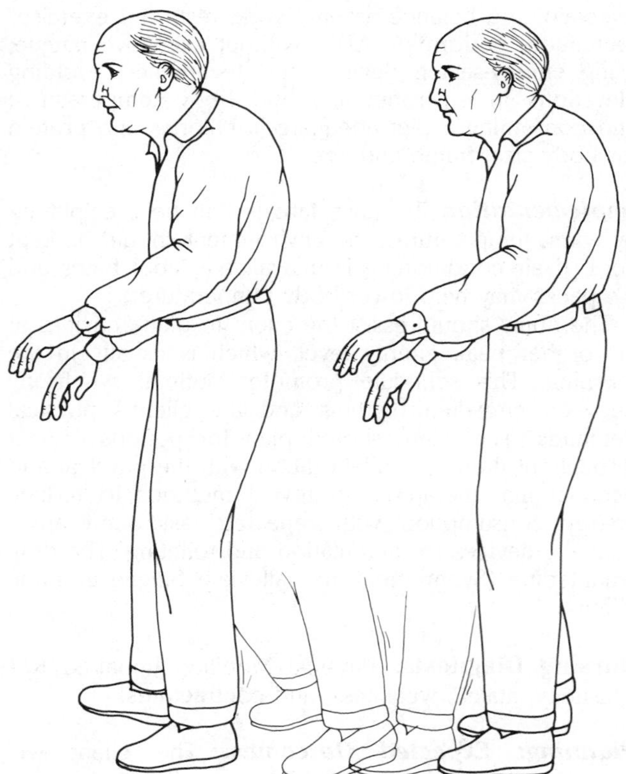

▲ **Figure 31-3**

Gait changes seen in Parkinson's disease. Some of the clinical manifestations of Parkinson's disease are stooped posture, bradykinesia, and a festinating gait.

Management

PHARMACOLOGIC MANAGEMENT

The symptoms of PD can be relieved by various medications, particularly levodopa and anticholinergic drugs. The purpose of these medications is to provide dopamine to the basal ganglia. The most common drug for this purpose is carbidopa/levodopa (Sinemet). Levodopa is a synthetic metabolic precursor of dopamine. Dopamine itself cannot be used because it cannot cross the blood-brain barrier. Carbidopa must be given with levodopa because it prevents peripheral metabolism of levodopa, allowing levodopa to reach the brain. Initiation of carbidopa/levodopa therapy is usually delayed until symptoms affect ADLs because the benefit of the drug seems to decline with prolonged use. The therapy is more effective in treating bradykinesia and rigidity than tremor. The dosage of levodopa is gradually increased until the optimal therapeutic response is achieved. This process may take several months. When the daily dose of levodopa approaches the desired level, the client often has involuntary dyskinesias (jerky, writhing movements), especially of the face, mouth, and tongue. Some clients prefer this state to being severely bradykinetic, because at least they can be mobile and perform voluntary movements more easily. Table 31-4 lists the drugs used in PD.

Occasionally, clients with PD experience parkinsonian crisis as a result of emotional trauma or sudden or inadvertent withdrawal of antiparkinson medication. Severe exacerbation of tremor, rigidity, and bradykinesia, accompanied by acute anxiety, sweating, tachycardia, and hyperpnea, occurs. Intervention for parkinsonian crisis includes respiratory and cardiac support. The person should be placed in a quiet room with subdued lighting. Barbiturates may be prescribed, as well as antiparkinson medication.

An "on-off response" (rapid fluctuation of symptoms) may occur in clients with PD. A person may be mobile and active ("on") one moment and akinetic and rigid ("off") the next. This transition may happen quickly, within 1 to 2 minutes. Initially, the "off" periods tend to occur 3 to 4 hours after a dose of antiparkinson medication. Later, the transition may happen at any time and be unrelated to medication ingestion. Apparently "off" periods are due to dopamine deficit, but this factor is not clear. A person experiencing on-off response may be temporarily helped by shortening the interval between medication doses or by gradually increasing the total dosage.

SURGICAL MANAGEMENT

Surgical intervention is not often used for PD. However, intractable tremor may be ameliorated by thalamotomy. Autologous transplantation of adrenal medullary tissue into the brains of PD clients, in the hope that these cells will produce dopamine, has yielded disappointing results. Fetal tissue transplantation conducted in the United States is very controversial for ethical reasons. Federal funding for this procedure has been put on hold, although some medical centers are doing this procedure with private funds.

NURSING MANAGEMENT

Nursing care for the PD client includes health assessment, medication instruction and monitoring, liaison with other members of the health care team, and client and family education.[28]

The client should be advised to maintain fluid intake of 2000 ml/24 h and increase intake of dietary fiber. Stool softeners and mild laxatives can be used. A regular time for bowel movements should be established, usually a half hour after the morning or evening meal.

The client should be taught various techniques to enhance voluntary movement. Clients often need to try different things on their own to find what helps most. Some clients grasp coins in the pocket to reduce embarrassing hand tremor. Others grip the arms of a chair. Mental thoughts, such as walking over imaginary lines, can aid ambulation. One client found that tossing small scraps of paper in front of him aided his walking. Another found that rocking back and forth helped initiate movement. Daily range-of-motion exercises should be encouraged to avoid rigidity and contractures. The client should be reminded to maintain good posture and to avoid flexion of the neck and shoulders. The client should sleep on a firm mattress. When resting, the client should avoid using a pillow to prevent flexion of the spine. Periodically lying prone also helps.

Because self-care activities are performed more slowly by the client with PD, extra time should be allowed for completion of tasks like dressing, bathing, and eating. Warming trays can keep food hot. Rest periods should be encouraged during meals to avoid aspiration.

As PD progresses, clients become rigid and unresponsive to verbal stimuli. During these stages, nurses continue to treat the client with dignity, speaking to the client rather than ignoring him or her.

The client should be taught about home safety. Loose carpeting should be removed. Grab bars should be placed in the bathroom. An elevated toilet seat should be installed. Clients with severe tremor should avoid carrying hot liquids. Walking aids such as a cane or walker can provide added stability.

The client and family need a lot of emotional support. Support groups are available in most major cities. The client and family can be referred to the American Parkinson Disease Association and Referral Centers by contacting the American Parkinson Disease Association, 116 John Street, New York, NY 10038, 1-800-223-APDA.

MYASTHENIA GRAVIS

Overview

Myasthenia gravis (MG) is an autoimmune disease that presents as muscular weakness and fatigue that worsens with exercise and improves with rest. It is caused by loss of acetylcholine (ACh) receptors in the postsynaptic neurons of the neuromuscular junction. The cause of MG is unknown, but 80 per cent of people with the generalized form of the disease have elevated

TABLE 31-4. Pharmacologic Management of Parkinson's Disease

Drug Classification and Example	Action	Indications	Common Side Effects	Nursing Implications
Anticholinergics				
Trihexphenidyl (Artane) Benztropine (Cogentin) Procyclidine (Kemadrin) Ethopropazine (Parsidol)	Inhibit action of endogenous acetylcholine and muscarine agonists to block the excitatory effect of the cholinergic system.	Tremor, rigidity, drooling	Dry mouth, constipation, blurred vision, confusion, hallucinations	Usually contraindicated in clients with acute-angle glaucoma and tachycardia. Monitor pulse and blood pressure during periods of dosage adjustment. Administer with meals. Do not withdraw medication suddenly.
Antihistamines				
Diphenhydramine (Benadryl)	Mild anticholinergic	Tremor, rigidity, insomnia	Dry mouth, lethargy, confusion	Use with caution in clients with seizures, hypertension, hyperthyroidism, heart and renal disease, and diabetes. Administer with meals or antacids.
Dopaminergics				
Amantadine (Symmetrel)	Cause the release of dopamine in the central nervous system.	Rigidity, bradykinesia	Dizziness, ataxia insomnia, leg edema	Monitor client for postural hypotension. Do not administer at bedtime.
Carbidopa/levadopa (Sinemet)		Tremor, rigidity, bradykinesia	Orthostatic hypotension, nausea, hallucinations, dystonia, dyskinesias	Monitor blood pressure. Use elastic stockings to increase venous return. Monitor client for urinary retention.
Dopamine Agonists				
Bromocriptine (Parlodel)	Activate dopamine receptors in the central nervous system.	Fluctuation of symptoms, dyskinesia, dystonia	Hallucinations, mental fogginess, orthostatic hypotension, confusion	Monitor blood pressure and mental status.
Pergolide (Permax)			Orthostatic hypotension, nausea, insomnia	Monitor blood pressure. Do not administer at bedtime.
Monoamine Oxidase Inhibitors				
Selegiline (Deprenyl)	Inhibit monoamine oxidase B, an enzyme that converts chemical by-products in the brain into neurotoxins that prevent substantia nigra cell death.	Adjuvant treatment	Being researched. Look up side effects	Being researched. Look up recent information on use.

titers of antibodies to the ACh receptor in their serum. MG may appear at any age, although there are two peaks of onset. In early-onset MG, at age 20 to 30 years, women are more often affected than men. In late-onset MG, after age 50, men are more often affected.

The primary feature of MG is increasing weakness with sustained muscle contraction. For instance, if the person is asked to hold the arms up, the power of muscle contraction diminishes and the arms gradually drift downward. After a period of rest, the muscles regain their strength. Muscle weakness is greatest after exertion or at the end of the day. Ocular symptoms are most common, with ptosis (drooping of the upper eyelid) or diplopia (double vision) occurring in the majority of clients. Ptosis is due to weakness of the levator palpebrae muscles of the eye. If not present at the time of examination, ptosis can be elicited by prolonged upward gaze, which creates fatigue of the muscle. Diplopia is a result of weakness and/or fatigue of the extraocular muscles. Other symptoms are weakness of the obicularis oculi muscles (which help close the eye), the facial muscles, the muscles of chewing and swallowing, and the limbs. Weakness of the facial and levator palpebrae muscles produces an expressionless face, with droopy eyelids, smoothed features, and a tendency for the mouth to hang open. An attempt to smile often turns into a snarl because of the weakness. A client may hold a hand under the jaw to keep it closed. Dysphagia and a nasal quality to speech occur when the muscles of chewing and swallowing are involved. In severe cases, respiratory muscle weakness may occur, which may necessitate intubation and mechanical ventilation (see discussion of myasthenic crisis in complications).

The course of MG varies, and there may be remissions and exacerbations. Clinical manifestations may progress quickly or slowly and may fluctuate from day to day. The severity of the disease varies greatly from person to person.

The diagnosis of MG is based on the clinical presentation. It can be confirmed by testing the client's response to anticholinesterase drugs. These drugs inhibit cholinesterase, an enzyme that breaks down ACh in the neuromuscular junction, thereby allowing more ACh to bind to the remaining ACh receptors. Edrophonium (Tensilon) is a short-acting drug that is given intravenously. A test dose of 2 mg (for adults) is injected first. If no untoward reaction occurs (such as increased weakness, change in heart rate or rhythm, nausea, or abdominal cramps), the remaining 8 mg is injected. The client is then observed for objective signs of improvement in muscle strength. The effect is transitory, wearing off after 3 to 5 minutes. Another drug, neostigmine methylsulfate (Prostigmin), may be used because the longer duration of effect on muscle strength (1 to 2 hours) allows better analysis of its effect. When either drug is used, atropine sulfate should be available to inject intravenously. This medication counteracts any severe cholinergic reactions (cardiac arrhythmias or abdominal cramping). Electromyography (EMG) helps confirm the diagnosis. Repetitive stimulation of the nerve with recording from the involved muscle shows a characteristic decrementing response of the muscle action potential.

Medical Management

There is no cure for MG. Pharmacologic intervention consists of two groups of medications: (1) short-acting anticholinesterase compounds and (2) corticosteroids. The most effective anticholinesterase drugs are pyridostigmine (Mestinon) and neostigmine (Prostigmin). Dosages are highly individualized, based on physiologic response to the medication. The goal is to achieve the maximum benefit (muscle strength and endurance) with the least side effects (excessive salivation, sweating, nausea, diarrhea, abdominal cramps, or tachycardia). Corticosteroids (usually prednisone) are directed toward reducing the levels of serum ACh receptor antibodies. However, clinical improvement can occur when there has been no significant decrease in antibodies, so this cannot be the sole mode of steroid action.[21] Corticosteroids may temporarily worsen symptoms; however, this is followed by gradual improvement in muscle strength. After a peak of improvement is reached and maintained for several weeks, the dosage of both prednisone and anticholinesterase medication may be gradually decreased. A low maintenance dose of alternate-day prednisone may be effective for many months or years. The precautions of any steroid therapy are important, including potassium supplements if indicated and liberal use of antacids. Potential complications of steroid use are cataracts, hypertension, diabetes, fluid retention, delayed wound healing, insomnia, and osteoporosis.

Complications

Two major complications of MG may occur. One is *myasthenic crisis*. Clients with moderate or severe generalized MG, especially those who have difficulty swallowing or breathing, may experience a sudden worsening of their condition. This is usually precipitated by an intercurrent infection, but it may occur spontaneously. If an increase in the dosage of the anticholinesterase drug does not improve the weakness, endotracheal intubation and mechanical ventilation may be required. In many instances, drug responsiveness returns in 24 to 48 hours, and weaning from the respirator can proceed.[22]

The other major complication of MG is *cholinergic crisis*. This occurs as a result of overmedication. The muscarinic effect of a toxic level of anticholinesterase medication causes abdominal cramps, diarrhea, and excessive pulmonary secretions. The nicotinic effect paradoxically worsens weakness and can cause bronchial spasm. If respiratory status is compromised, the client may need intubation and mechanical ventilation, and treatment is similar to that of the client in myasthenic crisis. Table 31-5 outlines the features and interventions of cholinergic and myasthenic crises.

TABLE 31–5. Myasthenic and Cholinergic Crises in Clients Experiencing Myasthenia Gravis

Myasthenic Crisis Is Caused by Undermedication

Clinical Manifestations

Sudden marked rise in blood pressure due to hypoxia
Increased heart rate
Severe respiratory distress and cyanosis
Absent cough and swallow reflex
Increased secretions, increased diaphoresis, increased lacrimation
Restlessness, dysarthria
Bowel and bladder incontinence

Intervention

Increased doses of cholinergic drugs as long as the person responds positively to Tensilon treatment
Possible mechanical ventilation if respiratory muscle paralysis is acute

Cholinergic Crisis Is Caused by Depolarization Block Resulting from Excessive Medications

Clinical Manifestations

Weakness with difficulty swallowing, chewing, speaking, and breathing
Apprehension, nausea, and vomiting
Abdominal cramps, diarrhea
Increased secretions and saliva
Sweating, lacrimation, fasciculations, blurred vision

Intervention

Discontinue all cholinergic drugs until cholinegric effects decrease
Provide adequate ventilatory support
1 mg IV of atropine may be necessary to counteract severe cholinegric reactions

IV, Intravenous.

Plasmapheresis is an adjunctive therapy for clients with refractory MG. It is a process by which plasma is separated from formed elements of blood. The plasma is discarded and the packed red cells are joined with albumin, normal saline, and electrolytes and returned to the client. The purpose is to remove plasma proteins containing antibodies that are believed to cause MG. Plasmapheresis produces transient improvement in clients who have actual or pending respiratory failure. Usually three to five treatments are required.[22] Potential complications include myasthenic or cholinergic crisis and, rarely, hypovolemia. Muscle strength should be assessed before and after the procedure, with particular attention paid to vital capacity, swallowing ability, diplopia, and ptosis to evaluate the effectiveness of the treatment.

Another intervention for MG is thymectomy. The thymus gland, located in the superior mediastinum, is important during fetal development for development of the immune system. It is usually atrophied and nonfunctioning in adulthood. The effect of thymectomy is not fully understood. It may alter some immunological control mechanism that affects the production of antibodies to the ACh receptor, or it may eliminate a trigger to antibody production.[21] Thymectomy is indicated for clients with thymoma, selected clients with generalized MG without thymoma, and selected clients with disabling ocular MG.[16]

Nursing Management

Clients with MG are usually managed in an outpatient setting. When they are hospitalized for diagnosis or during a crisis, the following nursing management procedure may be pertinent.

Because MG may involve the muscles of respiration, the client may experience dyspnea and ineffective cough and swallow mechanisms. This may lead to aspiration and pneumonia. Deep breathing and coughing should be encouraged. Suction equipment should be available at the bedside, and the client should be instructed on how to use it. When eating, the client should be instructed to sit bolt upright, swallow only when the chin is tipped downward toward the chest, and never speak while food is in the mouth. Oxygen and, in severe cases, mechanical ventilation may be required for some clients.

In MG, weakness is usually greatest following exertion and at the end of the day. Activities should be carefully planned to include rest periods so that energy is conserved and the muscles have a chance to regain their strength. Rearrangement of the home environment may help prevent unnecessary energy expenditure. Vocational retraining may be indicated for those who can no longer meet the physical demands of their jobs. Clients with severe disease or an acute exacerbation will be totally dependent on nursing care for ADLs. This level of care requires that complications of immobility be avoided.

The client and family should be provided with information about MG and its treatment. They should be aware of adverse reactions of both anticholinesterase drugs and steroids. They also should know how to recognize myasthenic and cholinergic crises and have a plan to seek medical intervention, if necessary. The Myasthenia Gravis Foundation, 15 East 26th Street, New York, NY 10010, publishes educational materials that can be helpful to the client and family. The toll free number is 1-800-541-5454.

AMYTROPHIC LATERAL SCLEROSIS

Overview

Amyotrophic lateral sclerosis (ALS) is the most common of the motor neuron diseases. The onset of ALS usually occurs in middle age. Men are affected more often than women. ALS involves degeneration of both the anterior horn cells and the corticospinal tracts. Consequently, both upper and lower motor neuron clinical manifestations are seen. Lower motor neuron clinical manifestations include weakness, atrophy, cramps, and fasciculations (irregular twitchings of muscle fibers or bundles). Upper motor neuron signs include spasticity and hyperreflexia. Involvement of the corticobulbar tracts causes dysphagia (difficulty swallowing) and dysarthria (slurred speech). The sensory system is not involved.

The course of the disease is relentlessly progressive. Death usually results from pneumonia due to respiratory compromise within 2 to 5 years. Weakness typically begins in the upper extremities and progressively involves the upper arms and shoulders and then the muscles of the neck and throat. The trunk and lower extremities are usually not affected until late in the disease. When the intercostal muscles and diaphragm become involved, respirations become shallow and coughing is ineffective. Cognition, as well as bowel and bladder sphincters, remain intact, even when the client is totally debilitated. In some cases, weakness begins in the brain stem, causing problems with speech and swallowing. This is called *bulbar ALS*.

Diagnosis of ALS is made by the clinical presentation and EMG. EMG criteria for the diagnosis of ALS include the presence of widespread anterior horn cell dysfunction with fibrillations, positive waves, fasciculations, and chronic neurogenic motor unit potential changes in multiple nerve root distribution in at least three limbs and the paraspinal muscles in the presence of normal sensory responses.[18]

Management

Supportive therapy is the only intervention for ALS. Results of therapeutic trials have been depressingly negative.[18] Clients with ALS are usually admitted to health care facilities only twice in their illness, first for diagnosis and later in the final stage of debilitation.

Supportive nursing care is an important aspect of managing the ALS client. In the outpatient arena, the nurse can provide ongoing assessment of daily living needs and make suggestions for modifications in activity level, clothing, and diet. Often, just allowing the client or family to talk about problems reduces anxiety and helps them find solutions to problems. Interventions should be aimed at conserving energy. Activities should be spaced during the day. Muscle stress, strenuous activity, and extremes of hot and cold should be avoided. Leg braces, canes, and walkers can prolong independence in ambulation. Hand braces, special utensils, and adaptive devices such as button hooks can enhance dressing and self-feeding. Pressure ulcers are not usually a problem because the sensory system remains intact and the client can feel when pressure on a body part is too great.

In the acute care setting, the nurse should gather information from the client and family about communication needs and what positions are best for respiration, handling secretions, eating, and turning routines.[27]

Fluid intake should be encouraged regularly, when the client is not fatigued. Proper positioning is imperative. Providing a cup with a spout may prevent liquid from running out of the corners of the mouth. Liquids may be given by using a large syringe with short tubing on the tip. The tube is placed at the back of the tongue, and gentle force is used to deliver small amounts of liquid.

Small, frequent, high nutrient feedings should be encouraged. The client should be told to sit bolt upright, with the head slightly flexed forward while eating. Papase tablets placed under the tongue 10 minutes before meals can make thick saliva less sticky. Plenty of time should be allowed for eating, and the client should not attempt to speak while food is in the mouth. Suction equipment should be available during meals to reduce the risk of aspiration, food and secretions that become lodged in the mouth and pharynx. The head may need to be stabilized by placing a soft cervical collar on the neck. The dietician should be consulted for special diet recommendations.

Although speech remains intelligible, the client can be trained to slow the rate of speech and exaggerate articulation. As symptoms progress, the client may need to repeat words or have an interpreter (usually the spouse). At this stage, it is important to eliminate extraneous noise, face the client when he or she is talking, and maintain eye contact. When speech contains only one-word phrases or is no longer possible, writing can be an effective means of communicating and should be encouraged. When writing is no longer possible, a speech pathologist can provide communication devices such as alphabet boards and portable memo writers.[9]

If the client is a smoker, he or she should be encouraged to stop. Exposure to people with respiratory infections should be avoided. The client should be reminded to use good posture. Pulmonary function tests should be performed regularly to assess ventilatory status. Clients generally experience respiratory fatigue when vital capacity is less than 1.5 liters. Some clients can be taught to use abdominal muscles to enhance respirations when the intercostal muscles and diaphragm become weak. A sign of pending respiratory insufficiency is shortness of breath while eating.

The client and family should be encouraged to talk about the losses they are experiencing and the feelings associated with them. Family members should be encouraged to take time for rest and activities away from the client. The client and family can be referred to an ALS support group. Kim[15] suggests the use of hope as a coping mechanism for ALS clients and describes nursing strategies to promote hope.

Eventually, clients face the difficult choice of deciding whether or not they will accept artificial ventilation. They should be encouraged to discuss this with family and friends and to seek input from ALS support groups. Information about these groups can be obtained from the ALS Society of America, 15300 Ventura Boulevard, Suite 315, Sherman Oaks, CA 91403, (818) 990-2151, or the Muscular Dystrophy Association, 810 Seventh Avenue, New York, NY 10019, (212) 586-0808.

Clients should be encouraged to complete advance

directives to indicate whether they desire life-sustaining treatments such as cardiopulmonary resuscitation, but this should be reassessed at regular intervals. Clients may change their minds on the basis of their experience with their illness, changes in their subjective appreciation of their quality of life, or changes in their evaluation of the benefits and burdens of life-sustaining measures as they realize the imminence of death.[26]

HUNTINGTON'S DISEASE

Overview

Huntington's disease (HD), also known as Huntington's chorea, is a genetically transmitted degenerative neurologic disease. It is characterized by abnormal movements (chorea), intellectual decline, and emotional disturbance. Clinical manifestations usually begin in the fourth and fifth decades, although occasionally they begin in young adulthood or even in children. Women and men are equally affected. The disease is relentlessly progressive, leading to disability and death within 15 to 20 years. Death usually results from respiratory complications due to aspiration.

The disease is autosomal dominant, meaning that offspring of an affected person have a 50 per cent chance of inheriting the disease. Because HD does not skip generations, offspring who have not inherited the disease will not pass it on to their offspring. New developments in molecular biology and linkage analysis of inherited diseases have identified that the abnormal gene for HD lies on the short arm of chromosome 4.[8]

The pathology of HD involves degeneration of the striatum (caudate and putamen) in the basal ganglia. Other subtle changes occur in the cortex and cerebellum, namely, loss of neurons and an increased number of glial cells (gliosis). The degeneration of the caudate nucleus leads to a reduction in several neurotransmitters, including gamma-aminobutyric acid, ACh, substance P, and met-enkephalin, and their synthetic enzymes. This leaves relatively higher concentrations of the other neurotransmitters, dopamine and norepinephrine. The relative excess of dopamine in HD, a disorder of excessive movement, can be contrasted to the lack of dopamine in PD, a disorder of lack of movement.

The abnormal movements in HD are subtle at first. The person may appear restless or fidgety. The person may be aware of these movements and try to mask them by making them seem to be parts of intentional movements, such as head scratching or leg crossing. As the disease progresses, the rapid, jerky choreiform movements become more pronounced and involve all muscles. The person is constantly in motion. Stress, emotional situations, and attempts to perform voluntary movement can aggravate the abnormal movements. During sleep, the movements diminish or disappear.

Emotional disturbances and mental deterioration may precede the abnormal movements. The person may become negative, suspicious, and irritable. This condition may progress to depression and psychosis. Temper outbursts and sexual promiscuity may also occur. Severe mood swings are common. Cognitive decline progresses, and eventually, the person becomes demented, unkempt, incontinent, and completely helpless.

The diagnosis of HD is made on the basis of clinical signs and symptoms and family history, because there is no specific diagnostic test for the disease itself. CT or MRI imaging of the brain may show atrophy of the head of the caudate, but this factor alone is not diagnostic of HD.

Management

There is no known treatment to cure or alter the course of HD. Halperidol (Haldol), a dopamine blocker, can control the abnormal movements and some behavioral manifestations. Diazepam (Valium) can be used to lower anxiety, aiding in control of movements. Antidepressants can help depression.

One of the most common and dangerous middle- to late-stage problems is dysphagia. Several interventions should be tried.[10] Medications need to be evaluated for their anticholinergic and sedative effects, which may impair swallowing. Mealtime should be free of stress and clutter and have an unhurried atmosphere. Use of adaptive eating utensils can encourage and extend independence in eating. The diet should include foods that are easy to swallow, those that form a bolus in the mouth (e.g., canned peaches, chopped meat in gravy and mashed potatoes, custards). Because many clients with HD require high caloric intake because of excessive movements, they should try eating frequent, small meals containing high-calorie foods. Clients should sit bolt upright while eating. While swallowing they should keep the chin down toward the chest. They can be trained to hold their breath before swallowing and cough after each mouthful is swallowed to clear the throat of any residual food.

If the client continues to have difficulty eating and loses weight despite dietary and environmental modifications, a feeding tube may become necessary. However, artificial feeding methods can often frighten families and represent ethical dilemmas about prolonging life. Nurses can help clients and their families make these difficult decisions by clarifying the issues and providing information on the types, risks, benefits, and long-term effects of artificial feeding methods.[10]

Poor control of oral and respiratory muscles can make communication difficult. The nurse can assist the family to develop signals such as raising a hand or keeping the eyes open or closed for yes/no responses. If physical signals are not an option, cards with printed words may be helpful. Keep communication simple and unstrained. Repeat words that are understood to let the client know that communication has been successful.

Excessive movements and falls may cause physical injury and can decrease independence. Pads on wheelchairs and beds, shin guards, and walking belts can prevent injury. Aids for ambulation (e.g., walking behind a wheelchair) can extend independence. Clothing should be light and simple to get on and off.

HD has a major impact on the family, not only because of the burden of care giving but also because of the risk to offspring of inheriting the disease (see Ethical Issues in Nursing). The discovery of linked polymorphic DNA markers for HD has led to the development of predictive testing programs. These programs can modify the risk of having inherited the gene, from 50 per cent to as high as 95 or as low as 5 per cent. However, the marker test requires blood samples from multiple family members and is costly.[11]

GUILLAIN-BARRÉ SYNDROME

Overview

Guillain-Barré syndrome (GBS) is an inflammatory disease of unknown etiology that involves degeneration of the myelin sheath of peripheral nerves. GBS is seen worldwide and affects people of all ages and races. Since the virtual elimination of poliomyelitis, GBS has become the most common cause of acute generalized paralysis, with an annual incidence of 0.75 to 2 cases per 100,000 population.[25] In one half to two thirds of cases, an upper respiratory or gastrointestinal infection precedes the onset of the syndrome by 1 to 4 weeks. Cytomegalovirus and Epstein-Barr virus have been implicated in these antecedent illnesses, as have mycoplasma pneumonia, *Salmonella typhosa,* and *Campylobacter jejuni.* An association between human immunodeficiency virus (HIV) and GBS has also been reported, so clients with GBS should be tested for HIV.

The characteristic feature of GBS is ascending weakness, usually beginning in the lower extremities and spreading, sometimes rapidly, to the trunk, upper extremities, and even the face. The weakness evolves over days to weeks, with maximal deficit by 4 weeks in 90 per cent of cases. Deep tendon reflexes are lost. Paresthesia (tingling sensation) in the limbs may occur early in the course of the illness. Deep, aching muscle pain in the shoulder girdle and thighs is common. The two most dangerous features of the disease are respiratory muscle weakness and autonomic neuropathy involving both the sympathetic and parasympathetic systems. The latter feature can involve orthostatic hypotension, hypertension, pupillary disturbances, sweating dysfunction, cardiac dysrhythmias, paralytic ileus, and urinary retention. Improvement and recovery occur with remyelination. However, if nerve axons are damaged, some residual deficits may remain. Recovery is usually maximal at 6 months, although severe cases may take up to 2 years for maximal recovery. Fortunately, 85 to 90 per cent of clients with GBS recover completely.

Diagnosis of GBS is based on history and physical examination, cerebrospinal fluid (CSF) examination, and electrophysiologic studies. The CSF contains increased protein, with few or no white blood cells. Nerve conduction velocity is slowed, although it may be normal in the early stage of the illness. "Conduction block," a diminution in amplitude or an absence of elicited muscle action potentials from stimulation of a peripheral nerve, also occurs.

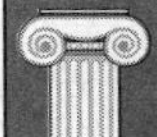

ETHICAL ISSUES IN NURSING

In Revealing Information about Huntington's Disease, which Should Take Precedence: Client Confidentiality or Beneficence?

Huntington's disease is a degenerative neurologic disorder that is autosomal dominant and afflicts 50 per cent of an affected parent's offspring. The disease usually appears in a person's 30s or 40s, bringing on irreversible dementia that leads to death within approximately 10 years after onset. The disease, at present, is incurable. Often a parent has had children before he or she knows he or she has the disease. Currently, there are diagnostic tests that detect the disease long before symptoms are present. Because offspring of a parent with Huntington's disease have a 50 per cent chance of developing it, early testing may assist them in their own decision to procreate. One dilemma that could surface from this would be whether or not the results of testing were positive, the person has a duty to disclose the results to his or her spouse, children, fiancé, or significant other.

There are several ethical principles that must be considered in this case. First, there is confidentiality. A person has the right not to have medical information disclosed to anyone unless he or she consents to do so. Is this right absolute even if it means that others may be harmed by such confidentiality? The American Nurses' Association code states that there is a duty of veracity, i.e., to tell the truth and not to deceive others. If a family member asks the nurse if another family member has a positive test for Huntington's chorea, what should the nurse do? Is there any duty of beneficence toward family members in disclosing information that could ultimately affect their own lives?

The profession of nursing is one that assists others in maintaining or improving their health status. Information gathered from diagnostic tests can greatly influence the treatment decisions of health care providers. Information regarding a positive test for Huntington's disease may assist in the counseling of those family members at risk for developing the disease. However, if information is withheld from those family members, counseling may not be given. Nurses must be sensitive to their clients' desire for confidentiality, but should also use this opportunity to teach their client about the effect the disease may have on other family members.

Management

The focus of therapy is supportive care. Respiratory or cardiovascular status must be monitored carefully. This includes vital signs, serial measurement of vital capacity, peripheral oxygen saturation, and electrocardiography. When vital capacity falls to 15 ml/kg of body weight, intubation and artificial ventilation are usually necessary. Plasmapheresis accelerates recovery, although the exact mechanism for this effect is not known (hypotheses include the removal of circulating antibodies or other humoral myelinotoxic or immunopathogenic factors[4]). Gamma-globulin infusion may prove to be the treatment of choice because of its ease and rapidity of administration and its relative safety, even in unstable patients.[25] However, further research must be performed.

Interventions to control infection and prevent complications of immobility are important. Proper body alignment should be maintained to prevent deformities and injury to paralyzed limbs. Once the client's condition has stabilized, rehabilitative interventions can be implemented.

The nurse also assists the client to cope with the progressive nature of GBS. During the early stages, clients are frightened because each day their paralysis has climbed upward. They are often admitted to an acute care agency with progressive weakness and within days are completely paralyzed. Clients fear they will never recover. Nurses assist clients in verbalizing their fears and offer support and encouragement that although the disorder is progressive, most clients gain full recovery. Encouragement is not hollow, however. The client is not taught to expect immediate resolution but is assisted to realize the usual time frames for recovery.

Summary

Degenerative neurologic disorders have many causes, including viruses, autoimmune responses, and heredity. Some have no known cause. Because of the many etiologies, these disorders are feared by both the client and family. In general, they are relentlessly progressive, slowly taking away both physical and mental ability. The nurse needs to focus care on the management of clinical manifestations and prevention of complications. Family support throughout the process of care is essential.

Bibliography

1. Acorn, S., & Andersen, S. (1990). Depression in multiple sclerosis: Critique of the research literature. *Journal of Neuroscience Nursing, 22*(4), 209-214.
2. Bartol, M. (1979). Nonverbal communication in patients with Alzheimer's disease. *Journal of Gerontological Nursing, 5*(4), 21-31.
3. Cummings, J. L., & Benson, D. F. (1992). *Dementia, a clinical approach*. Boston: Butterworth-Heinemann.
4. England, J. D. (1990). Guillain-Barré syndrome. *Annual Review of Medicine, 41*, 1-6.
5. Erickson, R. P., Lie, M. R., & Wineinger, M. A. (1989). Rehabilitation in multiple sclerosis. *Mayo Clinic Proceedings, 64*(7), 818-828.
6. Evans, D. A., et al. (1989). Prevalence of Alzheimer's disease in a community population of older persons. *Journal of the American Medical Association, 262*(18), 2552-2556.
7. Goodin, D. S. (1991). The use of immunosuppressive agents in the treatment of multiple sclerosis: A critical review. *Neurology, 41*(7), 980-985.
8. Gusella, J. F., et al. (1983). A polymorphic marker genetically linked to Huntington's disease. *Nature, 306*(5940), 234-238.
9. Hillel, A. D., & Miller, R. (1989). Bulbar amyotrophic lateral sclerosis: Patterns of progression and clinical management. *Head and Neck, 11*(1), 51-59.
10. Hunt, V. P., & Walker, F. O. (1989). Dysphagia in Huntington's disease. *Journal of Neuroscience Nursing, 21*(2), 92-95.
11. Hunt, V. P., & Walker, F. O. (1991). Learning to live at risk for Huntington's disease. *Journal of Neuroscience Nursing 23*(3), 179-182.
12. Hurley, A. C., et al. (1992). Assessment of discomfort in advanced Alzheimer patients. *Research in Nursing & Health 15*(5), 369-378.
13. Jones, P. S., & Martinson, I. M. (1992). The experience of bereavement in care givers of family members with Alzheimers disease. *Image: Journal of Nursing Scholarship 24*(3), 172-176.
14. Katzman, R., & Jackson, J. E. (1991). Alzheimer disease: Basic and clinical advances. *Journal of the American Geriatrics Society, 39*(5), 517-525.
15. Kim, T. (1989). Hope as a mode of coping in amyotrophic lateral sclerosis. *Journal of Neuroscience Nursing, 21*(6), 342-347.
16. Lanska, D. J. (1990). Indications for thymectomy in myasthenia gravis. *Neurology, 40*(12), 1828-1829.
17. McKhann, G., et al. (1984). Clinical diagnosis of Alzheimer's disease: Report of the NINCDS-ADRDA Work Group under the auspices of Department of Health and Human Services Task Force on Alzheimer's Disease. *Neurology, 34*(7), 939-944.
18. Mitsumoto, H., Hanson, M. R., & Chad, D. A. (1988). Amyotrophic lateral sclerosis: Recent advances in pathogenesis and therapeutic trials. *Archives of Neurology, 45*(2), 189-202.
19. Morris, R. G., Morris, L. W., & Britton, P. G. (1988 Aug). Factors affecting the emotional wellbeing of the caregivers of dementia sufferers. *British Journal of Psychiatry, 153*, 147-156.
20. Oger, J. J. F., & Aronson, B. G. W. (1984). Immunogenetics of multiple sclerosis. In G. N. Panayi & C. S. David (Eds.), *Immunogenetics* (pp. 177-206). Boston: Butterworth.
21. Pearlman, A. L. (1990). Neuromuscular junction. In A. L. Pearlman & R. C. Collins (Eds.), *Neurobiology of disease* (pp. 44-61). New York: Oxford University Press.
22. Perlo, V. P. (1988). Treatment of the critically ill patient with myasthenia. In A. H. Ropper & S. F. Kennedy (Eds.), *Neurological and neurosurgical intensive care* (pp. 247-252). Rockville, MD: Aspen Publications.
23. Pfeffer, R. I., Afifi, A. A., & Chance, J. M. (1987). Prevalence of Alzheimer's disease in a retirement community. *American Journal of Epidemiology, 125*(3), 420-424.
24. Rodriguez, M. (1989). Multiple sclerosis: Basic concepts and hypothesis. *Mayo Clinic Proceedings, 64*(5), 570-576.
25. Ropper, A. H. (1992). The Guillain-Barré syndrome. *New England Journal of Medicine, 326*(17), 1130-1136.
26. Silverstein, M. D., et al. (1991). Amyotrophic lateral sclerosis and life-sustaining therapy: Patients' desires for information, participation in decision making, and life-sustaining therapy. *Mayo Clinic Proceedings, 66*(9), 906-913.
27. Stone, N. (1987). Amyotrophic lateral sclerosis: A challenge for constant adaptation. *Journal of Neuroscience Nursing, 19*(3), 166-173.
28. Vernon, G. M. (1989). Parkinson's disease. *Journal of Neuroscience Nursing, 21*(5), 273-282.

Chapter 32

Nursing Care of Clients with Disorders of the Spinal Cord, Peripheral Nerves, and Cranial Nerves

DISORDERS OF THE SPINAL CORD

SPINAL CORD INJURY

Definition

Injury to the spinal cord can range in severity from mild flexion-extension "whiplash" injuries to complete transection of the cord with quadriplegia. Trauma to the cord can occur at any level but most commonly occurs in the cervical and lower thoracic–upper lumbar vertebrae.

Although this discussion focuses on nursing management of acute spinal cord injury, it should be remembered that there are approximately

200,000 spinal-cord-injured people living in America. Those nurses who do not routinely care for neurologically impaired individuals may find themselves caring for a client who has a spinal cord injury in addition to his or her presenting symptoms.

Incidence

Each year approximately 10,000 individuals sustain a spinal cord injury. Most of these individuals are males under the age of 40.

Etiology

Trauma is the most common cause of spinal cord injury. Traumatic spinal injury may be due to automobile or motorcycle accidents, gunshot or knife wounds, falls, or sporting mishaps. Disorders that may result in spinal cord injury include:

- Cervical spondylosis with myelopathy, producing spinal canal narrowing and causing progressive injury to the cord and roots;
- Myelitis (infective or noninfective inflammatory processes);
- Osteoporosis causing compression fractures of the vertebrae;
- Syringomyelia (central cavitation of the cord);
- Tumors, both infiltrative and compressive;
- Vascular diseases, usually infarction or hemorrhage (hematomyelia).

Whatever the cause, spinal cord injuries produce distinctive and debilitating syndromes. Nowhere else in the body can local insult produce such devastation in proportion to the extent of tissue involved.

Risk Factors

The feeling of immortality often held by adolescents and young adults contributes strongly to their risk for spinal cord injury. Young people may believe they can engage in dangerous behavior without being injured. The use of alcohol and illicit drugs can add to this belief. Primary prevention centers on public education. The hazards of drinking and driving or diving or jumping into water of uncertain depth must be stressed, particularly to teenagers. Encouraging the use of bicycle and motorcycle helmets is also a part of public education. This message may be best delivered by a young person who has experienced the devastation of spinal cord injury. There are several nationwide programs in which head-and-spinal-cord-injured people speak at school-sponsored educational programs. Nurses can assist with such educational programs, as well as sharing their knowledge of spinal cord injury prevention on a personal basis.

Secondary prevention involves preventing further damage to an already compromised spinal cord. Stabilization of the spine is essential to minimize neurologic deficits. Once the spine is stabilized, the nurse is responsible for maintaining the stabilization. This may involve the use of traction and specialized beds, a halo brace and/or a lumbar brace, or a corset. Care must be taken to prevent twisting of the spine during position changes or transfers.

Minimizing the complications of spinal cord injury is the goal of tertiary prevention. In the acute phase, this focuses on preventing respiratory and cardiovascular compromise. As the individual's medical condition stabilizes, nursing intervention is aimed at client and caregiver education. This must include maintenance of skin integrity, adaptive activities of daily living (ADLs), management of bowel and bladder function, and psychosocial adaptation to the lifestyle changes.

Pathophysiology

Spinal cord injuries most often occur as a result of injury to the vertebrae. The cord is injured due to acceleration, deceleration, or deformity that occurs from various forces (e.g., impact) applied to the spine. The forces injure the spinal cord by compressing, pulling, or tearing the tissues. The most common sites of injury are at the 1st to 2nd cervical, 4th to 6th cervical, and 11th thoracic to 2nd lumbar vertebrae. These segments of the spine are the most mobile and thereby injured more easily.

MECHANISM OF INJURY

Flexion-Rotation, Dislocation, or Fracture Dislocation. This type of injury most often occurs in the cervical spine, usually at C5 to C6. When it occurs in the thoracic-lumbar spine, it is commonly seen at T12 to L1. This form of injury ruptures supporting ligaments, fractures the vertebrae, damages blood vessels, and leads to ischemia of the spinal cord (Fig. 32 – 1*A*).

Hyperextension. This type of injury is commonly seen in elderly clients who have degenerative vertebral changes, young men who have been in an automobile accident in which they hit the windshield or steering wheel, and young people who sustained neck injuries while diving. This type of injury stretches the spinal cord against the ligamenta flava and can lead to dorsal column contusion and posterior dislocation of the vertebrae. Complete transection of the cord can follow a hyperextension injury. Complete lesions of the cord result in loss of all voluntary movement below the lesion and loss of reflex function in isolated segments of the cord (Fig. 32 – 1*B*).

Compression. Compression injuries are often caused by falls or jumps in which the individual lands on the feet or buttocks. The force of impact fractures the vertebrae and they compress the cord. Disc and bone fragments may be propelled backward into the spinal cord on impact. The lumbar and lower thoracic vertebrae are most commonly injured; about 50 per cent of these injuries result in incomplete lesions. Incomplete lesions occur when some of the spinal tracts are intact (Fig. 32 – 1*C*).

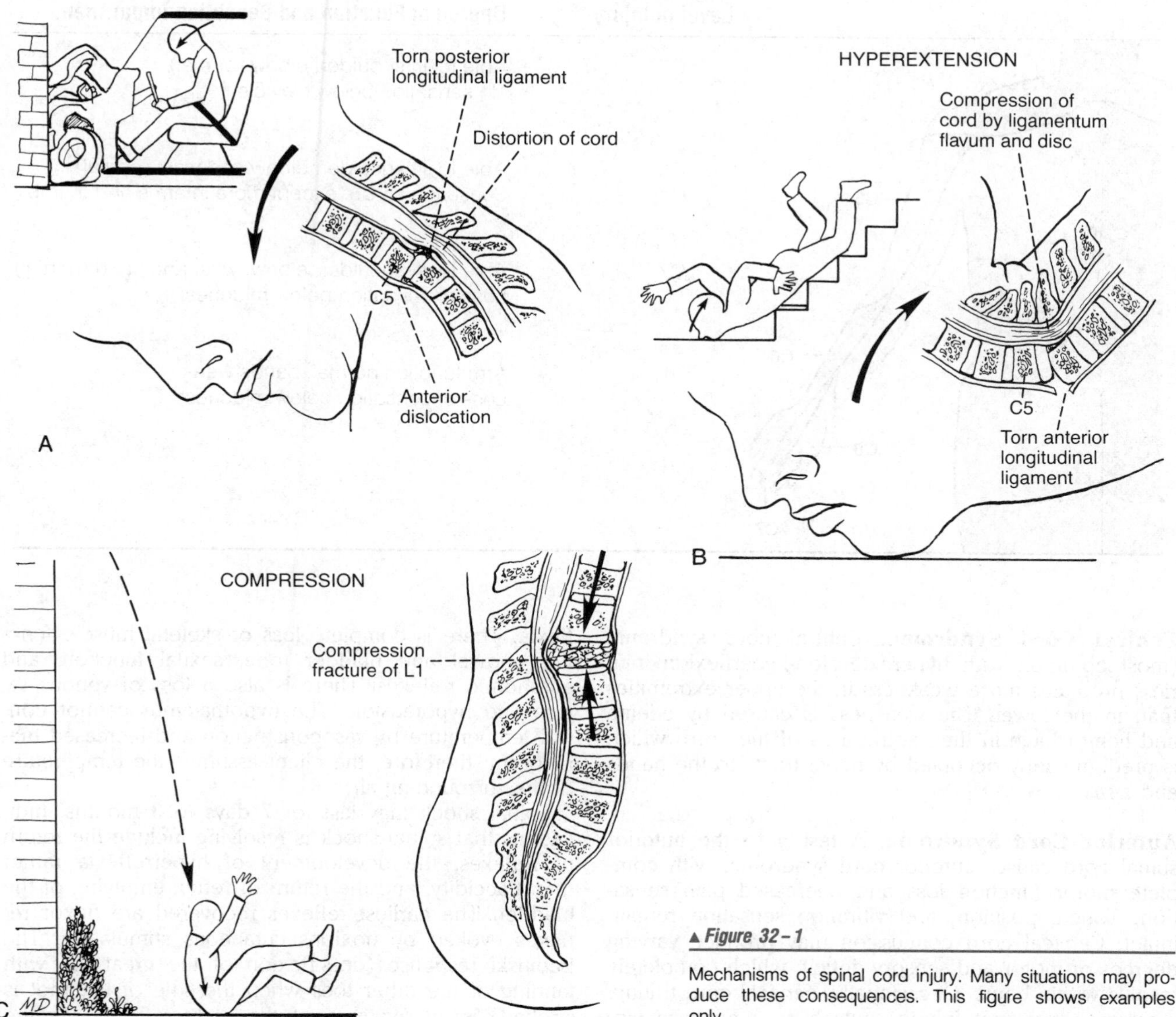

▲ *Figure 32-1*

Mechanisms of spinal cord injury. Many situations may produce these consequences. This figure shows examples only.

Edema and microscopic bleeding occur following injury. The site of injury has the most edema and bleeding, but there are some edema and bleeding for at least two cord segments to either side of the injury. The edema of the cord leads to temporary loss of sensation and function. Therefore, initially after injury it is not easy to determine the degree of permanent impairment. Following the edema and bleeding, there are massive necrosis and, finally, parenchymal and vessel destruction. The axon sheath begins to disintegrate within hours after injury.

LEVEL OF INJURY

Injury to the cervical spine and cord produces quadriplegia. Injuries above the fourth cervical vertebra (C4) may be fatal because of the loss of innervation to the diaphragm and intercostal muscles. Without immediate rescue breathing after the accident, the individual will die of respiratory failure. Today, due to the general public's knowledge of cardiopulmonary resuscitation, many people live after injuries to the cervical spine. Injuries to the remainder of the cervical spine create very specific patterns of motor loss (Table 32-1).

Injuries to the thoracic or lumbar spine produce paraplegia. Clients with such injuries have function of their upper extremities and can be mobile in a wheelchair or with crutches and braces. Table 32-1 describes the extent of paralysis according to the level of injury.

SYNDROMES CAUSING PARTIAL PARALYSIS

There are three spinal cord syndromes, each characterized by distinctive neurologic findings: central cord syndrome, anterior cord syndrome, and Brown-Séquard syndrome.

TABLE 32–1. Cervical Injury and Impairment

Level of Injury	Degree of Function and Sensation Impairment
C5	Able to lift shoulder, elbow (partial) No sensation below clavicle
C6	Able to lift shoulder, elbow and wrist (partial) Sensation as C5, except more in arms and thumb
C7	Able to lift shoulder, elbow, wrist and hand (partial) Loss of sensation below midchest
C8	Arm function normal, hands weak Loss of sensation below midchest

Central Cord Syndrome. Central cord syndrome (most common with hyperextension-hyperflexion injuries) produces more weakness in the upper extremities than in the lower. The weakness is caused by edema and hemorrhage in the central area of the cord, which is predominantly occupied by nerve tracts to the hands and arms.

Anterior Cord Syndrome. A lesion to the anterior spinal cord causes anterior cord syndrome, with complete motor function loss and decreased pain sensation. Touch, position, and vibration sensation remain intact. Cervical cord concussion may produce varying degrees of motor and sensory deficit, which completely resolve within hours. Occasionally, cervical cord trauma produces only root injuries, which may paralyze isolated muscles or muscle groups in the arms and shoulders. These deficits are usually permanent.

Brown-Séquard Syndrome. Brown-Séquard syndrome is caused by lateral hemisection of the cord (i.e., when a lesion cuts or affects half the cord) such as a bullet wound or knife wound. This results in ipsilateral motor paralysis, loss of vibratory and position sense, and contralateral loss of pain and temperature sensation.

COMPLETE TRANSECTION

Total transection of the spinal cord results in immediate loss of all sensation and voluntary movement in areas below the transection. Initially, all reflex activity is also lost, but it does recover; and sometimes reflexes may become hyperactive.

Spinal Shock. The immediate response to cord transection is called spinal shock or post-traumatic areflexia. There is complete loss of skeletal muscle function, bowel and bladder tone, sexual function, and autonomic reflexes. There is also a loss of venous return and hypotension. The hypothalamus cannot control temperature by vasoconstriction and increased metabolism; therefore, the client assumes the temperature of the surrounding air.

Spinal shock may last for 7 days to 3 months. Indications that spinal shock is resolving include the return of reflexes, the development of hyperreflexia rather than flaccidity, and the return of reflex emptying of the bladder. The earliest reflexes recovered are flexor reflexes evoked by noxious cutaneous stimulation. The Babinski response (dorsiflexion of the great toe with fanning of the other toes when the sole of the foot is stroked) is an example of the early reflexes. As the other flexor reflexes return, reflexes can be evoked from touching wider areas of skin.

Spasticity. As recovery progresses after cord transection, flexor responses are interspersed with extensor spasms. This ultimately develops into predominately extensor activity. The client's limbs spasm into extension with movement.

Spasticity is the increased tone or contraction of muscles, producing stiff movements. It may result from various central nervous system (CNS) injuries or diseases, such as spinal cord injuries, cerebrovascular accidents, and cerebral palsy. Spasticity may remain indefinitely or gradually decrease.

Spastic movements may be initiated by (1) emotion (e.g., anxiety, crying, anger, or laughing) or (2) cutaneous stimulation (e.g., tickling, stroking, or pinching). Although spastic movements may be annoying, a client may learn to recognize events that trigger such movements and use them to aid functional activities such as urination.

A certain amount of muscle spasm may help a paraplegic support the trunk or position an extremity. However, painful or recurrent spasms that forcibly flex or adduct lower limbs interfere with sitting and ambulation. Because these muscle spasms are reflex responses, the nurse should try to prevent them by removing sources of noxious stimulation that could trigger them. For example, bladder infections and pressure sores should be treated.

Following spinal cord transection, the brain can no longer influence the segmental spinal cord reflex movements, i.e., reflex movements built into the spinal cord. The lower part of the cord eventually works automatically on its own. Spinal automatisms are spinal reflex activities that occur automatically after spinal cord severance, such as flexor withdrawal reflex and reflex emptying of the bladder and bowel. These primitive, spinal mechanisms, normally kept inactive by higher centers, are "released" when the normal inhibitions of the higher centers are destroyed.

Clinical Manifestations

The initial clinical manifestations of acute spinal cord injury depend on the level and extent of injury to the cord. Below the level of injury or lesion, there is loss of (1) voluntary movement; (2) sensation of pain, temperature, pressure, and proprioception; (3) bowel and bladder function; and (4) spinal and autonomic reflexes.

Following a traumatic complete transverse spinal cord lesion, painful, intense muscular spasms of the lower extremities occur. The nurse should explain to the client and family that these muscle spasms are involuntary and do not mean that voluntary movement is returning. This may be very disappointing.

Muscle spasms vary from mild muscular twitchings to vigorous mass reflex states, depending on the posture. Violent, involuntary muscle spasms can actually throw a client off a bed. Bed side rails should be kept up and restraining straps kept comfortably secured over the client when lying on a stretcher. Muscle spasms are often aggravated by cold weather, prolonged periods of sitting, or emotionally upsetting events. Reflex spasms may become intolerable. They may be triggered by extrinsic or visceral stimuli, such as a distended bladder.

When the spinal cord is severed, blood pressure and temperature in the body part supplied by the isolated spinal cord fall markedly and respond poorly to reflex stimuli. Other functions may occur reflexively (e.g., control of the urinary bladder), but they lack integration with other visceral activities. Visceral activities may be initiated by atypical stimuli; e.g., scratching the skin may cause vasodilatation, sweating, and urination.

Nervous system lesions may produce defective urinary bladder functions known as cord bladder. For example, stimulation of the skin of the lower abdomen or thighs may cause reflex urination. This form of cord bladder is called an automatic bladder. Such stimulation may also cause reflex ejaculation and priapism, i.e., persistent abnormal penile erection without sexual desire in paralyzed men.

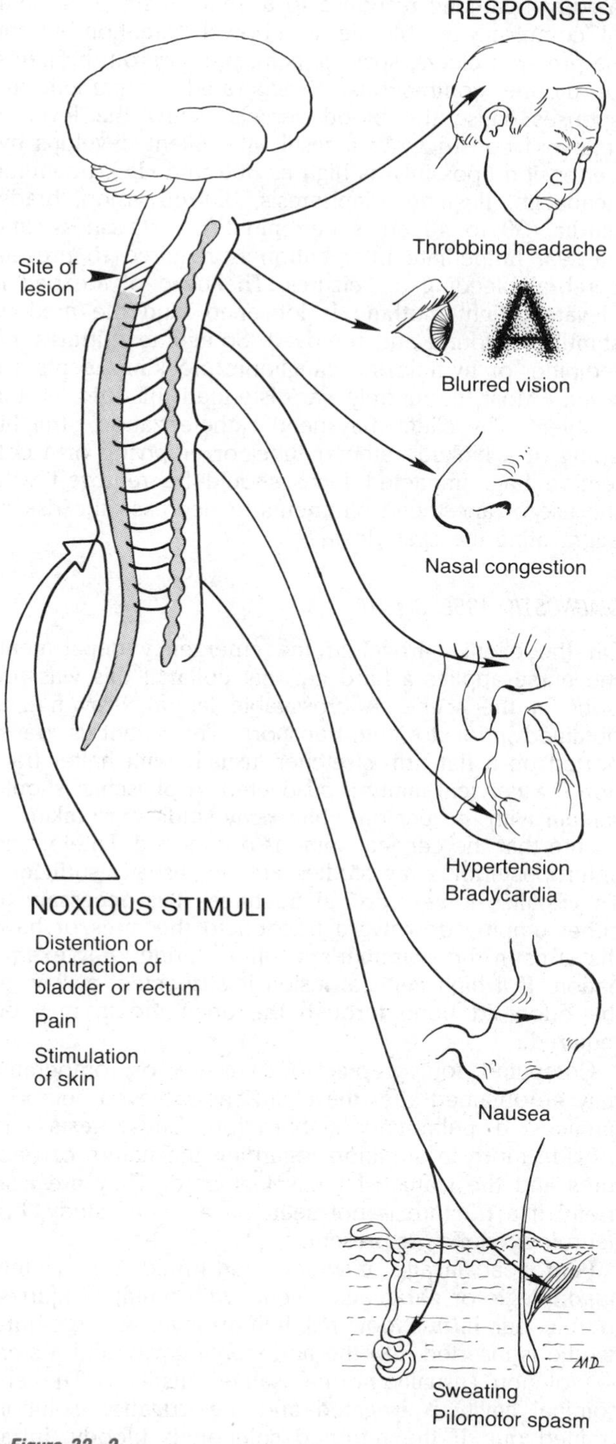

▲ *Figure 32-2*

Causes of hyperreflexia and assessment findings.

AUTONOMIC DYSREFLEXIA

Autonomic dysreflexia is a cluster of clinical manifestations that results when multiple spinal cord autonomic responses discharge simultaneously (Fig. 32-2). This syndrome occurs in clients with injury above T7 and can occur for up to 6 years after injury. The manifestations of autonomic dysreflexia result from an exaggerated sympathetic response to a noxious stimulus. Stimuli commonly are bladder and bowel distention but can be pressure ulcers, spasms, pain, pressure on the penis, or uterine contractions. Exaggerated sympathetic responses cause the blood vessels below the level of injury to constrict. As a result, the client develops hypertension (possibly as high as 300 mm Hg), pounding headache, flushing, diaphoresis, blurred vision, bradycardia (30 to 40 beats per minute), restlessness, and nausea. Immediate intervention is required to prevent cerebral bleeding or seizures. The head of the bed is elevated, tight clothing is loosened, and the noxious stimulus is found and removed. Sometimes nitrates, nifedipine, or hydralazine ganglionic blocking agents are given. Most commonly, a distended bladder is the problem. The client may need catheterization, straightening of a kinked catheter tube, or emptying of a collection bag. Impacted feces should be removed with the use of anesthetic ointments to decrease the risk of aggravating the dysreflexia.

DIAGNOSTIC ASSESSMENT

On the client's arrival in the emergency department, the nurse applies a hard cervical collar if this was not done at the scene. A cross-table lateral x-ray film is obtained prior to any transport. The client is transported on a flat firm stretcher, usually with halter traction if a cervical injury is suspected. A physician should remain with the person while x-ray studies are taken to ensure that the cervical spine is not moved. Lateral and anteroposterior x-ray studies are not usually sufficient. To visualize lower cervical fractures, it is necessary to either employ downward traction to the arms or have the arms in the swimmer's position during x-ray examination. If a high cervical lesion is suspected, a view of the odontoid bone through the open mouth may be required.

Computed tomographic (CT) scans or tomograms may be obtained after the client has achieved hemodynamic and pulmonary stabilization. These tests can provide more information regarding the nature of fractures and the status of the spinal cord. They are also useful if a fracture is not seen on an x-ray study, but neurologic deficit is present.

Peritoneal lavage may be performed for acutely quadriplegic or paraplegic clients with multiple injuries, to rule out intra-abdominal hemorrhage. A large-bore needle is inserted into the abdominal cavity and a sterile solution (usually normal saline) instilled. The abdominal cavity is irrigated and the irrigation solution drained out. If the returned solution is bloody, intra-abdominal bleeding is present.

Medical Management

IMMEDIATE CARE

Both the initial (especially during the first hour after injury) and long-term intervention provided for a client experiencing spinal cord injury significantly influences (1) the extent of the injury and associated deficits, (2) how well the person survives the acute phase of injury, and (3) the success of recovery and rehabilitation. People with spinal cord injury can lead productive and, in some cases, independent lives.

Spinal trauma is often associated with other injuries such as head and abdominal injuries. Anyone who has sustained multiple trauma should be handled as if there are spinal injuries until assessment procedures prove otherwise. When handling a client suspected of having a cervical spinal injury, the spine is kept in neutral alignment and flexion is prevented. If turning is required, a log-rolling maneuver is used. The client is placed in a supine position on a firm surface. The head is supported in alignment with the body and is immobilized by placing sandbags on either side of it or by taping it to the board, and a firm padded cervical collar is applied. Some physicians use halter traction immediately to keep the cervical spine aligned and prevent movement. Clothing is cut off rather than removed.

Cervical injury may produce respiratory distress. In this case, immediate action is taken to maintain a patent airway and provide adequate oxygenation. Damage at the C3 to C5 levels can involve the phrenic nerve, causing diaphragmatic paralysis and respiratory failure. It is important that the client's neck is not hyperextended during intubation; therefore, the jaw thrust technique is used. Suction is performed as necessary to maintain a patent airway. Mechanically assisted respiration may be required when definite loss or impairment of respiratory muscle function occurs.

Careful monitoring of hemodynamic parameters is essential. Heart rate, blood pressure, temperature, respirations, and fluid balance should be monitored continuously. Hypotension associated with spinal shock is initially treated with intravenous fluid. It is important to remember that hypotension with cervical injury is due to vasodilation and the inability to vasoconstrict, not volume depletion. Therefore, fluid resuscitation should be carefully monitored, to avoid fluid overload that can lead to pulmonary edema. Vasopressor agents are often employed in the acute phase of spinal cord injury to maintain adequate blood pressure.

A brief but thorough neurologic examination is made to assess the extent of injury and establish a baseline of function and involvement for later comparison.

If the client is conscious, the nurse asks where any pain is occurring. Sensation is tested by determining whether or not the person can feel touch or a pinprick in the feet, legs, trunk, hands, and arms. Levels of sensation are documented according to dermatomes. To assess motor function, the nurse asks the client to wiggle toes, move ankles, flex knees, and move hands and arms. The location, symmetry, and strength of muscle movement are documented (Table 32-2). The major reflexes, i.e., the ankle, knee, biceps, and triceps, are briefly tested. The nurse looks for areas of sensory sparing, such as sacral sparing, in which the perineum retains sensation.

If the client is unresponsive, assessment is more limited. The nurse observes for spontaneous movement

TABLE 32–2. Motor Assessment After Spinal Cord Injury

Spinal Nerve	Assessment Technique
C4 to C5	Shoulders are shrugged against downward pressure of examiner's hands
C5 to C6	Arm is pulled up from resting position against resistance
C7	From the flexed position, arm is straightened out against resistance
C7	Index finger is held firmly to thumb against resistance to pull apart
C8	Hand grasp strength is evaluated
L2 to L4	Leg is lifted from bed against resistance
L5 to S1	Knee is flexed against resistance
L2 to L4	From flexed position, knee is extended against resistance
L5	Foot is pulled up toward nose against resistance
S1	Foot is pushed down (stepping on the gas) against resistance

Modified from Marshall, S. B., et al. (1990). *Neuroscience critical care: Pathophysiology and patient management* (p. 327). Philadelphia: W. B. Saunders Company.

and to assess respiratory status, thorax expansion. Sensation and movement of extremities are assessed by watching the client for a few moments or by applying a painful stimulus (pinprick) and observing for withdrawal. The nurse obtains details of the injury and the client's condition immediately after the injury from anyone who observed the incident.

A person who has sustained a severe cervical injury should be placed immediately in skeletal traction to immobilize the cervical spine and reduce the fracture and dislocation. Various types of tongs may be used for this: Crutchfield, Barton, or Gardner-Wells. Tongs are inserted through the skull's outer table (Fig. 32–3). Traction is applied to the tongs via rope, pulleys, and weights. Weights begin with 10 to 20 lb (4.5 to 9.1 kg) and gradually increase to accomplish bony reduction. When proper alignment is obtained and verified by x-ray examination, the amount of traction may be reduced to that which is sufficient to maintain the position. Traction is not used to stabilize and immobilize thoracic or lumbar spinal fractures or fracture-dislocations because there is no effective way to provide it.

PHARMACOLOGIC MANAGEMENT

Vasoactive agents are commonly used to support blood pressure immediately after injury. High doses of methylprednisolone (15 mg/kg) started within 8 hours of injury have resulted in both improved motor and sensory function.

Long-term pharmacologic management may include urinary anti-infectives, anticoagulants, laxatives, and antispasmotics.

DIETARY MANAGEMENT

Nutritional intake may be compromised by respiratory impairment, position, emotional status, and/or gastrointestinal function. Intubation eliminates the possibility of oral intake, whereas a tracheostomy does not. Clients with a tracheostomy require time to adjust to swallow-

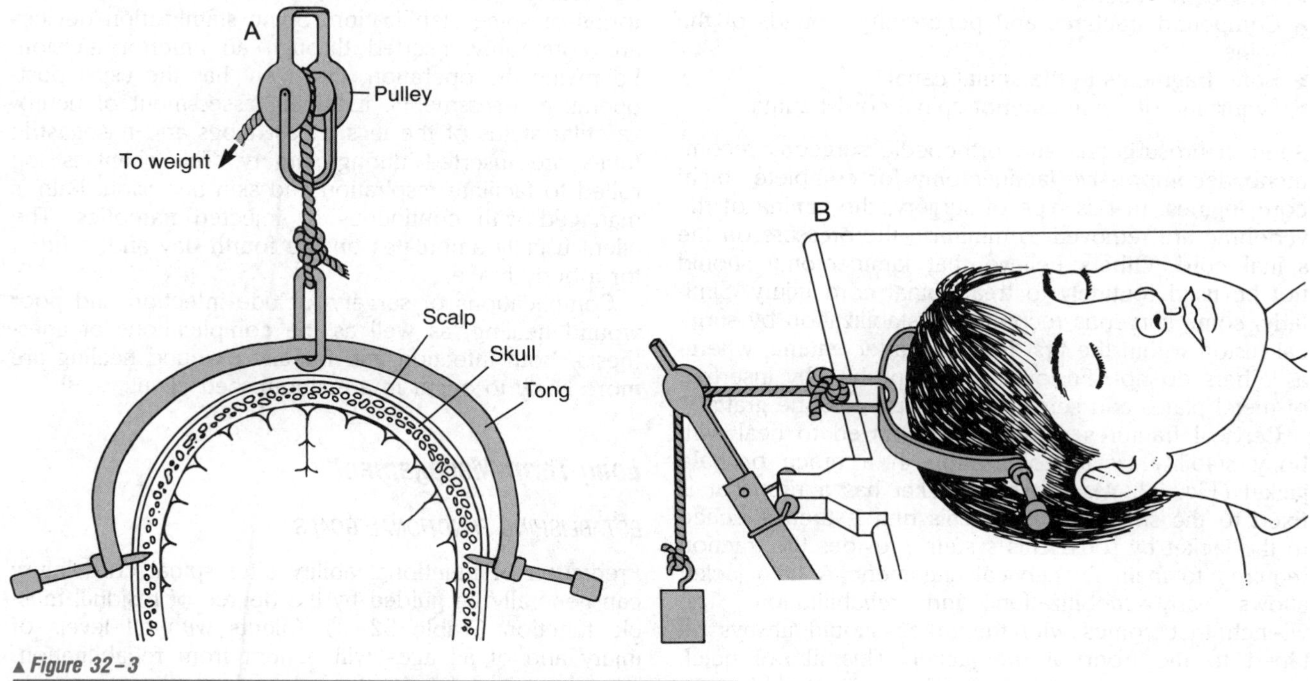

▲ ***Figure 32–3***

Skeletal traction for cervical injuries. *A*, Crutchfield tongs. *B*, Gardner-Wells tongs.

ing with the tube in place and must be carefully monitored to prevent aspiration.

Aspiration is also a risk for clients who must remain flat while in tongs and traction. Although these clients may be capable of swallowing, it is unlikely that they will be able to safely consume enough food to meet their metabolic needs. Clients in halo jackets often experience difficulty eating because their head is immobile. They should be encouraged to take small bites, eat slowly, and concentrate on swallowing.

Depression is a common reaction to spinal cord injury and may have an inhibitive effect on the appetite. Also, choosing when and what to eat may be one of the few areas of control left to an individual with spinal cord injury. As much free choice of dietary intake as is feasible should be encouraged.

Paralytic ileus is a common sequela of spinal cord injury. By frequently assessing bowel sounds and documenting the passage of stool, the nurse can determine when the parastasis has returned and the client is capable of digesting food.

Any of these conditions can severely limit a spinal-cord-injured client's oral intake at a time when a high-calorie, high-protein diet is needed. Enteral feeding and/or total parenteral hyperalimentation are often prescribed until oral intake is sufficient to meet body needs.

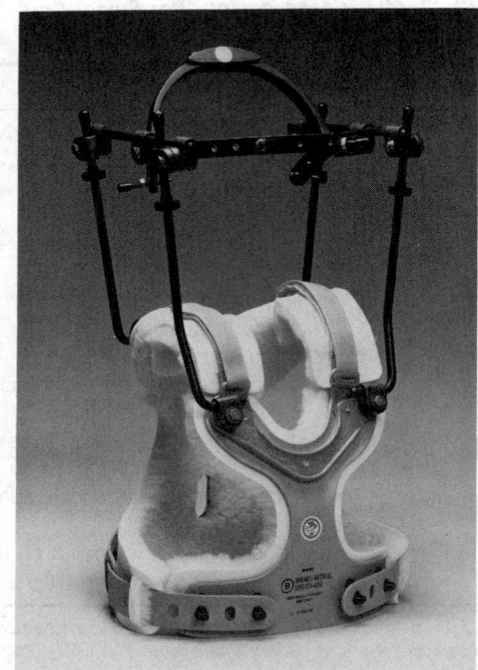

▲ Figure 32–4

Halo traction. This form of traction immobilizes the cervical spine and allows the client to move. Photo courtesy of Bremer Medical, Jacksonville, FL.

Surgical Management

Surgical intervention during the initial treatment of cervical spine injuries is controversial. Youmans[18] lists the following as the four major criteria for operative intervention:

- Progressive neurologic deficit
- Compound fractures and penetrating wounds of the spine
- Bone fragments in the spinal canal
- Syndrome of acute anterior spinal cord trauma

Some neurosurgeons and orthopedic surgeons recommend decompressive laminectomy for complete spinal cord injuries. In this type of surgery, the lamina of the vertebrae are removed to minimize the pressure on the spinal cord. Others believe that laminectomy should not be used routinely to treat spinal cord injury. Similarly, some surgeons recommend stabilization by surgical fusion within the first few days after trauma, whereas others do not. Fusion is accomplished by insertion of metal plates and screws and/or use of bone grafts.

Cervical fractures can also be allowed to heal with bony stability by immobilization in a brace or halo jacket (Fig. 32–4). The halo jacket has a ring that is fixed to the skull with pins. This ring is then attached to the jacket by rods. This system provides the traction required to maintain cervical alignment. A halo jacket allows early mobilization and rehabilitation. The wrench that comes with the brace should always be taped to the front of the jacket. This allows quick removal in case of emergency. The nurse should never grasp the rods to help in turning the client. If the client has some mobility remaining, the nurse always assists during the client's first attempt at any activity. The halo jacket changes the client's center of gravity and makes it easy for him or her to fall.

Burst fractures of the thoracic and lumbar spine can be treated with body casts, Harrington rods, or other forms of spine stabilization. Spine stabilization devices are commonly inserted through an anterior incision. Following the operation, the client has the usual postoperative assessments, including assessment of neurovascular status of the legs. Chest tubes and nasogastric tubes are inserted during surgery. The client is log rolled to faciliate respiration and skin perfusion. Pain is managed with continuous or injected narcotics. The client usually ambulates on the fourth day and is fitted for a body brace.

Complications of surgery include infection and poor wound healing, as well as the complications of anesthesia. Both infection and impaired wound healing are more likely to occur in a malnourished client.

Long-Term Management

ESTABLISHING FUNCTIONAL GOALS

Prediction of functional ability after spinal cord injury can generally be guided by the degree of residual muscle function (Table 32–3). Clients with all levels of injury and of all ages will benefit from rehabilitation. The client and family are involved in all phases. The client is taught skills that he or she cannot perform so

TABLE 32–3. Functional Goals in Spinal Cord Injury

Spinal Cord Level	Muscle Function	Functional Goals
C1–C2	Has no phrenic nerve function	Respirations managed with phrenic pacemaker
C3–C4	Neck control Scapular elevators Diaphragm function may be weak or absent	Manipulate electric wheelchair with breath control, chin control, or voice activation Limited self-feeding with ball-bearing feeders Operate environmental control units
C5	Fair-to-good shoulder control Functional deltoids and/or biceps Elbow flexion	Dress upper trunk Turn self in bed with or without arm slings Propel wheelchair with or without friction-surface handrims Self-feeding with handsplints or following tenodesis Assist getting to and from bed May learn to write or type
C6	Good shoulder control Wrist extension Supinators	Dress upper trunk, sometimes dress lower trunk Turn self in bed with arm slings Propel wheelchair with handrim projections Self-feeding with handsplints Transfer from wheelchair to bed with or without minimal assistance (e.g., sliding board) Assist getting to and from commode chair Self-catheterization
C7	May have weak shoulder depression Weak elbow extension Some hand function Triceps	Independent in transfer to bed, car, and toilet Total dressing independence Wheelchair without handrim projections Self-feeding with no assistive devices
T1–T4	Good-to-normal upper extremity muscle function Intrinsic muscles of the hand No trunk control	Independent in transfer to bed, car, and toilet Total dressing independence Wheelchair with standard handrims Self-feeding with no assistive devices Transfer from wheelchair to floor and return Wheelchair up and down curb Transfer from wheelchair to tub and return
T5–L2	Partial-to-good trunk stability	Total wheelchair independence Limited ambulation with bilateral long leg braces and crutches (injury at T12 or below)
L3–L4	All trunk-pelvic stabilizers intact Hip flexors Adductors Quadriceps	Ambulation with short leg braces with or without crutches, depending on level
L5–S3	Hip extensors Abductors, knee flexors, ankle control	No equipment needed if plantar flexion is strong enough for push off at end of stance

Modified from Rancho Los Amigos Hospital, Physical Therapy Department, Downey, CA.

that he or she can teach those who will provide this skill at home. Likewise, skills learned in a rehabilitation setting must be generalizable to a home environment and community setting prior to discharge. This process can be accomplished by the use of therapeutic weekend passes and participation in community activities as a part of the rehabilitation process.

In all phases of rehabilitation, it is imperative that a motivated client be given the opportunity to perform any skill, even if it can be accomplished more quickly by the nurse or physician. Allowing the client to attempt a complex skill demonstrates support of the client's self-care abilities. A description of functional outcomes for rehabilitation is provided in Table 32–3. It is intended to be a guide and may not represent the ability of all clients with various levels of injury.

Promoting Mobility. Wheelchairs provide mobility, and having the proper wheelchair is critical. The wheelchair design must provide the client the ability to propel the chair and prevent the development of spinal deformities and pressure ulcers. A high back and head support are needed for clients without arm function. Clients who can use their arms should have the back of the wheelchair at the level of the scapula. Cushions help decrease pressure and the risk of pressure ulcers. However, cushions do not prevent pressure ulcers, and the client still needs to shift weight every 10 to 15 minutes while in the chair.

Current emphasis is on strengthening muscles rather than using braces. However, back braces may be prescribed following lumbar spinal injury or intervertebral disc problems. A Taylor back brace (Fig. 32-5), splint, or heavy muslin corset with stays may be initially worn while the client is in bed. More frequently, a thoracic lumbar sacral orthosis (TLSO) is used. This is a custom-made plastic brace with front and back pieces that fasten together with Velcro straps. This brace provides stability for the healing spine.

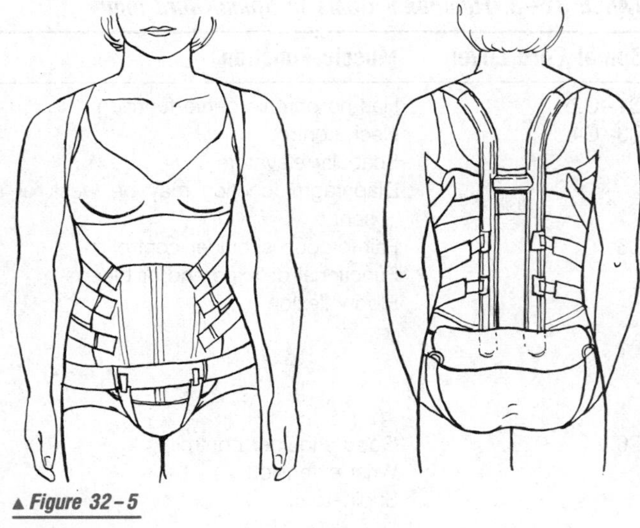

▲ Figure 32-5

Taylor splint.

LONG-TERM COMPLICATIONS

Long-Term Pain. Long-term pain occurs in almost all spinal-cord-injured clients. Dysesthetic pain, which is distal to the site of injury, is extremely disabling. It is similar to phantom pain seen after amputation. It is described as cutting, burning, piercing, radiating, or tightening. Usual treatment is with nonnarcotic analgesics and transcutaneous nerve simulators.

Spasticity. As discussed earlier, spasticity is a common complication of spinal cord injury. Spasticity is an increase in tonic stretch reflexes and often interferes with positioning and functional activities. Spasticity does maintain muscle bulk and venous return and serves as an aid for transfers. Treatment includes range-of-motion (ROM) exercises and pharmacologic agents such as baclofen, dantrolene sodium, and clonidine. Medications for the treatment of spasms are given only when the spasms cause discomfort or safety concerns.

Neurogenic Bladder. A neurogenic bladder occurs with both upper and lower motor neuron disorders. Upper motor neuron disorders produce a spastic or reflex bladder. Lower motor neuron disorders produce a flaccid bladder. There are many ways to manage the bladder, and treatment options must be tailored to fit the client's preferences and lifestyle as well as functional abilities.

Most clients with arm function are taught to empty their bladder using the Credés method to tap over the bladder and relax the sphincter (discussed later in the chapter). To ensure complete emptying, this method is often combined with other techniques such as catheterization and external catheters. Intermittent catheterization decreases the risk of infection and bladder stone formation caused by indwelling catheters. Clients with C6 and lower injuries can perform self-catheterization, although the technique requires adequate hand function and the ability to manage lower extremity clothing. External catheters are used for men who can void between catheterizations. Suprapubic catheters can also be inserted and seem to offer the advantages of decreased infection and urethral injury over indwelling catheters. Indwelling catheters are not ideal from a medical standpoint but are preferred by many clients because of the ease of management. Complications include infection, bladder stones, urethral damage, and a reported increased incidence of bladder cancer. A neurogenic bladder may also be treated with medications such as bethanechol (Urecholine) to stimulate bladder contraction. Urine acidifying agents may also be prescribed to reduce the risk of infection.

Neurogenic Bowel. A neurogenic bowel is similar to a neurogenic bladder because the client cannot defecate. The goal is to develop a bowel elimination method that is convenient, effective, and least expensive for the client. Sufficient fluid and fiber intake is essential. When fiber is added to or increased in the diet, it must be done slowly to avoid cramping and diarrhea. Stool softeners and bulk laxatives may also be used.

The bowel movements of clients with upper motor neuron damage are generally regulated with suppositories or digital stimulation every day or every other day. A lower motor neuron neurogenic bowel is more difficult to regulate, and often the client requires manual disimpaction.

Respiratory Dysfunction. Respiratory dysfunction is a significant cause of morbidity and mortality after spinal cord injury. The diaphragm is often the only functional muscle because the intercostal and abdominal muscles are paralyzed. Vital capacity and inspiratory reserve volume are markedly diminished. The client should be taught to use incentive spirometry and diaphragmatic breathing to enhance vital capacity. Glossopharyngeal breathing uses the muscles of the mouth, pharynx, and larynx to swallow air in to the lungs. This technique enhances vital capacity and promotes chest expansion.

Sexual Dysfunction. Sexual dysfunction in spinal-cord-injured males depends on the location of the lesion. Erection is possible in clients with upper motor neuron lesions. Reflex erections occur in lower motor neuron lesions. Ejaculation is possible with lower motor neuron lesions and if the lesion is more caudal. Unfortunately, fertility is about 5 per cent, but it is hoped that this rate will improve as technological developments progress.

Sexual dysfunction is approached from two avenues: (1) psychological counseling and (2) education about technological advances to facilitate sexual activity. Erection can be restored with external aids, an implantable penile prosthesis, and medications.

Female clients retain fertility after spinal cord injury. Problems with sexual function generally relate to positioning and the lack of vaginal lubrication. These problems can usually be addressed through client education.

Heterotopic Ossification. Heterotopic ossification is the formation of bone in abnormal locations, most often around the hips and knees after spinal cord injury. The client may develop swelling in the joint or loss of ROM. Heterotopic ossification is diagnosed by x-ray study or bone scan. Treatment includes the use of etidronate disodium (Didronel) and ROM exercises to the affected areas. Sometimes the bone is removed surgically.

Psychological Counseling. Psychological counseling is ongoing. Commonly, spinal-cord-injured clients participate in peer group sessions to share their experiences, help newly injured clients gain insight, and cope better with their situation. Vocational rehabilitation may help clients reach their maximum rehabilitation potential.

Nursing Management

ASSESSMENT

Rehabilitation begins on the client's admission to the health care facility. During the acute stage, nursing and medical attention appropriately focuses on immediate needs. However, it is also imperative to remember that the client probably has severe residual disabilities and must make major lifestyle changes. Care provided in the acute period can significantly affect the client's later life. Prevention of complications such as infection, pressure sores, and contractures facilitates rehabilitation and reduces suffering, disability, and expense.

A holistic assessment is essential when caring for clients with spinal cord injury. Every system of the body is affected in spinal cord injury. A complete baseline assessment is obtained initially. The results of subsequent serial assessments are then compared with the baseline.

The most important questions regarding spinal-cord-injured clients are the following:

- Is the client hemodynamically stable? Are vasopressor agents required to maintain adequate blood pressure? Is circulation adequate, as evidenced by palpable peripheral pulses and appropriate skin, nailbed, and mucous membrane color?
- Is respiration adequate? Are accessory muscles being used for respiration? Is the client exhibiting diaphragmatic breathing or nostril flaring? Does the client complain of shortness of breath? If pulse oximetry is available, are oxygen saturation levels adequate?

Other questions that may guide nursing assessment are: Are pupil responses, corneal responses, and eye movements normal? At what spinal cord level is sensation diminished or lost? At what level is motor function diminished or lost? Do the levels differ in different areas of the body? Is there any voluntary movement? Are normal reflexes, e.g., deep tendon, bulbocavernosus, and anal reflexes, absent? Is the client incontinent? Are there bowel sounds? Is the abdomen distended? Is the client edematous? Is the skin intact? What is the emotional condition of the client and family?

NURSING INTERVENTION

Collaborative Problem. High risk for ventilatory insufficiency or atelectasis.

Planning: Expected Outcomes. The client will show no signs of respiratory compromise, as evidenced by clear lung sounds, PaO_2, $PaCO_2$, and pH within normal limits, and unlabored respirations.

Implementation. Cervical spinal cord injury carries a high risk of respiratory compromise. Cord edema may temporarily impair respiratory function, requiring the use of mechanical ventilation. Intubation and ventilation can be frightening to a client who has been able to breathe independently. The nurse should provide reassurance that mechanical ventilation will probably not be permanent.

Chest physical therapy can help mobilize secretions and prevent pneumonia, as can suctioning and assisted coughing. Careful monitoring can prevent respiratory failure and emergency intubation. At the first sign of respiratory compromise, the nurse notifies the physician. The nurse explains the equipment used for intubation and mechanical ventilation to the client. Sedation is administered as needed after intubation, within the physician's orders.

For extended airway management, a tracheostomy may be required to (1) allow for long-term controlled ventilation, (2) facilitate the removal of tracheobronchial secretions, and (3) seal off the esophagus from the trachea to prevent aspiration.

Nursing Diagnosis: Aspiration, High Risk for R/T ineffective airway clearance and absent gag reflex.

Planning: Expected Outcomes. Client will exhibit no signs of aspiration, as evidenced by clear lung sounds; absence of stridor and fever; minimal amounts of clear mucus upon suctioning; and PaO_2, $PaCO_2$, and pH within normal limits.

Implementation. Aspiration is a common cause of morbidity in spinal-cord-injured clients. Suctioning equipment should be kept available, and breath sounds assessed every 1 or 2 hours in acutely ill clients. The results of arterial blood gases and pulse oximetry are monitored to determine the degree of oxygenation provided by ventilators or oxygen. Tracheobronchial suctioning is performed frequently to prevent or decrease the accumulation of secretions from immobility, the lack of a cough and sigh reflex, or pneumonia. The nurse should monitor the electrocardiogram for dysrhythmias (e.g., premature ventricular contractions [PVCs]) while suctioning due to hypoxia.

Nursing Diagnosis: Skin Integrity, Impaired, High Risk for R/T immobility and loss of protective reflexes.

Planning: Expected Outcomes. Client will have intact skin, as evidenced by no reddened areas over bony prominences, no areas or signs of skin irritation or dryness, and no signs of corneal irritation.

Implementation. When the client cannot respond to local tissue hypoxia resulting from being in one position for an extended period of time, the risk of pressure ulcers increases. Spinal-cord-injured clients should be placed on pressure-reducing beds or mattresses. However, the use of these special beds does not eliminate the need to assess the skin and rub the skin every 2 to 4 hours. In addition, the client's nutritional needs must be met to reduce the risk of pressure ulcers.

A client with spinal fractures may be placed on a Roto-Rest bed or a Stryker frame.

A Roto-Rest bed is currently popular for clients with spinal cord injuries or other disorders requiring prolonged immobilization (see Chapter 29, Fig. 29-8). It is equipped with supportive packs and straps that keep the body in alignment while it continuously oscillates from side to side. The continuous motion helps (1) prevent skin breakdown, (2) reduce urinary stasis, and (3) promote lung aeration. Unfortunately, the constant movement may also stimulate peristalsis, resulting in severe diarrhea. Some clients also experience disorientation from the constant movement. These clients also express fear of falling. Staff members should remain with the client during the initial rotations to provide emotional support and reassurance.

A Stryker frame has two metal frames (anterior and posterior) with taut canvas covers and a thin protective padding over each frame. The frames are supported on a movable cart with a pivot apparatus at each end. By securing one frame over the client while he or she lies on the other, two nurses can turn the client from back to abdomen and vice versa. During turning, the client is briefly sandwiched between the frames and is kept from falling or sliding by straps secured around both frames. Instruct clients who can use their arms to fold them around the anterior frame during turning. Strap the arms of clients who cannot use their arms alongside their body to prevent injury. Once the client is safely turned, the uppermost frame is removed. A small canvas strip across the posterior frame is removed for bedpan use. The anterior frame has space for the face so that, when lying prone, the person can rest, read, or eat without turning the head. Armrests may be fastened to the sides of the anterior frame if desired.

Clients on Stryker frames frequently express fear of falling. The frame is significantly narrower than a regular bed. Turning is very frightening for a client who does not have control of the body or the situation. The nurse should carefully explain the procedure before turning the client and be certain to have adequate experienced help to perform the turn. At least two experienced staff members are needed to use a Stryker frame. The nurse should be prepared to suction clients immediately after turning, because movement can mobilize respiratory secretions.

Once the client is able to be responsible for some ADLs, the nurse teaches the client about the risk of pressure ulcers and techniques to reduce risk. The client should shift body weight every 10 to 15 minutes while sitting in a wheelchair. Shifting weight promotes reactive hyperemia and vasodilation to bring blood into hypoxic tissues. Finally, the client should use a mirror to inspect for signs of pressure ulcers each evening before bedtime.

Nursing Diagnosis: Oral and Nasal Mucous Membranes, Altered, High Risk for R/T NPO status, inability to swallow, and mouth breathing.

Planning: Expected Outcomes. The patient will maintain intact oral and nasal mucous membranes, as evidenced by having oral and nasal mucous membranes pink, moist, and without lesions or bloody drainage.

Implementation. The client's teeth are brushed with a small toothbrush at least twice a day. The oral mucous membranes (especially the roof of the mouth), tongue, and gums are cleaned with toothettes. Agents containing lemon or alcohol should not be used for any length of time, because they dry the membranes. The mouth is then rinsed. Gauze wrapped around a tongue depressor or toothbrush and saturated with dilute mouthwash may help with aspects of oral care.

Nursing Diagnosis: Nutrition, Altered: Less Than Body Requirements, High Risk for R/T inability to eat and increased metabolic needs.

Planning: Expected Outcomes. Client will demonstrate signs of adequate nutrition, as evidenced by stabilization of weight; consumption of adequate calories for age, height, and weight; equal intake and output; healing of incisions/wounds within 12 to 14 days; and hemoglobin, blood urea nitrogen, lymphocyte, and albumin levels within normal limits for age and sex.

Implementation. Intravenous fluids are begun on admission for newly injured clients. Initially, the intravenous site provides access to the circulatory system for the administration of medications, but an intravenous infusion cannot be considered nutritional support.

The nutritional and fluid needs of comatose patients

are usually met through nasogastric feedings. If the client does not have paralytic ileus or delayed gastric emptying and if bowel sounds are audible and gastric residual volumes are less than 100 ml/h, nasogastric feedings are started.

Collaborative Problem. High risk for autonomic dysreflexia R/T spinal cord injury.

Planning: Expected Outcomes. The nurse will assess for, prevent, and respond to complications, as evidenced by assessing for clinical manifestations and intervening quickly to reduce dysreflexia.

Implementation. The nurse assesses the client for sudden indications of severe hypertension, severe throbbing headache, profuse diaphoresis, flushing of the skin above the level of the lesion, nasal stuffiness, pilomotor spasm, blurred vision, nausea, and bradycardia. If autonomic dysreflexia occurs, the nurse

- Monitors blood pressure closely,
- Elevates the head of the bed to a sitting position,
- Checks for possible sources of irritation (e.g., kinked or clogged catheter or distended bladder or lower bowel),
- Removes the stimulus. Once the source of irritation is removed, symptoms of autonomic dysreflexia usually subside and
- Notifies the physician if the above-mentioned measures do not correct the process

If blood pressure remains elevated, antihypertensive medication may be administered to lower blood pressure. Once symptoms have subsided, the client is observed closely for 3 to 4 hours. If medication has been given, the client may become hypotensive after the stimulus is removed. Autonomic dysreflexia may recur if the stimulus is not completely removed. If the identified source of irritation is bowel distention, the nurse must be very careful when disimpacting the client. An anesthetic lubricant is used, and another nurse must monitor the client's blood pressure every few minutes. The stimulation of trying to remove the impaction can increase the severity of the autonomic response.

Nursing Diagnosis: Injury, High Risk for R/T uncompensated sensory deficit.

Planning: Expected Outcomes. Client will be free of injury, as evidenced by no abrasions, reddened areas, ulcerations, or burns.

Implementation. Sensory loss poses serious problems for paralyzed clients because they cannot feel the pain or pressure that normally warns of tissue damage. These clients should not wear tight, restrictive clothing or ill-fitting shoes or braces. They need to develop the habit of preventive thinking to avoid potential danger. Dangerous situations include getting too close to heaters, radiators, and fireplaces and using heating pads or hot water bottles. Burns can be a serious problem, because impaired circulation delays healing. External heat should not be applied if there is a loss of sensation, and the bath water should not be too warm.

Regular foot and nail care is required to prevent nails rubbing or cutting the skin and prevent ingrown nails. Foot infections may be prevented by instructing the person not to cut corns or calluses.

Injections should be given above the level of the cord lesion whenever possible. Adequate absorption is not likely to occur in denervated areas of the body with impaired capillary and precapillary circulation.

Clients can also be injured from involuntary spasms. Avoid unnecessary stimulation of areas that elicit reflex spinal automatisms. When such reactions do occur, an unembarrassed, accepting response helps relieve the client's anxiety and embarrassment. The release of spinal automatisms makes people respond to stimuli in ways that may be puzzling to them and others unless the origin of such responses is explained. For example, stimulation of the limbs (perhaps toe flexion while the person's foot is being dried) may cause mass flexion of the upper and lower extremities. Mass flexion reactions may be accompanied by massive contractions of the abdominal wall; evacuation of the urinary bladder and bowel; and automatic response such as sweating, flushing, and pilomotor reactions below the level of the lesion.

Nursing Diagnosis: Incontinence, Total, R/T atonic bladder.

Planning: Expected Outcomes. The client will have improved bladder control, as evidenced by no infection and emptying of the bladder every 4 to 6 hours.

Implementation. Nursing intervention is planned to (1) prevent urinary tract infection, (2) preserve existing bladder capacity and muscle tone, and (3) establish and maintain a routine pattern of elimination requiring minimal artificial assistance.

The nurse observes the client carefully for indications of faulty bladder control and infection, including incontinence, retention, urgency, dribbling, frequency, enuresis, and precipitate micturition. The nurse documents such observations and informs the physician.

Urinary bladder atony (absence of tone) may last several weeks or months after spinal cord injury. In clients with upper motor neuron lesions, when spinal shock subsides and the reflex arc returns, as evidenced by increase in rectal tone, the bladder empties reflexively. During the period of atony, a retention catheter may be inserted to prevent bladder distention and keep the client dry and comfortable. Bladder overdistention causes stretching and fissure formation, a predisposition to infection, and may result in bladder rupture. When sensory pathways are damaged, the client does not feel the discomfort of bladder distention. However, prolonged catheter use also predisposes to infection.

Urinary complications may be avoided by (1) periodically examining the client for bladder distention, (2) accurately documenting fluid intake and output, (3) using aseptic technique when handling urinary catheters, and (4) observing for signs of bladder infection. The client should also be encouraged to drink cranberry juice to keep the urine acidic and decrease the possibility of infection. Urine acidifiers may be prescribed. Urinary complications occur because of incomplete emptying of the bladder, necessitating catheterization. Catheterization may predispose the client to infection and vesicoureteral reflux, which may lead to kidney complications. Renal calculi, pyelonephritis, and hydronephrosis are major causes of death and considerable disability in paralyzed clients.

To prevent development of renal calculi, the nurse encourages the client to drink about 3000 ml of fluid/day, unless contraindicated by other medical conditions. This is sufficient to maintain a minimal urinary output of 2000 ml/day. Drinking this much fluid may increase incontinence but is necessary to prevent renal calculi.

When the initial indwelling catheter is removed, a program of intermittent catheterization is commonly prescribed to empty the bladder regularly every 4 to 6 hours for several weeks. During this time, the client is taught methods of emptying the bladder without catheterization. Such methods promote urination by increasing intra-abdominal pressure on the bladder. Urinary flow may be initiated by Credés maneuver, Valsalva's maneuver, and the rectal stretch.

Credés Maneuver. The client makes a fist and presses it directly over the bladder and down toward the pubic bone with a kneading motion. Continue until the bladder is empty.

Valsalva's Maneuver. The client inhales deeply, holds the breath and bears down as hard as possible, as if for a bowel movement.

Rectal Stretch. The client inserts a finger into the rectum. When the anal sphincter is relaxed, the client maintains the relaxation by gently pulling on the sphincter. This relaxes the perineal floor. A Valsalva maneuver is performed at the same time.

Urination may also be stimulated by reflex stimulation. The following stimuli may be successful: tapping the suprapubic area; stroking the glans penis, thigh, or vulva; tugging pubic hairs; or flexing the toes. The stimulation may be applied by the client or care giver. As training continues, less stimulation is needed to initiate urination.

Catheterization may be required at home. Teach the client and/or care giver clean, rather than sterile, technique. This technique has the same infection rate as sterile insertion methods for home catheterization. Suprapubic catheters may be inserted for long-term bladder management. Occasionally, a surgical procedure such as sphincterotomy may be necessary. The bladder then empties continuously. An external, condom-type catheter connected to a straight closed drainage bag may be used to collect drainage in men. External appliances for females do not work as well.

Nursing Diagnosis: Bowel Incontinence or Constipation, High Risk for R/T paralysis.

Planning: Expected Outcomes. The client will have reduced risk of bowel incontinence/constipation, as evidenced by a bowel movement every 1 to 2 days, no signs of fecal impactions, and no incontinence.

Implementation. Nursing intervention is planned to (1) prevent constipation, distention, and impaction; (2) detect and treat these conditions if they occur; and (3) reestablish habitual, controlled bowel movements by conditioned reflex activity. The client is observed carefully for indications of constipation, diarrhea, or tenesmus (ineffective, painful straining at stool). If a client becomes impacted, a cleansing enema is usually prescribed to initially empty the lower bowel. However, enemas should be avoided for long-term bowel management. A paraplegic or quadriplegic client cannot retain enema solution; nor can the degree of intestinal distention be felt. Therefore, enemas must be administered carefully without overdistending the intestine with excessive fluid.

The client's intake of fluid and food and elimination pattern are documented. The routine daily pattern of bowel elimination is established, with the client using suppositories and other means of stimulating evacuation until reflex evacuation occurs.

A daily fluid intake of 3000 to 4000 ml/day is important for proper bowel function as well as bladder function. Also, the diet must be high in bulk and roughage such as bran, whole grains, fresh and dried fruits, and leafy green and raw vegetables. A stool softener such as docusate sodium (Colace) may be taken daily, but laxatives should be avoided. Metamucil is very effective for spinal-cord-injured clients if they drink enough fluid.

Bowel retraining is possible for most paraplegic and quadriplegic clients. It involves developing controlled bowel movements by conditioned reflex activity. Begin bowel retraining as soon as possible. Ensure privacy during the daily bowel routine, and if possible have the client sitting upright. When possible, include appropriate family members in the bowel retraining program as they may be involved in this aspect of long-term management. Always assess the family members' willingness to participate in such care. If the sexual partner is also responsible for hygiene and personal care, problems in role separation and intimacy may result. These issues should be openly discussed between partners.

With an effective bowel program, a client has a bowel movement once a day or every other day and is not incontinent at other times. Attaining continence may influence a paralyzed client's vocational future and positively affect his or her ability to have satisfying social relationships. It can also give the client the self-esteem to withstand other problems.

Nursing Diagnosis: Pain R/T spinal cord injury.

Planning: Expected Outcomes. The client will experience adequate pain relief, as evidenced by verbalization of improvement in comfort level, ability to rest without interruption by pain, and ability to participate in therapies without hindrance by pain.

Implementation. Clients with spinal injuries may experience pain at the level of the injury and radiating along spinal nerves originating in the area. Phantom pain may also be experienced. Pain usually occurs later than muscular spasms. Some paraplegic and quadriplegic clients experience both pain and spasm. Pain most often occurs in the lower extremities. Analgesics such as acetylsalicylic acid and nonsteroidal anti-inflammatory agents may be prescribed. Narcotics are seldom used after the initial injury and are contraindicated in clients with high cervical injuries because of the risk of respiratory depression.

Clients with thoracic injuries often tend to breathe shallowly to avoid pain. This can lead to respiratory complications. The nurse gives prescribed pain medication and encourages deep breathing and coughing to aerate the lungs and remove secretions from the respiratory tract.

Antispasmotics, nonsteroidal anti-inflammatory agents, and non-narcotic analgesics are prescribed for pain associated with spasticity. Surgery (e.g., neurectomy or chordotomy) is sometimes required for pain relief.

Collaborative Problem. High risk for thrombophlebitis R/T loss of muscle contraction in lower extremities and loss of venous return.

Planning: Expected Outcomes. The nurse will monitor for thrombophlebitis as evidenced by unilateral leg edema, erythema, and warmth.

Implementation. Muscular activity is a major factor in venous circulation. A paralyzed client experiences slowed venous return and pooling of blood in dependent limbs. These phenomena increase the risk of intravascular clotting. In the acute phase of spinal cord injury, antiembolic stockings, sequential compression devices, and subcutaneous heparin may be used prophylactically.

Education is vital to preventing vascular complications and minimizing their impact. Each time the nurse applies stockings and performs ROM exercises, the client is taught the importance of these activities. During assessment of the legs for signs of clot formation (i.e., redness and unilateral swelling and warmth), the nurse explains what is being done and why the client needs to incorporate this activity into daily routines. Clients are also taught not to cross their legs while sitting in a wheelchair.

Nursing Diagnosis: Impaired Physical Mobility R/T paralysis.

Planning: Expected Outcomes. Client will have maximum physical mobility, as evidenced by absence of tendon contractures, joint ankylosis, and muscle shortening, and effective use of adaptive devices.

Implementation. Spinal cord injury causing permanent mobility impairment produces problems with ambulation and potential complications arising from immobility.

Throughout the acute and rehabilitative phases of nursing care, every effort should be made to maximize the client's functional abilities and independence by encouraging the client to perform independently any ADLs for which capability remains.

Tendon Contractures, Joint Ankylosis, and Muscle Shortening. These problems are caused by improper positioning of a client in the bed or chair and lack of joint movements (e.g., because of spasticity or immobility). Intervention to prevent such problems includes (1) frequent position changes, (2) proper positioning of joints, (3) use of splints and removable casts, (4) intermittent turning to a prone position, (5) positioning of upper extremities away from the body, (6) draping of bedding over frames to keep pressure off feet, (7) keeping knee joints flexed 15 degrees when supine, and (8) use of active and passive conditioning exercises.

Passive exercises prevent contractures and painful reflex dystrophies of the hand and shoulder. Such exercises may be prescribed as soon as 48 to 72 hours after the injury. Active exercises, massage, and electrical stimulation may also be prescribed. Begin shoulder and arm exercises early. Strength in these areas and in the chest and back is essential for effective self-transfers and ambulation when the lower spine is stable enough to permit mobilization.

Muscle Weakness and Fatigue. Wristdrop and footdrop will develop in paralyzed extremities unless prevented. Footdrop may be prevented by keeping the client's feet firmly supported in dorsiflexion at right angles to the hips (high-topped athletic shoes are commonly used) to counteract the force of gravity on weakened muscles. Support a paralyzed arm in a sling when the client is out of bed, and a cock-up splint while in bed. Usually, the hand end of the splint is elevated 2 inches to support the wrist, and the fingers are maintained in a position of function. Posterior molded casts may be used instead of splints to support a paralyzed wrist while in bed. For some clients, pillows and a hand roll are adequate.

Rehabilitative programs often require strength and endurance. To prepare a client for ambulation, the unaffected parts of the body must be strengthened and suitable exercises started early. Tolerance for activity gradually increases. The nurse must take care not to fatigue the client. Periods of planned rest and recreation are important.

Physical therapy is essential for all clients with spinal cord injuries. Paraplegic clients need to learn various transfers to become self-sufficient. One transfer is illustrated in Figure 32–6. Learning to sit up precedes learning to transfer. Many paralyzed clients become mobile by using a wheelchair. Many types of wheelchairs are available, and selection needs to be made carefully, according to individual needs (Fig. 32–7). Prolonged, unrelieved periods of immobility can create

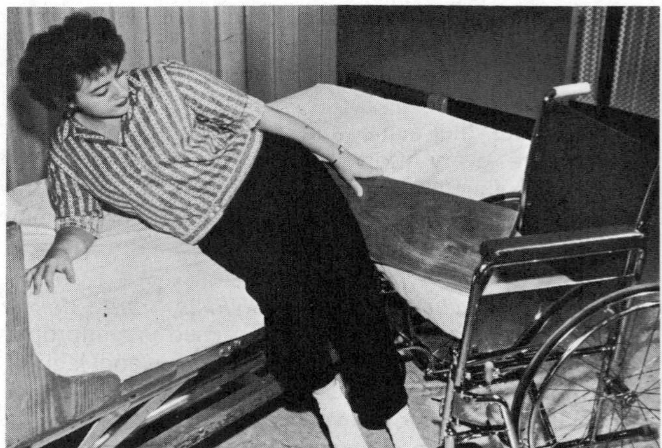

▲ Figure 32-6

Paraplegic bed-to-wheelchair lateral transfer using a sliding board. (From Ellwood, P. M., Jr. [1990]. Transfers—method, equipment, and preparation. In F. J. Kottke & J. F. Lehmann [Eds.], *Krusen's handbook of physical medicine and rehabilitation* [p. 540]. Philadelphia: W. B. Saunders Company.)

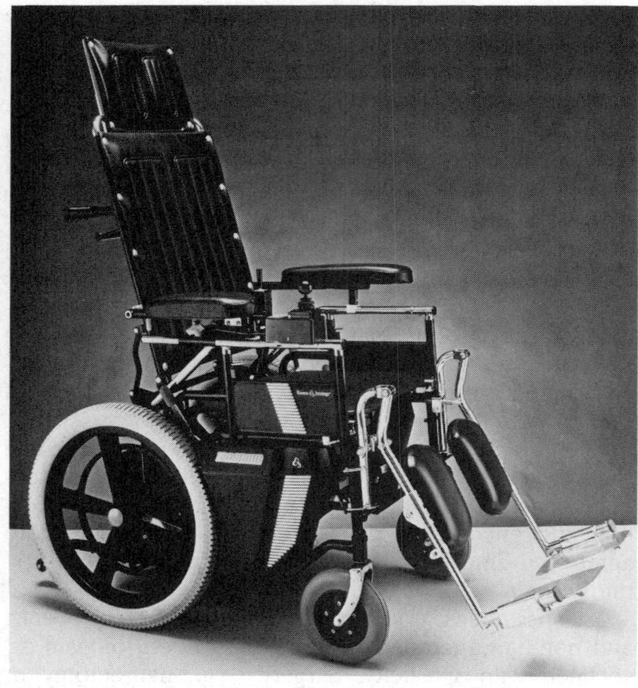

▲ Figure 32-7

C1-C3 spine injury wheelchair with power hand controls for clients with cervical injury. A respirator can be attached to the wheelchair. (Courtesy of Everett and Jennings, St. Louis, MO.)

renal calculi and pressure ulcers. When sitting up, a paralyzed client needs to shift body weight every 10 to 15 minutes and lift the body by pushing with the arms and hands against the chair arms or seat. This relieves pressure on the buttocks and prevents skin breakdown. By using a wheelchair, clients may become completely independent in all ADLs. Many clients drive and hold outside jobs.

Apply the brace or corset before helping the client out of bed. Following fracture of a cervical vertebra, cervical disc rupture, or whiplash injury (Fig. 32-8), the person may wear a neck brace (fitted so the chin rests on a cup and the neck is kept hyperextended), a hard collar (which extends up under the chin and prevents flexion of the neck), or a soft collar. Neck braces tend to limit vision, because people wearing them cannot look down at their feet. Safety awareness is important to prevent falls.

A thin, knitted undershirt is worn under the brace or corset to protect the skin and keep the appliance clean. To apply the brace or corset, the nurse turns the

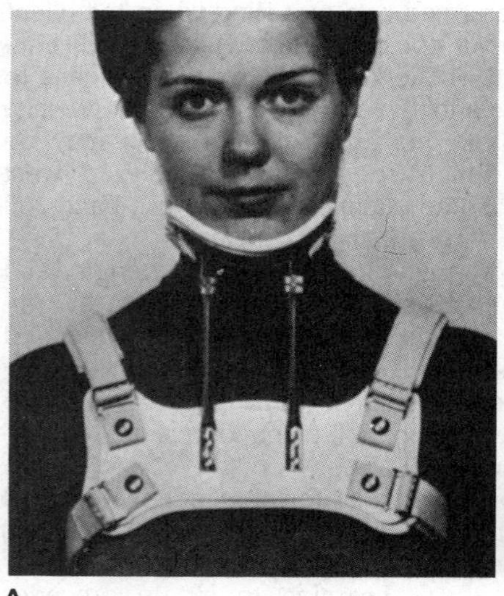

A

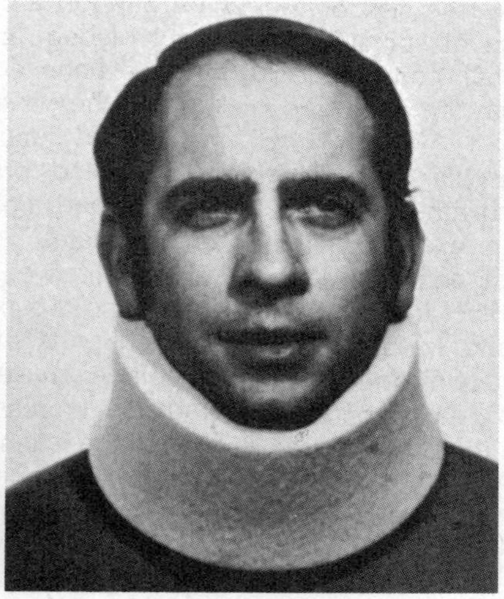

B

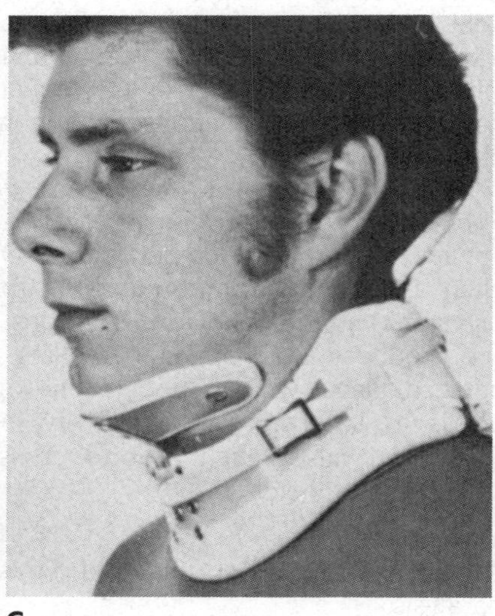

C

▲ Figure 32-8

Cervical appliances. *A*, Four-poster cervical orthosis. Such devices provide stability to the lower cervical spine. They are used for cervical instability without neurologic deficit. *B*, Simple (soft) cervical collar. Such collars support the head but do not restrict cervical motion. They are useful for acute neck sprains or radiculopathy. Some collars are designed to fasten at the back and others to fasten at the front. *C*, Cervical collar with chin piece. This orthosis provides additional support for the head and some restriction of cervical spine motion.

client to one side, places the appliance against the back, and then rolls the client back into it. The brace or corset is secured while the client lies supine. As recovery and rehabilitation progress, many clients learn to apply their own braces and corsets while in bed. Others continue to need help. The degree of the client's arm and hand function determines the ability to apply a brace.

Weight-bearing begins as early as possible after spinal cord injury. This stimulates osteoblastic activity and thus decreases the demineralization of bone (osteoporosis) that develops with prolonged immobilization. Standing boards or tilt tables assist the person gradually to a standing position. Having the person assume a standing position periodically each day also helps prevent contractures (e.g., hip contractures from long periods of sitting). Care must be taken when helping clients to stand or sit in a chair for the first time. Due to the loss of muscular activity on the peripheral venous system, these clients are very prone to orthostatic hypotension. Blood pressure should always be checked before and after transfers.

Clients easily lose their balance when wearing braces, particularly the halo brace, and must be very careful not to fall. A brace feels surprisingly heavy at first, especially if the client is weak. Some braces are now made from plastic and are considerably lighter. For safety, shoes, rather than slippers or just stockings, should be worn during ambulation. Shoes should tie or have Velcro straps for firm support and have a low heel. Hightop athletic shoes give added support. Slick soles, high or narrow heels, or stockinged feet are hazardous. Wearing shoes also helps prevent footdrop when the client lies down.

The fit, comfort, and appearance of braces, corsets, and shoes are important to the client. Try to assist clients who want to be as stylish as possible as well as benefit from therapeutic garments. Disabled clients are helped by (1) being encouraged to express their feelings concerning self-image and (2) having their feelings taken into consideration when fitting therapeutic garments. Some garments can be painful when first worn. The pain worsens if the garments do not fit properly. The client's skin should be inspected frequently, especially at first, because pressure sores can develop very quickly.

Nursing Diagnosis: Self-Care Deficit R/T loss of function secondary to spinal cord injury.

Planning: Expected Outcomes. The client will independently perform as many ADLs as possible. If the client is unable to independently perform an activity, he or she will be able to direct a care giver's performance. These goals will be evaluated by successful performance of an ADL by the client or at client's direction.

Implementation. Spinal cord injury is often accompanied by a feeling of powerlessness. Assisting the client to maximize independence can lessen this feeling. The client is assisted with muscle-strengthening exercises and use of adaptive devices. Clients with high cervical injuries are able to perform very few activities independently. Allow them adequate time to accomplish whatever tasks they can do. If the client is dependent in ADLs, nursing care should be adapted to the client's routine.

Nursing Diagnosis: Sexual dysfunction R/T spinal cord injury.

Planning: Expected Outcomes. The client will develop personally satisfying and socially acceptable means of expressing sexuality, as evidenced by interacting appropriately in social situations, verbalizing the effects of the injury on sexual function, discussing sexual issues with a team member, verbalizing methods of sexual expression, and verbalizing understanding of contraceptive implications.

Implementation. Spinal-cord-injured clients are often concerned about sexuality and their ability to achieve sexual fulfillment. They often worry about such concerns long before they express them to others. Nurses are often asked about sexuality issues before other professionals are approached, perhaps because nurses provide intimate care activities. Such care can promote a high degree of trust between those involved.

Some clients discuss their own sexual potential directly. Others refer to it obliquely or appear crude in the way they introduce the topic, e.g., by making inappropriate sexual comments or gestures. Such behaviors are attempts to acknowledge sexuality. Nurses try to look beyond the behavior to the underlying emotional concerns. They acknowledge the client's concerns and offer discussion, by saying, e.g., "You seem concerned about your sexuality, Janet. I understand that and I would like to talk with you about it if you want."

To be helpful, nurses need to be able to talk about sexuality without embarrassment. They also need accurate information about "normal" sexuality and how physiologic changes that occur because of injury affect sexual function.

The client can be referred to another person or an agency if appropriate. Referral should not be done too hastily, though. If someone talks with a nurse about this personal subject, it is probably because at that time that person feels most comfortable speaking with that nurse about it. The nurse should allow the client to lead the conversation, which may be difficult. Professionals often think they know what someone needs and wants, without listening to the person.

Generally, physiologic sexual response requires an intact nervous system. For example, psychogenic erection requires an intact spinal cord, second through fourth sacral nerve roots, and spinal reflexes; ejaculation is a function of skeletal muscle controlled by the somatic center in the pudendal nerve originating in the second through fourth sacral roots; and orgasm involves contraction of both smooth and skeletal muscle. It should be remembered, however, that there is more involved in sexual expression than physiologic response.

To some extent, sexual function can be predicted by the level of spinal cord lesion (Table 32–4). For example, psychogenic erection is often difficult or impossible after most spinal cord injuries. However, although physical limitations certainly occur, every individual is different. Many men do have erections after spinal cord injury. Many disabled people enjoy paraorgasm (phantom orgasm) by developing alternative erogenous zones. The genitals are not the only body areas that can be sexually excited, and intercourse is not the only means of sexual expression.

Some individuals find it disappointing, perhaps devastating, if they can no longer function sexually as they did before an injury. However, they can be helped to learn new ways of giving and receiving sexual pleasure. Sex and relationship counseling is sometimes helpful. The nurse's role is to facilitate expression of feelings and convey hope that new and real sexual enjoyment can be experienced. Some form of sexual expression is possible for anyone, regardless of disability. Before making specific suggestions of alternative expressions of sexuality, the nurse should interview the client regarding past sexual behavior and cultural taboos. Some clients may find specific methods of giving and receiving sexual pleasure unacceptable.

Society as a whole is becoming progressively more open about sexuality. Increasingly, the parenting potential of disabled people is receiving serious attention. Physical assessment is needed to determine a client's ability to reproduce. Male infertility is a frequent complication of spinal cord injury because of testicular atrophy, decreased sperm formation, and ejaculation infrequency. Most men are unable to ejaculate after spinal cord injury. Women usually remain fertile and can conceive and deliver a child. Adoption is a viable option, and conception by artificial insemination is possible.

Disabled people may have contraception concerns. Little is known about the effects of various kinds of contraceptives on disabled people. Oral contraceptives may be contraindicated. Paralyzed women often have slowed circulation, increasing the potential circulatory complications of oral contraceptives. To use an intrauterine device, a woman must have feeling in her

TABLE 32–4. Sexual Function in Clients with Spinal Cord Injury

Sexuality	Reproductive Functioning	Special Considerations for Contraceptive Methods
Females Lesions at C1–C3: Reflex lubrication is probable. Erogenous areas may develop above injury. Libido is intact. Lesions at C4–C6: Psychogenic lubrication is unlikely. Nongenital orgasm may be experienced. Lesions at C7: Able to use hands for holding and caressing. Lesions at T12–L5: Psychogenic stimulation of the clitoris, lubrication, labial swelling, and skin flush are possible but unlikely.	Menstruation and fertility unaffected. Pregnancy is not affected. Incidence of bladder infection during pregnancy increases. Risk of autonomic hyperreflexia during delivery and labor increases.	Birth control pills are contraindicated when circulatory problems present; thrombophlebitis could go undetected owing to lack of sensation in extremities. Intrauterine device may be contraindicated because pelvic inflammatory disease and other problems could remain undetected owing to lack of sensation. Client must be able to assess for vaginal bleeding.
Males Lesions at C1–C3: Reflex erection is caused by genital stimulation. Psychogenic erection is not possible. Erogenous areas above injury site may develop. Libido is intact. Lesions at C4–C6: Reflex erection is possible. Nongenital orgasm may be experienced; no ejaculation. Oral sex is possible. Libido is intact. Lesions at C7: Holding and caressing with hands are possible. Lesions at T12–L6: Psychogenic stimulation and erection are possible; no reflex erection. Lesions at S2–S4: Reflex erection is possible. Ejaculation is possible but may retrograde.	Semen can be obtained from the bladder of those clients who have retrograde ejaculation. For clients who cannot ejaculate, semen can be obtained through glandular vibratory stimulation. In general, semen quality is impaired, with poor motility the most common abnormality. Some clients are candidates for penile prosthesis.	Client or partner may apply condom.

pelvis. Then she can recognize early symptoms of pelvic inflammatory disease. Many paralyzed women do not have such feeling. Barrier devices, e.g., a diaphragm, a condom, or foam, may be used if at least one partner has enough manual dexterity to insert the diaphragm or foam or put on the condom.

Nursing Diagnosis: Anticipatory Grieving R/T sudden change in body image, loss of independence, and feelings of inadequacy.

Planning: Expected Outcomes. The client will progress through the grieving process and develop adaptive coping strategies, as evidenced by verbalizing feelings about the degree of injury and the future, participating in community activities, and expressing positive thoughts about the future.

Implementation. Adjusting to paralysis is difficult physically and psychosocially for the client and family. The family may experience the same reactions and need the same kind of help as the disabled client. Sudden paralysis in a previously healthy, active individual can be devastating. Typically, the sudden lifestyle changes brought about by serious spinal cord injury cause a grief reaction. This may involve initial shock and denial, leading to depression and anger. Crying and talking about the injury repeatedly may be helpful.

It takes time to accept disability and develop ways of coping. Psychological adjustment occurs when the client can accept and deal with reality.

A client may use psychological defense mechanisms in adjusting to paralysis. When caring for such a client, the nurse assesses the possible reasons for the behavior. Hostility, depression, anger, or withdrawal may be upsetting to the staff and family. These behaviors are coping mechanisms and should not be taken personally. Paralysis may cause complex changes in self-concept and body image. In the acute phase, immobilization can contribute to sensory deprivation, e.g., hallucinations. This may be minimized by providing visual, auditory, and tactile stimulation as desired by the client.

Paralyzed clients are often helped initially by being with others who are experiencing similar problems. Clients should be allowed to wear their own clothing as soon as possible and encouraged to be out of bed and out of their rooms. Planned social activities may reduce feelings of social isolation and help clients regain self-confidence. Peer counseling may be helpful, e.g., newly disabled clients talking with others who have adjusted to similar disabilities.

A sense of security is particularly important for a newly paralyzed client adjusting to enforced dependency. A paralyzed client should always have a means of summoning available help, yet needs to learn that it is safe to be alone at times. Gradually, trust develops in the client's abilities and resources, and some reliance on others is relinquished. These feelings and attitudes develop slowly as people experience truly trustworthy relationships.

To avoid unnecessary frustrations, the nurse should try to keep each person's environment comfortable, with necessary items conveniently placed. It is difficult and depressing for the client to have to ask for help repeatedly. Although recent advances have been made in the rehabilitation prognosis of paraplegic and quadriplegic people, it is important to be realistic as well as optimistic. The nurse needs to understand the tremendous lifestyle changes disabled clients must make. Some can be rehabilitated to a level of near independence, walking (maybe with braces or other appliances), driving a car, and coping with full-time employment outside their home. Quadriplegic individuals usually rely on a wheelchair and other devices and appliances.

Most paralyzed clients can become productive and happy. Even if some are unable to be "productive," all disabled clients have a right to satisfying, happy lives. Although many paralyzed clients achieve complete rehabilitation, others lead lives that are difficult, frustrating, and psychophysiologically complex. At times, severe mental depression may develop. Depression is assessed and professional counseling offered as indicated. Suicide frequently occurs.

Nursing Diagnosis: Family Coping, Ineffective, Compromised R/T spinal cord injury, loss of independence, perceived or actual change in future plans.

Planning: Expected Outcomes. The client and family identify areas of significant or potential loss and changes in family roles, work together to overcome obstacles, seek appropriate support services, and are able to restore a supportive family structure.

Implementation. Spinal cord injury has a devastating impact on the lives of the injured client and everyone connected with him or her. The injury affects not only physical functioning but also the psychological, vocational, educational, and social aspects of life. An organized team approach is vital to helping the injured client and family cope with lifestyle changes. Nurses are often the first professionals to assess client and family coping. An open, empathetic manner can allow these individuals to express their grief and uncertainty and ask questions. The nurse teaches the family about the normal grief response. The nurse also carefully probes about persistent denial of grief or lack of progression through grieving. Encouraging as much optimism as possible while remaining truthful and realistic may help spinal cord injury survivors to face the future.

The nurse assesses the previous roles of the client and other family members and how they handle stressful situations or losses. Sources of strength for the family are identified. The nurse assesses patterns of interaction between family members and the family's spiritual, social, and economic status, and usual lifestyle and cultural or ethnic influences. These variables often have an impact on grief responses.

Nursing Diagnosis: Health Maintenance, Altered R/T spinal cord injury.

Planning: Expected Outcomes. The client and/or family members will be able to successfully meet the client's needs, as evidenced by intact skin, bowel and bladder continence, ability to transfer in and out of wheelchair, absence of infection, maintenance of appropriate weight, and satisfying personal relationships.

Implementation. The learning needs of spinal-cord-injured clients and their family members are complex and ongoing. In the acute phase, information regarding spinal anatomy and physiology is needed. When the reality of the injury and the permanency of deficit are understood, coping skills may need to be taught. New means of performing activities and managing bodily functions must be learned. This teaching begins in the acute phase of hospitalization and should be incorporated into all aspects of care. Successful learning in this stage affects the client's entire life.

Teaching should be conducted in short sessions, using easily understood terms. Complex tasks should be taught in steps with return demonstrations.

EVALUATION

Spinal-cord-injured clients are hospitalized for a long time. Therefore, some expected outcomes need to be evaluated frequently, such as respiratory and cardiac functions. Other expected outcomes will not be met for months, such as independence in ADLs. The plan of care for each client needs to reflect these individual problems.

Modification in Plan of Care for the Elderly

For elderly clients, the most important modification of the nursing care plan is increased vigilance. Elderly people are more prone to the complications of immobility. A person with congestive heart failure may have difficulty breathing when lying flat. Elderly people are also more susceptible to sensory deprivation. The nurse must make sure the individual has his or her eyeglasses and hearing aid. If the person is not able to see a window or clock, he or she should be reoriented as needed. Discharge plans for elderly clients may be complicated if the care giver is also elderly. The spouse of an elderly spinal-cord-injured person may not have the physical strength to provide the needed care. Learning to provide the care may also be problematic.

Post-hospital Care

DISCHARGE TEACHING

Most spinal-cord-injured people are transferred from an acute care hospital to a rehabilitation facility. After functional capabilities have been maximized, the person is then discharged from the rehabilitation facility (see Bridge to Home Health Care). Paraplegic clients can usually live independently. Most quadriplegic people need some assistance with daily activities. Depending on the amount of assistance needed and the individual situation, this care may be provided by family members, a part-time paid attendant, or a full-time paid attendant. Ventilator-dependent individuals who cannot obtain in-home care or other individuals who do not have the personal and/or financial resources for in-home care may have no option except institutional living (see Ethical Issues in Nursing). Group living situations, especially for young adults, are becoming more available.

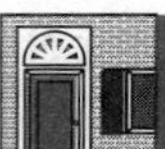

BRIDGE TO HOME HEALTH CARE

Rehabilitation of the Client with a Spinal Cord Injury

Prevention of skin breakdown in the desensitized and paralyzed areas of the body must be a top priority with clients and care givers. Pressure sores develop mainly over bony prominences that are exposed to unrelieved pressure in the lying or sitting position. Clients can use a mirror to examine areas they cannot view directly. Clients unable to inspect their own skin must take responsibility and ask for assistance from their care givers.

Frequent relief of skin pressure is necessary to prevent breakdown. Regular turning in bed not only relieves pressure but also aids renal function by preventing stagnation in the urinary tract. Using a special mattress such as a water bed or an alternating pressure pad can lengthen the time required between turning. Skin should be kept clean and dry. It is important that all wrinkles and debris are removed from bed linen. Removing pockets from clothing and selecting clothing with few seams also decrease skin pressure. Use pillows, foam rubber, blankets, or any other form of soft padding to protect vulnerable bony prominences.

Wheelchair cushions need to be inspected regularly for wear and replaced when necessary. Encourage clients who are able to lift up from the wheelchair seat to do so every 15 minutes. Clients unable to lift themselves will require a special cushion such as a Bye Bye Decubiti or ROHO Dry Flotation Cushion.

Passive movements of the paralyzed limbs are essential to stimulate circulation, maintain full mobility of joints and soft tissue, and prevent contractures. The client should have a daily range-of-motion program for the paralyzed limbs and a strengthening program for the uninvolved extremities.

Spasticity is a common complication that could prevent a client from performing some self-care activities. If a spasm occurs during a movement, hold the limb firmly and wait for the spasm to relax before completing the motion. Slow, steady movement works better than trying to hurry. Forced passive movement against spasticity may cause injury or even fracture a limb.

Clients with spasticity commonly have adductor spasticity. To prevent development of pressure sores, use a wedge large enough to keep thighs abducted. The core of the wedge can be made of an old blanket or other firm material covered with thick foam rubber and encased in stockinette. The wedge can be used in bed and in the wheelchair.

Provide clients with information about available community resources. Possibilities include transportation, care giver assistance, home adaptations, health services, financial assistance, and recreation.

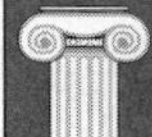

ETHICAL ISSUES IN NURSING

What Is the Government's Obligation to Put Care for Its Citizens Above Care for Noncitizens, Given Scarce Resources?

Rehabilitative nursing has become more specialized to meet the various needs of those clients who require physical rehabilitation. Clients who have spinal cord injuries often face long rehabilitative treatment regimes. Support is needed by these clients in several different areas of their life. Emotional, technical, and financial support are the three major areas in which rehabilitation clients have great need. Financing a long rehabilitation course can be quite expensive. For many clients, this cost must be picked up by government-sponsored insurance programs (i.e., Medicare or Medicaid).

There is usually no opposition to such governmental reimbursement programs, because such programs benefit those members of society who are in need of specialized health care. But what happens when those who take advantage of governmental resources, such as an expensive rehabilitation course, are not citizens of the society where the treatment is being rendered, in particular, the United States? This dilemma is further complicated when resources are limited. An example of this might be a situation where there are two available openings for rehabilitative treatment and there are three persons in need of such treatment. Two of the persons are citizens of the United States and one person is a citizen of another country. Should the United States citizens receive first chance at the rehabilitation spots? What if the individual who is not a United States citizen accepts treatment and then leaves the country halfway through the treatment course, thus wasting resources on an unfinished course and taking an opening that could have been given to someone who might have finished a course of treatment?

In larger metropolitan areas, the number of clients who are not United States citizens may be fairly high. Nurses who work in these areas often care for such clients and probably are not even aware of their citizenship status. Nursing care should be the same for all clients, regardless of citizenship. The ethical dilemma remains, however, regarding the allocation of governmental financial assistance to those who are not United States citizens. Is there not an obligation by government to care for its own citizens? Does this obligation include the exclusion of noncitizens? When resources become scarce, rationing takes place. No matter what governmental activity takes place regarding financial reimbursement, nurses should strive for justice in their nursing practice.

HERNIATED INTERVERTEBRAL DISC

Definition

Displacement of intervertebral disc material may be referred to as prolapse, herniation, rupture, or extrusion of the disc. These interchangeable terms indicate loss of integrity of the disc between two vertebrae. Ruptured intervertebral discs may occur at any level of the spine. As in spinal cord injury, thoracic involvement is the least common. Lumbar discs are more likely to rupture than cervical discs, due to the forces of gravity.

Incidence

Approximately 80 per cent of all individuals experience low back pain at some point in their lives. One third of these individuals also develop sciatica. This is inflammation of the sciatic nerve, usually caused by compression. The pain follows the course of the sciatic nerve down the leg. It is estimated that 10 per cent of individuals who seek medical attention for back pain have herniated discs.

Etiology

More than one half of the people with symptoms of a herniated disc give a history of a previous back injury. Flexing the back without bending the knees and making rotating movements create significant stress on the intervertebral disc. Repeated stress progressively weakens the disc, resulting in bulging and herniation. It is postulated that the pain is caused by stretching of the posterior annulus and the posterior longitudinal ligament.

Risk Factors

Heavy physical labor, strenuous exercise, and weak abdominal and back muscles all increase the risk of herniated disc. Use of proper body mechanics is the foundation of primary prevention of back injuries. Strengthening of the back and abdominal muscles provides a strong support for the spine. Bending the legs and keeping the back straight minimizes the stress of lifting. Shifting of positions is important for individuals with sedentary employment, such as truck drivers and office workers. Exercise should be encouraged and carried out in a planned and controlled fashion.

Secondary prevention addresses the individual who already has sustained a back injury and wishes to prevent recurrence. Slow, gentle exercise to strengthen muscles is helpful; this may be best supervised by a physical therapist. Weight reduction, if appropriate, reduces stress on the disc. A change in employment may be suggested if occupation is contributing to back pain.

Tertiary prevention focuses on minimizing the complications of a herniated disc. This involves careful monitoring of neurologic signs to detect further deterioration. Muscle strength and deep tendon reflexes are sequentially assessed. Spinal cord or nerve root compression is usually treated surgically.

Pathophysiology

The intervertebral disc is composed of three parts. The cartilaginous plates act as the superior and inferior limits of the disc. These are composed of hyaline cartilage and cover the top and bottom of the vertebrae.

The annulus fibrosus is the ring of tissue that gives size and shape to the disc and holds the nucleus pulposus in place. This semigelatinous material forms the center of the disc and provides the cushioning effect.

The annulus fibrosus is weaker in the back than in the front, which explains why most discs herniate in a retrograde fashion. In the case of a disc bulge, the annulus remains intact. With herniation, the annulus is usually torn, allowing extrusion of nucleus pulposus (Fig. 32-9).

Compression of spinal nerve roots may result from herniation of the disc. If compression remains untreated, weakness or paralysis of the innervated muscle group may result.

Clinical Manifestations

Assessment findings with a ruptured lumbar intervertebral disc include (1) lower back pain that radiates down the posterior thigh, (2) muscle spasm, (3) aggravation of pain by straining (coughing, defecation, bending, lifting, and straight-leg raising), (4) depression of deep tendon reflexes, and (5) hyperesthesia in the area of distribution of affected nerve roots.

Rupture of a small, laterally placed cervical disc typically causes (1) stiff neck, (2) shoulder pain that radiates down the arm into the hand, and (3) paresthesias and sensory disturbances in the hand. Electromyography or electrical testing of the peripheral nerves may localize the ruptured disc site.

DIAGNOSTIC ASSESSMENT

Plain x-ray studies may show spinal degenerative changes (at any level) that may indicate disc problems but usually do not show a ruptured disc. Osteophytes and narrowed disc interspaces are degenerative changes visible on plain x-ray films. Also, other spinal disorders (e.g., spinal tumors, vertebral fracture, rheumatoid arthritis, and osteoarthritis) that are useful in establishing an accurate diagnosis may be demonstrated.

Magnetic resonance image (MRI) may demonstrate spinal stenosis (narrowing of the spinal canal), extrusion of disc material into the spinal canal, and/or impingement of a spinal nerve root (Fig. 32-10).

Myelography may show narrowing of the disc space and/or impingement of a spinal nerve root. Myelography identifies the level of herniation and may rule out other spinal diseases. It is typically performed if the MRI is not conclusive. A CT scan is usually done following a myelogram. This sequence allows better imaging with only one administration of contrast material. CT scanning may demonstrate spinal stenosis or other changes associated with degenerative disc disease. CT scans are more useful at the thoracic or lumbar level than the cervical level.

Medical Management

Most cases of intervertebral disc herniation are initially treated conservatively unless there is progressive neurologic dysfunction. Then surgery is indicated.

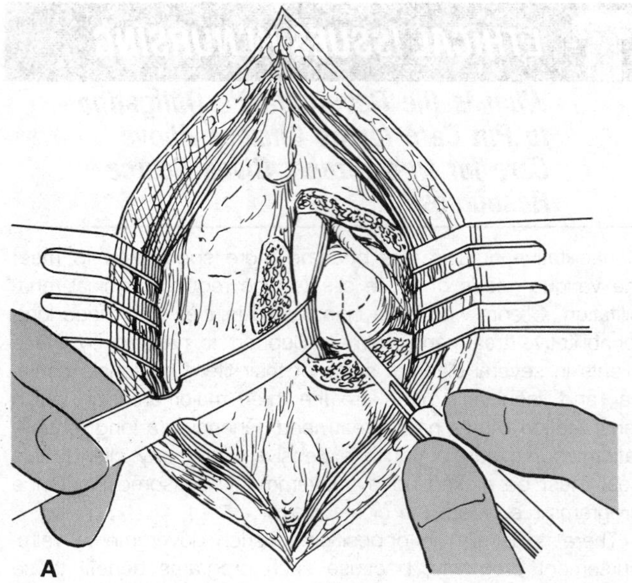

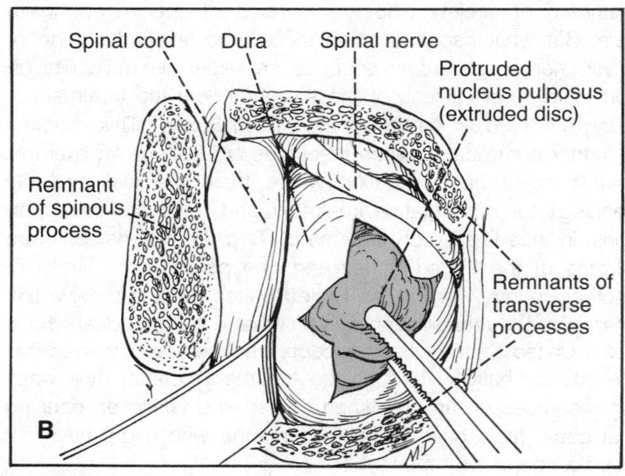

▲ *Figure 32-9*

Laminectomy for the interlaminal removal of a herniated disc.

Conservative intervention for disc problems at any spinal level includes prescribed medications such as anti-inflammatory agents, muscle relaxants, and analgesics. Muscle spasm (which often triggers a cycle of pain and increased muscle spasm) can be severe. Narcotics may be prescribed. Administer sufficient medication to achieve pain relief or adequate pain reduction. Deep ultrasonic heat treatment and moist local heat applications may also help. However, avoid prolonged heat, as it increases congestion. Recently, the use of ice has been found to reduce pain and spasm. Progressive muscle relaxation exercises and other stress reduction techniques can be helpful. Muscle stretching has also been effective for fascial pain.

Activities should be reduced during episodes of back or neck pain. Thus, conservative intervention also includes bed rest. Bed rest relieves back pain by relieving the back muscles and vertebrae of the stresses. The forces of gravity (e.g., weight of the head with cervical problems) and motion can increase back pain during activity. Lying in a prone position and sleeping with

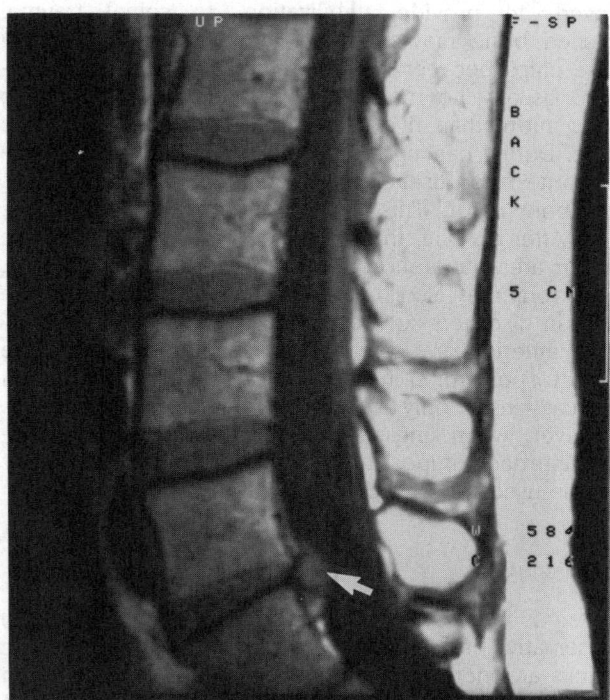

▲ Figure 32-10

A magnetic resonance image of the lumbar spine showing herniation of the disc between L_5 and S_1.

thick pillows under the head should always be avoided. For clients on bed rest, antiembolic stockings (applied by the nurse) and periodic flexion and extension of the feet are important to prevent thrombophlebitis. Bedside items (e.g., call light), should be placed conveniently to prevent the client from twisting the back to reach them.

Provide psychosocial support to the client and family. Disc problems often create fears and concerns related to pain, treatments, sexual activity, possible length of illness, and possible lifestyle changes. Socioeconomic considerations about employment and finances should be referred to a social worker.

Client education is an important aspect of back care. Back care is discussed in the Client Education Guide.

For severe lumbar disc problems, conservative intervention involves bed rest on a firm mattress. Use of traction for lumbar disc problems is controversial. The client should be encouraged to systematically change positions (unless in traction) while on bed rest. If the client requires assistance to turn, or when turning to place a bedpan, the nurse turns the client in a logrolling manner. Use of a fracture bedpan or a child's bedpan instead of a higher, regular-sized bedpan reduces back strain.

Sometimes, with severe lumbar disc pain, a semisitting position is prescribed to promote forward lumbar spine flexion and thus reduce back strain. A client with lumbar pain may be most comfortable when supine, with the bed's backrest elevated 10 to 30 degrees and the knees slightly flexed. Other positions of comfort include (1) the supine position with pillows under the legs or (2) the lateral position, in which the client lies

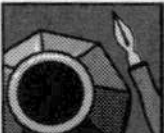

CLIENT EDUCATION GUIDE

Back Care

The following points should be included in client teaching about back care:

- Get out of bed by rolling onto one side near the edge of the mattress. Push up to a straight position by pushing off the bed with the arms while keeping the spine straight and swing the legs over the edge. Avoid twisting while getting up.
- Do not sleep while partially reclined or sitting in chair. Sleep on a bed with a firm (not hard) mattress. Avoid riding in or driving a car for a long distance or time. Sit erect without slouching. Avoid low couches and chairs, and use leg muscles when rising from a chair; a recliner chair is usually comfortable.
- When required to stand for a long time, bend one knee to reduce stress on the low back.
- Maintain a body weight that is close to ideal. Exercise and walk or swim to strengthen back muscles. Wear low-heeled shoes.
- Eat a diet high in fiber and fluids to soften bowel movements and reduce strain. (When adding fiber to the diet, add it slowly over days.)
- Use proper body mechanics when lifting. Get adequate help if the object is heavy. Use the muscles of the legs, not the back, by bending at the knees to get close to the object being lifted. Never turn and lift at the same time.

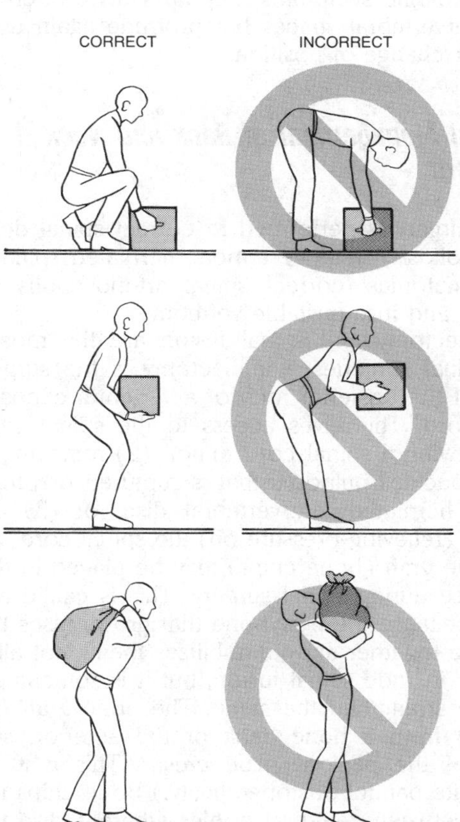

on the unaffected side with a thin pillow between the knees and the painful leg flexed to reduce tension on the sciatic nerve. Use of an over-bed trapeze is contraindicated.

A back brace or corset is often prescribed for a client with a ruptured lumbar disc. However, back supports are usually not recommended once symptoms are relieved, because restricted back motion progressively weakens musculature and causes further degeneration of spinal structures. Once the acute pain episode passes, progressive muscle strengthening exercises (usually William's flexion exercises or simple isometric exercises) may be prescribed. Strengthening the back and abdominal muscles helps prevent further problems if the exercises are done daily throughout life. See also the discussion of sciatic nerve injury.

Opinions differ concerning the advisability of performing head and neck ROM exercises in the presence of significant cervical disease. Teach the client to avoid activities that increase cervical disc pain. To prevent neck extension when in bed, only one flat pillow (to prevent neck flexion) is recommended in the presence of cervical disc problems. A soft cervical collar may be prescribed for mild-to-moderate cervical disc problems to keep the head slightly flexed. The neck should not be hyperextended. Intermittent traction may be applied for cervical disc herniation (5 to 8 lb weight) to relieve pain. The head of the bed may be slightly elevated with cervical traction. Otherwise, it is best kept flat when cervical pain is present.

Conservative intervention often produces satisfactory results in treating herniated disc unless there are obvious neurologic symptoms. Ruptured discs often recede into intervertebral spaces but protrude again upon exertion or change of position.

Surgical Management of Back and Neck Disorders

Spinal surgery is performed to correct spinal deformity (e.g., scoliosis); remove tumors, herniated spinal discs, and hematomas; correct spinal arteriovenous malformations; and fuse unstable vertebrae.

Laminectomy and spinal fusion are the most common spinal surgeries. Laminectomy is the surgical removal of the posterior arch of a vertebra, exposing the spinal cord. This gives access to the spinal canal for (1) removing a spinal cord tumor, (2) removing a portion of nucleus pulposus that is ruptured or protruding from a herniated intervertebral disc, or (3) decompressing (relieving pressure on) the spinal cord.

A bone graft (bone chips) may be placed in the disc interspace during spinal surgery. This is called a spinal fusion, because the new bone that grows fuses the two vertebrae together and immobilizes them. Not all spinal surgeries include spinal fusion, but it is sometimes indicated to strengthen the spine. The bone graft may be obtained from a bone bank or the anterior, superior region of the person's iliac crest. (This graft site is often quite painful postoperatively.) Bone chips may be placed between vertebral bodies where a disc was removed, to provide stabilization. In spinal trauma, crushed bone may be fused and stabilized by laying bone chips between the foramina of two to five vertebrae. Usually no more than five vertebrae are fused; fusing more than five causes loss of movement in the spine. During healing the graft gradually grows onto the vertebrae and fuses them permanently together in a firm, bony union. This causes permanent stiffness in the area. After a while, the stiffness is hardly noticed in the lumbar area but is more noticeable in the cervical area. Metal rods may also be used to straighten and fuse the spine in disorders such as scoliosis.

An anterior or posterior surgical approach may be taken to perform spinal fusions. The anterior approach is usually used only to perform cervical spine fusions. However, when unusual circumstances make a posterior approach impossible, the anterior approach may also be used for thoracic and lumbar fusions.

INDICATIONS

Surgery is indicated with spinal disc problems when (1) conservative intervention is ineffective, (2) neurologic deficits are increasing, and (3) repeated attacks of pain occur despite optimal treatment. Some surgeons use other criteria. A surgical approach is selected that gives the best exposure with the least risk.

Microsurgical techniques in disc removal cause less trauma to the surgical site than standard surgery and preserve more tissue integrity. Advantages of microsurgery include minimal nerve root retraction, preservation of an intact joint capsule (no bone is removed), improved hemostasis, and minimal stripping of the muscle and fascia from the spine. Sometimes foraminotomy is performed to enlarge the intervertebral foramen if it is narrowed and osteophytic processes (overgrowths of bone) entrap the nerve root and impinge on neural structures.

COMPLICATIONS

General potential complications following spinal disc surgery at any level include infection and inflammation; injury to nerve roots, the dural sac, the spinal cord, or other nearby structures; mechanical instability of the spine; inadequate disc removal; spinal cord compression; and hemorrhage.

Specific complications after posterior cervical surgery may include soft tissue hematoma, air embolism, and subcutaneous wound dehiscence. Specific complications following anterior cervical surgeries may include laryngeal nerve damage and injury to neck structures such as the carotid arteries, trachea, esophagus, and soft tissue. Following lumbar discectomy, chronic adhesive arachnoiditis, delayed epidural hematoma, or muscle spasms may occur. Also, severe pain may be experienced owing to improved sensation after nerve root decompression. The postoperative development of a spinal epidural hematoma is a surgical emergency because it may compress the spinal cord and cause irreversible damage.

Nursing Management

PREOPERATIVE MANAGEMENT

In today's economic climate, clients undergoing elective surgery are routinely admitted the day of surgery. This significantly decreases the amount of time nurses have for preoperative teaching.

The family is included in preoperative education. The nurse explains to the client that frequent turning follows surgery and that correct turning protects the back and helps the recovery process. The log-rolling method of turning is explained.

A baseline neurologic assessment is obtained for comparison after surgery. Assessment should include motor and sensory function of extremities, and psychological readiness for surgery.

The nurse explains that deep breathing, coughing, and turning after surgery help prevent pulmonary complications and that limitations of activity are necessary to prevent damage (flexion, extension, or twisting) to the surgical site and to eliminate straining. The client is also taught to roll onto the side and push the torso from the bed with his or her arms to rise from bed. This technique has often been used by clients with long-standing back pain and may be familiar to the client. In this case, the nurse reviews the client's technique for rising from bed. Clients with a recent injury may not be permitted to ambulate prior to surgery. For these clients, the nurse explains and demonstrates. The client is advised to ask for help rather than stretching to reach for objects. Stool softeners are given daily while the client is in the hospital to minimize straining at bowel movement.

The nurse encourages the client and family to express their concerns and fears about the spinal surgery. Many people fear postoperative problems such as paralysis and chronic pain. Concerns and fears should be allayed whenever possible.

When the client is being transferred to bed postoperatively, at least four people should assist. Transfer devices such as a sliding board may be used with adequate help. The client should be transferred gently and smoothly, with the spine supported and properly aligned at all times.

POSTOPERATIVE MANAGEMENT

Following spinal surgery, assessment is similar to that of other surgical clients. The respiratory and cardiovascular systems are assessed for stability. Dressings are checked for drainage. The level of pain and the response to analgesia are evaluated. Nutritional intake and elimination are assessed.

In addition, neurologic function is assessed, by asking the client to move all four extremities and comparing the results with those of the baseline evaluation. The client is questioned about the presence of numbness and/or tingling and changes in sensation or pain compared with preoperatively. Although there will be incisional pain, often the pain in an extremity associated with a herniated disc will be significantly decreased after surgery. In addition, many surgeons inject long-acting local anesthetics into disc spaces during surgery. This gives the client immediate relief from pain and promotes a positive attitude toward the outcome of surgery. Often the pain recurs on the second postoperative day. This is due to both the increase in swelling and the fact that the local anesthetic is wearing off. The nurse observes the client's movements in bed and reinforces preoperative teaching as needed.

Immediately after a posterior cervical discectomy, a soft cervical collar is worn. The client's head is kept flat except for a folded small blanket or folded sheet beneath the head to maintain spinal alignment while the client lies supine or on the side. Laryngeal nerve damage during surgery may cause permanent vocal impairment, such as a hoarse voice. Difficulty swallowing and throat discomfort are usually present for several days. A drain may be present and is usually removed by the surgeon on the first postoperative day. A hard cervical collar may or may not be prescribed following such a fusion. However, a postoperative x-ray study is typically taken before the client is permitted to assume an upright position, and follow-up x-ray studies are taken to assess healing. During recovery, jiggling movements such as from riding in a car should be avoided (except to go home initially). The graft could be displaced.

Positioning and Turning the Client. Postoperatively, immediately following lumbar discectomy, the person typically is not turned for an hour or so but remains flat to aid hemostasis. Side-to-side log-rolling then begins and is done every 2 hours. If a dural tear was repaired, the surgeon may order the person to remain flat longer to minimize the risk of cerebrospinal fluid leak or a tear in the dural sutures. Sometimes, around the third postoperative day, a temporary increase in pain occurs owing to muscle spasm or improved nerve root sensation.

Postoperative care, turning, and positioning after spinal fusion depend on whether the surgical approach was anterior or posterior and the surgeon's preference. The goal of nursing intervention is to prevent strain or flexion at the surgical site.

Following lumbar fusion, the bed is generally kept flat. Sometimes the head of the entire bed is elevated on 6-inch blocks, but the bed itself is not flexed, in order not to flex the client's spine. The mattress is firm and a bedboard may be placed under it. A client who will be in bed for a long time may be switched to an alternating air mattress bed or a bed that rocks from side to side. These beds aid turning and promote cardiopulmonary function and circulation. Use of special beds facilitates turning following spinal surgery.

Following microdiscectomy, in which the herniated fragment of disc is removed under microscopic visualization, the client may have the head of the bed elevated to whatever position is comfortable. Following cervical spine surgery, the surgeon often permits the head of the bed to be elevated slightly for comfort and to reduce edema.

If a client is lying supine following spinal surgery

(e.g., after removal of infection with an open incision remaining), the lower back muscles may be relaxed somewhat if pillows are placed under the entire length of the legs. This may also prevent possible thrombophlebitis in the femoral vessels. The nurse must not flex the client's knees by placing anything under the popliteal space; this is hazardous because it increases the risk of deep vein thrombosis.

When positioning a client in a side-lying position following spinal surgery, strain on the back may be prevented by (1) keeping the spine straight, (2) pulling the hips slightly back so the person is balanced, (3) flexing the upper leg and placing a pillow between the legs, and (4) placing a pillow to support the upper arm and prevent the upper shoulder from sagging. A client who has had cervical surgery is positioned in essentially the same manner. The nurse makes sure the spine is in line at the cervical area and places a small pillow under the head to keep the spine straight.

When turning a client to the side, the nurse uses a log-rolling maneuver. Twisting the client's spine or twisting at the hips must be avoided. Safety needs to be ensured during turning to prevent straining of the spine or rolling off the bed. It is beneficial to have extra help in turning a client the first few times after spinal surgery, and adequate help is advisable even after the client is able to participate in the turning process. Spinal bone grafts are delicate and heal slowly. Eventually, turning is permitted without help, while keeping the spine rigid.

During the first turning sessions, the client is generally apprehensive (e.g., he or she fears pain or damage to the spine during turning). If turning is not done smoothly, confidently, safely, and with a minimum of discomfort, this apprehension increases and impairs future turning sessions.

While the client is on the bedpan, the nurse supports the back and legs, so that all sections of the body are on the same plane. A fracture bedpan or a child's bedpan is used.

The call light is placed so the client can touch it without straining, and all calls are answered promptly so the client does not strain in trying to move. Once a client is allowed to reach for things, the objects needed should be conveniently placed.

Circulation in the client's back, head, and neck following spinal surgery is stimulated by giving frequent gentle back rubs, avoiding the area of surgery.

A sign is placed on the bed stating the prescribed position for the bed, which is discussed with the client. The nurse also instructs the client clearly about contraindicated activities and positions.

Progressive Activity. When helping the client up, the nurse uses the technique specified by the surgeon and has ample help to prevent a fall or other injury to the spine. Blood pressure is assessed before the move is begun. Postural hypotension may occur. The client is assessed carefully for dizziness, weakness, or fainting. If collapse occurs, proper spinal alignment is maintained, and the client is carefully returned to bed.

To prevent falls and enhance proper posture, the client should wear stockings and firm walking shoes when ambulating, rather than slippers or just stockings.

People with lumbar laminectomies or microdiscectomies are typically out of bed by the first or second postoperative day. Those with cervical fusions are usually out of bed by the first day postoperatively, normally wearing a cervical collar. A spinal fusion usually requires longer bed rest for healing. The surgeon should be consulted about permitted active or passive exercises. Some are contraindicated because they strain the back (e.g., toe touching and straight-leg raises).

Complications. The nurse continues to assess for clinical manifestations of complications and notifies the physician if they occur. The client's neurologic status is assessed and documented frequently, and the development or worsening of a neurologic deficit promptly reported to the surgeon. During the first 24 hours following an anterior cervical discectomy, the nurse assesses the client's ability to breathe, the operative site for excessive swelling, and the client's voice. A soft diet, throat lozenges, viscous Xylocaine, humidified air, minimal talking, and other comfort measures are appreciated. If a spinal fusion was performed with the anterior cervical discectomy, the surgeon is notified if radicular pain suddenly recurs. This could mean that the bone graft has moved out of place and surgery needs to be repeated.

Following surgery on the cervical spine, the nurse watches for indications of respiratory paralysis resulting from cord edema. Emergency tracheostomy equipment is kept readily available. Postoperatively, flexion of the neck is prevented.

Skin incisions for laminectomies and posterior spinal fusions are made directly over the spinous processes. The person is log-rolled for position changes to maintain skin integrity. The wound or dressing is observed for indications of hemorrhage or cerebrospinal fluid leakage. If present, the nurse notifies the surgeon. The dressing is reinforced as necessary with sterile compresses. The dressing must be changed if contaminated, e.g., with urine. Surgeons usually perform the first dressing change.

Every 2 to 4 hours during the first 48 postoperative hours, client's motor abilities and sensation in the extremities are assessed (see Chap. 28). Following lumbar surgery, the person focuses on moving the legs; if cervical, the shoulders and legs. The nurse checks pinprick and light touch with an alcohol wipe on the extremities. Progressive worsening of motor and sensory functions may indicate spinal cord edema or hemorrhage compressing the spinal cord. Assessment findings indicating cord damage or cord compression should be promptly documented and reported. If motor or sensory losses are present, injury from, e.g., falls or heat must be prevented.

The client is assessed for indications of postoperative improvement, e.g., "The tingling I had in my leg before surgery is gone now." These findings are documented.

Pain Management. Compression of various structures due to edema may cause pain for some time after spinal surgery. Muscle spasms may occur in the back and thigh as a result of irritation of nerves during surgery. Antispasmodics may be prescribed for muscle spasms. The area from which the bone was taken for a spinal fusion may also be painful for several days. Pain relief is provided as indicated. Pain medication is given readily. Narcotics are administered, commonly through epidural sites and patient-controlled analgesia devices. Then acetaminophen (Tylenol) with codeine (or an equivalent) is used. Eventually plain Tylenol is all that is required. The nurse should not wait until the client is in great pain. Appropriate nursing actions are taken to prevent or minimize pain. Keeping the operative leg and the spine correctly and comfortably positioned helps reduce pain and muscle spasms. Massage (not directly over the operated area) may also be relaxing and prevent or reduce pain. The client must always be kept in proper alignment.

Urinary Management. Following spinal surgery, urinary retention may occur. Most commonly, it occurs when the cauda equina is affected and not as often after thoracic surgery. Cervical surgery may affect the parasympathetic chain, causing urinary retention. If present, assessment typically reveals a urinary bladder that may feel distended and painful, or an inability to urinate. An indwelling catheter may be used for the first few days. Intermittent catheterization may also be used rather than indwelling catheters. When the client is able to void spontaneously, the use of a fracture pan allows the client to remain fairly flat. After 24 to 48 hours, bladder function usually resumes. It helps if the client is permitted to sit up when trying to urinate. After the client voids, the nurse checks residuals. If the bladder is full or cannot be emptied completely, the physician may order straight catheterization to check for residual urine. If the client cannot void voluntarily and the bladder is full, the excess urine will overflow. It may appear that the client is urinating, but actually the bladder remains full. Intermittent catheterization is required.

Men are accustomed to urinating standing up. Lying flat and using a urinal is an unnatural position. Their inability to pass urine does not necessarily indicate bladder dysfunction. Catheterization may be required for a full bladder until standing to void is permitted.

Bowel Management. The most common bowel problem after laminectomy and spinal fusion is paralytic ileus. This loss of bowel sounds and abdominal distention is due to lack of peristalsis from a sudden loss of parasympathetic function innervating the bowels. Assessment findings with paralytic ileus include nausea, vomiting, a hard abdomen, and absence of bowel sounds. Intervention typically includes insertion of a nasogastric tube on low suction and nothing by mouth. When bowel sounds return or the client passes gas or has a bowel movement, a clear fluid diet usually begins, progressing to a regular diet.

The client is assessed every 4 hours postoperatively for bowel distention. Bowel dysfunction may occur for several days postoperatively. Inactivity often causes problems with bowel elimination. Bowel movements are documented. Fluids are forced as ordered; a regular time for bowel movements and bowel care is encouraged; roughage is provided in the diet (when allowed); and medications and enemas as ordered (e.g., stool softeners, mild bulk laxative, or suppository) are administered. The client is instructed not to strain at bowel movement, because this increases pain and cerebrospinal fluid.

Often clients find it difficult or impossible to defecate when lying flat. A bowel movement may not occur until sitting up is possible.

Braces, Corsets, and Casts. Following spinal surgery, a brace or corset may be temporarily required to support the spine. Persons who have lumbar or thoracic spinal fusions wear a fiberglass brace. Initially, back braces or corsets may be worn all the time, whether the client is in or out of bed. As the client's muscles strengthen, decreased use of braces or corsets is usually recommended. Casts may be used for a while following any thoracic spinal surgery for clients with unstable thoracic spines (e.g., thoracic spinal cord trauma). This is not the only external method of stability for this region of the spinal cord.

Post-hospital Care

DISCHARGE TEACHING

Clients need clear instructions on ability to walk, lift, drive, and return to work. Most clients can resume activity 6 weeks after surgery. Specific physician instructions need to be followed.

Contraindicated activities vary. The person is instructed to ask the surgeon when it will be safe to perform activities that could damage the back, e.g., climbing stairs, lifting any weight greater than 5 lb, prolonged travel, sexual activity, sports, exercises, driving a car. See also Client Education Guide.

NEUROLOGIC DEVELOPMENTAL DISORDERS

Congenital neurologic disorders range from minor, practically unnoticeable defects (e.g., slight intelligence impairment from abnormal development) to striking, sometimes fatal, gross abnormalities (e.g., acrania [absence of the cranium], anencephaly [absence of the brain], microcephaly [extremely small brain], hydrocephaly [excessive enlargement of ventricular cavities of the brain], and spina bifida [various spinal closure defects]). Refer to pediatric and neurologic textbooks for discussions of these disorders.

Syringomyelia and Syringobulbia

OVERVIEW

These two conditions are relatively rare.

Syringomyelia. Syringomyelia is often associated with Arnold-Chiari malformation and/or spina bifida. Syringomyelia consists of abnormal cavities filled with yellow liquid in the spinal cord substance, especially the cervical cord. Scar tissue surrounds the cysts. Syringomyelia is characterized by (1) muscular weakness and wasting, (2) various sensory defects, and (3) indications of injury to the spinal cord's long tracts, such as hyperreflexia.

These disturbances may begin at any age but most often occur between ages 30 and 40. Syringomyelia often occurs with other developmental defects. Kyphosis (abnormal increased convexity in curvature of the thoracic spine when viewed from the side), scoliosis (lateral deviation in the normally straight vertical line of the spine), and club foot often occur with syringomyelia.

Early indications of cervical syringomyelia often include (1) atrophy, weakness, and fibrillations of the small muscles of the hands, (2) loss of pain sensation in the fingers or forearms, (3) weakness and atrophy of the shoulder girdle muscles, (4) Horner's syndrome (characterized by ptosis of the upper eyelid, constriction of the pupil, and anhidrosis and flushing of the affected side of the face, (5) nystagmus, and (6) vasomotor and trophic disturbances of the upper extremities. Although there is segmental loss or impairment of pain and temperature sensation, sensation for light touch remains. Segments of sensory loss may be separated by zones of normal sensation. Spasticity, ataxia, or paralysis of the lower extremities may occur as well as disturbed bladder control when the lumbosacral region of the spinal cord is involved.

Cranial nerve involvement may produce additional problems such as impairment of facial pain and temperature sensations, loss of the corneal reflex (necessitating protection of the eye), dysphagia, dysarthria, laryngeal stridor (possibly necessitating tracheotomy), nystagmus, and atrophy and fibrillation of the tongue muscles.

Syringomyelia may progress rapidly at first and then become stationary for many years. Some people live 40 years after onset. Others become incapacitated (from paralysis or sensory defects) or die within a few years.

Syringobulbia. Syringobulbia is the presence of similar cavities in the medulla oblongata. These cavities may occur in the medulla only, without involving the spinal cord, but they usually occur with cervical syringomyelia. Typical assessment findings include atrophy and fibrillation of the tongue, loss of pain and temperature sensation on one or both sides of the face, nystagmus, respiratory stridor, and dysphonia.

MANAGEMENT

Treatment of syringomyelia or syringobulbia includes relieving increased pressure on the cord from the fluid content of the cavities within the spinal canal by removing fluid buildup, either by direct surgical drainage or by shunt placement to restore cerebral spinal fluid outflow.

SPINAL TUMORS

Overview

Spinal tumors are similar in nature and origin to intracranial tumors but occur much less often. They are most common in young or middle-aged adults and most often involve the thoracic region. Spinal tumors may occur outside of the spinal cord (extramedullary) or within the substance of the spinal cord (intramedullary). Extramedullary tumors may be intradural, extradural, or extravertebral. Neurofibromas and meningiomas are the most common spinal cord tumors. Both are benign and operable and may not produce permanent damage if removed early enough.

Clinical manifestations of spinal tumors vary according to their location. Spinal cord compression is the common pathologic feature of all tumors within the spinal canal, because it has little room for expansion. Compression of the spinal cord interrupts the function of nerve fibers in the cord's peripheral portions.

Extramedullary tumors cause signs and symptoms by compressing the spinal cord or some of its nerve roots or by occluding blood vessels supplying the cord. Early characteristics of spinal cord compression include pain, sensory loss, muscle weakness, and wasting. Progressive cord compression is manifested by spastic weakness below the level of the lesion, decreased sensation, and increased reflexes. Severe cord compression destroys the cord and produces paraplegia or quadriplegia.

Intramedullary tumors produce more variable signs and symptoms. High cervical cord involvement causes spastic quadriplegia and sensory changes. Tumors in descending areas of the spinal cord produce motor and sensory changes appropriate to functions of that level.

Medical diagnosis is made after a complete general neurologic examination. The diagnostic tests that are used are x-ray study, CT scan, MRI, and myelogram.

Management

Intervention for spinal tumors is usually surgery, radiation therapy, or both. Immediate surgery is indicated if compression of the cord or nerve roots is evident. Often, marked improvement results or even complete restoration of function, especially if the tumor is encapsulated (e.g., meningioma or lipoma). However, surgery often does not have good results if cord necrosis is present, e.g., from compression or interrupted blood supply. Complete surgical removal of an intramedullary tumor is rare, but partial resection followed by radiation may clinically improve the client's condition. The course of the condition is usually gradually progressive.

VASCULAR SPINAL CORD LESIONS

Overview

Blood supply to the spinal cord occurs via the anterior and posterior spinal arteries and the radicular arteries (Fig. 32-11). The anterior spinal artery supplies most of the cord's cross-sectional area. The posterior spinal arteries supply the posterior white matter and part of the posterior gray matter. Various branches of the radicular arteries supply the superficial areas of white matter. A complex venous system drains the cord and empties into the anterior and posterior spinal veins and the two lateral veins.

As in the brain, spinal cord vascular lesions may be caused by rupture, thrombosis, or embolism. Trauma is the usual cause of hemorrhage into the spinal cord from cord or vessel injury. Arteriosclerosis of spinal vessels is not a common cause of thrombosis. Thrombosis of the spinal vessels is usually secondary to meningitis or to compression of the vessels by tumors, granulomas, or abscesses in the epidural space.

MYELOMALACIA

Myelomalacia (softening or infarction of the spinal cord) results from spinal artery occlusion. This serious condition has a poor prognosis. There is little or no return of normal function to involved areas. Myelomalacia is suspected when indications of transverse myelitis develop suddenly. Assessment findings of myelomalacia depend on the level of the lesion in the cord. There are always motor paralysis and dissociated sensory loss below the level of the lesion, accompanied by paralysis of bladder and bowel sphincters. Paralysis is usually bilateral but rarely complete. Initially, the limbs are flaccid and no deep tendon or superficial reflexes are elicited, as in spinal shock. After several weeks, spasticity, hyperreflexia, and clonus develop. Intervention focuses on maintaining body functions, preventing complications of immobility and providing pain relief. The person usually begins intensive rehabilitation 12 to 14 hours after onset of symptoms.

HEMATOMYELIA

Hematomyelia is hemorrhage into the substance of the spinal cord. It almost always follows trauma but may be caused by vascular malformation or a bleeding disorder. Clinical manifestations of hematomyelia usually develop suddenly, immediately after spinal injury, and depend on the size of the hemorrhage. Following trauma, it is important to differentiate between hematomyelia and a vertebral fracture dislocation. Immediate surgery to relieve cord compression is indicated if fracture dislocation is evident on x-ray film. Spinal angiography, spinal CT scans, and MRI enable visualization of vascular lesions. Some of these lesions are treated by ligating their feeding vessels, others by excising the entire malformation. Acute and chronic interventions are the same as for myelomalacia.

Management

Nursing care for individuals with vascular spinal cord lesions is the same as for other types of spinal surgery.

▼ INJURIES TO THE PERIPHERAL NERVES

Peripheral nerves can be injured in many ways—from bone fractures, stretching of the nerves, constriction by fascial bands, pressure, trauma associated with perforating wounds, or injection of drugs. The peripheral

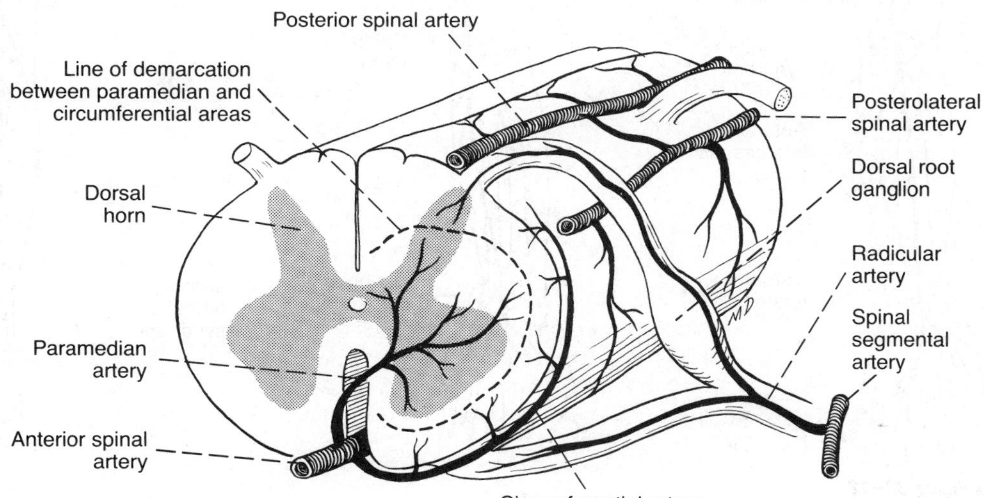

▲ **Figure 32-11**

Arterial supply of spinal cord.

nerves most commonly subjected to external pressure are the radial, common peroneal, ulnar, and long thoracic nerves. The median nerve is most often affected by constriction by fascial bands. The axillary nerve may be affected from an allergic reaction to serum injections. The sciatic nerve may be injured directly during medication injections. Any peripheral nerve can be injured by bone fractures or perforating wounds.

If a peripheral nerve is traumatically severed, the ends should be surgically anastomosed to enable healing. The nearer the site of injury occurs to the central nervous system, the poorer the chance of regeneration. When nerves are only slightly damaged, mild edema occurs at the injury site. This may cause temporary symptoms that recede in a few days or possibly weeks.

MEDIAN NERVE COMPRESSION AT THE WRIST

Carpal Tunnel Syndrome

Carpal tunnel syndrome is an entrapment neuropathy that occurs when the median nerve is compressed as it passes through the carpal tunnel in the wrist. This compression causes sensory and motor changes. Carpal tunnel syndrome typically produces increased pain and paresthesia at night, which may awaken the client. The syndrome may develop spontaneously without a known cause or may result from disease or injury. A common cause is trauma to the wrist involving the distal end of the radius and the carpal bones. Another common cause is repetitive movements of the hands and wrists, such as during typing or factory work (Fig. 32–12).

When the symptoms of carpal tunnel syndrome are mild and of short duration, or if the client does not want surgery, the wrist may be splinted in a neutral position with the hand resting to prevent mechanical irritation of the nerve. Temporary relief may be obtained by injection of a steroid suspension into the flexor tendons in the carpal tunnel. Pain relief may occur immediately but is usually transitory. Surgery is indicated with (1) severe symptoms of long duration, (2) muscle atrophy, or (3) progressive sensory loss in the fingers and hand. Usually, surgery for carpal tunnel syndrome involves decompression of the medial nerve by transecting the transverse carpal ligament.

Tarsal Tunnel Syndrome

Tarsal tunnel syndrome is the counterpart of the carpal tunnel syndrome in the lower extremity. In this syndrome, the posterior tibial nerve is trapped beneath the

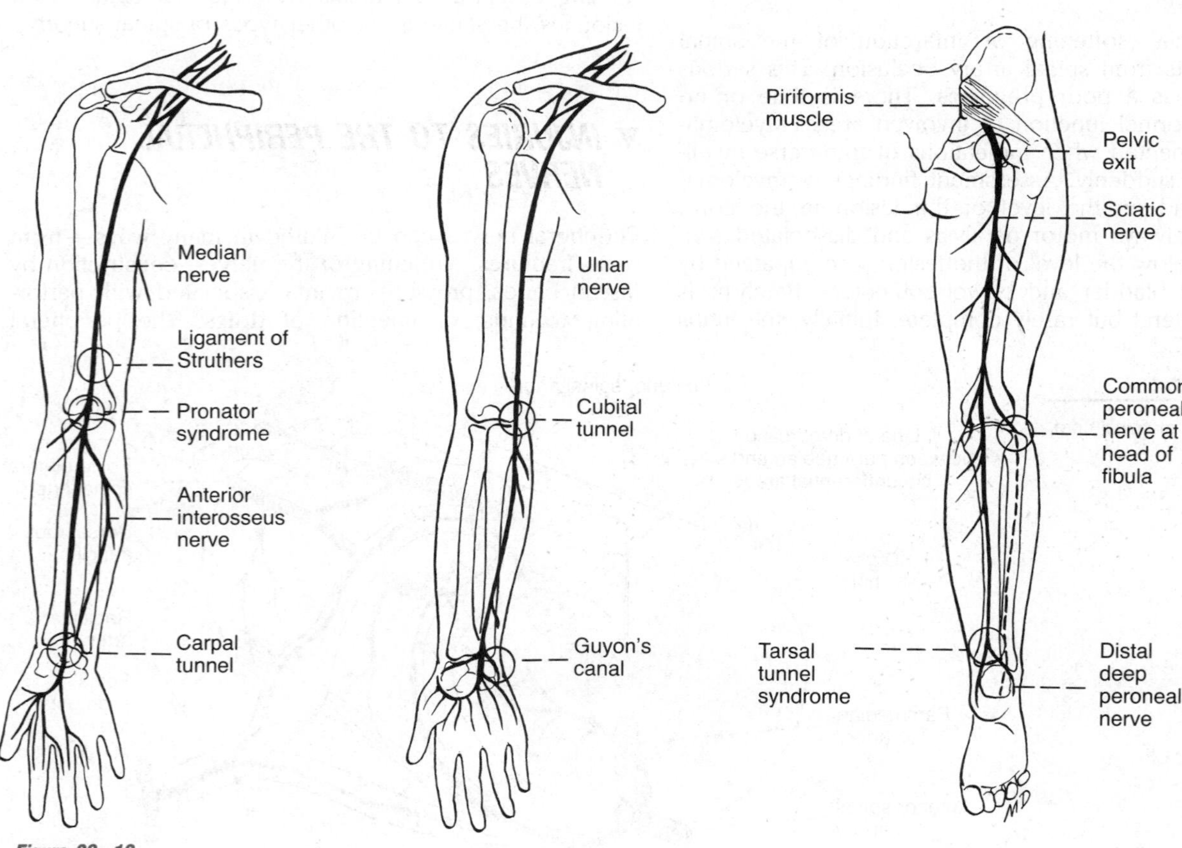

▲ **Figure 32–12**

Entrapment neuropathies.

flexor retinaculum and deep fascia along the foot's medial border.

ULNAR NERVE COMPRESSION AT THE ELBOW

Lying within a bony groove at the elbow, the ulnar nerve is susceptible to compression from direct trauma to the elbow (hitting the crazy bone) or from changes within the groove that gradually squeeze the nerve. Repeated mild trauma (e.g., habitual leaning on the elbows on a hard surface) can injure the ulnar nerve. Sensory changes occur in the ulnar aspect of the hand and wrist. The usual treatment for ulnar nerve compression at the elbow is surgical transplantation of the ulnar nerve.

SCIATIC NERVE INJURY

The sciatic nerve is the longest nerve in the body. The common peroneal nerve (a terminal branch of the sciatic) is injured more frequently than any other nerve. Because of its particular course and distribution, the sciatic nerve is exposed to internal and external trauma and inflammation more than any other nerve.

Sciatica is severe, usually constant pain in a lower extremity that occurs along the course of the sciatic nerve and its branches. There are many causes of sciatica. However, in about 90 per cent of people, the causes are ruptured intervertebral disc or osteoarthritis of the lumbosacral spine, producing mechanical pressure on the nerve or its spinal roots. Sciatic nerve injury can also result from incorrect medication injection technique.

Typically, the pain of sciatica begins in the buttocks and extends down the back of the thigh and leg to the ankle. Any movement of the lower extremities that stretches the nerve causes pain and involuntary resistance. Straight-leg raising on the affected side is limited. Complete extension of the leg is not possible when the thigh is flexed on the abdomen (Lasègue's sign). Treatment of sciatica is based on treating the underlying cause when possible. Laminectomy may be necessary.

▼ DISORDERS OF THE PERIPHERAL AND CRANIAL NERVES

Cranial and peripheral nerves may be damaged by tumors, infections, trauma, vascular and metabolic disturbances, and toxic agents. Neuritis is nerve damage from any cause. Mononeuritis is injury to a single nerve as a result of localized injury. Polyneuritis is diffuse damage to many nerves as a result of toxic agents or metabolic disturbances. Assessment findings with nerve damage depend on the type of nerve injured and the extent of damage.

Damaged motor nerves cause clinical manifestations such as flaccid paralysis, muscle wasting, and reflex loss in the muscle innervated by the injured nerve.

Damaged mixed nerves or sensory nerves cause vasomotor and trophic disturbances following either partial or complete interruption of the nerve. Following partial injury or incomplete division of a nerve, the person may experience stabbing pains, dysesthesias (pins-and-needles sensation), and occasionally the burning pains of causalgia. Damaged sensory nerves cause loss of sensation in the nerves' area of anatomic distribution.

PERIPHERAL NERVE TUMORS

Overview

Although solitary tumors (generally neurofibromas) may develop on any peripheral nerve, multiple tumors most often occur and are part of a syndrome known as neurofibromatosis (von Recklinghausen's disease). This hereditary disorder is characterized by multiple tumors of spinal and cranial nerves along with the involvement of many other systems. The disease is usually not life threatening, and lesions are excised only when they interfere with normal activity. Intracranial and intraspinal tumors are usually removed.

Management

Surgery for peripheral nerve entrapment is often done on an outpatient basis. In the recovery room, the dressings are checked for drainage and circulation, motion, and sensation to the extremity is assessed. Clients are encouraged to perform ROM exercises. Clients and family members are taught the signs of circulatory compromise and infection, medication management, and care of the dressing and/or incision.

CRANIAL NERVE DISORDERS

Cranial nerves can be affected in many ways by various nervous system disorders. For example, they may be secondarily affected by compression resulting from increased intracranial pressure or they may be directly damaged as a result of head injuries. In this section, diseases specific to the cranial nerves, not those associated with other disorders, are discussed. Regeneration of the first (olfactory) or second (optic) cranial nerve does not occur, because these nerves are actually part of the CNS.

TRIGEMINAL NEURALGIA

Definition

Trigeminal neuralgia is pain in the distribution of the fifth cranial nerve, the trigeminal nerve. The trigeminal nerve has three branches, the ophthalmic, maxillary, and mandibular (Fig. 32–13). Trigeminal neuralgia may occur in any one or more of these branches.

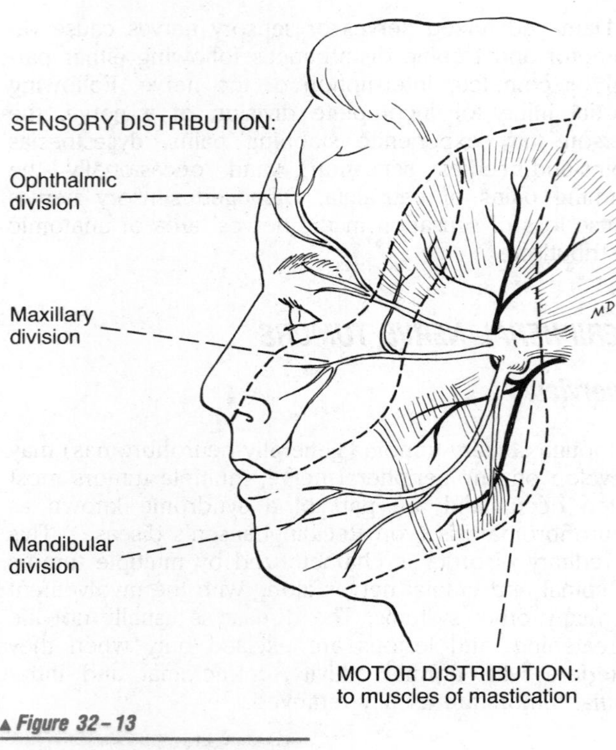

▲ *Figure 32-13*

Distribution of the trigeminal nerve.

Incidence

Trigeminal neuralgia occurs in about 1 of every 25,000 people. There are approximately 15,000 cases diagnosed each year in the United States. Trigeminal neuralgia can occur in adults of any age but is most common among the 50- to 70-year-old population. Approximately 60 per cent of clients are female.

Etiology

The causative mechanisms for trigeminal neuralgia can be divided into intrinsic and extrinsic lesions. Intrinsic lesions are those that occur within the nerve itself. These include gross abnormalities of the axon or myelin and multiple sclerosis.

Extrinsic lesions are outside the trigeminal root and cause distortion, stretching, or compression of the nerve. Mechanical compression is the most common extrinsic etiology. This compression may arise from a tumor or from vascular anomalies. Compression of the nerve by a blood vessel is a very common etiology. Dental abscesses may also result in irritation of the trigeminal nerve.

Risk Factors

There are no identified risk factors for trigeminal neuralgia. Consequently, there are no primary or secondary preventive measures. Tertiary prevention centers on minimizing the complications that can accompany any cranial pathology.

Pathophysiology

The current theory is that chronic irritation of the trigeminal nerve sets up a cascade of responses. The first response is that segmental inhibition within the trigeminal nucleus fails. This leads to hyperactivity of the primary afferent fibers because action potentials arise from ectopic foci. Tactile stimulation leads to paroxysmal neuronal discharges, triggering of nociceptive neurons, and a trigeminal neuralgia episode.

Clinical Manifestations

Trigeminal neuralgia is characterized by intermittent episodes of intense pain with sudden onset. This pain is not relieved by analgesics. Tactile stimulation, such as touch and facial hygiene, and even talking, may trigger an attack. Trigeminal neuralgia is more prevalent in the maxillary and mandibular distributions and on the right side of the face. Bilateral trigeminal neuralgia is rare but does occur.

DIAGNOSTIC ASSESSMENT

None of the diagnostic studies identifies trigeminal neuralgia as such. CT, MRI, and angiography can identify a causative lesion. The actual diagnosis is made on the basis of an in-depth history with attention paid to triggering stimuli and the nature and site of the pain.

Medical Management

The anticonvulsants carbamazepine (Tegretol) and phenytoin (Dilantin) are often prescribed as initial treatment for trigeminal neuralgia. The rationale for using these drugs is that they may dampen the reactivity of the neurons within the trigeminal nerve. For some clients, these medications are all the treatment that is ever needed. Liver impairment may result from administration of both Tegretol and Dilantin. Liver enzymes must be monitored before and during therapy. These medications should be used cautiously in clients with a history of alcohol abuse. Baclofen (Lioresal) is an antispasmodic that may be used alone or in conjunction with the anticonvulsants. Narcotics are not particularly effective in relieving trigeminal neuralgia pain.

Surgical Management

Surgical procedures can be categorized according to invasiveness. Less invasive procedures are nerve blocks using alcohol and glycerol, peripheral neurectomy, and percutaneous radiofrequency lesions. The relief obtained with these procedures is not always permanent. Complications include development of facial paresthesias and muscular weakness. These procedures, being less invasive, are often better tolerated by elderly or debilitated clients.

The more invasive techniques involve major surgical procedures. Microvascular decompression involves removing the vessel from the posterior trigeminal root. Rhizotomy is actual resection of the root of the nerve. These procedures require a craniotomy to allow access to the nerve. Complications include those of any surgical procedure as well as facial weakness and paresthesias.

Nursing Management

A careful history is obtained from the client regarding stimuli that trigger an attack. This information is used to plan care so as to minimize triggering events. The client's dental hygiene and nutritional intake are evaluated. These clients often do not eat enough to meet their daily nutritional needs and neglect their teeth because of the pain.

The nurse helps clients use and improve any pain control strategies they have developed. Individuals with trigeminal neuralgia need emotional support to help them deal with pain that has often been present for a long time.

Clients should be taught to use a water jet device instead of a toothbrush for dental hygiene, and a visit to the dentist as soon as possible after surgery should be recommended. If facial anesthesia is present following surgery, clients must learn to test the temperature of food before putting it into their mouth. They should chew on the unaffected side and inspect mucous membranes for irritation. The nurse assesses for aspiration and advances the diet slowly.

If the corneal reflex has been impaired, the client will need to be taught eye care. During the acute postoperative period, the nurse needs to apply eye drops and a protective shield. The client assumes these tasks with supervision and then independently.

BELL'S PALSY: SEVENTH CRANIAL (FACIAL) NERVE

Overview

This discussion concerns motor aspects of the facial nerve, the main motor nerve of the facial muscles. The facial nerve becomes paralyzed more often than any other. Facial paralysis may be central or peripheral in origin. Central facial palsy is an upper motor neuron paralysis or paresis. Sometimes it produces dissociation of motor function. In this situation, the client cannot voluntarily show the teeth on the paralyzed side, but can show them with emotional stimulation such as that causing smiles or laughter. This phenomenon is called voluntary emotional dissociation.

Bell's palsy is the most common type of peripheral facial paralysis. Bell's palsy is a unilateral paralysis of the facial muscles of expression with no evidence of a pathologic cause. Assessment findings on the affected side include (1) upward movement of the eyeball on closing the eye (Bell's phenomenon), (2) drooping of the mouth, (3) flattening of the nasolabial fold, (4) widening of the palpebral fissure, and (5) a slight lag in closing the eye. Eating may be difficult. Bell's palsy affects both women and men in all age groups. However, it is most common between ages 20 and 40 (Fig. 32-14).

Management

There is no known cure for Bell's palsy. Palliative measures include

- ▶ Analgesics if discomfort occurs from herpetic involvement;
- ▶ Corticosteroids to decrease nerve tissue edema;
- ▶ Physiotherapy, moist heat, gentle massage, stimulation of facial nerve with faradic current; and
- ▶ Corneal protection with artificial tear solution, sunglasses, eyepatch at night, and periodic gentle closure of the eye.

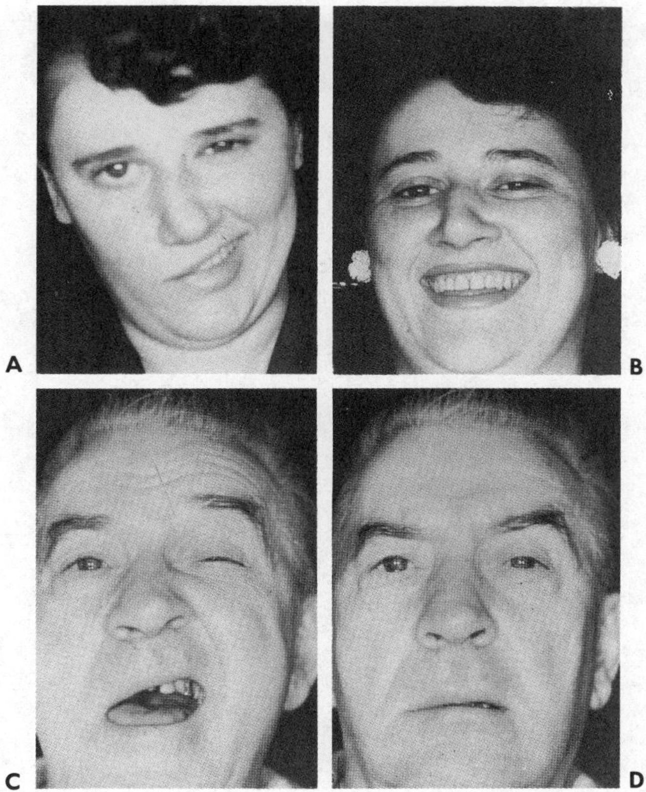

▲ **Figure 32-14**

A, Bell's palsy of 1 week's duration. *B*, After treatment, the paralysis of the seventh nerve disappeared. *C*, Bell's palsy following exposure to cold. Note right-sided paralysis and inability to close the right eye. *D*, Drooping of the right lip. (From Archer, W. H. [1975]. Oral and maxillofacial surgery [5th ed., pp. 1669, 1672]. Philadelphia: W. B. Saunders Company.)

Clients experiencing Bell's palsy often think they have had a stroke. Reassure the client that this is not true. Most clients recover from Bell's palsy within a few weeks without residual symptoms. If permanent complete facial paralysis occurs, surgery may be necessary. Anastomosis of the peripheral end of the facial nerve with the spinal accessory or the hypoglossal nerve allows closure of the eye during sleep and restores tone to the facial musculature.

Summary

Disorders of the peripheral nervous system range from life-threatening spinal cord injuries to temporary peripheral nerve compressions. This chapter focused on the spinal-cord-injured client. These clients have sustained a serious physical and psychological impairment. It is imperative that nurses comprehend the severity of the disorder and the impact it has on the client's life and livelihood.

Bibliography

1. Berard, E. J. (1989). The sexuality of spinal cord injured women: Physiology and pathophysiology. A review. *Paraplegia, 27*(2), 99.
2. Berard, E. J., et al. (1989). Effects of bethanechol and adrenoblockers on thermoregulation in spinal cord injury. *Paraplegia, 27*(1), 46.
3. Beretta, G., et al. (1989). Reproductive aspects in spinal cord injured males. *Paraplegia, 27*(2), 113–118.
4. Bodner, D. R., et al. (1989). The effect of verapamil on the treatment of detrusor hyperreflexia in the spinal cord injured population. *Paraplegia, 27*(5), 364.
5. Dunnum, L. (1989). Life satisfaction and spinal cord injury: The patient perspective. *Journal of Neuroscience Nursing, 21*(6), 43.
6. Frank, R. G., & Elliott, T. R. (1989). Spinal cord injury and health locus of control beliefs. *Paraplegia, 27*(4), 250–256.
7. Gaehle, K. E., et al. (1992). Thoracolumbar burst fractures. *AORN Journal 55*(3), 721–731.
8. Goldberg, S. (1986). *Clinical neuroanatomy made ridiculously simple.* Miami, FL: Medmaster.
9. Huang, C., et al. (1990). Anemia in acute phase of spinal cord injury. *Archives of Physical Medicine and Rehabilitation, 71,* 3.
10. Ingram, R. R., et al. (1989). Lower limb fractures in the chronic spinal cord injured patient. *Paraplegia, 27*(2), 133.
11. Kawamura, J., et al. (1989). The clinical features of spasms in patients with a cervical cord injury. *Paraplegia, 27*(3), 222.
12. Little, J. W., et al. (1989). Lower extremity manifestations of spasticity in chronic spinal cord injury. *American Journal of Physical Medicine and Rehabilitation, 68*(1), 32.
13. Marshall, S. B., et al. (1990). *Neuroscience critical care: Pathophysiology and patient management.* Philadelphia: W. B. Saunders Company.
14. Mitchell, M. (1989). *Neuroscience nursing: A nursing diagnosis approach.* Baltimore: Williams & Wilkins.
15. Presksto, D. (1992). The Kaneda device: A new anterior spine stabilization system. *AORN Journal, 55*(3), 734–746.
16. Rivara, F., et al. (1988). The public cost of motorcycle trauma. *Journal of the American Medical Association, 260*(2), 221–223.
17. Spica, M. M. (1989). Sexual counseling standards for the spinal cord-injured. *Journal of Neuroscience Nursing, 21*(1), 56.
18. Youmans, J. R. (1990). *Neurological surgery* (3rd ed.). Philadelphia: W. B. Saunders Company.

Unit 7

Sensory Disorders

To communicate is a basic human need. Essential to this interaction is the adequate functioning of our senses. A person unable to receive sensory input (e.g., through sight, sound, smell, taste, and touch) is disabled in communicating. For example, children born deaf or who develop hearing loss before learning speech not only have difficulty hearing sounds but also have difficulty learning to talk effectively. Likewise, people with impaired vision are limited in the amount of visual stimuli they can take in, interpret, and respond to. Both forms of sensory alterations increase the risk of injury.

Our senses are also a source of pleasure. Consider the joys of looking at the face of a loved one, hearing a bird sing, smelling the fragrance of a flower, tasting a favorite food, and stroking a companion animal. How would it affect you if you were to realize you would never again be able to enjoy the pleasures you derive from even one of your senses? Clients experiencing sensory disorders live with the reality and hardships of sensory deprivation.

We take our senses for granted, using them to function smoothly every moment of every day. Only when we lose sensory ability do we realize how we depended on it. This unit's chapters consider the problems experienced by people with sensory disorders of the eyes and ears. This unit also considers other problems of the eyes and ears.

Chapter 33 focuses on clients experiencing problems of the eyes and vision. Discussion includes basic structure and function, assessment, general care and protection of the eyes and vision, and appropriate nursing intervention related to eye disorders and their management. Chapter 34 discusses problems clients experience with their ears and hearing. Content pertains to basic structure and function, assessment, general care and protection of the ear and hearing, and appropriate nursing intervention related to problems of the ear, hearing, and management of these problems.

Chapter 33

Structure and Function; Assessment and Nursing Care of Clients with Eye Disorders

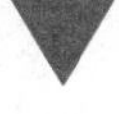

The eye is a complex organ that involves intricate microscopic structures capable of bringing the entire world into the mind. The visual pathway is a multidimensional system that transcends anatomic description. Although there have been great technologic advances in understanding ocular physiology, there remains an element of mystery regarding the science of vision.

The use of sight is an integral part of early life experiences. Most individuals are not consciously aware of the degree to which they depend on it for daily functioning. Once vision becomes significantly limited, the degree to which sight influences the activities of daily living becomes acutely apparent. Even simple tasks become difficult to perform. Seeing what food is being served at the table, selecting clothes for color and design, avoiding objects while walking, and reading books, magazines, or personal mail are no longer possible. The visually impaired person must adapt to this loss in order to maintain independence and control.

The role that vision plays in our lives is difficult to define. It is deeply personal and intimate. It is the connection between the mind and the body and the rest of the world. Leonardo da Vinci (1452 to 1519) best described this internal connection in his attempts to understand the human body. He wrote ". . . Now do you not see that the eye embraces the beauty of the whole world? It is the lord of astronomy and the maker of cosmography; it counsels and corrects all the arts of mankind; it leads men to the different parts of the world; it is the prince of mathematics, and the sciences founded on it are absolutely certain. It has measured the distances and sizes of the stars; it has found the elements and their locations; it . . . has given birth to architecture, and to perspective, and to divine art of painting. Oh excellent thing, superior to all others created by God! . . . What peoples, what tongues will fully describe your true function? The eye is the window of the human body through which it feels its way and enjoys the beauty of the world. Owing to the eye, the soul is content to stay in its bodily prison, for without it such bodily prison is torture."

Instinctively, various cultures throughout history have all placed an extremely high value on the eyes and vision. There are protocols for treatment of eye problems documented as early as 1500 BC in the Code of Hammurabi. However, in the modern Western world, the priorities of cost containment and convenience have become primary concerns in providing health care. Some types of eye surgery are inappropriately advertised as minor procedures, requiring little or no preparation, care, or concern. The challenges for the nurse are to assist the client in understanding these incomplete messages to the public and to provide quality ophthalmic health education.

▼ STRUCTURE AND FUNCTION OF THE EYE

STRUCTURE

The entire visual system is a complex group of structures that includes the eyeballs, muscles, nerves, fat, and bones. Although the eyes are intricate receptacles for light that adapt to varying conditions such as light intensity and object distance, the eyes do not actually see. The eyes are the external portion of the visual pathway to the brain. The pathway transmits and ultimately converts electrical impulses into vision. The eyes are often referred to as eyeballs or globes. They are not true spheres, however, but are actually a combination of two spheres with different curvatures.

Ocular Adnexa

The ocular adnexa are the accessory structures of the eye (muscles, fat, and bone) that support and protect it. Bony orbits and pads of fat surround each eye (Fig. 33-1).

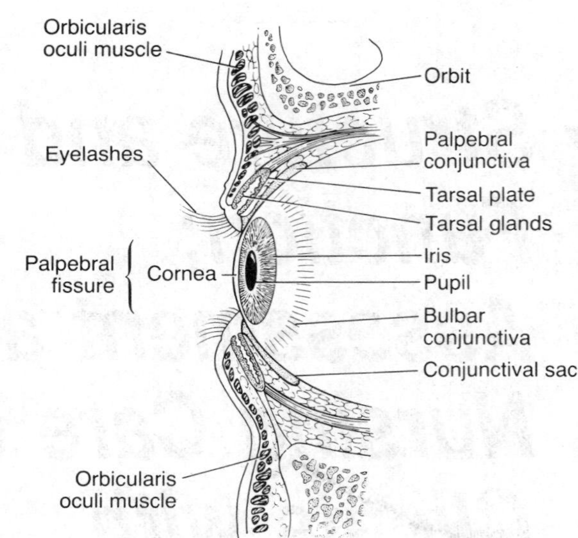

▲ Figure 33-1

Ocular adnexa.

OCULAR MUSCLES

The eyeball is moved by six ocular muscles, which are attached to the surface of the globe (Fig. 33-2). The four rectus muscles (the medial, lateral, superior, and inferior) move the eyes horizontally and vertically. The two oblique muscles (the superior and inferior) primarily rotate the eye in circular movements to allow vision at all angles.

EYELIDS

The eyelids (upper and lower) are elastic folds of skin that close to protect the anterior eyeball. When they close, the eyelids also distribute a film of tears, which prevents evaporation and drying of the surface epithelium.

The elliptic space between the two open lids is the palpebral fissure. The corners of the fissure are called the canthi. The medial or inner canthus is next to the nose and the lateral or outer canthus is the outside corner. (Fig. 33-3). Oil-secreting glands called the meibomian glands are embedded in both upper and lower lids.

LACRIMAL APPARATUS

The lacrimal gland is in the upper lid over the outer canthus and produces tears that reach the eyeball through secretory ducts. Tiny openings called puncti in both the upper and lower lids at the inner canthus direct tears to the lacrimal sac. The nasolacrimal duct directs the flow of tears into the nose (Fig. 33-4). The tear film is composed of lipids secreted by the meibomian glands, and dissolved salts, glucose, urea, protein, and lysozyme secreted by the lacrimal glands. Along with mucus secreted by goblet cells located in the lids, the tear film both lubricates and cleans the ocular surface.

Internal Eye

In the normal adult, the eye measures approximately 24 mm in diameter.

CONJUNCTIVA

The conjunctiva is a thin transparent layer of mucous membrane that lines the eyelids and covers the eyeball. The palpebral conjunctiva lines the eyelids and is contiguous with the bulbar conjunctiva which covers the eyeball. The elasticity of the bulbar conjunctiva allows the eye to move freely; however, the continuous sur-

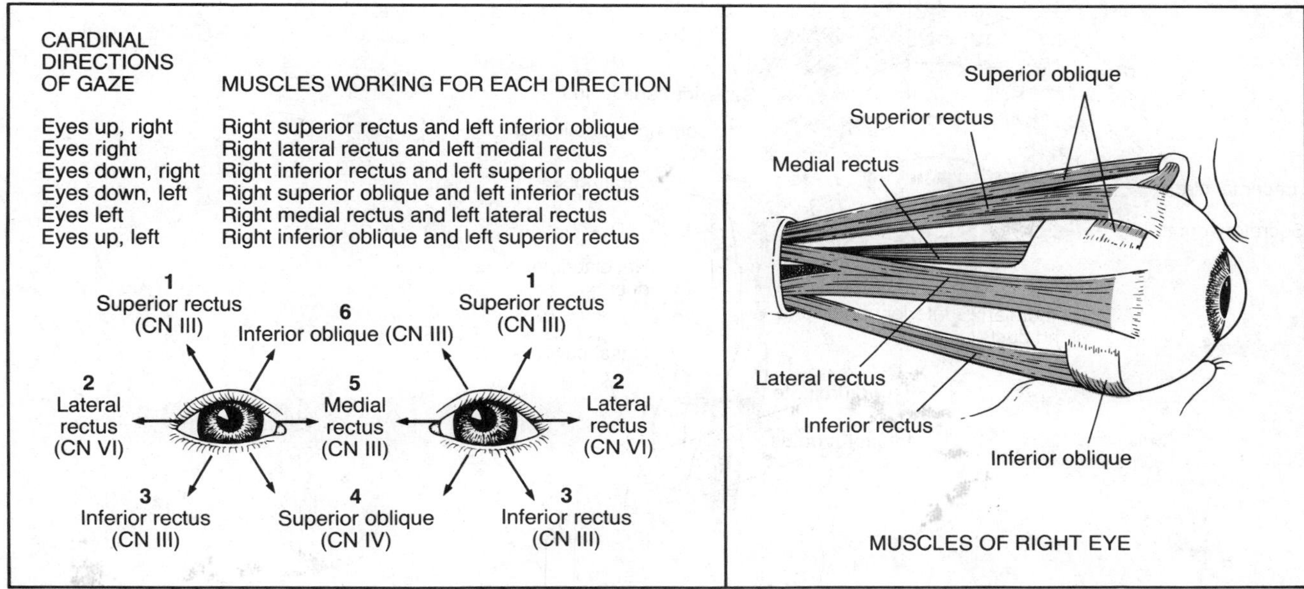

▲ *Figure 33-2*

The six cardinal directions of gaze and the muscles responsible for each. The six cardinal directions are (1) R—right, (2) L—left, (3) UR—up and right, (4) UL—up and left, (5) DR—down and right, and (6) DL—down and left.

face prevents the eye from coming out of its socket (see Fig. 33-1).

CORNEA

The cornea is a transparent avascular structure, with a brilliant, shiny surface (Fig. 33-5*A*). It is convex in shape and acts as a powerful lens to bend and direct (refract) rays of light to the retina. It is about 0.5 mm thick and composed of five layers. The cornea derives oxygen from the atmosphere (Fig. 33-5*B*). A rich network of nerve fibers in the outer layer (epithelium) produces a sensation of pain whenever the fibers are exposed.

SCLERA

The sclera is the fibrous protective coating of the eye. It is white, dense, and continuous with the cornea. In children, the sclera is thin and appears bluish because of the underlying pigmented structures. In old age, it may become yellowish because of degeneration.

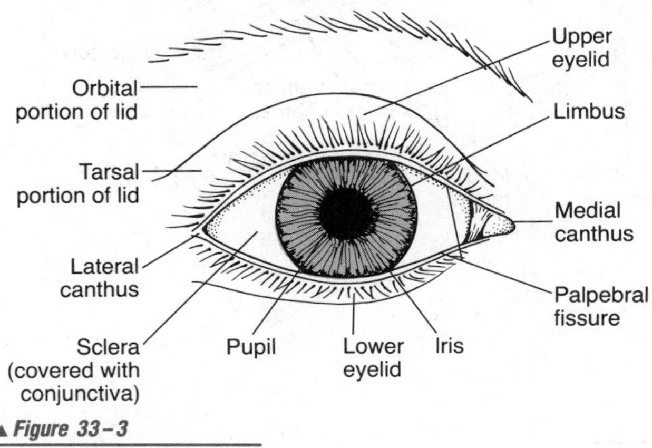

▲ *Figure 33-3*

Surface anatomy of the eye.

UVEAL TRACT

The uveal tract consists of three structures: (1) the iris, (2) ciliary body, and (3) choroid. The tract is the middle vascular layer of the eye and furnishes the blood supply to the retina.

Iris. The iris is a thin, pigmented diaphragm with a central aperture, the pupil. Iris color is determined by the degree of pigmentation in the stromal melanocytes. Pupil diameter is determined by the interaction of the two iris muscles—the sphincter and the dilator. Expansion and contraction of the iris regulate the amount of light entering the eye. As the iris contracts, it forms visible furrows on the surface. Between the iris and the cornea is a clear fluid called the aqueous humor. This fluid occupies the space called the anterior chamber of the eye.

Ciliary Body. The ciliary body is in direct continuity with the iris and is circular, surrounding the lens. It produces and secretes the aqueous humor, an alkaline fluid composed mainly of water. The ciliary body also supports the lens, because the lens' zonules insert into the ciliary body.

The aqueous humor is secreted by the ciliary body and circulates from the posterior chamber through the pupil into the anterior chamber (see Fig. 33-5*A*). The flow continues into the anterior chamber angle and is filtered out through the trabecular meshwork into Schlemm's canal (see Fig. 33-5*C*). From there aqueous is channeled into a capillary network and into

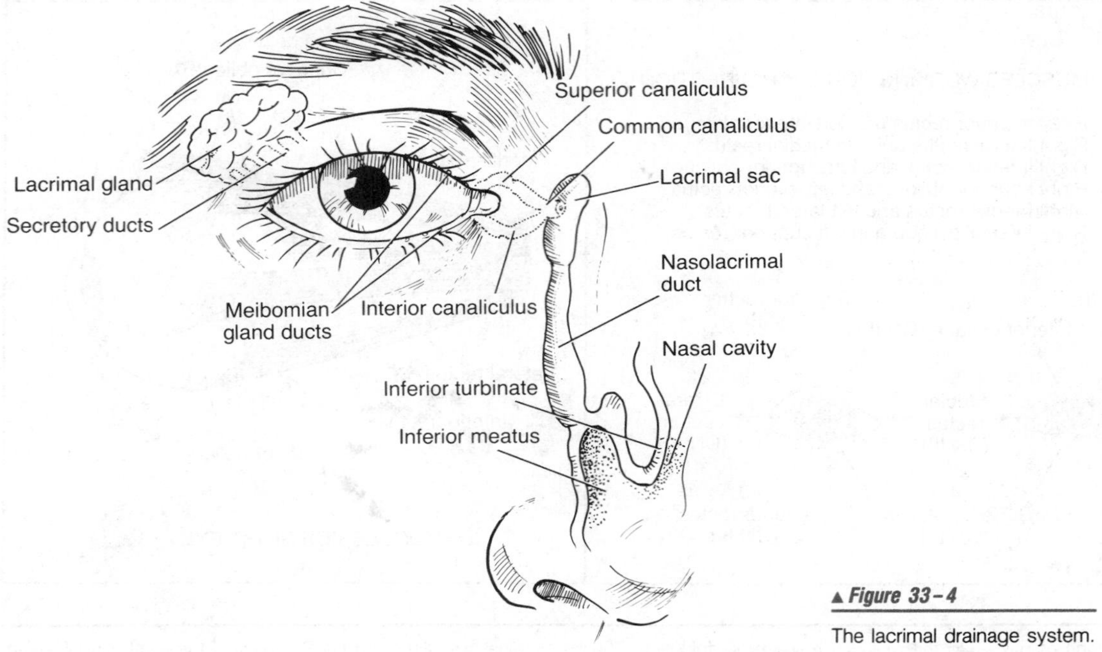

▲ ***Figure 33-4***

The lacrimal drainage system.

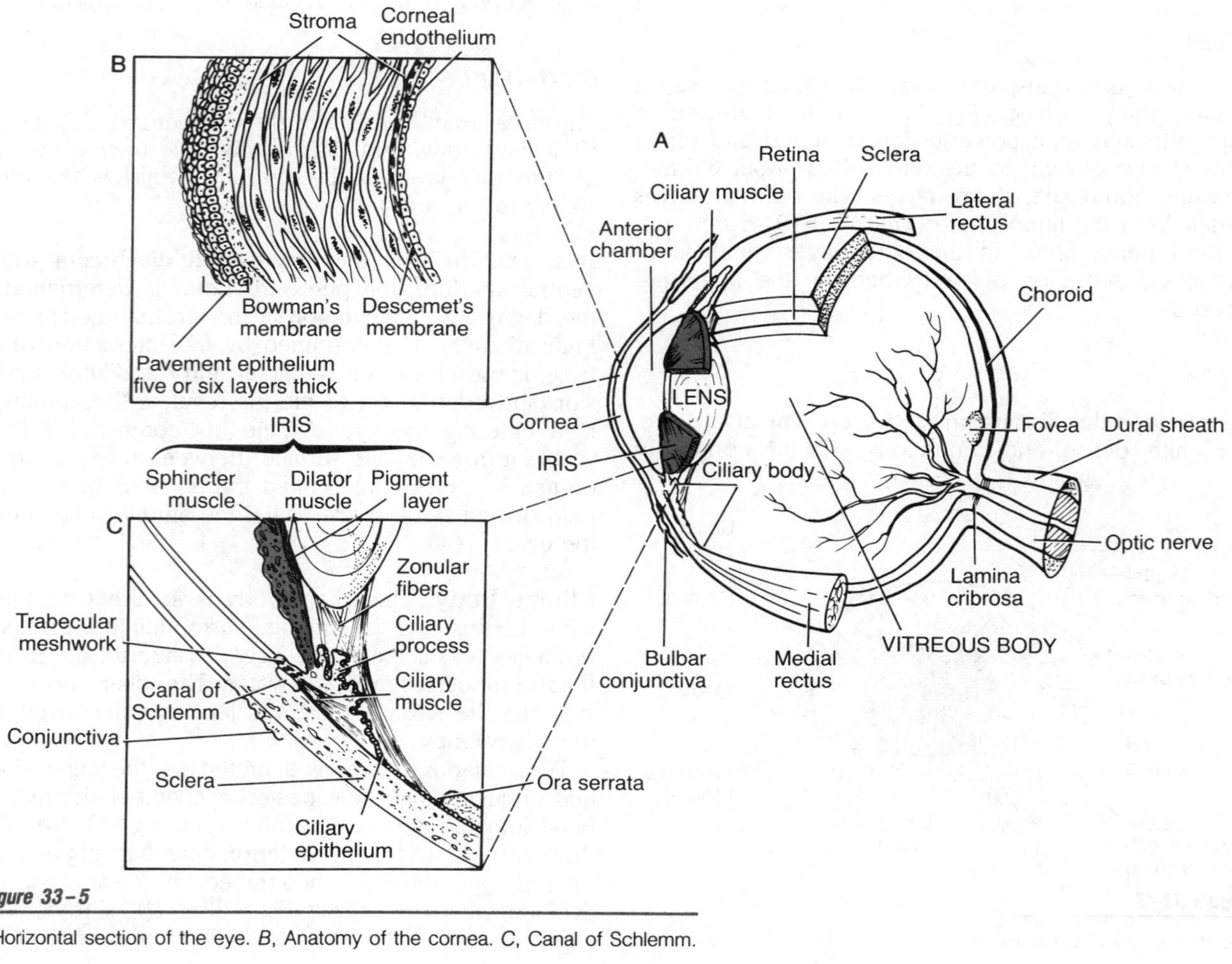

▲ ***Figure 33-5***

A, Horizontal section of the eye. *B*, Anatomy of the cornea. *C*, Canal of Schlemm.

episcleral veins. Normal intraocular pressure is maintained as long as there is a balance between the aqueous production and the aqueous outflow.

Choroid. The choroid is the posterior segment of the uveal tract between the retina and the sclera. It is composed of three layers of vessels and is attached to both the ciliary body and the optic nerve.

ANGLE STRUCTURES

Although the angle of the anterior chamber is not really a structure, it is a critical component of the eye. The angle is formed where the cornea and the iris meet. At the apex of the angle, a filtering system called the trabecular meshwork allows the outflow of the aqueous fluid. Aqueous is filtered out through the trabeculum into Schlemm's canal and then flows into the venous drainage system (see Fig. 33-5*C*).

LENS

The lens is a biconvex, avascular, colorless, and almost completely transparent structure, about 4 mm thick and 9 mm in diameter. It is suspended behind the iris by ligamentous fibers called zonules, which connect to the ciliary body. The sole purpose of the lens is to focus light on the retina. The physiologic interplay of the zonular fibers and elasticity of the lens allows for focusing on nearby or distant objects. The change of focus from distant to near is called accommodation. There are no pain fibers or blood vessels in the lens. The lens is surrounded by a transparent envelope called the capsule. The lens of the eye consists of about 65 per cent water and 35 per cent protein. The protein content is the highest of any tissue in the body. Potassium, ascorbic acid, and glutathione are also present in the lens.

VITREOUS HUMOR

The vitreous is a clear, avascular, jelly-like structure. The fluid is thick, viscous, and occupies a space called the vitreous chamber. It fills the largest cavity of the eye, accounting for two thirds of its volume. It helps maintain the shape and transparency of the eye.

RETINA

The retina is a thin, semitransparent layer of nerve tissue that forms the innermost lining of the eye. It consists of 10 distinct layers of highly organized, delicate tissue. The retina contains all the sensory receptors for the transmission of light, and is really part of the brain. There are two types of retinal receptors—the rods and the cones. The approximately 125 million rods are distributed in the periphery of the retina and function best in dim light. Damage to these structures results in night blindness. The cones, numbering about 6 million, provide for the resolution of small visual angles, resulting in perception of fine details. They are also responsible for color vision. The cones are concentrated in an area about 1.5 mm in the center of the retina. Damage to this area can severely reduce central vision. The center of the retina is an area about 5 mm in diameter called the macula. In an ophthalmoscopic examination, it appears as a yellowish spot with a depressed center (the fovea). The fovea, an area of 1.5 mm where only cones are present, is the point of finest vision.

The retina is composed of many fine layers of neural tissue attached to a single layer of pigmented epithelial cells. The photoreceptor cells in the retina are nourished by the capillaries of the choroid layer just beneath the pigment epithelial cell layer. Oxygen supply to these delicate structures is critical because the conversion of visual stimuli into impulses the brain records as images requires very active metabolic processes.

OPTIC NERVE

The optic nerve is located at the posterior portion of the eye and transmits visual impulses from the retina to the brain. The head of the optic nerve can be seen by ophthalmoscopic examination and is called the optic disc. The optic nerve contains no sensory receptors (rods or cones) and represents a blind spot in the eye. The nerve emerges from the back of the eye and extends for 25 to 30 mm, traveling through the muscle cone to enter the bony optic foramen and eventually joins the other optic nerve to form the optic chiasm. One half of the visual field of each eye is projected to the other side of the brain. For example, visual impulses from the right visual field of each eye are transmitted to the left occipital lobe (see Fig. 30-4).

FUNCTION

In human beings, the two eyes collaborate to work as though they were one, projecting to the same point in space and fusing their images so that a single mental impression is obtained. The ability of the eyes to fuse two images into a single one is called binocular vision.

Effects of Aging on the Eye

There are several age-related changes that occur in the structures of the eye and surrounding tissue.

EXTERNAL CHANGES

Eyebrows and eyelashes turn gray, and the skin around the eyelids becomes wrinkled and loosened due to loss of muscle tone and elasticity. Loss of orbital fat causes the eyes to sink deeper into the orbit and, sometimes, limits the upward gaze. Tear secretions may also diminish resulting in the condition of dry eyes.

CATARACT

The most frequent and significant age-related change in the eye is the formation of a cataract. With age, the thickness and density of the lens increase and the lens becomes progressively yellowed and opaque. Throughout the lifespan, the lens continues to grow by repeated formation of new fiber cells. The rate of growth, however, gradually diminishes. By the age of 70, formation of new fibers is considerably reduced, producing an age-related cell density. Loss of transparency is also due to molecular deterioration from the absorption of ultraviolet radiation. The yellow material is associated with the development of abnormal fluorescent substances in the aging lens. The lens also loses its accommodative power due to the atrophy of the ciliary muscles.

CORNEAL FUNCTION

The inner cell layer of the cornea (endothelium) decreases in numbers with age. Because this layer does not reproduce lost cells, the ability of this layer to heal after injury or surgery may be compromised. The corneal reflex also may be diminished or absent. Another phenomenon characteristic of aging is arcus senilis, which is a grayish yellow ring found on the periphery of the cornea surrounding the iris. This visible ring is thought to be the result of the accumulation of lipids.

UVEAL TRACT FUNCTION

The ciliary body produces less aqueous humor during the aging process, but there is less outflow, so the intraocular pressure remains relatively stable or increases just slightly. The ciliary muscle tends to atrophy with age, and sometimes, connective tissue replaces lost muscle tissue. The loss in muscle action, along with lens thickening, decreases the focusing ability of the lens. Decreasing ability to focus at near accommodation is called presbyopia.

VISUAL PERCEPTION

The major visual changes with aging include a decrease in visual acuity, tolerance of glare, ability to adapt to dark and light, and peripheral vision. All of these decreases are related to the changes in the eye structure, and all affect the quality and intensity of the light that is able to reach the retina.

GLARE TOLERANCE

Glare is a particular problem for the elderly. In combination with difficulty adjusting to dark and light, it is often the reason older people stop driving at night. The lights from oncoming traffic produce a glare from both the cornea and lens, which may make discernment of objects very difficult. In a similar manner, bright sunlight, either indoors or outdoors, causes an equally blinding glare. Indoor rooms should be lit with soft incandescent light and sheer curtains may be used to diffuse bright sunlight.

ADAPTATION TO DARK AND LIGHT

Because it takes longer to adapt to changes from dark to light and vice versa, older people are at a greater risk for falls and injuries. Any place where there is a sudden change from dark to light or light to dark can be dangerous. Entering theaters and getting up at night are two particularly hazardous situations that may be risky for older adults. It is interesting to note that eyes adapt to the dark by using the rod receptors, which are sensitive to short blue-green wavelengths. Red wavelengths are longer and are perceived by the cones. Thus, a red light in the bathroom at night allows for enough vision to function in the dark without the need for adaptation.

PERIPHERAL VISION

Peripheral vision also decreases with age and often interferes with social interactions and physical activities. Older adults suffering from peripheral vision loss may not notice someone sitting next to them and may also have difficulty finding objects out of their range of vision.

LIGHT PERCEPTION

The iris loses pigment with age so that many older people appear to have grayish or light blue eyes. The pupil becomes increasingly smaller with age. A decrease in pupil size results in a smaller amount of light reaching the retina, and the light must also pass through the densest and most opaque area of the lens.

VITREORETINAL FUNCTION

In the posterior chamber, the vitreous begins to liquefy and collapse. Small pieces of debris from separation and shrinkage may become visible as floaters, and although they may not obstruct vision, they are certainly an annoyance. Additionally, the retina also may degenerate due to local ischemia and loss of neural function.

▼ ASSESSMENT OF CLIENTS WITH EYE DISORDERS

One of the most important considerations in an ocular assessment is that many ophthalmic disorders are asymptomatic. The four most common preventable causes of permanent vision loss in developed nations are (1) amblyopia (reduced visual acuity that is uncorrectable with glasses in the absence of anatomic defects in the eye or visual pathways), (2) diabetic retinopathy, (3) age-related maculopathy, and (4) glaucoma. It is for these reasons that routine eye examinations are imperative.

The eye is a unique organ of the body in that the external anatomy of the eye may be easily assessed. Even the internal eye is visible through the cornea where blood vessels and central nervous system tissue (the retina and the optic nerve) may be visualized without the use of x-rays or invasive procedures. The effects of many systemic disorders, such as infections, neoplasms, vascular disorders, and autoimmune disorders, are detectable with an internal eye examination.

HISTORY

An ophthalmic history includes demographic data, the chief complaint, past medical history, family history, psychosocial history, and review of systems.

Demographic Data

Demographic data relevant to ocular assessment include age and sex. The incidence of cataracts, dry eye, retinal detachment, glaucoma, entropion, and ectropion increases with age. Males have hereditary color vision deficits. Women do not have as many hereditary visual problems.

Chief Complaint

The most common chief complaint is often a change or loss of vision but may also be less specific such as headache or eyestrain. It is common that the client is unable to verbalize a specific complaint. The chief complaint may be as vague as "Something is wrong with my eyes." Whenever possible, symptoms are characterized according to the rapidity of onset, the location, duration, and characteristics (such as frequency and severity). The associated circumstances surrounding onset are important, as well as the client's response to treatment. Current eye medications being used and all other current and past ocular disorders are recorded.

Ocular symptoms may be divided into three basic categories of abnormalities: (1) vision, (2) appearance, and (3) ocular sensation—pain and discomfort.

ABNORMAL VISION

Visual changes or loss of vision may be due to abnormalities in the eye or anywhere along the visual pathway. Considerations in this category include a refractive (focusing) error, lid ptosis (drooping of the eyelid), clouding or interference in the cornea, lens, aqueous or vitreous space, malfunction of the retina, optic nerve, or intracranial visual pathway.

Glare or halos may result from uncorrected refractive error, scratches on glasses, dilated pupils, corneal edema, or cataract. Flashing or flickering lights may indicate retinal traction or migraine. Floating spots may represent normal vitreous strands or the pathologic presence of blood, pigment, or inflammatory cells in the vitreous. Diplopia (double vision) may occur in one eye or both and may be due to refractive correction, muscle imbalance, or neuromuscular disorders.

ABNORMAL APPEARANCE

The most common abnormal appearance is the red eye. Causes of red eye include minor irritation, vascular congestion, subconjunctival hemorrhage, inflammatory disorders, infection, allergy, and trauma. Other external changes in appearance include growths or lesions, edema, redness, or abnormal position.

ABNORMAL SENSATION

Eye pain is often poorly localized. Nonspecific complaints may be eyestrain, pulling, pressure, fullness, or generalized headache. The pain may be periocular, ocular, or retrobulbar (behind the globe). Foreign body sensation produces a sharp superficial pain relieved by topical anesthesia. Deeper internal aching may indicate glaucoma, inflammation, muscle spasm, or infection. Reflex spasm of the ciliary muscle and iris sphincter that occurs with inflammation may produce brow ache and *photophobia* (sensitivity to light) or a constricted pupil (miosis). Itching is usually a sign of an allergic response. Dryness, burning, grittiness, and mild foreign body sensation can occur with dry eyes or mild corneal irritation. Tearing may be due to irritation or an abnormality of the lacrimal system. Increased ocular secretions usually indicate viral or bacterial infections and may also be present in allergic and noninfectious irritations.

Past Medical History

The past medical history focuses on the client's general state of health. Specifically, ask about systemic disorders commonly associated with ocular manifestations, such as diabetes mellitus, arthritis, hypertension, and thyroid disease.

CHILDHOOD AND INFECTIOUS DISEASES

Diseases occurring in childhood with possible ocular sequelae include diabetes mellitus, retinoblastoma, thyroid disorders, rheumatoid arthritis, exposure to sexually transmitted diseases such as syphilis and AIDS, and muscular dystrophy. Inquire about immunizations, particularly for measles (rubella).

MAJOR ILLNESSES AND HOSPITALIZATIONS

In addition to the above-mentioned systemic diseases, ask about hypertension and myasthenia gravis. Ocular diseases and structural problems include refractive errors (and corrective lenses used), strabismus, amblyopia, cataracts, glaucoma, and retinal detachment. If glasses or contact lenses are worn currently, ask when the last eye examination was and when the prescription was last changed. Inquire whether the client has been hospitalized or has had surgery related to the eyes or brain. Is there a history of head trauma or eye trauma related to motor vehicle accidents or sports injury? Has the client had surgery on the eyes such as laser treatment?

MEDICATIONS

Many medications affect the eyes. Prescription drugs include insulin, corticosteroids, oral hypoglycemics, and thyroid replacement hormones. Ask whether or not the client uses eye drops, and note the name, dose, and frequency taken. Specifically ask whether or not the client uses over-the-counter eye drops such as natural tears. Over-the-counter preparations that may dry the eyes include antihistamines and decongestants.

ALLERGIES

Note allergies to medications and other substances. Has the client ever had an allergic reaction to eye drops or other medications that have affected the eyes? Allergic symptoms include eye redness, tearing, and itching. Determine past allergic reactions not only to medications but also to inhalants (dust, chemicals, or pollens) and contactants (cosmetics or woolens).

Family History

Because there are many ocular disorders with familial tendencies, it is important to ask questions specifically about strabismus, glaucoma, myopia (nearsightedness), and hyperopia (farsightedness). Other common familial disorders include migraine, retinoblastoma, macular degeneration, retinitis pigmentosa, sickle cell anemia, keratoconus, and diabetes mellitus. Lack of a family history does not necessarily rule out the possibility of a genetic disorder. Some clients do not know the ocular history of family members, and some may be embarrassed or hesitant to share the information.

Psychosocial History and Lifestyle

Psychosocial history and lifestyle factors that influence ocular health include occupational hazards and leisure activities and hobbies. The nurse inquires about the nature of the client's work and hobbies. Is the client exposed to irritating fumes, smoke, or airborne particles? Are safety goggles worn in situations in which eye injury may occur from fragments of metal or sand? Is there a problem with insufficient lighting, leading to eyestrain or harsh, glaring lighting? Leisure and sports activities with increased incidence of eye injury include baseball, racquetball, and contact sports with potential for head trauma such as football. Participation in active outdoor activities such as gardening, hiking, and cross-country skiing increases risk of foreign body injury, abrasion, or penetrating injury. Does the client wear sunglasses or other protective eye gear when outdoors?

Health management behaviors related to the eyes are explored. If the client has a systemic disease that affects the eyes, are self-care measures practiced? For example, does the diabetic client aggressively manage the disease by attempting to regulate blood glucose levels with diet and ordered medication? If the client wears contact lenses, are the lenses cleaned and stored as recommended? Is the client capable of safely taking care of the lenses?

Review of Systems

The review of systems relevant to the eyes includes asking about symptoms such as headaches and problems with sinusitis. Specifically, ask whether symptoms occur in association with pain or discomfort, visual changes, swelling, redness, or drainage from the eye.

Detailed questions for the ROS are found in Chapter 11, Table 11–5.

PHYSICAL EXAMINATION

The role and scope of practice of the nurse in ophthalmic assessment and examination varies according to state nurse practice acts, institutions, and employer guidelines. Regardless of the level of responsibility in any practice situation, the nurse must be knowledgeable about ophthalmic clinical manifestations and diagnoses as they relate to the holistic approach in client care.

Examination of the eyes includes assessment of external structures, using inspection and palpation, extraocular movements (EOMs), visual acuity, and visual fields (peripheral vision). Nurses who have advanced clinical assessment skills may perform tonometry and examine the internal eye structures with an ophthalmoscope.

The client's body structure and features are observed for obvious deformities and apparent age. For example, the hand deformities or abnormal gait of an arthritic may be a clue to the diagnosis of an associated eye disorder of keratoconjunctivitis sicca (dry eye syndrome) in a client who complains of itching and burning eyes.

External Eye Examination

External eye structures include the eyebrows, eyelashes, eyelids, lacrimal apparatus, anterior portion of the eyeballs, conjunctivae, sclerae, corneas, anterior chambers, pupils, and irises. Inspect and palpate these structures while the client sits at eye level to the examiner.

EYE POSITION

Assess eye position for symmetry and alignment. Sunken or protruding eyes are abnormal findings, as is protrusion of one eye or both eyes as in exophthalmos.

EYEBROWS

Inspect the eyebrows for symmetry, hair distribution, skin condition, and movement. The eyebrows normally move up and down smoothly under control of the facial nerves. Hair loss of the lateral aspects occurs with aging. The skin may be dry and flaking (i.e., dandruff), which is abnormal.

EYELIDS AND EYELASHES

Examine the eyelids and eyelashes for placement and symmetry. When open, the upper lids rest at the top of the irises and the lower lids at the bottom so that the sclerae are not visible above or below the irises. Sagging of the upper lids that covers part of the pupil is abnormal and called ptosis. Ptosis may occur with aging but also results from edema, third cranial nerve disorders, and neuromuscular disorders. Check for effective closure by asking the client to close the eyes. Eyelids that turn inward (entropion) or outward (ectropion) can result in corneal irritation. Lid eversion and inversion are often due to aging tissues but may also be due to facial nerve paresis, scarring, or allergies. Elevate the eyebrows to inspect the upper lids for lesions. Inspect lower lids by asking the client to open the eyes and examine the skin. The eyelids and orbit are palpated for texture, firmness, mobility, and integrity of the underlying tissues.

BLINK RESPONSE

Blinking is an involuntary reflex that occurs bilaterally up to 20 times a minute. Rapid, infrequent, or asymmetric blinking is abnormal.

EYEBALLS

The eyeballs are palpated for symmetry and firmness. Instruct the client to close the eyes and look down. Place the tip of the index fingers on the upper eyelids, over the sclerae, and palpate gently. Normally, the eyeballs feel firm and symmetric, not asymmetric, hard, or soft. Nurses with advanced clinical skills may perform tonometry to measure ocular pressure. See the section on internal eye examination for discussion of tonometry.

LACRIMAL APPARATUS

The lacrimal apparatus is examined by retracting the upper lid and having the client look down so that part of the lacrimal gland may be visualized. Observe this area for swelling or tenderness. The eye surface should be moist, without excess tearing. Inspect the area between the lower lid and the nose, which should be free of edema. The area over the lower orbit rim near the inner canthus (over the lacrimal sac) is palpated gently. There should be no regurgitation of fluid from the sac or puncta.

CONJUNCTIVAE AND SCLERAE

The conjunctivae and sclerae are inspected for color changes, texture, vascularity, lesions, thickness, secretions, and foreign bodies. The bulbar conjunctivae are colorless and transparent, allowing the sclerae to be seen. Small blood vessels may be visible. In whites, the sclerae are white, whereas they may appear light yellow in clients with dark skin tones. To inspect the palpebral conjunctivae, the nurse may wish to wear gloves. Regardless of whether gloves are worn or not, meticulous handwashing is advised both before and after the conjunctivae are examined. The lower eyelids are retracted to expose the conjunctivae without applying pressure to the eyeballs. The nurse (or the client) gently pushes the lower lids down against the bony orbit while the client looks up. Healthy conjunctivae are pink to light red; paleness or bright red color are abnormal. If the lower palpebral conjunctivae are normal, the upper palpebral conjunctivae usually are not inspected. If examination is necessary, the upper eyelids are everted by gently pulling the upper lid down while the client looks down. A cotton-tipped applicator is placed just above the lid margin and the nurse pushes down on the upper lid, turning the eyelid inside out over the applicator. After the inspection, return the eyelid to its normal position by gently pulling the eyelashes forward while the client looks up.

CORNEA

Inspect the cornea from an oblique angle while shining a penlight on the corneal surface. The irises are easily visible. In the elderly, a thin, white ring around the corneas' edges may be seen (arcus senilis). Abnormalities include surface irregularity and cloudiness or opacity.

CORNEAL REFLEX

The corneal reflex test is performed to assess the function of the fifth (trigeminal) cranial nerves. The client is instructed to keep the eyes open and look straight ahead. A sterile cotton wisp is brought from behind the client and lightly touched to the cornea. The client should blink and tear, indicating that the nerves are intact. A separate wisp is used for each eye. An alternate method is to use a syringe or the bulb from an otoscope to gently puff air across the cornea, eliciting the blink and tear response. Clients who wear contact lenses may not respond to the same degree as clients who do not wear them because they become somewhat insensitive to the stimulus.

ANTERIOR CHAMBER

The anterior chamber is inspected with the cornea, using the same oblique angle and penlight. The chambers should appear clear and transparent with no cloudiness or shadows cast upon the irises. The chambers' depth between the corneas and irises normally is about 3 mm. Shallower or deeper chambers are abnormal and the client should be referred to an ophthalmologist.

IRIS AND PUPIL

The iris and pupil are inspected. The irises should light up with the oblique lighting from the penlight and have a consistent color. Bulging or uneven coloring are abnormal. When light shines into the eyes, the irises constrict as the optic nerves are stimulated, making the pupils smaller. Dim lighting causes the pupils to dilate. The nurse inspects the pupils for size, shape, equality, and ability to react to light and accommodation. Pupils are normally black, round, have smooth borders, and are equal in size to one another. Actual size depends on the level of lighting, effect of medications that alter iris contractility, changes in intracranial pressure, or lesions impinging on the optic nerve.

Dim the light to test pupil reactions to light and accommodation. Instruct the client to look straight ahead. To test direct response to light, bring the penlight in from the side to shine directly over the center of the pupil. The illuminated pupil should constrict briskly and evenly. This maneuver is repeated on the other eye. Both eyes should react to the same degree. Consensual response is tested by observing one pupil while the penlight is shined on the opposite pupil. Both pupils should constrict to the same degree, although the consensual response is slightly slower. Accommodation is tested by holding the penlight 4 to 6 in (10 to 15 cm) away from the client's nose. Instruct the client to look first at the penlight, then at the distant wall straight ahead, and then back at the penlight. While the client gazes from near to far and back again, observe the pupils' response to changes in distance. They should dilate when looking at the far point and constrict when looking at the near object. Then move the penlight toward the bridge of the client's nose and observe for the pupils to converge and constrict. Results of the pupil assessment that are normal are recorded as PERRLA (pupils equal, round, and reactive to light and accommodation). Abnormal results include light intolerance (photophobia), irregular or unequal pupils, or pupils that do not react to light or accommodation. Abnormalities of the pupil may be due to neurologic disease, intraocular inflammation, iris adhesions, the effect of systemic or ocular medications, or surgical alteration, or they may be benign variations of normal findings.

Examination of Ocular Motility

Evaluation of ocular motility provides information about the extraocular muscles; the orbit; cranial nerves III, IV, and VI; their brain stem connections; and the cerebral cortex. The client is asked to track a target with both eyes as it is moved in each of the six cardinal directions of gaze (see Fig. 33–2). The examiner notes the speed, smoothness, range, and symmetry of movements and observes for unsteadiness of fixation (nystagmus).

Extraocular Muscle Tests

The eyes normally move in parallel to each other, smoothly and in unison. To test the function of the oculomotor, trochlear, and abducens, ask the client to look straight ahead while standing directly in front, holding a penlight approximately 12 in (30 cm) from the eyes. Instruct the client to keep the head still and to follow the penlight's movements with the eyes only. Move the penlight slowly and smoothly through the six cardinal positions of gaze, being careful not to go beyond the client's field of vision. Move the penlight in an orderly manner from the center outward along each of the six directions, pause briefly to observe for nystagmus, then return to the center. Nystagmus is an involuntary rapid, oscillating movement of the eyeball and is considered an abnormal finding except for slight nystagmus in the extreme lateral gazes (i.e., endpoint nystagmus). If the eyes do not move in parallel motion or if the upper eyelid covers more than a tiny portion of the iris, the conditions are noted as abnormal findings.

CORNEAL LIGHT REFLEX TEST (HIRSCHBERG'S TEST)

The corneal light reflex test (Hirschberg's test) determines eye alignment. Shine a penlight at the bridge of the client's nose from a distance of 12 to 15 in (30 to 38 cm) while the client stares straight ahead. Observe where the light reflects from both corneas; the reflection should be symmetric. Asymmetric reflection is abnormal and may indicate strabismus. Strabismus is a disorder in which the eye axes cannot be directed to the same object. A constant deviation of ocular alignment is termed a tropia. Deviation toward the nose is called esoptropia, a deviation away from the nose is called exotropia, and a vertical (up or down) deviation is called hypertropia. Latent deviations are seen only when one eye is covered and are called phorias (esophoria and exophoria).

COVER-UNCOVER TEST

The cover-uncover test assesses eye muscle function and alignment for tropia and phoria. The client is asked to stare straight ahead at a fixed point approximately 20 in (51 cm) away. Cover one of the client's eyes with an opaque card while observing the uncovered eye for lateral or medial movement as it focuses on the fixed point. There should be none. Remove the eye cover and observe that eye for movement as it focuses on the fixed point. Again, there should be no movement. The maneuvers are repeated for the opposite eye. The test may need to be repeated several times to confirm abnormal findings of astigmatism.

Assessment of Vision

VISUAL ACUITY

Testing visual acuity is the standard and routine method used to determine the clarity of the ocular media (cornea, lens, and vitreous) and the function of the visual pathway from the retina to the brain. It is important to remember that while an abnormal acuity implies an uncorrected refractive error or pathologic process, normal acuity does not exclude disease of the visual system. Visual acuity is assessed in one eye at a time, then in both eyes together, with the client comfortably seated. Begin with the right eye while the left eye is covered by an occluder or an opaque card. Test visual acuity with and without corrective lenses. Visual acuity is traditionally measured with the Snellen chart (Fig. 33-6) at a distance of 20 ft; at this distance, rays of light from an object are practically parallel and little effort of accommodation is required. In rooms that are shorter than 20 ft, mirrors or projection may be used to achieve the required distance. Charts may also be reduced proportionately to compensate for distance. Adaptations may be needed for the client who is illiterate or does not speak English; variations of the Snellen chart are available for these instances. There must be adequate lighting for the client to see.

Begin by asking the client to read the smallest line of symbols or letters that are seen. The client is credited for the smallest line of print that is read with more than 50 per cent accuracy. Record the results according to the standardized numbers printed by the lines on the Snellen chart. The sizes of the symbols are identified according to the distances at which they are normally visible. For example, the largest symbols can be read 200 ft away by people with unimpaired vision. The results of visual acuity testing are expressed in a fraction. The numerator denotes the distance the client is from the chart letters, and the denominator denotes the distance from the chart at which a client with normal vision can see the chart letters. Vision that is 20/20 is normal, that is, the client is able to read from 20 ft what a person with normal vision can read from 20 ft.

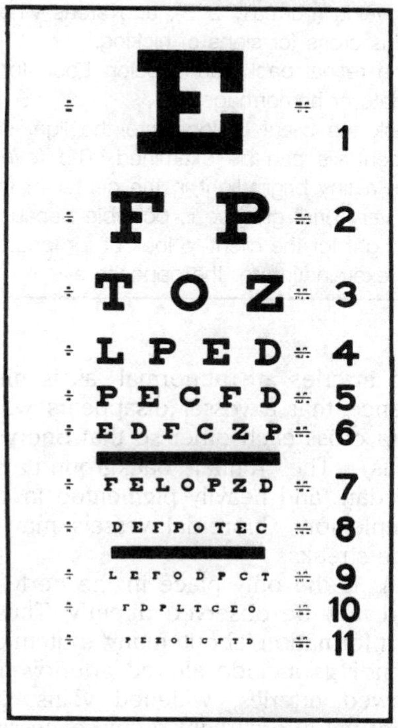

E 1
F P 2
T O Z 3
L P E D 4
P E C F D 5
E D F C Z P 6
F E L O P Z D 7
D E F P O T E C 8
L E F O D P C T 9
F D P L T C E O 10
P E Z O L C F T D 11

▲ *Figure 33-6*

A Snellen chart to assess visual acuity.

A client with a visual acuity of 20/60 sees at a distance of 20 feet to read what a client with normal vision can read at 60 feet. The client with myopia (i.e., nearsightedness) will have results of 20/30 or greater, signifying that the client can only read at 20 ft what a person with normal vision can read at 30 ft (or greater). Hyperopia (i.e., farsightedness) results are 20/15 or less, meaning the client can read at 20 ft what a person with normal vision can read at 15 ft (or less). It is not uncommon for a client to have a test result of 20/15, which indicates better than average visual acuity. Legal blindness is defined as 20/200 or less with corrected vision (glasses or contact lenses), or less than 20 degrees of visual field (see later) in the better eye.

When a client is unable to distinguish the largest letter on the chart, vision may be assessed by asking the client to read the number of fingers held up in front of him or her at a distance of 3 ft (CF = count fingers). If the client is unable to distinguish fingers, ask whether the client perceives hand movements (HM = hand motion). Finally, determine whether the client can perceive light (LP = light perception). NLP indicates no light perception.

Near vision is tested with a handheld card or newsprint 12 to 14 in (30 to 36 cm) from the client's eyes. Corrective lenses are worn if needed. The client with normal vision is able to read the material at that distance. Complaints of blurring or attempts by the client to move the card either closer or farther away signal abnormal near vision.

VISUAL FIELDS

Visual field testing evaluates peripheral vision. It may be accomplished by the confrontational method (Fig. 33-7) or with the use of a computerized instrument. The confrontational method assumes that the examiner has normal peripheral vision.

The client sits facing the nurse approximately 2 ft (60 cm) away. The eyes of the client and the nurse should be at the same level. Both the nurse and the client cover the eye directly opposite to one another with an opaque cover (e.g., the nurse's right eye and

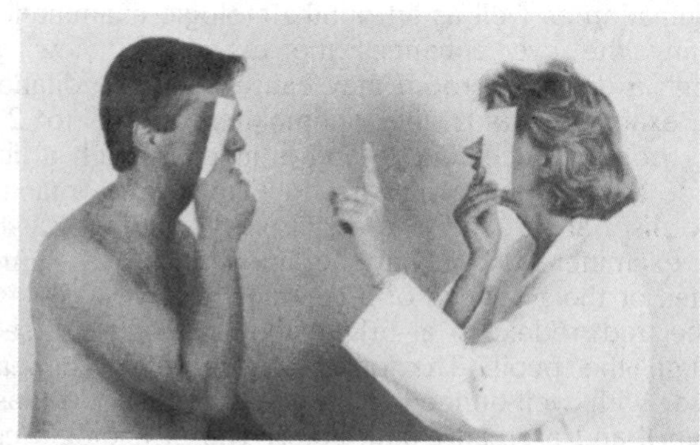

▲ *Figure 33-7*

Confrontational method of assessing visual fields. (From Jarvis, C. [1992]. *Physical examination and health assessment*. Philadelphia, W. B. Saunders.)

the client's left eye) and stare at each other's uncovered eye. The nurse holds a small object such as a penlight in the free hand and holds it equidistant between herself and the client, just out of view at the periphery of the visual field. Starting with the superior field, the nurse slowly brings the penlight down between the client and herself until the client states that he can see it (the nurse should be able to see the penlight at the same time). Repeat this maneuver at 45-degree angles, progressing through the superior, temporal, inferior, and nasal fields until all are tested. The nurse may need to position the penlight slightly behind the client to adequately test the client's temporal fields. The test is repeated for the other eye. Normal visual fields extend approximately 50 degrees superiorly, 90 degrees laterally, 70 degrees inferiorly, and 60 degrees medially. Gross visual field defects can be detected and, if found, the client is referred for further examination.

A variety of manual and computerized visual field testing equipment may be used to permit more accurate, reproducible detection and quantification of scotomas (areas of decreased visual function). Visual fields can be altered by central nervous system (CNS) disorders, such as a brain lesion or syphilis, and ocular disorders, such as glaucoma or retinal detachment.

Internal Eye Examination

Internal eye structures are visible only with illumination such as that provided by an ophthalmoscope. The ophthalmoscope is used to inspect the structures posterior to the iris, including the lens and fundus (which includes the retina, retinal vessels, choroid, optic disc, macula, and fovea). The ophthalmoscope requires considerable skill and practice.

DIRECT OPHTHALMOSCOPY

The handheld direct ophthalmoscope provides a magnified (15×) image of the fundus (posterior portion of the eye). It provides a detailed view of the disc and retinal vasculature and is a part of a general physical examination as well as an ophthalmologic examination. Dilating the eye enhances the examiner's view, although a darkened room may cause adequate dilation. The examiner holds the ophthalmoscope 1 to 2 in away from the client's eye and is able, through a light source and reflective mirrors, to examine the macula, optic disc, and retinal vessels (Box 33-1; Fig. 33-8). The examiner's view may be impaired by a cloudy cornea or the presence of a cataract.

The red reflex is a bright red-orange glow seen through the pupil. The optic disc normally appears round, with well-defined margins (except in the nasal margin), and a creamy pink color. The physiologic cup should be no larger than half the diameter of the optic disc. Retinal veins are darker than arteries and radiate from the disc. Veins are slightly thicker than arteries and should be free of pulsation. Tortuous vessels or straightened arteries are abnormal, as is nicking (i.e., the appearance that a vessel disappears where an artery and vein cross each other so that one vessel looks discontinuous). The retinal background is pink in whites, and dark and heavily pigmented in clients with a dark complexion. Choroidal vessels may appear as linear orange streaks.

The fundus is the only place in the body where the vascular bed may be observed directly. Thus examination yields information about many systemic diseases. Abnormal findings include altered arteriovenous (A/V) ratio, narrowed arteries, widened veins, pinched-off vessels, abnormal arterial light reflex, excessive tortuosity, numerous A/V nickings, exudates, white patches, and focal hemorrhage.

Box 33-1. Guidelines for Using Ophthalmoscope

1. Assemble ophthalmoscope by attaching the head to the handle
2. Darken room
3. Turn on ophthalmoscope light by depressing rheostat button and turning rheostat to the brightest light
4. Turn aperture selector to large round circle of light
5. Turn lens selector dial to zero
6. Instruct the client to stare straight ahead.
7. Leave both eyes open during the examination. The examiner learns to suppress visual stimulation from the eye that is not looking through the viewing aperture.
8. Hold the ophthalmoscope while steadying the client's head with the free hand
9. Approach the client from the side at an approximately 45-degree angle and a distance of 15 inches. Direct the light into the client's pupil.
10. Move slowly closer to the eye, keeping the light directed on the pupil. If the client blinks, hold position steady until the client's eye opens again. At approximately 15 inches, visualize the red reflex, then the anterior chamber. Moving closer, look at the lens. Finally, when very close (1-2 inches), vessels of the fundus may be seen.
11. Adjust the lens selector with index finger to focus on a blood vessel and follow it into the optic disc.
12. Focus on the disc, adjusting the lens selector as needed to correct for visual deficits of both the examiner and the client. Once focus is adjusted, examine the optic disc (color, margins, shape, presence of physiologic cup [see Plate 1]).
13. Follow the major blood vessels from the disc and look for evidence of tortuosity, pulsation, diameter, ratio of arteries/veins (normally 2:3), and areas where arteries and veins cross for signs of nicking.
14. Note the retinal background color. Look for presence of exudate or hemorrhage.
15. Last, ask the client to look into the light so that the fovea centralis can be examined. The fovea may be seen as a tiny bright light in the center of the macula. Only a very brief glimpse is possible because the light is too bright for the client to look at for long.
16. Repeat examination for the opposite eye.

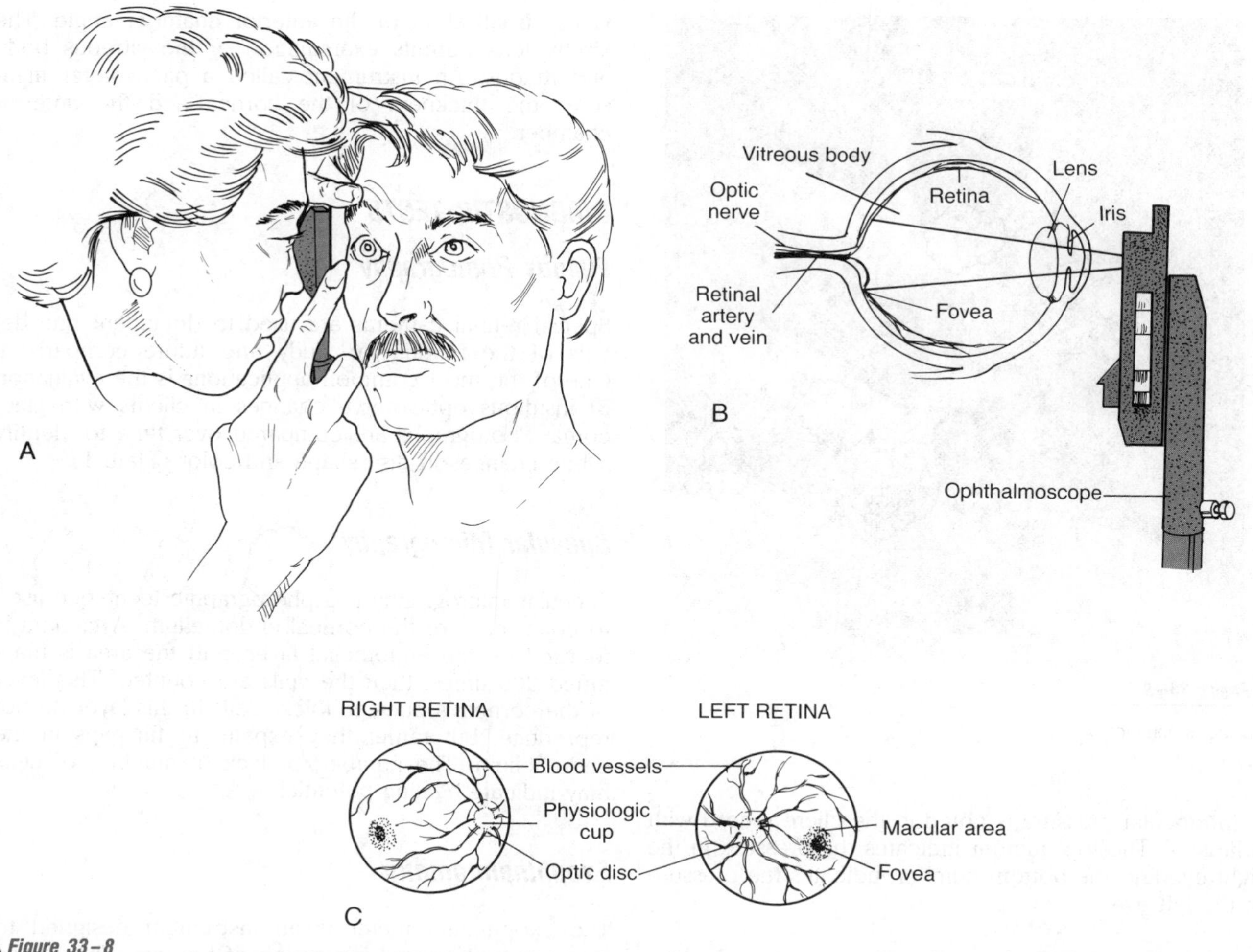

▲ ***Figure 33–8***

A, The examiner uses the right hand to hold the ophthalmoscope to the right eye to examine the client's right eye. The examiner uses the left hand and left eye when examining the client's left eye. Note the positioning of the examiner's free hand, which is placed to steady the client's head and to slightly retract the eyebrow. *B*, The examiner sees what appears in the angle of light through the viewing aperture. *C*, The actual area of retina visualized depends on the pupil dilation. Note structures that may be examined.

INDIRECT OPHTHALMOSCOPY

The indirect ophthalmoscope enables the examiner to obtain a stereoscopic picture over a large area of the retina. The light source comes from a head-mounted light. The examiner holds a convex lens in front of the client's eye, and through a viewing device attached to the headband, sees an inverted reversed image. The indirect ophthalmoscope has the advantage of binocular vision with depth perception for the examiner and permits a wider field of view.

TONOMETRY

Tonometry is the method of measuring the intraocular fluid pressure using calibrated instruments that indent or flatten the corneal apex. The eye can be thought of as an enclosed compartment through which there is a constant circulation of aqueous humor. The aqueous maintains the shape of the eye with a relatively uniform pressure within the globe. As the pressure increases, the eye becomes firmer and a greater force is required to cause the same amount of indentation. Pressures between 8 and 21 mm Hg are considered within the normal range.

The two most common types of tonometers are the Schiøtz and applanation. The Schiøtz tonometer (Fig. 33–9) is a portable handheld instrument that may be used in an office, clinic, emergency room, operating room, or at the bedside. It measures the amount of corneal indentation produced by a preset weight. The softer the eye, the more a given weight will be able to indent the cornea. The examiner first anesthetizes the cornea with a topical anesthetic eye drop. With the client in a supine position and looking straight upward, the Schiøtz tonometer is placed directly on the cornea. A conversion chart is used to translate the scale reading into millimeters of mercury.

The applanation tonometer is attached to a slit lamp microscope and measures the amount of force required to flatten the corneal apex by a standard amount. Anesthetic eye drops are also used prior to this examination method.

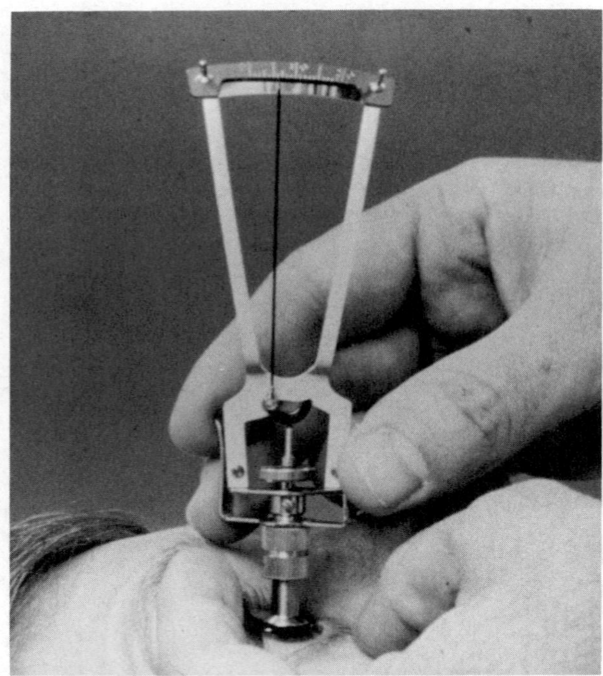

▲ Figure 33–9

Schiøtz tonometer.

Intraocular pressure is noted in the client record with a large T. The top number indicates the pressure in the right eye and the bottom number indicates the pressure in the left eye.

SLIT LAMP EXAMINATION

The slit lamp microscope is used to illuminate and examine the anterior segment of the eye under magnification. A linear slit beam of incandescent light is projected onto the globe, illuminating an optical cross section of the anterior chamber. The angle of illumination, length, width, and intensity of the light may be adjusted. The client is seated, and the head is stabilized by an adjustable chin rest and forehead strap. Details of the lid margins, lashes, conjunctiva, tear film, cornea, iris, lens, and aqueous can be studied. At the highest magnification setting, the abnormal presence of red or white blood cells in the aqueous may be visualized. The presence of protein (flare), called an anterior chamber reaction, that accompanies intraocular inflammation may also be detected. Normal aqueous is optically clear, without cells or flare.

Fluorescein dye is often used in a slit lamp examination to highlight corneal irregularities. Sterile paper strips containing fluorescein dye are wetted and touched against the inner surface of the lower lid, instilling the yellow dye into the tear film. A blue filter is attached to the light beam, causing the dye to fluoresce.

In addition to the applanation tonometer, several other devices may be attached to the slit lamp to expand the scope of the examination. A goniolens provides visualization of the anterior chamber angle. The Hruby lens permits examination of the vitreous body and fundus. An instrument called a pachymeter measures the thickness of the cornea and the anterior chamber.

DIAGNOSTIC TESTS

Fundus Photography

Special retinal cameras are used to document fine details of the fundus for study and future comparison. One of the most common applications is the evaluation of insidious optic nerve changes in clients with glaucoma. Photographs are compared over time to identify subtle changes in disc shape and color (Plate 1).

Specular Micrography

Specular micrography is a photographic technique used to count cells of the corneal endothelium. A camera is focused on the endothelial layer, and the area is magnified 200 times; then the cells are counted. This layer of the cornea is one-cell thick. Cells in this layer do not reproduce, but rather they expand to fill gaps in the endothelium. The number, or lack of number, of cells may indicate healing potential.

Exophthalmometry

The exophthalmometer is an instrument designed to measure the forward protrusion of the eye. This instrument provides a method of evaluating and recording the progression and regression of the prominence of the eye in disorders such as thyroid disease and tumors of the orbit.

Ophthalmic Radiology

X-ray study, tomography, and CT scan are useful in the evaluation of orbital and intracranial conditions. Common abnormalities evaluated by these methods include neoplasms, inflammatory masses, fractures, and extraocular muscle enlargement associated with Graves' eye disease. Radiology is also useful in the detection of foreign bodies.

Magnetic Resonance Imaging

Magnetic resonance imaging (MRI) has the advantage of not exposing the patient to ionizing radiation. Also, multidimensional views are possible without repositioning the patient (Fig. 33–10). MRI is used to image edema, areas of demyelination, and vascular lesions. However, the availability of MRI equipment is often limited and the examination takes longer. MRI may also cause movement of a metallic foreign body.

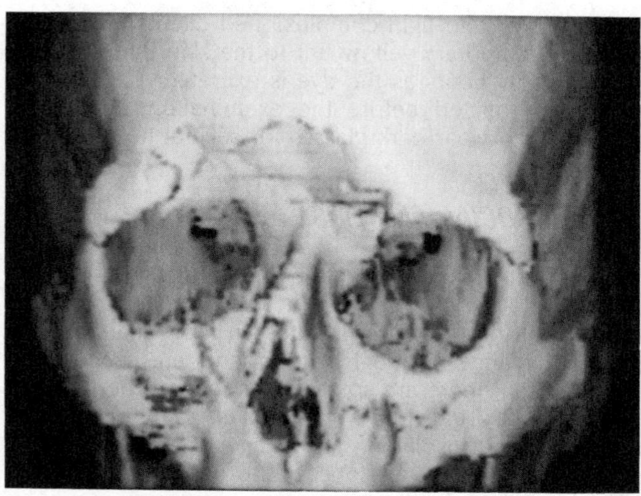

▲ Figure 33-10

MRI scan showing massive facial fractures. Note the three-dimensional appearance obtained with MRI.

Ultrasonography

Ultrasonography uses the principle of sonar to study structures not directly visible. High-frequency sound waves are transmitted through a probe placed directly on the eyeball. As the sound waves bounce back off the various tissue components, they are collected by a receiver that amplifies them on an oscilloscope screen. Sound waves derived from the most distal structures arrive last, having traveled the farthest (Fig. 33-11). Ultrasonography may be used to evaluate tissue characteristics of a lesion as well as size and growth over time. It may also be used to measure axial length (the distance from the cornea to the retina) in order to calculate the power for an intraocular lens implant in cataract surgery.

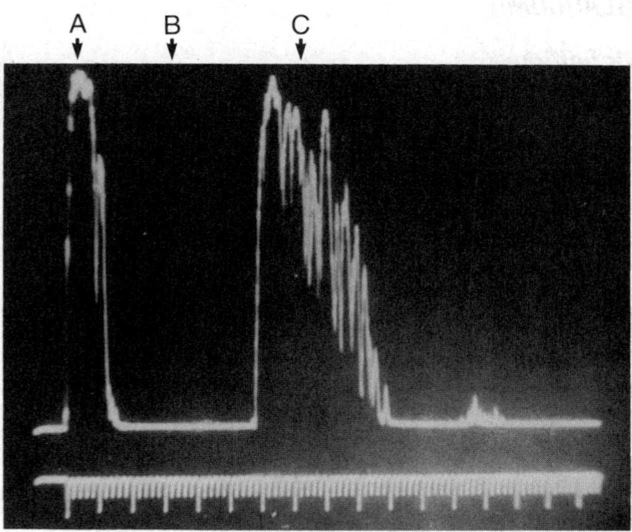

▲ Figure 33-11

Normal A-scan ultrasound of the eye. The sound beam is aimed in a straight line, and echoes are displayed as spikes. The amplitude depends on the density of the reflecting tissue and perpendicularity of the probe. *A*, cornea and lens; *B*, clear vitreous; and *C*, retina and choroid.

Ophthalmodynamometry

Ophthalmodynamometry is a test that consists of exerting pressure on the sclera with a spring plunger while observing the central retinal vessels emerging from the disc through an ophthalmoscope. This instrument gives an approximate measurement of the relative pressures in the central retinal arteries and is an indirect method of assessing carotid arterial flow on either side. Ophthalmodynamometry is indicated in the neurologic evaluation of patients who complain of "blacking out" of vision in one eye (amaurosis), spells of weakness on one side of the body, or other symptoms of cerebral ischemia. A difference of more than 20 per cent in the diastolic pressures between the two eyes suggests insufficiency of the carotid arterial system on the side with the lower pressure.

Electroretinography

An electrical potential exists between the cornea and retina of the eye. Because the retina is neurologic tissue, the normal retina exhibits certain electrical responses when stimulated by light. Electroretinography (ERG) measures the normal change in electrical potential of the eye caused by a diffuse flash of light. For this test, electrodes incorporated into a contact lens are placed directly on the eye. Eye movements disrupt the values of the test, so the client must be able to fixate on a target while keeping the eyes still. A normal ERG signifies functional integrity of the retina. Examples of retinal diseases that may be evaluated with ERG include retinitis pigmentosa (progressive degeneration of photoreceptor cells), massive ischemia, disseminated infection, or toxic effects from drugs or chemicals.

Visual Evoked Response

Visual evoked response (VER) is similar to ERG in that it also measures the electrical potential resulting from a visual stimulus. The entire visual pathway from the retina to the cortex may be evaluated in this examination through the placement of electrodes on the scalp. Reduced speed of neuronal conduction, such as with demyelination, results in an abnormal VER. Retinal or optic nerve disease may be diagnosed by stimulating each eye separately.

Fluorescein Angiography

Fundus photography is enhanced by the use of fluorescein dye whose molecules emit green light when stimulated by blue light. For this examination, the client is seated in front of a retina camera following pupillary dilation. A small amount of fluorescein dye is injected into an antecubital vein. The dye circulates throughout the body before eventually being excreted by the kidneys. As the dye passes through the retinal and choroidal circulation, it can be visualized and photographed because of its ability to fluoresce (Fig. 33–12). A rapid sequence of pictures captures the initial rapid perfusion of the retinal and choroidal vessels. Later photos may demonstrate the gradual leakage of dye from abnormal vessels. Changes in blood flow, ischemia, and hemorrhage may be detected. Because it can so precisely delineate areas of abnormality, it is an essential guide for planning laser treatment of retinal vascular disease.

Nurses may administer the intravenous flourescein dye injection under an ophthalmologist's direction. It is important to first assess the client's general health status and identify any allergies. Allergic reactions to other dye injections (i.e., for intravenous pyelogram [IVP] or cholangiogram) should be considered before the flourescein injection. Benadryl may be prescribed prophylactically. Although anaphylactic shock is a rare occurrence, emergency equipment should be located nearby. Occasionally, clients have a vasovagal response to the dye that includes vertigo, nausea, and momentary loss of consciousness. A consent for the procedure should be obtained. The nurse should explain that during the injection, the client may experience a warm sensation. The client will also hear the mechanics of the camera taking rapid-sequence photographs and experience the bright flashes of light. After the examination, the client should be encouraged to increase the intake of fluids because the dye is excreted through the kidneys. During the next 24 hours, the urine will be a yellow color and light-complexioned clients may experience a temporary yellow tint to the skin that will fade within a few hours as the dye is excreted. Because the pupils are dilated before the examination, it may be necessary to wear dark glasses for several hours.

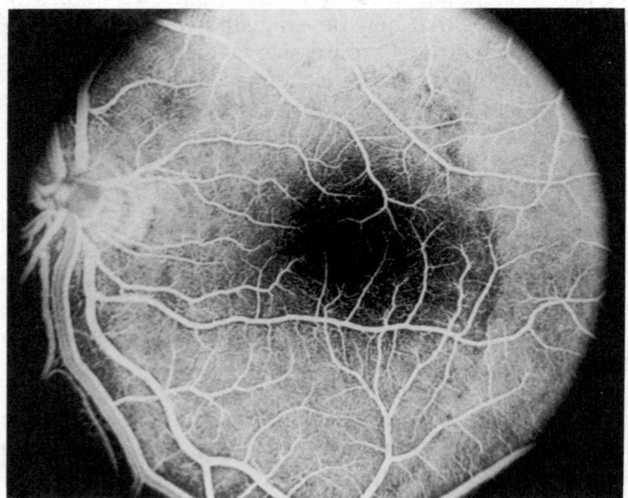

▲ **Figure 33–12**

Normal fluorescein angiography. The normal pattern of fluorescein angiography can be divided into three phases: The *filling phase* (pictured) takes 8 to 20 seconds. The *recirculation phase* starts 0.5 second after the filling phase and lasts 3 to 5 minutes. The *late phase* lasts 30 to 60 minutes. Photographs are taken prior to injection, at half-second intervals for 20 seconds, and then at intervals of 5 minutes.

PSYCHOSOCIAL FACTORS

The social stigma of blindness underlies the anxiety that clients experience with actual or potential vision loss. Total loss of vision isolates an individual within a different reality. Although most clients are successfully rehabilitated, there are some losses that are permanent. There are also individuals who, for a variety of reasons, remain socially isolated. The image of a blind person who is pitied and must accept the charity of others is disturbing.

Not all jobs and work environments are adaptable for a person who can no longer see. Clients with actual or potential vision loss may be faced with barriers in their vocations that force an unwanted change. Age may be a major factor in the client's ability to meet this challenge.

Self-esteem is closely related to the roles of the client in his particular lifestyle. Loss of control in personal, family, and work situations can be devastating. The issue of dependence versus independence for an individual may also be a factor in the client's ability to cope with the stressors of vision loss.

▼ NURSING CARE OF CLIENTS WITH EYE DISORDERS

GLAUCOMA

Definition

Glaucoma includes a group of ocular disorders characterized by increased intraocular pressure, optic nerve atrophy, and visual field loss. The individual response to intraocular pressure varies. Therefore, some people sustain damage from relatively low pressures and others sustain no damage from high pressure. The degree of increased pressure that causes ocular damage is not the same in every eye, and some individuals may tolerate a pressure for long periods of time that would rapidly blind another.

Incidence

It is estimated that over 50,000 persons in the United States are blind as a result of glaucoma. The incidence of glaucoma is about 1.5 per cent, and in blacks, between the ages of 45 and 65, the prevalence is at least 5 times that of whites in the same age group. In most cases, blindness can be prevented if treatment is begun early.

Pathophysiology

Intraocular pressure is determined by the rate of aqueous production in the ciliary body and the resistance to outflow of aqueous from the eye. Increased intraocular pressure (usually greater than 23 mm Hg) indicates the need for further evaluation. Intraocular pressure varies with diurnal cycles (the highest pressure is usually on awakening) and position of the body (increased when lying down). Normal variations do not usually exceed 2 to 3 mm Hg. Intraocular pressure and blood pressure are independent of each other, but variations in systemic blood pressure may be associated with corresponding variations in the intraocular pressure. Increased intraocular pressure may result from hyperproduction of aqueous or obstruction of the outflow. As aqueous fluid builds up in the eye, the increased pressure inhibits blood supply to the optic nerve and the retina. These delicate tissues become ischemic and gradually lose function.

Etiology/Risk Factors

Many terms are used to describe the various types of glaucoma. The terms primary and secondary refer to whether the etiology is the disease alone or due to another condition. Acute and chronic refer to the onset and or duration of the disorder. The terms open (wide) and closed (narrow) describe the width of the angle between the cornea and the iris (see Fig. 33–5*A*). Anatomically narrow anterior chamber angles predispose clients to an acute onset of angle-closure glaucoma.

PRIMARY OPEN-ANGLE GLAUCOMA

Approximately 90 per cent of primary glaucoma cases occur in clients with open angles. It is a multifactional disorder that is often genetically determined, bilateral, insidious in onset, and slow to progress. Symptoms appear late when vision is impaired by damage to the optic nerve. Because there are no early warning symptoms, it is imperative that regular ophthalmic examinations include tonometry and assessment of the optic nerve head (disc). This type of glaucoma is often referred to as the "thief in the night" because there are no early symptoms alerting the client that vision is being lost. The most common cause of chronic open-angle glaucoma is degenerative change in the trabecular meshwork, resulting in the decreased outflow of aqueous humor.

ANGLE-CLOSURE GLAUCOMA

An acute attack of angle-closure glaucoma can develop only in an eye in which the anterior chamber angle is anatomically narrow. The attack occurs due to a sudden blockage of the anterior angle by the base of the iris. When the aqueous flow is obstructed, intraocular pressure becomes markedly elevated, causing severe pain and blurred vision or vision loss. Some clients will see rainbow halos around lights, and some will experience nausea and vomiting.

LOW-TENSION GLAUCOMA

Low-tension glaucoma resembles primary open-angle glaucoma. The angle is normal, the optic nerves are cupped, and the visual fields show characteristic glaucomatous effects (peripheral vision deficits). These changes, however, develop in the presence of statistically normal intraocular pressures. The etiology of low-tension glaucoma is not known. Although the pressure readings are in the normal range, treatment is indicated to lower the pressure even further to avoid progressive optic nerve damage and visual field loss.

SECONDARY GLAUCOMA

Increased intraocular pressure may occur as a postoperative complication. Edematous tissue may inhibit the outflow of aqueous through the trabecular meshwork. Delayed healing of corneal wound edges may result in epithelial cell growth into the anterior chamber.

Glaucoma may occur as a result of trauma. Lens displacement, hemorrhage into the anterior chamber, lacerations, and contusions can disrupt the flow pattern of aqueous humor.

Inflammation of filtering structures in uveitis may cause increased intraocular pressure. Encroachment by a rapidly growing tumor and chronic use of topical corticosteroids may also produce the symptoms of open-angle glaucoma.

Clinical Manifestations

Clinical manifestations of glaucoma include

1. Increased intraocular pressure,
2. Cupping or indentation of the optic nerve head (disc), and
3. Visual field defects.

DIAGNOSTIC ASSESSMENT

An ophthalmoscopic examination shows atrophy (pale color) and cupping (indentation) of the optic nerve head. The visual field examination is used to determine the extent of peripheral vision loss (see the section on visual fields). In chronic open-angle glaucoma, a small crescent-shaped scotoma (blind spot) appears early in the disease. In acute angle-closure glaucoma, the fields demonstrate larger areas of significant vision loss.

In clients with angle-closure glaucoma, a slit lamp examination may demonstrate an erythematous conjunctiva and corneal cloudiness. The anterior chamber aqueous may also appear turbid and the pupil may be nonreactive. Slit lamp examination is used in open-angle glaucoma to look for any secondary causes and associated findings. Intraocular pressure is measured at the slit lamp with the applanation tonometer. Gonioscopy is performed to determine the depth of the anterior chamber angle and to examine the entire circumference of the angle for any abnormal changes in the filtering meshwork.

Medical Management

The goal of medical management is to facilitate the outflow of aqueous through remaining channels. This is achieved through the use of

- Topical miotics, which constrict the pupil and increase outflow;
- Topical epinephrine, which also increases the outflow;
- Topical beta-blockers or alpha-adrenergics, which suppress the secretion of aqueous humor; and
- Oral carbonic anhydrase inhibitors, which also reduce the production of aqueous humor.

When medical management is no longer effective, surgical intervention may be indicated.

Surgical Management

When maximum medical therapy has failed to halt the progression of visual field loss and optic nerve damage, surgical intervention is recommended. There are many procedures that are used to correct the aqueous outflow; however, there is no operation that is uniformly successful.

LASER TRABECULOPLASTY

The use of the laser to create an opening in the trabecular meshwork is often indicated before filtration surgery is considered. The laser produces scars in the trabecular meshwork, causing tightening of meshwork fibers. The tightened fibers allow increased outflow of aqueous. Intraocular pressure is reduced through improved outflow in about 80 per cent of cases. The effect of the laser treatment decreases with time, and the procedure may need to be repeated. Treatment with medications is usually continued.

FILTERING PROCEDURES

Operative procedures such as trephination, thermal sclerostomy, or sclerectomy create an outflow channel from the anterior chamber into the subconjunctival space. These are called filtering procedures. Aqueous is absorbed through the conjunctival vessels. In about 25 per cent of cases, the opening closes due to scar tissue formation, and reoperation is necessary.

A more common filtering procedure called trabeculectomy reduces some of the complications of surgery but achieves a somewhat lesser reduction in pressure. A half-thickness scleral flap is loosely sutured over the opening, through which the fluid escapes, again resulting in subconjunctival absorption of aqueous.

Glaucoma-filtering procedures differ from other surgical procedures in that the goal is to prevent the newly created opening for outflow from closing. Filtering procedures are less successful in young and black clients because of their increased ability to produce thicker fibroblastic healing tissue. Topical corticosteroids are used postoperatively because their anti-inflammatory action inhibits the proliferation of fibroblasts at the surgical site.

5-Fluorouracil (5-FU) and other antimetabolites are sometimes injected subconjunctivally because they also inhibit fibroblast proliferation and, thereby, reduce postoperative scarring.

Ocular implantation devices such as the Molteno implant are sometimes used to control the flow of aqueous in patients with complicated types of glaucoma. The device is sutured to the outer surface of the eyeball on the sclera between the ocular muscles. A tiny tube is inserted under the scleral flap directly into the anterior chamber, which directs the flow of aqueous more posteriorly than in the more common filtration procedures.

CILIODESTRUCTIVE PROCEDURES

When other surgical procedures have failed, cyclocryotherapy (the application of a freezing tip) or cyclophotocoagulation may be used to damage the ciliary body and decrease the production of aqueous.

Nursing Management

ASSESSMENT

The nursing assessment of the client includes establishing demographic data of age and race because open-angle glaucoma occurs most often in clients over 40 and in blacks. It is also important to determine whether there is a family history of glaucoma or other eye problems, or if the client has had ocular surgery, infections, or trauma. An accurate list of current medications is imperative since over-the-counter medications such as antihistamines may dilate the pupil, putting the client at risk for angle-closure glaucoma. A history of allergic reactions, particularly to medications or dye studies should always be noted.

The nurse should ask the client to describe any changes in vision. Although the symptoms of primary open-angle glaucoma are insidious, the client may describe blind spots in the periphery or an overall decreased visual acuity with loss of contrast sensitivity. Decreased uncorrectable visual acuity usually occurs when there has been irreversible damage to the optic nerve.

If it has been previously established that the client has visual loss from glaucoma, it is essential to assess how the client is coping with the loss of vision. Although individuals adapt to the loss of vision in different ways, clients usually experience stages of grief and loss and may be at any stage. Clients may be understandably anxious during examinations because it may be discovered that further vision loss has occurred. The nurse assesses the client's perception of glaucoma and the effect it has on the client's life. The nurse assists the client in identifying effective coping skills the client may have used in the past. Loneliness may be a significant finding (see Nursing Research).

NURSING INTERVENTION

Nursing Diagnosis: Visual Sensory/Perception Alterations R/T increased intraocular pressure.

Planning: Expected Outcomes. The client will maintain as much functional vision as possible, as evidenced by reporting no further loss of vision and adapting to any visual loss, demonstrate an ability to perform activities of daily living (ADLs), instill his or her own eye medications, and recognize clinical manifestations of complications.

Implementation. Since medications are an integral part of the treatment and care of a client with glaucoma, nursing interventions must be directed at the client's ability to understand and comply with prescribed therapy. The nurse must first determine the client's current level of knowledge and then provide necessary information about glaucoma and its treatment in understandable terms using diagrams. Because treatment for glaucoma is often complex, involving both oral and topical ophthalmic medications, a written plan of care in large print should be reviewed with the client and family. In order to maximize compliance, the plan of care must fit into the client's lifestyle. The nurse should reinforce that although some vision has been lost and cannot be restored, further loss may be prevented by adhering to the treatment plan.

The administration of eyedrops is a critical component of self-care for the client with glaucoma. After instructing the client and family on instillation technique, the nurse should validate the client or family's ability to properly instill eye drops by asking for a return demonstration. The discussion of side effects of medications is also very important (Table 33-1).

In emergent situations in which intraocular pressure must be brought under control, an oral osmotic agent may be administered in the form of glycerin (Osmoglyn). The agent is supplied in a variety of strengths, and the nurse must check the percentage of the solution ordered against what is supplied. The diuretic action of glycerin lowers intraocular pressure. Because the high sugar content effects some diabetic clients, a synthetic glycerin such as isosorbide (Ismotic) may be used. The average dose for an adult is 4 ounces, which may be repeated several times until the intraocular pressure is reduced to a tolerable level. The extreme sweetness and viscosity may be made more palatable by mixing the glycerin with equal parts of a tart juice such as lemon. Serving the solution over cracked ice also makes it more palatable. After 3 hours, the nurse should encourage the intake of water and other fluids to prevent mild to moderate dehydration and also make sure the client can get to the bathroom during the diuretic phase. Intravenous mannitol, a potent intravenous osmotic diuretic, may be used to arrest extremely high intraocular pressure. It should only be used for the management of a glaucoma crisis under close nursing and medical supervision. The client's cardiovascular and renal status should be carefully evaluated before treatment is begun. The nurse should document baseline vital signs before the treatment and frequently during the infusion. Because mannitol has a tendency to crystalize, the bottle may need to be warmed before it is administered. The vial should not be used while crystals are present. An in-line micropore filter should also be used to prevent infusion of any crystal particles.

Preoperative nursing care includes preparing the client for a surgical procedure that may be performed in either an outpatient or inpatient setting.

TABLE 33-1. Teaching the Client About Eye Drops for Glaucoma

Medication	Usual Frequency	Teaching Aspects
Pilocarpine hydrochloride	3 to 4 times/day	A miotic, causes pupillary constriction to open the canal of Schlemm Space out the administration, beginning upon awakening and ending at bedtime May cause blurred vision after instillation Brow ache has been reported Consider the use of thin gel strips (a timed release form) to improve compliance
Timolol maleate and other beta blockers such as levobunolol	Every 12 hours	Decreases production of aqueous humor Space out the administration Contraindicated in clients with asthma and COPD Assess for bradycardia prior to administration
Carbonic anhydrase inhibitors (acetazolamide/ Diamox)		Inhibits the production of aqueous humor Available as tablets and in sustained-release capsules Side effects include anorexia and tingling in the hands and feet

Outpatient Treatment. Laser therapy is most often performed in a clinic or office using topical anesthetic. It is important for the nurse to explain not only the expected outcome of the procedure, but also the popping sounds and flashing lights that the client will experience. The client should be informed that there will be a waiting period (usually 1 to 2 hours) after the procedure to evaluate a possible rise in intraocular pressure. Because of the instability of the intraocular pressure, the client should arrange to have a friend or family accompany him or her to provide transportation.

Inpatient Treatment. Preoperatively, the nurse should evaluate the level of the client's anxiety and knowledge about the procedure. Mild preoperative sedation is usually prescribed.

Postoperative nursing care may need to be accomplished in a matter of hours or days, depending on the expected length of stay. When the client returns from the operating room, the eye is covered with a patch and a metal or plastic shield for protection. The nurse should instruct the client not to lie on the operative side to avoid pressure on the operative site. When the effects of the perioperative sedation have diminished, the client may ambulate and eat as desired.

EVALUATION

The nurse determines the degree of expected outcome attainment. Generally the care of these clients is very short in the hospital setting. If long-term expected outcomes are important, other modes of quality assurance will be needed.

Post-hospital Care

DISCHARGE TEACHING

The plan for discharge must include client education, and evaluation of the home environment and available care.

Client and family education for postoperative eye care includes a review of

- Signs and symptoms of infection (redness, swelling, drainage, blurred vision, pain),
- Signs and symptoms of increased intraocular pressure (unrelieved pain, nausea, decrease in vision)
- The rationale for eye protection (shield or glasses at all times),
- Medications and eye drop instillation technique, and
- Return visit date and time.

Clients should be instructed to carefully cleanse the area around the eye with warm tap water and a clean wash cloth. Special eye wash solutions of balanced saline may be used, but are not necessary. The eye wash should not be applied directly to the eye. It is important that the client understand that rubbing or applying pressure over the closed eye could damage healing tissue. Although many clients with glaucoma may undergo repeated surgical procedures, the above-mentioned information should be carefully reviewed each time.

HOME HEALTH CARE NEEDS

Because the level of independence varies with individual clients, the nurse uses information supplied by the client and family or friends to assess how much support may be needed. Referrals may need to be made to visiting nurses for home health care or social services for assistance with rehabilitation or finances. The nurse assists the client and family to plan for housekeeping and meal preparation, safety in the home environment with decreased vision, transportation, and assistance with eye care.

CATARACTS

Definition

A cataract is an opacity of the lens.

Incidence

Although cataract formation is usually associated with aging, cataracts may be due to a variety of other causes. Some degree of cataract formation is to be expected in most persons over age 70. Over a million cataract operations are now being performed annually in the United States. A person with a normal lifespan is more likely to undergo a cataract operation than any other major surgical procedure.

Etiology/Risk Factors

AGE-RELATED CATARACTS

The most common cataract is age-related or senile cataract. Worldwide, it is the primary cause of reduced vision and blindness. Senile cataracts usually begin around the age of 50 and consist of cortical, nuclear, or posterior subcapsular opacities. These three forms may coexist in various combinations.

In cortical cataracts, spokelike opacifications are found in the periphery of the lens. They progress slowly, infrequently involve the visual axis, and often do not result in severe vision loss.

Nuclear sclerotic cataracts are a result of a progressive yellowing and hardening of the central lens (nucleus). Most individuals over the age of 70 have some degree of nuclear sclerosis.

Posterior subcapsular opacities occur centrally on the posterior lens capsule. They cause visual loss early in their development because they lie directly in the visual axis.

OTHER FORMS OF CATARACTS

Cataracts may develop as a result of many other ocular, systemic, and congenital disorders. Systemic disorders include diabetes, tetany, myotonic dystrophy, neurodermatitis, galactosemia, Lowe's syndrome, Werner's syndrome, and Down syndrome. Intraocular disorders that may be associated with cataract are iridocyclitis, retinitis, retinal detachment, and onchocerciasis. Blunt trauma, lacerations, foreign bodies, radiation, and exposure to infrared light, and chronic use of corticosteroids may also result in cataracts. Infections (German measles, mumps, hepatitis, poliomyelitis, chickenpox, infectious mononucleosis) during the first trimester of pregnancy may cause congenital cataracts.

Pathophysiology

Cataract formation is characterized chemically by a reduction in oxygen uptake and an initial increase in water content followed by dehydration. Sodium and calcium contents are increased. Potassium, ascorbic acid, and protein are decreased. The protein in the lens undergoes numerous age related changes including yellowing, which is from the formation of fluorescent compounds and molecular changes. These changes, along with the photoabsorption of ultraviolet radiation throughout life, suggest that cataracts may be due to a photochemical process.

Cataracts progress through the following clinical stages of development:

- *Immature* cataracts are not completely opaque, and some light is transmitted through them, allowing useful vision.
- *Mature* cataracts are completely opaque. The former term for this stage was ripe. Vision is significantly reduced.
- *Intumescent* cataracts are those in which the lens takes on water and increases in size. The lens may be mature or immature. The increase in size may result in glaucoma.
- *Hypermature* cataracts are those in which the lens proteins break down into short-chain polypeptides that leak out through the lens capsule. The pieces of protein are engulfed by macrophages, which may obstruct the trabecular meshwork, causing phacolytic glaucoma.

Clinical Manifestations

Clients experience blurred vision, sometimes monocular diplopia, photophobia, and glare. Clients usually see better in low-lit conditions when the pupil is dilated, which allows for vision around a central opacity. There is no complaint of pain. A cloudy lens can be observed (Plate 2).

DIAGNOSTIC ASSESSMENT

A cataract should be suspected when the red reflex seen with the direct ophthalmoscope is distorted or absent. Although cataracts can usually be diagnosed easily with the direct ophthalmoscope, an accurate determination of the type and extent of the lens change requires a slit lamp examination.

Medical Management

There is no known medical treatment that either prevents or reduces cataract formation.

Surgical Management

The objective of cataract surgery is to remove the opacified lens. Over the last two decades, cataract surgery has improved dramatically as a result of the operating microscope, new instrumentation, improved suture material, and refinement of the intraocular lens implant. The lens is surgically removed by an intracapsular or extracapsular procedure (Fig. 33–13).

Intracapsular cataract extraction (ICCE) consists of removing the lens including the lens capsule. Extracapsular cataract extraction (ECCE) consists of removing the lens and the anterior portion of the lens capsule. The posterior lens capsule is left intact. Although intracapsular surgery is highly successful and still performed, extracapsular extraction is by far the most common procedure in the United States. The primary reason for performing extracapsular surgery is to allow the insertion of a posterior chamber intraocular lens inside the remaining capsule, which results in fewer postoperative complications.

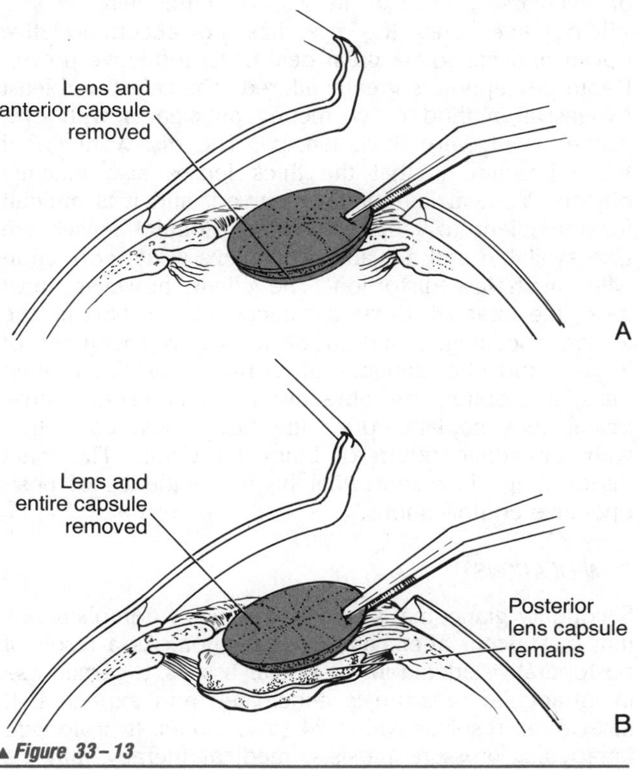

▲ **Figure 33–13**

Surgical approaches to lens removal for cataracts. *A*, Intracapsular cataract extraction. *B*, Extracapsular cataract extraction.

Phacoemulsification is an extracapsular technique that uses ultrasound vibrations to break up the lens material. Pieces of the anterior lens capsule and the lens are removed by suction through the phacoemulsifier tip. This technique requires a much smaller incision in the eye and is often called the small incision technique. These small incisions require only one to three sutures, and in some cases, none at all. Wound healing in small incision surgery occurs at the same rate as in larger incision techniques.

Cataract surgery is usually performed under local anesthesia with sedation. The client is given an intravenous injection of methohexital sodium (Brevital) or thiopental (Pentothol) to induce a few minutes of light anesthesia while the retrobulbar injection of local anesthetic is given.

INTRAOCULAR LENS IMPLANTATION

Following the extraction of the cataract, a new lens is inserted in the posterior chamber, or the client is left without a lens. Although there are many styles of lenses, they all consist of two basic parts: (1) a clear spherical optic usually made of polymethylmethacrylate (Plexiglas) and (2) footplates or haptics to hold the lens in place. Foldable lenses made of silicone or hydrogel material have been developed to fit through the smaller incisions, but data on long-term use are not available yet.

APHAKIA

Aphakia (absence of the lens) is corrected by the use of eyeglasses, contact lenses, or intraocular lenses. Without the lens, the eye has no accommodative power and has lost a great deal of its refractive power. Depth perception is greatly altered. The safest and least expensive method of correcting aphakia is with eyeglasses (with very thick lenses). The disadvantage of this correction is that the thick lenses also magnify objects. Vertical lines appear curved, and it is difficult for the client to judge distances. Contact lenses are also available and are able to achieve visual correction with much less distortion. The client, however, must have the manual dexterity necessary to handle the lenses. Cleaning, insertion of lenses, replacement of lenses, and the dangers of corneal abrasions often make this option less attractive to older clients. Intraocular lens implants offer the best visual correction with immediate return of binocular vision. The main disadvantage is a somewhat higher incidence of postoperative complications.

COMPLICATIONS

Secondary glaucoma is one of the major complications that may occur after cataract extraction. As a result of postoperative edema in the ocular tissues, a certain rise in intraocular pressure is anticipated and expected. It most often resolves within 24 to 72 hours. If prolonged intraocular pressure persists, medical therapy may be necessary. Postoperative infection, bleeding, macular edema and wound leaks, are also a possibility. The incidence of retinal detachment is higher in the first 12 months after cataract surgery.

Following extracapsular cataract extraction, the posterior capsule may become opacified and it is called an after cataract or secondary membrane. Subcapsular lens epithelial cells may regenerate lens fibers, which can obstruct vision. This postoperative complication occurs fairly frequently and, in the past, required a second operation to remove the opacified tissue. More recently, the neodymium-YAG laser is being used to create an opening in the capsule through pulses of laser energy that cause tiny "explosions" in the target tissue. Complications of this technique include a transient rise in intraocular pressure and possible damage to the intraocular lens.

Nursing Management

ASSESSMENT

During the history and physical examination, the nurse directs questions to the client about any predisposing factors (trauma, systemic diseases, medications such as corticosteroids, and other ocular problems). Visual acuity (both distant and near) in each eye is documented. It is important for the nurse to ask the client to describe visual disturbances. It is possible for the client's visual acuity to be relatively close to normal ranges, yet the client experiences difficulty in performing ADLs, for example. The client's individual perception of the quality of vision is an important factor in determining the need for surgery.

NURSING INTERVENTION

Nursing Diagnosis: Visual Sensory/Perceptual Alterations R/T cataract formation.

Planning: Expected Outcomes. The client will gain improved vision and will adapt to changes in visual correction.

Implementation. Adaptation is the key issue in caring for the client having cataract surgery. Nursing interventions are based on assisting the client to gain or maintain as much independence as possible. The client's lifestyle, abilities, and home environment must be evaluated. A 55-year-old client who is an architect and otherwise healthy may be having an early cataract removed because it interferes with his work in areas where bright light is used. A 75-year-old diabetic client who is retired and mainly watches television will have entirely different needs.

Unless there are other ocular complications or health factors, cataract surgery is performed on an outpatient basis. At the time of admission to the hospital or surgical facility, the nurse determines the client's current level of knowledge and understanding about the perioperative events. Preoperative sedation may include an oral sedative and/or medication to reduce intraocular pressure in the eye (a lower-than-normal intraocular pressure facilitates the surgical procedure). Preopera-

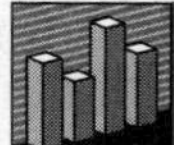

NURSING RESEARCH

The purpose of this descriptive, correlational study is to examine the level of loneliness in adults with limited vision to determine the relationship of loneliness to selected personal and social support factors. The sample consisted of 93 adults with limited vision. Limited vision was defined as a loss of vision that cannot be corrected by medical or surgical procedures or conventional eyeglasses. Several instruments were used to collect data on loneliness: the revised UCLA loneliness scale, the revised self-consciousness scale, the life orientation test, and the social support questionnaire.

Findings indicated that adults with limited vision rarely or sometimes felt lonely. Feelings of loneliness did not appear to have an impact on adjustment in this study group. Results of the regression analysis revealed that the best predictor of loneliness was social anxiety. Adults with limited vision have social anxiety with significantly higher levels of loneliness. Optimism and perceived social support had a negative correlation with loneliness. No doubt, a pessimistic outlook played a significant role in the loneliness of some adults in this sample. This study suggests that adults with limited vision who are pessimistic, socially anxious, and dissatisfied with existing social supports are at especially high risk for loneliness.

▼▼▼

Foxall, M. J., et. al. (1992). Predictors of loneliness in low vision adults. *Western Journal of Nursing Research, 14*(1), 86–99.

tive eye drops may include a dilating agent such as tropicamide (Mydriacyl) to dilate the pupil facilitating the surgery. A cycloplegic (Cyclogyl), may also be administered to paralyze the ciliary muscles.

Postoperative care includes observation of the ocular dressing, if present, and assessment of the client's ability to perform the activities of daily living at the preoperative level. The eye patch is usually removed the next morning but may be removed after a few hours if the client has limited vision in the other eye. The client is instructed to wear a metal or plastic shield to protect the eye from accidental injury or rubbing of the eye. Glasses may be worn during the day.

EVALUATION

The degree of expected outcome attainment should be assessed. Adaptation to restored normal vision is usually rapid. Adaptation to limited vision will require more time based on individual variations.

Post-hospital Care

DISCHARGE TEACHING

Discharge teaching includes client and family education regarding postoperative activities, eye care, medications, home care, and adaptation to visual correction.

Postoperative activity restrictions may vary among ophthalmologists. Generally, it is advisable for the client to avoid heavy lifting (over 5 pounds) or straining in the early postoperative period. The client should also avoid sleeping on the operative side.

Eye care for the client after cataract surgery is the same as that for glaucoma clients (see the section on glaucoma). Postoperative eye medications may include antibiotics and/or corticosteroids. The nurse should assess the client or family's ability to appropriately instill eye drops. The nurse should also review the rationale and schedule for the medications with the client and family. Postoperative discomfort should be minimal to moderate and is usually relieved by acetaminophen. Clients commonly experience an itching sensation after cataract surgery. However, the client should be instructed to report any pain that is unrelieved. The nurse should review the clinical manifestations of infection and increased intraocular pressure with the client and family.

Depending on the client's age, ability, and availability of assistance, the nurse should make a referral for home health care if it is indicated. Adjustment to changes in vision also varies with individual clients.

▼ Retinal Disorders

RETINAL DETACHMENT

Definition

Rhegmatogenous retinal detachment (secondary to a tear in the retina) is characterized by a retinal hole, liquid in the vitreous with access to the hole, and a subsequent fluid accumulation between the retina and the retinal pigment epithelium. The liquid seeps through the hole and separates the retina from its blood supply. Without intervention, the detachment continues to spread and the detached retina will lose the ability to function. It may become increasingly detached over a period of hours to years.

Incidence

Retinal detachment occurs mainly in the adult eye. The overall incidence is 1 in 10,000 people per year but the risk of detachment increases after the fourth decade and most often occurs between the ages of 50 and 70.

Etiology/Risk Factors

Predisposing factors to retinal detachment include cataract extraction, degeneration of the retina, trauma, and high myopia. Retinal holes and tears usually occur from spontaneous vitreous traction, but there may be abnormal adhesions between the retina and vitreous secondary to diabetic retinopathy, injury, or other ocular disorders. Atrophy of the vitreous may also result in a retinal tear.

Pathophysiology

When the retina is separated from its choroidal blood supply, it will die. The retinal tissues are at a high risk for avascular necrosis because they are delicate structures and have a high metabolic rate.

Clinical Manifestations

Characteristic symptoms of retinal detachment are described by clients as a shadow or curtain falling across the field of vision (Fig. 33–14). There is no pain associated with detachment of the retina. The onset is usually sudden and may be accompanied by a burst of black spots or floaters indicating that bleeding has occurred as a result of the detachment. Clients may also see flashes of light caused by separation of the retina.

Medical Management

Surgery is required to repair a detached retina because spontaneous reattachment of the retina is an uncommon occurrence. The indirect ophthalmoscope with a handheld magnifying lens is used to evaluate the extent and source of the detachment. A scleral depressor may also be used externally on the lid or conjunctiva to assist in rotating the eyeball and to indent the retina for increased viewing ability. Areas of detachment appear bluish gray as opposed to the normal red-pink color (Plate 3). Tears are most often horseshoe shaped but may be round.

Surgical Management

Surgical repair is required for retinal detachment. The goal is to place the retina back in contact with the choroid and to seal the accompanying holes and breaks. Often cryopexy (the use of a freezing probe) or laser photocoagulation is used to seal the hole if it has not progressed to detachment. Both methods create inflammation around the area, which scars and seals the hole.

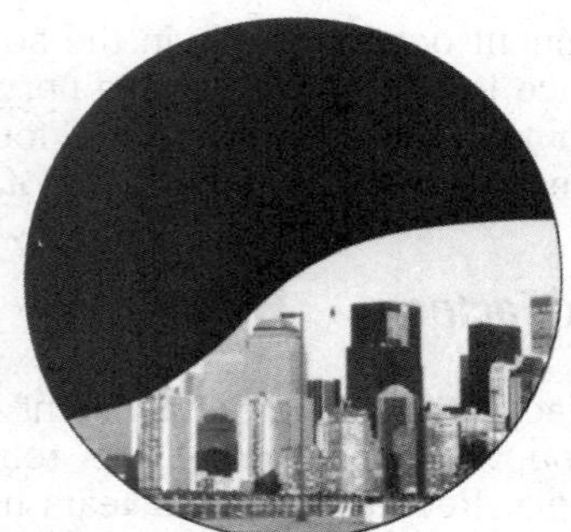

▲ **Figure 33–14**

Vision of a client with retinal detachment. (Courtesy of National Industries for the Blind, Wayne, NJ.)

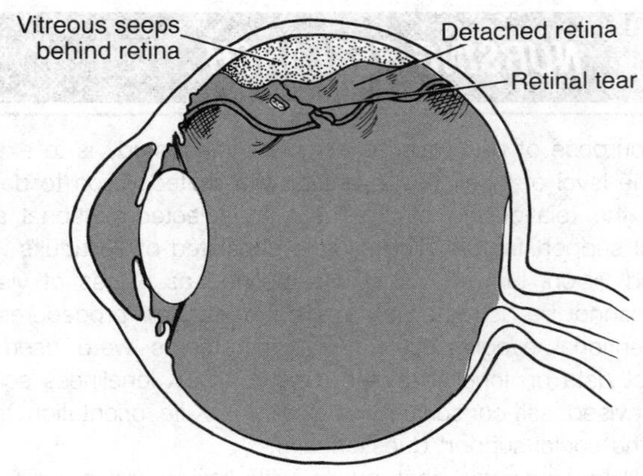

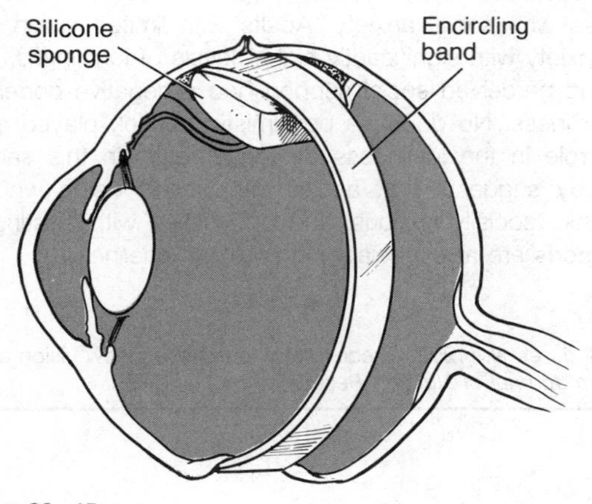

▲ **Figure 33–15**

Scleral buckling to repair a detached retina. A silicone sponge implant is placed over the tear and held in place with an encircling band. When the buckle is tightened, the implant indents the sclera, holding the choroid and retina together.

The surgical procedure to place the retina back in contact with the choroid is called scleral buckling (Fig. 33–15). The sclera is actually depressed from the outside by Silastic sponges or silicone bands that are sutured in place permanently. In addition to the buckling procedure, an intraocular injection of air and/or sulfahexafluoride (SF6) gas bubble may be used to apply pressure on the retina from the inside of the eye. This bubble holds the retina in place by gravitational force during the healing phase. Postoperative positioning of the client maximizes the tamponade effect of the air/gas bubble. The air/gas bubble is slowly absorbed.

COMPLICATIONS

Postoperative swelling of tissues and cells in the anterior chamber due to the inflammatory process or compromise of the venous drainage system may result in increased intraocular pressure. Because of the fragility of the tissues involved in the repair, redetachment of the retina may occur at any time. At times, the retina has been separated from its blood supply long enough so that, even when reattached, it no longer has useful function and the client's vision does not improve significantly. Postoperative infection is also a risk.

Nursing Management

ASSESSMENT

When the history is obtained and physical examination is performed, it is important for the nurse to assess the client's visual changes in both eyes. Visual field loss is seen by the client in the opposite quadrant of the actual detachment. For example, a tear in the temporal region, which is affected more frequently, creates a visual defect in the nasal area.

The pupil must be widely dilated for a retinal examination. The nurse explains that the client will experience an extremely bright light and be asked to change gaze frequently to facilitate the examination.

NURSING INTERVENTION

Nursing Diagnosis: Visual Sensory/Perceptual Alterations R/T compromised retinal function.

Planning: Expected Outcomes. The client will maintain as much functional vision as possible, as evidenced by reporting no further loss of vision and adapting to any visual loss, demonstrate an ability to perform activities of daily living (ADLs), instill his or her own eye medications and recognize clinical manifestations of complications.

Implementation. The focus of the care plan is assisting the client to cope with the fears and reality of vision loss and to adapt to changes in vision. The client must be aware of the clinical manifestations of further vision loss.

Preoperative nursing care involves preparing the client for a 1- to 3-day hospital stay; however, some retinal detachment surgery may be performed on an outpatient basis. The client may be placed on activity restrictions prior to surgery based on the size and location of the detachment. If the macula is threatened, the risk of further detachment is greater and the potential for vision loss is also greater. Most often, bathroom privileges are allowed.

The nurse should assess the client's current level of knowledge and understanding about the implications of retinal detachment and the expectations from the surgical procedure. Because retinal detachment repair may take several hours in the operating room, general anesthesia is used in many cases. The pupil must be widely dilated before the operation, and the client may be given a sedative.

Postoperatively, the nurse observes the eye patch for any drainage. Blood loss in retinal detachment surgery is minimal, and only serous drainage is expected on the postoperative dressing. Activity restrictions may be necessary if an air/gas bubble has been injected. The client will need to be positioned so that the bubble can apply maximal pressure on the retina by the force of gravity. The position is usually maintained for several days. The nurse provides comfort and support to assist the client with positioning and monitors the client during sleep.

Posterior segment surgery, such as scleral buckling procedures, results in considerably more discomfort than anterior segment procedures. Ocular muscles are separated, and the globe is manipulated to reach the posterior portions of the eyeball. Narcotics may be needed during the first 24 hours after surgery. Nausea and vomiting may also require management. Intravenous acetazolamide (Diamox) may be used to reduce increased intraocular pressure. The intraocular pressure is monitored closely during the first 24 hours. The client should be encouraged to resume a regular diet and fluids as tolerated.

The eye patch and shield are removed the next morning. Redness and swelling of the lids and conjunctiva should be expected from the surgical manipulation. After several days, the swelling and ecchymosis of the lids subsides, but the conjunctiva may remain red or pink for a few weeks.

Postoperative eye medications generally include an antibiotic-steroid combination drop to prevent infection and reduce inflammation. Cycloplegic agents are prescribed to dilate the pupil and relax the cilliary muscles, which decreases discomfort and helps prevent the formation of iris adhesions to the corneal endothelium (synechiae). The client should not expect immediate return of vision. Postoperative inflammation and the dilating drops interfere with vision. As healing takes place over weeks and months, vision may improve on a gradual basis. Either warm or cold compresses may be applied for comfort several times a day.

EVALUATION

The nurse evaluates the expected outcomes for the client. Revisions in the plan of care may be required.

Post-hospital Care

DISCHARGE TEACHING

The client is instructed to clean the eye with warm tap water using a clean wash cloth. Warm compresses may be continued at home. Either an eye shield or glasses should be worn during the day, and the shield should be worn during naps and at night. The client is usually instructed to avoid vigorous activities and heavy lifting during the immediate postoperative period. If an air/gas bubble has been injected, it may take several weeks to totally absorb. Clients are advised to avoid air travel during this time because the gas and air expand at high altitudes.

HOME HEALTH CARE NEEDS

Because retinal detachment surgery is often performed on an urgent basis, the client rarely has an opportunity to plan for the surgery. It is important for the nurse to evaluate the home environment and to assist the client and family in preparing for any necessary support. The home should be assessed for safety hazards, such as throw rugs, electrical cords, stairs, and poor lighting. Although the eye patch is usually removed early in the postoperative period, the client likely has decreased functional vision in the operative eye.

DIABETIC RETINOPATHY

Overview

Diabetic retinopathy is a progressive disorder of the retina characterized by microscopic damage to the retinal vessels, resulting in occlusion of the vessels. As a result of inadequate blood supply, sections of the retina deteriorate and vision is permanently lost.

Diabetic retinopathy is one of the leading causes of blindness in the United States and the world. All diabetics are prone to develop retinopathy, although studies indicate that there is a strong correlation between the incidence and severity of retinopathy with both the duration of the disease and erratic blood glucose control. Approximately 30 to 40 per cent of the diabetic population has some degree of retinopathy. Clients who have had diabetes for 15 to 20 years have an 80 to 90 per cent chance of developing retinopathy.

There are two types of retinopathy: (1) background, or nonproliferative diabetic retinopathy, and (2) proliferative diabetic retinopathy.

In background retinopathy, early pathologic changes demonstrate the hyperpermeability and weakening of the retinal vessels. The capillaries develop tiny dotlike outpouchings called microaneurysms, and the retinal veins become dilated and tortuous (Fig. 33-16*A*). Multiple hemorrhages occur from these defective vessels. Retinal edema is caused by leaking capillaries, and after the serous fluid is absorbed, a yellowish precipitate called a "hard exudate" remains. Hemorrhages, exudates, and ischemia contribute to impaired vision, particularly if these occur on or around the macula.

Progressive retinal ischemia stimulates the growth of new but ineffective blood vessels. These new and fragile blood vessels proliferate and grow into the vitreous. These vessels leak, hemorrhage, and undergo fibrous changes that may form bands that pull on the retina, causing detachment. This process is called proliferative retinopathy (Fig. 33-16*B*). With increasing ischemia, microinfarcts of the nerve fiber layer, called cotton-wool spots, appear.

Clients experience a wide range of visual disturbances and fluctuations. Retinal vessel hemorrhage into the vitreous space obstructs vision with black spots or floaters or may result in complete loss of vision. Areas of retinal ischemia become blind spots. Macular edema causes decreased central vision.

Management

In order to reduce the occurrence of hemorrhage and retinal detachment in progressive retinopathy, the argon laser is used to photocoagulate the blood vessels. Hundreds and even thousands of microscopic photocoagulation applications (burns) are systematically placed around the peripheral retina, avoiding the central area that includes the macula and the optic disc.

When a hemorrhage does not clear spontaneously over time, a vitrectomy (removal of a portion of the vitreous) may be performed. A vitrectomy may also need to be performed to release the traction of membranes on the retina.

Nursing interventions for the client with diabetic retinopathy are focused on assessment and management of diabetes. Because retinopathy is generally progres-

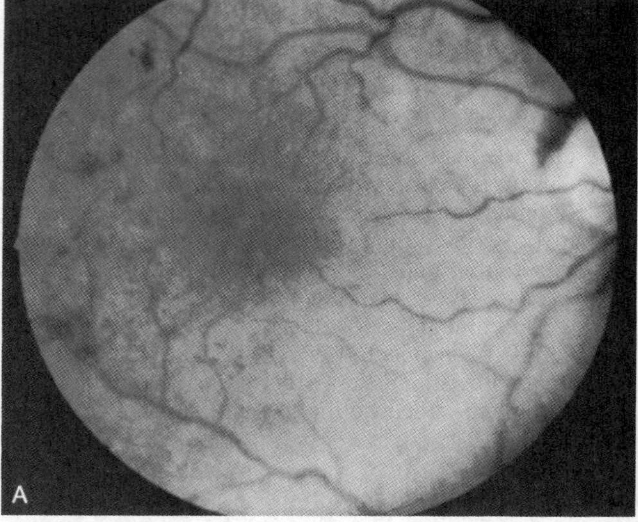

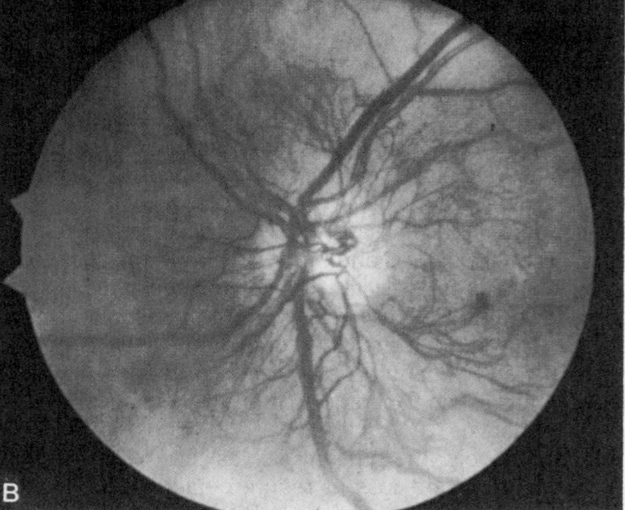

▲ **Figure 33-16**

Diabetic retinopathy. (From Smith, S. L. [1992]. Diabetic retinopathy. *Nursing Clinics of North America 27*(3), 745-759.)

sive, the client will need to cope with increasing visual deficits. Community referrals for rehabilitation and low vision aids often provide useful assistance. Visiting nurses often prepare insulin injections for the upcoming week, as the client cannot see clearly to aspirate correct amounts of the drug.

AGE-RELATED MACULAR DEGENERATION

Overview

Previously known as senile macular degeneration, age-related macular degeneration is an atrophic degenerative process that affects the macula and surrounding tissues, resulting in central visual deficits.

Age-related macular degeneration can be found to some degree in most adults over the age of 65. It is one of the most common causes of visual loss in the elderly. The exact etiology is unknown, but the incidence increases with each decade over 50. It may also be hereditary.

Age-related macular degeneration falls into two groups: (1) nonexudative and (2) exudative. Both are usually bilateral and progressive.

Also referred to as "dry" macular degeneration, nonexudative age-related macular degeneration is characterized by atrophy and degeneration of the outer retina and underlying structures. Yellowish round spots called drusen may be seen on the retina and macula with an ophthalmoscope. Drusen are deposits of amorphous material from the pigment epithelial cells of the retina. Over time, these spots increase, enlarge, and may calcify.

At this "wet," exudative stage of age-related macular degeneration, Bruch's membrane, which lies just beneath the pigment epithelial cell layer of the retina, becomes compromised and this results in serous fluid leaks from the choroid, with accompanying proliferation of choroidal blood vessels. A dome-shaped retinal pigment epithelium may be seen when examining the fundus. These leaks produce a visual effect called metamorphopsia, which is the blurred, wavy distortion of vision. The client may also notice a blurred scotoma or decreased central visual acuity (Fig. 33–17). Fundus photography and angiography may be performed on a regular basis to document and evaluate changes.

Management

There is no known means of medical treatment or prevention for age-related macular degeneration. Further damage from exudative macular degeneration sometimes may be arrested by the use of argon photocoagulation, even though laser damage to the retina in this area results in a blind spot. When the fovea is involved, central vision is lost and the only helpful measures are low-vision aids.

The client with age-related macular degeneration is threatened with the loss of central vision (see Bridge to Home Health Care). In order to evaluate changes in

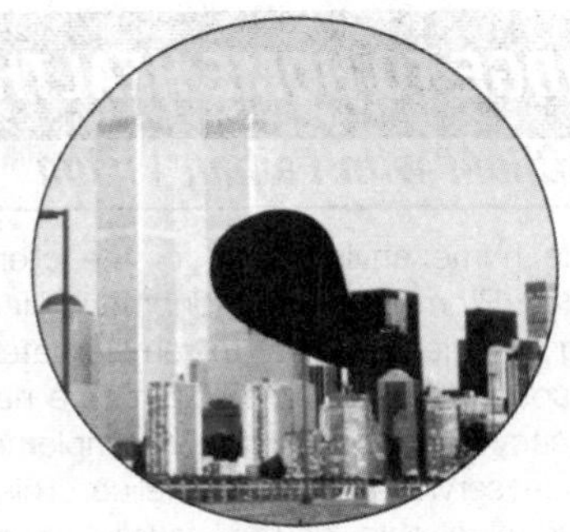
Macular Degeneration

▲ Figure 33–17

Vision of a client with macular degeneration. (Courtesy of National Industries for the Blind, Wayne, NJ.)

vision, the client is taught to use an Amsler grid at home. The nurse may be able to assist the client to maximize remaining vision with low-vision aids and community referral to a low-vision specialist and low-vision support groups.

▼ Corneal Disorders

CORNEAL DYSTROPHIES

Definition

Corneal dystrophies are a group of hereditary and acquired disorders of unknown etiology, characterized by deposits in the layers of the cornea and alteration of the corneal structure.

Risk Factors

Specific corneal dystrophies characteristically appear at different ages. They may be stationary or slowly progressive throughout life. The most common, Fuchs' dystrophy, usually begins in the third or fourth decade, affects more women than men, and is slowly progressive.

Pathophysiology

Corneal dystrophies are associated with all five layers of the cornea. Although the disease usually originates in the inner layers (Descemet's membrane, the stroma, and Bowman's membrane), the degeneration, erosion, and deposits affect all layers.

Clinical Manifestations

Fuchs' dystrophy is characterized by deposits in Descemet's membrane that look like warts. Descemet's membrane becomes thickened, and defects appear in

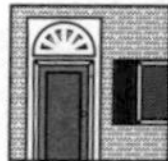

BRIDGE TO HOME HEALTH CARE

The Client with Failing Vision

Providing a safe home environment for the client with failing vision is essential. Promoting an autonomous lifestyle is desirable. Assessing the client's ability to remain safely at home is an important responsibility of home health care nurses.

Basic emergency procedures can be implemented by the use of nationwide services such as Lifeline. This service provides a portable electronic device usually worn around the client's neck or wrist. By simply pushing the button immediate contact is made with emergency personnel. Information can be obtained by calling toll-free 1-800-852-5433.

Local telephone companies can provide special adaptive equipment for 911 access. Phones that can be programed and have lighted and/or large numbers are available in most retail stores.

Home safety precautions can be simple. Burns can be prevented by color-coding water faucets. Use red for hot water and green for cold water. Marking the "Off" dials on stoves and microwaves with colored tape or paint will decrease the chance of injury.

Adequate lighting is essential. During the day, natural light is preferable. Open drapes or shades to provide ample light. Replace light bulbs with the highest wattage recommended.

Removal of hazards, such as throw rugs, clutter, and unnecessary furniture, will provide unrestricted ambulation. Handrails can be installed in hallways, bathrooms, and on steps to prevent falls. Equipment such as canes, walkers, raised toilet seats and tub rails promote safety. These items are available at medical supply stores.

Many commercial products are now marketed that can be of great assistance in the home. Pill organizers are clearly marked boxes with the day of the week and the times pills are to be taken. These can be filled by family members for a week at a time. Electronic lamp timers and voice activated switches will allow the client to function more independently.

Access to a television and a radio are important. Large print newspapers and reading materials will keep the client in touch with current events. The local library and the American Association for the Blind can provide assistance in obtaining needed items.

Creativity and planning can allow the client to remain at home in a safe environment for as long as possible.

the endothelial layer. Because the integrity of the cornea is compromised, it becomes edematous and cloudy. Vision is compromised not only by the corneal deposits but by the altered structure of the cornea secondary to the edema.

Medical Management

The cornea is evaluated by slit lamp examination. Fluorescein staining is used to enhance visualization of surface corneal defects. Corneal scrapings may be taken with a sterile spatula for further staining and microscopic evaluation. Specular micrography (see the section on diagnostic tests) may be used to evaluate the corneal endothelium.

Surgical Management

Corneal transplantation, or keratoplasty, may be indicated for a number of serious corneal conditions including corneal dystrophy. Penetrating keratoplasty denotes full-thickness corneal replacement; lamellar keratoplasty denotes a partial-thickness procedure.

Because there is a direct relationship between the age and health of the endothelial layer of the cornea, young donor tissue is preferred. Donor eyes are obtained from cadavers and must be enucleated soon after death due to rapid endothelial cell death, and the eyes must be stored in a preserving solution. Storage, handling, and coordination of donor tissue with surgeons is provided by a network of state eye bank associations around the country.

Corneal transplantation surgery is usually performed under local anesthesia (Plate 4). In surgery, the donor cornea is prepared first by using a trephine to cut a corneal button with a radius of usually 7.0 to 8.5 mm. The recipient cornea is prepared in the same manner; however, it is usually cut 0.5 mm smaller so that there is an overlap by the donor cornea, which is then sutured into place.

COMPLICATIONS

Graft rejection and/or failure may occur at any time after the transplantation. It can result from unsuitable storage of donor tissue, dystrophy of the donor's endothelium, surgical trauma, or immunologic rejection. Because the cornea is an avascular structure, bloodtyping, which is necessary for other types of grafts, is not necessary.

At the first sign of graft rejection, when the cornea becomes cloudy and edematous and when there is an anterior chamber reaction (presence of white blood cells or protein) (Plate 5), topical steroids are prescribed in frequent doses to control the inflammatory response and reverse the rejection reaction. In severe cases, a repeat transplantation may be necessary.

Wound leakage, bleeding into the anterior chamber, glaucoma, cataract, and infection are also complications that may occur.

Nursing Management

ASSESSMENT

It is important for the nurse to assist the client in describing symptoms. Because the cornea is extremely sensitive, pain is a common complaint. The type, onset, duration, and other associated factors document a clinical picture that results in the diagnosis.

NURSING INTERVENTION

Nursing Diagnosis: Visual Sensory/Perceptual Alterations R/T decreased corneal function.

Planning: Expected Outcomes. The client will have improved visual sensation and perception, as evidenced by functioning safely with current visual deficits and maintaining improved vision with corneal transplantation, recognizing clinical manifestations of graft failure, instilling eye drops correctly, and performing a daily check of vision.

Implementation. The focus of nursing care is to help the client adapt to the limitations in vision and to prepare the client to undergo surgery.

Because some corneal dystrophies and other disorders may progress slowly, the nurse assists the client in adaptation to vision loss (see nursing care for the client with cataracts). Corneal transplantation surgery is usually performed on an outpatient basis or may involve an overnight stay in the hospital.

Preoperative nursing care includes client and family education regarding perioperative events. The client is usually notified the day prior to the surgery that donor tissue has become available. Clients may be on a waiting list for several weeks or months. Receiving a call with short notice for the surgery usually produces a relatively high level of anxiety for the client and family. The nurse assists the client in coping with the rush of preoperative activities by using a calm and assured manner.

Postoperatively, the client returns from the operating room with an eye patch and protective shield in place. The nurse observes the patch for signs of drainage. There is no blood loss associated with this procedure. The client should experience only mild to moderate discomfort, which should be relieved by acetaminophen. Unrelieved pain may indicate a rise in intraocular pressure and is reported to the surgeon. Because the eye patch will be in place until the following morning, the nurse assesses the client's ability for self-care and teaches both the client and family the hazards of monocular vision (See postoperative care for the client with retinal detachment). The eye is examined the next morning with the slit lamp. Depending on the extent of preoperative visual limitations, most clients experience improved vision immediately. Clients are instructed, however, not to place their expectations too high. Vision continues to improve gradually because the healing process may take up to a year or more. Glasses or contact lenses are usually needed to obtain the best visual result.

EVALUATION

The expected outcomes are evaluated. Since many months may be required for visual restoration, revisions in the plan of care may be needed.

Post-hospital Care

DISCHARGE TEACHING

Postoperative eye drops usually include an antibiotic and a corticosteroid. Topical corticosteroid therapy may be needed indefinitely. Discharge instructions include the rationale for the medications and proper instillation technique. It is important for the client to wear eye protection in the form of regular glasses, sunglasses, or a protective shield to prevent any injury to the eye. The client is advised never to rub the eye. The area around the eye may be cleaned with warm tap water using a clean wash cloth.

Teaching the client and family to recognize the signs and symptoms of graft rejection is a critical component of discharge education. The following teaching tool may be useful in teaching the client to remember the signs of graft rejection. It involves the use of the letters RSVP which are familiar to most people:

R = redness
S = swelling
V = decreased vision
P = pain

The client is advised to evaluate the vision in the operative eye each day. A picture on the wall or some object in a well-lit room should be selected to use as a point of reference. If a change in vision from the day before is noted, the client should reevaluate his or her vision in a few hours. If no improvement is noted or if vision is worse, the client should notify the physician. Because graft rejection may occur at any time (even years) after the surgery, the client is advised to make the vision check a routine part of his or her ADLs for the rest of his or her life.

The nurse also teaches the client and family to recognize the signs of increased intraocular pressure and infection.

KERATITIS

Overview

The corneal epithelium is normally an effective barrier against microorganisms. Once it is compromised from disease or trauma, the underlying stromal layer becomes an excellent culture media for a variety of organisms.

Dry eyes or ineffective eyelid closure predispose the eye to keratitis. Clients who have a systemic collagen disorder such as rheumatoid arthritis are particularly susceptible to corneal infections and ulceration.

Tearing and photophobia are common, and blurred vision results from the inability of the cornea to provide the proper refractive surface. The client with a corneal defect from an infection will experience a great deal of discomfort, which is worsened by eyelid movement. The eye appears infected and indurated. Flourescein staining of the cornea outlines the affected area, which can be viewed through the slit lamp or with a handheld flashlight.

CORNEAL ULCERS

Corneal infections may develop into ulcerations (Plate 6) that severely compromise the integrity of the eye. Sources of infection include bacteria (e.g., *Staphylococcus aureus*, *Pseudomonas aeruginosa*, and *Strepto-*

coccus pneumoniae), fungi *(Candida, Aspergillus)*, viruses (adenovirus, herpes simplex, herpes zoster) and protozoa *(Acanthamoeba)*. Clinical findings under slit lamp examination are specific to particular organisms. Hypopyon (a layer of white cells in the anterior chamber) may accompany corneal ulceration.

MANAGEMENT

Topical antibiotic, antifungal, and antiviral therapy is prescribed, with the frequency of instillation based on the severity of the infection to prevent the progression to perforation and to promote healing. Maximal therapy includes the instillation of two broad-spectrum eye drops every 15 minutes around the clock. As the infection begins to respond to the medication, frequency is gradually decreased. Systemic intravenous medication may be prescribed as well.

In order to aid the healing process, surgical intervention may be necessary. Tarsorrhaphy (suturing the eyelid shut) promotes healing by decreasing eyelid blinking and by decreasing evaporation of the corneal tear film. For corneal perforation, a conjunctival flap may be performed to cover the defect. Tissue adhesive, a kind of super glue, may also be used to seal the perforation. A soft contact lens may be used as a bandage to maintain the seal. Large perforations may require either lamellar (partial-thickness) or penetrating (full-thickness) keratoplasty.

In cases in which medical and surgical interventions fail, enucleation (removal of the entire eyeball) may be necessary (see ocular melanoma for nursing care). In some cases, evisceration (removal of only the orbital contents) may be indicated. The scleral shell is left intact along with the ocular muscles, which allows for improved ocular prosthetic fit and function.

Although the early stages of corneal infection are often managed at home, the client may need to be hospitalized for the management of a severe corneal ulcer. If the client and family have been instilling frequent eye drops at home, the client may be fatigued from lack of sleep as well as anxious about possible vision loss. The nurse assesses the client's level of discomfort and methods of coping with the stress of pain and lack of sleep. Often at this stage, the client is not coping well at all.

Eye drops are given alternately every 15 minutes around the clock. This schedule is a challenge not only for the client but for the nurse as well. Handwashing is particularly important in this situation and is carried out even if gloves are worn to instill the drops. The threat of losing eyesight compels many clients to watch the clock for fear that the nurse will forget to administer an eye drop. The nurse can build the client's trust and reduce anxiety by maintaining the time schedule for the eye drops.

Effective sleep and rest are nearly impossible with interruptions every 15 minutes. The client rarely reaches the deeper stages of sleep and most experience restless light sleep in stage one and two. In addition to the eye pain the client may already be experiencing, some of the eye drops, such as fortified bacitracin, may cause stinging that lasts several minutes.

There are several comfort measures that can be instituted by the nurse. A daily routine of care should be outlined, based as much as possible on the client's normal routine at home. Because there are so many interruptions to the client's personal time and space, it is important to identify at least two periods of time during the day when the client may rest or nap with the only interruption being the nurse who comes in to administer the eye drop. A sign should be posted on the door to the client's room for privacy during these rest times. The nurse and client may also agree that the nurse will not open topics of conversation during this time but will quietly instill the eye drop. The nurse adopts this same routine during the client's normal nighttime. Some clients are actually able to sleep during the instillation of eye drops at night; however, the nurse should establish this routine with the client in advance. Older clients, who are accustomed to more stage two sleep than younger clients, are able to rest more effectively. Because younger clients tend to become confused and irritable more often, the nurse should speak to the client before touching him or her. Oral analgesics are given at regular intervals, and mild sleeping medications may be helpful at bedtime.

The client's eye may need to be cleansed frequently because the medications and excessive tearing will become dried and the lids will stick together. Warm tap water applied with soft gauze pads is used. The combination of tearing, medications, and cleaning may cause the skin of an elderly client to become excoriated. Antibiotic ophthalmic ointment may be applied to the lower lid margin and cheek to reduce irritation.

Clients usually become adapted to this regimen of interruptions after the first 48 hours. As the cornea begins to show signs of improvement, the eye drops may be reduced in frequency to every 30 minutes and then every hour. Most clients will not notice a great deal of difference in the every-30-minute routine, but when the routine is reduced to every hour, they will begin to sleep more heavily as the body attempts to compensate for lost sleep. At the end of an hour, the client may complain to the nurse that it has seemed like only a few minutes since the last drop. Intense dreaming may also be experienced during this time.

At discharge, the client should be able to demonstrate how to properly instill eye drops. The client will also understand the importance of complying with the medication regimen. The nurse should instruct both the client and family about the signs and symptoms of increasing infection. The eye may continue to be cleansed with warm tap water at home. The nurse also assesses the home environment if the client's vision is greatly reduced. Referrals for rehabilitation may be necessary as well.

KERATOCONUS

Keratoconus is a degenerative disease of the cornea characterized by a thinning and protrusion of the cornea in a cone shape (Plate 7). Blurred vision is the result of the change in the shape of the cornea, which may be corrected by contact lenses. Keratoconus is often slowly progressive between the ages of 20 and 60.

At some point, the conical shape of the cornea may no longer allow for contact lenses to correct vision. Corneal transplantation for keratoconus is highly successful.

▼ Uveal Tract Disorders

UVEITIS

Uveitis is an inflammation of the uveal tract that can effect one or more parts (iris, ciliary body, and choroid). Uveitis commonly occurs from a hypersensitivity reaction in its acute form or following microbial infection in its chronic form. Clients with this condition complain of pain, blurred vision, and photophobia. There is marked redness of the eye, and the pupil is usually constricted. Cells (white blood cells) and flare (protein), called an anterior chamber reaction, are seen in the anterior chamber fluid with the slit lamp.

The primary cause of discomfort in clients with uveitis is ciliary body muscle spasm. A cycloplegic medication such as atropine effectively relieves the spasm, and the dilation of the pupil prevents the inflamed iris from adhering to the lens and/or the corneal endothelium from forming synechiae. Topical steroid drops are prescribed to reduce the inflammation.

Photophobia (sensitivity to light) and eye discomfort are the chief complaints. The nurse should advise the client to wear dark glasses and to avoid bright light. Reduced lighting at home may be hazardous because the client's pupil is dilated, causing blurred vision. Oral analgesics usually relieve the ocular discomfort.

The nurse should be sure that the client and family understand the rationale for the prescribed medications. The client should also be able to recognize signs and symptoms of increased intraocular pressure.

▼ Malignant Ocular Tumors

CHOROIDAL MELANOMA

Overview

Although less than 1 per cent of the total population in the United States are affected by malignant ocular tumors, the treatment of these tumors can be a challenge to the client and nurse.

Choroidal melanomas are often detected during a routine ocular examination because there is no pain associated with the development of the tumor. By the time the tumor has grown large enough to obstruct vision, there may be involvement of the macula and metastasis.

Management

When ocular melanoma is discovered early, radiation therapy alone may be the treatment of choice. Radiation therapy to the eye is accomplished through the insertion of a tiny plate or plaque about the size of a dime that holds tiny seeds of radioactive iodine-125. The plaque is sutured to the sclera directly over the site of the tumor. It is left in place for several days, depending on the required dose, and then removed. Both insertion and removal are performed in the operating room. During the treatment, a lead shield is placed over the eye. Radiation exposure to the nurse who cares for the client is extremely minimal—a small fraction of a chest x-ray study. In spite of this extremely low exposure, the routine restrictions for hospital personnel and visitors are implemented for the sake of consistency.

During the client's hospitalization for this treatment, the nurse provides support and encouragement for the client. The plaque is only mildly to moderately uncomfortable, and discomfort should be relieved with acetaminophen. The difficult challenge for the client is confinement to the room with limitations on visitors at a time when support is essential. Eye medications include a cycloplegic and an antibiotic-steroid drop.

Enucleation (removal of the entire eyeball) has been the traditional method of treatment and may be combined with radiation treatments. Exenteration (removal of the eyeball and surrounding tissues and bone) may also be necessary.

Enucleation surgery is usually performed under general anesthesia. The ocular muscles are dissected from the eyeball which is removed by severing the optic nerve and vessels at the back. An acrylic sphere covered by donor scleral tissue is usually placed within the capsule of tissue that formerly held the eyeball. Scleral tissue encourages fibrovascular ingrowth, which prevents migration and extrusion of the implant. A soft plastic scleral shell is placed in the visible outer portion of the socket as a support until a permanent prosthesis (artificial eye; Plate 8) can be made. More recently, a new type of implant, hydroxyapatite, which is made of the same inorganic material present in human bone, is being used. Several weeks later, a central hole is drilled into the sphere and covering tissues. A peg (which will later be attached to the posterior surface of the artificial eye) is then fitted to the hole. The movement of the implant by the muscle cone is directly transferred to the prostheses. With the artificial eye being primarily supported by the peg instead of the lids and socket tissues, there are fewer cosmetic and structural complications.

The client undergoing enucleation for a malignant tumor is stressed not only with the threat of cancer but with disfigurement of the face. The nurse assesses the client's response, home, and family for support mechanisms.

The goal for the client following enucleation is that the client will adapt to monocular vision and return to his or her former level of independence. Nursing interventions are focused on assisting the client to grieve for the lost body part and for lost vision, and to identify coping mechanisms that will facilitate rehabilitation.

Preoperatively, the nurse assists the client in preparing for the surgical procedure. Most often, the client is made aware of the tumor at a routine office visit. Surgery is usually scheduled within a few days. Recognizing that the client is most appropriately in a stage of shock and denial, the nurse carefully explains the perioperative events. Although it is possible to have an enucleation as an outpatient procedure, the client may stay 24 to 48 hours in the hospital.

Routine postoperative care is provided. The client returns from the operating room with a pressure dressing over the eye. The nurse periodically assesses the dressing for bleeding because hemorrhage is a possibility in this surgery. Clients are understandably anxious about the removal of the dressing the next morning. The nurse prepares the client by explaining how the eye and conformer will appear. The socket and lids will be swollen, and the white plastic conformer is visible. The nurse also determines the client and or family's ability to care for the wound postoperatively.

Some clients are afraid that their appearance will frighten others, especially children. In this case, an eye patch may be worn for the 4 to 6 weeks before the prosthesis is fitted, but it should not be worn continuously.

The area around the lids may be cleansed with warm tap water using a clean wash cloth. Soap and water should be kept away from the socket. If the plastic conformer accidentally comes out, it should be washed and replaced. Antibiotic ophthalmic ointment is usually ordered to be instilled in the socket once or twice a day.

Adjustment to monocular vision is a challenge the client begins to face immediately. Depth perception is altered, and the client will need to exercise caution in walking, crossing streets, and driving. The nurse should advise the client to practice ADLs until visual and body adjustments are made.

The nurse also stresses the need for extra precaution with the remaining eye. Eye protection should be worn when engaging in any activity that might even remotely result in an injury. Many clients are advised to wear glasses even if no correction is needed.

▼ Eyelid, Lacrimal, and Conjunctival Disorders

HORDEOLUM

Hordeolum (stye) is an infection of the glands of the eyelids. It is most often caused by *Staphylococcus* infections, and clients complain of redness and pain due to the lid swelling. A localized swelling is noted on either the external or internal margin of the lid close to the lashes. As the hordeolum forms, it may fill with purulent material, becoming reddened and painful.

Warm compresses several times and antibiotics are prescribed. If the hordeolum does not resolve spontaneously, incision and drainage of the purulent material is indicated.

CHALAZION

A chalazion is a sterile chronic granulomatous inflammation of a meibomian gland. It is usually characterized by painless localized swelling along the lid margin without redness (Plate 9).

If the chalazion is large enough to distort vision or to be a cosmetic blemish, it may be surgically excised.

BLEPHARITIS

Blepharitis is a common chronic bilateral inflammation of the eyelid margins. Clients complain of itching and burning of the eyes and the eyes appear red, especially along the lid margins. Scales or granulations may be noted along the lashes of both the upper and lower lids.

Treatment is to keep the scalp as well as the eyebrows and lid margins clean. Scales should be removed with baby shampoo, water, and cotton-tipped applicators. Infected blepharitis may be treated with antibiotic ophthalmic ointment.

CONJUNCTIVITIS

Conjunctivitis is an inflammation of the conjunctiva due to bacterial, chlamydial (trachoma), viral, rickettsial, fungal, or parasitic infections; allergies; irritants; or secondary to systemic or other ocular diseases.

Generally, the first sign of conjunctivitis is hyperemia (redness), accompanied by tearing, and exudation (flaking and sticky substances on the lid margins). Other symptoms may include pseudoptosis (drooping of the upper lid), papillary hypertrophy, follicles, pseudomembranes, and granulomas. Conjunctivitis is treated with antibiotic eye drops or systemic medications.

BENIGN LID TUMORS

Benign tumors of the lids are very common and often increase in frequency with age. Melanocytic nevi (moles) and verrucae (warts) commonly appear on the lids and lid margins. Xanthelasma appears as yellow wrinkled patches, which are actually lipid deposits under the skin of the eyelids. These benign lesions may be removed for cosmetic reasons.

MALIGNANT LID TUMORS

Basal cell and squamous cell carcinomas of the lids are the most common malignant tumors of the eyelids.

These tumors do appear more frequently in individuals with fair complexions who have had chronic exposure to the sun. Malignant lid tumors are most often (90 to 95 per cent) of the basal cell type and frequently appear on the lower lid as nodules which gradually enlarge, becoming scaly and ulcerated.

Malignant tumors may be removed and treated by a variety of methods such as electrodessication, cryotherapy, or surgical removal. When the tumor is large, reconstruction may be required.

▼ Refractive Disorders

Light is bent (refracted) as it passes through the cornea and lens of the eye. Refractive errors exist when light rays are not focused appropriately on the retina of the eye.

There are three basic abnormalities of refraction that occur in the eye: (1) myopia, (2) hyperopia, and (3) astigmatism. Optical correction is important in order to distinguish between visual loss caused by disease and visual loss caused by refractive error. Refractometry is defined as the measurement of refractive error, and should not be confused with the term refraction. Refraction is defined as the methods used to determine which lens or lenses (if any) will most benefit an individual.

MYOPIA

Myopia, or nearsightedness, is a condition in which the light rays come into focus in front of the retina (Fig. 33-18*A*). In this case, the refractive power of the eye is too strong and a concave, or minus, lens is used to focus light rays on the eye. In the great majority of cases, myopia is caused by an eyeball that is longer than normal, which may be a familial trait. Transient myopia may occur with the administration of a variety of medications (sulfonamides, acetazolimide, salicylates, and steroids) and has been associated with other disorders, such as influenza, typhoid fever, severe dehydration, and large intakes of antacids (for stomach ulcers).

In some cases of myopia, surgical intervention (radial keratotomy) may be performed on the cornea to reduce or eliminate the need for myopic refractive correction. In one type of procedure, eight partial-thickness incisions are made in the cornea with a diamond blade in order to flatten the curvature of the cornea. Radial keratotomy is an elective procedure, and although it has been somewhat controversial over the past few years, it has been successful. Risks associated with this procedure include unsatisfactory correction, corneal glare, and postoperative infection. Currently, the excimer laser is under investigation for use in this type of corneal surgery. It can evaporate tissue cleanly, with almost no damage to adjacent cells. The excimer laser is able to make extremely precise incisions in the cornea and may be useful in refractive surgery as well as keratoplasty.

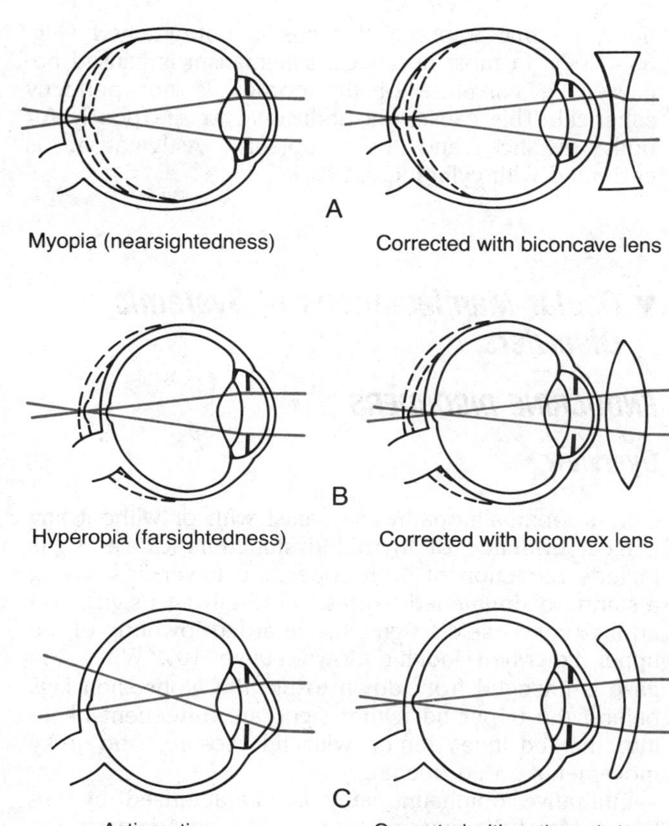

▲ **Figure 33-18**

Common refractive disorders and their correction. Dashed lines in *A* and *B* indicate normal eye contour.

HYPEROPIA

The hyperopic, or farsighted, eye is one that is deficient in its ability to focus light rays. The focal point falls behind the eye (Fig. 33-18*B*) and, consequently, the image that falls on the retina is blurred. Vision may be brought into focus by placing a convex, or plus, lens in front of the eye. The lens supplies the magnifying power that the eye is lacking. Hyperopia may be caused by an eyeball that is shorter than normal or a cornea that has less curvature than normal. Because children have a greater ability to accommodate, they are less often affected than adults. Demands for close work and reading usually bring on symptoms of headache or eyestrain. Correction is based on age and individual needs and complaints.

ASTIGMATISM

Astigmatism is a refractive condition in which rays of light are not bent equally by the cornea in all directions, so that a point of focus is not attained (Fig. 33-18*C*). In most instances, astigmatism is caused because the curvature of the cornea is not perfectly spherical. This causes the individual to see poorly for both distance and near objects. Astigmatism is corrected with cylindric lenses.

▼ Ocular Manifestations of Systemic Disorders

ENDOCRINE DISORDERS

Overview

Graves' ophthalmopathy may exist with or without any clinical evidence of thyroid dysfunction. Ocular signs include retraction of both upper and lower lids, giving a staring or frightened expression (Stellwag's sign), and lid lag (von Graefe's sign), the retarded lowering of the upper lid when looking down (Plate 10). When the gaze is changed from down to up, the globe then lags behind the upper lid. Other signs are infrequent blinking, marked fine tremor with lid closure, and jerky movements on lid opening.

Infiltrative ophthalmopathy is characterized by enlargement of the extraocular muscles and edema in the extracellular tissues. Subsequent degeneration of muscle tissue leads to fibrosis, which restricts muscle movement, resulting in double vision. Proliferation of orbital fat tissue along with the enlargement of muscle tissue and edema result in proptosis (the forward protrusion of the eyeballs), which is also called exophthalmos.

Management

As a primary measure, adequate control of thyroid abnormalities is essential. Diuretics as well as steroid therapy and radiotherapy may be indicated.

Surgical interventions include corrective lid surgery or tarsorrhapy for lid retraction in order to provide protection of the cornea. Decompression of the orbit, which usually involves the removal of the inferior and medial walls of the orbit, may be necessary to accommodate proliferative orbital fat and enlarged ocular muscles. Ocular muscle surgery may also be indicated.

The extent of the surgical procedure is likely to determine whether or not the client undergoing an orbital decompression will require a hospital stay. If the surgery is extensive, the operative sites may have suction drains. Drainage is usually serosanguineous. It will be important for the client to sleep with the head elevated to reduce postoperative swelling. The client is advised to expect redness, swelling, and ecchymoses around the eyes and lids. In the immediate postoperative period, the nurse checks the client's visual acuity every hour to monitor for the possibility of pressure on the optic nerve. The nurse should caution the client to modify normal activities for the first 2 weeks after surgery.

RHEUMATOID/CONNECTIVE TISSUE DISORDERS

Secondary Sjögren's syndrome is the presence of keratoconjunctivitis sicca, a common condition in which tear secretion is reduced, in association with a systemic disorder such as rheumatoid arthritis, psoriatic arthritis, connective tissue disorders, sarcoidosis, or Crohn's disease. Symptoms include ocular irritation and foreign body sensation. Frequent instillation of lubricating eye drops or ointment is effective in most cases.

Several ocular problems may be associated with systemic lupus erythematosus, a connective tissue disorder. The eyelids may be involved with the discoid lesions characteristic of the disease. Punctate epithelial keratopathy and secondary Sjögren's syndrome may also occur. Retinopathy of systemic lupus erythematosus produces cotton-wool spots and increased retinal vessel fragility as in diabetes. Optic neuropathy can also occur.

NEUROLOGIC DISORDERS

Approximately 90 per cent of clients with myasthenia gravis have ocular involvement. In the majority of cases, it is the presenting symptom. Ptosis (drooping of the eyelid) is bilateral, but may be asymmetric. Diplopia (double vision) is frequently in the vertical plane. Nystagmus is also present. Ocular myopathy and cranial nerve palsy may develop later, as can ophthalmoplegia (paralysis of all the extraocular muscles). Medical treatment is supportive and includes systemic steroids.

There is also a close association between optic neuritis and multiple sclerosis. Approximately three fourths of women and one third of men who develop optic neuritis will be diagnosed with multiple sclerosis when followed for 15 years. Typically, an attack of optic neuritis starts with an acute onset of vision loss in one eye, with periocular discomfort made worse by movement of the eye. Visual impairment is progressive over a 2-week period and usually recovers after 4 to 6 weeks. Recovery may take longer and may be incomplete. Medical treatment consists of oral, intravenous, and retrobulbar steroids.

CIRCULATORY DISORDERS

The primary response of retinal arterioles to hypertension is narrowing. In chronic hypertension, the blood-retina barrier is disrupted in small areas, resulting in increased vascular permeability. The fundus examination reveals vasoconstriction, leakage, and arteriosclerosis. Hypertensive retinopathy is graded for severity on a scale of 1 to 4, with 4 being the most severe. Systemic hypertension is also associated with an increased risk of retinal vein occlusion. There is no known treatment for retinal vein occlusion.

IMMUNOLOGIC DISORDERS

Ocular complications affect approximately 75 per cent of patients with acquired immune deficiency syndrome (AIDS). The conjunctiva and eyelids may be the first sites of Kaposi's sarcoma neoplasms. Another presenting manifestation is herpes zoster ophthalmicus. Cytomegalovirus (CMV) retinitis is the most frequent opportunistic infection involving the eye in AIDS. It is frequently bilateral and, if untreated, results in blindness. The most common eye findings are cotton-wool spots, similar to those seen in diabetes and hypertension. Medical treatment is intravitreal and intravenous ganciclovir in conjunction with oral zidovudine (AZT).

LYME DISEASE

Lyme disease, caused by the bite from a tick, has three stages. The initial stage involves a lesion and erythema around the bite, accompanied by regional lymphadenopathy, malaise, fever, headache, myalgia, arthralgia, and frequently conjunctivitis. Several weeks to months later during the second phase, there is a period associated with neurologic and cardiac problems. Along with these problems, there may also be cranial nerve palsies, uveitis, optic neuropathy, keratitis, choroiditis, and exudative retinal detachments.

Tetracycline and penicillin are effective in treating the initial infection and in preventing late complications.

Summary

It is essential for nurses to understand the complexity of ocular structures and the physiology of vision in order to provide comprehensive nursing care to their clients. The specialty practice of ophthalmic registered nursing is devoted to caring for clients with eye disorders. Ophthalmic registered nurses perform the roles of care giver, advocate, educator, counselor, technician, coordinator, and researcher. Ophthalmic nursing care is directed not only at those biologic systems that are affected by an actual or potential deficit, but it is an integration of how actual or potential visual deficits affect the individual as an entire being.

Bibliography

1. Anderson, W., et al. (1991). *Atlas of ophthalmic surgery* (Vol. 1). St. Louis: Mosby-Year Book.
2. Berkoben, R. (1988). The vital link: Home care for the patient after cataract surgery. *Quality Review Bulletin, 4*(5), 11-12.
3. Boyd-Monk, H. (1987). The structure and function of the eye and its adnexa. *Journal of Ophthalmic Nursing and Technology, 6*(5), 176-183.
4. Boyd-Monk, H., & Steinmetz, C. (1987). *Nursing care of the eye.* Norwalk, CT: Appleton & Lange.
5. Burlew, J. (1991). Preventing eye injuries—the nurse's role. *Journal of the American Society of Ophthalmic Registered Nurses, 16*(6), 24-28.
6. Carpenito, L. (1992). *Nursing diagnosis* (4th ed.). Philadelphia: J. B. Lippincott.
7. Catania, L. (1988). *Primary care of the anterior segment.* Norwalk, CT: Appleton & Lange.
8. Chan, D. (1989). *Clinical ocular oncology.* New York: Churchill Livingstone, Inc.
9. Chingnell, A. (1988). *Retinal detachment surgery.* New York: Springer-Verlag.
10. Clanton, C., & Means, M. (1988). Retinal reattachment—Quality and appropriateness of care. *Journal of Ophthalmic Nursing and Technology, 7*(4), 130-133.
11. Cullinan, T. (1986). *Visual disability in the elderly.* London: Croom Helm, Ltd.
12. deSmet, M., & Nussenbatt, R. (1991). Ocular manifestations of AIDS. *JAMA, 266*(21), 3019-3022.
13. Duane, T., & Jaeger, E. (1990). *Clinical ophthalmology* (Vol. 1). Philadelphia: J. B. Lippincott.
14. Duane, T., & Jaeger, E. (1990). *Clinical ophthalmology* (Vol. 2). Philadelphia: J. B. Lippincott.
15. Duane, T., & Jaeger, E. (1990). *Clinical ophthalmology* (Vol. 3). Philadelphia: J. B. Lippincott.
16. Duane, T., & Jaeger, E. (1990). *Clinical ophthalmology* (Vol. 4). Philadelphia: J. B. Lippincott.
17. Duane, T., & Jaeger, E. (1990). *Clinical ophthalmology* (Vol. 5). Philadelphia: J. B. Lippincott.
18. Friedlander, M. (Ed.) (1988). *Prevention of eye disease.* New York: Liebert, Inc. Publishing.
19. Gallagher, C. (1991). The young adult with recent vision loss: A pilot case study. *Journal of The American Society of Ophthalmic Registered Nurses, 16*(6), 8-14.
20. Garber, N. (1991). Basic ocular motility assessment. *Journal of Ophthalmic Nursing and Technology, 10*(5), 215-219.
21. Gardner, T., & Shoch, D. (1987). *Handbook of ophthalmology.* East Norwalk, CT: Appleton & Lange.
22. Gills, J., & Sanders, D. (1990). *Small incision cataract surgery.* Thorofare, NJ: Slack, Inc.
23. Goodman, D. F., et al. (1989). Complications of cataract extraction with intraocular lens implantation. *Ophthalmic Surgery, 20*(2), 132-140.
24. Hersh, P. (1988). *Ophthalmic surgical procedures.* Boston: Little, Brown & Co.
25. Hosein, A. (1989). Exenteration—the nursing approach. *Journal of Ophthalmic Nursing and Technology, 8*(3), 91-96.
26. Kaufman, H. (1989). Refractive surgery through the looking glass. *Acta Ophthalmologica 67* (Suppl), 192.
27. Kaye, G., et al. (1990). IOL implant patients need your help. *Journal of Ophthalmic Nursing and Technology, 4*(4), 18-23.
28. Legro, M. (1991). Quality of life and cataracts: A review of patient-centered studies of cataract surgery outcomes. *Ophthalmic Surgery, 22,* 431-443.
29. Lennerstrand, O., et al. (1988). *Strabismus and amblyopia.* Stockholm: Plenum Press.
30. Lichter, P. May (1988). Avoiding complications from local anesthesia. *Ophthalmology. 95*(5), 565-566.
31. Linberg, J. (1988). *Lacrimal surgery.* New York: Churchill Livingstone.
32. Machemer, R. Dec (1988). Proliferative vitreoretinopathy (PVR): A personal account of the pathogenesis and management. *Investigative Ophthalmology & Visual Science, 29*(12), 1771-1783.
33. Matteson, M., & McConnell, E. (1988). *Gerontological nursing: Concepts and practice.* Philadelphia: W. B. Saunders.
34. Mills, K. (Ed.) (1989). *Glaucoma.* Proceedings of the 4th International Symposium of the Northern Eye Institute, Manchester, UK, 14-16 July, 1988. Oxford, Pergamon Press.
35. Morgan, C., et al. (1988). Ocular complications associated with retrobulbar injections. *Ophthalmology, 95*(5), 660-665.
36. Newell, F. (1986). Ophthalmology: Principles and concepts (6th ed.). St. Louis; C. V. Mosby.
37. Obstbaum, S. (1991). *Glaucoma surgery atlas.* Norwalk, CT: Appleton & Lange.
38. Perkins, R., & Olson, R. (1991). A new look at postoperative instructions following cataract extraction. *Ophthalmic Surgery 22*(2), 66-68.

39. Perry, A. (1990). Integrated orbital implants. *Advances in Ophthalmic Plastic and Reconstructive Surgery, 8*, 75-81.
40. Petrowski, D. D. (1986). Care of an artificial eye after enucleation. *Journal of Ophthalmic Nursing and Technology, 5*(4), 135-139.
41. Portnoy, S., et al. (1989). Surgical management of corneal ulceration and perforation. *Survey of Ophthalmology, 34*(1), 47-58.
42. Rozakis, G. (1990). *Cataract surgery*. Thorofare, NJ: Slack, Inc.
43. Sardegna, J., & Paul, T. (1991). *The encyclopedia of blindness and vision impairment*. New York: Facts on File Publishing.
44. Servodidio, C. (1991). Teaching aids to patients diagnosed with choroidal melanoma. *Journal of American Society of Ophthalmic Registered Nurses, 16*(6), 21-23.
45. Sheffield, J., & Hilfer, S. (1987). *The microenvironment and vision*. New York: Springer-Verlag.
46. Singerman, L., & Jampol, L. (1991). *Retinal & choroidal manifestations of systemic disease*. Baltimore: Williams & Wilkins.
47. Skuta, G., & Parrish, R. (1987). Wound healing in glaucoma filtering surgery. *Survey of Ophthalmology, 32*(3), 149-170.
48. Smith, R. S. (1989). Refractive surgery. In R. D. Reincke (Ed.), *Ophthalmology annual* (p. 361-362). New York: Raven Press.
49. Smith, S. (1985). *Standards of ophthalmic nursing practice*. San Francisco: The American Society of Ophthalmic Registered Nurses.
50. Smolen, G., & Thoft, R. (1987). *The cornea* (2nd ed.). Scientific Foundations and Clinical Practice. Boston: Little, Brown & Co.
51. Stein, H., et al. (1988). *The ophthalmic assistant*. St. Louis: C. V. Mosby.
52. Tillman, W. (1987). *An eye for an eye*. Pittsburgh: Author.
53. Torento, C., & Sanchez, T. (1988). Pseudophakic bullous keratopathy and the nursing implications. *Ophthalmic Nursing Forum, 4*(3), 1-12.
54. Vine, A. K., et al. (1989). A new inexpensive customized plaque for choroidal melanoma iodine-125 plaque therapy. *Ophthalmology, 96*(4), 543-546.
55. Werner, E. (1991). *Manual of visual fields*. New York: Churchill Livingstone.
56. Wilson, S., & Kaufman, H. (1990). Graft failure after penetrating keratoplasty. *Survey of Ophthalmology, 34*(5), 325-356.
57. Young, R. (1991). *Age related cataract*. New York: Oxford University Press.

Chapter 34

Structure and Function; Assessment and Nursing Care of Clients with Ear Disorders

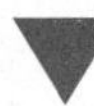

Hearing and balance problems can reduce the ability to communicate, limit social activities, and hinder the constructive use of leisure time. Career options, job opportunities, and financial security can also be compromised. Ear problems can interfere with the client's ability to remain independent, which can lead to isolation. Also, the aesthetic enjoyment of life and the ability to share human experiences can be temporarily or permanently diminished. All these situations can result in feelings of anger, anxiety, frustration, uncertainty, and loneliness, which ultimately may affect the quality of life.

STRUCTURE AND FUNCTION OF THE TEMPORAL BONE AND EAR

The ears are a pair of complex sensory organs for both hearing and balance. Their location on either side of the head produces binaural hearing, allows the detection of sound direction, and aids in maintaining equilibrium.

The ear and temporal bone can be divided into outer, middle, and inner ear. Sound is transmitted from the external ear, through the middle ear (which amplifies the sound), to the inner ear. The sound energy, after transformation, is carried by neural elements to the brain for decoding and, thus, hearing. The balance organs, located in the inner ear, also send impulses to the brain for normal balance. Hearing and balance are somewhat maintained with the loss of function of only one ear.

The internal ears are housed in the temporal bone of the skull. The bony anatomy of the temporal bone is the most detailed part of the skull. If a 50-cent coin were superimposed on the external auditory canal, the tympanic ring and tympanic membrane, the three ossicles, the jugular vein, the carotid artery, the facial nerve, and the auditory and vestibular parts of the inner ear would all be within the coin's circumference.

TEMPORAL BONE

The temporal bones that house the ear are two of the eight cranial bones that form part of the base and lateral wall of the skull. The temporal bone can be divided into four parts: squamous, mastoid, petrous, and tympanic portions. The petrous portion of the temporal bone houses the most dense bone in the body, the otic capsule. The temporal bone articulates with the sphenoid, parietal, and occipital bones (Fig. 34-1).

The temporal bone provides protection for the organs of hearing and balance. Therefore, the function of the temporal bone is to house the following structures: the external and internal auditory canals; the mastoid air cells, which serve to lighten the skull; the blood vessels; the facial and auditory nerves; the labyrinth; and the cochlea.

EXTERNAL EAR

The external ear is divided into the auricle, or pinna, and the external auditory canal or the ear canal. The ears are located on each side of the head at approximately eye level. If an imaginary line were drawn from the outer canthus of the eye to the top of the ear, this line should be parallel to the floor. The pinna is attached to the side of the head at approximately a 10-degree angle.

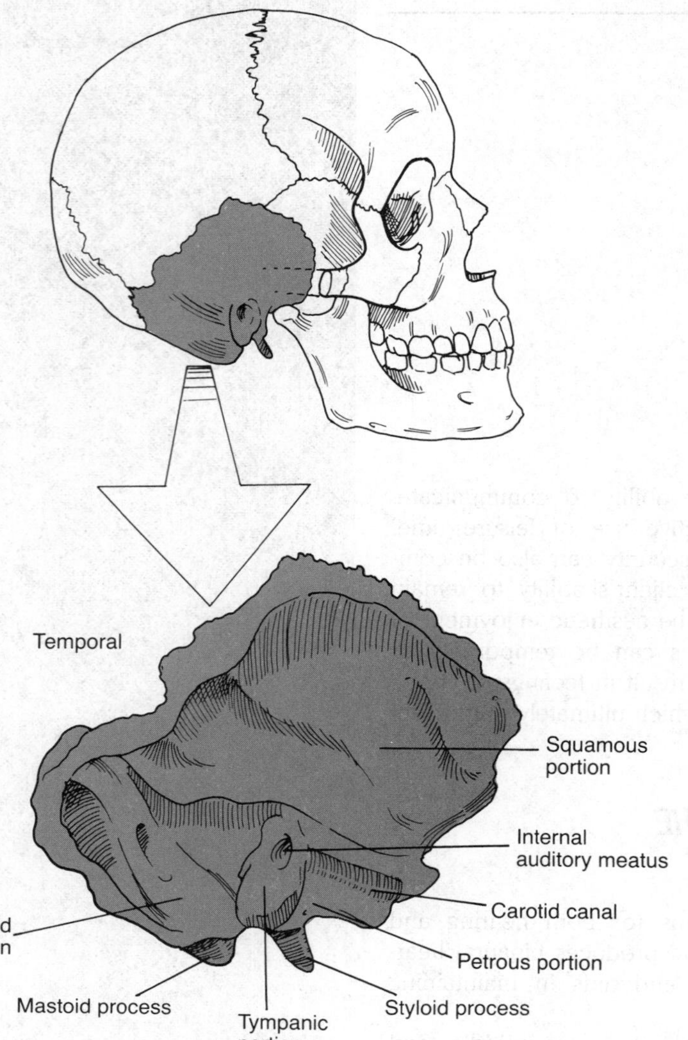

▲ **Figure 34-1**

Lateral view of temporal bone.

Pinna/Auricle

The conspicuous part of the ear that projects outward is called the pinna or auricle. The pinna is attached to the side of the head by skin. The pinna is composed mostly of cartilage, except for the fat and subcutaneous tissue in the lobule. The cartilage is held to the skull by small muscles and innervated by a branch of the facial nerve. The muscles are the posterior, anterior, and superior auricular muscles.

The parts of the pinna are illustrated in Figure 34-2. The concha is the deepest part and leads to the ear canal. The helix is the outer rim of the pinna and leads inferiorly to the lobule. The concha is bounded anteriorly by a triangular fold of cartilage called the tragus, which projects posteriorly over the entrance to the ear canal. Hair covers most of the ear but is usually rudimentary except in the region of the tragus and antitragus. Sebaceous glands are found on the skin surface also. The pinna functions to collect and direct sound.

In front of (anterior to) the external opening of the ear is the temporomandibular joint. The head of the mandible can be felt by the tip of a finger placed in the external meatus while the mouth is opened and closed. Very often, temporomandibular joint problems produce referred pain to the ear (otalgia) because of the same sensory nerve supply.

External Auditory Canal/Ear Canal

The ear canal extends from the concha of the pinna to the tympanic membrane. This S-shaped canal is approximately 2.5 cm (or 1 inch) in length and follows an inward, forward, and downward path. The lumen is irregular in shape; a skeleton of cartilage in the outer third is continuous with the cartilage of the pinna and a bony skeleton in the inner two thirds. The lumen of the ear canal is narrowest where the transition from cartilage to bone occurs. The skin covering the cartilage portion is thick; it contains sebaceous and ceruminous glands and hair follicles. The secretion of these cerumen glands and the fat from the sebaceous glands form a golden to black substance called cerumen (wax). The skin covering the bony portion is very thin.

The funnel shape of the external ear collects and directs sound to the eardrum. The head, pinna, and ear canal act as an integrated system to transmit sound vibrations on their way to the eardrum. The external ear actually amplifies certain frequencies.

The secretion of cerumen is a protective function for the ear. Wax is to the ear what tears are to the eyes. The sticky consistency of the wax, along with the fine hairs of the ear canal, helps cleanse the ear canal of foreign matter. The hairs become coarser during the aging process; thus, retention of wax is more of a problem to the elderly. Impacted cerumen can cause hearing losses in clients of all ages. At times, the wax must be mechanically removed.

TYMPANIC MEMBRANE

The tympanic membrane or eardrum, an oval disc approximately 1 cm in diameter, covers the end of the auditory canal and separates the canal from the middle ear. The eardrum is a thin, translucent, pearly gray membrane obliquely directed downward, and inward, so that the posterior part is more accessible than is the anterior part.

The eardrum consists of three tissue layers: an outer epithelial layer continuous with the skin of the ear canal, a fibrous supporting middle layer, and an inner

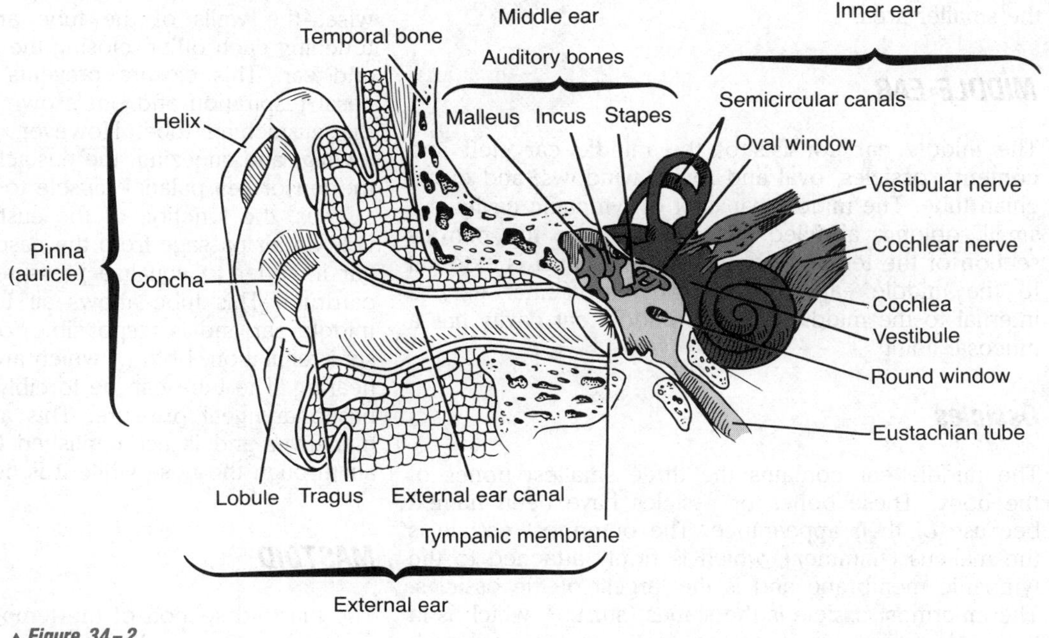

▲ Figure 34-2
Anatomy of external, middle, and inner ear.

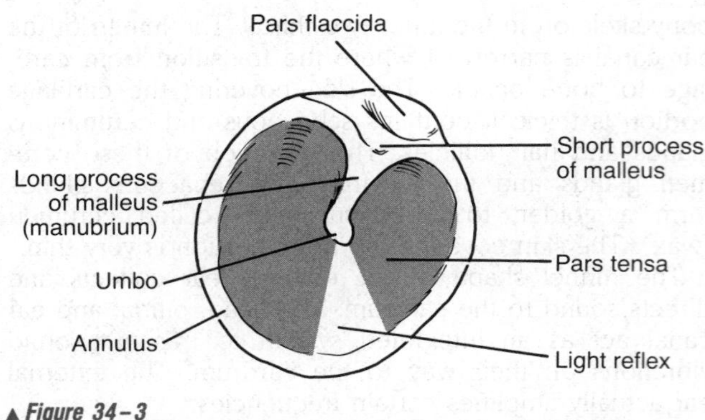

▲ **Figure 34-3**

Normal right eardrum (tympanic membrane).

mucosal layer continuous with the mucosal lining of the middle ear cavity.

Some distinguishing landmarks of the normal eardrum (Fig. 34-3) are the annulus, which is the fibrous border that attaches the eardrum to the temporal bone; the short process of the malleus, which protrudes into the eardrum superiorly; the long process of the malleus (manubrium); the umbo of the malleus, which is at the point of maximal concavity and attaches to the center of the eardrum; the pars flaccida, a small triangular area above the short process of the malleus; and the pars tensa, the remaining and largest portion of the eardrum.

The tympanic membrane serves as a common membrane between the external ear canal and the middle ear space. The tympanic membrane protects the middle ear and conducts sound vibrations from the external ear to the ossicles. The sound pressure applied to the stapes (smallest ossicle) in the oval window is 22 times greater than the sound pressure exerted on the eardrum. The pressure of the sound vibrations is increased as a result of transmission from a larger area to the smaller area.

MIDDLE EAR

The middle ear consists of the middle ear cleft and contents: ossicles, oval and round windows, and eustachian tube. The middle ear cleft or tympanic cavity is a small, oblong, air-filled space located in the petrous section of the temporal bone. The ear canal is external to the middle ear, and the labyrinth (inner ear) is internal to the middle ear. The middle ear cavity has a mucosal lining.

Ossicles

The middle ear contains the three smallest bones of the body. These bones or ossicles have been named because of their appearance. The outermost ossicle is the malleus (hammer), which is firmly attached to the tympanic membrane and is the largest of the ossicles. The innermost ossicle is the stapes (stirrup), which is in the oval window, in direct contact with the perilymph of the inner ear, and is the smallest of the ossicles. The incus (anvil) lies between the other two and has the same shape as a tooth with two roots (see Fig. 34-2).

The function of these ossicles is to transmit sound vibrations mechanically. The ossicles are held in place by joints, muscles, and ligaments, which also offer protective mechanisms from loud sounds. The light weight and configuration of the ossicles provide an efficient means of transmission of sound vibrations from the air molecules of the external ear to the fluid molecules of the inner ear. Fluids offer more resistance than air does and need more force to produce movement. The ossicular chain produces and magnifies this force necessary to move the inner ear fluids.

Windows

There are two windows in the middle ear, named because of their shape (see Fig. 34-2). The round window is an opening into the inner ear, where sound vibrations exit. The oval window also is an opening into the inner ear, where sound vibrations enter. The oval window is not a true window because the footplate of the stapes bone covers it.

Eustachian Tube

The eustachian tube is a narrow channel approximately 35 mm ($1\frac{1}{2}$ inch) in length and only 1 mm wide at its narrowest end. This tube connects the middle ear to the nasopharynx. The structure is mostly fibrous tissue, cartilage, and bone; it extends downward, forward, and inward from each middle ear. The lining of the eustachian tube is mucous membrane continuous with the lining of the middle ear at one end and the nasopharynx at the other end. Only a small section of this tube at the superior end remains permanently open. Otherwise, the walls of the tube are lightly opposing or touching each other, closing the tube to both the throat and ear. This closure prevents the sound of normal nasal respiration and one's own voice from passing up the eustachian tube. However, during yawning, swallowing, and sneezing, the eustachian tube is opened by the tensor veli palatini muscle to equalize pressure.

Thus, the function of the eustachian tube is to provide an air passage from the nasopharynx to the middle ear in order to equalize pressure on both sides of the eardrum. This tube allows air to enter and leave the middle ear and is responsible for ventilation and pressure regulation, both of which are necessary for normal hearing. The tube can be forcibly opened by increasing nasopharyngeal pressure. This act is called Valsalva's maneuver and is accomplished by attempting to blow air through the nose while it is held closed.

MASTOID

The mastoid section of the temporal bone includes the mastoid process, which is the cone-shaped part; the mastoid antrum, a large cavity posteriorly continuous with the middle ear; and the mastoid air cells that branch off the mastoid cavity.

The mastoid bone is located posterior to the pinna and can be felt as a bony protuberance behind the lower portion of the pinna. The mastoid cavity is close to several important cranial structures: the dura of the temporal lobe; the cerebellar dura; the sigmoid sinus; and the internal carotid artery. Therefore, infection of the middle ear and mastoid cavities can also involve these structures.

The cavity of the mastoid bone and the interconnected arrangement of the air-filled spaces aid the middle ear in adjusting to changes in pressure. The mastoid system acts as a buffer for the middle ear. The system of cavities and air cells also lightens the skull. The denseness of the temporal bone is necessary structurally for the protection of the delicate organs of hearing and balance.

INNER EAR (LABYRINTH)

The inner ear or labyrinth is located deep within the petrous section of the temporal bone; it contains the sense organs for hearing and balance and the eighth cranial nerve (Fig. 34–4). The inner ear is a complicated system of intercommunicating chambers and connecting tubes composed of two major structures: the bony labyrinth and the membranous labyrinth, which lies within but does not completely fill the bony labyrinth.

The bony labyrinth is the rigid capsule in which the membranous labyrinth lies. This otic capsule surrounds and protects the delicate membranous labyrinth. The vestibule connects the cochlea for hearing to the three semicircular canals for balance. The cochlea, which looks like a snail shell with $2\frac{1}{2}$ turns, is approximately 7 mm in diameter at the widest part and is structurally divided into two compartments. The upper compartment, the scala vestibuli, leads from the oval window to the apex of the cochlear spiral. The lower compartment, the scala tympani, leads from the apex of the cochlear spiral to the round window.

The three semicircular canals are at right angles to each other and, because of position, are named the superior, the posterior, and the lateral or horizontal canal. The horizontal canal lies closest to the middle ear.

The membranous labyrinth, within the bony labyrinth, is bathed in a fluid called perilymph, which communicates with the cerebrospinal fluid via the cochlear duct. The membranous labyrinth consists of the utricle; the saccule; the semicircular canals; the cochlear duct; and the end organ for hearing, the organ of Corti. The membranous labyrinth contains a different fluid called endolymph. This fluid also protects the end organ because it acts as a cushion against abrupt movements of the head (Fig. 34–5).

The utricle and saccule are vestibular receptors that position the head as it relates to the pull of gravity. The semicircular canals are arranged to sense rotational movements, such as movements or changes in position. Each of the semicircular canals connects with the utricle. Where the canals connect with the utricle, each canal has an enlarged portion called the ampulla. The ampulla contains a cluster of hair cells called the crista, which are concerned with dynamic balance. For example, when the head position is changed, movement of the endolymph stimulates the hair cells, which initiates increased impulses that travel over the vestibular division of the acoustic nerve to the brain.

Sound waves are transmitted by the ossicles to the delicate membrane of the oval window (Fig. 34–6). These vibrations move the perilymph in the scala vestibuli. The perilymph of the scala vestibuli is continuous with that of the scala tympani at the extreme tip of the snail shell called the helicotrema. The sound energy vibrations enter through the oval window and exit through the round window.

Vibrations in the perilymph of the scala vestibuli are transmitted through the vestibular membrane, or Reissner's membrane, to the endolymph that fills the cochlear duct. The cochlear duct is located between the scala vestibuli and scala tympani. The organ of Corti, which is bathed in the endolymph, lies on the basilar membrane in a spiral strip from the basal turn near the round window to the apex at the helicotrema. This structure transforms mechanical sound vibrations into neural activity and separates sound into different frequencies. This electrochemical impulse travels via the acoustic nerve to the temporal cortex of the brain. The acoustic nerve, or eighth cranial nerve, reaches the

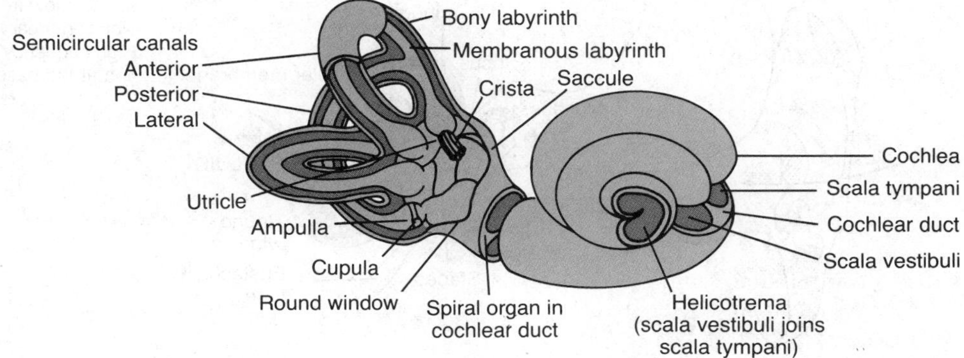

▲ **Figure 34–4**

Inner ear structures. (Adapted from Dorland's Illustrated medical dictionary [1981] [26th ed.]. Philadelphia: W. B. Saunders.)

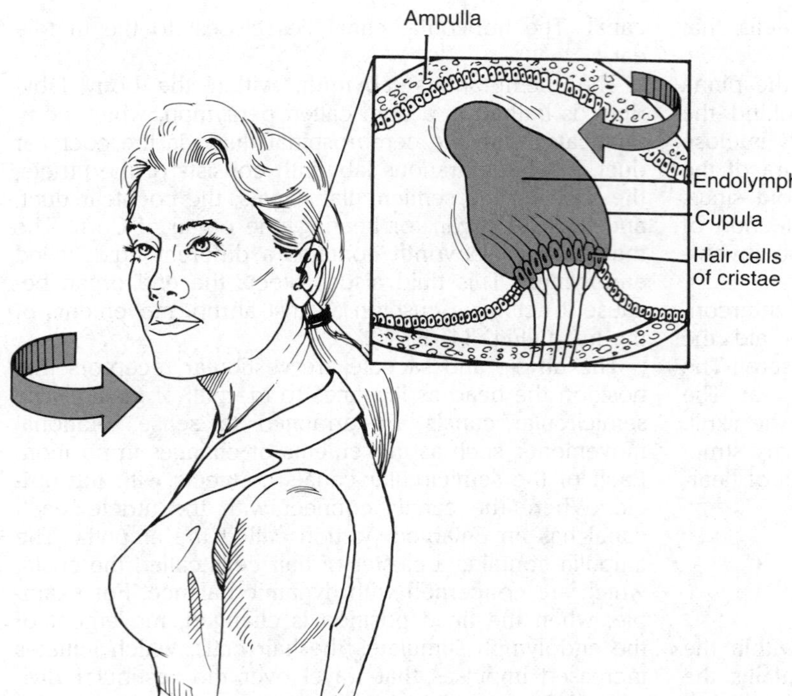

▲ *Figure 34-5*

The labyrinth of the inner ear assists with dynamic equilibrium to maintain balance and coordination.

cochlea and vestibule via the internal auditory canal. The facial nerve, or seventh cranial nerve, courses through the same canal.

CHANGES IN HEARING ASSOCIATED WITH AGING

Presbycusis is hearing loss in the elderly. Changes in the delicate labyrinthine structures over the decades cause a hearing loss predominantly in the higher frequencies. The reason for presbycusis is not yet fully understood but appears to be a stiffening of the tissues in the cochlea. Another factor is slow decreases in blood supply. The amount of hearing loss will have familial differences and can start in middle age. Tinnitus usually accompanies presbycusis. The majority of clients will eventually suffer from presbycusis during the aging process. In some of these clients, the amount of hearing loss warrants the use of a hearing aid. Presbycusis cannot be treated medically or with surgery.

Infections also cause a sensorineural hearing loss. Infections within the temporal bone are either viral or bacterial, usually associated with other ear problems. Systemic infections such as meningitis or syphilis can also cause a hearing loss.

▼ ASSESSMENT OF THE EAR

The otologic history can be the most important assessment tool and should be obtained before audiometric testing. Certain behavioral clues can suggest to the nurse that the client has a loss of hearing (Box 34-1).

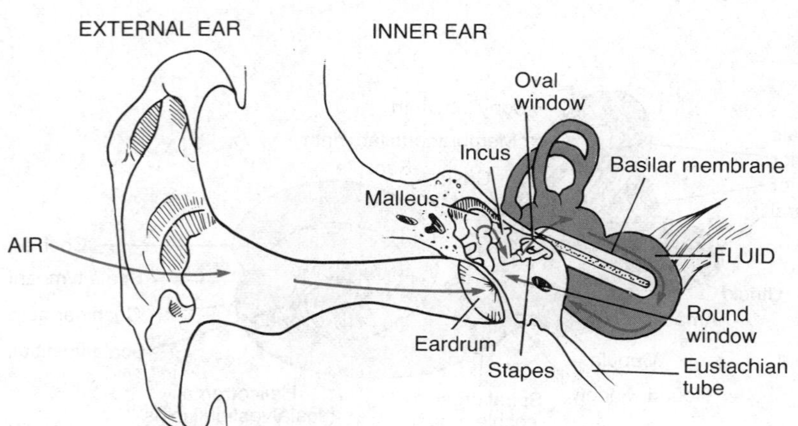

▲ *Figure 34-6*

Schematic representation of the transmission of sound. Low-frequency sound waves cause maximal vibration near the apex of the basilar membrane. High-frequency sound waves cause maximal vibration at the base of the basilar membrane.

Box 34–1. Clues Suggesting Loss of Hearing

Any adult who exhibits one or more of the following traits may be experiencing a loss of hearing.

Is irritable, hostile, hypersensitive in intercliental relations
Has difficulty hearing upper frequency consonants
Complains about people mumbling
Turns up volume on television
Asks for frequent repetition and answers questions inappropriately
Loses sense of humor, becomes grim
Leans forward to hear better
Shuns large- and small-group audience situations
Might appear aloof and "stuck up"
Complains of ringing in the ears
Has an unusually soft or loud voice

Significant data are collected by conducting a thorough interview. Specific items that should be included in the otologic history are identified in Box 34–2 (Otologic History Assessment Guide).

HISTORY

An otologic history includes demographic data, the chief complaint, past medical history, family history, psychosocial history, and review of systems. Ear problems often result from childhood illnesses or problems associated with adjacent structures. The history interview is essential for determining current problems related to the ear.

Demographic data relevant to otologic assessment include the client's age. Hearing loss occurs as a consequence of the aging process (presbycusis).

Chief Complaint

The most common chief complaints include hearing loss, pain, tinnitus, ear drainage, loss of balance, vertigo, and dizziness. The client may also complain of associated nausea or vomiting. The nurse completes a symptom analysis to determine onset, duration, frequency, and precipitating and relieving factors for the presenting symptom. The client's past medical history is explored carefully in order to determine the chronicity of the problem and to determine the cause.

Hearing loss may occur suddenly or gradually and vary according to whether loss is conductive, sensorineural, or related to a central nervous system disorder. The client may report inability to hear certain words or sounds or that sounds are muffled. *Pain* may be perceived by the client as a feeling of fullness in the ear. It may be intensified by movement and relieved by holding the head still or by application of heat. Ear pain may occur as a result of related problems of the nose, sinuses, oral cavity, or pharynx. *Ear drainage* can be bloody (sanguineous), clear (serous), mixed (serosanguineous), or pus (purulent). Drainage may also be accompanied by an odor. *Tinnitus* (ringing in the ears) may be reported as high- or low-pitched, roaring, humming, hissing, or loud and persistent. Tinnitus may occur more commonly at certain times of the day. *Loss of balance* may be accompanied by *vertigo* or *dizziness*.

Box 34–2. Otologic History Assessment Guide

1. Do you have any problems with your hearing?
2. How long have you had a hearing loss in the
   right ear? ____ yr
   left ear? ____ yr
3. Which is your worse ear? (circle) R L
4. Have you had extensive ear drainage since childhood?
5. Who in your family was hard-of-hearing before age 50?
   ____ mother ____ father ____ brother ____ sister
6. Have any of your blood relatives had ear surgery? If yes, who was the patient and surgeon? ________
7. Are you wearing hearing aids now?
   How old is the right aid? ____ yr
   How old is the left aid? ____ yr
8. Have you worked in loud noise?
   If so, please indicate the number of years. ____ yr
9. Are you still working in loud noise?
10. Were you around loud noise in the military? How many rounds have you shot outside the service? ________
11. Do you have head noise or ringing?
12. Do you have any of the following?

	right	left	both
Difference in pitch of sound	____	____	____
Distortion of hearing	____	____	____
Noise in your ear	____	____	____
Fullness or pressure in your ear	____	____	____
Pain in your ear	____	____	____
Drainage from your ear	____	____	____
Blurred vision	____	____	____
Double vision	____	____	____
Numbness in hands or feet	____	____	____
Weakness in arms or legs	____	____	____

	Yes	No
Tingling around the mouth or face	____	____
Loss of consciousness or blackouts	____	____
Fainting	____	____
Convulsion or seizure	____	____

13. Is vertigo or unsteadiness a major problem?
14. Have you had previous ear surgery?
15. If you have had previous ear surgery, please indicate which ear was operated, and the type of surgery and the physician who performed the surgery.

	Date	Surgery	Physician
Right ear	19 ___	________	________
	19 ___	________	________
Left ear	19 ___	________	________
	19 ___	________	________

16. If you are allergic to any medications, please list:
   ________ ________ ________

Past Medical History

CHILDHOOD AND INFECTIOUS DISEASES

Childhood diseases that commonly occur include acute middle ear infections (otitis media), eardrum perforations resulting from otitis media, complications of ear infections such as chronic otitis media, frequent upper respiratory tract infection, and acute and chronic sinus infections. Infectious diseases with ear problem sequelae include mumps, measles, and meningitis. Specifically inquire whether the client has been immunized for mumps, measles, and *Haemophilus influenzae* B (HIB). In utero exposure to maternal influenza or rubella may result in congenital hearing loss in the child. Premature birth is also associated with hearing problems.

MAJOR ILLNESSES AND HOSPITALIZATIONS

Inquire about a history of tonsillitis. Has the client had a tonsillectomy or adenoidectomy? Is there a history of ear surgery? Has the client had trauma to the head or ear, such as a severe blow or sustained loud noise exposure or concussion from sudden changes in air pressure (such as may occur in an explosion)? Is there a history of a chronic eardrum perforation?

MEDICATIONS

Certain medications can damage the vestibulocochlear nerve (eighth cranial nerve), with resultant hearing loss, tinnitus, or disturbances in equilibrium. Aspirin is a common cause of tinnitus. Other drugs include aminoglycosides, analgesics, salicylates, and antiprotozoal agents. (See Box 34-3 for a list of drugs causing ototoxic effects.) Inquire whether the client has taken or is currently taking medications and for how long.

ALLERGIES

In addition to asking about allergies to medications and other substances, inquire about allergies resulting in nasal stuffiness and congestion. Close proximity of the eustachian tubes may also result in edema, which obstructs the flow of air between the middle ear and nose so that air pressure cannot be equalized.

Box 34-3. Selected Ototoxic* Drugs

Aminoglycoside Antibiotics	**Other Drugs**
Streptomycin	Chemotherapeutic agents
Neomycin	Cisplatin
Gentamicin	Nitrogen mustard
Tobramycin	Salicylates
Amikacin	Quinine drugs
Kanamycin	Bleomycin
Netilmicin	Quinidine
Other Antibiotics	**Chemicals**
Vancomycin	Metals
Viomycin	Lead
Polymyxin B (Aerosporin)	Mercury
Polymyxin E	Gold
(colistin; Coly-Mycin)	Arsenic
Erythromycin	Alcohol
Minocycline	**Diuretics**
Capreomycin	Furosemide (Lasix)
	Ethacrynic acid (Edecrin)
	Acetazolamide (Diamox)

*Substances toxic to the ear.

Family History

The nurse asks about family members and whether there is a history of hearing loss. Age of onset for presbycusis is determined.

Psychosocial History and Lifestyle

Psychosocial and lifestyle factors that influence the occurrence of ear problems include occupational hazards, environmental exposure, and leisure activities and hobbies. Ask about exposure to loud noises (see Box 34-2): type, frequency, and duration. Is protective ear gear worn? Does the client swim, especially in water that may be contaminated? Has the client had problems with "swimmer's ear"? Does the client use ear plugs to prevent water from entering the ear canal?

Explore health management behaviors the client practices regarding ear hygiene. Does the client have a habit of putting objects into the ear, such as pencils, bobby pins, or cotton-tipped applicators?

Review of Systems

The review of systems related to the ear includes asking about problems with the nose, sinuses, mouth, pharynx, and throat. Ask whether the client has experienced head trauma, loss of balance, dizziness, or vertigo. Detailed questions for the review of systems are found in Chapter 11, Table 11-5.

PHYSICAL EXAMINATION

Physical examination of the ear includes assessment of hearing acuity, balance, and equilibrium. Because the external ear is completely visible, it is easy to identify anatomic landmarks and assess any abnormalities. The eardrum reveals significant information regarding the middle ear. However, much of the middle ear and inner ear is inaccessible to direct examinations, and inferences must be made by testing auditory and vestibular function.

Inspection and Palpation

EXTERNAL EAR

Gross examination of both ears should precede individual examination of either ear. Inspection and palpation are used for assessment of the external ear. The external ear should be inspected for size, configuration, and angle of attachment to the head. The configuration of the pinna is observed for gross deformity. Whether the ears protrude (and the degree), the color of the skin of the ear, and whether any additional skin tags are present are noted. The skin of the ear should be smooth and without breaks or inflammation, especially in the crevice behind the ear. Note any lumps, skin lesions, or cysts, and record approximate size and location.

Palpation and manipulation of the pinna produce information regarding tenderness, nodules, or tophi. Tophi are small, hard nodules in the helix that are deposits of uric acid crystals characteristic of gout. In palpation, move the pinna, feel the mastoid area, and press on the tragus. Note whether any of the manipulations produces pain or discomfort, which could indicate inflammation or infection.

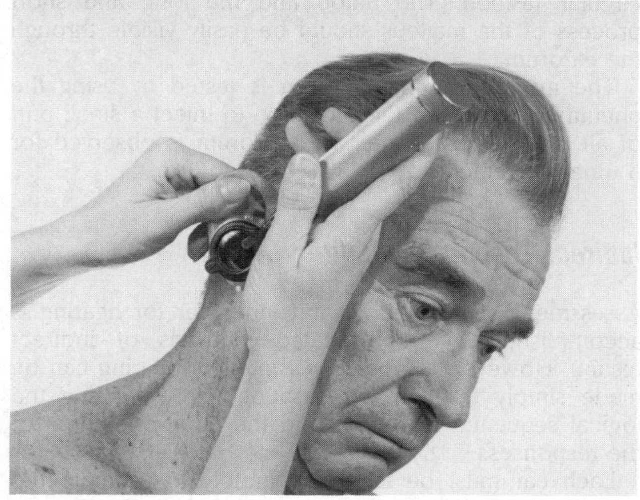

▲ *Figure 34–7*

Use of the otoscope. Hold the otoscope handle pointed up between the thumb and fingers. The pinna should be pulled back and up in the adult to straighten the auditory canal. (From Jarvis, C. [1992]. *Physical examination and health assessment*. Philadelphia, W. B. Saunders Company.)

EAR CANAL

Direct Observation. Inspection of the ear canal is carried out by direct observation, otoscopy, or microscopic examination. For direct observation, the adult is asked to tip the head slightly to the opposite side while the nurse pulls the pinna up, back, and out. A penlight is then used to inspect the ear canal for any abnormalities such as extreme narrowing of the ear canal, excessive wax, redness, scaliness, swelling, drainage, cysts, or foreign objects. Normally, none of these signs are present. Visualization of the eardrum with this method would be unlikely.

Otoscopy. The eardrum is located at the end of the only skin-lined canal in the body. Therefore, visualization is difficult and requires illumination and magnification for accurate assessment. An otoscope is portable, and otoscopic examination is the most common method used. An otoscope is a device (Fig. 34–7) consisting of a handle, a light source, a magnifying lens, and an attachment for visualizing the ear canal and eardrum. Some otoscopes have a pneumatic device for injecting air into the ear canal to test the mobility and integrity of the eardrum.

Specula for the otoscope come in a variety of sizes. The diameter of the meatus and the length of the ear canal vary; thus, the speculum with the largest diameter that fits comfortably into the ear canal should be selected. The light source must be checked for brightness. If the light appears yellowish or dim (like a flashlight with weak batteries), the batteries must be recharged or replaced.

The otoscope is held with the dominant hand, with the hand resting against the client's head. In this manner, should the client move suddenly, the otoscope will also move, so that the examination will be less likely to damage the external canal. With the nondominant hand, the pinna is pulled up, back, and out (in the adult); thus, the ear canal is straightened. While this is done, the client's head is gently tilted away from the nurse, and the speculum is inserted slowly and carefully into the ear canal. The nurse's eye is brought close to the magnifying lens in order to visualize the ear canal and eardrum. When a pneumatic bulb is present, the otoscope is advanced far enough to make a secure seal.

The ear canal is observed while the speculum is entering and leaving. The otoscope is moved in a circular fashion to visualize the entire ear canal; abnormalities such as extreme narrowing of the ear canal, nodules, redness, scaliness, swelling, drainage, cysts, foreign objects, or excessive wax are noted. Visualization of the eardrum will be impaired by most of these abnormalities. Sometimes the ear canal must be cleaned of wax, dead skin, and other debris. Wax and debris can be removed with a cerumen spoon (wax curet), suction aspirator, or irrigation.

Cerumen should not interfere with the examination when the amount is small. Cerumen is normally present in the external ear and varies in color from light yellow to black. Cerumen that is impacted in the ear canal is a cause of hearing loss. Therefore, assessment of the amount of cerumen is important.

The normal eardrum is slightly conical, quite shiny and smooth, and pearly gray in color. The position of the drumhead is oblique with respect to the ear canal. In the presence of disease, not only does the color of the eardrum change, but also other abnormalities such as retraction of the eardrum, bulging of the eardrum, perforation of the eardrum, or a white plaque (tympanosclerosis) in the eardrum can exist.

Carefully inspect the entire eardrum, including the border of the annulus, again rotating the otoscope in a circular fashion. The umbo and the long and short process of the malleus should be easily visible through the eardrum.

The mobility of the eardrum is tested by using the pneumatic device of the otoscope to inject a small puff of air into the ear canal. The eardrum is observed for normal movement.

Indirect Testing for Auditory Acuity

Assessment of the middle and inner ear for hearing is accomplished by sophisticated methods of indirect testing. However, a gross assessment of hearing can be made simply through conversation, by evaluating the logical sequence of replies and the appropriateness of the responses.

Each ear must be tested separately to estimate the hearing. Begin by occluding one of the client's ears with a finger. Then while standing 1 to 2 feet away, the nurse whispers two-syllable numbers softly toward the unoccluded ear, and the client is asked to repeat the numbers. The intensity of the nurse's voice can be increased from a soft, medium, or loud whisper to a soft, medium, or loud voice. If the nurse suspects that the client is lip reading, the client's face should be turned away. The client is asked whether hearing is better in one ear than in the other ear. If the auditory acuity is different, the ear that hears better should be tested first. Then, noise is produced in the better-hearing ear by rapidly but gently moving the finger in the client's ear canal while the other ear is tested.

A watch tick can also be used to test hearing. However, a watch tick produces a higher-pitched sound, which is less relevant to functional hearing than is the voice test.

The tuning fork also provides a general estimate of hearing loss. The three major tuning fork tests date from the 19th century and are named after their originators: Weber, Rinne, and Schwabach.

WEBER TEST

The tuning fork is set into vibration by striking the tines on the examiner's hand or knee. The rounded tip of the handle is placed on the center of the client's forehead or nasal bone (Fig. 34–8). Placement on the teeth (even if the client has false teeth) is a reliable option. The client is asked whether the tone is heard in the center of the head, the right ear, or the left ear. The Weber test is useful in identifying a hearing loss. Normally the sound is heard equally in both ears by bone conduction. If the client has a sensorineural hearing loss in one ear, the sound is heard in the other ear. If the client has a conductive hearing loss in one ear, the sound is heard in that ear.

RINNE TEST

The vibrating tuning fork is shifted between two positions: against the mastoid bone (bone conduction) and 2 inches from the opening of the ear canal (air conduction) (Fig. 34–8). As the position is changed, the client is asked to indicate which tone is louder (in front of the ear or behind the ear) or when one of the tones is no longer heard. The Rinne test is useful for differentiating between conductive and sensorineural hearing losses.

With conductive hearing loss, the pathways of normal sound conduction are blocked. However, vibrations against the mastoid bone can bypass the obstruction; therefore, bone conduction lasts longer or sounds louder than air conduction. With sensorineural hearing loss, the acoustic nerve has decreased ability to perceive vibrations from either route; therefore, normal patterns are reported by the client. Clients with normal hearing also report normal patterns.

Normally sound is heard twice as long or loud by air conduction than it is by bone conduction. Therefore, a normal response is one in which air conduction is greater than bone conduction, or a positive Rinne test finding. With a conductive hearing loss, a client hears bone conduction louder or longer than air conduction, or a negative Rinne test finding. With a sensorineural hearing loss, the client hears better by air conduction, or a positive Rinne test finding.

SCHWABACH TEST

This test is also used to detect a hearing loss. The Schwabach test compares the hearing of the examiner (who must have normal hearing) with the client's. When the client no longer hears the tuning fork, the examiner now listens.

Vestibular Acuity

ROMBERG TEST

To assess the inner ear for balance, perform a Romberg test. Have the client stand with feet together, arms out in front, and eyes open. Note the ability to maintain an upright posture. Perform the same test with the eyes closed. Normally, only a minimal amount of swaying exists. If the client loses balance, this may indicate a vestibular ear problem or cerebellar ataxia. A dysfunction is called a positive Romberg test finding.

A tandem Romberg should also be assessed. Instruct the client to walk forward and backward, heel to toe. A peripheral vestibular lesion may cause marked swaying or falling. A client without pathologic change is usually able to maintain balance, depending on age.

A past-pointing test can also indicate a labyrinthine disorder. With the client seated and facing the nurse, the nurse holds out an index finger at the client's shoulder level. The client is instructed to touch the nurse's finger with the right index finger. The client is asked to lower the arm, close the eyes, and touch the nurse's finger again. The procedure is repeated using the left index finger. The presence or absence, as well as the degree and direction of past-pointing, is observed and recorded. A labyrinthine disorder can lead to past-pointing when the eyes are closed. Cerebral lesions are indicated when past-pointing occurs whether the eyes are open or closed.

TEST FOR NYSTAGMUS

Nystagmus is the involuntary, rhythmic oscillation of the eyes, associated with vestibular dysfunction. Nystagmus occurs normally when a client watches a rapidly moving object or looks beyond 30 degrees laterally (end-point nystagmus). To check a client for gaze nystagmus, the nurse's finger is placed directly in front of the client at eye level. The client is asked to follow the finger without moving the head. The nurse's finger is moved slowly from the midline toward the right ear and left ear, but not more than 30 degrees. The eyes are observed for any jerking movements. For example, if the eyes jerk quickly to the left, and drift slowly back to the right, the client has left spontaneous (horizontal) nystagmus. Nystagmus can be horizontal, vertical, or rotary.

DIAGNOSTIC TESTS

Audiometric Tests

Audiology may be broadly termed the science of hearing. These tests can be performed at the bedside by the nurse to give some indication of the type and amount of hearing. More elaborate and specific audiometric hearing tests are performed to measure hearing. A hearing test is performed in a soundproof booth by an audiologist. An audiometer is an electronic instrument used to test the client's hearing by producing sounds of varying tones and loudness. Hearing is assessed by a special unit of measure called the decibel

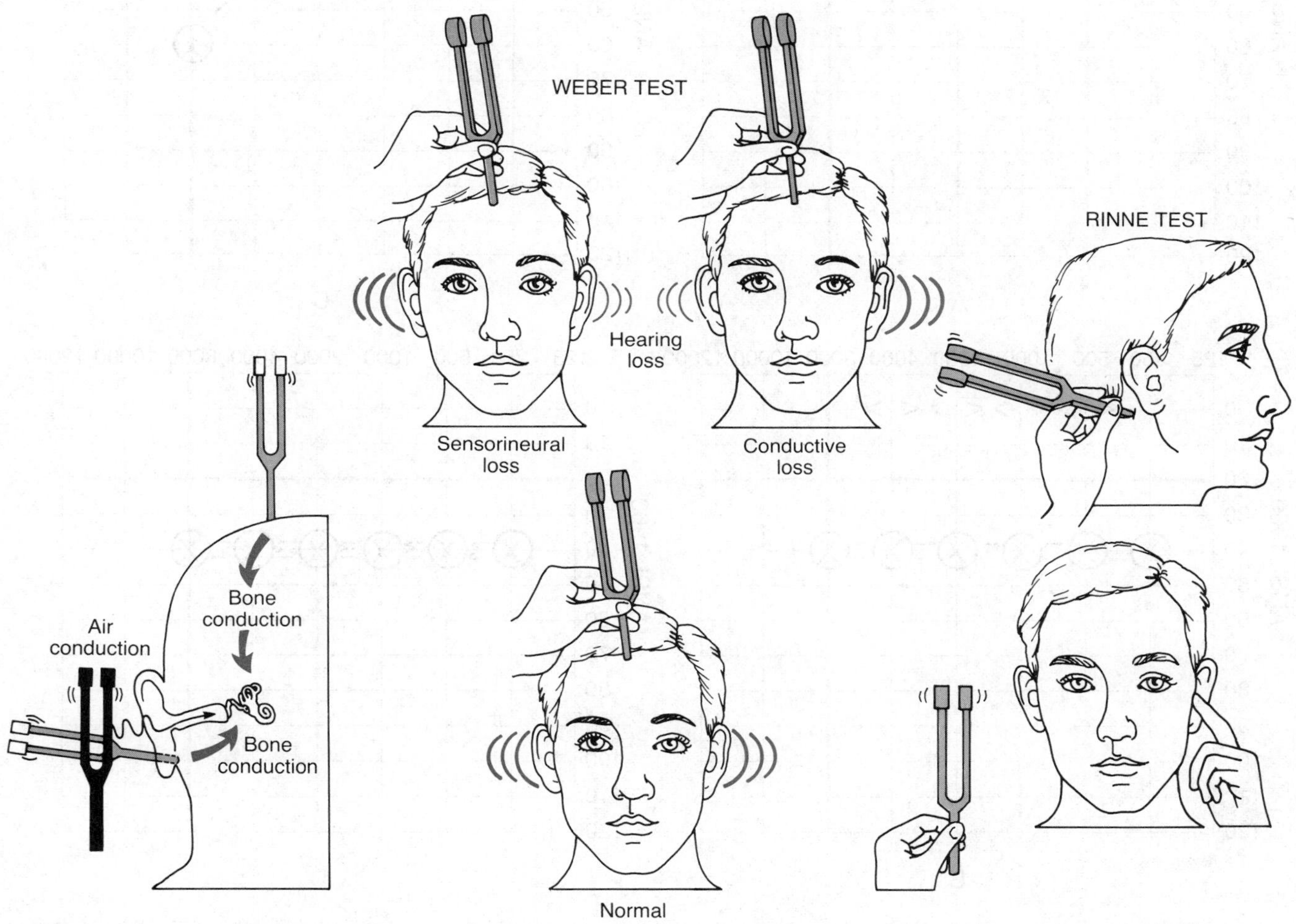

▲ *Figure 34–8*

The Weber and Rinne tests for hearing loss. The Weber test is used to detect lateralization of hearing damage; the Rinne test distinguishes between conductive hearing loss and sensorineural hearing loss. The two tests should be performed consecutively. The Weber test uses a vibrating tuning fork placed on the client's head or nose to produce a centrally located stimulus. The client should hear the sound equally in both ears. The tone is louder in an ear with unilateral conductive loss and quieter in unilateral sensorineural loss. The Rinne test then characterizes the unilateral hearing loss as conductive or sensorineural. The Rinne test is performed by holding a vibrating tuning fork about 2 inches from the external ear. When the client cannot hear the sound, the tuning fork is placed on the mastoid bone. When the tone is louder through air than through bone, the client has a positive Rinne finding, which indicates normal hearing or sensorineural hearing loss. A negative Rinne finding (louder bone conduction than air conduction) indicates a conductive loss.

(dB), a logarithmic function of sound intensity. Earphones are used for the audiogram. The client is asked to signal the audiologist by raising a hand or pressing a button when the tone is heard; the responses are plotted on a graph called an audiogram (Fig. 34–9).

The components of hearing are tested through assessment of air conduction, bone conduction, and speech. Air conduction is assessed by presenting tones through the earphones. By varying the loudness and frequency of tones, a hearing level is established. Bone conduction is assessed by presenting tones through a bone conduction oscillator placed behind the ear on the mastoid bone. The bone conduction level is the level at which the cochlea can hear, bypassing the middle ear structures, and is referred to as the nerve hearing level. A difference between air and bone conduction signifies a conductive hearing loss. When air and bone conduction are the same, either normal

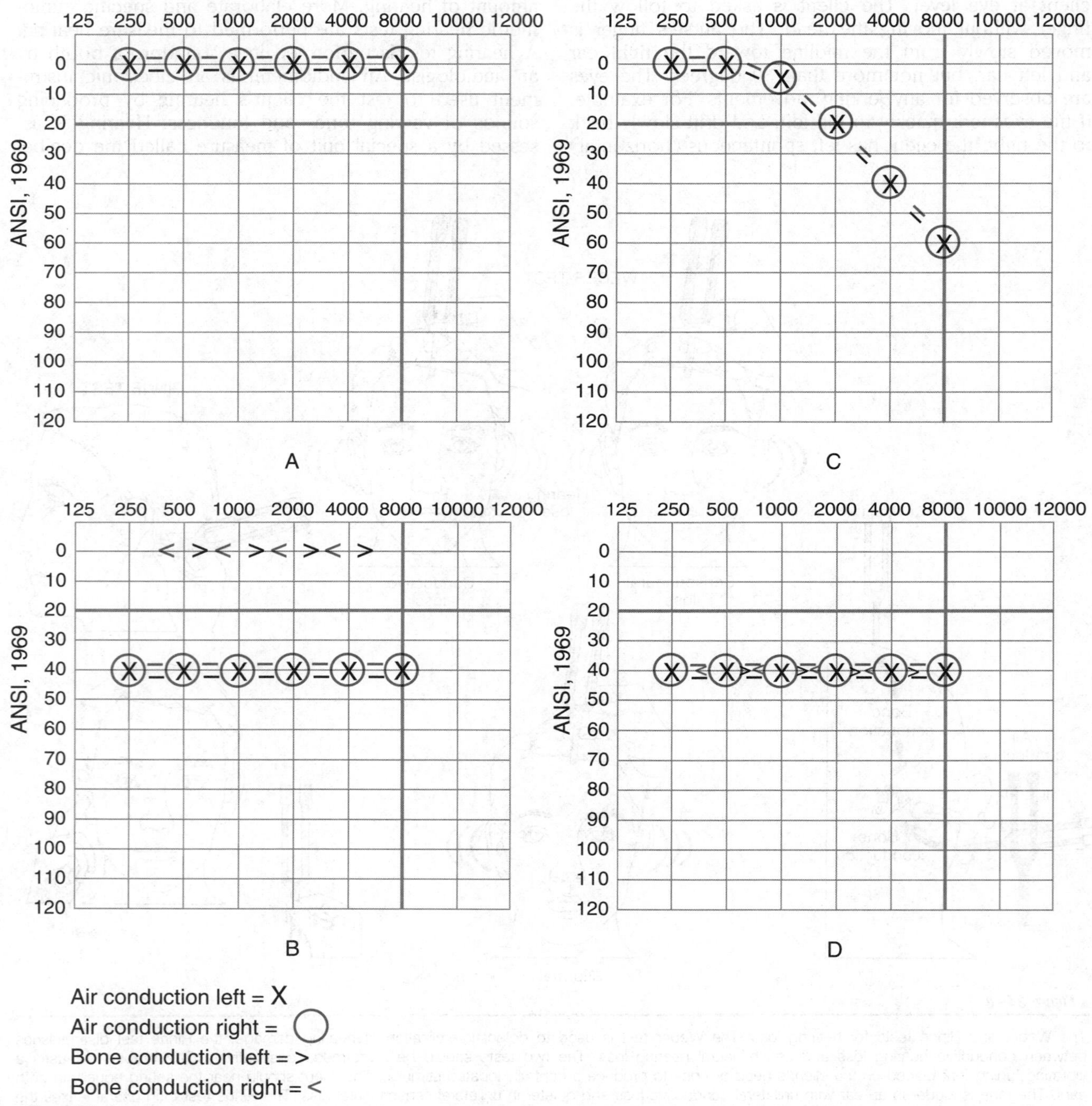

▲ **Figure 34–9**

Audiograms showing types of hearing. *A*, Normal hearing. *B*, Conductive hearing loss. *C*, High-frequency hearing loss. *D*, Sensorineural hearing loss. (Courtesy of Arnold G. Schuring, M.D.)

hearing or a nerve (sensorineural) hearing loss exists. Speech evaluation includes speech reception threshold and speech discrimination. Speech reception threshold is the level of speech hearing and serves as a check on the reliability of the air conduction test. Speech discrimination is the ability to understand the spoken word.

Normal hearing is a range of hearing established nationally by testing the hearing levels of people of all ages. A client with "normal hearing" has 80 per cent or more hearing, depending on age.

Some of these tests are performed by computer-assisted instruments. The object of these special tests is to differentiate whether a problem or lesion within the hearing system is located in the cochlea, in the acoustic nerve, or in the brain stem.

A popular test used for differentiating problems in the middle ear is tympanometry or impedance audiometry. This automatic test applies pressure to the tympanic membrane and measures the result; a distinctive tracing is created on a graft, called a tympanogram. Abnormalities of the tympanogram describe the function of the middle ear, eustachian tube, and ossicles. Tympanometry can also be used to measure the stapedial muscle reflex and its decay. This test also indicates the function of the acoustic nerve.

The auditory brain stem response test is currently one of the most popular approaches to the assessment of the auditory nervous system. By presenting a sound to the ear, and measuring the response (computer averaging) in the brain stem, specific diagnostic information can be obtained. Abnormal test results point to a lesion of the acoustic nerve or brain stem. Imaging tests of the head are usually ordered to confirm the abnormality.

Vestibular Tests

The vestibular system also can be tested by electrophysiologic means. Although the physical assessment of balance is important, the most common objective measurement of balance is accomplished by electronystagmography (ENG). The ENG instrument was developed to measure nystagmus (involuntary, rapid eye movement) in response to stimulation of the vestibular system. This stimulation includes testing the client at rest in different positions for both the eyes and the head, and with different temperatures of air or water in the ear canals, thus stimulating the semicircular canals. The different test results give a recording (electronystagmogram) that reflects the status of each labyrinth and can point to central nervous system disorders.

Platform posturography, which is performed while the client is standing, is one of the newest computerized balance tests. This test can help isolate the etiologic basis as vestibular, visual, or proprioceptive. This platform test helps to identify, quantify, and localize the source of balance disorders (Fig. 34-10).

Rotary chair or harmonic acceleration can also be used. Rotation of the client in a chair in darkness provides information about vestibular dysfunction and level of central compensation.

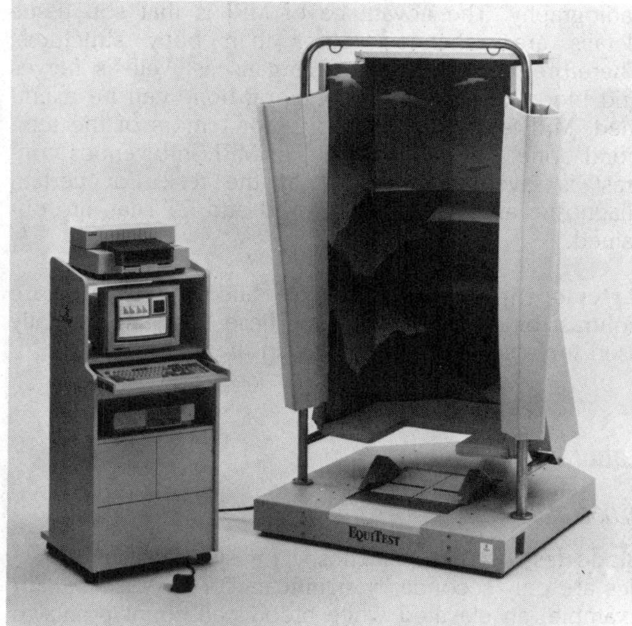

▲ *Figure 34-10*

Platform posturography to assess vestibular function. The client stands on a movable platform and has restricted vision by the panels with clouds. The platform is moved so that the client must compensate for the postural changes. Without visual cues, the vestibular system is tested for its ability to compensate. Because of the risk of falls, the client is strapped to the sides. (Photo courtesy of Neurocom International, Inc.)

Other Otologic Tests

IMAGING TESTS

The temporal bone and its structures are easily examined by x-ray study. The oldest but not necessarily most useful study is x-ray examination of the mastoid bone. More recent radiographic techniques have largely replaced plane film radiography.

Polytomography. Polytomography focuses on one plane and "opened up" the temporal bone for the first time. Very small structures within the temporal bone could be identified. In addition, the surgeon could assess the problems before surgery and anticipate the surgical treatment more closely.

Computed Tomography. The computer in a computed tomography (CT) scan mathematically reconstructs a cross section of the temporal bone from measurement of the radiographic film transmission. In order to show better soft tissue detail in the temporal bone, contrast is generally used. CT scan with contrast is the most commonly ordered CT scan for the ear.

Magnetic Resonance Imaging. Magnetic resonance imaging (MRI) is a completely different process from radiography. The advantage of MRI is that soft tissue details are enhanced rather than bony structures. Therefore, the membranous organs as well as nerves and blood vessels of the temporal bone can be examined. MRI is the test of choice for tumors of the temporal bone. For enhancement of MRI, intravenous contrast is given at the time of the test. For certain diagnostic assessments, both MRI and CT scan are obtained.

Arteriography. Arteriography and venography are contrast blood vessel studies. These tests are specially used for vascular abnormalities in the temporal bone.

Laboratory Tests

BLOOD TESTS

Blood tests that are diagnostic for systemic abnormalities are only secondarily significant for ear disease. For example, an elevated white blood cell count points to an infection but is not diagnostic of ear disease. However, in the presence of ear infection, and in the absence of other infection, blood tests are necessary for assessing acute ear infection. Other blood tests are useful for diagnosis of autoimmune diseases and other systemic illnesses that can affect hearing and balance.

EAR DRAINAGE CULTURES

Drainage from the ear canal or a surgical incision is usually cultured to identify the organism. This is especially necessary in acute infections in order to choose the appropriate antibiotic. When a long-term drainage is present, such as in chronic otitis media, cultures are less helpful because gram-negative bacillus growth covers up the original pathogen. In these cases, many physicians do not culture the drainage but begin broad-spectrum antibiotics.

TESTING FOR PRESENCE OF CEREBROSPINAL FLUID

When clear drainage is found in the ear, a dilemma is presented. Is this fluid cerebrospinal fluid or serous drainage? A fistula from the inner ear to the middle ear can drain cerebrospinal fluid. This pathway can also lead to meningitis by retrograde contamination. Therefore, an analysis of clear fluid drainage from the ear or nose is often helpful in diagnosing the problem.

TISSUE SPECIMENS

Biopsies of abnormal tissue from the ear canal, or from other tissue harvested during surgery, are necessary both to rule out a malignancy and to identify unusual problems. In an infected ear, abnormal tissue is readily identified with visual assessment. If the surgeon is in doubt about the findings, then a tissue sample is taken for pathologic examination.

▼ DISORDERS OF THE EXTERNAL EAR

OVERVIEW

Infections

The most common problems found in the external ear are infections, primarily bacterial or fungal. The most frequent infection, called external otitis, involves the external ear canal. This infection begins in the skin lining of the ear canal and can occlude the canal. External otitis occurs more frequently in the summer than in the winter. The most common form of external otitis is also called swimmer's ear, because it is prevalent when water remains in the ear canal. In addition, opportunistic fungal infections are common. When a debilitating systemic disease such as diabetes is present, the external otitis can spread wildly through cartilage and bone and is then named malignant external otitis.

Occasionally, infection can involve only the cartilage of the pinna (perichondritis), with resultant necrosis of the cartilage and loss of the distinctive shape of the pinna if the infection is not treated quickly. Frostbite of the pinna has findings similar to those of infection.

Another form of infection is seen as an ear canal furuncle or abscess.

Masses

Benign masses of the external ear canal are usually cysts arising from a sebaceous gland and more rarely from the cerumen glands. Cysts can also be congenital in nature. Bony protrusions seen in the lower bony portion of the ear canal are called exostosis. The skin covering the exostosis is normal. If the skin is red, the mass is usually an abscess. Infectious polyps found in the ear canal arise from either the tympanic membrane or, more commonly, the middle ear through a hole in the tympanic membrane. Malignant tumors are also found in the external ear. The cutaneous carcinomas are most often basal cell carcinoma on the pinna and squamous cell carcinoma in the ear canal. If not treated, these carcinomas can invade the underlying structures; squamous cell carcinoma may spread throughout the temporal bone. Rare tumors of the cerumen glands are of the adenoma cell type.

Trauma

Trauma, either sharp or blunt, is becoming a more common finding. A residual finding of repeated blunt trauma is a hypertrophic scar formation known as cauliflower ears, an occupational hazard for boxers. Acute trauma should be treated quickly to decrease the incidence of perichondritis. With prompt treatment, traumatic injuries seldom leave residual deformity.

Obstructions

On inspection of the external canal, the most frequent problem is impacted cerumen. Although the ear canal is self-cleaning, cerumen may become impacted from a disorder or improper cleaning. Removal of cerumen must be done carefully and may be necessary for examination of the tympanic membrane. The blind removal of earwax with an ear syringe should be done only when the ear is free of other abnormalities, such as an infection or perforation of the eardrum.

Surprisingly, a wide array of foreign bodies fit into the ear canal. The most common foreign body found in the adult ear is either a piece of cotton or, most annoying, an insect. Equally surprising is the difficulty that can be encountered in removing a foreign body. The least traumatic method of removing a foreign body is with the aid of an operating microscope. For removal of a live insect, the ear canal is filled with mineral oil, *not water,* to kill the insect. Water will cause the insect to swell, and it will become more difficult to remove.

Pain in the external ear is the most common symptom of infection. Pain is more intense when the ear canal is swollen. Painful sites are tender because of the close proximity of bone (a hard surface) when the ear is palpated. A clue to early external otitis is tenderness when the pinna is gently pulled on. A forerunner of pain in external otitis is itching in the ear canal. Inflammation (redness) is easily identified with an otoscope. At different stages of infection, drainage will be found from the ear canal. In early infectious disorders, the drainage may be clear and not discolored by pus.

A common complaint of clients with occlusion of the ear canal is loss of hearing. Both infection and cerumen can cause a sudden hearing loss. The client may also report a blocked ear.

MANAGEMENT

Medical Management

The most common external ear problems are infections, which are treated with both local and systemic antibiotics. However, the first rule of treating infection is meticulous cleaning of the site in order for the local antibiotic to reach the infected area. Thus, external otitis must be treated by microscopic cleaning before antibiotic drops or ointments are applied. If the ear canal is swollen shut, a wick must be inserted to allow the drops to penetrate the canal. If the infection is generalized or severe, systemic antibiotics are used. If debris accumulates in the ear canal, irrigations (with an ear syringe) can be used. Because external otitis is one of the most painful disorders of the ear, appropriate analgesics are required.

The removal of cerumen can lead to irritation from mild caustic commercial products. An infection that involves cartilage has to be treated aggressively and quickly with systemic antibiotics for avoidance of complications.

The surgical treatment of infections involves incision and drainage in the acute phase for abscesses and, at times, for perichondritis. The most common surgical treatment is excision of cysts and cutaneous carcinomas. For conditions that occlude the ear canal, more extensive surgery involving skin grafting, known as a canalplasty, is performed.

Nursing Management

The most frequent conditions of the external ear that are seen by the nurse are inflammation and infection. Pain is the most common subjective symptom, followed by decreased hearing, sense of fullness, throbbing sensation, and itching. The information to be collected includes the onset, duration, frequency, and intensity of symptoms, as previously described.

Observe the external ear for signs of redness, swelling, lumps, scaling, crusting, or drainage, either serous or purulent. In assessing the external ear, manipulation of the ear is important. If the client complains of pain when any part of the ear is palpated, an abscess, a lesion, or some kind of inflammation process of the ear canal is suspected. If an otoscopic examination is performed, care must be taken not to cause the client unnecessary pain. An abscess may be close to the opening of the canal, causing increased pain from the pressure of the speculum. Water in the ear canal from showering or swimming may aggravate the symptoms.

Clients with inflammations or infections of the external ear are usually diagnosed and treated on an ambulatory basis. These problems are not life-threatening or life-shortening and are easily treated with topical antibiotic solutions. During the infection, the client should avoid getting water in the ear while bathing or showering by using either earplugs or cotton coated with petroleum jelly.

Analgesics are often helpful. After the physician has prescribed the analgesic, instruct the client as to the amount, frequency, and duration. Ear pain usually results from the buildup of matter in the small ear canal, which leads to pressure and pain. Once the swelling and drainage are reduced by treatment, the pain subsides.

INSTILLATION OF MEDICATIONS

Eardrops. Antibiotics and anti-inflammatory agents are usually administered locally rather than systemically in problems involving the external ear. The procedure and directions for administration of eardrops and ointment can be found in a fundamentals textbook.

When a wick is used, the prescribed number of eardrops are placed directly on the wick. The wick serves not only as a bandage but also as an excellent vehicle to medicate the ear canal.

Commercially prepared wicks or single pieces of $\frac{1}{4}$-inch gauze can be used. The wick is gently inserted into the ear canal by means of forceps while the external ear is gently pulled upward and backward. The wick is usually slightly less than 1 inch in length.

SOFTENING AND REMOVAL OF CERUMEN

Eardrops. Wax visible in the ear canal can be removed with a cotton-tipped applicator. Do not put more than the cotton portion in the ear. Impacted accumulations of earwax may be softened and loosened for removal by alternate instillation of glycerin and hydrogen peroxide eardrops. The eardrops are warmed to body temperature and used daily as directed for 1 to 2 weeks. The ear is then irrigated gently with warm water for removal of the softened wax or cleaned under magnification with a cerumen spoon. Wax that is on the tympanic membrane should be removed by a physician or a clinical nurse specialist in otology.

Ear Irrigation. The ear is commonly irrigated to cleanse the external auditory canal or to remove impacted wax, debris, or foreign bodies. Irrigations are not used in clients with a history of or who are suspected of having a perforated eardrum. The irrigating solution (usually water) is warmed to body temperature and placed in the irrigating syringe. The client's clothes are protected with a plastic drape, and a kidney-shaped basin is placed below the ear to catch the irrigating solution. The client sits with the ear to be irrigated toward the nurse, with the head tilted toward the opposite ear. The external ear is pulled upward and backward for the adult, and the tip of the syringe is directed along the upper wall of the ear canal. The canal should not be completely obstructed by the syringe to allow the backflow of solution. When charting the ear irrigation, include the nature of returned solution regarding amount, texture, color of cerumen, or type of debris. Instruct the client to report pain, vertigo, or nausea during the procedure.

▼ DISORDERS OF THE TYMPANIC MEMBRANE, MIDDLE EAR, AND MASTOID

▼ Disorders of the Tympanic Membrane

OVERVIEW

Infections

Infections of the external ear canal can involve the surface of the tympanic membrane, and the tympanic membrane will be a "window" for infection of the middle ear. Infection can cause hard deposits in the tympanic membrane known as tympanosclerosis (see later). A specific viral infection of the tympanic membrane is bullous myringitis. This inflammatory disease forms blisters or bullae between the layers of the eardrum, which is extremely painful. Holes or perforations of the tympanic membrane can be caused by infection and can be accompanied by drainage.

Tumors

Both benign and malignant tumors can involve the tympanic membrane but seldom arise from it. However, an infectious glandular polyp can be isolated to the tympanic membrane. Tumors in the middle ear can be seen through or protrude through the tympanic membrane.

Trauma

The tympanic membrane is the most common ear structure damaged by trauma. Increased pressure from a hand slap or falling in water can rupture the thin membrane. Sports injuries, cleaning the ear with a sharp instrument, or industrial accidents involving welding sparks can also cause a perforation. When the tympanic membrane is perforated, infection is likely.

Because the tympanic membrane is a semitransparent membrane, it can reflect what lies underneath it as well as discoloration and displacement of the membrane. Therefore, both fluid in the middle ear and infection can be seen. The tympanic membrane may be dull or red instead of the normal pearly gray.

The tympanic membrane may be altered by either positive or negative pressure. The membrane may be bulging as a result of positive pressure in the middle ear that results from infection. This pressure is strong enough in some cases to "burst" the eardrum and cause drainage. A ruptured eardrum is more common in children than in adults and usually heals spontaneously. These disorders involving the tympanic membrane are painful, perhaps the most painful of all middle ear disorders. A negative pressure in the ear will cause a retraction of the tympanic membrane, outlining the ossicles. In these cases, fluid is usually found.

The major finding in tympanic membrane disorders is a perforation. A perforation may be either acute, as seen in trauma and acute infection, or chronic, as seen in repeated infection. An acute perforation has a better chance of healing spontaneously than does a chronic perforation. A perforation that is located away from the outside edge or annulus of the tympanic membrane is a central perforation. A perforation causes hearing loss, depending on its size and location. The largest hearing loss found with a perforation is approximately 35 dB (one third of the hearing). If a perforation is present, damage to the ossicles should be suspected, which will cause a greater hearing loss.

Medical Management

The medical management of tympanic membrane disorders involves both systemic and local antibiotics. Local antibiotics are used in the form of eardrops.

Surgery can be performed on the tympanic membrane with use of an operating microscope to magnify the area. The major surgical procedure performed is closure of a perforation. This procedure is called a myringoplasty if only the perforation is addressed, or a tympanoplasty if the middle ear is also involved. Sometimes the ossicles must also be reconstructed, which alters the type of tympanoplasty. A tympanoplasty may also be performed in conjunction with surgery involving the mastoid. The most common material that is used as a free graft to close the perforation is fascia taken from the temporalis muscle above the ear. Less commonly used tissue is perichondrium or vein. Tympanoplasty is a common surgical procedure with a high rate of success.

Other surgical treatments of the tympanic membrane include incision and drainage of vesicles, excision of polyps, and office patching of perforations. Myringotomy is discussed later.

▼ Disorders of the Middle Ear

OVERVIEW

Infections

OTITIS MEDIA

The most prevalent disorders of the middle ear are infections known as otitis media. Otitis media is caused by various types of bacteria, depending on the age of the client and type of infection. When the infection is sudden in onset and short in duration, the diagnosis is acute otitis media. When the infection is repeated, usually causing drainage and perforation, the problem is called chronic otitis media. In between bouts of otitis media, fluid may form in the middle ear, known as serous otitis media. This fluid is formed by a vacuum in the middle ear usually caused by a blocked eustachian tube. Infection can cause swelling of the mucosa throughout the middle ear and eustachian tube. When the swelling subsides, the fluid can then be too thick to drain. At times, serous otitis media is found in conjunction with upper respiratory infections or allergies. If the fluid remains over a period of years, it causes tympanic membrane retraction, or adhesive otitis media. Infection present over a long period of time can also cause necrosis of the tympanic membrane (perforations) or of the ossicles. Both problems create a conductive hearing loss. Necrosis of the bony covering of the facial nerve may cause facial paralysis. Because of the extraordinary anatomy of the temporal bone, middle ear infection can also lead to brain abscesses that are life-threatening if not treated properly. Cholesteatoma is a complication from otitis media but is also a problem of the mastoid and is discussed later.

TYMPANOSCLEROSIS

Tympanosclerosis is a result of repeated infection and deserves special emphasis. Tympanosclerosis is a deposit of collagen and calcium within the middle ear that can harden around the ossicles, causing a conductive hearing loss. Tympanosclerosis can also be found mounded up in the middle ear or as plaque in the tympanic membrane.

Otosclerosis

Otosclerosis or "hardening of the ear," which involves the stapes, is an important middle ear disorder. This bony disease of the otic capsule causes excess bone to form, which impedes normal movement of the stapes. The conductive hearing loss that results is one of the most common correctable middle ear disorders, second only to an infection of the ear. Another form of otosclerosis that does not fix the stapes is cochlear otospongiosis, which can cause a toxic sensorineural hearing loss.

Tumors

The most common benign growth in the middle ear is an infectious polyp. Next in frequency is a cholesteatoma, which is not a true tumor but acts like one. A facial nerve neuroma is found along the course of the facial nerve. Malignant tumors involving the middle ear can be primary or secondary in nature.

Trauma

Trauma to the tympanic membrane from a blast or blunt injury can involve the middle ear, causing a fracture or dislocation of the ossicles and tearing of the tympanic membrane. Also, the facial nerve is vulnerable to trauma. A basal skull fracture involves the temporal bone and, depending on the fracture site, causes ossicular damage as well as facial nerve paralysis and usually sensorineural hearing loss. Care of clients with facial fracture is discussed in Chapter 72.

Eustachian Tube Disorders

The eustachian tube is part of the middle ear but has separate problems. Because the eustachian tube connects the middle ear to the nasopharynx, pharyngeal disorders will also cause eustachian tube dysfunction and, thus, secondary middle ear problems. For example, the most common disorder is blockage of the eustachian tube by enlarged adenoid tissue in children. The most common blockage in adults is swelling of the mucosa in the eustachian tube during an upper respiratory infection that can lead to serous otitis media. In a persistent unilateral blocked eustachian tube, a malignant tumor must be ruled out as the cause. Acute blockage from barotrauma (altitude changes) caused by flying or underwater diving will also cause middle ear problems. The incidence of barotrauma is increased when an upper respiratory infection is present. Aerotitis media is a form of serous otitis media in which fluid or air is trapped in the middle ear because of the descent in an airplane. Any long-term blockage of the eustachian tube leads to serous otitis media and a hearing loss.

Because the middle ear is the transformer for hearing (transmitting sound vibrations from the tympanic membrane to the inner ear), a hearing loss is the most frequent symptom of middle ear disorders. Fortunately, a conductive hearing loss is found in 95 percent of hearing losses and is correctable by either medical or surgical treatment. Pain is also quite common because of pressure from infection or fluid behind the tympanic membrane. If the tympanic membrane perforates, pus, blood, and other material may drain from the ear. In chronic middle ear and mastoid problems, a thick yellow discharge is common. With acute otitis media, all three findings (hearing loss, pain, and discharge) can be present.

MANAGEMENT

With any form of otitis media, appropriate antibiotic therapy may be necessary. If drainage is present, culture and sensitivity study should be performed. However, most episodes of acute otitis media do not produce drainage, and the most probable bacterial cause need not be identified. In chronic ear discharge, the normal contaminants of the ear abound and unfortunately do not respond to the common antibiotics. Thus, local treatment involving ear irrigations, antibiotic drops, and antibiotic powders is used.

Blood coming from the ear canal usually points to a minor problem such as a scratch and not a major disease. Persistent hemorrhage must be checked by an otologist.

Because the eustachian tube is an integral part of middle ear disorders, decongestants and antihistamines are used to decrease the swelling and open the eustachian tube. Pain medication may be needed.

An incision into the tympanic membrane through which fluid is removed by suction is called myringotomy. To keep the incision open and prevent a recurrence of fluid, various types of transtympanic tubes can be inserted into the incision. These tubes extrude in 3 to 12 months by themselves and rarely have to be removed.

Reconstruction of the necrotic ossicles is not yet an exact science. Various methods of repositioning these tiny ear bones are now in use. The surgery is difficult to perform and, unfortunately, does not always remain successful over the long term. Therefore, various synthetic prostheses have been used to reconnect the ossicles to carry sound. In an attempt to prevent extrusion of the prostheses, tissue is combined with the prostheses in order to rebuild the ossicles. This semibiologic method is used in different forms by the majority of otologic surgeons (Fig. 34–11).

The surgical procedure of ossicular reconstruction is called ossiculoplasty. Other middle ear lesions are excised often in combination with other recognized middle ear procedures. For example, tympanosclerosis is removed routinely during tympanoplasty or ossiculoplasty.

Stapedectomy, removal and replacement of the stapes, was once a common middle ear procedure. The fixed stapes is replaced by an artificial stapes constructed of stainless steel or plastics. However, the pool of clients with otosclerosis is dwindling, and today stapedectomy is performed less and less.

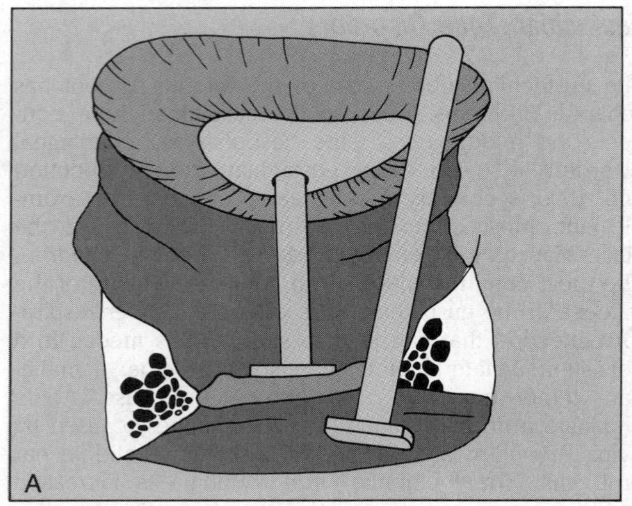

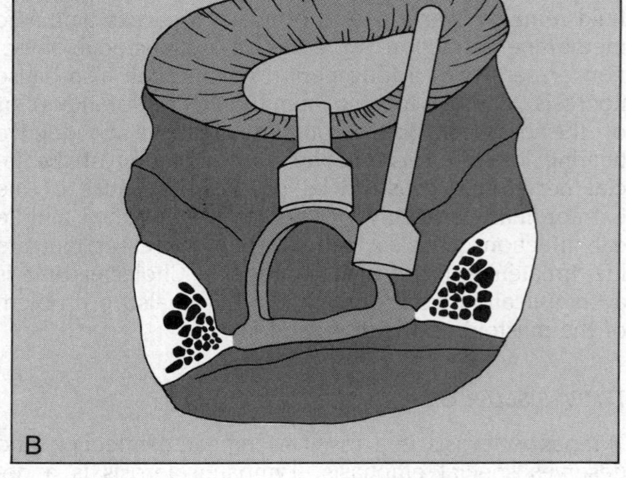

▲ **Figure 34–11**

Middle ear prostheses used for reconstruction. *A*, Ossicle columella prosthesis (total ossicular replacement). *B*, Ossicle cup prosthesis (partial ossicular replacement). (Courtesy of Arnold G. Schuring, M.D.)

▼ Disorders of the Mastoid

OVERVIEW

Infections

Before the discovery of antibiotics, a mastoid infection was a life-threatening event. Now, acute mastoiditis is indeed rare. Still, chronic mastoiditis is present. With repeated middle ear infections, the mastoid cavity becomes a significant part of the problem, which increases the amount of drainage. A chronic infection also leads to the development of cholesteatoma. Although a benign growth, the cholesteatoma causes erosion of the surrounding structures, which causes other problems. In the past, cholesteatoma has given rise to the "stories" of brain abscesses, vertigo, and facial paralysis. These complications are still seen today but, like acute mastoiditis, are infrequent. A cholesteatoma is a skin-lined sac that sheds debris into the center, thus enlarging in size. Often infection is present in the mass of the cholesteatoma. These chronic changes produce cholesterol granules, from which the term cholesteatoma was coined.

Tumors

The same tumors that arise in the middle ear can be found in the mastoid cavity. Because the mastoid cavity is connected to other air cells throughout the temporal bone and is close to the brain, malignant tumors in the mastoid carry a poor prognosis.

Today, drainage from the mastoid cavity is the most likely sign that appears. The drainage courses through the middle ear and out the tympanic membrane through a perforation. Tenderness over the mastoid cavity behind the ear points to an infection but usually is caused by an acute exacerbation of chronic mastoiditis rather than an acute mastoiditis. The protrusion of the pinna as a result of swelling over the mastoid may be part of this process.

Medical Management

Antibiotics are the most common medical therapy in use today. Because infection starts in the middle ear, the problems in the mastoid cavity are avoided by early use of antibiotics. Various irrigations of the mastoid and middle ear are used in chronic infections along with antibiotic eardrops or powders.

Radical mastoidectomy removes the mastoid bone for control of infection and cholesteatoma. However, because the radical mastoidectomy sacrificed hearing, a modified radical mastoidectomy was developed that saved the remaining middle ear structures. At the onset of the period of antibiotics, a simple mastoidectomy was performed, which maintained a normal-appearing ear canal. Because the radical and modified mastoidectomy exteriorize the mastoid cavity to the external ear canal, they are known as open mastoidectomies. Closed mastoidectomies are simple mastoidectomies with modifications, in conjunction with tympanoplasty and ossiculoplasty to retain or regain hearing. Today, even the open mastoidectomy is performed with various tympanoplasties.

Nursing Management

The nursing assessment of the client having problems with the tympanic membrane, the middle ear, or the mastoid cavity is the same, regardless of the need for surgery. A thorough history should precede the ear examination.

Hearing loss is the most frequent symptom of blockage of the tympanic membrane or the ossicles. Pain may also be present because of pressure from infection or fluid behind the tympanic membrane. Data are collected about the onset, duration, and severity of these symptoms.

The tympanic membrane is the only structure that can be visualized directly; the middle ear and mastoid cavity must be evaluated by indirect means. The eardrum may be normal, perforated, infected, retracted, or bulging according to the disease process involved. Pain is not usually elicited on palpation of the external ear; this phenomenon usually provides a differential diagnosis between problems of the external ear and middle ear structures. The mastoid prominences postauricularly may be tender or enlarged in acute mastoiditis (usually in children). Serous, purulent, or bloody drainage may be present.

Hospitalization is rarely necessary for the client with ear disorders not requiring surgery. For those clients having surgery, the hospital stay usually does not exceed 2 to 3 days. Surgical intervention normally follows unsuccessful attempts to treat the client medically.

Eardrops and ear ointment may be necessary for the client with problems of the tympanic membrane, middle ear, or mastoid cavity. In addition, oral antibiotics and analgesics may be needed. The client is instructed in the amount, frequency, and duration of medications. In addition to other treatment, the client may be asked to use a medicinal ear irrigation (Client Education Guide). The most common solution for ear irrigation is boric acid and alcohol, which is obtained by prescription. This solution cleanses the ear of debris and infection and provides a drying agent. A 2- or 3-ounce ear syringe will be needed. A family member performs the irrigation for the client. Usually, the ear irrigation is followed by the use of eardrops.

THE PERIOPERATIVE CLIENT

The responsibility of the nurse begins in the preoperative phase when the decision for surgical intervention is made. The scope of nursing activities for the client can be as broad as a preoperative assessment performed in an office or clinic or as limited as an assessment performed in the holding area of the surgical suite. Data are collected to assess (1) knowledge of events that

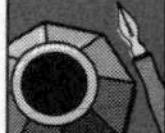

CLIENT EDUCATION GUIDE

Teaching for Clients with Infection of the Tympanic Membrane, Middle Ear, or Mastoid Cavity

Teaching for clients with infection of the tympanic membrane, middle ear, or mastoid cavity includes the following:

- Prevent further infections.
  Provide adequate treatment of allergic or upper respiratory infections.
  Avoid water in the ear (such as while showering, shampooing the hair, or swimming) with a tympanic perforation.
- During treatment for infection, avoid getting water in the ear. If the possibility exists, place two pieces of cotton in the ear, the first piece dry and the second piece saturated with petroleum jelly.
- Seek medical attention for signs of decreased hearing, pain in the ear, or drainage from the ear.

are going to occur, (2) mental readiness for surgery, and (3) physiologic status.

The client undergoing ear surgery should be told what to expect during surgery because frequently the client is given only local anesthesia. The client is awake but sedated during surgery. Instructions should be given about the length of the procedure, the estimated length of hospital stay, and immediate postoperative instructions. Very often, fear of the unknown can be decreased by understanding of events that will occur.

Immediate postoperative instructions may include the following:

- Specified positions, such as lying with operated ear up for several hours after surgery.
- If necessary, blow nose gently one side at a time.
- Sneeze or cough with mouth open.
- Normal occurrences in the initial period may include the following:

  Decreased hearing in operated ear from the packing (possibly, the sound of talking in a barrel)
  Noises in the ear such as cracking or popping
  Minor earache and discomfort in cheek and jaw
  Swelling of ear

Pain is not usually a major problem. Vertigo or lightheadedness may occur when the client ambulates for the first time; clients should be supervised when ambulating on the day of surgery to protect them from falling. Some clients who are quite vertiginous exhibit nystagmus from stimulation of the inner ear. The vertigo usually passes very quickly and seldom requires medication.

The ear rarely bleeds after surgery. A small amount of serosanguineous drainage on a cotton ball is expected. Most ear surgeries require only a cotton ball in the ear postoperatively, although a dressing over the ear may be necessary after tympanomastoidectomy. Postoperative client teaching is listed in the Client Education Guide.

▼ DISORDERS OF THE INNER EAR

HEARING IMPAIRMENT

Definition

Hearing impairment ranges from difficulty in understanding words or hearing certain sounds to total deafness. Up to 80 per cent of all hearing impairments are due to hearing nerve disorders, for which presently there is no cure.

Incidence

Hearing impairment is the nation's number one disability; 1 of every 15 Americans is affected. By the year 2050, approximately 1 of every 5 clients in this country will be 55 years of age or older. Of these estimated 58 million people, 26 million are expected to have hearing impairment.

Of the 10 million people in the United States with a hearing loss who are 65 years of age or older, over 90 per cent have a sensorineural hearing loss. Because of fear, misinformation, lack of information, and vanity, many clients do not admit that they have a hearing problem.

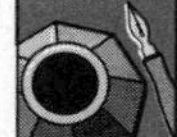

CLIENT EDUCATION GUIDE

Client Discharge Teaching After Ear Surgery

- Continue to blow nose gently one side at a time and to sneeze or cough with mouth open for 1 week after surgery.
- Avoid physical activity for 1 week and exercises or sports for 3 weeks after surgery.
- Return to work as recommended, usually 3 to 7 days after surgery (3 weeks if work is strenuous).
- Avoid heavy lifting, especially after stapedectomy.
- Change cotton ball in ear daily as prescribed.
- Keep ear dry for 4 to 6 weeks after surgery.

  Do not shampoo for 1 week after surgery.
  Protect ear when necessary with two pieces of cotton (outer piece saturated with petroleum jelly).

- Avoid airplane flights for first week after surgery. For sensation of ear pressure, hold nose, close mouth, and swallow to equalize pressure.
- Wear noise defenders for loud noise environments.
- Report any drainage other than a slight amount of bleeding to the physician.

Etiology

Factors that influence the type and amount of hearing loss include hereditary disease, toxic substances, trauma, age, and noise exposure. Infectious diseases (measles, mumps, and meningitis), arteriosclerosis, ototoxic drugs, neuromas of the eighth cranial nerve, otospongiosis, trauma to the head or ear, or degeneration of the organ of Corti are also etiologies of hearing loss and occur most commonly from age (presbycusis).

Conductive hearing loss may be caused by anything that blocks the external ear, such as wax, infection, or a foreign body; a thickening, retraction, scarring, or perforation of the tympanic membrane; or any pathophysiologic changes in the middle ear affecting or fixing one or more of the ossicles.

Noise-induced hearing loss can be traumatic, for example, a sudden loud noise such as a blast injury. More commonly, this hearing loss occurs over time from repeated injury from loud noise. The major cause is industrial noise, use of firearms, and listening to loud music.

Although the exact cause of sudden or fluctuating hearing loss is not known, it is thought to be vascular in nature. One cause that is not well understood is a fistula from the inner ear to the middle ear via the oval or round window.

Diseases that alter the central nervous system, such as cerebrovascular accidents and tumors, are the cause for central deafness, a rare form of sensorineural hearing loss.

Infection can also lead to hearing loss. An infection of the inner ear called labyrinthitis can be either viral or bacterial in origin. Viral labyrinthitis is usually isolated to the inner ear, whereas the rarer bacterial labyrinthitis is from infection in the middle ear and mastoid.

Both benign and malignant tumors of the temporal bone can involve the inner ear and lead to hearing loss. The most common benign tumor is an acoustic neuroma of the eighth nerve arising in the internal ear canal. Spread of this tumor out of the internal ear canal toward the brain stem will cause other neurologic problems and can be life-threatening. Other tumors in the cerebellar-pontine angle will likewise involve the seventh and eighth cranial nerves as they enter the internal acoustic meatus. Malignant tumors invade the entire inner ear, spreading from the middle ear and mastoid.

Pathophysiology

SENSORINEURAL HEARING LOSS

Sensorineural hearing loss is the most common inner ear disorder. It results from disease or trauma to the sensorineural structures or nerve pathways of the inner ear leading to the brain stem. The hearing loss may at times fluctuate, but usually a progressive hearing loss results. Sensorineural hearing losses are usually permanent and not correctable by medical or surgical treatment.

CONDUCTIVE HEARING LOSS

Any interference with the conduction of sound impulses through the external auditory canal, the eardrum, or the middle ear results in a conductive hearing loss. The inner ear is usually not involved in a conductive loss, and sound amplification can reach the inner ear. Most conductive hearing losses are correctable by medical or surgical treatment.

NOISE-INDUCED HEARING LOSS

Noise-induced hearing loss is characterized by a greater loss in the higher frequencies. The only treatment for noise-induced hearing loss is to prevent further injury by avoiding noise or by wearing ear protection.

SUDDEN OR FLUCTUATING HEARING LOSS

Sudden or fluctuating hearing loss is recognized as a separate hearing disorder because of the isolated finding and dramatic outcome. Because it is thought to be vascular in nature, attempted treatments are made to alter the vascular system in some way. Occasionally, the hearing may return to normal without the reason being understood. Unfortunately, most clients do not regain normal hearing. If a fistula is suspected, it is surgically closed by a tissue graft.

CENTRAL DEAFNESS

Central deafness is also known as central auditory dysfunction. With this phenomenon, the central nervous system cannot interpret normal auditory signals. Therefore, the hearing test findings are normal, although the client is "deaf."

OTHER TYPES OF HEARING LOSS

Different types of hearing loss are listed in Box 34–4. A client has a mixed hearing loss when both a conductive and sensorineural hearing loss are present simultaneously. A functional loss is a hearing loss for which no organic lesion can be found and special testing suggests normal hearing. A hearing loss may also be congenital or acquired. The majority of clients with ear problems have some degree of hearing loss.

Prevention

A major nursing responsibility is the identification of hearing impairment in clients in both hospital and community settings. Detection and referral of an ear problem are the first steps in limiting the client's disability. For maintaining normal ear function, adequate protection of the ears is important and involves several activities:

Early, adequate treatment of diseases
Prevention of trauma to the ear
Early detection of hearing losses
Monitoring side effects of ototoxic drugs
Monitoring noise pollution
Periodic ear examination

Box 34–4. The Types of Hearing Loss

Air conduction hearing loss: loss of hearing through the external and middle ears.
Bone conduction hearing loss: loss of hearing through the inner ear.
Central hearing loss: loss of hearing from damage to the brain's auditory pathways or auditory center.
Conductive hearing loss: loss of hearing in which air conduction is worse than bone conduction and involves the external and middle ear.
Fluctuating hearing loss: a sensorineural hearing loss that varies with time.
Functional hearing loss: loss of hearing for which no organic lesion can be found.
Mixed hearing loss: both sensorineural and conductive hearing loss occur.
Neural hearing loss: a sensorineural hearing loss originating in the eighth nerve or brain stem.
Sensorineural hearing loss: loss of hearing involving the cochlea and hearing nerve; bone and air conduction equal but diminished.
Sensory hearing loss: a sensorineural hearing loss in the cochlea and involving the hair cells and nerve endings.
Sudden hearing loss: a sensorineural hearing loss with a sudden onset.

Conductive hearing loss results from interference with conduction in the external and middle ear; sensorineural hearing loss, in the inner ear; and mixed hearing loss, in all three areas.

EARLY, ADEQUATE TREATMENT OF DISEASE

Secondary prevention of ear disorders includes seeing a physician for any disease that causes prolonged symptoms of the ear, such as pain, swelling, drainage, "plugged" feeling, or decreased hearing. The nurse must encourage clients with these symptoms to seek professional help. Many chronic problems such as perforations and necrotic ossicles can be prevented with adequate medical attention.

During upper respiratory infections (colds), the nose should be blown with at least one nostril open. Excessive pressure can force infected secretions up the eustachian tube into the middle ear.

PREVENTION OF TRAUMA TO THE EAR

Clients should be taught to avoid inserting hard instruments into the ear canal, obstructing the ear canal with objects, inserting unclean articles or solutions into the ear, or swimming in water identified as being polluted. These activities can lead to damage of the tympanic membrane or to ear infections. Also, adults often may insert cotton-tipped applicators too deeply into the ear canal in an attempt to remove cerumen or to scratch the ear canal.

EARLY DETECTION OF HEARING LOSS

The hearing nerve does not usually regain function; thus, early detection of hearing loss is important so the cause of the loss can be diagnosed and, it is hoped, the problem treated. However, the signs of a small loss of hearing are elusive.

A hearing loss in both ears may first be detected by a family member rather than by the client. The earliest sign is not hearing what was once heard. Another common sign is asking for a repetition of what was said. Usually the request is in the form of a question, such as "What did you say?" Sometimes the hard-of-hearing client may repeat the information, even incorrectly, to provoke a response and thus a repetition of the information.

A hearing loss in one ear is also difficult to detect. The client can notice the loss when using a telephone or by having difficulty with the direction of sounds.

MONITORING SIDE EFFECTS OF OTOTOXIC DRUGS

Some medicines can affect the cochlea, the vestibular labyrinth, or the eighth cranial nerve (Box 34–3). Clients taking ototoxic drugs need to know the signs and symptoms of side effects of these medicines so that the development of loss of hearing or balance can be prevented. If these symptoms (vertigo, decreasing hearing acuity, tinnitus) occur, the next dose of the drug should be omitted and the physician consulted. Audiometric and vestibular testing may be necessary.

MONITORING NOISE POLLUTION

Industrial and occupational noise is a primary cause of hearing loss in our society. The most common type of occupational hearing loss is caused by continuous loud noises. In the United States, the Occupational Safety and Health Administration (OSHA) has established acceptable levels of noise in work environments. The provisions regarding noise protection are complex; in general, exposure to noise levels in excess of 80 dB over an 8-hour day is considered excessive and should be avoided (Table 34–1). Ordinary speech level is heard at about 50 decibels (dB) and heavy traffic at about 70 dB; above 80 dB, noise becomes uncomfortable to the human ear. Exposure to levels greater than 85 to 90 dB for months or years will cause cochlear damage. The nurse must participate in teaching the proper use of protective ear devices or earplugs. Courses are available to educate nurses about industrial hearing conservation requirements.

A client firing guns who notices tinnitus (ringing in the ear), a sensation of fullness in the ear, or a temporary hearing loss should stop firing the guns or wear suitable ear protection. Sound in front of rock band speakers can reach up to 120 dB, and hearing losses have been measured in some members of rock bands. If proximity to the high noise level cannot be avoided, earplugs should be worn during exposure. Listening to music with regular speakers or earphones seldom causes hearing loss.

Earplugs are inserted into the external auditory canal and are capable of reducing the noise by 10 to 30 dB. Usually standardized plugs are effective, but custom-made plugs molded to the client's ear canal can also

TABLE 34-1. Decibel Ratings and Hazardous Time Exposure of Common Noises

Typical Level* (dB)	Example	Dangerous Time Exposure
0	Lowest sound audible to human ear	
30	Quiet library, soft whisper	
40	Quiet office, living room, bedroom away from traffic	
50	Light traffic at a distance, refrigerator, gentle breeze	
60	Air conditioner at 20 feet, conversation, sewing machine	
70	Busy traffic, office tabulator, noisy restaurant (constant exposure)	Critical level begins
80	Subway, heavy city traffic, alarm clock at 2 feet, factory noise	More than 8 hours
90	Truck traffic, noisy home appliances, shop tools, lawnmower	Less than 8 hours
100	Chain saw, boiler shop pneumatic drill	2 hours
120	Rock concert in front of speakers, sandblasting, thunderclap	Immediate danger
140	Gunshot blast, jet plane	Any length of exposure time is dangerous
180	Rocket launching pad	Hearing loss is inevitable

*Sound levels refer to intensity experienced at typical working distances. Intensity drops 6 dB with every doubling of distance from noise source. (Courtesy of American Academy of Otolaryngology-Head and Neck Surgery, Washington, DC.)

be purchased and are better tolerated. For noise levels reaching 120 dB and above, clients must wear both earmuffs and earplugs.

PERIODIC EAR EXAMINATIONS

Periodic ear examinations for evaluation of hearing are important in the adult because aging frequently causes degenerative changes in the ear as well as in other body tissues.

Clinical Manifestations

A sensorineural hearing loss is found with almost any inner ear disorder. The hearing loss is usually incomplete but can be progressive in some illnesses. A characteristic of a severe hearing loss is the loss of discrimination (understanding of words). To some clients, a hearing loss feels like a blockage in the ear.

Tinnitus accompanies most sensorineural hearing losses and is very annoying. Tinnitus actually can sound like a roaring, or crickets, and occasionally like music. In some clients, the tinnitus becomes the problem, and the underlying cause may be forgotten.

Clients with a hearing loss can also experience distorted or abnormal sounds. Sometimes a sound is heard at different pitches for each ear, which is called diplacusis. Or a sound causes a rapid increase in loudness, which is called recruitment. These abnormal sounds can cause the client discomfort.

Medical Management

AURAL REHABILITATION

If hearing loss is irreversible or not amenable to surgical intervention or if the client elects not to have surgery, aural rehabilitation may improve communication. The purpose of aural rehabilitation is to maximize the hearing-impaired client's communication skills.

The auditory sense is our primary mode of communication, and rehabilitation is directed toward teaching the client more effective use of the senses of vision, touch, and vibration plus maximizing the use of any remaining hearing ability. Rehabilitation is affected by all demographic variables and the severity of impairment. As with other forms of rehabilitation, success depends partly on the degree of motivation.

Hearing Aids. Because most hearing losses are permanent, the use of a hearing aid should always be considered. A client should undergo a trial period before purchasing the aid. Bilateral (binaural) aids are desirable.

The evolution in hearing aid development has led to smaller and more effective aids. Today, small hearing aids are available that fit into the ear canal. The latest advancement in hearing aids is the ability to produce digital hearing aids, some with remote control. Other advancements include microphones that enhance the voice of a speaker in front of the client, with suppression of background noise. Hearing aids will advance even further.

The maintenance of a hearing aid is becoming less of a problem today. Usually, the aid is returned to the dealer for factory repair while a loaner hearing aid is worn by the client.

Hearing aids are instruments made of miniature parts working together as a system to amplify sound in a controlled manner. They are used by both hearing-impaired clients (slight or moderate hearing loss) and deaf clients (severe or profound hearing loss). Hearing aids make sound louder but may not improve the ability to hear. Therefore, clients with decreased discrimination (the ability to understand what is spoken) benefit less from a hearing aid. The hearing aid amplifies all background noises, such as hospital machinery, footsteps, and department store noises, as well as speech. These noises may mask conversation or confuse the hearing-impaired client, especially the elderly.

There are several types of hearing aids, which vary according to the size to be worn and location. Hearing aids can be worn

- in the ear
- in the canal
- behind the ear (postauricular)
- in the temple of eyeglasses (eyeglasses aid)
- in the middle of the chest (body-worn aid)

Regardless of the type of aid, the hearing aid consists of the following parts:

- microphone to receive sound waves from the air and change sounds into electrical signals
- amplifier to increase the strength of electrical signals
- receiver (loudspeaker) to change the electrical signals back into sound waves
- battery to provide the electrical energy needed to operate the hearing aid

On all types of hearing aids but the body-worn type, all four components are housed in one small case. The louder sounds are then directed into the ear through a custom-fitted earmold (Fig. 34-12).

The hearing aid user should know how to care for the aid (Box 34-5) and what to do if the aid does not work. The nurse must also have a basic knowledge of the hearing aid to assist the client who is ill. The client is encouraged to use the hearing aid and to provide safe storage when it is not in use.

Implantable Hearing Devices. Three types of implantable hearing devices are either available for use or in the investigation stage. They are cochlear implants, bone hearing devices, and semi-implantable hearing devices.

Cochlear implants for those clients with no hearing at all are now available (Fig. 34-13). This device has a small computer that changes the spoken word to electrical impulses. The impulses are transmitted across the skin to an implanted coil that carries the impulse to the hearing nerve endings in the cochlea by an electrode introduced through the round window. The best of the cochlear implants use multichannels. The success of a cochlear implant varies widely and ranges from minimal improvement in auditory awareness to understanding of speech on the telephone.

In some cases of hearing loss, sound can be transmitted through the skull to the inner ear. For clients with a conductive hearing loss, a device is available in

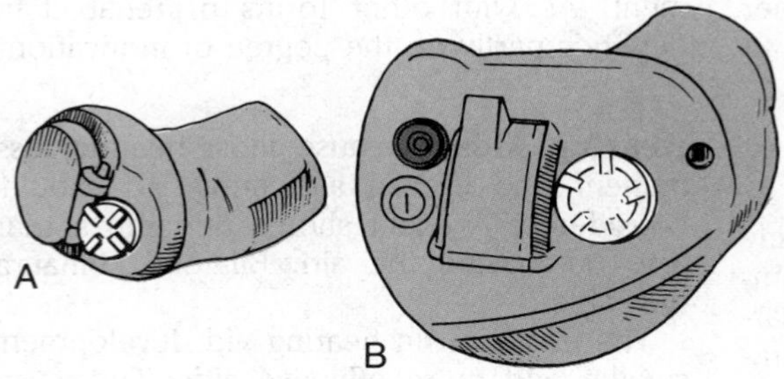

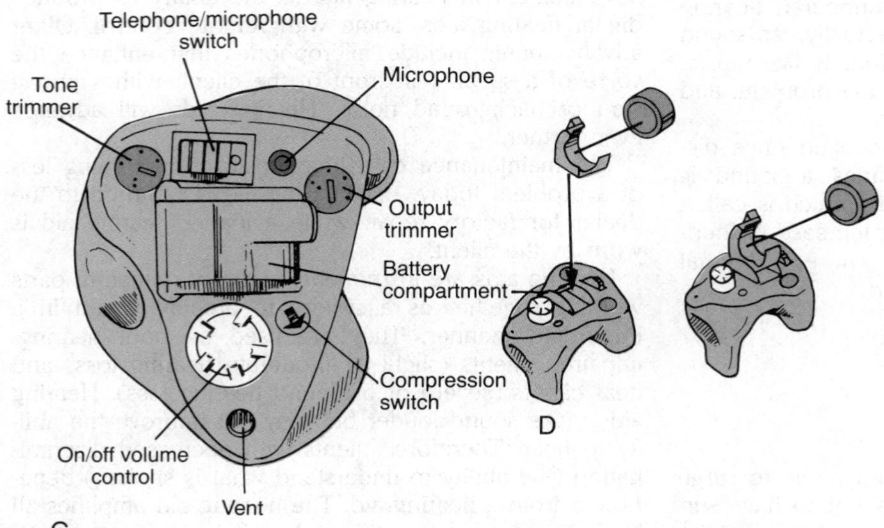

▲ *Figure 34-12*

Types of hearing aids and components. *A*, In-the-canal aid. *B*, In-the-ear aid. *C*, Hearing aid components. *D*, Battery compartment. (Courtesy of Arnold G. Schuring, M.D.)

Box 34–5. Care of a Hearing Aid

- Turn the hearing aid off when it is not in use.
- Open the battery compartment at night to avoid accidental drainage of the battery.
- Keep an extra battery available at all times.
- Wash the earmold frequently (daily if necessary) with mild soap and warm water with the use of a pipe cleaner to cleanse the cannula.
- Dry the earmold completely before reconnecting it to the hearing aid.
- Do not wear the hearing aid during an ear infection.

What to Do if Hearing Aid Fails to Work

- Check on-off switch.
- Inspect earmold for cleanliness.
- Examine battery for correct insertion.
- Examine cord plug for correct insertion.
- Examine cord for breaks.
- Replace battery, cord, or both, if necessary. The life of batteries varies according to amount of use and power requirements of the aid. Batteries last 2 to 14 days.
- Check the position of the earmold in the ear. If hearing aid "whistles," the earmold is probably not inserted properly into the ear canal, or the client needs to have a new earmold made.

which the receiver is implanted under the skin into the skull. The external device transmits the sound through the skin. This device is worn above the ear and not in the ear canal. Because some conductive hearing losses cannot be repaired, this device may provide an alternative rehabilitative method to conventional hearing aid potential.

The implantable device with the greatest potential usage will be for those clients now using a hearing aid. Clinical research has shown that a magnet implanted in the middle ear can be stimulated by an ear canal driver that changes sound to a magnetic force. This system eliminates several bothersome problems of hearing aids, such as feedback and hearing-in noise. A semi-implantable hearing device is the first step to a totally implantable device that would eliminate any external device. However, many challenges have to be met before this workable device is available. This method of hearing aid technology is still in the research stage.

Assistive Listening Devices. In addition to hearing aids, many practical devices are on the market that use hearing aid technology. These devices help the hard-of-hearing client hear the television or radio as well as use the telephone. For the client who cannot use a hearing aid, other assistive devices are available.

Hearing Education. Clients with a hearing loss need to have special education. Auditory training is an approach to enhance listening skills. The hearing-impaired client is initially exposed to gross differences in sound and then gradually "fine tuned" so that subtle differences in discrimination of two similar sounds can be made. The primary purpose of auditory training exercises is to help the client concentrate on the speaker. For some clients, only gross differences between sounds may be recognized.

Speech reading is the current term used for lip reading and is an important means of communication. Speech reading is the process of understanding vocal communication by the integration of lip movements with facial expressions, gestures, environmental clues, and conversation contexts. Speech reading is difficult without auditory cues. Many movements for speech are rapid, many sounds are similar (b, m, p), and certain sounds of any language are silent (the h in English). A high percentage of the words have to be guessed by the hearing-impaired client. Knowledge of this fact alone will help the nurse to be more understanding of the client using this approach.

Because of reduced auditory feedback (the inability of hearing-impaired clients to monitor their own speech), the clearness, pitch quality, or rate of the client's speech may deteriorate. These changes may alter the efficiency of communication and reduce the intelligibility of speech. The goal of speech training is to conserve, develop, or prevent deterioration of speech skills.

Last, but still important today, is sign language. Sign language allows communication by hand signals. Various hand signals represent different letters of the alphabet, words, or phrases.

Other than antibiotics for infections, the medical treatment of hearing loss is dismal. General modalities include steroids and vasodilators, but specific treatment is still lacking. The purpose of medication is to attempt to lessen the progressive hearing loss or, it is hoped, to reverse a sudden loss.

Surgical Management

When a sensorineural hearing loss occurs, surgery is usually not warranted. However, because mixed hearing loss exists (both conductive and sensorineural hearing loss), surgery may be performed to alleviate the conductive hearing loss component. Also, some surgery is performed today to try to stop progressive hearing loss. However, surgery for sensorineural hearing loss does not yet have a successful history.

The most common tumor of the acoustic and balance nerve complex is an acoustic neuroma. Because this slow-growing tumor can cause severe problems outside the temporal bone, it is eventually removed. The hearing loss remains, but the chance for further problems is less. Usually, the surgical technique for removal sacrifices the remaining hearing.

Nursing Management

ASSESSMENT

The nurse can identify clients with impaired hearing and encourage them to seek professional diagnosis and

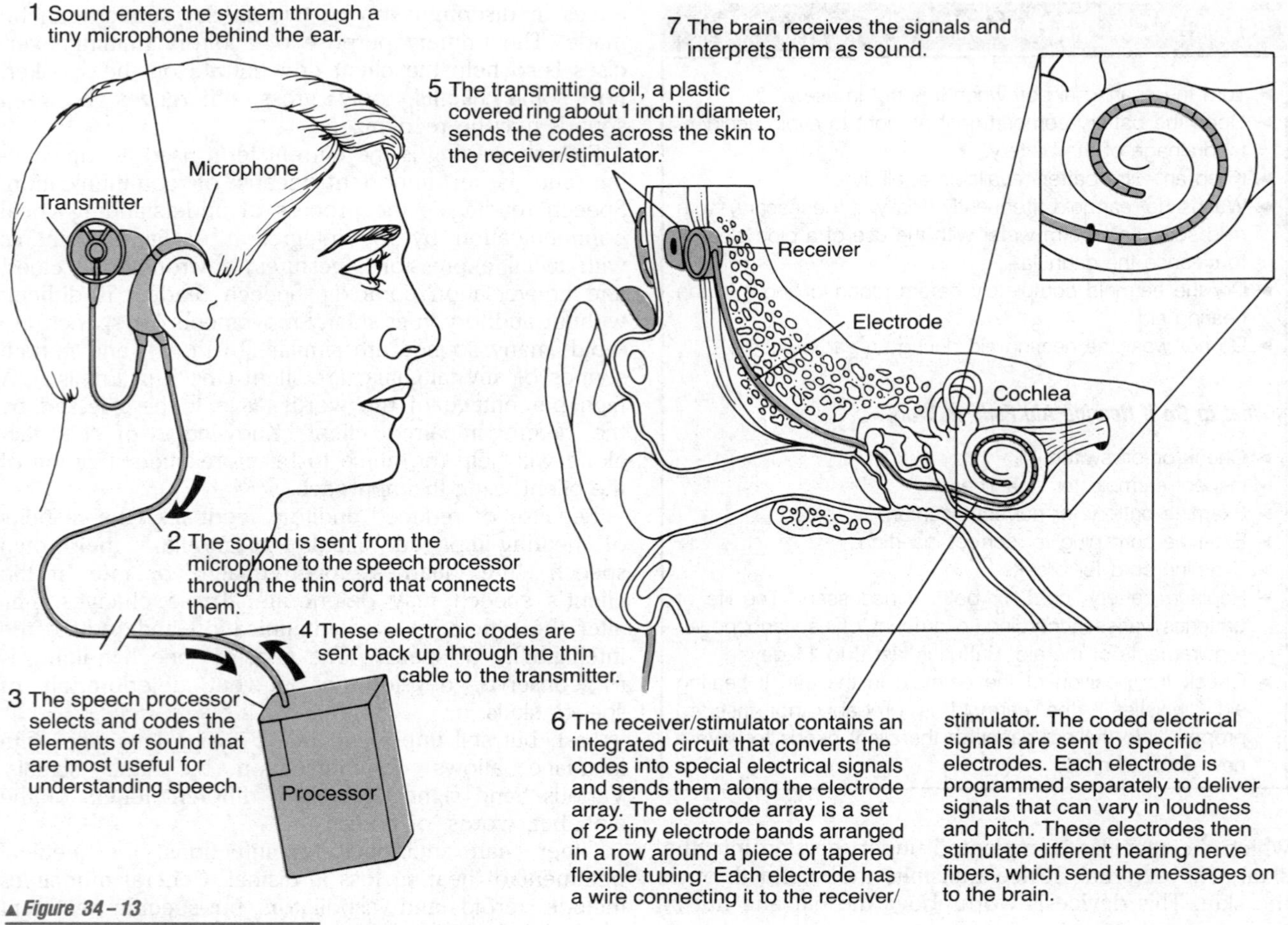

1 Sound enters the system through a tiny microphone behind the ear.
Microphone
Transmitter
2 The sound is sent from the microphone to the speech processor through the thin cord that connects them.
3 The speech processor selects and codes the elements of sound that are most useful for understanding speech.
Processor
4 These electronic codes are sent back up through the thin cable to the transmitter.
5 The transmitting coil, a plastic covered ring about 1 inch in diameter, sends the codes across the skin to the receiver/stimulator.
Receiver
Electrode
Cochlea
6 The receiver/stimulator contains an integrated circuit that converts the codes into special electrical signals and sends them along the electrode array. The electrode array is a set of 22 tiny electrode bands arranged in a row around a piece of tapered flexible tubing. Each electrode has a wire connecting it to the receiver/stimulator. The coded electrical signals are sent to specific electrodes. Each electrode is programmed separately to deliver signals that can vary in loudness and pitch. These electrodes then stimulate different hearing nerve fibers, which send the messages on to the brain.
7 The brain receives the signals and interprets them as sound.

▲ *Figure 34–13*

Cochlear implant to restore hearing.

treatment. Indications of a hearing loss may include the following:

Failure to respond to oral communication
Inappropriate response to oral communication
Excessively loud speech
Abnormal awareness of sounds
Strained facial expressions
Tilted head when listening
Constant need for clarification of conversation
Faulty speech articulation
Behavioral clues (see Box 34–1)

The impact of not hearing others may make some clients withdraw from social situations and become anxious and insecure. Clients with hearing losses can experience fears of inadequacy, feelings of inferiority, depression, and varying degrees of stress and isolation. Important nursing assessments include the extent and duration of the hearing loss, how the client has coped with stress previously, and what support systems are available (see Nursing Research).

The sensorineural hearing loss is assessed by history, physical examination, and audiometry. Occasionally, laboratory, radiologic, and vestibular examinations will be used. In an otology office, the nurse may have the responsibility of performing the history, otologic exami-

NURSING RESEARCH

A survey of 66 older women with impaired hearing examined the major influences on their quality of life. Deafness had occurred in early life in 27 and in older life in 39 women. The researchers recognized that regardless of age of onset, hearing impairment can have a profound impact on physiologic, psychological, and socioeconomic aspects of living. The stress-transactional framework by Lazarus and Launier was used to consider the relationships of variables.

The best predictors of quality of life were social hearing handicap (the degree of difficulty hearing social conversation), functional social support, and perceived health. Overall, the group of women who developed hearing loss later in life had a perception that the quality of their life was lowered because of their condition.

If hearing loss is perceived as a stressor, nurses need to find avenues in teaching to assist clients to overcome these problems. Content on social support, aural rehabilitation, and other adaptations to hearing loss should be incorporated into nursing practice.

▼▼▼

Magilvy, J. K. (1985). Quality of life of hearing-impaired older women. *Nursing Research 34*(3), 140–144.

nation, and screening audiometry. The history is often the most important part of the clinical assessment as previously described (see questionnaire in Box 34–2). The extent of the assessment of the sensorineural hearing loss by the nurse depends on the setting and the nurse's educational preparation and experience. All nurses, however, should be able to inspect the outer ear and grossly assess the auditory acuity.

Nursing Diagnosis: Social Isolation, High Risk for R/T perceived inability to interact with others secondary to hearing loss.

Planning: Expected Outcomes. The client will exhibit a willingness to be involved in social situations, as evidenced by attempting to become a part of social events, conversing with others, indicating less feelings of inadequacy, and responding appropriately to questions asked (not fabricating answers to cover hearing loss).

Box 34–6. Improving Communication with Hearing-Impaired Clients

- Get the client's attention by raising an arm or hand.
- Stand with a light on your face; this will help the client speech read.
- Talk directly to the client while facing him or her.
- Speak clearly, but do not overaccentuate words.
- Speak in a normal tone; do not shout. Shouting overuses normal speaking movements and may cause distortion and be too loud for the client with sensorineural damage. If the client has conductive loss only, sometimes making the voice louder without shouting is helpful.
- If the client does not seem to understand what is said, express it differently. Some words are difficult to "see" in speech reading, such as "white" and "red."
- Move closer to the client and toward the better ear.
- Write out proper names or any statement that you are not sure was understood.
- Do not smile, chew gum, or cover the mouth when talking.
- Inattention may indicate tiredness or lack of understanding.
- Use phrases to convey meaning rather than one-word answers. State the major topic of the discussion first and then give details.
- Do not show annoyance by careless facial expression. Clients who are hard-of-hearing depend more on visual clues for understanding.
- Encourage the use of a hearing aid if it is available; allow the client to adjust it before speaking.
- In a group, repeat important statements and avoid asides to others in the group.
- Avoid the use of the intercommunication system, because this may distort sound and cause poor communication.
- Do not avoid conversation with a client who has hearing loss. It has been said that to live in a silent world is much more devastating than to live in darkness, and clients with hearing loss appear to have more emotional difficulties than do those who are blind.

Implementation. Common nursing interventions to facilitate communication for clients with hearing loss are listed in Box 34–6. They can apply to all clients, regardless of the type or severity of hearing loss.

EVALUATION

The degree of outcome attainment should be evaluated at predetermined intervals. A client with a new hearing loss disorder will need frequent evaluation for determination of the degree of hearing regained as well as the coping strategies used. Because many forms of hearing loss are permanent or progressive, long-term evaluation should also be performed to be certain the client is adapting positively. The nurse will also want to determine whether the client has questions about the equipment used for hearing rehabilitation.

Post-hospital Care

The client should be taught to avoid restaurants that are noisy or crowded. When a hearing aid is used, it often amplifies *all* sounds; therefore, background noise is amplified also.

Because many health care professionals are adept at communicating with the hearing impaired, the client may find a transition into society overwhelming (also see Bridge to Home Health Care). The nurse will need to work with the client to enhance coping, encourage continued social involvement, and advocate the use of various organizations to their fullest extent. Many agencies and associations exist for the hearing-impaired client. Services are offered by audiology clinics sponsored by universities, hospitals, community programs, state or local departments of health, the Veterans Administration, and national organizations.

TINNITUS (HEAD NOISES)

Tinnitus literally means "ringing." However, not all ear noises are ringing sounds, but they fall under the broad classification of tinnitus. Tinnitus is not a disease but a very distressing symptom, and often a warning of hearing loss or other more serious problems. Ear noise that cannot be heard by an observer is classified as subjective tinnitus, which is the most common kind. Any ear noise that can be heard by someone other than the client is called objective tinnitus. In some cases, tinnitus is so severe or disruptive that clients have attempted suicide.

The major nursing responsibility should be to perform a thorough history and assessment about the onset, frequency, constancy, and level of intensity of the tinnitus. Unilateral tinnitus merits a complete neuro-otologic evaluation with the goal of ruling out the potential of a tumor, most likely an acoustic neuroma. The nurse should keep in mind that tinnitus is a symptom of an underlying pathologic process that warrants further referral.

Many approaches have been tried to alleviate this distressing symptom, such as biofeedback, electrostim-

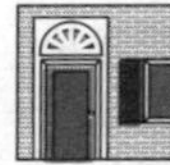

BRIDGE TO HOME HEALTH CARE

Clients with Severe Hearing Loss

Creative problem solving is required to communicate with clients who have severe hearing loss. To refer a client for a hearing test and hearing aid, check the yellow pages. Some companies offer free hearing test and in-home service, 30-day free trial, and repair. For severe hearing loss, written notes may be the only method of communication.

Background noise may make conversation between the nurse and client difficult. Therefore, turn the television or radio off and ask others involved in nonrelated conversations to use another room during your home visit.

Communicating over the phone may also be difficult. When calling a client, allow the phone to ring a long time. It may take four or five rings before the client realizes that the phone is ringing. Ten to 20 rings may be needed to allow time for the client to answer the phone. A TDD (telephone device for the deaf) transmits typed words over the phone line. One TDD is needed to call another one. Check the community section of the phone book for phone numbers that translate calls to a TDD.

Getting the client who is deaf to answer the door presents other problems. Often, clients do not hear doorbells or knocking. If you pound hard on the door, the client will feel the vibrations. The doorbell can also be connected to an electrical device that will cause the light of a room lamp to flicker on and off. Such a device can be purchased at an electronics store.

Remember that communication difficulties experienced by the home health nurse represent the client's generalized communication problems. Work with the client and his or her family and significant others to improve communication and the client's ability to function independently.

ulation, hypnosis, medication, hearing aids, and tinnitus maskers. Tinnitus maskers are quite similar to hearing aids except that they generate noise. The tinnitus masker can cause a phenomenon called residual inhibition. Residual inhibition is the absence of the tinnitus for a time period of 1 minute to a few weeks after treatment. However, every approach for the relief from tinnitus is only moderately successful, at best. Nurses need to educate clients to avoid unproven treatments for tinnitus.

BALANCE DISORDERS

Definition

Disorders of balance and coordination result from problems of the vestibular system and righting reflexes. Very few symptoms are more private than those involving one's sense of balance. Balance problems may be debilitating and also cause embarrassing gait problems, which can jeopardize safety.

Incidence

Over 90 million Americans, 17 years of age or older, have experienced vertigo or a balance problem.

Etiology

In considering the etiology of "vertigo," there are two major categories: disequilibrium, or lightheadedness, and vertigo. Vertigo is further subdivided to determine whether the disease is central or peripheral. Central disorders involve the central nervous system, whereas peripheral disorders are lesions of the eighth cranial nerve or inner ear. Although the cause of vertigo can be either central or peripheral, at least 70 per cent of all cases are due to labyrinthine/inner ear disorders.

VIRAL INFECTIONS

The most common balance disorder is a viral neuronitis characterized by a sudden onset of vertigo without a hearing loss. The first episode is usually the worst one, with subsequent episodes manifesting less and less vertigo. Many clients have experienced this self-limiting disorder, sometimes associated with influenza. In some clients, however, this disorder may extend for years, and the reason for this extension is not yet clear.

Another disorder is viral labyrinthitis, which affects both hearing and balance. These clients have extreme vertigo for longer periods plus varying degrees of hearing loss. Although most clients recover their balance, the hearing loss is usually permanent. In this same category of labyrinthitis are bacterial labyrinthitis and toxic labyrinthitis. Whereas bacterial labyrinthitis is self-explanatory, toxic labyrinthitis is caused by many different agents. The best understood cause is certain antibiotics. Other medicines can also cause this permanent disorder, which, unfortunately, is usually in both inner ears.

BENIGN PAROXYSMAL POSITIONAL VERTIGO

Another disorder causing vertigo without a hearing loss is benign paroxysmal positional vertigo (BPPV). This disorder is characterized by short bursts of vertigo precipitated by quick head movement or sudden changes in position. BPPV may also be a stage of viral neuronitis and occasionally is found with other types of balance disorders; often it is a result of head injury (car accident or fall).

PRESBYASTASIS

A disorder that is recognized more and more today is presbyastasis, or balance disorder of aging. Because of the generalized degenerative changes that occur in aging, balance and stability are also affected. Whereas the labyrinth has been focused on primarily, balance also depends on several other systems, namely, the visual system and the proprioceptive changes in the muscles. Because all three systems are involved in aging, the elderly have difficulty with stability, which causes falls and subsequent trauma.

MENIERE'S DISEASE

One of the best known balance disorders is Meniere's disease. This disorder is characterized by a triad of symptoms: vertigo, hearing loss, and tinnitus. The cause is unknown but is thought to be from an abnormality of either the formation or absorption of endolymph. Recurring episodic incapacitating bouts of vertigo and hearing loss characterize this disorder. Because of the violent nature of Meniere's disease, the diagnosis is usually dreaded. Initially, the associated hearing loss fluctuates, but it worsens in time.

OTHER BALANCE DISORDERS

Other balance disorders are found with associated problems, such as an acoustic neuroma of the eighth cranial nerve or autoimmune disease. Vertigo in these disorders is usually associated with hearing loss but may also be an early symptom.

Tumors rarely invade the balance system. When they do, vertigo is usually a late symptom because of the ability of the balance system to compensate.

Even if one labyrinthe is destroyed by trauma from a basal skull fracture, the balance system usually compensates, and the client will usually recover without vertigo. Acute trauma certainly causes extreme vertigo, which gradually recedes.

Pathophysiology

The ability to maintain balance depends on four systems being intact: the vestibular system (the labyrinth or inner ear); the visual system (the eyes); the proprioceptive system (the somatosensors of joints and muscles); and the cerebellar system (the coordinator). The sensations transmitted from the ears, the eyes, and the somatosensors are integrated in the brain stem and cerebellum and perceived in the cerebral cortex. Balance problems are most likely to occur when one or more systems are impaired or when the sensory information is contradictory.

Risk Factors

There is little that can be done to reduce the risk of balance disorders. Clients should be treated early for symptoms of ear problems. Clients at high risk of falling as a result of vertigo should arise slowly to prevent injury. Finally, situations that lead to vertigo should be avoided. Motion sickness occurs normally if the provocative stimulus is present. Special environmental situations such as deep-sea diving, high-speed flying, and space travel are situations for which humans have not been evolutionarily adapted.

Clinical Manifestations

Vertigo is the most common clinical manifestation in a client with a balance problem. The symptoms of balance disorders vary widely depending on the cause, the location (one or both ears), the client's age at onset, the extent of the loss, and the rapidity with which damage occurs. Clinical manifestations include, but are not limited to, spinning vertigo, sensation of falling, imbalance, staggering, giddiness, lightheadedness, disorientation, visual blurring, veering in one direction while walking, unsteadiness, reeling, faintness, wooziness, shakiness, instability, wobbly, bewildered, confused, dazed, clumsiness, floaty, falling, weak, or a vague feeling of uncertainty.

Vertigo is described in such varied terms that it is almost impossible to define. All descriptions should be accepted as vertigo. Because the balance system can compensate, and certain disorders recur, vertigo is usually not present constantly but is episodic in nature. Vertigo, like pain, is subject to psychological influences. Vertigo is second only to chronic pain as the most common symptom found in America today.

The close anatomic relationship between the balance and hearing systems sometimes causes the sensation of vertigo in conjunction with a hearing loss. However, in most instances, vertigo is present without a hearing loss.

Diagnostic Assessment

For the client with vertigo, the differential diagnosis may be accomplished by a thorough medical assessment, including audiometry, vestibular tests, imaging evaluation, and laboratory studies. The nurse may be involved in any or all of these procedures, according to the setting, and must be able to explain the procedure to the client to promote understanding and to gain trust. Clients may have a positive Romberg finding; a positive platform posturography examination is usually graded 1 to 6, with 6 being complete loss of balance. Nystagmus may also be evoked with electronystagmography.

Medical Management

The treatment of acute vertigo involves several medicines, which are called antivertiginous medicines. These medicines tend to suppress the balance system or the central nervous system. In chronic vertigo, vasodilators are used. Other medicines used for specific disorders include antibiotics, steroids, diuretics, tranquilizers, and vitamins. The nonspecific medical treatment mentioned points to the fact that a curative approach does not yet exist.

Vestibular rehabilitation is now a recognized form of control for vertigo. Whereas certain forms of exercises for balance disorders have been available for decades, only now has this treatment modality been formalized. Because the balance system can compensate for a partial or complete absence, head and total body exercises are performed by the client to hasten compensation. Usually, physical therapists are involved in structuring this treatment. Vestibular rehabilitation uses all three organ systems that provide balance.

Control of Meniere's episodes is usually possible, although a cure is not yet available. Clients are treated with low-sodium diets, diuretics, and balance exercises.

Surgical Management

The delicate inner ear does not lend itself to surgical treatment, except for procedures that destroy the balance system on purpose. Nonetheless, surgeons have gingerly developed surgical techniques involving the inner ear in an attempt to alleviate vertigo and save hearing. The endolymphatic sac procedures include decompression and various forms of shunts to the central nervous system or mastoid cavity. The intent of these procedures is to lessen the fluid pressure within the labyrinth and control the vertigo of Meniere's disease. Other attempts to do the same are performed through the oval or round window. A destructive procedure to remove the membranous labyrinth, either subtotally through the oval window or totally through the mastoid bone, is called labyrinthectomy. Of course, any remaining hearing is sacrificed. Also, vestibular nerve resection can be performed to alleviate vertigo. Vestibular nerve resection can be performed through the labyrinth (sacrificing hearing) or around the labyrinth (saving hearing). The retrolabyrinthine surgical choice is the most common form of surgical control for vertigo today. Alleviation of the client's vertigo is usually immediate. Because of the compensation by all of the other structures related to maintaining balance, a client can function with only one labyrinth.

The necessity of removing tumors of the inner ear and internal auditory canal has also led to various approaches through and around the temporal bone.

Nursing Management

Because vertigo is only a symptom, the diagnosis and treatment of the underlying disease are frustrating to both the client and health care providers. The nurse's role becomes even more important because psychological factors complicate the illness. The nurse's ability to understand and assess the client with vertigo aids in providing care that will contribute toward the client's recovery.

The major nursing responsibilities to the client with a balance problem include insight, evaluation, and education. Unlike vision or hearing, there is no single organ responsible for balance problems. The balance system is composed not only of vestibular (ear) input but also of visual and proprioceptive information. Therefore, the diagnosis, treatment, and rehabilitation of the client with a balance problem can be difficult as well as frustrating. The complexity of the client with a balance problem presents many challenges to the nurse, who requires an empathetic attitude.

ASSESSMENT

Nursing assessment of the client with a balance problem should include the following:

- ► A client interview obtaining a health history and specific information about the onset and characteristics of the balance problem and associated hearing problems.
- ► An interview with a family member to identify the effect of the client's balance problem on others.
- ► Physical examination with specific emphasis on eyes, ears, thyroid, heart, and lungs, including a specific neurologic examination.
- ► Review of laboratory tests.

The importance of the history and interview cannot be overemphasized. An adequate description about vertigo should include information about the onset, exacerbating and alleviating factors, associated symptoms, and predisposing factors in the medical history as previously described. All clients bring some degree of anxiety regarding this illness to the examination. Balance problems can have devastating effects on the client's behavior. The disruption of the client's routine, the severity of the "attacks," and the fear of the unknown can make the client agitated, anxious, or depressed. The nurse must be aware of these feelings and demonstrate self-confidence, patience, courtesy, and gentleness.

A structured questionnaire such as the one shown in Box 34–7 should be completed by the client. These questions can also be used to facilitate the interview. However, the interview should be guided by client cues. A gross assessment of the client's balance can be made by watching the client's gait. Evidence of instability may be noted if the client touches the wall or walks with a wide-based gait.

The same inspection, palpation, and otoscopic examination should be performed for the client with a balance problem as was performed for the client with a hearing loss (see earlier). The client should be assessed for the loss of hearing and tinnitus, symptoms that can accompany a balance problem.

NURSING INTERVENTION

Nursing Diagnosis: Injury, High Risk for R/T tendency to fall and lose balance.

Planning: Expected Outcomes. The client will reduce the risk of injury, as evidenced by moving slowly, remaining immobile when dizzy, and using aids for ambulation if gait and balance are unstable.

Implementation. Responsibilities of the nurse caring for a client with vertigo include the promotion of comfort and safety. Clients who are experiencing vertigo are sometimes reluctant to move because movement aggravates the symptoms. Specific nursing care activities include the following:

- ► Encourage the client to move slowly.
- ► Encourage and facilitate eating by providing the

Box 34–7. Assessment Guide for Clients with Balance Disorders

I. When you are dizzy, do you experience any of the following sensations? Please read the entire list first. Then circle the numbers of those that describe your feelings most accurately.
   1. Lightheadedness
   2. Tendency to lose balance or to fall
   3. Objects spinning or turning around you
   4. Sensation that you are turning
   5. Headache
   6. Nausea or vomiting
   7. Pressure in the head

II. Please fill in the blank spaces.
   1. When did the dizziness first occur? ______
   2. Is your vertigo constant? ______
   3. Does it come in attacks? ______
   4. How often do attacks occur? ______
   5. How long are the attacks? ______
   6. Does vertigo occur only in certain positions? ______
      when upright? ______
      when lying flat? ______
      turning to the right? ______
      turning to the left? ______
   7. Have you ever stumbled or fallen because of vertigo? ______
   8. Do you know of anything that will stop the vertigo or make it better? ______
      make your vertigo worse? ______
      bring on an attack? ______
   9. Did you ever injure your head? ______
   10. Do you take any medications regularly (i.e., tranquilizers; oral contraceptives; barbiturates; a course of antibiotics, such as streptomycin, neomycin)? ______
   11. Do you use tobacco in any form? ______
       alcohol? ______
   12. Have you worked for long in a noisy environment? ______
   13. Do you suffer easily from motion sickness? ______

client with desired foods and fluids (vertigo may cause nausea and vomiting).

- Assist the client with hygiene as needed while encouraging independence.
- Keep side rails up when the client is in bed.
- Assist the client as needed in ambulation.
- Encourage the client to verbalize specific problems created by the vertigo.
- Teach the client:

Nature of the disorder

Diagnostic tests and planned medical or surgical therapy for the vertigo

Ways to protect self from injury when dizzy, such as remaining immobile or using an aid for walking

Information about prescribed medications

Symptoms requiring medical attention

Approximately 5 per cent of all clients with vertigo undergo surgical intervention at present. However, an increasing number of clients will undergo surgical procedures in the future because of new surgical developments and advanced technology. The care of the client experiencing surgery of the inner ear was described earlier.

EVALUATION

The degree of goal attainment should be assessed every day. If vertigo is increasing, the client may need to remain at bed rest to reduce the risk of falls.

Post-hospital Care

Most clients with vertigo are managed as outpatients. Therefore, the client needs adequate information for self-care, such as ways to protect self from inadvertent injury, medications, and follow-up evaluations.

Summary

Disorders of the ear include disorders due to infection in the outer, middle, or inner ear. The risk of infection of the meninges is present, and infection requires antibiotic treatment. Hearing loss is a common disorder that often leads to social isolation. Nurses should be skilled in both psychosocial and physical aspects of care. It is essential that the client has a functional hearing aid. Balance disorders increase the client's risk of injury from falls. Nursing care of clients with vertigo is directed at education.

Bibliography

1. Adams, R., & Victor, M. (1985). *Principles of neurology* (3rd ed.). New York: McGraw-Hill.
2. Alberti, P. M., & Ruben, R. J. (1988). *Otologic medicine and surgery* (vol. I). New York: Churchill Livingstone.
3. Alberti, P. M., & Ruben, R. J. (1988). *Otologic medicine and surgery* (vol. II). New York: Churchill Livingstone.
4. Bates, B. (1991). *A guide to physical examination* (4th ed.). Philadelphia: J. B. Lippincott.
5. Brinkman, K. (1991). Why can't your patient hear you? *RN, 54*(1), 46–48.
6. Bulechek, G. M., & McCloskey, J. C. (1985). *Nursing interventions, treatments for nursing diagnosis*. Philadelphia: W. B. Saunders.
7. Campbell, S. L. (1984). Some sound advice for managing a hearing impaired patient. *Nursing 84, 14*(12), 46. *Core curriculum for neurosurgical nursing* (1984). Chicago, IL: The American Association of Neuroscience Nurses.
8. Cleveland, P., & Morris, J. (1990). Meniere's disease. *RN, 53*(8), 28–32.
9. Counter, R. T. (1980). *Color atlas of temporal bone surgical anatomy*. England: Year Book Publishers.
10. DeWeese, D. D., & Saunders, W. H. (1988). *Textbook of otolaryngology* (7th ed.). St. Louis: C. V. Mosby.

11. Goldstein, J. C., et al. (1989). *Geriatric otolaryngology*. Philadelphia: B. C. Decker.
12. Hahn, A. B., et al. (1982). *Pharmacology in nursing* (15th ed.). St. Louis: C. V. Mosby.
13. Hanawalt, A., & Troutman, K. (1984). If your client has a hearing aid. *American Journal of Nursing, 84,* 900.
14. Hawke, M., et al. (1984). *Clinical otoscopy*. New York: Churchill Livingstone.
15. Hughes, G. B. (1985). *Textbook of clinical otology*. New York: Thieme-Stratton.
16. Jahn, A. F., & Santos-Sacchi, J. (1988). *Physiology of the ear*. New York: Raven Press.
17. Lee, K. F. (1983). *Comprehensive surgical atlas in otolaryngology and head and neck surgery*. New York: Grune & Stratton.
18. Magilvy, J. K. (1985). Quality of life of hearing-impaired older women. *Nursing Research, 34*(3), 140–144.
19. Programmed instruction: Patient assessment: examination of the ear (1975). *American Journal of Nursing, 75*(3), 457–476.
20. Reiner, A. (1988). *Manual of patient care standards*. Rockville, MD: Aspen Publishers.
21. *Report of the task force on the National Strategic Research Plan of the National Institute on Deafness and Other Communication Disorders* (1989). Bethesda, MD: Institute of Health.
22. Riley, M. A. K. (1987). *Nursing care of the client with ear, nose and throat disorders*. New York: Springer.
23. Rudy, E. B. (1984). *Advanced neurological and neurosurgical nursing*. St. Louis: C. V. Mosby.
24. Schuring, L. T. (1991). Assessment of the ear. In Phipps, et al. (Eds.), *Medical-surgical nursing concepts and clinical practice* (4th ed., pp. 1947–1958). St. Louis: Mosby Year Book.
25. Schuring, L. T. (1991). Management of clients with problems of the ear. In Phipps, et al. (Eds.), *Medical-surgical nursing concepts and clinical practice* (4th ed., pp. 1959–1982). St. Louis: Mosby Year Book.
26. Serra, A. M., et al. (1986). *Ear, nose and throat nursing*. Oxford, England: Blackwell Scientific Publications.
27. Tortorelli, B. (1981). Acoustic neuroma: an overview of the disorder and nursing care of these clients. *Journal of Neurosurgical Nursing, August,* 170–171.
28. Voke, J. (1984). Aspects of hearing, physiology of the ear. *Nursing Times, August 15, 80*(33), 28–30.
29. Voke, J. (1984). Aspects of hearing, functions of the cochlea. *Nursing Times, August 22, 80*(34), 60–62.
30. Wilson, W. R., & Nadol, J. R. (1983). *Quick reference to ear, nose and throat disorders*. Philadelphia: J. B. Lippincott.

Unit 8

Respiratory Disorders

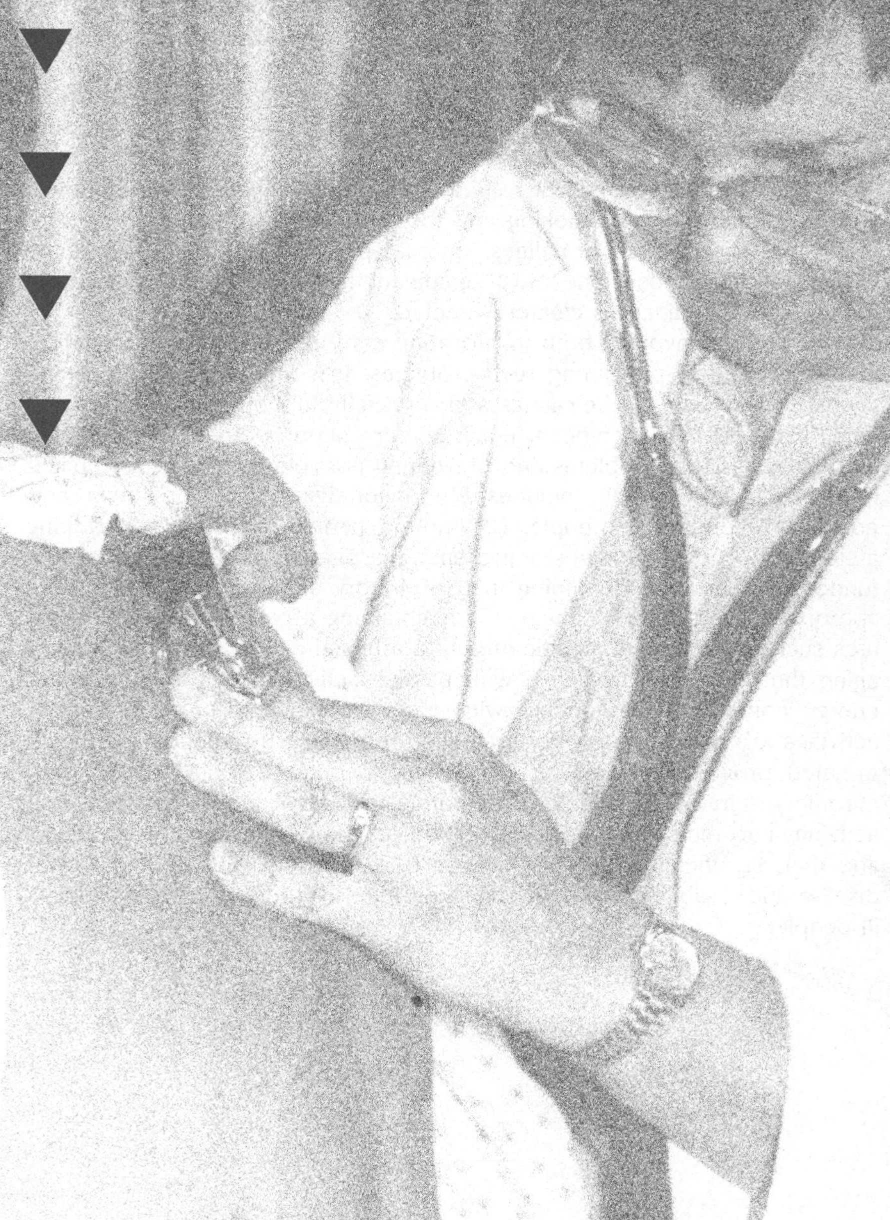

Breathing is a basic human need that we tend to ignore unless we have some difficulty with it. Only then are we aware of the process. Breathing is a physiologic function that is almost synonymous with being alive. We experience difficulty in breathing as a threat to life itself. People with respiratory disorders are often very anxious, fearing they may die and perhaps uncomfortably. Whether death is a real possibility often has nothing to do with the fear.

Respiratory problems are widespread. They may be acute (short term) or chronic (long term). Acute disorders range from minor inconveniences such as colds or flu to more life-threatening problems such as asthma, some types of pneumonia, and chest trauma. Chronic respiratory problems are widespread, causing significant disability. People who experience them often have to make radical lifestyle changes, often retiring from work earlier than they wish. Such disabling conditions include chronic obstructive pulmonary disease (COPD), now called chronic airflow limitation, and certain restrictive lung diseases.

There are many causes of respiratory problems: allergies, occupational factors, genetic factors, smoking and tobacco use, infection, neuromuscular disorders, chest abnormalities, trauma, pleural conditions, pulmonary vascular abnormalities. The most significant factor in chronic respiratory illness and lung cancer is cigarette smoking.

Nurses are involved both in providing care for clients with respiratory conditions and in preventing such problems. It is important to encourage clients to take care of their lungs and especially to stop smoking. In acute health care settings, significant nursing intervention is directed at relieving existing respiratory problems and preventing possible respiratory complications. Such intervention includes (1) encouraging deep breathing and coughing in immobile people; (2) turning people at risk of developing atelectasis or pneumonia; (3) preventing aspiration in paralyzed or obtunded people; (4) determining that respiratory therapy is given in a safe, appropriate, and timely manner; (5) maintaining a patent airway by measures such as suctioning, positioning, and artificial airway care; (6) encouraging the alternation of active with passive activities and other forms of energy conservation in people with chronic problems; (7) coordinating activities of daily living with breathing retraining techniques and goal-oriented progressive exercise; (8) helping people (especially those with chronic respiratory problems) incorporate relaxation and stress reduction activities into their daily lives; (9) helping people with respiratory problems and their significant others learn ways to lessen the likelihood of further disease and disability; and (10) providing intensive nursing care for acutely ill people.

Chapter 35

Structure and Function of the Respiratory System

Gas exchange is the primary function of the respiratory system. The respiratory system takes oxygen from the atmosphere, transports oxygen to the lungs, exchanges oxygen for carbon dioxide in the alveoli, and returns carbon dioxide to the air. This chapter reviews the anatomy and physiology of the respiratory system so the student can see the relationship between alterations in the structure or function and disease (Fig. 35-1).

Because gas exchange is the primary function of the lungs, structure of the airways and lung tissue involved with gas exchange are described first, followed by the actual process of gas exchange. Next, the gross anatomy of the lung, thorax, and pleural space that influences movement of the air is discussed. Many of the common lung diseases have an effect on these mechanical factors of air movement. Control of ventilation is next. The final section is defense mechanisms of the lungs. The delicate structure of the lungs requires special protective mechanisms.

STRUCTURE OF THE AIRWAYS

Upper Airway

The upper airway consists of the nasal cavities, pharynx, and larynx. Major functions of the upper airway are (1) air conduction to the lower airway for gas exchange; (2) protection of the lower airway from foreign matter; and (3) warming, filtration, and humidification of inspired air.

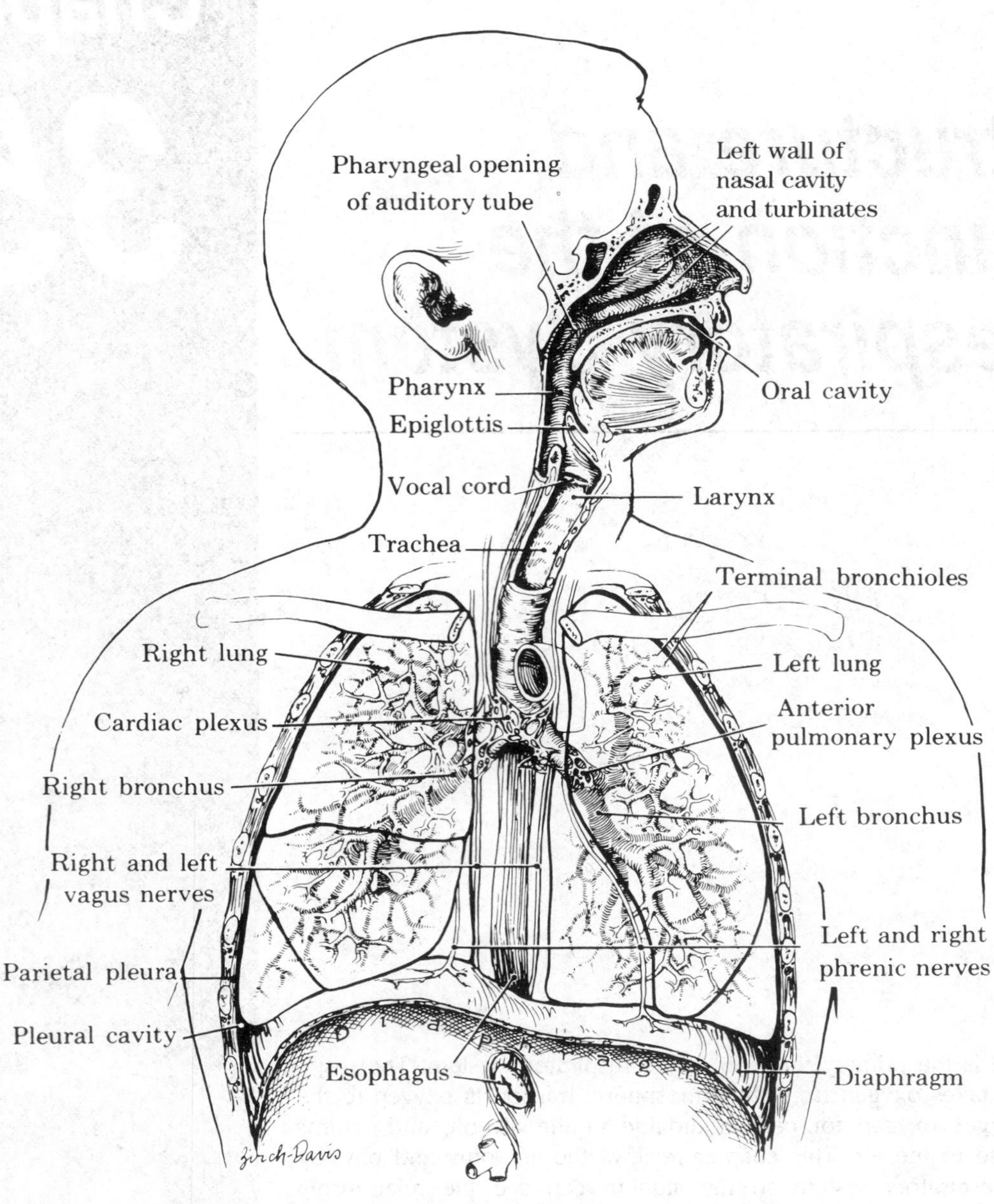

▲ *Figure 35–1*

Structure of the respiratory system. (From *Dorland's Illustrated Medical Dictionary* [27th ed.] [1988]. Philadelphia: W. B. Saunders.)

NOSE

The nose is formed from both bone and cartilage. A very small portion of the nose is bone; the nasal bone only forms the bridge of the nose. The remainder of the nose is composed of cartilage and connective tissue. The nasal cartilages form the shape of the nose (Fig. 35–2).

The openings of the nose on the face are called nostrils or nares. Each nostril leads to a cavity, called a vestibule. The vestibule is lined anteriorly with skin and hair (called vibrissae). The vibrissae filter foreign objects and prevent them from being inhaled. The posterior vestibule is lined with mucous membrane. This membrane is composed of columnar epithelial cells, which secrete mucus. Along the sides of the vestibule are turbinates. The turbinates are mucous membrane–covered projections. They contain a very rich blood supply (from the internal and external carotid arteries), and they warm and humidify inspired air. Regardless of the temperature of air inspired, by the time the air reaches the lung (in about 0.25 second) the air has been warmed to 36° to 37° C (96.8° to 98.6° F) and humidified to 70 to 80 per cent. The mucus also helps trap foreign particles. The cilia of the membrane assist in moving the particles down into the pharynx. The posterior part of the nasal cavity opens into the internal nares and the nasopharynx. The two nasal vestibules are divided by the septum.

The nose also provides for the sense of smell and is

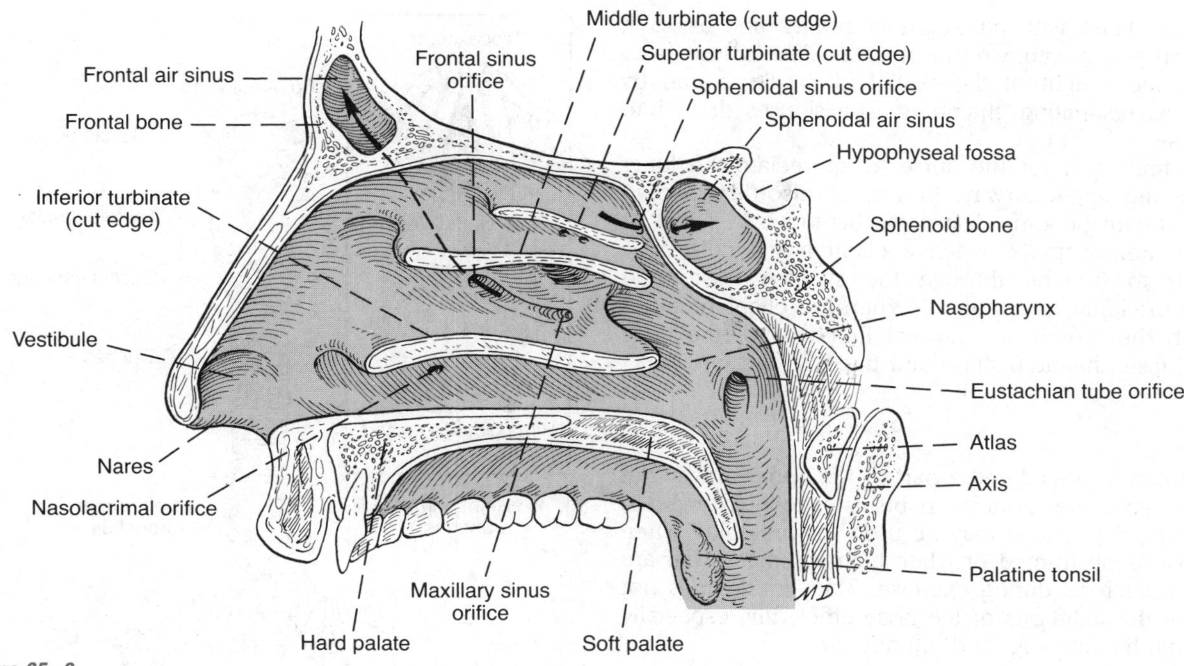

▲ *Figure 35–2*

Structure of the nose and sinuses.

an adjunct to taste. The part of the mucous membrane covering the cribriform plate is modified for olfaction.

The nasolacrimal glands, which produce tears, are connected to the nose via the nasolacrimal duct. Excess tears are excreted through this duct.

The nose provides a sneeze reflex, which is similar to the cough reflex. Irritation of the nasal passages causes receptors in the trigeminal nerve (cranial nerve V) to stimulate the respiratory center in the medulla. The medulla stimulates a blast of air through the nose that carries foreign matter out the nose and mouth.

SINUSES

Paranasal sinuses are open areas within the skull. They are named for the bones in which they lie—frontal, ethmoid, sphenoid, and maxillary (Fig. 35-3). These

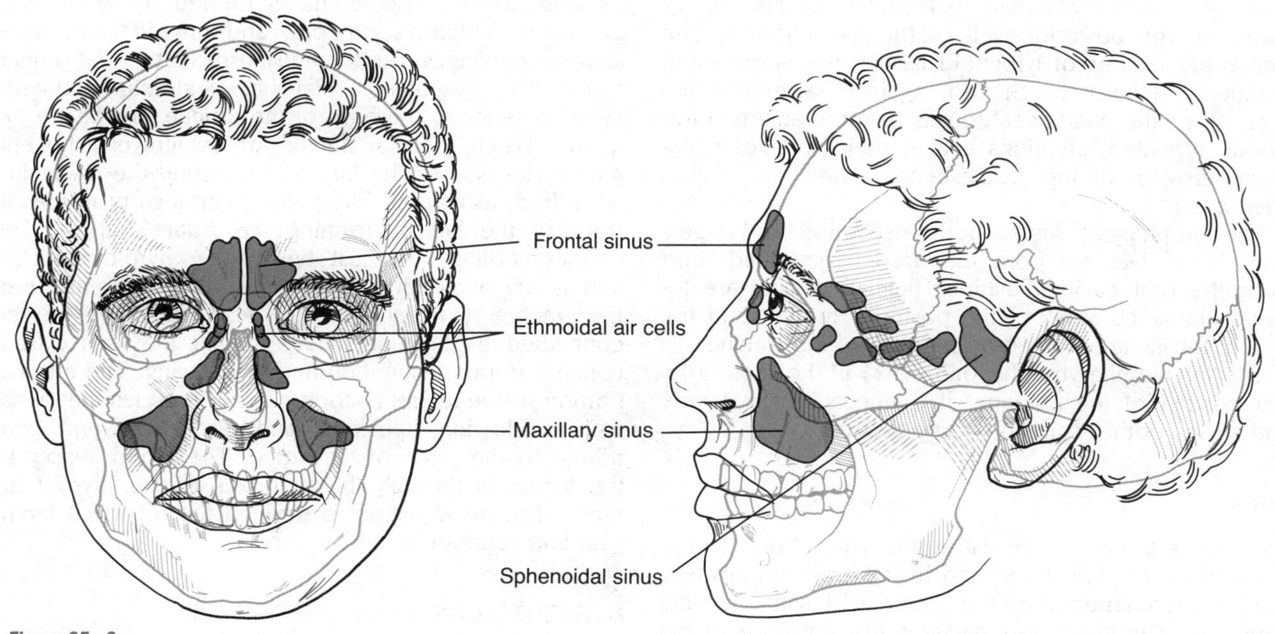

▲ *Figure 35–3*

Location of the sinuses.

areas are lined with mucous membranes and assist in warming and humidifying inspired air. The sinuses also lighten the weight of the skull and modify sound by acting as resonating chambers. The sinuses drain into the nose.

It is important for the nurse to appreciate the function of the upper airway. In various disorders and in the treatment of some disorders, this function is lost or altered. For example, when a client has a cold, it is difficult to breathe through the swollen nose, and mouth breathing is common. When the client breathes through the mouth, the normal functions of the nose (smell, taste, humidification and filtering) are lost.

MOUTH

The mouth is considered a part of the upper airway but only because the mouth can be used to deliver air to the lungs. The mouth may be used for breathing when the nose is obstructed or when high volumes of air are needed, such as during exercise. The mouth does not perform the functions of the nose efficiently, especially warming, humidifying, and filtering air.

PHARYNX

The pharynx is a funnel-shaped tube that extends from the nose to the larynx. It is commonly divided into three sections: (1) the nasopharynx, located above the margin of the soft palate; (2) the oropharynx, that part of the pharynx visible when the tongue is depressed with a tongue depressor; and (3) the laryngopharynx, located below the base of the tongue. The nasopharynx is the upper section and receives air from the nasal cavity. The nasopharynx is lined with ciliated columnar epithelium. From the ear, the eustachian tubes open into the nasopharynx. The pharyngeal tonsils are located on the posterior wall of the nasopharynx. The tonsils are masses of lymphoid tissue; they serve as an additional defense mechanism against bacterial infection. When the pharyngeal tonsils become enlarged following repeated infections and at their point of maximum growth during adolescence, they are called adenoids.

The oropharynx serves both respiration and digestion. It receives air from the nasopharynx and food from the oral cavity. Palatine (faucial) tonsils are located along the sides of the posterior mouth, and the lingual tonsils are located at the base of the tongue.

The laryngopharynx (hypopharynx) is the most inferior portion of the pharynx. It connects to the larynx and serves both respiration and digestion.

LARYNX

The larynx is commonly called the voice box. It connects the upper (pharynx) and lower (trachea) airways. It is located anterior to the fourth and sixth cervical vertebrae. The upper esophagus is just posterior to the larynx. The larynx consists of the endolarynx and a surrounding triangular-shaped bone and cartilage. The endolarynx is formed by two pairs of folds of tissue, which form the false vocal cords and the true vocal cords. The slit between the vocal cords forms the glottis (Fig. 35-4). The larynx is formed by three large cartilages (epiglottis, thyroid, and cricoid) and three smaller cartilages (arytenoid, corniculate, and cuneiform). The epiglottis, a leaf-shaped structure immediately posterior to the base of the tongue, lies above the larynx. When food or liquids are swallowed, the epiglottis closes over the larynx, protecting the lower airways from aspiration. The thyroid cartilage protrudes in front of the larynx, forming the Adam's apple. The cricoid cartilage lies just below the thyroid cartilage and is the anatomic site for an artificial opening into the trachea (tracheostomy). These cartilages are all connected by ligaments that prevent the larynx from collapse during inspiration and swallowing. The internal portion of the larynx is composed of muscles that assist with swallowing, speaking, and respiration, and contribute to the pitch of the voice. The blood supply to the larynx is through the branches of the thyroid arteries. The nerve supply is through the recurrent laryngeal and superior laryngeal nerves.

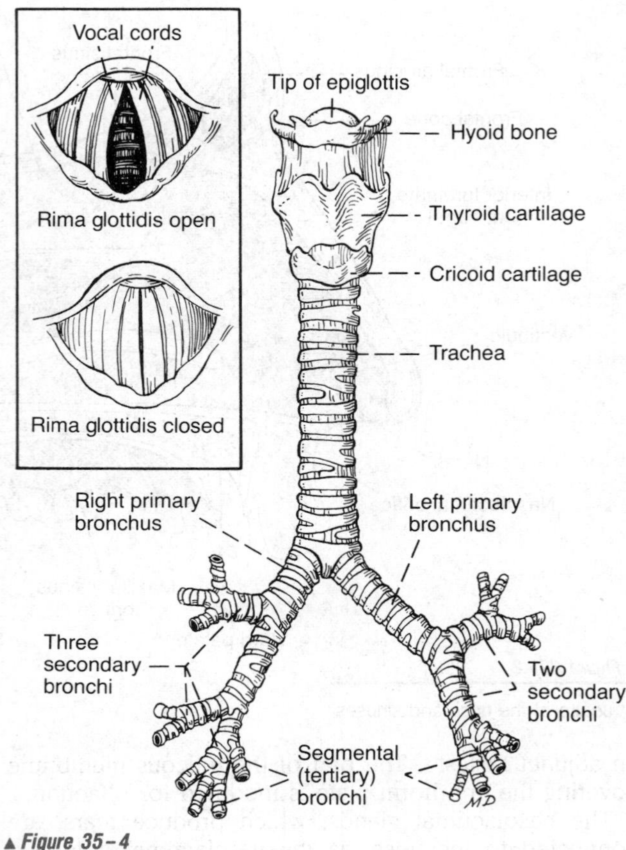

▲ ***Figure 35-4***

Upper airway structure.

EFFECTS OF AGING ON THE UPPER AIRWAY

Most of the changes that occur with aging are seen in the lower airway. The movement of the cilia of the upper airway slows and becomes less effective. This change predisposes the aged client to increased respiratory infections.

Lower Airway

The lower airway (tracheobronchial tree) is composed of the (1) trachea, (2) right and left mainstem bronchi, (3) segmental bronchi, (4) subsegmental bronchi, and (5) terminal bronchioles (see Fig. 35-1.) Smooth muscle, wound in overlapping clockwise and counterclockwise helical bands, is found in all of these structures.

TRACHEA

The trachea or windpipe passes from the larynx to the two main bronchi (also called primary bronchi) that enter the lungs. The trachea is a flexible, muscular, 4- to 5-inch long air passage with C-shaped cartilaginous rings. The point at which the trachea divides into the right and left mainstem bronchi is called the carina.

MAIN BRONCHI

The right mainstem bronchus is shorter and wider, and extends more vertically downward than the left. Thus, foreign bodies are more likely to lodge in the right mainstem bronchus than in the left mainstem bronchus.

SEGMENTAL AND SUBSEGMENTAL BRONCHI

The segmental and subsegmental bronchi are subdivisions of the main bronchi and are spread in an inverted, treelike formation through each lung. Cartilage surrounds the airway in the bronchi. This structure contrasts with the bronchioles, the final pathway to the alveoli, which contain no cartilage and thus can collapse and trap air.

TERMINAL BRONCHIOLES

The terminal bronchioles are the last airways of the conducting system, and they branch into the respiratory zone, where gas exchange takes place (Fig. 35-5). The respiratory zone consists of the respiratory bronchioles, the alveolar ducts, and alveolar sacs.

ALVEOLI

The lung parenchyma is the working area of the lung tissue, consisting of millions of alveolar units. Alveoli, small air sacs at the end of the respiratory bronchioles, permit exchange of the oxygen and carbon dioxide. The entire alveolar unit (respiratory zone) is made up of respiratory bronchioles, alveolar ducts, and alveolar sacs.

It is estimated that there are 24 million alveoli at birth. By the time a person is 8 years old, the number of alveoli has increased to the adult number of 300 million. The total working alveolar surface area is approximately 750 to 860 square feet. The large number of alveoli and the large surface area are necessary to meet both resting and exercise oxygen requirements. Each alveolar unit is supplied with 9 to 11 prepulmonary and pulmonary capillaries. The blood supply for these capillaries comes from the right ventricle of the heart. The major function of the alveolar unit is the exchange of oxygen and carbon dioxide between pulmonary capillaries and alveoli.

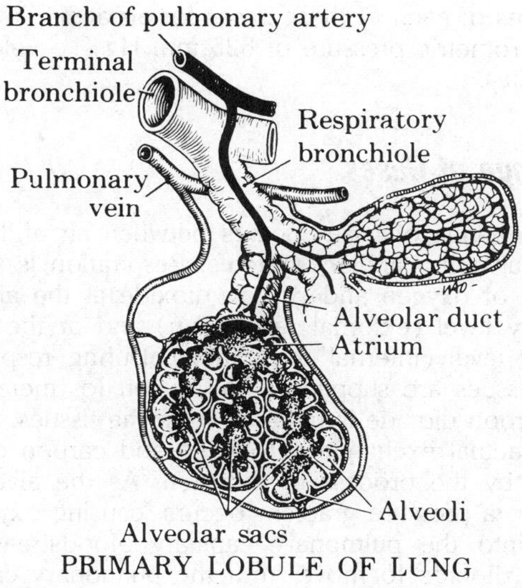

▲ Figure 35-5

Gas exchange occurs in the respiratory zone, which consists of the respiratory bronchioles, alveolar ducts, and alveolar sacs.

GAS EXCHANGE

Concentration of Atmospheric Gases

The make-up of the air passing through the conducting system is based on the barometric pressure. In the earth's atmosphere, air contains 20.84 per cent oxygen, 78.62 per cent nitrogen, 0.04 per cent carbon dioxide, and 0.50 per cent water vapor. Each gas exerts a pressure, called its partial pressure, as if it were the only gas present. The sum of the partial pressures is the barometric pressure. Table 35-1 shows the partial

TABLE 35-1. Partial Pressure (PP) of Atmospheric Gases

Components of Air		PP at Sea Level 760 mm Hg	PP One Mile Up 625 mm Hg
Nitrogen	78.62%	597.0	491.37
Oxygen	20.84%	159.0	130.26
Carbon dioxide	0.04%	0.3	0.25
Water vapor	0.50%	3.7	3.12

Partial pressure (PP) may be calculated for any atmospheric pressure by multiplying the concentration of a gas by the atmospheric or barometric pressure.

pressures of each of these gases for air at sea level and at a barometric pressure of 625 mm Hg (i.e., elevation of 1 mile).

Exchange of Gases

The exchange of gases occurs between air and blood in the alveolar-capillary systems. Respiration is the exchange of oxygen and carbon dioxide at the alveolar-capillary level (external respiration) and at the tissue-cellular level (internal respiration). During respiration, body tissues are supplied with oxygen for metabolism and carbon dioxide is released from the tissues.

The actual exchange of oxygen and carbon dioxide occurs by the process of diffusion. As the alveoli fill with air, a pressure gradient occurs, causing oxygen to move into the pulmonary capillary bloodstream and carbon dioxide to move from the pulmonary capillary bed into the alveolus, where it is exhaled. Oxygen concentrations in the alveoli rise higher than the oxygen concentration in the pulmonary capillaries. Conversely, carbon dioxide concentration in the alveoli is lower than that in blood. These differences in concentration result in differences in partial pressures. Because gases move from an area of greater partial pressure to areas of less partial pressure, gas exchange occurs. See Figure 35-6 for partial pressures of gases during normal respiration.

Ventilation and Perfusion Relationships

Two per cent of the cardiac output enters the bronchial circulation. This blood supplies the metabolic needs of the lungs. The remaining volume of cardiac output enters the pulmonary circulation, an extensive vascular network delivering unoxygenated or desaturated blood from the right side of the heart to the pulmonary capillaries. Each alveolar unit is covered with a network of pre-pulmonary and pulmonary capillaries. Oxygen and carbon dioxide are exchanged through this intricate system.

The relationship between ventilation (air flow) and perfusion (blood flow) determines the efficiency of gas exchange. When there is ventilation without perfusion, a unit of deadspace exists. An example is a pulmonary embolus preventing blood flow through a pulmonary capillary. When there is no ventilation of an alveolar unit but perfusion continues, a shunt exists. This occurs

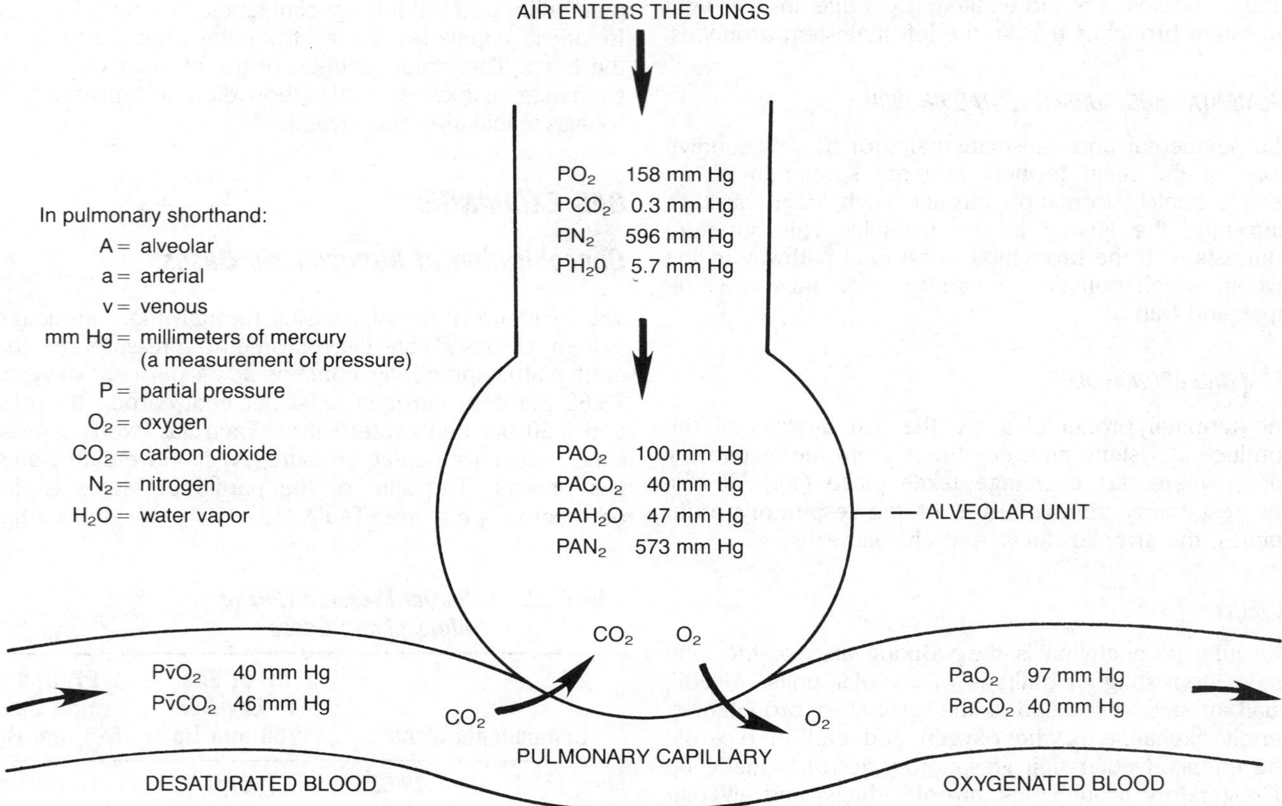

▲ *Figure 35-6*

Partial pressures of gases during normal respiration.

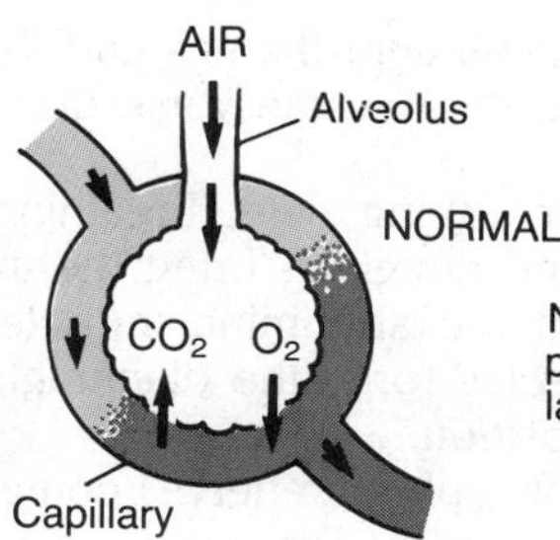
AIR
Alveolus
NORMAL
CO_2 O_2
Capillary
Normal functioning alveolus and pulmonary capillary flow. Ventilation and perfusion match.

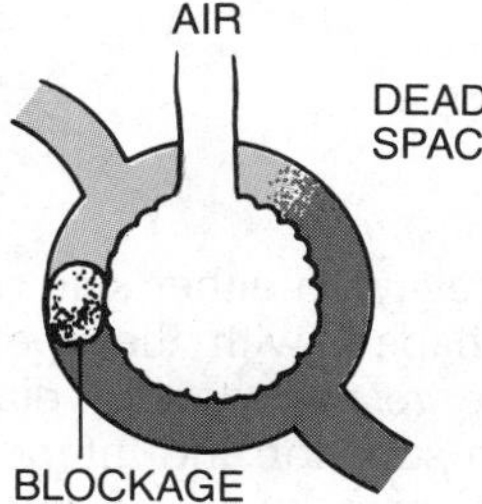
AIR
DEAD SPACE
BLOCKAGE
When there is ventilation without perfusion a deadspace unit exists, e.g., pulmonary embolus preventing blood flow through pulmonary capillary.

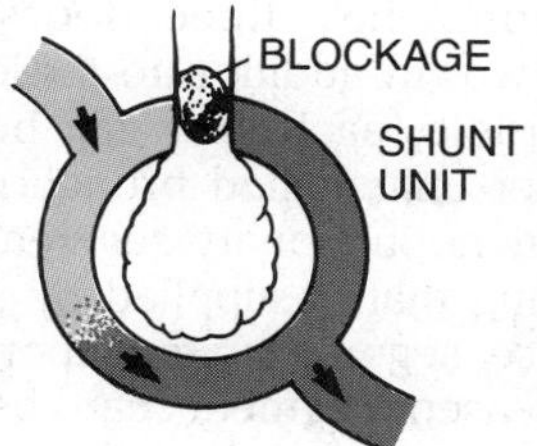
BLOCKAGE
SHUNT UNIT
When there is no ventilation to an alveolar unit but perfusion continues, a shunt unit exists and unoxygenated blood continues to circulate, e.g., atelectasis, pneumonia. The alveoli collapse.

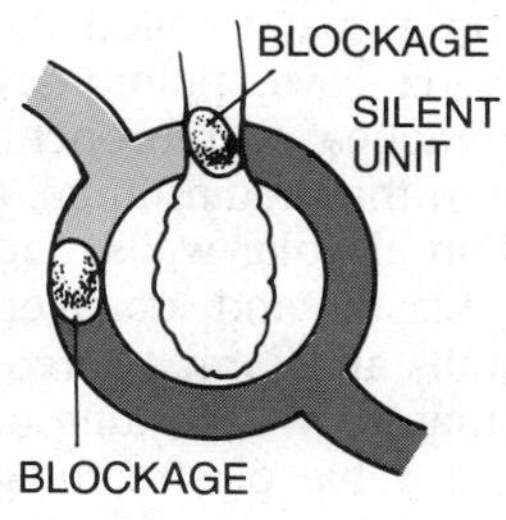
BLOCKAGE
SILENT UNIT
BLOCKAGE
When there is neither ventilation or perfusion a silent unit develops, e.g., pulmonary embolus combined with ARDS (adult respiratory distress syndrome). The alveoli collapse.

▲ *Figure 35-7*

Relationships between ventilation (air flow) and perfusion (blood flow).

with collapse of alveoli (atelectasis). Low ventilation/perfusion ratios (V/Q) and high V/Q ratios both result in lower oxygen levels in the blood. See Figure 35-7 for the relationship between ventilation and perfusion.

Gravity also affects ventilation and perfusion. Blood flows to more dependent lung segments. Air flows more easily to the upper lung segments because air is less dense than blood.

Oxygen Transport

After oxygen diffuses into the pulmonary capillaries, it is transported throughout the body by the circulatory system. The oxygen is dissolved in the plasma (3 per cent) or bound with hemoglobin (97 per cent) in ferrous iron. The combination of ferrous iron and oxygen forms oxyhemoglobin, which releases oxygen to tissues having a low partial pressure of oxygen. Tissues take up oxygen at varying rates. The most metabolically active tissues receive it first. Methemoglobin, carbon monoxide, and other chemicals impair the uptake of oxygen by tissues.

The oxyhemoglobin dissociation curve represents the relationship between the partial pressure of oxygen in the arterial blood (PaO_2) and the saturation of hemoglobin. This relationship is represented in Figure 35-8 as an S-shaped curve. Changes in the PaO_2 at the flat, top portion of the curve result in small changes in oxygen saturation. The opposite is true as the slope of the curve steepens. At the steepest portion of the curve, with the PaO_2 below 60 mm Hg, small changes in the PaO_2 result in large drops in oxygen saturation.

The oxyhemoglobin curve is affected by a number of factors, including temperature, pH, PCO_2, and the concentration of 2,3-diphosphoglycerate in the red blood cells. A shift of the curve to the right indicates a release of oxygen at the tissue level. The increased unloading of oxygen at a given PO_2 in the tissue capillary is a useful adaptive mechanism for the body. This occurs when the hemoglobin has less affinity for the oxygen. With a shift to the left, the hemoglobin has a high affinity for oxygen, inhibiting its release at the tissue level.

Carbon Dioxide Transport

Carbon dioxide is the waste product of tissue metabolism. It is carried by the blood three ways: (1) in

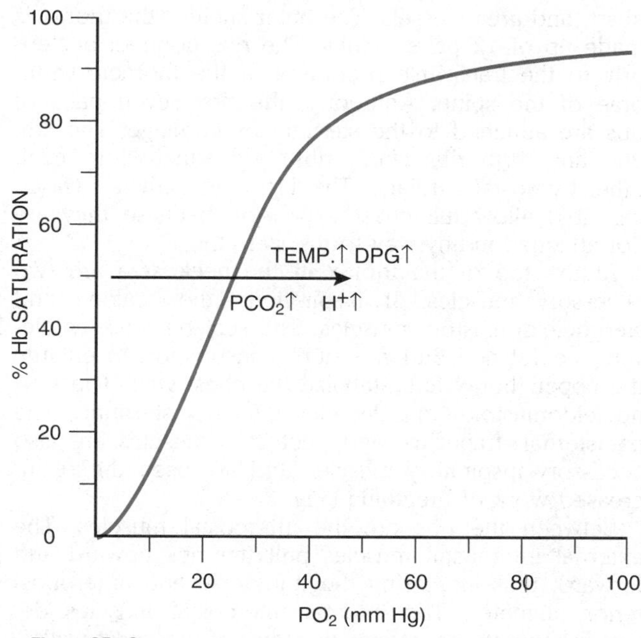
100
80
60
40
20
0
% Hb SATURATION
TEMP.↑ DPG↑
PCO_2↑ H^+↑
20
40
60
80
100
PO_2 (mm Hg)

▲ *Figure 35-8*

Rightward shift of the O_2 dissociation curve by increase of H^+, P_{CO_2}, temperature, and 2,3-diphosphoglycerate (DPG). (Modified from West, J. B: [1989]. Respiratory physiology: The essentials [4th ed.]. Baltimore: Williams & Wilkins.)

plasma; (2) coupled with hemoglobin; or (3) combined with water as carbonic acid. Most carbon dioxide is carried by red blood cells as carbonic acid. It rapidly breaks down into hydrogen ions and bicarbonate ions. As venous blood enters the lungs for gas exchange, these chemicals form carbon dioxide, which is exhaled from the lungs.

Acid-Base Disturbance

Thus, the lungs, through gas exchange, have a key role in regulating the acid-base balance of the body. Pulmonary disorders that change the carbon dioxide level in the blood cause either respiratory acidemia or respiratory alkalemia. Hypercapnia (retention of excessive amounts of carbon dioxide) causes respiratory acidemia, and hypocapnia (low amounts of carbon dioxide in the blood) results in respiratory alkalemia.

The effectiveness of ventilation is best measured by the partial pressure of carbon dioxide in the arterial blood ($PaCO_2$). Because the respiratory system is normally set to maintain a $PaCO_2$ between 35 and 45 mm Hg at sea level, a $PaCO_2$ above this range represents hypoventilation. Anesthetic agents, sedatives, and narcotics all tend to increase the resting $PaCO_2$. (For a complete discussion of acid-base balance, see Chap. 14).

MECHANICS OF BREATHING

Thorax

The bony thorax provides protection for the lungs, heart, and great vessels. The outer shell of the thorax is made up of 12 pairs of ribs. The ribs connect posteriorly to the transverse processes of the thoracic vertebrae of the spine. Anteriorly, the first seven pairs of ribs are attached to the sternum by cartilage. The 8th, 9th, and 10th ribs (false ribs) are attached to each other by costal cartilage. The 11th and 12th ribs (floating ribs) allow full chest expansion because they are not attached in any way to the sternum.

At the top of the thorax in the neck area are two accessory muscles of inspiration—the scalene and sternocleidomastoid muscles. The scalene muscles elevate the 1st and 2nd ribs during inspiration to enlarge the upper thorax and stabilize the chest wall. The sternocleidomastoid muscle elevates the sternum. The parasternal, trapezius, and pectoralis muscles are also accessory inspiratory muscles and are used during increased work of breathing (Fig. 35–9.)

Between the ribs are the intercostal muscles. The external intercostal muscles pull the ribs upward and forward, thus increasing the transverse and anteroposterior diameter. The internal intercostal muscles decrease the anteroposterior diameter of the chest wall.

The diaphragm serves as the lower boundary of the thorax. The diaphragm is dome shaped in the relaxed position, with central muscular attachments to the xiphoid process of the sternum and the lower ribs. On inspiration, the dome of the diaphragm flattens and the rib cage lifts. This action increases the transverse diameter of the thorax.

Expiration is usually passive during quiet breathing. However, forced expiration and coughing bring the internal intercostal muscles and the abdominal muscles into play. The abdominal muscles force the diaphragm upward to its dome-shaped position.

The diaphragm's nerve supply (phrenic nerve) comes through the spinal cord at the level of the third, fourth, and fifth cervical vertebrae. Thus, spinal injuries at this level impair ventilation.

Lungs

The lungs lie within the thoracic cavity on either side of the heart. The lungs are cone shaped, with the apex above the first rib and the base resting on the diaphragm. Each lung is divided into superior and inferior lobes by an oblique fissure. The right lung is further divided by a horizontal fissure, which bounds a middle lobe. The right lung, therefore, has three lobes, whereas the left lobe has only two. In addition to these five lobes that are externally visible, each lung can be subdivided into about 10 smaller units called bronchopulmonary segments. Each bronchopulmonary segment represents the portion of the lung that is supplied by a specific tertiary bronchus. These segments are important surgically, because a diseased segment can be resected without having to remove the entire lobe or lung.

The two lungs are separated by a space called the mediastinum. The heart, aorta, vena cava, pulmonary vessels, esophagus, part of the trachea and bronchi, and the thymus gland are located in the mediastinum.

The lungs contain gas, blood, thin alveolar walls, and support structures of the lung. Elastic and collagen fibers contribute to the alveolar walls and form a three-dimensional basket-like structure that allows the lung to inflate in all directions. They are capable of stretching if a pulling force is exerted on them from outside the body or if they are inflated from within. The elastic recoil helps return the lungs to their resting volume.

Pleural Space

The pleural space is a potential space between two serous membranes—the visceral pleura and the parietal pleura. The visceral pleura covers the lung and the fissures between the lobes of the lung. The parietal pleura covers the inside of each hemithorax, the mediastinum, and the top of the diaphragm. The parietal pleura joins the visceral pleura at the hilus (a notch in the medial surface of the lung, where the mainstem bronchi, pulmonary blood vessels, and nerves enter the lung).

Normally, there is no space between the pleurae. A thin film (only a few milliliters) of serous fluid acts as a lubricant in the potential space. The fluid also causes the moist pleural membranes to adhere, creating a

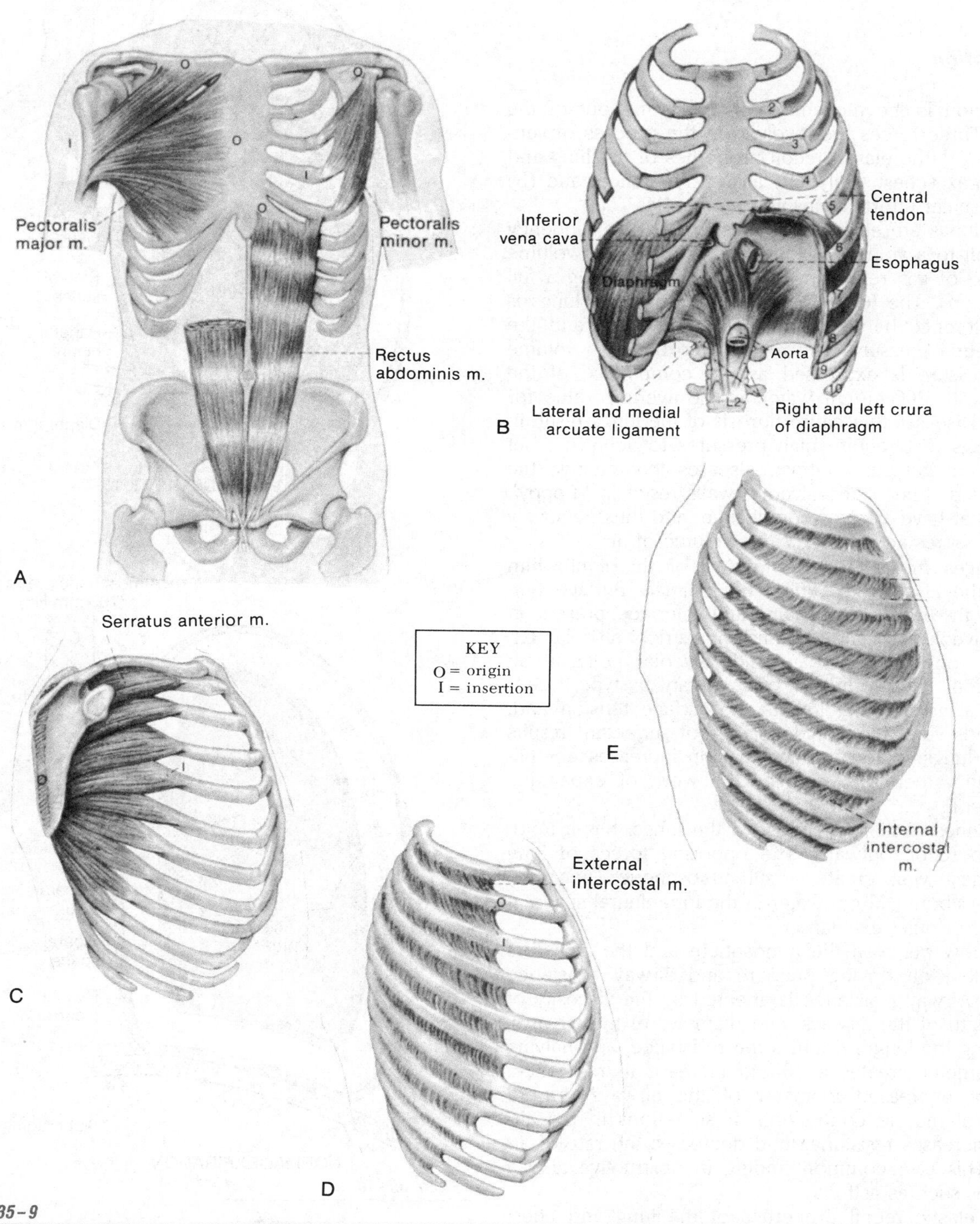

▲ *Figure 35–9*

Muscles of respiration. (From Jacob, S., & Francone, C. A. [1989]. *Elements of Anatomy and Physiology* [2nd ed.]. Philadelphia: W. B. Saunders.)

pulling force that helps hold the lungs in an expanded position. If air or increased amounts of serous fluid, blood or pus accumulate in the space, the lungs are compressed and respiratory difficulties follow.

Ventilation

Ventilation is the movement of air in and out of the lungs. Three forces are involved in the process of ventilation: (1) the elastic recoil properties of the lung and the thorax (chest wall), (2) airway resistance, and (3) the muscular efforts of inspiratory muscles.

The lungs are elastic structures that have a tendency to recoil to a volume slightly less than residual volume (volume of gas remaining in the lungs following a full exhalation). The force required to distend the lungs is the difference between the alveolar pressure and the intrapleural pressure. The relationship between volume and pressure is expressed as the compliance of the lungs, with 200 ml/cm water as the average value for adults. Diseases that cause fibrosis of the lungs result in stiff lungs that require high pressures to achieve a set volume of gas. In contrast, diseases that change the elastic structure of the alveolar walls result in "floppy" lungs that have a larger compliance, and thus, relatively low pressures achieve the same volume of air.

Changes in the surface tension of the liquid film lining the alveoli also affect compliance. Surface tension is the result of the air-liquid interface present in each alveoli. The surface tension restricts alveolar expansion on inspiration and aids alveolar collapse on expiration. The production of surfactant by type II cells in the alveolar lining lowers the surface tension and, thus, aids ventilation. A deficiency of surfactant results in stiff lungs. A low surface tension increases compliance and, therefore, reduces the work of expanding the alveoli.

The chest wall, in contrast to the lungs, has a tendency to recoil outward. The opposing forces of lung and chest wall create a sub-atmospheric (negative) force of about −5 cm water in the intrapleural space at the end of quiet exhalation.

Air flow between the atmosphere and the alveoli is dependent on driving pressure and airway resistance (Raw). Airway resistance is affected by the viscosity of air, length of the airways, and diameter of the airways. Doubling the length doubles the resistance, and halving the diameter creates a 16-fold increase in resistance. Thus, a decreased diameter of the airways due to bronchial muscle contraction or secretions in the airways increases resistance and decreases the rate of air flow. This is a common finding in obstructive airway diseases such as asthma.

The elastic recoil properties of the lung and chest wall, coupled with the muscular effort required to overcome the recoil of the lungs and airflow resistance, make air movement possible. The pressure within the lungs (alveolar pressure) and between the pleura (intrapleural or intrathoracic pressure) must be less than atmospheric pressure for inspiration to occur. As the diaphragm and the external intercostal muscles work to enlarge the size of the thorax, the intrapleural and alveolar pressures decrease below atmospheric pressure. The expanding thorax creates a more negative intrapleural pressure, which expands the lungs. The alveolar pressure then becomes lower than the atmo-

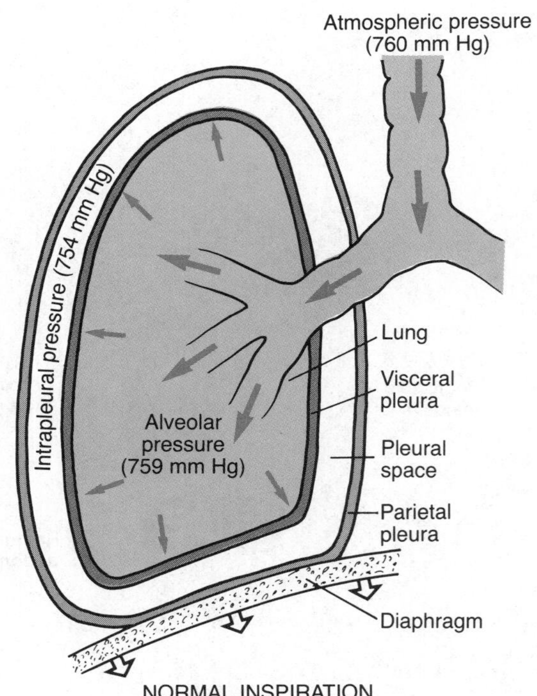

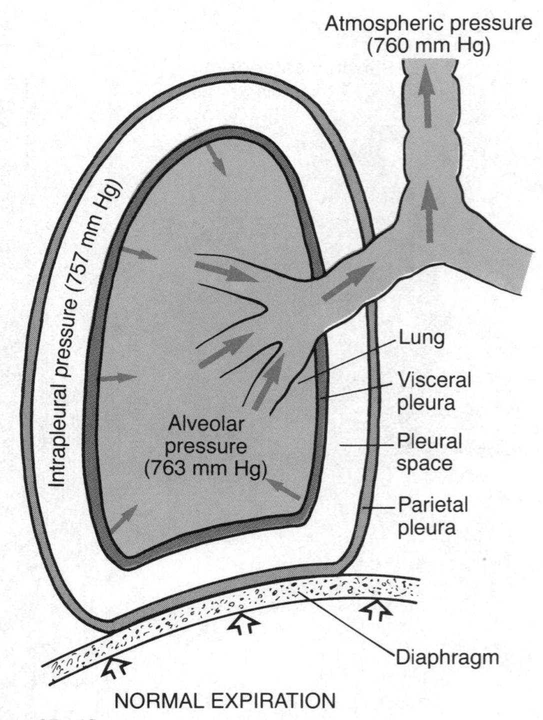

▲ *Figure 35-10*

Normal inspiration and expiration.

spheric pressure, and air flows into the lungs. During exhalation, the inspiratory muscles relax. The elastic recoil of the lung tissue, along with a rise (less negative) in intrapleural pressure, causes air to move out of the lungs. The stopping of airflow is the point at which the recoil pressure of the lungs balances the muscular and elastic forces of the chest. See Figure 35-10 for an illustration of normal inspiration and expiration.

CONTROL OF VENTILATION

The pacemaker of the lungs is located in the pons and medulla of the central nervous system. Output from the respiratory neurons, located in the medulla, descends via the ventral and lateral columns of the spinal cord to phrenic motor neurons of the diaphragm and intercostal motor neurons of the intercostal muscles. The result is rhythmic respiratory movements. Output from the respiratory neurons located in the pons (pneumotaxic center) affects the ventilatory phases of expiration and inspiration.

Ventilation may be modified by neural reflexes. The neural reflexes are stimulated by mechanical and chemical stimuli.

Mechanical Stimuli. One example of a neural reflex stimulated by mechanical stimuli is the cough reflex. Inhaled irritants and mucus (mechanical stimuli) can excite rapidly adapting pulmonary stretch receptors concentrated in the region of the carina and the large bronchi. The stimulation of the receptors results in high-velocity expiratory gas flow (cough).

Chemical Stimuli. Chemical stimuli are the partial pressures of oxygen (PO_2) and carbon dioxide (PCO_2) in the blood. Receptors responsive to changes in oxygen, carbon dioxide, and pH are located in two areas. One area is the carotid body receptors, located close to the carotid sinus, and the aortic bodies, located near the aortic arch. The second area for the chemical receptors is on the brain side of the blood-brain barrier. Low PaO_2 levels cause high receptor output from the carotid bodies to the medulla and increase the rate and depth of ventilation. The arterial pH is another major stimulus. A decrease in pH with acidemia increases the output from the carotid body to the central nervous system and stimulates ventilation. The $PaCO_2$ also stimulates peripheral receptors. Chemoreceptors on the brain side of the blood-brain barrier are sensitive to the hydrogen ion content of brain extracellular fluid as well as to CO_2 levels.

THE LUNGS

Defense Mechanisms of the Lung

The respiratory gas-exchanging membrane has a surface area almost the size of a tennis court. The size of the membrane of the lungs and the daily exposure of the lungs to atmospheric pollutants requires efficient protective mechanisms. The elaborate defense mechanisms of the lungs fall into three categories: (1) clearance mechanisms, (2) immunologic responses in the lung, and (3) pulmonary reaction to injury. An intact respiratory epithelium and mucociliary system are necessary for the efficient functioning of the lung defense mechanisms.

RESPIRATORY EPITHELIUM

The predominant cell of the upper respiratory tract (trachea and bronchi) is a one-cell layer thick squamous ciliated cell. The cilia are microscopic, hairlike projections that protect the airways with a rapid, coordinated, unidirectional sweeping motion toward the mouth. The movement of the cilia propels a mucus blanket toward the mouth. This blanket is produced by goblet cells located on the mucosal surface (Fig. 35-11). The mucociliary system propels debris (pollutants and infectious agents) to the mouth within 30 minutes for the large bronchi, 2.5 hours for most of the bronchial tree, and 5.6 hours for the peripheral airways. At the mouth, the debris is removed from the airways by swallowing or coughing. Sputum is mucus removed by coughing.

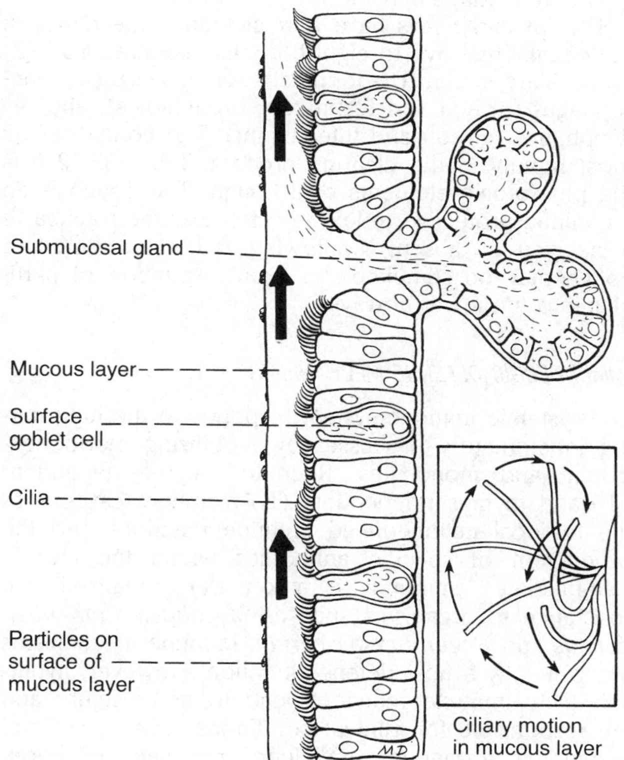

▲ Figure 35-11

The mucociliary blanket is an important respiratory defense mechanism. Mucus is secreted by surface goblet cells. About 100 ml of mucus is normally secreted each day by the submucosal glands. Mucus covers the epithelial lining of the tracheobronchial tree in two layers—the watery sol layer close to the mucosal surface and the thicker gel layer. The cilia (hairlike projections) beat in an upward direction toward the upper airway. Particulate matter is trapped on the mucous layer and moved upward by the cilia. Debris-laden mucus is then either swallowed or expectorated as sputum.

The alveolar lining is made up of flat membranous pneumocytes (type I cells). Rounded granular cells (type II) are found in the alveolar corners. These type II cells are resistant to injury and cover most of the alveolar surface after exposure to infectious agents. Alveolar macrophages, derived from blood monocytes that migrate into the lungs, are also found over the surface of the alveoli. Alveolar macrophages are active phagocytes that remove dead cells and protein. Macrophages are also metabolically active cells that synthesize and secrete substances that regulate the immune system. They leave the lung by either the mucociliary system or the lymphatic system.

CLEARANCE DEFENSE MECHANISMS

The upper airways filter particles. Inhaling air through the nose is more effective in air cleaning and conditioning than inhaling air through the mouth. The nose has a larger surface-volume ratio and a much more tortuous pathway for airflow than the mouth. Thus, particle deposition on the mucociliary system is more efficient when the client breathes by nose rather than by mouth. The larger particles (greater than 10 μ) are generally trapped, but the smaller particles (less than 1 μ) may readily enter the lower airways.

The lower airways have four clearance mechanisms: (1) cough (first five to eight bronchial generations), (2) mucociliary system (to terminal bronchioles), (3) macrophages (alveoli and respiratory bronchioles), and (4) lymphatics (alveoli and interstitium). The cough occurs most rapidly in the clearing process. Table 35-2 lists the physiologic elements of a cough. The cough is an automatic protective reflex used to clear the trachea. If a delayed or absent swallowing reflex is present, a cough may be stimulated to avoid aspiration of particles into the lower airways.

TABLE 35-2. Physiologic Elements of a Cough

Deep inspiration	Inhaled volume of air must be sufficient to (1) increase lung volume, (2) increase diameter of bronchi and bronchioles, and (3) move mucus up and out of airways
Inspiratory pause	A pause (inspiratory pause) allows a buildup and distribution of air and pressure distal to mucus
Closed glottis	Requires intact muscles and nerves supplying larynx. A closed glottis allows the development of high intrapleural pressures, resulting in a high air flow velocity to propel mucus out of airway
Abdominal muscles	These muscles increase intra-abdominal pressure, which forces the diaphragm upward to increase intrapleural pressure against the closed glottis
Open glottis	After intrapleural pressures increase, the glottis opens suddenly and allows a high velocity of air to leave the lungs; flow rates may be as high as 300 L/min
Mucus is expelled	Occurs because of high velocity of air leaving the airway

IMMUNOLOGIC DEFENSE MECHANISMS

The systemic immune system responds to the lung during inflammatory processes by mobilizing blood neutrophil and monocytes. Recruited thymus-dependent (T) and thymus-independent (B) lymphocytes contribute to local cell-mediated immune reactions and the production of specific antibodies within the alveoli. Cell-mediated immunity is a key determinant in the resistance to organisms such as *Mycobacterium tuberculosis* and *Pneumocystis carinii.* Immune mechanisms are generally a host defense function. However, hypersensitivity immune reactions lead to tissue injury and are responsible for clinical conditions such as asthma, granuloma formation, and lung transplant rejection. (See Chap. 24 for a detailed discussion of type I, type II, type III, and type IV hypersensitivity reactions.)

PULMONARY REACTION TO INJURY

Injury to the lung barrier, inflammation, and repair are the three components of responses of the lung to injury. Any injury to the lung affects the barrier between the atmosphere and the bloodstream. This barrier is within the alveolar septum and is made up of epithelial (type I and type II pneumocytes) and vascular endothelial cells. Injury, due to airborne and blood-borne agents, may increase vascular permeability and cause pulmonary edema. Inflammatory cells such as neutrophils arrive soon after acute injury. Then, the proportion of lymphocytes, monocytes, and macrophages increase.

The basic lung repair processes include lymphatic drainage of excess fluid and phagocytic removal of protein and debris. This action generally restores lung function and structure. More severe injury requires endothelial and epithelial cell regeneration, and proliferation of interstitial cells (fibroblasts). The lung's ability to re-create alveolar septa determines the degree that normal lung function and structure are restored.

Effects of Aging on the Lungs

Changes in lung structure occur with age. One change is the actual shape of the lung. The lungs become rounder as a result of an increase in the anteroposterior diameter, circumference, area, and height of the lung. There is an increase in the proportion of the lung formed by alveolar duct air and a relative decrease in alveolar air. Loss of alveolar wall tissue and elastic tissue fibers in the alveolar walls occurs. The result is a deterioration of lung function.

The frequency of emphysema and the prevalence of a chronic cough and sputum production is higher in the elderly population. This suggests that environmental or occupational pollutants as well as the normal aging process may be a component in the decline of lung function.

Summary

The primary function of the lungs is gas exchange. The physical structure of the airways allows air to be warmed, filtered, and humidified as it enters the body. In the alveolar sacs, oxygen is exchanged for carbon dioxide. The mechanics of breathing are coordinated by the ribs, diaphragm, pleural space, elastic recoil of the lungs, and nervous system. In addition to respiration, the respiratory system provides one form of acid-base balance. When these processes of structure and function are altered, various disorders can occur.

Bibliography

1. Guyton, A. (1991). *Textbook of medical physiology* (8th ed.). Philadelphia: W.B. Saunders.
2. Kersten, L. D. (1989). *Comprehensive respiratory nursing*. Philadelphia: W.B. Saunders Company.
3. McCance, K., & Huerter, S. (1989). *Pathophysiology*. St. Louis: C.V. Mosby.
4. Shapiro, B., et al. (1991). *Clinical applications of respiratory care* (4th ed.). Chicago: Year Book Medical Publishers.
5. Solomon, E., et al. (1990). *Human anatomy and physiology* (2nd ed.). Philadelphia: W.B. Saunders College Publishing.
6. Spence, A., & Mason, E. (1983). *Human Anatomy and Physiology* (2nd ed.). Menlo Park, CA: Benjamin Cummings Publishing Company.
7. West, J. (1989). *Respiratory physiology: The essentials* (4th ed.). Baltimore: Williams & Wilkins.
8. Wilson, S., & Thompson, J. (1990). *Respiratory disorders*. St. Louis: C. V. Mosby.

Chapter 36

▼ Assessment of Respiratory Disorders

▼ GENERAL RESPIRATORY ASSESSMENT

Nurses caring for clients experiencing respiratory disorders perform and interpret a variety of assessment procedures. This chapter discusses the respiratory physical assessment and diagnostic procedures. The data obtained during the respiratory assessment are used to plan client care.

HISTORY

A respiratory history gathers information about a client's present condition and previous respiratory problems. The nurse interviews the client or family and focuses on the clinical manifestations of the chief complaint, events leading up to the current condition, past medical history, family history, and psychosocial history.

The detail and time taken for a respiratory history depend on the client's condition (e.g., acute, chronic, or emergency). State questions simply, using short, easy-to-understand sentences. Whenever necessary, reword questions to clarify statements the client seems not to understand. Ask questions in the context of the client's daily activities (e.g., "Are you able to carry the groceries in from the car?" or "Are you able to make your bed, vacuum, bathe, or dress yourself without stopping to rest and catch your breath?").

The history begins with obtaining biographic data from the client. Included are the client's name, age, sex, and living situation. The living situation, whether it is alone or with children or disabled significant others, will be important in planning for discharge.

Chief Complaint

The chief complaint is determined to establish priorities for intervention and to assess the client's level of understanding of the current condition. Common respiratory complaints include cough, sputum production, dyspnea, hemoptysis, wheezing, and chest pain. The nurse focuses on the symptoms and prioritizes questions to elicit a symptom analysis. The following questions are included in the initial respiratory history.

What are the client's current respiratory symptoms?
When did each symptom start?
What is the perceived cause of the symptom (after exercise, a respiratory infection)?
When do the symptoms affect the client?
What helps to relieve the symptoms?

In emergency or acute situations, these questions are all that may be asked until the client is stabilized and comfortable. Whenever possible, seek further details from significant others.

Take an extensive respiratory history as the client's condition allows. Detailed questioning provides valuable clues to the (1) client's symptoms, (2) degree of existing respiratory dysfunction, (3) client's (and family's) understanding of the condition and its management, and (4) client's (and family's) support system and ability to cope with the symptoms and management of the condition on an ongoing basis.

SYMPTOM ANALYSIS

The following symptom analysis is performed to evaluate respiratory symptoms.

In what setting does the symptom occur most often? The setting refers to the time and place or the particular situation—physical setting and psychological environment—present when the client experiences the complaint. An example is a morning cough after the client has had a cigarette, or the employee who complains of respiratory distress at work.

Onset refers to the gradual or sudden appearance of the symptom. The nurse asks the client whether there is a specific time of day during which the complaint occurs most frequently, for example, the morning cough or the shortness of breath associated with bedtime.

The client is asked to identify a time period during which the complaint has occurred—days, weeks, or months. Identify any previous occurrence, frequency, and recurrence rate.

Ask the client to describe the complaint in his or her own words and any unique properties of the complaint. The use of direct quotes is helpful in documenting the quality of the complaint.

The nurse asks the client to describe the amount, size, number, and extent of the chief complaint. Especially with sputum production, the client is asked to estimate how much sputum is produced a day—cup, tablespoon, or teaspoon. Avoid using terms such as a "little" or a "lot" because they have different meanings for different clients.

If possible, ask the client to identify the exact location of the complaint. Location is important when the client is complaining of chest pain.

Can the client identify factors that precipitate the symptom or make it worse, for example, dust, cats, dogs, dry winds, or stress? Does the symptom occur during exercise, after eating, while coughing? Did onset awaken the client from sleep? Do symptoms seem associated with any time of year, place, or specific events?

Ask the client if any other signs and symptoms occur in conjunction with the chief complaint, for example, chills, fever, night sweats, anorexia, weight loss, excessive fatigue, anxiety, or hoarseness.

The nurse asks the client what relieves the signs and symptoms. Identify ways the client obtains symptom relief (e.g., medication [prescription and over-the-counter], sitting upright, lying down, resting, coughing, physical therapy, increased humidification, oxygen).

DYSPNEA

Dyspnea is one of the most common symptoms experienced by clients with pulmonary and cardiac disorders. Dyspnea is difficulty breathing. It is a subjective symptom and a reflection of the client's assessment of his or her degree of work of breathing for a given task and/or effort. Clients may define dyspnea as shortness of breath, suffocation, tightness, being winded, or breathless. According to Gift and Nield,[4] the most supported objective sign of dyspnea is accessory muscle use. The nurse asks the client to identify when dyspnea is felt—with exercise/activity, all the time, even at rest? What activities does the client avoid because they cause dyspnea? Tools used to evaluate the level of dyspnea are the Borg scale (Table 36-1) and the visual analog scale (Fig. 36-1).[9] Ask about other events that may occur with dyspnea (e.g., pain, sweating, dizziness, cough, wheezing, chest tightness). Nonrespiratory conditions may also cause dyspnea (e.g., heart disease, anemia, obesity, excessive exercise, fever, metabolic acidosis).

TABLE 36-1. The Modified Borg Category-Ratio Scale for Estimation of Respiratory Effort Sensation

0	Nothing at all
0.5	Very, very slight
1	Very slight
2	Slight
3	Moderate
4	Somewhat severe
5	Severe
6	
7	Very severe
8	
9	Very, very severe
10	Maximal

From Burden, J., et al. (1982). The perception of breathlessness. *American Review of Respiratory Diseases, 126*, 825-828.

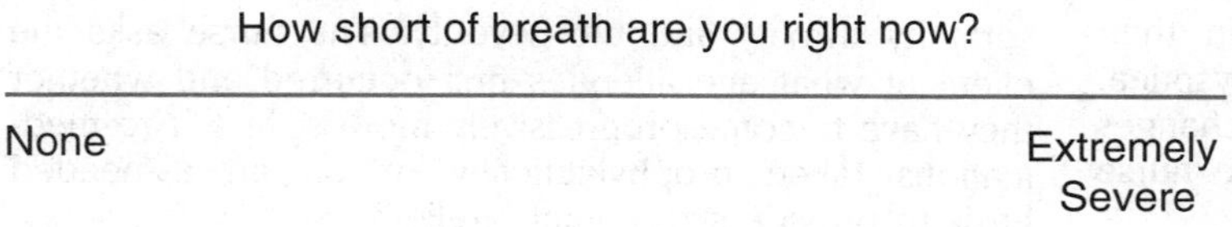

How short of breath are you right now?

None — Extremely Severe

▲ *Figure 36-1*

Visual analog scale of dyspnea. (From Hayes, M., & Patterson, D. [1921]. Experimental development of the graphic rating method. *Psychological Bulletin, 18,* 98–99.)

COUGH

The nurse asks the client when the cough started. How long has the cough been present? Is it painful? The nurse also asks whether the client is having any sputum production and, if so, how much and how many times a day. Has the client tried any products that may have alleviated the cough? Further questioning helps determine whether the cough is associated with bronchitis, asthma, cigarette smoking, or some other stimulus.

SPUTUM PRODUCTION

Sputum is the substance expelled by coughing or clearing the throat. The tracheobronchial tree normally produces about 3 ounces of mucus a day as part of the normal cleansing mechanism. However, sputum production with coughing is *not normal.* The nurse questions the client about the color (clear, yellow, green, rust, bloody), odor, quality (watery, stringy, frothy, thick), and quantity (teaspoon, tablespoon, or cup). Changes in color, odor, quality, or quantity are important to document in the client's medical record. Is sputum produced only after lying in a certain position? The nurse also considers whether there is a possibility that the sputum could actually be secretions from the oral or nasopharyngeal area or sinuses rather than from the tracheobronchial tree? For example, draining sinuses may produce a productive cough.

HEMOPTYSIS

Hemoptysis is blood expectorated from the mouth in the form of gross blood, frankly bloody sputum, or blood-tinged sputum. The nurse attempts to identify the source of the blood—lungs, nosebleed, stomach. Blood from the lungs is usually bright red because blood in the lungs stimulates an immediate cough reflex. However, if the blood remains in the lungs for any period of time, it may turn dark red or brown. Most hemoptysis is associated with frothy bright red blood. The nurse asks the client if the hemoptysis was produced as a result of forceful coughing. Also, an estimate of the amount of blood expectorated is obtained. Pulmonary causes of hemoptysis include chronic bronchitis, bronchiectasis, pulmonary tuberculosis, cystic fibrosis, upper airway necrotizing granulomas, pulmonary embolism, pneumonia, lung cancer, and lung abscesses. Cardiovascular abnormalities, anticoagulants, and immunosuppressive drugs that cause parenchymal bleeding may also cause hemoptysis.

WHEEZING

Wheezing sounds are produced when air passes through partially obstructed or narrowed airways on expiration. Clients with advanced disorders may also have inspiratory wheezing. Wheezing may be audible or heard only via a stethoscope. The client may not complain of wheezing but may complain of chest tightness or chest discomfort instead. The client is asked to identify when the wheezing occurs and if the wheezing relieves itself or if medication is required for relief. Wheezing is not necessarily asthma. Other causes include bronchospasm, mucosal edema, airway secretions, collapsed airways due to loss of elasticity, and foreign objects or tumors partially obstructing airflow.

STRIDOR

Stridor sounds are produced when air passes through partially obstructed or narrowed upper airways on inspiration. Inquire about changes in voice character, hoarseness, difficulty swallowing, sleep-related disorders such as insomnia, degree of snoring (has sleep partner moved to another room?), hypersomnolence in the morning, early morning headaches, weight gain, fluid retention, apnea, and restlessness. Aspiration of a foreign body into the upper airway may lead to stridor.

CHEST PAIN

Chest pain may be associated with pulmonary and cardiac problems, and differentiation between the two is important. Coughing and pleuritic infections can cause chest pain. Retrosternal pain (behind the sternum) is usually burning, constant, and aching in nature. Pleuritic chest pain is commonly a sharp, stabbing pain that increases with movement or deep breathing. Pain can also originate in the bony and cartilaginous parts of the thorax. The location of the chest pain is important to obtain from the client. The nurse must differentiate pleuritic pain from cardiac pain or angina. Cardiac chest pain usually presents itself as an aching, heavy, squeezing sensation with pressure or tightness in the substernal area. Further evaluation of this presentation of chest pain is necessary. (See Chap. 41, Table 41-1, for comparison of selected causes of chest pain.) Ask whether there are other symptoms, problems, or situations related to the chest pain (e.g., occurs only with deep breathing or with certain body movements).

Past Medical History

The past medical history examines the health history of the client and family members for data related to the upper and lower respiratory systems (upper respiratory history and physical examination are discussed later). These systems are common sources of health problems, both acute and chronic. The nurse assesses clients with chronic conditions for changes in their chronic respiratory symptoms (e.g., cough, dyspnea, sputum production, or wheezes) because these changes provide clues to the new problem's cause. The nurse includes questions about the following areas.

CHILDHOOD AND INFECTIOUS DISEASES

In addition to obtaining data regarding common childhood diseases and immunizations, ask the client about past occurrence of tuberculosis, bronchitis, influenza, asthma, pneumonia, and frequency of lower respiratory infections after upper respiratory infection. Determine the existence of congenital problems such as cystic fibrosis or premature birth history that are associated with respiratory complications such as obstructive or restrictive pulmonary disease.

IMMUNIZATIONS

Inquire about immunization against pneumonia (Pneumovax) and influenza. Ask the client for the dates of these immunizations. Pneumovax provides lifelong immunity against pneumococcal pneumonia, whereas "flu shots" must be received annually in the fall.

MAJOR ILLNESSES AND HOSPITALIZATION

The client is asked about previous hospitalizations or treatment for respiratory problems. Determine dates of illnesses or hospitalization, the specific respiratory problem, medical treatment (including surgery, use of a ventilator, and inhalation or oxygen therapy), and the present status of the problem. Ask whether a chest radiograph was taken or other types of pulmonary diagnostic tests were performed. These test results can provide baseline data for the evaluation of the current problem. The nurse also inquires about previous injuries to the mouth, nose, throat, or chest (such as blunt trauma, fractured ribs, or collapsed lung [pneumothorax]).

MEDICATIONS

Detailed information is obtained regarding both prescribed and over-the-counter medications because many affect the respiratory system. The client may have taken antibiotics for respiratory infections, bronchodilators, or steroids.

ALLERGIES

The nurse questions the client about a history of allergies in an attempt to identify a possible allergic basis for the condition. Ask about precipitating factors such as foods, medications, pollens, smoke, fumes, dust, and animal dander. Sources of molds that may cause allergic symptoms include the water reservoir of a furnace humidifier, air conditioners, and plant soil. The client is asked to describe the allergic symptoms experienced (e.g., chest tightness, wheezing, rhinitis, watery eyes, scratchy throat) and the severity. The nurse asks the client at what age allergies first occurred and whether they have become progressively more severe. Are medications taken prophylactically or on an as-needed basis to provide symptomatic relief?

Family History

The nurse questions the client about the family history of respiratory diseases. Blood relatives (genetically transmitted diseases) and family members (infectious conditions) experiencing asthma, cystic fibrosis, emphysema or chronic obstructive pulmonary disease (COPD), lung cancer, respiratory infections, tuberculosis, or allergies are identified. List the age and cause of death of each deceased family member including mother, father, brothers, sisters, children, grandparents, aunts, and uncles. Ask whether household members smoke; tobacco products may precipitate or aggravate respiratory symptoms.

Psychosocial History and Lifestyle

Respiratory status is affected by numerous factors that may lead to acute problems or affect the client's coping with chronic problems such as COPD. Areas to assess include the following.

HABITS

The client is asked to report any history of smoking cigarettes, cigars, or pipes. The nurse calculates the pack years, which helps quantify the smoking history. Use this formula: years of smoking × packs smoked per day = pack years. Also ask the client about the use of smokeless tobacco (such as snuff, chewing tobacco) and smoking nontobacco substances (such as marijuana and clove cigarettes). Ask about alcohol use. Ciliary action is slowed by alcohol, which reduces mucus clearance from the lungs. Profound alcohol ingestion depresses the cough reflex so that risk of aspiration is increased. Clients who use and abuse recreational drugs are at risk for drug overdose and respiratory failure. If the client shares needles, the risk of human immunodeficiency virus infection is increased, along with the development of acquired immunodeficiency syndrome and opportunistic infections such as *Pneumocystis carinii.*

OCCUPATION

Any possible environmental agents that may contribute to the client's condition are identified. Ask specifically about the work environment and hobbies; focus on exposure to dust, asbestos, beryllium, silica, or other toxins or pollutants. Farmers are exposed to airborne particles that may be inhaled, such as grain dust, fertilizers, and animal dander. Hobbies may involve chemicals, heat, dusts, grinding, soldering, or welding.

GEOGRAPHIC LOCATION

Ask questions related to recent travel to areas where respiratory diseases are prevalent, such as Asia, where tuberculosis is common; the Ohio River valley (histoplasmosis); or the San Joaquin valley (valley fever). Living in cities with polluted air has also been related to asthma.

ENVIRONMENT

Ask about the client's living conditions, such as number of people sharing the household. Crowded living conditions increase exposure risk to infectious respiratory diseases such as tuberculosis, cold viruses, and the like. If the client has a chronic respiratory condition, inquire whether mobility within the home is impaired by obstacles such as stairs.

EXERCISE

Clients with chronic respiratory conditions often do not have the lung capacity to sustain even mild forms of exercise and become dyspneic. Ask whether tolerance for activity has decreased or remained stable. The client is asked to describe typical activities such as walking, light housekeeping chores, or grocery shopping that either are tolerated or conversely result in shortness of breath.

NUTRITION

Chronic respiratory diseases result in decreased lung capacity and greater workload for the lungs and cardiovascular system. Weight loss occurs as protein stores are depleted and may be compounded by anorexia from medications and fatigue from the increased work of breathing. The client may not have enough energy to consume the needed calories to maintain body weight.

Review of Systems

The client is asked to describe other symptoms associated with the respiratory system. In addition to cough, dyspnea, sputum production, hemoptysis, wheezing, and chest pain, these include breathlessness, fever, hoarseness, night sweats, anorexia, weight loss, and dependent edema. Upper respiratory symptoms include colds, nasal discharge, epistaxis, postnasal drip, sinus pain and swelling, and sinus headaches. Hypoxia may be seen as subtle neurologic changes such as restlessness, disorientation, or personality changes. Tachycardia usually accompanies respiratory problems. Stomach upset, nausea, and vomiting can result from accumulation of excess mucus swallowed from draining sinuses. Anorexia and weight loss are seen in chronic respiratory conditions.

Detailed questions for the review of systems are found in Chapter 12, Table 12–5.

PHYSICAL EXAMINATION

Physical examination follows the health history. The techniques of inspection, palpation, percussion, and auscultation are used. Successful examination requires that the nurse be familiar with the anatomic landmarks of the posterior, lateral, and anterior thorax (Fig. 36–2). These landmarks are used by the nurse to locate and visualize the underlying structures, particularly the lobes of the lungs, the heart, and major vessels.

It is essential to compare the findings on one side of the thorax with the other side. Palpation, percussion, and auscultation proceed in a back-and-forth or side-to-side manner so that the nurse is continually evaluating findings by using the opposite side of the client as the standard for comparison.

The condition of the client's skin is noted throughout the examination of the thorax. Abnormalities are noted and recorded. Respiratory rate and rhythm, if not assessed previously with the vital signs, are assessed during inspection of the thorax (see Chap. 12).

Inspection

The physical examination actually begins during the history taking as the nurse observes the client and his or her response to questions. Signs and symptoms of respiratory distress are noted at this time: tachypnea, gasping, grunting, central cyanosis, open mouth, flared nostrils, dyspnea, color of facial skin and lips, and use of accessory muscles. The nurse notes the inspiratory to expiratory ratio; the normal ratio is 1:2. The client's speech pattern is observed. How many words or sentences can be said before another breath is taken? Clients who are short of breath may be able to say only three or four words before taking another breath. During the physical examination, the client should be undressed to the waist while privacy and warmth are maintained. Inspection and palpation are often performed together but are discussed separately here.

HEAD AND NECK

The key to any assessment technique is to develop a systematic approach. Logically, it is easiest to start with the head and work down. Inspection begins with observation of the head and neck area for any gross abnormalities that would interfere with respiration. The examiner also notes the odor of the breath and whether any sputum is present.

CHEST WALL CONFIGURATION

Inspection continues as the nurse observes the chest wall configuration. Chest size and contour are observed while the anteroposterior (AP) diameter is noted. The AP-transverse diameter refers to the ratio of the side view compared with the front view. The transverse diameter is generally twice the size of the AP diameter. Increased AP diameter or barrel chest is a characteris-

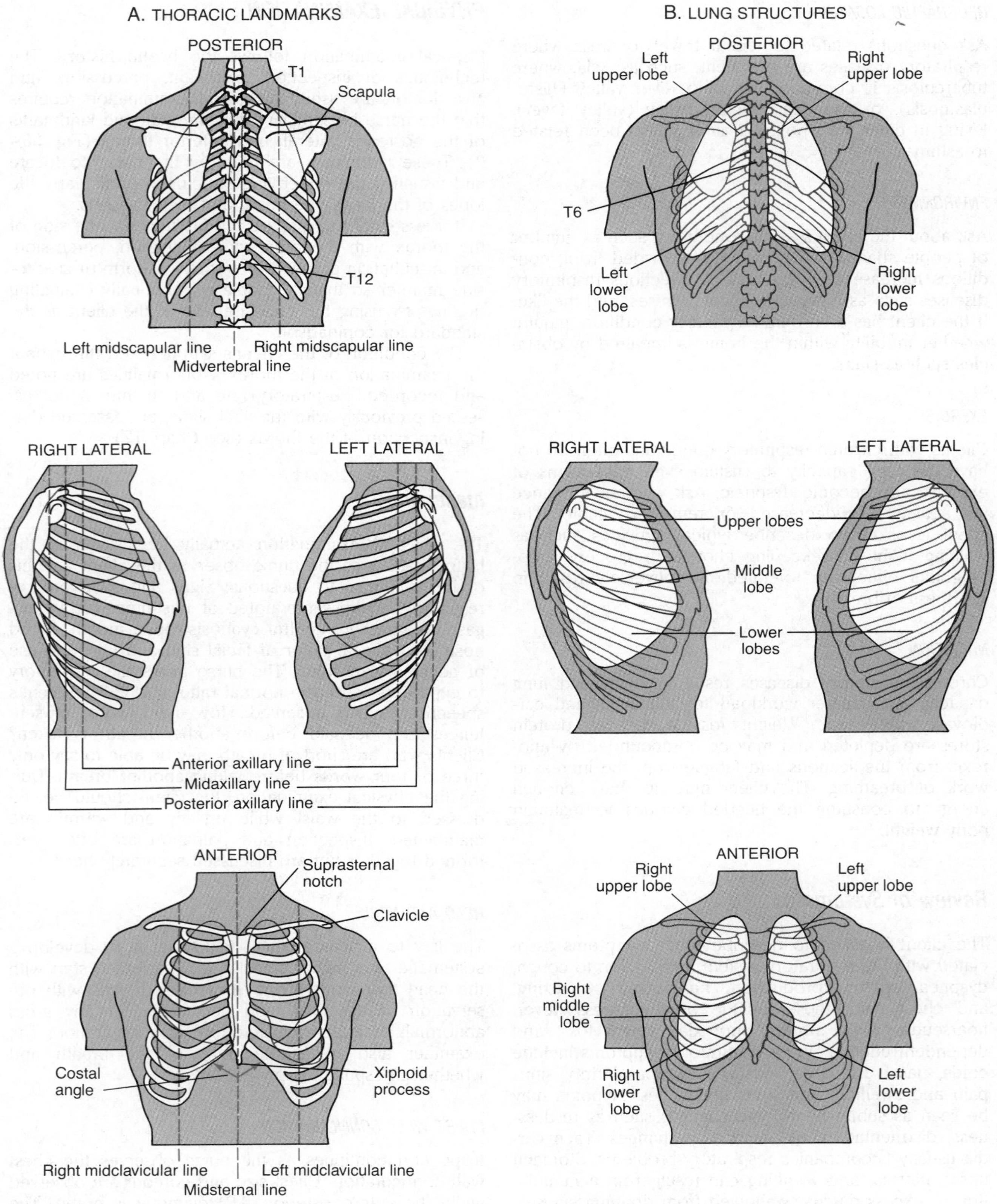

A. THORACIC LANDMARKS
POSTERIOR
T1
Scapula
T12
Left midscapular line
Right midscapular line
Midvertebral line
RIGHT LATERAL
LEFT LATERAL
Anterior axillary line
Midaxillary line
Posterior axillary line
ANTERIOR
Suprasternal notch
Clavicle
Costal angle
Xiphoid process
Right midclavicular line
Left midclavicular line
Midsternal line
B. LUNG STRUCTURES
POSTERIOR
Left upper lobe
Right upper lobe
T6
Left lower lobe
Right lower lobe
RIGHT LATERAL
LEFT LATERAL
Upper lobes
Middle lobe
Lower lobes
ANTERIOR
Right upper lobe
Left upper lobe
Right middle lobe
Right lower lobe
Left lower lobe

▲ *Figure 36–2*

Respiratory examination. *A*, Thoracic landmarks; *B*, underlying lung structures. During chest examination, it is important to document the location of unusual or abnormal findings in a universally understood manner. Use the thoracic landmark and lung structure terminology shown.

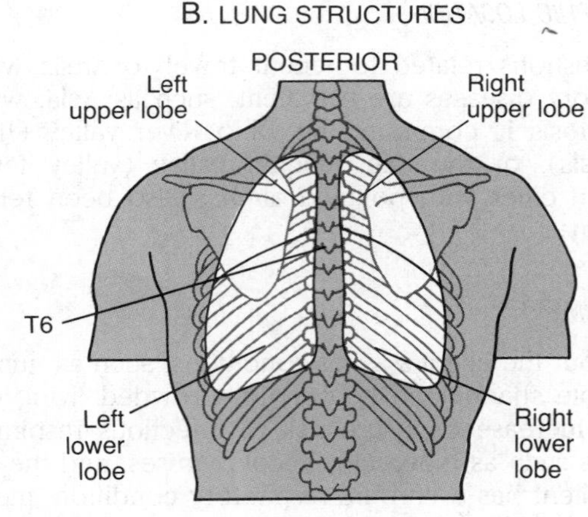

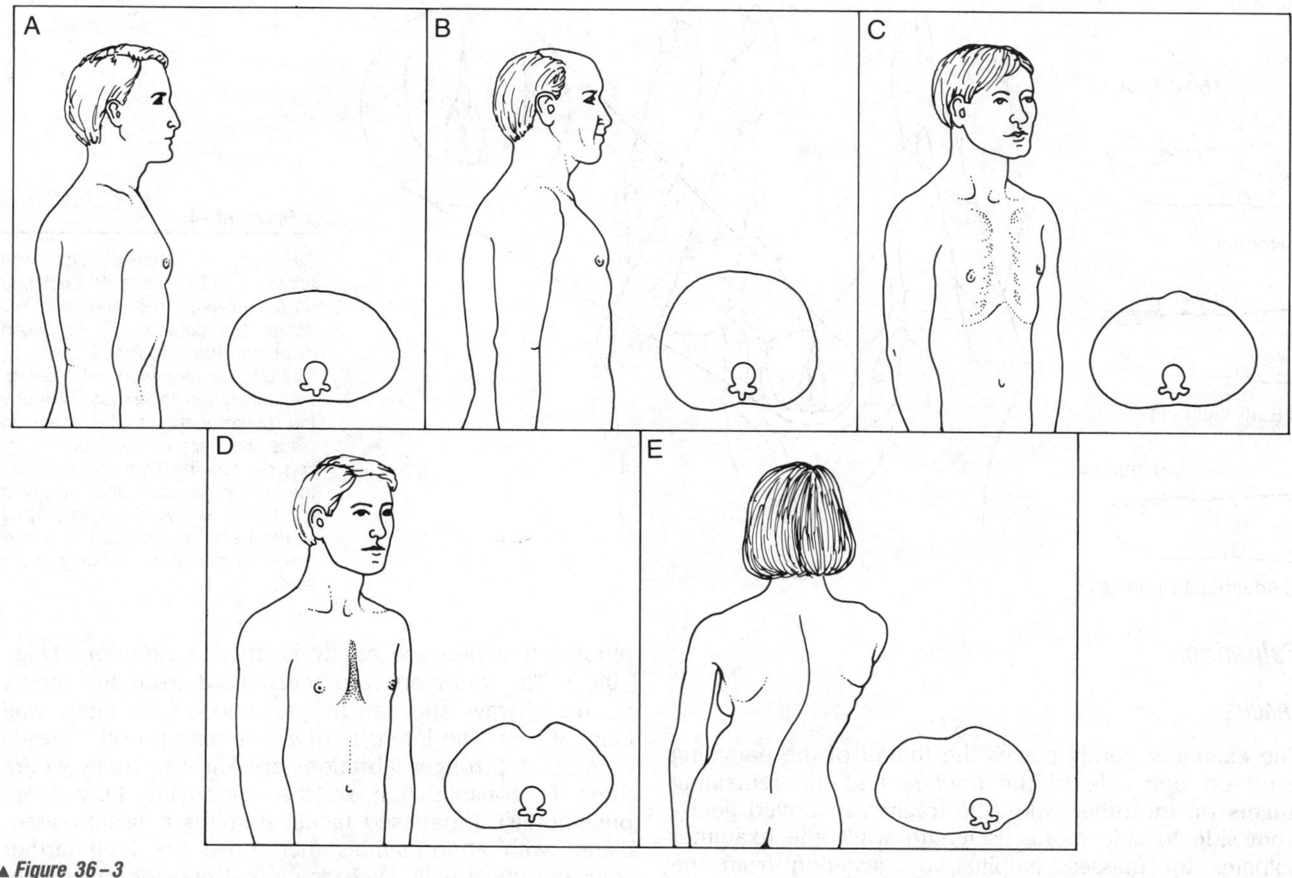

▲ *Figure 36-3*

Chest deformities. *A,* Normal adult, for comparison. *B,* Barrel chest. *C,* Funnel chest (pectus excavatum). *D,* Pigeon chest (pectus carinatum). *E,* Thoracic kyphoscoliosis.

tic finding in clients with COPD. Figure 36-3 contains drawings of the various chest deformities.

CHEST DEFORMITIES

Funnel Chest. Funnel chest (pectus excavatum) is a deformity in which the sternum is depressed and the organs that lie below it are compressed. In severe cases, the sternum may touch the spinal column. Causes of funnel chest include Marfan's syndrome and congenital connective tissue disorders.

Pigeon Chest. Pigeon chest (pectus carinatum) is the opposite of funnel chest. The sternum juts forward and increases the AP diameter. Congenital atrial or ventricular septal defects are the most common causes of pigeon chest, but rickets, Marfan's syndrome, and severe primary kyphoscoliosis may contribute to pigeon chest.

Thoracic Kyphoscoliosis. Thoracic kyphoscoliosis is the accentuation of the normal thoracic curve. The client takes on a hunched over or hunchback appearance. Causes include osteoporosis secondary to aging, spinal tuberculosis, rheumatoid arthritis, and poor posture over a long period of time. The underlying lungs are distorted, which can make interpretation of lung findings difficult.

CHEST MOVEMENT

Chest movement is observed during respiration. Normal respiratory rate is 12 to 22 breaths per minute. Rate is observed for amplitude, or depth of expansion, and rhythm. Abdominal breathing is more apparent in men, whereas women are more thoracic breathers. Use of accessory muscles, retractions, symmetry, and any paradoxic movements are noted.

FINGERS AND TOES

Examination of the fingers and toes may reveal clubbing, which may be present in clients with pulmonary fibrosis, lung cancer, or bronchiectasis. With clubbing, the nail bed loses its normal angle of 160 degrees between the nailplate and the finger, and the angle increases to 180 degrees. The base of the nail bed may also feel spongy and soft. With advanced clubbing, the finger takes on a bulbous or spoon-like appearance. Early clubbing may be assessed by use of the Schamroth technique (Fig. 36-4). The physiologic cause of clubbing has not yet been identified.

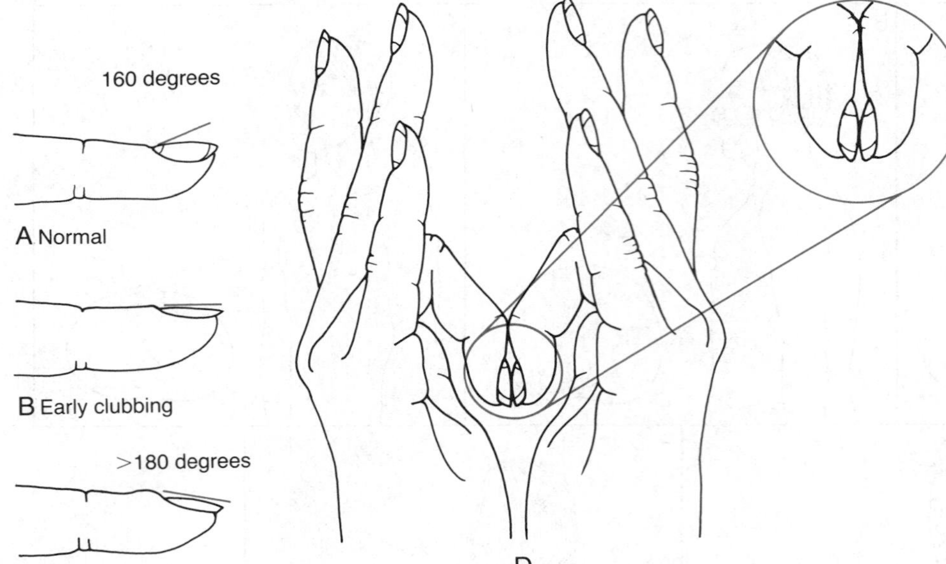

▲ *Figure 36–4*

Clubbing. *A,* Normal digit with angle of 160 degrees. *B,* Flattened angle between nail and skin exceeds 180 degrees. *C,* Advanced clubbing with rounded nail. *D,* Clubbing is assessed with use of the Schamroth technique, whereby the nurse instructs the client to place the nails of the fourth (ring) fingers together while extending the other fingers and to hold the hands up. A diamond-shaped space between the nails is a normal finding, that is, clubbing is absent.

Palpation

TRACHEA

The examiner gently places the thumb of the palpating hand on one side of the trachea and the remaining fingers on the other side. The trachea is moved gently from side to side along its length while the examiner palpates for masses, crepitus, or deviation from the midline. The trachea is usually slightly movable and quickly returns to midline position after displacement.

CHEST WALL

The chest wall is palpated with the heel or ulnar aspect of the examiner's hand held against the client's chest. Abnormalities found on inspection are further investigated during palpation. Palpation combined with inspection is particularly effective in assessing whether the movements, or thoracic excursion of the chest during inspiration and expiration, are symmetric and equal in amplitude. During palpation, the nurse assesses for any crepitus, tenderness of the chest wall, muscle tone, swelling, and tactile fremitus.

THORACIC EXCURSION

For evaluation of thoracic excursion, the client is in a sitting position, and the examiner's hands are placed on the client's posterior chest wall (Figs. 36–5 and 36–6). The thumbs meet midline over the spine, and the fingers face upward and out like a butterfly. As the client inhales, the examiner's hands should move up and out symmetrically. Any asymmetry may be indicative of a disease process in that region.

TACTILE FREMITUS

Tactile fremitus is the transmission of the vibration of air movement through the chest wall during phonation. Palpate the posterior chest wall while the client says phrases that produce relatively intense vibrations (e.g., "99"). The vibrations are transmitted from the larynx via the airways and can be palpated on the chest wall (Fig. 36–6). The intensity of vibrations on both sides is compared. Stronger vibrations are felt over areas where there is consolidation of the underlying lung (e.g., pneumonia). Decreased tactile fremitus is usually associated with abnormalities that move the lung farther from the chest wall, such as pleural effusion and pneumothorax.

Percussion

Percussion is an assessment technique of producing sounds by tapping on the chest wall with the hand. Percussion technique is discussed in Chapter 12. Tapping on the chest wall between the ribs produces

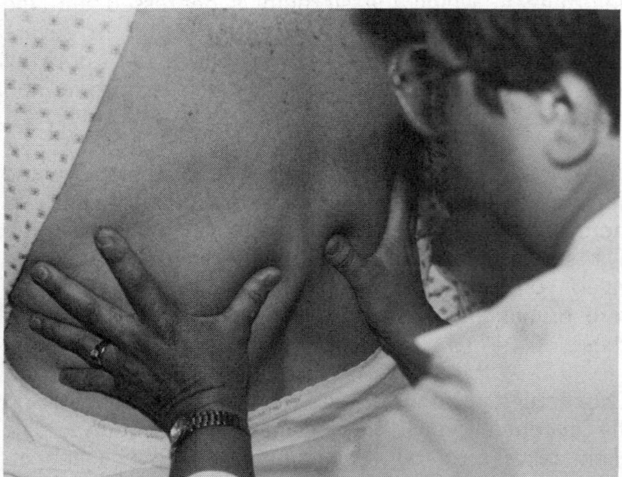

▲ *Figure 36–5*

Thoracic excursion assesses the degree and symmetry of chest movement.

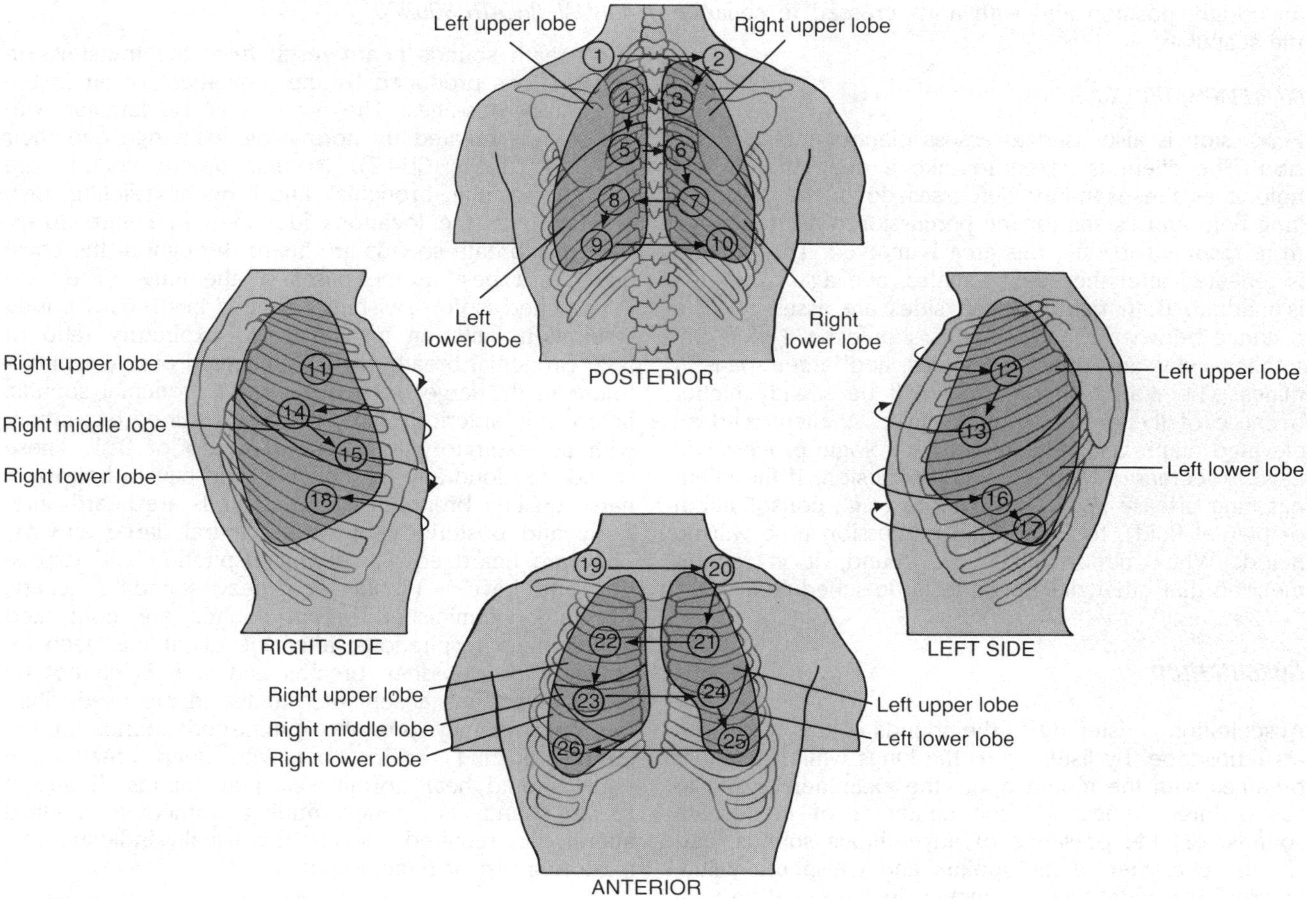

▲ *Figure 36-6*

Lung assessment. Sequence for palpation, percussion, and auscultation of the thorax (posterior, lateral, and anterior).

various sounds that are described in regard to their acoustic properties—resonant, hyperresonant, dull, flat, or tympanic. Resonant sounds are low-pitched, hollow sounds heard over normal lung tissue. Hyperresonant sounds indicate an increased amount of air in the lungs or pleural space. These sounds are louder and lower-pitched than are resonant sounds. Emphysema and pneumothorax produce hyperresonant sounds. Hyperresonant sounds are normally heard in children and very thin adults. Percussion over dense lung tissue, such as a tumor or consolidation, results in a dull percussion note. Dull sounds are thudlike, medium-pitched, and normally heard over the liver and heart. Flat percussion notes are soft, high-pitched, and the result of percussion over airless tissue. This sound can be replicated with percussion of the thigh or bony structures. Tympanic notes are high, hollow, drumlike sounds heard with percussion over the stomach, a large tension pneumothorax, or a large air-filled chamber. Percussion sounds of the chest are described in Figure 36-7.

Percussion begins at the apices and proceeds to the bases, moving from the posterior areas to the lateral areas and then to the anterior areas (see Fig. 35-6). The posterior chest is best percussed with the client in

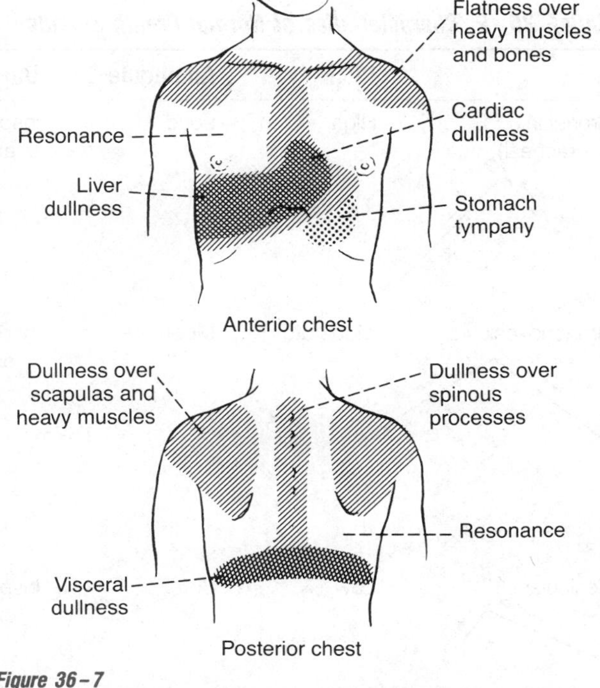

▲ *Figure 36-7*

Location of thoracic percussion tones and their associated structures.

an upright position and with arms crossed to separate the scapulae.

DIAPHRAGMATIC EXCURSION

Percussion is also used to assess diaphragmatic excursion. The client is asked to take a deep breath and hold it as the examiner percusses down the posterior lung field and listens for the percussion note to change from resonant to dull; this area is marked. The process is repeated after the client exhales, and again the area is marked. Both right and left sides are assessed. The distance between the two marks should be 3 to 6 cm; smaller spans are found in females, and larger spans in males. The marks on the right will be slightly higher because of the presence of the liver. A client with an elevated diaphragm related to a pathologic process will have a decreased diaphragmatic excursion. If the client has lung disease in the lower lobes (e.g., consolidation or pleural fluid), the same dull percussion note will be heard. When abnormalities are found, it is recommended that other diagnostic tests be scheduled.

Auscultation

Auscultation is listening to the sounds of the chest with a stethoscope. By listening to the lungs while the client breathes with the mouth open, the examiner is able to assess three things: (1) the character of the breath sounds, (2) the presence of adventitious sounds, and (3) the character of the spoken and whispered voice. Figure 36-6 identifies a sequence for auscultation with comparison of sounds from right to left. At each position, listen with the diaphragm for a full respiratory cycle of inspiration and expiration as the client breathes through the mouth.

NORMAL BREATH SOUNDS

The breath sounds heard result from the transmission of vibrations produced by the movement of air in the respiratory passages. The nurse must be familiar with the sounds created by normal air exchange and their location (Table 36-2). Normal breath sounds are termed vesicular, bronchial, and bronchovesicular; they are heard in the locations identified in Figure 36-8. Vesicular breath sounds are heard throughout the chest and heard best in the bases of the lungs. They are low-pitched, soft, "swishing" sounds best heard during inspiration, with an inspiratory to expiratory ratio of 5:2. Bronchial breath sounds are heard over the manubrium in the large tracheal airways. Bronchial sounds, heard only anteriorly, are best heard during expiration, with an expiratory to inspiratory ratio of 2:1. These sounds are loud and high-pitched and have a hollow or harsh quality. Bronchovesicular sounds are heard anteriorly and posteriorly over the central, large airways. They are heard equally during inspiration and expiration and have a tubular or breezy sounding quality. Absent or diminished breath sounds are confirmed during deep respirations; after the client has been instructed to take deep breaths and sounds cannot be heard, the terms absent or diminished are used. Shallow breaths may produce diminished sounds in the peripheral lung regions, but with deep breaths the nurse should hear normal vesicular sounds. If absent breath sounds are a new finding, immediate medical attention is required because this usually indicates respiratory arrest or pneumothorax.

ADVENTITIOUS BREATH SOUNDS

Adventitious sounds are abnormal sounds superimposed on normal breath sounds (Table 36-3 outlines

TABLE 36-2. Characteristics of Normal Breath Sounds

	Pitch	Amplitude	Duration	Quality	Normal Location
Bronchial (tracheal)	High	Loud	Inspiration < expiration	Harsh, hollow, tubular	Trachea and larynx
Bronchovesicular	Moderate	Moderate	Inspiration = expiration	Mixed	Over major bronchi where fewer alveoli are located: posterior, between scapulae especially on right; anterior, around upper sternum in first and second intercostal spaces
Vesicular	Low	Soft	Inspiration > expiration	Rustling, like the sound of the wind in the trees	Over peripheral lung fields where air flows through smaller bronchioles and alveoli

From Jarvis, C. (1992). *Physical examination and health assessment*. Philadelphia: W. B. Saunders.

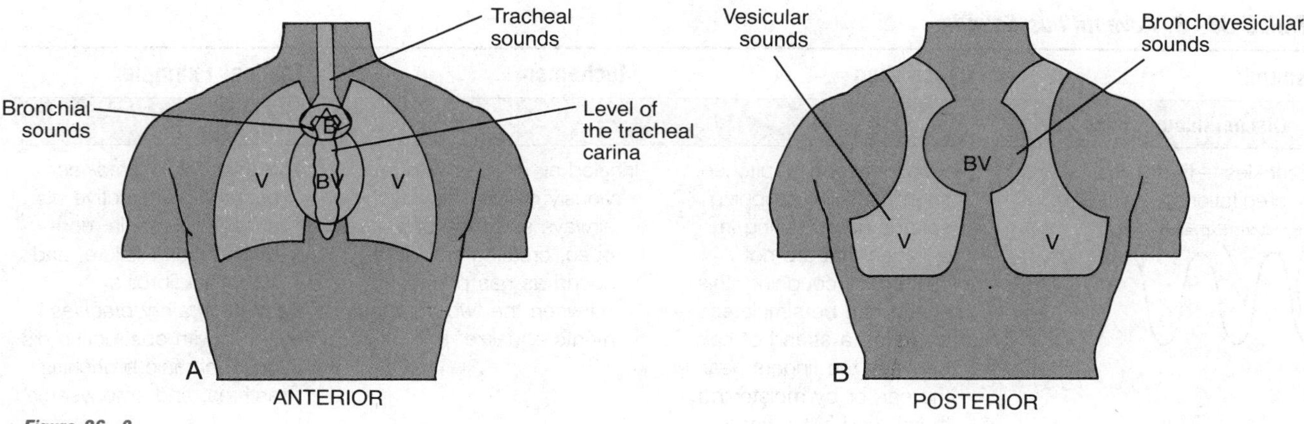

▲ *Figure 36–8*

Location of normal breath sounds.

adventitious sounds). The current American Thoracic Society nomenclature for adventitious sounds is used throughout this chapter. Adventitious sounds are described as (1) crackles, (2) rhonchi, (3) wheeze, or (4) pleural friction rub.

Crackles. Crackles are audible when there is a sudden opening of small airways that contain fluid. In the past, crackles were called rales. The sound of a crackle can be reproduced by rubbing a lock of hair between the thumb and finger close to the ear. Crackles are usually heard during inspiration and do *not* clear with a cough. Crackles can be found in clients with pulmonary edema, pulmonary fibrosis, or pneumonia.

Rhonchi. Rhonchi occur as the result of the passing of air through fluid-filled, narrow passages. Rhonchi sometimes are referred to as gurgles. Diseases with excess mucus production, such as pneumonia, bronchitis, or bronchiectasis, are associated with rhonchi. Rhonchi are usually heard on expiration and may clear with a cough.

Wheezes. A wheeze is a musical or hissing noise that results from the passage of air through a narrowed airway. Wheezes are heard during inspiration and expiration and, if severe, are audible without a stethoscope. Wheezing is commonly associated with asthma and its bronchoconstriction and edema, but foreign bodies can also cause airway narrowing and wheezing.

Pleural Friction Rub. Pleural friction rubs are the result of pleural inflammation often associated with pleurisy, pneumonia, or pleural infarct. A rub is described as a creaking, grating noise similar to that of two pieces of leather rubbing together. A rub is audible on inspiration and expiration over the area of the inflammation. Chest wall splinting can be associated with a pleural friction rub.

VOICE SOUNDS

The nurse assesses voice sounds (vocal resonance) by auscultation if tactile fremitus is abnormal. Auscultation while the client speaks normally reveals muffled and indistinct sounds. The sound is louder medially over the larger airways and softens toward the periphery. Consolidation results in *bronchophony* or increased resonance so that when the client says "99," it is heard clearly. If bronchophony is present, the nurse assesses for *egophony*, or a change in the sound of the letter *e* to *a* that has a nasal or bleating quality. A third voice test for consolidation is *whispered pectoriloquy*. The client is asked to whisper "one-two-three." If the words are distinct, whispered pectoriloquy is present. Consolidation enhances the transmission of sound vibrations and results from lung tumors, pneumonia, or pulmonary fibrosis.

▼ ASSESSMENT OF NOSE AND SINUSES

HISTORY

Upper respiratory problems can occur alone or progress to lower respiratory complications, such as in viral infections.

Chief Complaint

The client may present with a current complaint of nosebleeds (epistaxis), sinus infection, hayfever, postnasal drip, rhinitis, sneezing, or nasal, facial, or referred ear pain. Obstruction from engorged mucous membranes or nasal polyps may occlude the upper airway. A loss or decreased sense of smell may accompany symptoms of the common cold and allergies or may signal a more serious neurologic problem. The nurse inquires whether the client has experienced these symptoms previously and, if so, when and how often. The client is asked to describe self-treatment measures such as nasal sprays, decongestants, antihistamines, and other over-the-counter cold and allergy medications. A complete symptom analysis is performed to determine the nature of the problem including onset, duration, and severity. Ask the client to relate factors that alleviate or aggravate the symptoms such as increased humidity, sitting upright, lying supine, weather and season changes, or allergies.

TABLE 36-3. Adventitious Sounds

Sound*	Description	Mechanism	Clinical Example
Discontinuous Sounds			
Crackles—fine (rales, crepitations) Inspiration Expiration	Discontinuous, high-pitched, short crackling, popping sounds heard during inspiration that are not cleared by coughing; this sound can be simulated by rolling a strand of hair between the fingers near the ear, or by moistening thumb and index finger and separating them near the ear	Inhaled air collides with previously deflated airways; airways suddenly pop open, creating crackling sound as gas pressures between the two compartments equalize	*Late inspiratory crackles* occur with restrictive disease: pneumonia, congestive heart failure, and interstitial fibrosis *Early inspiratory crackles* occur with obstructive disease: chronic bronchitis, asthma, and emphysema
Crackles—coarse (coarse rales)	Loud, low-pitched, bubbling and gurgling sounds that start in early inspiration and may be present in expiration; may decrease somewhat by suctioning or coughing but will reappear shortly; sound like opening a Velcro fastener	Inhaled air collides with secretions in the trachea and large bronchi	Pulmonary edema, pneumonia, pulmonary fibrosis, and in the terminally ill who have a depressed cough reflex
Atelectatic crackles (atelectatic rales)	Sound like fine crackles, but do not last and are not pathologic; disappear after the first few breaths; heard in axillae and bases (usually dependent) of lungs	When sections of alveoli are not fully aerated, they deflate and accumulate secretions; crackles are heard when these sections reexpand with a few deep breaths	In aging adults, bed-ridden persons, or in persons just aroused from sleep
Pleural friction rub	A very superficial sound that is coarse and low-pitched; it has a grating quality as if two pieces of leather are being rubbed together; sounds just like crackles, but *close* to the ear; sounds louder if the stethoscope is pushed harder onto the chest wall; sound is inspiratory and expiratory	Caused when pleurae become inflamed and lose their normal lubricating fluid; their opposing roughened pleural surfaces rub together during respiration; heard best in anterolateral wall where there is greatest lung mobility	Pleuritis, accompanied by pain with breathing (rub disappears after a few days if pleural fluid accumulates and separates pleurae)
Continuous Sounds			
Wheeze—high-pitched (sibilant rhonchi) 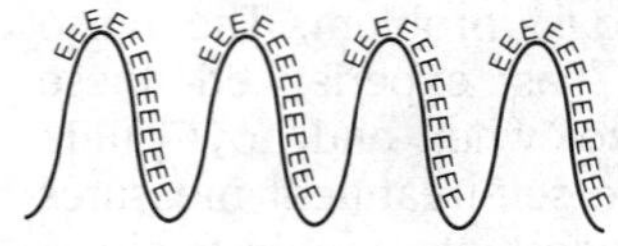	High-pitched, musical squeaking sounds that predominate in expiration but may occur in both expiration and inspiration	Air squeezed or compressed through passageways narrowed almost to closure by collapsing, swelling, secretions, or tumors; the passageway walls oscillate in apposition between the closed and barely open positions; the resulting sound is similar to a vibrating reed (Forgacs, 1978)	Obstructive lung disease such as asthma or emphysema

TABLE 36-3. Adventitious Sounds Continued

Sound*	Description	Mechanism	Clinical Example
Continuous Sounds *Continued*			
Wheeze—low-pitched (sonorous rhonchi)	Low-pitched, musical snoring, moaning sounds; they are heard throughout the cycle, although they are more prominent on expiration; may clear somewhat by coughing	Airflow obstruction as described by the vibrating reed mechanism above; the pitch of the wheeze cannot be correlated to the size of the passageway that generates it	Bronchitis

*Although nothing in clinical practice seems to differ more than the nomenclature of adventitious sounds, most authorities concur on two categories: (1) discontinuous, discrete crackling sounds and (2) continuous, coarse, or musical sounds.

From Jarvis, C. (1992). *Physical examination and health assessment.* Philadelphia: W. B. Saunders.

Nasal and sinus problems may be allergy-related and provoked by pollen, fumes, smoke, animal dander, or dust particles. Epistaxis episodes may increase during the winter months if insufficient humidity dries mucous membranes. A foul taste in the mouth, unpleasant breath odor (halitosis), nasal obstruction, and facial pain (particularly over the frontal and maxillary sinuses) accompany sinusitis. Chronic sinusitis may be accompanied by headache or facial pain present on awakening and diminishing during the day.

Past Medical History

The nurse asks about past problems with frequent colds, sinus infections, nasal stuffiness, or trauma (fracture). Episodes of epistaxis are explored for cause (such as hypertension), frequency, and treatment (such as cauterization or nasal packing).

PHYSICAL EXAMINATION

The nurse uses inspection and palpation to examine the nose and sinuses. The structures assessed include the external nose, vestibule, nasal mucosa, septum, turbinates, nasal canals, and sinuses. Function of the first cranial nerve (olfactory) is usually not tested unless a deficit in the sense of smell is reported or suspected.

Nose

EXTERNAL NOSE

The external nose is inspected and palpated for deviations from normal alignment, symmetry, color, discharge, nasal flaring, lesions, and tenderness. Normal findings are listed. The skin color over the nose is the same as that of the facial skin. Alignment is straight and symmetric without deviation from midline. Discharge from the nares should be absent, and the nares should not flare (spread) with respirations. The client is able to breathe quietly through the nose rather than mouthbreathe. Masses, lesions, and tenderness are absent. The nurse checks the nasal canals for patency by asking the client to occlude one naris with a finger and to breathe through the open naris while closing the mouth. This is repeated for the opposite naris. The client should be able to breathe without difficulty through both nares. The nurse asks the client to tip the head back and inspects the outer nares for crusting, bleeding, or dryness, which should be absent.

INTERNAL NOSE

The nurse next inspects the vestibules with use of a penlight while the client's head is tipped back. Normal findings include the presence of coarse hairs, a clear passage without discharge, and a midline septum. Further examination of the internal nose requires use of a nasal speculum; this is not done unless it is indicated.

If detailed examination of the internal nose is done, the nurse either attaches a nasal speculum tip to the otoscope head or uses a metal nasal speculum (Fig. 36-9) and penlight for illumination. The client tips the head back, and the nurse gently inserts the speculum into one naris with care being taken not to scrape the mucosa. One naris is inspected at a time.

Hold the speculum correctly and insert the blades gently about $\frac{1}{2}$ inch into the nostril. Gain additional control of the speculum by resting the index finger of the dominant hand on the side of the client's nose. Steady the client's head with the nondominant hand. Open the blades gently and vertically, avoiding pressure on the septum and turbinates. Slowly move the head to inspect all areas of the nasal chamber. Observe the condition of the mucous membrane (e.g., pallor, redness, swelling.) Normally, the mucosa is moist and dark pink without sign of inflammation, pallor, or blue color. Presence of discharge is abnormal. The septum is midline without deviation, masses, perforation, or exudate. The turbinates (only the inferior and part of the middle turbinates are visible, the superior is not) have the same color as the mucosa and should be free of exudate, swelling, or inflammation. Look for polyps and other masses. Observe plugs of mucus for color, consistency, amount, and odor.

Inspection may be hampered by nasal congestion. It may be necessary to shrink the nasal mucosa with a topical vasoconstrictor (e.g., ephedrine, cocaine,

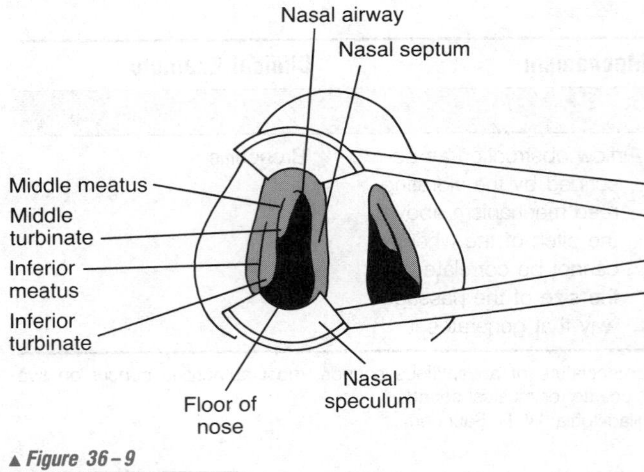

▲ *Figure 36–9*
Nasal speculum insertion.

phenylephrine hydrochloride) for adequate inspection. When these agents are instilled into the nose, the client should be instructed to say *e* and hold the sound. This technique raises the posterior tongue, occludes the upper airway, and prevents the fluid from running into the pharynx.

Nasopharynx

The nasopharynx is best examined with a mirror with the tongue depressed with a tongue blade or gauze. Prevent the mirror's fogging by warming it before putting it into a mouth. Hold the mirror to one side of the uvula and focus light on it. A small part of the nasopharynx can be observed with a nasal speculum. Specialists may use a nasopharyngoscope to examine the nasopharynx.

Paranasal Sinuses

Assess the paranasal sinuses by (1) inspecting and palpating the soft overlying tissues, (2) observing any nasal secretions (it is possible to determine which sinus is infected according to where purulent discharge appears), and (3) transillumination of the maxillary and frontal sinuses.

The nurse palpates and percusses the frontal and maxillary sinuses to assess for swelling and tenderness, which should be absent. The *frontal sinuses* are palpated simultaneously by placing the thumbs above the eyes, just under the bony ridge of the orbits, and applying gentle pressure. The *maxillary sinuses* are palpated by use of either the index and third fingers or thumbs to gently press on each side of the nose just under the zygomatic bones. Direct percussion is used over the eyebrows for the frontal sinuses and on either side of the nose below the eyes in line with the pupils for the maxillary sinuses.

TRANSILLUMINATION

Transillumination is a technique to further assess the sinuses if tenderness is present. Either a penlight or the otoscope handle fitted with a transilluminator head (Chap. 12) is used. The room is darkened. The light is placed against the orbital bones immediately below the eyebrows and directed upward. The nurse shields the light source with one hand. Normally, a reddish glow appears above the frontal sinus area. Lack of illumination may indicate sinus congestion and pus accumulation. The maxillary sinuses are assessed by placing the light beneath the center of the eyes and the zygomatic bones and directing it down and in toward the roof of the mouth. The nurse asks the client to open the mouth. A glow should appear on the hard palate on the side being illuminated.

For more completely assessing sinus conditions, sinus radiographs may be used. Air, normally present in the sinuses, appears as dark areas on a developed film.

Smell

The senses of taste and smell are closely related. Many conditions affect taste and smell, such as viral infections, normal aging, head injuries, and local obstruction. Some medications can affect smell and taste, such as metronidazole (Flagyl), local anesthetics, clofibrate (Atromid-S), some antibiotics, some antineoplastics, allopurinol, phenylbutazone, levodopa, codeine, morphine, carbamazepine (Tegretol), lithium, and trifluoperazine (Stelazine).

Smell impairment may be (1) hyposmia (decrease in smell sensitivity) or (2) anosmia (bilateral and complete absence of smell sensitivity). Smell assessment is done by having the client identify various odors. Various substances are placed in individual test tubes (covered to eliminate visual cues). Testing each nostril separately, have the client sniff the tubes (first with eyes closed and then with eyes open). Document whether the client (1) can perceive each odor and (2) can identify each odor accurately. Smell is perceived mainly via the olfactory nerves, although some are perceived via the trigeminal nerves. Trigeminal irritants are perceived even by clients experiencing anosmia. (Therefore, a client who claims not to smell trigeminal irritants has a hysterical loss of smell rather than hy-

TABLE 36–4. Substances Used in Assessing Smell

Olfactory stimulants	Trigeminal stimulants
Coffee (instant powder)	Ammonia
Phenylethyl alcohol	Acetone
Almond oil	Menthol
Peppermint	Distilled water
Musk	

From Gordon, C. B. (1982). Practical approach to the loss of smell. *American Family Physician*, *26*, 191.

posmia or anosmia.) Olfactory stimulants and trigeminal stimulants commonly used to assess smell are listed in Table 36-4.

DIAGNOSTIC TESTS

Diagnostic procedures augment the assessment of clients experiencing respiratory disorders. In order to help the new nurse remember which diagnostic test is used when and for what purpose, the tests are discussed in the framework of what is being evaluated—functional status, anatomy, or specimens. The diagnostic test may be used for one or all three of these reasons. This listing is by no means all-inclusive but identifies the most commonly used diagnostic tests.

Diagnostic Tests for Function

The diagnostic tests that evaluate the functional status of the pulmonary system include (1) arterial blood gas analysis, (2) pulmonary function tests, (3) pulse oximetry, (4) capnography, and (5) ventilation/perfusion studies.

ARTERIAL BLOOD GAS ANALYSIS

Arterial blood gas (ABG) analysis directly measures the partial pressures of oxygen (PaO_2), carbon dioxide ($PaCO_2$), and pH. Other data are calculated such as oxygen saturation and HCO_3. PaO_2 reflects the efficiency of gas exchange (ventilation/perfusion), whereas $PaCO_2$ reflects the effectiveness of ventilation. The acid-

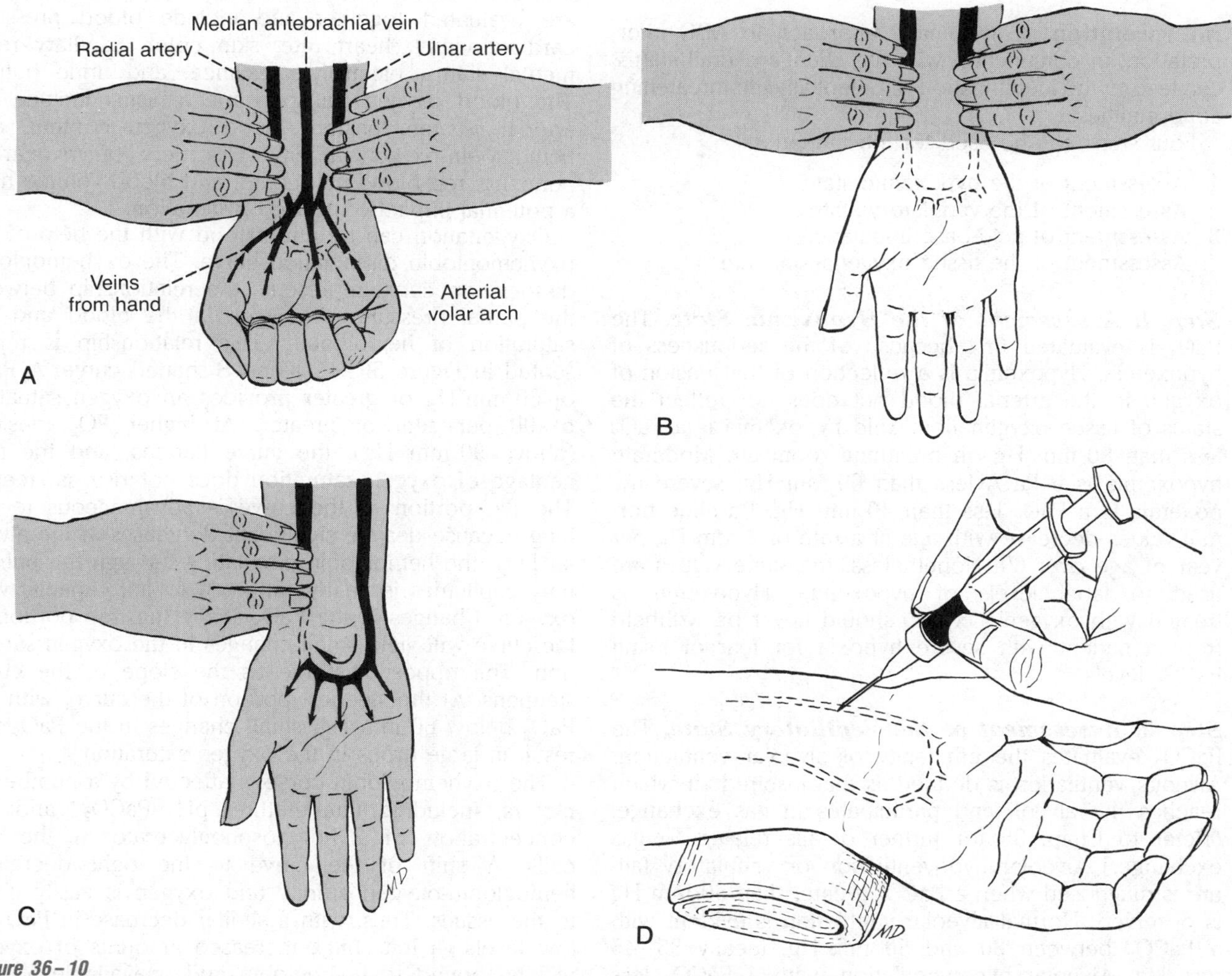

▲ *Figure 36-10*

Allen test is a quick assessment of collateral circulation in the hand, and is essential before performance of a radial artery puncture, for example, for collecting an arterial blood gas sample. *A*, Both radial and ulnar arteries are occluded by the examiner's fingers. The client closes the hand into a fist. *B*, When the hand is opened and arteries are still occluded, the client's hand is pale. *C*, When either the ulnar or radial artery is released the entire hand should become pink due to collateral circulation. Patency of both arteries is assessed one at a time. *D*, Arterial blood gas sample is drawn from the radial artery with a heparinized needle and syringe.

base status of the body (Chap. 15) is indicated by the pH of arterial blood.

ABGs are essential for the assessment of clients who are acutely ill with pulmonary and nonpulmonary disorders, require artificial airways, are dependent on mechanical ventilation, and are experiencing chronic respiratory diseases.

A sample of arterial blood is obtained by arterial puncture. This procedure is done by inserting a sterile needle (connected to a heparinized syringe) into one of the percutaneous arteries (i.e., radial, brachial, or femoral). The radial artery is most commonly used because it is readily accessible, is easily palpated, and is not associated with as severe complications as the other two sites are. Low complication rates are related to ease of access and presence of collateral circulation via the ulnar artery. For serial ABG analyses or ongoing respiratory monitoring, multiple punctures may be avoided by using an arterial line (i.e., a sterile cannula inserted into one of the arteries) (Fig. 36-10).

Interpretation. A systematic approach to ABG interpretation, in conjunction with the client's overall status, can lead to the identification of potentially life-threatening abnormalities.

Four steps can be used for interpretation:

1. Assessment of the hypoxemic state
2. Assessment of the ventilatory state
3. Assessment of acid-base imbalance
4. Assessment of the tissue oxygenation state

Step 1: Assessment of the Hypoxemic State. The PaO_2 is evaluated first because of the seriousness of hypoxemia. Hypoxemia is a reflection of the tension of oxygen in the arterial blood but does not reflect the status of tissue oxygenation. Mild hypoxemia is a PaO_2 less than 80 mm Hg on breathing room air. Moderate hypoxemia is a PaO_2 less than 60 mm Hg; severe hypoxemia is a PaO_2 less than 40 mm Hg. Baseline normal values decrease with age at a rate of 1 mm Hg per year of age over 60. Nonetheless, the same values are used to label levels of hypoxemia. Hypoxemia is treated with oxygen. Oxygen should never be withheld from a patient with severe hypoxia for fear of rising $PaCO_2$ levels.

Step 2: Assessment of the Ventilatory State. The $PaCO_2$ evaluates the efficiency of alveolar ventilation. Alveolar ventilation is defined as that inspired air which reaches the alveoli and participates in gas exchange. (Refer to Chap. 35 for further details related to gas exchange.) Alveolar hypoventilation or ventilatory failure is diagnosed when a $PaCO_2$ greater than 50 mm Hg is observed. Normal alveolar ventilation is evident with a $PaCO_2$ between 30 and 50 mm Hg, ideally 35-45 mm Hg, Alveolar hyperventilation, with a $PaCO_2$ less than 30 mm Hg, is the result of overbreathing.

Step 3: Assessment of Acid-Base Balance. The pH-acid-base balance is evaluated next. The lungs play a major role in acid-base balance. Changes in the retention or elimination of carbon dioxide will directly affect pH. However, the lungs may act in a compensatory manner to correct metabolic acid-base disorders with hypoventilation or hyperventilation as the compensatory mechanism. Changes in the pH that correlate with changes in carbon dioxide indicate primary respiratory abnormalities. For example, an increase in the $PaCO_2$ will result in a decrease in the pH, as in ventilatory failure. The lungs are not able to remove carbon dioxide, and the ABG reflects a decrease in ventilation with an increase in $PaCO_2$ and decrease in pH. The reverse is also true; as the $PaCO_2$ decreases, the pH will increase, as in a hyperventilatory state. Deep, rapid respirations "blow off" carbon dioxide, and the ABG reveals a low $PaCO_2$ level with an increased pH.

Step 4: Assessment of the Tissue Oxygenation State. Step 4 includes the evaluation of the cardiac status, peripheral perfusion status, and blood oxygen transport. Cardiac status and peripheral perfusion status are evaluated together and include blood pressure, cardiac output, heart rate, skin color, capillary refill, mental status, electrolyte balance, and urine output. The blood oxygen transport mechanisms include the arterial oxygen tension, blood oxygen content, and hemoglobin-oxygen affinity. Disorders of myocardial pumping, red blood cell count, and blood volume have a potential impact on tissue oxygenation.

Oxygenation can be understood with the help of the oxyhemoglobin dissociation curve. The oxyhemoglobin dissociation curve represents the relationship between the partial pressure of oxygen in the blood and the saturation of hemoglobin. This relationship is represented in Figure 36-11 as an S-shaped curve. A PaO_2 of 60 mm Hg or greater provides an oxygen satuation of 90 per cent or greater. At higher PO_2 tensions (above 90 mm Hg), the curve flattens, and the percentage of oxygen saturation does not rise as steeply. The flat portion of the curve is advantageous to the lung because despite significant decreases in the alveolar PO_2, the hemoglobin circulating through the pulmonary capillaries is nearly saturated to full capacity with oxygen. Changes in the PaO_2 at the flat, top portion of the curve will yield small changes in the oxygen saturation. The opposite is true as the slope of the curve steepens. At the steepest portion of the curve, with the PaO_2 below 60 mm Hg, small changes in the PaO_2 will result in large drops in the oxygen saturation.

The oxyhemoglobin curve is affected by a number of factors, including temperature, pH, $PaCO_2$, and the concentration of 2,3-diphosphoglycerate in the red cells. A shift of the curve to the right decreases hemoglobin-oxygen affinity and oxygen is easily given to the tissues. Thus, with a similar decrease in PaO_2 to low levels (a left shift), increased amounts of oxygen will be bound to hemoglobin and unavailable for tissues. During a left shift, hemoglobin has a high affinity for oxygen, so less oxygen is available for tissues. The body's tissues benefit from the steep portion of the curve. As even a small decrease in the oxygen tension occurs, oxygen is rapidly released to the tissues by the

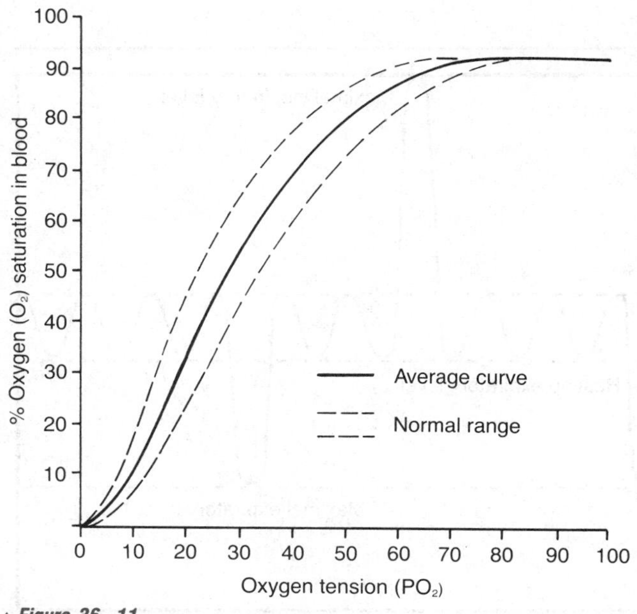

▲ *Figure 36-11*

Oxyhemoglobin dissociation curve. This curve represents the relationship between the partial pressure of oxygen (PO_2) in the blood and the saturation of hemoglobin with oxygen (O_2).

hemoglobin. This is illustrated by the way the curve quickly drops off as the saturation curve reflects the lower saturation of hemoglobin. The oxyhemoglobin saturation curve shifts upward to the left when conditions occur that cause oxygen and hemoglobin to bind more tightly, so that less oxygen is actually released to the tissues. The curve shifts down and to the right when conditions occur that cause hemoglobin to be released more readily to the tissues.

Nursing Management. The physician or other clinician skilled in arterial puncture must collect the blood sample. In most hospitals, physicians are the only personnel allowed to draw from the femoral artery, whereas nurses with special training can draw radial or brachial samples.

Before the sample is drawn, the site must be treated with a disinfectant and allowed to dry. The client should be told the stick will be painful for a moment. If the client is quite anxious about the test or other problems and hyperventilating, the results of the test may be altered. If the client is not likely to cooperate, the nurse may need to hold the client's arm still during the stick in order to avoid inadvertent injury to nerves, vessels, and tendons. The amount of blood needed for the sample varies with each laboratory but may be as small as 0.5 ml or as large as 10 ml. After the sample is drawn, continuous pressure should be applied to the site for 5 minutes for radial and brachial sites and 10 minutes for femoral sites. Pressure bandages are commonly used. If the client has a tendency to bleed, pressure will be needed for a longer period of time.

It is important to note whether the client is receiving oxygen; the amount and source of oxygen should be recorded on the laboratory request form. The results will be examined in light of the degree of oxygen needed. For example, if a client's PaO_2 is 85 on 50 per cent oxygen, this client has a more significant problem with oxygen transport than does the client who is at 85 on room air (21 per cent oxygen).

Complications from arterial sampling include bleeding or hematoma formation at the site and injury to the artery and surrounding structures. The nurse should report any of these signs to the physician.

PULMONARY FUNCTION TESTS

Pulmonary function tests (PFTs) help the practitioner further evaluate the lungs. PFTs can provide information related to lung volumes, lung mechanics, and diffusion capabilities of the lung. The obtained data allow the practitioner to determine the

- presence of pulmonary disease or abnormality of lung function
- extent of abnormalities
- severity of impairment
- progression of the disorder
- appropriate treatment

Preparation for PFTs includes education about the purpose of the test, how the tests are done, and what to expect during the tests. Explicit instructions will be given during the testing, and complete patient cooperation is important. The nurse should instruct the clients that they may feel short of breath after the test. Also instruct clients not to smoke or use a bronchodilator 6 hours before undergoing a PFT.

PFTs done in a pulmonary function laboratory cover the entire range of respiratory volumes. On the other hand, PFTs done outside of a laboratory are modified to ventilation tests of forced expiratory volume, vital capacity, and maximal voluntary ventilation measures.

Lung Volumes and Capacities. Lung volumes are measured with a dilutional technique using helium or body plethysmography.

The body plethysmograph, or the body box (Fig. 36-12), is a device used to measure lung volumes. While sitting in the airtight box, the client is instructed to perform a panting maneuver. The changes in the box pressure reflect changes in the thoracic volume. Clients who cannot "pant," who cannot tolerate closed spaces, or who have equipment that would interfere with the test cannot be tested by this method.

To use helium to test the lungs, the client inhales a mixture of air with a known concentration of helium. Helium will not significantly diffuse into the pulmonary bed. The helium will diffuse throughout all the air in the breathing box and lungs. The client exhales and is disconnected from the box. Changes in helium concentration in the box can be computed to determine total lung volume. Table 36-5 defines common lung volumes. Lung capacities are figures calculated from two or more lung volumes. They include the inspiratory capacity, functional residual capacity, and vital capacity (see Table 36-5).

TABLE 36–5. Pulmonary Function Test (PFT) Components

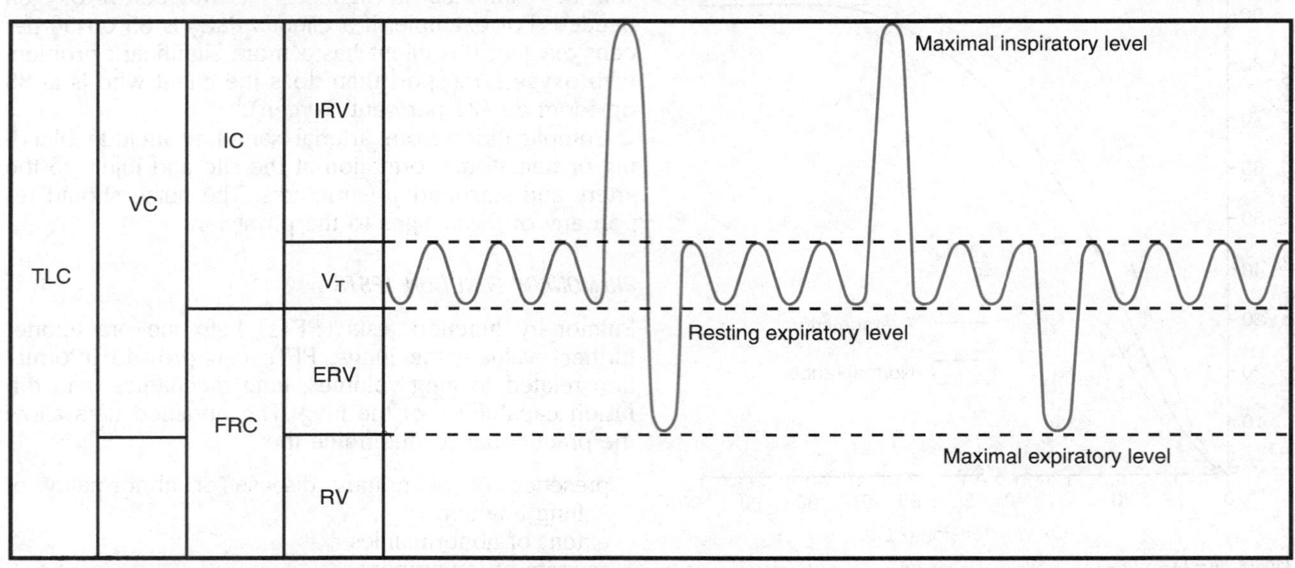

Lung Volumes and Capacities		
VC	*Vital capacity*	Volume of air that is measured during a slow, maximal expiration after a maximal inspiration; normal range varies with age, sex, and body size
IC	*Inspiratory capacity*	Largest volume of air that can be inhaled from resting expiratory volume
ERV	*Expiratory reserve volume*	Largest volume of air exhaled from resting end-expiratory level
FRC	*Functional residual capacity*	Volume of air remaining in lungs at resting end-expiratory level
RV	*Residual volume*	Volume of air remaining in the lungs at the end of maximal expiration
TLC	*Total lung capacity*	Volume of air contained in the lungs after maximal inspiration
V_T	*Tidal volume*	Volume of air inhaled or exhaled during each respiratory cycle; normal range is 400 to 700 ml
f	*Respiratory rate*	Frequency of breathing is the number of breaths per minute; normal range is 12 to 22
Lung Mechanics		
FVC	*Forced vital capacity*	Maximal volume of air that can be forcefully expired after a maximal inspiration to total lung capacity
FEV_t	*Forced expiratory volume*	Volume of air expired during a given time interval (t in seconds) from the beginning of an FVC maneuver
$FEF_{25\%-75\%}$	*Forced expiratory flow*$_{25\%-75\%}$	Average of flow during the middle half of an FVC maneuver
PEFR	*Peak expiratory flow rate*	Maximal flow rate attained during an FVC maneuver
MVV	*Maximal voluntary ventilation*	Largest volume that can be breathed during a 10- to 15-second interval with voluntary effort
MIP	*Maximal inspiratory pressure*	Greatest negative or subatmospheric pressure that can be generated during inspiration against an occluded airway
MEP	*Maximal expiratory pressure*	Highest positive pressure that can be generated during a forceful expiratory effort against an occluded airway

Clients with obstructive and restrictive diseases will have disease-specific changes in lung volumes and capacities. Table 36–6 categorizes the diseases and outlines the differences in the PFTs. Clients with obstructive lung diseases have air trapping and associated symptoms. The total lung capacity will be increased with severe disease along with lung hyperinflation as seen on the chest radiograph. Restrictive disorders are characterized by decreased total lung capacity, a decreased residual volume, and usually difficulty taking a deep breath.

Lung Mechanics. Lung mechanics evaluate the flow of gas in and out of the lung. These measurements evaluate the respiratory muscles, lung and chest wall compliance, and airway resistance, which is sometimes called the lung's bellow function. The flow rates are measured during the exhalation phase of the respiratory cycle. Depending on the test, the client may be asked to exhale forcefully or to the maximal expiratory level. See Table 36–6 for definitions of maneuvers that test lung mechanics. Lung mechanics are measured with a spirometer. The client exhales or inhales into a mouth-

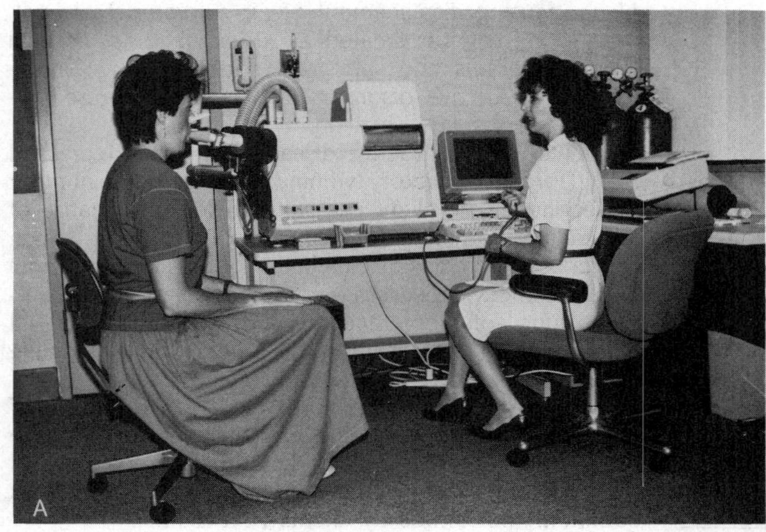

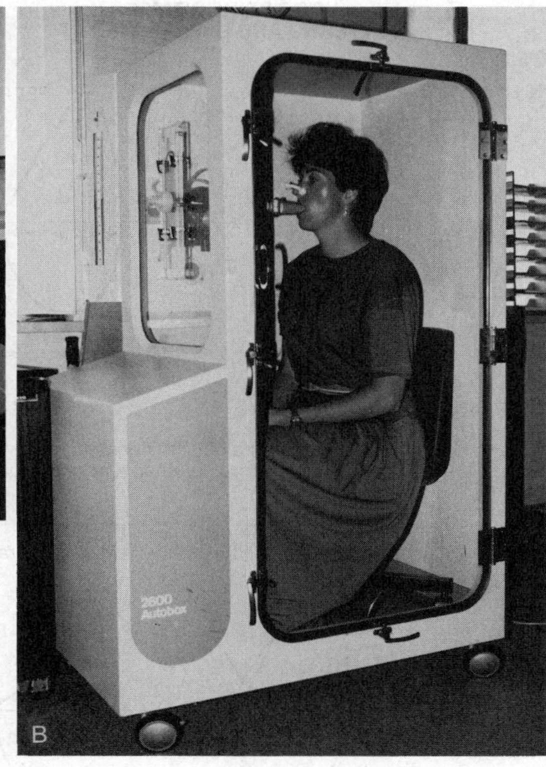

▲ *Figure 36–12*

Two different types of equipment used to assess pulmonary function are pictured. *A,* Computerized pulmonary function test machine. *B,* Body plethysmography unit, often called a body box. (Note the client being assessed is inside the "box.") (Photographs courtesy of Sharp Memorial Hospital Pulmonary Physiology Laboratory, San Diego, CA.)

TABLE 36–6. Categorization of Obstructive and Restrictive Pulmonary Disorders and PFT Findings

	Obstructive	Restrictive
	Disorders or diseases affecting the patency or elasticity of the airways, leading to an increase in airway resistance; expiration primarily affected	Disorders or diseases causing interference or change in chest wall or lung parenchyma; inspiration primarily affected
		Examples include
		Kyphoscoliosis
	Emphysema	Abdominal distention/obesity
	Chronic bronchitis	Pulmonary fibrosis
	Asthma	Neuromuscular diseases and disorders
	Bronchiectasis	Chest wall trauma
	Airway inflammation in response to irritants, infections, or allergies	Congenital chest wall changes
		Inflammatory changes of the lung tissue or pleura
		Tumors
		Pulmonary edema
PFTs and Findings		
VC (vital capacity)	Decreased	Normal or decreased
FEV_t (forced expiratory volume)	Decreased	Decreased, but not as severe as in obstructive disease
FEV_t/VC ratio	Decreased	Normal to increased
RV (residual volume)	Increased	Decreased
FRC (functional residual capacity)	Increased	Decreased
TLC (total lung capacity)	Increased	Decreased

LOOP SPIROGRAM PATTERNS AND EXPLANATION

NORMAL PATTERN

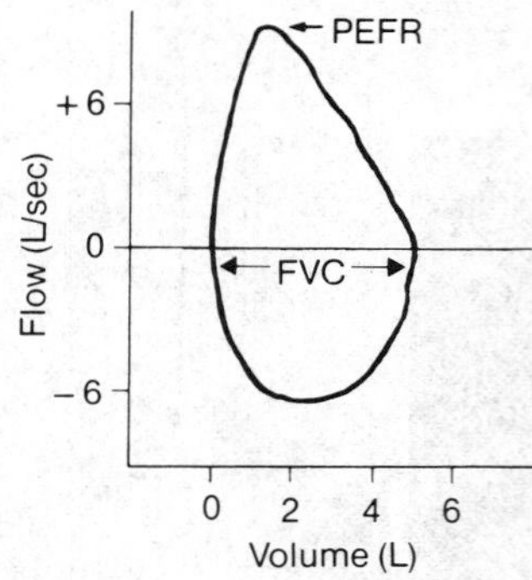

The expiratory curve shows a straight line decrease in flow after peak flow (PEFR). The inspiratory curve has a normal rounded pattern.

OBSTRUCTIVE PATTERN

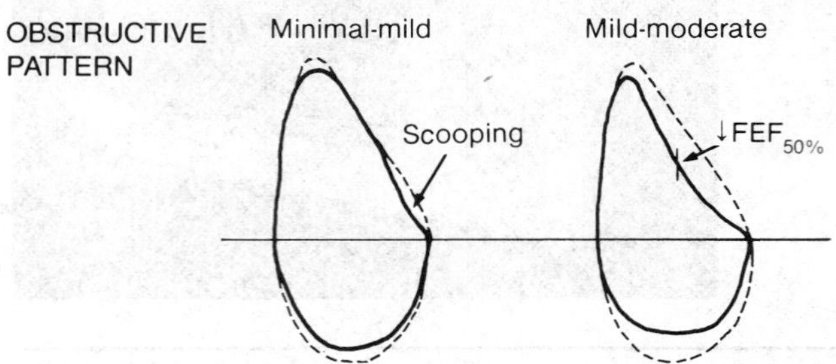

The expiratory curve shows scooping at low lung volumes (minimal to mild obstruction). As obstruction increases, the scooping becomes more marked and is accompanied by a decreased $FEF_{50\%}$ (mild to moderate obstruction).

Severe (e.g., emphysema)

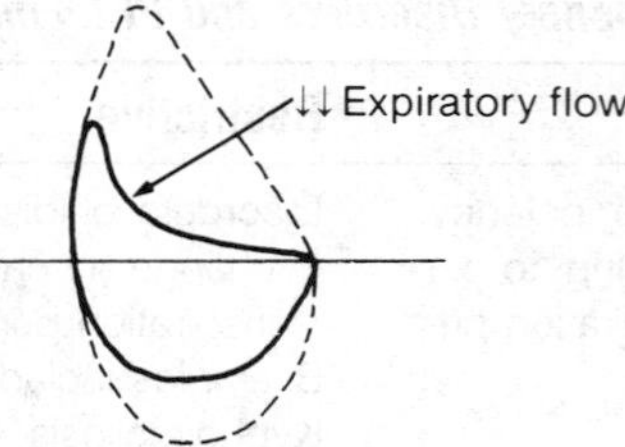

The expiratory curve shows a sudden decrease in PEFR in an "index finger" pattern, followed by a nearly horizontal line.

The inspiratory curve is normal, except for absolute decreases in flow rates.

RESTRICTIVE PATTERN

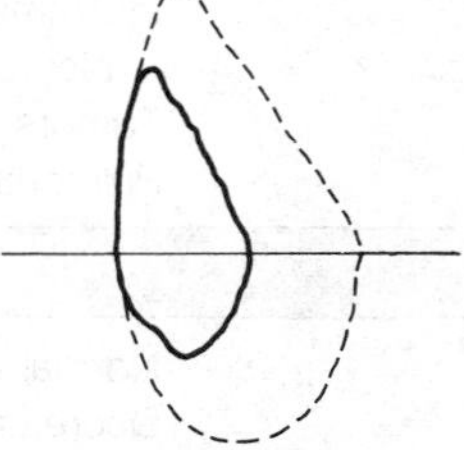

The entire loop resembles a miniature normal flow-volume loop. The FVC is markedly reduced. The expiratory curve shows a straight line decrease in flow with decreasing lung volumes. Peak flow rates may be normal, increased, or decreased, depending on the degree of respiratory impairment.

*The dotted lines represent the boundaries of the normal flow-volume loop.

◄ ***Figure 36–13***

Flow volume loop patterns for obstructive and restrictive disease. (From Kersten, L. D., et al. [1989]. *Respiratory nursing* [p. 382]. Philadelphia: W. B. Saunders.)

piece, causing displacement of air or water. Flow volume loops can be created as visual patterns. Normal loop spirograms and spirogram patterns with obstructive and restrictive disorders are shown in Figure 36–13.

Clients with obstructive diseases will have decreased FEV_t (forced expiratory volume; subscript *t* is number of seconds). The client can still exhale, but because of the nature of the disease, exhalation takes much longer, compared with exhalation of air from a normal lung. Restrictive diseases cause a decreased FEV, because lung volumes are decreased. The FEV_t/FVC will be normal to increased in the client with restrictive disorders.

Lung mechanics are a reflection of the efficacy of the lung's bellow function. Typically with obstructive lung disorders, chest bellow function is impaired and the client is dyspneic. Home testing of peak flow is commonly performed by clients with asthma.

Lung mechanics are measured before and after administration of beta-adrenergic agents. Reversible lung disease is said to be present if a 15 per cent change in the FVC, FEV_t, and $FEF_{25-75\%}$ is noted.

Diffusion. Studies of the diffusing capacity of the lung (DL or DLCO) measure gas transfer of carbon monoxide across the alveolar capillary membrane. The DL indicates the ease with which carbon monoxide diffuses across the alveolar capillary membrane and can bind with hemoglobin. (Remember that hemoglobin has 210 times greater affinity for carbon monoxide than for oxygen.) With a normal hemoglobin and normal ventilatory function, the only limiting factor to diffusion of carbon monoxide is the alveolar capillary membrane.

A single breath method is most commonly used. The client inhales a mixture of gases, holds the breath for 10 seconds, and exhales; a sample of the exhaled air is collected for analysis. The equipment necessary to perform the diffusion test is expensive and therefore not commonly used, even though useful information is obtained.

Decreases in the DL indicate the presence of a diffusion defect. Disorders such as pulmonary fibrosis, anemia, and chronic airflow limitations (emphysema) decrease the DL. An increased DL is found during exercise, polycythemia, and hypervolemia.

PULSE OXIMETRY

Pulse oximetry combines the principles of plethysmography and spectrophotometry to measure arterial oxygen saturation noninvasively. The pulse oximeter (Fig.

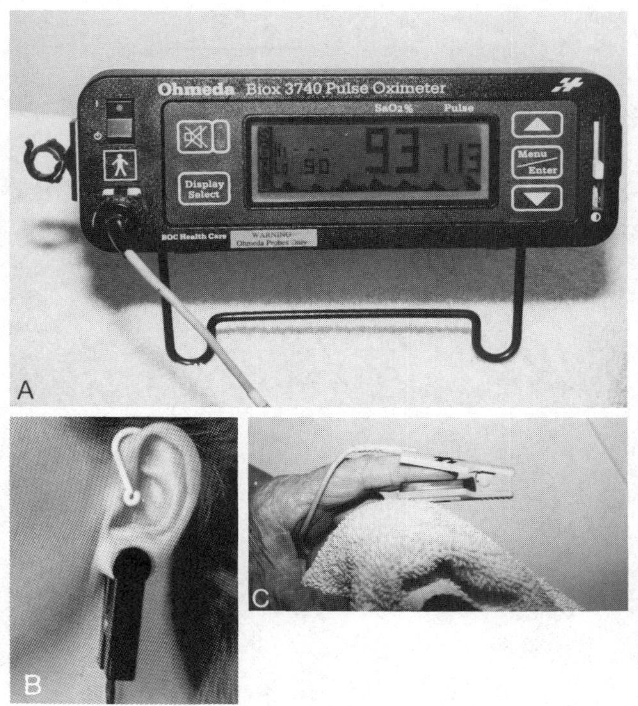

▲ **Figure 36-14**

Oximetry. Noninvasive monitoring of SaO_2 (oxygen saturation) is done with a pulse oximeter. This unit (*A*) has an ear probe and a finger probe. The ear probe (*B*) is used during measurements of oxygen saturation while exercising. The finger probe (*C*) is most frequently used for stationary measurements. (Courtesy of Ohmeda, Boulder, CO.)

36-14) passes a beam of light through the tissue, and a sensor measures the amount of light absorbed by the oxygen-saturated hemoglobin. Arterial saturations have a close correlation with the saturations obtained from the pulse oximeter if the arterial saturation is above 70 per cent. The following provides a quick guide for comparison of oxygen saturation and PaO_2:

Oxygen saturation	PaO_2
50%	25 mm Hg
75%	40 mm Hg
90%	55 mm Hg

Limitations with pulse oximetry are still present despite the advancement of the technology. Hypotension, hypothermia, and vasoconstriction reduce arterial blood flow, and movement of the finger interferes with the interpretation of the oxygen saturation.

CAPNOGRAPHY

Capnography, another noninvasive procedure, is the measurement of exhaled carbon dioxide concentrations. The amount of carbon dioxide found in exhaled air—end tidal carbon dioxide ($etCO_2$)—correlates very closely with the arterial carbon dioxide ($PaCO_2$) in clients with normal respiratory, cardiovascular, and metabolic function. The normal gradient of $PaCO_2$–$etCO_2$ is approximately 5 mm Hg. As the $PaCO_2$ increases with hypoventilation, or decreases with hyperventilation, associated changes will be noted in the $etCO_2$. Capnography requires a continuous sampling of exhaled air.

VENTILATION/PERFUSION SCANNING (LUNG SCAN)

Ventilation/perfusion scanning is used to assess lung ventilation and lung perfusion. This scan is often called a V/Q scan. V/Q scans are valuable in diagnosing pulmonary embolism, pulmonary infarction, emphysema, fibrosis, or bronchiectasis. Quantitative perfusion scans may be helpful in preoperative assessment of clients for surgical resection of thoracic malignancy. The test has two parts (done together or separately): (1) assessing the pulmonary vasculature (perfusion scan) and (2) assessing the distribution of ventilation (ventilation scan).

- *Perfusion scan.* Radioactive dye is injected intravenously and carried into the pulmonary vasculature. Decreased blood flow to any part of the lung is revealed as a decrease in the amount of radioactivity shown on either x-ray film with use of a rectilinear scanner or on Polaroid film with use of a gamma or scintillation camera. Scanning is done in both the anterior and posterior views.
- *Ventilation scan.* Radioactive gas is inhaled, which produces an image of the areas where ventilation is occurring. Assessment of the pattern of deposition of radioactive gas in the alveoli is also possible.

Ventilation images are compared with the pictures taken during the perfusion scan. There should be an equal amount of radioactivity discernible on both ventilation and perfusion pictures. If there are areas in which there is ventilation but little or no perfusion, a pulmonary embolus is suspected (Fig. 36-15). Further assessment may be needed. If there is doubt as to the cause of impaired perfusion, pulmonary angiography may be needed.

There is no specific preparation for a lung scan. With the exception of local discomfort from the injection of radioactive dye, the procedure is painless.

Diagnostic Tests to Evaluate the Anatomy

The following diagnostic procedures are used to assess the anatomy: (1) chest radiography; (2) ultrasonography; (3) fluoroscopy; (4) computed tomography (CT scan); (5) bronchoscopy; (6) pulmonary angiogram; and (7) gallium scan.

CHEST X-RAY STUDIES

Chest x-ray studies provide information about the chest that may not be available through other assessment means. Also, they often graphically illustrate the cause of respiratory dysfunction. Chest films may reveal abnormalities when there are no physical signs or symptoms of pulmonary disease.

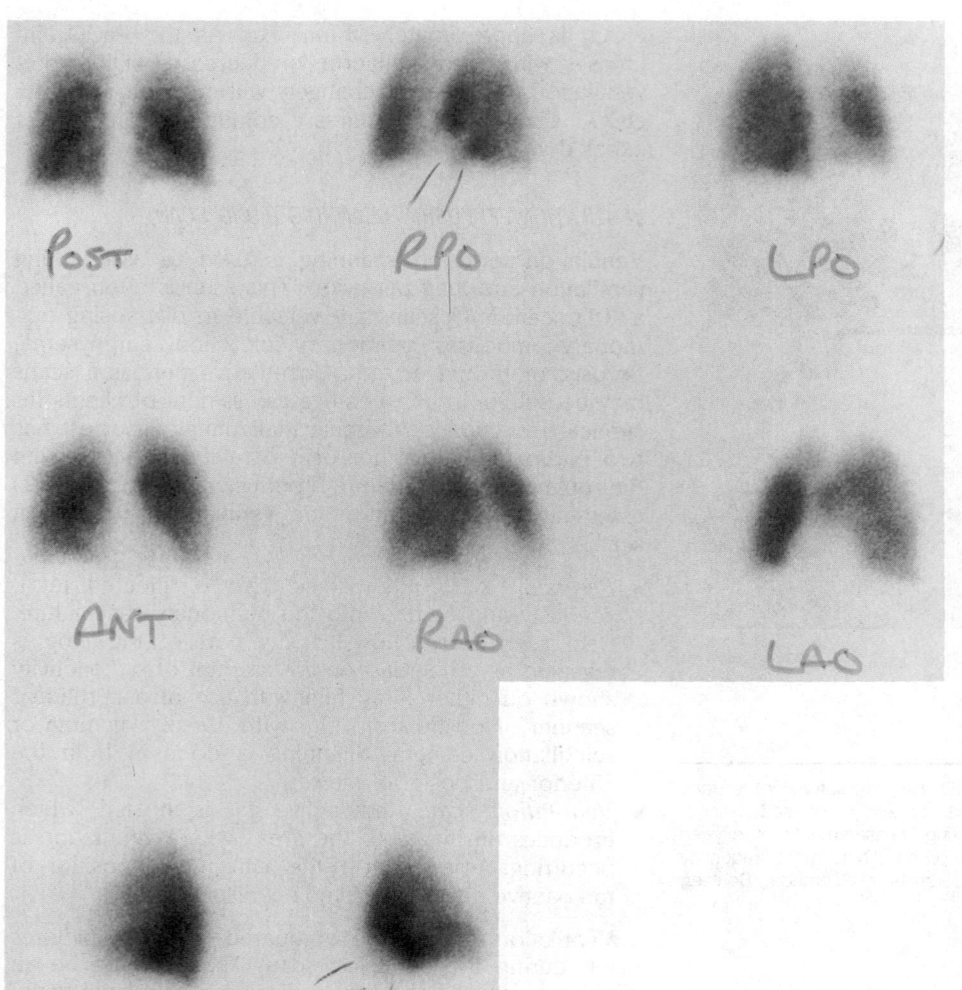

▲ *Figure 36 – 15*

Ventilation-perfusion scan with technetium 99m. Upright radionuclide pulmonary perfusion study indicating perfusion deficit of the right posterior basilar segment, suggesting a pulmonary embolism or pneumonia. This client had a pulmonary venogram (see Fig. 39–19 of venogram in Chap. 39) that did document a PE.

Chest films show the bony structures (e.g., ribs, sternum, clavicles, scapulae, and upper portion of the humerus). The vertebral column is visible vertically through the middle of the thorax. The two hemidiaphragms normally appear rounded, smooth, and sharply defined, with the right hemidiaphragm slightly elevated above the left. The junction of the rib cage and the diaphragm, called the costophrenic angle, is normally clearly visible and angled. Heart tissue is dense and appears white but less intensely white than bony structures. The heart shadow is normally clearly outlined and extends primarily onto the left side of the thorax and occupies no more than one third of the chest width. Close observation shows the trachea in the upper middle chest almost superimposed over the cervical and thoracic vertebrae. The trachea bifurcates at the level of the fourth thoracic vertebra into the right and left mainstem bronchi. The pulmonary blood vessels, bronchi, and lymph nodes are located in the hilum on both the right and left sides of the midthorax. Lung tissue appears black on x-ray film. Vascular lung structures are visible as white, thin, wispy strings fanning out from the hilum (Fig. 36 – 16).

Chest x-ray studies may be taken (1) as part of routine screening procedures, (2) when pulmonary disease is suspected, (3) to monitor the status of respiratory disorders and abnormalities (e.g., pleural effusion, atelectasis, and tuberculous cavitary lesions), (4) to confirm endotracheal or tracheostomy tube placement, (5) after traumatic chest injury, or (6) in any other situation in which radiographic information helps the management of a respiratory problem.

Standard Radiographic Positions. Routine adult chest x-ray studies are taken with the client standing or sitting facing the x-ray film, with the chest and shoulders in direct contact with the film cassette. The shoulders are rotated forward to pull the scapulae away from the lung field. The x-ray cathode penetrates from the posterior. This position is called the posteroanterior (PA) position. The radiograph is usually taken at full inspiration, which causes the diaphragm to move downward. Radiographs taken on expiration are sometimes requested for demonstrating the degree of diaphragm movement or for assisting in the assessment and diagnosis of pneumothorax.

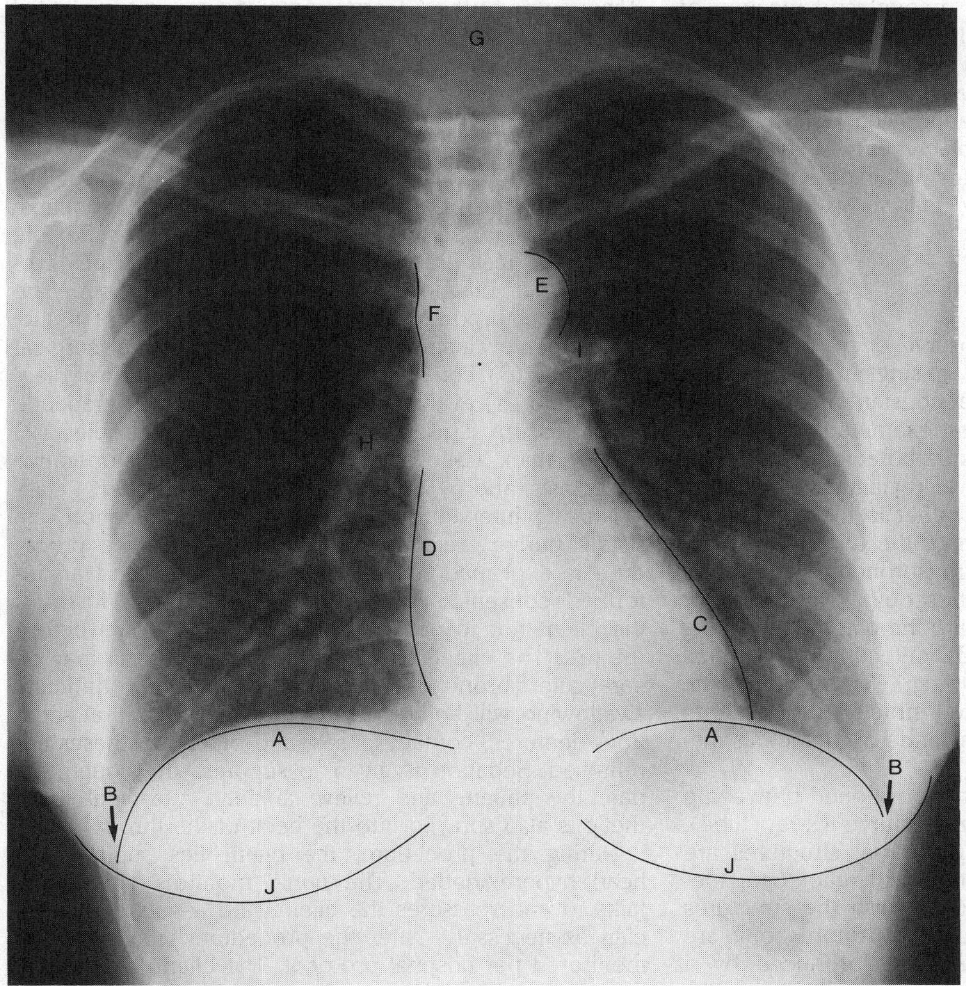

▲ **Figure 36–16**

This is a normal chest x-ray study taken from a posteroanterior view (PA). The backward L in the upper right corner is placed on the film to indicate the client's left side of the chest. Some anatomic structures can be seen on the x-ray study. A, diaphragm; B, costophrenic angle; C, left ventricle; D, right atrium; E, aortic arch; F, superior vena cava; G, trachea; H, right bronchus; I, left bronchus; and J, breast shadows.

For clients unable to be transported to the radiology department, a portable chest radiograph may be taken. Portable radiographs are usually taken with the film placed behind the client, and the x-ray beam penetrates from the front of the chest—the anteroposterior (AP) position. Because the x-ray beam enters from the anterior chest, the heart will appear larger than it really is and larger than on a PA view.

Other positions include

- lateral view, which usually accompanies a standard PA view. It is taken from either the right or left side of the chest. The arms are raised above the head, and the side of the chest is placed against the film. The lateral view allows better visualization of the heart and the diaphragm dome. When used in conjunction with a PA film, a lateral position gives a three-dimensional view, allowing more specific identification of an abnormality's location.
- lateral decubitus position, which may be used when it is necessary to determine whether opaque areas on the pleura are due to solid or liquid media. This view is taken with the client lying on either the right or left side, depending on which side of the chest is being assessed. In a left lateral decubitus position, the client is lying on the left side. The term "decubitus" refers to a "lying-down" position.
- oblique position, which is used to see behind and around underlying structures. The shoulders are rotated either to the right or left of the film. By turning the client, the angle at which the x-ray beam passes through the chest is shifted. In a right oblique position, the right side is closest to the film. The view may be taken from either an anterior or posterior position.
- lordotic positions, which are useful if clearer visualization of the upper lung fields is needed. The angle of the x-ray cathode is lowered and the beam directed at an upward angle. This angle removes the clavicles and first and second ribs from the field of vision.

ULTRASONOGRAPHY

Ultrasonic waves (sound waves too high in frequency for a human ear to detect) are used diagnostically to assess various body structures. The waves are directed at the organ or structure, and as they vibrate back from the target, they are transduced into oscilloscope tracings. Sonography may be used in conjunction with other pulmonary diagnostic procedures such as thoracentesis or pleural biopsy to assess fluid or fibrotic abnormalities. Ultrasonography is especially helpful and very accurate in detecting the amount and location of 50 ml or less of pleural fluid. In comparison, a positive detection by chest radiography requires at least 500 ml of liquid. If the technique is used in combination with thoracentesis, the ultrasonographer can determine the best location for the needle placement as well as the depth of the fluid. This facilitates obtaining an adequate amount of fluid for laboratory analysis without unnecessary puncturing and probing.

FLUOROSCOPY

Fluoroscopy uses x-rays to observe deep structures in motion. Instead of producing a single, still image, a fluoroscopy screen registers a constant image of the chest (or other body part) being examined. This makes it possible for the chest and intrathoracic structures to be observed while they function dynamically. Fluoroscopy is not used routinely but rather in those situations in which continual observation of the thorax is an advantage (e.g., to observe the transbronchial passage of biopsy forceps during a bronchoscopy). Other uses for fluoroscopy include (1) observing the diaphragm during inspiration and expiration, (2) detecting mediastinal movement during deep breathing, (3) assessing the heart, blood vessels, and related structures, (4) identifying esophageal abnormalities, and (5) detecting mediastinal masses.

In a darkened room, a client is positioned between a fluorescent screen and an x-ray source (x-ray tube), and the images of the moving internal structures are projected on a screen. Sometimes a radiopaque medium is administered to help distinguish the structures being assessed. Images projected by fluoroscopy are not as clear and definitive as those produced by a standard chest film. However, if abnormalities are discovered, still photographs and cinefluorography may be done for a permanent record. Cinefluorographs are motion pictures that allow more leisurely study and re-study of the area photographed, without exposure of either radiology personnel or the client to unnecessary radiation.

COMPUTED TOMOGRAPHY

Computed tomography (CT), also called CAT scan, provides more sophisticated tomography than is possible with conventional x-ray equipment. By using a computer to regulate the layers or "slices" of tissue examined, the camera rotates in a circular pattern, and three-dimensional assessment of the thorax (or other body area) is possible. Still photographs are taken at each level. CT is able to visualize most abnormalities, but small early lesions may be missed.

Often CT studies are done before and after the intravenous administration of a contrast containing a radioactively tagged iodine isotope. If a contrast is used, it is extremely important to find out whether the client is allergic to iodine or shellfish.

CT scans are particularly helpful in diagnosing peripheral (e.g., pleural) or mediastinal disorders. Special techniques can be used to view pulmonary nodules. "Thin cuts" of the CT are used in diagnosing interstitial lung disorders such as pulmonary fibrosis and bronchiectasis.

BRONCHOSCOPY

Bronchoscopy is the passage of a lighted bronchoscope into the bronchial tree (Fig. 36-17). Bronchoscopy may be performed with rigid steel or flexible fiberoptic instruments. Bronchoscopy may be performed for diagnostic or therapeutic purposes. The diagnostic purposes include (1) examination of tissue, (2) further evaluation of a tumor for potential surgical resection, (3) collection of tissue specimens for diagnosis, and (4) evaluation of bleeding sites. Therapeutic bronchoscopy is used to (1) remove foreign bodies, (2) remove thick, viscous secretions, (3) treat postoperative atelectasis, and (4) destroy and remove lesions.

Nursing interventions include client preparation, assisting during the study, and observation. The procedure is explained to the client and family and an informed consent is obtained. The nurse also instructs the client not to eat or drink anything 6 hours before the test. The client is told that his or her throat may be sore after bronchoscopy, and some initial difficulty swallowing will be present. Before preprocedural sedation, dentures, contact lenses, and other prostheses are removed. Sedation is given to suppress the cough, sedate the patient, and relieve anxiety. A topical anesthetic is also sprayed into the back of the throat.

During the procedure, the client lies supine with head hyperextended. The nurse monitors vital signs, talks to and reassures the client, and assists the physician as necessary. After the procedure, vital signs are monitored per hospital protocol. The client is observed for signs of respiratory distress including dyspnea, changes in respiratory rate, use of accessory muscles, and changes in or absent lung sounds. Expectorated secretions are inspected for evidence of any hemoptysis. Nothing is given by mouth until the cough and swallow reflexes have returned, which is usually in 1 to 2 hours. Once the client can swallow, feeding may begin with ice chips and small sips of water. Lung sounds are monitored for 24 hours. Development of adventitious sounds should be reported to the physician.

ALVEOLAR LAVAGE

Sterile saline can be injected during bronchoscopy to wash tissues. The saline is aspirated and examined for atypical cells. Alveolar lavage may be used in the diagnosis of interstitial lung disease, sarcoidosis, hypersensitivity pneumonitis, and *Pneumocystis carini* pneumonia.

THORASCOPY

Thorascopy is a new diagnostic procedure that is an alternative to open lung biopsy and thoracotomy for pleural surface disorders. Typically, three small incisions are made into the middle chest wall. A camera is

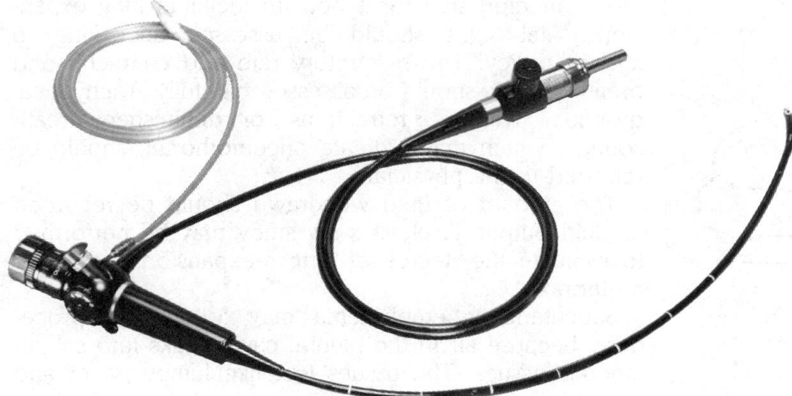

▲ Figure 36-17

A flexible fiberoptic bronchoscope. (Courtesy of The Olympus Corporation, New Hyde Park, NY.)

inserted through the first incision to inspect tissue, and tissues are manipulated and biopsied through the other incisions. A chest tube is inserted to promote lung reexpansion.

Advantages of the procedure include reduced anesthesia time, less pain, and shortened hospital stay. In addition, biopsies may be obtained from the lower lobes, which are not routinely biopsied during open lung biopsy procedures.

PULMONARY ANGIOGRAPHY

Sometimes the vascular structure of the thorax may need to be assessed. Angiography and other procedures designed to examine specific vascular structures (i.e., aortography for the aorta) all use similar techniques. A contrast is injected into the vascular system through an indwelling catheter. During pulmonary angiography, the catheter may be inserted either peripherally or directly into the main pulmonary artery or one of its branches. The contrast is injected while cinefluorographs or still photographs are taken. (Pulmonary angiography is shown in Fig. 39-19.)

Pulmonary angiography may be done to (1) detect congenital abnormalities of the pulmonary vascular tree, (2) detect abnormalities of the pulmonary venous circulation, (3) assess acquired diseases of the pulmonary arterial and venous circulation (e.g., primary pulmonary arterial hypertension), (4) assess the destructive effects of emphysema, (5) investigate the potential benefit of resection for bronchogenic carcinoma, (6) assess peripheral pulmonary lesions, and (7) assess the extent of thromboembolism in the lungs.

As with any procedure in which a catheter is inserted into the peripheral or central vasculature, it is important after the procedure to observe the site of catheter entry for infection, hematoma formation, or local reaction to contrast media. Continue to observe for signs of adverse reaction to contrast media (e.g., increasing respiratory distress, hypotension, stridor, and other indications of anaphylaxis).

MAGNETIC RESONANCE IMAGING

Magnetic resonance imaging (MRI) is the use of magnetic fields rather than radiation to create images of body structures. MRI has limited usefulness in pulmonary assessment. It may be used to diagnose chest wall invasion by peripheral lung cancer.

GALLIUM SCAN

This type of scan is usually done 24 to 48 hours after an intravenous injection of radioactive gallium citrate is administered. Many organs take up radioactive gallium, and so do some tumors and inflammations. An example of the use of gallium scan is in differentiating embolism from pneumonitis as the cause of infiltrate on a chest radiograph. Gallium has an affinity for areas of inflammation such as those caused by pneumonia. However, there is little inflammation involved in a nonseptic pulmonary embolism. Therefore, gallium accumulates around pneumonitis but not around a pulmonary embolism. The usefulness of gallium scanning in clinical pulmonary assessment is limited.

Specimens

The following procedures are used for the recovery and analysis of pulmonary specimens: (1) thoracentesis, (2) biopsy, and (3) sputum collection.

THORACENTESIS

Thoracentesis is the drainage of fluid or air found in the pleural space. Therapeutic thoracentesis will remove an accumulation of pleural fluid or air that has caused lung compression and respiratory distress. When the main goal is to determine the cause of an infection or empyema, diagnostic thoracentesis is performed. The fluid collected is sent to the laboratory and assessed for specific gravity, glucose, protein, pH, culture, sensitivity study, and cytology. The color and consistency of the pleural fluid are also documented.

Before thoracentesis, the client is prepared and positioned. The client is instructed about the importance of holding still during the procedure. Sudden movement may force the needle through the pleural space and injure the visceral pleura or lung parenchyma.

Figure 36-18 is an example of appropriate position-

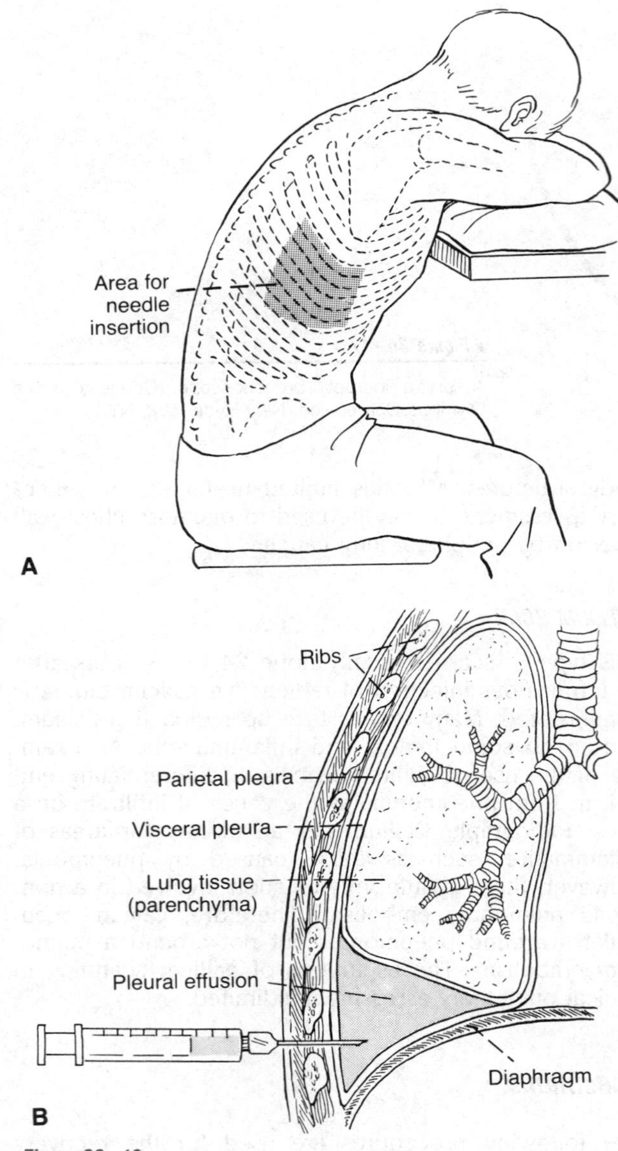

▲ *Figure 36–18*

A, Thoracentesis position. Arms are raised and crossed. Head rests on folded arms. This position allows the chest wall to be pulled outward in an expanded position. If an overbed table is not available, the arms may be left down but positioned forward of the hips or crossed in front of the chest. *B* shows the usual site for the insertion of a thoracentesis needle for a right-sided effusion. The actual site varies with each client, depending on the location and volume of the effusion. The physician tries to keep the needle as far away from the diaphragm as possible while at the same time inserting the needle close to the base of the effusion so that gravity can help with drainage.

ing during thoracentesis. With the client in the upright position, pleural fluid accumulates in the base of the thorax. An alternative is to place the client in a recumbent position with his or her arm resting under the head. During the procedure, assist the physician; monitor vital signs; and observe for dyspnea, complaints of difficulty breathing, nausea, or pain.

After the procedure, the client is usually turned onto the unaffected side for 1 hour to facilitate lung expansion. Vital signs should be assessed according to agency policy. The respiratory rate and character and breath sounds should be assessed carefully. Tachypnea, dyspnea, cyanosis, retractions, or diminished breath sounds, which may indicate pneumothorax, should be reported to the physician.

The amount of fluid withdrawn should be recorded as fluid output. A chest x-ray study may be performed to evaluate the degree of lung reexpansion and pneumothorax.

Subcutaneous emphysema may follow this procedure, because air in the pleural cavity leaks into subcutaneous tissues. The tissues feel like lumpy paper and crackle when palpated (crepitus). Usually subcutaneous emphysema causes no problem unless it is increasing and constricting vital organs (e.g., trachea). The client often needs reassurance about this disorder.

If the client has pleural effusion due to a malignancy, cytotoxic medications may be inserted into the pleural space after thoracentesis. Some of these agents burn, and others require the client to roll about in order to have the medication coat the entire pleural space. The nurse will need to review the interventions used with the various medications.

BIOPSY

Biopsy specimens may be taken from various respiratory tissues for assessment. As previously mentioned, biopsy of tracheobronchial structures may be performed during bronchoscopy. Biopsies of scalene and mediastinal nodes may be done (with local anesthesia) to obtain tissue for pathogenic analysis by culture or cytologic assessment.

Pleural biopsies may be performed surgically through a small thoracotomy incision or during thoracentesis, with use of a Cope needle. Needle biopsy is a relatively safe, simple diagnostic procedure useful in determining the cause of pleural effusions. The needle removes a small fragment of parietal pleura, which is used for microscopic cellular examination and culture. If bacteriologic studies are needed, the biopsy specimen should be obtained before chemotherapy is begun.

The preparation and positioning of a client for pleural biopsy is similar to that for thoracentesis. Rare complications include (1) temporary pain from intercostal nerve injury, (2) pneumothorax, and (3) hemothorax. After the biopsy procedure, observe for indications of complications (e.g., dyspnea, pallor, diaphoresis, excessive pain). There is a possibility of the development of pneumothorax associated with needle biopsy. Chest tubes and chest drainage equipment must be available. Follow-up chest x-ray studies are usually taken after the procedure. The development of hemothorax is indicated by a substantial increase in fluid in the pleural space and requires immediate thoracentesis.

As with pleural biopsy, lung biopsy may be done by (1) surgical exposure of the lung (open lung biopsy) or (2) using a needle designed to remove a core of lung tissue. Tissue is then examined for abnormal cellular structure and bacteria. Lung biopsies are most often done to identify pulmonary tumors or parenchymal changes (e.g., sarcoidosis).

Needle puncture (aspiration) biopsy of chest lesions is done under fluoroscopy. After a lesion is found on a chest x-ray study and localized under fluoroscopy, topical anesthesia is administered, and the needle is inserted through the chest wall into the lung tissue and lesion. A small sample of cells is aspirated for microscopic study, and the needle is withdrawn. Aspiration biopsy may enable definitive diagnosis of malignant neoplasms, granulomas, or other nonmalignant growths. Possible complications of needle aspiration lung biopsy are hemoptysis, hemothorax, and pneumothorax. After the procedure, examine any sputum closely for evidence of blood. Observe for respiratory distress (may indicate pneumothorax). Monitor vital signs, breath sounds, skin color, and temperature.

SPUTUM COLLECTION

Normally, the goblet cells produce 100 ml of mucus a day, but an infectious process can lead to excessive mucus production, commonly called sputum. Assessment of sputum for bacteria, fungus, or cellular elements assists the practitioner in treating the underlying infection. The sputum is initially inspected for color, quantity, quality, presence of blood, food particles, or other unusual contents. If possible, sputum should be collected before antimicrobial treatment is begun. Acid-fast smear and culture specimens are collected in the morning, at which time it is more plentiful and concentrated from pooling through the night. Sputum can be collected by the direct method or the indirect method, or by gastric lavage.

To obtain a specimen by the direct method the client first brushes the teeth to reduce contamination, then he or she coughs into a sputum specimen container. The client should be encouraged to cough and not spit so as to obtain sputum. Sputum can be thinned by inhaling nebulized saline or water.

Indirect techniques to obtain sputum use a sterile suction catheter with a sputum trap attached to the catheter. Sputum can be obtained by transtracheal aspiration also. A puncture is made with a needle through the cricothyroid membrane into the trachea, and sputum is aspirated.

Gastric lavage is not a common technique to obtain sputum but can be used in uncooperative or extremely ill clients. Lavage is based on the assumption that sputum is swallowed while sleeping and sometimes after coughing. A nasogastric tube is inserted using appropriate techniques. Gastric juice is aspirated with a syringe and sent to the laboratory. The tube is then removed.

Once collected, the sputum is sent to the laboratory for Gram stain, culture, and sensitivity study. The Gram stain classifies the bacteria as gram-positive or gram-negative and provides guidelines for appropriate antimicrobial therapy, along with the sputum culture. After the Gram stain, the sputum is incubated for 24 hours on the appropriate culture medium and studied by a microbiologist. The culture allows further identification of the infecting organism. Once the organism is identified, its sensitivity to antibiotic treatment will be tested and appropriate antibiotic therapy prescribed.

Identification of organisms that cause tuberculosis and similar diseases (acid-fast bacilli) requires tests other than the Gram stain, culture, and sensitivity study. Regardless of the technique used to obtain the specimen, the nurse notes the color, consistency, odor, and amount of sputum obtained.

NOSE AND THROAT CULTURES

Bacteria in the nose and throat can be identified by culture during assessment of the upper airway. Some bacteria are normally present (e.g., streptococci, staphylococci, pneumococci, *Haemophilus influenzae,* and *Klebsiella pneumoniae*). Other organisms are abnormal (e.g., those causing diphtheria or tuberculosis).

Take a swab from the nose and throat using a sterile cotton swab. Place the swab in a sterile culture tube. Some laboratories require the swab to be suspended in a tube containing 2 ml of fluid (to keep air in the tube moist and prevent evaporation and drying of the specimen). The fluid is not a culture medium, so the swab should *not* touch the fluid. If Loeffler's medium is used in the tube (i.e., if diphtheria is suspected), the medium should touch the swab. When culture tubes without fluid are used, take the specimen to the laboratory immediately, where the swab is streaked across a culture plate.

Summary

Respiratory assessment begins with obtaining a thorough client history. One of the most essential aspects of history taking is to determine the degree of dyspnea and the impact it has on activities of daily living. The client's smoking history should also be noted, because it is a common risk factor for respiratory disorders. The chest is inspected for obvious deformity and shape. Percussion, palpation, and auscultation assist in locating areas of possible fluid accumulation or consolidation that interfere with breathing.

Chest x-ray studies, bronchoscopy, pulmonary function tests, and arterial blood gases are common diagnostic assessments. The nurse teaches the client about the diagnostic assessment and monitors for potential complications after the study.

Bibliography

1. Bates, B. (1991). *A guide to physical assessment and history taking* (5th ed.). Philadelphia: J. B. Lippincott.
2. Cherniack, R. M., & Cherniack, L. (1983). *Respiration in health and disease* (3rd ed.). Philadelphia: W. B. Saunders.
3. Comroe, J. H. (1974). *Physiology of respiration* (2nd ed.). Chicago: Year Book.
4. Gift, A. G. & Nield, M. D. (1991). Dyspnea: A case for nursing diagnosis status. *Nursing Diagnosis, 2* (2), 66–71.

5. Guyton, A. C. (1986). *Textbook of medical physiology* (7th ed.). Philadelphia: W. B. Saunders.
6. Jarvis, C. (1992). *Physical examination and health assessment.* Philadelphia: W. B. Saunders.
7. Kersten, L. D. (1989). *Comprehensive respiratory nursing.* Philadelphia: W. B. Saunders.
8. Loudon, R., & Murphy, R. L. (1984). State of the art: lung sounds. *American Review of Respiratory Diseases, 130* (4), 663–673.
9. McCord, M., & Cronin-Stubbs, D. (1992). Operationalizing dypsnea: Focus on measurement. *Heart & Lung, 21* (2), 167.
10. Mikami, R., et al. (1987). International symposium on lung sounds. *Chest, 92* (2), 342–345.
11. Murray, J. F. (1986). *The normal lung* (2nd ed.). Philadelphia: W. B. Saunders.
12. Murray, J. F., & Nadel, J. A. (1988). *The textbook of respiratory medicine.* Philadelphia: W. B. Saunders.
13. Pontoppidan, H., et al. (1973). *Acute respiratory failure in the adult.* Boston: Little, Brown.
14. Ruppel, G. (1991). *Manual of pulmonary function testing* (4th ed.). St. Louis: Mosby.
15. Rutherford, K. A. (1989). Principles and application of oximetry. *Critical Care Nursing Clinics of North America, 1* (4), 649–657.
16. Sanchez, F. (1986). Fundamentals of chest x-ray interpretation. *Critical Care Nurse, 6* (5), 41–61.
17. Shapiro, B. A., et al. (1991). *Clinical application of respiratory care* (4th ed.). Chicago: Year Book.
18. Shapiro, B. A., et al. (1989). *Clinical application of blood gases* (4th ed.). Chicago: Year Book.
19. University of Washington, School of Medicine (1989). *The respiratory system.* Seattle, WA: Health Sciences Academic Services.
20. Von Rueden, K. T. (1990). Noninvasive assessment of gas exchange in the critically ill. *AACN Clinical Issues in Critical Care Nursing, 1* (2), 239–247.
21. West, J. B. (1990). *Respiratory physiology* (4th ed.). Baltimore: Williams & Wilkins.

Chapter 37

Common Respiratory Interventions

Some interventions to help clients experiencing respiratory problems are implemented by nurses. Others are performed by specifically trained therapists (who may or may not be nurses). It is important for nurses to understand the interventions administered by other health care professionals as well as the interventions that are specifically nursing procedures.

Intervention for respiratory problems is based on careful assessment (see Chap. 36). The most appropriate intervention is chosen for each client after consideration of both physical and psychosocial factors. Usually, the least invasive interventions, such as coughing and deep breathing, are tried before more invasive procedures (e.g., endotracheal suctioning). The sequence of this chapter moves from the least invasive respiratory interventions (e.g., positioning, hydration) to the most invasive interventions (e.g., endotracheal intubation, mechanical ventilation).

GENERAL INTERVENTIONS

Positioning and Posture

Clients with respiratory problems can usually breathe more comfortably if they are positioned so that the head and chest are elevated. Elevating the chest and head promotes expansion of the lungs and increases the efficiency of the respiratory muscles. Instructing the client to rotate the shoulders backward will enable unrestricted movement of the diaphragm, thus facilitating diaphragmatic breathing. A semi-Fowler's position may be suitable for those clients with moderate respiratory distress. To position a dyspneic client correctly in bed, place a pillow lengthwise behind the back and head. Do not flex the head forward with another pillow. A client who is weak or severely dyspneic is often most comfortable sitting upright leaning on a padded overbed table (Fig. 37-1 *A* to *C*). By resting the arms on the table, the client will increase the effectiveness of the secondary inspiratory muscles. While standing, clients with chronic respiratory disorders can often breathe most effectively by maintaining a straight posture leaning slightly forward (Fig. 37-1*D*).

Environmental Control

The single most important cause of respiratory irritation is cigarette smoke. Chronic pulmonary diseases (e.g., chronic bronchitis, pulmonary emphysema) and lung cancer are major health problems that are adversely affected by air pollution and cigarette smoking. When caring for clients with respiratory disorders, keep the environment as pollutant-free as possible. This intervention has been greatly aided with the promotion of "smoke free" health care facilities.

Activity and Rest

Some respiratory problems force clients to alter their normal activities of daily living (ADLs). Certain acute disorders (e.g., influenza) require bed rest for several days before normal activity is resumed. Clients experiencing chronic respiratory disorders may need to permanently modify their ADLs, change to sedentary work, or even retire. Remaining active for as long as possible is physically as well as psychosocially helpful for clients who suffer from chronic respiratory disorders. Encourage and facilitate activity and ambulation within the limits of the client's abilities and the physician's recommendations.

Adequate rest is extremely important but may be difficult to obtain because of distressing symptoms (e.g., dyspnea, coughing). When possible, identify and correct conditions that are disturbing rest (e.g., positioning, humidification, sleep interruptions [awakened to cough, void, take medications]). Cough suppressant medication may be prescribed to help ensure a restful night.

Oral Hygiene

Most clients with breathing difficulty breathe through their mouth. Mouth breathing dries the oral mucosa, and dry mucosa increases the risk of stomatitis. Coughing is common in this population of clients, and sputum

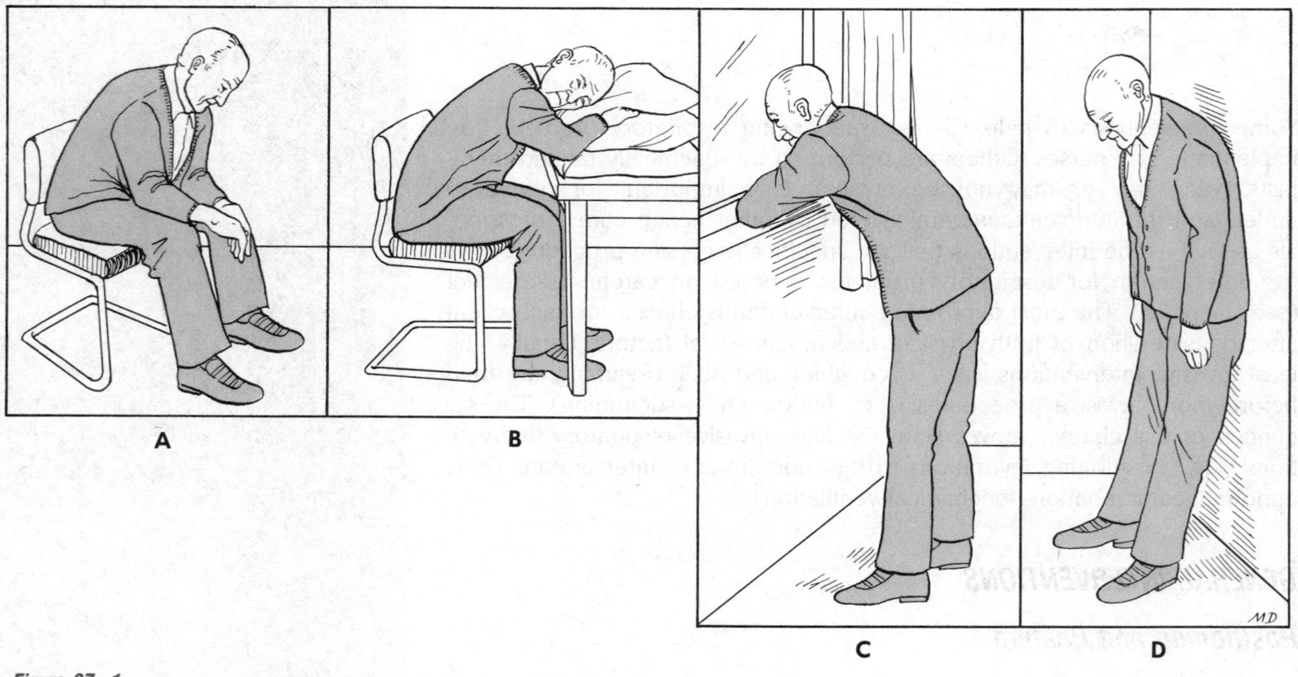

▲ **Figure 37-1**

Dyspnea positions, which facilitate breathing and conserve energy. They can be easily assumed anywhere without causing undue notice. *A*, Relaxed sitting position leaning over knees. *B*, Sitting and leaning forward (important to keep thoracic and lumbar spine straight and not "collapse" chest). *C*, Forward lean in a standing position. *D*, Relaxed standing position with weight placed on hips and legs.

may dry to the oral mucosa. For these reasons, thorough oral hygiene is important for clients with respiratory problems. It may improve appetite and promote a general feeling of well being. Cleaning the mouth temporarily removes the unpleasant taste and odor of sputum. The use of antiseptic mouthwash helps to reduce the number of pathogens in the oral cavity, thus helping to prevent infection. Oral hygiene is essential after the administration of aerosolized mucolytics, steroids, antibiotics, and enzymes because these medications may interfere with the balance of normal flora that prevents infection. Gas-forming foods (e.g., beans, cabbage) are undesirable because they produce abdominal distention, which may lead to decreased ventilation.

Hydration

Optimal hydration (1) helps liquefy bronchopulmonary secretions for easier removal (thick, tenacious secretions are difficult to cough up and expectorate) and (2) prevents constipation and fluid imbalances. Encourage a client with tenacious secretions to take 3000 to 4000 ml of fluid a day. Before encouraging a client to drink this much water, be certain the client has no pre-existing cardiac or renal disorders that might impair fluid excretion. A client confined to bed needs fresh fluids that are within easy reach. Document fluid intake and output.

Infection Prevention and Control

Opportunistic infections are of increasing importance. These may be drug-induced or nosocomial. Superinfections occur when drugs used to treat an infection also destroy the body's normal flora. In the absence of this natural protection, a secondary or superinfection may develop. Also, infection may develop in clients receiving drugs that suppress the immune system, such as corticosteroids or chemotherapeutic agents. Nosocomial infections include those acquired from contaminated equipment, e.g., suction catheters, aerosol generators, room humidifiers, and other respiratory equipment. Nosocomial infections from contaminated equipment indicate serious error in technique. To control infection or prevent its development, employ prophylactic measures such as

- using proper handwashing with a bacteriostatic soap
- observing universal precautions to prevent cross-contamination
- turning and repositioning clients confined to bed
- encouraging activity, coughing, and deep breathing to mobilize secretions
- maintaining a clear airway
- changing respiratory therapy equipment daily (e.g., aerosol tubes, humidifiers)
- restricting contact with clients having respiratory or other infections
- isolating clients with infectious disorders to reduce spread
- maintaining resistance to disease in clients with respiratory problems by adequate rest, nutrition, and hydration
- providing client education on how to prevent the spread of airborne infections; e.g., cover nose and mouth with disposable tissues when sneezing or coughing, dispose of tissues carefully, wash hands frequently
- assessing for indications of infection in clients receiving chemotherapeutic agents or corticosteroids and for development of superinfections in clients receiving antibiotics
- administering antibiotics as prescribed. Specific antibiotic prescriptions are based on bacteriologic culture and sensitivity reports. Sometimes broad-spectrum antibiotics are prescribed before culture sensitivity reports are available.

Clients with chronic respiratory problems can try to avoid repeated respiratory infections by

- wearing warm, dry, protective clothing while outside in cold or damp weather
- avoiding excessive exertion in very cold or humid environments
- balancing work, rest, and recreation
- avoiding crowded places when respiratory infections are prevalent
- avoiding smoke-filled environments and not smoking
- taking influenza shots and antibiotics as prescribed
- observing sputum for signs of infection (e.g., increased amounts, change in color)
- consulting a physician if a new infection seems to be developing. Even infections that appear "minor" need vigorous treatment to prevent progressive, serious superinfections.

Psychosocial Support

Reducing anxiety is very important because anxiety worsens symptoms such as dyspnea and bronchospasm. Some respiratory conditions produce frightening feelings such as suffocation or choking, causing the client to panic and fight for air. While performing physical interventions, nurses can support and help calm fearful clients. Remember that a client's behavior may be influenced by physical factors. For example, metabolic imbalances such as acid-base imbalances or hypoxia may also cause confusion. Fatigue and physical discomfort caused by the effort of breathing or lack of sleep may make a client irritable and depressed. It is important that the nurse understand this common reaction to stress. Helping families and other significant persons deal appropriately with these coping mechanisms is also important.

Some respiratory symptoms may be disturbing for the client, significant others, and nurses. For example, a client coughing up foul-smelling sputum may feel unclean and embarrassed. Significant others and nurses may feel repulsed when handling contaminated articles or when the client expectorates. This is understandable, but it is important not to express these feelings outwardly in front of the client. Teach the client to dispose of tissues properly and to cover the mouth and nose when coughing.

Many respiratory conditions are difficult to accept and live with (e.g., lung cancer, emphysema). Support the client and significant others in making realistic future plans. For example, whereas the function of severely damaged lungs cannot be permanently or markedly improved, the client may be helped to feel better and become more active. An attitude of hopelessness is self-defeating. With encouragement, symptomatic relief may be achieved even though the prognosis is limited.

Chronic respiratory disease necessitates many changes and adaptations. The goal of care is to preserve and make the most of existing lung function. These limitations are often hard for clients to accept. The acceptance process is an individual one. It may be facilitated by effective therapeutic relationships with nurses and other health care professionals (within health care facilities and in the community). Direct nursing care may be needed as well as referrals to other support services (e.g., social workers, respiratory therapists).

Denial of respiratory symptoms is not unusual until the severity of symptoms eventually forces recognition of the illness by the client and significant others. Even when professional help is sought, some clients resist recommended treatment. Such clients may need extra education to obtain information and planning sessions to experience some control in decision making.

Self-care is essential with respiratory disorders and should start with relieving specific self-care problems in daily living. For example, clients may need to learn more effective ways to control breathing before they can learn about postural drainage and exercises. Self-care activities may include (1) performing postural drainage and breathing exercises, (2) increasing daily fluid intake, (3) taking prescribed medication, and (4) performing specific respiratory therapies. Praise clients who faithfully follow their recommended regimens and encourage those who are unable to do so and who feel discouraged.

Allow clients to develop their own daily routine. Dyspneic clients often need frequent rest periods and usually know when they can be most comfortably active during the day. Clients producing sputum usually know when postural drainage is most effective (e.g., before getting out of bed). Some clients develop ritualistic and apparently compulsive patterns around their daily routines. Do not interfere with these patterns. The client perceives them as useful and necessary.

Whenever possible, include the family in teaching and planning sessions on long-term respiratory intervention. Remember that family members are experiencing stress also and may become tired, despondent, and frustrated. They too may need professional support.

RESPIRATORY PHARMACOLOGIC AGENTS

Various pharmacologic agents are used to treat clients with respiratory disorders. Some of the more common classifications are presented in Table 37–1. Medications are discussed further throughout the unit in relation to specific respiratory conditions.

Antimicrobials (Antibiotics)

Antibiotics, commonly ampicillin and tetracycline, can be used to treat pulmonary infection. Even though the most common causes of respiratory infection are viruses, there are few antiviral medications. Treatment for viral infection is symptomatic (e.g., decongestants). At times, antibiotics may be prescribed because the virus lowers the client's resistance to bacterial infection.

Bronchodilators

Bronchodilators act directly on bronchial smooth muscle to relieve bronchospasm. They are commonly divided into two groups: (1) beta-adrenergics, e.g., albuterol (Ventolin); and (2) theophylline preparations, e.g., aminophylline. Common side effects that may be noted during bronchodilator therapy are increased heart rate, palpitations, nervousness, skeletal muscle tremors, nausea, and anorexia.

Some of the newer bronchodilators are beta-adrenergics (stimulators), which have a very limited alpha effect. These medications provide better bronchodilation than the earliest drugs (e.g., epinephrine). Side effects are minimal and include tachycardia, tremors, and nausea.

Adrenal Glucocorticoids

Adrenal glucocorticoids (e.g., prednisone) reduce inflammation, which thickens bronchial walls and decreases the size of the bronchial lumina. Beclomethasone (Vanceril) and triamcinolone are available in a metered dose inhaler. They provide topical steroid therapy and prevent bronchospasm. Glucocorticoids decrease the responsiveness of the cells to allergic stimuli, thereby reducing bronchoconstriction. They are used frequently in the treatment of asthma. Because steroids can reduce the immune response, aerosolized doses are often preferred to oral doses because less of the drug is required to obtain the desired effect. Clients with acute, serious respiratory disorders are commonly treated with high doses, intravenous steroids, or both. Glucocorticoids are prescribed with caution because of their wide variety of side effects.

Antitussives

Antitussive agents inhibit the cough reflex in the cough center. Examples are benzonatate (Tessalon), codeine phosphate, dextromethorphan hydrobromide (Robitussin DM), and hydrocodone bitartrate (Hycodan). Many antitussives are prepared in syrup form that coats and protects the mucous membranes. By reducing local irritations, these soothing syrups reduce afferent nerve im-

Text continued on page 949

TABLE 37-1. Pharmacologic Management of Respiratory Disorders

Class	Example	Action	Use	Common Side Effects	Nursing Implications
Antimicrobials					
Penicillins	Penicillin G sodium Procaine penicillin G (Wycillin) Potassium penicillin V (Pen-Vee K) Nafcillin (Unipen) Ampicillin Amoxicillin Carbenicillin Ticarcillin		Bactericidal against a wide variety of gram-positive and some gram-negative organisms Most effective in the treatment of bacterial pneumonia	Allergic reactions (skin rashes, anaphylaxis) Gastrointestinal disturbances (nausea and vomiting, epigastric distress) Central nervous system toxicity manifested by hallucinations, hyperreflexia, seizures when administered in very large doses to patients with neurologic reactions (thrombocytopenia, agranulocytosis, anemia) Impaired renal function	Check for history of penicillin allergy before administration of drug Observe for allergic manifestations and other side effects Evaluate effects of drug especially when given concurrently with drugs that may increase or decrease its action, e.g., gentamicin is synergistic to penicillin; probenecid decreases its renal excretion; tetracycline and erythromycin both inhibit bactericidal activity of penicillin Monitor for development of resistant organisms; susceptibility testing should be done before and during the course of therapy
Cephalosporins	Cephalexin (Keflex) Cefamandole (Mandol) Cefazolin (Ancef, Kefzol) Cephalothin (Keflin) Cefoxitin (Mefoxin) Cephapirin (Cefadyl)		Effective against numerous infections but used primarily for *Klebsiella pneumoniae* along with aminoglycoside	Gastrointestinal disturbances Nephrotoxicity (decreased urine output and creatinine clearance, hematuria, proteinuria) Phlebitis with intravenous administration	Assess for allergic reactions to cephalosporins and penicillins; it is controversial whether cephalosporins can be given without causing allergic reactions when there is a known hypersensitivity to penicillin Monitor for toxic side effects Assess effectiveness when administered with bacteriostatic antibiotics, e.g.,

Table continued on following page

TABLE 37–1. Pharmacologic Management of Respiratory Disorders Continued

Class	Example	Action	Use	Common Side Effects	Nursing Implications
					tetracyclines and erythromycins, which may decrease or destroy their effects
Aminoglycosides	Kanamycin (Kantrex) Neomycin Amikacin sulfate Gentamicin (Garamycin) Tobramycin Streptomycin		Bactericidal against a wide range of gram-positive and gram-negative bacteria and mycobacteria; however, they differ in clinical uses Streptomycin: used in the treatment of tuberculosis in combination with other tuberculostatic drugs Neomycin: used for reducing intestinal flora and thereby decreasing blood ammonia levels Gentamicin: used to treat bacteremia caused by *Proteus*, *Pseudomonas*, *Escherichia coli*, and *Klebsiella* Amikacin and tobramycin: used to treat gentamicin-resistant infection	Ototoxicity Nephrotoxicity Neuromuscular blockade Peripheral neuritis Resistant infection	Assess client for beginning auditory and vestibular damage, e.g., vertigo, ataxia, roaring in the ears, hearing loss Monitor renal function, especially when administered to elderly clients or to those with renal insufficiency Monitor peak and trough levels and drug dosages Assess neuromuscular effects, especially when administered with muscle relaxants and sedatives
Tetracyclines	Chlortetracycline HCl (Aureomycin) Demeclocycline HCl (Declomycin) Doxycycline hyclate (Vibramycin)		Bacteriostatic for many gram-negative and gram-positive organisms, including mycobacteria, rickettsiae, mycoplasma, and agents of psittacosis	Gastrointestinal disturbances Allergic reactions Hepatotoxicity Enamel hypoplasia Permanent staining of teeth when used during tooth development	Avoid use in children, during pregnancy, and when there is impaired hepatic or renal function Do not administer with food, milk, milk products, antacids because they inhibit tetracycline absorption Monitor client for a developing superinfection

TABLE 37-1. Pharmacologic Management of Respiratory Disorders Continued

Class	Example	Action	Use	Common Side Effects	Nursing Implications
					Monitor liver function in long-term therapy Instruct client to avoid direct sunlight because sunburn reaction or erythema is likely to occur
Bronchodilators					
Beta-adrenergics	Albuterol (Ventolin) Isoproterenol (Isuprel) Terbutaline (Brethine)	Relaxation of constricted airways by stimulating beta-adrenergic receptors	Symptomatic relief of asthma and bronchial spasms	Gastrointestinal upset Nausea Nervousness, anxiety Frequency Diarrhea Insomnia Tachycardia Palpitations Esophageal reflux Tremors	Use with caution in clients with hypertension, tachycardia, hypoxemia, glaucoma, hyperthyroidism, benign prostatic hypertrophy, diabetes Monitor for central nervous system symptoms Give with food or antacids; avoid smoking
Theophylline	Theophylline (Theo-Dur)	Bronchial relaxation by inhibition of the breakdown of cyclic adenosine monophosphate			
Adrenal glucocorticoids	Prednisone Beclomethasone (Vanceril)	Reduce inflammation and inflammatory response in bronchial walls	Symptomatic relief and preventive care of asthma	With systemic agents—gastrointestinal upset, gastric irritation and ulceration, euphoria, hunger, insomnia, adrenal shutdown	Administer in morning if dosage is 4 times daily; give with food Plan to supplement clients with cortisone agents during periods of stress
Antitussives	Narcotics: any product with codeine Non-narcotics: dextromethorphan	Suppress cough reflex Act centrally on the cough center or peripherally within the tracheobronchial tree to decrease sensitivity to irritant receptors	To treat dry, nonproductive coughs that interfere with sleep or other activities	Dizziness Sedation Sweating Nausea Dry mouth Constipation Urinary retention Palpitations	Caution client about possible sedation Administer with caution to patients with asthma, COPD, cardiac disease, convulsions, renal or hepatic disease, central nervous system depression, benign prostatic hypertrophy, alcoholism, or hypothyroidism
Mucolytics	Water Acetylcysteine (Mucomyst)	Thin mucus	Chronic pulmonary conditions that lead to thick, dry sputum	Bronchospasm with Mucomyst	Administer Mucomyst by aerosolized bronchodilator

Table continued on following page

TABLE 37-1. Pharmacologic Management of Respiratory Disorders Continued

Class	Example	Action	Use	Common Side Effects	Nursing Implications
Antiallergenics	Cromolyn sodium (Intal)	Stabilizes mast cell	Asthma, especially due to exercise or allergen exposure	Headache Rash Cough Worsening of asthma	Require 3 weeks of continuous therapy before they are effective Use in decreased dosages for clients with liver or renal disorders
Antihistamines	Diphenhydramine hydrochloride (Benadryl)	Block action of histamine at H_1-receptor sites, smooth muscles of the blood vessels, bronchioles, and gastrointestinal tract	Relieve symptoms of allergies Adjunct in treatment of anaphylaxis	Sedation Epigastric distress Hypotension Palpitations Tachycardia Thickening of bronchial secretions Vertigo Urinary frequency	Warn about sedation Use carefully in clients with convulsions, hyperthyroidism, cardiovascular and renal disease, hypertension, diabetes Avoid use with alcohol Monitor for dry mucous membranes Give with meals or antacids
	Terfenadine (Seldane)	Specific, selective histamine H_1-receptor antagonist		Dryness of nose, mouth Dysrhythmias when used to toxic levels	Do not use in conjunction with ketoconazole or levamisole (Ergamisole). Use cautiously with erythromycin
Cough preparations Expectorants	Guaifenesin (Robitussin)	Facilitate removal of thick mucus from lungs and act as soothing demulcent by stimulating secretion of a lubricant	Facilitate productive cough	Nausea and vomiting Gastrointestinal irritation Drowsiness	Instruct client not to use more than 1 week without seeing physician Use high fluid intake and humidity to loosen secretions Do not follow with water, except potassium iodide
Decongestants	Ephedrine sulfate (Efedron)	Dry mucous membranes and reduced mucus production	Reduce allergy and cold symptoms	Rebound inflammation of mucous membranes	Instruct client not to use for more than 1 week without seeing physician

Adapted from Matassarin-Jacobs, E. (1990). *Saunders review for NCLEX-RN*. Philadelphia: W. B. Saunders.

pulses arising in the respiratory tract. Advise the client not to take anything by mouth for a while after swallowing a cough medication. Swallowing water (or other liquids, foods, or medications) washes the medication off the pharyngeal mucosa, thus causing the desired local soothing effect to be lost. Many antitussives contain narcotics or alcohol and have a sedative effect. They therefore are sometimes abused, and psychic dependency may develop. In general, cough suppressants are avoided.

Mucolytics

Mucolytics help liquefy pulmonary secretions so that they can be expectorated. They are prescribed for clients with abnormal, viscid, or inspissated (dry) mucous secretions in acute and chronic disorders such as pneumonia, bronchitis, tuberculosis, or cystic fibrosis. Acetylcysteine (Mucomyst) may be aerosolized to reduce the viscosity (thickness) of secretions. Because acetylcysteine can cause bronchospasm, it may be used with an aerosolized bronchodilator.

Antiallergenics

Cromolyn sodium (Intal) has a unique antiallergenic effect that helps clients with asthma. It stabilizes mast cells, inhibiting the release of mediators of type I allergic reactions (histamine and slow-reacting substance of anaphylaxis [SRS-A]), thereby reducing pulmonary reactiveness. Cromolyn sodium requires 2 to 3 weeks of continuous therapy before effective levels can be achieved. If bronchospasm occurs, cromolyn sodium is not effective in relieving the acute bronchospastic attack. Unlike steroids, cromolyn sodium has few side effects. Cromolyn sodium is available in a "spinhaler" that aerosolizes a powder for inhalation, as a liquid that can be nebulized for inhalation, or in a metered dose form. Antihistamines may also be used to relieve symptoms of allergies.

Vasoconstrictors and Decongestants

Medications in this classification may be used to treat allergic reactions. They are administered by various routes: (1) topically (e.g., nose drops, sprays, and aerosols); (2) parenterally; and (3) orally. Examples of decongestants are ephedrine sulfate and phenylephrine hydrochloride (Neo-Synephrine). These drugs must be used for short periods only (less than 1 week) because they can produce nasal irritation and cause a rebound effect, worsening nasal congestion.

RESPIRATORY THERAPY

Administering Oxygen

Oxygen (O_2) is administered to treat the harmful and possibly lethal effects of hypoxemia (lowered blood oxygen). The need for oxygen is assessed by arterial blood gases (ABGs), oxygen saturation measuring devices (oximeters), and monitoring for indications of hypoxemia. Oxygen, used for both acute and chronic conditions, does not cure a disease. Examples of pulmonary and nonpulmonary disorders that may cause hypoxemia and the need for supplemental oxygen include airway obstruction, pulmonary edema, acute respiratory failure, chronic respiratory insufficiency, cardiac disorders, metabolic disorders, and shock.

Never withhold oxygen from a hypoxic client. However, like any drug, oxygen is prescribed in dosages safe for the client. Oddly, sometimes high concentrations of oxygen can be fatal, whereas low concentrations can be lifesaving.

INDICATIONS

Oxygen administration is required whenever hypoxemia occurs or is expected to occur. With the relief of hypoxemia, hypoxia (reduced oxygen in tissues) can be prevented.

There are three major indications for oxygen administration: reduced arterial blood oxygen, increased work of breathing, and need for decreased myocardial workload.

Reduced Arterial Blood Oxygen. Tissue hypoxia is impossible to measure accurately because levels vary greatly in different body parts. Hypoxemia, however, may be assessed by measuring the amount of oxygen in a sample of arterial blood (ABG analysis). Normal arterial blood oxygen levels range from 80 to 100 mm Hg. If arterial blood oxygen (PaO_2) falls below normal, supplemental oxygen usually corrects the hypoxemia if the hypoxemia is caused by hypoventilation or small ventilation/perfusion defects. If the hypoxemia is caused by ventilation/perfusion mismatch that is greater than 25 per cent, such as in adult respiratory distress syndrome (ARDS) or pneumonia, other methods of oxygen administration may be needed.

Increased Work of Breathing. The body responds to hypoxemia by increasing the rate and depth of respirations in an effort to bring more oxygen into the blood. Consequently, a hypoxemic client shows signs of respiratory distress (e.g., use of accessory muscles, diaphoresis, cyanosis). A vicious cycle develops as respiratory effort increases, the body requires more and more oxygen to support the effort, and oxygen consumption increases accordingly. The result is fatigue and possibly respiratory arrest or cardiac complications. Hypoxemia can be relieved when supplemental oxygen is administered to a client with signs of increased work of breathing. As hypoxemia is relieved, the client no longer requires additional respiratory effort and resumes a normal breathing pattern.

Need for Decreased Myocardial Workload. When the body becomes hypoxemic, the heart attempts to compensate for the lack of oxygen by increasing the cardiac output. Whereas the heart's increased output circulates the available oxygen to the tissues quicker and more efficiently, the myocardial workload increases. Administering supplemental oxygen increases the amount of oxygen available to the tissues, thus decreasing hypoxemia and myocardial workload. Because hypoxemia stresses the myocardium, oxygen is prescribed for clients experiencing myocardial infarction, congestive heart failure, coronary artery disease, or other cardiac problems.

COMPLICATIONS

There are few complications of oxygen therapy, and generally it is safely used. Oxygen-induced hypoventilation, oxygen toxicity, atelectasis, and ocular damage are important to understand.

Oxygen-Induced Hypoventilation. A normal respiratory drive occurs when blood carbon dioxide rises slightly and stimulates the primary respiratory centers in the medulla and pons. Secondary respiratory centers in the carotid bodies and the arch of the aorta are activated by decreases in blood oxygen tension (e.g., lower than 60 mm Hg). Clients with chronic respiratory dysfunction may retain carbon dioxide. When carbon dioxide is retained over a long period of time, the medullary center in the brain is no longer stimulated by the increased level of carbon dioxide in the blood. In these clients, respiration is stimulated by low levels of oxygen in the blood (PaO_2). Administration of unspecified and unmonitored doses of oxygen may depress ventilation (hypoventilation) or even cause apnea. Serial ABGs alert the nurse to increasing $PaCO_2$ levels. However, the risk of oxygen-induced hypoventilation in clients with suspected chronic pulmonary disease should not prevent the administration of oxygen in life-threatening situations. Chronic carbon dioxide retention is diagnosed by a baseline $PaCO_2$ above 45 mm Hg with a compensated pH (pH in the normal range or slightly acidotic).

Oxygen Toxicity. Oxygen toxicity is a medically induced, potentially fatal, progressive condition in which ventilatory failure occurs in clients who inspire a high concentration of oxygen for a prolonged period of time. A high concentration of oxygen can be defined as a fraction of inspired oxygen (FIO_2) of greater than 60 per cent. The development of oxygen toxicity is related to both time and dose. Pathophysiologic changes begin within the lungs after 24 to 48 hours of exposure to high oxygen concentrations.

Early indications of oxygen toxicity may include a mild tracheobronchitis that begins as a substernal soreness, nasal congestion, pain on inspiration, and increased coughing. As the condition worsens, the cough becomes more severe, substernal soreness increases, and dyspnea develops. Prolonged exposure to oxygen in high concentrations may cause structural damage to the lung tissue (e.g., interstitial edema, thickening of the alveolar capillary membranes, intra-alveolar hemorrhage, and atelectasis). Exudates of protein, fibrin, and cellular debris bind together to form hyaline membranes in the alveoli. These changes impair the transport of oxygen. Clients at risk for oxygen toxicity are those on bleomycin or steroids and those with hyperthermia, hyperthyroidism, protein deficiency, vitamin E deficiency, and adrenergic stimulation.

Assessment findings at the end stage of oxygen toxicity include progressive atelectasis, consolidation, and fibrosis of the lung. Chest films show progressive opacification of the lungs. Oxygenation is greatly impaired and breathing is difficult owing to decreasing compliance. Auscultation may reveal diminished breath sounds and audible rales.

ABG analysis is monitored to prevent oxygen toxicity. If a client develops oxygen toxicity, ABG values show a decreasing PaO_2 with an increased FIO_2 requirement. At the same time, an increase in the pressure required to deliver a mechanical ventilator breath is noted. This increased pressure may indicate a decrease in lung compliance or the ability of the lung to stretch or distend.

Intervention for oxygen toxicity is aimed at maintaining adequate oxygenation and treating the underlying, precipitating disease. The best intervention is to prevent oxygen toxicity from occurring. This can be done by using positive end-expiratory pressure in conjunction with mechanical ventilation (see section on mechanical ventilators) to maintain oxygenation and avoid FIO_2 values greater than 0.6.

Decreasing the client's work of breathing as well as oxygen consumption is an area that also needs to be addressed. This may be accomplished by promoting rest, using sedation, and decreasing oxygen consumption (e.g., controlling hyperthermia and hyperthyroidism and limiting activity).

Even when a client demonstrates oxygen toxicity, oxygenation must still be supported. Unfortunately, a dangerous cycle occurs because the "stiff" or noncompliant lungs require high levels of oxygen for hypoxemia to be prevented, and yet the oxygen itself is the cause of the problem.

Nursing assessment and intervention for clients with oxygen toxicity include

- emotional support for the client and family
- assessment of fluid and electrolyte status
- monitoring and documenting ABG response to changes in treatment (ABGs are usually taken every 3 to 4 hours or as needed)
- assessing and documenting inspired oxygen concentration after any change in FIO_2
- aseptic airway care (lung damage increases the risk of infection)
- prevention of any further damage or complications by using positive end-expiratory pressure to reduce FIO_2

Atelectasis. As a result of increased oxygen concentrations in the inspired air, alveoli may collapse. The mechanism for this oxygen-induced side effect is the elimination of nitrogen from the lungs. Nitrogen, which makes up 78 per cent of room air, is absorbed in small amounts by the blood. Most nitrogen remains in the alveoli, adding volume to the alveoli, which in turn helps to prevent alveolar collapse. When the level of inspired oxygen rises, the oxygen molecules replace the nitrogen molecules. However, oxygen molecules are readily absorbed into the bloodstream, leaving the alveoli empty and thus predisposing them to collapse. This phenomenon is known as nitrogen washout. In addition to the loss of intra-alveolar volume, hyperoxia retards the production of surfactant. Loss of surfactant also allows the forces of surface tension to collapse the affected alveolar units. These collapsed alveoli continue to be perfused with blood, which leads to hypoxemia. Hypoxemia results from unoxygenated blood passing these closed alveolar units without receiving oxygen. This condition is called intrapulmonary shunting.

Carefully assess clients receiving high concentrations of oxygen for indications of atelectasis, including vague discomfort, anxiety, tachypnea, fever, cough, tachycardia, shortness of breath, and substernal retractions. Assessment findings vary, depending on the extent of atelectasis. ABG analysis is essential, and chest X-ray studies are taken during the course of administration of high concentrations of oxygen. Serial chest films are necessary if atelectasis develops. Auscultation demonstrates diminished or absent breath sounds in the affected areas. Serial parameter checks of vital capacity, inspiratory force, and tidal volume indicate the degree of impairment.

Nursing interventions appropriate for clients with atelectasis may include early ambulation, coughing, deep breathing, incentive spirometry, hydration, and frequent position changes. Watch for changes in oxygenation with position changes. Gravitational effects on the blood flow can result in hypoxemia owing to the intrapulmonary shunting. ABG analysis with supplemental oxygen administration may be necessary if hypoxemia occurs.

Atelectasis may occur in other situations, including hypoventilation, impingement of a portion of the lung by space-occupying lesions, mucous plugs, effects of anesthesia, immobility, pleural effusion, and pneumothorax.

Ocular Damage. Retinal injury can occur in adults exposed to 100 per cent oxygen. Arterial oxygen tensions of 150 mm Hg for a period of greater than 4 hours can cause retrolental fibroplasia. Clients with previous retinal disease (e.g., retinal detachment) are especially vulnerable. Tearing, edema, and visual impairment result from the toxic effects of high concentrations of oxygen on the cornea and lens of adults.

NURSING MANAGEMENT

Become familiar with the various methods of oxygen administration. Nurses must be knowledgeable about oxygen therapy so that they can administer as well as detect equipment malfunction. The percentages of oxygen delivered by most equipment are approximate. When oxygen concentration must be closely governed, monitor the gas delivered to a client at least every 8 hours with an oxygen analyzer (Fig. 37–2).

A nurse responsible for oxygen therapy must know

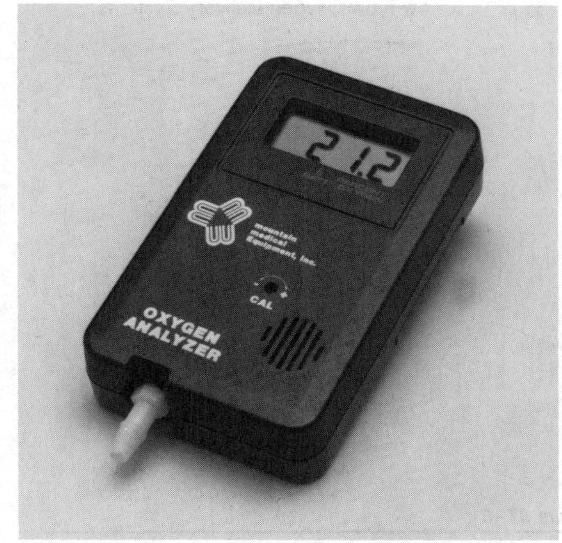

▲ *Figure 37–2*

An oxygen analyzer is essential to the accurate determination of inspired O_2 concentrations. This model may be placed in line in the delivery system of many high-flow oxygen systems. (Courtesy of Mountain Medical Equipment, Inc., Littleton, CO.)

about the (1) hazards of oxygen therapy and (2) clinical indications of hypoxia, respiratory acidosis, carbon dioxide narcosis, respiratory alkalosis, and oxygen toxicity. (Respiratory acidosis and alkalosis are discussed in Chap. 15.)

Nursing intervention during oxygen administration includes (1) correctly administering the prescribed amount of oxygen; (2) maintaining a patent airway by correct positioning, suctioning, and productive coughing; (3) giving mouth and nose care every 3 to 4 hours; (4) changing the client's position periodically and providing skin care; (5) changing equipment as necessary (e.g., changing tanks before they become empty); (6) providing appropriate education; and (7) offering psychosocial support to the client and family.

When oxygen is administered for the first time, explain the process to the client, demonstrate the equipment, and explain the expected outcomes of the oxygen therapy. Oxygen administration may frighten some clients. Be sensitive to these feelings and offer emotional support and reassurance. A dyspneic person may initially remove an oxygen administration device if the equipment increases the feeling of suffocation. An oxygen nasal cannula is usually more comfortable than a mask is (Fig. 37–3). Stay with clients until they adjust to the equipment and begin to feel the benefits of the oxygen. Careful assessment of clients on oxygen systems is important, especially during the first 30 to 60 minutes when oxygen-induced hypoventilation can develop.

Some clients become dependent on oxygen and are afraid to have it discontinued even when it is no longer necessary. Stay with such clients and gradually withdraw the oxygen. Sometimes it helps to keep oxygen available for 2 to 3 days to be used only for respiratory distress. When clients realize that most activities are

Low-Flow Oxygen Delivery Systems

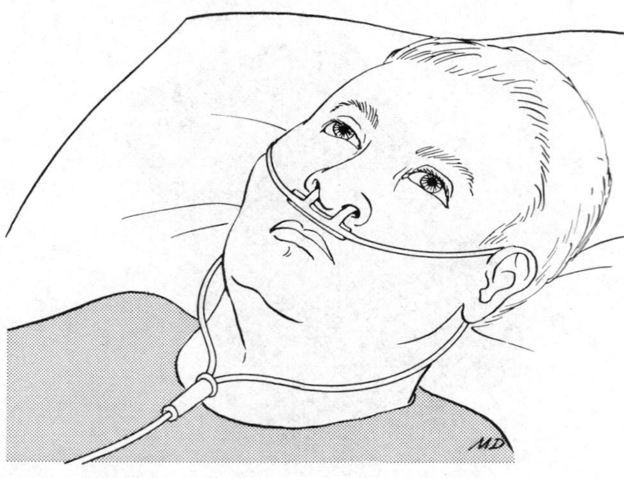

▲ *Figure 37-3*

Nasal cannula (nasal prongs) as a means of delivering oxygen.

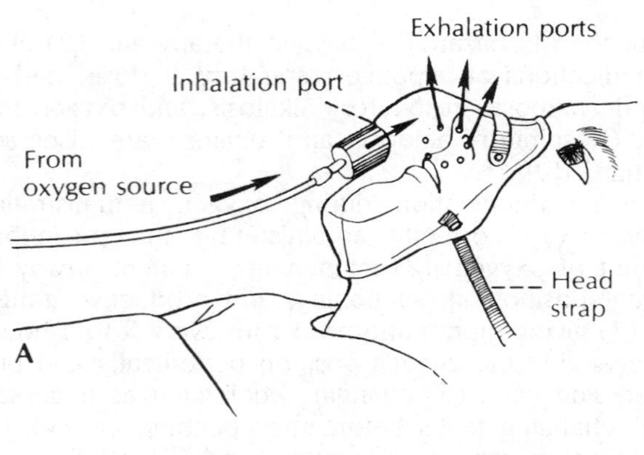

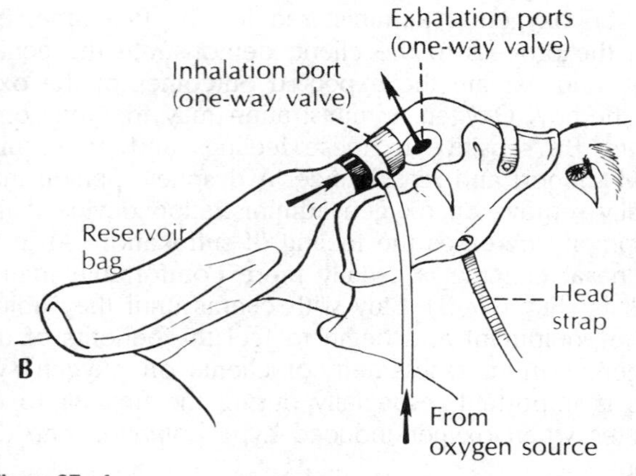

▲ *Figure 37-4*

Oxygen masks. *A*, Standard oxygen mask used to administer moderate ranges of oxygen. *B*, Partial rebreathing oxygen mask used for short-term, high concentration of oxygen. Oxygen fills the reservoir bag. During inhalation, oxygen flows through the one-way valve. During exhalation, the valve closes, exhalation ports open, and the air passes into the atmosphere. Oxygen masks must fit securely and snugly.

possible without oxygen, the dependency on it diminishes.

OXYGEN DELIVERY SYSTEMS

Oxygen is supplied for administration from either a portable tank (cylinder) or a wall outlet (which leads via pipes to large stores of oxygen). Oxygen can be administered by masks, nasal cannula, face tent, ventilator, or nebulizer. The equipment used to administer oxygen is divided into two categories: low-flow and high-flow systems. The terms *low-flow* and *high-flow* refer to the rates of oxygen delivered by the equipment. Low-flow systems deliver oxygen at flow rates that supplement the oxygen contained in ambient (room) air. High-flow systems meet or exceed the client's inspiratory flow rate, allowing an accurate delivery of inspired oxygen.

Low-Flow Systems. These systems deliver a wide range of oxygen concentrations, i.e., from 21 to 90 per cent. Variables controlling the fraction of inspired oxygen (FIO_2) include (1) capacity of the anatomic reservoir (nasopharynx, oropharynx, and nose); (2) type of oxygen reservoir system (nose, mask, or reservoir bag); (3) oxygen flow rate (liters per minute); and (4) client's ventilation pattern. Low-flow systems (e.g., nasal cannulas, masks, and masks with reservoir bags) are the most common and are easy to use. However, the determination of oxygen concentration is not precise and cannot be readily measured with an oxygen analyzer.

Table 37-2 shows the concentrations of oxygen available at various liter flows with the five standard low-flow systems. A regular ventilatory pattern is assumed. Oxygen (100 per cent) comes from a wall outlet. The actual inspired oxygen concentration is determined by (1) the amount of air entrained (drawn in) by the client and (2) the dilution of the oxygen with room air. FIO_2 in a low-flow system varies significantly with tidal volume and ventilatory pattern changes. In a low-flow system, (1) the larger the tidal volume, the lower is the FIO_2, or (2) the smaller the tidal volume, the higher is the FIO_2.

A nasal cannula requires patent nasal passages (see Fig. 37-3). Advantages of this system include ease of use, comfort, and that it does not need to be removed for eating or taking medications. The main disadvantage of this system is that the oxygen concentration delivered cannot be closely controlled as a result of variations in tidal volume and rate of breathing. Oxygen flow rates administered via nasal cannula range from 1 to 6 liters per minute (L/min). Flow rates above 6 L/min are uncomfortable and rarely increase total oxygen delivery because much of the extra oxygen is flushed out of the nose and mouth. Mouth breathing, however, does not affect the FIO_2 as much as might be thought because oxygen in the nose is drawn into the trachea by air in the oral cavity.

Simple masks (Fig. 37-4*A*) provide oxygen concentrations of 35 to 55 per cent with flow rates between 6 and 10 L/min. Because oxygen concentration is variable, these masks are rarely used clinically. However, it has been noted that in those clients who breathe pri-

TABLE 37-2. Oxygen Concentration in Various Delivery Systems

Type of Face Mask	Flow System	L/min	0.%
a. Nasal cannula	Low flow	1 to 6 L/min	24 to 44%
b. Simple face mask	Low flow	5 to 8 L/min	40 to 60%
c. Partial rebreather mask	Low flow	6 to 10 L/min	60 to 80%
d. Non-rebreather mask*	Low flow	6 to 15 L/min	95 to 100%
e. Venturi mask†	High flow	4 to 15 L/min	24 to 40 or 50%
f. Face tent	Low flow	4 to 8 L/min	30 to 55%

* The non-rebreather mask gives the highest oxygen concentration possible other than intubation or mechanical ventilation. 6-15 L/min will give 95-100%.

† The Venturi mask delivers oxygen concentrations precise to within 1%. This mask can deliver a very controlled amount of oxygen e.g., 4 L/min blue adapter = 24%; 8 L/min green adapter = 35%.

When the O_2 is jetted into the tube, air is pulled from the room and oxygen is mixed, providing a precise mixture within 1% accuracy. When using the Venturi mask, prevent occlusion of air entrainment ports by bed linen, clothing, or other objects. Obtain an order from physician for O_2 per nasal cannula while client is eating. If the client is on Venturi O_2 concentration of 24%, he or she should receive O_2 by nasal cannula at 1-L flow (20% atmospheric oxygen + 4% O_2 = 24%), 28% Venturi = 2-L flow per n.c. The Venturi mask is replaced when client is finished eating.

marily through their mouths, this method of oxygen administration is more effective than is a nasal cannula. Any mask, when used, should be removed when the client is eating. In order to maintain adequate oxygen delivery during mealtimes, a nasal cannula with flow rates up to 6 L/min may be utilized. The face mask should be returned after the client has finished eating or if the client is abnormally short of breath.

Partial rebreathing masks (Figure 37-4*B*) are used to deliver oxygen concentrations up to 80 per cent. The reservoir bag does not have a one-way valve between it and the mask. Approximately one third of the client's exhaled air goes back into the reservoir bag. The oxygen flow rate through the system must be maintained at a minimum of 6 L/min to ensure that the client does not rebreathe large amounts of exhaled air. This liter flow allows the reservoir to remain full so that a sufficient volume of gas is available if the client decides to take a larger tidal volume.

Face tents are another method for delivering oxygen via a low-flow system. The major advantage of this system is the ability to deliver high humidity. The disadvantage, as with other low-flow methods, is that the oxygen cannot be closely controlled. Oxygen flow rates of 4 to 8 L/min usually provide an oxygen concentration of 40 per cent with normal respirations. Face tents have a wide variation in oxygen delivery and therefore are seldom used.

High-Flow Systems. High-flow systems provide a flow rate and reservoir capacity adequate to meet total inspired-air needs. A client using a high-flow system breathes only the gas supplied by the apparatus. For this reason, a high-flow system provides a consistent and accurate FIO_2 as long as inspiratory flow requirements do not exceed the total liter flow delivered by the apparatus.

High-flow systems have three major advantages: (1) consistent FIO_2; (2) control of the entire inspired atmosphere, including temperature and humidity; and (3) easy analysis of FIO_2 with an oxygen analyzer (see Fig. 37-2). This is a significant advantage for critically ill people.

High-flow systems can deliver either high or low oxygen concentrations. A Venturi device (Fig. 37-5*A*) is used to blend oxygen and air at the desired FIO_2. Oxygen moves through a connecting tube to a channel in the mask that has one diameter on the distal side and a smaller diameter on the proximal side. Oxygen flows through this channel. As the oxygen passes through the proximal end, a pressure drop occurs that creates a suction or entrainment (drawing-in) effect. The degree of entrainment gives a specific dose (percentage) of oxygen. This mechanism entrains a specific amount of room air for each liter flow of oxygen. The air:oxygen entrainment ratio provides a specific oxygen percentage and large total flow rates of air and oxygen. For example, if a Venturi system set for 40 per cent oxygen is used, it has an air:oxygen entrainment ratio of 3:1. If the flowmeter is set at 10 L/min, and for each liter of oxygen, 3 liters of air are entrained, the total liter flow is 40 L/min. Each FIO_2 has its own air:oxygen entrainment ratio. Thus, each FIO_2 has a different total liter flow. The higher the FIO_2, the lower is the total liter flow.

To facilitate clinical use of the Venturi device, various colored adapters exist that can be used to deliver exact oxygen concentrations (Fig. 37-5*B*).

A mask with a reservoir and a one-way valve (non-rebreathing) is used if oxygen concentrations of greater than 60 per cent are required (Fig. 37-5*C*). The bag is an oxygen reservoir. When the client exhales, the one-way valve closes and all of the expired air is deposited into the atmosphere, not the reservoir bag. In this way, the client is not rebreathing any of the expired gas. When a non-rebreathing mask is used, observe the bag during inhalation. It must not collapse by more than half its full capacity with each breath. Flow rates of 6 to 15 L/min are used to ensure that the reservoir bag remains full. Oxygen concentrations of 60 to 99+ per cent can be obtained with this system depending on the pattern, depth, and rate of ventilation. All oxygen masks must fit securely to provide the highest percentage of oxygen.

Humidity and Aerosol Therapy. Humidity is water vapor in the air. An aerosol is a suspension of solid or liquid particles in a flow of gas. Because oxygen and

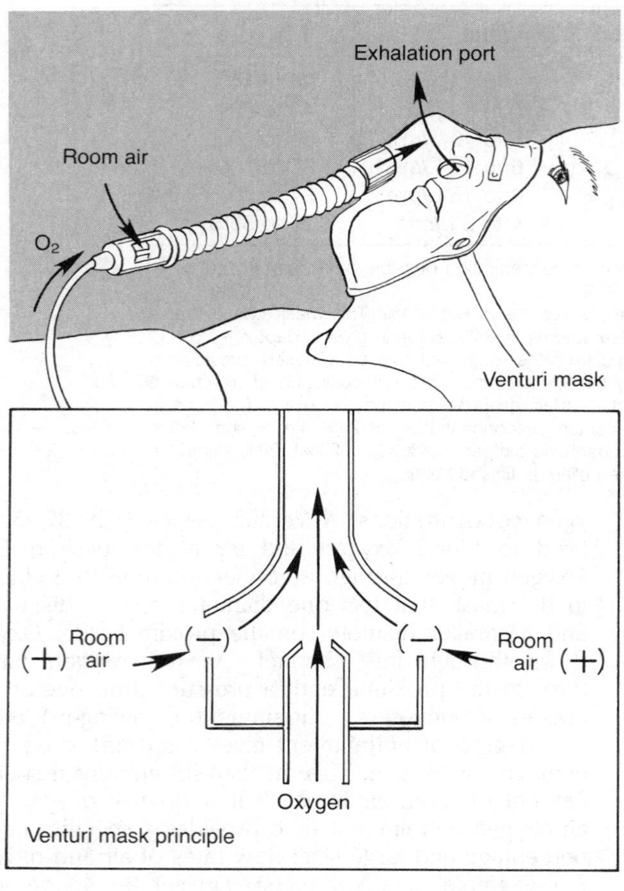

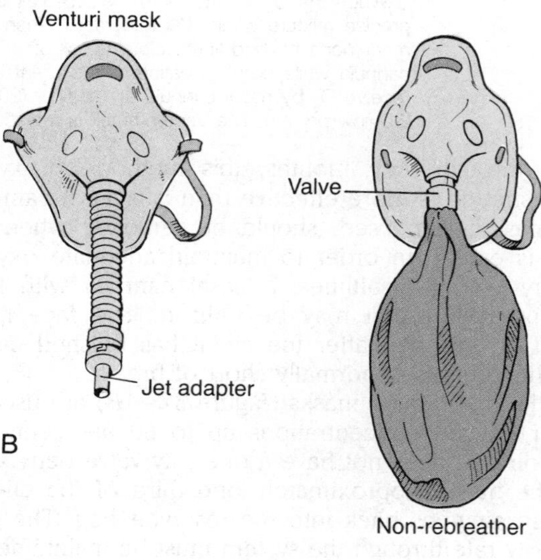

▲ *Figure 37-5*

The Venturi system provides high-flow delivery of precise percentages of oxygen.

other compressed gases are dry (contain no water vapor), humidity may be added to them before they are inhaled. If an inhaled mist is needed to prevent mucosal drying and secretion retention, an aerosol is indicated.

Humidification. Humidifiers are devices that add water vapor (humidity) to inspired gas. Humidity is needed to decrease the drying effects of the gases and increase comfort. Moist air (1) prevents drying and irritation of respiratory mucous membranes, (2) prevents drying and thickening of respiratory tract secretions, and (3) loosens secretions, making them more easily removed. Dry, thick secretions form plugs and crusts within the tracheobronchial tree. Mucous plugging may result in inadequate ventilation and obstruction.

Generally, humidification of oxygen delivered by nasal cannula at flow rates of less than 4 L/min or by a Venturi mask is not required because adequate amounts of humidified room air are inspired. If higher flow rates are required, the use of a bubble humidifier is encouraged. A bubble humidifier causes the oxygen to pass through water before reaching the client, thus increasing the humidity of the gas inspired (Fig. 37-6).

Nebulization (Aerosolization). A nebulizer mechanically produces an aerosol by means of a Venturi device that entrains liquid and breaks it up into droplets. These droplets are then further broken down into a mist by a baffle device. The size of the solid or liquid particles dispersed in the gas will vary widely depending on the type of baffle used. Nebulizers such as the metered dose inhaler produce particles ranging from 2 to 5 μm. This is the ideal range for penetration of the pulmonary tree. However, the size of the particles when they initially leave the inhaler may be as large as 40 μm. These particles will shrink with evaporation, but if they are inhaled too quickly, they may be too large to reach the lower airways. Typically, metered dose inhalers disperse only 10 per cent of the delivered medication into the pulmonary tree.

Nebulizers are used (1) for airway hydration, (2) for administration of aerosolized medication, and (3) as an adjunct therapy for the mobilization of retained secretions. Water, isotonic saline, and 0.25 to 0.45 per cent saline may be nebulized to hydrate the airways and liquefy inspissated secretions that occlude the airway. However, bronchospasm can be induced by aerosolization of any substance. Clients who develop bronchospasm from nebulized saline are probably better treated with bronchodilator therapy.

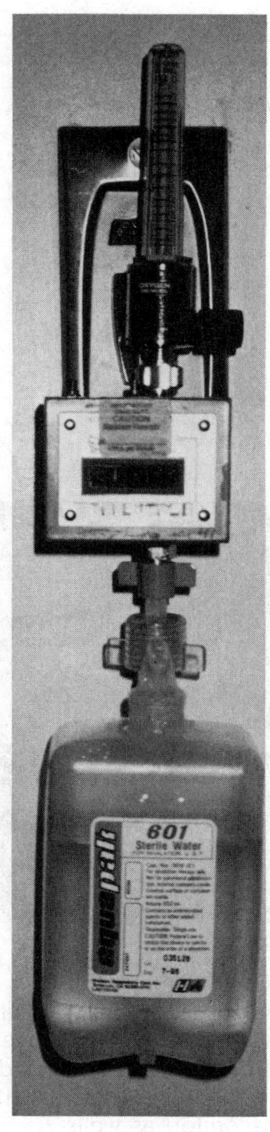

▲ *Figure 37-6*

A humidifier for use in oxygen administration with oxygen administration devices over 4 liters/minute.

Nebulizers used for hydration, large-volume nebulizers, are most often used for continuous aerosol therapy. Small-volume nebulizers (e.g., bronchodilators, mucolytics) are used to administer medication to the respiratory system.

A jet nebulizer uses the force of the gas powering the nebulizer to draw the solution up into a tube where it is eventually broken up by a stream of gas (Fig. 37-7*A*). Larger particles are then baffled out and fall back into the solution reservoir. Usually the nebulizer entrains (draws in) air from the room to provide a large gas flow rate. This is necessary to meet a client's inspiratory demands, to reduce the work of breathing, and to ensure a stable concentration of oxygen. Small-volume and large-volume nebulizers are powered in various ways: (1) by a pocket-sized metered dose inhaler, (2) by compressors (see Fig. 37-7*B*), (3) by compressed gases (e.g., oxygen or compressed air), or (4) by an intermittent positive-pressure breathing machine.

Ultrasonic nebulization (mist therapy) produces particles small enough to reach the respiratory bronchioles. These minute particles are produced when high-frequency sound waves vibrate through water or isotonic saline. Ultrasonic mists can be fanned as a "cold fog" into tents (high-humidity tent therapy) or attached to oxygen masks or face tents.

Mist therapy is sometimes ordered before or during intermittent positive-pressure breathing treatments or postural drainage. Prepare clients carefully for mist treatments. Stay with them throughout the treatment to ensure that they are familiar with the procedure and benefit from it. Teach them to cough effectively during and after the mist treatment. Document tolerance of the procedure (emotionally and physically) and the effectiveness of the treatment (e.g., amount of sputum produced). Some clients do not tolerate mist therapy well. The high water content in the air used may produce bronchospasm and a feeling of shortness of breath. Such a client is usually relieved by clearing the airways of water-laden secretions. If bronchospasm occurs, a bronchodilator may be administered. Because of these potential airway problems, mist therapy is used only for selected clients.

Nebulization may be prescribed as a continuous or intermittent procedure. Nebulized medication is specifically prescribed, including amount and frequency. If metered dose inhalers are used, a specific number of inhalations is prescribed. If other types of aerosol generators are used, treatment may take 10 to 20 minutes.

Assess the client carefully, documenting the effectiveness of treatment and any adverse reactions. For example, if bronchospasm was evident before therapy, did a nebulized bronchodilator improve the quality of breath sounds?

Nebulized air is also used in clients with tracheostomy. Tracheostomy creates an artificial air passage that bypasses the upper airway (see Chap. 38). Thus, the "new airway" is exposed to air that is not warmed, moistened, or filtered by upper respiratory mucosa. Nebulization or a cool mist is therefore used immediately after tracheostomy is established. A relative humidity of 100 per cent is desirable. The temperature of the nebulized mist may need to be monitored to prevent possible hyperthermia.

For preventing infection, it is important to use sterile nebulized solution and to change and sterilize the tubings, nebulizer, and connections at least every 24 hours. The water reservoir and moist tubing are an excellent breeding ground for bacterial colonization and infection.

After aerosol treatments, postural drainage, chest percussion, and expulsive coughing may be carried out. Nasal and oral hygiene should be performed to remove the secretions from the mucous membranes.

Facilitating Effective Coughing

Effective coughing is of utmost importance. An effective cough augments the body's own ciliary clearance

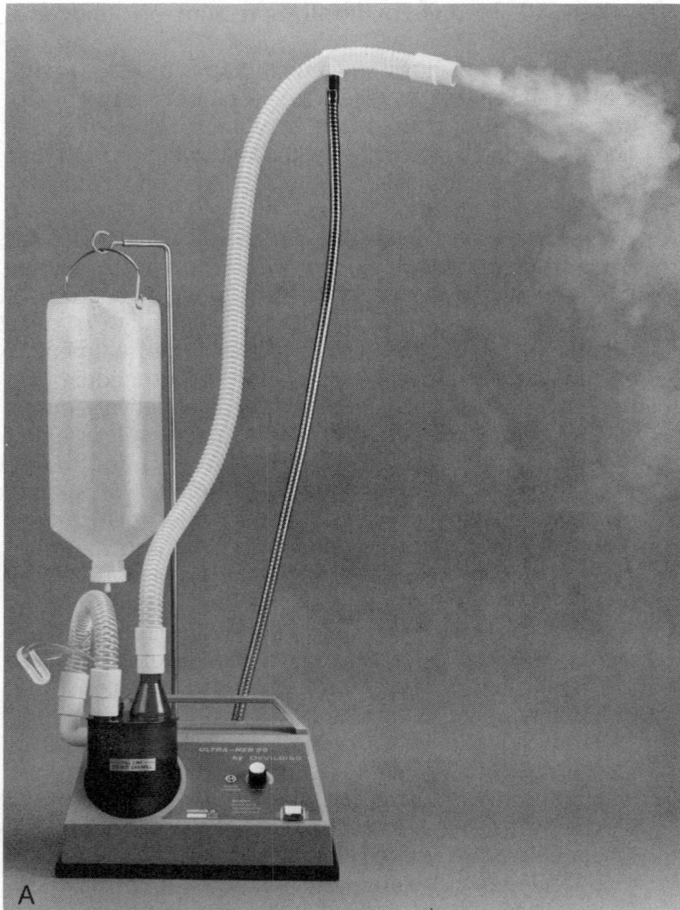

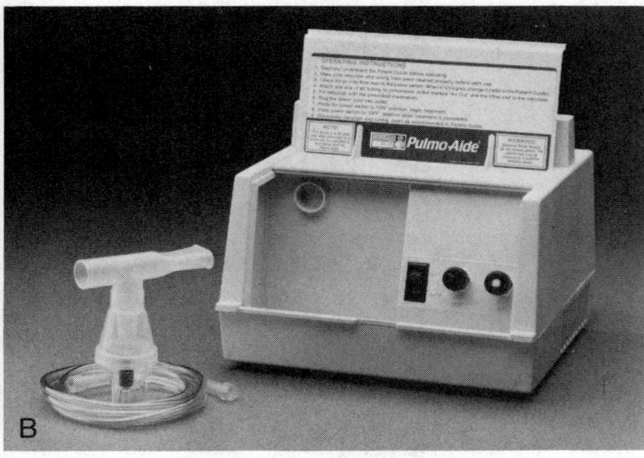

▲ *Figure 37–7*

Aerosalized medications can be administered through nebulizers. *A*, Medi-Mist (Courtesy of Mountain Medical Equipment, Inc. Littleton, CO) *B*, Pulmo-Aide (Courtesy of DeVilbis, Somerset, NJ)

mechanisms, thus helping to maintain patent airways. Ineffective (forced) coughing may cause adverse effects in clients with severe chronic lung disease. It may (1) collapse airways, producing air trapping; (2) rupture thin-walled alveoli (blebs); or (3) cause pneumothorax. Ineffective coughing is especially dangerous for clients with unstable cardiac and cerebral function. An effective cough is one in which the client uses (1) the diaphragm; (2) posture; (3) slow, deep, stacked breaths; and (4) short expulsive blasts of air to mobilize and expectorate secretions.

Five steps that create an effective cough while ensuring that muscular energy is not wasted are to

- assume a position that will facilitate effective use of the abdominal muscles. Assume a sitting position with the knees slightly flexed. If sitting in a chair or on the side of the bed is not possible, sit with the head of the bed raised and flex the knees with the feet planted firmly on the mattress.
- take slow, deep inspirations, using diaphragmatic breathing
- bear down against the glottis to produce a Valsalva-type maneuver. When the pressure inside the thorax peaks, a cough will be produced.
- exhale through pursed lips. Prolonged exhalation will move secretions to one of the tracheobronchial cough reflex centers.
- learn coughing technique before it is needed. Preoperative teaching about proper coughing techniques has been shown to be very effective. Coughing and pain medication administration should be maximized. Splinting of the operative site may help to alleviate some of the discomfort as well.

Modifications of the coughing technique are needed in those clients with chronic obstructive pulmonary disease (COPD) and early airway collapse. Effective coughing can be produced if smaller amounts of air are inspired before coughing. This technique creates less change in the intrathoracic pressure, which may help to prevent early airway collapse.

When helping clients learn effective coughing, nurses can use phrases such as "get air behind the mucus," "cough from your boots," and "build a pillar of air" to help clients understand what to do. The following nursing interventions also facilitate effective coughing:

- Position change. Roll the client from side to side to cause secretions to drain into large airways.
- Increased level of activity. Have the person sit in a chair or walk about. Encourage deep, diaphragmatic breathing with slow exhalation during ambulation.
- Vibrations/end-expiratory assist. Place your hands around the client's lower ribs. As the client exhales or coughs, apply firm, upward vibrating pressure.

This often supports the thorax enough to achieve an expulsive cough.

- Sips of water. A few sips of water or a cup of hot tea or coffee may stimulate coughing.
- Manually stimulated cough. Use a manual, self-inflating resuscitation bag to give a client with a tracheostomy or endotracheal tube a deep inflation. This often loosens secretions and promotes a cough in a client with an artificial airway.
- Splinting with a pillow over the client's abdomen.
- As a last resort, consider alternatives to coughing, such as suctioning.

INCENTIVE SPIROMETRY

When performed properly, deep breathing plays a key role in preventing and treating atelectasis. A deep breath is a very potent bronchodilator and is essential for effective coughing.

Incentive spirometry is used to encourage maximal deep breathing; it is a form of goal-directed therapy. The incentive to perform is provided by visualizing the amount of volume that is being achieved with each inspiration. The goal or volume to be achieved with each inspiration is set by the practitioner. The goals are individualized for each client. The nurse should consider the client's probable (or known) tidal volume and forced expiratory effort in setting the goal for incentive spirometry exercises. The goals set should be obtainable but only after some reasonable effort. Incentive breathing devices affect the inspiratory capacity and work on the principle of sustained, voluntary, maximal inflation (Fig. 37-8).

Incentive spirometry is most effective if taught to the client before it is needed (e.g., preoperatively) rather than when a client is sedated or in pain. It is often used to encourage deep breathing after surgery. People with pneumonia and neuromuscular weakness, and those on prolonged bed rest are also helped by incentive spirometry. Teach the client to perform a minimum of 8 to 10 sustained, voluntary, maximal inflation maneuvers an hour. Leave the device near the client. Supervise the client and increase the goals frequently. The incentive spirometry procedure is shown in the Client Education Guide.

Some clients may be overzealous and, unless told not to rush, may develop indications of hyperventilation (e.g., dizziness, lightheadedness). Incentive therapy requires the client's cooperation. It is not effective for a client unable to take deep breaths because of pain, uncoordinated breathing, weakness, obtundation, senility, or lack of motivation or cooperation.

Other types of respiratory therapy that may be used with incentive spirometry to optimize bronchopulmonary hygiene include (1) hydration; (2) aerosolized medications; (3) mobilization maneuvers such as turning, position changes, and ambulation; (4) chest physiotherapy; (5) breathing retraining; (6) assistance with and encouragement in effective coughing techniques; and (7) postural drainage.

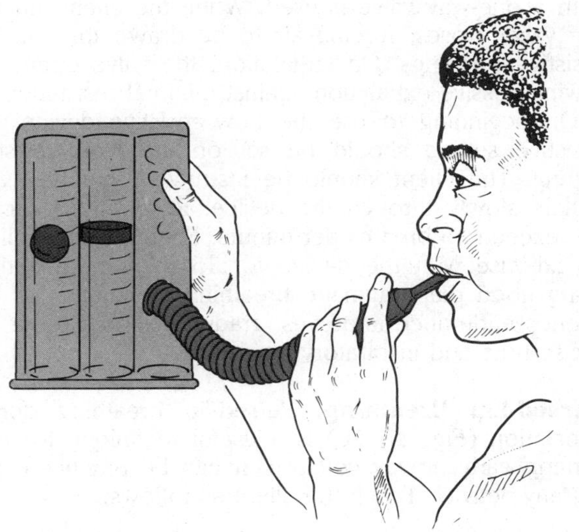

▲ **Figure 37-8**

Incentive spirometer encourages voluntary deep breathing by providing a visual cue to the client about the efficiency of deep breathing.

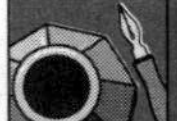

CLIENT EDUCATION GUIDE

Incentive Spirometry

1. Set attainable goals for the client.
2. Instruct the client to exhale slowly to a point of comfort.
3. Next, tell the client to place the mouthpiece between the teeth and place the lips around the mouthpiece.
4. Inhaling through the mouth only (a noseclip may be necessary), take in a slow, deep breath (using the diaphragm, not the accessory muscles), until the preset goal is attained.
5. Hold the breath for 3 to 5 seconds.
6. Exhale normally.
7. Rest between attempts.
8. Repeat steps 3, 5, 6, and 7.

BREATHING RETRAINING

Acute or chronic respiratory dysfunction often predisposes to ineffective breathing habits. Breathing retraining involves various methods to improve breathing patterns and ensure maximal use of the available respiratory function. It allows clients to "get the most out of what they have" and teaches them how to control breathing.

To be effective, breathing retraining must be correctly learned and performed constantly as a part of the client's way of life. It is not effective if practiced only periodically, e.g., a few minutes several times a day. For breathing exercises to be most helpful, good general body muscle tone that is maintained by following a program of regular exercises is also encouraged.

Breathing retraining must be adapted to a client's needs and not cause undue stress or increase dyspnea. Teach the client to do the following before beginning breathing exercises:

- Clear the respiratory tract of secretions by coughing. Suctioning may be necessary.
- Use an aerosolized bronchodilator to open the air passages and loosen tenacious mucus, then cough.
- Perform postural drainage to help remove secretions.
- Clear nasal passages. If blowing the nose does not bring relief, decongestant medications may be prescribed.

Diaphragmatic Breathing (Abdominal Breathing). The major muscles of respiration are the diaphragm and the intercostals. The diaphragm is a potentially strong, dome-shaped muscle separating the thorax and the abdomen. Clients with COPD (e.g., emphysema) have lost much of the elastic tissue in the lung. These clients use accessory muscles to breathe, such as the shoulder muscles, which are much less effective. This change results in pulmonary distention, gas trapping, and inefficient use of the respiratory muscles. By learning diaphragmatic breathing, the diaphragm is used more effectively, thereby decreasing the use of accessory muscles and the work of breathing. Expected benefits of diaphragmatic breathing include an increased tidal volume, a decreased respiratory rate, an increased exercise tolerance, and an increase in alveolar ventilation. Normally, during inspiration the diaphragm descends, enlarging the thorax, and air rushes into the lungs. During exhalation the diaphragm relaxes, recoils, and moves upward, forcing air out of the lungs.

When performed properly, diaphragmatic breathing causes the abdomen to rise visibly during deep inhalation and contract during exhalation. Tightening the abdominal muscles during exhalation helps the diaphragm squeeze air out of the lungs. By placing one hand on the abdomen and the other on the chest, the client can feel if breathing is correct while sitting up or reclining. Guidelines for teaching diaphragmatic breathing are in the Client Education Guide.

Diaphragmatic breathing requires practice to become part of one's normal breathing. Gradually the client adjusts this controlled breathing pattern to the rhythm of body movements (e.g., walking) and develops rhythm in which exhalation takes at least twice as long as inhalation. A metronome may help establish this rhythm.

Some breathing exercises emphasize forced exhalation to force "trapped" air out of the lungs while using a diaphragmatic breathing pattern. One method is to push on the chest with the flattened palms of the hands while exhaling (Fig. 37-9). Another exercise is to pull a band of material snugly around the chest while exhaling and relax the band when inhaling. Using a piece of tightly woven fabric at least 3 inches wide (e.g., drapery pleating tape) and maintaining even tension are important during this exercise.

Inspiratory Resistive Breathing. Inspiratory resistive breathing is simply imposing additional work on the inspiratory muscles during diaphragmatic breathing. With use of this method, over time, inspiratory muscle strength as well as endurance will be improved. Exercise tolerance will be enhanced with stronger, more efficient inspiratory muscles.

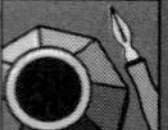

CLIENT EDUCATION GUIDE

Diaphragmatic Breathing

1. Help the client get comfortable, both physically and mentally.
2. Help the client assume a comfortable semi-Fowler's position with shoulders rotated slightly inward and with the knees bent.
3. Place your thumbs in the client's epigastric notch, i.e., just below the xiphoid process (Fig. 37-9). Comfortably spread your fingers around the lower ribs. Maintain this position.
4. Ask the client to inhale through the nose while relaxing the abdomen and pushing your thumbs "out" with the abdominal wall. The practitioner should provide gradual abdominal pressure during inspiration.
5. Instruct the client to pause naturally and briefly at the end of inspiration. This creates a smooth ventilation pattern and an even distribution of air in and out of the lungs.
6. Ask the client to exhale gently as you press inward and upward on the epigastric notch with your thumbs. Have the client contract the abdominal muscles and purse the lips during exhalation.
7. Ideally, the length of exhalation should be two to three times that of inhalation. This is especially important for clients who have difficulty breathing out effectively, e.g., those with chronic lung disease. However, do not overemphasize the length of exhalation time. If the client places undue effort on counting, anxiety and dyspnea may occur, defeating the purpose of breathing retraining.
8. When diaphragmatic breathing has been mastered in a semi-Fowler's position, the client should practice it in other positions (lying, standing, and sitting) and then during exercise. A hand or a weighted object, e.g., 5-lb sandbag or a book, placed on the upper abdomen may remind the client to use the diaphragm.

To strengthen inspiratory muscles, a flow resistor with a one-way valve is used. When the client inhales, the valve closes, forcing air to be drawn through the resistive openings. On exhalation, the valve opens, allowing passive exhalation against minimal resistance.

On beginning to use the flow resistive device, the resistive setting should be set on the least resistive setting. The client should be instructed to inhale and exhale slowly through the device. Respirations should not exceed 15 breaths per minute. Encourage the client to exercise with the device for 15 minutes at a time using good diaphragmatic breathing technique. As the client's endurance improves, gradually increase the exercise time and inspiratory resistance.

Pursed-Lip Breathing. Pursed-lip breathing during exhalation (Fig. 37-10) is a useful technique for preventing early airway collapse. It can be practiced during any activity. Teach the client as follows:

- Encourage the client to relax and breathe in through the nose.
- Next, instruct the client to exhale slowly and completely through pursed lips for a comfortable length of time.

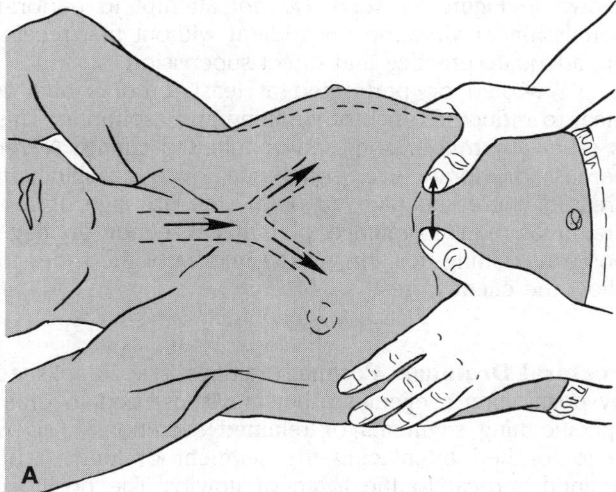

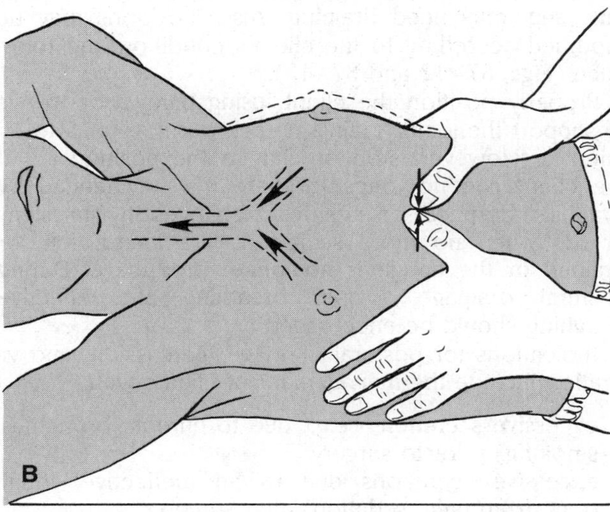

▲ *Figure 37-9*

Assessing diaphragmatic excursion during diaphragmatic breathing. Place your thumbs on the epigastric notch and spread your fingers around the lower ribs. *A*, As the client breathes in, your thumbs should spread out. *B*, As the client breathes out, your thumbs should move together again. (See text for discussion.)

With chronic lung disorders, airways lose their elasticity and may collapse during exhalation (especially during forced or labored exhalation). This traps air beyond (distal to) the point of collapse. The client is unable to exhale efficiently and becomes short of breath, anxious, and increasingly dyspneic. Pursing the lips slows or retards the flow rate of exhaled air. This (1) creates a back pressure in the airways, which keeps the "flabby" airways open and prevents airway collapse, and (2) helps empty the lungs more completely.

Coaching Breathing Retraining. Breathing retraining helps a client with respiratory dysfunction develop a sense of normality without creating undue respiratory distress. Coaching is a very important component of any breathing retraining technique. It improves instruction, demonstration, discussion, and practice. During teaching sessions, discuss the ways the technique will help the client (e.g., increased activity without shortness of breath). The technique is demonstrated, and the client practices it while the nurse observes and offers support. Genuine encouragement and praise help keep a client committed to an exercise routine. As the clients become proficient in controlled breathing, they often learn to reduce and control anxiety-produced dyspnea and thus prevent disease from controlling their lives.

It is important that the client develop a habit of using the breathing techniques all the time rather than just "practicing" them periodically. Pursed-lip and diaphragmatic breathing can be used during all activities of daily living.

Relaxation. To develop maximal breathing control, the client must learn to relax. When helping a client learn to relax, the nurse must assume an unhurried and calm manner. Have the client wear loose clothing. Teach the client the dyspnea positions (see Fig. 37-1), which facilitate diaphragmatic breathing without increasing the work of other muscle groups. These positions can be assumed at any time or place and facilitate relaxation, which may allow the client to gain control of the breathing pattern. Instruct the client to use diaphragmatic breathing and slow, relaxed, pursed-lip exhalation. Various relaxation exercises may be used. Many self-relaxation tapes and books are available. Meditation is also a powerful means of relaxation. In addition, the following exercises may promote relaxation.

- Slow head rolling to the left and right in a circular pattern coordinated with breathing. Inhale as the head goes from left to right. Exhale as the head swings from right to left.
- Shoulder rolling (backward and forward) coordi-

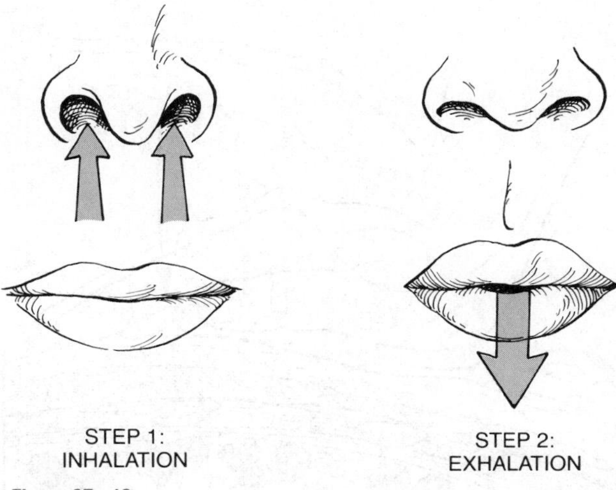

▲ *Figure 37-10*

Breathing retraining, pursed-lip breathing. Step 1: Inhale slowly through nose, keeping mouth closed. Count "one and two." Pause briefly. Step 2: Exhale through pursed lips as if gently blowing a candle flame. Count "one, two, three, four." Because exhalation is a passive process, allow adequate time to empty lungs and reduce air trapping. Exhalation should take at least twice as long as inhalation. Learning to breathe with this technique helps clients control respiration when excited, anxious, or exercising or during respiratory distress.

nated with breathing. Inhale while rolling the shoulders backward. Exhale while bringing them forward.

- Arm swinging (backward and forward) coordinated with breathing. Inhale while the arms swing upward and forward. Exhale on the downward and backward swing.
- Tightening all muscle groups from head to toe while inhaling and relaxing all muscle groups while exhaling.

During these exercises, have the client inhale through the nose and exhale through pursed lips. Teach the client to make a conscious effort to exhale slowly and as completely as possible. The ventilation pattern must be relaxed, unhurried, and comfortable.

CHEST PHYSIOTHERAPY

Chest physiotherapy (CPT) is a combination of percussion over the chest wall, vibration, coughing, and deep breathing. CPT combined with postural drainage is an effective method of mobilizing secretions.

The goals of CPT may include mobilization and clearance of sputum, an increase in exercise tolerance, improving ventilation, and restoring effective breathing patterns.

Percussion and Vibration. Percussion (Fig. 37–11*A*) is performed by clapping on the chest wall with a cupped hand over an affected area of the lung. A cupped hand "captures" a pocket of air as it strikes the chest. Do not slap the chest wall. Place a towel on the chest of the client over the area in which the percussion is being performed. A hollow, deep sound is produced when percussion is done correctly.

Vibration is applied to the chest; energy waves from the hand are used to move secretions from affected lung areas during the expiration phase of respiration, as shown in Figure 37–11*B*. *Do not* attempt to perform percussion or vibration on a client without first receiving adequate practice and direct supervision.

CPT should be performed at least 2 hours after a meal to reduce the risk of vomiting and aspiration. This is especially true in confused or tube-fed clients. Never percuss or vibrate over soft tissue, over the spine, in areas of increased pain, or below the rib cage. If several areas require drainage, plan apical section drainage positions (sitting position) in the middle of the series to allow the client to rest.

Postural Drainage. Postural drainage is accomplished by positioning a client so that gravity is used to drain specific lung segments of retained secretions. This is accomplished by placing the segment of lung to be drained vertical to the force of gravity. The positions used for postural drainage differ, depending on which lung segments need draining. Also, positions may be modified according to the client's condition and tolerance (Figs. 37–12 and 37–13).

Properly position the client, using pillows or towels to support the joints. Maintain each position for 5 to 10 minutes. However, stop or change the position (1) if the client can no longer tolerate it as evidenced by cyanosis, dyspnea, or significant changes in vital signs or (2) when no more secretions are heard, felt, or drained or the cough is no longer productive. During postural drainage, proper breathing and effective coughing should be encouraged.

Indications for postural drainage, percussion, and vibration include the management of clients with

- excessive secretions (e.g., due to chronic bronchitis, smoking) prior to surgery
- excessive secretions due to an ineffective cough (e.g., from pain, sedation) after surgery

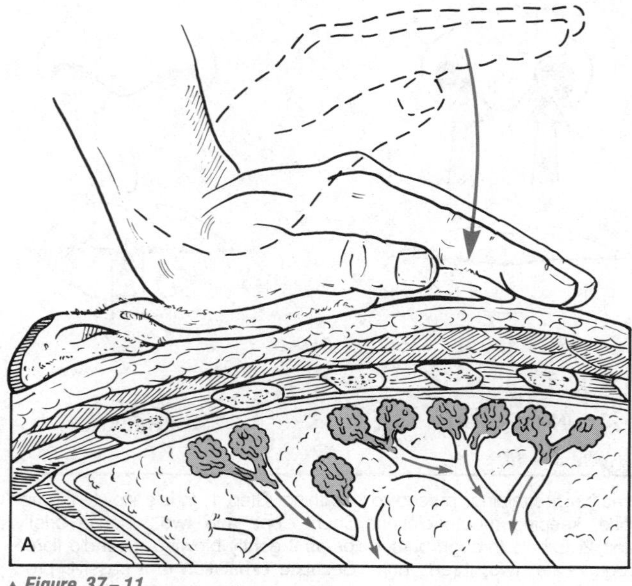

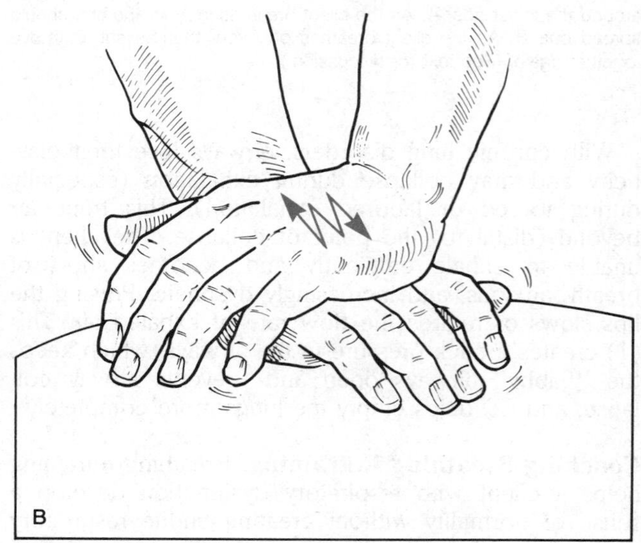

▲ Figure 37–11

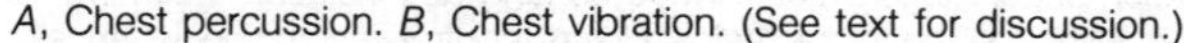

A, Chest percussion. *B*, Chest vibration. (See text for discussion.)

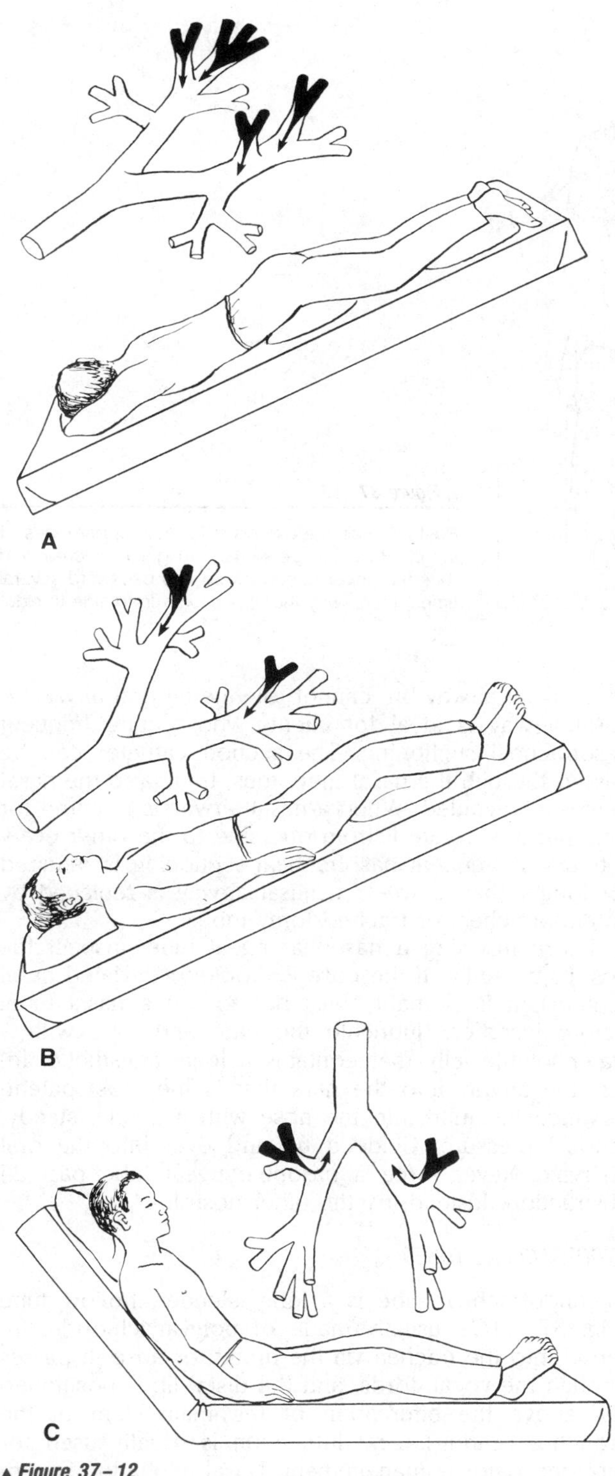

▲ Figure 37-12

Commonly used postural drainage positions. *A* drains posterior basilar segments, *B* drains middle lobes, and *C* drains upper lobes.

- any chronic disease process producing abnormal sputum that increases the risk of recurrent infection (e.g., cystic fibrosis, bronchiectasis, chronic bronchitis); also, for bronchial or lobar pneumonia that is productive of secretions and lung abscess (if abscess does not involve the vascular system)
- bronchospasm or extreme sputum tenacity that makes it difficult or exhausting to raise secretions (e.g., asthma, bronchiectasis)
- musculoskeletal abnormalities that interfere with effective coughing (e.g., scoliosis, quadriplegia, "barrel chest")

Contraindications for postural drainage include the presence of

- increased cyanosis or exhaustion after its use
- secretions that, once mobilized, could obstruct the airway, especially when suction equipment is not available
- unstable vital signs, including increased intracranial pressure
- any pre-emergent medical or surgical situation

Contraindications for percussion and vibration include the presence of

- known or suspected carcinoma or metastatic disease in the area to be treated
- bronchospasm that increases by their use
- pain during the treatment
- possible hemorrhage or seizure activity a predisposition to pathologic rib fractures (use percussion judiciously)

Client Teaching. It is important to teach clients who have respiratory problems (and their significant others) these techniques so that they can participate in their care. In large health care facilities, CPT is usually performed by respiratory therapists. In smaller settings, it is often a nursing responsibility. Even when respiratory therapists are available, nurses often become involved in the program by continuing teaching, supervision, and support. Education and supervised practice are essential for anyone administering CPT and postural drainage.

CPT is used in various respiratory disorders (e.g., bronchiectasis, COPD) and after chest surgery and chest injury. It often takes several weeks of treatment for a client with a chronic respiratory problem to experience any benefit. Help clients understand the length of time needed so they do not become discouraged.

Artificial Airways

Comatose or obtunded clients often require an artificial airway to maintain airway patency. There are various kinds of artificial airways: oral airway, nasal airway, endotracheal tube, tracheostomy tube. It is often necessary to quickly select an appropriate airway that will only minimally traumatize the client.

ORAL (OROPHARYNGEAL) AIRWAYS

An oral airway (Fig. 37-14*A*) is a hollow, curved, rubber or plastic tube that lies between the posterior pharynx and the root of the tongue. There are various sizes of oral airways. It is essential to select the proper airway. The length of an airway should match the dis-

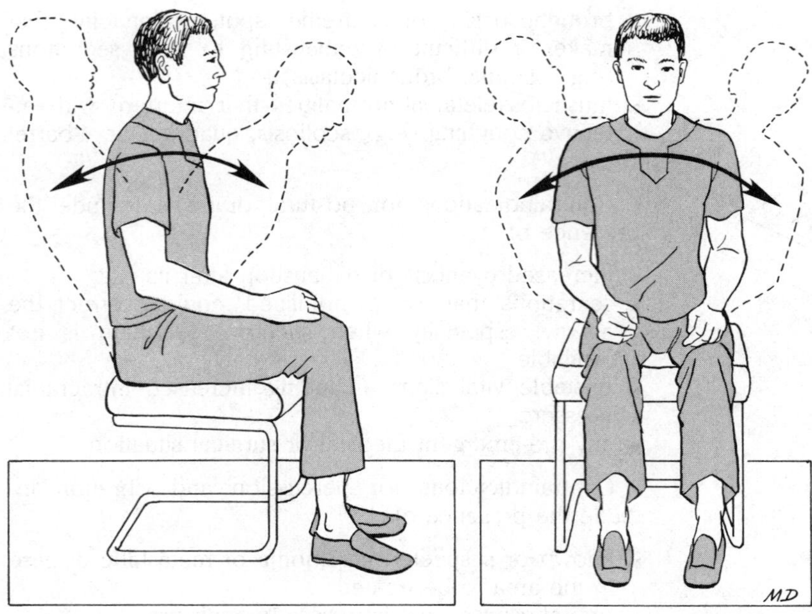

▲ *Figure 37–13*

Postural drainage exercises to drain upper lobes of lungs. Have the person sit upright in a chair and rock the upper torso forward and backward several times, then sway the upper torso from side to side.

tance between the lips and the angle of the jaw. Too long an oral airway causes gagging or coughing. Too short an airway may push the tongue back into the throat and increase airway obstruction. Contraindications for the use of oral airways may include a conscious person, facial fractures, or a foreign body in the oral cavity.

To insert an oral airway, hyperextend (tilt back) the neck and carefully open the mouth. Pass the airway through the teeth with its tip directed toward the roof of the mouth. Rotate the airway while advancing it toward the back of the oral cavity. It will slide into place and hold the tongue up and forward. The end of the tube should lie at the base of the tongue, and the outer flange should be positioned with the bite block between the teeth. Once inserted, an oral airway prevents the tongue from obstructing the airway of an unconscious client.

A conscious client or someone with an intact gag reflex cannot tolerate an oral airway. Hence, a client who can expel an airway probably does not need one. If gagging occurs, remove the airway. An oral airway is a temporary, short-term device. If a client requires an artificial airway for an extended period, an endotracheal tube is more appropriate.

NASAL AIRWAYS (NASOPHARYNGEAL AIRWAYS, NASAL TRUMPETS)

The nasal airway (Fig. 37–14*B*) is a hollow, soft rubber tube that fits into the nasal passage. When inserted correctly, the nasopharyngeal airway provides a passageway from the nares to the base of the tongue. In selecting the airway, length is more important than diameter. The proper length can be estimated by measuring the distance from the nose to the earlobe. Airway diameter should be slightly smaller than the nostril. A nasal airway may be appropriate for clients who require an artificial airway but cannot tolerate an oral airway. A nasal airway is ideal for clients who require frequent nasotracheal suctioning. The suction catheter can be passed through the nasal tube; thus, trauma to the nasal mucosa is avoided. When a nasal airway is required for long periods, rotate it from one side to the other every 8 hours. If frequent nasotracheal suctioning is required for longer than a week, a nasal airway is replaced by an endotracheal or tracheostomy tube.

Before inserting a nasopharyngeal tube, inspect the nostrils carefully. If the nose is crooked (deviated nasal septum), it is probably best not to use a nasal tube. Before insertion, lubricate the nare and tube with a water-soluble jelly that contains a local anesthetic. Insert the airway into the nare that is the most patent. Advance the tube into the nose with a gentle, steady, upward pressure. Guide it up and over into the oral pharynx. Never force a nasopharyngeal tube past an obstruction. Instead, try the other nostril.

ENDOTRACHEAL TUBES

An endotracheal tube is a long, slender, hollow tube (Fig. 37–14*C*), usually made of polyvinylchloride, inserted into the trachea via the mouth or nose. It passes through the vocal cords, and the distal tip is positioned just above the bifurcation of the main stem of the bronchus (carina). Oral intubation is usually used for short-term airway management. Nasal intubation is generally more secure and is believed to be more comfortable because it does not move as much in the airway. However, many institutions are not using nasal intubation owing to the risk of sinusitis. If a client requires prolonged intubation, a tracheostomy may be performed (Fig. 37–14*D*).

Indications for endotracheal intubation include

- relief of airway obstruction
- prevention of aspiration

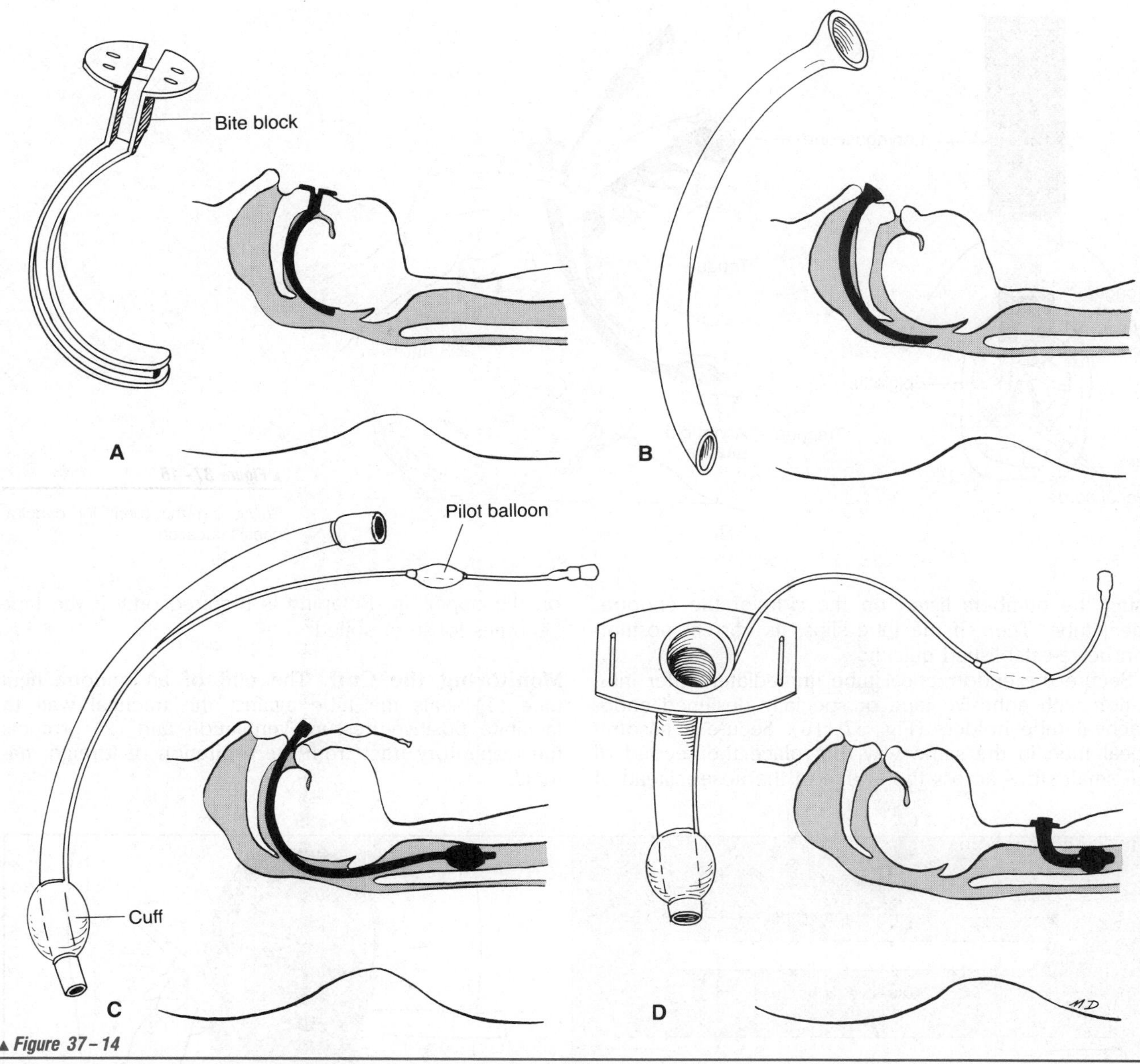

▲ *Figure 37-14*

Artificial airways. *A*, Oral airway; *B*, nasal airway; *C*, endotracheal tube; *D*, tracheostomy tube. Endotracheal tubes have several parts: 15-mm adapter on the proximal end, pilot balloon, radiopaque pilot line, and cuff. All respiratory therapy and anesthesiology equipment is designed to connect with a 15-mm adapter. Consequently, a client can easily be manually ventilated, mechanically ventilated, or anesthetized via the same endotracheal tube.

- facilitation of tracheal suctioning
- facilitation of artificial ventilation

Inserting the Tube. The client is positioned supine with all dental bridgework and plates removed. Loose teeth should be identified. These items can be jarred loose and aspirated during intubation. The client's head is hyperextended, the lower aspect of the neck flexed, and the mouth opened (Fig. 37-15). This position brings the mouth, pharynx, and larnyx into a straight line. A laryngoscope is used to hold the airway open, expose the vocal cords, and serve as a guide for the tube into the trachea. Endotracheal tubes are inserted only by fully trained health care team members.

Intubation should not cause or exacerbate hypoxia. If the client's neck and mandible are mobile, the procedure usually takes about 30 seconds. Certain pre-existing conditions, such as rheumatoid arthritis of the neck, can make intubation difficult. For clients with expected difficulty of intubation, an oxygen mask can be used to provide oxygen through the mouth. An oxygen saturation monitor is also used to warn of hypoxemia.

Immediately after an endotracheal tube has been inserted, tube placement is verified by auscultation and chest x-ray examination to ensure aeration of both sides of the chest. Record in the nurses' notes and on the respiratory flow sheet the point at which the tube meets the lips or nostrils. This position can be noted by

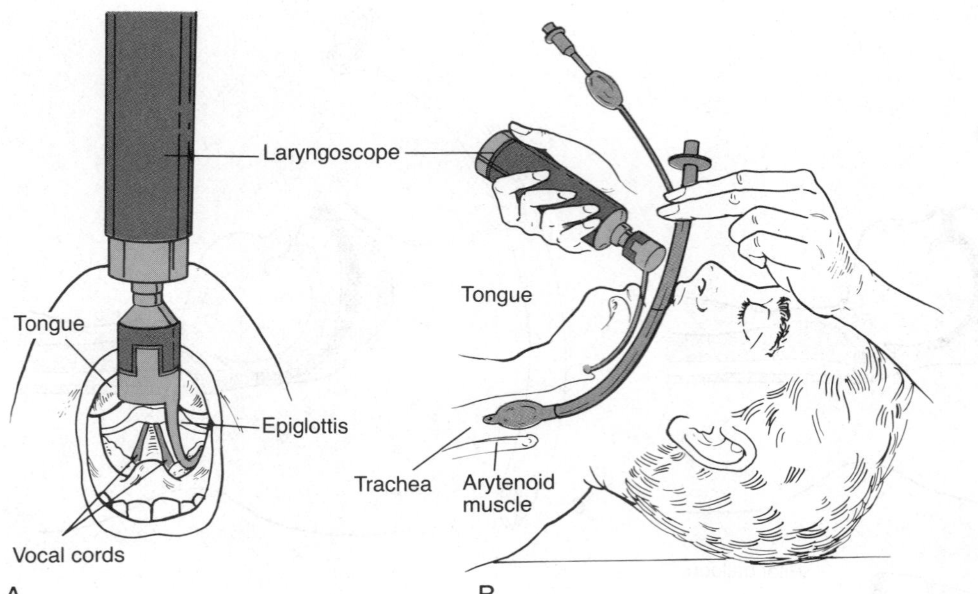

▲ **Figure 37-15**

Positioning the client for endotracheal intubation.

using the numbers listed on the side of the endotracheal tube. Then, if the tube slips, its correct position can be re-established quickly.

Secure the endotracheal tube immediately after intubation with adhesive tape or specially designed endotracheal tube holders (Fig. 37-16). Secure a nasotracheal tube in the same way, but place the second of the small strips across the bridge of the nose instead of on the upper lip. Retaping is required only if the tape becomes loose or soiled.

Monitoring the Cuff. The cuff of an endotracheal tube (1) seals the tube against the tracheal wall to facilitate positive-pressure ventilation and (2) protects the respiratory tract from the aspiration of foreign material.

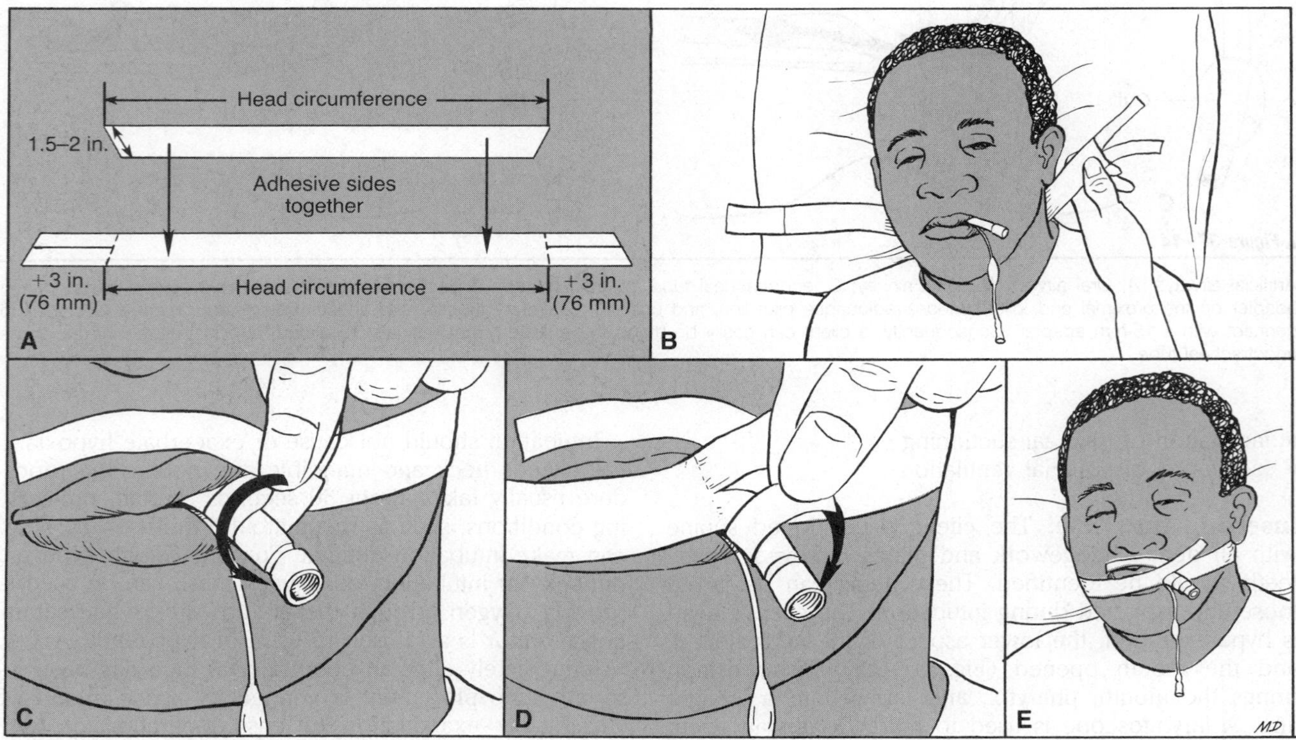

▲ **Figure 37-16**

Securing a cuffed endotracheal tube with tape. *A,* Two strips of tape are torn, one measuring head circumference and the other 6 inches longer. They are placed with adhesive sides together to form a strip. *B,* Place the strip behind the head and tear one end of the strip in half. *C,* Secure the tube to the upper lip with the untorn end. *D,* Wrap the torn segments around the tube to secure it.

The amount of air required to seal an endotracheal (or tracheostomy) tube cuff is reflected by the cuff pressure, which is usually maintained at less than 20 mm Hg. Cuff pressure, measured with a manometer, is important because it reflects the pressure the cuff is exerting on the tracheal wall. Too high a cuff pressure impedes circulation to the tracheal mucosa. This decrease in blood flow may lead to stenosis and necrosis of the trachea.

Cuff Inflation and Deflation. Most endotracheal tubes are designed with soft plastic cuffs to use high volumes at low pressures. They are inflated with a high enough volume of air to seal the trachea while exerting the lowest possible pressure on the tracheal wall.

Low cuff pressure is necessary to prevent damage to the tracheal mucosa. Circulatory pressures in the tracheal wall are arterial pressures of 30 mm Hg and venous pressures of 18 mm Hg. Therefore, a cuff pressure of around 18 mm Hg will compromise venous pressure. A cuff pressure of approximately 30 mm Hg will stop all circulation to the tracheal mucosa, and necrosis may develop.

The most common method of cuff inflation is the minimal leak technique. The aim of this technique is to provide an adequate seal in the trachea at the lowest possible cuff pressure. This is attained by slowly injecting air into the cuff while auscultating the neck area over the cuff during a positive-pressure breath. Minimal leak has been achieved when only a very small leak is noted at the peak inflation pressure.

Generally, endotracheal cuffs should remain inflated at all times. Tracheostomy cuffs are occasionally deflated when the client is no longer on mechanical ventilation and has begun to eat. Swallowing effectiveness is improved with the cuff down in some clients. Also, fenestrated tracheostomy tube cuffs are always deflated when the inner cannula is removed and the outer opening is closed or "plugged." This decreases the amount of airway resistance by allowing air to move around the tracheostomy tube as well as providing for adequate sputum clearance. If cuff deflation is required for any reason, use the following procedure:

1. Suction the trachea (remember to hyperventilate and hyperoxygenate before and during this procedure).
2. Clean the area above the cuff of secretions by gently suctioning deep into the oropharynx.
3. Advance the suction catheter to the end of the endotracheal or tracheostomy tube. Deflate the cuff while applying suction to the suction catheter, so that any secretions lying above the cuff will be removed.
4. Repeat pharyngeal suctioning.

Cuff Leaks. Cuff leaks are a major problem. They may be caused by a rupture or tear in the cuff or pilot system and by the endotracheal tube's changing positions in the trachea. Signs of a leak in or around the endotracheal tube cuff include (1) the pilot balloon's not filling when air is injected, (2) the client's ability to talk when the cuff is inflated, (3) air heard leaking during positive-pressure breathing, and (4) food suctioned up through the tube. Because the system is not functional, the endotracheal tube is replaced. Before replacement, increasing tidal volume may help maintain ventilation by compensating for the escaping gas. The client is at high risk for aspiration while the cuff is leaking.

Removing the Tube (Extubation). Extubation is the removal of the endotracheal tube. The client's respiratory function is monitored throughout the time of intubation (heart rate, ABGs, lung sounds, and lung expansion). When the client demonstrates adequate arterial oxygen levels, tidal volume, vital capacity, and negative inspiratory force as well as a level of consciousness to sustain spontaneous respiration, the endotracheal tube may be removed. Endotracheal tubes are removed with physician's orders and only by health care team members qualified to reintubate if necessary. The occurrence of laryngospasm and tracheal edema after extubation may occlude the airway and require reintubation. If the client has been on mechanical ventilation, weaning from the ventilator is accomplished before extubation; this process is discussed later (see Mechanical Ventilators).

The endotracheal tube is suctioned, the cuff deflated, and the tube removed. Immediately after extubation, the client is usually placed on oxygen. The client is also assessed for signs of respiratory distress and hypoxia as evidenced by restlessness, irritability, tachycardia, tachypnea, and decreased PaO_2 or increased $PaCO_2$. If these signs are noted, the physician should be notified, and the nurse should prepare for reintubation.

Some clients are restless and extubate themselves. Because the cuff is not deflated, there can be damage to the tracheal wall and bleeding. In most cases, the client requires reintubation, and this is done swiftly to prevent hypoxia and to avoid having to insert the endotracheal tube through swollen tissues. Sometimes, however, the client will be monitored and not reintubated, especially if the client was nearing the time for extubation. To prevent this problem, clients with endotracheal tubes are restrained.

Complications. Endotracheal intubation can lead to complications. Tracheal necrosis from cuff pressures over 20 mm Hg, tracheal trauma from self-extubation, and aspiration from inability to seal the airway are the most common complications.

Nursing Management

Suctioning. Suctioning secretions is a common nursing intervention used to (1) remove secretions from the nose, mouth, and tracheobronchial tree and (2) stimulate productive coughing. Suctioning the nose and mouth is a relatively simple, safe procedure. (The technique is discussed in a fundamentals textbook.)

The goal of all suctioning procedures is to remove secretions and to stimulate productive coughing without creating complications.

The trachea may be suctioned by passing a sterile catheter through the mouth or nose or via an endotracheal or tracheostomy tube. Effective tracheal suctioning is a gentle yet swift procedure in which timing is very important. When properly performed, it is relatively painless and promotes comfort for a client experiencing respiratory distress. Suctioning can save a client's life, but if improperly performed, it can be painful, detrimental, and even fatal.

Oral and nasal tracheal suctioning should not be the first-line therapy for removal of secretions. Try other techniques to stimulate productive coughing before using tracheal suctioning for this purpose. Tracheal suctioning is needed only for clients (1) with tenacious secretions that require suction removal, (2) with impaired pulmonary function that interferes with the cough reflex, or (3) with debilitation and weakness who cannot bring up secretions even after vigorous coughing.

Many complications may be avoided by hyperinflating a client's lungs and providing oxygen before, during, and after tracheal suctioning. Possible complications from tracheal suctioning include infection, hypoxemia, mechanical trauma to the mucosa, alveolar collapse (atelectasis), bradycardia, tachycardia, rupture of a bronchial suture line, and cardiac arrhythmias. Complications and nursing precautions are presented in Table 37-3 and Figure 37-17.

Nursing Precautions

Assessment. Assess for clinical manifestations of airway obstructions requiring suctioning. These include noisy, wet respirations; restlessness; increased pulse and respirations; visible mucus bubbling into an artificial airway; rhonchi identified by auscultation; an increase in peak airway pressure visible on a manometer if the client is on continuous mechanical ventilation. Cyanosis is a late sign of upper airway obstruction. A conscious client is usually aware of airway obstruction and can ask for help. Obtunded clients need careful and constant assessment with prompt suctioning when indicated.

TABLE 37-3. Complications of Tracheal Suctioning

Complication	Pathophysiologic Basis	Nursing Precautions
Hypoxemia	Suctioning removes the oxygen from the airways	Preoxygenate the client with manual ventilation or ventilator sighing, to $1\frac{1}{2}$ the usual tidal volume and with a high FIO_2 (0.6-1.0)
Dysrhythmias (premature ventricular contractions, tachycardia, bradycardia, asystole)	Hypoxemia can be caused by prolonged suctioning, stimulating pacemaker cells within the heart; a vasovagal response may also occur, causing bradycardia	Limit suctioning to 10 seconds, preoxygenate Monitor the electrocardiogram during suctioning Use extra caution in clients (1) with PaO_2 below 70 mm Hg (suctioning further reduces PaO_2), (2) with a large alveolar-arterial gradient (indicating very low cardiopulmonary reserve), and (3) in generally poor condition, e.g., with inadequate oxygenation, hypotension, arrhythmias, acid-base imbalances
Bronchospasm	Respiratory reflex caused by irritation of the tracheal membranes, improper ventilation, and coughing	Be certain to time the inflation stage of mechanical ventilation with the client's own inspiratory effort Do not forcibly inflate the bag against the client's exhalation May require bronchodilators
Airway trauma	Direct trauma to the airway or excessive pressures used to suction	Keep the suction level below 120 mm Hg Suction only as the client needs it, usually no more often than every hour
Infection	Introduction of pathogens into the sterile airway	Use sterile technique for suctioning procedures Change reservoirs of water for humidification daily Assess the color and quantity of sputum
Atelectasis/lobar collapse	Use of excessive wall suction pressure and a suction catheter that is too large for the airway causes a vacuum, collapsing the lung units distal to the tip of the catheter	Use suction catheter that does not exceed one third to one half of the diameter of the airway being suctioned A 12- to 14-French catheter is used in the average adult Use smaller catheters if the endotracheal tube size is less than a 7-French Suction pressure is kept at less than 120 mm Hg

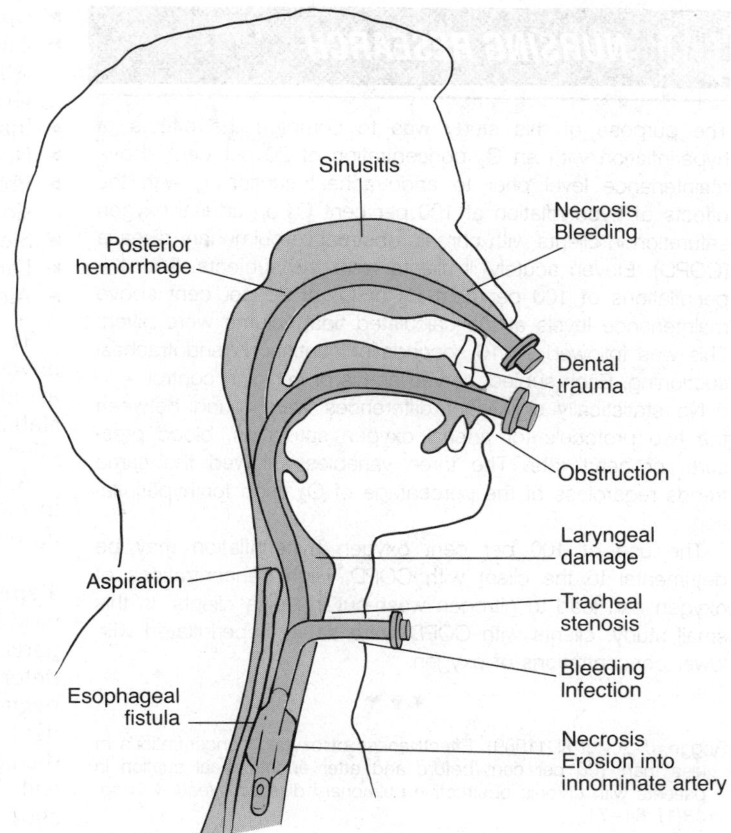

▲ *Figure 37-17*

Complications of endotracheal intubation and tracheostomy. (From Marino, P. [1991]. *The ICU book*. Philadelphia: Lea & Febiger.)

Thinning Secretions. Clients with excessive tracheobronchial secretions are often helped by humidification of their inspired air to loosen secretions. Tracheobronchial hydration may be done by (1) parenteral or oral methods, (2) aerosolization of liquid, or (3) direct instillation of liquefying agents. To loosen thick, tenacious mucus, 3 to 5 ml of sterile normal saline may be instilled directly into the trachea via the catheter or endotracheal tube, just before suctioning. Distribute the normal saline throughout the lungs by manually hyperinflating with a self-inflating resuscitation bag, or have the client take two to three deep breaths.

Providing Oxygenation. Before suctioning, oxygenate the client with use of a manual resuscitation bag. Hyperinflate the lungs with 100 per cent oxygen for five or six breaths to increase the PaO_2 before suctioning. Tracheal suctioning removes oxygen and therefore lowers the PaO_2, which may trigger cardiac dysrhythmias. When possible, assess pulse and heart rhythm before and during suctioning. Tachycardia is a result of agitation and hypoxemia. If tachycardia occurs during tracheal suctioning, assess its severity and proceed only if it is mild. Bradycardia results from vagal stimulation of the larynx and carina. If bradycardia develops, discontinue suctioning immediately and ventilate the client with 100 per cent oxygen. Report and document untoward effects of suctioning immediately. The use of less than 100 per cent oxygen for hyperinflation in clients with COPD is discussed in Nursing Research.

Performing Psychosocial Interventions. Tracheal suctioning can be an uncomfortable, often frightening procedure. Once the catheter passes between the vocal cords, the client cannot talk because the cords cannot approximate. Naturally, the client may become very anxious and restless. Explain the procedure and gently tell the client what to do throughout the procedure, e.g., not to swallow while the catheter is being inserted, and not to cough or talk. Reassure the client that the procedure will be very quick, 15 seconds at most. Your skill and competence will be the most reassuring of all.

Sometimes during tracheal suctioning a client instinctively wants to pull at the catheter, especially when the cough reflex is stimulated. Explain this tendency and ask the client to try to control this desire. Occasionally it is necessary to spray the nasopharynx with a topical anesthetic in clients with very active gag reflexes. However, this is generally avoided because it depresses the cough reflex and increases the risk of aspiration.

Loss of a sense of personal dignity may accompany tracheal intubation or tracheostomy. The whole experience is very frightening. The client cannot speak or breathe normally, and the presence of the tube may limit physical mobility. Spend time with the client (encourage significant others to do the same); communicate concern and understanding, both verbally and nonverbally.

Helping Clients Cope with Inability to Speak. An en-

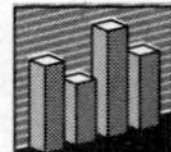

NURSING RESEARCH

The purpose of this study was to compare the effects of hyperinflation with an O_2 concentration of 20 per cent above maintenance level prior to endotracheal suctioning with the effects of hyperinflation at 100 per cent O_2 on arterial oxygen saturation in clients with chronic obstructive pulmonary disease (COPD). Eleven acutely ill clients were the subjects. Four hyperinflations of 100 per cent O_2 or O_2 at 20 per cent above maintenance levels at the calculated tidal volume were given. This was followed by 10 seconds of continuous endotracheal suctioning. Each subject served as his or her own control.

No statistically significant differences were found between the two protocols for arterial oxygen saturation, blood pressure, or heart rate. The three variables followed the same trends regardless of the percentage of O_2 used for hyperinflation.

The use of 100 per cent oxygen hyperinflation may be detrimental to the client with COPD. High concentrations of oxygen can lead to nitrogen wash-out in these clients. In this small study, clients with COPD were safely hyperinflated with lower concentrations of oxygen.

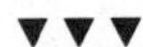

Rogge, J. A., et al. (1989). Effectiveness of oxygen concentrations of less than 100 per cent before and after endotracheal suction in patients with chronic obstructive pulmonary disease. *Heart & Lung, 18*(1), 64–71.

dotracheal tube passes through the vocal cords. A tracheostomy bypasses them altogether. Therefore, a client with either cannot cough effectively or speak. Create a means of communication. For example, keep a pencil and paper pad readily available. Be patient and willing to spend time communicating with the client so that feelings of frustration are avoided.

Providing Oral Hygiene. Careful oral hygiene is essential every few hours for a client requiring suctioning or with an endotracheal tube. Secretions pool in the oropharynx because of the inflated tracheal cuff. Frequent oral suctioning above the cuff is highly recommended. The client's teeth should be brushed and oral mucosa moistened with solutions without alcohol or lemon because these solutions dry mucous membranes.

TRACHEOSTOMY

A *tracheotomy* is a surgical opening made into the trachea for airway management (see Figure 37–14*D*). A *tracheostomy* is the surgical creation of a stoma from the trachea to the overlying skin. Even though the terms indicate different procedures, they are often used interchangeably. Realizing the difference in terms, but for the benefit of simplicity, the term tracheostomy is used in the text.

Indications for tracheostomy are

- Need for long-term artificial airway
- Upper airway obstruction
- Upper airway bleeding
- Altered level of consciousness, such as increasing lethargy or obtundation, producing inability to protect the lower airway
- Inability to clear lower airway secretions
- Need for continuous mechanical ventilation
- Prolonged endotracheal tube insertion, causing erosion or pain
- Sleep apnea
- Laryngeal or tracheal fracture
- Airway burns

Tracheostomy is by far the most satisfactory artificial airway. It totally bypasses the upper airway and glottis, avoiding complications in those areas. It is easier to stabilize, suction, and attach respiratory equipment. The client can eat and, with some adjustments, can talk.

A tracheostomy is performed by making an incision in the lower neck (Fig. 37–18). It can be performed as an emergency or elective procedure.

Types of Tracheostomy Tubes. Tracheostomy tubes vary in their (1) composition, (2) number of separate parts, (3) shape, and (4) size. The type to be used is determined before the tracheostomy procedure is begun. Incorrectly fitting tubes can precipitate permanent or life-threatening damage. A tracheostomy tube's diameter should be smaller than the trachea so that it will lie comfortably within the tracheal lumen. Air should be able to pass between the outer wall of the tracheostomy tube and the tracheal mucosa. There is no standard tracheostomy tube–sizing system, but all packages indicate the inner and outer diameter in millimeters.

The length and curve of a tracheostomy tube are important. Tracheostomy tubes may be long (e.g., Hollinger tube, Shiley single-channel tube), or short. They may be angled from 50 to 90 degrees. Short to moder-

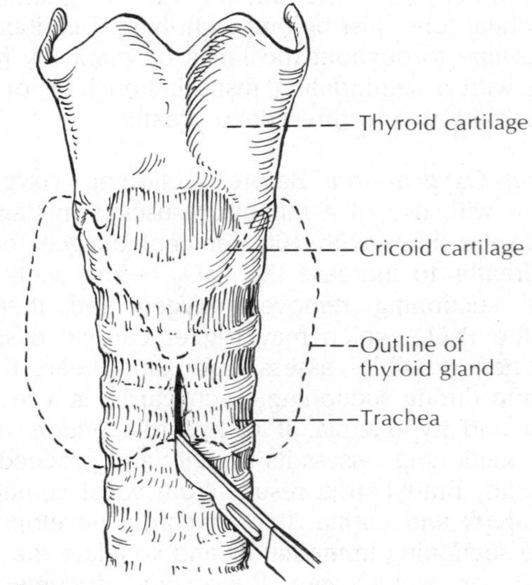

▲ **Figure 37–18**

Incision for a tracheostomy is made vertically through the second, third, or fourth tracheal ring.

ately short tubes with an angle of about 60 degrees are most often used. A tube must be long enough to avoid dislodgement into paratracheal tissue when the person coughs or turns the head. The lower end of a tracheostomy tube should be located above the carina. The tube's curve must allow the tip to be in a straight line with the trachea rather than to press on the anterior or posterior tracheal wall.

Tracheostomy tubes may be cuffed or uncuffed. Inflated cuffs permit mechanical ventilation and protect the lower airway by creating a seal between the upper and lower airways. Tracheostomy cuffs do not hold the tube in place. Rather, when inflated, they seal the area between the outer cannula and the tracheal wall. To inflate a tracheostomy cuff, inject air with a syringe through the one-way valve into the pilot line and pilot tube. Once the syringe is removed, the one-way valve prevents air's escaping from the inflated cuff. A pilot balloon reflects the presence or absence of air in the cuff. However, it cannot be considered an absolute indicator of cuff inflation.

Most tracheostomy tube cuffs are designed to exert a low pressure against the tracheal wall through use of an easily distensible cuff that accepts a high volume of air without generating excessive force (i.e., high volume-low pressure cuffs). See Table 37-4 for cuff inflation/deflation technique. Low cuff pressure is necessary to prevent tracheal mucosa damage. The volume of air in the cuff determines the pressure exerted on the tracheal mucosa. Cuff pressures should not exceed 20 cm H_2O. Cuff pressure above 42 cm H_2O stops circulation to the tracheal mucosa and precipitates necrosis. This is because the normal pressure within tracheal arteries is 42 cm H_2O. In the veins and lymphatics the normal pressures are 24 cm H_2O and 7 cm H_2O, respectively.

Tracheostomy tubes are made of various substances (e.g., nonreactive plastic, stainless steel, sterling silver). Plastic tubes are used for only one person. Metal tubes may be reused for different people following sterilization. The most common "trach" tube is a universal, or standard, tracheostomy tube (Fig. 37-19) with three parts: (1) outer cannula, (2) inner cannula, and (3)

TABLE 37-4. Inflation and Deflation of Tracheostomy Tube Cuff*

Inflation (Minimal Leak Technique)

Objective

Inflate the cuff with the minimum volume of air required to adequately seal the trachea during positive pressure ventilation and to prevent aspiration of foreign material while exerting the lowest possible cuff-to-tracheal wall pressure.

Intervention

1. Withdraw all residual air from the cuff
2. Place 6 ml air in a syringe
3. Place the diaphragm of a stethoscope over the person's neck in the area of the tracheostomy tube cuff
4. On inhalation, slowly inject air through the one-way valve into the pilot line in 1-ml increments
5. Auscultate the neck area over the cuff
6. Apply positive pressure to the tracheostomy tube with a manual self-inflating bag. An audible air leak will be heard via the stethoscope unless the cuff is inflated
7. Continue slowly injecting air until the air leak is no longer present during inhalation
8. When a leak is no longer auscultated, withdraw a small amount of air from the cuff until a very small leak is heard. This is called a *minimal* leak
9. Note the amount of air necessary to achieve the minimal leak. This is the *minimal occluding volume (MOV)*
10. Once minimal leak is attained, measure the cuff pressure with a manometer
11. Routinely measure and document cuff pressures

Deflation

Objective

Allow air to flow around tracheostomy tube to (a) permit phonation and (b) provide opportunity to blow secretions above the cuff into the oropharynx where they may be removed by suctioning

Intervention

Routinely deflating the cuff is not necessary provided safe cuff inflation and cuff pressure measurements are performed

1. Remove ventilator assembly (if present), and attach a self-inflating bag to the 15-mm adapter on the inner cannula
2. Hyperoxygenate, hyperinflate, and suction trachea to remove secretions below the cuff. Remove secretions above the cuff by gently applying suction deep into the oropharynx
3. Insert an empty syringe into the one-way valve, and pull back on the plunger to remove the air in the cuff. At the same time, apply positive pressure with the manual self-inflating bag. This will blow secretions lying directly above the cuff into the mouth, which will prevent secretions accumulated above the cuff from draining into trachea and lower airway
4. Suction oropharynx again
5. If the person is ventilator dependent, remember that with the cuff "down" or deflated, a portion of ventilation volume will not reach the lungs. Air will escape through the upper airway and may compromise the person's ventilatory status. This volume loss will create an audible leak. Phonation is possible during the exhalation phase of the ventilator

*The same procedure is used for inflation and deflation of endotracheal tube cuffs.

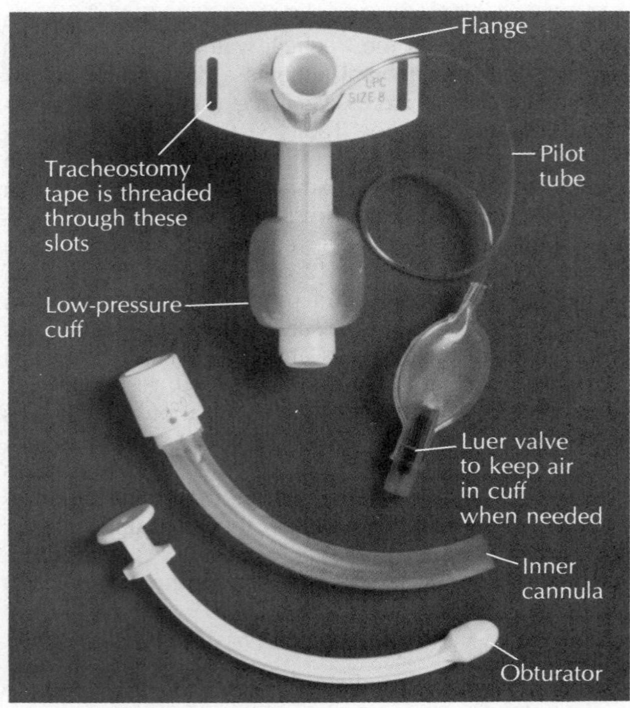

▲ **Figure 37–19**

Parts of a tracheostomy tube. (Courtesy of Shiley, Inc., Irvine, CA.)

obturator. The parts fit together as one unit and may not be interchanged with other units. Therefore, all three parts of each individual set are kept together.

The outer cannula fits in the person's tracheostomy stoma to keep it open. The outer cannula has a flange or neck plate that fits flush with the neck and has holes on each side to attach the securing tapes. A tracheostomy tube must be secured to prevent accidental extubation, excessive motion, or misalignment. Cloth tape is most often used.

The obturator fits in the outer tube before insertion. Its rounded tip smooths the end of the cannula and facilitates nontraumatic insertion of the tube into the stoma. The obturator is immediately removed after insertion to open the tube. Place the obturator in a plastic wrapper and tape it to the head of the client's bed in a conspicuous place. Then, if the tracheostomy tube is accidentally displaced, the obturator can be immediately placed into the outer cannula for quick reinsertion.

Once a tracheostomy tube's obturator is removed, the inner cannula fits into the outer cannula. Lock it into place to prevent accidental removal (e.g., when coughing). The inner cannula maintains airway patency. It is removed easily for cleaning. At the distal end, most inner cannulas have a standard 15-mm adapter that fits respiratory therapy and anesthesiology equipment. Some manufacturers make an optional disposable inner cannula. Some health care facilities believe it is more cost effective to replace a used inner cannula with a new one. This procedure may be appropriate for clients with excessive secretions who require frequent inner cannula cleansing.

Single-Cannula Tracheostomy Tube. This tube is slightly longer than a double-cannula tube. Because it does not have an inner cannula, it requires less tube care. However, it is not appropriate for clients producing secretions, because maintaining airway patency is difficult. This tube requires optimal airway humidification.

Fenestrated Tracheostomy Tube. A fenestrated tracheostomy tube differs from a universal tracheostomy tube, in that it has an opening (*fenestration*) on the curvature of the posterior wall of the outer cannula. This tube may be used (a) while a client is being weaned from a tracheostomy and (b) for a client needing long-term tracheostomy. When the inner cannula is in place, the tube functions as a universal tracheostomy tube. When the inner cannula is removed, however, the fenestration permits air to flow through both the upper airway and the tracheostomy opening. This permits speech, more effective coughing, and other uses of the upper airway. When the inner cannula is replaced with a *short decannulation stopper (tracheostomy plug)*, all airflow passes through the upper airway. When plugged, the person can speak, cough normally, breathe deeply, and breathe through the upper airway. If oxygen is required through the tracheostomy, administer nasal oxygen when a tracheostomy tube is plugged with a decannulation stopper. Fenestrated tracheostomy tubes may be cuffed or cuffless. If a fenestrated tube has a cuff, it is imperative to deflate it before plugging the tracheostomy. If the cuff is left inflated, sufficient air cannot pass in or out of the lungs and asphyxiation results.

Talking Tracheostomy. This is a one-way valve in a plastic T-piece attached to the 15-mm end of the inner cannula of a universal tracheostomy tube. It permits talking without the need to plug the tracheostomy tube. The one-way valve allows air (and supplemental humidification and oxygen) to flow into the arm of the T-piece during inspiration. Then on exhalation, the one-way valve closes, directing air from the lungs up through the vocal cords and upper airway. Phonation and effective coughing are facilitated by this normal passage of air.

A talking tracheostomy is *never* used unless there is enough room around the tracheostomy tube to permit sufficient airflow for breathing. Always deflate a cuffed tracheostomy tube before using a talking tracheostomy adapter. Cuff inflation prevents exhalation, causing suffocation.

Communitrach. This tube allows speech but requires coordination. It functions similarly to a universal tracheostomy tube, with some modifications. An airflow tube (which looks like a second pilot tube) runs outside the Communitrach and opens just above the cuff. There is a port at the distal end of the airflow tube. When occluded, compressed air or oxygen flow is directed through the airflow tube, generating an airflow up through the vocal cords. This airflow enables speech, although it does not sound "normal."

The flow of air or oxygen through a Communitrach does not create the same airflow as occurs with natural phonation. The air or oxygen flow rate is controlled by a flowmeter that is too far away for the person to control when trying to speak. Mucosal irritation may develop from air or oxygen flowing into the upper airway. The small holes in the air supply tube that direct gas flow upward may become occluded, thus reducing the flow and limiting intelligible speech.

A Communitrach may be successful for a person who can coordinate occluding the airflow with speech. Before inserting the tube, it is important for the person to realize that speech with a Communitrach will not sound normal.

Tracheostomy Button. This button is sometimes used during weaning as an intermediate device between using a standard tracheostomy tube and complete extubation. A button is a short, straight tracheostomy tube that fits into the stoma of a tracheostomy but is not deep enough to enter the tracheal lumen. It has a removable cap with a one-way flap inside that permits inhalation but not exhalation. When the cap is on the tube, the person can talk. Remove the cap for suctioning.

A button cannot be used with a ventilator. It replaces (once the tracheostomy tract is well established) a standard tracheostomy tube, for people with retained secretions who do not require ventilatory assistance. A button creates less airway resistance than a plugged standard tracheostomy tube. Hence, breathing is easier. Artificial humidification of inspired air is necessary with a button (as with any tracheostomy tube), since the natural airway is bypassed.

Permanent Tracheostomies. Many people with permanent tracheostomies lead a full life (see Chap. 38). Uncuffed tracheostomy tubes are most often recommended for these individuals. To minimize the tracheostomy's appearance, many persons prefer a low-profile inner cannula. This does not have a 15-mm adapter incorporated. Instead, it fits into the outer cannula and lies flush with the neck. "Breathable" (i.e., not plastic or rubber) clothing may be arranged to conceal the tracheostomy. Sometimes, the margins of the entire tracheal opening are sutured to the skin, creating a permanent stoma. This is often performed when a permanent opening, such as after laryngectomy, is necessary. However, a permanent stoma is not satisfactory for people with chronic pulmonary disorders. They need a tracheostomy tube so that secretions can be removed.

Metal Tracheostomy Tube. These tubes are made of sterling silver or stainless steel. The most popular type is the Jackson tracheostomy tube. It does not have a cuff. Metal tubes are most often used following a permanent tracheostomy or laryngectomy. The inner cannula locks together with the outer cannula. Because metal tubes do not have a standard 15-mm adapter, rapid adaptation to respiratory or anesthesia equipment is impossible unless a specific adapter is available. The Hollinger tube is of metal and similar to the Jackson tube.

Potential Problems Associated with Tracheostomy Tubes and Cuffs. Problems develop from prolonged contact between tube cuffs at high pressure and the tracheal wall. These include (1) obstruction, (2) cuff inflation problems, (3) tracheoesophageal fistula, and (4) malposition of the tube.

Factors contributing to tracheal wall breakdown include (1) long-term ventilation requiring a cuffed tracheostomy tube, (2) infection, (3) misalignment of the tracheostomy tube such that the tube's tip lies directly against the tracheal wall, (4) incorrect tracheostomy tube size (e.g., too small a tube not only compromises airway patency but also necessitates high cuff pressures to obtain an adequate seal), and (5) the person's general poor condition. Shock, hypoxemia, general debilitation, impaired defense mechanisms, use of immunosuppressive agents and/or radiation, anemia, and malnutrition all affect tissue well being.

When long-term tracheostomy is required, uncuffed tracheostomy tubes are usually used. Even people requiring long-term mechanical ventilation tolerate uncuffed tracheostomy tubes. Tidal volumes and respiratory rates are adjusted on the ventilator to produce satisfactory ventilation and arterial blood gases while eliminating the risks associated with tracheostomy tube cuffs.

Other possible complications associated with tracheostomy tubes include tube displacement, accidental extubation, airway obstruction, and infection.

Tube Displacement. A tracheostomy tube's tip should lie 1 to 2 cm above the carina. If the tube is too long or the stoma was placed too low, intubation of the right main bronchus may occur, allowing ventilation in the right lung only. If the person's neck is short and thick, a tube may be accidentally inserted into the soft tissues of the neck.

Accidental Extubation (Tube Removal). A tracheostomy tube that is not properly secured may be accidentally dislodged from the stoma. This may occur while changing the tube-securing ties. Manipulation of a tracheostomy tube often produces vigorous coughing. Coughing can expel the tube from the stoma unless it is held firmly. Hold the tube with two fingers placed on the flange or neck plate on either side of the adapter. With accidental extubation, if the stoma is less than 4 days old, it may close because a tract is not yet formed. If this occurs, call for help immediately. Maintain ventilation and oxygenation by bag and mask. If ventilation is impossible you must reinsert the tube. To do so, deflate the cuff; remove the tube's inner cannula; insert the obturator in the outer cannula; elevate the person's shoulders with a pillow and gently hyperextend the neck. You may need to use tracheal dilators (spreaders) to hold the stoma open (Fig. 37–20). Insert the obturator into the outer cannula. Insert the outer cannula into the client's neck and immediately remove the obturator. Auscultate for breath sounds. If present, insert the inner cannula and reconnect to oxygen and ventilation equipment. *If the tracheostomy tube cannot be reinserted in 1 minute, call a code for*

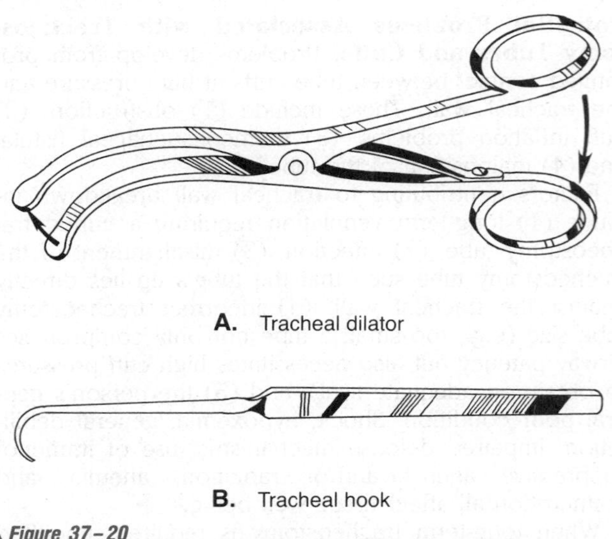

▲ **Figure 37-20**

Equipment for emergency reinsertion of a tracheostomy tube. The tracheal dilator (*A*) and the tracheal hook (*B*) are often kept at the bedside during the first few days following a tracheostomy. They are used to hold the stoma open to facilitate quick and safe reinsertion of the tube should accidental extubation occur. Once the stoma is well established, they are not required.

respiratory arrest. Unless the client is breathing adequately, an emergency cricothyroidotomy will be necessary (see Chap. 80).

If accidental extubation occurs 4 days following a tracheostomy, the same procedure is used. It is generally easier to reinsert the tube. However, if bleeding occurs or the airway is obstructed, use emergency measures, as indicated earlier.

Airway obstruction. The flow of air through a tracheostomy tube may become occluded for several reasons. The tracheostomy tube may be misaligned so its opening lies against the tracheal wall, preventing airflow. Cuff overinflation causes the cuff to herniate over the tip of the tube, obstructing airflow. Without adequate airway care, the inner cannula can occlude with dried secretions or excessive bronchial secretions.

Infection. Tracheostomies increase the risk of bronchopulmonary infection because (1) they bypass upper airway protective mechanisms (i.e., filtering, warming, and humidifying) and (2) cuffs decrease mucociliary transport and coughing, thus increasing retained secretions. Stoma site infection may also occur. Nosocomial infection is also a potential problem. The lower airway (below the larynx) is normally sterile. Therefore, all solutions, devices, and so forth entering the trachea must be sterile. Organisms (e.g., *Pseudomonas aeruginosa* and other gram-negative bacteria) grow readily in respiratory equipment and contaminate the lower airway. Some bacteria may colonize a tracheostomy without causing infection.

Nursing Management. Following tracheostomy, frequent assessment is required, including (1) monitoring vital signs; (2) assessing mucous membrane color; and (3) observing for indications of shock, hemorrhage, respiratory insufficiency, or complications from the client's general condition or the surgical intervention.

Nursing Diagnosis: Airway Clearance, Ineffective R/T secretion accumulation. A client with a tracheostomy is unable to perform the Valsalva maneuver and therefore has a limited ability to cough and deep breathe. Thus, the client's ability to maintain a clear airway is compromised. Intervention to promote airway clearance and pulmonary aeration includes (1) changing the client's position frequently, (2) providing humidification and hydration, (3) eliminating factors that impair airway clearance (e.g., reduce fever, use sedatives cautiously), and (4) performing frequent manual ventilation, hyperinflation, and suctioning to promote lung expansion and reduce the risks of atelectasis, pulmonary infection, and ineffective gas exchange. Hyperinflation creates an "artificial sigh," improving lung aeration and facilitating removal of tracheobronchial secretions by enhancing the cough effort. When the client's condition is stabilized sufficiently, coughing may be enhanced by having the client place a finger over the tracheostomy tube opening while attempting to cough. It is important that the client's hands be washed before doing this. Have the person cough into paper tissues and carefully dispose of them.

When a cuffed tracheostomy tube is used, secretions collect above the cuff. It is difficult to reach such secretions by oropharyngeal suctioning. However, the secretions can be "blown" into the mouth by simultaneously deflating the cuff and giving a deep manual inflation. If secretions above the cuff are not "blown up," they will fall into the lower airway when the cuff is deflated. Infection from oral contaminants and/or impaired gas exchange can result.

Suction the airway as needed. Careful technique reduces mucosal trauma, which can lead to tracheal infection. Mucosal trauma is indicated by (1) tracheal irritation and tracheitis, and (2) bloody tracheal secretions.

If tracheal secretions are thick and not easily removed, directly instill a small amount of sterile normal saline into the trachea to try to reduce the viscosity of the secretions. Instill the saline directly into the tracheostomy tube during inhalation. Immediately inflate the lungs manually with a self-inflating bag. If the inner cannula is encrusted, soak it in hydrogen peroxide (H_2O_2) and rinse it with sterile distilled water or normal saline to remove the crusts. This increases airway patency (Table 37-5).

Provide adequate hydration. The normal hydrating mechanisms of the upper airway are bypassed by a tracheostomy. Hydration can be ensured by oral, parenteral, or inhalation routes. Inhalation may be provided by (1) increasing the humidity of room air (room humidifier) or of dry gases (e.g., oxygen) or (2) administering aerosols.

If humidification is insufficient, the body tries to make up the deficit by taking fluid from body water. The result is inspissated mucus, which compromises airway patency and increases the risk of secretion

TABLE 37–5 Tracheostomy Care

Pre-procedure

- Auscultate chest to assess need for suctioning
- Assemble *equipment:* tracheostomy care kit* or individual supplies (i.e., hydrogen peroxide [H_2O_2], scissors, fresh tracheostomy tape or other type of tracheostomy-securing device, sterile normal saline, two sterile basins, plastic or paper bag for disposal of used items)

Prepare Person

- Tell the person what you are going to do
- If teaching self-care, describe the items you have assembled and the purpose of each
- Loosen the caps on the hydrogen peroxide and normal saline
- Open tracheostomy kit on a firm surface
- Pour H_2O_2 into one basin and normal saline into the other
- Close the caps on the H_2O_2 and normal saline
- Remove used tracheostomy dressing and discard
- Wash hands and clean under fingernails

Tracheostomy Care

- Put on sterile gloves
- Dip cotton-tipped applicator into H_2O_2 and clean skin around stoma. Repeat as many times as needed to remove mucus from the skin. Clean area behind the neck plate. Observe the condition of the skin
- Dip another applicator into normal saline. Rinse H_2O_2 and mucus from skin
- Use a dry 4 × 4 gauze sponge to wipe area if necessary
- Hold neck plate steady with the fingers of one hand and remove inner cannula with the other. Tracheostomy tube motion may stimulate a cough or produce an uncomfortable sensation similar to strangling or choking
- Place inner cannula in H_2O_2. Use small brush or pipe cleaners to scrub mucus from the inside of the inner cannula. If the mucus is very thick, let the inner cannula soak at least 3 minutes. Repeat process until the inner cannula is clean
- Carefully reinsert inner cannula and lock it in place
- If a tracheostomy dressing is needed, use pre-cut one in the trach care kit, use a pre-cut drain dressing, or fold a 4 × 4 dressing into a V. *Do not cut standard 4 × 4's unless they are tightly woven and do not fray or leave gauze filaments when cut*

Changing Tracheostomy Ties

- Changing tracheostomy ties always requires two people. At least one person must be experienced in this procedure and capable of handling accidental extubation. The tube is easily dislodged by coughing when the tracheostomy tube is manipulated
- One person holds the tracheostomy tube in place by placing two fingers directly on the neck plate. Apply firm pressure. Never remove fingers until the new ties are tied and secured
- 3/4-inch twill tape is most comfortable for ties
- Always tie the twill with a square knot
- Never position knots directly over the carotid artery or the spinal cord
- Tie knots with tension that allows two fingers to slip between the skin and the tapes
- Change tracheostomy ties when soiled and at least every 8 hours, initially. People with permanent tracheostomies usually need them changed once a day

Post-activity

- Discard soiled disposable supplies, solutions, and equipment. Send nondisposable items for decontamination
- Note the size and type of the tracheostomy tube. Make sure there is an identical tube placed at the head of the bed
- Make sure the obturator is taped in an easily visible place
- Replace equipment used
- Document procedure. Note quality and quantity of any blood or mucus, and the skin integrity. Document any unusual observations and notify physician
- If the person or significant others are being taught the procedure, document their progress
- Ensure that emergency situations may be handled appropriately, e.g., a tracheal dilator or tracheal hook kept in the room to assist in emergency tracheostomy tube replacement. (This is not usually needed when the stoma has become well established)

*Prepackaged tracheostomy care kits are expensive for prolonged or permanent use. People discharged from the hospital with a tracheostomy often find it more cost-effective to assemble individual items. Most United States third-party payers do not provide an unlimited supply of packaged tracheostomy care kits.

pooling and subsequent infection. Many factors can impair the mucociliary mechanisms of the lungs, e.g., dehydration, fever, anesthesia, anticholinergic drugs, sedatives, and immobility. All of these factors may be experienced by a person with a tracheostomy. Dried mucus occludes air passages and leads to atelectasis, pneumonia, and potentially severe gas exchange abnormalities. Nursing intervention for insufficient hydration includes careful monitoring of fluid intake and output and administering prescribed additional hydration, e.g., parenterally.

Nursing Diagnosis: Gas Exchange Impaired, High Risk for. Following tracheostomy, impaired gas exchange may occur because of various factors.

- Factors affecting oxygen delivery include (1) aspiration of blood, oral secretions, or gastric contents, (2) restricted lung expansion from immobility, (3) excessive tracheobronchial secretions, (4) inability to cough and deep breathe, and (5) pre-existing medical conditions (e.g., obesity, fever, inadequate hydration, pneumonia, tracheal injury such as from burns).
- Factors affecting the removal of carbon dioxide include (1) sedatives or anesthesia, (2) deteriorating level of consciousness, and (3) any other condition potentially affecting ventilation efficiency and leading to hypoventilation and retention of carbon dioxide.

Assessment of gas exchange by ABG analysis is important immediately following tracheostomy and whenever there is a change in the person's condition or a change in treatment. Noninvasive monitoring is appropriate once baseline values are established by ABG. Remember, if shock or hypotension exists, or if peripheral vasoconstrictive drugs are used, data provided by transcutaneous monitoring will be incorrect because an accurate reading is not possible.

Nursing Diagnosis: Infection, High Risk for R/T tracheostomy's bypassing normal upper airway protective mechanisms and to surgical incision. Nursing intervention is required to prevent respiratory infection as well as oral and skin infection following tracheostomy. Use aseptic technique for all intervention directly involving the tracheostomy. Careful handwashing, appropriate use of gloves, use of sterile supplies and solutions, and changing and decontaminating respiratory equipment every 24 hours are essential. Clean and inspect the skin around the stoma and the stoma itself. Observe for indications of irritation, inflammation, skin breakdown, and purulent drainage. If skin or stomal infection does occur, a topical antibacterial ointment may be prescribed.

Tracheostomy dressings (Fig. 37–21) are often used, especially in the early postoperative stage. Damp blood-and-mucus–soaked dressings are a perfect medium for the growth of microorganisms. They also promote tissue irritation and breakdown. Change dressings whenever they are damp. Using H_2O_2 and cotton-tipped applicators, carefully clean the skin each time the dressing is changed. Rinse with normal saline and dry the area. Do not use plastic-backed or water-proofed dressings. Moisture, secretions, and blood may seep behind them, and these dressings hold warmth and moisture in. Skin then becomes irritated and macerated.

Nursing Diagnoses: Fluid Volume Deficit and Nutrition, Altered: Less Than Body Requirements, High Risk for. Intravenous fluids are usually given during the first 24 hours following tracheostomy. Then, if the person is alert and swallowing and if gag mechanisms are intact, oral fluid and food may be attempted.

If a cuffed endotracheal tube was used before the tracheostomy, assess for tracheoesophageal fistula before permitting oral feedings. The risk of a tracheoesophageal fistula increases if both a cuffed endotracheal tube and a nasogastric feeding tube were used. To assess for the presence of such a fistula, give the person a "test swallow" of water (room temperature and colored blue with vegetable dye) before giving fluid or food. Severe coughing or blue fluid suctioned from the tracheostomy tube indicates a fistula. Withhold oral food and fluid, and continue feeding by nasogastric tube or other methods.

If the client's swallowing mechanism is impaired following tracheostomy, intravenous fluid may be prescribed for a short time. A client with a long-term or permanently impaired swallowing mechanism (e.g., following a cerebrovascular accident) requires a permanent feeding tube or gastrostomy feedings (G-tube) (Chap. 53). G-tube feedings may cause reflux and be aspirated into the trachea. Before administering G-tube feedings, inflate the tracheostomy tube's cuff. Leave it inflated for at least 1 hour after feeding. Suction above the cuff before deflating it to remove any tube-feeding material.

When feeding someone with a tracheostomy, have the client sit upright. Often, food and fluids with texture (e.g., pudding) are easier to swallow than water. Tipping the chin toward the chest narrows the airway and helps food enter the esophagus. Overinflation of a tracheostomy tube's cuff causes swallowing difficulty. If oral fluid intake is limited, continue intravenous fluids to make up the deficit.

Nursing Diagnosis: Communication, Impaired verbal R/T bypassing of vocal cords by tracheostomy. Make sure the client can always reach an emergency call system to summon help. Do not use an intercom system because the person cannot talk. Be sure all personnel know this. Make a written list of common needs, words, and phrases so the client can point on the list to communicate needs (e.g., "I want to pass urine"; "I need a drink"; "I have pain"). Use a paper and pencil to facilitate communication.

Nursing Diagnosis: Injury, High Risk for. Secure a tracheostomy tube properly. If tracheostomy tube–securing tapes require knotting, always tie a square knot. Avoid placing the knot over the person's carotid artery or spine. Make sure the tapes are not too tight (i.e., allow room for two fingers to slide comfortably under the tape). Inspect the skin under the securing

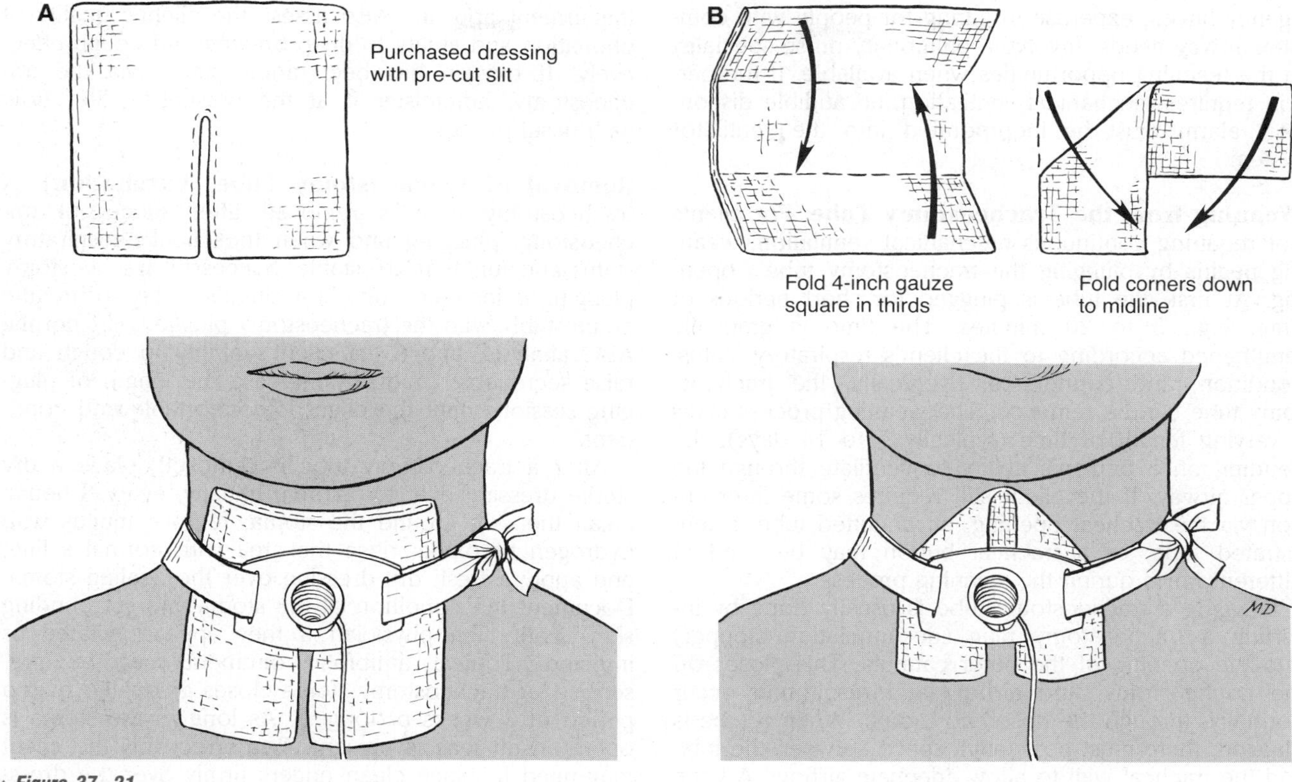

▲ *Figure 37–21*

Tracheostomy dressings. If there is significant bleeding or tracheal secretions, cleaning the skin and changing the dressing frequently may prevent infection and skin breakdown. *A*, Manufactured dressing with precut slit has no fine threads that could unravel and enter the stoma. Place dressing around the tracheostomy tube with the slit downward (*as shown*) or upward. *B*, 4 × 4 gauze pad folded and placed under tracheostomy tube. Do not have any cut edges that could unravel.

tape for skin irritation. People requiring a long-term tracheostomy may use more comfortable securing devices (e.g., padded straps with Velcro fasteners). Secure the tube in midline tracheal alignment. Create a "loop" in aerosol or ventilator tubing assembly; i.e., let the tube loop down to catch condensate. Drain water and condensate in the tubing away from the tracheostomy. Support ventilator and aerosol tubing to prevent pulling on the tracheostomy tube. Be careful not to disconnect tubing when turning the person.

Do not allow smoking in the room of a person who has a tracheostomy. Do not use aerosol spray cans (e.g., room deodorizers) near the person. Do not shake bedding or create dust clouds. Be careful when shaving or tending the person's hair that whiskers or hair do not fall into the trachea. Cover the tracheostomy with a thin cloth towel during shaving.

Nursing Diagnosis: Oral Mucous Membrane, Altered. Oral hygiene is important to prevent (1) oral infection and (2) lower airway infection from oral bacteria passing downward. Frequent oral hygiene also makes a person more comfortable. Provide oral hygiene (e.g., brushing teeth, using mouthwash) every 2 hours, especially for people who are not taking any food or fluid by mouth, or who are obtunded or unconscious.

Nursing Diagnosis: Constipation R/T absence of Valsalva maneuver. When the glottis and vocal cords are bypassed (as with tracheostomy), a person cannot perform a Valsalva maneuver. This impairs the person's ability to defecate. Use prescribed stool softeners, laxatives, and even enemas as necessary.

Nursing Diagnosis: Anxiety and Fear. These problems due to various factors affecting individuals with tracheostomies, e.g., inability to talk, fear of suffocating, anxiety about diagnosis, fear that the tracheostomy tube will come out. Frequent observation is essential. Your presence and skillful nursing care are most reassuring.

Nursing Diagnosis: Health Maintenance, Altered R/T knowledge deficit regarding permanent or long-term tracheostomy care. When a person's tracheostomy is long term or permanent, begin teaching during routine care as appropriate. Use a mirror to allow the person to observe procedures. Include family members and significant others. Before discharge from the health care facility, the person and significant others need to be confident in performing tracheostomy care, suctioning, preoxygenating, safety measures, aerosol therapy, and other aspects of the individual's airway maintenance. Arrange home follow-up by a home health agency having expertise in caring for people with complex airway needs. Involve a pulmonary nurse specialist in the teaching opportunities when available. If the person requires mechanical ventilation, an audible disconnect alarm must be incorporated into the ventilator system.

Weaning from the Tracheostomy Tube. For clients not requiring continuous mechanical ventilation, weaning begins by plugging the tracheostomy tube's opening. At first, the tube is plugged for short periods of time, e.g., 5 to 20 minutes. The time is gradually lengthened according to the client's respiratory status, condition, and confidence. Eventually, the tracheostomy tube can be removed. The weaning process takes a varying length of time (typically 7 to 14 days), depending on a person's ability to ventilate through the upper airway. If the client still requires some intervention via the tracheal opening, an uncuffed tube, a fenestrated tube, or a tracheal button may be used at different times during the weaning process.

Plugging a tracheostomy tube is usually done by inserting a tracheostomy plug (decannulation stopper) into the opening of the outer cannula. This closes off the tracheostomy, and airflow and respiration occur normally, through the nose and mouth. When a tube is plugged, there must be enough space between the tube and the tracheal wall to allow adequate airflow. A large tracheostomy tube may need to be replaced with a smaller one to allow sufficient airflow past the tracheostomy tube. When plugging a cuffed tracheostomy tube, the cuff must be deflated. If the cuff remains inflated, ventilation cannot occur, and respiratory arrest could result.

Ideally, tracheostomy plugging is attempted only when an uncuffed or fenestrated tracheostomy tube is in place.

Explain the process to the client and family. Naturally, most clients are anxious about weaning because they fear they may not be able to breathe. Constant, supportive observation during weaning is necessary and reassures the client. Encourage the client to begin to think about breathing through the nose again. This breathing is a strange sensation for people who have used a tracheostomy tube for a long time. Explain to them ways to facilitate optimal respiration and to maintain control of breathing (e.g., inhale slowly and completely through the nose; avoid holding the breath).

ABG analysis and measurement of spontaneous respiratory mechanics (respiratory rate, tidal volume, vital capacity, inspiratory effort, expiratory effort) are important assessments during weaning. Oximetry and other noninvasive assessment may also be used once baseline ABGs are established.

During weaning from tracheostomy, assess for indications of respiratory distress or ventilation impairment. Findings may include (1) abnormal respiratory rate and pattern, (2) use of accessory muscles to assist breathing, (3) abnormal pulse and blood pressure, (4) abnormal skin and mucous membrane color, and (5) abnormal ABGs. Remove the tracheostomy plug immediately if any indication of respiratory distress or ventilation impairment appears. Also assess the client's quality of phonation and ability to deep breathe and cough effectively. If oxygen has been administered via the tracheostomy, administer it at the prescribed liter flow with nasal prongs.

Removal of Tracheostomy Tube (Extubation). A tracheostomy tube is removed after successful tracheostomy plugging and when the client's respiratory status and function are stable. Successful tracheostomy plugging is indicated by (1) a client's ability to breathe comfortably with the tracheostomy plugged, (2) normal ABG analysis, and (3) a client's ability to cough and raise secretions. Gradually increase the length of plugging sessions until the client is comfortable and confident.

After a tracheostomy tube is removed, place a dry sterile dressing over the stoma. Initially, every 8 hours, clean the skin around the stoma; remove mucus with hydrogen peroxide; rinse the area with normal saline; and apply a fresh dry dressing over the healing stoma. Document the condition of the stoma and surrounding skin. Notify the physician if they appear irritated or infected. Topical antibiotic ointment may be prescribed. A tracheostomy stoma closes gradually (over a period of 2 weeks or longer). As long as the stoma is open, an air leak is present. To correct this the client may need to place clean fingers firmly over the dressing to facilitate normal speech and coughing.

Following extubation, ongoing respiratory function assessment is necessary. Some complications of tracheostomy do not appear for months following tracheostomy tube removal, e.g., tracheal stenosis.

Permanent Tracheostomy. Most clients with a permanent tracheostomy use a universal, or fenestrated, cuffless, tracheostomy tube or an Olympic trach button. However, some do not need a tracheostomy tube (e.g., a "laryngectomee" with a permanently constructed stoma). Care of a client who has had a laryngectomy is discussed in Chapter 38. The same principles apply to a client with a permanent tracheostomy.

Learning self-care is important for individuals with permanent tracheostomies. It provides a sense of self-control and reduces dependency on others. However, significant others must also be able to provide tracheostomy care and other aspects of airway management. The client and significant others are often anxious about home management. Careful preparation before discharge reduces this anxiety. Close follow-up is essential. Home health services are necessary. Order home health care equipment from medical suppliers who employ respiratory therapists or nurses. Ideally, have the equipment initially delivered to the hospital, so the client and significant others can learn its use with the supervision of professionals.

Tracheostomy Tube Changes. Recommendations for changing tracheostomy tubes vary. Most physicians and health care facilities have established protocols. Although some facilities change tracheostomy tubes as often as every month, others wait longer. Ideally, the tube should be changed every 6 to 8 weeks, or more frequently if the person is at risk of recurrent tracheobronchial infections. Each person has a unique set of circumstances that may dictate the frequency of tracheostomy tube changes.

Emergency Resuscitation. Emergency mouth-to-neck (mouth-to-tracheostomy or mouth-to-stoma) resuscitation may be necessary if a person with a tracheostomy or laryngectomy experiences respiratory depression or respiratory arrest. If the person has a tracheostomy tube, provide ventilation by attaching a manual self-inflating bag to the standard 15-mm adapter on the inner cannula. Some volume is lost from an uncuffed tube. Adequate ventilation can often be compensated for by altering the usual method of manual inflation (e.g., compress the bag more forcefully and quickly). If the tracheostomy tube is cuffed, inflate the cuff and maintain ventilation at the correct rate, i.e., 12 to 16 breaths a minute for an adult. If inflation of the cuff impedes ventilation, immediately deflate the cuff and attempt to compensate for volume loss by compressing the bag more forcefully or quickly. If ventilation continues to be impaired or prevented and you determine the cause is a malfunction in the tube, remove the tube immediately and provide mouth-to-stoma ventilation. Keep the nose and mouth closed during mouth-to-stoma breathing to prevent air from escaping through the upper airway (see also Chap. 38.)

Mechanical Ventilators

Some clients are not able to adequately ventilate their lungs because of various disorders resulting in respiratory insufficiency or failure. These clients require immediate intervention, including the establishment of an artificial airway (e.g., by endotracheal intubation or tracheostomy) and mechanical lung ventilation with a positive-pressure ventilator.

INDICATIONS

The decision to use mechanical ventilation is a separate issue from the decision to intubate. In emergency situations, however, mechanical ventilation nearly always follows intubation, at least until a more complete assessment of the client can be performed.

The two main indications for mechanical ventilation include inadequate ventilation and hypoxemia. Inadequate ventilation from apnea or alveolar hypoventilation may lead to a decreasing pH (acidosis) and a stable or rising $PaCO_2$. A gradually rising $PaCO_2$ usually indicates a need for ventilatory support, but it is not used as a single criterion. Many variables, such as mixed acid-base disorders, can have an impact on $PaCO_2$ levels. The pH is the most important indicator of the need for ventilatory support. Mechanical ventilation is usually needed for clients with respiratory acidosis with a pH of less than 7.2. The physician may decide to intubate at more normal pH levels depending on the client's situation. If a client is in acute ventilatory failure that is worsening by the minute, extubation is warranted regardless of pH values.

Hypoxemia may be severe and not controllable by non-rebreathing face masks. Mechanical ventilation allows the client to inhale high percentages of oxygen (FIO_2). In many cases, once the oxygen debt is paid off or the underlying disorder stabilized, the FIO_2 can be reduced below 0.50.

A group of clients who are an exception to these guidelines are those clients with COPD (emphysema). Mechanical ventilation is delayed for as long as possible. These clients can tolerate higher $PaCO_2$ levels, and acute respiratory failure is likely to reverse with bronchodilator therapy, respiratory therapy, and other supportive measures.

Common clinical indications and disorders that frequently require mechanical ventilation are presented in the Bridge to Critical Care.

Positive-pressure ventilators may be broadly categorized as (1) those for short-term use (intermittent positive-pressure breathing) and (2) those for continuous supportive use (continuous mechanical ventilation), which provide for all aspects of ventilation and oxygen administration.

INTERMITTENT POSITIVE-PRESSURE BREATHING

Intermittent positive-pressure breathing (IPPB) uses a pressure-cycled ventilator (Fig. 37-22) to deliver pressurized breaths to a spontaneously breathing client in 10- to 20-minute treatments. Possible indications for IPPB include (1) atelectasis, (2) impaired or ineffective cough, (3) delivery of aerosolized medications into the respiratory tree in people unable or unwilling to deep breathe, and (4) reversal of acute hypoventilation.

Contraindications to IPPB include (1) tension pneumothorax, (2) undiagnosed hemoptysis, (3) exacerbation of undesired cardiovascular and other physiologic effects, (4) inability of the client to use the IPPB correctly, (5) chronic carbon dioxide retention, and (6) increased intracranial pressure.

Currently IPPB is infrequently prescribed. IPPB is uncomfortable, and its benefits have not been substantially proved. IPPB can be an effective therapy if the candidates are carefully screened and goals and outcomes are clearly understood.

CONTINUOUS MECHANICAL VENTILATION

The use of continuous mechanical ventilation (CMV) is now an ordinary level of care for clients managed in critical care and on general care units. The client on CMV is a challenge to the nurse providing care. The nurse must be familiar with the equipment, complications of CMV, and nursing management. The goals of CMV are to (1) maintain adequate ventilation, (2) deliver precise concentrations of FIO_2, (3) deliver adequate tidal volumes in order to obtain an adequate minute ventilation and oxygenation, and (4) decrease the work of breathing in those clients who cannot sustain adequate ventilation on their own. Continuous mechanical ventilators can be either pressure-cycled or

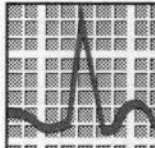

BRIDGE TO CRITICAL CARE

The Ventilator-Dependent Client

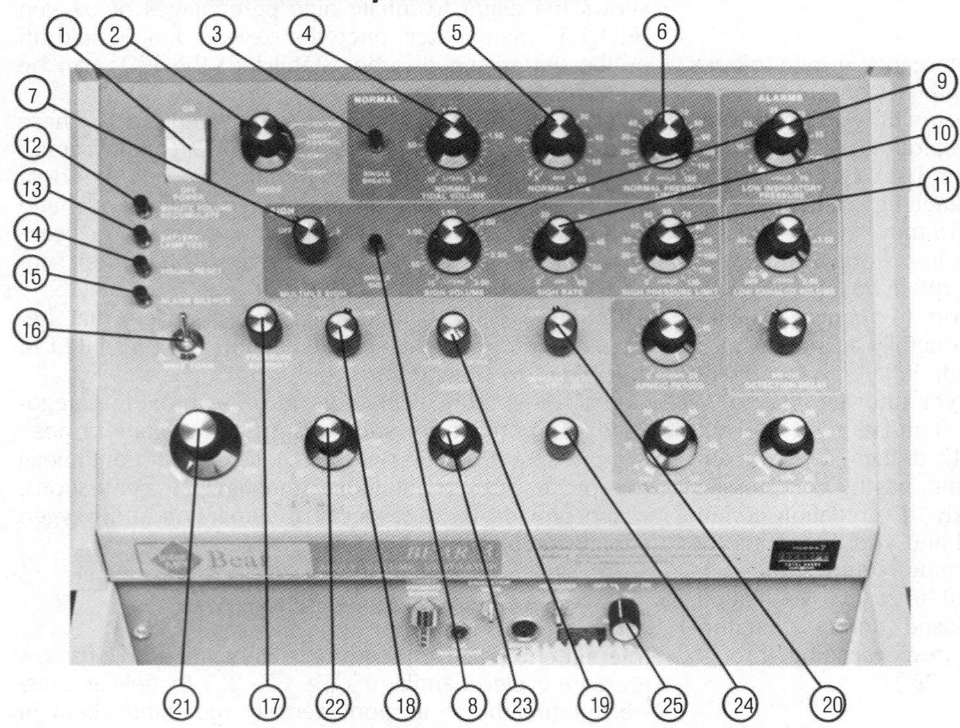

① **POWER ON/OFF** — Controls electrical power to the ventilator.

② **MODE CONTROL** — Selection of mode of operation.

③ **NORMAL SINGLE BREATH** — Manual breath; operable 350 milliseconds after the end of exhalation. Operates in all modes.

④ **TIDAL VOLUME** — 100–2000 ml. When tidal volume is delivered, inspiration ends. (Exhaled tidal volume and minute volume are displayed.)

⑤ **NORMAL RATE** — 0.5–60 BPM. (Rate display indicates the sum of the machine and patient breaths.)

⑥ **NORMAL PRESSURE LIMIT** — 0–120 cmH_2O. When the selected pressure is reached, inspiration ends and terminates volume delivery. (Audio-visual alert, PRESSURE LIMIT on display panel shows that pressure limit was reached.)

⑦ **MULTIPLE SIGH** — Number of sighs to be delivered in succession at preset intervals. (CONTROL and ASSIST-CONTROL modes only.)

⑧ **SINGLE SIGH** — Manual sigh; operable 350 milliseconds after the end of exhalation when MULTIPLE SIGH is set at 1, 2 or 3 position.

⑨ **SIGH VOLUME** — 150–3000 ml. When sigh volume is delivered, sigh breath ends.

⑩ **SIGH RATE** — 2–60 sighs per hour (CONTROL and ASSIST-CONTROL modes only.)

⑪ **SIGH PRESSURE LIMIT** — 0–120 cmH_2O. When the selected sigh pressure is reached, inspiration ends and terminates volume delivery. (Audio-visual alert, PRESSURE LIMIT on display panel shows that pressure limit was reached.)

⑫ **MINUTE VOLUME ACCUMULATE** — Tidal volume accumulates for one minute, displays for second minute and then automatically returns to tidal volume. (MINUTE VOLUME ACCUMULATE indicator blinks during accumulation and remains lit during the display of minute volume.)

⑬ **BATTERY/LAMP TEST** — Activates all digital and LED displays, as well as testing the battery powered, power-loss sensing circuit.

⑭ **VISUAL RESET** — All activated visual alarm/alert indicators remain on, until the VISUAL RESET button is pushed.

⑮ **ALARM SILENCE** — Allows silencing of all audible alarms except the VENT INOPERATIVE alarm. The alarm system will reset automatically in 60 seconds or can be reset manually by depressing the ALARM SILENCE pushbutton (display panel light shows ALARM SILENCE on).

⑯ **WAVE FORM** — Control Flow Pattern delivered during positive pressure breaths.

⑰ **PRESSURE SUPPORT** — Adjusts pressure support levels during spontaneous breaths only in SIMV and CPAP. Range 6–65 cmH_2O pressure.

⑱ **PSV** — Activates pressure support in SIMV and CPAP modes only. *Note: if on during Assist/Control or Control Ventilation, PSV indicator on display panel will flash.*

⑲ **ASSIST-SENSITIVITY** — Adjustable from LESS (2.5cmH$_2$O) to MORE (2.1cmH$_2$O). Senses patient effort in ASSIST-CONTROL and SIMV modes to deliver synchronized positive pressure breaths (Display light shows inspiratory source.)

⑳ **INVERSE RATIO ALERT/LIMIT** — OFF: Allows INVERSE I:E RATIO (visual alert only; display panel light indicates INVERSE RATIO is OFF). ON: Prevents inverse ratio, 1:1 ratio terminates inspiration (Audio-Visual alert).

㉑ **OXYGEN %** — 21–100% oxygen (63%). Connect to 30–100 psig oxygen source for concentrations higher than 21%. Audio-Visual alert on display panel shows oxygen source pressure less than 30 psig with OXYGEN % control setting higher than 21%.

㉒ **PEAK FLOW** — 10–120 LPM. Controls initial flow rate during positive pressure breaths, no effect on spontaneous flow.

㉓ **INSPIRATORY PAUSE** — 0–2.0 seconds. Delays the beginning of exhalation.

㉔ **PEEP** — 0–40 cmH_2O. Leak compensated in all modes except CONTROL (effective lead compensation is the available flow less the patient demand, as long as PEEP exceeds 1 cmH_2O to keep the demand valve open. NOTE: ASSIST sensitivity may be compromised if excessive leak compensation is required.)

㉕ **NEBULIZER** — Allows intermittent administration of medication during positive pressure breaths (14psig @ 11 LPM). Does not alter oxygen concentration or tidal volume (display panel light shows NEBULIZER ON).

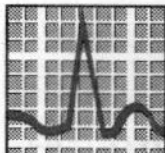

BRIDGE TO CRITICAL CARE

The Ventilator-Dependent Client Continued

Parameters for Weaning

Inspiratory force (IF)	>-20 cm Hg
Tidal volume (V_T)	10–15 ml/kg
Vital capacity (VC)	$>$10–15 ml/kg
Expiratory force (EF)	$>+60$ cm H_2O
Resting minute ventilation (VE)	$>$10 L/min
$PaCO_2$	Within normal range
PaO_2	Minimally 70–80 mm Hg on 0.5 FIO_2
Dead space to tidal volume (V_D/V_T)	0.55–0.60
PaO_2 on 100% O_2	$>$300 mm Hg
Shunt fraction	$<$15%

Parameters Indicating an Unsuccessful Weaning Attempt

Change in blood pressure: a rise or fall of 20 mm Hg systolic and/or 10 mm Hg diastolic
Pulse rate: increase of 20 beats/min or pulse $>$ 110
Respiratory rate: an increase of 10/min or a rate of more than 30 to 35/min
Tidal volume: less than 250 to 300 ml (adult)
Significant electrocardiographic changes

PaO_2	60 mm Hg	Acceptable values in clients with COPD may be lower PaO_2 and pH and higher $PaCO_2$
$PaCO_2$	55 mm Hg	
pH	7.35	

Troubleshooting Mechanical Ventilator Alarms

High Pressure Alarms

1. Check to see whether the client is biting on the ETT.
2. Check to see whether the ventilator tubing is kinked.
3. Listen to lung sounds. Is there bronchospasm or pulmonary embolus?
4. Question the possibility of mucus plugging. Suction vigorously.
5. Is the client coughing?
6. Check for water in the tubing.
7. Is the client out of rhythm with the ventilator? The client may be breathing against an incoming mechanical breath.

Low Pressure/Low Exhaled Tidal Volume Alarms

1. Check for disconnected tubing.
2. Listen for a cuff leak.
3. Is the client on an IMV mode of ventilation? If so, he or she may need small spontaneous breath tidal volumes.

Minute Ventilation Alarms

1. Assess the client's respiratory rate. If it is rapid, this may produce a larger minute ventilation than normal, especially if he or she is on an assist/control mode of ventilation.
2. The alarms may not have been reset after a rate or volume change on the ventilator.

Oxygen Alarms

1. Check the oxygen to ensure that it is set on the proper amount.
2. Check to make sure that the alarms were changed after a change in FIO_2 on the ventilator.

NOTE: If at any time an alarm is sounding and the nurse cannot quickly ascertain the problem, the client should be disconnected from the ventilator and a manual resuscitation bag should be used to support him or her until the problem can be corrected.

Common Clinical Indications and Disorders Requiring Mechanical Ventilation

Disorders	Clinical Indications
Lung or airway disorders or trauma (pneumonia, ARDS, rib fractures, asthma, pulmonary edema)	PaO_2 below 60 mm Hg with $FIO_2 > 0.4$ $PaCO_2$ above 45 mm Hg pH below 7.3 Hemodynamic instability
Circulatory disorders (myocardial infarction, cardiogenic shock)	Same as for lung and airway disorders
Acute exacerbations of COPD	PaO_2 below 35 to 45 on oxygen pH below 7.2 to 7.25 Respiratory rate above 30 to 40 per min
Neuromuscular disorders and trauma (Guillain-Barré syndrome, myasthenia gravis, head injury)	Maximum inspiratory pressure per 25 cm H_2O Vital capacity less than 10 to 15 ml/kg body weight Respiratory rate above 30 to 40 per min
Airway obstruction (facial trauma, aspiration)	Presence of inspiratory stridor
Prophylactic management following surgery	Major cardiac, pulmonary or gastrointestinal surgery. Hemodynamic instability during surgery.

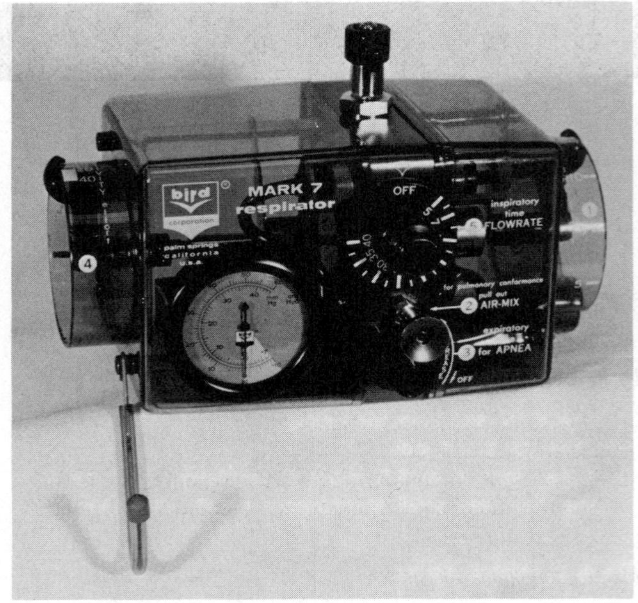

▲ **Figure 37-22**

An intermittent positive-pressure breathing apparatus (IPPB). This is used to facilitate lung expansion. The IPPB is a pressure-sensitive respirator that is attached to oxygen and given to the client via a mouthpiece.

volume-cycled ventilators (Fig. 37-23). Pressure-cycled ventilators deliver a volume of gas to the airway using positive pressure during inspiration. This positive pressure is delivered until the preselected pressure has been reached. When the preset pressure is reached, the machine cycles into exhalation. Pressure-cycled ventilators are currently used in only a small portion of those clients who require CMV.

Volume-cycled ("volume-controlled" or "volume-limited") ventilators deliver a preset tidal volume of inspired gas. The tidal volume that has been preselected is delivered to the client regardless of the pressure required to deliver this volume. A pressure limit can be set to prevent dangerously high airway pressures from occurring. An artificial airway is necessary for CMV.

PHYSIOLOGIC EFFECTS

Decreased cardiac output is the most common physiologic effect of positive pressure, with either intermittent or continuous mechanical ventilation. Normal, unassisted respiration begins with subatmospheric pressure. Negative pressure increases during inhalation and decreases during exhalation. Positive pressure applied to the airway has the opposite effect. As positive pressure inflates the lungs, pressure in the thorax builds, decreasing the flow of blood to the vena cava, and reducing blood flow to the right atrium of the heart. Exhalation is passive, and pressures return to their normal, resting, subatmospheric level. Positive pressure also briefly affects the left side of the heart by increasing filling and output. This increase is due to the displacement of blood from the pulmonary system into the left ventricle. However, this effect is noted only immediately after the institution of positive-pressure ventilation. If positive-pressure ventilation is continued for more than a few minutes, the blood flow to and from the right ventricle is decreased. This in turn decreases the filling of the left ventricle, leading to a lowered cardiac output. The lowered cardiac output will be reflected in the hypotension that clients commonly exhibit immediately after being placed on mechanical ventilation. It is imperative that nurses monitor blood pressure closely.

Other body systems are also affected by positive pressure. As the diaphragm descends into the abdomen during the inspiratory phase, blood flow to the splanchnic area decreases. This decrease in splanchnic blood flow may lead to ischemia of the gastric mucosa. Ischemia of the gastric mucosa may be one of the reasons that clients who receive positive-pressure ventilation for an extended period of time have a high incidence of gastrointestinal bleeding and stress ulcerations. Decreasing blood flow to the splanchnic region also results in a decreased blood flow to the kidneys. This decrease in blood flow signals the posterior pituitary gland to increase secretion of vasopressin or antidiuretic hormone. Elevated vasopressin levels lead to reabsorption of free water in the renal tubular cells, thereby increasing water retention. Lymphatic flow also decreases as a result of positive pressure.

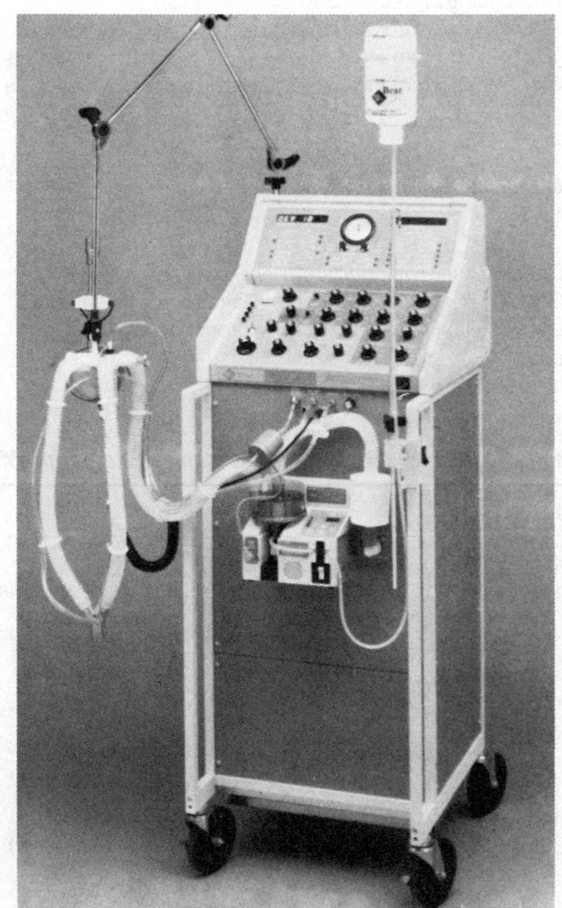

▲ **Figure 37-23**

A volume-cycled mechanical ventilator.

Positive pressure can cause neurophysiologic changes. When ABG values improve in acute, uncompensated respiratory failure, improved cerebral oxygenation results. A client with compensated respiratory acidosis (chronic carbon dioxide retention) may be adversely affected by positive-pressure breathing owing to "blowing-off" of carbon dioxide. Acute alkalosis may occur, producing faintness, dizziness, lightheadedness, and anxiety. If severe alkalosis persists, convulsions, cardiac arrhythmias, and cerebral edema may occur. Cerebral edema may contribute to intensive care unit psychosis.

ASSISTED AND CONTROLLED VENTILATION

Ventilators cycle as a result of either inspiration effort, i.e., assisted (person-cycled) ventilation, or an automatic, preset number of breaths, i.e., controlled (machine-cycled) ventilation.

With assisted (person-cycled) ventilation, the client's own inspiratory effort turns on ("trips") the ventilator, thus initiating the mechanical inspiratory phase. When the inspiratory effort has been sensed, the ventilator delivers a preset tidal volume and FIO_2. Some clients are able to make only weak inspiratory efforts. However, because the ventilator can be adjusted to respond to the respiratory abilities of each client, even a slight inspiratory effort may activate the positive-pressure phase, inflating the lungs at a preset flow rate. When the flow of gas stops, the client passively exhales without assistance from the machine. Some machines can be programmed (assist/control) to trigger another inspiration automatically if, after a period of delay, the client does not spontaneously trigger the machine. This ensures continued ventilation if the inspiratory efforts cease or the client becomes too weak to trigger the machine regularly. Assist/control ventilation allows the clients to take as many breaths as they desire. Every breath that they receive will be delivered by the machine at the same preset tidal volume and FIO_2. Assisted ventilation is indicated for clients who can control their own respiratory rate and pattern.

Controlled (machine-cycled) ventilation governs a client's rate of ventilation by automatically cycling the ventilator at a predetermined number of cycles per minute; the ventilator does all of the work of breathing, and the client does none. The respiratory cycle allows an expiratory time conducive to the return of blood flow to the right side of the heart. This mode is independent of the client's efforts or pattern of breathing. This mode of ventilation is the only mode that allows consistent physiologic results, but only if the client is chemically paralyzed with neuromuscular blocking agents, such as vecuronium bromide (Norcuron) or pancuronium bromide (Pavulon).

Clients who are on controlled mechanical ventilation and have spontaneous respirations may "fight" or "buck" the ventilator because they cannot synchronize their respirations with the machine's cycle. If the client continues to fight the ventilator, exhaustion and ineffective alveolar ventilation will result. If the nurse is unable to help such a client relax and breathe in cycle with the machine, the physician should be notified. With an artificial airway in place, the client who is fighting the ventilator may be safely sedated to reduce ventilatory efforts, and thus ventilatory control can be maintained. Medications that can be prescribed for this include morphine and diazepam (Valium). If additional control is required, the use of neuromuscular blocking agents may be indicated. These agents include pancuronium bromide (Pavulon), curare, vecuronium bromide (Norcuron), and atracurium besylate (Tracrium). These drugs block the transmission of nerve impulses, resulting in muscle paralysis. Because these agents do not affect sensorium, or perception of pain, they should *always* be used in conjunction with sedation or analgesics. These clients are not comatose or deaf, and the nurse should talk to them and explain what is happening. These clients are in great need of reassurance and support because of their helplessness.

Muscle-paralyzing agents may be administered in continuous intravenous drip, with the rate of infusion titrated to control the prolonged paralytic effects. Reversal of these effects is accomplished by drugs that inhibit acetylcholinesterase and allow an excess of acetylcholine to accumulate at the myoneural junction, e.g., neostigmine (Prostigmin) and edrophonium (Tensilon). Serial doses may be needed because recurrence of paralysis is possible. Careful assessment is important.

Controlled respiration and muscle paralysis are often used if a client (1) has muscle spasms, (2) is confused or tachypneic, or (3) is making respiratory efforts out-of-phase with the mechanical ventilator. Paralyzing agents may also be used to ensure effective mechanical ventilation for clients who have sustained head injury, flail chest, seizure disorders, or tetanus.

POSITIVE END-EXPIRATORY PRESSURE AND CONTINUOUS POSITIVE AIRWAY PRESSURE

Positive end-expiratory pressure (PEEP) and continuous positive airway pressure (CPAP) are ventilator techniques applied during expiration whereby intrathoracic pressures are not allowed to return to ambient pressure. This increased pressure helps to keep the alveoli open, increase functional residual capacity (FRC), and enhance oxygenation as a result of the enlarged surface area that is available for diffusion. With the implementation of PEEP or CPAP, oxygenation is improved, thus allowing the use of lower levels of FIO_2. In this way, the body's metabolic oxygen requirements are met without the toxic effects of higher concentrations of oxygen.

CPAP is usually applied to a client with spontaneous respiration. PEEP, on the other hand, is applied during mechanical ventilation in conjunction with controlled, assist/controlled, or intermittent mandatory ventilation. Figure 37–24 illustrates the differences among PEEP, CPAP, and CMV.

Weaning clients from PEEP is accomplished by reducing the oxygen level by 2- to 5-cm decrements. Careful monitoring of PaO_2 is ongoing.

Physiologic Effects. FRC is the volume of air remaining in the lung after normal expiration. If end-expira-

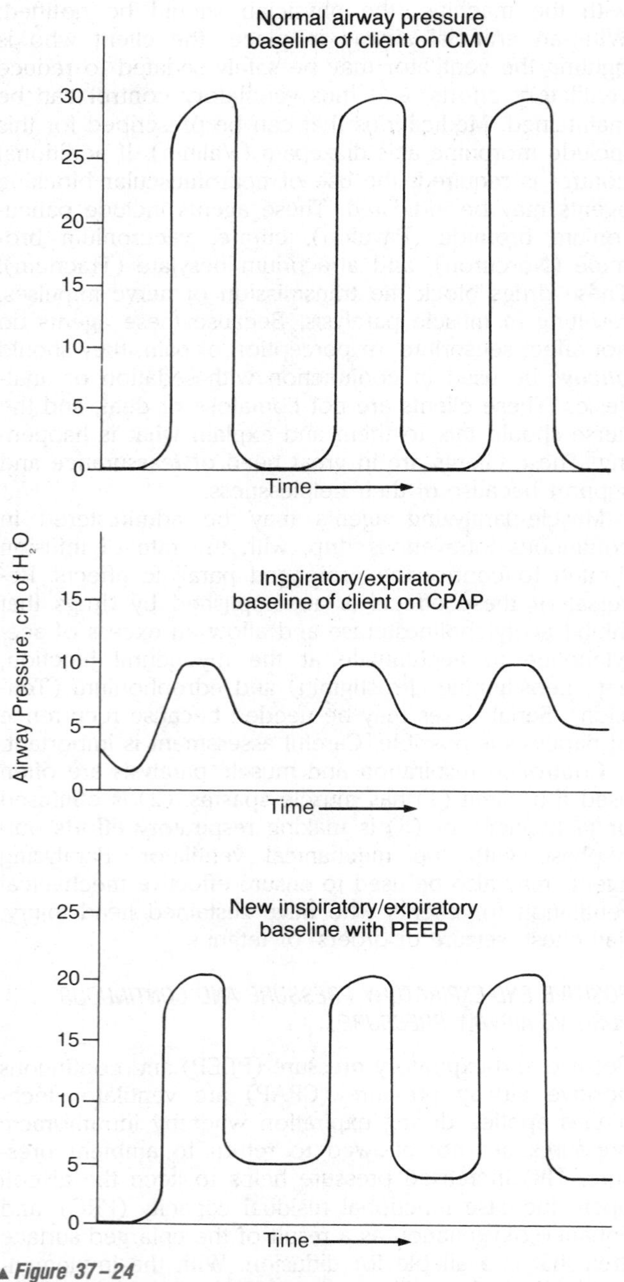

▲ *Figure 37-24*

The reset resting inspiratory/expiratory levels for CMV, CPAP, and PEEP. Zero represents ambient pressure.

tory alveolar volumes remain above their critical closing point, the alveoli remain open and functioning. However, if they fall below the closing point, the alveoli have a tendency to collapse. If alveolar collapse occurs, the volume of FRC also decreases. When alveoli collapse, hypoxemia results, and the lungs become "stiffer" or less compliant.

When alveoli collapse, pulmonary blood flow continues. Although perfusion (blood flow) continues, oxygenation of blood flow to that alveolus does not occur (Fig. 37-25). As alveoli collapse, the residual volume is decreased. A decreased residual volume also causes reduced FRC. This results in a true intrapulmonary shunt (perfusion without oxygenation). Lung compliance is also affected. Once alveolar collapse occurs, reinflation requires very high opening pressures, the generation of which significantly increases the work of breathing. The hypoxemia resulting from alveolar collapse and the increased oxygen consumption caused by the increased work of breathing may severely compromise the client.

Hazards. The physiologic effects of positive airway pressure on inspiration/expiration are basically the same as those effects discussed for IPPB and CMV. There are a few added risks, such as (1) rupture of the lung from increased intrathoracic and intra-airway pressures (barotrauma), (2) pneumothorax, (3) subcutaneous emphysema, (4) pneumomediastinum, and (5) cardiovascular embarrassment. Cardiovascular embarrassment results from the increased intrathoracic pressure caused by the PEEP, which leads to a decrease in cardiac output. If cardiac output cannot be improved with vasopressor or increased blood volume, hepatic and renal function become compromised. CPAP and PEEP also increase intracranial pressure. In neurologically injured clients, this is an added risk.

Assessment of clients on CPAP and PEEP includes

- blood pressure and heart rate
- breath sounds
- urinary output
- signs of increased heart failure
- chest films (before and after institution of CPAP and PEEP)
- observing for subcutaneous emphysema (palpate both the posterior and anterior subcutaneous tissue)
- ABGs

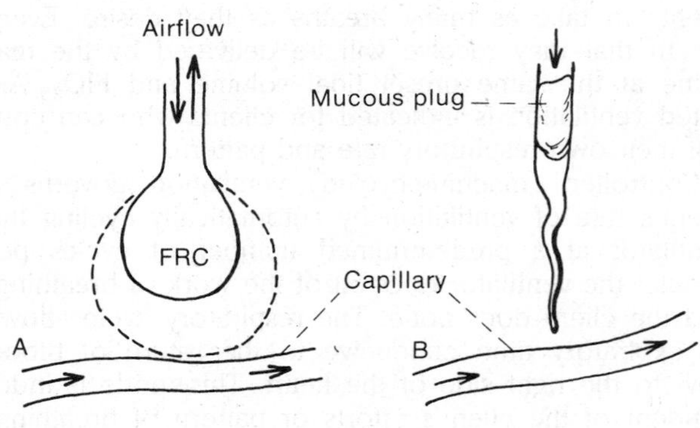

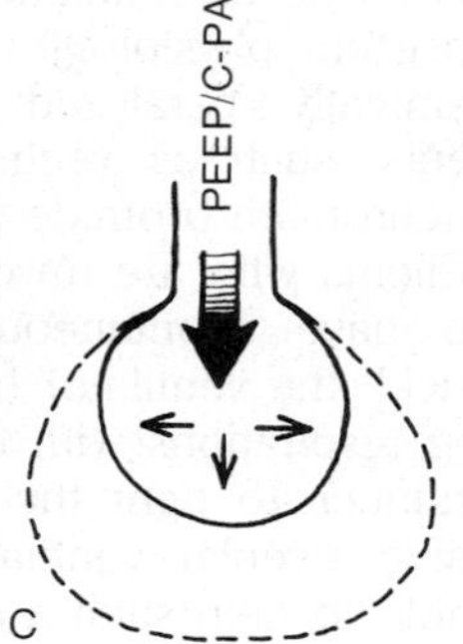

▲ *Figure 37-25*

Effects of positive airway pressure on alveolus. *A*, Normal alveolus. Dotted line represents expansion during inspiration. *B*, Collapsed alveolus. Perfusion continued. *C*, Alveolus opened by positive pressure. Dotted line indicates alveolus during inspiration and solid line indicates end-expiratory alveolar volume.

The aim of CPAP or PEEP therapy is to find the amount of pressure that produces the best PaO_2 and reduces the amount of shunt without producing adverse effects (e.g., hypotension). This value is called Best PEEP. Positive airway pressure may be applied in adult levels of +5 to +20 cm H_2O. Pressures greater than +20 cm H_2O are often referred to as Super PEEP.

INTERMITTENT MANDATORY VENTILATION

Intermittent mandatory ventilation (IMV) is a popular method of weaning a client from mechanical ventilation in which the ventilator is set to deliver a specific respiratory rate. If a client breathes at a rate higher than the machine rate, the breaths will not be positive-pressure ventilations. For example, if a ventilator is set on the IMV mode, rate of 8, and tidal volume of 800 ml, then it will deliver 8 breaths each minute at a volume of 800 ml. However, if the client breathes two additional breaths in that minute, these breaths open a flow of humidified, oxygenated gas from the machine at whatever tidal volume the client can obtain. As the client is increasingly able to breathe on his or her own, the IMV rate is slowly reduced until all breaths are spontaneous and ABGs are within the normal range for that client.

Nearly all mechanical volume ventilators are equipped with an IMV mode. Rather than being put on assisted or controlled ventilation, an intubated client may be immediately placed on IMV. This may facilitate a more rapid progression through the weaning process. Disconnecting the ventilator can then be considered. Extubation is done when all the initial criteria for intubation and mechanical ventilation are reversed. Some physicians use a T-piece before extubation. One end of the T-piece attaches directly to a flow of aerosolized oxygen from a large-volume nebulizer. The opposite end attaches to a small length of large-bore tubing that acts as an oxygen reservoir to maintain a constant FIO_2. The flow rate of oxygen should be fast enough to flush exhaled gas from the circuit to prevent rebreathing of exhaled air.

PRESSURE SUPPORT VENTILATION

Pressure support is a recent ventilation method that has been adapted to most modern volume ventilators. Pressure support ventilation (PSV) is a form of ventilation that augments spontaneous inspiratory effort with a preset level of positive airway pressure. When the client on PSV initiates a breath, the machine is triggered and delivers a flow of gas at the preset pressure. The flow rate remains constant until the inspiratory flow rate drops to one fourth the original rate. PSV cannot be used with assist/control ventilation because of the fact that every time the machine senses a spontaneous breath it will deliver a machine breath at the preset tidal volume.

PSV allows the client to set his or her own tidal volume, respiratory rate, and rhythm. PSV can be used in either a "mixed" or "stand alone" method. The mixed method uses two modes of mechanical ventilation at the same time. Usually, IMV and PSV are used together. The IMV mode is set for a particular rate, tidal volume, and FIO_2. If no spontaneous breaths are initiated, then the PSV is not used. However, if the client wants to breathe above the set IMV rate, the breaths above the IMV rate are augmented by the preset PSV. In the stand alone mode, PSV is used without another mode of ventilation as a back-up. The client must have a documented intact ventilatory drive before the stand alone mode may be used. If possible, the stand alone mode is preferable, because the client has complete control of the respiratory pattern. This is by far the more comfortable of the two methods.

Pressure support is useful for clients who are difficult to wean from mechanical ventilation. If the mixed method is used, gradually wean the IMV rate down until the IMV rate is zero before beginning to decrease the PSV. At this point, the stand alone method is being used. Slowly decrease the amount of pressure support until the PSV is at 5 cm H_2O. At this point, if the client is capable of total spontaneous respiration and the respiratory rate is less than 25, extubate and apply a cool mist face mask or tent.

HIGH-FREQUENCY VENTILATION

High-frequency ventilation (HFV) is another mode of mechanical ventilation used for clients who cannot be adequately ventilated with conventional techniques. HFV is often useful for clients with severe noncompliant lungs. HFV uses respiratory rates of 60 to 100 breaths per minute with considerably lower tidal volumes than those used in CMV. Although the results are not completely understood, apparently with HFV air moves in and out of the lungs by a force similar to diffusion. The overall advantage of HFV over conventional forms of ventilation is that with HFV there is a reduction in peak and mean airway pressure, resulting in better ventilation of noncompliant lungs, e.g., as in ARDS.

UNILATERAL LUNG VENTILATION

Unilateral lung ventilation (ULV) requires tracheal intubation with a special tube that permits the separate ventilation of each lung. A separate ventilator is used for each lung. In this way, one lung can be ventilated at a different volume and rate from the other lung. A client with a bronchopulmonary fistula who requires mechanical ventilation can benefit from ULV. For example, an undamaged lung can be ventilated with high volumes and pressures, whereas a damaged lung is ventilated with low volumes and pressures and allowed to heal.

Nursing Management. Because clients with respiratory difficulties are usually tense and apprehensive, the transition to mechanical ventilation needs to be done in as smooth and calm a fashion as possible. A common fear that clients have is that the machine will fail and they will be unable to breathe or summon help in time. Careful preparation of clients receiving ventilator therapy may help to relieve these fears and also contribute to successful treatment. (A client receiving CMV who is inadequately prepared may panic and offset the positive effects of mechanical ventilation.) Explain the basic mechanics of the ventilator, how the machine will help breathing, what it will feel like, and how to cooperate. Never leave clients on CMV unattended. Around-the-clock nursing care by nurses experienced in the care of clients on CMV is essential.

Assessment. Assessment is essential to maintain effective breathing patterns with CMV.

- Monitor the respiratory status by ABG analysis, chest films, auscultation, and tracheal aspirate cultures.
- Ensure that ordered arterial blood samples are taken for regular ABG analysis. Document and inform the physician of ABG results.
- Assess and document vital signs for cardiovascular depression, inspiratory pressures, breath sounds, arterial oxygen tension, and ventilatory parameters hourly. Report trends or abnormal findings to the physician.

CMV is almost entirely automatic, but there are some nursing problems: maintaining prescribed inspired oxygen concentrations and the patency of endotracheal and tracheostomy tubes; supplying adequate humidification; and preventing trauma, infection, and mechanical problems such as loose connections and kinks in tubing.

Nursing care for clients with inadequate ventilation requires skill in assessing for indications of respiratory distress, i.e., restlessness, apprehension, irritability, wakefulness, use of the accessory muscles of respiration, pallor, increasing pulse rate, and labored respirations.

Nursing Intervention. When surrounded by machines, health care providers may sometimes overlook the client and focus on the machines exclusively. Clients on ventilators are highly dependent and need comprehensive, holistic care with meticulous attention to detail. They need health care providers who are not only skillful in managing the machines but also understanding and supportive during stressful experiences.

CMV is used when clients have an ineffective breathing pattern. Mechanical ventilators are an external, temporary means of maintaining an effective breathing pattern. Be familiar with the ventilator and with signs of malfunction (see Bridge to Critical Care). Check the machine frequently to ensure proper functioning and the adequate operation of all alarm systems. Check the electrical cords frequently to avoid disconnection. Safely place them so that they cannot be pulled loose or cause falls.

Always have a self-inflating resuscitation bag readily available. Manual ventilation may be used during tracheobronchial suctioning, if it is necessary to disconnect the ventilator temporarily for tests or treatments, to change apparatus on the machine, or to ventilate the client if the ventilator fails.

When clients are initially placed on a ventilator, they must be closely observed so that the effectiveness of the therapy can be evaluated and complications can be prevented from occurring. Serious complications that may arise during initial mechanical ventilation include rapid electrolyte changes, severe alkalosis (frequently with convulsions), and hypotension due to decreases in cardiac output.

A Nursing Care Plan on the care of the client on mechanical ventilation discusses other interventions.

Ethical Implications. Placing a client on CMV involves ethical considerations. CMV does not necessarily "save life," but it may prolong life. For some, it allows the body time to heal. For others (those with terminal illness), it may prolong suffering.

If a situation arises in which a client requires CMV, the overall clinical picture needs to be considered before initiation of CMV. Discuss possibilities of the client's recovery with the physician and consult with the family if possible. Once a client is placed on CMV, legal issues may make it difficult to discontinue CMV (see Ethical Issues in Nursing).

Weaning. The physician decides when to begin weaning a client from CMV. The decision is often based on assessments made by nurses and respiratory therapists. Weaning may cause psychological and physiologic changes. The length of time required for successful weaning generally relates to the underlying disease process and to the client's state of health before a ventilator is used. For example, a young client who has had an overdose of drugs usually weans rapidly. However, a client with COPD who develops acute respiratory failure and has little or no pulmonary reserve often takes longer and requires much professional patience and skill.

Criteria for a weaning trial are

- improvement, correction, or stabilization of the active disease process
- nutritional and fluid status sufficient to maintain the increased metabolic needs and demands of spontaneous respiration
- adequate physical strength and mental alertness
- afebrile status, i.e., any infections controlled
- stable cardiovascular, renal, and cerebral status
- optimal levels of ABGs, electrolytes, hemoglobin, and other laboratory tests
- achievement of the physiologic parameters listed in the Bridge to Critical Care

Careful assessment of ventilatory status before and during weaning is necessary, including spontaneous tidal volume; vital capacity; maximal voluntary ventilation; inspiratory effort; breath sounds; cardiovascular, renal, and cerebral status; and ABGs.

Weaning from mechanical ventilation can be accomplished in two ways. The first is called the "rapid" wean. This technique is used when mechanical ventilation has been instituted for prophylaxis (e.g., surgery). First, the client must meet all of the requirements in the Bridge to Critical Care. Start in the morning after the client has had a good night's rest. Place the client in a semi-Fowler's position. Reduce the mechanical ventila-

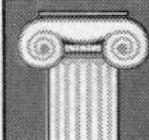

ETHICAL ISSUES IN NURSING

How Should the Decision to End Continuous Mechanical Ventilation Be Made?

Continuous mechanical ventilation (CMV) is used for many different reasons. Ventilator support may be needed for short-term care, as in certain cases of severe pneumonia, or for more long-term care, as in some stroke patients. In some emergency cases, ventilator support is required to stabilize a client's condition. No matter why CMV is initiated, there are degrees of benefit it offers to the patient. A positive benefit is that CMV allows the lungs to rest in order that healing may take place (such as in severe pneumonia). However, CMV may produce an unwanted effect such as artificially prolonging death and causing suffering, as with severe stroke patients and/or patients in terminal states.

The decision to place a person on CMV is made by the client, or his or her surrogate, and the medical team. This decision may be a very difficult one, e.g., when a client is in a persistent vegetative state, and the wishes of the client regarding CMV are not known. However, it is even more difficult for persons to decide for another whether to discontinue CMV. To many persons, this decision is viewed as somehow causing the person's death and this is very uncomfortable for them.

The best alternative to this dilemma is for all persons, while in a state of health, to decide what they would want done should a situation arise requiring resuscitative measures, including CMV. Advance directives such as a living will or a health care power of attorney can help people guide their own treatment should certain health care situations arise. In fact, as of December 1991, all health care facilities who take Medicare and/or Medicaid reimbursement must include, on admission, an advance directive assessment of all their clients.

Nurses have a great deal of influence over the health care teaching of their clients. Information about advance directives may be shared with clients, community members, family members and friends. The more the public is made aware of such directives, the easier it is for health care professionals to guide their care. In many cases, people have strong feelings about the initiation of certain treatments, such as CMV. Advance directives allow all persons to decide, in advance of crisis situations, what they wish to have done in such situations. By allowing all persons to exercise advance directives, health care providers may avoid many legal/ethical dilemmas which occur in the initiation, continuation, or discontinuation of certain treatments.

---

tor's respiratory rate to one half the original rate. Obtain ABGs in 30 minutes. If the ABGs are at or near the client's baseline, place the client on a T-piece or "blow by" at the same FIO_2. Obtain ABGs in 30 minutes. If the ABGs are again at or near the baseline and the respiratory rate is below 25 to 30 breaths per minute, extubate. Place on a face tent for high humidity.

The second method for weaning is called a "gradual" or "slow" wean. This technique is utilized when prolonged mechanical ventilation has been used or a neuromuscular disorder is present. The first step in this technique is to ascertain whether or not spontaneous breathing is present. Once spontaneous breathing has been established, slowly decrease the amount of ventilatory support. Continue to decrease ventilatory support until the client is able to accept full responsibility for his or her own ventilatory requirements. This technique may take weeks or even months. Patience is critical.

A first weaning attempt may not be successful. Failure in weaning may be due to (1) decreased muscular strength caused by protein-carbohydrate malnutrition or certain disease processes, or uncoordination of respiratory muscles due to disuse from prolonged CMV; (2) increased work of breathing due to increased airway resistance, abdominal distention, a small-diameter artificial airway, upper airway obstruction, and unresolved acute lung diseases; and (3) increased ventilation requirements (see Bridge to Critical Care). If the first attempt at weaning is not successful, it is important to determine the reasons and try to eliminate them in subsequent attempts. The client must be returned to CMV.

RESPIRATORY HOME CARE

Clients with chronic respiratory diseases often require frequent hospitalization because of the recurrent nature of their diseases (e.g., COPD). However, whenever possible, it is desirable to help clients manage at home rather than in an acute care facility.

Respiratory home care can require a range of intervention from simple oxygen therapy to CMV. The principles for intervention are the same whether at home or in a health care facility. Some modifications are necessary, however, for a home environment.

Multidisciplinary Approach

Before a client with respiratory disease is discharged from a health care facility, it is important to assess the type of care needed at home. A team of allied health professionals meets to assess specific needs. A typical team consists of nurse, physician, respiratory therapist, physical therapist, occupational therapist, dietician, discharge coordinator, home health nurse, social worker, and pastoral services person. Consultants from other health care services may also be present. (See Bridge to Home Health Care.)

Many criteria must be met before instituting "home care" to ensure safety and optimize the person's quality of life. Much depends on (1) the client's attitude and motivation and (2) the attitude and resources of significant others. The following areas are among those assessed for determining the feasibility of providing home care:

- availability of a strong, positive support system
- motivation and trainability of family or other care providers

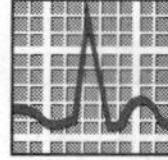

BRIDGE TO CRITICAL CARE

The Mechanically Ventilated Client

Nursing Diagnosis/ Collaborative Problem	Planning: Expected Outcomes	Implementation: Nursing Interventions	Rationales
Altered Respiratory Function (Airway Clearance, Ineffective; Gas Exchange, Impaired; Breathing Pattern, Ineffective) R/T pathologic processes in the lung, trauma, anesthesia, surgery on the chest or abdomen, neuromuscular disorders	Client will have improved respiratory function as evidenced by • less crackles and rhonchi • ventilation in both lungs • no signs of hypoxia • ABGs returning to preintubation level or normal parameters	Auscultate lung sounds every hour and as needed	Indicates the amount of fluid and secretion in the lungs; validates that endotracheal tube (ETT) is placed correctly so that both lungs can be ventilated
		Suction as needed, provide pre- and post-hyperinflation and hyperoxygenation	Suctioning removes airway secretions, facilitating ventilation; oxygen and inflation reduce hypoxia during suctioning
		Instill normal saline into artificial airway as needed	Promotes coughing and loosens secretions
		Provide adequate humidity via the ventilator or nebulizer	Replaces the function of the upper airway to warm and humidify the inspired air; thins secretions to facilitate their removal
		Turn and reposition every 2 hours	Allows both lungs to be fully ventilated, mobilizes secretions
		Position with affected lung upper most	Facilitates drainage into large airways
		Secure ETT properly	Prevents accidental dislodgement
		Use a bite block or oral airway	Prevents ETT compression If the client is biting it; bite block is more comfortable for the conscious client
		Assist in changing ETT prn	Assures adequate ventilation
		Monitor ABG values and arterial oxymetry	Indicates the degree of oxygenation; lack of improvement in ABGs may require a change in interventions
		Perform range-of-motion exercises; ambulate to chair when feasible	Immobility leads to decreased respiration muscle strength
Individual Coping, Ineffective R/T dependency while on CMV	Client will exhibit positive coping strategies as evidenced by • reduction in the level of stress or anxiety • decreased feelings of powerlessness	Develop a means of communication	Allows client to have needs met
		Place nurse call device within reach	Allows client to contact nurse
		Be available and visible	Reduces anxiety in client
		Provide distractions (e.g., TV, radio)	Reduces anxiety because client does not focus on ventilator and noises
		Explain all procedures	Allows client to feel respected
		Medicate prn	Antianxiety medications and narcotics may be needed but use with caution in clients being weaned because these drugs suppress respiratory drive
		Provide privacy	Demonstrates client respect
		Respect client's rights and opinions	Demonstrates client respect and maintains dignity
		Provide a calm environment	Anxiety is contagious, and if the client becomes anxious, ventilation will be more difficult and oxygen needs will increase

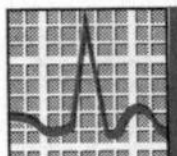

BRIDGE TO CRITICAL CARE

The Mechanically Ventilated Client Continued

Nursing Diagnosis/ Collaborative Problem	*Planning: Expected Outcomes*	*Implementation: Nursing Interventions*	*Rationales*
		Explain to client and family that vocal cords have been bypassed, which prevents talking; encourage them to use other modes of communication	Clients can hear and respond even though they cannot talk
Collaborative Problem, High Risk for complications of continuous mechanical ventilation positive-pressure ventilation	The nurse will monitor the client for pulmonary barotrauma, cardiovascular depression, inadvertent extubation, and malposition of endotracheal tube	Assess for acute, increasing, or severe dyspnea, agitation, panic, decreased or absent breath sounds, localized hyperresonance, increased breathing effort, tracheal deviation away from the side with abnormal findings, subcutaneous emphysema, and decreasing PaO_2 levels	Barotrauma is damage to the lungs from extrapulmonary air changing intrapleural pressures during positive-pressure ventilation.
		Have a high index of suspicion for clients' pre-existing lung lesions, high positive end-expiratory pressure, and invasive thoracic procedures; contact the physician if symptoms occur	Barotrauma can lead to pneumothorax or tension pneumothorax
		Assess for acute or gradual fall in blood pressure, tachycardia (early sign), bradycardia (late sign), dysrhythmias, weak peripheral pulses, acute or gradual increase in pulmonary capillary wedge pressure, and respiratory "swing" (depression) in arterial or pulmonary artery waveforms during inspiration	Cardiovascular depression can occur after an increase in tidal volume, PEEP, CPAP, or with hyperinflation; the positive pressure decreases venous return and afterload due to an increase in intrathoracic pressure
		Monitor for signs of inadvertant extubation: vocalization, low-pressure alarm, bilateral decrease in upper lobe airway sounds, gastric distention, clinical manifestations of inadequate ventilation; inadvertent extubation occurs, notify physician, because reintubation is necessary; manage ventilation and oxygenation with a self-inflating resuscitation bag	Inadvertent extubation can be obvious, such as when the tube is found in the client's hand; it can also be obscure, such as when the tube slips into the hypopharynx or esophagus

Care Plan continued on following page

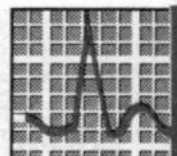

BRIDGE TO CRITICAL CARE

The Mechanically Ventilated Client Continued

Nursing Diagnosis/ Collaborative Problem	*Planning: Expected Outcomes*	*Implementation: Nursing Interventions*	*Rationales*
Infection, High Risk for R/T impaired primary defenses in respiratory tract	Client will remain free of infection AEB: • clear sputum • no fever • lung sounds clearing • no increased difficulty with ventilation • white blood cell count within normal limits	Wash hands thoroughly	Proper handwashing will decrease the spread of infection
		Use sterile technique for: • suctioning • changing dressings	The respiratory tract is considered sterile
		Monitor for increased breathing effort, localized changes in auscultation, and changes in PaO_2	Infected lung segments transmit sound differently (more solid) and do not permit O_2/CO_2 exchange
		Provide oral care every 2 hours	The client's mouth becomes dry, and stomatitis may develop from the lack of oral secretions
		Drain water from ventilator tubing; do not drain water back into the humidifier	Water may become a source of contamination, especially with *Pseudomonas*
		Monitor laboratory values, white blood cell count	White blood cell increases may indicate pulmonary infection
		Monitor sputum for changes in color, consistency, amount, and odor	Infection may cause sputum to increase, darken, thicken, and become malodorous
Nutrition, Altered: Less than Body Requirements R/T lack of ability to eat while on ventilator	Client will exhibit adequate nutritional intake AEB: • stable weight, or weight appropriate to height • intake of 1200 kcal/day per nasogastric tube • no signs of catabolism • wounds healing • no infection	Provide adequate nutrition	Intake of 1200 kcal (approx.) is adequate to maintain weight; inadequate nutrition decreases diaphragmatic muscle mass, decreases pulmonary function performance, and increases mechanical ventilation requirements
		Begin tube feeding as soon as it is evident that client will remain on CMV for a length of time	The client should not be allowed to develop a catabolic state
		Avoid excessive carbohydrate loads	Carbohydrate loads may increase carbon dioxide production to the point of producing hypercapnia
		Weigh daily	Changes in body weight are a reliable indicator of nutritional balance
		Monitor intake and output	Fluids are still required, and output should match intake
		Assess for complications of tube feeding: • aspiration • diarrhea • constipation	Feed client sitting upright, with cuff inflated Check for residual tube feeding every shift or before beginning another feeding Diarrhea is most often due to osmotic changes from a too-high concentration of tube feeding or the use of sorbitol-based elixirs; consider decreasing the concentration or changing to crushed pills

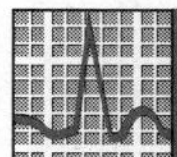

BRIDGE TO CRITICAL CARE

The Mechanically Ventilated Client Continued

Nursing Diagnosis/ Collaborative Problem	*Planning: Expected Outcomes*	*Implementation: Nursing Interventions*	*Rationales*
			Constipation is due to a lack of free water within the feeding; add 100 ml of water every 4–6 hours if allowable
		Monitor laboratory values (calcium, magnesium, phosphorus, total protein, and albumin)	These trace elements and proteins may not be adequately supplied by a tube feeding
		Monitor bowel sounds	Bowel obstruction and ileus present as changes in bowel sounds
		Before tube feeding or between bolus feedings, test pH and guaiac every shift	Changes in pH may indicate an increased risk of gastric stress ulcers; positive guaiac tests indicate bleeding

- financial resources
- physical resources of the home, e.g., access to electrical outlets, accessibility of bathroom and bedroom, absence of long flights of stairs
- client's physiologic needs and status, e.g., dyspnea and exercise tolerance, and psychosocial status and needs
- client's maximal capabilities
- specific professional support needed, e.g., personnel, equipment, services

Many respiratory devices require electricity, and electrical outlets must be readily available. The supplier of the equipment usually helps to arrange for all necessary equipment and home adaptations. Duplicate equipment and circuits must be available so that when one piece of equipment is being cleaned and dried the other can be used.

An important aspect of home respiratory care is cleaning and disinfecting equipment. Contaminated respiratory care equipment is a serious potential source of infection.

Providing education and ongoing support for the client and family is probably the most essential component of respiratory home care. Motivation is key to the success of the plan. Goals include developing skills and habits to ensure overall safety and a self-determined, quality lifestyle in the home.

Plan education according to the established attainable short- and long-term goals. For success, the client and significant others must be involved in goal setting because they are often most aware of what they need. The amount and type of training required depend on the client's condition and capabilities, the intervention needed, and the capabilities of the significant others. For example:

- A client with a tracheostomy and significant others need to learn how to clear the airway by suctioning and how to care for the stoma.
- A client needing oxygen therapy and the family must know the required technique and the precautions necessary when using pressurized gas cylinders.
- A client requiring CMV and the family need in-depth training about the mechanics and management of the ventilator.

All education must be individually designed for each unique home situation. When mechanical skills are involved, it is important to explain a procedure, then demonstrate it, and have clients perform the procedure under supervision. The client and family must practice all necessary skills with professional support (probably in the health care facility) before they are expected to perform them without supervision at home. Be sure they know how to get professional help if needed.

Respiratory intervention that may be required at home by clients experiencing chronic respiratory conditions includes oxygen therapy, aerosolization and humidification, chest physiotherapy, IPPB, and mechanical ventilation.

Oxygen Therapy. Home oxygen administration uses the same delivery systems as in health care facilities (e.g., cannulas, masks). The oxygen source is different, however. Clients who require continuous oxygen may purchase or rent an oxygen concentrator to extract oxygen from room air (Fig. 37–26). This may be more cost effective than large oxygen cylinders. Cylinder oxygen is also used in the home, and lightweight liquid oxygen systems are available for clients requiring oxygen while ambulatory.

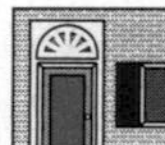

BRIDGE TO HOME HEALTH CARE

The Ventilator-Dependent Client

Good communication between the ventilator-dependent client, family members and/or caregivers, and the home health nurse, the physician, and specific community resources is essential. As soon as the nurse obtains physician's orders and establishes a plan of care, the nurse calls the DME (durable medical equipment) supplier. All the equipment and supplies that will be required in the home are reviewed. The nurse may want to plan a shared home visit with the equipment supplier. Next, the nurse needs to check with the local electric company to make sure if the community has a list of persons, who in case of an electrical failure, receive priority to get their service turned back on immediately. It's very important to have a portable, battery-operated ventilator in the home in case of a power failure.

Plan to spend several hours with the family and caregivers on initial visits. They need to be taught about the equipment, ventilator alarms, suctioning, dressing changes, and other care requirements. Be certain they give satisfactory return demonstrations. Often, the equipment is very intimidating to the family. Write as much information down as possible such as phone numbers of the home health nurse, the equipment suppliers, and the physician. Also write instructions about the use of the equipment. Writing this information on a large piece of paper in large print is helpful. Ask the family to keep it close to the client. This will prevent the family or caregivers from shuffling through various papers or pamphlets to obtain pertinent information. It is not unusual to have families or caregivers forget everything the nurse has said once she/he leaves. Remember the client is probably happy to be home in his own environment, but the family may be very anxious and frightened. The nurse also addresses the use of help to provide periods of rest for the family.

Equipment noise may be quite a nuisance for clients and caregivers. Suggest a radio, TV, or cassette player with earphones. If clients can communicate through writing, make sure they have a small chalkboard or dry erase board in which to communicate messages or needs to others. The family or client may want to hire a tutor to teach sign language, but most persons learn to read lips. Keep the room light and open; a bed by a window serves as extrasensory stimuli. Be sure to caution the family to avoid irritants or pollutants such as smoke, animal fur or dander, bird feathers, and/or heavy dust in the environment.

Mechanical Ventilation. CMV is being increasingly used outside of health care facilities. Small, portable, electrically powered ventilators are available for home use. Some models can be adapted to a 12-volt car battery and attached to a wheelchair. Supplemental oxygen must be bled into the inspiratory side of the circuit to provide an FIO_2 greater than 0.21. Family members need to learn daily maintenance checks and how to manage machine problems. The nurse should develop emergency plans with the client and family in case machines fail. A second ventilator must always be readily available.

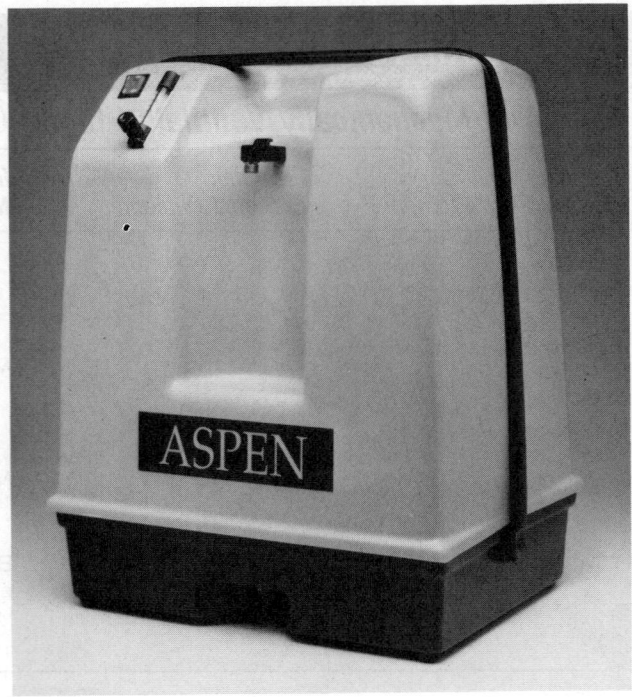

▲ *Figure 37–26*

Oxygen concentrator, which extracts oxygen from room air. (Courtesy of Mountain Medical Equipment, Inc., Littleton, CO.)

Aerosolization and Humidification. Humidification may be provided at home by steam from boiling water or a hot shower, and mist therapy can be provided by vaporizers or room humidifiers. The latter are usually available over-the-counter at pharmacies and are often useful for upper airway disorders. They are not so helpful for lower airway disorders, however. Humidifiers produce an aerosol output that is typically restricted to particles of a larger size that are unable to penetrate deep within the lungs. Small-volume medication nebulizers and metered dose inhalers are easily used at home. Small air compressors can be rented or purchased to power small-volume nebulizers.

Chest Physiotherapy. The client's family can learn the techniques of chest physiotherapy, percussion, vibration, and diaphragmatic breathing. If the client has an adjustable "hospital" bed at home, the various positions required are easier to assume. If not, pillows can be used for positioning.

Intermittent Positive-Pressure Breathing. Intermittent positive pressure breathing (IPPB) is seldom used, but if necessary, portable, electrically powered IPPB units are available. Disposable incentive spirometers can be used at home but are rarely necessary.

Summary

Respiratory interventions begin with proper positioning and smoking cessation, as well as prevention of complications by keeping the client hydrated, nourished, and free from infection. Because many chronic respiratory disorders lead to a loss of activity tolerance and anxiety, the clients often need psychosocial support to comply with techniques that facilitate coughing and airway management. Oxygen therapy can include nasal prongs at a low flow of oxygen to support the client. Continuous mechanical ventilation can provide for all needed ventilation. Nurses must be skilled clinicians in assessment and in the use of the various devices used in airway management.

BIBLIOGRAPHY

1. Barnes, T. A., & Lisbon, A. (Eds.) (1988). *Respiratory care practice.* Chicago: Year Book.
2. Brown, L. H. (1990). Pulmonary oxygen toxicity. *Focus on Critical Care, 17*(1), 68-75.
3. Bolgiano, C. S., et al. (1990). Administering oxygen therapy: What you need to know. *Nursing 90, 20*(6), 47-51.
4. Burton, G., et al. (1991). *Respiratory care: A guide to clinical practice.* Philadelphia: J. B. Lippincott.
5. Cerniack, N. S. (Ed.) (1991). *Chronic obstructive pulmonary disease.* Philadelphia: W. B. Saunders.
6. Clark, A. P., et al. (1990). Effects of endotracheal suctioning on mixed venous oxygen saturation and heart rate in critically ill adults. *Heart and Lung, 19*(5) (Suppl), 552-557.
7. Deshpande, V., et al. (1988). *A comprehensive review in respiratory care.* Norwalk: Appleton and Lange.
8. Dettenmeier, P. A. (1990). Planning for successful home mechanical ventilation. *AACN Clinical Issues in Critical Care Nursing, 1*(2), 267-279.
9. Dolan, J. T. (Ed.) (1991). *Critical care nursing: Clinical management through the nursing process.* Philadelphia: F. A. Davis.
10. Dunleap, E. (1987). Safe and easy ways to secure breathing tubes. *RN, 50*(8), 26-27.
11. Fedorovich, C., & Littleton, M. T. (1990). Chest physiotherapy: evaluating the effectiveness. *Dimensions of Critical Care Nursing, 9*(2), 68-74.
12. Ferland, P. (1991). Are you ready for ventilator patients?*Nursing 91, 21*(1), 42-47.
13. Frost, G. F. (1988). An evaluation of incentive spirometry for bronchodilator therapy. *The Canadian Journal of Respiratory Therapy, 24*(5), 11, 14-16.
14. Gray, J. E., et al. (1990). The effects of bolus normal saline instillation in conjunction with endotracheal suctioning. *Respiratory Care, 35*(8), 785-790.
15. Gregg, B. L. (1989). Inspiratory muscle training with a weighted incentive spirometer in subjects with chronic airways obstruction. *Respiratory Care, 34*(10), 860-867.
16. Hee, M. K., et al. (1992). Intubation of critically ill patients. *Mayo Clinic Proceedings, 67*(6), 569-576.
17. Hudak, C. M., et al. (Eds.) (1986). *Critical care nursing: A holistic approach* (4th ed.). Philadelphia: J. B. Lippincott.
18. Jeffrey, A. A., et al. (1989). Accuracy of inpatient oxygen administration. *Thorax, 44*(12), 1036-1037.
19. Kersten, L. (1989). *Comprehensive respiratory nursing.* Philadelphia: W. B. Saunders.
20. Kinney, M. R., et al. (Eds.) (1988). *AACN's clinical reference for critical-care nursing* (2nd ed.). New York: McGraw-Hill.
21. Kirby, M. J., et al. (Eds.) (1990). *Clinical applications of ventilatory support.* New York: Churchill Livingstone.
22. Lehner, B. E., & Schachter, E. N. (1980). *The pharmacology of respiratory care.* St. Louis: C. V. Mosby.
23. MacIntyre, N. R. (1989). Pressure support in perspective. *Respiratory Care, 34*(2), 134-135.
24. MacIntyre, N. R. (1988). Weaning from mechanical ventilatory support: volume-assisting intermittent breaths versus pressure-assisting every breath. *Respiratory Care, 33*(2), 121-125.
25. Majors, M. (1988). Nutritional support of the mechanically ventilated patient. *Critical Care Nursing Quarterly, 11*(3), 50-61.
26. Marino, P. (1991). *The ICU book.* Philadelphia: Lea and Febiger.
27. Massaro, D. (1986). Oxygen: toxicity and tolerance. *Hospital Practice, 21*(7), 95-101.
28. Mathews, P. J., et al. (1992). Airway monitoring and ventilation. *Nursing 92, 22*(2), 48-51.
29. McPherson, S. P., & Spearman, C. B. (Eds.) (1990). *Respiratory therapy equipment* (4th ed.). St. Louis: C. V. Mosby.
30. McSweeny, A. J., & Grant, I. (Eds.) (1988). *Chronic obstructive pulmonary disease: A behavioral perspective.* New York: Dekker.
31. *Physicians desk reference* (1991). Oradell, NJ: Medical Economics Data.
32. Rapoport, D. M. (1987). Techniques for administering nasal CPAP. *Respiratory Management, 17*(4), 17-18, 21.
33. Scanlan, C. L. (Ed.) (1990). *Egan's fundamentals of respiratory care* (5th ed.). St. Louis: C. V. Mosby.
34. Shapiro, B., et al. (1991). *Clinical applications of respiratory care.* St. Louis: C. V. Mosby.
35. Sonnesso, G. (1991). Are you ready to use pulse oximetry? *Nursing 91, 21*(8), 60-64.
36. Spearing, C., & Cornell, D. J. (1987). Incentive spirometry: inspiring your patient to breathe deeply. *Nursing, 17*(9), 50-51.
37. Spearman, C. B., & Sanders, H. G. (1987). The new generation of mechanical ventilators. *Respiratory Care, 32*(6), 403-418.
38. Stiesmeyer, J. K. (1991). What triggers a ventilator alarm? *AJN, 91*(10), 60-65.
39. Stone, K. S., & Turner, B. (1989). Endotracheal suctioning. *Annual Review of Nursing Research, 7*(1), 27-49.
40. Sutton, P. P. (1988). Chest physiotherapy: time for reappraisal. *British Journal of Diseases of the Chest, 82*(2), 127-137.
41. Weilitz, P. B. (1991). *Pocket guide to respiratory care.* St. Louis: C. V. Mosby.
42. Wyngaarden, J. B., et al. (1992). *Cecil textbook of medicine.* Philadelphia: W. B. Saunders.

Chapter 38

Nursing Care of Clients with Upper Airway Disorders

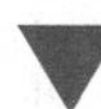

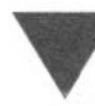

TUMORS

CANCER OF THE LARYNX

Cancers of the larynx account for only 2 to 3 per cent of all malignancies. However, clients with these tumors present a unique challenge to the nurse because of the cosmetic and functional deformities commonly seen with this disorder and its treatment. Benign and early malignant tumors may be treated with limited surgery, and the client recovers with little functional loss. Advanced tumors require extensive surgery. At times the operation may render the client unable to speak, breathe through the nose or mouth, or eat normally. In addition, the defect left by the operation and its reconstruction may cause a significant deformity and a need for more than one operation to restore appearance.

Definition

Cancer of the larynx is cancer of the voice box. It commonly occurs on the glottis (true vocal cords), the supraglottic structures (above the vocal cords), or the subglottic structures (below the vocal cords). Laryngeal cancer is classified and treated by its anatomic site. Supraglottic tumors occur on the posterior surface of the epiglottis to the vocal cords, including the false vocal cords. Glottic tumors are tumors of the true vocal cords. Subglottic tumors occur on the undersurface of the true vocal cords.

Incidence

There will be an estimated 12,500 cases of laryngeal cancer each year. Eighty per cent of those cases will be in men. Over the past 30 years, the incidence of cancer of the larynx has remained steady in men; it is up 150 per cent in women.[1] If untreated, cancer of the larynx is inevitably fatal; 90 per cent of untreated clients die within 3 years. Like other cancers, however, it is potentially curable if discovered early enough.

Etiology

Considerable data indicate that the etiologic agent of laryngeal cancer is cigarette smoking. Three of four clients who develop laryngeal cancer have smoked or currently smoke. The inhalation of other noxious fumes, such as polluted air, may contribute to the risk. Chronic laryngitis and voice abuse may also contribute to the disorder.

Risk Factors

The risk of laryngeal cancer is increased in clients who smoke tobacco. This risk of laryngeal cancer is increased even more in clients who smoke and abuse alcohol. In this regard, laryngeal cancer is one of the most preventable cancers. Primary prevention is to decrease the number of people who smoke and drink to excess. Secondary prevention is through the early detection of signs of laryngeal cancer, as shown in Box 38-1. Tertiary prevention, the reduction of morbidity, is discussed throughout this section.

Box 38-1. Clinical Warning Signs of Laryngeal Cancer

- Change in voice quality
- A lump anywhere in the neck or bod
- Persistent cough, sore throat, or earache
- Hemoptysis
- Sores within the throat do not heal
- Difficulty swalling or breathing

Pathophysiology

Cancer of the larynx is most often squamous cell carcinoma. It begins as a small hard patch, and in time it ulcerates and abscesses. Cancer of the glottis grows slowly owing to limited lymphatic supply. Cancer elsewhere in the larynx spreads more quickly because there are abundant lymphatic vessels. Metastatic disease often may be palpated as neck masses. Distant metastasis occurs in the lungs. Patterns of spread of laryngeal cancer are shown in Figure 38-1.

Tumors on the glottis prevent it from closing during speech, which causes hoarseness or a voice change. Supraglottic tumors cause pain in the throat especially with swallowing, a sensation of a foreign body in the throat, neck masses, and pain radiating to the ear by way of the glossopharyngeal and vagus nerves. Subglottic tumors have no early symptoms; symptoms do not appear until the tumor grows to obstruct the airway.

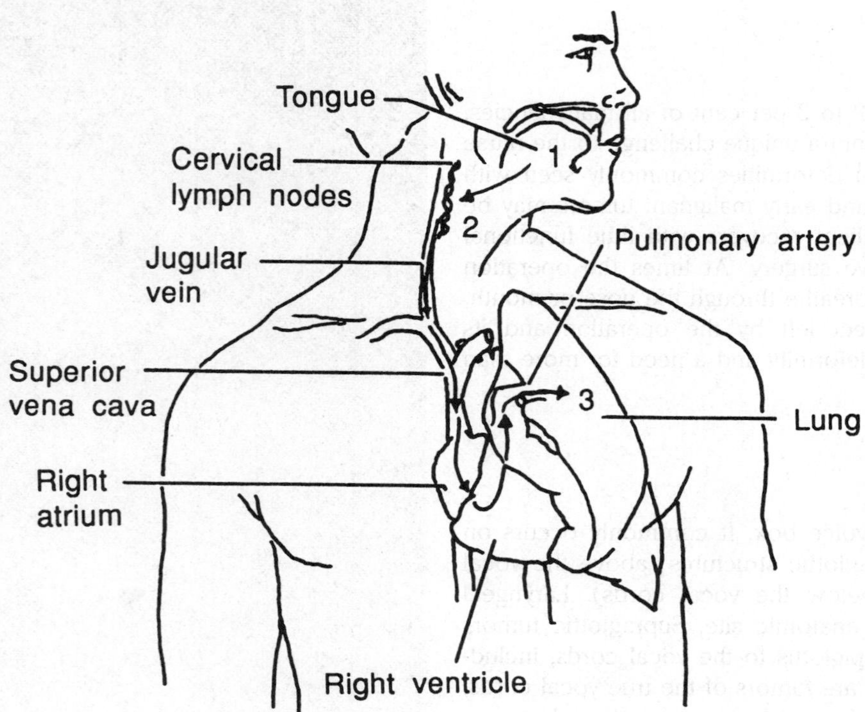

▲ **Figure 38-1**

The pattern of spread of head and neck cancer. (From Black, J. [1991]. Reconstructive surgery in the elderly. *Plastic Surgical Nursing, 11*[4], 157.)

Clinical Manifestations

The earliest symptoms of laryngeal cancer are dependent on the location of the tumor (Table 38-1). In general, hoarseness that lasts longer than 2 weeks should be evaluated. Unfortunately, most clients wait before seeking a diagnosis for chronic hoarseness.

DIAGNOSTIC ASSESSMENT

The diagnosis of laryngeal cancer is made from visual examination of the larynx with direct or indirect laryngoscopy (Fig. 38-2*A*). The nasopharynx and posterior soft palate are inspected indirectly with a small mirror or an instrument resembling a telescope. While the mirror is inserted, slight pressure is applied to the tongue, and the client is instructed to say "uh-hah," which elevates the soft palate. The instrument should not touch the tongue or the client will gag. The nasopharynx is then inspected for drainage, bleeding, ulceration, or masses.

Direct visualization of the larynx may be accomplished with use of several different instruments; most are lighted scopes. The client is instructed to protrude the tongue, and the examiner *gently* pulls the tongue forward with a gauze sponge. A laryngeal mirror or telescopic rod is inserted into the oropharynx; again, contact with the oral cavity is avoided. The client is instructed to breathe in and out rapidly through the mouth or to "pant like a puppy." Panting decreases the gagging sensation caused by the examination. During quiet respiration, the base of the tongue, epiglottis, and vocal cords are examined for signs of infection or tumor (Fig. 38-2*B*). The client is instructed to say a high-pitched *e* to approximate (close) the vocal cords. The examiner observes the movement of the cords, the color of the mucous membrane, and the presence of any lesions. If the client is unable to cooperate with this examination, it may be performed with a fiberoptic endoscope inserted through the nose.

Before any definitive treatment for tumor is initiated, a panendoscopy and biopsy should be performed to determine exact location, size, and extent of the primary tumor. Sometimes computed tomography or magnetic resonance imaging is used to assist with this process. Laboratory analysis includes a complete blood count, electrolytes, serum calcium levels, and kidney and liver function tests. These data help determine the physiologic state of the client for surgery. Because the airway will be altered after surgery, the client requires a thorough pulmonary assessment with arterial blood gas determinations for identification of any pre-existing pulmonary disorders that would interfere with breathing. Clients who will have a partial laryngectomy must have an adequate pulmonary reserve in order to produce an effective cough. The surgery places clients at increased risk of aspiration, and they must be able to cough to rid the airway of aspirated secretions. Finally, for ascertaining possible tumor spread or other primary tumors, a chest radiograph and barium swallow or esophagogram are performed.

Medical Management

Once the tumor has been located and a biopsy performed, the tumor can be staged. Staging has important implications for treatment choice and outcome. It is essential to determine the extent of the primary tumor in order to select the most appropriate intervention. Staging is accomplished by (1) measuring the size of the primary tumor, (2) determining the presence of enlarged lymphatic nodes, and (3) determining the presence of distant metastasis. Data obtained are called the TNM classification (T, tumor; N, nodes; and M, metastasis). The TNM classification system for laryngeal cancers is shown in Box 38-2. See also Chapter 21 for more information on staging.

Treatment of glottic cancer depends on the degree of tumor involvement. If the tumor is limited to the true vocal cord, without causing a limitation of the cord's movement, radiation therapy is usually the best treatment, with cure rates of 85 to 95 per cent. The dosage of radiation therapy depends on the size and location of the tumor; it is usually a minimal dose of 5500 to 6000 cGy (cGy is a more accurate term for rads) over 5 to 7 weeks. During radiation therapy, the client needs to be assessed for signs of destruction of normal tissue, ability to eat, and other side effects.

Supraglottic tumors may be treated with radiation therapy or a partial laryngectomy with or without lymph node dissection. Subglottic tumors are usually more advanced carcinomas in which the tumor has spread to surrounding tissues. Metastasis is common. Treatment requires a total laryngectomy with or without radical neck dissection on the same or both sides. The operative site may require reconstruction with pectoralis myocutaneous flaps (see Chap. 72).

PHARMACOLOGIC MANAGEMENT

Chemotherapy is generally not effective in advanced laryngeal cancer, but it may have the ability to control the development of new primary tumors through a process called chemoprevention.

DIETARY MANAGEMENT

Most clients with advanced laryngeal cancer also have malnutrition from not being able to eat, as well as from the effects of the cancer. Before surgery, the client should be fed via the nasogastric or intestinal route.

Surgical Management

The goals for surgical intervention for laryngeal cancer are to (1) remove the cancer, (2) maintain adequate physiologic function of the airway, and (3) achieve a personally acceptable physical appearance.

An option for small tumors is the use of laser to eradicate them. Laser surgery for vocal cord tumors can preserve much of the normal glottis and leave the client with a usable voice. Sometimes laser is combined

TABLE 38–1. Clinical Manifestations of Laryngeal Cancer

Area	Symptoms
Glottic Tumor 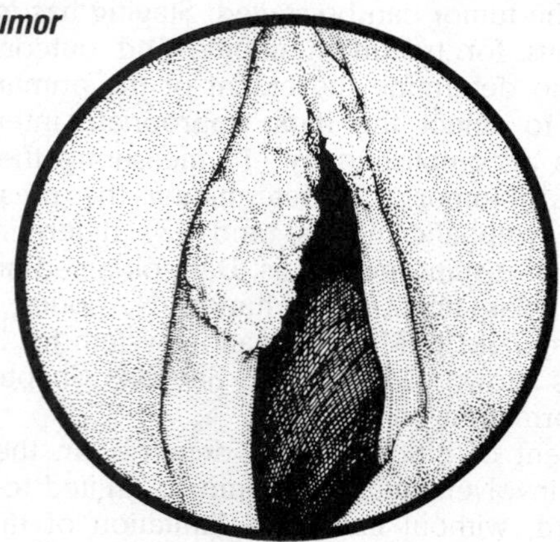 True glottic tumors interfere with normal closure and vibration of the vocal cords	*Early:* voice change hoarseness, hemoptysis *Late:* dyspnea, respiratory obstruction, dysphagia, weight loss, pain *Metastasize:* through regional lymph nodes (rare except in superior or inferior tumors)
Supraglottic Tumor 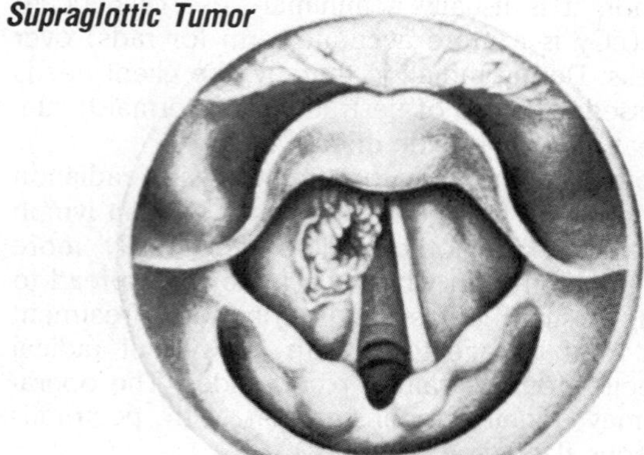 Carcinoma of false cord partially hiding true cord	*Early:* aspiration on swallowing (especially liquids), persistent unilateral sore throat, foreign body sensation, dysphagia, weight loss, neck mass, hemoptysis *Late:* dyspnea, pain in the throat or referred to the ear
Subglottic Tumor 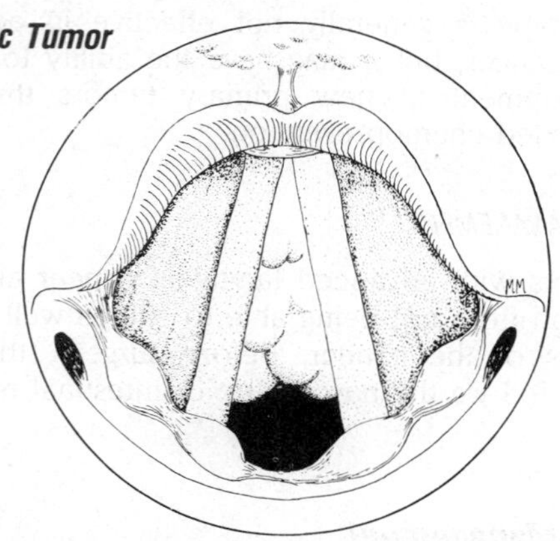 Subglottic polyp; this type of polyp can be single and smooth or lobulated as shown	*Early:* None *Late:* dyspnea, airway obstruction, dysphagia, weight loss, hemoptysis

Top and bottom figures from DeWeese, D. F., & Saunders, W. H. (1982). *Textbook of otolaryngology* (6th ed.). St. Louis: C. V. Mosby; middle figure from Del Regato, J. A., et al. (1985). *Ackerman and Del Regato's Cancer* (6th ed.). St. Louis: C. V. Mosby.

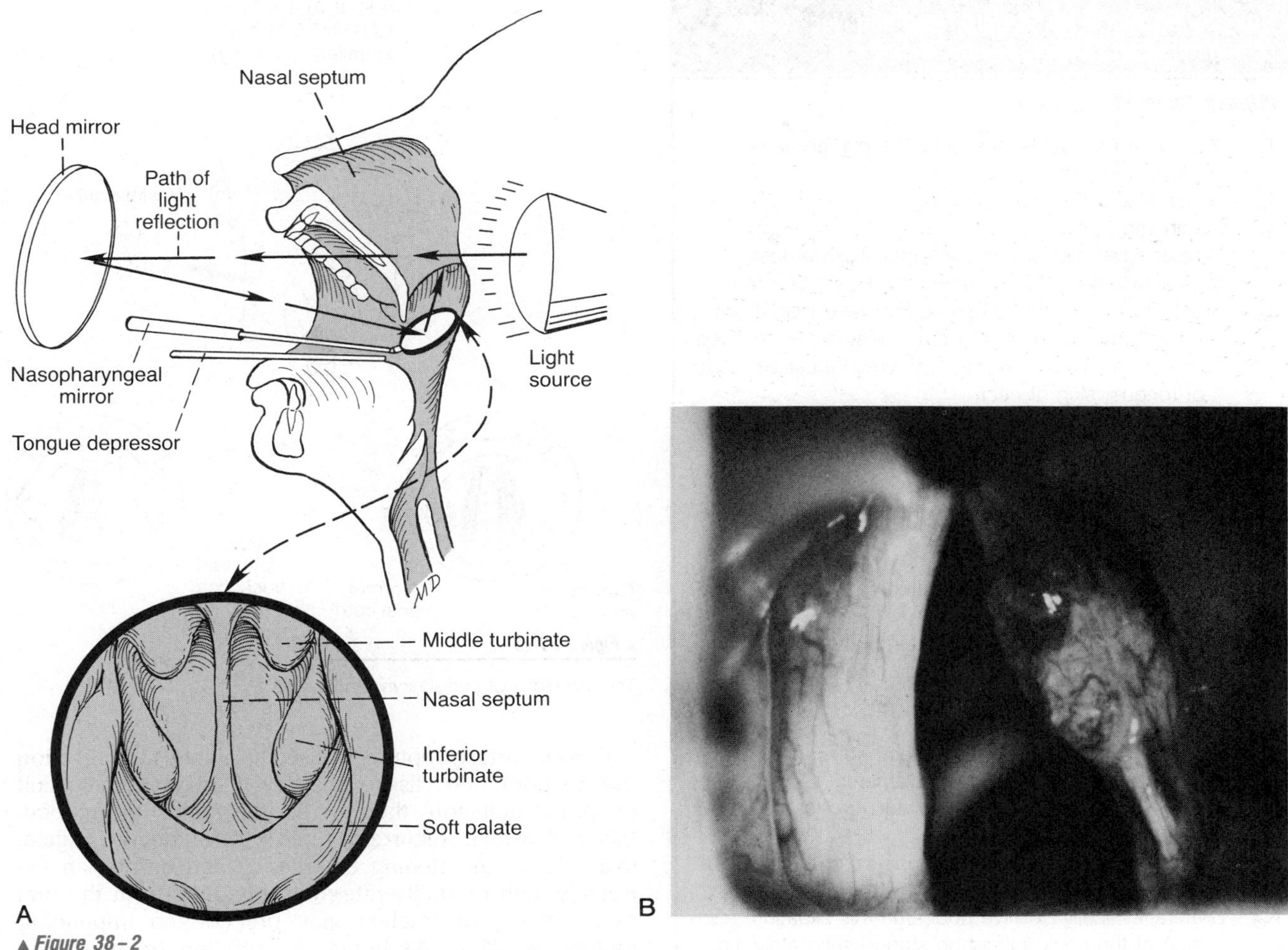

▲ *Figure 38–2*

A, Indirect laryngoscopy. Enables assessment of the pharynx and buccal cavity and some visualization of the larynx. (Laryngeal structure and function are best assessed by direct visualization, such as flexible or rigid laryngoscope or flexible fiberoptic bronchoscopy.) Indirect laryngoscopy is performed using a head mirror, tongue depressor, light source, and a small examining mirror. The mirror is positioned behind the soft palate after the tongue is depressed. To visualize the larynx, the tongue is gently grasped with a gauze sponge and pulled forward. A mirror is placed against the soft palate in front of the uvula and moved gently until the cords are visualized. The sound "eee" will cause the larynx to move. The larynx is assessed for symmetric cord motion. *B*, Squamous cancer of right vocal cord as seen during laryngoscopy.

with radiation therapy. Nursing considerations for the use of laser are in Chapter 19.

PARTIAL LARYNGECTOMY

For cancer of one true vocal cord or one true vocal cord and a portion of the other, a partial laryngectomy is feasible. This operation is also called a vertical partial laryngectomy and is the removal of half or more of the larynx (Fig. 38–3). A horizontal neck incision is made, and the diseased portion of one vocal cord is removed. Sometimes up to one third of the contralateral cord is also removed. This operation is generally well tolerated, and the client has only mild difficulty swallowing and an altered, but adequate, voice.

Another form of partial laryngectomy is the supraglottic laryngectomy. This surgery is performed for cancer of the supraglottis. The operation removes the superior portion of the larynx from the false vocal cords to the epiglottis and may extend upward to remove a portion of the base of the tongue. Lymph node dissection also may be performed. Because the true vocal cords are preserved, the voice quality is excellent. The major postoperative problem is risk of aspiration because the epiglottis, which closes over the larynx, has been removed. Airway is managed with a tracheostomy after surgery; when the edema subsides in surrounding tissues, it can usually be removed. The client will need to be taught how to swallow to avoid aspiration.

Possible complications after laryngeal surgery are airway obstruction, hemorrhage, carotid artery rupture, fistula formation, and tracheostomy stenosis.

Airway obstruction is due to edema in the surgical site, bleeding into the airway, or loss of airway from a plugged tracheostomy tube. These problems constitute an emergency and require immediate intervention for restoration of the airway. See care of the obstructed airway.

Hemorrhage is usually the result of inadequate he-

Box 38-2. Criteria for Staging Head and Neck Cancer (American Joint Committee on Cancer)

Primary Tumor (T)

T_x Minimal requirements to assess the primary tumor cannot be met
T_0 No evidence of primary tumor
T_{is} Carcinoma *in situ*
T_1 Greatest diameter of primary tumor 2 cm or less
T_2 Greatest diameter of primary tumor less than 4 cm
T_3 Greatest diameter of primary tumor more than 4 cm
T_4 Massive tumor more than 4 cm in diameter with deep invasion to involve antrum, pterygoid muscles, base of tongue, skin of neck

Nodal Involvement (N)

N_x Minimal requirements to assess the regional nodes cannot be met
N_0 No clinically positive node
N_1 Single clinically positive homolateral node 3 cm or less in diameter
N_2 Single clinically positive homolateral node more than 3 cm but less than 6 cm in diameter of multiple clinically positive homolateral nodes, none more than 6 cm in diameter
N_{2a} Single clinically positive homolateral node more than 3 cm but less than 6 cm in diameter
N_{2b} Multiple clinically positive homolateral nodes, none more than 6 cm in diameter
N_{3a} Clinically positive homolateral node(s), one more than 6 cm in diameter
N_{3b} Bilateral clinically positive nodes (in this situation, each side of the neck should be staged separately, i.e., N_{3b}: right, N_{2a}; left, N_1)
N_{3c} Contralateral clinically positive node(s) only

Tumor Metastasis (M)

M_0 No metastases present
M_1 Metastases clinically demonstrable

Stage Grouping

Stage I	$T_1N_0M_0$
Stage II	$T_2N_0M_0$
Stage III	$T_3N_0M_0$
	$T_1T_2T_3$; N_1M_0
Stage IV	T_4N_0 or N_1M_0
	Any T, N_2 or N_3, M_0
	Any T, any N, M_1

mostasis during surgery. Some blood-tinged sputum is expected in the tracheal secretions for the first 48 hours, but frank bleeding from the tracheotomy site or tube is a sign of hemorrhage and must be reported to the physician immediately. The nurse should also assess the client for other signs of bleeding such as evident hematoma or unilateral swelling, tachycardia, hypotension, and changes in respiratory patterns.

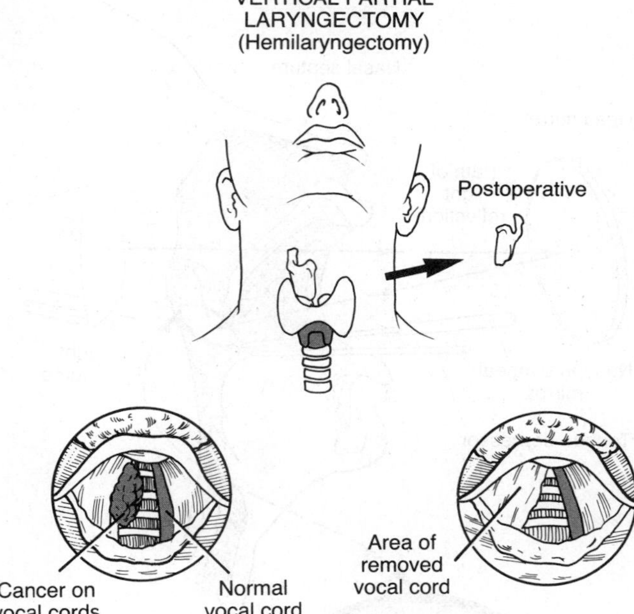

▲ **Figure 38-3**

The technique of partial laryngectomy.

Carotid artery rupture is usually a late complication due to poor neck tissue integrity. It may be the result of prior radiation therapy to the area, bronchocutaneous fistula, recurrent tumor, or infection. Again, this is a life-threatening emergency and carries an extremely high mortality rate. Mild bleeding from the oral cavity, neck, or trachea may precede an impending rupture by 24 to 48 hours. A pulsating tracheostomy tube may indicate that the tip of the tube is resting on the innominate artery and may cause injury to the artery.

A fistula is an abnormal opening between two body cavities. Fistulas between the hypopharynx and the skin are the most common. Many fistulas heal on their own, but surgery may be required, depending on the location and size.

Tracheostomy stenosis is the scarring and narrowing of the ostomy site in the neck. It usually occurs weeks or months after surgery. In some clients, it may lead to a narrowed airway and difficult breathing. The stenotic stoma may be stretched open by use of increasingly larger tracheostomy tubes.

TOTAL LARYNGECTOMY

For large glottic tumors with fixation of the vocal cords, a total laryngectomy is required. The larynx is the connection of the pharynx (upper airway) and the bronchus (lower airway). When the larynx is removed, a permanent opening is made into the trachea for breathing and the voice is lost. The esophagus remains attached to the pharynx (Fig. 38-4). Because no air can enter the nose, the client loses the sense of smell. The biggest problem for the client after laryngectomy is loss of voice. The client should be made aware that

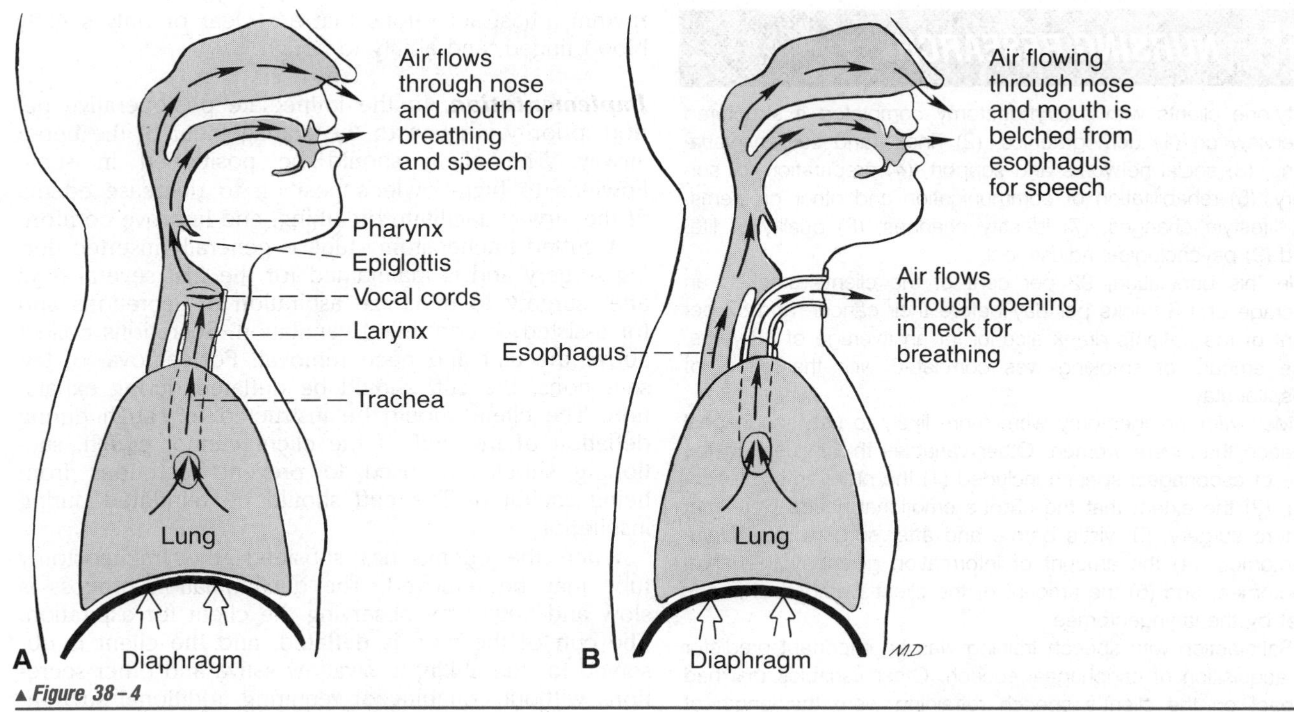

▲ *Figure 38-4*

Prior to laryngectomy, air flow is through the nose and mouth. Surgical removal of the larynx requires that a new opening be made for air passage. The trachea and esophagus are separated.

without surgery, the voice quality will worsen as the tumor spreads, but in any case the loss of voice is a serious psychological problem. Because the trachea and pharynx are permanently separated by surgery, there is no risk of aspiration, unless a fistula forms from the trachea to the esophagus. Besides this, the potential complications of the total laryngectomy are the same as for the partial laryngectomy (see earlier).

NECK DISSECTION

Metastasis to the cervical lymph nodes is common with tumors of the upper aerodigestive tract. Surgical management of laryngeal tumors often includes neck dissection. Radical neck dissection (also called en bloc) is the removal of lymphatic drainage channels and nodes, sternocleidomastoid muscle, spinal accessory nerve, jugular vein, and submandibular area. A modified radical neck dissection leaves various structures in the neck to minimize deformity.

Nursing Management

The Client Undergoing Partial Laryngectomy

ASSESSMENT

Before Surgery. In addition to usual preoperative assessments, the nurse should assess the client's nutritional status. The nurse should assess current body weight to ideal body weight, usual caloric intake, lymphocyte levels, and hemoglobin and hematocrit. The client's state of dentition and oral care should also be assessed. Because many of these clients have abused tobacco and alcohol, their dentition and oral cavity are frequently in poor repair. In addition, if the client is still an active alcoholic, plans should consider support through the period of alcohol withdrawal. The ideal plan would allow some nutritional support and oral care before surgery. Unfortunately, today few clients can be admitted before surgery and therefore this must be accomplished in an outpatient setting before the operation.

The client's work history and financial concerns should also be investigated during this initial assessment. A lack of medical insurance or money may account for the client's lack of personal and medical care.

The client's usual coping strategies and family support should also be noted. There will be some degree of disfigurement after surgery and a period of time during which the client is unable to speak. Preoperative plans should consider alternative methods of communication and family support networks. The psychosocial impact of laryngectomy is discussed in Nursing Research.

Because of the multiple problems common in these clients, a team approach to their care is used. Members of the team usually include physician/surgeon, nurses, social worker, dietician, speech/swallowing therapist, physical therapist, and home health care coordinator. If extensive surgery is required, a plastic surgeon and maxillofacial prosthodontist may also care for the client during reconstruction.

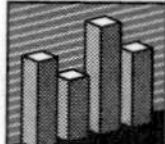

NURSING RESEARCH

Fifty-one clients with a laryngectomy completed a structured interview on (1) demographics, (2) illness and surgery variations, (3) social networks and support, (4) preparation for surgery, (5) rehabilitation of communication and other problems, (6) lifestyle changes, (7) identity changes, (8) quality of life, and (9) psychological adjustment.

In this population, 92 per cent of the clients smoked an average of 1.3 packs per day before their cancer, and 86 per cent of the patients drank alcohol for an average of 35 years. The amount of smoking was correlated with the length of hospital stay.

Men with laryngectomy were more likely to use esophageal speech than were women. Other variables that influenced the use of esophageal speech included (1) the preoperative teaching, (2) the extent that the client's emotional needs were met before surgery, (3) visits before and after surgery by a laryngectomee, (4) the amount of information given by the laryngectomee, and (5) the amount of the client's emotional needs met by the laryngectomee.

Satisfaction with speech training was an important predictor of acquisition of esophageal speech. Other variables that had impact on the client's speech retraining were the length of hospitalization and number of supports. The extent of surgery was significantly higher in the electrolarynx users and the writers and gesturers than in the clients who learned esophageal speech. Those clients who learned esophageal speech and used writing or gesturing to communicate were more satisified with their training than were the clients who used the electrolarynx.

Quality of life was most affected by a visit from a previous laryngectomee and having needs met before surgery. Adjustment as a whole was higher if the client received preoperative counseling, stayed in the hospital as brief a time as possible, and was satisfied with social supports.

▼▼▼

Stam, H., Koopmans, J., & Mathieson, C. (1991). The psychosocial impact of laryngectomy: a comprehensive assessment. *Journal of Psychosocial Oncology, 9* (3), 37–57.

After Surgery. In addition to the routine assessments of any postoperative client, after a partial laryngectomy the client needs to have careful assessment of the airway, lung sounds, position of the tracheostomy tube, and potential complications of the surgery (see earlier).

NURSING INTERVENTION

Nursing Diagnosis: Aspiration, High Risk for R/T loss of normal reflexes and excessive secretions secondary to surgery.

Planning: Expected Outcomes. The client will not aspirate, as evidenced by clear breath sounds throughout the chest, normal (for age) respiratory rate and rhythm, chest secretions that are clear or only slightly blood tinged, and ability to cough.

Implementation. In the immediate postoperative period, priority is given to the management of the upper airway. The client should be positioned in semi-Fowler's to high-Fowler's position to decrease edema of the airway, facilitate breathing, and improve comfort.

A cuffed tracheostomy tube is generally inserted during surgery and is maintained for the first several days after surgery to minimize aspiration of secretions and for assisted or controlled ventilation. Secretions collect above the cuff and need removal. For removal of the secretions, the cuff should be deflated during exhalation. The client should be instructed to cough during deflation of the cuff. If the client cannot cough, suctioning should be used to prevent secretions from being aspirated. The cuff should be reinflated during inspiration.

When the edema has subsided, the tracheostomy tube may be removed. The decannulation process is slow and begins by observing the client for aspiration. The cuff of the tube is deflated, and the client is observed for the ability to swallow saliva and other secretions without coughing or requiring additional suctioning. If there are increased secretions through and around the tracheostomy tube, aspiration is occurring and the cuff should be reinflated. If no aspiration is occurring, the tracheostomy tube can be replaced with a smaller uncuffed tube (Fig. 38–5). If this is tolerated without aspiration, the tube is capped to determine the

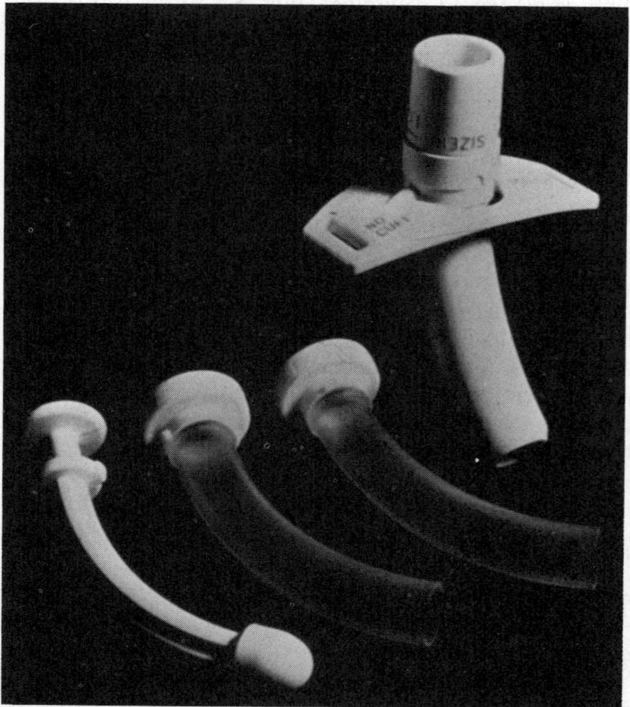

▲ **Figure 38–5**

Parts of an uncuffed tracheostomy tube (L-R obturator, two inner cannula, outer cannula).

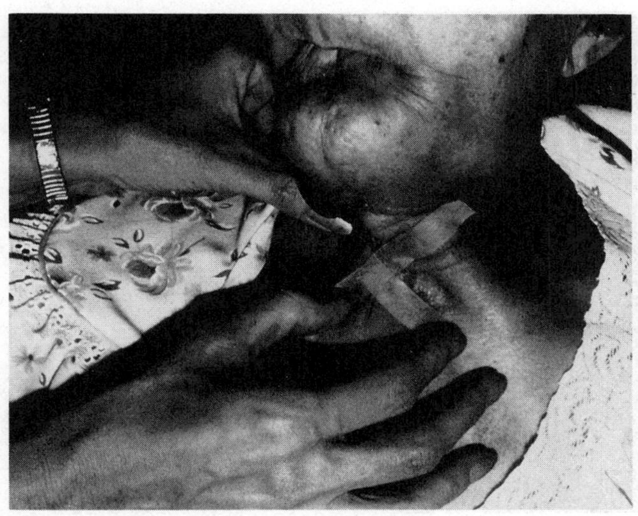

▲ Figure 38-6

Closing stoma after decannulation. The skin is cleansed with hydrogen peroxide and protected with tincture of benzoin. The skin edges are pulled together and taped in an X. An occlusive dressing is applied.

client's ability to breathe through the upper airway. If the client can breathe through the upper airway for 24 hours, the tracheostomy tube is removed, and the stoma is taped closed and covered with an occlusive dressing (Fig. 38-6).

Nursing Diagnosis: Airway Clearance, Ineffective R/T physical alteration in airway and presence of tracheostomy tube.

Planning: Expected Outcomes. The client will have improved airway clearance, as evidenced by effortless, quiet respirations at baseline rate and clear breath sounds.

Implementation. The client may have copious secretions because of the presence of the tracheostomy tube, history of chronic obstructive lung disease, and aspiration. There may also be oral secretions that cannot be swallowed. In the alert and conscious client, coughing and deep breathing will mobilize and eliminate many of these secretions. However, in the client having head and neck surgery and just emerging from anesthesia, this may not be possible. Suctioning of the trachea will be needed for the first 24 to 48 hours after surgery. The frequency of suctioning depends on the client's needs, but suctioning every hour is common for the first 24 hours. Sterile technique must be used to avoid introducing microorganisms into the tracheobronchial tree in a client with impaired immune defenses due to malignancy and surgery. (Suctioning techniques can be found in a fundamentals of nursing textbook.)

A tracheostomy tube with an inner cannula is commonly used in these clients. Mucous collects in the inner cannula, which can be removed and cleaned without removing the entire tube. The inner cannula should be cleaned as often as necessary to provide a clear airway for the client. In the immediate postoperative phase, the inner cannula is cleaned after suctioning. Once the client is ambulatory and handles secretions safely, it can be cleaned as necessary but at least three times a day.

To remove and clean the inner cannula, the nurse puts on gloves and removes the inner cannula from the tracheostomy tube. The neckplate of the outer cannula should be held in place to avoid moving it while the inner cannula is removed. Disposable inner cannulas are available; the inner cannula is disposed of, and a new one is inserted. If the inner cannula needs to be cleaned, it is placed in hydrogen peroxide to loosen the secretions. Then a small brush is used to remove the accumulated secretions, and the cannula is rinsed with water or saline. The clean inner cannula can be reinserted and anchored (Fig. 38-7).

Chest physiotherapy, ultrasonic nebulization, or aerosol administration of medications in addition to ambulation, coughing, and deep breathing is recommended to prevent pulmonary complications. These treatments are performed every 4 hours for the first few days after surgery and then usually decreased to four times a day once the client can ambulate.

Collaborative Problem. High Risk for Acute Airway Distress R/T accidental decannulation.

Planning: Expected Outcomes. The nurse will monitor for a patent airway, as evidenced by clear breath sounds; quiet, effortless respirations; and a patent, intact cannula.

Implementation. Tracheostomy tube displacement or accidental decannulation may result in acute airway distress. To prevent this emergency, many surgeons are

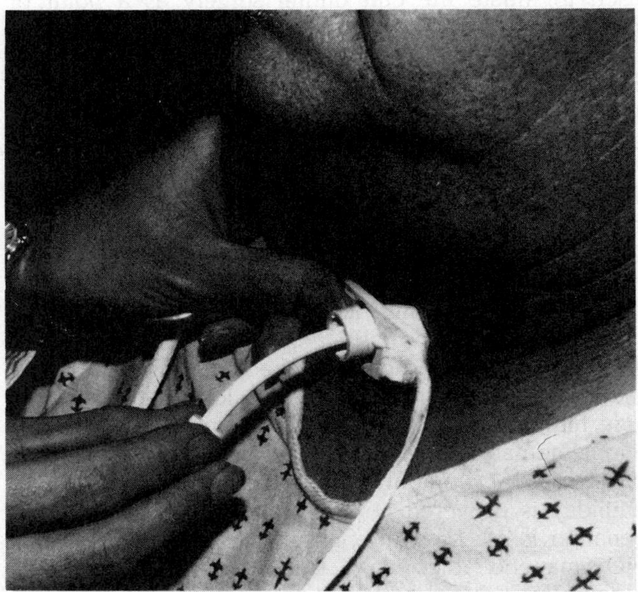

▲ Figure 38-7

Reinserting a cleaned inner cannula.

attaching long sutures (called stay sutures) from the tracheal wall to the client's chest. If the tube is accidentally removed, the sutures can be loosened on the chest and pulled upward and outward to open the stoma for tube reinsertion. If stay sutures are not used and the tracheostomy tube is displaced or removed, a tracheal dilator and an emergency tracheostomy tray must be available for reinsertion of the tube. After approximately 72 hours, a tract will form between the skin and trachea, and the tube can be reinserted with little difficulty (Fig. 38-8).

Collaborative Problem. High Risk for Tracheal Necrosis and Stenosis.

Planning: Expected Outcomes. The risk of tracheal necrosis or stenosis will be reduced, as evidenced by use of a high-volume, low-pressure tracheostomy cuff, routine deflation of the cuff, and avoidance of the minimal leak technique to reinflate the cuff.

Implementation. A high-volume low-pressure cuff should be used to prevent excess pressure on the tracheal mucosa. Excessive pressure can result in tracheal ischemia with eventual necrosis and stenosis. Although low-pressure cuffs are used, cuffs should be deflated every shift to improve circulation to the cuff site and remove accumulated secretions. Only a minimal amount of air should be used to reinflate the cuff to prevent overinflation and excess pressure. The minimal occlusion volume technique should be used to seal the space between the tracheal wall and the cuff. The minimal leak technique should not be used; it is not effective in clients who have had head and neck surgery because of edema of the airway. (These techniques are discussed in Chapter 37.) To assist with the minimal occlusion technique, the nurse should ascertain and document on the medical record the amount of air used to inflate the cuff during surgery as a point of reference.

Nursing Diagnosis: Infection, High Risk for (Respiratory) R/T loss of normal filtration systems in the mouth and nose with use of an artificial airway.

Planning: Expected Outcomes. The client will not develop clinical manifestations of a respiratory infection, as evidenced by afebrile state, clear or slightly blood-tinged secretions, white blood cell count remaining within normal limits, and clear lung sounds.

Implementation. Once a tracheostomy is performed, the nose and upper airway are no longer able to provide filtration, warming, and moistening of inspired air. Supplemental humidification and airway protection will be required. Commonly, 40 per cent oxygen with high humidity is delivered at 4 to 6 liters per minute. Oxygenation is assessed through arterial blood gases, and FIO_2 may be adjusted. If the client has pre-existent chronic lung disease, oxygen may have to be delivered at lower percentages or not at all. Compressed air with high humidity may be substituted for these clients. Humidified oxygen or compressed air is administered through a tracheostomy mask or universal adaptor to a cuffed tracheostomy tube. The supplemental humidification is usually given for the first 48 hours and then on a supplemental basis.

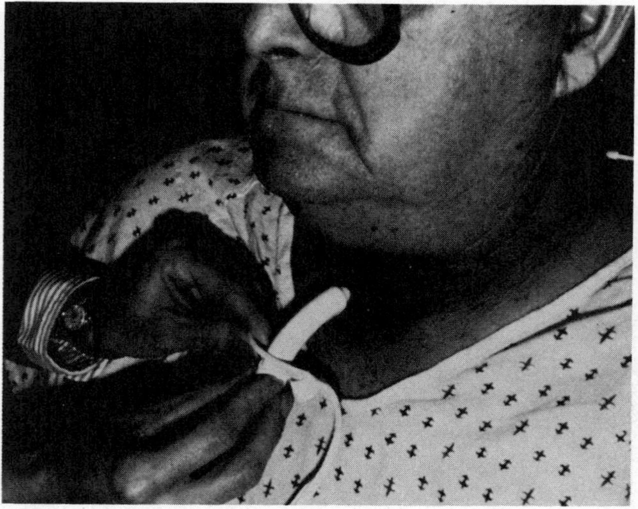

▲ *Figure 38-8*

Insertion of laryngectomy tube into permanent tracheostoma. The obturator or guide is inserted into the outer cannula. After the tube is lubricated with water-soluble ointment, the client is instructed to take a deep breath, and the lubricated tube is inserted. The obturator is removed, and the tube is tied in place.

Nursing Diagnosis: Nutrition, Altered: Less than Body Requirements R/T malignancy and swallowing difficulties.

Planning: Expected Outcomes. The client will have an improved nutritional status, as evidenced by maintaining baseline body weight or losing less than 5 pounds; consuming adequate fluid, protein, fat, and carbohydrate each 24 hours; swallowing without aspirating or choking; hemoglobin, hematocrit, and lymphocyte count remaining within normal limits.

Implementation. Immediately after surgery, it is likely the client will have a nasogastric tube for removal of gastric secretions until postoperative ileus subsides. The nurse should assess for bowel sounds, passing of flatus, and hunger as signs of returning gastrointestinal function. Some clients will be tube fed with commercial supplements. The nurse must continually ascertain the correct presence of the tube before each feeding. (Techniques to check tube placement can be found in a fundamentals of nursing textbook.) The tube feeding can be administered by pump, slow drip, or bolus feeding depending on the client's tolerance. Aspiration remains a high risk with partial laryngectomy, and precautions to guard the client from it are critical.

Because the epiglottis has been removed, when to begin oral feeding after a partial laryngectomy is controversial. One approach is to begin oral feedings with the tracheostomy tube in place, when edema has subsided and the client is able to swallow secretions. The advantage of this technique is that aspirated liquid can be suctioned. A second technique is to delay oral feeding until the client has been decannulated and the stoma has healed. The advantage of this technique is that with a closed stoma, the client will be able to increase intrathoracic pressure and remove any aspirated material through an effective cough.

Whenever the client eats, eating should begin with a nonpourable pureed diet; liquids are reserved until swallowing has been relearned. One technique for swallowing is presented in the Client Education Guide. Once swallowing can be accomplished without aspiration, carbonated beverages may be added. Thin liquids should be held until the risk of aspiration is minimal.

Nursing Diagnosis: Infection (Wound), High Risk for R/T loss of primary defenses (incision) and malignancy.

Planning: Expected Outcomes. The client will develop no clinical manifestations of wound infection, as evidenced by incisional edges remaining approximated; amounts of wound drainage decreasing; absence of redness, swelling, tenderness, or warmth beyond the suture lines; remaining afebrile; and white blood cell count remaining within normal limits.

Implementation. During surgery, a wound drain is placed into the surrounding tissues of the neck and attached to constant suction. A common mechanism for collecting the drainage is a Hemovac container, which is attached to the client's gown to prevent accidental dislodgement. Using universal precautions, the amount and color of the drainage should be assessed by the nurse every 4 hours for the first 24 hours. The wound should be assessed for signs of hematoma or seroma formation by noting whether the amount of drainage is increasing or there is change in the color or consistency of the drainage. The color of the incision lines should also be assessed. If the drainage is subsiding, the drain may be removed by the physician. Dressings are placed over the drain puncture sites on the skin. Small to moderate amounts of serosanguineous drainage should be expected for another 48 to 72 hours.

The suture lines should be cleansed at least twice daily with hydrogen peroxide followed by water or saline rinse. A thin film of antibiotic ointment may be applied to the suture line to prevent crusting of secretions and promote healing.

EVALUATION

The degree of goal attainment is evaluated, and revisions are made in the interventions as needed to meet the revised goals. Depending on the client's preoperative condition (e.g., malnourished), additional time may be required to meet the various goals.

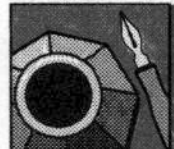

CLIENT EDUCATION GUIDE

Swallowing Technique After a Partial Laryngectomy

1. Have the client begin with soft or semisolid foods.
2. Stay with the client during meals until the technique of swallowing is mastered without choking.
3. Offer encouragement; learning to reswallow is frustrating.
4. Guide the client in the following steps:
   a. Take a deep breath.
   b. Bear down to close the vocal cords.
   c. Place food into your mouth.
   d. Swallow.
   e. Cough to rid the closed cord of accumulated food particles.
   f. Swallow.
   g. Cough.
   h. Breathe.

The Client Undergoing Total Laryngectomy

The nursing management of the client after a total laryngectomy is the same as the care given a client with a partial laryngectomy except for feeding and teaching about the permanent stoma care. Clients who have a total laryngectomy will have a permanent tracheostomy and need to learn how to speak using alternative methods.

Immediately after surgery, the client's nutrition is supplemented with nasogastric feedings. When the client exhibits signs of swallowing his or her own secretions, the edema has subsided and feeding can begin. The diet usually begins with soft or semisoft foods and progresses as healing occurs.

Communication. For the first few days after surgery, the client should communicate by writing. If the client is very fatigued, common client requests such as "I need something for pain" may be written on a pad of paper, and the client can just point to the statement. Even though the client cannot speak, conversation should still include the client's input through nodding and pointing and not be directed only to others such as the family. Avoiding conversation with the client because of the difficulty in communication is demeaning and leads to client frustration.

An artificial larynx may be used as early as 3 to 4 days after surgery. These electronic devices are held alongside the neck, or a plastic tube is inserted in the mouth; vibration produces mechanical speech (Fig. 38-9). The air inside the mouth is vibrated, and the client articulates as usual. The speech quality is monotone and artificial, but it is better than no speech at all.

Esophageal speech is a technique that requires the client to swallow and hold air in the upper esophagus. By controlling the flow of air, the client can pronounce as many as 6 to 10 words before stopping to reswallow air. The voice is deep but it is loud and entirely effective once the technique is mastered.

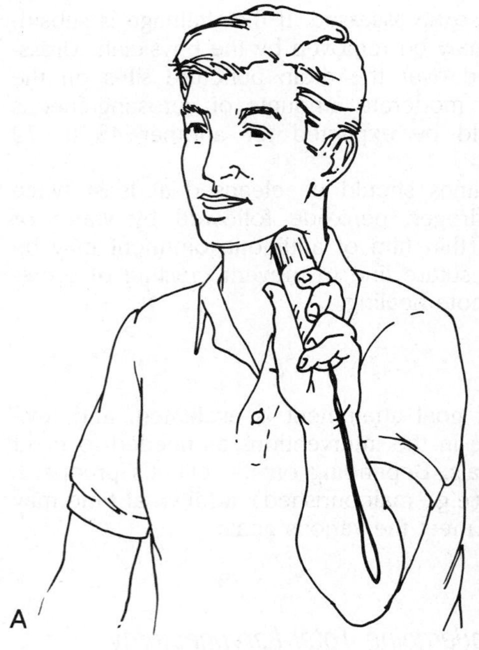

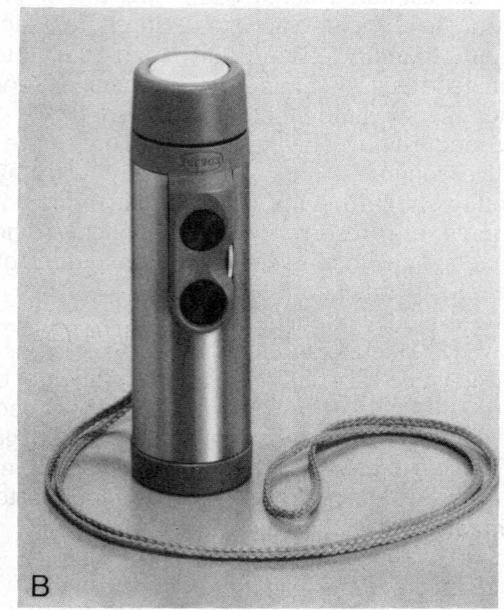

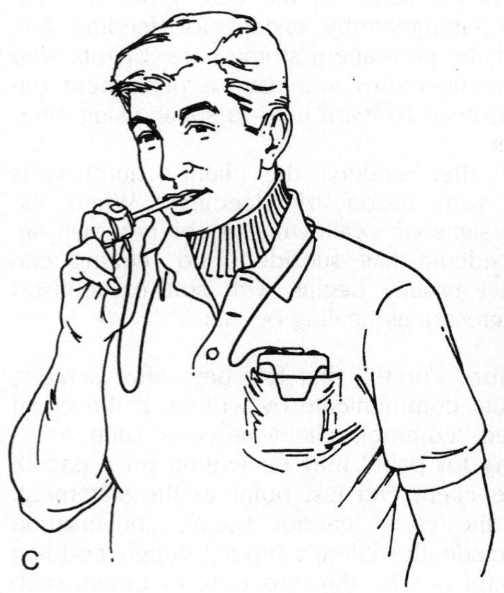

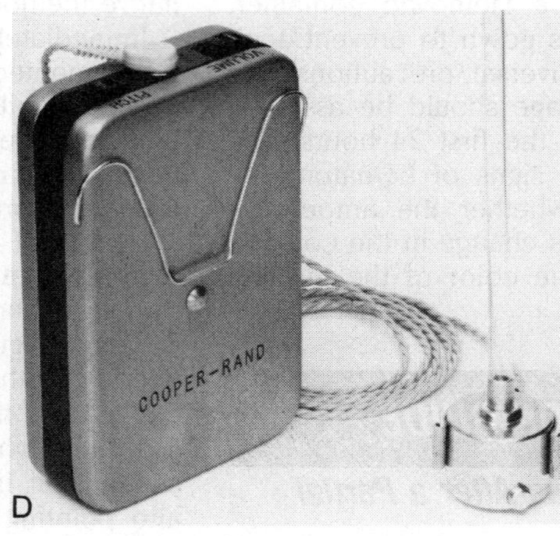

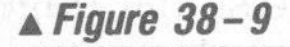

▲ **Figure 38–9**

A and *B*, Artificial larynx (electrolarynx). This handheld, battery-powered speech aid is placed against the neck. *A*, When activated, it creates a vibration that is transmitted to the neck and into the mouth. Words silently formed by the mouth become sounds from the vibrations emitted by the device. Any type of artificial larynx requires muscle and tongue control and hand strength. It normally is not used until immediate postoperative neck tenderness has subsided. (*B*, Courtesy of Servox Electrolarynx Mfg. by Siemens Hearing Instruments, Inc., Union, NJ.) *C* and *D*. Electronic speech aid (Cooper Rand). Allows the person to adjust tone, pitch, and volume. An oral connector permits speech without the necessity for placing the device against the neck. This is an advantage immediately after surgery, when the neck is too sensitive for a neck-vibrating device. (*D*, Courtesy of Luminaud, Inc., Mentor, OH.)

Tracheoesophageal puncture is a surgical technique that may also restore speech. A small puncture is made into the upper tracheostoma to the cervical esophagus for creation of a fistula. Once the fistula is healed, a small one-way valve in inserted, called a voice button or trapdoor prosthesis. By occlusion of the valve, air can be shunted into the esophagus, producing speech. These devices require maintenance; therefore, only clients who are highly motivated, are able to perform self-care, and have good manual dexterity are eligible for this procedure.

The techniques to restore speech require much time for mastery; the client is seen by a speech therapist after dismissal from the hospital (Fig. 38–10). There are community support groups for clients after laryngectomy, called the Lost Cord Club and International Association of Laryngectomees, that may offer needed reassurance.

Much patience is required by the client and family while the client is relearning to speak. The process is time-consuming and frustrating and requires more time to speak. The family should be encouraged to give the client enough time to formulate the words and not speak for the client.

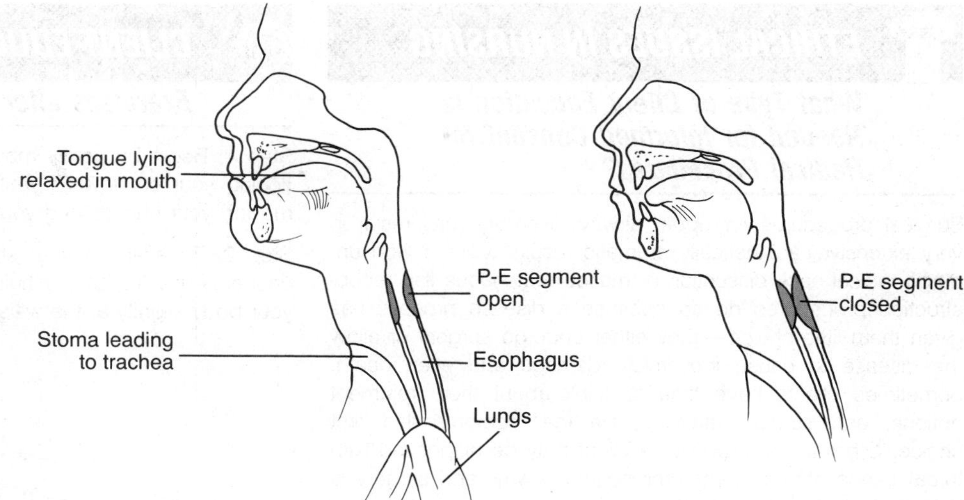

▲ *Figure 38-10*

Tracheoesophageal puncture for voice rehabilitation after laryngectomy. A prosthesis is inserted into a created fistula in the neck. The prosthesis has a one-way valve that permits air to pass into the esophagus but prevents accidental aspiration. To speak, the client occludes the prosthesis with a finger or attachment. Exhaled air is then shunted through the prosthesis, where it vibrates, and exits the mouth as spoken word.

The Client Undergoing Neck Dissection

ASSESSMENT

Before surgery, the client's understanding of the plans for surgery should be assessed. The nurse should determine what the surgeon has told the client and how much information has been retained or lost because of anxiety. In addition, the fears the client has about the diagnosis of cancer and fears of deformity after surgery should be addressed (Ethical Issues in Nursing). The nurse can explain to the client and family what to expect after surgery (e.g., placement in the intensive care unit, tracheostomy, drainage tubes) and review postoperative care (e.g., communication technique if a tracheostomy will be placed).

The client's support systems and degree of coping should be assessed. If the client is an alcoholic, the use of alcohol may be the usual coping tool. Because alcohol will not be available, the nurse should assess the other coping mechanisms available to the client and encourage the client to motivate them. Sources include friends, family, and insurance and other finances. If new support systems are needed, these should be identified as soon as possible, such as use of other clients who have had the same surgery or diagnosis.

After surgery, the usual postoperative assessments are performed with special attention given to the airway. Airway patency can be lost as a result of edema of the neck or bleeding within the area. If the surgical defect was repaired with musculocutaneous flaps, the flap should be assessed for arterial inflow and venous outflow. The temperature, color, and blanching should be noted every hour for the first 24 hours and every 4 hours after that time.

NURSING INTERVENTION

Collaborative Problem: Airway obstruction, High Risk for R/T to edema or bleeding.

Planning: Expected Outcomes. The client will have no airway distress, as evidenced by normal breathing patterns, no cyanosis or pallor, no stridor, and no hematoma formation.

Implementation. Assess the client for signs of airway edema or bleeding. Auscultate lung sounds every 2 hours for the first 24 hours. Report signs of airway obstruction immediately.

Place the client in a semi-Fowler's position to minimize postoperative edema. Neck drainage catheters, inserted into the surgical wound, are monitored for amount of drainage. The drains should be aspirated under strict aseptic technique by use of a blunt-tipped needle at least every 4 hours to maintain patency of the drains and allow drainage of blood or serum from the wound. Sanguineous or serosanguineous drainage is expected for the first 72 hours after surgery. Once drainage has stopped, the catheters are removed.

Pressure dressings may be used in the immediate postoperative period, depending on physician preference. If a dressing is used, it should be reinforced as needed and observed for any drainage. If musculocutaneous flaps are needed for coverage, pressure dressings will not be used, and special flap care will be required. (See Chap. 72 for specific care of flaps.)

Nursing Diagnosis: Physical Mobility, Impaired R/T shoulder dysfunction.

Planning: Expected Outcomes. The client will retain usual shoulder function, as evidenced by full (or previously normal) range of motion in shoulder and maintenance of shoulder strength.

Implementation. Most clients will report only minimal pain in the surgical site due to the disruption of the sensory nerve fibers from the incisions used. If an en bloc radical neck dissection has been performed, clients will experience shoulder dysfunction resulting in

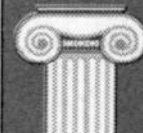

ETHICAL ISSUES IN NURSING

What Type of Client Education Is Needed for Informed Consent to Radical Procedures?

Surgical procedures for upper airway disorders may result in very extensive, aesthetically dramatic results. Clients who undergo radical neck dissection or musculocutaneous flap reconstruction procedures do so because a disease process has given them little choice—they either undergo surgery or allow the disease to cause irreversible damage and even death. Sometimes clients have time to think about their treatment options, and surgery may not be the recommended first choice. Other times, however, a client may be diagnosed with throat cancer that is compromising the airway, and surgery is indicated as soon as possible.

The question here is not what treatment is best for the client, but rather what information is given to and processed by the client in order that he or she might make an informed consent to such a radical procedure. Clients who are candidates for radical neck procedures are most likely aware of the severity of their condition. The physician explains the diagnosis, treatment options, and treatment recommendations. Again, there are times when surgery, however radical, may be the only treatment option (unless the client opts for no treatment). Do clients really understand how their body image will change after such a procedure? Can they really understand that they may never speak in the normal way that they have spoken their whole life (as with a total laryngectomy)? Do they understand that without treatment, they may not speak either? Is there anything that can help them understand all the psychosocial implications of a radical neck procedure? Finally, is their consent to such procedures really informed if they do not have an understanding of these issues?

Client education is of paramount importance to these clients. Nurses who work in a surgical setting in which these kinds of clients are seen have a large responsibility in helping their clients understand the possible results of such radical procedures. Our current society places great importance on the physical components of our body, in particular the face, and clients need to understand the physical changes that will take place as a result of surgery. Nurses can help their clients work through their feelings by offering supportive services such as social work, support groups, or psychiatric counseling. If possible, all of these aspects should be explored before surgery. Only through such teaching efforts in which nurses play a vital role can clients truly make informed decisions regarding life-altering surgery.

a forward rotation and dropping of the shoulder. Sectioning of the spinal accessory nerve during neck dissection will also interrupt the innervation to the upper trapezius muscle.

Exercises to increase range of motion and muscle strength, shown in the Client Education Guide, are encouraged to prevent a frozen shoulder and restore full movement. If a selective or modified neck dissection has been performed, minimal change will occur.

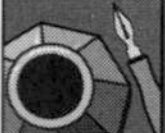

CLIENT EDUCATION GUIDE

Exercises after Radical Neck Surgery

Step 1: Begin by gently moving your head from side to side, tipping your ear toward your shoulder on the same side and moving your chin toward your chest.

Step 2: To exercise your shoulders using the hand on your unoperated side, lean or hold onto a low table or chair. Bend your body slightly at the waist and:

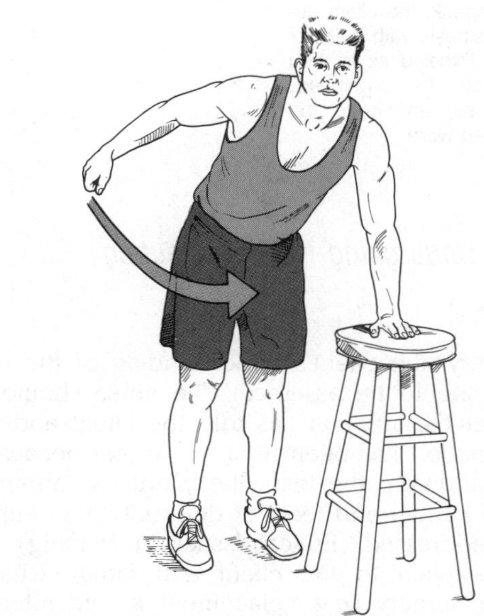

a. Swing shoulder and arm from left to right.

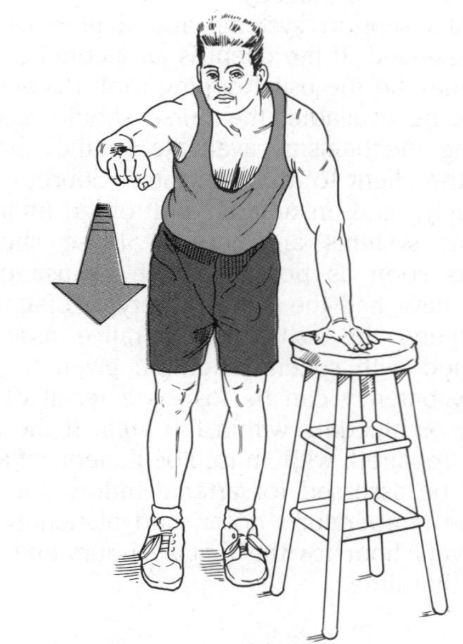

b. Swing shoulder and arm from front to back.

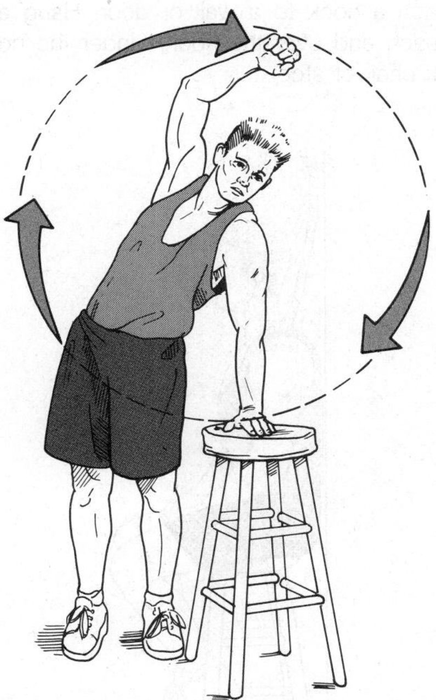

c. Swing shoulder and arm in a wide circle, gradually bringing your arm all the way over your head.

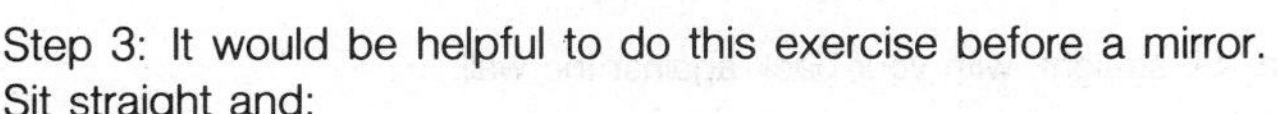

Step 3: It would be helpful to do this exercise before a mirror. Sit straight and:

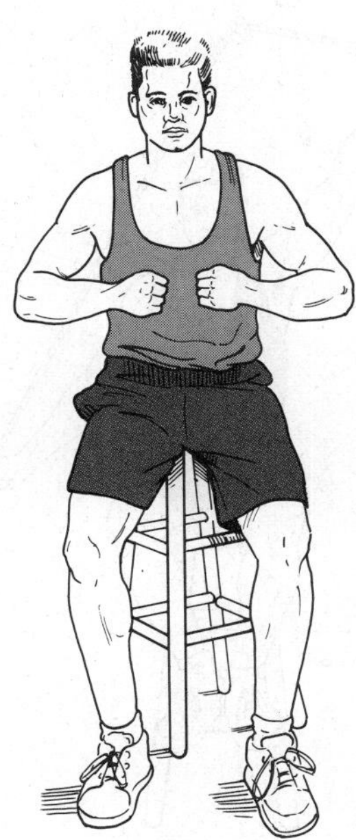

a. Place hands in front of you with your elbows at right angles, sticking out from your body.

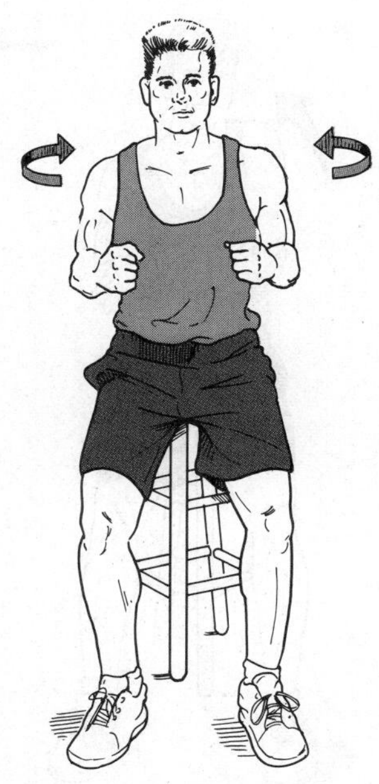

b. Rotate your shoulders back, bringing elbows to your side.

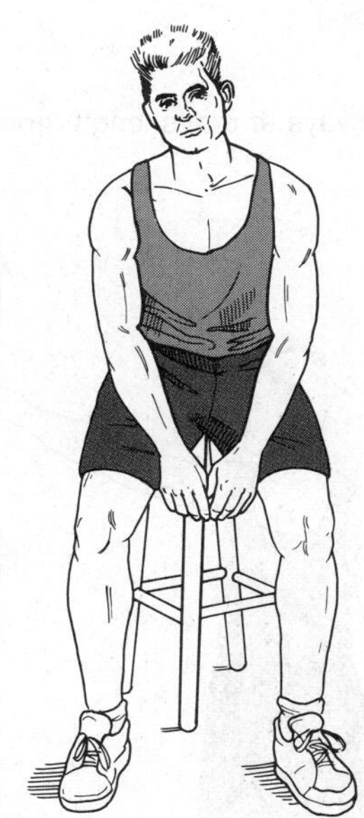

c. Relax your whole body.

Client Education Guide continued on following page

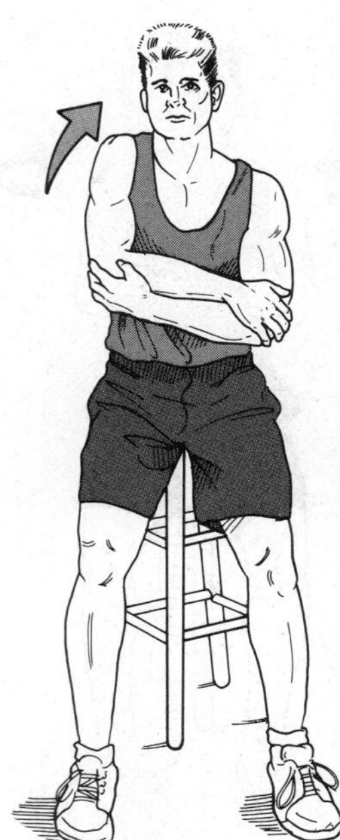

d. With arms crossed in front of you, support the elbow on the operated side with your opposite hand, and help lift the arm and shoulder while shrugging.

Step 4: Stand sideways at arm's length from the wall.

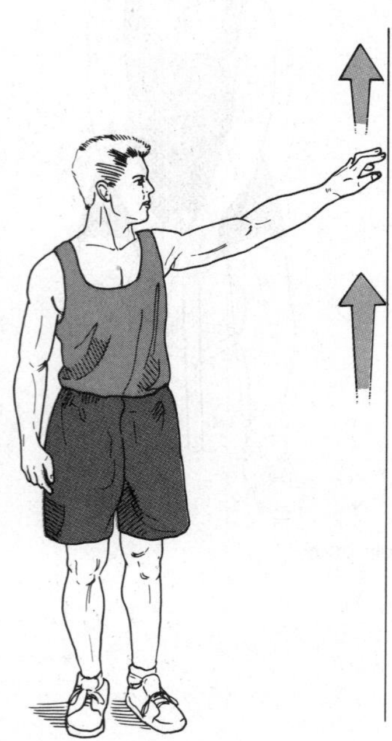

a. Walk your fingers slowly up the wall.

b. As your fingers climb up, begin to move your body closer to the wall.

c. Continue until your arm is high above your head and shoulder.

Step 5: Attach a hook to a wall or door. Hang a short rope knotted at each end over the hook. Under the hook, place a straight-back chair or stool.

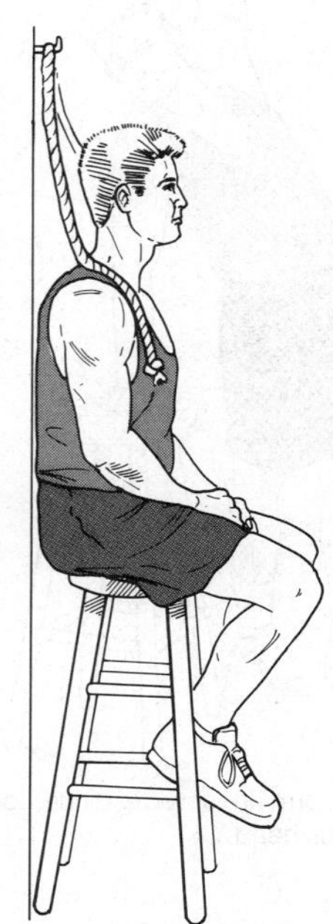

a. Sit straight, with your back against the wall.

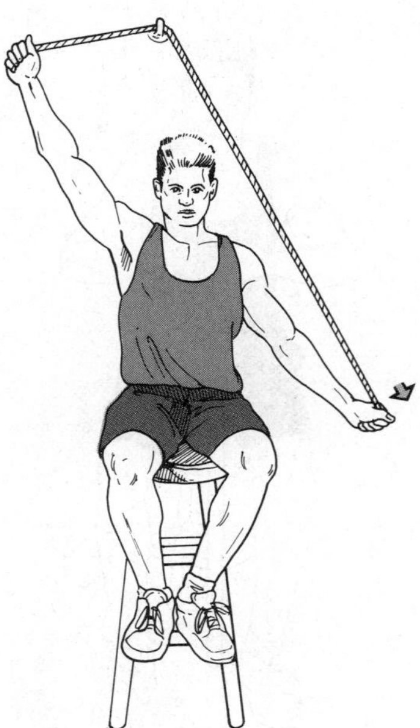

b. Pull one arm and shoulder up with the rope by bringing the other arm and shoulder down. Repeat with the other arm. It is important in this exercise not to bend your body. Keep the motion in the shoulder.

Post-hospital Care

The Client Undergoing Partial Laryngectomy

After dismissal from the hospital, therapy may be needed for swallowing and sometimes for speech. If the client needs to continue wound care until full healing occurs, instructions should be given in writing. Ongoing assessment for potential malignancy will be required.

The Client Undergoing Total Laryngectomy

Discharge Teaching. Clients should be dismissed with an extra tracheostomy tube to allow daily changes at home. To provide humidified air, normal saline may be instilled into the stoma several times each day to stimulate coughing, moisten the mucosa, and loosen dried secretions and crusts. A bedside humidifier or vaporizer will also aid in humidifying the inspired air. So that foreign bodies are prevented from entering the stoma, a stoma bib or covering should be worn. These coverings can be purchased, or the client may improvise by using a scarf, necktie, or turtleneck shirt.

The client should be encouraged to continue speech therapy as begun in the hospital (see Bridge to Home Health Care).

Once the incision has completely healed, the tracheostomy tube will not be required (Fig. 38-11). This process varies but usually takes about 6 to 8 weeks. Occasionally, the tube will be required at night, if the stoma is small or the client does not get adequate air exchange during sleep. Once the tracheostomy has been removed, the client will be able to disguise the stoma with clothing and begin to regain a sense of normalcy.

Tub baths or showers are permitted, but the client must use caution to prevent introduction of water into the stoma. Commercial stoma shower covers are available, and the water spray should be aimed at midchest. Water sports are prohibited. If the client fishes, a life preserver will need to be worn at all times on the boat.

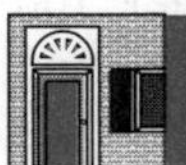

BRIDGE TO HOME HEALTH CARE

The Laryngectomy Client

Trouble shooting problems is vital in bridging from hospital to home care of the laryngectomy client. When learning esophageal speech, the client may experience indigestion from excessive air intake. Decreased appetite may result from air in the digestive tract. The client should be encouraged to speak slowly and practice correct technique. The client may also experience an inability to maintain adequate air intake due to mucous buildup in the tracheostomy and stoma site. Routine cleaning of the tracheostomy helps eliminate this problem.

Remember that the client will not be able to eat and talk at the same time. Follow the communication techniques learned to converse with any communicatively impaired client.

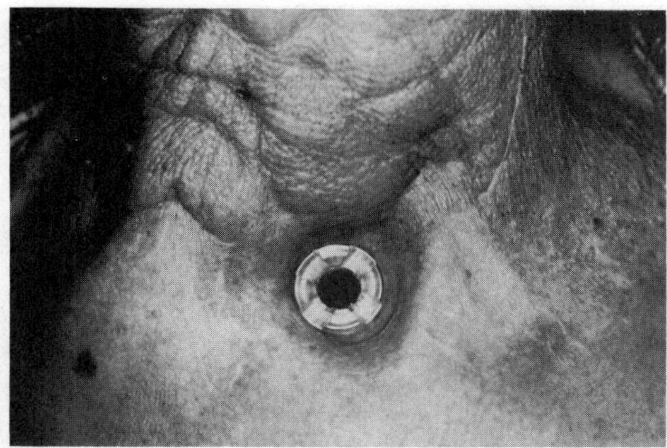

▲ *Figure 38-11*

Healed tracheostomy incision.

The client should wear a Medic Alert bracelet to identify the fact that resuscitation cannot be performed through the mouth. The client will need mouth-to-stoma rescue breathing (Fig. 38-12).

The client may require a nutritional plan for the first few weeks at home. The dietician should work with the client and family to determine the consistency of food easiest to swallow as well as the kinds of foods required to obtain needed protein and calories.

It is essential that the client not smoke so that lung function is preserved and the formation of other aerodigestive tract tumors is prevented. For some clients after laryngectomy, the process of smoking cessation seems pointless. Some clients continue to smoke by inhaling the cigarette smoke through the stoma. The attitude is one of "Why quit now? What else could happen to me?" The nurse should use extra support and encouragement with the client, remembering to be an advocate of the client's choice as well as providing assurance that the quality of life after smoking cessation improves.

Follow-up Care. Follow-up care is important to assess the healing process, evaluate coping mechanisms, and examine the client for possible metastasis or new tumors. The client should be taught to report any of these signs or symptoms to the physician:

- a lump anywhere in the neck or body
- persistent cough, sore throat, or earache
- hemoptysis
- sores around the stoma or within the trachea that do not heal
- difficulty swallowing or breathing

The Client Undergoing Neck Dissection

Clients should be cautioned about potential injury to the neck tissue because of lack of sensation. The use of a heating pad or exposure to temperature extremes may result in tissue injury (burns, frostbite) in a client who cannot feel these temperatures. Clients with tra-

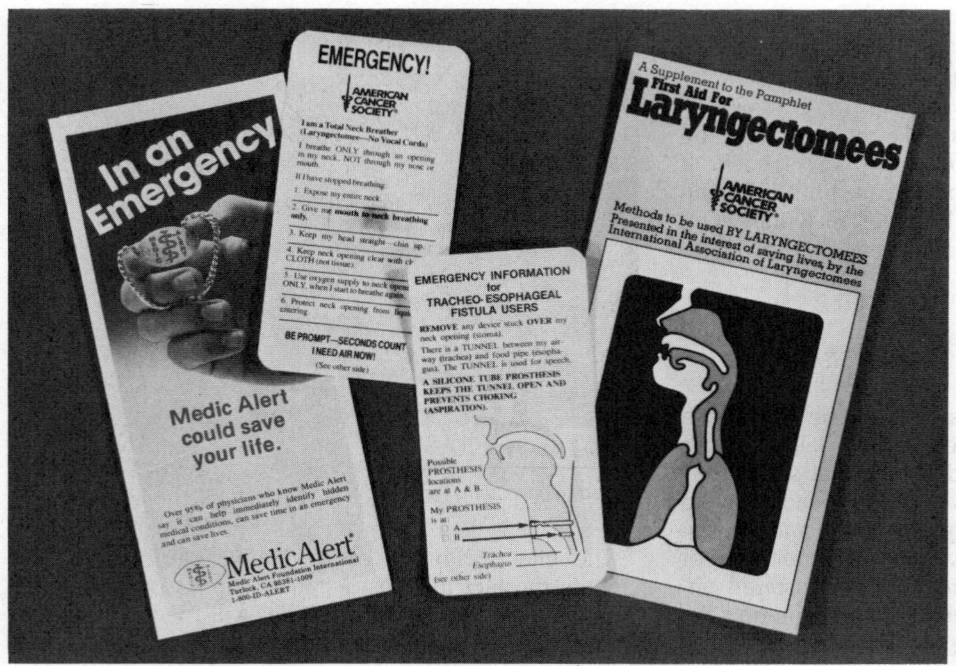

▲ **Figure 38–12**

This emergency wallet card is available from the American Cancer Society. It provides vital information to a rescuer who finds a person with a laryngectomy in either respiratory or cardiac arrest. People who have had a total laryngectomy, and breathe only through a stoma in the neck, cannot be ventilated by mouth-to-mouth or mouth-to-nose ventilation. Mouth-to-stoma artificial ventilation is necessary.

cheostomy will need specific instructions for its management. Ongoing malignancy care should be explained.

BENIGN TUMORS OF THE LARYNX

Papillomas are one type of benign tumor of the larynx. They are small wartlike growths believed to be viral in origin. Papillomas may be removed by surgical excision or laser. Surgery must be exact, because the nondiseased portion of the vocal cords needs to be retained for function. Other types of benign tumors of the larynx include nodules and polyps. Nodules and polyps frequently occur in singers and cheerleaders who project their voice.

▼ OBSTRUCTIONS OF UPPER AIRWAY

▼ Acute Airway Obstruction

ACUTE LARYNGEAL EDEMA

This may be associated with inflammation, injury, or anaphylaxis. It is manifested by hoarseness and dramatic shortness of breath. Dyspnea progresses rapidly, and unless a patent airway is established, respiratory arrest occurs. Endotracheal intubation may be very difficult because the larynx is edematous and is likely to bleed. Emergency tracheostomy may be required. If anaphylaxis is the precipitating cause, subcutaneous epinephrine, 1 : 1000, is given. Intravenous corticosteroids are also used.

CHRONIC LARYNGEAL EDEMA

This may occur when lymph drainage is obstructed owing to infection or tumor. If the edema is significant, an artificial airway may be required (either a tracheostomy or an endotracheal tube). The choice of route depends on the severity of edema.

LARYNGOSPASM

This is a spasm of laryngeal muscles. This may occur (1) after administration of some general anesthetic agents, (2) after repeated and traumatic attempts at endotracheal intubation, (3) as a response to some inhaled agents and foreign material, such as industrial fumes and dusts, and chemicals, and (4) hypocalcemia.

Management is directed at reestablishing the airway as quickly and efficiently as possible. Administer 100 per cent oxygen until the airway is fully reestablished and the larynx relaxes and stops spasming. Titrate FIO_2 according to pulse oximetry values. If the laryngospasm persists, paralysis with neuromuscular blocking agents, such as succinylcholine, may be required to allow intubation until the spasm breaks. Manual or mechanical ventilation is then necessary until the effects of the paralyzing agent have worn off. Occasionally, emergency cricothyroidotomy or tracheotomy may be necessary, and should not be delayed.

LARYNGEAL PARALYSIS

Laryngeal paralysis is usually due to surgery on the neck, peripheral disorders, and occasionally, to CNS disorders. One of the most common causes of laryngeal paralysis is trauma to the recurrent laryngeal nerve during thyroidectomy. Among the peripheral causes of laryngeal paralysis are aortic aneurysm; mitral stenosis; thoracic surgery; thyroid gland carcinoma; neck injuries; tuberculosis; tumors of the bronchi, lungs, and mediastinum; metallic poisons (e.g., lead); and infection (e.g., diphtheria). CNS disorders that may lead to laryngeal paralysis include cerebrovascular accident (CVA, or stroke) and myasthenia gravis. Complete laryngeal paralysis is rare.

Unilateral or bilateral vocal cord paralysis may occur. If one vocal cord is affected, the airway is usually not impaired and the primary symptom is hoarseness. When both vocal cords are affected (1) the voice is weak (though adequate); (2) the airway is compromised; and (3) dyspnea, intercostal muscle retraction, and stridor occur when the person is active. If the paralyzed cords are bilaterally adducted, an emergency tracheotomy may be required. Surgery, such as *arytenoidectomy*, in which one or both arytenoid cartilages are removed and the vocal cords are held in an open position, may be used to open the glottis.

LARYNGEAL INJURY

Laryngeal injury most often results form trauma during a motor vehicle accident, such as when the driver's neck strikes the steering wheel. Other causes include the inhalation of hot gases or aspiration of caustic liquids. If complete airway obstruction does not occur, carefully assess for post-traumatic edema, which may lead to complete obstruction. Few outward signs may be present. It is often easy to overlook potential problems in the neck structures while focusing on other, possibly more dramatic injuries. Observe for increased dyspnea, intercostal muscle retraction, stridor, inability to speak, and change in respiration patterns.

The thyroid cartilage may be fractured. This problem leads to soft tissue and laryngeal edema as well as hematoma. If airway obstruction occurs, tracheostomy may be necessary. Indications of a fractured thyroid cartilage include (1) tender, swollen ecchymotic neck; (2) stridor; (3) possible cyanosis; and (4) possible subcutaneous emphysema.

Damage to the larynx above the cricoid cartilage may lead to tracheal stenosis. The cricoid cartilage forms the only complete circle of cartilage in the upper airway, and it maintains the open lumen of the upper end of the airway.

▼ Chronic Airway Obstruction

NASAL POLYPS

Nasal polyps are outpouchings of mucous membrane lining the nose or paranasal sinuses. Polyps are most commonly seen in clients with severe allergies and may be single or multiple. Most clients seek medical attention for obstruction to nasal breathing.

The medical management for clients with nasal polyps is symptomatic. Attempts are made to decrease the size of the polyps by eliminating or treating the causative factor (i.e., allergy). In many clients, surgery is needed to remove nasal polyps in order to restore nasal breathing before allergy treatment. Nasal polypectomy (removal of nasal polyps) can be done in the physician's office or in the operating room. Nasal polypectomy is usually performed with use of a local anesthetic. The anesthetic (commonly lidocaine with epinephrine) is sufficient to eliminate discomfort while also producing vasoconstriction to minimize bleeding during the procedure. A snarelike instrument is used to remove the polyps. The bleeding sites are cauterized, and intranasal packing is inserted. In some instances, intranasal splints will be used to prevent formation of adhesions. The nasal packing is maintained for several hours to minimize the possibility of postoperative bleeding and is generally removed before client discharge.

Because of the presence of nasal packing and edema, clients will breathe through the mouth for the first 24 to 48 hours. The use of humidification, frequent mouth care, and increasing oral fluids will help to minimize the dryness and oropharyngeal discomfort. The nurse should frequently inspect the oral cavity to evaluate the effectiveness of these measures. Clients with polyps frequently also have asthma. Asthmatic symptoms may be exacerbated after surgery.

The client is placed in a semi- to high-Fowler's position after surgery to minimize edema. In addition, continuous ice compresses are recommended for the first 48 hours to decrease edema and control bleeding. With the proper application of nasal packing at the time of surgery and the use of ice compresses in the immediate postoperative period, nasal bleeding should be minimal. However, the client should be assessed for changes in vital signs and the oropharynx inspected for the presence of blood. Because the nasal packing absorbs anterior bleeding, it is essential to observe the client for posterior nasal bleeding. If active posterior bleeding occurs, the client will swallow frequently and blood will be present in the throat.

Most clients have only minimal discomfort after a nasal polypectomy. Mild analgesics may be used for any postoperative discomfort. The use of aspirin and aspirin-containing products should be avoided because of the anticoagulant effects in these medications. In addition, some clients have nasal polyps, asthma, and aspirin allergy. This syndrome is called triad disease. The client may not be aware of the aspirin allergy. The client should be taught not to try to clean the nose or sneeze. If the client needs to sneeze, the client should sneeze through an open mouth.

DEVIATED NASAL SEPTUM AND NASAL FRACTURE

The nasal septum, the dividing structure of the nose, is usually straight and divides the nose into two equal chambers. After trauma, the septum may become deviated, creating asymmetric breathing passages (Fig. 38-13). For some clients, the deviation may cause an obstruction to nasal breathing, dryness of the nasal mucosa causing bleeding, and occasionally a cosmetic deformity.

If a nasal fracture occurs, immediate medical management is advised. Within several hours of nasal injury, severe edema may occur, which causes difficulty in reducing the fracture. Immediately after the injury, ice should be applied. A simple nasal fracture may be reduced in an emergency facility with use of local anesthesia. If immediate reduction of the nasal fracture is not possible, it is advisable to wait several days until edema subsides but before healing begins.

Surgical management of a client for correction of a deviated nasal septum, reconstruction of a cosmetic deformity of the nose, or reduction of a nasal fracture is similar. All three procedures are usually performed under local anesthesia with use of mild sedation in conjunction with the anesthesia. Because of the vasoconstrictor properties of local anesthetics, they appear to decrease the bleeding during and immediately after surgery. Surgery to correct a deviated nasal septum is known as a nasal septoplasty and consists of making an incision on either side of the septum, elevating the mucous membrane, and straightening or removing the offending portion of the cartilage. If a cosmetic deformity is also of concern or if the deformity interferes with septal reconstruction, a rhinoplasty (reconstruction of the external nose) may be done in conjunction with the nasal septoplasty or as a separate procedure. (See also Chap. 72.)

After these three procedures, intranasal packing and internal splints may be used to maintain the position of the septum as well as to control bleeding and prevent hematoma formation. If the patient has had rhinoplasty or reduction of a nasal fracture, an external splint and a small dressing may also be applied. Some clients may return directly to the nursing unit after surgery because of the local anesthesia, whereas others may be observed in the recovery area until the effects of intraoperative medications are minimized. Areas of concern for the nurse regardless of the location of recovery include airway management, edema, hemorrhage, and pain control. Because of the presence of bilateral nasal packing, after nasal septoplasty, rhinoplasty, and nasal fracture reduction, clients will require the same care as that for the patient after nasal polypectomy.

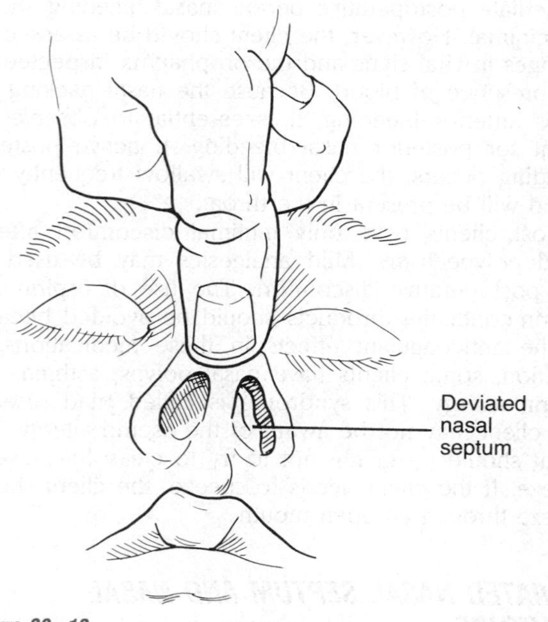

▲ *Figure 38-13*

Deviated nasal septum, as viewed when tip of nose is pushed back. Dislocation of the columellar end of the septal cartilage has occurred, causing deflection of that portion of cartilage into left nostril. Note obstruction of nasal airway on that side.

▼ HEMORRHAGIC, INFECTIOUS, AND INFLAMMATORY CONDITIONS

EPISTAXIS

Epistaxis (nosebleed) may result from irritation, trauma, infection, or tumors. In addition, epistaxis may also be the result of systemic disease (such as atherosclerosis, hypertension, blood dyscrasias) or systemic treatment (such as chemotherapy or anticoagulants).

The initial treatment of epistaxis is application of pressure by pinching the anterior portion of the nose for a minimum of 5 to 10 minutes. This is often successful because most common epistaxis occurs in the anterior part of the septum. In addition, the application of ice compresses to produce vasoconstriction may also decrease bleeding. If these initial measures do not stop bleeding, nasal packing may be necessary. Once the location of the bleeding vessel is located, cauterization of the bleeding vessel with silver nitrate is attempted, and nasal packing may be inserted. For a client with anterior nasal bleeding, anterior nasal packing may be all that is required. Antibacterial ointment such as bacitracin or Neosporin is applied to half-inch gauze and gently, but firmly, inserted into the anterior nasal cavities to apply pressure to the bleeding vessels. Petrolatum gauze packing should be avoided because it has no antimicrobial properties, and a malodorous discharge may develop within 1 to 2 days with its use. Nasal packing should remain in place for a minimum of 48 to 72 hours.[14]

Posterior Plugs. For those clients with posterior epistaxis, a posterior plug may be necessary in addition to the anterior nasal packing (Fig. 38-14). Insertion of a posterior plug is very uncomfortable for clients, and a mild analgesic may be required to reduce anxiety and discomfort. A small, red rubber catheter is passed through the nose into the oropharynx and mouth. A gauze pack is tied to the catheter, and the catheter is withdrawn; this moves the pack into proper placement in the nasopharynx and posterior nose to apply pressure. The nasal cavity is packed with half-inch gauze, and the strings from the posterior pack are tied around a rolled gauze or bolus for maintaining its position. The

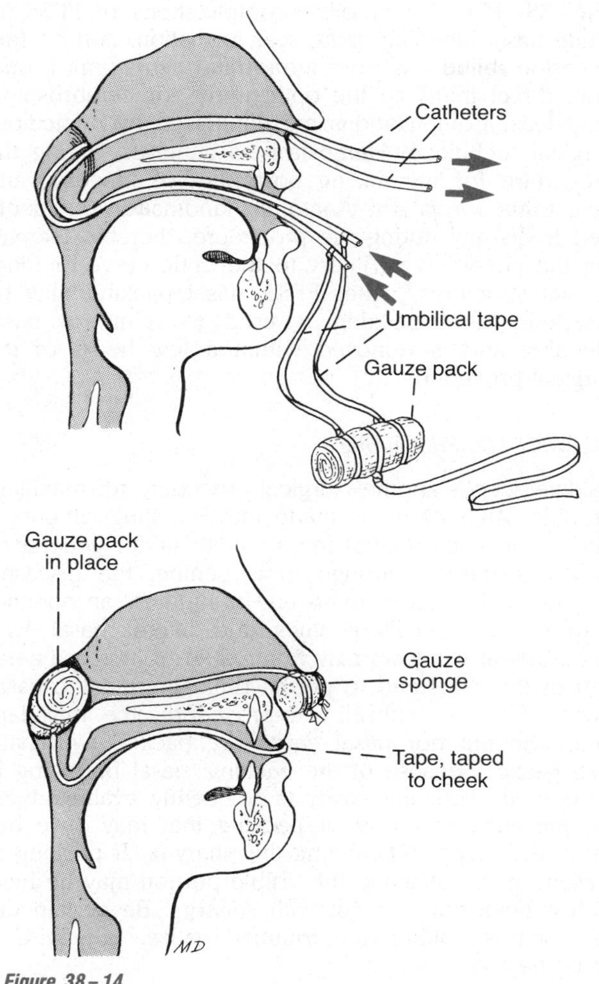

▲ *Figure 38–14*

Instillation of posterior nasal pack (plug) (typically used in emergency). (See text.)

ties from the oral cavity are taped to the client's face in order to prevent loosening or dislodgement of the plug. Clients with posterior plug and anterior nasal packing are admitted to the hospital. Clients with nasal packing and posterior plugs are monitored closely for hypoxia. General comfort measures, such as humidification, the use of a drip pad to collect bloody drainage and mucus, and the use of water-soluble ointment around the nares to provide lubrication will alleviate some discomfort. The client should be monitored closely for any signs of bleeding from the anterior or posterior nares. The nurse must inspect the oral cavity for the presence of blood and proper placement of the posterior plug. If the posterior plug is visible, the nurse should notify the physician for readjustment of the packing. Posterior nasal packs remain in place for 5 days.[14] Prophylatic antibiotics are employed to prevent toxic shock syndrome and sinusitis.

Arterial Ligation. If medical measures are not sufficient to eliminate epistaxis, surgical interventions may be necessary. Internal maxillary or ethmoid artery ligations may be required to control nasal bleeding. An incision is made in the gumline above the incisor on the affected side, and the maxillary sinus is entered. The artery that supplies the area of bleeding is identified, and a metal clip or suture is used to ligate the artery. Clients will have nasal packing inserted for a minimum of 24 hours, during which time they must be observed for additional bleeding, hyper- or hypotension, and infection. Upon discharge, the client is instructed to minimize activity for approximately 10 days. This is most frequently accomplished by avoiding strenuous exercise; not blowing the nose; sneezing with the mouth open; and no lifting, stooping, or straining. The use of water-soluble ointment at the entrance of the nose and around the nares may provide comfort, and mouth rinses of half-strength hydrogen peroxide mixed with water or saline should be provided for oral hygiene. The use of a humidifier or vaporizer will add supplemental moisture to prevent dryness and crusting of secretions.

SINUSITIS

Definition and Incidence

Sinusitis is an infection of one of the paranasal sinuses. Pansinusitis is infection of more than one sinus. It is a common medical condition that affects an estimated 35 million people a year.[24]

Pathophysiology

The sinuses are protected against infection by mucociliary action. The normal mucus produced by the sinuses is removed through small openings into the nose called ostia. When the ciliary action is impaired or the ostia are obstructed, mucus can accumulate in the sinus and become infected.

Clinical Manifestations

Sinusitis is considered by evaluation of the client's symptoms and confirmed by x-ray study. Generalized symptoms of fever and chills with local symptoms of pain in the sinuses exacerbated with bending, pain or numbness in the upper teeth, and a purulent or discolored nasal discharge may be present.

DIAGNOSTIC ASSESSMENT

Sinus radiographs or computed tomography may show opacification of the sinus, thickened mucous membranes, and an air-fluid level, all indicative of sinusitis.

Medical Management

The medical management of sinusitis includes use of the appropriate antibiotic to manage the bacterial infection; decongestants to reduce edema; steroid nasal sprays to reduce mucosal inflammation; and humidification by way of normal saline solution irrigations or a vaporizer/humidifier to prevent nasal crusting and to moisten secretions.

Antral Irrigation. Antral irrigation or sinus lavage may be performed in clients who are not responding to treatment or who have increased purulent exudate in the maxillary sinus. Antral irrigation is performed with the use of a local anesthetic. A trocar is inserted through the ostium in the lateral wall of the nose into the sinus. The client should be prepared for the procedure with thorough explanations of the anesthetic, the sensation of the trocar passing through the ostium, and feelings of pressure. Normal saline solution is then injected through the cannula to rinse the sinus of purulent exudate. The client is placed in a sitting position, leaning slightly forward with the mouth open to allow drainage of the irrigating solution through the nose and mouth. A culture of the exudate may be made to determine the causative organism in order to prescribe an appropriate antibiotic.

Surgical Management

FUNCTIONAL ENDOSCOPIC SINUS SURGERY

If nonoperative measures fail, functional endoscopic sinus surgery (FESS) may be necessary. The major objective of FESS is the reestablishment of sinus ventilation and mucociliary clearance.[7] Small sinus endoscopes are passed through the nasal cavity and into the sinuses to allow direct visualization of the sinuses in order to remove diseased tissue and enlarge sinus ostia (Fig. 38-15). The possible complications of FESS include nasal bleeding, pain, scar formation, and on rare occasion, blindness from intraorbital hematoma formation, direct injury to the optic nerve, or cerebrospinal fluid leak. Complications are minimized by meticulous surgical technique. Hemostasis is achieved during the procedure for minimizing postoperative bleeding and hematoma formation. Anatomic landmarks are identified frequently during the procedure, thereby decreasing the possibility of injury to the optic nerve or intracranial structures.[7] After FESS, nasal packing may be inserted. Nasal packing is used to minimize nasal bleeding and is removed within a few hours of the surgical procedure.

CALDWELL-LUC PROCEDURE

Caldwell-Luc is another surgical procedure for maxillary sinusitis. An incision is made into the gingival buccal sulcus above the lateral incisor teeth under general or local anesthesia. Through this opening, the diseased mucous membrane is removed. In addition, an opening between the maxillary sinus and lateral nasal wall (nasal antral window) may be created to increase aeration of the sinus and to permit drainage into the nasal cavity. After a Caldwell-Luc procedure, the maxillary sinus and anterior nasal cavity are packed with half-inch gauze. Because of the packing, nasal breathing is obstructed. The oral cavity is frequently evaluated for the presence of blood or packing that may have become dislodged, obstructing the pharynx. If packing is present in the pharynx, the visible portion may be held with a hemostat and cut with scissors. Be certain the hemostat is holding the trimmed gauze, otherwise it could be aspirated.

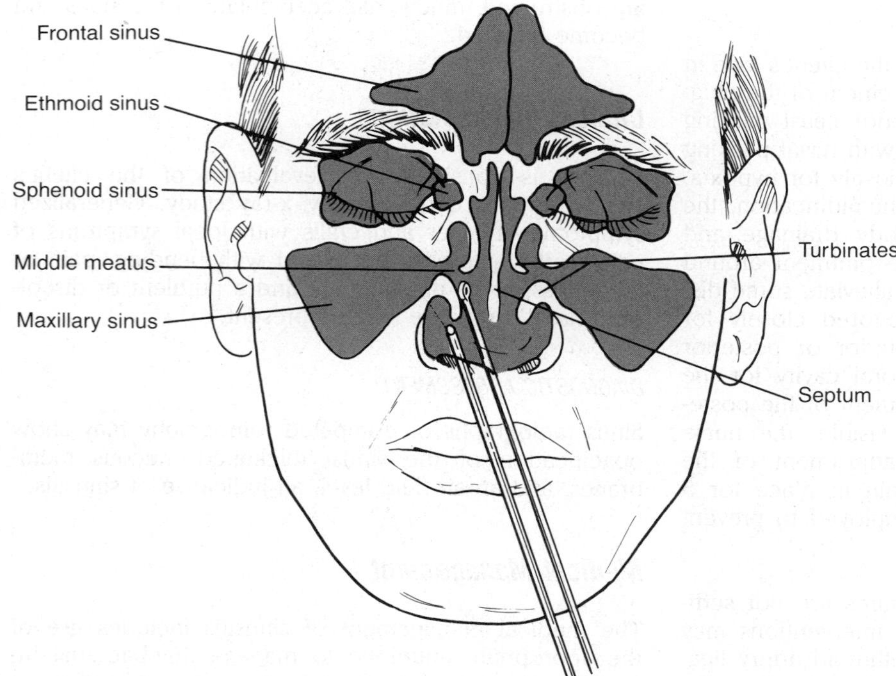

▲ **Figure 38-15**

Functional endoscopic surgery. The middle meatus is the site where most of the sinuses drain and if plugged obstructs drainage. With an endoscope the sinuses can be seen and obstructions removed.

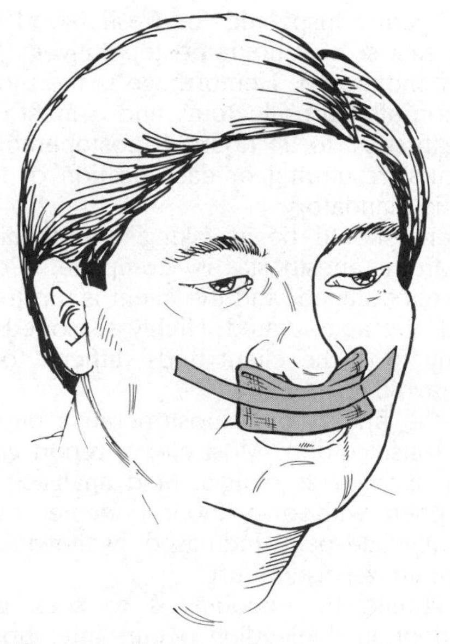

▲ *Figure 38–16*

A nasal drip pad is taped beneath the nares to absorb drainage after nasal or sinus surgery. The usual technique is to fold 3 × 3 dressings into thirds and tape in place. These dressings can be changed at the nurse's discretion.

EXTERNAL SPHENOETHMOIDECTOMY

External sphenoethmoidectomy is a surgical procedure to remove diseased mucosa from the sphenoid or ethmoid sinuses. A small incision is made over the ethmoid sinus on the lateral nasal bridge, and the diseased mucosa is removed. The client will have nasal and ethmoid packing inserted. In addition to the instructions given after a Caldwell-Luc operation (see later), an eye pressure patch is usually applied to decrease periorbital edema.

Nursing Management

Following sinus surgery, the client is observed for an increase in bleeding, respiratory distress, and edema for the first 24 hours after surgery. Ice compresses are applied to the nose and cheek to minimize edema and control bleeding. The client is placed in a semi- to high-Fowler's position for 24 to 48 hours after surgery to minimize postoperative edema. The nasal packing is generally removed the morning after surgery; however, antral packing remains in place for 36 to 72 hours. Mild analgesics should be given to the patient to minimize discomfort after surgery and before removal of the packing.

After a Caldwell-Luc procedure, the client receives the same instructions as after FESS. Postoperative sequelae include numbness of the upper teeth due to interruption of sensory nerves from the mucosal incision. This sensation may remain for several weeks.

DISCHARGE TEACHING

Clients are instructed to increase fluids to moisten secretions. Although there may be some pain, a mild analgesic is all that is required. Minimal nasal bleeding is expected for 24 to 48 hours after surgery. A "drip pad" under the nose may eliminate the need to be constantly wiping the nose (Fig. 38–16). Clients are instructed to avoid blowing the nose for 7 to 10 days after surgery; clients are told to sniff backwards or spit, not blow. Nasal saline sprays may be started 3 to 5 days after surgery to moisten the nasal mucosa. Clients are requested to have minimal physical exercise and avoid strenuous activity, lifting, and straining for approximately 2 weeks. After FESS, clients will be required to return to the physician's office for removal of crusts and debris and examination of the nose.

PHARYNGITIS

Pharyngitis is inflammation of the pharynx and may be viral or bacterial in origin. A culture of the pharyngeal mucosa is sometimes indicated before treatment. Clients may complain of a sore throat, difficulty swallowing, fever, malaise, and cough, and have an elevated white blood cell count. Treatment of pharyngitis depends on the causative agent. Both viral and bacterial pharyngitis are contagious by droplet spread. Good handwashing technique is essential, and the use of a mask may prevent spread. Antibiotics are used to treat the bacterial pharyngitis; comfort measures are required for viral types. Bed rest, fluids, warm saline irrigations or gargles, analgesics, and antipyretics are recommended until the symptoms are alleviated.

Chronic pharyngitis (chronic pharyngeal inflammation) is most common in people who (1) habitually use tobacco and alcohol, (2) have a chronic cough, (3) are employed or live in dusty environments, or (4) use their voices excessively. Clinical manifestations vary according to the degree of irritation and inflammation.

TONSILLITIS

Overview

Tonsillitis is an acute infection of the tonsils, almond-shaped lymphoid tissue located in the tonsillar fossa of the oropharynx. Streptococcus is the most common infecting organism, although tonsillitis can be caused by *Haemophilus influenzae, Streptococcus pyogenes,* and other organisms.

The client with tonsillitis will complain of throat pain, difficulty in swallowing, otalgia (referred pain to the ear), and generalized malaise. Examination will disclose an acutely inflamed mucous membrane around the tonsillar area with or without the presence of purulent exudate. In some clients, lymphadenopathy of the cervical lymph nodes may also be present.

The adenoids, lymphoid tissue located in the nasopharynx, are larger in children and begin to atrophy at puberty. In some children who have repeated infections, adenoid hypertrophy may occur, which leads to nasal obstruction, obstructive sleep apnea, and eustachian tube dysfunction with resultant middle ear effusion.

Complications from streptococcal tonsillitis include pneumonia, nephritis, osteomyelitis, and rheumatic fever. Acute tonsillitis may become chronic. Acute otitis media, acute rhinitis, acute sinusitis, and peritonsillar abscess or other deep-neck abscesses may also develop.

Management

Antibiotics are used to treat acute tonsillitis. In addition, the client is instructed to minimize activity; bed rest is encouraged, and fluid intake is increased. Saline throat irrigations or gargles may relieve the discomfort. Mild analgesics such as acetaminophen, with or without codeine, may be prescribed.

Surgical removal of the tonsils (tonsillectomy) and the adenoids (adenoidectomy) is collectively called adenotonsillectomy, or T&A. The tonsils and adenoids may be removed separately but are most often removed in the same procedure. Removal of chronically diseased tonsil or adenoid tissue is indicated (1) when there are recurrent, incapacitating episodes of acute or chronic tonsillitis; (2) when tonsillar or adenoid hypertrophy causes obstruction of the airway and impairs swallowing; (3) following resolution of a peritonsillar abscess; (4) when ear problems related to eustachian tube obstruction occur; or (5) when there are sinus complications. T&A is most often done in children. Tonsillectomy may also be indicated for a carrier of diphtheria, because tonsils may "seed" the infection. Adults with recurrent sore throats, ear pain, or hearing dysfunction or who snore because of hypertrophied adenoid or tonsil tissue may also benefit from this procedure. Although tonsillectomy and adenoidectomy are not as routine as in the past, they are indicated in clients who have repeated episodes of infection. Tonsillectomy may be performed under general or local anesthesia, although general anesthesia is most commonly used.

Surgical intervention is not used during an acute infection, that is, upper respiratory infection. Other contraindications for T&A include hematologic disorders such as hemophilia, aplastic anemia, purpura, or leukemia.

A snarelike or blunt dissection instrument is used to remove the tonsillar tissue, and cautery is applied to bleeding vessels. Potential hazards associated with T&A include (1) failure to secure obscure, hard-to-reach, or hard-to-visualize bleeding points; (2) airway obstruction due to blood and secretions collecting in the airway during surgery; and (3) aspiration of blood and secretions. Because of the risk of perioperative bleeding, preoperative assessment includes a complete blood count, urinalysis, and coagulation studies. Atropine may be administered to control secretions during surgery.

After tonsillectomy, the client is placed in a lateral decubitus position until awake and alert. This will provide for drainage of blood and other secretions through the nose and mouth. The oropharynx and mouth should be gently inspected for fresh blood frequently during the first several hours postoperatively. Vital signs are closely monitored. Hemorrhage is the most serious complication after tonsillectomy and is most often seen during the first 12 to 24 hours. If postoperative hemorrhage occurs, resuturing or cauterization of the bleeding vessel is mandatory.

The client should begin taking oral feedings once recovery from anesthesia is complete. Cool fluids should be encouraged, and the client is progressed to a soft, bland diet as tolerated. Highly seasoned foods, as well as any food the client finds difficult to swallow, should be avoided.

Pain in the first 7 to 10 postoperative days is common after tonsillectomy. Most clients report generalized throat pain as well as otalgia. Mild analgesics such as acetaminophen with or without codeine may be required to alleviate pain. Increased swallowing of fluids will also minimize discomfort.

Clients should be encouraged to seek immediate medical attention if bleeding occurs after hospital dismissal. Delayed bleeding may occur once the healing membrane separates from the underlying tissue (7 to 10 days). The surgical site is usually well healed in 14 to 21 days, and the client should have minimal if any difficulty after this time.

CHRONIC TONSILLITIS

Chronic tonsillitis is not as common as once believed. The most frequent symptom is recurrent sore throat. Between episodes of acute tonsillitis, the throat remains uncomfortable. The tonsils are often enlarged, and if they are infected, a sharp line may be seen between the color of the buccal mucosa and that of the tonsillar pillar. The most reliable indication of chronic tonsillitis is the expression of purulent material from the tonsil crypts with a wooden tongue blade. Once chronic tonsillitis is diagnosed, surgical removal is recommended. Surgery is contraindicated during acute tonsillar infection, although tonsillectomy may be performed in a person with acute peritonsillar abscess.

PERITONSILLAR ABSCESS (QUINSY)

Peritonsillar abscess may arise from acute streptococcal or staphylococcal tonsillitis. The tissue between the tonsils and the fascia covering the superior constrictor muscles becomes infected, causing extensive swelling of the soft palate. The uvula may be pushed to one side, and up to half of the pharyngeal opening may be occluded. Pus formation in the fascial space pushes the tonsil forward toward the midline of the throat (Fig. 38-17).

Peritonsillar abscesses typically occur several days after the onset of acute tonsillitis. As the symptoms of tonsillitis begin to resolve, increasing pain develops on one side of the throat and ear. Inflammation creates a partial obstruction to swallowing. Often, the client keeps the mouth partially open to allow drooling,

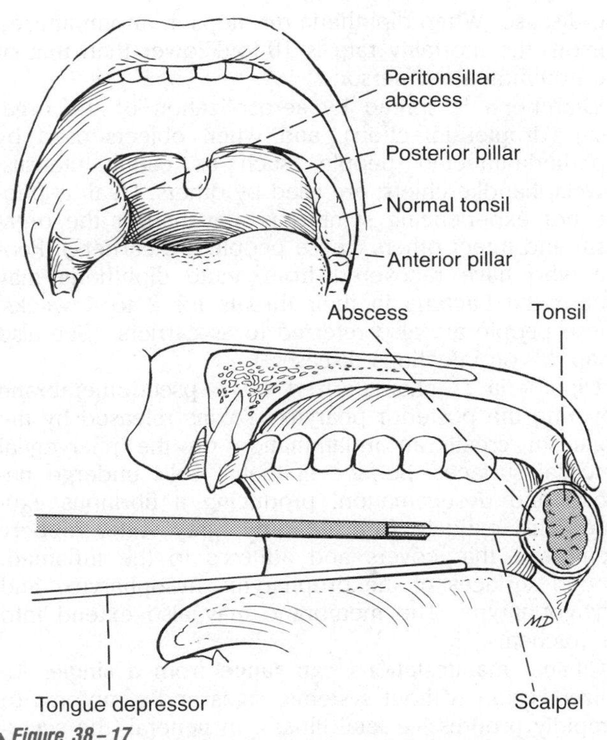

▲ *Figure 38–17*

Peritonsillar abscess, which may rupture spontaneously or require surgical incision. The incision is made near the anterior pillar at the point of greatest fluctuance.

rather than attempting painful swallowing. The voice takes on a characteristic "hot potato," or muffled, sound. Thick secretions are raised with difficulty.

A peritonsillar abscess may rupture spontaneously, allowing pus to drain through the anterior pillar. If spontaneous rupture does not occur, surgical intervention may be necessary. With the person in a sitting position (to allow expectoration of pus and blood), an incision is made and the abscess drained.

Topical anesthetic throat sprays, analgesic agents, hot saline throat irrigations (40.5°–43.3° C [105°–110° F]), saline or alkaline mouthwashes or gargles, and ice collars may be used to make the throat more comfortable. Local anesthetic injections may be prescribed for severe pain. The person may be able to swallow more easily by standing up and having someone stand behind him or her to pull upward on the sides of the neck while trying to swallow. Cool and room-temperature fluids are most easily tolerated. The person may be able to take cool to warm soft foods. High-dose antibiotics are often prescribed early to avoid the need for incision and drainage. It takes at least one month for the infection of a peritonsillar abscess to subside. Usually, a tonsillectomy is performed following resolution of the abscess and infection, to prevent recurrence.

RHINITIS

Rhinitis is inflammation of the nasal mucosa. Symptoms of rhinitis include increased nasal drainage. Normally this drainage is clear mucus. If the infection spreads to the sinuses, however, drainage may become yellow or green. Rhinitis may be classified as acute, allergic, or vasomotor. Acute rhinitis is also known as the common cold or coryza. Acute rhinitis may be bacterial or viral in origin; it is treated symptomatically. Acute rhinitis usually lasts 5 to 7 days, with or without treatment. Common interventions for acute rhinitis are symptomatic and include supplemental humidification, decongestants to reduce the edema of the nasal mucosa, increased fluids to prevent dehydration, and analgesics to relieve the generalized myalgia. Sometimes antibiotics are given, not to treat the virus but to prevent a secondary infection by bacteria.

Allergic rhinitis is most often seen as a seasonal disorder. In addition to obstruction to nasal breathing, the client with allergic rhinitis may also experience irritation of other mucous membranes (i.e., the conjunctiva, causing tearing and edema of the eyelids). Treatment of allergic rhinitis is also symptomatic. A complete allergy evaluation may be required to determine the offending allergen. Most clients are placed on a desensitization program, told to avoid the antigen, and treated symptomatically with antihistamines, steroids or mast cell–stabilizing sprays.

Vasomotor rhinitis causes the same symptoms as do acute and allergic rhinitis but has no known specific cause. Clients complaining of vasomotor rhinitis who have a negative culture and negative allergy evaluation are treated symptomatically. If medications have been prescribed for clients with rhinitis (especially nasal sprays), the client must be taught about the use of the medications, including side effects and possible interactions with other medications.

LARYNGITIS

Laryngitis is inflammation of the larnyx, or hoarseness. Hoarseness is a common symptom that may be due to inflammation of the vocal cords, abnormal movements of the vocal cords, or a benign or malignant tumor of the vocal cords. All of these interfere with normal mobility of the vocal cords, which produces an abnormal sound.

Laryngitis, inflammation of the vocal cords, may be due to an inflammatory process or vocal abuse. The laryngeal membrane is continuous with the lining of the upper respiratory tract, and infections in other areas of the nose and throat may include the larynx. Edema of the vocal cords caused by the chronic irritation of an upper respiratory tract infection inhibits the normal mobility of the vocal cords, which causes an abnormal sound.

Laryngitis may also be the result of gastroesophageal reflux disorder (GERD). In this syndrome, the sphincter between the stomach and esophagus relaxes, and gastric acid is allowed to enter the esophagus. Reflux of gastric secretions, especially during sleep, may result in the aspiration of gastric secretions into the larynx, causing a chemical irritation or burning of the mucous membrane lining the larynx.[13] Clients with gastroesophageal reflux may complain of hoarseness from the chemical irritation of the gastric acid on the vocal cords, increased mucus production from the body's natural tendency to protect the irritated membrane, foreign body sensation, or sore throat. Chronic cough and asthma may also be associated symptoms of GERD.

Abnormal voice may also be the result of vocal abuse. Screaming, shouting, and loud speaking over a period of time may produce edema of the vocal cords and the formation of nodules or polyps, outpouchings of inflamed mucous membranes.

The initial treatment of laryngitis is to treat the causative factors. If inflammatory laryngitis is suspected, the inflammation should be treated. Antibiotics may be used if a bacterial infection is suspected. In severe cases, systemic steroids (such as Medrol Dosepak) may be prescribed to reduce inflammation and edema. Supplemental humidification may add increased moisture to liquefy secretions, and mucolytic agents may be prescribed to thin and mobilize mucus. Clients with laryngitis may also be placed on voice rest to allow the edema of the vocal cords to subside without added strain. The client should be cautioned to avoid whispering, which will also cause excessive vocal cord strain.

Gastroesophageal reflux is initially treated symptomatically. The client is instructed to elevate the head of the bed to minimize reflux; to avoid eating or drinking for 2 to 3 hours before going to sleep; to avoid caffeine, alcohol, and tobacco, which are known to increase gastric secretions; and to use antacids and hydrogen inhibitors (famotidine [Pepcid], ranitidine [Zantac]) to neutralize and decrease acid production.[13]

Chronic laryngitis may stem from repeated infections, allergy, chronic irritant exposure, long-term voice abuse, and reflux esophagitis of acidic gastric contents.

Chronic laryngitis is manifested by a tickling sensation in the throat, voice huskiness, and painful or difficult phonation. Management involves correction or removal of the irritation, in addition to the measures to increase comfort (see acute laryngitis). Long-term voice retraining may be necessary if improper use or overuse of the voice is the main cause of chronic laryngitis. This retraining includes (1) learning to use the voice without straining and (2) forming and projecting words to use the diaphragm without shouting.

DIPHTHERIA

Overview

Diphtheria is an acute, toxin-mediated infectious disease by the toxinogenic bacteria *Corynebacterium diphtheriae*, which is a small, rod-shaped, gram-positive aerobic pathogen. Over recent years, there has been a resurgence in the incidence of diphtheria, even in developed nations. Diphtheria is a highly contagious disease that is spread easily in areas with poor personal hygiene, crowding, and limited access to medical care. Immunization reduces the susceptibility and severity of the disease. When diphtheria develops in an immunized person, the mortality rate is 10-fold lower than that of the nonimmunized person.

Diphtheria is spread by aerosolization of the organism (droplet infection), and when objects used by diphtheria-infected people, such as eating utensils, towels, handkerchiefs, are used by others. Healthy people not experiencing symptoms may harbor the organism and infect others (these people are carriers). People who have recovered from acute diphtheria may harbor the bacteria in their throats for 2 to 4 weeks. These people are also referred to as carriers. (See also Chap. 25 on infectious diseases.)

Diphtheria is characterized by a pseudomembrane covering the posterior pharynx. Toxins released by the organism create an inflammation on the pharyngeal mucosal surfaces. Surface epithelial cells undergo necrosis and desquamation, producing a fibrinous exudate. This exudate forms a dirty, gray-white, rubbery membrane that covers and adheres to the inflamed, eroded surfaces of the oropharynx, nasopharynx, and laryngopharynx. The membrane may also extend into the trachea.

Clinical manifestations can range from a single, localized lesion without systemic signs and symptoms to a rapidly progressive fatal illness. In general, the severity of diphtheria is correlated with the site of the local lesion. Anterior nasal lesions tend to be chronic, but clients have few symptoms. People with chronic lesions are most often carriers, especially in developed countries.

Tonsillar diphtheria is seldom life threatening, although it can be associated with severe complications. A low-grade fever, fatigue, headache, and sore throat are common manifestations. Tonsillar diphtheria can progress rapidly to more fatal forms.

Pharyngeal diphtheria, especially that with a membrane covering the larnyx or bronchus, is the most serious form of diphtheria. The client is gravely ill, with a weak pulse, restlessness, and confusion. Fever may or may not be present. Because of the location of the membrane, the airway is often obstructed and the client has stridor and cyanosis. The neck may also be swollen and warm.

Diphtheria is diagnosed by culture of the material with the ELISA or Elek test. Gram-stain or fluorescent antibody stains may also be performed, and these tests are more quickly performed. Although cultures are used to identify the organism, treatment begins while waiting for the definitive results.

Complications include disorders of nervous and cardiac tissues, including congestive heart failure, dysrhythmias, and paralysis.

Management

The goals of treatment for clients with presumed or known diphtheria are to neutralize the free toxins, eliminate further toxin production, control the local infection, provide physiologic support during the course of the disease, and prevent transmission. These goals are met through the use of equine diphtheria antitoxin, antibiotics, and respiratory support as well as management of congestive heart failure, cardiac dysrhythmias, neuropathies, renal failure, and bleeding.

All contacts should be cultured. Those persons immunized 5 or more years previously should receive a booster dose. Those persons who were never immunized should be treated with immunization and antibiotics.

Nursing management focuses on management of the airway obstruction. Suction equipment and a tracheotomy tray should be kept at the bedside. Oxygen is administered.

Clients experience pain, especially with swallowing. In addition to analgesia, pain can be reduced by limiting the diet to liquids and soft foods. Throat irrigation and fluids may also help control pain.

During antitoxin administration, the nurse observes the client for anaphylaxis; epinephrine is kept at the bedside.

To prevent transmission of the disease, the client is placed in strict isolation. Contacts need to be identified, screened, immunized, and treated.

Summary

Disorders of the upper airway can range from the simple cold to cancer of the larynx. This chapter has presented care of those clients most commonly hospitalized with upper airway disorders. Nursing management can also range from assessment of life-threatening airway obstruction to teaching techniques that reduce the spread of infection.

Bibliography

1. American Cancer Society. (1992). *Cancer facts and figures.* New York: Author.
2. Anthony, C. P., & Thilodeau, G. A. (1979). *Textbook of anatomy and physiology* (10th ed.). St. Louis: C. V. Mosby.
3. Feinstein, D. (1987). What to teach the patient who's had a total laryngectomy. *RN, 50* (4), 53-57.
4. Griffin, C., & Lockhart, J. (1987). Learning to swallow again. *American Journal of Nursing, 87* (3), 314-317.
5. Harris, L. L., & Kraege, J. (1986). After T-E puncture: relearning to speak. *American Journal of Nursing, 86* (1), 55-58.
6. Hillel, A., et al. (1989). Radical neck dissection: A subjective and objective evaluation of postoperative disability. *Journal of Otolaryngology, 18* (1), 53-61.
7. Kennedy, D. W., & Zinreich, S. J. (1989). Functional endoscopic surgery. In E. N. Myers, et al. (Eds.), *Advances in otolaryngology—Head and neck surgery* (vol. 3, pp. 1-27). Chicago: Year Book.
8. Krakoff, I. (1991). Cancer chemotherapeutic and biologic agents. *CA: A Cancer Journal for Clinicians, 41* (5), 264-278.
9. Lavertu, P., et al. (1989). Secondary tracheoesophageal puncture for voice rehabilitation after laryngectomy. *Archives of Otolaryngology—Head and Neck Surgery, 115* (3), 350.
10. Litwack, K. (1991). Managing postanesthetic emergencies. *Nursing 91, 21* (9), 49-51.
11. Lockhart, J., Troff, J., & Artim, L. (1992). Total laryngectomy and radical neck dissection. *AORN Journal, 55* (2), 458-479.
12. Logemann, J. A. (1983). *Evaluation and treatment of swallowing disorders.* San Diego: College-Hill Press.
13. Olson, N. R. (1986). The problem of gastroesophageal reflux. *Otolaryngologic Clinics of North America, 19* (1), 119-113.
14. Petruzzelli, G. J., & Johnson, J. T. (1989). How to stop a nosebleed. *Postgraduate Medicine, 86* (4), 44-56.
15. Romm, S. (1986). Cancer of the larynx: current concepts of diagnosis and treatment. *Surgical Clinics of North America, 66* (1), 109-118.
16. Sabiston, D. (1991). *Textbook of surgery.* Philadelphia: W. B. Saunders.
17. Sigler, B. A. (1987). Nursing care for head and neck tumor patients. In S. E. Thawley & W. R. Panje (Eds.), *Comprehensive management of head and neck tumors* (pp. 79-100). Philadelphia: W. B. Saunders.
18. Sigler, B. A. (1989). Nursing care of patients with laryngeal carcinoma. *Seminars in Oncology Nursing, 5* (3), 160-165.
19. Sigler, B. A. (1988). Nursing care of the head and neck cancer patient. *Oncology, 8* (2), 49-59.
20. Sigler, B. A. (1982). Solid neoplasms: Neoplasms of the head and neck. In D. A. Jones, et al. (Eds.), *Medical-surgical nursing: A conceptual approach* (pp. 241-265). New York: McGraw-Hill.
21. Sigler, B. A., & Hooper, J. A. (1989). Nursing care of the head and neck cancer patient. In E. N. Myers & J. Y. Suen (Eds.), *Cancer of the head and neck* (pp. 1045-1071). New York: Churchill Livingstone.
22. Singer, M. I. (1988). Surgical restoration of the voice after total laryngectomy. In E. N. Myers, et al. (Eds.), *Advances in otolaryngology—Head and neck surgery* (vol. 2, pp. 141-165). Chicago: Year Book.
23. Singer, M. I., & Blom, E. D. (1990). Medical techniques for voice restoration after total laryngectomy. *CA: A Cancer Journal for Clinicians, 40* (3), 166-173.
24. Slavin, R. G. (1991). Recalcitrant asthma: Could sinusitis be the culprit? *The Journal of Respiratory Diseases, 12* (2), 182-194.
25. Wyngaarden J., et al. (1992). *Cecil textbook of medicine* (19th ed.). Philadelphia: W. B. Saunders.
26. Yoshida, G. Y., et al. (1989). Primary voice restoration at laryngectomy: 1989 update. *Laryngoscope, 99,* 1093-1095.

Chapter 39

Nursing Care of Clients with Lower Airway Disorders

AIRWAY DISORDERS

ASTHMA

Definition

Asthma is a disorder of the bronchial airways characterized by periods of bronchospasm (spasms of prolonged contraction of the airway). Asthma is a complex disorder involving biochemical, immunologic, endocrine, infectious, autonomic, and psychological factors.

Incidence

Asthma affects about 2 to 3 per cent of the United States population, and its incidence is rising. It is the most common chronic disease in children and adults.

Etiology

Asthma occurs in families, which indicates that it is an inherited disorder. Apparently environmental factors (e.g., viral infection) interact with inherited factors to produce disease.

Risk Factors and Prevention

Methods of primary prevention include reduction of air pollution and cigarette smoking. Secondary smoke inhalation is known to increase the incidence of respiratory disorders. Secondary prevention through early detection in known asthmatics is through the daily monitoring of peak airflow volumes. In many clients, peak airflow volume decreases about 24 hours before asthma symptoms begin. Tertiary prevention in clients who are known asthmatics mainly consists of avoiding known allergens. Clients who develop asthma along with respiratory infections can begin early treatment when clinical manifestations of upper respiratory infection begin.

Pathophysiology

Asthma can be divided into two main categories: extrinsic (allergic) and intrinsic (nonallergic). Extrinsic asthma is caused by agents such as dust, lint, pollen, insects, mold spores, smoke, medications, and foods. The client with extrinsic asthma is allergic to these items. This form of asthma usually begins in childhood. In contrast, intrinsic asthma does not have easily identifiable allergens and is triggered by many internal disorders, such as the common cold or upper respiratory infection, or even exercise. This form of asthma usually begins in adults over the age of 35 years. Both forms of asthma can be triggered by changes in environmental temperature, strong odors (perfumed soaps and cosmetics), stress, emotion, exercise, and exposure to specific allergens (mold spores, pollen). Clients with intrinsic asthma may also have nasal polyps and aspirin allergy (called triad disease).

In both forms of asthma, the airway is hyperreactive. Extrinsic asthma is an example of type I hypersensitivity reaction (see Chap. 24). When the client comes in contact with an allergen, the B lymphocytes are stimulated and differentiate into plasma cells, which produce IgE antibodies. IgE antibodies attach to the mast cells and basophils in the bronchial walls. Mast cells and basophils release chemical mediators (i.e., histamine, bradykinin, prostaglandins, and slow-releasing substance of anaphylaxis [SRS-A]. SRS-As are also called leukotrienes). These chemical mediators cause bronchial smooth muscle to contract and close the airways. These substances also increase vascular permeability, which leads to airway edema.

Intrinsic asthma begins with both a parasympathetic and a sympathetic response. The parasympathetic nervous system causes a release of acetylcholine, which leads to bronchoconstriction. The sympathetic nervous system stimulates the mast cells (see preceding).

Both alpha- and beta-adrenergic receptors of the sympathetic nervous system are found in the bronchi. Stimulation of the alpha-adrenergic receptors causes bronchoconstriction; conversely, stimulation of the beta-adrenergic receptors causes bronchodilation. Cyclic adenosine monophosphate (cyclic AMP) balances the two receptors. Some theories on the cause of asthma suggest that the client lacks beta-adrenergic stimulation.

Once the airway is in spasm, mucus plugs the airway, trapping distal air. Ventilation/perfusion (V/Q) mismatch, hypoxemia, and increased workload of breathing follow (V/Q mismatch is discussed in Chap. 37). Hyperventilation eventually occurs as the lung attempts to respond to the increased volume and pressure.

Asthma symptoms commonly worsen at night. In the normal population, the best lung function is at 1600 hours, the worst at 0400 hours. In the asthmatic, the same circadian rhythm exists, but it is combined with greater bronchial reactivity during the nighttime. The mechanisms of nighttime asthma are not fully understood, but more than being exposed to bedding or bedroom allergens is involved. Some possible mechanisms include decreased levels of epinephrine, cyclic AMP, and cortisol. Clinical manifestations may also be due to increased levels of histamine, increased inflammatory cells in the airway, airway cooling, and airway secretions.

Complications

Status asthmaticus is a severe, life-threatening complication of asthma. It is an acute episode of bronchospasm that tends to intensify. With severe bronchospasm, the workload of breathing increases 5 to 10 times, which can lead to acute cor pulmonale. When air is trapped, a severe paradoxic pulse develops as venous return is obstructed. This condition is seen as a blood pressure drop of over 10 mm Hg during inspiration. Pneumothorax commonly develops. If status asthmaticus continues, hypoxemia worsens, and acidosis begins. If the condition is untreated or not reversed, respiratory or cardiac arrest will ensue.

Clinical Manifestations

During asthma attacks, clients are dyspneic and have marked respiratory effort. At the beginning of an attack, there is a sensation of chest constriction, inspiratory and expiratory wheezing, nonproductive coughing, prolonged expiration, tachycardia, and tachypnea (Box 39-1).

The severity of asthma can be classified as mild, moderate, or severe, depending on the symptoms. A scoring system is depicted in Table 39-1.

DIAGNOSTIC ASSESSMENT

Spirometry reveals decreased peak expiratory flow rate, forced expiratory volume (FEV_1), and forced vital ca-

Box 39-1. Clinical Manifestations of Bronchial Asthma

General Appearance

Anxious: as asthma becomes more severe, $PaCO_2$ rises, and central nervous system depression occurs

Age Range

All ages; is a component of CAL

Assessment Findings

Nasal flaring as respiratory distress increases
Lips pursed in an effort to exhale
Use of accessory muscles as work of breathing increases
Paradoxic pulse increases as bronchospasm worsens
Wheezing, cough, or dyspnea; if no breath sounds, status asthmaticus (life-threatening), intubation, and mechanical ventilation are urgent
Cyanosis is late development

Cardiac Involvement

Tachycardia
Electrocardiogram may show right-sided heart strain

Smoking History

Uncommon; smoke is often an allergen that triggers bronchospasm

Diagnostic Findings

Pulmonary Function

Increased FRC; FEV_1 decreased; peak flow decreased

Arterial Blood Gases

If untreated, asthma progresses in severity; $PaCO_2$ goes from below normal to normal and finally elevates
A normal $PaCO_2$ indicates tiring; elevated $PaCO_2$ indicates significant tiring leading to respiratory arrest
As $PaCO_2$ rises, PaO_2 falls; effects of hypercapnia and hypoxia are noticeable
If $PaCO_2$ rises and remains uncorrected, pH falls, causing respiratory acidosis

Chest Film

Hyperinflation

Overview

Swollen mucous membranes of bronchioles and surrounding tissue
Muscles of bronchioles become spastic, causing narrowing
Thick mucus fills bronchioles and alveoli; breathing becomes labored; expiration difficult

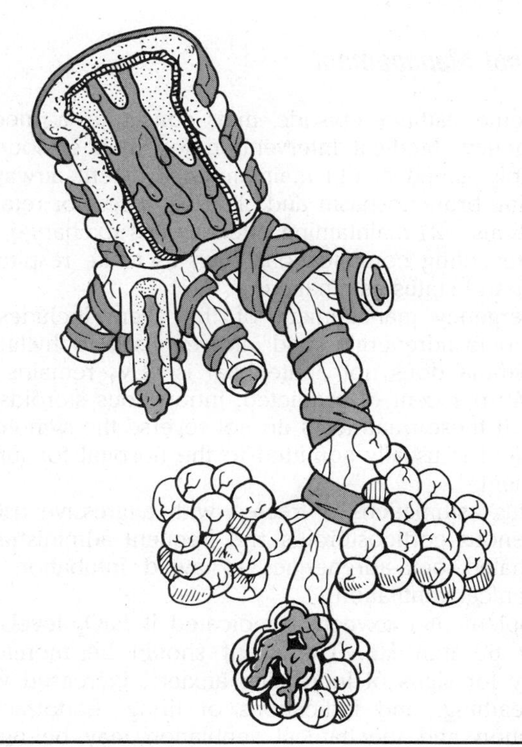

pacity (FVC). Functional residual capacity (FRC), total lung capacity (TLC), and residual volume (RV) are increased. Blood gas analysis reveals hypoxemia and respiratory alkalosis. Chest radiography may reveal hyperinflation.

Baseline assessment of pulmonary status will include arterial blood gas (ABG) analysis (Table 39-2 for typical ABG changes during an asthma attack) and essential pulmonary function studies (i.e., peak flow rate and forced expiratory volume, measured with spirometry or peak flowmeter). A 20 per cent improvement in FVC, FEV, and PEFR following inhaled administration of a beta-agonist bronchodilator implies a reversible airflow obstruction, i.e., asthma.

Auscultation of breath sounds will usually reveal wheezing, especially during expiration. The inability to auscultate wheezing in an asthmatic client with acute respiratory distress may be an ominous sign. It may indicate that the small airways are too constricted to allow any airflow. This client may require immediate, aggressive medical intervention.

TABLE 39-1. Assessing the Severity of Asthma

Clinical Manifestations	Score 0	Score 1
Loss of exercise tolerance, capable of work?	Yes	No
Using accessory muscles, tracheal tug and intercostal retraction present?	Absent	Present
Wheezing?	Absent	Present
Respiratory rate per minute	Under 25	Over 25
Pulse rate per minute	Under 120	Over 120
Palpable pulsus paradoxus	Absent	Present
Peak expiratory flow rate (L/min)	Over 100	Under 100

Score the client in each area. A score of 4 or more suggests severe asthma, and the client will require careful observation to determine whether there is a response to therapy or hospitalization is necessary.

From Cochrane, G., & Rees, P. (1989). *A colour atlas of asthma.* London: Wolfe Medical Publications.

TABLE 39-2. Alterations in Arterial Blood Gases Associated with Asthma

	Mild	Moderate	Severe	Status Asthmaticus
PaO_2	Slightly elevated	Normal to mild hypoxemia	Hypoxemia	Severe hypoxemia
$PaCO_2$	Decreased	Decreased to normal	Elevated	Significantly elevated
pH	Alkalosis	Alkalosis	Alkalosis	Acidosis

A problem with the use of diagnostic tests for asthma is that when the client is not having an acute attack, blood gases, pulmonary function tests, and chest film are often normal.

Medical Management

An acute asthma episode may constitute a medical emergency. Medical intervention for such episodes is primarily aimed at (1) maintaining a patent airway by relieving bronchospasm and clearing excess or retained secretions, (2) maintaining effective gas exchange, and (3) preventing complications such as acute respiratory failure and status asthmaticus.

Emergency management of the client includes inhaled beta adrenergics and intravenous theophylline. If the asthma does not abate, that is FEV_1 remains less than 40 per cent of predicted, intravenous steroids are given. If these treatments do not reverse the symptoms, the client is usually admitted to the hospital for further treatment.

Status asthmaticus is treated with aggressive use of intravenous corticosteroids and frequent administration of inhaled beta-adrenergics to avoid intubation and mechanical ventilation.

Supplemental oxygen is indicated if PaO_2 levels fall below 60 mm Hg. The client should be monitored closely for signs of increasing anxiety, increased work of breathing, and indications of tiring. Endotracheal intubation and mechanical ventilation may be necessary. Medically induced paralysis may be necessary in rare cases.

After the acute asthma attack is over, the client is assessed for determination of the precipitating event or factors and is instructed in self-care activities.

PHARMACOLOGIC MANAGEMENT

Beta-adrenergic agents are the mainstay of bronchodilator therapy. Beta-adrenergic agents with varying degrees of beta-2 selectivity are used by nebulizer or metered-dose inhaler. Some beta-adrenergic agents can be administered parenterally also. The use of parenteral agents in adults is not common because inhaled agents have equal effect and do not have systemic side effects that accompany parenteral agents. Common agents include albuterol (Proventil) and isoetharine (DeyLute).

Clients with very mild asthma (less than 3 to 4 attacks per year) can use the inhalers on an as-needed basis. Clients with moderate asthma (6 to 8 attacks annually) should use inhalers on a regular, daily basis. Clients with severe asthma combine inhalers with other agents.

Treatment with metered-dose inhalers consist of two puffs about 3 to 5 minutes apart. The first dose dilates the narrowed airways, allowing the second breath to extend further. The client begins by exhaling fully and then inhaling with a slow sustained breath attempting to reach total lung capacity (TLC). Aerosol "spacers," extensions that collect the medication in a chamber from which the client inhales, are available for clients who have difficulty coordinating inhalation with the spray.

In addition to beta-adrenergic agents, theophylline and aminophylline are moderately potent bronchodilators used to manage asthma. The use of theophylline is limited by its toxicity and by the wide variations in the rate of metabolism. Theophylline levels are monitored to evaluate the effectiveness of the drug.

Antihistamines had been ineffective in the treatment of asthma until recently. In the past decade, more potent H_1-receptor agonists, such as terfenadine (Seldane), have emerged with fewer central nervous system side effects. Early clinical trials indicate that they produce bronchodilation and alleviate asthmatic symptoms. It is likely that H_1-receptor agonists will become part of the treatment of asthma.

Anticholinergics, corticosteroids, and mast cell stabilizers have also been used in treating asthma. Medications used in management of respiratory disorders are discussed in Chapter 37.

Nursing Management

ASSESSMENT

Initially, the client should be assessed for signs or symptoms of airway distress. If the client is having acute airway distress, this emergency must be managed before a detailed history of the disease is performed. Known medication allergies should be determined so that these medications are avoided in treatment. In addition, ascertaining whether the client has a history of cardiac disease is important initially, because the medication used to treat the asthma may worsen a diseased heart.

Once the asthma is controlled, the history of the client's asthma should be explored. The nurse should assist the client to determine if there is a pattern to the symptoms. These data may help identify a trigger to the asthmatic symptoms. If an extrinsic trigger can be identified, then many times it can be reduced or eliminated. For example, if the client is allergic to mold,

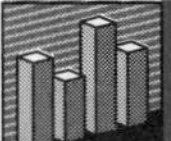

NURSING RESEARCH

The purpose of this study (Gift, 1991) was to compare selected psychological and physiologic variables during periods of intense dyspnea with those at times of no or low dyspnea in clients with asthma. Thirty-six adults ranging from 19 to 76 years old were tested when they first came to the emergency department in acute dyspnea and again when they had no or low dyspnea just before discharge. Anxiety, depression, hostility, and somatic complaints were found to be higher when clients were experiencing acute dyspnea, whereas peak expiratory flow rates and oxygen saturation were significantly lower. Respiratory rate, pulse, wheezing, and accessory muscle use were greater during acute dyspnea in these asthmatics, whereas in a similar study of COPD patients (Gift & Cahill, 1990), only accessory muscle use was found to be higher during acute dyspnea.

The findings of this study indicate that acute dyspnea in the asthmatic patient is accompanied by various psychophysiologic changes. This offers the clinician a variety of indicators for monitoring dyspnea onset and for evaluating the effectiveness of clinical interventions in this patient population.

▼▼▼

Gift, A. G. (1991). Psychologic and physiologic aspects of acute dyspnea in asthmatics. *Nursing Research, 40:*196–199.

Gift, A. G., & Cahill, C. A. (1990). Psychophysiologic aspects of dyspnea in chronic obstructive pulmonary disease: a pilot study. *Heart and Lung, 19:*252–257.

common sources of mold can be avoided. The nurse should also ask about current medications, especially those used to treat other illnesses. Some clients are inadvertently placed on medications that may induce bronchospasms. For example, if a noncardioselective beta-blocker, such as propranolol (Inderal), is prescribed for hypertension, it may cause bronchospasm.

Within the psychosocial domain, the nurse can ask about the client's ability to manage the asthma and general adaptation to the illness. Denial of the illness can lead to a lack of treatment of early symptoms. It is important to determine whether the client feels control over the illness and feels capable of managing it. Clients who have this feeling of control, called an internal locus of control, may have improved compliance with treatments. Other psychological correlates to asthma symptoms are discussed in Nursing Research.

Another area of assessment includes determining whether the client is experiencing an increased number of stressors. Stressful lifestyles may increase the number of asthmatic symptoms.

The attitude of the family should also be assessed. The family can be a great source of support and assist the client to recognize early symptoms. In contrast, an unsupportive family may contribute to denial or be an additional source of stress to the client.

The client with a new diagnosis of asthma may be asked to assess the home and work environment for likely triggers to the symptoms. The presence of pets that shed hair or dander, cigarette smoke, or occupational exposure may require some lifestyle changes. Elimination of irritants is generally performed in a reasonable fashion. Improvements in a client's symptoms that may result from a major lifestyle change, such as job change or loss of a pet, may be quickly offset by the stress felt from such a move.

NURSING INTERVENTION

Nursing Diagnosis: Breathing Pattern, Ineffective R/T impaired exhalation and anxiety.

Planning: Expected Outcomes. The client will have improved breathing patterns, as evidenced by a decreasing respiratory rate to within normal limits; decreased signs of dyspnea, nasal flaring, and use of accessory muscles; decreased signs of anxiety; ABG levels returning to normal limits; and vital capacity measurements within normal limits or greater than 40 per cent of predicted, including FEV_1, TLC, and RV.

Implementation. The nurse should assess the client frequently, observing the respiratory rate and depth and the breathing pattern for shortness of breath, pursed-lip breathing, nasal flaring, sternal and intercostal retractions, and a prolonged expiratory phase. In acute asthma, these assessments may be needed continually or every hour.

ABGs should be monitored to determine the effectiveness of treatments. Pulmonary function test results should be compared with normal levels. The degree of dysfunction will assist the nurse to plan for activity.

The client should be placed in Fowler's position and given oxygen as ordered. Bronchodilators and steroids are commonly prescribed. Tachycardia and tremors are common side effects of bronchodilator therapy. The nurse should monitor for therapeutic levels of theophylline (8 to 20 μg/mL).

Nursing Diagnosis: Airway Clearance, Ineffective R/T increased production of secretions and bronchospasm.

Planning: Expected Outcomes. The client will have an effective airway clearance, as evidenced by decreased inspiratory and expiratory wheezing; decreased rhonchi; PaO_2 over 60 mm Hg, $PaCO_2$ equal or less than 40 mm Hg, and pH greater than 7.35; and decreasing dry, nonproductive cough.

Implementation. Lung sounds should be assessed every hour during acute episodes for determining the adequacy of gas exchange. If the airway is compromised, the client may require suctioning. Some clients develop asthma as a result of pulmonary infection. The nurse should monitor the color and consistency of the sputum and assist the client to cough effectively. Fluids should be encouraged to thin the secretions and replace fluids lost through rapid respirations. The humidity in the room may be increased slightly. If chest secretions are thick and difficult to expectorate, the client may benefit from chest physiotherapy (postural drainage, percussion, and vibration) and frequent position changes. The client should be given frequent oral care, every 2 to 4 hours, to remove the taste of the secretions.

Refer to the care plan for the client with COPD when working with clients with diagnoses of Activity Intolerance; Anxiety; Nutrition, Altered; or Sleep Pattern Disturbance.

EVALUATION

The degree of expected outcome attainment should be evaluated. Revisions in the plan of care may be necessary. Generally, asthma can be reversed quickly, if there is no underlying problem such as infection.

Post-hospital Care

The client with asthma should be taught about prescribed bronchodilators and steroids, including side effects and precautions for administration. Bronchodilators can cause difficulty sleeping and should be given at a time when the client is tired. They must be taken close to bedtime to alleviate increased symptoms of asthma during the night. Steroids can cause gastric irritation and must be taken with food. Many inhaled medications require an understanding of how to manipulate the equipment. The nurse should ask the client to perform a return demonstration with the equipment.

Assist the client and family to understand the early symptoms of asthma, how to treat it at home, and when to seek additional help. Known allergens should be avoided. Pollution indexes and pollen counts should be monitored and outdoor activities avoided during times of high counts.

CHRONIC AIRFLOW LIMITATIONS

Definition

Chronic obstructive pulmonary disease (COPD), also called chronic obstructive lung disease (COLD), refers to a number of disorders that affect movement of air in and out of the lungs. The most important of these disorders are obstructive bronchitis, emphysema, and asthma.

Whereas bronchitis, emphysema, and asthma may occur in a "pure form," they most commonly coexist, and assessment findings overlap. Although the term COPD is commonly used, to specialists in pulmonary medicine it is not completely accurate, and the nurse may see the term "chronic airflow limitation" (CAL) in its place.

CAL may occur either as a result of increased airway resistance secondary to luminal narrowing as a result of bronchial mucosal edema or smooth muscle contraction, or as a result of decreased elastic recoil (seen in emphysema). Decreased elastic recoil results in a decreased driving force to empty the lung.

Incidence

CAL is a widespread disorder; it affects 1 of 14 people over the age of 45 years.[28] The disorder usually begins in the fifth or sixth decade of life and is predominant in the elderly. CAL is more common in men, although the incidence in women is increasing. It is more frequent in clients living in urban environments and among the socioeconomically disadvantaged. Morbidity and mortality rates for CAL are increasing as the effects of chronic irritation and pollution increase.

Etiology

The specific causes of CAL are not clearly understood. However, the effects of numerous irritants found in cigarette smoke (i.e., stimulation of excess mucus production and coughing, destruction of ciliary function, and inflammation and damage of bronchiolar and alveolar walls) make smoking the leading risk factor for the development of the disorder.

Chronic respiratory infections, including sinusitis, contribute to the development of CAL, as does the aging process. In addition, heredity and genetic predisposition seem to have a role.

Risk Factors

The primary prevention for COPD is smoking cessation or never starting in the first place. In addition, the control of air pollution will reduce the incidence of COPD. Secondary prevention consists of early treatment and diagnosis of diseases that cause COPD, such as pneumonia. Early COPD detection in high-risk clients through lung function studies is beginning to be used. Longitudinal research studies are being conducted to determine if cigarette smokers will show excessive declines in pulmonary function tests as they age.

Pathophysiology

In order to understand COPD, each of its components are discussed.

Chronic Obstructive Bronchitis. Chronic obstructive bronchitis is inflammation of the bronchi, which causes increased mucus production and chronic cough. In order to diagnose chronic bronchitis as opposed to acute bronchitis, the symptoms must continue for 3 months of the year and for 2 consecutive years. Additionally, if the client has a decreased FEV_1/FVC ratio less than 75 per cent and chronic bronchitis, then the client is said to have chronic *obstructive* bronchitis. This term implies that the client has obstructive lung disease combined with chronic cough.

This disorder is caused by exposure to irritants, especially cigarette smoke. Clients with chronic bronchitis have (1) an increase in the size and number of submucous glands in the large bronchi, which increases mucus production; (2) thicker, more tenacious mucus; and (3) impaired ciliary function, which reduces mucus clearance. Therefore, the lung's mucociliary defenses are impaired, and there is increased susceptibility to infection. When infection occurs, the mucus production is even greater, and the bronchial walls inflame and thicken. Chronic bronchitis initially affects only the larger bronchi, but eventually all airways are involved. The thick mucus and enlarged bronchi obstruct airways, especially during expiration. The airways collapse, and air is trapped in the distal portion of the lung. This obstruction leads to reduced alveolar ventilation, hypoxia, and acidosis. The client has poor tissue oxygenation; an abnormal V/Q (ventilation-perfusion) ratio develops, with a corresponding fall in PaO_2. Impaired ventilation may also result in increased levels of $PaCO_2$ (V/Q ratio is discussed in Chap. 37). The client appears cyanotic. As compensation for the hypoxemia, polycythemia (an overproduction of erythrocytes) occurs. Cyanosis and peripheral edema have led to the slang term "blue bloater" for the client with chronic bronchitis (Fig. 39-1).

As the disease progresses, copious amounts of sputum are produced; pulmonary infection is common. During infections, the client has marked reduction in FEV_1 with increased RV and FRC. If these problems are not reversed, hypoxemia will lead to cor pulmonale (see Chap. 43) and congestive heart failure (see Chap. 42).

Emphysema. Emphysema is a disorder in which the alveolar walls are destroyed, which leads to permanent overdistention of the air spaces. Air passages are obstructed as a result of these changes, rather than from mucus production as in chronic bronchitis. Difficult expiration in emphysema is due to the destruction of the walls (septa) between the alveoli, partial airway collapse, and loss of elastic recoil. As the alveoli and

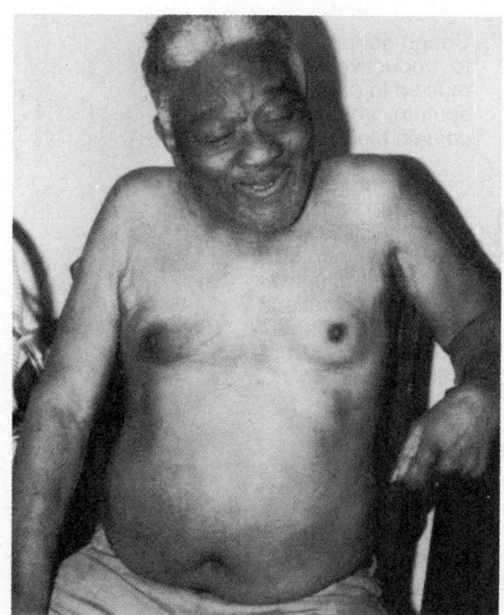

▲ *Figure 39-1*

Client with chronic bronchitis and all the classic findings of the "blue bloater." In addition, slight gynecomastia and petechiae are present in the midsternal area, both side effects of large-dose oral corticosteroid therapy. The patient's shoulders are raised, and muscles are tensed, from shortness of breath and increased work of breathing. (From Kersten, L. D. [1989]. *Comprehensive respiratory nursing.* Philadelphia: W. B. Saunders.)

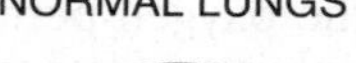

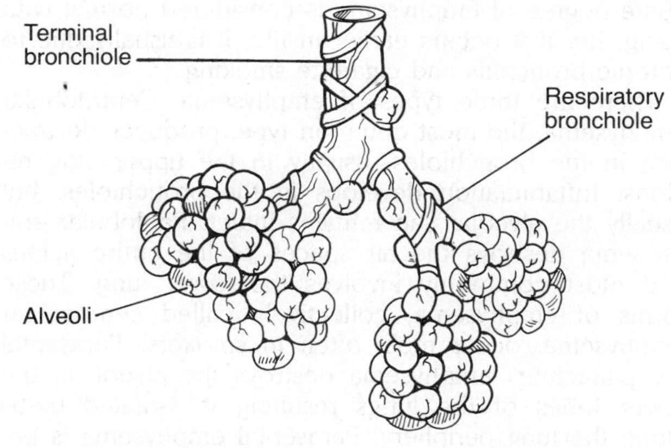

CENTRIACINAR EMPHYSEMA

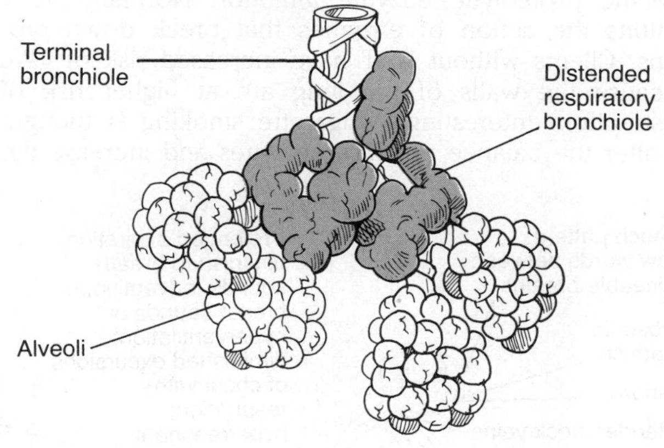

PANACINAR EMPHYSEMA

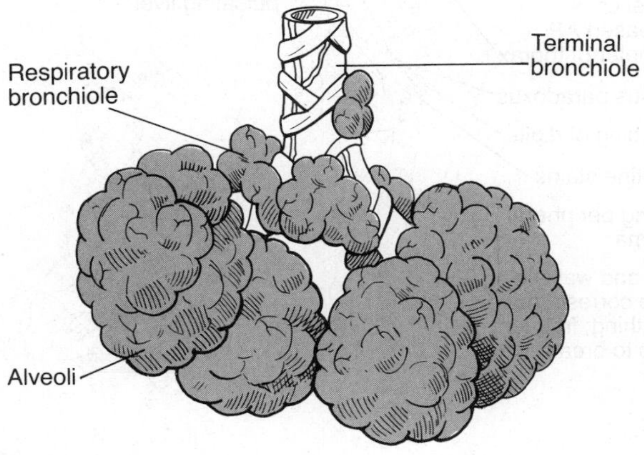

▲ *Figure 39-2*

Types of emphysema.

septa collapse, pockets of air form between the alveolar spaces (called blebs) and within the lung parenchyma (called bullae). This process leads to increased ventilatory "dead space," or areas that do not participate in gas or blood exchange. The work of breathing is increased because there is less functional lung tissue to exchange oxygen and carbon dioxide. Emphysema also causes destruction of the pulmonary capillaries, further decreasing the oxygen perfusion and ventilation. Some degree of emphysema is considered normal with aging, but if it occurs earlier in life, it is usually due to chronic bronchitis and cigarette smoking.

There are three types of emphysema. Centrilobular emphysema, the most common type, produces destruction in the bronchioles, usually in the upper lung regions. Inflammation develops in the bronchioles, but usually the alveolar sac remains intact. Panlobular emphysema destroys the air spaces of the entire acinus and most commonly involves the lower lung. These forms of emphysema, collectively called centriacinar emphysema, occur most often in smokers. Paraseptal (or panacinar) emphysema destroys the alveoli in the lower lobes of the lungs resulting in isolated blebs along the lung periphery. Paraseptal emphysema is believed to be the likely cause of spontaneous pneumothorax. A small number of clients with CAL have an inherited deficiency of alpha$_1$-antitrypsin (AAT), a nonspecific proteolytic enzyme inhibitor. Normally, AAT inhibits the action of enzymes that break down proteins. Clients without AAT have increased risk of CAL because the walls of the lung are at higher risk of destruction. Interestingly, cigarette smoking is thought to alter the balance of these enzymes and increase the destruction of the lung tissue. Panacinar emphysema occurs in the elderly and in clients with alpha$_1$-antitrypsin deficiency (Fig. 39–2).

As the disease progresses, there is increasing dyspnea and pulmonary infection. Eventually cor pulmonale (right-sided congestive heart failure) develops.

Clinical Manifestations

Recall that all three disorders, asthma, chronic bronchitis, and emphysema, are present to some degree in the client with CAL. Figure 39–3 illustrates the common physical findings in the client with CAL.

Chronic Bronchitis (Box 39–2). Clients who have chronic obstructive bronchitis as their major disease experience productive cough, decreased exercise tolerance, wheezing, and shortness of breath. Spirometry shows airway obstruction (decreased FEV$_1$). The clients will have prolonged expiration and an elevated hematocrit level. A history of smoking, cyanosis, and symptoms of cor pulmonale are also common.

Emphysema (Box 39–3). Clients who have primary emphysema have marked dyspnea on exertion that later progresses to dyspnea at rest. Cough is uncommon. The client is often thin, has tachypnea with prolonged expiration, and uses the accessory muscles for respiration. The client often leans forward with arms braced on the knees to support the shoulders and chest for breathing. The anteroposterior diameter of the chest is enlarged (Fig. 39–4) and the chest has hyper-

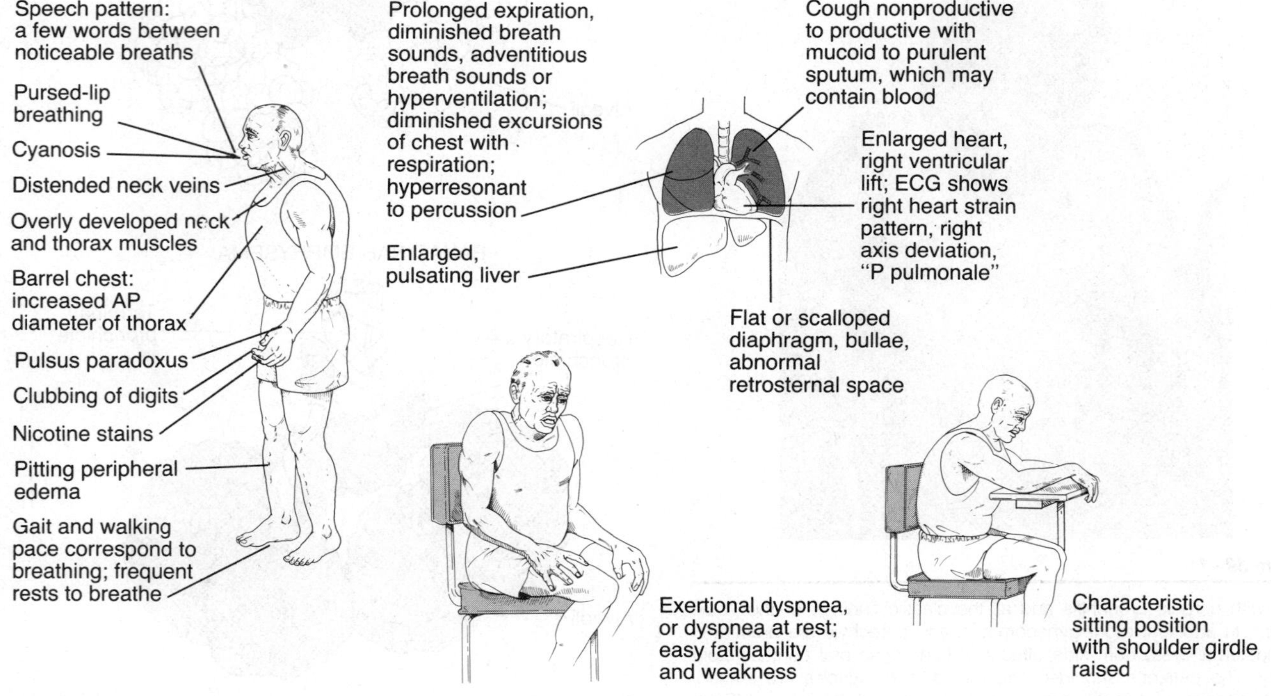

▲ *Figure 39–3*

Clinical manifestations associated with CAL (COPD).

Box 39–2. Clinical Manifestations of Chronic Bronchitis

General Appearance

Tendency to overweight; cyanotic secondary to polycythemia; dependent edema secondary to right-sided heart failure; barrel chest

Age Range

45–65 years

Assessment Findings

Persistent cough, copious sputum production; variable levels of dyspnea; variable wheezing on expiration; frequent respiratory infections

Symptoms usually occur over a long period of time.

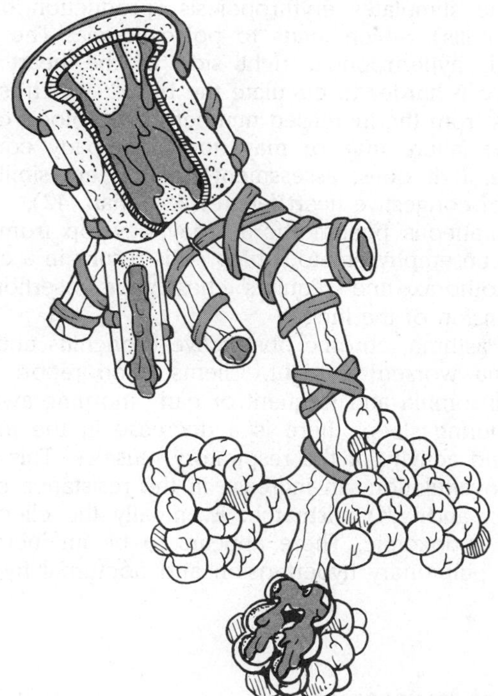

Cardiac Involvement

Enlarged heart; cor pulmonale; hematocrit > 60%.

Smoking History

Invariably, a long history of smoking

Diagnostic Findings

Pulmonary Function

Small airways affected early (reduced $FEF_{25-75\%}$); FEV_1 reduced later as airway damage progresses; normal to variable diffusion capacity

Arterial Blood Gases

Increased $PaCO_2$ common; hypoxemia usually present and increasing in severity as disease progresses

Chest Film

Chest film shows normal or "dirty" chest with increased bronchovascular markings

Overview

Bronchioles narrowed as a result of thickened mucous membrane; surrounding tissue inflamed

Mucus and pus impede action of respiratory cilia

Box 39–3. Clinical Manifestations of Emphysema

General Appearance

Thin; pink skin color; flattened hemidiaphragms

No signs of right-sided heart failure with dependent edema until end stage

Age Range

65–75 years

Assessment Findings

Persistent shortness of breath with gradual progressive exertional dyspnea

Infrequent respiratory infections

On auscultation, diminished breath sounds even with deep breathing.

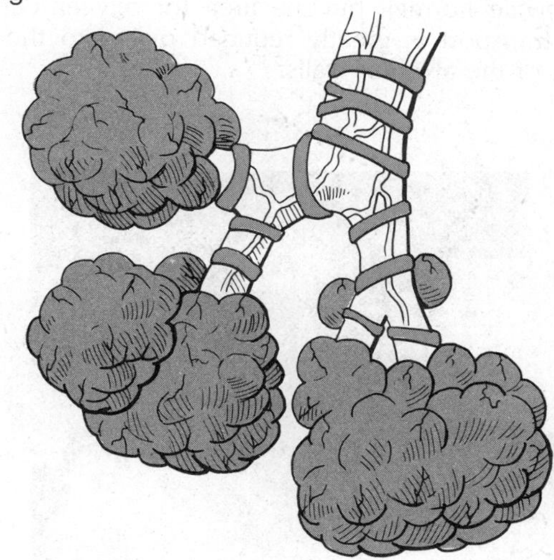

Expiratory wheezing not a prominent finding

Rare sputum production and cough

Cardiac Involvement

No cardiac enlargement; cor pulmonale late; hematocrit < 60%

Smoking History

Usually, but not always, a smoking history

Diagnostic Findings

Pulmonary Function

Reduced $FEF_{25-75\%}$ and FEV_1; reduced diffusion capacity due to destruction of alveoli

Arterial Blood Gases

$PaCO_2$ usually low or normal until end stage; mild to moderate hypoxemia

Chest Film

Chest film shows overinflation, flattened diaphragms, increased retrosternal air space, and increased lucency of lower lung fields

Overview

Walls of individual air sacs torn; repair not possible

Small bronchioles collapse, trapping air; exhalation difficult

Lung tissue becomes inelastic; lungs enlarged

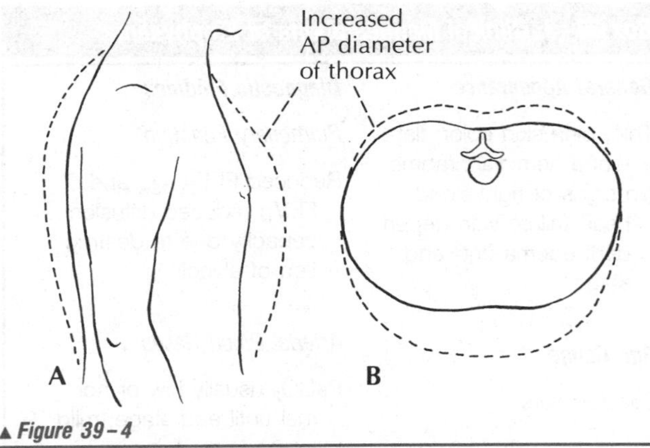

▲ *Figure 39-4*

Chest wall changes associated with COPD. Heavy lines indicate a normal thorax. Dotted lines indicate changes occurring with COPD. The chest becomes barrel shaped.

resonant sounds to percussion. ABGs are usually normal until later stages. These clients have come to be known as "pink puffers" because of their normal arterial oxygen levels and dyspnea (Fig. 39-5).

Pulmonary function tests reveal decreased FVC and FEV_1. There is an increase in FRC, RV, and TLC. TLC can be twice normal, but the area for oxygen/carbon dioxide transport is greatly reduced owing to the destruction of the alveolar walls.

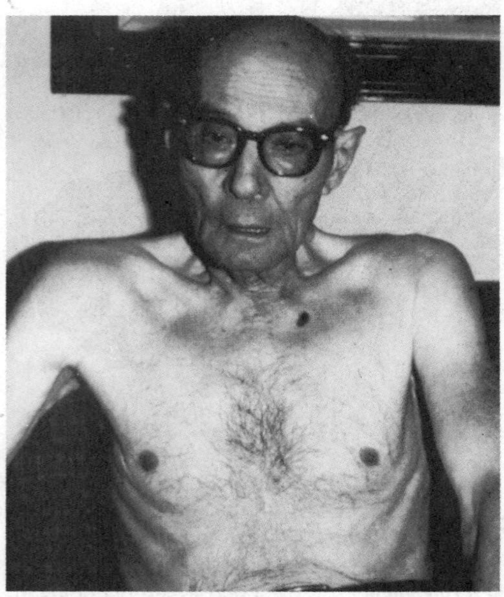

▲ *Figure 39-5*

Client with emphysema and all the classic findings of the "pink puffer." Use of accessory muscles of respiration (intercostal, neck, and shoulder muscles) and the cachectic appearance reflect two factors: (1) shortness of breath, client's most disturbing complaint, and (2) the tremendous increased work of breathing necessary to increase minute ventilation and maintain normal arterial blood gases. (From Kersten, L. D. [1989]. *Comprehensive respiratory nursing.* Philadelphia: W. B. Saunders.)

Asthma. Asthma is one component of the triad of CAL. Asthma is a reactive airway disorder because allergens cause the airways to react in bronchospasm. Reactive airways increase mucus production (bronchitis). The two disorders of bronchospasm and increased mucus are called asthmatic bronchitis. Many clients with CAL have some degree of asthma in that they have wheezing and bronchospasm. Asthma can also occur alone.

Complications

Respiratory infections commonly develop in clients with CAL as a result of alterations in the normal respiratory defense mechanisms and decreased immune resistance. Because respiratory status is already compromised, infection frequently leads to acute respiratory failure and is a common reason for hospitalization.

The client often develops cor pulmonale (chronic enlargement of the heart's right ventricle) owing to increased cardiac workload. As CAL progresses, hypoxemia leads to pulmonary vasoconstriction. To pump blood through the narrowed vessels, the right side of the heart must generate high pressures; over time, the right ventricle enlarges and thickens. Additionally, hypoxemia stimulates erythropoiesis (production of red blood cells), which leads to polycythemia. The overworked, hypertrophied right side of the heart must work even harder to circulate the blood, which is now viscous from the increased number of red blood cells.

Heart failure may or may not accompany cor pulmonale. If it does, assessment findings are similar to those of congestive heart failure (see Chap. 42).

Spontaneous pneumothorax may develop from rupture of an emphysematous bleb. This results in a closed pneumothorax and requires chest tube insertion for reexpansion of the lung.

Like asthma, chronic obstructive bronchitis and emphysema worsen at night. Clients often report sleep onset insomnia and frequent or early morning awakenings. During sleep, there is a decrease in the muscle tone and activity of the respiratory muscles. This leads to hypoventilation, an increase in the resistance of the airways, and V/Q mismatch. Eventually the client becomes hypoxemic. There appears to be an increased risk of pulmonary hypertension and nocturnal hypoxemia.

Medical Management

The main goals for the client with CAL are to improve oxygenation and decrease carbon dioxide retention. These are accomplished by (1) relieving the portion of the airway obstruction that is reversible (asthma), (2) facilitating the elimination of bronchial secretions, (3) preventing and treating respiratory infection, (4) increasing exercise tolerance, (5) controlling complications, (6) avoiding airway irritants/allergens, and (7) relieving anxiety and treating depression that often accompany CAL.

PHARMACOLOGIC MANAGEMENT

Common classifications of medications used in the treatment of CAL include bronchodilators, antihistamines, steroids, antibiotics, expectorants, and mast cell membrane stabilizers. In addition, Pneumovax and the flu vaccines should be taken yearly. The medications are listed in Table 37-1. Narcotics, tranquilizers, and sedatives are used with caution in treatment of CAL because they depress the respiratory center.

There are some ongoing studies examining the effect of alpha$_1$-antitrypsin replacement therapy. The future looks promising for the treatment of early emphysema with the replacement of this protective enzyme inhibitor.

Oxygen is used when the client has severe exertional or at rest hypoxemia (PaO_2 below 40 mm Hg). One to 3 L oxygen by nasal cannula is required to raise PaO_2 to 60 to 80 mm Hg. Oxygen is used cautiously in clients with emphysema; the normal respiratory drive is obliterated because of the long-standing hypercapnia, and carbon dioxide retention can occur. Cautions for use of oxygen are discussed in Chapter 37.

PULMONARY HYGIENE

Pulmonary hygiene is used to rid the lungs of secretions and thereby improve ciliary action and reduce the risk of infection. In the hospital, the client may be treated with nebulized bronchodilators and the use of positive-pressure airflow or positive end-expiratory pressure devices to increase the caliber of the airways. In addition, postural drainage and chest physiotherapy may be prescribed to move the secretions from the small to the large airways, from which they can be expelled.

EXERCISE

Exercise does not improve lung function. Instead, it is used to enhance cardiovascular fitness and train skeletal muscles to function more effectively. Progressively increased walking is the most common form of exercise. Before a walking program is begun, ABGs should be assessed and compared with resting levels. Supplemental oxygen should be used during exercise if the client becomes severely hypoxemic.

Breathing exercises may also be prescribed. Diaphragmatic breathing should be encouraged, and the client should be discouraged from rapid, shallow "panic" breathing.

CONTROLLING COMPLICATIONS

Edema and cor pulmonale are treated with diuretics and digitalis for improving cardiac function. Phlebotomy may be used to reduce blood volume in clients with marked elevations in hematocrit (over 60 percent). Phlebotomy reduces blood volume and thereby reduces cardiac workload. At times, the client must receive continuous mechanical ventilation (CMV) for adequate oxygenation, although it is usually difficult to wean the client from CMV.

AVOIDING IRRITANTS

Known allergens should be avoided. Smoking should cease. All clients with CAL should avoid high altitudes, and supplemental oxygen may be required for air travel. No specific climate has been shown to alter the course of the disorder.

PSYCHOLOGICAL SUPPORT

Clients with CAL often continue to deteriorate despite the medical care given. It is difficult to cope with failing health that limits activity and employment. As much as possible, the client should be encouraged to live an active life with daily exercise.

DIETARY MANAGEMENT

Clients with CAL often have difficulty eating because of dyspnea. The client should be offered frequent small meals, rather than large meals. Oxygen delivery devices should be adjusted so that the mouth is not obstructed but oxygen is delivered through the nose during eating.

Surgical Management

Surgery is uncommon for the treatment of CAL. At times, bullectomy may benefit clients who have repeated spontaneous pneumothorax. Bullectomy is the removal of large bullae that compress the lung and add to dead space.

Nursing Management

ASSESSMENT

Nursing History. The nursing history can assist the nurse in determining many aspects about the client. The nurse can ascertain whether the client's symptoms are those of chronic bronchitis, emphysema, or asthma. In addition, the nurse can determine the ability of the client to recognize the signs and symptoms that require further care. For example, if a client says "I knew I was developing an infection and went to the doctor," the statement indicates an understanding of the disorder. In contrast, if another client does not fully understand the reasons for hospitalization, the nurse will need to teach the client about CAL. A review of past medical history will help determine whether the client has other disorders that have impact on treatment (such as heart disease) and the current medications.

A thorough history may need to be delayed until the client is able to breathe comfortably, or it may be taken over short periods of time or obtained through the family.

Physical Assessment. The nurse should collect data with an emphasis on the respiratory and cardiac system. The degree of dyspnea, amount of activity, and signs of congestive heart failure should be noted. ABGs should be analyzed to determine the adequacy of oxygenation and possible need for oxygen.

Psychosocial Assessment. When assessing the client with CAL, the nurse should consider the possible effects of decreased oxygenation on the central nervous system. Hypoxemia may result in impaired cognition.

The nurse should consider the impact of stressors that may have led to exacerbations of CAL. Possible factors may include the progressive illness itself, marital problems, or financial concerns. Another portion of the psychosocial assessment is reviewing coping strategies that the client normally uses. It is important to determine whether these strategies are working now and if not, why not. Support systems, such as friends and family, are also important components of psychosocial stability. The reliability of the client's support system should be determined.

NURSING INTERVENTION

There are several nursing diagnoses that can occur in the client with CAL. They are listed in the Care Plan for the client with CAL (see also Bridge to Home Health Care).

Modification of Plan of Care for the Elderly

The elderly client frequently has other problems that influence the treatment of CAL. For example, the client may have decreased exercise tolerance, impaired nutrition, or a long-standing habit of smoking that retards rehabilitation. The nurse should also consider the possibility of drug-drug interactions.

Post-hospital Care

Home oxygen therapy may be required by the client with COPD. Clients and their families should be instructed in the proper use of this therapy, including potential hazards and complications (see discussion in Chap. 37).

DISCHARGE TEACHING

In order to facilitate self-care and adherence, the client and significant others need thorough information about the disease process and prescribed medications and treatments. The signs and symptoms of impending respiratory problems (e.g., increased confusion or drowsiness) and right-sided heart failure (e.g., peripheral edema, distended neck veins) should be reviewed so that prompt intervention can be obtained should complications develop. Teaching should include a discussion of the hazards of infection and ways to decrease personal risk (i.e., avoid crowds during flu and cold season, obtain immunization against influenza and pneumococcal organisms, cleanse respiratory equipment well). Emphasis should also be placed on the avoidance of exposure to respiratory irritants such as smoke, dust, mold, and severe air pollution, which can increase mucus production and cause bronchospasm.

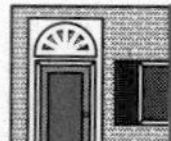

BRIDGE TO HOME HEALTH CARE

Oxygen Conservation Activities for the CAL Client

At home, the client with CAL needs to think of himself or herself as an active person. At the same time, he or she must choose activities that will conserve oxygen, improve breathing, and prevent infection.

Activity balanced with rest will conserve oxygen. Teaching pursed-lip breathing will immediately assist the client through activities of daily living. Smaller, more frequent, balanced meals will decrease shortness of breath when eating. Air pollution should be avoided. Cigarette smoking irritates the lung tissue by causing an increased secretion of mucus, which leads to infection and long-term damage. Other irritants to avoid are hair sprays, dust, and cold weather. Gradually increasing exercise builds strength and endurance; walking is an ideal form of exercise.

After leaving the hospital environment, infection control becomes the client's responsibility. Keeping mucus thin by increasing fluid intake to 8 to 10 glasses of water daily makes coughing and expectoration of mucus easier and avoids pooling of mucus in the lungs. Avoiding crowds and smoke-filled environments lessens exposure to upper respiratory infections. Teaching the client to report changes in the color of his or her sputum to the home health care nurse or the physician will ensure early treatment of infection. The client who thinks of himself or herself as an active person will make the most successful transition to the home environment.

FOLLOW-UP

Ongoing respiratory assessment is essential. Annual ABG analysis, pulmonary function tests, and noninvasive monitoring (see Chap. 37) are often required.

TRACHEOBRONCHITIS

Overview

Acute tracheobronchitis is an inflammation of the mucous membranes of the trachea and the bronchial tree. This disorder commonly follows viral infections of the upper respiratory tract. However, it may also result from inhalation of noxious or irritating gases and particulate matter (including cigarette smoke), bacterial

Text continued on page 1038

CARE PLAN

The Client with CAL

Nursing Diagnosis/ Collaborative Problem	Planning: Expected Outcomes	Implementation: Nursing Interventions	Rationales
Gas Exchange, Impaired R/T decreased ventilation and mucus plugs	The client will maintain adequate gas exchange, AEB blood gas values (i.e., PaO_2 of at least 60 mm Hg, pH within normal limits, and $PaCO_2$ at baseline)	1. Regularly monitor respiratory rate and pattern, ABG results, and signs of hypoxia/hypercapnia. Report significant changes promptly.	1. Prompt recognition of deteriorating respiratory function can reduce potentially lethal outcomes.
		2. Administer low-flow oxygen therapy (1–3 L/min 24–31% FIO_2) as needed via nasal prongs or high-flow venturi mask (24 to 31 per cent FIO_2).	2. Oxygen corrects existing hypoxemia. Excessive increases in oxygen (55 to 70 per cent FIO_2) may diminish respiratory drive and further increase carbon dioxide retention.
		3. Assist client into high-Fowler's position.	3. The upright position allows full lung excursion and enhances air exchange.
		4. Administer bronchodilators if ordered. Monitor for side effects.	4. Bronchodilators relax bronchial smooth muscle, facilitating airflow. Common side effects include tremor, tachycardia, and other cardiac dysrhythmias.
		5. Use caution when administering narcotics, sedatives, and tranquilizers.	5. These medications are respiratory depressants and can further impair ventilation.
Airway Clearance, Ineffective R/T excessive secretions and ineffective coughing	The client will have improved airway clearance, AEB effective coughing techniques and maintaining patent airways	1. Teach client to maintain adequate hydration by a. drinking at least 8–10 glasses of fluid/day (if not contraindicated) b. increasing humidity of environmental air	1. Hydration helps to thin secretions.
		2. Teach and supervise effective coughing techniques (Chap. 37)	2. Proper coughing techniques conserve energy, reduce airway collapse, and lessen client frustration.
		3. Perform chest physical therapy, if needed, and instruct client/significant others in these techniques (Chap. 37).	3. Chest physical therapy techniques utilize forces of gravity and motion to facilitate secretion removal.
		4. Assess breath sounds before and after coughing episodes.	4. This assessment will help in the evaluation of coughing effectiveness.

Care Plan continued on following page

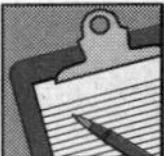

CARE PLAN

The Client with CAL Continued

Nursing Diagnosis/ Collaborative Problem	Planning: Expected Outcomes	Implementation: Nursing Interventions	Rationales
Activity Intolerance R/T inadequate oxygenation and dyspnea	The client will have improved activity tolerance, AEB maintaining a realistic activity level and demonstrating use of energy conservation techniques	1. Advise client to avoid conditions that increase oxygen demand, such as smoking, temperature extremes, excess weight, and stress.	1. These factors increase peripheral vascular resistance, which increases cardiac workload and oxygen requirements.
		2. Instruct client in energy conservation techniques such as pacing activities throughout the day, interspersed with adequate rest periods, and alternating high- and low-energy tasks.	2. Conservation techniques allow the client to accomplish more tasks, with a limited energy supply.
		3. Assist client to schedule a gradual increase in daily activities and exercise.	3. Gradual increases in physical activity improve respiratory and cardiac conditioning, thus improving activity tolerance.
		4. Teach the client to use pursed-lip and diaphragmatic breathing techniques during activities (Chap. 37).	4. Breathing retraining ensures maximal use of available respiratory function. Pursed-lip breathing leaves positive end-diastolic pressure in the lungs and helps keep airways open.
		5. Schedule active exercise after respiratory therapy or medication (e.g., bronchodilator in metered dose inhaler).	5. Lung function is maximized during peak periods of treatment/drug effect.
		6. Maintain supplemental oxygen therapy, as needed.	6. Supplemental oxygen helps alleviate exercise-induced hypoxemia, thus improving activity tolerance.
		7. Assess patient for signs of a negative response to activity (e.g., significant change in respiratory rate, failure of pulse to return to near resting rate within 3 minutes of activity, changes in mental status).	7. Significant changes in respiratory, cardiac, or circulatory status signal activity intolerance.
Anxiety R/T acute breathing difficulties and fear of suffocation	The client will express an increase in psychological comfort and demonstrate use of effective coping mechanisms	1. Remain with client during acute episodes of breathing difficulty and provide care in a calm, reassuring manner.	1. Reassure the client that competent help is available, if needed. Anxiety can be contagious. The nurse must remain calm.
		2. Provide a quiet, calm environment.	2. Reduction of external stimuli helps promote relaxation.

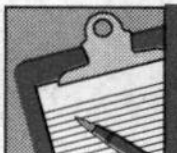

CARE PLAN

The Client with CAL Continued

Nursing Diagnosis/ Collaborative Problem	*Planning: Expected Outcomes*	*Implementation: Nursing Interventions*	*Rationales*
		3. During acute episodes, open doors and curtains and limit number of people and unnecessary equipment in client's room.	3. Environmental changes may lessen the client's perceptions of suffocation.
		4. Encourage the use of breathing retraining and relaxation techniques (Chap. 37).	4. A feeling of self-control and success in facilitating breathing will help reduce anxiety.
		5. Use sedatives and tranquilizers with extreme caution. Nonpharmaceutical methods of anxiety reduction are more useful.	5. Oversedation may cause respiratory depression.
Nutrition, Altered: Less than Body Requirements R/T reduced appetite, decreased energy level, and dyspnea	The client will maintain body weight within normal limits for sex and body build and hemoglobin and albumin levels within normal range	1. Promote mouth care before meals and as needed.	1. Coughing and sputum production may impair appetite. Mouthbreathing dries mucous membranes.
		2. Advise client to eat small, frequent meals (e.g., six meals a day).	2. Large meals may create an excessive feeling of fullness that may make breathing uncomfortable and difficult.
		3. Advise client to avoid gas-producing foods, such as beans and cabbage.	3. Gas-forming foods may cause abdominal bloating and distention and thus impair ventilation.
		4. Instruct client in the use of high-calorie liquid supplements, if indicated.	4. Increased calorie intake is needed to provide energy for increased work of breathing. Liquid supplements provide high-calorie concentrations in a relatively small volume.
		5. Advise hypoxemic clients to use oxygen via nasal cannula during meals.	5. Adequate oxygenation increases energy available for eating.
		6. Suggest methods to make meal preparation more convenient (e.g., Meals on Wheels program).	6. Reducing energy expenditure on preparation will maximize energy availability for eating.
		7. Monitor food intake, weight, and serum hemoglobin and albumin levels.	7. Changes in body weight reflect the degree of nutrition or malnutrition. Hemoglobin and albumin levels reflect protein intake.

Care Plan continued on following page

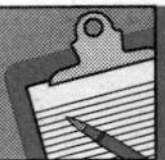

CARE PLAN

The Client with CAL Continued

Nursing Diagnosis/ Collaborative Problem	Planning: Expected Outcomes	Implementation: Nursing Interventions	Rationales
Sleep Pattern Disturbance R/T dyspnea and external stimuli	The client will report feeling adequately rested	1. Promote relaxation by providing a darkened, quiet environment; ensuring adequate room ventilation; and following bedtime routines, as possible.	1. The hospital environment can interfere with relaxation and sleep. Using established bedtime rituals increases relaxation.
		2. Schedule care activities to allow periods of uninterrupted sleep.	2. For most people, completing four to five complete sleep cycles (60–90 minutes) per night promotes a feeling of being rested.
		3. Instruct client in measures to promote sleep:	3.
		a. Plan physical exercise during the day and passive, nonstimulating activities in the evening.	a. Activity increases the need for sleep and contributes to a feeling of "tiredness."
		b. Avoid stimulants, such as caffeine.	b. Stimulants increase metabolism and inhibit relaxation.
		c. Maintain a consistent bedtime and a regular bedtime routine.	c. Consistency promotes relaxation and prevents disruptions of the biologic clock.
		d. Eat a high-protein snack before bedtime.	d. Protein digestion produces tryptophan, an amino acid that has a sedative effect.
		e. Use relaxation techniques (e.g., meditation, massage, warm bath, warm beverage).	e. Sleep is difficult unless the client is relaxed.
		4. If the client awakens during the night, suggest the use of a quiet, diverting activity, such as reading, in another room.	4. Frustration over being awake will further deter sleep efforts. The bedroom should be mentally associated with sleep to enhance future sleep promotion.
		5. If dyspnea is severe, a recliner chair or hospital bed may be more comfortable than a regular bed.	5. The upright position facilitates ventilation.

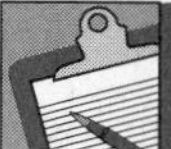

CARE PLAN

The Client with CAL Continued

Nursing Diagnosis/ Collaborative Problem	Planning: Expected Outcomes	Implementation: Nursing Interventions	Rationales
Family Processes, Altered R/T chronic illness of a family member	The family will verbalize their feelings, participate in the care of the ill family member, and seek external resources as needed	1. Plan intervention considering the client and significant others as the unit of care. Encourage participation in the planning process.	1. CAL affects not only the client experiencing the condition but also the client's significant others.
		2. Assess family communication patterns and intervene if ineffective. Family counseling may be needed.	2. Effective communication helps each member to understand their own and others' feelings. Counseling may facilitate healthy interaction.
		3. Encourage as wide a social support system as feasible.	3. The use of various support people prevents a few family members from being overloaded with responsibility.
		4. Encourage the client and family to seek support from other sources (e.g., self-help groups and support groups such as Better Breathers Clubs sponsored by the American Lung Association).	4. Clients may benefit from opportunities to share common experiences and learn from others in similar situations.
		5. Provide the family with anticipatory guidance as client's CAL progresses.	5. Knowing what to expect facilitates family adjustment.
High Risk for Sexual Dysfunction, R/T dyspnea, reduced energy, and changes in relationships	The client will report increased satisfaction with sexual function	1. Provide opportunity for client to discuss concerns.	1. Many people are embarrassed or reluctant to talk about their sexual concerns.
		2. Suggest measures that may facilitate sexual activity (e.g., alternative positions, use of bronchodilator therapy before beginning sexual activity).	2. Such measures can reduce physical exertion and maximize available oxygen levels.
		3. Encourage client and partner to consider other forms of sexual expression (e.g., hugging, cuddling, stroking, kissing).	3. Alternative methods require less energy expenditure than does intercourse.
		4. Refer to a professional skilled in sexuality, if appropriate.	4. Talking with a skilled professional may further assist client with constructive problem solving.

pneumonia, overvigorous tracheobronchial suctioning, and harsh paroxysms of coughing.

Clinical manifestations of tracheobronchitis include a raw burning pain over the upper anterior chest wall over the midsternum. Pain is increased with exposure to very cold environments, cigarette smoke, cough, and tracheobronchial suctioning. In addition, the client may have a cough that progresses from dry to productive as the irritation increases. Fever, headache and malaise may also be present.

Management

Treatment is focused on the cause of the cough. Cough suppressants are rarely effective. Antibiotics, bronchodilators, corticosteroids (inhaled and systemic), and anticholenergics are the mainstream of treatment. Sinusitis is a common accompanying finding, as well as the etiology of tracheobronchitis

Priority nursing goals include the relief of pain and elimination of the tracheal irritation. Strongly advise the client to stop smoking. Whenever possible, eliminate other irritating gases or substances from the environment. Promote airway clearance by encouraging effective coughing (Chap. 37), increasing fluid intake, changing positions, and increasing inspired humidity. Inspired humidity may be increased through the use of aerosols. Administer prescribed medications. Cold environmental air should be avoided if possible, or the client should cover the mouth and nose before going outdoors and enter a warmed car.

Observe for cough-related syncope. Lightheadedness or fainting may occur with forceful coughing spells. This is due to prolonged elevation of intrapulmonary pressure during the compressive phase of a cough. The increased pressure impairs venous return to the thorax, causing a decrease in cardiac output. Cerebral ischemia and fainting may result.

BRONCHIECTASIS

Bronchiectasis is a form of obstructive lung disease. It is an extreme form of bronchitis. This disorder causes permanent, abnormal dilation and distortion of bronchi and bronchioles. It develops when bronchial walls are weakened by chronic inflammatory changes in the bronchial mucosa.

Bronchiectasis most often develops after recurrent inflammatory conditions, following infection or obstruction. However, any condition producing a narrowing of the lumen of the bronchioles may create bronchiectasis, including tuberculosis, adenoviral infections, and pneumonia. Some forms of bronchiectasis are congenital and are associated with cystic fibrosis, sinusitis, dextrocardia (heart located on right side of chest), and alterations in ciliary activity (Kartagener's syndrome). Bronchiectasis is usually localized to a lung lobe or segment rather than generalized throughout the lungs. At times, however, persistent, nonresolving infection may cause the disorder to spread to other parts of the same lung. Diagnosis may be confirmed through chest X-ray study, bronchogram or chest CT scan.

Clinical manifestations vary according to the etiologic agent. The main manifestations are cough and purulent sputum production in voluminous quantities. Fever, hemoptysis, nasal stuffiness, and drainage from sinusitis are also common. The client may complain of fatigue and weakness, and clubbing may be found on physical assessment.

Medical and nursing management of bronchiectasis are the same as for CAL. Most cases are managed medically to prevent progression of the disorder and control symptoms. Antibiotics, chest physical therapy, hydration, bronchodilators, and oxygen are commonly prescribed. Severe cases may be treated by surgical resection if the pathologic process is well localized in one lobe or two adjacent lobes and when no contraindications to surgery exist.

▼ PARENCHYMAL DISORDERS

ATELECTASIS

Overview

Atelectasis denotes the collapse of lung tissue at any structural level (e.g., segmental, basilar, lobar, microscopic). It develops when there is interference with the natural forces that promote lung expansion. Such interference may result from a reduction in lung distending forces, localized airway obstruction, insufficient pulmonary surfactant, or increased elastic recoil. Examples of each of these causes are given in Box 39–4. It is

Box 39–4. Causes of Atelectasis

- Decreased lung distention forces
  - Pleural space encroachment (e.g., pneumothorax, pleural effusion, pleural tumor)
  - Chest wall disorders (e.g., kyphoscoliosis, flail chest)
  - Impaired diaphragmatic movement (e.g., ascites, obesity)
  - Central nervous system dysfunction (e.g., coma, neuromuscular disorders, oversedation)
- Localized airway obstruction
  - Mucus plugging
  - Foreign body aspiration
  - Bronchiectasis
- Insufficient pulmonary surfactant
  - Respiratory distress syndrome
  - Inhalation anesthesia
  - High concentrations of oxygen (oxygen toxicity)
  - Lung contusion
  - Aspiration of gastric contents
  - Smoke inhalation
- Increased elastic recoil
  - Interstitial fibrosis (e.g., silicosis, radiation pneumonitis)

particularly common in postoperative clients, especially those undergoing high abdominal or thoracic surgeries.

Atelectasis may be diagnosed by physical examination, although it is usually detected first by chest x-ray examination. Some clients are asymptomatic. If significant hypoxemia is present, dyspnea, tachypnea, tachycardia, and cyanosis may occur. Chest auscultation may reveal diminished breath sounds or crackles over the involved area. In severe forms, physical assessment findings may include (1) tracheal shift toward the side of the atelectasis, (2) decreased tactile fremitus over the affected lung area, (3) decreased percussion note over the atelectatic region, and (4) a decrease in size of the chest and decreased movement on the involved side. However, none of these signs is specific for atelectasis, and the entire clinical picture must be considered.

Management

One of the primary goals of nursing intervention is to prevent atelectasis in the high-risk client. Frequent position changes and early ambulation help promote drainage of all lung segments. Deep breathing and effective coughing enhance lung expansion and prevent airway obstruction. Hyperinflation therapy with use of an incentive spirometer (see Chap. 37) may also be helpful.

If atelectasis develops, treatment is directed toward the underlying cause. If the client becomes hypoxic, oxygen should be administered as prescribed. More aggressive measures to maintain airway patency, such as postural drainage, chest physiotherapy, or tracheal suctioning, may also be ordered. If an airway obstruction is causing atelectasis, bronchoscopy may be used to remove the material.

INFLUENZA

Overview

The term "flu" is often used inappropriately to describe many symptoms and disorders. Influenza actually refers to acute viral respiratory tract infections accompanied by fever. Influenza usually occurs seasonally in epidemic form. Clients most at risk for influenza include (1) very young children, (2) the elderly, (3) clients living in institutional situations, (4) clients with chronic diseases, and (5) health care personnel.

Influenza differs from a common cold primarily by its sudden onset and widespread occurrence within the population. Assessment findings with influenza include fever, myalgias (muscular pain), and cough. Influenza predisposes clients to complications such as viral bronchitis or pneumonia, bacterial pneumonia, and superinfections. Chest findings are usually negative unless pneumonia results. Clients with colds (1) are usually afebrile, (2) have malaise as a major systemic symptom, and (3) commonly produce nasal symptoms.

Management

Influenza is a communicable disease spread by droplet infection. Prevent the spread of this infection by encouraging clients with influenza to remain at home, practice frequent handwashing, and cover the nose and mouth when sneezing or coughing.

Encourage clients at risk for influenza to obtain annual immunization before the start of the "flu season," in the winter. Immunization controls influenza for many clients (e.g., elderly, clients with chronic illnesses, clients living in crowded environments). Those who have not been immunized and are exposed to influenza should obtain inoculation immediately. Clients allergic to eggs or who have a history of Guillain-Barré syndrome should not receive an influenza immunization. Additional protection may be prescribed by the daily short-term administration of the antiviral agent amantadine hydrochloride. This is effective against type A influenza virus only and does not replace immunization.

Intervention for influenza is based on assessment findings as they arise (e.g., supportive measures to relieve fever, myalgia, and cough).

PNEUMONIA

Definition

Pneumonia (pneumonitis) is an inflammatory process of lung parenchyma usually associated with a marked increase in interstitial and alveolar fluid.

Incidence

Little over a century ago, pneumonia was the leading cause of death in the United States. Whereas advances in antibiotic therapy have significantly improved disease outcomes, pneumonia still remains a major cause of morbidity and mortality, especially among the elderly. It accounts for more than 10 per cent of hospital admissions and occurs in about 5 per cent of clients who are admitted with other diagnoses.

Etiology

There are many causes, including bacteria, viruses, mycoplasmas, fungal agents, and protozoa. Pneumonia may also result from (1) aspiration of food, fluids, or vomitus or (2) inhalation of toxic or caustic chemicals, smoke, dusts, or gases. Pneumonia may complicate immobility and chronic illnesses. It often follows influenza.

Risk Factors

Pneumonia is most likely to occur when normal defense mechanisms are weakened or overcome by the

Box 39-5. Risk Factors Predisposing a Client to Pneumonia

- Smoking
- Air pollution
- Upper respiratory infection
- Altered consciousness: alcoholism, head injury, seizure disorder; drug overdose; general anesthesia
- Tracheal intubation (bypassing the upper airway)
- Prolonged immobility
- Immunosuppressive therapy: corticosteroids; cancer chemotherapy
- Nonfunctional immune system: AIDS
- Severe periodontal disease
- Prolonged exposure to especially virulent organisms
- Malnutrition
- Dehydration
- Chronic diseases: diabetes mellitus; heart disease; chronic lung disease; renal disease; cancer
- Prolonged debilitating disease
- Inhalation of noxious substances
- Aspiration of oral/gastric material
- Aspiration of foreign material (e.g., petroleum products)
- Chronically ill, elderly clients who generally have poor immune systems, often residing in group-living situations where there is an increased probability of disease transmission, especially through the respiratory system

virulence, quality, or number of organisms. Box 39-5 lists risk factors predisposing a client to pneumonia. Young or otherwise healthy clients may develop pneumonia as a consequence of upper respiratory or viral infections. Group living or working conditions may facilitate wide transmission.

General measures to reduce the incidence of pneumonia involve decreasing the proliferation and spread of pneumonia-causing organisms. Adequate nutrition and fluid intake and proper hygiene measures help maintain normal defenses. Resistance is also enhanced by avoiding cigarette smoke, which decreases the ciliary clearance of secretions. Clients at risk for the development of pneumonia, especially those with chronic diseases, should avoid exposure to infected clients.

In the hospital, rigorous handwashing by medical personnel is essential for reducing the transmission of infectious agents. Proper infection control measures of respiratory equipment are vital. Effective airway clearance and mobilization (e.g., coughing, turning, early ambulation) should be promoted, particularly in clients at risk.

Pathophysiology

The common feature of all types of pneumonia is an inflammatory pulmonary response to the offending organism or agent. Infectious agents are usually introduced by inhalation. The defense mechanisms of the lungs lose effectiveness and allow organisms to penetrate the lower airways, in which inflammation develops. Organisms may also be introduced into the pulmonary system via the bloodstream. Circulating organisms that are too large to flow through the pulmonary capillary bed become lodged in the lungs, leading to a potential source of infection.

BACTERIA ASSOCIATED WITH PNEUMONIA

Gram-Positive Bacteria

Streptococcus pneumoniae (Pneumococcal Pneumonia). This is the most common cause of community-acquired pneumonia. Pneumococcal pneumonia often follows influenza and is frequently seen in clients with chronic diseases, immunosuppression, and alcohol abuse. Immunization is available and is effective against at least 23 strains of the pneumococcal organism. A single dose is usually protective for a lifetime.

Staphylococcus aureus. This organism usually reaches the lungs through the blood or by aspiration. Incidence is highest among hospitalized adult clients, but it is also common in diabetics, drug abusers, and clients on hemodialysis. The organism can be quite virulent, causing considerable morbidity and mortality despite appropriate antibiotic therapy. Toxins associated with the staphylococcus organism can cause extensive parenchymal tissue necrosis.

Gram-Negative Bacteria

Haemophilus influenzae. This organism is a common cause of infection in children and in clients with chronic debilitating diseases, chronic airway limitations, or immune defects. *H. influenzae* may affect multiple lobes of the lungs and has a high mortality rate, especially among the elderly. It may also cause infections at other sites (e.g., epiglottitis, endocarditis, meningitis).

Pseudomonas aeruginosa. *Pseudomonas* is the most common cause of hospital-acquired gram-negative pneumonia. This organism thrives in warm, moist environments such as respiratory therapy equipment and liquid soap dispensers. It is common in the respiratory tract of hospital employees and in clients with cystic fibrosis. In addition to the lungs, *Pseudomonas* may infect wounds, burns, tracheostomies, and the urinary tract.

Klebsiella pneumoniae (Friedländer's Bacillus). This is the most common gram-negative organism encountered outside the hospital setting. The incidence of *Klebsiella* pneumonia is increased among the elderly and those with chronic debilitating disease. It is also common in hospitalized clients with complicated or prolonged illnesses. The organism reaches the lung most frequently through aspiration of oropharyngeal secretions. Necrosis, abscess formation, hemoptysis, and permanent fibrotic lung changes may occur, leading to a high mortality rate.

Anaerobic Bacteria. Anaerobic bacterial pneumonias are commonly caused by anaerobic streptococcus, *Fusobacteria*, and *Bacteroides* species. Infection usually develops after aspiration of oropharyngeal secretions. Altered consciousness (from alcohol, coma, or seizures), impaired swallowing mechanisms, or poor dentition are often the precipitating causes. The infection is commonly insidious in onset. Sputum is usually foul smelling but may not appear for 7 days after infection. The chest film typically reveals lung abscess, empyema, and necrotizing pneumonia, with primary involvement in dependent lung zones (especially the right lung, in which aspirated secretions tend to settle). Accurate culture identification may require the use of a sheathed brush to obtain a specimen during fiberoptic bronchoscopy. This device allows the maintenance of an environment that is as anaerobic as possible and reduces cross-contamination with other upper airway flora.

Atypical Bacteria

***Legionella pneumophila* (Legionnaires' disease).** This organism was first identified in 1976 after a major outbreak of pneumonia at an American Legion convention in Philadelphia that resulted in 29 deaths. The organism was traced to a contaminated air conditioning system but has also been isolated from soil; construction workers and those living near soil excavations are at risk. Legionnaires' disease is most commonly seen in older adults, smokers, or others with impaired lung defenses. Diagnosis may be made through serologic testing.

Mycoplasma pneumoniae. This organism has characteristics of both bacteria and viruses. It is transmitted by droplet infection and spreads rapidly in settings where people live or work closely together (e.g., dormitories, military units). *M. pneumoniae* accounts for about 20 to 40 per cent of the pneumonias affecting ambulatory clients. Onset is often insidious, with slowly rising fever, headache, malaise, and nonproductive cough.

VIRUSES ASSOCIATED WITH PNEUMONIA

Many different viruses are responsible for pneumonias in adults, including influenza, parainfluenza, and adenovirus. Most are community acquired; the resulting infection follows an insidious course, which is similar to the one seen in atypical pneumonias. Viral pneumonias are usually self-limiting and are treated symptomatically. However, they will frequently lower the client's resistance, which increases the risk of a secondary bacterial pneumonia.

FUNGI AND PROTOZOA ASSOCIATED WITH PNEUMONIA

Fungi and protozoa are opportunistic organisms; they become pathogenic only when the client's physiologic state is altered and normal bacterial flora are suppressed. Opportunistic pneumonias are commonly seen after extended antibiotic use and in clients who are immunosuppressed (e.g., clients taking corticosteroids or antineoplastics; clients with acquired immunodeficiency syndrome [AIDS]) or severely debilitated. These forms of pneumonia are not spread by person-to-person contact. Common fungal infections include candidiasis, histoplasmosis, aspergillosis, coccidioidomycosis, and cryptococcosis. Protozoan infection is most common with *Pneumocystis carinii* pneumonia, typically seen in the client with AIDS.

Clinical Manifestations

The onset of all pneumonias is generally marked by any or all of the following: fever, chills, sweats, pleuritic chest pain, cough, sputum production, hemoptysis, dyspnea, headache, or fatigue. The elderly client, however, may present not with fever or respiratory symptoms but with altered mental status and volume depletion.

Chest auscultation reveals bronchial breath sounds over areas of consolidation (i.e., dense areas on the chest film). Consolidated lung tissue transmits bronchial sound waves to outer lung fields. Crackling sounds (from fluid in interstitial and alveolar areas) and whispered pectoriloquy may be heard over affected areas. Tactile fremitus is usually increased over areas of pneumonia. Percussion is dulled over affected areas. Unequal chest wall expansion may occur during inspiration if a large area of lung tissue is involved. This is due to decreased distensibility in the affected area.

Assessment findings with specific types of pneumonia are shown in Table 39-3.

DIAGNOSTIC ASSESSMENT

Definitive diagnosis is usually determined through sputum culture and sensitivity or serologic testing. At times, fiberoptic bronchoscopy or transcutaneous needle aspiration or biopsy may be necessary for confirmation. Additional diagnostic testing may include (1) skin tests, if tuberculosis or coccidioidomycosis is suspected; (2) blood and urine cultures to assess systemic spread; and (3) ABG analysis to assess the need for supplemental oxygen.

Chest x-ray examination provides information about the location and extent of pneumonia. On the chest film, areas of pneumonia appear as white opacification, that is, consolidation. At times, the outline of bronchi can be seen within the consolidation, which indicates that the bronchi are surrounded by water density. This is known as the air bronchogram sign.

Pneumonia may involve one or more lobe segments of the lungs (segmental pneumonia), one or more entire lobes (lobar pneumonia) (Fig. 39-6*A*), or entire lobes or segments of lobes in both lungs (bilateral pneumonia). On the basis of location and radiologic appearance, pneumonias may be classified as bronchopneumonia, interstitial pneumonia, alveolar pneumonia, or necrotizing pneumonia.

Bronchopneumonia (bronchial pneumonia) (Fig. 39-6*B*) involves the terminal bronchioles and alveoli. The radiologic appearance of bronchopneumonia is scat-

TABLE 39-3. Assessment and Treatment of Pneumonias

Common Name	Clinical Manifestations	Management
Pneumococcal pneumonia (caused by *Streptococcus pneumoniae*)	Sudden onset with a single shaking chill, high fever, stabbing, pleuritic chest pain, malaise, weakness, occasional vomiting, tachypnea, dyspnea, and elevated white blood cell count; single or multiple lobar consolidation on the chest film; cough productive of rusty brown or blood-streaked purulent sputum that turns yellow and mucoid	Primary: penicillin G intravenously or penicillin V orally Alternative: cephalosporins or erythromycin Prevention: vaccine available
Staphylococcal pneumonia (caused by *Staphylococcus aureus*)	Sudden onset with fever, multiple chills, pleuritic pain, dyspnea, rales, decreased breath sounds, elevated white blood cell count, and exaggerated cough productive of purulent golden-yellow or blood-streaked sputum; chest film may show patchy infiltrates, empyema, abscesses, and pneumothorax; disease may start with headache, cough, and myalgia	Primary: nafcillin or oxacillin Alternative: cephalosporins or vancomycin if client is sensitive to penicillin
H. flu pneumonia (caused by *Haemophilus influenzae*)	Similar to pneumococcal pneumonia; cough productive of apple- or lime-green purulent sputum, which may be blood-tinged	Primary: ampicillin or third-generation cephalosporins such as cefotaxime and moxalactam Alternative: chloramphenicol
Gram-negative bacterial pneumonia (most commonly caused by *Klebsiella pneumoniae*)	Sudden onset with high fever, multiple chills, pleuritic pain, dyspnea, cyanosis, and elevated white blood cell count; lobar consolidation and cavitation on the chest film; cough productive of red sputum resembling currant jelly—mucoid, sticky, and difficult to expectorate	Cephalosporins such as cefotaxime and aminoglycosides such as tobramycin
Anaerobic bacterial pneumonia, hypostatic pneumonia (caused by normal oral flora)	Insidious onset with low-grade fever, dyspnea, rales, cyanosis, hypertension, tachycardia, and elevated white blood cell count; patchy infiltrates in dependent lung segments on the chest film; cough productive of purulent greenish-yellow, foul-smelling sputum	Primary: third-generation cephalosporins (such as cefotaxime) or penicillin G Alternative: cefoxitin, clindamycin, or chloramphenicol
Legionnaires' disease (caused by *Legionella pneumophila*)	Prodrome of 24-48 hours with fever, headaches, and malaise followed by high fever with pulse-temperature dissociation, dyspnea, hypoxia, pleuritic pain, nausea, vomiting, diarrhea, confusion, and elevated white blood cell count; single or multilobar consolidation and small pleural effusions on the chest film; dry cough productive of scant mucoid or blood-tinged sputum	Primary: erythromycin Alternative: tetracycline or rifampin
Mycoplasma pneumonia (caused by *Mycoplasma* microorganisms)	Insidious onset with slowly rising fever, headache, myalgia, malaise, and normal white blood cell count; pulmonary infiltrate—sometimes extensive—on the chest film; cough productive of scant mucoid sputum; client may show only minimal signs and symptoms	Primary: erythromycin in severe cases Alternative: tetracycline

TABLE 39–3. Assessment and Treatment of Pneumonias Continued

Common Name	Clinical Manifestations	Management
Viral pneumonia (caused by influenza A virus)	Prodrome with headache and myalgia followed by high fever, dyspnea, normal breath sounds with occasional wheezing and rales, and normal or slightly elevated white blood cell count; diffuse, patchy infiltrates on the chest film; dry cough with initial mucoid sputum that later turns purulent; cough may be unproductive	None indicated

From Coleman, D. A. (1986). Pneumonia: where nursing care really counts. *RN*, *49*:23.

tered and fluffy with patchy shadows that follow the pathway of a lung's central conducting air passages but do not visibly outline the bronchi (i.e., no air bronchogram sign).

Interstitial (reticular) pneumonia involves inflammatory responses within lung tissue surrounding the air spaces or vascular structures, rather than the air passages themselves. Lacy networks of linear markings, often indicating chronic pulmonary changes (e.g., fibrosis), may be evident radiologically.

In alveolar (acinar) pneumonia, fluffy shadows are caused by fluid accumulation in a lung's distal air spaces. The shadows are small, are difficult to distinguish singly, and often coalesce (i.e., unite into a single group).

Necrotizing pneumonia causes the death of a portion of lung tissue, surrounded by viable tissue; x-ray examination may reveal cavity formation at the site of necrosis. Necrotic lung tissue, which does not heal, constitutes a permanent loss of functioning parenchyma.

Medical Management

The primary treatment for most forms of pneumonia is antibiotic therapy. Table 39–3 lists the drugs of choice for each form.

Hospitalization is not always necessary for clients with pneumonia. If the client has intact defense mechanisms and good general health, recuperation can often take place at home with rest and supportive treatment. The term "walking pneumonia" is sometimes used to describe this situation.

Clients who are ambulatory but have an ongoing health problem that predisposes them to pneumonia may require hospitalization. Similarly, clients who are already hospitalized for other reasons are at risk for developing nosocomial (hospital-acquired) pneumonias because of their decreased ability to combat infection and their potential exposure to resistant strains of organisms.

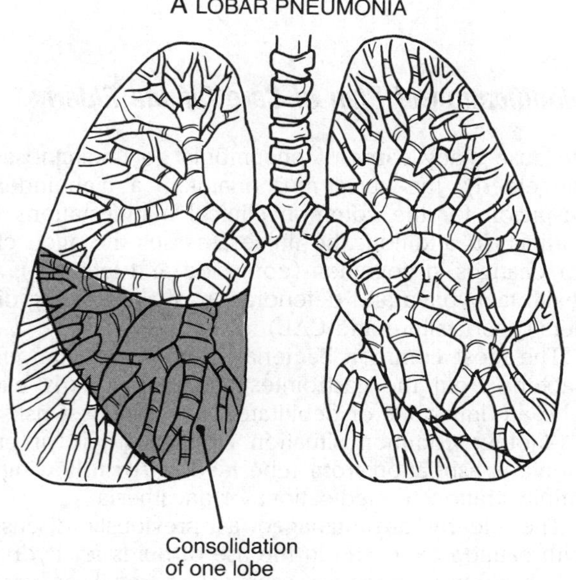

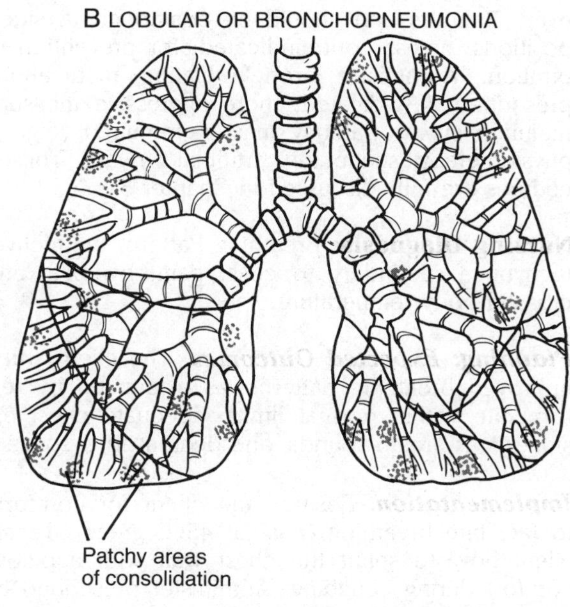

▲ *Figure 39–6*

Two types of pneumonia. *A*, Lobar pneumonia with consolidation in one lobe of one lung. *B*, Lobular or bronchopneumonia with patchy consolidation throughout both lungs.

Nursing Management

ASSESSMENT

The following should be determined through the nursing history:

- contact with other clients experiencing similar symptoms (suggests viral or mycoplasma pneumonia)
- factors suggesting the presence of noninfectious diseases that produce symptoms similar to those of pneumonia (e.g., pulmonary embolism, allergic or hypersensitivity reaction to drugs or other substances, neoplasm)
- presence of tuberculosis or contact with others who have active tuberculosis
- exposure to animals or birds (suggests certain diseases such as histoplasmosis or cryptococcosis)
- travel to areas where certain pulmonary diseases are common (e.g., Asia, Africa, South America)

Assess and monitor the client for possible hypersensitivity reactions, superinfections, altered renal function, and blood dyscrasias.

NURSING INTERVENTION

Nursing Diagnosis: Airway Clearance, Ineffective R/T inflammation and increased secretions.

Planning: Expected Outcomes. The client will maintain effective airway clearance, as evidenced by maintaining patent airway and effectively clearing secretions.

Implementation. Measures should be taken to promote airway patency. These may include increasing fluid intake, effective coughing and deep-breathing techniques, and frequent turning. Clients with an altered level of consciousness should be turned at least every 2 hours and should be positioned in side-lying positions, unless contraindicated, for prevention of aspiration. Administer bronchodilating medications as prescribed. If indicated, more aggressive measures to maintain airway patency may be required (e.g., chest physiotherapy, suctioning, artificial airway). These procedures are fully discussed in Chapter 37.

Nursing Diagnosis: Breathing Pattern, Ineffective R/T tachypnea secondary to chest pain, hypoxia, and increased body temperature.

Planning: Expected Outcomes. The client will have improved breathing patterns, as evidenced by respiratory rate within normal limits, adequate chest expansion, clear breath sounds, and decreased dyspnea.

Implementation. Position the client for comfort and to facilitate breathing (e.g., at 45 degrees). Teach the client how to splint the chest wall with a pillow for comfort during coughing. Administer prescribed cough suppressants and analgesics. Be cautious, however, because such medications may depress respirations. Routinely auscultate the chest and document findings. Monitor ABGs and observe for signs of hypoxia or hypercapnia.

Nursing Diagnosis: Activity intolerance R/T depleted energy reserves and impaired oxygen/carbon dioxide transport.

Planning: Expected Outcomes. The client will have improved activity tolerance, as evidenced by ability to perform activities of daily living and demonstrating progressively increasing physical activities.

Implementation. Assess the client's baseline of activity and response to activity. Note whether client tolerates any activity by assessing for changes in respiratory and pulse rate, marked dyspnea, pallor or cyanosis, and dysrhythmias. Schedule activity after treatments or medications. Use oxygen as needed. Gradually increase activity on the basis of tolerance.

Teach the client to avoid conditions that increase oxygen demand such as smoking, temperature extremes, weight gain, and stress. Pursed-lip and diaphragmatic breathing as well as techniques to decrease energy use should be reinforced. High-energy activities should be interspersed with rest.

Provide psychosocial support and a quiet environment to reduce anxiety and promote rest. Pace nursing care and visitors, as warranted by the client's condition.

EVALUATION

The degree of expected outcome attainment is monitored every 2 to 3 days. Elderly clients may require additional time to fully recover.

Modification of Plan of Care for the Elderly

Because many cases of pneumonia go undiagnosed in the elderly, the nurse must maintain a high index of suspicion for the common clinical manifestations (see earlier). In addition, the nurse assesses the aged client for changes in cognition (confusion and lethargy), anorexia, tachypnea and deterioration of pre-existing disorders (heart failure and CAL).

The most common bacterial source of pneumonia is bacteria from the gastrointestinal tract. Elderly clients who are immobile or debilitated are at highest risk.

Another common situation increasing risk of pneumonia is aspiration from tube feeding, or following the administration of medications or anesthesia.

The elderly are managed as previously discussed, with caution exercised in the use of fluids for hydration so as to not aggravate pre-existing renal or cardiac disorders. Likewise, oxygen is used as needed in clients with CAL to maintain blood oxygen levels without impairing the drive to breathe.

Post-hospital Care

DISCHARGE INSTRUCTIONS

The client and family are taught techniques of deep breathing and coughing. Chest physical therapy may be prescribed until the chest clears. The client is taught the importance of completing prescribed antibiotics. Plans for rest and gradual resumption of activity should be discussed. A list of complications that require physician notification (return of fever, chest pain, hemoptysis, chills) should be provided.

Follow-Up Care

The client is followed in a clinic setting until the chest clears according to x-ray study and clinical manifestations abate. The client is encouraged to plan for immunization the next winter. Contacts that live with the client are also monitored for the onset of pneumonia.

LUNG ABSCESS

Overview

A lung abscess is a collection of pus within lung tissue. In its early stages, it resembles a localized pneumonia. If lung abscess is undiagnosed and untreated, tissue necrosis may occur.

Single lung abscesses occur most often behind a bronchial obstruction. They nearly always create putrid (foul) material. The bronchial obstruction may be due to

- aspirated foreign material (e.g., vomitus, teeth, blood, or food, or tissue during upper airway surgery)
- benign or malignant tumors
- inspissated (thickened through evaporation or absorption) mucus in bronchial tree
- accumulated mucus due to impaired airway clearance during unconsciousness (e.g., during oversedation, alcohol-induced unconsciousness, or epileptic seizure)

Multiple lung abscesses follow pneumonia caused by necrotizing bacteria (i.e., bacteria that create necrotic lung tissue). These organisms spread through the bloodstream. Bacteria may also arise from septic emboli from infected foci such as septic phlebitis (especially with chronic, debilitating conditions such as congestive heart failure, cirrhosis, malnutrition, or alcoholism). Lung abscesses frequently occur in immunosuppressed clients (e.g., after organ transplantation). Multiple abscesses are usually not putrid.

Early assessment findings in a client with a lung abscess are the same as with bronchopneumonia (i.e., chills, fever, pleuritic pain, cough). The body attempts to wall off the abscess with fibrous tissue. If the attempt is unsuccessful, the abscess ruptures into a bronchus, causing a cough producing copious amounts of sputum. With a single abscess, the sputum is purulent, foul smelling, and foul tasting. After bronchial rupture, hemoptysis often occurs.

Chest auscultation reveals decreased breath sounds and dullness to percussion over the affected area. Rales may be present when the abscess drains.

Management

Antibiotics are used to treat lung abscesses, most commonly penicillin. If performed early, bronchoscopy may be helpful in removing foreign matter and promoting the drainage of abscess contents. In severe cases, surgical removal of a portion of the lung, or of the entire lung, may be indicated.

Caring for a client with a lung abscess is similar to caring for a client experiencing pneumonia (e.g., hydration, effective cough techniques, and postural drainage). Lung abscesses produce copious volumes of sputum. Nursing intervention focuses on removing sputum from the lungs through drainage, expectoration, and antibiotic therapy. The nurse notes the color, quantity, quality, and smell of the expectorated material, including the presence of blood. Expectorated material is sent for microbiologic assessment. Gloves are used when handling sputum-contaminated articles.

The sputum may have a foul taste. Provide frequent opportunities to use mouthwashes and to perform tooth brushing and flossing. Because long-term antibiotic administration is usually necessary, observe oral mucous membranes for indications of *Candida albicans* overgrowth (i.e., white, cheesy patches). Encourage long-term dental care.

Antibiotic therapy for lung abscess may be necessary for up to 6 weeks. Clients with lung abscesses must understand the importance of compliance with the medication schedule. The entire course of antibiotics must be taken. Teaching regarding medications includes (1) reasons for taking them; (2) specific directions such as time of day, frequency, and when to take in relation to food; (3) potential side effects; and (4) what to do if side effects occur. Reassessment after antibiotics are completed (e.g., reculture of sputum, chest films) is essential to evaluate treatment effectiveness.

PULMONARY TUBERCULOSIS

Definition

Tuberculosis (TB) is a chronic, infectious disease that is characterized by the formation of tubercles, or granulomas, in the lungs.

Incidence

Despite improved methods of detection and treatment, TB remains a worldwide health problem with an estimated 3 million new cases diagnosed each year.[47]

Before the development of anti-TB drugs in the late

1940s, TB was the leading cause of death in the United States. Drug therapy, along with improvements in public health and general living standards, resulted in a marked decline in incidence. However, recent influxes of immigrants from developing third world nations, along with the emergence of the human immunodeficiency virus (HIV) epidemic, led to an increase in reported cases in 1986, reversing a 40-year period of decline.

Etiology

TB is a reportable communicable disease caused by *Mycobacterium tuberculosis*. This aerobic organism is an acid-fast bacillus that produces niacin. The tubercle bacillus is airborne, transmitted by aerosolization. Droplet nuclei (1 to 5 μm in size) are emitted during coughing, laughing, sneezing, or singing. Infected droplet nuclei may then be inhaled by a susceptible client (host). Before pulmonary infection can occur, the inhaled organisms must resist the lung's defense mechanisms and actually penetrate lung tissue.

Brief exposure to TB does not usually cause infection. Clients most commonly infected are those having repeated close contact with an infected individual who is not yet diagnosed. When a client is diagnosed as having TB, public health officials (often nurses) talk with the client and develop a contact list. Everyone with whom the client has had contact is then assessed with a tuberculin skin test and chest radiograph to determine whether they have been infected with TB.

In countries that do not have public health programs and those in which TB commonly occurs in cattle, humans may develop bovine TB from drinking raw milk from infected cattle. This form of TB can be prevented by pasteurizing milk and maintaining tuberculin skin-testing programs for cattle.

Risk Factors

Although TB may affect anyone, certain segments of the population have an increased risk of contracting the disease. These high-risk groups include

- the elderly, who constitute nearly half of the newly diagnosed cases of TB in the United States
- racial and ethnic groups such as Native Americans, Eskimos, and blacks, especially the economically disadvantaged or homeless; also, immigrants from Southeast Asia, Ethiopia, Mexico, and Latin America
- clients dependent on alcohol or other chemicals because of malnutrition, debilitation, and generally poor health; older alcoholics who are of minority races are at even greater risk
- infants and children under the age of 5 years
- clients with reduced immunity, including those with HIV infection, with malnutrition, on cancer chemotherapy, or on steroid therapy

Pathophysiology

PRIMARY (FIRST) INFECTION

The first time a client is infected with TB, it is said to be a "primary infection." Only a small proportion of clients infected with TB (about 5 per cent of North Americans) actually develop active, clinical disease. Primary TB infections are usually located in the apices of the lungs or near the pleurae of the lower lobes. Although a primary infection may be only microscopic in size (and hence never even appear on x-ray film), the following sequence of events typically occurs.

A small area of bronchopneumonia develops in the lung tissue (primary, or Ghon, focus). Many of the infecting tubercle bacilli are phagocytized by wandering macrophages. However, before the development of hypersensitivity and immunity, many of the bacilli may survive within these blood cells and be carried into regional bronchopulmonary (hilar) lymph nodes via the lymphatic system. The bacilli may even spread throughout the body. Thus, the infection, although small, rapidly spreads.

The primary infection site may or may not undergo a process of necrotic degeneration (caseation), which produces cavities filled with a cheeselike mass of tubercle bacilli, dead white blood cells, and necrotic lung tissue. In time, this material liquefies and may drain into the tracheobronchial tree and be coughed up as sputum. The air-filled cavities remain and may be detected radiologically.

Most primary tubercles heal over a period of months through the formation of fibrous scars and, ultimately, calcified lesions (calcified primaries or Ghon tubercles). These lesions may contain living bacilli that can reactivate (even after many years) and can cause reinfection or secondary TB (see later).

Primary TB infections cause the body to develop a state of sensitivity (allergic reaction to tubercle bacilli or their proteins). This cell-mediated immune response appears in the form of sensitized T cells and is detectable by a positive reaction to a tuberculin skin test (see Chap. 36). The development of this tuberculin sensitivity occurs in all body cells 2 to 6 weeks after the primary infection. It is maintained as long as living bacilli remain in the body (perhaps for life). This acquired immunity usually inhibits the further growth of the bacilli and the development of active infection (discussed later).

The term "tuberculin converter" refers to a client who does not show radiologic or bacteriologic evidence of pulmonary TB but whose tuberculin skin test converts from a known negative reaction to a known positive reaction (i.e., from less than 5 mm of induration with a Mantoux skin test to 10 mm or more with the same test). It is important to know that the absence of a positive (reactive) tuberculin test does not always mean that TB is absent.

Primary TB infections are often not recognized because usually they are relatively asymptomatic. Calcified lesions and a positive skin test are frequently the only reminders that a primary TB infection has occurred.

Most clients harbor tubercle bacilli for life and never develop actual disease. Usually, their body defenses are adequate to arrest primary infection, and they heal by fibrosis and calcification. However, a primary TB infection is occasionally not controlled, and progressive primary disease develops. In this situation, the primary complex sites progress and worsen, possibly causing cavitation and the spread of active infection, and the client becomes clinically ill.

The reason active TB disease develops in some clients (instead of being controlled by the acquired immune response) is poorly understood. However, factors that seem to play a role in the progression from TB infection to active disease include (1) advancing age, (2) immunosuppression, (3) hormonal changes, (4) malnutrition, (5) alcoholism, (6) presence of other disease states (e.g., poorly controlled diabetes mellitus, chronic renal failure, or silicosis), and (7) gastrectomy.

REINFECTION

In addition to progressive primary disease, reinfection (or secondary disease) may also lead to a clinical form of active TB. Primary sites of infection containing TB bacilli may remain latent for years and then reactivate if the client's resistance is lowered. Because reinfection is possible (infection does not provide total immunity) and because dormant lesions may reactivate, it is extremely important for clients who have had a TB infection to be reassessed periodically for evidence of active disease.

Clinical Manifestations

Typical findings with pulmonary TB include fatigue; anorexia; weight loss; persistent, long-term, low-grade fever; chills and sweats (often at night); nonresolving bronchopneumonia; dyspnea; hemoptysis; persistent, progressive, and often productive cough; chest pain that may be pleuritic or dull in nature; and chest tightness.

The detection and diagnosis of TB is achieved by objective tests and subjective assessment findings. The diagnosis can be difficult because TB mimics many other diseases. Also, TB may occur concurrently with other diseases. Often, a diagnosis of TB is not considered or obtained until a client with pulmonary symptoms fails to improve after treatment for other pulmonary disorders such as pneumonia.

History includes assessing the probability of recent or past exposure to TB as well as the client's occupation, other usual activities, and travel or residence in countries with a high incidence of TB. A history of exposure to TB is certainly significant, but most clients are not aware of exposure. Also, during assessment for TB, it is advisable to determine whether the client has been previously tested for TB and to obtain the results of that testing.

DIAGNOSTIC ASSESSMENT

Culture of *M. tuberculosis* from sputum or other body secretions or tissue is the only method of confirming the diagnosis. If TB is disseminated throughout the body or is suspected in another organ system, an acid-fast smear and culture is performed on appropriate tissue or fluid (e.g., urine for suspected TB of kidney).

Tuberculin test results, of which a Mantoux test is most reliable, are also used in diagnosis.

Chest x-ray examination is valuable for detecting old lesions or new ones once they are large enough to be seen. Cavities may be present with far-advanced disease. Inflammation that accompanies a new infection may also be apparent.

Medical Management

Figure 39-7 summarizes detection, diagnosis, and medical intervention related to TB.

Clients with active TB must be identified and properly treated not only for their own welfare but also to

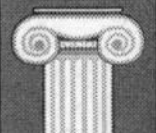

ETHICAL ISSUES IN NURSING

How Should the Federal Government Regulate Testing for Tuberculosis?

In the recent past, tuberculosis (TB) has been a disease that has not commanded much attention (at least in the United States). Gone are the TB sanatoriums that were once so prolific across the country. During the 18th and 19th centuries, TB was the leading cause of death in young people all over the world. The rate of infection in the modern United States has been low in recent times, but an upsurge has been noted in the past few years that is thought to be related to the acquired immunodeficiency syndrome (AIDS).

TB is transmitted from person to person by the inhalation of infected droplets through respiratory secretions. The infecting bacterium, *Mycobacterium tuberculosis*, remains a medical problem in many developing countries. In the United States, TB is commonly associated with overcrowding and poverty conditions. Testing may not be done in these areas, frequently because of a lack of health care services provided to these areas. Immigration, either permanent or through university programs, is also a cause of TB reintroduction. Undetected, this disease can be fatal.

How are public health agencies supposed to regulate such an infectious and possibly fatal disease? A person can be infected with TB without knowing it simply by breathing in the bacterium. Should there be massive testing campaigns in which all persons must be tested? How can the United States government be responsible for testing all foreign students? What about illegal aliens who, for fear of deportation, would not seek testing even if it were legislated?

With the rise of tuberculosis in America and the ease by which it is transmitted, health care workers need to take special caution in their care of all clients. Health care providers need to think about routine testing of clients and themselves for TB. Government agencies can make rules and set guidelines, but many of the infected may slip through the cracks. Nurses need to keep up with current public health care concerns in order to protect themselves and also to better serve their clients.

prevent the transmission of TB to others (see Ethical Issues in Nursing). Screening programs can effectively detect the presence of TB infection. However, they are cost-effective only for groups at high risk of developing or having TB. In addition to the groups previously discussed, these may include (1) health care providers at risk of exposure to TB, (2) children entering schools in areas where TB is prevalent, (3) food handlers (not because TB is food-borne, but because immigrants from countries with prevalent TB often work in food-related occupations where they have numerous contacts), and (4) clients living or working in institutions, if there is an increased risk or a high prevalence of TB in the population, environmental factors that facilitate TB transmission, or the potential for infecting young children or immunosuppressed clients.

PHARMACOLOGIC MANAGEMENT

Preventive Measures. Prevention of active TB with isoniazid preventive therapy (IPT) consists of taking 300 mg of isoniazid daily for 9 to 12 months. IPT stops the growth of the bacilli, thus preventing active pulmonary or extrapulmonary TB. IPT is recommended for clients who (1) are newly infected (have converted tuberculin skin tests but no other indication of active disease), (2) live or closely associate with others who have active TB, (3) have significant tuberculin skin test reactions and abnormal chest films compatible with inactive TB, (4) have positive tuberculin skin tests and conditions (e.g., steroid therapy, diabetes mellitus, AIDS) placing them at increased risk for TB, and (5) are less than 35 years old and have significant tuberculin skin test reactions, even though they may have a normal chest film and no other risk factors (because of the cumulative risk, over time, of reactivation).

Therapeutic Measures. Clients with diagnosed active TB are usually started on three or more medications to be certain the resistant organisms are eliminated. The dose of some drugs may initially be large because the bacilli are difficult to kill. Treatment continues long enough to eliminate or substantially reduce the number of dormant or semidormant bacilli. Long-term, uninterrupted chemotherapy is important.

Medications used for TB may be divided into first- and second-line drugs. Table 39–4 lists and discusses medications in these categories. First-line drugs are almost always initially prescribed until culture and sensitivity laboratory reports are available. Clients with a previous history of incomplete TB chemotherapy may have developed resistant organisms.

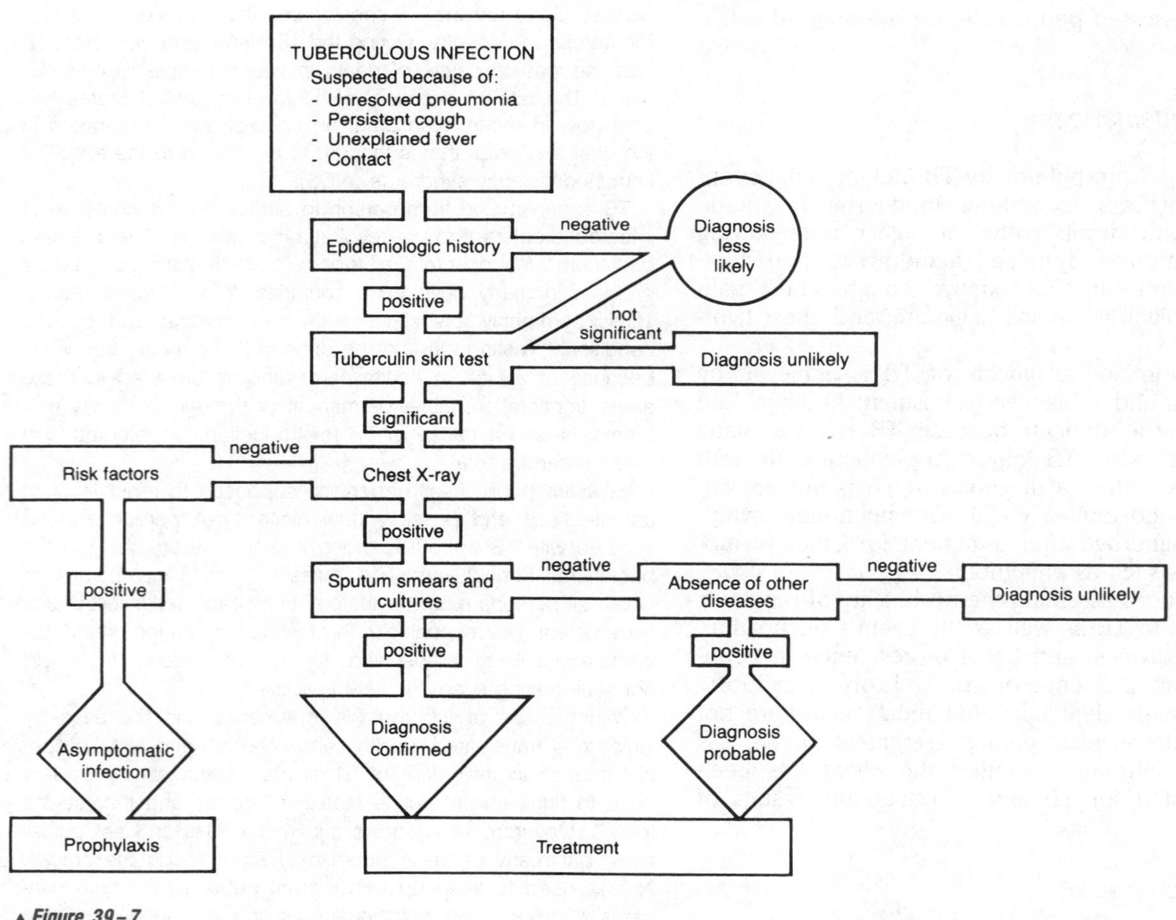

▲ **Figure 39–7**

Algorithm for diagnosis and management of tuberculosis: a logical progression. (American Lung Association, The Christmas Seal People ©.)

TABLE 39-4. Tuberculosis Medication

	Dosage*				
	Daily	**Twice Weekly**	**Most Common Side Effects***	**Tests for Side Effects***	**Comments/Intervention**
First-Line Drugs					
Isoniazid	5-10 mg/kg up to 300 mg PO or IM	15 mg/kg PO or IM	Peripheral neuritis, nausea, hepatitis, hypersensitivity	AST/ALT (not as a routine)	Bactericidal; pyridoxine 10 mg/day as prophylaxis for neuritis; 50-100 mg as treatment; take at bedtime if nausea occurs
Ethambutol	15-25 mg/kg up to 2.5 g PO	50 mg/kg PO	Optic neuritis (reversible with discontinuation of drug; very rare at 15 mg/kg), skin rash	Red/green color discrimination and visual acuity†	Use with caution with renal disease or when eye testing is not feasible; check red/green discrimination with each follow-up visit
Rifampin	10-15 mg/kg up to 600 mg PO	600 mg PO	Hepatitis, febrile reaction, purpura (rare)	AST/ALT (not as a routine)	Bactericidal; orange urine color; affects action of other drugs (e.g., inactivates birth control pills)
Streptomycin	15 mg/kg up to 1 g IM	25-30 mg/kg IM	Eighth nerve damage, nephrotoxicity	Vestibular function, audiograms†; blood urea nitrogen and creatinine	Use with caution in older clients or those with renal disease
Pyrazinamide	25 mg/kg up to 2 g PO	50 mg/kg, up to 3.5 g PO	Hyperuricemia, hepatotoxicity	Uric acid, AST/ALT	Rapidly bacteriostatic and slowly bacteriocidal, thus kills bacilli not attacked by other anti-TB drugs
Second-Line Drugs					
Capreomycin, kanamycin	12-15 mg/kg up to 1 g IM		Auditory toxicity, nephrotoxicity, vestibular toxicity (rare)	Vestibular function, audiograms†; blood urea nitrogen and creatinine	Use with caution in older clients; rarely used with renal disease
Ethionamide	15 mg/kg up to 1 g PO		Gastrointestinal disturbance, hepatotoxicity, hypersensitivity	AST/ALT	Divided dose may help reduce gastrointestinal side effects; antinausea drugs may be prescribed
Para-aminosalicylic acid (aminosalicylic acid)	200-300 mg/kg up to 12 g PO		Gastrointestinal disturbance, hypersensitivity, hepatotoxicity, sodium load	AST/ALT	Gastrointestinal side effects very frequent, making compliance difficult
Cycloserine	15 mg/kg up to 1 g PO		Psychosis, personality changes, convulsions, rash	Psychological testing	Very difficult drug to use; side effects may be blocked by pyridoxine, ataractic agents, or anticonvulsant drugs; monitor closely

AST/ALT, aspartate aminotransferase/alanine aminotransferase; IM, intramuscularly; PO, orally.
* Check product labeling for detailed information on dose, contraindications, drug interaction, adverse reactions, and monitoring.
† Initial levels should be determined on start of treatment.
Modified from Pérez-Stable, E. J., & Hopewell, P. C. (1989). Current tuberculosis treatment regimens: choosing the right one for your patient. *Clinics in Chest Medicine, 10*:323-337.

The duration of treatment varies. Some programs have a two-phase approach: (1) an intensive phase using two or three drugs, aimed at destroying large numbers of rapidly multiplying organisms, and (2) a maintenance phase, usually with two drugs, directed at eliminating most remaining bacilli. The length of each phase depends on the success of treatment and the client's compliance. Some courses are as short as 6 months; others last 24 months. The average is 9 to 12 months. Some TB protocols call for medication two or three times a week rather than daily. These programs are often used for noncompliant clients, and the drugs are administered in a clinic or physician's office to ensure that they are received.

If the medication regimen does not seem effective (e.g., worsening symptoms, continued acid-fast bacilli in sputum, increasing infiltrates, or cavity formation), the program needs reevaluation, and the client's compliance should be assessed. At least two medications (never just one) are added to a failing TB chemotherapy program.

Because medications used to treat TB have potentially serious side effects (see Table 39–4), baseline studies (depending on the specific drugs prescribed) are performed. Drug toxicity can limit the treatment of TB. Drug tolerance, drug effect, and drug toxicity depend on factors such as age, medication dosage, time since last dosage, the medication's chemical formula, renal and intestinal function, and compliance with chemotherapy program.

HOSPITALIZATION

If pulmonary TB is diagnosed in the hospitalized client, the client is often kept in the hospital for 1 to 2 weeks until therapeutic drug levels are established. The newly diagnosed client should be cared for in a private room that has fresh, circulating air and is irradiated with ultraviolet light, if possible. Further hospitalization is not usually necessary.

Some clients with active TB may be hospitalized if (1) they are acutely ill, (2) their living situation is considered a high risk, (3) they are suspected of noncompliance, (4) there is a history of previous TB and noncompliance and the disease has reactivated, (5) concomitant diseases are present and acute, (6) improvement does not occur after chemotherapy, or (7) their organisms are highly resistant to usual treatment, requiring second- or third-line drugs. In this last situation, brief hospitalization is necessary to monitor the effects and side effects of the drugs.

Clients whose TB is not improving or who are unable to tolerate medication may require assessment and treatment at medical facilities specializing in the treatment of complicated pulmonary TB and other forms of mycobacterial disease.

Nursing Management

Nursing management of the client with TB may include many of the interventions discussed earlier in this chapter and in Chapter 37, depending on the specific nursing diagnoses identified. Possible nursing diagnoses for the client with TB include Anxiety; Airway Clearance, Ineffective; Gas Exchange, Impaired; Pain; Individual Coping, Ineffective; Family Coping, Ineffective; Altered Health Maintenance; Noncompliance; and Sleep Pattern Disturbance.

Post-hospital Care

FOLLOW-UP

TB treatment is a long process. Nurses in clinics and public health facilities are often responsible for follow-up assessment and monitoring. Determining medication compliance, understanding the pharmacologic actions of medications, monitoring unwanted side effects, collecting sputum specimens for acid-fast smear and culture, obtaining serial chest films, and observing for reversal or worsening of initial assessment findings are all part of the ongoing follow-up of clients with TB.

DISCHARGE TEACHING

As recently as the 1960s, clients with TB were often confined for treatment for months or years in sanatoriums. Many clients are not familiar with current treatments and still have perceptions of TB as a "shameful" disease. It is essential that clients experiencing TB, and their significant others, receive the information in the Client Education Guide.

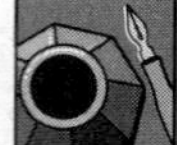

CLIENT EDUCATION GUIDE

Pulmonary Tuberculosis

Teach the client as follows:

- TB is infectious, but it may be cured or arrested if you take your medication as prescribed.
- TB is transmitted by droplet infection and is not carried on articles such as clothing, books, or eating utensils. You do not need to dispose of any possessions.
- Cover your nose and mouth when coughing, laughing, or sneezing.
- Wash your hands very carefully after any contact with body substances, masks, or soiled tissues. Sputum is highly contaminated. Cough into paper tissues and dispose of them properly.
- Wear masks in appropriate situations when advised. Make sure they are tight-fitting, and change them frequently.
- People with TB are usually not restricted in their activities for more than 2 to 4 weeks after medication is begun, and they are not isolated from others, as long as compliance is maintained. TB is no longer treated by isolation in sanatoriums.
- Treatment may be necessary for a long time. Take your medication exactly as prescribed and report all side effects to your doctor. Do not stop the medication for any reason without the doctor's supervision. Keep an adequate supply of medication available at all times to avoid running out. Compliance with treatment is essential.

Provide information regarding side effects of prescribed medications, as indicated in Table 39–4.

Suspicion of noncompliance is dealt with in various ways. In the United States, public health departments have regulations that may be enforced regarding noncompliance with TB treatment. In some cities, a noncompliant client can be arrested, taken to court, and even jailed as a public health hazard. Less drastic means usually ensure compliance. Providing complete information, as outlined in the Client Education Guide, and ongoing support helps. The more information clients have, and the more personal control they perceive, the more likely they are to comply with treatment. Each client should be treated as an individual.

EXTRAPULMONARY TUBERCULOSIS

Overview

Extrapulmonary tuberculosis (XPTB) is TB occurring anywhere outside the lungs. Although TB of the lungs is the most common form of the disease, after initial invasion, tubercle bacilli can spread throughout the body via the blood and lymph.

Proportionally, XPTB is high among Caucasians, although recent trends indicate increases in nonwhite people. The mean age of persons with XPTB is in the 40s, except for meningeal TB, which is more common in clients aged 20 to 30 years.

Mycobacterium tuberculosis thrives in oxygen-rich areas. In XPTB, it most commonly grows in highly aerobic sites, such as the renal cortex, bone growth plates, and meninges. It may also occur in the genitourinary tract, lymph nodes, pleurae, pericardium, abdomen, and endocrine glands.

Despite the severity of the disease, XPTB is often difficult to detect. Assessment findings are frequently nondistinct. Weight loss, fatigue, malaise, fever, and sweats may or may not be present. "Cold" abscesses and draining sinuses frequently occur with XPTB of bones and joints.

Miliary Tuberculosis. Widespread dissemination throughout the body is termed miliary tuberculosis. It is more common in clients aged 50 years or older and in very young children with unstable or underdeveloped immune systems. In the very young, miliary TB spreads rapidly after primary infection. Older clients infected with TB many years earlier may develop miliary tuberculosis from delayed or late dissemination after immune system compromise.

Assessment findings with miliary TB are usually nonspecific (e.g., anorexia, weakness, fatigue, weight loss, fever, chills, sweats, headache, and abdominal pain). Signs and symptoms may precede changes in the chest film. Some people never develop the classic radiographic pattern of diffuse, finely nodular shadows of millet-seed size.

Management

The diagnosis and treatment of XPTB proceed in a similar manner to that of pulmonary TB. However, the treatment period may be longer, and more medications may be used. Treatment will depend on the extent, severity, course, and complications of the disease. Sometimes corticosteroids are used in treating XPTB. They are not usually indicated for pulmonary TB.

NONTUBERCULOUS MYCOBACTERIA

Nontuberculous mycobacteria (NTM), also known as MOTT (mycobacteria other than tuberculosis), are responsible for increasing numbers of mycobacterial infections. Although this infection is still relatively uncommon (i.e., approximately 1.8 cases per 100,000 in the United States), changing disease patterns have recently appeared: more cases; wider geographic distribution; and new groups of vulnerable hosts, most notably AIDS clients. If current trends continue, NTM disease incidence may exceed that of TB by the early 21st century.[42]

NTM are widely distributed in nature (i.e., in water, soil, animals, and birds), and most clients acquire their infections from environmental sources rather than from other diseased clients. Whereas NTM diseases occur worldwide, there is marked geographic variation in disease rate.

The most commonly occurring NTM diseases are caused by *Mycobacterium avium* complex, *Mycobacterium kansasii*, and *Mycobacterium fortuitum*. The primary site for NTM disease is the lungs, although extrapulmonary sites (e.g., lymph nodes, skin, joints) may occur. Disseminated disease with multiple organ involvement is also possible, most commonly in immunosuppressed clients (e.g., clients with AIDS). Pulmonary NTM disease is very similar to TB, although the signs and symptoms may be less severe. Clients with pre-existing bronchopulmonary disease (e.g., bronchiectasis, COPD, or healed pulmonary TB) are at highest risk for pulmonary involvement.

Diagnosis of NTM disease is often difficult because of the widespread distribution in the environment of the organisms, which frequently occur in sputum from clients with normal lungs. Definitive diagnosis of disease is possible only if NTM are isolated from normally sterile sites (e.g., blood, cerebrospinal fluid, lymph nodes) or through biopsy. However, NTM disease is strongly suspected when a client presents with a clinical syndrome that is compatible with NTM, no other pathogens can be identified, and repeated sputum cultures reveal large numbers of NTM.

The same medications used to treat TB are prescribed for NTM disease. However, NTM are considerably more resistant to drugs than is *M. tuberculosis*. Consequently, combined drug regimens and longer treatment periods are necessary. Treatment typically includes three to six different medications and lasts for a minimum of 24 months, continuing until there are no acid-fast bacilli in the sputum in consecutive collections taken over a period of 1 year. As a result, medication adherence is critical.

Unsuccessful treatment may result in further lung damage and general debilitation. Regular, daily medication is essential. The more clients understand about the condition and its management, the more likely they will be to complete the full medication course.

Other aspects of the nursing management of NTM disease are the same as for pulmonary TB (see preceding discussion). However, because these diseases are not believed to be transmitted from person to person, beyond good hygiene, isolation and other measures to control infection are not necessary.

FUNGAL PULMONARY DISEASES

Overview

Most fungi that are pathogenic to humans limit their activities to the skin. However, the spores of some fungi become airborne and can be inhaled into the respiratory tract, causing pulmonary diseases that, in their chronic forms, produce granulomatous conditions similar to TB. The most common of these are coccidioidomycosis and histoplasmosis. Each has a specific geographic distribution and occurs in people living or traveling in the regions where these fungi are found. Person-to-person transmission is virtually unknown.

Coccidioidomycosis is found in the Western Hemisphere, primarily in California (the San Joaquin Valley), New Mexico, Arizona, western Texas, and northern Mexico. The disease is most likely to develop in those engaging in desert recreational activities or working in construction or other occupations that involve digging (e.g., archaeology). The disease is mild and self-limiting in 60 per cent of those affected. Such clients are either symptomatic or have only mild upper respiratory assessment findings. The remaining 40 per cent develop a syndrome similar to influenza with cough, fever, pleuritic chest pain, myalgias, and arthralgias. Erythema multiforme (a flat, red rash that erupts with dark red papules) occurs in a few people.

The causative organism of *histoplasmosis*, the fungus *Histoplasma capsulatum*, is endemic to the central and eastern portions of North America, most notably in the Ohio, Missouri, and Mississippi River valleys. It is also found in South and Central America, India, and Cyprus. This fungus lives in moist soil of appropriate chemical composition, in mushroom cellars, on the floors of chicken houses and bat caves, and in bird droppings (especially from starlings and blackbirds). As with coccidioidomycosis, histoplasmosis infections are usually asymptomatic or mild.

The diagnosis of fungal pulmonary diseases is usually based on history and clinical assessment findings. Skin testing is also used for coccidioidomycosis. Chest films may show hilar adenopathy, small areas of infiltrates, or signs of pneumonia. Sometimes, cavities and calcified nodules may form, usually remaining in the lungs as permanent indicators of previous infection.

A few clients may develop disseminated or chronic forms of pulmonary fungal diseases. When disseminated disease occurs, central nervous system, liver, spleen, gastrointestinal tract, or musculoskeletal involvement may be present. Chronic disease may result in progressive cavitary changes similar to those seen with TB. Emphysema-like pulmonary structural changes may also occur.

Management

Mild, primary forms of fungal pulmonary disease usually do not require treatment. Progressive, disseminated, or chronic forms are treated with intravenous amphotericin B. This fungicidal antibiotic is quite toxic, and acute reactions (e.g., seizures, anaphylaxis, headache, or decreased renal function) may occur during infusion. Antiemetics, antihistamines, antipyretics, or hydrocortisone may be prescribed as premedications. In order to reduce the incidence of thrombophlebitis at the intravenous site (a common problem), a small amount of heparin may be added to the infusion. Ketoconazole, a less toxic oral medication, may also be used. However, the long-term effectiveness of this medication has not yet been determined. If the disorder is not responsive to drug therapy, surgical removal of affected areas (e.g., lung cavities) may be necessary.

Nursing management includes providing (1) preventive education to minimize exposure of clients to infectious fungi (i.e., teach to avoid high-risk situations and to recognize early indications of infection) and (2) appropriate support and education for infected clients and their significant others, along with symptomatic management of the disease. Education involves teaching about not only the disease and intervention measures but also reportable indications of complications.

OTHER FUNGAL AND FUNGUS-LIKE INFECTIONS

In addition to the pathogenic fungi, other common fungi spores may cause serious, potentially fatal pulmonary disease in immunocompromised clients (e.g., clients with AIDS, clients receiving cancer chemotherapy). These fungi include *Aspergillus*, *Blastomyces dermatitidis*, *Candida*, and *Cryptococcus neoformans*. Treatment of these infections is also with amphotericin B.

Pulmonary infections caused by actinomycetes (gram-positive organisms), once classified as fungi, may also be seen. Nocardiosis is caused by the *Nocardia* species and is treated with sulfadiazine. Surgical drainage may be required. Actinomycosis (caused by *Actinomyces israelii*) develops from dental, facial, or neck infections. Pulmonary disease may result if the organism is aspirated; treatment with penicillin is required.

NONCARDIOGENIC PULMONARY EDEMA

Pulmonary edema is the abnormal accumulation of fluid in the interstitial and alveolar spaces of lung tissue. It results from an imbalance between hydrostatic and colloidal osmotic pressures within the respiratory circulation. When the normal balance between these two forces is interrupted (i.e., hydrostatic pressure increases or colloidal osmotic pressure decreases), fluid leaves the pulmonary capillaries and enters interstitial spaces.

Some fluid in the interstitial spaces of the lungs is not uncommon. It normally escapes from the microcirculation and enters the interstitium, providing nutrients for the cells. The lymphatic system drains excess interstitial fluid volume. Additional fluid in the pleura drains into the hilar lymph nodes. However, if this pathway becomes overwhelmed, fluid moves from the interstitium into the alveolar walls. If the alveolar epithelium is damaged, the fluid accumulates in the alveoli. Alveolar edema is a serious sign late in the progression of fluid imbalance.

Pulmonary edema most commonly results from left-sided heart failure (see Chap. 42). Noncardiogenic pulmonary edema may result from a variety of conditions (Box 39-6). Sometimes, the precipitating event has occurred 12 to 24 hours earlier (e.g., smoke inhalation). At other times, noncardiogenic pulmonary edema develops rapidly, as with neurogenic causes.

Pulmonary manifestations of pulmonary edema are the same, regardless of the cause. In the noncardiogenic form, however, no signs of cardiac involvement (i.e., cardiac enlargement, presence of S_3 heart sound, jugular vein distention, and elevated pulmonary wedge pressures) will be seen.

Dyspnea will be present, usually accompanied by a cough. As fluid fills the interstitium and alveolar spaces, lung compliance decreases and oxygen diffusion is impaired. Cyanosis may be present, and ABGs will reveal progressive hypoxemia. Chest auscultation reveals rales and occasional diffuse wheezing.

Medical and nursing management of noncardiogenic pulmonary edema are essentially the same as for adult respiratory distress syndrome (see later). Overall, intervention is aimed at reversing the precipitating event and providing supportive respiratory measures.

Box 39-6. Common Causes of Noncardiogenic Pulmonary Edema

- Aspiration of gastric contents, especially if significant amount of hydrochloric acid is present
- Drug-induced (e.g., after administration of narcotics)
- Fluid overload from intravenous fluids
- Hypoalbuminemia (e.g., nephrotic syndrome, hepatic disease, malnutrition)
- Smoke inhalation (e.g., in people or firefighters trapped in a building)
- Inhalation of toxic chemicals (e.g., sulfur dioxide, paraquat, phosgene, chlorine, nitrogen oxides)
- High altitudes (i.e., greater than 8000 ft)
- Neurogenic stimulus (e.g., conditions causing increased intracranial pressure, epileptic seizures, head trauma, profound infection)
- Near-drowning syndrome (i.e., inhalation of large quantities of fresh or sea water)
- Mechanical ventilation, oxygen toxicity, Adult respiratory distress syndrome (ARDS)
- Malignancies blocking outflow of lymph within the lungs
- Unilaterally, after reexpansion of collapsed lung (pneumothorax)

ACUTE RESPIRATORY FAILURE

Respiratory failure is a broad, nonspecific clinical diagnosis used to indicate that the respiratory system is unable to supply the oxygen necessary to maintain metabolism or cannot eliminate sufficient carbon dioxide. Acute respiratory failure is defined as a PaO_2 of 50 mm Hg or less or a $PaCO_2$ of 50 mm Hg or more. In clients with chronic hypercapnia, $PaCO_2$ elevations of 5 mm Hg or more from their previously stable levels indicate acute respiratory failure superimposed on chronic respiratory failure. Various factors may precipitate respiratory failure. If these factors are not recognized and corrected, other organ systems are affected. Box 39-7 lists some causes of acute respiratory failure.

Classically, a client in acute respiratory failure has an elevated arterial carbon dioxide. Elevated $PaCO_2$ di-

Box 39-7. Causes of Acute Respiratory Failure

Factors Decreasing Ventilatory Drive

- Depression of respiratory drive with drugs (e.g., barbiturates, sedatives, narcotics, tranquilizers)
- Brain disorders (e.g., stroke, brain tumor, brain trauma)
- Obstructive sleep apnea syndrome
- Obesity

Chest Wall Dysfunction and Neuromuscular Factors

- Anesthetic blocking agents
- Cervical spinal cord injury
- Neuromuscular disorders (e.g., muscular dystrophy, Guillain-Barré syndrome, amyotrophic lateral sclerosis, polio, and post-polio effects)
- Neuromuscular blocking agents (e.g., curare)
- Kyphoscoliosis

Factors in Lung Parenchyma

- Near-drowning
- Pneumonia
- Interstitial lung diseases
- Pulmonary edema
- Chronic airflow limitation
- ARDS
- Inhalation of toxic chemicals, gases, or smoke
- Pulmonary contusion

Other Factors

- Carbon monoxide inhalation
- Upper airway obstruction (e.g., foreign body, tumor, micrognathia)
- Abdominal distention due to intestinal obstruction
- Ascites

rectly relates to alveolar hypoventilation from either (1) decreased minute ventilation with normal dead space ventilation or (2) normal or increased minute ventilation with increased dead space ventilation. In the first category are clients with normal lungs whose respiratory status is impaired by drugs or diseases affecting respiration (e.g., neuromuscular disorders). In the second category are clients with intrinsic lung diseases such as COPD or severe pneumonias. Lung damage in these clients increases the amount of dead space (wasted ventilation). Thus, even with normal or increased minute ventilation, they cannot blow off a sufficient amount of carbon dioxide.

Diagnosis of respiratory failure is sometimes difficult. Assessment findings indicating hypoxemia and hypercapnia often occur subtly. By the time abnormalities are recognized, an emergency may exist. If respiratory failure is suspected, confirmation with ABG analysis is essential. Diagnosis is made by clinical observation and blood gas analysis.

Management

Intervention for acute respiratory failure is directed to (1) treating the underlying cause of the respiratory failure and (2) restoring gas exchange to maintain physiologic function.

Nursing intervention focuses on (1) promoting effective airway clearance and effective gas exchange, (2) preventing complications of immobility, (3) monitoring and documenting indications of altered tissue perfusion, (4) monitoring and promoting effective breathing patterns, (5) reducing anxiety and fear, and (6) promoting comfort. If endotracheal intubation and mechanical ventilation are required, the client must communicate nonverbally. When acute respiratory failure is superimposed on chronic respiratory disease or chronic respiratory failure, nursing intervention is directed to (1) promoting self-care and (2) performing teaching activities to prevent complications and to increase treatment compliance. Discussions earlier in this chapter and in Chapter 37 outline interventions appropriate for clients with acute respiratory failure.

ADULT RESPIRATORY DISTRESS SYNDROME

Definition

Adult respiratory distress syndrome (ARDS) is a sudden, progressive pulmonary disorder characterized by severe dyspnea, hypoxemia, and diffuse bilateral infiltrates. It follows acute and massive lung injury that results from a variety of clinical states, often occurring in previously healthy individuals. The syndrome was first described in 1967 and has been alternatively referred to by a variety of terms, including shock lung, wet lung, Da Nang lung (in reference to the high number of cases observed during the Vietnam era), post-traumatic lung, congestive atelectasis, capillary leak syndrome, and adult hyaline membrane disease.

Incidence

It is estimated that at least 150,000 cases of ARDS occur each year in the United States.[6] Despite major advances in intensive pulmonary care, mortality rates are still greater than 50 per cent. Furthermore, 90 per cent of deaths from ARDS occur within 2 weeks of disease onset.[42]

Etiology

ARDS develops as a result of an insult, condition, or noxious event that traumatizes the lung tissue. The insult may be directly to lung tissue or indirect, occurring in other body areas.

Risk Factors

Conditions at high risk of leading to ARDS are listed in Box 39-8.

Pathophysiology

The initial insult is followed by a period of apparently normal lung function that may last from 1 to 96 hours. Then, hypoxemia rapidly develops and progresses, along with decreasing lung compliance and the development of diffuse lung infiltrates.

Box 39-8. Clinical States that May Lead to ARDS

Direct Pulmonary Trauma

- Viral, bacterial, or fungal pneumonias
- Lung contusion
- Fat embolus
- Aspiration (e.g., foreign material, drowning, vomitus)
- Massive smoke inhalation
- Inhaled toxins
- Prolonged exposure to high concentrations of oxygen

Indirect Pulmonary Trauma

- Sepsis
- Shock
- Multisystem trauma
- Disseminated intravascular coagulation
- Pancreatitis
- Uremia
- Drug overdose
- Anaphylaxis
- Idiopathic
- Prolonged cardiobypass surgery
- Massive blood transfusions
- Pregnancy-induced hypertension
- Increased intracranial pressure
- Radiation therapy

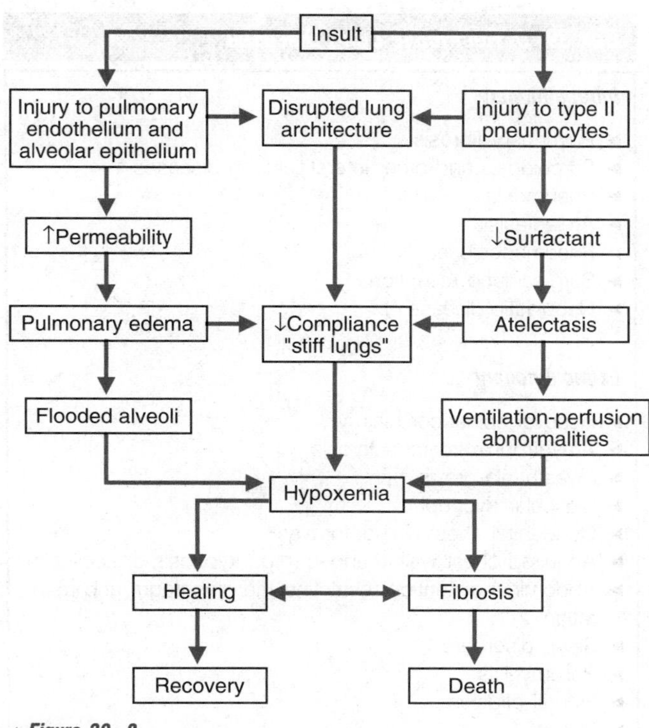

▲ **Figure 39-8**

Pathophysiology of ARDS. (From Bradley, R. B. [1987]. Adult respiratory distress syndrome. *Focus on Critical Care, 14*:48.)

The hallmark of ARDS is increased permeability of the pulmonary endothelium and alveolar epithelium, with resultant movement of fluid into the interstitial and alveolar spaces. This leads to the development of pulmonary edema, which decreases lung compliance and impairs oxygen transport. The alveolar cells, which produce pulmonary surfactant (type II), are also damaged, which leads to atelectasis and further impairment in lung distensibility and gas exchange. This pathophysiologic chain of events is shown in Figure 39-8.

There are several possible courses that the ARDS client may follow: (1) full healing and recovery; (2) mild pulmonary fibrosis followed by healing and recovery; (3) healing initially, followed by severe fibrosis and death; or (4) rapid progression to fibrosis and death. The client's final outcome is difficult to predict at disease onset.

In addition to lung fibrosis, a number of other complications may arise during supportive management of the client with ARDS. These include cardiac dysrhythmias due to hypoxemia, oxygen toxicity, renal failure, thrombocytopenia, gastrointestinal bleeding secondary to stress ulcers, sepsis from invasive lines, and disseminated intravascular coagulation (see Chap. 46).

Clinical Manifestations

The earliest clinical sign of ARDS is usually an increased respiratory rate. Breathing becomes increasingly labored; the client may exhibit air hunger, retractions, and cyanosis. Chest auscultation may or may not reveal the presence of adventitious sounds. If present, abnormal sounds may range from fine inspiratory crackles to widespread rales.

DIAGNOSTIC ASSESSMENT

Blood gas analysis reveals increasing hypoxemia (PaO_2 <70 mm Hg when FIO_2 >0.4) that does not respond to increased FIO_2 levels and compensatory hypocapnia. In the early stages, respiratory alkalosis is present because of hyperventilation. Later metabolic acidosis develops from increased work of breathing and hypoxemia. The chest film usually demonstrates diffuse, bilateral, and rapidly progressing interstitial or alveolar infiltrates (Fig. 39-9).

Medical Management

The key to the successful management of ARDS is early detection and initiation of treatment. The goals of therapy are respiratory support, treatment of the underlying cause when possible, and prevention of complications.

Endotracheal intubation, mechanical ventilation, and positive end-expiratory pressure are usually required to maintain adequate blood oxygen levels. Sedation may be necessary to reduce anxiety and restlessness during ventilator management. If tachypnea, restlessness, or respirations out of phase with the ventilator (''bucking'') cannot be managed by sedation, pharmacologic paralysis (e.g., pancuronium bromide, curare) may be induced (see Chap. 37).

The use of pharmacologic agents in the treatment of ARDS will vary according to the client's underlying disease process. Inotropic agents (e.g., dopamine) may be indicated to improve cardiac output and increase systemic blood pressure. Antibiotics are administered if

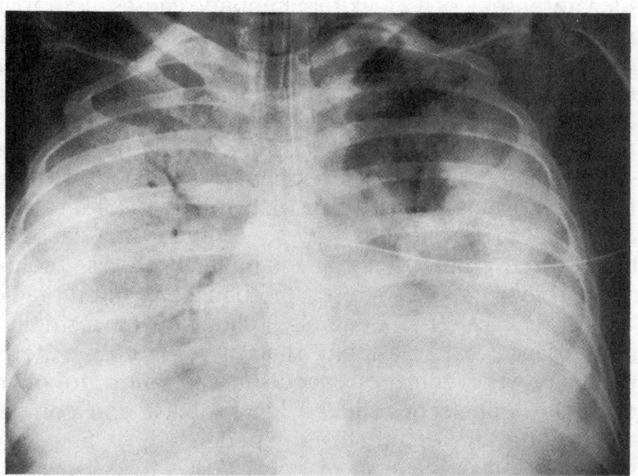

▲ **Figure 39-9**

Adult respiratory distress syndrome (ARDS). This chest x-ray study shows massive consolidation from pulmonary edema following multisystem trauma. (From Fraser, R. G., Paré, J. A., & Paré, P. D., et al [1990]. *Diagnosis of diseases of the chest,* 3rd ed. Philadelphia: W. B. Saunders.)

suspected or confirmed infection is present. Although it remains controversial, the use of large doses of corticosteroids is also common. The rationale for steroid administration is to reduce inflammatory response and promote pulmonary membrane stability. However, controlled clinical trials of corticosteroid use have failed to demonstrate their effectiveness in ARDS.[42]

Nursing Management

The principles of nursing management of clients with pneumonia, pulmonary edema, and other pulmonary disorders that affect gas exchange are also appropriate in the care of the client with ARDS. In addition, nursing interventions associated with continuous mechanical ventilation will also be used. Evaluation of the client's response to treatment, as well as careful monitoring for potential complications, is essential.

Emotional support for the client's family or significant others is also important. The disease can progress very rapidly, leaving family members unprepared for the severity of the client's condition. Clear communications and frequent condition updates are essential for keeping the family adequately informed.

RESTRICTIVE LUNG DISORDERS

Overview

Restrictive lung disorders are a major category of pulmonary problems. The category includes any disorder that limits lung expansion and produces a pattern of abnormal function on pulmonary function tests characterized by a decrease in lung volume (TLC).

There are many causes of restrictive lung diseases. They may result from (1) conditions affecting interstitial lung tissues (there are over 100 identified interstitial lung diseases) or (2) extrapulmonary causes. Extrapulmonary causes include neurologic and neuromuscular disorders and disorders affecting the thoracic cage, pleura, and diaphragm movement. Obesity may also lead to restrictive lung disorders. Peripheral (obstructive) sleep disorders may also be categorized as restrictive lung diseases (see Chap. 17). See Box 39-9 for a representative list of restrictive lung disorders.

Clinical manifestations vary according to the cause of the restrictive disorder. For example, kyphosis, scoliosis, and kyphoscoliosis result in changes in the thoracic cage (Fig. 39-10). Generally, clients with restrictive lung disease exhibit a rapid, shallow respiratory pattern. Chronic hyperventilation occurs in an effort to overcome the effects of reduced lung volume and compliance. Shortness of breath is experienced, at first only with exertion but later at rest also. ABGs reveal alveolar hyperventilation (i.e., reduced $PaCO_2$) during the initial and intermediate phases of the disease process. As the disease progresses, respiratory muscle fatigue may occur, leading to inadequate alveolar ventilation and carbon dioxide retention. Hypoxemia is a common finding, especially in the later stages of restrictive lung disease.

Box 39-9. Restrictive Lung Diseases

Intrapulmonary

- Pulmonary fibrosis
- Sarcoidosis and other interstitial lung diseases
- Pneumonia
- Atelectasis
- Pneumoconioses
- Surgical lung resection
- Neoplastic disease

Extrapulmonary

- Head or spinal cord injury
- Amyotrophic lateral sclerosis
- Myasthenia gravis
- Muscular dystrophy
- Congenital chest wall deformity
- Acquired chest wall changes (e.g., kyphosis or scoliosis)
- Abdominal distention restricting the diaphragm and respiration
- Sleep disorders
- Poliomyelitis
- Pleural effusion
- Pleurisy
- Excessive obesity

These are representative of the many disorders affecting lung volumes and compliance of either chest wall or lung tissue (i.e., restrictive lung diseases).

Pulmonary function tests demonstrate impairment of the lungs' bellows action. Commonly, the FEV_1/FVC ratio will be normal or increased (i.e., 75 per cent or more of expected values). The FEV_1/FVC ratio by itself is not an absolute indicator of restrictive lung disorders. The TLC is the primary indicator of the disease. TLC is less than 80 per cent of expected values in these clients. Some clients have a mixture of restrictive and obstructive lung disorders.

Often, a specific diagnosis of restrictive lung disease is made only after extensive testing, including biopsy, immunologic testing (e.g., blood studies to determine increased globins and autoantibodies), and tests to differentiate neurologic dysfunction such as electromyography or spinal fluid analysis.

Interstitial lung diseases cause characteristic chest x-ray findings. Terms such as reticular or interstitial pattern, nodular pattern, reticulonodular pattern, honeycomb pattern, ground-glass pattern, miliary pattern, or Kerley's lines are used to describe the specific appearance of various forms of interstitial lung disease. Chest films may also show extrapulmonary disorders (e.g., large abdominal tumor restricting diaphragm movement).

Management

The management of the client is based on the degree of impairment and the ability to reverse the condition. Clients with spinal deformities may be helped with spi-

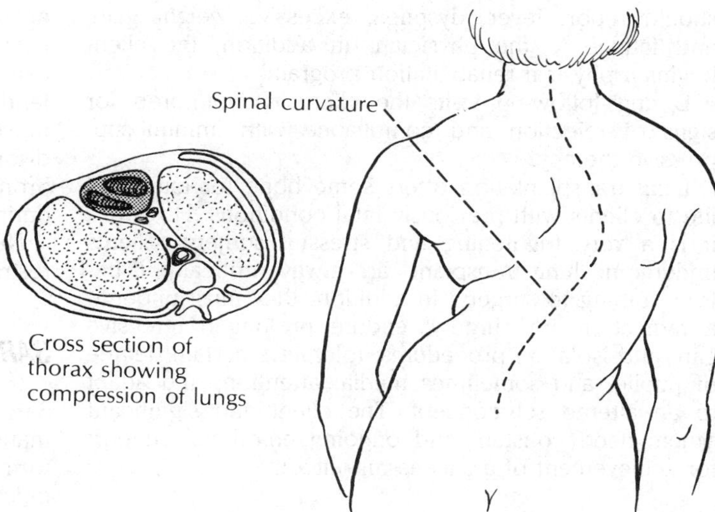

▲ *Figure 39-10*

Thoracic kyphoscoliosis. Note the S shape of the spine. These thoracic deformities alter the chest cage space. Lung tissue may be compressed, producing altered lung function (restrictive lung disease).

nal surgery. Likewise, obese clients will breathe better after weight loss. Clients with restrictive lung disorders due to interstitial disease are discussed later. Selected clients may benefit from the use of transtracheal oxygen administration and/or nocturnal mechanical ventilation with a mask, especially those clients with post-poliomyelitis syndrome.

The primary goals for nursing management of the client with restrictive lung disease are (1) promotion of adequate oxygenation, (2) maintenance of a patent airway, and (3) achievement of the highest possible functional level. Interventions to attain these goals are similar to those used in the treatment of COPD (see earlier). ABG analysis is important for monitoring oxygen needs and assessing the effects of physical activity. $PaCO_2$ levels should be monitored because rising carbon dioxide levels are an indicator of impending respiratory failure.

Most restrictive lung disorders are not reversible. End-stage disease is characterized by the development of pulmonary hypertension, cor pulmonale, severe oxygenation problems, and eventual ventilatory failure. Efforts should be made to maintain the client's functional status and quality of life at as high a level as possible.

LUNG TRANSPLANTATION

Some clients with end-stage disease may be candidates for single-lung transplantation. This procedure involves replacement of one of the diseased lungs with a lung from a cadaver donor. Although the procedure is still relatively uncommon, the success of lung transplantation is increasing with advanced surgical techniques and antirejection medications (immunosuppressives).

The surgical procedure involves removal of the diseased lung and attachment of the donor lung at three major anastomosis sites. First, the donor bronchus is sutured to the recipient's bronchial stump. A pedicled omental graft from the abdomen is wrapped around the bronchial anastomosis to protect the site and provide additional blood flow to the transplanted bronchus. Second, the two major pulmonary veins from the donor lung are attached to the recipient's left atrium. Last, the pulmonary artery is anastomosed. A portion of the pericardium may be wrapped around the pulmonary artery for extra support.

Following surgery, the client is observed for excessive bleeding. The nurse monitors vital signs, hemodynamic pressures, ECG and chest tube drainage. Pulmonary edema may develop in the denervated transplanted lung. Therefore, the client is placed on continuous mechanical ventilation with positive end-expiratory pressure (PEEP) for 24 to 48 hours. Fluids are restricted, lung sounds are auscultated and the degree of peripheral edema is monitored. Following extubation, the client is assisted to cough and deep breathe and use incentive spirometry to expand the lung.

The client is at high risk of infection and transplant rejection. Protective isolation (reverse isolation) is used to decrease inadvertent exposure to pathogens. The client is also monitored for clinical manifestations of infection such as changes in vital signs, local infections at intravenous access sites and incision lines, and changes in respiratory status (excessive secretions, tachypnea, dyspnea, fatigue). Rejection of the lung may present as dyspnea, changes in chest x-ray (the development of white-out on the film), a need for ventilatory support, and fatigue.

Following the initial surgery, the client may develop alterations in self-concept related to changes in appearance from the side effects of medications such as steroids and immunosuppressants, a change in lifestyle, or a change in work ability and role performance. The nurse is sensitive to these issues and encourages the client and family to discuss their feelings and explore options.

Prior to discharge, the client is taught about the medication regimen and the nurse stresses the need for daily medication despite a lack of symptoms. The client should report fever, dyspnea, excessive weight gain, and fatigue to the physician. In addition, the client begins a physical rehabilitation program.

During follow-up visits the client is monitored for signs of rejection and compliance with immunosuppressive therapy.

Lung transplantation offers some hope for extended life to clients with previously fatal conditions. However, it is a very frightening and stressful surgery. Clients undergoing lung transplants are always critically ill before coming to surgery. In addition, they must undergo a radical, major surgery; endure prolonged intensive care and isolation procedures; tolerate a certain degree of public, and sometimes media, attention; and adapt to an altered self-concept. The client and significant others need constant and ongoing emotional support for achievement of a successful outcome.

INTERSTITIAL LUNG DISEASE

Overview

Interstitial lung diseases (ILDs) are a group of diffuse, inflammatory lower respiratory tract disorders. The term interstitial is used to describe the fact that the interstitium of the alveolar walls is thickened and usually fibrotic. The alveolar walls thicken as a result of the accumulation of inflammatory cells. The thick alveolus becomes nonfunctional.

The etiology of ILD is not clearly defined. It most commonly develops from idiopathic pulmonary fibrosis, sarcoidosis, and collagen vascular disorders. ILD can also result from the inhalation of inorganic dust, such as crystalline silica, asbestos and coal dust, and organic dust from organisms encountered in farming, air conditioner use, and animal husbandry.

Clinical manifestations are insidious and nonspecific, such as dyspnea and nonproductive cough. Because the symptoms are nonspecific, ILD may go undiagnosed for years.

The diagnosis of ILD can be complex, because many other disorders can produce similar clinical manifestations. The client history plays a major part in diagnosis, because it is important to determine to what agents the client has been exposed. Clients report progressive dyspnea and often have dyspnea at rest. Chest expansion is normally reduced, reflecting a decreased TLC. Inspiratory and expiratory crackles are frequently heard. The crackles have a characteristic sound, like the sound of Velcro being pulled apart. Clubbing of the finger tips may be evident. Diagnostic assessment may include gallium ventilation perfusion scans. These scans usually reveal impaired perfusion in the lower lobes and multiple areas of impaired ventilation. Bronchoscopy and biopsy may also be used to confirm ILD.

Management

The management of a client with ILD is based on the degree of impairment. The inflammation is controlled with corticosteroids. The client is taught that corticosteroids reduce further impairment, but previously damaged alveolar-capillary units are lost forever. Many clients have subjective improvement on steroids and can eventually be tapered off of the drugs. If the offending agent is known, the initial treatment is to remove the client from exposure to the agent. As the disorder progresses, clients are usually treated with bronchodilators to help mobilize secretions and oxygen during periods of exercise.

Nursing management is the same as for clients with restrictive lung disorders.

SARCOIDOSIS

Sarcoidosis is an inflammatory condition that affects many body systems. The disease is characterized by the formation of widespread granulomatous lesions. In addition to lung involvement, which occurs in over 90 per cent of cases, clients may present with clinical manifestations involving the peripheral lymphatic system, skin, liver, eyes, spleen, bones, salivary glands, joints, and heart. The onset of sarcoidosis is generally between the ages of 20 and 40 years. The incidence in the United States ranges from 11 to 40 per 100,000 people. The disorder is approximately 14 times more common in blacks than in whites, and although the male:female ratio is about even in the nonblack population, black females develop sarcoidosis twice as frequently as do black males.[27]

The exact cause of sarcoidosis remains unknown. However, the disease itself is becoming more fully understood. There is now evidence that a triggering agent, which may be genetic, infectious, immunologic, or toxic, stimulates enhanced cell-mediated immune processes at the site of involvement.[27] A series of interactions between T lymphocytes and monocytes/macrophages leads to the formation of noncaseating (i.e., do not undergo necrotic degeneration) granulomas, which are characteristic of the disease. Granuloma formation may regress with therapy or as a result of the disorder's natural course but may also progress to fibrosis and restrictive lung disease.

About a third of the clients with sarcoidosis are asymptomatic; diagnosis is made by chest x-ray study findings of hilar adenopathy and pulmonary fibrosis. Clients with pulmonary manifestations usually present with a dry cough and shortness of breath. Chest pain, hemoptysis, or pneumothorax may also be present. Systemic symptoms may include fatigue, weakness, malaise, weight loss, and fever. A definitive diagnosis of sarcoidosis is made by tissue biopsy. When lung involvement is suspected, bronchoscopy, bronchoalveolar lavage, mediastinoscopy, or open lung biopsy may be performed.

Medical management is primarily determined by the degree to which the client's life is disturbed by the symptoms experienced. If the client with sarcoidosis is asymptomatic, management involves ongoing assessment for further disease progression. Repeat chest films at 6-month intervals are often indicated. When symptoms are present, medical treatment usually consists of systemic corticosteroids. When corticosteroids are administered, dramatic improvement may occur.

Nursing intervention for clients with sarcoidosis is the same as that for other restrictive lung diseases and hypoxemia. The nurse should assess for drug side effects, especially adverse responses to corticosteroids. The nurse should also assess for signs of improvement, such as (1) increased exercise tolerance, (2) disappearance of initial assessment findings, (3) improved pulmonary function studies, (4) side effects of steroids (weight gain, change in mood, development of diabetes mellitus), and (5) improved oxygenation. If assessment findings worsen, the nurse should document them and notify the physician.

OCCUPATIONAL LUNG DISEASES

Lung diseases are among the most common occupational health problems. They are caused by the inhalation of various chemicals, dusts, and other particulate matter that are present in certain work settings. Not all clients exposed to occupational inhalants will develop lung disease. Harmful effects depend on the (1) nature of the exposure; (2) duration and intensity of the exposure; (3) particle size and water-solubility of the inhalant (the larger the particle, the lower the probability of its reaching the lower respiratory tract; highly water-soluble inhalants tend to dissolve and react in the upper respiratory tract, whereas poorly soluble substances may travel as far as the alveoli); (4) smoking history; and (5) presence of underlying pulmonary disease.

The most commonly encountered occupational lung diseases are described in Table 39–5. Acute respiratory irritation results from the inhalation of chemicals such as ammonia, chlorine, and nitrogen oxides in the form of gases, aerosols, or particulate matter. If such irritants reach the lower airways, alveolar damage and pulmonary edema can result. Although the effects of acute

TABLE 39–5. Characteristics of Occupational Lung Diseases

	Onset of Symptoms	Diagnosis	Treatment	Clinical Course
Acute respiratory irritation	Usually within minutes of exposure to irritant, but pulmonary edema may be delayed several hours	Consistent history; physical findings of respiratory tract irritation and damage	Prevention of exposure; respiratory support as needed	Upper respiratory tract signs resolve in hours to days; pulmonary edema resolves in days to weeks; residual damage rare
Occupational asthma	Usually within minutes of exposure to precipitant but possibly delayed 4 to 6 hours or more	Pulmonary function tests showing obstructive pattern during exacerbations; chest film usually normal; skin tests, IgE measurement, and history of atopy helpful only if the disorder is IgE-mediated	Prevention of exposure; asthma medications	Usually resolves within hours; airways may remain persistently hyperreactive
Hypersensitivity pneumonitis	Usually 4 to 8 hours after exposure to antigen; possible subacute or chronic presentation	Specific IgG antibodies; radiographic findings ranging from normal to pulmonary edema to interstitial fibrosis; pulmonary function tests giving restrictive or restrictive/obstructive pattern	Prevention of exposure; respiratory support as needed; steroids helpful in some cases	Symptoms usually resolve in several days; radiographic and pulmonary function findings normalize in a few weeks; however, there may be permanent lung damage
Pneumoconioses	Requires long-term exposure; first symptom often cough progressing to dyspnea	Restrictive pattern on pulmonary function tests; on chest film, asbestosis is associated with interstitial markings in lower lobes and silicosis with opacities in upper lobes	Prevention of exposure; cessation of smoking	Gradual worsening

From Mandel, J. H., & Baker, B. A. (1989). Recognizing occupational lung disease. *Hospital Practice, 24*:21.

irritants are usually short-lived, some may cause chronic alveolar damage or airway obstruction.

Occupational asthma is defined as variable airflow obstruction caused by a specific agent in the workplace. By far the greatest number of occupational agents causing asthma are those with known or suspected allergic properties, such as plant and animal proteins (e.g., wheat flour, cotton, flax, and grain mites). In most cases, the asthma will resolve after exposure is terminated. However, hyperreactivity of the airways may persist for years.

Hypersensitivity pneumonitis, or allergic alveolitis, is most commonly due to the inhalation of organic antigens of fungal, bacterial, or animal origin. The nature of the exposure and the client's immunologic reactivity will determine the pulmonary response. Nonatopic people (i.e., those with no history of allergies) develop a pulmonary response to organic dusts more often than do atopic individuals, although they too may exhibit pulmonary reactions.

Pneumoconioses, or the "dust diseases," result from inhalation of minerals, notably silica, coal dust, or asbestos. These diseases are most commonly seen in miners, construction workers, sandblasters, potters, and foundry and quarry workers. Pneumoconioses usually develop gradually over a period of years, eventually leading to diffuse pulmonary fibrosis that diminishes lung capacity and produces restrictive lung disease. Early symptoms may include cough and dyspnea on exertion. Chest pain, productive cough, and dyspnea at rest develop as the condition progresses.

Early detection is one way to prevent progression of the disease process. When the nurse takes a respiratory history, it should include a complete occupational history and questions about (1) the actual job performed rather than title or job description, (2) past as well as current occupations, and (3) exposure to organic and inorganic substances in each job. Assess dyspnea, cough, chest tightness, or other symptoms indicating potential lung disease. Some employers support ongoing assessment programs (e.g., routine pulmonary function studies or chest films) for workers at risk for occupational disorders.

Exposure precautions are essential for avoiding permanent pulmonary disability. Safety measures include adequate ventilation, wearing masks, and using care when handling garments worn in dusty environments.

Nursing intervention for clients experiencing occupational lung diseases is similar to that for clients with other restrictive lung disorders (see Restrictive Lung Disease). Supportive measures can help these clients to adjust their lifestyles to their condition.

If occupational lung disease is significant, the client may qualify for disability allowances. Nurses can refer clients to community resources, such as federal or state departments of labor, if they have questions concerning eligibility. Because of legal problems that may surround compensation claims, the nurse may have to deal with much hostility and resentment aimed toward the employer and the legal system. These clients may also experience much anxiety and uncertainty about their future health status. A calm, positive approach is often needed.

MALIGNANT LUNG TUMORS

Definition

Lung cancer is malignancy in the epithelium of the respiratory tract. At least a dozen different cell types of tumors are included under the classification of lung cancer. The four major types of lung cancer include small cell carcinoma (oat cell carcinoma), squamous cell carcinoma, adenocarcinoma, and large cell carcinoma. Clinically, lung cancers are grouped into two divisions—small cell lung cancer, and non-small cell lung cancer. The term lung cancer excludes other disorders such as sarcomas, lymphomas, blastomas, and mesotheliomas.

Incidence

The incidence of lung cancer is rising at a faster rate than that of any other cancer type. In 1986, lung cancer exceeded breast cancer as the leading cause of death from cancer in American women. It continues to be the number one cause of cancer deaths in men, as it has been for the past 30 years. Mortality rates are similar for white and nonwhite women but greater in nonwhite versus white men. The incidence of specific types of cancer is discussed later.

Etiology

The most common cause of lung cancer is cigarette smoking. Cigarette smoke contains several organ-specific carcinogens. Genetic predisposition to the development of lung cancer also plays a role in the etiology. Other carcinogens include inhaled toxins, such as asbestos, and pollutants.

Risk Factors

Cigarette smoking is the leading risk factor for the development of lung cancer; as many as 80 to 90 per cent of lung malignancies occur in clients who smoke. Heavy smokers (i.e., those who smoke more than 25 cigarettes a day) have 20 times the risk of developing lung cancer than do nonsmokers. Whereas smoking cessation lowers the risk, the decrease is gradual and does not approach that of a nonsmoker until 15 to 20 years later. Recent studies have also suggested that passive smoke (i.e., smoke inhaled from the environment surrounding an active smoker) may be responsible for up to 5 per cent of all lung cancers (see Ethical Issues in Nursing).[51]

The risk of lung cancer is increased even further in the smoker who is also exposed to other carcinogenic agents, such as radioactive isotopes, polycyclic hydrocarbons, vinyl chloride, metallurgical ores, and mustard gas. Whether these occupational factors increase the risk of cancer development in the nonsmoker is still unclear. The inhalation of asbestos fibers, however, is

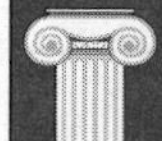

ETHICAL ISSUES IN NURSING

Is It a Nurse's Responsibility to Educate Clients and Others on the Dangers of "Second-Hand Smoke"?

Since the 1960s, research has supported the claim that smoking cigarettes is dangerous to one's health. Smoking assaults the respiratory structures and with repeated assaults, may even lead to lung cancer. In more recent times, however, research has introduced the ill effects of "second-hand smoke." These ill effects are the result of one person's smoke from cigarettes on another person's lungs. Second-hand smoke has been linked to altered respiratory function and even to cancer.

People may have a right to do whatever they will to their own bodies, but is this right valid when, perhaps, some of their actions adversely affect the health of others? The concept of nonmaleficence applies to all persons, not just to health care workers. One should not engage in activities that may bring harm to another (i.e., second-hand smoke, driving while intoxicated, and the like).

Many health care facilities are designated as "smoke free" in order to promote a more healthy environment for their workers and their clients. Nursing care of those who smoke should reinforce the damage that second-hand smoke can do. Nurses may assist their clients who smoke to better health by giving them information on hospital or local stop-smoking programs. Nurses act beneficently toward their clients when assisting them to better health through the encouragement of their participation in stop-smoking programs. People who smoke may act beneficently toward others by not subjecting them to the effects of their second-hand smoke.

associated with higher cancer risks for both smokers and nonsmokers.

Air pollution has also been implicated in increasing the risk of lung cancer, although its exact role is not known. The rate of lung cancer in clients who live in urban areas is 2.3 times greater than in those living in rural areas.

Pathophysiology

Lung cancers are divided into two major categories: small cell lung cancers (SCLC) and non-small cell lung cancers (NSCLC), which include epidermoid or squamous cell, adenocarcinoma, and large cell. The characteristics of each of these types are described in Table 39-6. In general, survival rates are best for NSCLC, especially with treatment in its early stages. Despite increasing knowledge and technology, however, overall survival from lung cancer remains low, especially for clients with small cell carcinomas.

Metastatic spread of pulmonary tumors is usually to the long bones, vertebral column (especially the thoracic vertebrae), liver, and adrenal glands. Brain metastasis is also common, occurring in as many as 50 per cent of cases.

Paraneoplastic syndromes (i.e., remote effects of a malignancy) occur in 10 to 20 per cent of lung cancer clients. These usually result from the secretion of substances (e.g., hormones) by the tumor itself. These substances then act on target organs, producing a variety of symptoms, such as hypercalcemia, mental changes, gynecomastia, and Cushing's syndrome. Occasionally, symptoms of paraneoplastic syndrome may occur before detection of the primary lung tumor.

Clinical Manifestations

The warning signals of lung cancer are presented in Box 39-10. In many instances, lung cancer may mimic other pulmonary conditions. Lung cancer may also be manifested by extrapulmonary symptoms that occur before pulmonary symptoms appear. Specific clinical assessment findings vary according to tumor type, location, and extent as well as pre-existing pulmonary health.

Centrally located pulmonary tumors usually obstruct airflow, producing symptoms such as coughing, wheezing, stridor, and dyspnea. As obstruction increases, bronchopulmonary infection often occurs distal to the obstruction. Chest, shoulder, and back pain may develop as the tumor invades the perivascular nerves. Squamous and small cell tumors often cause hemoptysis. Small cell tumors may also extend into the pericardium, causing pericardial effusion and, possibly, tamponade. Cardiac rhythm disturbances are also likely. Centrally located pulmonary tumors are easiest to locate and identify with fiberoptic bronchoscopy and sputum cytologic study. Positive tissue diagnosis is possible 90 per cent of the time.

Peripheral pulmonary tumors often do not produce assessment findings initially. In time, pleural pain develops that increases on inspiration, is sharp and severe, and is usually localized. Pleural effusion also develops and, along with the pain, limits lung expansion. Only 30 per cent of peripheral lung tumors are successfully categorized by bronchoscopic and cytologic examination.

Pancoast's tumors occur in the apices of the lungs in both squamous cell and adenocarcinomatous cancers. Assessment findings do not occur until the tumor growth extends into surrounding structures. Pancoast's tumors often involve the first thoracic and eighth cervical nerves within the brachial plexus. This causes arm

Box 39-10. Warning Signals of Lung Cancer

- Any change in respiratory patterns
- Persistent cough
- Sputum streaked with blood
- Frank hemoptysis
- Rust-colored or purulent sputum
- Chest, shoulder, or arm pain
- Recurring episodes of pleural effusion, pneumonia, or bronchitis
- Dyspnea, unexplained or out of proportion

TABLE 39-6. Overview of Malignant Pulmonary Neoplasms

Cell Type	Approximate Incidence	Specific Characteristics	Growth Rate
Epidermoid (squamous cell)	30-35% of lung cancer	Arises from bronchial epithelium; as growth occurs, cavitation may develop in lung distal to tumor. Pancoast's tumors arise in apex and upper lung zones Abundant keratin formation noted microscopically Secondary infections distal to obstructive tumor in bronchioles frequently occur	Slow growth, metastasis not common If tumor metastasizes, usually to lymph, adrenals, and liver (in that order)
Adenocarcinoma	25-30% of lung cancer	May arise proximally but more often peripherally (60-70%); arises from bronchial mucus gland Often subpleural; often difficult to distinguish from other tumors in the body; rarely cavitates; often arises in previously scarred lung tissue Incidence strongly linked to cigarette smoking Increasing incidence in women Bronchiolo-alveolar cell carcinomas are a subtype	Slow growth May metastasize throughout lung or to other organs of the body
Large cell	10-20% of lung cancer	More often peripheral mass, either single or multiple masses Cavitation common May be located centrally, midlung, or peripherally Rare hilar involvement Often grows to large tumor mass before diagnosis	Slow; metastasis may occur to kidney, liver, and adrenals, in that order
Small cell (oat cell)	20-25% of lung cancer	65-75% present with hilar or central mass May narrow bronchi through compression Involvement of diaphragm through paralysis of phrenic nerve and hoarseness through paralysis of recurrent laryngeal nerve Pleural, pericardial effusions and tamponade Does not form cavities	Rapid growth Metastasis to mediastinum, thoracic and extrathoracic structures occurs early

and shoulder pain on the affected side and atrophy of the arm and hand muscles on that side. With continuing tumor growth, the ribs over the tumor (usually the first and second ribs) may be invaded. Bone pain and later involvement of the sympathetic nerve ganglia lead to Horner's syndrome. This syndrome consists of miosis (pupil contraction), partial eyelid ptosis, and anhidrosis (absence of sweating) on the affected side of the face.

The primary assessment finding with pleural tumors (malignant mesotheliomas) is chest pain. Dyspnea, cough, weight loss, and fever may also be present. Thoracotomy is usually required for a definitive diagnosis.

Metastasis. Tumor spread, by either direct extension or metastasis, may produce further clinical symptoms. Direct extension to the recurrent laryngeal nerve produces hoarseness. Compression of the esophagus may produce dysphagia. Invasion or compression of the superior vena cava produces superior vena cava syndrome, a potentially life-threatening emergency. Obstruction of venous blood flow leads to clinical manifestations that may include shortness of breath;

facial, arm, and trunk swelling; distention of the thoracic veins; chest pain; and venous stasis. Immediate, palliative surgical treatment may be necessary.

Regional lymph node involvement may produce symptoms due to impaired lymph drainage. Involvement of the mediastinal lymph nodes may result in vocal cord paralysis, dysphagia, diaphragm paralysis on the affected side (due to phrenic nerve compression), vena cava compression, and malignant pleural effusion. When mediastinal lymph nodes are involved, surgical excision of the pulmonary tumor is usually no longer possible.

DIAGNOSTIC ASSESSMENT

Numerous diagnostic tests may be used to determine the presence and extent of the disease. Sputum cytology and chest radiography are most commonly used. Tomograms and computed tomographic (CT) scans may be used when visualization on standard chest radiographs is unclear or suggests a pulmonary lesion. Bronchoscopy may be performed with centrally located lesions; bronchial washing/brushing is done to obtain tumor cells for cytologic and pathologic assessment. In addition, percutaneous needle biopsy, mediastinoscopy, or direct surgical biopsy may be required to confirm the diagnosis. Radionuclide scans may be used to detect metastasis to the bone, liver, or brain (see Chap. 21).

Staging is performed to provide a guideline for the selection of appropriate therapies and the estimation of prognosis. Staging information is valuable for helping clients and their families to make treatment decisions and to set appropriate short- and long-term goals.

The TNM classification scheme is used for lung cancer staging (Box 39-11 and Fig. 39-11). The definitions and stage groupings were recently revised to provide more descriptive information for classifying limited versus extensive disease for SCLC as well as for NSCLC. This revised system appears to provide a better basis for predicting 5-year survival rates than did previously used systems.[42]

Box 39-11. Classification of Pulmonary Malignancies

Primary Tumor (T)

- T_x Tumor proven by presence of malignant cells in bronchopulmonary secretions but not visualized roentgenographically or bronchoscopically, or any tumor that cannot be assessed as in a retreatment staging
- T_0 No evidence of primary tumor
- T_{is} Carcinoma in situ
- T_1 A tumor that is 3 cm or less in greatest dimension, surrounded by lung or visceral pleura and without evidence of invasion proximal to a lobar bronchus at bronchoscopy
- T_2 Tumor more than 3 cm in greatest dimension or a tumor of any size that either invades the visceral pleura or has associated atelectasis or obstructive pneumonitis extending to the hilar region; at bronchoscopy, the proximal extent of demonstrable tumor must be within a lobar bronchus or at least 2 cm distal to the carina; any associated atelectasis or obstructive pneumonitis must involve less than an entire lung
- T_3 A tumor of any size with direct extension into the chest wall (including superior sulcus tumors), the diaphragm, or the mediastinal pleura or pericardium without involving the heart, great vessels, trachea, esophagus, or vertebral body; or a tumor in the main bronchus within 2 cm of the carina without involving the carina
- T_4 A tumor of any size with invasion of the mediastinum or involving the heart, great vessels, trachea, esophagus, vertebral body, or carina in the presence of malignant pleural effusion

Nodes (N)

- N_0 No demonstrable metastases to regional lymph nodes
- N_1 Metastasis to lymph nodes in the peribronchial or the ipsilateral hilar region or both, including direct extension
- N_2 Metastases to ipsilateral mediastinal lymph nodes and subcarinal lymph nodes
- N_3 Metastasis to contralateral mediastinal, contralateral hilar, ipsilateral or contralateral scalene, or supraclavicular lymph nodes

Distant Metastasis (M)

- M_0 No (known) distant metastasis
- M_1 Distant metastasis present, specify site(s)

From Mountain, C. F. (1986). A new international staging system for lung cancer. *Chest, 89*:225s-233.

Medical Management

The key to increasing the survival rate of clients with lung cancer is early detection. When premalignant changes begin, dysplastic cells are identifiable with fiberoptic bronchoscopy and sputum cytologic studies. At this stage, lesions are potentially curable. However, a tumor must be at least 1 cm in diameter before it is detectable on chest film. Unfortunately, invasion and metastasis have usually already occurred.

Management of the client with lung cancer depends on tumor type and stage as well as the client's underlying health status. Primary treatment modalities include radiation therapy, chemotherapy, and surgery.

RADIATION THERAPY

Radiotherapy may be used as a potentially curative treatment in clients with locally advanced disease who are poor surgical risks, who have technically inoperable tumors, or who refuse thoracotomy. Radiation therapy may also be used in combination with surgery or chemotherapy to improve treatment outcomes. Radiotherapy is administered over a period of 5 to 6 weeks,

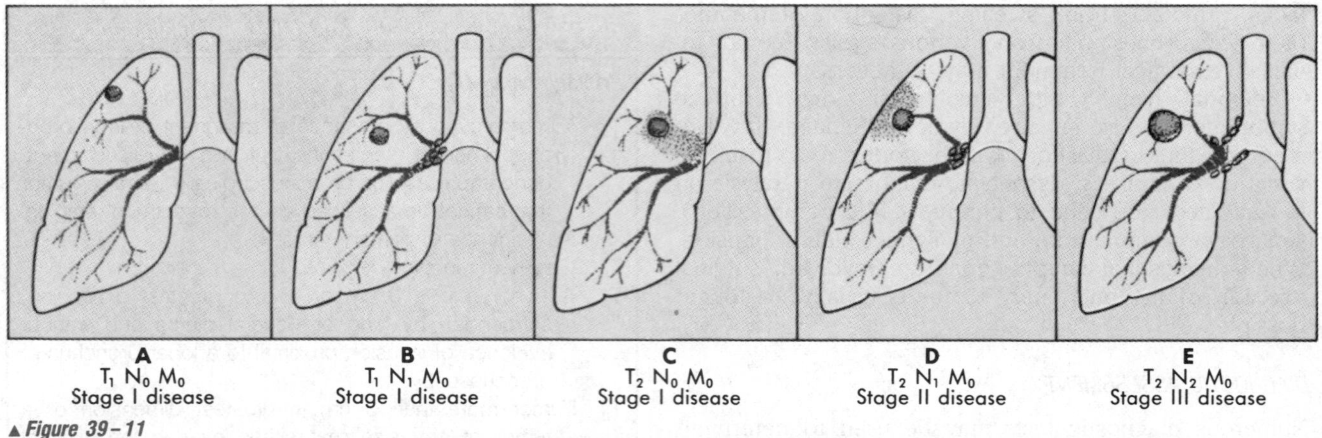

▲ *Figure 39-11*

Staging of lung cancer by the TNM classification system. *A* and *B*, Stage I disease includes tumors classified as T_1, with or without metastasis to the lymph nodes in the ipsilateral hilar region. *C*, Also included in Stage I are tumors classified as T_2 but having no nodal or distant metastases. *D*, Stage II disease includes those tumors classified as T_2, with metastasis only to the ipsilateral hilar lymph nodes. *E*, Stage III includes all tumors more extensive than T_2, or any tumor with metastasis to the lymph nodes in the mediastinum or with distant metastasis. (From McCance, K. L., & Huether, S. E. [1990]. *Pathophysiology: The biologic basis for disease in adults and children.* St. Louis; C. V. Mosby Co.)

either consecutively or in split courses. Doses are limited by other structures in the treatment area and by normal tissue tolerance. Irreversible fibrotic changes and other pulmonary side effects may occur. To delineate the area to be irradiated precisely, CT scanning is often performed before treatment begins. This method also minimizes tissue damage to surrounding areas.

Radiotherapy may also be used for palliation of symptoms such as hemoptysis and obstruction or compression of bronchi, blood vessels, or esophagus. Irradiation of metastases to the brain and bone may reduce the distressing symptoms associated with these sequelae as well.

CHEMOTHERAPY

The response of lung cancer to chemotherapy depends on the tumor's cell type. SCLC responds well to chemotherapeutic agents because of its rapid growth rate. However, this rapid growth pattern also causes metastasis to occur readily. As a result, long-term survival rate for SCLC is still low.

Chemotherapy's effectiveness in the treatment of NSCLC remains controversial. It is commonly used in clients treated with surgery or radiation who experience recurrent disease or distant metastasis. However, large-scale studies have failed to demonstrate a significantly improved overall survival rate for these clients.[20] As a result, the decision to use chemotherapy is usually made on an individual basis, depending on the client's previous history, current condition, and acceptance of the risks and side effects involved.

Surgical Management

Surgical intervention is the treatment of choice in early stage NSCLC. Cure is possible if the disease is still localized to the thoracic cavity and no distant metastases are present. However, only 20 to 25 per cent of clients with NSCLC meet these criteria at time of diagnosis. Surgical survival rates (over a 5-year period) drop from 50 per cent survival for stage I to 15 per cent survival for stage III cancers.

The role of surgical resection in the treatment of SCLC remains under investigation. Surgery may be effective for clients in the early stages of SCLC, after chemotherapy. For clients with more advanced disease, surgery causes unnecessary risk and stress, with no valid benefits.

The primary aim of surgical resection is to remove the tumor completely while as little of the surrounding lung tissue as possible is removed. The extent of the surgery will depend on the location and size of the pulmonary tumor and the degree of the underlying pulmonary pathologic process. Clients with pre-existing pulmonary disease may not be able to tolerate extensive lung tissue removal.

Pulmonary Resection. Common pulmonary resection procedures are shown in Figure 39-12.

Wedge Resection. This procedure involves the removal of a small, localized area of diseased tissue near the surface of the lung. Because the resected area is small, pulmonary structure and function are relatively unchanged after healing.

Segmental Resection. This procedure involves the removal of one or more lung segments (a bronchiole and its alveoli). The remaining lung tissue overexpands to fill the space previously occupied by the removed segment.

Lobectomy. Lobectomy refers to removal of an entire lobe of the lung. After lobectomy, some compensatory nonpathologic emphysema occurs as the remaining lung tissue overexpands to fill in that portion of the thoracic space previously occupied by the resected tissue.

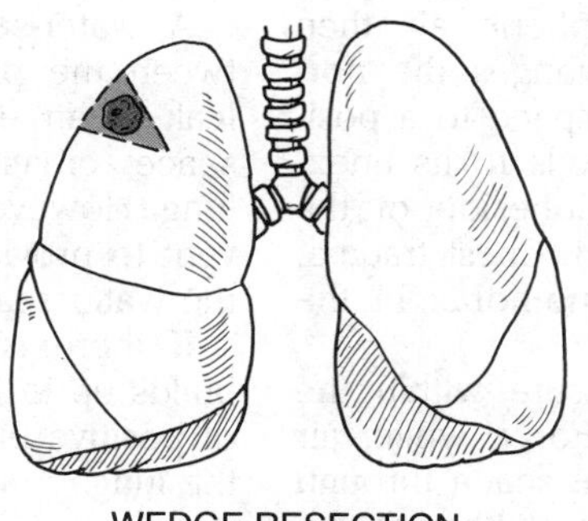

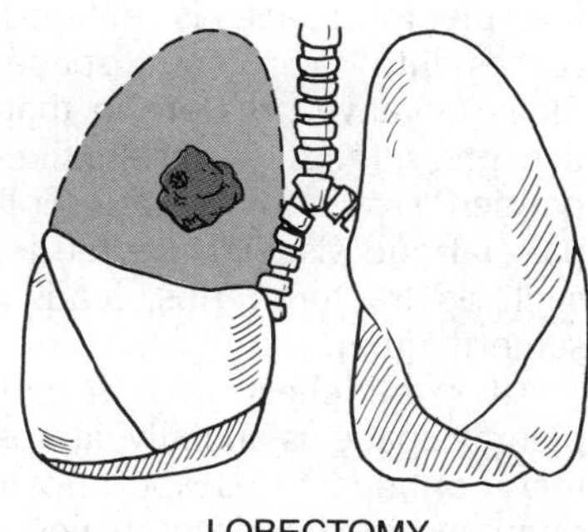

SEGMENTAL RESECTION

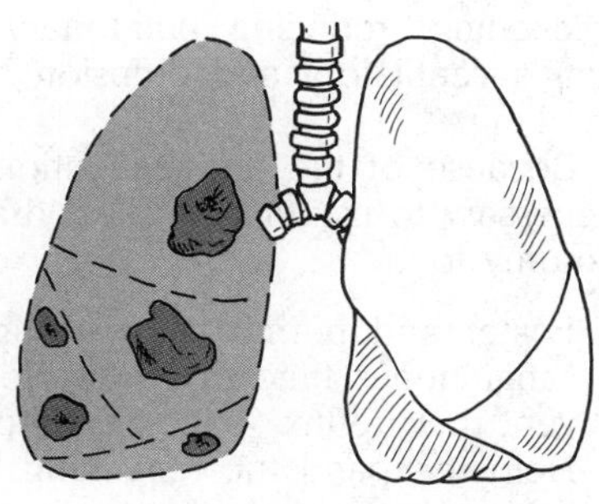

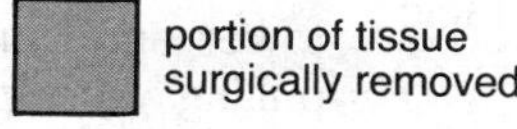

▲ *Figure 39-12*

Pulmonary resections.

Pneumonectomy. This procedure involves removal of an entire lung. Once the lung is removed, the involved side of the thoracic cavity is an empty space. In order to reduce the size of this cavity, the phrenic nerve is severed on the affected side to paralyze the diaphragm in an elevated position. A thoracoplasty may also be performed, which is removal of several ribs or portions of ribs to further reduce the thoracic space.

Closed chest drainage is usually not used after pneumonectomy. The serous fluid that accumulates in the empty thoracic cavity, and eventually consolidates, prevents extensive mediastinal shift of the heart and remaining lung.

LASER THERAPY

Another surgical treatment modality is laser therapy. Currently, laser use is palliative for the relief of endobronchial obstructions caused by nonresectable lung tumors. Lasers do not produce systemic or cumulative toxic effects and are well tolerated. Laser therapy may be done in the outpatient setting. However, in order to use the laser, the tumor mass must be accessible by bronchoscope. Therefore, tumors pressing on bronchial tissue from outside the bronchial lumen are not amenable to laser therapy. The use of laser as an operative modality is discussed in Chapter 19.

CLOSED CHEST DRAINAGE

Closed chest drainage is commonly used after chest surgery. It is also used to treat empyema or pneumothorax (spontaneous or following injuries). This section discusses the principles and purpose of chest drainage, the specific apparatus used, guidelines for assessing the functioning of closed chest drainage systems, precautions, and indications of complications.

Closed chest drainage means that the chest drainage system is closed to atmospheric pressure. Various equipment may be used. Historically, closed chest drainage was performed using a glass bottle water-seal apparatus (one or two bottle set-ups) with or without controlled mechanical suction. Most health care facilities have replaced glass bottle water-seal drainage systems with disposable single units (e.g., Pleur-evac). However, an understanding of the principles of bottle chest drainage is basic to understanding any type of closed chest drainage. A clear understanding of normal ventilation mechanisms (structure and function) is also essential to understand the principles of closed chest drainage (see Chap. 35).

Purposes of Closed Chest Drainage. Chest surgery actually causes a pneumothorax on the operated side. During thoracotomy, the parietal pleura is incised and the pleural space is entered. Atmospheric air then rushes into the pleural space. This changes the normally negative pressure in that pleural space to a positive pressure. As a result, the lung recoils to its unexpanded size and remains collapsed. Cohesion of the parietal and visceral pleurae is disrupted. Chest trauma, such as fractured ribs, leads to pneumothorax in the same manner.

After the chest wall is closed, pressure within the pleural space is initially atmospheric. For a while, air may continue to escape into the pleural space through openings in the visceral pleural incision. Although the pleura is sutured, it takes time to heal. The trauma of surgery causes serosanguineous fluid to collect in the thoracic cavity until healing occurs. Unfortunately, such fluid is a good culture medium and predisposes the client to infection. Also, the fluid may cause pleural thickening, reducing pulmonary compliance and the lung's ventilatory and diffusion capacities by stiffening the lung.

Because of the above-mentioned factors, it is often necessary to use closed chest drainage following thoracotomy to

- Foster and permit the drainage of air and/or serosanguineous fluid from the pleural space and to prevent their reflux (back-, or return, flow)
- Help reexpand the remaining lung tissue by reestablishing normal negative pressure in the pleural space
- Prevent mediastinal shift and lung tissue collapse by equalizing pressures on both sides of the thoracic cavity (operated and nonoperated sides)

Principles Used in Closed Chest Drainage Systems. Three principles are used in all closed drainage systems: gravity, water seal, and suction.

Gravity. Air and fluid flow from a higher level (pressure) to a lower level (pressure). Therefore, always keep chest drainage apparatus below the level of the person's chest.

Water Seal. A water seal provides a barrier between atmospheric pressure (pressing on the outside of the body) and subatmospheric (negative) intrapleural pressure (normal, 754 to 758 mm Hg).

On expiration, air and fluid in the pleural space travel through the drainage tubing into the first compartment. The air bubbles up through the bottle and enters atmospheric air.

On inspiration, the water seal prevents atmospheric air from being sucked back into the pleural space (which would collapse the lung). The fluid in the water-seal compartment is not drawn into the chest cavity, because the fluid is heavier than air.

As air and fluid drainage commences, the pressure in the pleural space becomes more negative. The greater this negative pressure is, the more the lung expands. Lung expansion, in turn, forces more fluid and air out of the pleural space. This cycle continues until the lung is fully expanded and intrathoracic negative pressure returns to its normal (subatmospheric) level.

A water-seal drainage system must be airtight between the pleural space and the water seal. Any air leak is an entry for atmospheric air into the pleural space, creating a positive pressure that collapses the lung. However, a water-seal chamber MUST have an air vent to provide an escape route for air passing through the water seal from the pleural space.

If there is no air vent, air from the pleural space builds up in the water-seal chamber, creating a buildup of positive pressure in the pleural space and collapsing the lung.

Suction. Suction is a pull force of less than atmospheric pressure (760 mm Hg). A suction of 20 cm H_2O creates a subatmospheric pressure of 746 mm Hg. Again, air or fluid moves from higher to lower pressure. Suction of 10 to 20 cm H_2O may be applied to a chest drainage system if gravity drainage is not adequate or if a person's cough and respirations are too weak to force air and fluid out of the pleural space through the chest catheters. Additionally, suction may be applied to closed chest drainage (1) if air is leaking into the pleural space faster than it can be removed by a water-seal apparatus or (2) to speed up the removal of air from the pleural space. Never apply suction to the same chamber as the drainage and/or water-seal chambers. A separate suction chamber is needed.

Suction may be applied to a two- or three-bottle water-seal system. A suction chamber contains a long tube with its top end open to atmospheric air and its lower end immersed in water. Suction is regulated by pulling atmospheric air through the long tube that is immersed in 10 to 20 cm of water. The immersed tube provides a barrier between the atmospheric air and the water. The deeper the tube is immersed in water, the more suction (subatmospheric pressure) is created. With suction, air travels from the person's pleural cavity via the water seal, through the air vent, into the suction chamber, and then to the suction source.

If the long tube in the suction bottle were not immersed in water, atmospheric air would go straight from the air vent into the suction source as fast as the suction was applied. Passing through water slows the air, and the suction force is controlled. Increasing the source of suction only causes more air to travel through the air vent. The suction applied to the person remains stable. An occluded atmospheric air vent is dangerous because it would cause the suction to be directly applied to the pleural cavity. Suction force greater than 50 cm H_2O may cause lung damage.

Insertion of Chest Catheters. Chest catheters are usually inserted in an operating room during chest surgery. However, in some emergencies or to treat problems such as empyema, a chest catheter may be inserted in a treatment room or at the bedside. (Chest catheters are also called chest drains, chest tubes, or thoracotomy tubes.)

Two catheters are usually placed in the chest following resectional surgery (except pneumonectomy). One of these (the upper, or anterior, tube) is placed anteriorly through the second intercostal space to permit the escape of air rising in the pleural space. The other catheter (the lower, or posterior, tube) is placed posteriorly through the eighth or ninth intercostal space in the midaxillary line to drain off serosanguineous fluid accumulating in the lower portion of the pleural space. The lower tube may have a larger diameter than the upper tube, to enhance fluid drainage.

Chest catheters are brought out of the chest wall through stab wounds or through the incisional line. The catheters are secured to the person's skin with sutures. However, also tape the tubes to the outside of the dressing for extra security against tube displacement.

The two chest catheters may be joined to each other with a plastic Y-junction (and then attached to one closed chest drainage system). However, it is preferable to leave them separate and to attach them to separate drainage systems. This makes it possible to monitor air and fluid drainage from each tube and later to remove a nondraining tube without disrupting the rest of the system. Flexible drainage tubing connects the chest catheter to the drainage apparatus. Usually, chest catheters are connected to a closed chest drainage apparatus before the person leaves surgery.

Three-bottle Water-seal Apparatus (Fig. 39-13). The first bottle collects drainage from the pleural cavity, the second bottle acts as the water seal, and the third bottle is the suction control. The three-bottle system allows for separate drainage collection and measurement, a stable water-seal system, and controlled suction. A disadvantage is that the system can be cumbersome. A Pleur-evac is a common commercially made three-bottle system (see Fig. 39-14).

Nursing Management

Assessing Chest Drainage. It is important to measure *and* document the amount of drainage coming from the pleural space. This record helps determine the amount of blood loss and the flow rate of drainage from the pleural space. Pleur-evac systems are manufactured with a marked strip to record the amount of

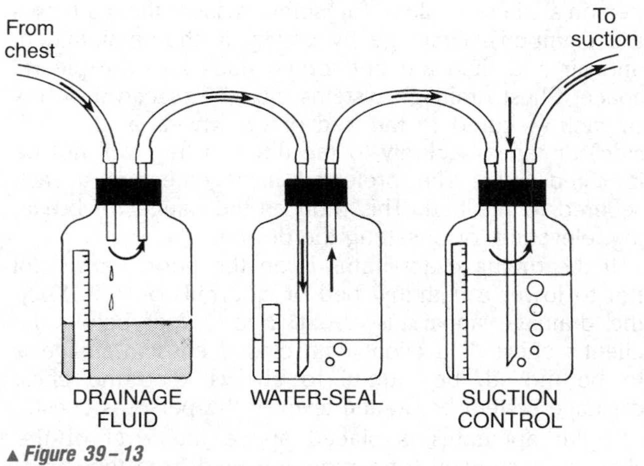

▲ *Figure 39-13*

Three-bottle system for chest drainage.

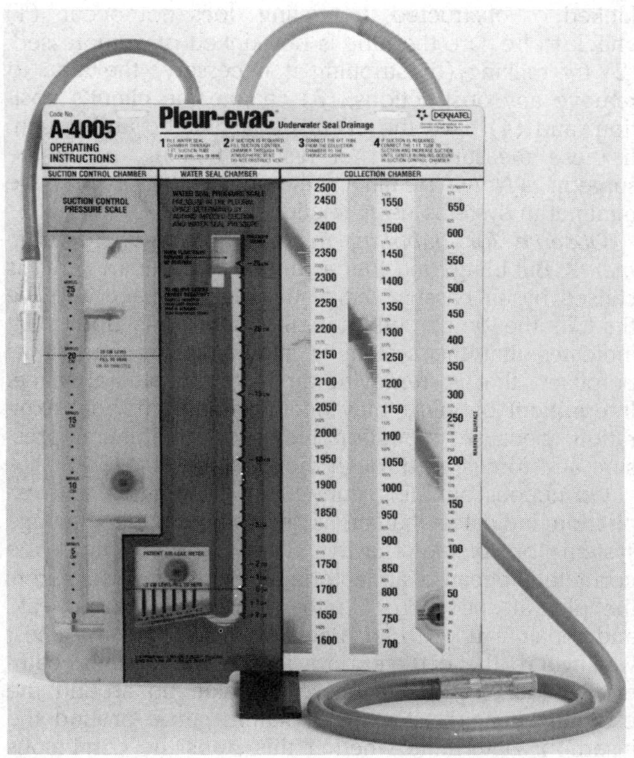

▲ *Figure 39-14*

Pleur-evac, a commercially manufactured, three-chambered system for closed chest drainage. (Courtesy of Deknatel, Division of Howmedica, Floral Park, NY.)

drainage. This is important in planning blood replacement therapy and assessing the client's status. Usually as much as 500 to 1000 ml of drainage occurs in the first 24 hours after chest surgery. Between 100 and 300 ml of drainage may accumulate during the first 2 hours. After this, the drainage should lessen. Excessive drainage may require further surgery to determine its cause.

Chest drainage is normally grossly bloody immediately following surgery. However, it should not continue to be so for more than several hours. Assess blood loss by monitoring the rising fluid level in the collection bottle. Suspect hemorrhage if the BP drops and the pulse is rapid. Check fluid in the drainage collection bottles. If the fluid level has not risen, check the tubes for patency. Notify the surgeon if the drainage remains frankly bloody for longer than the first few postoperative hours, if bleeding recurs after it has stopped, or any other signs of hemorrhage. The client may be bleeding rapidly within the chest.

Assessment of Water-Seal Functioning

Observe the water seal. Fluid in the water-seal compartment rises with inspiration and falls with expiration. This process is sometimes called tidaling. When tidaling occurs, the drainage tubes are patent, and the apparatus is functioning properly. Tidaling stops when the lung has reexpanded or if the chest drainage tubes are kinked or obstructed. If tidaling does not occur, (1) check to be sure the tube is not kinked or compressed, (2) try milking (or stripping if necessary) the tube to remove any obstructions, (3) change the client's position, and (4) have the client deep breathe and cough. If these measures do not restore tidaling, notify the surgeon. (*Note:* Tidaling may not occur or may be minimal in systems using suction.)

Observe for bubbling in the water-seal compartment. Bubbling in the water-seal compartment is caused by air passing out of the pleural space into the fluid in the bottle. Intermittent bubbling is normal. It indicates that the system is accomplishing one of its purposes, that is, removing air from the pleural space. Intermittent bubbling may occur with the normal expiration, because expiration increases intrapleural pressure and forces air through the tube.

Continuous bubbling during both inspiration and expiration indicates that air is leaking into the drainage system or pleural cavity. This situation must be corrected, because air entering the system also enters the pleural space. Locate the source of the air leak, and repair it if you can. Begin by inspecting the chest wall where the catheters are inserted. If a chest catheter is loose, gently squeeze the skin up around the catheter or apply sterile petrolatum gauze around the insertion. Determine whether this stops the continuous bubbling in the bottle. If this does not stop it, check the tubing, inch by inch, and all the connections. A break in the tubing or a loose connection may be found that can be sealed with tape. If the leak still cannot be located, it may be necessary to replace the water-seal bottle.

Rapid bubbling in the absence of an air leak indicates considerable loss of air, such as from an incision or tear in the pulmonary pleura. Notify the physician *immediately* so that appropriate intervention is taken to prevent collapse of the lung or mediastinal shift. Suction may be needed, or the amount of suction may need to be increased, or thoracotomy may be necessary.

When caring for a person on water-seal drainage, find out whether this particular person's water-seal bottle should be "bubbling." Knowing this facilitates accurate assessment of the drainage pattern (e.g., if intermittent bubbling changes to constant bubbling or if the apparatus that has not been "bubbling" begins to bubble).

Assessment of Suction Apparatus Function. Because most suction motors can create potentially damaging amounts of suction, the degree of suction in the system (and thus in the pleural space) must be controlled. To control the amount of pressure exerted by a wall suction outlet, a suction valve or meter is inserted between the wall outlet and the water-seal bottle. A suction control compartment sometimes is not used so that higher suction pressures can be obtained via a wall suction outlet. In these circumstances, it is essential to maintain the exact pressure prescribed. When portable suction machines are used, a suction control bottle is used to govern the amount of negative pressure permitted to build up within the system.

Proper functioning of a suction control compartment is indicated by continuous bubbling. Vigorous bubbling does not increase the amount of suction, it just causes the water in the bottle to evaporate more rapidly.

Absence of bubbling in a suction control bottle means that the system is not functioning properly and that the correct level of suction is not being maintained. Possible reasons for malfunction of a mechanical suction apparatus include (1) large amounts of air leaking into the pleural space or into the drainage apparatus and (2) mechanical problems in the pump or suction power source. The most serious problem is air leaking into the pleural space.

If bubbling in the suction control bottle stops, check for air leaks by briefly clamping the chest drainage tube and observing the suction control bottle. If bubbling begins in the suction control bottle, there is nothing wrong with either the drainage apparatus or the pump. The problem is therefore an air leak into the pleural space around the chest tubes. If the air leak cannot be sealed off (e.g., with petrolatum gauze), notify the surgeon immediately. If bubbling does not begin in the suction control bottle when the chest catheter is clamped, the problem is in the drainage connections or the pump. Check the system carefully, looking for loose connections, air leaks around bottle tops, or air leaks in the tubing (e.g., split tubing). Also, make sure that the tubing is not kinked, is correctly positioned, and has no dependent loops. If the suction power source appears to be causing the problem (i.e., bubbling in the suction control bottle does not recommence after all the tubing and all connections are checked), obtain another pump or power source immediately.

Because the chest catheter remains clamped during this inspection, observe the client closely for indications of tension pneumothorax. As soon as the problem is corrected, the fluid in the suction control bottle will begin to bubble. Immediately remove the clamps on the chest catheter.

Promoting Chest Drainage. Apparatus for closed chest drainage must always be placed lower than the person's chest (unless for some reason the catheters are clamped). Drainage by gravity is thus maintained, and air and fluid are not forced back into the pleural space. Chest drainage systems must be placed in a box or rack (secured to the bed or on wheels at the bedside) or taped securely to the floor so they will not be knocked over. The preferred arrangement is a rack secured to the bed. This reduces the danger of breaking, elevating, or upsetting the device.

If the drainage apparatus is on the floor, be careful not to lower a high-low bed or side rails onto it. Keep the drainage apparatus about 2 to 3 feet below the client's chest. If a client with closed chest drainage is to be moved, be careful to always keep the chest drainage system below the level of the person's chest.

If the apparatus is placed above the level of the client's chest, even for a moment, fluid from the drainage bottle is siphoned back into the pleural cavity. If absolutely necessary, chest tubes may be double-clamped very briefly during momentary movement of the apparatus above the level of the person's chest (e.g., when moving drainage apparatus from one side of the bed to the other if the tubing is not long enough to allow movement around an end of the bed).

Follow positioning orders carefully. If an individual can be positioned on the side that has chest catheters, be sure the person is not lying on (compressing or kinking) the catheters or tubing. This could (1) impair drainage and cause retrograde pressure (forcing drainage back into the pleural cavity) and (2) increase the client's discomfort. When the client is in a lateral position, place small sandbags or folded towels on either side of the tubing, to prevent the client's body weight from compressing the tubing.

Drainage tubing (connecting the chest catheters to the drainage apparatus) should be neither too short nor too long. Excessive tubing length causes tangling and kinking. Attach the drainage tubing to the edge of the client's mattress so it falls straight to the drainage apparatus, with no dependent loops. Dependent loops of tubing that contain fluid obstruct fluid flow and create back-pressure, thus impairing air or fluid drainage. Drainage tubing may be secured to bedding in various ways.

- Place a rubber band or strip of adhesive tape around the drainage tubing, then pin the other end of the band or tape to the mattress.
- Coil the tubing near the client's side on the bed.

Make sure the tubing is long enough to allow the person to turn and sit up without pulling on the chest catheters. Each time the client is turned or moved, check chest catheters to be sure they are not being pulled or displaced, and check drainage tubing to be certain it is properly positioned.

Check the patency of drainage tubing and chest catheters frequently. Observe the fluid collecting in the drainage bottles. Be sure the person is not lying on the tubing and that it is not kinked or compressed. Ensure that the tube is not internally plugged, such as with blood clots. The flow of drainage fluids can be observed easily through clear plastic tubing. If the tubing is not patent, drainage of air and fluid from the pleural space is impossible.

Routine milking or stripping chest tubes is not performed because it creates excessive negative pressure. To "strip" a chest drainage tube (Fig. 39-15*A*), the nurse gently compresses it and slides the hand over the tubing in a direction away from the person's chest and toward the drainage system. The nurse should be sure the tubing is stabilized with the other hand so that the tube will not be pulled on or displaced while stripping. Stripping is performed to remove air, fluid, or blood clots. Because stripping can be painful if performed too vigorously, do it as gently as possible. Using hand lotion makes it possible to slide more easily down the length of tubing.

To "milk" a chest drainage tube (Fig. 39-15*B*), clasp one hand around the tube as close to the chest as possible and squeeze the tube against the palm of the hand. Then proceed similarly, hand-over-hand, toward the drainage apparatus. Some plastic chest tubes have a built-in bulb device for milking. Milking is a much safer procedure than stripping, because it causes only a mild, intermittent increase in intrathoracic pressure.

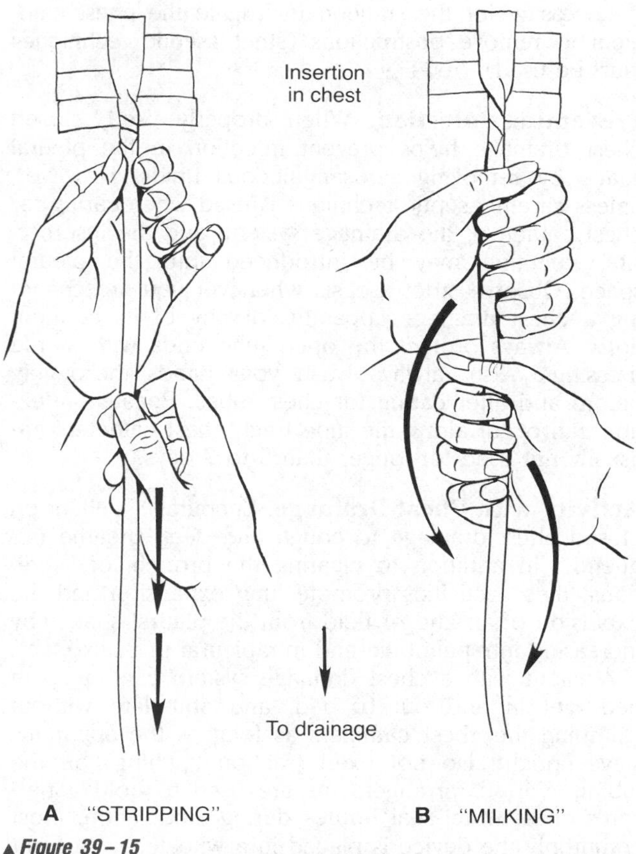

▲ ***Figure 39-15***

Stripping and milking chest tubes is performed carefully to remove blood clots. These procedures are not performed routinely.

Stripping a chest tube may cause complications because it creates excessive negative intrapleural pressure (over −100 cm H_2O). Stripping is only appropriate when a chest tube is clogged and milking the tube is unsuccessful or the drainage has many clots.

Accumulations of blood, fluid, or air in the pleural space may eventually compress the lung, precipitating tension pneumothorax or mediastinal shift. Therefore, if the drainage apparatus malfunctions, correct the problem immediately, and observe the person closely for indications of complications. Early detection of tension pneumothorax, for example, can prevent mediastinal shift if appropriate treatment is given promptly.

Notify the surgeon immediately if complications are suspected. While waiting for the surgeon, try to locate and correct the cause of any problems within the drainage system. A relatively simple action may correct a malfunctioning system, such as straightening a kinked tube or setting upright a water-seal bottle that has been knocked over. Sometimes milking or stripping a tube will dislodge an obstructing blood clot. Occasionally, it is necessary for the surgeon to irrigate the chest catheters to remove obstructions (strict aseptic techniques must be used).

Preventing Infection. When properly used, closed chest drainage helps prevent infection in the pleural space by removing serosanguineous fluids. However, unless careful aseptic technique is used when caring for chest catheters, the drainage system, and the insertion site, infection may be introduced into the pleural space. Observe strict asepsis whenever you are changing a chest drainage apparatus or any of its connections. Always protect the open tube ends with sterile dressings. Also, always wash your hands thoroughly before and after caring for chest tubes. Because infection can occur along the tube tract, chest catheters are usually not used for longer than 5 to 7 days.

Activity with Chest Drainage. Encourage a client on closed chest drainage to cough and deep breathe frequently. In addition to clearing the bronchi of secretions, these activities promote lung expansion and the expulsion of air and/or fluid from the pleural space (by increasing intrapulmonic and intrapleural pressure).

A client with a chest drainage system can sit up in bed, get in and out of bed, and ambulate without clamping the chest catheters as long as the apparatus stays upright. Do not exert traction (pulling) on the tubing. Various arrangements are used to hold a person's chest water-seal bottles during ambulation. Most commonly the device is placed in a wheelchair in front of the client. If suction is to be maintained, the person can walk only those few steps permitted by the length of tubing.

Clamping Chest Drainage Tubing. Always keep rubber-shod clamps at the bedside of a person on closed chest drainage. The clamps are 6- to 8-inch, strong forceps with protective rubber on the tips. Keep 2 clamps available for each chest catheter so that each can be double-clamped (for extra safety) if clamping is required. When not in use, keep the clamps in a visible, readily available place, for example, at the head of the bed. Do not tape the clamps to the bed, or they will be too difficult to release for emergency use. Do not leave the clamps lying on the bedside stand or in a drawer. They are likely not be there when the nurse needs them, or they may be hidden by other articles.

Except for those emergencies in which clamping is clearly indicated, NEVER clamp chest drainage tubes without an order to do so.

If clamps must be used, the best time to apply them to a chest catheter is following an expiration. Remove the clamps as soon as possible.

Potential Emergencies

Intervention if Water-Seal Bottle Is Accidentally Elevated Above the Level of the Person's Chest. Immediately lower the bottle and contact the surgeon. This serious accident causes fluid in the bottle to be siphoned or to flow by gravity into the pleural space, precipitating collapse of the lung and/or mediastinal shift.

Intervention if Apparatus Is Broken. If the chest drainage device is broken, atmospheric air enters the pleural space through the drainage tubing. Intervention depends on whether the person has been "bubbling" or not. If the person has not been "bubbling," immediately clamp the chest catheter, wipe the exposed ends of the catheter with an antiseptic solution, reconnect it to another chest drainage apparatus, and unclamp.

In such an emergency, rapid assessment is necessary to determine (1) the extent to which exposing the pleural space to atmospheric air would disrupt the treatment and (2) the pros and cons of shutting off air flow into and out of the chest cavity with clamps. Such decisions must be made quickly. Knowing whether the person was "bubbling" or not before the accident is important, because there is no way to observe this after a device has broken.

Intervention if the Chest Tube Is Accidentally Removed. Cover the insertion site with sterile petroleum gauze and notify the surgeon. Observe the client for respiratory distress.

If clamps have been applied to a chest tube and it is noticed that the person is beginning to experience respiratory distress before being reconnected to another apparatus, tension pneumothorax (and possibly mediastinal shift) is probably occurring. (Indications of respiratory distress include rapid, shallow breathing, apprehension, chest pain, and cyanosis.) Immediately release the clamps on the chest catheter and call for the surgeon. It is best to open the clamps and create an open pneumothorax. Then at least air can move both in and out of the pleural space and is not trapped there, building up pressure.

Alternative Chest Drainage Equipment

Flutter Valve. A flutter valve may be used instead of water-seal drainage bottles in closed chest drainage setups. The *B-P Heimlich Chest Drainage Valve* (Fig. 39–16) is pre-sterilized, disposable, and about 7 inches long. When inserted between a chest catheter and a drainage collecting apparatus, the valve permits the unidirectional flow of air and fluid from the pleural space into a collection apparatus and prevents the reflux of air or fluid back into the chest.

A flutter valve is a single piece of wide, thin rubber tubing. It is open at the end that attaches to a chest catheter and is compressed at the other end so that its flattened sides (valve leaflets) remain in contact with each other. Air and fluid draining from the intrapleural space enter the "open" end and pass out through the valve's flattened ends. The air and fluid cannot reenter the flattened sides of the tubing because these two sides remain in contact with each other. A flutter valve offers minimal resistance to air or fluid leaving the intrapleural space. The valve is enclosed in a clear plastic case that (1) protects the tubing from being kinked and (2) facilitates assessment of the passage of fluid and blood through the valve. Expansion and contraction of the valve leaflets (caused by changes in intrapleural pressure associated with ventilatory chest movements) can also be observed.

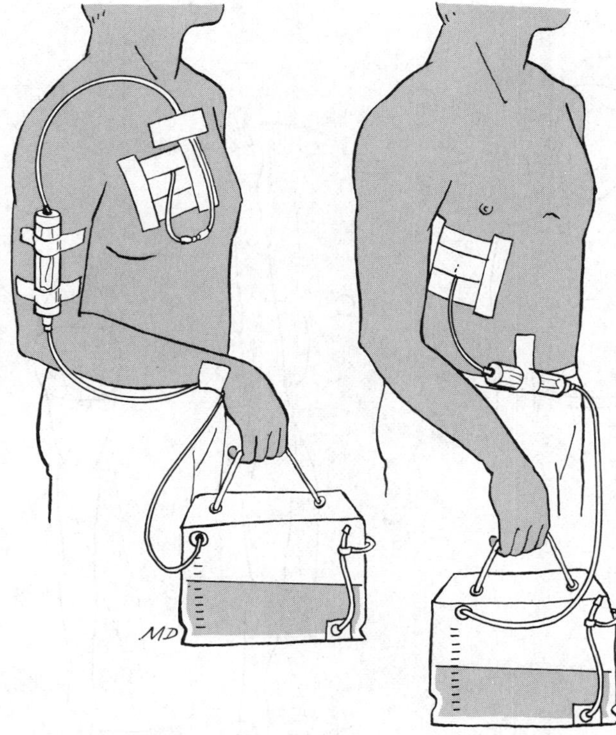

▲ **Figure 39-16**

Heimlich flutter valve: an alternative to water-seal drainage. A valve allows chest drainage while preventing reflux of air and fluid back into the chest. It allows ambulation and greater mobility than other systems. The valve may be attached to the arm or body, and the drainage bag may be carried at any level, because reflux is prevented.

A flutter valve functions in any position, allowing the person to assume any position desired. It allows greater freedom of movement than a water-seal system. The person can be comfortably ambulatory if the drainage tube is connected to a vented portable plastic bag or even a rubber glove. Because a flutter valve functions in the same way as a water-seal bottle, it can be attached to controlled chest suction if necessary.

McSwain's Dart System. This system may replace water-seal drainage bottles for people with a pneumothorax. A McSwain's dart system is a pre-sterilized, disposable small-bore catheter with built-in PVC tubing and a molded, one-way injection valve. It operates on the same principle as a flutter valve (see earlier). Air from the intrapleural space can escape out through the catheter, but the one-way valve prevents air from being sucked back into the chest. Controlled suction may be applied to the end of the tubing for rapid evacuation of air from the pleural space. As with the flutter valve, the McSwain's dart system functions in any position and allows the person to move freely.

Removal of Chest Catheters. A physician determines when to remove water-seal chest drainage. As mentioned earlier, one indication that the evacuation of intrapleural air and fluid is completed and that the lung has reexpanded is the cessation of fluctuation in the long tube of the water-seal bottle (if suction is not applied). The reexpanded lung blocks the catheters' openings into the pleural space. Thus, fluctuations of intrapleural pressure during inspiration and expiration are no longer transmitted to the water-seal apparatus. When the lung is completely reexpanded, no air or fluid passes through the chest catheters.

Usually, a lung is fully reexpanded after 2 to 3 postoperative days of chest drainage. Generally, chest catheters are left in place connected to drainage bottles for 24 hours after all air drainage and significant fluid drainage have stopped. Sometimes, the catheters are temporarily clamped to see how the person will tolerate their removal. Chest catheters may not be removed if the chest is draining more than 50 to 70 ml of fluid daily. The sooner the chest catheters can be removed, the better. Their presence often contributes to postoperative pain and inactivity. Also, the longer the catheters are in place, the greater the risk of infection. When treating empyema, chest catheters may be used longer than when following chest surgery.

Chest auscultation, chest percussion, and chest x-ray study confirm lung reexpansion. The surgeon removes the chest catheter when convinced it is safe to do so. Although both chest catheters may be removed at the same time, it is more common for the upper one to be left in place longer than the lower.

Removal of chest catheters can be moderately painful. The prescribed premedication for pain relief should be administered about one-half hour before the procedure. Assemble equipment as necessary, such as sterile scissors, knife or suture set to cut sutures securing the catheter(s), sterile petrolatum gauze, 4 × 4 gauze to cover the wound, and three strips of tape 2 inches wide and about 6 inches long.

Nursing Management

Diagnostic Phase

The client who is undergoing diagnostic tests for lung cancer faces an uncertain future. If the diagnosis is confirmed, the client can anticipate a variety of physical difficulties, potentially extensive medical treatment, and many emotional changes. The nursing assessment plays a critical role in developing a plan of care that will provide needed support.

The nursing history should include an exploration of the client's chief complaints, particularly cough (productive or nonproductive), dyspnea, pain, or recurrent infection. The client should be asked about the presence of risk factors, including a smoking history, exposure to occupational respiratory carcinogens, or a family history of the disease. Socioeconomic situation and available social support should also be assessed because these factors will affect subsequent management options.

Nursing management during the diagnostic phase will focus on emotional support and client education, along with required physical care. The nurse can help clients maintain a sense of control by keeping them informed

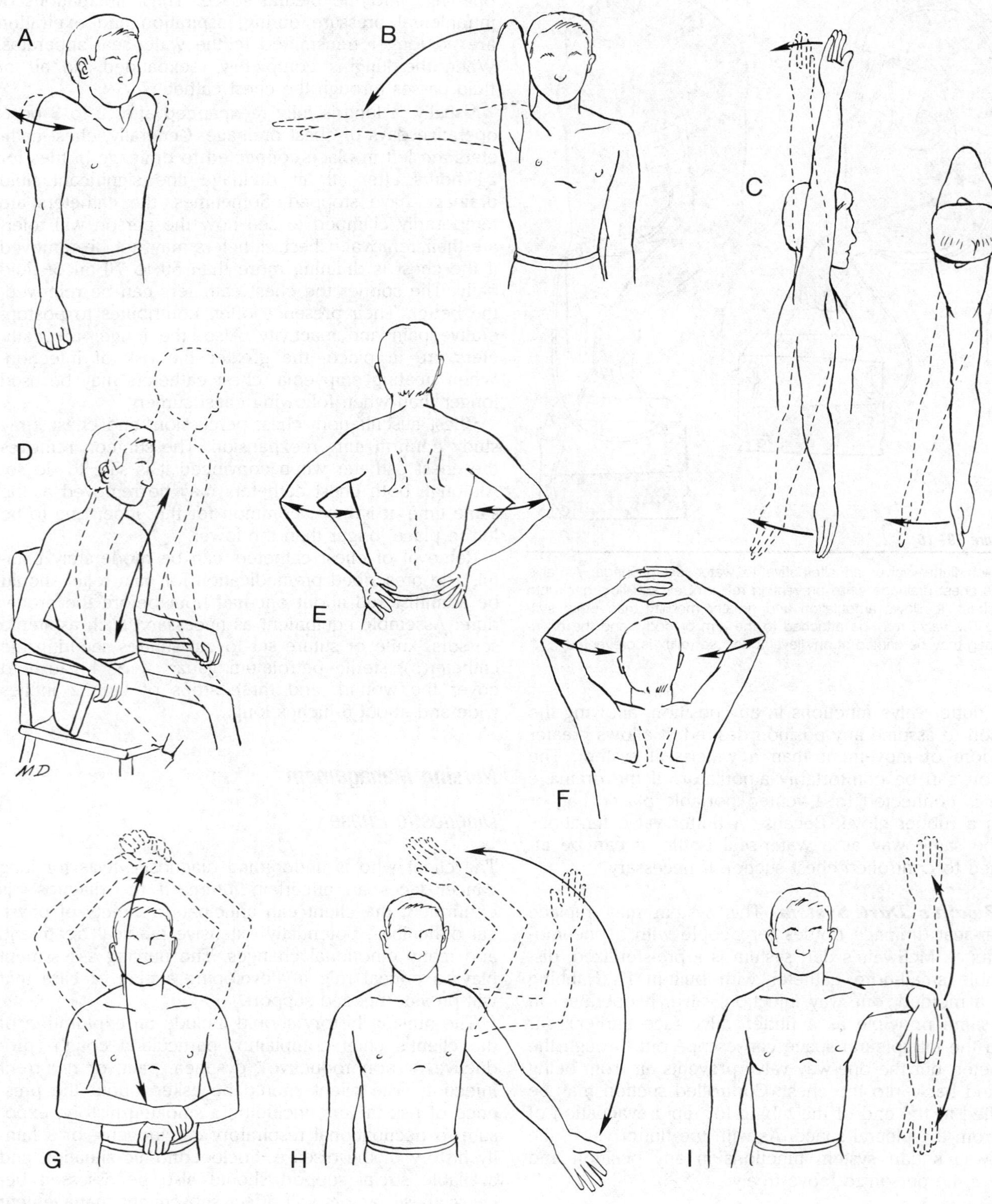

▲ Figure 39–17

Arm and shoulder exercises often prescribed after chest surgery.

about all scheduled tests. Once a diagnosis of lung cancer is confirmed, nursing care must incorporate aspects of assisting the client to cope with anxiety and fear, family responses, financial considerations, absence from work and social activities, and possible changes in life goals.

Treatment Phase

PREOPERATIVE ASSESSMENT

Preoperative preparation is the same as for any surgical client but with greater emphasis on assessment and preparation of the respiratory system (see Chap. 19 for discussion of preoperative nursing care). Extensive pulmonary function testing may be ordered before chest surgery for determining the client's ability to tolerate the proposed surgical intervention. Clients with impaired pulmonary function may be treated with antibiotics, bronchodilating medications, intermittent positive-pressure breathing procedures, and supervised breathing exercises to improve respiratory efficiency. Clients are encouraged to refrain from smoking during the preoperative period, because smoking will increase pulmonary secretions and decrease blood oxygen saturation.

PREOPERATIVE NURSING INTERVENTION

Nursing interventions during the preoperative period are primarily aimed at reducing the client's anxiety level. Anxiety results from fear of cancer and its prognosis, as well as from fear of the surgical procedure and insufficient knowledge of surgical routines and postoperative self-care activities. The client and family are taught about

- the anticipated surgical procedure. Assess the client's (and family's) understanding and give further information as needed.
- the early postoperative period. Talk specifically about what will be happening to the client and how he or she can participate in recovery activities. Specific explanations should be given about the presence of chest tubes (except with pneumonectomy) and drainage tubes, intubation and mechanical ventilation, oxygen therapy, and available pain relief measures.
- postoperative exercises (Figs. 39-17 and 39-18). These include (1) respiratory exercises to maintain effective pulmonary function; (2) leg exercises to prevent thrombophlebitis; and (3) arm/shoulder exercises to maintain normal range of motion and correct posture. These exercises should be demonstrated, and opportunity should be given for practice and return demonstration.

POSTOPERATIVE ASSESSMENT

During the immediate postoperative period, thorough assessment is essential. Make observations as often as the client's condition warrants. This will be determined by factors such as (1) amount of anesthesia received and the client's reaction to it, (2) amount of intraoperative blood loss, (3) preoperative client condition (e.g., presence of pre-existing medical conditions such as diabetes, heart disorders), (4) client's response to pain, and (5) facility protocols. In general, make assessments every 15 minutes until the client is stable, then every 30 minutes for several hours. Hourly assessment is usually indicated throughout the first postoperative night. More frequent assessments may be required if the client's condition changes.

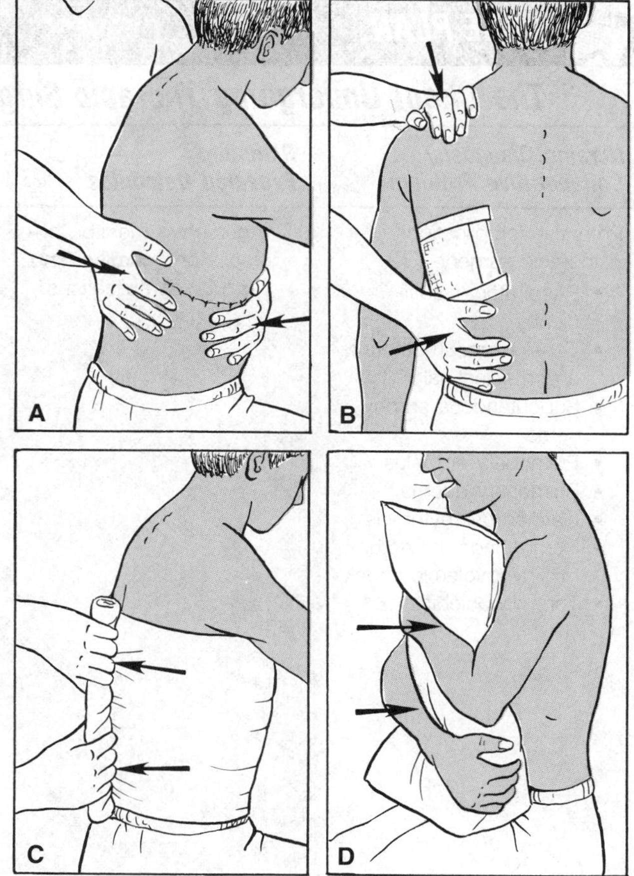

▲ **Figure 39-18**

Splinting techniques to promote effective coughing and deep breathing. Apply firm, even pressure after the person has taken a deep breath and during forced expiratory cough. Do not squeeze the chest or interfere with chest inspiratory expansion. *A*, Place one hand around the person's back and the other around the incisional area. *B*, Support the area below the incision with one hand while exerting downward pressure on the shoulder on the affected side with the other. *C*, Place a towel or draw sheet snugly (but not tightly) around the chest. *D*, Have the person hug a pillow during forced expiratory cough.

POSTOPERATIVE NURSING INTERVENTION

Nursing interventions are based on careful assessment and appropriate nursing diagnoses. General postoperative nursing measures will be applicable (see Chap. 19). Nursing management specific to thoracic surgery is dis-

Text continued on page 1081

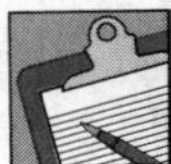

CARE PLAN

The Client Undergoing Thoracic Surgery

Nursing Diagnosis/ Collaborative Problem	Planning: Expected Outcomes	Implementation: Nursing Interventions	Rationales
Potential complications of thoracic surgery: • Respiratory insufficiency • Tension pneumothorax and mediastinal shift • Subcutaneous emphysema • Pulmonary embolus • Pulmonary edema • Cardiac dysrhythmias • Hemorrhage, hemothorax, hypovolemic shock • Thrombophlebitis	The nurse will monitor for respiratory, cardiac, and vascular complications.	1. Monitor for signs and symptoms of respiratory failure: a. increased respiratory rate b. dyspnea c. use of accessory muscles and/or retractions d. cyanosis e. decreased PaO_2 levels and increased $PaCO_2$ levels f. restlessness g. increase in adventitious breath sounds	1. Postoperatively, respiratory insufficiency may result from an altered level of consciousness due to anesthesia and pain medications, incomplete lung reinflation, decreased respiratory effort due to chest pain, and inadequate airway clearance.
		2. Monitor for signs and symptoms of tension pneumothorax: a. severe dyspnea b. tachypnea and tachycardia c. extreme restlessness and agitation d. progressive cyanosis e. laryngeal and tracheal deviation to unaffected side f. PMI (point of maximal impulse) shift laterally or medially	2. Postoperative tension pneumothorax can result from air leaking through pleural incision lines if closed chest drainage fails to function properly.
		3. Observe for subcutaneous emphysema around incision and in the chest and neck. a. Assess progression by periodically marking the chest with a skin-marking pencil at outer periphery of emphysematous tissue. b. If neck involvement occurs, measure neck circumference at least every 2–4 hours.	3. Subcutaneous emphysema may result from air leakage at pulmonary incision site. a. Rapid progression (i.e., an increase of more than a hand's width in 1 hour) may indicate leakage through bronchial stump. b. Severe subcutaneous emphysema in the neck may compress the trachea and may require tracheostomy.
		4. Monitor for signs and symptoms of pulmonary embolus: a. chest pain	4. Pulmonary embolism is a serious potential complication after chest surgery and a

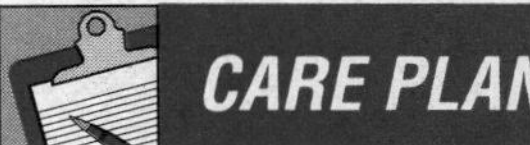

The Client Undergoing Thoracic Surgery Continued

Nursing Diagnosis/ Collaborative Problem	Planning: Expected Outcomes	Implementation: Nursing Interventions	Rationales
		b. dyspnea and tachypnea c. fever d. hemoptysis e. indications of right-sided heart failure	significant cause of postoperative hypoxemia.
		5. Monitor for signs of acute pulmonary edema: a. dyspnea b. rales c. persistent cough d. frothy sputum e. cyanosis	5. Circulatory overload may result from the reduced size of the pulmonary vascular bed due to surgical removal of pulmonary tissue and delayed reexpansion of the operated lung. Additionally, hypoxia increases capillary permeability, causing fluid to enter pulmonary tissue.
		6. Monitor intravenous flow rates. Consult physician if fluid amounts (maintenance plus intermittent medications [e.g., antibiotics]) exceed 125 ml/hr.	6. After chest surgery, intravenous fluids should not exceed 125 ml/hr because of possible circulatory overload.
		7. Assess cardiac monitor for the development of cardiac dysrhythmias, particularly atrial fibrillation, atrial flutter, and paroxysmal atrial tachycardia.	7. Cardiac dysrhythmias are fairly common after chest surgery. Rhythm disturbances result from a combination of factors, including increased vagal tone, hypoxia, mediastinal shift, and abnormal blood pH.
		8. Assess dressing/incisional area every 4 hours for evidence of bleeding (increase to every 1–2 hours if bleeding develops). 9. Assess drainage in closed chest drainage system for signs of bleeding.	8 & 9. Blood loss may be great with major thoracic surgery because a. blood vessels in the thorax are of large caliber b. the incision is often large and produces considerable capillary oozing c. adhesion and tissue planes within the thorax are generally quite extensive and vascular

Care Plan continued on following page

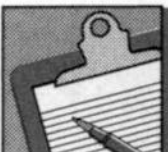

CARE PLAN

The Client Undergoing Thoracic Surgery Continued

Nursing Diagnosis/ Collaborative Problem	Planning: Expected Outcomes	Implementation: Nursing Interventions	Rationales
		10. Monitor for signs of hypovolemic shock: a. increased pulse b. decreased blood pressure c. restlessness and decreased level of consciousness d. decreased urine output (<30 ml/hr) e. cool, pale, clammy skin f. increased respirations	10. The body compensates for lost blood volume by increasing blood flow (through increased heart rate) to vital organs and decreasing peripheral circulation.
		11. Monitor for thrombophlebitis: a. unilateral leg edema b. calf tenderness, redness, unusual warmth	11. Anesthesia and immobility reduce vasomotor tone, leading to decreased venous return and peripheral pooling of blood.
		12. Encourage client to perform leg exercises. Discourage placing pillows under knees, crossing the legs, or prolonged sitting.	12. These measures prevent venous stasis, thus reducing the risk of thrombophlebitis.
Airway Clearance, Ineffective R/T increased secretions and decreased coughing effectiveness due to pain	The client will demonstrate effective airway clearance, as evidenced by clear breath sounds, effective coughing and adequate air exchange in the lungs	1. Once the vital signs are stable, place client in semi-Fowler's position.	1. The upright position enhances lung expansion and facilitates ventilation with minimal effort.
		2. Assist client to cough and deep breathe at least every 1 or 2 hours during the first 24 to 48 postoperative hours.	2. Coughing helps to move tracheobronchial secretions out of the lung. Deep breathing dilates the airways, stimulates surfactant production, and expands lung tissue.
		3. When possible, schedule coughing and deep breathing sessions at times when pain medication is maximally effective (i.e., 15–20 minutes after intravenous administration and 30–45 minutes after intramuscular or subcutaneous administration). (If client-controlled analgesia is used, timing is not	3. The less postoperative pain a client experiences, the more effective are coughing and deep breathing.

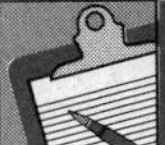

CARE PLAN

The Client Undergoing Thoracic Surgery Continued

Nursing Diagnosis/ Collaborative Problem	Planning: Expected Outcomes	Implementation: Nursing Interventions	Rationales
		as crucial because analgesia level is more consistent).	
		4. Assess breath sounds before and after coughing.	4. This will help in evaluation of coughing effectiveness.
		5. Provide support and reassurance:	5.
		a. Explain that breathing exercises will not damage lungs or suture line.	a. Fear of "splitting open" the incision may hamper coughing efforts.
		b. Manually splint the incision area during coughing and deep breathing	b. Physical support of the incision is both comforting and reassuring.
		c. Offer sips of warm water.	c. Warm water can aid relaxation and produce more effective coughing.
		6. Maintain adequate level of hydration and adequate humidity of inspired air.	6. Fluids and moisture help to thin secretions, making them easier to expectorate.
		7. Monitor results of chest x-ray examination.	7. Frequent chest films help detect atelectasis and infection.
		8. Evaluate need for suctioning.	8. If coughing is ineffective, suctioning may be required to remove pulmonary secretions. Suctioning should be performed cautiously so that disruption of pulmonary suture lines is avoided.
Pain R/T surgical procedure	The client will have improved comfort, as evidenced by verbalizing that discomfort is reduced, using less narcotics, moving in bed with less pain.	1. Administer pain medication as ordered.	1. After chest surgery, the client's chest will be quite painful because of the trauma of surgery and the presence of chest tubes. The severance of intercostal nerves during surgery may also produce sensations of pain, numbness, or heaviness in the operative area.
		2. Offer pain medication before pain becomes severe.	2. A preventive approach to pain control provides a more consistent level of relief and reduces client anxiety.

Care Plan continued on following page

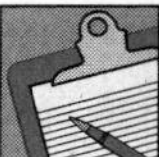

CARE PLAN

The Client Undergoing Thoracic Surgery Continued

Nursing Diagnosis/ Collaborative Problem	Planning: Expected Outcomes	Implementation: Nursing Interventions	Rationales
		3. Assess medication effectiveness and avoid overmedication.	3. A delicate balance with pain management is essential. Adequate pain relief must be obtained. However, overmedication can depress respirations and the cough reflex.
		4. Use nonpharmacologic pain relief measures, concurrently.	4. Proper positioning, relaxation techniques, and the like can augment effects of medications.
Physical Mobility, Impaired R/T pain and muscle dissection and restricted positioning	The client will maintain physical mobility in arm and shoulder, as evidenced by regaining preoperative arm and shoulder function	1. Position client as indicated by phase of recovery and surgical procedure.	
		a. Nonoperative side-lying position may be used until consciousness is regained.	a. This position promotes hemodynamic stability in the immediate postoperative period and prevents aspiration.
		b. Semi-Fowler's position (head of bed elevated 30 to 45 degrees) is recommended once vital signs are stable.	b. The upright position enhances lung expansion and facilitates chest tube drainage.
		c. Avoid positioning client on operative side if a wedge resection or segmentectomy has been performed.	c. Lying on the operative side hinders expansion of remaining lung tissue.
		d. Avoid complete lateral positioning after pneumonectomy.	d. Because the mediastinum is no longer held in place on both sides by lung tissue, extreme turning may cause mediastinal shift and compression of the remaining lung.
		2. Gently turn the client every 1 to 2 hours, unless contraindicated.	2. Frequent turning promotes mobilization and drainage of air and fluid from the pleural space. Turning also improves circulation, promotes lung aeration, and enhances comfort.

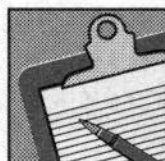

CARE PLAN

The Client Undergoing Thoracic Surgery Continued

Nursing Diagnosis/ Collaborative Problem	Planning: Expected Outcomes	Implementation: Nursing Interventions	Rationales
		3. Avoid traction on chest tubes while changing client position. Check for kinking or compression of tubing.	3. Traction may dislodge the chest tubes. Kinking or compression inhibits drainage and reestablishment of negative intrapleural pressure.
		4. Encourage regular ambulation, once client's condition is stable. Maintain supplemental oxygen, if ordered.	4. Early ambulation improves ventilation, circulation, and morale. Oxygen therapy should be maintained during activity to avoid hypoxia.
		5. Begin passive range-of-motion (ROM) exercises of the arm and shoulder on the affected side 4 hours after recovery from anesthesia. Exercises should be performed two times every 4 to 6 hours through the first 24 postoperative hours, with progression to 10 to 20 times every 2 hours.	5. ROM exercises help prevent adhesion formation in the operative area, which can lead to dysfunction syndrome (i.e., "frozen" shoulder).
		6. Active ROM exercises are begun once the client's condition permits (see Fig. 39–13).	6. Active ROM exercises prevent adhesions of the incised muscle layers.
		7. Encourage client to use arm on affected side in daily activities (e.g., eating, reaching, grooming). Keep bedside stand on operative side to encourage reaching. Teach importance of continued use after discharge.	7. Regular use of the affected arm and shoulder reduces the possibility of contractures.
		8. Carefully assess client's response to activity and exercise. Observe for signs of dyspnea, shortness of breath, and fatigue.	8. It may take time for client's activity tolerance to increase, because the body must adjust to reduced respiratory capacity after resectional surgery.
		9. Allow adequate rest periods between activities.	9. Adequate rest will allow the client to cooperate more fully with activities.
Individual Coping, Ineffective High Risk for R/T temporary dependence and loss of full respiratory function	The client will use adaptive coping mechanisms, as evidenced by verbalizing feelings related to emotional state and taking	1. Provide opportunity for client to ventilate feelings.	1. Loss of normal body function and self-care capabilities can lead to feelings of powerlessness, anger, and grief.

Care Plan continued on following page

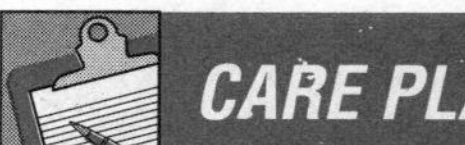

CARE PLAN

The Client Undergoing Thoracic Surgery Continued

Nursing Diagnosis/ Collaborative Problem	Planning: Expected Outcomes	Implementation: Nursing Interventions	Rationales
	appropriate actions to regain self-care capabilities		Open expression of these feelings can help client to begin the coping process.
		2. Encourage use of positive coping strategies that have been successful in the past.	2. The use of effective coping actions can decrease feelings of hopelessness and helplessness.
		3. Allow client to have as much control over daily activities and decision making as is possible.	3. Active involvement in the plan of care gives the client a sense of control and promotes return to independence.
		4. Support and praise all independent activities that promote recovery.	4. Emotional support and encouragement helps motivate client to continue progress toward independence.
Altered Health Maintenance R/T self-care after discharge	Client will be able to maintain health, as evidenced by stating or demonstrating discharge plans	5. Provide thorough instruction and preparation for hospital discharge:	5. Thorough understanding promotes compliance and enhances self-care capabilities.
		a. proper wound care	a. Wound care will vary according to condition of incision and client.
		b. continuation of exercise program	b. Continued exercise increases activity tolerance and prevents complications.
		c. precautions regarding activity and environmental irritants	c. Heavy lifting should be avoided. Return to work will depend on client's condition and type of job. However, it is usually possible within 4 to 6 weeks. Environmental irritants can cause severe coughing episodes.
		d. Clinical manifestations to be reported to health care professional	d. Evidence of infection, deteriorating respiratory status, or other complications should be reported promptly.
		e. importance of regular follow-up care	e. The client should be followed closely for signs of surgical complications, recurrence of malignancy, and metastasis.
		f. community agencies that can provide resources, as needed	f. Community resources can facilitate home management.

cussed in the Care Plan. Chest tubes are placed to facilitate drainage and lung reexpansion in all clients having chest surgery, except following pneumonectomy.

Terminal Phase

During the end stage of lung cancer, the emphasis of nursing care is on physical and emotional support of the client and family. Effective physical care and comfort for the terminally ill client can greatly contribute to a peaceful death. Extensive measures may be required to control the client's pain, including epidural or intrathecal analgesia. Measures should be taken to enhance the therapeutic effects of pain-relieving medications as well as to minimize potential side effects.

Clients in the terminal phase of the disease can be expected to experience some degree of anger or depression. These emotions may be expressed through abusive or aggressive behavior toward family and care givers, thus adding to stress and anxiety levels. The nurse should find ways to help the client to ventilate thoughts and feelings as well as to assist significant others in understanding and coping with the situation.

BENIGN LUNG TUMORS

Benign pulmonary neoplasms account for less than 10 per cent of all primary pulmonary tumors. The term "benign" may be misleading, because although they are not directly harmful to the body, some of these tumors may still have serious physiologic effects. Mechanical interference with lung function (e.g., obstruction of a major bronchus) may occur, depending on the tumor's location. In addition, some of these tumors may become malignant over time.

The most common benign lung tumor is the hamartoma, which usually arises in peripheral lung parenchyma. This tumor is more common in older men. Other benign tumor types include the fibroma, hemangioma, lipoma, and papilloma.

Benign tumors may also arise from pleural (mesothelial) tissue. Benign mesotheliomas occur in both sexes, usually between the ages of 40 and 60 years. They may be a postinflammatory response (i.e., subsequent to pulmonary infections), although their specific cause is unknown.

Benign lung tumors are often difficult to diagnose because clients may be asymptomatic. Unless there is pre-existing lung disease or major airway obstruction, pulmonary function studies and ABGs are usually within normal limits. The tumor may be first detected through chest radiography. Confirmatory diagnosis usually requires bronchoscopy or, more commonly, thoracotomy.

Until the diagnosis is confirmed, most clients will be quite anxious and fearful of the possibility of cancer. Emotional support is an important adjunct to the physical preparation required for diagnostic procedures.

Surgical intervention is the treatment of choice for all benign neoplasms. Tumor removal promptly alleviates any respiratory symptoms that may be present. Postoperative management is the same as that used with the surgical treatment of malignant lung disease.

▼ DISORDERS OF THE PULMONARY VASCULATURE

PULMONARY EMBOLISM

Definition

Pulmonary embolism (PE) is an occlusion of a portion of the pulmonary blood vessels by an embolus. An embolus is defined as a detached intravascular solid, liquid, or gaseous mass that is carried by the bloodstream from its point of origin to a distant site. A PE is an acute and potentially lethal disorder.

Incidence

PE is one of the four most common causes of sudden death in the United States. Over 600,000 people develop pulmonary emboli each year and half of these individuals will die within 2 hours after embolization.[39] Several autopsy studies indicate that major pulmonary emboli occur in as many as 25 per cent of hospitalized patients. The diagnosis of pulmonary embolism is often difficult to make because of the vagueness of the clients' clinical symptoms. The importance of making the diagnosis is confirmed by studies revealing the mortality rate for untreated PE is between 20 per cent and 35 per cent; the mortality rate is 8 per cent when the condition is recognized and appropriately managed.[58]

Etiology

Virtually 99 per cent of all emboli develop from thrombi (clots).[22] Other sources of emboli include tumors, air, fat, bone marrow, amniotic fluid, septic thrombi, and vegetations on heart valves that develop with endocarditis. The most common source of pulmonary emboli is venous thrombosis in the thigh and pelvis.

Risk Factors

Clients at the highest risk of developing pulmonary embolism are those who have had surgery on the pelvis or legs, have had trauma to the pelvis or lower legs, are immobile for other reasons, are obese, require estrogen therapy, or have clotting abnormalities.

Measures to reduce the risk of PE include early ambulation of all clients, leg exercises in bedridden clients, and avoidance of smoking. Prophylactic heparin is often administered.

Clients with deep vein thrombosis must be carefully assessed for early clinical manifestations of PE (see later). Clients with a past history of deep vein thrombosis or a previous occurrence of PE also have an increased risk. These clients should avoid restrictive clothing on the legs and prolonged sitting or standing.

Pathophysiology

Emboli travel to the lungs and lodge in the pulmonary vasculature. The size and number of emboli determine the location. Blood flow is obstructed, leading to decreased perfusion of the section of lung supplied by the vessel. The client continues to ventilate the lung portion but because the tissue is not perfused, a ventilation perfusion mismatch occurs and hypoxemia develops.

If the emboli lodges in a large pulmonary vessel, it increases proximal pulmonary vascular resistance, causes atelectasis, and eventually decreases cardiac output. If the emboli is in the smaller vessels, less dramatic clinical manifestations follow but perfusion is still altered.

The arterioles constrict due to platelet degranulation, accompanied by a release of histamine, serotonin, catecholamines, and prostaglandins. The chemical agents result in bronchial and pulmonary artery constriction. This vasoconstriction probably plays a major role in the hemodynamic instability that follows a PE.

Clinical Manifestations

Chest pain is the most common symptom of pulmonary embolism, but it is not diagnostic of the condition. The pain most often associated with PE is pleuritic. Pleuritic pain is caused by an inflammatory reaction of the lung parenchyma or by pulmonary infarction or ischemia caused by obstruction of small pulmonary arterial branches. Typical pleuritic chest pain is sudden in onset and aggravated by breathing. The client is also dyspneic, especially if the embolus has occluded major arteries or major portions of lung tissue. Apprehension, cough, diaphoresis, syncope, and hemoptysis may occur. The presence of hemoptysis indicates that the infarction or areas of atelectasis have produced alveolar damage.

Respirations typically increase, the client also develops crackles, an increased physiologic split of the second heart sound, tachycardia, and fever. Less common findings include heart gallops, edema, heart murmur, and cyanosis.

DIAGNOSTIC ASSESSMENT

The diagnosis of pulmonary embolism is suggested by chest pain, especially pleuritic in nature; hemoptysis; dyspnea; a low arterial PO_2; and a wedge-shaped density on chest x-ray study.

ECG patterns suggestive of pulmonary emboli include inverted T waves on leads V_1 to V_4, transient right bundle branch block axis deviation, right ventricular hypertrophy, and tall P waves in leads II, III, and AVF.

Arterial blood gas analyses indicate arterial hypoxemia (low PO_2) and hypocapnia (low PCO_2) in massive pulmonary embolism. There may be a severe respiratory alkalosis.

A radioisotope lung scan is performed by intravenously injecting particles of human serum albumin that have been labeled with radioactive iodine (^{131}I) or technetium (^{99m}Tc). These macroaggregated particles are trapped in the pulmonary microvasculature and are distributed according to pulmonary flow. Both lungs are scanned with a scintillation counter, and the amount of radioactivity counted gives an indication of obstruction to flow.

Pulmonary angiograms provide the most effective means of diagnosing pulmonary emboli (Fig. 39-19). This procedure is performed by injecting radiopaque contrast agent into the right atrium and pulmonary artery via a catheter threaded through a peripheral vein. Visualization of any filling defects of the heart and right pulmonary artery is achieved by taking sequential x-ray studies.

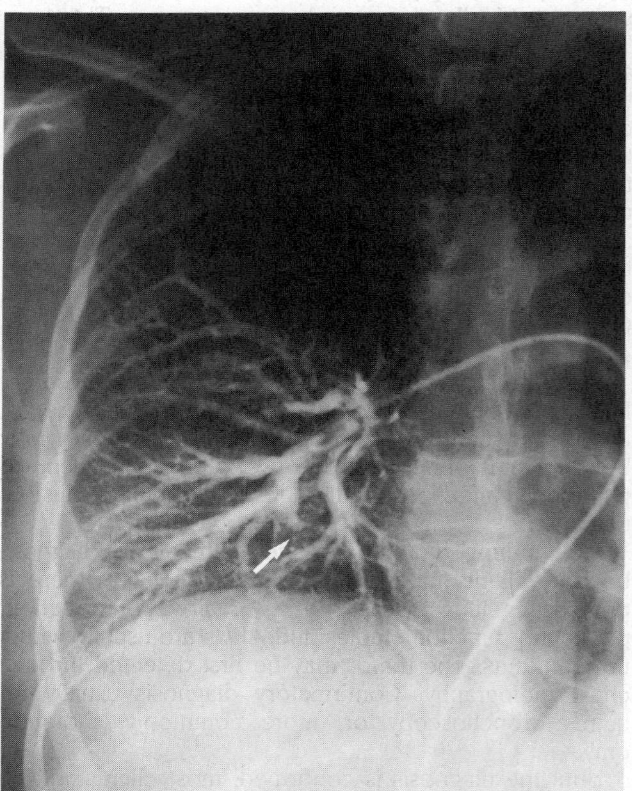

▲ **Figure 39-19**

Angiogram showing pulmonary thrombus *(arrow)*.

Medical Management

Successful management of PE depends on the prompt recognition of the condition and immediate treatment. Medical management focuses on anticoagulation to reduce the size of future thrombi, slow the development of emboli from thrombi, and maintain cardiopulmonary stability.

Anticoagulation is begun with intravenous heparin sodium. The client is administered anticoagulants until the partial thromboplastin time is 2 to 2.5 times the normal value. Administration of sodium warafin (Coumadin) is begun about 3 days before heparin is stopped to provide a transition, because the half-life of heparin is very short. Clients are maintained on warfarin for 3 to 6 months.

Cardiopulmonary support varies with the client's symptoms. Sometimes hypoxemia can be reversed with low-flow oxygen by nasal cannula. Other clients require endotracheal intubation to maintain PaO_2 over 60 mm Hg.

Hypotension is treated with fluids. If fluids do not raise the preload (right ventricular end-diastolic pressure) enough to raise blood pressure, inotropic agents may be required.

Chest pain and apprehension are usually treated with intravenous analgesics (e.g., morphine sulfate). Because the usual cause of PE is thrombus from the lower legs, the legs are usually elevated with caution to avoid severe flexure of the hips. Such flexure will again slow blood flow and increase the risk of new thrombi.

The use of fibrinolytic therapy in the management of massive PE is not clear. Some clinicians have found that although the treatment dissolves the clot, it does not improve the mortality rate.

Surgical Intervention

There are three surgical interventions for pulmonary embolus: (1) vein ligation to prevent the embolus traveling to the heart; (2) vena cava plication, or insertion of an umbrella filter to allow blood flow while trapping emboli (Figure 39–20); and (3) embolectomy.

An embolectomy involves surgical removal of emboli from the pulmonary arteries. Before the advent of the cardiopulmonary bypass, the procedure had an extremely high mortality rate. Even now, embolectomy during anticoagulant therapy carries a high risk, partly because of possible misdiagnosis and partly because operating on clients in profound shock is dangerous.

Nursing Management

The client is closely monitored for hypoxemia and respiratory compromise. Vital signs are assessed every 15 minutes until they are stable. Lung sounds are auscultated every 2 to 4 hours. Blood gas values are monitored. To facilitate breathing, the client is placed in semi-Fowler's position, and oxygen is applied per doctor's orders.

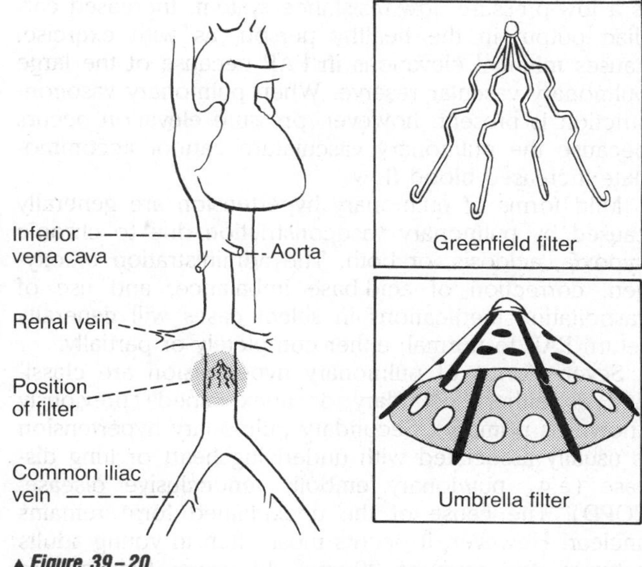

▲ **Figure 39–20**

Inferior vena cava (IVC) filters, such as Greenfield and umbrella filters, prevent emboli from traveling to the lung.

The client is also monitored for clinical manifestations of right-sided heart failure. Heart sounds are ascultated every 4 hours, assessing for murmurs or extra heart sounds. The nurse monitors for right-sided heart failure (e.g., peripheral edema, distended neck veins, liver engorgement).

The nurse assesses for effectiveness by monitoring the partial thromboplastin time (PTT). The usual goal is 2 to 2.5 times the control (normal) value. The nurse also monitors for manifestations of excess anticoagulation, bleeding (evidenced by blood in the urine, stool, and along the gums or teeth), subcutaneous bruising, or flank pain. When invasive studies are necessary, such as arterial blood gases, pressure is applied for 30 minutes to the puncture site.

The client typically experiences fear associated with the sudden onset of severe chest pain and inability to breathe. The person becomes anxious, restless, and apprehensive. Many times, the client will not reveal his or her innermost fears. The nurse's firm emotional support can be a stabilizing factor at this time. This support can effectively be shown by staying with the person. In addition, the nurse should give intensive care efficiently but should not display fear.

Analgesics are given as needed to reduce pain and anxiety. Anxiety and pain increase oxygen demand and dyspnea. Oral care is given while oxygen is in use, especially if the client breathes through the mouth.

PULMONARY HYPERTENSION

Pulmonary hypertension is defined as a prolonged elevation of the mean pulmonary artery pressure (PAP) above 18 mm Hg (norm, 10 to 20 mm Hg) and systolic PAP above 30 mm Hg (norm, 20 to 30 mm Hg) at rest or during exercise. Normally, the pulmonary circulation is a low-pressure, low-resistance system. Increased cardiac output in the healthy person, as with exercise, causes minimal elevations in PAP because of the large pulmonary vascular reserve. When pulmonary vasoconstriction is present, however, pressure elevation occurs because the pulmonary vasculature cannot accommodate increased blood flow.

Mild forms of pulmonary hypertension are generally caused by pulmonary vasoconstriction due to chronic hypoxia, acidosis, or both. The administration of oxygen, correction of acid-base imbalance, and use of vasodilating medications in select cases will generally return PAP to normal, either completely or partially.

Severe forms of pulmonary hypertension are classified as either secondary or unexplained (previously known as primary). Secondary pulmonary hypertension is usually associated with underlying heart or lung disease (e.g., pulmonary emboli, venocclusive disease, COPD). The cause of the unexplained form remains unclear. However, it occurs most often in young adults between the ages of 20 and 40 years; females are affected more often than are males. The condition is progressive, leading to right-sided heart failure and severe dyspnea.

Clients with mild pulmonary hypertension may be relatively asymptomatic. In moderate to severe forms, the main (and occasionally only) symptom is dyspnea. Fatigue, syncope, angina-like chest pain, palpitations, and muscular weakness may also occur. Chest x-ray examination reveals right ventricular hypertrophy, enlarged pulmonary arteries, prominent hilar vessels, and normal or reduced intrapulmonary vascular markings. Cardiac catheterization provides the most valuable diagnostic measurements. Typical findings include elevated PAP and increased arteriovenous oxygen differences accompanied by normal systemic blood pressure and normal to low cardiac output. Pulmonary wedge pressures remain normal because left ventricular function is typically unchanged.

The overall prognosis in severe pulmonary hypertension is poor. There is no known cure for the disorder, although treatment of the underlying cause of secondary forms may slow its progression. Vasodilator therapy may also be employed with some success. Additionally, supportive intervention will be used to reduce hypoxemia. A few clients with severe, unexplained pulmonary hypertension have undergone heart-lung transplantation, but data regarding long-term effectiveness are not yet available.[33] Interventions appropriate for underlying diseases and preparation for diagnostic procedures are incorporated into nursing care.

▼ DISORDERS OF THE PLEURA AND PLEURAL SPACE

PLEURAL PAIN

Pleural pain is a common pulmonary symptom associated with a variety of disorders. It arises from the parietal pleura, which is richly supplied with sensory nerve endings. Pleuritic pain indicates the presence of pleural inflammation (pleurisy) due to pneumonia, pulmonary infarction, or other cause; pleural effusion; or pneumothorax. It is often accompanied by a pleural friction rub that is discovered during chest auscultation.

Pleuritic chest pain often develops abruptly and is usually severe enough that the client seeks medical attention. It frequently occurs only on one side of the chest, usually in the lower lateral portions of the chest wall, and is aggravated by deep breathing or coughing. Most of the time, the client can point directly to the exact location of the pain. However, pleural pain may also be referred to the neck, shoulder, or abdomen. Because other types of chest pain (e.g., cardiac pain, chest wall pain) may be misinterpreted as pleuritic pain, careful assessment is necessary.

Pleuritic chest pain may restrict normal respiratory efforts, leading to problems with gas exchange and airway clearance. If pain-relieving measures, including administration of prescribed analgesics, do not relieve the pain, the physician may perform an intercostal nerve block (Chap. 16).

PLEURAL EFFUSION

Overview

A pleural effusion is an accumulation of fluid in the pleural space. Pleural fluid normally seeps continually into the pleural space from the capillaries lining the parietal pleura and is reabsorbed by the visceral pleural capillaries and lymphatics. Any condition that interferes with either the secretion or drainage of this fluid will lead to pleural effusion.

Causes of pleural effusion can be grouped into four major categories:

- conditions that increase subpleural capillary pressure (e.g., congestive heart failure)
- conditions that decrease capillary oncotic pressure (e.g., liver or renal failure)
- conditions that cause inflammation of the pleura, pleural spaces, or underlying structures (e.g., infections or tumors)
- conditions that impair lymphatic function (e.g., lymphatic obstruction)

Clinical manifestations of pleural effusion will depend on the amount of fluid present and the degree of lung compression. If the effusion is small (i.e., <250 ml), its presence may be discovered only by chest x-ray examination. With large effusions, lung expansion may be restricted and the client may experience dyspnea, primarily on exertion. Tactile fremitus may be decreased or absent, and percussion notes may be dull or flat.

Management

PRIMARY PLEURAL EFFUSION

Thoracentesis (see Chap. 36) is used to remove excess pleural fluid. The fluid is then analyzed to determine if it is transudate or exudate. Transudates are substances that have passed through a membrane or tissue surface. They occur primarily in conditions in which there is protein loss and low protein content (e.g., left ventricular failure, cirrhosis, nephrosis). Transudative effusions are sometimes referred to as hydrothorax. Exudates are substances that have escaped from blood vessels. They contain an accumulation of cells, have a high specific gravity and a high lactate dehydrogenase (LDH), and occur in response to malignancies, infections, or inflammatory processes. Exudates occur when there is an increase in capillary permeability. Differentiating between transudates and exudates helps establish a specific diagnosis. Diagnosis may also require analysis of the fluid for (1) white and red blood cells, (2) malignant cells, (3) bacteria, (4) glucose content, (5) pH, and (6) LDH.

Pleural fluid may be (1) hemorrhagic, or bloody (e.g., if tumor is present, after trauma, or after pulmonary embolus with infarction), (2) chylous, or thick and white-colored (e.g., after lymphatic obstruction or trauma to the thoracic duct), or (3) rich in cholesterol (e.g., chronic, recurrent effusions due to tuberculous rheumatoid arthritis).

If there is a high white cell count and the pleural fluid is purulent, the effusion is called an empyema. An empyema of any amount requires drainage and treatment for the infection. If the pus is not drained, it may become thick and almost solidified or loculated (containing cavities). This is called fibrothorax. Fibrothorax may significantly restrict lung expansion and may require surgical intervention. The procedure, known as decortication, involves the removal of the restrictive mass of fibrin and inflammatory cells. Decortication is usually not performed until the fibrothorax is relatively solid, so it can be easily removed. After the procedure, closed chest drainage with suction (see Chap. 37) is used to reexpand the lung rapidly and fill the pleural space. If the fibrous material has restricted the lung for some time, the lung may not reexpand effectively, and further intervention (usually thoracoplasty), may be needed.

RECURRENT PLEURAL EFFUSION

In some cases, pleural effusions may recur despite repeated thoracenteses (e.g., malignancy-induced effusions), with resultant compromise of lung function or persistent pleural pain. Treatment of recurrent effusions is accomplished through obliteration of the pleural space. Methods of obliterating the pleural space include

- pleurectomy (pleural stripping). This procedure consists of surgically stripping the parietal pleura away from the visceral pleura. This produces an intense inflammatory reaction that promotes adhesion formation between the two layers during healing.
- pleurodesis. This involves the instillation of a sclerosing substance (e.g., unbuffered tetracycline, nitrogen mustard, talc) into the pleural space via a thoracotomy tube. This creates an inflammatory response that scleroses tissue together.

Because pleural space obliteration creates permanent changes, the client's existing and predicted postprocedure respiratory status must be carefully determined. If a large area is involved, significant alterations in ventilatory mechanics (e.g., deep breathing, coughing) may occur, leading to compromised respiratory function.

After the procedure, closely monitor lung function, including respiratory rate and ventilation pattern. Document alleviation or persistence of pleural pain and watch for indications of a return of the pleural effusion. Pulmonary function studies (see Chap. 36) and ABGs should also be evaluated.

BRONCHOPLEURAL FISTULA

A bronchopleural fistula is a connection between the pleural space and a bronchus. It may occur when (1) an undrained empyema erodes into a bronchus or (2) the pleural space does not heal spontaneously after chest tube removal (see Chap. 37). A bronchopleural fistula increases the risk of pleural infection. It may also compromise ventilation and oxygenation.

The management of a client with a bronchopleural fistula is often complex, requiring a critical care setting. Bronchopleural fistulas may be slow to heal. The client may be discharged home with a chest tube connected to a collection system. It is important that the client and family understand how to care for the chest tube and collection system, signs and symptoms of irritation at the chest puncture site, and changes in chest drainage that require the physician to be notified (e.g., blood).

METASTATIC PLEURAL TUMORS

Primary tumors in the lungs and other organs often metastasize to the pleura. The primary tumor is usually in a lung but may occur in the breast, ovaries, liver, kidneys, uterus, testicles, or larynx, or it may result from leukemia or lymphoma. Metastatic pleural disease causes about half of all pleural effusions.

Assessment findings with malignant pleural effusion are the same as for pleural effusion from other causes. Diagnosis of pleural effusion is by chest x-ray examination. The source of the effusion is determined by cytologic examination of pleural fluid obtained by thoracentesis. Intervention is the same as for pleural effusion and the primary malignancy. (See previous discussion.)

▼ DISORDERS OF THE DIAPHRAGM

SUBDIAPHRAGMATIC ABSCESS

A subdiaphragmatic abscess may develop as a result of (1) gastrointestinal perforation; (2) surgery on the upper gastrointestinal system, liver, or biliary tract; (3) abdominal trauma; or (4) other intra-abdominal surgery. A subdiaphragmatic abscess produces abdominal and thoracic symptoms, which potentially compromise respiratory status (see Restrictive Lung Disease).

Thoracic assessment findings may include pleuritic pain or pain referred to the shoulder on the affected side. Dyspnea and poor or no diaphragmatic movement are common. Abdominal assessment findings may include flank pain or tenderness and a palpable abdominal mass in the region of the abscess. Generalized assessment findings include fever, anorexia, weight loss, and vomiting.

A subdiaphragmatic abscess is diagnosed by chest x-ray examination. The diaphragm is almost always elevated on the affected side. Fluoroscopic studies of diaphragmatic movement reveal limited or absent diaphragmatic movement on the affected side. Pleural effusion also commonly occurs. Thoracentesis and analysis of the pleural fluid reveal an exudate. Subdiaphragmatic abscesses may erode and perforate the diaphragm.

Intervention for subdiaphragmatic abscess includes (1) antibiotic administration, (2) draining the abscess, and (3) supportive measures to maintain ventilation and respiratory status. An untreated subdiaphragmatic abscess is nearly always fatal. With treatment, the mortality rate is still high but drops to approximately 25 per cent.

DIAPHRAGMATIC PARALYSIS

Overview

Many situations may affect diaphragm function and result in paralysis, either unilateral or bilateral.

Unilateral diaphragmatic paralysis is more common than is bilateral. Causes of unilateral diaphragmatic paralysis include (1) severing of the phrenic nerve during surgery; (2) bronchogenic or metastatic tumors; (3) neurologic disorders such as poliomyelitis, encephalitis, herpes zoster, and diphtheria; (4) accidental or birth trauma; (5) mechanical obstruction (e.g., from aortic aneurysm); (6) infectious processes such as tuberculosis, pneumonia, pleuritic disorders, or subdiaphragmatic abscess; and (7) other disorders (e.g., pulmonary infarction, congenital abnormalities). Causes of bilateral diaphragmatic paralysis include (1) many neuromuscular disorders, including amyotrophic lateral sclerosis, muscular dystrophy, and Guillain-Barré syndrome; (2) alcohol and lead neuropathy; (3) closed chest trauma; and (4) anatomic causes (such as congenital absence of phrenic nerve, eventration, traumatic diaphragmatic rupture, and spinal injuries).

Although the diaphragm is the primary muscle of respiration, its role can be assumed in part by the accessory and abdominal muscles. As a result, diaphragmatic paralysis is often difficult to detect.

Unilateral diaphragmatic paralysis is diagnosed by fluoroscopy. The person is asked to "sniff" during fluoroscopy. If paralysis is present, the nonparalyzed side of the diaphragm descends during inspiration (the "sniff"), and the paralyzed side paradoxically rises during this maneuver. Clients with unilateral diaphragmatic paralysis usually experience dyspnea when lying on the affected side. Dyspnea on exertion is not usual unless there is underlying lung disease. Both TLC and VC are reduced by about 20 per cent. There is also less ventilation to the affected side and mild hypoxemia because of shifts of ventilation and blood flow. Pre-existing lung disease combined with unilateral diaphragmatic paralysis may be disabling, depending on the extent of the lung disease.

The effects of bilateral diaphragmatic paralysis are potentially much more severe than those of unilateral paralysis. However, the problem is often subtle and overlooked, especially if the client has a neuromuscular disorder. Fatigue, disturbed sleep, and morning headache are frequently the only assessment findings. A classic manifestation of bilateral paralysis of the diaphragm is increased dyspnea when lying flat on the back (supine). Paradoxic inward abdominal movement during inspiration when supine and active use of the accessory muscles of inspiration also occur. The pulmonary effects of bilateral paralysis include reduced VC and TLC when the client is upright, which are even more reduced when the client is supine. The FRC is also decreased, as is lung compliance. In the side-lying position, ventilation is preferentially distributed to the uppermost lung tissue and away from blood flow, which leads to a significant mismatch of ventilation and perfusion. Severe hypoxemia results. Reduced tidal volume leads to retention of carbon dioxide and respiratory acidosis. Respiratory muscle function decreases during rest and sleep, further compromising respiratory status.

Management

There is little that can be done to treat diaphragmatic paralysis. Management is aimed, instead, at supporting ventilatory function, as needed. If the phrenic nerve is intact, a phrenic nerve pacer may be surgically inserted. However, this is possible only if the phrenic nerve can be stimulated (this is tested by a fluoroscopic procedure). This procedure is useful only for clients with spinal cord injuries.

Assess the client for subjective indications of hypoxemia or hypercapnia. Monitor ventilatory mechanics (e.g., inspiratory effort, spontaneous VC) and ABGs, observing for deteriorating trends.

Nursing management focuses on maintenance of a patent airway and detection of deteriorating gas exchange. Because inspiration is impaired, the client may need assistance to cough and deep breathe effectively (see Chap. 37). Position the client on the unaffected side in semisitting or sitting position. Suction as necessary. Increase hydration to liquefy secretions. Administer oxygen, if prescribed. If respiratory function declines significantly, the physician and client (or possibly significant others) must decide whether to place a permanent tracheostomy and to use mechanical ventilation or other assistance devices (e.g., rocking bed, chest cuirass).

▼ CONGENITAL DISORDERS

CYSTIC FIBROSIS

This inherited disorder of the exocrine (mucus-producing) glands affects the (1) sweat glands; (2) respiratory system; (3) digestive tract, particularly the pancreas; and (4) reproductive tract. Cystic fibrosis is the most common inherited genetic disease in the Caucasian population, affecting approximately 1 in 2000 white newborns in the United States. Previously, this condition was considered a "pediatric problem" because it was fatal in childhood. However, advances in treatment, including antibiotics, chest physiotherapy, and nutrition programs, have extended the average life expectancy for cystic fibrosis into the early 20s, with maximum survival estimated at 30 to 40 years. Diagnosis of cystic fibrosis is established by an abnormal sweat test, that is, an abnormally high concentration (>60 mEq/L) of chloride in the sweat.

Pulmonary involvement is the most common and most severe manifestation of cystic fibrosis. Over 90 per cent of cystic fibrosis clients die with severe pulmonary disease. The disease process causes tracheobronchial secretions to become thick and viscous, leading to (1) interference with normal ciliary action, (2) plugging of airways, and (3) creation of a reservoir for bacterial growth and infection. Bronchiectasis may also develop, which compounds the infection risk. (Pediatric texts completely discuss all facets of cystic fibrosis.)

The goal of pulmonary therapy is to prevent infections by removing secretions, improving aeration, and administering antimicrobial agents. Effective clearing of tracheobronchial secretions is promoted by (1) ensuring adequate hydration; (2) administering prescribed mucolytic aerosols; and (3) teaching and supervising effective coughing techniques, postural drainage, and chest percussion. These techniques are discussed in Chapter 37. The chest should be auscultated before and after therapy, noting quality of respiration.

Adequate aeration is maintained by (1) following the techniques for maintaining clear airways, (2) administering oxygen if hypoxemia is present, and (3) maintaining correct body position to facilitate breathing (e.g., sitting up). Recent studies have also shown that exercise can improve pulmonary function in these clients.[49] The client should be assessed for signs of hypercapnia and indications of respiratory failure.

Antimicrobial therapy has played a significant role in extending the life expectancy of cystic fibrosis clients. Oral antibiotics may be given prophylactically on a routine basis. Intravenous antibiotics are essential during acute infections. The specific choice of antibiotic should be determined by sputum culture and sensitivity. Infections are most commonly caused by *Staphylococcus aureus* and *Pseudomonas aeruginosa.* Sputum should be assessed for color, quality, and quantity. All respiratory equipment should be thoroughly cleaned on a routine basis for preventing reinfection from contaminated equipment.

Recently, a new treatment for cystic fibrosis has been developed. This treatment uses a virus to carry DNA into the lung cells. The DNA is able to produce functional proteins; the treatment must be repeated in order to keep working.

Treatment of end-stage disease is primarily concerned with the management of severe complications. Obstruction of the airways leads to a state of hyperinflation. In time, fibrosis develops, and restrictive lung disease is superimposed on the obstructive disease. Pneumothorax may develop, requiring lung reinflation with chest tubes.

Persistent pulmonary infection with *Pseudomonas* organisms is common in the end stages of cystic fibrosis. Treatment with continuous, large doses of intravenous antibiotics is usually indicated. Moderate to severe hemoptysis can occur if the infection causes erosion of pulmonary blood vessels. Blood replacement and temporary cessation of postural drainage may be required.

Over time, pulmonary obstruction leads to chronic hypoxia, hypercapnia, and acidosis. Pulmonary hypertension and, eventually, cor pulmonale may result. Treatment may include digitalis, diuretics, and oxygen therapy.

Attention to psychosocial concerns is a nursing priority throughout the disease course. In the adult cystic fibrosis client, psychosocial concerns center around three major areas: disease management (e.g., treatment compliance, sleep disturbance, hemoptysis, nutrition, and hospitalizations); growth and development (e.g., daily activities, school/work, and sex and reproduction); and family relations (e.g., substance abuse, depression, anxiety, and marital problems).[8] Nursing intervention involves assisting clients to cope with these problem areas as well as providing emotional support to both the client and family.

Summary

Pulmonary disorders can be classified as acute or chronic, obstructive or restrictive, infectious or noninfectious, and those caused by cardiac disorders. Because of the potential morbidity and mortality with these disorders, nursing assessment and intervention are critical to successful client management.

Bibliography

1. Aberman, A. (1986). Managing asthmatics. *Emergency Medicine, 18*:26.
2. Armstrong, D. A. (1987). Lung cancer: the diagnostic workup. *American Journal of Nursing, 87*:1433.
3. Belman, M., Thomas, S., & Lewis, M. (1986). Resistive breathing training in patients with chronic obstructive pulmonary disease. *Chest, 90*:662.
4. Bernard, G. R., & Bradley, R. B. (1986). Adult respiratory distress syndrome: diagnosis and management. *Heart and Lung, 15*:250.
5. Bordow, R. A., & Moser, K. M. (1985). *Manual of clinical problems in pulmonary medicine* (2nd ed.). Boston: Little, Brown.
6. Bradley, R. B. (1987). Adult respiratory distress syndrome. *Focus on Critical Care, 14*(10):49.

7. Brandstetter, R. D. (1986). The adult respiratory distress syndrome. *Heart and Lung, 15*(3):155.
8. Brissette, S., et al. (1987). Nursing care plan for adolescents and young adults with advanced cystic fibrosis. *Issues in Comprehensive Pediatric Nursing, 10*:87.
9. Burrows, B. (1990). Airways obstructive diseases: pathological mechanisms and natural histories of the disorders. *Medical Clinics of North America, 74*(3):547–560.
10. Carpenito, L. J. (1992). *Nursing diagnosis: Application to clinical practice* (4th ed.). Philadelphia: J. B. Lippincott.
11. Carpenito, L. J. (1991). *Nursing care plans and documentation.* Philadelphia: J. B. Lippincott.
12. Caruthers, D. D. (1990). Infectious pneumonia in the elderly. *American Journal of Nursing, 90*(2):56.
13. Cassingham, B. (1985). The silent epidemic: asbestosis and related diseases. *Occupational Health Nursing, 33*(7):360.
14. Chan-Yeung, M. (1988). Occupational asthma update. *Chest, 93*(2):407.
15. Clinical highlights: infection and ventilatory failure in emphysema. *Hospital Medicine, 22*(8):95, 1986.
16. Coleman, D. A. (1986). Pneumonia: where nursing care really counts. *RN, 49*(2):23.
17. Davidson, P. T. (1989). The diagnosis and management of disease caused by M. avium complex, M. kansasii, and other mycobacteria. *Clinics in Chest Medicine, 10*(9):431.
18. DeVito, A., & Kleven, M. (1987). Dyspnea. *RN, 50*(6):38–46.
19. Eggland, E. T. (1987). Teaching the ABC's of COPD. *Nursing 87, 17*(1):60.
20. Engelking, C. (1987). Lung cancer: chemotherapy. *American Journal of Nursing, 87*(11):1438.
21. Engelking, C. (1987). Lung cancer: the language of staging. *American Journal of Nursing, 87*(11):1434.
22. Fahey, V. A. (1988). *Vascular nursing.* Philadelphia; W. B. Saunders.
23. Feinsilver, S. H. (1988). Respiratory failure in asthma and COPD. *Emergency Medicine, 21*(4):90.
24. Greifzu, S., Crebase, C., & Winnick, B. (1987). Lung cancer: by the time it's detected, it may be too late. *RN, 50*(3):52.
25. Hahn, K. (1989). Sexuality and COPD. *Rehabilitation Nursing, 14*(7):191.
26. Haylock, P. J. (1987). Lung cancer: radiation therapy. *American Journal of Nursing, 87*(11):1441.
27. Johns, C. J., Scott, P. P., & Schonfeld, S. A. (1989). Sarcoidosis. *Annual Review of Medicine, 40*:353.
28. Johnson, A. P. (1988). The elderly and COPD. *Journal of Gerontological Nursing, 14*(12):20.
29. Johnson, N. T., & Pierson, D. J. (1986). The spectrum of pulmonary atelectasis: pathophysiology, diagnosis, and therapy. *Respiratory Care, 31*(11):1108.
30. Kersten, L. D. (1989). *Comprehensive respiratory nursing: A decision making approach.* Philadelphia: W. B. Saunders.
31. Krokosky, N. J. (1985). Black lung and silicosis. *American Journal of Nursing, 85*(8):883.
32. Krull, K., & Hatswell, E. (1988). Single-lung allograft: a nursing perspective. *Critical Care Nurse, 8*(9):35.
33. Lareau, S., & Larson, J. (1987). Ineffective breathing pattern related to airflow limitation. *Nursing Clinics of North America, 22*(1):179.
34. Ledger, S. D. (1986). Management of a patient in respiratory failure due to chronic bronchitis. *Intensive Care Nursing, 2*:30.
35. Lekander, B. J. (1988). Preventing complications for the heart and lung transplant recipient. *Dimensions of Critical Care Nursing, 7*(1):18.
36. Mandel, J. H., & Baker, B. A. (1989). Recognizing occupational lung disease. *Hospital Practice, 24*(1):21.
37. Martin, R. (1990). The sleep-related worsening of lower airways obstruction: understanding and intervention. *Medical Clinics of North America, 74*(3):701–714.
38. Masden, L. A. (1990). Tuberculosis today. *RN, 53*(3):44–50.
39. McCance, K., & Huether, S. (1990). *Pathophysiology.* St. Louis: C. V. Mosby.
40. McNaull, F. W. (1987). Lung cancer: what are the odds? *American Journal of Nursing, 87*(11):1428.
41. Meredith, J. W. (1988). Emergency management of chest injury, including complications and immediate life-threatening injury. *Topics in Emergency Medicine, 10*(7):60.
42. Mitchell, R. S., Petty, T. L., & Schwarz, M. I. (1989). *Synopsis of clinical pulmonary disease* (4th ed.). St. Louis: C. V. Mosby.
43. Naccarato, M., & Kresevic, D. (1989). Caring for adults who have cystic fibrosis. *American Journal of Nursing, 89*(11):1462.
44. National Consensus Conference on Tuberculosis (1985). Preventive treatment of tuberculosis. *Chest, 87*(2):128s.
45. O'Brien, R. J. (1989). The epidemiology of nontuberculous mycobacterial disease. *Clinics in Chest Medicine, 10*(9):407.
46. O'Byrne, C. (1985). Postoperative care and complications in the thoracotomy patient. *Critical Care Quarterly, 7*(3):53.
47. Perez-Stable, E. J., & Hopewell, P. C. (1989). Current tuberculosis treatment regimens: choosing the right one for your patient. *Clinics in Chest Medicine, 10*(3):323.
48. Raffin, T. A. (1986). Pancoast syndrome. *Hospital Medicine, 22*(5):218.
49. Rose, J., & Jay, S. (1986). A comprehensive exercise program for persons with cystic fibrosis. *Journal of Pediatric Nursing, 1*(10):323.
50. Rostad, M. (1990). Advances in nursing management of patients with lung cancer. *Nursing Clinics of North America, 25*(2):393.
51. Sexton, D. L. (1990). *Nursing care of the respiratory patient.* Norwalk, CT: Appleton and Lange.
52. Sheehy, S. B. (1985). *Emergency nursing: Principles and practice.* St. Louis: C. V. Mosby.
53. Shuey, K. M. (1989). Case studies in thoracic surgery. *Dimensions in Oncology Nursing, 3*(4):14.
54. Timberlake, G. A., et al. (1986). Trauma rounds. Problem: deceleration thoracic trauma. *Emergency Medicine, 18*(4):52.
55. Votava, K. M., & Bartock, B. S. (1990). Home rehab for cardiopulmonary patients. *RN, 53*(10):79.
56. Walker, C. L. (1988). The clinical challenge of cystic fibrosis. *Journal of Intravenous Nursing, 11*(11):373.
57. Wyngaarden, J. B., Smith, L. H., & Bennett, J. C. (1992). *Cecil textbook of medicine* (19th ed.). Philadelphia: W. B. Saunders.
58. Young, J. R., Olin, J. W., & Bartholomew, J. R. (1991). *Peripheral vascular disease.* St. Louis: C. V. Mosby.

Unit 9

Cardiovascular Disorders

The heart is one of the few truly vital organs. Disorders related to the heart are currently the leading cause of death throughout the western world. Within the United States alone, nearly 1 million people die every year from cardiovascular (CV) ailments.

Fortunately, heart disease as a cause of death as been gradually declining since the early 1970s. Heart disease was the cause of only 10 per cent of deaths at the turn of the century, rising to 39 per cent of deaths in the 1960s. Since 1970, deaths from heart disease have begun to decline, primarily because of detection, prevention, and intervention. During the 1980s, several advances have been made in diagnostic assessments, pharmacologic intervention, and public awareness of cardiopulmonary resuscitation and preventive interventions. With continued advances in research and clinical practice, the coming decades may see additional breakthroughs in preventing and treating cardiovascular disorders worldwide.

Through research, the understanding of cardiovascular disease continues to grow hourly. As a result, the care of people with heart disease is currently one of the most progressive areas in nursing.

Nurses caring for clients with cardiac disorders must understand cardiac structure and function. They must be able to swiftly identify life-threatening dysrhythmias on an electrocardiogram, and be ready to initiate emergency intervention when appropriate. Because cardiovascular disorders are long term, another important component of nursing care is education of the client about self-management of his or her disorder. Caring for individuals with cardiovascular disorders is not confined to the critical care unit but is common throughout the scope of nursing practice, on medical-surgical units, in pediatric wards, on obstetric units, in surgery, and in the community.

Chapter 40

Structure and Function of the Cardiovascular System

The human heart beats approximately 72 times per minute, 100,000 times a day and 22.5 billion times in a lifetime. This small pump, weighing approximately 11 ounces, pumps approximately 5 quarts of blood each minute and 75 gallons an hour. With computer-like efficiency, it pumps oxygen rich blood into the arterial system. This pump contracts every second of every day throughout a lifetime, resting only 0.4 second between beats.

The heart beats continuously, and unlike other muscles of the body, it cannot stop to rest when tired and worn from work. Instead, it must keep pumping continuously with sufficient force to circulate blood properly to all parts of the body. And, amazingly, it must increase its work output by four or five times its resting level if it is to sustain the body during periods of stress, that is, hard exercise, emotions, and illness.

When the heart does not work efficiently, the client's life may be threatened. This normally efficient and remarkably durable structure can develop structural defects and functional disturbances. What happens to the body when this mechanism begins to weaken and fail? What happens to the tissues and cells when the heart cannot pump oxygenated blood to them in adequate amounts? To understand cardiac disease, one must first examine normal cardiac function.

This chapter reviews normal cardiovascular structure, function, and control as a basis for understanding pathologic conditions presented in the following chapters.

▼ CARDIOVASCULAR STRUCTURE AND FUNCTION

The cardiovascular system consists of the heart, arteries, capillaries, veins, and lymphatics.

The functions of the heart are to pump oxygenated blood into the arterial system, which carries it to the cells, and to collect deoxygenated blood from the venous system and deliver it to the lungs for reoxygenation (Fig. 40-1).

The function of the arteries, capillaries, veins, and lymphatics is to carry blood to and from tissues and cells throughout the body.

STRUCTURE OF THE HEART

The heart is located within the mediastinum, which is the space between the lungs in the thoracic cavity. The heart is cone shaped and lies on the diaphragm. It is tilted forward and to the left. The apex of the heart is at the bottom (tip of the cone) and is left of the midline. The base is at the top of the heart, where the great vessels enter the heart, and is posterior to the sternum.

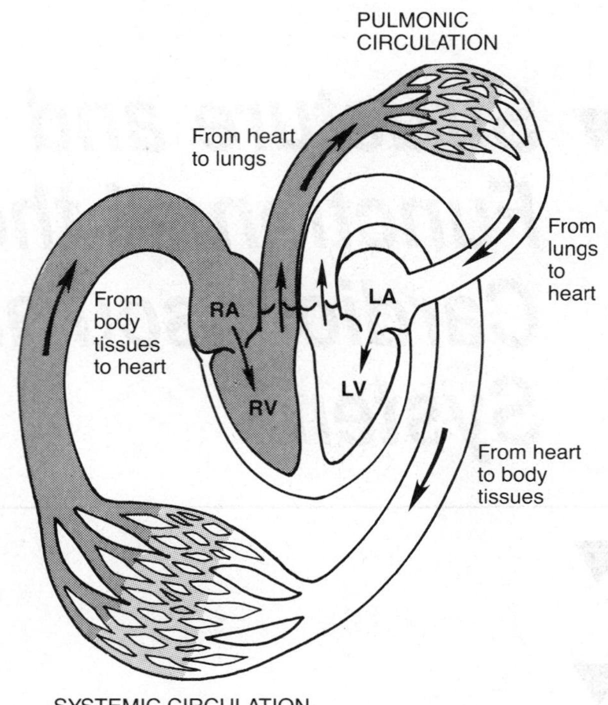

▲ *Figure 40-1*

Schematic circulation. In the peripheral capillaries, blood oxygen is exchanged for carbon dioxide. The deoxygenated blood returns to the right atrium *(RA)* and right ventricle *(RV),* to be pumped into the lungs where carbon dioxide is exchanged for oxygen. Oxygenated blood from the lungs enters the left atrium *(LA)* and left ventricle *(LV)* of the heart to be pumped into the systemic circulation once again.

Layers

The heart consists of three distinct layers of tissue: epicardium, myocardium, and endocardium. The *epicardium* covers the outer surface of the heart. It has the same thin, transparent structure as the visceral pericardium. The *myocardium,* the middle layer, consists of striated muscle fibers interlaced into bundles. It is the actual contracting muscle of the heart. The *endocardium,* the innermost layer, consists of thin endothelial tissue. It lines the inner chambers and the heart valves (Fig. 40-2).

Chambers

Each side of the heart consists of two chambers, an upper collecting chamber (atrium) and a lower pumping chamber (ventricle). A muscular wall, the septum, separates the chambers of the right side of the heart from those of the left side of the heart. The *right atrium* receives deoxygenated blood from the body via the superior and inferior vena cava. The blood then flows into the right ventricle. The *right ventricle,* a flat muscular pump, receives blood from the right atrium and pumps it to the lungs against low resistance, via the pulmonary artery. The *left atrium* receives oxygenated blood from the lungs via the four pulmonary veins. The blood then flows into the left ventricle. The *left ventricle,* the heart's largest, most muscular chamber, receives oxygenated blood from the lungs via the left atrium and pumps it out into the systemic circulation via the aorta. The left ventricle pumps against high systemic pressure.

The heart is actually two pumps working in unison. The right side receives deoxygenated blood from the body and pumps it to the lungs via the pulmonary arteries. At the same time, the left side receives oxygenated blood from the lungs and pumps it out through the aorta to all parts of the body (Fig. 40-3).

Pericardium

Encasing the heart is the pericardium, a loose-fitting covering that protects the heart from trauma and infection. It consists of two layers, one sac inside another: the parietal pericardium and the visceral pericardium. The *parietal pericardium* is the tough, fibrous outer membrane that is attached anteriorly to the lower half of the sternum, posteriorly to the thoracic vertebrae, and inferiorly to the diaphragm. It provides an effective barrier to infection from surrounding structures. The *visceral pericardium* is the thin, inner layer, which closely adheres to the heart and to the first several centimeters of the pulmonary artery and aorta.

The pericardial space is between the visceral and parietal layers and holds 5 to 20 ml of pericardial fluid. The fluid lubricates the pericardial surfaces as they slide over each other when the heart beats, and it cushions the heart against external trauma.

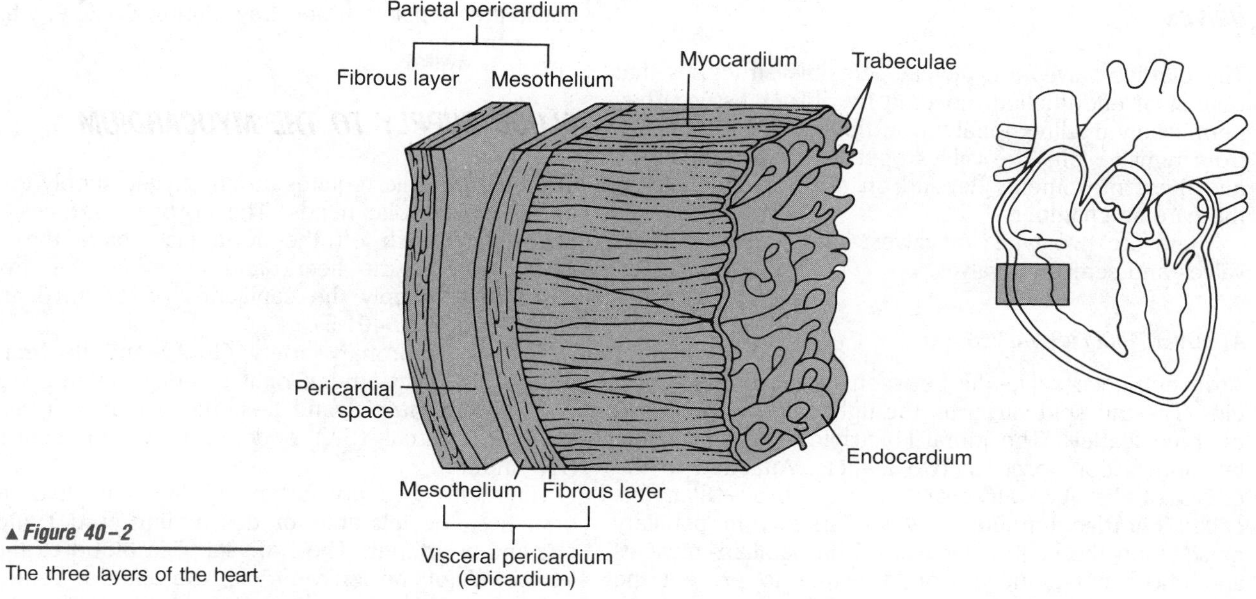

▲ *Figure 40-2*

The three layers of the heart.

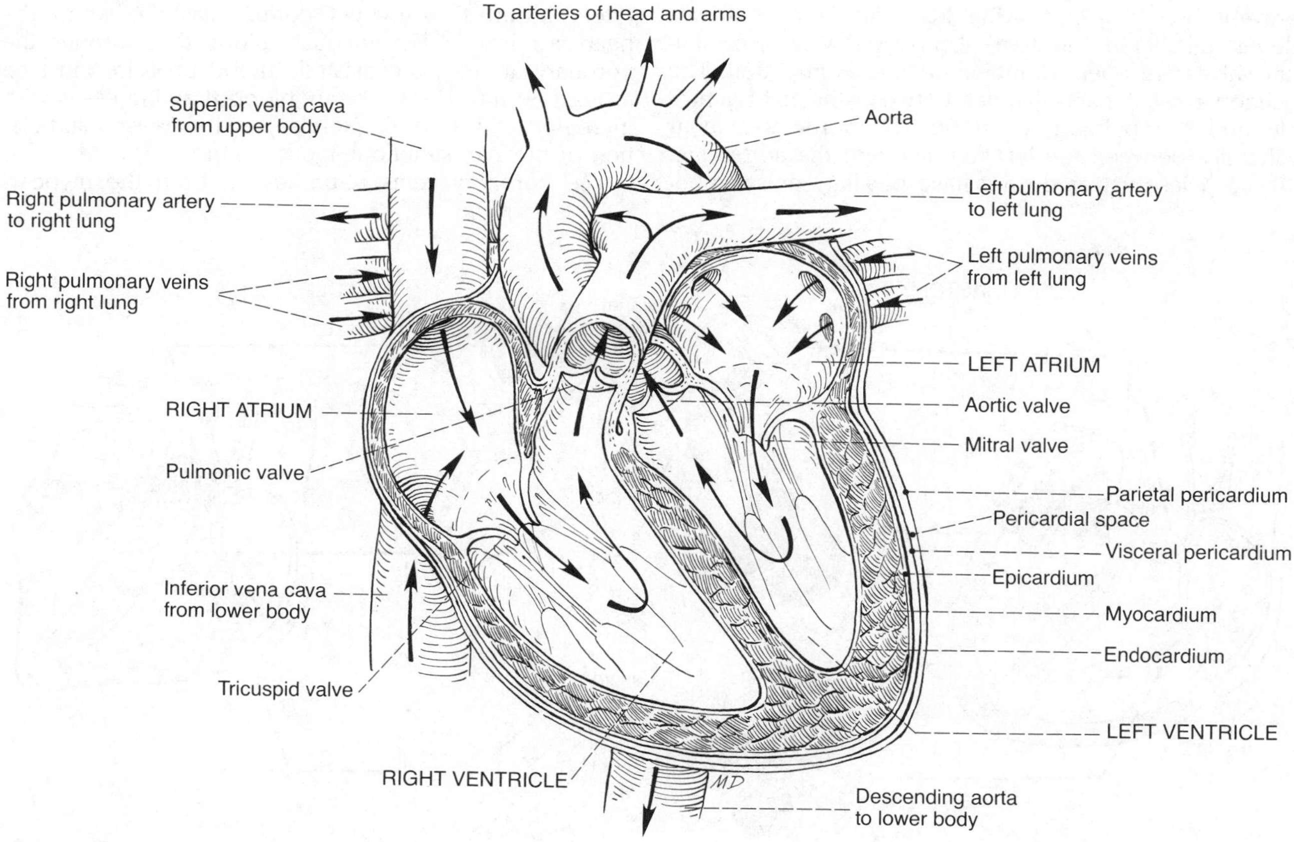

▲ *Figure 40-3*

Structure and circulation of the heart. Blood entering the left atrium from the right and left pulmonary veins flows into the left ventricle. The left ventricle pumps blood into the systemic circulation through the aorta. From the systemic circulation, blood returns to the heart through the superior and inferior venae cavae. From there, the right ventricle pumps blood into the lungs through the right and left pulmonary arteries.

Valves

The cardiac valves are delicate, flexible structures that consist of endothelium covered by fibrous tissue. They permit only unidirectional blood flow through the heart, from right to left. The valves open and close passively, and these movements depend on pressure gradients in the cardiac chambers.

There are two types of valves: atrioventricular (AV) valves and semilunar valves.

ATRIOVENTRICULAR VALVES

Atrioventricular valves lie between the atria and ventricles. The tricuspid valve, on the right side, is composed of three leaflets. The mitral (bicuspid) valve is on the left and is composed of two leaflets. Attached to the edges of the AV valves are strong, fibrous filaments called chordae tendineae, which arise from papillary muscles on the ventricular walls. The papillary muscles and chordae tendineae work together to prevent the AV valves from opening during ventricular contraction (systole). These valves prevent backflow of blood during periods of high pressure blood flow.

SEMILUNAR VALVES

The semilunar valves consist of three cuplike cusps that prevent blood from flowing back into the ventricles during relaxation (diastole). Unlike AV valves, semilunar valves are open during ventricular contraction. The pulmonic semilunar valve lies between the right ventricle and the pulmonary artery. The aortic semilunar valve lies between the left ventricle and the aorta (Fig. 40-4). These valves do not have papillary muscles because they regulate blood flow during diastole, which is a low pressure flow.

BLOOD SUPPLY TO THE MYOCARDIUM

The heart muscle requires a rich oxygen supply to meet its own metabolic needs. The coronary arteries (right and left) branch off the aorta just above the aortic valve, encircle the heart, and penetrate the myocardium. They supply the capillaries of the myocardium with blood (Fig. 40-5).

The right coronary artery (RCA) and its branches perfuse the right atrium, right ventricle, inferior portion of the left ventricle, and posterior septal wall, as well as the sinoatrial (SA) node and the atrioventricular (AV) node.

The left coronary artery (LCA) has two major branches, the left anterior descending (LAD) and the circumflex arteries. The LAD supplies blood to the anterior wall of the left ventricle, the anterior ventricular septum, and the apex of the left ventricle. The circumflex artery provides blood to the left atrium, the lateral and posterior surfaces of the left ventricle, and occasionally the posterior interventricular septum. In some clients, the circumflex artery supplies the SA and AV nodes.

Unlike other arteries, 75 per cent of the coronary artery blood flow occurs during diastole, when the heart is relaxed.[2] For adequate blood flow through the coronary arteries, the diastolic blood pressure must be at least 60 mm Hg. Coronary blood flow increases with increased activity (i.e., exercise) and increased stimulation of the sympathetic nervous system.

The coronary veins return blood from the myocar-

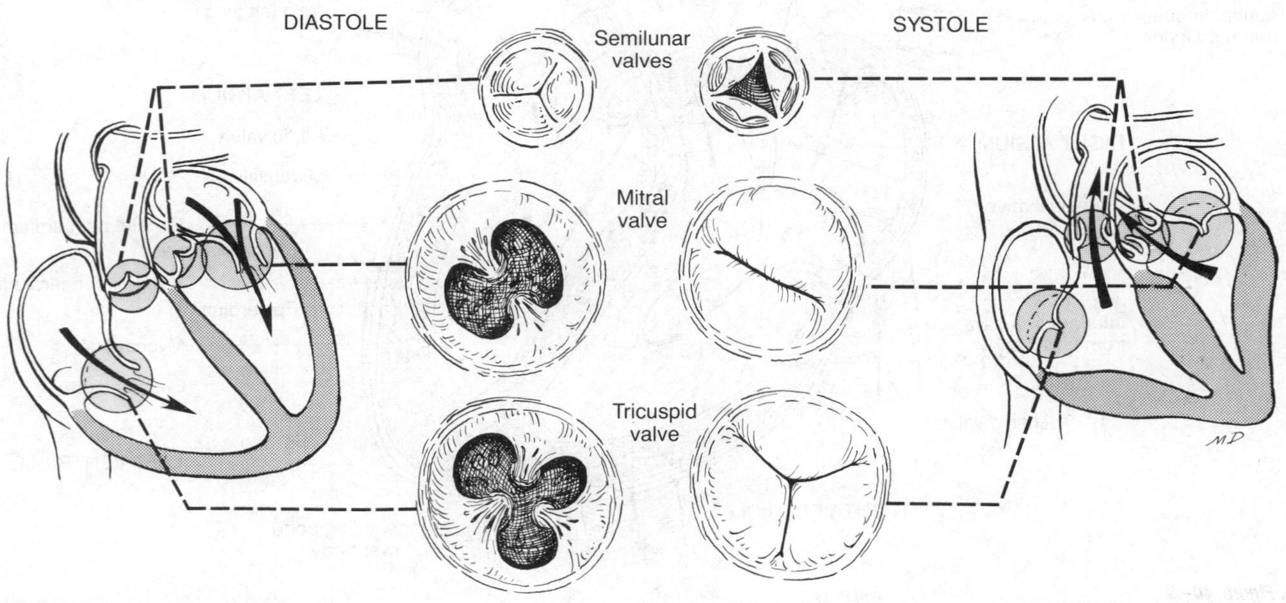

▲ **Figure 40-4**

Valves of the heart. The semilunar, mitral, and tricuspid valves are shown here as they appear during diastole (ventricular filling) and systole (ventricular contraction).

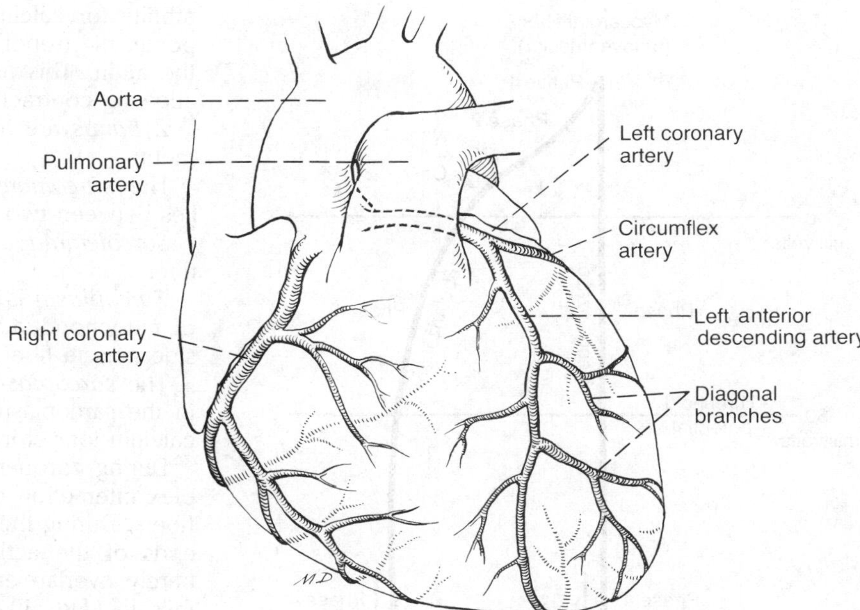

▲ *Figure 40-5*

Coronary arteries. The right and left coronary arteries branch off the aorta just above the aortic valve and normally supply the myocardium with oxygenated blood.

dium to the right atrium. These veins usually run parallel to the arteries.

ELECTROPHYSIOLOGIC PROPERTIES OF THE HEART

The electrophysiologic properties of cardiac muscle regulate the heart rate and rhythm. These properties include excitability, automaticity, conductivity, and refractoriness.

Excitability

The ability of cardiac muscle cells to depolarize in response to a stimulus is called excitability. Once stimulated, the whole heart muscle contracts. In contrast, skeletal muscle contracts partially to produce a graded force. If the heart contracted only partially, it would not effectively pump blood. Excitability is influenced by hormones, electrolytes, nutrition, oxygen supply, medications, infection, and nerve characteristics.

In myocardial cells, as in neurons, differences in intracellular and extracellular ion concentrations create electrical and concentration gradients for ionic movement across the semipermeable cell membrane. At rest, the inside of a myocardial cell is more negative than the outside. This "resting membrane potential" primarily results from the differences in concentrations of sodium (Na^+) and potassium (K^+). Although both ions are present on either side of the cell membrane, potassium has a greater intracellular concentration and sodium has a greater extracellular concentration. A lowered intracellular concentration of cations (positive ions) results when the cell membrane allows movement of potassium out of the cell, yet remains relatively impermeable to sodium.

When the cardiac cell is stimulated to a certain threshold, the transmembrane potential undergoes a dramatic change known as an action potential (Fig. 40-6). The action potential consists of depolarization and repolarization phases. The electrocardiogram reflects these waves of depolarization and repolarization sweeping over the heart.

Stimulation of the cardiac cell initiates depolarization and the subsequent change in transmembrane potential. The intracellular electrical potential shifts from negative to positive. This change results from an increase in cell membrane permeability to sodium, with resultant rapid influx of sodium ions. The wave of depolarization spreads to adjacent cells and through the whole heart.

The cell returns to its resting (relaxed) state during repolarization. Sodium permeability drops sharply, and potassium and chloride move out of the cell, returning the membrane to resting potential. In the process of depolarization and repolarization, small amounts of sodium leak into the cell and potassium leaks outward. The cell membrane monitors this balance, actively pumping sodium back out and potassium inward.

Other ions, such as calcium, chloride, and magnesium, also play a role in the action potential and the contraction it causes. The most important ion is calcium. During depolarization, myocardial cell membrane permeability to calcium increases and calcium moves into the cell. As the intracellular concentration of calcium increases, calcium reacts with contractile elements and myocardial muscle fibers contract.

The heart muscle is composed of long, narrow cells called fibers (Fig. 40-7). Coronary muscle fibers contain myofibrils, Z bands, sarcomere, sarcolemma, sarcoplasm, and sarcoplasmic reticulum.

Myofibrils consist of myosin filaments and actin filaments. *Myosin filaments* are dark bands that contain cross-bridges (similar to arms and hands) that protrude

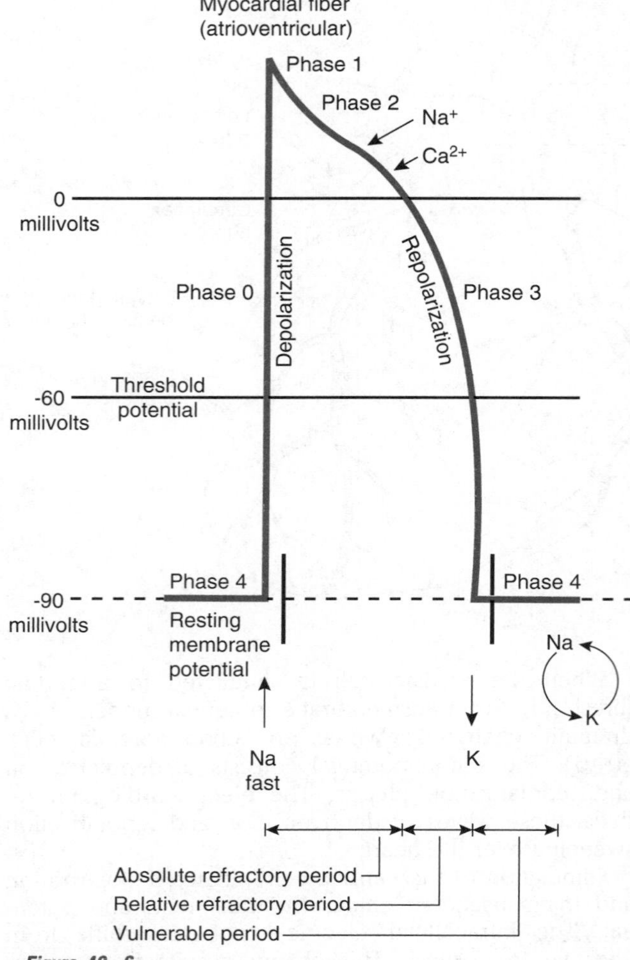

▲ **Figure 40–6**

Action potential of cardiac cells. The action potential of cardiac cells has five phases:

Phase 0: Sodium rapidly enters the cell through fast sodium channels, and cell depolarization (contraction) begins
Phase 1: The fast sodium channels close
Phase 2: Sodium continues to enter, along with calcium, but more slowly
Phase 3: Potassium enters the cell
Phase 4: The cell returns to its resting potential, sodium is pumped out of the cell, and potassium is pumped into the cell through the cell's sodium-potassium pump.

There is a period in all cardiac cells during which time they cannot be stimulated to fire another action potential. During the end of the action potential, the membrane is relatively refractory and can be reexcited only by a larger than usual stimulus. Immediately after the action potential, the membrane has transitory hyperexcitability and is said to be in a "vulnerable state."

from the side of the myosin. *Actin filaments* consist of three parts: actin, a tropomyosin strand, and troponin. The actin portion is composed of light bands containing active sites. The second part, the tropomyosin strand, is a loosely attached covering that physically covers the active sites of the actin strand. This covering prevents the interaction of actin and myosin that will cause contraction. The third part, troponin, attaches the tropomyosin to the actin. But troponin has a strong affinity for calcium. When calcium combines with troponin, the troponin no longer holds the tropomyosin in the actin. This uncovers the active sites on the actin, allowing contraction to proceed.

Z bands are attached at each end of the actin filament.

The *sarcomere* is the portion of the myofibril that lies between two successive Z bands.

Sarcolemma is the cell membrane of the muscle fiber.

Sarcoplasm is a matrix of fluid and a large number of mitochondria in which myofibrils are suspended inside muscle fiber.

The *sarcoplasmic reticulum* is a network of channels in the sarcoplasm. It contains a high concentration of calcium ions stored in the T tubules of the sarcoplasm.

During coronary muscle contraction, there is a complex interaction of all the intricate parts of the muscle fibers. During the relaxed state of the heart muscle, the ends of the actin filament in between two Z bands barely overlap each other but completely overlap the myosin (Fig. 40–8). During muscle contraction, actin filaments are pulled inward among the myosin. The actin filaments now overlap each other. The Z bands are smaller, too, as they are pulled up by the action of the actin and myosin. Muscle contraction occurs as a result of this sliding filament mechanism.

The action potential initiates the muscle contraction by releasing calcium through the T channels of the sarcoplasm. The calcium diffuses to the myofibrils, where it binds with troponin. As soon as the actin filaments become activated by calcium, the heads of the cross-bridges from the myosin filaments immediately become attracted to the active sites of the actin. Contraction then occurs.

After contraction, free calcium ions are actively pumped out of the cell back into the sarcoplasmic reticulum and muscle relaxation begins.

Automaticity

The ability of cardiac cells to initiate an impulse spontaneously and repetitively, without external neurohormonal control, is known as automaticity, or rhythmicity. Given the proper laboratory conditions, the heart can continue to beat outside of the body by means of its intrinsic control system. In contrast, skeletal muscle must be stimulated by a nerve in order to depolarize and contract. Heart muscle can depolarize spontaneously and stimulate its own contraction. Pacemaker cells have the highest rate of automaticity of all cardiac cells. The conduction tissue area with the highest automaticity, or rate of spontaneous depolarization, assumes the role of pacemaker. In normal circumstances, this is the SA node. Electrophysiology of the heart is discussed in more detail in Chapters 41 and 42.

Conductivity

Conductivity is the ability of heart muscle fibers to propagate electrical impulses along and across cell

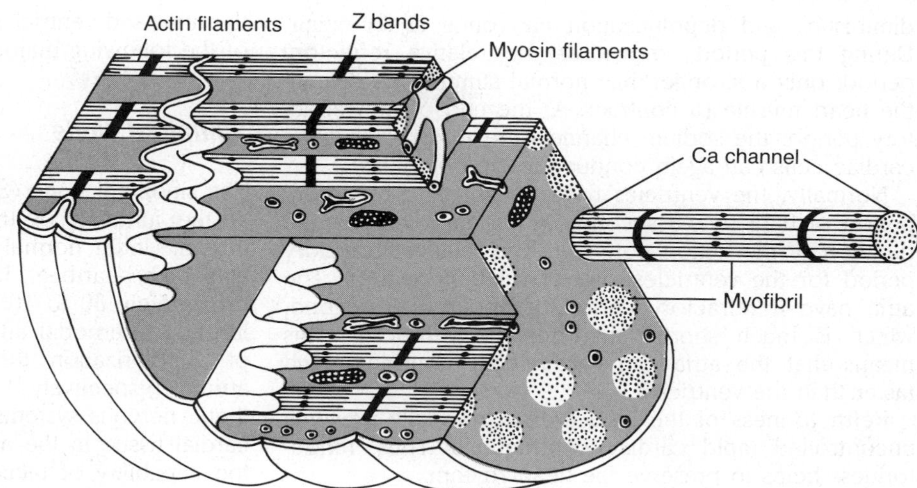

▲ Figure 40–7

The sarcomere, the functional unit of the cardiac muscle. Ca^{2+} enters through calcium ion channels on surface.

membranes. The heart muscle must conduct the action potential from its origin throughout the heart rapidly and in a coordinated manner so that the heart will contract as a unit. Intercalated discs join adjacent myocardial cells, allowing the action potential to travel over the entire muscle mass.

Refractoriness

Refractoriness is the heart's inability to respond to a new stimulus while still in a state of contraction due to an earlier stimulus. Thus, the heart muscle does not respond to restimulation during the action potential, preventing the possibility of tetanic contractions seen in skeletal muscle. Such sustained contractions of the heart would be fatal because there would not be enough time for ventricular filling. Refractoriness develops because the sodium channels of the cardiac cell membrane become inactivated during an action potential (depolarization).

Refractoriness occurs in two periods. The absolute refractory period occurs during depolarization and the first part of repolarization. During this period, cardiac cells do not respond to any stimuli, however strong. Then, in the final stages of repolarization, refractoriness

▲ Figure 40–8

During coronary muscle contraction, the actin filaments are pulled along the myosin, and the heart muscle contracts.

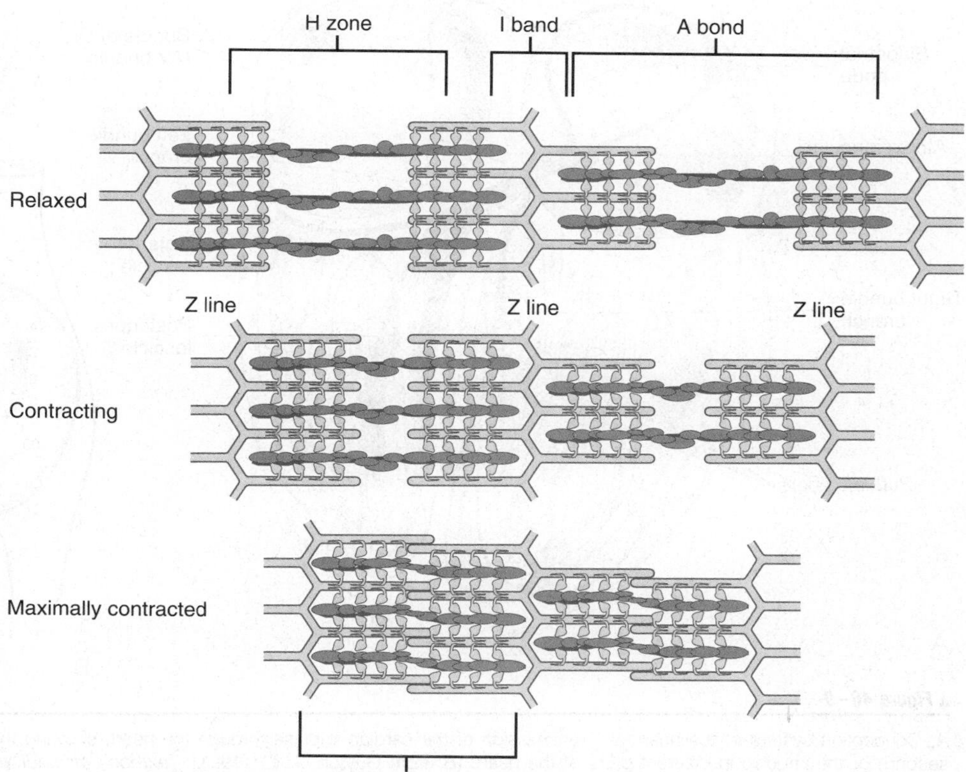

diminishes and depolarization can once again occur. During this period, known as the relative refractory period, only a stronger-than-normal stimulus can excite the heart muscle to contract. At the end of the refractory period, the sodium channels are restored and the cardiac cells can again conduct action potentials.

Normally, the ventricles have an absolute refractory period of 0.25 to 0.3 second, which approximates the duration of the action potential. The relative refractory period for the ventricles lasts about 0.05 second. The atria have a refractory period of about 0.15 second, which is much shorter than for the ventricles. This means that the atria can rhythmically contract much faster than the ventricles.[1]

Refractoriness of the myocardium normally prevents uncontrolled rapid cardiac contractions. Thus, refractoriness helps to preserve the heart rhythm.

CARDIAC CONDUCTION SYSTEM

The cardiac conduction system (Fig. 40-9) consists of modified cardiac muscle cells. These cells are characterized by their ability to conduct electrical impulses very rapidly. The conduction system acts to spread the action potential, initiated in one area of the myocardium, rapidly through the whole heart. Spread of the action potential stimulates synchronized contraction of the atria and ventricles. The conduction system consists of the following major parts.

Sinoatrial Node

The sinoatrial node (SA node) or pacemaker is located at the junction of the superior vena cava and right atrium. Under normal circumstances, the SA node initiates each heartbeat. It generates electrical impulses approximately 60 to 100 times per minute but can adjust its rate. Internodal and interatrial tracts carry the wave of depolarization through the right atrium and left atrium, respectively.[11] The sympathetic and parasympathetic nervous systems control the SA node. Any myocardial tissue in the atria, AV bundle, or ventricles has the capability of taking over the role of pacemaker if that tissue generates impulses at a higher rate than the SA node.

Atrioventricular Node

The AV node, or AV junction, is located in the lower aspect of the atrial septum. The AV node receives electrical impulses from the SA node. Within the AV node, the impulse is delayed 0.07 seconds while the atria contract. This delay enables atrial contraction to

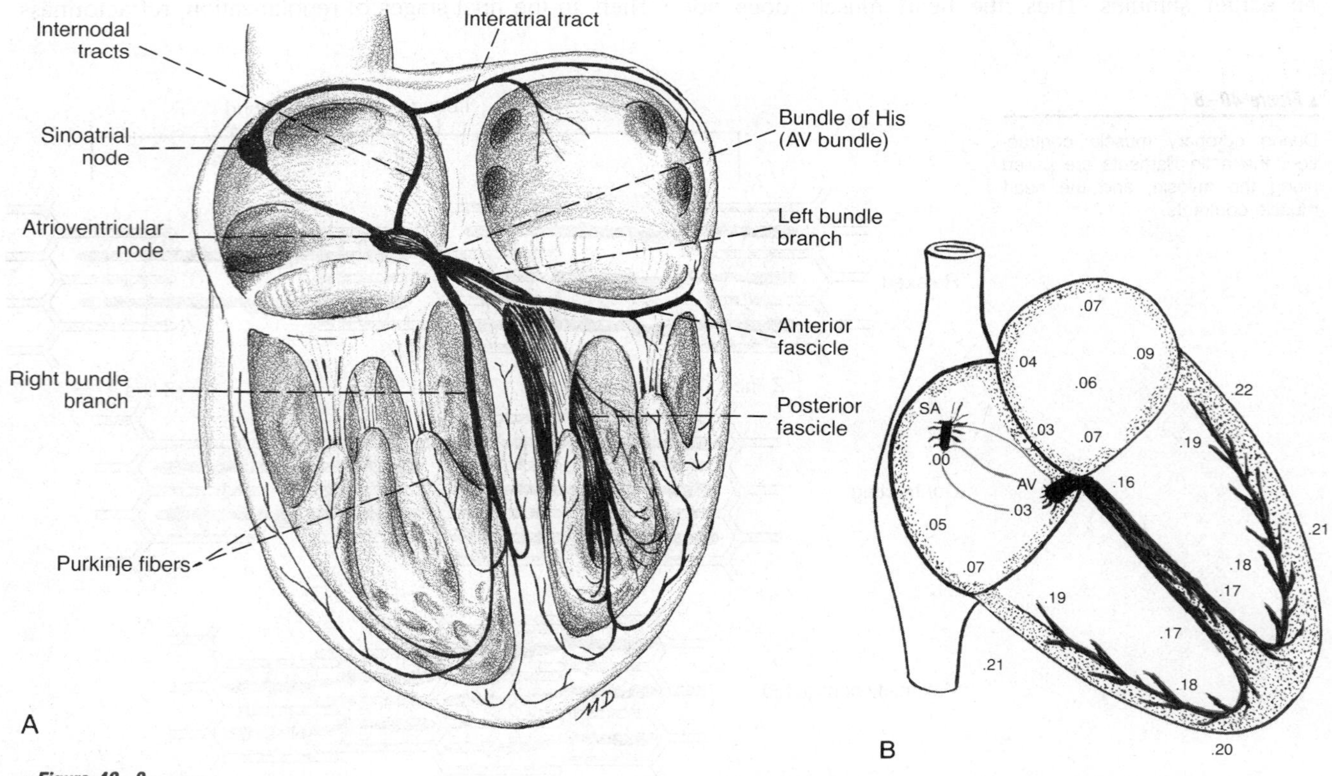

▲ **Figure 40-9**

A, Conduction system of the heart. *B*, Transmission of the cardiac impulse through the heart, showing the time of appearance (in fractions of a second) of the impulse in different parts of the heart. (*B*, from Guyton, A. C. [1991]. *Textbook of medical physiology* [8th ed.]. Philadelphia: W. B. Saunders.)

complete before the ventricles are stimulated and contract.

Bundle of His

The bundle of His (AV bundle) fuses with the AV node to form another pacemaker site. If the SA node fails, the bundle of His can initiate and sustain a heart rate of 40 to 60 beats/min. The bundle of His is relatively short, branching into right and left segments. The right bundle branch (RBB) courses down the right side of the interventricular septum. The left bundle branch (LBB) bifurcates into anterior and posterior fascicles, both of which extend into the left ventricle. The right and left bundle branches terminate in Purkinje's fibers.

Purkinje's Fibers

Purkinje's fibers are a diffuse network of conducting strands beneath the ventricular endocardium; they rapidly spread the wave of depolarization through the ventricles. Activation of the ventricles begins in the septum and then moves from the apex of the heart upward. Within the ventricular walls, depolarization proceeds from endocardium to epicardium. Repolarization is a passive event that occurs in each cell and does not involve the conduction system. Repolarization occurs in reverse order, so that the last cells to depolarize are the first ones to repolarize.

THE CARDIAC CYCLE

One cardiac cycle (Fig. 40-10) is equivalent to one complete heartbeat. The sequence of events in the cardiac cycle is divided into two parts: (1) systole (contraction) and (2) diastole (relaxation).

Ventricular Systole

In the isovolumetric contraction phase, the ventricles begin to contract, closing the AV valves and building up pressure within the ventricles. As the aortic and pulmonic valves also remain closed at this point, no blood leaves the ventricle. As the AV valves close, the first heart sound (S_1) is heard. The ejection phase begins when pressure in the ventricles exceeds the aortic and pulmonic pressures. The semilunar valves open, and the ventricles pump blood into the systemic and pulmonary circulations.

Ventricular Diastole

In early diastole, as the ventricles begin to relax, aortic and pulmonic pressures exceed ventricular pressures, and the semilunar (aortic and pulmonic) valves close. The valve closure causes the second heart sound (S_2). The AV valves remain closed, and again all four valves are closed and no blood moves in or out of the ventricles. This is called isovolumetric relaxation. As the ventricles continue to relax, the AV valves open and blood rushes into the ventricles, initiating the rapid ventricular filling phase.

Extra Heart Sounds

Because blood rapidly fills the ventricles, the ventricular wall must expand suddenly to accommodate it. If ventricular wall compliance is decreased (as in conges-

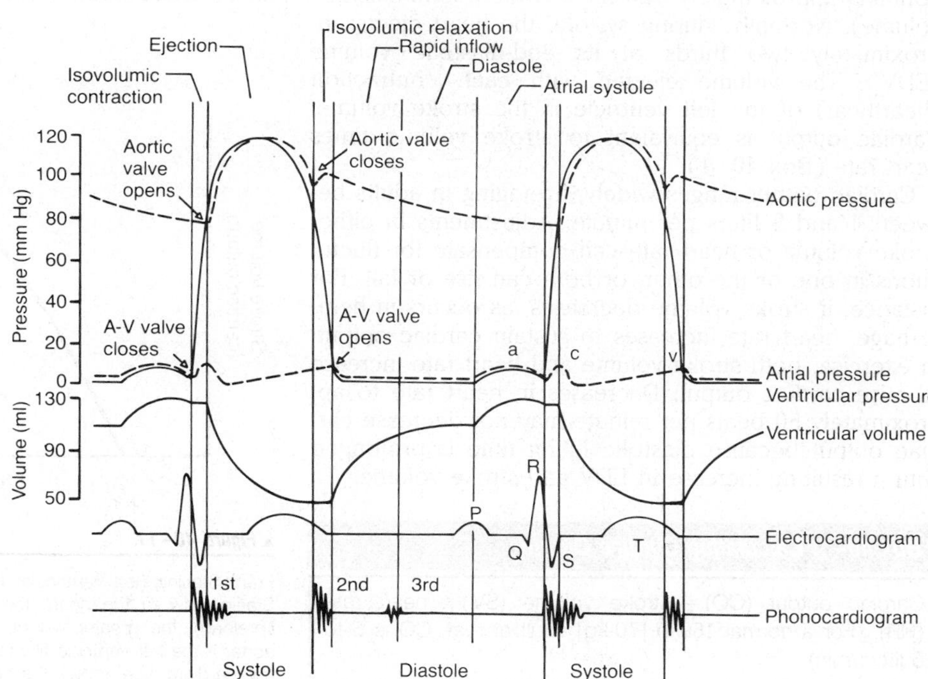

▲ *Figure 40-10*

The events of the cardiac cycle, showing changes in left atrial pressure, left ventricular pressure, aortic pressure, ventricular volume, the electrocardiogram, and the phonocardiogram. (From Guyton, A. C. [1991], *Textbook of medical physiology* [8th ed.]. Philadelphia: W. B. Saunders.)

tive heart failure or valvular regurgitation), structures within the ventricular wall vibrate and a third heart sound (S_3) may be heard. An S_3 heart sound may be a normal finding in individuals younger than 30 years of age. During the last phase of ventricular diastole, atrial contraction (atrial systole or atrial kick) occurs, contributing 20 to 30 per cent more blood volume to the ventricles. A fourth heart sound (S_4) may be heard on atrial systole if resistance to active ventricular filling is present. This is not a normal finding, and its causes include hypertrophy, disease, or injury of the ventricular wall.

MECHANICAL PROPERTIES OF THE HEART

The heart propels blood throughout the body. It can perform this task because it is able to contract. Myocardial contraction, as stated earlier, occurs in response to depolarization and the diffusion of calcium into myocardial cells, where it combines with troponin to activate contractile elements. Proper contractility depends on intact electrophysiologic stimuli and conduction and on a functional myocardium. If the heart muscle is damaged (e.g., following a myocardial infarction), contractile units fail to function properly. Hence, the strength of contraction decreases. One way to measure myocardial contractility is by the cardiac output.

Cardiac Output and Cardiac Index

Cardiac output is the volume of blood ejected by each ventricle into the pulmonic and systemic circulations per minute by rhythmic ventricular contraction. At the end of ventricular diastole (filling phase), each ventricle contains approximately 120 ml of blood (end-diastolic volume). Normally, during systole, the heart ejects approximately two thirds of its end-diastolic volume (EDV). The volume ejected with each contraction (heartbeat) of the left ventricle is the stroke volume. Cardiac output is equivalent to stroke volume times heart rate (Box 40-1).

Cardiac output ranges widely, averaging in adults between 4 and 8 liters per minute. Adjustments in either stroke volume or heart rate can compensate for fluctuations in one or the other, or both can rise or fall. For instance, if stroke volume decreases, as occurs in hemorrhage, heart rate increases to sustain cardiac output. In exercise, both stroke volume and heart rate increase to raise cardiac output. Decreases in heart rate to approximately 50 beats per minute may not decrease cardiac output because diastolic filling time is prolonged with a resulting increase in EDV and stroke volume.

Box 40-1. Calculating Cardiac Output

Cardiac output (CO) = stroke volume (SV) × heart rate (HR). (For a normal 150-lb [70-kg] adult at rest, CO is 5 to 6 liters/min)

Clinicians compute the cardiac index (CI) from the cardiac output to compensate for individual differences in body size. The cardiac index is the cardiac output divided by the body surface area. Therefore, the cardiac index describes the cardiac output in terms of liters per minute per square meter of body surface (liters/min/m^2). The cardiac index gives a better indication of how well the tissues are being perfused than does the cardiac output alone. Normal cardiac index is 2.5 to 4.0 liters/min/m^2.

Stroke Volume

Stroke volume has a major influence on cardiac output. There are several determinants that influence stroke volume; these factors include preload, afterload, and the contractile state of the heart.

PRELOAD

Preload is the myocardial fiber length of the left ventricle at end diastole. It is determined by the end-diastolic volume. The Frank-Starling law of the heart states that the greater the myocardial fiber length, or stretch, the greater will be its force of contraction. This phenomenon is similar to the increased recoil of a rubber band when subjected to greater stretching. Preload, therefore, increases when increased end-diastolic blood volume (e.g., from increased venous return) subjects myocardial fibers to greater stretch. The ventricles respond with a greater force of contraction, producing a larger stroke volume and increased cardiac output. There are, however, limits to this phenomenon. After a point, further stretching of the myocardium does not improve stroke volume and, indeed, may actually decrease it (Fig. 40-11).[4] This concept may be seen in an overstretched rubber band.

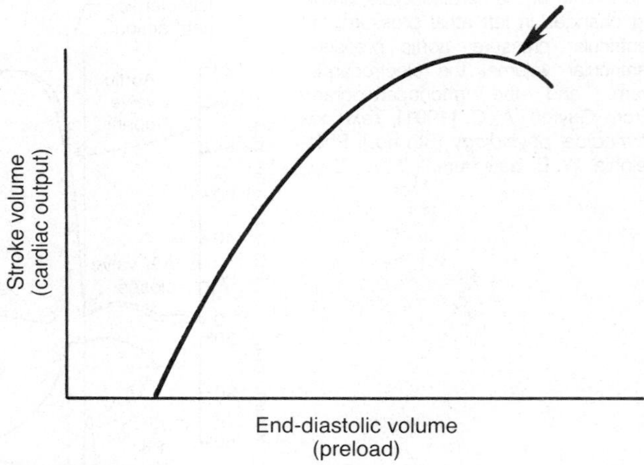

▲ Figure 40-11

Frank-Starling (left ventricular function) curve. According to the Frank-Starling law of the heart, the more the left ventricle fills with blood (preload), the greater will be the quantity of blood ejected into the aorta. If the left ventricle fills to such an extent that it overdistends the myocardium *(see arrow)*, the heart (cardiac output) will fail.

AFTERLOAD

Afterload is the resistance to left ventricular ejection. More specifically, it is the amount of tension required by the left ventricle to open the aortic valve during systole and eject blood. Afterload directly relates to arterial blood pressure, left ventricular size, and the characteristics of the valves.[7] A low degree of afterload is analogous to pumping air into a bicycle tire that is flat; the tire has low pressure inside and, thus, you need to apply little pumping force. One must push much harder to pump air into a full tire with high inner pressure. Likewise, if arterial blood pressure is high, the heart must work harder to pump blood into the circulation. The stroke volume is inversely related to afterload. For example, if afterload increases owing to peripheral vasoconstriction (thus increasing arterial blood pressure), there will be reduced shortening of the myocardial fibers. Thus, the ventricles, with less effective contractions, cannot eject a normal stroke volume.

CONTRACTILE STATE

The contractile state (or inotropic state) refers to the vigor of contraction generated by the myocardium regardless of its blood volume (preload). The ability to alter contractile force and velocity is an inherent property of the myocardium. Sympathetic stimulation increases myocardial contractility and ventricular pressure, thereby ejecting blood more rapidly, and increasing stroke volume. Metabolic abnormalities such as hypoxemia and metabolic acidosis decrease myocardial contractility, reducing stroke volume.

Cardiac Pressures

With the use of a pulmonary artery pressure catheter (Swan-Ganz), pressures inside the cardiac chambers can be measured. These pressures are useful in determining factors such as preload, afterload, volume, filling pressures, and resistance. Normal cardiac pressures are shown in Figure 40-12. The technique and nursing implications are discussed in the Bridge to Critical Care in Chapter 42.

Heart Rate

The normal heart rate is 60 to 100 beats/min. Sinus tachycardia is a rate of more than 100 beats/min; it can follow exercise or emotional upset. Sinus bradycardia is a rate of less than 60 beats/min. Variations in heartbeat are normally caused by exercise, size of the individual, age, gender, hormones, temperature, blood pressure, anxiety and stress, and pain.

Exercise causes increased need for oxygen and elimination of CO_2, which, in turn, causes increased heart rate. The conditioned athlete, however, usually has a lower heart rate at rest. The size of the individual also affects heart rate. A larger person has a slower heart rate. *Age* affects heart rate, which is fastest in the fetus (120 to 160 beats/min) and lowest in adults (65 to 80 beats/min). *Gender* affects heart rate. Women have a faster rate than men. The hormones epinephrine and thyroxine cause increased heart rate. Temperature also affects heart rate. Fever causes an increased heart rate;

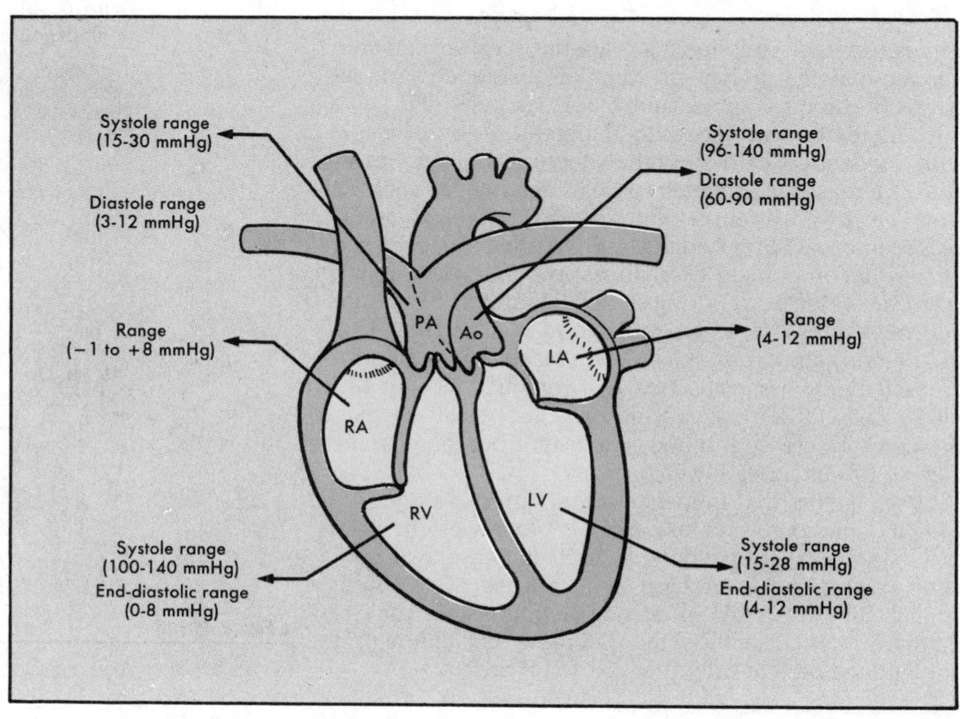

▲ **Figure 40-12**

Normal intracardiac pressures. RA, Right atrium; LA, left atrium; RV, right ventricle; LV, left ventricle; PA, pulmonary artery; Ao, aorta. (From McCance, K. L., & Huether, S. E. [1990]. *Pathophysiology: The biologic basis for disease in adults and children.* St. Louis: CV Mosby.)

hypothermia causes a decreased heart rate. Blood pressure, too, affects the heart rate. Hypotension causes increased heart rate. Finally, anxiety and stress as well as *pain* can cause increased heart rate.

Arterial Pressure

Arterial pressure is the pressure of blood against arterial walls. Types of arterial pressure include systolic pressure, diastolic pressure, pulse pressure, and mean arterial pressure. Systolic pressure is the maximum pressure of the blood exerted against the artery walls when the heart contracts. It is normally 100 to 140 mm Hg. Diastolic pressure is the force of blood exerted against the artery walls during the heart's relaxation (or filling) phase. It is normally 60 to 90 mm Hg. Blood pressure (BP) is expressed as systolic/diastolic (e.g., 120/80). Pulse pressure is the difference between systolic and diastolic pressures. It is normally 40 to 60 mm Hg and reflects stroke volume and arterial elasticity. Mean arterial pressure (MAP) is equivalent to one third of the pulse pressure (PP) plus the diastolic blood pressure (DBP):

$$\text{MAP} = \tfrac{1}{3}\,\text{PP} + \text{DBP}$$

MAP may be used in hemodynamic monitoring.

The two determinants of BP are cardiac output (CO) and peripheral vascular resistance (PVR), and can be shown through the formula

$$\text{BP} = \text{CO} \times \text{PVR}$$

Circulatory factors influencing arterial pressure include: cardiac output, peripheral vascular resistance, arterial elasticity, blood volume, and blood viscosity (Fig. 40–13). Increased cardiac output increases arterial pressure. Decreased cardiac output decreases arterial pressure. Increased peripheral vascular resistance, such as from narrowed arterioles, increases BP. Dilated arterioles decrease BP. Arterial elasticity affects BP. Elastic vessels accommodate to changes in blood flow. Rigid, sclerotic vessels cause increases in systolic pressure and pulse pressure. Decreased blood volume (e.g., due to hemorrhage) results in decreased pressure. Increased blood viscosity, due to overabundance of red blood cells (RBCs) or plasma proteins, results in high pressure. Decreased blood viscosity from anemia or lack of RBCs causes lower pressure.

Other factors that influence arterial pressure are age, weight, emotions, and exercise. BP is lowest in neonates and highest in older adults. It increases with excess weight, and it increases with release of catecholamines in response to strong emotions or stress. Extreme physical activity may increase BP, although a conditioned athlete often has a low BP at rest.

Venous Pressure

Venous pressure is the pressure exerted by blood in the veins. In small veins and venules, there are no pulsations; venous pressure is about 12 to 15 mm Hg. In large veins leading to the heart (e.g., jugular veins), pulsations reflect back from right atrial contractions. Blood flows back to the heart via the venous system with assistance from (1) vessel wall tone, (2) the pumping action of skeletal muscles, and (3) the negative thoracic pressure during inspiration.

Capillary Pressure

Capillary (hydrostatic) pressure is the pressure exerted by the blood against the capillary wall. It is 25 to 30 mm Hg at the arterial end of the capillaries and 10 to 15 mm Hg at the venous end. Capillary pressure and

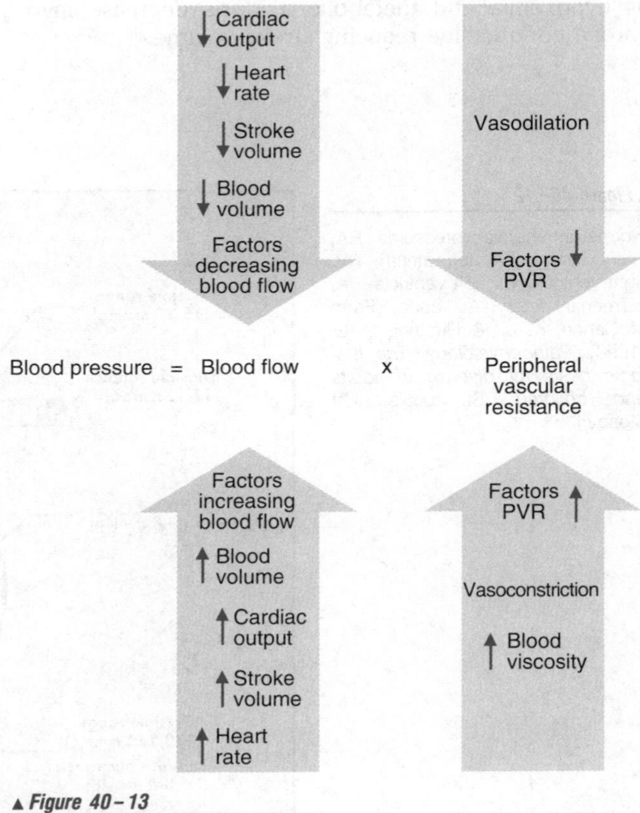

▲ **Figure 40–13**

Factors affecting blood pressure.

its relationship to plasma oncotic pressure contribute to the balance of interstitial fluid. Capillary BP and filtration are discussed in Chapter 44.

A high capillary pressure causes capillary filtration to increase and fluid to shift from the vascular system into the interstitium (edema). Low capillary pressure causes capillary filtration to decrease and draws fluid from the tissues into the circulatory system, which may raise BP.

REGULATION OF CARDIAC FUNCTION AND BLOOD PRESSURE

The ability of the circulatory system to adapt to internal and external changes depends on the proper function and integration of several factors. Among the most important regulatory mechanisms are the autonomic nervous system; peripheral baroreceptors, stretch receptors, and chemoreceptors; and several hormones.

Autonomic Nervous System

The autonomic nervous system (ANS) plays an important role in regulating

- Heart rate (chronotropic effect),
- Myocardial contractility (inotropic effect),
- Conduction velocity, and
- Peripheral vascular resistance (arterial and venous constriction and dilation).

The two subdivisions of the ANS are the sympathetic and parasympathetic nervous systems. These systems, with opposing influences, balance their activities to promote cardiovascular adaptation to internal and external demands. ANS responses are involuntary. These responses occur without thinking about them.

Parasympathetic nerves arise from the dorsal motor nucleus of the vagus nerve, located in the medulla oblongata. They innervate the atria, ventricles, and conduction system. When stimulated, parasympathetic nerve endings release the neurotransmitter acetylcholine, which produces inhibitory effects opposite to those of norepinephrine. Parasympathetic stimulation decreases the rate of SA node firing, thus lowering heart rate. Atrial and ventricular contractility and conductivity lessen as well.

Sympathetic nerve fibers originate between the first thoracic and second lumbar vertebrae and terminate in all areas of the heart. With stimulation, the nerve endings release the neurotransmitter norepinephrine, producing the following acceleratory effects on the heart: (1) increased heart rate, (2) increased conduction speed through the AV node, (3) increased atrial and ventricular contractility, and (4) peripheral vasoconstriction.

The sympathetic nervous system influences adrenal activity. The adrenal medulla responds to stimulation by secreting catecholamines (norepinephrine and epinephrine) into the circulation. Norepinephrine and epinephrine exert their influences by interacting with adrenergic receptors found within cell membranes of the heart and blood vessels. The response to stimulation depends on the type and location of adrenergic receptors involved. There are three types of receptors: (1) alpha-1, (2) alpha-2, (3) beta-1, and (4) beta-2.

Alpha (α)-adrenergic receptors are located in peripheral arteries and veins. When stimulated, alpha receptors produce a dramatic vasoconstrictive response.

Beta-1 (β_1)-adrenergic receptors are predominantly located in the heart. When stimulated, beta-1 receptors cause an increase in heart rate, AV node conduction, and myocardial contractility. This may result in increased cardiac output and BP.

Beta-2 (β_2)-adrenergic receptors are found in the arterial and bronchial walls. Stimulation of beta-2 receptors causes smooth muscles to dilate, producing vasodilation of arterial vessels and bronchodilation.

In general, epinephrine influences alpha-2 and beta-2 receptors, whereas norepinephrine predominantly affects alpha-1 and beta-1 receptors.

Baroreceptors, Stretch Receptors, and Chemoreceptors

Changes in sympathetic and parasympathetic activity occur in response to messages sent from sensory receptors involved in various parts of the body. Important receptors involved in cardiovascular reflexes include the baroreceptors, the stretch receptors, and the chemoreceptors.

Baroreceptors (also called pressoreceptors) are specialized nerve endings affected by changes in arterial blood pressure. They are located in the walls of the aortic arch and carotid sinuses. Increases in arterial pressure stimulate baroreceptors, which send impulses to the medulla oblongata. As a result, heart rate and arterial pressure decrease (also called the vagal response). When arterial pressure decreases, baroreceptors receive less stimulation and thus send fewer impulses to the medulla oblongata. Then, sympathetic-mediated vasoconstriction occurs and heart rate increases.

Stretch receptors are located in terminal sections of the vena cava and the right atrium. These receptors respond to pressure changes, which reflect circulatory volume status. When BP decreases in the vena cava and the right atrium (e.g., hypovolemia), stretch receptors send fewer impulses than usual to the central nervous system (CNS). This process results in a sympathetic response causing increased heart rate and blood vessel constriction. Hypervolemia produces opposite effects.

Chemoreceptors, found in the aortic arch and carotid bodies, are primarily sensitive to hypoxemia and secondarily to increased CO_2 and decreased arterial pH (acidemia). These changes stimulate chemoreceptors that transmit impulses to the CNS.

Hormonal Influences

In addition to epinephrine and norepinephrine from the adrenal medulla, several other hormones regulate cardiovascular activity. The most important hormones include antidiuretic hormone (ADH) and the renin-angiotensin-aldosterone mechanism.

Several studies have shown that increases in central venous volume (such as those that occur with hypervolemia) result in decreased ADH release from the posterior pituitary gland.[2, 4] Inhibition of ADH secretion, in turn, increases diuresis, decreasing blood volume. Hence ADH influences BP indirectly by regulating vascular volume.

Renin is an enzyme that is synthesized, stored, and released from the kidney. It is secreted in response to a decrease in renal blood flow and to sympathetic stimulation. The major function of renin is the conversion of angiotensinogen to angiotensin I. Angiotensin I is then converted to angiotensin II in the lungs. This last substance, a potent vasoconstrictor, causes BP to increase. Angiotensin II also stimulates the release of aldosterone, which promotes water and sodium retention by the kidneys. Blood volume and BP increase as a result.

Other hormonal regulators of blood pressure include histamine, which is a potent vasodilator of small blood vessels, although it may also constrict the large arteries. Bradykinin, which is one of a group of vasoactive peptides and is a powerful vasodilator, especially of cutaneous vessels. Muscle metabolites (lactic acid), which have a strong vasodilator action. Serotonin, which is liberated from platelets that stick to the vessel wall in the injured area. Although a powerful constrictor of cutaneous arterioles, it dilates capillaries.

Other factors also influence cardiac activity and blood pressure. For example, cerebral cortical input from anger, fear, pain, or excitement can augment the effects of the sympathetic nervous system. Increased activity and exercise cause an increased need for oxygen and the elimination of metabolic wastes, which, in turn, cause an increased heart rate and force of contraction. The conditioned athlete, however, usually has a lower heart rate. Body temperature can also affect heart activity. Fever increases the metabolic needs of the body, thereby necessitating an increase in heart rate to increase blood flow to the tissues. The opposite is true in hypothermia, when metabolic needs of tissues decline. Other factors influencing cardiac activity and BP include serum electrolyte levels and medications.

EFFECTS OF NORMAL AGING ON THE CARDIOVASCULAR SYSTEM

Persons over 65 years of age show changes in their cardiovascular system. These changes include the development of disease processes such as coronary artery disease as well as the physiologic aspects of aging.

The older adult loses elasticity of the aorta, which leads to aortic dilation. Coronary arteries become rigid and thickened. This condition increases the likelihood of coronary artery disease and hypertension.

The heart muscle also undergoes changes with aging that lead to dilation of the cardiac chambers and less contractility. The conduction system loses pacemaker cells and, thus, conduction abnormalities can arise. Heart valves thicken and become calcified causing a systolic ejection murmur.

Cardiovascular diseases common to the elderly include coronary artery disease, hypertension, valvular disease, dysrhythmias, and syncope.

Summary

Although the heart can be viewed as simply a pump, this remarkable, durable organ is much more than just a pump. The heart is a continuously beating organ that never rests. It moves blood throughout the body to oxygenate cells for energy, thinking, digestion, and movement. Blood is propelled through the four chambers of the heart in one direction, from right to left. It is then delivered to the body through a system of arteries. In the capillaries, nutrients are exchanged for waste, and the deoxygenated blood returns through the veins to the right side of the heart. Heart disease remains the major cause of death and is due to disorders of structure or function of the heart. These disorders are studied in the following chapters.

Bibliography

1. Abrams, J. (1987). *Essentials of cardiac physical diagnosis.* Philadelphia: Lea & Febiger.
2. Ahrens, T., & Taylor, L. (1992). *Hemodynamic waveform analysis.* Philadelphia, W. B. Saunders.
3. Berne, R. M., & Levy, M. N. (1988). *Physiology.* St. Louis: C.V. Mosby.
4. Braunwald, E., et al. (1991). Normal and abnormal circulatory function. In E. Braunwald (Ed.), *Heart disease.* Philadelphia: W. B. Saunders.
5. Guyton, A. C. (1991). *Medical physiology* (8th ed.). Philadelphia: W. B. Saunders.
6. Hollenberg, N. K., & Hollenberg, I. B. (1989). *The heart facts.* Glenview, Illinois: Scott, Foresman Co.
7. Hurst, J. W. (1990). *The heart.* New York: McGraw-Hill.
8. Hurst, J. W., et al. (1988). *Atlas of the heart.* New York: McGraw-Hill.
9. Jarvis, C. (1992). *Physical examination and health assessment.* Philadelphia, W. B. Saunders.
10. McCance, K. L., & Richardson, S. J. (1990). Structure and function of the cardiovascular and lymphatic systems. In K. L. McCance & S. E. Huether (Eds.), *Pathophysiology.* St. Louis: C. V. Mosby.
11. Sanderson, R. C., & Kurth, C. L. (1983). *The cardiac patient: A comprehensive approach* (2nd ed.). Philadelphia: W. B. Saunders.
12. Solomon, E. P., Schmidt, R. R., & Adragna, P. J. (1990). *Human anatomy and physiology* (2nd ed.). Philadelphia, Saunders College.

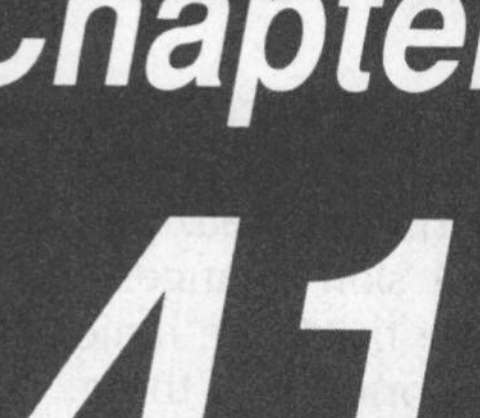

Chapter 41

Assessment of Clients with Cardiovascular Disorders

Cardiovascular disease remains the most common cause of death in the United States. Because of the high incidence of heart disease and the seriousness of its complications, nurses must know how to assess the cardiovascular system. Assessment of the cardiovascular system incorporates data obtained from history taking, physical examination, and diagnostic studies. From these data, nursing and medical diagnoses are derived and the approach to client management is formulated.

ASSESSMENT OF THE HEART

HISTORY

Assessment is a dynamic process. It begins with the initial visit with the client and continues throughout the course of intervention. A health history includes information about the following three areas: the client's chief complaint, current health status, and past medical history.

Chief Complaint

The nurse inquires about the client's chief complaint(s) to establish priorities for intervention and also to evaluate how well the client understands the presenting condition.

Common clinical manifestations of cardiovascular disorders include shortness of breath, chest pain or discomfort, dyspnea, palpitations, fainting, fatigue, and peripheral skin changes, such as edema. A client may have more than one major symptom. When this occurs, the nurse prioritizes them.

A symptom analysis is performed on the chief complaint, using the following questions:

- How long has the symptom been experienced?
- How much does the symptom bother the client?
- Does any particular type of incident or episode trigger the symptom?
- What activities or interventions alleviate the symptom?
- What is the perceived cause of the symptom (heart attack, heartburn, indigestion)?
- What impact does the symptom have on the client's lifestyle?

CHEST PAIN

Pain in the chest is a common symptom, occurring in such cardiac disorders as angina, myocardial ischemia, myocardial infarction, and pericarditis. Chest pain may also be present in pulmonary diseases such as pleurisy, pneumonia, and pulmonary embolism. Cardiac pain most often results from myocardial ischemia, i.e., lack of blood supply to the myocardial tissues. Because chest pain is caused by a number of different conditions, it is highly variable in nature. To evaluate chest pain and its causation, the nurse obtains sufficient descriptive data about the pain in the following areas.

Characteristics. Chest pain may be described as a "strange feeling," indigestion, dull heavy pressure, burning, crushing, constricting, aching, stabbing, or tightness.

Location. Chest pain occurs in the substernal or precordial areas. It may be diffuse or localized. The pain may also radiate to the jaw, teeth, neck, one or both shoulders, arms, elbows, or the back. If the pain radiates down the arm, it may cause a sensation of numbness or tingling. Sometimes the client feels only the radiated pain and no precordial (in the chest) pain.

Duration. The nurse notes the time pain begins and ends to determine the duration of discomfort. Several intermittent small episodes of chest pain are not considered as one long period of pain. Generally, the pain of myocardial infarction lasts longer than one half hour, or until intervention is instituted. Conversely, anginal pain typically lasts less than 20 to 30 minutes.

Severity. To assist the client in better quantifying the chest pain, the nurse may use a scale of 1 (least severe) to 10 (most severe). This recorded scale can then be used to compare future episodes of chest pain. For example, the client may report 10/10 pain on admission and then report 3/10 pain the following day.

Precipitating or Aggravating Factors. The pain may sometimes be associated with certain factors or conditions. Such factors as emotional excitement, temperature extremes, exertion, deep sleep, position changes, deep breathing, straining during bowel movements, and eating may trigger the onset of chest pain.

Associated Symptoms. The nurse asks the client whether other symptoms accompany the onset of chest pain, i.e., anxiousness, shortness of breath, nausea, diaphoresis, vertigo, or palpitations.

Alleviating Factors. Anginal pain may be relieved by resting, sublingual nitroglycerin, oxygen, and a change in position. Pain that is not relieved with these interventions and lasts 20 minutes or longer highly suggests myocardial infarction.

Table 41–1 compares selected cardiac, pulmonary, gastrointestinal, musculoskeletal, neurologic, and anxiety-related conditions in relation to the assessment of chest pain.

SHORTNESS OF BREATH

Labored breathing, or shortness of breath, is termed dyspnea. Like chest pain, this common symptom affects clients with cardiac and pulmonary disorders. Dyspnea also may occur in clients experiencing anxiety, depression, and various psychosomatic conditions.

Although dyspnea can develop in any form of heart disease, it usually occurs in conjunction with cardiac enlargement and other pathologic cardiovascular structural and physiologic changes. Dyspnea develops when the left ventricle fails and the lungs become congested and edematous.

There are several forms of dyspnea: exertional dyspnea, orthopnea, and paroxysmal nocturnal dyspnea.

Exertional Dyspnea. This is the most common form of cardiac-related dyspnea. Exertional dyspnea occurs during mild to moderate exercise or activity and disappears with rest. If severe, exertional dyspnea can greatly limit activity tolerance. The nurse asks the client to describe the degree of activity that typically precipitates the onset of dyspnea, e.g., walking up one flight of stairs, or walking to the mailbox. Noncardiac conditions such as obesity, poor physical conditioning, anemia, asthma, and obstructions of the nasal passages may also lead to dyspnea with mild exercise. This form of dyspnea is abbreviated DOE (dyspnea on exertion).

Orthopnea. Orthopnea is difficult breathing that occurs when the client is resting flat in bed and is relieved when the client assumes an upright or semivertical position. The nurse asks clients what actions they take to facilitate breathing: Do they sit up in a chair or dangle their feet at the bedside? What position do they sleep in? The nurse records the degree of head elevation the client requires to breathe. Orthopnea usually indicates a more serious compromise of the cardiovascular system than does exertional dyspnea.

Paroxysmal Nocturnal Dyspnea. This is a form of difficult breathing that occurs in terrifying "attacks" during the night, waking the individual from sleep. Paroxysmal noctural dyspnea is associated with severe left ventricular failure.

FATIGUE

Easy fatigability on mild exertion is a frequent problem for clients experiencing cardiac disease. Progressive deterioration in activity tolerance results from the heart's inability to pump an effective volume of blood to meet the varying metabolic demands of the body.

PALPITATIONS

The term palpitation is derived from the Latin word *palpitare*, meaning "to throb." Palpitation is a common symptom in heart disease. It is a sensation of rapid heartbeats, skipping, irregularity, thumping, or pounding, and may be accompanied by anxiousness. Tachycardia (rapid heart rates), increased force of myocardial contraction (as can occur with ingestion of caffeine or with emotional or physical stress), or premature ventricular beats may cause palpitations. The onset and termination of palpitations are often abrupt.

SYNCOPE

Syncope, or fainting, is a momentary loss of consciousness resulting from a reduction in cerebral blood flow. Certain cardiac disorders, especially cardiac dysrhythmias (irregular heart rhythm), can precipitate a sudden decrease in cardiac output. Valvular disorders may also cause an adverse change in circulatory hemodynamics and cause syncope or vertigo. Clients who are prone to syncopal episodes (e.g., those with Stokes-Adams syndrome) should wear medic-alert bracelets to inform emergency health care providers.

WEIGHT GAIN

Due to fluid accumulation, an expanded blood volume may result when the heart fails. An increase in body weight of 3 pounds or more within 24 hours results from fluid rather than body mass changes. The nurse asks the client about trends in weight changes. Body weight is a sensitive indicator of water and sodium retention and will increase even before edema occurs. Methods to ensure accurate measurement of weight are discussed in fundamentals textbooks.

Past Medical History

The past medical history explores the health history of both the client and family members. Information acquired here reveals the lifelong health record of the client, past experiences within the health care system, attitudes regarding health, and nonmodifiable and modifiable risk factors that may have contributed to the development of cardiovascular symptoms. The client is asked questions about the following areas.

CHILDHOOD AND INFECTIOUS DISEASES

In addition to the usual data regarding common childhood diseases and immunizations, the nurse asks about the client's experiences with rheumatic fever and severe streptococcal infections. These two conditions are associated with structural heart diseases. The presence of known congenital anomalies is also ascertained.

MAJOR ILLNESSES AND HOSPITALIZATIONS

The history or presence of any major illness is determined. Particular attention is paid to those conditions that have the greatest influence on the client's current cardiovascular performance, i.e., diabetes mellitus, chronic obstructive lung disease, kidney disease, anemia, hypertension, stroke, gout, thrombophlebitis, collagen diseases, and bleeding disorders. Previous hospitalizations, pregnancies, or outpatient intervention are also of interest. The nurse inquires about previously performed cardiovascular diagnostic studies, such as an electrocardiogram (ECG) or an exercise stress test. Results of such studies provide baseline data for comparative analysis when later studies are performed.

MEDICATIONS

Prescription as well as over-the-counter and recreational drug use is evaluated. Whenever possible, brand names or simple descriptors should be used instead of generic names. For example, the nurse asks if the client is currently taking "water-pills," "heart pills," or "blood pressure" medications. Numerous medications can affect the overall performance of the cardiovascular system. The nurse asks specifically about the use of the following agents: antihypertensives, diuretics, vasodilators (nitroglycerin), cardiotonic drugs (digoxin), anticoagulants, bronchodilators, contraceptives, and steroids. Noncardiac medications can also have profound secondary effects on cardiovascular performance. For example, tricyclic antidepressants and other psychotropic medications can potentiate dysrhythmias. Oral contraceptives increase the incidence of thrombophlebitis. Steroid use may cause hypertension and increases fluid retention. Various antineoplastic agents may be cardiotoxic, causing dysrhythmias and cardiomyopathy.

The nurse discusses the use of recreational drugs with the client. Cocaine toxicity is a major threat to the cardiovascular system. Its systemic sympathomimetic effects result in a "fight or flight" response that increases heart rate, contractility, blood glucose levels, and peripheral vasoconstriction. Cocaine also potentiates the effects of the circulating catecholamines (epinephrine and norepinephrine).

Finally, the use of over-the-counter drugs like aspirin and cold remedies is discussed. While investigating use of these drugs, the nurse notes the dose and times of administration.

TABLE 41–1. Assessment of Chest Pain

Condition	Location	Quality	Severity	Course	Aggravating or Relieving Factors	Symptoms or Signs
Angina	Retrosternal region; radiates to neck, jaw, epigastrium, shoulders, arms—left common	Pressure, burning, squeezing, heaviness, indigestion	Moderate to severe	<10 minutes	Aggravated by exercise, cold weather, emotional stress, or after meals; relieved by rest or nitroglycerin; atypical (Prinzmetal's) angina may be unrelated to activity and caused by coronary artery	S_4, paradoxical split S_2 during pain
Intermediate syndrome or coronary insufficiency	Same as angina	Same as angina	Increasingly severe	>10 minutes	Same as angina, with gradually decreasing tolerance for exertion	Same as angina
Myocardial infarction	Substernal; may radiate like angina	Heaviness, pressure, burning, constriction	Severe, sometimes mild (in 25% of patients)	Sudden onset; lasting longer than 15 minutes	Unrelieved	Shortness of breath, sweating, weakness, nausea, vomiting, severe anxiety
Pericarditis	Usually begins over sternum and may radiate to neck and down left upper extremity	Sharp, stabbing knifelike	Moderate to severe	Lasts many hours to days	Aggravated by deep breathing, rotating chest or supine position; relieved by sitting up and leaning forward	Pericardial friction rub, syncope, cardiac tamponade, pulsus paradoxus (Kussmaul's sign)
Dissecting aortic aneurysm	Anterior chest; radiates to thoracic area of back; may be abdominal; pain shifts in chest	Tearing	Excruciating, tearing, knifelike	Sudden onset, lasts for hours	Unrelated to anything	Lower blood pressure in one arm, absent pulses, paralysis, murmur of aortic insufficiency, pulsus paradoxus, stridor; myocardial infarction can occur
Mitral valve prolapse syndrome	Substernal; sometimes radiates to the left arm, back, jaw	Stabbing, sharp	Variable; generally mild but can become severe	Episodes are paroxysmal, may be prolonged	Not related to exertion, not relieved by nitroglycerin or rest	Variable palpitations dizziness, syncope, dyspnea
Pulmonary embolism (most pulmonary emboli do not produce chest pain)	Substernal "anginal"	Not pleuritic unless infarction exists	Can be severe	Sudden onset; lasts minutes to <hour	May be aggravated by breathing	Fever, tachypnea, tachycardia, hypotension, elevated jugular venous pressure, right ventricular lift, accentuated P_2, occasional murmur of tricuspid insufficiency and right ventricular S_4; with in-

						farction usually in the presence of congestive heart failure, rales, pleural rub, hemoptysis, clinical phlebitis present in minority of cases
Pulmonary hypertension	Substernal	Pressure; oppressive	Variable		Aggravated by effort	Pain usually associated with dyspnea; right ventricular lift, accentuated P_2
Spontaneous pneumothorax	Unilateral	Sharp, well localized		Sudden onset; lasts many hours	Painful breathing	Dyspnea, hyperresonance, and decreased breath and voice sounds over involved lung
Pneumonia with pleurisy	Localized over area of consolidation	Pleuritic, well localized	Moderate		Painful breathing	Dyspnea, cough, fever, dull to flat percussion, bronchial breathing, rales, occasional pleural rub
Gastrointestinal disorders	Lower substernal area, epigastric, right or left upper quadrant	Burning, colic-like aching			Precipitated by recumbency or meals	Nausea, regurgitation, food intolerance, melena, hematemesis, jaundice
Musculoskeletal disorders	Variable	Aching		Short or long duration Prolonged period of time	Aggravated by movement, history of muscle exertion	Tender to pressure or movement Rash appears in area of discomfort with herpes
Neurologic disorders (herpes zoster)	Dermatomal in distribution			Unassociated with external events		
Anxiety states	Usually localized to a point	Sharp burning; commonly location of pain moves from place to place	Mild to moderate	Varies; usually very brief	Situational anger	Sighing respirations, often chest wall tenderness

Note. P_2, pulmonic second sound.
From Andreoli, K., et al. (1987). *Comprehensive cardiac care* (6th ed., pp. 54–55). St. Louis: C. V. Mosby.

PSYCHOSOCIAL HISTORY AND LIFESTYLE

Information in this area provides abundant data about risk factors for the development of cardiovascular disease. From this background information, the nurse formulates a plan to assist the client in making necessary lifestyle adaptations to promote health and lessen disease.

The client's age, sex, race, and family history are nonmodifiable risk factors. These factors are discussed in Chapter 42 as risk factors for coronary artery disease. Nevertheless, the relationship of these risk factors to cardiovascular disease is sensitively discussed when the client asks, "Why did my heart condition happen?" Information about marital status, household members, children, living environment, employment, spiritual orientation, and hobbies helps in the identification of support systems and coping mechanisms.

Include information about the following modifiable risk factors in history taking.

Stress. Research indicates a strong correlation between stress response and the manifestations of various cardiac disorders. Common stressors include change in job, residence, health, or marital status. Chapter 3 discusses stress response in detail.

Personality Type. Much has been written about the relationship between personality traits and the development of coronary artery disease. Researchers have identified a positive correlation between the two, although precise proof has remained elusive. Clients identified as having a "type A personality" are thought to be more vulnerable to the development of coronary artery disease. These clients are described as being highly competitive, rapid of speech and action, impatient, and high achievers.

Exercise. The client is asked about the type and amount of exercise routinely engaged in during an average week before and after the onset of current symptoms. Several studies suggest that effective, routine aerobic exercise may decrease the likelihood of a coronary event. Research confirms that a sedentary lifestyle potentiates the lethality of a myocardial infarction, and it is considered a significant risk factor in the development of coronary artery disease. To be effective, aerobic exercise should raise the heart rate from 50 to 100 per cent of baseline (depending on age and prior physical conditioning) for at least 20 to 30 minutes. Such exercise must be performed at least three times a week to be beneficial. The prevailing thought is that aerobic exercise, along with general body conditioning, makes the heart more efficient in its use of oxygen. Examples of aerobic exercises include swimming, jogging, brisk walking, bicycling, and rowing.

Diet. A dietary history assesses excess or deficit caloric intake and the approximate intake of foods high in sodium, cholesterol, saturated fat content, and caffeine. Although these are elements common to the average American diet, they have been linked to the development of atherosclerosis and hypertensive disease. The nurse examines not only the individual's daily food habits, but also the his or her attitudes toward food and resistance toward therapeutic alterations in diet. Cultural beliefs and economic status can greatly affect the choice of foods. Therefore, clinicians must consider these factors before prescribing changes in diet. In addition, the primary food purchaser and preparer are identified for inclusion in dietary instruction.

Habits. If the client smokes, the nurse inquires about the duration of this smoking habit and the number of cigarettes smoked daily. Cigarette smoking increases the risk of coronary artery disease and worsens hypertension. Nicotine, a major ingredient in cigarettes, probably causes peripheral vasoconstriction, increasing resistance to left ventricular emptying and thus increasing myocardial workload. Smoking increases the mortality rate of middle-aged clients with diagnosed coronary artery disease and greatly potentiates the development of peripheral vascular disease.

There is no conclusive evidence to show that caffeine and alcohol intake increase the risk of developing atherosclerosis. Nevertheless, caffeine is a stimulant that, in excessive amounts, can increase heart rate and blood pressure (BP), both of which can raise the myocardial work load and precipitate angina pectoris, heart failure, and some dysrhythmias. Therefore, the nurse assesses the intake of caffeine and cautions those with known heart disease to limit the use of caffeine to the equivalent of two 8-oz. cups of coffee per day.

Researchers state that only excessive alcohol intake has deleterious effects on the cardiovascular system and its performance. An intake of 100 g of pure (100 per cent) alcohol may slightly increase BP and heart rate. This amount is approximately equal to three beers or one mixed drink. Alcoholism, in contrast, has been associated with the development of hypertension and damage to the heart muscle, leading to congestive cardiomyopathy. The nurse asks the client to approximate daily and weekly alcohol consumption, bearing in mind that the client may minimize the estimated consumption if addicted to alcohol.

Review of Systems

The client is asked about past problems involving the cardiovascular system, including paroxysmal nocturnal dyspnea, chest pain, palpitations, shortness of breath, fatigue, edema, orthopnea, wheezing, fainting (syncope), weight gain, heart murmurs, hypertension, and history of rheumatic fever.

Cardiovascular problems also affect the pulmonary, renal, and neurologic systems. The nurse asks about productive cough, decreased urination, dark or concentrated urine, edema of the legs, dizzy spells, and memory loss.

Detailed questions for the review of symptoms are found in Chapter 11, Table 11–4.

PHYSICAL EXAMINATION

Nurses, especially those who care for the critically ill or who are family nurse practitioners, should be able to perform a basic cardiovascular examination. Assessment of the client's cardiovascular status must be ongoing, because the underlying condition can change dramatically within minutes. A physical examination involves obtaining objective data via observation, palpation, and auscultation. Percussion is rarely performed to assess cardiovascular status.

The order of the examination proceeds in logical fashion from head to foot. It is often performed routinely along with vital signs.

General Appearance

Much may be learned through simple observation. Before beginning the examination, the nurse looks at the client and considers:

- Does the client lie quietly in bed or is he or she restless and moving about continuously?
- What is the client's posture? Can he or she lie flat in bed or tolerate only an upright and erect position?
- What is the facial expression? Are there grimaces of pain or obvious signs of respiratory distress?
- Are there signs of significant cyanosis or pallor?
- Can the client answer questions without dyspnea during the interview?

Level of Consciousness

The client's general level of consciousness is noted. This important assessment reflects the adequacy of cerebral perfusion and oxygenation. The nurse also assesses whether the client is manifesting appropriate behavior based on the surroundings:

- What is the client's affect?
- Are there obvious signs of anxiety, fear, depression, or anger?
- How does the client react to those in the immediate vicinity, including significant others?

Assessment of general appearance and level of consciousness provides an initial composite picture of the client and indicates the level of comfort and distress.

Blood Pressure

The nurse measures the BP of both arms during the initial examination to rule out dissecting aortic aneurysm, coarctation of the aorta, vascular obstruction, vascular outlet syndromes, and errors in measurement. If the client's arms are inaccessible, pressures are obtained using the thighs and popliteal artery or the calves and posterior tibial artery. If pressures are difficult to auscultate, systolic pressures can be determined through palpation or by using a Doppler.

When recording BP measurements, the nurse notes both systolic and diastolic pressures, e.g., 120/70. However, the muffling of Korotkoff's sounds may also be included and recorded as 120/80/70. The American Heart Association recommends recording the point at which the sound disappears (fifth Korotkoff's sound) as the diastolic pressure in adults. The nurse records in which arm the BP measurement was taken and the position of the client at the time of the BP reading.

POSTURAL BLOOD PRESSURE

A postural BP reading is taken when an extracellular volume depletion or decreased vascular tone is suspected. BP is recorded in relation to the client's position (Fig. 41 – 1).

PARADOXICAL BLOOD PRESSURE (PULSUS PARADOXUS)

Paradoxical BP is frequently found in clients with pericardial tamponade constrictive pericarditis and pulmonary hypertension. It is an abnormal fall in systolic BP of greater than 10 mm Hg during inspiration. To check for a paradoxical pulse, the nurse places a sphygmomanometer on the client's arm and a stethoscope over the brachial artery and instructs the client to breathe normally. The cuff is inflated 20 mm Hg above the systolic BP. The nurse slowly deflates the cuff (1 to 2 mm Hg/sec) and listens for Korotkoff's sounds to appear only during expiration. (Sounds are first heard during expiration and then during inspiration.) The cuff is then deflated until Korotkoff's sounds are heard equally well during inspiration and expiration. The degree of paradoxical BP is the difference between the level of BP when sounds are first heard during expiration and the level of BP when sounds are heard on both expiration and inspiration. Normally, this difference is less than 10 mm Hg. If the client has normal breathing and a systolic difference of greater than

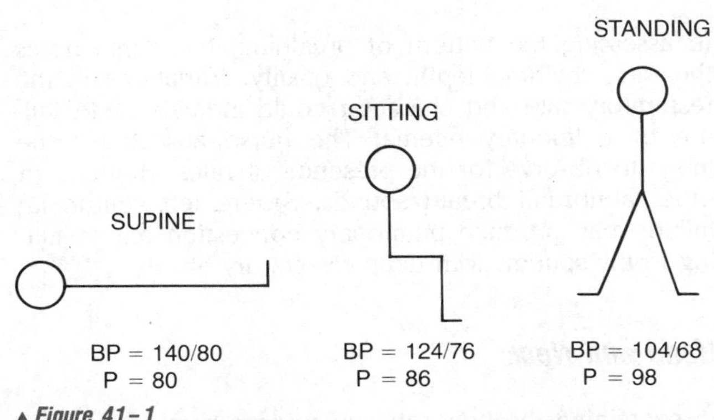

▲ **Figure 41 – 1**

Recording postural blood pressure (BP). After measuring person's BP and pulse in the supine position, leave the BP cuff in place and assist the client to sit. Then measure the BP within 15 to 30 seconds. Assist the client to stand, and measure again. A BP drop of more than 10 to 15 mm Hg systolic and more than 10 mm Hg diastolic indicates postural hypotension. Postural hypotension is typically accompanied by a 10 to 20 per cent increase in heart rate (pulse). Sample measurements given earlier indicate postural hypotension.

10 mm Hg, possible cardiac compression including a cardiac tamponade is considered.

Pulse

Pulses can have varying characteristics. If the pulse is irregular, the nurse assesses for a pulse deficit by taking apical and radial pulses simultaneously, noting differences in rate. Peripheral pulse assessment is discussed in Chapter 44.

Water-hammer pulse is a large, bounding pulse with a rapid rise and fall. It is associated with an increased stroke volume and widened pulse pressure, such as occurs with emotional excitement. It may be seen in aortic regurgitation and patent ductus arteriosus.

Pulsus tardus is a weak and feeble pulse, with a slow upstroke and prolonged peak. It is associated with a decrease in stroke volume and diminished pulse pressure, as seen in hypovolemic shock.

Pulsus alternans has a regular rhythm along with alterations in pulse amplitude. Strong beats alternate with weak ones. This type of pulse may be seen in myocardial infarction and/or congestive heart failure when the left ventricle function is depressed.

Bigeminal pulse primarily results from an underlying rhythm disturbance, which is most commonly associated with premature ectopic beats. A strong beat alternates with a premature (early), weak beat. The irregularity of the pulse differentiates this type of pulse from pulsus alternans.

Pulsus bisferiens is characterized by a rapid upstroke and has two systolic peaks. This pulse may be present in aortic regurgitation (with or without stenosis), and large left-to-right shunts, idiopathic hypertrophic subaortic stenosis (hypertrophic obstructive cardiomyopathy). This pulse is best felt in the carotid artery.

Respirations

In assessing the pattern of breathing, the nurse notes the rate, rhythm, depth, and quality. Variations in the respiratory rate and character could indicate heart failure or pulmonary edema. The nurse auscultates the lungs to observe for the presence of rales, rhonchi, or other abnormal breath sounds. Severe left ventricular failure may produce pulmonary congestion and resulting frothy sputum with deep respiratory efforts.

Head and Neck

In examining the head, the nurse pays particular attention to the lips, ear lobes, and buccal mucosa. The presence of a bluish tinge or duskiness is indicative of central cyanosis. Central cyanosis implies serious heart or lung disease in which the hemoglobin is not able to fully saturate with oxygen. Peripheral cyanosis usually accompanies this condition.

EXAMINATION OF NECK VEINS

The nurse examines the neck veins to estimate central venous pressure (CVP). The distensibility of the neck veins reflects the pressure and volume changes within the right atrium. The internal jugular veins, although harder to detect than the external jugular veins, are more reliable indicators of CVP. The external jugular vein can be easily engorged with only slight provocation, i.e., breath-holding, twisting the neck, and constrictive clothing. Exceptions are weight-lifters, football players, and professional speakers and singers, who have over-developed neck muscle tendons. The vessels are prominent and visible, but soft and compressible.

To measure jugular vein distention, the following protocol is suggested.

1. Have the client assume a relaxed supine position with the head of bed at an angle of comfort. Ideally, the head of bed should be inclined between 15 and 30 degrees to maximize jugular vein prominence. In clients with greatly increased right atrial pressure, head elevations from 45 to 90 degrees may be required.
2. Use a small pillow to support the client's head, avoiding sharp neck flexion. The head should be turned slightly away from the examiner. Remove any clothing that compresses the neck or upper thorax.
3. Use tangential (oblique) lighting so that small shadows are cast on the neck, making the veins more apparent. Observe both sides of the neck. The internal jugular vein lies deep to the sternocleidomastoid muscle and runs in the same direction along its length to the jaw and ear lobe (Fig. 41-2). Identify the pulsations of the internal jugular. The external jugular may be used if the internal jugular is not visible.

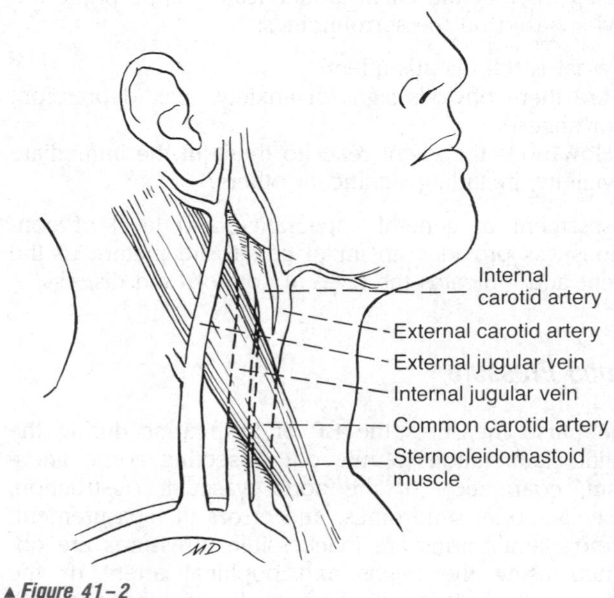

▲ **Figure 41-2**

Location of internal jugular vein.

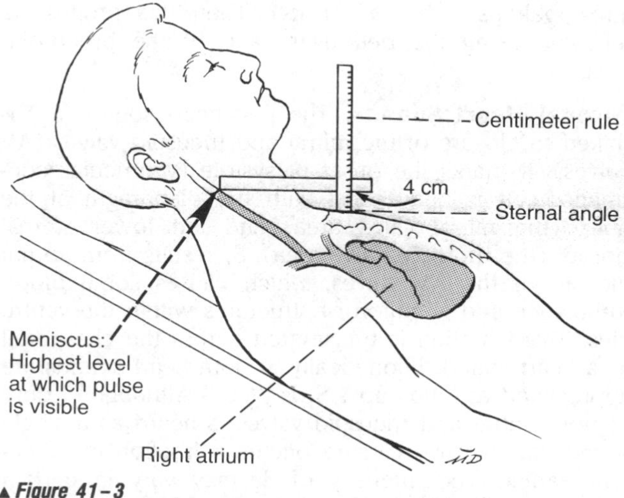

▲ *Figure 41-3*

Estimation of jugular vein measurement to assess central venous pressure.

4. Note the highest point at which the internal jugular pulses can be seen (the meniscus). Use the sternal angle (manubrial joint) as a reference point to measure the height of venous pulsation. This point is approximately 4 to 5 cm above the center of the right atrium. Using a centimeter ruler, measure the vertical distance between the sternal angle and the point of highest venous pulsations. Figure 41-3 demonstrates the method of jugular vein measurement.
5. Normally, the value is less than 3 or 4 cm above the sternal angle with the head of the bed elevated at 30 to 40 degrees. Higher values indicate increased right atrial or right ventricular pressure as seen in right ventricular failure, tricuspid regurgitation, or pericardial tamponade. Flat jugular veins noted with the client lying supine may suggest extracellular volume depletion. Unilateral distention may indicate vessel obstruction on that side.

The timing and amplitude of the jugular vein pulsations may also be assessed to evaluate right-sided heart function, tricuspid valve performance, and the presence of certain dysrhythmias.

EXAMINATION OF CAROTID ARTERIES

Examining the carotid arteries provides evidence regarding the adequacy of stroke volume and the patency of the arteries. With the fingertips, the nurse gently palpates the carotid arteries one side at a time, checking and comparing the rate, rhythm, and amplitude of the pulse. A bruit (a blowing sound) may be heard by listening to the carotid arteries with the diaphragm of a stethoscope while the client holds his or her breath. Tracheal breath sounds are heard if respiration is ongoing. A bruit generally indicates that the carotid artery has narrowed. Bruits typically result from atherosclerosis or radiation of sounds from an aortic valve murmur.

Chest

INSPECTION AND PALPATION OF THE PRECORDIUM

Inspection and palpation of the precordium are performed together to determine the presence of normal and abnormal pulsations. For more efficient assessment of the precordium, the client should be supine with the chest exposed. The left lateral position may also be used as it allows the heart to move closer to the chest wall. This position accentuates precordial movements and certain heart sounds. The examination area should have good lighting and be warm and quiet. The nurse stands on the client's right side and observes the anterior chest for size, shape, symmetry of movement, and any apparent pulsations. The location of pulsation in relation to the intercostal space and the midclavicular line is recorded. Palpation is used to confirm the observed phenomenon. When palpating, the fingers and palmar aspect of the hand are used.

Normally, the point of maximum intensity (PMI) or apical impulse is seen at the apex. The PMI is associated with left ventricular contraction and should appear at the fifth intercostal space medial to the left midclavicular line. It is most prominent in thin clients and may be obscured in those who are obese or who have large breasts. It is palpated as a single, faint, instantaneous tap beneath the examiner's fingers and is no more than 2 cm in diameter. Turning the client to the left side may assist in locating the PMI, but this maneuver will displace its location. With left ventricular enlargement and aneurysm, the PMI is more diffuse, sustained, and displaced downward and to the left of the midclavicular line.

Right ventricular enlargement can produce an abnormal pulsation that is viewed as a sustained thrust along the left sternal border. Termed heaves or lifts, these pulsations may be found in association with various disorders, such as valvular disease and pulmonary hypertension. Thrills represent turbulent blood flow through the heart, especially across abnormal heart valves. The best way to feel thrills is to use the heel or ulnar surface of the hand to palpate the precordium over each of the five cardiac landmarks (Fig. 41-4). Thrills are perceived as a rushing vibration, much like feeling the throat of a purring cat. Thrills are associated with significant heart murmurs. They may also be palpated over partially obstructed blood vessels.

AUSCULTATION OF HEART SOUNDS

Auscultation of the precordium yields valuable information about the presence of normal or abnormal heart rate and rhythm, ventricular filling, and blood flow across heart valves. Assessment of heart sounds is a sophisticated skill, requiring study of heart sound characteristics and extensive clinical practice. It is important that the nurse become thoroughly familiar with the techniques of auscultation of the normal cardiac sounds. With practice and experience, abnormal heart sounds will be detected.

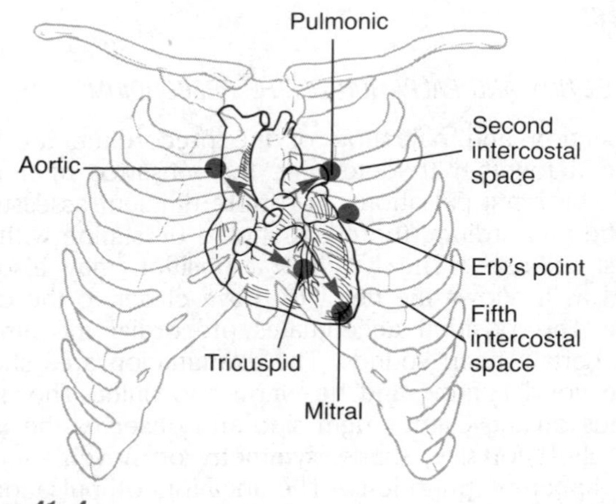

▲ *Figure 41–4*

Precordial locations for cardiac palpation and auscultation of heart sounds. Closure of mitral and tricuspid valves produces the S_1 heart sound; closure of pulmonic and aortic (semilunar) valves produces the S_2 heart sound.

Discerning abnormal heart sounds is difficult even for skilled practitioners under ideal circumstances. The sensitivity of the human ear falls sharply when the frequency of sound vibrations is below 1000 Hz. Most cardiac murmurs and sounds range below that frequency. Therefore a reliable stethoscope is a must, and the nurse should take care when selecting one (see discussion of auscultation and choice of a stethoscope in Chapter 12).

The environment is key to successful auscultation. The surroundings should be warm and quiet. An exposed chest is ideal, but the nurse should prevent shivering, which can greatly distort heart sound transmission. The nurse instructs the client to breathe through the nose while resting in a supine position. Again, use of the left lateral position may facilitate auscultation. Having the client assume an upright position, lean forward, and hold the breath after exhalation helps when assessing for early diastolic murmurs and pericardial friction rubs.

A systematic approach should always be used in evaluating heart sounds. Methods vary, and examiners should develop their own routine to ensure a thorough assessment each time cardiac auscultation is performed.

Examination of heart sounds may progress from the base (right second intercostal space) of the heart to the apex, or from the apex to the base. Whichever approach is used special attention must be paid to each of the precordial locations diagrammed in Figure 41–4. Each area corresponds to a specific valvular outflow tract. In auscultating each area, the nurse concentrates on one component of the cardiac cycle at a time, i.e., the first heart sound (S_1) and then the second heart sound (S_2). It is difficult to assess everything at one time. As many as three or four abnormalities may be occurring simultaneously. Several complete cardiac cycles are listened to at each of the five precordial areas. The nurse listens carefully, noting the quality (crisp or muffled), intensity (loud or soft), rhythm (irregular or regular), and presence of extra sounds (murmurs, gallops, rubs, or clicks). Then this process is repeated using the bell over each of the precordial areas.

Normal Heart Sounds. The first heart sound (S_1) is linked to closure of the mitral and tricuspid valves (AV valves). It marks the onset of systole (ventricular contraction). It is heard best with the diaphragm at the apex (the mitral valve area) and left lower sternal border (the tricuspid valve area). S_1 results from abrupt closure of the AV valves, which causes some blood turbulence and vibration of structures within the ventricles. This vibration is transmitted across the chest wall as a heart sound. Phonetically, if both heart sounds are appreciated as "lub-dup," S_1 is "lub." Although closure of both mitral and tricuspid valves is heard as a single sound, mitral valve closure occurs a fraction of a second earlier. The intensity of S_1 may vary in certain pathologic conditions. Diseased and stiffened AV valves (as seen in rheumatic heart disease) may augment S_1, while rhythms of asynchrony between the atria and ventricles (as in atrial fibrillation and AV block) will cause varying intensity to the first heart sound.

The second heart sound (S_2) relates to closure of the pulmonic and aortic (semilunar) valves and is heard best with the diaphragm at the base of the heart. Phonetically, it is the "dup" of the heart sound. It signifies the end of systole and the onset of diastole (ventricular filling). At the base of the heart, normal S_2 is always louder than S_1, whereas both sounds usually are of nearly equal intensity at the left sternal border over Erb's point. Usually S_1 is the louder of the two sounds at the apex and occurs just after or along with the carotid pulse.

Knowing the usual quality of sound at various points on the precordium can help in the differentiation of S_1 and S_2 during rapid heart rates. Likewise, simultaneous palpation of the carotid pulse during auscultation is helpful to discern sounds. Carotid pulsation occurs with systole or S_1. Figure 41–5 illustrates the relationship of heart sounds to events during the cardiac cycle.

Physiologic (normal) splitting of S_2 occurs during inspiration. Normal splitting results from delayed closure of the pulmonic valve. Both aortic and pulmonic components of S_2 (A_2 and P_2) can be heard. Inspiration creates negative pressure within the thoracic cavity, "pulling" blood from the periphery into the right side of the heart. Because of this transient augmentation in venous return, right ventricular volume increases and emptying is delayed, delaying pulmonic valve closure. The "split-second heart sound" is best heard over the pulmonic area. The two components of S_2 occur so close together that the pause between them produces a phonetic gap similar to the "pl" sound in the word "split."

Abnormal Heart Sounds. There are many abnormal heart sounds that may indicate a serious heart disorder or change in cardiac function. The nurse may not be able to label each abnormality, but with a thorough understanding of the normal sounds, the nurse should be able to recognize the various abnormal sounds and refer the problem to the physician.

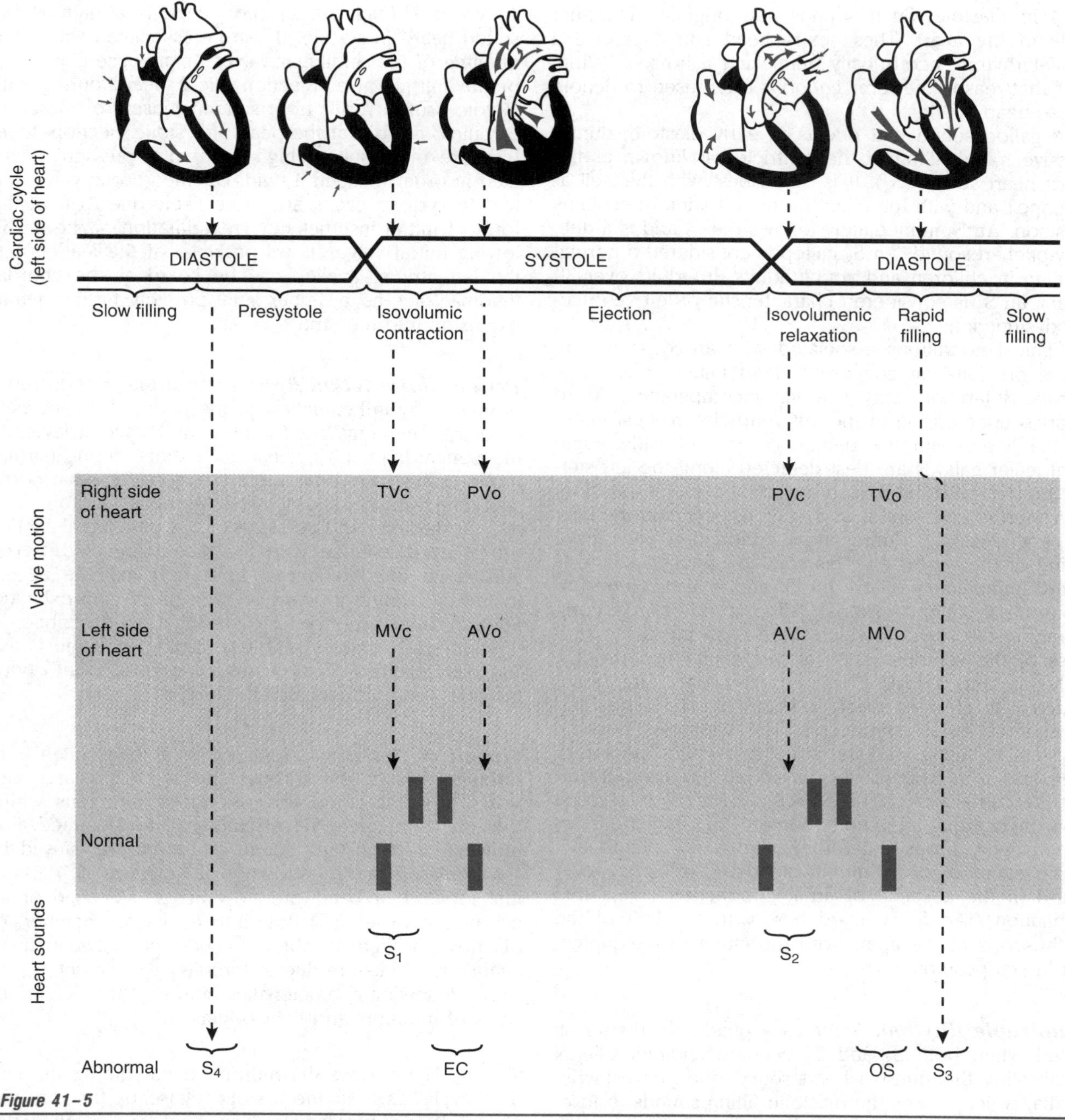

▲ **Figure 41-5**

Relationship of heart sounds to events during the cardiac cycle. Understanding heart sounds is facilitated when they are correlated with cardiac cycle events and valvular movements. KEY: MVc, mitral valve closing; TVc, tricuspid valve closing; PVo, pulmonic valve opening; AVo, aortic valve opening; AVc, aortic valve closing; PVc, pulmonic valve closing; TVo, tricuspid valve opening; MVo, mitral valve opening; EC, ejection click; OS, opening snap.

Pathologic Splitting of S_2. A wide splitting of S_2 may be heard during both inspiration and expiration, with an increase during inspiration. This form of splitting occurs in right bundle branch block, due to delay in the depolarization of the right ventricle and late closure of the pulmonic valve. Fixed splitting is a hallmark sign of atrial septal defect. This form of S_2 split is continuous and does not vary with respirations. Fixed splitting occurs because the emptying of the right ventricle is prolonged. Paradoxical splitting occurs from a delay in the closure of the aortic valve due to aortic stenosis, left bundle branch block, or patent ductus arteriosus. In paradoxical splitting, the S_2 split is heard during expiration rather than inspiration.

Gallops. Diastolic filling sounds or gallops (S_3 and S_4) occur during the two phases of ventricular filling. Sudden changes of inflow volume cause vibrations of the valves and ventricular supporting structures, producing low-pitched sounds that occur either early (S_3) or late

(S_4) in diastole. Such sounds can originate in either side of the heart. These extra heart sounds create a triplet rhythm, acoustically mimicking a horse's gallop. For that reason the term *gallop* is often used to denote these heart sounds.

A gallop sound that occurs in early diastole, during passive, rapid filling of the ventricles, is known as the third heart sound (S_3). It is heard best with the bell at the apex and with the client in the left lateral decubitus position. An S_3 immediately follows the S_2 and is a dull, low-pitched sound. An S_3 gallop is considered a normal finding in children and young adults. In adults over 30 years, an S_3 is considered characteristic of left ventricular dysfunction.

Clinical conditions associated with an S_3 gallop are those precipitating congestive heart failure, e.g., myocardial infarction and valvular incompetence. Third heart sounds arising in the left ventricle are best heard at the apex, with the person on the left side. Right ventricular gallops are best detected along the left sternal border, with the person assuming a supine position.

A fourth heart sound, or S_4 gallop, occurs in the later stage of diastole, during atrial contraction and active filling of the ventricles. This soft, low-pitched sound is heard immediately before the S_1 and is also referred to as an atrial gallop. An atrial gallop is found most commonly in disorders in which there is an increased stiffness of the ventricle; such as ventricular hypertrophy, ischemia, and fibrosis. These conditions are often associated with elevated diastolic ventricular pressures and a vigorous atrial contraction. The ventricles become resistant to filling, and the structures within the ventricles vibrate in response to the added blood input during the "atrial kick." The presence of an S_4 may result from myocardial infarction (transient S_4), hypertension, hypertrophy, fibrosis, cardiomyopathy, cor pulmonale, aortic stenosis, or pulmonic stenosis. An S_4 is never heard in the absence of atrial contraction (i.e., atrial fibrillation). An S_4 is heard best with the bell of the stethoscope at the apex, with the client in the supine, left lateral position.

Quadruple Rhythm. At times a quadruple rhythm is noted when both S_3 and S_4 become audible. Clients manifesting this unusual heart sound often have tachycardia, which causes the diastolic filling sounds to fuse, forming a summation gallop that may be louder than the first or second heart sounds. It can be heard best at the apex and resembles the sound of a galloping horse.

Opening Snaps. These high-pitched sounds heard in diastole are produced by the opening of certain stenosed valves. Valves normally open silently, but when they become calcified or rigid from disease, greater pressure is required to force them open. When they do "pop" open, they produce a characteristic sound. Opening snaps occur with the opening of a stenotic mitral and (rarely) tricuspid valve. The resulting sound is brief, high pitched, and of a snapping quality. It is heard early in diastole at the apex using a diaphragm.

Ejection Clicks. An ejection click is a high-pitched sound heard in systole. It can be associated with either opening of the semilunar valves or prolapse (inversion) of the mitral valve. Ejection clicks heard during early systole usually result from sudden tensing of the aortic or pulmonic root at the peak of systolic ejection. Often they are the result of high ventricular pressure generated in order to open a rigid, calcified aortic valve. Mid to late systolic clicks are more likely due to a benign form of mitral insufficiency (regurgitation). When a billowing mitral valve allows prolapse of the leaflets into the left atrium, a click can be heard as the chordae tendinae act as a tether and prohibit further leaflet excursion into the atria.

Pericardial Friction Rub. A pericardial friction rub is produced by inflammation of the pericardial sac (pericarditis). The roughened parietal and visceral layers of the pericardium rub against each other during cardiac motion. This sound has three components, each corresponding with cardiac activity: ventricular systole, ventricular diastole, and atrial systole. A pericardial friction rub is best detected with the diaphragm at the apex and along the left sternal border. It may be accentuated by leaning forward or lying prone and exhaling. Friction rubs produce a sound that is described as "to-and-fro," scratchy, grating, rasping, and much like "squeaky leather." Friction rubs may be present during the first week of myocardial infarction.

Murmurs. Murmurs are heard as a consequence of turbulent blood flow through the heart and large vessels. Turbulent blood flow produces vibrations within the heart and great vessels that can be detected as a blowing or swooshing sound. Murmurs are caused by (1) increased rate or velocity of blood flow, (2) abnormal forward or backward flow across stenosed or incompetent valves, (3) flow into a dilated chamber, or (4) flow through an abnormal passage between heart chambers. Bruits are due to turbulence in vessels.

The following characteristics help identify the various types of murmurs and their origins.

Timing. When does the murmur occur during the cardiac cycle? Is it in the systolic phase or the diastolic phase? It is imperative to identify S_1 and S_2 to determine the phase. The murmur is then described as occurring in early, mid-, or late systole or diastole. A murmur that is heard throughout the systolic phase is described as pansystolic or holosystolic.

Quality. What is the quality or sound of the murmur? Is it blowing, harsh, rumbling, or musical? For example, the murmur of mitral stenosis is described as rumbling, whereas the murmur of mitral regurgitation creates a blowing sound.

Pitch. What is the frequency (pitch) of the murmur? Is it high and heard best with the diaphragm or low and heard best with the bell?

Location. Where is the murmur loudest? Murmurs, like all sounds, are loudest at their point of origin. Is the murmur of highest intensity over the aortic, pulmonic, tricuspid, or mitral valve outflow tract? The location is usually described in terms of its position in relation to intercostal spaces.

Radiation. The sound of the murmur is transmitted in the direction of blood flow. It may be transmitted upstream, as with regurgitant murmurs, or downstream, as noted in stenotic murmurs. Therefore, the sound may be transmitted to the axilla, neck, back, and other locations on the chest.

Configuration. Note the shape of the sound. Does the sound begin soft and become louder (crescendo)? Does it do just the opposite (decrescendo)? Does it seem to have a "diamond shape" (crescendo-decrescendo)? The sound may be fairly constant (plateau). Table 41-2 compares selected heart murmurs.

Intensity. The degree of intensity (loudness) is typically measured using a rating system that does not necessarily reflect the seriousness of disease. Six grades (I to VI) of intensity are noted (Box 41-1). A grade II murmur would be recorded as II/VI.

EXAMINATION OF THE LUNGS

Because of the intimate relationship between the cardiovascular and respiratory systems, assessment of the cardiovascular system must include evaluation of the respiratory system. A more thorough discussion of respiratory assessment is in Chapter 36. Some common respiratory findings related to cardiovascular disease are as follows.

Tachypnea. Tachypnea, or rapid respirations, is often associated with the pain and anxiety that may accompany myocardial ischemic pain. Tachypnea also commonly occurs as a compensatory mechanism in congestive heart failure and pulmonary edema.

Crackles. Rales or crackles are a frequent sign of left ventricular failure and usually occur just after the onset of an S_3 gallop. As pulmonary capillary pressure rises from the backward pressure of left ventricular failure, fluid shifts into the intra-alveolar spaces and crackles can be auscultated. Crackles may also result from atelectasis due to limited chest wall excursion from prolonged bed rest, chest splinting from pain, and the effects of sedatives and narcotics. Crackles are best heard at the lung bases (gravitational effects on the fluid) and occur during late inspiration.

Blood-Tinged Sputum. A pink frothy sputum may indicate acute pulmonary edema. This symptom accompanies diffuse pulmonary crackles and denotes very serious left ventricular failure. Frank hemoptysis may be associated with pulmonary embolus. A cough frequently occurs in association with hemoptysis.

Cheyne-Stokes Respirations. These abnormal respirations are characterized by abnormal periods of deep breathing alternating with periods of apnea. This is a common finding in heart failure, anemia, and brain damage (from anoxic encephalopathy).

Abdomen

Examination of the abdomen provides data regarding cardiac competency. It is, however, of less value than other assessment parameters discussed in this section. Abdominal assessment is discussed in Chapter 52.

INSPECTION AND PALPATION

Upon inspection, the nurse may note abdominal distention. Palpation may confirm the presence of ascites (fluid accumulation within the peritoneal cavity) and an enlarged liver. Both of these findings indicate liver failure, which can be a sequela of chronic right ventricular failure.

AUSCULTATION

Auscultation can yield the following clues about cardiovascular function:

- Decreased bowel tones can accompany potassium (K^+) depletion. K^+ depletion can complicate chronic diuretic use without sufficient K^+ replacement.
- Increased bowel tones, indicative of hypermotility, may result from laxative use or may be a side effect of certain antiarrhythmics (such as quinidine).
- Loud bruits, heard with the bell just over or above the umbilicus, may herald the presence of an aortic obstruction or aortic aneurysm (the latter can be detected by a palpable abdominal pulsation). Bruits heard over the upper midline or toward the back typically arise from renal arterial stenosis.

DIAGNOSTIC TESTS

The four most common types of diagnostic procedures used to diagnose cardiovascular disease are graphic procedures, laboratory tests, x-ray studies, and hemodynamic studies.

Nursing responsibilities in diagnostic testing include

- Explaining the purpose and procedure and answering any questions,
- Scheduling the test,
- Performing any necessary preliminary (e.g., adjustments in medications and special diets) care, and
- Promoting maximum emotional and physical comfort.

Laboratory Tests

Data obtained from laboratory tests are used to diagnose a variety of cardiovascular ailments (e.g., myocar-

Box 41–1. Grading of Heart Murmurs

Grade I	Faint; heard after listener has "tuned in"
Grade II	Faint murmur heard immediately
Grade III	Moderately loud, with accompanying thrill
Grade IV	Loud
Grade V	Very loud; heard only with the stethoscope
Grade VI	Very loud; heard without the stethoscope

dial infarction), to screen individuals considered at risk for cardiovascular disease, to determine baseline values, to identify the presence of concurrent conditions (e.g., diabetes mellitus, electrolyte imbalance) that may affect the course of intervention, and to evaluate the effectiveness of intervention. We consider here only those tests that are more commonly used to determine cardiovascular function and disease.

COMPLETE BLOOD CELL COUNT (CBC)

The erythrocyte red blood cell count usually decreases in rheumatic fever and infective endocarditis. It usually increases in heart diseases characterized by inadequate oxygenation of tissues, e.g., right-to-left congenital shunts and heart conditions accompanied by obstructive lung disease.

Measuring the packed cell volume, or hematocrit, is the easiest way to ascertain the concentration of red cells in the blood. An elevated hematocrit can result

TABLE 41–2. Heart Murmurs

Type of Heart Sound	Origin	Preferred Method of Auscultation
Systolic murmurs Ejection type 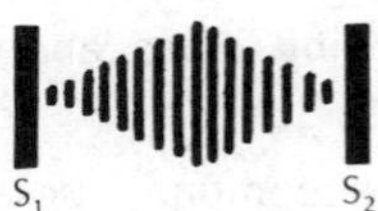	Systolic ejection murmurs are associated with forward blood flow during ventricular contraction across stenotic aortic or pulmonic valves.	Use of the stethoscope diaphragm is indicated. Ejection murmurs are typically of medium pitch and harsh quality and may be associated with an early ejection click. Aortic ejection murmurs are best heard over the aortic valve with radiation into the neck, down the left sternal border, and occasionally to the apex. They may be accompanied by a decreased S_2. Pulmonic ejection murmurs are heard best over the pulmonic valve, with radiation toward the left shoulder and left neck vessels. These murmurs may be accompanied by a wide-split S_2.
Pansystolic regurgitant murmurs 	Pansystolic murmurs occur when blood regurgitates through incompetent mitral and tricuspid valves (AV valves) or a ventricular septal defect as pressures rise during systole and blood seeks chambers of lower pressure. Damage to valve leaflets, papillary muscles, and chordae tendineae results in mitral valve insufficiency (blood regurgitates from left ventricle to left atrium) and tricuspid valve insufficiency (blood regurgitates from the right ventricle to right atrium). A ventricular septal defect results in blood regurgitation from the left ventricle to the right ventricle.	All regurgitant murmurs are high pitched, and those of AV valve incompetence have a blowing quality. Mitral regurgitant murmurs are heard at the apex with radiation into the left axilla and may be accompanied by an ejection click and signs of left ventricular failure. Tricuspid regurgitant murmurs are heard loudest over the tricuspid area, with radiation into the sternum. Ventricular septal defects are usually loud, harsh, and heard best over the left sternal border in the fourth, fifth, and sixth intercostal spaces with radiation over the precordium but not the axilla.
Early systolic murmurs 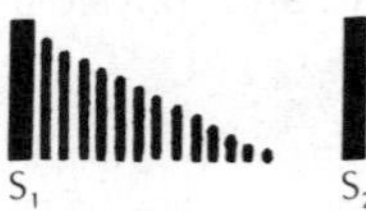	Early systolic murmurs (innocent murmurs) are associated with high cardiac outputs, as there is increased blood flow velocity across normal semilunar valves. Causes include anemia, tachycardia, thyrotoxicosis, and fever. The murmur disappears with correction of the underlying condition. These are a normal variant in children.	These murmurs are best heard with the bell over the base of the heart or along the lower left sternal border. They are usually no greater than a grade II, are of medium pitch, and have a blowing quality. Intensity may increase during inspiration with the patient in a left recumbent position or with increased heart rates.

TABLE 41–2. Heart Murmurs Continued

Type of Heart Sound	Origin	Preferred Method of Auscultation
Late systolic murmurs S_1 EC S_2	Late systolic murmurs imply mild mitral regurgitation as the mitral valve balloons into the left atrium late in ventricular systole.	These are best heard with the diaphragm of the stethoscope over the apex and is often preceded by a mid or late systolic ejection click.
Diastolic murmurs Early diastolic murmur S_1 S_2 S_1	Early diastolic murmurs (decrescendo murmurs) are usually caused by semilunar valve insufficiency, with regurgitation due to valvular deformity or dilation of the valvular ring. They are heard immediately following the second heart sound and then diminish in intensity as the pressure in the aorta or pulmonary artery falls and the ventricles fill.	These murmurs are heard best with the diaphragm at the base of the heart with the patient leaning forward in deep expiration. They are high-pitched and blowing and radiate down the left sternal border, perhaps to the apex or down the right sternal border. Accompanying signs of heart failure may be present.
Diastolic filling rumbling S_1 S_2 S_1	Diastolic filling rumbles are caused as blood flows across stenotic AV valves (more often mitral). They may also occur during augmented blood flow across normal AV valves. The murmur has two phases, becoming louder as the blood flow from the atrium to the ventricle increases with passive ventricular filling just after AV valve opening and again during atrial contraction (presystole).	With the bell, this murmur is heard over only a small area at and just medial to the apex. Exercise and a left lateral position of the patient increase the intensity of the sound. It is a low-pitched, rumbling sound often accompanied by an augmented S_1 and an opening snap.

Note. AV, atrioventricular.
From Huang, S. L., et al. (1989). *Coronary care nursing* (2nd ed., p. 19). Philadelphia: W. B. Saunders Company.

from obstructive lung disease and conditions of vascular volume depletion with hemoconcentration (e.g., hypovolemic shock and excessive diuresis). Decreases in hematocrit and hemoglobin indicate anemia, which is commonly caused by hemorrhage, hemolysis (from prosthetic valves), and chronic disease states. Patients with anemia have a significant reduction in red cell mass and a decrease in the oxygen-carrying capacity. Anemia can manifest as angina or aggravate congestive heart failure and produce heart murmurs.

The leukocyte (white blood cell) count elevates in infectious and inflammatory diseases of the heart (e.g., infective endocarditis and pericarditis). It is also elevated following myocardial infarction because large numbers of white cells are necessary to dispose of the necrotic tissue resulting from the infarction.

CARDIAC ENZYMES

Enzymes are special proteins that catalyze chemical reactions in living cells. Cardiac enzymes are organ-specific enzymes that are present in high concentrations in myocardial tissue. Tissue damage causes a release of enzymes from their intracellular storage areas. For example, myocardial infarction causes cellular anoxia, which alters membrane permeability and causes spillage of enzymes into the surrounding tissue. This leakage of enzymes can be detected by rising plasma levels.

The enzymes most commonly used to detect myocardial infarction are creatine kinase (CK) and lactic acid dehydrogenase (LDH). Serum elevations of these two enzymes following myocardial insult occur in sequence. Because these enzymes are also found in other organs and tissues (e.g., skeletal muscle and liver), cardiac specificity must be determined by measuring isoenzyme activity. Isoenzymes are the various forms of CK and LDH, identified only by a process known as electrophoresis. There are three isoenzymes of CK: CK-MM (skeletal muscle), CK-MB (myocardial muscle), and CK-BB (brain). An elevated CK-MB, then, indicates myocardial damage. Elevation of CK-MB may occur within 4 to 6 hours and peaks 18 to 24 hours after the acute ischemic event. Of particular importance is the fact that up to a threefold elevation of CK may follow an intramuscular injection. Intramuscular injections should be avoided when treating a suspected myocardial infarction.[11]

There are five isoenzymes for LDH (numbered 1 to 5), of which only LDH_1 and LDH_2 are cardiac-specific. If the serum concentration of LDH_1 is higher than the concentration of LDH_2, the pattern is said to have flipped, signifying myocardial necrosis. Eighty per cent of individuals demonstrate elevations in LDH within 48 hours after myocardial infarction.

As well as indicating the presence of myocardial damage, these elevations in serum cardiac enzymes can reveal the timing of the acute cardiac event. This is discussed in further detail in Chapter 42.

BLOOD COAGULATION TESTS

Blood coagulation tests are used to examine the ability of the blood to clot. It is important to evaluate coagulation tests such as prothrombin time and partial thromboplastin time in individuals with a greater tendency to form thrombi, e.g., people with atrial fibrillation, infective endocarditis, or prosthetic valves. Research has shown an increase in coagulation factors during and after a myocardial infarction. Therefore, the client is at greater risk of thrombophlebitis and extension of clots in the coronary artery. Chapter 45 discusses coagulation tests in detail.

SERUM LIPIDS

Serum lipids play a major role in the development of atherosclerosis. Serum lipids are composed of fatty substances that are insoluble in water. They are derived from dietary intake of fats or synthesized in the liver. The lipid profile measures serum cholesterol, triglycerides, and lipoprotein levels and is used to assess a client's degree of risk for developing coronary artery disease. Serum lipids are discussed in Chapter 42.

SERUM ELECTROLYTES

Cardiovascular disorders may impact on fluid and electrolyte regulation. In addition, certain medications alter electrolyte balance.

Potassium. The serum potassium level lowers as a result of diuretic therapy, vomiting, diarrhea, and alkalosis. Cardiac effects of hypokalemia include increased electrical instability, ventricular dysrhythmias, and increased risk of digitalis toxicity. Characteristic changes on the ECG include flattening and inversion of the T wave, the appearance of a U wave, and sagging of the ST segment.

A high serum potassium level is usually associated with kidney and endocrine disorders. The cardiac effects of hyperkalemia include asystole and ventricular dysrhythmias.

Sodium. The serum sodium level reflects water balance and may decrease (indicating water excess) in congestive heart failure, stress, excessive intravenous infusion of hypotonic fluids, and vomiting. Extensive use of diuretics and severely restricted sodium intake also lower serum sodium.

Calcium. The serum calcium level lowers as a result of multiple transfusions of citrated blood, renal failure, alkalosis, and laxative and antacid abuse (phosphate excess). Cardiac manifestations of hypocalcemia include serious ventricular dysrhythmias, prolonged QT interval, and cardiac arrest. Hypercalcemia occurs in thiazide diuretic use, acidosis, adrenal insufficiency, immobility, and vitamin D excess. A high serum calcium level shortens the QT interval and causes AV block, tachycardia, bradycardia, digitalis hypersensitivity, and cardiac arrest.

BLOOD UREA NITROGEN

Blood urea nitrogen (BUN) is a test of renal function, specifically, the ability of the kidney to excrete urea and protein. The BUN level elevates in kidney diseases, during water and saline depletion, and heart disorders that adversely affect renal circulation, e.g., congestive heart failure and cardiogenic shock.

BLOOD GLUCOSE

Diabetes mellitus is a major risk factor in the development of atherosclerosis. In addition, the stress of an acute cardiac event can greatly elevate blood glucose, causing unstable hyperglycemia in clients with latent diabetes mellitus. For these reasons, blood glucose is routinely assessed in all clients with acute cardiovascular disorders.

Electrocardiogram

Each heartbeat is the result of an electrical impulse. This impulse, which begins in the sinoatrial node of the right atrium, is conducted through a network of fibers (the conduction system) within the heart and causes the heart to contract. This same electrical impulse spreads outward from the heart to the skin, where it can be detected by electrodes attached to the skin. The ECG (or EKG) is a display of the electrical action of the heart. There are several types of ECG: continuous monitoring, 12 lead, and signal averaged ECG. Through analysis of the ECG wave forms, any disorder of cardiac rate, rhythm, or conduction can be identified.

ECG is a common test. It is performed on clients over the age of 40 prior to surgery to assess for unknown heart disease and is a frequent noninvasive diagnostic test in almost all clients with known or suspected heart disease.

CONTINUOUS ELECTROCARDIOGRAM MONITORING

Four steps are required for ECG monitoring: (1) attaching the electrodes to the client's skin, (2) connecting the electrodes to the monitor by way of a cable, (3) adjusting the monitor to obtain a readable ECG, and (4) setting the alarms for desired high and low rates. The client should be reassured that the ECG does not cause electrical shock and does not hurt.

Attaching the Electrodes. Electrodes pick up the electrical impulses from the heart on the skin. It is apparent that unless the signal is detected accurately, the remaining phases of ECG monitoring have little value. The most common form of electrodes are disc-type or floating electrodes, which are deliberately separated from direct contact with the skin by a spacer filled with conductive gel. The gel is used to improve the signal by reducing local electrical interference on the skin. The gel is surrounded by a ring of adhesive. By peeling a paper backing off the pad, the electrode can be immediately applied to the skin. Three electrodes are required for continuous ECG monitoring. Two of these serve to detect the heart's activity; the third is an electrical ground.

The electrodes should be attached to the lead wires before they are applied to the chest wall. This process avoids applying pressure to the electrode, which could hurt the client and squeeze the gel outward, reducing contact.

Some clients require special preliminary steps before the electrodes are attached. If the client has a lot of hair on the chest, it should be shaved to provide contact. If the client is wet or has been sweating, the sites should be dried off before the electrodes are applied.

In positioning the electrodes on the chest wall, locations are selected that will provide the clearest ECG wave forms. The two most common positions are the conventional position and the modified chest lead position (Fig. 41-6). Electrodes should be changed if the tracing is not clear or if they become dry or lose skin contact.

Connecting the Monitor. The electrodes are connected to the monitor by lead wires. These wires are 12 to 18 inches in length. One end snaps on to the electrodes, and the other end is attached to a cable that is connected to the monitor. At the cable is a cable receptacle for the attachment of each wire. The receptacle and lead wires are color coded to facilitate connection.

Adjusting the Monitor. If the electrodes were applied properly and the wires are secure, the ECG pattern should be clear and distinct. If the pattern is not clear, the first steps should be checked. If the client's chest is large, the pattern may appear small and the gain (degree of magnification) should be adjusted until the pattern is clear.

Setting the Alarms. If the client's heart rate is between 60 and 100 beats per minute (bpm), it is customary to set the low alarm at 50 bpm and the high alarm 140 bpm.

At times, false alarms may occur due to poor electrode contact. The nurse may be tempted to set the alarm limits widely apart (e.g., 40 to 180 bpm) or, worse, to turn the alarm off completely. This practice defeats the purpose of the alarm system and should never be adopted.

ELECTROCARDIOGRAM TRACINGS

Once the client is attached to continuous ECG monitoring, the heart rhythm is assessed hourly. Rhythm strips are logged into the medical record routinely as well as when dysrhythmias are noted. Dysrhythmias are discussed in Chapter 42.

The impulse waves, recorded by the ECG machine onto graph paper, are arbitrarily designated by the letters P, Q, R, S, and T. The QRS letters are generally referred to as the QRS complex. Figure 41-7 depicts the typical ECG pattern formed by these waves.

The components of the ECG are defined as follows:

The P wave represents depolarization of the atria.

The PR interval represents the time it takes for the impulse to spread from the atria to the ventricles.

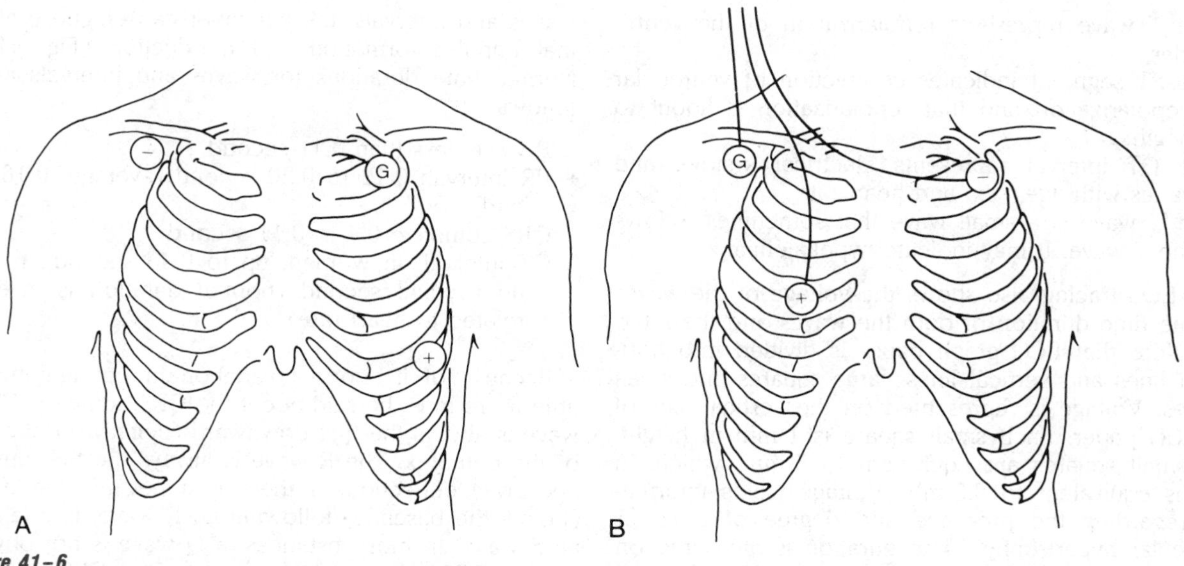

▲ *Figure 41-6*

Common positions for continuous monitoring lead placement. Use lead II (A) or lead V_1 (B). (From Phillips, R. E., & Feeney M. K. [1990]. The cardiac rhythms: A systematic approach to interpretation (3rd ed.). Philadelphia, W. B. Saunders.)

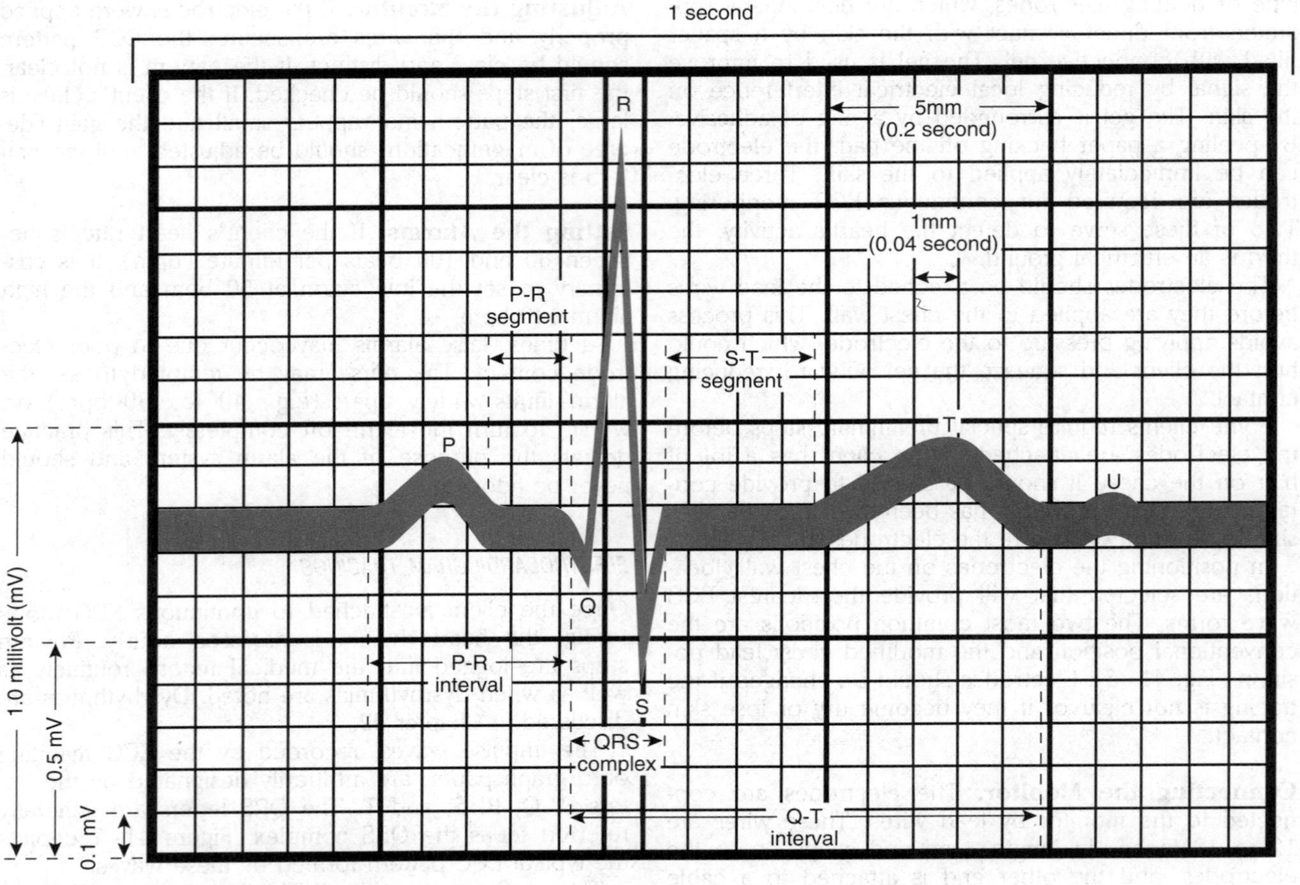

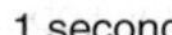

▲ *Figure 41–7*

Normal ECG pattern. The P wave represents depolarization of the atria to the ventricles. The QRS complex represents depolarization of the ventricles, and the T wave represents repolarization of the ventricles. The small U wave is sometimes seen following the T wave. Time and voltage lines of ECG paper: vertically, 1 mm = 0.1 millivolt (mV) mV; 5 mm = 0.5 mV and 10 mm = 1.0 mV. Horizontally, 1 small box = 0.04 second; 5 small boxes = 0.20 second, and 25 small boxes = 1 second.

The T wave represents repolarization of the ventricles.

The ST segment indicates completion of ventricular depolarization and that repolarization is about to begin.

The QT interval represents electrical systole, and varies with age, sex, and heart rate.

The U wave is a small wave that sometimes follows the T wave. It may indicate hypokalemia.

An ECG tracing also shows the voltage of the waves and the time duration of both the waves and the intervals. Note that ECG graph paper is divided into horizontal lines and vertical lines, large squares and small squares. Voltage is represented on the vertical axis of the ECG paper. Each small square is 1 mm in height. Five small squares are equivalent to 5 mm, which, in turn, is equivalent to 0.5 mV. Voltage yields information regarding the presence and degree of atrial or ventricular hypertrophy. Time duration is measured on the horizontal axis. Each small square signifies the passage of 0.04 second. Each large square indicates the passage of 0.20 second. By studying the duration of the waves and intervals, the examiner can diagnose abnormal impulse formation and conduction (Fig. 41–8). Normal time durations for waves and intervals are as follows:

P wave: less than 0.11 second

PR interval: 0.12 to 0.20 second (average, 0.16 second)

QRS complex: 0.4 to 0.11 second

QT interval: in women, up to 0.43 second; in men, up to 0.42 second (normal duration is inversely related to heart rate)

Because of its normal variation in configuration, a little more must be said about the QRS complex. The Q wave is always the first downward (negative) deflection of the complex. The R wave is always the first upward (positive) deflection. If there is a negative deflection (below the baseline) following an R wave, it is labeled an S wave. In most instances, a Q wave is not obvious on the ECG of the normal heart. The QRS complex may appear as a mostly positive or mostly negative deflection, depending on the recording electrode used.

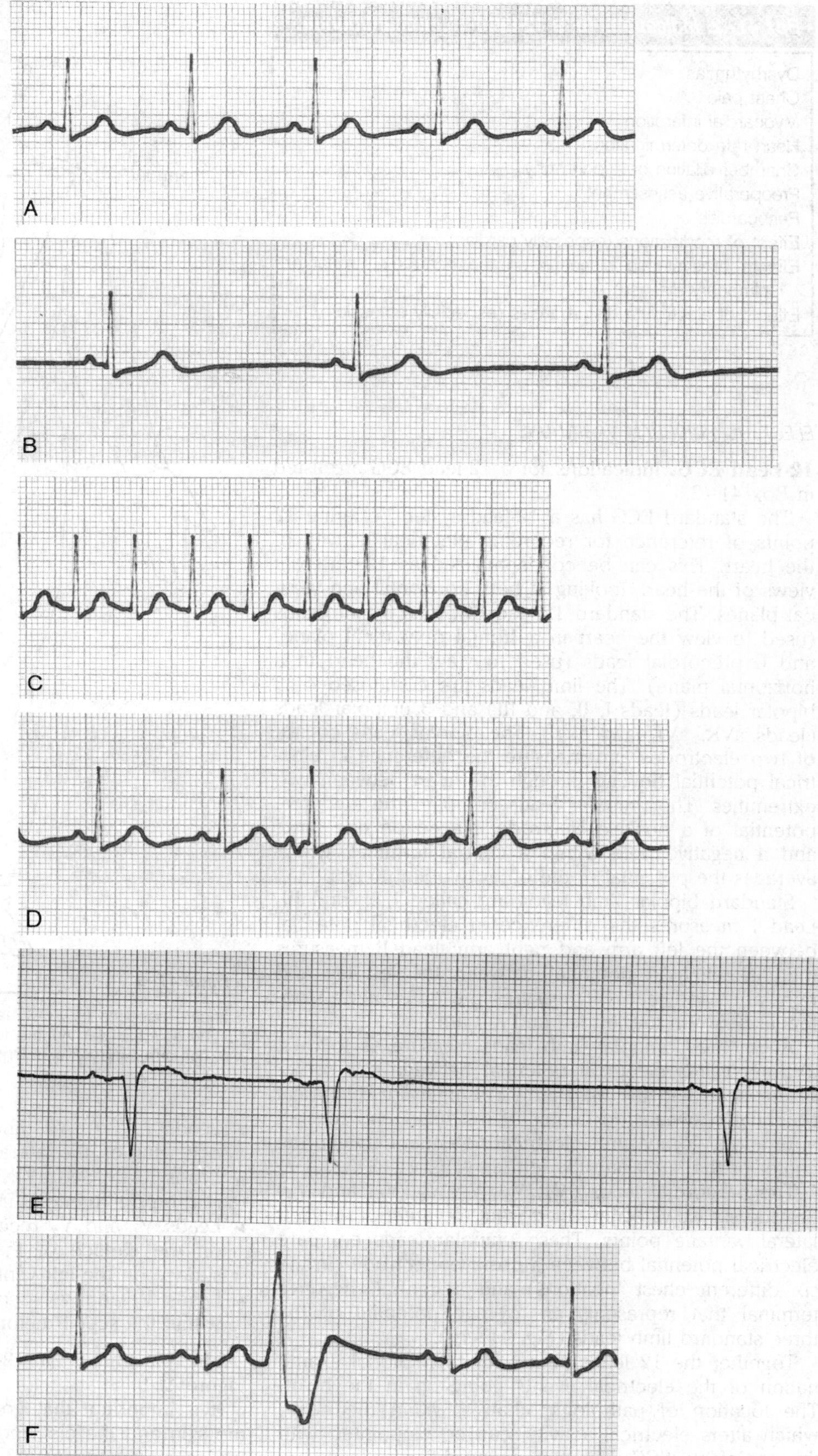

▲ *Figure 41–8*

Electrocardiogram. *A*, Normal sinus rhythm; *B*, sinus bradycardia; *C*, sinus tachycardia; *D*, normal sinus rhythm with a premature atrial contraction (PAC); *E*, sinus rhythm with sinus arrest; and *F*, sinus rhythm with a premature ventricular contraction (PVC).

Box 41-2. Indications for a 12-Lead Electrocardiogram

- Dysrhythmias
- Chest pain
- Myocardial infarction
- Heart rate determination
- Chamber dilation or hypertrophy
- Preoperative assessment
- Periocarditis
- Effect of medications (especially cardiac)
- Effects of systemic diseases on the heart (i.e., renal or pulmonary disease)
- Effects of electrolyte disturbances (especially potassium)

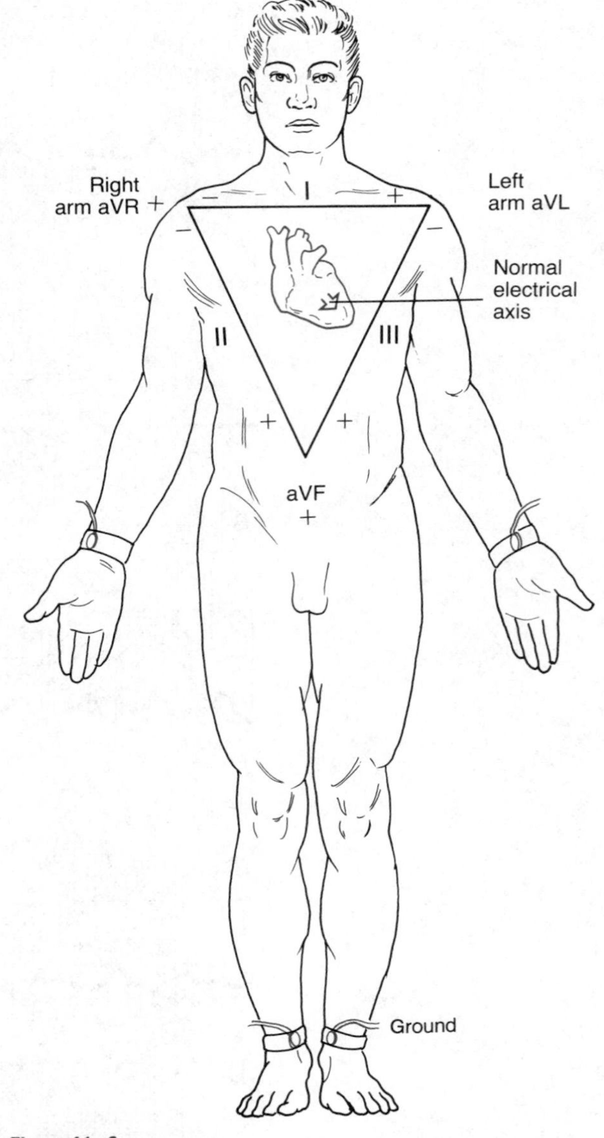

▲ *Figure 41-9*

Standard positions for ECG leads. Bipolar limb leads are I, II, and III (Einthoven's triangle). Augmented unipolar limb leads: aVR (right arm), aVL (left arm), and aVF (left leg).

ELECTROCARDIOGRAM VARIATIONS

12-Lead ECG. Indications for a 12-lead ECG are listed in Box 41-2.

The standard ECG has a 12-lead system, offering 12 points of reference for recording electrical activity of the heart. This can be conceptualized as 12 different views of the heart, looking in both horizontal and vertical planes. The standard 12-lead ECG has 6 limb leads (used to view the heart in a frontal or vertical plane) and 6 precordial leads (used to view the heart in a horizontal plane). The limb leads are composed of 3 bipolar leads (leads I, II, and III) and 3 unipolar leads (leads aVR, aVL, and aVF). The bipolar leads consist of two electrodes and measure the difference in electrical potential flowing through the heart between two extremities. The unipolar leads compare the electrical potential of a positive electrode, placed on one limb, and a negative pole within a central terminal, which averages the potential of the other two limb leads.

Standard bipolar limb leads are called I, II, and III. Lead I measures the difference in electrical potential between the left arm and right arm; lead II measures the difference in potential between the left leg and right arm; and lead III measures the difference in potential between the left leg and left arm.

Augmented unipolar limb leads measure as follows: aVR measures electrical potential between the center of the heart and the right arm; aVL measures electrical potential between the center of the heart and the left arm; and aVF measures electrical potential between the center of the heart and the left leg (Fig. 41-9).

The precordial leads (V_1, V_2, V_3, V_4, V_5, and V_6) provide six views of the heart from the anterior and left lateral vantage points. These unipolar leads compare electrical potential between a positive electrode (in the six different chest locations) and a central, negative terminal that represents an average potential of the three standard limb leads (Fig. 41-10).

Together the 12 leads permit multidirectional examination of the electrical events going on in the heart. The location of pathologic change within the heart, which alters electrical activity, can be pinpointed with the use of the ECG. Views from the different leads are oriented to various surfaces of the myocardium:

- Leads I, aVL, V_5, and V_6 record electrical events occurring on the lateral surface of the left ventricle.
- Leads II, III, and aVF record electrical events occurring on the inferior surface of the left ventricle.
- Leads V_1 and V_2 record electrical events occurring on the surface of the right ventricle and anterior surface on the left ventricle.
- Leads V_3 and V_4 record electrical events occurring within the septal region of the left ventricle.

The placement of 12-lead electrodes is shown in Figure 41-9.

It is important that good contact be made between the skin and the electrodes. To facilitate this, the electrodes are placed firmly on the flat surface just above the wrists and ankles. There are many varieties of elec-

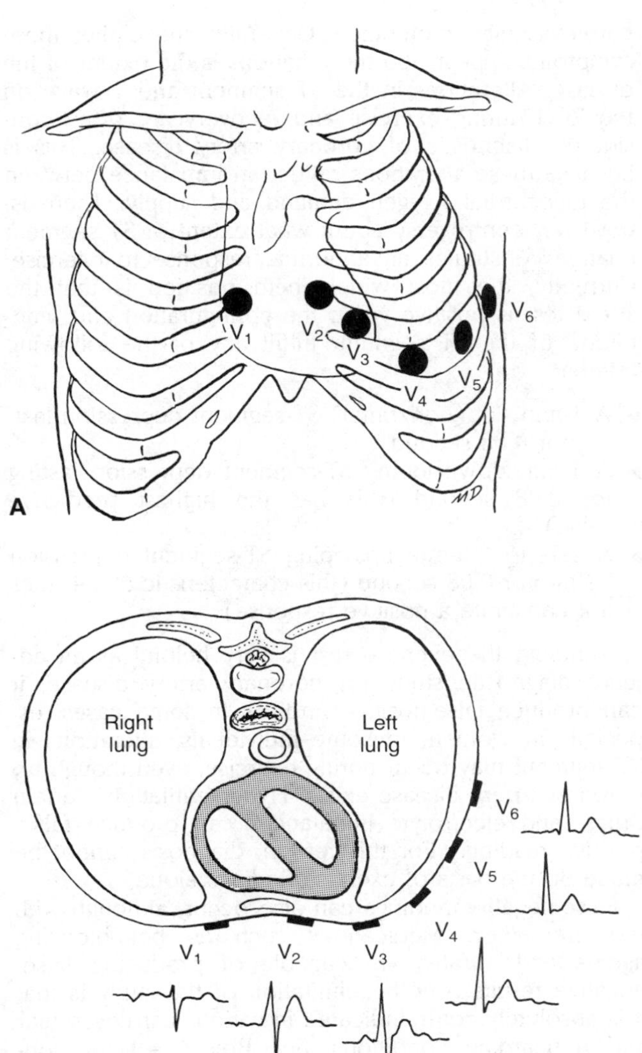

▲ **Figure 41-10**

Placement of chest (*V*) leads. *A*, Precordial (chest) lead placement. *B*, Normal ECG findings with corresponding chest leads to cross section at fourth rib level.

trodes: adhesive back, foam, cloth, plastic, and suction cups. In clients with an amputation, the electrodes are applied to the stump of the affected extremity. Note that the leg and arm electrodes must remain attached in order to obtain the precordial leads. Some ECG machines are able to record only one lead at a time, while others can record 3, 6, or all 12 leads simultaneously.

The nurse notes any unusual chest deformities, respiratory distress, or tremors that may account for alterations in the recording and whether the client experiences angina pectoris or chest discomfort at the time of the ECG.

Signal-Averaged ECG. A signal-averaged ECG is used to identify the presence of electrical impulses called late potentials. These impulses occur during diastole late into the QRS and ST segment. This noninvasive test may be done at the bedside and is used to predict which clients may be prone to ventricular tachycardia resulting in sudden death. In a signal-averaged ECG, a computer is used to record and process low-level signals that are not detected by a traditional ECG. This technique allows detection of signals that may otherwise be masked by noise that conceals the small electrical events of the heart. Late potentials are multiphasic, low-amplitude, high-frequency spikes that appear after the terminal portion of the QRS complex and extend into the ST segment. They are thought to be generated by delayed activation in an abnormal area of the heart. The presence of late potentials in patients with normal sinus rhythm identifies the risk for ventricular tachycardia and sudden cardiac death.[15]

Holter Monitoring. When the client wears a portable Holter monitor, an ECG tracing may be recorded continuously over a period of a day or longer on an outpatient basis. Whereas a standard ECG is obtained over a relatively short time period, Holter monitoring continues for an extended period. Thus, Holter monitoring is done to determine which dysrhythmias may be causing clinical manifestations that may not occur during a routine ECG but do occur when the client is ambulating at home or work. The monitoring system records at preset time intervals and when it senses an unusual event.

To prepare the client, the examiner places two to three electrodes on the chest and attaches them to the telemetry unit. This unit is not much larger than a beeper and is worn in a sling fashioned about the chest or waist. The client is encouraged to go about his or her daily activities as normal and keep a written account of these activities along with any symptoms that may develop. These data are extremely useful in documenting transient dysrhythmias and correlating the client's perceived symptoms to the underlying rhythm. Holter monitoring also helps clinicians evaluate the effectiveness of pacemaker and pharmacologic antiarrhythmic therapy.

Exercise ECG (Stress Testing). Exercise ECGs, referred to as stress testing, are valuable tools in detecting and evaluating coronary artery disease. Stress testing involves (1) using controlled and carefully supervised exercise to increase myocardial oxygen demands and (2) evaluating the coronary arteries' ability to meet the increased demands successfully. Its greatest advantage is that it provides information about the cardiovascular system in a dynamic state. A study of the heart during activity cannot be duplicated by the resting, recumbent position typically used in routine physical examination. Stress testing may be used in conjunction with myocardial radionuclide testing.

Exercise testing may have single or multiple stages. A single-stage test is one in which exercise workload is constant throughout. Multiple-stage testing involves increasing the exercise workload in increments until a desired point is reached. These incremental increases in workload may occur every 1 to 5 minutes. The duration of testing varies with the type of test being used and the client's tolerance for testing.

The two major modes of exercise used for stress testing in the United States are bicycle ergometry and treadmill. Bicycle ergometry uses a device equipped with a wheel operated by pedals that can be adjusted to increase the resistance to pedaling (multistage testing). It can be used for arm cranking, foot pedaling, or both. Bicycle ergometry has the advantage of being a relatively inexpensive test and portable. It does, however, require frequent recalibration and can induce localized muscle group fatigue.

Treadmill testing is the most commonly used mode of stress testing, especially when used in conjunction with thallium-201 imaging. The treadmill is a motorized device that has an adjustable conveyor belt able to reach speeds of 1.0 to 10 miles per hour. The conveyor belt can be adjusted from a horizontal position to a 20 per cent gradient, allowing the client to walk or run on slopes at all different angles.

Prior to stress testing, the nurse informs the client of the purposes and risks of exercise testing and obtains a signed consent for testing. The client must have a detailed physical examination before testing. In addition, the examiner must take a baseline, resting ECG immediately before testing begins. During the exercise test, the client's BP (using an automatically inflating cuff) and ECG are closely monitored by a physician or appropriately trained individual.

A multilead monitoring system is most often used to provide maximal views of the heart wall. The examiner makes frequent observations throughout testing for any untoward manifestation related to impaired cardiovascular performance. These symptoms include chest pain, ventricular arrhythmia, extreme dyspnea, claudication (leg pain due to peripheral vascular disease), vertigo, and a sudden drop in BP. Reasons for terminating the test are as follows:

- Chest pain or fatigue
- Greatly increased heart rate (age-related):

  20–29 years: 170 bpm
  30–39 years: 160 bpm
  40–49 years: 150 bpm
  50–59 years: 140 bpm
  60–69 years: 130 bpm

- Untoward signs and symptoms of myocardial ischemia or heart failure
- Failure of systolic BP to rise or a drop in BP (below resting levels)
- Sudden development of bradycardia
- Serious cardiac dysrhythmia
- Severe hypertension
- Severe dyspnea
- ST-segment depression (greater than 2 to 4 mm)
- A sudden loss of coordination (cerebral ischemia)

Because these symptoms occur with some frequency, an emergency cart containing cardiac drugs and resuscitation equipment is kept close at hand at all times. Clients rarely die from this procedure.

A positive exercise test is one that must be terminated before the predicted maximal (or submaximal) limits have been achieved owing to manifestations of cardiovascular intolerance. Generally, the earlier these symptoms appear, the more serious is the extent of the disease. Alterations in the ST segment and T wave on the ECG during exercise and recovery are often considered diagnostic of coronary artery disease. This is because these alterations reflect an imbalance between the myocardial oxygen demand and supply. There is, however, controversy about what extent of ST segment change constitutes an abnormal response to exercise. Currently, the most widely held position is that the stress test is positive when the configuration and magnitude of the ST segment fulfill any of the following criteria:

- A 1-mm flat (horizontal) ST-segment depression lasting for 0.08 second
- A 1-mm downsloping ST-segment depression lasting for 0.08 second (this has the highest predictive value)
- A 1.5- to 2.0-mm upsloping ST-segment depression lasting for 0.08 second (this characteristic alone does not constitute a positive response)

Although the exercise test is very helpful as an adjunct diagnostic study for coronary artery disease, it can produce false-positive findings in some cases, especially in women. In some individuals, alterations in ST segment may occur during exercise, even though no coronary artery disease exists. Hyperventilation, certain drugs, and electrolyte imbalances can produce false-positive readings. For this reason, diagnosis cannot be made on the basis of exercise findings alone.

False-negative findings can also occur, although with less frequency. Medications such as beta-blocking agents and nitrates are capable of producing false-negative results. Another limitation of the study is that it is absolutely contraindicated in various cardiovascular and noncardiac conditions. See Box 41–3 for contraindications to exercise testing.

Nurses need to be familiar with the stress testing procedure to provide clear teaching guidelines to clients scheduled to undergo exercise testing. Many clients harbor misconceptions and unnecessary fears about the procedure. Although the procedure is not painful, it can produce a great deal of fatigue. The nurse warns the client that this test may trigger chest pain and dyspnea. Along with this warning, the nurse points out that the procedure is performed in a controlled environment with prompt nursing and medical attention close at hand. It is very important that the client arrive for the exercise testing appointment relaxed and well rested. Teaching guidelines for stress testing are given in the Client Education Guide.

Electrophysiologic Studies

The electrophysiologic study is an invasive method of recording intracardiac electrical activity. It is used to shed light on the mechanisms of dysrhythmias, to differentiate between supraventricular and ventricular dysrhythmias, to evaluate sinoatrial (SA) or AV node dysfunction, to determine the need for a pacemaker, and

Box 41–3. Contraindications to Exercise Testing

Acute Cardiovascular Disease

Acute myocardial infarction (usually avoided in those individuals less than 2 weeks post-infarction)
Unstable angina pectoris
Heart failure
Pericarditis
Myocarditis
Endocarditis
Life-threatening dysrhythmias
Thrombophlebitis
Recent systemic embolus
Thrombophlebitis
Dissecting or enlarging aneurysm

Severe Diseases Restricting Mobility

Renal failure
Severe pulmonary disruptions
Orthopedic disorders affecting the spine or lower extremities
Neurologic impairment (e.g., stroke or paralysis)
Systemic infection

Left ventricular outflow obstruction (aortic stenosis, hypertension, or hypertrophic cardiomyopathy)

to evaluate the effect of anti-arrhythmic agents used to prevent the occurrence of tachycardias.

An electrophysiologic catheter has four electrodes at the distal tip that record or stimulate (pace). Under fluoroscopy, the catheter is threaded into the heart via the femoral, basilic, or subclavian vein. The catheter sites selected depend on the purpose of the examination. One catheter is left at the bundle of His just beneath the AV node as a point of reference. An additional catheter is introduced high in the right atrium. If Wolff-Parkinson-White syndrome is suspected, a catheter may be placed in the coronary sinus. A catheter may also be placed in the right ventricle. During mapping of ventricular tachycardia, a catheter may be introduced into the left ventricle via an artery.

The procedure is designed to reproduce any dysrhythmia so that its origin may be isolated. Ventricular tachycardia is induced by using programmed stimulation to fire an impulse at different times during the cardiac electrical cycle. If the dysrhythmia is induced, the person's BP and hemodynamic responses are observed. It is possible for arterial pressure, surface ECGs, and ECGs from intracavitary catheters to be recorded simultaneously. The morphology and rate of the induced tachycardia are compared with the morphology and rate of the patient's own spontaneous ventricular tachycardia. The ventricular tachycardia is often terminated by rapid ventricular decremental pacing. If the tachycardia cannot be stimulated, intravenous isoproterenol may be infused to simulate stress or exercise, which may produce the tachycardia.

Antiarrhythmic drugs may be administered during the study to evaluate their effect. After the initial anti-arrhythmic has been given, induction of ventricular tachycardia is attempted. If ventricular tachycardia is induced, the dosage may be increased or other drugs administered and the electrophysiologic studies are repeated in several days to determine the effectiveness of the anti-arrhythmic drug therapy.

Frequently when the irritable focus has been identified (e.g., accessory pathway or bundle of His), an ablation may be performed. Ablation of the irritable focus may be accomplished by the use of radiofrequency, direct current, ethyl alcohol, or cryosurgery. Radiofrequency ablation is the most popular method because its effect may be localized, with less damage to surrounding tissue.

Chest X-Ray Studies

The physician routinely orders posteroanterior, lateral, and oblique chest x-ray films to determine the size, silhouette, and position of the heart. In the acutely ill client, an anteroposterior x-ray film is taken at the bedside. Specific pathologic changes of the heart are difficult to determine on x-ray examination, but anatomic changes in the heart and pulmonary sequelae of various cardiac conditions can be seen. Valvular and pericardial calcifications; pulmonary congestion (from heart failure); pericardial effusion; and placement of central lines, endotracheal tubes, hemodynamic monitoring devices, and intra-aortic balloon catheters are all assessed on x-ray film.

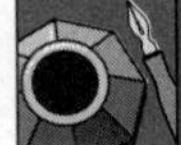

CLIENT EDUCATION GUIDE

Stress Testing

Get sufficient rest the night before the test.

- Avoid eating a heavy meal just prior to the test, although it is advisable to eat a light meal 1 to 2 hours before the test.
- Avoid smoking (if possible), alcohol, and beverages containing caffeine during the day of testing.
- Wear nonconstrictive, comfortable clothing and rubber-soled, supportive shoes during testing. Only a loose-fitting, front-buttoning shirt (or blouse) should be worn. (Women should wear a bra.)
- Continue all usual medications unless specified otherwise by the physician. (An inquiry about this should be made to the physician.)
- Following the test, rest and keep the physician informed of any lingering symptoms of cardiovascular distress, i.e., chest pain, shortness of breath, or dizziness.
- Avoid taking a hot shower for 1 to 2 hours following the test because this may potentiate hypotension, resulting in a fainting episode. If bathing is desired, use only tepid water.

Magnetic Resonance Imaging

Although magnetic resonance imaging (MRI) is the most expensive noninvasive diagnostic option, a variety of information may be obtained in a single image. MRI provides the best information on chamber size, wall motion, valvular function, and great vessel blood flow.[23] The MRI is commonly used for examination of the aorta, detection of tumors/masses, cardiomyopathies, and pericardial disease. In MRI, a strong magnetic field and radiowaves are used to detect and define the differences between healthy and diseased tissue. MRI is able to image over three spatial dimensions and over time. It can actually show the heart beating and the blood flowing in any direction. All standard quantitative functional indexes can be obtained from an MRI study with the exception of transstenotic gradients.

Information obtained from MRI includes

- Normal morphology and structural pathology;
- Wall thickness, chamber volumes, valve areas, vessel cross sections, and extent, location, and size of lesions;
- global and regional biventricular function, including ejection fractions, stroke volumes, and cardiac outputs;
- blood flow quantifications within vessels over the cardiac cycle; and
- tissue characterization of para- and intracardiac masses, pericardial effusions, and myocardial infarction.

The average length of the procedure ranges from 45 minutes to 1 hour. The client should remove all metal items such as watch, zippers, and eyeglasses prior to the procedure. Clients with pacemakers, prosthetic valves, or recently implanted clips or wires are not eligible for MRI scans. The nurse prepares the client for the fact that lying on the table inside the MRI is very confining and that the scanner makes a loud knocking noise. Any client who is claustrophobic may need sedation. The client may choose to wear mirrored glasses that allow visualization outside the magnet. A family member may remain in the room during the procedure if the client is particularly apprehensive.

Positron Emission Tomography

The positron emission tomographic (PET) scanner is a diagnostic imaging tool that allows visualization of regional physiologic function and images the biochemistry that often separates normal from diseased myocardium. Cellular metabolic information is obtained by mapping regional myocardial glucose metabolism. Combining information from the perfusion and the metabolism images provides a thorough assessment of regional cardiac viability.

Compounds found normally in the body are radiolabeled with cyclotron-produced isotopes of carbon, nitrogen, oxygen, or fluorine (a substitute for hydrogen). After infusion, the radiopharmaceuticals travel through the patient's bloodstream, serving as tracers of normal physiologic activity. These tracer isotopes have a very short half-life and deliver only a very low radiation dose. The circular array of scanning around the body detects these paired gamma rays, which are associated with positron decay events. A computer then reconstructs images of the radionuclide distribution within the body.

The scanner looks like a standard computed tomographic unit and is silent. The scanning procedure takes about 2 to 3 hours. An intravenous radiopharmaceutical, *(N)*-ammonia, is administered and a 20-minute bloodflow image is begun. Next an intravenous injection of 2-[18F]fluoro-2-deoxy-D-glucose follows. It takes this about 40 minutes to localize in the myocardium. Final uptake of this tracer is proportional to the glucose metabolic activity of myocardial cells and provides an excellent indication of regional tissue viability.

The following are clinical indications for PET scanner use:

- Detection of coronary artery disease
- Assessment of myocardial viability
- Assessment of progression of coronary artery stenosis
- Documentation of collateral coronary circulation
- Differentiation of ischemia and dilated cardiomyopathy

The terms "match" and "mismatch" describe the relationship between the perfusion and the metabolism study. A perfusion study that shows similarities between a perfusion study with poor blood flow and a metabolic study showing decreased glucose uptake of necrotic tissue is described as a "match." A perfusion study that shows poor blood flow and a metabolic study that shows only stunned viable myocardium that has survived the initial insult is described as a "mismatch."

Echocardiography

The echocardiogram, a noninvasive diagnostic procedure based on the principles of ultrasound, is used to evaluate structural and functional changes in a wide variety of heart ailments. It is one of the mainstays of diagnostic cardiology because it is totally noninvasive, can be used at the bedside, and provides accurate information at no risk to the client.

An echocardiogram is performed by placing a transducer on several areas of the chest wall. This transducer emits short pulses of high-frequency sound through the chest wall and heart. Wave pulses bounce off tissues of varying densities and are reflected back to the transducer as a series of echoes, thus creating an image via an oscilloscope graph. The bursts of ultrasound are directed at the part of the heart under investigation. The echocardiogram records the structure and motion of that area in relation to its distance from the anterior chest wall (Fig. 41–11). An electrocardiogram

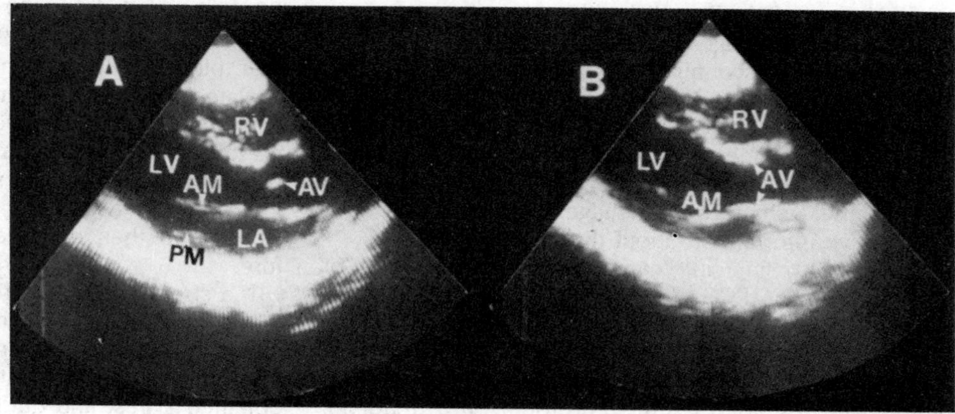

▲ *Figure 41–11*

Long-axis cross-sectional echocardiographic images of the left ventricle (LV), right ventricle (RV), mitral valve, aortic valve, and left atrium (LA) during diastole *(A)* and systole *(B)*. During diastole, the anterior (AM) and posterior (PM) mitral leaflets are apart and the aortic valve leaflets (AV) come together as a single echo in the midportion of the aorta *(A)*. With systole, *(B)* the mitral leaflets come together and the aortic valve leaflets separate. (From Braunwald, E. [1992]. *Heart disease,* [4th ed., p. 67]. Philadelphia, W. B. Saunders, p. 67.)

is recorded simultaneously on the graph. Two-dimensional echocardiography generates a continuous picture of the beating heart. These images are recorded on videotape for analysis.

Echocardiograms are used to help assess and diagnose pericardial effusion, cardiomyopathy, valvular disorders (including prosthetic valves), cardiac shunts, myocardial ischemia, chamber size, left ventricular function, ventricular aneurysms, and cardiac tumors (atrial myxoma). In addition, they are very useful during heart biopsies because the physician can view the heart on a monitor while taking tissue samples.

Nursing intervention for clients undergoing echocardiography involves explaining the procedure and reassuring the client that the study is noninvasive, painless, and without complication. An echocardiogram can be performed at the bedside, although it is preferrable to send the client to the echocardiography laboratory.

Transesophageal Echocardiography

Transesophageal echocardiography (TEE) gives a higher quality picture of the heart than does a regular echocardiogram. It is especially useful in clients who have thickened lung tissue or thick chest walls or are obese. The procedure may also be used intraoperatively where conventional echocardiography is ineffective. The client needs to be in bed or on a table with ECG leads attached. ECG and BP are monitored. The throat is anesthetized and sedation is given. An esophageal scope is inserted through the mouth and passed into the esophagus by the physician. Because the probe is placed behind the heart, it allows the left atrium to be viewed. TEE allows clearer visibility of the heart and its structures and is most useful in diagnosis of cardiac masses, prosthetic valve function, and aneurysm.

The procedure lasts approximately 15 minutes to 1 hour. No food or liquids should be taken or 8 to 10 hours before the procedure. The client is not to eat or drink anything following the procedure for at least 2 hours or until the effects of the anesthetic wear off.

Phonocardiography

Phonograms are recordings of audible vibrations coming from the heart and great vessels. Phonograms are used to assist in diagnosing the timing of cardiac sounds and murmurs. Microphones are placed under elastic straps, usually at the base and apex of the heart. No preparation is required for this assessment.

Myocardial Scintigraphy

Myocardial function, motion, and perfusion may be studied by a method called scintigraphy, which involves the intravenous injection of a radioactive isotope. As the isotope is absorbed by the blood cells of the heart muscle, photons are emitted. These photons are detected by an external gamma camera, which produces a radionuclide image. Because these nuclear imaging techniques are relatively noninvasive, they are frequently used diagnostic tools.

Thallium-201 Scintigraphy. Thallium-201 is the most widely used isotope for myocardial perfusion due to its short (73 hours) half-life and low total body radiation dose. Thallium-201 is a radioactive analogue of potassium, which is easily extracted by smooth skeletal and cardiac muscle fibers that possess the potassium active-transport system. Eighty-eight per cent of blood-borne thallium-201 is taken up on its first pass through the heart. The amount of thallium-201 found in the myocardium after an intravenous injection depends on the regional myocardial perfusion and the efficiency of cellular extraction. Regional perfusion is dependent on coronary artery patency. Areas of the myocardium that receive less blood flow also receive less thallium.

A high concentration of thallium-201 is present in well-perfused cells, and a lower concentration remains in the blood, setting up a concentration gradient for the diffusion of thallium-201. Infarcted or scarred myocardium does not extract any thallium-201, showing up as "cold spots." If the defective area is ischemic, the cold spots fill in or become "warm" on the delayed images. Infarcts continue to appear cold with little or no perfusion of thallium-201 either during a stress test or with delayed images.

The perfusion scanning is performed with a special camera that is capable of showing the source of emitted low-energy photons on a screen. Each photon detected by the camera is recorded on film and a computer screen over a half-hour period. The computer refines and enhances the images and then provides quantitative information about the myocardial walls.

Thallium-201 imaging can be performed before or after an exercise ECG study or as a resting study only. Ischemic myocardium may show up on a resting thallium-201 study. Two sets of images are taken 3 hours apart and compared. The thallium-201 stress test begins with a graded exercise protocol on a treadmill. The client has a slow infusion of intravenous normal saline. The ECG is monitored continuously. About 1 minute before the peak of the stress test, thallium-201 is injected intravenously. The client should exercise for the last minute to ensure thallium-201 distribution to the heart during 85 per cent maximum stress. The client then cools down and reclines on an examination table for the perfusion scan. Continuous imaging in a 180-degree arc over the chest is obtained. The client then waits for 3 hours and returns for repeat films. Before the delayed images are obtained, the client receives additional thallium-201 by intravenous injection. The two sets of images are then carefully compared.

Persantine Thallium-201 Test. This test may be used as an alternative to standard treadmill exercise when the client is not able to achieve a vigorous level of exercise. Persantine (dipyridamole) serves as a pharmacologic stress agent. It is given intravenously to dilate the coronary arteries, which would normally dilate during the stress of exercise. Arteries that are narrowed as a result of coronary artery disease do not expand as much as normal arteries. Infusion of Persantine for 5 minutes is followed by an injection of thallium-201. Thallium-201 travels easily through normal arteries that have dilated and travels less freely through narrowed arteries. At 7 minutes, images are taken.

Any form of caffeine as well as medications for asthma, such as theophylline or aminophylline, should be omitted prior to this test. Aminophylline is the antagonist to Persantine and may be given slowly intravenously to reverse any adverse side effects.

Technetium-99m Ventriculography (Gated Blood Pool Imaging or "MUGA"). This test studies the motion of the left ventricle wall and measures the ventricle's ability to eject blood (ejection fraction). If a coronary artery is narrowed, causing ischemia, the segment of the myocardium it serves exhibits diminished wall motion or contractility. In addition, hemodynamic changes may be measured by observing the actual filling and emptying of the cardiac chambers. Changes in cardiac output as well as ejection fraction may be obtained. Gated blood pool images represent the blood pool within the ventricular and atrial chambers.

Intravenous stannous pyrophosphate (PYP) is given to allow the red blood cells to tag onto the technetium-99m. Approximately 20 minutes after the PYP is injected, the technetium-99m is injected. The client is then placed on a heart monitor and images are begun.

Gated blood pool scans use counts from any one of a number of consecutive beats. Multiple serial images are obtained using a gamma camera. The cardiac cycle is broken into intervals, with counts taken during these intervals for a number of beats. These counts are stored and then displayed in a weighted average picture.

If a stress gated blood pool study is to be performed, the client is put on a bicycle ergometer with a gamma camera positioned to project the right and left blood pools. The ECG is monitored continuously. Images are obtained at rest and during each stage of exercise.

First-Pass Cardiac Study. During a first-pass study, a single intravenous injection of technetium-99m is administered intravenously and traced as it passes through the heart. Only the initial pass of the technetium-99m is recorded as it passes through the cardiac chambers. Ejection fraction and information about ventricular wall motion are obtained. A first-pass study may be performed during exercise or rest.

NURSING RESPONSIBILITIES FOR MYOCARDIAL SCINTIGRAPHY

1. Ask female clients if they are pregnant or suspect pregnancy, because these studies involve radiation exposure (although minimal).
2. Explain the purpose of the procedure to the client and tell him or her what to expect during the procedure. Explain that electrodes will be placed on the chest and an intravenous line will be inserted for the administration of the radioisotope. Generally, total exposure to radiation during these scans is less than or equal to that of one chest x-ray study.
3. Instruct the client to wear walking shoes if exercise on the treadmill or bicycle is anticipated.
4. Encourage the client to notify the nurse or technologist of any signs of ischemia (chest pain) during or after the procedure.
5. Follow the diet protocol of the institution. Some tests may require fasting. A light meal is preferred over a heavy meal if the scan will be taken during exercise. This prevents nausea and stomach cramping during exercise and allows for better uptake of the radioisotope.
6. Check the physician's orders for omission of any medications. Usually beta-blockers, calcium channel blockers, and xanthines are prohibited prior to the procedure.

Cardiac Catheterization

This complex procedure involves the insertion of a catheter into the heart and surrounding vessels to obtain detailed information about the structure and performance of the heart, valves, and circulatory system. Specifically, cardiac catheterization is performed to:

- Confirm a diagnosis of heart disease and to determine the extent to which the disease has affected the structure and function of the heart (Fig. 41-12).
- Determine congenital abnormalities.
- Obtain a clear picture of cardiac anatomy prior to heart surgery.
- Obtain pressures within the heart chambers and the great vessels (aorta and pulmonary artery).
- Measure blood oxygen concentration, tension, and saturation within the heart chambers.
- Determine cardiac output.
- Perform angiography for better coronary artery visualization.
- Obtain endocardial biopsies.
- Allow infusion of fibrinolytic agents directly into an occluded coronary artery in the hope that coronary blood flow may be restored.

Cardiac catheterization is usually performed in the controlled environment of a cardiac catheterization laboratory. Typically, only one side of the heart is catheterized, although it is sometimes necessary to insert the catheter into both sides of the heart.

Right-Sided Catheterization. For a right-sided cardiac catheterization, the physician inserts a sterile, radiopaque catheter through the antecubital or femoral vein. Under fluoroscopic guidance, the catheter is advanced slowly to the right atrium and right ventricle and is finally wedged in a small branch of the pulmonary artery. Clinicians continuously monitor the ECG during the procedure. Premature ventricular contractions may occur as the catheter is being passed through the ventricles. If they occur frequently, cardiac output falls, and the physician may need to withdraw the catheter temporarily or order administration of lidocaine (an antiarrhythmic).

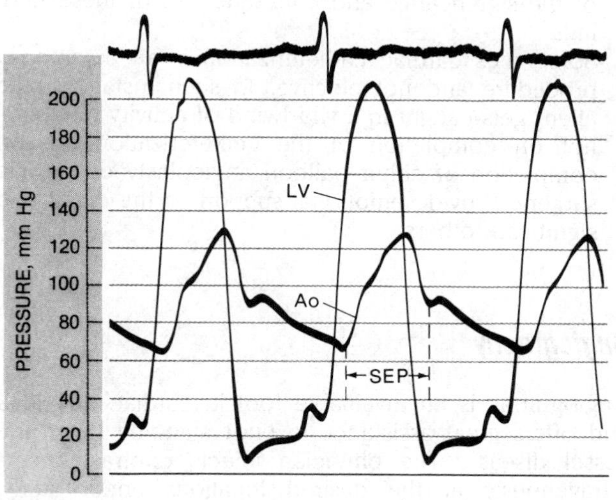

▲ *Figure 41-12*

Left ventricular (LV) and aortic (Ao) pressure tracings in aortic stenosis. During systole, there is a large pressure gradient between LV and Ao, and the rate of rise of the aortic pressure is slow. The systolic ejection period (SEP) is the period of time in each cycle during which blood is being ejected from the left ventricle into the aorta. The vertical time lines are 1 second apart. (From Grossman, W.: Profiles in valvular heart disease. In W. Grossman and D. S. Baim [Eds.], *Cardiac catheterization, angiography, and intervention* (4th ed.). Philadelphia, Lea and Febiger, 1991.)

Left-Sided Catheterization. This procedure is far more difficult to perform than right-sided catheterization. There are two major methods of catheter introduction: (1) The catheter can be passed retrograde (backwards) from the brachial or femoral artery into the aorta and then to the left ventricle, or (2) rarely during right-sided catheterization, the middle or lower third of the atrial septum is punctured and the catheter is passed transseptally into the left atrium.

As the catheter is passed through the venous or arterial system and into various heart chambers, the desired studies are performed. The catheter has several end or side holes that allow blood withdrawal for oxygen analysis from the various cardiac chambers. Pressures can be obtained by attaching the catheter to a transducer with its connecting amplifier and recording device. Radiopaque contrast materials and indicator solutions can be injected via the catheter into the left ventricle to examine the mitral valve, the left ventricular outflow tract, wall motion and thickness, left ventricular end diastolic volume, and ejection fraction.[7]

COMPLICATIONS

Although cardiac catheterization has become a safer and more useful diagnostic tool in recent years, it is far from innocuous and has inherent complications. Most complications are related to the puncture site. Clot formation during catheterization is prevented by administering moderate amounts of anticoagulant (usually 4000 to 5000 U of heparin), which increases the risk of bleeding at the insertion site or into the retroperitoneal area. In addition, trauma from arterial cannulation may potentiate vasospasm or clot formation, causing temporary or permanent arterial occlusion to the affected extremity. Dysrhythmias frequently develop during catheterization owing to direct catheter stimulation of the atrium and ventricle. In addition, the client may experience anginal pain. Pain occurs when contrast dye replaces the blood flowing through the coronary arteries under study. Lack of blood flow causes a painful regional cardiac hypoxia. Occasionally, clients may have an allergic reaction to the iodine-based contrast media. Allergic symptoms include flushing, nausea and vomiting, tingling and numbness, weakness, and urticaria. Fortunately, anaphylactic shock is rare. Osmotic diuresis following injection of the hypertonic radiographic contrast agents can produce significant dehydration. Finally, myocardial and aortic perforations are rare but potentially deadly complications of cardiac catheterization.

NURSING ASSESSMENT AND INTERVENTION

Prior to cardiac catheterization, the client must be physically and emotionally prepared. Cardiac catheterization is both an important and frightening procedure. Major steps in preparing the person are as follows:

1. Explain the procedure, its purpose, and its hazards to the client.
2. Explain that the procedure will be carried out in a special cardiac catheterization room and that the client will be lying on an x-ray examination table with ECG leads attached to the extremities. The physician and cardiac nurses will be wearing scrub gowns and masks and the room will be darkened at some point to take x-ray films.
3. Tell the client that there is little or no pain associated with the procedure, because a local anesthetic is used to numb the catheter insertion site. However, the client may feel fatigue and various aches, because it will be necessary to lie quietly for up to 2 hours on a hard table. The client may also, at times, experience certain sensations: a fluttery feeling as the catheter passes through the heart; a flushed, warm feeling when the dye is injected; a strong desire to cough (with right heart angiography); and palpitations due to transient heart irritability. The client should also be forewarned about the sound made by the x-ray apparatus during the procedure.
4. Have the client sign a consent for the procedure after the client has been carefully informed and questions have been answered satisfactorily.
5. Ask if there is any history of allergies, particularly to iodine-containing substances or shellfish. The physician may order a skin test with an iodine-containing solution the day before the procedure.
6. Withhold solid food for 6 to 8 hours and liquids for at least 4 hours prior to the procedure to prevent vomiting and aspiration.
7. Be sure that the client's height and weight are recorded in the chart. This is needed for calculating the amount of dye that will be administered.
8. Mark the peripheral pulses distal to the probable cannulation sites with a felt-tipped pen and record the quality of the pulses in the chart. This will aid in locating the pulses after the procedure. Pulses are checked at this time for post-procedure comparisons and to detect possible occlusion of the vessel that will be undergoing cannulation.
9. Administer the prescribed medications (often a sedative and, sometimes, an antibiotic). The insertion site may be prepared by shaving and cleansing it with an antiseptic solution.
10. Insert an intravenous line.

Following cardiac catheterization, assessment, prevention, and early detection of complications are the primary goals. Post-catheterization care varies, depending on the institution, but the following are basic points:

1. Assess vital signs every 30 minutes for 2 hours initially and then less frequently, as specified by the institution policy.
2. Keep the extremity in which catheter insertion occurred straight for 4 to 6 hours after the procedure. If the antecubital vessel was used, immobilize the arm on an armboard. If the femoral artery was used, enforce strict bed rest for 6 to 12 hours following the procedure. The client may turn from side to side. However, to keep the leg straight at the groin and prevent arterial occlusion, do not elevate the head of the bed more than 15 degrees.
3. Check the pressure dressing over the puncture site for intactness and for evidence of bleeding. Occasionally a sandbag is applied to the insertion site for 4 to 6 hours. Monitor the site for hematoma formation and ask the client about the presence of increasing pain or tenderness.
4. Check the pulses, color, warmth, and sensation of the extremity distal to the insertion site every 30 minutes during the first hour and then as specified by health care facility policy. Notify the physician at once if the client experiences numbness or tingling. Also note if the extremity becomes cool, pale, or cyanotic or if sudden loss of peripheral pulses occurs. These manifestations represent serious impairment of circulation.
5. Monitor cardiac rhythm for the occurrence of dysrhythmias. Also assess the client for chest pain. If either is found, notify the physician and intervene per ordered protocols.
6. Encourage fluid intake (if the underlying condition allows) for adequate fluid replacement and renal elimination of the contrast.
7. Observe for nausea, vomiting, rash development, and other signs of hypersensitivity to the contrast.
8. Because the procedure is lengthy as well as a psychological drain on the client, institute supportive measures to promote comfort. Whatever the findings of the procedure, the client needs clear explanations of the significance and consequences of these findings.
9. Sometimes cardiac catheterization is an emergency procedure and not elective. In such instances, the client gets caught in a whirlwind of activity that ends not on completion of the catheterization but on completion of either balloon angioplasty or cardiac surgery. Provide emotional support to the client and significant others.

Angiography

Angiography is an invaluable tool in cardiac diagnosis and offers great assistance in understanding heart and vessel disease. The physician injects contrast agents intravenously at the desired locations under study. These contrast materials, which are usually iodinated water-soluble compounds, are given in doses determined by the client's weight.

Angiocardiography is the intravenous injection of contrast into the heart during cardiac catheterization. Immediately after the contrast is injected, a series of x-ray films are taken that reveal the course of the contrast as it circulates through the heart, lungs, and great vessels.

Cineangiography involves taking moving pictures during cardiac catheterization. This is particularly valuable because the examiners can view the film at both rapid and slow speeds, permitting detailed and unlimited review of the study.

Coronary angiography refers to the injection of contrast directly into the coronary arteries (via the coronary ostia) during cardiac catheterization. Table 41-3 outlines the various forms of angiocardiography.

Hemodynamic Studies

Four important parameters are used to assess hemodynamic status: CVP, pulmonary artery (PA) pressure, cardiac output, and intra-arterial pressure. All of these parameters require invasive procedures. Critical care nurses perform all of these routinely at the bedside. Hemodynamic studies provide a wealth of information reflecting the earliest changes in the circulatory system that are not yet clinically detectable.

The monitoring of hemodynamic pressures provides information about blood volume, fluid balance, and how well the heart is pumping. Current technology allows us to measure right atrial pressure (CVP), PA pressures during systole and diastole (reflecting right and left ventricular pressures), and pulmonary capillary wedge pressure (PCWP) (a direct indicator of left ventricular pressure).

The Pulmonary Artery Catheter. Development of the balloon-tipped, flow-directed catheter has enabled continuous direct monitoring of PA pressure.

The most commonly used PA flow-directed catheter is the Swan-Ganz catheter (see Bridge to Critical Care). This catheter has four lumens. The proximal lumen terminates in the right atrium, allowing CVP measurement, fluid infusion, and venous access for blood samples. The distal lumen terminates in the PA and measures PA systolic pressure, PA diastolic pressure, PA mean pressure, and PCWP. There is a small lumen that is used for inflation and deflation of the balloon. The fourth lumen is the thermistor port and permits the measurement of cardiac output. In addition, some catheters have an additional port for the infusion of fluids and capabilities for cardiac pacing and measuring of the oxygen saturation of the blood. Five-lumen catheters also exist.

TABLE 41-3. Major Types of Angiocardiography

Angiocardiography Procedure	Method Employed
Right-sided angiocardiography	Contrast medium is injected into the right heart chambers and pulmonary artery by means of a catheter threaded up a vein and into the heart during cardiac catheterization.
Left-sided angiocardiography	Contrast medium is injected into the left side of the heart through a transvenous catheter passed through the atrial septum during cardiac catheterization or via a catheter passed retrograde through an artery into the left heart.
Selective coronary artery angiocardiography	Contrast medium is injected directly into the ostium of each coronary artery via a catheter that is placed retrograde through an artery into the aorta.

Inserting the Catheter. Insertion of a Swan-Ganz catheter is not risk free for the client. The potential complications of the catheter are PA infarction, pulmonary embolism, injury to the heart valves, and injury to the myocardium. In addition, while the catheter is in place, the heart valves have less ability to close completely.

PA monitoring must be carried out in a critical care unit under careful scrutiny of an experienced nursing staff. Prior to insertion of the catheter, the nurse should explain to the client that (1) the procedure may be uncomfortable but not painful, and (2) a local anesthetic will be given at the catheter insertion site. The nurse's support of the critically ill client at this time helps promote cooperation and lessens the client's anxiety.

Using sterile technique, the physician inserts the PA flow-directed catheter at the bedside via percutaneous puncture of the brachial, subclavian, jugular, or femoral vein. The catheter has been previously flushed with heparinized solution and attached to pressure tubing, which in turn is connected to a transducer. The transducer monitors pressure fluctuations at the catheter tip and converts them to electrical signals, resulting in a digital and wave-form readout on an oscilloscope (monitor). Once in the vein, the catheter is advanced into the right atrium. The balloon is then inflated. Inflation of the balloon facilitates propulsion of the catheter through the heart and provides a cushion at the catheter tip that helps prevent ventricular irritability upon contact.

The inflated balloon follows the direction of blood flow through the right ventricle into the pulmonary artery, where it finally wedges in the right or left branch of the pulmonary artery. Clinicians can follow the path of the balloon by observing wave forms and pressure readings on the monitor (see Bridge to Critical Care).

When wedged, the catheter is "pointing" indirectly at the left end-diastolic pressure. The inflation of the balloon (wedging) blocks blood flow from the right heart in that vessel so that the PCWP is not influenced by existing pressure within the PA. Elevations in PCWP (greater than 18 to 20 mm Hg) therefore indicate increased left ventricular pressure, as seen in left ventricular failure, and they may coincide with onset of pulmonary congestion. Pressures climbing to more than 30 mm Hg generally herald the onset of pulmonary edema. Conversely, low PCWP suggests insufficient volume and pressure in the left ventricle, as seen in hypovolemic shock. Pressure changes commonly related to

BRIDGE TO CRITICAL CARE

Swan-Ganz Monitoring

Positioning the Swan-Ganz Catheter

Measuring Cardiac Output by Thermodilution

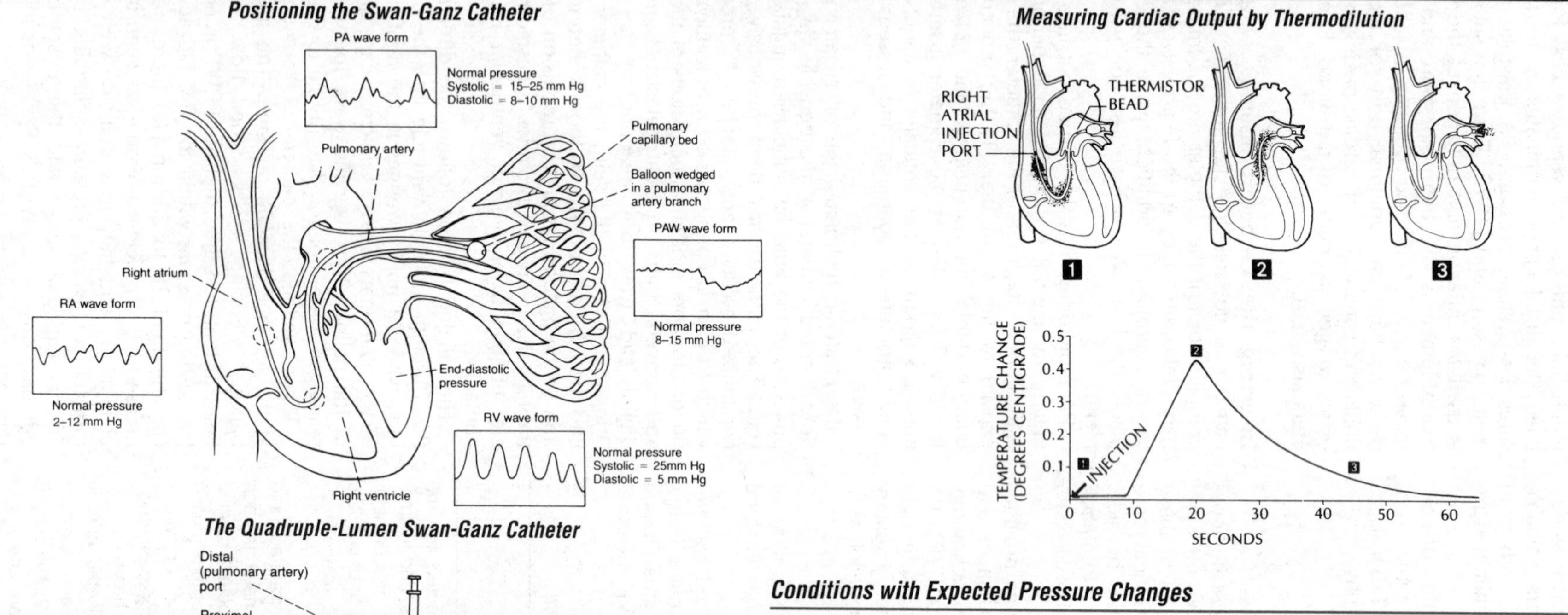

The Quadruple-Lumen Swan-Ganz Catheter

Conditions with Expected Pressure Changes

Condition	Pressure Changes* RA	RV	PAP	PAWP	
Heart failure (volume overload)	↑	↑	↑	↑	
Hypovolemia	↓	↓	↓	↓	
Cardiogenic shock†	— or ↑	— or ↑	— or ↑	— or ↑	(Diastolic)
Pulmonary hypertension	↑	↑	↑	— or ↑	
Cardiac tamponade	↑	↑	↑	↑	(Diastolic)
Pulmonary emboli	↑	↑	↑	↑	(Systolic)
Mitral valve stenosis/insufficiency‡	↑	↑	↑	↑	

*RA, right atrial pressure; RV, right ventricular pressure; PAP, pulomonary artery pressure; PAWP, pulmonary artery wedge pressure.

†Pressure readings depend on the heart's ability to handle circulating volume. Chronic lung disease elevates all readings.

‡Mitral valve disease produces unreliable pressure readings.

various cardiac conditions are discussed in the Bridge to Critical Care.

Obtaining Measurements. The nurse takes PA and PCWP measurements at routine intervals with the client in a supine position and the head of the bed at an angle of no more than 25 degrees. The transducer is kept at the level of the right atrium. Also, measurements should be taken on end expiration, especially if the client is on a mechanical ventilator.

Measurements of the PA systolic and diastolic pressures are taken with the balloon deflated. PA systolic pressure indicates the peak pressure generated by the right ventricle. PA diastolic pressure indicates the lowest pressure in the pulmonary artery. Mean PA pressure is an average of the systolic and diastolic pressures. The normal adult PA systolic and diastolic pressure is 20 to 30/10 mm Hg.

The balloon is inflated to measure PCWP. PCWP reflects the pressure in the distal branches of the PA, thus estimating pressures within the left atrium or the end-diastolic pressure in the left ventricle. The normal PCWP is 8 to 13 mm Hg. The only time the balloon should be inflated after it is in place is to obtain further PCWP readings. Leaving the catheter in a wedged position can lead to infarction of the lung tissue being supplied by that vessel. A fixed-wedge wave form requires immediate notification of the physician for repositioning of the catheter. From the PCWP, the function of the left ventricle is known. The client can be given fluids, inotropic agents, or other treatments to support and improve peripheral circulation.

Obtaining Blood Samples. The PA catheter also provides a means of readily obtaining samples of mixed venous blood from the PA. Mixed venous blood refers to blood from both the inferior and superior vena cava and the coronary veins. The normal oxygen saturation of mixed venous blood is 75 per cent, whereas the normal oxygen saturation for arterial blood is 95 per cent. The difference between the arterial and venous oxygen saturation signifies the amount of oxygen extracted by the tissues of the body. In heart failure, the oxygen saturation of mixed venous blood may fall considerably, even though the arterial oxygen saturation may remain the same. This indicates that less blood is reaching the tissues owing to a decrease in the cardiac output. Therefore, more oxygen is extracted in the periphery to compensate for the decreased blood flow.

CENTRAL VENOUS PRESSURE

CVP is the pressure within the superior vena cava, reflecting the pressure under which the blood is returned to the superior vena cava and right atrium. CVP is determined by vascular tone, blood volume, and the ability of the right heart to receive and pump blood. When the tricuspid valve is open at the end of diastole, the atrium and ventricle are, in effect, one chamber. At this time, the CVP is equal to the pressure in the right ventricle and is a good indicator of right ventricular function (Table 41-4).

CVP can also be seen as a measurement of preload on the right side of the heart. Preload is the amount of blood presented to the heart, or when the ventricle is full prior to the next ejection. Preload is the right ventricular end diastolic pressure. (Preload is also discussed in Chapter 42).

CVP can be measured with a central venous line placed in the superior vena cava or a balloon flotation catheter in the PA. Normal CVP pressure is 2 to 12 mm Hg. A drop in CVP pressure indicates a decrease in circulating volume, which may result from fluid imbalance, hemorrhage, or severe vasodilation and pooling of blood in the extremities with limited venous return. A rise in CVP indicates an increase in blood volume due to a sudden shift in fluid balance, excessive intravenous fluid infusion, renal failure, or sodium and water retention.

For an accurate CVP measurement, a baseline must be established for the transducer position. The zero point on the transducer needs to be at the level of the right atrium. The right atrium is located at the midaxillary line at the fourth intercostal space. The client should be supine and flat in bed for the most accurate reading.

If the client has orthopnea or another condition that prohibits lying flat or supine, a CVP reading can be obtained by placing the client in a 45-degree position and the zero point of the transducer adjusted to the

TABLE 41-4. Indications for Central Venous Pressure (CVP) and How They May Affect the Readings

To Assess	↑ CVP (>11 cm H_2O)	↓ CVP (<3 cm H_2O)
Right-sided heart hemodynamics	Right heart failure (including chronic CHF, LVF) Constrictive pericarditis Cardiac tamponade Valvular stenosis Pulmonary hypertension	Early LVF
Blood volume	↑ Circulating volume	↓ Circulating volume
Vascular tone	Vasoconstriction Hypertension	Vasodilation/peripheral pooling Septic shock

Note. CHF, congestive heart failure; LVF, left ventricular failure.
From Huang, S. H., et al. (1989). *Coronary care nursing* (2nd ed., p. 101). Philadelphia: W. B. Saunders Company.

level of the right atrium. To obtain a comparison of the data, the nurse must be certain with any CVP reading that the client is in the same position as he or she was for previous measurements.

In measuring CVP, the nurse makes certain that the client is relaxed at the time of the measurement. Straining, coughing, or any other activity that increases the intrathoracic pressure causes falsely high measurements. If the CVP is measured while the client is on a ventilator, the readings should always be taken at the point of end expiration for greatest accuracy.

The connections between the catheter and the attachments must be checked frequently to make certain that they are secure (in order to prevent air embolism). The dressing at the insertion site is changed according to health care facility policy to prevent infection. Complications of the procedure include pneumothorax, phlebitis, air emboli, pulmonary emboli, fluid overload, dysrhythmia, sepsis, and microelectric shock.

In order to maintain patency of the system, a small amount of heparinized fluid is delivered under pressure at a constant rate of flow.

PULMONARY ARTERY PRESSURE

The CVP is not a satisfactory means of determining the status of left-sided heart function, especially in critically ill persons, e.g., those who are immediately recovering from cardiac surgery, have experienced myocardial infarction, have cardiomyopathy, or are in cardiogenic shock. Significant changes can occur in the left side of the heart without being reflected for some time in the right side of the heart. This can lead to a delay in intervention or even inappropriate intervention.

During diastole, blood flows freely from the PA through the pulmonary capillaries, left atrium, and open mitral valve to the left ventricle. Therefore, the pressure in the left ventricle at the end of diastole approximates the diastolic pressure in the PA, pulmonary capillaries, and left atrium.

Starling's principle tells us that the heart muscle contracts most effectively when under slight stretch. PA pressure measurements can assist in determining whether the ventricle is understretched and the client needs fluids, overstretched and the client needs diuretics, or appropriately stretched and at maximum function.

CARDIAC OUTPUT MEASUREMENT

As detailed in Chapter 40, cardiac output is the amount of blood pumped out of the left ventricle into the arterial system every minute: i.e., cardiac output is equal to the stroke volume (volume of blood pumped out with each beat) multiplied by the heart rate. Therefore, if the stroke volume of the left ventricle is between 50 and 90 ml (average, 70 ml), and the heart rate is 80 bpm, the normal cardiac output of the left ventricle is roughly between 4 and 8 L. Table 41–5 lists the conditions that change cardiac output. The cardiac output of the right ventricle is considered equal to that of the left. This is because the right ventricle,

TABLE 41–5. Conditions That Cause a Change in Cardiac Output

Conditions That Decrease Cardiac Output	Conditions That Increase Cardiac Output
Acute congestive heart failure	Hypoxia
Pericarditis with effusion	Hyperthyroidism
Old age	Excitement
Arterial hemorrhage	Exercise
Standing motionless, which decreases the venous return to the heart	Food intake
	Oral and intravenous fluid intake
Myxedema	Early stage of septic shock
Shock	Pregnancy
Valvular heart disease	
Myocardial ischemia	
Dysrhythmias	
Paroxysmal atrial tachycardia (PAT)	
Atrial fibrillation	
Heart block	
Ventricular tachycardia	
Heat stroke	

although not as muscular as the left ventricle, pumps against less resistance.

Currently, the most common method for determining cardiac output is thermodilution. This method requires a cardiac output computer and a quadruple-lumen PA catheter and can be obtained by the nurse at bedside. One lumen terminates in a right atrial injection port, and another lumen terminates in a temperature electrode (thermistor) bead. A known amount of iced or room-temperature solution (saline or 5 per cent dextrose in water) is rapidly injected into the right atrial port. The cool injectate mixes with blood in the right atrium, quickly dropping the "mixed blood" temperature. This mixture travels with the flow of blood, and the change in blood temperature is detected by the thermistor bead at the distal end of the catheter in the PA and recorded as a time-temperature curve in the computer. The area under this curve is used to calculate cardiac output. Three to five cardiac output measurements are obtained and averaged to calculate cardiac output.

Normal cardiac output in adults ranges widely from 4 to 8 L/min. However, these values do not take into account individual needs, which vary according to body size. To compensate for size differences, the nurse often calculates a cardiac index (CI). The CI is determined by dividing cardiac output (CO) by body surface area (BSA). Using the client's height and weight, the BSA may be calculated on the DuBois Body Surface Chart. Normal CI for a person at rest is 2.5 to 4 L/min/m^2.

INTRA-ARTERIAL PRESSURE MONITORING

Systemic intra-arterial monitoring has become a common method for obtaining BP measurements in the acutely ill individual. This method provides continuous detection of arterial BP via an indwelling catheter. It is of greatest benefit in the client with low cardiac output, fluctuating hemodynamic status, and excessive peripheral vasoconstriction and in whom cuff BP measurements are undetectable or unreliable. (Note that intra-arterial pressure readings are at least 10 mm Hg higher than cuff BP readings.) The intra-arterial line offers one other advantage: it simplifies obtaining blood samples for arterial blood gas and blood studies, minimizing the need for arterial or venous punctures.

The physician introduces a short, nonreactive Teflon catheter into an artery (radial, brachial, axillary, femoral, or even the dorsalis pedis) using sterile technique.

Prior to catheter insertion, the examiner must assess the adequacy of circulation in the chosen extremity. If the radial artery is chosen as the site for insertion, the physician evaluates blood flow to the hand by performing an Allen test. The examiner first instructs the person to hold out the hand, then checks for obstruction of the ulnar artery by placing one thumb lightly over the radial artery and one thumb over the ulnar artery. The client is then instructed to make a tight fist for 1 minute. After 1 minute, the client is directed to open the hand and extend the fingers. The examiner releases the pressure over the ulnar artery. If the fingers become pink rapidly (within 6 seconds), adequate ulnar circulation exists. If pallor of the hand persists, the examiner should suspect ulnar artery obstruction, and thus not perform cannulation of the radial artery. Radial artery patency may be checked in the same method, but by releasing pressure over the radial, rather than ulnar, artery.

The major complications of intra-arterial monitoring include hemorrhage caused by loose connections of the monitoring system, hematoma at the insertion site, infection (local or systemic), and embolization of the artery that supplies the distal portion of the cannulated extremity.

Besides accurate monitoring and recording of arterial pressure, nursing responsibilities focus on preventing complications of arterial cannulation. The nurse should

- ▶ Check all connections frequently to ensure that they remain tight and secure. Accidental blood loss from a disconnected catheter can be as much as 200 ml in 4 to 5 minutes.
- ▶ Evaluate the cannulated extremity for neurovascular function every 2 hours. Assess color, temperature, capillary filling, and sensation distal to the site of cannulation.
- ▶ Check the insertion site for redness or signs of infection daily and change dressing per institutional policy.

Summary

Cardiovascular assessment can range from taking BP to the insertion of hemodynamic monitors. Even though the use of invasive diagnostic tests is increasing, the nurse needs to be able to accurately assess heart sounds, BP, and client history. These data are just as important as the invasive studies, and frequently it is the nurse who identifies early signs of heart disease in the client through routine screening.

Bibliography

1. Adler, L., Brundage, B., & Shapiro, B. (1991). Tomorrow's cardiac imaging—today. *Patient Care, 25*(11), 143–161.
2. Ahrens, T. & Taylor, L. (1992). *Hemodynamic waveform analysis*. Philadelphia: W.B. Saunders.
3. American Heart Association (1991). *Heart and stroke facts*. Dallas: Author.
4. Andreoli, K., et al. (1987). *Comprehensive cardiac care* (6th ed.). St. Louis: C. V. Mosby.
5. Bates, B. (1991). *A guide to physical exam and history taking* (5th ed.). Philadelphia: J. B. Lippincott.
6. Bentley, L. (1987). Radionuclide imaging techniques in the diagnosis and treatment of coronary heart disease. *Focus on Critical Care, 14*(6), 27–31.
7. Braunwald, E., et al. (Ed.) (1990). *Harrison's principles of internal medicine* (12th ed.). New York. McGraw-Hill.
8. Canobbio, M. (1990). *Cardiovascular disorders*. St. Louis: C. V. Mosby.
9. Dennison, R. (1990). Understanding the four determinants of cardiac output. *Nursing 90, 20*(7), 35–42.
10. Ehman, R. L. & Julsrud, P. R. (1989). Magnetic resonance imaging of the heart: Current status. *Mayo Clinic Proceedings 64*(9), 1134–46.
11. Fahey, V. (1988). *Vascular nursing*. Philadelphia: W. B. Saunders Company.
12. Huang, S., (1989). *Coronary care nursing* (2nd ed.). Philadelphia: W. B. Saunders Company.
13. Izor-Povenmire, K., & House, M. A. (1989). Acute crack cocaine intoxication: A case study. *Focus on Critical Care, 16*(2), 112–119.
14. Lamb, J., & Carlson, V. (1986). *Handbook of cardiovascular nursing*. Philadelphia: J. B. Lippincott.
15. Loveys, B., & Woods, S. (1986). Current recommendations for thermodilution cardiac output measurements. *Progress in Cardiovascular Nursing, 1*(4), 242–247.
16. Nelson, S. (1989). Clinical utility of signal averaged electrocardiography. *Practical Cardiology, 15*(3), 59–72.
17. Purcell, J. (1990). Advances in treatment of dilated cardiomyopathy. *AACN Clinical Issues in Critical Care Nursing, 1*(1), 31–45.
18. Sadler, D. (1984). *Nursing for cardiovascular health*. Norwalk, CT: Appleton-Century-Crofts.
19. Schelbert, H. (1989). Myocardial ischemia and clinical applications of positron emission tomography. *American Journal of Cardiology, 64*, 46–52.
20. Stein, E. (1987). *Clinical electrocardiography: A self-study course*. Philadelphia: Lea & Febiger.
21. Thelan, L. A. et al. (1990). *Critical care nursing*. St. Louis: C.V. Mosby.
22. Underhill, S., et al. (1989). *Cardiac nursing* (2nd ed.). Philadelphia: J. B. Lippincott.
23. Weeks, L. (Ed.). (1986). *Advanced cardiovascular nursing*. Boston: Blackwell Scientific Publications.
24. Wolf, G. (1989). Magnetic resonance imaging and the future of cardiac imaging. *American Journal of Cardiology, 64*, 60–63.

Chapter 42

Nursing Care of Clients with Disorders of Cardiac Function

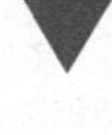

DISORDERS OF CARDIAC FUNCTION

CORONARY ARTERY DISEASE

Definition

The heart muscle must have an adequate blood supply to contract properly. The coronary arteries carry oxygen and blood to the myocardium. When a coronary artery is narrowed or blocked, the area of the heart muscle supplied by that artery becomes ischemic and injured, and infarction may result. The major disorders due to insufficient blood supply to the myocardium are angina pectoris, congestive heart failure (CHF), and myocardial infarction (MI). These disorders are collectively known as coronary artery disease (CAD), also called coronary heart disease or ischemic heart disease.

Incidence

CAD is the leading cause of death in Americans today. Nearly 1 million Americans died in 1989 from cardiovascular diseases.[4, 70] Someone dies from cardiovascular disease every 34 seconds! As high as these figures may seem, mortality from cardiovascular disease, including coronary heart disease and stroke, has declined over the last 40 years. Contributing to this decline in mortality are factors such as improved technologies and therapies for treatment of cardiovascular disease, use of thrombolytic drugs in acute MI, improved surgical techniques, and successful modification of risk factors in populations at risk.

Etiology

Although CAD claims more lives each year than does any other disease, its causes are poorly understood. CAD results from the development of obliterative atherosclerotic lesions within the coronary arteries that narrow or obstruct these vessels. Atherosclerosis, a disorder of lipid metabolism, is characterized by (1) deposits of fat-containing substances along the intima of blood vessels and (2) smooth muscle cell proliferation. It underlies most causes of cardiovascular disease and death.

Risk Factors

Although all the causes of CAD are not known, clinical evidence suggests that many factors contribute to the onset of atherosclerosis. The concept of risk factors helps categorize these causes and prevent CAD. Risk factors that precipitate CAD can be presented in three categories: (1) nonmodifiable risk factors, (2) modifiable risk factors, and (3) contributing factors (Table 42-1).

NONMODIFIABLE RISK FACTORS

Heredity. Genetic factors contribute to four traits that increase the incidence of atherosclerosis: hypertension, dyslipidemia, diabetes, and obesity. In the Framingham study, a longitudinal study of CAD, a family history of heart disease was found to be an independent predictor for CAD in men but not in women.[4, 67]

Age. Symptomatic CAD appears predominantly in clients over age 40 years. However, clients in their 30s, and even their 20s, sometimes suffer anginal attacks or MI.

TABLE 42-1. Risk Factors and Coronary Artery Disease

Personal Risk Factors that Cannot Be Changed	Personal Risk Factors that Can Be Changed	Contributing Factors
Heredity	Smoking	Obesity
Age	Hypertension	Physical inactivity
Male sex	Elevated serum cholesterol	Stress response
		Diabetes

Data from Guidelines for cardiopulmonary resuscitation (CPR) and emergency cardiac care (ECC) (1962). *Journal of the American Medical Association, 268*(16), 2205-2211. Copyright 1992, American Medical Association.

Gender. Women of childbearing age display one fourth the risk of developing CAD, compared with men of the same age. This obvious difference in susceptibility diminishes after menopause; however, even after age 65 years, women continue to be less likely than are men to develop CAD.[67] Women who take oral contraceptives are more likely to develop CAD. This risk is particularly significant in women who smoke. Once oral contraceptives are discontinued, the increased risk of CAD does not continue.[67] Women with an early menopause face three times the risk of CAD as do women with a normal or late menopause.

Two lifestyle changes during the past decade may increase the incidence of CAD among women. More women (many with the full responsibility of the household and children) have entered the work force. Also, more women begin smoking at an earlier age.

Race. White men die more frequently from CAD than do nonwhites. On the other hand, the death rate for white women is generally a little lower than that for nonwhite women. Among elderly women, death rates tend to be about the same for all races.

MODIFIABLE RISK FACTORS

Environment, smoking, hypertension, elevated serum cholesterol levels, and diabetes constitute other major risk factors.

Environment. CAD is seven times more prevalent in North America, Australia, Europe, and New Zealand than in Japan, Switzerland, and Italy. Also, urban populations have a higher incidence of CAD than do rural populations. In developing countries, CAD is most prevalent in the affluent; in Great Britain and the United States, the opposite is true.[67]

Cigarette Smoking. One of the three major risk factors in CAD is cigarette smoking. How smoking causes CAD remains unknown. Male adult smokers have a 70 per cent higher mortality rate than do male nonsmokers, and all smokers have more than twice the risk of heart attack than do nonsmokers. Clients who smoke have two to four times the risk of sudden cardiac death.

The three substances thought to increase the prevalence of CAD are tar, nicotine, and carbon monoxide. Tar contains hydrocarbons and other carcinogenic substances. Nicotine increases the release of epinephrine and norepinephrine, which results in peripheral vasoconstriction, elevated blood pressure and heart rate, greater oxygen consumption, and increased likelihood of dysrhythmias. In addition, nicotine activates platelets and stimulates smooth muscle cell proliferation in the arterial walls. Clients who quit smoking will lose their increased risk in 24 months.[71]

Hypertension. High blood pressure afflicts nearly 60 million American adults and children. Men over 45 years of age with blood pressure exceeding 140/90 and all adult women with pressures above 160/95 have a 50 per cent higher chance of mortality. As blood pressure increases, the risk for cardiovascular events also escalates. Although hypertension cannot always be prevented, it can and should be treated in order to lower the risk of CAD and premature death.

Elevated Serum Cholesterol. An elevated serum cholesterol level definitely increases the risk of developing CAD. A client with a serum cholesterol level greater than 259 mg/dl is three times more likely to develop CAD than is one with a serum level of 200 mg/dl.

Cholesterol, a sterol found in animal tissue, circulates in the blood in combination with triglycerides and protein-bound phospholipids. This complex is called a lipoprotein. There are four basic groups of lipoproteins, all produced in the intestinal wall. Elevation of lipoproteins is called hyperlipoproteinemia. Elevation of lipids, a component of lipoproteins, is called hyperlipidemia.

Lipoproteins and their functions are listed in the following.

- Chylomicrons primarily transport dietary triglycerides and cholesterol.
- Very-low-density lipoprotein (VLDL) mainly transports the triglycerides synthesized by the liver.
- Low-density lipoprotein (LDL) has the highest concentration of cholesterol and transports endogenous cholesterol to body cells.
- High-density lipoprotein (HDL) has the lowest concentration of cholesterol and transports endogenous cholesterol to body cells.

Recent investigations have documented how the presence of lipoproteins may predispose the body to development of CAD. Clients with high levels of HDL in proportion to LDL are less likely to develop CAD than are clients with low HDL. High concentrations of HDL seem to have a protective effect against the development of CAD. Experts believe that the cholesterol in HDL does not become incorporated into the fatty plaques that develop in the lining of the artery wall, as does LDL. The ratio of total cholesterol to HDL or of LDL to HDL is the best test for predicting the risk of CAD.[67] Exercise and low-fat, low-cholesterol diets increase the amount of HDL in the blood.

Diabetes. Diabetes frequently appears in middle-aged, overweight clients. A fasting blood sugar of more than 120 mg/dl, or a routine blood sugar of 180 mg/dl and evidence of sugar in the urine, signals the presence of diabetes and represents an increased risk of CAD. Diabetes leads to early atherosclerosis. For women in particular, diabetes is a contributing factor to the development of CAD.[71]

CONTRIBUTING FACTORS

Obesity, lack of exercise, and response to stress also increase the risk of CAD. Obesity places an extra burden on the heart, requiring the muscle to work harder to pump enough blood to support added tissue mass. In addition, obesity is often associated with a sedentary lifestyle, elevated serum cholesterol, and high blood pressure.

Researchers have still not established the relationship between exercise and CAD. However, the Framingham Study demonstrated an inverse relationship between exercise and the risk of CAD. Exercise may reduce the risk of CAD by decreasing weight, reducing blood pressure, and elevating the protective lipoprotein HDL.[71]

Stress appears to be associated with elevated blood pressures. Although moderate stress plays a role in modern life, excessive response to stress can be a health hazard. Significant stressors include major changes in residence, occupation, or status.

Type A behavior is characterized by aggressiveness, ambition, competitiveness, and a preoccupation with deadlines. Although type A behavior has not been correlated with an increased incidence of CAD in men, it may be a significant factor in working women.[67] The anger component in the stress response is also important. Recent studies question type A behavior as a risk factor. Because the behavior still appears, perhaps it needs new descriptions.[18]

It has recently been reported that the electrocardiographic (ECG) abnormality seen with left ventricular hypertrophy is independently associated with CAD. The mechanism that accounts for this fact is unknown.[71]

The role that some of the modifiable risk factors have in precipitating heart disease is controversial. Hypertension, hyperlipidema, and cigarette smoking have been objectively identified as predictive of CAD.[17]

Pathophysiology

The broad term arteriosclerosis, or hardening of the arteries, encompasses the following conditions: atherosclerosis, Mönckeberg's sclerosis, and arteriolar sclerosis.

Atherosclerosis is an occlusive arterial disease most commonly involving the aorta and the femoral, coronary, and cerebral arteries. The process of atherosclerosis includes the accumulation and deposit of cholesterol and lipids in the arterial wall. Electron microscopic studies also document that structural changes occur in the layers of the arterial wall.

Mönckeberg's sclerosis involves calcium accumulations in the medial layer of the arteries. Arteriolar sclerosis is thickening of the small artery walls.

ALTERATIONS IN THE ARTERIAL WALL DUE TO ATHEROSCLEROSIS

There are three layers in the arterial wall separated by elastic laminae: the intima, the media, and the adventitia (Fig. 42–1*A*). The intima, a single layer of cells on the inner surface of the artery, normally provides an impermeable barrier to proteins in the blood. The media (middle layer) is made up almost entirely of smooth muscle cells. The adventitia consists mainly of a few smooth muscle cells, fibroblasts, and loose connective tissue.

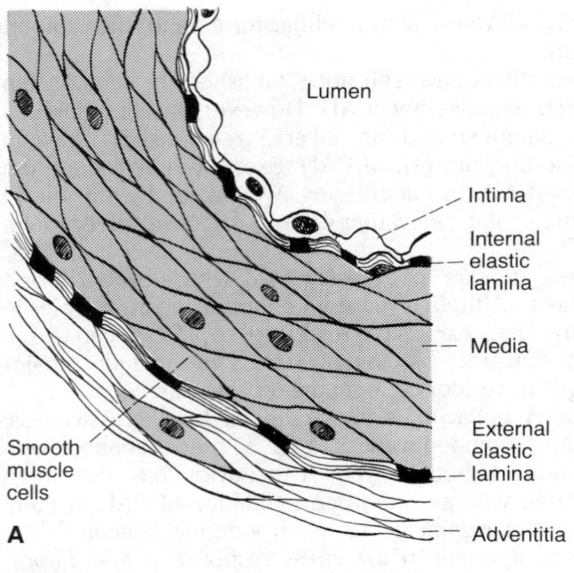

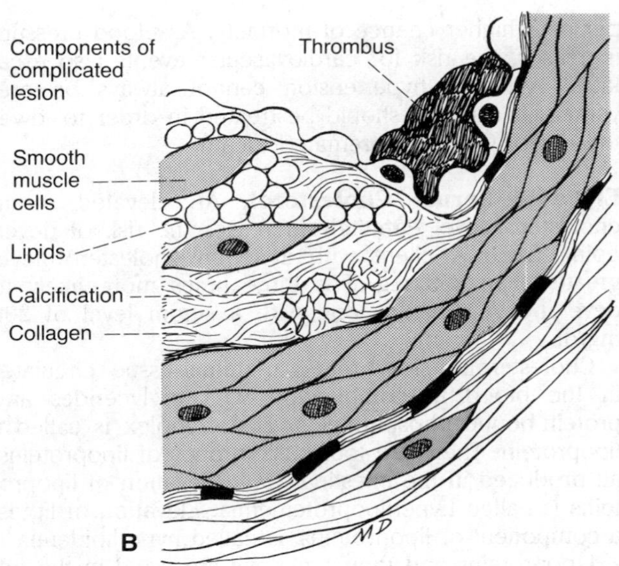

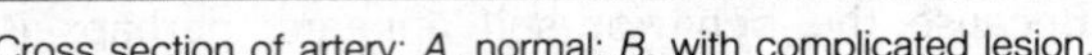
▲ *Figure 42-1*

Cross section of artery: *A*, normal; *B*, with complicated lesion.

Atherosclerosis primarily affects the intima of the arterial wall. The lesions affecting this layer and commonly seen in atherosclerosis are the fatty streak, the fibrous plaque, and the complicated lesion.

The fatty streak appears as a smooth, yellowish, slightly raised streak on the inner surface of the artery. It is characterized by the presence of lipoprotein deposits (mostly cholesterol). These deposits are located in the intima of the artery, inside smooth muscle cells and macrophages. Fatty streaks have been seen in infants as young as 1 month old. Researchers have not yet determined whether they are reversible or are a precursor to plaque formation.

The raised fibrous plaque appears as a yellowish-gray bump on the surface of the artery. The plaque is made up of three types of material: (1) smooth muscle cells from the medial layer, (2) collagen, and (3) accumulated lipid within the intimal layer.

A complicated lesion, as shown in Figure 42-1*B*, contains the fibrous plaque, calcium deposits, and a thrombus due to hemorrhage into the plaque.

THEORIES OF PATHOGENESIS

Over the last 10 years, our understanding of the atherosclerotic process has changed. A number of currently popular theories attempt to explain the development of atherosclerosis. These theories, although still controversial, endeavor to trace the formation of the fatty streak and raised fibrous plaque. Many of these theories have been integrated into the response-to-injury hypothesis. This theory suggests that certain changes occur in response to a nonspecific injury to the inner surface of the arterial wall. These changes then produce a classic lesion (Fig. 42-2). Nonspecific injury (mechanical, chemical, hormonal, or immunologic) may arise from such diverse causes as hypertension, hydrocarbons from smoking, cholesterol, catecholamines, angiotensin, or hormones. In turn, nonspecific injury results in the shedding or desquamation of the superficial layer of the artery. Continued exposure to the source of intimal injury results in continued lipid deposit and proliferation of smooth muscle cells.

Other theories for explaining the development of CAD include the monoclonal hypothesis, the senescence hypothesis, the thrombogenic hypothesis, the lipid-irritation hypothesis, and the hemodynamic hypothesis.

According to the monoclonal hypothesis, the primary process of proliferation of smooth muscle cells arises from the unchecked multiplication of a single cell.

The senescence hypothesis suggests that the development of atherosclerosis occurs with age. Smooth muscle cell proliferation results from an age-dependent decline in control over replication of intimal smooth muscle cells. This results in the characteristic increase in smooth muscle cell proliferation.

According to the thrombogenic hypothesis, the aggregation of platelets at the injury site converts into connecting tissue. This conversion results from the migration of smooth muscle cells and fibroblasts from the arterial wall into the thrombus.

The lipid-irritation hypothesis holds that the deposit of lipids in the arterial wall from the blood acts as an irritant that induces proliferation of smooth muscle cells.

The hemodynamic hypothesis attempts to explain why plaques commonly appear in arterial branchings. According to the hemodynamic hypothesis, plaque formation results from turbulence, pressures, and stresses that all act as irritants on the endothelial wall.

In general, most theories include the following major events in the development of atherosclerotic plaque:[71]

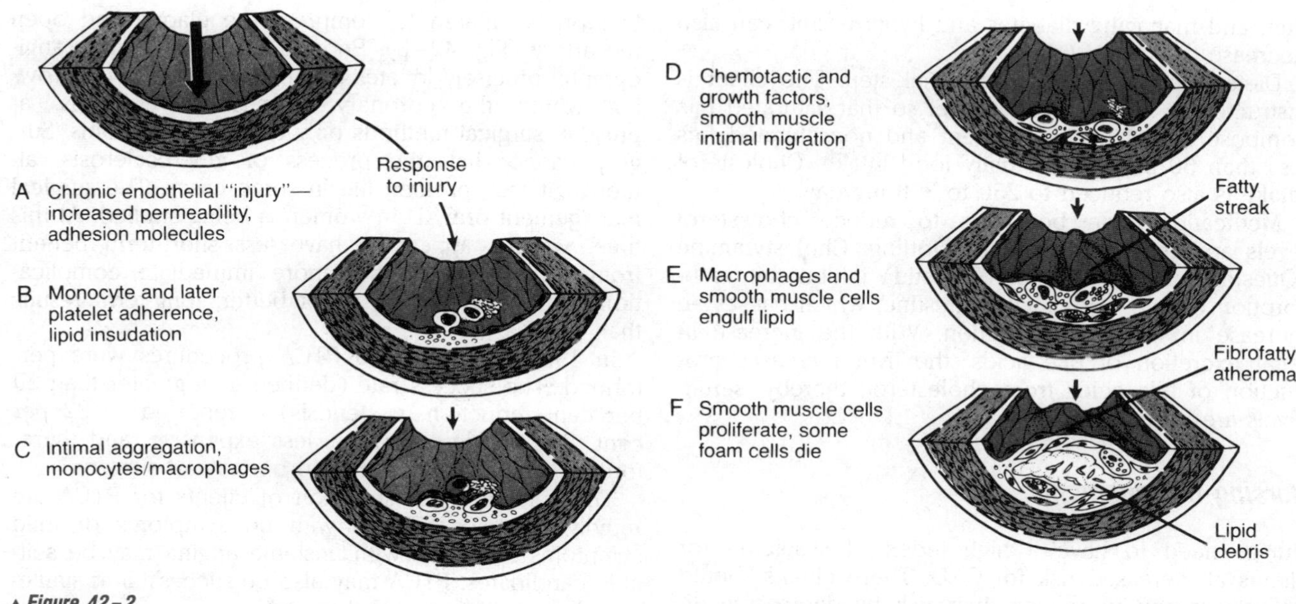

▲ *Figure 42-2*

The response to injury theory of atherogenesis. *A*, The process begins with focal areas of endothelial injury, usually very subtle, that result in increased endothelial permeability. *B*, Lipids and platelets assimilate into the area. The lipoproteins commonly include low density lipoproteins (LDLs) and very low density lipoproteins (VLDLs). *C*, Oxidized LDL attracts monocytes and macrophages to the cite. *D*, Plaques begin to form foam cells which imbed in the endothelium. *E*, Lipids are engulfed by the cells, and smooth muscle cell develops leading to a fatty atheroma *(F)*. (From Kumar, V., et al. [1992]. *Basic pathology* [p. 281]. Philadelphia: W. B. Saunders.)

- endothelial injury
- platelet/fibrin interaction
- smooth muscle cell proliferation
- lipid entry and accumulation
- fibrosis
- thrombus formation
- ulceration and calcification

SEQUELAE OF CORONARY ARTERY DISEASE

It is important to recognize that CAD is a progressive disorder; if not prevented or treated in early stages, it will progress to more severe forms of cardiac disorders. Common sequelae of CAD include sudden cardiac death, angina pectoris, and MI. In addition, clients may develop heart failure, chronic arrhythmias, conduction disturbances, and unstable angina. Sudden cardiac death is presented here; the other sequelae are the focus of the rest of this chapter.

Sudden cardiac death is not a clinical diagnosis but a descriptive term to identify clients who die from cardiac causes within 24 hours of the onset of symptoms. CAD makes up 75 per cent of all causes of cardiac death. Other risk factors of sudden cardiac death include hypertrophic and dilated cardiomyopathies, Wolff-Parkinson-White syndrome, long QT syndrome, valvular abnormalities, and electrolyte abnormalities (hypomagnesemia and hypokalemia).

Primary ventricular fibrillation is the major cause of sudden cardiac death. Dyspnea and fatigue are the most commonly reported symptoms experienced immediately preceding sudden cardiac death. Angina is a primary symptom in less than 35 per cent of cases.[21]

Clinical Manifestations

Atherosclerosis, by itself, does not necessarily produce symptoms. For manifestations to develop, there must be a critical deficit in blood supply to the heart in proportion to the demands of the myocardium for oxygen and nutrients. In other words, there must be a supply and demand imbalance. When atherosclerosis progresses slowly, the collateral circulation that develops generally can meet the heart's demands. Thus, whether symptoms of CAD develop depends on the total blood supply to the myocardium (by way of coronary arteries and collateral circulation) and not solely on the condition of the coronary arteries (see the discussion of angina, which appears later in this chapter). Often, symptoms of CAD do not appear until the lumen of the coronary artery narrows by 75 per cent.

DIAGNOSTIC ASSESSMENT

Techniques to determine the extent of CAD and identify the affected vessels include electrocardiogram, nuclear scanning, and angiography. (See Chap. 41 for complete discussion.)

Medical Management

Prevention, rather than treatment, is the goal for clients with CAD. Fatty streaks are capable of regressing and disappearing entirely if cholesterol and fat intake are reduced. Cessation of cigarette smoking, controlling diet, and managing diabetes and hypertension can also decrease the risk of CAD.

Dietary modification is an initial step. The client is instructed to alter his or her diet so that saturated fats compose less than 10 per cent and nonsaturated fats less than 30 per cent of daily food intake. Cholesterol intake is also reduced to 250 to 300 mg/day.

Medications can be given to reduce cholesterol levels and reduce the risk of clotting. Cholestyramine (Questran) and colestipol (Colestid) inhibit the reabsorption of bile acids in the intestine, which causes an increase in the fecal excretion. With the increase in fecal excretion of bile acids, the liver increases production of bile acids from cholesterol; thereby, serum levels are lowered.

Nursing Management

Nurses need to have a high index of suspicion for clients at increased risk for CAD. These clients should be encouraged to reduce their risk by decreasing dietary intake of fats and cholesterol, increasing exercise, controlling diabetes and hypertension, keeping body weight at near-ideal levels, and ceasing smoking. The risk and incidence of CAD are so pervasive that many clients are doing these activities on an ongoing basis. The nurse should reinforce these behaviors.

The level of motivation sustained by a client to reduce cardiovascular risk factors is the primary predictor of success. Nursing researchers are studying methods to improve motivation.

Surgical Management

PERCUTANEOUS TRANSLUMINAR CORONARY ANGIOPLASTY

Percutaneous transluminar coronary angioplasty (PTCA) is a surgical technique in which a balloon-tipped catheter is inserted into a blocked coronary artery. The balloon is inflated to compress the plaque and open the artery (Fig. 42-3). Prior to surgery coronary angiography precisely locates lesions and points of narrowing within the coronary arteries. Nevertheless, at present, surgical methods only ease the symptoms. Surgery cannot halt the process of atherosclerosis, although it may prolong life in some cases. The surgical management of CAD in women is being studied. At this time, women appear to have less short-term benefit from surgery (i.e., suffer more immediate complications) but have similar, if not better, long-term results than men.[23]

In 1990, over 330,000 PTCA procedures were performed. The success rate (defined as a greater than 20 per cent reduction in stenosis) is reported as 82 per cent. PTCA is less invasive, less expensive, and therefore an attractive alternative to open-heart surgery.

The guidelines for selection of clients for PTCA are rapidly changing. Clients with no symptoms or mild symptoms to clients with unstable angina may be suitable candidates. PTCA may also be successful in single-vessel or multiple-vessel disease.[24]

In addition to PTCA, new therapeutic devices for coronary application continue to evolve as alternatives to bypass surgery. Atherectomy is a procedure that uses a device consisting of a balloon and motorized cutter. The cutter is positioned against the blockage and mechanically débrides the plaque.

An intravascular stent is a coilspring tube, placed in the coronary artery, that acts as a mechanical scaffold to reopen the blocked artery. Materials ranging from stainless steel to bioabsorbable compounds are being tested as intravascular stents. Clients with intravascular stents are placed on anticoagulation and antiplatelet agents.

Lasers are currently being used with balloon angioplasty to vaporize atherosclerotic plaque. After the initial balloon angioplasty, a brief burst of laser radiation is administered, and additional remaining plaque is removed.[35]

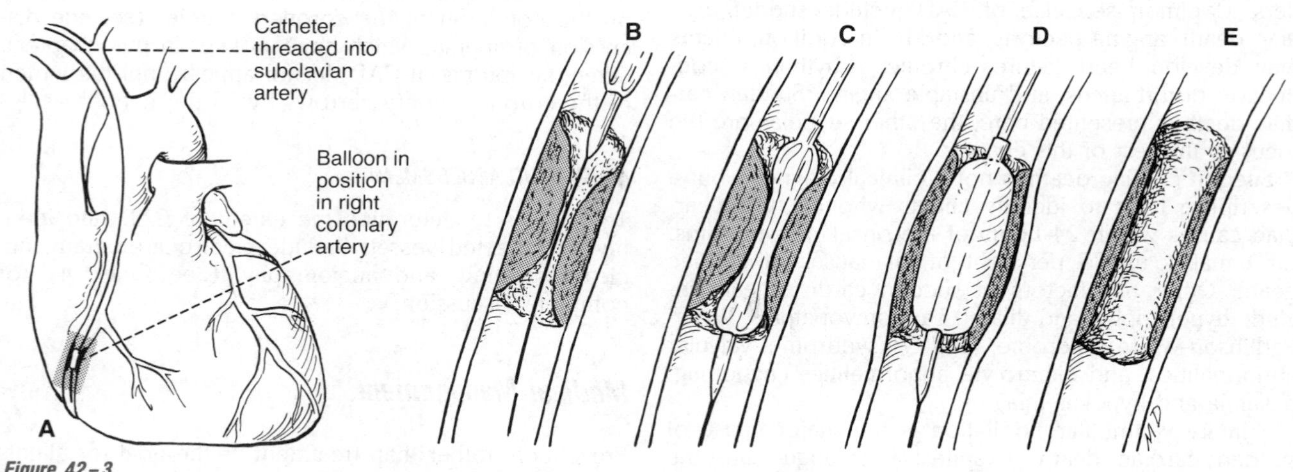

▲ Figure 42-3

Percutaneous transluminar coronary angioplasty (PTCA). *A*, Balloon-tipped catheter positioned in blocked artery. *B*, Balloon is centered. *C*, Balloon expands to (*D*) compress blockage. *E*, Artery diameter opened.

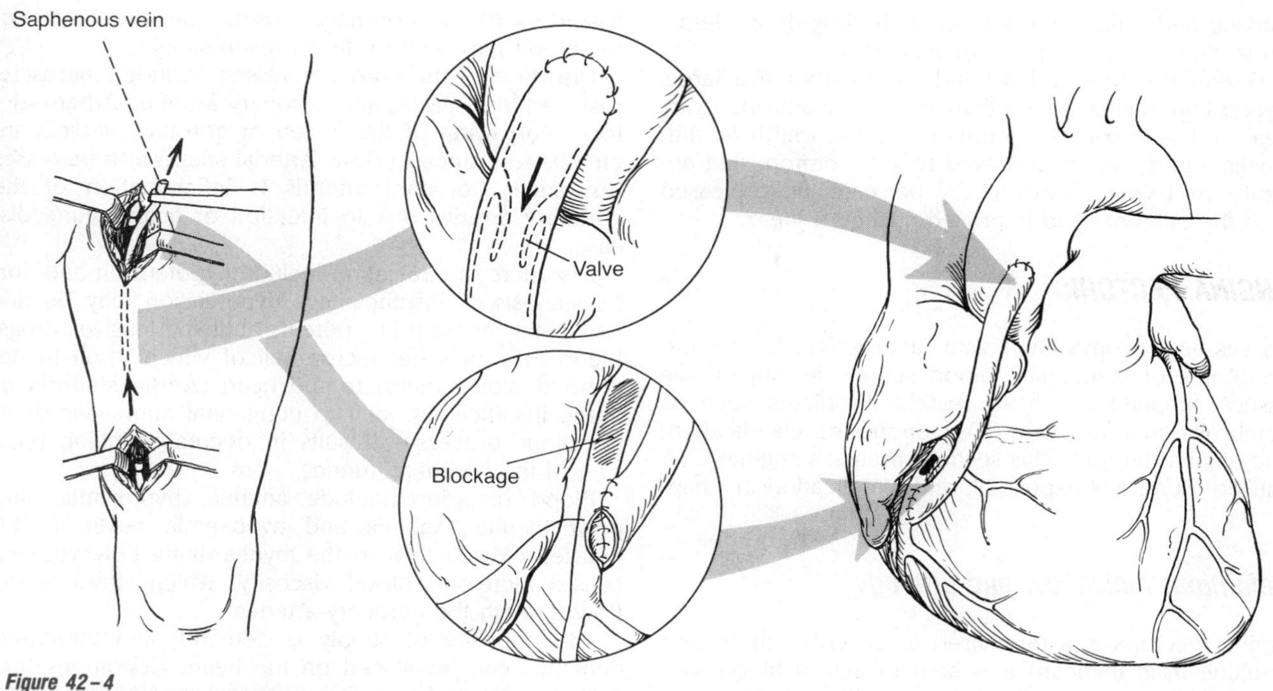

▲ *Figure 42-4*

Coronary artery bypass graft (CABG). A section of saphenous vein is harvested from the leg and anastomosed to coronary artery to bypass the obstruction.

Nursing Management

Prior to PTCA the client is usually given an anticoagulant. Aspirin is a common drug used. This protocol helps reduce the risk of occlusion of the artery during the procedure. During the procedure, the client is given heparin (an anticoagulant) and/or calcium agonists or nitrates to reduce coronary artery spasm.

The client is also typed and crossmatched for blood in the event that emergency coronary artery bypass grafting is needed. A consent is signed for angioplasty and surgery if required for spasm, perforation of the artery, or occlusion.

Following PTCA, the client is monitored for changes in vital signs, especially the quality and rhythm of pulse and EKG. Fluids are forced, orally or by intravenous routes; they assist with excretion of contrast and because contrast causes diuresis. The puncture site is monitored for hematoma, and pulses are palpated to assess peripheral perfusion. Complications include acute myocardial infarction resulting from perforation of an artery, refractory arterial spasm, or occlusion.

CORONARY ARTERY BYPASS GRAFT

Coronary artery bypass graft (CABG) surgery involves the bypass of a blockage in one or more of the coronary arteries using the saphenous or mammary veins as replacement vessels.

Advances such as the development of calcium channel blockers, and nonsurgical techniques such as PTCA, have reduced the number of CABG surgeries performed. Also, survival rates of people with CABGs have not been found to be significantly better than survival rates of medically treated people. The CABG nevertheless remains a common surgery, and because it can reduce angina in 80 to 90 per cent of patients refractory to medical management, it will continue as an important intervention in the management of coronary heart disease.

During CABG surgery, the surgeon harvests a length of saphenous vein from the thigh or lower leg. The heart is accessed through an median sternotomy. While the person is on cardiopulmonary bypass and the heart is not beating, the surgeon sews the distal end of the vein to the aorta and the proximal end to the coronary vessel distal to the blockage (Fig. 42-4). In some cases, the internal mammary artery (IMA) can be grafted to a coronary artery. The disadvantage of the IMA is that more time is required to remove it and it is shorter. It is used only to revascularize the portion of the myocardium supplied by the left anterior descending artery. IMA grafts have a greater chance of remaining patent. The veins are reversed so that their valves do not interfere with blood flow.

Nursing management of the client following heart surgery is discussed in Chapter 43.

Over half of all CABGs are performed on people over 65, and 75 per cent of them on men.[4] Elderly clients have a similar postoperative recovery as do younger clients, but the pace is slower. Each client remains hospitalized for 4 more days on the average. They also have a higher mortality rate.[30]

Postoperative complications that are more prevalent in the elderly include dysrhythmias related to aged sinoatrial node cells, drug toxicity related to impaired hepatic and renal perfusion, multiple drug-drug interactions, and decreased physical stamina.

During the first and second weeks after discharge, depression, fatigue, incisional chest discomfort, dyspnea, and anorexia are common. By the fourth to fifth weeks, elders report improved mood, comfort, and appetite. At 1 year, almost all (93 per cent) were pleased with the outcome and improved quality of life.[30]

ANGINA PECTORIS

As vessels become lined with atherosclerotic plaques, symptoms of inadequate blood supply develop in the tissues supplied by these vessels. Problems such as cerebrovascular accident (CVA or stroke), claudication, and angina develop. This section discusses angina; CVA can be found in Chapter 29, and claudication in Chapter 44.

Definition, Incidence, and Etiology

Angina pectoris is a term used to describe chest pain resulting from myocardial ischemia (lack of blood supply). Angina pectoris is common, although its exact incidence is not recorded. The cause of angina pectoris is CAD (discussed in the preceding section). Angina can occur in clients with normal coronary arteries also, but it is less common. Clients with aortic stenosis, hypertension, and hypertrophic cardiomyopathy can have angina pectoris.

Risk Factors

Exertion, emotion, and exposure to cold precipitate angina. Primary prevention is through the lifelong commitment to decreasing the risk factors of CAD (see earlier). Secondary prevention is through the recognition and early treatment of anginal attacks. Tertiary prevention is the resolution of angina before myocardial damage occurs, which is discussed in this chapter.

Pathophysiology

The coronary arteries normally supply the myocardium with blood to meet its metabolic needs during varying workloads. The coronary vessels are usually quite efficient and perfuse the myocardium during diastole. When the heart needs more blood, the vessels dilate. As the vessels become lined, and eventually occluded, with atherosclerotic plaques, the vessels lose their ability to dilate in order to supply the heart with extra blood. As the vessels become occluded, they cannot supply the myocardium with blood for normal workloads. A growing mass of plaque in the vessel collects platelets, fibrin, and cellular debris. Platelet aggregations are known to release prostaglandin capable of causing vessel spasm. This in turn promotes platelet aggregation, and a vicious cycle begins.

Myocardial ischemia develops if the blood supply through the coronary vessels or oxygen content of the blood is not adequate to meet the metabolic demands. Disorders of the coronary vessels, the circulation, or the blood may lead to decreases in supply.

Disorders of the coronary vessels include atherosclerosis, arterial spasm, and coronary arteritis. Atherosclerosis, narrowing of the lumen of coronary vessels, increases resistance to flow. Arterial spasm also increases resistance. Coronary arteritis is inflammation of the coronary arteries due to infection or autoimmune disease.

Disorders of circulation include hypotension and aortic stenosis or insufficiency. Hypotension may be due to spinal anesthesia, potent antihypertensive drugs, blood loss, or other factors, all of which result in decreased blood return to the heart. Aortic stenosis or aortic insufficiency, due to congenital anomalies or to infectious processes, results in decreased filling pressure of the coronary arteries.

Blood disorders include anemia, hypoxemia, and polycythemia. Anemia and hypoxemia result in decreased oxygen flow to the myocardium. Polycythemia causes increased blood viscosity, which slows blood flow through the coronary arteries.

The opposite of supply is demand, and increased demands can be placed on the heart. Conditions that increase demands on the myocardium include conditions that increase cardiac output and conditions that increase myocardial need for oxygen.

Conditions that increase cardiac output include exercise, emotion, digestion of a large meal, anemia, and hyperthyroidism.

Conditions that increase myocardial need for oxygen include damage to the myocardium, hypertrophy of the myocardium, aortic stenosis, aortic insufficiency, diastolic hypertension, thyrotoxicosis, strong emotion, and heavy exertion. Damaged myocardium is unable to utilize oxygen properly. Hypertrophied myocardium has "outgrown" its normal blood supply and requires added supplies of oxygen. Aortic stenosis or insufficiency and diastolic hypertension cause the heart to work harder. Thyrotoxicosis increases oxygen consumption. Finally, strong emotions and heavy exertion increase the heart's and the body's need for oxygen.

Myocardial ischemia occurs when either supply or demand is altered. In some clients, the coronary arteries can supply adequate blood when the client is at rest; but when the client attempts activity or becomes taxed in some other manner, angina develops. Myocardial cells become ischemic within 10 seconds of coronary artery occlusion. After several minutes of ischemia, the heart pumping function is reduced. The reduction of pumping deprives the ischemic cells of much needed oxygen and glucose. The cells convert to an anaerobic metabolism, which leaves lactic acid as a waste product. As lactic acid accumulates, pain develops. Angina pectoris is transient, lasting for only 3 to 5 minutes. If blood flow is restored, no permanent myocardial damage occurs.

Clinical Manifestations

Characteristics. Angina pectoris produces transient paroxysmal attacks of substernal or precordial pain that may radiate to the left shoulder and down the inner side of the left arm. Less frequently, pain may be referred to the right shoulder and arm, epigastrium, jaw, neck, or left scapula region. The pain of angina usually has the following characteristics.

Sensation. The sensation of anginal pain is described as squeezing, burning, pressing, choking, aching, or bursting. The client often says the pain feels like "gas" or "heartburn" or "indigestion." Clients do not describe anginal pain as sharp or knifelike.

Severity. The pain of angina is usually mild or moderate in severity. Rarely is the pain described as severe.

Location. Eighty to 90 per cent of clients experience the pain as retrosternal or slightly to the left of the sternum.

Radiation. The pain usually radiates to the left shoulder and upper arm. It may then travel down the inner aspect of the left arm to the elbow, wrist, and fourth and fifth fingers. The pain may also radiate to the right shoulder, neck, jaw, or epigastric region. On occasion, the pain may be felt only in the area of radiation and not in the chest. The client rarely experiences the pain localized to any one single small area over the precordium.

Duration. Anginal attacks usually last a short time, typically less than 5 minutes. However, attacks precipitated by a heavy meal or extreme anger may last 15 to 20 minutes.

Relief. Most anginal attacks quickly subside with the administration of nitroglycerin and with rest.

The typical "exertion-pain-rest-relief" symptom pattern is the major clue to the diagnosis of angina pectoris. Other symptoms accompanying the pain include dyspnea, pallor, sweating, faintness, palpitations, dizziness, and digestive disturbances.

Patterns. Classic angina pectoris may be subdivided into the following basic patterns.

Stable Angina. Stable angina is paroxysmal chest pain or discomfort triggered by a predictable degree of exertion or emotion. Stable angina characteristically has a stable pattern of onset, duration, and intensity of symptoms.

Unstable Angina. Unstable angina (preinfarction angina, crescendo angina, or intermittent coronary syndrome) is paroxysmal chest pain triggered by an unpredictable degree of exertion or emotion, which may occur at night. Unstable angina attacks characteristically increase in number, duration, and intensity over time.

Variant Angina. Variant angina (Prinzmetal's angina) is chest discomfort that is similar to classic angina but is of longer duration and may occur while at rest. These attacks tend to happen in the early hours of the day. Variant angina may result from coronary artery spasm and may be associated with elevation of the ST segment on the ECG.

Nocturnal Angina. Nocturnal angina occurs only during the night and is possibly associated with the REM sleep that accompanies dreaming.

Angina Decubitus. Angina decubitus is paroxysmal chest pain that occurs when the client reclines and lessens when the client sits or stands up.

Intractable Angina. Intractable angina is chronic incapacitating angina unresponsive to intervention.

Postinfarction Angina. Postinfarction angina occurs after MI, when residual ischemia may cause episodes of angina.

DIAGNOSTIC ASSESSMENT

Electrocardiogram. The ECG tracings remain normal in 25 to 30 per cent of clients with angina pectoris. An ECG taken in the presence of pain may document transient ischemic attacks. An ECG taken during an episode of pain may also suggest the coronary artery involved and the amount of cardiac muscle affected by the ischemic event.

Exercise Electrocardiogram ("Stress Test"). An ECG may also be taken while the client exercises on a treadmill or stationary bicycle. The client increases exercise performance according to a defined program until reaching 85 per cent of maximal heart rate. ECG or vital sign changes may indicate ischemia.

Radioisotope Imaging. Various nuclear imaging techniques are used as diagnostic tools to evaluate the myocardial muscle. Regions of poor perfusion or ischemia appear as areas of diminished or absent activity ("cold" spots).[35]

Coronary Angiography. Angiography provides the most accurate information about the patency of the coronary arteries. This diagnostic assessment allows visualization of the artery and any partial or complete blockages.

These diagnostic assessments are fully described in Chapter 41.

Medical Management

Medical management of clients with angina pectoris focuses on two goals: the relief of the acute attack and prevention of further attacks for reducing the risk of MI.

Angina pectoris is diagnosed by history and various diagnostic assessments. A complete history of the pain and its pattern is taken. Clients are encouraged to describe the pain in their own words. A complete symptom analysis is recorded. This description provides a baseline that can be used in ongoing care.

Most physical findings are transient. The client ex-

TABLE 42–2. Antianginal Agents

Class	Example	Action	Common Side Effects	Nursing Implications
Opiate analgesic	Morphine sulfate	Opiate analgesic used to relieve severe pain and anxiety associated with acute MI Also reduces venous return: thereby, myocardial workload is decreased	Sedation, confusion, hypotension, nausea and vomiting, constipation, dry eyes, and respiratory depression	When administering IV, administer slowly over 3 to 5 minutes; monitor closely for hypotension and respiratory depression
Vasodilators	Nitrates/nitrites: nitroglycerin SL and nitroglycerin IV Long-acting: isosorbide dinitrate (Isordil, Sorbitrate, and other manufacturers) Nitroglycerin topical (Nitrobid, Transderm-Nitro, and other manufacturers)	Relax smooth muscle of coronary and peripheral blood vessels, causing an increase in their diameter: thereby, blood flow is improved and resistance is decreased As peripheral resistance decreases, workload on heart is reduced, and oxygen demand to supply ratio improves	Flushing, headache, dizziness, hypotension	Assess baseline cardiac function, heart rate, and blood pressure Postural hypotension may occur; caution clients to change position slowly, to sit or lie down, especially when taking nitroglycerin tablets SL Can take up to 3 SL nitroglycerin at 5-minute intervals if necessary; if pain is not relieved after 15 minutes, physician should be contacted immediately or client should report to hospital Tablets are inactivated by light, heat, air, and moisture; store at room temperature, in tight-fitting amber glass container A potent nitroglycerin tablet should produce a burning sensation under tongue when taken SL: check expiration date
Calcium channel blockers	Diltiazem (Cardizem) Nifedipine (Procardia)	Reduce vascular smooth muscle tone by interfering with the ability of free calcium ions to initiate muscular contraction Act on coronary and peripheral arteries, causing vasodilation, increased myocardial oxygen supply, and decreased peripheral resistance	Dizziness, hypotension, bradycardia with diltiazem, diarrhea, abdominal cramps, nausea, vomiting, rash, dermatitis	Assess baseline cardiac function, ECG, heart rate, and blood pressure Monitor hepatic and renal function Food delays absorption and decreases plasma levels Decrease dosage gradually Administer slowly by IV

IV, intravenously; SL, sublingually; MI, myocardial infarction.

hibits pallor or has cold and clammy skin. Tachycardia and hypertension may be recorded. Pulsus alternans may be present at the onset of ischemia attacks. On auscultation, an S_3 or S_4 gallop or a paradoxic split of S_2 may be noted. If the client has a mitral regurgitation from ischemia of the papillary muscle, a murmur will be heard.

PHARMACOLOGIC MANAGEMENT

The primary goal of pharmacologic treatment of angina is to reduce myocardial oxygen consumption by altering the various components of the process. The components of myocardial oxygen consumption that can be pharmacologically treated are blood pressure, heart rate, contractility, and left ventricular volume. The agents used in the treatment of angina are listed in Table 42-2.

The three major types of medications used in angina pectoris are vasodilators, beta-adrenergic blocking agents (e.g., propranolol), and calcium channel blockers.

Vasodilators. Nitroglycerin, a short-acting nitrate, has been the medication of choice against anginal attacks since 1867. Today, nitroglycerin remains the major weapon against acute attacks. Administered sublingually, nitroglycerin acts to relieve the pain of angina within 1 to 2 minutes.

Nitroglycerin decreases the oxygen requirements of the myocardium by causing coronary and systemic vasodilation and a decrease in blood pressure, which consequently decreases the cardiac workload. Side effects of nitroglycerin include headache, hypotension, dizziness, and flushing.

Long-acting nitrates act to maintain coronary artery vasodilation, thereby promoting a greater flow of blood and oxygen to heart muscle. Currently, the most frequently prescribed nitrates are isosorbide dinitrite (Isordil) and long-acting nitroglycerin preparations (e.g., nitroglycerin ointment).

Nitroglycerin is also available as a slow-release concentrated patch that can be worn for 24 hours. In addition, clinicians can administer nitroglycerin intravenously in the acute care setting. Monitor the client carefully while the medication is titrated to reduce symptoms of chest pain. Long-acting nitrates produce the same general side effects as nitroglycerin (i.e., severe headache, flushing of the skin, nausea and vomiting, hypotension, vertigo, and syncope). Approximately two thirds of clients on long-acting nitrates develop a tolerance to the medication. Therefore, it is generally suggested that a 12-hour drug-free interval be maintained to preserve responsiveness to the nitrate. For most clients, this drug-free time is at night.[13]

Beta-Blocking Agents. Administration of a beta-adrenergic blocking agent (e.g., propranolol) will reduce the workload of the heart and may decrease the number of anginal attacks. Propranolol reduces the oxygen requirements of the myocardium by blocking beta-receptors and slowing heart rate. This, in turn, raises the exercise tolerance of clients with reduced coronary blood flow. Because propranolol interferes with the pumping action of the heart, use extreme caution when administering this drug to clients with any degree of heart failure. Do not administer propranolol to clients with a history of bronchial asthma, significant mitral or aortic valvular disease, allergic rhinitis during the pollen season, or brittle diabetes. Never give propranolol in conjunction with monoamine oxidase inhibitors.

Side effects of propranolol include nausea, vomiting, mental depression, mild diarrhea, fatigue, and impotence. Propranolol given in combination with nitrates on an around-the-clock schedule appears to be superior to either type of medication given alone.

Because of the adverse effects of propranolol on the bronchial tree, pharmaceutical companies have developed other beta-blockers that act more specifically on the heart (cardioselective). Examples of beta-blocking agents that are cardioselective are metoprolol (Lopressor) and atenolol (Tenormin). In small doses, these medications can induce full cardiac beta-blockage without causing wheezing in clients with pulmonary disease. At larger doses, cardioselective beta-blockers may become nonselective and block both the heart and bronchial beta-receptors.

Calcium Channel Blockers. Calcium plays a major role in the electrical excitation of cardiac cells and in the contraction of vascular and cardiac muscle cells. The Food and Drug Administration has accepted three calcium channel blockers for use in the United States: nifedipine, verapamil, and diltiazem. The clinical use of each medication varies with the way each agent affects the heart. Physicians usually order nifedipine (Procardia) to treat angina. Nifedipine appears to complement the antianginal action of the vasodilators and beta-blockers. Common side effects include flushing, dizziness, headache, and pedal edema. Verapamil (Calan, Isoptin) primarily acts as an antiarrhythmic. Because of verapamil's effect of decreasing heart rate and blood pressure, give it with caution when it is combined with beta-blockers that have a similar effect. Diltiazem (Cardizem) has become popular because it has effects similar to verapamil and nifedipine with a lower incidence of side effects.

DIETARY MANAGEMENT

In the average American diet, approximately 45 per cent of the total calories come from fat, a level in excess of the prudent diet recommended by the American Heart Association. Dietary fat comes in many forms and disguises. A high intake of cholesterol and saturated fats is associated with the development of coronary heart disease, whereas a proportional intake of polyunsaturated and monounsaturated fats is linked with lower risk. The prudent diet should include no more than 30 per cent of calories from fat, 55 per cent from carbohydrate (at least half of these should be complex carbohydrates), and 15 per cent from protein. When fat intake does not exceed 30 per cent of total calories, the expected rise in triglycerides from a high carbohydrate diet is minimal. Saturated fats should account for no more than 10 per cent of the caloric intake.

Nursing Management

In addition to documenting the clinical manifestations of angina, the nurse should attempt to determine how long the client has had angina, risk factors of CAD, and emotional reaction to the chest pain. Cardiac monitoring should be started, a 12-lead ECG obtained, and ongoing angina controlled. Until the angina is controlled and coronary blood flow reestablished, the client is at risk of myocardial damage from myocardial ischemia. If the client reports angina, the nurse should assess the pain and ask the client whether it is the same pain experienced in the past. New characteristics or increased pain should be noted. Sublingual nitroglycerin should be given as prescribed. Because nitroglycerin causes vasodilation and hypotension, blood pressure should be monitored. If the pain is not relieved after three nitroglycerin tablets 5 to 10 minutes apart or morphine, the physician should be notified. In addition, an environment that provides rest and security as well as decreases fear and anxiety will help reduce pain.

Post-hospital Care

The client must be knowledgeable in the care of episodes of angina and how to reduce the risk factors that exacerbate the process.

The following information should be used as needed to help clients control risk factors of angina pectoris.

First, educate the client to avoid activities or habits that precipitate angina, such as eating large meals, drinking coffee, smoking, excessive strenuous exercise, going out in cold weather, or excess stress.

If an attack begins, the client should stop the activity and sit down.

Antianginal medication, e.g., nitroglycerin, should be used. Three pills can be taken sublinguinally 5 to 10 minutes apart. If the pain does not subside, worsens, or radiates, the client should be taken to an emergency department (not drive himself or herself).

Second, explain the importance of daily management of hypertension. It is important that the client take daily medication even though no clinical manifestations are evident (see also Chap. 44).

Third, encourage and help plan a regular program of daily exercise to promote improved coronary circulation and weight management.

Fourth, instruct clients who smoke to quit smoking at once. Smoking cigarettes raises carboxyhemoglobin in the blood, which reduces the amount of oxygen available to the myocardium and can precipitate an anginal attack. Also teach clients to avoid "passive smoking" (e.g., being with a smoker or in a smoke-filled room) in order to reduce the risk of anginal attacks. Clients with angina pectoris exposed for 2 hours to cigarette smoke suffered elevations in carboxyhemoglobin concentrations, decreased exercise time, and increased heart rate and blood pressure.

Fifth, urge overweight clients to lose excess weight. Encourage them to eat small meals, avoid high-calorie and high-cholesterol diets, abstain from gas-forming foods, and rest for short periods after meals. In addition, suggest a high-fiber diet, which may not only prevent constipation and other intestinal tract ailments but also decrease the number and severity of anginal attacks. Diets high in fiber may also lower serum cholesterol and triglyceride levels. CAD is less common among clients with high intake of dietary fiber than in those with low intake. High-fiber diets have also been shown to decrease hypertension.

Finally, help the client who leads an active, hectic life to adjust activities to a level below that which precipitates anginal attacks. Encourage brief rest periods throughout the working day, an early bedtime, and longer or more frequent vacations.

Advise clients who are anxious and nervous to perhaps seek counseling. The nurse may also suggest that the physician prescribe a mild tranquilizer. Relaxation techniques may also be used.

ACUTE MYOCARDIAL INFARCTION

Acute myocardial infarction (MI), also known as a heart attack, coronary occlusion, or just "a coronary," is a life-threatening condition characterized by the formation of localized necrotic areas within the myocardium. MI usually follows the sudden occlusion of a coronary artery and the abrupt cessation of blood and oxygen flow to the heart muscle.

Because heart muscle must function continuously, blockage of blood to the muscle and the development of necrotic areas within the myocardium represent a serious event, which may claim the client's life. Indeed, even if the client survives the initial attack, complications may arise, and the likelihood of suffering a subsequent fatal heart attack increases.

Incidence, Etiology, and Risk Factors

Every year approximately 1,500,000 Americans fall victim to heart attacks. MI is the leading cause of death in America. Heart attacks will cause an estimated 500,000 deaths each year.[70] Approximately 300,000 clients die each year before they reach the hospital. Studies indicate that, unfortunately, half of all heart attack victims wait more than 2 hours before getting help. On the basis of data from the Framingham study, approximately 45 per cent of all heart attack clients are under the age of 65 years, and 5 per cent are under age 40 years.

The risk factors that predispose a client to heart attack are the same as for all forms of CAD (see earlier).

The most common cause of MI is complete or nearly complete occlusion of a coronary artery due to ongoing atherosclerosis. The vessel lumen slowly occludes and is often blocked with a thrombus. When blood flow ceases abruptly, the myocardial tissue supplied by that artery dies and becomes necrotic. Other causes of acute occlusion include coronary artery spasm and hemorrhage into a plaque.

Pathophysiology

MI can be considered the endpoint of CAD. Unlike the temporary ischemia that occurs with angina, prolonged unrelieved ischemia causes irreversible damage to the myocardium. Cardiac cells can withstand ischemia for about 20 minutes before cellular death occurs. Because the myocardium is very metabolically active, signs of ischemia can be seen within 8 to 10 seconds of decreased blood flow. When the heart is not sustained with blood and oxygen, it converts to anaerobic metabolism. This form of metabolism creates less ATP and lactic acid as a byproduct. Myocardial cells are very sensitive to changes in pH and become less functional. Acidosis makes the myocardium more vulnerable to the effects of the lysosomal enzymes within the cell. Acidosis leads to conduction system disorders, and dysrhythmias develop. Contractility is also reduced, decreasing the heart's ability to pump. As the myocardial cells necrose, certain intracellular enzymes are introduced into the bloodstream, where they can be detected by laboratory tests.

The infarcted site is called the zone of infarction and necrosis. Around it is a zone of hypoxic injury. This zone is able to return to normal but may also necrose if blood flow is not restored. The outermost zone is called the zone of ischemia; damage to this area is reversible.

The most common site for myocardial infarction is the anterior wall of the left ventricle near the apex. Infarction of the anterior left ventricle results from thrombosis of the descending branch of the left coronary artery (Fig. 42-5).

Other common sites for a myocardial infarction are (1) the posterior wall of the left ventricle near the base and behind the posterior cusp of the mitral valve and

▲ **Figure 42-5**

Areas of myocardium affected by arterial insufficiency of specific coronary arteries.

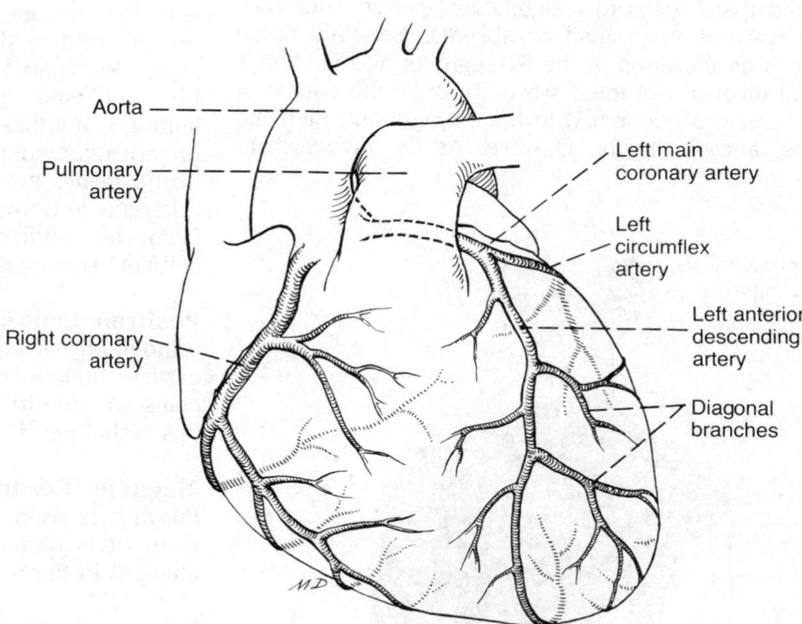

AREA OF MYOCARDIUM INVOLVED	CORONARY ARTERY SUPPLY
Anterior	Left coronary artery, left anterior descending branch
Posterior	Right coronary artery
Inferior	Right coronary artery
Anteroseptal	Left coronary artery, left anterior descending branch
High lateral	Circumflex artery, marginal branch, or LCA, diagonal branch
Apical	Usually LCA, left anterior branch, may be RCA, posterior descending branch

(2) the inferior (diaphragmatic) surface of the heart. Infarction of the posterior left ventricle results from occlusion of the right coronary artery or circumflex branch of the left coronary artery. An inferior infarction occurs when the right coronary artery occludes. In nearly one fourth of inferior wall MIs, the right ventricle has been infarcted. Atrial infarctions develop less than 5 per cent of the time.

Clinical Manifestations

The major symptom of MI is chest pain (Fig. 42-6), similar to angina pectoris but more severe in character and duration and unrelieved by nitroglycerin. The pain may radiate to the neck, jaw, shoulder, back, or left arm. Also, the pain may present near the epigastrium, simulating that of indigestion.

Table 42-3 outlines clinical manifestations of MI along with pathophysiologic bases.

DIAGNOSTIC ASSESSMENT

ECG Changes. Ischemia and myocardial infarction cause changes in the Q wave, ST segment, and T wave. Infarcted tissue leads to a significant Q wave (normally the Q wave is very small or absent). Ischemic tissue produces an elevation in the ST segment and peaked T wave or inversion of the T wave. Through the course of an MI, changes occur first in the ST segment, then the T wave, and finally the Q wave. As the myocardium heals the ST segment and T waves return to normal, but the Q wave remains evident. (See Fig. 42-7.)

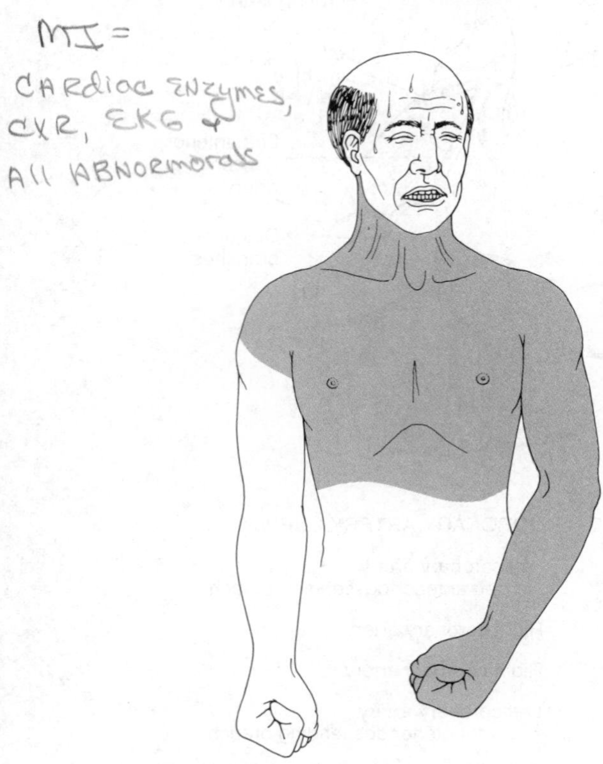

▲ Figure 42-6

Possible extent of pain from myocardial infarction.

Laboratory Studies. Laboratory findings include elevated serum CPK-MB, elevated LDH_1 isoenzyme, leukocytosis, and elevated erythrocyte sedimentation rate.

Serum levels of CPK-MB (an isoenzyme of CPK found only in cardiac muscle) increase 4 to 6 hours after the onset of chest pain, reach a peak in 12 to 18 hours, and return to normal levels in 3 to 4 days.

LDH_1 is plentiful in the heart muscle and is released into the serum when myocardial damage occurs. LDH_1 elevates 12 hours after onset of myocardial damage, peaks within 24 to 48 hours, and slowly returns to normal over the next 10 days.

Leukocytosis of 10,000 to 20,000 cells/mm^3 appears on the second day after MI and disappears in 1 week.

Radionuclide Imaging. Radionuclide imaging is a new method for diagnosing MI. A scintigram or scintiscan visually represents gamma rays emitted by a radioisotope. Technetium-99m-tagged pyrophosphate binds with calcium in areas of myocardial necrosis. Areas of uptake ("hot" spots) seen on nuclear imaging indicate areas of infarction.[72] However, because this test does not give positive results for 24 hours, it cannot be used to diagnose an acute MI during the early stage. Radiolabeled antimyosin is another agent used for "hot" spot imaging.[72] As mentioned earlier, thallium-201, another radioisotope, produces a "cold spot" on an infarcted or ischemic area. It has limited diagnostic value, however, because it cannot be used to differentiate between a new infarcted area and old scar from an earlier infarct. Multiple-gated acquisition (MUGA) scanning is also used.

Positron Emission Tomography. Positron emission tomography is an imaging technique used to evaluate cardiac metabolism and assess tissue perfusion. Clinicians are able to assess the severity of CAD with use of this technique.[72]

Magnetic Resonance Imaging. Magnetic resonance imaging is used to evaluate structural defects of the heart. It is particularly valuable in depicting structural changes in the myocardium and pericardium.[72]

Echocardiography. Echocardiography is useful in assessing the ability of the heart walls to contract and relax. The transducer is placed externally on the chest, and images are relayed to a monitor screen. In addition, echocardiography is useful in evaluating valvular function.[72]

Transesophageal Echocardiography. Transesophageal echocardiography is a new technique in imaging in which the transducer is placed against the wall of the esophagus. The image of the myocardium is clearer because no air is between the transducer and the heart. This technique is particularly useful in viewing the posterior wall of the heart.[72]

TABLE 42-3. Myocardial Infarction: Clinical Manifestations and Pathophysiologic Bases

Clinical Manifestations	Pathophysiologic Bases
Pain	
Crushing, severe, prolonged, unrelieved by rest or nitroglycerin; often radiating to one or both arms, the neck, and back	Cessation of blood supply to myocardium caused by thrombotic occlusion causes accumulation of metabolites within ischemic part of myocardium; this affects nerve endings
Shock	
Systolic blood pressure below 80 mm Hg, gray facial color, lethargy, cold diaphoresis, peripheral cyanosis, tachycardia or bradycardia, weak pulse	In some cases, shock caused primarily by severe pain; in others, by severe reduction in cardiac output and by inadequate tissue perfusion resulting in tissue hypoxia
Oliguria	
Urine flow of less than 30 ml/hr	Indicates renal hypoxia due to inadequate tissue perfusion resulting from hypotension. Cardiogenic shock is seen with damage to more than 40 per cent of left ventricle
Fever	
Temperature rises within 24 hours and lasts 3 to 7 days; usually 37.5° to 39.5° C (100° to 103° F), accompanied by leukocytosis and elevated sedimentation rate	Fever and elevated white blood cell counts result from destruction of myocardial tissue and ensuing inflammatory process; fever drops when fibroblasts begin to replace leukocytes and scar tissue starts to form
Apprehension	
Great fear of death, restlessness	Severe pain of a heart attack is terrifying; also, most clients are aware of the significance of a heart attack; restlessness results from shock and pain
"Indigestion"	
"Gas pains around the heart," nausea and vomiting	Client may prefer to believe that pain is caused by "gas" or "indigestion" rather than by heart disease; nausea and vomiting may result from severe pain or from vagovagal reflexes conducted from area of damaged myocardium to gastrointestinal tract
Acute Pulmonary Edema	
Sense of suffocation, dyspnea, orthopnea, gurgling; bubbling respirations	In some cases, left ventricle becomes severely crippled in pumping action owing to infarction; severe pulmonary congestion results

Prognosis

Since the advent of coronary care units and devices that aid in promptly recognizing and treating life-threatening arrhythmias, 70 to 80 per cent of those suffering from an acute MI survive the initial attack. Chances for survival greatly diminish with the presence of the following:

- old age (80 years or older has a 60 per cent mortality rate)
- evidence of other cardiovascular diseases, respiratory diseases, or uncontrolled diabetes mellitus (presence of angina or previous MI results in a chance of mortality greater than 30 per cent)
- anterior location of MI (anterior MI has a 30 per cent mortality rate)
- hypotension (systolic blood pressure of less than 55 mm Hg on admission has a 60 per cent mortality rate)

Deaths generally result from severe dysrhythmias, cardiogenic shock, congestive heart failure, rupture of the heart, and recurrent MI.

Clients fortunate enough to avoid developing complications after MI still require a period of 6 to 12 weeks for complete recovery. Unfortunately, however, 50 per cent of those who completely recover from their first coronary will die within 5 years; 75 per cent will die within 10 years from massive infarctions.[66]

Medical Management

Major goals of care for clients with acute MI are (1) successful treatment of the acute attack and prompt alleviation of manifestations, (2) prevention of complications and further attacks, and (3) rehabilitation and education of the client and significant others.

MANAGEMENT OF THE ACUTE ATTACK

The client who suffers an acute MI needs immediate admission to a hospital with a coronary care unit, if possible. The first 24 hours after an MI is the time of highest risk for sudden death. Invasive monitoring (arterial and pulmonary artery pressure lines) are commonly used. (See Bridge to Critical Care on arterial lines and Chap. 41 for Bridge to Critical Care on pulmonary artery pressure lines.)

The first 6 hours after the onset of pain is the crucial time frame for the salvage of the myocardium. Pain control is a priority. Continued pain is a symptom of myocardial ischemia. Pain also stimulates the autonomic nervous system and preload, increasing myocardial demands. Oxygen is used to treat tissue hypoxia. Because dysrhythmias are common, ECG monitoring is essential. Anti-arrythmics are begun. Anticoagulants are begun to decrease the risk of embolism. Stool softeners are used to decrease constipation and the risk of bradycardia from straining.

Recently clinicians have treated acute MIs with medications that lyse or dissolve the clot that forms part of the blockage of the coronary artery. Thrombolytic therapy includes streptokinase, urokinase, tissue-plasminogen activator (t-PA), and acylated plasminogen streptokinase activator complex (APSAC). It is generally recommended that to be most effective, thrombolytic agents must be given within 3 to 6 hours after the onset of chest pain.[31] After the thrombolytic agent is administered, intravenous heparin therapy is usually continued for 5 to 7 days. All of these thrombolytic agents can be given intravenously, and some clinicians are initiating the infusions at the scene of the infarction.

Not all clients with MI are suitable candidates for thrombolytic therapy. Complications of thrombolytics include bleeding, allergic reactions, and stroke.[31] Successful reperfusion of the coronary arteries is evidenced by return of the ECG changes to normal; relief of chest pain; presence of reperfusion dysrhythmias (usually ventricular); and a rapid, early peak of the CK-MB enzymes ("washout").

PREVENTION OF COMPLICATIONS

The possibility of death from complications always accompanies an acute MI. Thus, prime collaborative goals include prevention of life-threatening complications or at least recognition of them.

Dysrhythmias. Specifically, these are ventricular premature beats, ventricular tachycardia and fibrillation, supraventricular tachycardia, and heart block.

Dysrhythmias are the major cause of death after an MI; 40 to 50 per cent of deaths occur because of dysrhythmias. Ectopic rhythms arise in or near borders of intensely ischemic and damaged myocardial tissues. Damaged myocardium may also interfere with the conduction system, causing dissociation of the atria and ventricles (heart block). Supraventricular tachycardia sometimes occurs as a result of heart failure. Spontaneous or pharmacologic reperfusion of a previously ischemic area may also precipitate ventricular arrhythmias.

Provide continuous cardiac monitoring and frequent counts of premature ventricular contractions (PVCs) (many monitoring systems count continuously). Notify the physician if more than three PVCs occur per minute. Provide prompt intervention for dysrhythmias per protocol or orders. For frequent PVCs, administer procainamide (Pronestyl) or lidocaine intravenously. For ventricular tachycardia, administer lidocaine or procainamide or provide elective cardioversion. For ventricular fibrillation, provide immediate defibrillation. For supraventricular fibrillation, administer digitalis or quinidine, treat heart failure, and provide elective cardioversion. For heart block, administer atropine or isoproterenol (with caution) and use a temporary pacemaker. Dysrhythmias are discussed later in this chapter.

Cardiogenic Shock. Cardiogenic shock results in 9 per cent of the deaths from MI. An estimated 80 per cent of clients who develop shock die from the complications. Causes include decreased myocardial contraction and diminished cardiac output, undetected dysrhythmias, and sepsis.

Clinical manifestations include systolic blood pressure significantly below a client's normal blood pressure, diaphoresis, rapid pulse, restlessness, cold clammy skin, and gray skin color.

Shock can be prevented with rapid relief of pain and sufficient intravenous fluids to prevent circulatory collapse. It is also vital to identify dysrhythmias rapidly.

Administer vasopressors such as levarterenol, dopamine, dobutamine, and metaraminol (Aramine) as prescribed to raise blood pressure by increasing peripheral resistance. In other cases, vasodilators such as nitroprusside promote better blood flow in the microcirculation. Positive inotropic agents such as dopamine increase cardiac contractility and cardiac output and improve tissue perfusion. Administer oxygen therapy and antiarrhythmic agents as prescribed, and continuously monitor interarterial and pulmonary artery pressures. Chapter 20 discusses shock in detail.

Heart Failure and Pulmonary Edema. The most common cause of in-hospital death for clients with cardiac disorders is congestive heart failure (CHF). CHF is responsible for one third of deaths after an MI.[66]

Heart failure may develop at the onset of the infarction, or it may occur weeks later. Clinical manifestations include dyspnea, orthopnea, weight gain, edema, enlarged tender liver, distended neck veins, and crackles. CHF is managed by correcting the underlying etiology, relieving symptoms, and enhancing cardiac

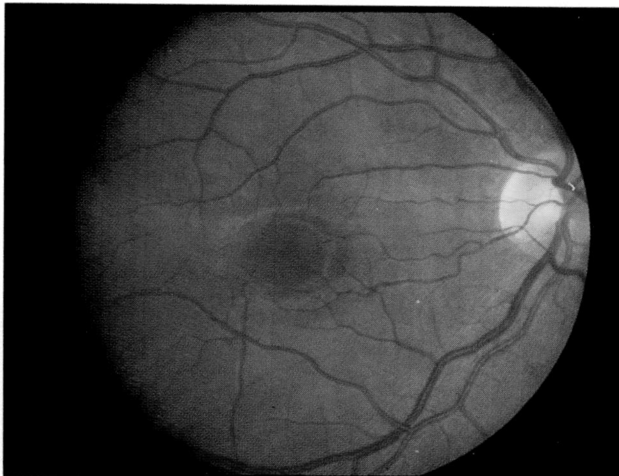

▲ ***Plate 1.*** The normal fundus. (Courtesy of Ophthalmic Photography at the University of Michigan W. K. Kellogg Eye Center.)

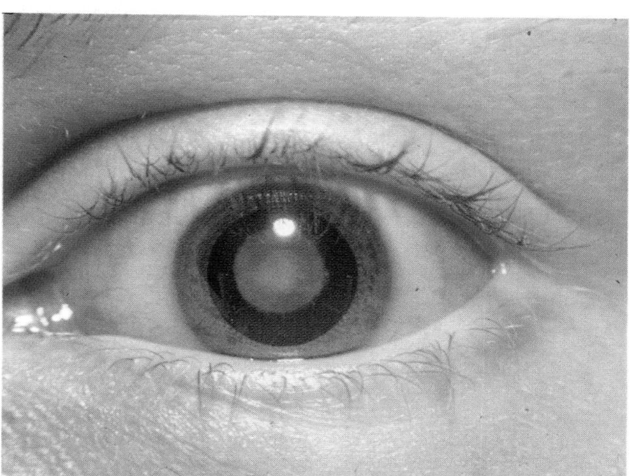

▲ ***Plate 2.*** Cloudy appearance of the lens affected by cataract. (Courtesy of Ophthalmic Photography at the University of Michigan W. K. Kellogg Eye Center.)

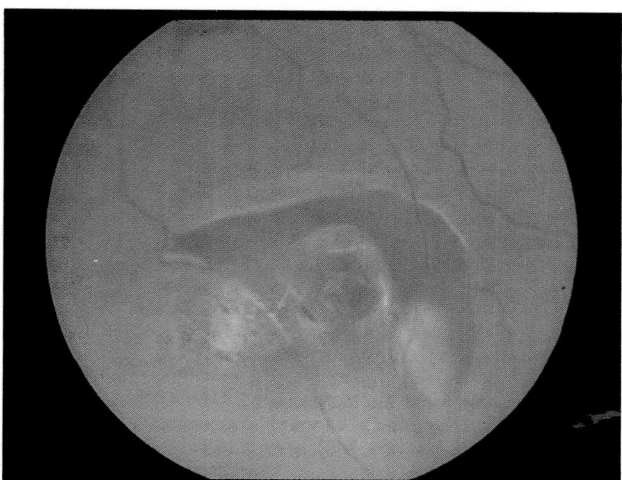

▲ ***Plate 3.*** Bluish gray appearance of areas of retinal detachment. (Courtesy of Ophthalmic Photography at the University of Michigan W. K. Kellogg Eye Center.)

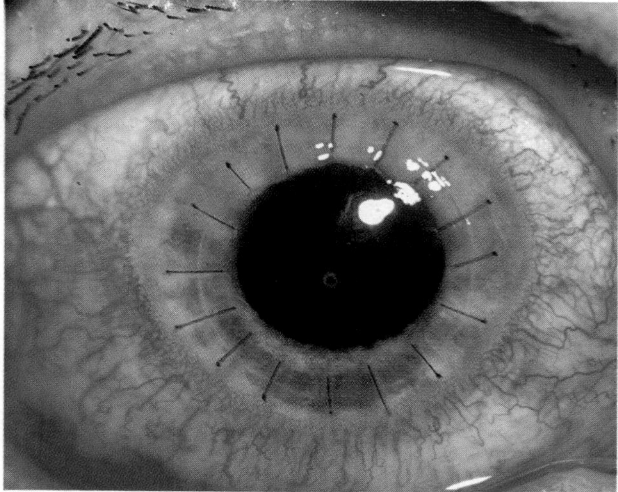

▲ ***Plate 4.*** Keratoplasty. (Courtesy of Ophthalmic Photography at the University of Michigan W. K. Kellogg Eye Center.)

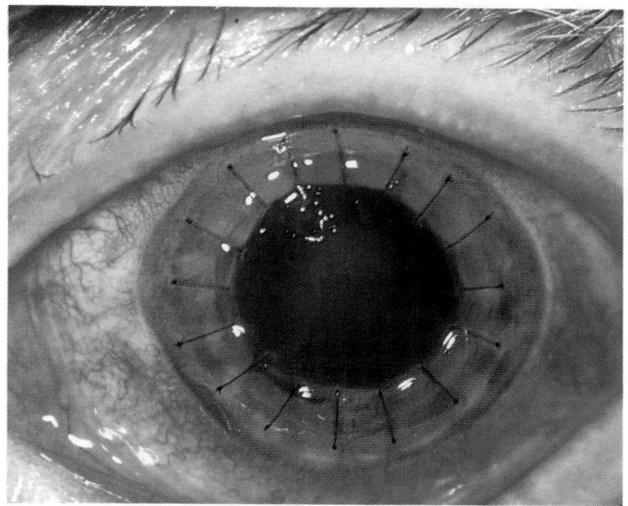

▲ ***Plate 5.*** Acute graft rejection. (Courtesy of Ophthalmic Photography at the University of Michigan W. K. Kellogg Eye Center.)

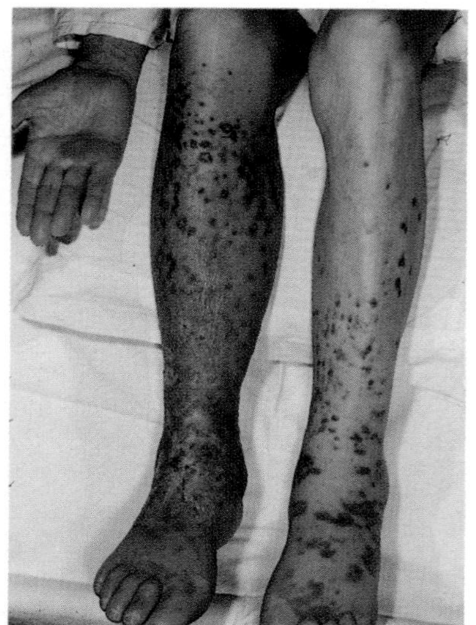

▲ ***Plate 16.*** Kaposi's sarcoma.

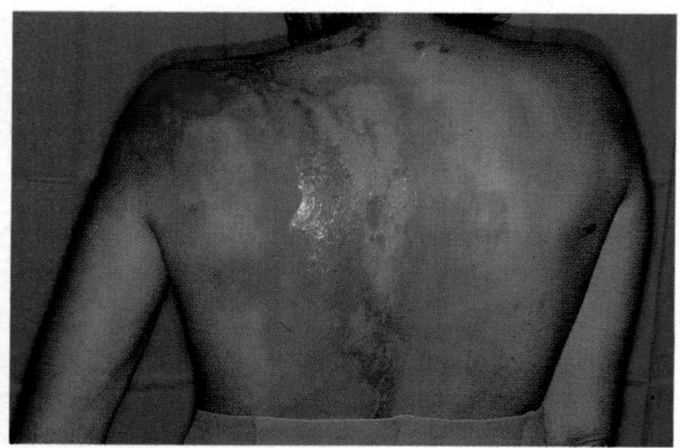

▲ ***Plate 17.*** Partial-thickness burn injury.

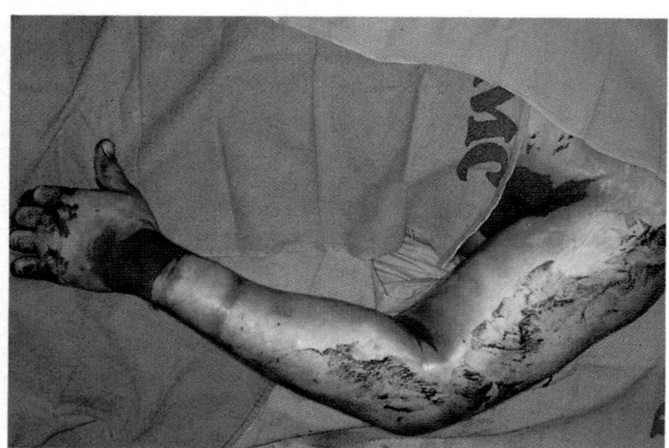

▲ ***Plate 18.*** Full-thickness burn injury.

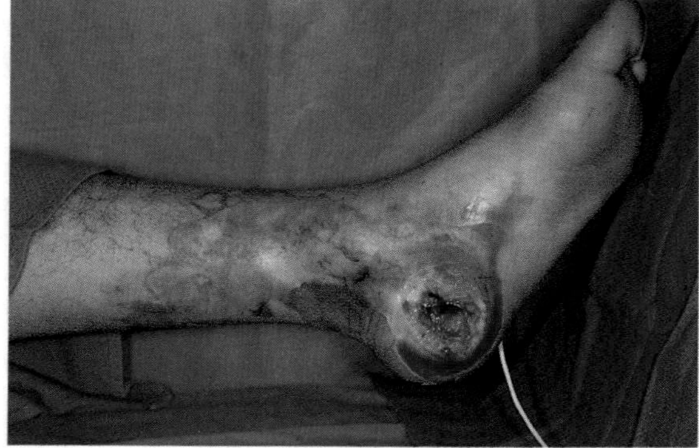

▲ ***Plate 19.*** Full-thickness burn injury with underlying subcutaneous tissue damage at the heel from contact with an electrical source.

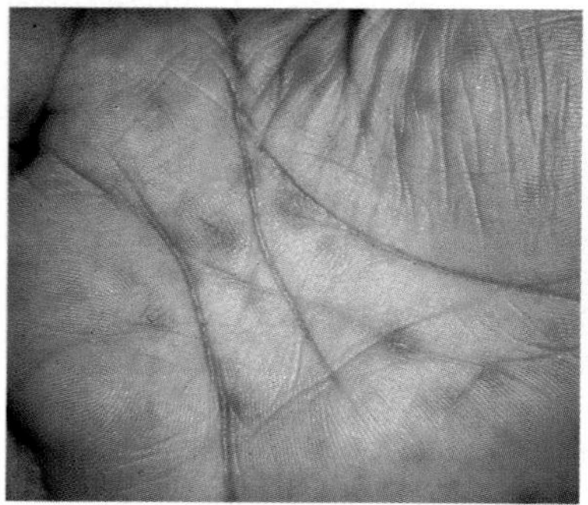

▲ ***Plate 20.*** Rash seen in secondary syphilis. (From Lookingbill, D. P., & Marks, J. G. [1986]. *Principles of dermatology.* Philadelphia: W. B. Saunders.)

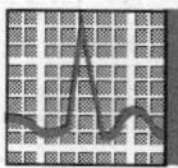

BRIDGE TO CRITICAL CARE

Arterial Lines

Insertion of a catheter into an artery for direct measurement of systolic, diastolic, and mean blood pressure readings.

Insertion sites include

- Radial
- Brachial
- Axillary
- Femoral
- Dorsalis pedis

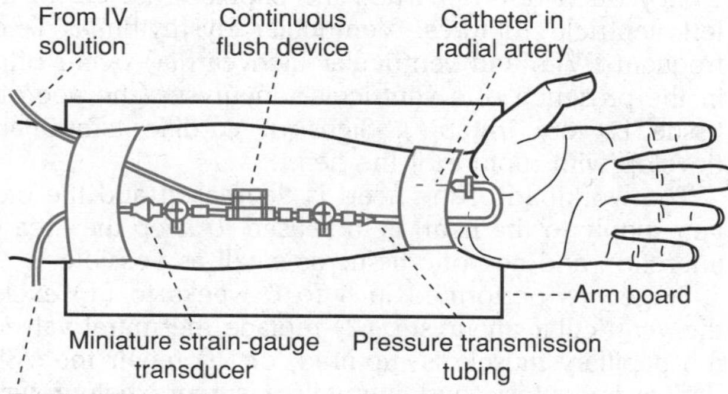

Indications For Use

- Monitoring any major medical or surgical condition that compromises cardiac output or fluid volume status
- Continuous assessment of arterial perfusion to the major organ systems
- Continuous measurement of systole, diastole, and mean arterial blood pressure
  MAP = (2 x diastolic + systolic) divided by 3
- Direct arterial access — blood gas measurements
- Assessment of arterial compliance and stroke volume
  Pulse pressure = (systolic - diastolic)

Nursing Precautions

- Access collateral circulation prior to arterial cannulation
- Allen's test to access radial and ulner arteries
- Continued assessment of tissue perfusion at arterial site
- Maintenance of arterial line patency (pressure tubing, heparinized solution, pressure bag)

Complications

- Blood back up from improper set-up
- Thrombus formation
- Embolization
- Arterial spasm
- Ischemic damage
- Amputation
- Hemorrhage
- Infection

Typical Arterial Waveform

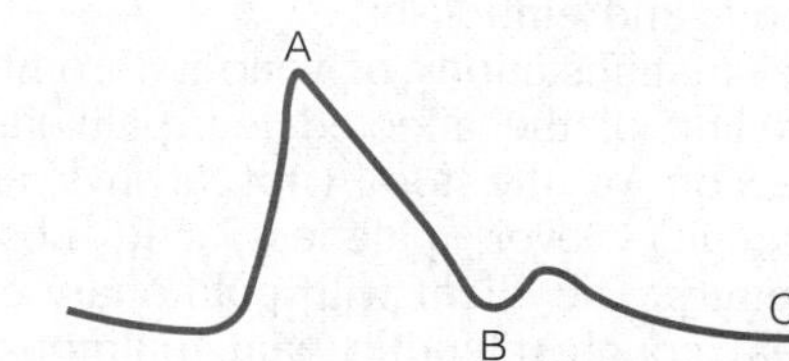

The three components of a typical waveform: A, systolic peak; B, dicrotic notch; and C, end-diastole.

Effect of PVCs on Arterial Pressure

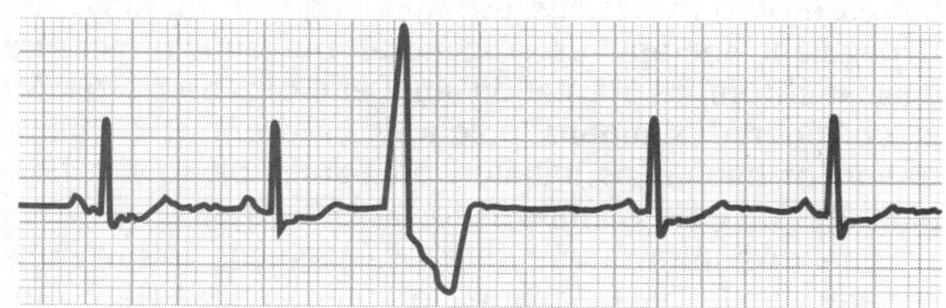

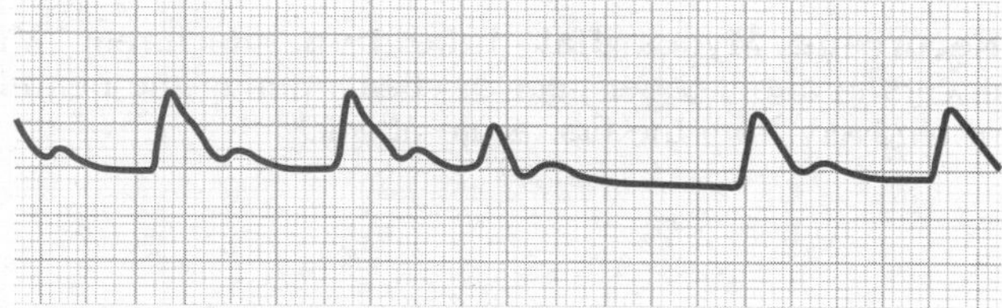

…cussed later in this chap-

… Embolism. Pulmonary embolism (PE) … develop secondary to phlebitis of the leg or pelvic veins (venous thrombosis). Pulmonary embolism occurs in 10 to 20 per cent of clients at some point either during the acute attack or in the convalescent period.

Prolonged bed rest, increased blood viscosity, increased blood coagulability, hemostasis, and decreased circulation due to positioning in bed all increase the risk of thrombus and embolism.

The clinical manifestations of venous thrombosis are pain and swelling of the affected leg, pain in the calf upon dorsiflexion of the foot (not always a reliable indicator, though), fever, paleness, and absence of pulse in extremity. The client with pulmonary embolism has tachypnea, cough, pleuritic pain, pulmonary rales, cyanosis, fever, sometimes shock, and cardiac arrest.

Prevention is the best treatment for PE. Encourage the client to move legs and feet frequently. Avoid placing pressure under the knees with pillows or Gatch bed. Apply Ace bandages or elastic stockings to legs. Administer sufficient fluids to prevent dehydration and increase blood viscosity; use anticoagulant therapy. Anticoagulant therapy as a general preventive measure against thrombus formation and embolization after MI is considered standard practice. Intravenous administration of heparin is initiated on admission to the hospital and may be continued for 3 to 7 days.

Sedation, intravenous therapy, oxygen, intravenous heparin, oral anticoagulants, or pulmonary artery embolectomy may be required.

Recurrent Myocardial Infarction. Recurrent MI occurs in about 5 per cent of clients during the period of recovery from the first acute attack.[66]

Possible causes include overexertion, embolization, or further thrombotic occlusion of a coronary artery by an atheroma. The clinical manifestation is the return of angina. Management is the same as for the acute MI.

Complications Due to Necrosis of the Myocardium. Complications due to necrosis of the myocardium include ventricular aneurysm, rupture of the heart, ventricular septal defect (VSD), and ruptured papillary muscle. These problems are infrequent but serious complications that usually occur 7 to 10 days after an MI. Weak, friable necrotic myocardial tissue increases vulnerability to these complications (Fig. 42–7).

Manifestations of CHF develop with ventricular aneurysm, rupture of the ventricular septum, and rupture of the papillary muscle. Symptoms of severe mitral insufficiency often develop when the papillary muscle of the left ventricle ruptures. Ventricular dysrhythmias (e.g., frequent PVCs and ventricular tachycardia) occur often in the presence of a ventricular aneurysm (the necrotic tissue is very irritable). Signs of cardiac tamponade develop with rupture of the heart.

The workload of the heart is decreased and the oxygen supply to the heart is increased to keep the area of infarction and necrotic tissue as small as possible.

Surgery is performed in 4 to 6 weeks to (1) excise the ventricular aneurysm, (2) replace the mitral valve if the papillary muscle is ruptured, or (3) repair the VSD. Pericardiocentesis and immediate surgery help relieve cardiac tamponade occurring after rupture of the heart. Also, the surgeon repairs the rupture.

Pericarditis. Up to 28 per cent of clients suffering an acute transmural MI will develop early pericarditis (within 2 to 4 days). The inflamed area of the infarction rubs against the pericardial surface and causes it to lose its lubricating fluid. A pericardial friction rub can

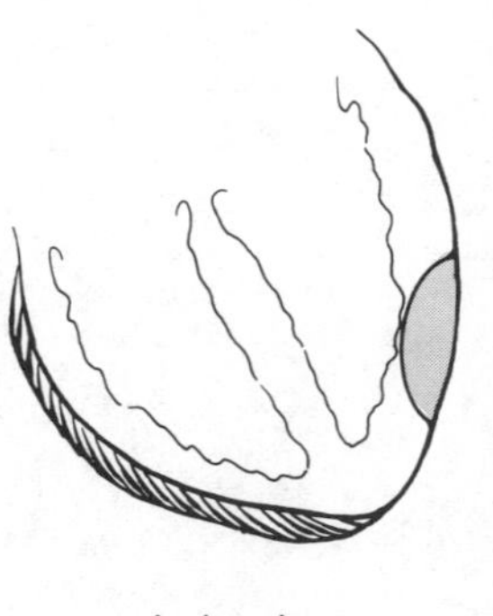

Ischemia

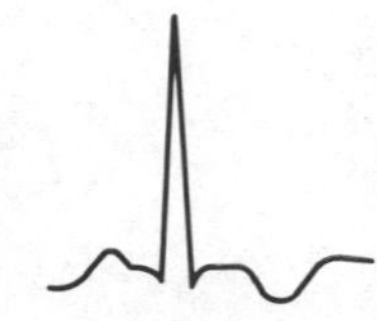

Injury

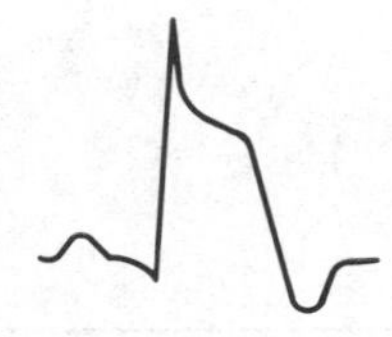

Infarction

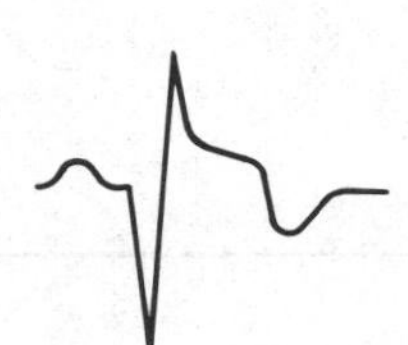

▲ *Figure 42–7*

Areas of change and ECG patterns that accompany these changes during myocardial infarction.

be auscultated across the precordium. The client complains of chest pain that is aggravated with movement, deep inspiration, and cough. The pain of pericarditis is relieved when the client sits up and leans forward.

Frequent assessment may lead to early identification and intervention. Relieve pain with analgesics, such as acetaminophen, or other anti-inflammatory agents. Reduce the client's anxiety by differentiating the pain of pericarditis from the pain of MI.[74]

Dressler's Syndrome (Late Pericarditis). The form of pericarditis known as Dressler's syndrome can occur as late as 6 weeks to months after an MI.[75] Although the etiologic agent is unknown, current research suggests an autoimmune causation. The client usually presents with a fever lasting 1 week or longer, pericardial chest pain, pericardial friction rub, and occasionally pleuritis with pleural effusions. This is a self-limiting phenomenon, and no prevention is known. Treatment includes aspirin, prednisone, and narcotic analgesics for pain. Anticoagulation therapy may precipitate cardiac tamponade and should be avoided in these clients.[74]

REHABILITATION

A successful rehabilitation program begins the moment a client with a "coronary" enters the coronary care unit for emergency care and continues for months and even years after discharge home from the health care facility (see Bridge to Home Health Care).

Goals of Rehabilitation. The overall goal of rehabilitation is twofold: to help the client (1) live as full, vital, and productive a life as possible and (2) remain within the limits of the heart's ability to respond to increases in activity and stress. Although the myocardium must rest, bed rest puts the client at risk for developing hypovolemia, hypoxemia, muscle atrophy, and pulmonary embolus. Thus, the client must avoid both invalidism and reckless overexertion.

Six important subgoals of the rehabilitation process are to (1) develop a program of progressive physical activity; (2) teach the client and significant others concerning cause, prevention, and treatment of CAD; (3) help the client accept the limitations imposed by illness; (4) aid the client in adjusting to changes in occupational goals; (5) lessen avoidable risk factors; and (6) change the psychosocial factors adversely affecting recovery from CAD.

Program of Physical Activity. Clients who have suffered a heart attack usually remain on bed rest for only 24 hours unless complications such as CHF or dysrhythmias develop. Remember that protracted bed rest produces severe problems. The client loses 10 to 15 per cent of skeletal muscle and contractile strength within the first week of bed rest, and 20 to 25 per cent in 3 weeks of bed rest.

The client must increase activities gradually to avoid overtaxing the heart as it pumps oxygenated blood to the muscles. The METs (metabolic equivalents) system provides one way of measuring the amount of oxygen needed to perform an activity: 1 MET equals 3.5 ml of oxygen per kilogram of body weight per minute. One MET is approximately equivalent to the oxygen uptake a client requires when resting. Early mobilization activities after an acute MI should not exceed 1 to 2 METs

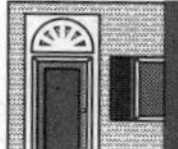

BRIDGE TO HOME HEALTH ...

Myocardial Infarction Rehabilitation

Successful cardiac rehabilitation can be done in the home setting. Bridging hospital care to home care involves continuing the exercise program and nursing assessments implemented in the hospital; the home health nurse serves as a facilitator and communicator.

Cardiac assessment of the client includes but is not limited to vital signs, lung sounds, peripheral pulses, and auscultation of heart sounds. Other important assessments include diet history and current weight and height measures. The home health nurse should possess knowledge of basic arrhythmias, murmurs, and extra heart sounds. The detection of an S_3 or S_4 heart sound is critical for detecting impending complications. Some clients are discharged with a Holter monitor in place, but most are not. Orthostatic blood pressure readings are assessed because of side effects precipitated by antihypertensive drugs, vasodilators, and antianginal agents. Occasionally, portable electrocardiograms and chest films are done by home radiology companies.

Teaching medication actions, side effects, and methods of administration is more successful in the home, where stress levels are usually lower. Written medication sheets can be individualized for each client, with dosage of medication and time of administration written in by the nurse.

Ambulation in the home should be equivalent to levels achieved at the hospital. If exercise equipment is absent in the home, creative ideas are necessary for bridging the gap between hospital and home care. The client and family are taught to measure blood pressure and pulse before and after each exercise program. The home health nurse teaches when to stop exercise, what signs and symptoms are critical, and when to schedule rest periods and pace daily activities. Recording vital signs, activities, and tolerance is essential. Perhaps most important of all is to establish goals with the client according to lifestyle and needs.

The home health nurse often refers clients to community resources such as the American Heart Association and the Red Cross. Encouraging participation in lifeline services can increase the sense of security of those clients who live alone. When possible, a family member should be encouraged to take courses in cardiopulmonary resuscitation.

Finally, the home health nurse is in a unique position to reinforce teaching about healthy heart strategies. These include reducing weight, continuing lifelong exercise programs, decreasing dietary sodium and fats, reducing stress levels, and ceasing smoking. Family members should be included in the teaching when appropriate. A written contract can be used as a tool for help in establishing goals with the client and identifying steps toward these goals. These goals are still the cornerstone of any successful cardiac rehabilitation program.

eeding). Later activi- 11 METs (e.g., cycling, (e.g. ctivity level increase, monitor heart rate, pressure, and fatigue and adjust the client's activity level accordingly. During early activities, the heart rate should not rise more than 25 per cent above resting level. Blood pressure must not rise more than 25 mm Hg above normal.

The typical program of activity for clients recuperating from an acute MI is designated by phases.

Phase I (In-Hospital). Phase I begins with admission to the coronary care unit. Provide complete bed rest for the first day or so with use of bedside commode for bowel movements. Provide a liquid diet for the first 24 hours.

Clinicians may allow the client to shave and feed himself or herself, move around in bed, and brush his or her teeth once blood pressure and vital signs stabilize. A coronary care nurse or physiotherapist should start passive exercises.

As strength is regained, have the client sit for brief periods on the side of the bed and dangle the feet. Allow the client to ambulate to a bedside chair for 15 to 20 minutes if permissible after the first day.

When the client is transferred from the coronary care unit to an intermediate or regular unit, bathroom privileges and self-care activities are encouraged. Wireless heart monitoring may continue. Allow brief walks in the hall with supervision. The length and duration of these walks progressively increase according to the client's endurance.

Help the client avoid fatigue. Dyspnea, chest pain, tachycardia, and a sense of exhaustion warn that the client is attempting to do too much. Instruct the client regarding these warning signs of overexertion.

Client education during phase I should include anatomy and physiology of the heart and CAD, risk factors and management of CAD, behavioral counseling, and home activities.

Phase II (Intermediate). If no complications arise, the physician will discharge the client home by the end of the second week. Nearly 50 per cent of the million clients who suffer an acute MI have an uncomplicated hospital course without evidence of angina, heart failure, or major arrhythmias. There is a growing trend toward early discharge of clients with uncomplicated myocardial infarcts. A team at one health care facility discharges post-MI clients at the end of the first week. However, they allow clients to go home early only if their households have adequate help and are conducive to rest. Also, such clients are followed carefully by trained nurse-clinicians who come to their homes and supervise their physiologic status, exercise, and diet on an alternate-day basis. Researchers hope that earlier discharge after MI will reduce depression as well as the expense of hospitalization.

Resuming sexual activity may be one of the most difficult phases of returning to normal life after an MI. One study reports that over 50 per cent of a group of women reported fear of returning to normal sexual activity after an MI (44 per cent of their husbands reported similar concerns). The physician may allow sexual intercourse 4 to 8 weeks after an MI. Caution clients not to eat or drink alcoholic beverages immediately before intercourse. Taking nitroglycerin before intercourse may help prevent exertional angina.

Advise the client to stop smoking completely. Encourage frequent walks, but the client must avoid strenuous activities such as shoveling snow. The walking program aims toward a goal of 2 miles in less than 60 minutes. A monitored group program may be useful to assist the client in achieving the best possible physical conditioning. These programs offer a variety of training devices, such as treadmills, stationary bicycles, and rowing machines, to facilitate fitness. In addition, clients are trained in warm-up and stretching exercises.

After an acute MI, many clients will be instructed to take one aspirin daily. Aspirin decreases platelet aggregation and may be useful in preventing MIs. Side effects include epigastric distress, gastrointestinal bleeding, and nausea.

Some clients may be able to return to work at the end of 8 or 9 weeks if they remain asymptomatic. Clients with less physically strenuous jobs can sometimes work full-time, but manual laborers may have to work part-time or find more sedentary work.

Between the eighth and tenth weeks, the client requires a complete physical examination, including ECG, exercise stress tests, lipid analysis, and chest radiography. Clinicians need to correct pre-existing health problems that might have contributed to the development of CAD (e.g., hypertension, anemia, hyperthyroidism, aortic valvular disease).

Encourage the client to schedule additional examinations as necessary. Clients with recurrent indigestion, "heartburn," chest pain, or above-the-waistline pain associated with activity or emotional stress need to see their physician.

Phase III (Long-Term). Clinicians trained in cardiac rehabilitation may provide detailed, written instructions for a long-term exercise program. Various methods are used to determine the appropriate exercise routines. Periodic evaluation is necessary to assess the client's endurance and tolerance to the prescribed exercise program.

Nursing Management

The focus of the plan of care for the MI client includes (1) recognizing and treating potentially life-threatening dysrhythmias; (2) monitoring for complications from decreased cardiac output; (3) maintaining a therapeutic critical care environment; (4) identifying the psychosocial impact of the MI on the client and family; and (5) educating the client in lifestyle changes and rehabilitation after the MI.

Nursing diagnoses or collaborative problems that may apply to the client after an acute MI are discussed in the care plan.

Text continued on page 1164

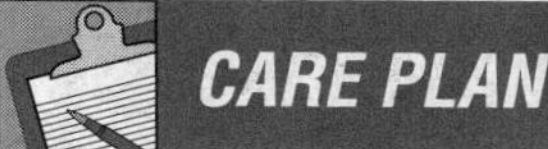

CARE PLAN

The Client with a Myocardial Infarction

Nursing Diagnosis/ Collaborative Problem	Planning: Expected Outcomes	Implementation: Nursing Interventions	Rationales
Pain, Acute (Chest) R/T myocardial ischemia resulting from coronary artery occlusion with loss/restriction of blood flow to an area of the myocardium and necrosis of the myocardium • typically substernal pain, tightness, pressure, or heaviness • pain radiating to arms, especially on the left side • complaints of neck, shoulder, back, and arm pain • nausea and vomiting • diaphoresis • weakness • anxiety • shortness of breath • dysrhythmias • palpitations	Client will have improved comfort in chest, as evidenced by • states a decrease in the rating of the chest pain • is able to rest, displays reduced tension, sleeps comfortably • requires decreased analgesia or nitroglycerin	Assess characteristics of chest pain, including location, duration, quality, intensity, presence of radiation, precipitating and alleviating factors, and associated symptoms; have client rate pain on a scale of 1 to 10 and document findings in nurses' notes	Pain is an indication of myocardial ischemia. Assisting the client in quantifying pain may differentiate preexisting and current pain patterns as well as identify complications
		Assess respirations, blood pressure, and heart rate with each episode of chest pain	Respirations may be increased as a result of pain and associated anxiety; release of stress-induced catecholamines will increase heart rate and blood pressure
		Obtain a 12-lead ECG on admission, then each time chest pain recurs for evidence of further infarction	Serial ECG and stat ECGs record changes that can give evidence of further cardiac damage and location of myocardial ischemia
		Monitor response to drug therapy. Notify physician if pain does not abate	Pain control is a priority, as it indicates ischemia
		Provide care in a calm, efficient manner that will reassure the client and minimize anxiety; stay with client until discomfort is relieved	Decreases external stimuli, which may aggravate anxiety and cardiac strain and limit coping abilities
		Limit visitors	Prevention of overstimulation and promote rest
Dysrhythmias R/T electrical instability or irritability secondary to ischemia or infarcted tissue • increase or decrease in heart rate • change in rhythm • dysrhythmias	Client will have no dysrhythmias, as evidenced by • normal sinus rhythm • normotension	Teach client/family about need for continuous monitoring; keep alarms on and limits set at all times	Continued monitoring keeps staff aware of myocardial changes. Family anxiety decreased
		Assess apical heart rate; auscultate for change in heart sounds (murmurs, rub, S_3 and S_4)	Indicative of early cardiac decompensation and potential loss of cardiac output
		Document rhythm strip every shift and PRN if dysrhythmias occur; measure pulse rate and QRS segments with each strip; note and report any deviations from the client's baseline	Dysrhythmias are the most common complication after an MI
		Report three or more multifocal PVCs per minute to physician	Indicate ventricular irritability, which decreases cardiac output and may lead to life-threatening dysrhythmias
		Administrator antidysrhythmics as ordered	Antidysrhythmics reduce myocardial irritability

Care Plan continued on following page

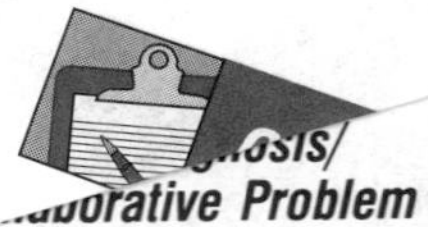

... Myocardial Infarction Continued

...gnosis/ ...aborative Problem	Planning: Expected Outcomes	Implementation: Nursing Interventions	Rationales
		Monitor effects of antidysrhythmic agents	Desired result is increased diastolic threshold potential and decreased action potential duration
		Monitor serum potassium levels	Altered potassium levels can affect cardiac rhythms
		Maintain a patent intravenous line or heparin lock at all times	Administration of intravenous cardiac medications in emergency
Decreased Cardiac Output R/T negative inotropic changes in the heart secondary to myocardial ischemia, injury, or infarction • change in level of consciousness • weakness/dizziness • loss of peripheral pulses • abnormal heart sounds • hemodynamic compromise • cardiopulmonary arrest	Client will have improved cardiac output, as evidenced by • cardiac rate, rhythm, and hemodynamic parameters within normal limits • dysrhythmias controlled or absent • absence of angina	Assess for and document the following as evidence of myocardial dysfunction with decreasing cardiac output 1. Mental status—be alert to restlessness and decreased responsiveness 2. Lung sounds—monitor for crackles and rhonchi 3. Heart sounds—note the presence of gallop, murmur, and increased heart rate 4. Urinary output—be alert to output <30 ml/hr 5. Peripheral perfusion—monitor for pallor, mottling, cyanosis, coolness, diaphoresis, and peripheral pulses 6. Vital signs—note any abnormalities in client's vital signs 7. Presence of jugular neck vein distention 8. Dependent edema (sacral) 9. Weakness, fatigue 10. Decreased activity level 11. Shortness of breath with activity 12. Monitor arterial blood gases	Cerebral perfusion is directly related to cardiac output and aortic perfusion pressure and is influenced by hypoxia and electrolyte and acid-base variations; crackles may develop, reflecting pulmonary congestion related to alterations in myocardial function; hypotension related to hypoperfusion, vagal stimulation, or ventricular dysfunction may occur; hypertension may be related to pain, anxiety, catecholamine release, or pre-existing vascular problems; urinary output less than 30 ml/hr may reflect reduced renal perfusion and glomerular filtration as a result of reduced cardiac output
		If client has pulmonary artery catheter, record hemodynamic parameters every 2 to 4 hours and PRN; be alert to pulmonary capillary wedge pressure greater than 18 mm Hg, cardiac output less than 4 L/min, and cardiac index less than 2.5 L/min	Hemodynamic pressures reflect intravascular responses and ventricular function; use to assess drug therapy and for prevention or early detection of complications of myocardial infarction (i.e., extension, heart failure, cardiogenic shock)
		Maintain hemodynamic stability by monitoring the ef-	Assess effect of drug therapy on myocardial contrac-

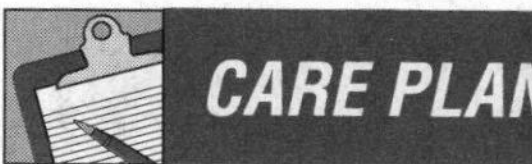

CARE PLAN

The Client with a Myocardial Infarction Continued

Nursing Diagnosis/ Collaborative Problem	Planning: Expected Outcomes	Implementation: Nursing Interventions	Rationales
		fects of beta-blockers and inotropic agents	tility and function
Gas Exchange, Impaired R/T decreased cardiac output • increased or decreased heart rate • decreased blood pressure • decreased temperature • dusky color • impaired capillary refill • reduced arterial PaO_2 • dyspnea	Client will have improved gas exchange, as evidenced by • vital signs within normal limits for client • absence of cyanosis • absence of dyspnea • arterial blood gases within normal limits	Administer oxygen as ordered; continuous oximetry	Increases amount of oxygen available for myocardial uptake; oximetry measures peripheral oxygenation
		Monitor arterial blood gases as ordered	Presence of hypoxia indicates need for supplemental oxygen
		Continue to assess client's skin, capillary refill, level of consciousness, and vital signs every 2 to 4 hours and PRN	Provides data on adequacy of tissue perfusion and oxygenation
		Prepare for intubation and mechanical ventilation if hypoxia increases	With increasing hypoxia, mechanical ventilation may be necessary to oxygenate the client adequately
Powerlessness R/T hospital environment and anticipated lifestyle changes • withdrawn • verbalizes "feelings of doom" • crying • anger	Client will have an improved feeling of control, as evidenced by • verbalizing feelings of powerlessness • verbalizing a sense of control over present situation and future outcomes	Provide opportunities for the client to express feelings about self and illness	Creates supportive climate, sends message that care givers are willing to help
		Explore reality perceptions and clarify if necessary	Listening to the feelings as well as to the words of the client can help client see a more hopeful outlook
		Eliminate unpredictability of events by allowing adequate preparation for tests/procedures	Information can help client or family feel more hopeful about situation and more willing to participate in care
		Reinforce the client's right to ask questions	Keep a supportive climate to let client feel free to ask questions or have information repeated
		Allow choices when possible	Allows client to feel independent
		Provide positive reinforcement for increased involvement in self-care	When clients participate in planning for care, they are more apt to feel a sense of control and to follow through with actions
		Help client identify strengths and areas of control	Self-confidence and security come with a sense of control; allow full client participation
Anxiety/Fear R/T hospital admission and fear of death • client/family appear restless, hostile; or withdrawn • client/family verbalize fatalism or act extremely emotional as if in grieving process	Client will have reduced feelings of anxiety/fear, as evidenced by • demonstrates appropriate range of feelings and initial signs of effective coping, such as participation in treatment regimen	Limit nursing personnel; provide continuity of care	Continuity of care promotes security and development of rapport with and trust of health care providers
		Allow and encourage client/family to ask questions; do not avoid questions. Bring up common concerns	Accurate information about the situation reduces fear, strengthens client-nurse relationship, assists client and family to deal realisti-

Care Plan continued on following page

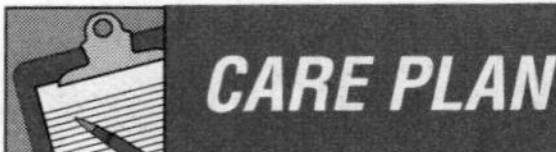

CARE PLAN

The Client with a Myocardial Infarction Continued

Nursing Diagnosis/ Collaborative Problem	*Planning: Expected Outcomes*	*Implementation: Nursing Interventions*	*Rationales*
	• ability to rest • client/family ask less questions		cally with situation
		Allow client/family to verbalize fears	Sharing information elicits support and comfort and can relieve tension and unexpressed worries
		Stress that frequent assessments are routine and do not necessarily imply a deteriorating condition	Client may feel reassured to know that frequent assessments may prevent development of more serious complications
		Repeat information as necessary because of reduced attention span of client/family	Attention span is short, and time perception may be altered. Anxiety decreases learning and attention
		Provide a comfortable, quiet environment for client and family	Enhances coping mechanisms as well as reduces myocardial workload and oxygen consumption
Constipation, High Risk for R/T bedrest, pain medications, and NPO/soft diet • subjective feeling of fullness • abdominal cramping • painful defecation • palpable impaction	Client will have improved bowel elimination, as evidenced by eliminating a stool without straining or having a vasovagal response	Ensure adequate bulk in diet and adequate fluid intake	Bulk and fluid within the colon prevent straining
		Monitor effectiveness of softeners or laxatives; instruct on prevention of straining and avoiding Valsalva's (vasovagal) maneuver	Stool softeners decrease myocardial workload of straining; Valsalva's maneuver causes bradycardia, decreasing cardiac output
		Use bedside commode rather than bedpan	Bedpan use requires more straining and increases vasovagal response
Health Maintenance, Altered R/T myocardial infarction and implications for lifestyle changes	Client/family will have improved knowledge of medical regimen and lifestyle changes, as evidenced by verbalizing an understanding of a heart attack and the necessary lifestyle changes regarding diet, medications, stress reduction, quitting smoking, and cholesterol, weight, and blood pressure reduction	Discuss the following with clients and family, providing both oral instructions and written materials: • anatomy and functions of the heart muscle • coronary arteries and the atherosclerotic process • definition of "heart attack" • healing process of the heart and the role of collateral circulation	Use of multiple learning methods enhances retention of material; information helps client understand the underlying problems or overall heart functions
		Assist client with identifying his or her own risk factors	Risk factor identification is the first step before changes can be implemented
		Assist client in devising a plan for risk factor modification (e.g., diet; smoking cessation; cholesterol, stress, and blood pressure reduction)	Information helpful in providing opportunity for client to identify risk factors, assume control, and participate in a treatment regimen
		Provide guidelines for a diet low in cholesterol and saturated fat; arrange for di-	Consultation with other health professionals enhances client learning from others;

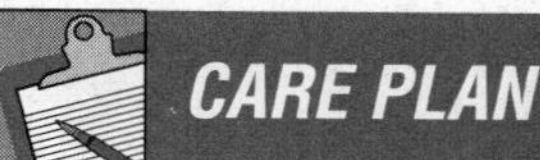

CARE PLAN

The Client with a Myocardial Infarction Continued

Nursing Diagnosis/ Collaborative Problem	Planning: Expected Outcomes	Implementation: Nursing Interventions	Rationales
		etary consultation before client is discharged from hospital	guidelines developed with the client and family before discharge will help once they are home
		Discuss post–myocardial infarction activity progression; arrange for cardiac rehabilitation consultation	Continued follow-up will let client know how he or she is doing; outpatient cardiac rehabilitation will support and assist client in the lifestyle changes necessary for a healthy recovery and life
		Teach client/family about medications that will be taken after hospital discharge, including name, purpose, dosage, schedule, precautions, and potential side effects	The more the client understands the medical regimen and potential side effects, the more adept he or she will be in monitoring for them
Activity Intolerance, High Risk for R/T imbalance between oxygen supply and demand • weakness, fatigue • change in vital signs • dysrhythmias • dyspnea • pallor • diaphoresis	Client will have improved activity tolerance, as evidenced by • participating in desired activities • meeting own activities of daily living • reduced fatigue and weakness • vital signs within normal limits during activity • absence of cyanosis, diaphoresis, and pain	Monitor vital signs before, immediately after activity, and 3 minutes later	Trends determine client's response to increase in activity. Vital signs should return to baseline in 3 minutes. Pulse rate over established limits and development of chest pain or dyspnea may indicate need for alterations in exercise regimen or medication changes
		Monitor for tachycardia, dysrhythmias, dyspnea, diaphoresis, or pallor after activity	Indicators of myocardial oxygen deprivation that may require decrease in activity, changes in medications, or use of supplemental oxygen
		Encourage verbalization of feelings or concerns regarding fatigue or limitations	Knowing limitations prevents exertion and increasing myocardial workload
		Provide assistance with self-care activities and provide frequent rest periods, especially after meals	Large meals may increase myocardial workload and cause vagal stimulation, with resultant bradycardia or ectopic beats; caffeine, a direct cardiac stimulant, increases heart rate
		Increase activity per cardiac rehabilitation nurse and physician orders	Gradual increase in activity increases strength and prevents overexertion, enhances collateral circulation, and restores normal lifestyle as much as possible

PVCs, premature ventricular contractions; PRN, pro re nata.

Post-hospital Care

Recovery after having an MI may be lengthy and difficult. The client may have undergone surgery or managed medically, but regardless, a serious threat to integrity occurred. Four stages of recovery have been documented:[40] (1) "Defending oneself" occurs for up to 7 days after the MI. During this period, clients attempt to prove that they are not seriously ill. Coping strategies include denial and minimization. Some clients conceal the recurrence of chest pain. (2) "Coming to terms" with MI is a process of comprehending that a heart attack really occurred, understanding why it happened, and considering its impact on the future. Clients face their own mortality during this phase, which takes place over 3 to 8 days. (3) "Learning to live" is the process of life adjustment to find a lifestyle that can be tolerated and maintained while preserving a sense of self-worth. A variety of strategies are used to regain self-control, such as gauging progress, seeking reassurance, learning about health, and being cautious. (4) "Living again" is the last stage when clients come to terms with the fact that they will not be living life to its fullest. Clients learn to accept limitations and to refocus on other aspects of life. Some clients are unable to adjust. They are caught between stages 2 and 3. Sometimes the client finds he or she has had too many setbacks and is powerless to make changes or gain control.

CONGESTIVE HEART FAILURE

Definition

Heart failure can be defined as a physiologic state in which the heart is unable to pump enough blood to meet the metabolic needs of the body (determined as oxygen consumption) at rest or during exercise even though filling pressures are adequate. The heart fails when, owing to intrinsic disease or structural defects, it cannot handle a normal blood volume or, in the absence of disease, it cannot tolerate a sudden expansion in blood volume (e.g., during exercise). Heart failure is not a disease itself; instead, the term denotes a group of manifestations related to inadequate pump performance from either the cardiac valves or myocardium. Whatever the cause, pump failure results in hypoperfused tissue followed by pulmonary and systemic venous congestion. Because heart failure causes vascular congestion, it is often called congestive heart failure (CHF). Other terms used to denote heart failure include cardiac decompensation, cardiac insufficiency, and ventricular failure.

Incidence

Estimates from the American Heart Association[4] indicate that between 2.3 and 3 million Americans have CHF and are alive. The incidence of those developing the condition is around 400,000. Annually, 37,371 clients die from CHF.

Etiology

The performance of the heart depends on two essential components: fiber length (Frank-Starling mechanism) and the inherent contractility (inotropic state) of the muscle. The normal heart automatically responds to maintain the cardiac output. In health and disease, a complicated interplay automatically adjusts the extent of shortening of myocardial fibers and, consequently, the stroke volume and the cardiac output. Five interrelated factors are involved: preload, afterload, contractility, the coordinated pattern of contraction, and heart rate (Table 42-4). Adverse changes in these determinants of myocardial performance ultimately cause the heart to fail. The causes of heart failure can be divided into three subgroups: (1) abnormal loading conditions, (2) abnormal muscle function, and (3) conditions or diseases that precipitate or exacerbate heart failure. CHF results from damaged heart muscle. This damage can result from atherosclerosis, a congenital heart defect, high blood pressure, pulmonary hypertension, MI, or valvular disorders.

ABNORMAL LOADING CONDITIONS

The workload of the myocardium greatly increases with abnormal "loading" (or work) of the ventricles. Preload refers to the length of the ventricular myocardial fibers just before ventricular contraction. The load or stretch placed on the ventricular fibers corresponds to the end-diastolic ventricular volume and pressure. Preload is determined by the condition of the heart valves (especially the mitral valve), blood volume, ventricular wall compliance, and venous tone. Whereas an increase in preload usually precipitates an increase in myocardial contractility (Starling's law), filling pressures may rise beyond the capabilities of the normally compliant heart. Suddenly, or over time, this expansion in preload lessens the force and efficiency of ventricular contraction. Cardiac output decreases. Under the strain of this load, the heart will fail. Table 42-5 lists conditions that may result in increased preload.

TABLE 42-4. Terms Used to Describe Cardiac Function

Term	Function
Afterload	Force that the ventricle must develop during systole in order to eject the stroke volume
Cardiac output	Stroke volume × heart rate
Diastole	The normal period in the heart cycle during which the muscle fibers lengthen, the heart dilates, and cavities fill with blood
Inotropic state	A measure of contractility
Preload	Stretch of myocardial fibers at end diastole
Stroke volume	The amount of blood ejected from the ventricle with each contraction
Systole	That part of the heart cycle in which the heart is in contraction; the myocardial fibers are tightening and shortening

TABLE 42-5. Abnormal Loading Conditions of the Heart

Increased Preload	Increased Afterload
Regurgitation of any of the four valves	Aortic valvular stenosis
Hypervolemia	Mitral valvular stenosis
Congenital defects (left to right shunts)	Pulmonic valvular stenosis
Ventricular septal defect	Systemic hypertension
Atrial septal defect	Pulmonary hypertension
Patent ductus arteriosus	High peripheral vascular resistance
Congestive heart failure	

Afterload corresponds to the amount of intramyocardial wall tension that the heart must generate to overcome systemic pressure and allow adequate ventricular emptying. In other words, afterload indicates how "hard" the heart must pump to force blood into the circulation. The tone of systemic arterioles, the elasticity of the aorta and large arteries, the size and thickness of the ventricle, the presence of aortic stenosis, and the viscosity of the blood all determine afterload. High peripheral vascular resistance and a high blood pressure force the ventricle to work harder to eject blood. Subjected to prolonged high pressures, the ventricle will eventually fail. Table 42-5 lists conditions that increase afterload.

ABNORMAL MUSCLE FUNCTION

There are certain conditions that directly interfere with myocardial contractility. Intrinsic conditions are inherent in the cardiac muscle and include MI, myocarditis, cardiomyopathy, and ventricular aneurysm. Such disorders impair the contractile function of the myocardial fibrils, which reduces ventricular emptying and stroke volume.

After MI, some of the heart muscle is replaced by noncontracting scar tissue, and the ventricles pump less efficiently. Some degree of heart failure, either chronic or transient, appears in over half of clients after MI.

Sometimes certain conditions externally compress the heart, thereby hampering ventricular filling and myocardial contractility. Disorders that greatly restrict cardiac chamber filling and myocardial fiber stretch include constrictive pericarditis, which is an inflammatory and fibrotic process of the pericardial sac, and cardiac tamponade, which involves the accumulation of fluid or blood within the pericardial sac. Because the pericardium encloses all four heart chambers, compression of the heart (1) decreases diastolic relaxation and thereby elevates diastolic pressure and (2) hampers forward blood flow through the heart.

Risk Factors

Some clients have pre-existing mild to moderate heart disease with no evidence of CHF. In these clients, adequate cardiac output depends on functional compensatory mechanisms. When the heart undergoes undue stress, these compensatory mechanisms may prove inadequate, and the heart fails. Careful assessment helps identify precipitating causes for the great increase in cardiac workload. Recognition of these factors allows prompt treatment and long-term prevention.

Conditions that Precipitate or Exacerbate Heart Failure

Physical or Emotional Stress. Strenuous physical exercise and strong emotions (fear, excitement, anxiety) increase sympathetic nervous tone and catecholamine release. This increases myocardial work by increasing heart rate, myocardial contractility, and blood pressure.

Dysrhythmia. Cardiac dysrhythmias, most notably tachycardia (rapid heart rate), are the most common factors precipitating heart failure. A rapid heart beat shortens the time for ventricular filling (diastole), which in turn reduces cardiac output. In addition, the workload and oxygen requirements of the myocardium increase.

Infection. Any systemic infection increases the oxygen demands of the body tissues. The heart must keep pace with these demands. Fever and hypoxemia, which occurs in some pulmonary infections, further tax the ailing heart and may precipitate failure.

Anemia. Reduction in the oxygen-carrying capacity of the blood, as in anemia, necessitates increased cardiac output to meet the body's need for oxygen. Whereas a normal heart may adjust to the increased workload, a compromised heart cannot, and failure ensues.

Thyroid Disorders. Thyrotoxicosis, associated with hyperthyroidism, augments the metabolic needs of the body, accelerating heart rate and the workload of the heart. If thyrotoxicosis is untreated, heart failure may occur. In hypothyroidism, the thyroid produces an inadequate amount of thyroxine (thyroid hormone). This can indirectly lead to heart failure by predisposing the client to coronary atherosclerosis.

Pregnancy. Heart failure ranks high among causes of death during pregnancy. Like anemia and hyperthyroidism, pregnancy increases the metabolic needs of the body, thereby increasing the workload of the heart. Pregnant women with rheumatic valvular disease are particularly prone to heart failure.

Paget's Disease. In some cases, Paget's disease also increases myocardial workload. This disease causes vascular proliferation in the bones. When the disease involves over one third of the skeleton, a high cardiac output state exists and may tax the compromised heart (see Chap. 67).

Nutritional Deficiency. Thiamine (vitamin B_1) deficiency causes beriberi. It occurs in cultures in which polished rice constitutes the primary food source. Alcoholism (especially with Wernicke's syndrome) is also associated with thiamine deficiency. Thiamine deficiency interferes with cardiac function by reducing myocardial contractility and causing tachycardia and ventricular dilation.

Pulmonary Disease. Increased pressure in the pulmonary system due to chronic obstructive lung disease, severe pulmonary embolization, or primary pulmonary artery hypertension can produce sizable resistance to right ventricular emptying. Such resistance may lead to right ventricular hypertrophy and failure.

Hypervolemia. An excess in circulating blood volume can result from poor renal function, cardiac disease, medications (such as steroids), or excessive intake of sodium (promoting water retention). Iatrogenic causes include overadministration of intravenous fluids. Expanded circulatory volume augments venous return, increasing preload. A diseased heart may not be able to pump the increased load, and cardiac decompensation occurs.

Pathophysiology

The myocardium of the left ventricle may either (1) be diseased and unable to meet normal circulatory demands or (2) be intrinsically normal but unable to meet increased circulatory needs. When failure first begins, the left ventricle fails to eject a sufficient amount of blood. At this point, the compensatory mechanisms of sympathetic nervous system activation (tachycardia, dilation, and hypertrophy) come into play. When these mechanisms fail, the amount of blood remaining in the left ventricle at the end of diastole increases. This increase in residual blood in turn decreases the ventricle's capacity to receive blood from the left atrium. The left atrium, having to work harder to eject blood, dilates and hypertrophies. It is unable to receive the full amount of incoming blood from the pulmonary veins, and left atrial pressure increases. This leads to subsequent pulmonary congestion, pulmonary edema, and respiratory symptoms (Fig. 42–8).

The right ventricle, because of the increased pressure in the pulmonary vascular system, must now dilate and hypertrophy in order to meet its increased workload. It too eventually fails. Engorgement of the venous system then extends backward to produce congestion in the gastrointestinal tract, liver, viscera, kidneys, legs, and sacrum, with edema as the main manifestation. Right ventricular failure thus results.

Right ventricular failure usually follows left ventricular failure. Occasionally, right ventricular failure develops independently of left ventricular failure. Some causes are

- pulmonary diseases (e.g., pulmonary hypertension, recurrent pulmonary embolism, chronic obstructive pulmonary disease, and cor pulmonale), which force the right ventricle to pump against increased pressure within the lungs
- constrictive pericarditis, which obstructs the inflow of blood to the heart from the venous system
- tricuspid and pulmonic valvular disorders, which produce greater demands on the right ventricular myocardium
- right ventricle infarction (rare)

The healthy heart can meet the demands of life through the use of cardiac reserve. Cardiac reserve is the heart's ability to increase output in response to stress. The normal heart has the ability to increase its output up to five times resting level. However, the failing heart, even at rest, is pumping near its capacity and thus has lost much of its reserve. The compromised heart has a limited ability to respond to the body's needs for increased output in situations of stress.

The heart in failure has recourse to three main compensatory mechanisms to meet the body's demands: (1) ventricular dilation, (2) ventricular hypertrophy, and (3) increased sympathetic nervous system stimulation (tachycardia). The last, however, is an adaptive mechanism available only to the chronically failing heart.

VENTRICULAR DILATION

Ventricular dilation refers to lengthening of the muscle fibers, which increases the volume of the heart chambers. Dilation causes an increase in preload and thus cardiac output, because a stretched muscle contracts more forcefully (Starling's law). However, dilation has limits as a compensatory mechanism. Muscle fibers, if stretched beyond a certain point, cease to increase the ventricular contractility. Second, a dilated heart requires more oxygen. Thus, the dilated heart with a normal coronary blood flow can suffer from a lack of oxygen. Hypoxia of the heart further decreases the muscle's ability to contract.

VENTRICULAR HYPERTROPHY

Ventricular hypertrophy refers to an increase in the diameter of the muscle fibers. The walls of the heart chamber thicken, and the weight of the heart increases. Hypertrophy generally follows persistent dilation, further increasing the contractile power of the muscle fibers. Like dilation, hypertrophy has limits as a compensatory mechanism. A hypertrophied heart does far greater work than does a normal-sized heart and, as a consequence, has a greater demand for oxygen. Unfortunately, as the heart's muscle mass increases, the number of capillaries supplying the muscle fibers remains the same. Thus, the hypertrophied heart may simply outgrow its coronary blood supply and become hypoxic. As the myocardium becomes hypoxic, the contractile force of the heart decreases. Ventricular hypertrophy may also impede ventricular emptying if the enlarged muscle blocks the valve areas.

INCREASED SYMPATHETIC NERVOUS SYSTEM STIMULATION

Increased sympathetic nervous system stimulation is the least effective compensatory mechanism and often

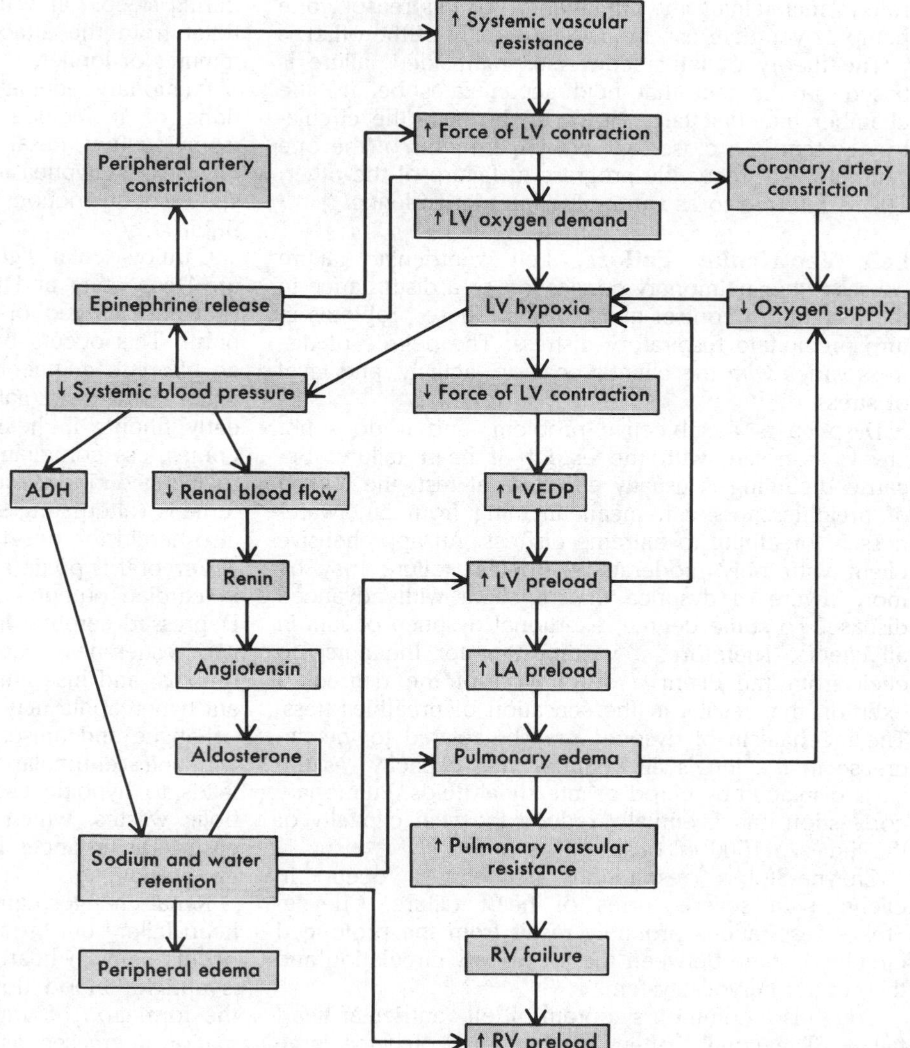

▲ *Figure 42-8*

Left-sided congestive heart failure from elevated peripheral vascular resistance. Left heart failure leads to right heart failure. In addition, peripheral vascular resistance and afterload are further impaired by adrenal and renal responses. Key: LV, left ventricle; LVEDP, left ventricle end-diastolic pressure; LA, left atrium; ADH; anti-diuretic hormone; RV; right ventricle. (From McCance, K., & Huether, S. [1990]. *Pathophysiology*, St. Louis, C. V. Mosby [p. 972].)

proves to be more of a burden than a blessing. Sympathetic activity produces venous and arteriolar constriction, thus increasing peripheral vascular resistance (afterload) and myocardial workload. In addition, sympathetic stimulation reduces renal blood flow, and the kidneys respond by retaining water and sodium. The expanded blood volume increases the load on an already compromised heart. Interestingly, sympathetic activity does not greatly affect the failing inotropic (contractile) state of the myocardium. Finally, tachycardia occurs as a cardiac response to distention of the great veins at their atrial attachment (Bainbridge reflex).

Cardiac compensation exists when these three mechanisms—ventricular dilation, ventricular hypertrophy, and sympathetic nervous system stimulation—succeed in maintaining an adequate cardiac output and blood flow to the tissues in the presence of pathologic changes. Cardiac decompensation occurs when the heart, despite these mechanisms, fails to cope with the demands put on it and must expend most of its reserve. At this point, symptoms of CHF develop because the heart cannot maintain adequate circulation.

Clinical Manifestations

Heart failure may be categorized as left versus right ventricular, backward versus forward, high versus low output, and systolic versus diastolic.[41]

LEFT VERSUS RIGHT VENTRICULAR FAILURE

The heart is composed of two pumps, a right and a left. Each pump bears its own stressors and has its own role in maintaining the circulation. For this reason, one pump or ventricle can fail independently of the other.

The theory of left-sided versus right-sided failure is based on the fact that fluid accumulates behind the chamber that first fails. However, because the circulatory system is a closed circuit, impairments of the one ventricle will frequently progress to failure of the other. This is referred to as ventricular interdependence.

Left Ventricular Failure. Left ventricular failure causes either pulmonary congestion or a disturbance in the respiratory control mechanisms. These problems in turn precipitate respiratory distress. The degree of distress varies with the client's position, activity, and level of stress.

Dyspnea is a subjective problem, and it does not always correlate with the extent of heart failure. Because breathing is usually effortless at rest, the feeling of breathlessness can mean anything from an awareness of breathing to extreme distress. An apprehensive client with only moderate ventricular failure may be more aware of dyspnea than a client with advanced disease. To some degree, exertional dyspnea occurs in all clients. Therefore, it is important for the nurse to elicit from the client a description of the degree of exertion that results in the sensation of breathlessness. The mechanism of dyspnea may be related to the decrease in the lung's air volume (vital capacity) as the air is displaced by blood or interstitial fluids. Pulmonary congestion can eventually reduce the vital capacity of the lungs to 1500 ml or less.

Cheyne-Stokes respirations sometimes occur in clients with severe forms of heart failure. Cheyne-Stokes respirations probably result from the prolonged circulation time between the pulmonary circulation and the central nervous system.

Cough is a common symptom of left ventricular heart failure. The cough, often hacking, may produce large amounts of frothy, blood-tinged sputum. The client coughs because a large amount of fluid is trapped in the pulmonary tree, irritating the lung mucosa. On auscultation, bilateral crackles may be heard.

Orthopnea is a more advanced stage of dyspnea. The client often assumes a "three-point position," sitting up with both hands on the knees and leaning forward. Orthopnea develops because the supine position increases the amount of blood returning from the lower extremities to the heart and lungs (preload). This gravitational redistribution of blood increases pulmonary congestion and dyspnea. The client learns to avoid respiratory distress at night by supporting the head and thorax on pillows. In severe heart failure, the client may resort to sleeping upright in a chair.

Paroxysmal nocturnal dyspnea (PND) resembles the frightening sensation of suffocation. The client suddenly awakens with the feeling of severe suffocation and seeks relief by sitting upright or opening a window for a breath of "fresh air." Respirations may be labored and wheezing (cardiac asthma). PND represents an acute aggravation of pulmonary congestion. It stems from (1) a combination of increased venous return to the lungs due to recumbency and (2) suppression of the respiratory center to sensory input from the lungs during sleep. Once the client is in the upright position, relief from the attack of PND may not occur for 30 minutes or longer.

Pulmonary edema may develop. Clinical manifestations of it include extreme breathlessness, anxiety, frothy sputum, nasal flaring, use of accessory breathing muscles, tachypnea, noisy and wet breathing, diaphoresis, vasoconstriction, and hypoxia in arterial blood gas findings.

Cardiovascular signs also denote left ventricular failure. Inspecting and palpating the precordium may reveal an enlarged or left laterally displaced apical impulse. This occurs because the left ventricle dilates in an effort to augment ventricular contraction and emptying. Also, heart gallop (S_3 or S_4) sounds may be an early finding in heart failure as the left ventricle becomes less compliant and its walls vibrate in response to filling during diastole. The appearance of pulsus alternans (alternating strong and weak heart beats) may also herald the onset of left ventricular failure.

Cerebral hypoxia may occur as a result of a decrease in cardiac output causing inadequate brain perfusion. Depressed cerebral function can cause anxiety, irritability, restlessness, confusion, impaired memory, bad dreams, and insomnia. Impaired ventilation with resultant hypercapnia may also be a precipitant.

Fatigue and muscular weakness are often associated with left ventricular failure. Inadequate cardiac output leads to hypoxic tissue and slowed removal of metabolic wastes, which in turn causes the client to tire easily. Disturbances in sleep and rest patterns may aggravate fatigue.

Renal changes can occur in both right- and left-sided heart failure but are more striking in the latter. Nocturia occurs early in heart failure. During the day, the client is upright, blood flow is away from the kidneys, and the formation of urine is reduced. At night, urine formation increases as blood flow to the kidneys improves. Nocturia may interfere with effective sleep patterns, which may contribute to fatigue. As cardiac output falls, decreased renal blood flow may result in oliguria, a late sign of heart failure.

In addition, if renal artery pressure falls, lowered glomerular filtration increases retention of sodium and water. In response to a continued reduction in renal blood flow, the renin-angiotensin-aldosterone mechanism activates. Aldosterone, released from the adrenal cortex, promotes further retention of sodium and water by the renal tubule. This results in an expansion in blood volume of up to 30 per cent and edema. As the sodium concentration in the extracellular fluid increases, so also does the osmotic pressure of the plasma. The hypothalamus responds to the higher osmotic pressure by releasing antidiuretic hormone (ADH) from the posterior pituitary. This, in turn, promotes renal tubular reabsorption of water. However, aldosterone is more important than is ADH in the production of edema.

RIGHT VENTRICULAR FAILURE

When the right ventricle fails, peripheral edema and venous congestion of the organs develop. Liver enlargement (hepatomegaly) and abdominal pain occur as the liver becomes congested with venous blood. If this occurs rapidly, stretching of the capsule surrounding the liver causes severe discomfort. The client may notice either a constant aching or a sharp pain in the right upper quadrant. In chronic heart failure, abdominal tenderness generally disappears.

In severe CHF, lobules of the liver may become so congested with venous blood that they become anoxic. Anoxia leads to necrosis of the lobules. In long-standing CHF, these necrotic areas may become fibrotic and then sclerotic. As a result, a condition called cardiac cirrhosis develops, manifested by ascites and jaundice, which are symptoms of liver damage.

In chronic heart failure, the increased workload of the heart and the extreme work of breathing increase the metabolic demands of the body. Anorexia, nausea, and bloating develop secondary to venous congestion of the gastrointestinal tract. The combination of increased metabolic needs and decreased caloric intake results in a marked wasting of tissue mass and cardiac cachexia.[41] Anorexia and nausea may also result from digitalis toxicity. This is a common problem because digitalis is usually prescribed for CHF.

Dependent edema is one of the early signs of right ventricular failure. Venous congestion in the peripheral vascular beds causes increased capillary hydrostatic pressure. Capillary hydrostatic pressure overwhelms the opposing pressure of plasma proteins, and fluid shifts out of the capillary beds into the interstitial spaces, with resultant pitting edema. Edema is usually symmetric and occurs in the dependent parts of the body where venous pressure is the highest. In ambulatory clients, edema begins in the feet and ankles and ascends up the lower legs. It is most noticeable at the end of a day and often decreases after a night's rest. In the recumbent client, pitting edema may develop in the presacral area and, as it worsens, progress to the genital region and medial thighs. Concurrent jugular vein distention differentiates the edema of CHF from that of lymphatic obstruction, cirrhosis, and hypoproteinemia. Anasarca, a late sign in heart failure, is substantial and generalized edema. It can involve the upper extremities, genital area, and thoracic and abdominal walls. Cyanosis of the nail beds appears as venous congestion reduces peripheral blood flow.

Clients with CHF often feel anxious, frightened, and depressed. Almost all clients realize that the heart is a vital organ and that when the heart begins to fail, health also fails. As the course of the disease progresses and symptoms worsen, the client may develop an overwhelming fear of permanent disability and death. Clients express their fears in varying ways: experiencing frightening nightmares, insomnia, acute anxiety states, depression, or withdrawal from reality.

BACKWARD VERSUS FORWARD FAILURE

The clinical presentation of heart failure arises from inadequate cardiac output or the pooling of blood behind the failing chamber, or both. Backward failure is the term used to refer to the venous congestion arising from the damming of blood behind the failing chamber. Forward failure refers to the problems of inadequate perfusion. It results when reduced contractility produces a decrease in stroke volume and cardiac output. As cardiac output falls, blood flow to vital organs and peripheral tissue diminishes. This causes mental confusion, muscular weakness, and renal retention of sodium and water. Extracellular fluid retention increases circulating blood volume, further taxing the ailing heart.

Backward failure may develop concurrently with forward failure. Forward failure may result when reduced contractility produces a decrease in stroke volume and cardiac output. As the ventricles fail to expel their contents, blood accumulates and pressure rises in the ventricles and in the atria and venous systems that empty into them. A rise in blood volume within the venous systems causes hydrostatic pressure to exceed capillary oncotic pressure; thereby, fluid is forced out of the vascular beds and into the interstitium. The fluid shift results in pulmonary edema, peripheral (dependent) edema, and serous effusion.

HIGH VERSUS LOW OUTPUT FAILURE

High output failure occurs when the heart, despite normal to high cardiac output levels, is simply not able to meet the accelerated needs of the body. A diseased heart, unable to handle the increased strain, may eventually fail, manifesting signs of low output failure. Causes of high output failure include sepsis, Paget's disease, beriberi, anemia, thyrotoxicosis, arteriovenous fistula, and pregnancy.

Low output failure occurs in most forms of heart disease, including congenital, valvular, rheumatic, coronary, and cardiomyopathic heart diseases. Because the heart is unable to pump an adequate supply of blood to the body, low output failure results in hypoperfused tissue cells. The underlying disorder is related not to increased metabolic needs of the tissues but to poor ventricular pumping action and a low cardiac output.

SYSTOLIC VERSUS DIASTOLIC FAILURE

Heart failure may be caused by the inability of a ventricle to eject an adequate volume of blood (systolic failure) or the inability of the ventricle to accept sufficient blood (diastolic failure).[41]

Systolic heart failure refers to a decrease in the ability of the ventricle to contract forcefully and maintain an adequate forward cardiac output. Situations in which the inotropic state is impaired include MI, coronary atherosclerosis, dilated cardiomyopathy, and massive pulmonary embolus.

Diastolic heart failure occurs when ventricular relaxation is incomplete and the chamber is unable to accept sufficient blood. The ventricle's compliance, or ability to relax, may be impaired because of an injured or ischemic myocardium. Examples of heart diseases in which diastolic dysfunction may occur include coronary atherosclerosis, amyloidosis, restrictive cardiomyopathy, or subendocardial fibrosis.

Complications

The symptoms of heart failure depend on the specific ventricle involved, the precipitating causes of failure, the degree of impairment, the rate of progression, the duration of the failure, and the client's underlying condition. Symptoms of pulmonary congestion and edema dominate the clinical picture of left ventricular failure. Right ventricular failure is associated with signs of abdominal organ and peripheral edema (Table 42-6).

ACUTE PULMONARY EDEMA

Acute pulmonary edema, a medical emergency, usually results from left ventricular failure. In clients with severe cardiac decompensation, the capillary pressure within the lungs becomes so elevated that fluid is pushed from the circulating blood into the interstitium, then into the alveoli, bronchioles, and bronchi. The resulting pulmonary edema, if untreated, may cause death from suffocation. Clients with pulmonary edema literally drown in their own fluids.

The dramatic symptoms of acute pulmonary edema terrify the client and significant others. Typical manifestations include severe dyspnea; orthopnea; pallor; tachycardia; expectoration of large amounts of frothy, blood-tinged sputum; fear; wheezing; sweating; bubbling respirations; and cyanosis.

REFRACTORY HEART FAILURE

Heart failure is termed refractory or intractable when recommended diet, medications, and interventions fail to alleviate symptoms and restore partial cardiac reserve. To treat refractory heart disease, the physician usually (1) reviews the client's entire course, (2) reassesses the medical intervention, and (3) prescribes the following interventions:

- a prolonged period of complete bed rest in a health care facility
- severe sodium restriction (e.g., 250-mg sodium diet)
- fluids restricted to less than 500 ml/day
- diuretic therapy using several different types of diuretics

Prognosis

The prognosis for the client with CHF depends on (1) the degree of cardiac hypertrophy, (2) the amount of cardiac reserve, and (3) the presence of other heart or associated disorders. The prognosis can generally be predicted by the client's response to therapeutic measures. A very slow or inadequate response to prescribed medications, special diets, activity limitations, and so forth signals a poor prognosis. Nevertheless, thorough ongoing assessments, early intervention, therapeutic compliance, and prevention of complications can control this disorder.

TABLE 42-6. Clinical Manifestations of Right and Left Ventricular Failure

Left Ventricular Failure	Right Ventricular Failure
Weakness	Weight gain
Fatigue	Ankle or pretibial swelling and pigmentation
Mental confusion	Abdominal distention
Insomnia	Anorexia, nausea, gastric distress
Anorexia	Subcostal pain
Diaphoresis	Pitting edema (in dependent areas; sacral, ankle, pretibial)
Anxiety	Ascites
Breathlessness	Jugular vein distention
Cough	Neck vein pulsations
Orthopnea or paroxysmal nocturnal dyspnea	Hepatomegaly
Tachycardia, premature atrial contractions	Parasternal life (heave)
Gallop heart sounds (S_3, S_4)	Increased central venous pressure
Diminished S_3	
Pulmonary crackles	
Enlarged point of maximal impulse	
Pulsus alternans	
Elevated pulmonary artery wedge pressure	

Adapted from Michaelson, C. (1983). *Congestive heart failure.* St. Louis: C.V. Mosby.

Diagnostic Assessment

The diagnosis of CHF rests primarily on presenting manifestations and pertinent data from the client's health history. Diagnostic studies assist in determining the underlying cause and the degree of heart failure. Such studies include a chest radiography, ECG, and echocardiogram.

Chest radiography can be very helpful in diagnosing left ventricular failure. Typically, an enlarged cardiac silhouette, pulmonary, venous congestion, and interstitial edema are noted. Interstitial edema is called Kerley-B lines on x-ray study. Pleural effusions may develop and generally reflect biventricular failure.

Arterial blood gases are drawn. Early CHF with pulmonary edema may lead to respiratory alkalosis because of hyperventilation. However, as the disorder progresses and oxygenation becomes more impaired, acidosis will develop.

Liver enzymes document the degree of liver failure. Elevated blood urea nitrogen and creatinine levels reflect decreased renal perfusion.

An ECG provides little help in determining the presence or extent of heart failure but may give clues to its cause. Abnormalities in the ECG arise from the underlying cardiac disorder and from therapeutic agents. For instance, cardiac dysrhythmias may occur because of myocardial ischemia or electrolyte imbalance induced by diuretics or digitalis excess. Therefore, the ECG plays an important role in the management of heart failure.

Echocardiography, a noninvasive diagnostic technique, uses ultrasound to assess cardiac function. This procedure provides information about cardiac chamber size and ventricular function and aids in assessing myocardial, valvular, congenital, and pericardial heart diseases.

Medical Management

Clients with acute CHF are usually admitted to an intensive care unit where they receive continuous assessment and intervention. Those with chronic CHF require continuing assessment, emotional support, and assistance.

The goals in the management of CHF are to improve ventricular pump performance and reduce myocardial workload.

Positioning. The client is placed in a high Fowler's position or chair to reduce pulmonary venous congestion and ease dyspnea. The legs are maintained in a dependent position as much as possible.

Oxygen Administration. Administer oxygen in high concentrations by mask or cannula to (1) relieve hypoxia and dyspnea and (2) lessen pulmonary capillary permeability. For hypoxemia, the physician may order a partial-rebreather mask with a flow rate of 8 to 10 L/min to deliver oxygen concentrations of 40 to 70 per cent. A non-rebreather mask can achieve higher oxygen concentrations. If these methods fail to raise the arterial oxygen tension above 60 mm Hg, the client may need intubation and ventilatory management. Intubation provides a route for removing secretions from the bronchi. Should severe bronchospasm or bronchoconstriction present, bronchodilators are given. Some bronchodilators also stimulate the myocardium and may lead to dysrhythmias.

PHARMACOLOGIC MANAGEMENT

Improving Ventricular "Pump" Performance

Digitalis. Digitalis exerts a direct and beneficial effect on myocardial contraction in the failing heart. Digitalis acts to

- increase ventricular contractility (inotropic effect)
- increase ventricular emptying and the capacity of the heart for work
- slow conduction of impulses through the atrioventricular (AV) node and Purkinje fibers
- increase the AV nodal refractory period
- augment stroke volume
- increase cardiac output

Improved cardiac output enhances kidney perfusion, which may create a mild diuresis of sodium and water.

A number of different digitalis preparations are available, and all have approximately the same effect on the heart. However, digitalis medications differ significantly in their potency, speed of action, elimination from the body, and gastrointestinal irritation. Table 42-7 lists digitalis preparations and their distinguishing characteristics.

The effectiveness of digitalis in heart failure depends on the severity and underlying cause of the condition. It is most effective in heart failure associated with low cardiac output caused by ischemic, rheumatic, hypertensive, or congenital heart disease. Digitalis may also be initiated to control the ventricular response in atrial fibrillation, which is the most common dysrhythmia in heart failure.[13] Digitalis is not given for heart failure associated with high cardiac output states, such as anemia and thyrotoxicosis. Digitalis is contraindicated in heart failure due to constrictive pericarditis or cardiac tamponade. Digitalis should be used with caution in acute MI because it increases myocardial oxygen demand.

When administering digitalis, assess for signs of digitalis toxicity. Clients most prone to the toxic effects of digitalis include the elderly and those with advanced heart disease, severe arrhythmias, or acute MI. Also, clients with cor pulmonale, hypothyroidism, hepatic disease, renal disease, metabolic alkalosis, or hypokalemia (lowered serum potassium) more readily develop toxic effects. Digitalis toxicity occurs in approximately one of every five clients. It may present with systemic or cardiac manifestations.

The major signs and symptoms of digitalis toxicity are outlined in Table 42-8. Any of these manifestations should be reported to the physician, digitalis should be withheld, and interventions to abate the undesirable symptoms should be initiated.

Digitalis toxicity may be a life-threatening condition. The guidelines in Box 42-1 should be carefully followed.

Dopamine and Dobutamine. Other inotropic agents (e.g., dopamine, dobutamine, and amrinone) may be ordered for clients with severe low output heart failure.

TABLE 42-7. Pharmacologic Properties of Selected Cardiac Glycosides

Agent	Absorption	Excretion	Onset of Action	Peak Effect	Half-life	Therapeutic Plasma Level	Toxic Plasma Levels
Digoxin	55-75% gastrointestinal	Principally renal; some hepatic	5-30 min	1-5 hr (IV)	30-40 hr	0.5-2.0 ng/ml	2.4 ng/ml
Digitoxin	90-100% gastrointestinal	Principally hepatic; some renal excretion	30 min-2 hr	4-12 hr	5-7 days	14-26 ng/ml	35 ng/ml

Based on data in Kuhn, M. (1991). *Pharmacotherapeutics*. Philadelphia: F.A. Davis.

TABLE 42-8. Signs and Symptoms of Digitalis Toxicity

Gastrointestinal tract	Anorexia, nausea, vomiting, diarrhea, abdominal cramps (these symptoms are common in 50 per cent of clients with digitalis toxicity and are often the first indication of toxicity)
Central nervous system	Headache, fatigue, lethargy, depression, restlessness, irritability, drowsiness; profound symptoms may include convulsions, neuralgia, delusions, hallucinations, aphasia, memory loss
Cardiovascular system	Bradycardia, ventricular bigeminy or trigeminy, ventricular tachycardia, atrioventricular conduction block, and atrial tachycardia with block
Eyes	Flickering flashes of light; "colored vision" usually yellow or blue, halo vision, photophobia, blurring; diplopia, scotomata (blind spots in visual field)

These medications facilitate myocardial contractility and enhance stroke volume.

Dopamine is a naturally occurring catecholamine with alpha-adrenergic, beta-adrenergic, and dopaminergic activity. When given in small doses (less than 4 μg/kg/m), dopamine stimulates the dopaminergic receptors in the renal, mesenteric, cerebral, and coronary vascular beds, which causes vasodilation. The primary result is an increase in renal blood flow, glomerular filtration rate, and sodium excretion. The alpha- and beta-adrenergic receptors in the vasculature and myocardium are affected with moderate doses of dopamine (4 to 8 μg/kg/m). The results are increases in heart rate, stroke volume, and cardiac output. Alpha-adrenergic effects, such as intense vasoconstriction, dominate when dopamine is given in doses larger than 8 μg/kg/m.[16, 59] Although dopamine may effectively improve cardiac output, it may do so at the expense of the myocardium. An increase in heart rate may increase myocardial oxygen demands and decrease myocardial oxygen supply, which may prove costly to the already ischemic myocardium.

Box 42-1. Guidelines for Digitalis Preparations

1. Read the labels of all digitalis preparations with care. Digitalis preparations have similar names but different strengths and dosages.
2. Always take the client's pulse for one full minute *apically* before giving a dose of digitalis.
3. Carefully note both the rate and rhythm of the pulse and chart them.
4. If the heart beat is very rapid, below 60, or irregular (if it is normally regular), withhold the drug and notify the physician.
5. Observe the client carefully for signs of digitalis toxicity. When severe symptoms present, call the physician before administering the drug.
6. Advise the client and significant others to monitor the pulse rate daily. Also reinforce the importance of taking prescribed potassium supplements.

Another inotropic agent is dobutamine, a synthetic derivative of dopamine that has strong beta-stimulatory effects within the myocardium; it increases heart rate, AV conduction, and myocardial contractility. Dobutamine is capable of increasing the cardiac output without increasing the myocardial oxygen demands or reducing coronary blood flow.[59]

Amrinone is also used to increase cardiac output in clients with severe heart failure. In addition to the positive inotropic effects, amrinone increases renal blood flow and glomerular filtration rate.[59]

Reducing Myocardial Workload

Reduce Preload. Diuretic therapy plays an integral part in the successful management of CHF. Diuretics enhance renal excretion of sodium and water, which reduces circulating blood volume, diminishes preload, and lessens systemic and pulmonary congestion. Table 42-9 describes characteristics of osmotic diuretics.

Although they are effective, diuretics should be administered cautiously because they have side effects. First, diuretics can produce mild to severe electrolyte imbalance. Hypokalemia, a particularly dangerous problem, potentiates digitalis toxicity and can cause myocardial weakness and cardiac arrhythmias. Second, vigorous diuresis may produce hypovolemia and hypotension, jeopardizing cardiac output.

Reduce Afterload. Vasodilating agents have become an increasingly important intervention for CHF. Vasodilators vary in their mechanisms of action, which include (1) direct dilation of veins, (2) dilation of arterioles, (3) combined action on veins and arterioles, and (4) inhibition of angiotensin-converting enzyme. Closely assess the client receiving vasodilators because they can cause rapid drops in blood pressure.

Venous dilators relax venous smooth muscle and increase the capacity of the systemic venous bed; thereby, blood is "trapped" in the veins, and blood return to the heart is decreased. This increased venous capacity reduces preload. Examples of venous dilators include nitroglycerin and isosorbide dinitrate.

Arteriolar dilators reduce systemic arteriolar tone, which decreases peripheral vascular resistance and afterload. Reduction in afterload reduces the left ventricular workload and increases cardiac output. Improved renal perfusion may initiate diuresis. Hydralazine is the most commonly used arterial dilator. Be aware that hydralazine may precipitate reflex tachycardia.

Combined venous and arteriolar dilators decrease both preload and afterload. Sodium nitroprusside helps manage severe heart failure. A potent vasodilator, sodium nitroprusside relaxes the smooth muscles of both

TABLE 42-9. Characteristics of Some Commonly Used Osmotic Diuretics

Diuretic	Site of Action	Effects on Serum Electrolytes	Action: Onset (hr)	Action: Peak (hr)	Action: Duration (hr)
Thiazides					
Chlorothiazide (Diuril)	Act in the distal tubule to inhibit absorption of sodium and chloride	↓ Cl^- ↓ K^+ ↑ HCO_3^-	2 (PO) ¼ (IV)	4 ½	6-12 2
Hydrochlorothiazide (Hydro-Diuril)			2 (PO)	4	6-12
Chlorthalidone (Hygroton)			2 (PO)	6	48-72
Loop Diuretics					
Furosemide (Lasix)	Act in distal tubule to inhibit absorption of sodium and chloride	↓ Cl^- ↓ K^+ ↑ HCO_3^- ↓ Na^+	1 (PO) 5 min (IV)	1-2 ½	6-8 2
Ethacrynic acid (Edecrin)			½ (PO) 5 min (IV)	2 ½	6-8 2
Potassium-Sparing Diuretics					
Spironolactone (Aldactone)	Act in distal convoluted tubule to inhibit absorption of sodium	↑ K^+	Gradual (PO)	3 days after starting therapy	2-3 days after ending therapy
Triamterene (Dyrenium)			2-4 (PO)	6-8	7-24

IV, intravenously; PO, orally.
Adapted from Kuhn, M. M. (1991). *Pharmacotherapeutics*. Philadelphia: F. A. Davis.

veins and arterioles. It does not directly affect the heart muscle or heart rate. Prazosin, an oral agent, provides another example of this class of medication. Physicians often prescribe prazosin for clients with advanced, chronic CHF.

Angiotensin-converting enzyme (ACE) inhibitors suppress the renin-angiotensin-aldosterone system; thereby, the production of the potent vasoconstrictor angiotensin II is blocked. This results in an increase in renal blood flow and a decrease in renal vascular resistance, which enhances diuresis. ACE inhibitors, such as captopril, improve hemodynamic status and have been shown to prolong the survival of clients with CHF.[9, 22]

Researchers are studying the use of beta-adrenergic receptor antagonists in heart failure. Traditionally, these agents were contraindicated in heart failure. However, recent studies have shown that administration of beta-blockers in heart failure may result in improved symptomatic and functional status.[9]

DIETARY MANAGEMENT

The two major objectives in the treatment of CHF are to improve cardiac efficiency and to control sodium-water retention. Sodium restrictions are placed on the diet to prevent, control, or eliminate edema. Two- to four-gram sodium diets are usually prescribed (Table 42-10).

From the use of some loop diuretics, potassium is lost via the kidneys, which can lead to dysrhythmias and electrolyte imbalances. Hypokalemia sensitizes the myocardium to digitalis and therefore predisposes the client to digitalis toxicity. Potassium supplements and a dietary potassium can keep the client's potassium in balance.

It is usually not necessary to restrict fluid intake in clients with mild or moderate heart failure. However, with more advanced failure, it is beneficial to limit water to 1000 ml daily. The reason for this restriction is that excessive water intake tends to dilute the amount of sodium in the body fluids and may produce a low-salt syndrome (hyponatremia). Hyponatremia is characterized by lethargy and weakness. It results more often from the combination of a restricted sodium diet, increased sodium loss during diuresis, and excessive water intake.

OTHER MEASURES

In addition to improving ventricular pump performance and reducing myocardial workload, the client also needs to reduce physical and emotional stress. Sometimes clinicians overlook rest to diminish the workload of the heart as an intervention. The client must rest both physically and mentally. The proper use of rest as the initial step in the management of CHF offers many

TABLE 42-10. Sodium Content of Selected Foods

Foods Low in Sodium	
Dairy products	Skim milk, eggs, cottage cheese, cream cheese, ice cream
Meats*	Turkey, chicken, veal, lamb, liver, fresh fish, tuna packed in water (meats should be unprocessed)
Fruits and vegetables*	Any fresh or frozen food in this group
Beverages	Any juice (except tomato or V-8), coffee, tea, Perrier water
Breads	Some breads and cereals
Seasonings	Garlic, onion, bay leaf, pepper, dill, nutmeg, rosemary, allspice, thyme, sage, caraway, cinnamon, almond and vanilla extract, fresh dried herbs
Fats	Margarine, oils, shortening, unsalted salad dressings
Desserts	Sherbet, fruit ice, gelatin, fruit drinks
Miscellaneous	Unbuttered, unsalted popcorn; unsalted nuts; vinegar
Foods High in Sodium	
Milk and dairy products	Aged, hard cheese; pasteurized-processed cheese; buttermilk
Meats	Sausage, wieners, ham, bacon, corned beef; all smoked, pickled, or cured meats; canned meats, "TV dinners," salami, most luncheon meats, beef jerky
Fruits and vegetables	Pickled or canned fruits and vegetables, olives, sauerkraut, pickles
Breads and cereals	Salted crackers, macaroni (and cheese), pretzels, rye rolls, pizza, commercial pancake mixes
Beverages	Tomato juice, V-8 juice, beef broth, bouillon
Fats	Commercial salad dressings, dips and party spreads, peanut butter
Seasonings	Garlic, celery, or onion salt; Accent, monosodium glutamate (MSG), meat tenderizer, soy sauce, catsup, steak sauce, mustard, canned soup
Desserts	Fruit pies, doughnuts, cake, commercial puddings
Miscellaneous	Baking soda, baking powder, salted popcorn, salted nuts, potato chips

*Food sources high in potassium.

benefits. Rest can promote diuresis, slow the heart rate, and relieve dyspnea, all of which allow more conservative use of pharmacologic agents (e.g., digitalis, diuretics, and vasodilators).

Whether the physician prescribes complete bed rest or a program of modified bed rest depends on the seriousness of the client's condition. Clinicians may use the functional and therapeutic classifications of heart disease as a guide for activity prescription (Box 42-2).

The physician may prescribe a mild sedative or small doses of barbiturates and tranquilizers to promote rest and overcome problems of restlessness, insomnia, and anxiety.

The client may also be at risk for injury due to immobility. The client should be confined to bed only long enough to regain cardiac reserve, but not so long as to promote the complications of immobility. The client confined to bed rest should be given specific teaching/learning guidelines for preventing the harmful effects of immobility. Passive leg exercises should be performed several times daily to prevent venous stasis, which may lead to the formation of venous thrombi and pulmonary emboli. The physician may also initiate anticoagulant therapy to prevent these potentially deadly complications.

Surgical Management

The use of a variety of drugs is typically the mode of therapy in treatment of CHF. However, attempts are under way to provide respite for the heart in acute failure, for example, after MI. The common feature of the different approaches is to unload the heart for hours to days while it is recuperating. The most popular

Box 42-2. Functional and Therapeutic Classification of Heart Disease

Class I

No limitation on physical activity. Ordinary physical activity does not cause undue fatigue, palpitation, dyspnea, or anginal pain.

Class II

Slight limitation of physical activity. Comfortable at rest, but ordinary physical activity results in fatigue, palpitation, dyspnea, or anginal pain.

Class III

Marked limitation of physical activity. Comfortable at rest, but less than ordinary physical activity causes fatigue, palpitation, dyspnea, or anginal pain.

Class IV

Unable to carry on any physical activity without discomfort. Symptoms of cardiac insufficiency or of the anginal syndrome may be present even at rest. If any physical activity is undertaken, discomfort is increased.

Classifications by the Criteria Committee, New York Heart Association.

devices are (1) venoarterial bypass, which assists the heart by diverting blood to a pump that returns it to the arterial tree, and (2) counterpulsation, which operates in synchrony with the heart beat to adjust the aortic blood pressure by rhythmically changing either the volume of blood in the aorta (with use of an external pump) or the capacity of the aorta (with use of an internal balloon). All methods aim to reduce the external work of the heart and the tension that it develops during systole and to decrease myocardial oxygen consumption at the same time as coronary arterial perfusion is improved.

When the heart is irreversibly damaged and can no longer adequately function and the client is at risk of dying, cardiac transplantation and the use of an artificial heart to assist or replace the failing heart are also being pursued as last measures for heart failure. With the development of cyclosporine and with improvements in the procurement and myocardial protection of the donor heart, cardiac transplantation has become an accepted therapeutic procedure. One-year survival rates after transplantation are greater than 85 per cent. Although transplantation may not be appropriate for all clients, it may be the only option available to some.[56]

Nursing Management

ASSESSMENT

The nurse should assess the client for the clinical manifestations of CHF, especially in the high-risk client.

Nursing Diagnosis: Cardiac Output, Decreased R/T heart failure and/or dysrhythmias.

Planning Expected Outcomes. The client will have increased cardiac output, as evidenced by regular cardiac rhythm, heart rate within normal limits, hemodynamic parameters within normal limits.

Implementation. Assess vital signs and heart rhythm every 15 minutes to 1 hour, depending on the stability of the client's vital signs. Tachycardia is a common compensatory mechanism, but it further taxes the myocardial oxygen supply. Monitor dysrhythmias hourly. Most intensive care units have a central area of monitors for all clients in the unit. Common dysrhythmias include premature atrial contractions, premature ventricular contractions, and paroxysmal atrial tachycardia. Dysrhythmias reduce ventricular filling time, decrease myocardial contractility, and increase myocardial oxygen demands. All of these conditions further compromise cardiac output. Respirations are usually rapid and labored, and the client is orthopneic. Hypotension, if present, is due to decreased perfusion, vagal stimulation, and dysrhythmias. Hypertension is usually due to pain, anxiety, or previous history of hypertension.

Monitor lung and heart sounds every 2 to 4 hours. Crackles are common, and respirations may be wet and frothy as pulmonary congestion develops. Heart sounds may be distant and include an S3 or S4 as filling and ejection times are delayed. Administer oxygen as prescribed to improve tissue hypoxia.

Monitor urine output hourly, noting changes in color and volume of output. Oliguria may reflect decreased renal perfusion. Diuresis is expected and promoted once the client is digitalized and given diuretics. Fluid balance and left ventricular function for many clients are managed with a pulmonary artery catheter. The catheter and nursing responsibilities are discussed in Chapter 41.

Assess for changes in mental status every 4 hours. Adequate cerebral perfusion requires adequate cardiac output. The client may exhibit changes in problem solving as an early indicator of cerebral hypoxia.

Feed the client small meals, and provide a rest period after meals. Large meals increase myocardial workload and cause vagal stimulation, which results in bradycardia. If caffeine causes tachycardia or ectopic beats, it should be avoided.

Nursing Diagnosis: Fluid Volume Excess R/T reduced glomerular filtration, decrease cardiac output, increases antidiuretic production, and sodium water retention.

Planning: Expected Outcomes. The client will have an adequate fluid balance, as evidenced by output exceeding intake if on diuretics, clearing breath sounds, stable vital signs, decreasing weight, and resolving edema.

Implementation. Monitor intake and output every 2 hours during acute phases of CHF. Maintain Fowler's position to facilitate breathing. Provide frequent oral care, at least every 4 hours. Clients need oral care more often if they are breathing through the mouth. Weigh the client daily to monitor response to diuretic therapy. Body weight is a more sensitive indicator of fluid balance than is intake and output.

Monitor for signs of increasing peripheral edema. Assess jugular neck vein distention, peripheral edema in the legs or sacrum, and hepatic engorgement or pain in the right upper quadrant.

Provide the client with a low sodium diet. Physicians commonly order a 2- to 4-g diet. Fluid restrictions may also be used until diuresis is achieved.

Nursing Diagnosis: Gas Exchange, Impaired R/T fluid in alveoli.

Planning: Expected Outcomes. The client will have improved gas exchange, as evidenced by vital signs within normal limits for client's age and condition, skin and mucous membranes without cyanosis or pallor, decreased dyspnea, and arterial blood gases within normal limits.

Implementation. Auscultate breath sounds every 2 to 4 hours, noting adventitious sounds indicating congestion. Encourage the client to turn, cough, and deep breathe to clear to the airway and to facilitate oxygen delivery. Maintain Fowler's position to facilitate diaphragmatic expansion and ventilation. Administer oxygen as ordered to improve tissue oxygenation. Monitor arterial blood gas results; changes may reveal severe hypoxia or acidosis. If respiratory failure develops, the client will require intubation and continuous mechanical ventilation.

Nursing Diagnosis: Peripheral Tissue Perfusion, High Risk for Decreased R/T decreased cardiac output and vasoconstriction.

Planning: Expected Outcomes. The client will have adequate peripheral tissue perfusion, as evidenced by warm, dry skin, peripheral pulses present, and rapid blanching.

Implementation. Monitor the client's peripheral pulses every 4 hours. Note the color and temperature of the skin. Keep the extremities warm to promote vasodilation to decrease preload. Be alert for the development of thrombophlebitis, because the legs are commonly kept flat or dependent to decrease venous return. Encourage active range of motion or provide passive range of motion to decrease venous pooling. Clinical manifestations of thrombophlebitis include unilateral swelling, calf pain, pallor. Homan's sign, which is pain in the calf with dorsiflexion of the foot, is not a reliable indicator of thrombophlebitis.

Nursing Diagnosis: Activity Intolerance, High Risk for R/T decreased cardiac output.

Planning: Expected Outcomes. The client will have improved tolerance of activity, as evidenced by having increased levels of activity without dyspnea.

Implementation. Intersperse nursing care activity with rest periods. Monitor the client's response to each activity, noting the development of dyspnea, tachycardia, angina, hypotension, diaphoresis, and dysrhythmias. Vital signs are assessed prior to any major activity (i.e., getting into a chair, walking), immediately after and 3 minutes later. The length of time required for vital signs to return to baseline indicates the degree of cardiac deconditioning. Increase activity levels according to the cardiac rehabilitation nurse or physician orders.

Instruct the client to avoid activities that increase cardiac workload during acute stages of care. Activities that precipitate fatigue may demand more cardiac output than the ailing heart can supply.

During the acute stages of CHF, the nurse provides all self-care activity for the client and allows the client to participate as dyspnea allows.

Nursing Diagnosis: Skin Integrity, Impaired, High Risk for R/T decreased peripheral tissue perfusion and immobility.

Planning: Expected Outcomes. If possible, turn the client from side to side every 2 hours. If the client is too dyspneic to turn, provide a pressure reduction mattress. Use heel protectors or elevate the client's calf. Wash the lower legs carefully, and apply lotion to maintain skin integrity.

Collaborative Problem. High Risk for digitalis toxicity R/T impaired drug excretion from hepatic and renal involvement.

Planning: Expected Outcomes. The nurse will monitor the client for signs of digitalis toxicity.

Implementation. Assess the client for decreased heart sounds, hypokalemia, and first-degree heart block. Monitor serum digitalis levels and potassium.

Nursing Diagnosis: Anxiety, High Risk for R/T to decreased cardiac output, hypoxia, and fear of death or serious consequences.

Planning: Expected Outcomes. The client will have few signs of anxiety, as evidenced by being able to rest calmly in bed, being able to ventilate fears, and vital signs becoming stable.

Implementation. Provide for psychological rest by maintaining a calm environment; anxiety is contagious. Explain in advance the routine regimens and management strategies. Allow the client to ask questions. If the client seems reluctant, the nurse can state common fears and questions elicited from other clients. This strategy often encourages the client to ask questions that were thought but not spoken.

Anxiety often develops as a result of the diagnosis of CHF, presenting symptoms, and fear of death. Emotionally support both the client and significant others. Intervention for CHF involves a long, often difficult period of adjustment. The initial fear of death, brought on by the dramatic symptoms of acute heart failure, can evolve into a long-term strain on coping resources (see Ethical Issues in Nursing). Remember that anxiety and fear further tax the client's failing heart. Take time to talk about the client's concerns and anxieties. Many clients with CHF fail to cope with their condition. They need the nurse's skill and emotional support as well as the additional support of a cardiovascular clinical specialist, counselor, social worker, religious leader, or other appropriate person.

EVALUATION

CHF is not resolved slowly. The client will often make initial strides once diuresis begins, being able to breathe more easily. But the disorder is usually chronic, and much more time is required for complete resolution. Many times, the eventual goal must be accepted as less than full resolution.

Modification of the Plan of Care for the Elderly

Heart failure is becoming increasingly a disorder of the very old. Cardiac decompensation can be triggered by seemingly minor illnesses and dietary indiscretions.

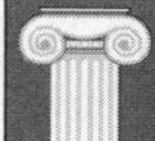

ETHICAL ISSUES IN NURSING

What Is the Nurse's Role in a "Do Not Resuscitate" Decision?

Cardiac disorders come in varying degrees of severity. "Simple" problems such as hypertension may be controlled by medication. More severe interventions may include open-heart surgery. In the most severe cases, the heart muscle may have experienced such injury that there may be no more procedures that can be done to correct the disorder. At this point, medication and perhaps behavioral modification are the only things that may prolong life, because the next cardiac insult will most likely be fatal.

With regard to hospitalized clients, in such serious cases, the institution of cardiopulmonary resuscitation (CPR) upon cardiac arrest may prolong life, if it is successful; but with no corrective treatment options left for such a client, should CPR be performed at all? When medical-surgical science and technology can no longer ward off death, a "do not resuscitate" (DNR) order by the physician appears to be the logical course. Should the client need to consent to such a DNR order? Should the client or family members have a right to refuse a DNR order even if the physicians believe that all resuscitative measures would be futile? What is the nurse's role in a DNR decision?

All clients have a right to autonomy, that is, they have a right to direct their care as they wish. This right, however, may be limited by the options given them by their medical staff. If certain treatment choices are considered futile, should clients be allowed to choose them? Health care providers have an obligation to act beneficently toward their clients. Could the withholding of CPR or other resuscitative measures ever be of benefit to the client?

Nurses see their clients in all stages of health and illness. The dying process is perhaps the most difficult stage to deal with. Dealing with clients who are not to be resuscitated can be very stressful for the nurses caring for them. The natural defense mechanism is to keep distance between yourself and the client. This may make you feel better but may also make the client feel alienated. Nurses must come to terms with their own feelings about DNR clients and death and dying issues. In doing so, nurses can help make such natural processes less painful for their clients and their families and also for themselves.

Medications commonly used by the elderly may have an impact on heart performance even though they pose little risk of interaction with cardiovascular medications. Nonsteroidal anti-inflammatory agents tend to worsen heart disease because they promote sodium retention; tricyclic antidepressants and neuroleptic agents lead to orthostatic hypotension. Conversely, cardiac performance can have an impact on the medication's action also. The development of right ventricular failure can markedly increase the prothrombin time and thereby increase the acton of anticoagulants.

Serum potassium is closely monitored. The combination of hypokalemia and digitalis therapy can lead to lethal dysrhythmias.

Sodium is controlled in the diet, whereas the intake of cholesterol in the elderly usually is not reduced. Trace elements lost in diuresis are usually replaced with a multivitamin.

Post-hospital Care

When the client leaves the health care facility and returns home, schedule adjustments to help avoid overexhaustion. The client may require a nap in the afternoon, shorter working hours, more sleep at night, and frequent vacations. With growing strength and improvement, the client may gradually undertake mild exercise (e.g., walking short distances on level ground, playing a few holes of golf, and simple calisthenics). Such exercises, when performed sensibly, can strengthen the heart muscle and improve its performance.

The client will need instruction before discharge on measures to prevent the recurrence of CHF. Such measures include

- Take digitalis and all other medications exactly as prescribed.
- Stay on the sodium-restricted diet.
- Adhere to the program of diuretic therapy.
- Treat all infections promptly.
- Have medical follow-up as ordered, usually every 2 weeks until stable.

DYSRHYTHMIAS

Definition

The heart has its own intrinsic conduction system that allows the orderly depolarization of cardiac muscle tissue. Normal conduction and depolarization via this system result in adequate cardiac output and tissue perfusion. Also, this normal pattern of depolarization produces normal sinus rhythm.

Dysrhythmias, also called arrhythmias, are disorders of the heart rate and rhythm caused by disturbances in the conduction system. Dysrhythmias can lead to dramatic changes in circulatory dynamics, such as hypotension, heart failure, and shock.

Incidence

Dysrhythmias are common in clients with cardiac disorders but also occur in other clients with normal hearts. The most serious complication of dysrhythmia is sudden death. It is estimated that there are 300,000 deaths from dysrhythmias in the United States each year. Sixty per cent of deaths in the first hour after an MI are due to dysrhythmias.

Etiology

Dysrhythmias are caused by (1) the abnormal rhythmicity of the sinus node (the internal pacemaker) of the heart; (2) a shift of the pacemaker function from the sinus node to another part of the atrium; (3) a block in transmission of the impulse through the heart; (4) abnormal pathways of conduction through the heart; and (5) the spontaneous generation of impulses from any place along the conduction system.

ABNORMAL RHYTHMICITY OF THE SINUS NODE

Rhythms that begin in the sinus node can have normal rates, that is, between 60 and 100 beats per minute, or the rate can decrease or increase.

Tachycardia, a rate above 100 beats per minute, has transmission of impulse through the conduction system that is normal, except that there is a shortened time between each QRS complex. Tachycardia can result from increased metabolic demands that occur with fever, sympathetic stimulation, and toxic conditions. When the myocardium is weakened, such as with MI or CHF, tachycardia also occurs because the heart is not effective as a pump. Blood flow to the extremities is decreased, and this triggers reflexes to increase heart rate.

Bradycardia, a heart rate below 60 beats per minute, occurs normally in athletes because their heart is an effective pump with a greater than normal stroke volume. Because cardiac output is the product of stroke volume and heart rate, the heart rate decreases and yet cardiac output is adequate. Bradycardia can also occur from vagal nerve stimulation.

The sinus node can also be affected by respiration. During inspiration, venous return to the right atrium is delayed because of increased intrathoracic pressure. In quiet respiration, heart rate can decrease about 5 per cent. It can decrease up to 30 per cent with deep respiration.

SHIFT OF THE PACEMAKER FUNCTION TO ANOTHER PART OF THE ATRIUM

Although the sinus node in the right atrium is the usual impulse generator, impulses can develop in other points along the atrium, within the atrioventricular (AV) junction, or even within the ventricle conduction systems. Atrial conduction changes most commonly occur from localized reentry phenomena, which are discussed under pathophysiology.

BLOCK IN TRANSMISSION OF THE IMPULSE THROUGH THE HEART

Blocks that slow or stop an impulse can occur in the atrium, in the AV junction, or within the Purkinje fibers of the ventricles. Blocks develop as a result of ischemia of the tissues, scarring of conduction pathways, compression of the AV bundle by scar tissue, inflammation of the AV node, extreme vagal stimulation of the heart, electrolyte imbalances, increased atrial preload, digitalis toxicity, beta-blocking agents, impaired cellular metabolism, MI (especially inferior), and valvular surgery.

ABNORMAL PATHWAYS OF CONDUCTION THROUGH THE HEART

The pathway of conduction can be altered by the size of the heart, blocks in transmission, ischemia, and hyperkalemia and in response to various medications such as epinephrine. The alteration of pathways in the heart can cause serious dysrhythmias and is more fully explained under pathophysiology.

SPONTANEOUS GENERATION OF IMPULSES FROM ANY PLACE ALONG THE CONDUCTION SYSTEM

The entire conduction system is capable of generating impulses for causing the heart to contract. These impulses occur when the heart is ischemic; has areas of calcification along different points in the heart; or has toxic irritation of the AV node, Purkinje system, or myocardium from drugs, nicotine, or caffeine.

Risk Factors

Dysrhythmias may occur from a primary problem within the heart, a secondary response to systemic disorders, electrolyte disorders, or drug toxicity.

Pathophysiology

Reentry and abnormal automaticity are the pathophysiologic mechanisms that lead to tachydysrhythmias. Conduction disorders lead to bradydysrhythmias.

REENTRY MECHANISMS

Normally, when the cardiac impulse has traveled throughout the heart, it has no place to go, so it simply dies off. Then the heart remains quiet until a new impulse begins in the sinus node.

There are some circumstances in which this mechanism does not occur. Instead, the impulse travels around and around in the cardiac muscle without stopping. This phenomenon is called reentry and sometimes circus movement. Because reentry can cause some serious dysrhythmias, it is important to understand the problem fully.

An impulse can be imagined to occur in a circle. If the impulse starts at the top of the circle and travels around, it will stop when it reaches the top again. In the heart, the cardiac muscle is the circle, and it is refractory to further stimulation during repolarization. Three conditions impair this process and allow the impulse to reenter the circle.

First, if the length of the pathway is long, by the time the impulse returns to the top, the muscle will no longer be in a refractory state. Therefore, the impulse can travel around the circle again.

Second, if the distance is the same but the velocity is slowed, there will be an increased time interval, and the impulse can reenter the circle.

Third, if the refractory time for the cardiac cell is shortened, the impulse can reenter it.

All three conditions occur in clients. Clients with dilated hearts can have enlongated pathways. Clients with hyperkalemia, ischemia, and blockage of the Purkinje fibers have slowed velocity. Finally, various medications, such as epinephrine, cause shortened refractory times. Clinical problems such as fibrillation and flutter are due to reentry phenomena.

ABNORMAL AUTOMATICITY

Normal automaticity occurs in specialized cells in the AV node and Purkinje fibers. Once the action potential of the cell is reached, the muscle fiber contracts, and the wave of depolarization spreads over the myocardium.

Abnormal automaticity develops when the resting potential of the cell membrane is reduced from −90 mV to −70 mV. This reduction makes the membrane unstable and subject to abnormal conduction patterns and ectopic beats. Abnormal automaticity is commonly caused by ischemia, hyperkalemia, hypoxia, or medications.

CONDUCTION DELAYS

Delay in the transmission of impulse can occur in the AV node or within the bundle of His and Purkinje fibers in the ventricle. Blocks can produce slowed rhythms because of a reduction in the action potential amplitude and excitability at long diastolic intervals. Blocks can also be progressive (e.g., Mobitz type II). In this type of block, the properties of the impulse-carrying fiber change along its length, so that the action potential loses its efficacy as a stimulus to excite the fiber ahead of it.

Clinical Manifestations

The clinical manifestations of dysrhythmias include palpitations, anginal pain, fainting, shortness of breath, or swelling of the extremities. Physical assessment findings may reveal a heart rate below 50 or above 140 beats per minute; an extremely irregular heart rhythm or pulse; a first heart sound that varies in intensity; sudden appearance of symptoms of CHF, shock, and angina pectoris; and a slow, regular heart rate that does not change with activity.

DIAGNOSTIC ASSESSMENT

The electrocardiogram (ECG) is a recording of the electrical activity in the heart through electrodes on the skin. ECGs can be recorded on ruled paper as a permanent record or seen on a visual monitor.

Each heart beat produces a complex on the screen or paper. Waves of the segment are named P, Q, R, S, and T and represent specific actions within the heart (Fig. 42-9). The P wave shows contraction of the atria; the QRS complex represents contraction of the ventricles; the T wave indicates repolarization of the heart muscle; the PR interval is the time between atrial contraction and the beginning of ventricular contraction during which the impulse is traveling through the AV node; and the ST segment marks the return of the ECG wave to isoelectric line or its gradual sloping to baseline. Elevations or depressions of the ST segment occur with myocardial ischemia, injury, and infarction.

A normal sinus rhythm is a heart rhythm that begins in the sinoatrial (SA sinus) node and is between 60 and 100 beats per minute, with normal intervals and no aberrant or ectopic beats. Assessment of the ECG is described in Box 42-3.

Management of Disorders Arising in the Atria

DISTURBANCES IN AUTOMATICITY

Sinus Tachycardia. Sinus tachycardia is characterized by a rapid, regular rhythm at a rate of 100 to 180 beats per minute with a normal P wave and QRS complex (Fig. 42-10*A*). It often occurs in response to an increase in sympathetic tone or decreased vagal tone. Causes of sinus tachycardia include fever; emotional and physical stress; heart failure; hyperthyroidism; hypercalcemia; medications including caffeine, atropine, nitrates, epinephrine, isoproterenol, and nicotine; and exercise. Most clients do not experience symptoms except for occasional palpitations. Those with underlying heart disease may not tolerate the increased myocardial workload and reduced ventricular and coronary artery filling time that accompanies the increased heart

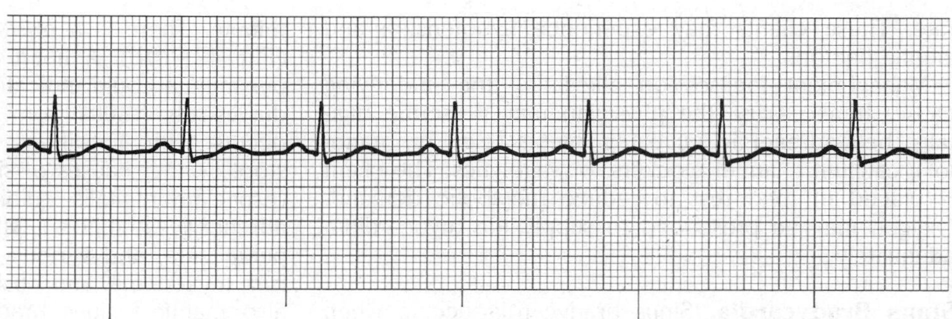

▲ Figure 42-9

Normal sinus rhythm as it appears on an ECG strip.

Box 42–3. Interpretation of Dysrhythmias from the Electrocardiogram

There are seven basic steps that assist you in the identification of dysrhythmias. The electrocardiogram should be studied in an *orderly* fashion in the following manner.

Step 1

Calculate the heart rate. The simplest method for obtaining the rate is to count the number of R waves in a 6-inch strip of the electrocardiographic tracing (which equals 6 seconds). Multiply this sum by 10 to get the rate per minute. Because the electrocardiographic paper is marked into 3-inch intervals (at the top margin), the approximate heart rate can be rapidly calculated.

Another method is to count the number of large squares between R waves. Find an R wave crossing a large square. Count the number of large squares until the next R wave. The approximate heart rate is

1 large square	300 beats per minute
2 large squares	150 beats per minute
3 large squares	100 beats per minute
4 large squares	75 beats per minute
5 large squares	60 beats per minute
6 large squares	50 beats per minute
7 large squares	43 beats per minute
8 large squares	37 beats per minute
9 large squares	33 beats per minute
10 large squares	30 beats per minute

Step 2

Measure the regularity (rhythm) of the R waves (ventricular rhythm). This can be done by gross observation or actual measurement of the intervals (R-to-R). If the R waves occur at regular intervals (with a variance of less than 0.12 second between beats), the ventricular rhythm is normal. When there are differences in R-to-R intervals (greater than 0.12 second), the ventricular rhythm is said to be irregular. The division of ventricular rhythm into regular and irregular categories assists in identifying the mechanism of many dysrhythmias.

Note atrial regularity and measure the atrial rate. Measure the regularity (rhythm) of the P waves (P-to-P). Use the above method, but calculate the distance between the same point on two consecutive P waves.

Step 3

Examine the P waves. If P waves are present and precede each QRS complex, the heart beat originates in the sinus node, and a sinus rhythm exists. The absence of P waves or an abnormality in their position with respect to the QRS complex indicates that the impulse started outside the sinoatrial node and that an ectopic pacemaker is in command.

Step 4

Measure the PR interval. Normally, this interval should be between *0.12 and 0.20 second.* Prolongation or reduction of this interval beyond these limits indicates a defect in the conduction system between the atria and the ventricles.

Step 5

Measure the duration of the QRS complex. If the width between the onset of the Q wave and the completion of the S wave is greater than *0.12 second* (three fine lines on the paper), an intraventricular conduction defect exists.

Step 6

Examine the ST segment. Normally this segment is isoelectric, meaning it is neither elevated nor depressed because the positive and negative forces are equally balanced during this period. Elevation or depression of the ST segment indicates an abnormality in the onset of recovery of the ventricular muscle, usually because of injury (e.g., acute myocardial infarction).

Step 7

Examine the T wave. Normally the T wave is upright and one third the height of the QRS complex. Any condition that interferes with normal repolarization (e.g., myocardial ischemia) may cause the T waves to invert. An abnormally high serum potassium level will cause the T wave to become very tall—sometimes the height of the QRS complex.

rate. These clients may experience hypotension and angina pectoris.

Management focuses on alleviating the underlying cause. If necessary, the physician may prescribe digitalis, beta-adrenergic inhibiting agents (e.g., propranolol), calcium channel blockers, or vagolytics. The client is placed on bed rest to reduce metabolic demand. Oxygen may be prescribed to supply the myocardium adequately.

Sinus Bradycardia. Sinus bradycardia occurs when the SA node fires at a rate less than 60 times per minute. There is a normal P wave and QRS complex (Fig. 42–10*B*). A heart rate that falls below 40 beats per minute could indicate an SA block. Sinus bradycardia usually results from increased vagal tone such as occurs with Valsalva's maneuvers (e.g., straining at stool). Other causes of sinus bradycardia include drugs (especially digitalis, quinidine, procainamide, and beta-adrenergic inhibitors), MI (most often inferior MI), hyperkalemia, and various diseases such as hypothyroidism, myxedema, and obstructive jaundice. Athletes may also manifest sinus bradycardia because of their improved stroke volume.

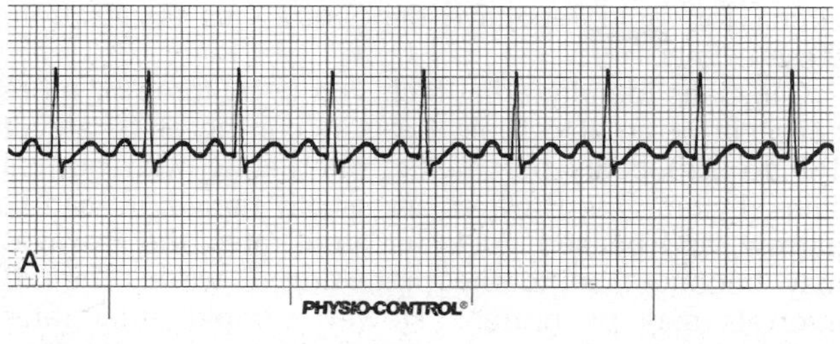

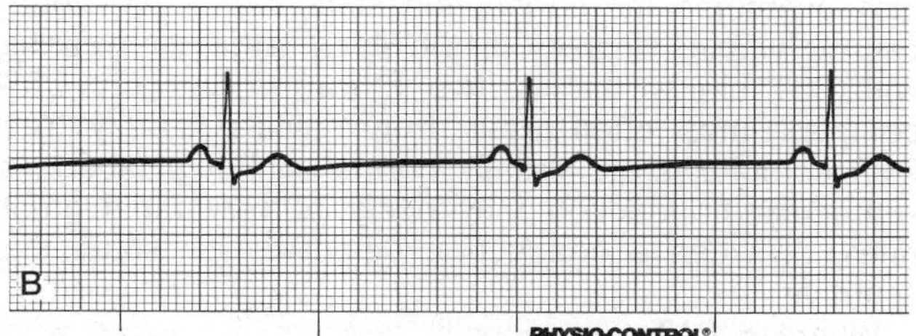

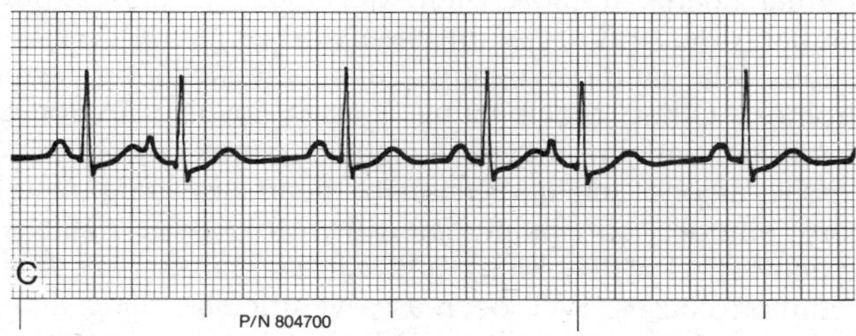

▲ *Figure 42–10*

ECG strips of disorders due to disturbances in atrial automaticity. *A*, Sinus tachycardia. *B*, Sinus bradycardia. *C*, Premature atrial contractions.

Sinus bradycardia may be asymptomatic. In symptomatic clients, a subsequent fall in cardiac output may precipitate fatigue, lightheadedness, or syncope. The slowed rate of SA discharge may force junctional or ventricular pacemakers to take over, thereby producing ectopic beats.

Intervention focuses on relief of symptoms and aims to correct the underlying causes of sinus bradycardia. The goal of intervention is to increase the heart rate just enough to relieve symptoms but not enough to cause tachycardia. Beta-adrenergic agonists (isoproterenol) and vagolytics (atropine) may be used, or a temporary transvenous pacemaker may be used.

Premature Atrial Contractions. Premature atrial contractions (PACs) most often result from enhanced automaticity of the atrial muscle. They occur in normal and diseased hearts. PACs are associated with stress, fatigue, alcohol, smoking, coronary artery disease, cardiac ischemia, heart failure, cardioactive medications (digitalis, quinidine, procainamide), pulmonary congestion, and pulmonary hypertension. Frequent PACs may mark the onset of atrial fibrillation, CHF, and atrial irritability.

PACs usually interrupt an underlying sinus rhythm. They characteristically cause P waves that occur early (premature P waves) and differ from the normal sinus P wave in direction, size, and/or shape. Also, a noncompensatory pause usually follows a PAC (Fig. 42–10*C*). To determine the noncompensatory pause, the clinician compares two uninterrupted normal sinus intervals with the P-to-P intervals between two normal sinus beats containing the PAC. The P-to-P interval will be shorter than two normal sinus intervals. This corresponds with early depolarization and rate resetting of the SA node. Sometimes the PAC occurs early within the refractory period of the ventricles, becoming buried within the preceding T wave. The PAC cannot be conducted to the ventricles at that time and therefore presents as a pause that may mimic SA conduction defects. If the PR interval (from the premature P wave) is less than 0.12 second, the premature beat is of junctional origin and is not a PAC.

For detecting PACs, palpate the pulse and auscultate the heart. An early beat will be heard or felt, but it may be difficult to differentiate a PAC from premature beats of other origins (e.g., premature junctional or premature ventricular contractions). The client who experiences numerous PACs may note palpitations or "missed beats." By themselves, PACs are usually benign. However, the client should seek evaluation of the condition. Intervention usually focuses on correcting the underlying cause and may include quinidine or procainamide.

Sinus Dysrhythmia. Sinus dysrhythmia is characterized by phasic changes in the automaticity of the SA node, which cause it to fire at varying speeds. The ECG has a normal P wave, PR interval, and QRS complex. Considered a normal variant, sinus dysrhythmia most frequently develops in conjunction with alterations in vagal tone. SA node firing, and thus heart rate, speeds up during inhalation and slows down during exhalation. The heart rate generally ranges between 60 and 100 beats per minute. This dysrhythmia appears most often in children, although it occurs at all ages. In older clients with underlying CAD, there is often no correlation between phasic rate changes and respiratory pattern. Sinus dysrhythmia does not usually require intervention other than alleviation of the underlying cause.

DISTURBANCES IN CONDUCTION

SA Conduction Defects. Under certain circumstances, the impulse from the SA node is either (1) not generated in the SA node (SA arrest) or (2) not conducted from the SA node (sinus exit block). Causes of SA node conduction abnormalities include conditions that increase vagal tone, CAD, MI, digitalis and quinidine toxicity, and hypertensive disease. These dysrhythmias may also occur from tissue hypoxia, scarring of intra-atrial pathways, or electrolyte imbalances.

During SA arrest, neither the atria nor the ventricles are stimulated, which produces a pause in the rhythm. An entire PQRST will be missing for one or more cycles. After the pause of sinus arrest, a new pacemaker focus assumes the pacing responsibility. The new pacer paces the heart at its inherent rate, which is usually slower than the original SA node rate. The most likely new pacer site is another atrial focus, but the junction or ventricle can also escape to assume pacing responsibility.

In sinus exit block, there is a conduction delay between the sinus node and the atrial muscle. Unlike SA arrest, the rhythm of SA node discharge in sinus exit block remains constant and uninterrupted. The ECG characteristically displays a normal sinus rhythm that is interrupted intermittently by pauses. This creates a pattern of pauses that, when measured, are multiples of the underlying P-to-P interval. Sinus arrest differs from SA exit block in that the SA node intermittently fails to fire at all. The result is the occurrence of pauses that are longer and not a multiple of the underlying P-to-P interval. These pauses are also frequently terminated by escape ectopic beats. Sinus arrest often has a more serious prognosis.

With SA conduction abnormalities, the clinician can palpate or auscultate an irregular pulse. Clinicians can only infer impulse formation within the SA node from the appearance of P waves, which reflect atrial depolarization.

The client usually remains asymptomatic, depending on the duration and frequency of the pauses. However, lengthy pauses can cause lightheadedness or syncope.

Intervention is unnecessary unless the client becomes symptomatic and exhibits signs of decreased cardiac output. Intervention may include administration of vagolytics (atropine) or sympathomimetics (isoproterenol) to increase the rate of the SA node firing. If pharmacologic measures fail, a pacemaker may be required. Finally, the physician needs to determine and treat the underlying cause of the dysrhythmia.

DISTURBANCES IN IMPULSE GENERATION

Atrial dysrhythmias are caused by ectopic foci that develop in one of the atrial walls and act to "take over" pacemaker function from the SA node.

Atrial and junctional dysrhythmias are sometimes called supraventricular dysrhythmias because the abnormal foci for ectopic beats originate at a site above the ventricles. An atrial focus may release an impulse before the SA node is due to discharge its normal impulse. This single premature impulse produces a PAC. On the other hand, an atrial ectopic focus may become so irritable that it produces impulses in rapid succession, thereby totally taking over the role of pacemaker. Such rapid rates of impulse formation occur in paroxysmal atrial tachycardia, atrial flutter, and atrial fibrillation.

Paroxysmal Atrial Tachycardia. Paroxysmal atrial tachycardia (PAT) is the sudden onset of a rapid firing from an ectopic atrial pacemaker (Fig. 42–11*A*). PAT is due to the reentry phenomenon. In this instance, the supraventricular conducting fibers vary in their degree of refractoriness. This (1) allows the atrial impulses to travel down less refractory conduction pathways to the bundle of His and (2) permits retrograde conduction through previously refractory parallel fibers. An open circuit for rapid repetitive depolarizations results from these events.

Clinicians identify atrial tachycardia by three or more consecutive atrial ectopic beats occurring at a rate of 160 to 230 beats per minute alternating with normal sinus rhythm. The P waves are usually upright in lead II, narrow, and peaked. At faster atrial rates, the P waves may become lost in the preceding T wave. The PR intervals may be normal. However, rapid atrial rates may overcome the conduction limits of the AV node, causing varying degrees of AV block. Atrial tachycardia with 2:1 block (that is, two P waves for every QRS complex) most often results from digitalis toxicity. The QRS complexes are usually normal, although aberrant ventricular conduction may occur at very rapid atrial rates, or when a conduction defect exists within the ventricle.

Whereas PAT occasionally appears in clients with normal hearts, it most often develops in clients with cardiac disease. Cardiac problems precipitating PAT include MI, cardiomyopathy, and preexcitation syndromes. Other precipitating causes involve extreme emotions, caffeine ingestion, fatigue, smoking, and excessive alcohol intake. Rheumatic heart disease, pulmonary emboli, cor pulmonale, thyrotoxicosis, digitalis toxicity (PAT with block), and cardiac surgery are less common causes. PAT decreases ventricular filling time and mean arterial pressure. PAT also increases myocardial oxygen demand.

Management of PAT varies with the severity of symptoms. Clients experiencing this dysrhythmia may note palpitations and lightheadedness. Clients with extremely rapid heart rates or significant underlying cardiovascular disease may develop syncope and heart failure. The client's heart rate must be immediately reduced. Any maneuver that stimulates the vagus nerve can successfully terminate PAT or increase AV block. Vagotonic maneuvers include carotid sinus massage and Valsalva's maneuvers (bearing down as with bowel movements). Useful pharmacologic agents include propranolol, edrophonium, and verapamil. Sedatives may also be used to reduce sympathetic stimulation. The physician may also employ synchronous cardioversion as an effective means of terminating PAT if medications and vagal stimulation are not effective.

Atrial Flutter. Atrial flutter is an accelerated rhythm resulting from rapid firing of an ectopic atrial focus. Probably this focus is quite close to the AV junction and, like PAT, sets up a reentry pattern of fast, consecutive depolarizations. Atrial flutter differs from PAT in that it produces a much more rapid atrial rate. The P waves are actually inverted or bidirectional, producing a "picket fence" or "saw-toothed" pattern of "flutter waves" (Fig. 42–11*B*). Atrial rate generally ranges from 250 to 350 beats per minute. The AV node cannot conduct all of the atrial impulses that bombard it; that is, it cannot produce a 1:1 conduction. Therefore, the ventricular rate will always be slower than the atrial rate. Thus, the pulse, which reflects ventricular rate, may be normal even though the atrial rate is quite rapid.

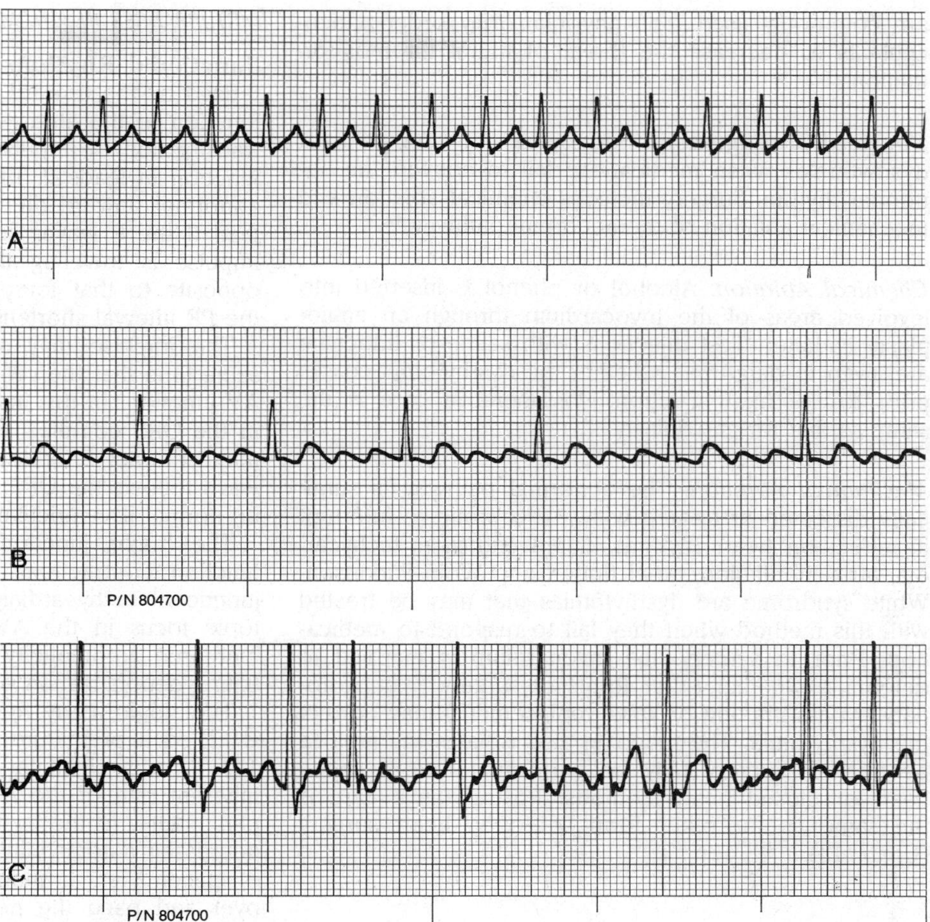

▲ *Figure 42–11*

Disturbances in atrial impulse generation. *A*, Paroxysmal atrial tachycardia. *B*, Atrial flutter (note sawtoothed pattern of P waves). *C*, Atrial fibrillation (note irregularly occurring R waves).

The ratio of atrial to ventricular beats may be constant (2:1, 3:1, 4:1, 7:1, and so forth), or it may vary. A variable degree of block produces an irregular pulse.

Atrial flutter most commonly occurs in association with organic diseases such as CAD, mitral valve disease, pulmonary embolus, and hyperthyroidism. In addition, it may follow cardiac surgery. The client may sense occasional palpitations and chest pain, especially when rapid ventricular rates exist.

Intervention aims at controlling rapid ventricular rates. Cardioversion is used. Medications used to treat atrial flutter include digitalis, quinidine, verapamil, propranolol, and procainamide, especially if cardioversion is not successful. Carotid sinus massage helps temporarily slow the ventricular response so that flutter waves can be identified.

Atrial Fibrillation. Atrial fibrillation is characterized by rapid, chaotic atrial depolarization. The atrial tissue responds to impulses of more than 500 per minute. Atrial fibrillation is a disorder due to the reentry phenomenon. However, at extremely rapid rates, the entire atrium may not be able to recover from one depolarization wave before the next begins. This results in mechanical and electrical disorganization of the atria. As with atrial flutter, the AV node is bombarded with more impulses than it can conduct. Most of these impulses are blocked, which results in a very irregular ventricular rhythm. The ventricular rate ranges from less than 50 to more than 200 per minute. Examination of the ECG reveals erratic or no P waves and a baseline that appears to be irregular and undulating (Fig. 42–11*C*).

Atrial fibrillation most often affects older clients. The causes are similar to those of atrial flutter and include CHF, restrictive pericarditis, organic heart disease, and cor pulmonale. Clients may be asymptomatic, or they may note an irregular pulse and palpitations. The client may have a pulse deficit between apical and radial pulses. Because of atrial disorganization, there is no "atrial kick." This can decrease cardiac output by as much as 20 to 30 per cent. With increasing ventricular rates, cardiac output falls even further and may result in angina pectoris, heart failure, and shock.

Mural thrombi formation can severely complicate atrial fibrillation. Blood pools in the "quivering" atria because of lack of adequate contraction of atrial muscle. This blood can clot, which increases the potential for cerebral and pulmonary vascular emboli.

Atrial fibrillation is managed with cardioversion if the client has a rapid ventricular response. Digoxin, calcium channel blockers, quinidine, and procainamide are commonly used. The physician may order anticoagulants to decrease the threat of mural thrombi formation.

Surgical Management. Surgery can be used to treat dysrhythmias when medications fail to convert the abnormal rhythm. Surgery includes chemical ablation and mechanical ablation of the abnormal pathway.[42, 74]

Chemical Ablation. Alcohol or phenol is inserted into involved areas of the myocardium through an angioplasty catheter. Test injections with saline or lidocaine are given to determine whether the dysrhythmia ceases prior to the final injection. Postoperative care is the same as that for angioplasty.

Mechanical Ablation. The abnormal pathway is surgically dissected or treated with a cryoprobe to interrupt its effect on heart rhythms. Supraventricular tachycardia, atrial fibrillation, atrial flutter, and Wolff-Parkinson-White syndrome are dysrhythmias that may be treated with this method when they fail to respond to medication. Prior to surgery, the myocardium is mapped to determine whether other forms of surgery (e.g., coronary bypass grafting or valve replacement) may correct the dysrhythmia. The mapping also isolates the area to be treated. Surgery may be performed through open heart or closed heart methods. Postoperative care is the same as for other forms of open heart surgery (Chap. 43).

Management of Disorders Arising Within the Atrioventricular Junction

Two major types of dysrhythmias arise in the AV junction: (1) disturbances in automaticity, that is, the AV junctional tissue assumes the role of the pacemaker; and (2) disturbances in conduction, that is, the AV junction blocks impulses journeying from the atria to the ventricles. Both of these types of dysrhythmias may result from ischemia or trauma in the area of the AV junction, that is, after MI or cardiac surgery. Digitalis toxicity and hyperkalemia may also cause junctional dysrhythmias.

DISTURBANCES IN AUTOMATICITY

Junctional Rhythms. Junctional rhythms are characterized by the upward spread of impulses from the AV junction to the atria rather than the normal downward transmission of impulses from the SA node to the AV junction in leads II, III, and aVF. The ECG reveals the abnormal upward direction of impulse spread (e.g., in lead II the P waves are inverted). This is because the impulse is traveling through the atria in a direction opposite to that found in normal sinus rhythm. Also, the PR interval shortens to less than 0.12 second.

The impulse may spread through the atria at the same time that the ventricles are being activated by the AV junction. In this instance, the P wave will be buried in the QRS complex and not observed. Also, the atria may contract after the ventricles. In this case, the P wave follows the QRS complex. The QRS complex will be normal if ventricular conduction is normal.

The major junctional dysrhythmias are premature junction contractions, junctional escape rhythm, and junctional tachycardias. As occurs with PACs, an ectopic focus in the AV junctional tissue may develop increased automaticity and discharge prematurely, initiating depolarization of the heart.

The single, early firing of a junctional ectopic focus is called a premature junctional contraction (Fig. 42–12). It has a significance similar to that of a PAC. The inherent rate of the AV junction is 40 to 60 impulses per minute. In the event that the SA node experiences decreased automaticity and fails to function in the role of pacemaker, a junctional escape rhythm will take over and pace the heart at its own inherent rate. A junctional rhythm with a rate that exceeds 60 beats per minute is termed a junctional tachycardia.

Usually, clients can tolerate junctional rhythms. However, clients with severe forms of cardiac disease may not tolerate junctional rhythms when atrial contraction fails to occur before ventricular contraction because cardiac output decreases.

Management for rapid junctional rhythms centers on pharmacologic agents and electrical cardioversion. Clients with a junctional escape rhythm do not require intervention unless they are symptomatic. Then, heart rate may be boosted with the administration of atropine or pacemaker insertion. Premature junctional contractions may be treated with quinidine.

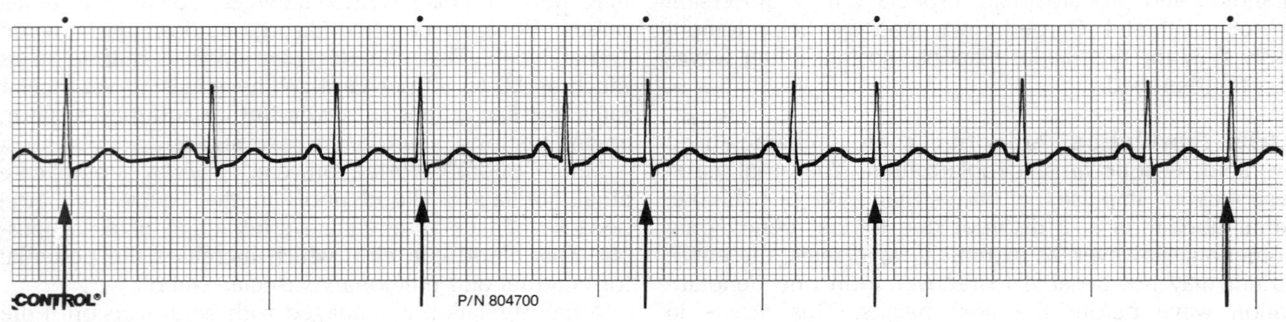

▲ **Figure 42–12**

Junctional escape rhythm.

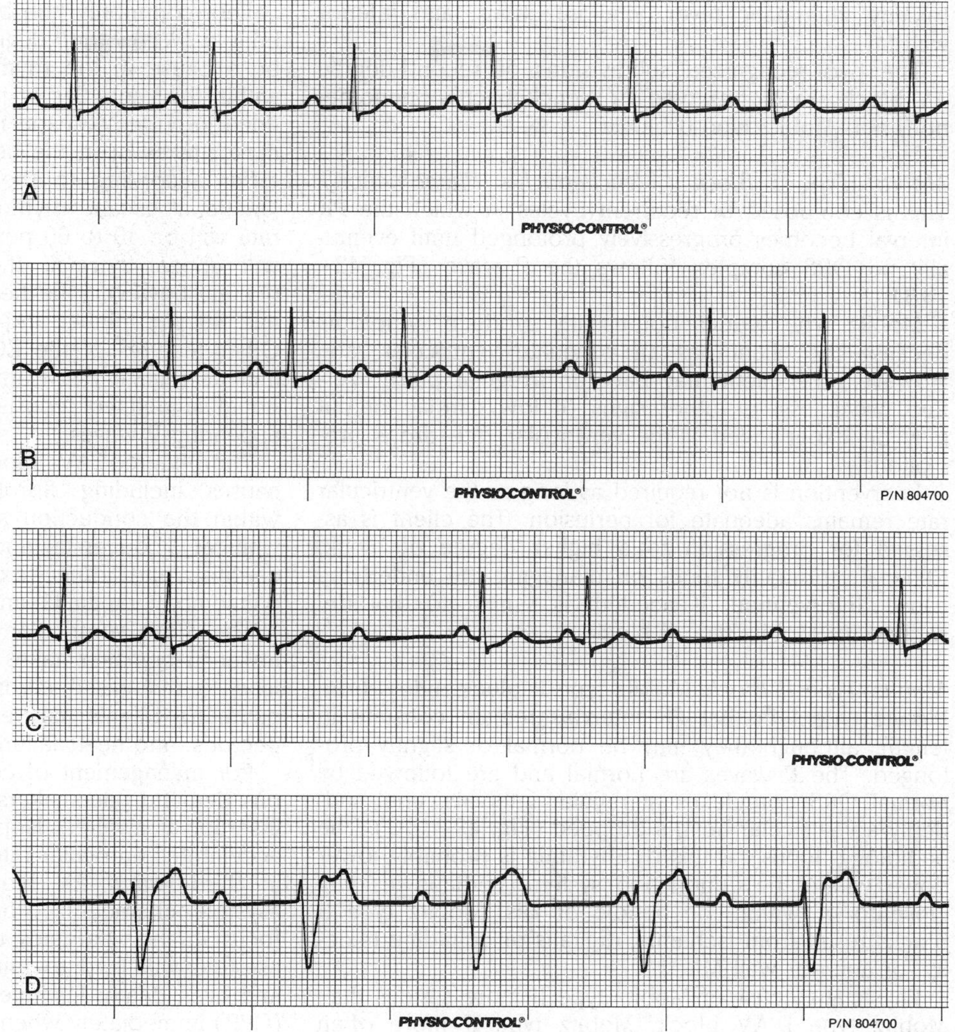

▲ *Figure 42–13*

Disturbances in junctional conduction. *A*, First-degree AV block. *B*, Second-degree AV block (Mobitz type I, Wenckebach's; note regularly occurring P waves and increasing PR intervals). *C*, Second-degree AV block (Mobitz type II). *D*, Third-degree AV block (note variable PR interval and lack of association of P wave with QRS complex).

DISTURBANCES IN CONDUCTION

AV Block. AV block comprises the second group of disturbances arising in the area of the AV junction. Impulses passing through the AV junction are blocked in varying degrees. Therefore, the conduction of impulses from the atria to the ventricles slows or stops entirely, depending on the degree of the AV block. Normally the impulse coming from the SA node is delayed at the AV junction for less than 0.20 second before traveling on to the bundle of His. However, when the AV junction has been damaged by ischemia, rheumatic fever, or drug toxicity, impulses are delayed at the AV junction for abnormally long periods of time.

First-Degree AV Block. This disturbance occurs when conduction in the AV node slows so that the PR interval is longer than 0.20 second (Fig. 42–13*A*). This block is often associated with CAD, increased vagal tone, and congenital anomalies. It may also result from digitalis administration.

First-degree AV block does not describe a distinct and separate rhythm. Rather, it describes the dominant rhythm more completely (e.g., sinus bradycardia with first-degree AV block). First-degree AV block, existing alone as the only abnormal feature of a client's ECG, produces no symptoms and requires no intervention. If the block is due to digitalis, the medication may be discontinued.

Second-Degree AV Block. This dysrhythmia indicates increased conduction disruption at the AV junction. An intermittent block of supraventricular impulses at the AV junction delays or prevents the depolarization wave through the bundle of His. This results in intermittently dropped QRS complexes. Atrial depolarization continues without disturbance, and normal-appearing P waves occur at regular intervals. The degree of AV block and the number of dropped QRS complexes vary. Every second, third, or fourth (or more) impulse from the atria may be fully blocked, with creation of a discrepancy between the atrial and ventricular rates. Second-degree AV block does not usually affect conduction through the ventricles, and QRS complexes appear normal in configuration.

Second-degree AV block occurs with CAD, digitalis

toxicity, rheumatic fever, viral infections, and inferior wall MI.

The two recognized subdivisions of second-degree AV block are Mobitz type I (Wenckebach's phenomenon) and Mobitz type II block.

Mobitz Type I Block (Wenckebach's Phenomenon). This is composed of recurrent cycles in which the PR interval becomes progressively prolonged until eventually no QRS complex follows the P wave (Fig. 42-13*B*).

Mobitz type I does not usually produce symptoms because the client has an adequate ventricular rate. However, the client may have an irregular pulse. Vertigo, weakness, or other signs of low cardiac output may be experienced if the ventricular rate drops precipitously.

Intervention is not required as long as the ventricular rate remains adequate for perfusion. The client is assessed for progression to a higher degree of block. Clinicians primarily focus on managing the underlying cause. Intervention, if needed, is similar to that described for Mobitz type II block.

Mobitz Type II Block. Mobitz type II block differs from Mobitz type I in that PR intervals remain constant in length, although they may be normal or slightly prolonged. The P waves are normal and are followed by normal QRS complexes at regular intervals, until suddenly a ventricular beat is dropped (Fig. 42-13*C*). The pathologic focus for this dysrhythmia is probably lower down within the conduction system, perhaps residing close to or within the bundle of His. Mobitz type II blocks result from ischemia, digitalis or quinidine toxicity, or anterior wall MI.

Physicians consider Mobitz type II more serious than Mobitz type I AV block. Mobitz type II more often progresses to a higher degree of AV block, especially in clients with an anterior wall MI. This is dangerous because a complete heart block (third-degree AV block), a potentially life-threatening dysrhythmia, may suddenly occur.

Clients with second-degree AV block require close ECG monitoring for possible progression to complete heart block (third-degree). Intervention includes (1) administration of atropine and isoproterenol (which speed the rate of impulse conduction), (2) insertion of a temporary or permanent pacemaker, and (3) withholding cardiac depressant drugs (e.g., digitalis). Second-degree block, which occurs after MI, particularly an inferior MI, may be reversible as the injury of ischemia heals. If Mobitz type II develops after MI, transvenous demand pacing may be required.

Third-Degree AV Block. In third-degree heart block, all impulses from the atria are blocked, and the action of the atria and the ventricles becomes completely disassociated; that is, the atria and the ventricles each have their own pacemaker and beat completely independently of each other (Fig. 42-13*D*). The site of block may occur in the AV node or in the bundle branches.

Less commonly, the block may occur within the His bundle. When third-degree block develops, there may be a pause in the rhythm before a lower pacemaker within the ventricles or junctional tissues begins to produce impulses (escape rhythm). Once the lower pacemaker takes over, the heart rate and QRS duration will differ according to the site of the pacemaker. If a junctional escape rhythm occurs, the ventricular heart rate will be 40 to 60 per minute and the QRS complex will appear normal. If a ventricular escape rhythm occurs, however, the heart rate will range between 20 and 40 per minute and the QRS complex will widen. Other features of the ECG in third-degree heart block include regular P-to-P intervals, regular R-to-R intervals, no meaningful or consistent PR intervals, and normal-appearing P waves.

Third-degree AV block results from a variety of causes including fibrotic or degenerative changes within the conduction system, MI (especially anterior wall MI), congenital anomalies, cardiac surgery, myocarditis, and drug toxicity (digitalis, procainamide, quinidine, verapamil), and trauma.

The slow ventricular rate that develops once the lower pacemaker takes over impulse formation may lead to decreased cardiac output and circulatory impairment. Clients may experience hypotension, angina pectoris, and heart failure.

For management of complete heart block, transvenous demand pacemakers are inserted while pacemaker insertion is awaited. Isoproterenol may also be used to accelerate ventricular rate. The greatest danger inherent in third-degree AV block is ventricular standstill or asystole, characterized by the Stokes-Adams attack. If a focus in the ventricles does not initiate a heart beat, asystole will lead to immediate loss of consciousness and even death. Institute cardiopulmonary resuscitation (CPR) immediately when asystole occurs!

Management of Disorders Arising in the Ventricles

Disorders of ventricular origin can be divided into the following two groups:

- dysrhythmias that result from ventricular ectopics or a ventricular escape rhythm
- disturbances of impulse conduction through the ventricles as a result of (1) injury to either the right or left bundle branches or (2) pre-excitation syndrome

DISTURBANCES IN VENTRICULAR AUTOMATICITY

Ventricular dysrhythmias arise below the level of the AV junction. These dysrhythmias are characterized by ectopic impulses, which result from either myocardial irritability or the phenomenon of reentry. The three ventricular dysrhythmias are (1) premature ventricular contractions, (2) ventricular tachycardia, and (3) ventricular fibrillation.

Ventricular dysrhythmias are generally more serious and life-threatening than are atrial or junctional dysrhythmias. This is because ventricular dysrhythmias more often develop in association with intrinsic heart disease. Conversely, atrial dysrhythmias frequently arise in normal hearts affected by emotions, fatigue, and so forth. Also, ventricular dysrhythmias usually cause greater hemodynamic compromise (e.g., hypotension, heart failure, and shock). The independent contraction of the ventricles results in a reduced stroke volume and therefore a reduced cardiac output. Rapid ventricular rates prevent optimal filling of the ventricular chambers and reduce stroke volume even further. At rates less than 40 per minute, cardiac output is simply not sufficient to support the body's vital functions.

The ECG tracing of ventricular dysrhythmias reveals wide and bizarre QRS complexes. Normally, impulses traverse the ventricles via the shortest, most efficient route. This normal pathway results in a narrow QRS complex. When an impulse originates in the ventricles, however, the impulse follows an abnormal pathway through the ventricular muscle tissue. This abnormality appears as a wide (greater than 0.10 second) complex on the ECG.

Premature Ventricular Contractions. Premature ventricular contractions (PVCs), also called ventricular premature beats, are the most common of all dysrhythmias other than those of the sinus node. They are usually caused by the firing of an irritable focus in the ventricle. A ventricular impulse forms before the next expected impulse from the SA node and takes the place of the normal beat. On the ECG, a wide and bizarre QRS appears, interrupting the underlying rhythm (Fig. 42–14*A*).

PVCs result from enhanced ventricular automaticity or reentry. Factors promoting PVCs include hypoxia, hypokalemia, hypocalcemia, acidosis, CAD, heart failure, toxic agents (e.g., digitalis, tricyclic antidepressants), exercise, hypermetabolic states, and intracardiac catheters. Also, prolonged sinus arrest or sinus bradycardia may invite the formation of ventricular ectopy. PVCs, innocuous as long as they remain infrequent or isolated, do not require intervention. PVCs are dangerous when they are (1) frequent (more than six per minute), (2) coupled with normal beats (bigeminy), (3) multiform (Fig. 42–14*B*), (4) occurring in pairs (Fig. 42–14*C*), (5) occurring as a result of acute MI, and (6) falling on the T wave.

Clinicians refer to "falling on the T wave" as the R-on-T phenomenon. The downward slope of the T wave is the most vulnerable period of the cardiac cycle. If the heart is stimulated at this time, it often cannot respond to the stimulus in an organized fashion because the muscle fibers are in various stages of repolarization. Therefore, PVCs occurring during this vulnerable period can precipitate the more life-threatening dysrhythmias of ventricular tachycardia and ventricular fibrillation (Fig. 42–14*D*). Intervention for dangerous PVCs involves administration of antidysrhythmic agents that have myocardial depressant actions. In acute situations, the clinician may administer class I and class II antidysrhythmic agents intravenously, followed by a continuous intravenous drip. Table 42–11 describes a variety of antidysrhythmic agents.

Ventricular Tachycardia. This dysrhythmia occurs when an irritable ectopic focus in the ventricles takes over the recurrent role of pacemaker. All factors that cause PVCs can initiate ventricular tachycardia, but it develops most frequently after MI.

Ventricular tachycardia is characterized by rapidly occurring series of PVCs (three or more) with no normal beats in between (Fig. 42–14*E*). P waves are absent, and PR interval is absent. QRS complex is wide (greater than 0.12 second) and bizarre. The ventricular rate ranges between 100 and 250 beats per minute, usually 130 to 170 beats per minute. The ventricular rhythm is slightly irregular. Ventricular tachycardia, an extremely dangerous dysrhythmia, produces a very low cardiac output that can quickly lead to cerebral and myocardial ischemia. At any time, ventricular tachycardia can develop into ventricular fibrillation.

Ventricular tachycardia that causes loss of consciousness must be terminated immediately with electroshock therapy. The physician may also order intravenous administration of antidysrhythmic agents, usually lidocaine.

Torsades de Pointes. Torsades de pointes is a form of ventricular tachycardia. It has delayed repolarization of the ventricle revealed as a prolonged QT interval and a broad flat T wave in preceding sinus rhythm. The rhythm is regular or irregular with a ventricular rate of 150 to 300 beats per minute. The QRS complex is wide and bizarre. Torsades de pointes is usually due to drug toxicity (procainamide, quinidine, amiodarone) or electrolyte imbalances (hypokalemia or hypomagnesemia). Clinical manifestations begin with palpitations and syncope. This rhythm often precedes ventricular fibrillation and sudden death. Torsades de pointes is treated only if the QT interval is prolonged with temporary overdrive ventricular or atrial pacing. Intravenous magnesium sulfate may also be used.

Ventricular Fibrillation. Ventricular fibrillation is characterized by extremely rapid, erratic impulse formation and conduction. It usually results from severe myocardial damage, hypothermia, R-on-T phenomenon, hypoxia, contact with high-voltage electricity, electrolyte imbalance, and toxicity from quinidine, procainamide, or digitalis. The ECG tracing displays bizarre, fibrillatory wave patterns, and it is impossible to identify P waves, QRS complexes, or T waves (Fig. 42–14*D*). Ventricular fibrillation may be either coarse or fine. This lethal dysrhythmia causes abrupt cessation of effective blood flow. Death results within minutes without immediate intervention.

When ventricular fibrillation appears, the clinician must immediately initiate CPR and defibrillation. The physician may prescribe epinephrine for fine ventricular fibrillation in order to increase myocardial responsiveness to intervention.

DISTURBANCES IN CONDUCTION

Bundle Branch Block. Bundle branch block means that conduction is impaired in one of the bundle

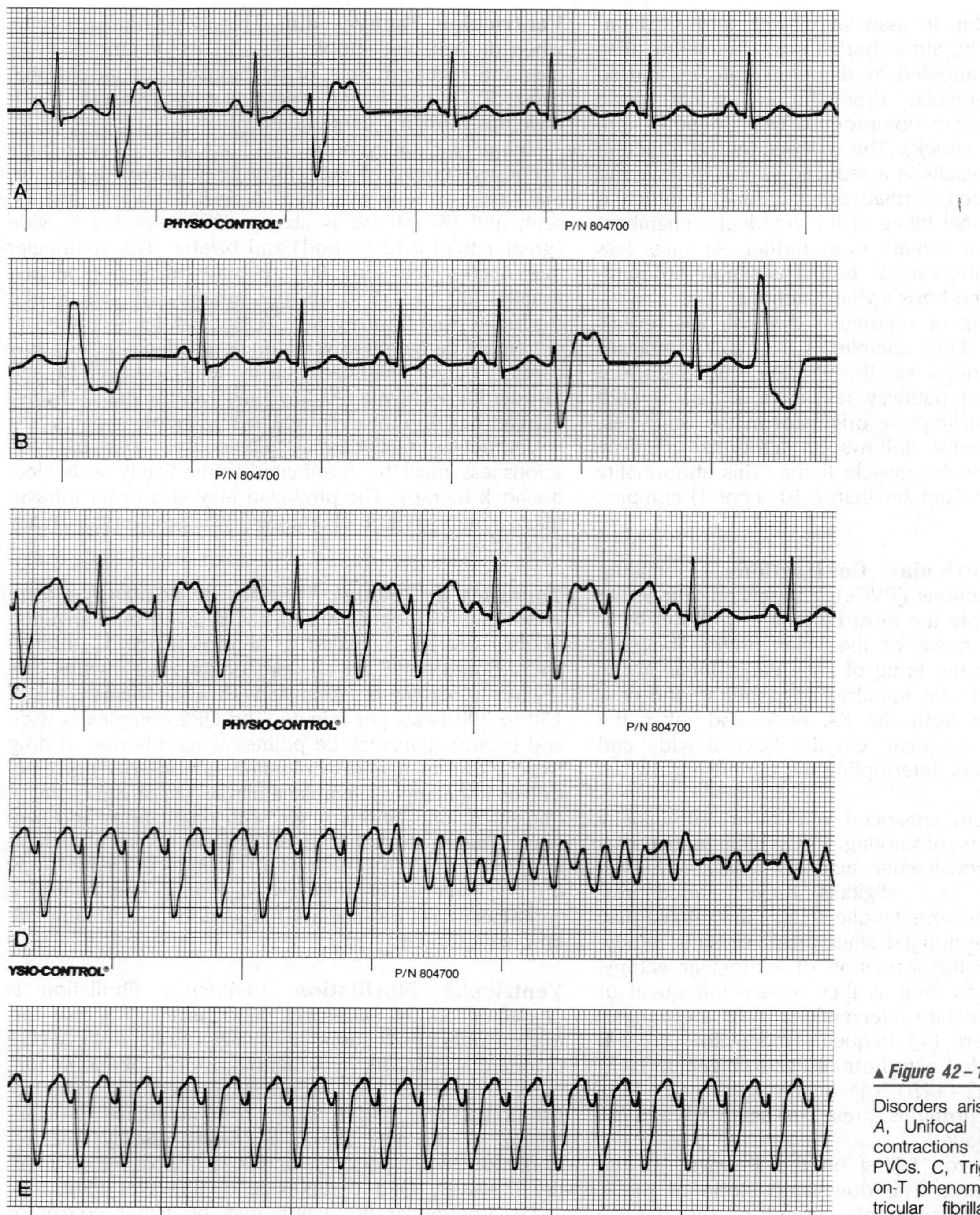

▲ *Figure 42-14*

Disorders arising in the ventricles. *A*, Unifocal premature ventricular contractions (PVCs). *B*, Multifocal PVCs. *C*, Trigeminal PVCs. *D*, R-on-T phenomenon leading to ventricular fibrillation. *E*, Ventricular tachycardia.

branches (distal to the bundle of His), and thus the ventricles do not depolarize simultaneously. In bundle branch block, the abnormal conduction pathway through the ventricles causes a wide and notched QRS complex. The defect may result from myocardial fibrosis, chronic CAD, MI, inflammation, pulmonary embolism, or congenital anomalies.

These disturbances of conduction through the ventricles result in either a right bundle branch block (RBBB) or a left bundle branch block (LBBB). Because of its association with left ventricular disease, LBBB has a worse prognosis than does RBBB. The left bundle branch is composed of anterior and posterior fascicles (little bundles) of which one or both may be involved. There is no specific intervention for this conduction defect. However, if RBBB exists along with block in one of the fascicles of the left bundle, the one remaining fascicle represents the only conduction pathway to the ventricles. Therefore, in this situation the physician may elect to insert a pacemaker.

TABLE 42-11. Medications Used to Manage Dysrhythmias

Class	Example	Action	Common Side Effects	Nursing Implications
Class IA antidysrhythmics	Quinidine	Prolongs refractoriness and slows conduction velocity Decreases membrane responsiveness by increasing effective refractory period in Purkinje fibers to decrease automaticity and reentry disturbances Used in treatment of atrial fibrillation, PVCs, and ventricular tachycardia	Prolongs QRS complex or QT interval, which increases vulnerable period in ventricle Can cause tinnitus, vertigo, visual disturbances, loss of hearing, confusion, delirium, and gastrointestinal symptoms May also cause sinus arrest, SA block, and AV block	Monitor vital signs and ECG, especially QT interval Give with meals Monitor plasma levels Avoid excessive citrus fruits, which increase urine pH and decrease excretion
Class IB antidysrhythmics	Lidocaine (Xylocaine)	Depresses the phase 4 stage of the action potential and increases the ventricular fibrillation threshold In the Purkinje fibers, action potential, effective refractory period, and automaticity are decreased Use in treatment of reentry disturbances, including PVCs and ventricular tachycardia	Because lidocaine is an anesthetic, it can cause paresthesias, numbness, agitation, and disorientation May lead to hallucinations, decreased hearing, twitching, seizures, confusion, and respiratory arrest	Monitor vital signs and ECG continuously Therapy usually initiated with a bolus and then maintained with an IV infusion Common infusion rate is 1–4 mg/min Monitor kidney and liver function tests
Class IC antidysrhythmics	Tambocor (Hecainide acetate)	Depresses sinus node automaticity and prolongs conduction in the atria, AV node, ventricle, and Purkinje fibers	Can aggravate existing dysrhythmias and precipitate new ones May lead to dizziness, visual disturbances, headache, fatigue, palpitations, chest pain, and gastrointestinal distress	Monitor vital signs and ECG continuously Use cautiously in clients taking digitalis and propranolol Usual blood level is 0.2–1 mg/ml
Class II antidysrhythmics	Propranolol (Inderal)	Blocks sympathetic stimulation at the sinus node Reduces automaticity in Purkinje fibers Used to treat atrial fibrillation, atrial flutter, and supraventricular tachycardia	Can cause bronchospasm Contraindicated in bronchial asthma, bronchospasm, and chronic obstructive pulmonary disease	Monitor vital signs and ECG Administer with food
Class III antidysrhythmics	Bretylium tosylate (Bretylol)	Increases action potential duration and refractory period in Purkinje fibers Increases threshold for developing ventricular fibrillation	Hypotension, nausea, and vomiting Neurologic symptoms	Monitor vital signs and ECG closely Potentiates effects of digoxin and warfarin Hypotension more common in clients receiving quinidine or procainamide Monitor liver enzymes Clients on amiodarone need pulmonary function tests with diffusion capacity
Class IV antidysrhythmics	Verapamil (Calan)	Blocks slow calcium channel and has slight nonspecific sympathetic depressant effect	Hypotension, syncope, peripheral edema, constipation, bradycardia, AV blocks	Monitor vital signs and heart rhythm Monitor lung sounds and liver function tests

Table continued on following page

TABLE 42-11. Medications Used to Manage Dysrhythmias Continued

Class	Example	Action	Common Side Effects	Nursing Implications
		Increases relative refractory period through AV node Interferes with reentry of impulses at AV node Used in treating paroxysmal supraventricular tachycardia, atrial fibrillation, and atrial flutter	May precipitate or worsen congestive heart failure Reduces clearance of digitalis	Administer with food Monitor blood pressure and PR interval
Anticholinergics, which compete with receptors for acetylcholine at the para-sympathetic neuronal terminals; this increases the sympathetic tone	Atropine	Accelerates impulse formation in the sinus and AV nodes by inhibiting vagal tone Used to treat SA block, Mobitz I, and complete heart block	Vasodilation; may allow the emergence of junctional pacemakers Depresses exocrine glands (salivary, bronchial mucosa, and sweat glands) Inhibits motor tone of the viscera, leading to distention of the gastrointestinal tract and urinary bladder, dilation of the pupils, and cerebral excitability at high doses and cerebral depression at toxic levels	Monitor vital signs and heart rhythm closely Common rate of administration is 0.4-1 mg every 1-2 hr
Beta-adrenergics (catecholamines); these medications stimulate the heart; they bind to specific receptor sites on the membrane of excitable cells and act directly on automatic and conducting cells by augmenting their sympathetic tone	Isoproterenol (Isuprel)	Stimulates impulse formation and conduction Augments myocardial contraction Produces vasodilation Used to manage symptomatic sinus bradycardia, to increase impulse conduction in SA or AV block, to stimulate escape pacemaker activity in complete AV block	Increases myocardial oxygen demands Generates ectopic beats, especially PVCs Causes central nervous system excitation, facial flushing Action potentiated by antihistamines, tricyclic antidepressants, and thyroid hormone	Assess vital signs closely Common rate of administration is 1-2 mg of a 1:5000 solution via an infusion pump Used as a temporary measure with atropine
	Norepinephrine (Levophed)	Stimulates automatic and conductive myocardial fibers (beta-adrenergic) Also has alpha-adrenergic properties, which cause powerful vasoconstriction of the skin, skeletal muscles, kidneys, liver, and intestinal tract Increases heart rate, myocardial contraction, and blood pressure	Ischemia of the splanchnic organs or digits Cardiac and central nervous system effects, like isoproterenol	Assess vital signs closely Common rate of administration is 0.5-3 ml/min in a 0.004 mg/ml dextrose solution Monitor closely for extravasation
	Epinephrine	Like isoproterenal and norepinephrine, it increases heart automaticity, conductivity, and contractility	Hypoglycemia/hyperglycemia, dangerously high blood pressure, mental excitation	Assess vital signs closely Usual dose is 0.1 mg IV or transbronchially

TABLE 42–11. Medications Used to Manage Dysrhythmias Continued

Class	Example	Action	Common Side Effects	Nursing Implications
		Causes dilation of skeletal muscle blood vessels and constriction of the vessels in the skin, mucous membranes, and splanchnic bed Stimulates breakdown of glycogen to raise blood sugar Inhibits histamine release from mast cells, relaxes smooth muscle in the larynx and bronchial tree	Ischemia of the splanchnic organs or digits	
	Dopamine hydrochloride (Intropin)	The immediate chemical precursor to the natural production of norepinephrine, it triggers the release of norepinephrine and therefore produces the same effect as norepinephrine Dilates renal vessels through specific receptors in the kidney, uniquely responsive to dopamine (this is an advantage over norepinephrine)	See rorepinephrine, except that renal perfusion remains intact	Monitor vital signs closely Infuse by pump with microdrip Usual rate of infusion is 0.5–2.0 μg/kg/min; may be increased to 20 μg/kg/min
	Dobutamine (Dobutrex)	Synthetic catecholamine that acts like dopamine except that it produces a more potent effect on myocardial contractility, a lesser effect on increasing sinus node function, and a slight constriction of peripheral vessels Reduces ventricular preload and afterload Does not increase myocardial oxygen demand as much as the other adrenergics Used in left ventricular failure and cardiogenic shock		Same as dopamine Usual dose is 2.5–2.0 μg/kg/min

AV, atrioventricular; ECG, electrocardiogram; IV, intravenous; PVCs, premature ventricular contractions; SA, sinoatrial.

Hemiblocks. A hemiblock occurs in the anterior limb of the left bundle branch. These blocks can be found in the left anterior or left posterior branch.

Pre-excitation Syndromes. Pre-excitation syndromes occur when part or all of the ventricle is reentered by a depolarization wave traveling down a congenital or acquired accessory conducting pathway between the atrium and ventricle. There are several types of disorders in this category, of which Wolff-Parkinson-White syndrome (WPW) appears most frequently. Clients with WPW frequently develop sudden attacks of very rapid supraventricular dysrhythmias. Most adults with WPW have normal hearts. However, if the tachydysrhythmias occur persistently, clients with WPW may develop myocardial fatigue and ventricular failure. Clients with WPW do not require intervention unless they experience recurring tachydysrhythmias. In this instance, the physician may elect to use vagotonic maneuvers, cardioversion, or propranolol administration.

Electrical Management of Dysrhythmias

Dysrhythmias are electrical disturbances within the heart muscle and conduction system. These disturbances can often be effectively managed with exogenously delivered currents of electricity. Electrical intervention can (1) bring abrupt order to erratic electrical discharge or (2) resume the flow of electrical current where there is none. Methods of electrical therapy include defibrillation and synchronous countershock (cardioversion).

DEFIBRILLATION

Defibrillation is an emergency procedure in which the clinician delivers an electrical current to the heart to terminate a life-threatening dysrhythmia. The most crucial element for survival after cardiac arrest is the time interval from collapse to care, especially defibrillation. If ventricular fibrillation is reversed with defibrillation in 6 minutes, the client is three times more likely to survive than if care is delayed.

Defibrillation delivers an electrical current (shock) of preset voltage to the heart through paddles placed on the chest wall (closed chest procedure). This causes the entire myocardium to completely depolarize at the very moment of shock. It may also allow restoration of organized cardiac action. Defibrillation is always indicated in ventricular fibrillation. It is also used in ventricular tachycardia when the client is unconscious and pulseless. Specially trained nurses, emergency medical technicians, and physicians perform this procedure in emergency settings. Computer-driven defibrillators are now available that automatically interpret the rhythm and advise the clinician whether electroshock is needed. An algorithm for ventricular fibrillation is shown in Figure 42-15.

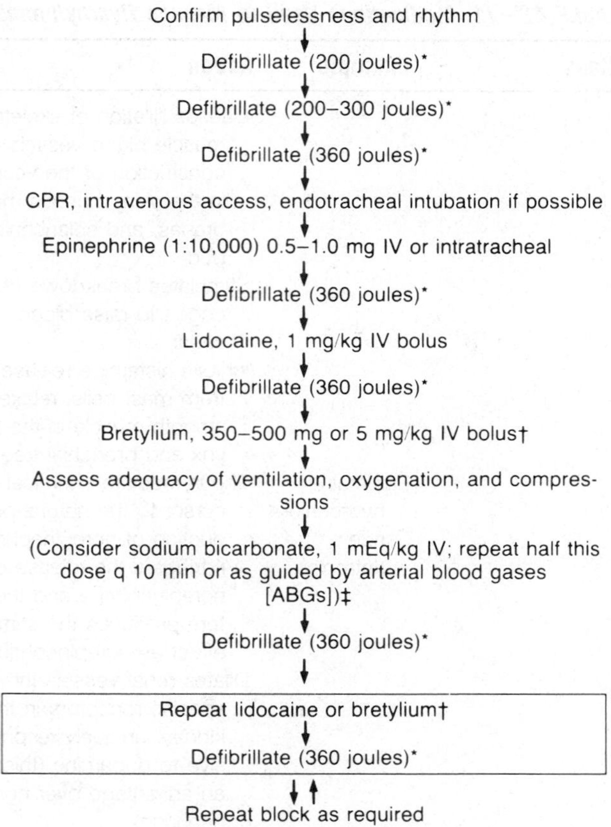
Confirm pulselessness and rhythm
Defibrillate (200 joules)*
Defibrillate (200–300 joules)*
Defibrillate (360 joules)*
CPR, intravenous access, endotracheal intubation if possible
Epinephrine (1:10,000) 0.5–1.0 mg IV or intratracheal
Defibrillate (360 joules)*
Lidocaine, 1 mg/kg IV bolus
Defibrillate (360 joules)*
Bretylium, 350–500 mg or 5 mg/kg IV bolus†
Assess adequacy of ventilation, oxygenation, and compressions
(Consider sodium bicarbonate, 1 mEq/kg IV; repeat half this dose q 10 min or as guided by arterial blood gases [ABGs])‡
Defibrillate (360 joules)*
Repeat lidocaine or bretylium†
Defibrillate (360 joules)*
Repeat block as required
*Assess pulse and rhythm after each shock.
†Repeat bretylium at 700 to 1000 mg or 10 mg/kg IV bolus; lidocaine at 0.5 mg/kg q 8 min to a total dose of 3 mg/kg may be substituted for bretylium.
‡Sodium bicarbonate is of questionable value during cardiac arrest.

▲ **Figure 42-15**

Algorithm for ventricular fibrillation and ventricular tachycardia. Pulseless ventricular tachycardia is treated identically to ventricular fibrillation. (From Rakel, R. E. [1992]. *Conn's current therapy.* Philadelphia: W. B. Saunders.)

Before Defibrillation. Immediately before defibrillation, do the following:

- Check the ECG to verify the presence of ventricular fibrillation or tachycardia on the ECG.
- Check the client's pulse.
- Check leads for any loose connections.
- Remove any topical nitroglycerin patches (causes a burn).

On confirmation of the emergency, the code alarm is given over the health care facility intercom system to summon the emergency team (e.g., "Code 99," "Dr. Blue"). In the meantime, CPR measures are started by the first person on the scene. The clinician turns on the defibrillator and sets it at 200 to 360 watt-seconds (joules) unless the client has digitalis toxicity or is small in stature (in this case, a lower setting is used). Then the clinician turns the machine's synchronizer switch to off. In the presence of fibrillation, the synchronous mode must not be used. The nurse starts an intravenous line as needed for administration of resuscitation medications.

Open chest defibrillation occurs in an operating room setting where electrical current may be applied directly to the heart.

During Defibrillation. When ventricular fibrillation develops, clinicians must attempt defibrillation at the earliest opportunity. The paddles are lubricated with electrode paste or conducting pads to enhance conduction and prevent burning of the skin. The paste should not extend beyond the paddles, and the paddles must lie flat against the body in order to avoid burns. The clinician places the paddles firmly against the chest, using approximately 25 to 30 pounds of pressure. Clinicians often use a transverse (anterolateral) position for paddle placement. One paddle is placed at the second intercostal space, at the right of the sternum, and the other paddle is positioned at the fifth intercostal space, anterior axillary line (Fig. 42-

16*A*). If it is convenient, clinicians may attempt placing the paddles in an anteroposterior position. Because electricity is carried along metal devices and the client, all personnel, including the clinician administering the shock, must stand back from the bed.

After Defibrillation. The clinician immediately assesses the ECG and pulse after defibrillation. If the first countershock is unsuccessful, then the client must be immediately defibrillated again at the same energy level. Most of the cardiac monitors and ECG machines that are connected to the client being defibrillated can withstand the shock. Some monitors, however, may not record the ECG for several seconds after the shock has been administered. Defibrillators are frequently equipped with paddles that are capable of monitoring the ECG, even immediately after defibrillation. Therefore, if the paddles are left in place after the shock has been delivered, the cardiac response can be quickly evaluated.

CPR should be continued if the second defibrillation is not successful. The nurse administers appropriate medications again before the next defibrillation attempt. A successful response is indicated by cessation of fibrillation, restoration of sinus rhythm, and palpation of a regular pulse. After successful defibrillation, the client requires continuous ECG monitoring. The nurse must also continually assess vital signs along with neurologic status.

In documenting the outcome of defibrillation, the nurse must record the following points:

- preprocedure rhythm
- times and voltage of shocks delivered
- postdefibrillation rhythm pattern
- names, times of administration, and doses of administered medications
- other hemodynamic data available before, during, and after the defibrillation

Termination of Resuscitation. In general, if an organized rhythm and pulse have not returned after 15 to 20 minutes of CPR and advanced cardiac life support, success with further treatment is extremely unlikely. Many times the client has other noncardiac disorders that make resuscitation attempts futile.

Advances in Defibrillation

Current-Based Approach. Defibrillation has potential hazards, particularly myocardial damage. Research has shown that the higher the amount of energy or frequency of the shocks, the greater the risk of injury. Advances in defibrillators allow measurement of transthoracic impedance. Once impedance is determined, the defibrillator automatically selects the amount of current needed that can restore rhythm and cardiac output. It is hoped this mode of defibrillation will reduce the risk of complications.[2]

Automatic Implantable Cardioverter Defibrillator. A recent advance in coronary care is the development of the automatic implantable cardioverter defibri-

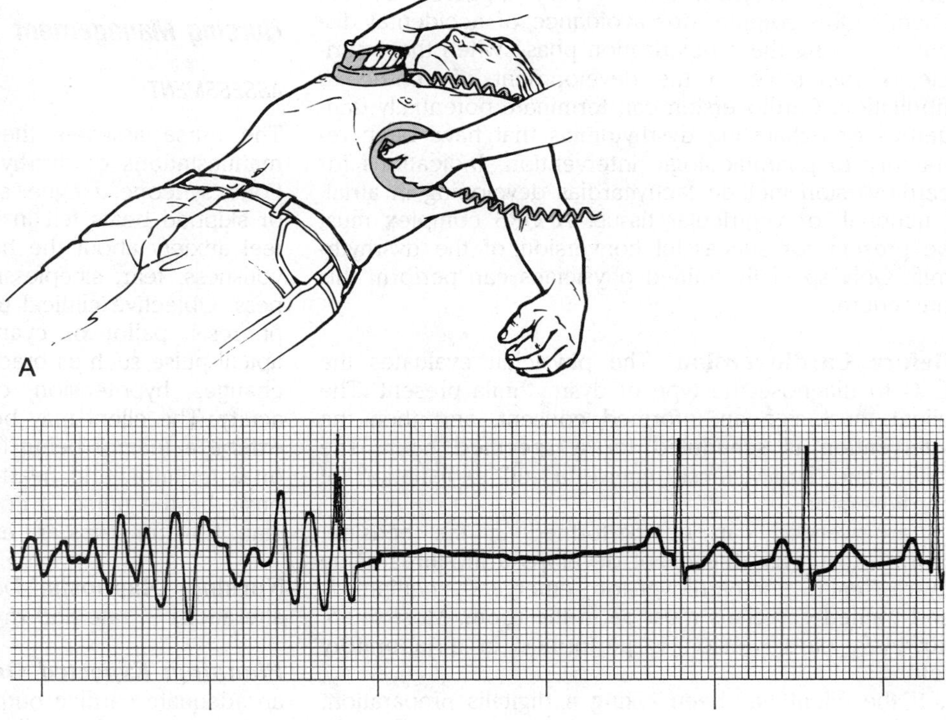

▲ *Figure 42–16*

A, Anterolateral paddle placement for external countershock. External paddles are placed at the second right intercostal space and at the anterior axillary line in the fifth left intercostal space. *B*, Ventricular fibrillation converted to normal sinus rhythm with external countershock.

llator (AICD). It is a system that consists of a pulse generator and a sensor that continuously monitors the heart rhythm. When it detects a dysrhythmia, it automatically delivers a countershock. For ventricular fibrillation, the AICD will give an electrical countershock within 15 to 20 seconds. It can also detect and treat ventricular tachycardia with cardioversion. This implanted system does not require as much energy as external defibrillation does because less energy is lost when the impulse is directly applied to the heart.

The AICD is implanted surgically into a pouch into the abdominal wall through a thoracotomy incision. It has been approved by the Food and Drug Administration for two types of conditions: (1) survival of one or more episodes of sudden cardiac death resulting from ventricular tachycardia or ventricular fibrillation; and (2) recurrent, refractory, life-threatening ventricular dysrhythmias that can develop into ventricular tachycardia or ventricular fibrillation, or both, despite antidysrhythmic therapy.

Clients who require AICDs have a great deal of anxiety. Anxiety can develop from past episodes of near-death as well as from feelings of not ever being able to die. Other patients fear that the AICD will not be able to reverse their dysrhythmia. The nurse is sensitive to these thoughts and facilitates their discussion.

CARDIOVERSION

Cardioversion, most often an elective procedure, is the use of electricity to convert a cardiac dysrhythmia to a normal sinus rhythm that is capable of sustaining improved cardiac output. Cardioversion is not used for ventricular fibrillation. The cardioverter (or defibrillator) delivers an electrical current to the heart. The electrical discharge is synchronized with or triggered by the client's QRS complex for avoidance of accidental discharge during the repolarization phase when the ventricle is vulnerable to the development of ventricular fibrillation. Cardioversion can terminate potentially dangerous or exhausting dysrhythmias that have been refractory to pharmacologic intervention. Indications for cardioversion include tachycardias developing in atrial, junctional, or ventricular tissue. A QRS complex must be present for successful conversion of the dysrhythmia. Only specially trained physicians can perform this procedure.

Before Cardioversion. The physician evaluates the ECG to diagnose the type of dysrhythmia present. The client must sign an informed consent, and then the intervention is scheduled for a specified hour. The client and family must receive a full explanation of cardioversion.

Cardioversion can be performed at the bedside. However, in case the client develops a life-threatening dysrhythmia after cardioversion, emergency equipment and trained clinicians must be in the room. Most often, however, cardioversion is performed in a laboratory setting.

If the client has been taking a digitalis preparation, hold the drug for 2 days before the procedure. Digitalis may predispose the client to the development of ventricular dysrhythmias during cardioversion. A low serum potassium level also increases the risk of lethal dysrhythmias. Therefore, administer potassium replacement therapy as prescribed before cardioversion. Premedicate the client with prescribed antidysrhythmics to ensure maintenance of postconversion rhythms. Administer oxygen, if prescribed, before cardioversion and discontinue afterward. Keep the client NPO for several hours before cardioversion. Start an intravenous line. To reduce fear and promote amnesia, administer diazepam (Valium) intravenously as prescribed.

During Cardioversion. The physician (1) sets the machine within a range of 50 to 200 watt-seconds (more or less voltage depending on the underlying circumstances); (2) turns the synchronizer switch to on in order to deliver the shock during the QRS complex and not on the downslope of the T wave; (3) lubricates the paddles and places them exactly as described for defibrillation; (4) calls for all health care personnel to stand back from the bed; and (5) while standing back from the bed, depresses and holds the buttons on the paddles until the shock is delivered.

After Cardioversion. Clinicians immediately assess the ECG and pulse after cardioversion. In some cases, ventricular fibrillation or tachycardia occurs, demanding emergency action. Monitor the client's ECG rhythm continuously for at least 2 hours and carefully assess for complications.

A successful response to cardioversion resolves the dysrhythmia and restores normal sinus rhythm. With a good response and no complications, the client may be discharged the following day.

Nursing Management

ASSESSMENT

The nurse assesses the client for subjective clinical manifestations of dysrhythmias. These include palpitations, syncope, fatigue, shortness of breath, chest pain, or skipped beats felt in the chest. The client may also feel anxiety about the heart disorder and express nervousness, fear, sleeplessness, uncertainty, or hopelessness. Objective clinical manifestations may include diaphoresis, pallor or cyanosis, variations in radial and apical pulse such as bradycardia or tachycardia, rhythm changes, hypotension, crackles, or decreased mental acuity. The client may be demanding of the nurse and exhibit a fear of being left alone. The client is placed on a monitor, and heart rhythm is monitored continuously by the nurse, a computer, and a monitor technician. Rhythm strips are examined at least every shift.

Nursing Diagnosis: Decreased Cardiac Output R/T alterations in rate and rhythm of the heart.

Planning: Expected Outcomes. The client will have an adequate cardiac output, as evidenced by heart rate and rhythm and blood pressure returning to baseline; level of consciousness returning to baseline; skin is warm and dry; lung sounds are clear; no S_3 or S_4 and no dysrhythmias.

Implementation. The nurse monitors heart rate and rhythm and vital signs continuously, many times with the aid of the computer. Skin temperature, lung sounds, heart sounds, and peripheral pulses are assessed every 4 hours. Laboratory studies are monitored, especially if the client is suspected of having an MI. Antidysrhythmic medications are given according to orders. Blood levels may be used as a guide for dosages. Many medications, especially antidysrhythmics, can rise to toxic levels, especially if the client has pre-existing liver or renal disorders.

The nurse maintains a quiet atmosphere and administers analgesics to control pain. Stimulation can lead to increased levels of catecholamine release and trigger tachycardias and increased oxygen demand.

Oxygen is applied with nasal prongs to supplement serum levels. Hypoxia can lead to further myocardial ischemia and dysrhythmias.

If life-threatening dysrhythmias develop, many nurses are trained to defibrillate the client. Other emergency interventions include CPR, various medications, and preparation of the client for pacemaker insertion.

Nursing Diagnosis: Anxiety R/T sudden onset of life-threatening disorder and risk of death.

Planning: Expected Outcomes. The client will have a reduced level of anxiety, as evidenced by stating a decreased level of anxiety and discussing feelings of helplessness or hopelessness; increased ability to sleep or rest; return of heart rate to baseline; and reduction of dyspnea.

Implementation. The nurse identifies the client's anxiety and assists the client in discussing sources of fear. Misconceptions are clarified. Commonly, the client or a member of the family has had a heart condition and the client's ability to cope may be directly influenced by that experience. The nurse also explains the equipment present in the room. Most rooms are stocked with various equipment, and its presence does not always indicate the severity of the client's condition. The nurse remains with the client and tells the client and family what is happening to the client and what will be happening, such as blood will be drawn soon. Finally, the nurse explores the usual coping methods with the client. Positive coping methods are usually supported; maladaptive coping mechanisms are discussed, and substitutions are suggested. For example, smoking may be a common coping mechanism, but it is not permitted with cardiac disorders, nor is it permitted in most hospitals. Therefore, if smoking is the client's coping mechanism when stressed, a substitution will need to be found such as nicotine patches or chewing gum.

EVALUATION

The degree of expected outcome attainment is assessed hourly (or more often) if the client has life-threatening dysrhythmias. Anxiety can sometimes be abated quickly, but commonly it requires several days for abatement. Some clients remain anxious for their entire hospital stay.

Post-hospital Care

DISCHARGE TEACHING

Clients who have experienced cardiac dysrhythmias while at a health care facility may be apprehensive about leaving the facility. Those who have experienced innocuous dysrhythmias may need only calm reassurance and an explanation of the cause of their disorder. Clients with recurring life-threatening dysrhythmias such as ventricular tachycardia will require comprehensive and specialized attention. These clients may have experienced many frightening events in the course of their hospitalization. Teaching about the nature of the disorder is done several times, because the client may have an attention span shorter than normal as a result of severe anxiety. Before discharge, make certain clients appreciate the importance of taking antidysrhythmic agents as prescribed. Include details concerning medication administration, dosage, and side effects in the discharge plan.

When a client is at risk of developing a life-threatening dysrhythmia, check if the client's housemates and significant others know how to perform CPR techniques. Refer these individuals to community agencies that provide CPR training (e.g., the American Heart Association, the American Red Cross, local fire departments, and some local hospitals).

Sometimes clients with serious, chronic, or potential dysrhythmias use portable telemetry units for monitoring themselves at home after discharge. This allows the resumption of daily activities while providing continuous 24-hour surveillance of cardiac rhythm. Nurses are often responsible for instructing clients in the use of these units. Ask these clients to keep a diary of their daily activities so that clinicians can correlate factors in the client's life that may be contributing to the development of rhythm disturbances.

Finally, instruct clients concerning the importance of regular medical follow-up. Advise them to keep regular appointments with their physician after discharge. Also, the client and significant others should know how to obtain emergency medical attention if necessary.

Living under the constant threat of sudden death provokes anxiety, depression, and, occasionally, dependent behavior in the client. In some cases, psychosocial counseling may bolster coping resources. Significant others also benefit from counseling. The nurse can recommend community and private counseling services for the client and significant others.

▼ PACEMAKERS

A pacemaker is a device that delivers battery-supplied electrical stimuli over leads with electrodes in contact with the heart. A pacemaker initiates the heartbeat when the heart's intrinsic conduction system fails or is unreliable. Problems with the conduction system develop when (1) the SA node is damaged and unable to promote a reliable rhythm; (2) impulses from the SA node and atria are not adequately transmitted through the AV junction to the ventricles; or (3) dysrhythmias from ectopic foci are present.

Sophisticated pacemakers use computers that allow multiple programs. They can send out appropriately timed signals, sense cardiac activity, and preserve normal atrial and ventricular sequence (synchrony). Future pacemakers will be able to respond, as the heart does, to changing metabolic requirements by responding to changes in blood pH, oxygenation, respirations, temperature, or muscle activity.[32] The artificial pacemakers control the heart beat by means of direct electrical stimulation of the ventricles or atria. Table 42–12 outlines the indications for pacemaker insertion.

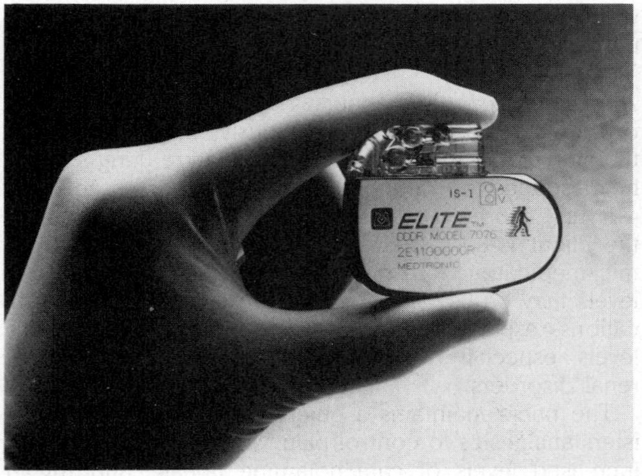

▲ Figure 42–17

Permanent pacemaker (pulse generator). (Courtesy of Medtronics.)

ARTIFICIAL PACEMAKER DESIGN

Whereas there are numerous pacemaker models, each with unique capabilities, every pacemaker consists of a pulse generator and a lead-electrode system.

The pulse generator is essentially the pacemaker's power source. It houses the electronic circuitry responsible for sending out appropriately timed signals and for sensing cardiac activity. The output circuit controls the current pulse delivery rate, pulse duration, and refractory period. The sensing circuit is responsible for identifying and analyzing any spontaneous intrinsic electrical activity and responding appropriately.

The pulse generator can be external or internal. The external unit is designed for temporary pacing, primarily for support of critical bradycardias. The unit is the size of a small transistor radio and operates by dry-cell batteries (Fig. 42–17). The unit has dials for adjustment of both power and rate of discharge. The pulse generator can also be permanently implanted. A small incision is made in the anterior chest wall. The pacemaker is about the size of a stethoscope head and can be reprogrammed after insertion as needed.

The lead delivers the electrical impulse from the pulse generator to the myocardium. The leads consist of flexible conductive wires enclosed by insulating material. The electrode is the end of the lead that delivers the impulse directly to the myocardial wall. It is usually made of platinum-iridium, a highly conductive material that also deters the adherence of platelets. Not only does this system deliver electrical impulses, but it relays information about spontaneous intracardiac signals back to the sensing circuit within the pulse generator. Electrodes can be unipolar or bipolar. Unipolar designs incorporate the cardiac electrode as the negative terminal of the electrical circuit with the metallic shell or second wire of the impulse generator as the positive electrode. Bipolar systems use two wires, each ending in an electrode a short distance apart.

TABLE 42–12. Indications for Artificial Pacemakers

Dysrhythmias from depressed impulse formation
- Asystole
- Sick sinus syndrome
  - Sinus arrest
  - Symptomatic sinus bradycardia

Dysrhythmias from blocked conduction
- Third-degree AV block with slow ventricular rate or syncope (Stokes-Adams attack)
- Mobitz II AV block in a client with an MI
- Right bundle branch block with left hemiblock
- New left bundle branch block in a client with an MI

Dysrhythmias from reentry phenomenon
- Atrial tachydysrhythmias
- Ventricular tachydysrhythmias
- Atrial fibrillation with a slow ventricular rate

Prophylactically before surgery in clients with a history of cardiac arrest or AV blocks

AV, atrioventricular; MI, myocardial infarction.

TYPES OF PACEMAKERS

Pacemakers are classified by uniform codes according to a classification system. The classification originally used a three-letter code: the first letter denoted the cardiac chamber to be paced (the atrium [A], ventricle [V], or both [dual] chambers [D]); the second letter reflected the chamber to be sensed (the atrium [A], ventricle [V], dual [D], or none); and the third letter indicated the type of response to occur, that is, sensed myocardial electrical activity will cause the pacemaker's impulse to be "triggered" (T) or "inhibited" (I) or both (D). For example: AVVI pacemaker: V, the ventricle is paced; V, the ventricle is sensed; and I, the pacemaker will inhibit pacing when the client's own impulse (e.g., ectopic beat) is sensed. Later, two more categories were added: programmability and rate modulation, and antitachydysrhythmia functions. The fourth and fifth categories are infrequently stated in practice, except for R, which indicates a rate-adaptive pulse generator driven by a sensor. The basic three-letter code nomenclature is used in this text.

PACEMAKER FUNCTION

Because there are so many types of pacemakers, general function of pacemakers is discussed first. A simple demand pacing system (VVI or AAI) functions in the following manner. The cardiac cycle normally begins with the client's own beat. The pacemaker has a sensor that senses if the intrinsic beat has occurred; if not, the pacer sends out an impulse to begin myocardial depolarization through a pulse generator. The impulse generator is said to capture the myocardium and thereby maintain heart rhythm.

For a predetermined amount of time after the pacemaker impulse, the pacemaker is incapable of sensing incoming signals. This process prevents the pacer from sensing its own generated electrical current and acting again. The refractory period is followed by the noise sampling period. If any electromagnetic interference is sensed during this phase, the pacemaker goes into a fixed-rate mode of operation and remains in this mode until the source of interference is removed. At the end of the noise-sampling period, the alert period begins, and the cycle starts over again. If a PCV or PAC occurs during the alert period, the pacemaker will sense it and start its cycle over again without emitting any impulse.

PACING MODES

Asynchronous (Fixed Rate) Pacing (AOO, VOO, DOO)

This pacing mode delivers an electrical impulse to the heart at a preset fixed rate regardless of intrinsic cardiac pacemaker action. Because there is no sensing mechanism, the pacing mechanism virtually ignores the client's own intrinsic heart rhythm. This single mode style is the earliest form of pacemaker first used in 1958. Although infrequently used today, this mode of pacing is appropriate for clients with a natural heart rate below 60 beats per minute and without a tendency to develop dysrhythmias. Its circuitry is simpler than others, which reduces the chance of pacemaker failure. The major disadvantages of fixed rate pacing use are

- Potential tachycardia when both the pacemaker and SA node fire.
- Atrial and ventricular synchrony does not occur.
- There is increased risk that a ventricular pacemaker stimulus may occur during the vulnerable period (the peak and early downslope of the T wave), producing ventricular tachycardia or ventricular fibrillation.
- The mechanism does not allow the heart to vary its rate so that it can accommodate variation in the client's activity levels.

Noncompetitive (Demand) Pacing (VVI, VVT, AAI, AAT)

With demand pacing, the pacemaker fires only on demand or when needed to stimulate atrial or ventricular contraction. Demand pacemakers are advantageous in clients with AV block, SA arrest, severe sinus bradycardia, or dysrhythmias requiring electrical overdrive. These clients have their own beats; the pacemaker senses for beats. If intrinsic beats are sensed, the pacemaker is inhibited. If a spontaneous P wave or QRS complex does not occur, the pacemaker discharges at a preset delay interval. Noncompetitive pacing can adjust to the heart's underlying rhythm.

To set up demand pacing, the physician must first preset a heart rate into the unit that is suitable for the client. For example, the clinician may program a preset rate of 60 into the demand pacemaker unit. When the client's heart rate falls below 60 beats per minute, artificial pacing ensues. If the natural heart rate increases to greater than 60 beats per minute, the unit will not fire a stimulus (Fig. 42-18).

Typically, the pacemaker is programmed only to sense ventricular activity and to elicit a ventricular depolarization. If AV node conduction remains intact, then the physician may use atrial demand pacing. In this case, absence of P waves will elicit a pacemaker stimulus to the atrium.

ATRIAL DEMAND PACING

The atrium is paced and the ventricle is allowed to depolarize following the usual pathways (AV node, Purkinje fibers). Atrial demand pacing is used for clients with symptomatic sinus bradycardia (Fig. 42-19).

VENTRICULAR DEMAND PACING

The ventricle is paced in clients with AV block. The pacemaker senses for ventricular depolarization. When it does not occur at a preset rate, the pacer fires. A

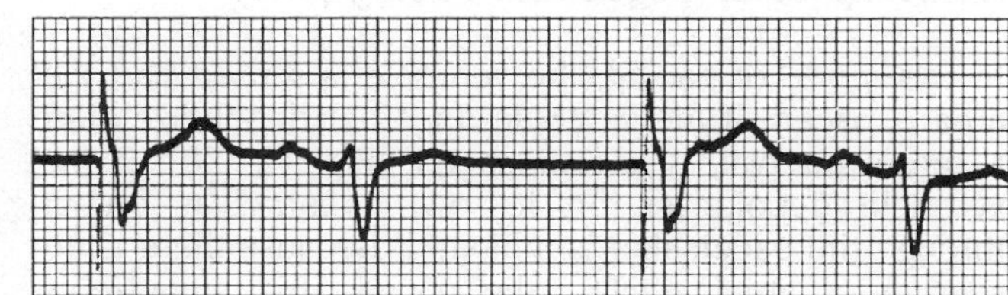

▲ **Figure 42-18**

Demand pacing. Pacemaker initiates electrical impulse when sinus fails to pace. (From Phillips, R. E., & Feeney, M. K. [1989]. *The cardiac rhythms* [3rd ed, p. 457]. Philadelphia, W. B. Saunders.)

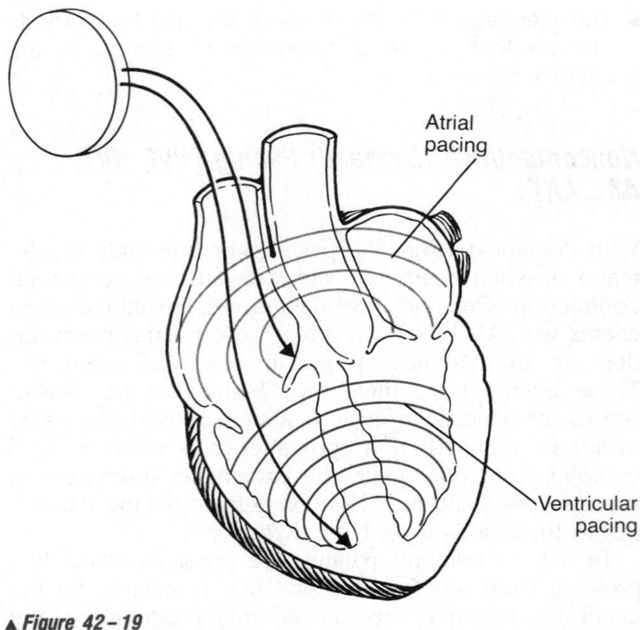

▲ *Figure 42-19*

Atrioventricular (AV) pacing. Atrial pacing is done first, followed directly by ventricular pacing.

disadvantage of this mode is that atrial and ventricular contractions are not synchronous. This loss of "atrial kick" filling the ventricles may lead to hypotension, chest pain, and CHF (called pacemaker syndrome) (Fig. 42-19).

Synchronous Pacing (VAT, VDD)

Synchronous pacing operates in a manner similar to that of the demand mode. In synchronous pacing, the sensing electrode is placed in the atrium and the pacing electrode is placed in the ventricle. Thus, the pacemaker unit senses atrial activity and elicits a stimulus to prompt a ventricular depolarization. A major benefit is that it permits the heart rate to vary, and atrial-ventricular synchrony occurs, depending on the physiologic demands of the body. A built-in safety mechanism causes ventricular depolarizations to occur at a fixed rate should atrial rates become too fast.

Atrioventricular Sequential Pacing (DVI)

In this mode of pacing, the ventricle is sensed and the atria is paced. If the ventricle does not depolarize after a preset interval, it is also paced (Fig. 42-20). If the ventricle depolarizes on its own, ventricular output through the pacemaker is inhibited. Because there is no sensing of atrial activity, the paced atrial impulse is preset at a specific interval to follow a sensed or paced QRS complex. The atria is paced regardless of its own intrinsic activity; therefore, competition may occur, leading to atrial fibrillation.

Universal Atrioventricular Pacing (DDD)

Universal or physiologic pacemakers are the most sophisticated pacemakers currently available. They consist of both atrial and ventricular circuits that sense and pace their respective chambers. If spontaneous atrial activity does not occur, the atrium is paced. Any sensed atrial activity inhibits the pacing function. If ventricular depolarization does not occur in the preset time limit, the ventricle is paced. This type of pacing is used in the management of clients with atrial bradydysrhythmias with or without abnormal AV node conduction and in normal sinus node function with AV block. The advantage of this mode of pacemaker is that it more closely mimics the normal heart. Atrial kick occurs, which increases cardiac output by 30 per cent, and the heart rate can be changed to meet metabolic demands. The major risk of this mode of pacing is the development of pacemaker-induced tachycardia. If a skeletal muscle activity is sensed, a ventricular beat may be triggered.

METHODS OF PACING

Temporary Pacing

Temporary pacing may be used in emergent or elective situations that require limited, short-term pacing (under 2 weeks). In this form of pacing, the pulse generator is external. Temporary pacemakers can be inserted by transthoracic and, most commonly, transvenous, transesophageal, and transcutaneous routes (Fig. 42-21).

Nursing Management

Before the procedure, the nurse explains the purpose of the temporary pacemaker to the client and family. The nurse ascertains that a permit for the procedure has been signed and that all questions have been answered. Necessary equipment is gathered, and the functioning of the external generator is checked (battery and sense and pace modes). The client's vital signs are assessed, and a rhythm strip is obtained.

During the procedure, the nurse reassures the client while monitoring the ECG and vital signs continuously. When the pacing catheter is in the vein, alligator clips can be used to connect the exposed tip of the catheter to an ECG machine for monitoring the progression of the catheter through the heart. Large P waves are seen as the catheter passes through the atrium, and larger QRS complexes are seen in the ventricles. The stimulus and sensitivity settings are set and maintained according to the physician's orders. The electrode is taped or sutured at the insertion site.

After the procedure, the vital signs are assessed routinely along with heart rhythm and emotional reactions to the procedure and pacing. All connections are secured and routinely checked. Battery and control settings are also monitored. The incision site is cleaned and dressed according to protocols. The nurse keeps

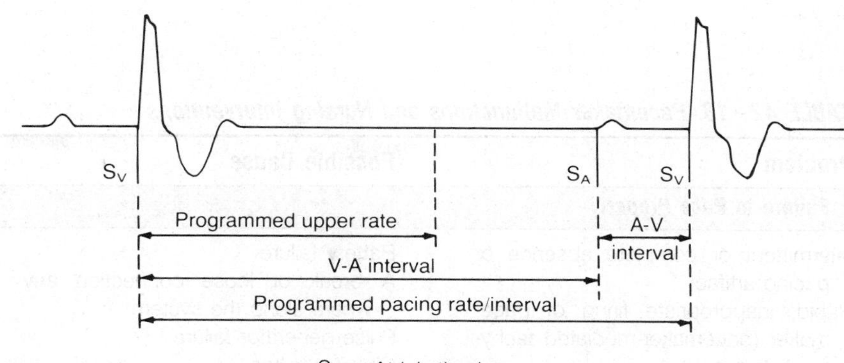

▲ **Figure 42–20**

Physiologic timing cycles. The A-V (delay) interval can be thought of as an artificial PR interval. The programmed pacing rate/interval is also called the V-V interval. Ventricular pacing will occur if intrinsic ventricular activity does not occur within the V-V interval. (From *Symbiotics series: selecting the DDD patient* [1984]. Minneapolis: Medtronics.)

the generator dry and the controls protected from mishandling. The client must be protected from electromicroshocks and electromagnetic interference. There are several interventions that protect the client. Exposed wires are covered with rubber gloves or electrical tape. The pulse generator is enclosed in a rubber glove to keep it dry. Rubber gloves are worn when exposed wires are handled. Electrical equipment is checked for adequate grounding.

In addition to protecting the client from injury, the nurse monitors the pacemaker function. The location and type of pacing lead is documented. The pacing mode, stimulus threshold, sensitivity setting, pacing rate and intervals, and intrinsic rhythm are noted. Pacing intervals are shown in Figure 42–20.

Pacemaker complications can occur from insertion. They include phlebitis at the site, pneumothorax, atelectasis, pericardial fluid accumulation, diaphragmatic stimulation (seen as hiccupping or twitching at the pacemaker site), and dysrhythmias. Complications can also occur from malfunctioning of the pacemaker (Table 42–13).

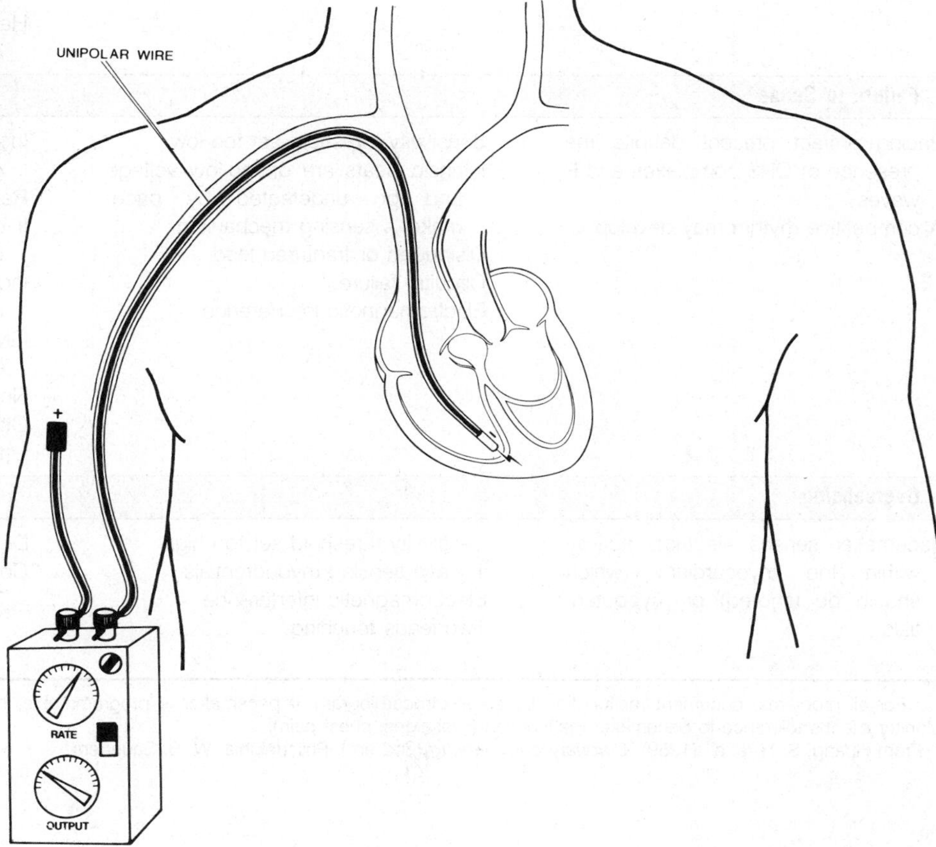

▲ **Figure 42–21**

Endocardial electronic pacemaker with temporary external power pack. (From Phillips, R. E., & Feeney, M. K. [1989]. *The cardiac rhythms* [3rd ed.]. Philadelphia: W. B. Saunders.)

TABLE 42–13. Pacemaker Malfunctions and Nursing Interventions

Problem	Possible Cause	Nursing Interventions*
Failure to Pace Properly		
Intermittent or complete absence of pacing artifact Rapid, inappropriate firing of pacemaker (pacemaker-mediated tachycardia)	Battery failure A break or loose connection anywhere along the system Pulse generator failure Circuitry failure "Oversensing" or "undersensing" by the pacemaker	Replace pulse generator Replace battery unit Check and tighten all connections between pulse generator and leads Reduce or increase sensitivity threshold of pacemaker unit Assess client's tolerance of pacemaker failure; have emergency drugs on hand; perform CPR as indicated
Failure to Capture		
Pacing artifact present but is not followed by a QRS complex or P wave	Decreased conductivity by the myocardial tissue due to electrolyte imbalance, infarction, drug toxicity, perforation, or excessive fibrosis of tissue at electrode site Lead displacement due to migration, or idle manipulation of pulse generator ("twiddler's syndrome")	Increase voltage by 1–2 mA (temporary pacemaker) Increase amplitude of pacemaker output (and/or pulse width) Reposition client to either side in attempt to improve contact of electrode with endocardium; in temporary pacemaker, try moving arm if lead wire is inserted in antecubital area Obtain chest film to determine pacemaker position Have emergency drugs on hand; initiate CPR if necessary
Failure to Sense		
Pacing artifact present despite the presence of QRS complexes and P waves A competitive rhythm may develop	Sensitivity threshold set too low Intrinsic beats are of too-low voltage and go undetected by pacemaker's sensing mechanism Dislodged or fractured lead Circuitry failure Electromagnetic interference	Increase sensitivity threshold on pulse generator Reposition client If client's intrinsic rhythm/rate is adequate, turn off pacemaker Increase pacing rate to overdrive client's intrinsic heart rate Give antidysrrhythmics to decrease ectopy Notify physician Obtain chest film to determine electrode placement
Oversensing		
Pacemaker senses electrical activity within the myocardium (which should be ignored) or myopotentials	Sensitivity threshold set too high T wave sensing myopotentials Electromagnetic interference Two leads touching	Decrease sensitivity threshold Correct conditions that produce large T waves

* For all problems, document malfunction by an electrocardiogram. If pacemaker is programmable, have reprogramming machine available. Monitor client's tolerance to pacemaker malfunction (vital signs, chest pain).

From Huang, S. H, et al. (1989). *Coronary care nursing* (2nd ed.). Philadelphia: W. B. Saunders.

Transvenous (Endocardial) Pacing

Transvenous pacing provides the most common means for pacing the heart in emergency situations. The surgeon (1) inserts the pacing electrode via the transvenous route (via the antecubital, femoral, jugular, or subclavian veins) and (2) threads the electrode into the right atrium or right ventricle so that it comes into direct contact with the endocardium. This procedure can be done at the bedside under fluoroscopic control or in a cardiovascular laboratory. Major drawbacks include thrombophlebitis, infection at the insertion site, sepsis from unsterile technique, increased chance of lead displacement as the client changes position, and the discomfort of having the extremity nearest the insertion site immobilized (Fig. 42-22).

Permanent Pacing

Permanent pacing is indicated in long-term management of symptomatic or life-threatening dysrhythmias. The surgeon inserts the pacing electrode either via the transvenous route or by direct application to the epicardial surface during thoracotomy. The surgeon places the permanent pulse generator into a small tunnel burrowed within the subcutaneous tissue below the right clavicle or, less often, the left clavicle. The pulse generator is a small, hermetically sealed (to prevent ingress of body fluids) lithium battery.

THE USE OF PERMANENT PACEMAKERS

The client and family are taught about the purpose for the pacemaker and the experience of having a pacemaker inserted. Most permanent pacemakers are inserted transvenously. The nurse tries to keep the ECG leads off the possible insertion site. The insertion site is prepared according to hospital policy. A preoperative ECG is obtained, and a patent intravenous line is maintained. Prophylactic antibiotics may be given.

After the insertion, the nurse monitors vital signs and pacemaker function. Pain can usually be managed with oral analgesics if the transvenous approach was used. Initially the client is taught to avoid excessive extension or abduction of the arm on the operative side. The nurse performs passive range-of-motion exercises on the arm.

Paced and nonpaced ECGs are obtained. A magnet may be placed over the pulse generator, converting it to a fixed rate pacing mode, so that the client's intrinsic rhythm can be determined. The location of the pacemaker electrodes is determined by x-ray examination. The model and serial numbers of the pulse generator and leads are recorded along with the date of implantation and programmed functions of the initial implant.

The client and family are taught how to care for the pacemaker and precautions to follow (see Client Education Guide).

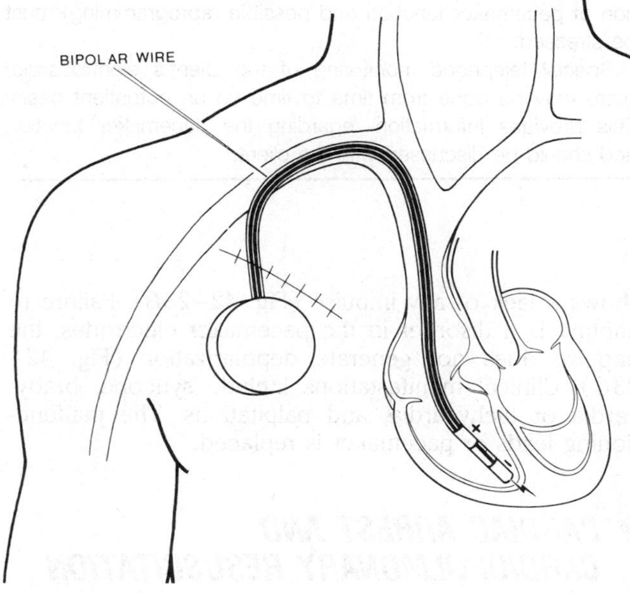

▲ *Figure 42-22*

Transvenous catheter placement, dual-chamber pacing. Separate electrodes in the atrium and ventricle allow synchronized contraction, and thus stroke volume is improved. (From Phillips, R. E., & Feeney, M. K. [1990]. *The cardiac rhythms. A systematic approach to interpretation.* [3rd ed.]. Philadelphia, W. B. Saunders.)

DEFIBRILLATING PACEMAKER CLIENTS

Because pacemakers are vulnerable to extraneous electromagnetic interference, newer models possess components to suppress input. These safety mechanisms may fail, however. Therefore, during defibrillation, certain precautions are taken:

- Use anteroposterior type paddles if available.
- When using anterior paddles, place them at least 4 to 5 inches away from the pulse generator and leads.
- Use the lowest defibrillator current possible or the ACLS standard of 200 to 300 joules for the first two shocks.
- If a temporary pacing system is in use, disconnect the pacing lead from the pulse generator immediately before defibrillation and reconnect it after the shock.
- A pacemaker programmer-analyzer should be readily available to examine the pacing system for damage and erroneous reprogramming after defibrillation.
- Monitor for pacemaker malfunction for at least the next 24 hours.[37]

ELECTROCARDIOGRAM OF PACED BEATS

The ECG of a paced rhythm appears different from that of a normal sinus rhythm. A pacing artifact is seen. With atrial pacing, a P wave follows the artifact but may be hidden in some leads. Leads II and V1 are best for deciding whether a P wave follows a pacer spike. The QRS complex appears normal with atrial pacing; the impulse travels through usual conduction systems.

The ECG with ventricular pacing shows an abnormal QRS complex, because the impulse begins in the ven-

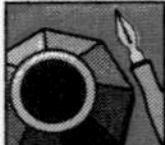

CLIENT EDUCATION GUIDE

The Client with a Permanent Pacemaker

Wound Care

Assess wound daily; report any signs of inflammation (redness, tenderness, discharge) to the physician. Avoid constrictive clothing (e.g., tight bra straps), which puts excessive pressure on the wound and the pulse generator.

Avoid extensive "toying" with the pulse generator, because this could cause pacemaker malfunction.

Pacemaker Management

Take pulse daily, either radial or carotid (this should be demonstrated by the nurse); notify physician if pulse is slower than the set rate; also report excessive palpitations, vertigo, or syncope.

Avoid being near areas with high voltage, magnetic force fields, or radiation; this can cause pacemaker malfunction. Things to avoid include large running motors (gas or electric), standing near high-tension wires, power plants, radio transmitters, large industrial magnets, and arc welding machines (riding in a car is safe, but avoid bringing pacemaker 6 to 12 inches from distributor coil of running engine).

Although pacemakers are less likely to be affected by the newer models of microwave ovens, the client with a pacemaker should maintain a safe distance from them (at least 5 feet). Contact with such equipment can cause a sudden return of prepacemaker symptoms.

Carry a pacemaker identity card (along with programming information—the pacemaker manufacturer and emergency phone numbers) at all times; a special ALERT bracelet is also recommended.

The airport's metal detector may be triggered by the pacemaker's metal casing and the programming magnet. This should be mentioned to the security guards. (The metal detector itself will not harm the pacemaker.) While traveling on planes, avoid sitting near the galley, because the flight meals are typically heated in a microwave oven.

Avoid engaging in activity that can produce blunt trauma over the pulse generator; such activities would include playing football or firing a rifle with the butt end against the affected shoulder.

Some stores have antitheft devices that may affect pacemaker function. If symptoms suddenly arise, move away from the area and notify the store clerk about the pacemaker.

If radiation therapy has been prescribed to the area in which the pulse generator was implanted, a relocation of the pulse generator will be necessary.

Activity Levels

Avoid vigorous movement of the arms and shoulders and lifting weights greater than 5 to 10 pounds for the first 6 weeks after surgery; this could increase risk of electrode dislodgement. Normal activities can be resumed in 6 weeks, including sexual activity.

Medications

The purpose, dose, schedule, and possible side effects of prescribed medications should be thoroughly discussed; written information sheets can reinforce learning.

Follow-up Care

The importance of regular physician or clinic visits (for evaluation of pacemaker function and possible reprogramming) must be stressed.

Special telephone monitoring of the client's electrocardiogram may be done from time to time on an outpatient basis. This provides information regarding the pacemaker function and should be discussed with the client.

---

tricle. With right ventricular endocardial pacing, a pseudo-LBBB ECG wave is created. If the left ventricle is paced, a pseudo-RBBB is created.

The nurse assesses the ECG strip for pacer spikes followed by the expected appearance of a P wave or QRS complex. Spikes not followed by depolarization waves or paced beats that appear too early or too late may signal pacemaker failure.

PACEMAKER FAILURE

Pacemakers can develop malfunctions in the sensor or pulse generator. Failure to sense is the inability of the sensor to detect intrinsic beats, and the pacemaker sends out impulses too early (Fig. 42–23*A*). Failure to pace is a malfunction of the pulse generator. The ECG shows a lack of any impulse (Fig. 42–23*B*). Failure to capture is a disorder in the pacemaker electrodes; the impulse does not generate depolarization (Fig. 42–23*C*). Clinical manifestations include syncope, bradycardia or tachycardia, and palpitations. The malfunctioning leads or pacemaker is replaced.

▼ CARDIAC ARREST AND CARDIOPULMONARY RESUSCITATION

CPR techniques are used to restore circulation and ventilation artificially during cardiopulmonary arrest. In cardiopulmonary arrest, the client's heart, circulation, and respiration suddenly cease. Box 42–4 lists principal causes.

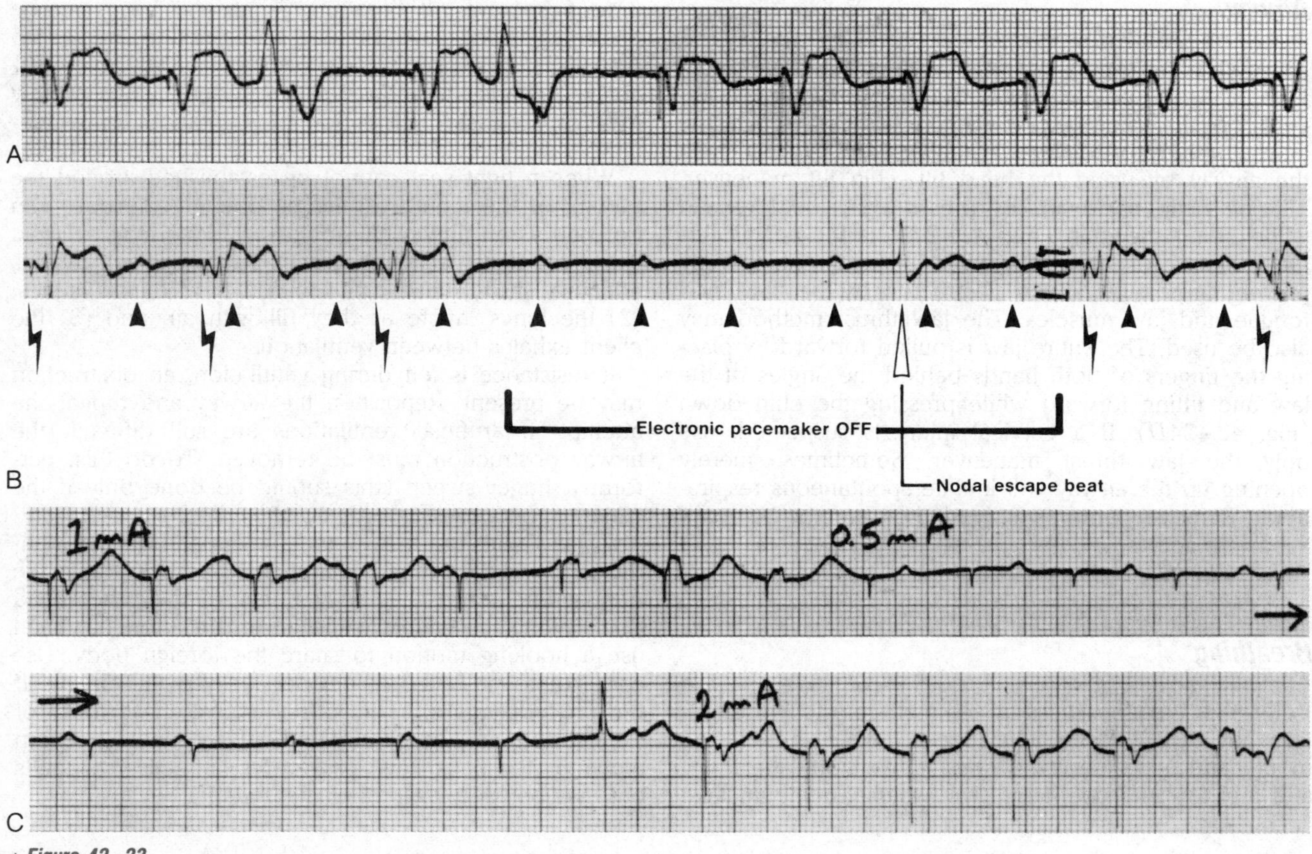

▲ *Figure 42-23*

Pacemaker failures. *A*, Failure to sense. *B*, Failure to pace. *C*, Failure to capture. (From Phillips, R. E., & Feeney, M. K. [1989]. *The cardiac rhythms* [3rd ed.]. Philadelphia: W.B. Saunders.)

Box 42-4. Various Causes of Cardiopulmonary Arrest

Cardiac arrest can result from
- Ventricular fibrillation
- Ventricular tachycardia
- Asystole
- Electromechanical dissociation

Respiratory arrest can result from
- Coma
- Electrocution
- Airway obstruction
- Injuries (auto accidents, lightning)
- Drowning
- Smoke inhalation
- Suffocation
- Myocardial infarction
- Drug overdose
- Stroke
- Epiglottitis

From Standards and guidelines for cardiopulmonary resuscitation (CPR) and emergency cardiac care (ECC) (1992). *Journal of the American Medical Association, 268*(16), 2185. Copyright 1992, American Medical Association.

Clinical manifestations of cardiopulmonary arrest are as follows:

- abrupt and complete unconsciousness (no response to tap or gentle shaking while asking, "Are you OK?")
- apnea or gasping (agonal) respirations
- absence of heart beat (no carotid, femoral, or radial pulsations) and blood pressure
- development of pallor or cyanosis
- dilation of the pupils (may occur after several minutes of pulselessness)
- ECG reveals asystole or ventricular fibrillation

GENERAL PROCEDURE FOR CPR

Of highest priority are the ABCs — *a*irway, *b*reathing, and *c*irculation — of basic resuscitation. Each should begin with an assessment phase. The assessment phases and ABCs occur in the following sequence: (1) determine unresponsiveness, (2) open airway, (3) determine breathlessness, (4) perform rescue breathing, (5) determine pulselessness, and (6) provide circulation.

Airway

As soon as unresponsiveness has been determined, deliver air to the lungs. Exhaled air adds oxygen (16 per cent) to the client's blood as it passes through the lungs, thereby providing oxygen for the tissues. Open the airway by using the head tilt-chin lift maneuver. Tilt the head backward by pressing on the forehead while lifting the chin (Fig. 42-24*B* and *C*). This lifts the tongue away from the back of the throat, thereby preventing possible airway obstruction by the slackened tongue and jaw muscles. The jaw thrust method may also be used. The entire jaw is pulled forward by placing the fingers of both hands behind the angles of the jaw and lifting forward while pressing the chin down (Fig. 42-24*D*). If a cervical injury is suspected, use only the jaw thrust maneuver. Sometimes, merely opening up the airway will initiate spontaneous respirations. Remove dentures only if they cannot be managed in place.

Breathing

Determine breathlessness by remembering to "look, listen, and feel." Place your cheek above the client's mouth and nose. Look for chest movement, and listen and feel for air movement. This evaluation should take 3 to 5 seconds. If breathing is absent, begin rescue breathing. Use an Ambu bag and provide breaths to make the chest rise (usually a volume of 800 ml) for 1 to $1\frac{1}{2}$ seconds' duration. Delivering ventilations rapidly may cause gastric distention, regurgitation, or aspiration.

When a tight seal cannot be established around the mouth, or the mouth cannot be opened, the nose can be used as an airway. A stoma technique may be used if the client has a tracheostomy. Artificial ventilation is adequate if (1) the chest is seen to rise 1 to 2 inches, (2) the lungs inflate as they fill with air, and (3) the client exhales between ventilations.

If resistance is felt during ventilation, an obstruction may be present. Reposition the airway and repeat the attempt. If artificial ventilations are still difficult, the airway obstruction must be removed. To do this, perform a finger sweep (this should be done only if the client is unconscious). Grasp the client's tongue and lower jaw with the thumb and fingers and lift the mandible. This action may be enough to partially clear the obstruction. Insert the index finger of the other hand down along the cheek to the base of the tongue. Then use a hooking motion to snare the foreign body. Use care not to push the object deeper into the airway. If this procedure fails, perform the manual chest thrust, or the abdominal thrust (Heimlich maneuver). Sharp blows to the back have proved less effective in adults but may be used if all other methods fail.

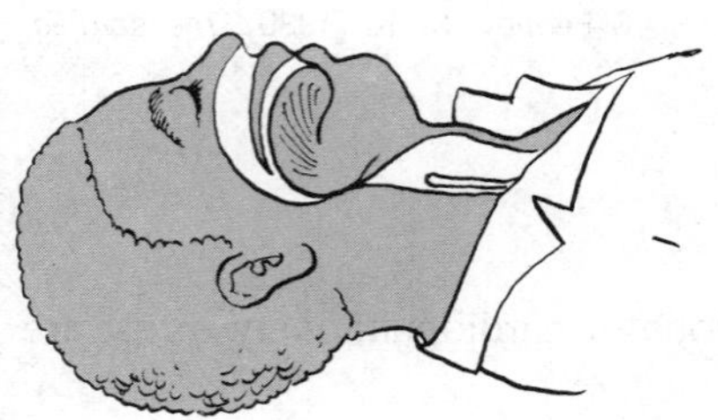

A. Airway obstructed by tongue

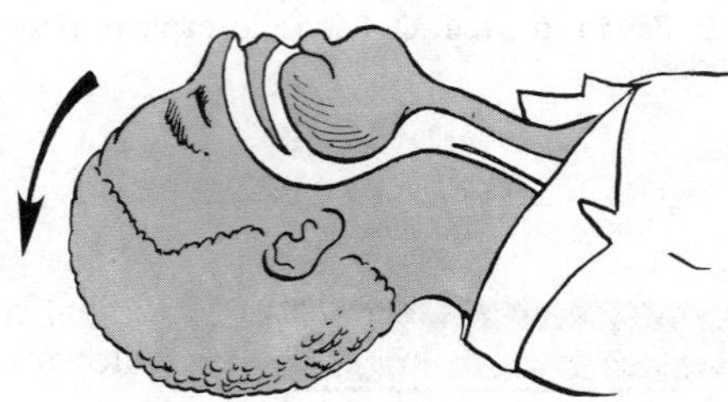

B. Obstruction relieved by head tilt

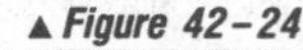

▲ Figure 42-24

Opening the airway. The most common cause of airway obstruction during resuscitation is the tongue *(A)*. Open the airway by tilting the head *(B)*, and using the head tilt-chin lift *(C)*, or the jaw thrust maneuver *(D)*.

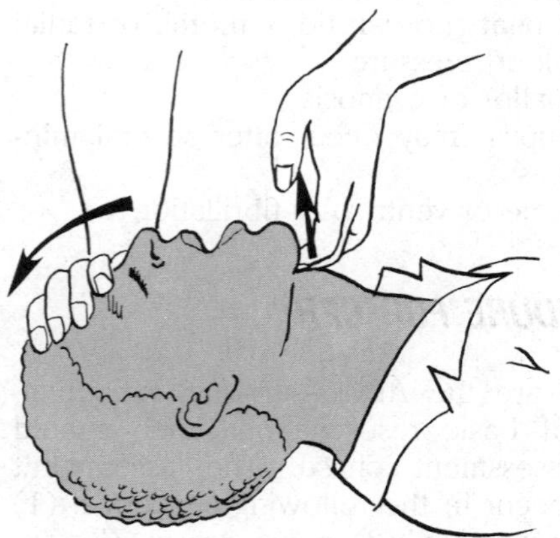

C. Head tilt-chin lift maneuver

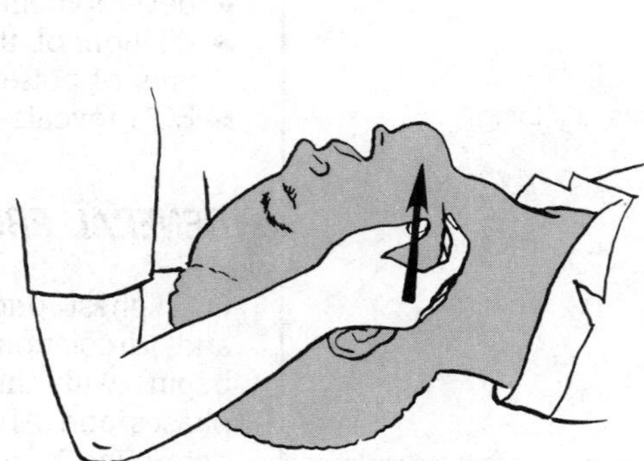

D. Jaw thrust maneuver

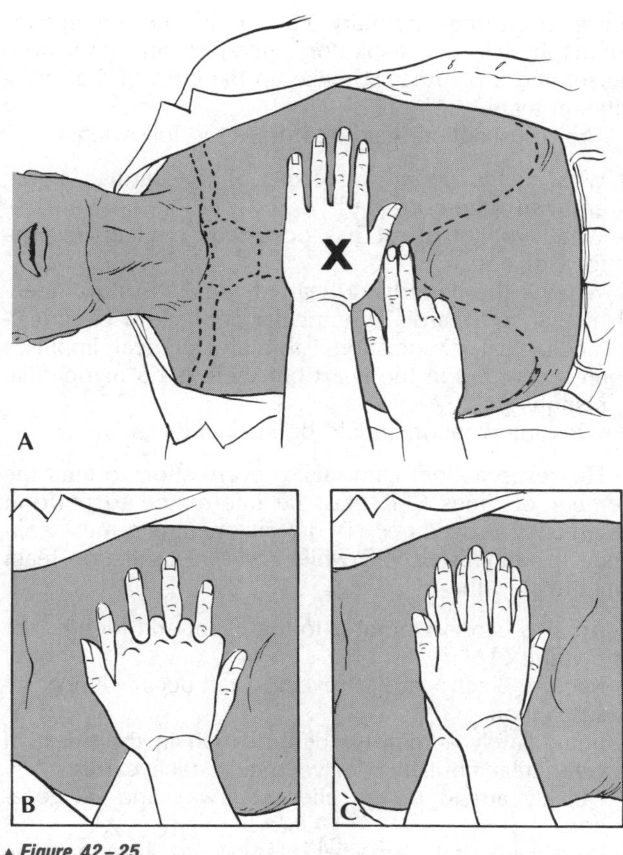

▲ **Figure 42-25**

Hand placement for chest compressions. *A*, Slide fingers (of the hand closest to the client's feet) along the costal margin to the xiphoid process. With the middle finger on the xyphoid process, place the first finger next to it and the heel of the opposite hand along the first finger as shown. The heel of the hand should rest firmly on the sternum. The other hand is placed on top, and the fingers may be interlaced *(B)*, or extended *(C)*, during compressions.

Circulation

Determine pulselessness by measuring the carotid pulse for a full 5 to 10 seconds. If the pulse is absent or questionable, shout for help. Direct the individual who responds to activate the emergency medical system by phoning the appropriate number and providing necessary information about the emergency. Immediately begin external cardiac compressions. Place the client's body, at least from hips to shoulders, on a hard, horizontal surface to establish optimal cardiac compressions. In health care facilities, a cardiac board is often placed beneath the client on a bed.

As soon as the client is positioned, expose the chest. Note sternal landmarks by marking off two fingerbreadths above the xyphoid process. Place the heel of the hand nearest the client's head alongside the index finger on the lower half of the sternum. The long access of the heel of your hand should be placed along the long access of the sternum (Fig. 42-25). Then, place the other hand on top of the first hand and interlace or extend the fingers, being careful to keep the fingers off the chest wall. This position prevents rib fracture.

Perform cardiac compressions by maintaining the elbows in a straight, locked position, with the shoulders directly over the client's sternum so that the thrust for compressions is straight down on the sternum (Fig. 42-26). This method uses body weight rather than arm muscles and facilitates smooth, easy compressions. Avoid sharp, jerking motions, which are less effective. Allow the chest to return to its normal position after each compression. The time for release should equal the time of compression. For preventing position migration, the hands should not be removed between compressions. Lightly maintain hand position on the lower half of the sternum. Compress the sternum 3.8 to 5 cm (1.5 to 2 inches) at a ratio of two breaths to 15 cardiac compressions (one rescuer) or one breath to five cardiac compressions (two rescuers). In two-

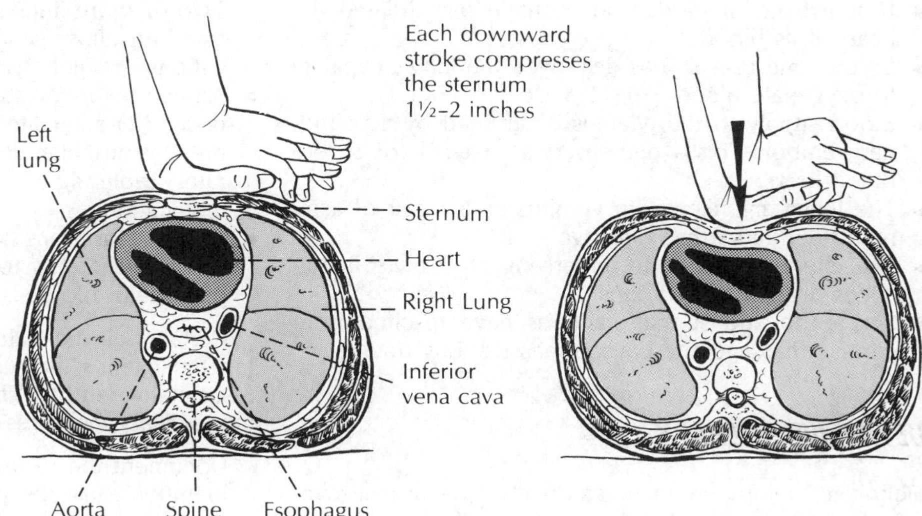

▲ **Figure 42-26**

Cross section of the thorax during chest compression. Note that compressions are straight down through the heels of the hands.

rescuer resuscitation, pause briefly (1 to 1.5 seconds) to allow ventilations to occur.

Optimal external chest compressions can produce systolic pressure peaks of more than 100 mm Hg. For maximal effect, it is recommended that external chest compression be delivered at a rate of 80 to 100 per minute. Using a cadence such as "one and two and three and four and one and . . ." will help maintain this rate.

Assess for a return of the carotid pulse (for 5 seconds) after four cycles of compressions and ventilations. Resume CPR within 7 seconds if the carotid pulse is absent, and reassess the pulse every few minutes. If the carotid pulse is present, check for spontaneous breathing (for 3 to 5 seconds). If the client is breathing, stop CPR but continue to monitor the client closely until professional help arrives. If breathing is absent, continue to monitor the pulse as rescue breathing is performed (12 times per minute).

Carry out CPR until one of the following occurs: (1) the client regains a satisfactory intrinsic pulse, (2) the client is pronounced dead, or (3) the rescuer is exhausted and unable to continue, and no one else is available to perform CPR.

A precordial thump, a direct blow with a closed fist over the precordium, is no longer recommended during resuscitation. Precordial thump was thought to create enough electrical energy to "shock" the heart into a more satisfactory heart rhythm. However, it is effective only in a well-oxygenated heart and thus is rarely used today.

When a cardiac arrest is recognized within 10 to 15 seconds after onset, cough CPR can prolong consciousness if the client is able to cough forcefully. Vigorous coughing raises intrathoracic pressure, providing blood flow to the brain, and can be seen as "self-induced CPR."

Despite heroic resuscitation efforts, CPR does not always revive the client. Factors responsible for ineffective resuscitation include the following:

- Incorrect resuscitation techniques have been used.
- Too much time has elapsed before initiation of CPR.
- Hemorrhage or cardiac tamponade has drained the heart of its blood.
- Severe lung disease has destroyed the lung's capacity to oxygenate blood.
- Blood supply to the heart is obstructed by a pulmonary embolus or is decreased as a result of severe blood loss.
- The lungs are filled with vomitus as a result of aspiration during cardiac massage.
- The client has extreme underlying electrolyte imbalances or circulating toxins.
- Severe rib and sternal fractures have resulted from cardiac massage and caused massive lung trauma.

DEFINITIVE THERAPY

Definitive therapy commences once a special resuscitation team has arrived to take over CPR. Typically, a nurse from the coronary care unit, the emergency room physician, a respiratory therapist, an intravenous nurse, and a pharmacist make up the core of the resuscitation team.

The resuscitation team addresses the following:

- What is the underlying cause of the cardiac arrest, and can it be corrected?
- What type of arrest has occurred (cardiac, respiratory, or both)?
- What is the underlying heart rhythm? Asystole? Ventricular tachycardia? Ventricular fibrillation? Electrical-mechanical dissociation (normal electrical impulses are occurring in the heart but there is no myocardial response)?
- What intervention should be instituted?

The resuscitation team makes every effort to limit the number of times CPR must be interrupted to perform emergency procedures. Two team members must continue to administer CPR while some resuscitation team members do the following:

- Apply a cardiac monitor to the client and identify the rhythm.
- Record electrocardiac events that occur during resuscitation.
- Immediately administer defibrillation in the event of ventricular fibrillation or ventricular tachycardia.
- Quickly attend to the client's airway and oxygenation.
- Insert an oral (artificial) airway to maintain the tongue in a forward position.
- Administer 100 per cent oxygen.
- Insert an endotracheal tube as soon as possible to achieve maximal airway clearance and oxygenation.
- Suction the client as necessary to maintain a patent airway. Suction can also facilitate gastric decompression if the stomach fills with air during artificial ventilation. A distended abdomen may compromise respirations.
- Start an intravenous line for administration of resuscitation medications. Large-bore catheters are preferable, because they allow more rapid infusion rates. Two or more lines help ensure access to the circulation and allow simultaneous administration of medications or solutions that are incompatible.
- Administer medications to (1) correct metabolic acidosis, (2) stimulate myocardial contraction, (3) suppress ventricular ectopy, and (4) accelerate cardiac rate. Table 42-14 lists the more commonly used medications.
- Prepare for transthoracic or transvenous pacing in the event of asystole, severe bradycardia, or complete heart block.

Certain activities, although not directly related to saving the client's life, can improve the efficiency of the resuscitative efforts. The team must perform the following ancillary measures as soon as possible:

- Document the resuscitation. The nurse or other team member must keep an accurate, ongoing record, documenting all procedures and medications given

TABLE 42-14. Resuscitation Medications

Medication	Indications
Oxygen	Hypoxemia
IV fluids	Expansion of circulating blood volume
Morphine sulfate	Pain of acute myocardial infarction
Lidocaine	Ventricular ectopy, including ventricular tachycardia and fibrillation
Procainamide hydrochloride	Ventricular ectopy and ventricular tachycardia when lidocaine is contraindicated or has failed to suppress ventricular ectopy
Bretylium tosylate	Resistant ventricular tachycardia and ventricular fibrillation
Beta-adrenergic receptor blocking medications	Reduce rate of nonfatal infarction and recurrent ischemia after thrombolytic therapy
Atropine sulfate	Symptomatic sinus bradycardia
Isoproterenol hydrochloride	Bradycardia that is refractory to atropine and torsades de pointes
Verapamil/diltiazem	Reentrant dysrhythmias that use atrioventricular nodal conduction
Adenosine	Reentrant dysrhythmias
Magnesium	Dysrhythmias due to hypomagnesemia
Epinephrine hydrochloride	Increases myocardial and cerebral blood flow
Norepinephrine	Severe hypotension and low peripheral resistance
Dopamine hydrochloride	Severe hypotension with bradycardia
Dobutamine hydrochloride	Heart failure
Amrinone	Heart failure
Calcium	Hyperkalemia, hypocalcemia, or calcium channel block toxicity
Digitalis preparations	Atrial flutter, atrial fibrillation, or paroxysmal supraventricular tachycardias
Nitroglycerin	Heart failure or unstable angina
Sodium nitroprusside	Heart failure and hypertension
Sodium bicarbonate	Severe acid-base imbalance
Diuretics	Cerebral edema or acute pulmonary edema
Thrombolytic agents	Coronary artery occlusion

Data from Guidelines for cardiopulmonary resuscitation (CPR) and emergency cardiac care (ECC) (1992). *Journal of the American Medical Association, 268*(16), 2205-2211. Copyright 1992, American Medical Association.

during the resuscitative effort. Use of a flowsheet format that includes the times of each intervention provides an immediate reference for the number of medications given and the length of time elapsed between procedures (e.g., defibrillation). This document should be kept as a permanent record of the event.

- Provide information. The client's record (if there is one) and the primary care giver, who either knows the client or has witnessed the precipitating event, should remain close by to provide information to the resuscitation team.
- Reduce environmental overcrowding. Remove excess furniture from the area. If appropriate, ask people to leave the room, because excess personnel can also interfere with emergency activities.
- Reassure individuals nearby. People within hearing or viewing distance of the resuscitation effort are often distressed by what they observe. Pull curtains and have available health care providers sit with anxious individuals until activities calm down. People in the immediate vicinity are usually aware of the gravity of the situation and will appreciate an honest, reassuring manner.
- Notify family members. Family members should be notified of the critical nature of events if they are not present at the time of the emergency. Arrange to have a nurse meet them when they arrive and inform them of changes in the client's condition. The client's spiritual adviser may also be notified to render additional support.

FOLLOW-UP INTERVENTION

Diagnostic tests are often made during and after resuscitation to determine precipitating causes, evaluate the effectiveness of resuscitation, and detect complications. Tests commonly performed are (1) chest radiograph, (2) ECG, (3) hemodynamic monitoring, and (4) laboratory studies (including arterial blood gases, electrolytes, blood urea nitrogen, creatinine, blood glucose, and cardiac enzymes). Table 42-15 summarizes postresuscitation complications.

Clients who survive cardiopulmonary arrest are admitted to a critical care unit, where they receive continuous cardiac monitoring and have vital signs taken every 15 minutes until stable. Postresuscitation assessment provides important information regarding the effectiveness of the resuscitation. Common disorders include recurrent dysrhythmias, coma, other neurologic disorders, and renal failure.

After the client regains consciousness, profound anxiety often appears. Remember that clients need psychological support when they have undergone such a catastrophic physiologic event. Many clients have a very clear recall of the events surrounding the resuscitation, including the verbal communication that occurred. For this reason, members of the resuscitation team should be careful about what they say.

Take time to assess the client's coping mechanisms. Dismay at perceived betrayal by the body and fear of

TABLE 42-15. Postresuscitation Complications

Complications	Etiology	Clinical Manifestations
Trauma		
Fractured ribs and sternum	Improper chest compressions (increased risk in elderly and those with chronic lung disease)	Chest pain that increases with inspiration; asymmetric chest wall movement; crepitus noted over fracture site; "floating" sternum
Pneumothorax	Improper chest compressions; improper central venous line insertion	Chest pain; dyspnea, hypoxemia, cyanosis, decreased or absent breath sounds over affected area, tracheal deviation (tension pneumothorax); noted on chest film
Ruptured spleen	Improper chest compressions	Upper left quadrant pain, hypotension, failing hematocrit
Aspiration pneumonia	Vomiting of the client who is in a semiconscious state	Respiratory distress, hypoxemia, tracheal suctioning of gastric contents; noted on chest film
Anoxic encephalopathy	Prolonged cerebral hypoperfusion during time of unattended arrest or from poorly managed resuscitation	Prolonged coma; confusion; short-term memory lapses; behavioral changes
Renal failure	Prolonged hypoperfusion of kidneys causing acute tubular necrosis	Within 24 hours after resuscitation, urine output will fall below 30 ml/hr; elevated BUN (>20 ml/100 ml) and creatinine (>1.5 mg/100 ml)
Congestive heart failure	Overly vigorous use of sodium bicarbonate and intravenous fluids during resuscitation	Increased heart rate, increased respiratory rate; heart gallops; pulmonary crackles (rales), increased pulmonary artery wedge pressure; noted on chest film
Cardiac tamponade	Perforation of cardiac structures from intracardiac injections or transvenous/transthoracic pacemaker lead insertion	Dyspnea; distended neck veins; narrowing pulse pressure; decreased blood pressure, pulsus paradoxus >10 mm Hg
Skin burns	Repeated defibrillation or delivery of high voltages	Erythema and blistering of skin beneath site of defibrillator paddle placement
Oral, tracheal, and laryngeal damage	Improper or repeated endotracheal intubation causing breakage of teeth and soft tissue injury	Broken teeth, bloody mouth, respiratory distress, hoarseness, stridor
Cervical neck injury	Hyperextension of neck during attempts to open airway can result in cervical nerve trauma	Decreased sensory or motor movement below level of cervical injury

BUN, blood urea nitrogen.

sudden death can bring on overdependency, withdrawal, and anger. Encourage expression of such feelings and concerns, not only by the client but by significant others who are equally stressed by the sudden, serious nature of the disorder. Clear explanations and clarification of misconceptions about what has happened help move the client forward to optimal physiologic and psychological recovery.

Summary

Cardiovascular disorders are the nation's number one killer. In 1989, nearly one million people died of cardiovascular disease according to the American Heart Association. The seriousness of these disorders makes the nurse's role in management critical. Nursing care can range from client education about medications and reducing risk factors to defibrillating a client with a lethal dysrhythmia.

Bibliography

1. ACC/AHA Task Force Report (1990). Guidelines for the early management of patients with acute myocardial infarction. *Journal of the American College of Cardiology, 16*(2), 249-292.
2. Allard, K. S. (1992). Current trends in defibrillation. *Med-Surg Nursing Quarterly, 1*(1), 27-43.
3. Allen, J. K. (1990). Physical and psychosocial outcomes after coronary artery bypass graft surgery: review of the literature. *Heart and Lung, 19*(1), 49-54.
4. American Heart Association. *1992 Heart and Stroke Facts,* Dallas TX: American Heart Association.
5. Baas, L. S. (1992). Nursing responsibilities during CPR. *Med-Surg Nursing Quarterly, 1*(1), 1-26.
6. Becker, D. M., et al. (1989). Cholesterol: interpreting the new guidelines. *American Journal of Nursing, 89*(12), 1621-1633.

7. Berry, S. L., & Schleicher, C. A. (1992). Adjusting the beat: what to teach about antiarrhythmics. *American Journal of Nursing, 92*(6), 28-33.
8. Biggers, V. T. (1992). Codes for a code. *American Journal of Nursing, 92*(5), 56-61.
9. Borek, M., et al. (1989). Angiotensin-converting enzyme inhibitors in heart failure. *Medical Clinics of North America, 73*(2), 315-338.
10. Boykoff, S. L. (1989). Strategies for sexual counseling of patients following a myocardial infarction. *Dimensions of Critical Care Nursing, 8*(6), 368-373.
11. Calhoun, D. A., & Oparil, S. (1990). Treatment of hypertensive crisis. *The New England Journal of Medicine, 323*(17), 1177-1183.
12. Canobbio, M. (1990). *Cardiovascular disorders*. St. Louis: C.V. Mosby.
13. Chatterjee, K. (1989). Digitalis and non-ACE inhibitor vasodilators in heart failure. *Cardiology Clinics, 7*(1), 99-118.
14. Christman, N. J., et al. (1988). Uncertainty, coping, and distress following myocardial infarction: transition from hospital to home. *Research in Nursing and Health, 11*(2), 71-82.
15. Cimini, D. M. (1992). Indium-111 antimyosin antibody imaging. *Critical Care Nurse, 12*(6), 44-51.
16. Colucci, W. S. (1989). Positive inotropic/vasodilator agents. *Cardiology Clinics, 7*(1), 131-144.
17. Criqui, M. H. (1986). Epidemiology of atherosclerosis: An updated overview. *American Journal of Cardiology, 57*(5), 18C-23C.
18. Dimsdale, J. E. (1988). A perspective on type A behavior and coronary disease. *New England Journal of Medicine, 318*(2), 110-112.
19. Disler, L., et al. (1987). Cardiogenic shock in evolving myocardial infarction: treatment by angioplasty and streptokinase. Part 1. *Heart and Lung, 16*(6), 649-651.
20. Drew, B. J. (1992). Using cardiac leads: the right way. *Nursing 92, 22*(5), 50-54.
21. Dunn, F. G. (1990). Prevention of sudden cardiac death. *Cardiovascular Clinics, 20*(3), 95-109.
22. Dzau, V. J., & Creager, M. A. (1989). Progress in angiotensin-converting enzyme inhibition in heart failure. *Cardiology Clinics, 7*(1), 119-130.
23. Eysmann, S. B., & Douglas, P. S. (1992). Reperfusion and revascularization strategies for coronary artery disease in women. *Journal of the American Medical Association, 268*(14), 1903-1907.
24. Faxon, D. P. (1991). Percutaneous coronary angioplasty in stable and unstable angina. *Cardiology Clinics, 9*(1), 99-113.
25. Fleury, J. (1992). The application of motivational theory to cardiovascular risk reduction. *IMAGE: The Journal of Nursing Scholarship, 24*(3), 229-239.
26. Folta, A., & Metzger, B. L. (1989). Exercise and functional capacity after myocardial infarction. *Image, 21*(4), 215-219.
27. Gawlinski, A. (1989). Saving the cardiogenic shock patient. *Nursing 89, 19*(12), 34-41.
28. Gifford, R. W. (1991). Management of hypertensive crises. *Journal of the American Medical Association, 266*(6), 829-835.
29. Gleeson, B. (1991). Loosening the grip of anginal pain. *Nursing 91, 21*(1), 33-40.
30. Gortner, S. R., et al. (1992). Elders after CABG. *American Journal of Nursing, 92*(8), 44-49.
31. Gruppo Italiano per lo Studio della Streptochinasi nell' Infarto Miocardico (GISSI) (1986 Feb 22). Effectiveness of intravenous thrombolytic treatment in acute myocardial infarction. *Lancet, 1*(8748), 397-401.
32. Hayes, D. L. (1992). The next 5 years in cardiac pacemakers: A preview. *Mayo Clinic Proceedings, 67*(4), 379-384.
33. Henneman, E. A., & Henneman, P. L. (1989). Intricacies of blood pressure measurement: reexamining the rituals. *Heart and Lung, 18*(3), 263-271.
34. Higgins, C. A. (1990). The AICD: a teaching plan for patients and families. *Critical Care Nurse, 10*(6), 69-74.
35. Holmes, D. R., & Bresnahan, J. F. (1991). Interventional cardiology. *Cardiology Clinics, 9*(1), 115-134.
36. Hopson, J. R., et al. (1989). The role of energy and current in successful defibrillation and cardioversion. *Cardiology Board Review, 6*(5), 31-45.
37. Huang, S., et al. (1989). *Coronary care nursing* (2nd ed.). Philadelphia: W. B. Saunders.
38. Jessup, M., et al. (1992). CHF in the elderly: Is it different? *Patient Care, 26*(18), 40-61.
39. Jessup, M., et al. (1992). Managing CHF in the older patient. *Patient Care, 26*(18), 65-88.
40. Johnson, J. L., & Morse, J. M. (1990). Regaining control: The process of adjustment after myocardial infarction. *Heart & Lung, 19*(2), 126-135.
41. Kannel, W. B. (1989). Epidemiological aspects of heart failure. *Cardiology Clinics, 7*(1), 1-9.
42. Kater, K. M., et al. (1992). Corralling atrial fibrillation with "maze" surgery. *American Journal of Nursing, 92*(7), 34-38.
43. Kerber, R. E., et al. (1988). Energy, current and success in defibrillation and cardioversion: clinical studies using an automatic impedance-based method of energy adjustment. *Circulation, 77*(5), 1038-1046.
44. King, K. B., et al. (1992). Patient perceptions of quality of life after coronary artery surgery: Was it worth it? *Research in Nursing & Health, 15*(5), 327-334.
45. Letterer, R. A., et al. (1992). Learning to live with congestive heart failure. *Nursing 92, 22*(6), 34-42.
46. Mailis, A., et al. (1989). Chest wall pain after aortocoronary bypass surgery using the internal mammary artery graft: A new pain syndrome? *Heart & Lung, 18*(11), 553-558.
47. Manson, J. E., et al. (1990). A prospective study of obesity and risk of coronary heart disease in women. *The New England Journal of Medicine, 322*(13), 882-889.
48. Meek, J. (1991). The dreaded defibrillator. *American Journal of Nursing, 91*(5), 32-33.
49. Miller, P., et al. (1988). Influence of a nursing intervention on regimen adherence and societal adjustments postmyocardial infarction. *Nursing Research, 37*(5), 297-302.
50. Miller, P., et al. (1990). Marital functioning after cardiac surgery. *Heart & Lung, 19*(1), 55-61.
51. Gruppo Italiano per lo studio della Streptochinasi nell' Infarto (1986). Effectiveness of intravenous thrombolytic treatment in acute myocardial infarction. *Lancet, 1*(8478), 397-402.
52. Moss, A. J., & Benhorin, J. (1990). Prognosis and management after a first myocardial infarction. *The New England Journal of Medicine, 322*(11), 743-752.
53. Nara, A. R., et al. (1989). *Biophysical measurement series: blood pressure*. Redmond, WA: SpaceLabs Inc.
54. Niemann, J. T. (1992). Cardiopulmonary resuscitation. *New England Journal of Medicine, 327*(15), 1075-1080.
55. Packa, D. R. (1989). Quality of life of cardiac patients: A review. *The Journal of Cardiovascular Nursing, 3*(2), 1-11.
56. Pifarre, R., et al. (1989). Cardiac transplantation. *Cardiology Clinics, 7*(1), 183-194.
57. Rakel, R. E. (1992). *Conn's current therapy*. Philadelphia: W. B. Saunders.
58. Rossi, L. (1984). Nursing care for survivors of sudden cardiac death. *Nursing Clinics of North America, 19*(3), 411-425.
59. Sanders, M. J., et al. (1989). The use of inotropic agents in acute and chronic congestive heart failure. *Medical Clinics of North America, 73*(2), 283-314.
60. Shah, P. K. (1991). Pathophysiology of unstable angina. *Cardiology Clinics, 9*(1), 11-26.
61. Sica, D. A., & Gehr, T. (1989). Diuretics in congestive heart failure. *Cardiology Clinics, 7*(1), 87-97.
62. Sirles, A. T., & Selleck, C. S. (1989). Cardiac disease and the family: Impact, assessment, and implications. *The Journal of Cardiovascular Nursing, 3*(2), 23-32.
63. Sommers, M. S. (1992). The near-death experience after cardiopulmonary arrest. *Med-Surg Nursing Quarterly, 1*(1), 55-62.
64. Sommers, M. S. (1992). Preventing complications of CPR. *Med-Surg Nursing Quarterly, 1*(1), 44-54.
65. Standards and guidelines for cardiopulmonary resuscitation (CPR) and emergency cardiac care (ECC) (1986). *Journal of the American Medical Association, 255*(21), 2843-2959.
66. Stewart, S. L. (1992). Acute MI: A review of pathophysiology, treatment, and complications. *The Journal of Cardiovascular Nursing, 6*(4), 1-25.
67. Stokes, J. 3d (1990). Cardiovascular risk factors. *Cardiovascular Clinics, 20*(3), 3-20.
68. Stuart, J. V., & Sheehan, A. M. (1991). Permanent pacemakers:

The nurse's role in patient education and follow-up care. *The Journal of Cardiovascular Nursing, 5*(3), 32–43.
69. Sytkowski, P. A., et al. (1990). Changes in risk factors and the decline in mortality from cardiovascular disease. *The New England Journal of Medicine, 322*(23), 1635–1640.
70. *Vital statistics of the United States 1988 (vol. II, part B)*. U.S. Department of Health and Human Services, Hyattsville, MD, 1990.
71. Waller, B. F. (1989). Atherosclerotic and nonatherosclerotic coronary artery factors in acute myocardial infarction. *Cardiovascular Clinics, 20*(1), 29–104.
72. Wolfe, C. L. (Ed.) (1989). Cardiac imaging: diagnosis and assessment of cardiac disorders. *Cardiology Clinics, 7*(3), 483–737.
73. Wright, S. M. (1990). Pathophysiology of congestive heart failure. *The Journal of Cardiovascular Nursing, 4*(3), 1–16.
74. Zipes, D. P. (1992). Management of cardiac arrhythmias: Pharmacological, electrical and surgical techniques. *In* Braunwald, E., (Ed.) *Heart disease* (4th ed.) Philadelphia: W. B. Saunders.
75. Zwerner, P. L., & Gore, J. M. (1985). Differentiating periinfarction pericarditis from recurrent ischemia in acute myocardial infarction. *Practical Cardiology, 11*(12), 94–111.

Chapter 43

Nursing Care of Clients with Cardiac Structure Disorders

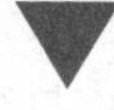

Bacteria and other microbes are found in abundance in our environment. The heart can become infected by these microbes, with the initiation of an inflammatory response. Involvement of the heart can be lethal during the acute stage or lead to structural damage that can impair heart function.

RHEUMATIC FEVER

Definition, Incidence, and Etiology

Rheumatic fever is a diffuse inflammatory disease. It is a delayed response to an infection by group A beta-hemolytic streptococcus. Although these infections remain common, the incidence of rheumatic fever has declined dramatically in the United States. In many parts of the world, rheumatic heart disease is still the leading cause of death from heart disease in the 5- to 24-year-old group.

Risk Factors

Rheumatic fever develops in only a relatively small percentage of clients (3 per cent) after even a virulent bout of streptococcal infection; there is, therefore, some evidence of host predisposition. Genetic links have been studied with no clear correlation to the incidence of disease.[79] Once rheumatic fever is acquired by clients, they become more susceptible to a recurrent infection than the general population is. Poor hygiene and crowding are risk factors for acute rheumatic fever in underprivileged areas. If appropriate antibiotic therapy for group A beta-hemolytic streptococcal infections is given within the first 9 days of the infection, rheumatic fever will usually be prevented.[56]

Prevention of rheumatic fever is most important. The most effective measures against rheumatic fever are probably socioeconomic. In the affluent sections of Western world cities where there is spacious housing and noncrowding, there is also a very low incidence of rheumatic fever. Nevertheless, it is of course quite important to treat streptococcal infections with an adequate antimicrobial regimen.

Pathophysiology

Rheumatic fever produces a diffuse, proliferative, and exudative inflammatory process. In rheumatic fever, there is involvement of the heart, joints, subcutaneous tissue, central nervous system, and skin. Although the exact pathogenesis is not clear, it is probably through an abnormal humoral and cell-mediated response to streptococcal cell-membrane antigens. These antigens bind to receptors on the heart, tissues, and joints, which begins the autoimmune response. The inflammatory process often produces permanent and severe heart damage.

Rheumatic fever produces carditis, or inflammation of the heart. This carditis affects the pericardium, epicardium, myocardium, and endocardium. There may be Aschoff bodies, which are minuscule nodules with localized fibrin deposits surrounded by areas of necrosis in the myocardium that are due to the inflammation of rheumatic fever. Endocardial inflammation causes swelling of the valve leaflets, which leads to valve dysfunction and murmurs. Small bacterial vegetations form on the valve tissues. Rough eroded areas of the valves attract platelets, which adhere and form platelet-fibrin clumps that eventually cause scarring and shortening. The valves lose their elasticity, and cardiac function is impaired. First, the damaged valve may become narrowed or stenosed. This increases the cardiac workload, because higher pressure must be generated to propel blood through the narrow valve. Second, the valve leaflets may become so short that they cannot close securely. As a result, blood regurgitates (leaks backward) through the damaged valve into the chamber from which it was ejected. Both valvular stenosis and regurgitation eventually cause heart failure from the high workload (Table 43–1).

Complications of rheumatic fever include valvular disorders, cardiomegaly, and congestive heart failure. These complications may be fatal.

Clinical Manifestations

Rheumatic fever almost always follows a streptococcal infection of the nasopharynx. Clinical manifestations usually include arthritis, carditis, fever, subcutaneous nodules, erythema marginatum, chorea, abdominal pain, weakness, malaise, weight loss, and anorexia.

Arthritis. Arthritis, a prominent finding, is very painful and migratory. It most often affects the larger joints, such as ankles, knees, elbows, shoulders, and wrists. The arthritis may or may not be symmetric. If the client takes aspirin early in the course of the disease, these symptoms may not be as apparent. Joint symptoms may last hours or days.

Carditis. Carditis, one of the most common manifestations of rheumatic fever, is the most destructive consequence of this disease. Characteristics include a significant murmur, cardiomegaly, pericarditis that produces a significant friction rub, and congestive heart failure. Chest pain due to pericardial inflammation may be present. Sometimes there is myocardial involvement that produces atrioventricular (AV) conduction defects or atrial fibrillation.

TABLE 43–1. Effects of Rheumatic Fever on the Myocardium, Endocardium, and Pericardium

Condition	Characteristic Lesion	Cause of Lesion	Significance of Pathophysiologic Involvement
Rheumatic myocarditis	Aschoff bodies, minute nodules, in connective tissue around small arteries in myocardium	Formed by leukocytes that mass in inflamed tissues	Nodules may eventually become fibrotic; damage from fibrosis may eventually damage arteries in myocardium; myocarditis may cause temporary loss in contractile power of heart; permanent damage rarely results
Rheumatic endocarditis	Tiny vegetations resembling little beads form along line of closure of valve leaflets (primarily mitral and aortic valves)	Probably result from inflammation, ulceration, and erosion of valve leaflets	Progressive fibrosis, scarring, and calcification of valve leaflets result in valvular incompetency and stenosis
Pericarditis	Nonspecific lesions	Result from diffuse, nonspecific fibrinous or serofibrinous inflammatory reaction	May cause pericardial friction rub; usually no serious sequelae

Fever. Fever, with a temperature of 38° C (100.4° F) or higher, alternates with periods when temperature returns to normal.

Subcutaneous Nodules. Subcutaneous nodules are small, painless, firm nodules that adhere loosely to the tendon sheaths (especially in knees, knuckles, and elbows). They are usually evident only during the first week or so of the disease and usually only in children.

Erythema Marginatum. Erythema marginatum is an unusual rash seen primarily on the trunk. The lesions are crescent-shaped and have clear centers. The rash is transitory and may change in appearance in minutes or hours.

Chorea. Chorea (St. Vitus' dance) is a disorder of the central nervous system. It is manifested by sudden, irregular, aimless, involuntary movements. The chorea disappears without treatment and has no permanent sequelae.

Abdominal Pain. Abdominal pain, a common symptom, varies in site and severity. The pain may be related to engorgement of the liver.

Weakness, Malaise, Weight Loss, and Anorexia. Weakness, malaise, weight loss, and anorexia probably develop as a result of fever, pain, and the general debilitation associated with serious illness.

No single diagnostic feature identifies rheumatic fever. Many of the common clinical manifestations are associated with other disorders as well as rheumatic fever. The Jones criteria were developed to assist in diagnosis (Table 43-2). The symptoms of rheumatic fever may last 3 months.

DIAGNOSTIC ASSESSMENT

A positive throat culture for group A beta-hemolytic streptococci can help with the diagnosis. An elevated white blood cell count, erythrocyte sedimentation rate, and C-reactive protein indicate inflammation and may also be increased.

Medical Management

The medical therapy for acute rheumatic fever depends on the manifestations and severity of the attack. The first priority is to eradicate the streptococcal infection. Usually this can be accomplished with oral administration of penicillin or erythromycin. Clients with arthritis symptoms are greatly relieved with salicylates; however, because these drugs can confuse the diagnosis, a firm diagnosis should be in place before the administration of salicylates.

Corticosteroids are used to treat carditis, especially if there is evidence of congestive heart failure. If congestive heart failure develops, treatment including cardiac glycosides and diuretics is effective.

Bed rest is usually prescribed to reduce cardiac work until evidence of inflammation has subsided. For clients with rheumatic valvular heart disease, bacterial endocarditis prophylaxis is necessary (see Infective Endocarditis).

TABLE 43-2. Guidelines for the Diagnosis of Initial Attack of Rheumatic Fever (Jones Criteria, 1992 Update)*

Major Manifestations
Carditis
Polyarthritis
Chorea
Erythema marginatum
Subcutaneous nodules
Minor Manifestations
Clinical findings
Arthralgia
Fever
Laboratory findings
Elevated acute phase reactants
Erythrocyte sedimentation rate
C-reactive protein
Prolonged PR interval
Supporting Evidence of Antecedent Group A Streptococcal Infection
Postive throat culture or rapid streptococcal antigen test
Elevated or rising streptococcal antibody titer

* If supported by evidence of preceding group A streptococcal infection, the presence of two major manifestations, or of one major and two minor manifestations indicates a high probability of acute rheumatic fever.

From Diagnosis of Rheumatic Fever—Special Writing Group (1992). *Journal of the American Medical Association, 268*(15), 2069-2073. Copyright 1992, American Medical Association.

Nursing Management

ASSESSMENT

Nursing assessment involves gathering subjective and objective data concerning the client's

- cardiac function
- tolerance to activity and feelings regarding activity restrictions
- support systems
- coping strategies
- nutritional status
- level of discomfort
- knowledge (of the client and significant others) concerning the nature of and intervention for rheumatic fever

NURSING INTERVENTION

Nursing Diagnosis: Pain R/T inflammatory response.

Planning: Expected Outcomes. The client will experience increased comfort, as evidenced by reports of restful sleep and reduced discomfort; reports of joint pain relief; reduced use of pain medications; and a relaxed body posture and calm facial expression.

Implementation. Obtain a clear description of the pain or discomfort. Identify the source of greatest discomfort as a focus for interventions. Administer analgesics as needed. Balance rest and activity based on degree of pain and activity tolerance. Other pain interventions are discussed in Chapter 16.

Nursing Diagnosis: Activity Intolerance R/T reduced cardiac reserve and enforced bed rest.

Planning: Expected Outcomes. The client will demonstrate progression toward an optimal level of physical activity tolerance, based on underlying cardiovascular status and psychosocial readiness, as evidenced by ability to pace activity; to verbalize improvement in fatigue; to express acceptance of any imposed activity restrictions; and to steadily increase activity level to include one flight of stairs without chest pain, or electrocardiographic (ECG) changes, while heart rate remains under 90 beats per minute.

Implementation. Bed rest is important in the acute phase because it reduces myocardial oxygen demand. Bed rest usually continues until the following criteria are met:

- Temperature remains normal without the use of salicylates.
- Resting pulse remains under 100.
- ECG tracings show no signs of myocardial damage.
- Sedimentation rate returns to normal.
- There is no pericardial friction rub present.

Once ambulatory, the client must still be careful not to overdo. The nurse should assess the client's stamina and response to exercise to gauge the degree of gradual activity progression. Take vital signs before and after exercise. After 3 to 5 minutes of rest, repeat vital signs. The client should decrease or discontinue activity if chest pain, vertigo, dyspnea, confusion, a drop in blood pressure, or an irregular pulse rate develops. The length of activity restriction depends on whether carditis develops and the extent of permanent heart damage. Restrictions may extend for months. In severe cases of rheumatic carditis, clients may be forced to undergo restrictions on a permanent basis. Encourage a gradual increase in activity within the limits of the client's condition.

The client experiencing chorea requires sedatives, bed rest, and protection from self-injury. A carefully planned and supervised activity schedule should be maintained and evaluated.

Nursing Diagnosis: Nutrition, Altered: Less than Body Requirements R/T fever and infection associated with rheumatic fever.

Planning: Expected Outcomes. The client will maintain or restore adequate nutritional balance, as evidenced by resumption of ideal weight (based on premorbid status), no further weight loss, normal serum albumin, and a positive nitrogen balance.

Implementation. A high-protein, high-carbohydrate diet helps maintain adequate nutrition in the presence of fever and infection. Hypermetabolic states (fever and infection) can induce a catabolic state, thus delaying healing. Vitamin and mineral supplements may also benefit the client. Oral hygiene every 4 hours, small attractive meal servings, and foods that are not overly rich, sweet, or greasy promote the appetite. Adequate fluid intake prevents dehydration due to fever. If the client shows signs of severe carditis or congestive heart failure, sodium and fluids must be restricted. Daily weights can serve as an indication of nutritional status and effectiveness of nursing interventions.

Nursing Diagnosis: Altered Health Maintenance R/T preventive measures against initial and recurring attacks of rheumatic fever.

Planning: Expected Outcomes. The client and family will demonstrate adequate knowledge of rheumatic fever and its cause, course, and therapy, as evidenced by the ability to accurately describe the causes and process of rheumatic fever, its clinical manifestations, its prevention, and rationale for prescribed interventions.

Implementation. Today, streptococcal infections do not have to develop into rheumatic fever if the client seeks immediate assessment and begins antibiotics. Also, clients who have recovered from an attack of rheumatic fever may prevent subsequent attacks by taking prophylactic doses of antibiotics and observing good health practices. Because repeated attacks may lead to serious heart disease and permanent cardiac disability, the importance of avoiding subsequent attacks of rheumatic fever must be stressed.

Penicillin is the prophylactic medication of choice. For penicillin-allergic clients, the physician will usually prescribe erythromycin.

The client typically takes prophylactic agents for rheumatic fever for 5 years after the initial attack. After 5 years, recurrences rarely occur. Clients who have had rheumatic fever remain vulnerable to bacterial endocarditis. Therefore, in addition to the antibiotics they take to prevent rheumatic fever recurrence, they must take prophylactic medications before and after any surgical procedure or dental work. Advise clients that they must adhere to this practice permanently.

EVALUATION

The degree of expected outcome attainment is evaluated. Revisions in the plan of care may be required.

Post-hospital Care

DISCHARGE TEACHING

If a client has been hospitalized for rheumatic fever, discharge teaching becomes a necessary intervention for prevention of future illness. These guidelines should be stressed during teaching:

- Take good care of teeth and gums and obtain prompt dental care for cavities and gingivitis. Prophylactic medication may be needed before teeth are cleaned by a dentist.
- Avoid people who have an upper respiratory infection or who have had a recent streptococcal infection.
- Notify the physician if any of the symptoms of streptococcal sore throat (pharyngitis) develop. It is extremely important to begin antibiotic therapy promptly for any infection. The clinical manifestations include an elevated temperature (102° to 104° F); chills; sore throat; and enlarged, painful lymph nodes. Instruct clients who have had rheumatic fever that they must guard against infections for the rest of their lives to avoid possible development of heart disease.

INFECTIVE ENDOCARDITIS

Definition

Endocarditis is an inflammatory process of the endocardium, especially the valves. This disorder was once lethal, but morbidity and mortality have been greatly reduced with the use of antibiotics and advanced diagnostic procedures.

In the past, many different terms and classifications have been used to describe infective endocarditis. The nurse may still see these terms used or find them in old medical records. Some are defined here.

Subacute bacterial endocarditis develops gradually over several weeks or months and is usually caused by organisms of low virulence, such as *Streptococcus viridans,* which has a limited ability to infect other tissues.

Acute bacterial endocarditis develops over days or weeks with an erratic course and earlier development of complications. It is frequently caused by *Staphylococcus aureus,* which is capable of infecting other body tissues.

Native valve endocarditis is an infection of a previously normal or damaged valve.

Prosthetic valve endocarditis is an infection of an artificial valve.

Nonbacterial thrombotic endocarditis is caused by sterile thrombotic lesions (frequently aggregates of platelets), which may develop in clients with malignancies or other chronic diseases.

Incidence

Changes in the susceptible population are currently altering the classic picture of endocarditis. The proportion of acute cases is rising. Five of every 1000 patients admitted to a hospital have endocarditis. Overall mortality is 20 to 30 per cent and as high as 70 per cent in the aged.[21] Fewer patients are developing the classic physical signs of advanced endocarditis, such as Osler's nodes, finger clubbing, or Roth's spots (see Clinical Manifestations). The proportion of cases due to streptococci has fallen slightly. The proportion of cases caused by gram-negative bacilli, fungi, and other unusual microbes is increasing.

The changes are traced to several notable alterations in the population. The increase in the incidence of endocarditis caused by yeasts and fungi is attributable to the increased number of clients with valve prostheses, to the increased number of clients addicted to intravenous drugs, and to long-term antimicrobial therapy or immunosuppression.

The decrease in the incidence of rheumatic fever lowers the incidence of endocarditis, whereas the number of children surviving congenital heart disease raises the incidence of endocarditis. The growing elderly population also increases the number of endocarditis episodes.

Etiology

Circulating microorganisms in the bloodstream attach to the endocardial surface and multiply. Usually the multiplication of these organisms requires a rough or abnormal endocardium. Intravenous drug abusers may be injecting particulate matter into the bloodstream, with damage to the previously normal endocardium that allows the organism to adhere, thereby initiating acute bacterial endocarditis.

Defective heart valves causing changes in blood flow and pressures encourage the proliferation of vegetations. Open heart surgery to replace damaged valves increases the risk of endocarditis. Fortunately, coronary artery bypass grafting, one of the most frequently performed surgeries in the United States, carries a low risk for infective endocarditis. This is because the endocardium is not invaded during the operation.

Risk Factors

Most clients who develop endocarditis have a preexisting heart condition, but some cases develop even though there is no known heart disease. Acquired valvular disease (especially mitral valve prolapse) and heart valve prostheses can lead to infective endocarditis. In some cases, endocarditis follows an invasive procedure, such as minor surgery, dental procedures, or insertion of renal shunts, urinary catheters, or long-term indwelling catheters (for dialysis, hemodynamic monitoring, or hyperalimentation). Factors that place clients at high risk are listed in Box 43–1.

Secondary prevention in high-risk clients includes the use of prophylactic antibiotics in an attempt to prevent bacterial endocarditis. Bacteremias frequently occur during dental or surgical procedures. Clients at risk (those with a previous case of endocarditis and those with congenital heart defects or prosthetic valves) should follow a specific antibiotic regimen before certain dental or surgical procedures. Tertiary prevention

Box 43-1. Factors that Place Clients at High Risk for Infective Endocarditis

Congenital heart disease
Rheumatic heart disease
Degenerative heart disease
Mitral valve prolapse
Cardiac structural and valve lesions
Heart valve replacement
Cardiac surgery
Chronic debilitating disease
Intravenous drug abuse
Immunosuppression related to
- Cancer
- Collagen vascular disease
- Hepatitis
- Burn injury
- Diabetes mellitus
- Radiation therapy
- Prolonged drug therapy (antibiotic, cytotoxic, or steroid medications)
- Invasive procedures

Adapted from Guzzetta, C., & Dossey, B (1984). *Cardiovascular nursing: bodymind tapestry*. St. Louis: C. V. Mosby.

(the reduction of complications) is discussed within the text.

Pathophysiology

Microorganisms are able to enter the bloodstream in many ways. Once the colonization process begins on the endothelium, replication occurs, and bacterial colonies form within layers of platelets and fibrin. As the colonies become entangled within the tight layers of fibrin and platelets, the colony becomes less and less vulnerable to the body's defense mechanisms. The bacteria stimulate the humoral immune system to produce nonspecific antibodies, but the bacteria are protected by the fibrin-platelet aggregation. It is not uncommon for these vegetations to form thromboses and to then travel to other organs, forming abscesses (Fig. 43-1).

The vegetations can severely damage heart valves by perforating and deforming the valve leaflets. Extensions of the bacteria may invade the aorta or pericardium. The amount of damage depends on the type and virulence of organisms causing the infection.

There are many possible complications. Congestive heart failure may develop due to structural valvular damage. Arterial emboli can occur from the vegetation. Systemic embolization occurs in 30 per cent of clients with left-sided infective endocarditis (Fig. 43-2). Common infarction sites are the kidney, spleen, and brain. Pulmonary embolus is associated with right-sided infective endocarditis. Emboli can also travel to the brain and produce a myriad of symptoms. Occasionally, a client will develop renal disease in the form of immune complex glomerulonephritis. Renal function will usually return to normal after the infection has been controlled.

Clinical Manifestations

Clinical manifestations of infective endocarditis vary according to its acute or subacute nature, but many symptoms are common to all types.

Clinical manifestations can be divided into three groups:

- ► Evidence of systemic infection includes fever, chills, rigors, sweats, malaise, weakness, anorexia, weight loss, backache, and splenomegaly.
- ► Evidence of an intravascular lesion includes dyspnea, chest pain, murmurs, cold and painful extremities, petechiae, Roth's spots, Osler's nodes, splinter hemorrhages, and stroke.
- ► Evidence of an immunologic reaction to infection includes arthralgia, proteinuria, hematuria, casts, and acidosis.[14]

General malaise, fatigue, weakness, and anorexia are quite common. Headaches and musculoskeletal complaints are frequent. Clients with infective endocarditis often feel as if they have the flu.

In the acute type of infective endocarditis, the clinical manifestations occur more quickly and are more severe. Clients appear very ill. Symptoms of fever, rigors, and prostration are so severe that admission to a hospital usually occurs within a few days.

Symptoms of cardiac failure may develop suddenly in either acute or subacute endocarditis. Mechanical complications include perforation of a valve leaflet, rupture

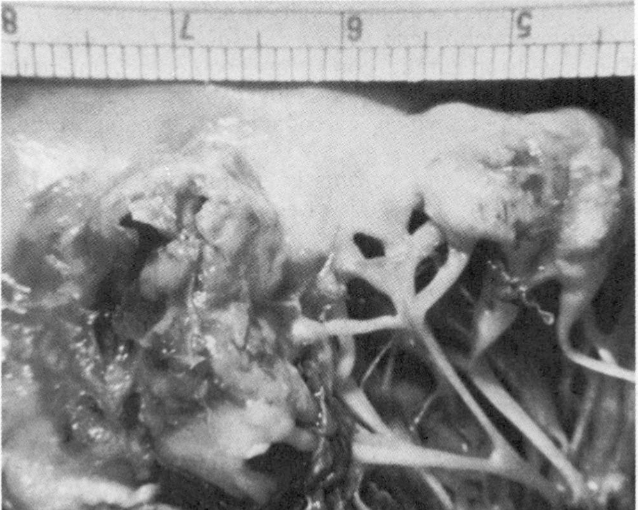

▲ **Figure 43-1**

Infective endocarditis can lead to vegetations of the heart valves. This client had large vegetations of the mitral valve leaflets. (From Braunwald, E. [1992]. *Heart disease: A textbook of cardiovascular medicine* [4th ed.]. Philadelphia: W. B. Saunders.)

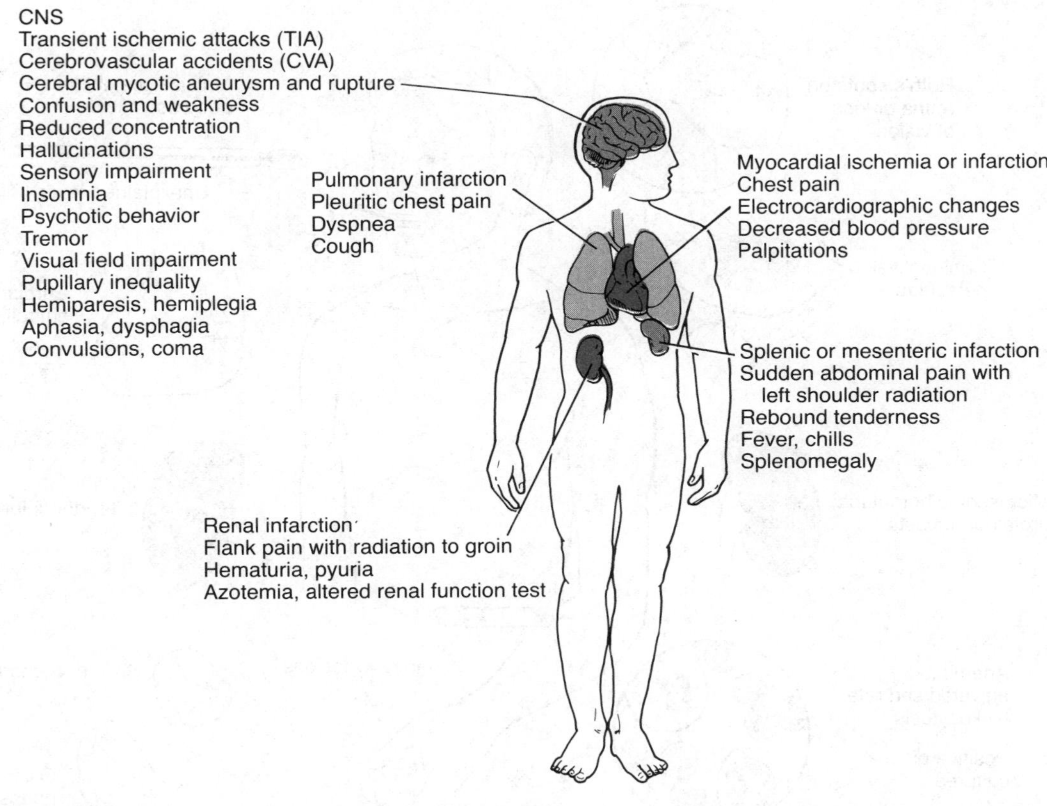

▲ *Figure 43–2*

Locations and clinical manifestations of emboli of infective endocarditis. (Data from Guzzetta, C., & Dossey, B. [1984]. *Cardiovascular nursing: Bodymind tapestry*. St. Louis: C. V. Mosby.)

of one of the chordae tendineae, or development of a functional stenosis from obstruction of blood flow by large vegetations. Myocardial infarction may develop as a result of coronary artery embolism.[14]

Unusual physical examination findings may be present (Fig. 43–3), including splinter hemorrhages, Osler's nodes, finger clubbing, Janeway lesions, ocular signs, and splenomegaly.

Splinter hemorrhages are caused by microembolization and are characterized by linear subungual hemorrhages that appear similar to tiny splinters under the nail.

Osler's nodes are painful, erythematous, pea-sized nodules in the skin of the extremities, usually on the fingertips. They are due to inflammation around a small, infected embolus.

Finger clubbing is found less frequently now but is common in long-standing infective endocarditis. The pathogenesis continues to remain unclear.

Janeway lesions are flat, small, nontender red spots that are found in the palms of the hands and the soles of the feet.

Ocular signs are sometimes present, including

- conjunctival petechiae—small, bright red hemorrhages that are easily seen if the upper and lower eyelids are everted
- Roth's spots, visualized by funduscopic examination as a white or yellow center surrounded by a bright red, irregular halo
- loss of vision, which can occur during the course of endocarditis from embolization to the brain or to the retinal artery

Splenomegaly is an enlarged spleen that is soft and may or may not be tender.

DIAGNOSTIC ASSESSMENT

Blood cultures for bacteria, fungus, and yeast are the most important diagnostic tests. ECG, complete blood count, and other routine diagnostic procedures are helpful.

Because the clinical manifestations of endocarditis are numerous and often nonspecific, several modalities are employed for differential medical diagnosis. Blood cultures should be obtained for all clients with both fever and heart murmur. ECGs should be done on admission to the hospital and repeated during the hospital stay. Although a negative ECG does not rule out endocarditis, echocardiography can be helpful. Transesophageal echocardiography can be useful in diagnosis. Chest radiography is useful for determining early congestive heart failure.

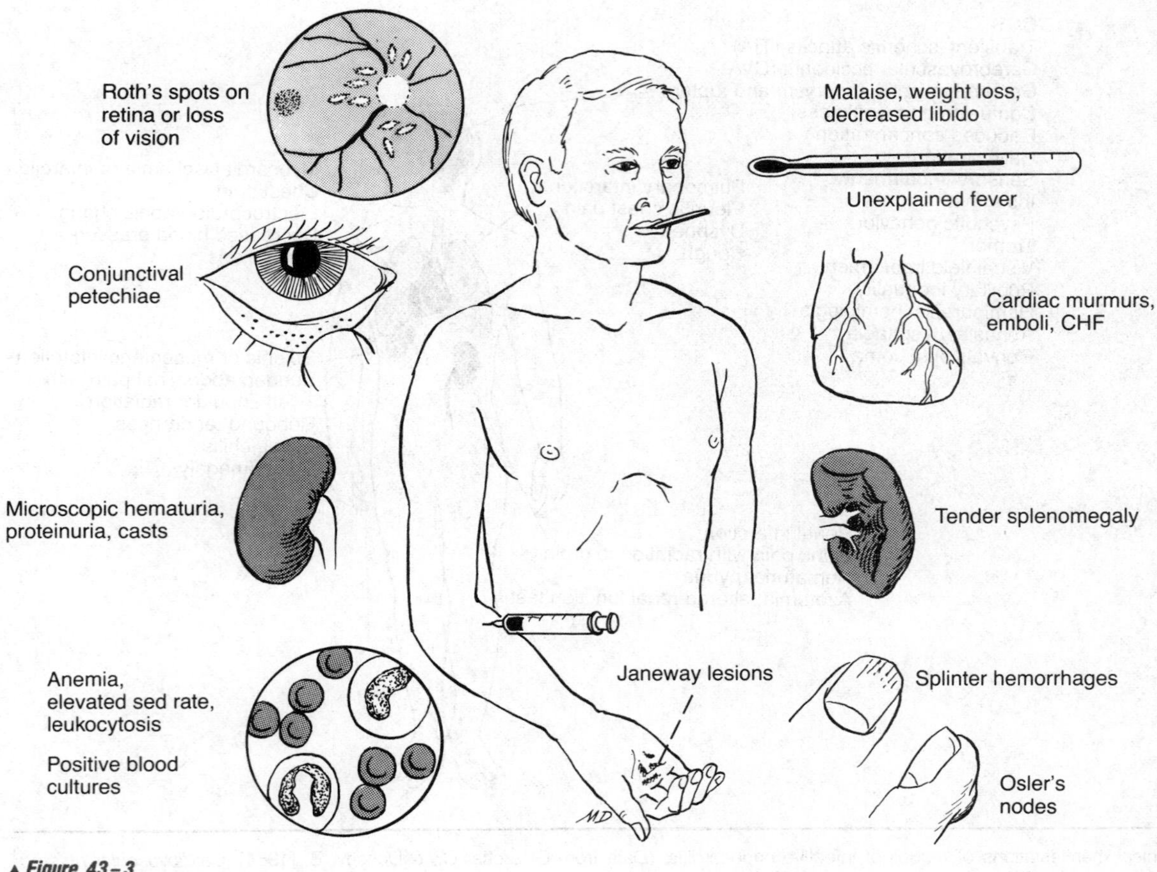

▲ *Figure 43–3*

Manifestations of subacute bacterial endocarditis.

Medical Management

The chief aims of management are to eradicate the infecting organism and to treat complications. Antimicrobial therapy has changed this disease from one that was almost always fatal to one that is rarely fatal. The choice of antibiotic depends on the organism involved. Penicillin and streptomycin are commonly used. Therapy is usually continued intravenously for 4 to 6 weeks. This is usually begun in the hospital but is occasionally continued at home with extensive discharge planning and education. Occasionally, it is necessary for the client to undergo heart valve replacement for reversal of newly developed congestive failure.

Nursing Management

ASSESSMENT

In infective endocarditis, nursing assessment focuses on gathering data about the client's hemodynamic stability (particularly the presence of a new heart murmur and embolic complications), level of comfort, coping ability, support from significant others, and potential for self-care.

NURSING INTERVENTION

Nursing Diagnosis: Pain R/T fever and malaise.

Planning: Expected Outcomes. The client will be as comfortable as possible, as evidenced by reporting restful sleep, demonstrating behavior associated with comfort and relaxation, decreased use of analgesia, and reporting reduction of discomfort after comfort measures.

Implementation. Administer antibiotics intravenously as prescribed. Antibiotics will relieve most discomfort within a few days. Treat fever, when present, with rest, cooling measures, forced fluids, and sometimes salicylates. As with most infectious processes, the client should be encouraged to eat a nutritious diet, to drink sufficient fluids, and to rest mentally and physically.

Nursing Diagnosis: Decreased Cardiac Output R/T cardiac valve dysfunction.

Planning: Expected Outcomes. The client will have restoration and maintenance of hemodynamic status, as evidenced by stable blood pressure and pulse, adequate urine output (>30 ml/hr), no new heart murmur development, clear lung fields with no reports or evidence of dyspnea, increased levels of activity, and alertness and orientation.

Implementation. The client may need to be hospitalized for 2 to 6 weeks. Do not enforce complete bed rest unless fever or signs of heart damage develop. Auscultate every 8 hours for heart murmurs. Assess for rapid pulse, easy fatigability, dyspnea, restlessness, signs of heart failure, and embolic manifestations. Document these manifestations if they occur and report them to the physician.

When the client's condition improves, plan and implement a progressive activity schedule. As activity increases, monitor the client's physical response to exercise. For example, assess blood pressure, heart rate, diaphoresis, vertigo, and weakness.

EVALUATION

The degree of goal attainment is evaluated. Revisions in the plan of care may be required.

Post-hospital Care

DISCHARGE TEACHING

The nurse teaches the client and family about:

- the cause of infectious endocarditis
- the purpose of long-term antibiotic administration and need to comply with the entire course of therapy
- the need for prophylactic antibiotics when undergoing dental procedures and surgical interventions or instrumentation
- the importance of ongoing assessments to determine the efficacy of treatment and to identify the early signs of complications (see Client Education Guide)

HOME HEALTH CARE

Recently, there has been a trend toward allowing some clients requiring prolonged intravenous antibiotic therapy to return home while they are still receiving therapy. Clients who are alert, cooperative, and reasonably stable and who wish to return home may be allowed to do so. Typically, the nurse, pharmacist, and physician teach the techniques of self-administered intravenous antibiotics. Before discharge, the client must demonstrate the knowledge and technique required for antibiotic administration. The physician's office or home health care nurses often monitor the client's progress.

Home intravenous antibiotic therapy offers many benefits. It is less costly, motivates clients to become active participants in their own care, reestablishes a more normal lifestyle, and promotes a sense of control that aids in psychosocial and physiologic recovery. To be effective, this program requires exceptional communication and cooperation between health care team members and the client.[24]

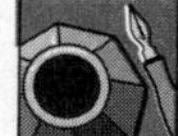

CLIENT EDUCATION GUIDE

Infective Endocarditis

Plan to begin discharge teaching well in advance of the anticipated discharge date. By the time of discharge, the client should be prepared for the following:

- Self-administration of intravenous antibiotics with the help of a significant other if the client is to be discharged before therapy is concluded.
- An activity program that will allow gradual return to the former lifestyle. Clinicians usually recommend about a month of convalescence at home before a full schedule is resumed.
- Compliance with antibiotic prophylaxis when dental or surgical procedures become necessary. Clients need to inform their dentists and physicians of their endocarditis.
- Self-administration of careful oral hygiene to help prevent bacteremia and further endocarditis. Suggest daily flossing and use of a soft toothbrush. The client's dentist should be consulted before water-jet devices are used because they may cause gum bleeding.
- Self-monitoring for the manifestations of endocarditis. Have clients monitor their temperature daily for a month and document it. Instruct them to report fever, chills, malaise, anorexia, weight loss, and increased fatigue to the physician.

MYOCARDITIS

Overview

Myocarditis is an inflammation of the myocardial wall. It can be caused by almost any bacterial, viral, rickettsial, or parasitic organism as well as radiation, toxic agents such as lead, and drugs such as lithium and cocaine. Myocarditis affects clients of all ages and may be acute or chronic. An immune-deficient client is at greater risk of myocarditis. Frequently, the inflammation is not limited to the myocardium itself but extends to the pericardium, with production of an associated pericarditis. The incidence of myocarditis is not possible to ascertain. The incidence varies with the age of clients and various etiologic agents.

In the United States, most cases of myocarditis are due to viral infections. Viruses associated with this disorder include coxsackieviruses A and B, mumps, influenza groups A and B, rubella, rubeola, adenoviruses, echoviruses, variola, cytomegalovirus, and Epstein-Barr virus.[49] Other causes of myocarditis include

- bacterial infections: diphtheria, typhoid fever, staphylococcal, pneumococcal, tetanus, and tuberculosis
- hypersensitive immune reactions: acute rheumatic fever and postcardiotomy syndrome
- toxins and chemicals: alcohol
- radiation: large doses of radiation therapy to the chest for the treatment of malignancy
- parasitic infections: Chagas' disease and toxoplasmosis

Myocardial damage from acute myocarditis is usually the result of the direct invasion or the toxic effects of the microorganism in cardiac myocytes. This can cause an alteration in cellular energy systems and cellular damage. Actual virus is only rarely isolated from human hearts in acute myocarditis; even in the laboratory during experimental infections, it is never isolated after 3 weeks. This does not prevent the infection from becoming subacute or chronic or from causing dilated cardiomyopathy.[76] Usually myocarditis involves both ventricles. If there is impairment of myocardial contractility, there may be an elevation of ventricular diastolic pressures and volumes in order to maintain stroke volume. Disruptions leading to cardiac dysrhythmias can cause a decrease in cardiac output.

Complications that may develop from myocarditis include congestive heart failure, dilated cardiomyopathy, and sudden death from lethal arrhythmias or rupture of a myocardial aneurysm.

Myocarditis displays a wide variation in clinical manifestations. There may be no signs or symptoms at all. The health history may reveal a recent upper respiratory infection, a viral pharyngitis, or tonsillitis. The most frequent symptoms, however, include fatigue, dyspnea, palpitations, and chest pain. The client often experiences chest pain as a mild continuous pressure or soreness in the chest. Thus, the chest pain of myocarditis can be distinguished from the effort-induced pain of angina pectoris. Tachycardia, if present, may be disproportionate to the degree of fever, exertion, or illness. Dysrhythmias can also occur, sometimes producing a fatal circulatory collapse. There may be a pericardial friction rub if the client has pericarditis.

In most cases, myocarditis is self-limiting and uncomplicated. If myocardial involvement becomes extensive or prolonged, myofibril degeneration can produce heart failure, with pulmonary congestion, dyspnea, neck vein distention, peripheral edema, and cardiomegaly. Recurrent myocarditis can produce cardiomyopathy.

The chest radiograph may show an enlarged cardiac silhouette due to ventricular enlargement or pericardial effusion. Routine blood tests may show a moderate leukocytosis and elevated cardiac enzymes. Echocardiography is helpful in determining heart chamber size and ventricular functioning. Gallium scan shows regional wall abnormalities, dilated ventricles, and hypokinesis of the left ventricle.

ECG abnormalities and elevated serum levels of cardiac enzymes are helpful to the physician diagnosing this illness. The ECG may show a bundle branch block or complete AV heart block.

Management

Clients with acute myocarditis are usually admitted to the hospital for observation. Clients with pericardial effusion, dysrhythmias, congestive heart failure, or hypotension are usually admitted to the intensive care unit (ICU). Medical management begins with specific therapy for the underlying infection. Bed rest is suggested to decrease cardiac work. Supplemental oxygen may be prescribed for clients with low cardiac output or dysrhythmias. Immunosuppressive therapy is currently being investigated; initial reports are favorable in the treatment of myocarditis.[76] Antipyretic agents are helpful for the fever and the hemodynamic effects of fever that increase myocardial work. Clients who remain at home may use telemetry (Holter) monitoring of the heart. This monitoring provides continuous surveillance of the client's heart rhythm. Household members may need training in cardiopulmonary resuscitation (CPR) in case a serious complication occurs.

The outlook for clients with myocarditis is generally good. Most patients recover rapidly. Some have recurrent or chronic myocarditis, and some become very ill and die.

Nursing management for the client experiencing myocarditis is essentially the same as that provided to clients with infective endocarditis and rheumatic fever. Review those sections within this chapter.

Teaching begins when acute symptoms have subsided and the client has demonstrated physical and emotional readiness. Teach clients with myocarditis how to monitor their pulse rate and rhythm. Instruct them to immediately report any sudden changes in heart rate, rhythm, or palpitations. Encourage family members to take CPR training. They can obtain this training from groups such as the local fire department, the American Red Cross, or the American Heart Association.

Because the myocardial infectious process resolves slowly and late complications can occur, advise clients to continue self-monitoring and to schedule clinical follow-up appointments, even after apparent recovery.

The potential of lethal arrhythmias may frighten the client and significant others. The client who is experiencing extreme anxiety, fear, and ineffective coping may manifest insomnia, tearfulness, somatic complaints, inability to problem solve, and agitation. Determine with the client (and family) the specific focus of anxiety. Clarify any misconceptions that arise. Speak slowly and calmly and focus on the present situation, giving feedback about current reality. Encourage the use of relaxation techniques to help allay stress. Schedule activities around periods of undisturbed sleep. Educating family members about CPR can enhance their sense of preparedness for an emergency.

PERICARDITIS

Overview

Acute pericarditis is a syndrome that is caused by inflammation of the parietal and visceral pericardium. This inflammatory process may develop either as a primary condition or secondary to a number of diseases and circumstances (Box 43–2).

Pericarditis may be either acute or chronic (recurring). It is not known why pericarditis may be a single illness in some clients and recurring in others. The chronic pericarditis is usually called constrictive pericarditis. Constrictive pericarditis is present when a fibrotic, thickened, and adherent pericardium restricts diastolic filling of the heart.[57] This eventually results in cardiac failure.

Box 43–2. Causes of Pericarditis

Infections
- Viral: coxsackie, influenza
- Bacterial: tuberculosis, staphylococcus, streptococcus, meningococcus, pneumococcus
- Parasitic
- Fungal

Myocardial injury
- Myocardial infarction (Dressler's syndrome)
- Cardiac trauma: blunt or penetrating
- Post cardiac surgery

Hypersensitivity
- Collagen diseases: rheumatic fever, scleroderma, systemic lupus erythematosus, rheumatoid arthritis
- Drug reaction: procainamide, methysergide, hydralazine
- Radiation therapy
- Cobalt therapy

Metabolic disorders
- Uremia
- Myxedema
- Chronic anemia

Neoplasm: lymphoma

Aortic dissection

Acute pericarditis may be either dry (fibrinous) or exudative. The exudate that is present with acute pericarditis may be serous, purulent, or hemorrhagic. This exudate can accumulate in the pericardial sac, causing a cardiac tamponade that restricts cardiac filling and emptying. Without prompt treatment, shock and death can result from decreased cardiac output.

Dry pericarditis can follow a common viral infection, myocardial infarction, tuberculosis, bacteremia, or renal failure. Delicate adhesions form within the pericardial space along with serous fibrin deposition, hemorrhage, and calcification. Adhesions may eventually obliterate the pericardial sac. Inflammation of the pericardium frequently penetrates the myocardium to some degree, which produces myopericarditis.

The characteristic symptom of pericarditis is chest pain. The nature of this pain varies with the client. Sometimes the pain is quite similar to the pain of myocardial infarction; at other times, it mimics the pain of pleurisy. The pain is exacerbated with respirations and rotating the trunk but usually does not radiate to the arms. Sitting up frequently relieves the pain.

The pericardial friction rub is a classic sign of acute pericarditis. The rub is produced by inflamed, roughened pericardial layers that create friction as their surfaces rub together during heart movement. Auscultation over the precordium reveals a scratchy, leathery, or creaky sound that is heard anywhere over the precordium but most frequently at the left mid to lower sternal border. The rub is best heard with the diaphragm of the stethoscope and with the client holding his or her breath. In some clients, it is best heard with the client sitting up. Pericardial friction rubs vary with intensity from hour to hour and from day to day.

Fever is another common finding in pericarditis. The client's temperature may rise to 39.4° C (103° F). Chills, malaise, joint pain, anorexia, nausea, and weight loss accompany the fever. Dyspnea and chest pain can potentiate anxiety. An increase in heart rate usually corresponds to the degree of fever and anxiety.

Chest x-ray studies help little in detecting acute pericarditis. ECG changes provide more distinctive evidence of the underlying inflammatory process. The ECG frequently shows a decrease in the amplitude of the QRS complex and changes in the ST-segment elevation and the T wave.[47]

Laboratory studies show an elevated erythrocyte sedimentation rate and may show an elevated white blood cell count. Cardiac enzymes are usually normal but may be elevated.

Management

When acute pericarditis is of known etiology, treatment of the underlying cause is indicated. If no causal agent is known, symptomatic intervention for acute dry pericarditis will be provided. Pain and fever, usually self-limited, may be eased by aspirin given in maximally tolerated doses. The physician may prescribe a nonsteroidal anti-inflammatory agent. Stronger analgesia, such as morphine sulfate, may be necessary if chest pain becomes severe.

The focus of nursing care related to pericarditis is the same as that described for the other inflammatory cardiac diseases discussed in this chapter. Nursing assessment of the client with pericarditis also includes scrutiny for the presence of pericardial tamponade (pulsus paradoxus, distended neck veins). Vigilant assessment is necessary. Provide reassurance concerning the temporary nature of the disease.

ACUTE PERICARDITIS WITH EFFUSION

Overview

Acute pericarditis with effusion results when fluid accumulates within the pericardial sac. Rapid or excessive fluid accumulations may compress the heart and reduce ventricular filling and cardiac output. When fluid accumulates slowly, the fibrous pericardium is better able to stretch and accommodate its presence. One to 2 L of fluid can be tolerated without increase in intrapericardial pressure if accumulation is slow. However, the normal unstretched pericardial sac can accommodate the rapid addition of only 80 to 200 ml of fluid without decrease in cardiac output.

Pericardial effusion may be asymptomatic. If dry pericarditis precedes the condition, the friction rub will often disappear. Fever may develop. Heart sounds may be muffled because the pericardial fluid further separates the stethoscope and the heart chambers.

Pulsus paradoxus can be present. If the client has normal breathing and a systolic difference of greater than 10 mm Hg, evaluation for cardiac compression and possibly cardiac tamponade should be done.[24]

Echocardiography is the most accurate technique for evaluating pericardial effusion. The test is sensitive enough to detect as little as 20 ml of pericardial fluid.[47, 57] Pericardiocentesis is not indicated unless there is evidence of cardiac compression caused by cardiac tamponade.[12, 47] (See the next section.)

Management

Care of the client with pericardial effusion is similar to the plan of intervention for dry pericarditis. Bed rest, analgesia, and proper positioning can help alleviate symptoms. Psychological support is very important.

CARDIAC TAMPONADE

Overview

Cardiac tamponade is a life-threatening complication. It exists when accumulated fluid in the pericardial cavity restricts diastolic ventricular filling. This fluid can be blood, pus, or air in the pericardial sac that accumulates fast enough and in sufficient quantity to compress the heart and restrict blood flow in and out of the ventricles. This is a cardiac emergency! Large or rapidly accumulating effusions raise the intrapericardial pressure to a point at which venous blood cannot flow into the heart, which decreases ventricular filling. As a result, venous pressure rises, and cardiac output and arterial blood pressure fall. A narrowing pulse pressure signals cardiac tamponade. The heart attempts to compensate by beating rapidly (tachycardia). Tachycardia cannot sustain the cardiac output for very long. Prompt intervention is necessary to prevent shock and death.

In cardiac tamponade, assessment reveals hypotension, tachycardia, jugular venous distention, cyanosis of lips and nails, dyspnea, muffled heart sounds, diaphoresis, and paradoxic pulse. The client may be comfortable and quiet one minute and then very restless with a feeling of impending doom the next minute. Clients may panic when fluid accumulates rapidly. Slowly developing tamponade has symptoms resembling congestive heart failure: nonspecific ECG changes, decreased voltage, and visualization of fluid in the pericardial sac on echocardiogram (Box 43-3).

Box 43-3. Pathophysiologic Changes in Cardiac Tamponade and Clinical Manifestations

Impaired right-sided cardiac filling
- Elevated venous pressure (increased central venous pressure)
- Distended neck veins
- Kussmaul's sign (distended neck veins on inspiration)

Distended pericardial sac
- Muffled heart sounds
- Pulsus paradoxus
- Decreased friction rub
- Decreased QRS voltage and electrical alternans
- Enlarged cardiac contour on chest film

Reduced cardiac output
- Hypotension
- Narrowed pulse pressure
- Tachycardia
- Dyspnea
- Restlessness, anxiety

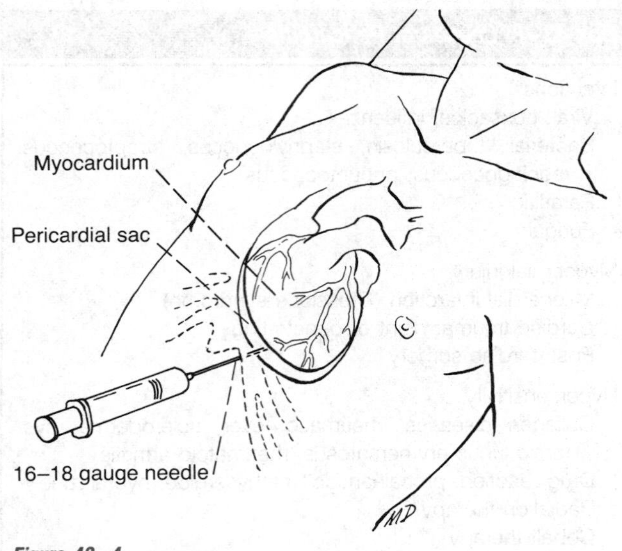

▲ Figure 43-4

Subxiphoid approach to pericardiocentesis.

Management

Cardiac tamponade requires immediate intervention. The emergency intervention of choice is pericardiocentesis, which involves aspirating the fluid or air from the pericardial sac (Fig. 43-4). This procedure relieves the pressure on the heart, thereby improving cardiac function and perhaps saving the client's life.

CHRONIC CONSTRICTIVE PERICARDITIS

Chronic constrictive pericarditis is a chronic inflammatory condition in which the pericardium changes into a thick, fibrous band of tissue. This tissue encircles, encases, and compresses the heart, which prevents proper ventricular filling and emptying. Cardiac failure eventually results from this slow compression.

Chronic constrictive pericarditis usually begins with an initial episode of acute pericarditis characterized by fibrin deposition, often with a pericardial effusion. In the majority of cases, the visceral and parietal layers become completely fused. Constrictive pericarditis is usually symmetric scarring that causes uniform constriction of all heart chambers. The heavily fibrosed pericardium restricts diastolic filling in all chambers and decreases systolic ejection.

Symptoms include right ventricular failure first, and decreased cardiac output that is manifested by fatigue on exertion, dyspnea, leg edema, ascites, low pulse pressure, distended neck veins, and delayed capillary refill time.

Constrictive pericarditis is a progressive disease without spontaneous reversal of symptoms. A minority of clients survive for many years with minor symptoms. The majority of clients become progressively more disabled over time. Treatment is both surgical and medical. Medical treatment includes digitalis preparations, diuretics, and sodium restriction to relieve symptoms of right ventricular failure. Surgical intervention involves the excision of the damaged pericardium (pericardiectomy) and should be performed early in the course of the disease.[1, 47, 65]

▼ STRUCTURAL ABNORMALITIES OF THE HEART

Structural abnormalities of the heart may be either congenital or acquired. Congenital heart disorders result from faulty development of the heart's structures in utero. Acquired defects arise from disease processes that develop after birth. Congenital disorders include septal defects, vessel stenosis, abnormally positioned vessels, and postnatal patency of the ductus arteriosus. Cardiomyopathies are acquired disorders in which disease of the cardiac muscle fibers reduces myocardial contractility or distensibility. Valvular disorders may be either congenital or acquired.

CARDIOMYOPATHY

Definition

Cardiomyopathy is a heart muscle disorder of unknown etiology (idiopathic). The dominant feature of cardiomyopathies is the involvement of the heart muscle itself. The definition excludes structural and functional abnormalities due to valvular disorders, coronary artery disease, and systemic and pulmonary vascular disorders.[76] Idiopathic cardiomyopathies can be classified according to the ventricular changes they cause (Fig. 43-5).

The three major classes are

- idiopathic dilated (congestive) cardiomyopathy
- idiopathic hypertrophic cardiomyopathy (also called idiopathic hypertrophic subaortic stenosis)
- idiopathic restrictive cardiomyopathy

Table 43-3 compares diagnostic data for the three classifications of idiopathic cardiomyopathy. The incidence of cardiomyopathies has not been recorded.

DILATED CARDIOMYOPATHY

Dilated cardiomyopathy is a syndrome characterized by cardiac enlargement. The first abnormality noticed is

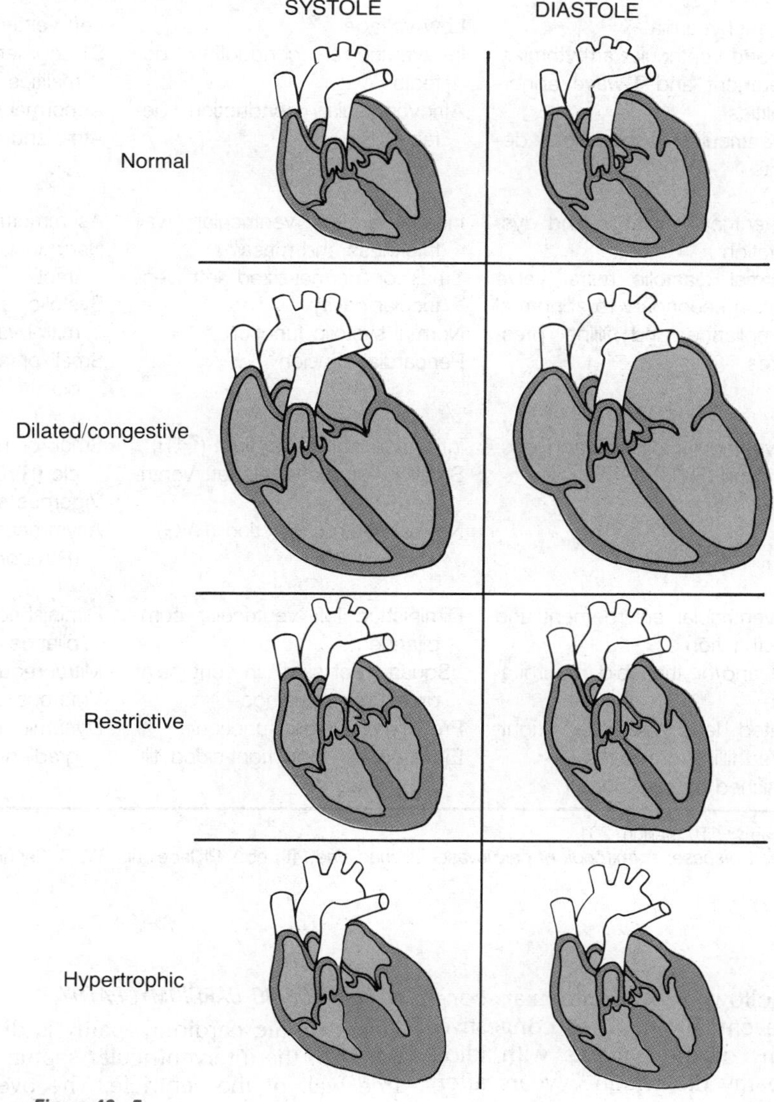

▲ *Figure 43-5*

Types of cardiomyopathy.

TABLE 43–3. Diagnostic Data for the Three Types of Cardiomyopathy

	Dilated	Restrictive	Hypertrophic
Symptoms	Congestive heart failure, particularly left-sided Fatigue and weakness Systemic or pulmonary emboli	Dyspnea, fatigue Right-sided congestive heart failure Signs and symptoms of systemic disease: amyloidosis, iron storage disease, etc.	Dyspnea, angina pectoris Fatigue, syncope, palpitations
Physical examination	Moderate to severe cardiomegaly; S_3 and S_4 Atrioventricular valve regurgitation, especially mitral	Mild to moderate cardiomegaly: S_3 or S_4 Atrioventricular valve regurgitation; inspiratory increase in venous pressure (Kussmaul's sign)	Mild cardiomegaly Apical systolic thrill and heave; brisk carotid upstroke S_4 common Systolic murmur that increases with Valsalva's maneuver
Chest roentgenogram	Moderate to marked cardiac enlargement, especially left ventricular Pulmonary venous hypertension	Mild cardiac enlargement Pulmonary venous hypertension	Mild to moderate cardiac enlargement Left atrial enlargement
Electrocardiogram	Sinus tachycardia Atrial and ventricular arrhythmias ST-segment and T-wave abnormalities Intraventricular conduction defects	Low voltage Intraventricular conduction defects Atrioventricular conduction defects	Left ventricular hypertrophy ST-segment and T-wave abnormalities Abnormal Q waves Atrial and ventricular arrhythmias
Echocardiogram	Left ventricular dilation and dysfunction Abnormal diastolic mitral valve motion secondary to abnormal compliance and filling pressures	Increased left ventricular wall thickness and mass Small or normal-sized left ventricular cavity Normal systolic function Pericardial effusion	Asymmetric septal hypertrophy Narrow left ventricular outflow tract Systolic anterior motion of the mitral valve Small or normal-sized left ventricle
Radionuclide studies	Left ventricular dilation and dysfunction (RVG)	Infiltration of myocardium (^{201}Tl) Small or normal-sized left ventricle (RVG) Normal systolic function (RVG)	Small or normal-sized left ventricle (RVG) Vigorous systolic function (RVG) Asymmetric septal hypertrophy (RVG or ^{201}Tl)
Cardiac catheterization	Left ventricular enlargement and dysfunction Mitral and/or tricuspid regurgitation Elevated left- and often right-sided filling pressures Diminished cardiac output	Diminished left ventricular compliance "Square root sign" in ventricular pressure recordings Preserved systolic function Elevated left- and right-sided filling pressures	Diminished left ventricular compliance Mitral regurgitation Vigorous systolic function Dynamic left ventricular outflow gradient

RVG, Radionuclide ventriculogram; ^{201}Tl, thallium-201.
From Braunwald, E. (1992). *Heart disease: A textbook of cardiovascular medicine* (4th ed.). Philadelphia: W. B. Saunders.

ventricular enlargement followed by ventricular contractile dysfunction. This eventually leads to congestive heart failure. Three fourths of the patients with idiopathic dilated cardiomyopathy die within 5 years after the onset of symptoms.[42, 78]

HYPERTROPHIC CARDIOMYOPATHY

Hypertrophic cardiomyopathy is disproportionate thickening of the interventricular septum, compared with the free wall of the ventricle. The overgrowth of the wall leads to rigidity in the wall and thereby increases resistance to blood flow from the left atrium. There is also obstruction of left ventricular outflow.

Clients with hypertrophic cardiomyopathy can lead long, relatively asymptomatic lives. In many clients, symptoms will stabilize, or even improve, over a period of years. However, an otherwise stable course is often interrupted by sudden death. Sudden death appears more often in younger clients and may be avoided by eliminating strenuous exercise if the diagnosis is known.

RESTRICTIVE CARDIOMYOPATHY

Restrictive cardiomyopathy is the least common form of cardiomyopathy. This form is characterized by excessively rigid ventricular walls. The rigid walls impair filling during diastole; however, contractility with systole is usually normal.

Etiology

DILATED CARDIOMYOPATHY

Dilated cardiomyopathy associated with pregnancy can disappear. There may be spontaneous rapid improvement in some women and early fatality in others. Other etiologic factors are listed in Box 43-4.

HYPERTROPHIC CARDIOMYOPATHY

Hypertrophic cardiomyopathy appears to be a genetically transmitted disease of the heart muscle, but its exact cause remains a mystery. It appears most often in young adults, both men and women.[39]

Although this disease is also known as idiopathic hypertrophic subaortic stenosis, many clients do not have the obstructive or stenotic component of the disease. Therefore, it is more accurate to use the term hypertrophic cardiomyopathy to describe this disease.

The predominant feature of hypertrophic cardiomyopathy involves unexplained myocardial hypertrophy, which typically appears with disproportionate thickening of the interventricular septum. The term asymmetric septal hypertrophy is sometimes used to describe the disorder.

RESTRICTIVE CARDIOMYOPATHY

Any infiltrative process of the heart that results in fibrosis and thickening can cause restrictive cardiomyopathy. The most frequently associated disease is amyloidosis (deposition of eosinophilic fibrous protein in the

Box 43-4. Etiology of Cardiomyopathy and Myocarditis

Inflammatory

- Infective
  - Viral
  - Rickettsial
  - Bacterial
  - Mycobacterial
  - Fungal
  - Parasitic
- Noninfective
  - Collagen diseases
  - Granulomatous
  - Kawasaki's disease

Metabolic

- Nutritional
  - Thiamine
  - Scurvy
  - Obesity
  - Carnitine deficiency
- Endocrine
  - Acromegaly
  - Thyrotoxicosis
  - Myxedema
  - Uremia
  - Cushing's disease
  - Pheochromocytoma
  - Diabetes mellitus
- Altered metabolism
  - Gout
- Electrolyte imbalance

Toxic

- Cobalt
- Alcohol
- Bleomycin and doxorubicin
- Phenothiazines and antidepressants
- Carbon monoxide
- Lead
- Chloroquine
- Lithium
- Cyclophosphamide
- Hydrocarbons
- Catecholamines
- Phosphorus
- Insect stings and snake bites
- Reserpine
- Corticosteroids
- Cocaine

Infiltrative

- Amyloidosis
- Hemochromatosis
- Neoplastic
- Glycogen storage disorders
- Sarcoidosis

Fibroplastic

- Endomyocardial fibrosis
- Endocardial fibroelastosis
- Carcinoid

Hematologic

- Sickle cell anemia
- Polycythemia vera
- Thrombotic thrombocytopenic purpura
- Leukemia

Hypersensitivity

- Hypersensitivity to medications
- Giant cell myocarditis
- Cardiac transplant rejection

Genetic

- Hypertrophic cardiomyopathy
  - With gradient
  - Without gradient
- Neuromuscular
  - Duchenne's muscular dystrophy
  - Kearns-Sayre syndrome
  - Nemaline cardiomyopathy
  - Multicore cardiomyopathy

Miscellaneous Acquired

- Postpartum cardiomyopathy
- Obesity

Idiopathic

- Idiopathic dilated cardiomyopathy
- Idiopathic restrictive cardiomyopathy
- Idiopathic hypertrophic cardiomyopathy
- Idiopathic right ventricular cardiomyopathy

Physical Agents

- Heatstroke
- Hypothermia
- Radiation
- Tachycardia

Modified from Braunwald, E. (1992). *Heart disease: A textbook of cardiovascular medicine* (4th ed.). Philadelphia: W. B. Saunders.

heart). Other disorders include glycogen storage disease, hemochromatosis, and sarcoidosis.[66]

Risk Factors

Four conditions seem to lower the threshold for the development of cardiomyopathy: (1) chronic ingestion of excessive alcohol, (2) pregnancy, (3) systemic hypertension, and (4) a variety of infections.

Pathophysiology

DILATED CARDIOMYOPATHY

Whatever the cause of congestive cardiomyopathy, it results in a diffuse degeneration of myocardial fibers, with a decrease in contractile function. There is enlargement and dilation of all four chambers. Left ventricular filling pressures are generally elevated because of poor contractile function.

HYPERTROPHIC CARDIOMYOPATHY

In its severest form, the left ventricular myocardium reaches tremendous dimensions and encroaches on the left ventricular chamber, which becomes small and elongated. Septal hypertrophy may obstruct the left ventricular outflow tract during systole. Frequently, there is diastolic dysfunction in the form of stiffness of the left ventricle during diastolic filling. This stiffness raises left ventricular end-diastolic pressure, which eventually results in elevation of left atrial, pulmonary venous, and pulmonary capillary pressures.

RESTRICTIVE CARDIOMYOPATHY

In restrictive cardiomyopathy, the ventricular walls are excessively rigid and impede ventricular filling. Myocardial contractility is usually unaffected. Fibrotic infiltrations into the myocardium, endocardium, and subendocardium cause the ventricles to lose their ability to stretch. The tight heart muscle hampers ventricular diastolic filling. Filling pressures increase, and cardiac output falls. Eventually, cardiac failure and mild ventricular hypertrophy occur.

Clinical Manifestations

DILATED CARDIOMYOPATHY

Clinical manifestations usually develop gradually in clients with congestive cardiomyopathy. Fatigue and weakness are common. Chest pain may be present and may be associated with ischemic heart disease. Right-sided heart failure is a late and ominous sign.

Systemic blood pressure is usually normal or low. Symptoms often reveal signs of congestive heart failure, such as dyspnea, orthopnea, tachycardia, palpitations, and peripheral edema. Jugular veins are frequently enlarged. The liver can be engorged. An S_4 gallop often precedes the development of congestive heart failure, and an S_3 gallop generally occurs with heart failure. If the heart rate is rapid, both S_4 and S_3 may fuse to form a summation gallop sound. There may be a systolic murmur of mitral or tricuspid insufficiency, because ventricular dilation prevents sufficient closure of those valves. Gallop sounds and regurgitant murmurs may be intensified by an isometric handgrip exercise because of the increase it causes on systemic vascular resistance. Pulmonary crackles become audible as failure progresses.

Diagnostic tests including ECG, echocardiography, chest radiography, and blood chemistries are useful for the physician's diagnosis. ECG findings include sinus tachycardia, ventricular dysrhythmias, ST-segment changes, and left bundle branch block.

HYPERTROPHIC CARDIOMYOPATHY

Clients with hypertrophic cardiomyopathy most commonly present with clinical manifestations in late adolescence or early adulthood, but symptoms may appear at any age. Many clients with hypertrophic cardiomyopathy are asymptomatic and often have relatives with incapacitating symptoms of the disease. Sadly, sudden death is frequently the first clinical manifestation of the disease in asymptomatic clients.

The most common symptom of the disease is dyspnea. Dyspnea is due to the high pulmonary pressures produced by the elevated left ventricular end-diastolic pressure. Angina pectoris, fatigue, and syncope are also common symptoms. Cardiac dysrhythmias are frequently present. Palpitations, paroxysmal nocturnal dyspnea, and frank congestive heart failure are less common. Many clients complain of dizzy spells. Exertion tends to worsen most symptoms.

Physical examination may be normal in asymptomatic clients. The appearance of a fourth heart sound may be the only sign of the disease. ECG, chest film, echocardiogram, and radionuclide scanning are very useful to the physician in diagnosing hypertrophic cardiomyopathy.

RESTRICTIVE CARDIOMYOPATHY

Restrictive cardiomyopathy causes clinical manifestations related to decreasing cardiac output. As cardiac output falls and intraventricular pressures rise, signs of congestive heart failure appear. The earliest manifestations may include exercise intolerance, fatigue, and shortness of breath followed by neck vein distention, peripheral edema, and ascites. In severe or end-stage disease, the clinical manifestations of restrictive cardiomyopathy are indistinguishable from chronic constrictive pericarditis. (See preceding text for a more complete discussion of pericarditis.) Cardiac murmurs are usually minimal or absent. Congestive heart failure without cardiac enlargement indicates restrictive cardiomyopathy.

DIAGNOSTIC ASSESSMENT

Specific diagnostic assessments for the various forms of cardiomyopathy are listed in Table 43–3.

Medical Management

DILATED CARDIOMYOPATHY

Because the cause of idiopathic dilated cardiomyopathy is not known, there is no specific therapy. Treatment is similar to that for congestive heart failure. Only transplantation and specific vasodilator therapy (hydralazine plus nitrates) have prolonged life.[63, 76, 78] Heart transplantation shows a 1-year survival rate of over 80 per cent and a 3-year survival of 70 per cent in appropriate clients. The 1-year survival in nontransplanted clients is 5 per cent.[40, 79]

Rest improves cardiac function and reduces heart size. Most clients experience severe activity intolerance during the later stages of the disease, which automatically limits their activities. However, during the earlier stages of the disease, most clients find it difficult to accept rigidly imposed activity restrictions. Clients should avoid poorly tolerated activities. Advise clients that physical and emotional stress exacerbates the disease. Because alcohol depresses myocardial contractility, the client should abstain from drinking alcoholic beverages.

Pharmacologic Management. Intervention in dilated cardiomyopathy focuses on controlling congestive heart failure by enhancing myocardial contractility and unloading the heart. Digitalis preparations, vasodilators, diuretics, and sodium-restricted diets provide the major means for achieving these objectives. Antiarrhythmic agents may help suppress ventricular irritability. In appropriate candidates, the implantation of the automatic internal cardiac defibrillator may be used to prevent sudden cardiac death.[50, 78] (See Chap. 42.)

The combined problem of ventricular dilation and ineffective myocardial contractility also increases the risk of pooled blood within the heart and subsequent clot formation. Therefore, the physician may prescribe anticoagulants to help prevent clots and emboli.

HYPERTROPHIC CARDIOMYOPATHY

Goals of intervention are to reduce ventricular contractility and to relieve left ventricular outflow obstruction. Beta-adrenergic blocking agents, such as propranolol, provide the mainstay of medical intervention for hypertrophic cardiomyopathy. These medications reduce myocardial contractility. With decreased vigor of ventricular contraction, outflow obstruction diminishes. Beta-adrenergic blockade also reduces heart rate (which further reduces myocardial workload) and prevents arrhythmias. Calcium channel blocking agents such as verapamil are also being used to relieve symptoms and improve exercise tolerance.

RESTRICTIVE CARDIOMYOPATHY

Currently there are no specific interventions for restrictive cardiomyopathy. Intervention aims at diminishing congestive heart failure. Diuretics, vasodilators, and salt restriction help accomplish this goal. Digitalis may help in some forms of restrictive cardiomyopathy.

Death due to dysrhythmia from restrictive cardiomyopathy may occur suddenly; or a more progressive course may be followed with eventual, intractable heart failure. The prognosis largely depends on the underlying cause. Unfortunately, intervention for these clients rarely brings about long-term improvement.

Surgical Management

Surgical intervention for hypertrophic cardiomyopathy may become necessary if medical management is ineffective. Several surgical procedures have been developed to reduce the outflow gradient. The most popular surgical treatment consists of excising a portion of the hypertrophied septum, called myotomy or myectomy.

The excision of fibrotic endocardium is successful in a limited number of clients with restrictive cardiomyopathy. Cardiac transplantation is becoming increasingly common surgery for clients with dilated cardiomyopathy. Valve replacement may also be required, but it is not commonly performed. Cardiac surgery is discussed later in this chapter.

Nursing Management

ASSESSMENT

Nursing assessment for cardiomyopathy focuses on

- the duration and extent of symptoms
- limitations on activity and lifestyle
- coping strategies employed
- the client's and family's understanding of, perception of, and reaction to the illness
- genetic counseling

NURSING INTERVENTION

The management of the client with cardiomyopathy is outlined in the care plan. In addition, clients who are acutely or chronically ill with cardiomyopathy require strong psychosocial support. The uncertain and serious consequences of the disease create fear and anxiety. The chronic nature of the disorder can deplete coping resources, leaving those afflicted with feelings of helplessness and hopelessness. As physical capabilities diminish, feelings of inadequacy, frustration, and poor self-esteem grow. Clients may become irritable, angry, withdrawn, or dependent.

Even though their prognosis is often poor, help those who suffer from this debilitating disorder maintain hope and dignity. Encouragement, a caring touch, a listening ear, and attainable goals can promote a high quality of life. Create an environment in which clients can openly

CARE PLAN

The Client with Cardiomyopathy

Nursing Diagnosis/ Collaborative Problem	Planning: Expected Outcomes	Implementation: Nursing Interventions	Rationales
Congestive Heart Failure, High Risk for R/T mechanical dysfunction of the heart	The nurse will monitor for clinical manifestations of CHF: • Peripheral edema • Pulmonary edema • Decreased renal perfusion • Decreased CO • Diaphoresis • Dyspnea/orthopnea • Anxiety • Frothy, pink sputum	Assess the client every 4–8 h for • Neck vein distention • Peripheral edema • Altered lung sounds • Dyspnea or orthopnea • Tachycardia • Hypotension • Confusion • Urine output > 30 ml/hr	To detect early signs of CHF; as the heart muscle fails to pump effectively, falling cardiac output stimulates the adrenergic system and the renin-angiotensin-aldosterone system. These changes lead to tachycardia and oliguria. Increased preload and afterload lead to neck vein distention, peripheral edema, altered lung sounds, dyspnea and orthopnea. Hypoxia may lead to confusion
		Monitor BUN, bilirubin, liver enzymes, and creatinine	These laboratory studies indicate liver failure from congestion of blood
		Monitor fluid balance every 8–24 hr Daily weights	Clients are treated with potent diuretics to reduce pulmonary and peripheral edema. Accurate assessment of fluid balance and weight assist in determining the effectiveness of the treatment
Decreased Cardiac Output R/T alterations in cardiac structure and function	The client will demonstrate improved cardiac output, as evidenced by • Clear lung sounds • Vital signs WNL • Warm, dry skin • Normal sinus rhythm • Absence of S_3 or S_4 • Stable body weight • Urine output > 30 ml/hr • Decreased peripheral edema, neck vein distention, and ascites	Monitor for clinical manifestations of decreasing CO	Early detection of decreasing CO improves treatment options
		Encourage bed rest during acute phase, limit self-care	Decreases oxygen consumption and demand on myocardium
		Avoid Valsalva's maneuvers (with hypertrophic cardiomyopathy)	Valsalva's maneuvers decrease the inflow of venous blood and impair outflow
		Observe and record dysrhythmias q 4–8 hr	Dysrhythmias may further impair CO
		Monitor intake and output q 1–8 hr	Fluid retention may occur with decreased CO and CHF
		Restrict intravenous and oral fluids as ordered	Decreases the amount of circulating fluids
		Administer unloading and inotropic agents	Used to improve ejection, reduce preload, and improve contractility
		Administer calcium antagonists as ordered	Decreases LV outflow obstruction and increases LV compliance to improve ventricular filling

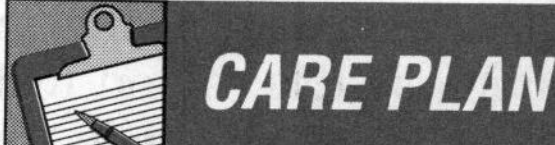

CARE PLAN

The Client with Cardiomyopathy Continued

Nursing Diagnosis/ Collaborative Problem	Planning: Expected Outcomes	Implementation: Nursing Interventions	Rationales
		In hypertrophic: avoid nitrates, beta-adrenergics, and cardiac glycosides	These agents increase contractility and increase obstruction
		Hemodynamic monitoring: monitor arterial pressure, RAP, PAP, PCWP, CO/CI q 2–4 hr as indicated	Monitors the degree of CHF and the response to therapy
Activity Intolerance R/T mechanical dysfunction of the heart and decreased cardiac reserve	The client will have an improved activity tolerance, as evidenced by	Assess tolerance to activities in bed before ambulating	Provides a baseline to plan activity
	• Demonstrating a progression of activity appropriate ot the disorder	During activity, monitor pulse, respirations, color, and ECG	Provides early detection of orthostatic changes as well as data on the ability of the diseased myocardium to meet oxygen demand
	• Showing a willingness to combine rest and activity • Demonstrating minimal change in pulse or BP during activities	Discontinue activity if chest pain, dyspnea, cyanosis, dizziness, hypotension, sustained tachycardia, or dysrhythmias develop	Evidence of myocardial hypoxia
	• Demonstrating minimal fatigue after activity	Monitor pulse, respirations, and BP 3 minutes after activity	Evaluate tolerance of activity
	• Having pulse, respirations, and BP return to normal range within 3 minutes of the activity • Accepting any imposed restrictions	Explore which sedentary activities client may enjoy	May provide diversion, if activity is not permitted; these activities do not place a demand on the diseased myocardium

BP, blood pressure; BUN, blood urea nitrogen; CHF, congestive heart failure; CO, cardiac output; CO/CI, cardiac output/cardiac index; ECG, electrocardiogram; LV, left ventricular; PAP, pulmonary artery pressure; PAWP, pulmonary artery wedge pressure; RAP, right atrial pressure; WNL, within normal limits.

express concerns and acknowledge fears. Acceptance, empathy, and kindness can help clients with cardiomyopathies adopt more successful coping strategies.

The poor prognosis for these disorders need not lead to frustration and despair. With optimism and conscientious effort, the nurse can assist the client with cardiomyopathy to maintain a realistic level of health and achieve a quality of life that reflects personal fulfillments.

Post-hospital Care

With hypertrophic cardiomyopathy, syncope or sudden death may follow physical exertion. Therefore, warn the client with hypertrophic cardiomyopathy to avoid strenuous physical exercise such as running or active competitive sports. In addition, encourage household members to learn CPR. Although chest pain often accompanies this disease, nitroglycerin can worsen obstruction. Instead, clinicians treat chest pain with reduced activity and beta-blocking agents.

Hypertrophic cardiomyopathy predisposes the client to the risk of infective endocarditis. Advise clients with this cardiomyopathy always to take prophylactic antibiotics before and after dental and surgical procedures. (See earlier discussion of prevention of and intervention for infective endocarditis.) Also relay this vital information to the client's family.

All clients with cardiomyopathy need clear, honest education concerning the disease and its cause and intervention. Both the nurse and the client must be vigilant for untoward effects of therapy. Clients with restrictive cardiomyopathy are especially prone to digitalis toxic effects.

VALVULAR HEART DISEASE

Definition

The four heart valves maintain the one-way flow of blood. When the valves are healthy, the blood flows through the heart and lungs in a unilateral direction (see Figs. 40-3 and 40-4). Dysfunction occurs when the heart valves are unable to fully open or fully close. A stenosed valve may impede the flow of blood from one chamber to the next. An insufficient valve may allow blood to regurgitate back into the chamber from which blood is being pumped (Fig. 43-6).

MITRAL VALVE DISEASE

Disorders of the mitral valve obstruct the flow of blood from the atrium to the ventricle (stenosis) or allow blood to leak back from ventricle to atrium (regurgitation). Mitral regurgitation overworks the left atrium and left ventricle; mitral stenosis overworks the left atrium.

Mitral Stenosis. Mitral stenosis is a block in blood flow resulting from an abnormality of the mitral valve leaflets, which prevents proper opening of the valve during diastole.

Mitral Regurgitation. Mitral regurgitation occurs when blood from the left ventricle is ejected back into the left atrium during systole because of abnormalities of the mitral valve. Regurgitation of the mitral valve sometimes occurs with mitral stenosis.

Mitral Valve Prolapse. In mitral valve prolapse, one or both of the valve leaflets bulge into the left atrium during ventricular systole. Various names have been given to the disorder: late apical systolic murmur, Barlow's syndrome, and floppy mitral valve syndrome. Usually a benign disorder, it may progress to a stage of pronounced regurgitation and ventricular dilation. Although it is often an isolated abnormality, this syndrome is associated with a number of other conditions, such as endocarditis, myocarditis, atherosclerosis, systemic lupus erythematosus, muscular dystrophy, acromegaly, and cardiac sarcoidosis. In addition, there may be a genetic component. It tends to be more common in young women.[43]

AORTIC VALVE DISEASE

Aortic valve disease is far less common than mitral valvular disease. However, it often occurs in conjunction with mitral disease. Aortic stenosis obstructs the forward flow of blood from the left ventricle into the aorta and systemic circulation. Aortic regurgitation allows blood to leak back from the aorta into the left ventricle. Both aortic stenosis and regurgitation overwork the left ventricle.

Aortic Stenosis. Aortic stenosis is an obstruction to flow across the aortic valve during systole. This obstruction to flow creates a resistance to ejection and increased pressure in the left ventricle.

Aortic Regurgitation. Aortic regurgitation is due to an incompetent aortic valve. During systole, blood that is ejected into the aorta reenters the left ventricle. In order to maintain normopressures, the left ventricle hypertrophies.

TRICUSPID VALVE DISEASE

The tricuspid valve sits between the right atrium and the right ventricle. Pure lesions of the tricuspid valve are uncommon. Tricuspid stenosis or regurgitation usually develops in combination with other structural disorders of the heart. Lesions of the tricuspid valve are relatively rare occurrences that stress the right side of the heart and produce right ventricular failure.

PULMONIC VALVE DISEASE

Abnormalities of the pulmonic valve are usually congenital defects. Few lesions develop after birth. Pulmonary hypertension, caused by mitral stenosis, pulmonary emboli, or chronic lung disease, can precipitate functional pulmonary regurgitation.

Incidence

Valvular heart disease remains fairly common in the United States, even though the incidence is steadily decreasing as the incidence of rheumatic fever decreases. Mitral valve prolapse syndrome is one of the most common cardiac abnormalities; as much as 5 to 10 per cent of the population is affected.[43] The incidence of the other forms of valvular heart disease is not recorded.

Etiology

Mitral Stenosis. The most common cause of mitral stenosis is rheumatic valvulitis that leads to fibrotic thickening and fusion of the valve. However, only 50 per cent of clients with recognized mitral stenosis recall a history of acute rheumatic fever. Nonrheumatic causes of mitral stenosis include malignant carcinoid, systemic lupus erythematosus, rheumatoid arthritis, and certain viruses.

Mitral Regurgitation. Mitral valve prolapse, coronary artery disease, and rheumatic fever are the most common causes of mitral regurgitation.[58] Regurgitation can occur even in a structurally sound valve from left ventricular failure and dilation causing an enlargement of the valve orifice.

Mitral Valve Prolapse. Mitral valve prolapse appears to be due to connective tissue abnormalities in the valve leaflets. Mitral valve prolapse can also occur in clients with connective tissue disorders, such as Marfan's syndrome and Ehlers-Danlos syndrome.

Aortic Stenosis. Aortic stenosis can be caused by several congenital defects of the aortic valve. It can

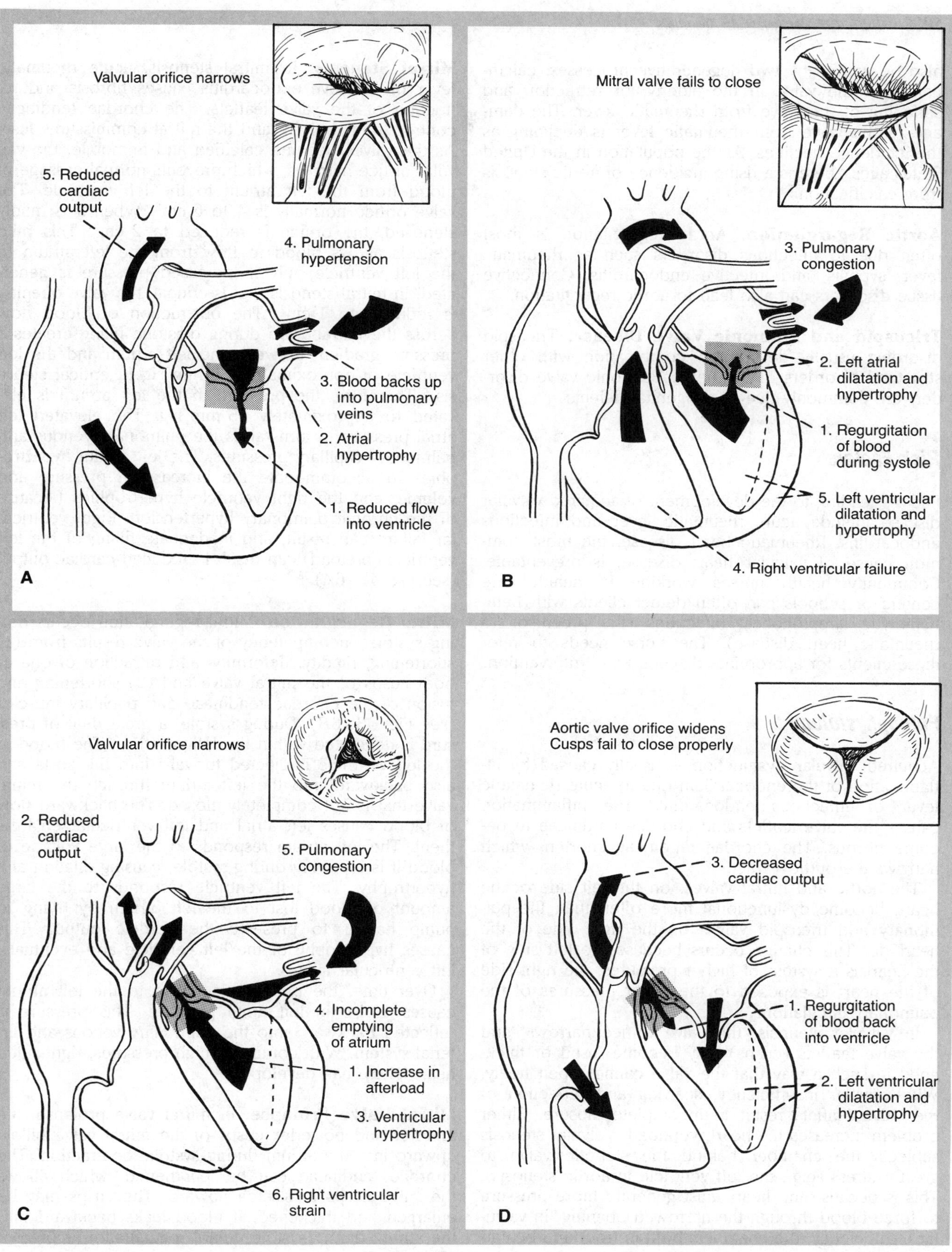

▲ *Figure 43–6*

Cardiac valve disorders. *A*, Mitral stenosis. *B*, Mitral insufficiency. *C*, Aortic stenosis. *D*, Aortic insufficiency.

also be caused by two degenerative processes: calcification of the valve in the elderly, or retraction and stiffening of the valve from rheumatic fever. The damage to the valve from rheumatic fever is declining as the incidence declines. As the population in the United States ages, there is a rising incidence of aortic stenosis from calcification.[59]

Aortic Regurgitation. Aortic regurgitation is most often due to infectious disorders such as rheumatic fever, syphilis, and infective endocarditis. Connective tissue disorders can also lead to aortic regurgitation.

Tricuspid and Pulmonic Valve Disease. Tricuspid disorders usually develop in combination with other structural disorders of the heart. Pulmonic valve disorders are commonly due to congenital defects.

Risk Factors

Factors leading to the development of acquired valvular disease include acute rheumatic fever and infectious endocarditis. Rheumatic heart disease, the most common cause of valvular heart disease, is preventable. Community health nurses working in health care centers or schools can often detect clients with beta-hemolytic streptococcal infections (the precursor to rheumatic heart disease). The nurse needs to refer these clients for appropriate diagnosis and intervention.

Pathophysiology

Acquired valvular dysfunction is usually caused by inflammation of the endocardium due to acute rheumatic fever or infectious endocarditis. The inflammation causes the valve leaflets and chordae tendineae to become fibrous. The chordae tendineae shorten, which narrows the outflow tract.

The aortic and mitral valves, on the left side of the heart, become dysfunctional more often than the pulmonary and tricuspid valves on the right side of the heart do. This change occurs because the left side of the heart is a system of higher pressures; the right side of the heart is exposed to the lower pressures of the pulmonary circulation.

In valvular stenosis, the valve orifice narrows, and the valve leaflets (cusps) may become fused or thickened in such a way that the valve cannot open freely. With valvular insufficiency, scarring and retraction of the valve leaflets result in incomplete closure. Either problem increases the heart workload. Valvular stenosis subjects the chamber behind the stenotic valve to greater stress (e.g., the left ventricle in aortic stenosis). This is because the heart must generate more pressure to force blood through the narrowed opening. In valvular insufficiency, the chambers both in front and behind the valve are taxed.

For a time, the heart may be able to compensate for the additional strain through dilation and eventual hypertrophy. However, if valvular damage worsens, without intervention the heart will eventually fail.

Mitral Stenosis. In mitral stenosis, acute rheumatic fever or infective endocarditis causes fibrosis and retraction of the valve leaflets. The chordae tendineae contract and shorten, and the mitral commissures fuse. As the valves become calcified and immobile, the valvular orifice narrows, which prevents normal passage of blood from the left atrium to the left ventricle. The valve orifice normally is 4 to 6 cm^2. When it is mildly stenosed, the orifice is reduced to 2 cm^2. This mild stenosis allows blood to flow from the left atrium to the left ventricle only if increased pressure is generated. In mitral stenosis that is critical, the valve opening is reduced to 1 cm^2. The obstruction of blood flow across the mitral valve during diastolic filling creates a pressure gradient between the left atrium and the left ventricle of approximately 20 mm Hg in critical stenosis.[7] Therefore, the pressure in the left atrium is elevated to approximately 25 mm Hg. The elevated left atrial pressure in turn raises the pulmonary venous and pulmonary capillary pressures. The left atrium hypertrophies to accommodate the increase in pressure and volume, and the right ventricle hypertrophies because of the chronic pulmonary hypertension. Right ventricular failure can result, and inadequate filling of the left ventricle (preload) can result in reduced cardiac output (see Fig. 43–6*A*).[58]

Mitral Regurgitation. Mitral regurgitation occurs during systole. Incompetency of the valve results from (1) shortening, rigidity, deformity, and retraction of one or both cusps of the mitral valve and (2) shortening and fusion of the chordae tendineae and papillary muscles (see Fig. 43–6*B*). During systole, a great deal of pressure is generated within the left ventricle. The blood in the left ventricle is ejected forward into the aorta and also backward into the left atrium through the mitral valve that is not completely closed. The backward flow of blood causes left atrial and left ventricular enlargement. The left atrium responds to the large volume of blood it is receiving during systole, causing dilation and hypertrophy. The left ventricle responds to the large amount of blood lost to the left atrium by trying to pump harder to preserve the cardiac output. This causes hypertrophy of the left ventricle and eventually left ventricular failure.

Over time, the increase in blood to the left atrium causes a rise in left atrial pressure. This pressure is reflected backward into the pulmonary venous and arterial system. With continued high pressures, right-sided heart failure can develop.

Mitral Valve Prolapse. In mitral valve prolapse, the anterior and posterior cusps of the mitral valve billow upward into the atrium during systolic contraction. The chordae tendineae can be lengthened, which allows the valve cusps to stretch upward. The cusps may be enlarged and thickened. If blood leaks backward into the atrium during systole, mitral regurgitation is present (Fig. 43–7).

Aortic Stenosis. In aortic stenosis, the orifice of the aortic valve becomes narrowed, which causes a decrease in the blood flow from the left ventricle into the

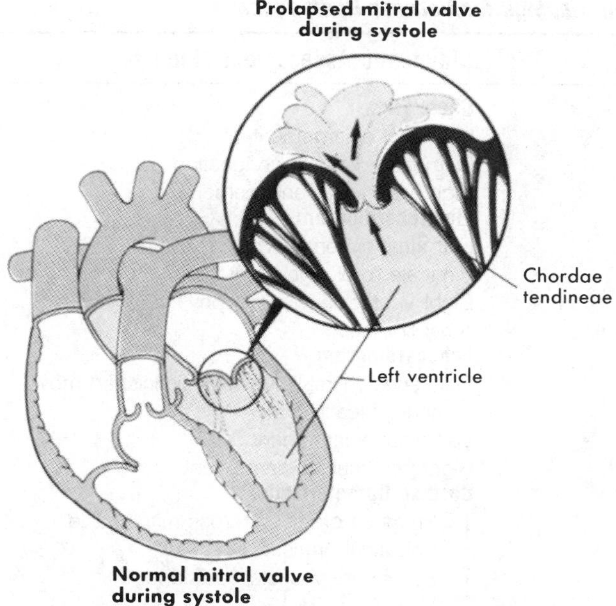

▲ *Figure 43-7*

Mitral valve prolapse. Normal mitral valve *(left)* and prolapsed mitral valve *(inset)*. Prolapse permits the valve leaflets to billow back into the atrium during left ventricular systole. The billowing causes the leaflets to part slightly, permitting regurgitation into the atrium. (From McCance, K., & Huerther, S. [1990]. *Pathophysiology: The biologic basis for disease in adults and children.* St. Louis: Mosby-Year Book.)

aorta. The pressure within the left ventricle rises as the blood is ejected through the narrowed opening. A pressure gradient develops between the left ventricle and the aorta. The elevation of the pressure in the left ventricle during systole causes the ventricle to hypertrophy. Dilation of the left ventricle occurs over time when there is a deterioration of the contractility of the hypertrophied muscle. Eventually, dilation and hypertrophy of the left ventricle are unable to maintain adequate cardiac output. There is a rise in left ventricular end-diastolic pressure, decrease in cardiac output, and increase in pulmonary hypertension (see Fig. 43-6*C*).

Aortic Regurgitation. Aortic regurgitation (aortic insufficiency) is a diastolic event in which blood that is propelled forward into the aorta is allowed to regurgitate backward into the left ventricle through an incompetent valve. This causes abnormal filling and a volume overload of the left ventricle. The magnitude of the overload depends on the severity of the incompetence. However, a small incompetent area can result in a significant aortic regurgitation over time.

Because the left ventricle receives blood from both the atrium and the systemic circulation, aortic regurgitation will gradually increase left ventricular end-diastolic volume. Left ventricular stroke volume is increased to produce an effective forward moving stroke volume into the systemic circulation. There is a compensatory dilation in the left ventricle but minimal increase in left ventricular end-diastolic pressure.[59] As much as 60 per cent of the stroke volume can be regurgitated, markedly increasing left ventricular workload. The compensatory mechanisms of dilation and hypertrophy help maintain an adequate cardiac output. However, as the condition progresses and the contractile state of the myocardium declines, cardiac output falls (see Fig. 43-6*D*).

Tricuspid and Pulmonic Valve Disease. Because the tricuspid valve is on the right side of the heart, the major hemodynamic alterations with tricuspid stenosis are decreases in cardiac output and increased right atrial pressures. The inability of the right atrium to propel blood across the stenosed valve explains these changes. Likewise, with tricuspid regurgitation, the pressures in the right atrium are elevated. In this situation, however, it is due to regurgitation of the blood volume in the right ventricle back into the right atrium during systole.

Pulmonic stenosis and regurgitation lead to decreases in cardiac output because blood does not reach the left side of the heart in adequate supply for metabolic demands. Right-sided heart failure can also develop.

Clinical Manifestations

Mitral Stenosis. The symptoms of mitral stenosis may appear gradually or suddenly (Table 43-4).

On auscultation, a loud first heart sound and then an opening snap that ushers in a low-pitched, rumbling diastolic murmur will be heard. The opening snap is best heard at the apex with the diaphragm of the stethoscope. The diastolic murmur is best heard at the apex using the bell of the stethoscope while the client is in a left lateral recumbent position.[5]

Atrial fibrillation is a common finding in clients with mitral stenosis. During episodes of atrial fibrillation, the pulse becomes irregular and faint, and the blood pressure often drops.

Up to 20 per cent of clients with mitral stenosis will develop systemic embolization.[58] Ineffective atrial contractions allow some stagnation of blood in the left atrium and encourage the formation of mural thrombi. These thrombi easily break away and travel as emboli throughout the arterial system, causing tissue infarction.

Mitral Regurgitation. Clients with mitral regurgitation may be asymptomatic, but if the cardiac output falls, symptoms will develop. When cardiac output falls, fatigue and dyspnea are the first symptoms. Symptoms gradually increase to include orthopnea, paroxysmal nocturnal dyspnea, and peripheral edema. Pulmonary symptoms are less severe than in mitral stenosis because changes in the mean pulmonary capillary pressure are less exaggerated. However, when the right side of the heart is affected, the symptoms are the same as in mitral stenosis (see Table 43-4).

Auscultation reveals a blowing, high-pitched systolic murmur with radiation to the left axilla, heard best at the apex. The first heart sound may be diminished, and often a splitting of the second sound will be heard. Severe regurgitation is associated with a third heart sound (S_3).

TABLE 43-4. Clinical Manifestations and Diagnostic Assessment Findings for Valvular Heart Disease

Valve Disorder	Clinical Manifestations	Diagnostic Assessment Findings
Mitral stenosis	Diastolic, rumbling, low-pitched murmur—at apex Loud snapping S_1 Dyspnea, orthopnea, PND Fatigue Palpitations Pulmonary crackles Hemoptysis Cough Neck vein distention Narrowed pulse pressure Hoarseness Peripheral edema	**Chest Film** Left atrial enlargement Pulmonary venous congestion Right ventricular enlargement **Electrocardiogram** Left atrial hypertrophy P-mitrale (prolonged, notched P wave) Right ventricular hypertrophy Atrial fibrillation **Echocardiogram** Thickened mitral valve with diminished movement of leaflets Left atrial enlargement Right ventricular enlargement **Cardiac Catheterization** ↑ Pressure gradient across mitral valve ↑ Left atrial pressure ↑ Pulmonary vascular resistance ↑ LVEDP, ↑ PAWP ↓ Cardiac output
Mitral regurgitation (insufficiency)	Pansystolic, blowing, high-pitched murmur—at apex, radiating to axilla Weakness, fatigue Left ventricular failure: dyspnea, orthopnea, PND, pulmonary crackles, S_3 and S_4 Palpitations Right ventricular failure: neck vein distention, peripheral edema, hepatomegaly	**Chest Film** Left atrial and ventricular enlargement Pulmonary vascular congestion **Electrocardiogram** Left atrial hypertrophy P-mitrale Atrial fibrillation Left ventricular hypertrophy **Echocardiogram** Bizarre motion of mitral leaflets Hyperdynamic left ventricle Enlarged left atrium and ventricle **Cardiac Catheterization** ↑ Left atrial pressure ↑ Amount of regurgitant flow Rule out prolapse and congenital disorders ↑ LVEDP (preload), ↑ PAWP ↓ Cardiac output
Aortic stenosis	Systolic, harsh, crescendo-decrescendo murmur—right sternal border radiating to neck Dyspnea, orthopnea, PND S_3 and S_4 Fatigue Vertigo and syncope Chest pain Ventricular tachycardia Bradycardia Low pulse pressure Palpable thrill at second right intercostal space	**Chest Film** Calcification of aortic valve Left ventricular enlargement Prominent ascending aorta **Electrocardiogram** Left ventricular hypertrophy Sinus tachycardia, atrial fibrillation Atrioventricular conduction delay Left and right bundle branch block **Echocardiogram** Limited aortic valve movement Thickened left ventricular wall **Cardiac Catherization** ↑ Pressure gradient in systole across aortic valve ↓ Size of aortic orifice ↑ LVEDP

TABLE 43-4. Clinical Manifestations and Diagnostic Assessment Findings for Valvular Heart Disease Continued

Valve Disorder	Clinical Manifestations	Diagnostic Assessment Findings
Aortic regurgitation (insufficiency)	Diastolic, blowing, decrescendo murmur—left sternal border, increases with inspiration Loud S_2 Dyspnea, orthopnea, PND Fatigue, weakness Syncope Palpitations (water-hammer pulse) Pulmonary congestion, S_3 and S_4 Sinus tachycardia, PVCs Wide pulse pressure Large and diffuse diastolic thrill, left sternal border Neck vein distention, ankle edema, hepatomegaly, ascites	**Chest Film** Calcification of aortic valve Left ventricular enlargement Dilation of ascending aorta **Electrocardiogram** Left ventricular hypertrophy Sinus tachycardia, PVCs **Echocardiogram** Dilated and hyperdynamic left ventricle Enlargement of aortic root and left atrium Early closure of mitral valve Diastolic fluttering of aortic valve **Cardiac Catheterization** ↓ Aortic diastolic pressure ↑ LVEDP ↑ Regurgitant flow Reflux through aortic valve
Tricuspid stenosis	Diastolic, rumbling murmur—left sternal border, increases with inspiration Signs of right ventricular failure: neck vein distention, peripheral edema, hepatomegaly, right upper quadrant pain	**Chest Film** Right atrial enlargement **Electrocardiogram** Tall, peaked P wave—right atrial hypertrophy Atrial arrhythmias **Echocardiogram** Thickening and abnormal motion of tricuspid valve **Cardiac Catheterization** ↑ Pressure across tricuspid valve
Tricuspid regurgitation (insufficiency)	Same as for tricuspid stenosis	**Chest Film** Right atrial and ventricular enlargement **Electrocardiogram** Tall, peaked P wave Right ventricular hypertrophy **Echocardiogram** Right ventricular dilation Paradoxic septal motion Tricuspid valvular thickening and abnormal motion

LVEDP, left ventricular end-diastolic pressure; PAWP, pulmonary artery wedge pressure; PND, paroxysmal nocturnal dyspnea; PVCs, premature ventricular contractions.

Vital signs are usually normal unless the client has severe mitral regurgitation. Atrial fibrillation is common in clients with this condition. However, emboli and hemoptysis occur far less often than in mitral stenosis.

Mitral Valve Prolapse. It is not uncommon for many clients with mitral valve prolapse to be completely asymptomatic. In a healthy client, a physical examination may reveal a regurgitant murmur or a midsystolic click on auscultation. If symptoms are present, they may include tachycardia, lightheadedness, syncope, fatigue, weakness, dyspnea, chest discomfort, anxiety, and palpitations related to dysrhythmias.[56] Symptoms may be vague. Mitral valve prolapse has recently been associated with an autonomic dysfunction in which large quantities of catecholamines are produced, with or without adrenergic stimulation. This may help explain the vague and various symptoms.[11] There is minimal morbidity and mortality associated with mitral valve prolapse. Clinically, clients have no physical limitations.[56]

Aortic Stenosis. Symptoms of aortic stenosis tend to occur gradually and late in the course of the disease. There is usually a long latent period in which the client is asymptomatic. Symptoms begin to appear as the obstruction and ventricular pressure increase to critical levels. Angina pectoris is a frequent symptom in approximately 60 per cent of clients. The character of the angina is similar to that in clients with coronary artery disease. The angina commonly is brought on by exertion and relieved by rest. Myocardial oxygen consumption is higher in clients with aortic stenosis because of the hypertrophy of the left ventricle, and this probably accounts for the angina.[59]

Syncope is another frequent clinical manifestation. It also occurs during exertion because of a fixed cardiac output and an increased demand.[7] Syncope at rest may be due to arrhythmias. Exertional dyspnea, paroxysmal nocturnal dyspnea, and pulmonary edema occur with increasing pulmonary venous hypertension due to left ventricular failure.

In severe aortic stenosis, additional symptoms may include palpitations, fatigue, and visual disturbances. Sudden death occurs in 15 to 20 per cent of symptomatic clients as a result of dysrhythmias and myocardial ischemia.[59]

On auscultation, the systolic murmur may be associated with a diminished second heart sound and an early ejection click. There will be systolic thrill over the aortic areas (see Table 43–4).

Aortic Regurgitation. Clients with chronic severe aortic regurgitation may have a long period of time with no symptoms. During this time, the left ventricle gradually enlarges. Clients may complain of an uncomfortable awareness of the heart beat and palpitations. These symptoms are due to the large left ventricular stroke volume with rapid diastolic runoff. This is also apparent with prominent pulsations in the neck and even head bobbing with each heart beat. Sinus tachycardia or premature ventricular contractions may make palpitations more pronounced.

On physical examination, the client may have an increased systolic blood pressure due to the large stroke volume and a decreased diastolic blood pressure due to the regurgitation and distal runoff. Carotid artery pulsations may be exaggerated. The arterial pulse pressure widens, and palpable pulse amplitude increases. This may be noted as a sudden sharp pulse, followed by a swift collapse of the diastolic pulse (Corrigan's or water-hammer pulse). Auscultation reveals a soft, high-pitched, blowing decrescendo diastolic murmur heard best at the second right intercostal space and radiating to the left sternal border (see Table 43–4).

Tricuspid and Pulmonic Valve Disease. Clinical manifestations of tricuspid stenosis are dyspnea and fatigue, pulsations in the neck, and peripheral edema. Physical assessment reveals prominent waves in the neck veins as the atrium is vigorously contracting against the stenotic valve. A diastolic murmur is heard best along the left lower sternal border. The murmur increases with inspiration. The ECG reveals tall, tented P waves in leads II, III, and aV (see Table 43–4).

Tricuspid insufficiency causes hepatic congestion and peripheral edema. The client often has atrial fibrillation and evident jugular waves. The murmur is holosystolic along the left sternal border.

Pulmonic regurgitation may lead to dyspnea and fatigue. The murmur is a high-pitched diastolic blow along the left sternal border. There are no significant changes in the ECG. Pulmonic stenosis causes similar clinical manifestations except that the murmur is often a crescendo-decrescendo type.

DIAGNOSTIC ASSESSMENT

Various diagnostic assessments are used to detect valvular lesions or structural heart changes. These studies include echocardiography, chest radiography, or cardiac catheterization. Table 43–4 summarizes clinical manifestations and diagnostic assessment findings for valvular disorders.

Medical Management

Mitral Stenosis. Untreated mitral stenosis can progress from mild disability to severe disability in about 5 years.[58] Improvement of symptoms can be achieved with oral diuretics and a diet restricted in sodium. Digitalis is useful in clients with atrial fibrillation for slowing the ventricular heart rate. Beta-blockers may decrease the heart rate and therefore increase exercise tolerance. Anticoagulants are helpful in clients who are not anticipating surgical intervention.

Mitral Regurgitation. Symptom reduction is the aim of nonsurgical treatment of mitral regurgitation. The client should restrict physical activities responsible for producing fatigue and dyspnea. Reducing sodium intake and promoting sodium excretion with diuretics will lessen the work of the heart. Nitrates and angiotensin-converting enzyme inhibitors have demonstrated hemodynamic improvement and symptom relief in clients with chronic mitral regurgitation.[58]

Mitral Valve Prolapse. Treatment of mitral valve prolapse depends on the symptoms. Beta-blockers are helpful in relieving syncope, palpitations, and chest pain. For preventing infective endocarditis, the client is given antibiotics prophylactically before any invasive procedures.

Aortic Stenosis. Noninvasive assessment of clients with Doppler echocardiography should be done. Those clients with known or suspected critical obstruction of the aortic valve should be told to avoid vigorous athletic and physical activity. Clients with mild obstruction may continue exercise if it is tolerated.

Prophylactic antibiotics should be given for invasive medical or dental procedures for prevention of infective endocarditis. Digitalis and diuretics that are usually used for ventricular failure will not help in aortic stenosis because the mechanical obstruction to outflow will not be reduced.[56] Beta-blockers will usually not be used because they can depress myocardial function and induce left ventricular failure. Cardiac dysrhythmias should be treated pharmacologically.

Aortic Regurgitation. Medical intervention for aortic regurgitation is the same as for aortic stenosis: to relieve the manifestations of congestive heart failure and to prevent infection of the already deformed aortic cusps.

Tricuspid and Pulmonic Valve Disease. Surgery is common in the management of clients with tricuspid stenosis. However, before surgery on the tricuspid valve can be performed, the diseased mitral valve (stenosis) must often be corrected.

Tricuspid stenosis usually responds well to diuretics and digitalis therapy. If the leaflets are severely stenotic, surgery may be required.

Treatment of pulmonic valve disorders is usually symptomatic and, again, surgery may be required.

Surgical Management

When conservative medical intervention fails to improve hemodynamics in valvular disorders, surgical intervention is indicated. The surgeon usually performs valve repair or replacement for severe valvular defects that are accompanied by left ventricular dysfunction and heart failure. Valvular surgery must be performed at an appropriate time during the course of the disease. The projected natural history of the condition, the degree of impact on the client's lifestyle, and the projected performance of the artificial valve are factors that the surgeon and the client consider before valvular surgery is performed. Valvular repairs are discussed later in the chapter.

Mitral Stenosis. Because medical management cannot reduce the obstruction through the valve in mitral stenosis, surgery is frequently the treatment of choice. Surgical intervention is divided into two types, valve replacement and valve reconstruction. Replacement of the valve is associated with more complications than are reconstructive procedures. Mitral commissurotomy is frequently the reconstructive procedure of choice if the mitral valve is pliable. Clients with mitral valves that are not pliable usually must have the mitral valve replaced.

Mitral Regurgitation. Surgical intervention should be done before severe left ventricular dysfunction develops. Surgical intervention is of two types: repair or replacement. Repair or reconstruction of the mitral valve is now the treatment of choice if the natural valve is not thickened, severely deformed, or calcified. Replacement of the valve is considered if the reconstructive procedure is not likely to be sufficient.[7, 13, 48]

Mitral Valve Prolapse. Surgical intervention is not usually needed for mitral valve prolapse.

Aortic Stenosis. Surgical intervention should be considered for aortic stenosis when the pressure gradient is greater than 50 mm Hg or the valve orifice is less than 0.8 cm^2. Clients with symptomatic aortic stenosis have a poor prognosis without surgical intervention. There is an increase in sudden death once myocardial failure develops.[48]

Aortic Regurgitation. Surgical replacement of the incompetent valve provides the only effective long-term intervention for aortic regurgitation. The surgeon's critical concern involves the proper timing of the surgery. In clients with acute, severe aortic regurgitation and left ventricular failure, early valve replacement can be lifesaving. A high percentage of patients with aortic regurgitation and aortic stenosis show striking clinical improvement with valve replacement.[7]

Tricuspid and Pulmonic Valve Disease. Intervention for tricuspid valve disorders involves correction of the valvular deformity, usually with annuloplasty and alleviation of the heart failure. Interventions for pulmonic valve disease focus on ameliorating the underlying cause and the presenting signs of right-sided heart failure.

Nursing Management

ASSESSMENT

Nursing assessment involves gathering subjective and objective data concerning (1) the type, severity, and progress of the valvular disorder; (2) the degree of heart failure; (3) the client's tolerance to activity; (4) the client's support systems; and (5) the degree of knowledge that the client and family have concerning the nature of and intervention for the disorder.

NURSING INTERVENTION

Nursing Diagnosis: Decreased Cardiac Output R/T valvular abnormalities and arrhythmias.

Planning: Expected Outcomes. The client will maintain or restore a normal cardiac output, as evidenced by clear lungs on auscultation, maintenance of stable weight, urine output averaging greater than 30 ml/hr, no reported (or observed) dyspnea or orthopnea, vital signs within normal limits, regular heart rhythm, absence of S_3 and S_4 heart sounds, and decreased or absent peripheral edema.

Implementation. The main focus of nursing intervention for valvular heart disease is to help the client maintain a normal cardiac output, thereby preventing manifestations of heart failure, venous congestion, and inadequate tissue perfusion. To evaluate the effectiveness of therapeutic interventions, perform ongoing hemodynamic assessment. Monitor vital signs closely every 1 to 4 hours. A decrease in cardiac output is manifested in a compensatory rise in heart rate, a drop in blood pressure, or a decrease in urinary output. Carefully auscultate the chest to identify the presence of adventitious breath sounds (crackles, rhonchi) or heart gallops (S_3, S_4) every 4 hours.

Nursing Diagnosis: Individual Coping, Ineffective R/T chronic nature of valvular disease and activity limitations.

Planning: Expected Outcomes. The client will use adaptive coping strategies, as evidenced by the ability to recognize personal coping patterns and identify appropriate support systems and personal strengths.

Implementation. Clients may find it difficult to cope physically and psychosocially after discharge. The chronicity of valvular heart disease and its potential complications can create an atmosphere of uncertainty, fear, and frustration. Take time to help the client identify support persons, personal strengths, and coping strategies. Assess how the client handles frustration or anger and what activities are particularly relaxing. Address the client's fears and misconceptions. In some instances, counseling referrals may help. Stress the importance of follow-up physical examinations and intervention.

Valvular heart disease requires lifelong management. Having a sincere desire to understand and accept each client's response to chronic illness, the nurse can help the client with valvular heart disease adapt to difficult lifestyle changes and achieve a positive sense of well-being.

EVALUATION

The degree of attainment of expected outcomes should be evaluated on an ongoing basis. Because valvular disorders are chronic, extended time frames may be needed for goal attainment. Revisions in the plan of care may be required.

Post-hospital Care

DISCHARGE TEACHING

Before discharge, prepare detailed teaching material for the client and family concerning the therapeutic regimen, the disease process, factors contributing to symptoms, and the rationale for intervention.

Give information concerning prescribed medications. Medications frequently prescribed include digoxin, quinidine, diuretics, beta-blockers, potassium supplements, anticoagulants, and prophylactic antibiotics. Clearly explain their rationale, dosages, side effects, and special considerations in their use.

Review exercise prescriptions with the client. Clients with aortic stenosis often require activity restrictions. The client should demonstrate the ability to pace activity, verbalize improvement in fatigue, and express acceptance of any imposed activity restrictions.

Address dietary restrictions and plan interdisciplinary follow-up. Make sure the client knows whom to call when questions arise.

CARDIAC SURGERY

Cardiac surgery is performed when the probability of survival with a useful life is greater with surgical treatment than with nonsurgical treatment. The first heart surgery was performed in 1923 by Cutler and Levine.[27] That procedure was repair of a stenosed mitral valve. Since that time, heart surgery has been revolutionized by the development of open-heart techniques that allow surgeons to visualize the heart directly while they explore, incise, repair, and suture. These improved operating conditions have enabled today's surgeons to replace diseased valves with prosthetic valves, repair severe congenital lesions, and perform heart transplants. Today, under ideal conditions, cardiac surgery should have a hospital mortality approaching zero. However, a description of the results of cardiac surgery by hospital mortality alone is not sufficient. The preoperative condition of the client's heart and other body systems greatly influences the results of cardiac surgery. The identification of incremental risk factors will continue to improve results.

Types of Heart Surgery

There are three types of cardiac surgery: (1) reparative, (2) reconstructive, and (3) substitutional. Reparative surgeries are likely to produce cure or excellent and prolonged improvement. These operations include closure of patent ductus arteriosus, atrial septal defect, and ventricular septal defect; repair of mitral stenosis; and simple repair of tetralogy of Fallot. Reconstructive procedures are more complex. They are not always curative procedures, and reoperation may be needed. Reconstructive procedures include coronary artery bypass grafting and reconstruction of an incompetent mitral, tricuspid, or aortic valve. Substitutional surgeries are not usually curative because of the preoperative condition of the client. Examples of substitutional surgeries include valve replacement, cardiac replacement by transplantation, ventricular replacement or assistance, and cardiac replacement by mechanical devices.

Valvular Surgery

The repair or replacement of cardiac valves with acquired stenosis or incompetence is not considered curative, but generally good and long-lasting palliation results. Cure is usually unable to be obtained because of the preoperative condition of the heart or other body systems. Indications for surgery include

- progressive impairment of cardiac function due to scarring and thickening of the valve with either (1) impaired narrowing of the valvular opening (stenosis) or (2) incomplete closure (insufficiency, regurgitation)
- gradual enlargement of the heart with symptoms of decreased activity, shortness of breath, and congestive heart failure.

Surgical therapy for mitral valve stenosis can include valve commissurotomy or valve replacement. Commissurotomy or valve reconstruction can be accomplished if the preoperative assessment indicates that the valve is quite pliable. If the valve is nonpliable, valve replacement is necessary. In clients with mitral regurgitation, valve reconstruction or annuloplasty may be done. This may include the use of a flexible ring that is sewn into the valve for stabilization. Clients experiencing aortic stenosis may be surgically treated with valve replace-

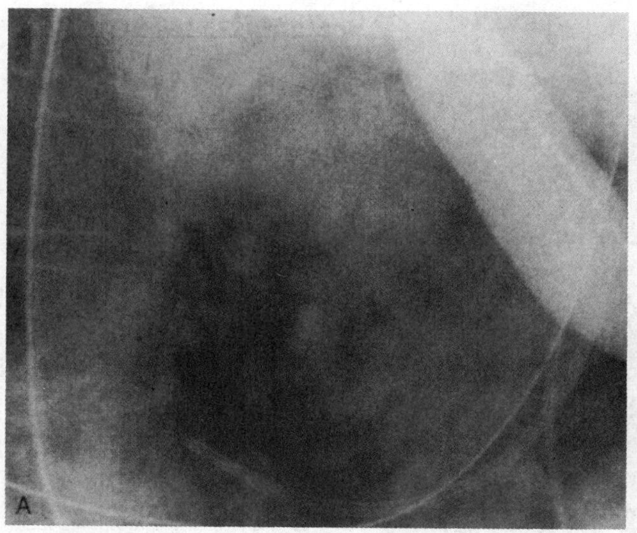

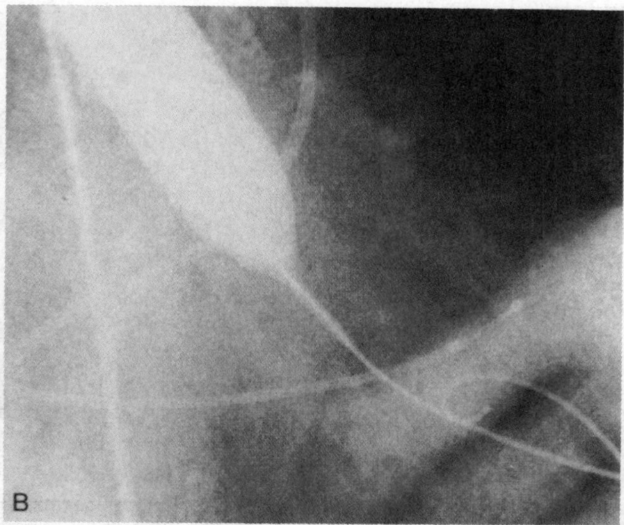

▲ *Figure 43-8*

A, Valvuloplasty balloon inflated across the aortic valve. Note the indentation ("waist") in the balloon. *B*, Valvuloplasty balloon inflated across the aortic valve after dilation. Note the disappearance of the indentation seen in *A*. (From Barden, C., et al. [1990]. Balloon aortic valvuloplasty: Nursing care implications. *Critical Care Nurse, 10*(6), 26.)

ment or balloon aortic valvuloplasty. The valvuloplasty procedure uses a catheter with a balloon to dilate the valve orifice (Fig. 43-8).[4] Surgical treatment for the client with aortic regurgitation is not always the treatment of choice but may be considered.

Artificial cardiac valves are continuing to show improvements in design, safety, function, and durability. Mechanical and tissue prosthetic valves are currently available. The type of valve prosthesis used is based on a number of considerations. The surgeon primarily considers the client's tolerance of anticoagulation and the durability of the valve. Clients with mechanical valves require continuous anticoagulation therapy for the remainder of their lives. Therefore, if the client has a preoperative history of bleeding or noncompliance with pharmacologic regimens, the surgeon may decide to use a tissue valve. The overall advantages and disadvantages of tissue and mechanical valves are almost equal. The mechanical valves are very durable but require anticoagulant therapy; the tissue valves may not require anticoagulation therapy but are less durable. Some physicians generally recommend mechanical valves in clients under 65 or 70 years of age and tissue valves in clients 70 years or older.[7] Artificial valves are shown in Figure 43-9.

Potential complications of heart valves include a risk of thrombus formation, especially in mechanical valves. Newer types of heart valves have reduced rates of thrombus. Most clients require long-term anticoagulation. The major risk with tissue valves is durability. The leaflets of these valves may degenerate, calcify, or develop structural abnormalities. Mitral valves tend to fail most often because of the higher stress on the valve. The rate of tissue valve failure is 2 to 5 per cent for the first 6 years, and then the rate accelerates. Almost every client with a tissue valve will require replacement eventually.[51]

Management of the client after heart surgery is discussed later in this section.

Heart Transplantation

Cardiac transplantation is now a standard and effective treatment for clients with end-stage cardiac disease. The clinical use of transplantation is now in its third decade. The first successful human heart transplant was performed in 1967 in South Africa by Dr. Christiaan Barnard. Much publicity and discussion throughout the world has surrounded heart transplantation since that time. Between 1967 and 1970, about 150 heart transplantations were performed with a dismal 85 per cent mortality rate.[73] Almost all institutions stopped performing the operation for several years while advances in the laboratory continued.

In the 1980s, heart transplants were being performed on a routine basis (see Ethical Issues in Nursing). The survival rate has improved dramatically as a result of advances in technique and better control of the rejection process. At Stanford University, the mean life expectancy for clients awaiting transplantation (surgery not performed) is about 3 months. More than 80 per cent of clients who receive transplanted hearts survive for at least 1 year. Approximately 60 per cent of these clients are alive at 5 years. Another important statistic is that 85 per cent of those 1-year survivors have been rehabilitated and have returned to work or school (Fig. 43-10).[37]

Technique. The current orthotopic technique for heart transplant retains a large portion of the right and left atrium in the recipient and implants the donor heart to the atria (Fig. 43-11*A,B,C*). Cardiopulmonary bypass is used during the operation (see later discussion). Tem-

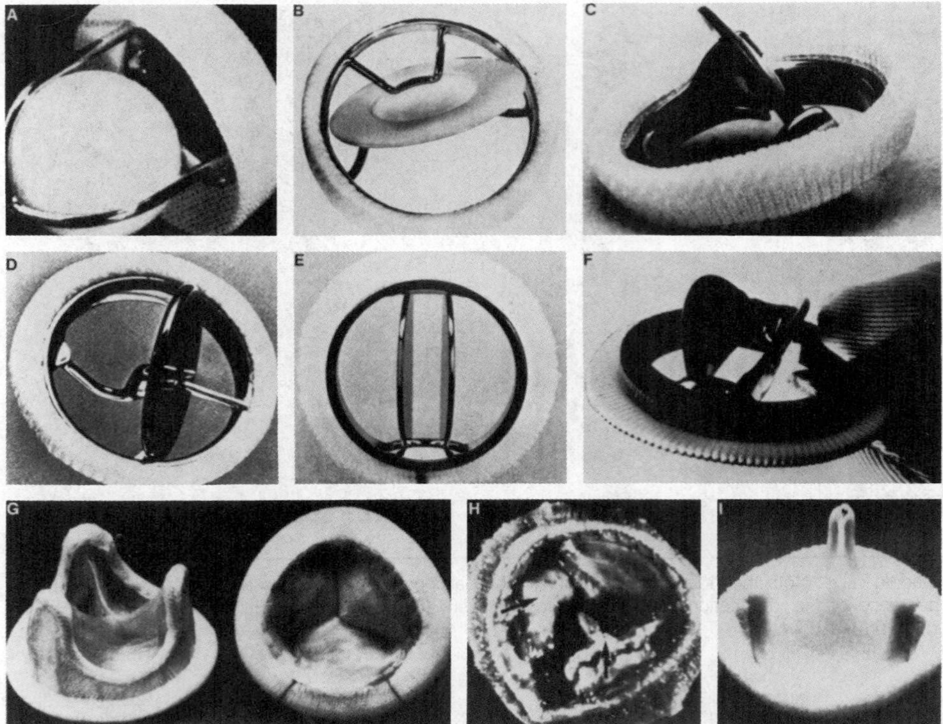

▲ **Figure 43–9**

Prosthetic cardiac valves. *A*, Starr-Edwards caged-ball valve with cloth sewing ring and bare struts. *B*, Björk-Shiley tilting disc valve. *C*, Omniscience tilting disc valve. *D*, Medtronic-Hall tilting disc valve. *E*, St. Jude medical bileaflet valve as viewed end on. Note the large size of the effective orifice area compared with the potential orifice area and the minimal obstruction to flow by the leaflets. *F*, Duromedics bileaflet valve. *G*, Carpentier-Edwards prosthetic valve. *H*, Porcine valve removed several years after implantation because of primary valve failure; arrows point to areas of calcification and destruction of leaflets. *I*, Ionescu-Shiley pericardial valve. (*A* from Starek, P. J. K., and *F* from Clark, R. E. [1987]. *In Heart valve replacement and reconstruction*. Chicago: Year Book Medical Publishers; *B* from Björk, V.; *C* from Austin, E. H., III; *E* and *I* from Crawford, F. A., Jr.; *G* and *H* from Magilligan, D. J., Jr., [1987]. *In* F. A. Crawford [Ed.], *Cardiac surgery: Current heart valve prostheses* [vol. 1]. Philadelphia: Hanley and Belfus; *D* from Cobanoglu, A., & Brockman, S. K. [1986]. *In* W. S. Frankl & A. N. Brest [Eds.], *Valvular heart disease: Comprehensive evaluation and management*. Philadelphia: F. A. Davis.)

ETHICAL ISSUES IN NURSING

Is it Ethical to Keep Dying Post-Transplant Clients Alive Mechanically in Order to Skew Survival Statistics?

Cardiac transplant procedures are becoming more and more common. As technology and scientific knowledge progress, the field of cardiac transplant surgery continues to mature, giving clients with cardiac structure problems hope for a cure from their disorders. Although such procedures are performed with greater frequency, the transplant candidate must meet rigorous standards. Standards for acceptance of a client into a cardiac transplant program vary from institution to institution and from surgeon to surgeon. Clients with the greatest promise for success are the most logical candidates for heart transplants.

Criteria for the selection of such transplant clients may appear unjust in that not all candidates have equal access to the procedure. All candidates do, however, have equal opportunity to qualify. The qualification factors allow that the most promising candidates receive the transplants. Once the most promising of candidates receives a transplant, all activity revolves around the continued success of the operation. The client is monitored very closely, and nursing care is very intense. The most important goal is the client's survival. When complications arise and serious situations compromise the transplant, all efforts are put forth to reverse such complications. There may be situations, however, when all efforts to ward off organ rejection fail and death is imminent.

Although the primary goal of cardiac transplant surgery is in the best interest of the client, could secondary goals be in the best interest of the health care providers or of the institution at which such transplants are performed? Could such secondary goals include the attainment of favorable transplant statistics? Such secondary goals are not, in and of themselves, unethical. On the other hand, is it unethical for transplant clients who have no hope for survival to be kept alive mechanically without further treatment options in order to skew the survival statistics?

Nurses who care for cardiac transplant clients must be very alert to their client's condition, perhaps from moment to moment. When a transplant client has been given every treatment appropriate to the condition and does not respond positively, the nursing staff is acutely aware of the client's prognosis. If futile treatments are continued without hope for survival, nurses should investigate alternative actions with the health care team. Nurses have a responsibility to their clients to question treatment plans that do not benefit their clients.

porary pacemaker wires and chest drainage catheters are inserted.

Another type of heart transplant is the heterotopic transplant. In this form the donor heart is placed parallel to the recipient's heart (Fig. 43–10*D*). The right side of the client's heart can continue to function while the dysfunctional left side of the heart is bypassed.

▲ *Figure 43-10*

Actuarial survival after orthotopic heart transplantation at Stanford University, January 1968 to September 1987. (From Hurst, J. W. [1990]. *The heart* [7th ed.]. New York: McGraw-Hill.)

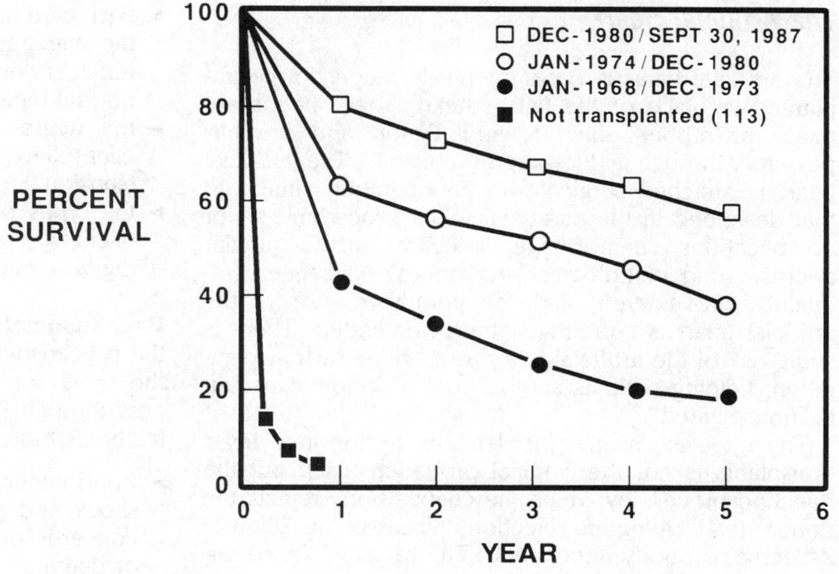

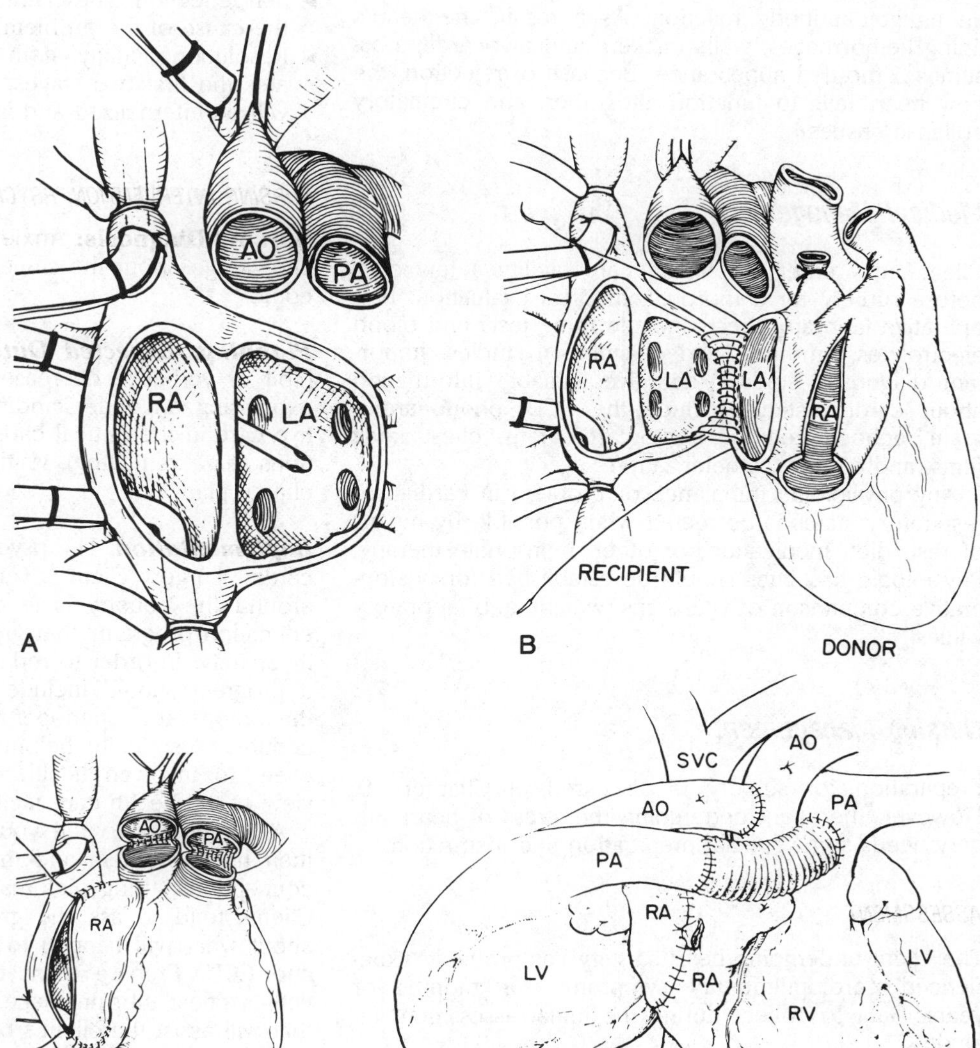

▲ *Figure 43-11*

Cardiac transplantation. *A* to *C*, Orthotopic transplantation. *D*, Heterotopic transplantation. (From Bolman, R. M. [1990]. Cardiac transplantation: The operative technique. *In* M. E. Thompson (Ed.), *Cardiac transplantation*. Philadelphia: F. A. Davis.)

The Artificial Heart

The artificial heart is a commercially made device implanted in place of the failing heart. These hearts are made of rubber, silicone, and Teflon and are air-powered through a life-support console. The artificial heart is attached surgically in an operation similar to that described in the heart transplant procedure. Major complications (hemorrhage, infection, acute tubular necrosis, and neurologic disturbances) have been frequently encountered, and the permanent use of the artificial heart is currently not recommended. There is some use of the artificial heart as a bridge to transplantation, helping patients survive until a donor heart can be transplanted.

The greatest single problem in performing heart transplants is not the surgical procedure itself but the rejection process by which the client's body rejects the donor heart. Allograft rejection, discussed in Chapter 24, remains poorly understood. The recipient forms antibodies against the foreign heart tissue, which leads to an antigen-antibody reaction. As a result, the heart's lining hemorrhages, walls thicken, and myocardium assumes a mottled appearance. Because of rejection, the new heart fails to function altogether, and circulatory collapse ensues.

Medical Management

Clients may enter the health care facility a few days before surgery for a thorough medical evaluation. Preoperative laboratory tests include urine tests and blood electrolytes, enzymes, and coagulation studies. Important diagnostic studies that give valuable information about cardiac status include the ECG, phonocardiogram, echocardiogram, vectorcardiogram, chest x-ray films, and cardiac catheterization.

Any physiologic imbalance or problem in cardiac or respiratory status is corrected when possible by means of rest, diet, medication, or other appropriate therapy. Physiologic baselines should be established for postoperative comparison of vital signs, weight, and laboratory values.

Nursing Management

Preparation for surgery is discussed in Chapter 19. However, the client undergoing the stress of heart surgery needs some special preparation and instruction.

ASSESSMENT

The client undergoing heart surgery has probably experienced cardiopulmonary symptoms for months or years. Data to collect during the initial assessment include

- the primary cardiovascular problem that requires surgical correction and its duration
- the purpose of the surgery and the risk involved
- past cardiopulmonary illnesses that may predispose the client to postoperative complications (e.g., bacterial endocarditis, pulmonary embolus, allergy, abnormal bleeding)
- the degree of cardiac impairment (e.g., does the client have symptoms when at rest or only during exertion?)
- the types of medications and interventions that the client has received or is currently receiving (e.g., digitalis, quinidine, oxygen)

Psychosocial Assessment. The nurse should note the psychosocial readiness for surgery and reactions to the need for heart surgery. Typically, the client will pass through three psychosocial stages when preparing for heart surgery:

- Confrontation. The client may initially experience shock and grief about the impending surgery. Chief concerns may be helplessness and fear of disability or death.
- Self-reflection. The client may try to explain or justify the cause of the problem.
- Resolution. Finally, if the client successfully negotiates the first two stages, the meaning of the surgery will be internalized and incorporated into the "self."

NURSING INTERVENTION: PSYCHOLOGICAL PREPARATION

Nursing Diagnosis: Anxiety, High Risk for R/T lack of knowledge about the surgery and possible fear of outcome.

Planning: Expected Outcomes. The client will exhibit or verbalize decreased anxiety, as evidenced by expressing an understanding of immediate postoperative care in the critical care unit (CCU), usual interventions (e.g., ventilator), visiting hours, and probable discharge plans.

Implementation. The psychological preparation of the cardiac surgery client is very important. Many hospitals around the country have quite extensive preoperative education programs that greatly reduce client and family anxiety. In order to reduce this preoperative anxiety, a program should include a thorough explanation of the preoperative, perioperative, and postoperative procedures. Also quite helpful is the introduction of the client to involved health care team members and a view of the health care facility environment.

Allow clients to tell you in their own words about their heart problem and the surgery. Correct any misconceptions, using pictures and a model of the heart. Clients tend to ask the greatest number of questions about what will happen to them in the recovery room and CCU. Prepare them to awaken from anesthesia with a chest tube in place. Also discuss the ventilator that will assist the client's breathing for the first 8 to 24 hours. Remind clients that during this time they will be unable to talk. Explain that an intravenous line for fluid or blood will be inserted in an arm, and various equipment that continuously monitors vital signs will be attached to the skin. Questions concerning the necessity of using blood products should be answered. Use these facts to respond to concerns about transfusion. Blood transfusions postoperatively are used only as needed; blood is screened carefully, so there is very little risk of contracting acquired immunodeficiency syndrome (AIDS). Family members can be screened for possible donation. Emphasize that although the client will experience pain, the pain will be swiftly relieved by medication and comfort measures.

Finally, explain that the client will be awakened frequently in the CCU for vital nursing assessments and interventions. Give examples of scheduled activities: vital signs every 15 minutes; temperature every 2 hours; frequent turning, coughing, and deep breathing; blood draws for tests every morning.

Clients also need information concerning discharge from the CCU and health care facility. Explain the average length of stay in the CCU, the room to which the client will return from the CCU, the average length of stay in the health care facility, and the diet and activities permitted once the client is back home. Be general in the discussion. Remember that many unforeseen events can arise and greatly alter the postoperative course.

Nursing Diagnosis: Anxiety, High Risk for R/T lack of knowledge regarding the health care facility.

Planning: Expected Outcomes. The client will reduce risk for anxiety as evidenced by verbalizing decreased anxiety and an understanding of the services and visiting policies of the CCU.

Implementation. Give verbal and written information concerning (1) health care facility services, rules, and regulations; (2) visiting hours; (3) the chaplain's name and visitation hours (if appropriate); and (4) names of clinical nurse specialists and other health care professionals who can be contacted for information.

Most clients benefit from a tour of the recovery room and CCU. (If they are not physically able to participate in a tour, audiovisual material is helpful.) Familiarize the client with the equipment that will be used in the CCU (e.g., chest drainage tubes, oxygen apparatus, ventilators, cardiac monitors, and intravenous set-ups). Reassure the client that lights and alarm noises are part of the critical care environment and do not indicate that something is wrong.

NURSING INTERVENTION: PREOPERATIVE CARE

Preparation the evening before and the day of surgery is essentially the same as the preparation of clients for any thoracic surgery (see Chap. 39). The client may often take several showers with an antimicrobial soap; skin prep (shaving) for a thoracotomy is performed in the operating room. If the surgeon plans a coronary artery bypass graft, the legs may also be prepared in the operating room (see Chap. 19).

NURSING INTERVENTION: INTRAOPERATIVE CARE

Cardiopulmonary Bypass. Cardiopulmonary bypass is used during cardiac surgery to divert the client's unoxygenated blood and to return reoxygenated blood to the client's circulation. This technique is called extracorporeal circulation (ECC) and is accomplished with a pump oxygenator (heart-lung machine). The diversion of the client's blood allows the surgeon to visualize the heart directly during the operation. The pump oxygenator, more than any other device, has made sophisticated open-heart surgery possible (Fig. 43-12).

The four purposes of the pump oxygenator are to (1) divert circulation from the heart and lungs, providing the surgeon with a bloodless operative field; (2) perform all gas exchange functions for the body while the client's cardiopulmonary system is at rest; (3) filter, rewarm, or cool the blood; and (4) circulate oxygenated, filtered blood back into the arterial system.

Briefly, the procedure for ECC is as follows.[6] The machine must be primed (filled) before the procedure begins. Historically, this was done with 3 to 4 L of heparinized blood, but today it is usually done with a physiologic crystalloid solution (e.g., Ringer's lactate). After opening the client's chest, the surgeon inserts two large-bore cannulas through the right atrium into the superior and inferior venae cavae and suction catheters into the thoracic cavity and ventricles. Blood is next pumped from the venae cavae, the thoracic cavity, and the ventricles into the pump oxygenator. In the machine, a heat exchanger rewarms (or cools, if the surgeon desires hypothermia) the blood. An oxygenator then removes carbon dioxide from the blood and adds oxygen. Finally, the blood passes through a filter that

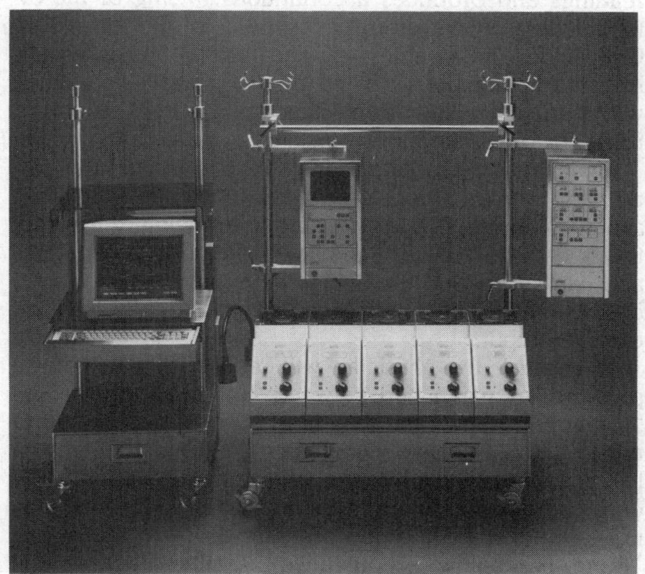

▲ **Figure 43-12**

A Stöckert heart-lung bypass machine with computer-aided perfusion system. During open heart surgery, circulation of oxygenated blood is obtained by using a heart-lung bypass machine. (Courtesy of Sorin Biomedical, Irvine, CA.)

removes air bubbles and other emboli before returning to the body via either the aorta or the femoral artery.

Although the pump oxygenator is considered safe, it does have risks. The pump can crush and destroy blood cells; sludging of cells can lead to thrombus formation; or air emboli can form. Other complications related to ECC are shock, hemorrhage, hemolysis, and kidney or lung damage.

The extracorporeal membrane oxygenator is a more expensive but improved method of ECC. The advantages include decreased trauma to blood cells and prolonged pump time (up to several days). However, the clinical benefits are still being evaluated.[35]

POSTOPERATIVE ASSESSMENT

The most reliable measures of cardiovascular function and tissue perfusion are the vital signs, including arterial blood pressure, pulses, venous and left heart filling pressures, temperature. Heart sounds and continuous ECG monitoring are also performed. Stabilization of vital signs after heart surgery usually indicates adequate cardiovascular function. Conversely, severe deviations indicate complications such as hemorrhage, shock, cardiac tamponade, or infection. The normal ranges for each vital sign after cardiac surgery and the meaning of deviations follow.

Arterial Blood Pressure. To obtain an accurate blood pressure reading postoperatively, the physician (1) places an 18- or 20-gauge Teflon catheter intra-arterially, usually into the radial artery, and (2) attaches this catheter to a strain-gauge transducer via stiff connecting tubing called pressure transmission tubing. This is connected to an electronic pressure monitor and oscilloscope. The monitor provides numerical pressure readings and produces a continuous tracing of the arterial pressure waveform as shown in the Bridge to Critical Care in Chapter 42. The arterial line is usually irrigated (continuously or at intervals) with heparinized water or saline. The arterial line is sometimes used as a route for obtaining blood for laboratory studies.

Most pressure monitors are able to monitor the pulmonary artery, arterial pressures, and ECG tracing simultaneously. This assists in determining the effect that the surgery may have had on hemodynamic status and cardiac output. It can also demonstrate the effect a dysrhythmia or body temperature change may have on cardiac output.

In general, the physician will request that the blood pressure be maintained between 20 mm Hg above and 20 mm Hg below the baseline blood pressure. After mitral and aortic valve surgery, clients may tolerate a low systolic blood pressure of 90 mm Hg without difficulty. After surgery on coronary arteries, clients may not tolerate systolic blood pressure drops of more than 10 mm Hg below preoperative baseline because the myocardium may not be adequately perfused. Maintaining a sufficient diastolic blood pressure is also very important because the myocardium receives 70 per cent of its blood supply during this phase of the cardiac cycle. Careful assessment and monitoring of the client's hemodynamic status is essential.

Pulses. Check radial pulse for rate, rhythm, and volume. Rapid radial pulse may indicate dysrhythmias, shock, fear, fever, hypoxia, congestive heart failure, or hemorrhage. Slow radial pulse may indicate heart block or severe anoxia.

Check apical-radial pulse for a pulse deficit. Pulse deficit may indicate atrial fibrillation, a frequent complication of mitral stenosis.

Assess peripheral pulses. Absence of pedal pulses may indicate presence of peripheral emboli blocking a blood vessel in the extremity. Report this finding immediately to the surgeon. If pulses are absent, assess all pulses in the extremity and check the lower extremities for coldness, pallor, or cyanosis.

Venous and Left Heart Filling Pressures. The central venous and pulmonary artery pressures are usually monitored postoperatively. A pressure higher than normal may be acceptable after open-heart surgery. This is because a heart that has been diseased and then is subjected to surgical trauma is weak and needs a higher filling pressure to (1) strengthen the force of myocardial contraction and (2) maintain an adequate cardiac output. Therefore, the surgeon will usually specify parameters for venous and pulmonary artery pressures that address this problem.

If the client has a Swan-Ganz catheter in place, a pulmonary artery wedge pressure (PAWP) can be obtained and a cardiac output measured by the thermodilution method. The PAWP is a reflection of the left atrial filling pressure (see Bridge to Critical Care for a discussion of the Swan-Ganz catheter and these parameters).

Causes of abnormally elevated central venous pressure and left heart filling pressure include hypervolemia and ineffective myocardial contractions. Abnormally decreased central venous pressure and left heart filling pressure result from hypovolemia.

Body Temperature. Initially, the client has a low temperature of 35° to 36° C (95° to 96.8° F) because of hypothermia induced during surgery. With careful warming in a heating blanket, the client may reach a normal temperature within 4 hours. Be aware that the blood pressure may drop as body temperature elevates.

The temperature may rise 1° to 1.5° C (2° or 3° F) above normal during the first or second day postoperatively and may remain elevated for 3 to 4 days. Treat this with acetaminophen suppositories as prescribed and minimal bed covering. For persistent elevations, apply ice bags or use a hypothermia blanket if prescribed.

Report abnormal findings, such as an elevated temperature to 38.5° C (101° F) or higher or an elevation that persists for more than 4 or 5 days. Abnormal temperature elevation may result from infection, dehydration, hemolysis due to transfusion reaction, or atelectasis. The untoward effects of the elevated temperature include increased metabolic demands (which increase the work of the heart), dehydration, and hypovolemia.

Abnormally low temperatures ranging from 34.4° C (94° F) to 36° C (96.8° F) result from shock or car-

Intra-Aortic Balloon Pumping (IAPB) — Counterpulsation

When the left ventricle fails to support adequate circulation and perfusion, intra-aortic balloon pumping can be used in both medical and surgical settings to support the injured or ischemic myocardium. The device consists of a polyethylene balloon that is inserted via the femoral artery into the descending thoracic aorta distal to the left subclavian artery, and is connected to an external pneumatic pumping system.

The pump inflates the balloon with helium or carbon dioxide during diastole, and deflates it during systole. The inflation-deflation cycle is triggered by the client's ECG, specifically by the R wave which signals the beginning of systole. Balloon deflation during diastole augments coronary artery filling. Systolic balloon deflation decreases afterload.

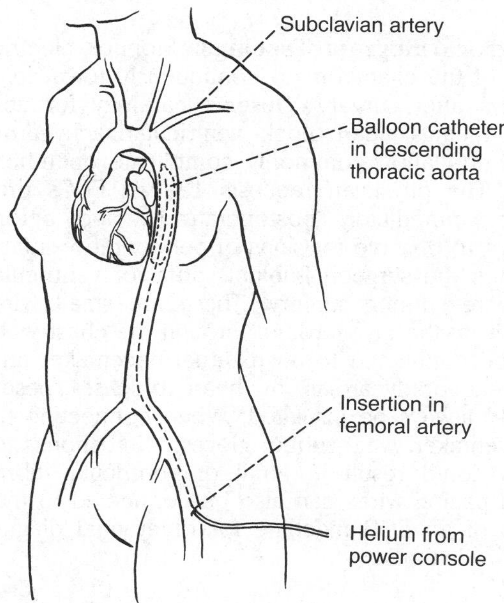

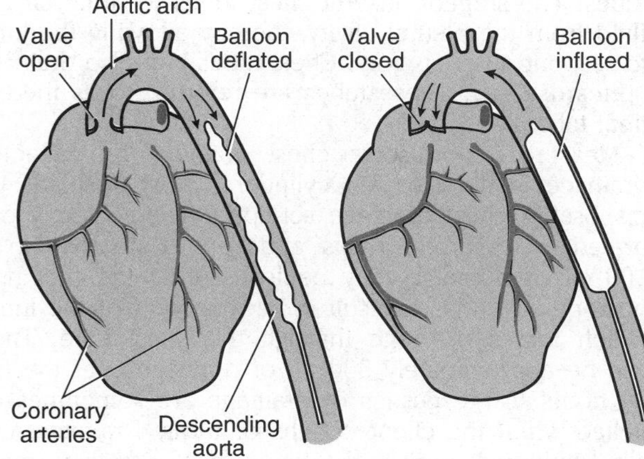

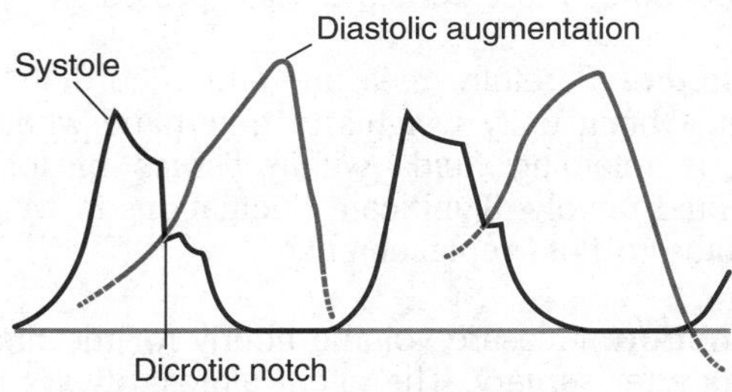

IABP inflating at end of systole (dicrotic notch)
Blood pressure waves

Guidelines For Management of IAPB

Major Goals

- Aids left ventricular ejection
- Improves cardiac output by reducing myocardial (ventricular) workload
- Increases coronary artery perfusion, decreasing myocardial ischemia
- Reduces the amount of myocardial damage
- Provides hemodynamic stability until definitive treatment can be initiated

Indications for Use

- Complications of acute myocardial infarction
  - Cardiogenic shock
  - Papillary muscle rupture or dysfunction with severe mitral valve regurgitation
  - Ventricular septal defect
  - Refractory ventricular arrhythmias related to ischemia
- Left ventricular failure
- Unstable angina refractory to medications
- Preoperative open heart surgery or cardiac transplantation
- Prophylaxis, noncardiac surgeries, high-risk PTCA
- Septic shock
- Low cardiac output syndromes

Complications

- On insertion, dissection of the arterial system (femoral, iliac, aorta)
- Dislodge plaque causing embolization
- Balloon rupture
- Arterial occlusion
- Mechanical destruction of RBCs
- Inability to wean from IABP
- Hematoma at insertion site

Nursing Precautions

- Assessing for alterations in tissue perfusion
- Impair physical mobility
- High risk for alterations in cardiac output
- Anxiety (client and family)
- High risk for sensory perceptual overload
- High risk for infection
- High risk for bleeding

Contraindications

- Aortic aneurysm
- Aortic insufficiency
- Central or peripheral atherosclerosis
- Age
- Severe left ventricular dysfunction
- Multisystem failure
- Chronic debilitating disease
- Bleeding disorder
- History of emboli

diac decompensation. The physician may order a warming blanket to increase temperature.

Respirations. To assess respiratory function, prevent respiratory complications, and provide appropriate intervention, closely monitor the rate and depth of respirations, presence of dyspnea, and presence of wheezing.

Make certain the ventilator is set at a rate that adequately ventilates the client and delivers an appropriate tidal volume and oxygen percentage. A conscious client may initiate respirations in addition to those delivered by the ventilator (usually the assist light will come on). Adjust the rate, tidal volume, and oxygen level so that adequate ventilation of the lungs and oxygenation of the blood are ensured. Adjustments are usually determined by arterial blood gas analysis and the assessments by the physician and the nurse.

Assessment of depth of respiration may reveal shallow respirations, which may be due to pain. Give a narcotic provided vital signs are stable.

Assessment of dyspnea may reveal that the client is "fighting" the ventilator, in other words, breathing against instead of with the machine. This can lead to inadequate ventilation. The client may feel short of breath. Airway obstruction (possibly due to excessive secretions), pain, fear, anoxia, acidosis, hemorrhage, and improper placement of the tube may cause the client to have difficulty in breathing and must be investigated immediately. The physician usually orders arterial blood gas studies and a chest film. The ventilator settings may need adjustment, and the client may require sedation. (See Bridge to Critical Care for ventilators in Chap. 37.) While the client is on the ventilator, make sure the ventilator alarms are functioning. Never turn off the alarms, not even during suctioning.

Wheezing results from pulmonary edema, bronchospasm, or airway obstruction. It may be treated with bronchodilators.

Assess amount of pulmonary secretions: copious or scant.

Assess color. Sputum is normally white and translucent. Yellow color suggests infection and represents the presence of white blood cells. Green represents old retained secretions with the breakdown of white blood cells. Green and foul-smelling secretions usually suggest *Pseudomonas* infection. Red denotes fresh blood. Streaking with red suggests upper airway or tracheal bleeding. Brown represents old blood residue.

Assess for accompanying signs of retained secretions: apprehension, perspiration, rapid pulse, dyspnea, cyanosis, and gurgling respirations.

Assessment of respiration in the preextubation period involves drawing blood for arterial blood gas analysis and measuring respiratory parameters including inspiratory effort and tidal volume. The client is ready for extubation if these values are within normal limits.

Respiratory assessment in the postextubation period begins with careful assessment of clinical manifestations of respiratory distress. Check the rate, depth, and character of respirations frequently. Note the client's skin color and vital signs; changes may indicate inadequate ventilation and the need for reintubation. Arterial blood gases should be analyzed for determining whether the client is breathing adequately after extubation.

Heart Sounds. For the first two days postoperatively, assess heart sounds at least every 4 hours. Pericardial rubs are commonly caused by the irritation and inflammation from surgery. A new murmur may indicate valve problems. Notify the physician if one develops. A gallop probably indicates hypervolemia. See cardiovascular assessment in Chapter 41.

Electrocardiogram Tracings. Monitor electrical activity of the client's heart continuously for at least 3 or 4 days after surgery. Observe carefully for abnormal ECG tracings; heart block, ventricular tachycardia, and atrial fibrillation commonly complicate open-heart surgery. The physician requests 12-lead ECGs preoperatively, immediately postoperatively, and before discharge to observe for signs of perioperative infarction.

Often the surgeon implants atrial or ventricular pacing wires during surgery. These are small wires that lead from the myocardium through the chest wall. They can be connected to an external pacemaker and used to treat bradycardias or heart blocks. These wires should always be insulated. When connecting them to a pacemaker, wear rubber gloves. Microshocks to these wires could result in atrial or ventricular fibrillation. Atrial pacing wires can also be connected to the chest leads of an ECG machine for differential diagnosis of atrial arrhythmias.

Chest Drainage. Check chest drainage from chest tubes. The surgeon inserts chest tubes to drain air and fluid from the pleural cavity, thereby allowing the lungs to respond after surgery. Chest tubes can also drain the pericardial sac. These tubes are referred to as mediastinal tubes.

Measure and observe chest drainage by collecting drainage in a calibrated cylinder. (Most hospitals use disposable chest drainage set-ups that are clearly calibrated). Measure findings and record hourly. Up to 100 ml of drainage may be lost during the first hour postoperatively as a result of reexpansion of the lungs, which forces drainage through the chest tube. There will be approximately 500 ml of drainage over the first 24 hours. Large gushes of drainage are sometimes expelled when the client coughs or turns. Drainage, usually dark red during the early postoperative phase, gradually becomes more serous as time passes.

Fluid Balance. Carefully measure and record intake and output. Obtain daily weights to determine whether the client is retaining fluids within tissues or losing excessive fluid rapidly. Significant fluctuations in weight act as a guide to fluid replacement.

Renal Function. Measure volume hourly for the first 8 to 12 hours after surgery. The client almost always has an indwelling urinary catheter. Normal output is greater than 30 ml/hr. Urine may be bloody as a result of hemolysis of erythrocytes during ECC.

The specific gravity should be assessed. Normal findings are 1.015 to 1.020. Specific gravity may rise because of oliguria or presence of red blood cells. Lowered specific gravity results from overhydration or inability of kidney tubules to filter waste products.

Electrolyte Balance. Daily electrolyte studies are performed to determine blood levels of sodium, potassium, and chloride. The physician replaces electrolytes parenterally if they are deficient. When diuretics are given to reduce volume overload, monitor potassium closely and replace as prescribed. The heart may be particularly sensitive to hypokalemia soon after surgery. Obtain hematocrit, hemoglobin, and prothrombin time daily to determine extent of blood loss or hemorrhage, and daily blood gases to determine the pH, PCO_2, and PO_2 of arterial blood (see Chap. 15).

Neurologic Response. After heart surgery, carefully observe the client's level of consciousness, pupil size and reaction, orientation, and ability to move extremities.

Monitoring Level of Consciousness. The client should awaken within 1 to 2 hours after surgery. Failure to awaken may result from embolization of air, calcium, fat, or thrombotic particles to the brain. Slow return to consciousness (over 2 to 4 days) may result from a diffuse neurologic deficit due to poor cerebral capillary perfusion during ECC.

Monitoring Pupil Size and Reaction. Check pupils hourly during the early postoperative period for size, equality in size, and reaction to light. Pupils dilate when blood contains excess carbon dioxide.

Monitoring Orientation. Disorientation and restlessness may indicate anoxia or embolization to the brain. Also, fatigue or fear can produce mental confusion.

Monitoring Ability to Move Extremities. Hemiplegia, inability to move an extremity, or extreme weakness of an extremity may indicate embolization to the motor area of the brain.

After cardiac surgery, clients may become disoriented, delusional, and psychotic. Severe depression is not uncommon.

Causes of confusion, hallucinations, and psychotic behavior include (1) isolation within the ICU, (2) sensory deprivation, (3) lack of rest and sleep over an extended period, (4) fear and anxiety, (5) an impersonal environment if care providers are preoccupied with monitors and machines, and (6) desynchronization of circadian rhythm (CCUs are active and well-lighted 24 hours a day).

Causes of postoperative depression include (1) fatigue and debility after surgery and (2) resumption of responsibilities.[60]

Nursing Diagnosis: Decreased Cardiac Output, High Risk for R/T heart failure, metabolic acidosis, weakening of the left ventricle, dysrhythmias, and cardiac tamponade.

Planning: Expected Outcomes. The client will have improved cardiovascular function, as evidenced by adequate tissue perfusion, stabilization of vital signs, clear lung sounds on auscultation, stable body weight, adequate urine output (30 ml/h or greater), no reported or observed dyspnea or orthopnea, regular heart sounds without S_3 or S_4 and decreased or absent peripheral edema (blood pressure within 20 mm Hg of baseline values).

Implementation. Intervention for a failing heart muscle often involves administration of inotropic agents (e.g., dopamine, isoproterenol, or epinephrine), which increase cardiac contractility. Administer inotropic agents cautiously because they also increase the work of the heart and its need for oxygen.

Complications resulting from persistent hypotension are cerebral ischemia, renal shutdown, myocardial infarction, and shock. To correct these complications, the surgeon may use some mechanical device to support the failing heart if medications are unsuccessful.

The intra-aortic balloon pump is a counterpulsation device that supports the failing heart by increasing coronary artery perfusion and reducing afterload. It consists of a sausage-shaped balloon catheter that is passed through the femoral artery and positioned in the descending thoracic aorta just distal to the subclavian artery. This catheter is attached to a power console that inflates and deflates the balloon in time with the heart. The balloon is inflated during diastole; blood is pushed back into the aorta, and coronary artery perfusion is improved. The balloon is deflated during systole; resistance is decreased, and thereby the workload of the heart is reduced (see Bridge to Critical Care). The timing of the balloon inflations and deflations is critical. A registered nurse with specific education in the use of the balloon pump is assigned to care for this client. Monitoring the effects of the pumping on the client's vital signs requires special skills.

Collaborative Problem. Hypertension R/T epinephrine release.

Planning: Expected Outcomes. The nurse will monitor the client for hypertension, as evidenced by blood pressure 20 mm Hg over baseline for sustained periods.

Implementation. Hypertension is also dangerous in a client who has undergone a coronary artery bypass graft because the high blood pressure may cause the new graft to break loose or leak. Vasoactive medications can be used to improve cardiac functioning (e.g., vasodilators such as sodium nitroprusside).

Nursing Diagnosis: Airway Clearance, Ineffective, High Risk for R/T retained secretions.

Planning: Expected Outcomes. The client will exhibit improved airway clearance, as evidenced by clear lung sounds, afebrile state, strong nonproductive cough, and arterial blood gas values within normal limits.

Implementation. Frequently turn and suction the intubated client. Help the nonintubated client turn, take deep breaths, and cough every 1 to 2 hours; suction the trachea if the temperature rises above 38.5° C (101° F) and the client is coughing ineffectively. In addition, the client can wear a high-humidity oxygen mask after removal of the endotracheal tube for help in loosening secretions. Chest physiotherapy may be used to loosen secretions. In rare cases, bronchoscopy may be indicated for removal of secretions. Complications of retained secretions include atelectasis, pneumonia, and subsequent inadequate oxygenation of the tissues.

Collaborative Problem. Dysrhythmias, High Risk for R/T potassium imbalance, trauma to the conduction system during surgery, hypoxia, decreased cardiac output, or acidosis.

Planning: Expected Outcomes. The nurse will monitor the client for dysrhythmias, as evidenced by changes in heart rhythm on the ECG.

Implementation. Most dysrhythmias can be effectively treated with antiarrhythmic medications. These medications are listed in Chapter 42. Some life-threatening dysrhythmias require defibrillation or cardioversion (see Chap. 42).

Collaborative Problem. Hemorrhage R/T surgical trauma or slipped ligature.

Planning: Expected Outcomes. The nurse will monitor the client for amounts of drainage in excess of 2 ml/kg body weight/hr or a sustained period of bleeding through the chest tube (over 1 minute).

Implementation. The physician should be notified because the client may need to be returned to the operating room for repair of the bleeding sites.

Replace blood by transfusion as prescribed. The chest drainage may be autotransfused back into the client from the chest drainage system through an intravenous line. The use of blood transfusions has decreased dramatically since the onset of the AIDS virus. However, sometimes it is necessary to replace blood lost during surgery. If the client's hematocrit is adequate, albumin or high-molecular-weight plasma expanders, such as hetastarch, may be prescribed in place of blood.

Collaborative Problem. Cardiac tamponade R/T occlusion in the pericardial drainage system.

Planning: Expected Outcomes. The nurse will monitor the client for sudden cessation of chest drainage with an increase in venous pressure, pulsus paradoxus, dyspnea, oliguria, distant or inaudible heart sounds, or lowered left atrial pressure.

Implementation. Chest tube stripping is no longer performed. Gentle milking of the chest tube to express clots that could block drainage may be performed. If clots cannot be removed by gentle milking of the tube, the physician may need to declot the tube using a long catheter with an inflatable balloon on the end. The client may need to be returned to the operating room or have a pericardial tap for removal of fluid.

Chest wound infection can be prevented with prophylactic administration of antibiotics. The physician orders portable chest films daily until the lungs have reexpanded.

Collaborative Problem. Renal Failure, High Risk for R/T hypovolemia, decreased cardiac output, or hemolysis of erythrocytes during cardiopulmonary bypass.

Planning: Expected Outcomes. The client will have urinary output greater than 30 ml/hr.

Implementation. A client with decreased urine output may be treated with extra fluids (sometimes called a fluid challenge) if dehydration is the probable etiologic factor. Other interventions may include correcting shock or low output failure and administering a diuretic (e.g., furosemide) intravenously. The client who develops renal failure requires peritoneal dialysis or hemodialysis.

Nursing Diagnosis: Fluid Volume Excess, High Risk for R/T fluid volume overload.

Planning: Expected Outcomes. The client will maintain normal hemodynamic parameters and urine output and demonstrate no signs of overhydration.

Implementation. During the course of surgery, the client typically receives 3 to 4 L of extra fluid. Often this fluid accumulates as edema and does not increase the vascular volume very much. However, the fluid does place the client at high risk for circulatory overload. Because of this, intravenous fluids are administered judiciously for the first 3 days postoperatively to avoid overwork of the heart. Typically, 500 to 700 ml/m^2 body surface/24 hr including oral intake (normal surface area is 1.5 to 2.0 m^2) will be given. Administer sodium-containing fluids cautiously to prevent circulatory overload and heart failure.

Collaborative Problem. Paralytic Ileus R/T shunting of blood from the gastrointestinal tract during surgery, side effects of anesthesia and narcotics, immobility, and sympathetic responses.

Planning: Expected Outcomes. The nurse will monitor the client for clinical manifestations of ileus, as evidenced by hypoactive or absent bowel sounds, abdominal distention, nausea, vomiting, lack of appetite, and no passing of flatus.

Implementation. Give sips of water 4 hours after extubation if the client is fully responsive and not nauseated. The client may have clear liquids next, followed by solid foods. Watch for signs of abdominal distention and paralytic ileus (see Chap. 19). If either of these conditions develops, stop oral fluids at once and notify the physician.

Nursing Diagnosis: Pain, High Risk for R/T sternal and leg incision.

Planning: Expected Outcomes. The client will have increased comfort, as evidenced by normal heart rate, no restlessness, normal respiratory rate, reports of comfort, decreasing use of narcotics, and periods of rest.

Implementation. Give narcotic analgesics for pain postoperatively as ordered. Avoid overmedicating a client who is recovering from hypothermia because narcotic metabolism is slowed and the medication may not be excreted.

Attempt to relieve the pain and restlessness with comfort measures before administering a narcotic (see Chap. 16).

Nursing Diagnosis: Tissue Perfusion, Altered Cerebral, High Risk for R/T surgical procedure and hemodynamic stability.

Planning: Expected Outcomes. The client will demonstrate adequate cerebral tissue perfusion, as evidenced by continuous progress toward an alert level of consciousness.

Implementation. To prevent mental confusion, undue fear, anxiety, and tension:

- Always address the client by name and introduce yourself by name.
- Place a calendar and clock at the bedside to orient the client to the date and time of day.
- Take an interest in the client. Do not ignore the client while working with monitors and equipment.
- Position the cardiac monitor so that it is out of the client's view. Many clients are nervous when watching their own heart action.
- Schedule the day so that periods of nursing intervention alternate with periods of rest and relaxation.
- Encourage the client to freely discuss fears and anxieties.
- Prepare significant others for changes in the client's sensorium after surgery. Before visiting times, warn visitors if the client is hallucinating or is severely depressed so that they know what to expect.
- Explain all interventions to the client and allow time for questions.

Nursing Diagnosis: Physical Mobility, Impaired, High Risk for R/T prolonged bed rest after surgery.

Planning: Expected Outcomes. The client will demonstrate postoperative mobility, as evidenced by having mobility that is equal or greater than preoperative mobility.

Implementation. Prolonged periods of bed rest after heart surgery (or any surgery) may cause weakness, pooling of respiratory secretions, atelectasis, thrombophlebitis, osteoporosis, urinary retention, renal calculi, and a negative nitrogen balance. Planned activity is the most important single factor in preventing the complications of bed rest. The type and amount of activity allowed for each client depend on the type of surgery and the client's general postoperative condition.

Turning and Exercising. If the client is stable, turn from side to side at intervals for back care. Perform passive exercises and leg flexion every 2 hours to prevent thrombosis of lower extremities.

Typical Ambulation Schedule. The day after surgery, the client usually dangles her or his legs over the side of the bed for a short period. That evening or on the second postoperative day, the client usually sits in a chair for a brief time. The third to fifth day postoperatively, the client begins to ambulate in the room and down the hallway. By the eighth to tenth day, the client is usually fully ambulatory. Cardiac monitors are used to evaluate the client's response to increasing activity.

It usually takes 8 to 10 weeks for clients to fully regain strength after surgery. On discharge home, the client gradually increases activity until moderate walks and climbing stairs do not cause undue fatigue. The client usually returns to work 2 months after surgery.

Collaborative Problem. Rejection of the Transplanted Heart R/T immune reaction after surgery.

Planning: Expected Outcomes. The nurse will monitor for clinical manifestations of rejection, as evidenced by decreases in oxygenation, fever, malaise, anxiety, and infiltrates on chest film.

Implementation. Rejection and infection are the most common complications of cardiac transplantation. The prevention of rejection with immunosuppression is continually being examined (see immunosuppressive protocol, Box 43-5). Cyclosporine has been helpful in preventing rejection but is quite toxic. Renal failure, hypertension, liver toxic effects, and neurologic disturbances are not uncommon.

Nursing Diagnosis: Infection, High Risk for R/T loss of primary defenses and use of immunosuppressive agents in clients with transplant.

Planning: Expected Outcomes. The client will exhibit no clinical manifestations of infection, as evidenced by remaining afebrile and having white blood cell levels within normal limits, no malaise, and no abnormal heart sounds.

Implementation. Infection remains the major cause of death in the early postoperative period as well as a major cause of death after 1 year. Clients are treated prophylactically with antibiotics. Nonhealing sternal

Box 43–5. Stanford University Immunosuppressive Protocol for Heart Transplantation—1988

- Cyclosporine
  Loading dose 2–8 mg/kg 2–3 hours preoperatively (dose according to preoperative renal function)
  Target serum level (first month) 100–150 ng/ml
  Target serum level (thereafter) 50–150 ng/ml
- Steroids
  Methylprednisolone 500 mg intraoperatively
  Methylprednisolone 125 mg intravenously every 8 hours × 3
  Prednisone beginning 0.6 mg/kg/day + tapering
- Azathioprine
  Loading dose 4 mg/kg intravenously 2–3 hours preoperatively
  Maintenance 1–2 mg/kg/day (to white blood cell tolerance)
- OKT_3
  5 mg intravenously every day × 14 days beginning postoperative day 1

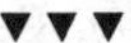

From Hurst, J. W. (1990). *The heart* (7th ed.). New York: McGraw-Hill.

wounds are promptly treated. Omental grafts may be required (see Chap. 72).

EVALUATION

The degree of expected outcome attainment should be examined frequently. Some of the problems discussed in the care of the client after heart surgery require prompt treatment (e.g., dysrhythmias); others can be evaluated over longer periods of time. Revisions in the plan of care may be required.

Post-hospital Care

As the client returns home, the activity level will continue to increase. It takes approximately 6 weeks postoperatively for the sternum to heal. During that time, advise the client to lift nothing heavier than 5 pounds. Also, the client must not drive, because driving can strain the incision. As the client gets into and out of bed or a chair, the client's arms should not bear weight; the arms may be used only for balance.

Some cities have developed exercise rehabilitation programs for clients who have had heart attacks or heart surgery. These programs involve supervised, closely monitored exercise sessions and teaching.

Low-sodium and low-cholesterol diets are often prescribed for clients after cardiac surgery. In order for the client to be able to comply with dietary instruction, the diet must be carefully planned. Diets for clients with heart disease are discussed in Chapter 42.

Teach the client or a significant other to check the pulse daily for rate and regularity and to call the physician about a resting heart rate rise of more than 20 beats per minute or a new irregularity. The client can also use heart rate to monitor responses to exercise. Authorities usually recommend a rise of not more than 20 beats per minute for the immediate postoperative period.

If the client needs to wear antiembolism hose at home, teach a household member how to apply them. The client usually wears these hose on the venectomy limb during the daytime for several weeks.

Teach the client and significant others to inspect the incision daily. Care of the incision may include swabbing with povidone-iodine and applying dry dressings over oozing areas.

Make sure the client knows how and when to schedule follow-up appointments. Instruct the client to report the following to the primary health care provider:

- signs or symptoms of infection, including fever, and increased redness, tenderness, or swelling of incisions
- palpitations, tachycardia, or irregular pulse (if normally regular)
- dizziness or increased fatigue
- sudden weight gain or peripheral edema
- shortness of breath

Modification of Plan of Care for the Elderly

Elderly clients often have many other disorders that interfere with or delay their ability to respond to the hemodynamic changes with surgery and during recovery. The elderly client is also more prone to problems with skin breakdown and renal impairment. Fluids must be closely titrated because there are often pre-existent heart disorders.

THE ADULT CLIENT WITH A SURGICALLY CORRECTED DEFECT

Because of the dramatic advances in surgical treatment of children with congenital heart defects in the 1960s, many of these children are living into adulthood. Many of these clients have residual or potential problems, sequelae, or complications that may require medical care. Some clients purposefully forego some surgical intervention. There are also unavoidable consequences of some successful surgical repairs.[53] The only surgery that is not likely to have any long-term problems is the repair of a patent ductus.

There may be only a minor problem that remains after surgical repair. A residual murmur may be found. Proper assessment is crucial for proper diagnosis. Noninvasive diagnostic procedures like color-flow Doppler echocardiography are helpful.

The risk of infective endocarditis is increased in those with artificial valves or with suture repair of atrial septal defect.

It is not uncommon for a client with a repaired coarctation of the aorta to find that the aorta has gradually become narrowed again. Frequently, these clients may develop idiopathic hypertension.

Clients who have had cyanotic defects repaired as children are likely to have sequelae and complications in adulthood.[53] There may be some degree of exercise intolerance that can be better managed after proper stress testing.

Arrhythmias frequently present a lifelong complication. Clients who have had intraventricular repairs may present with ventricular arrhythmias or complete heart block. A 24-hour Holter monitor and stress testing may help evaluate the client's activity tolerance.

Most clients who have had previous congenital heart repairs do well in adulthood. They can be relatively asymptomatic and come to the attention of the health care team only when they present for an unrelated injury or illness.

Summary

The client with a cardiac disorder frequently has activity intolerance, decreased cardiac output, and ineffective coping due to the seriousness of the disorder. Nurses must be skilled in physical and psychosocial aspects of disease when providing care.

Bibliography

1. Aagaard, M. T., & Haraldsted, V. Y. (1984). Chronic constrictive pericarditis treated with total pericardiectomy. *Thoracic and Cardiovascular Surgeon, 32*(5), 311-314.
2. Antunes, M. J., et al. (1987). Valvuloplasty for rheumatic mitral valve disease. *Journal of Thoracic and Cardiovascular Surgery, 94*(1), 44-56.
3. American Heart Association, Committee on Rheumatic Fever and Bacterial Endocarditis (1984). Prevention of rheumatic fever. *Circulation, 70,* 1118A.
4. Barden, C., et al. (1990). Balloon aortic valvuloplasty: nursing care implications. *Critical Care Nurse, 10*(6), 22-30, 86.
5. Bates, B. (1987). *A guide to physical examination and history taking.* Philadelphia: J. B. Lippincott.
6. Blanche, C., et al. (1990). Technical aspects of cardiopulmonary bypass. In R. J. Gray & J. M. Matloff (Eds.), *Medical management of the cardiac surgery patient.* Baltimore: Williams and Wilkins.
7. Braunwald, E. (1988). Valvular heart disease. In E. Braunwald (Ed.), *Heart disease.* Philadelphia: W. B. Saunders.
8. Breu, C., et al. (1982). Treatment of patients with congestive cardiomyopathy during hospitalization: A case study. *Heart and Lung, 11*(3), 229-236.
9. Carceller, A. M., et al. (1986). Wall thickness, cavity dimensions, and myocardial contractility of the left ventricle in patients with simple transposition of the great arteries. *Circulation, 73*(4), 622-627.
10. Carpenito, L. J. (1989). *Nursing diagnosis.* Philadelphia: J. B. Lippincott.
11. Cornell, L. V. (1985). Mitral valve prolapse syndrome: etiology and symptomatology. *Nurse Practitioner, 10*(4), 25-34.
12. Craig, R. J., et al. (1968). Pressure and volume changes of the left ventricle in acute pericardial tamponade. *American Journal of Cardiology, 22*(1), 65-74.
13. Craver, J. M. (1990). Surgical reconstruction for regurgitant lesions of the mitral valve. In J. W. Hurst (Ed.), *The heart.* New York: McGraw-Hill.
14. Durack, D. T. (1990). Infective and noninfective endocarditis. In J. W. Hurst (Ed.), *The heart.* New York: McGraw-Hill.
15. Engle, M. A. (1985). A long look at surgery for coarctation of aorta. *Journal of the American College of Cardiology, 6*(4), 887-888.
16. Evans, R. W., et al. (1986). Donor availability as the primary determinant of the future of heart transplantation. *Journal of the American Medical Association, 255*(14), 1892-1898.
17. Fragomeni, L. S., et al. (1990). Donor identification and organ procurement for cardiac transplantation. In M. E. Thompson (Ed.), *Cardiac transplantation.* Philadelphia: F. A. Davis.
18. Friedman, W. F. (1988). Congenital heart disease in infancy and childhood. In E. Braunwald (Ed.), *Heart disease.* Philadelphia: W. B. Saunders.
19. Funk, M. (1986). Heart transplantation: postoperative care during the acute period. *Critical Care Nurse, 6*(2), 27-46.
20. Gonzalez-Lavin, L., et al. (1983). Endomyocardial fibrosis: diagnosis and treatment. *American Heart Journal, 105*(4), 699-705.
21. Gregoratos, G., & Karlinger, J. (1979). Infective endocarditis: diagnosis and management. *Medical Clinics of North America, 63*(1), 173-199.
22. Guzzetta, C. E. (1984). The person with infective endocarditis. In C. E. Guzzetta & B. M. Dossey (Eds.), *Cardiovascular nursing.* St. Louis: C. V. Mosby.
23. Guzzetta C. E., et al. (1989). *Clinical assessment tools for use with nursing diagnosis.* St. Louis: C. V. Mosby.
24. Guzzetta, C. E., & Dossey, B. M. (1990). Cardiovascular assessment. In Dossey, B. M., et al. (Eds.), *Essentials of critical care nursing.* Philadelphia: J. B. Lippincott.
25. Guyton, A. C. (1991). *Textbook of medical physiology.* Philadelphia: W. B. Saunders.
26. Guyton, R. A., & Hatcher, C. R. (1990). Techniques of valvular surgery. In J. W. Hurst (Ed.), *The heart.* New York: McGraw-Hill.
27. Hancock, E. W. (1984). Congenital heart disease. In E. Rubenstein (Ed.), *Scientific American Medicine.* New York: Scientific American.
28. Hastillo, A., & Hess, M. L. (1990). Selection of patients for cardiac transplantation. In M. E. Thompson (Ed.), *Cardiac transplantation.* Philadelphia: F. A. Davis.
29. Heyman, S. (1985). Effects of cardiopulmonary bypass on coagulation. *Dimensions in Critical Care Nursing, 4*(2), 70-80.
30. Hosier, D. (1987). Resurgence of rheumatic fever. *New York State Journal of Medicine, 88*(7), 352-353.
31. Huang, S., et al. (1983). *Coronary care nursing.* Philadelphia: W. B. Saunders.
32. Hudak, C. M., et al. (1990). *Critical care nursing.* Philadelphia: J. B. Lippincott.
33. Hurst, J. W. (1990). *The heart* (7th ed.). New York: McGraw-Hill.
34. Ikaheimo, M. J., & Takkunen, J. T. (1986). Echocardiography in acute infectious myocarditis. *Chest, 89*(1), 100-102.
35. Ingram, R. H., & Braunwald, E. (1988). Pulmonary edema: cardiogenic and noncardiogenic. In E. Braunwald (Ed.), *Heart disease.* Philadelphia: W. B. Saunders.
36. Ivert, T. S., et al. (1984). Prosthetic valve endocarditis. *Circulation, 69*(2), 223-232.
37. Johnston, J. (1991). A new beginning: current trends in pediatric heart transplantation. *Focus on Critical Care, 18*(1), 23-28.
38. Kaplan, E. L. (1990). Acute rheumatic fever. In J. W. Hurst (Ed.), *The heart* (7th ed., p. 1524). New York: McGraw-Hill.
39. Kereiakes, D. J., et al. (1983). Apical hypertrophic cardiomyopathy. *American Heart Journal, 105*(5), 855-856.
40. Kirklin, J. W., et al. (1988). Cardiac surgery. In E. Braunwald (Ed.), *Heart disease.* Philadelphia: W. B. Saunders.
41. Lababidi, Z., et al. (1984). Percutaneous balloon aortic valvuloplasty: results in 23 patients. *American Journal of Cardiology, 53*(1), 194-197.
42. Lang, R. M., et al. (1985). Adverse cardiac effects of acute alcohol ingestion in young adults. *Archives of Internal Medicine, 102*(6), 742-747.
43. Lavie, D., & Savage, D. (1987). Prevalence and clinical features of mitral valve prolapse. *American Heart Journal, 113*(5), 1281.
44. Lee, M. E., & Gray, R. J. (1990). Low output states following cardiac surgery. In R. J. Gray & J. M. Matloff (Eds.), *Medical management of the cardiac surgery patient.* Baltimore: Williams and Wilkins.
45. Lee, R. E., & Ramos, R. (1990). Nursing care of the cardiac surgical patient. In R. J. Gray & J. M. Matloff (Eds.), *Medical management of the cardiac surgery patient.* Baltimore: Williams and Wilkins.

46. Lock, J., et al. (1986). The use of catheter intervention procedures for congenital heart disease. *Journal of the American College of Cardiology, 7*(6), 1420-1423.
47. Lorell, B. H., & Braunwald, E. (1988). Pericardial disease. In E. Braunwald, (Ed.), *Heart disease*. Philadelphia: W. B. Saunders.
48. Magilligan, D. J. (1987). Advantages and disadvantages of tissue valves. In P. J. Starek (Ed.), *Heart valve replacement and reconstruction*. Chicago: Year Book.
49. Matsumori, A., & Abelmann, W. (1984). Viral myocarditis: highlighting a condition that too often "travels incognito." *Consultant, 24,* 109.
50. Miller, D., & Borer, J. (1983). Cardiomyopathies: a pathophysiologic approach to therapeutic management. *Archives of Internal Medicine, 143,* 2157.
51. Murdock, D. K., et al. (1987). Rejection of the transplanted heart. *Heart and Lung, 16*(3), 237-245.
52. Nottingham, A., & Rambo, A. (1987). Electrocardiographic phenomena in the transplanted heart. *Focus on Critical Care, 13*(6), 41-46.
53. Nugent, E. W., et al. (1990). The pathology, abnormal physiology, clinical recognition, and medical and surgical treatment of congenital heart disease. In J. W. Hurst (Ed.), *The heart* (7th ed.). New York: McGraw-Hill.
54. O'Rourke, R. A., & Crawford, M. H. (1980). Timing of aortic valve replacement in patients with chronic aortic regurgitation. *Circulation, 61*(3), 493-495.
55. Packer, D. L., et al. (1986). Tachycardia-induced cardiomyopathy: a reversible form of left ventricular dysfunction. *American Journal of Cardiology, 57*(8), 563-570.
56. Parker-Cohen, P. D., et al. (1990). Alterations of cardiovascular function. In K. L. McCance & S. E. Huerther (Eds.), *Pathophysiology*. St. Louis: C. V. Mosby.
57. Permanyer-Miralda, G., et al. (1985). Primary acute pericardial disease: a prospective series of 231 consecutive patients. *American Journal of Cardiology, 56*(10), 623-630.
58. Rackley, C. E., et al. (1990). Mitral valve disease. In J. W. Hurst (Ed.), *The heart* (7th ed.). New York: McGraw-Hill.
59. Rackley, C. E., et al. (1990). Aortic valve disease. In J. W. Hurst (Ed.), *The heart* (7th ed.). New York: McGraw-Hill.
60. Raymond, M., et al. (1984). Coping with transient intellectual dysfunction after coronary bypass surgery. *Heart and Lung, 13*(5), 531-539.
61. Schakenbach, L. H. (1987). Physiologic dynamics of acquired heart disease. *Journal of Cardiovascular Nursing, 1*(3), 1-17.
62. Scheld, W. M., & Sande, M. A. (1984). Endocarditis and intravascular infections. In G. L. Mandell, et al. (Eds.), *Principles and practice of infectious diseases*. New York: John Wiley and Sons.
63. Seifert, F. C., et al. (1985). Surgical treatment of constrictive pericarditis: analysis of outcome and diagnostic error. *Circulation, 72,* (Suppl. II), 264-273.
64. Shabetai, R. (1983). Cardiomyopathy: how far have we come in 25 years, how far yet to go? *Journal of the American College of Cardiology, 1*(1), 252-263.
65. Shapiro, B. A., et al. (1985). *Clinical application of respiratory care* (3rd ed.). Chicago: Year Book.
66. Siegel, R. J., et al. (1984). Idiopathic restrictive cardiomyopathy. *Circulation, 70*(2), 165-169.
67. Starek, P. J. (1987). Technical aspects of uncomplicated valve replacement. In P. J. Starek (Ed.), *Heart valve replacement and reconstruction*. Chicago: Year Book.
68. Stephenson, L. W., et al. (1984). Combined aortic and mitral valve replacement: changes in practice and prognosis. *Circulation, 69*(3), 640-644.
69. Stollerman, G. H. (1986). Autoimmunity and rheumatic fever. In I. R. Cohen (Ed.), *Perspectives in autoimmunity*. Boca Raton, FL: CRC Press.
70. Stollerman, G. H. (1988). Rheumatic and heritable connective tissue diseases of the cardiovascular system. In E. Braunwald (Ed.), *Heart disease*. Philadelphia: W. B. Saunders.
71. Swartz, M. H., & Dack, S. (1982). Mitral valve prolapse syndrome. *Hospital Medicine, 18,* 49.
72. Tamer, D., et al. (1983). Hemodynamics and intracardiac conduction after operative repair of tetralogy of Fallot. *American Journal of Cardiology, 51*(3), 552-556.
73. Thompson, M. E. (1990). *Cardiac transplantation*. Philadelphia: F. A. Davis.
74. Topol, E. J., et al. (1985). Hypertensive hypertrophic cardiomyopathy of the elderly. *New England Journal of Medicine, 312*(5), 277-283.
75. Weiland, A. P., & Walker, W. E. (1986). Physiologic principles and clinical sequelae of cardiopulmonary bypass. *Heart and Lung, 15*(1), 34-39.
76. Wenger, N. K., et al. (1990). Cardiomyopathy and specific heart muscle disease. In J. W. Hurst (Ed.), *The heart* (7th ed.). New York: McGraw-Hill.
77. Wilson, W. R., et al. (1984). Treatment of streptomycin-susceptible and streptomycin-resistant enterococcal endocarditis. *Annals of Internal Medicine, 100*(6), 816-823.
78. Wynne, J., & Braunwald, E. (1988). The cardiomyopathies and myocarditides. In E. Braunwald (Ed.), *Heart disease*. Philadelphia: W. B. Saunders.
79. Zabriskie, J. B. (1985). Rheumatic fever: The interplay between host, genetics and microbe. *Circulation, 71*(6), 1077-1086.

Chapter 44

Nursing Care of Clients with Peripheral Vascular Disorders

STRUCTURE AND FUNCTION OF THE VASCULAR SYSTEM

The flow of blood is essential for sustaining human life. The vascular system provides conduits for blood to travel from the heart to nourish body tissues, to carry away cellular wastes to the excretory organs, to allow lymphatic flow to drain tissue fluid back into the circulation, and to return blood to the heart for recirculation (Fig. 44–1).

Blood flow depends on the efficiency of the heart as a pump and the patency of the blood vessels. Circulation is influenced by viscosity, hydration, mechanisms affecting coagulation and fibrinolysis, and local changes in the size of the vessels as well as by inflammatory, neurogenic, and iatrogenic processes.

STRUCTURE OF BLOOD VESSELS

There are three types of blood vessels: arteries, veins, and capillaries. Arteries carry blood away from the heart after it has been oxygenated in the pulmonary circulation. Arteries are composed of three distinct layers (Fig. 44–2):

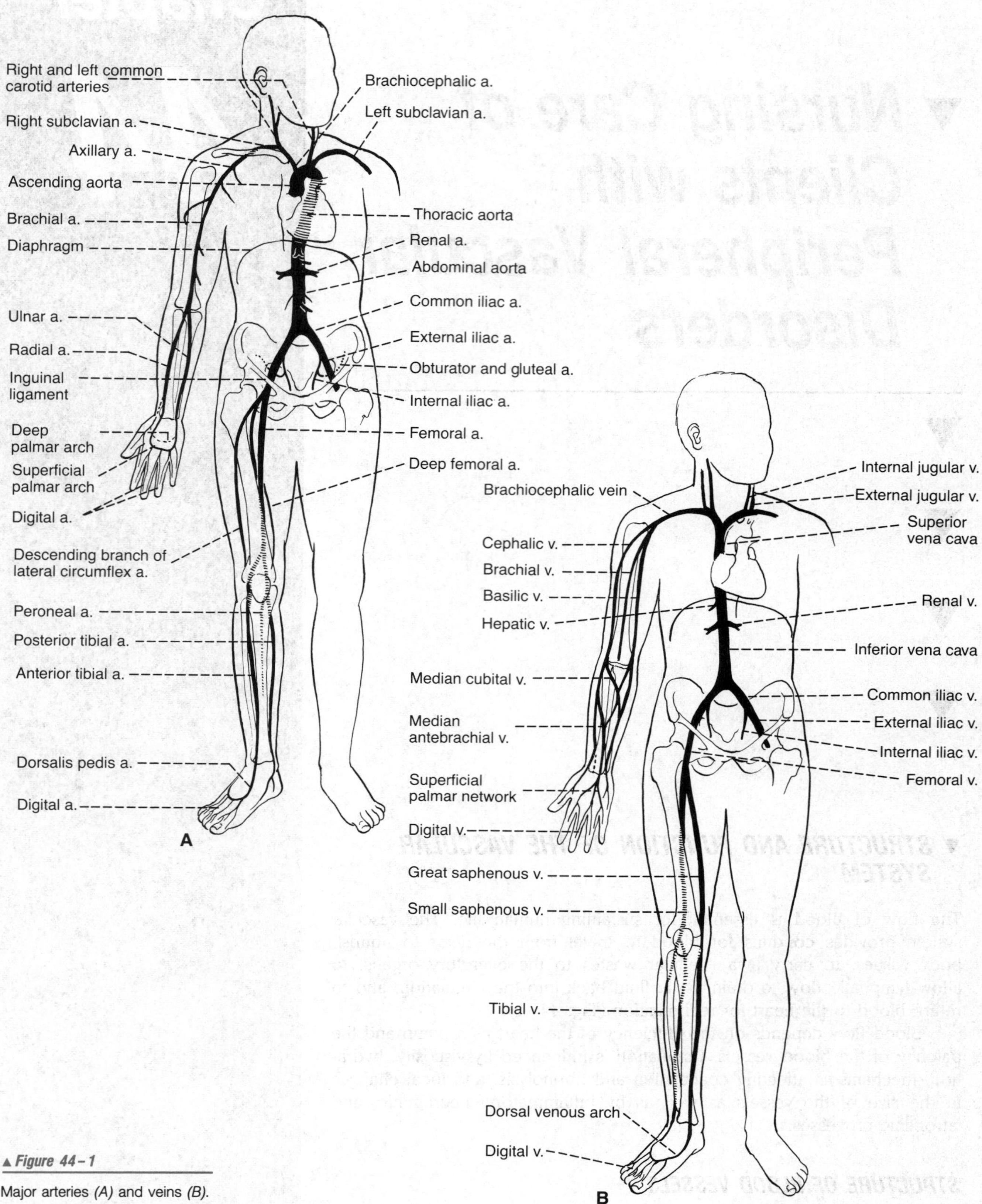
Right and left common carotid arteries
Brachiocephalic a.
Left subclavian a.
Right subclavian a.
Axillary a.
Ascending aorta
Brachial a.
Thoracic aorta
Renal a.
Diaphragm
Abdominal aorta
Common iliac a.
Ulnar a.
External iliac a.
Radial a.
Obturator and gluteal a.
Inguinal ligament
Internal iliac a.
Deep palmar arch
Femoral a.
Superficial palmar arch
Deep femoral a.
Digital a.
Descending branch of lateral circumflex a.
Peroneal a.
Posterior tibial a.
Anterior tibial a.
Dorsalis pedis a.
Digital a.
A
Internal jugular v.
Brachiocephalic vein
External jugular v.
Superior vena cava
Cephalic v.
Brachial v.
Basilic v.
Renal v.
Hepatic v.
Inferior vena cava
Median cubital v.
Common iliac v.
Median antebrachial v.
External iliac v.
Internal iliac v.
Femoral v.
Superficial palmar network
Digital v.
Great saphenous v.
Small saphenous v.
Tibial v.
Dorsal venous arch
Digital v.
B

▲ *Figure 44–1*

Major arteries *(A)* and veins *(B)*.

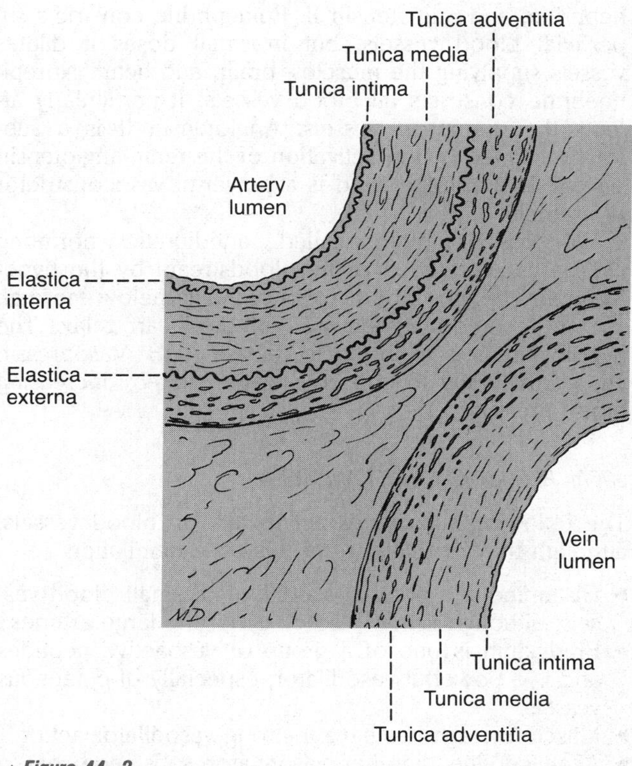

▲ *Figure 44-2*

Cross sections of artery and vein. Note thickness of arterial wall, compared with the venous wall.

1. tunica intima, the innermost layer that provides a smooth passageway through which blood flows;
2. tunica media, the middle layer composed of elastic connective tissue and circular smooth muscle; this layer is responsible for regulating the diameter of the vessel by dilation and constriction;
3. tunica adventitia, composed of elastic and collagen fibers; this outermost layer gives support to the vessel and maintains its shape.

Arteries can be classified into two categories. First are the conductive arteries, including the major vessels. These conduits are elastic and are able to stretch and recoil in order to accommodate the flow of blood. They expand with each surge of blood ejected from the heart and then resume their original diameter. It is this recoil that propels blood forward to all parts of the body and that is the basis of the pulse felt on palpation. Conductive arteries follow relatively straight courses and have comparatively few branches. Conductive arteries are most severely affected by atherosclerosis, particularly at branch points.

The second category includes distributive arteries that provide nutrients. These are branches of larger arteries and primarily function as suppliers of oxygen and essential nutrients. Each branch gives off further branches of arteries of smaller caliber until the blood passes from the smallest arteries into the arterioles and then into capillaries, where it nourishes the tissues. Arterioles are small, thick-walled vessels with an overall diameter of about 0.2 cm. They are important regulators of the peripheral circulation because they are innervated with sympathetic nerves in the muscle of the tunica media. Therefore, the arteriole constricts and dilates to regulate peripheral vascular resistance, a component of blood pressure.

Before blood enters the capillary network, it passes through structures called precapillary sphincters. These sphincters work in conjunction with the autonomic nervous system to relax and constrict capillary openings. The precapillary sphincters can also be influenced by local changes in temperature, pH, and oxygen.

The capillaries are the functional units of the vascular system because they are the vessels that allow substances to diffuse to and from the blood into the interstitial space (Fig. 44-3). The capillary network is composed of a single layer of endothelial cells. Constriction of the capillary network increases peripheral vascular resistance and increases systolic and diastolic pressure. Dilation decreases peripheral vascular resistance and diastolic blood pressure.

From the capillaries, blood flows into venules. Venules are tiny veins that have extremely thin walls that allow the passage of substances and serve to remove waste products from capillaries. The venules merge to form veins that eventually combine to form larger veins that carry deoxygenated blood back to the heart. Approximately 75 per cent of the total blood volume at any given time can be found in the venous system. Veins are also known as capacitance vessels because of their ability to stretch.

Veins lie closer to the skin's surface than arteries do, and although they still contain three walls, their walls are thinner and contain less smooth muscle and less elastic tissue. Most veins also contain valves that prevent the backflow of venous blood (Fig. 44-4). Valves break the hydrostatic column of blood into small units, thereby reducing the hydrodynamic load in the propulsion of blood toward the heart. A valve consists of two

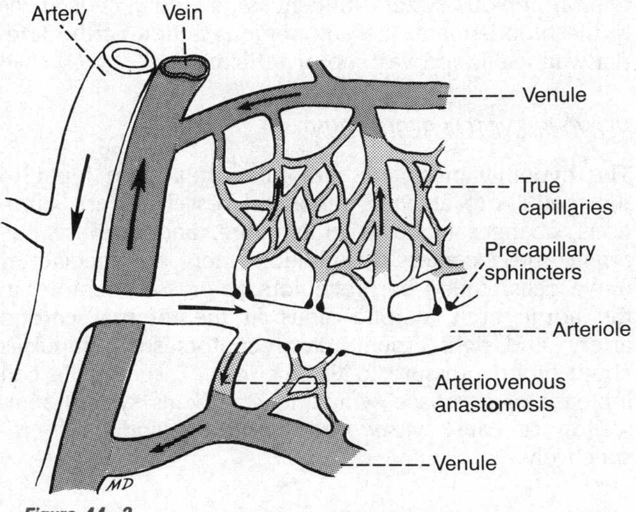

▲ *Figure 44-3*

Capillary bed. Food, fluids, and gases are delivered to tissues through the capillaries and collected from the capillaries for recycling or excretion. Precapillary sphincters help regulate the flow.

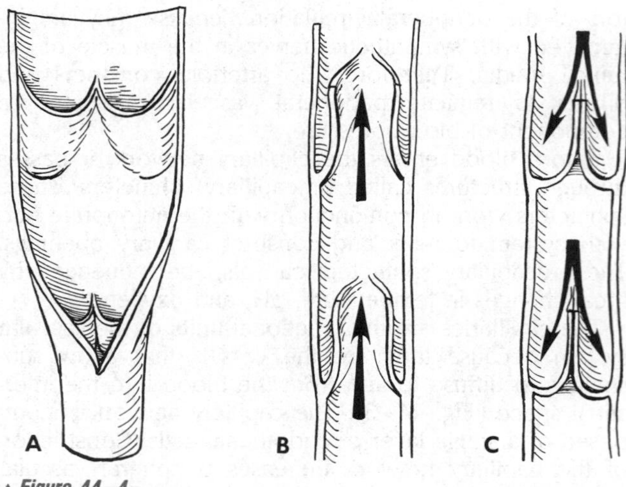

▲ Figure 44–4

One-way venous valves. *A*, Split vein shows valve shape. *B*, Valves allow blood to be pumped back to heart, but prevent it from draining back into periphery *(C)*.

frail cusps composed of endothelial folds. Valve competence depends on the integrity of the vein wall. The valve becomes incompetent when the cusps no longer meet at the midline. Valvular incompetence develops when veins have been overstretched by excess venous pressure for a prolonged period of time, as occurs during pregnancy or when the person is standing still for long periods.

FUNCTION OF BLOOD VESSELS

Factors Regulating the Arteries

All normal arteries are contractile in that they can decrease (vasoconstrict) or increase (vasodilate) their diameter in response to appropriate stimuli. The complex mechanisms regulating vasomotor activity consist of central nervous system influences, chemical substances in the bloodstream, the autonomous action of the arterial wall itself, and vasomotor reflexes.

NERVOUS SYSTEM REGULATION

The hypothalamus and cerebral cortex send input to the medulla to activate peripheral vessels. Stress, emotions, changes in body temperature, and exercise can trigger these centers. In addition, there are specialized nerve cells, called baroreceptors or pressoreceptors, in the aortic arch, carotid sinus in the internal carotid artery, and right atrium. Baroreceptors send impulses about blood pressure to the medulla. The medulla can increase or decrease sympathetic nervous system stimulation to cause vasoconstriction or vasodilation, respectively.

HORMONAL AND CHEMICAL REGULATION

Three powerful substances within the blood help control the diameter of blood vessels: epinephrine, norepinephrine, and angiotensin II. Epinephrine constricts superficial blood vessels, but in small doses it dilates vessels supplying the muscles, brain, and heart. Norepinephrine constricts all blood vessels. It particularly affects the peripheral vessels. Angiotensin II is a substance formed by the activation of the renin-angiotensin system of the kidney and is a powerful vasoconstrictor of arteries.

Vasopressin, often called antidiuretic hormone (ADH), is secreted into the bloodstream by the hypothalamus. When blood pressure falls below normal, stretch receptors in the wall of the heart relax. The hypothalamus is triggered to release ADH. Vasopressin causes the body to conserve water, thereby increasing blood pressure.

LOCAL REGULATORY MECHANISMS

The following substances act locally on blood vessels, although they circulate in the systemic circulation.

- Histamine is a potent vasodilator of small blood vessels, although it may also constrict the large arteries.
- Bradykinin is one of a group of vasoactive peptides and is a powerful vasodilator, especially of cutaneous vessels.
- Muscle metabolites have a strong vasodilator action.
- Acetylcholine, another vasodilator substance, has a transient action. It causes vasodilation in muscles.
- Serotonin is liberated from platelets that stick to the vessel wall in the injured area. Although a powerful constrictor of cutaneous arterioles, it dilates capillaries.
- Tissue oxygen levels, carbon dioxide tension, and potassium and lactic acid levels affect arterial flow.

VASOMOTOR REFLEXES

Principal vasomotor reflexes observed in the limbs are those concerned with regulation of body temperature. After application of heat, it is possible to measure the degree of vasodilation by recording the skin temperature of fingers or toes. However, measurements of blood with use of a plethysmograph provide more accurate data. In a normal client, placement of the trunk or the legs in warm water always causes indirect vasodilation in the hands.

Factors Affecting Venous Pressure and Volume

In the recumbent position, the pressure gradient between the peripheral venous circulation and right atrium provides the major driving force for propulsion of the blood. The valves allow blood flow in one direction only. Inspiration facilitates blood flow into the right atrium by creating an intrathoracic vacuum and, hence, distention of the vena cava lumen. Expiration decreases the inflow. If intrathoracic pressure is increased by contraction of the thoracic muscles (as in forced expiration, lifting a heavy weight, or Valsalva's maneuver), the intrathoracic pressure rises enough to compress the vena cava. Initially, intrathoracic pressure increases venous return to the right atrium. Later, it inhibits return.

In the upright position, blood return from the lower limbs to the heart depends almost entirely on contraction of the calf muscles and competency of the valves. When a leg muscle contracts, it presses against the veins in the leg, thus compressing them and pumping blood toward the heart. On standing still, this "muscle pump" does not work, and the venous pressures in the lower part of the leg rise to about 90 mm Hg. When sitting or lying in bed, the calf muscle pump is not activated, especially if the client does not flex the calf muscles.

Factors Affecting Blood Flow

PERIPHERAL VASCULAR RESISTANCE

Blood flows because a blood pressure gradient exists within the vascular system. Because fluid always flows from a high- to a low-pressure area, blood flows from the aorta (in which the blood pressure is around 100 mm Hg) to veins (which have a blood pressure of only 1 to 6 mm Hg). The maintenance of regional blood flow depends on peripheral vascular resistance in the muscular arteries and arterioles. The resistance is affected by the local regulatory mechanisms discussed earlier.

Within the venous system, blood flow (which is against gravity) depends not only on the blood pressure gradient but also on (1) valves located within the veins and (2) the pumping action of muscles surrounding the veins.

METABOLIC NEEDS OF TISSUES

The needs of the tissues for blood and oxygen are constantly changing, depending on the client's activity level, thermal environment, and state of health. When the metabolic needs of the body increase, more blood flow to tissues is needed, and the arteries normally dilate. When the metabolic needs of the tissues decrease, the needs of the tissue for blood also decrease, and the vessels constrict.

Normally, by dilating and constricting, blood vessels are able to vary the amount of blood that the tissues of the extremities receive. However, sclerosed, obstructed, damaged, inelastic blood vessels are unable to dilate and constrict normally. Consequently, these vessels fail to supply tissues with the additional blood they require during increased physical exercise, with the application of heat, or in infection.

AUTOREGULATION

The capacity of tissues to regulate their own blood flow is called autoregulation. The myogenic theory of autoregulation suggests that regulation probably results from the intrinsic contractile response of smooth muscle to stretch. As the blood pressure rises, the blood vessels distend, and the vascular smooth muscle fibers that surround the vessel contract. The blood vessel closes when the pressure of blood flowing through it falls below 70 mm Hg.

The Effects of Aging on the Vascular System

Changes in intima and media resulting from age most often affect the larger and medium-sized vessels. The most prominent changes are intimal thickening, loss of elasticity, and an increase in both diameter and calcium content. These changes are referred to as arteriosclerosis, or hardening of the arteries. Thickened intima inhibits the diffusion of nutrients from the vessel.

STRUCTURE AND FUNCTION OF THE LYMPHATIC SYSTEM

The lymphatic system returns interstitial fluids to the general circulation and assists with immune reactions and fat digestion. The lymphatic system consists of plexuses of small, thin, veinlike vessels (lymphatics) that empty lymph into the left and right brachiocephalic veins (Fig. 44–5). Also, certain lymphatic organs that resemble lymph nodes, such as tonsils, spleen, and thymus, are part of the lymphatic system. Lymph is a fluid similar to plasma and tissue fluid except that it contains no high-molecular-weight proteins. Lymph nodes are small, oval bodies situated so that lymph flows through them on its way to the veins. Finally, there are collections of lymphoid tissue situated in the walls of the intestinal tract and in the spleen and thymus as well as circulating lymphocytes.

The lymphatic vessels tend to lie near the veins. The peripheral lymphatics join larger lymphatics and pass through regional lymph nodes before entering the bloodstream. Ultimately, all lymphatics converge into two main trunks, the thoracic duct and the right lymphatic duct, which empty into the junction of the subclavian and internal jugular veins of the left and right sides, respectively. The thoracic duct drains most of the lymph vessels of the body: lower extremities, pelvis, abdominal cavity, left thorax, and left head, neck, and upper extremity. The right lymphatic duct is the common trunk for lymph flow from the right side of the head, neck, thorax, and upper arms.

Active and passive mechanisms transport the lymph along the lymphatic vessels. Valves in the lymphatics promote proximal flow. Lymph flow results from a combination of interstitial pressure, negative and positive pressures in the thoracic and abdominal cavities, compression of adjacent muscles, and arterial pulsation.

The three fundamental functions of the lymphatic system are (1) development and maintenance of the immune system, (2) transport of fluids and proteins (and other colloid substances) from the interstitial spaces back to the veins, and (3) reabsorption of fats from the small intestine. Each function is discussed separately.

Macrophages within the lymph nodes trap antigens

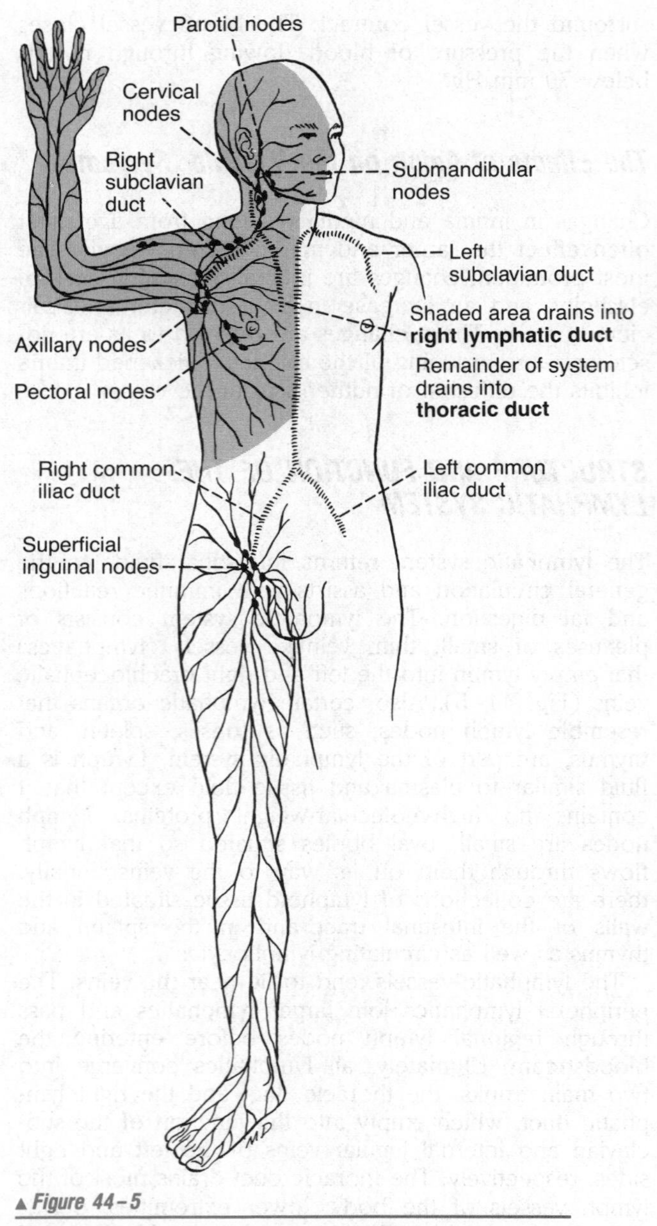

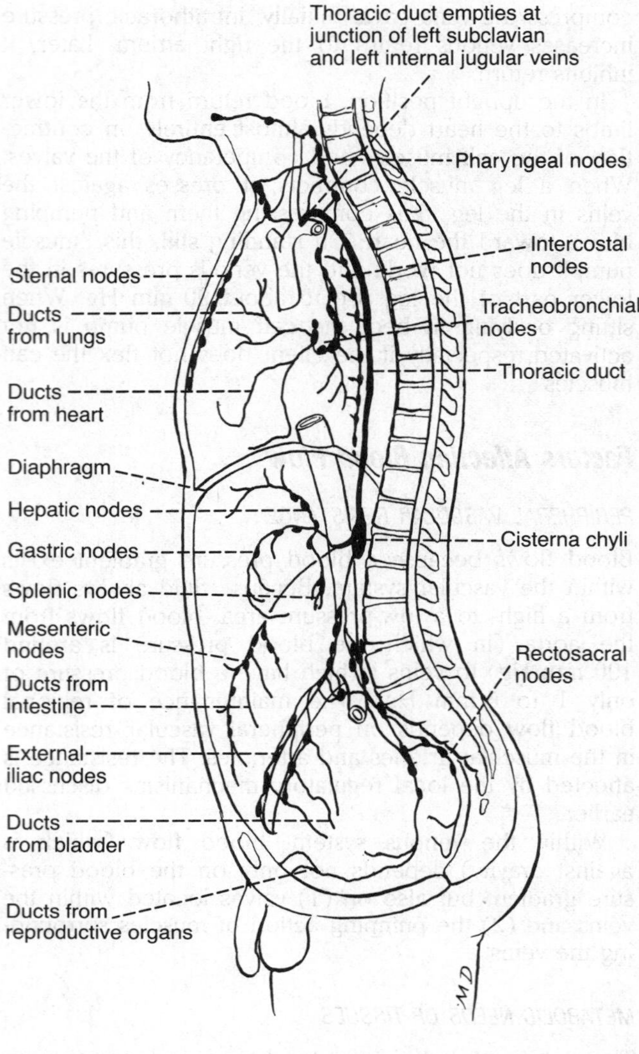

▲ **Figure 44–5**

Superficial and deep lymphatic collecting channels and nodes.

for destruction by lymphocytes. These immunologically competent cells respond by generating clones of specifically reactive (sometimes called killer) lymphocytes. Phagocytosis of antigen by macrophages or mononuclear phagocyte cells in the lymph nodes can also occur.

The lymphatics are an important element in the fluid exchange and protein transport between blood and tissue. Lymphatic capillaries permit free entry of fluid, small and large molecules, and cellular elements from the interstitial space. During infections, bacteria and leukocytes with phagocytized bacteria are transported into the lymphatic system. Unfortunately, neoplastic cells are also transported into the lymphatics. From here, cancer cells can invade lymph nodes and distant organs.

The mechanisms of transport for fluid and other substances between the lymphatics and the interstitial spaces are explained by Starling's hypothesis (Fig. 44–6). Hydrostatic pressure in the lymphatic capillaries (1 to 2 mm Hg) measures about the same as the hydrostatic pressure in the interstitial space. The wall of a lymphatic capillary is similar to a blood capillary except that it has larger "pores," that is, there are larger spaces between the endothelial cells through which large molecules can pass. This wall structure, coupled with the equal pressures in the interstitial spaces and the lymphatic capillaries, suggests that there is relatively free communication between the interstitial spaces and the lymph capillaries. Thus, any increase in the interstitial pressure will increase lymph flow, as will any agent or procedure that increases the rate of filtration from

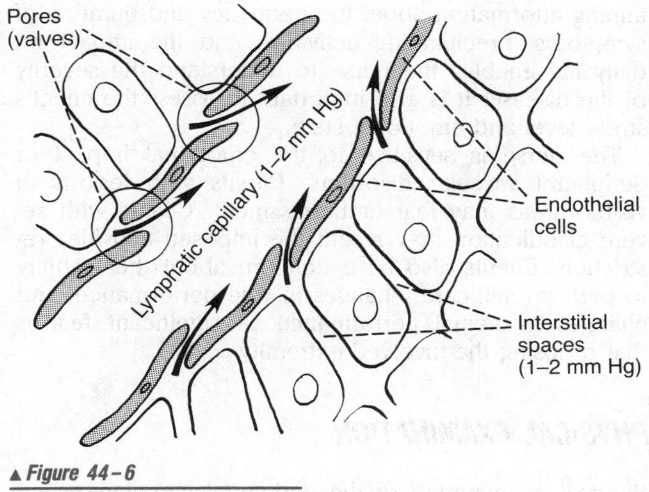

▲ **Figure 44-6**

Structure of lymphatic capillaries.

the blood capillaries. Interstitial pressures and lymphatic flow can be increased by raising venous pressure, reducing plasma oncotic pressure, or altering capillary permeability. A general increase in systemic arterial pressure does not significantly increase lymph flow, but hypotension decreases or stops lymph flow. Ordinarily, the volume of lymph represents the difference between capillary filtration and reabsorption, which is approximately 2 to 4 L daily.

Finally, the third function of the lymphatic system is involved in the reabsorption of digested fat. This function is performed by the lymph capillaries of the intestine, called lacteals. Lymph that is laden with fat is called chyle.

The Effects of Aging on the Lymphatic System

Lymphatic tissue diminishes in older people, which results in a decrease in the number of lymph nodes and in the size of the remaining nodes. The lymph nodes in the elderly may also tend to be fatty and fibrotic, compared with those in the young; thus, the ability to fight infection is reduced.

▼ ASSESSMENT OF THE PERIPHERAL VASCULAR SYSTEM

Peripheral vascular disease is common among the elderly and clients with diabetes. It is characterized by disturbances of blood flow through the peripheral vessels. These disturbances eventually result in damage to tissues of the extremities and organs as a result of (1) ischemia and (2) excessive accumulation of waste and fluid due to venous or lymphatic stasis.

Any factor that narrows, obstructs, or damages blood vessels and thus impedes blood flow is dangerous. When the blood flow slows, tissue nutrition decreases, cellular waste products accumulate, ischemia develops, and the danger of thrombus and embolus formation escalates. Without intervention, tissue damage may advance to the point of ulceration or gangrene. The limb may have to be amputated.

Peripheral vascular nursing assessment includes the collection of data through history and physical examination of the arterial and venous circulation. The focus of assessment is on whether the peripheral vascular system is intact and functional.

HISTORY

While assessing the history of the client, the nurse should be alert to risk factors of cardiovascular disease (see Chap. 41). In addition, the current medications the client receives may give the nurse cues to those medications that increase the risk of vascular disease (e.g., birth control pills) as well as those agents currently being taken for circulatory disorders (e.g., vasodilators). Some clients are reluctant to mention what they believe to be minor symptoms. Consequently the nurse performs a careful assessment, asking specific questions skillfully, to obtain important information concerning the early manifestations of these insidious conditions.

Chief Complaint

When assessing for vascular disease, the nurse asks for specific data in order to determine whether the client has arterial or venous disease and the frequency and duration of clinical manifestations. Vascular changes may be associated with extremity discomfort of varying characteristics and intensity. Some clients experience burning and stinging in the involved extremities. Some may report cramping and numbness, intolerance of local heat and cold, or inability to sense temperature changes. Clients may also lack sensation to touch or to the position of the involved part. The client is asked about the presence of edema and about changes in pain or edema associated with changes in position. Color changes in the extremities are also common (e.g., dependent cyanosis or rubor), as is the presence of lesions, especially lesions that are difficult to heal.

With arterial disorders, the chief complaint is usually leg pain with walking, called intermittent claudication. Intermittent claudication results from inadequate oxygenation of the tissues due to occlusion of the vessels. It is a pathologic process similar to angina. As the ischemia becomes more severe, the pain also becomes more severe to the point that the client has leg and foot pain at rest or during the night (known as rest pain). This pain is due to ischemia of the nerves and is called lancinating or shooting pain. Elevation of the legs decreases blood flow and increases pain. Clients often report that they sleep upright with legs dangling in order to control pain.

The description of intermittent claudication varies with each client but generally includes cramping, and/or aching. Rarely, clients limp. The pain increases with activity, especially walking and climbing stairs, and decreases with rest. Unless the ischemia is severe, the client is typically distressed only with walking and is relieved within 1 to 2 minutes after stopping and standing in place.

Information regarding the sequence, duration, and persistence of the discomfort, manner of onset, and associated symptoms is obtained from the client. The nurse documents the amount of activity required to cause pain, called claudication distance. The extensiveness of the disease can be gauged by the distance the client can walk without pain. For example, one client may develop claudication after walking one block, whereas another can walk six blocks before developing pain.

Clients may also report impotence. Aortoiliac disorders can lead to impotence. If the client is suspected of having aortoiliac disease, the nurse asks about sexual changes.

Pain in clients with chronic venous disease, by contrast, has a slow onset and not associated with exercise or rest. These clients have typically worked at a job involving many hours of standing in one place, had multiple pregnancies, or abdominal obesity. In these situations, the leg veins have been subjected to increased pressure gradients and obstruction to the return of venous blood. The vein wall eventually loses its competency, and the client has leg edema, ulcerations of the lower third of the leg. The client may also have varicose veins and a history of phlebitis. The client will often report feeling heaviness in the legs and nighttime cramping. Exercise and elevation generally relieve the pain and swelling as venous return is improved.

Past History

Any medical history of vascular impairment is also noted. The nurse asks specifically whether the client has had a history of hypertension, phlebitis, extremity blood clots, pulmonary emboli, cerebrovascular accidents, edema, varicose veins, stasis ulcers, leg cramps, or extremities that are cold, pale, or blue. The client is asked about any past medical tests, surgery, or treatments involving the cardiovascular system and about prior treatment for diabetes mellitus or hypertension.

The nurse assesses for adequacy of proper nutrient and fluid intake. Clients should be assessed for dietary intake, including cholesterol and sodium. A social history is taken to determine use of tobacco, alcohol, and drugs.

Occupational history should be recorded. If the clients' occupation is unfamiliar to the nurse, the client is questioned on the number of hours in various positions (e.g., standing, walking).

Family history helps determine risk factors and provides clues to the reported and observed alterations. A family history of diabetes, hypertension, coronary artery disease, and known peripheral vascular disease is assessed.

The client's activity, rest, and sleep habits need to be assessed. The nurse also assesses the degree to which symptoms interfere with activities of daily living. Obtaining information about the frequency and duration of symptoms, precipitating activities, and the impact on daily life enables the nurse to understand the severity of the disease. It is also important to assess the client's stress level and emotional state.

The nurse is sensitive to the emotional impact of peripheral vascular disorders. Clients with lesions in visible areas may fear embarrassment. Clients with severe claudication may resent the imposed activities restriction. Clients also have concern about the inability to perform self-care, changes in role performance, and changes in sexual performance. A significant fear is that of losing the involved extremity.

PHYSICAL EXAMINATION

Physical examination of the peripheral vascular system for discovering signs of vascular disorders follows the three steps of inspection, palpation, and auscultation. Table 44–1 compares and contrasts the signs of arterial and venous disorders. The client should be examined in a well-lighted and warm room for minimizing cutaneous and small artery vasoconstriction.

Inspection

The nurse observes the lower extremities, noting skin color, hair distribution, venous pattern, swelling, or atrophy. Lack of hair growth may indicate inadequate circulation to an area. Varicosities indicate venous insufficiency. Angiomas (benign tumors of blood and lymph vessels) and petechiae (small, purplish, hemorrhagic spots on the skin from several causes, including hemorrhage) are also noted. If atrophy is suspected, it may represent long-standing arterial insufficiency, and so the nurse measures the muscle in centimeters and compares it with the opposite side. The presence of skin lesions, ulcerations, or scar tissue indicating healed ulcers is also noted; ischemic fissures of the feet and ulcers of ankles and heels are reliable signs of arterial insufficiency. Scars indicating healed ulcers over the medial malleolus can indicate chronic venous insufficiency.

CAPILLARY REFILL

The capillary bed is the portion of the vascular system that is farthest from the heart. Capillary refill time is an evaluation of peripheral perfusion and cardiac output. This assessment is usually completed while pulses are assessed. The nail bed of the toe or finger is depressed until it blanches (becomes pale). The area is released, and the nurse observes the length of time required for usual skin color to return. Normal capillaries refill in a fraction of a second, but "normal" findings include up to 3 seconds. With diminished blood flow, the return to normal color is delayed, and a refill time of more than 3 seconds is sometimes called "sluggish." Note whether the environment is cold, because external temperatures can delay capillary refill.

TABLE 44–1. Clinical Manifestations in Arterial and Venous Disorders

Manifestation	Arterial Disorders	Venous Disorders
Pain	Intermittent claudication Cramping Worse with elevation	Aching pain Exercise improves pain Better with elevation Nocturnal cramping Pruritus, paresthesias Heaviness in the legs at end of day Positive finding of Homans' sign common
Skin	Absence of hair Small, painful ulcers on pressure points, especially lateral malleolus Thin, shiny skin Thick toenails	Brown discoloration Broad, shallow, painless ulcers of the ankle and lower leg Normal toenails
Color	Pale, dependent cyanosis	Brown discoloration Dependent cyanosis
Temperature	Cool	May be warm if thrombophlebitis is present
Sensation	Decreased; sometimes itching, tingling numbness	Pruritus
Pulses	Decreased to absent Possible systolic bruit over involved arteries	Usually unaffected, but may be difficult to palpate if legs edematous
Edema	May be present	Present, worse at end of day, improved with elevation
Muscle mass	Reduced	Unaffected

EDEMA

Edema of the leg is assessed by the examiner's thumb pushing on the skin over the foot or tibia for 5 seconds. Edematous skin may leave an indentation called a pit—thus, the name pitting edema. The degree of edema is often graded; however, the scale used to grade pitting edema is variable. It may be based on the time for the pitting to resolve and the skin surface to return to baseline or on the depth of indentation created by the thumb's pressure. A commonly used scale is as follows:

- 0 No edema
- 1+ Barely detectable depression accompanied by normal foot and leg contours
- 2+ A deeper depression (less than 5 mm) accompanied by normal contours
- 3+ Deep depression (5 to 10 mm) accompanied by foot and leg swelling
- 4+ An even deeper depression (more than 1 cm) accompanied by severe foot and leg swelling

Edema resulting from cardiac disease is generally bilateral and occurs in dependent areas. These areas are the legs when a client is ambulatory and may include the sacrum if the client is bedridden. Edema tends to be unilateral when the client has chronic venous obstruction, traumatic injury, or lymphatic obstruction. This type of edema is hard and nonpitting and is called brawny edema.

ELEVATION PALLOR

In clients with arterial occlusion, the foot becomes gray and pale when elevated. When the leg is placed in a dependent position, it becomes dusky and red over 30 to 60 seconds. The changes in color are a result of a loss of vasomotor tone due to tissue hypoxia—the arterial system cannot pump adequate blood into the capillary system through the arterial blockages against gravity. The degree of pallor is tested by elevating the leg 30 to 45 degrees and observing for pallor over 60 seconds. The results can be graded:

- 0 No pallor in 60 seconds
- 1 Definite pallor in 60 seconds
- 2 Definite pallor in 30 seconds
- 3 Definite pallor in less than 30 seconds
- 4 Definite pallor with leg flat in bed

Because the leg elevation with this test can cause the client pain from further decrease of arterial supply to the leg, it should be performed only as needed. The nurse notes the degree of pallor at rest and uses the test only to assist with determining the severity of ischemia.

CLUBBING

Clubbing is a condition in which the nail bed angle increases to 180 degrees or more. It is related to a long-standing lack of oxygen to the peripheral tissues and is commonly associated with pulmonary disease.

The nurse assesses the nail bed angle by inspecting the nails from the side or using the Schamroth method to check for clubbing. Clubbing is classified as early, late, or prolonged, as described in Chapter 36.

TRENDELENBURG'S TEST

Superficial varicose veins are usually easy to recognize. They appear as dilated, tortuous (twisting) veins. At times, however, the client may have dilated veins from other causes, and further assessment is needed. The client lies down with the leg elevated until the veins are empty. A tourniquet is applied at midthigh, snugly enough to occlude the superficial veins. With the tourniquet in place, the client stands. The examiner then notes the time required for the veins to fill from below. Normally, veins fill in about 35 seconds. The tourniquet should be released after 60 seconds. Usually, when the tourniquet is released, no further blood fills the vein from above. If additional blood flows into the vein from above, the valve is incompetent, and allows backflow of blood. The vein normally fills from below; a varicose vein would fill from above because of incompetent valves.

Palpation

TEMPERATURE

The temperature of the legs is palpated with the dorsal surface of the hand. The temperature and vascular tone should be the same in both legs. Vasoconstriction produces cold, pale, moist skin with collapsed superficial veins. Bilateral vasoconstriction may be due to environmental factors such as smoking, room temperature, apprehension, or generalized arterial disease. Unilateral or localized vasoconstriction indicates peripheral vascular disease.

Skin turgor may also be noted at the time skin temperature is being assessed. Turgor refers to the normal tension found in the skin. Dehydrated skin is loose and easily lifted off the extremity surface. Taught, shiny skin indicates edema. "Tenting" of the skin is an unreliable sign of dehydration in older clients, owing to a loss of subcutaneous tissue.

PULSES

The nurse palpates the pulse by placing the first three fingers along the length of the selected artery (Fig. 44-7). Gentle pressure is used against the bone or firm surface followed by a gradual release. The nurse palpates radial, carotid, axillary, brachial, and ulnar pulses (upper extremities) and femoral, popliteal, posterior tibial, and dorsalis pedis pulses (lower extremities). The carotid pulse can be included in the examination for completeness, but is not commonly assessed as part of the peripheral vascular system. Pulses should be palpated bilaterally and simultaneously except for the carotid pulse. Carotid pulses should be palpated sequentially to avoid stimulation of the carotid sinus, which could produce bradycardia or sinus arrest. The temporal pulse is usually assessed as part of the head and neck examination (see Chap. 38). Ulnar pulse assessment is performed during Allen's test (see following).

Always note rhythm, amplitude, and symmetry of pulses. The rate of peripheral pulses is not counted. Peripheral pulses should be compared for rate, rhythm, and quality. Pulses are graded as follows:

0	Absent
+1	Weak and thready
+2	Normal
+3	Full and bounding

The nurse records the scale used to assess pulse quality. Several scales are used in practice.

Note whether a pulse is absent or feels unequal bilaterally. The dorsalis pedis pulse is congenitally absent in approximately 10 to 17 per cent of the normal adult population. The posterior tibial pulse is absent congenitally in 9 per cent of the black adult population.

ALLEN'S TEST

There are times when it is important to test blood flow in the upper extremity. Blood flow to the hand is normally supplied by both the ulnar and radial arteries, which join at the volar arch in the palm. Allen's test is used to assess the patency of the radial and ulnar arteries distal to the wrist. It is a common test performed before arterial blood gases are drawn (see Chap. 36) or an arterial line is inserted (see Chap. 42).

Compress the radial and ulnar arteries. Ask the client to clench the fist, then have the client open the hand, which should be pale and mottled. The radial artery is released, assessing patency of the ulnar artery. The hand should regain full color promptly (less than 6 seconds). Repeat the process, this time releasing the ulnar artery to assess the patency of the radial artery. If the hand remains pale, either the radial or ulnar artery (depending on the one being tested) is possibly occluded.

HOMANS' SIGN

The nurse assesses for signs of phlebothrombosis by gently compressing the gastrocnemius muscle of the calf and asking the client whether this movement causes pain or tenderness. The test can also be performed quickly by dorsiflexing the foot. Calf pain that occurs with this maneuver is a positive finding of Homans' sign and should be reported to the physician.

The reliability of Homans' sign is being questioned. Studies indicate that about 50 per cent of people with deep venous thrombosis (DVT) have a negative response to Homans' test, and 50 per cent of people have a positive response to Homans' test when they do not have DVT. Doppler studies are more accurate.

Auscultation

Auscultation of the peripheral vascular system is done with a stethoscope, but best results are obtained with a

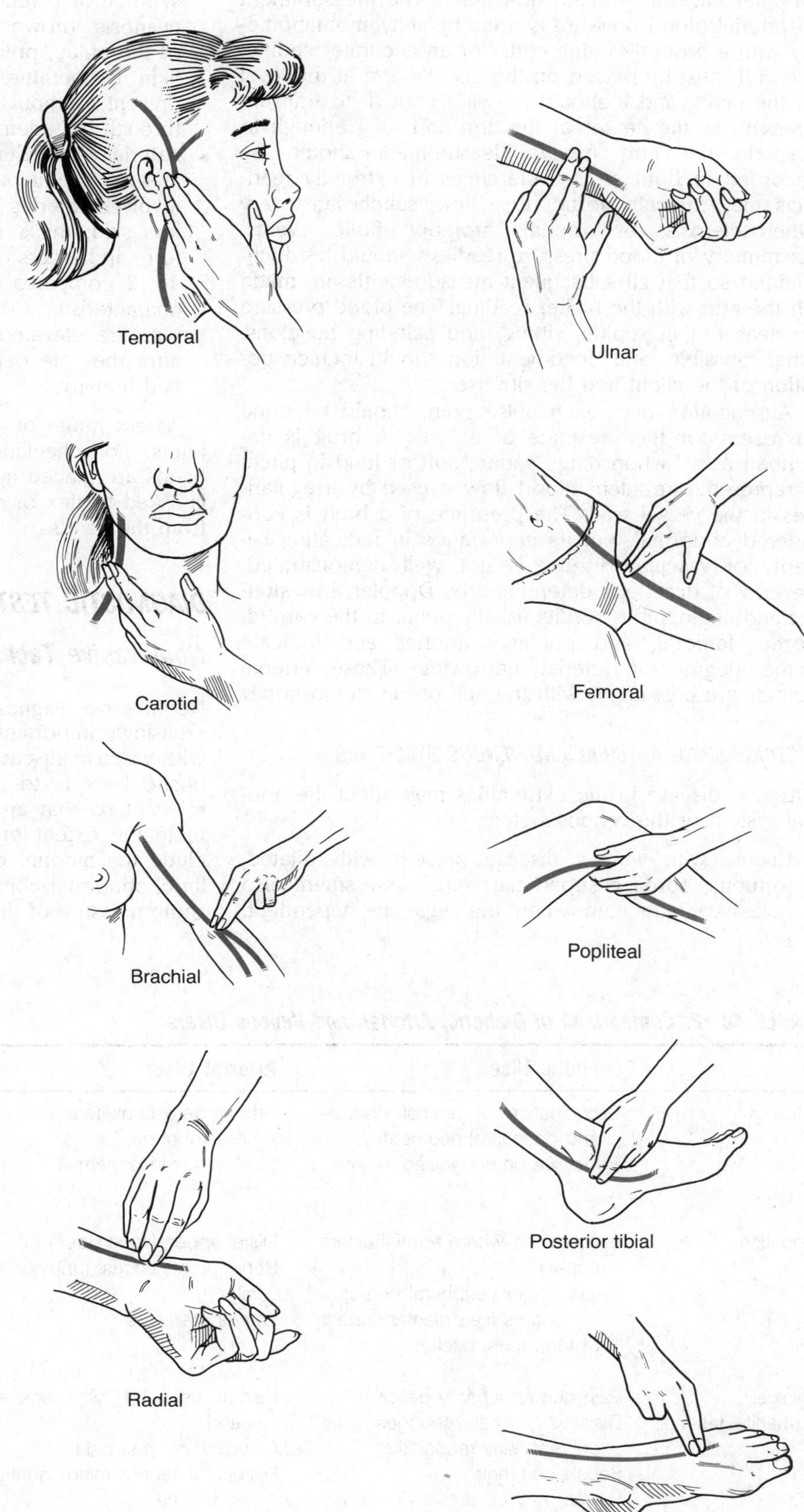

▲ *Figure 44–7*

Peripheral pulses are assessed bilaterally from head to toe and rated for amplitude, rhythm, and symmetry.

Doppler ultrasonographic flowmeter. The measurement of arterial blood pressure is done by sphygmomanometry with a properly fitting cuff. For an accurate reading, the cuff must be placed on the client's arm at the level of the heart, and it should be wide enough to transmit pressure to the center of the arm and long enough to encircle the arm firmly. Measurement should be recorded in both arms. Differences in extremity readings may indicate aortic dissection, subclavian artery atherosclerosis, or arterial thromboembolic events. Asymmetry of blood pressure readings should be documented so that all subsequent measurements are made on the arm with the higher reading. The blood pressure is measured in supine, sitting, and standing positions, when possible, and documentation should include position of the client and the site used.

Auscultation over each pulse point should be done to assess for the presence of a bruit. A bruit is described as a "whooshing" sound, soft or loud in pitch; it represents turbulent blood flow caused by irregularities in the vessel wall. The presence of a bruit is considered abnormal, but its importance in indicating severity of vascular disease is not well demonstrated. Severity of disease is determined by Doppler flow studies and angiography. Bruits usually occur in the carotid, aortic, femoral, and popliteal arteries and indicate some degree of arterial narrowing. These arterial sounds are best heard with the bell of the stethoscope.

DISTINGUISHING ARTERIAL AND VENOUS SYMPTOMS

Vascular disease in the extremities may affect the arterial system or the venous system.

- Clients with venous disease present with dilated, tortuous, cordlike superficial veins. Assessment also reveals aching pain when the legs are dependent. With chronic venous insufficiency, edema, dependent cyanosis, brown skin discolorations, possible ulcers of the ankle, pruritus, and paresthesia will be noted. Skin temperature remains normal, and pulses are present, although they may be hard to palpate through the edema.
- Arterial insufficiency is hallmarked by decreased or absent arterial pulses; a possible systolic bruit over involved arteries; muscular atrophy; thin, shiny, hairless skin; thick, ridged toenails; cool skin temperature; and ulcers on pressure points of the feet. Table 44–2 compares diabetic, arterial, and venous ulcer characteristics. The skin color is pale gray when the legs are elevated above heart level and dusky red after they are dependent. Edema, if present, is mild and brawny.

Assess range of motion of the hip, knee, and ankle joints. For checking muscle strength, the examiner's hands are placed against the lower legs, and the client is asked to flex or extend the knees against opposition from the hands.

DIAGNOSTIC TESTS

Noninvasive Techniques

Noninvasive diagnostic techniques have assumed an increasingly important role in the management of clients with vascular disease. The purpose of noninvasive diagnostic tests is to provide data that are reliable and relevant so that an evaluation can be made to determine the extent of the disease process. Variables include the amount of blood flow through the affected limb, abnormal compared with normal blood flow, and some measure of the degree of functional limitations.

TABLE 44–2. Comparison of Diabetic, Arterial, and Venous Ulcers

	Diabetic Ulcer	Arterial Ulcer	Venous Ulcer
Etiology	Combination of arterial disease and peripheral neuropathy Repetitive unrecognized trauma	Arteriosclerosis obliterans Atheroembolism (Both result in ischemia)	Valvular incompetency Incompetent perforators History of deep vein thrombosis Venous hypertension
Location	Same areas where arterial ulcers appear Areas where peripheral neuropathy occurs (i.e., plantar aspect of foot, toes, heels)	Distal appendages (toes) Bone prominences (anterior tibial) Lateral malleolus	Medial aspect of distal third of lower extremity Behind medial malleolus
Clinical manifestations	Pain due to sensory deficit Diabetic retinal changes that prevent early recognition Sepsis common Pulses may be present or diminished (arteries become calcified)	Painful, especially with legs elevated Claudication, rest pain History of recent minor nonhealing trauma Atrophic changes Pulses poor quality or absent	Not often painful Dark pigmentation Eczema or stasis dermatitis Edema Comfortable with legs elevated Normal arterial pulses

LIMB BLOOD PRESSURE

The measurement of blood pressure is the most commonly applied noninvasive test of cardiovascular function. It may be the best single indicator of how well perfusion is being maintained. Acute and chronic arterial occlusion produces regional hypotension.

ANKLE-BRACHIAL INDEX

The measurement of the ankle-brachial index (ABI) is the most commonly used parameter for overall evaluation of extremity status. A regular arm blood pressure cuff is applied above the malleoli, and the arterial pulse is found at either the dorsalis pedis or posterior tibial site. With a Doppler probe placed over the pulse, the cuff is inflated to above systolic pressure. The cuff is deflated until the pulse returns. This represents systolic endpoint. The usual procedure is to measure the pressure in both the dorsalis pedis and posterior tibial branches; the higher of the two pressures is used as the indication of leg status. This number is then divided by the higher of the two branchial artery pressures. (For example, an ankle pressure of 60 mm Hg with a brachial pressure of 120 mm Hg gives an index of 0.5.) Ankle pressure is normally the same or higher than the brachial systolic pressure. Normal foot arteries have an index of 1.0 to 1.2. Indexes below 1.0 suggest arterial obstruction has lowered ankle pressure. An ABI of 0.8 to 1.0 suggests mild obstruction, 0.5 to 0.8 is moderate obstruction, and less than 0.5 is severe obstruction.

DOPPLER ULTRASONOGRAPHY

Hand-held Doppler instruments permit assessment of peripheral arterial disease by audible evaluation of arterial signals or measurement of limb blood pressures (Fig. 44–8). This test is simple and inexpensive, but the technique may not detect minor disease and is less accurate than duplex scanning.

Brightness mode (B-mode) ultrasound is the creation of a two-dimensional image from ultrasound waves. It can be used to assess vein size, compressibility, flow patterns, thrombus and valve function.

ULTRASONIC DUPLEX SCANNER

Ultrasonic duplex scanners are used to localize the site of vascular disease and to estimate its hemodynamic significance. The technique is the most sensitive and specific noninvasive modality for detecting deep vein thrombosis. This device provides both an ultrasonographic image of the vessel and a Doppler signal characterizing the flow pattern at a given site. The anatomic data allow more specific localization of the level of stenosis than is possible with simple pressure or waveform techniques. The major limitations to these devices are their cost, complexity, and lack of portability.

PLETHYSMOGRAPHY

Plethysmographs record a biologic change in volume in a portion of the body associated with cardiac contractions or respirations or in response to pneumatic venous occlusion. These instruments detect and quantify vascular disease on the basis of changes in pulse wave contour, blood pressure, or arterial or venous blood flow.

COMPUTERIZED TOMOGRAPHY

Computerized tomography (CT) allows visualization of the arterial wall and its structures. CT scans can be used in the diagnosis of abdominal aortic aneurysms and postoperative complications, such as graft infection, graft occlusion, hemorrhage, and abscess.[25]

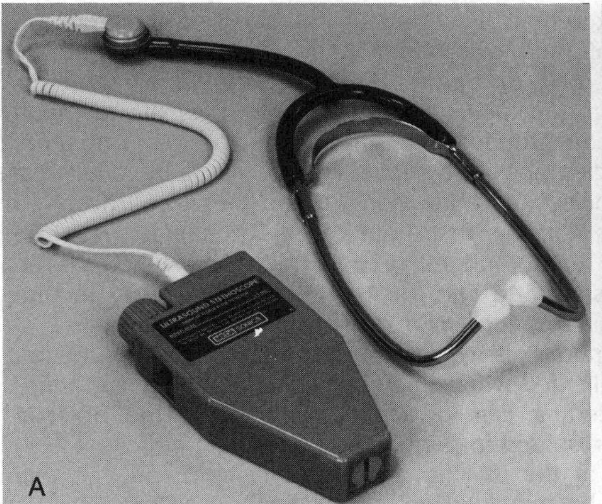

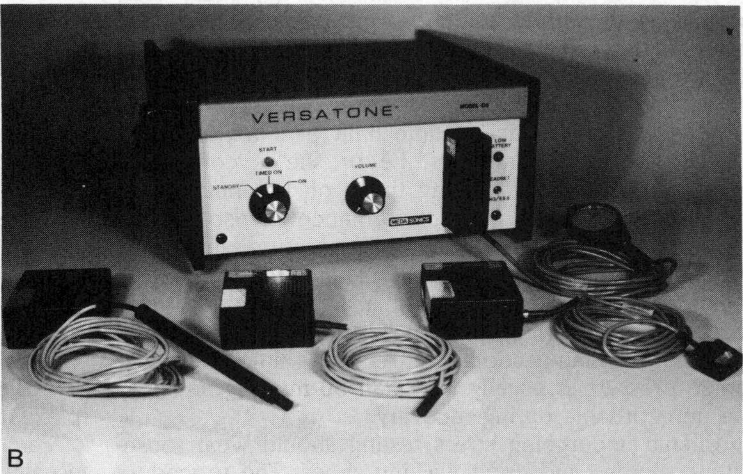

▲ *Figure 44–8*

The Doppler ultrasound flowmeter detects blood flow. *A*, Ultrasound stethoscope. *B*, Multipurpose ultrasound instrument with interchangeable probes. (Courtesy of MedaSonics, Inc., Mountain View, CA.)

Clients must lie still while a long tube passes over them. If the client cannot lie still or is claustrophobic, sedation may be necessary.

MAGNETIC RESONANCE IMAGING

Magnetic resonance imaging (MRI) is the use of magnetic fields, rather than radiation, to obtain cross-sectional images of the client. MRI is used to detect deep vein thrombosis from the pelvic iliac veins and leg veins. Clients with implanted metal devices, such as aneurysm clips or iron or steel in their body (e.g., shrapnel) cannot undergo MRI. The client is placed in a long magnetic tube. Clients who cannot lie still or have claustrophobia may require sedation.[25]

IMPEDANCE PLETHYSMOGRAPHY

Impedance plethysmography is also used to measure venous blood volume changes in the extremities. It is used to diagnose deep vein thrombosis. It is based on the assumption that blood is a good conductor of electricity and a small change in blood volume will result in a change in resistance. During the procedure, electrodes from a plethysmograph are applied to a limb, along with a pressure cuff. As pressure is increased, electrical resistance is increased; thus, the quality of venous blood flow is indicated.

The client is informed about the purpose of the procedure, that a technique similar to blood pressure measurement will be used, and that the procedure lasts 30 to 60 minutes. Clients must be able to assume a supine position with the involved extremity elevated above the level of the heart.

EXERCISE TESTING

Exercise testing provides an objective measurement of the severity of intermittent claudication and how much it interferes with the client's lifestyle. The most commonly used method for stress testing is the treadmill exercise test. The treadmill test is similar to that used for coronary clients except that walking speed is usually 1.5 to 2 miles per hour, with a grade elevation of 10 to 20 per cent and a time limit of 5 minutes. If a client can walk 5 minutes, he or she is considered mildly symptomatic; walking times of 1 minute represent severe disease. Test performance is also gauged by measurement of ankle systolic pressure. In normal clients, the time required for return to preexercise ankle pressure is usually less than 3 minutes with a 20 per cent (or less) drop from baseline. In clients with intermittent claudication, the recovery time is longer; ankle pressure is usually less than 50 mm Hg and may be unrecordable during recovery.

Clients undergoing stress testing should wear loose-fitting clothes and good walking shoes. The procedure should be explained so the client knows what to expect. The client should also know that exercise will be stopped at the maximal level of exertion or when symptoms become disabling.

Invasive Techniques

CONTRAST ANGIOGRAPHY AND VENOGRAPHY

Contrast angiography is the most invasive of the diagnostic procedures for arterial disorders and has the greatest risk for the client. It is frequently performed before vascular surgery and can be used intraoperatively to evaluate an operation. The procedure involves injecting contrast into the arterial system and performing radiographic studies. Angiography is performed in a catheterization laboratory or a special procedures room of the radiology department. The client is given nothing by mouth 2 to 6 hours before the procedure. A mild sedative may be used. Angiography is performed under sterile conditions. Local anesthesia is given at the injection site, and a catheter is placed percutaneously. Contrast is injected through the catheter, and then fluoroscopy may be done. Serial pictures of the movement of the dye are taken by cameras positioned over the study field. Most angiograms take 30 to 90 minutes.

Venography is performed in a similar manner except that the venous system is examined. Venograms can be used to detect deep vein thrombosis or other abnormalities such as incompetent valves.

Before the procedure, the client is informed of the indications for the test and of potential risks. Informed consent is needed from the client. It is important to document the presence and quality of peripheral pulses before the procedure. During the procedure, the injection contrast may cause a burning or flushing sensation and the client may experience some nausea. Because radiopaque dye is being used, the client's possible allergy to the dye or shellfish (which contain iodine) should be assessed before the diagnostic test. Clients with known dye allergies can often be premedicated for reducing the incidence and severity of allergic reactions to the dye.

After the procedure, a pressure dressing is placed on the injection site. Pulses distal to the site are monitored for the next 4 to 6 hours. Intravenous fluids are continued for 8 to 24 hours after the procedure for help with dye excretion. Fluid status is assessed; observe for signs of fluid overload. On the client's return to the nursing unit or before discharge, the nurse monitors vital signs, palpates pulses, and observes the insertion site frequently for bleeding or hematoma formation. Postangiography protocols vary, but generally vital signs, pulses, and insertion site are monitored every 15 minutes for the first hour, every 30 minutes for the second hour, and every hour for 2 to 6 hours. The client is on bed rest for 4 to 8 hours and may require analgesia, especially for relief of back discomfort.

The nurse also assesses motor and sensory function especially following angiography of the upper extremity. Bleeding can cause compression of the brachial plexus resulting in permanent neurologic deficits.

Pain at the injection site is fairly common and can usually be managed with mild analgesics. More severe pain or pain distal to the puncture site requires further assessment of peripheral pulses, neurovascular assessment, and palpation for masses. The physician should be notified of abnormal assessment data.

Complications of angiography in addition to allergic reaction to the contrast media include thrombi, perforation of the vessel, emboli, and renal failure. Creatinine levels should be monitored. Pseudoaneurysm is a significant complication and may extend hospital stay. Pseudoaneurysm is a contained arterial wall outpouching with persistent communication between the artery and the fluid component of an adjacent mass. Pseudoaneurysms generally result from arterial trauma (after arterial puncture) or occur at the surgical site. They are a site of infection, a source of emboli, and associated with intravascular thrombosis. They can enlarge, compress an adjacent structure, and even rupture, although rupture is rare.

OTHER RADIOGRAPHIC IMAGING

Contrast angiography has been the diagnostic standard for arterial disorders for years. Because of improved techniques, the client risk and discomfort have decreased. It is likely, however, in the future, that MRI techniques will supply much of the information currently available only with angiography. MRI has the double advantage of not requiring ionizing radiation and not using any form of injection into the arterial system. The expense and time required for the procedure will make it a less than optimal technique for routine screening and follow-up.

Vascular Endoscopy (Angioscopy). Vascular endoscopy permits imaging of intra-arterial disease in color and in three dimensions with use of fiberoptic technology. Equipment consists of a flexible fiberoptic angioscope, a light source, irrigation system, camera, video recorder, and monitor. The angioscope's major asset is to permit visualization of the surface of the vessel for identifying thrombus, plaque, hemorrhage, ulceration, or embolus. Angioscopes can be used to remove debris from a vessel and to check the integrity of an anastomosis from within a vessel. They may also be used to remove the valves from veins to prepare them for use as bypass grafts. Complications are rare but may include intimal damage, vessel spasm, thrombosis or embolism, perforation, and fluid overload. The incidence of infection is also very low.

Intravascular Ultrasonography. Intravascular ultrasonography provides information about the atherosclerotic intima beneath the luminal surface. It can thus determine the thickness of the arterial wall and can distinguish thrombus and calcium from vascular tissue, allowing more exact removal of lesions. One current limiting factor is the need for specialized interpretation of the scans.

▼ HYPERTENSION

Definition

Arterial hypertension, or high blood pressure, is generally defined as a persistent elevation of systolic blood pressure above 140 mm Hg and of diastolic pressure above 90 mm Hg. The published 1988 Report of the Joint National Committee on Detection, Evaluation and Treatment of High Blood Pressure notes the remarkable changes in the control of hypertension over the past 20 years.[38] The public is more knowledgeable about high blood pressure, more likely to visit a physician for hypertension, and more likely to follow medical advice. These practices have contributed to a 50 per cent decrease in the national age-adjusted stroke mortality since 1972 and a 35 per cent decline in coronary artery disease mortality. Hypertension remains, however, a major contributor to morbidity and mortality in our society.

CLASSIFICATION OF HYPERTENSION

Hypertension may be classified according to type (systolic and diastolic), cause, and degree of severity.

Systolic and Diastolic Hypertension. Systolic hypertension is systolic pressure greater than 140 mm Hg. Clients over age 65 frequently have systolic pressure over 140 mm Hg and diastolic pressure over 90 mm Hg. For these clients, hypertension is defined as systolic pressure over 160 mm Hg and/or diastolic pressure over 95 mm Hg.

Diastolic hypertension is diastolic pressure greater than 90 mm Hg.

Primary and Secondary Hypertension. Primary hypertension, also known as essential or idiopathic hypertension, constitutes more than 90 to 95 per cent of all cases of hypertension. The etiology of primary hypertension is multifactorial; a number of interacting homeostatic forces are involved. Characteristics include either a gradual onset and prolonged course (benign hypertension) or an abrupt onset and a short dramatic course that proves rapidly fatal without swift intervention (malignant or accelerated hypertension). Secondary hypertension results from an identifiable cause. A variety of specific disease states or problems are responsible. Five to 10 per cent of the hypertensive population have secondary hypertension. The importance of identifying clients with secondary hypertension centers on the fact that sometimes the disorder creating the hypertension can be corrected with medications or surgery.

Borderline Hypertension. Borderline or labile hypertension is defined as intermittent elevation of blood pressure interspersed with normal readings. Clients with borderline hypertension still carry an increased risk of developing cardiovascular disease.

White Coat Hypertension. White coat hypertension is defined as hypertension in a population of clients who have normal blood pressures except when blood pressure measurements are taken by a health care professional, especially a physician. The cause of this response is thought to be anxiety. The significance of white coat hypertension is not clear.

Malignant Hypertension. Malignant hypertension is a syndrome of markedly elevated BP (diastolic BP over 140 mm Hg) associated with papilledema. Accelerated hypertension is a syndrome of markedly elevated BP with retinal hemorrhage and exudate. Accelerated hypertension presumably develops into malignant hypertension if not well managed.

Benign Hypertension. Benign hypertension is a term used to describe uncomplicated hypertension, usually of long duration and mild to moderate severity. Benign hypertension may be primary or secondary.

Incidence

Arterial hypertension affects nearly 60 million clients in the United States. Prevalence of hypertension increases with advancing age, and blacks are affected more than whites are. Hypertension is the most common public health problem in the United States. In addition, hypertension is the single most important predictor of cardiovascular risk. Blood pressure level is related to severity of atherosclerosis, stroke, nephropathy, peripheral vascular disease, aortic aneurysms, and congestive heart failure.

Alarmingly, a significant portion of the hypertensive population remains undiagnosed, and only a small number of those who have been diagnosed receive adequate intervention. Among those being treated, many do not follow their recommended treatment regimen. Unfortunately, primary hypertension remains a sizable health problem and a challenge for health care practitioners.

Etiology

Primary hypertension has no single or specific cause but is multifactorial. It develops in response to increased cardiac output or to a rise in peripheral resistance. Factors that affect these two forces include

- genetic propensity (1) to a heightened neurologic response to stress or (2) for a defect in renal excretion or cellular transport of sodium
- obesity associated with high levels of insulin (hyperinsulinemia) that lead to raised blood pressure
- environmental stress
- loss of elastic tissue and arteriosclerosis of aorta and other large arteries

Secondary hypertension can result from a variety of identifiable primary causes (Table 44–3).

TABLE 44–3. Causes of Secondary Hypertension

Renal
- Renal parenchymal disease
  - Acute glomerulonephritis
  - Chronic nephritis
  - Polycystic disease
  - Connective tissue diseases
  - Diabetic nephropathy
  - Hydronephrosis
- Renovascular
- Renin-producing tumors
- Renoprival
- Primary sodium retention (Liddle's syndrome, Gordon's syndrome)

Endocrine
- Acromegaly
- Hypothyroidism
- Hyperthyroidism
- Hypercalcemia
- Adrenal
  - Cortical
    - Cushing's syndrome
    - Primary aldosteronism
    - Congenital adrenal hyperplasia
  - Medullary: pheochromocytoma
- Extra-adrenal chromaffin tumors
- Carcinoid
- Exogenous hormones
  - Estrogen
  - Glucocorticoids
  - Mineralocorticoids: licorice
  - Sympathomimetics
  - Tyramine-containing foods and monoamine oxidase inhibitors

Coarctation of the aorta

Pregnancy-induced hypertension

Neurologic disorders
- Increased intracranial pressure
  - Brain tumor
  - Encephalitis
  - Respiratory acidosis
- Sleep apnea
- Quadriplegia
- Acute porphyria
- Familial dysautonomia
- Lead poisoning
- Guillain-Barré syndrome

Acute stress, including surgery
- Psychogenic hyperventilation
- Hypoglycemia
- Burns
- Pancreatitis
- Alcohol withdrawal
- Sickle cell crisis
- Postresuscitation
- Postoperative

Increased intravascular volume

Alcohol, drugs, and so on

Adapted from Braunwald, E. (1992). *Heart disease: A textbook of cardiovascular medicine* (4th ed.). Philadelphia: W. B. Saunders.

Risk Factors

PRIMARY PREVENTION

Prevention of hypertension involves the identification of nonmodifiable risk factors and the identification and management of modifiable risk factors. Risk factors serve to determine a client's risk for this chronic illness. The relative risk for hypertension depends on the number and severity of modifiable risk factors.

Nonmodifiable Risk Factors

Family History. The genetic predisposition that makes certain families more susceptible to hypertension seems to be associated with elevated intracellular sodium levels and lowered potassium to sodium ratios. This is found more often in blacks. Clients with parents who have hypertension have a greater risk of developing hypertension at a younger age. This has not been demonstrated to be solely genetic; environmental factors may also be involved.

Age. The incidence of hypertension increases with age; 50 to 60 per cent of clients over 50 years of age have a blood pressure over 140/90 mm Hg. However, epidemiologic studies have shown a poorer prognosis in clients whose hypertension began at a young age.

Gender. Men experience hypertension at higher rates and at an earlier age than do women until after age 60 years. Men also have greater risk of cardiovascular morbidity and mortality. After age 50, hypertension is more prevalent in women. The reasons are not clear.

Ethnic Group. Hypertension is the most serious health problem for blacks in the United States. Hypertension is more prevalent in blacks, and at any given blood pressure, blacks have a greater mortality rate in comparison with whites. The reason for the increased prevalence of hypertension among blacks is unclear, but it has been attributed to heredity, greater salt intake, and greater environmental stress.

Modifiable Risk Factors

Stress. Stress has been shown to cause increased peripheral vascular resistance and cardiac output and to stimulate sympathetic nervous system activity. Stress may be associated with occupational factors, socioeconomic levels, and personality characteristics.

Obesity. Obesity, in particular that located in the upper body with increased amounts of intra-abdominal fat, is an important cause of hypertension; the combination may be related to hyperinsulinemia secondary to insulin resistance.

Nutrients. Sodium is an important etiologic factor in essential hypertension. A high-salt diet may induce excessive release of natriuretic hormone, which may indirectly increase blood pressure. Sodium loading has also been shown experimentally to stimulate vasopressor mechanisms within the central nervous system. Potassium deficiency has been implicated as a cause of hypertension. Also, calcium intake may be lower among hypertensive than among normotensive clients. The impact of caffeine is controversial. It raises blood pressure acutely but does not have sustained effects.

Prevention in the Community. The incidence of hypertension presents a national problem that individual interventions alone cannot counter. Prevention of hypertension and early discovery of new cases depend on a national public health effort. To be successful, this national effort needs to enlist governmental support and involve such nationwide structures as business and industry, labor organizations, health care institutions, voluntary associations, and local communities.

Because the exact cause of primary hypertension remains unknown, if has been difficult for public health services to develop a comprehensive primary prevention program. However, several risk factors associated with the development of hypertension are known. Once high-risk clients are identified, clinicians can teach them how to modify certain risk factors such as diet, sodium intake, exercise, and so forth.

Hypertensive clients usually find out about their condition through incidental screening in health care facilities or organized community screening in public settings (e.g., shopping malls, schools, the workplace). Nurses are actively involved in both approaches. About 80 per cent of Americans come into contact with some aspect of the health care system at least once a year (i.e., in a physician's office, clinic, or hospital). Each encounter with the health care system presents an opportunity for incidental blood pressure screening. Blood pressure measurement should be a routine procedure at every initial encounter with a health care practitioner and annually thereafter.

Organized community screening programs help assess the remaining 20 per cent of Americans not in contact with any part of the health care system. Such programs identify not only untreated hypertensive clients but also those who have discontinued intervention or who are not adequately controlled on current intervention. In addition, screening programs provide an opportunity to educate the public. It is particularly important to screen high-risk "target groups" such as black and elderly populations. Community services need to keep "target groups" in mind when choosing the setting for blood pressure screenings. Those who take blood pressure readings need to inform clients in writing of their blood pressure, its significance, and, if necessary, the importance of follow-up evaluation.

SECONDARY PREVENTION

Because the beginnings of adult hypertension often lie in childhood and adolescence, children over the age of 3 years need yearly blood pressure determinations. Asymptomatic youngsters who, on three separate occasions, have an elevated blood pressure reading require a careful work-up and follow-up program.

Of national concern is the rise in childhood obesity. In the past 20 years, obesity among 6- to 11-year-old

American children increased 54 per cent; among the 12- to 17-year-old population, the increase was 39 per cent. Obese teenagers have an 80 per cent chance of becoming obese adults. In that obesity in children is a major cause of hypertension, these statistics dramatically demonstrate the need for attention to this issue.[38]

TERTIARY PREVENTION

Once diagnosed, hypertension requires ongoing management despite the absence of symptoms. The many sequelae of unmanaged hypertension (i.e., stroke and myocardial infarction) could be prevented or their severity reduced if hypertension were well managed. Because of the cost of antihypertensives, side effects, and lack of symptoms, unfortunately many clients do not manage the disorder well.

Pathophysiology

PRIMARY (ESSENTIAL) HYPERTENSION

The actual pathogenesis of hypertension remains unknown. Arterial blood pressure is a product of cardiac output and total peripheral resistance. Cardiac output is determined by stroke volume and heart rate. Control of peripheral vascular resistance is maintained by the autonomic nervous system and circulating hormones. Therefore, any factor producing an alteration in peripheral vascular resistance, heart rate, or stroke volume affects systemic arterial blood pressure.

Four control systems play a major role in maintaining blood pressure. These include the arterial baroreceptor system, regulation of body fluid volume, the renin-angiotensin system, and vascular autoregulation. It is probable that no single defect causes essential hypertension in all clients.

Arterial baroreceptors are found in the carotid sinus, aorta, and wall of the left ventricle. These baroreceptors monitor the level of arterial pressure and counteract rises through vagally mediated cardiac slowing and vasodilation with decreased sympathetic tone. The role of the arterial baroreceptors in hypertension is not well understood. It may be that the sensitivity of the baroreceptors is reset so that pressure rises are inadequately sensed; or the mechanism may be excessive central nervous system–mediated stimulation of adrenergic nerves.

Changes in fluid volume affect systemic arterial pressure. Thus, an abnormality in the transport of sodium in the renal tubules may cause essential hypertension. When there is an excess of sodium and water, total blood volume increases, thereby increasing blood pressure. In functional kidneys, a rise in pressure leads to diuresis. Pathologic changes that alter the pressure threshold at which kidneys excrete salt and water alter systemic blood pressure. In addition, the overproduction of sodium-retaining hormones has been implicated in hypertension.

Renin and angiotensin play a role in blood pressure regulation. Renin is an enzyme produced by the kidney that catalyzes a plasma protein substrate to split off angiotensin I, which is removed by a converting enzyme to the lung to form angiotensin II, then angiotensin III (Fig. 44–9). Angiotensin II and III act as vasoconstrictors and control aldosterone release. With increased sympathetic nervous system activity, angiotensin II and III also seem to inhibit sodium excretion, which results in elevated blood pressure. Increased renin secretion has been investigated as a cause of increased peripheral vascular resistance in primary hypertension.

Clients may also develop hypertension from deficiencies in vasodilators such as prostaglandins or congenital abnormalities in resistance vessels.

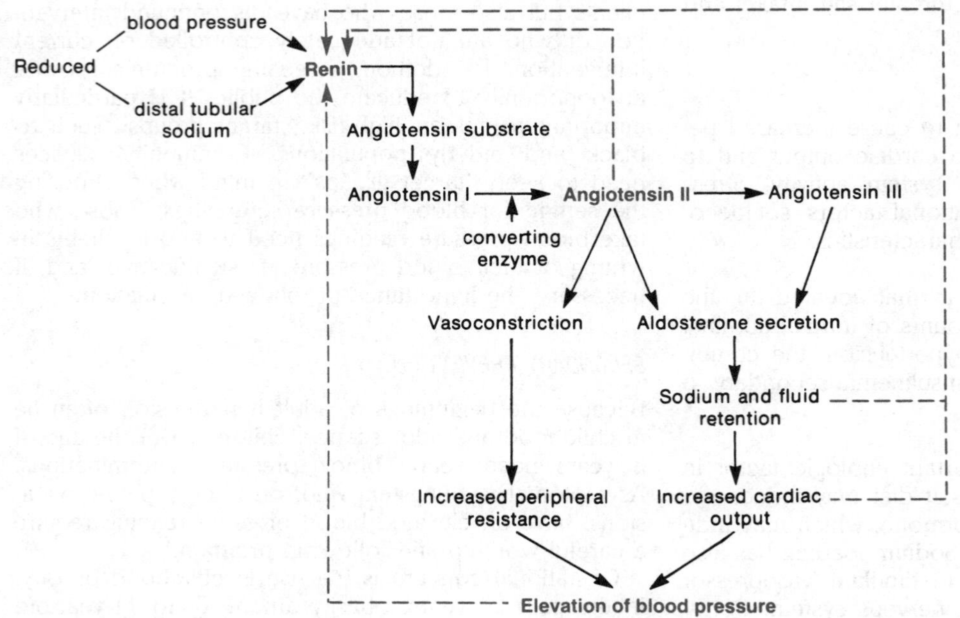

▲ **Figure 44–9**

Role of renin-angiotensin-aldosterone system in regulation of blood pressure. Solid lines represent positive interactions; broken lines show negative interactions or feedback inhibition. (From Kumar, V., Cotran, R. S., & Robbins, S. L. [1992]. *Basic pathology* [5th ed.]. Philadelphia: W.B. Saunders.)

SECONDARY HYPERTENSION

The primary mechanisms involved in producing secondary hypertension include (1) increased secretion of catecholamines (e.g., pheochromocytoma), (2) increased release of renin (e.g., renal artery stenosis), and (3) expansion of sodium and blood volume (e.g., Cushing's syndrome).

Among the causes listed, the use of estrogen-containing oral contraceptive pills remains the most common cause of secondary hypertension. Most women demonstrate a slight elevation in blood pressure with their use, and approximately 5 per cent develop hypertension that persists after discontinuation of the pill.

Renal parenchymal disease, mainly chronic glomerulonephritis, constitutes the next most common form of secondary hypertension. Any serious insult to the kidney that interferes with sodium excretion, renal perfusion, or the renin-angiotensin-aldosterone mechanism may elevate blood pressure.

The adrenal glands cause secondary hypertension as a result of primary excesses of aldosterone, cortisol, and catecholamines. Primary aldosteronism usually arises from solitary benign adenomas of the adrenal cortex that release excess aldosterone. Excess aldosterone causes renal retention of sodium and water, expands blood volume, and elevates blood pressure. Other adrenal cortical problems can result in excess production of cortisol (Cushing's syndrome). Clients with Cushing's syndrome have an 80 per cent risk of developing hypertension. Cortisol increases blood pressure by increasing renal sodium retention, angiotensin II levels, and vascular reactivity to norepinephrine. Pheochromocytoma, a small tumor of the adrenal medulla, can cause hypertension owing to the release of excessive amounts of epinephrine and norepinephrine.

VESSEL CHANGES

Early in the course of primary or secondary hypertension, there may be no obvious pathologic changes in the blood vessels and organs. The client may experience few or no symptoms other than intermittent elevations of blood pressure (labile hypertension). Slowly, widespread pathologic changes take place in both the large and small blood vessels and in the heart, kidney, and brain.

The large vessels such as the aorta, coronary arteries, basilar artery to the brain, and peripheral vessels in the limbs become sclerosed and tortuous. Their lumens narrow, with resultant decreased blood flow to the heart, brain, and lower extremities. As the damage continues, large vessels may occlude or hemorrhage.

Small vessel damage, equally dangerous, causes structural changes in the heart, kidneys, and brain. Elevated diastolic blood pressure damages the intima of the small vessels. Because of intimal damage, fibrin accumulates in the vessels, local edema develops, and intravascular clotting may occur. The net result of these changes involves (1) a decreased blood supply to the tissues of the heart, brain, kidneys, and retina and (2) progressive functional impairment of these organs.

In the development of hypertensive cardiovascular disease, a vicious circle of pathologic changes occurs in which each new manifestation of the disease complicates other manifestations of the disease. When arterioles are constricted, the heart must increase its contractility to maintain normal cardiac output and overcome elevations in "afterload." This chronic overwork leads to hypertrophy of the heart, primarily the left ventricle. Hypertrophy may lead to coronary insufficiency and myocardial infarction if the enlarged heart muscle outgrows its blood supply. If the hypertrophied heart cannot maintain sufficient cardiac output, left ventricular failure ensues. Left ventricular hypertrophy is a major risk factor for cardiac arrhythmias and sudden death.

As diastolic pressure rises in the failing left ventricle and atrium, the congestion extends back to involve the entire pulmonary tree; this, in turn, may lead to right ventricular failure. Blood may back up into the systemic circulation, causing systemic venous pressure to rise. Venous congestion and reduced arterial blood flow decrease renal perfusion. The kidneys may then fail, which further aggravates the hypertension. The increased arterial pressure in the arteries, coupled with arteriosclerotic weakening of the blood vessels, can cause aneurysms to develop and blood vessels to rupture.

Clinical Manifestations

The early stages of hypertension have no clinical manifestations, other than elevations in blood pressure. This unfortunate fact means that there are no signs or symptoms to lead a person to seek health care. As hypertension advances, without treatment clients may report morning occipital headache, fatigue, dizziness, palpitations, flushing, blurred vision, and epistaxis.

Prognosis

The advent of effective antihypertensive agents has dramatically reduced the mortality rate associated with hypertension. Still, if untreated, nearly one half of hypertensive clients die of heart disease, a third die of stroke, and the remaining 10 to 15 per cent die of renal failure. Hypertension may also be a silent factor in many deaths attributed to stroke or heart attacks. When hypertension arises as a secondary process, death usually results from the primary disease.

Resources for materials on high blood pressure are available to health care professionals. Materials include bibliographies, brochures, posters, medical management research, catalogs for audiovisual aids, and guides for organizing local programs.

Medical Management

DIAGNOSIS OF HYPERTENSION

The diagnosis of hypertension in the adult is determined when the average of two or more diastolic blood pressure readings, on at least two separate visits at least 2 weeks apart, is 90 mm Hg or higher, or when the average of multiple systolic blood pressure readings over several visits is greater than 140 mm Hg. Because blood pressure is variable and can be affected by multiple factors, it should be measured so that readings are representative of the client's usual level. The following techniques are strongly recommended.

1. Clients should be seated with their arm bared, supported, and positioned at heart level. They should not have smoked tobacco within the past 15 minutes or ingested caffeine within the past hour.
2. Measurement should begin after 5 minutes of quiet rest. The back should be supported, and both feet should be flat on the floor with the legs uncrossed. The client should not speak while blood pressure is being monitored.
3. The appropriate cuff size is used to ensure an accurate measurement. The rubber bladder should encircle at least two thirds of the limb being measured. The bladder's width should be one third to one half the circumference of the limb. Several sizes of cuffs (e.g., child, adult, and large adult) should be available. If the cuff is too wide, the blood pressure reading will be falsely low. If the cuff is too narrow, the reading will be falsely high. Inaccurate cuff size is the most common error in taking blood pressure measurement.
4. Measurements should be taken with a mercury sphygmomanometer, a recently calibrated aneroid manometer, or a validated electronic device. Aneroid gauges should be calibrated every 6 months against a mercury manometer.
5. Both the systolic and diastolic blood pressure should be recorded. The disappearance of sound (phase V) should be used for the diastolic reading.
6. Two or more readings should be averaged. If the first two readings differ by more than 5 mm Hg, additional readings should be obtained.

Clients should be informed of their blood pressure reading and advised of the need for periodic remeasurement. When working with lay clients, the examiner should refer to hypertension as "high blood pressure" to help allay confusion associated with the term "hypertension." Many clients unfamiliar with medical terms may believe that hypertension denotes a state of being "hypertense," that is, being worried or agitated. For these clients, the term "high blood pressure" more accurately conveys the nature of the health problem.

Categorization of Severity. The 1988 Joint National Committee on Detection, Evaluation and Treatment of High Blood Pressure has developed a classification of diastolic and systolic blood pressure readings (Table 44-4). Clinicians can use this classification to categorize blood pressure readings and to diagnose hypertension in clients aged 18 years or older. Risk related to hypertension continues to increase as systolic and diastolic pressures rise. Classifying hypertension according to blood pressure readings reflects the degree of risk and helps determine intervention. The 1984 Joint National Committee used these same classifications to develop follow-up criteria for first-occasion measurement (Table 44-5).

TABLE 44-4. Classification of Blood Pressure in Adults Aged 18 Years or Older*

Range (mm Hg)	Category†
DBP	
<85	Normal BP
85-89	High-normal BP
90-104	Mild hypertension
105-114	Moderate hypertension
≥115	Severe hypertension
SBP, when DBP is < 90	
<140	Normal BP
140-159	Borderline isolated systolic hypertension
≥160	Isolated systolic hypertension

From 1988 Joint National Committee: The 1988 report of the Joint National Committee on Detection, Evlauation, and Treatment of High Blood Pressure. *Archives of Internal Medicine, 148,* 1023, 1989. Copyright 1989, American Medical Association.

*Classification based on the average of two or more readings on two or more occasions; BP indicates blood pressure; DBP, diastolic blood pressure; and SBP, systolic blood pressure.

†A classification of borderline isolated systolic hypertension (SBP 140 to 159 mm Hg) or isolated systolic hypertension (SBP ≥160 mm Hg) takes precedence over high-normal BP (DBP 85 to 89 mm Hg) when both occur in the same client. High-normal BP (DBP 85 to 89 mm Hg) takes precedence over a classification of normal BP (SBP <140 mm Hg) when both occur in the same client.

TREATMENT OF HYPERTENSION

The goal of treating clients with hypertension is to prevent morbidity and mortality associated with high blood pressure. The objective is to achieve and maintain arterial blood pressure below 140/90 mm Hg, if possible.

Normalizing high blood pressure may involve psychosocial and economic stressors for the client. These stressors are considered when intervention is initiated. As mentioned earlier, most hypertensive clients do not have symptoms and are not aware that they have hypertension. The long-term nature of intervention along with the high costs and untoward side effects of pharmacologic interventions promote poor adherence with therapeutic regimens. Poor adherence has great impact on the effectiveness of intervention.

Intervention for secondary hypertension rests on treating the underlying disorder, whereas intervention for primary hypertension aims directly at reducing blood pressure. Careful differential diagnosis of primary versus secondary causes of high blood pressure must precede any intervention.

Nonpharmacologic Intervention. Nonpharmacologic intervention is widely advocated as initial therapy for most clients, at least for the first 3 to 6 months after

TABLE 44-5. Follow-up Criteria for First-Occasion Measurement

Range (mm Hg)	Recommended Follow-up
Diastolic	
<85	Recheck within 2 years*
85-89	Recheck within 2 years
90-104	Confirm promptly (not to exceed 2 months)
105-114	Evaluate or refer promptly to source of care (not to exceed 2 weeks)
≥115	Evaluate or refer immediately to source of care
Systolic, when diastolic is ≤90	
<140	Recheck within 2 years*
140-199	Confirm promptly (not to exceed 2 months)
≥200	Evaluate or refer promptly to source of care (not to exceed 2 weeks)

*Rechecking within 1 year is recommended for clients at increased risk of progressing to higher blood pressures (family history of hypertension, cardiovascular event, weight gain, obesity, black race, use of an oral contraceptive, or excessive ethanol consumption).

From *The 1984 Report of the Joint National Committee on Detection, Evaluation, and Treatment of High Blood Pressure* (NIH Publication No. 88-1088). Washington, DC: U.S. Government Printing Office.

initial diagnosis. This therapy may be effective for many of the 40 per cent of clients with mild hypertension (diastolic levels between 90 and 94 mm Hg). For the remainder of the population of clients with hypertension, nonpharmacologic therapy may aid in reducing blood pressure such that less drug therapy is needed.

Weight Reduction. The relationship between obesity and blood pressure has been clearly established from numerous studies. Weight reduction to within 15 per cent of ideal body weight is recommended for all obese hypertensive clients. Those who are able to maintain weight loss usually achieve significant falls in blood pressure.

Sodium Restriction. Studies demonstrating the antihypertensive efficacy of moderate sodium restriction to a level of approximately 1 to 2.5 g of sodium or 4 to 6 g of salt have been reported since the early 1970s. These studies also demonstrate the ability of most clients to adhere to such a regimen. Moderate sodium restriction is not hazardous and may reduce the degree of potassium depletion accompanying diuretic therapy.

Modification of Dietary Fat. Modification of dietary intake of fat by decreasing the fraction of saturated fat and increasing that of polyunsaturated fat may decrease blood pressure and will decrease the cholesterol level, which is an important risk factor for coronary artery disease. The use of fish oil supplements to lower cardiovascular risk has been shown to lower blood pressure in preliminary studies, but fish oil supplementation may cause deficient blood clotting and excessive bleeding in some clients. Therefore, this therapy is not recommended until long-term results are known.

Exercise. A regular program of aerobic (isotonic) exercise facilitates cardiovascular conditioning, can aid the obese hypertensive client in weight reduction, and may provide some benefit in reducing blood pressure. Heavy isometric exercises such as weightlifting may be harmful; blood pressure often rises to very high levels because of vasovagal reflexes that occur during an isometric contraction. Advise hypertensive clients to initiate exercise programs gradually and receive ongoing professional surveillance of their condition.

Restriction of Alcohol. The consumption of more than 1 to 2 ounces of alcohol per day is associated with a higher prevalence of hypertension, poor adherence to the antihypertensive therapy, and, occasionally, refractory hypertension. Alcohol intake needs to be carefully assessed; those who do drink should be advised to do so in moderation (i.e., less than 1 to 2 ounces of ethanol per day). There is 1 ounce (28 g) of ethanol in 2 ounces of 100-proof whiskey, 8 ounces of wine, or 24 ounces of beer.

Caffeine Restriction. Although acute ingestion of caffeine may raise blood pressure, chronic moderate caffeine ingestion appears to have no significant effects on blood pressure. Instruct clients to limit caffeine to 250 mg (the amount in two to three cups of brewed coffee) because it probably raises blood pressure by activating the sympathetic nervous system. This sympathetic response particularly affects those not used to drinking coffee.

Relaxation Techniques. A variety of relaxation therapies, including transcendental meditation, yoga, biofeedback, and psychotherapy, have been shown to reduce blood pressure in hypertensive clients at least transiently. Although each has its advocates, none has been conclusively shown to be either practical for the majority of hypertensive clients or effective in maintaining a significant long-term effect.

Smoking Cessation. Smoking has not been statistically linked to the development of hypertension. However, nicotine definitely increases heart rate and produces peripheral vasoconstriction, which does raise arterial blood pressure for a short time. Smoking cessation is strongly recommended, however, to reduce the client's risk for cancer, pulmonary disease, and cardiovascular disease. Smokers appear to have a higher frequency of malignant hypertension and subarachnoid hemorrhage. In addition, risk reduction brought about by antihypertensive therapy may not be as great in smokers as in nonsmokers.

Potassium Supplements. The high ratio of sodium to potassium in the modern diet has been held responsible for the development of hypertension. However, even though potassium supplements may lower blood pressure, they are too costly and potentially hazardous for routine use. A reduction of high-sodium, low-potassium processed foods with an increase of low-sodium, high-potassium natural foods may be all that is needed to achieve the potential benefits.

Calcium Supplements. The most recent studies examining the antihypertensive effects of calcium supplements demonstrate that this therapy may be helpful for a small portion of the population with hypertension. Clients should ensure a reasonable dietary calcium intake rather than using potassium for preventing or treating hypertension.

Magnesium Supplements. The antihypertensive effect of supplemental magnesium has been less well studied than that of potassium or calcium. Lower magnesium levels have been noted in hypertensive clients, and diuretic therapy may induce hypomagnesemia. In the presence of documented hypomagnesemia, supplementation may be considered.

Pharmacologic Intervention. Considerable debate continues regarding the appropriate time and circumstances for the initiation of pharmacologic management of hypertension. Clinicians sometimes question whether the benefits of medications outweigh their risks and inconveniences, particularly in mildly hypertensive clients. However, antihypertensive agents do decrease cardiovascular mortality and morbidity associated with hypertension.

Once a decision has been made to use pharmacologic intervention, one of several drugs can be used. If therapy is chosen carefully, more than half of those with mild hypertension can be controlled with a single drug, and more than 90 per cent should be controlled with no more than two drugs. Long-term compliance has emerged as an essential element in reducing morbidity and mortality associated with hypertension. Several factors related to specific drug use, including side effects, interference with lifestyle, cost, and inconvenience of use, play an important role in noncompliance. Thus, drug selection is a critical part of the management of the client with hypertension. The ultimate factors in determining whether a correct choice has been made are that the medication controls the blood pressure, is tolerated, is safe, and is a drug the client is willing to take long term.

Antihypertensive medications can be classified by mode of action into the following categories: diuretics, adrenergic inhibitors, vasodilators, angiotensin-converting enzyme (ACE) inhibitors, and calcium antagonists. Table 44-6 outlines major antihypertensive agents.

Diuretics are used to initiate and maintain antihypertensive therapy. Thiazide diuretics have been used for more than 30 years in the treatment of hypertension. Their efficacy and safety are well demonstrated. They are most effective in older and in black clients who tend to have a low renin type of hypertension. Diuretics lower blood pressure by reducing extracellular fluid volume.

The Stepped-Care Approach. The goal of antihypertensive therapy is to control blood pressure with a minimum of side effects. The Joint National Committee on Detection, Evaluation and Treatment of Hypertension has recommended the stepped-care approach to the treatment of hypertension (Table 44-7). The 1988 report expands the pharmacologic choices available for initial and subsequent therapy and encourages substituting drugs as well as adding or reducing drugs to improve blood pressure control or reduce side effects. Clinicians are encouraged to adopt an individualized approach to drug therapy, considering demographic concerns, the presence of concomitant diseases or therapies, and quality of life in selecting drugs for individual clients.

Step-Down Therapy. Once a client with mild hypertension has been controlled for one year or more, medications can be titrated down slowly. Regular follow-up is essential.

Combination Therapy. More than 50 per cent of clients with mild hypertension can be controlled with one drug; the rest will require combination therapy. If more than one drug is necessary, several combination therapies have proved effective. The combination of a diuretic with a beta-adrenergic blocker or other adrenergic inhibitor has been effective in both blacks and whites, unlike the responses to the individual drugs. The combination of diuretic and ACE inhibitor is synergistic because diuretics create high-renin hypertension, a milieu in which ACE inhibitors are effective. Orthostatic hypertension can be a problem, especially in older clients or those with acute volume depletion. The combination of a diuretic and calcium channel blocker has additive effects on blood pressure.

Complications: Malignant Hypertension

OVERVIEW

Malignant (accelerated) hypertension is an emergency characterized by diastolic pressures above 120 mm Hg, retinal hemorrhage and exudates with papilledema, acute renal failure, and rapid vascular deterioration. Malignant hypertension has a peak incidence at age 40 to 50 years; its occurrence in clients below 30 or over 60 years of age should raise the suspicion of a secondary cause of hypertension. Without treatment, malignant hypertension results in a 90 per cent mortality rate within 1 year secondary to renal or congestive heart failure, cerebrovascular accident, myocardial infarction, or aortic dissection. Blood pressure control reduces the chances of these complications.

The most common cause of malignant hypertension is untreated hypertension. Other causes include eclampsia, dissecting aortic aneurysms, pyelonephritis, sudden catecholamine release (pheochromocytoma), drug or toxic substance ingestion/exposure, or food and drug interactions (monoamine oxidase inhibitors and aged cheeses).

The presenting manifestations of malignant hypertension include hypertensive retinopathy. The retinopathy is characterized by arteriolar constriction, flame-shaped hemorrhages resulting from damaged capillary endothelium, and soft exudates secondary to transudation of protein from ischemic infarction of nerve fibers. Papil-

TABLE 44-6. Antihypertensive Medication Therapy

Medication	Actions	Comments	Contraindications	Side Effects	Nursing Considerations
Diuretics					
Thiazide and Related Sulfonamides					
Bendroflumethiazide (Naturetin) Benzthiazide (ExNa, Aquatag) Chlorothiazide (Diuril) Chlorthalidone (Hygroton) Hydrochlorothiazide (Esidrex, Hydro-Diuril, Oretic) Methyclothiazide (Naturon) Polythiazide (Renese) Trichlormethiazide (Metahydrin, Naqua) Metolazone (Zaroxolyn) Quinethazone (Hydromox)	Promote renal excretion of sodium, water, and potassium Blood volume and cardiac output are decreased at first; with continued therapy, levels rise to normal Peripheral vascular resistance is increased at first, then drops below normal	All thiazides have a comparable effect on blood pressure, differing mainly in potency and duration Alone, thiazides can control hypertension in 40% of clients; in combination, they permit smaller doses of other antihypertensive agents Inexpensive	Known sensitivity to sulfonamide-derived drugs; renal insufficiency or failure; hepatic disease; lactation; blood urea nitrogen 40% or higher	Hypokalemia, hyperglycemia, hyperuricemia, hypercalcemia, lethargy, dry mouth, thirst, restlessness, muscle cramps, hypotension, polyuria, fatigue, tachycardia, gastrointestinal disturbances, vertigo, gout, leukopenia, and agranulocytosis Sexual dysfunction may occur May increase cholesterol, low-density lipoprotein, and triglyceride levels	Warn client that orthostatic hypotension may be potentiated by alcohol, barbiturates, and narcotics Monitor serum electrolytes, blood urea nitrogen, uric acid Teach client which foods are high in potassium and low in sodium Daily weight monitoring Resulting hypokalemia can potentiate digitalis toxicity Monitor diabetic clients closely
Loop Diuretics					
Furosemide (Lasix) Ethacrynic acid (Edecrin) Bumetadine (Bumex)	Comparable to thiazides Act on loop of Henle to minimize sodium and water reabsorption	Drug of choice in clients with renal failure	Comparable to thiazides; not recommended in pregnant women	Same as thiazides, hyponatremia, plus dehydration, vascular thrombosis, and embolism in elderly Can cause side effects, oral and gastric burning, and a sweet taste	Comparable to thiazides May avoid taking drug before bedtime to prevent frequent urination and loss of sleep May need to increase dose of hypoglycemic agents
Potassium-Sparing Diuretics					
Spironolactone (Aldactone) Triamterene (Dyrenium)	Block action of aldosterone in distal loop, promoting excretion of sodium and water and retention of potassium Action of triamterene is unknown	These are weak diuretics that potentiate other antihypertensive drugs	Acute renal insufficiency, rapidly progressing impaired renal function, and hyperkalemia Avoid concomitant use with calcium channel blocking agents	Hyperkalemia, hyponatremia, elevated blood urea nitrogen, gynecomastia, menstrual irregularity, hirsutism, headache, urticaria, impotency, and ataxia (with spironolactone) Blood dyscrasias with triamterene	Administer after meals to reduce nausea Potassium supplementation not required Closely monitor potassium, especially in those with renal insufficiency

Table continued on following page

TABLE 44–6. Antihypertensive Medication Therapy Continued

Medication	Actions	Comments	Contraindications	Side Effects	Nursing Considerations
Vasodilators					
Hydralazine (Apresoline)	Direct action on smooth muscle walls of arterioles causing arteriolar vasodilation Cardiac output increases initially, then returns to normal Peripheral vascular resistance is decreased There is also some vasodilation	Most commonly used in combination with a beta-blocking agent and a diuretic with good results. Antihypertensive effects can be counteracted by the increase in cardiac output	Coronary artery disease, mitral valvular rheumatic heart disease, and hypersensitivity to drug	Minimal side effects Headache, palpitation, flushing, dyspnea, angina pectoris, and lupus-like syndrome (after prolonged use)	Monitor for reflex tachycardia Treat headache with acetaminophen, cold packs, or relaxation techniques
Adrenergic Inhibiting Agents					
Beta-adrenergic Inhibitors (beta-blockers)					
Propranolol (Inderal) Metoprolol (Lopressor) Nadolol (Corgard) Atenolol (Tenormin) Timolol (Blocadren) Pindolol (Visken) Labetalol (Trandate, Normodyne)	Block beta-receptors in the heart and peripheral vessels to reduce peripheral vascular resistance	These agents vary in their effects on beta-receptors: some (i.e., propranolol) affect $beta_1$- and $beta_2$-receptors; others (e.g., atenolol, metoprolol, and pindolol) are cardioselective, affecting only $beta_1$-receptors	Bronchial asthma, allergic rhinitis, chronic obstructive pulmonary disease, bradycardia, heart block, pulmonary hypertension, congestive heart failure Do not give with (or less than 2 weeks after) therapy with monoamine oxidase inhibitors	Bradycardia, congestive heart failure, bronchospasm, hypoglycemia, fatigue, vivid and colorful dreams, insomnia, Raynaud's phenomenon, depression, nausea, vomiting, diarrhea, fluid retention, and (rarely) impotence	Avoid use in clients with bronchial asthma Assess for signs of heart failure Instruct client to take own pulse daily for evidence of bradycardia or irregularity Warn diabetics that these medications may mask signs of hypoglycemia Do not stop abruptly; this may exacerbate myocardial ischemia Toxic effects are reversed with isoproterenol or dopamine
Alpha-adrenergic Inhibitors					
Prazosin hydrochloride (Minipress)	Vasodilation occurs with a decrease in peripheral vascular resistance Cardiac output and heart rate are usually unchanged	Most effective in combination with a diuretic or other sympatholytic agent	Not recommended for pregnant women	First-dose syncope; postural hypertension, dizziness, lightheadedness, headache, drowsiness, nausea, lethargy, palpita-	Monitor closely after drug administration (especially first dose) because postural hypotension and syncope may occur

TABLE 44-6. Antihypertensive Medication Therapy Continued

Medication	Actions	Comments	Contraindications	Side Effects	Nursing Considerations
Adrenergic Inhibiting Agents					
				tions, rash, nervousness, diphoresis, impotence, urinary frequency, and depression	30 to 90 minutes after dose is initiated Used cautiously in the elderly because postural hypotension is more pronounced
Central-Acting Adrenergic Inhibitors					
Clonidine (Catapres)	Suppress central nervous system sympathetic outflow Cardiac output decreases at first, then returns to normal Peripheral vascular resistance and heart rate decrease	An extremely effective medication, especially in clients with severe hypertension or reninde-pendent disease	Not recommended for pregnant women Tricyclic antidepressants may block drug's effect	Dry mouth, sedation, dizziness, constipation, headache, fatigue, bradycardia, and some sodium and water retention (transient), hyperglycemia	Action potentiated by alcohol, sedatives, digitalis, propranolol, and guanethidine Diabetics may require more insulin Drug should be discontinued over 2 to 4 days to prevent rebound hypertension Recommended periodic eye examinations Chewing gum or hard candy may relieve dry mouth
Calcium Channel Blocking Agents					
Nifedipine (Procardia) Verapamil hydrochloride (Calan, Isoptin) Diltiazem (Cardizem) Nicardipine (Cardene)	Block entry of calcium into smooth muscle cells and may interfere with the intracellular release of calcium Cause arteriolar vasodilation and decreased peripheral vascular resistance	Nifedipine has the most potent vasodilating effect Nifedipine and diltiazem are preferred agents in this group	Severe congestive heart failure, sick sinus syndrome, or progressive heart block Avoid use with beta-blocking agents	Headache, dizziness, palpitations, weakness, nausea, flushing, hypotension, arrhythmia, constipation, diarrhea, rash, fluid retention, and edema Verapamil can cause bradycardia	Watch for sudden hypotension, especially with the administration of nifedipine; this can occur 5 minutes after sublingual administration and 20 minutes after the oral route Monitor pulse for bradycardia with use of verapamil May exacerbate asthma, peripheral vascular disease, and diabetes

Table continued on following page

TABLE 44–6. Antihypertensive Medication Therapy Continued

Medication	Actions	Comments	Contraindications	Side Effects	Nursing Considerations
Adrenergic Inhibiting Agents					
Angiotensin-converting Enzyme Inhibitors					
Captopril (Capoten) Enalapril (Vasotec) Lisinopril (Zestril, Prinivil)	Inhibits conversion of angiotensin I to angiotensin II May also inactivate the vasodepressor bradykinin Reduces peripheral vascular resistance without changing cardiac output	Extremely effective in clients with high-renin, severe hypertension Most effective when given in conjunction with a diuretic	Use with caution in clients with preexisting renal insufficiency and renal artery stenosis	Fever, rash, stomatitis, taste loss, tongue ulceration, hyperkalemia, granulocytopenia, hemolytic anemia, renal damage with proteinuria	Monthly urine protein analysis recommended along with a leukocyte count to detect renal damage Taste loss is a frequent side effect and may decrease desire for eating Hypotension may accompany first dose
Peripheral-Acting Adrenergic Inhibitors					
Reserpine (Serpasil)	Depletes brain and peripheral nerve tissues of norepinephrine Decreases peripheral vascular resistance, heart rate, and standing blood pressure	Has same actions as other rauwolifa alkaloids Seldom used alone but in combination with a diuretic or other symptholytic agent	Mental depression, especially with suicidal tendencies; peptic ulcer disease, ulcerative colitis	Depression, weight gain, nasal stuffiness, peptic ulceration, postural hypotension, drowsiness, constipation, bizarre dreams, bradycardia, and impotence	Observe for signs of depression; instruct client to notify physician or nurse if "low mood" sets in Depletes catecholamines, so stop reserpine 2 weeks before elective surgery Concurrent use with digitalis and quinidine may potentiate arrhythmias

ledema results from obstruction of venous outflow from the optic discs because of intracranial hemorrhage.

Additional clinical manifestations include hypertensive encephalopathy manifested by restlessness, changes in level of consciousness (confusion, somnolence, lethargy, memory defects, coma, seizures), blurred vision, dizziness, headache, nausea, and vomiting. Assessment may also reveal renal insufficiency, proteinuria, hematuria, urinary sediment casts, hemolytic anemia, left ventricular failure, and pulmonary edema. Severe headache may be occipital or anterior in location, is steady and throbbing in quality, and is often worse in the morning. Visual blurring, reduced visual acuity, and even blindness can occur.

MANAGEMENT

Malignant hypertension constitutes a true medical emergency, and any delay in initiating intervention can be catastrophic. The seriousness of the crisis correlates not so much with the level of blood pressure elevation as with the extent of target organ damage. Intervention relies almost entirely on parenteral administration of medications. Most often, the physician orders the concurrent administration of two or three agents (Table 44–8).

These clients require monitoring in an intensive care unit. Parameters requiring close scrutiny include urinary output, blood pressure (via an intra-arterial catheter), central venous pressure, and pulmonary capillary wedge pressure. Continuous electrocardiographic monitoring helps assess for ischemic myocardial changes and arrhythmias.

The treatment goal is to lower blood pressure, but as blood pressure lowers, evidence of target organ impairment (especially of kidneys) may appear. Consequently, restoration of blood pressure must be done slowly and with care. Once the client is out of immediate danger,

TABLE 44-7. Stepped-Care Approach to Drug Therapy of Hypertension

Step 1	The physician starts with less than a full dose of a thiazide diuretic, beta-blocker, calcium channel blocker, or angiotensin-converting enzyme inhibitor and adjusts the dosage as necessary.
Step 2	If blood pressure control is not obtained, the physician increases the dose of the first drug or adds a drug of a different class.
Step 3	If blood pressure control is not obtained, the physician substitutes a second drug or adds a third drug of a different class.
Step 4	If blood pressure control is not obtained, the physician adds a third or fourth drug and evaluates further.

From U.S. Department of Health and Human Services (1988). *The 1988 Report of the Joint National Committee on Detection, Evaluation, and Treatment of High Blood Pressure* (NIH Publication No. 88-1088). Washington, DC: U.S. Government Printing Office.

oral medications are administered while continuously monitoring vital signs. The physician typically prescribes a combination of diuretic, beta-blocker, and hydralazine. With better surveillance and control of hypertensive clients, hypertensive crisis is becoming less common.

The nurse monitors blood pressure frequently (every 15 minutes) and titrates the medications to manage the blood pressure. The clients' head is raised to decrease risk of cerebral bleeding. Anxiety is reduced, and urinary output is also closely monitored.

Nursing Management

NURSING ASSESSMENT

The assessment of the client with hypertension involves three main objectives: (1) to determine the extent of target organ involvement, (2) to ascertain the presence of other cardiovascular risk factors, and (3) to identify the type of hypertension (primary or secondary) in-

TABLE 44-8. Parenteral Drugs for Treatment of Hypertensive Emergency (in Order of Rapidity of Action)

Drug	Dosage	Onset of Action	Adverse Effects
Vasodilators			
Nitroprusside (Nipride, Nitropress)	0.25-10 μg/kg/min as IV infusion	Instantaneous	Nausea, vomiting, muscle twitching, sweating, thiocyanate intoxication
Nitroglycerin	5-10 μg/min as IV infusion	2-5 min	Tachycardia, flushing, headache, vomiting, methamoglobinemia
Diazoxide (Hyperstat)	50-100 mg/IV bolus repeated, or 15-30 mg/min by IV infusion	2-4 min	Nausea, hypotension, flushing, tachycardia, chest pain
Hydralazine (Apresoline)	10-20 mg IV 10-50 mg IM	10-20 min 20-30 min	Tachycardia, flushing, headache, vomiting, aggravation of angina
Enalaprilat (Vasotec IV)	1.25-5 mg every 6 hr	15 min	Precipitous fall in blood pressure in high renin states; response variable
Nicardipine (Cardene)	5-10 mg/hr IV	10 min	Tachycardia, headache, flushing, local phlebitis
Adrenergic Inhibitors			
Phentolamine (Regitine)	5-15 mg IV	1-2 min	Tachycardia, flushing
Trimethaphan (Arfonad)	0.5-5 mg/min as IV infusion	1-5 min	Paresis of bowel and bladder, orthostatic hypotension, blurred vision, dry mouth
Esmolol (Brevibloc)	500 μg/kg/min for 1 min then 50-300 μg/kg/min IV for 4 min; if effect inadequate, repeat loading dose and increase dose of maintenance infusion	1-2 min	Hypotension
Propranolol (Inderal)	1-10 mg load; 3 ng/hr	1-2 min	Beta-blocker side effect (e.g., bronchospasm, decreased cardiac output)
Labetalol (Normodyne, Trandate)	30-80 mg IV bolus every 10 min 2 mg/min IV infusion	5-10 min	Vomiting, scalp tingling, burning in throat, postural hypotension, dizziness, nausea

IM, intramuscular; IV, intravenous.
From Kaplan, N.M. (1992). Hypertension. In R.E. Rakel, *Conn's current therapy 1992.* Philadelphia: W.B. Saunders.

volved. Clinicians can obtain information relevant to these areas from the history, physical examination, and laboratory studies.

History. Note the following points when interviewing the hypertensive client:

- Family history of hypertension, diabetes mellitus, or cardiovascular disease.
- Previous documentation of high blood pressure, including age of onset and currently prescribed medical regimen.
- History of any disease or trauma to target organs.
- Results and side effects of previous antihypertensive therapy.
- Clinical manifestations of cardiovascular disorders, such as angina, dyspnea, or claudication.
- History of weight gain, exercise activities, sodium intake, fat intake, and alcohol use.
- Psychosocial and environmental factors (e.g., emotional stress, cultural food practices, and economic status) that may influence blood pressure control.
- Presence of other cardiovascular risk factors, including smoking, obesity, hyperlipidemia, and exercise levels.
- History of all prescribed and over-the-counter medications. Medications that may either raise blood pressure or interfere with the effectiveness of antihypertensive medications include oral contraceptives, steroids, nonsteroidal anti-inflammatory agents, cold remedies, appetite suppressants, cyclosporine, tricyclic antidepressants, and monoamine oxidase inhibitors.

Physical Examination. Physical assessment should include determination of blood pressure as well as evaluation of target organs.

Evaluation of target organs typically includes the following data: (1) funduscopic examination for retinal arteriolar narrowing, hemorrhages, exudates, and papilledema; (2) examination of the neck for distended veins, carotid bruits, and enlarged thyroid; (3) examination of the heart for increased heart rate, arrhythmias, enlargement, precordial impulses, murmurs, and S_3 and S_4 heart sounds; (4) examination of the abdomen for bruits, aortic dilation, and enlarged kidneys; (5) examination of extremities for diminished or absent peripheral pulses, edema, and bilateral inequality of pulses; and (6) neurologic evaluation for signs of cerebral thrombosis or hemorrhage.

Be especially alert to assessment findings suggesting secondary hypertension. These include headache, palpitations, and excessive perspiration (pheochromocytoma); leg claudication and diminished or absent lower extremity pulses (aortic coarctation); truncal obesity with pigmented striae (Cushing's syndrome); and polyuria, fatigue, and muscle cramps (hyperaldosteronism).

Laboratory Studies. A few general laboratory tests are usually done before intervention begins. These tests provide useful information in determining the severity of vascular disease, the extent of target organ damage, and the possible causes of hypertension. Studies used in the routine evaluation of hypertension include a complete blood count, urinalysis, determinations of serum potassium and sodium, fasting blood sugar, serum cholesterol, blood urea nitrogen, serum creatinine, electrocardiogram, and chest radiograph. Clients with potential for secondary hypertension may need more extensive studies.

Nursing Intervention

Nursing Diagnosis: Health Maintenance, Altered R/T knowledge deficit about the disease process, its consequences, and the rationale for intervention and proper administration of prescribed medications.

Planning: Expected Outcomes. The client and significant others will demonstrate knowledge required for self-care, as evidenced by their ability to describe the disease process, factors contributing to its symptoms and risks, and reasons that management of this disease is important; their ability to describe the proper administration of prescribed medication therapy, including drug name, rationale for use, dosage, frequency, potential side effects, and measures to minimize side effects; their demonstration of proper blood pressure measurement technique for home blood pressure monitoring; and their ability to discuss the importance of lifelong medical follow-up for hypertension control.

Implementation. Because of the chronicity of hypertension and its dangerous complications, clients with this condition need clear, practical, and realistic learning guidelines concerning effective handling of high blood pressure. Guidelines should include information concerning the disease and its management. The nurse uses written materials with clear illustrations to introduce the subject of hypertension to the newly diagnosed client. Teach the client to monitor and record his or her own blood pressure at home at least once a week and record the findings in a diary.

Nursing Diagnosis: Nutrition, Altered: More than Body Requirements R/T high sodium, calorie, and fat intake.

Planning: Expected Outcomes. The client will demonstrate knowledge of and adherence to the nutritional regimen by describing specific dietary modifications including sodium, fat, and calorie restrictions and their rationale; listing common foods to be avoided; reduced levels of urine sodium and blood cholesterol; and weight loss.

Implementation. The two most important aspects of dietary intervention for hypertension are weight reduction (for overweight clients) and mild to moderate sodium restriction. It is important, therefore, to advise the client with hypertension to eat a diet low in salt, calories, cholesterol, and saturated fat. Discuss the prescribed diet with those in the household who prepare food. If possible, enlist the aid of a dietician to provide detailed dietary instruction. Before dietary intervention begins, the client's patterns of food intake, lifestyle, food preferences, and ethnic, social, cultural, and financial influences are assessed. A highly individualized approach to dietary counseling is critical.

Sodium. Sodium is a hidden ingredient in many processed foods, beverages (including water), and over-the-counter drugs (particularly antacids, cough remedies, and laxatives). It cannot be seen and is often not tasted. Whereas the average adult daily intake of salt is 5 to 15 g, the therapeutic effects of sodium reduction on blood pressure do not occur until salt intake is reduced below 5 g/day. Low-salt diets can be very difficult to adhere to, at least initially. The nurse can reassure the client that it becomes easier as the palate adjusts to decreased salt over a period of several weeks to months. When someone becomes fully accustomed to the low-salt diet, unsalted foods usually cease to taste bland. Research has suggested a relationship between lower blood pressure and increased intake of the minerals calcium, potassium, and magnesium, but the data are not yet conclusive.[41] Guidelines for teaching clients about sodium reduction are presented in the Client Education Guide.

Fat and Cholesterol. Hypertension and high serum cholesterol (greater than 250 mg/dl) seem to be linked risk factors in the development of coronary artery disease. The level of serum cholesterol is partly determined by the consumption of cholesterol, saturated and polyunsaturated fats, and total calories. Because the body produces its own cholesterol, extra cholesterol in the diet is not necessary. Saturated fats are animal fats, including dairy products and beef and chicken fats, and also solid vegetable fats such as shortening, avocados, and coconut oils. Unsaturated fats are other vegetable fats. A diet low in saturated fats and high in polyunsaturated fats is beneficial in reducing blood pressure. Guidelines for teaching clients about fat and cholesterol reduction are presented in the Client Education Guide.

Calories and Weight. Weight reduction in the overweight hypertensive client can significantly reduce blood pressure and decrease workload of the heart. Ideally, weight loss should be no more than 0.5 kg (1 lb) a week. The average adult with hypertension is advised to reduce caloric intake by at least 250 calories per day. The overall goal should be achievement and maintenance of a weight that is within 15 per cent of desirable weight.

Nursing Diagnosis: Health Maintenance, Altered R/T lack of exercise regimen.

Planning: Expected Outcomes. The client will begin and maintain an appropriate exercise program, as evidenced by self-report, demonstration of ability to monitor heart rate during exercise, sensation of reduced physical and emotional stress, and reduced blood pressure.

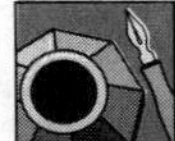

CLIENT EDUCATION GUIDE

Low-Sodium Diet

Avoid Foods High in Sodium

1. Read labels of foods carefully for "sodium," "Na+," "salt," "NaCl," "bicarbonate of soda," and "MSG" because these are all sources of sodium. If these words appear in the first four to five ingredients listed on the package, avoid the food item.
2. Sodium is present in large amounts in common commercial preparations such as baking powder, baking soda, monosodium glutamate, meat tenderizer, and soy sauce.
3. Sodium is often added to canned, boxed, and some frozen foods. (Frozen fruits and vegetables are okay.)
4. Avoid eating canned, smoked, pickled, or cured meat and fish products (canned tuna in water is okay). Pickled or preserved vegetables always contain salt.
5. Not all dietetic foods are sodium-free.
6. In restaurants, choose foods that are baked, broiled, boiled, or roasted and without salted gravies or juices. Avoid soups and salted or cheesy dressings. Carry your own salt substitute if desired. "Fast foods" also tend to be high in sodium.
7. "Lite" salt has half the sodium of table salt per unit. Non-sodium salt substitutes have a high potassium content and may be used to help prevent potassium deficiency if the client is taking a thiazide diuretic.

Preparing Low-Sodium Meals

1. Do not add salt at the table.
2. Use no salt during food preparation (2-g sodium diet); or use only half the salt called for in the recipe (4-g sodium diet).
3. Prepare canned vegetables (if they are to be eaten at all) by draining off the canned liquid and heating the food in tap water.
4. Natural spices, herbs, and condiments like pepper, parsley, chili, horseradish, lemon, and cloves contain negligible amounts of salt. These can be used liberally. Onion or garlic powder (dehydrated or pulverized) is also useful in low-salt cooking. Steak sauce, catsup, marinade, and soy sauce are all high in sodium.
5. Herb salts (celery, onion, garlic) contain salt and are not recommended.
6. Low-sodium cookbooks are available in bookstores and from heart associations.
7. Foods high or low in sodium are listed in Chapter 14.

Implementation. Exercise programs may heighten the client's sense of well-being, provide an outlet for emotional tensions, and raise the levels of high-density lipoproteins relative to total blood cholesterol. Elevated high-density lipoprotein levels are associated with a decreased risk of cardiovascular morbidity and mortality. The client should be instructed, however, to avoid heavy weightlifting, isometric exercises, and other activities inappropriate to the client's physical limitations.

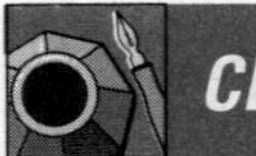

CLIENT EDUCATION GUIDE

Low-Fat, Low-Cholesterol Diet

Avoid Foods High in Saturated Fats and Cholesterol

1. Use margarine and vegetable oils instead of butter.
2. Avoid gravies, creams, and cheese sauces.
3. Avoid fried foods; broil, bake, or boil instead.
4. Use skim or low-fat milk and milk products.
5. Choose lean cuts of meat. Trim off all visible fat. Remove all poultry skin.
6. Use a wire rack when roasting, broiling, or baking meats so that the fat can drip off.
7. Fish, poultry, and veal have lower fat content. Breast of chicken and turkey are the leanest poultry available. Avoid duck and goose. Haddock, cod, and water-packed tuna are the leanest fish available.
8. Use Teflon-coated pans when cooking to reduce need for shortening.
9. Meat stews, soups, and gravies can be prepared in advance and chilled until the fat hardens. The fat is then skimmed off.
10. Eat no more than three egg yolks per week. Egg whites are low in cholesterol, as are many egg substitutes.
11. Limit the use of organ meats and shellfish.

A modest but consistent exercise program provides greater benefits than do spurts of strenuous activity mixed with periods of inactivity. A gradually increasing program of aerobic activity such as walking, jogging, or swimming can thus be recommended. Current recommendations include aerobic exercise, maintaining 70 to 80 per cent of maximal heart rate for 20 to 30 minutes, three times a week. Maximal heart rate is calculated by subtracting age from 220.

Nursing Diagnosis: Noncompliance, High Risk for R/T lack of understanding about the seriousness of high blood pressure, cost of therapy, side effects of medications.

Planning: Expected Outcomes. The client will demonstrate understanding of the seriousness of high blood pressure and accept the treatment plan, as evidenced by active participation in creating treatment plan, description of underlying causes of hypertension and self-care strategies, adherence to scheduled follow-up appointments, description of actions and side effects of current medications, and expression of commitment to and self-responsibility for controlling hypertension.

Implementation. The greatest problem in the management of chronic hypertension involves the client's lack of adherence to nonpharmacologic and pharmacologic intervention. An estimated 40 to 60 per cent of clients with hypertension fail to comply with prescribed therapy. There are several reasons that hypertensive clients fail to follow prescribed regimens. The asymptomatic nature of the disease tends to minimize the perceived seriousness of the problem and importance of intervention. Also, therapeutic regimens often demand difficult lifestyle changes, such as low-sodium diets, weight loss, and smoking cessation. Many hypertensive agents have annoying side effects, and those who require antihypertensive medication may consider the intervention worse than the disease. The high cost of prescribed medications and the inconvenience of obtaining health care also contribute to noncompliance. Nursing interventions for promoting compliance with the antihypertensive treatment regimen include individualizing care, assuring adequate follow-up, communicating often with the client, and teaching the client and family. Compliance usually improves dramatically when the client understands the causative factors underlying hypertension as well as the consequences of inadequate intervention and health maintenance.

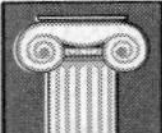

ETHICAL ISSUES IN NURSING

What Is the Responsibility of Health Care Providers in the Care of Noncompliant Hypertensive Clients?

Hypertension is a major predisposing factor to heart disease. Although it can many times be easily treated with medication, many clients are not aware that they have high blood pressure. There are many behavioral activities one can practice to safeguard against hypertension, including exercise; eating a low-fat, low-sodium diet; limiting alcohol consumption; and avoiding high-stress activities. Sometimes clients need medication along with their healthy lifestyle adjustments in order to keep their hypertension under control.

Teaching hypertensive clients the importance of proper medication use is vital. Often, because they may not feel any physical symptoms of hypertension, clients may forget to take their medication or feel that there is no need to take it regularly. Reinforcement from health care providers that medications must be taken as ordered no matter what symptoms they may or may not have is vital. Teaching clients about behavioral changes as described is also very important for health care providers to do. What do health care providers do with clients who, even after the most intense teaching has been done, are not compliant with their treatment? Should the nurses and doctors give up treating such clients? What is the responsibility of hypertensive clients regarding the following of their treatment guidelines? If such noncompliant clients receive public funds for their health care, should they have to pay back the public programs for treatments rendered as a result of their noncompliance?

Because hypertension is oftentimes not indicated by physical symptoms, clients with hypertension can easily ignore their treatment regimen. Not until their high blood pressure causes more severe cardiac and peripheral vascular problems do clients realize the negative aspects of their noncompliance. Not all hypertensive clients, of course, are noncompliant. It is the noncompliant clients, however, who present great challenges to the nursing staff. Again, client teaching is one of the greatest services nurses can offer their clients with high blood pressure.

Antihypertensive medications may cause emotional lability, sleep disturbances, and sexual changes including impotency. Discuss these potential problems with the hypertensive client and significant others. Counseling may help the client cope.

EVALUATION

The nurse evaluates the attainment of expected outcomes. Hypertension is a long-term disorder, and goal attainment should be evaluated after several months.

Modification of Plan of Care for the Elderly

Hypertension is one of the most prevalent cardiovascular diseases among the elderly. Research has provided conflicting findings on the effectiveness of treating hypertension in older adults. Because of this disagreement, there is a wide range of therapy given to elderly hypertensives, who consequently require extensive support, detailed advice, and careful follow-up. Older adults are also more likely to experience adverse reactions to antihypertensive drugs and therefore need to be monitored more closely.[46] Blood pressure readings in older adults may show greater variability from one reading to the next than do those of younger clients. The examiner must thus guard against making a diagnosis based on too few readings.[12]

▼ NURSING CARE OF CLIENTS WITH ARTERIAL DISORDERS

CHRONIC ARTERIAL OCCLUSION

Overview

Peripheral arterial occlusive disorders are conditions that involve narrowing of the arterial lumen or damage to the endothelial lining. They are sometimes classified according to duration of the problem, acute or chronic.

Peripheral arterial occlusive diseases can be caused by atherosclerosis, embolism, thrombosis, trauma, vasospasm, inflammation, or autoimmunity. The cause of some disorders remains unknown.

Most of the pathologic changes that occur in peripheral arterial occlusive disease are due to atherosclerosis. Atherosclerosis is considered in detail in Chapter 42.

It is the responsibility of the peripheral arterial system to deliver oxygen-rich blood to the peripheral vascular beds. Any alteration in blood flow will disrupt the balance between oxygen supply and demand. Prolonged reduction in blood flow or the involvement of large areas of decreased perfusion initiates the compensatory mechanisms of vasodilation, collateralization, and utilization of anaerobic pathways for metabolic demands to be met. These compensatory mechanisms are useful in protecting blood supply to the peripheral vascular bed but are limited by certain factors. Vasodilation has a limited effect because arteries that become oxygen-deprived quickly dilate fully. The diffuse network of collateral vessels needed to protect blood supply develops slowly over time. Cellular anaerobic metabolism tries to meet the basic requirements, but the waste products of lactic acid and pyruvic acid build up quickly, are extremely toxic, and are excreted slowly. Significant increases in these two acids will change the body's acid-base balance. As the compensatory mechanisms prove inadequate to meet peripheral vascular needs and without medical or surgical intervention, the eventual result is peripheral gangrene.

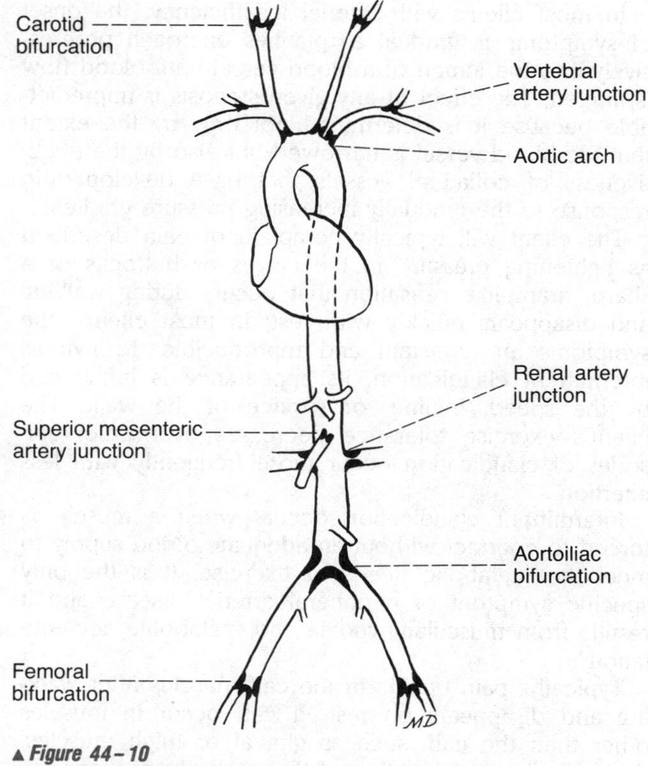

▲ **Figure 44–10**

Major sites of peripheral atherosclerotic occlusive disease.

Clinical Manifestations

Clinical manifestations of chronic arterial occlusion due to peripheral vascular disease may not appear for 20 to 40 years. The lower limbs are far more susceptible to arterial occlusive disorders and atherosclerosis than are the upper limbs. The most common locations for stenosis in a lower extremity are the aortoiliac bifurcation and the femoral bifurcation (Fig. 44–10). These lesions cause narrowing of the arterial lumen and critically reduce blood flow, possibly producing thrombosis or aneurysm.

The most important manifestations of chronic arterial occlusive disease are intermittent claudication and rest pain.

In most clients with arterial insufficiency, the onset of symptoms is gradual as plaques encroach progressively into the lumen of a blood vessel until blood flow is limited. The effect of any given stenosis is unpredictable because it is determined not only by the extent that the blood vessel is narrowed but also by the effectiveness of collateral vessels that have developed in response to the gradually increasing pressure gradient.

The client will typically complain of pain described as tightening pressure in the calves or buttocks or a sharp, cramplike sensation that occurs during walking and disappears quickly with rest; in most clients, the symptoms are constant and reproducible. Known as intermittent claudication, its appearance is influenced by the speed, incline, or surface of the walk. The client's exercise tolerance decreases over time; episodes of claudication occur more frequently with less exertion.

Intermittent claudication occurs when a muscle is forced to contract without an adequate blood supply to meet the metabolic needs of exercise. It is the only specific symptom of peripheral arterial disease and it results from muscular hypoxia and metabolite accumulation.

Typically, pain occurs in the calf muscles after walking and disappears on rest. It can occur in muscles other than the calf, such as gluteal or thigh muscles, depending on the location of the occlusive process.

One classic characteristic of intermittent claudication is that it is reproducible; that is, the same situation produces the same response almost every time. The client who cannot walk the length of a house because of leg pain one day but is able to walk indefinitely the next does not have intermittent claudication.

Nearly half of clients who experience claudication have associated severe coronary artery disease. Claudication, usually insidious in onset, generally occurs in men, although there is an increased incidence in women after menopause. Usually, claudication strikes males in their sixth or seventh decade.

The development of pain at rest, usually occurring at night when the client lies supine, indicates progressive disease. Usually described as a dull aching in the toes or forefoot, this sensation may awaken the client from sleep and cause him or her to hang the foot over the side of the bed or get up and walk around for relief. As symptoms progress, the client may start to sleep in a chair with legs dependent. This often results in a moderate degree of lower extremity edema. The affected foot usually demonstrates dependent rubor.

Other symptoms of arterial insufficiency involve the cutaneous circulation and are nonspecific. Their presence, however, in combination with claudication indicates advanced disease. Skin and subcutaneous tissues require little blood flow for maintenance of normal nutrition. Coldness of feet is an unreliable sign, but a sudden onset of coldness is indicative of arterial insufficiency or occlusion. Clinical signs associated with arterial insufficiency include weak or absent peripheral pulses, color changes associated with position changes, hypertrophied toenails, tissue atrophy, ulceration, and gangrene. Paresthesias with exertion indicate ischemia of the peripheral nerves because of the phenomenon of "arterial steal." This phenomenon occurs as arterioles of the muscles are maximally dilated because of hypoxia. In order to meet muscular metabolic needs, these arterioles steal from cutaneous and peripheral nerve vessels, which results in coldness and "pins and needles" sensation.

Lower extremity pain may also appear in a number of other disorders unrelated to arterial disease. Other conditions that cause a similar type of pain include arthritis, lumbar disc protrusion, neuritis, venous stasis, and muscle cramps. Other forms of chronic arterial disease include aortoiliac and aortofemoral disorders.

Aortoiliac disorders are a form of chronic arterial occlusive disease characterized by aortoiliac stenosis and occlusion. Assessment reveals hip, thigh, and buttock claudication with absent or diminished femoral and distal pulses. Dependent rubor is common when aortoiliac and femoropopliteal disorders are combined.

A femoropopliteal disorder refers to an occlusion in the chief arteries of the proximal leg or thigh. The most common symptom of superficial femoral artery and popliteal disease is calf claudication that will either improve or develop into rest pain. Popliteal artery disease and stenosis in the anterior or posterior tibial artery results in claudication in the distal leg and foot.

Diagnostic Assessment

During the past decade, the use of noninvasive methods of circulatory assessment has increased dramatically. Techniques range from simple measurement of ankle/arm blood pressure index to the use of MRI to measure arterial blood flow. Whereas the recording of ankle/arm index provides information at the bedside, segmental Doppler systolic blood pressures and pulse waveform analysis, via plethysmography, provide more objective information about the level and severity of occlusive disease. Arteriography is the definitive examination when surgery is being considered. Arteriography reveals the lumen of the blood vessels. It is not a measurement of actual blood flow like the noninvasive assessment.

Medical Management

Medical management of clients with chronic arterial occlusive disease is recommended for those with intermittent claudication and, in general, mild to moderate disease. Surgical intervention has been reserved for clients who develop rest pain, non-healing ulcers, or disabling claudication.

Smoking cessation is strongly recommended because cigarette smoking is highly correlated with chronic arterial occlusive disease. Clients who are able to stop smoking successfully have been shown to improve their treadmill walking distance.

VASCULAR REHABILITATION

Daily walking exercise has been shown to be beneficial to clients with intermittent claudication, although the mechanism by which it improves symptoms is controversial. It probably combines "training effect" and an increase in collateral blood supply to the extremity. Many clients can significantly increase their walking distance, and most can avoid surgery if they exercise regularly and stop smoking.

DIETARY MANAGEMENT

Interventions for lowering blood lipid levels are recommended for those clients with hyperlipidemia. The initial steps for lowering cholesterol involve dietary intervention. For obese clients, the first goal is to reduce calories to achieve ideal body weight. The next major step is to reduce the total fat intake in the diet to 30 per cent or less of total calories. Saturated fat intake should be reduced. The most common sources of saturated fat in the American diet are hamburger meat and other red meats, fried foods, and dairy products, especially whole milk and cheese. Increasing the quantity of fish and poultry and changing to skim milk and nonfat cheese may be sufficient in order to meet saturated fat recommendations. The third major goal is to reduce the amount of sources of cholesterol, including egg yolks, organ meats, shellfish, and animal meats. Increasing dietary fiber, especially soluble fiber such as that found in oats, lentils, and beans, has a beneficial effect on lipid levels. Fast foods, snack foods, and restaurant dinning account for a large amount of the increased fat intake in the United States. Dietary counseling by a registered dietician is a helpful intervention in helping clients and families change eating habits.

PHARMACOLOGIC MANAGEMENT

Pharmacologic intervention may be needed for those clients with high levels of hyperlipidemia and in those for whom dietary changes have been less than successful. The major drug groups include nicotinic acid, fibrin acid derivatives, bile acid resins, meglutol (HMG), CoA-reductase inhibitors, and probucol. These medications have varying degrees of effectiveness, and each has important side effects.

Vasodilators have been popular in the past, although there are no convincing studies to support their use. Pentoxifylline (Trental) has been introduced and shown to be effective in some clients in combination with conditioning exercise. Pentoxifylline is reported to act by reducing blood viscosity and enhancing oxygen delivery to the muscle of the affected limb. The major side effect is gastrointestinal upset, which may be avoided by taking the medication with meals.

ENDOVASCULAR INTERVENTIONS

During the 1980s, an entirely new field of treatment for atherosclerotic vascular disease arose called endovascular interventional therapies. This is a new multidisciplinary field that applies recently innovated techniques of angioscopy, intraluminal ultrasonography, balloon angioplasty, laser, mechanical atherectomy, thrombolytic therapy, and stents. This field can be defined as a diagnostic and therapeutic discipline that uses catheter-based systems to treat vascular disease. The goal is to operate from within the artery to remove partial or total blockages. Most of the procedures can be done in the radiology department or cardiac catheterization suites. Additional benefits of these therapies include (1) a puncture wound replaces long incisions; (2) significant reduction in postoperative care; (3) reduction in cardiac and pulmonary complications from general anesthesia, because most of these procedures are done under local or regional anesthesia; and (4) reduction in hospital costs and hospital stay.

Percutaneous Transluminal Angioplasty. Percutaneous transluminal angioplasty (PTA, balloon angioplasty) is a procedure that uses a catheter with a distal inflatable balloon to mechanically dilate vessel stenoses. Originally it was thought that angioplasty worked by compressing plaque against the vessel wall. Recent studies show angioplasty causes a controlled injury to the vessel wall by stretching the artery, thereby enlarging the lumen. Observation of a segment of an arterial wall that has undergone PTA reveals rupture of the plaque at the thinnest place, stretching of the artery wall away from the plaque, and rupture of the media with the lumen of the artery being maintained by the adventitia. The enlarged vessel's new dimensions are maintained by the hydrostatic pressure of the increased luminal blood flow (see Fig. 42-3).

PTA has been used successfully, in varying degrees, for treatment of hemodynamically significant stenoses in the coronary, aortic, iliac, femoral, popliteal, tibial, mesenteric, and renal circulations as well as stenoses in arteriovenous shunts for dialysis.

Complications of balloon angioplasty include bleeding, hematoma and thrombus formation at the insertion site, perforation, and dissection of the artery. Reocclusion that occurs over a longer period of time is due to accelerated cell growth of the intima (intimal hyperplasia) that occurs in response to injury.

Major nursing concerns are acute reocclusion and bleeding. Clients are anticoagulated with heparin during the procedure; thus, the arterial puncture site requires frequent assessment of swelling, bleeding, ecchymosis, or hematoma formation. Peripheral pulses are assessed usually every 15 to 30 minutes during the first post-procedure hour, then hourly for the next 4 to 8 hours. Clinical manifestations of circulatory compromise, such as sudden change in limb color or temperature, increasing muscle discomfort, pain at rest, and motor or sensory paresthesia, should be reported immediately. PTA clients will take aspirin or dipyridamole long term.

Laser-Assisted Balloon Angioplasty. Laser-assisted balloon angioplasty (LABA) uses laser energy and balloon catheters to reverse ischemia by reforming the diseased artery. LABA is used for high-grade and total occlusions that are difficult or impossible to cross. In these situations, laser recanalization is used to cross lesions to allow subsequent balloon angioplasty. After access is gained to the artery in the same fashion as for PTA, the laser probe or fiber is advanced to the obstructing lesion under fluoroscopy. The catheter tip is placed as close to the center of the occlusion as possible. Very gentle pressure is then applied to the catheter until the occluding lesion has been crossed. Standard balloon angioplasty is then used to enlarge the channel to its full diameter. After the procedure is completed, antiplatelet or anticoagulant therapy is given.

LABA carries a higher incidence than PTA of arterial wall perforation or dissection. Nursing responsibilities are much the same as in the care of the client after PTA.

Peripheral Atherectomy. Atherectomy selectively removes atheroma from atherosclerotic diseased arteries. The advantages of this technique over PTA are (1) decreased risk of arterial rupture because the vessel is not stretched as much and (2) decreased risk of thrombus formation because the arterial surface is smoother after the procedure.

Many atherectomy devices have been devised, and each offers its own unique features with advantages and disadvantages. The devices use various high-speed rotating drills, circular cutters or blades, or a football-shaped metal burr studded with diamond chips that serve as microblades. The plaque is pulverized into small particles. Most of the devices provide for particle retrieval, which allows examination for determining whether the occlusion was plaque or thrombus. Atherectomy devices require fluoroscopy and contrast for visualization of the lesion. The restenosis rate is about the same as for angioplasty. The major complications are perforation and arterioembolization.

Nursing care for the atherectomy client is the same as for an angioplasty client.

Intravascular Stents. The recognized problem of restenosis after PTA has led to the development of intravascular stents. Stents are designed to provide a scaffold to maintain the intraluminal structure and patency of the artery. So far, stents have been used mostly to treat residual stenoses or dissections after balloon angioplasty. Several types of stents have been developed, including flexible, rigid, balloon-expandable, and self-expanding. After a stent has been in place for about 8 months, it becomes covered by a thin neointimal layer. After the procedure, clients are treated with aspirin and dipyridamole.

Nursing care includes client education regarding medications as well as information about the procedure and the stent.

Thrombolytic Therapy. Thrombolytic therapy is an important aspect of management of extensive venous or arterial thrombosis. Streptokinase and urokinase are used to treat acute arterial emboli and arterial graft occlusion. Contraindications to therapy include surgery within the past 10 days, including arteriogram, lumbar puncture or paracentesis, recent trauma, renal or liver biopsy, and pregnancy. Thrombolytic agents are given through a peripheral vein or through an intra-arterial catheter. The agents have a half-life of 16 to 18 minutes. A loading dose is given followed by continuous infusion. Thrombin times or fibrinogen levels or both may be monitored to be certain that the thrombolytic system has been activated. Major adverse reactions include hemorrhage, allergic reactions, and fever.

Nursing management is related to the stage of fibrinolytic therapy—preinfusion, intrainfusion, and postinfusion. Prior to infusion, the client is monitored closely (commonly in intensive care). Baseline values are obtained for partial thromboplastin time, prothrombin time, thrombin time, platelet count, hematocrit, and white blood cell count. Because of the risk of hemorrhage, if data reveal a bleeding disorder, the physician is notified. A history of recent streptococcal infection may diminish the drug's effects. Baseline pulses and assessments are performed in each extremity, using Doppler ultrasonography if needed.

During infusion, vital signs, pulses, skin color, movement, and sensation are assessed frequently. The nurse assesses for clinical manifestations of bleeding and hematoma formation. If bleeding does occur, direct pressure is applied, the infusion is stopped, and the physician is notified. Bleeding typically is from the gastrointestinal or genitourinary tract, intramuscular, intracerebral, or retroperitoneal.

No intramuscular injections are given for 24 hours after infusion, and any medications that have side effects of bleeding are used with caution. There is also a chance that a partially lysed thrombus will embolize. After infusion, pressure is continued on the puncture site. The involved extremity is positioned in straight alignment to facilitate perfusion. The client's leg remains immobile. Heparin therapy in low doses is also begun. Streptokinase is administered from glass bottles because it is inactivated by plastic containers. Administration is regulated by a volume control pump.

NURSING MANAGEMENT OF CLIENTS WITH ARTERIAL DISORDERS

Assessment

The client with arterial disorders should be assessed for a past history of arterial problems, surgery, medications, and ulcerations. Because of the chronic nature of the problem, a psychosocial assessment should also be performed. Feelings of powerlessness may exist.

Nursing Intervention

Nursing Diagnosis: Tissue Perfusion, Altered Peripheral R/T interruption of blood flow secondary to arterial occlusion.

Planning: Expected Outcomes. The client will maintain normal peripheral tissue perfusion to affected extremities, as evidenced by warm, dry skin with normal peripheral pulse, color, temperature, motor and sensory function, and capillary filling.

Implementation

Position the Client. For safely positioning a client with peripheral vascular disease, first learn whether the disorder is arterial or venous in nature.

Because blood flows to dependent parts of the body (i.e., parts lower than the heart), position clients with arterial disease so that blood flows toward their legs and feet. In severe cases of arterial insufficiency, the physician may order the head of the client's bed to be elevated on 6-inch blocks so that blood from the heart flows more easily to the extremities whenever the client sleeps or rests. When placing the client in reverse Trendelenburg's position, watch for dependent edema. In milder cases, clients can benefit from simply sitting for periods of time with their feet flat on the floor. Remind clients with arterial insufficiency to avoid raising their feet above heart level unless the physician has specifically prescribed this as an exercise. Authorities vary in their opinion as to the best position for enhancing arterial flow to the feet.

Provide Warmth. Warmth can be both a blessing and a curse for clients with vascular disease. Warmth is beneficial for clients only when it acts as insulation against cold and chilling. For example, encourage the client with vascular disease to set the thermostat at home at around 70° to 72° F (21° to 22° C). If possible, keep the client's room comfortably warm. Teach the client to enter warmed cars in the winter.

Applying any source of heat directly to the extremities is especially dangerous. Heat increases tissue metabolism. If the arteries are unable to dilate normally, blood flow to the extremities becomes inadequate, and the tissues in turn become ischemic. The use of hot water bottles, heating pads, and hot foot soaks is strictly contraindicated unless specifically ordered by the physician, especially for diabetics with peripheral neuropathies and paraplegics.

Prevent Vasoconstriction. Factors that cause vasoconstriction include nicotine and caffeine (cause vasospasm), high emotion (stimulates the sympathetic nervous system), and chilling. The nurse can help clients avoid the damaging effects of prolonged vasoconstriction in the following ways.

- Explain the dangers of smoking to the client who uses tobacco. Encourage the client to stop smoking completely. The client who realizes that smoking literally threatens life and limbs may develop sufficient motivation to abstain permanently. Help the client locate therapy groups or biofeedback training.
- Protect the client whenever possible from upsetting, emotionally charged situations. Encourage the client to try to relax, both mentally and physically. Counseling services may be indicated for nervous, high-strung clients. Offer information regarding stress reduction classes. Remember to involve significant others.
- Prevent the client from becoming chilled, using the methods previously described.

Nursing Diagnosis: Skin Integrity, Impaired, High Risk for R/T decreased peripheral circulation.

Planning: Expected Outcomes. The client will maintain intact skin surfaces, as evidenced by healed skin surfaces, freedom from signs of infection, and signs of wound healing.

Implementation

Arterial Ulcers. Because of poor circulation, clients with chronic ischemic limbs are highly prone to ulcerations and infection of the extremities. Moreover, once a lesion develops, it tends to heal poorly or not at all (especially in diabetics). Without normal vessels and adequate blood flow, the damaged tissues fail to receive needed oxygen, nutrients, antibodies, and protective leukocytes, and the process of tissue damage continues. Eventually, the client may be forced to undergo limb amputation.

Although skin grafting may ultimately be required to cover the site of arterial ischemic leg ulcers (once the ulcerated area is free from infection and granulation tissue is evident), it should be remembered that intervention for the skin lesion does not cure the underlying disease. Most ulcers require revascularization to heal. Arterial bypass surgery improves circulation when the client has an aortoiliac or femoropopliteal occlusion. For this surgery to be successful, however, the arteries in the leg must be healthy enough to carry sufficient blood to the foot once the block has been removed or bypassed.

General intervention involves keeping the area of ulceration clean and free from pressure and irritation. Bed rest reduces the oxygen needs of the impaired tissues. Débridement followed by application of wet-to-damp saline dressings is also a standard intervention for leg ulcers. Whirlpool treatments also provide good débridement. If the ulcer does not become infected, granulation then is enhanced with wet-to-wet dressings or a moist occlusive dressing such as DuoDerm.

Foot Care. Lesions resulting from peripheral artery disease increase the danger of injury to the extremities. Prevention of injury to the extremities, particularly the feet, is an important component of care. Excellent foot care should be an integral part of the daily routine of clients with peripheral vascular disorders, because prevention is easier to initiate and maintain than is correction. Foot problems can result in added hospital costs, increased hospitalization for diabetics, increased morbidity, vascular bypass operations, and amputations.

Important points concerning foot care include the following.

1. There are no minor foot problems for clients with peripheral vascular disease, especially clients with diabetes mellitus.
2. Ascertain whether the client is wearing adequate footwear and hosiery and whether nails and skin on the feet are properly cared for.
3. Be careful when referring clients to a podiatrist. Not all podiatrists are vascular specialists.
4. Refer the client with corns, calluses, and ingrown toenails to a physician who specializes in peripheral vascular disease.

Guidelines for correct foot care of clients with vascular disorders are presented in the Client Education Guide.

Nursing Diagnosis: Pain R/T ischemia.

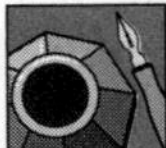

CLIENT EDUCATION GUIDE

Foot Care

Daily Hygiene

Don't soak; use mild soap and a washcloth.
Dry well between toes.
Check water temperature with a bath thermometer or elbow, not toes, to prevent burns; 32.2° to 35° C (90° to 95° F) is safe.
Gently rub corns or calluses. Avoid cutting, digging, or using harsh commercial products.

Daily Inspection and Lubrication

Use good lighting.
Put on glasses.
Report ulcerations, redness, calluses, blisters, cracking of skin on the feet, thickening of nails, and so on to physician promptly.
Rub soothing lotions or lanolin on hands, feet, legs, and arms to prevent dryness.
Do not use lotion on sores or in between toes.
Do not use perfumed lotions.
Dust feet lightly with cornstarch if they sweat.

Care of Toenails

Use clippers, not scissors.
Cut straight across.
No bathroom surgery.
Do not use razor blades.
If eyesight is poor or you are unable to reach toes, find qualified assistance.
Use lamb's wool between overlapping toes.

Proper Shoes and Socks

Never go barefoot, not even at the beach or in the home.
Avoid high heels and shoes with pointed toes.
Make sure nothing is in shoes before putting them on feet.
Avoid tight socks and shoes.
Wear cotton socks for absorbency. Change socks daily.
Alternate the use of several comfortable, firm, well-made shoes during the week.
Avoid shoes that cause feet to perspire (canvas shoes do).
Make sure shoes and slippers fit well and are sturdy enough to prevent foot injury.

Safety

Avoid sunburn.
Avoid scratching insect bites on legs to prevent creation of open lesions.
Do not use heating pads.
Wear adequate foot protection on cold days.
Turn lights on in dark hallways and rooms.
Do not sit with legs crossed.
Use a cane or walker, if indicated.
When in doubt, ask for help. Have phone numbers handy.

Activity

Walking is good, but ask physician first.
Do not walk if there are open ulcerations.
Walk until pain begins, stop and rest, then begin again.
Elevate feet if they swell.
Find a nurse and a physician who will get to know you and your feet and will take the time to talk with you when you need help.

Planning: Expected Outcomes. The client will experience abatement or absence of pain, as evidenced by self-report and demonstrated knowledge of pain relief measures, both pharmacologic and nonpharmacologic.

Implementation. The pain of ischemia is usually chronic, continuous, and difficult to relieve. Leg ulcers are also typically very painful. Because of pain, clients with arterial disorders are often depressed and irritable. Pain limits their activities, disturbs their sleep, saps their energy, and demoralizes them emotionally. Thus, pain must be relieved if the client is to rest and improve.

Any measure that increases circulation to the extremities will help alleviate ischemic pain (e.g., bypass surgery, warmth, proper positioning, vasodilators, and tobacco avoidance). Whereas pain can also be subdued by analgesics, interventions that augment circulation are best. For more information on pain control, see Chapter 16.

When strong analgesics such as morphine are necessary "around the clock," the client may come to accept amputation. Amputation can improve the quality of life by diminishing pain and improving mobility with a prosthesis.

Nursing Diagnosis: Health-Seeking Behaviors, R/T exercise, weight reduction, and smoking cessation.

Planning: Expected Outcomes. The client will begin and maintain the chosen health promotion program, as evidenced by demonstrated knowledge of the specific activities of the program, regular evaluation of goals against performance, and verbalized feelings of increased well-being.

Implementation

Exercise. A prescribed moderate program of exercise and rest helps increase circulation. For example, the client often benefits from taking short walks followed by periods of rest. The nurse instructs the client to walk as much as possible every day, provided there are no ulcerations. The exercise program should begin judiciously and progress gradually until the client has substantially lengthened walking distances. For obese and chronically ill clients, it is important that (1) an exercise program be individually tailored to the client's abilities, goals, interests, and resources and (2) it be written with specific instructions.[20]

Several studies have shown that clients involved in an exercise program generally feel better and can slowly improve their walking distance. Clients should be reminded that at first it may be painful to walk any distance, and they may need to stop frequently to rest. They should also be encouraged to walk in enclosed shopping malls in the winter for safety from falls due to icy pavements and to avoid vasoconstriction from the cold outdoors.

Some clients are not aware of chest pain, shortness of breath, or fatigue because their attention is focused on leg discomfort. Question them carefully about these discomforts. Medical or surgical intervention may reduce pain and thus improve walking ability.

Weight Reduction. Obesity is a risk factor of arterial disorders. However, there is no evidence that a special diet will alter the course of atherosclerosis once it has appeared. Nevertheless, overweight clients should be encouraged to reduce and improve dietary habits in conjunction with activity as tolerated. The nurse encourages clients to follow a low-fat, low-cholesterol diet with more fruits and vegetables. Weight management and dietary reduction of fat and cholesterol are included in the discussion of hypertension (see earlier).

Smoking Cessation. Cigarette smoking influences vascular disability. It is a potent vasoconstrictor. Clients who stop smoking and start exercising may improve their walking capacity, among other things. Smoking cessation is extremely difficult, because nicotine is a highly addictive chemical. Social support, especially of friends and family members, seems to be an important factor in assisting smokers to quit their habit.[21] Nurses can educate their clients about the dangers of cigarette smoke, encourage them to stop, act as role models for nonsmoking, and support policies to prohibit smoking in the workplace.

Nursing Diagnosis: Activity Intolerance, High Risk for R/T pain (intermittent claudication).

Planning: Expected Outcomes. The client will tolerate appropriate levels of activity free from pain and excess fatigue, as evidenced by normal vital signs, absence of pain, and verbalized understanding of benefits of gradual increase in activity and exercise.

Implementation. Although exercise helps the majority of clients with vascular disorders, there are some clients *who must not exercise,* for example, clients with leg ulcers, pain at rest, cellulitis, deep vein thrombosis (see later), or gangrene. Exercise and activity increase the metabolic needs of tissues and, consequently, tissue requirements for oxygenated blood. For this reason, clients with tissue breakdown or necrosis must remain for a period on complete bed rest. Even minimal activity raises the oxygen requirements of their tissues above that which their damaged arteries can provide.

When assisting the client with a walking program, the nurse makes clear that *pain* should be the guide to the amount of activity to be undertaken. Intermittent claudication signals that the muscles and tissues of the legs are not receiving enough oxygen. Before the client begins a walking program, the nurse takes a careful history and performs a physical assessment. It is important to establish a cardiopulmonary profile and to carefully examine the client's feet and legs to locate open ulcerations or anatomic deformities. The client should have sturdy shoes for prevention of foot trauma. It bears repeating that a client with open ischemic ulcerations should not walk.

A popular form of exercise for clients with vascular disorders is the Buerger-Allen routine. These exercises are divided into three parts as shown in Figure 44-11.

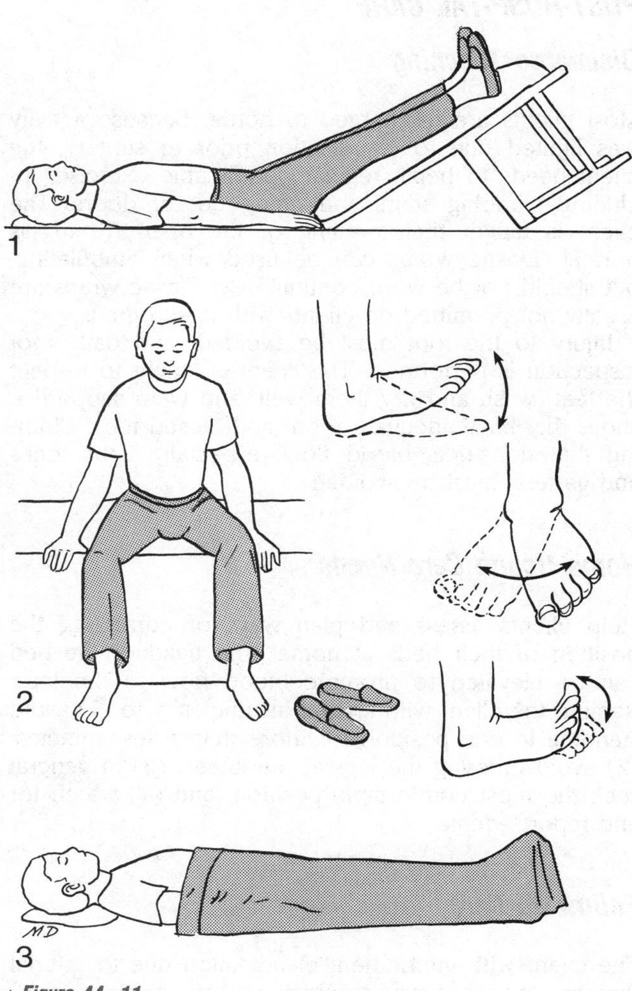

▲ **Figure 44-11**

Buerger-Allen exercises. *1,* Elevate feet on padded chair or board for ½ to 3 minutes. *2,* Sit in relaxed position while you flex and extend, then pronate and supinate each foot for 3 minutes. Your feet should become entirely pink. If feet are blue or painful, elevate them and relax as necessary. *3,* Lie quietly for 5 minutes, keeping legs warm with a blanket.

Evaluation

The nurse monitors the attainment of expected outcomes. The care of the client is long term, and adequate time should be allowed for goal attainment.

MODIFICATION OF PLAN OF CARE FOR THE ELDERLY

Age-related changes and impairments of physiologic function concomitant with arterial disease will affect the nursing diagnoses of activity intolerance (possibly increased), altered peripheral tissue perfusion (possibly reduced), and pain. Recognition of pain may be complicated by physical or cognitive impairments, ongoing drug therapy, and psychosocial factors such as depression or social isolation.[46]

POST-HOSPITAL CARE

Discharge Teaching

Most clients are discharged to home. Because activity was limited due to claudication prior to surgery, the client needs to begin regular permissable exercise, including climbing stairs and going out of doors. The client is taught that swelling of the operative leg is normal. Elastic wraps can be used when ambulating, but should not be worn continuously. Elastic wraps are usually not permitted on clients with in situ grafts.

Injury to the foot must be avoided, and daily foot inspection is performed. The client is taught to inspect the feet, wash and dry them well, and wear supportive shoes that have adequate room and closed toes. Clothing that constricts blood flow, especially tight socks and garters, must be avoided.

Home Health Care Needs

Help clients assess and plan ways of correcting the position of their beds at home. The head of the bed can be elevated to promote blood flow to the legs. Remind the client with arterial insufficiency to (1) avoid standing in one position for more than a few minutes; (2) avoid crossing the legs at the knees; (3) in general seek the most comfortable position; and (4) watch for and report edema.

Follow-up Care

The client with intermittent claudication due to arterial disease should have a check-up at least every 3 months. At this time, document the (1) extent of claudication, (2) impact on lifestyle, (3) manifestations of ischemia, (4) pulses, (5) ankle/arm indices, (6) condition of the feet, and (7) venous filling time to determine improvement, stability, or progression of the disease.

Surgical Management of Arterial Disorders

Arterial obstruction can be reconstructed with bypass operations. Selecting the client for surgery follows careful assessment of history, physical assessment, and diagnostic assessments including arteriography. Arteriography provides a necessary road map indicating the level of obstruction, because it is essential to reconstruct the arterial inflow to the legs before correcting the outflow. This process prevents newly placed bypass grafts from thrombosing because of inadequate blood supply to the graft. During the operation the surgeon assesses inflow, and after it is ascertained that inflow to the femoral system is adequate, a distal site is chosen for outflow.

Various locations along the arterial system can be reconstructed. If the aortoiliac segment is obstructed, clients can have aortofemoral bypass grafting or axillofemoral reconstruction. If the person is a good surgical risk, the option of choice is aortofemoral bypass (Fig. 44–12). The operative mortality is 1 per cent. The patency rates of aortofemoral grafts are 80 to 90 per cent at 5 years.

Axillofemoral grafting is reserved for people who have increased operative risk, usually because of their

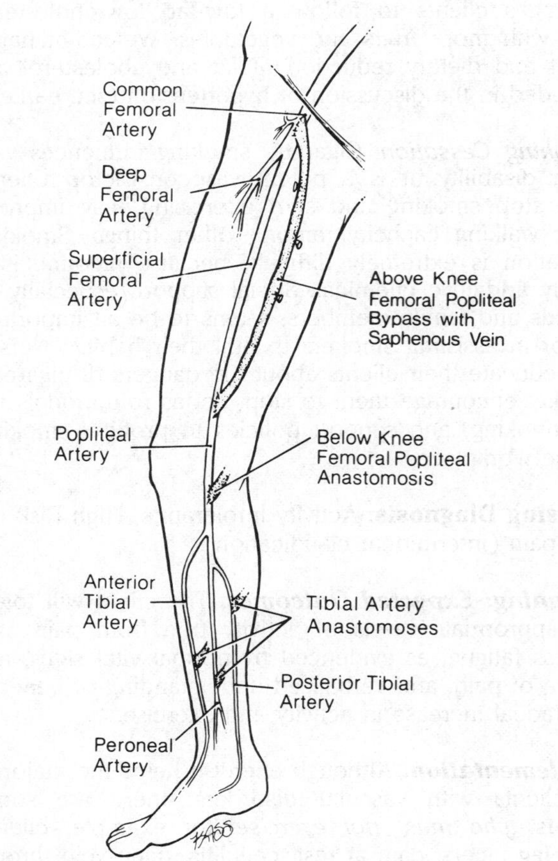

▲ **Figure 44–12**

Femoral artery bypass grafts. The anastomosis can be to any one of three tibial arteries. (From Fahey, V. A. [1988]. *Vascular Nursing*. Philadelphia: W.B. Saunders.)

cardiopulmonary status. The graft starts at the axillary artery and travels subcutaneously along the lateral chest wall to the femoral artery. It may then be combined with a femorofemoral graft to revascularize both extremities.

Axillofemoral grafts have a higher incidence of occlusion than aortofemoral grafts and carry a mortality rate of 4 to 5 per cent, but the necessary anesthesia time is greatly reduced. The patency rates are 60 to 70 per cent at 5 years, in part because thrombi are easily removed from axillofemoral grafts. Almost all patients will take one aspirin every day as an antiplatelet intervention.

The femoral artery can be bypassed with grafts anastomosed (surgically connected) to any one of three lower leg arteries (posterior tibial, anterior tibial, or peroneal artery).

The success of bypass grafts of the legs depends largely upon what material is used for grafting. The client's own saphenous vein remains the most successful grafting material used today. Seventy-five per cent of saphenous vein grafts are patent after 5 years; in contrast, only 12 per cent of synthetic material (polytetrafluorethylene, PTFE) is patent after the same length of time. (Goretex is a common brand name for this material.) Unfortunately, the client's own saphenous vein is not always large enough or long enough for the surgery or may have been removed during another operation. In these cases, PTFE is used. In situ grafts can also be used for reconstruction. In situ grafts are the use of the client's own vein for a bypass of the artery. A section of vein is anastomosed proximally and distally and then stripped of its valves. The vein then becomes an artery for the client.

Postoperative care includes the initial use of anticoagulants (heparin sodium) in clients who have had previously thrombosed femoral bypass grafts. The client is eventually placed on warfarin sodium (Coumadin) based on coagulation studies, especially prothrombin and partial thromboplastin times. Dextran is sometimes used to improve blood flow in the microcirculation. Medications that decrease platelet aggregation, aspirin and dipyridamole (Persantine) are also used to increase the length of graft patency. Oxygen saturation monitors may also be used to measure tissue perfusion.

Broad-spectrum antibiotics are used before and after surgery. Clients are carefully monitored for clinical manifestations of infection (e.g., elevated white blood cell count, fever, changes in wound appearance).

It is also possible to treat some clients with fibrinolytics. Three drugs, streptokinase, urokinase, and tissue plasmogen activator, are in current clinical use. All three drugs convert the client's plasminogen to the active molecule plasmin that instigates fibrinolysis.

The client is placed at bed rest for the evening after surgery, with the leg flat in bed. The leg is wrapped with light dressings or a vascular boot. Boots are commonly used in clients who had a loss of sensation prior to surgery or who are risk of pressure ulcers. Elastic wraps are not used if vein grafts have been used for reconstruction. Leg swelling is common after revascularization related to the reperfusion of ischemic muscles and surgical dissection around lymphatic drainage systems in the leg. If edema worsens when the client's leg is dependent, elastic wraps and a mild diuretic can be used. Edema usually resolves within 4 to 8 weeks.

COMPLICATIONS

Reclotting of the graft is possible. Peripheral tissue perfusion is monitored and noninvasive follow-up studies are performed to assess patency.

Infection is not a common complication after bypass surgery, but it can occur especially when synthetic grafting material is used. Because infection in a synthetic graft requires its removal, infection often results in the loss of a limb. Poorly nourished clients appear to be a highest risk of infection and delayed healing.

Bleeding may develop along the suture line and can indicate a disruption in the suture line, pseudoaneurysm formation, or a slipped ligature (suture). These problems require additional surgery.

Compartment syndrome may also develop from swelling around the fascial compartments of the leg. In addition to loss of sensation and function, muscle cells can die and release myoglobin, which can cause acute tubular necrosis in the kidney.

LUMBAR SYMPATHECTOMY

Surgical lumbar sympathectomy has been used as treatment for lower extremity occlusive disease since the early 1900s. Its effectiveness, however, has always been controversial. Studies demonstrate that this procedure increases blood flow primarily to the skin rather than to the muscle. Lumbar sympathectomy may be useful in clients who have ischemic skin ulceration related to arterial insufficiency and local trauma rather than for relief of symptoms of intermittent claudication. Since the advent of bypass surgery, lumbar sympathectomy is rarely used.

Nursing Management

PREOPERATIVE PREPARATION

Preoperatively, the nurse obtains baseline vital signs and documents the character of peripheral pulses comparing one side to the other. Know exactly which pulses are palpable and which pulses can be assessed only with the Doppler. Mark the sites where peripheral pulses can be palpated with ink to assist with postoperative assessment.

Before the client goes to surgery, it is common to begin intravenous fluids, insert a urinary catheter and weigh the client. Just before surgery, arterial and central venous pressure lines may be inserted.

In addition, broad-spectrum antibiotics normally are prescribed for 48 hours preoperatively. All infections (e.g., tooth abscesses, urinary tract infections, respiratory infections) must be resolved, especially if the surgeon plans to use a synthetic graft. Adequate circulating blood volume must be maintained to permit good perfusion throughout the period of arterial repair.

As with any preoperative assessment, it is vital to perform careful cardiac and pulmonary evaluation. Even though the incision for a femoral artery bypass is peripheral and major complications are infrequent, remember that the client probably has other manifestations of atherosclerosis (such as heart and kidney disease) that may complicate the surgery. If the operation is not an emergency, malnutrition can be reversed and open wounds cleaned.

The client and family are taught the various procedures involved and are offered psychological support. The nurse first assesses readiness and desire to learn about the surgery.

Postoperative care of the client after bypass surgery is described in the Nursing Care Plan.

POSTOPERATIVE MANAGEMENT

Postoperative care of the client after bypass surgery is described in the Nursing Care Plan.

DISCHARGE PLANNING

The client with intermittent claudication due to arterial disease should have a check-up at least every 3 months. At this time, document the (1) extent of claudication, (2) pulses, (3) ankle/arm indices, (4) condition of the feet, and (5) venous filling time to determine improvement, stability, or progression of the disease.

ACUTE ARTERIAL OCCLUSION

Overview

Acute occlusion of a limb's main artery may be caused by trauma, embolism, or thrombosis and may occur in a healthy or diseased artery. About 90 per cent are in the lower limbs.

It is important to differentiate between arterial thrombosis and arterial embolism. Acute arterial thrombosis is usually due to arterial obstruction by a blood clot that forms in an artery damaged by atherosclerosis. Arterial thrombosis may also develop in an arterial aneurysm, especially aneurysms that form in the popliteal artery.

In arterial embolism, the wall of the artery is often healthy; the obstruction in the artery arises most frequently from a thrombus within the heart. Causative factors include atrial fibrillation, myocardial infarction, prosthetic heart valves, and rheumatic heart disease. Sometimes, portions of a blood clot, such as platelet emboli, form at points of turbulence, lodge at a bifurcation, and initiate a thrombus. Atheromatous emboli sometimes block small arteries. In the lower extremity, over half the emboli lodge in either the superficial femoral or the popliteal artery. Other noncardiac causes of emboli are abdominal aortic aneurysm, peripheral aneurysm, and diabetes mellitus. Most of these emboli lodge in the lower extremities. About 15 per cent travel to the arms. Arterial thrombosis is usually superimposed on atherosclerosis and consequently develops in a damaged vessel.

The circulatory changes that follow arterial occlusion and that predict the outcome are complex and depend on a variety of factors. Acute occlusion produces a fall in mean and pulse pressures in the distal arteries and a decrease in tissue perfusion and oxygenation. In a normal artery, blood flow is restored by collateral channels, but with acute emboli, there is no time for collateral vessels to develop.

The classic manifestations of acute ischemia due to thrombus or embolism are known as the six Ps:

1. pain or loss of sensory nerves secondary to ischemia
2. paresthesias and loss of position sense. The client is unable to detect pressure or sense a pinprick. The client cannot tell if toes are flexed or extended.
3. poikilothermia (coldness)
4. paralysis
5. pallor due to empty superficial veins and no capillary filling. Pallor can progress to a mottled, cyanotic, cadaverous cold leg.
6. pulselessness

Muscle necrosis may start as early as 2 to 3 hours after occlusion. Complete paralysis with stiffness of muscles and joints (rigor mortis) indicates irreversible damage. The leg must be amputated in order to prevent systemic reaction to the products of massive muscle destruction and systemic sepsis.

Management

Surgery is required to correct arterial embolism. Surgery for thrombosis usually involves an arterial reconstructive procedure for revascularization of the leg. Arterial emboli can be removed by an embolectomy.

If the decision is made to remove the occluding embolus or thrombus, surgery should be performed as quickly as possible, generally under local anesthesia. If hours have elapsed since the occlusion occurred, the viability of the limb will determine whether embolectomy should be attempted.

While decisions about surgery are being made, put the client to bed in a comfortable, warm room. Protect the limb from pressure and other trauma and keep it at room temperature, neither warm nor chilled. The best position for the limb is level or slightly dependent.

If medical intervention is selected or the surgeon is delayed, anticoagulants are generally started. Heparin is usually continued for a minimum of 2 to 7 days, after which a change to an oral anticoagulant may be made. The prevailing practice is to treat all clients who have a definite source of embolism and who have satisfactorily recovered from the acute episode of occlusion with long-term anticoagulant therapy.

Aside from surgery, fibrinolytic agents may be used to dissolve a thrombus or embolus.

ANEURYSMS

Definition

An aneurysm may be defined as a permanent localized dilation of an artery. A 50 per cent increase in the size

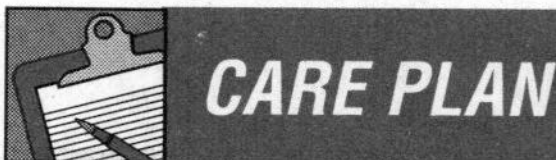

CARE PLAN

The Client Undergoing Arterial Bypass Surgery of the Lower Extremity

Nursing Diagnosis/ Collaborative Problem	Planning: Expected Outcomes	Implementation: Nursing Interventions	Rationales
Fluid Volume Deficit, High Risk for R/T hemorrhage, hematoma, third spacing of fluid, or diuresis from contrast given during angiography	Client will maintain adequate vascular fluid volume as evidenced by hemodynamic stability; urine output ≥ 30 ml/h; warm, dry skin; alert, awake; no excess drainage on dressings; intake equals output; stable hemoglobin and hematocrit	Observe for increase in pulse, decrease in blood pressure, anxiety, restlessness, pallor, cyanosis, thirst, oliguria, clammy skin, venous collapse, and level of consciousness	Hemorrhagic shock can develop from surgical or postoperative blood loss
		Check dressings for excessive drainage	Incision drainage first appears on dressings
		Assess pulmonary artery pressures and/or cardiac output if parameters are available	Pulmonary artery pressures and cardiac output parameters are reliable indicators of hemodynamic stability
		Check daily weights; monitor intake and output closely	Intake should equal output. Weight is a reliable indicator of fluid balance
		Check lab values, i.e., hematocrit, hemoglobin, and notify doctor if abnormal	Hematocrit and hemoglobin normally fall slighty because of surgical blood loss. Transfusion may be required
		Check creatinine level after angiography	Contrast is excreted by kidneys
Tissue Perfusion, Altered, R/T graft thrombosis, compartment syndrome, progressive arterial disease, or inadequate anticoagulation	Patient will maintain adequate tissue perfusion to lower extremities, as evidenced by full pedal pulses, intact sensory and motor function; minimal swelling	Check pedal pulses every hour for 24 hours, then every shift, unless otherwise ordered. Obtain Doppler pressures per doctor's orders	Pedal pulses indicate graft patency
		Check sensory and motor function of extremities	Compartment syndrome may develop because of bleeding
		Check leg for hematoma or severe swelling	Severe swelling may impede flow through graft
		Monitor CPK levels when appropriate	Enzymes are released from ischemic muscle
		Observe for change in color and presence of red blood cells in urine	Due to release of myoglobin, secondary to ischemic muscle
		Avoid raising knee gatch and placing pillows under the knees	Pressure may increase possibility of thrombosis
Skin Integrity, Impaired, High Risk for R/T altered circulation, altered nutritional state, presence of infection, multiple surgical procedures	Patient will maintain adequate skin integrity	Inspect lower extremities on daily basis	Early detection of ulcerations will improve chances of healing
		Provide proper skin care using lanolin creams	Soft skin does not crack open
		Protect lower extremities from trauma	Tissue perfusion is decreased, injured sites heal poorly
		Use sheepskin, bed cradle or heel protectors when appropriate	These are devices used to protect the skin from breakdown

Care Plan continued on following page

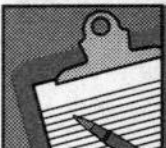

CARE PLAN

The Client Undergoing Arterial Bypass Surgery of the Lower Extremity Continued

Nursing Diagnosis/ Collaborative Problem	Planning: Expected Outcomes	Implementation: Nursing Interventions	Rationales
		Check sensory and motor function of extremities	Compartment syndrome may develop because of bleeding or edema
		Avoid tape on the skin below the knee	Tape burns from tape removal may be slow to heal
		Monitor nutritional status and albumin level. Obtain dietician consultation, if necessary	Malnutrition is the most common cause of delayed healing
		Observe strict aseptic technique during dressing changes	Reduces risk of infection
		Monitor for low-grade fever, elevated white blood cell count, any drainage from wound, and graft exposure each shift	These are clinical manifestations of wound infection
		Apply 4-inch Ace bandages below the knee to the affected extremity when out of bed, if ordered	Edema can inhibit wound healing
Physical Mobility, Impaired, R/T surgical procedure, pain, or nerve injury, secondary to ischemia	Client will maintain intact motor function, will avoid potential complications of immobility, and demonstrate use of adaptive devices to increase mobility	Assess causative factors for immobility, and patient's range of motion and ability to ambulate	Mobility can be facilitated once cause is known
		Encourage progressive ambulation and range of motion while in bed	These activities promote venous return and muscle strength
		Request physical therapy consult when appropriate	
		Encourage independence in activities of daily living	
Pain R/T surgical incision	Client verbalizes and/or demonstrates increased level of comfort	Assess patient's level of pain: type, duration, and location	Provides baseline data to evaluate effectiveness of treatment
		Provide comfort measures and means of distraction	Distraction is a nonpharmacologic method of pain management
		Medicate with prescribed analgesics prn	
		Evaluate effectiveness of pain medication after each administration	Determines adequacy of analgesics
Body Image Disturbance, R/T change in body image from surgery	Client demonstrates movement toward reconstruction of altered body image	Establish a trusting relationship with patient	Initial step of therapeutic communication
		Encourage patient to verbalize feelings	Allows unexpressed concerns to be addressed
		Promote social interaction	Encourages client to return to previous lifestyle
		Make appropriate referrals if indicated	

Adapted from Fahey, V. A. (1988). *Vascular nursing.* Philadelphia, W. B. Saunders.

of a vessel is the usual criterion. Once initiated, an aneurysm tends to enlarge gradually, and this, along with the thrombus that develops within the aneurysm, leads to the usual complications of aneurysms: rupture, pressure on surrounding structures, thrombosis, and distal embolization.

Incidence

Atherosclerotic aneurysms occur about 10 times more often in men than in women and, for the most part, occur after the age of 50 years.

Etiology

The most common cause of arterial aneurysm is atherosclerosis. Less common causes include congenital defects of the arterial wall (e.g., Marfan's disease), trauma (both blunt and penetrating types), infection including syphilis, polyarteritis, and hereditary abnormalities of connective tissue. Hypertension seems to enhance aneurysm formation.

A combination of factors, such as "wear and tear" and impaired nutrition, over time results in weakening of the arterial wall, which leads to tortuosity, dilation, and aneurysm formation in atherosclerotic arteries. Atherosclerotic aneurysms tend to develop where the artery is not supported by skeletal muscle or is subject to frequent bending with physical activity. The most common locations for arteriosclerotic aneurysms are the thoracic and abdominal aorta, the iliac arteries, and the femoral and popliteal arteries.

Classification

Aneurysms may be classified according to the following.

Location. Aneurysms are designated either venous or arterial. They are also described according to the specific vessel in which they develop (e.g., aortic, iliac artery) and, more precisely, according to the exact area of the vessel that they affect (e.g., thoracic aortic aneurysm, abdominal aortic aneurysm).

Etiology. Aneurysms can be classified according to the cause, such as atherosclerotic aneurysm, mycotic aneurysm (due to bacterial infection), hypertensive aneurysm, or syphilitic (luetic) aneurysm.

Gross Appearance. Classification of aneurysms is sometimes based on their shape, anatomic features, and size. Fusiform aneurysms are localized, rather uniform dilations of an artery; the term saccular is used to describe an outpouching of an artery at a point where the medial coat is thinned (Fig. 44–13). A dissecting aneurysm occurs as the hematoma in the arterial wall forms a localized enlargement of the involved artery, separating the layers of the arterial wall. A dissecting aneurysm may be either acute or chronic. A pseudoaneurysm, or false aneurysm, results from the development of a sac around a hematoma that maintains a communication with the lumen of an artery whose wall has been ruptured or penetrated.

Abdominal Aortic Aneurysm

OVERVIEW

Abdominal aortic aneurysms (AAA) occur about four times more often than thoracic aneurysms. The natural course of untreated AAA is to expand and rupture.

The aorta is under greater stress than the rest of the arterial system because of its large diameter and its exposure to high pressure during each systolic ejection of blood. Abdominal aneurysms may extend into the iliac arteries. When the aneurysm reaches about 5 cm

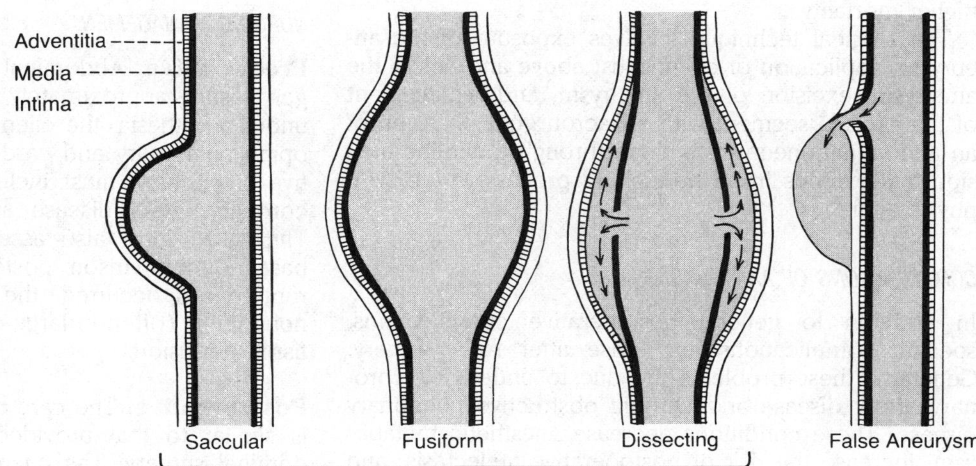

▲ *Figure 44–13*

Classification of aneurysms. In a true aneurysm, layers of the vessel wall dilate in one of the following ways: *saccular,* a unilateral outpouching; *fusiform,* a bilateral outpouching; or *dissecting,* a bilateral outpouching in which layers of the vessel wall separate, with creation of a cavity. In a false aneurysm, the wall ruptures, and a blood clot is retained in an outpouching of tissue.

in diameter, it can usually be palpated. An abdominal aneurysm measuring 6 cm or greater in diameter has a 20 per cent chance of rupturing in 1 year.

CLINICAL MANIFESTATIONS

Most abdominal aneurysms are asymptomatic; discovery is usually made on physical or x-ray examination of the abdomen or lower spine for other reasons. The most common symptom is awareness of a pulsating mass in the abdomen, with or without pain, followed by abdominal pain and back pain. Groin pain and flank pain may be experienced because of increasing pressure on other structures.

The most frequent complication of AAA is rupture, which occurs most often in those aneurysms 5 cm in diameter or greater. Rupture causes intense pain, typically in one or both flanks with radiation to the lower abdomen, groin, or genitalia. Rupture is also accompanied by a decrease in hemoglobin and signs of hemorrhage, shock, and abdominal distention.

Ninety per cent of large abdominal aneurysms can be diagnosed on physical examination; however, smaller aneurysms and aneurysms in obese clients may be more difficult to confirm. Ultrasonography and computed tomographic scan are the most accurate diagnostic tools. Abdominal aortography is not essential for making the diagnosis but helps identify circulatory anomalies important at the time of resection. Therefore, angiography should not be performed until surgery is contemplated.

Surgery is usually not performed on clients with an asymptomatic AAA smaller than 4 to 5 cm. Every 6 months, an ultrasonographic examination is indicated to determine whether there is any change in the size. Antihypertensives are usually prescribed.

SURGICAL MANAGEMENT

Surgical management of an aneurysm may be performed as an emergency or an elective procedure. Elective resection and graft replacement has a surgical mortality of less than 5 per cent; emergency surgical treatment after the aneurysm has ruptured has a much higher mortality.

The surgical technique involves exposure of the aneurysm, application of clamps just above and below the aneurysm, excision of the aneurysm, and replacement of the excised segment with a Dacron graft. Excision of an abdominal aneurysm is done through a midline incision that extends from the xiphoid process to the symphysis pubis.

COMPLICATIONS OF AAA SURGERY

In addition to general postoperative complications, specific complications may arise after AAA surgery. Generally, these problems are due to underlying coronary artery disease and chronic obstructive pulmonary disease. These conditions decrease anesthetic metabolism, increase the risk of postoperative atelectasis, and decrease the client's tolerance of hemodynamic changes from blood loss and fluid shifts. Proper preoperative screening with stress testing and pulmonary function testing help reduce the incidence of complications, which include the following.

Abdominal aortic aneurysm repair is considered a major operation, and a number of specific postoperative complications can develop. One of the most serious complications is acute myocardial infarction. To reduce the risk of this complication, many clients undergo coronary artery bypass prior to aneurysm repair.

Changes in sexual function may also develop following repair of abdominal aortic aneurysm. Retrograde ejaculation occurs in about two thirds of clients, and loss of potency occurs in one third.

Renal failure can develop for several reasons. The kidney can sustain ischemia from decreased aortic blood flow, decreased cardiac output, emboli, inadequate hydration, or the need for clamps on the aorta above the renal arteries during surgery.

Emboli can also develop and lodge in the arteries of the lower extremities or mesentery. Clinical manifestations include those of acute occlusion in the leg. Bowel necrosis is exhibited as fever, leukocytosis, ileus, diarrhea, and abdominal pain.

The spinal cord can also become ischemic, resulting in paraplegia, rectal and urinary incontinence, or loss of pain and temperature sensation. Spinal cord ischemia tends to occur more commonly when a AAA has ruptured.

About 4 per cent of all ruptured AAAs rupture into the inferior vena cava, producing aortocaval fistula. Manifestations include intractable congestive heart failure (CHF) because of the right-to-left shift, massive lower extremity edema, acute abdominal pain, ascites, pleural effusions, and hepatomegaly. The AAA may rupture into the duodenum, producing aortoenteric fistula. Gastrointestinal bleeding that may progress to shock is the presenting sign.

Respiratory, cardiac, and renal complications discussed earlier cause additional problems for the person with a ruptured AAA. Other complications are more common to abdominal surgery and include bleeding, infection, and rupture of the suture line.

NURSING MANAGEMENT

Preoperative. Abdominal aortic surgery is major surgery lasting approximately 4 hours. During these hours under anesthesia, the client faces a great risk of developing pulmonary and cardiac complications. Preoperative assessment must include detection of concurrent coronary artery disease and cerebrovascular disease. The nurse must also assess all peripheral pulses for baseline comparison postoperatively. If dissection or rupture has occurred, the client may receive intravenous fluids (often in large volumes) for maintenance of tissue perfusion.

Postoperative. The care of the client after AAA repair is similar to that provided for clients with other abdominal surgery. The client is generally admitted to a critical care area for 24 to 48 hours, where clinicians

(1) monitor vital signs and other hemodynamic parameters, (2) manage fluid and electrolytes, and (3) obtain daily weights. Clients are often maintained on a ventilator, at least overnight, to facilitate respiratory exchange. The nurse assesses circulation at least hourly, with assessment of pulses distal to the graft site. Any signs of occlusion, including changes in pulses, severe pain, cool to cold extremities below the graft, and pale or cyanotic extremities, are reported to the physician immediately.

Objective signs of a successful operation include (1) return to normal color, sensation, and warmth of the limb; (2) elevated ankle/arm index; and (3) reduction or elimination of pain. The nurse ensures that the client will have help at home and arranges for follow-up with an individualized risk factor modification program to prevent further disorders caused by atherosclerosis.

Ruptured Abdominal Aortic Aneurysm

The abdominal aneurysm may rupture (1) into the peritoneal cavity (usually with fatal results), (2) into the mesentery, (3) behind the peritoneum (the most common type of rupture with the best prognosis), (4) into the inferior vena cava (which results in shock and heart failure due to massive arteriovenous fistula), or (5) into the duodenum or rectum, causing severe gastrointestinal hemorrhage.

Ruptured AAA presents with a triad of manifestations, including (1) abdominal pain combined with intense back and flank pain and possible scrotal pain, (2) a pulsating abdominal mass; and (3) shock, with systolic blood pressure below 100 and apical pulse rate over 100. Other manifestations include ecchymosis in the flank and perianal area; severe sudden pain in the abdomen, paravertebral area, or flank; lightheadedness; and nausea with sudden hypotension. In addition, the red blood cell count falls and the white blood cell count rises. These are also the signs of a ruptured postoperative abdominal bypass graft.

There is a period after the initial rupture in which the blood is walled off in the retroperitoneal space, or tamponaded. If the ruptured AAA can be identified during this phase, the client has a much greater chance of survival. Once the aorta ruptures anteriorly into the peritoneal cavity, death is almost certain.

Surgery is the only intervention for clients with ruptured AAA. New surgical and grafting techniques and faster methods for transport (e.g., helicopters) now permit rapid resection of ruptured AAA and sometimes save the client's life. The operative mortality rate for repair of ruptured abdominal aneurysms may be as high as 35 per cent.

The client who has undergone aneurysm repair is taught activity restrictions, wound care, and pain management. Activities that involve lifting heavy objects, usually more than 15 to 20 pounds, are not permitted for 6 to 12 weeks postoperatively. Activities that involve pushing, pulling, or straining may also be restricted. Driving may also be restricted because of postoperative weakness.

Peripheral Aneurysms

OVERVIEW

Aneurysms are found more commonly in the lower than in the upper extremities. The most common site is the popliteal space.

Popliteal aneurysms cause ischemic manifestations in the lower limbs and an easily palpable pulse. Although the client may be aware of an enlarged area behind the knee, there is seldom discomfort. Peripheral aneurysm is differentiated from other swellings by the presence of expansile pulsation. Thrombosis may occur and possibly result in severe ischemia with gangrene and loss of the limb.

MANAGEMENT

Bypass operations are the only satisfactory intervention for aneurysms of the popliteal artery and must be performed before emboli develop. Results are excellent in uncomplicated cases.

THROMBOANGIITIS OBLITERANS (BUERGER'S DISEASE)

Overview

Thromboangiitis obliterans is a vasculitis of small and medium-size veins and arteries in the extremities of young adults. The disease process starts distally and progresses cephalad, involving both upper and lower extremities. It is a disease of the second through fourth decades, seen predominantly in men, although the incidence in women is increasing.

The cause of Buerger's disease remains unknown. Almost all clients are moderate to heavy smokers. Many clients have a hypersensitivity reaction to intradermal injection of tobacco products. Therefore, the probable etiology is an exaggerated autoimmune reaction.

Pain is the outstanding symptom. Intermittent claudication is a common problem that occurs in almost all clients at some stage of the disease. It is often the first symptom noted by the client, usually in the arch of the foot. It is somewhat less common in the calf of the leg but may be noted in both sites. Rest pain with persistent ischemia of one or more digits and coldness or cold sensitivity may be early symptoms. Various types of paresthesias may occur. Pulsations in the posterior tibial and dorsalis pedis arteries are weak or absent. In advanced cases, the extremities may be abnormally red or cyanotic, particularly when dependent. Advanced forms of the disorder occur when color or temperature changes involve only one extremity, only certain digits, or only portions of digits.

Ulceration and gangrene are frequent complications and may occur early in the course of the disease. These lesions can appear spontaneously but often follow trauma. Gangrene usually occurs in one extremity at a time. Edema of the legs is fairly common in advanced cases. Changes in the nails and skin appear, and segmental thrombophlebitis affects the smaller veins in about 40 per cent of clients. The primary diagnostic study is leg arteriography. Biopsy may also be used; inflammatory lesions are usually noted.

Thromboangitis is usually not life threatening. It does, however, result in disability from pain and amputation.

Management

Intervention is generally the same as for atherosclerotic peripheral arterial disease: (1) arresting progress of the disease, (2) producing vasodilation, (3) relieving pain, and (4) providing emotional support.

The need for smoking cessation must be clearly and unequivocally conveyed to the client and family. Information about programs to promote abstinence from tobacco should be provided.

For clients with rest pain and ischemic lesions, adequate pain control is essential. Vasodilation by calcium channel blockers or prazosin may be helpful for a small number of clients. Regional sympathetic ganglionectomy also produces vasodilation and may be recommended. Because of vasoconstriction, the client should be taught to avoid exposure to cold. Ulcerations will need wound care to facilitate healing.

Amputation should be deferred until conservative interventions have failed. However, it is unwise to delay amputation of the leg when (1) gangrene extends well into the foot, (2) pain is severe and cannot be controlled, or (3) severe infection or toxic effects occur. Amputation above the knee is seldom necessary.

RAYNAUD'S DISEASE

Overview

The term "Raynaud's phenomenon" refers to intermittent episodes during which small arteries or arterioles in extremities constrict, causing temporary pallor and cyanosis of the digits and changes in skin temperature. These episodes occur in response to cold temperature or strong emotion. As the episode passes, the changes in color are replaced by redness. These local changes are not necessarily related to the status of the peripheral vascular system as a whole. "Raynaud's disease" is a primary vasospastic disorder. If the disorder is secondary to another disease or underlying cause, the term "Raynaud's phenomenon" is used.

Raynaud's disease appears to be caused by (1) a hypersensitivity of digital arteries to cold, (2) release of serotonin, and (3) congenital predisposition to vasospasm. Eighty per cent of clients with Raynaud's disease are women between the ages of 20 and 49 years. Primary Raynaud's disease rarely leads to tissue necrosis. Secondary Raynaud's phenomenon is often associated with connective tissue or collagen vascular diseases such as scleroderma, systemic lupus erythematosus, or rheumatoid arthritis. Raynaud's phenomenon may occur after trauma, or it may also be related to various neurogenic lesions and certain occlusive arterial diseases.

The typical progression of Raynaud's phenomenon is pallor in the digits; followed by cyanosis accompanied by feelings of cold, numbness, and occasionally pain; and finally intense redness accompanied by tingling or throbbing. The pallor is caused by vasoconstriction of the arterioles in the extremity, which leads to decreased capillary blood flow. Blood flow becomes sluggish, and cyanosis appears. The intense redness or rubor results from the end of vasospasm and a period of hyperemia as oxygenated blood rushes through the capillaries.

Criteria for diagnosing primary Raynaud's disease include

- intermittent attacks of pallor or cyanosis of the digits by exposure to cold or from emotional stimuli
- bilateral or symmetric involvement
- no evidence of occlusive disease in the digital arteries or of any systemic disease that might be causing the changes
- gangrene, which (when it occurs) is limited to the skin of the tips of the digits
- a history of manifestations for at least 2 years

Management

Conservative measures will be helpful for the majority of clients with primary or secondary Raynaud's disease. These measures include keeping hands and feet warm and dry; protecting all parts of the body from cold exposure to prevent reflex sympathetic vasoconstriction of the digits; and cessation of tobacco use. Biofeedback has been of help to some clients.

Pharmacologic management is begun when the vasospastic attacks interfere with the client's ability to work or perform activities of daily living or when trophic lesions develop. The aim of drug therapy is to induce smooth muscle relaxation, to relieve spasm, and to increase arterial flow. Calcium antagonists, such as nifedipine are currently the drugs of first choice because they have been shown to decrease the frequency, duration, and intensity of vasospastic attacks. Other categories of drugs used in treatment include alpha-adrenergic receptor blockers, vasodilators, and those that interfere with sympathetic nerve activity.

Sympathectomy is sometimes performed. Its effectiveness seems to be mainly in primary Raynaud's and in the treatment of lower extremity disease. The long-term results of sympathectomy are disappointing. The duration of benefit is limited as peripheral nerves regenerate.

The symptoms of Raynaud's phenomenon may be alarming, so the nurse reassures the client that the condition is not likely to lead to a serious disability. Advise the client to stay warm by wearing wool gloves and turtleneck sweaters, turning up the thermostat at home if necessary, and staying out of drafts. Central heating is important to prevent chilling and the shunting of blood from the extremities to the trunk. Encourage clients to limit their intake of caffeine or chocolate. They must stop smoking in order to control the disease. Stress can also bring on vasospasm, so stress management workshops and biofeedback programs may prove beneficial. The nurse also teaches the client about any prescribed medications.

SUBCLAVIAN STEAL SYNDROME

Subclavian steal syndrome produces arm ischemia arising from subclavian artery blockage. The arm is perfused from the carotid artery as blood is taken from the brain to supply the arm. The most prevalent physical finding is a significant difference in blood pressure of the right and left arm. Other manifestations include dizziness, syncope, and arm paresthesias.

Intervention is surgical with carotid-subclavian bypass, transluminal dilation of the subclavian artery, or endarterectomy of the subclavian artery.

THORACIC OUTLET SYNDROMES

Thoracic outlet syndromes are a group of disorders that produce symptoms affecting the neck, shoulder, and upper extremities by compression or mechanical irritation of the brachial plexus, subclavian artery, or subclavian vein as these structures pass through the thoracic outlet. There are three types of syndrome: neurologic, which accounts for 95 per cent of all thoracic outlet clients; arterial, which makes up 1 to 2 per cent of clients but is the most serious form; and venous, which accounts for 3 to 4 per cent of clients.

Aching or throbbing pain and paresthesias of the neck and upper limb are the most prominent symptoms of the neurologic type syndrome. In more than half of the clients, the symptoms appear to follow a hyperextension injury to the neck or upper back. Intervention is usually nonsurgical and involves physical therapy. Some clients will be managed with the surgical removal of the first rib, but this intervention is controversial.

Arterial thoracic outlet syndromes result from chronic compression of the subclavian artery. This leads to the formation of intimal and mural thrombus and eventually peripheral embolization. This type of syndrome is more serious because it frequently results in severe ischemia of the upper extremity. Diagnosis is made by arteriography; treatment is the surgical excision of the anatomic abnormality and removal of the emboli.

Venous thoracic outlet syndrome is caused by external compression of the axillosubclavian vein that results in thrombosis. The primary symptoms are sudden swelling, pain, and cyanosis of the upper extremity. Treatment choices are conservative and include arm elevation and anticoagulation, thrombectomy, or thrombolytic therapy.

▼ NURSING CARE OF THE CLIENT EXPERIENCING AMPUTATION

Extremity amputation is the surgical removal of all or part of an extremity. Clients with peripheral vascular disease are the most frequent candidates for amputation of the lower extremities. Diabetes mellitus is a major etiology of arterial occlusion and has been associated with more than 50 per cent of major amputations in clients with lower extremity occlusive disease.

Amputations are classified as primary or secondary. Primary amputations are undertaken as definitive surgical treatment for lower extremity ischemia. Secondary amputations are those that follow a previous vascular reconstructive procedure. Amputations may also be required for acute limb-threatening conditions, mainly trauma, and for malignant tumors and congenital deformities.

Amputation of a limb is an emotional issue for clients and families. To many clients the word "amputation" like the word "cancer" is thought more often than spoken. Some clients will endure multiple attempts at revascularization or extended periods of intense pain in an effort to avoid amputation. The nurse can play an integral role in assessing client and family fears and concerns, in promoting the use of positive coping mechanisms, and in coordinating efforts of the rehabilitation team toward a positive outcome. The rehabilitation team must design a total care plan tailored to the client's personality and needs. Intervention focuses on the whole client rather than on a diseased or missing limb.

ASSESSMENT BEFORE AMPUTATION

Before amputation, the surgeon and rehabilitative team consider (1) the client's physical condition, (2) the type of amputation to be performed (i.e., closed or open), (3) the level of amputation required, (4) peripheral vascular function test results, (5) the client's general attitude toward amputation, (6) the client's rehabilitation potential, and (7) the type of postoperative prosthetic-fitting and rehabilitative program.

Client's Physical Condition

The following physical conditions may determine the need for amputation: ischemic gangrene, rest pain, infection, and massive injury.

Type of Amputation

There are two types of amputation procedure: the open, or guillotine, amputation; and the closed, or "flap," amputation (Fig. 44-14). The major indication for guillotine amputation is infection. In open amputation, the surgeon does not close the stump with a skin flap immediately but leaves it open, allowing the

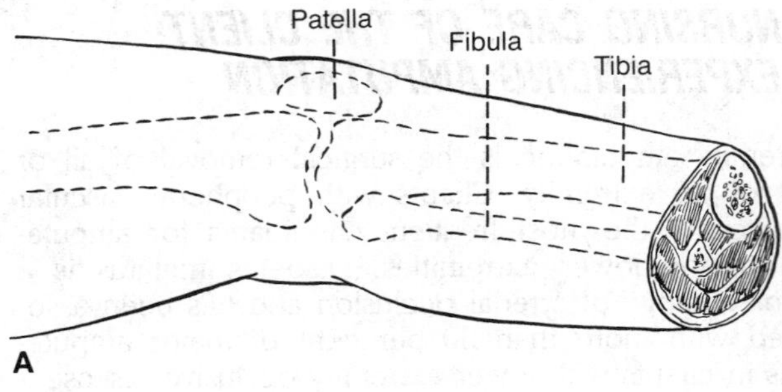

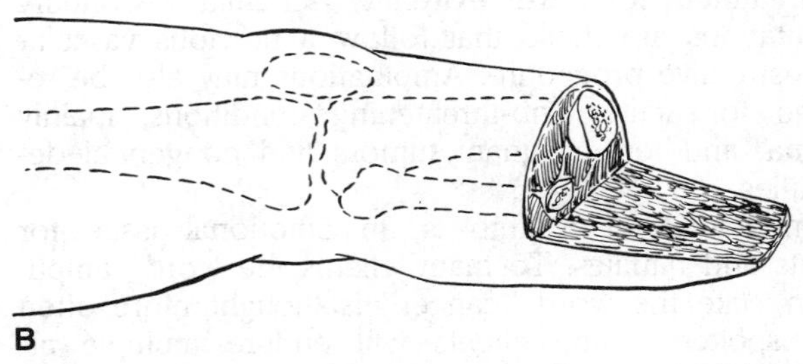

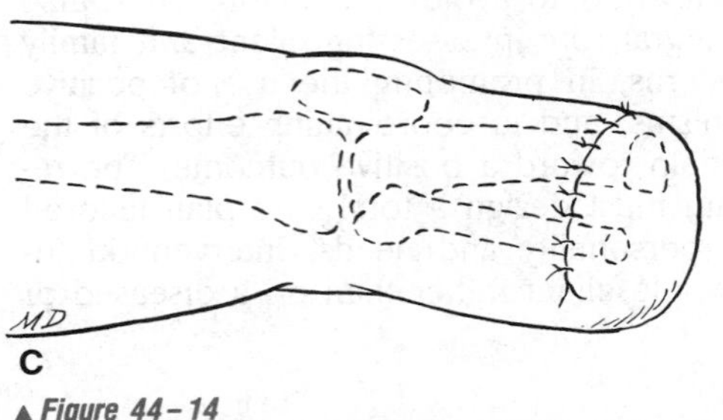

▲ *Figure 44 – 14*

Open and closed amputations. *A*, Step 1 of open amputation; this technique is used when infection complicates amputation. *B*, Closed amputation (or step 2 of open amputation, performed when infection has resolved). *C*, Stump closure.

wound to drain freely. The infected wound is treated with antibiotics and bed rest.

Once the infection is completely eradicated, the client undergoes another surgery for stump closure.

During a "flap" amputation, the surgeon closes or covers the stump with a flap of skin sutured over the end of the stump. This type of amputation is performed when there is no evidence of infection and, consequently, no need for open drainage. However, the surgeon may insert small drains to promote wound healing.

Improvements in vascular surgery have provided outstanding examples of long-term limb salvage in clients who in the past would have required amputation. Current data indicate that revascularization should be the first option considered in clients with critical limb ischemia. This recommendation is based on observations that (1) prior revascularization does not raise the level of amputation, (2) mortality rates for amputation are at least as high as for arterial bypass, and (3) there is no difference in cost between amputation and successful bypass.

Levels of Amputation

The level of amputation for any extremity should be as distal as possible. Clients with below-knee amputations (even bilateral) more successfully achieve independent function with a prosthesis than do those with above-knee amputations (Fig. 44 – 15).

DIAGNOSTIC ASSESSMENT

Angiography is the most common diagnostic study used to determine vascular patency. It commonly reveals a range of problems, from marked reductions to the absence of blood flow.

Client's Attitude Toward Amputation

Attitude toward amputation depends to a large degree on the client's age and maturity. Young clients may resist amputation even though it would greatly improve their function. For some, the thought of amputation dramatically conflicts with their ideal self-image.

Conversely, some clients who suffer from the agonizing pain of chronic ischemia may welcome amputation. These clients are more concerned with removing the source of their pain than they are with altering their body image or function.

Evaluation of Rehabilitative Potential

Ideally, clients should attain independent function with the use of a prosthesis. However, prosthetic rehabilitation requires cooperation, commitment, good coordination, and a tremendous amount of energy. A majority of clients may be expected to regain ambulatory status after ischemic amputation.

Not all amputees, however, are candidates for prostheses. General contraindications may involve concurrent medical conditions (i.e., chronic and progressive mental deterioration; advancing neurologic problems; chronic obstructive pulmonary disease; cardiac disease with congestive heart failure or angina). The use of a prosthesis increases energy requirements and workload.

Postoperative Prosthetic Fitting and Rehabilitative Program

Clients are either (1) fitted immediately with a prosthesis or (2) fitted a week or two later when the stump wound has healed and the sutures have been removed. The surgeon decides on the type of prosthetic fitting

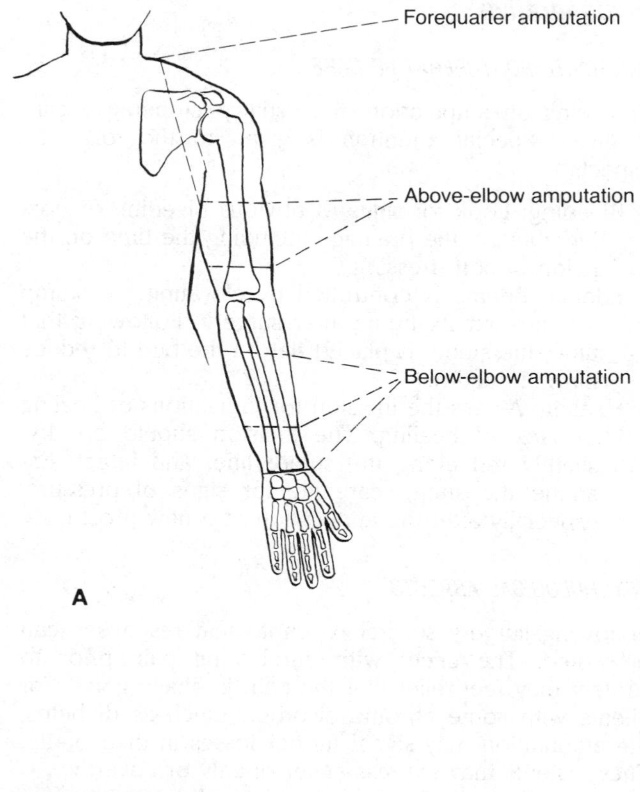

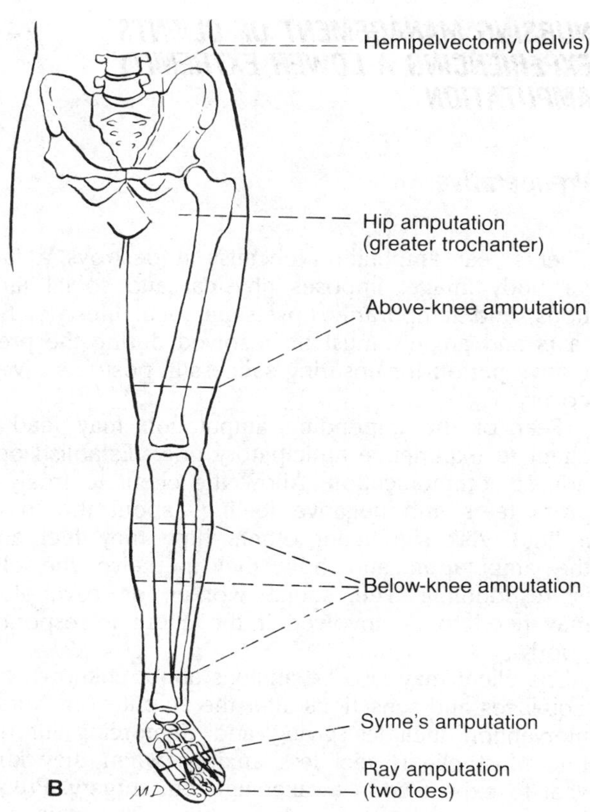

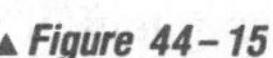
▲ **Figure 44–15**

Common sites of amputation: *A*, upper extremity; *B*, lower extremity.

before surgery. Ideally, the client facing amputation goes to surgery expecting some functional restoration of the limb. Carefully describing the prosthesis to the client helps pave the way to successful rehabilitation.

IMMEDIATE POSTOPERATIVE PROSTHESIS FITTING

Application of the total-contact rigid dressing to the stump in the operating room is one of the most important aspects of immediate prosthetic fitting. After suturing the skin, the surgeon applies an occlusive dressing (such as silk or Telfa) and places a small amount of fluffed gauze over the end of the stump. The surgeon or prosthetist then applies the rigid dressing, carefully distributing pressure evenly over the end of the stump. The rigid dressing protects the stump from injury and prevents swelling by gently compressing the tissues. Controlling edema enhances wound healing, comfort, and freedom of movement. In below-knee amputations, the surgeon immobilizes the knee; thereby, joint flexion is eliminated.

The socket of the distal end of the rigid dressing is designed to connect to a pylon. A pylon is an adjustable rigid support, the proximal end of which attaches to the below-knee socket or to the knee unit of an above-knee prosthesis. The distal end connects to a foot-ankle assembly.

The rigid dressing is usually changed three to four times before application of a permanent prosthesis. Cast changes are necessary because the stump tends to shrink as it heals and, consequently, is no longer compressed by the original cast.

DELAYED PROSTHESIS FITTING

Immediate prosthetic fitting is not always possible. However, anyone with a new amputation who is capable of ambulating should receive a temporary prosthesis as soon as possible after surgery. When a conventional delayed prosthesis fitting is anticipated, the client returns from surgery with the stump dressed and covered with Ace bandages or stump socks.

Soft dressing may be used whenever the wound requires frequent inspection. The dressings may be accompanied by external anteroposterior splints for prevention of joint contractures. However, soft dressings poorly control wound pressure and pain. Also, some health care professionals believe soft dressings risk greater wound contamination because of repeated wound inspections.

When the sutures are removed 2 to 3 weeks after surgery, the surgeon or prosthetist fits the client with a provisional temporary prosthesis made of plaster of Paris or plastic.

NURSING MANAGEMENT OF CLIENTS EXPERIENCING A LOWER EXTREMITY AMPUTATION

Preoperative

Clients fear amputation because it destroys a familiar body image, imposes physical and social limitations, and temporarily upsets personal lifestyle. Such fears and anxiety must be resolved during the preoperative period for ensuring successful postoperative recovery.

Fear of the impending amputation may lead the client to experience anticipatory grief. Establish open, honest communication. Allow the client to freely express fears and negative feelings about the loss of a limb. Ask significant others how they feel about the amputation and how they perceive the client is responding. The social worker or psychologist may need to be involved if the client is responding poorly.

The client may also be anxious about unknown consequences and sensations after the amputation. Nursing intervention includes giving and reinforcing information. Most clients feel less anxious when they know what to expect upon awakening from surgery. Prepare the client for phantom limb sensation. The majority of clients with new amputations experience the peculiar sensation that their missing limb is still present. This "phantom limb" sensation may or may not be painful. Also, it may either disappear within hours after surgery or persist for years. Its cause is unknown. For avoidance of misunderstandings, inform clients that phantom limb sensations occur and are normal.

Establish expectations. Clients want to know what to expect after surgery and what health care professionals will expect of them. Emphasize that the client is the most important member of the rehabilitation team. To achieve independence, the client will need to (1) exercise several times a day, (2) strictly limit weight-bearing (if the client is losing part of a leg) until instructed otherwise, (3) learn all the intricacies of stump and prosthesis care, and (4) master the use of the prosthesis.

Clients with diabetes mellitus are a high-risk surgical group and require careful preoperative assessment of their metabolic status. Clients with ulcerated legs or osteomyelitis may be treated with antibiotics and bed rest. Debilitated clients need nourishment with foods high in protein. They also may benefit from vitamin and mineral supplements. Severely anemic clients may require iron preparations and blood transfusions. Dehydrated clients should receive preoperative intravenous fluids for correction of fluid imbalances.

The client may experience very severe to moderate pain before surgery. Intervene with supportive measures. For example, use footboards and cradles to avoid pressure on injured or ischemic limbs. Also administer prescribed analgesics as necessary to relieve pain.

Postoperative

IMMEDIATE POSTOPERATIVE CARE

Following an amputation, the usual postoperative care is given. Special attention is given to the following aspects:

Bleeding: Look for signs of obvious bleeding or oozing. Outline the drainage including the time on the pylon or soft dressing.

Edema: Edema is controlled by elevating the stump for the first 24 hours after surgery. Following that time, the stump is placed flat on the bed to reduce hip contracture.

Healing: Assess the incision for indications of healing or lack of healing. The incision should be dry, slightly red along the suture line, and intact. Examine the stump carefully for signs of pressure, especially after the application of a new prosthesis.

PSYCHOLOGICAL ASPECTS

Following surgery several psychological responses can be noted. The client with unrelenting pain prior to surgery may feel relief that the pain is finally gone. For clients with some chronic disorders, such as diabetes, the amputation may signal further losses in their battle. These clients may express anger openly or covertly.

Many clients express depression after amputation. The client may cry easily, eat little, sleep poorly, sleep more, or avoid interactions with others. Many times depression is a reaction to the fear that the client will never walk again, and therefore, early ambulation is therapeutic.

Phantom pain is the feeling of pain in the amputated extremity. It commonly follows traumatic amputation, especially of the upper extremity. Phantom pain has been used for years to describe the normal perception of the missing extremity that all amputees feel. For example, when the leg is amputated, the client will feel the presence of the missing foot for many weeks. This perception is due to intact peripheral nerves proximal to the amputation site that used to carry messages between the brain and the now amputated part. This sensation is normal, and the client should be prepared for it. Phantom pain is abnormal and tragic. It is difficult to treat and requires both physical and emotional care.

REHABILITATION AND PROSTHESIS TRAINING

The most common prosthesis for clients with a below-the-knee amputation is a patellar tendon-bearing limb prosthesis. The interior of the prosthesis contacts all surfaces of the stump and weight bearing is on several areas. Clients with above-the-knee amputation are fitted with either a quadrilateral socket or ischial containment prosthesis. Weight is borne on the ischial tuberosity and soft tissues of the proximal stump, respectively.

Prostheses for the upper extremity consist of a hook or hand device, a harness to supply force to the hand, and a socket for attachment.

The client coping with an upper extremity amputation must be highly motivated to master the prosthesis and achieve independence. For successful rehabilitation, the client must integrate the prosthetic arm and hand into the total body image.

Cosmetic prostheses are primarily used to enhance self-esteem and make reentry into society minus a limb more tolerable for clients who are not candidates for a functioning prosthesis. Because the construction of cosmetic prostheses does not allow weight-bearing, caution the client never to attempt transfers or ambulation with a cosmetic prosthesis.

ADJUSTMENT TO A PROSTHESIS

The client coping with a new amputation must adjust to the prosthesis physically as well as psychologically. Physically, the client increases strength and endurance with regularly scheduled exercise; controls weight-bearing until the wound completely heals; and practices ambulating with the new prosthesis until a skillful, automatic gait is developed.

Psychologically, these clients must integrate the new prosthesis into their self-image if they are to become truly independent again. Psychological adjustment to a prosthesis is often more difficult and may take longer than physical adjustment. Some clients may benefit from talking with others who have mastered the use of their prostheses and have attained independent function. Support groups may be helpful in this endeavor.

STUMP AND PROSTHESIS CARE

After lower limb amputation, provide clients with client education guidelines concerning how to care for their stump and prosthesis in the health care facility or at home (see Client Education Guide).

Physical mobility will be compromised for the client who has just experienced an amputation. Amputating a limb displaces the center of gravity, normally located just below the umbilicus. A client coping with an amputation must relearn balance because the prosthesis, however similar, will not be an exact replica in weight and movement of the lost limb. Adapting to a change in the center of gravity occurs slowly but progressively until the conscious effort of maintaining balance comes under unconscious control.

When the prosthesis is not worn (e.g., during the night), turning also requires a readaptation in body balance. Consequently, the client may need assistance while turning until the new center of gravity is comfortable.

DISCHARGE PLANNING AND SELF-CARE

When making discharge plans for the client with a new amputation (and probably a prosthesis), consider the client's ambulatory level and the tasks with which the client may need help. Frequently, by the time clients with amputations are aware of their changed circumstances, they are at home, alone, and without the informed and professional advice that can prepare them for their altered lives. Schedule home visits from community health care nurses until such clients have adjusted to their new situation and feel reasonably comfortable and confident in their ability to provide self-care.

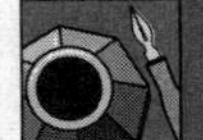

CLIENT EDUCATION GUIDE

Stump and Prosthesis Care

Stump

- Inspect the stump daily for redness, blistering, or abrasions.
- Use a mirror to examine all sides and aspects of the stump. Skin breakdown on the stump is extremely serious because it interferes with prosthesis training and may prolong hospitalization and recovery. Clients with diabetes mellitus are particularly susceptible to skin complications, because changes in sensation may obliterate the awareness of stump pain.
- Perform meticulous daily stump hygiene. Wash the stump with a mild soap, and then carefully rinse and dry it. Apply nothing to the stump after it is bathed. Alcohol dries and cracks the skin, whereas oils and creams soften the skin too much for safe prosthesis use.
- Wear woolen stump socks over the stump for cleanliness and comfort. Woolen socks must be washed in cool water and mild soap to prevent shrinkage. To prevent stretching, wash socks gently. Dry stump socks flat on a towel.
- Torn socks should be replaced because mending creates wrinkles that irritate the skin.
- Put on the prosthesis immediately when arising and keep it on all day (once the wound has healed completely) to reduce stump swelling.
- Continue prescribed exercises to prevent weakness.

Prosthesis

- Instruct the client to remove sweat and dirt from the prosthesis socket daily by wiping the inside of the socket with a damp soapy cloth. To remove the soap, use a clean damp cloth. Remind the client to dry the prosthesis socket thoroughly.
- Never attempt to adjust or mechanically alter the prosthesis. If problems develop, consult the prosthetist.
- Schedule a yearly appointment with the prosthetist.

▼ NURSING CARE OF CLIENTS WITH VENOUS DISEASE

Venous disorders can be separated into acute and chronic conditions. Chronic venous disorders can be further separated into varicose vein formation and chronic venous insufficiency. Acute venous disorders include thromboembolism. Acute venous disorders will be discussed first.

ACUTE VENOUS DISORDERS

Definition

Acute venous disorders are due to thrombus (clot) formation. Thrombus formation obstructs venous flow. Blockage may occur in both the superficial and deep veins.

SUPERFICIAL THROMBOPHLEBITIS

Superficial thrombophlebitis is usually an easily diagnosed condition; it is often iatrogenic, resulting from careless insertion of intravenous catheters or inattentive care of intravenous sites. Symptoms are local and include a raised, red, slightly indurated, warm tender cord along the course of the involved vein. Comfort is promoted and symptoms are relieved by the application of heat.

DEEP VEIN THROMBOSIS

Deep vein thrombosis refers to thrombophlebitis of the deep veins. Veins and valves permanently damaged by deep vein thrombosis increase the risk for another deep vein thrombosis, pulmonary embolism, and venous stasis ulcers.

Incidence

Deep vein thrombosis is a common disorder, more so in women than in men, and more so in adults than in children. It is particularly common among hospitalized clients. Around one third of clients over 40 years of age who have had either major surgery or an acute myocardial infarction develop deep vein thrombosis.[58]

Etiology

Thrombus formation is usually attributed to (1) venous stasis, (2) hypercoagulability, or (3) injury to the venous wall. This is known as Virchow's triad. It is thought that at least two of the three conditions must be present for thrombi to form.

VENOUS STASIS

Immobilization or absence of the calf muscle pump causes venous stasis. Other conditions that may cause stasis are surgery, immobility, obesity, pregnancy, paralysis, and congestive heart failure.

HYPERCOAGULABILITY

Hypercoagulability often accompanies malignant neoplasms (especially visceral and ovarian tumors). Dehydration and blood dyscrasias may raise the platelet count, decrease fibrinolysis, increase the clotting factors, or increase the viscosity of the blood. Oral contraceptives and hematologic disorders may also increase the coagulability of the blood.

VEIN WALL TRAUMA

Conditions that may cause vein wall trauma are intravenous injections, thromboangiitis obliterans (Buerger's disease), fractures and dislocations, chemical injury from sclerosing agents, opaque mediator radiography, and certain antibiotics (such as chlortetracycline). The resulting damage to the vein wall attracts platelets and accumulation of blood debris. This in combination with low blood flow and a hypercoagulable state results in thrombus formation.

Risk Factors and Prevention

Common clinical risk factors for venous thrombosis and pulmonary thromboembolism are presented in Table 44-9. In addition to those listed, varicose veins (see later) seem to be associated with the development of thrombosis.[18]

Immobile clients with deep vein thrombosis have a decreased risk of developing into pulmonary embolism versus those clients who are ambulatory. This has been shown to underestimate the risk of pulmonary embolism after hospital discharge in clients who have "low-risk" surgery. Presumably, hospitalized clients are treated prophylactically with anti-embolism stockings and anticoagulants. Clients discharged to their homes seldom receive this prophylaxis.

Prevention is geared toward promoting venous return, avoiding injury to the endothelial wall, and maintaining normal coagulability. Prevention methods generally used for the high-risk hospitalized client have included mechanical methods such as devices that elevate the foot of the bed, compression stockings, motorized foot movers, and intermittent calf muscle compressors. Pharmacologic prevention has included warfarin, platelet antiaggregation agents (aspirin being the most common), heparin, and dextran.

Additional nursing measures generally recommended for prevention of venous stasis include the following.

TABLE 44-9. Common Conditions Associated with Venous Thrombosis and Pulmonary Thromboembolism

Surgery, especially orthopedic surgery, gynecologic cancer surgery, major abdominal surgery, coronary artery bypass grafting, renal transplantation, and splenectomy
Congestive heart failure, myocardial infarction, cardiomyopathy
Immobolization (bed rest, stroke, prolonged travel, and so forth)
Malignancy
Previous deep vein thrombosis
Pregnancy, particularly in the puerperium and after cesarean section
Trauma
Estrogen therapy or oral contraceptives
Age over 50 years
Obesity

VARICOSE VEINS

- Facilitate active and passive range-of-motion exercises for postoperative, postpartum, and immobilized clients.
- Encourage early ambulation, especially for postoperative and postpartum clients.
- Encourage postoperative deep-breathing exercises to promote thoracic pumping action.
- Avoid use of pillows under legs postoperatively to facilitate venous return.
- Teach client to avoid sitting or standing in one position for prolonged periods of time.

Nursing interventions for preventing injury to the vein wall include the following:

- Administer prophylactic, preoperative, low-dose heparin therapy for (1) elderly clients with hip fractures, (2) obese clients undergoing surgery, (3) all clients undergoing major surgery, or (4) clients on bed rest.
- Teach clients about risk of oral contraceptives.
- Maintain adequate hydration.

Nursing interventions for preventing injury to the vein wall include the following:

- Avoid infiltration during intravenous therapy.
- Use heel cushions during surgery to elevate the calves, thereby avoiding damage to the intima of the vein.

Pathophysiology

Thrombus development is a local process. It begins by platelet adherence to the endothelium. Where the platelets adhere to collagen, adenosine diphosphate (ADP) is released. ADP is also released from the damaged tissues and disrupted platelets. ADP produces platelet aggregation that results in a platelet plug.

Deep vein thrombi vary from 1 mm in diameter to long tubular masses filling main veins. Small thrombi are found commonly in the pocket of deep vein valves.

Newly formed thrombi may become pulmonary emboli. Probably 24 to 48 hours after formation, thrombi undergo lysis or become organized and adhere to the vessel wall. This diminishes the risk of embolization.

As thrombi become larger in diameter and length, they obstruct the veins. The resulting inflammatory process can destroy the valves of the veins; thus, venous insufficiency and postphlebitic syndrome are initiated.

If a thrombus occludes a major vein (e.g., femoral, vena caval, axillary), the venous pressure and volume rise distally. Conversely, if a thrombus occludes a deep small vein (e.g., tibial, popliteal), collateral venous channels usually relieve the increased venous pressure and volume.

COMPLICATIONS

Pulmonary emboli, most of which start as thrombi in the large deep veins of the legs, are an acute and potentially lethal complication of deep vein thrombosis. Pulmonary embolism is discussed in Chapter 39.

Clinical Manifestations

The presence of superficial thrombophlebitis is easily ascertained by finding the inflamed vein. In contrast, the clinical manifestations of deep vein thrombosis (DVT) are less distinctive; about one half of clients are asymptomatic. The most common signs and symptoms are pain in the region of the thrombus and unilateral swelling distal to the site. Other clinical manifestations include redness or warmth of the leg, dilated veins, or low grade fever. Unfortunately, the first clinical manifestation may be pulmonary embolism. Frequently, clients have thrombi in both legs even though the symptoms are unilateral.

Homans' sign—discomfort in the upper calf during forced dorsiflexion of the foot—is commonly assessed during physical examination. Unfortunately, it is insensitive and nonspecific. It is present in less than one third of clients with documented deep vein thrombosis. In addition, more than 50 per cent of clients with a positive finding of Homans' sign do not have venous thrombosis.

Diagnostic Assessment

NONINVASIVE TECHNIQUES

The Doppler ultrasonographic flowmeter determines blood flow in the larger blood vessels as well as the patency of vessels. Reliability of the test is directly related to the skill of the examiner; its accuracy is affected by inability to detect partially or totally occluded veins, inaccessibility of deep pelvic and thigh veins, and inability to distinguish collateral circulation from native veins.

Venous duplex scanning has become the primary diagnostic test of DVT because it allows visualization of the vein, which provides an extremely reliable diagnosis of venous thrombus.

Plethysmographic examination of the venous system entails the recording of volume changes in a limb during venous filling and emptying. Impedance plethysmography measures maximal venous filling capacity by applying a pneumatic cuff at thigh level and then recording the rate of venous emptying after cuff release. The rate of venous emptying correlates well with the degree of venous obstruction and is also a very good indicator of deep vein thrombosis.

Plethysmography may produce false-negative results if the client (1) cannot sustain deep inspiration long enough to cause pooling of blood in the deep veins, (2) is unable to lie flat and laterally rotate hip and bend knee, (3) is in congestive heart failure, or (4) has peripheral arterial occlusion. The client must lie perfectly still during plethysmography because any movement can cause distortion and false readings.

INVASIVE TECHNIQUES

Venography, discussed earlier under assessment of the peripheral vascular system, was previously viewed as the diagnostic standard but is now being replaced with

Table 44–10. Clinical Assessment of Thrombophlebitis

Veins	Causative Factors	Clinical Manifestations	Edema	Pulmonary Embolism	Chronic Venous Insufficiency/ Postphlebitic Syndrome
Superficial					
Saphenous, median cephalic, median basilic	Varicose veins, intravenous injections. Buerger's disease, blood dyscrasias, cancer	Tender, indurated, red, visible, palpable cord along vein Ovoid nodules in skin	Rare	Rare	Rare
Deep Veins					
Femoral, iliac, axillary, subclavian, superior and interior vena cava, tibial and popliteal	Immobility, congestive heart failure, blood dyscrasias, cancer, oral contraceptives, fractures, dislocations, obesity, dehydration	Increased muscle turgor and tenderness over affected vein Possible superficial venous distention Deep muscle tenderness, increased warmth in affected limb, occasionally with fever (rarely over 38.3° C or 101° F) Positive finding of Homans' sign Cyanosis of occlusion is severe	Common	Possible	Possible; deep vein thrombosis is leading cause of pulmonary embolism and postphlebitic syndrome

duplex scanning. Venography is done on most clients before vascular surgery. Complications of this procedure include thrombophlebitis and clot formation.

Ventilation-perfusion (V-Q) scan or pulmonary artery arteriography may be used to assess pulmonary embolism.

Medical Management

Superficial thrombophlebitis can be managed with local measures, such as warm packs and elevation of the extremity. Sometimes, anti-inflammatory medications are required. Bed rest with leg elevation is usually prescribed for clients with DVT until local signs of inflammation subside. After 7 to 15 days, the client is usually allowed to ambulate wearing elastic stockings.

PHARMACOLOGIC MANAGEMENT

Anticoagulant therapy is based on the premise that the initiation or extension of thrombi can be prevented by inhibiting the synthesis of clotting factors or by accelerating their inactivation. The anticoagulants heparin and warfarin do not induce thrombolysis but effectively prevent clot extension.

Heparin is the drug of choice for the treatment of thromboembolic disease. Heparin prevents the activation of clotting factor IX and inhibits the action of thrombin in forming fibrin threads. An intravenous bolus of 5000 to 10,000 units followed by 750 to 1000 units per hour can be given via continuous intravenous infusion. Heparin's effect is measured by partial thromboplastin (PTT) levels. Therapeutic PTT values are usually $1\frac{1}{2}$ to 2 times normal control levels.

The specific antidote to heparin is protamine sulfate. Unfortunately, an excessive dose of protamine may actually prolong clotting. Heparin is contraindicated in the following conditions: severe hypertension; cerebrovascular hemorrhage; active gastrointestinal ulceration; overt bleeding from the gastrointestinal, genitourinary, or respiratory tract; recent neurosurgery; or heparin allergy.

Coumarin Derivatives. Coumarin derivatives inhibit hepatic synthesis of the vitamin K–dependent clotting factors. The most common coumarin is warfarin sodium (Coumadin). The coumarins are used to prevent and treat venous thrombosis.

The effect of the coumarin derivatives is determined by measurement of the prothrombin time (PT). PT must be measured every day before coumarin is administered. Generally, a PT of 1½ to 2 times the normal reading is desired. The antidote for the coumarin derivatives is vitamin K (Mephyton). If bleeding occurs, the physician will discontinue the medication for a period.

The coumarin derivatives require 24 to 48 hours to take effect. Therefore, heparin, which is fast-acting, is used initially with coumarin and discontinued when the coumarin begins to take effect. Anticoagulation is usually continued about 3 to 6 months after an acute venous thrombosis and after pulmonary embolism.

Fibrinolytic Agents. Fibrinolytic medications (e.g., streptokinase and urokinase) dissolve thrombi by stimulating the conversion of plasminogen to plasmin, an enzyme that decomposes fibrin. Fibrinolytic therapy was discussed earlier in this chapter.

Surgical Management

Surgical measures for DVT fall into two categories: (1) intervention for the thrombus itself and (2) surgical prophylaxis against pulmonary embolism involving ligation or interruption of the inferior vena cava with a filter or an "umbrella."

Venous Thrombectomy. The direct removal of venous thrombi was previously recommended. Now it is rarely performed because there is a high incidence of recurrent postoperative thrombosis.

Umbrella Procedure. During this procedure, a filter on an umbrella is inserted in the vena cava to trap large emboli. Some types of umbrellas can be inserted under local anesthesia by threading the device through the femoral or jugular vein. A rare complication of this technique is the migration of the filter into the iliac vein, renal vein, right atrium, right ventricle, or pulmonary artery. Such migrations may be fatal.

Nursing Management

Goals of nursing management are to prevent existing thrombi from becoming emboli and to prevent new thrombi from forming. When caring for the client with deep vein thrombosis, (1) protect the client from thromboemboli and bleeding due to anticoagulant therapy, (2) teach the client about deep vein thrombosis and anticoagulation therapy, (3) provide analgesia, (4) assess for pulmonary embolism, and (5) reduce anxiety.

Bed Rest. Bed rest is indicated to prevent emboli. Bed rest also prevents pressure fluctuations in the venous system that occur with walking.

Because clients with thrombi will be on bed rest for about 5 to 7 days, provide them with orthoframe and trapeze, pressure-reduction mattress, and heel protectors. Remember to have nightstand, over-the-bed table, call light, and telephone in easy reach. Stool softeners and coughing and deep-breathing exercises are also recommended.

Elevate Legs. Elevation of the legs above the level of the heart facilitates blood flow by the force of gravity. The increase of blood flow prevents venous stasis and the formation of new thrombi. Elevation of the legs also decreases venous pressure, which thus relieves edema and pain. Elevate the foot of the bed 6 inches (Trendelenburg's position), with a slight knee bend to prevent popliteal pressure. The veins of the legs should be level with the right artrium. The head of the bed may be raised to facilitate eating and bathing. Apply elastic wraps snugly from toe to groin. Rewrap them every 4 to 8 hours.

Continuous Warm Packs. Administer warm packs around the involved area. The heat relieves venospasm, produces analgesia, and hastens resolution of inflammation.

Relieve Discomfort. Bed rest, elevation of the extremity, and application of warm packs usually relieve discomfort. Some clients need a mild sedative or analgesic.

Monitoring Anticoagulant Therapy. Intravenous heparin followed by oral anticoagulation is used to decrease the risk of new thrombi. The nurse assesses for effectiveness by monitoring the PTT. The usual goal is 2 to 2.5 times the control (normal) value. The nurse also monitors for manifestations of excess anticoagulation; bleeding, evidenced by blood in the urine, stool, and along the gums or teeth; subcutaneous bruising; or flank pain. When invasive studies are necessary (e.g., arterial blood gases), 30 minutes of pressure is applied to the puncture site.

Monitor for Development of Pulmonary Embolism. Pulmonary embolism is an acute and potentially lethal complication of deep vein thrombosis.

Chest pain is the most common symptom of pulmonary embolism, but it is not diagnostic of the condition. The pain most often associated with pulmonary embolism is pleuritic. Pleuritic pain is caused by an inflammatory reaction of the lung parenchyma or by pulmonary infarction or ischemia caused by obstruction of small pulmonary arterial branches. Pleuritic chest pain is typically sudden in onset and is aggravated by breathing.

Hemoptysis occurs in about 30 per cent of clients. The presence of hemoptysis indicates that pulmonary infarction or atelectasis has produced alveolar hemorrhage. Other clinical manifestations may include cough, diaphoresis, dyspnea, and apprehension. Because of the seriousness of pulmonary embolism, the physician is prompty notified of these clinical manifestations. Pulmonary embolism is fully discussed in Chapter 39.

DISCHARGE TEACHING

When teaching clients about deep vein thrombosis, first assess their learning abilities. Many clients with thrombophlebitis are older and may suffer from sensory loss or limited mobility.

The nurse begins teaching the first day of heparinization, discussing reasons for anticoagulants and bed rest. The nurse also informs the client about the complications of therapy and emphasizes manifestations to report. Prevention is the key to DVT. Therefore the nurse teaches risk factors of deep vein thrombosis and how to avoid them. Continue teaching with explanations of medications the client is taking, actions, doses, timing, adverse effects, and importance of monitoring coagulation status. Clients need to know who to contact and how to reach a health care practitioner in case problems develop.

CHRONIC VENOUS INSUFFICIENCY

Overview

Chronic venous insufficiency, also known as postphlebotic syndrome, is marked by (1) chronic swollen limbs; (2) thick, coarse, brownish skin around the ankles (referred to as the "gaiter" area); and (3) venous stasis ulceration. Chronic venous insufficiency results from dysfunctional valves that reduce venous return, which thus increases venous pressure and causes venous stasis. Skin ulcerations also occur. Because existing valves are destroyed, venous blood flow is bidirectional, resulting in inefficient venous outflow. The net effect of this change is that the weight of the venous blood column from the right atrium is transmitted along the full length of the veins. Very high venous pressure is exerted at the ankle and the venules become the final pathway for the highest venous pressure.

Chronic venous insufficiency follows most severe cases of deep vein thrombosis but may take as long as 5 to 10 years to manifest. However, about 20 per cent of clients with chronic venous insufficiency have no history of deep vein thrombosis. Within 5 years of a known deep vein thrombosis, almost 50 per cent of clients develop chronic induration and stasis dermatitis, and 20 per cent suffer from venous stasis ulcer. Therefore, clients with a history of deep vein thrombosis must be monitored periodically for life. Alert them to observe for the slightest skin changes. Once the skin is broken and a venous ulcer develops, the client faces a frustrating chronic problem. Venous stasis ulcers do not heal well.

Management

Important goals are to increase venous blood return and to decrease venous pressure. Antigravity measures increase blood return to the heart. They include elevating the legs above the heart level and avoiding prolonged standing or sitting. Advise the client to avoid (1) crossing legs, (2) chairs that are too high for feet to touch the floor or too deep (and press on the popliteal area), (3) garters, and (4) sources of pressure above the legs (e.g., tight girdles). Encourage the client to sleep with the foot of the bed elevated 6 inches. At least one third of every 24 hours should be spent with the feet and legs elevated above the heart.

Increased venous pressure on the tissues of the leg can be counteracted by the compression of elastic support hose. Ideally, this support should just balance the increased venous pressure. Thus, hose should be fitted individually to the client's legs. Measurements of the ankle and calf circumference and from 1 inch below the knee or 1 inch below the groin to the bottom of the foot are usually taken. Measure after the client has been recumbent and leg edema is minimal. Stockings that extend above the knee often bind the popliteal space and act as a tourniquet, especially when the knee is bent. Knee-length elastic stockings are preferable.

After thrombosis of a deep calf vein, clients should wear elastic support for at least 6 to 8 weeks and probably for life. Elastic support compresses the superficial veins when the client walks and, with walking, increases blood flow in the veins while keeping venous pressure to a minimum. Standing and sitting are not allowed during the acute phase because they increase the hydrostatic pressure in the capillaries, which promotes edema. Once the threat of embolization is over, encourage walking and exercises in bed to decrease venous pressure and to promote blood flow. Also recommend that the client on bed rest dorsiflex the feet against a footboard for exercise.

Sometimes pneumatic vascular compression leggings are ordered to aid blood flow. These leggings or boots are attached by polyethylene tubing to an electric pump. Air is pumped into each legging alternately for 1 minute at a time at a pressure of 40 to 45 mm Hg. Use of these leggings is usually discontinued when the client starts walking.

VENOUS STASIS ULCERATION

Overview

Venous stasis ulcer represents the end stage of chronic venous insufficiency. Over a period of years, the excess venous pressure causes small skin veins and venules to rupture, with creation of stasis ulcers. Subcutaneous fibrosis, cutaneous atrophy, and lymphatic obstruction contribute to the development of stasis ulcers, characteristically located in the malleolar area. Once the skin is broken, infection occurs, usually due to either *Staphylococcus* or *Streptococcus*.

Management

When ulcers are present, cultures are taken. Antibiotics may be required to treat infection or cellulitis. Local wound care begins. Some ulcers require débridement of eschar, whereas others require protection. Transparent, moisture-permeable dressings are used to promote epithelialization. Solutions such as povidone-iodine (Betadine) can be used to control infection, but it is important to realize that any solution other than normal saline retards healing. (Wound care is discussed in Chap. 18). Skin grafting may be necessary to achieve healing. Surgery to remove incompetent, varicose veins or improve perfusion may also be necessary. Once the ulcer has healed, the client is measured for elastic stockings and taught the precautions discussed in the previous section on chronic venous insufficiency.

Unna's boot represents a popular form of bandage impregnated with calamine, zinc oxide, and glycerin. When wrapped snugly around the leg, it provides excellent compression during ambulation and applies minimal pressure during limb elevation. Unna's boot is a permeable dressing that can be applied directly over skin ulcers, thereby allowing drainage of exudate. It creates a moist and warm interface between the ulcerated skin and the bandage. It can be changed on a weekly or biweekly basis, which forces the client to wear it without interruption and thereby improves compliance (Bridge to Home Health Care). Disadvantages of Unna's boot include skin irritation, discomfort, difficulty in bathing, and pain while changing the boot. Unna's boot has been shown to achieve healing rates of 70 per cent.

VARICOSE VEINS

Overview

Varicose veins are a common complaint of clients with venous insufficiency. The loss of valvular competence and the constant elevation of venous pressure cause distention and tortuosity of the superficial veins. The greater and lesser saphenous veins and perforator veins in the ankle are common sites of varicosities.

Varicose veins may be either primary or secondary. Primary varicose veins often result from a congenital or familial predisposition that leads to loss of elasticity of the vein wall. Secondary varicosities occur when trauma, obstruction, deep vein thrombosis, or inflammation damages valves.

Varicose veins are a prevalent problem that continues to rise in incidence and affects a large percentage of the adult population. It has been estimated that 24 million Americans have varicose veins. The prevalence increases with age and peaks between the fifth and sixth decades of life. Varicose veins are more common in women; however, the gender ratio decreases with advancing age and almost disappears in clients over 70 years old. Prolonged standing has been implicated as an etiologic factor of varicose veins, but epidemiologic studies have not demonstrated an association between standing at work and increased incidence of varicose veins.

Clients with varicose veins often complain of aching, heaviness, itching, moderate swelling, and, frequently, unsightly appearance of their legs. Severity of discomfort is difficult to assess and does not seem related to the size of varicosities. A superficial inflammation may develop along the path of the varicose vein and may be associated with complaints of fever and malaise.

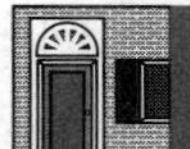

BRIDGE TO HOME HEALTH CARE

The Client with Peripheral Vascular Disease

An important aspect of home health care of a client with peripheral vascular disease is prevention of further complications. Specifically, the client needs to learn how to prevent edema and to avoid trauma. Properly fitted anti-embolic hose or Jobst stockings can reduce edema in the lower extremities. The measurements required for anti-embolic hose are the ankle, calf, thigh, and length from heel to thigh. A regular tape measure can be used, and the measurement is reported to the supply company or pharmacy to obtain the correct size. Jobst stockings are specially fitted; the client needs to be measured by the company that supplies the stockings.

An assessment of the lower extremities should be performed on each home visit to observe for stasis ulcers and the condition of the extremities. The nurse should observe for pain in the extremities; color changes of the skin or nails; impaired growth of nails; shiny, taut skin; discrepancy in size of one extremity; enlarged veins; temperature variations; and ulcerations. The lower extremities can be measured on each home visit.

When a stasis ulcer is detected, no matter how small, treatment needs to begin. Some examples of treatments that can be used are Unna's boot, wet-to-dry dressings, Duoderm, and Duoderm compression wraps. An open and draining wound should be cleansed with saline and dried well; an appropriate dressing is applied. Each physician may have a preference for which dressing procedure to start.

Usually a client cannot change the dressing because of its location on the lower extremities. Treatment of stasis ulcers is a long process, and healing is slow. Duoderm compression wraps help keep the edema to a minimum and promote quicker healing.

Duoderm compression wraps can be applied to an open, draining wound. Cleanse the open wound with saline, dry well, apply Duoderm cut in pieces to fit, wrap the extremity with Kling or Kerlix, then wrap with Duoderm compression dressing. Kling helps prevent the Duoderm compression wrap from sticking to the skin. The frequency of home visits for changing the dressing depends on the amount of drainage.

Duoderm compression dressings are expensive but heal a wound more quickly by keeping edema to a minimum. A wet-to-dry dressing with saline can be used for a smaller wound if edema is not a problem.

Clients sometimes forget to let the nurse know about edema or a change in the condition of an extremity. Clients should be instructed when to call the nurse about their condition.

Remember, prevention is the key for a client with peripheral vascular disease. The client should be taught prevention measures of limiting smoking, avoiding constrictive clothing, avoiding excessive heat to extremities (hot water bottle and heating pad), daily hygiene, and proper care of feet. Health education is important for preventing further complications of a disease process that does not have a cure.

To assess for varicose veins, carefully examine both legs in good lighting. Varicosities appear as dilated, tortuous skin veins (Figure 44–16). Check for patency by use of the Doppler flowmeter.

Incompetency of the deep and superficial veins can be diagnosed by (1) noting venous pressure changes during walking, (2) Trendelenburg's test, (3) phlebography, (4) Doppler flowmeter, and (5) plethysmography. (See assessment section in this chapter.)

Surgical Management

Sclerotherapy is the injection of a sclerosing agent into varicosed veins. The agent damages the vein and endothelium, causing an aseptic thrombosis that closes the vein. Sclerotherapy is palliative, not curative, and is usually performed for cosmetic reasons. It is most effective in closing small, residual varicosities after surgical intervention for varicose veins. (Sclerotherapy is contraindicated before such surgery, because it makes vein stripping more difficult.) Within minutes after injection of the sclerosing agent, elastic compression and active walking should commence. Elastic bandages are worn for about 6 weeks.

Surgical management of varicose veins consists of ligation (tying off) of the greater saphenous vein with its tributaries at the saphenofemoral junction, combined with saphenous vein stripping and ligation of incompetent perforater veins. Removal of the vein is performed through multiple, short incisions. An incision is made at the ankle over the saphenous vein and a nylon wire is threaded up the vein to the groin. The wire is brought out through the groin, capped, and then the wire and vein are pulled out through the ankle incision.

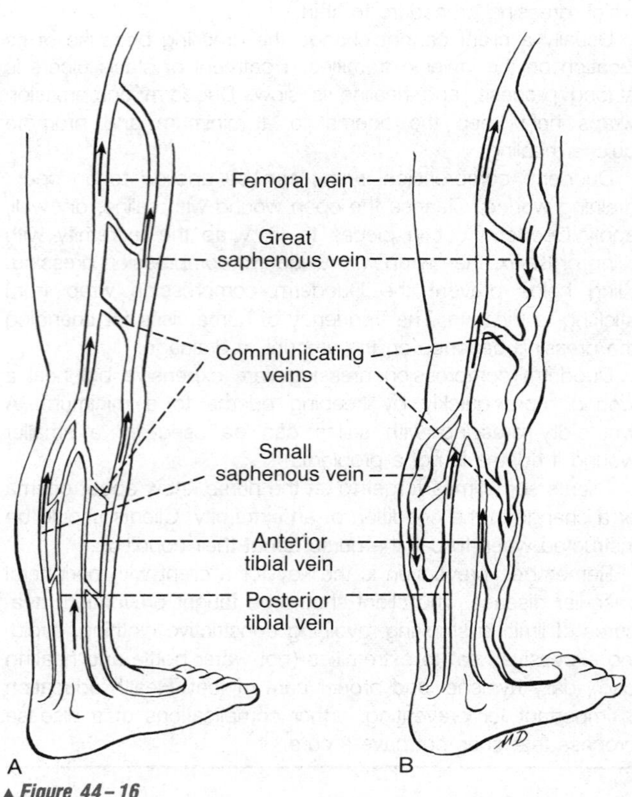

▲ *Figure 44–16*

Venous return from the legs. *A*, Normal flow. *B*, Varicosities and retrograde venous flow.

Elastic compression bandages are applied from foot to groin. The client is usually hospitalized overnight. Complications are rare. They include the usual surgical complications, bleeding, infection, and nerve damage. Hemorrhage most commonly occurs at the surgical wound site in the groin. Bleeding comes primarily from the stripped canal. The risk of serious bleeding can be decreased by carefully wrapping the leg from foot to groin and by applying compression, especially to the upper thigh and groin. Some discoloration and bruising along the stripped track are normal. One week after stripping, the client's leg looks ecchymotic.

Saphenous nerve damage may occur with surgery. In the distal third of the leg, the saphenous nerve runs close to the saphenous vein. Thus, risk of nerve injury increases when the distal part of the vein is involved.

Deep vein thrombosis, embolism, and infection are rare following varicose vein surgery, especially if postoperative precautions (bandaging, movement, exercise) are taken.

Postoperative Nursing Management

Three important postoperative nursing objectives are to (1) maintain firm elastic pressure over the whole limb, (2) promote regular movement and exercise of the legs, and (3) elevate the foot of the bed 6 to 9 inches so that the legs are above the heart level when the client is in bed. The client ambulates for short periods, starting 24 to 48 hours after surgery. Instruct clients to walk rather than to stand or sit. After ambulation, elevate the legs again.

Nurses must also assess for complications after varicose vein surgery. The major problems are hemorrhage, infection, nerve damage, and deep vein thrombosis.

▼ NURSING CARE OF CLIENTS WITH LYMPHATIC DISORDERS

LYMPHEDEMA

Overview

Lymphedema is swelling due to impaired transcapillary fluid transport and transportation of lymph. Failure of lymph transport allows the plasma proteins in the interstitial fluid to accumulate. The increase in fluids increases interstitial colloid osmotic pressure. The osmotic pressure is reduced by drawing water into interstitial areas. In addition, as the lymph channels dilate, valves become incompetent. The fluid seeks new pathways through the tissues, which causes inflammation, lymphatic thrombosis, and eventually fibrosis. Lymphedemas are best classified into primary and secondary forms.

PRIMARY LYMPHEDEMA

Primary lymphedema may be classified according to age of onset: congenital (present at birth), praecox (early in life), or tarda (late in life). Congenital and familial lymphedema is also called Milroy's disease. It is inherited as an autosomal dominant trait.

Of the primary forms, lymphedema praecox is the largest group; it peaks in the second decade and is more common in females than in males. The edema usually appears spontaneously and without known cause (Fig. 44-17*B*).

SECONDARY LYMPHEDEMA

Secondary lymphedema occurs because of some damage or obstruction to the lymph system by another disease process or by a procedure: trauma, neoplasms (primary or metastatic), filariasis, inflammation, surgical excision, or high doses of irradiation.

Postsurgical lymphedema is usually seen after surgical excision of axillary, inguinal, or iliac nodes usually performed as a prophylactic or therapeutic measure for metastatic tumor. For example, lymphedema of the arm is encountered after mastectomy (Fig. 44-17*A*).

Filariasis, caused by the filarial nematode *Wuchereria bancrofti* (and others), is one of the most common diseases of the world; it is transmitted by mosquitoes from human to human. The living embryos (microfilariae) of the adult worms are found in the bloodstream. The larvae migrate to the lymphatics, where they mature into adult worms. Adult worms in the lymph nodes and lymphatics lead to obstruction, lymphedema, and elephantiasis. Most clients have intermittent attacks of high fever, chills, malaise, fatigue, tender regional lymphadenopathy, severe muscle pain, and areas of erythema with increased edema. For clients with advanced disease, there is little that can be offered in terms of cure.

Lymphedema secondary to neoplasms in the lymph nodes is common. The malignant disease may be primary (a lymphoma or Hodgkin's disease) or metastatic from some other site.

Chronic lymphedema secondary to inflammation is relatively uncommon, probably as a result of early control with antibiotics. Chronic lymphedema due to recurrent lymphangitis and cellulitis is caused by bacterial organisms.

Radiation in moderate amounts does not appear to damage the lymph vessels. However, heavy radiation for a particularly resistant tumor usually leads to lymphatic obstruction.

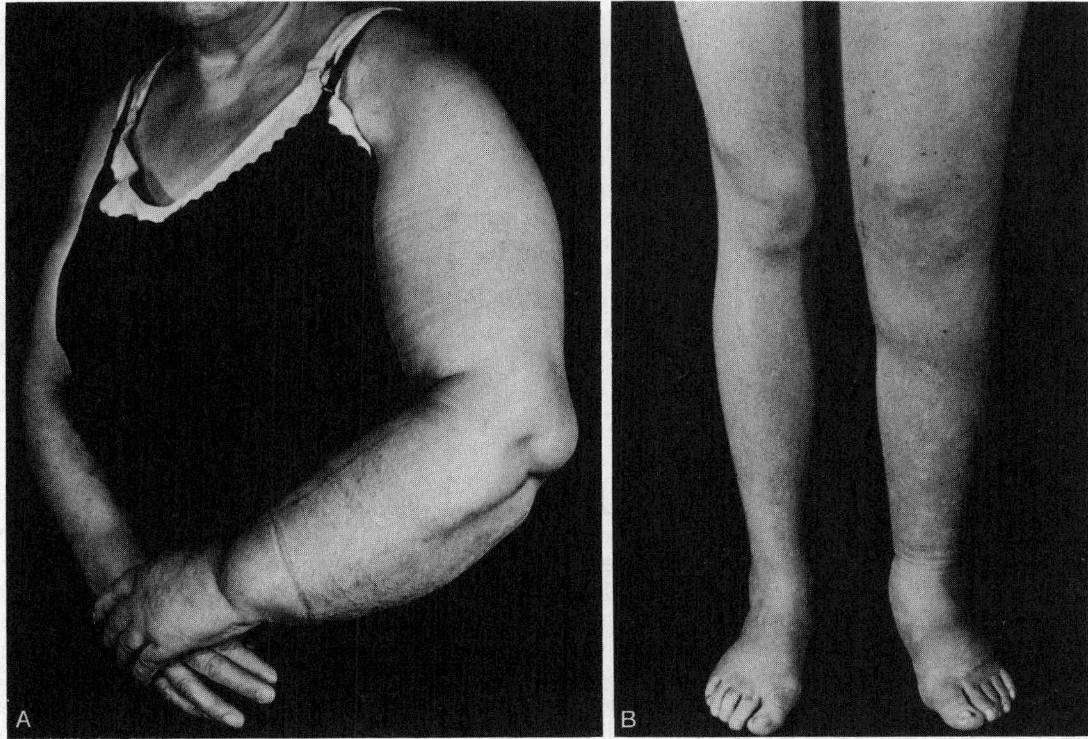

▲ **Figure 44-17**

Types of lymphedema. *A*, Secondary lymphedema of the arm following mastectomy. *B*, Primary lymphedema.

Prevention

Clients at high risk of lymphedema have the extremity elevated to improve lymphatic drainage. Range-of-motion exercises also decrease edema by activating the muscle pump.

Clinical Manifestations

Primary lymphedema presents as (1) bilateral mild edema of ankles and legs in women at puberty or shortly after, (2) unilateral edema of the entire leg in men and women (Fig. 44-17), and (3) bilateral edema present at birth or early age. The skin of clients with congenital lymphedema contains vesicles (blisters) filled with lymph.

A dull, heavy sensation is present, but actual pain is absent. Elevation of the limb and rest in bed cause a reduction but not disappearance. Smooth skin becomes roughened; the edema is nonpitting. Acute lymphangitis and cellulitis are infrequent. Ulceration of the skin does not occur. However, the limb becomes greatly enlarged, uncomfortable, and unsightly.

Lymphedema can be diagnosed with isotopic lymphography, lymphangiography, and phlebography.

Management

There is no known cure for lymphedema once the swelling appears. The goal of treatment is to remove as much fluid as possible from the affected extremity and to maintain as normal-appearing an extremity as possible.

Physical therapy for arm or leg lymphedema involves a mechanical or manual squeezing of the tissue in order to press the stagnant lymphatic fluid to the proximal part of the limb. This is followed by specific active and passive exercises to transport the lymph farther into the lymphatic system and finally into the bloodstream. A number of pneumatic pumping devices for intermittent compression are available. Diuretics may also be prescribed. Elastic stockings are used to maintain the effects of the pneumatic pump.

SURGICAL INTERVENTION

When lymphedematous limbs are massively swollen to the point that compression devices or stockings are no longer beneficial, surgery may be required. The most common surgical procedure for lymphedema is excisional, in which all skin, subcutaneous tissue, and deep fascia in the leg are removed. The leg is covered with skin grafts. Scarring is evident, and the cosmetic appearance may not be acceptable to all clients. Another form of surgery is the removal of the bulk of edematous tissues. This form of surgery is not curative, but the final appearance may be more acceptable.

Nursing Management

The client with lymphedema is at high risk for infection. Therefore, the nurse monitors the affected extremity for clinical manifestations of infection such as redness, warmth, pain, and fever. Meticulous skin care is given to the extremity using mild soaps and lotions. Nails are kept trimmed.

To reduce the swelling, the extremity is elevated above the right atrium. Pneumatic pumps may be used to reduce the extremity size. If pumps are used, the nurse teaches the client how to apply the device, and the frequency and reasons for its use. When stockings are used, the nurse ascertains that the stockings fit and do not gather behind the knee. Activity such as walking should be promoted rather than sitting or standing. For bedridden clients, the nurse teaches bed exercises to promote venous and lymphatic return and maintain muscle strength.

Clients with lymphedema may suffer from disturbances in self-concept due to the visibility of their deformity. The nurse encourages the client to discuss these feelings and helps the client understand that such feelings are normal. Variations in clothing style may be suggested to disguise the deformity.

Finally, when caring for clients with lymph disorders, remember that these clients must cope with difficult, chronic diseases. Take time to give emotional support to the client and family. Emphasize the possible need for lifelong follow-up.

LYMPHADENITIS

Lymph nodes act as defense barriers and are secondarily involved in virtually all systemic infections and in many neoplastic disorders arising elsewhere in the body. Generalized lymphadenopathy (enlargement of two or three regionally separated lymph node groups) is usually due to inflammation, neoplasm, or immunologic reactions.

The infections that lead to lymphadenitis are so numerous and varied that a detailed description would involve a list of all systemic microbiologic diseases. The specific node or nodes affected in an infectious disease depend on the location of the infection, the nature of the invading organism, and the severity of the disease. Lymphadenitis can be classified nonspecifically as either acute or chronic.

Acute Lymphadenitis

Acute lymphadenitis usually follows one of two pathologic patterns: (1) suppuration in lymph nodes that drain infections, caused by pyogenic organisms, or (2) reticuloendothelial hyperplasia, edema, and leukocyte infiltration of the nodes caused by nonpyogenic organisms such as spirochetes, rickettsiae, and viruses.

Acutely inflamed lymph nodes are most common locally in the cervical region in association with infections of the teeth or tonsils or in the axillary or inguinal regions secondary to infections of the extremities. Generalized lymphadenopathy is characteristic of the secondary stage of syphilis, viral infections, and bacteremia. Clinically, in acute lymphadenitis, the lymph nodes are enlarged, tender, warm, and reddened.

Chronic Lymphadenitis

In the course of long-standing infection, the lymph nodes frequently become scarred with fibrous connective tissue replacement. Clinically, these nodes are enlarged, firm to palpation, and not tender or warm. The management of lymphadenitis is treatment of the underlying disorder.

Summary

Clients with vascular diseases can challenge a broad range of the nurse's capability and skill—from monitoring a client with malignant hypertension in an intensive care unit, to performing and teaching meticulous foot care, to educating and counseling a client to make significant lifestyle changes. Vascular diseases involve a broad spectrum of arterial, venous, and lymphatic problems. Nursing care for clients with arterial disorders centers on promoting circulation and adequate tissue perfusion, protecting against skin breakdown and injury, managing pain, and encouraging positive lifestyle changes. Nursing care for clients with venous disorders focuses on monitoring therapeutic regimens such as thrombolytic therapy, controlling and preventing thrombus formation, and promoting circulation by increasing venous blood return and decreasing venous pressure. Nursing care for clients with infectious lymphatic processes targets the primary infection; nursing care for lymphedema is palliative. Limb amputation requires particularly sensitive assessment, teaching, and counseling skills. The unique nursing care needs of clients with vascular disorders along with the exploding knowledge base that nurses need to command has led to the growth of vascular nursing as a recognized area of specialty practice. The Society for Peripheral Vascular Nursing was founded in 1982.[25]

Bibliography

1. Baker, J. D. (1991). Assessment of peripheral arterial occlusive disease. *Critical Care Nursing Clinics of North America, 3*(3), 493–498.
2. Barnes, R. W. (1991). Noninvasive diagnostic assessment of peripheral vascular disease. *Circulation, 83* (Suppl. I), I-20–I-27.
3. Beal, K., & Danzig, B. (1990). Lasers in vascular surgery. *Nursing Clinics of North America, 25*(3), 711–717.
4. Beaver, B. M. (1986). Health education and the patient with peripheral vascular disease. *Nursing Clinics of North America, 21*(2), 265–272.
5. Becker, G. J., et al. (1991). High-tech options for leg ischemia. *Patient Care, 25*(11), 61–68.
6. Bergan, J. J., & Yao, J. S. T. (1991). *Venous disorders*. Philadelphia: W. B. Saunders.
7. Beven, E. G. (1991). Thoracic outlet syndromes. In J. R. Young, et al. (Eds.), *Peripheral vascular disease* (pp. 497–510). St. Louis: Mosby–Year Book.
8. Blank, C. A., & Irwin, G. H. (1990). Peripheral vascular disorders. *Nursing Clinics of North America, 25*(4), 777–794.
9. Braunwald, E. (1992). *Heart disease: A textbook of cardiovascular medicine* (4th ed.). Philadelphia: W. B. Saunders.
10. Bright, L. D., & Georgi, S. (1992). Peripheral vascular disease: Is it arterial or venous? *AJN 92*(9), 34–43.
11. Bondy, B. (1987). An overview of arterial disease. *Jounal of Cardiovascular Nursing, 1*(1), 1–11.
12. Chenitz, W. C., et al. (1991). *Clinical gerontological nursing: A guide to advanced practice.* Philadelphia: W. B. Saunders.
13. Chobanian, A. V., & Gavras, H. (1991). Hypertension. *Clinical Symposia, 42*(5), 2–32.
14. Cisar, N. S., & Pifarre, R. (1990). Traumatic descending thoracic aneurysms: discussion and nursing care. *Progress in Cardiovascular Nursing, 5*(1), 13–20.
15. Coffman, J. D. (1991). Raynaud's phenomenon: an update. *Hypertension, 17*(5), 593–602.
16. Collins, J. W. (1991). The treatment of mild to moderate hypertension in patients with diabetes mellitus. *Nurse Practitioner, 16*(6), 28–40.
17. Creamer-Bauer, C., & Webber, M. (1990). Patient teaching strategies for peripheral laser procedures. *Progress in Cardiovascular Nursing, 5*(2), 50–58.
18. Dantzger, D. (1991). *Cardiopulmonary critical care* (2nd ed.). Philadelphia: W. B. Saunders.
19. Dennis, K. E., et al. (1991). Beta-blocker therapy: identification and management of side effects. *Heart and Lung, 20*(5), 459–463.
20. Edmunds, M. W. (1991). Strategies for promoting physical fitness. *Nursing Clinics of North America, 26*(4), 855–866.
21. Eells, M. A. W. (1991). Strategies for promotion of avoiding harmful substances. *Nursing Clinics of North America, 26*(4), 915–927.
22. Ekers, M. A. (1986). Psychosocial considerations in peripheral vascular disease: cause or effect. *Nursing Clinics of North America, 21*(2), 255–264.
23. Eton, D., & Ahn, S. S. (1991). Trends in endovascular surgery. *Critical Care Nursing Clinics of North America, 3*(3), 535–547.
24. European Working Group on Critical Leg Ischaemia (1991). Second European consensus document on chronic critical leg ischaemia. *Circulation, 84*(Suppl. I), I-1–I-22.
25. Fahey, V. A. (1988). *Vascular nursing*. Philadelphia: W. B. Saunders.
26. Fellows, E., & Jocz, A. M. (1991). Getting the upper hand on lower extremity arterial disease. *Nursing 91, 21*(8), 34–42.
27. Fuster, V., & Verstraete, M. (1992). *Thrombosis in cardiovascular disorders*. Philadelphia: W. B. Saunders.
28. Gold, M. E. (1991). Pharmacology of the nitrovasodilators: antianginal, antihypertensive and antiplatelet actions. *Nursing Clinics of North America, 26*(2), 437–450.
29. Graor, R. A. (1991). Deep vein thrombosis. In J. R. Young, et al. (Eds.), *Peripheral vascular disease* (pp. 403–422). St. Louis: Mosby–Year Book.
30. Hall, L. T. (1990). Endovascular surgery: an overview. *Progress in Cardiovascular Nursing, 5*(2), 43–49.
31. Herman, J. A. (1986). Nursing assessment and nursing diagnosis in patients with peripheral vascular disease. *Nursing Clinics of North America, 21*(2), 219–231.
32. Herron, D. G. (1991). Strategies for promoting a healthy dietary intake. *Nursing Clinics of North America, 26*(4), 875–884.
33. Hockenberry, B. (1991). Multiple drug therapy in the treatment of essential hypertension. *Nursing Clinics of North America, 26*(2), 417–436.
34. Houston, M. C. (1989). New insights and new approaches for the treatment of essential hypertension: selection of therapy based on coronary heart disease risk factor analysis, hemodynamic profiles, quality of life, and subsets of hypertension. *American Heart Journal, 117*(4), 911–943.
35. Houston, M. C. (1989). Pathophysiology, clinical aspects and treatment of hypertensive crises. *Progress in Cardiovascular Diseases, 32*(2), 99–148.
36. Huber, C., et al. (1992). Postoperative pulmonary embolism after hospital discharge. *Achives of Surgery, 127*(3), 310–313.

37. Itskovits, H. D. (1991). The role of adrenergic drugs in antihypertensive therapy. *Cleveland Clinic Journal of Medicine, 58*(1), 79-92.
38. Joint National Committee (1988). The 1988 Report of the Joint National Committee on detection, evaluation and treatment of high blood pressure. *Archives of Internal Medicine, 148,* 1023-1038.
39. Kaplan, N. (1991). Long term effectiveness of non-pharmacological treatment of hypertension. *Hypertension, 18*(3), I-153-I-160.
40. Leon, A. S. (1991). Recent advances in the management of hypertension. *Journal of Cardiopulmonary Rehabilitation, 11*(3), 182-191.
41. Mahan, L. K., & Arlin, M. (1992). *Krause's food, nutrition and diet therapy* (8th ed.). Philadelphia: W. B. Saunders.
42. Mancia, G., & Parati, G. (1990). Clinical significance of "white coat" hypertension. *Hypertension, 16*(6), 624-626.
43. Mannick, J., et al. (1991). Aortofemoral bypass for atherosclerotic aortoiliac disease. In C. B. Ernst & J. C. Stanley, *Current therapy in vascular surgery* (pp. 391-393). Philadelphia: B. C. Decker.
44. Markel, A., et al. (1992). Pattern and distribution of thrombi in acute venous thrombosis. *Achives of Surgery, 127*(3), 305-309.
45. Massey, J. A. (1986). Diagnostic testing for peripheral vascular disease. *Nursing Clinics of North America, 21*(2), 207-218.
46. Matteson, M. A., & McConnell, E. S. (1988). *Gerontological nursing: Concepts and practice.* Philadelphia: W. B. Saunders.
47. Monreal, M. et al. (1992). Deep venous thrombosis and the risk of pulmonary embolism. *Chest, 102*(3), 677-681.
48. Moore, W. S. (1991). *Vascular surgery: A comprehensive review* (3rd ed.). Philadelphia: W. B. Saunders.
49. Pickering, T. G., et al. (1988). How common is white coat hypertension? *Journal of the American Medical Association, 259*(2), 225-228.
50. Schumann, D. (1991). Sublingual nifedipine controversy in drug delivery. *Dimensions of Critical Care Nursing, 10*(6), 314-320.
51. Schwartz, G. L. (1990). Initial therapy for hypertension—individualizing care. *Mayo Clinic Proceedings, 65,* 73-87.
52. Schwartz, L. L., et al. (1991). Hypertension: role of the nurse-therapist. *Mayo Clinic Proceedings, 65*(1), 67-72.
53. Setara, J. F., & Black, H. R. (1992). Refractory hypertension. *New England Journal of Medicine 327*(8), 543-547.
54. Stason, W. B. (1991). Opportunities to improve the cost-effectiveness of treatment for hypertension. *Hypertension, 18*(3), I-161-I-165.
55. Thacker, H. L., & Jahnigen, D. W. (1991). Managing hypertensive emergencies and urgencies in the geriatric patient. *Geriatrics, 46*(10), 26-36.
56. Ting, M. (1991). Wound healing and peripheral vascular disease. *Critical Care Nursing Clinics of North America, 3*(3), 515-522.
57. Winer, N. (1990). Hypertensive crisis. *Critical Care Nursing Quarterly, 13*(3), 23-33.
58. Wyngaarden, J. B., et al. (1992). *Cecil textbook of medicine* (19th ed.). Philadelphia, W. B. Saunders.
59. Young, J. R., et al. (1991). *Peripheral vascular disease.* St. Louis: Mosby-Year Book.

Unit 10

Hematologic Disorders

Within each of us, a sea of fluid bathes, nourishes, and protects our internal environment. Moreover, an internal river—a river of blood with a million tributaries—branches through every organ and tissue, transporting life-sustaining fluid to and from each cell. Disorders of the blood affect our entire body, resulting in tissue hypoxia, infection, or hemorrhage.

Tissue hypoxia results from an alteration in the blood's oxygen-carrying capacity. It also is discussed in Unit 9. Susceptibility to infection results from alterations in the immune system that cannot function normally with some hematologic abnormalities. Infection is discussed in the next chapter of this unit and in Chapter 25. Hemorrhage can result when blood elements decrease or malfunction. It also is discussed throughout this chapter and in Chapter 20.

This unit introduces basic concepts of hematology and then covers the care of clients with hematologic disorders. The first chapter, on the basic concepts, includes information about the components, functions, characteristics, and formation of blood. An overview of hematologic abnormalities, the problems these abnormalities create, and the major diagnostic studies is presented. The assessment of clients with hematologic disorders also is discussed. In addition, the first chapter discusses the various blood types and the exacting procedures that underlie safe blood administration. This information will help the nurse develop skill in administering blood and blood products and in assessing clients for transfusion reaction and other complications.

The second chapter in this unit includes information on disorders of the red and white blood cells and platelets. Disorders such as anemia, leukemia, lymphoma, infectious mononucleosis, polycythemia, and clotting disorders are described; and the nursing care of clients with these problems is discussed.

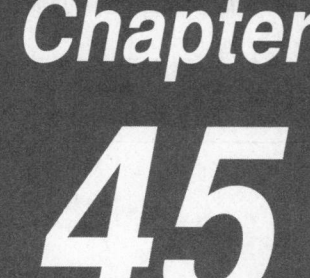

Basic Concepts of Hematology

STRUCTURE AND FUNCTION

DEFINITION AND FUNCTIONS OF BLOOD

Blood is a mixture of cells (red blood cells, white blood cells, and platelets) and plasma. It circulates continuously through the heart and vascular system. Propelled through the body by the heart's pumping action, the blood performs many vital functions (Table 45-1), such as

- Supplying oxygen from the lungs and absorbed nutrients from the gastrointestinal tract to cells;
- Removing waste products from tissues to the kidney, skin, and lungs for excretion;
- Transporting hormones from their origin in the endocrine glands to other parts of the body;
- Protecting the body from dangerous microorganisms;
- Promoting hemostasis (the arrest of bleeding); and
- Regulating body temperature by heat transfer.

CHARACTERISTICS OF BLOOD

The major characteristics of blood are color, viscosity, pH, volume, and composition.

Color. Arterial blood is bright red due to the oxygen bound to hemoglobin and oxygen within red blood cells. Venous blood is dark red because it has a lower oxygen content than arterial blood.

TABLE 45-1. Functions of Blood

Component	Function	Diagnostic Tests	Survival
Red blood cells	Mediate the exchange of oxygen and carbon dioxide between lungs and tissue	Red blood cell count Hemoglobin Hematocrit Reticulocyte count Blood indices: mean corpuscular hemoglobin concentration, mean corpuscular volume, mean corpuscular hemoglobin Red cell fragility Morphologic description in stained smear	120 days
Platelets	Form platelet plug to arrest bleeding Promote thrombin production	Platelet aggregation Platelet count Bleeding time	7-10 days
White blood cells	Protection from bacteria and other foreign substances	White blood cell count with differential	
Granulocytes	White cells containing granules broken down into three subcategories		6-8 h circulating in the blood and 2-3 days in the tissues
Neutrophils	Phagocytosis		
Eosinophils	Allergic and inflammatory reactions		
Basophils	Prevention of clotting in microcirculation Allergic reactions		
Lymphocytes	Formation of immunoglobins Cellular immunity	Immunoglobins Cell markers (T cell, B cell, etc.) Mixed lymphocyte culture	
Monocytes	Phagocytosis	White blood cell count with differential	
Plasma			
Water	Liquid in which cells circulate		
Proteins		Total protein	
Albumin	Maintains colloidal osmotic pressure	Albumin level	
Gamma globulins	Contains antibodies for body's defense	Quantitative immunoglobulins	
Fibrinogen	Blood coagulation	Fibrinogen level	

Viscosity. Blood is three to four time more viscous than water. Blood has a specific gravity of 1.048 to 1.066.

pH. Blood is slightly alkaline, with a pH of 7.35 to 7.45 (neutral is 7.0).

Volume. An adult has about 70 to 75 ml of blood/kg of body weight. Thus, the average adult body contains about 4 to 5 liters of blood.

Composition. Plasma makes up about 55 per cent of the blood, and solid suspended particles (blood cells and platelets) compose the other 45 per cent (Fig. 45-1).

Plasma is the liquid portion of the blood. Its major function is to maintain the blood volume within the vascular compartment. A straw-colored, watery substance, plasma is composed of 92 per cent water; 7 per cent proteins; and less than 1 per cent nutrients, metabolic wastes, respiratory gases, enzymes, hormones, clotting factors, and inorganic salts. The proteins include serum albumin (alpha-1 globulin, alpha-2 globulin, beta globulin, and gamma globulin) as well as fibrinogen, prothrombin, and protein essential for blood coagulation. Serum albumin and gamma globulin are necessary for maintaining colloidal osmotic pressure (see Chap. 14). Gamma globulin also contains the antibodies (immunoglobulins) IgM, IgG, IgA, IgD, and IgE, which are essential in the body's defense against microorganisms (see Chaps. 23 and 24).

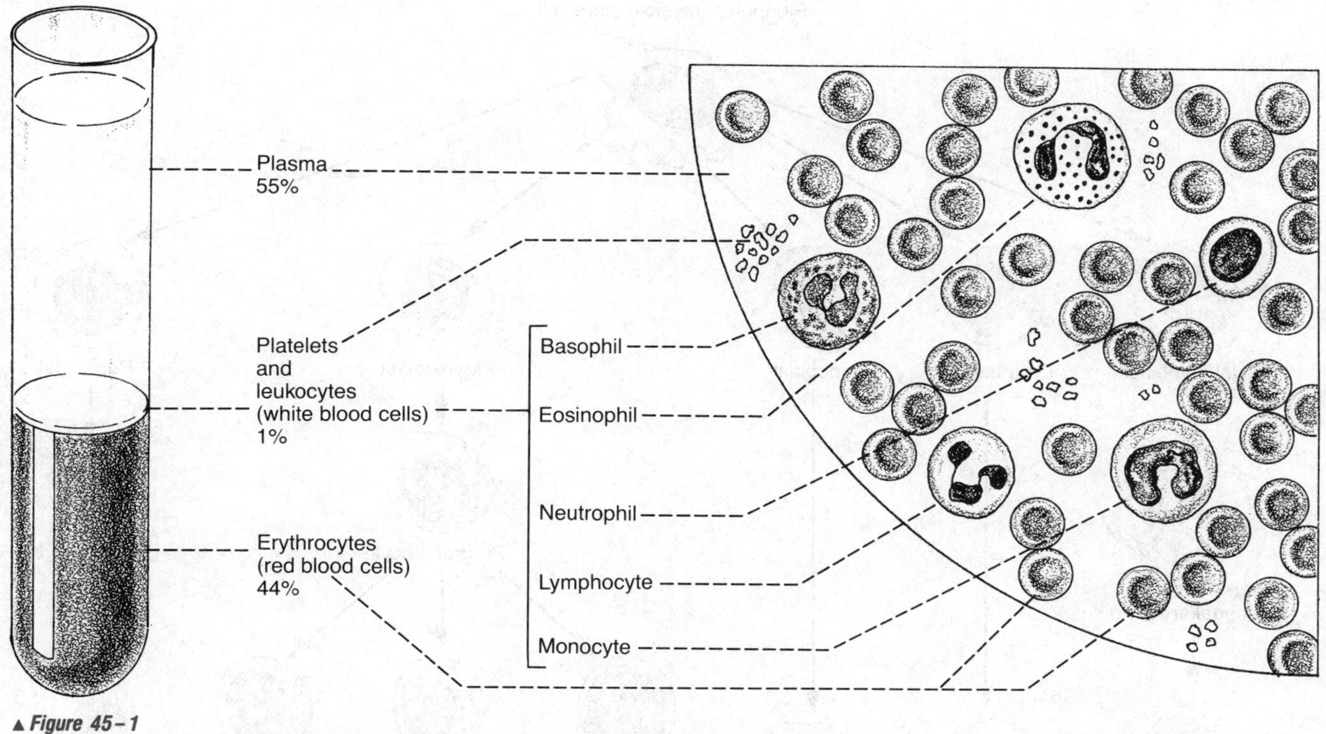

▲ **Figure 45-1**

Blood is composed of plasma (about 55 per cent) and cellular elements, including leukocytes, thrombocytes (platelets), and erythrocytes (about 45 per cent). There are 600 times as many erythrocytes as leukocytes.

HEMATOPOIESIS: FORMATION OF BLOOD

Because normal blood cells have a limited life span, constant formation of the blood cells is required throughout life. This process by which blood cells are formed is called hematopoiesis. In adults, this function is primarily performed in the red (functioning) bone marrow. An abundance of data suggests that blood cells derive from one pluripotent stem cell. The pluripotent stem cell is capable of differentiating to produce the mature cells found in the circulating blood (Fig. 45-2).

Pluripotent stem cells have the property of self-renewal (proliferation) or of differentiating into a specific cell line. When a stem cell differentiates, it loses its capacity for self-renewal and becomes committed to a specific cell line, such as the erythrocyte, myeloid, megakaryocyte, and lymphocyte lineages. Hematopoiesis is regulated by hematopoietic growth factors, which include colony-stimulating factors and erythropoietin.[2, 6]

Most lymphocytes are formed in lymph nodes, thymus, and spleen from precursor cells (lymphoblasts) that migrated there from the bone marrow. Cells that evolve from the thymus are called T lymphocytes and are responsible for cellular immunity (reactions that do not require an antibody). Cells from other tissues become B lymphocytes, which provide humoral immunity through the production of the circulating antibodies IgM, IgA, IgG, IgE, and IgD. Each of the cellular elements of the blood is discussed in more detail throughout this unit.

ERYTHROCYTES (RED BLOOD CELLS)

The structure of the red blood cell (RBC) ideally suits it to carry out its most important function, transporting oxygen. A normal erythrocyte has the shape of a biconcave disc, with a unique ability to undergo cellular deformation. The ability of the RBC to undergo deformation is essential to its negotiation through capillaries and splenic channels, because the diameter of the human RBC (8 μm) far exceeds that of the capillaries (2 to 3 μm).[2] One cubic millimeter of blood contains about 5 million erythrocytes.

Formation

The production of erythrocytes is termed erythropoiesis. The bone marrow produces about 200 billion erythrocytes daily. Normal production depends on three factors: (1) genetically normal precursor cells; (2) functioning bone marrow; and (3) an adequate intake of iron, vitamin B_{12}, folic acid, protein, pyridoxine, and traces of copper. If any of these factors is missing, erythrocytes may be fragile, misshapen, abnormally large or small, deficient in hemoglobin, or too few in number.

Erythrocytes arise from a undifferentiated progenitor cell in the bone marrow called a pluripotent stem cell in response to erythropoietin, a factor within the plasma that is primarily produced in the kidneys. Before becoming erythrocytes, young cells leave the bone

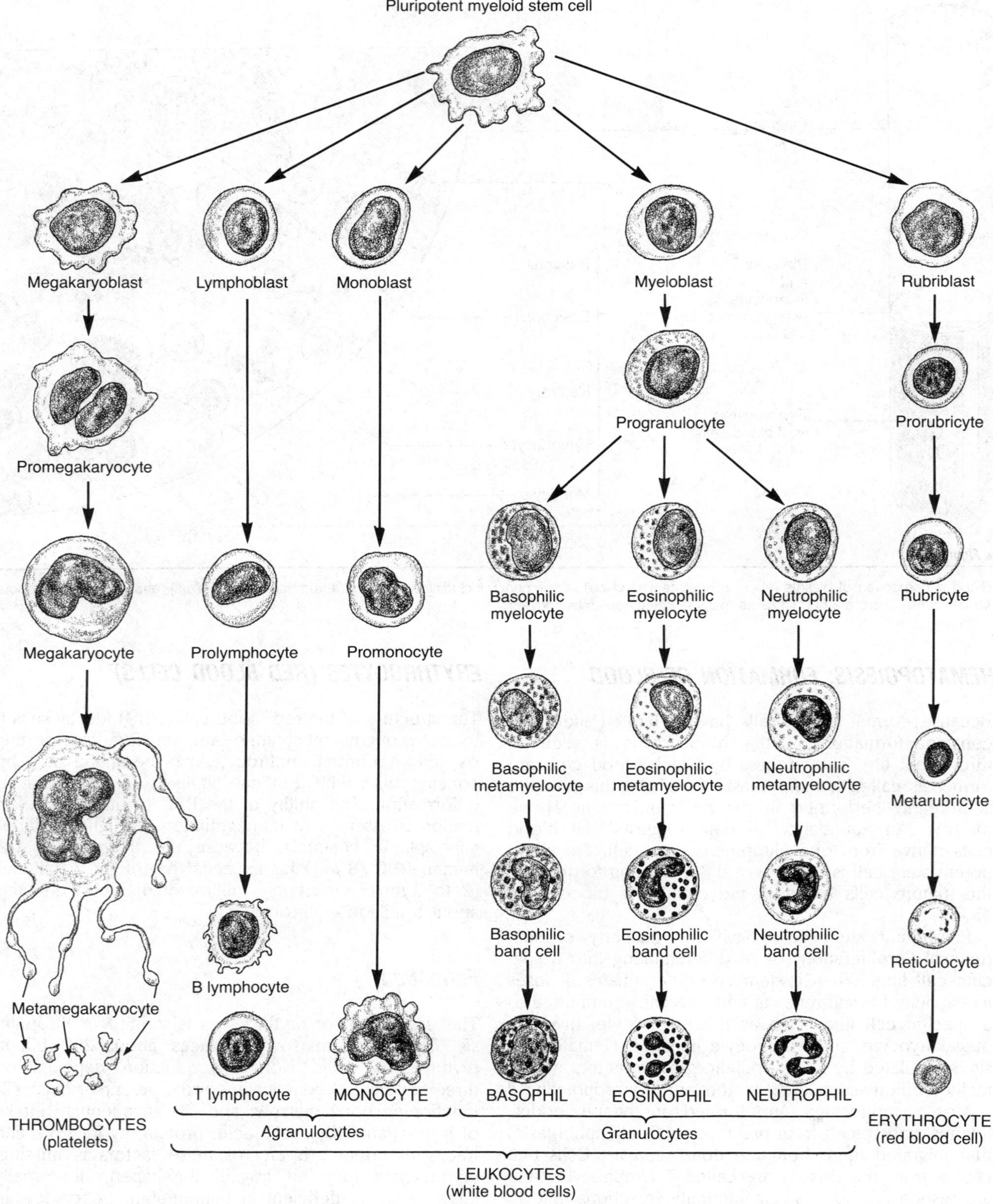

▲ ***Figure 45-2***

Origin, development, and structure of thrombocytes, leukocytes, and erythrocytes from pluripotent stem cells.

marrow by a venous route and enter the general circulation as reticulocytes. Reticulocytes evolve into mature erythrocytes during the first 2 to 4 days in the bloodstream. Typically, about 1 per cent of circulating RBCs are reticulocytes. A reticulocyte count can be used to estimate the production of RBCs, because the reticulocyte fraction increases when erythropoiesis is accelerated.[11]

The spleen sequesters some of these erythrocytes. This reserve corps of erythrocytes enters the circulation whenever the RBC count drops significantly below normal levels (e.g., during pregnancy and emergencies such as hemorrhage or carbon monoxide poisoning).

As erythrocytes age, they become fragile and worn, eventually rupturing. At this point, the hemoglobin escapes. Macrophages within the liver, spleen, lymph nodes, and bone marrow quickly phagocytize both hemoglobin and the empty membrane (called a ghost cell). The hemoglobin breaks down into its heme (iron and porphyrin) and globin (polypeptide chain) fractions. Iron of the heme fraction returns to the liver, spleen, and bone marrow to be reused in making hemoglobin. The liver converts the porphyrin of the heme fraction into bilirubin, an orange pigment, and secretes it into the bile to be excreted from the body in the feces and urine. During periods of increased RBC destruction (e.g., in hemolytic anemia), excessive amounts of bilirubin form and may accumulate in the body's tissues.

Normally, about 180 million aged erythrocytes are destroyed each minute, giving way to 180 million young erythrocytes. As a result, the number of RBCs remains constant. If the erythrocyte loss exceeds erythrocyte production, however, the abnormally low number of erythrocytes cannot pick up an adequate amount of oxygen from the lungs to deliver to the tissues. The resulting hypoxia (low blood oxygen) stimulates the kidneys to release erythropoietin, which then induces the bone marrow to produce more RBCs. Because the healthy bone marrow can increase its RBC production six to eight times over the normal rate, it usually keeps pace with increased destruction or loss. This hemostatic mechanism maintains a remarkably constant number of erythrocytes.

Vitamin B_{12} is essential for normal RBC maturation and normal nervous system function. Because it is not synthesized in the body, vitamin B_{12} must be supplied in the diet. Animal products such as meat and dairy products are the only sources. For this reason, vitamin B_{12} is called the extrinsic factor (meaning outside the body). When released from food during gastric digestion, vitamin B_{12} binds with a glycoprotein called intrinsic factor (inside the body) in the duodenum and is transported to the distal ileum, where specific receptors in the mucosa bind the B_{12} for absorption into the blood.

Folic acid, a B-group vitamin, is necessary for red cell formation and maturation but, unlike vitamin B_{12}, does not play a role in nervous system function. Synthesized by many plants and bacteria, the major dietary sources of folic acid are vegetables and fruits. Cooking destroys some forms of folic acid.

Function

Red blood cells are composed of an encircling membrane and hemoglobin, a protein that combines with oxygen and carbon dioxide. Hemoglobin itself is composed of globin (four polypeptide chains) and heme, iron-containing organic structures. Heme contains the red pigment porphyrin. About 200 to 300 million molecules of hemoglobin inhabit each erythrocyte, making up 95 per cent of its weight.

The most important characteristic of hemoglobin is its ability to combine chemically with oxygen in a loose and easily reversed connection. The compound resulting from this union is termed oxyhemoglobin. The ability of hemoglobin to bind depends in part on the blood's pH and temperature.[5] A decrease in pH (acidosis) reduces oxygen saturation, allowing the oxygen to dissociate from hemoglobin to the tissue. Oxygen saturation also is decreased with hypothermia.

Oxyhemoglobin causes arterial blood to be bright red and is formed as the erythrocytes pass through the alveoli of the lungs. As oxygenated blood enters tissue capillaries, 25 per cent of the oxyhemoglobin releases its oxygen, which diffuses out of the blood vessels into the interstitial spaces. Deoxygenated, or reduced, hemoglobin gives venous blood its dark red color.

In addition to combining with oxygen, hemoglobin also can combine with carbon dioxide. Carbon dioxide, released from the body's cells, diffuses into the interstitial spaces and then into the capillaries, where it is picked up by deoxygenated hemoglobin and carried to the lungs. In the lungs, carbon dioxide separates from the hemoglobin and diffuses into the alveoli, where it is exhaled.

A third gas with which hemoglobin readily combines is carbon monoxide. Whereas oxygen forms a bond that is easily reversed, carbon monoxide remains bound to hemoglobin. Hemoglobin combined with carbon monoxide cannot transport oxygen to cells and tissues. Consequently, carbon monoxide poisoning results in tissue hypoxia.

Iron is essential for hemoglobin production. The adult human body contains about 50 mg of iron/100 ml of blood. Total body iron ranges between 2 and 6 g, depending on the size of the client and the amount of hemoglobin contained in the client's cells. Hemoglobin holds about two thirds of this iron (called essential iron). The other third resides in the bone marrow, spleen, liver, and muscle. If a client develops an iron deficiency, these iron stores are depleted first, followed by a reduction in the iron contained in hemoglobin.

BLOOD GROUPS AND BLOOD TYPING

Human RBCs display antigens that are either glycoproteins or glycolipids on the surface of the red blood cell membrane. Together the various blood group systems contribute more than 400 characterized antigens. Antigens are inherited from the parents. Less than a dozen of these blood group antigens attract frequent clinical notice, and of these only the ABO and Rhesus (Rh) systems are major determinants of compatibility testing.[15]

Antibodies are proteins (immunoglobulins) that float freely in the plasma. Antibodies are usually produced following exposure to an antigen that the client does not have. The body recognizes the antigen as foreign, and the immune system responds by producing an antibody. Combining an antigen on the surface of a cell with an antibody initiates a series of immune responses that can result in the destruction of the cell.[7, 15]

The ABO Blood Group System

The ABO blood type is inherited as an autosomal trait. The four major blood types of clinical importance in this genetic system are A, B, AB, and O. Blood is typed according to the antigens found on the RBC and the antibodies found in the serum.

Usually, for the antibodies to be formed, there must be exposure to foreign or homologous red cell antigens through pregnancy or transfusion. The major exceptions are the A and B antigens, for which there are structurally similar proteins in the environment, resulting in antibody formation against the missing A and/or B antigen by the age of 3 months.

The two major antigens within the blood group system are antigens A and B. A client may have one (type A or type B), both (type AB), or neither (type O) antigen on his or her RBCs. There also are two major antibodies found in the serum, anti-A and anti-B. A client with type A blood has anti-B antibodies; a client with type B blood has anti-A antibodies, a client with type O blood has anti-A and anti-B antibodies, and group AB has neither antibody (Table 45-2).

The Rh System

The Rh blood groups are nearly equal in clinical importance to the ABO groups. The Rh factor was named for the rhesus monkey used in the initial experiments by Landsteiner and Weiner in 1940. Although Rh serology involves more than 20 different antigens, the D antigen has the most clinical significance because of the high risk of formation of an anti-D in an Rh-negative recipient. The term Rh positive means the client has the D antigen, whereas the Rh-negative client has no D antigen.

TABLE 45-2. The ABO Blood Group System

Blood Type	Antigen	Antibody in Serum	Frequency in United States
A	A	Anti-B	41%
B	B	Anti-A	10%
AB	A and B	None	4%
O	None	Anti-A and anti-B	45%

The incidence of Rh antigens varies widely among different populations. About 85 per cent of Caucasians are Rh positive, and about 95 per cent of African Americans are Rh positive.[11]

The most striking difference between the ABO and Rh systems is that in the ABO system, there is spontaneous development of antibodies directed against A and/or B antigens not present on the RBC. In the Rh system, antibody formation is never spontaneous. Instead, a client must first be exposed to the Rh antigen, for example, through a blood transfusion or pregnancy. This means that clients with Rh-negative blood, transfused for the first time with Rh-positive blood, do not experience a reaction because their blood does not yet contain anti-Rh antibodies (anti-D). About 50 per cent of people, however, develop sensitivity and form antibodies against the D as a result of exposure to the D antigen from transfusion or pregnancy. Should a sensitized client receive a second transfusion or have a second pregnancy with exposure to the D antigen, some degree of RBC destruction will occur. However, it is usually possible to prevent sensitization from occurring the first time by administering a single dose of anti-Rh antibodies in the form of Rh immune globulin (RhoGAM) immediately following the exposure to the D antigen.

The Human Leukocyte Antigens System

Human leukocyte antigens (HLAs) also are called histocompatibility antigens because the antigens (glycoproteins) are found on the surface of most cells in the body except RBCs (including circulating and tissue cells). The HLA system is a series of closely linked genes located on the short arm of chromosome 6. The major function of the HLA antigen is regulation of the immune response, distinguishing self from non-self. This plays a major role in the rejection of transplanted tissues when donor and recipient HLA antigens do not match.[15] There also is an association between HLA antigens and some diseases. For example, in ankylosing spondylitis, the association with HLA factor is so strong that HLA typing can be used diagnostically.

HEMOSTASIS

Normal hemostasis is a process that repairs vascular breaks to reduce blood loss from blood vessels while maintaining the flow of blood through the vascular system. The three components of the hemostatic mechanism are the blood vessels, platelets (or thrombocytes), and coagulation factors. These components accomplish hemostasis in three phases (Fig. 45-3): (1) the vascular phase, in which there is vasoconstriction of the vessels; (2) the formation of a platelet plug; and (3) the coagulation or formation of a fibrin clot. Once the fibrin clot has served its purpose, it is balanced by fibrinolysis (clot dissolution), thus preventing thrombosis.

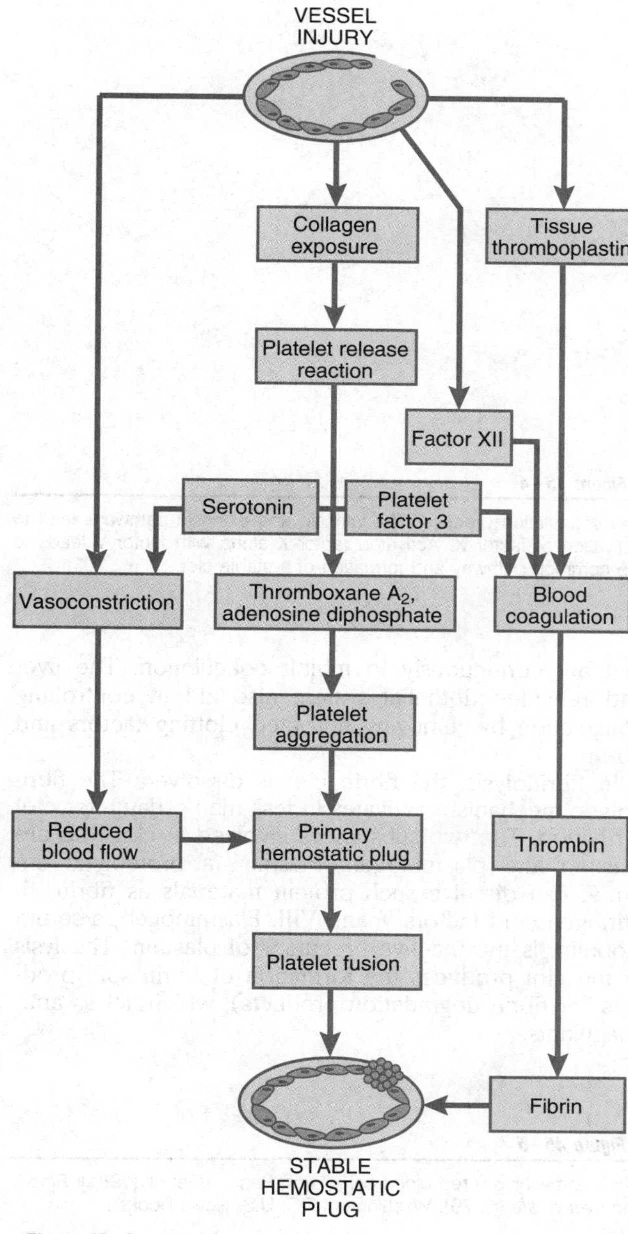

▲ *Figure 45-3*

Mechanism of normal hemostasis.

Blood Vessels

Whenever bleeding results from injury or disease, the blood vessels supplying the damaged site constrict. This is helpful because vasoconstriction slows the flow of blood to the injured area, decreasing blood loss. Vasoconstriction results from muscular tissue and reflex nervous system reactions. Serotonin is a potent local vasoconstrictor that is secreted by cells in the small intestine and promotes blood vessel constriction upon injury.

Platelets (Thrombocytes)

Platelets are small, anucleated cell fragments derived from giant cells called megakaryocytes in the bone marrow. Adequate numbers of cells (150,000 to 400,000/mm^3) are required in the peripheral blood to play the role of hemostasis. When platelets come into contact with an alteration of the endothelial cell lining of a blood vessel, they become sticky and adhere to one another, thus sealing the surface of the vessel lining. Along with these adhesive reactions, the platelets have a secretory response resulting in the release of intracellular storage granules from within the platelet. Granule constituents include substances that can stimulate circulating platelets and cause them to acquire new adhesive properties. These platelet constituents can activate additional platelets that aggregate to form a thrombus.

Platelets control hemostasis unless large blood vessels have been damaged. If bleeding is severe, coagulation factors must join with platelets to form a permanent clot.

Blood Coagulation

The coagulation system consists of a series of interactions that result in the formation of a fibrin clot. The system consists of clotting proteins (except factor IV), that is, factors that circulate in the plasma (except factor III, which is released from damaged cells) in an inactive state (see Table 46-12).

The formation of a fibrin clot can result from activation of one of two pathways: the intrinsic or the extrinsic pathway. Various factors are needed by these two pathways for completion of a final common pathway that results in a fibrin clot (Fig. 45-4).

The extrinsic pathway is initiated when there is tissue injury, outside the vessels, such as a burn. Damaged tissues release factor III (tissue thromboplastin), which initiates the clotting cascade to form activated factor X, which leads to the final common pathway of clot formation.

The intrinsic pathway involves the blood itself (i.e., antigen-antibody reactions and endotoxins) or damage to the blood vessels. All factors for the intrinsic system are present in the plasma. This pathway is initiated when factor XII is exposed to a foreign surface, which initiates a cascade of enzymatic reactions to activate factor X, leading to the common pathway.

Activated factor X is responsible for the conversion of prothrombin to thrombin and soluble fibrinogen to an insoluble fibrin clot. The protein fibrin forms dense interlacing threads that entrap erythrocytes and platelets (Fig. 45-5). The platelets then release a contractile protein, which causes shrinkage and retraction of the clot into a firm, insoluble fibrin mass. The process of retraction squeezes out the clear yellow serum. Serum differs from plasma in that it does not contain clotting factors.

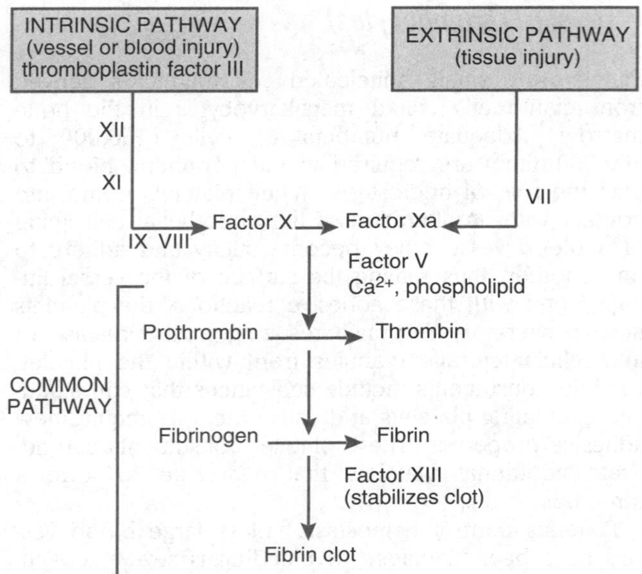

▲ *Figure 45-4*

The coagulation process. The intrinsic and extrinsic pathways lead to activation of factor X. Activated factor X along with factor V leads to the common pathway and formation of a stable clot.

In some cases, the formation of a fibrin clot is unnecessary because hemostasis occurs at an early stage. Temporary clots are sometimes insufficient. For example, bleeding from a small pinprick can normally be ended by a platelet plug, while more serious cuts require the interaction of the various coagulation factors.

Fibrinolysis and Anticoagulants

The coagulation system is controlled by several mechanisms to maintain a flow of blood through the vascular space. The blood carries natural anticoagulants, for example, heparin, antithrombin, and antithromboplastin, that act continuously to inhibit coagulation. The liver and reticuloendothelial system also aid in controlling coagulation by removing activated clotting factors and fibrin.

In fibrinolysis, the fibrin clot is dissolved. The fibrinolytic mechanism activates in less than a day after clot formation. The two substances involved in clot lysis are plasmin and plasminogen. Plasmin, a proteolytic enzyme, can dissolve such protein materials as fibrin, fibrinogen, and factors V and VIII. Plasminogen, a serum globulin, is the inactive precursor of plasmin. The lysis of the clot produces the formation of fibrin split products (or fibrin degradation products), which act as anticoagulants.

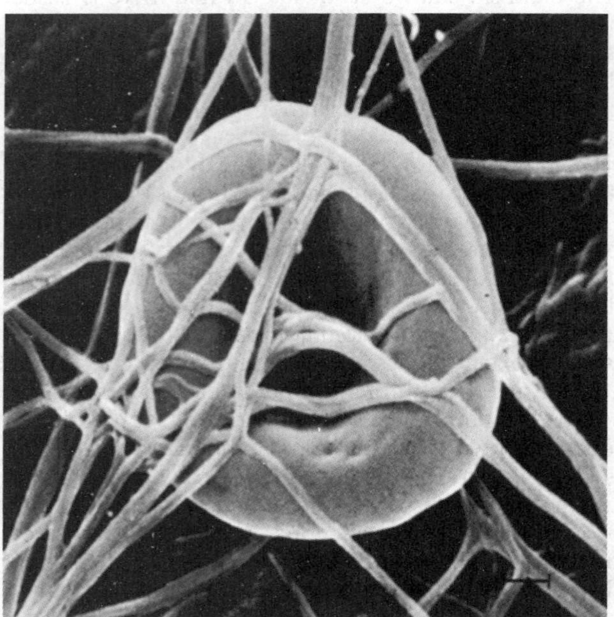

▲ *Figure 45-5*

Fibrin enmeshing a red blood cell. (From Page, J., et al. [1981]. *Blood: The river of life* [p. 79]. Washington, DC: U.S. News Books.)

THE FUNCTION OF THE SPLEEN AND LIVER IN HEMATOPOIESIS

The spleen and liver both have important roles in the hematopoietic system. The spleen, located in the upper part of the abdominal cavity on the left side of the body, is the largest lymphatic organ (Fig. 45-6). It is composed of a fibrous tissue capsule surrounding a network of fiber. It functions to purify the blood and protect the body from various stressors. The spleen separates the plasma from the cellular components. The components are filtered through three types of matter within the spleen. Soluble antigens in the plasma are delivered to the white pulp, where phagocytic cells process the antigens and initiate antibody production.[11] The hemoconcentrated fraction of blood is delivered to the red pulp that phagocytizes unwanted cells. Many cells are processed in the marginal pulp: damaged erythrocytes are detained and phagocytized or modified, monocytes are held and permitted to differentiate into macrophages, platelets are stored, and granulocytes are detained or destroyed.[11]

Other functions of the spleen include (1) acting as a reservoir for erythrocytes (less than 2 per cent of the red cell mass), (2) metabolizing iron by capturing hemoglobin released from destroyed red cells, and (3) performing pitting (removal of particles from an RBC without destroying the cell itself).

The liver contributes to the hematopoietic system in many ways. It (1) synthesizes plasma proteins and clotting factors; (2) decomposes hemoglobin into bilirubin, which is converted into bile, which helps with fat digestion; and (3) stores iron in the form of ferritin.

EFFECTS OF AGING ON THE HEMATOLOGIC SYSTEM

A review of the research on the effects of aging in the hematologic system finds few well-documented and clinically significant direct effects of aging on the blood and bone marrow. Age is associated, however, with an increased prevalence of chronic disease states known to affect the hematopoietic system.

The function of the T cells is diminished, although the total leukocyte count usually remains unchanged. The resulting deficiency is one of cellular immune competence, which gradually develops throughout the lifespan. Hemoglobin concentration remains unchanged or minimally changed by age, and platelet counts remain unchanged. Bone marrow cellularity decreases, but this may reflect only an increase in adipose tissue resulting from decreased bone mass in the elderly.[3, 14]

HEMATOLOGIC ABNORMALITIES

Overview

Disorders of the blood and blood-forming organs are usually divided into categories that involve primarily (1) erythrocytes, (2) leukocytes, (3) platelets, (4) clotting mechanisms, and (5) hematopoiesis. General factors involved as either the primary or secondary cause of hematopoietic disorders include hemorrhage, malabsorptive disorders, drug and chemical toxicity, genetic predisposition, metabolic disturbances, malignant overproduction of cells, increased destruction of cells by an overactive spleen, dietary deficiencies, infections, radiation, immunologic defects, autoimmune response, and idiopathic (unknown) factors.

There are four basic pathophysiologic disturbances that characterize hematopoietic disorders: (1) a decrease in the number of cells, (2) overproduction of normal or defective cells, (3) defects in the coagulation mechanism, and (4) disorders of the spleen.

A decrease in the number of erythrocytes results in anemia. Anemia is a condition characterized by a reduction in the oxygen-carrying capacity of the blood. Hypoxia produces fatigue, among other problems.

A decrease in all types of leukocytes is termed leukopenia. A reduction in granulocytes is called granulocytopenia. The granulocytes (composed of neutrophils, eosinophils, and basophils) work with monocytes and lymphocytes to guard the body against invasion by foreign materials. Therefore, granulocytopenia and neutropenia (decrease in the number of neutrophils) predispose a client to severe infections.

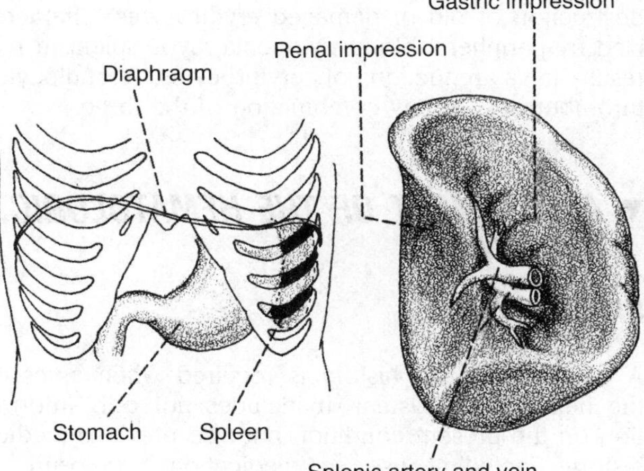

▲ Figure 45-6

The spleen.

A decrease in the thrombocyte, or platelet, count is called thrombocytopenia. Because thrombocytes are an important component in the clotting mechanism, hallmarks of thrombocytopenia are easy to spot: bruising; petechiae (fine red hemorrhagic rash); and a tendency to bleed readily from the perianal area, gastrointestinal tract, and mucous membranes.

Polycythemia

An abnormal increase in erythrocyte production is called polycythemia. Increased manufacture of abnormal, immature leukocytes is termed leukemia. The abnormal malignant proliferation of plasma cells results in plasma cell myeloma or multiple myeloma. These conditions (polycythemia, leukemia, and plasma cell myeloma) are usually classified as myeloproliferative diseases because the malignant overproduction of cells takes place within the bone marrow.

Cellular overproduction within the lymphatic tissues results in lymphoproliferative disorders. Examples include (1) Hodgkin's disease and non-Hodgkin's lymphomas, characterized by malignant proliferation of lymphocytes and other cells within the lymph nodes, and (2) lymphocytic leukemia, characterized by an overproduction of lymphoblasts within the lymph nodes and bone marrow that are released into the blood.

Defects in the Coagulation System

Caused by depletion or absence of one or more clotting factors, disorders of the coagulation system can result in hemorrhage. They include hemophilias, hypoprothrombinemia, and disseminated intravascular coagulation.

Disorders of the Spleen

Enlargement of the spleen (splenomegaly) occurs in association with many blood dyscrasias. Hypersplenism, a clinical syndrome that affects the spleen, arises from either overactivity of the spleen or exaggeration of one or more of the splenic functions, such as excessive destruction of old or damaged erythrocytes. Characterized by peripheral blood cytopenia, hypersplenism may result in a reduction of erythrocytes, granulocytes, thrombocytes, or any combination of the three.

▼ ASSESSMENT OF THE HEMATOLOGIC SYSTEM

HISTORY

A complete health history is required when assessing the hematologic system. It includes not only information on the present condition but also previous medical history, including use of medications, exposure to chemicals or radiation, family history, psychosocial history and lifestyle data, and review of systems (ROS).

Chief Complaint

Clients present with many vague and nonspecific symptoms, including chills, fever, chronic fatigue, weight loss, and physical discomfort. The nurse conducts a symptom analysis (see Chap. 11) to determine whether the onset was sudden or gradual and whether it was associated with trauma or a known disease. Disorders of the hematologic system often affect all organs and tissues throughout the body, resulting in widespread pathophysiologic manifestations. The ROS outlines the systems and their common hematologic findings as well as their possible pathophysiologic bases.

Past Medical History

MAJOR ILLNESSES AND HOSPITALIZATION

The nurse asks the client about previous hematologic problems that may provide clues for the current problem. This entails inquiring about problems such as anemia, recurrent infections, delayed wound healing, thrombophlebitis, deep vein thrombosis, liver disease, or excessive bleeding. Has the client been diagnosed previously with a hematologic disorder?

Surgical procedures that may affect the hematologic system include splenectomy, tumor removal, cardiac valve replacement, and resections of the gastrointestinal tract. For example, loss of duodenal tissue results in decreased iron absorption, partial or total gastrectomy reduces intrinsic factor production and vitamin B_{12} absorption, and loss of the terminal portion of the ileum leads to inability to absorb vitamin B_{12}.

The client is asked whether he or she has received a blood or blood product transfusion. If so, what was the reason for the transfusion? Were there any problems or reactions to the blood or blood products? Does the client know his or her blood type, including Rh factor? This information is particularly important for the client who may be pregnant and is Rh negative (see earlier discussion of the Rh system).

Health problems involving the liver, such as cirrhosis or hepatitis, can disrupt production of several clotting factors. This increases the client's risk for bleeding disorders. Other causes of bleeding disorders include genetic factors and chemical toxicity. The nurse asks the following questions when assessing the client with a bleeding disorder.

- How long has the client had a bleeding problem? Was it present in childhood, or has it appeared only recently? Do any members of the family have a history of bleeding disorders?
- Is the bleeding linked with any specific event or procedure? For example, does severe bleeding occur with menses or following minor trauma, a tooth extraction, minor surgery, shaving, or participation in contact sports? Does the client have frequent nose-

bleeds (epistaxis)? Is there a history of bleeding into the joints or cavities? Does the client bruise easily? Does the client report petechiae?

- How severe are any bleeding episodes, and what is their duration? More precisely, is there prolonged oozing of blood from a site or sudden massive bleeding? (Sudden bleeding is far less common than prolonged slow hemorrhage.)
- Does the client have a history of hepatic, splenic, or renal disease? These three conditions are often characterized by hemorrhagic manifestations. Has the client recently taken either anticoagulants or medications that may suppress the bone marrow activity (e.g., chloramphenicol or antineoplastic agents) or medications that interfere with platelet functions?

MEDICATIONS

The nurse asks the client what medications are being used, as a treatment for either a hematologic condition or some other disorder. This includes over-the-counter medications; for example, aspirin or aspirin-containing compounds can interfere with platelet aggregation and cause prolonged bleeding.

ALLERGIES

The nurse specifically inquires about known allergies and allergic reactions, particularly anaphylaxis. If not previously determined, the client is asked for a history of blood or blood product transfusions, as well as any complications from the transfusions such as fever, chills, back or flank pain, shock, wheezing, headache, vomiting, or urticaria (hives).

FAMILY HISTORY

A family history of bleeding disorders can be important. A family history of jaundice, anemia, bleeding disorders (hemophilia or polycythemia), malignancies, or congenital blood dyscrasias, such as sickle cell disease, is investigated.

Psychosocial History and Lifestyle

Hematologic disorders can result in many physiologic changes that affect the client's psychosocial status and ability to perform activities of daily living (ADLs). Areas to assess include the following.

OCCUPATION

The nurse asks the client about previous exposure to toxic chemicals or radiation as a result of occupational exposure or as a treatment. Radiation and chemicals such as benzene, lead, and phenylbutazone can increase the incidence of hematologic problems, particularly anemia. Does the client have sufficient energy to perform ADLs and occupational tasks? Are there problems with fatigue, dyspnea, or other symptoms that interfere with a productive lifestyle? Has the client missed time from work or school, resulting in financial loss or other economic concerns, such as health or life insurance eligibility?

HABITS

Nutritional habits have a significant effect on the hematologic system. The nurse carefully explains to the client the importance of asking about the use or abuse of alcohol and other recreational drugs. Chronic substance abuse is often accompanied by malnutrition and vitamin deficiency. Many substances, most notably alcohol, damage the structure and function of liver cells, resulting in decreased clotting factor production and bleeding tendencies.

A dietary history also is important when assessing whether there may be any vitamin deficiencies causing anemia. Weight loss may indicate hematologic alterations or deficits in nutrients. The nurse asks the client whether he or she is eating foods that contain iron, folic acid, and vitamin B_{12}, all necessary for the development of red cells.

Review of Symptoms

Symptoms related to disorders of the hematologic system can be general as well as specific. The nurse conducts a symptom analysis and a focus assessment (see Chap. 11) for all reported symptoms.

General symptoms include fatigue, apathy, lethargy, malaise, weakness, heat intolerance (anemia), chills, fever, night sweats (infection, particularly recurrent infections), and delayed wound healing (leukopenia).

Integumentary symptoms may be pruritus (Hodgkin's disease and lymphoma), jaundice (hemolytic anemia and pernicious anemia resulting in bile pigment accumulation), pallor, flushing (iron deficiency anemia), petechiae, ecchymoses, and prolonged bleeding (thrombocytopenia and clotting disorders).

Delayed wound healing, lymph node swelling, and infections (leukopenia) may be immunologic manifestations.

Sensory effects on the eyes include visual disturbances (anemia and polycythemia), blindness (thrombocytopenia and retinal hemorrhage related to anemia), and yellowed sclera (jaundice). Regarding effects on the ear, the client might experience vertigo or tinnitus (severe anemia). Symptoms affecting the nose include epistaxis (thrombocytopenia and clotting disorders). Oral manifestations include smooth tongue (pernicious anemia, iron deficiency anemia, and nutritional deficiencies), gingival bleeding (thrombocytopenia and clotting disorders), sores, and ulcerations (leukemia and neutropenia).

The client may exhibit neck lymphadenopathy, particularly if painful (lymphoma).

Respiratory symptoms include fatigue, dyspnea, and orthopnea (anemia).

Cardiovascular symptoms include tachycardia, palpitations (compensatory mechanism to increase cardiac output secondary to anemia); murmurs, particularly systolic (increased volume and velocity of blood through valves related to anemia); and angina (decreased oxygen supply to the heart related to rapid-onset anemia).

The client's gastrointestinal system may be affected by dysphagia (mucous membrane atrophy related to iron deficiency anemia), abdominal pain (intestinal obstruction related to lymphoma, retroperitoneal bleeding, acute hemolysis, allergic purpura, and sickle cell disease), hepatomegaly, splenomegaly (hemolytic anemia resulting in increased need for removal of erythrocytes), hematemesis, and melena (thrombocytopenia and clotting disorders).

Urinary symptoms include hematuria (hemolysis and clotting disorders).

Reproductive symptoms are amenorrhea and menorrhagia (iron deficiency and clotting disorders).

The client may experience musculoskeletal back pain (hemolysis), sternal tenderness (leukemia and sickle cell disease), bone pain (blast crisis in leukemia and multiple myeloma resulting in pathologic fractures), and joint pain (hemarthroses or bleeding into joints, often related to hemophilia).

Systemic neurologic symptoms are confusion (severe anemia and malignant process or infections in the brain), headache (anemia, polycythemia, invasion or compression of brain related to leukemia, lymphoma, infection, or brain hemorrhage related to thrombocytopenia or clotting disorder), syncope (severe anemia and polycythemia), and paresthesias (peripheral neuropathy secondary to pernicious anemia or hematologic malignancy and side effect of vincristine therapy). In addition, the client may experience mental depression (hematologic disorders resulting in fatigue, discomfort, and acute and chronic problems related to disease process or coping difficulties related to a diagnosis of cancer).

PHYSICAL EXAMINATION

The physical examination for the hematologic system can entail both a complete head-to-toe examination and examinations of specific systems, depending on the nature of the client's problem. For example, the client who presents with abdominal pain and absent bowel sounds related to intraluminal hemorrhage needs a complete gastrointestinal examination as well as a hematologic assessment. Similarly, the client with hemarthrosis needs a complete examination of the affected joint as well as a hematologic assessment.

The portions of the physical examination specifically related to the hematologic system include the lymphatic system, liver, and spleen. Lymph node assessment is discussed in Chapter 23, and assessment of the liver and spleen is described in Chapter 57. Findings from the history and physical examination are supplemented by laboratory tests and specific diagnostic studies.

DIAGNOSTIC TESTS

Diagnosis of a blood disorder depends primarily on laboratory analysis. Although dozens of specific tests are used to diagnose individual disorders, all cases generally call for (1) a complete blood count (CBC) to determine the number of leukocytes and erythrocytes; (2) a total differential count to indicate the relative percentages of the different leukocytes; (3) coagulation studies such as prothrombin time (PT) or partial thromboplastin time (PTT) and bleeding time; (4) a bone marrow aspiration and biopsy to determine both the cellularity of the bone marrow and the morphology of the cells present; and (5) a peripheral blood smear (a study of the morphology of blood cells to help differentiate various anemias and blood dyscrasias). The results of laboratory tests also guide therapy for, for example, the client receiving chemotherapy or radiation therapy.

Hematologic Tests

COMPLETE BLOOD COUNT

The CBC includes the RBC count, hemoglobin, hematocrit, red cell indices, white blood cell (WBC) count with or without differential, and platelet count. Table 45-3 presents the normal values for the CBC. In Table 45-4 the effects of blood dyscrasias on the CBC are reviewed.

TABLE 45-3. Normal Values for Adult Complete Blood Counts

Measure	Value*
Erythrocytes	
Hemoglobin (oxygen-carrying pigment of the red blood cells)	Women: 12.0-15.5 g/dl of blood Men: 13.0-16.5 g/dl of blood
Red blood cell count	Women: 4.0-5.0 million/mm³ of blood Men: 4.8-5.5 million/mm³ of blood
Hematocrit (% volume of red cells in whole blood)	Women: 37-45% of blood volume Men: 40-45% of blood volume
Leukocytes	
White blood cell (WBC) count (number of cells/mm³ of blood)	4-9 thousand/mm³ of blood
Differential count	
Granulocytes	
Neutrophils	60-70% of total WBCs
Eosinophils	0-5% of total WBCs
Basophils	0-3% of total WBCs
Agranulocytes	
Lymphocytes	30-40% of total WBCs
Monocytes	0-5% of total WBCs
Thrombocytes	
Platelets (number of cells/mm³ of blood)	150-450 thousand/mm³ of blood

*Normal values may differ significantly between laboratories.

TABLE 45-4. How Blood Dyscrasias Affect the Complete Blood Count

Increased by	Decreased by
Red blood cell count	
Polycythemia vera, cardiac and pulmonary disorders characterized by cyanosis, dehydration, acute poisoning	Anemia, fluid overload, recent hemorrhage, leukemia
Hemoglobin	
Hemoconcentration from polycythemia or dehydration	Hemodilution (fluid overload), anemia, recent hemorrhage
Hematocrit	
Hemoconcentration from loss of fluid, dehydration, polycythemia	Hemodilution, anemia, acute massive blood loss
Mean corpuscular volume	
Pernicious anemia, macrocytic anemia, folic acid or vitamin B_{12} deficiency anemias	Microcytic anemia, iron deficiency anemia, hypochromic anemias, thalassemia, lead poisoning
Mean corpuscular hemoglobin	
Macrocytic anemia	Microcytic anemia
Mean corpuscular hemoglobin concentration	
Spherocytosis	Microcytic, hypochromic anemia, thalassemia, iron deficiency anemia
White blood cell count	
Infection, leukemia, tissue necrosis	Bone marrow depression
Neutrophils	
Inflammatory disease or response, tissue necrosis (burns, myocardial infarction), granulocytic leukemia and other malignancies, acute stress response, bacterial infection	Bone marrow depression, viral diseases, drugs (chemotherapy, some antibiotics, psychotropics)
Eosinophils	
Allergic reactions, parasitic infestations, skin diseases, neoplasms, pernicious anemia	Stress response, Cushing's syndrome
Basophils	
Leukemia, some hemolytic anemias, polycythemia vera	Corticosteroids, allergic reactions, acute infections (note: decline is unlikely to be detected because normal count is 0–2%)
Lymphocytes	
Viral infections (infectious mononucleosis, pertussis, tuberculosis), lymphocytic leukemia, chronic bacterial infections	Acquired immune deficiency syndrome (AIDS), adrenal corticosteroids, immunosuppressive drugs
Monocytes	
Infections (tuberculosis, malaria, Rocky Mountain spotted fever), collagen vascular diseases, monocytic leukemia	Drug therapy, prednisone
Platelet count	
Malignancies, polycythemia vera, splenectomy	Idiopathic thrombocytopenia purpura, viral infection, AIDS, anemias, hemolytic disorders, chemotherapeutic drugs or radiation, hypersplenism or splenomegaly, infiltrative bone marrow disease, disseminated intravascular coagulation

RED BLOOD CELL COUNT

The RBC count measures the number of RBCs per cubic millimeter (mm^3) of blood. These values are useful in verifying findings from other hematologic tests used to diagnose anemia and polycythemia. Normal values vary with age and sex.

HEMOGLOBIN

The hemoglobin determination evaluates the hemoglobin content of erythrocytes by measuring the number of grams of hemoglobin/100 ml of blood. This measurement helps indicate anemias and polycythemia in clients. Normal hemoglobin levels vary with age and sex.

HEMATOCRIT

Often used in place of the RBC count, hematocrit measures the per cent volume of RBCs in whole blood. This test is useful in the diagnosis of anemia, polycythemia, and abnormal hydration states. The hematocrit value is roughly three times the hemoglobin concentration. Normal values also vary with age and sex.

RED BLOOD CELL INDICES

RBC indices measure erythrocyte size and hemoglobin content. These values derive from the RBC count and hemoglobin level. The three RBC indices — mean corpuscular volume, mean corpuscular hemoglobin, and mean corpuscular hemoglobin concentration — are de-

TABLE 45-5. The Erythrocyte Indices

Mean Corpuscular Volume (MCV)	Mean Corpuscular Hemoglobin (MCH)	Mean Corpuscular Hemoglobin Concentration (MCHC)
Measures average size or volume of individual erythrocytes	Measures hemoglobin content within erythrocyte of average size	Measures average hemoglobin concentration within 100 ml of packed red cells
Formula: $\frac{Hct}{RBC}$	Formula: $\frac{Hb}{RBC}$	Formula: $\frac{Hb}{Hct}$
Normal value: $87 \pm 5\ \mu^3$	Normal value: $29 \pm 2\ \mu\mu g$ (pg)	Normal value: 30–36 g/100 ml of packed red cells
MCV <80 means abnormally small (i.e., *microcytic*) cells MCV >94 means abnormally large (i.e., *macrocytic*) cells	MCH <27 indicates hemoglobin deficiency (*hypochromic* cells) MCH >32 indicates *macrocytic* cells with abnormally large volume of hemoglobin	MCHC <32 indicates hemoglobin deficiency MCHC remains normal when MCH >32 because cells are oversized (i.e., fewer cells can be packed together within 100 ml)

Note. Hct, hematocrit; Hb, hemoglobin; $\mu\mu g$, micromicrogram (also known as pg [picogram]); RBC, red blood cells.

scribed in Table 45-5. The indices are helpful in assessing the various anemias.

WHITE BLOOD CELL COUNT

The WBC count measures the number of WBCs in a cubic millimeter (mm^3) of blood. It helps detect infection of inflammation and is useful in monitoring a client's response to chemotherapy or radiation therapy.

WHITE BLOOD CELL DIFFERENTIAL

This test determines the proportion of each of the five types of WBCs in a sample of 100 WBCs. To figure the actual (absolute) number of a specific cell, multiply the percentage of the cell by the total WBC count. The differential helps in evaluating the body's capacity to resist and overcome infection and in detecting and identifying leukemias.

PLATELET COUNT

The platelet count evaluates thrombocyte (platelet) production, which has a role is in blood clotting. The count is valuable in assessing the severity of thrombocytopenia (abnormally low platelet count), which could result in spontaneous bleeding.

PERIPHERAL BLOOD SMEAR

A peripheral blood smear is an examination of the peripheral blood to determine variations and abnormalities in erythrocytes, leukocytes, and platelets. Cells of normal size and shape are termed normocytes. Cells of normal color are called normochromic. Abnormalities of erythrocyte size, shape, and color usually indicate some form of anemia (Table 45-6).

TABLE 45-6. Abnormalities of the Erythrocyte

Abnormality	Characteristics of Abnormal Cell	Conditions Characterized by Abnormality
Anisocytes	Vary from normal in size	Any of the anemias
Poikilocytes	Abnormally shaped (e.g., tear- or club-shaped)	Any of the anemias; most bizarre shapes seen in the severe anemias
Microcytes	Abnormally small (<6 μ)	Microcytic anemias (e.g., iron deficiency anemia, thalassemia major)
Macrocytes	Abnormally large (>9 μ)	Macrocytic anemias (e.g., pernicious anemia, folic acid deficiency anemia)
Hypochromic cells	Appear pale because of abnormally low hemoglobin content	Any of the anemias
Spherocytes	Relatively small and round rather than biconcave in shape	Hereditary spherocytosis, warm antibody-induced immunohemolytic disease
Schistocytes	Fragmented, with bizarre shapes (e.g., triangles, spirals)	Hemolytic anemia (e.g., thrombotic thrombocytopenic purpura)
Sickle cells	Crescent- or sickle-shaped owing to presence of abnormal hemoglobin (Hb S)	Sickle cell anemia
Target cells	Thin with small amount of hemoglobin in center	Hemoglobin C diseases, thalassemia major, sickle cell anemia
Metarubricytes	Nucleated	Severe anemia

TABLE 45-7. Laboratory Tests Used in the Diagnosis of Hemorrhagic Disorders

Name of Test	Purpose	Normal Values	Interpretation of Findings
Bleeding time (Bl time)	Measures the ability to stop bleeding after a small puncture wound	3-8 min in adults (varies with test method)	Prolonged bleeding time occurs in vascular maladies, and after aspirin ingestion
Platelet count	Measures number of circulating platelets in venous or arterial blood	150,000-450,000	Low count results in prolonged bleeding time and impaired clot retraction; diagnostic of thrombocytopenia
Partial thromboplastin time (PTT)	Complex method for testing normalcy of intrinsic coagulation process; employed to identify deficiencies of coagulation factors, prothrombin, and fibrinogen; monitoring heparin therapy	25-38 sec	Prolongation of time indicates coagulation disorder due to deficiency of a coagulation factor; not diagnostic for platelet disorders
Prothrombin time (Pro time)	Determines activity and interaction of factors V, VII, X, prothrombin, and fibrinogen; used to determine dosages of oral anticoagulant drugs	11-15 sec (one-stage)	Prolongation of time indicates person receiving anticoagulants; abnormally low fibrinogen concentration; deficiencies of factors II, V, VII, and X; presence of circulating anticoagulants as seen in lupus erythematosus; impaired prothrombin activity
Activated clotting time	Crude measure of coagulation process in venous blood; used to control heparin therapy; commonly used during cardio-vascular surgery and in ICU	7-120 sec (depends on type of activator used)	Prolonged time occurs in severe coagulation problems; therapeutic administration of heparin
Thrombin time	Measures functional fibrinogen available, as shown by time needed to form fibrin clot after thrombin is added	10-15 sec	Prolonged time indicates DIC or hypofibrinogenemia; presence in blood of excess heparin or other anticoagulants
Thromboplastin generation test (TGT)	Measures generation of thromboplastin; if result abnormal, second stage is done to identify missing coagulation factor	12 sec or less (100%)	Abnormal values found in hemophilia
Fibrinogen level	Measures level of fibrinogen	200-400 mg/100 ml	Abnormally low values may indicate liver disease, congenital afibrinogenemia, or acquired afibrinogenemia, DIC
Clot retraction	Indicates function and number of platelets; measures time needed for contraction of an undisturbed clot	50-100% in 24 hr	Clot retraction retarded in thrombocytopenia; clot is small and soft in thrombasthenia (functional disturbance of platelets)
Capillary fragility test (Tourniquet test, Rumpel-Leede test)	Crude test of vascular resistance and platelet number and function; done by placing blood pressure cuff on arm for 5 min and then counting petechiae	No petechiae	Petechiae appear in thrombocytopenia and vascular purpura
Fibrin split products (FSP) test	Measures the products that result from the breakdown of fibrin clots	Screening assay <10 mcg/ml of FSP Quantitative assay <3 mcg/ml	Abnormally high levels helpful in diagnosis of DIC; monitoring of fibrinolytic therapy

Note. ICU, intensive care unit; DIC, disseminated intravascular coagulation.

DIRECT AND INDIRECT ANTIGLOBULIN TESTS

Direct antiglobulin test (Coombs' test) is used to (1) detect certain antigen-antibody reactions between serum antibodies and RBC antigens, (2) differentiate between various forms of hemolytic anemia, (3) determine unusual blood types, and (4) test for hemolytic diseases in newborns. The direct antiglobulin test examines erythrocytes for the presence of antibodies (agglutinins) that damage erythrocytes without causing clumping or hemolysis. It is used to crossmatch blood for blood transfusions, test umbilical cord blood for erythroblastosis fetalis, and diagnose acquired hemolytic anemia.

The indirect antiglobulin test identifies antibodies to erythrocyte antigens in the serum of clients who have a greater than normal chance of developing transfusion reactions. Both tests are agglutination procedures that use a suspension of RBCs.

RETICULOCYTE COUNT

A reflection of RBC production, the reticulocyte count measures the responsiveness of the bone marrow to a diminished number of circulating erythrocytes. Specifically, this test measures the number of reticulocytes released from the bone marrow into the blood. An increase in the reticulocyte count indicates an increase in erythrocyte production, probably due to excessive RBC destruction (e.g., hemolytic anemia) or loss (e.g., hemorrhage). A decrease in the reticulocyte count may indicate bone marrow failure or pernicious anemia. In addition, it is employed to evaluate the effectiveness of therapy for pernicious anemia and bone marrow failure.

BONE MARROW ASPIRATION

This important procedure is used to assess and diagnose most blood dyscrasias (e.g., aplastic anemia, the leukemias, pernicious anemia, and thrombocytopenia). Examination of the bone marrow reveals the number, size, and shape of the red cell, white cell, and platelet precursors. Hematologists study the marrow cells for various maturational abnormalities. Bone marrow samples are most commonly taken from the posterior iliac crests. Other possible sites for sampling include the sternum and the anterior iliac crests. To prepare the client for a bone marrow aspiration, the nurse

- Explains the purpose and procedure of the examination,
- Makes sure the client has signed an informed consent form before aspiration,
- Obtains an order for sedation if the client is extremely apprehensive, and
- Positions the client according to health care facility policy.

The procedure for a bone marrow aspiration is as follows:

- The nurse cleanses the skin with an antiseptic solution such as betadine.
- The physician anesthetizes the skin and subcutaneous tissue down to the periosteum with a local anesthetic.
- A short, sharp, beveled needle containing a stylus is inserted through the bone cortex into the marrow space. Once the needle is in the marrow space, the stylus is removed. A syringe is then attached to the needle and about 1 ml of marrow is withdrawn. Because the marrow space itself cannot be anesthetized, removal of the marrow usually produces moderate to severe pain of short duration. It stops as soon as suction on the marrow space is stopped.
- The marrow is ejected onto slides.
- Slides must be labeled and sent to the laboratory immediately.

Following the procedure, the nurse applies pressure until the bleeding stops. Most clients require only a small bandage over the site because there is usually minimal bleeding. However, many clients who require bone marrow aspiration are thrombocytopenic and may need a longer period of pressure to stop bleeding. A pressure dressing and sandbag also may need to be applied in these cases. The nurse observes the site frequently on the day of the procedure and for several days following for clients with an increased risk of bleeding. There may be some discomfort or pain that requires a mild analgesic.

A biopsy of the bone may be taken at the time of marrow aspiration. This bone specimen is ejected into a jar containing a preservative and is sent to the laboratory with the marrow.

Coagulation Screening Tests

Laboratory studies provide the most crucial evidence for pinpointing the type and cause of a bleeding disorder (Table 45-7). Initially, four basic laboratory tests are performed to discern whether the bleeding problem is due to a vascular, coagulation, or platelet defect. These tests include (1) bleeding time, (2) PT, (3) platelet count, and (4) PTT. Ninety-nine per cent of all bleeding disorders are diagnosed by the PT and PTT.

Summary

Understanding the structure, function, and assessment of the hematologic system will help the nurse care for clients with any of the wide variety of disorders that affect this highly complex system. Once this complex system is understood, the nurse should be better able to provide complete care for clients with hematologic disorders.

Bibliography

1. Adams, S. (1992). The HLA system: Seminar, 1992.
2. Alkire, K., & Collingwood, J. (1990). Physiology of blood and bone marrow. *Seminars in Oncology Nursing, 6,* 99-107.
3. Baldwin, J.G. (1988). Hematopoietic function in the elderly. *Archives of Internal Medicine, 148,* 2544-2546.
4. Carlson, K., & Golub, A. (1987). *Autologous and directed blood programs.* Arlington, VA: American Association of Blood Banks.
5. Corbett, J.V. (1992). *Laboratory tests and diagnostic procedures with nursing diagnoses.* East Norwalk, CT: Appleton & Lange.
6. DiJulio, J. (1991). Hematopoiesis: An overview. *Oncology Nursing Forum, 18,* 3-6.
7. Duguid, J.K.M. (1990). Developing techniques in blood transfusion. *Bailliere's Clinical Haematology, 3* (1), 999-1017.
8. Ganong, W.F. (1985). *Review of medical physiology.* Los Altos, CA: Lange Medical Publications.
9. Hoffbrand, A.V. (1988). *Recent advances in hematology.* Edinburgh: Churchill Livingstone.
10. Hoffbrand, A.V., & Pettit, J.E. (1988). *Sandoz atlas of clinical hematology.* London: Gower Medical Publishing.
11. Hoffman, R., et al. (1991). *Hematology: Basic principles and practice.* Edinburgh: Churchill Livingstone.
12. Jandel, J.H. (1991). *Blood: Pathophysiology.* Cambridge, England: Blackwell Scientific Publications.
13. Perez, W.E., & Viets, J.L. (1990). Transfusion and coagulation:

An overview and recent advances in practice modalities. *Nurse Anesthetist, 1,* 149–161.

14. Read, E.J., & Klein, H.G. (1986). Hematological effects of aging: Considerations for clinical trials. In N.R. Cutler & P.K. Narang (Eds.), *Drug studies in the elderly* (pp. 123–144). New York: Plenum.
15. Salmon, C., et al. (1984). *The human blood groups.* New York: Masson.
16. Sherman, J.L. (1988). *Guide to patient evaluation: History taking, physical examination, and the nursing process.* New York: Medical Examination.
17. Williams, W.J., et al. (1983). *Hematology* (3rd ed.). New York: McGraw-Hill.

Chapter 46

Nursing Care of Clients with Hematologic Disorders

This chapter discusses disorders affecting red blood cells (erythrocytes), white blood cells (leukocytes), primarily the lymph system and spleen, and platelets and clotting factors.

Red blood cell disorders include anemias and polycythemias. Major disorders that affect white blood cells are (1) the leukemias (acute and chronic), (2) agranulocytosis, and (3) multiple myeloma (plasma cell myeloma). Disorders primarily affecting the lymph nodes and spleen are the lymphomas, classified as either (1) Hodgkin's disease or (2) non-Hodgkin's lymphoma. Disorders affecting platelets and clotting factors include (1) hemorrhagic disorders, (2) purpura, and (3) coagulation disorders.

DISORDERS AFFECTING RED BLOOD CELLS

The Anemias

Definition

Anemia is a reduction in red blood cells (erythrocytes), which in turn decreases the oxygen-carrying capacity of the blood. Not a disease in itself, anemia reflects an abnormality in red blood cell number, structure, or function.

Anemia is the principal manifestation of many abnormal conditions, such as (1) deficiency states caused by a dietary lack of iron, vitamin B_{12}, and folic acid; (2) hereditary disorders of red blood cells; (3) disorders involving the hematopoietic tissues (bone marrow damage or a hyperactive spleen); and (4) bleeding from the gastrointestinal tract or any organ secondary to cancer or trauma. Increased destruction of red blood cells can also result from extrinsic sources, physical causes such as prosthetic heart valves, or thrombotic thrombocytopenic purpura. It can also result from antibodies, as in immune thrombotic thrombocytopenia; from infectious agents and toxins; or from other causes, such as hypersplenism, vasculitis syndromes, or osmotic and physical injury.

Incidence

Studies suggest the prevalence of anemia increases with age; an estimated average of 20 per cent of the elderly are anemic.[5] However, anemia cannot be assumed to be caused simply by aging without the exclusion of reversible causes. The elderly client should be fully assessed for an underlying cause of anemia.

The incidence of anemia is high, especially in underdeveloped countries where nutrition is poor and in tropical regions where the hookworm (a parasite that extracts blood from the intestinal wall of its host) is endemic. Some epidemiologists calculate that at least one half of the world's population suffers from anemia sometime in their lives.

Etiology

Major causes of anemia are (1) excessive blood loss, (2) deficiencies and abnormalities of red blood cell production, and (3) excessive destruction of red blood cells.

Risk Factors

Poor nutrition, blood loss, and conditions that cause excessive red blood cell destruction are risk factors for the development of anemia. Proper nutrition will obviously help prevent anemia. With the other risk factors, early detection can help decrease the severity of the anemia.

Pathophysiology

Two basic pathophysiologic alterations underlie all red blood cell disorders:

1. a decrease in the hemoglobin concentration or the number of functional red blood cells (anemia) due to one or more of the following:
   - insufficient production of red blood cells by the bone marrow
   - defective synthesis of red blood cells due to the absence of an essential factor
   - increased destruction of red blood cells caused by hereditary factors or an acquired condition
   - increased loss of red blood cells caused by acute or chronic bleeding
2. an increased number of circulating red blood cells (polycythemia) due to one of the following:
   - a disorder of unknown etiology, similar to cancer
   - a compensatory mechanism that develops in response to tissue hypoxia (secondary polycythemia)

Anemias are classified according to either the morphologic features of the red blood cells (e.g., normocytic, microcytic) or the cause of the condition (e.g., hemolytic, hemorrhagic). It is important to be familiar with the more accurate and commonly used morphologic classification system. However, it is more practical to relate nursing assessment, diagnosis, and treatment of an anemia to the classification in Table 46-1

TABLE 46-1. Classification of Anemias

Acquired Anemias
Anemias resulting from reduced red blood cell production
Anemias due to deficiencies of factors necessary for red blood cell production
Iron deficiency anemia
Anemias due to deficiencies of vitamin B_{12} and folic acid (megaloblastic anemias)
Pernicious anemia
Other anemias due to vitamin B_{12} deficiency
Anemia due to folic acid deficiency
Anemias of bone marrow failure
Aplastic anemia
Hemolytic anemias
Anemias resulting from excessive red blood cell destruction
Hemolysis due to trauma
Hemolysis due to chemical agents and medications (toxic hemolytic anemia)
Hemolysis due to infectious agents
Hemolysis due to systemic diseases (secondary hemolytic anemia)
Hemolysis due to isoimmune hemolytic reactions
Hemolysis due to autoimmune disorders
The paroxysmal hemoglobinurias
Secondary anemias
Anemias Due to Excessive Blood Loss
Acute posthemorrhagic anemia
Anemia due to chronic blood loss
Congenital Anemias
Hemoglobinopathies
Sickle cell anemia and sickle cell trait
Thalassemia
Hemolytic anemias due to intrinsic red blood cell defects
Glucose-6-phosphate dehydrogenase (G6PD) deficiency
Hereditary spherocytosis

than to its cellular characteristics. Table 46-1 divides the anemias into acquired (common to uncommon), anemias due to excessive blood loss, and congenital categories.

Clinical Manifestations

Symptoms accompanying anemia differ, depending on the severity and chronicity of the anemia, the age of the client, and the presence of other disorders.

Tissue hypoxia is the underlying cause of all symptoms accompanying anemia. Respiratory and cardiovascular compensatory mechanisms produce many of the symptoms. Clients with mild anemia (hemoglobin of 10 to 12 g/100 ml) are usually asymptomatic. If symptoms do occur, they typically follow strenuous exertion.

Clients with moderate anemia also suffer from dyspnea, palpitations, diaphoresis with exertion, and chronic fatigue.

Severely anemic clients appear pale and always feel exhausted. They may have severe palpitations, sensitivity to cold, loss of appetite, profound weakness, dizziness, and headaches. Severely anemic clients, particularly the elderly, can eventually develop serious cardiac complications. Congestive heart failure may arise as a result of increased demands on the heart to beat faster and harder (to transport more oxygen to the tissues). Angina pectoris may also develop, either alone or with congestive heart failure. In severe anemia, angina pectoris results from insufficient oxygenation of the myocardium. Clients with pre-existing heart conditions, in addition to anemia, are particularly vulnerable to circulatory and pulmonary complications.

Other signs and symptoms of anemia associated with specific systems include

- *integumentary:* pallor (particularly of palm lines, nail beds, conjunctiva, and circumoral area), delayed wound healing, sore mouth and tongue, sensitivity to cold, jaundice, spider angiomas
- *respiratory:* shortness of breath, dyspnea on exertion, orthopnea
- *cardiovascular:* palpitations, angina, tachycardia, cardiomegaly, claudication, dependent edema, bruits, tachypnea, fatigue, weakness
- *gastrointestinal:* anorexia, nausea, dietary change (clay-eating, pica), tarry stool, constipation, diarrhea, hemorrhoids, hematemesis, weight loss
- *genitourinary:* hematuria, menstrual irregularity, loss of libido, impotence
- *neurologic:* headache, dizziness, sternal tenderness, numbness, tingling of extremities, irritability, paralysis
- *general:* chronic fatigue, malaise

DIAGNOSTIC ASSESSMENT

The diagnosis of anemia relies on blood tests, physical assessment and examination, psychosocial assessment, and the health history. The red blood cell count, hemoglobin level, and hematocrit confirm the presence of anemia. To determine the specific type of anemia present, the hematologist examines a bone marrow specimen and a peripheral blood smear and calculates red cell indices and, in some cases, the rate of red blood cell destruction.

A thorough history, physical examination, observation, and review of records are essential in evaluating the client suspected of having a red blood cell abnormality. Elicit a data base from the client that provides information about the possible cause of the disease process, the symptoms, and the pathophysiologic mechanism. Specifically ask about the history of the present illness, significant past medical history, and current medications.

Medical Management

The goals of care for clients with anemia include (1) alleviating or controlling the causes, (2) relieving the symptoms, and (3) preventing complications.

Management of the anemias ranges from specific treatments to symptomatic care. Treatment also varies in intensity and duration because some anemias resolve within a few weeks or months whereas others require lifelong intervention.

The anemias caused by deficiency states respond best to specific intervention. For example, iron preparations and diet can cure iron deficiency anemia; injections of vitamin B_{12} control pernicious anemia.

Other anemias (e.g., aplastic anemia due to bone marrow failure and some of the acquired hemolytic anemias) may be successfully treated by stopping a cytotoxic medication or avoiding a dangerous chemical agent.

Oxygen therapy may be prescribed for clients with severe anemia, because their blood has a reduced capacity for oxygen. Oxygen helps prevent tissue hypoxia and lessens the workload of the heart as it struggles to compensate for the lower hemoglobin levels.

Blood transfusions are valuable in treating anemia due to acute blood loss. They may also benefit clients with severe chronic anemia (hemoglobin less than 6 g/100 ml) who have responded poorly to other forms of therapy. Transfusion therapy, in which the specific blood components required are transfused, supports clients until they spontaneously recover or respond to treatment.

Long-term red blood cell support, however, carries with it the potentially fatal complication of iron overload. The normal iron level of 2 to 3 g usually remains constant because iron is metabolized at a fixed rate. Each unit of red blood cells contains an additional 200 mg of iron. Clients who receive more than 100 units of red blood cells frequently develop excess iron stores in major organs.

Complications of iron overload include cardiac myopathies (pericarditis, arrhythmias, congestive heart failure), thyroid insufficiency, endocrine and pancreas malfunction (glucose intolerance), liver fibrosis, profound anemia, and skin discoloration. Cardiomyopathies related to iron overload are a frequent cause of death in the chronically transfused client.

PHARMACOLOGIC MANAGEMENT

Deferoxamine (Desferal) is an iron chelating agent that can prevent iron overload when it is properly administered. However, the short half-life of this agent requires intravenous infusion over a prolonged period. A common treatment regimen is a continuous pump infusion 12 hours a day, 5 days a week. In addition to the high cost of this therapy, it is difficult for clients to maintain a normal lifestyle, and compliance is a major problem.

Iron and vitamin B_{12} can be given when the client has anemia due to deficiency of these elements.

DIETARY MANAGEMENT

When the anemia is related to poor nutrition, or when the cause is blood loss, proper nutrition can improve red blood cell production. A diet high in iron, vitamin B_{12}, and folic acid will help increase red blood cell production if a deficiency of these nutrients is present.

▼ Acquired Anemias

As stated in Chapter 45, effective erythropoiesis depends on the adequate intake and proper assimilation of iron, vitamin B_{12}, folic acid, protein, pyridoxine, and traces of copper. The most common deficiency state is iron deficiency. In addition, deficiencies of vitamin B_{12} and folic acid are prevalent. Protein deficiency is also frequently seen. Pyridoxine (vitamin B_6) and copper deficiencies occur infrequently in humans.

IRON DEFICIENCY ANEMIA

Definition

Iron deficiency is defined as anemia associated with either inadequate absorption or excessive loss of iron; it is chronic, microcytic, hypochromic anemia.

Incidence

The worldwide incidence of iron deficiency anemia is high. It is common in countries where nutrition is poor; it is also prevalent in tropical zones and in the southern United States, Mexico, and Puerto Rico, where blood-sucking parasites such as the hookworm are endemic. The poor of all nations suffer far more frequently from iron deficiency than do the middle and upper classes.

Menstruating women and young children also are vulnerable to iron deficiency, whereas adult men and postmenopausal women rarely develop this problem. Iron deficiency anemia also occurs with chronic blood loss.

Etiology

Iron deficiency anemia is caused by an inadequate supply of iron needed to synthesize hemoglobin. This results in a decreased supply to the developing red blood cells of a crucial component of hemoglobin—iron—essential to the oxygen-carrying function of heme. When these disorders of heme synthesis become severe, the marrow produces red blood cells that are deficient in hemoglobin concentration and that are hypochromic and microcytic.

Risk Factors

The major risk factor for iron deficiency anemia is inadequate nutrition. An adequate intake of iron, with normal absorption of the iron, should prevent the disorder.

Pathophysiology

An average diet supplies the body with about 12 to 15 mg/day of iron, of which only 5 to 10 per cent (0.6 to 1.5 mg) is absorbed. The amount of iron normally absorbed daily is sufficient for meeting the needs of women past childbearing age and healthy men. However, it does not meet the greater needs of menstruating and pregnant women, adolescents, children, and infants. These five groups of clients must have a higher daily intake of iron for prevention of deficiency. Economic constraints, poor dentition, and lack of interest in food preparation commonly lead to iron deficiency in elderly clients. Fortunately, the gastrointestinal tract can increase its absorption of iron from 10 per cent daily to about 20 to 30 per cent daily. In this way, the body often compensates for diminishing iron stores due to inadequate iron intake or excessive iron loss.

Iron is stored in the form of ferritin, an iron-phosphorus-protein complex that contains about 23 per cent iron. It is formed in the intestinal mucosa when ferric iron joins with the protein apoferritin. Ferritin is stored in the tissues, primarily in the reticuloendothelial cells of the liver, spleen, and bone marrow.

Normal iron excretion is less than 1 mg/day. Iron is excreted in urine, sweat, bile, and feces and from the skin as desquamated cells. The average woman loses another 0.5 mg of iron daily or 15 mg monthly during menses. Menstruation is the most common cause of iron deficiency in women. Gastrointestinal tract bleeding is a common etiologic factor in men; it may result from peptic ulcers, hiatal hernia, gastritis, cancer, hemorrhoids, diverticula, ulcerative colitis, or salicylate poisoning.

Bleeding from the gastrointestinal tract is usually chronic and occult (obscure or not readily apparent). A chronic blood loss of as little as 2 to 4 ml/day can result in iron deficiency anemia, because every 2 ml of blood contains 1 mg of iron. The body can compensate for such losses to some degree by excreting less than 0.5 mg of iron daily rather than the normal 1 mg.

Alteration in the mucosa of the duodenum and proximal jejunum (as in chronic diarrhea, malabsorption syndromes such as celiac disease, and gastrectomy) affects iron absorption, predisposing clients to iron deficiency states. Tannates (in tea), carbonates, the food preservative EDTA, and the medicinal antacid magnesium trisilicate all hinder nonheme iron absorption. Clay-eating (pica), a practice of women and children in socioeconomically disadvantaged areas, causes iron to precipitate as an insoluble substance within the intestinal tract.

Clinical Manifestations

In mild cases of iron deficiency anemia, the client is asymptomatic. However, in more severe cases, assessment reveals the general symptoms of anemia (e.g., palpitations, dizziness, and sensitivity to cold).

Later during the disease, hair and nails usually become brittle. In severe cases, dysphagia (difficulty in swallowing), stomatitis (inflammation of the mucosa of the mouth), and atrophic glossitis (tongue is inflamed and smooth owing to atrophy of papillae) may appear. This triad of symptoms is known as the Plummer-Vinson syndrome, a condition that primarily affects middle-aged women who have recently had their teeth extracted. Despite the weakness and discomfort associated with iron deficiency anemia, death rarely occurs unless severe cardiac complications develop.

DIAGNOSTIC ASSESSMENT

Examinations of the blood and bone marrow form the basis for diagnosing iron deficiency anemia. Because they are deficient in hemoglobin, the red blood cells are small (microcytic) and pale (hypochromic), a morphologic characteristic of iron deficiency. Other characteristics of anemia are hemoglobin level decreased to as low as 3.6 g/100 ml; total red blood cell count moderately reduced, rarely dropping below 3 million cells/100 mm^3; mean cell volume (MCV), mean cell hemoglobin (MCH), and mean cell hemoglobin concentration (MCHC) reduced; serum iron level (normally between 50 and 150 μg/100 ml of blood) may be decreased to 10 μg; total iron-combining capacity elevated to 350 to 500 μg/100 ml (normal is 250 to 350 μg/100 ml); hemosiderin (an insoluble form of storage iron) completely absent from the bone marrow; immunoradiometric serum ferritin assay below normal.

Once the diagnosis of iron deficiency anemia is confirmed, studies are conducted to find the cause of the anemia. If gastrointestinal tract bleeding is suspected, approximate the amount of blood lost daily and the site of bleeding.

X-ray studies (gastrointestinal tract series), stool examination for occult blood, esophagoscopy, gastroscopy, and sigmoidoscopy are commonly done.

Medical Management

Therapeutic goals for clients with iron deficiency anemia are to (1) diagnose and correct the underlying cause of the anemia and (2) correct the iron deficit through diet and supplemental iron preparations.

PHARMACOLOGIC MANAGEMENT

Supplemental iron is usually administered to increase iron available in the blood. The medications of choice are ferrous sulfate (Feosol), 0.2 g orally, three times a day, with meals; ferrous gluconate (Fergon), 0.3 g orally, twice a day; and iron-dextran (Imferon), 100 to 250 mg intramuscularly. Figure 46-1 illustrates the Z-track technique for administration of iron-dextran. Clients usually receive iron supplements for at least 6 months for repletion of the body stores.

Parenteral iron therapy is administered to clients who (1) have an intolerance to oral iron preparations, (2) habitually forget to take their medications, or (3) continue to suffer blood losses. Iron-dextran is the parenteral drug of choice. The client typically feels more energetic and has an increased appetite within 48

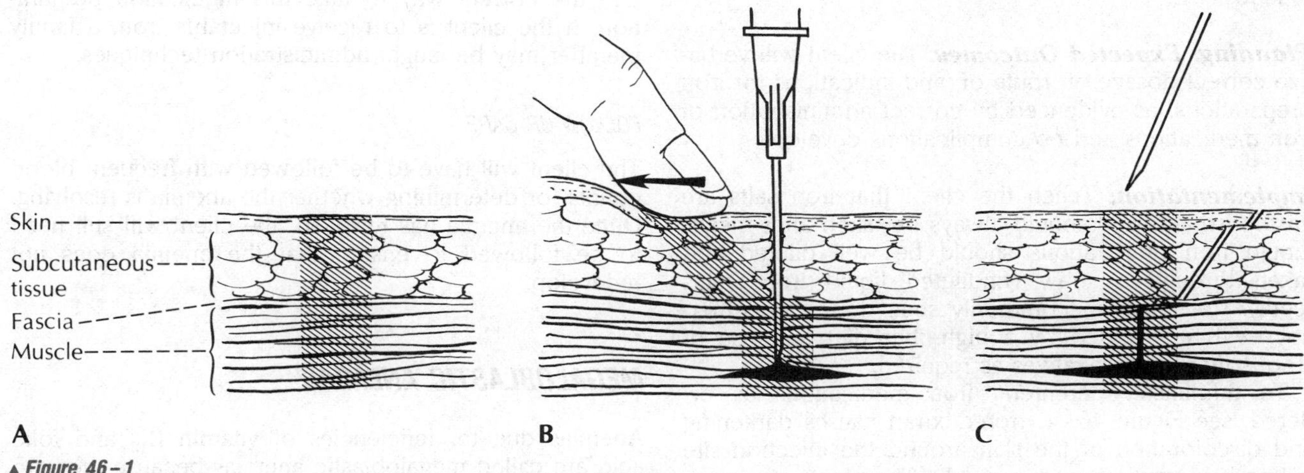

▲ Figure 46-1

Z-track technique used for administration of iron-dextran. *A*, Normal tissue relationships before injection. *B*, Altered tissue relationships during injection. Retract tissue, insert needle, administer medication, remove needle, and release tissue. *C*, Normal tissue relationships after injection. Note angled Z-track left by needle.

hours. Peak reticulocytosis occurs about day 10. Red blood cell indices and hemoglobin content gradually return to normal.

Nursing Management

ASSESSMENT

Nursing assessment for iron deficiency anemia focuses on data collection of causative factors and risk factors, dietary history, family history, psychosocial problems, and medications. Common physical symptoms are stomatitis, smooth red tongue, cold sensitivity, brittle hair, and spoon-shaped brittle nails (integumentary); dyspnea on exertion (respiratory); tachycardia (cardiovascular); and dizziness, dysphagia, numbness, tingling, decreased concentration, headache, and fatigue (neurologic).

NURSING INTERVENTION

Nursing Diagnosis: Nutrition, Altered: Less than Body Requirements R/T disease, treatment, and lack of knowledge of adequate nutrition.

Planning: Expected Outcomes. The client will have nutritional deficiencies corrected and optimal nutrition will be achieved, as evidenced by blood tests reaching normal range, activity tolerance improved, and anemia resolved.

Implementation. Teach basics of good nutrition; encourage diet high in protein, iron, and vitamins with frequent small meals. Encourage foods cooked in iron pots and ingestion of foods such as liver (the richest source), oysters, lean meats, kidney beans, whole wheat bread, kale, spinach, egg yolk, turnip tops, beet greens, carrots, apricots, and raisins. Document client's weight. Encourage good oral hygiene.

Nursing Diagnosis: Knowledge Deficit R/T iron preparations.

Planning: Expected Outcomes. The client will verbalize correct dosage of, route of, and indications for iron preparations, as evidenced by correct administration of iron medications and no complications developing.

Implementation. Teach the client that iron salts are gastric irritants and should always be taken after meals. Liquid iron preparations should be well diluted and taken through a straw (undiluted liquid iron stains teeth). Constipation, commonly seen during iron therapy, will be avoided by a high-fiber diet and use of stool softeners or laxatives as required.

To administer parenteral iron medications as ordered, see Figure 46–1. Iron-dextran causes darkening and discoloration of the skin around the injection site unless it is administered properly. Therefore, when administering this medication:

- Use one needle to withdraw iron-dextran and another needle to administer it; thus, staining from iron that adheres to the needle is avoided.
- Give the injection with a 2- or 3-inch, 19- or 20-gauge needle, deep into the upper outer quadrant of the buttock. Never use the arm or any other exposed area.
- Use the Z-track and air-lock injection techniques to prevent medication leakage.
- Never massage the site of injection.
- Throughout therapy, observe for pain at the injection site, abscesses, lymphadenitis, fever, headache, urticaria, hypotension, or anaphylactic shock. Anaphylaxis rarely occurs.

EVALUATION

The nurse must evaluate client outcomes on the basis of the established plan of care. If these goals have not been achieved, the plan and interventions must be revised to meet the client's needs.

Modification of Plan of Care for the Elderly

The older client is more prone to iron deficiency anemia because of poor nutritional intake and a decreased absorption of iron in the intestine. Older clients will also require complete assessment for diagnosis of the cause of the anemia. They often experience chronic blood loss from a variety of diseases that also may cause the anemia, so differential diagnosis will be required.

Post-hospital Care

DISCHARGE TEACHING

Proper nutritional intake is one of the most important areas for client teaching. The client can often easily correct the problem simply by improving intake.

The client must be taught about iron preparations and the correct way to take this medication preparation. If the client is to receive injectable iron, a family member may be taught administration techniques.

FOLLOW-UP CARE

The client will have to be followed with frequent blood counts for determining whether the anemia is resolving. Once the anemia has resolved, the client will still need to be followed to ensure that the anemia does not redevelop.

MEGALOBLASTIC ANEMIAS

Anemias due to deficiencies of vitamin B_{12} and folic acid are called megaloblastic anemias because they are characterized by the appearance of megaloblasts (large primitive red blood cells) in the blood and bone marrow.

Other common features of the megaloblastic anemias are leukopenia and thrombocytopenia (decrease in platelets); oral, gastrointestinal, and neurologic symptoms; and favorable response to injections of either vitamin B_{12} or folic acid.

The underlying defect in the megaloblastic anemias is disturbed DNA synthesis. Deficiencies of either vitamin B_{12} or folic acid impede the formation of DNA precursors, which causes abnormal maturation of red blood cells, leukocytes, and platelets. The same basic etiologic factors—dietary inadequacies, impaired absorption, and metabolic disturbances—underlie both vitamin B_{12} and folic acid deficiency. In the former, the diet is deficient in meat and dairy products; in the latter, vegetables are lacking.

The principal cause of impaired vitamin B_{12} absorption is intrinsic factor deficiency. The small intestine cannot absorb vitamin B_{12} (the extrinsic factor) unless the intrinsic factor (i.e., a substance of internal origin) combines with it. When the intrinsic factor is missing, pernicious anemia develops. Conditions such as tapeworm, overgrowth of intestinal bacteria, or intestinal diverticula may also impair vitamin B_{12} absorption. Folic acid antagonists, anticonvulsants, or liver disease may inhibit folic acid absorption and use. Intestinal malabsorption of both vitamins may result from any of a group of disorders such as sprue, celiac disease, steatorrhea, or surgical resection of the small intestine. Metabolic changes, such as those that occur in hyperthyroidism, pregnancy, or cancer, can lead to additional requirements for both vitamin B_{12} and folic acid.

PERNICIOUS ANEMIA

Definition

Pernicious anemia refers to anemia due to decreased absorption of vitamin B_{12}.

Incidence

Pernicious anemia is the most prevalent form of vitamin B_{12} deficiency in the United States and Canada. The most common megaloblastic anemia, pernicious anemia, occurs in only 0.1 per cent of the population. It mainly strikes men and women over the age of 50 years and primarily affects people of northern European origin. Occasionally, it develops in southern European, Asian, and African Americans. Although rare, juvenile pernicious anemia has been found in children under 10 years of age. Juvenile pernicious anemia is a congenital disorder in which the stomach secretes abnormal intrinsic factor.

Etiology

This chronic, progressive, megaloblastic anemia of adults is caused by a deficiency of intrinsic factor. Lack of intrinsic factor due to atrophy of the stomach's glandular mucosa is the basic defect in pernicious anemia.

Although heredity may play a role, the exact reason for mucosal atrophy and associated hypochlorhydria remains unknown. Pernicious anemia may be inherited as a single dominant autosomal factor. Prolonged iron deficiency, which may cause gastric atrophy, is a second possible predisposing factor. However, pernicious anemia may also be an autoimmune disorder. Ninety per cent of clients with pernicious anemia have autoantibodies that react specifically against parietal gastric cells, and 60 per cent have anti-intrinsic factor antibody.

Risk Factors

One major risk factor for the development of pernicious anemias is gastric resection. The parietal cells in the stomach secrete the intrinsic factor required for vitamin B_{12} absorption. The disease can also be congenital as a result of absence of the intrinsic factor.

Pathophysiology

The four major characteristics of pernicious anemia are

- abnormally large red blood cells (macrocytic anemia)
- hypochlorhydria (deficiency of gastric hydrochloric acid)
- neurologic and gastrointestinal symptoms
- a fatal outcome unless the client receives lifelong injections of vitamin B_{12}

Unless it is controlled with vitamin B_{12}, pernicious anemia inevitably develops after total gastrectomy. Also, 15 per cent of clients develop pernicious anemia after partial gastrectomy or gastrojejunostomy for a peptic ulcer.

Pathologic consequences of vitamin B_{12} deficiency are macrocytic anemia and gastrointestinal disorders. Both problems respond to injections of vitamin B_{12}. Lack of vitamin B_{12} also alters the structure and disrupts the function of the peripheral nerves, spinal cord, and brain. Thus, the third major consequence of this disorder is disturbed nervous system function and, in extreme cases, permanent neurologic damage unresponsive to vitamin B_{12} therapy. Central nervous system symptoms develop in three quarters of clients with pernicious anemia. Clients with this anemia tend to be fair-haired or prematurely gray.

Clients with pernicious anemia have a high incidence of benign gastric polyps and gastric carcinoma; they require routine assessment for gastric bleeding and tumor growth obstruction.

Untreated pernicious anemia causes death; delayed intervention results in permanent disabilities. In addition to the nervous system damage already mentioned, severe macrocytic anemia of long duration can trigger congestive heart failure and angina pectoris in the elderly.

Clinical Manifestations

The major symptom of pernicious anemia is low hemoglobin, hematocrit, and red blood cell levels. Diagnosis of pernicious anemia is based on the presence of anemia, gastrointestinal symptoms, and neurologic disorders; laboratory blood and bone marrow tests; the absence of gastric hydrochloric acid; and a favorable response to a vitamin B_{12} "therapeutic trial."

Low hemoglobin levels and consequent hypoxemia may trigger congestive heart failure because of increased demands on the heart to transport oxygen to the tissues. Angina pectoris also may develop from insufficient oxygenation of the myocardium.

DIAGNOSTIC ASSESSMENT

Laboratory findings that confirm a diagnosis of pernicious anemia include the following.

- Red blood cells are usually reduced to fewer than 3 million/mm^3; MCV and MCHC are likely to be elevated, with white blood cells and MCH decreased.
- On peripheral blood smear, red blood cells are oval, macrocytic, and hyperchromic.
- The bone marrow contains high numbers of megaloblasts (an abnormal form of red blood cell maturation).
- Unconjugated bilirubin (a product of hemoglobin breakdown) is usually elevated owing to hemolysis of defective red blood cells.
- Serum lactate dehydrogenase is extremely high. (Lactate dehydrogenase is an enzyme present in many tissues that is released into the circulation when tissues are damaged).
- Schilling's test measures the absorption of orally administered, radioactive vitamin B_{12} (tagged with cobalt-60) before and after parenteral administration of the intrinsic factor. This procedure detects lack of intrinsic factor and is the definitive test for pernicious anemia.
- Gastric secretion analysis to check for the presence of free hydrochloric acid is another important test; most clients with pernicious anemia have low-volume gastric secretions with a high pH and free hydrochloric acid. Furthermore, these findings do not change even after the administration of histamine, which normally stimulates gastric secretion.

Medical Management

Clients with pernicious anemia need both immediate care and lifelong therapy with maintenance vitamin B_{12}. During the acute phase of illness, the client may be treated with vitamin B_{12} injections.

The response to vitamin B_{12} injections is usually quick and dramatic, often occurring within 24 to 48 hours. Within 72 hours, reticulocytes begin to increase; by the end of the first week, the total red blood cell count rises significantly. Cardiovascular involvement usually lessens with improved hematopoiesis. Although peripheral nerve function may improve with treatment, spinal cord and brain damage usually persist.

Additionally, the client may need oral iron supplementation if the hemoglobin level fails to rise in proportion to an increased red blood cell count. As stated earlier, iron deficiency may be an etiologic factor in pernicious anemia and must be corrected if it is present. Iron deficiency anemia can also develop during treatment of pernicious anemia. Injections of vitamin B_{12} may cause a rapid regeneration of red blood cells that depletes iron. As a result, the hemoglobin level remains low although the total red blood cell count rises.

Folic acid is sometimes given with vitamin B_{12} to clients with a history of poor nutrition. Folic acid can be dangerous, however, because it may intensify neurologic problems. Clients who are taking large doses of folate may obscure a vitamin B_{12} deficiency. Therefore, a therapeutic trial of folate should never be given without pernicious anemia first being ruled out.

PHARMACOLOGIC MANAGEMENT

Prescribed medications are

- vitamin derivatives (to correct nutritional or metabolic deficiency): cyanocobalamin (Berubigen, Cyanabin, vitamin B_{12}, and others); folic acid (Folvite)
- Hematinic agents (to correct nutritional deficit): ferrous sulfate (Feosol) or ferrous gluconate (Fergon)
- Digestants (to enhance metabolism of vitamins): hydrochloric acid diluted in water with meals during the first few weeks of vitamin B_{12} therapy

Blood transfusions are usually unnecessary, because clients with pernicious anemia respond to vitamin B_{12} injections. Occasionally, however, blood transfusions may be lifesaving.

Nursing Management

Once the acute stage of the illness is past, the client with pernicious anemia must undertake a lifelong program of maintenance therapy. Monthly injections of vitamin B_{12} are needed to avoid relapse. The nurse plays a vital role in educating clients with this disorder about the importance of continuous care.

In addition to medications, clients with permanent neurologic disabilities need an intensive program of physical therapy and rehabilitation. Because clients with pernicious anemia are at risk for developing gastric carcinoma, also encourage them to see their physician at least twice a year for a complete physical examination.

If therapy remains adequate and uninterrupted, the client with pernicious anemia can expect a life free of anemic symptoms, without further symptoms of neuropathy.

OTHER ANEMIAS DUE TO VITAMIN B_{12} DEFICIENCY

Whereas pernicious anemia arises from lack of the intrinsic factor, another group of anemias results from lack of the extrinsic factor (vitamin B_{12}). This problem may be caused by faulty diet, defective absorption due to intestinal disease, or metabolic disturbances. The megaloblastic anemia that characterizes these conditions is the same as that seen in pernicious anemia. However, hypochlorhydria and degenerative neurologic changes do not occur.

Treatment for vitamin B_{12} deficiency depends on the specific cause. The oral administration of 25 μg of vitamin B_{12} daily, with a more balanced diet, corrects inadequate dietary intake.

Extremely deficient diets are rarely seen in developed countries except among the very poor who cannot afford meat and among some vegetarians. However, inadequate diets are common in India and other countries with large populations of poor people.

Poor absorption of vitamin B_{12} results from (1) an overgrowth of intestinal bacteria due to intestinal stasis, (2) infestation with the fish tapeworm, or (3) one of the malabsorption syndromes. Bacteria that proliferate within intestinal blind loops and diverticula (small blind pouches that form in the walls of the colon) compete with the host for available vitamin B_{12}. This problem can be corrected by (1) surgical removal of the pouches or blind loops and (2) administration of broad-spectrum antibiotics to control infection. The fish tapeworm eaten in raw fish also competes with its host for vitamin B_{12}. Treatment involves removal of the tapeworm and the temporary administration of vitamin B_{12} until the anemia resolves.

Treatment for anemia caused by malabsorption syndromes (e.g., sprue and celiac disease) consists of administering 100 μg of vitamin B_{12} intramuscularly daily for 10 days followed by 100 μg of vitamin B_{12} monthly until the absorption dysfunction clears.

Clients who have an increased need for the vitamin due to metabolic changes (e.g., in pregnancy or hyperthyroidism) may take oral vitamin B_{12} as a supplement.

ANEMIA DUE TO FOLIC ACID DEFICIENCY

Anemia associated with folic acid deficiency is very common. This condition has many causes, most of which are the same as the causes of vitamin B_{12} deficiency. Usually, folic acid deficiency results from a poor diet lacking in such foods as green leafy vegetables, liver, citrus fruits, and yeast. Clients with chronic alcoholism, because of their typically inadequate diets, are particularly susceptible to this problem. High levels of alcohol in the blood also partially block the response of the bone marrow to folic acid, which thereby interferes with erythropoiesis.

Folic acid deficiency, like vitamin B_{12} deficiency, can develop with malabsorption syndromes (e.g., sprue, celiac disease, steatorrhea). Certain medications can also impede folic acid absorption and utilization. For example, a serious anemia may develop with (1) the long-term use of anticonvulsant medications (e.g., primidone, diphenylhydantoin, and phenobarbital), (2) the administration of antimetabolites (e.g., folic acid antagonists, purine analogs, and pyrimidine analogs) to clients with cancer and leukemia, or (3) the administration of certain oral contraceptives.

Finally, folic acid deficiency may occur with increased demands for folate, such as during the growth spurts of infancy and adolescence. During the third trimester of pregnancy, expectant mothers need six times the normal amount of folic acid because of the increased demands of the developing fetus.

Folic acid, like vitamin B_{12}, is necessary for DNA synthesis. Both vitamin B_{12} and folic acid deficiencies cause symptoms of megaloblastic anemia (fatigue, cardiac symptoms, slight jaundice) and gastrointestinal tract disturbances (e.g., dyspepsia; smooth, beefy tongue). However, unlike pernicious anemia, a folic acid deficiency does not cause neurologic manifestations.

Anemia due to folic acid deficiency has a slow and insidious onset. The client, often thin and emaciated, usually appears quite ill. The client's malnourished and debilitated state frequently leads to other deficiencies, for example, of iron, protein, minerals, and other vitamins. Some clients may also have an electrolyte imbalance and may develop neurologic symptoms as a result of thiamine, calcium, or magnesium deficiencies (problems frequently linked with alcoholism). Cirrhosis of the liver and bleeding varices further complicate anemia for the alcoholic client.

The megaloblastic anemia caused by folic acid deficiency is the same as that seen in pernicious anemia. It is diagnosed by blood smear and bone marrow examinations. On confirmation of macrocytic anemia, the physician must decide whether it results from folic acid or vitamin B_{12} deficiency. In folic acid deficiency, the serum folate level is less than 4 ng (normal is 7 to 20 ng); Schilling's test is normal; hydrochloric acid is probably present in the gastric juice; neurologic symptoms are absent; and the client responds favorably to a therapeutic trial of 50 to 100 μg of folic acid administered intramuscularly daily for 10 days.

For correction of anemia due to folate deficiency, the client receives oral doses of folic acid (0.1 to 5 mg) daily until the blood picture improves or until the cause of intestinal malabsorption is corrected. Clients with malabsorption syndromes may need parenteral folic acid initially, followed by maintenance therapy with oral doses.

Folic acid is administered intramuscularly in the form of folinic acid (Calcium Leucovorin injection). Additionally, vitamin C is sometimes prescribed because it increases the role of folic acid in promoting erythropoiesis.

ANEMIAS OF BONE MARROW FAILURE

Definition

The anemias of bone marrow failure have several names, each of which is descriptive of some aspect of the disease (aplastic, hypoplastic, regenerative, or primary refractory anemia). Aplastic anemia, the most commonly used term, describes bone marrow that is severely hypoplastic ("empty"), that is, devoid of erythroid, myeloid, and megakaryocytic cell lines. Hypoplastic bone marrow results in anemia, leukopenia, and thrombocytopenia. When all three cellular elements are suppressed, the condition is known as pancytopenia.

Incidence

Pancytopenia affects clients of all ages, and both sexes are equally susceptible. The incidence of aplastic anemia is about four cases per million population. Congenital aplastic anemia (Fanconi's anemia) usually occurs in childhood.

Etiology

In about one half of cases, the cause of aplastic anemia is unknown. Acquired aplastic anemia may result from either an autoimmune mechanism or a direct injury by myelotoxins. Three groups of myelotoxins are (1) agents that always cause marrow damage when received in sufficiently large doses, such as radiant energy (x-rays, radium, and radioactive isotopes of gold or phosphorus), benzene and its derivatives, alkylating agents, and antimetabolites used to treat malignant tumors; (2) agents that occasionally cause marrow failure, such as chloramphenicol (Chloromycetin, the drug most commonly linked with aplastic anemia), sulfonamides, quinacrine, phenylbutazone, the anticonvulsants diphenylhydantoin and mephenytoin, and gold compounds; and (3) agents that have been linked with aplastic anemia in only a few cases, such as streptomycin, tripelennamine, DDT, meprobamate, hair and aniline dyes, and carbon tetrachloride.

Risk Factors

Clients treated with the etiologic agents are at increased risk of developing aplastic anemia. If clients are receiving any of these agents, they must have their blood count monitored at frequent intervals.

Pathophysiology

The etiologic agents cause the bone marrow to stop producing blood cells when radiant energy inhibits mitosis, or cell division, and antimetabolites used in cancer therapy block the synthesis of purines or nucleic acids. Usually, however, the exact mechanism of marrow failure from these agents is unknown. Why certain drugs and chemicals cause pancytopenia in some clients and not in others also is mysterious. Current thought is that some clients are hypersensitive to certain agents, and the development of bone marrow failure in these cases is an idiosyncratic reaction.

The onset of aplastic anemia may be insidious or rapid. In idiopathic or hereditary cases, the onset is usually gradual. When bone marrow failure results from a myelotoxin, however, the onset may be explosive, with quickly developing symptoms. If the condition does not reverse itself when the offending agent is removed, the condition can prove to be fatal.

Clinical Manifestations

Symptoms of pancytopenia are particularly severe. Not only does the red blood cell count fall, but so do the leukocyte and platelet counts. The client consequently develops the following three conditions: normocytic anemia, granulocytopenia, and thrombocytopenia.

NORMOCYTIC ANEMIA

The red blood cell count is usually below 1 million/mm^3, with a low reticulocyte count. The client reports progressive fatigue, lassitude, and dyspnea.

GRANULOCYTOPENIA

The leukocyte count may be less than 2000/mm^3 (normal is 6000 to 9000/mm^3). The client, therefore, suffers from an increased susceptibility to infection, because without leukocytes, the body cannot adequately battle bacteria and other invading organisms. If the granulocyte count drops below 500/mm^3, the client may develop a fulminating bacterial infection.

THROMBOCYTOPENIA

The platelet count may fall below 20,000/mm^3 (normal is 150,000 to 450,000/mm^3), which usually causes bleeding into the skin and mucous membranes. If platelets are severely reduced, the client will hemorrhage.

DIAGNOSTIC ASSESSMENT

The diagnosis of aplastic anemia and pancytopenia is based on the differential blood count, the client's symptoms, history of exposure to a myelotoxin, and bone marrow examination. In pancytopenia, the bone marrow is fatty and contains very few developing blood cells.

Medical Management

The client with pancytopenia is often critically ill. Prompt medical attention and skillful nursing care are necessary. The first step in halting the process of aplastic anemia is immediate withdrawal of an offending agent or drug.

Any client undergoing radiotherapy or receiving a medication that is a suspected myelotoxin must be monitored for marrow failure by frequent hemograms. A significant drop in the red blood cell, leukocyte, or platelet count signals the need to stop the drug. Usually, stopping a suspicious agent is followed by a rise in the blood count. Unfortunately, chloramphenicol marrow failure may progress despite discontinuation of the drug.

If aplastic anemia develops from a suspected myelotoxic agent, blood transfusions are the mainstay of therapy until bone marrow activity signals recovery. If the marrow fails to recover and long-term red blood cell support is required, iron overload often results. This complication was a leading cause of death before iron chelating therapy became available.

Bone marrow transplantation is now the treatment of choice for aplastic anemia when (1) an autoimmune phenomenon is suspected or (2) the bone marrow fails to regenerate after discontinuation of myelotoxic agents. Currently, transplantation can take place only if the client has an HLA (human leukocyte antigen) identical donor.

Because the marrow of the aplastic client is so severely depressed, all transfusions of cellular blood components must be irradiated in order to inactivate lymphocytes and prevent transfusion-associated graft-versus-host disease (GVHD) (see Chap. 24).

Comparing the results of clients treated by bone marrow transplantation with conventional therapy of steroids and androgens reveals a 2-year survival rate of 60 to 80 per cent with bone marrow transplantation, whereas those treated conventionally had a 25 per cent survival rate.

PHARMACOLOGIC MANAGEMENT

Corticosteroids and androgens are sometimes prescribed to stimulate bone marrow activity; unfortunately, these drugs often fail to work as desired.

Nursing Management

Preventing and treating complications resulting from pancytopenia is of major importance in caring for the client with aplastic anemia. The two main complications of this anemia are infection and bleeding.

HEMOLYTIC ANEMIA

Major hallmarks of hemolytic anemia are

- a shortening of the red blood cell life span
- an abnormal increase in the number of red blood cells destroyed by macrophages
- failure of the bone marrow to replace destroyed red blood cells

Premature hemolysis of red blood cells results from either (1) an intracorpuscular defect within the erythrocyte itself, a defect that is sometimes triggered by an extracellular agent (e.g., drugs, plasma components, or splenic hyperactivity), or (2) an extracorpuscular factor (e.g., infections and chemical or physical agents).

Hemolytic anemia may be acute or chronic. Severe, acute episodes of hemolysis, known as hemolytic crises, punctuate some chronic forms of hemolytic anemia. The client with hemolytic anemia suffers from all the general manifestations of anemia discussed earlier (lassitude, fatigue). The specific signs and symptoms that characterize hemolytic anemia are listed and explained in Table 46-2. Renal failure may be a complication of severe hemolysis. It is caused by excretion of an increased load of red blood cell degradation products.

Laboratory findings indicative of hemolytic anemia usually include normocytic anemia, reticulocytosis due to increased efforts of the bone marrow to compensate for excessive erythrocyte destruction, increased red blood cell fragility, shortened erythrocyte lifespan, hyperbilirubinemia, increased fecal and urinary urobilinogen, and (in cases of massive intravascular hemolysis) hemoglobinemia.

Treatment for hemolytic anemia includes the following steps.

1. Pinpoint and eliminate, whenever possible, causative factors that precipitate episodes of hemolysis (e.g., infections, exposure to certain chemicals).
2. Maintain fluid and electrolyte balance.
3. Administer oxygen, because a decreased number of red blood cells may cause hypoxia.
4. Maintain renal function. In cases of severe hemolysis, infusions of either sodium bicarbonate or sodium lactate are administered to alkalize the urine.
5. Combat anemia and shock with the cautious administration of blood transfusions. Caution is necessary because the transfused cells will be rapidly destroyed in the presence of autoimmune hemolytic disease.
6. If corticosteroids fail to halt hemolytic reactions in autoimmune disorders, splenectomy is usually the treatment of choice.

The major extracorpuscular factors that cause hemolytic anemia include trauma, chemical agents and medications, infectious agents, systemic diseases, isoimmune reactions, and autoimmune disorders.

TABLE 46-2. Hemolytic Anemia: Assessment Data and Pathophysiologic Bases

Assessment Data	Pathophysiologic Bases
Jaundice	Accumulation of bilirubin within the blood due to excessive destruction of erythrocytes
Splenomegaly, hepatomegaly	Macrophages within the spleen and liver become hyperactive because of increased demands to phagocytize defective erythrocytes
Cholelithiasis (pigment gallstones)	Excessive accumulation of bilirubin within the gallbladder due to erythrocyte destruction

HEMOLYSIS DUE TO TRAUMA

When red blood cells are exposed to excessive turbulence in the circulation, they may fragment. Fragmented erythrocytes (schistocytes) are quickly destroyed by phagocytes, which results in anemia.

Hemolytic anemia may develop after external trauma or severe burns. In addition, hemolysis sometimes occurs after prosthetic cardiac valve replacement or cardiac septal defect repair.

Clinical findings include hemoglobinemia, hemoglobinuria, and a drop in the erythrocyte count. Treatment is directed toward correcting the underlying problem.

TOXIC HEMOLYTIC ANEMIA (HEMOLYSIS DUE TO CHEMICAL AGENTS AND MEDICATIONS)

Chemicals and medications can cause hemolysis. Hemolytic reactions are usually due to one of the following factors: the oxidant effects of the medication or chemical, or an immune reaction caused by the medication.

Chemical oxidants vary in their potency and in their ability to destroy red blood cells. Some mild chemical oxidants cause hemolytic reactions in only a small segment of the world population (e.g., clients with G6PD deficiency). Other very potent oxidants cause hemolytic reactions in every client exposed to a sufficient amount (e.g., benzene, phenylhydrazine, nitrites, potassium chlorate, arsenic, colloidal silver, and lead). These powerful compounds can damage the red blood cell membrane, resulting in a fragile cell that is quickly destroyed.

A common example of hemolysis due to contact with a chemical agent is lead poisoning (plumbism). Lead poisoning causes characteristic changes in the brain, nervous system, spinal cord, and digestive tract. Industrial workers who are daily exposed to lead vapors, mist, or dust may become victims of plumbism. Also, small children can develop lead poisoning when they are allowed to chew on furniture or windowsills covered with lead-based paint. Flakes of lead-based paint found in older, deteriorating buildings also are a hazard.

Between 1976 and 1980 in the United States, the mean blood lead level declined by about 35 per cent, apparently because of the decreased use of leaded gasoline, stricter controls in industry, and the growth of widespread screening programs. Nevertheless, researchers estimate that 1.5 million Americans are exposed to potentially dangerous levels of lead while on the job. Clinicians have also discovered that blood lead levels once thought safe and even normal are dangerous and result in many metabolic and neurologic disorders. A lead level higher than 40 μg/100 ml in adults and 25 μg/100 ml in children now is considered unsafe.

Treatment in this condition usually involves the administration of chelating agents such as calcium disodium edetate.

An immune response, the second major cause of toxic hemolysis, is the result of an antigen-antibody reaction (see Chap. 24). Medications that can precipitate antigen-antibody reactions in susceptible clients are quinine, quinidine, methyldopa, sulfonamides, phenacetin, and penicillin.

The most common example of an immune response to a drug is the "penicillin reaction." Penicillin is a potentially dangerous drug because it is a hapten. A hapten is a substance that is normally nonantigenic but can combine with a body protein. When penicillin combines with a body protein, the protein is modified so it can act as a foreign antigen. The body builds antibodies that react with the altered body protein in an antigen-antibody reaction. Because of the danger of triggering an immune response, always take a careful medication history before administering any medication (e.g., penicillin) that is a hapten.

Finally, certain snake and spider venoms as well as some vegetable poisons (e.g., some mushrooms) cause hemolytic reactions that frequently are fatal.

HEMOLYSIS DUE TO INFECTIOUS AGENTS

Bacterial endocarditis, malaria, miliary tuberculosis, infectious hepatitis, infectious mononucleosis, and meningococcemia may be complicated by hemolytic anemia. Infectious organisms can cause hemolytic anemia in three ways: (1) by releasing toxins that cause hemolysis; (2) by entering the red blood cell and destroying it; and (3) by promoting antigen-antibody reactions. For example, an organism may attach itself to the surface of a red blood cell, so altering it that it acts as a foreign antigen. In response, antibodies form against the altered red blood cells, and an immune reaction takes place.

SECONDARY HEMOLYTIC ANEMIA (HEMOLYSIS DUE TO SYSTEMIC DISEASES)

Hemolytic anemia sometimes complicates the following systemic conditions: Hodgkin's disease, leukemias, renal cortical necrosis, lymphomas, and systemic lupus erythematosus.

HEMOLYSIS DUE TO ISOIMMUNE HEMOLYTIC REACTIONS

An isoimmune hemolytic reaction is an antigen-antibody reaction that destroys red blood cells. The client develops antibodies in response to antigens from another individual of the same species. One example is a transfusion reaction due to ABO incompatibility. The most severe transfusion reactions involve the hemolysis of the donor's red blood cells by the recipient's antibodies. Erythroblastosis fetalis, a disorder of the newborn, is an example of a hemolytic isoimmune reaction resulting from incompatibility between the blood of an Rh-positive fetus and an Rh-negative mother.

HEMOLYSIS DUE TO AUTOIMMUNE DISORDERS

Autoantibodies, like isoantibodies, can destroy red blood cells. Unlike isoantibodies, they arise in response to autoantigens that have developed within the client's own body (see Chap. 24).

Autoimmune hemolytic anemia is a disorder of the immune mechanism in which the immune system produces antibodies that agglutinate the client's own red blood cells in an antigen-antibody reaction. As a result, the agglutinated cells clump together and are phagocytized within the spleen.

This condition arises in two ways. First, it may develop secondary to other autoimmune disorders or follow the administration of certain drugs. Autoimmune conditions such as systemic lupus erythematosus and the lymphoproliferative diseases (leukemia, lymphoma) are sometimes complicated by hemolytic anemia. Medications that can precipitate autoimmune hemolytic anemia include penicillin (which acts as a hapten), quinidine, quinine, and methyldopa.

Second, this disease can develop spontaneously without a history of prior autoimmune disease. This form, known as idiopathic autoimmune anemia, is characterized by a mild to moderate hemolysis; the red blood cells become coated with IgG antibodies that arise spontaneously or after ingestion of one of the above-mentioned medications.

The manifestations of autoimmune hemolytic anemia differ little from those of other hemolytic anemias. Profound, sporadic, and sometimes fatal hemolytic crises are common. Other complications include gallstones and thrombocytopenic purpura. Autoimmune hemolytic anemia is diagnosed by a positive direct antiglobulin test. The direct antiglobulin test detects whether the client's red blood cells are coated with antibodies.

Treatment for secondary autoimmune hemolytic anemia includes treating the underlying autoimmune condition and stopping the use of any suspicious medications. The idiopathic form of the disease is treated with steroids, transfusions, and splenectomy when indicated. The steroid of choice is prednisolone. Recently, clients refractory to steroids have been treated with immunosuppressive agents (e.g., cyclophosphamide and azathioprine) with some success.

Transfusion may give temporary relief from symptoms. However, special crossmatching is required because clients often have developed sensitivities to many blood antigens, and donor cells may be rapidly destroyed by the client's antibodies. Administer red blood cells slowly, and be aware of the chance of immediate transfusion reaction (see section on transfusion reactions).

Splenectomy is indicated if medications fail to produce a remission or if steroid therapy produces severe side effects. Once the spleen is removed, recurrences of hemolytic anemia may develop, but they are less severe and can be controlled with steroid therapy.

PAROXYSMAL HEMOGLOBINEMIAS

Paroxysmal hemoglobinuria is a rare but serious condition involving acute episodes of intravascular hemolysis that result in passing of hemoglobin into the urine.

Attacks of paroxysmal hemoglobinuria can be caused by sleep (paroxysmal nocturnal hemoglobinuria), exposure to cold temperatures (paroxysmal cold hemoglobinuria), and extreme exertions, as in marching for long distances (march hemoglobinuria).

Paroxysmal nocturnal hemoglobinuria (PNH), the most common of these three conditions, produces severe symptoms (e.g., jaundice, chronic fatigue, scleral icterus, and splenomegaly). In addition, the client's urine often has a dark brown or port wine hue after sleep. If hemoglobinuria continues for days or weeks, substantial iron losses eventually result in iron deficiency anemia.

Laboratory results in PNH include the following: red blood cell count indicating normocytic anemia, increased reticulocyte count, increased red blood cell fragility, and shortened lifespan; increased bilirubin; increased fecal and urinary urobilinogen; and bone marrow hyperplasia.

Treatment for PNH is symptomatic. Most clients with PNH eventually require blood transfusions. Donor red blood cells initially survive normally and suppress the production of the client's abnormal red blood cells, with resultant marked clinical improvement. After repetitive transfusions, however, alloimmunization is likely to occur, which makes further transfusion therapy difficult. If evidence of increased hemolysis follows transfusion of packed donor red blood cells, administration of washed or frozen red blood cells may stop this problem. Clients with iron deficiency anemia also receive iron.

The course of PNH is exceedingly variable. Clients experience waxing and waning hemolysis, which may be exacerbated by infection, transfusion, and immunization. Although a client with PNH may have a normal lifespan, debilitating attacks of hemolytic anemia can occur at any time. Many clients lead an active, normal life between attacks.

▼ Secondary Anemias

The secondary anemias, as the name implies, arise in association with other conditions, such as (1) chronic systemic diseases (e.g., rheumatoid arthritis, malnutrition, leukemia), (2) the lymphomas and multiple myeloma, (3) chronic infections (lung abscess, empyema, pelvic inflammatory disease), (4) acute and chronic renal disease complicated by uremia, (5) cirrhosis of the liver, (6) endocrine disorders (myxedema), and (7) cancer.

The anemia accompanying cancer results from chronic blood loss, cell hemolysis, or the development of space-occupying lesions within the bone marrow (myelophthisic anemia).

Although the cause of the secondary anemias varies

with the underlying condition, all have two factors in common: the red blood cells have a shortened lifespan, and the bone marrow fails to produce enough red blood cells to compensate for losses.

The anemia that develops in these conditions may be moderate to severe, depending on the underlying cause. Treatment involves correcting the underlying condition. Packed red blood cell transfusions are sometimes given when hemoglobin levels fall below 8 to 9 g/100 ml.

▼ Anemias Due to Excessive Blood Loss

ACUTE POSTHEMORRHAGIC ANEMIA

Definition

Acute posthemorrhagic anemia is a normocytic, normochromic anemia that develops after the rapid loss of red blood cells during a massive hemorrhage.

Etiology

Common causes of acute bleeding are severed blood vessels due to trauma, spontaneous rupture of an aneurysm, hemorrhagic disorders, and erosion of an artery by a cancerous growth or ulcerative lesion.

Pathophysiology

The adverse effects of acute hemorrhage result from a rapid decrease in blood volume and red blood cells; thereby, the oxygen-carrying capacity of the blood is reduced. The severity of symptoms of and the prognosis for acute hemorrhage depend on (1) the rate of bleeding, (2) the site of the hemorrhage, and (3) the volume of blood lost. A gradual loss of even a large amount of blood is usually less threatening than is the rapid loss of a smaller volume.

Clinical Manifestations

Signs and symptoms of acute blood loss are restlessness, dizziness, syncope, thirst, pallor, diaphoresis, rapid thready pulse, a dramatic drop in blood pressure, rapid deep respirations that later become shallow, and disorientation or coma that is indicative of cerebral anoxia.

In addition to these symptoms, internal hemorrhage into body organs and tissues causes fever, pain in the area of bleeding due to distention of tissues, and symptoms of organ displacement (e.g., hemothorax can result in a mediastinal shift). If internal or external hemorrhage remains uncontrolled, the blood pressure continues to drop, and hypovolemic shock develops (see Chap. 20).

DIAGNOSTIC ASSESSMENT

After hemorrhage, red blood cell count, hematocrit, and hemoglobin results may be high (although they are actually low) because of vasoconstriction and loss of plasma volume. These tests return to normal after infusion of intravenous fluid and restoration of intravascular volume from extracellular fluids.

ANEMIA DUE TO CHRONIC BLOOD LOSS

Definition

Anemia due to chronic blood loss is a chronic, microcytic, hypochromic anemia secondary to a chronic loss of blood.

Etiology

The major causes of chronic blood loss are bleeding peptic ulcers, prolonged or excessive menses, bleeding hemorrhoids, and cancerous lesions within the gastrointestinal tract.

Pathophysiology

The results of chronic bleeding are (1) continuous loss of small numbers of erythrocytes, usually replaced by the bone marrow, and (2) continuous loss of iron, which results in a total depletion of iron stores.

Because of this iron loss, the anemia of chronic bleeding closely resembles iron deficiency anemia. Correction of the anemia involves locating and controlling the site of bleeding and replacing iron with a proper diet and iron supplements.

Clinical Manifestations

Signs and symptoms of anemia due to chronic blood loss are the same as those associated with iron deficiency anemia. In mild cases of anemia, the client is asymptomatic. However, in more severe cases, assessment reveals the general symptoms of anemia (palpitations, dizziness, and sensitivity to cold).

Medical Management

Intravenous infusions of fluids, electrolytes, and packed red blood cells should be administered if symptoms of anemia cannot be managed with oxygen therapy, sedation, and rest. Oral fluids should be encouraged for maintenance of tissue hydration and renal perfusion.

PHARMACOLOGIC MANAGEMENT

Iron intake may be supplemented by the administration of ferrous sulfate (Feosol), 200 mg orally three times daily with meals.

DIETARY MANAGEMENT

A diet high in iron and protein is needed.

Surgical Management

Surgery may be needed to stop the chronic loss of blood.

Nursing Management

ASSESSMENT

Assessment of the client with either acute or chronic anemia due to blood loss usually shows pallor, diaphoresis, and coolness (integumentary); rapid, thready pulse and hypotension (cardiovascular); rapid, deep respirations, which later become shallow (respiratory); and restlessness, dizziness, syncope, severe headache, and disorientation (neurologic). Pain in the bleeding area is caused by tissue distention.

NURSING INTERVENTION

Nursing Diagnosis: Fluid Volume Deficit R/T blood loss.

Planning: Expected Outcomes. The client will maintain optimal fluid volume, as evidenced by absence of signs of hypovolemia such as hypotension, thirst, or decreased urine volume.

Implementation. General supportive measures, including fluid replacement and maintenance of adequate oxygenation and blood pressure, will be effective. Administer intravenous fluids and blood components as ordered. Measure intake and output, estimate blood loss, and increase oral fluid intake as tolerated. Monitor the complete blood count (CBC).

▼ Congenital Anemias

HEMOGLOBINOPATHIES (ANEMIAS DUE TO DEFECTIVE HEMOGLOBIN)

In abnormal hemoglobin synthesis, the globin portion of the hemoglobin molecule is defective. Any deviation in the polypeptide chain results in a disorder of hemoglobin synthesis.

Hemoglobinopathies are a group of conditions characterized by the formation of abnormal hemoglobin. Specifically, they result from abnormalities of the alpha and beta polypeptide chains in the globin molecule. Usually, the beta chains are defective. The abnormalities resulting in defective hemoglobin usually consist of minute variations in the amino acid residue sequence.

The three major forms of normal hemoglobin are hemoglobin A, hemoglobin A_2, and fetal hemoglobin (hemoglobin F). Ninety-seven per cent of normal hemoglobin is composed of hemoglobin A, and 2 to 3 per cent is hemoglobin A_2 and F. Variants of hemoglobin A number over 100, including hemoglobin C, D, E, G, H, I, J, K, L, M, N, O, P, Q, and S. Fortunately, most of these abnormal hemoglobins are not detrimental and cause neither anemia nor any symptoms.

In the United States, the only abnormal hemoglobins of consequence are hemoglobin S (sickle cell hemoglobin), hemoglobin C, and hemoglobin D. These forms of abnormal hemoglobin produce a mild disorder in clients who are heterozygous carriers of the trait (those who inherit the gene from only one parent) but cause a profound, sometimes fatal anemia in homozygous carriers (those who inherit the gene from both parents).

The only other abnormal hemoglobins (see section on congenital conditions for discussion of sickle cell anemia) that produce anemias of consequence within the United States are hemoglobin C and D. Homozygous hemoglobin C disease (Hb CC disease) occurs in 1 of every 6000 blacks. Two to 3 per cent of blacks carry the hemoglobin C trait only. Although their erythrocytes do not assume a sickle shape, clients with Hb CC disease suffer from a severe anemia accompanied by symptoms similar to those of sickle cell anemia. Clients who carry the trait (i.e., they have A-C hemoglobin) usually remain asymptomatic.

Treatment consists of relief of symptoms. Occasionally, blood transfusions are required.

S-C hemoglobin disease is more common than Hb CC disease because so many blacks are heterozygous carriers of the sickle cell trait. Manifestations of this condition include sicklemia, anemia, and splenomegaly. Hematuria, retinal hemorrhages, and aseptic necrosis of the femoral head may also be present.

Hb S-D disease is uncommon. Apparently, it affects all races alike. Symptoms are similar to those of sickle cell anemia but less severe.

THE THALASSEMIAS

Definition

The thalassemias are a group of inherited, chronic, hemolytic anemias.

Incidence

These anemias predominantly affect clients of Mediterranean or southern Chinese ancestry; they were first discovered among people living around the Mediterranean, hence the name *thalassos,* meaning "sea." Other names are Mediterranean anemia and Cooley's anemia. The thalassemias also affect American blacks and people from central Africa and southern Asia.

Etiology

The production of extremely thin, fragile erythrocytes called target cells characterizes the thalassemias.

Risk Factors

Clients from Mediterranean, central African, American black, southern Chinese, or southern Asian backgrounds are at risk for these inherited anemias.

Pathophysiology

The severity of the anemia produced by the thalassemias depends on whether the afflicted client is homozygous or heterozygous for the thalassemia trait. Thalassemia major and intermedia, both characterized by a profound anemia, appear in homozygotes. Thalassemia minor, characterized by a mild anemia, develops in heterozygotes.

Unlike the alpha and beta polypeptide chains in sickle cell anemia, the polypeptide chains in the thalassemias are completely normal in structure but insufficient in number because of a genetic alteration.

Either alpha or beta chains can be affected by diminished synthesis. In alpha-thalassemia, alpha-chain synthesis slows. In beta-thalassemia, beta-chain synthesis diminishes. Because beta-thalassemia is more common, it is called classic thalassemia, or simply thalassemia.

The outlook for clients with thalassemia major is usually poor. Children are retarded in their growth and development. Many fail to live through puberty. Thalassemia minor, on the other hand, does not affect life expectancy.

Clinical Manifestations

The symptoms of thalassemia major resemble those of other hemolytic anemias (e.g., jaundice, cholelithiasis, leg ulcers, and enlarged spleen). In addition, thalassemia is characterized by a pronounced bone hyperactivity that causes a thickening of the cranium and a mongoloid appearance or facies.

Thalassemia minor is usually asymptomatic, except for a mild anemia. Blood smears of clients with this condition contain small, defective red blood cells.

DIAGNOSTIC ASSESSMENT

Laboratory findings in thalassemia (beta form) include the following: target cells (abnormally thin, fragile cells) and other bizarrely shaped red blood cells appear in the circulation; the serum bilirubin and fecal and urinary urobilinogen are elevated because of the severe hemolysis of abnormal cells; an elevated fetal hemoglobin is present, in some cases as high as 90 per cent; and elevated Hb A (a normal variant of Hb A), as high as 6 per cent instead of the normal 1.5 to 3 per cent, is found.

The high percentages of Hb F and HbA_2 result from the decrease in beta chains characteristic of this anemia. The bone marrow compensates by producing abnormally large numbers of alpha chains, gamma chains (normally made only during fetal life), and delta chains. Fetal hemoglobin (Hb F) results from the combination of alpha and gamma chains. Hb A_2 results from the combination of alpha and delta chains.

Medical Management

Transfusion therapy is the only treatment available. Clients with thalassemia major receive packed red blood cells, which may be given (1) on a monthly or bimonthly basis (regular transfusion regimen), (2) whenever the hemoglobin falls below 3 to 4 g/100 ml (nonsystemic transfusion), or (3) every 15 days to maintain the hemoglobin at 12 to 15 g/100 ml (hypertransfusion regimen). When it becomes clear that transfused cells are being rapidly destroyed by the spleen (causing a severe hemolytic anemia), splenectomy is necessary.

Because clients with thalassemia must receive many transfusions, they can develop an iron overload, which may eventually cause myocardial hemosiderosis and cardiac arrhythmias. Excessive iron can be somewhat removed from the blood by chelating agents such as deferoxamine.

Thalassemia minor is usually so mild that treatment is not required. However, clients who carry the thalassemia trait need genetic counseling.

▼ Hemolytic Anemias Due to Intrinsic Red Blood Cell Defects

GLUCOSE-6-PHOSPHATE DEHYDROGENASE DEFICIENCY

Definition and Etiology

Glucose-6-phosphate dehydrogenase (G6PD) is an important red blood cell enzyme. G6PD deficiency can be classified as an enzymopathy, a genetic defect that involves the partial or complete deficiency of certain essential enzymes.

Risk Factors

A deficiency of G6PD makes red blood cells more susceptible to hemolysis after ingestion of medications and foods classified as chemical oxidants.

Incidence

An inherited sex-linked disorder, G6PD deficiency is a common problem affecting at least 100 million people in the world. Among Americans, G6PD deficiency affects about 20 per cent of blacks and about 1 to 2 per cent of whites. It is common among Sephardic Jews, Greeks, Italians, and Arabs.

Pathophysiology

G6PD helps use about 10 per cent of the glucose metabolized by red blood cells. When exposed to oxidative medications and foods, red blood cells require even more glucose for energy. If a G6PD deficiency exists, the red blood cells cannot adequately metabolize more glucose and so cannot cope with the oxidative effects of certain substances. As a result, hemolysis occurs. Because young, newly released red blood cells contain a large amount of G6PD, only aging red blood cells are destroyed upon exposure to oxidative agents.

Clinical Manifestations

Clients with this enzymopathy may remain completely asymptomatic throughout their lives. Typically, symptoms develop only after a stressor, such as viral or bacterial infection or certain medications or toxins. Occasionally, however, spontaneous attacks of hemolytic anemia develop that are not precipitated by a known external factor.

More than 40 oxidative medications and foods produce hemolytic anemia in clients with G6PD deficiency (e.g., primaquine, quinine, aspirin, sulfonamides, phenacetin, vitamin K derivatives, chloramphenicol, thiazide diuretics, and the fava bean). After exposure to any of these agents, the client with G6PD deficiency develops acute intravascular hemolysis lasting about 7 to 12 days. During this acute phase, the client suffers from anemia and jaundice.

DIAGNOSTIC ASSESSMENT

Laboratory findings include moderate hemoglobinemia and hemoglobinuria, an elevated serum bilirubin, reticulocytosis, and the appearance of Heinz bodies (small particles of oxidized hemoglobin) within the red blood cell. After the acute hemolytic stage, the blood picture begins to improve whether the offending drug is stopped or not. The hemolytic reaction is self-limiting, because only older red blood cells in contact with a chemical oxidant are destroyed. However, if drug exposure continues for a long period, the client will develop chronic hyperhemolysis until contact with the offending agent ceases.

Medical Management

Correcting the anemia primarily involves identifying and removing the medication or food precipitating the hemolytic reaction. Care of the client during the week of acute hemolysis is purely symptomatic (rest, fluids, and nutritious diet).

Because medications that precipitate hemolytic reactions in G6PD deficiency are common (e.g., aspirin), and because G6PD has a high worldwide incidence, screening tests for this enzymopathy should be a part of every public health program. Careful screening is particularly important for the black population. Tests performed during hemolytic episodes may be falsely negative owing to the increased proportion of young red blood cells.

HEREDITARY SPHEROCYTOSIS (CONGENITAL HEMOLYTIC JAUNDICE, CONGENITAL SPHEROCYTIC ANEMIA)

Definition, Incidence, and Etiology

Hereditary spherocytosis is a common form of chronic hemolytic anemia found in all races and ages. A simple mendelian dominant trait, spherocytosis can be inherited even if only one parent carries the abnormal gene. In about 20 per cent of cases, hematologic abnormalities are absent in other family members, which suggests that a spontaneous mutation in the client caused the illness.

Pathophysiology

The two most distinctive characteristics of hereditary spherocytosis are (1) the appearance of large numbers of spherical red blood cells (spherocytes) and (2) an enlarged spleen. Spherocytosis develops because the red blood cells have a defective cellular membrane that is extremely permeable to the influx of sodium ions. To curtail the flow of sodium ions through its defective membrane, the red blood cell must increase its metabolic work and, so, its use of glucose.

When glucose and cellular energy become depleted, sodium ions flow through the cellular membrane without resistance. Thus, the red blood cell interior becomes hypertonic; water is drawn into the cell, which causes the red blood cell to swell and become spherical. Spherocytes, thick and rigid, are easily trapped within the splenic venous sinusoids, where they are devoured by phagocytes. As a result, the spleen becomes enlarged, and the client suffers from anemia and jaundice because of the massive red blood cell hemolysis within the spleen.

Clinical Manifestations

Symptoms of hereditary spherocytosis are the same as symptoms of hemolytic anemia discussed earlier (e.g., malaise, mild anemia, jaundice, gallstones, and splenomegaly). Splenomegaly is particularly pronounced, and clients may experience left upper quadrant fullness and abdominal pain. In the presence of systemic infection, the hemolytic rate may increase, inducing further splenic enlargement. Occasionally, acute abdominal pain results from splenic infarction. Such severe hemolytic crises are sometimes fatal.

DIAGNOSTIC ASSESSMENT

Laboratory findings are distinctive and include spherocytes in the blood smear; reticulocytosis; lowered red blood cell count and hemoglobin values; positive direct antiglobulin test; and increased osmotic fragility.

Osmotic fragility is increased (greater than 0.5 per cent) because the spherocyte, already swollen and hypertonic, cannot tolerate a further influx of water, and it ruptures quickly when placed in hypotonic saline solutions.

Surgical Management

Although blood transfusions may benefit a client in hemolytic crisis, the only treatment indicated in all cases of hereditary spherocytosis is splenectomy. Ninety per cent of clients who undergo splenectomy experience complete reversal of symptoms. Although spherocytes continue to circulate, these misshapen cells usually have a longer lifespan once the spleen is removed.

Nursing Management

ASSESSMENT

See each section under anemia for the appropriate assessments.

NURSING INTERVENTION

Collaborative Problem. Iron overload R/T chronic infusion of iron through red blood cell transfusions.

Planning: Expected Outcomes. The nurse will recognize potential for iron overload, as evidenced by implementation of preventive therapy and monitoring of treatment compliance.

Implementation. Monitor for signs of iron overload by performing routine assessment of cardiac status and observing for symptoms of liver dysfunction, diabetes related to pancreatic malfunction, and thyroid insufficiency. Because there is no effective means for removal of the iron stores causing these complications, the primary goal is early detection, treatment of symptoms, and prevention.

The nurse must teach the client the importance of iron chelation therapy, which will prevent this complication. An opportune time for routinely assessing treatment compliance is during periodic clinic visits for red blood cell transfusions. Referrals to home health care agencies and other groups who may help with financial aide and emotional support may also be appropriate.

Collaborative Problem. Alteration in oxygen-carrying capacity of blood R/T anemia.

Planning: Expected Outcomes. The client will have maintained adequate organ oxygenation, as evidenced by limiting activities or by receiving supplemental agents to enhance red blood cell function, production, or replacement.

Implementation. The nurse will administer blood according to policy and teach indications and possible side effects (see section on blood transfusions). Instruct the client in the cause of anemia, preventive and treatment measures, diet therapy, and proper administration of iron supplements and their effect on stools. Provide oxygen therapy if ordered. Pace activities and schedule rest periods to prevent fatigue.

Nursing Diagnosis: Tissue Perfusion, Altered R/T deficit or malfunction of red blood cells.

Planning: Expected Outcomes. The client will experience optimal peripheral tissue perfusion, as evidenced by warm, pink extremities; adequate pulses noted in extremities; and no complaints of tingling or numbness.

Implementation. Monitor for signs of oxygen deprivation: increased pulse and respirations, decreased blood pressure, and shortness of breath. Report symptoms immediately to the physician and start appropriate medical support. Keep the extremities warm to prevent vasoconstriction. Bathe the client in warm, *not* hot, water.

Nursing Diagnosis: Nutrition, Altered: Less than Body Requirements R/T anorexia, stomatitis, knowledge deficit, and inability to get proper foods (physical/financial problems).

Planning: Expected Outcomes. The client will maintain proper nutrition, as evidenced by maintenance of or increase in the body weight and improved intake of proper nutrients.

Implementation. Assess the client's usual diet and eating pattern. Make referrals when necessary (e.g., social worker, dietician, home health care aide). Provide symptom management for the anorexia. Administer vitamin B_{12} and other medication as ordered. Encourage a diet high in iron, protein, and vitamins.

Nursing Diagnosis: Individual Coping, Ineffective, High Risk for R/T chronic status of disease.

Planning: Expected Outcomes. The client will cope effectively with the chronic nature of the illness, as evidenced by client's statements and demonstration of effective coping behaviors such as maintaining usual activities and ability to establish positive relationships.

Implementation. Provide the client with opportunities to express concerns, fears, feelings, and expectations. Encourage the client to develop realistic goals and activity levels. Instruct the client in the need for rest periods and adequate diets. Collaborate with the client to establish follow-up appointments that enable the client to lead a more normal life. Use other resource persons such as support systems, clinical specialists, social workers, and psychiatric liaison personnel.

EVALUATION

The nurse must evaluate client outcomes on the basis of the established plan of care. If these goals have not been achieved, the plan and interventions must be revised to meet the client's needs.

Modification of Plan of Care for the Elderly

The nursing care plan for the aged client should include consideration of problems related to poor dentition, economic constraints, and lack of interest in food preparation.

Post-hospital Care

DISCHARGE TEACHING

The client will need to be taught about the particular type of anemia and the implications of that disease. Commonly, the client will need to learn about a diet high in iron, protein, folic acid, and other elements essential to the improved production of red blood cells.

FOLLOW-UP CARE

The client will need to be followed at regular intervals to have the CBC checked.

▼ Polycythemias (Overproduction of Red Blood Cells)

Polycythemia is defined as an increase in both the number of circulating erythrocytes and the concentration of hemoglobin within the blood. Red blood cells may number as high as 8 to 12 million/mm³, and the hemoglobin concentration rises to 18 to 25 g/100 ml.

POLYCYTHEMIA VERA

Definition/Incidence

Polycythemia vera is classified as a myeloproliferative disorder (meaning overgrowth of bone marrow). It usually develops in middle age, particularly among Jewish men.

Etiology

Although the precise cause remains unknown, it is possibly a form of malignancy similar to leukemia and is often considered a premalignant condition.

Pathophysiology

The three major hallmarks of the condition are (1) relentless, unrestrained production of erythrocytes; (2) production of excessive myelocytes (leukocytes within the bone marrow); and (3) overproduction of platelets.

Clinical Manifestations

The inordinate mass production of these three cell lines results in the following pathologic consequences: (1) an increase in the blood viscosity; (2) an increase in the total blood volume, which may be twice or even three times greater than normal; and (3) severe blood congestion of all tissues and organs. Because of these problems, the client suffers many symptoms.

Diagnostic Assessment

Laboratory findings include red blood cell count as high as 8 to 12 million/mm³; hemoglobin level of 18 to 25 g/100 ml; hematocrit level greater than 54 per cent in men and greater than 49 per cent in women; platelet count usually increased in polycythemia vera; normal arterial blood gases; hyperplastic bone marrow; and serum uric acid three to four times normal.

SECONDARY POLYCYTHEMIA

When the body's demand for oxygen increases for any reason, the bone marrow must produce more red blood cells in order to prevent tissue hypoxia. This compensatory response to tissue hypoxia is called secondary polycythemia.

Hypoxia that is sufficiently prolonged to cause polycythemia results from chronic lung disease (particularly emphysema), congenital heart disease, and prolonged exposure to altitudes of 10,000 feet or more. People who live in mountainous areas are not hypoxic because their blood has "thickened." These mountain dwellers produce high numbers of red blood cells, which increases the oxygen-carrying capacity of their blood and enables them to live at an altitude that would incapacitate a newcomer.

The symptoms and laboratory findings for clients with secondary polycythemia are the same as those for clients with polycythemia vera, except the white blood cell and platelet counts are normal and splenic enlargement is absent.

RELATIVE POLYCYTHEMIA

Whenever the body loses plasma without losing red blood cells, the concentration of red blood cells increases relative to the amount of plasma remaining in the vascular system. Some causes of relative polycythemia are fluid loss and dehydration as a result of not enough fluid intake, diarrhea, vomiting, burns, and excessive administration of diuretics.

Medical Management

POLYCYTHEMIA VERA

The goals of care in polycythemia vera are twofold: (1) reduction of blood volume and viscosity and (2) reduction of bone marrow activity. These are accomplished through phlebotomy, the administration of myelosuppressive agents, and radiation therapy.

Phlebotomy. Emergency treatment involves removing 500 to 2000 ml of blood until the hematocrit reaches 45 per cent. Once the hematocrit has been reduced, subsequent phlebotomies should be carried out as frequently as necessary for maintaining the hematocrit at about 45 per cent. As iron deficiency supervenes, red blood cell production will be retarded, so that clients managed by phlebotomy alone may require as few as two or three phlebotomies a year.

Myelosuppressive Agents. These include administration of radioactive phosphorus, which sometimes produces remissions that last from 6 months to 2 years (see Chap. 22). Other drugs useful for combating polycythemia are chlorambucil, busulfan, and hydroxyurea.

Radiation Therapy. Radiation therapy may be used to decrease the production of red blood cells in the marrow.

Thrombotic complications claim the lives of about 30 per cent of those affected with polycythemia vera; another 10 to 15 per cent die from hemorrhage. Finally, for obscure reasons, about 15 per cent die from either myelogenous leukemia or myelofibrosis accompanied by pancytopenia. Prognosis depends on age at diagnosis, treatment used, and complications.

SECONDARY POLYCYTHEMIA

Medical management for secondary polycythemia involves treating the underlying disease or condition causing hypoxia.

RELATIVE POLYCYTHEMIA

Treatment simply involves the reestablishment of fluid and electrolyte balance.

Nursing Management

ASSESSMENT

In its early stages, polycythemia usually remains asymptomatic (increased hematocrit level may be an incidental finding). However, as altered circulation secondary to increased red blood cell mass leads to hypervolemia and hyperviscosity, the client may complain of a feeling of fullness in the head, dizziness, headache, tinnitus, visual disturbances, and other symptoms, depending on the body system affected. Symptoms include ruddy complexion and dusky, red mucosa (integumentary); hypertension (with dizziness, headache, and a sense of fullness in the head) and congestive heart failure (shortness of breath, orthopnea), which causes increased clotting leading to cerebrovascular accident, myocardial infarction, or peripheral gangrene; bleeding (hemorrhage in capillaries, venules, and arterioles), which causes rupture of vessels (cardiovascular function); enlargement of liver and spleen, peptic ulcer (gastrointestinal function); and gout (painful swollen joints, usually big toe) secondary to increased uric acid (skeletal).

NURSING INTERVENTION

Nursing Diagnosis: Tissue Perfusion, Altered R/T hypervolemia and hyperviscosity.

Planning: Expected Outcomes. The client will experience optimal peripheral tissue perfusion, as evidenced by warm, pink extremities; adequate pulses noted in extremities; and no complaints of tingling or numbness.

Implementation. Administer medications as prescribed. Monitor vital signs and breath sounds. Notify the physician immediately if any signs of a thrombotic event are present. For reducing the blood viscosity, encourage intake of oral fluids. Monitor intake and output. Administer anticoagulants as ordered and monitor for signs of bleeding. Monitor blood studies. For preventing the development of thrombi from circulatory stasis, encourage the client to ambulate if possible, elevate the feet when seated, and wear support hose. Turn bedridden clients frequently, and provide passive exercise to their extremities. Caution clients undergoing phlebotomy to avoid foods high in iron (clams, oysters, liver, legumes), because a high iron intake somewhat counteracts the therapeutic effects of phlebotomy.

EVALUATION

The nurse must evaluate client outcomes on the basis of the established plan of care. If these goals have not been achieved, the plan and interventions must be revised to meet the client's needs.

▼ DISORDERS AFFECTING WHITE BLOOD CELLS

White blood cells (leukocytes) are divided into two groups: granulocytes (polymorphonuclear leukocytes) and agranulocytes (mononuclear cells). Granulocytes, in turn, are divided into three groups: neutrophils, basophils, and eosinophils. The three names derive from the color of these cells after staining.

Agranulocytes include lymphocytes (B and T) and monocytes. Plasma cell, or plasmacyte, is another name for B lymphocyte. Plasma cells, formed within the bone marrow and lymph nodes, are probably the primary producers of immunoglobulins (antibodies). Pathologic conditions involving plasma cells are called plasma cell dyscrasias.

Major defects that affect leukocytes and plasma cells are (1) the leukemias, acute and chronic; (2) agranulocytosis; and (3) multiple myeloma (plasma cell myeloma).

▼ The Leukemias

Definition

Leukemia is a malignant disease of the blood-forming organs.

Incidence

Leukemia accounts for 8 per cent of all human cancers and is the most common malignancy in children and young adults. One half of all leukemias are classified as acute, with rapid onset and progression of disease resulting in 100 per cent mortality within days to months without appropriate therapy. The remaining leukemias are classified as chronic, which have a more indolent course.

Etiology

Although the exact cause of leukemia is unknown, there are several host factors associated with leukemia. These include exposure to radiation and chemicals, congenital abnormalities (i.e., Down syndrome), presence of primary immune deficiency, and infection with the human leukocyte virus HTLV-1.

Acute leukemia is caused by the neoplastic proliferation of large numbers of abnormal, immature leukocytes in the bone marrow that infiltrate the lymph nodes, liver, spleen, and eventually all body systems. In addition, the production of other blood cells (i.e., red blood cells, platelets, neutrophils) is inhibited by a mechanism not clearly understood, which results in inadequate oxygen transport, thrombocytopenia, and immune system malfunction (Fig. 46-2).

The French-American-British (FAB) Cooperative Group has developed a system for classifying acute leukemias based on morphologic characteristics and the percentage of immature cells in the bone marrow (Table 46-3).

For the leukemic process to be termed acute, at least 50 per cent of the marrow cells must be immature. Acute leukemias are most common in children aged 2 to 4 years. The incidence declines by age 8, then rises again among clients age 65 years and over.

Chronic leukemias have a gradual onset and a more protracted course than do the acute forms. In some cases, the client lives for 5 or more years, with or without treatment. The white blood cells produced are more mature and thus can better defend the body against invading microorganisms. Chronic leukemia occurs in clients between the ages of 25 and 60 years.

Risk Factors

Overexposure to radiation is a major risk factor for the development of leukemia, often years after the initial exposure. Alkylating agents used to treat other cancers, especially in combination with radiation therapy, also increase the client's risk for the development of leukemia. Care in the client's exposure to radiation can help decrease the risk.

Pathophysiology

ACUTE LEUKEMIA

There are two major forms of acute leukemia: *lymphocytic leukemia,* which involves the lymphocytes and lymphoid organs; and *nonlymphocytic leukemia,* which involves hematopoietic stem cells that differentiate into myeloid cells: monocytes, granulocytes, erythrocytes, and platelets.

From these two broad categories, leukemias are further classified according to the specific malignant cell line. Ninety per cent of acute leukemia is acute lymphoblastic leukemia (ALL), caused by the malignant proliferation of precursor lymphocytes called lymphoblasts. ALL presents most often in children 2 to 10 years of age. Advances in therapy during the last several decades have significantly improved the chances for remission and even a cure. However, the prognosis for clients with ALL is less favorable if any of the following factors exist:

- presentation in younger or older age groups
- male sex
- high leukocyte count (over 100,000) at time of diagnosis
- central nervous system involvement
- chromosomal abnormalities
- some cell subclass types (i.e., T-cell ALL, pre-B cell ALL)

ALL was one of the first human cancers to be cured by combination chemotherapy.

Acute nonlymphocytic leukemia (ANLL, formerly known as acute myelogenous leukemia or AML) is characterized by aberrations in the growth of megakaryocytes, monocytes, granulocytes, and erythrocytes. Typically, however, aberrations in one cell type predominate. The most common type of ANLL involves maturational arrest and proliferation of cells in the myeloblastic and monoblastic stages of development. The prognostic factors are less clearly defined in ANLL, and long-term prognosis is usually poor. Bone marrow transplantation is currently the best treatment option.

CHRONIC LEUKEMIA

Chronic leukemia is classified as chronic myelogenous leukemia (CML) or chronic lymphocytic leukemia

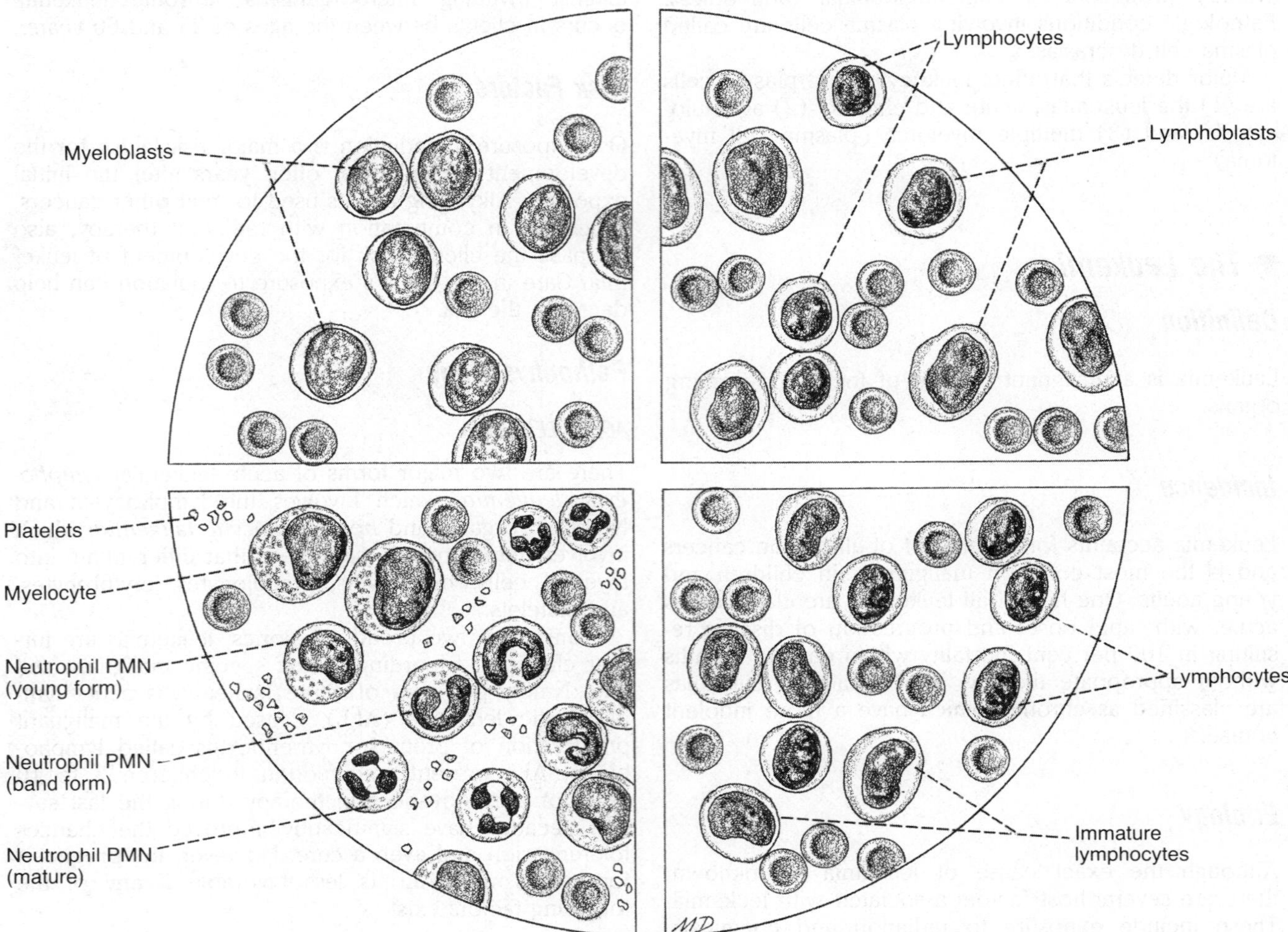

▲ *Figure 46-2*

Types of leukemia: a comparison.

TABLE 46-3. FAB Classification of Acute Leukemia

Acute lymphocytic leukemia	
L1	Common childhood leukemia
L2	Adult ALL
L3	Rare subtype, blasts resembling those in Burkitt's lymphoma
Acute myeloblastic leukemia	
Granulocytic	
M1	Myeloblastic leukemia without maturation
M2	Myeloblastic leukemia with maturation
M3	Hypergranular promyelocytic leukemia
Monocytic	
M4	Myelomonocytic leukemia
M5	Monocytic
Erythroid	
M6	Erythroleukemia

(CLL). CML originates in the pluripotent stem cell (see Fig. 45-2). Initially, the marrow is hypercellular with a majority of normal cells. Typically, the peripheral blood smear reveals leukocytosis and thrombocytosis. There is increased production of granulocytes. Ninety per cent of the time, examination of the bone marrow cells during metaphase shows a chromosome translocation called the Philadelphia chromosome. After a relatively slow course for a median of 4 years, the client with CML invariably enters a blast crisis that resembles acute leukemia (Fig. 46-3).

CLL is a form of leukemia characterized by the proliferation of early B lymphocytes. CLL is an indolent form of leukemia most often seen in men over 50 years of age. It is also the only leukemia with a possible genetic predisposition. It is usually discovered when the CBC is performed as part of a routine physical examination. A peripheral blood smear reveals increased

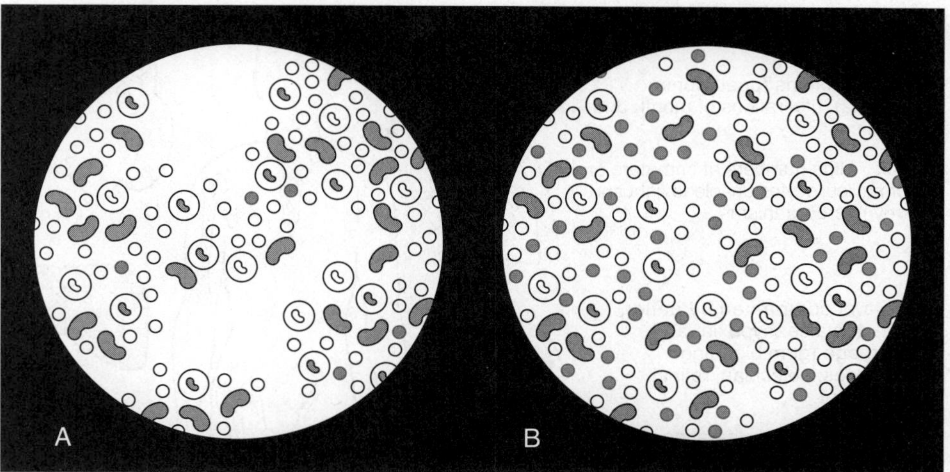

▲ *Figure 46–3*

A, This microscopic view of a normal bone marrow specimen shows a normal distribution of blood cell types and fatty spaces. Blast cells appear as round, black circles. *B*, During blast crisis, the number of blast cells increases, and fatty spaces shrink.

number of both mature and slightly immature lymphocytes.

As the disease progresses, lymphocytes infiltrate the lymph nodes, the liver, the spleen, and ultimately the bone marrow. A staging system has been developed that correlates stage with the extent of lymphocyte infiltration. Progression of the disease may take as long as 15 years.

Blast crisis results in the death of more than 70 per cent of clients with CML. During this phase, increasing numbers of blasts (immature myeloid precursor cells, especially myeloblasts, the most primitive granulocyte precursors) proliferate in the blood and bone marrow. Blast crisis is diagnosed when blasts and promyelocytes (another myeloid cell precursor type) exceed 20 per cent in the blood and 30 per cent in the marrow. Increased fibrotic tissue in the marrow is another sign of blast crisis. Leukopenia, thrombocytopenia, and anemia are also evident. Death usually occurs within 6 months of onset.

Clinical Manifestations

The signs and symptoms of all types of leukemia are similar. The clinical history will usually reveal symptoms characteristic of anemia, thrombocytopenia, and leukopenia. Clients often complain of fatigue, weakness, easy bruising, bleeding gums, epistaxis, fever, headache, and generalized pain. In some types of leukemia (most frequently CML), the client may have the feeling of abdominal fullness and early satiety as a result of splenomegaly. On physical examination, pallor, scattered petechiae and ecchymoses, generalized lymphadenopathy, hepatosplenomegaly, bone and joint pain, and fever may be found. Assessment data for leukemia with the pathophysiologic basis can be found in Figure 46–4.

DIAGNOSTIC ASSESSMENT

A comprehensive evaluation of all body systems is necessary for establishing the treatment plan. Tests most often included in the initial evaluation are CBC values, bone marrow aspiration, lumbar puncture, radiographic tests, and lymphangiograms.

CBC Values. CBC values vary greatly. The total white blood cell count may be normal, abnormally low (less than 1000/mm^3), or extremely high (greater than 200,000/mm^3). The differential may reveal that one type of leukocyte is overwhelmingly predominant. There may be abnormal leukocytes, including immature blast forms, noted on the peripheral smear. The platelet count and hemoglobin level are usually low.

Bone Marrow Aspiration. Bone marrow aspiration or biopsy is a key diagnostic tool for confirming the diagnosis and identifying the malignant cell type. If an adequate sample of marrow cannot be obtained by aspiration, a fragment of bone can be removed for a bone marrow biopsy. Typical findings on the bone marrow aspirate and biopsy are an overall increase in the number of marrow cells with an increase in the proportion of earlier forms.

Lumbar Puncture. Lumbar puncture determines the presence of blast cells in the central nervous system; 5 per cent of cases present with this abnormality.

Radiographic Tests. Radiographic tests may include radiographs of the chest and skeleton; magnetic resonance imaging and computed tomographic scans of the head and body detect lesions and sites of infection.

Lymphangiogram. Lymphangiogram or lymph node biopsy may be performed to locate malignant lesions and accurately classify disease.

The treatment of all classifications of leukemia is targeted at destroying neoplastic cells and maintaining a sustained remission. During each phase of therapy, the medical treatment may vary, but the basic nursing principles are the same.

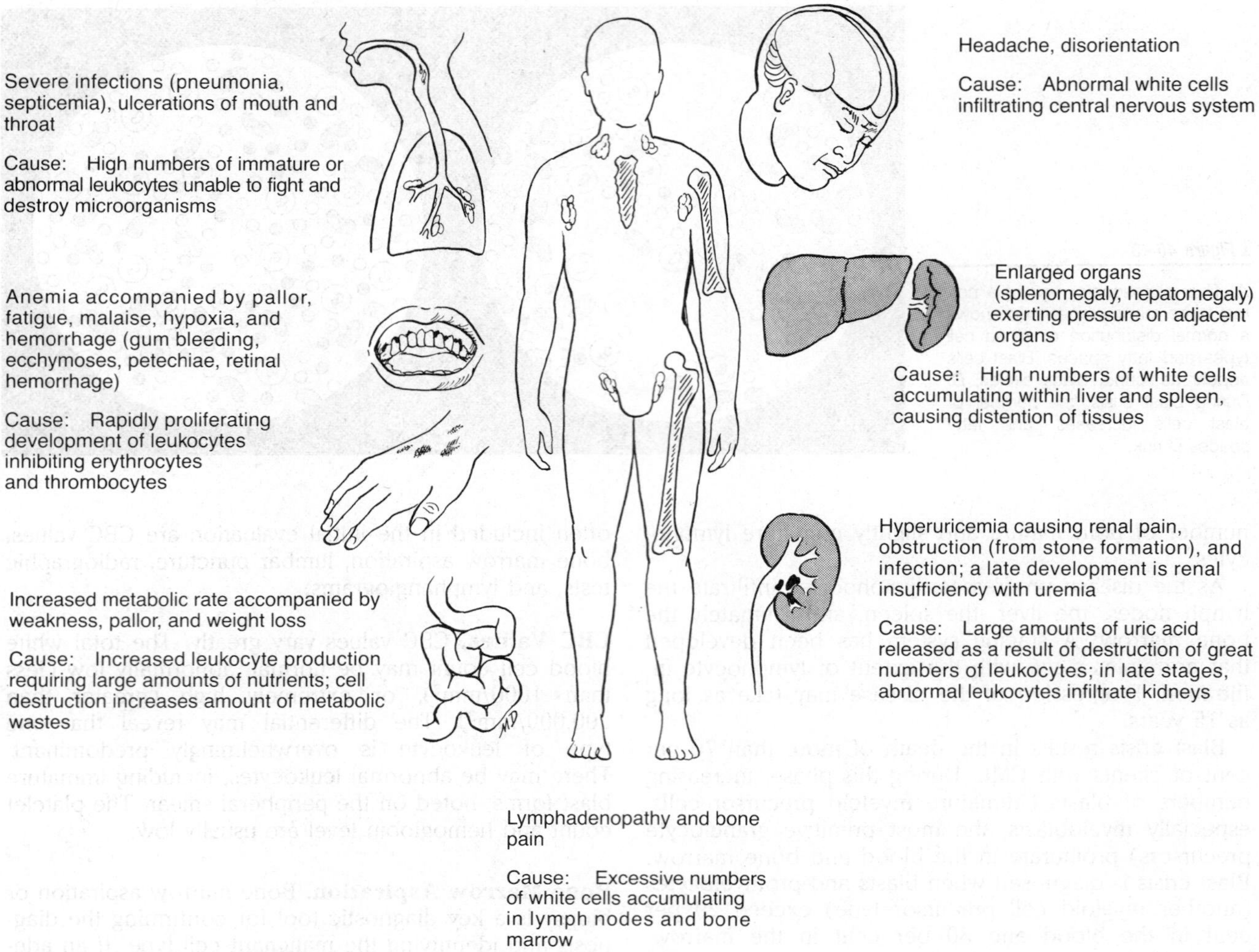

Severe infections (pneumonia, septicemia), ulcerations of mouth and throat

Cause: High numbers of immature or abnormal leukocytes unable to fight and destroy microorganisms

Headache, disorientation

Cause: Abnormal white cells infiltrating central nervous system

Anemia accompanied by pallor, fatigue, malaise, hypoxia, and hemorrhage (gum bleeding, ecchymoses, petechiae, retinal hemorrhage)

Cause: Rapidly proliferating development of leukocytes inhibiting erythrocytes and thrombocytes

Enlarged organs (splenomegaly, hepatomegaly) exerting pressure on adjacent organs

Cause: High numbers of white cells accumulating within liver and spleen, causing distention of tissues

Hyperuricemia causing renal pain, obstruction (from stone formation), and infection; a late development is renal insufficiency with uremia

Cause: Large amounts of uric acid released as a result of destruction of great numbers of leukocytes; in late stages, abnormal leukocytes infiltrate kidneys

Increased metabolic rate accompanied by weakness, pallor, and weight loss

Cause: Increased leukocyte production requiring large amounts of nutrients; cell destruction increases amount of metabolic wastes

Lymphadenopathy and bone pain

Cause: Excessive numbers of white cells accumulating in lymph nodes and bone marrow

▲ **Figure 46-4**

Leukemia: assessment data and pathophysiologic bases.

Medical Management

ACUTE LEUKEMIA

The treatment plan for leukemia is determined by disease classification, presence or absence of prognostic factors, and disease progression.

Radiation therapy may be administered as an adjunct to chemotherapy when leukemic cells infiltrate the central nervous system, skin, rectum, and testes or when a large mediastinal mass is noted at diagnosis (as may occur in ALL).

Current treatment modalities for acute leukemia destroy both normal and aberrant cells. Therapy is aimed at preventing and resolving complications of acquired and induced pancytopenia, which are anemia, bleeding, and infection. Transfusions of red blood cells and platelets are required until the marrow can produce mature ones.

Reduced exposure to microorganisms helps prevent infection, but laminar flow rooms and reverse isolation have minimal benefits. The client must be watched closely for signs of infection, which may be inhibited because of the severely compromised state of the immune system. Therefore, broad-spectrum antibiotics and antifungals must be started at the first signs of infection.

It is important to note that if the client requires intravenous infusions of red blood cells and amphotericin B, an antifungal agent, they should be separated by at least 1 hour so that serious pulmonary complications are prevented.

CHRONIC MYELOGENOUS LEUKEMIA

The goal of therapy in the chronic phase of CML is to control leukocytosis and thrombocytosis. Leukapheresis may be performed to lower an extremely high peripheral leukocyte count quickly and prevent acute tumor lysis syndrome, but results are temporary. Likewise, thrombocytosis as high as 2 million may require plateletpheresis. Apheresis is usually performed with use of automated blood cell separators designed to selectively remove the desired blood element and return remaining cells and plasma to the client (Fig. 46-5). If painful

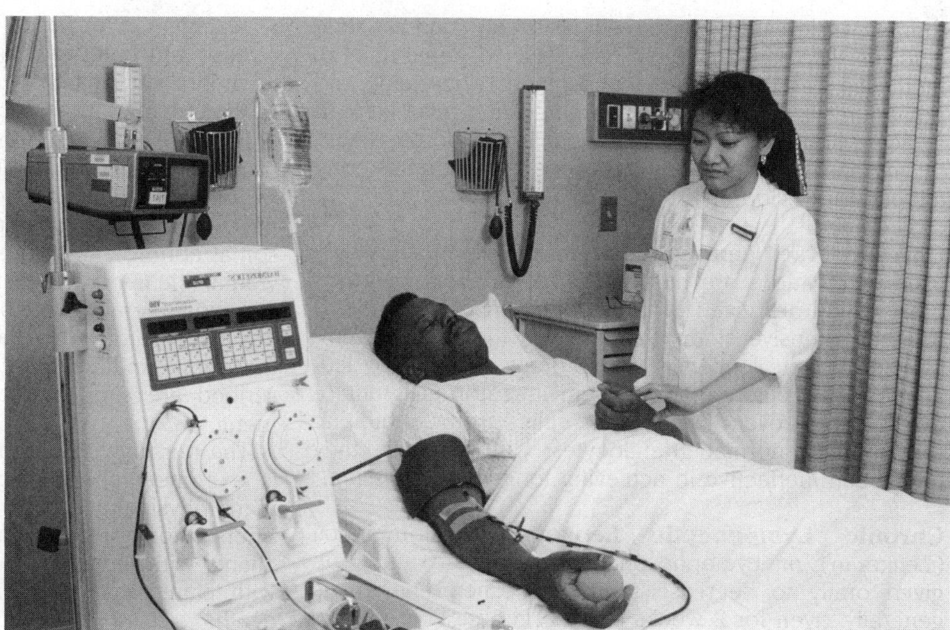

▲ *Figure 46–5*

The white blood cell level can be temporarily lowered by leukapheresis. Several automated blood cell separators effectively remove large numbers of white cells and return red cells and plasma to the client. The Haemonetics V50 is a cell separator commonly used to perform this procedure.

splenomegaly develops, irradiating or removing the spleen relieves this symptom.

CHRONIC LYMPHOCYTIC LEUKEMIA

The goal of therapy in CLL is palliation. Total body irradiation or local radiation to the spleen may also be given as a palliative treatment to reduce complications. Two complications seen during later stages are hemolytic anemia due to autoimmune disorder and hypogammaglobulinemia that further increases susceptibility to infection. Antibiotics, transfusions of red blood cells, and injections of gamma globulin concentrates may be required for these clients.

PHARMACOLOGIC MANAGEMENT

Acute Leukemia. The treatment protocol for acute leukemia involves three phases: induction, consolidation, and maintenance.

Induction. During the induction phase, the client receives an intensive course of chemotherapy designed to induce a complete remission of the disease. The usual criteria for complete remission are less than 5 per cent of the bone marrow cells are blast cells and peripheral blood counts are normal. Both conditions must be sustained for at least 1 month. Once remission is achieved, the consolidation phase begins.

Consolidation Phase. During the consolidation phase, modified courses of intensive chemotherapy are given to eradicate any remaining disease.

Maintenance Phase. During the maintenance phase, small doses of different combinations of chemotherapeutic agents are given every 3 to 4 weeks. This phase may continue for a year or more and is, therefore, structured to allow the client to live as normal a life as possible.

Table 46–4 lists the various chemotherapeutic agents used to treat leukemia. Note that these drugs are also used in the treatment of Hodgkin's disease and other lymphomas.

If the white blood cell count is high when chemo-

TABLE 46–4. Chemotherapeutic Agents Commonly Used to Treat Leukemia

Type of Leukemia	Agent
Acute nonlymphocytic	Cytarabine in combination with 6-thioguanine or mercaptopurine; with vincristine, prednisone, and cyclophosphamide; with daunorubicin and 6-thioguanine; or with doxorubicin or daunorubicin
Acute lymphocytic	Vincristine, prednisone, L-asparaginase, cyclophosphamide, and daunorubicin
Chronic lymphocytic	Chlorambucil, prednisone, cyclophosphamide, and vincristine
Chronic myelogenous	Busulfan, hydroxyurea, cytosine arabinoside, daunorubicin, methotrexate, prednisone, vincristine, and L-asparaginase
Hairy cell	Chlorambucil, zorubicin, cytarabine, cyclophosphamide, and large-dose methotrexate with folinic acid–SF (leucovorin) rescue

therapy is initiated, rapid cell lysis can increase uric acid in the blood, which can lead to renal failure; increased levels of serum phosphate, uric acid, and potassium; and decreased serum calcium. This can lead to acute tumor lysis syndrome, which can be prevented by increasing intravenous hydration and administering allopurinol (Zyloprim).

Chronic Myelogenous Leukemia. The most widely used medications are busulfan (Myleran) and hydroxyurea, which are given orally. A blast crisis (Fig. 46–3) requires intensive chemotherapy with those agents employed in acute leukemia. These drugs can destroy leukemic blast cells, transform them into normal granulocytes, or prevent leukemic cells from inhibiting formation of normal granulocytes. Unfortunately, they have been ineffective in achieving long-term remission.

Chronic Lymphocytic Leukemia. Chlorambucil (Leukeran) or cyclophosphamide (Cytoxan) may be given orally to decrease symptoms. Chemotherapy is generally given for 2 weeks of every month (i.e., on the medication for 2 weeks and off the medication for 2 weeks). When anemia (stage III) and thrombocytopenia (stage IV) develop, daily oral prednisone is given as an adjunct to the alkylating agents. Prednisone has a marked lymphocytolytic effect and may stimulate the production of red blood cells and platelets.

Surgical Management

ACUTE LEUKEMIA

Bone marrow transplantation presents a treatment option for clients under about 40 years of age who have a suitable HLA-matched donor. Studies indicate that transplant performed during the first remission has a higher success rate than does transplant performed during repeat remissions or the blast phase of chronic leukemia. See Chapters 22 and 24 for a detailed discussion of this aggressive form of therapy.

CHRONIC MYELOGENOUS LEUKEMIA

Bone marrow transplantation before blast crisis offers the best treatment option.

CHRONIC LYMPHOCYTIC LEUKEMIA

Splenectomy is an option if marked splenomegaly and thrombocytopenia present a serious risk of hemorrhage.

Nursing Management

ASSESSMENT

Nursing care for leukemia focuses on

- obtaining a thorough health history to aid in diagnosis and treatment
- recognizing, preventing, and treating complications of ablative chemotherapy and radiation therapy
- teaching in order to increase understanding of disease and compliance with treatment
- supporting psychosocial needs of clients with a life-threatening illness

It is imperative to obtain a thorough health history from the client and family members. A family history of exposure to chemical toxins (e.g., benzene and arsenic), viral infection (Epstein-Barr, HTLV-1), chromosomal abnormalities, use of medications such as phenylbutazone and chloramphenicol, chemotherapy, or radiation therapy may provide key information regarding the type of leukemia. The severity and longevity of the signs and symptoms of leukemia previously described are also important facts to obtain and document.

The nursing role during the acute phases of leukemia is extremely challenging because the client will have many physical and psychosocial needs. Modern therapy offers hope for remission and possibly cure for some clients with leukemia, but it is still a diagnosis equated with pain, expensive long-term therapy, and potential death.

NURSING INTERVENTION

Collaborative Problem. Sepsis, high risk for R/T neutropenia or leukocytosis secondary to leukemia or treatment.

Planning: Expected Outcomes. The health care team will prevent infection or will diagnose infection early and treat it effectively, as evidenced by neutrophil count greater than $1000/mm^3$, no evidence of fever or respiratory difficulty, and decrease of symptoms and increase of neutrophil count with treatment.

Implementation. The nurse should institute good handwashing technique for everyone coming in contact with the client. The client should be in a private room with reverse isolation or laminar flow if the neutrophil count is less than $500/mm^3$. Visitors with possible communicable diseases should be limited.

The client should be on a low-bacteria diet that excludes raw fruits and vegetables. The nurse should assist the client with a daily bath using antimicrobial soap. The client, or nurse if the client is unable, should practice meticulous oral hygiene several times a day.

Female clients should douche per physician orders and avoid the use of tampons. Daily stool softeners are ordered to reduce the risk of anal fissures. Rectal suppositories, rectal temperatures, and other invasive procedures should be avoided whenever possible.

The nurse should provide meticulous skin decontamination before venipunctures. Maintain sterile occlusion of central venous catheters and perform routine dressing care according to institutional policy. Intravenous tubing should be changed daily.

Oral temperature should be taken every 4 hours and the physician notified of a temperature over 38° C (100° F). Assess the cause of fever before initiation of therapy by obtaining cultures of blood, urine, central line sites, and other potential sources of infection. Administer antibiotics as ordered. Therapy usually consists of multiple broad-spectrum antibiotics administered intravenously on alternating schedules. Administer antipyretics as ordered for relief of discomfort, avoiding aspirin if the client is thrombocytopenic.

Monitor the client closely for signs and symptoms of fungal or viral infections (i.e., increased respirations, rales, dyspnea, changed oral mucosa). Monitor respiratory rate and auscultate breath sounds regularly. Viral and fungal pneumonia is a common cause of death in the neutropenic client (also see Bridge to Home Health Care).

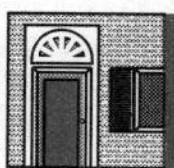

BRIDGE TO HOME HEALTH CARE

The Immunosuppressed Client

Bridging the care of the immunosuppressed client from the hospital environment to that of the home is a challenge. However, the home environment can often be safer and easier to control than that of the hospital and provides the client with a feeling of participation rather than isolation. Identifying sources of infection and practicing infection control in the home can allow the immunosuppressed client to remain independent.

The importance of good personal hygiene must be stressed for both the client and family members for preventing spread of infection. Handwashing before preparing or eating meals and after elimination must be practiced by all family members. Use of antibacterial soap is preferred. Daily bathing and good oral hygiene should also be stressed. Use of a soft toothbrush and lotion will prevent skin complications.

Diet and exercise must also be monitored closely. A balanced diet that is high in protein will promote the client's ability to fight infection and increase energy levels. Activity must also be balanced with periods of rest for avoiding fatigue and lowered resistance. Fresh fruits and vegetables that harbor bacteria must also be avoided. All meat must be cooked for removal of microorganisms.

The home environment must also be altered to eliminate sources of infections. Contact with family and friends should be monitored, and those who are infectious should be avoided; small children are a particular concern. Crowds are a common source of infection, and if one must go out in public, a mask should be worn.

Animals including household pets carry many types of germs. Although the family pet need not be removed from the home, close contact should be avoided. Animal licks, bites, and scratches are all sources of infection. Care of the family pet should be assigned to a family member other than the client. Birdcages, litter boxes, and fish tanks all harbor bacteria.

Additional sources of bacteria in the home include standing water, such as that found in fish tanks, flower vases, plants, and humidifiers. The presence of these items in the home should also be avoided; however, if they are present, changing the water daily is recommended. In the case of furnaces and air conditioners, the filters should be changed weekly.

The last and perhaps most important responsibility of the home health care nurse is to teach the family members to recognize the signs and symptoms of infection and report them to the health care team.

Collaborative Problem. Bleeding, high risk for R/T thrombocytopenia secondary to either leukemia or treatment.

Planning: Expected Outcomes. Bleeding as a result of injuries such as falls, punctures, cuts, or other environmental hazards, will be prevented or will be diagnosed and treated successfully, as evidenced by absence of bleeding and platelet count greater than 30,000/mm³.

Implementation. Institute bleeding precautions:

- Use cotton swabs or sponges for oral hygiene, avoiding flossing or hard toothbrushes.
- Instruct the client to avoid blowing or picking the nose, straining at bowel movements, douching or using tampons, or using razors.
- Do not give any injections, intramuscularly or subcutaneously, or insert rectal suppositories.
- Do not give aspirin or medications containing aspirin. Instruct the client not to take these products.
- Avoid catheters whenever possible. If catheters must be inserted, lubricate them well and insert them gently. Avoid mucosal trauma during suctioning.
- Pad the bed rails and remove all hazards and sharp objects from the environment.
- Use an air mattress and turn the client frequently to avoid pressure areas. Use bed cradles to protect extremities.
- Avoid overinflation of the blood pressure cuff and rotate cuff to different sites. Avoid prolonged use of tourniquets.
- Use only paper tape, avoiding all strong adhesives.

The client and significant others should be taught to institute bleeding precautions during periods of thrombocytopenia.

Monitor the client every 4 hours for signs of bleeding, such as ecchymoses, petechiae, epistaxis, gingival bleeding, hematuria, occult positive stools, enlarged abdominal girth, disorientation, confusion, and changes in level of consciousness. All urine, stool, and emesis should be tested for blood. The nurse should routinely take and record vital signs, noting symptoms of altered tissue perfusion related to anemia (increased respirations and pulse; decreased blood pressure).

Check the platelet count, hemoglobin level, and hematocrit daily. Report hemoglobin level of less than 10 g/100 ml and platelet count of less than 20,000/mm³. Administer packed red blood cells and platelet concentrates as ordered. Keep a current blood sample in the laboratory for crossmatching if needed in an emergency.

Nursing Diagnosis: Nutrition, Altered: Less than Body Requirements R/T gastrointestinal tract effects of radiation therapy and chemotherapy.

Planning: Expected Outcomes. The client will maintain body weight and adequate nutritional status, as evidenced by stable weight, adequate caloric intake, and maintenance of fluid and electrolyte balance.

Implementation. Administer antiemetics as ordered for nausea and vomiting. Premedicate the client before meals to encourage food and fluid intake. Administer local and intravenous analgesics as ordered to relieve pain caused by mucositis. Allow the client to make food selections. Small, frequent feedings may be tolerated better than three large meals a day. Monitor weight daily. If the client cannot tolerate food for an extended period, begin total parenteral nutrition as ordered and monitor intake.

Nursing Diagnosis: Body Image Disturbance R/T alopecia, weight loss, and fatigue.

Planning: Expected Outcomes. The client will not develop disturbance of body image, as evidenced by client's understanding of disease condition and temporary nature of changes in body image and energy.

Implementation. Inform the client of the potential for hair loss before treatment. Encourage the use of scarves, hats, or wigs as desired. Explain the temporary nature of alopecia, although the hair may be a different color or texture when it returns.

Encourage the client to balance rest with exercise and activities so that muscle tone can be maintained without the client's developing severe fatigue. Discuss daily dietary requirements with the client and provide high-carbohydrate meals and oral supplements.

Nursing Diagnosis: Sexual Dysfunction, High Risk for R/T effects of chemotherapy or radiation therapy on reproductive organs.

Planning: Expected Outcomes. The client will understand the potential for sterility that may result from therapy, as evidenced by client's ability to state outcomes from therapy and the effect on sexuality.

Implementation. Describe to the client the normal cellular destruction that might lead to temporary or permanent destruction of reproductive functions. Inform the client that sexual libido will not be altered after the acute phase of the illness. Provide the client with emotional support and references to support groups. In appropriate cases, inform the client of reproductive alternatives, such as sperm banking and artificial insemination.

Nursing Diagnosis: Individual Coping, Ineffective, High Risk for R/T denial of terminal prognosis.

Planning: Expected Outcomes. The client will cope effectively with the potentially fatal prognosis, as evidenced by appropriate verbalization of fears and concerns and maintenance of effective communication with significant others.

Implementation. Offer the client the opportunity to discuss fears and concerns about the disease process and potentially fatal prognosis. Use other members of the health care team (clergy, social workers) to provide emotional support throughout the disease process. Include significant others in client education and care. Inform the client of support groups, financial aid resources, and other sources of assistance.

EVALUATION

The nurse must evaluate client outcomes on the basis of the established plan of care. If these goals have not been achieved, the plan and interventions must be revised to meet the client's needs.

Modification of Plan of Care for the Elderly

Elderly clients, as stated earlier, are more prone to chronic leukemia. The use of chemotherapy is less vigorous than with acute leukemia. Bone marrow transplantation is not an option with the elderly client.

Post-hospital Care

After the induction phase of therapy has been successfully completed, the client frequently returns home to recover and await subsequent courses of therapy that may be given on an outpatient basis if no serious complications arise. It is not uncommon, then, for clients to return home with anemia and thrombocytopenia. They may also suffer from residual effects of chemotherapy or radiation therapy such as loss of appetite, nausea, and mucositis. Most clients find it difficult to leave the hospital setting because of a significantly altered body image.

DISCHARGE TEACHING

The client and significant others should be taught how to recognize symptoms of complications as well as appropriate actions. It is imperative that they are well informed of measures to ensure safety and reduce risks of bleeding and infection.

HOME HEALTH CARE NEEDS

Discharge planning for clients with these complex needs should include many members of the multidisciplinary team such as nutritionists, home health care agencies, clergy, and cancer support groups.

FOLLOW-UP CARE

The client will be closely followed at regular intervals for many years after treatment in order to monitor for exacerbation of the leukemia. Clients undergoing bone marrow transplantation will also need follow-up care for the variety of complications that may occur, such as premature cataracts or reproductive failure.

BONE MARROW TRANSPLANTATION

In the last 25 years, bone marrow transplantation has progressed from a treatment of last resort to a viable therapeutic modality for a variety of hematologic, malignant, and nonmalignant disorders. Whereas the basic procedures involved in transplantation are well established, many of the techniques used to purify bone marrow to decrease complications and improve prognosis are still investigational.

Indications

Bone marrow transplant may be considered the treatment of choice for clients with the following conditions:

- aplastic anemia
- malignant disorders, specifically leukemia (certain types of acute, chronic, and preleukemic states), lymphoma, multiple myeloma, neuroblastoma, and selected solid tumors (metastatic breast cancer, small cell lung cancer, advanced ovarian cancer, poor-risk germ cell tumors)
- nonmalignant hematologic disorders, such as Fanconi's anemia, thalassemia, and sickle cell anemia
- immunodeficiency disorders, such as severe combined immunodeficiency disease and Wiskott-Aldrich syndrome

Bone Marrow Harvesting

HISTOCOMPATIBILITY TESTING

Immunologic recognition of the differences in HLA antigens is the first step in host transplant rejection. As described in Chapters 23 and 24, the HLA system antigens are a complex set of protein structures found on the surface membrane of all human nucleated cells, solid tissues, and circulating blood cells except red blood cells. This genetically inherited mixture of antigens is considered representative of the tissue type of each client.

Siblings have a one in four chance of having identical sets of HLA antigens. This would provide the optimally matched allogeneic bone marrow donor. Because of the complexity of the HLA system, nonrelated clients have less than a 1 in 5000 chance of having identical HLA types. The establishment of the National Bone Marrow Donor Registry in 1987 has given hope to many clients who do not have a compatible relative donor. More than 100,000 donors have now been typed as potential bone marrow donors for unrelated clients who require transplant.

SOURCES OF BONE MARROW

There are three classifications of bone marrow donors: allogeneic, syngeneic, and autologous.

Allogeneic Bone Marrow. Allogeneic bone marrow is obtained from a relative or unrelated donor having an identical HLA type. This has been the most common type of marrow transplant, but it has the highest rate of morbidity and mortality because of complications of incompatibility such as GVHD (see later).

Syngeneic Bone Marrow. Syngeneic marrow is donated by an identical twin. Although syngeneic marrow is a perfect HLA match, which eliminates the risks of marrow rejection, the incidence of leukemic relapse is higher than when an allogeneic donor is used.

Autologous Bone Marrow. Autologous marrow is removed from the intended recipient during the remission phase to allow another course of ablative therapy to be given if a relapse occurs. Whereas autologous marrow eliminates the risk of adverse immunologic responses such as GVHD and graft rejection, relapse after autologous bone marrow transplant is a frequent occurrence. This may be due to contamination of the harvested bone marrow by malignant cells. Techniques to purge residual tumor cells from marrow (chemotherapy, monoclonal antibodies) are currently under investigation.

DONOR PREPARATION

An extensive work-up is performed for ensuring compatibility and the mental and physical well-being of the prospective donor. This evaluation includes histocompatibility testing, medical history and physical examination, chest film, electrocardiogram, laboratory evaluation (CBC, chemistry profile, viral testing, RPR [syphilis], ABO and Rh, coagulation studies, cytomegalovirus status), and psychological evaluation (may include psychiatric consultation).

Before marrow harvest, an informed consent, including potential donor complications (pain, fever, hematoma), must be obtained. In rare instances, the donor may experience serious adverse effects of general anesthesia. Because of the significant loss of red blood cells during the harvesting process, syngeneic and allogeneic donors are required to donate autologous blood before the procedure.

MARROW COLLECTION

The donor is given general or spinal anesthesia in the operating room. The marrow is obtained in 2- to 5-ml aliquots from the marrow spaces of the posterior and, occasionally, anterior iliac crests and sternum. Only two to three skin punctures are required; the aspiration needle is redirected to various marrow spaces without being withdrawn (Fig. 46–6). A total of 400 to 800 ml of marrow is obtained. The blood is placed in heparinized tissue culture media and filtered for removal of fat and bone particles. Marrow can be infused immediately or frozen in a solution containing dimethyl sulfoxide (DMSO), which preserves stem cells in the frozen state.

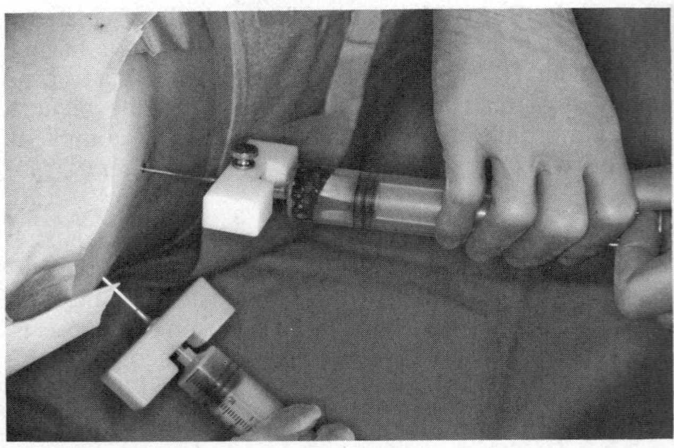
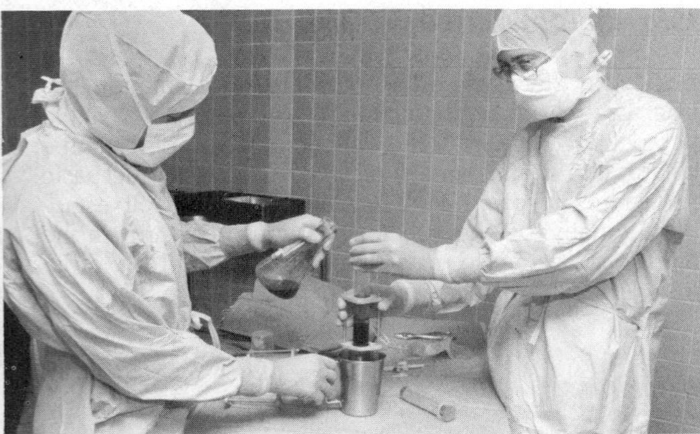

▲ Figure 46-6

Bone marrow aspiration for bone marrow transplant. *A*, Aspiration. *B*, Collection and preservation of marrow.

The Transplant

RECIPIENT PREPARATION

The physical and psychological evaluation of the recipient is similar to that of the donor. Additional testing may be required to stage existing disease accurately. The recipient must receive immunoablative therapy before transplant. This serves three purposes: malignant cells are destroyed; the immune system is inactivated, which thereby reduces the risk of GVHD; and the marrow cavities are emptied to provide space for implantation of the transfused stem cells.

Common protocols combine total body irradiation and very high doses of a single chemotherapeutic agent or fractionated doses of multiple agents. A small catheter is inserted to provide suitable access for marrow infusion as well as for antibiotics, blood products, hyperalimentation, and frequent blood sampling.

BONE MARROW INFUSION

The infusion of the marrow is often anticlimactic after the client has undergone the rigorous preparatory chemotherapy and radiation therapy. The marrow is usually administered immediately after the conditioning regimen is complete. Marrow is administered from a large blood infusion bag equipped with a standard blood filter. Small volumes may also be prefiltered and given by intravenous push by a physician.

Potential immediate adverse reactions are allergic (urticaria, chills, fever), volume overload, and pulmonary complications secondary to fat emboli. The period immediately after transplant is critical. Multisystem failure related to the ablative therapy is common, as are immune reactions caused by the transplanted cells.

The most common and potentially disastrous complication of bone marrow transplant is GVHD, which may occur acutely 7 to 30 days after the infusion of viable lymphocytes. The exact mechanism of GVHD is not clearly understood, but it appears that T lymphocytes from the donor attack and destroy vulnerable host cells. Once the engrafted cells mount this immune response against the host, little can be done to alter the course. The most likely organs to be affected are skin, gut, and liver. Acute GVHD is staged according to the organ system affected. Maculopapular rash involving less than 25 per cent of the body surface, moderate increase in liver function studies, and mild gastrointestinal symptoms are classified as stage I. This occurs in the majority of allogeneic transplant clients. Stage II to stage IV are classified by increasing degrees of erythema with bullous formation and desquamation, hepatic coma, and more than 200 ml of stool per day. These clients seldom recover because there is no effective therapy for severe GVHD. Localized skin involvement may resolve without treatment. Systemic complications may be treated with immunosuppressive drug therapy.

Chronic GVHD, a long-term form of the disease with less acute symptoms, may occur even if the client has not experienced acute GVHD. Chronic GVHD resembles autoimmune collagen vascular disorders, such as systemic lupus erythematosus. It is characterized by scleroderma-like skin fibrosis and Sjögren's syndrome, in which the mucosa and lacrimal ducts are abnormally dry.

Diagnosis of chronic GVHD is confirmed by skin and oral mucosal biopsy. Chronic GVHD appears approximately 100 days after transplantation; it may affect the liver, gastrointestinal system, oral mucosa, and lungs as well as the skin.

Whereas severe GVHD is usually fatal, researchers believe that a complete absence of this immune reaction increases the risk of leukemic relapse. This may be due to a beneficial graft-versus-leukemic reaction that mild GVHD stimulates. Studies are in progress for determining the number of T cells that must be purged from the marrow to reduce the risk of severe GVHD but not destroy the antileukemic effects of mild disease.

Nursing Management

The client will remain pancytopenic until the transplanted stem cells make their way to the medullary cavities, where subsequent growth and reconstitution of the marrow are confirmed. Indications of successful engraftment are an increase in platelets and red blood cells in the peripheral blood count. This may occur as early as 14 days after marrow infusion. Each day that recovery is delayed places the client at added risk. Graft rejection is evident if the bone marrow fails to produce peripheral blood cells after several weeks.

Nursing management of bone marrow transplant clients follows the plan of care for any completely immunosuppressed client. In addition, those receiving allogeneic transplant must be closely observed for signs of GVHD. Because no therapy effectively prevents or treats this complication, nursing care focuses on symptom management, pain relief, and emotional support.

AGRANULOCYTOSIS

Definition

Agranulocytosis (granulocytopenia, malignant neutropenia) is an acute, potentially fatal blood dyscrasia characterized by profound neutropenia. Neutropenia is a reduction in the number of circulating neutrophils. Because neutrophils make up roughly 93 per cent of all granulocytes, the terms neutropenia and agranulocytosis are often used interchangeably.

Incidence

Agranulocytosis is a fairly rare condition. For unknown reasons, women are much more susceptible to this condition than are men. However, even among females, agranulocytosis is relatively rare.

Etiology

The most common cause of agranulocytosis is drug toxicity or hypersensitivity. Two groups of agents are capable of suppressing granulocyte production:

- agents that always produce neutropenia when given in sufficiently large doses over time, such as many cancer chemotherapeutic agents, ionizing radiation, and benzene
- agents that produce neutropenia only in clients particularly sensitive to the drug, such as tranquilizers (chlorpromazine), antithyroid agents (propylthiouracil), anticonvulsants (phenytoin), antibiotics (chloramphenicol), and phenylbutazone

Agranulocytosis can occur in clients who have anemias related to diminished erythropoiesis (such as aplastic anemia, megaloblastic anemia). It may also accompany certain diseases, such as tuberculosis, typhoid fever, malaria, and uremia.

Risk Factors

Exposure to any of the etiologic factors increases the client's risk of developing agranulocytosis. Avoidance of these agents, whenever possible, helps prevent the development of the condition.

Pathophysiology

Agranulocytosis results either from the failure of neutrophil production to keep pace with destruction of the cells or from increased destruction of neutrophils, which removes them from circulation. Chemotherapy, radiation, and aplastic anemia all decrease or stop neutrophil production through interference with granulopoiesis.

Accelerated destruction of the neutrophils can result from infection, autoimmune disease, and idiosyncratic reactions to many drugs. The destruction may be so rapid that production can not keep up with it.

Agranulocytosis may reverse when the cause is removed, or the client will require a bone marrow transplant for survival.

Clinical Manifestations

The symptoms of agranulocytosis result from the neutropenia. Neutrophils constitute a swift and powerful defense against invading microorganisms. Consequently, decreases in their number result in a greater susceptibility to bacterial invasion, especially when the client's white blood cell count drops below 500/mm^3. The mucous membranes of the throat and mouth are particularly vulnerable.

Typically, the onset of this acute disease is rapid. For the first 2 or 3 days, there is severe fatigue and weakness. Next, the client develops a sore throat, ulcerations of the pharyngeal and buccal mucosa, dysphagia, high fever, weak and rapid pulse, and severe chills. Without prompt antibiotic treatment, the disorder usually causes death within a week.

DIAGNOSTIC ASSESSMENT

Diagnosis of agranulocytosis rests on the following:

- leukopenia evidenced by white blood cell counts of 500 to 3000/mm^3 with extreme reduction in polymorphonuclear cells (0 to 2 per cent)
- bone marrow examination revealing an absence of granulocytes, a maturational arrest of young developing cells, or an increased number of myeloid precursors (signifying peripheral granulocyte destruction)
- cultures of the urine, blood, and ulcerative lesions in the throat and mouth that are positive for bacteria (usually gram-positive cocci)
- a history of exposure to an offending agent, plus all the above findings. Because many clients medicate themselves with potentially dangerous drugs, investigate all drugs taken within the past 6 to 12 months.

Medical Management

Treatment for clients with agranulocytosis involves eliminating potentially toxic agents that may be responsible for marrow suppression. Agranulocytosis caused by toxic substances usually reverses within 2 to 3 weeks after their elimination.

Surveillance cultures of blood, throat, sputum, urine, and stool should be taken at frequent intervals for monitoring the status of infections.

Granulocyte transfusions may be done if the client develops antibiotic-resistant sepsis. Lymphocyte and monocyte infusions are under investigation for the treatment of immune diseases and genetic disorders. Once removed from the client or an HLA-matched donor (preferably an identical twin), the cells are treated or altered and then reinfused.

PHARMACOLOGIC MANAGEMENT

Pharmacologic treatment includes antimicrobial therapy in the event of positive cultures, fever, or signs and symptoms of impending shock. Combinations of broad-spectrum antibiotics are usually administered until the offending organism is identified. Untreated infectious processes in this situation carry a mortality rate of 80 per cent. Treatment includes marrow stimulation with daily dosage of oxymetholone or lithium carbonate.

Nursing Management

ASSESSMENT

Physical assessment should include vital signs with attention paid to a high fever or a weak, rapid pulse. Any complaints of a sore throat, dysphagia, or mouth sores should be examined. The client's history should include names of all drugs the client has taken or is presently taking (prescription or nonprescription).

NURSING INTERVENTION

Nursing Diagnosis: Knowledge Deficit R/T toxic agents that cause agranulocytosis.

Planning: Expected Outcomes. The client will understand the cause of agranulocytosis, as evidenced by the client's verbalization of understanding of the cause of the disorder, the need to avoid self-medication, and the importance of follow-up examinations.

Implementation. An important aspect of nursing management is to prevent agranulocytosis by providing clients with teaching regarding potentially dangerous medications and chemicals. To enhance awareness, encourage the client to avoid self-medication without a physician's order, to schedule frequent follow-up by a physician when medications known to cause granulocytopenia are prescribed, and to realize that repeated exposure to toxic chemicals such as benzene may cause agranulocytosis.

MULTIPLE MYELOMA (PLASMA CELL MYELOMA)

Definition

Multiple myeloma is a neoplastic condition characterized by abnormal malignant proliferation of plasma cells secreting a monoclonal paraprotein, accumulation of mature plasma cells in the bone marrow, and complications throughout the body as a result of dissemination of the disease (such as lytic bone lesions and osteoporosis, hematopoietic suppression, hypercalcemia, proteinuria, and renal failure).

Incidence

The condition commonly occurs in clients over 40 years of age; the average age is 60 years. It is more common in men and blacks. Multiple myeloma is considered a lymphoid malignancy. Its incidence is about 1 per cent of all malignant diseases.

Etiology/Risk Factors

There are no particular etiologic factors or risk factors identified for multiple myeloma.

Pathophysiology

Multiple myeloma is characterized by an abnormal proliferation of plasma cells. With this overproduction of plasma cells, bone destruction also occurs. In addition to bone destruction, multiple myeloma is characterized by disruption of red blood cell, leukocyte, and platelet production, which results from plasma cells crowding the bone marrow. Impaired production of these cell forms causes anemia, increased vulnerability to infection, and bleeding tendencies, respectively.

Complications of multiple myeloma include hypercalcemia, renal problems, and neurologic disorders. Hypercalcemia resulting from the release of calcium during bone destruction is present in 30 per cent of newly diagnosed clients with multiple myeloma. It causes confusion, anorexia, nausea, vomiting, constipation, abdominal pain, ileus, and impairment of renal concentrating mechanisms that can eventually lead to irreversible renal failure. In addition, renal disease results from particles of coagulated protein that block the convoluted tubules. The major neurologic complications entail compression of the spinal cord, sometimes followed by paraplegia.

Clinical Manifestations

The onset of multiple myeloma is usually gradual and insidious. Most clients pass through a long presymptomatic period that lasts 5 to 20 years. The client is usually asymptomatic; only 10 per cent of clients will be diagnosed at this stage. Diagnosis at this stage is usually made only by chance as a result of an elevated serum protein level during a screening examination.[3]

Once symptoms appear, they typically involve the skeletal system, particularly the pelvis, spine, and ribs. Some clients have backache or bone pain that worsens with movement. Others suffer sudden pathologic fractures accompanied by severe pain. In time, skeletal destruction increases, and the client may develop sternum and rib cage deformities. Diffuse osteoporosis usually appears, accompanied by a negative calcium balance. The skull shows multiple osteolytic lesions. Drainage of calcium and phosphorus from damaged bones eventually leads to the development of renal stones, particularly in immobilized clients.

DIAGNOSTIC ASSESSMENT

Diagnosis of multiple myeloma rests on x-ray studies, bone marrow biopsy, and blood and urine examination. X-ray studies reveal diffuse lesions in the bone, widespread demineralization, and osteoporosis. The bone marrow contains large numbers of immature plasma cells. Normally, plasma cells constitute 5 per cent of the bone marrow cellular population. Because of the abnormal number of plasma cells producing immunoglobulins, peripheral blood samples sent for plasma electrophoresis reveal a large amount of abnormal immunoglobulin. Another diagnostic sign of multiple myeloma is the appearance of light-chains from the abnormal immunoglobulin in the urine called Bence-Jones protein.

Medical Management

Not all clients diagnosed with multiple myeloma should be treated. Symptoms, physical findings, and laboratory data must be considered. In some cases, treatment might be withheld, and the client is reevaluated in 2 to 3 months. If overt symptoms are present, chemotherapy is the preferred initial treatment. Palliative radiation should be limited to clients with disabling pain from a well-defined location that has not been responsive to chemotherapy.

Management is also aimed at early recognition and treatment of complications of the disease. Clients with hypercalcemia often become anorexic, nauseated, drowsy, confused, and disoriented and may require hospitalization.

PHARMACOLOGIC MANAGEMENT

There is some controversy over the most effective chemotherapy regimen. Melphalan and prednisone or a combination of alkylating agents have both shown objective responses. Prednisone and melphalan given orally for a period of 7 days and repeated at 6-week intervals produces positive results in 50 to 60 per cent of the clients. Leukocyte and platelet counts should be monitored regularly and doses adjusted until modest cytopenia occurs. Combination chemotherapy, commonly melphalan, cyclophosphamide (Cytoxan), carmustine (BCNU), vincristine (Oncovin), and prednisone, has shown a 70 to 75 per cent response rate. This therapy may continue for 1 to 2 years, but relapse almost always occurs when chemotherapy is discontinued. Interferon appears to be beneficial in prolonging the duration of remission.

Corticosteroids, mithramycin, furosemide, and intravenous hydration were commonly prescribed for hypercalcemia; however, newer agents now exist. Etidronate disodium (Didronel) or gallium nitrate (Ganite) and intravenous hydration are now used to effectively treat the hypercalcemia.

In addition, be alert to the possibility of spinal cord compression, another complication of multiple myeloma. Treatment usually consists of radiation therapy and large doses of steroids, although a laminectomy may be indicated.

Nursing Management

ASSESSMENT

Clients with multiple myeloma must be closely assessed for the development of hypercalcemia so that it can be treated adequately. The client's pain should also be monitored so that pain medications can be administered to control the pain.

NURSING INTERVENTION

Nursing Diagnosis: Injury, High Risk for R/T hypercalcemia secondary to bone destruction.

Planning: Expected Outcomes. The client will not suffer injury from hypercalcemia, as evidenced by initiation of treatment before serum calcium levels are excessively elevated; absence of renal stones; no permanent renal damage; absence of nausea, vomiting, constipation, abdominal pain, or ileus; and no evidence of confusion or disorientation.

Implementation. Administer fluids in adequate amounts to maintain an output of 1.5 to 2 L daily. Clients with multiple myeloma usually require about 3 L of fluid per day. The client needs sufficient fluid not only to dilute the calcium overload but also to prevent protein from precipitating in the renal tubules, even after being effectively treated with chemotherapy. Administer medications to increase calcium excretion and decrease calcium loss from bone such as furosemide (Lasix), steroids and mithramycin, Didronel, or Ganite.

Antiemetics may be required for relief of nausea and vomiting. Small, frequent feedings may be better tolerated, and stool softeners may be routinely required. Closely monitor intake, output, and blood studies to determine effectiveness of treatment. The client should be weighed daily so that any significant loss is noted and can be corrected.

If disorientation or confusion occurs, remove sharp

objects and other potentially hazardous items from the environment. The side rails should be raised, and light restraints may be required. The nurse should monitor the client's mental status closely.

Nursing Diagnosis: Pain R/T bone degeneration and possible pathologic fractures.

Planning: Expected Outcomes. The client will have pain controlled and fractures will be prevented, as evidenced by client's report of pain relief and absence of pathologic fractures.

Implementation. Clients with multiple myeloma suffer from bone pain and pathologic fractures. Administer adequate amounts of ordered analgesics to control the client's pain. The client may be referred to the physical therapist for establishing an exercise and activity plan that will reduce the incidence of fractures. Braces may be prescribed to help control pain, especially a brace for the spine.

EVALUATION

The nurse must evaluate client outcomes on the basis of the established plan of care. If these goals have not been achieved, the plan and interventions must be revised to meet the client's needs.

Post-hospital Care

DISCHARGE TEACHING

Significant others should be taught the signs and symptoms of hypercalcemia and to report these immediately to the physician. They should also be taught how to institute safety measures for preventing falls and injuries.

HOME HEALTH CARE NEEDS

The client may need some assistive devices at home, such as a toilet riser and handhold bars in the bathroom.

FOLLOW-UP CARE

The client's calcium level will need to be measured at regular intervals for assessment of the development of hypercalcemia.

▼ DISORDERS OF THE LYMPHOIDAL SYSTEM

Lymphoma is a diverse group of lymphoid neoplasms that results in uncontrolled proliferation of lymphocytes. It arises in the lymphoid tissues, that is, lymph nodes, thymus, spleen, and lymphoid tissue of the gastrointestinal tract. Lymphomas include a number of diseases that have different manifestations, treatments, and prognoses, depending on the lymphocyte type and stage of differentiation. Lymphomas are classified as either (1) Hodgkin's disease or (2) non-Hodgkin's lymphoma. Lymphomas that contain the Reed-Sternberg cell (multinucleated giant cells) are termed Hodgkin's disease; those without it are called non-Hodgkin's lymphoma.

HODGKIN'S DISEASE

Definition

Hodgkin's disease is a chronic, progressive, neoplastic disorder of lymphatic tissue characterized by the painless enlargement of lymph nodes with progression to extralymphatic sites such as the spleen and liver. The pathologic involvement of tissues and organs throughout the body follows.

Incidence

A disorder of young adults, Hodgkin's disease principally occurs between the ages of 20 and 40 years. Among those affected, men outnumber women, and boys are stricken five times more often than are girls. Hodgkin's disease involves the proliferation of abnormal histiocytes called Reed-Sternberg cells, which are part of the tissue macrophage system. As these atypical glial cells multiply, they replace other cellular elements normally found within the lymph nodes.

Etiology

The cause of lymphoma is unknown. However, clients who develop long-term immunosuppression due to illness, therapeutic treatment, or drug abuse suffer an increased incidence of the disease. There appears to be a higher risk of Hodgkin's disease in clients with high titers of Epstein-Barr virus or a history of mononucleosis.

Risk Factors

Immunosuppression due to therapy or as a result of disease is a major risk factor for the development of Hodgkin's disease. This risk is usually not preventable, so clients should be carefully monitored for the development of this disease. Drug abuse is the most preventable cause of the disease.

Pathophysiology

The exact mechanism of growth and spread of Hodgkin's disease remains unknown. Some have suggested that the disease progresses by extension to adjacent structures. It may also disseminate via the lymphatics, because lymphoreticular cells inhabit all tissues of the body except the central nervous system. Hematologic spread may also occur, possibly by means of direct infiltration of blood vessels.

Hodgkin's disease is divided into categories or stages according to the microscopic appearance of the involved lymph nodes, the extent and severity of the disorder, and the prognosis. Table 46-5 shows one method of staging.

The complete remission rate for clients with Hodgkin's disease is 75 to 90 per cent. The recurrence rate varies with the stage of disease and is 10 to 20 per cent. When untreated, clients with Hodgkin's disease have a life expectancy of 5 years.

Clinical Manifestations

Hodgkin's disease usually presents as a painless enlarged lymph node, often in the cervical region. The client may experience unexplained fevers, night sweats, and weight loss. Many clients also experience pruritus. Hepatosplenomegaly may be present, although it usually does not cause symptoms. Likewise, although disease may be present in the bone marrow, it often does not cause pancytopenia.

In addition, some clients with Hodgkin's disease experience pain over the involved nodes after ingesting alcohol. Others may have a nonproductive cough, and the chest film may reveal a mediastinal mass. Other symptoms arise when enlarged lymph nodes obstruct or compress an adjacent structure (e.g., edema of the face, neck, and right arm secondary to superior vena cava compression; or renal failure secondary to urethral obstruction). Figure 46-7 outlines the major assessment data for Hodgkin's disease.

TABLE 46-5. Modified Ann Arbor Staging Classification

Stage	
I	Involvement of a single lymph node region (I) or of a single extralymphatic organ or site (I_E)
II	Involvement of two or more lymph node regions on the same side of the diaphragm (II) or localized involvement of an extralymphatic organ or site and of one or more lymph node regions on the same side of the diaphragm (II_E)
III	Involvement of lymph node regions on both sides of the diaphragm (III), which may also be accompanied by involvement of the spleen (III_S) or by localized involvement of an extralymphatic organ or site (III_E) or both (III_{SE})
III_1	Involvement limited to the lymphatic structures in the upper abdomen, that is, spleen, or splenic, celiac, or hepatic portal nodes, or any combination of these
III_2	Involvement of lower abdominal nodes, that is, para-aortic, iliac, inguinal, or mesenteric nodes, with or without involvement of the splenic, celiac, or hepatic portal nodes
IV	Diffuse or disseminated involvement of one or more extralymphatic organs or tissues, with or without associated lymph node involvement

E, extralymphatic site; S, splenic involvement.
From Glick, J. H. (1992). Hodgkin's disease. *In* J. B. Wyngaarden, et al. (eds.), *Cecil textbook of medicine* (19th ed.). Philadelphia: W. B. Saunders.

DIAGNOSTIC ASSESSMENT

Lymph node biopsy provides a definitive test for diagnosing Hodgkin's disease. With peripheral lymph node enlargement, one entire node is removed and examined for the presence of Reed-Sternberg cells. Some clients do not have enlarged peripheral lymph nodes but may simply notice pruritus, intermittent fever, and weakness. In these cases, chest films or computed tomographic scans may contain evidence of mediastinal or hilar adenopathy. However, Hodgkin's disease can be definitely diagnosed only by pathologic examination of tissues. Also, because of immune system disturbances, clients with Hodgkin's disease usually react abnormally to tuberculin skin testing.

Medical Management

Treatment for Hodgkin's disease varies according to its stage at diagnosis. Stage I and stage II are treated with radiation therapy and supplemental chemotherapy. Clients with stage III disease may receive radiation coupled with an aggressive multiagent chemotherapy regimen.

PHARMACOLOGIC MANAGEMENT

In stage IV disease, a multiagent drug regimen is the treatment of choice. MOPP, a combination of chemotherapeutic agents, is the most widely used regimen (Table 46-6). Other chemotherapeutic regimens have also been used with success.

The most distressing and immediate side effect of the chemotherapeutic agents used to treat Hodgkin's disease is severe nausea and vomiting. Symptoms may be severe enough to force a client to discontinue therapy. Pancytopenia, a toxic effect of these agents, usually occurs 10 to 14 days after intravenous therapy. Any degree of anemia, leukopenia, or thrombocytopenia indicates that treatment must be delayed or medication dosage adjusted.

Nursing Management

Caring for the client with Hodgkin's disease revolves around control of complications associated with the client's pancytopenia. Supportive measures to prevent or control bleeding and infection are important. If these complications can be avoided during the treatment regimen for Hodgkin's disease, the client has a good chance for long-term survival.

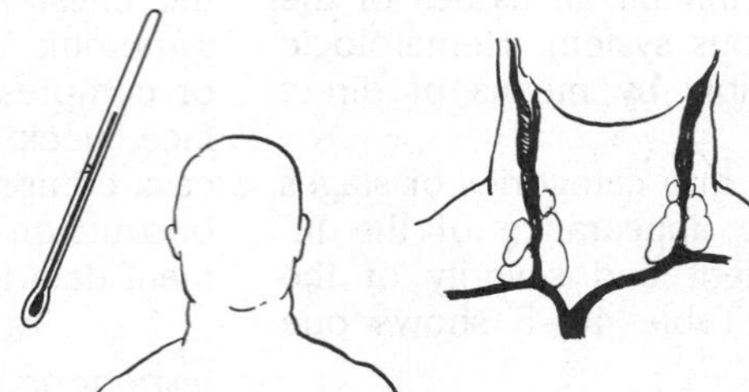
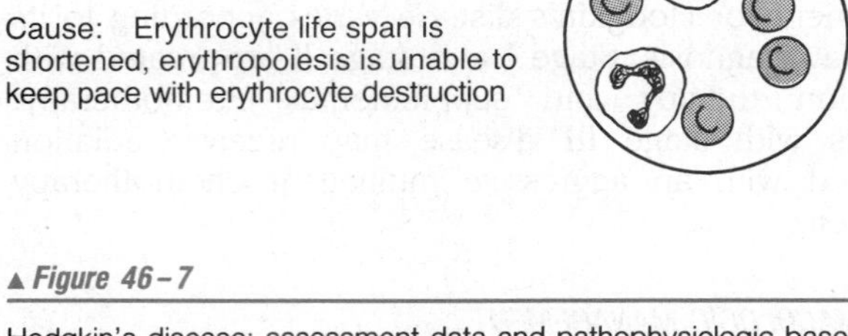

Severe pruritus is an early sign
Cause: Unknown
Irregular fever usually present; temperature is elevated for a few days, then drops to normal or subnormal for several days; continuous high fever may indicate impending death
Cause: Apparently related to neoplastic involvement of internal nodes or viscera
Jaundice
Cause: Obstruction of bile ducts as a result of liver damage causes bilirubin to accumulate in the blood and discolor the skin
Hepatosplenomegaly
Cause: Dissemination of the disorder from lymph nodes to other organs
Renal failure
Cause: Ureteral obstruction by enlarged lymph nodes
Progressive anemia accompanied by fatigue, malaise, anorexia
Cause: Erythrocyte life span is shortened, erythropoiesis is unable to keep pace with erythrocyte destruction
Edema and cyanosis of face and neck
Cause: Enlarged lymph nodes place pressure on veins, obstructing drainage of this area
Pulmonary symptoms including nonproductive cough, stridor, dyspnea, chest pain, cyanosis, and pleural effusion
Cause: Mediastinal lymph node enlargement, involvement of lung parenchyma, and invasion of pleura
Alcohol-induced pain in bone, in involved lymph nodes, or around the mediastinum occurs immediately after drinking alcohol and lasts for 30 to 60 minutes
Cause: Unknown
Bone pain, vertebral compression
Cause: Dissemination of disease from lymph nodes to bones
Paraplegia
Cause: Compression of spinal cord resulting from extradural involvement
Nerve pain
Cause: Compression of nerve roots of brachial, lumbar, or sacral plexuses
M.D.

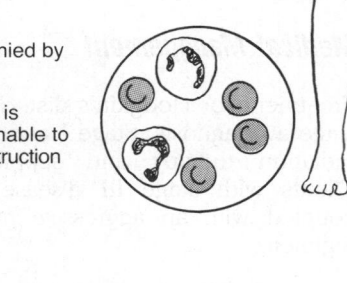

▲ ***Figure 46–7***

Hodgkin's disease: assessment data and pathophysiologic bases.

NON-HODGKIN'S LYMPHOMA

Non-Hodgkin's lymphomas are a group of lymphoid disorders. Involvement of the disease starts in the lymph nodes, although a significant number arise outside the lymphatic system more than in Hodgkin's disease. Non-Hodgkin's lymphoma is more common in adults in their middle and older years; it is more common in males than in females in a ratio of 5:3. Many classification systems are used to differentiate non-Hodgkin's lymphoma according to histologic type and cytologic characteristics. Treatment protocols and prognosis for clients with non-Hodgkin's lymphoma vary greatly. Without effective treatment, non-Hodgkin's lymphomas are very quickly fatal.

TABLE 46–6. MOPP Combination Chemotherapy Regimen for Hodgkin's Disease*

	M	O	P	P
Day of Cycle	***Mustargen (nitrogen mustard)***	***Oncovin (vincristine)***	***Procarbazine***	***Prednisone†***
1, 8	IV	IV	PO	PO
2, 9			PO	PO
3, 10			PO	PO
4, 11			PO	PO
5, 12			PO	PO
6, 13			PO	PO
7, 14			PO	PO

* Therapy consists of at least *six* 14-day *cycles* with 14-days' rest between cycles. Intravenous (IV) or oral (PO) medication doses are adjusted according to laboratory test results of white blood cells and platelets.

† In first and fourth cycle only.

Treatment consists of radiation therapy, chemotherapy, or a combination of both. Overall, the prognosis of non-Hodgkin's lymphoma is poorer than that of Hodgkin's disease. Stage I is rarely observed, because it is not usually diagnosed at this stage. If the disease is detected during this early stage, remissions have been achieved by use of involved field radiotherapy alone. In stage II disease, if the involved areas are continuous and together, radiotherapy proves effective. Clients with stage III and stage IV disease will probably benefit more from combination chemotherapy with or without radiation therapy.

The cure rate for aggressive tumors with treatment is significantly better than for the slower-growing, low-grade type, presumably because rapidly growing cells are more susceptible to chemotherapy and radiation therapy. In some clients with large masses, surgical removal or debulking of the mass may be required before chemotherapy or radiation therapy.

INFECTIOUS MONONUCLEOSIS

Definition

Infectious mononucleosis (also known as glandular disease and the "kissing disease") is a self-limiting condition characterized by painful enlargement of the lymph nodes, lymphocytosis, sore throat, and fever.

Incidence

Primarily a disease of the young, infectious mononucleosis usually strikes children between the ages of 3 and 5 years and young adults between the ages of 15 and 25 years. The greatest incidence occurs among college students, medical students, and nurses. Although this disease usually occurs sporadically, epidemic forms may sweep through colleges and children's homes.

Etiology

The cause of infectious mononucleosis is a herpesvirus, the Epstein-Barr virus. Although the exact mode of transmission remains unknown, the disease may be transmitted through the oropharyngeal route during close contact, such as with kissing.

Pathophysiology

Infectious mononucleosis is a relatively mild disorder but has widespread effects on the body. For example, the lymph nodes enlarge, lymphocytosis occurs, the spleen may swell to two to three times its normal size, liver function is sometimes impaired, and both peripheral and central nervous system involvement can develop.

Clinical Manifestations

The onset of infectious mononucleosis follows an incubation period of 2 to 6 weeks. Before frank clinical symptoms present, the client may experience fatigue, headaches, malaise, and myalgias. Subsequently, assessment reveals temperatures up to 39° C (102.2° F), pharyngitis, and lymphadenopathy that is more pronounced in the cervical regions. Ten to 15 per cent of those affected develop a maculopapular rash that closely resembles the rash of rubella. Splenic enlargement causes left upper quadrant pain. Nervous system involvement may lead to severe headache. In rare cases, liver involvement may develop into a hepatitis-like syndrome. When infectious mononucleosis is severe, the client may develop the following two complications:

- splenic rupture resulting from the infiltration of the spleen by massive numbers of lymphocytes
- streptococcal pharyngitis or Vincent's angina secondary to bacterial invasion of the throat

DIAGNOSTIC ASSESSMENT

The diagnosis of infectious mononucleosis is based on three criteria: physical assessment, laboratory tests, and a positive heterophil or Monospot test.

History and Physical Examination. Physical assessment typically reveals fever, lymphadenopathy, sore throat, and splenomegaly.

Laboratory Tests. The white blood cell count usually ranges from 12,000 to 20,000/mm³, of which 50 per cent are lymphocytes and monocytes and 10 to 20 per cent are large, atypical lymphocytes.

Positive Heterophil (Monospot) Test. In 1932, Paul and Bunnell discovered that the blood of clients with infectious mononucleosis contained heterophil antibodies that would agglutinate the red blood cells of sheep. Human beings normally do not produce agglutinins against sheep erythrocytes. Consequently, a positive heterophil test helps confirm a diagnosis of infectious mononucleosis; clients usually test positive within 5 to 7 days of acute onset. However, positive tests sometimes occur in other conditions.

Medical Management

No specific intervention either mitigates or shortens the disease process. Because infectious mononucleosis must simply run its course, treatments are directed at symptom control. Bed rest is recommended until fever is resolved. Salicylates, cool sponge baths, and a large fluid intake help control fever. Warm saline throat irrigations may relieve the sore throat.

PHARMACOLOGIC MANAGEMENT

Steroids do not in any way alter or accelerate the course of the disease. Physicians may prescribe them, however, to promote a sense of well-being.

Nursing Management

In addition to providing symptomatic relief, the nurse works toward preventing complications and administering treatment. When caring for clients with infectious mononucleosis, the nurse should do the following:

- Caution the client against engaging in excessive activity, especially contact sports, for a period of at least 1 month, which could result in splenic rupture or lowered resistance to infection.
- Watch closely for and report the two signs of splenic rupture: abdominal pain and shock.
- If throat pain worsens, report it immediately so that appropriate antibiotic therapy can be started.

Although complications sometimes develop, the prognosis for clients with infectious mononucleosis is generally excellent. The febrile phase of this disorder typically lasts 2 to 4 weeks. During the long convalescence, the client slowly regains strength and energy.

SPLENECTOMY

Despite the important functions of the spleen, it can be removed (splenectomy) without harm in adults. Its role can be taken over completely by other organs (e.g., liver, lymph nodes, and bone marrow). The most frequent indication for splenectomy is rupture of the spleen complicated by severe hemorrhage. Splenic irradiation may achieve a reversal in cytopenia without the risk of surgery.

Causes of splenic rupture include (1) trauma (e.g., automobile accidents, bullet or knife wounds, severe blows to the spleen), (2) accidental tearing of the splenic capsule during surgery on neighboring organs, and (3) disease of the spleen that causes softening or damage (e.g., infectious mononucleosis and malaria).

In hypersplenism, a second important indication for splenectomy, the spleen destroys, in excessive numbers, one of the blood cell types (i.e., erythrocytes, leukocytes, or platelets). Signs of hypersplenism include moderate to massive splenomegaly, anemia, leukopenia, or thrombocytopenia and a compensatory increase in the production of the affected cell line by the bone marrow. Overactivity of the spleen develops either as a primary condition of unknown origin or as a condition secondary to another disease.

Primary hypersplenism occurs in idiopathic thrombocytopenic purpura and congenital spherocytosis. Some etiologic factors associated with secondary hypersplenism include lymphomas (including Hodgkin's disease), leukemias, polycythemia vera, acute infections (including infectious mononucleosis), chronic infections, malaria, syphilis, the hemoglobinopathies, and cirrhosis of the liver.

Primary hypersplenism can be alleviated by splenectomy. Splenectomy is only palliative for clients with secondary hypersplenism, because the surgery has little or no effect on the course of the primary illness. When hypersplenism is diagnosed, it is important to teach the client to prevent complications associated with the specific cytopenia.

Laboratory indications for splenectomy include granulocytopenia of less than $500/mm^3$ and thrombocytopenia of less than $20,000/mm^3$. The surgery itself is relatively simple unless the spleen is greatly enlarged or surrounded by adhesions.

The spleen has an important role in the phagocytosis of circulating opsonized organisms. After splenectomy, young children are at high risk for fulminant infections due to *Streptococcus pneumoniae, Haemophilus influenzae, Neisseria meningitidis,* and other encapsulated organisms. Continuous prophylactic antibiotics may be advisable during the early years. Adults are also at increased risk of infection, especially during the first 3 years after surgery. The splenectomized client should be advised to seek medical treatment at the earliest signs of infection.

Nursing Management

ASSESSMENT

The unique functions performed by the spleen will eventually be taken over by other organs. However, the loss of the spleen due to cessation of function or splenectomy does require the client to be monitored for potentially serious complications. The nursing care of the client undergoing splenectomy is generally the same as that discussed in Chapter 19.

Nursing Diagnosis: Tissue Perfusion, Altered, High Risk for R/T bleeding.

Planning: Expected Outcomes. The client will not suffer from hemorrhage or will have hemorrhage detected early, as evidenced by normal blood pressure and pulse, no evidence of bleeding, and absence of signs of shock.

Implementation. The client should be carefully monitored for the development of hemorrhage by frequently taking and recording the client's vital signs and measuring the abdominal girth. Clients undergoing splenectomy for thrombocytopenia are still at increased risk for hemorrhage in the postoperative period. Platelet transfusions may be given both before or after surgery if the platelet count is less than $100,000/mm^3$.

Nursing Diagnosis: Infection, High Risk for R/T loss of macrophage activity after splenectomy.

Planning: Expected Outcomes. The client will not develop an infection or will have infection detected and treated early, as evidenced by absence of fever, no rales or symptoms of pneumonia, and wound healing without difficulty.

Implementation. Teach the client to recognize early signs and symptoms of infection (fever, chills, productive cough, shortness of breath, myalgia, neck stiffness) and to seek medical treatment immediately. Be sure the client and significant others understand the importance of prophylactic antibiotics; monitor compliance. If prophylactic antibiotics are not being taken routinely, advise the client to obtain a limited supply when traveling to locations where medical care is not immediately available. Routine immunizations against influenza and pneumococci are also recommended.

EVALUATION

The nurse must evaluate client outcomes on the basis of the established plan of care. If these goals have not been achieved, the plan and interventions must be revised to meet the client's needs.

▼ DISORDERS OF PLATELETS AND CLOTTING FACTORS

Disorders of hemostasis affecting platelets and clotting factors include (1) hemorrhagic disorders, (2) purpura, and (3) coagulation disorders. The three components of the hemostatic mechanism are the blood vessels, platelets (thrombocytes), and coagulation factors.

▼ Hemorrhagic Disorders

OVERVIEW

Normal clot formation and lysis depend on intact blood vessels, an adequate number of functioning platelets, sufficient amounts of the 12 clotting factors, and a well-controlled fibrinolytic system. Consequently, the four basic problems underlying hemorrhagic (bleeding) disorders are

- weak, damaged vessels that rupture easily or spontaneously
- platelet deficiency (thrombocytopenia) due to hypoproliferation, excessive pooling of platelets in the spleen, or excessive platelet destruction
- deficiency or total lack of one of the clotting factors
- excessive or insufficient fibrinolysis

Disorders of hemostasis fall into two major categories: purpura and coagulation disorders. Table 46-7 outlines the types of bleeding disorders in these two categories.

TABLE 46-7. Classification of Disorders of Hemostasis

Purpura
Vascular defect purpura
Familial hemorrhagic telangiectasia
Anaphylactoid purpura (allergic purpura)
Toxic purpura
Platelet disorder purpura
Idiopathic thrombocytopenic purpura
Secondary thrombocytopenias
Coagulation Disorders
Hemophilia
Hypoprothrombinemia
Disseminated intravascular coagulation (DIC)

The diagnosis of hemorrhagic disorders depends on a complete health and family history, physical examination, and laboratory tests for platelet and clotting defects. The history usually offers numerous clues to the type of bleeding problem and its cause.

If the history indicates a bleeding disorder, examine the client for overt signs of bleeding. Petechiae (tiny hemorrhagic spots caused by intradermal or submucosal bleeding) are usually present in vascular and thrombocytopenic purpuras. The presence of ecchymoses (large, blotchy, subcutaneous hemorrhagic areas), hematomas (subdermal hemorrhage), and hemarthrosis (blood within the joints) points to hemophilia. However, ecchymoses may develop in any hemorrhagic disorder. Clients who hemorrhage severely from several areas during childbirth or a major surgical procedure may have a fibrinogen deficiency. In addition to any evidence of bleeding, search for signs of hepatic cirrhosis (hepatomegaly, jaundice, and so forth) and splenomegaly.

Laboratory studies provide most crucial evidence for pinpointing the type and cause of a bleeding disorder (see Table 45-8).

Clients with hemorrhagic disorders need to understand (1) why they are at risk of bleeding, (2) the signs and symptoms of bleeding, and (3) preventive measures to avoid bleeding. Those who can be managed by home health care should be referred to appropriate health care agencies. Clients with bleeding disorders should carry an identification card at all times that indicates their diagnosis, name of physician or health care agency, and blood type. It is important to assess each client before even minor invasive procedures, such as dental extractions, to rule out a history of bleeding disorders.

▼ Purpura

IDIOPATHIC THROMBOCYTOPENIC PURPURA

Definition

Purpura is defined as the extravasation of small amounts of blood into the tissues and mucous membranes. Bleeding results from either vessel damage (vascular purpura) or a platelet deficiency (thrombocytopenic purpura).

The term thrombocytopenia means a reduction in platelets below 100,000/mm^3. The two major problems that characterize thrombocytopenia are (1) spontaneous bleeding into any part of the body (such as the central nervous system, muscle, joints) when the platelet count is less than 20,000/mm^3 and (2) prolonged oozing from sites despite local measures to curtail bleeding. The two principal types of thrombocytopenia are idiopathic thrombocytopenic purpura (ITP) and secondary thrombocytopenia.

ITP refers to thrombocytopenia caused by an unknown, possibly autoimmune cause.

Incidence

Ninety per cent of adults with ITP are under 40 years of age; the ratio of women to men is 3 to 4:1. In children, 85 per cent of whom are under 8 years of age, the disease is self-limiting.

Etiology and Risk Factors

Childhood ITP is usually acute and follows recovery from a viral infection. In adults, the onset of ITP is usually gradual, without a preceding illness, and with a chronic course. In a small percentage of adult cases, the disease has an acute onset.

Pathophysiology

This disorder is characterized by the premature destruction of platelets. Normally, platelets survive 8 to 10 days within the circulation. However, platelet survival in ITP is as brief as 1 to 3 days or less.

ITP is an autoimmune bleeding disorder characterized by the development of antibodies to one's own platelets, which are then destroyed by phagocytosis in the spleen and, to a lesser extent, in the liver.

In adults, indications for treatment depend on severity of bleeding and the degree of thrombocytosis.[83]

Clinical Manifestations

In most cases, ITP takes a course of remissions and exacerbations that, in untreated cases, may continue for years. Assessment reveals petechiae, ecchymosis, epistaxis, bleeding from the gums, and easy bruising. Women may have extremely heavy menses or bleeding between periods.

Complications of ITP include cerebral hemorrhage, which proves fatal in 1 to 5 per cent of clients with ITP; severe hemorrhages from the nose, gastrointestinal tract, and urinary system; bleeding into the diaphragm, which can result in pulmonary complications; and nerve pain, extremity anesthesia, or paralysis resulting from the pressure of hematomas on nerves or brain tissues.

DIAGNOSTIC ASSESSMENT

Laboratory findings that confirm the presence of ITP include (1) a platelet count below 100,000/mm^3, (2) prolonged bleeding time with normal coagulation time (all coagulation factors are present and normal), (3) increased capillary fragility as demonstrated by the tourniquet test, (4) positive platelet antibody screening, and (5) bone marrow aspirate containing normal or increased megakaryocytes.

Clients with ITP have a good prognosis: 80 per cent of children and 10 to 20 per cent of adults recover spontaneously without treatment.

Medical Management

The three basic interventions for ITP are steroid therapy, splenectomy, and platelet transfusions.

PHARMACOLOGIC MANAGEMENT

Clients suffering from severe bleeding of short duration receive steroids (such as prednisone). The purpose of steroid therapy in ITP is to suppress the phagocytic response of splenic macrophages. However, steroids rarely produce a permanent cure. Clients also receive steroids before splenectomy. Plasmapheresis is sometimes used as short-term therapy until the steroid therapy takes effect. Intravenous infusion of gamma globulin in combination with plasmapheresis is under investigation for clients whose condition is refractory to other treatments. Danazol (Danocrine) has recently been used with success in some clients. Immunosuppressive therapy used in refractory cases includes vincristine (Oncovin), vinblastine (Velban), azathioprine (Imuran), and cyclophosphamide (Cytoxan).

Surgical Management

The treatment of choice for clients with ITP is splenectomy (see earlier). In 60 to 80 per cent of cases, removal of the spleen results in complete and permanent remission. The effectiveness of the splenectomy is believed to be related to the removal of the site of premature destruction of the antibody-sensitized platelets. Because young children often recover spontaneously from ITP, pediatricians do not usually recommend splenectomy until the child is over 6 years of age.

Nursing Management

ASSESSMENT

Clients with ITP usually present with easy bruising, petechiae, and purpura. Platelet counts are well below normal limits.

NURSING INTERVENTION

Nursing Diagnosis: Injury, High Risk for R/T increased risk of bleeding secondary to low platelet count.

Planning: Expected Outcomes. The client will not

suffer injury, as evidenced by absence of bleeding or bleeding that is diagnosed early and treated effectively.

Implementation. During the acute phase, teach the client oral hygiene measures to prevent gum bleeding. The client should not use a hard toothbrush and should refrain from flossing during this phase. The client should not receive any injections, aspirin, or nonsteroidal anti-inflammatory drugs. The nurse should monitor the client's platelet count, vital signs, and signs of bleeding or increased intracranial pressure. Teach the client to avoid Valsalva's maneuver and to use stool softeners.

Nursing Diagnosis: Tissue Integrity, Impaired R/T intradermal bleeding, petechiae, and purpura.

Planning: Expected Outcomes. The client will not develop impaired tissue integrity, as evidenced by early detection and treatment of any bleeding and no apparent alteration in tissue integrity.

Implementation. The nurse should carefully inspect and monitor the client's skin condition, noting petechiae, purpura, and bruising. Apply an ice bag or manual pressure over any bleeding site to promote hemostasis. Teach the client and significant others to implement bleeding precautions when the platelet count is low and how to institute immediate medical care for hemorrhage.

Nursing Diagnosis: Pain R/T bleeding into the tissues.

Planning: Expected Outcomes. The client will have pain controlled or eliminated, as evidenced by the client's statements of relief.

Implementation. The nurse should position the client comfortably, using pillows, a bed cradle, lightweight blankets, and other measures to decrease pressures on the tissues. Ask the client what pain is being felt and use that information to determine the need for analgesics as ordered.

EVALUATION

The nurse must evaluate client outcomes on the basis of the established plan of care. If these goals have not been achieved, the plan and interventions must be revised to meet the client's needs.

Modification of Plan of Care for the Elderly

Elderly clients are less likely to develop ITP. When they do develop it, bleeding can be more severe because of their already fragile capillaries. Steroids are used, and surgery is avoided unless necessary.

Post-hospital Care

DISCHARGE TEACHING

The client should be taught about long-term steroid therapy. It is important that the client learn methods to avoid bleeding. The client who has had splenectomy should be taught to avoid close contact with people with infections.

FOLLOW-UP CARE

The client will need to be seen at regular intervals for monitoring of platelet levels. Clients will need continued follow-up until the problem resolves or for the rest of their lives.

OTHER PURPURAS

Vascular Defect Purpura

The major characteristic of vascular purpura is easy rupture of the smaller blood vessels upon any undue pressure, with resultant bleeding into the tissues. The causes of vascular purpura are many (e.g., heredity, allergy, exposure to poisons, drug hypersensitivity, poor nutrition, infection, and hypertension). Major forms of vascular purpura are (1) familial hemorrhagic telangiectasia, (2) anaphylactoid purpura (allergic purpura), and (3) toxic purpura.

FAMILIAL HEMORRHAGIC TELANGIECTASIA

This hereditary condition is characterized by multiple, thin, dilated capillaries and arterioles. These fragile vessels are usually found on the oral and nasal mucosa and in the gastrointestinal and renal tracts. Fragility of the vessels leads to spontaneous bleeding or bleeding with minimal trauma. Small red-to-violet lesions (telangiectasia) are often seen on the lips, oral and nasal mucosa, tongue, toes, and fingertips. These lesions blanch when pressed and bleed spontaneously.

Diagnosis is make solely by identification of characteristic lesions. Treatment is symptomatic. Treatments include topical hemostatics and administration of estrogens. Severe gastrointestinal tract hemorrhage warrants treatment with iron therapy and transfusions. Because this condition is hereditary, genetic counseling is advisable.

ANAPHYLACTOID PURPURA (ALLERGIC PURPURA)

This form of vascular purpura arises from an allergic reaction that damages the vascular epithelium. It causes acute or chronic inflammation of blood vessels supplying the skin, joints, gastrointestinal tract, and kidneys. Typically, attacks of the disease spontaneously subside within 1 to 6 weeks. However, episodes of bleeding tend to recur over the years.

Assessment reveals arthritic pains, abdominal pain, hematuria, gastrointestinal tract hemorrhage, fever, and malaise. Skin lesions occur in the form of erythema, urticaria, and pruritus.

Treatment primarily involves elimination of possible allergens and alleviation of symptoms. Immunosuppressive therapy (such as steroids, cyclophosphamide) and exchange plasmapheresis have been tried with some success.

TOXIC PURPURA

This condition is characterized by damage to blood vessels after exposure to certain medications and poisons (such as snake venom).

Treatment involves identification of the offending agent when possible.

Symptomatic or Secondary Purpura

These disorders arise secondary to other disorders and are not caused by intrinsic or inherited disorders of the vasculature. Such conditions include

- serious tissue trauma arising from a blow or a burn
- arterial hypertension resulting in increased capillary pressure
- bloodstream infections that damage the vascular epithelium, such as subacute bacterial endocarditis
- scurvy (the result of vitamin C deficiency), which causes increased capillary fragility
- uremia and cachexia, which for unknown reasons result in vessel weakness

Treatment of the purpura involves treating the primary disorder.

Unlike idiopathic (primary) thrombocytopenic purpura, the secondary thrombocytopenias have identifiable causes. For example, these types of purpura may arise secondary to viral infections, bone marrow failure, the defibrination syndrome, disseminated lupus erythematosus, lymphoproliferative disorders, infectious mononucleosis, and drug hypersensitivity. Common offending drugs include quinidine, quinine, the sulfonamides, phenylbutazone, and chlorothiazide derivatives. Assessment data and laboratory findings are the same as those found in ITP.

Treatment focuses on mitigating the underlying causes as well as controlling any bleeding. All potentially toxic drugs must be identified and discontinued. The platelet count usually begins to rise within a few days, reaching normal values within a week after removal of toxic agents. To control bleeding, the physician may order the administration of corticosteroids.

Platelet transfusions are given when the platelet count falls below 20,000 to 30,000/mm³ or as needed for treatment of hemorrhage. Clients can be supported with platelet transfusions for weeks to years. Although transfused platelets have a shortened lifespan, they may function effectively for 5 to 6 days. Long-term platelet therapy leads to the development of platelet antibodies. Platelet counts obtained 10 to 60 minutes after transfusion that show no rise in the peripheral platelet count, or even a decrease, indicate the presence of platelet antibodies. Platelet therapy can be continued only by finding specially matched donors who are able to provide HLA-matched platelets. Premedication with diphenhydramine hydrochloride (Benadryl), acetaminophen, or hydrocortisone may decrease the possibility of reactions to platelet transfusions.

HLA-MATCHED PLATELETS

Clients who have been repeatedly exposed to foreign HLA antigens may develop antibodies. Should this occur, the client usually becomes nonresponsive or refractory to platelet concentrates possessing those antigens. If testing confirms the presence of HLA antigens, single-donor platelets obtained by apheresis from a donor with identical HLA antigens may improve platelet responsiveness. Because the HLA system consists of a large number of potential antigens, the chance of locating an identical match from an unrelated donor pool is remote (1 in 5000 to 20,000). A family member, such as a sibling, is the most likely suitable match; however, transfusion should be avoided if there is any chance that this donor may be needed as a bone marrow donor for this client.

Clients undergoing immunosuppressive treatment who may require platelet therapy should have samples collected for HLA typing (30 ml of heparinized blood) before the onset of leukopenia. Identifying a donor and performing apheresis can be a labor-intensive process that usually requires advanced planning.

▼ Coagulation Disorders

The coagulation disorders stem from a defect in the clotting mechanisms. One or more of the clotting factors is depleted or absent. The three important coagulation disorders discussed here are hypoprothrombinemia, disseminated intravascular coagulation, and the hemophilias (see section on congenital conditions).

HYPOPROTHROMBINEMIA

The term hypoprothrombinemia refers to a deficient amount of circulating prothrombin. Prothrombin is a protein produced in the liver and normally found in the blood. For prothrombin synthesis to take place, vitamin K (a fat-soluble vitamin) must be present in the liver to act as a catalyst. Hypoprothrombinemia develops from a vitamin K deficiency or liver disorder or from an overdose of aspirin, coumarin, or coumarin-derivative anticoagulant (such as warfarin), which antagonizes the action of vitamin K.

The fat-soluble vitamin K is generally obtained in a balanced diet and is also synthesized by certain gastrointestinal tract bacteria. Because it is fat-soluble, vitamin K depends on the presence of bile for absorption. Once absorbed, vitamin K catalyzes prothrombin synthesis within the liver cells. Vitamin K deficiency results from improper diet; gastrointestinal tract disorders interfering with the absorption of vitamin K, such as malabsorption syndrome and jaundice due to bile duct obstruction; liver damage so extensive that liver cells cannot produce bile or synthesize prothrombin; and prolonged sulfonamide or antibiotic administration that sterilizes the bowel, thereby halting vitamin K manufactured by gastrointestinal tract bacteria.

Dicumarol is an effective anticoagulant used to reduce clot formation in clients with heart disease and peripheral vascular disorders. It acts by interfering with vitamin K in prothrombin synthesis. In excessive doses, the prothrombin time is prolonged (usually below 40 or 50 percent). If the prothrombin time drops below 10 to 15 per cent, the danger of bleeding or spontaneous hemorrhage increases.

The major manifestations of hypoprothrombinemia are ecchymosis after minimal trauma, epistaxis, postoperative hemorrhage from the incision, hematuria, gastrointestinal tract bleeding, and prolonged bleeding from a venipuncture. The outstanding laboratory finding is a prolonged prothrombin time.

Treatment for hypoprothrombinemia aims at the underlying cause. For example, vitamin K deficiency resulting from malabsorption is corrected through intramuscular or intravenous administration of vitamin K, such as menadione sodium bisulfite (Hykinone) or menadiol diphosphate (Synkayvite).

If overdosage with a coumarin anticoagulant is the underlying problem, anticoagulant therapy is stopped. In order to normalize the prothrombin time, phytonadione (fat-soluble vitamin K) is administered orally for minor bleeding problems or intravenously for hemorrhage.

Finally, if prothrombin deficiency results from liver disease, concentrates of prothrombin or of prothrombin and factors VII, IX, and X may be transfused.

DISSEMINATED INTRAVASCULAR COAGULATION

Definition

The term disseminated intravascular coagulation (DIC) means diffuse or widespread coagulation within arterioles and capillaries all over the body. The syndrome of DIC is known by many titles including consumption coagulopathy, defibrination syndrome, diffuse intravascular clotting, and intravascular coagulation, but most commonly it is referred to as DIC.

Etiology

DIC is a complex and important coagulation disorder characterized by two apparently conflicting manifestations: (1) diffuse fibrin deposition within arterioles and capillaries all over the body, with resultant widespread clotting, and (2) hemorrhage from the kidneys, brain, adrenals, heart, and other organs.

The causes of DIC are many, and there is considerable overlap among syndromes that precede its occurrence. Four categories of causative factors are (1) introduction of tissue coagulation factors into the circulation, (2) damage to vascular endothelium, (3) stagnant blood flow, and (4) infection.

Risk Factors

Table 46-8 lists conditions that may precipitate DIC. Be alert for signs of DIC in caring for clients with any of these conditions.

Pathophysiology

The pathologic chain of events characterizing DIC is as follows.

1. Certain disease states (Table 46-9) cause the release of thromboplastic substances that result in activation of thrombin, which in turn activates fibrinogen and results in deposition of fibrin throughout the microcirculation.
2. Platelet aggregation or adhesiveness is increased; this enables fibrin clots to form and microthrombi to form in the brain, kidneys, heart, and other organs, causing microinfarcts and tissue necrosis.
3. Red blood cells become trapped in the fibrin strands and are destroyed (hemolysis). The resultant sluggish circulation of blood reduces the flow of nutrients and oxygen to the cells.
4. Platelets, prothrombin, and other clotting factors are consumed in the process, which compromises coagulation and predisposes to bleeding.
5. Excessive clotting activates the fibrinolytic mechanism, which causes the production of fibrin split products.
6. Fibrin split products act to inhibit platelet clotting functions, which causes further bleeding.
7. Ultimately, with clots being lysed and clotting factors being depleted, the blood loses its ability to clot.

The prognosis for clients with DIC varies. The condition may be self-limiting. On the other hand, hemorrhage, organ damage, or even death may occur within a few days.

Clinical Manifestations

The onset of DIC is usually acute and develops within days to hours after an initial assault to the body system,

TABLE 46-8. Conditions That May Precipitate DIC

Shock
Cirrhosis
Purpura fulminans
Glomerulonephritis
Acute fulminant hepatitis
Acute bacterial and viral infections
Conditions that may cause the release of platelet factor III
- Fat emboli
- Snake bites
- Hemolytic processes due to
  - infection
  - transfusion reactions
  - immunologic disorders
- Tissue damage due to
  - trauma
  - heat stroke
  - extensive burns
  - transplant rejections
  - surgery—particularly if extracorporeal circulation was used

Conditions that may cause the release of thromboplastin from the tissues
- Neoplastic growths
  - acute leukemias
  - prostatic cancer
  - bronchogenic cancer
  - giant cavernous hemangioma
- Obstetric conditions
  - abruptio placentae
  - retained dead fetus
  - amniotic fluid embolism

such as shock syndrome. Subacute DIC may not be apparent initially but may fulminate as the clinical course progresses. Chronic cases of DIC characteristically develop in clients with cancer or in mothers carrying a dead fetus. Manifestations may be mild or extremely severe.

Assessment of clients with DIC reveals purpura, petechiae, and ecchymoses on the skin, mucous membranes, heart lining, and lungs; prolonged bleeding from a venipuncture; severe, uncontrolled hemorrhage during surgery or childbirth; oliguria and acute renal failure; and convulsions and coma, which may terminate in death.

DIAGNOSTIC ASSESSMENT

Laboratory findings in severe cases of DIC indicate that the hemostatic mechanism has failed totally. A prolonged prothrombin time, very low platelet count, and incoagulable blood are typical findings. Table 46-9 lists the laboratory tests used in the diagnosis of DIC.

Medical Management

The treatment of DIC is currently under investigation as researchers attempt to validate the most suitable means of managing this dangerous syndrome. To prevent DIC successfully, clinicians must correct the basic problem (such as shock, delivery of a fetus, surgery, or irradiation for cancer), reverse the pathologic clotting, control bleeding and shock, detect occult bleeding, prevent further bleeding, accurately measure blood loss, administer blood products and medication as prescribed, and observe for and report transfusion reactions and medication side effects.

Manifestations of thrombosis are treated with intravenous heparin, although its use in the treatment of DIC is still controversial. It should be reserved for clients who continue to bleed in spite of vigorous treatment with fresh frozen plasma and platelets. Heparin therapy, which interrupts the clotting cascade by blocking thrombin activity, causes the fibrinogen level to increase and the number of fibrin degradation products to decrease. Packed red blood cells are administered to replace blood volume lost through hemorrhage.

PHARMACOLOGIC MANAGEMENT

Cryoprecipitate is given for depletion of factors V and VIII. Administration of antithrombin III (in fresh frozen plasma) shortens the course of the disorder and decreases the complications of DIC. In cases in which bleeding cannot be controlled with heparin, aminocaproic acid (Amicar) is given. Cardiac, renal, and electrolyte studies should be followed closely during its use.

Several new agents to control bleeding and reverse laboratory signs of DIC are being studied. Protease inhibitors gabexate and aprotinin (Trasylol) have been used with some success. These drugs are still considered investigational.

Nursing Management

It is important to assess all body systems for the effect DIC has had: bleeding or oozing of blood from venipuncture sites or mucosal surfaces and wounds, pallor,

TABLE 46-9. Laboratory Tests Used in Diagnosis of DIC

Test	Results
Prothrombin time	Prolonged
Partial thromboplastin time	Usually prolonged
Thrombin time	Usually prolonged
Fibrinogen level	Usually depressed
Platelet count	Usually depressed
Fibrin split products	Elevated
Protamine sulfate test	Strongly positive
Factor assays II, V, VII	Reduced

petechiae, ecchymoses, and hematomas (integumentary); tachypnea, hemoptysis, orthopnea, and basilar rales (respiratory); tachycardia and hypotension (cardiovascular); abdominal distention, guaiac-positive stools or nasal aspirate (gastrointestinal); hematuria and oliguria (genitourinary); and vision changes, dizziness, headache, changes in mental status, and irritability (neurologic).

Nursing care of clients with DIC will vary, depending on the severity of the process. Generally, the goal of care is to monitor and quantify blood loss and provide supportive therapy with blood components in order to resolve symptoms of hemorrhage and control further bleeding. Monitor appropriate laboratory values to determine treatment effectiveness and observe for signs of thrombosis. For avoidance of further complications, avoid injections, apply pressure to bleeding sites, and turn and reposition the client frequently and gently. This condition sometimes results in overt bleeding from body orifices and other clinical symptoms that are very frightening to the client and significant others. They will all require strong emotional support.

▼ CONGENITAL CONDITIONS IN WHICH SURVIVAL INTO ADULTHOOD IS EXPECTED

SICKLE CELL ANEMIA AND SICKLE CELL TRAIT

Definition

Sickle cell anemia (Hb SS disease) is a chronic hereditary hemolytic disorder.

Incidence

Sickle cell anemia primarily affects the world's black population (see Fig. 46-8). In Nigeria, up to 30 per cent of the population carries the sickle trait (see Fig. 46-8).

Etiology and Risk Factors

As shown in Figure 46-8, whether a client will have sickle cell anemia, sickle cell trait, or neither depends on the genes for hemoglobin inherited from each parent.

Pathophysiology

In sickle cell anemia, the red blood cells contain an abnormal hemoglobin, that is, hemoglobin S (Hb S) instead of hemoglobin A (Hb A). These abnormal cells assume a sickle, or crescent, shape when oxygen in the blood decreases (Fig. 46-9). Once they "sickle," the red blood cells become rigid and may obstruct capillary blood flow, causing further hypoxia and, consequently, more sickling.

Sickle cell trait, generally a relatively mild condition, may produce few or no symptoms. It is present in clients who are heterozygous for sickle cell hemoglobin.

Hb S results when valine replaces glutamic acid on each beta chain of the hemoglobin molecule. Valine is an amino acid that tends to form strong hydrophobic bonds. This valine substitution causes an abnormal bonding between Hb S molecules when oxygen in the blood decreases.

The exact mechanisms that precipitate the various forms of sickling crises or "attacks" remain somewhat unclear. However, two major factors are definitely linked with the sickling of cells: (1) hypoxia, due to low oxygen tensions, and (2) an increased blood viscosity, due to an increased concentration of sickled cells.

Exposure to low oxygen tensions (as a result of climbing to high altitudes, flying in nonpressurized planes, exercising strenuously, or undergoing anesthesia without receiving adequate oxygenation) results in hypoxia. Although both Hb S and Hb A have the same solubility when oxygenated, deoxygenation of the blood drastically affects Hb S.

When normal hemoglobin gives up its oxygen, it becomes only half as soluble as when it is oxygenated, whereas sickle cell hemoglobin becomes 50 times less soluble. The decreased solubility of Hb S causes it to crystallize, thereby deforming the cell's shape. The heavy concentration of misshapen cells during a sickling crisis makes the blood abnormally viscous, which results in an extremely sluggish circulation. The pathologic situation is compounded if dehydration is present.

Owing to the increased viscosity and the irregular shape of the cells, the sickle cells tend to pack together or "log jam" within the smaller blood vessels. Occlusion of the microcirculation increases hypoxia, which causes more erythrocytes to sickle. Thus, a vicious cycle ensues. The organs most vulnerable to infarction and necrosis are the brain and kidneys, because of their constant demand for oxygen, and the bone marrow and spleen, because of their normally sluggish circulation.

Clinical Manifestations

Sickle cell anemia usually manifests itself during childhood but occasionally does not appear until adulthood. Young children who develop the disease fail to grow properly. They typically have spindly legs, a short trunk, and a tower-shaped skull because of bone marrow hyperactivity.

Symptoms, whenever they occur, are due to three underlying factors:

- hemolytic anemia from the destruction of sickle cells; hemoglobin values usually lie in a range of 7 to 10 mg/100 ml

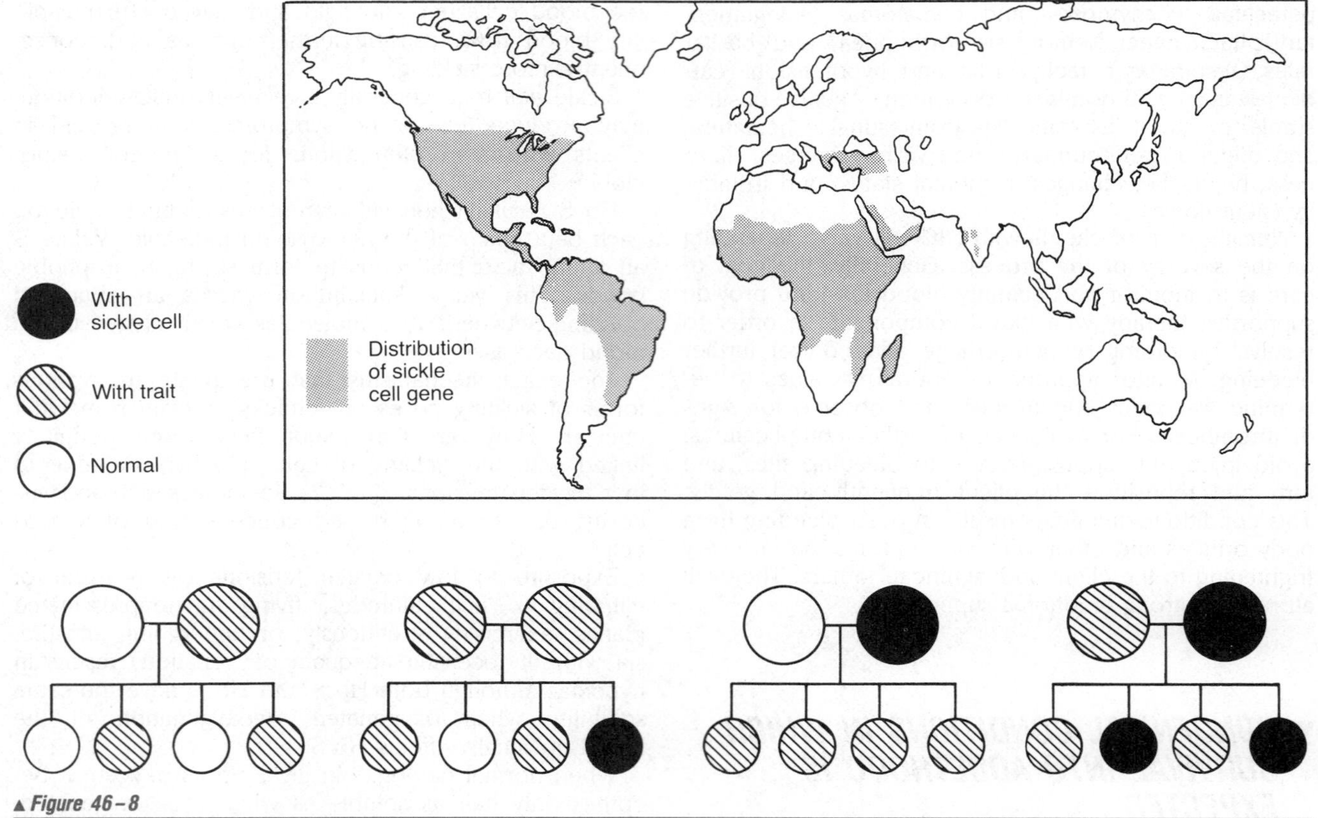

▲ *Figure 46–8*

Geographic distribution and inheritance pattern of sickle cell gene. (Redrawn from Page, J., et al. [1981]. *Blood: the river of life.* Washington, DC: Torstar Books.)

- thrombosis and infarction from the occluded microcirculation
- an elevated bilirubin from the released hemoglobin that may result in gallstone formation (cholelithiasis)

These three problems profoundly affect all organs and tissues with severe, often fatal consequences. Infarctions in the spleen are so common that, after childhood, the spleen of most sickle cell anemia clients is small and scarred.

Other clinical manifestations include necrosis of the head of the femur possibly leading to osteomyelitis, necrotic bone marrow with development of infection, renal medullary ischemia resulting in diminished capacity to concentrate urine, priapism, pulmonary infarctions, myocardial infarctions, and cerebrovascular accidents. Leg ulcers are found in about 75 per cent of older children or adults with the disease.

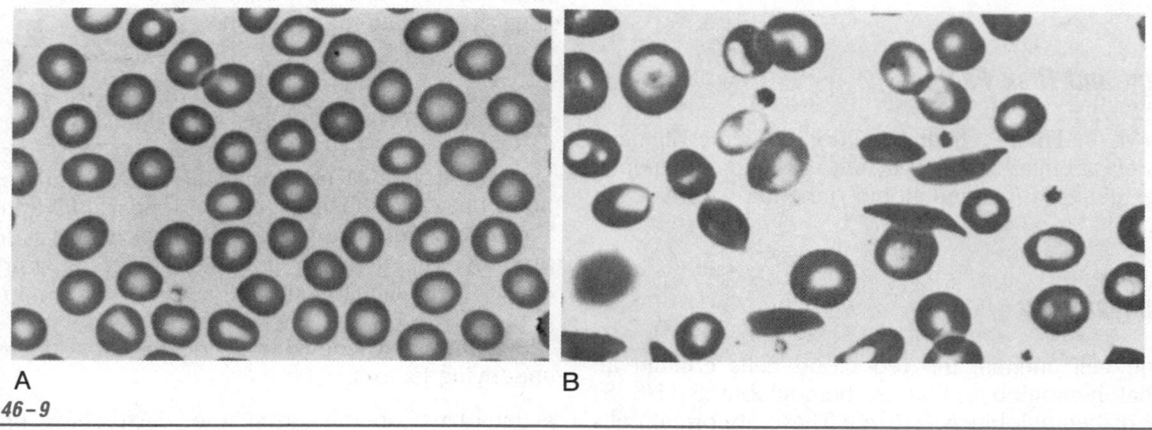

▲ *Figure 46–9*

Erythrocytes. Comparison of normal red blood cells *(A)* and sickled cells *(B)* (magnification ×875). Sickled cells in *B* are indicated by arrows. (From Henry, J. B. [1991]. *Clinical diagnosis and management* [18th ed.]. Philadelphia: W. B. Saunders.)

Thrombotic episodes often cause moderate to severe pain of the extremities, joints, and abdomen. Proliferation of the bone marrow, in an attempt to compensate for the chronic anemia, leads to osteoporosis and, later, osteosclerosis. These are only a few of the possible complications of sickle cell anemia.

Cerebral hemorrhage, or shock, claims the lives of many children with this disorder. However, some clients survive until age 50 years or older. Death usually results from uremia caused by progressive renal damage.

DIAGNOSTIC ASSESSMENT

Four laboratory procedures currently indicate the presence of sickle cell hemoglobin in either homozygous or heterozygous carriers: stained blood smear; sickle cell slide preparation; sickle-turbidity tube test (Sickledex); and hemoglobin electrophoresis.

Stained Blood Smear. A stained blood smear is examined for the presence of sickle cells.

Sickle Cell Slide Preparation (Sickle Prep). A blood specimen is observed for the sickling phenomenon after deoxygenation of the blood. This test is accurate but time-consuming.

Sickle-Turbidity Tube Test (Sickledex). This is an excellent mass screening test that detects sickle cell hemoglobin. After a finger prick, blood is mixed with Sickledex solution in a test tube. Five minutes later, the specimen is observed for cloudiness, which demonstrates the presence of Hb S. Solutions mixed with normal hemoglobin remain clear. Although indicative of Hb S, this test does not differentiate between sickle cell disease and the trait.

Hemoglobin Electrophoresis. Hemoglobin electrophoresis differentiates between sickle cell anemia and sickle cell trait. By means of an applied electric field, the various types of hemoglobin within a blood specimen are separated. If a blood specimen contains both Hb S and Hb A, the client has sickle cell trait. If only Hb S is present, the client has sickle cell anemia.

Many blacks are unaware that they carry the sickle cell trait and that they can transmit this trait to their offspring. Consequently, researchers are perfecting mass screening tests for the detection of Hb S among the black population. Clients having only the sickle cell trait may never be detected unless they are exposed to extremely low oxygen tensions (e.g., mountain climbing or flying in a nonpressurized plane), extremely hard work or exercise, or pregnancy. When exposed to extreme stressors, the client with the trait may develop symptoms of sickle cell disease.

Medical Management

Treatment for sickle cell anemia consists chiefly of supportive care (e.g., rest, oxygen, intravenous administration of fluids and electrolytes to ensure adequate hydration, sedation, and the prescription of analgesics).

In some cases, the slow administration of packed red blood cells or partial exchange transfusion helps relieve severe anemic symptoms. During episodes of increased risk (e.g., surgery, pregnancy), some clients benefit from hypertransfusion (transfusions until more than 50 per cent of the circulating red blood cells are of donor origin).

PHARMACOLOGIC MANAGEMENT

Anticoagulants, steroids, and cobalt treatments have all been used to reverse the sickling process without success. Clients with sickle cell disease have an increased need for folic acid and therefore usually receive a daily oral supplement to prevent increased anemia from folate deficiency.

Hydroxyurea and erythropoietin are being used in clinical trials in an attempt to increase fetal hemoglobin in those clients diagnosed with sickle cell disease.

Nursing Management

ASSESSMENT

Assessment findings include jaundice or pallor and ulceration (integumentary); joint swelling, disproportionately long arms and legs, fragility, and bone pain (skeletal); delayed sexual maturity and retarded growth (developmental status); enlargement of liver and spleen (gastrointestinal); and self-esteem disturbance, ineffective family coping, altered family processes, anticipatory grieving, noncompliance with health regimen, powerlessness, hopelessness, self-care deficit in activities of daily living, and altered thought processes (psychoemotional status).

Assessment findings during *sickle cell crisis* include systolic murmurs, arrhythmias, and enlargement (cardiac function); dyspnea and acute respiratory distress, that is, shortness of breath, chest pain, and cyanosis (respiratory); signs and symptoms of increased intracranial pressure due to cerebral hemorrhaging (sensory and motor function); and signs and symptoms of uremia, such as decreased urinary output and edema (renal function).

NURSING INTERVENTION

Nursing Diagnosis: Pain R/T sickling crisis.

Planning: Expected Outcomes. The client will have pain relieved, as evidenced by verbalization of pain relief.

Implementation. Assess for pain every 2 to 4 hours and administer analgesics as needed according to orders; monitor for effectiveness of analgesia. Apply heat to joints as ordered. Provide rest periods. Administer fluids to prevent dehydration and recurrence of pain crisis. Increase oral fluid intake. Monitor intake and output. Provide the client with information on how to prevent crises, such as (1) warn the client to avoid high altitudes and flying in nonpressurized planes, because oxygen tension is lowered under these conditions; and (2) caution the client against becoming dehydrated and advise the client to call a physician if vomiting, diarrhea, high fever, or any other cause of water loss develops.

Nursing Diagnosis: Knowledge Deficit R/T disease, treatment, and prevention of crises.

Planning: Expected Outcomes. The client will understand the disease, treatment, and prevention of crises, as evidenced by client's statements and absence of crises.

Implementation. When teaching clients about sickle cell anemia or sickle cell trait, include the following points in the discussion:

- Explain the nature of the disease, and give the client a chance to express feelings and ask questions.
- Encourage black parents to have themselves and their children tested for the presence of Hb S.
- Encourage the client to have routine medical examinations that include a red blood cell count.
- Encourage young adults who carry Hb S to ask their physician for genetic counseling before marrying or having children.
- Warn young women with sickle cell anemia that pregnancy carries a very high risk for them. They may develop pulmonary or renal complications, or both.

HEMOPHILIAS

Definition

There are three major types of hemophilia: A (classic hemophilia), B (Christmas disease), and von Willebrand's disease. Their major characteristics are compared in Table 46-10. Because classic hemophilia makes up 80 per cent of all hemophilias, the discussion of symptoms and treatment refers only to this type.

Incidence

The hemophilias are relatively common disorders. Within the United States alone, an estimated 25,000 clients are afflicted with a form of hemophilia. The hemophilias are characterized by prolonged bleeding, particularly after accidental, surgical, or dental trauma.

Etiology

It is genetically transmitted in a sex-linked (X chromosome) recessive pattern. Females usually transmit the defective gene, but males develop the bleeding disorder. Females rarely have hemophilia. Female hemophilia carriers transmit the gene to half of their daughters. They transmit the disorder to half of their sons. Males with hemophilia transmit the gene to all of their daughters but to none of their sons.

TABLE 46-10. Comparison of the Three Forms of Hemophilia

Form of Hemophilia	Etiology	Transmission	Major Laboratory Findings
Hemophilia A (classic hemophilia)	Inherited factor VIII (antihemophilic globulin) deficiency	Transmitted as sex-linked *recessive* trait; transmitted by females; occurs in males and, rarely, homozygous females	Coagulation time prolonged but bleeding time normal; factor VIII missing from plasma
Hemophilia B (Christmas disease)	Inherited factor IX (plasma thromboplastin component) deficiency	Transmitted as sex-linked *recessive* trait; transmitted by females; occurs in males and, rarely, homozygous females	Laboratory findings and symptoms same as in hemophilia A; factor IX missing
Von Willebrand's disease	Inherited factor VIII deficiency and defective platelet dysfunction	Transmitted as autosomal *dominant* trait to both sexes; occurs in both males and females	Both coagulation time and bleeding time prolonged; low factor VIII levels; platelet adhesiveness decreased

Risk Factors

Because this is a hereditary disease, the only way to control the risk is through genetic testing and counseling for decreasing the transmission.

Pathophysiology

Hemophilia A, the most common of the congenital coagulation disorders, is due to a deficiency in the procoagulant protein factor VIII (Table 46-11).

TABLE 46-11. Coagulation Factors

Factor	Name	Source	Function	Comments
I	Fibrinogen	Liver	Produces fibrin	Protein found in plasma at average level of 300 mg/100 ml
II	Prothrombin	Liver (requires vitamin K)	Produces thrombin	Glucoprotein found in plasma
III	Thromboplastin			Requires factors V, VII, X
	Incomplete form	Tissues and platelets		
	Complete form	Plasma	Acts on prothrombin to produce thrombin	A product of interaction between factors VIII, IX, and XI
IV	Calcium	Diet	Activates enzymes	Inorganic ion required in all stages of coagulation; normal plasma level 4.8–5.2 mEq/L
V	Labile factor	Plasma	Accelerates conversion of prothrombin to thrombin	Deteriorates rapidly at room temperature; used up in clotting process
VI	Unassigned			In early studies was thought to be the active form of factor V
VII	Stable factor	Liver	Accelerates conversion of prothrombin to thrombin	Stable to heat and storage; not consumed in clotting
VIII	Antihemophilic globulin	Plasma globulin	Essential to thromboplastin formation and conversion of prothrombin to thrombin	Unstable at room temperature; completely consumed in clotting
IX	Plasma thromboplastin component (Christmas factor)	Liver	Influences amount of thromboplastin made	Not consumed during clotting
X	Stuart-Prower factor	Liver? (requires vitamin K)	Essential to thromboplastin formation and conversion of prothrombin to thrombin	Stable at room temperature; similar to factor VII
XI	Plasma thromboplastin antecedent	Unknown	Essential to thromboplastin formation	Stable at room temperature
XII	Hageman factor	Unknown	Uncertain	Relatively stable; activated on contact with glass
XIII	Fibrin stabilizing factor	Unknown	Maintains clot after formation	High levels in plasma; deficiency associated with mild bleeding tendency, poor wound healing

Clinical Manifestations

Hemophilia may be mild or severe, depending on the level of factor VIII or IX coagulant activity. Usually diagnosed in childhood, this disorder is manifested in the following ways: slow persistent bleeding from cuts, scratches, and other minor traumas; delayed hemorrhage that follows minor injuries—bleeding may not start from a site until hours or even days after the moment of trauma; severe hemorrhaging from the gums after dental extraction or even brushing the teeth with a hard toothbrush; severe, sometimes fatal, epistaxis after injury to the nose; overwhelming gastric hemorrhage, which may be linked with gastric disorders such as ulcers; recurrent hematoma formation in the deep subcutaneous tissue, in the intramuscular tissues, and around the peripheral nerves. If nerves are compressed by hematomas, the client suffers severe pain, anesthesia of the innervated part, nerve damage, and paralysis. In addition, muscular atrophy sometimes results. Finally, there is recurrent hemarthrosis (bleeding into the joints), which is common in untreated cases and may result in serious joint deformity and permanent crippling. Hemarthrosis affects the knees, ankles, elbows, wrists, fingers, hips, and shoulders, in that order. All of this bleeding can be controlled with the administration of the missing factor (VIII or IX).

DIAGNOSTIC ASSESSMENT

Platelet function, platelet count, bleeding time, and prothrombin time are normal. The activated partial thromboplastin time will be prolonged. Quantitative assays for factor VIII will determine the severity of the disease.

Medical Management

The goals of care for clients with hemophilia are to stop topical bleeding as quickly as possible; to raise the level of antihemophilic factor (AHF) in the plasma, thereby temporarily supplying the missing factor causing hemorrhage; and to prevent complications leading to and caused by bleeding.

Immediate transfusion of factor VIII or IX concentrate is the primary treatment. Although plasma and cryoprecipitate contain factor VIII, concentrates have a known AHF content and carry less risk of blood volume overload. Hepatitis and HIV infection represent the major infectious risks, but improved purification techniques now used routinely in the preparation of concentrated factors have virtually eliminated this risk. Because the procoagulant activity of AHF disappears rapidly, clients need transfusions every 12 hours until bleeding stops.

Transfusion of packed red blood cells or white blood cells are used only to replace blood volume when there has been severe loss. Prophylactic transfusion of factor VIII to a level of 50 per cent above normal is recommended in cases of minor injury, surgery, and dental extractions.

One major complication is linked with repeated transfusions and AHF therapy. About 5 per cent of hemophiliacs become sensitized to AHF and develop autoimmune anti-AHF antibodies. In clients with low titers of factor VIII antibodies, major and life-threatening hemorrhages are treated with massive doses of factor VIII from animal sources (bovine and porcine), inactivated prothrombin complex concentrates (Konyne, Proplex), or activated prothrombin complex concentrates (FEIBA, Autoplex). Clinicians are using various experimental treatments such as immunosuppressive therapy to combat this problem. Topical bleeding can usually be temporarily controlled by applying pressure to the injured site, packing the area with a fibrin foam, and applying topical hemostatics such as thrombin.

Hemarthrosis may be controlled if the client receives AHF in the early stages of bleeding. Joint immobilization and local chilling (such as packing ice around the joint) may bring relief. If pain is severe, it may be necessary to aspirate blood from the joint. Once bleeding stops and swelling subsides, the client should perform active range-of-motion exercises without weight-bearing to prevent further complications, such as deformity and muscle atrophy.

The prognosis for clients with hemophilia has greatly improved since the discovery of AHF. Before this, 50 per cent of hemophiliacs died before they reached their fifth birthday. Today, death rarely occurs after minor trauma. Home infusion of AHF ensures that treatment is instituted at the first sign of bleeding, and complications are thus prevented. Clinicians have developed training programs for hemophiliacs with strict guidelines. When these guidelines are carefully followed, clients with hemophilia lose less time from work or school and need fewer emergency room visits. Fatalities mainly follow the development of autoimmune antibodies (anti-AHF) and retroperitoneal bleeding after internal hemorrhage.

PHARMACOLOGIC MANAGEMENT

Analgesics and corticosteroids often reduce joint pain and swelling. In mild hemophilia, the use of intravenous desmopressin may eliminate the need for AHF. Desmopressin acts by causing an increase in plasma factor VIII activity.

Nursing Management

ASSESSMENT

Although most clients with hemophilia are successfully maintained with home health care, they may be seen in the hospital during acute bleeding episodes or for nonrelated treatments. If even a minor invasive procedure is planned, it is crucial to assess the factor VIII level and administer a sufficient quantity of factor concentrate before the procedure.

During routine medical examinations, these clients should be assessed for frequency of bleeding episodes and effectiveness of home therapy. Examine joints for signs of bleeding and related atrophy.

NURSING INTERVENTION

Nursing Diagnosis: Knowledge Deficit R/T potential for bleeding.

Planning: Expected Outcomes. The client will understand how to prevent or immediately treat bleeding, as evidenced by the client's ability to describe precautions, absence of injury, or rapid treatment of unavoidable injury.

Implementation. Provide teaching about bleeding precautions for prevention of injury or trauma that may precipitate a bleeding episode. Effective and prompt administration of factors to reduce the incidence of bleeding episodes and resultant complications, such as joint atrophy, is a priority. The client should avoid activities that may induce bleeding. Genetic counseling (if the client has the hereditary form of hemophilia) and teaching of the client and significant others should be done.

During client teaching, review routine situations that increase the client's risk of bleeding, such as contact sports, minor invasive procedures, falls, and cuts. Teach the client to recognize early symptoms and why it is critical to intervene with treatment immediately. Discuss situations that require medical consultation.

EVALUATION

The nurse must evaluate client outcomes on the basis of the established plan of care. If these goals have not been achieved, the plan and interventions must be revised to meet the client's needs.

Post-hospital Care

DISCHARGE TEACHING

The client requires a great deal of teaching for managing the disease independently at home. The client will need to learn self-intravenous infusion administration techniques to control the bleeding.

FOLLOW-UP CARE

Clients will need to be followed closely for the rest of their lives so the disease can be controlled.

▼ BLOOD TRANSFUSIONS

Hematologic disorders or the aggressive ablative therapy used to treat some hematologic diseases can require acute or chronic support with a variety of blood components. Technologic advances to improve the quality and safety of transfusions have caused a revolution in blood banking. This field has evolved into a broader specialty of transfusion medicine wherein the administration of blood components is considerably more complex and tightly regulated. The Joint Commission on Accreditation of Healthcare Organizations requires that all blood transfusions be evaluated in order to confirm that clear medical indications for the transfusion exist and that the client responds as expected. The transfusionist plays a critical role in this process. It is the nurse's responsibility to administer appropriate blood components in a manner that will ensure safety and efficacy.

PREPARING FOR TRANSFUSION

Assessment of the Client

The physician's order for transfusion should specify blood component, volume, and rate of infusion. However, as with all potentially hazardous biologics, the nurse must confirm that the drug being given is safe and appropriate in the present clinical situation. Table 46–13 describes each blood component, appropriate and inappropriate uses, and other pertinent information.

Informed Consent and Client Teaching

In recent years, failure to disclose information and obtain consent for transfusion has resulted in litigation when transfusion complications occurred. Informed consent involves explaining medical indications for transfusion, benefits, risks, and alternatives.

Two alternatives to homologous (random) blood transfusion should be considered: autologous and directed (or designated) donation. Clients who do not have leukemia or bacteremia should be offered the option of donating their own blood before a scheduled surgical procedure if there is a reasonable expectation that blood will be required. Although the risk/benefit ratio should be evaluated, experience to date indicates that even clients with heart disease and other high-risk conditions tolerate the procedure well. The elimination of disease transmission, alloimmunization, and other potential transfusion complications makes this a reasonable option for many surgical clients.

Autologous donations can be made every 3 days if the donor's hemoglobin remains at or above 11 g/100 ml. For the blood to be maintained in a liquid state, donations should begin within 5 weeks of the transfusion date. Red blood cells can be stored frozen for 10 years, but the expense involved and time required for final preparation limit this practice to those who have extremely rare blood types. Donations should cease at least 3 days before the date of transfusion.

Another frequently used method of autologous blood collection is intraoperative, postoperative, or posttraumatic blood salvage. This procedure involves suctioning blood from body cavities, joint spaces, and other closed operative or trauma sites. Tissue debris and other sterile contaminants may necessitate special processing such as washing. Salvaged blood must be reinfused within 6 hours of collection.

A second option is for transfusion recipients to designate their own donors. Directed donations have not been shown to decrease the risk of contracting human immunodeficiency virus (HIV). In fact, some evidence indicates that directed donors have a higher incidence of hepatitis. This is probably due to the fact that a large percentage of directed donors are giving blood for the first time, and it is well documented that first-time donors more frequently test positive for hepatitis surrogate markers. In spite of this evidence, clients frequently feel more comfortable identifying their donors. It is essential to discuss all of these options with the client in sufficient time for permitting donation and blood testing.

Documentation of informed consent may consist of a form in the medical record stating that this information was presented in a manner understandable to the client (that is, "Risks of and alternatives to blood transfusion were explained, and the client consented.") If the client is clinically unable to consent to transfusion, a reasonable effort should be made to secure consent from a family member. If no family member is available or time does not allow, a note to this effect should be placed in the chart. Institutional policy will vary regarding who is permitted to obtain consent (see Ethical Issues in Nursing). Some facilities restrict this responsibility to the physician; others allow both nurses and physicians to perform this procedure. Regardless of the degree of nursing involvement in the formal process, the nurse is the client's most readily available source of information.

The client's understanding of the transfusion should be assessed and accurate responses should be made to questions and concerns. If questions are outside the nurse's area of expertise, transfusion medicine staff can serve as a valuable resource.

It is also the transfusionist's responsibility to describe the details of the transfusion procedure. Venous access, length of transfusion, and expected outcomes should be explained. The client should be informed of normal physiologic responses to transfusion and symptoms to be reported immediately. Clients released from care after transfusion should be given written information, including the name and phone number of a contact person.

Pretransfusion Testing

In today's climate, the client's major concern is likely to be the safety of the transfusion, specifically the risk of contracting AIDS. The transfusionist should dispel misconceptions and provide factual information. Efforts to ensure a safe and effective transfusion begin before the blood or component is collected. For many decades, prospective donors have been asked two categories of questions: those intended to protect the donor from possible risks of donation, and those intended to protect the recipient from risks of transfusion.

In order to decrease the risk of HIV transmission to blood recipients, there has been a marked increase in the second group of questions. In addition, donors are required to read information about behaviors known to increase the risk of HIV infection and, in most collection centers, they are questioned directly about their involvement in such activities.

Finally, a method must be made available for donors to indicate anonymously that their unit is or is not safe for transfusion. In addition to obtaining a thorough donor history, many serologic and infectious disease tests are routinely performed on the donor's blood. Table 46–13 provides an overview of these tests.

When a need for blood is identified, several tests are done to confirm that the client's blood is compatible with that of the donor. First, the recipient's ABO and Rh type are identified. To determine the presence of antibody other than anti-A or anti-B, an antibody screen is performed. This test is done by adding the recipient's serum to donor red blood cells known to have a certain set of minor blood group antigens. Coombs' sera are added to facilitate visibility of cellular agglutination, an indicator of antigen-antibody complex formation (also referred to as an indirect antiglobulin test). The results are viewed macro- and microscopically. More than 400 minor red cell antigens have been identified on red blood cells, each of which can stimulate the production of an antibody. However, only the few (approximately 30) that are of sufficiently potent antigenicity to be clinically significant are included in the routine antibody screen.

It is not uncommon for chronically transfused clients to develop multiple antibodies. Identifying the antibodies and obtaining blood from donors who do not possess the antigens can significantly complicate the testing procedure and lengthen the time required for blood preparation.

Blood products containing red blood cells may be further tested for compatibility to crossmatch testing. For this procedure, donor red blood cells are combined with the recipient's serum and Coombs' sera. After an inoculation period, the results are viewed microscopically. If no red blood cell agglutination has occurred, the crossmatch is compatible. Studies indicate that crossmatching adds very little to the safety of transfusion (0.01 to 0.1 percent) if a negative antibody screen is initially obtained.[16] In these situations, the Coombs' phase can be eliminated to shorten the procedure and reduce cost.

Text continued on page 1393

TABLE 46–12. Blood Components

	Whole Blood	Red Blood Cells	Platelet Concentrates	Fresh Frozen Plasma	Cryoprecipitate	Granulocyte Concentrates	Plasma Derivatives	Coagulation Factor Concentrates
Composition	RBC, plasma, plasma proteins (globulins, antibodies), 63 ml of anticoagulant-preservative	RBC with CPDA-1 solution (anticoagulant-preservative only), final hematocrit no higher than 80% (80% RBC, 20% plasma) RBC with 100 ml additive solution, final hematocrit about 55–60%	Single-unit platelets contain a minimum of 5.5×10^{10} (1 unit) platelets in 50–70 ml of plasma obtained by separating platelet-rich plasma from 1 unit of fresh whole blood; 6–10 units may be pooled for 1 transfusion Single-donor platelets contain a minimum of 3.0×10^{11} platelets (6 units) obtained from single donor by use of automated cell separator during apheresis; recipient exposed to fewer donors, which decreases complications	91% water, 7% protein (globulin, antibodies, clotting factors), and 2% carbohydrates Freezing within 8 hr of collection preserves all clotting factors	Each unit contains about 80–120 units of factor VIII (antihemophilic factor) that represents 50% of antihemophilic factor originally present in unit, von Willebrand's factor, 250 mg of fibrinogen, and 20–30% of factor XIII present in a unit of whole blood, suspended in 10–20 ml of plasma	Unit obtained by granulocytapheresis contains a minimum of 1.0×10^{10} granulocytes, variable amounts of lymphocytes (usually <10%), 30–50 ml of RBC and 100–400 ml of plasma, and 6–10 units of platelets; the platelets can be separated from the unit if the granulocyte recipient is not thrombocytopenic	*Albumin:* 96% albumin, 4% globulin and other proteins extracted from plasma; available as a 5% solution, oncotically equivalent to plasma, and also a concentrated 25% solution *Plasma protein fraction:* 83% albumin and 17% globulins extracted from plasma; less pure than albumin and has higher degree of contamination with other plasma proteins; in 5% solution only	*Factor VIII:* Lyophilized concentrate containing large quantities of factor VIII; prepared from large pools of donor plasma, but heat treatment during fractionation process significantly reduces risk of transmitting viral disease *Factor IX:* Lyophilized concentrate containing large quantities of factor IX; also contains factors II, VII, and X; product prepared from large pools of donor plasma, but heat treatment during fractionation process significantly reduces risk of transmitting viral disease
Volume	500 ml/unit	250–350 ml/unit 350–400 ml/unit	50–70 ml/unit 200–400 ml/unit	200–250 ml	5–10 ml/unit	200–400 ml with platelets 100–200 ml without platelets	Albumin: 250 and 500 ml (5%); 50 and 100 ml (25%)	Multiple-dose vial

Table continued on following page

TABLE 46-12. *Blood Components* Continued

	Whole Blood	Red Blood Cells	Platelet Concentrates	Fresh Frozen Plasma	Cryoprecipitate	Granulocyte Concentrates	Plasma Derivatives	Coagulation Factor Concentrates
Use	Acute, massive blood loss with hypotension, tachycardia, shortness of breath, pallor, and low hemoglobin/hematocrit	Acute or chronic blood loss with tachycardia, shortness of breath, pallor, low hemoglobin/hematocrit, and fatigue	To control or prevent bleeding associated with deficiencies in platelet number or function Used prophylactically for platelet counts <10,000–20,000/mm³ Administered if evidence of bleeding with platelet count <50,000/mm³	To increase level of clotting factors in clients with demonstrated deficiency If PT and PTT are <1.5 times normal, FFP is rarely indicated	To correct deficiencies of factor VIII (hemophilia A), von Willebrand's factor, factor XIII, and fibrinogen Occasionally used to control bleeding in uremic clients	To treat clients with acquired neutropenia or congenital WBC dysfunction, who have serious infections unresponsive to conventional antibiotics Granulocytes are not currently licensed by FDA Long-term therapeutic benefit of granulocyte transfusion still questionable and continues to be evaluated	To provide volume expansion in situations in which crystalloid solutions are not adequate, such as plasma exchange, shock, and massive hemorrhage Also used for treatment of acute liver failure, burns, and hemolytic disease of the newborn	*Factor VIII:* To treat moderate to severe congenital factor VIII deficiency (hemophilia A) *Factor IX:* To treat factor IX deficiency (hemophilia B or Christmas disease); may be used to treat congenital factor VII or factor X deficiency
Inappropriate Use	Volume expansion; enhancement of wound healing	Volume expansion; enhancement of wound healing to improve general well-being	Treatment of ITP (unless life-threatening bleeding); prophylactically with massive transfusion; prophylactically after cardiopulmonary bypass surgery	Volume expansion; nutritional supplement; prophylactically with massive blood transfusion; prophylactically after cardiopulmonary bypass surgery	Any other use	Any other use	Any other use	Dose calculated to body weight and desired level of factor activity Factor VIII coagulant activity level of 30–50% commonly endpoint of therapy Lyophilized concentration provided with sterile diluent for reconstitution

Average Adult Dose and Rate	Determined by blood loss As rapidly as needed to stabilize hemodynamics	2–4 units; 1 unit over $1\frac{1}{2}$–2 hr, not to exceed 4 h	6–10 units given over 30–90 min (determined by volume tolerance)	Determined by situation; 200 ml/h or more slowly if circulatory overload a potential problem	Dose calculated on plasma volume; 8–10 bags supply 2 g fibrinogen Amount of factor VIII required for transfusion calculated as follows: 1. Blood volume (ml) = weight (kg) × 70 ml/kg 2. Plasma volume (ml) = blood volume (ml) × (1.0 − hematocrit) 3. Units factor VIII required = plasma volume (ml) × (desired factor VIII level U/ml − initial factor VIII level U/ml) 4. Bags of cryoprecipitate = units factor VIII/100 To achieve the desired therapeutic level, this dose may need to be repeated in 8–12 h; administer at 1–2 ml/min	1 unit (1×10^{10} granulocytes) daily given slowly over 1–2 h (based on 200-ml volume)	Dependent on client situation Albumin given at 1–10 ml/min (5%) or more rapidly if client is in shock; 0.2–0.4 ml/min (25%) PPF must not exceed 10 ml/min	Given IV push

Table continued on following page

TABLE 46-12. Blood Components Continued

	Whole Blood	Red Blood Cells	Platelet Concentrates	Fresh Frozen Plasma	Cryoprecipitate	Granulocyte Concentrates	Plasma Derivatives	Coagulation Factor Concentrates
Equipment	19-gauge needle, standard straight or Y-type blood administration set with minimum 170 μm filter, 0.9% saline	19-gauge needle, standard straight or Y-type blood administration set with minimum 170 μm filter, 0.9% saline	19- to 21-gauge needle, component administration set with standard 170 μm filter, 0.9% saline	19- to 23-gauge needle, component administration set with standard 170 μm filter, 0.9% saline	19- to 21-gauge needle, component administration set with standard 170 μm filter, 0.9% saline	19- to 21-gauge needle, component administration set with standard 170 μm filter, 0.9% saline *Never* use a leukocyte-depleting filter to infuse granulocytes	19- to 21-gauge needle and standard IV infusion set A filter may be required by some manufacturers; check product insert for specific instructions Administration set with filter may be supplied with the albumin	IV push through filtered needle or IV drip using component recipient set
ABO/Rh Compatibility	The ABO type of the donor should be identical with the recipient's Rh− blood can be given to an Rh− or Rh+ recipient	A can match with A or O; B can match with B or O; O can match only with O; AB can match with A, B, or O Rh− blood can be given to either Rh+ or Rh− recipient	Whereas platelets have no ABO or Rh antigens, they are suspended in 200–400 ml of plasma containing donor antibodies and a small number of RBC There is evidence that platelet survival decreases if donor plasma is incompatible, and large volumes of incompatible plasma may cause a positive direct Coombs' test	A can match with A or AB; B can match with B or AB; AB can match only with AB; O can match with A, B, AB, or O Rh− and Rh+ can be given to either Rh+ or Rh− recipient	Cryoprecipitate contains no RBC and a small volume of plasma ABO cross-matching not needed, and plasma compatibility preferred but not required	Granulocytes contain a significant number of RBC and plasma; therefore, ABO of donor should be identical with recipient's Rh− components may be transfused to an Rh+ recipient	Antibodies destroyed during processing; therefore, compatibility not a factor	Antibodies destroyed during processing, so compatibility not a factor

			It is also possible for even a small number of Rh+ RBC to stimulate anti-D in an Rh− recipient; therefore, plasma ABO and Rh compatibility is recommended					
Special Considerations	Whole blood transfusion is rarely indicated Treatment with specific blood components is usually recommended	RBC may be viscous, so 0.9% saline may be added to achieve optimal flow rates	Because platelet concentrates contain few RBC, crossmatch testing is not required Plasma ABO and Rh compatibility is recommended especially when the total volume of the transfusion exceeds 150–200 ml For some clients, a leukocyte depletion filter may be used to prevent complications Only filters specially designed for platelet transfusion should be used	Plasma carries same risk of disease transmission as does whole blood If only volume expansion is required, products of choice are crystalloid or colloid solutions, such as saline or albumin Plasma contains no RBC, and Rh compatibility and crossmatching are not required ABO compatibility must be confirmed before administration	Single units of cryoprecipitate may be pooled into 1 container by the blood collection center If individual bags are issued, 0.9% saline may need to be added to rinse residual cryoprecipitate from bags and tubing	Granulocytes have short survival (<24 hr); infuse as soon as possible Granulocyte concentrates contain a significant number of RBC; pretransfusion testing ordinarily the same as for RBC transfusion Increased incidence of febrile, nonhemolytic reactions with granulocyte transfusions; infuse slowly, observe client closely; premedication with an antihistamine, acetaminophen, steroids, or meperidine may be indicated to prevent repeat reactions	PPF and albumin cannot transmit hepatitis or HIV infection; the pasteurization process used to prepare the products destroys such viruses Hypotension has been associated with rapid infusion of PPF; 25% albumin can cause a significantly increased blood pressure because of its ability to draw fluid into the intravascular space	Factor VIII and factor IX assays should be performed at appropriate intervals to assess response Factor VIII concentration lacks vWF and should not be used in treatment of von Willebrand's disease

Table continued on following page

TABLE 46–12. *Blood Components* Continued

	Whole Blood	Red Blood Cells	Platelet Concentrates	Fresh Frozen Plasma	Cryoprecipitate	Granulocyte Concentrates	Plasma Derivatives	Coagulation Factor Concentrates
						Do *not* administer amphotericin B within 4 hr of granulocyte transfusion (pulmonary insufficiency seen with concurrent administration)		
Expected Outcomes	Prevention or resolution of hypovolemic shock and anemia In a nonbleeding adult, 1 unit of whole blood should increase hematocrit by 3% and hemoglobin by 1 g/100 ml	Resolution of symptoms of anemia In a nonbleeding adult, 1 unit of RBC should increase hematocrit by 3% and hemoglobin by 1 g/100 ml	Prevention or resolution of bleeding due to thrombocytopenia or platelet dysfunction 1 unit should raise peripheral platelet count 5000 to 10,000/mm^3 if underlying cause is resolved or controlled Efficacy of platelet transfusion can be determined by obtaining platelet counts at 1 hr and 18–24 hr after infusion	Treatment effectiveness is assessed by monitoring coagulation function that is measured by the PT and PTT or by specific factor assays	Correction of factor VIII, von Willebrand's factor, factor XIII, and fibrinogen deficiency; cessation of bleeding in uremic clients Laboratory values required to assess effectiveness of treatment	Improvement in or resolution of infection No increase in peripheral WBC count usually seen after granulocyte transfusion in adults, although increase may be seen in children An improvement in clinical condition due to resolving infection is the only measure of treatment effectiveness	The client will acquire and maintain adequate blood pressure and volume support	The client will develop hemostasis due to increased levels of factor VIII and factor IX activity

FFP, fresh frozen plasma; HIV, human immunodeficiency virus; ITP, idiopathic thrombocytopenic purpura; IV, intravenous; PPF, plasma protein fraction; PT, prothrombin time; PTT, partial thromboplastin time; RBC, red blood cells; WBC, white blood cells.

TABLE 46-13. Routine Donor Infectious Disease Testing

Test	Purpose	Confirmatory Test	Follow-up/ Deferral
RPR (rapid plasma reagin)	Determines presence of *Treponema pallidum* infection (syphilis)	FTA (fluorescent antitreponemal antibody)	Blood discarded; donor deferred for 1 year; treponemes die in blood after 5 days of refrigeration
ALT (alanine aminotransferase)	Surrogate test for hepatitis C	None	Blood discarded if ALT out of range; donor deferred for repeat mild elevations or single gross abnormality
Anti-HBc	Surrogate test for hepatitis C; high incidence in HIV-positive donors	None	Blood discarded; donor may be permanently deferred
Anti-HCV	Determines presence of antibody to hepatitis C virus	None	Blood discarded; donor permanently deferred
HBsAg	Determines presence of hepatitis B surface antigen	Repeat test procedure after neutralization of HBsAg in sample with anti-HBs; results unaffected if false-positive, at least 50% reduction if true-positive	On confirmation, blood discarded; donor permanently deferred
Anti-HIV	Determines presence of antibody to human immunodeficiency virus	Western blot, 0.5% false-positive rate	Blood discarded if enzyme-linked immunosorbent assay (ELISA) positive twice; donor permanently deferred if repeat ELISA positive, Western blot positive or indeterminant
Anti-HTLV-1	Determines presence of antibody to human T-cell lymphotropic virus, type 1	Western blot and RIPA (radioimmunoprecipitation assay)	Infection may cause T-cell leukemia in 10–15 years; confirmed positive donors permanently deferred

Routine serologic testing requires a 10-ml clotted sample and a 7-ml citrated sample. Approximately 1 hour will be required for testing in routine situations. In the event of a medical emergency, O-negative red blood cells and AB plasma can be safely administered to most clients without serologic testing.

Failure to correctly label the samples used for blood bank testing resulted in 13 reported transfusion deaths from 1976 to 1985.[16] Several precautionary measures should be taken to reduce this risk. Samples must be labeled at the bedside after asking clients to state their name and comparing it with that on the identification bracelet. If clients are unable to state their name, identity should be confirmed by a family member or other familiar person whenever possible. The date and initials of the phlebotomist must be written on the sample label. Many institutions have adopted a secondary identification system. Several commercial systems are available; each is designed to ensure that the sample used for crossmatch has been drawn from the client who receives the transfusion.

Obtaining Venous Access

Suitable venous access for transfusion varies with the product being infused. When packed red blood cells weighing less than 300 g are infused, a 19-gauge or larger needle will be needed to achieve maximal flow rate. If a smaller gauge needle must be used, the red blood cells can be diluted with 0.9 per cent saline. No solution other than normal saline should be added to blood components.

Components containing a significant volume of plasma or other diluent can be safely infused at a rapid rate through smaller gauge needles or catheters. A central catheter is an acceptable venous access option for blood transfusion. It should be noted, however, that a large volume of refrigerated blood infused rapidly into the ventricle of the heart has been known to cause cardiac arrhythmias. Warming the blood can reduce the risk of this complication. Another issue of concern is the use of multilumen catheters that may allow blood to mix with incompatible solutions and medications as

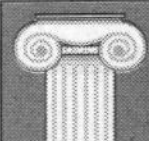

ETHICAL ISSUES IN NURSING

Should Parents Who Are Jehovah's Witnesses Have the Right to Refuse a Lifesaving Transfusion for Their Child?

Blood transfusions are a common and effective treatment for many disorders that may be life-threatening. In the past, there was never much controversy over the transfusion of blood products. Currently, however, because of acquired immunodeficiency syndrome (AIDS), transfusions are a little more risky even though testing is done on all donor blood for the AIDS virus and for hepatitis. Even so, transfusions are common, and although concern over safety remains, the receiving of blood products is not considered highly controversial.

Controversy does exist regarding blood component therapy for those who are members of the Jehovah's Witnesses church. The belief among these members is that they should receive no blood components donated from another person. There is hardly a dilemma when a competent adult Jehovah's Witness refuses blood component therapy (although there might be some issues that could cause controversy). However, should a Jehovah's Witness parent have the right to refuse perhaps a lifesaving transfusion for a minor child? Minors are not legally competent to make most health care decisions and, thus, rely on their parents as surrogate decision makers. These paternal decisions in most cases are thought to be out of beneficence in the best interest of the child. Is the refusal of a lifesaving treatment for a child, such as a blood transfusion, on the basis of religious beliefs of the parents ethical? Should these parents have such a surrogacy right regarding their own beliefs when the children may or may not wish to exercise the same beliefs of their Jehovah's Witness parents?

Nurses need to be aware of their clients who hold such religious restrictions on certain treatments. In dealing with competent adults, such decisions may not be truly understood by the health care providers, but they should be respected as a right of freedom of religion. The ethical and legal issues arise in dealing with minor children of parents who refuse physically beneficent treatments for their children on the basis of their religious beliefs. All nurses should be aware of their institution and state policies regarding such situations. In life or death situations, the nurse can truly make a difference by being informed of such policies and by acting responsibly no matter what personal feelings may be at hand.

---

they exit the catheter tips. Experience indicates that the circulation achieved through a blood vessel suitable for central line placement results in rapid mixing of fluids. As a result, no harmful effects have been reported.

Requesting Blood Release

Blood banking regulations state that refrigerated components may not be returned to inventory if they have been warmed to more than 10° C (50° F). To meet this requirement, most transfusion medicine services consider 30 minutes to be the maximal allowable time out of monitored storage. For avoiding delays that may result in the waste of a scarce commodity, certain procedures should be performed before blood is requested.

An intravenous catheter appropriate for transfusing the requested component should be functional, flushed with normal saline, and maintained at a keep vein open (KVO) rate. Vital signs should then be taken and recorded. Fever may be a cause for delaying the transfusion. In addition to masking a possible symptom of an acute transfusion reaction, fever can also compromise the efficacy of platelet transfusions.

Premedication may also be required if the client has a history of adverse reactions. In many cases, febrile reactions can be prevented by administering acetaminophen or diphenhydramine hydrochloride (Benadryl). Steroids have been used to avoid severe fever, rigors, and chills that accompany granulocyte transfusions. A history of allergic reactions may require prophylactic administration of antihistamines. For effectiveness to be ensured, oral medication should be administered 30 minutes before the transfusion is started. Intravenous medication may be given immediately before the transfusion is initiated.

Blood should be released from the blood bank only to adequately trained personnel. The name and identification number of the intended recipient must be provided and a permanent record of this information maintained in the blood bank. So that delivery to the wrong client is avoided, blood should be transported to only one client at a time.

BEGINNING THE TRANSFUSION

Confirming Blood Acceptability

The most critical phase of transfusion is confirming product compatibility and verifying client identity. A summary was recently compiled of transfusion-associated deaths reported to the Food and Drug Administration from 1976 through 1985. It revealed that the number of deaths resulting from noninfectious complications of transfusion occurred with the same frequency as HIV transmission (1 per 10,000); 158 of the 355 deaths reported resulted from acute hemolysis. In 69 of the deaths, the cause was traced to sample collection or laboratory processing error. However, in 77 cases, the wrong unit of blood was given to the client on the nursing unit ($n = 55$) or in the operating suite ($n = 22$).[69] The transfusionist can prevent this tragedy through meticulous adherence to the procedures described in this chapter.

Before going to the client's bedside, the nurse should verify ABO and Rh compatibility. This can usually be done by comparing the bag label with the medical record and forms issued from the blood bank. The bag label should also be checked to ensure that the correct component has been issued and for date of expiration. Components expire at midnight of the day marked on the bag unless otherwise specified.

Inspect the unit for leaks, abnormal color, clots, excessive air, and bubbles. Check carefully for important labels (such as autologous, directed) or instructions (such as "use leukocyte-depleting filter"). Cellular components (whole blood, red blood cells, and platelets) for a specific client population should be clearly marked *irradiated.* Clients with Hodgkin's or non-Hodgkin's lymphoma, acute leukemia, or congenital immunodeficiency disorders and bone marrow transplant recipients may develop posttransfusion GVHD if lymphocytes contaminating cellular components engraft and divide. Transfusions from first-degree family members have also been known to cause fatal GVHD. A small dose of radiation delivered to the component before release from the blood bank renders the lymphocytes incapable of mitotic action without presenting a radiation risk to the recipient or transfusionist.

At the bedside, ask clients to state their name and compare it with the name on the identification bracelet. As with sample collection, clients unable to state their name should be identified by a person who knows them well. Compare the name and number on the identification bracelet with the tag on the blood bag. If applicable, check the secondary identification system. The American Association of Blood Banks recommends that two qualified individuals perform this critical step.

Blood Infusion Equipment and Devices

Most blood products should be infused through administration sets designed specifically for this use. The set usually contains a 170 μm filter designed to trap fibrin clots and other debris that accumulates during blood storage. Most standard filters have a four-unit capacity. Tubing is available in two basic configurations: straight or Y-type. The use of Y-type tubing simplifies the process of adding normal saline to red blood cells and provides ready access to a saline flush if the transfusion must be interrupted. Straight tubing usually has a medication injection site a few inches from the needle. If an adverse reaction develops, a KVO saline drip initiated at this site will maintain patency of the intravenous line but avoid exposure to the 30 to 50 ml of blood remaining in the tubing and filter. The administration set should be changed every 4 to 6 hours, or according to institution policy, to reduce the risk of septicemia.

Many devices are available to increase the safety of the transfusion. Special filters, electromechanical devices, and blood warmers are frequently used at the bedside. The transfusionist should be familiar with how and why special equipment is used.

Nonstandard Filters

The physician or nurse may determine that the standard 170 μm filter is not adequate in certain clinical situations. The transfusion medicine service may also recommend the use of a nonstandard filter in order to decrease the risk of transfusion complications. Several types of specialty filters are described in Table 46-14. Although each is technically easy to use, inappropriate use can significantly compromise desired results. It is, therefore, critically important to follow the manufacturer's instructions exactly. An insert may be found inside the package, or instructions may be printed on the exterior of the packaging container.

Electromechanical Infusion Devices

Several types of infusion devices are available to regulate and monitor the flow of intravenous solutions. There are basically two types: infusion controllers, which monitor flow by gravity, and infusion pumps, which deliver solutions under pressure. Infusion controllers may be used with all blood products if they are designed to function with opaque solutions. However, the negative pressure exerted by the peristaltic or syringelike cassette action of infusion pumps could cause red blood cell hemolysis. If the transfusion product contains a significant number of red blood cells, the manufacturer should be consulted before a pump designed for crystalloid and colloid solutions is used.

Many studies have been done to determine the effect of mechanical devices on red blood cells. They clearly indicate that in addition to pump action, there are other factors that affect the degree of red blood cell hemolysis. These include length of tubing, diameter of tubing, type of filter, infusion rate, needle gauge, blood age, temperature, and viscosity. Therefore, it is imperative that machines tested and approved for the infusion of red blood cells be used exactly as recommended by the manufacturer.

If manual pressure cuffs are used to increase red blood cell flow rate, the pressure should not exceed 300 mm Hg. Standard sphygmomanometers should not be used for this purpose because they do not exert uniform pressure against all parts of the bag.

Blood Warmers

Blood warmers may be used to prevent hypothermia, which can be induced by rapid infusion of large volumes of refrigerated blood. Neonatal exchange transfusion, plasma exchange, surgery, and trauma are all clinical situations that may require the use of a blood warmer. Other clients of concern are those with cold agglutinin disease. These clients have antibodies that react at temperatures under 37° C (98.6° F). Systemic circulatory cooling can cause intravascular agglutination. This condition may be detected during serologic testing. Once this client has been identified, the transfusion service may recommend the use of a blood warmer for all transfusions.

There are two types of devices approved by blood bank regulatory agencies for warming blood. For dry heating, a bag is placed between two aluminum heating

TABLE 46–14. Nonstandard Filters

Filter	Design Features	Recommended Use	Special Considerations
High-flow filter	Standard pore size, large surface area; filters up to 10 units at high-flow rate	For massive transfusions primarily in critical care units, operating and emergency rooms	Appropriate for adults only
Pediatric filter	Standard pore size; small surface area reduces priming volume; may contain intermediate storage container for precise volume control	For small-volume transfusions; primarily neonates, children, geriatric clients	
Microaggregate filter	Plastic chamber containing mesh or fiber that effectively removes particles 20–40 μm in size	For preventing fibrin, leukocytes, or platelets from migrating to lungs during massive transfusion; marginally effective for preparation of leukocyte-reduced red blood cells	Instruction for use varies with manufacturer; follow priming and flushing instructions exactly to optimize effectiveness
Leukocyte-reducing filter	Chamber containing synthetic fibers treated to capture leukocytes; priming volume 20–40 ml; expensive ($20–60/filter)	For removal of 95–99+% of leukocytes from red blood cells or platelets to reduce incidence of febrile reactions, HLA alloimmunization, cytomegalovirus infection	Platelet and red blood cell filters are *not* interchangeable; follow manufacturer's instructions for priming, flushing, and rinsing, because failure to do so can severely compromise efficacy

plates, or a disposable cuff-style bag is wrapped around a cylindric aluminum heating element. A second type uses warm water to increase the temperature of the blood. Water baths containing water warmed to 37° C (98.6° F) may be used only if they have been specifically designed for warming blood. The blood bag should never be fully immersed in water. Studies indicate that water baths create an optimal medium for the growth of harmful organisms, which can contaminate the blood bag port and cause septicemia. Two transfusion-related deaths were traced to a water bath contaminated with *Pseudomonas*.

Conventional blood warmers have some limitations. The rate of infusion can be impeded by the additional tubing and blood warming bags required for conventional warming devices. Standard blood warmers also require substantial priming volume, which makes them inappropriate for small-volume transfusions. Devices have been designed specifically for these situations but care must be taken to use only equipment tested and approved for use with blood components. Acceptable devices must have a visible thermometer and an audible or visible alarm to alert the user if the temperature exceeds 38° C (100.4° F).

DURING TRANSFUSION

Monitoring the Client and Documenting Signs and Symptoms of Transfusion Reaction

The first 10 to 15 minutes of any transfusion are the most critical. If a major ABO incompatibility exists or a severe allergic reaction such as anaphylaxis occurs, it is usually evident within the first 50 ml of the transfusion. Therefore, it is recommended that the transfusion begin slowly, under close observation of medical personnel. If no evidence of a reaction is noted within the first 15 minutes, flow can be increased to the prescribed rate. Before leaving the client unattended, instruct the client to report anything unusual immediately. It is advisable to take and record vital signs before the transfusion begins, after the first 15 minutes, and every hour until 1 hour after the transfusion has been discontinued. The vital signs should be checked immediately if the client displays any untoward symptoms.

The recommended rate of infusion varies with the blood component being transfused. Components containing few red blood cells, such as platelets, plasma, and cryoprecipitate, may be infused rapidly, but care

Box 46–1. Possible Signs and Symptoms of a Transfusion Reaction

General

- Fever (rise of 1° C or 2° F)
- Chills
- Muscle aches, pain
- Back pain
- Chest pain
- Headache
- Heat at site of infusion or along vein

Nervous System

- Apprehension, impending sense of doom
- Tingling, numbness

Respiratory System

- Respiratory rate
  - Tachypnea
  - Apnea
- Dyspnea
- Cough
- Wheezing
- Rales

Gastrointestinal System

- Nausea
- Vomiting
- Pain, abdominal cramping
- Diarrhea (may be bloody)

Cardiovascular System

- Heart rate
  - Bradycardia
  - Tachycardia
- Blood pressure
  - Hypotension, shock
  - Hypertension
- Peripheral circulation
  - Color cyanosis, facial flushing
  - Temperature: cool/clammy; hot/flushed/dry
  - Edema
- Bleeding
  - Generalized (DIC)
  - Oozing at surgical site

Renal System

- Changes in urine volume
  - Oliguria, anuria
  - Renal failure
- Changes in urine color
  - Dark, concentrated
  - Shades of red, brown, amber
  - May indicate the presence in urine of red blood cells (hematuria) or of free hemoglobin (hemoglobinuria)

Integumentary System

- Rashes, hives (urticaria), swelling
- Itching
- Diaphoresis

should be taken to avoid circulatory overload. This is of particular concern in neonatal, pediatric, and geriatric clients and in clients with cardiac disease. For avoiding the risk of septicemia, infusions should not exceed 4 hours. If the client's size or medical condition does not allow infusion within 4 hours, the unit may be split into smaller aliquots in the blood bank.

Regulatory agencies require complete documentation of the transfusion, including identification of personnel starting and ending the transfusion, unique product number, and outcome (that is, "no reaction noted"). If an adverse reaction does occur, the symptoms, actions taken, and future recommendations should also be recorded in the client's medical record.

Nursing Management

Exposure to foreign blood elements may mediate immunologic and nonimmunologic reactions affecting all major body systems as described in Box 46–1. Any unusual sign or symptom occurring during or immediately after a transfusion should be considered a potential reaction. Unconscious clients should be monitored closely because signs of a reaction may be inhibited in the unconscious state (Box 46–2). The most frequently seen acute reactions are described in Table 46–15.

Whereas treatment may vary depending on the signs and symptoms, certain standard procedures should be followed when a reaction is suspected. In all cases,

Box 46–2. Signs of Transfusion Reaction in an Unconscious Patient

- Weak pulse
- Fever
- Hypotension
- Visible hemoglobinuria
- Increased operative bleeding (oozing at surgical site)
- Vasomotor instability (tachycardia, bradycardia, or hypotension)
- Oliguria/anuria

TABLE 46–15. Acute Transfusion Reactions

Reaction	Cause	Clinical Manifestations	Management	Prevention
Immunogenic				
Allergic Incidence: 1%	Sensitivity to foreign proteins in plasma	Urticaria, hives, flushing, itching (no fever)	Administer antihistamines as directed If symptoms mild and transient, transfusion may resume	Treat prophylactically with antihistamines
Febrile, nonhemolytic Incidence: 0.5–1.0%	Sensitization to donor white blood cells, platelets, or plasma proteins	Sudden chills and fever (rise in temperature of more than 1° C, 1.8° F), headache, flushing, anxiety, muscle pain	Give antipyretics as prescribed; avoid aspirin in thrombocytopenic clients	Consider leukocyte-poor blood products (filtered, washed, or frozen) if fever occurs more than once
Acute hemolytic Incidence: 1 : 25,000 Fatal: 2 : 1,000,000	Infusion of ABO incompatible red blood cells	Chills, fever, low back pain, flushing, tachycardia, tachypenia, hemoglobinuria, hemoglobinemia, hypotension, vascular collapse, bleeding, acute renal failure, shock, cardiac arrest, death	Treat shock Maintain blood pressure with IV solutions Give diuretics as prescribed to maintain urine flow Insert indwelling catheter or measure hourly output Dialysis may be needed	Meticulously verify recipient from sample collection to transfusion
Anaphylactic Incidence: 1 : 150,000	Infusion of IgA proteins to IgA-deficient recipient who has developed anti-IgA antibodies	Anxiety, urticaria, wheezing progressing to cyanosis, shock, and possible cardiac arrest	Initiate CPR if indicated Have epinephrine ready for injection (0.4 ml of a 1 : 1000 solution subcutaneously)	Give blood components from IgA-deficient donors or remove *all* plasma by washing
Nonimmunogenic				
Circulatory overload Estimated Incidence: 1 : 10,000 (not usually reported to blood bank)	Infusion of blood at a rate too rapid for the size, cardiac status, or clinical condition of the recipient	Cough, dyspnea, pulmonary congestion (rales), headache, hypertension, tachycardia, distended neck veins	Place client in upright position with feet in dependent position Administer diuretics, oxygen, and morphine as prescribed Phlebotomy may be required	Adjust transfusion volume and flow rate on basis of client size and clinical status If slow transfusion will exceed 4 h, request that unit be aliquoted into smaller volumes
Septicemia Incidence: very rare	Transfusion of component contaminated with microorganism	Rapid onset of chills, high fever, vomiting, diarrhea, marked hypotension and shock	Treat symptoms and administer antibiotics, IV fluids, vasopressors, and steroids as directed Obtain culture of client and blood containers	Collect, process, store, and transfuse blood according to industry standards Infuse within 4 h of starting time

IV, intravenous; CPR, cardiopulmonary resuscitation.

stop the transfusion and keep the intravenous line open with normal saline. Treat life-threatening symptoms, such as respiratory or circulatory failure, immediately. Contact the client's physician and the blood bank. According to institutional policy, obtain appropriate laboratory samples. Samples used to evaluate a reaction include blood and urine. Free hemoglobin found in either indicates that red blood cells have hemolyzed, the most serious serologic finding. To avoid clouding the diagnostic picture by venous trauma, obtain blood samples from a large peripheral vein using at least a 19-gauge needle. The blood sample is also used to repeat ABO and Rh type, antibody screen, and direct antiglobulin testing. A discrepancy between initial and repeat testing may indicate that incompatible blood was transfused. After laboratory testing, a physician specialized in transfusion medicine will evaluate the clinical and laboratory evidence for determining whether the client's symptoms were caused by the transfusion. The physician may then make recommendations for reducing the risk of complication in the future.

Transfusion services are required to maintain records of reaction evaluations and future transfusion restrictions. These records are consulted when future transfusions are required. Special processing, such as washing, may then be performed in the blood bank to reduce the risks of another adverse reaction. In some cases, instructions may be placed on the unit informing the transfusionist that a special filter or infusion device should be used at the bedside.

DELAYED TRANSFUSION COMPLICATIONS

Complications can occur days to years after a transfusion. Fever, mild jaundice, and decreased hematocrit may indicate a delayed hemolytic reaction. Hemolysis of red blood cells may occur 3 days to several months after the transfusion if an antibody was undetected during crossmatch testing and red blood cells containing that antigen were transfused. Usually no medical treatment is required. Iron overload may occur in clients receiving more than 100 units of blood over a period of time, such as in clients with aplastic anemia.

Clinical manifestations are congestive heart failure, arrhythmias, impaired thyroid and gonadal function, diabetes, and cirrhosis. Deferoxamine (Desferal), which chelates and removes accumulated iron via the kidneys, may be administered intravenously or subcutaneously to prevent this potentially fatal complication. Post-transfusion GVHD can occur if donor lymphocytes engraft and divide in the marrow spaces of an immunocompromised recipient. Symptoms are fever, rash, diarrhea, and hepatitis. This frequently fatal complication can be prevented by irradiation of all cellular components.

Many diseases can be transmitted through blood transfusion. The most common is hepatitis C. Although symptoms are milder than those seen with hepatitis B, chronic liver disease and cirrhosis may develop. Hepatitis B should be considered if the recipient develops anorexia, malaise, nausea, vomiting, dark urine, and jaundice within 4 to 6 weeks of transfusion. An elevated alanine aminotransferase and aspartate aminotransferase are frequently seen, indicating liver damage that may be permanent. Hepatitis B and C are treated symptomatically. With advances in donor testing and screening in the United States, the risk of hepatitis has decreased to about 3 per cent.

On rare occasions, HIV-1 is transmitted from an infected donor to a blood recipient. The client may be asymptomatic for several years or develop flulike symptoms in 2 to 4 weeks. Whereas more than 25,000 cases of transfusion-associated AIDS were reported before routine donor testing in 1985, the incidence has decreased to 1 per 100,000 to 150,000 as a result of careful donor screening and testing.[84] Other infectious diseases that may be transmitted through blood transfusion are HIV-2, HTLV-1, Chagas' disease, Lyme disease, babesiosis, syphilis, Epstein-Barr virus, cytomegalovirus, and malaria. Blood donors are questioned or tested for potential exposure to these diseases.

Summary

Hematologic diseases are complex disorders that require the nurse to understand the hematopoietic system. The nurse is often involved in the administration of blood and blood products for treatment of a wide variety of these disorders. Many of the blood disorders are life-threatening (such as acute blood loss and leukemia), whereas others are easily controlled with proper nutrition or regular medication (such as pernicious anemia or iron deficiency anemia).

Because blood and blood product transfusions are used so commonly in the treatment of hematologic disorders, it is vital that the nurse understand this procedure. The nurse must understand the implications of these procedures and the proper techniques of administration so the client will receive safe and effective care.

Bibliography

1. Adams, S. (1992). The HLA system. *Seminar.*
2. Afessa, B., et al. (1992). Outcome of recipients of bone marrow transplants who require intensive-unit care support. *Mayo Clinic Proceedings, 67,* 117–122.
3. Alexanian, R., & Barlogie, B. (1990). New treatment strategies for multiple myeloma. *American Journal of Hematology, 35,* 194–198.
4. Anderson, K. C., & Braine, H. G. (1990). Specialized cell component therapy. *Seminars in Oncology Nursing, 6,* 140–149.
5. Baldwin, J. G. (1988). Hematopoietic function in the elderly. *Archives of Internal Medicine, 148,* 2544–2546.
6. Bell, T. (1990). Disseminated intravascular coagulation and shock. *Critical Care Nursing Clinics of North America, 2,* 255–268.

7. Brandy, B. (1990). Nursing protocol for the patient with neutropenia. *Oncology Nursing Forum, 17,* 9-15.
8. Brunner, L., & Suddarth, D. (1991). *The Lippincott manual of nursing practice* (pp. 270-275). Philadelphia: J. B. Lippincott.
9. Buchsel, P. C., & Keller, J. (1989). Bone marrow transplantation. *Nursing Clinics of North America, 24,* 907-938.
10. Cain, J., et al. (1991). Myelodysplastic syndromes: a review for nurses. *Oncology Nursing Forum, 18,* 113-117.
11. Carlson, K., & Golub, A. (1987). *Autologous and directed blood programs* (pp. 9-16). Arlington, VA: American Association of Blood Banks.
12. Carpenito, L. J. (1991). *Nursing care plans and documentation: Nursing diagnoses and collaborative problems.* Philadelphia: J. B. Lippincott.
13. Dicke, K. A. (1990). Modern trends in the treatment of multiple myeloma. *Current Opinion in Oncology, 2,* 277-284.
14. DiJulio, J. (1991). Hematopoiesis: an overview. *Oncology Nursing Forum, 18,* 3-6.
15. Dolan, J. T. (1991). *Critical care nursing: Clinical management through the nursing process.* Philadelphia: F. A. Davis.
16. Duguid, J. K. M. (1990). Developing techniques in blood transfusion. *Bailliere's Clinical Haematology, 3*(1), 999-1017.
17. Epstein, C., & Bakanauskas, A. (1991). Clinical management of DIC: early nursing interventions. *Critical Care Nursing, 11,* 42-54.
18. Folkes, M. E. (1990). Transfusion therapy in critical care nursing. *Critical Care Nursing, 13,* 15-28.
19. Freedman, S., et al. (1990). Nursing considerations in the administration of blood component therapy. *Seminars in Oncology Nursing, 6,* 155-162.
20. Freireich, E. H., et al. (1978). *Leukemia and lymphoma.* New York: Grune and Stratton.
21. Froberg, J. H. (1989). The anemias: causes and courses of action. *RN, 52*(1), 24-30.
22. Fuller, A. K. (1990). Platelet transfusion therapy for thrombocytopenia. *Seminars in Oncology Nursing, 6,* 123-128.
23. Garry, P. J., et al. (1991). A prospective study of blood donations in healthy elderly persons. *Transfusion, 31,* 686-697.
24. Gilyon, K., & Kuzel, T. (1991). Cutaneous T-cell lymphoma. *Oncology Nursing Forum, 18,* 901-908.
25. Gloe, D. (1991). Common reactions to transfusions. *Heart and Lung, 20,* 506-512.
26. Gobel, B. H. (1990). Plasma and plasma derivative therapy for coagulation disorders. *Seminars in Oncology Nursing, 6,* 129-135.
27. Goodnough, L. T., et al. (1989). Red cell mass in autologous and homologous blood units. *Transfusion, 29,* 821-824.
28. Graham, D. L., et al. (1992). Cytogenetic and molecular detection of residual leukemic cells after allogeneic bone marrow transplantation in chronic granulocytic leukemia. *Mayo Clinic Proceedings, 67,* 123-127.
29. Greifzu, S. (1991). Helping cancer patients fight infection. *RN, 54,* 24-29.
30. Griffin, K. B. (1990). Postoperative bleeding, current nursing management. *Critical Care Nursing Clinics of North America, 2,* 549-557.
31. Guyatt, G. H., et al. (1990). Diagnosis of iron-deficiency anemia in the elderly. *American Journal of Medicine, 88,* 205-209.
32. Hahn, K. (1989). Monitoring a blood transfusion. *Nursing 89, 19,* 20-22.
33. Harmening, D. (1992). *Clinical hematology and fundamentals of hemostasis.* Philadelphia: F. A. Davis.
34. Hoffbrand, A. V. (1988). *Recent advances in hematology.* Edinburgh: Churchill Livingstone.
35. Hoffbrand, A. V., & Pettit, J. E. (1988). *Sandoz atlas of clinical hematology.* London: Gower Medical Publishing.
36. Hoffman, R., et al. (1991). *Hematology: Basic principles and practice.* New York: Churchill Livingstone.
37. Huff, N. L. (1990). Sickle cell anemia: an I.V. nursing challenge. *Journal of Intravenous Nursing, 12,* 245-250.
38. Illott, S. (1990). Infection control in general practice. *Nursing Standards, 5,* 25-28.
39. Iserson, K. V., & Huestis, D. W. (1991). Blood warming: current applications and techniques. *Transfusion, 31,* 558-568.
40. Kinney, M. R., et al. (1988). *AACN's clinical reference for critical-care nursing.* New York: McGraw-Hill.
41. Kotwas, L., et al. (1990). Blood collection techniques. *Seminars in Oncology Nursing, 6,* 109-116.
42. Letendre, L., et al. (1992). Mayo Clinic experience with allogeneic and syngeneic bone marrow transplantation, 1982 through 1990. *Mayo Clinic Proceedings, 67,* 109-116.
43. Linden, J., et al. (1988). In vitro and in vivo evaluation of an electromechanical infusion pump. *Laboratory Medicine, 19,* 574-576.
44. Litwack, K. (1991). Bleeding and coagulation in the PACU. *Critical Care Nursing Clinics of North America, 3,* 121-127.
45. Litwack, K. (1992). Practical points for transfusion therapy. *Journal of Post Anesthesia, 2,* 257-261.
46. Maloney, P. A., & Ryan, L. (1990). Hyperviscosity-polycythemia syndrome: a case study. *Journal of Perinatology Neonatal Nurse, 4,* 64-70.
47. Mansouri, A. (1990). Acquired hemostatic abnormalities in the elderly. *Journal of the American Gerontologic Society, 38,* 809-816.
48. Mark, R., et al. (1985). Rapid warming by blood bag immersion. *Anesthesia, 40,* 74-78.
49. Martinelli, A. M. (1991). Sickle cell disease. *AORN Journal, 53,* 716-724.
50. Masorrli, S. T., & Piercy, S. (1984). A lifesaving guide to blood products. *RN, 47,* 32-37.
51. McVay, P. A., et al. (1991). Probable reasons that autologous blood was not donated by patients having surgery for which crossmatched blood was ordered. *Transfusion, 31,* 810-813.
52. Meyer, C. (1991). New drugs: the class of 1991. *American Journal of Nursing, 91,* 40-43.
53. Napier, J. (1987). *Blood transfusion therapy: A problem-oriented approach* (pp. 54-66). New York: John Wiley and Sons.
54. Oniboni, A. C. (1990). Infection in the neutropenic patient. *Seminars in Oncology Nursing, 6,* 50-59.
55. Parsons, L., & Klopovich, P. (1990). Immune globulin therapy. *Seminars in Oncology Nursing, 6,* 136-139.
56. Pavel, J. (1990). Red blood cell transfusions for anemia. *Seminars in Oncology Nursing, 6,* 117-122.
57. Pavel, J. N., et al. (1990). *Transfusion therapy guidelines.* Bethesda, MD: National Blood Resource Education Program, NHLBI, NIH.
58. Perez, W. E., & Viets, J. L. (1990). Transfusion and coagulation: an overview and recent advances in practice modalities. *Nurse Anesthetist, 1,* 149-161.
59. Picard, V. T., et al. (1990). Transfusion therapy: associated risks and alternative approaches. *American Nephrology Nurses' Association, 17,* 457-464.
60. Querin, J. J., & Stahl, L. D. (1990). 12 simple, sensible steps for successful blood transfusions. *Nursing 90, 20,* 68-81.
61. Rahr, V., & Tucker, R. (1990). Non-Hodgkin's lymphoma: understanding the disease. *Cancer Nursing, 13,* 56-61.
62. Rayfield, S., & Theriot, B. L. (1990). Maximizing safe blood transfusions. *Advances in Critical Care, 5,* 17-19.
63. Rivers, R., & Williams, N. (1990). Sickle cell anemia: complex disease nursing challenge. *RN, 53,* 24-29.
64. Rostad, M. (1990). Management of myelosuppression in the patient with cancer. *Oncology Nursing Forum, 17,* 4-8.
65. Rosvoll, R. V., et al. (1990). *Accreditations requirements manual* (pp. 4-59). Arlington, VA: American Association of Blood Banks.
66. Rutman, R., et al. (1990). The transfusion service and nursing. *Seminars in Oncology Nursing, 6,* 152-154.
67. Rutman, R., et al. (1990). Home transfusion for the cancer patient. *Seminars in Oncology Nursing, 6,* 163-167.
68. Sander, S. G., et al. (1987). Alternative approaches to transfusion: autologous blood and directed blood donations. *Progress in Hematology, XV,* 183-219.
69. Sazama, K. (1990). Reports of 355 transfusion-associated deaths: 1976-1985. *Transfusion, 30,* 583-590.
70. Scherer, J. C. (1991). *Introductory medical-surgical nursing.* Philadelphia: J. B. Lippincott.
71. Schlossberg, D. (1989). *Infectious mononucleosis.* New York: Springer-Verlag.
72. Schultz, B. M., & Freedman, M. L. (1987). Iron deficiency in the

elderly. *Bailliere's clinical haematology, 1,* 291–313.

73. Shulman, I. A. (1989). Adverse reaction to blood transfusion. *Blood Transfusion, 85,* 35–42.
74. Snyder, E. L. (1982). *Blood transfusion therapy: A physician's handbook* (pp. 14–16). Arlington, VA: American Association of Blood Banks.
75. Swearingen, P. L. (1991). *Manual of critical care: Applying nursing diagnoses to adult critical illness.* St. Louis: Mosby-Year Book.
76. Toy, P. T., et al. (1987). Predeposited autologous blood for elective surgery, a national multicenter study. *New England Journal of Medicine, 316,* 517–520.
77. Tucker, R., & Rahr, V. (1990). Nursing care of the patient with non-Hodgkin's lymphoma. *Cancer Nursing, 13,* 229–234.
78. Urden, L. D., et al. (1992). *Essentials of critical care nursing.* St. Louis: Mosby-Year Book.
79. Urlich, S. P. (1987). Preventing post splenectomy complications. *Nursing 87, 17,* 98–100.
80. Widmann, F. K., et al. (1992). *Standards for blood banks and transfusion services* (pp. 1–58). Arlington, VA: American Association of Blood Banks.
81. Williams, W. J., et al. (1983). *Hematology* (3rd ed.). New York: McGraw-Hill.
82. Wood, L., & Jacobs, P. (1989). Myeloma—the integral role played by the professional nurse. *Curationis, 12,* 67–71.
83. Wyngaarden, J. B., et al. (1992). *Cecil textbook of medicine* (19th ed.). Philadelphia: W. B. Saunders.
84. Yap, P. L. (1990). Transfusion transmitted viral infections—recent developments in blood donor screening. *Postgraduate Medical Journal, 66,* 906–909.
85. Yardley, J. (1989). Multiple myeloma. *Nursing 89, 3,* 4–7.
86. Yeomans, A. C., & Harle, M. T. (1990). Myelodysplastic syndromes. *Seminars in Oncology Nursing, 6,* 9–16.
87. Young, L. M. (1990). DIC: the insidious killer. *Critical Care Nursing, 10,* 26–33.

Unit 11

Urinary Disorders

Proper kidney function is vital, and because the bladder is connected to the kidneys, it is crucial to provide skillful care for both upper and lower urinary tract disorders. The care of clients with short-term, easily managed urinary disorders such as bladder infections is as important as the maintenance care of clients with long-term or terminal disorders such as chronic renal failure.

Include significant others in your nursing care planning to help ensure continuity of care between the health care facility and the client's home. This is particularly important for people with long-term urinary problems. Total care planning requires consideration of the physical, sexual, emotional, social, spiritual, and cognitive needs of the individual and significant others. Remember to use all resources of the health care team, the health care facility, and the community.

This unit consists of four chapters. Chapter 47 reviews the structure and function of the urinary system. Chapter 48 describes the assessment of people experiencing urinary disorders. Specific disorders of the ureters, bladder, and urethra are discussed in Chapter 49. Disorders of the kidneys are covered in Chapter 50. As mentioned previously, disorders of the lower urinary tract can affect the kidney and vice versa.

As dialysis and renal transplants have become more successful, increasing numbers of clients are being treated for end-stage renal disease. Thus, more people with renal disorders and their significant others are asking questions and seeking support. Nurses, therefore, must clearly understand (a) the interventions affecting the urinary tract, and (b) the needs of people with these disorders and their significant others.

This unit provides information regarding important nursing interventions and the specific needs of people with urinary tract disorders. It will enable you to plan and intervene effectively to meet these needs.

Chapter 47

Structure and Function of the Urinary System

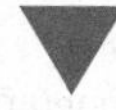

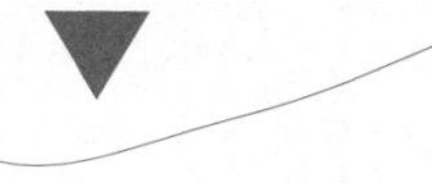

STRUCTURE

The urinary tract is composed of four organs: (1) kidneys, (2) ureters, (3) bladder, and (4) urethra. Figure 47-1 illustrates the anatomic location of these four organs.

Kidneys

The kidneys are located retroperitoneally, in the posterior aspect of the abdomen, on either side of the vertebral column. They lie between the twelfth thoracic and the third lumbar vertebrae. The left kidney is usually positioned slightly higher than the right. Adult kidneys average approximately 11 cm in length and 5 to 7.5 cm in width and are 2.5 cm thick. Affixing the kidneys in position behind the parietal peritoneum are a mass of perirenal fat (adipose capsule) and connective tissue called Gerota's (subserosa) fascia. A fibrous capsule (renal capsule) forms the external covering of the kidney itself, except the hilum. The kidney is further protected by layers of muscle of the back, flank, and abdomen, as well as layers of fat, subcutaneous tissue, and skin.

Each organ is shaped like a kidney bean, with the distal edge being convex and the medial boundary being concave. In the innermost part of the concave section is the hilus, through which pass the renal artery, renal vein, lymphatics, and nerves, and the renal pelvis, the natural upper extension of the ureter. A firm, tough, fibrous capsule surrounds and adheres to the renal parenchyma. Inside this capsule, each kidney is divided into three major areas: (1) the cortex, (2) medulla, and (3) pelvis. Figure 47-2 demonstrates the anatomy of the kidney.

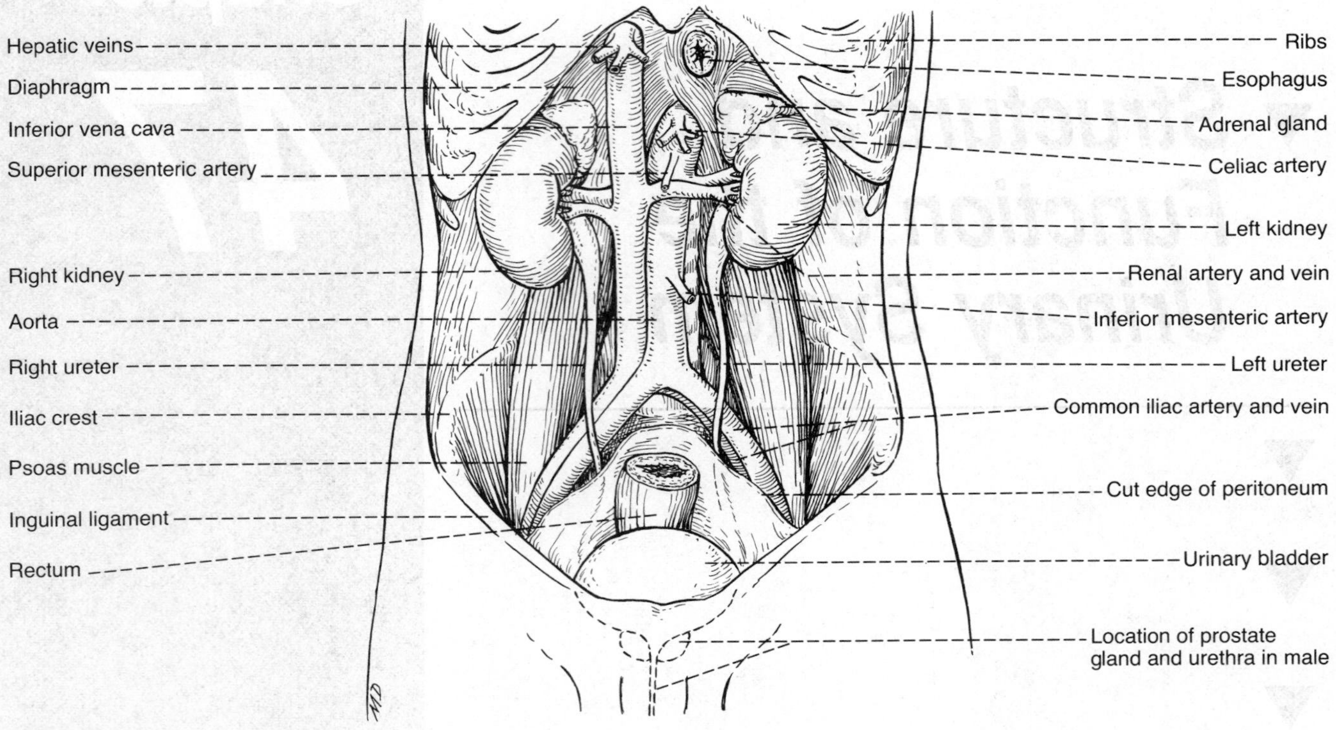

▲ *Figure 47–1*

Anatomic relationships of kidneys and related structures.

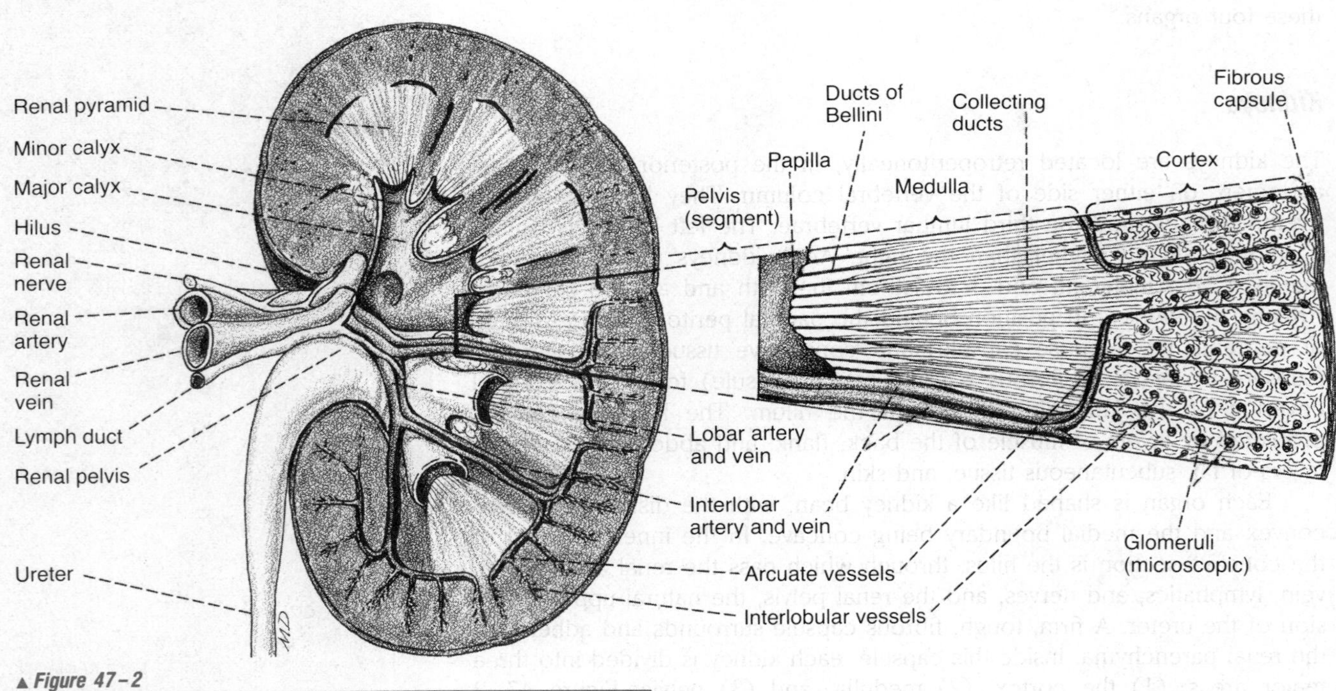

▲ *Figure 47–2*

Anatomy of the kidney. *Inset,* Enlargement of a segment of the kidney.

The cortex of the kidney lies just under the fibrous capsule, and portions of it extend down into the medullary layer to form the renal columns (columns of Bertin) or cortical tissue that separates the pyramids. The medulla is divided into 8 to 18 cone-shaped masses of collecting ducts called renal pyramids. The bases of the pyramids are positioned on the corticomedullary boundary. Their apices extend toward the renal pelvis, forming papillae. The *papillae* each have 10 to 25 openings on the surface, through which the urine empties into the renal pelvis. The inset in Figure 47-2 shows the anatomy of a renal pyramid. There are eight or more groups of papillae in each pyramid, each emptying into a minor calix, and several minor calices join to form a major calix. The two to three major calices are outpouchings of the renal pelvis. They serve to channel the urine from the pyramids to the renal pelvis. The inner area of the kidney, or renal pelvis, is a cavity lined with transitional epithelium. The combined volume of the pelvis and calices is approximately 8 ml. Volumes in excess of this amount damage the renal parenchymal tissue. The renal pelvis narrows as it reaches the hilus and becomes the proximal end of the ureter.

The functioning unit of the kidney is the nephron. Each kidney contains more than one million of these units! A nephron is a microscopic structure consisting of a glomerular (Bowman's) capsule and tubular system that empties into the renal pelvis and the ureter. Figure 47-3 illustrates a functioning nephron.

Located in the cortex of the kidney is a double-walled cup, called the glomerular or Bowman's capsule (Fig. 47-3). It is lined with a simple squamous epithelium to allow easy filtration from the blood. Inside the capsule is the glomerulus, a tuft of nonanastomosing capillaries fed by an afferent arteriole and drained by an efferent arteriole. The proximal tubule is a convoluted portion with millions of microvilli lining its lumen, forming a brush border, thereby vastly increasing its membrane surface area. As it nears the medullary layer, the tubule abruptly narrows and forms the descending loop of Henle. This then turns back on itself as the ascending limb of the loop of Henle, the latter being larger in diameter than the descending limb. The loop of Henle, as it moves back into the cortex of the kidney, becomes the distal convoluted tubule, which joins a collecting duct. Each collecting duct receives the terminal end of several nephrons as it courses through the cortex and medulla of the kidney. As the collecting ducts within a renal pyramid get closer to the apex of the pyramid, several coalesce to form a larger duct of Bellini, which opens onto the surface of a papilla (see Fig. 47-2).

The macula densa lies between the afferent arteriole and the distal convoluted tubule, where it passes close to the arteriole. These closely packed cells, which are located in the distal tubular epithelium of each nephron, may function as chemoreceptors. The juxtaglomerular cells are found between the macula densa and the afferent arteriole just before it enters the glomerular capsule. Together these two cellular structures form the juxtaglomerular apparatus, which is thought to

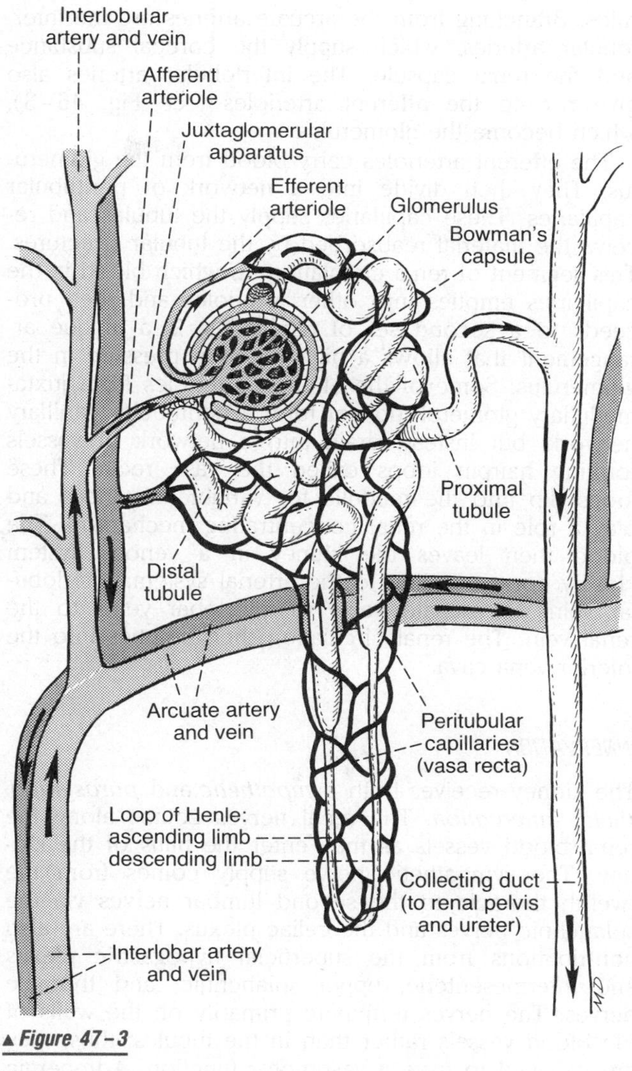

▲ *Figure 47-3*

Nephron.

play a major role in the renin-angiotensin system. The enzyme renin helps to regulate water and sodium retention and, consequently, blood pressure.

CIRCULATION

The kidneys receive 20 to 25 per cent of the cardiac output under resting conditions, averaging more than 1 liter of arterial blood per minute. The renal arteries (see Fig. 47-2) branch from the abdominal aorta at the level of the second lumbar vertebra. Passing laterally to the hilus of the kidney, each artery usually divides into the anterior and posterior branches, which supply the anterior and posterior portions of the kidney, respectively. Further subdivisions of the primary branches of the renal artery are called lobar arteries. These vessels supply the papillae. The lobar arteries further divide into interlobar arteries, which run between the renal pyramids until they reach the corticomedullary zone. Here, they form incomplete arches called arcuate arteries around the bases of the pyramids. Branching from the arcuate arteries are the interlobular arteries, which supply the cortical substance and the renal capsule. The interlobular arteries also give rise to the afferent arterioles (see Fig. 46-3), which become the glomerulus.

The efferent arterioles carry blood from the glomerulus. They then divide into a network of peritubular capillaries. These capillaries supply the tubules and receive the material reabsorbed by the tubular structures. This segment of renal circulation, in which blood in the capillaries empties into other arterioles and then proceeds to a second set of capillaries, is a unique arrangement that allows a high filtration pressure in the glomerulus. Some of the efferent arterioles from juxtamedullary glomeruli do not form a peritubular capillary network, but instead drain into a network of vessels forming hairpin loops called the vasa recta. These loops dip into the medulla for variable distances and play a role in the renal concentrating mechanism. The blood then leaves the kidney in a venous system closely corresponding to the arterial system: interlobular veins to arcuate veins to interlobar veins to the renal vein. The renal circulation then empties into the inferior vena cava.

INNERVATION

The kidney receives both *sympathetic* and *parasympathetic innervation*. The renal nerves course along the renal blood vessels as they enter the hilus of the kidney. The sympathetic nerve supply comes from the twelfth thoracic to the second lumbar nerves via the splanchnic nerves and the celiac plexus. There are also contributions from the superficial hypogastric plexus and intermesenteric, upper splanchnic, and thoracic nerves. The nerves terminate primarily on the walls of the blood vessels rather than in the tubules; thus, they are believed to have a vasomotor function. Adrenergic fibers also end in close proximity to the juxtaglomerular cells and renal tubes. A completely denervated kidney continues to form urine.

Ureters

The ureters form the medial tapering of the renal pelvis at the hilus of the kidney. They are 25 to 35 cm long in the adult. Ureters lie in the extraperitoneal connective tissue and descend vertically along the psoas muscle toward the pelvic cavity (see Fig. 47-1). After dipping into the pelvic cavity, the ureters course anteriorly to join the bladder in its posterolateral aspect. At each ureterovesical junction, the ureter runs obliquely through the bladder wall for about 1.5 to 2 cm before opening into the lumen of the bladder. There are three points of potential obstruction: (1) at the ureteropelvic junction, (2) the pelvic brim (where ureters cross iliac arteries), and (3) at the ureterovesical junction. The ureter is much narrower at these points. Calculi typically lodge here because it is difficult for them to pass through this narrow passageway. This anatomic arrangement usually functions as a valve that prevents the backward flow, or reflux, of urine into the kidney.

Each ureter has definite elastic characteristics and is made of three tissue layers: (1) an inner mucosa (transitional epithelial membrane) lining the lumen, (2) a muscular layer, and (3) a fibrous outer layer. When cancer of the bladder or ureter is diagnosed, there is potential for recurrence in either structure. Half of clients with ureteral cancer experience spread of the cancer to the bladder. Only about 3 per cent of clients with bladder cancer have spread of the cancer to the ureter.[33] The musculature is generally designated as inner longitudinal and outer circular. However, along most of the ureter, the muscle fibers actually run obliquely and blend with one another to form a meshlike tissue. The muscle arrangement allows urine to be propelled down the ureter by peristaltic action. This peristalsis is probably regulated by a myogenic pacemaker located near the renal calices.

Blood is supplied to the ureters by one or more vessels that run longitudinally along the tube. The number and assortment of arteries anastomosing with the ureteric vessels vary with each individual. Because the ureters travel through several anatomic areas, the ureteral vessels are fed by several of the following arteries: (1) renal (frequently), (2) testicular or ovarian, (3) aorta and common iliac, (4) internal iliac (frequently), (5) vesical, (6) umbilical, and (7) uterine.

The ureter's innervation comes from the eleventh thoracic to the first lumbar nerves. The network of nerves becomes progressively more dense toward the terminal end of the ureters.

Bladder

The urinary bladder is a hollow organ located in the anterior half of the pelvis behind the symphysis pubis. Figures 47-4 and 47-5 illustrate the position in the female and male, respectively, of the bladder and urethra in relation to the other anatomic structures of the pelvis. The space between the bladder and the symphysis pubis is filled with a loose connective tissue that allows the bladder to stretch cranially as it fills. The peritoneum covers the top border of the bladder, while the base is held loosely in place by the true ligaments. The bladder is also enveloped by a loose fascia.

The bladder wall has several tissue layers. The internal lining of the vesical is transitional epithelium with some mucus-secreting glands. Then there are three ill-defined muscle layers. The inner and outer layers tend to have fibers running longitudinally, whereas those of the middle layer are circular. The fibers from these layers exchange with each other frequently so that the result is a meshlike muscle layer called the detrusor muscle. This arrangement allows the bladder wall to be elastic while maintaining strength. Bundles of these smooth muscle layers come together at the base of the bladder to form the internal sphincter, or opening into the urethra. The trigone describes the triangular area cornered by the ureterovesical junctions and the internal sphincter.

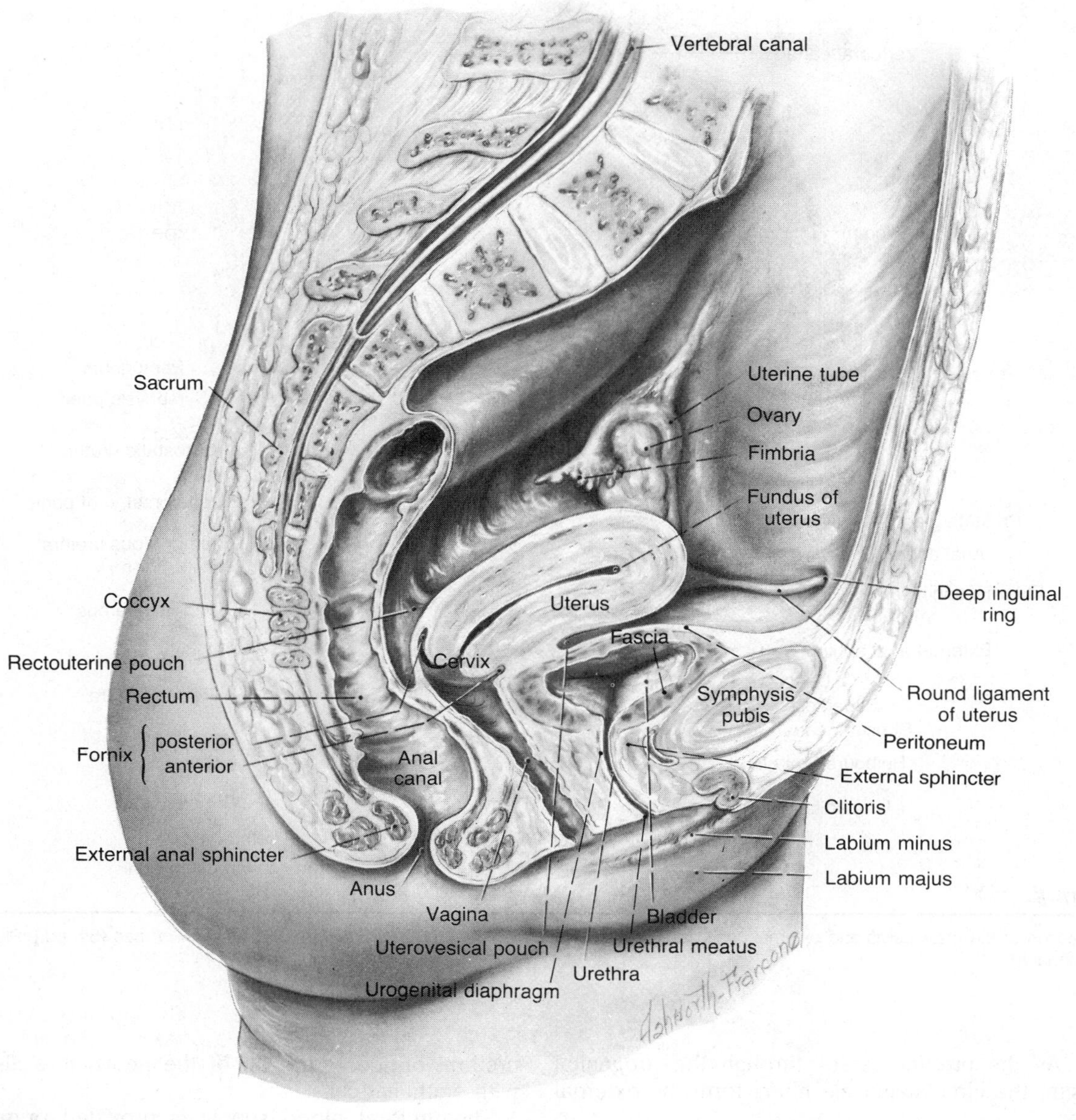

▲ *Figure 47-4*

Sagittal section of the female pelvis. (From Jacob, S. W., et al. [1982]. *Structure and function in man* (5th ed.). Philadelphia: W. B. Saunders.)

The superior and lateral aspects of the bladder are served by the superior vesical artery, branching from the umbilical artery and internal iliac artery. The inferior vesical artery, supplying the underside of the bladder, may arise independently or in common with the middle rectal artery. The veins draining the bladder pass to the internal iliac trunk.

Innervation for the bladder comes from the hypogastric sympathetic, pelvic parasympathetic, and pudendal somatic nerves. Ganglia are most commonly found in the bladder base and around the urethral orifice. These areas tend to act in continuity with each other, and their functions seem to be coordinated by both the sympathetic and parasympathetic nervous systems.

Urethra and Meatus

The urethra is a tube that starts at the base of the bladder and extends to the surface of the body. There is a great difference between the female and male urethra. The female urethra is approximately 4 cm in length and curves slightly forward as it reaches the external opening or meatus. The meatus is located between the clitoris and the vaginal orifice. It is lined with epithelium, which contains some mucus-secreting glands. The longitudinal muscle layer is a continuation of longitudinal layer of bladder muscle. The circular muscle fibers encircle the urethra and meet with the circular bladder muscle. This muscle thins out near the

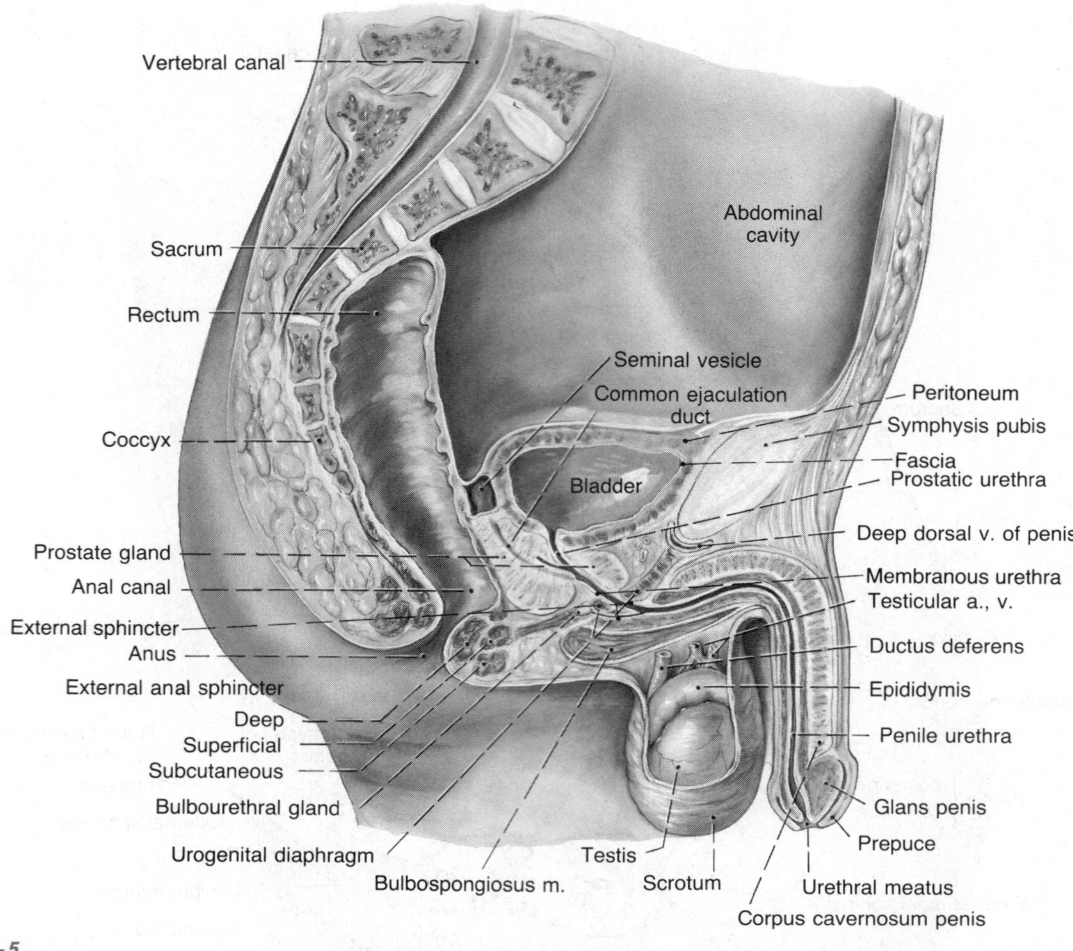

▲ *Figure 47–5*

Sagittal section of the male pelvis and external genitalia. (From Jacob, S. W., et al. [1982]. *Structure and function in man* [5th ed.]. Philadelphia: W. B. Saunders.)

meatus. As the urethra passes through the urogenital diaphragm, the circular muscle fibers form the external sphincter.

In males, the reproductive system is anatomically connected to the urinary tract. Both systems share the same outlet from the body, the urethra. The prostate gland, although not a direct part of the urinary system, is a major cause of urinary dysfunction in men. This gland is located below the bladder neck and completely surrounds the urethra. Normally, this relationship causes no problem, but if the gland enlarges, it constricts the urethra and obstructs the outflow of urine. Further discussion of the male reproductive system is found in Chapter 75. The male urethra is about 20 cm long and is divided into three main sections. The prostatic urethra extends about 3 cm below the bladder neck, through the prostate gland, to the pelvic floor. The ejaculatory ducts of the reproductive system empty into its posterior wall. The membranous urethra is about 1 to 2 cm in length and ends where the muscle layer forms the external sphincter. The distal portion is the cavernous, or penile, urethra. It is approximately 15 cm long and travels through the penis to the urethral orifice at the tip of the penis. It is also lined with epithelial cells.

The urethral blood supply is provided primarily by the internal pudendal artery and urethral artery. This supply of blood is supplemented by those vessels feeding the surrounding anatomic structures. Innervation arises from sources similar to those supplying the bladder.

FUNCTION

The urinary tract plays a major role in the maintenance of homeostasis. The main functions of the kidneys are to (1) remove waste products from the body and (2) regulate fluids, electrolytes, blood pressure, and pH within the body. The main functions of the lower urinary tract are the storage and elimination of formed urine. These functions are accomplished through the formation of urine, a complex task involving the processes of filtration, reabsorption, and secretion. Once formed, urine is excreted from the body.

The kidneys also have several nonexcretory metabolic and endocrine functions. In this section, we consider their role in blood pressure regulation, red blood cell production, insulin degradation, prostaglandin synthesis, calcium and phosphorus regulation, vitamin D metabolism, and regulation of other substances in the body.

Kidneys

FORMATION OF URINE

Urine is formed in the nephrons by three processes: (1) filtration, (2) reabsorption, and (3) secretion. Filtration is the passage of a liquid through a filtering membrane as the result of a pressure differential. In the kidney, this takes place in the glomerulus. The tubular portion of the nephron is the site for (1) reabsorption, which is the taking back of fluids and other substances through body tissues, and (2) secretion, which involves the active transport of certain chemicals from the bloodstream into the tubules. Figure 47–6 shows how different anatomic portions of the nephron use each of these processes to regulate the amount and constituents of the urine being formed.

Glomerular Filtration. The glomerulus is a semipermeable membrane that allows free passage of water and electrolytes across it. However, it is usually impermeable to molecular substances, such as albumin and other plasma proteins, which are too large to pass through the membrane. The fluid that is filtered through this glomerular membrane is called glomerular filtrate. The glomerular filtration rate (GFR) is the amount of glomerular filtration that occurs within a given period of time. The GFR for a normal adult male of average size is approximately 125 ml/min.

Several factors can influence the GFR. These include (1) hydrostatic and oncotic pressure gradients between the glomerular capillaries and Bowman's capsule, (2)

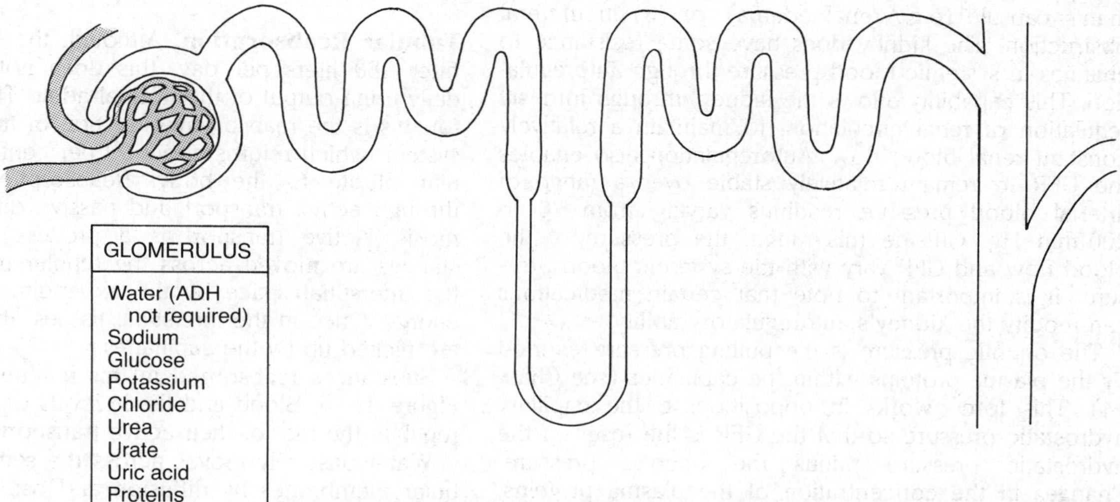

	GLOMERULUS	PROXIMAL TUBULE	LOOP OF HENLE	DISTAL TUBULE	COLLECTING DUCT
FILTRATION (from blood)	Water (ADH not required) Sodium Glucose Potassium Chloride Urea Urate Uric acid Proteins Amino acids Bicarbonate Creatinine Phosphate Inulin PAH	Isotonic filtrate	Hypertonic filtrate	Isotonic or hypotonic filtrate	Hypertonic or hypotonic filtrate
REABSORPTION (into blood)		Water (ADH not required) Sodium Glucose Potassium Chloride Urea Urate Uric acid Proteins Amino acids Carbon dioxide	Water Sodium Chloride Urea Urate Carbon dioxide	Water (ADH required) Sodium Chloride Urea Urate Carbon dioxide	Water (ADH required) Sodium Chloride Urea Urate Carbon dioxide
SECRETION (from blood)		Creatinine Hydrogen PAH		Potassium Uric acid Hydrogen	Potassium Hydrogen

▲ Figure 47–6

Normal physiologic function of the nephron in urine formation. Although inulin and para-aminohippuric acid (PAH) are not normally present, they are important test substances.

rate of renal blood flow, (3) permeability of the glomerular membrane, and (4) changes in the total area of the glomerular capillary bed. Most important is the amount and pressure of the blood supply reaching the glomerulus, because without blood flow there is no glomerular filtration.

Pressure within the glomerular capillaries is usually higher than that in other capillary beds in the body. Whereas hydrostatic pressure in other capillaries is normally 15 to 20 mm Hg, glomerular capillary pressure is 70 mm Hg. The higher pressure is caused by the unique anatomic structure of the afferent arterioles and the high resistance in the efferent arterioles. The "pushing out" of fluid from the glomerular capillaries through the semipermeable membrane into Bowman's capsule results from this high pressure. Since filtration occurs under exceedingly high pressure and is a result of the hydrostatic pressure differential, this process is called ultrafiltration.

Changes in the GFR occur when this pressure gradient is altered (1) in the glomerular capillaries (e.g., changes in the systemic blood pressure), (2) in Bowman's capsule (e.g., renal edema), or (3) in ureteral obstruction. The kidney does have some resistance to changes in systemic blood pressure through autoregulation. This capability allows the kidney, through intrinsic regulation of renal circulation, to maintain a relatively constant renal blood flow. Autoregulation also enables the GFR to remain relatively stable over a range of arterial blood pressure readings varying from 70 to 200 mm Hg. Outside this range, the pressure of the blood flow and GFR vary with the systemic blood pressure. It is important to note that certain medications can modify the kidney's autoregulatory ability.

The oncotic pressure is the pulling pressure exerted by the plasma proteins within the capillaries (see Chap. 14). This force works in opposition to the capillary hydrostatic pressure so that the GFR is the result of the hydrostatic pressure minus the oncotic pressure. Changes in the concentration of the plasma proteins, such as with fluid depletion and hypoproteinemia, alter the influence of this force.

Closely allied with the pressures affecting GFR is the amount of renal blood flow reaching the glomerulus. Anything enhancing or interfering with renal circulation alters the GFR. The list of influential factors is long. Such things as direct trauma to, or obstruction of, blood vessels interrupts this flow. Medications may alter blood flow. For instance, glucagon (a protein substance produced by the islands of Langerhans in the pancreas) and low levels of dopamine (a catecholamine precursor of norepinephrine) produce direct renal vasodilation without apparent effect on the systemic blood pressure. Other vasopressors, such as norepinephrine bitartrate (Levophed), cause renal vasoconstriction and, at high rates, may drastically reduce GFR and cause acute renal failure. Some diuretics cause vasoconstriction, whereas others increase renal blood flow. Activation of the adrenergic nervous system (e.g., by a stressful event) may decrease blood flow through release of either norepinephrine from the renal sympathetic nerves or epinephrine from the adrenal medulla. Bacterial pyrogens, as in sepsis, prompt vasodilation. Also, a high-protein diet increases renal blood flow.

As mentioned earlier, normal capillary permeability interferes with the passage of plasma proteins into the filtrate. Any pathologic process that changes this relationship interferes with the normal oncotic pressure gradient. For example, if plasma proteins escape across the membrane, such as nephrotic syndrome, the oncotic "pull" is reduced, resulting in increased water filtration.

Changes in the total area of the capillary glomerular bed modify the structures filtering the blood. These changes usually involve a reduction in the functioning area and they result from glomeruli-destroying diseases or partial nephrectomy.

The results of the filtration process represent the first stage in the formation of urine. The composition of this ultrafiltrate is approximately 94 per cent water and 6 per cent solutes. The list of normal solutes is shown in Figure 47-6.

Tubular Reabsorption. Although the kidneys initially filter 180 liters per day, this does not represent the daily urine output of the normal adult. The main reason for this is the reabsorptive function of the renal tubular system, which returns about 99 per cent of the glomerular filtrate to the body. Reabsorption takes place through active transport and passive diffusion and osmosis. Active transport is a process in which substances are moved across the tubular membranes into the interstitial space by the expenditure of metabolic energy. Once in the interstitial tissues, these substances are picked up by the capillaries.

Substances reabsorbed in this manner are shown in Figure 47-6. Blood and tissue levels of these elements regulate the rate of their active transport.

Water passively moves across the semipermeable tubular membranes by diffusion and osmosis, according to the concentration gradient. As solutes are transported into the interstitial spaces, the concentration of solutes outside the tubules rises, causing water to shift out of the tubular system. This obligatory water reabsorption is thus not dependent on the body's state of hydration, but rather on the osmotic forces. The process of reabsorption occurs without the aid of antidiuretic hormone (ADH) in the proximal tubules. However, as illustrated in Figure 47-6, ADH is required in the distal tubule and collecting duct. ADH increases the permeability of these membranes, allowing the water to move more freely along its concentration gradient.

Some substances are poorly reabsorbed through the tubular membranes. These include urea, phosphate, sulfate, uric acid, nitrate, and phenols, all waste products that need to be excreted from the body. As water is reabsorbed by osmosis, the concentration of these substances inside the tubule rises, causing some of the molecules to pass through to the interstitial spaces. However, because this process is very inefficient, the body is able to excrete these metabolic wastes.

Tubular Secretion. In addition to reabsorption, tubular cells are also capable of secretion. Secretion is a chemical activity allowing transport of substances from the blood into the tubules. The two physiologic elements most involved in this process are potassium and hydrogen, although ammonia and uric acid are also included. Some drug metabolites are excreted through this mechanism, such as acetaminophen, probenecid, and penicillin.

REGULATION OF FLUIDS AND ELECTROLYTES

The regulation of fluids and electrolytes in the body occurs primarily because of the feedback systems between the nephrons and the body fluids and tissues. These systems alter the processes described earlier—filtration, reabsorption, and secretion—thereby determining the amount and composition of the urine excreted from the body.

Assuming that the renal blood flow is adequate, the fluid volumes are maintained principally through the diluting and concentrating mechanisms of the nephrons. Dilution occurs as a result of reabsorbing solute without water, and concentration is produced by reabsorbing water without solute. The process allowing the production of hyperosmolar urine is called the "countercurrent" mechanism. This mechanism arises from the anatomic arrangement of the loop of Henle and the peritubular capillaries. A countercurrent system occurs when a tube or vessel makes a hairpin turn and one section travels parallel to, opposite to, and in close proximity to the other section over some distance. There continues to be debate about how this mechanism works, but the end result is concentration of the urine. Physiologists hypothesize that as the filtrate travels through the ascending loop of Henle, where the membrane is impermeable to water, sodium and chloride are moved out into the interstitial space by active transport. This reduces the salt concentration in the distal tubule and increases the concentration in the interstitium. Because of the concentration gradient, some of the interstitial salt diffuses back into the descending loop of Henle, where it moves around the hairpin turn and is again actively transported into the interstitial tissues. Since the medullary salt concentration was already slightly higher than before, the additional transport of salt raises the osmolarity even more. This continuing process is known as countercurrent multiplication.

The resulting hypertonicity of the interstitial fluid is maintained because the vasa recta, tiny capillaries that ascend and descend with the loop of Henle, operate as countercurrent exchangers. Solutes move out of the blood vessels going toward the cortex and into vessels descending into the pyramids. At the same time, water diffuses out of the descending vessels and into the ascending vessels. This recirculation preserves the solute concentration in the interstitium.

If this process were to continue unmediated, the urine produced would be very dilute. This is because the membranes of the distal tubule and collecting ducts are relatively impermeable to water without the activity of ADH. The excretion of dilute urine is desirable when body fluid volume is too high. In the presence of ADH, however, these membranes become permeable to water and allow water reabsorption to take place freely. Thus, the hypo-osmolar fluid delivered to the distal tubule becomes iso-osmolar with the interstitial spaces by the time it reaches the papillae. The fluid reabsorbed in this manner diffuses into the vasa recta and is returned to the general circulation through the renal circulation. Therefore, the presentation of dilute urine to the distal tubule allows regulation of water balance in the body. If the body needs to conserve fluids, such as in dehydration, ADH is released and water is reabsorbed.

Because of this influence of ADH on the concentrating and diluting abilities of the nephrons, anything that affects the release of ADH also affects the amount of urine produced. ADH release is regulated by variation in serum osmolality (state of hydration) and blood volume. As osmolality increases, ADH release increases. As osmolality decreases, ADH release decreases. The effect of changes in circulating ADH occurs within a matter of minutes.

Of lesser influence is the loss of blood volume. Usually, ADH is not released until there is a serious loss of circulating blood volume that then stimulates a stress response. The stress response usually causes a release of ADH, leading to water conservation. One example is the release of ADH in postoperative individuals; this is caused by surgical stress and some anesthetic agents. Alcohol intake and a cold environment also may cause ADH release.

Urea augments the concentration of urine. As water is reabsorbed from the tubule, the concentration of urea increases. The inner medullary portion of the collecting duct is permeable to urea and thus reabsorbs it freely along the concentration gradient into the interstitium. This helps maintain the high osmolarity of the interstitial space so that more water is reabsorbed in the presence of ADH.

Electrolyte excretion by the kidney is influenced by a variety of factors including hydrostatic and osmotic pressures and the circulating effect of aldosterone and other adrenocortical hormones. The movement of sodium also affects the regulation of several other electrolytes. For instance, the active reabsorption of sodium causes passive reabsorption of chloride and bicarbonate. The reabsorption of potassium usually decreases the reabsorption of sodium. If body levels of potassium are too high, excess potassium is secreted into the tubules. Chapter 14 further discusses the role of the kidney in water and electrolyte regulation.

REGULATION OF HYDROGEN ION BALANCE

Regulation of pH within the body is performed primarily by the kidney. Metabolic acids such as phosphoric, keto, uric, and sulfuric acids are normally excreted as they are formed. Then, in the presence of acid-base imbalances, the kidneys excrete either hydrogen or bicarbonate ions to restore balance. In response to acidotic states, the kidneys may also form new bicarbonates that are released in the blood.

Normally, the cells of the renal tubules secrete equivalent amounts of hydrogen and bicarbonate. Hydrogen ions are secreted into the proximal and distal tubules and the collecting ducts through the hydration of carbon dioxide in the presence of carbonic anhydrase. The carbonic acid then splits into carbon dioxide and water. The carbon dioxide is reabsorbed from the tubules, carried through the body, and excreted by the lungs. The water is excreted in the urine.

In acidosis, excess hydrogen ions are secreted into the proximal and distal tubules and collecting ducts and excreted in the urine. There is a limit to the hydrogen gradient and, without buffers to tie up the free hydrogen in the urine, this limit is reached rapidly. As mentioned earlier, hydrogen reacts with bicarbonate to form carbon dioxide and water. It also reacts with diphasic phosphate to form monobasic phosphate and with ammonia to form ammonium ion. The formation of these compounds allows the secretion of more hydrogen. The excess acid is excreted in the urine.

When needed, the kidneys can also regenerate new bicarbonate. Carbon dioxide is converted into carbonic acid, which dissociates into hydrogen and bicarbonate. The hydrogen ion is excreted in the urine and the bicarbonate is reabsorbed into the interstitial fluid.

With alkalosis, the excretion of hydrogen ions ceases. At higher levels of bicarbonate concentrations in the body, bicarbonate may actually be excreted in the urine, resulting in increased systemic pH levels. Further discussion of the kidney's contribution in hydrogen ion regulation is included in Chapter 14.

REGULATION OF BLOOD PRESSURE

Recall from Chapter 14 that in the event of blood volume depletion, the renin-angiotensin-aldosterone system works to maintain the blood pressure. As arterial blood pressure drops, reflex vasoconstriction in the splanchnic circulation effectively reduces renal blood flow and thus GFR. This stimulates the release of renin from the juxtaglomerular cells.

The mechanisms regulating the release of renin may be classified as (1) intrarenal, which includes baroreceptors in the afferent arterioles and natrioreceptors in the macula densa that are sensitive to changes in sodium concentration; (2) sympathetic, which includes renal nerves as well as the action of catecholamines; and (3) humoral, which includes the effects of sodium, potassium, vasopressin, and angiotensin II. The renin is released into the bloodstream, where it acts on *angiotensin I.* This substance is produced in the liver, and it has a weak vasoconstrictive effect on peripheral vessels. As angiotensin I passes through the lungs, it is converted by an enzyme into angiotensin II, a powerful vasoconstrictor that exerts its effects on the smooth muscle of arteriolar walls. *Vasoconstriction* increases the peripheral resistance, and thus the blood pressure, which in turn causes a drop in renin secretion in the kidney.

In addition, aldosterone production may be stimulated by angiotensin I. It may raise the blood pressure by facilitating the reabsorption of sodium and water from the distal tubule, resulting in increased blood volume.

Kallikrein, an enzyme found in the urine, catalyzes the formation of vasodilator hormones. Urinary kallikrein may be produced in the kidney and thus is different from plasma kallikrein. No one knows exactly what role kallikrein plays in blood pressure regulation. Levy and associates, in studying normotensive and hypertensive black and white males, found that although all groups had increased urinary kallikrein activity when put on a low-sodium diet, black males with hypertension had the smallest gain. They also found a direct correlation between urinary kallikrein activity and renal blood flow. These studies not only seem to indicate that kallikrein is important in blood pressure regulation, but they also account for some of the racial differences in the resistance of the renal vasculature.

OTHER METABOLIC AND ENDOCRINE FUNCTIONS

In addition to the production of renin, the kidney has several other metabolic and endocrine functions. These include the synthesis of 1,25-dihydroxycholecalciferol, biogenesis of erythropoietin, degradation of insulin, synthesis of prostaglandins, and provision of the energy required to perform its own functions.

1,25-dihydroxycholecalciferol *(DHCC)* is a hormone derived from vitamin D. It helps stimulate absorption of calcium from the intestine and works with parathyroid hormone to encourage osteoclastic bone activity. Thus, DHCC helps maintain calcium homeostasis in the body. Cholecalciferol, obtained through diet or from ultraviolet light, is first hydroxylated in the liver and then again in the kidney to form DHCC.

Erythropoietin is a glycoprotein that induces the production of red blood cells in the bone marrow. Since the 1950s there has been debate as to the source of this hormone. The current theory reestablishes the kidney as the point of origin. The synthesis of erythropoietin seems to be stimulated by an *oxygen deficit* in the kidney. Scientists hypothesize that anemia, hypoxia, renal ischemia, and circulatory alterations caused by vasoconstrictors prompt the synthesis of the enzyme erythrogenin. This enzyme, in turn, acts as a catalyst in the formation of erythropoietin from a circulating substrate. Although there may be extrarenal oxygen sensors in the pituitary gland, hypothalamus, and carotid bodies, the principal sensors are probably located in the cortex or medulla of the kidney.

Insulin is deactivated by the renal tubular cells. Approximately 20 per cent of the insulin secreted by the pancreas is removed from the circulation by the kidneys and then degraded in the tubules.

Prostaglandins are a series of closely related fatty acids that have a great variety of proven and hypothesized physiologic actions. They are formed in most, if not all, organs of the body. In the kidney, prostaglandins are synthesized in the collecting tubules and medullary interstitial cells, and removed from the kidney through the renal vein and in the urine. Their synthesis is stimulated by a number of factors, including angiotensin, vasopressin, bradykinin, alpha-adrenergic catecholamines, calcium, loop diuretics, renal ischemia, unilateral ureteral obstruction, cirrhosis with ascites, glomerulonephritis, hypertension, and acute renal failure. They are inhibited by anti-inflammatory agents, especially nonsteroids.

Medullary prostaglandins regulate urine concentration by increasing sodium excretion, inhibiting sodium and urea reabsorption, and antagonizing the action of ADH. Cortical prostaglandins regulate GFR, vascular resistance, and the secretion of renin. It appears that prostaglandins are not essential for renal function in healthy people, but that their actions become important when renal function is compromised. For instance, renal prostaglandins contribute to the excretion of excess sodium in hypertensive, but not normotensive, people.

The active transport system of the kidney requires significant energy production. The provision of this energy is probably the major metabolic activity of the kidney. Because the active transport of sodium is the primary cause for energy use in the kidney, there is a close correlation between the (1) sodium reabsorption rate, (2) renal blood flow rate, (3) GFR, and (4) renal oxygen consumption rate. The kidneys extract relatively little oxygen from the renal blood flow, and this rate remains stable even in states of low blood flow.

MOVEMENT OF URINE THROUGH THE KIDNEYS

As the above-mentioned functions are carried out, the forming urine moves through each nephron. It travels through the collecting ducts toward the apex of the pyramids, where it flows through the openings in the papillae into the renal pelvis. As the urine enters and distends the pelvis, the muscle wall contracts, propelling the urine across the ureteropelvic junction into the ureter. This movement of urine into the ureter is a relatively constant process, because the maximum safe capacity of the adult renal pelvis is 3 to 5 ml. Amounts greater than this level cause renal tissue damage due to pressure.

Ureters

The chief function of the ureter is to transport urine from the renal pelvis to the bladder. Peristaltic waves occurring from one to five times per minute move the urine down the ureter into the bladder through the ureterovesical junction. Although there is controversy about the mechanism that initiates these contractions, it appears that there are pacemaker sites located in the calices, and that waves are propagated along the ureters from muscle cell to muscle cell by means of intracellular junctions. Generally, these contractions move from the kidney toward the bladder, but retrograde peristalsis can occur.

Recall that the main function of the ureterovesical junction is to prevent the backflow of urine to the kidney during voiding or when the bladder becomes overdistended. Thus, this structure prevents damage to renal tissue from pressure and from the implantation of microorganisms that would ordinarily be washed out of the bladder. In addition to its anatomic placement, the valve works because of the lack of smooth muscle in its wall just proximal to its entry into the bladder. Thus, the usual intravesical pressure tends to keep the valve collapsed except when urine is spurting through it. During micturition, the ureters are closed off by the muscular contractions of the bladder.

Bladder

The bladder stores urine received from the ureters until it is passed from the body. There is a slight increase in the intravesical pressure for approximately the accumulation of the first 25 ml. Then the pressure stays relatively stable until about 400 to 500 ml have been collected. This accommodation occurs because of the slow stretching of the detrusor muscle. The pressure curve rises markedly as the bladder fills with more than 500 ml and soars as micturition is initiated.

Electromyographic (EMG) tracings do not measure or demonstrate activity of the bladder muscle related to filling; but rather the increased electrical response of the urethral sphincter to increased bladder pressure and volume. The bladder is composed of smooth muscle, whereas the urethral sphincter is composed of striated muscle and is the only area commonly monitored by the EMG.

Micturition, also called urination and voiding, is the act of emptying the bladder. As the bladder fills and the muscle fibers expand, stretch receptors in the bladder wall are stimulated. The first urge to void is felt at about 150 ml and a marked feeling of fullness usually occurs around 400 ml, although this level can be increased or decreased through habit patterns. Impulses are sent to the sacral portion of the spinal cord, where the micturition reflex is initiated, causing the bladder to contract and the urethral sphincters to open. As the bladder musculature contracts, the pressure forces the urine out through the urethra. The bladder muscle fibers extend longitudinally down the urethra, and as they contract, they shorten the urethra and pull the bladder down toward a point of fixation at the distal portion of the pubis. Unless the reflex is mediated at this point, urination occurs immediately.

The impulses initiating the micturition reflex are also sent to the cerebral cortex. After a period of successful toilet training in early childhood, the external sphincter is usually under voluntary control. If the client feels that environmental conditions are not right for urination, the external sphincter contracts, stopping the flow of urine. The micturition reflex also can be initiated by the cerebral cortex.

Voluntary contraction of the abdominal muscles (in addition to contraction of the detrusor muscle and relaxation of the sphincters) facilitates micturition by increasing pressure on the bladder wall. During urination, the perineal muscles must be relaxed. Voluntary contraction (or exercising) of the perineal muscles assists the external sphincter to resist the outflow of urine. In essence, this voluntary contraction is the Valsalva maneuver.

Urethra and Meatus

The urethra is the pathway through which the urine normally leaves the body. The detrusor contraction during micturition is preceded for about 5 seconds by a significant fall of pressure within the urethra. This facilitates movement of urine from the bladder, with its higher pressure, into the urethra. Following the act of micturition, the female urethra empties by gravity, whereas the male urethra empties by several contractions of the bulbocavernosus muscle.

The female urethra is about 3.5 to 4.0 cm long, exiting the urinary bladder through the pelvic floor. The urethral meatus is located anterior to the vagina and slightly below the clitoris.

The male urethra is about 15 to 20 cm long, with the urethral meatus located at the tip of the penis. The male urethra is divided into three sections. The prostatic urethra is about 3.75 cm long and passes through the prostate gland after leaving the bladder. The next portion is the membranous urethra, about 1.25 cm in length, which passes along the wall of the pelvic floor. The remainder of the urethra is called the bulbar cavernous urethra, and it extends the length of the penis, ending in the urethral meatus.

The urethra ends in the meatus, which is under voluntary control in the adult. When voiding is not appropriate, the external sphincter contracts, holding back the flow of urine until the reflex stimulation ceases.

EFFECTS OF AGING ON URINARY FUNCTION

As a part of the natural aging process, the kidney becomes smaller. The cause of this loss of tissue, which occurs especially in the renal cortex, is unknown. It may be focal, as the result of scarring, or diffuse, owing to renal blood vessel changes.

Because of this loss of functioning nephrons and generalized circulatory changes, renal function decreases with advancing age. Affected are the glomerular filtration rate, tubular reabsorption, and ability to concentrate the urine. All normal regulatory and metabolic functions of the kidney become less efficient, and there is little or no reserve with which to respond to periods of increased stress.

The aging process also affects the act of micturition. The bladder becomes funnel shaped owing to alterations in the connective tissue and weakening of the pelvic floor muscles. Irritability of the bladder wall often increases, adding more urgency to the normal desire to void. Finally, impairment of the detrusor muscle's ability to elongate results in decreased bladder capacity. Because of these changes, the elderly person may have problems with incontinence, frequency, retention, and dysuria.

Summary

An understanding of the structure and function of the renal and urinary system is needed before the nurse can adequately care for clients experiencing disorders in this system. Once the nurse has a thorough understanding, appropriate interventions can be taken to provide comprehensive client care.

Bibliography

1. Avoiding a voiding problem. (1983). *Transition, 1,* 55.
2. Bagley, D., et al. (1985). *Urologic endoscopy: A manual and atlas.* Boston: Little, Brown & Co.
3. Beck, L. H. (1990). Kidney function and disease in the elderly. *Hospital Practice, 26,* 75–90.
4. Bertani, T., et al. (1986). *Drugs and the kidneys (vol. 33).* New York: Raven Press.
5. Bower, A., & Thompson, J. (1992). *Clinical manual of health assessment (3rd ed.).* St. Louis: C. V. Mosby.
6. Brenner, B. M., & Rector, F. C., Jr. (1986). *The kidney.* Philadelphia: W. B. Saunders.
7. Brown, W. W. (1989). Geriatric nephrology and urology—1989. *Peritoneal Dialysis International, 9,* 27–28.
8. Charlton, C. A. (1983). *The urological system.* New York: Churchill Livingston.
9. Cummings, N., & Klahr, S. (1985). *Chronic renal disease: Causes, complications, and treatment.* New York: Plenum Medical Book Co.
10. Dunn, M. (1984). Clinical effects of prostaglandins in renal disease. *Hospital Practice, 19,* 99.
11. Epstein, M. (1985). Aging and the kidney: Clinical implications. *American Family Physician, 31,* 123.
12. Goldberg, E. (1986). *A primer of water, electrolyte, and acid-base syndromes. (7th ed.).* Philadelphia: W. B. Saunders.
13. Gosling, J., et al. (1982). *Functional anatomy of the urinary tract.* Baltimore: University Park Press.
14. Groer, M. W., & Shekleton, M. E. (1989). *Basic pathophysiology: A holistic approach (3rd ed.).* St. Louis: C. V. Mosby.
15. Guyton, A. C. (1991). *Textbook of medical physiology (8th ed.).* Philadelphia: W. B. Saunders.
16. Hald, T., & Bradley, W. (1982). *The urinary bladder: Neurology and dynamics.* Baltimore: Williams & Wilkins.
17. Henrich, W., & Campbell, W. (1983). The systemic β-adrenergic pathway to renin secretion relationships with the renal prostaglandin system. *Endocrinology, 113,* 2247.
18. Jard, S., et al. (1984). The mechanisms of action of antidiuretic hormone. *Advances in Nephrology, 113,* 163.
19. Javadpour, N. (1984). *Cancer of the kidney.* New York: Thieme-Stratton.
20. Lapides, J. (1976). *Fundamentals of urology.* Philadelphia: W. B. Saunders.
21. Marsh, D. (1983). *Renal physiology.* New York: Raven Press.
22. Massary, S. G., & Gassock, R. J. (Eds.) (1988). *Textbook of nephrology.* Baltimore: Williams & Wilkins.
23. Matteson, M. A., & McConnell, E. S. (1988). *Gerontological nursing: Concepts and practice.* Philadelphia: W. B. Saunders.
24. Porth, C. (1990). *Pathophysiology (3rd ed.).* Philadelphia: J. B. Lippincott.
25. Re, R. N. (1987). The renin-angiotensin systems. *Medical Clinics of North America, 71,* 877–895.
26. Rebensen-Piano, M. (1989). The physiologic changes that occur with aging. *Critical Care Nursing Quarterly, 12*(1), 1–14.
27. Sabiston, D. C. (1991). *Textbook of surgery: The biological basis of modern surgical practice.* Philadelphia: W. B. Saunders.
28. Schrier, R., & Gottschalk, C. (1988). *Diseases of the kidney (4th ed.).* Boston: Little, Brown & Co.
29. Slate, W. (1982). *Disorders of the female urethra and urinary incontinence.* Baltimore: Williams & Wilkins.
30. Smith, D. R. (1988). *General Urology (12th ed.).* Norwalk, CT: Appleton & Lange.

31. Stanton, S. (1984). *Clinical gynecologic urology*. St. Louis: C. V. Mosby Co.
32. Vander, A. J. (1985). *Renal physiology (3rd ed.)*. New York: McGraw-Hill.
33. Walsh, P. C., et al. (Eds.) (1992). Campbell's urology (6th ed.). Philadelphia, W. B. Saunders.
34. Wyngaarden, J. B., & Smith, L. H. (1988). *Cecil textbook of medicine (18th ed.)*. Philadelphia: W. B. Saunders.
35. Zawada, E. (1982). The aging bladder: A source of many clinical problems. *Hospital Medicine, 18,* 101.

Chapter 48

Assessment of Clients with Urinary Disorders

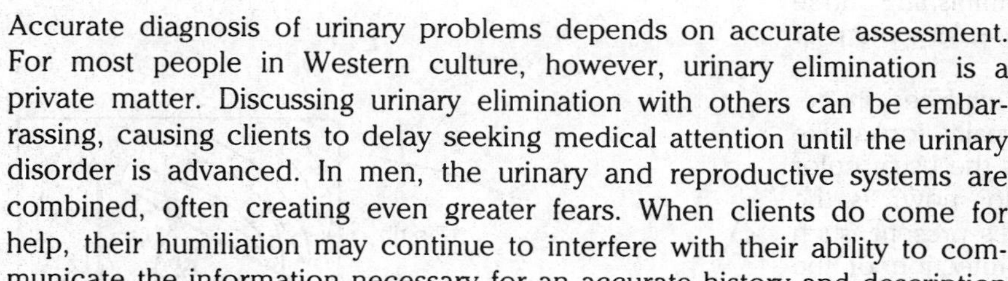

Accurate diagnosis of urinary problems depends on accurate assessment. For most people in Western culture, however, urinary elimination is a private matter. Discussing urinary elimination with others can be embarrassing, causing clients to delay seeking medical attention until the urinary disorder is advanced. In men, the urinary and reproductive systems are combined, often creating even greater fears. When clients do come for help, their humiliation may continue to interfere with their ability to communicate the information necessary for an accurate history and description of their current problem.

The physical examination and specific diagnostic studies used to assess urinary function can also be distressing. For example, providing a urine specimen may be embarrassing, especially if the client has to carry the full container down the hall or bring it from home. Some studies require the client to urinate in front of others as with a voiding cystogram or urinary flow rate. When assessing the client, keep in mind the client's likely embarrassment or discomfort and be understanding. Provide as much privacy as possible.

Use of good communication skills is the key to obtaining complete and accurate information. Allow the client to express anxiety and, in turn, try to make the client comfortable and at ease. Be aware of what the client communicates nonverbally, because subtle clues may be crucial to diagnosing the client's problem.

HISTORY

As with other systems, history taking is probably the most important part of the assessment process. Most problems usually are discovered at this point.

A urologic history consists of the chief complaint and current health history, past medical history, family history, psychosocial history and lifestyle, and review of systems (ROS). If the client reports urologic symptoms, a detailed symptom analysis is performed (see Chap. 11).

Chief Complaint

Common major symptoms in urologic disorders include a change in the usual patterns of voiding, urine incontinence, pain, and associated gastrointestinal symptoms. There may be more than one symptom present, and each is explored with the client.

CHANGE IN URINARY PATTERNS

The client is asked to describe his or her usual patterns of voiding, including frequency, amounts, and usual times of the day or night. Ask if there are any particular methods the client uses to stimulate urination, such as listening to running water, applying pressure over the lower abdomen, or performing the Valsalva maneuver. Does the client experience difficulty starting or maintaining the urine stream (hesitancy)? Has there been a change in the force or shape of the stream? Does the client have feelings of urgency or difficulty controlling micturation? If so, is the urgency associated with a known factor such as consuming caffeine or, for women, following pregnancy and vaginal delivery? Older men may report gradually diminishing urine stream force and hesitancy if they have enlargement of the prostate gland.

Changes in urine characteristics are explored in detail. Ask the client what the urine usually looks like before symptoms were present. What is the usual color and odor? What is the color and odor now? Is the urine clear or cloudy? Are there particles present, such as clots, mucus, or shreds of tissue? Infection of the urinary tract results in inflammation so that the urine becomes cloudy with debris.

URINE INCONTINENCE

Urine incontinence is the loss of control over the release of urine from the bladder. There are several types of urine incontinence, such as stress incontinence, urge incontinence, total incontinence, and reflex incontinence. The nurse asks the client to describe the onset and associated symptoms that occur with incontinence. How often does it occur? Is there dribbling of urine between voidings? If so, how much? Does incontinence occur at predictable times, such as with coughing, sneezing, and laughing? Does the client have an awareness of the need to void prior to incontinent episodes? How long has the client had difficulty with incontinence? Is the problem getting worse? What methods does the client use to cope with incontinence? The client may have concerns about strike-through wetness on clothing or odor being noticeable to others and may resort to using pads or shields for protection.

PAIN

The client is asked to describe any pain associated with the urinary tract, including its location, type, severity, and duration. Is the pain getting worse or better? Is the client able to relate factors that may have precipitated the pain? What makes the pain better? What makes it worse? Is the pain accompanied by uncomfortable or painful urination (dysuria)? If dysuria is present, when during voiding does it occur?

A careful description of any pain may help pinpoint the source of the problem. Kidney pain, which is usually caused by sudden distention of the renal capsule, produces a dull, constant ache in the costovertebral angle (CVA) lateral to the sacrospinalis muscle just below the twelfth rib. This pain often spreads along the subcostal area to the umbilicus.

Radiculitis often mimics renal pain, so it is important to differentiate between the two. Radicular pain is a hyperesthesia of the skin supplied by the irritated peripheral nerve. This nerve can be stimulated by pinching both the skin and fat of the abdominal and flank regions. Exerting pressure over the CVA with the thumb may elicit local tenderness of the involved peripheral nerve at its point of emergence, whereas gentle percussion over the angle may be necessary to elicit renal pain, indicating a deeper, more visceral sensation. Figure 48-1 illustrates percussion over the costovertebral angle (Murphy's percussion).

Ureteral pain is exhibited as back pain from capsular distention and as colicky pain caused by spasm of the renal pelvis and ureteral muscle. It radiates from the

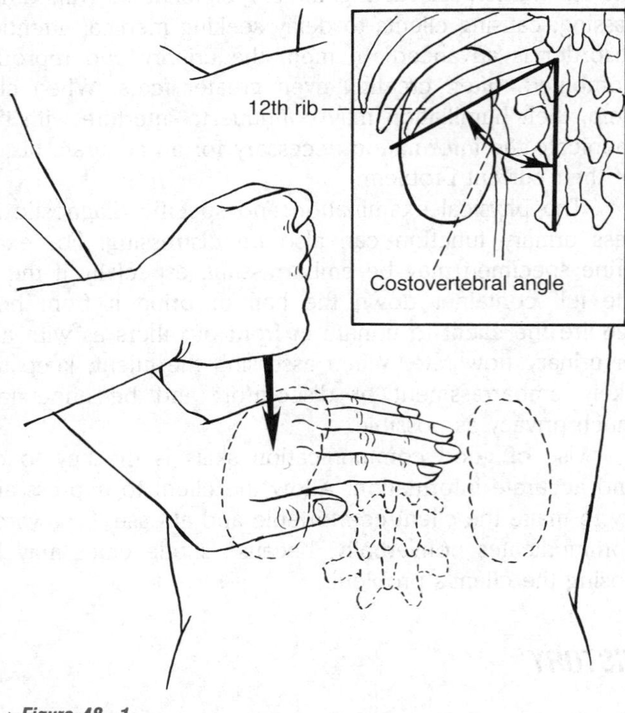

▲ ***Figure 48-1***

Percussion over the costovertebral angle (CVA).

costovertebral angle down across the abdomen to the genital area. In males, pain originating in the upper ureter is referred to the scrotal wall. Females describe ureteral pain in the ipsilateral labium. Ureteral pain is often sharp and excruciating and may result in a generalized systemic shock syndrome.

The most common bladder discomfort arises from overdistention and is felt in the suprapubic area. Bladder infection causes urgency spasms and/or a burning pain during micturition in the distal urethra for females and in the prostatic urethra for males. Urethral pain is usually felt along the course of the urethra or meatus.

Determining precisely when during the act of micturition burning occurs helps differentiate between bladder and urethral origins. Burning at the beginning of urination (as the bladder contracts the inflamed tissue where the bladder drains into the urethra) indicates urethritis. Suspect bladder infection when the burning occurs during and after the voiding process.

GASTROINTESTINAL SYMPTOMS

Urinary tract disorders may be accompanied by gastrointestinal symptoms, such as anorexia, nausea, vomiting, diarrhea, or a metallic taste in the mouth. The unpleasantness of these symptoms may lead the client to alter the amount and type of fluids consumed. Ask the client to describe how much fluid is consumed in a day and the types of liquids that are drunk. How does the fluid intake compare with the urinary output? Does the client have unusual fluid loss from diarrhea, vomiting, or excess perspiration? Have there been weight changes (loss or gain) of 2 pounds or more within a 24-hour period? Such weight fluctuations are usually related to a change in fluid balance.

Renointestinal reflexes may cause gastrointestinal and renal symptoms to occur simultaneously. Afferent stimuli originating in the renal capsule or pelvic musculature may cause pylorospasm or other changes in the smooth muscle of the enteric tract and adnexa. Additionally, the anatomic proximity of the kidneys and gastrointestinal structures may mean that intestinal disturbances will mimic renal disorders. The right kidney lies close to the hepatic flexure of the colon, duodenum, head of the pancreas, common bile duct, liver, and gallbladder, whereas the left kidney is bordered by the splenic flexure of the colon, stomach, pancreas, and spleen. This partially explains why clients experience nausea and vomiting, anorexia, diarrhea, and abdominal discomfort concomitantly with urinary tract symptoms. Renal inflammation may also produce signs of peritoneal irritation.

Past Medical History

The past medical history explores the client's experiences with disorders of the urinary tract. These data may be linked to current health problems or may be associated with increased risk for the client to develop urinary tract disorders.

CHILDHOOD AND INFECTIOUS DISEASES

Ask the client to relate incidences of urinary tract infection (UTI), particularly in females, during childhood. Frequent UTIs can result in structural changes from chronic inflammation and strictures. Chronic or inadequately treated infections can lead to more serious sequelae such as hydronephrosis. Skin or upper respiratory infection of streptococcal origin can result in acute glomerulonephritis, as can infectious mononucleosis, mumps, measles, cytomegaloviral infection, and other primary infections.

MAJOR ILLNESSES AND HOSPITALIZATIONS

The client is asked about previous hospitalizations or treatment for urinary problems. Determine the date of illnesses or hospitalization, the specific urinary problem, medical treatment (including surgery or manipulation of the urinary tract such as catheterization), and the present status of the problem. Ask if the client has had diagnostic studies of the urinary tract such as an intravenous pyelogram (IVP) or cystogram. Results of these studies can provide baseline data for assessment of the current problem.

Ask the client whether there has been trauma to the urinary tract such as a direct blow to the flank or falls with resulting contusion over the lower posterior thorax. How was the problem treated and what was the result? Specific surgical procedures to inquire about include any type of urinary diversion. Why was the surgery necessary? Is the diversion temporary or permanent? How does the client manage the diversion or are there problems with its management?

Major illnesses and diseases that are linked to urinary tract problems include hypertension, diabetes mellitus, gout, and connective tissue disorders (e.g., scleroderma, systemic lupus erythematosus). Ask the client about problems with urinary tract stones (calculi) as well as the previously mentioned UTIs and systemic infections.

MEDICATIONS

A complete medication history is obtained, including past use, because many drugs are nephrotoxic. Determine the quantity and length of use for medications because the nephrotoxic effects of certain drugs are dose specific. Diuretics alter the quantity of urine output. Phenazopyridine (Pyridium) and nitrofurantoin (Macrodantin) alter urine color. Anticoagulants can cause hematuria. Other medications that can affect the urinary tract include antibiotics, narcotics, cholinergics, rifampin, aminophylline, and oncologic agents. Over-the-counter medications that can affect the urinary tract include nonsteroidal anti-inflammatory agents (NSAIDs) (ibuprofen), phenacetin, and salicylates.

ALLERGIES

The nurse asks the client about allergies to foods, dyes, and medications. Specifically, inquire about allergies to shellfish, seafood, to iodine. Has the client ever had a diagnostic test in which a contrast medium was used? What was the result?

Family History

A family history of certain renal and urinary disorders increases the risk of the client developing similar problems. In addition to hypertension, diabetes mellitus, gout, and recurrent UTIs, ask about congenital urinary tract disorders, polycystic kidney disease, nephritis (Alport's syndrome), and urinary calculi.

Psychosocial History and Lifestyle

Urinary tract disorders affect many aspects of the client's life, including his or her psychological, social, and occupational, as well as physical factors.

PSYCHOSOCIAL FACTORS

Psychological Factors. Assess the client's emotional reaction to the history-taking process and to the physical examination. Just as people are emotionally affected by the performance of the urinary system, so is the urinary system affected by emotions in a number of ways, such as by (1) past experiences, (2) the power of suggestion, (3) anxiety and fear, (4) depression, (5) changes in body image, and (6) the fear of death.

Past Experiences. A client's past experiences produce various effects on the process of voiding. As mentioned earlier, cultural teachings lead most people to consider the act of micturition a private matter. Western society and childrearing practices support this viewpoint by providing locks on bathroom doors, separate public restrooms for men and women, and so forth. This attitude may inhibit the micturition reflex if the client is in an environment where privacy is missing, such as, a commode behind the curtain in a multibed hospital room.

Experiences linked with childhood toilet training can have long-lasting effects. A client's negative or positive attitudes toward bladder elimination can sometimes be traced back to this developmental period. Reinforcement for positive behavior tends to result in continued, problem-free elimination patterns. Punishment as the primary motivator during toilet training, however, may carry over into adulthood, producing guilt or anxiety that is exhibited in micturition problems. The guilt or shame from prolonged enuresis (involuntary discharge of urine, usually during sleep at night or bed-wetting) may cause voiding dysfunction long after the enuresis has been cured. In addition, to punish their parents, children may not use the toilet and this behavior may appear again in adult life.

Power of Suggestion. The micturition control center is connected to the various sensory portions of the brain, allowing micturition to be initiated by any number of auditory, visual, or somesthetic stimuli, such as running water in a sink. In fact, the mere act of thinking about voiding may be enough to stimulate the reflex.

Anxiety and Fear. Anxiety may stimulate or hinder micturition. The most noticeable effect of anxiety is to increase the frequency of voidings and produce urgency. Very commonly, people have a strong urge to void when facing stressful situations even though they may have urinated just moments before. Conversely, anxiety characterized by general muscle tension can interfere with urination, because relaxing the perineal muscles is essential to completing micturition. Anxiety also may intensify the manifestations of urinary tract disorders. Fear of the unknown or concern about the disorder's prognosis, for instance, makes pain seem worse. Also, moderate to severe burning pain on urination will cause the client to inhibit micturition in order to avoid discomfort.

Depression. Incontinence is not the result of depression; rather depression is the result of long-standing, untreated, unmanaged urinary incontinence. Urinary incontinence is a sign of an underlying physiologic problem. The isolation and changes in the client's social patterns caused by incontinence can easily lead to a sense of worthlessness and depression. It is not the depression, however, that needs to be treated; but rather the incontinence needs to be corrected so that the depression will disappear.

Changes in Body Image. Many urinary disorders necessitate a change in body image and lifestyle, which, in turn, may lead to anxiety, depression, or anger. Changes that affect body image include an inability to control body functions such as urination, a dependence on others, and a dependency on machines or devices. Anatomic alterations that alter the way urine leaves the body are sometimes surgically created. If the client is unable to produce urine at all, a machine must perform this vital blood-cleansing function. These dramatic and often permanent alterations can destroy a client's healthy body image.

Adapting to a serious disruption of body image often leads the client and significant others along a path of denial, anger, and depression before they finally accept the new self-concept. During this time, the client who has the dysfunction can suffer a loss of self-esteem. Additional conflicts involve dependence and independence. Changes in life role and responsibilities, lifestyles, and interpersonal relationships may develop. The client and significant others may need long-term psychosocial counseling.

Fear of Death. The possibility of impending death is a real concern for clients with urinary tract problems because most realize that a functioning urinary system is necessary for life. Urinary tract cancers, such as bladder or renal, and renal failure are problems that are most likely to cause fear of death. Whether the problem is large or small, it is always possible that a urinary disorder may become terminal. Some clients may be able to discuss this fear openly, whereas others may not be able to admit such a possibility. Many times, this fear is suggested by behavior such as acting out, denial, and social withdrawal.

Learn as much as you can about the client's psychological disposition. Carefully listen to conversation and observe behavior patterns. In some cases, a client may voice fear directly, by openly saying, "I'm afraid of dying." On the other hand, some people are unable to express their fears directly. In this case, look for indirect cues in the way the client answers questions or initiates conversation. Subtle cues may be camouflaged in seemingly unconscious statements.

Whatever communication techniques the nurse uses, the nurse should consciously assess the client's emotional state, because no one else on the health care team may be assisting the client and significant others in this crucial realm.

LIFESTYLE

Urinary problems may cause a change in lifestyle. To assess the kind and extent of changes that may occur, baseline data are collected in the following areas.

Living Conditions. Does the client live alone or with others? How many people live in the household? How many bathrooms are there, and where are they located? For example, does the client have to negotiate stairs to gain access to the toilet? Does this present a physical limitation to the client with impaired mobility? Does the client have need for a bedside commode or a bedpan to facilitate urinary elimination?

Support Systems. Are there others available to assist the client who is dependent for help with urinary elimination? Can the client rely on family members, or is a referral needed to a community agency?

Financial Status. If the client has need of special equipment (e.g., ostomy supplies), are there resources to help pay for it? Is a source for supplies accessible?

Occupation. What kind of work does the client do? Are there barriers in the workplace to allowing the client to take time for urinary elimination? Are there hazards in the workplace setting that increase the client's risk for developing urinary problems such as exposure to nephrotoxic chemicals (e.g., carbon tetrachloride, phenol, and ethyl glycol)?

Hobbies and Leisure Activities. Does the client participate in hobbies or recreational activities, or has a urinary problem resulted in a reluctance to participate? Has the client had to give up favorite activities because of incontinence?

Habits. Ask about diet, activity and exercise, smoking, and use of recreational drugs. A diet high in calcium and with low fluid intake can contribute to calculi formation. Dehydration also increases the client's risk of UTI and renal failure. The client's activity level may indicate a risk of developing urinary stasis if the client is sedentary. Urinary stasis, in turn, predisposes the client to UTI and calculi formation. The client with impaired physical mobility is at even greater risk if bone demineralization is an accompanying factor. Cigarette smoking has been linked to the occurrence of bladder tumors, particularly in women. Drug use may expose the client to nephrotoxic agents and subsequent renal damage.

Review of Systems

Urinary function affects and is affected by other body systems. The nurse asks questions about the general status as well as specific body systems because the resulting data may reveal related renal problems. For example, assessing the neuromuscular system provides information about the client's ability to control urination. Gastrointestinal symptoms (bleeding or a metallic taste in the mouth) may indicate renal disease. Assessing the client's immune system, for example, for the presence of allergies, can help determine which diagnostic tests and medication will cause allergic reactions and are thus contraindicated.

Specifically, ask the client about fatigue, headaches, blurred vision, changes in mentation, elevated blood pressure, changes in body weight, itching, numbness or tingling of the extremities, excess thirst, chills, bleeding tendencies, anorexia, nausea and vomiting, and edema of the face or extremities.

Additional questions for the ROS may be found in Chapter 11, Table 11–5.

PHYSICAL EXAMINATION

The physical examination is based on the information obtained during the history-taking process. Although most of the data needed come directly from examining the urinary system, consider other systems, too.

Urinary Tract Organs

KIDNEYS

Inspect for masses in the upper abdomen and flank areas. Typically, because of the location of the kidneys, only the lower poles of the right kidney can be felt on deep palpation. With the client lying supine on a hard surface, deep palpation is accomplished in the following manner: For the right kidney, stand on the right side of the client, place the right hand on the abdomen between the rib cage and the iliac crest, and position the left hand posteriorly in the costovertebral angle (Fig. 48–2). Support the area from below in the left hand and have the client take a deep breath. As the client inhales, use the right hand to compress the tissue in deep palpation. Instruct the client to exhale and then hold the breath. Slowly release the pressure with the

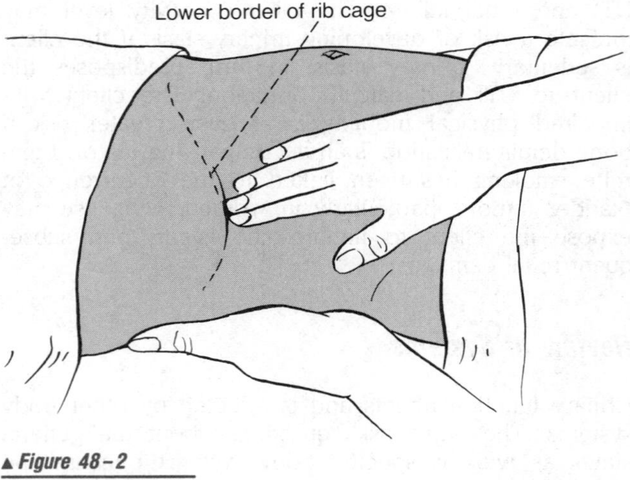

▲ Figure 48-2

Palpating the kidneys.

right hand; the pole, if felt, is a smooth, firm rounded mass that descends on inspiration and slips upward and away on exhalation. Instruct the client to breathe normally and remove both hands. Palpate the left kidney standing on the client's right side reaching across with the left hand under the client and using the right hand to palpate. The left kidney should not be felt because it lies higher up in the rib cage. In older adults, the muscles lose tone and elasticity, so the kidneys drop and may be palpated more readily.

Depending on the size of the client and the skill of the examiner, it may be possible to outline both kidneys anteriorly and posteriorly by percussion (see Fig. 48-1). This technique is particularly helpful when pain and muscle spasm prevent proper palpation. Assess costovertebral angle tenderness by placing the left hand over the area and striking it with the right fist. Ordinarily, this percussion would produce a dull sound and no discomfort. With inflammation, there is exquisite tenderness.

Auscultation is performed in the costovertebral angle and upper abdominal quadrants. There is normally no sound unless aortic pulsations are heard. A systolic bruit is often associated with stenosis or aneurysm of the renal artery.

BLADDER

As the bladder distends, it rises out of the pelvic cavity above the pubic symphysis. In a very thin client or one with a very distended bladder, it may be visible on inspection and palpated. When a distended bladder is palpated, it is felt as a smooth, round, and rather tense mass. The adult bladder can be percussed if it contains at least 150 ml of urine. Percussion is accomplished in the normal manner, with the sound of bowel often being hollow and the sound of the distended bladder being duller. The bladder can be outlined, which may extend as high as the umbilicus. After the initial assessment, have the client void and then palpate and percuss again to distinguish the bladder from a possible mass. Residual urine also could be measured at this point. This test is discussed later in this chapter.

URETHRA

Urethral examination primarily involves inspecting the external meatus and the perineal area for signs of discharge, abnormal tissue growth, cleanliness, and anatomic integrity. Note any aberrant location of the meatus. Palpate the penis for masses along the distal portion of the male urethra, and palpate the perineal area for tenderness. In the female, the posterior urethra is examined vaginally for masses, tenderness, or expressed discharge from the urethra.

The size and patency of the meatus and the urethra may be evaluated by the urologist passing instruments of varying diameter through the urethra. This evaluation is performed with different sizes of rubber or plastic catheters or, if preferred, special urologic instruments. A *sound* is a smooth, cylindric rod with a rounded tip. Its size ranges from 8 to 32 French. Figure 48-3 illustrates examples of sounds. The urethra and meatus may be dilated using the sounds. Xylocaine jelly or other local anesthetic is applied before the sound is passed under aseptic conditions, beginning with a small size and increasing in diameter until the largest caliber is found that can be easily inserted. Strictures, which will be discussed in Chapter 49, may make insertion more difficult.

ALTERNATIVE URINARY OUTLET

The client who has had a urinary diversion procedure, such as an ileal conduit or continent urinary reservoir, will have an opening in the abdominal wall. Assess this stoma, and note its location, size, shape, color, intactness, and odor. Observe the quality and quantity of the drainage. In addition, evaluate the condition of the periostomal skin for color, cleanliness, intactness, and the absence of lesions such as maceration and irritation. For the client with the ileal conduit, observe the cleanliness and appropriateness of the urine collection system, to assess the client's teaching and learning needs. Finally, the client's responses during this part of the examination may indicate the client's acceptance of the altered urinary function.

The client may have a catheter that partially or completely drains the urine from the body. The catheter may be inserted into the bladder, a ureter, or a kidney,

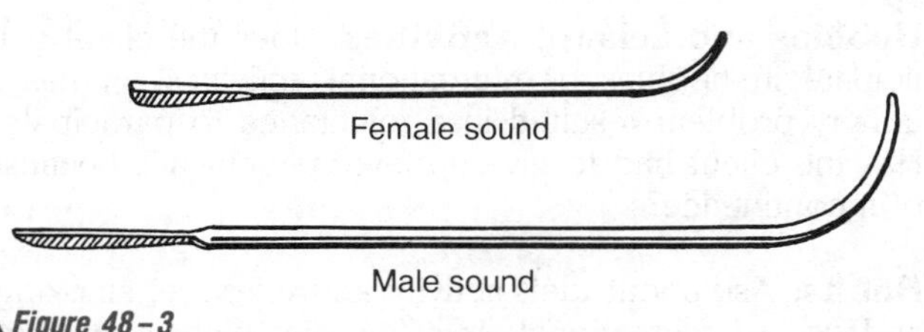

▲ Figure 48-3

Sounds used to calibrate the diameter of the urethra, determine patency, and (if necessary) dilate strictures.

and may come out of the body through the urethra, the abdomen, or flank wall. Inspect these catheters during the examination, checking them for patency, location, and cleanliness. Palpate the tubing for sedimentation by rolling it between the thumb and fingers and feeling for a gravelly sensation. Observe the tissues around the catheter where it enters the body for cleanliness and the absence of lesions such as inflammation and ulceration.

Related Body Systems

Selected information from other body systems is crucial for correctly assessing urinary tract problems and planning interventions.

FLUID STATUS

An accurate *intake* and *output* measurement helps determine the client's fluid status. Intake or output of disproportionate amounts of fluid may indicate volume excess or depletion. Keeping track of intake and output helps identify the presence of important signs of abnormal kidney function, such as oliguria, anuria, and polyuria.

The normal adult on a regular diet who takes in about 1200 to 1500 ml of measurable fluids daily should excrete 1200 to 1500 ml of urine plus insensible fluid loss in a 24-hour period. When determining the presence of oliguria, anuria, or polyuria, remember that the output is in relation to normal intake. *Oliguria* is a urine volume significantly below this amount, usually 400 ml/24 h (134 ml/8 h). *Anuria* means the absence of urine production (or less than 100 ml/24 h). These two conditions may indicate shock, poisoning, or any other process that would interfere with urine formation in the kidney. Anuria would, of course, be a normal finding in clients undergoing renal dialysis. *Polyuria* implies significantly larger than normal amounts of urine output. It can be caused by disorders such as acute or chronic renal failure, diabetes mellitus, diabetes insipidus, or by interventions such as diuretic administration.

When polyuria is present, it is important to discriminate between water diuresis and solute diuresis. *Water diuresis* is characterized by a low urine specific gravity, a low urine osmolality, and a normal to elevated serum sodium level. It indicates either a lack of antidiuretic hormone (ADH), as after trauma to the posterior pituitary gland, or unresponsiveness of the renal tubules, as with hypokalemia or hydronephrosis. *Solute diuresis* results from impaired tubular absorption of a particular solute, as may accompany diabetes mellitus or relief of an acute bladder obstruction. It is characterized by a high urine specific gravity, an elevated urine osmolality, and a normal or low serum sodium level.

Body weight is a good indicator of fluid gains and losses, provided it is carefully measured daily and compared with previous findings. A gain or loss of more than 2 pounds in 24 hours is considered related to fluid loss or retention. Dry mucous membranes may signal volume depletion, whereas the presence of edema may be a sign of volume excess. In assessing edema, it is important to determine its progression or recession. Measuring the girth of edematous parts daily provides accurate, objective documentation.

NEUROLOGIC STATUS

Renal dysfunction may interfere with normal activity within the nervous system, as when a buildup of calcium causes tetany, decreased calcium produces weakness, or toxins accumulate in chronic renal failure. Conversely, the urinary tract depends on an intact nervous system in order to carry out its main function: removing waste from the body. Any abnormality in nervous stimulation to the urinary organs or their surrounding tissue interferes with the propulsion and expulsion of urine. In addition to assessing gross nervous function (e.g., the ability to walk and maintain balance), the examiner may test the intactness of innervation specific to urinary tract function. Because the anal and urinary sphincters are supplied by branches of the same nerve, the intactness of one may indicate that the other sphincter functions as well. Stroke the perianal skin to test for sensation.

To initially evaluate anal sphincter tone, insert a gloved, lubricated finger into the anus and notice the amount of resistance felt. With the finger still in the rectum, test the bulbocavernous reflex if instructed in this procedure: Squeeze the glans penis or clitoris or gently jerk on an indwelling catheter. This will contract the external anal sphincter and bulbocavernous muscle when the S2 to S4 reflex is intact. Other tests evaluating relevant neurologic activity are described later in this chapter.

INTEGUMENTARY STATUS

Note the color of the skin when assessing renal dysfunction. For instance, erythropoietin deficiency anemia may cause pallor. Deposits of a carotene-like substance, caused by renal excretion failure, may give the skin a yellowish gray cast. *Dry skin* may indicate chronic renal failure and may also suggest volume depletion. Bruises or petechiae may represent bleeding tendencies. Crystal deposits on the skin (found primarily in areas of concentrated perspiration) is a secondary sign of severe, prolonged renal failure.

MUSCULOSKELETAL STATUS

Assess the client's movements during examination to (1) determine general body tone and (2) judge the client's physical ability to handle urinary elimination needs. Specific muscle groups involved in micturition are the perineal and abdominal muscles. To assess their strength, have the client consciously contract or tighten the perineal and abdominal muscles. Changes in tautness can then be seen and palpated. The ability to purposely interrupt the flow of urine midstream by perineal muscle contraction also indicates adequate perineal musculature.

CARDIOVASCULAR STATUS

Monitoring the cardiovascular system can identify fluid and electrolyte imbalances. Most specific to the urinary tract is blood pressure measurement. Hypertension is a finding in many renal diseases and may result from fluid volume overload or disturbance of the renin-angiotensin system. *Increasing* hypertension can possibly lead to irreversible renal shutdown, and thus requires immediate medical action.

RESPIRATORY STATUS

To some extent, the quality of respirations reflects the client's fluid and acid-base balances. Respiratory assessment is discussed further in Chapter 36. In addition, during renal failure, the breath may have an odor of urine or fruit-flavored gum, which is the result of toxins built up in the bloodstream.

OTHER SYSTEMS

A vaginal and rectal examination are routinely performed to assess urinary problems. If appropriate, inspect and palpate these two orifices to help identify fistulas, masses, prolapses, and diverticula. In the male, because of the proximity to the rectum, the posterior lobe of the prostate can be examined for enlargement, tenderness, or masses. In the female, a vaginal examination can detect prolapse of the bladder.

DIAGNOSTIC TESTS

A number of diagnostic tests are available to evaluate the status of the urinary system. They include laboratory tests; x-ray, ultrasound, and radioisotope studies; pressure profiles; endoscopy; and surgical exploration. The history, physical examination, and results of previous studies determine which procedures to use.

During diagnostic testing, the nurse has many roles. The nurse may be directly involved in collecting and testing specimens and in assisting the examiner during certain procedures. Specific studies require particular post-test care, such as watching for hemorrhage after a kidney biopsy. The nurse also allows the person to express concerns and answers questions about the test. Finally, the nurse must be able to use test results appropriately in the person's care plan.

Laboratory Tests

URINE STUDIES

Collection of Specimens. The accurate outcome of any laboratory test depends on collecting the right kind of specimen in the proper manner, in the right container, and at the right time. Once the specimen has been collected, it must be stored properly until the correct testing procedure is performed and the findings are accurately interpreted. The nurse and appropriate others — the individual, people in the household, laboratory personnel — all share this responsibility.

The types of urine specimens include random, clean-catch (midstream), catheter, 12-hour, 24-hour, and double voided.

Random Specimens. A random specimen is one that can be collected at any time. However, an *early morning* specimen gives more definitive results for some values. Generally, the person needs no special preparation, although the female may be asked to wash the perineal area to clean away any collected debris. The specimen is then collected in any clean container. This type of specimen cannot be used for culture and sensitivity tests, because the lack of specific perineal cleaning and the use of an unsterile container contaminate the specimen.

Clean-Catch Specimens. The goal of a clean-catch, or midstream, specimen is to reduce as much as possible the contamination of the specimen by external organisms. This type of specimen is usually collected if the urine is to be cultured. Circumcised men, however, may not need to follow this procedure because there is little difference in urine collected in this way versus a simple voided urine. Uncircumcised men are asked to withdraw the foreskin before voiding to decrease the risk of contamination.

Catheter Specimens. A catheterized specimen may be used for culture. Avoid this procedure when possible because of the increased risk of introducing organisms into the urethra or bladder during the catheterization. In renal failure especially, there may not be enough urine produced to wash out these bacteria, thus increasing the risk of urinary tract infection. When catheterization is used, a straight catheter of the smallest size is inserted into the bladder under aseptic conditions, either through the urethra or as a suprapubic tap, allowing urine to flow directly from the end of the catheter into a sterile specimen container.

A specimen also may be collected from an indwelling catheter. Urine standing in the collection bag undergoes several chemical changes, may be contaminated with bacteria, and does not reflect the client's current urinary status. For these reasons, it should never be used for urine specimens. Instead, obtain the specimen from the catheter or drainage tubing. Opening the drainage system to the air can introduce microorganisms. Most urinary drainage systems have a specimen collection port built into the top of the drainage tubing. This self-sealing rubber-covered area is cleansed, and the urine is aspirated with a sterile needle and syringe. The tubing may need to be clamped for 15 to 20 minutes below the port to allow enough urine to build up. If there is no collection port and the catheter is not Silastic, use a small-gauge (25) needle and syringe to aspirate urine from the catheter itself. Using aseptic technique, insert the needle into the catheter distal to the sleeve leading to the balloon, slanting the needle tip toward the drainage tubing and avoid entering the balloon lumen. Puncture the catheter at an angle to allow resealing after the needle is withdrawn. This cannot be performed with a Silastic catheter because it will not reseal after being punctured.

A special procedure is used to obtain a specimen for culture from a person with an ileal conduit, a type of urinary diversion created from segments of the ileum. It is virtually impossible to insert a catheter directly into the conduit without contaminating it with organisms from the stoma or from the first few centimeters of the ileum. Therefore, cleanse the stomal area with soap and water and rinse it with sterile water. Next, don sterile gloves and cut an 18 French rubber whistle-tip catheter to about 10 cm in length. Cut a pediatric feeding tube approximately 30 cm from the connector end. Lubricate the rubber catheter and insert it into the stoma about 2 to 5 cm (1 to 2 in), gently rotating it if you feel any resistance. Holding the outer catheter in place, thread the feeding tube through it for about 7.5 cm (3 in). Put the connector end of the inner tube into a test tube or specimen container and allow the urine to flow by gravity. If there is no urine flow within several minutes, have the person move around or apply gentle suction on the catheter with a 5-ml syringe. When the specimen is collected, remove both catheters and replace the collection bag.

12- or 24-Hour Specimens. A 12- or 24-hour specimen is usually collected in one large container. Some of the specimens may need a chemical preservative in the container and refrigeration during the collection process. If appropriate refrigeration is not available, the specimen container may be packed in ice or insulated ice packs. In this case, make sure the cooling agent is replaced frequently enough to maintain the specimen at the necessary temperature. When the specimen collection begins, the person voids and this specimen is discarded. All urine voided in the next 12 or 24 hours, as appropriate, is placed in the container. Twelve or 24 hours from the time of the first voiding, instruct the client to void again and add this urine to the specimen. One of the major needs during this collection process is careful communication among all persons involved. If any single urine specimen is inadvertently discarded, the entire procedure must begin again.

Double-Voided Specimens. A double-voided specimen is sometimes used when the urine is being tested for glucose and ketones. Traditionally, clinicians thought the second voided sample was more accurate. However, two recent studies demonstrate that 94 per cent of the second voided specimens contain the same amounts of glucose as, or lesser amounts than, the first voided specimen.[58] Also, with the advent of self-monitoring of blood glucose, single-voided specimens for glucose and ketones appear to be better indicators of overall control. However, double-voided specimens are necessary when giving supplemental insulin based on urinary glucose results.

When a double-voided specimen is needed, the person empties the bladder. This specimen may be tested in case a second sample cannot be obtained. The person is then instructed to urinate again, 20 to 30 minutes after the first voiding. The person may drink a glass of water after the first voiding to facilitate producing the second sample.

Examination of the Urine. The urine can be examined by direct visualization, microscopy, or laboratory tests. The results of these examinations may indicate pathologic changes in the urinary tract as well as in other parts of the body.

Routine Urinalysis. A routine urinalysis is usually performed on a single, random specimen, although a midstream or catheter specimen may be used. Table 48-1 summarizes the usual observations made during this test and the normal findings.

Color. The color of urine normally ranges from pale yellow to deep amber, depending on its concentration. Some color changes occur because of medications or food ingested, whereas other colors may indicate pathologic processes. Foods that often cause red urine include blackberries, rhubarb, beets, and foods containing red dyes. Ingesting large amounts of carotene causes a bright yellow urine. Table 48-2 shows some common medications producing urinary color changes.

The most common significant color change indicating a pathologic disorder results from bleeding in the urinary tract. Bleeding in the upper tract produces dark red or smoky gray urine, whereas bleeding in the lower tract appears as red urine. Other color changes from pathologic conditions include red-brown or tea-colored urine, due to the release of myoglobin from severely damaged muscle tissue, dark yellow or green urine indicating the presence of urobilinogen or bilirubin, and green urine produced by *Pseudomonas* organisms.

Opacity. Freshly voided urine is normally transparent. It becomes cloudy on standing, but this can be reversed by adding a few drops of acid. Increases in opacity denoting a pathologic condition usually results from the presence of bacteria, crystals, or other foreign material in the urine.

Specific Gravity. Specific gravity indicates the concentration of the urine. This test can be used to estimate the client's general fluid status. Because one of the major functions of the kidney is to maintain fluid bal-

TABLE 48-1. Normal Findings in a Routine Urinalysis

Component	Normal Values
Color	Pale yellow to deep amber
Opacity	Clear
Specific gravity	1.002-1.035
Osmolality	275-295 mOsm/L
pH	4.5-8
Glucose	Negative
Ketones	Negative
Protein	Negative
Bilirubin	Negative
Red blood cells	None to 3
White blood cells	None to 4
Bacteria	None
Casts	None
Crystals	None

TABLE 48-2. Common Medications Producing Urinary Color Change

Medication	Color Change in Urine
Amitriptyline	Blue
Anthraquinone laxatives	Reddish brown in acid urine; red in alkaline urine
Chloroquine	Rusty-yellow
Chlorzoxazone	Orange or purple-red
Levodopa or methyldopa	Red or brown in hypochlorite toilet bleach
Methylene blue	Green
Multiple vitamins (with riboflavin)	Bright yellow
Phenazopyridine	Orange-brown, orange-red, or red
phenolphthalein	Pink-red in alkaline urine
phenothiazines	Red, red-brown, or pink
phenytoin	Red, red-brown, or pink
rifampin	Bright orange-red
sulfasalazine	Orange-yellow

ance, typically the more concentrated the urine, the more fluid depleted the person. Conversely, well-hydrated clients have more dilute urine, with specific gravities as low as 1.005. Typically, clients with a history of infections or other problems are encouraged to be very well hydrated to maintain dilute urine and a high output. For renal function, this measurement primarily indicates the ability of the client's kidneys to concentrate and dilute urine. When the kidneys lose these abilities, the urine no longer reflects physiologic stimuli and the specific gravity becomes fixed at a level equal to that of the plasma, usually 1.010 (isosthenuria). This occurs with tubular disease or endocrine disease involving ADH insufficiency. Contrast media used during x-ray procedures can produce readings above 1.040. Other substances in the urine, such as molecules of glucose or protein, also can cause high values.

Osmolality. Urine osmolality is a more precise way to measure the concentrating ability of the kidneys than is specific gravity. This is because the latter is a constant weight-to-weight relationship and is not unduly affected by the presence of glucose or protein. Urine osmolality increases in hypernatremia, acidosis, and shock. It decreases in diabetes insipidus, hypercalcemia, excessive fluid intake, renal tubular acidosis, severe pyelonephritis, and sometimes, hyperglycemia.

pH. Urinary pH usually reflects the plasma pH, with alkalinization or additional acidification occurring in order to maintain the body's acid-base balance. Metabolic alkalosis, low-protein diets high in vegetables and citrus fruits, alkalinizing medications such as soda bicarbonate and acetazolamide, and ammonia-splitting bacteria all produce alkaline urine. Urinary pH also indicates renal tubular acidosis in which tubular reabsorption is impaired. Strongly acid urine results from metabolic acidosis, metabolic alkalosis in potassium deficiency, a high-protein diet, uncontrolled diabetes, and some medications, such as ammonium chloride and mandelic acid.

Glucose. Glucosuria depends on the plasma glucose level and the renal threshold. The level of sugar in the urine indicates the point at which the blood sugar level exceeds the reabsorptive capacity of the kidney and glucose is excreted. Glucosuria normally may result from eating a heavy meal or from emotional stress. Intravenous solutions containing glucose may also raise the serum glucose level above the renal threshold. Hyperalimentation solutions always breach this threshold, so people who receive this form of nutrition need supplemental insulin. Abnormal findings of glucose in the urine appear with uncontrolled diabetes, other pancreatic disorders, and impaired proximal tubular reabsorption.

Urine glucose testing is performed in the home or health care facility using one of a variety of available tests including copper reduction (e.g., Clinitest) or enzyme glucose oxidase (e.g., Testape, Clinistix, Keto-Diastix). The most important factor in successful urine testing for glucose is meticulous adherence to test directions.

In evaluating the test results, remember that many outside factors can cause false-negative or false-positive readings. Such factors include ascorbic acid, cephalosporins, chemotherapy metabolites, chloramphenicol, ethanol, levodopa, metaxalone, methyldopa, nalidixic acid, paraldehyde, phenazopyridine, probenecid, salicylates, sulfonamides, and tetracyclines. Pregnant women, especially those in their third trimester, and lactating women should use enzyme testing rather than copper reduction methods, because the latter reacts to the lactose in their urine and may yield possible false findings.[49, 58]

Ketones. Ketones are found in the urine when the body's fat stores are metabolized for energy, thus producing an excess of metabolic end products. This occurs with uncontrolled diabetes and other states of altered carbohydrate metabolism, fasting, pregnancy and lactation, excessive lipid metabolism, and severe infections accompanied by vomiting and diarrhea. False-positive findings may be caused by levodopa and phenolphthalein as well.[57]

Protein. The protein usually measured during a routine urinalysis is albumin. Although frequently a benign finding, proteinuria often denotes abnormal glomerular permeability, decreased tubular reabsorption, or an overflow of protein in the plasma. Factors influencing glomerular basement membrane permeability include exercise, vasoactive substances such as norepinephrine, and diseases that hinder normal renal microarchitecture. Examples of systemic diseases that may cause proteinuria are diabetes mellitus, systemic lupus erythematosus, lymphoma, solid tumors, hypertension, preeclampsia, hepatitis, sickle cell disease, secondary syphilis, febrile diseases, and stress, such as trauma or surgery. Medications that may cause a false-positive result include penicillamine, gold, captopril, probenecid, and fenoprofen.[56, 63]

One of the proteinurias not attributed to albumin is Bence Jones protein, which is found in multiple myeloma. Bence Jones protein is not included in a routine urinalysis but is detected either by heating the specimen or by electrophoresis (Chap. 47). Other protein components may be found in macroglobulinemia and various tubular defects.

There are three main categories of *benign proteinuria:* (1) functional (associated with high fever, exposure to cold, emotional stress, and strenuous exercise), (2) idiopathic transient, and (3) orthostatic (protein appears in the urine only when the person is standing). Proteinuria usually disappears as soon as the predisposing factor is removed.

Pathologic proteinuria usually indicates serious renal disease. In the absence of other abnormal findings, the follow-up of an isolated instance of proteinuria may consist of serial urinalyses to make sure the proteinuria does indeed disappear. However, if proteinuria persists, there may be further evaluation of the urinary system.

Bilirubin. Bilirubinuria usually indicates extrahepatic biliary tract obstruction. Other causes include hepatitis, portal inflammation, and hepatocellular damage. Use a fresh urine specimen for this test. When a urine specimen containing bilirubin is shaken, a yellow foam is produced. A false-positive finding may occur in a person taking chlorpromazine.

Red Blood Cells. Hematuria, or the presence of red blood cells, can be either microscopic (seen only under the microscope) or gross (obviously bloody). Hematuria is sometimes accompanied by other symptoms. Asymptomatic hematuria often presents a challenging diagnostic problem and requires meticulous evaluation. The cause may be benign or may indicate a pathologic condition. Although, the cause of the hematuria may never be found, rigorous investigation is required. Hematuria is always considered to be a sign of urinary tract carcinoma until proved otherwise.

A study involving 200 clients with asymptomatic hematuria found that 20 per cent had significant lesions, usually low-stage, low-grade vesical neoplasms; renal parenchymal disease, or ureteral calculus; 32 per cent had moderately significant findings such as renal calculi, bacterial cystitis, vesicoureteral reflux, and vesical diverticulum; and 55 per cent had insignificant lesions, with their hematuria resulting from prostatic hyperplasia, urethrotrigonitis, renal cyst, and cystocele.[18]

Hematuria also may appear in renal tuberculosis, sickle cell anemia (or sickle cell trait), IgA and IgG nephropathy, systemic lupus erythematosus, and polyarteritis nodosa.

Hemolytic anemia and hemolytic transfusion reactions produce detectable hemoglobin in the urine. Anticoagulants and the use of analgesics leading to papillary necrosis also can produce red blood cells in the urine. Hematuria following trauma, especially in the abdominal and pelvic area, may indicate injury to the urinary tract. Long-distance runners frequently exhibit hematuria (often with clots), which disappears as they recover from the run.

When collecting urine from a woman, note whether she is menstruating, because contaminating the specimen with menstrual blood will give a false-positive result. Povidone-iodine washed into the urine specimen will give a false-negative result for occult blood. Finally, it is helpful to determine when during voiding blood appears: (1) bleeding only at the onset of micturition usually indicates lesions below the bladder; (2) constant bleeding throughout voiding denotes bladder or upper urinary tract lesion; and (3) terminal bleeding, occurring only during the last few drops of voiding, locates the site as the bladder neck or prostate. As with proteinuria, asymptomatic hematuria probably will be monitored initially with repeat urinalyses to determine whether or not the finding is indeed transient. If bleeding persists, further evaluation is necessary.

White Blood Cells. White blood cells in the urine usually designate an *infectious process* somewhere in the urinary tract. When accompanied by casts, renal epithelial cells, a few red blood cells or bacteria, the leukocytosis is usually the result of a kidney infection. Bladder infections give rise to leukocytosis with red blood cells and bladder epithelial cells, but no casts. Noninfectious inflammatory diseases of the urinary tract may also produce white blood cells in the urine.

Pyuria means pus, or a large collection of white blood cells, in the urine. A quantitative determination of more than 5 clumps of white blood cells per high powered field indicates urinary pathogens. A large collection of pus may make the urine turbid and foul smelling. Although most pyuria is caused by urinary tract infection, it also may result from renal calculi, obstruction, irritation of the urothelium by a foreign body, tumors, or renal tuberculosis.

Bacteria. Because urine is normally sterile, bacteriuria represents infection within the urinary tract or contamination of the specimen. Bacteria in the urine, whether or not accompanied by physical signs and symptoms of urinary tract infection, needs further evaluation with urine cultures.

Casts. Casts are formed elements organized in the nephrons (especially the tubules) by agglutination of protein. They most likely are formed in the distal tubules and the collecting ducts. Casts usually indicate tubular or glomerular disease. There are several varieties of casts and the identification of the specific type helps pinpoint the contributing problem.

A few hyaline casts can be found normally, especially after strenuous exercise. However, some experts hypothesize that their presence in people at rest may indicate future renal or cardiovascular disease. They also are found in acute glomerulonephritis, acute pyelonephritis, malignant hypertension, chronic renal disease, congestive heart failure, and diabetic nephropathy. Contrary to expectations, they may not be present in advanced renal disease.

Red cell casts denote bleeding within the nephron as

the result of glomerulonephritis, acute renal allograft rejection, or acute tubular necrosis. Red cell casts may be the only manifestation of renal involvement in pathologic conditions such as systemic lupus erythematosus, subacute bacterial endocarditis, arteritis, and diabetic nephropathy.

White cell casts, or leukocyte casts, indicate bacterial infection and noninfective inflammatory disease. They often are hard to distinguish from epithelial casts, which denote, among other conditions, sloughing of renal tubular epithelium due to eclampsia, poisoning with heavy metals, amyloidosis, and acute renal allograft rejection. White cell casts and epithelial casts are frequently intermixed.

Granular casts indicate conditions such as renal parenchymal disease, acute renal rejection, pyelonephritis, chronic lead poisoning, and viral disease. Granular casts also may be found in the urine after strenuous exercise. The final stages of tubular inflammation and degeneration produce waxy casts. Chronic renal failure and chronic and acute renal allograft rejection cause the formation of waxy casts. Fatty casts represent the degeneration of cellular casts incorporated with fat droplets or cholesterol esters. They indicate a nephrotic syndrome or diabetic nephropathy.

Crystals. Crystalluria may or may not indicate disease. Common findings are calcium oxalate, uric acid, and urate crystals in acid urine, and phosphate, carbonate, and amorphous crystals in alkaline urine. The presence of crystals in the urine is an important predisposing factor in *calculus formation.*

In addition to the routine urinalysis, several other tests may be performed to examine the urine. Twelve- and 24-hour urine specimens determine the secretion rate of a number of elements. Tests measuring urinary levels of sodium, potassium, calcium, chloride, phosphorus, and uric acid, and quantitative determination of proteins help diagnose and treat renal problems.

Serial Urine Tests. Serial urines are collected on clients with hematuria to determine whether it is increasing or decreasing. The procedure is simple. When the client voids, save a sample of the urine in a cup labeled #1. Do the same for the next two voidings, labeling the cups #2 and #3 respectively. When the client voids a fourth time, discard sample #1 and the new sample becomes #3. In this way, the nurse or physician can examine the samples and note any change in the hematuria over time and voidings. The voidings are usually collected on a daily basis.

An alternative way to obtain serial urines is by collecting three specimens from the same voiding. The initial voiding goes in cup #1, the midstream urine in cup #2, and the remainder of urine in cup #3. Urine collection in this manner permits an assessment of the source of bleeding (i.e., kidney, bladder, or urethra).

Bacteriologic Studies. Because the kidneys, ureters, and bladder normally are sterile, the urine formed and transported in them also is sterile. Organisms typically colonize the distal portion of the urethra, but these bacteria ordinarily do not reach further up the urinary tract. Therefore, the presence of organisms in the urine is an abnormal finding. Any signs and symptoms reported by the person and/or the presence of significant bacteriuria or urinary leukocytosis indicate the need to examine the urine further.

Significant bacteriuria initially may be determined by using dipsticks that measure leukocyte esterase, an enzyme released from the leukocytes when the client has pyuria. In a study of 203 persons, this dipstick method proved to be 100 per cent sensitive with no false-negative findings and 76 per cent specific with 24 per cent false-positive findings in its predictive capability.[13] Therefore, a negative dipstick finding requires no further evaluation, but any positive findings need to be confirmed by culture of the specimen.

Pathogens in the urine are most specifically determined by culture. The urine specimens used for this testing are collected by catheterizing the bladder or by obtaining a clean-catch specimen, as described previously. The main goal in obtaining urine for culture is to provide the laboratory with a specimen uncontaminated by organisms outside the urinary tract.

Many authorities suggest that this specimen should be obtained early in the morning to allow adequate accumulation of organisms within the urine being cultured. Once you receive the specimen, immediately transport it to the laboratory. If the urine will not be examined within 30 minutes, refrigerate it because the bacteria will multiply more rapidly at room temperature.

Frequently, the first screening test performed is a Gram stain in the uncentrifuged urine. This is done so if any organisms are found, this stain will differentiate between the broad classifications of gram-positive and gram-negative organisms. This differentiation can help the physician decide which broad-spectrum antibiotic to start the client on until the final cultures are available. The treated urine is then examined under a microscope, and an initial report of the type and gross amount of organisms may be given. Whether or not a Gram stain is performed, identifying the specific pathogens must be done by culturing the urine.

The urine is swabbed onto media plates or onto agar-coated paddles that are placed into an appropriate growth environment for 24 to 72 hours. Any colonies present are studied further to name and quantify the specific organisms present. Merely finding organisms does not signify clinical infection. Each colony seen represents 1000 organisms per ml, and levels below 10,000 organisms per ml usually represent contamination of the specimen. Concentrations of 100,000 organisms per ml generally constitute significant infection. If the client is symptomatic, however, a culture of a single organism at a level of 10,000 organisms per ml may be significant and require treatment.

Once the causative organisms are identified, sensitivity tests are performed to designate the proper antibiotics to combat their growth. Once the urine has been obtained for the culture and sensitivity, the client may be started on a broad-spectrum antibiotic until the final sensitivity report is available. The determination of sensitivity tests is becoming even more important as the number of resistant organisms increases. Treatment with an ineffective antibiotic is costly in terms of lost time and money and of continued discomfort and possible injury to the client. Be aware of culture and sensitivity reports. If these reports are overlooked, treatment with nonspecific broad-spectrum antibiotics may continue longer than necessary.

Clearance Studies. Although direct examination of the urine gives a gross estimate of renal function, more definitive measures such as clearance studies sometimes are necessary. Clearance is defined as the amount of plasma totally cleared of a given substance in 1 minute.

The kidneys clear the blood of certain substances by means of filtration and excretion. Clearance studies determine the glomerular filtration rate and tubular excretory ability by measuring clearance rates of creatinine, urea, inulin, para-aminohippuric acid, phenolsulfonphthalein, and radioactive isotopes (Fig. 48-4). Quantitative renal excretory function is the difference between the filtration rate of any given substance across the glomerular wall and the rate at which the substance is then excreted in the urine.

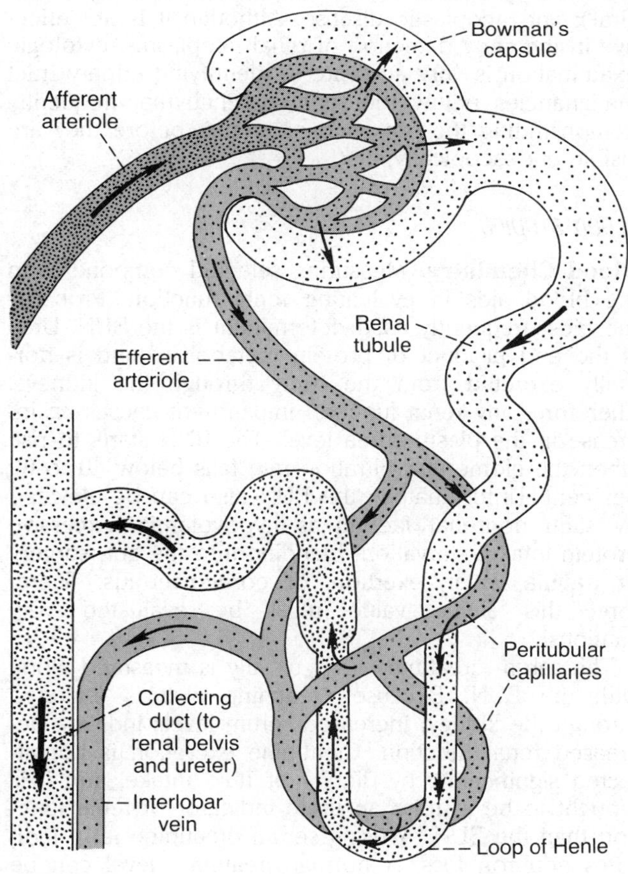

▲ *Figure 48-4*

Renal clearance measures the kidney's ability to remove a substance from the plasma in 1 minute. It is measured by assessing the quantity of the substance in urine collected over a specific amount of time.

For a substance to measure the glomerular filtration rate, it must be one that is filtered freely in the glomerulus but is unable to pass through the tubular epithelium in any direction. Creatinine and urea clearance tests are generally used because both substances are endogenous, which eliminates the need to establish and maintain a plasma level.

Creatinine clearance is currently the most accurate measure of glomerular filtration rate. Virtually all formed creatinine, a product of muscle metabolism, is filtered by the glomerulus, and as the glomerular filtration rate falls, the serum creatinine rises. Urine for this test is collected over a 12- or 24-hour period, although a 24-hour specimen is preferred. The test may begin at any time, although it is best to begin and end the test in the early morning. A fasting blood sample is drawn sometime during the collection period. An adult female normally excretes 0.8 to 1.7 g/24 h and a male excretes 1.0 to 1.9 g/24 h. Take care when applying these values to people older than 40 years of age. Longitudinal studies demonstrate declining creatinine clearance rates after age 34, with the rate of decline speeding up after age 65. This decline probably is due to reduced muscle mass and renal blood flow.[45]

Urea clearance is used sometimes. Because the rate of tubular secretion varies with the rate of urine flow, it is not as useful as creatinine clearance. To perform this procedure, ensure a urine flow of at least 2 ml/min. Have the client fast for several hours before the test. The client empties the bladder and then drinks two or more glasses of water. Exactly 1 hour later, the client voids and a blood sample for a blood urea nitrogen (BUN) is taken. At this point, the client drinks another two or more glasses of water, and in exactly 1 hour, voids again. At each voiding, the entire specimen is kept, carefully labeled with the time, and sent to the laboratory. If necessary, the bladder is catheterized to obtain an accurate specimen. The normal clearance is 65 to 99 ml/min or 40 to 69 ml/min if the urine flow rate is below 2 ml/min.

Phenolsulfonphthalein (PSP) is secreted by the proximal tubule at a rate proportional to the renal blood flow. After the person empties the bladder, 6 mg of PSP is injected intravenously and urine specimens are collected at specified intervals. Various laboratories have different time intervals, but all require the client to void 15 minutes after the injection of PSP—this is the most crucial specimen. To make sure the client is able to void when necessary, encourage fluids before and during the test. Also, inform clients that the dye may turn the urine red and reassure them that they are not bleeding. The dye begins to appear in the bladder 3 to 6 minutes after its administration; 20 to 30 per cent of it is excreted in 15 minutes, and 65 to 75 per cent is excreted within an hour. Chlorothiazide, penicillin G, and hypoproteinemia may cause false-positive findings.

Radioisotopes frequently are used to determine clearance rates. This procedure, called a renogram, involves the intravenous injection of a minute amount of a radioactive compound. The client is positioned supine, prone, or sitting with a scintillation camera placed posterior to the kidneys. A third radiation counter may be placed over the chest to monitor the disappearance of the isotope from the blood. The radioactive emission rate is recorded on videotape over a period of 15 to 30 minutes. A recording also may be made over the bladder just prior to and just after voiding at the end of the test. The test does not require special preparation of the individual. Also, because the dose of radioactivity is so low, there are no special precautions to observe in caring for the client or the urine specimen.

This test measures renal blood flow and active tubular transport, glomerular filtration, tubular secretion, and excretion. Each kidney can be compared with the other in terms of these measurements. There is no particular follow-up care. The client can void into a commode or toilet. Although a small amount of radiation may be present, it is not dangerous.

Other techniques using radioisotopes to measure renal function use blood determination to calculate clearance rates; for example, a radioisotope is injected and plasma samples are drawn to determine the amount of remaining isotope.

Concentration and Dilution. The loss of the kidney's ability to concentrate and dilute urine indicates significant renal tubular damage. Normally, as the body becomes fluid depleted, larger volumes of water are reabsorbed, resulting in more concentrated urine with a specific gravity over 1.020. Conversely, with increased fluid intake, more water is excreted, causing more dilute urine with a specific gravity often as low as 1.005. One of the first kidney functions to be lost is this ability to concentrate and dilute urine. In severe renal damage, the specific gravity may become fixed at a level of 1.008 to 1.012, regardless of the amount of fluid intake.

Several tests can be performed to evaluate this aspect of renal function. The Fishberg and Addis tests frequently are used to measure concentration ability. The Fishberg concentration test (a 12-hour test) involves withholding all food or fluid after the evening meal. Early morning specimens are collected, and their specific gravity is determined. A reading of less than 1.024 suggests renal function impairment. The Addis concentration test calls for severe fluid restriction for 24 hours. The amount of fluid allowed the client differs with each laboratory. A 12-hour specimen is collected during the last half of the fluid-restricted period. A possibility of vascular collapse exists during the period of water deprivation, so observe the client closely. Because of the risk to already compromised kidneys, clients with renal failure are not submitted to these tests. Factors that can interfere with the kidney's normal concentrating ability include decreased sodium intake, low-protein diet, and glucosuria.

For dilution tests, the client first empties the bladder and then receives a measured amount of fluid either (1) by drinking 1200 ml of water or fruit juice within 30 minutes or (2) through a rapid intravenous infusion. Physical activity is kept to a minimum during the test to prevent fluid losses through other routes. Urine specimens are collected at specified intervals — usually every 30 minutes — for 3 hours. The volume is measured and the specific gravity determined for each specimen. With normal renal function, the entire 1200 ml should be voided, and the specific gravity will be about 1.002. This test is risky for people with compromised cardiac systems because of the large volume of fluid taken.

Cytologic Examination. Examining cells exfoliated from the urinary tract can be useful in diagnosing cellular problems. The specimen needs good cellular content, so an early morning specimen is preferred. If the specimen is obtained through catheterization, be sure to note this information on the specimen container, because epithelial cells from the urethra or bladder may have been added to the urine by the catheter. If the specimen will not be examined immediately, it may be refrigerated for up to 48 hours or mixed with an appropriate fixative agent. Usually, three random specimens are collected for cytologic evaluation and compared before concluding the presence or absence of disease in the urinary tract. The three specimens may be obtained from three different times within one day, three days in a row at the same time, or three times in the course of a month.

Cytologic examination may help in identifying and monitoring the progress of inflammatory processes resulting from chemical toxins, autoimmune disease, or bodily substances (e.g., hemoglobin and myoglobin); infectious processes (including bacterial, fungal, and viral); and neoplastic disease. Although it is not effective in the early detection of renal neoplasms, cytologic examination is very accurate in identifying urinary tract malignancies below the renal parenchyma, frequently demonstrating the presence of tumors before they are visible endoscopically.[15, 50]

BLOOD STUDIES

Blood Chemistry. Measuring selected components in the blood aids in evaluating renal function. Probably the most frequently used determinant is the BUN. Urea is the end product of protein metabolism and is normally excreted from the body through the kidneys. Therefore, any renal function impairment causes an increase in the plasma urea level. The BUN starts to rise when the glomerular filtration rate falls below 40 to 60 per cent. Unfortunately, the BUN also can be elevated by such nonrenal factors as hypovolemia, excessive protein intake, starvation, bleeding into the gut, surgery or trauma, fever, exertion, or corticosteroids. Therefore, this single value must be evaluated very cautiously.

The serum creatinine level usually is measured along with the BUN. Because creatinine also is excreted through the kidney, increased serum levels indicate decreased renal function. Creatinine excretion is not affected significantly by dietary or fluid intake, and it is thought to be a more accurate indicator of renal function than the BUN. A rising serum creatinine level indicates nephron loss. A normal creatinine level can be found with up to a 25 per cent nephron loss. Twice the normal creatinine level signifies a 50 per cent nephron loss and the beginning of diminished renal reserve. A creatinine level eight times the normal value indicates a

75 per cent nephron loss with definite renal insufficiency. A creatinine level ten or more times normal signals at least a 90 per cent nephron loss and indicates end-stage renal disease.[54]

Sometimes a BUN creatinine ratio is used as a renal function indicator, with the normal ratio being 20/1. BUN elevations in relation to serum creatinine denote renal impairment due to prerenal causes such as blood loss, severe diarrhea, heart failure, and liver disease.

There are specific tests associated with other portions of the urinary tract. Prostatic enzymes and testicular markers are discussed in Chaps. 74 and 75.

Hematology. Inspecting a random blood sample provides some data about renal function as well as the progress of disease processes within the urinary tract. Decreased red blood cells, hemoglobin, and hematocrit may indicate bleeding from the urinary tract or may signal reduced erythropoietic function by the kidney. An increased white blood cell count with increased neutrophils may denote an infectious process, whereas a return to normal values represents recovery from infection.

Radiologic Studies

In most diagnostic protocols, examining the urinary tract by x-ray study is the next step in identifying actual or potential malfunction. These studies may be performed with or without the use of contrast material and may involve static or dynamic films, or both. Because these examinations are performed in the x-ray department, the nurse's primary responsibility is to adequately prepare the client physically and mentally for the procedure. This helps ensure accurate results.

KIDNEYS, URETERS, AND BLADDER

An x-ray study of the kidneys, ureters, and bladder (KUB) is a simple film of the lower abdomen. It involves no contrast medium, poses no risk to the client, and can be performed without considering the remaining kidney function. The outline of these organs demonstrates their size, shape, and location. This helps identify soft tissue masses, malformations, and radiopaque calculi.

INTRAVENOUS PYELOGRAM

An intravenous pyelogram (IVP) involves the intravenous injection of a radiopaque contrast medium that is filtered by the kidney and excreted through the urinary tract. This examination helps identify the absence or presence, location, size, and configuration of the kidneys, ureters, and bladder. The IVP also helps determine filling of the renal calices and pelvis. A postvoiding film is obtained to assess the efficiency of bladder emptying. If bladder emptying is incomplete, a voiding cystourethrogram (VCUG) would help determine the cause of retention.

Physical preparation of the client for an IVP generally involves restricting fluids and cleaning out the bowel. Food and fluids are withheld after midnight before the examination. This relative fluid depletion allows the radiopaque contrast medium to be more concentrated when it enters the kidney, thus providing clearer films. If the person is receiving intravenous fluids, the infusion rate may be slowed for several hours before the study. Fluid depletion is contraindicated in clients with multiple myeloma, severe diabetes mellitus, or uric acid nephropathy. These conditions can seriously compromise the renal function of these clients, with reduced renal perfusion due to decreased renal blood flow, predisposing the client to the development of acute renal failure. If these clients must have an IVP, they should be well hydrated.

Because the kidneys are located retroperitoneally, the bowel must be cleared of gas and fecal material that may partially or totally obscure the kidneys. Cathartics are usually administered the evening before the examination. This part of the preparation, however, may be omitted in clients with suspected or known inflammatory bowel disease, or when vigorous colonic activity is otherwise contraindicated. If cathartics were not effective or not given for any reason, administer enemas or a rectal suppository early in the morning before the x-ray study.

The combination of fasting and cathartics may cause weakness, especially in clients already debilitated by age and illness. Take care to ensure the comfort and safety of the client. Omit bedtime sedation and keep the call light handy. Instruct the client to call for assistance with ambulation, and keep the side rails up, if necessary. Alert care providers to heed and answer the client's call light promptly.

During the examination, the client is placed supine on the x-ray table. Initially, a KUB film is taken as a scout film. This helps to ensure the bowel is clear enough to continue with the procedure. It also screens for calculi in the renal collecting system. Because the contrast medium in the collecting ducts is the same density as any calcification in this area, some types of stones can be missed easily during the IVP. The radiopaque contrast medium is injected intravenously as a bolus or through an infusion drip. The contrast medium normally produces a flushed face, a warm feeling in the body, nausea, and a salty taste in the mouth. These are transitory effects and do not mean the study should be stopped.

The iodine in the substance, however, may cause severe allergic reactions in hypersensitive clients. Before the examination begins, carefully question the client about any allergic history. A known sensitivity to iodinated contrast media is an absolute contraindication to continuing the procedure unless the client has been premedicated with a steroid infusion. If the client is unsure about an iodine allergy, ask the client about an allergy to shellfish. The presence of allergy to shellfish requires skin testing before intravenous injection.

A negative skin test or history, however, does not guarantee there will be no reaction. If any signs of allergic responses such as itching, hives, wheezing, or other signs of respiratory distress appear, call for immediate discontinuation of the injection. Antihistamine, epinephrine, vasopressors, oxygen, and cardiopulmonary resuscitation equipment must be available to halt the anaphylactic response.

In addition to possible anaphylactic reactions from the contrast medium, cases of acute renal failure following injection of the contrast medium have been documented. Although the incidence is low, assess carefully for this adverse effect. Predisposing factors include vascular disease, multiple myeloma, diabetes mellitus, and preexisting renal insufficiency. These factors, in addition to the fluid depletion, markedly increase the risk of renal failure. Following the test, the nurse should force fluids while carefully monitoring renal function and output.

After the contrast medium is injected, films are taken at regular intervals, usually at 2 minutes, 5 minutes, 15 minutes, 20 minutes, 30 minutes, and 60 minutes. The client is usually kept supine throughout this time, although upright, oblique, and lateral films may be obtained as well. Ureteric compression is frequently performed to enhance distention of the collecting system and upper ureters. A compression band with inflatable balloons or sandbags is applied across the client's lower abdomen after the 5-minute film and is left in place until the 10-minute films are obtained. Sometimes, with delayed renal functioning, additional x-ray studies may be needed 1 to 2 hours later.

In advanced renal failure or with a unilateral, nonvisualized kidney, a large bolus of undiluted contrast medium may be used to better visualize the urinary system. This technique is called high-bolus urography. In preparing the client for this examination, it is usually unnecessary to restrict fluids. Risk increases somewhat with this technique. Potentially serious electrocardiographic abnormalities have occurred in older people with evidence of previous heart disease. Identified risk factors include previously abnormal electrocardiogram, coronary artery disease, and congestive heart failure.

When the client has completed the examination, continue to observe for reactions to the contrast medium. Counteract the fasting and fluid depletion with food and increased fluids.

RETROGRADE PYELOGRAM

A retrograde pyelogram involves passing a small-caliber catheter through a cystoscope into the ureters and into the renal pelvis. (Cystoscopy is described later in this chapter.) A small amount of contrast medium is injected into the kidney through the catheters, and x-ray films are taken to delineate the collecting system. The client may feel some discomfort in the kidney region when the contrast medium is injected, but there is no actual pain unless the renal pelvis has been overdistended. As the catheters are withdrawn, more contrast medium is injected, and films are taken to record the outline of the ureters. Preparing and caring for the client during and after this procedure is the same as that for the client undergoing an IVP and a cystoscopy.

Performing a retrograde pyelogram is indicated when the renal collection system or ureters have not been satisfactorily visualized during the IVP. It is also helpful in assessing the degree of ureteral obstruction. It can be used in clients who are hypersensitive to intravenous contrast media because the contrast medium is not absorbed through the mucous membranes.

There are no particular contraindications to this procedure, although it does carry some risk. Entering the urinary tract occasionally causes primary urinary tract infection or aggravates pre-existing infections. Manipulating the ureters also may cause edema, resulting in temporary obstruction to urine flow.

COMPUTED TOMOGRAPHY

This procedure, also called a CT or CAT scan, involves an x-ray beam sweeping around the body and taking multiple, thin, cross-sectional pictures of the internal structure. This procedure allows measurement of various tissue densities. The computer then uses these density readings to reconstruct visual images of the body structures. Intravenous administration of contrast medium, using either bolus technique or intravenous infusion, may be used to enhance the image. This contrast medium is the same used in the intravenous pyelogram, so the potential for anaphylactic reaction or for acute renal failure exists. Other than preparing for potential complications, there is no special preparation or post-procedure care for the client.

There are several indications for CT scanning. These include examining the renal and urinary tract when excretory urogram and ultrasound have been unsatisfactory; characterizing renal retroperitoneal and pelvic masses; staging and monitoring renal tumors; evaluating a nonfunctioning kidney, urinary tract trauma, a transplanted kidney, suspected renal calculi, or gas-forming infections; and CT-guided procedures.

CYSTOURETHROGRAPHY

X-ray examination of the bladder and urethra can be performed separately or together. During cystography, contrast medium is injected into the bladder through a catheter. When the bladder is full, films are taken to profile the size and shape of the bladder and to detect the presence of any vesicoureteral reflux. The client is frequently asked to void, and a follow-up x-ray is performed to measure the amount of residual urine.

URETHROGRAPHY

Urethrography outlines the inner size and shape of the urethra and checks for extravasation and strictures. In males, x-ray studies are performed after a thick, jelly-like radiopaque substance is injected via a wide-mouth syringe into the urethral meatus. This material usually reaches only as far as the urogenital diaphragm. In females, the procedure requires a less viscous contrast media and a special catheter.

VOIDING CYSTOURETHROGRAPHY

Voiding cystourethrography provides visualization of urethral lesions, vesicoureteral reflux, and bladder and urethral obstructions. The radiopaque material is instilled into the bladder through a urethral catheter. Then the catheter is removed and the client is asked to void. Films are taken during the voiding process to observe the contrast medium flow. The micturition process may be recorded on film to better visualize the movement of the contrast medium. Voiding in the presence of other people can be very embarrassing for the client and may even interfere with the ability to void. Giving emotional support and judiciously placing screens may help put the client at ease.

RENAL ANGIOGRAPHY

Renal angiography makes it possible to visualize renal vasculature. It is used to (1) diagnose renal artery stenosis or renal vein thrombosis, (2) study renovascular hypertension, (3) demonstrate vascular damage after trauma, (4) investigate causes of acute renal failure, and (5) differentiate highly vascular tumors from avascular cysts.

Renal angiography involves injecting a radiopaque contrast medium into the renal vascular tree and taking serial x-ray films to outline blood vessels. Access to the circulation is usually through the femoral artery. A guide wire is threaded into the artery through an arterial needle. The needle is then removed, leaving the guide wire in place, and a radiopaque flexible catheter is passed over the guide wire. Using fluoroscopy, the catheter and wire are advanced through the femoral and iliac arteries into the aorta. When the catheter is in position at the renal arteries, the guide wire may be removed and contrast medium injected; or the wire and catheter may be guided into the renal artery itself before the contrast medium is injected. The latter procedure is called selective renal arteriography. Once the contrast medium has been injected, films are taken at the rate of two to three per second for several seconds to show filling and emptying of the renal artery tree. Delayed films are usually performed to visualize the function of the renal veins.

There are alternative sites for vascular access. A translumbar aortogram involves direct puncture of the aorta at the renal arteries with a long needle. Puncturing the axillary artery or antecubital vein also may be done.

In addition to anaphylactic reactions and possible renal damage due to the radiopaque contrast medium, several other serious potential complications may result from this procedure. Hemorrhaging along the route of the vessel puncture may be external or, especially with a translumbar aortogram, internal. Vascular injury may occur at the puncture site or anywhere along the path of the guide wire and catheter. Thrombosis or embolism can occur as a result of plaque dislodging from the vessel walls during the procedure.

Pre-examination preparation is the same as for the IVP, including testing the client for hypersensitivity to the contrast medium. This procedure is usually performed under local anesthesia, although pre-procedure sedation frequently is given.

One of the chief potential side effects of this examination is post-vessel puncture hemorrhage. Pressure dressings are applied over the puncture site immediately after the catheter is removed. Observe the area frequently for several hours for signs of fresh bleeding. The client usually is placed on bed rest for several hours to allow complete sealing of the puncture site. If a femoral puncture has been performed, check pedal pulses frequently to detect any reduced circulation to the feet that may result from vascular injury. Monitor vital signs closely to check for the presence of internal hemorrhage, particularly after a translumbar aortogram.

RENAL PHLEBOGRAPHY

One way to study the venous system of the kidneys is renal phlebography. Because of the small caliber of the renal artery and the copious blood flow in the renal veins, renal arteriography is often inadequate to satisfactorily visualize these vessels. During renal phlebography, the femoral vein is punctured and a catheter is threaded through the inferior vena cava and into the renal veins. The rest of the procedure, as well as caring for the person, is the same as for renal arteriography.

Radioisotope Studies

In addition to renal function tests performed with radioisotopes as described earlier, radioactive compounds can be used to evaluate renal structures, ureters, and the bladder. For renal studies, as with clearance studies, a radioisotope is injected intravenously and a scintillation camera or probe and/or computer is used to record the size and shape of the kidneys. The isotope compounds used are retained in the kidneys for several hours or days. Lesions in the kidney, such as tumors or infarcts, do not absorb the radioactivity and thus appear as "cold" or "blank" spots on the scanner. In this case, the diagnostician needs to investigate further to determine the actual cause of the cold spot. Indications for this procedure include renal hypertension, renal masses, trauma, obstruction, and evaluating transplanted kidneys.

To evaluate the effectiveness of the vesicoureteral valves and the bladder, the radioactive agent is instilled into the bladder through a catheter. Recording the radioactivity is conducted as described earlier. This procedure is performed primarily to evaluate vesicoureteral reflux, but it may also be used to detect large bladder defects.

Ultrasonography

Ultrasound, or sonography, projects high-frequency waves into the abdomen. These waves are reflected back from the surfaces of retroperitoneal structures and converted into electrical energy that are shown on an oscilloscope. Instant-developing pictures are taken of the oscilloscope image to record the outline of the structures. The person lies on a table, and a lubricant, such as mineral oil, is applied to the skin over the area to be examined. This oil promotes good contact between the skin and the transducer used to administer and receive the ultrasonic waves.

Ultrasonography of the kidneys has many uses. Its prime value may well be in differentiating between fluid-filled cysts and solid masses. Other applications include localizing and mapping out the kidney before biopsy by percutaneous aspiration, evaluating transplanted kidneys, determining hydronephrosis in nonfunctioning kidneys, demonstrating papillary necrosis, identifying calculi, describing diverticula, estimating residual urine, and demonstrating changes resulting from urinary tract infections.

An ultrasound study of the bladder is frequently done to determine post-void residuals. Ultrasonography is entirely safe. It is noninvasive, involves no contrast media, and has produced no ill effects in anyone, including the offsprings of women pregnant at the time of the examination. The technique is also considered highly accurate, although several factors can cause scanning artifacts. For instance, sound waves penetrate bone and gas very poorly, so the ribs, bowel, and lung limit the amount of kidney that can be scanned effectively.

Urodynamic Studies

Urodynamic studies are a series of procedures that evaluate the motor and sensory functioning of the bladder and the efficiency of micturition. These tests are used primarily to diagnose voiding problems or loss of bladder control, such as with incontinence, and to evaluate the effectiveness of reconstructive bladder surgery. A series of measurements provide diagnostic information about bladder capacity, pressure profiles before and during micturition, and the dynamics of the urinary stream.

UROFLOWMETRY

Uroflowmetry is a simple, noninvasive procedure in which the client voids into a special commode chair equipped with a load cell mechanism that measures weight over time and records the findings on graph paper. This information can be used to calculate the urine flow rate. The client should have a full bladder for the test or, if this is not possible, a catheter can be inserted and the bladder filled. The client is then asked to void and the measurements retaken. Figure 48-5 depicts the normal urinary flow rate and the parameters used to describe and assess the flow of urine during voiding.

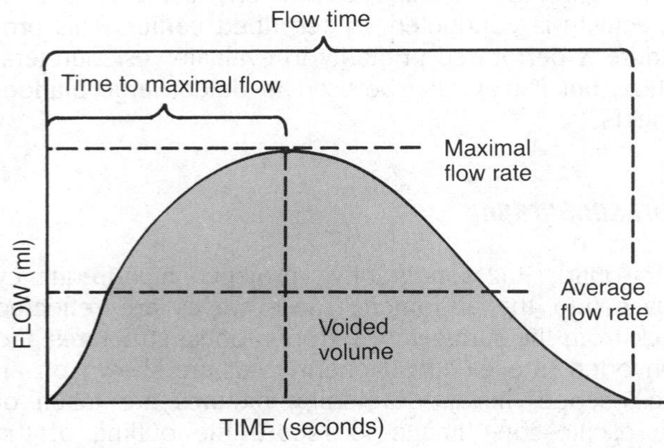

▲ *Figure 48-5*

Diagram of terminology used in urodynamic studies. Shaded area shows voided volume. Dotted lines show how voided volume is divided into time and flow rate.

A residual urine test may be performed after voiding. A residual urine test is obtained by having the client attempt to empty the bladder completely. The client can then be catheterized, with the amount of urine obtained recorded as the residual volume. More recently, bladder ultrasonography is being performed to determine residual urine after measurement of the urinary flow rate so that this urodynamic procedure may remain totally noninvasive.

CYSTOMETROGRAPHY

A cystometrogram measures bladder pressure during filling and voiding. No pre-procedure preparation is needed other than client teaching.

In some institutions, at the beginning of the examination, the client voids while the examiner notes (1) the time and effort needed to initiate voiding; (2) size, force, and continuity of the stream; and (3) whether dribbling occurs after voiding ceases. A catheter is then passed into the bladder, usually through the urethra. Any residual urine is removed and measured. The distal end of the catheter is attached to an apparatus that will deliver saline or carbon dioxide to the bladder while measurements of the intravesical pressures are recorded. Figure 48-6 illustrates one type of setup of this equipment (there is also special equipment used to perform the test). The distending agent is infused into the bladder at a constant rate. The intravesical pressure is continuously recorded, and the client is asked when the urge to void is first felt, then when the bladder feels full, and when they feel they must absolutely void. The pressures at which these sensations are noted are recorded on the intravesical pressure tracing.

The client may be asked to cough or perform other maneuvers at specified points during the examination to evaluate the resulting pressure changes. Bladder filling also may be repeated in several different positions in order to reproduce the client's symptoms, including sitting or standing. When filling has been completed, the catheter is removed and the client allowed to empty the bladder while the examiner makes the same observations as during the initial voiding. The amount of residual urine is again determined. To measure bladder pressure during voiding, a tiny urethral catheter may be inserted and left in place during voiding. Intra-abdominal pressure can be measured using a small rectal catheter.

After the procedure, the client is monitored for the development of a urinary tract infection. The nurse also should monitor the client's voiding to make sure that the client does not develop urinary retention.

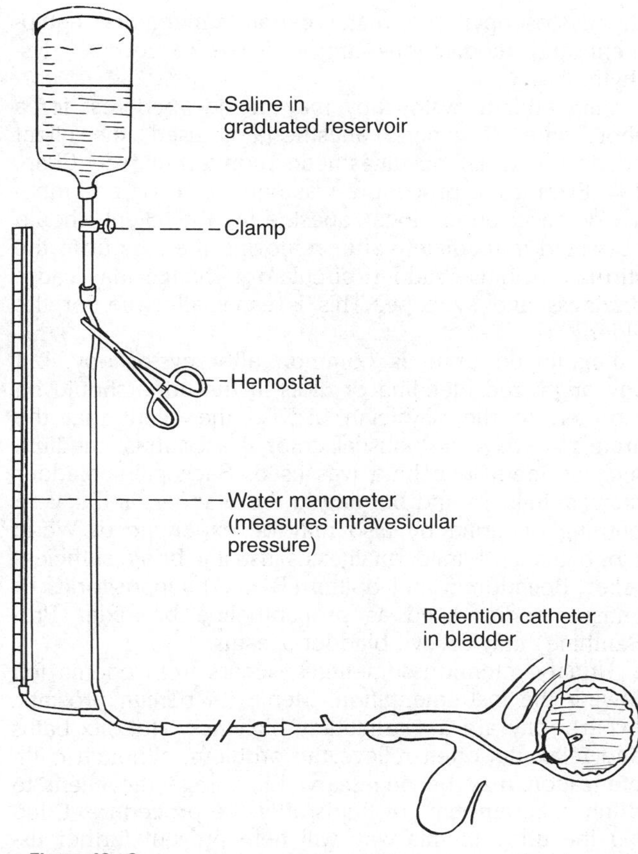

▲ *Figure 48-6*

Equipment for manual cystometrography. A pressure transducer may be used in place of the water manometer.

Electromyography

An *electromyogram (EMG)* measures striated perineal muscle activity, including the sphincters, during bladder filling and micturition. Several methods can measure this activity, including anal plug, urethral and anal catheter electrodes, paste-on electrodes, or needle electrodes. Because the purpose of the study is to compare perineal muscle activity with detrusor contractions, EMG is not performed alone but usually in conjunction with cystometrography or other pressure profile studies.

Urethral Pressure Profile Studies

Urethral pressure profile studies primarily determine the resistance to urine flow in the urethra and, particularly, evaluate stress incontinence. The three main methods used for determining urethral pressures are (1) resistance to fluid or gas infusion; (2) small, inflated intraluminal balloons, which provide pressure on the urethral walls; and (3) catheter tip transducers, which directly measure pressure resistance. In the infusion method, a small catheter with multiple holes is inserted into the urethra with the distal end connected to a pressure transducer. As the catheter is very slowly withdrawn, fluid or gas is instilled into the urethra. Urethral pressures are determined at several levels of bladder fullness, including maximum capacity. The main factors measured are the intraluminal closing forces and effective urethral length.

Direct Visualization

RIGID CYSTOSCOPY

The oldest method of direct visualization of the urinary tract is cystoscopy, which involves inserting a cystoscope into the bladder via the urethra. This procedure may be useful for diagnostic as well as therapeutic purposes. Its five major diagnostic uses include (1) directly inspecting the bladder, making it possible to see tumors, calculi, ulcers, or other defects; (2) collecting urine directly from the kidney pelvis and separately from each kidney; (3) x-ray visualization through retrograde pyelogram, as described earlier; (4) measuring bladder capacity and evidence of vesicoureteral reflux; and (5) biopsy of the ureters, bladder, and urethra. It also provides endoscopic access to the upper urinary tract. The cystoscope is used in intervention to (1) resect tumors, (2) remove stones and foreign bodies, (3) fulgurate bleeding areas, (4) dilate the ureters, (5) empty the renal pelvis, and (6) implant radium seeds.

Today's rigid cystoscope consists primarily of a sheath and an optical lens system. The sheath is a solid metal tube which, when the obturator (a core that prevents trauma) is in place, can be passed through the urethra into the bladder. Once the cystoscope is in position, the obturator is removed from inside the sheath and the lighted lens system is introduced. Figure 48-7 shows a cystoscope in place.

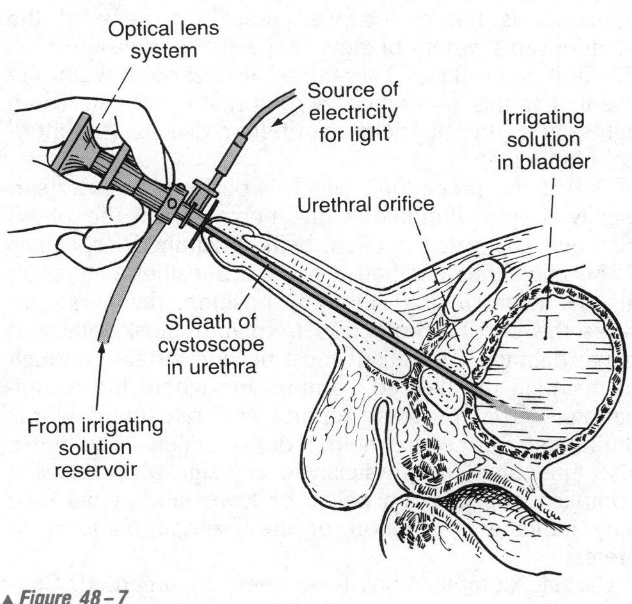

▲ *Figure 48-7*

Cystoscope in the male bladder.

Several attachments accomplish various functions. Forceps may be passed through the sheath to get tissue samples for biopsy or to remove foreign bodies. A guide can be used to help direct small catheters into and up the ureters to the renal pelvis so that specimens can be obtained from each kidney separately. Scissors, needles, and electrodes also may be introduced into the bladder or urethra as needed.

Cystoscopy may be performed in the hospital or in the physician's office. It also may be performed under local or general anesthesia. The client must remain very still during the examination to avoid urinary tract trauma. Therefore, the type of anesthesia used may depend on whether or not the client can maintain the necessary position.

Physiologic and psychosocial preparation is needed before a cystoscopy. Cathartics or enemas, or both, may be given before the procedure to clear the bowel, especially if a retrograde pyelogram is also being performed. Some clients, especially those receiving general anesthesia, may be required to fast for several hours beforehand. Clients having a local anesthesia may be instructed to maintain an adequate fluid intake to ensure an effective urine flow for specimen collection and for retrograde pyelography, if it is to be performed. Clients who cannot have anything by mouth may receive intravenous fluids. A sedative or narcotic, and sometimes an anticholinergic, typically is administered before the procedure.

As with any procedure, effective teaching helps to alleviate anxiety and ensure optimum cooperation. This is particularly important if the cystoscopy is performed under local anesthesia. Because the procedure is usually performed with the client in the lithotomy position, it can be very tiring and uncomfortable, but it is essential to remain still throughout the examination. You can help the client with deep breathing and general relaxation exercises to decrease discomfort as the cystoscope is introduced. The desire to void will be pronounced as the cystoscope passes the neck of the bladder and when bladder capacity is measured by filling it with fluid. The nurse also should warn the client that this procedure is performed with the room lights off so the physician can better visualize the internal bladder.

During the procedure, which is performed under surgically aseptic conditions, the nurse assists the physician and supports the client being examined, especially if the client has not had a general anesthesia. In placing the client in the lithotomy position, the nurse ensures the client's protection from musculoskeletal and nerve damage. The client must be comfortable enough to maintain the desired position throughout the examination. Verbal progress reports and reassuring words during the procedure help reduce anxiety. The nurse also must alert the physician to any sign of developing complications. Sudden pelvic or lower abdominal pain may indicate perforation of the urethra, bladder, or ureters.

Cardiac complications have been documented. Consequently, monitor high-risk clients continuously during the cystoscopy, and make certain emergency equipment and medications are available to reverse dysrhythmias.

Care after a cystoscopy may include bed rest for a short time. If general anesthesia is used, the client needs the usual postanesthetic monitoring (see Chap. 19). Even if the procedure was performed on an ambulatory basis under local anesthesia, the client should not stand immediately after removing the legs from the stirrups, because sudden circulatory change may cause dizziness and syncope. This is especially true for the elderly.

Pink-tinged urine is common after cystoscopy, but any bright red bleeding or clots in the urine should be reported to the physician. Advise the client that the urine may have an unusual color if a contrast medium such as methylene blue was used. Back pain, bladder spasms, fullness and burning in the bladder, and severe burning on urination also may be experienced. Warm tub baths and mild analgesics usually bring sufficient relief. Belladonna and opium (B & O) suppositories or antispasmodics such as propantheline bromide (Pro-Banthine) may relieve bladder spasms.

Urinary retention sometimes occurs from edema following the instrumentation. Men with benign prostatic hypertrophy are at particularly high risk. Hot sitz baths and relaxants often relieve the problem, although catheterization may be necessary. Encourage the client to drink large amounts of fluids after the procedure. Diluting the urine in this way will help prevent further tissue irritation and will decrease the burning sensation when the client voids. Some chilling and a rise in temperature often occur following cystoscopy. If these symptoms do not subside readily after providing extra warmth and offering frequent fluids, investigate the client's condition further. Cystoscopy may spread infection in the urinary tract and can cause bacteremia. Although the method is controversial, some authorities recommend using prophylactic antibiotics after urinary tract instrumentation because of the risk of infection.

Clients are often discharged almost immediately or within several hours after cystoscopy. Give the client written instructions as well as verbal instructions, because clients may not remember the instructions later, after they have gone home.

Flexible Fiberoptic Cystourethroscopy

The rigidness of the standard cystoscope often prevents the examiner from visualizing some parts of the bladder. The evolution of flexible endoscopic instruments has helped solve this problem. The client being examined may be positioned supine or prone. In a study of 80 men, flexible endoscopy was found to be equivalent or more accurate than rigid cystoscopy 94 per cent of the time. Preparation and positioning were simpler, discomfort was less, and the length of the examination was unchanged.[14]

Ureteroscopy and Nephroscopy

Ureteroscopes have been developed to examine the ureter and kidneys. Ureteroscopy evaluates tumors, obstruction, calculi, and the presence of foreign bodies. General or regional (spinal or epidural) anesthesia is used for these procedures because the dilation of the ureteral orifice causes considerable discomfort.

Performed under strict aseptic technique, nephroscopy allows the physician to observe the renal pelvis, calices, fundus, and collecting system. It can be performed to (1) locate and remove calculi; (2) diagnose the cause of hematuria; and (3) biopsy, fulgurate, and resect tumors. Nephroscopy is a safe procedure that is not associated with any significant complications except possible infection. Nursing care for the client before and after the procedure are similar to those needed by clients having a renal biopsy (discussed later).

Renal Biopsy

A renal tissue specimen for biopsy may be obtained using an open or closed technique. For open biopsy, the surgeon performs a nephrostomy. This incision through the flank allows direct visualization of the kidney, and the tissue obtained is adequate 100 per cent of the time. However, the procedure has a prolonged recuperation period, and therefore, it increases direct costs and time lost from work. Chapter 50 discusses caring for the client having a renal biopsy.

One method of *closed* biopsy is the retrograde renal and ureteral brush procedure. This technique collects tissue specimens from the renal pelvis and ureters, particularly from areas of radiolucent filling defects found during excretory urogram. The initial part of the procedure is conducted as a cystoscopy under general anesthesia. A whistle-tip ureteral catheter is introduced, and its proper positioning is guided by fluoroscopy or multiple x-ray films. A biopsy brush is then passed through the catheter, and the lesion is brushed several times. The brush is removed and any tissue adhering to its bristles is sent to the laboratory. If no tissue is found on the brush, 24- to 48-hour urine specimens may be collected to catch any cells that may have been dislodged by the bristles.

Postoperatively, the client may be given intravenous fluids at a rapid rate to reduce the possibility of clots forming at the biopsy site and to foster specimen collection. Some oozing of blood may be expected for 24 to 48 hours. Moreover, some people experience severe renal colic, which is usually relieved by narcotics and fluids.

The percutaneous renal biopsy is perhaps the most frequently used procedure. During this examination, a specially designed needle pierces the skin and enters the kidney to obtain a small sample of tissue. Fluoroscopy and ultrasound techniques allow more precise localization of the biopsy needle.

This important diagnostic tool is helpful either as a one-time examination or when performed serially to monitor the progress of a disease, especially in any disease process that is evenly distributed throughout the kidney. Contraindications to percutaneous biopsy include a single functioning kidney, infection, tumors (because of the danger of dissemination), hydronephrosis, severe hypertension, coagulation disorders, and an uncooperative client. Severe renal failure has previously been regarded as a contraindication. However, better procedures for localizing the kidney have reduced the dangers associated with this technique. Pregnancy usually is considered a contraindication because of the high doses of radiation that may be necessary during localization of the needle. Using ultrasound instead eliminates this risk.

Before the biopsy begins, a battery of x-ray and laboratory studies is done. These usually include excretory urogram, urine culture, hematocrit and blood urea nitrogen determinations, and bleeding and coagulation studies. If an aneurysm is suspected, renal arteriography is mandatory to avoid puncture of this vascular defect. Replacement blood may be ordered as standby.

The procedure usually is performed under local anesthesia with little or no premedication. The client is placed in a prone position with a firm pillow or sandbag under the abdomen to straighten the spine's natural lordosis. The kidney to be biopsied is located with ultrasound and/or fluoroscopy and contrast medium is injected intravenously. After careful skin preparation, the skin is infiltrated with the anesthetic. The client is instructed to take in as deep a breath as possible and hold it. The probe needle then is (1) inserted through the skin, midway between the last rib and the iliac crest (Fig. 48-8), and (2) positioned inside of the

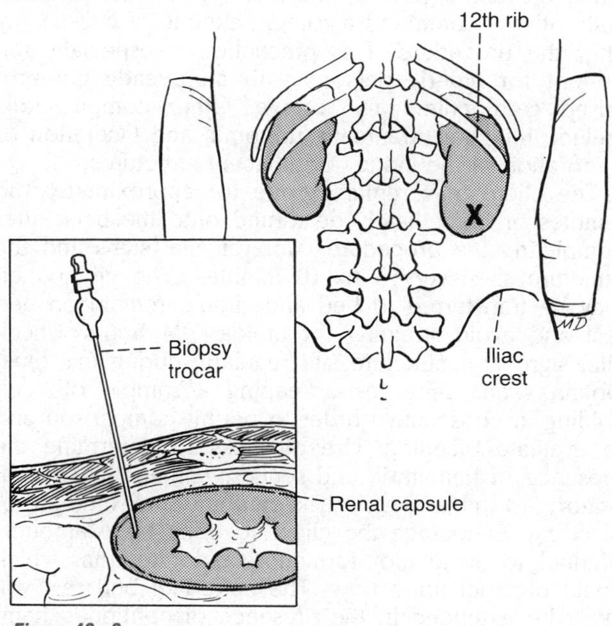

▲ *Figure 48-8*

Percutaneous renal biopsy showing trocar location.

renal (fibrous) capsule slightly lateral to the midline of the kidney. After the correct position of the distal end of the needle has been confirmed, the probe needle is removed and the biopsy trocar inserted. The client may now be allowed to breathe normally, but he or she must inspire deeply each time a tissue specimen is taken. When enough tissue is obtained, the trocar is removed and firm pressure immediately applied to the site. After several minutes, a pressure dressing is applied.

The incidence of complications ranges from 0.75 per cent for major complications to 10 per cent for minor ones, which include microscopic hematuria, pain, fever, or extravasation of the contrast medium.[27a] An increased heart rate and hypotension occasionally develop during the procedure. This problem probably is the result of sympathetic stimulation by the needle or pressure of the pillow or sandbag against the abdominal vessels or sympathetic nerves. The condition is transient, and vascular stability is usually restored as soon as the person moves into a supine position.

Hemorrhage is a major complication. It may be suggested by gross or microscopic hematuria, flank or abdominal pain, hypotension, and a decreasing hematocrit. However, low hematocrit and hypotension alone are not sufficient indicators of hemorrhage, because some people develop these conditions without significant bleeding. Hemorrhage may occur because of hemodilution or as a result of massive sympathetic stimulation caused by penetration of the needle.[8a]

Continued bleeding or the resulting hematoma may require surgical exploration, and these problems may necessitate removal of the involved kidney. Intrarenal arteriovenous fistulas may occur, causing an audible bruit over the kidneys, and may lead to hypertension. Because of the chances of pneumothorax, especially when the upper pole of the kidney is biopsied, some authorities recommend a routine expiratory chest x-ray after the procedure. This precaution is especially important for elderly persons with an already compromised cardiopulmonary reserve. Other complications include infection, traumatic urinoma, and laceration or perforation of the kidney or adjacent structures.

The client may remain prone for approximately 30 minutes or immediately be turned onto the back after completing the procedure. Monitor vital signs and the puncture site every 5 to 10 minutes. The client then may be transferred to bed and should remain on bed rest and avoid straining for at least 24 hours. Check vital signs and puncture site regularly during this time. Obtain serial urine tests, keeping a sample of each voiding in consecutive order to permit comparison and to evaluate bleeding. Use dipsticks to determine the presence of hematuria and send specimens to the laboratory to more precisely determine the amount of bleeding. Encourage the client to drink large amounts of fluid to avoid clot formation and retention, which could obstruct urine flow. The period of bed rest will likely be extended in the presence of continued hemorrhage. A hematocrit and hemoglobin study is usually performed within 8 to 10 hours to test for anemia. The client may also need emotional support while waiting for the diagnosis and its implications.

On discharge, advise the client to avoid strenuous activity for approximately 2 weeks. Also, instruct the client about the signs of hemorrhage and what to do if hemorrhage occurs. Bleeding may develop several days after the biopsy.

The mortality rate for percutaneous renal biopsy is 0.2 per cent.[12a] Thus, biopsy usually is not performed unless the knowledge to be gained is likely to affect intervention.

Summary

In order to care for a client with disorders of the urinary and renal system, the nurse must be aware of the assessments needed to determine proper functioning of the system. Clients may find some of the assessment embarrassing, so sensitive care is required to reassure them. The nurse must carefully explain the diagnostic tests to the client and prepare them adequately for each of the diagnostic examinations. The nurse also provides the client with emotional support to complete the diagnostic process so that appropriate treatment may be initiated.

Bibliography

1. Abraham, P., & Smith, C. (1984). Medical evaluation and management of calcium nephrolithiasis. *Medical Clinics of North America, 68,* 281.
2. Abramson, A. (1983). Neurogenic bladder: A guide to evaluation and management. *Archives of Physical Medicine and Rehabilitation, 64,* 6.
3. Adler, S. (1980). An approach to diagnosis and treatment of pyelonephritis. *Consultant, 20,* 207.
4. A quick check for UTI. (1984). *Emergency Medicine, 16,* 60.
5. Bagley, D., et al. (1985). *Urologic Endoscopy: A manual and atlas.* Boston: Little, Brown & Co.
6. Beck, L. H. (1990). Kidney function and disease in the elderly. *Hospital Practice, 26,* 75–90.
7. Benejam, R., & Narayana, A. (1985). Urinanalysis: The physician's responsibility. *American Family Physician, 31,* 103.
8. Bertani, T., et al. (1986). *Drugs and the kidneys (Vol. 33).* New York: Raven Press.

8a. Bolton, W. (Sep, 1977). Nonhemorrhagic decrements in hematocrit values after percutaneous renal biopsy. *Journal of the American Medical Association, 238,* 1266.

9. Bower, A., & Thompson, J. (1992). *Clinical manual of health assessment (3rd ed.).* St. Louis: C. V. Mosby.
10. Brenner, B. M., & Rector, F. C., Jr. (1986). *The kidney.* Philadelphia: W. B. Saunders.
11. Cella, J. H., & Watson, J. (1989). *Nurse's manual of laboratory tests.* Philadelphia: F. A. Davis.
12. Chadwick, A. T. (1989). BV 2000: A noninvasive technique to assess bladder function. *Journal of Neuroscience Nursing, 21,* 256–257.

12a. Chambers, J. (1983). Bowel management in dialysis patients. *American Journal of Nursing, 83*(7), 1051.

13. Chernow, B., et al. (1984). Measurement of urinary leukocyte esterase activity: A screening test for urinary tract infections. *Annals of Emergency Medicine, 13,* 150.
14. Clayman, R., et al. (1984). Flexible fiberoptic and rigid-rod lens endoscopy of the lower urinary tract. A prospective controlled comparison. *Journal of Urology, 131,* 715.

15. Colon, V., & Schumann, G. (1980). Urine cytology: Urinary tract cytology. *American Family Physician, 21,* 92.
16. Fritz, M. (1988). Noninvasive bladder volume measurement. *Urologic Nursing, 9,* 8–9.
17. Goldberg, E. (1986). *A primer of water, electrolyte, and acid-base syndromes (7th ed.).* Philadelphia: W. B. Saunders.
18. Greene, L. (1980). Management of gross and microscopic hematuria. *Consultant, 20,* 95.
19. Groer, M. W., & Shekleton, M. E. (1989). *Basic pathophysiology: A holistic approach (3rd ed.).* St. Louis: C. V. Mosby.
20. Guyton, A. C. (1991). *Textbook of medical physiology (8th ed.).* Philadelphia: W. B. Saunders.
21. Hald, T., & Bradley, W. (1982). *The urinary bladder: Neurology and dynamics.* Baltimore: Williams & Wilkins.
22. Hargiss, C., & Larson, E.: How to collect specimens and evaluate results. *American Journal of Nursing, 81,* 2166.
23. Histaminuria (1984). *American Family Physician, 29,* 355.
24. Huffman, J., et al. (1983). Extending cystoscopic techniques into the ureter and renal pelvis. *Journal of the American Medical Association, 250,* 2002.
25. Kee, J. L. (1986). *Laboratory and diagnostic tests with nursing implications (2nd ed.).* Norwalk, CT: Appleton-Century-Crofts.
26. Kulberg, A.: Urinanalysis and urine culture. *Topics in Emergency Medicine, 5,* 47.
27. Kunin, C. M. (1987). *Detection, prevention, and management of urinary tract infections (4th ed.).* Philadelphia: Lea & Febiger.
27a. Lang, E. (Apr, 1977). Renal cyst puncture and aspiration: A survey of complications. *American Journal of Roentgenology, 128,* 723.
28. Mackety, C. J. (1990). Lasers in urology. *Nursing Clinics of North America, 25,* 697–709.
29. Mariani, A., et al. (1984). Dipstick chemical urinanalysis: an accurate cost-effective screening test. *Journal of Urology, 132,* 64.
30. Marrie, T., & Costerton, J. (1983). A scanning electron microscopic study of urine droppers and urine collecting systems. *Archives of Internal Medicine, 143,* 1135.
31. Massary, S. G., & Gassock, R. J. (Eds.) (1988). *Textbook of nephrology.* Baltimore: Williams & Wilkins.
32. McConnell, E., & Zimmerman, M. (1983). *Care of Patients with Urologic Problems.* Philadelphia: J. B. Lippincott.
33. McGuckin, M. (1981). Getting better urine specimens with the clean-catch mid-stream technique. *Nursing 81, 11,* 72.
34. Melchior, H. (1975). Urodynamics. *Urological Research* 3.51.
35. Menon, M., & Krishnan, S. (1983). Evaluation and medical management of the patient with calcium stone disease. *Urologic Clinics of North America, 10,* 595.
36. Metheny, N. (1987). *Fluid balance: Nursing considerations (3rd ed.).* Philadelphia: J. B. Lippincott.
37. Mitchell, J. (1981). Diagnosis: Acute renal failure. *Hospital Medicine 17,* 87.
38. Murray, R., & Zentner, S. (1989). *Nursing assessment and health promotion through the life span.* Englewood Cliffs, NJ: Prentice-Hall.
39. Pagana, K. D., & Pagana, T. J. (1985). *Diagnostic testing and nursing implications (2nd ed.).* St. Louis: C. V. Mosby.
40. Porth, C. (1990). *Pathophysiology (3rd ed.).* Philadelphia: J. B. Lippincott.
41. Re, R. N. (1987). The renin-angiotensin systems. *Medical Clinics of North America, 71,* 877–895.
42. Rebensen-Piano, M. (1989). The physiologic changes that occur with aging. *Critical Care Nursing Quarterly, 12*(1), 1–14.
43. Resnick, I., & Older, R. (1982). *Diagnosis of genitourinary disease.* New York: Thieme-Stratton.
44. Resnick, N. M. (1989). Diagnosis and treatment of the institutionalized elderly. *Seminars in Urology, 7,* 117–123.
45. Rowe, J., et al. (1976). The effect of age on creatinine clearance in men: A cross-sectional and longitudinal study. *Journal of Gerontology, 31,* 155.
46. Rubenstein, E. (Ed.). (1984). Evaluation of renal morphology. *Scientific American Medicine, 7,* 1.
47. Sabiston, D. C. (1991). *Textbook of surgery: The biological basis of modern surgical practice.* Philadelphia: W. B. Saunders.
48. Schrier, R., & Gottschalk, C. (1988). *Diseases of the kidney (4th ed.).* Boston: Little, Brown & Co.
49. Schumann, D. (1976). Tips for improving urine testing techniques. *Nursing 76, 6,* 23.
50. Schumann, G., & Colon, V. (1980). Urine cytology: Renal cytology. *American Family Physician, 21,* 102.
51. Shelter, M. (1984). Excretory urogram and pyelogram. *RN, 47,* 95.
52. Shelter, M. (1984). Renal arteriogram and cystourethrogram. *RN, 47,* 89.
53. Smith, D. R. (1988). *General Urology (12th ed.).* Norwalk, CT: Appleton & Lange.
54. Stark, J. (1980). BUN/creatinine: Your keys to kidney function. *Nursing 80, 10,* 33.
55. Stark, J. L. (1988). A quick guide to urinary tract assessment. *Nursing 88, 18,* 57–58.
56. Stewart, D., et al. (1984). Evaluation of proteinuria. *American Family Physician, 29,* 218.
57. Swerdlow, M., & Jao, W. (1981). Urinanalysis: The "poor man's biopsy," rich with clues. *Consultant, 21,* 265.
58. Valenta, C. (1983). Urine testing and home blood-glucose monitoring. *Nursing Clinics of North America, 18,* 645.
59. Vander, A. J. (1985). *Renal physiology (3rd ed.).* New York: McGraw-Hill.
60. Walsh, P. C., et al. (Eds.) (1992). Campbell's urology (6th ed.). Philadelphia: W. B. Saunders.
61. Ware, F. (1981). Renal function tests: A guide to interpretation. *Hospital Medicine, 17,* 77.
62. Weber, J. (1988). *Nurses' handbook of health assessment.* Philadelphia: J. B. Lippincott.
63. Whittier, F. (1982). Proteinuria: incidental finding or tip of an iceberg? *Consultant, 22,* 151.
64. Wilburn, R. (1982). Diagnosis: Hematuria. *Hospital Medicine* 18:65.
65. Wilkinson, G. B. (1988). Clean catch urodynamic studies: A balloon teaching device. *Urologic Nursing, 9,* 18–19.
66. Wyngaarden, J. B., & Smith, L. H. (1988). *Cecil textbook of medicine (18th ed.).* Philadelphia: W. B. Saunders.

Nursing Care of Clients with Disorders of the Ureters, Bladder, and Urethra

The principal function of the ureters, bladder, and urethra is to transport urine from the kidneys. The bladder, urethra, and, sometimes, ureters are called the lower urinary tract. The ureters are sometimes classified, with the kidneys, as the upper urinary tract. Anything that obstructs the flow or interferes with the neuromuscular ability to move and expel urine reduces the ability of these organs to fulfill their role. A disorder can cause psychosocial as well as physiologic problems, which then influence the severity of the disorder and healing progress. The nurse must consider both realms in identifying problems and implementing interventions to solve these problems.

BLADDER DISORDERS

URINARY TRACT INFECTION (CYSTITIS)

Definition

Urinary tract infection (UTI) refers to an infection within the lower urinary tract, usually affecting the bladder, although the urethra and ureters may be involved. *Cystitis* is an inflammation of the bladder wall, usually caused by ascending bacteria. The term "cystitis" is often used to refer to a UTI that is symptomatic. Abacterial or interstitial cystitis is an inflammation of the bladder mucosa that occurs without an infection. This disorder is discussed later.

Incidence

UTIs are a very common problem. The bladder is the most frequent site of infection within the urinary tract. Studies show that at least 25 per cent of all women develop UTI or cystitis sometime in their lives. Men rarely develop UTIs before the age of 50 years because of the length of their urethra and the antibacterial properties of prostatic fluid.

Acute UTIs account for 6 to 7 million office visits a year for young women.[49] Recurrence is common after treatment for an initial UTI; about 20 per cent of women with UTIs have frequent recurrences.

Etiology

The most common UTI-causing organisms are *Escherichia coli, Enterobacter, Pseudomonas,* and *Serratia.* These organisms, normally found in the gastrointestinal tract, contaminate the urine because of the proximity of the urethral orifice and the anus. *E. coli* itself is responsible for about 90 per cent of UTIs in women. *Staphylococcus saprophyticus,* an organism that has been recognized in Europe for some time, is now drawing more attention in the United States. It especially affects young women, occurs most often in the summer and early autumn, and has a high propensity for ascending into the upper urinary tract.

Candida is another growing cause of UTIs. It is associated with sepsis and death, especially in debilitated clients who are already experiencing one or more of these conditions: blood dyscrasia, diabetes mellitus, cancer, drug addiction, immunosuppression, and persistent UTI treated with a variety of antibiotics. Any *Candida* found in the urine is significant, although the laboratory must determine that the organism is actually colonized and not simply a contaminant.

Risk Factors

There are many risk factors associated with UTIs. Women are more susceptible to this disorder because of the female urethra and perineum; sexually active and pregnant women are the most vulnerable. The short female urethra reduces the distance between the bladder and the external environment. The location of the external meatus makes it very vulnerable to vaginal and fecal contamination. Colonization of the vaginal introitus and urethra with *E. coli* is a significant variable characteristic of women who suffer recurrent UTIs.

There are several ways women can compensate for the female anatomy, especially the proximity of the urethra and anus and the short urethra. Proper wiping, front to back, is the easiest way to accomplish this. Women who suffer frequent UTIs are also encouraged to shower rather than take a tub bath, because a bath is more likely to cause irritation and contamination of the urethra. Avoiding bubble baths is another way to decrease the irritation. Wearing cotton underpants, which are more absorbent, and avoiding pantyhose with slacks, which traps more moisture in the perineal region, are also ways to decrease a woman's risk of UTI.

Sexual intercourse increases the risk of UTIs in women; the motion during coitus "milks" the organisms up the urethra and into the bladder. "Honeymoon cystitis" is a term frequently used to describe this phenomenon. Poorly fitting diaphragms used for contraception are also linked to UTI because of the pressure against the bladder, which prevents complete bladder emptying. Spermicide is also associated with an increase in UTIs. These agents appear to increase the vaginal pH, alter the normal vaginal flora, and be associated with increased colonization of *E. coli.*

In order to help decrease the risk associated with sexual intercourse, a woman should wash well before intercourse and void immediately after. She should also drink at least 3000 ml of fluid per day, preferably fluids that acidify the urine. An acid-ash diet is one that increases the acidity of the urine. Cranberry juice is the most common fluid; however, medications such as methenamine hippurate (Hiprex) or vitamin C in large doses will also decrease the urine pH. Proper fitting of a diaphragm and correct use of spermicide also help decrease the risk.

About 10 per cent of all pregnant women experience UTIs. The mechanical compression of the ureters and the hormonal changes apparently cause hydroureters, hydronephrosis, and bladder hypotonia, which then lead to urinary stasis and reflux, the two prime facilitators of organism growth.

For decreasing the risk during pregnancy, a woman should increase her fluid intake and void at least every 2 hours. She should also be monitored frequently for the development of an infection and have that infection treated immediately.

Hormonal changes in aging women alter the vaginal pH and thus vaginal flora. Decreased vaginal lubrication also increases the risk of urethral irritation during intercourse. The use of estrogen vaginal creams can restore vaginal pH. The use of water-soluble lubricants for intercourse can decrease the urethral irritation and thereby decrease the risk of UTIs.

In women, clothing can contribute to the development of cystitis, such as synthetic underwear and pantyhose, tight jeans, and lounging in wet bathing suits. Allergens or irritants, such as feminine hygiene spray, bubble baths, perfumed toilet paper and sanitary napkins, and soaps, contribute to the development of cystitis in some women. Women with a history of infections should avoid as many of the risk factors as possible.

A previous UTI increases vulnerability to recurrence. The convalescent bladder is less resistant to bacterial invasion than is a healthy bladder. Studies show that this susceptibility increases with each successive infection. It is vital, therefore, that UTi's be treated adequately and completely for sterilization of the urine and avoidance of recurrence. Clients should have the cause of infection identified and be taught all possible preventive measures to avoid recurrence.

The presence of an indwelling catheter dramatically increases the risk of UTI. UTIs are the most frequent nosocomial infection. The rates in most hospitals are well above 50 per cent for UTIs in catheterized clients, with some reports as high as 100 per cent. Strict asepsis is vital in decreasing the incidence of UTI with catheterized clients. Nurses must maintain a closed urinary system in all clients unless it is absolutely necessary to disrupt the system. Most specimens can be obtained from the system by use of sterile technique without opening the system. Daily, meticulous perineal care is also important, although the agent to be used is controversial. Many authorities feel that soap and water is still the best agent to use for this.

In older male clients, obstructive uropathy, loss of the bactericidal properties of prostatic secretions, poor bladder emptying, and other medical disorders contribute to the development of UTIs. It is estimated that the incidence of UTI in older men is approximately 15 per cent.

Pathophysiology

Several pathophysiologic mechanisms are involved in the development of UTIs. The principal factor is the host's loss of resistance to invading organisms. The bladder is normally resistant to infection. The lining of the bladder is composed of mucin-producing cells, which help maintain the integrity of the bladder lining and prevent cellular inflammation and damage. Although numerous pathogens reach the bladder, the sterility of the urine is quickly reestablished. The bladder's resistance to infections is due to the antibacterial properties of the bladder mucosa and urine as well as to phagocytosis. Also, voiding washes organisms out of the lower urinary tract, helping to prevent infection.

Anything that breaks down these defenses opens the way to possible infection. Loss of the integrity of the mucosal lining may be caused by an indwelling catheter, calculus, tumor, or parasites. Also, standing urine is very susceptible to organism growth. Therefore, anything that contributes to urinary stasis significantly increases the risk for development of UTI. Distention of the bladder leads to many UTIs. As the bladder wall expands, blood flow decreases. Ischemic tissue becomes more vulnerable to organism invasion. Common causes of bladder distention include urethral obstruction and suppression of voiding. Infection also can occur from the client's own colon via the hematogenous or lymphatogenous routes.

Undertreated cystitis predisposes to the recurrence of infection. It is vital that UTIs be adequately treated for eradication of the bacteria present in the urine. If cystitis is not adequately treated, it can predispose to the development of upper UTIs, including pyelonephritis. As stated previously, even adequate treatment does not prevent recurrence.

Clinical Manifestations

The cardinal symptoms of cystitis are burning on urination, frequency, urgency, inability to void, incomplete emptying of the bladder, and voiding in small amounts. Low back pain is also a common problem, as is suprapubic pain. Assessment may reveal hematuria, cloudy urine, abdominal and flank pain, malaise, chills, fever, and nausea and vomiting. Remember that about 10 per cent of clients with bacteriuria will be asymptomatic. Lack of assessment findings, therefore, should not preclude the diagnosis of UTI.

Most of the symptoms are due to the irritation of the bladder and urethral mucosa. The bacteriuria causes the inflammation, fever, and chills. If the ureters become inflamed also, abdominal symptoms may occur.

DIAGNOSTIC ASSESSMENT

Definitive diagnosis is usually based on a urine culture. However, the dipstick test for leukocyte esterase activity is increasingly used to determine bacteriuria early so interventions can begin promptly. This method is 100 per cent sensitive and 76 per cent specific.

A urine culture is essential for positive diagnosis because dipsticks alone can give false-positive results. The specific causative organism must be accurately identified. Follow-up cultures are also used to determine the effectiveness of medications used to treat the infection. Because the potential is high for contamination and false-positives during specimen collection, some individuals require serial cultures before organisms can definitively be identified. Asymptomatic clients should have three consecutive positive cultures before a final diagnosis of UTI is established.

Some authorities indicate that the traditional 100,000/ml bacterial count benchmark, for voided specimens, may not be appropriate. Some feel that bacterial counts as low as 1000 to 10,000/ml (for voided specimens) may indicate an active infectious process in the lower urinary tract, especially if the client has symptoms of cystitis. This area is still unclear, and further research is needed. A colony count of 10,000/ml indicates an active infectious process in a catheterized specimen. Even a low colony count in a catheterized specimen, however, is significant and should be investigated.

Sensitivity tests are also done routinely on the urine specimens for identifying the antibiotics that can be used to treat the infection successfully.

In some cases of severe or recurrent cystitis, an intravenous pyelogram (IVP), retrograde pyelogram, or cystoscopy might be done to detect any abnormalities. Congenital anomalies, foreign bodies, calculi, and tumors can be detected as well as abnormalities the repeated infections may have caused. These tests will also detect obstruction within the urinary tract; a common cause of UTI, especially in older men.

Medical Management

Management of UTI is multifaceted, and an initial, acute infection may be treated differently from recurrent infections. The principal intervention of an initial infection is the administration of antibiotics specific to the causative organisms.

PHARMACOLOGIC MANAGEMENT

Pharmacologic intervention begins with a broad-spectrum antibiotic even before the culture and sensitivity results are known, because medication should start as soon as possible. Later, on the basis of sensitivity reports, the exact medication for this infection can be given. Commonly used pharmacologic agents include trimethoprim-sulfamethoxazole (Bactrim, Septra), nitrofurantoin (Macrodantin), sulfisoxazole (Gantrisin), ciprofloxacin (Cipro), ampicillin, methenamine mandelate (Mandelamine), and cephalosporins (Table 49-1). Medications containing azo dyes are believed to have an anesthetic effect on the urinary tract mucosa and are used to treat the burning sensation often felt with cystitis (such as Pyridium or Azo-Gantrisin).

For pregnant women, certain medications must be avoided because of the risk to the fetus. Do not administer trimethoprim-sulfamethoxazole (Bactrim) or sulfonamides in the last trimester of pregnancy. Tetracycline should not be given at all during pregnancy or to children under 12 years of age. Care must also be taken in treating the elderly because many suffer from compromised renal function.

The typical course of antibiotic therapy is 10 to 14 days. However, a single *large* dose, although not accepted by all authorities, is effective in many clients, especially women with an initial uncomplicated infection of the lower urinary tract. Large single-dose therapy does not suppress the client's normal flora to the same degree as does long-term therapy and reduces the development of resistant organisms.[49]

A urine culture must be obtained approximately 1 week after discontinued pharmacologic therapy for determining whether the medication has eradicated the bacteriuria. When urine is not yet sterile, the physician will continue antibiotic therapy with the same or another antibiotic. Sometimes the course of antibiotics may need to be extended a few additional weeks. Persistent infections may require therapy for months. When the infection flares up each time therapy is discontinued, suppression therapy may be prescribed to keep the urine sterile. This consists of small doses of antibiotics that the client takes daily or several times a week, often for years.

For some clients, frequent recurrent infections are a frustrating problem. Three or more UTIs a year is considered frequent, whether they involve the same or different organisms. Each infection period must be treated with antibiotics. Caution the client against self-diagnosis and treatment of recurrent UTIs. Each infection requires culture and sensitivity and specific treatment. The physician may prescribe continuous suppression therapy or episodic administration of antibiotics.

There is a growing trend to give the client control over the medication regimen when identical recurrent infections have occurred. For example, women whose occurrences relate to sexual activity may be provided with a supply of antibiotics, with instructions to take a prescribed dose after intercourse. Others with frequent recurrences are (1) given a prescription for medication, (2) taught to recognize early signs of UTI, (3) instructed to begin antibiotic therapy at the first hint of infection, and (4) advised to come in 1 week after completing the regimen for a follow-up urine culture.

Treating the client with asymptomatic bacteriuria is yet another problem. In general, physicians currently suggest that an asymptomatic infection be treated only if it is certain that intervention will prevent further morbidity.

Antibiotics can cause some problems. They have the potential for destroying the normal flora, which leads to problems such as vaginal yeast infections in women. There is also the possibility that resistant organisms can develop.

Complications can also occur if the infection is not completely eradicated. An ascending infection can migrate from the bladder to the kidneys, resulting in the development of pyelonephritis. Recurrent pyelonephritis can predispose the client to the development of chronic renal failure if the damage to the kidneys is severe enough.

DIETARY MANAGEMENT

Acidifying the urine decreases the rate of bacterial multiplication. Traditionally, cranberry juice and ascorbic acid (vitamin C) have been used to do this. However, current studies indicate that neither adequately reduces the urinary pH and, therefore, is not as reliable as was previously thought. Although cranberry juice can acidify the urine, commercial products do not contain a sufficiently high concentration of pure juice to reduce the pH unless the client can drink a prodigious amount.

An acid-ash diet is more effective in acidifying the urine (Box 49-1). Encourage a diet of meats, eggs, cheese, prunes, cranberries, plums, and whole grains. Foods not included on the diet include carbonated beverages, anything containing baking soda or powder, fruits other than those listed, all vegetables except corn and legumes, olives, pickles, and nuts other than peanuts.

Remember that acidifying the urine may or may not be advantageous, depending on the specific antiseptic or antibiotic being used. For instance, methenamine mandelate (Mandelamine) and methenamine hippurate (Hiprex) require acid urine to be effective. On the other hand, the action of aminoglycosides, nitrofurantoin (Macrodantin), and sulfonamides is diminished by acidic urine.

Fluid intake should also be increased to at least 2 to 3 L/day so that a good output is ensured. The increased fluid is extremely important when the client is taking sulfa drugs because these can form crystals in concentrated urine.

TABLE 49-1. Medications Used to Treat Cystitis and Other Urinary Disorders

Agent	Action	Dosage	Side Effects	Nursing Implications
Urinary Antiseptics				
Cinoxacin (Cinobac)	Effective against *E. coli, Klebsiella, Enterobacter, Proteus, Serratia,* and *Citrobacter*	1 g daily in two to four divided doses for 7-14 days	Dizziness, headache, photosensitivity, nausea and vomiting, abdominal pain, diarrhea, rash	Contraindicated in clients who are hypersensitive to nalidixic acid; warn client about photophobic effect; give with meals to decrease gastrointestinal side effects
Nalidixic acid (NegGram)	For acute and chronic UTIs, especially gram-negative bacterial infections	1 g qid for 7-14 days for acute or 2 g daily for long-term use	Drowsiness, weakness, headache, photophobia, diplopia, abdominal pain, nausea and vomiting, rash, angioedema	Use with caution in clients with liver or renal disorders; contraindicated in clients with a history of convulsions; instruct client to report visual disturbances; encourage fluids and closely monitor output; avoid sunlight
Norfloxacin (Noroxin)	For complicated and uncomplicated UTIs caused by gram-negative organisms, including *Pseudomonas;* especially useful for clients allergic to penicillin, cephalosporin, and sulfa drugs	400 mg PO bid for 7-10 days for mild infections and for 10-21 days for severe infections	Fatigue, somnolence, headache, nausea, constipation, elevated liver function tests, rash	Encourage high fluid intake to ensure high urine output; advise client to take medication 1 hr before or 2 hr after meals because food may hamper absorption
Nitrofurantoin (Macrodantin)	To treat acute and chronic UTIs in clients with adequate creatinine clearance	For acute UTI, 50-100 mg PO qid for 10-14 days, after meals Chronic therapy, 50-100 mg PO as needed; IV, 180 mg bid for adults over 120 lb	Nausea and vomiting, gastrointestinal upset, diarrhea, rash, asthma, peripheral neuropathies, anaphylaxis, dizziness, hypotension	Maintain adequate intake and output; use cautiously in clients with anemia, diabetes, vitamin B deficiency, electrolyte imbalances, or debilitating diseases; watch for hypersensitivity; keep urinary pH in acid range with vitamin C and cranberry juice; give with food; warn client that drugs may discolor urine
Methenamine mandelate (Mandelamine)	Effective in acid urine against gram-positive and gram-negative organisms for chronic UTIs	1 g PO qid after meals	Nausea and vomiting, diarrhea, elevated liver enzymes, rash, dysuria, and frequency in large doses	Contraindicated in clients with renal or hepatic disease or severe dehydration; maintain high urine output; warn client to limit intake of alkaline foods and increase intake of cranberry juice and foods that acidify urine; adminis-

Table continued on following page

TABLE 49-1. Medications Used to Treat Cystitis and Other Urinary Disorders Continued

Agent	Action	Dosage	Side Effects	Nursing Implications
				ter with food or after meals, but avoid antacids
Sulfonamides				
Co-trimoxazole, sulfamethoxazole-trimethoprim (Bactrim, Septra)	To treat acute UTIs	160 mg trimethoprim/800 mg sulfa or double with double-strength tablet for 10 to 14 days	Gastrointestinal distress, agranulocytosis, allergic reactions, headache, glossitis, stomatitis, hepatitis, pruritus, photosensitivity, arthralgia, peripheral neuritis, hearing loss, crystalluria, hypoglycemia	Administer with large amounts of fluid; monitor serum glucose levels; monitor for allergies, which occur more commonly in AIDS clients; maintain alkaline pH—more soluble in alkaline urine
Sulfisoxazole (Gantrisin)	To treat acute UTIs	Initially 2-4 g PO, then 1-2 g qid for 10-14 days	Agranulocytosis, aplastic anemia, headache, depression, nausea and vomiting, diarrhea, toxic nephrosis, crystalluria, erythema multiforme, epidermal necrolysis, exfoliative dermatitis, hypersensitivity, anaphylaxis, serum sickness	Monitor closely for allergy; give each dose with full glass of water; maintain high fluid intake; monitor intake and output; more soluble in alkaline urine; monitor CBC; instruct client to take full dose; if Azo-Gantrisin is given, urine will be dark brown to red in color
Urinary Analgesics				
Phenazopyridine (Pyridium)	To treat pain of urinary tract irritation or infection	100-200 mg PO tid until pain disappears, usually about 2-3 days	Nausea, headache, vertigo	Warn client that urine will be red to orange in color; contraindicated in clients with renal or hepatic disease; always given with antibiotic—does not treat infection, only pain
Cholinergics				
Bethanechol chloride (Urecholine)	To treat acute postoperative or other nonobstructive urinary retention and for neurogenic atony of bladder with retention	2.5-10 mg sc, never IM or IV; 10-30 mg PO tid or qid; all doses should be individually determined	Cardiac arrest and vascular collapse if given IM or IV, headache, hypotension, abdominal cramps, diarrhea, nausea and vomiting, urinary urgency, flushing, bronchoconstriction	Never used in clients with any possibility of bladder obstruction; never give IM or IV, can lead to circulatory collapse; watch closely for cholinergic overdose; atropine antidote; have bedpan readily available, works within 15 min after injection or 60 min after oral dose; given on empty stomach to decrease nausea and vomiting

TABLE 49–1. Medications Used to Treat Cystitis and Other Urinary Disorders Continued

Agent	Action	Dosage	Side Effects	Nursing Implications
Anticholinergics				
Propantheline bromide (Pro-Banthine)	To decrease bladder muscle spasms	Up to 60 mg PO qid	Palpitations, blurred vision, confusion in elderly clients, dry mouth, constipation, urinary hesitancy and retention, decreased sweating	Do not use in clients with narrow angle glaucoma, obstructive uropathy or gastrointestinal disease, or ulcerative colitis; monitor urine output closely; provide gum or hard candy for dry mouth
Antibiotics				
Ciprofloxacin (Cipro)	To treat severe or complicated UTIs	250 mg PO every 12 hr	Headache, restlessness, tremor, lightheadedness, seizures, nausea, diarrhea, vomiting, oral candidiasis, crystalluria	Contraindicated in clients allergic to quinolone antibiotics, in pregnancy, and in children; give 2 hr after meals; may cause control nervous system stimulation and seizures; have client drink plenty of water with medication; prolonged use may result in overgrowth of resistant organisms
Cephalexin monohydrate (Keflex)	To treat genitourinary infections	250 mg to 1 g PO every 6 hr	Transient neutropenia, anemia, pseudomembranous colitis, nausea, anorexia, diarrhea, dyspepsia, urticaria, hypersensitivity	Use carefully in clients with a history of renal insufficiency, previous hypersensitivity to penicillin or cephalosporins; prolonged use may lead to overgrowth of resistant organisms; take with food to decrease gastrointestinal distress; be sure client takes full dose of medication; obtain cultures before starting medication

bid, twice daily; CBC, complete blood count; IM, intramuscularly; IV, intravenously; PO, orally; qid, four times daily; SC, subcutaneously; tid, three times daily; UTIs, urinary tract infections.

Surgical Management

Surgery is done to treat any anomalies that may be present and are causing the repeated infections. Bladder neck strictures and ureteral pelvic junction abnormalities are the most common problems. Benign prostatic hypertrophy (BPH), the common cause of cystitis in older men, can also be treated surgically. Urinary calculi may also require surgical intervention. Once these disorders are corrected, the infections should stop.

Nursing Management

ASSESSMENT

The nurse should start by assessing the client's risk factors for the development of cystitis. This involves obtaining a detailed history and physical examination. The nurse should have the client describe the symptoms present in detail.

The nurse must also collect the necessary urine culture and sensitivity specimen. The nurse should instruct

Box 49–1. Acid-Ash Diet

Foods Allowed

Meat, fish, poultry, shellfish, cheese, and eggs
Grains: bread, cereals, crackers, rice, whole grain, pasta, and corn
Vegetables: corn and lentils
Fruits: cranberries, prunes, plums, and their juices
Foods with large amounts of chlorine, phosphorus, and sulfur

Foods Prohibited (Basic Foods)

All milk and milk products
All vegetables except corn and lentils
All fruits except cranberries, plums, and prunes
Foods containing large amounts of potassium, sodium, calcium, and magnesium.

Neutral Foods

Coffee and tea
Butter, margarine, oils
White sugar and honey
Cornstarch and tapioca
All pure fats
All pure carbohydrates

the client on the proper procedure for collection so that contamination from other organisms is minimized.

NURSING INTERVENTION

There are several appropriate nursing diagnoses for the client with UTI.

Nursing Diagnosis: Urinary Elimination, Altered (a variety of specifiers such as retention, urgency, and so on) R/T irritation of the bladder mucosa.

Planning: Expected Outcomes. The client will have urinary elimination return to normal within 3 days of the start of treatment, as evidenced by absence of fever, normal white count, and absence of pain, burning, frequency, and urgency.

Implementation. The nurse should monitor the client's voiding, noting problems such as frequency, urgency, retention, and dysuria. The symptoms need to be treated immediately so the client can return to normal urinary function.

Nursing Diagnosis: Pain, Acute R/T irritation of bladder and urethral mucosa.

Planning: Expected Outcomes. The client will be able to urinate without discomfort within 24 hours of treatment, as evidenced by absence of pain and burning on urination.

Implementation. The nurse should also administer any medications prescribed specifically to treat pain, such as Pyridium or Azo Gantrisin. Again, forcing fluids will also help relieve the pain by diluting the urine and making it less irritating to the mucosa. A warm sitz bath may also help the pain, especially if the urethra is also irritated. Baking soda can be added to the water to produce a greater soothing effect. Some clients find that a heating pad applied to the suprapubic area helps reduce bladder spasms and suprapubic pain.

Nursing Diagnosis: Infection, High Risk for R/T urinary stasis, pregnancy, or other risk factors.

Planning: Expected Outcomes. The client will not develop UTI or will have infection treated effectively, as evidenced by sterile urine culture.

Implementation. The nurse can help the client to reestablish a normal urinary pattern. One of the best ways to do this is through administration of the prescribed anti-infective agents listed in Table 49–1. The problems of urgency, frequency, and possible incontinence will decrease within 24 hours of the beginning of medication. The nurse should also check the culture and sensitivity report to be sure that the proper anti-infectives are being administered.

Nursing Diagnosis: Knowledge Deficit R/T prevention, medications, hygiene, and fluid intake.

Planning: Expected Outcomes. The client will be able to describe ways to prevent UTI, the correct method for taking medication, the proper way to wipe after voiding, and the required fluid intake.

Implementation. The nurse can do much to help the client learn to prevent cystitis. After analyzing the client's risk factors, the nurse can devise specific ways to help the client prevent cystitis from occurring or treat it if it has occurred. Increased fluid intake to wash bacteria out of the bladder is one of the simplest ways to help prevent the infections. The nurse should instruct the client to drink at least eight 8-ounce glasses of water a day and to avoid caffeine and alcohol, which can seriously irritate the bladder. Remember, coffee, tea, chocolate, and some over-the-counter medications contain caffeine.

Many nursing interventions are directed at preventing the initial infection or recurrences. The nurse should teach all clients at risk to maintain a high daily fluid intake of at least 2000 ml a day unless otherwise contraindicated. Remind the client to void at the first urge (unless the bladder program is planned otherwise) and at least every 2 to 3 hours during the day and one or two times at night to prevent bladder distention. Encourage women to void immediately after sexual intercourse and to drink at least two glasses of water as soon as possible. Recommend that women use a position for sexual intercourse that minimizes pressure on the anterior vaginal wall. The nurse should emphasize the need for women to maintain good perineal hygiene and teach them to wipe the labia from front to back. Advise the use of tampons rather than sanitary pads.

The nurse should teach all high-risk clients the signs and symptoms of cystitis, pointing out that the client should seek health care assistance as soon as possible if these occur. When administering medication, make sure that the client understands the drug and its side effects, emphasizing the importance of taking the full course of the drug, even if the symptoms of infection disappear.

Finally, because of the high risk for more serious or recurrent infection and the possible need to begin further intervention early, emphasize the importance of complying with the recommended schedule of follow-up urine cultures.

EVALUATION

The nurse can evaluate the effectiveness of the interventions on the basis of the expected outcomes identified for this client. If interventions were not successful, the goals and interventions should be modified so that goals can be met.

Modification of Plan of Care for the Elderly

In older adults, cystitis may occur more often, but for different reasons. In older women, the changes in the aging vagina and bladder increase the risk for cystitis. The atrophy of the vagina, decreased vaginal secretions, and muscle weakness in the vagina and bladder predispose this group to infection. In older men, BPH is one of the main risk factors for UTI, and the incidence of BPH increases with age.

The causes of UTIs in this group will alter both prevention and treatment. In men, the best treatment for recurrent UTI is to treat the BPH. Once this problem is eliminated, the infections should be eliminated. In women, use of vaginal lubricants before intercourse can help decrease infections. The Kegel exercise, which helps tighten the vaginal and bladder muscles, is also helpful in women, particularly if women practice these exercises routinely throughout their lives. If the weakness in the muscles is severe, surgery such as an anterior colporrhaphy and bladder suspension can be done.

When administering medications to older adults, the nurse must consider the renal and hepatic function of the client. Many of the drugs used to treat UTIs require the client to have good renal and hepatic function. There are often changes in the cardiovascular system. Forcing fluids is contraindicated in clients with congestive heart failure.

Post-hospital Care

DISCHARGE TEACHING

The discharge teaching revolves around helping the client learn methods of preventing the initial infection or recurrence of infections. We must teach clients the proper method of treating the infections, such as correct medication procedures, and other associated activities, such as forcing fluids and measuring their own output.

HOME HEALTH CARE NEEDS

The client has few home health care needs associated with this condition. As long as the client follows the discharge instructions, there should be no particular needs.

FOLLOW-UP CARE

The major need for clients is a follow-up culture. It is important that the client's urine is documented to be sterile again. The client also needs to be reminded of those measures that will help prevent recurrence and the importance of the early reporting of any symptoms that suggest recurrence.

INTERSTITIAL CYSTITIS

Cystitis may also be noninfectious. Interstitial cystitis (IC) can be caused by chemical agents, such as medications like cyclophosphamide. Other causes can include radiation therapy and possibly autoimmune responses. This disorder is also called painful bladder disease (PBD). If it is associated with hemorrhage, as with radiation therapy and drugs like cyclophosphamide, it is called hemorrhagic cystitis.

This disorder occurs mainly in women (90 to 95 per cent). Although at one time it was considered a disease of menopause, it actually occurs more frequently in younger women.

IC is a poorly understood disorder with an unclear pathophysiology. One factor that is clear, however, is that in spite of the symptoms, the urine is sterile. There seems to be some change in the permeability of the glycosaminoglycan layer of the bladder mucosa, which is usually impermeable to urea and other substances.

On cystoscopy and hydrodilation of the bladder, glomerulations in the bladder wall, Hunner's ulcers, and a severely decreased bladder capacity are noted. The presence of these findings is considered diagnostic by many physicians, whereas others believe the condition is present even without these findings. This second group bases the diagnosis on the absence of any other disease of the bladder that could cause the symptoms.

The clinical manifestations of PBD are severe lower abdominal or pelvic pain, urgency, frequency (up to 60 times a day in some clients), nocturia, and, in some women, dyspareunia. Some clients may exhibit only the frequency and pain; others will have all symptoms. In the past, especially when this condition occurred in menopausal women, physicians often felt that it was a psychosomatic disorder. This is much less prevalent today, but the nurse should guard against this type of assumption.

Because this problem is not caused by infection, the prevention and treatment are different from those of infective cystitis. Antibiotics may actually cause further bladder irritation. The treatment for IC is controversial, with no one accepted treatment. Drugs such as anti-inflammatories, antispasmodics, tricyclic antidepressants, and antihistamines are used, as well as tranquilizers and occasionally narcotics.

Other treatments include instillation of a variety of agents into the bladder to promote healing and pain relief. These include agents such as sodium oxychlorosene (Clorpactin), silver nitrate, and dimethyl sulfoxide (DMSO). Oral sodium pentosan polysulfate (Elmiron), a heparin analog, is given possibly to create a mucin layer in the bladder.

The major nursing responsibility associated with this syndrome is supporting the client through diagnosis and treatment. Because the cause of this disorder is unclear, there is little the nurse can teach the client about preventive measures. It is a chronic disorder requiring long-term client support. Clients require a great deal of reassurance because the diagnosis and treatment are so uncertain. The nurse should become familiar with the national and local resources for clients with IC/PBD and refer clients to these as appropriate.

URINARY INCONTINENCE

Definition

Incontinence has been defined by the International Continence Society for the Standardization of Terminology as "a condition in which involuntary loss of urine is a social or hygienic problem and is objectively demonstrable."[49] There are a number of different types of incontinence, such as enuresis, stress, urge, paradoxic (overflow), reflex, environmental, and psychological (Table 49-2). The International Continence Society for the Standardization of Terminology divides it into four categories on the basis of anatomic or physiologic dysfunction. These are stress, urge, overflow, and reflex incontinence.

Incidence

Wide ranges of figures are available on the prevalence of incontinence. These estimates range from about 10 per cent to more than 30 per cent of all older clients with stress and urge incontinence, both alone and combined, seemingly the most common. There are few accurate estimates of the incidence of this problem in adults other than the elderly.

Etiology

Incontinence is often caused by interference with sphincter control. This includes anatomic, physical, physiologic, psychosocial, and pharmacologic factors.

Anatomic and physiologic incontinence results from sphincter weakness or damage, urethral deformity, alteration of the urethrovesical junction, detrusor instability, and weak abdominal and perineal muscle tone.

Sphincter weakness or *damage* is often caused by obstetric trauma, postoperative weakness, and congenital weakness. After a suprapubic prostatectomy, men often experience temporary incontinence for several days once the postoperative catheter is removed. A transurethral prostatectomy may cause more damage, with a longer period of incontinence or possibly permanent incontinence. A radical perineal or retropubic prostatectomy may cause permanent incontinence if the sphincter is partially damaged during the operation.

Urethral deformity is often caused by recurrent UTIs, previous gynecologic surgery, trauma, and estrogen deficiency vulvitis.

Alteration of the *urethrovesical junction* occurs in women. This angle, between the bladder and the posterior proximal urethra, is important to continence in women. Common causes of the loss of this angle include multiple pregnancies, aging, and surgical procedures resulting in abdominal perineal weakness. Figure 49-1 shows how the alteration of the urethrovesical angle from 90 to 100 degrees to less than 90 degrees reduces the competency of the internal sphincter.

TABLE 49-2. Types of Incontinence

Type of Incontinence	Description
Stress	Increased intra-abdominal pressure caused by activities such as coughing, laughing, sneezing, walking, or running leads to an involuntary loss of urine; the intravesicular pressure increases to overcome the resistance of the internal sphincter in the urethra
Enuresis	Nighttime incontinence or "bed-wetting" is usually associated with childhood, although the problem can extend into adulthood
Urge	Inability to hold back the flow of urine when feeling the urge to void; spasmodic bladder contractions accentuate the problem
Overflow (paradoxic)	Retention with overflow of small amounts of urine; occurs when the intravesicular pressure exceeds maximal urethral pressure without detrusor activity
Reflex	Abnormal activity of the spinal cord reflex leading to involuntary loss of urine
Psychological	Client aware of need to urinate, but unable to respond appropriately to urge because of dementia or confusion
Environmental	Client aware of need to urinate, but physically unable to either reach the toilet on own or receive adequate assistance to do so

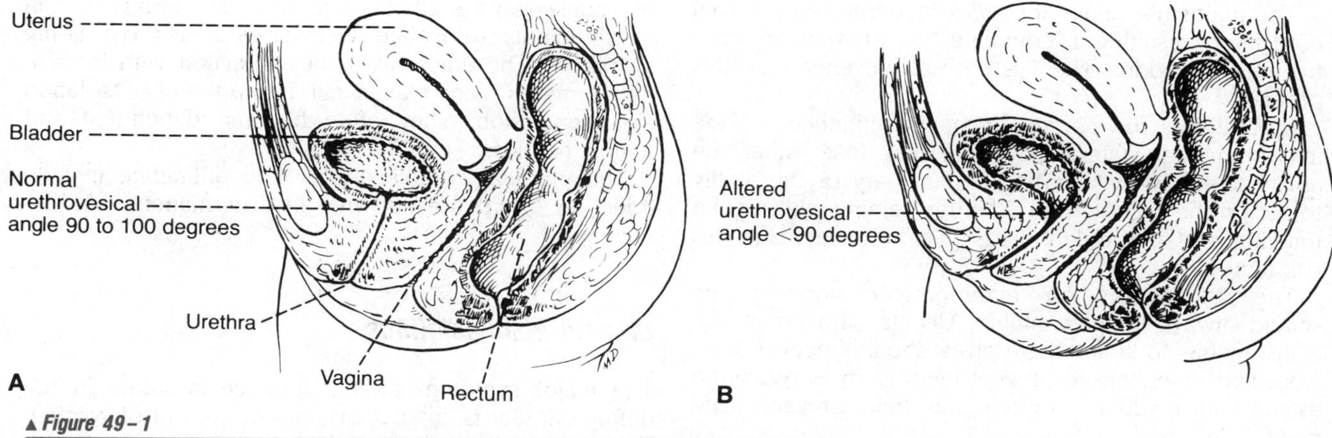

▲ **Figure 49-1**

Alteration in the normal urethrovesical angle contributes to incontinence in women. *A*, Normal angle. *B*, Altered angle.

Detrusor instability is commonly caused by

- bladder lesions (e.g., infection, neoplasms, and senile trigonitis)
- lower motor neuron lesions (e.g., tumor, prolapsed disc, complication of pelvic surgery, and osteoarthritis of the spinal cord)
- upper motor neuron lesions (e.g., tumor, cerebrovascular accident, multiple sclerosis, and transection of the spinal cord)
- large bowel diseases, spastic colon, and diverticulosis

Weak abdominal and *perineal muscle tone* is caused by obesity, lack of exercise, and loss of tone after childbirth or prostatectomy.

Physical causes of incontinence are those independent of the urinary tract. These are related to physical immobility, often of the elderly. These clients are often physically unable to get to the toilet or bedpan independently because of causes such as strokes, fractures, and weakness. Failing vision can also contribute to this if the client is unable to see the commode or bedpan.

Psychosocial causes of incontinence range from true psychological problems such as dementia to simple confusion. Clients may be unaware of the need to void or simply unable to know what to do when they feel the urge. Other possible causes include regression, dependence, rebellion, insecurity, manipulative attention seeking, sensory deprivation, and the disturbance of conditioned reflexes.

Various medications also contribute to incontinence, especially overflow incontinence. These include (1) narcotics, tranquilizers, sedatives, and hypnotics, all of which affect bladder fullness cues and the ability to attend to them; (2) alcohol; (3) rapid-acting diuretics; (4) antihistamines; (5) atropine and atropine-like substances; (6) hypotensives; (7) alpha-adrenergic blockers; (8) beta-adrenergics; and (9) ganglionic blockers.

Other factors contributing to the development and maintenance of incontinence include fecal impaction, bladder scarring, urethral adhesions, diabetes mellitus, and obesity. Incontinence may also be a sign of "giving up." Frequent voiding by clients who fear "accidents" leads to decreased bladder capacity, increased detrusor tone, and thickening of the bladder wall, which results in a vicious cycle of dysfunction.

Risk Factors

The risk factors for each type of incontinence vary. The main risk factor for *stress* incontinence is the loss of the correct posterior urethrovesical junction angle in women. This weakness can be caused by anything that decreases the muscle tone surrounding the bladder. Muscle exercises that increase the muscle tone help prevent this from happening.

In men, the major risk factor for stress incontinence is urethral irritation from infection, from radiation damage to the bladder, or after a prostatectomy. Preventing infection is one way to avoid this. Muscle exercises, the Kegel exercises, improve control and muscle tone after the prostatectomy.

There are a variety of diseases that are risk factors for *urge* incontinence; multiple sclerosis is common because of the severe bladder muscle spasms. Other conditions that increase the risk of developing urge incontinence include UTIs, arthritis that may interfere with movement, and strokes. There is little to be done to help clients avoid these risk factors.

Medications such as hypnotics, tranquilizers, sedatives, and diuretics can cause urge incontinence by interfering with mobility. Careful monitoring of clients on these drugs, keeping bedpans handy, and frequent toileting can help decrease this risk.

The major risk factor for *overflow* incontinence is retention with bladder distention. The causes can be a nervous system lesion, obstruction of the bladder outlet, or even a fecal impaction. Because the usual cause of bladder outlet obstruction is BPH, this incontinence can be prevented by early treatment. Fecal impaction is preventable by helping the client maintain regular bowel habits.

The major risk factor for *reflex* incontinence is spinal cord injury resulting in complete loss of voluntary control of the bladder. There is no real prevention for this problem.

Risk factors for *psychological* incontinence include altered mental states; the client may lose either the ability to know that voiding is necessary or the ability to act on the urge to void. Bladder training with regular toileting and controlled fluids can help decrease this risk factor.

The risk factors for *environmental* incontinence should always be preventable. Clients who are physically unable to toilet themselves should receive sufficient and timely aid to prevent incontinence. Again, an established bladder program can help prevent accidents.

Pathophysiology

The pathophysiologic changes associated with incontinence are related to the specific causes. *Stress* incontinence occurs when the intravesical pressure exceeds the maximum urethral pressure in the absence of detrusor activity. This increased vesical pressure is often associated with activities such as sneezing, coughing, and laughing. There may be some weakness in the urethral sphincter or, in women, changes in the urethrovesical angle. Normally, in the first stage of voiding, the urethrovesical angle is lost as the bladder descends. The muscle weakness experienced by women as a result of childbirth, aging, or other problems causes weakness of the pelvic floor that helps to destroy the critical angle. With the loss of the angle, there is descent and funneling of the bladder neck with the bladder rotating down and back. This places them in the anatomic position for the first stage of voiding, so any activity that causes downward pressure on the bladder leads to voiding. In men, the pathophysiologic change is usually BPH causing retention, overflow, and stress incontinence.

Urgency incontinence is associated with several pathophysiologic changes. One problem is uninhibited detrusor contraction associated with motor disorders. Another cause is decreased mobility from an upper motor neuron lesion combined with the inability to stop voiding once the impulse is felt.

Overflow incontinence is related to a problem with retention and overdistention of the bladder with an overflow of the excessive amount of urine. The pathophysiologic cause of the retention is usually obstruction at the bladder outlet such as with BPH.

Reflex incontinence is related to abnormal spinal cord activity associated with the absence of the sensation to void. Bladder contraction occurs without direct stimulus for the central nervous system.

Psychological incontinence has as its basic pathophysiologic mechanism changes in the client's mental status; *environmental* incontinence is a problem with impaired mobility.

If incontinence is not controlled, it can lead to both psychological and physical problems. The psychological consequences of incontinence are serious. It can cause clients to isolate themselves and avoid going anywhere. The embarrassment associated with incontinence makes many clients sink into a world of isolation and depression. They often become dependent and almost helpless.

The physical complications of incontinence include infection, skin breakdown, and permanent bladder changes.

Clinical Manifestations

The major symptom of incontinence is stated in the definition, that is, involuntary loss of control of voiding. If it is urge incontinence, it may be associated with bladder spasms. The amount of urine expelled can help differentiate whether it is overflow or stress incontinence, because these usually produce small amounts of urine.

DIAGNOSTIC ASSESSMENT

Urodynamic evaluation is the major diagnostic test for incontinence. In order to determine the precise cause of the client's incontinence, the incontinence should be reproduced during the examination. These tests can also assess detrusor function and the likelihood that treatment will be successful. The degree of pelvic floor prolapse can be assessed by physical examination and radiologic tests.

The variety of urodynamic examinations, including cystometrogram and electromyogram, are described in Chapter 48. Ultrasonography of the bladder or kidneys can detect residual urine. A cystoscopy with cystography may also be useful in diagnosing this problem.

Medical Management

The goals of treatment for the client with incontinence include the following: (1) incontinence must be carefully evaluated and treatment based on this evaluation; (2) treatment decisions must be based on the specific abnormalities identified for each client; (3) the client's personality, expectations, environment, and clinical status are determinants of the treatment modalities; (4) plans to circumvent environmental constraints should be part of the treatment plan; and (5) the client must be able to make an informed choice among treatment options.

There are many noninvasive therapies that may be effective in controlling some types of incontinence. Pelvic muscle exercises, the Kegel exercises designed for postpartum women, have long been the technique used to improve control. Reports of success range from 30 to 90 per cent with the use of these. Recently, a new device, the Femina cones, has improved the success of these exercises. These cones are weighted and inserted into the vagina. Correct muscle contraction is required to keep them in place. Early reports are that

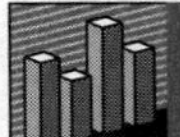

NURSING RESEARCH

A study was conducted on older women who were experiencing incontinence to determine whether pelvic muscle strength can be measured objectively. This is important because pelvic muscle exercises, like the Kegel exercises, are believed to increase pelvic muscle strength and thereby to improve stress incontinence.

This study compares the accuracy of digital palpation done by the primary care nurses with vaginal myography (perinometry). The nurses were able to accurately measure the muscle strength.

The finding of this study supported the validity of a digital measure of pelvic muscle strength in incontinent older women. A scale describing these measures was developed and validated. This scale can then be used to assess improvement in muscle strength after exercises, leading to improved continence.

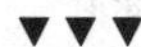

Brink, C. A., Smapselle, C. M., Wells, T. J., et al. (1989). A digital test for pelvic muscle strength in older women with urinary incontinence. *Nursing Research, 38*(4), 196–199.

they dramatically improve the effectiveness of pelvic muscle exercises.

Behavioral techniques to increase the client's awareness of the need to void can also be initiated. Biofeedback has been used with clients experiencing stress or urge incontinence. Clients are trained to control sphincter, detrusor, and abdominal muscles. It is not a technique that all clients are comfortable with and does require extensive training. The use of biofeedback has been shown to be successful in eliminating incontinence in about 20 to 25 per cent of clients and provided significant improvement in another 30 per cent of clients.

Bladder training is another approach that is used for incontinence. With this technique, the client first voids at short intervals throughout the day, usually hourly or less if necessary. The client then tries to lengthen the time between voiding to intervals up to 3 hours. This seems to eliminate the problem in about 10 to 15 per cent of clients with urge and stress incontinence, and most clients find at least some improvement.

Institutionalized clients can also use a form of bladder training. With these clients, health care workers check the clients at hourly intervals, urging use of the bedpan and praising success. The time between voiding can often be increased to every 2 hours with success.

UTIs must be eliminated for irritation to the detrusor muscle to be reduced. In the case of stress incontinence, it is important to suppress a chronic cough.

PHARMACOLOGIC MANAGEMENT

Pharmacologic intervention for incontinence is primarily guided by the following. During the urine collection phase, the detrusor relaxes because of beta-adrenergic activity. At the same time, the bladder outlet contracts in response to alpha-adrenergic stimulation. When these actions are insufficient to maintain urine storage in the bladder, medications can be prescribed as supplements or replacements for these physiologic activities.

A variety of medications have been tried to control incontinence. Table 49–3 summarizes these medications. Medications are used mainly with urge incontinence to relax the bladder and possibly increase bladder capacity and sometimes stress incontinence. These medications are contraindicated in clients with bladder outlet obstructions or weak detrusor muscles.

Propantheline, dicyclomine, imipramine, flavoxate, or oxybutynin chloride may decrease detrusor hyperactivity. Alpha-adrenergic agents that increase urethral resistance include phenylephedrine, ephedrine, phenylpropanolamine, or imipramine. Calcium channel blockers, which antagonize transmembrane movement of calcium, are being used with some success. If external sphincter spasticity or dyssynergia is the problem, the physician may order baclofen, dantrolene, or diazepam. Topical and systemic estrogens help relieve estrogen deficiency urethral problems in postmenopausal women.

DIETARY MANAGEMENT

The major nutritional alteration involves controlling fluid intake especially after dinner, so the client will have less incontinence during the night. For obese clients, weight reduction programs may help decrease stress incontinence. The client should avoid bladder stimulants such as alcohol, chocolate, and coffee.

Surgical Management

Electrical inhibition of the micturition reflex has been successful for many clients. These devices, which deliver barely perceptible electrical stimulation, effect improved urethral closure by direct and reflexogenic contraction of the striated paraurethral musculature. They also may increase bladder volume through bladder inhibition and may stabilize detrusor activity. Figure 49–2 shows the three main types of electrical devices. Electrodes may be implanted surgically within the pelvic muscles for direct stimulation; indirect stimulation may be achieved by using either intravaginal or anal devices. The intravaginal device or anal plugs can be removed and reinserted as necessary. The anal plug must be removed for defecation and frequent cleaning. Once chosen, the apparatus is attached to a control box. The client can then activate the system as desired to relieve incontinence.

The implantation of an artificial urinary sphincter may help some clients achieve continence. This surgical procedure is usually reserved until after all else has

TABLE 49-3. Medications Used to Treat Incontinence

Agent	Action	Dosage	Side Effects	Nursing Implications
Propantheline bromide (Pro-Banthine)	Anticholinergic that inhibits detrusor contraction and may increase bladder capacity; delay and decrease in amplitude of involuntary contractions	15 mg PO tid; larger doses produce too much drying	Dry mouth, dry eyes, constipation, confusion or excitement in elderly; precipitation of glaucoma, blurred vision, mydriasis, palpitations, urinary retention	Do not use in clients with narrow angle glaucoma, obstructive uropathy or obstructive gastrointestinal disease, ASHD, hypertension, hiatal hernia, and hepatic or renal disease; monitor vital signs and urinary output; use gum or hard candy to alleviate dry mouth
Oxybutynin chloride (Ditropan)	Direct smooth muscle relaxant that works directly on bladder muscle; helps with detrusor instability	Up to 5 mg PO qid	Drowsiness, dry mouth, palpitations, tachycardia, blurred vision, mydriasis, constipation, urinary hesitancy or retention	Contraindicated in clients with myasthenia gravis, gastrointestinal obstruction, obstructive uropathy; use cautiously in elderly; stop therapy at intervals to see if problem has resolved; rapid onset of action, peaks at 3-4 hr and lasts 6-10 hr; monitor with periodic cystometry; store in tightly closed container
Verapamil hydrochloride (Calan)	Depressant effect on bladder muscles; use for incontinence not well documented	80 mg PO tid	Dizziness, hypotension, heart failure, constipation, nausea, urinary retention, peripheral edema	Use with incontinence not well studied; use cautiously in elderly and clients with existing heart disease; monitor urinary output; check pulse and blood pressure regularly
Imipramine hydrochloride (Tofranil)	Anticholinergic and direct relaxant effect on detrusor and contracting effect on bladder outlet (alpha-adrenergic effect)	25-75 mg PO daily	Drowsiness, dizziness, orthostatic hypotension, tachycardia, urinary retention, sweating, blurred vision, mydriasis	Do not use in clients recovering for myocardial infarction, with BPH, or with history of glaucoma or seizure disorders; decrease dose in elderly or debilitated clients; monitor for urinary retention or constipation; warn client to avoid alcohol
Phenylpropanolamine hydrochloride (Acutrim)	Alpha- and beta-adrenergic antagonist used to treat stress incontinence; produces smooth muscle contraction at bladder outlet	25 mg every 4 hr	Hypertension, tachycardia, palpitation, insomnia, nervousness, restlessness	Monitor effectiveness; check blood pressure frequently; warn against use of over-the-counter drugs that may interact, especially pseudoephedrine; maintain in

TABLE 49-3. Medications Used to Treat Incontinence Continued

Agent	Action	Dosage	Side Effects	Nursing Implications
				light-resistant, tight container
Estrogens	For postmenopausal women with urge incontinence, but ineffective against stress incontinence	Dosage varies with particular agent used	Headache, increased risk of thromboembolism, nausea and vomiting, breakthrough bleeding, hyperglycemia, hypercalcemia, urticaria	Do not use in clients with history of thromboembolic disease of any kind; monitor effectiveness in reducing incontinence; warn client about possible increased risks of cancer

ASHD, arteriosclerotic heart disease; BPH, benign prostatic hypertrophy; PO, orally; qid, four times daily; tid, three times daily.

failed. Figure 49-3 shows a sphincter device consisting of an inflatable cuff, a reservoir, and a control pump. The surgeon implants the cuff around the bladder neck or urethra, a deflation (or control) pump in the scrotum or labia, and a fluid reservoir in the abdomen. The cuff keeps the urethra closed until the client manually squeezes the pump, thereby moving the fluid from the cuff to the reservoir. The client can then void. The cuff automatically refills afterward, again occluding the urethra. This method has been successful with many clients. However, candidates must have an unobstructed lower urinary tract, no detrusor hyperreflexia, no progressive neurologic disease affecting bladder function, and the manual dexterity and motivation to manage the system. Failure of the device poses a long-term risk for reoperation.

Other surgical procedures are used to correct or compensate for anatomic defects contributing to incontinence. The most common surgical procedures are intended to restore the normal urethrovesical angle or to lengthen and support the urethra. Reestablishing the urethrovesical angle allows the internal sphincter to function normally. Lengthening the urethra increases its resistance.

In the Marshall-Marchetti-Krantz procedure, one of several common older techniques, the bladder neck and urethra are sutured to the perichondrium of the symphysis pubis or the periosteum of the superior pubic ramus. Newer procedures such as the Raz are now being done transvaginally. This repair process involves elevation and suspension of the bladder with the use of tissue or inorganic materials for support. Postoperatively, clients undergoing this surgery need a suprapubic or urethral catheter for 5 to 8 days. During this time, they require a high fluid intake to prevent infection. Also, the drainage system must always be patent, because the pressure of a filling bladder inhibits the healing process.

Once healing occurs, a reconditioning or clamp and release program is then initiated to help the detrusor

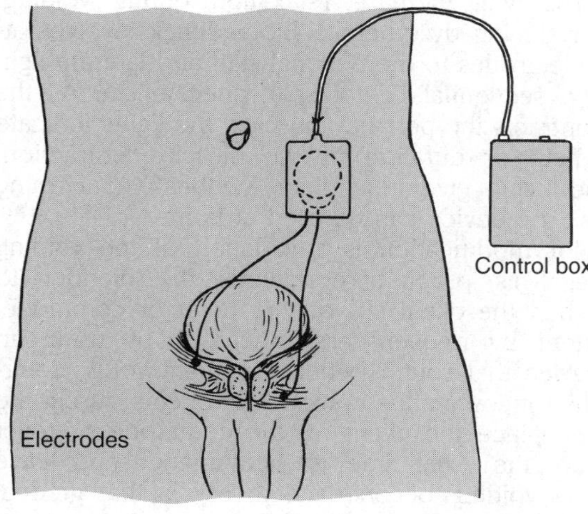

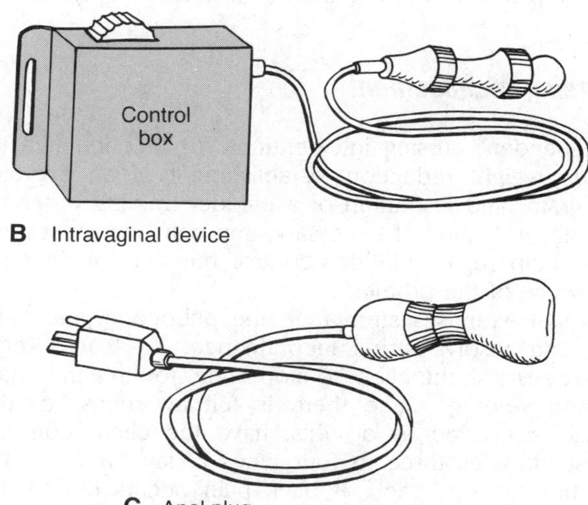

▲ *Figure 49-2*

Electrical devices used to control incontinence.

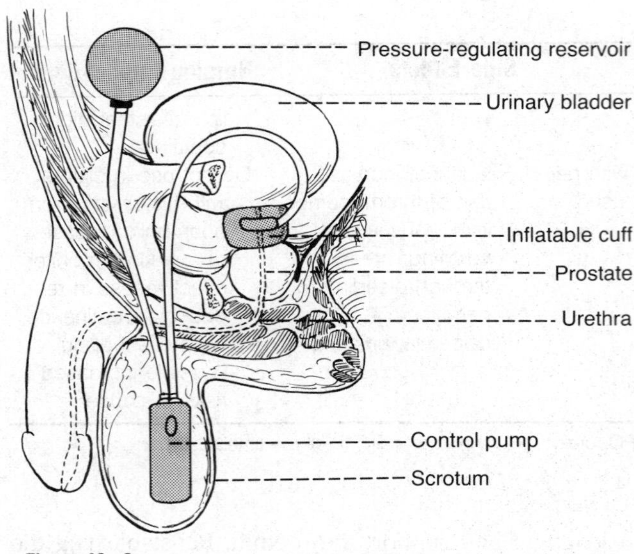

▲ *Figure 49-3*

Artificial urinary sphincter. This surgically implanted urethral sphincter restores continence. To urinate, the client deflates the cuff around the bladder neck by squeezing the control pump within the scrotum. The cuff reinflates automatically.

muscle regain tone. Clamp the catheter for lengthening intervals while urine collects in the bladder. If the client begins to experience severe pressure, the catheter should be unclamped immediately. Otherwise, the catheter is unclamped periodically to empty the bladder. If a suprapubic catheter is used, the client should try to void when the bladder is filled; then, if the client is unable to void, the catheter can be emptied. After voiding, measure the residual urine to determine the effectiveness of bladder emptying.

Other surgical procedures aim to provide an intact, patent route for the transport of urine. Scar tissue that interferes with normal bladder neck function must be removed. If urethral or sphincter narrowing contributes to the problem of incontinence, it must be dilated.

Nursing Management

Independent nursing interventions for incontinence include weight reduction, establishment of an exercise program, and institution of a bladder training program. Weight reduction, if necessary, and pelvic exercises not only help regain bladder control but may prevent recurrence of the problem.

Kegel exercises strengthen the pubococcygeal muscle and resolve stress incontinence. To teach Kegel exercises, ask the client to stop urine flow several times during voiding. Once there is full awareness of the muscles needed to do this, have the client contract these muscles three to four times a day for 5- to 10-minute sessions each. If back pain occurs during the exercises, the client is probably contracting the wrong muscles and thus needs to go back to step 1 of the exercise program.

A successful bladder training program requires a great deal of patience on everyone's part. The first step in instituting the program is to discuss all procedures and the expected outcome with the client. The sensitive nurse tries to inspire a sense of hope and the knowledge that something indeed can be done about incontinence.

A bladder training program involves (1) adequate fluid intake, (2) muscle-strengthening exercises (as described in the preceding), and (3) carefully scheduled voiding times. To implement this program, you will need to plan well-organized teaching guidelines. If the program involves behavioral modification or intermittent catheterization, refer to the following discussion. During the program, although the bed and clothing may be padded to protect them from becoming wet, avoid diapering, because this further demeans the client and may give "permission" to be incontinent.

Many clients suffering from incontinence reduce their fluid intake, thinking this will decrease urine production and result in better control. Actually, adequate urine production is necessary to stimulate the micturition reflex. Therefore, unless it is contraindicated by the client's physical status, encourage a daily fluid intake of 2000 to 2500 ml. Carefully space these fluids throughout the day and limit them in the evening to allow longer sleep periods at night. Have the client avoid beverages containing caffeine, because they contribute to bladder irritability.

Meanwhile, develop a voiding schedule with the client. Determine how often the client urinates during the day by maintaining a voiding record. Check frequently for wetness and document results. Depending on the voiding pattern, conduct the client to the toilet or commode every 30 minutes to 2 hours. As the program progresses, encourage the client to hold the urine longer and thus increase voiding intervals.

Biofeedback and behavior modification may be included in this bladder training program. Use biofeedback techniques to help the client regain control over the external urethral sphincter and pelvic floor musculature. This will increase relaxation during voiding, thereby reducing dyssynergia. Biofeedback involves attaching electrodes to the perianal skin and lateral thigh, then to a sequential light display mechanism. As the client contracts the perianal muscles, the lights indicate the strength or duration of the muscle contraction. Thus the lights give immediate feedback concerning progress. The device can be used at home.

Behavior modification is a variation of the voiding schedule. This program conditions the bladder to empty when the client sits on the toilet or commode. First, either by frequent assessment or by using an alarm device that sounds when the client voids, determine when incontinence consistently occurs during the day. Then place the client on the commode or toilet just before the usual time of incontinence and leave there until voiding occurs. The theory is that gradual conditioning through use of the commode or toilet stimulates micturition. Once a stimulus-response pattern has been established, it can help achieve continence throughout the day. Programs are more successful when bladder capacity is at least 150 to 200 ml. With a capacity below this level, the client voids too frequently to achieve an optimal outcome.

Mechanical pressure is sometimes used to interfere with the outflow of urine. For example, a pessary is inserted into the vagina, where it exerts pressure on the bladder neck area. Some of these devices have inflatable balloons that are periodically released to permit voiding. However, the use of pessaries is linked with complications, including discomfort, leukorrhea, ulceration, fistulas, and malignancy. A penile clamp, as illustrated in Figure 49-4, is used to compress the urethra in the male. The use of this appliance is controversial. It must be removed and repositioned frequently to prevent pressure sores and ischemic necrosis of the penis.

Psychotherapy and hypnosis also help manage incontinence. Psychotherapy may aid the client whose incontinence has a psychogenic origin as well as assist clients in dealing with embarrassment, increased dependence, and self-image problems that may accompany incontinence.

Sometimes none of these measures is effective. Nursing intervention must then be aimed at protecting the client's skin, clothing, bed linen, and so on. Adult-sized disposable pads or briefs help protect and increase the social mobility of clients experiencing chronic incontinence. These commercially available undergarments, with elasticized legs, have a cellulose padding that draws fluid away from the skin by capillary action. Some brands include an odor-reducing agent. If the skin does become wet, it must be meticulously cleaned and dried to prevent serious rashes and skin breakdown resulting from maceration and ammonia production. Use indwelling catheters to drain urine only as a last resort because they contribute to UTIs.

External condom drainage involves putting a thin rubber or plastic sheath over the penis and connecting it to either a leg bag or a bedside drainage bag. When the bladder releases urine, the urine runs down the tube into the collecting device. Problems with this system include leakage (with or without detachment of the condom), twisting of the condom, and stasis of urine, which can macerate the penis. Attach the condom sheath so that it stays in place without compromising circulation to the distal penis. Make sure that the condom is not too tight, particularly at the ring. You may need to remove the pubic hair before prepping the skin. Wash the penis with soap and water and allow it to dry thoroughly. Remove skin oils from the penis with alcohol and, if appropriate, apply an adhesive paste or commercial skin barrier. Many commercially prepared condom systems contain a double-sided adhesive liner that is applied to the penis before the condom. Many newer devices are self-adhesive. When rolling the condom sheath over the penis, take care to allow at least 1.5 cm between the distal end of the penis and the internal end of the sheath. This will reduce skin irritation. Make sure the foreskin is over the glans. Use only elastic tape (to allow expansion or erections). Apply this tape in a spiral only.

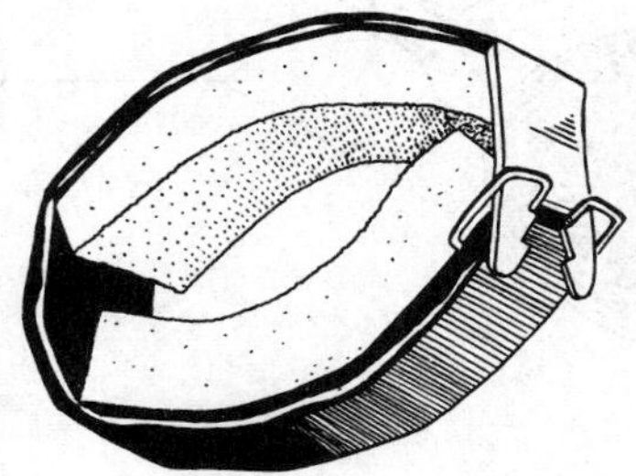

▲ *Figure 49-4*

A penile clamp compresses the urethra to prevent incontinence.

To avoid impaired circulation, never encircle the penis completely with tape. Frequently monitor the patency of the system and remove the condom at least daily to clean and dry the skin.

Modification of Plan of Care for the Elderly

Incontinence is a common problem among the elderly. They can be treated with any of the previously mentioned treatments. The elderly are more sensitive to many medications, so care should be used when administering them to older adults. The nurse should also remember that muscle weakness, with external factors such as decreased mobility and dependency, is a major cause of incontinence.

Post-hospital Care

DISCHARGE TEACHING

The teaching will be based on the specific interventions chosen to help the client handle the incontinence. If it is muscle weakness, the nurse should reinforce the Kegel exercises and be sure the client knows how to use the Femina cones, if ordered. If it is bladder training, make sure the client understands the routine.

HOME HEALTH CARE NEEDS

The client's home should be assessed for barriers that may interfere with easy access to the toilet facilities. If the toilet is not easily accessible, suggest that the family get a bedside commode.

FOLLOW-UP CARE

The client needs to be followed at regular intervals to be sure that the interventions are working and the incontinence remains under control. Referral to continence clinics may be appropriate for some clients in order to ensure close follow-up of continuing problems. Help for Incontinent Persons (HIP) and the Simon Foundation for Continence both publish newsletters containing important information for the incontinent client and family.

URINARY RETENTION

Definition

Urinary retention means that the urine is retained in the bladder. Urine production continues, but accumulated urine is not released.

Incidence

The incidence of retention varies with the cause. More than 50 per cent of men over 50 years of age experience BPH, a common cause of retention. Neurologic injury may also cause retention, and most spinal cord injuries occur in young adults. In postoperative clients, 10 to 15 per cent of those receiving general anesthesia require catheterization because of an inability to void, and 20 to 25 per cent of those who receive spinal anesthesia require a catheter.

Etiology

Obstruction at or below the bladder outlet is the most common cause of urinary retention. This retention can be caused by a variety of disorders including BPH, urethral strictures, urethral valves (now considered to be congenital diaphragms in the urethra), phimosis, meatal stenosis, fibrosis, calculi, blood clots, tumors, and bladder neck contractures.

Retention may also be caused by decreased sensory input to and from the bladder, muscle tension, and anxiety. Surgery has traditionally been a factor; spinal anesthesia causes retention more than does general anesthesia.

Other causes include medication that may interfere with the micturition reflex and neurologic injuries due to diabetes, strokes, and spinal cord injuries that also interfere with this reflex. Anorectal problems predispose to retention by applying pressure on the urethra. Decreased intake can also lead to retention through slowed production of urine and failure of normal detrusor reflexes.

Risk Factors

One of the major risk factors for retention is BPH. This is not a preventable problem, although the client with an enlarged prostate should be monitored closely for the development of an obstruction secondary to the enlargement.

Clients with a history of chronic UTIs that may have caused scarring of the bladder neck or urethra are also at greater risk.

Pathophysiology

Retention is a hazardous condition because the resulting urinary stasis contributes to the evolution of UTI and stone formation. There is also the potential for long-term structural damage in the bladder, ureters, or kidneys. Continued bladder distention may lead to loss of bladder tone.

The pathologic effects of any obstruction produce a snowballing effect; retained urine increases hydrostatic pressure against the bladder wall. This results in hypertrophy of the detrusor muscle, formation of trabeculae (development of connective tissue in the bladder wall), or development of diverticula. At the same time, peristalsis in the ureteral musculature increases against the pressure of the accumulating urine. The ureter gradually becomes elongated, tortuous, and fibrotic. The increasing pressure is also transmitted through the renal pelvis and calices into the renal parenchyma. The resulting hydronephrosis also exerts pressure on the blood vessels, causing ischemia and adding to the renal damage. If the process is not interrupted, it can proceed to renal failure and death. Figure 49-5 demonstrates the sequence. Even after the retention is relieved, in later stages of pressure-related damage, there may be permanent damage.

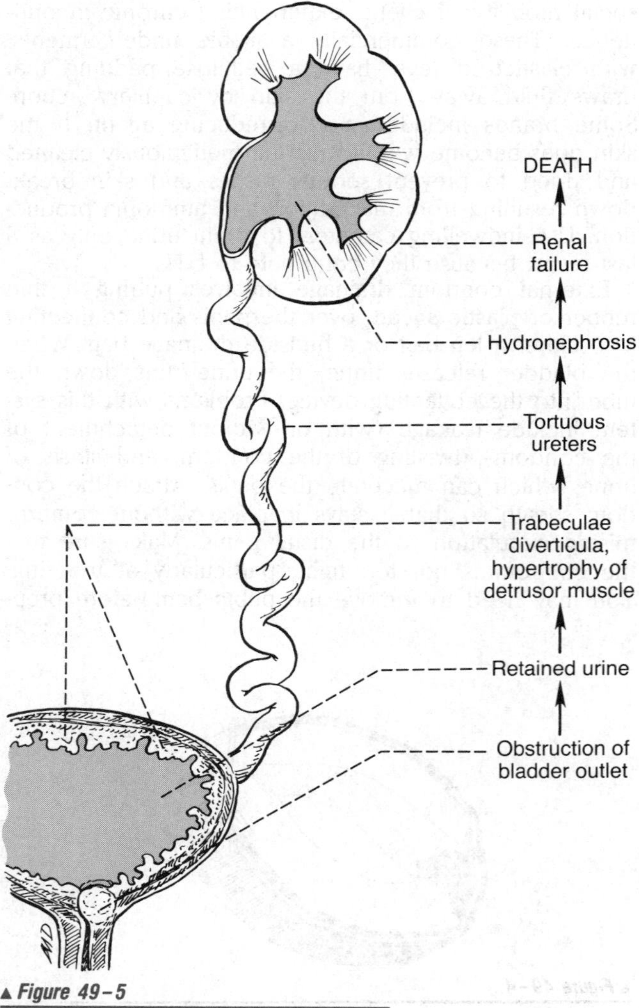

▲ **Figure 49-5**

Potential effects of urinary tract obstruction.

Medications, such as opiates, sedatives, antispasmodics, antiparkinsonians, beta-adrenergic blockers, and psychotropic agents, can interfere with normal neurologic function and the micturition reflex. Diseases with neurologic impact, such as diabetes mellitus, tabes dorsalis, and spinal cord lesions, also interfere with the micturition reflex.

Anorectal problems, such as hemorrhoids, abscess, or fecal impaction, contribute to urinary retention, either from obstruction or from secondary spasms of the perineal musculature, hampering the ability to relax.

Decreased fluid intake, either oral or intravenous, reduces glomerular filtration rate, and very slow urine production causes the bladder to fill as slowly. This may allow the detrusor muscle to accommodate the increased volume until the muscle's fibers are stretched beyond their ability to contract. When this happens, micturition cannot occur.

Retention with overflow results from the following events. As the bladder continues filling, the intravesical pressure rises. Eventually, this pressure overcomes the restraint of the sphincter. Urine flows out of the bladder until it reduces the intravesical pressure, but only to the level at which the external sphincter can again control the flow of urine. The client reports that the bladder does not feel really empty. The bladder overfills again, and the cycle is repeated.

Prolonged obstruction leads to high pressures in the urinary tract and may predispose to the development of bladder diverticula. A diverticulum is a pouch or sac resulting from the herniation of the mucous membrane lining due to a weakness in the muscular wall of an organ. Many diverticula are asymptomatic and found only accidentally during investigation of other conditions. Bladder diverticula can cause two major problems: (1) UTIs due to stasis of the urine and (2) malignancies probably related to chronic irritation from a persistent infection. Intervention involves removing the obstruction and relieving the retention, followed by surgical excision of the pouch and reestablishing normal patency of the urinary tract. Postoperatively, the client requires catheter drainage of urine to allow complete tissue healing. Because these clients have had long-term infection, they will probably require medication for months after surgery.

Clinical Manifestations

The primary manifestation of urinary retention is a distended bladder and the client's inability to void. A high fluid intake but low urinary output record documents that fluid either is not being converted to urine (oliguria or anuria) or is being retained in the bladder.

If the client voids more than once per hour, and releases only 25 to 50 ml at any one time, the problem may be retention with overflow.

DIAGNOSTIC ASSESSMENT

The major diagnostic test for retention is catheterization. If there is more than 250 to 500 ml of urine in the bladder and the client has not been able to void, retention is present. If the cause is thought to be an obstruction, cystoscopy may be done to determine the cause of that obstruction.

Medical Management

If obstruction causes the urinary retention, the urethra will need to be dilated or the occlusion removed for long-term relief. For dilation of the urethra, progressively larger indwelling catheters may be inserted each day. The urethra can be dilated more quickly with size-graded sounds, filiforms, followers, or other dilating instruments, usually under local or sometimes general anesthesia.

The insertion of sounds should be performed only by trained professionals because perforation of the urethra could occur.

Urinary catheterization with either a straight catheter or a retention catheter is commonly used to treat retention.

PHARMACOLOGIC MANAGEMENT

Cholinergic medications help stimulate bladder contraction, but these drugs must never be used if a mechanical obstruction is present. In this instance, intravesical pressure increases against an obstructed outlet, which may cause ureterovesical reflux or a ruptured bladder. Although their effect is somewhat controversial, bethanechol (Urecholine) and neostigmine (Prostigmin) are often administered. Bethanechol improves detrusor tone but also increases bladder outlet and urethral resistance. In order to counteract this, it is sometimes combined with phenoxybenzamine (Dibenzyline), prazosin (Minipress), and terazocrin (Hytrin), potent alpha-adrenergic blockers.

Surgical Management

Surgical intervention is sometimes necessary for obstructions below the bladder. If the bladder neck becomes rigid owing to inflammation, cystoplasty may be done to insert an elastic wedge into the area. A transurethral incision of the bladder neck might also be done. Excising urethral strictures, sometimes with plastic repair of the urethra (urethroplasty), helps return it to proper functioning. A meatotomy may be done to better open the urethral meatus.

Suprapubic catheterization is sometimes used to relieve urinary retention, especially in instances in which urethral catheterization is difficult or dangerous, such as with severely enlarged prostates, with urethral strictures, or in quadriplegics. The suprapubic catheter is inserted by the physician, often under local anesthesia and frequently in the client's room. General anesthesia may be used if another surgical procedure is also performed. To facilitate proper placement of the catheter, the bladder must be distended with fluid before the catheter is inserted. If the bladder is insufficiently distended with urine, additional fluid is instilled through a catheter or cystoscope.

The suprapubic skin is prepped. With use of sterile technique, the catheter may be inserted through a small surgical incision or by passing a trocar through the skin into the bladder. Once the trocar is in place, the pointed core of the cannula is removed. The catheter then is threaded through the cannula and attached to a closed drainage system. It may be sutured in place or secured with a commercially made retention seal.

When the suprapubic catheter is removed, the muscle layers of the bladder immediately contract over the puncture site and shrink the surface wound, precluding any need for sutures.

Advantages of the suprapubic over the urethral catheter include a lower rate of UTIs, ease in evaluation of the client's ability to void normally, and increased comfort.

Potential complications of the suprapubic catheter include dislodgement of the catheter, hematuria (especially after the use of a large bore catheter), bowel perforation during trocar insertion, and failure of the wound to close with the development of a urinary fistula.

Nursing Management

It is important for the nurse to distinguish retention from oliguria and anuria. Oliguria means that the kidneys are producing less than 400 ml of urine per 24 hours, whereas anuria means that the kidneys are producing less than 100 ml of urine per 24 hours. In urinary retention, the kidneys are producing a normal amount of urine, but it is not voided. Thus, the bladder fills with urine and is raised above the level of the pubic symphysis, sometimes being displaced to either side of midline. Any percussion over the bladder produces a "kettledrum" sound. The client may experience increasing discomfort and the need to urinate. Assessment may reveal restlessness and diaphoresis.

Nursing interventions may be used initially to treat retention. Provide privacy, warm the bedpan, and place the client in a normal sitting or standing position, using gravity and increased intra-abdominal pressure to help relieve the problem. Make use of the "power of suggestion" by running water or flushing the toilet within earshot of the client. Tape-recorded aquatic sounds may be effective. A warm bath, or pouring warm water over the perineum, often promotes muscle relaxation. Immersing the hands in water sometimes works, as does blowing bubbles with a straw in a glass of water. Applying ice to or stroking the inner thigh with light pressure will stimulate trigger points that may activate the micturition reflex. Anal dilation with a gloved finger is sometimes helpful. If the client is very tense and anxious, any measure that induces relaxation may aid in relieving the situation (e.g., a backrub or soothing music).

The client with a suprapubic catheter requires care similar to that needed with a urethral catheter. The most frequent problem is catheter obstruction due to (1) twisting or kinking or (2) sediment or clots. Disconnecting the catheter from the drainage tubing can disrupt the siphon drainage.

When the suprapubic catheter is removed, frequent dressing changes may be needed to control the urinary leakage from the site. As the site of the suprapubic catheter heals, less drainage will occur.

With appropriate training and a physician's prescription, a straight or retention catheter is inserted through the external meatus, into the urethra beyond the internal sphincter, and into the bladder. Use the straight catheter when it will be removed as soon as the bladder is drained. Use the retention, or indwelling, catheter for undetermined time periods, keeping it in place by inflating the balloon near the catheter's tip. Regardless of the type of catheter, use strict aseptic techniques for insertion. One exception is the use of a clean technique for those clients on an intermittent self-catheterization program. (See further discussion under Neurogenic Bladder Dysfunction.)

The retention catheter is attached to either a bedside drainage bag or a leg bag. A leg bag is frequently used with long-term catheterization, especially for the client going home with an indwelling catheter. This device allows the client more mobility and eliminates the embarrassment of carrying a drainage bag in public view. Figure 49-6 shows a leg bag in position. Because of the bag's small capacity, it must be emptied frequently. At night, a conventional drainage system is used so that the client can sleep through the night without needing to empty the leg bag. Instruct the client to avoid attaching the leg bag too tightly because the rubber straps can lead to skin irritation, thrombophlebitis, and

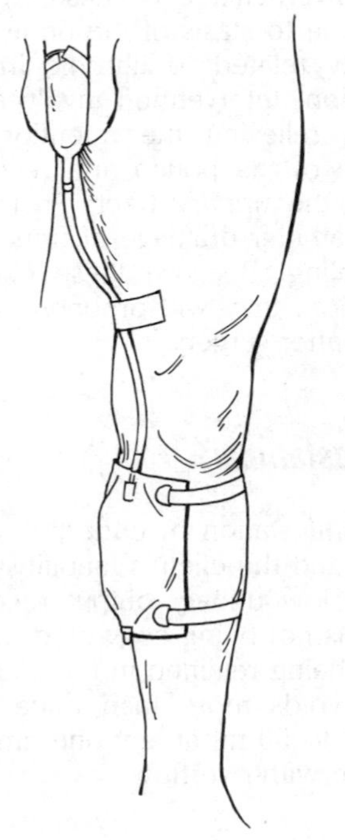

▲ **Figure 49-6**

Condom drainage and leg bag. The bag may be attached to the calf of the leg, as shown, or to the thigh.

ulcer formation. Even loose straps tend to tighten as the bag fills. Newer models have Velcro leg straps for clients with circulatory problems, those allergic to latex, or those at high risk for skin breakdown. Meticulous skin care and periodic removal of the bag help prevent these problems. Cleanliness and odor control are managed by washing the apparatus with soap and water and soaking it in a 1 per cent acetic acid (white vinegar) solution overnight.

Using indwelling catheters involves several physical hazards, including urinary tract infection and tissue trauma. Over 80 per cent of people who develop nosocomial UTIs have undergone urologic instrumentation of some kind. It is well documented that bacteriuria increases in direct relationship to duration of catheter placement. Although exact infection rates differ, estimates range between 4 per cent (within 24 hours) and 95 per cent (within 4 weeks). The most common causative organisms are *Escherichia coli, Proteus, Klebsiella, Aerobacter, Pseudomonas aeruginosa, Streptococcus, Staphylococcus, Providentia,* and *Serratia marcescens*. These organisms may enter the urinary drainage system when it is opened for any reason, or they may intrude via the thin layer of fluid and exudate that forms around the exterior of the catheter. The development of and intervention for UTI are discussed in this chapter.

Probably the most important weapon in preventing infection is conscientious handwashing before and after any handling of the catheter or drainage system.

To aid in preventing infection:

- Maintain a closed drainage system.
- Avoid backflow of urine.
- Avoid unnecessary manipulation of the catheter during perineal cleansing.
- Prevent microbial invasion and colonization in the urine collection bag.
- Maintain patency of the catheter.
- Encourage a high fluid intake.
- Provide urine acidification.

Because of the potential development of resistant organisms and possible adverse reactions, antibiotics should not be used prophylactically to prevent bacteriuria.

Tissue trauma may occur during the catheterization procedure. Tissue irritation or necrosis may result from (1) using an oversized catheter or (2) continuous pressure, for example, not enough slack is left in the catheter between the meatus and the site of taping on the leg or abdomen. An indwelling catheter that continually moves in and out of the distal urethra can cause tissue breakdown, enhancing encrustation on the outside of the catheter.

There is still some misunderstanding about what is referred to as bladder decompression drainage. This is really an older concept based on a faulty assumption that emptying a distended bladder rapidly through a catheter could result in bladder hemorrhage and hypotension. This procedure involved clamping the catheter after 1000 ml had been drained and then reopening it after an hour to drain another 1000 ml, until the bladder was decompressed. This has not been found to be true, and most physicians do not require the catheter to be clamped after 1000 ml have been drained. If the client's catheter does drain large amounts of urine, over 3000 ml, fluid replacement to balance output is important. Cystometric studies have shown that this problem does not occur with retention. The current thinking is that any amount can be drained. Drainage does not occur rapidly because the usual size of a catheter does not allow rapid drainage.

Modification of Plan of Care for the Elderly

The older clients are more prone to retention because of chronic decrease in bladder tone. Retention leading to infection may also be worse in older clients. The treatments, however, remain the same.

Post-hospital Care

DISCHARGE TEACHING

The client who goes home with an indwelling suprapubic or urethral catheter needs to know how to care for the catheter at home. The family and significant others should learn the proper ways to empty the drainage bag and ways of preventing infection, such as forcing fluids and an acid-ash diet. They should also be taught the signs and symptoms of UTI and instructed to call the physician if one occurs.

HOME HEALTH CARE NEEDS

The client may need an extra leg bag or drainage bag. The client's home should be assessed for the availability of toilet facilities for when the catheter is removed.

Follow-up Care

The client who goes home with a catheter in place will need to be seen later for removal of the catheter; this varies depending on the cause of the retention. The nurse should check with the physician for the timing of a follow-up visit.

URINARY REFLUX

Definition

Urinary reflux, or the backward flow of urine within the urinary tract, usually begins at the vesicoureteral junction so urine flows back into the ureter and frequently upward into the renal pelvis.

Incidence

The incidence of reflux is related to the incidence of the causes. If BPH is the cause, then the incidence increases in men over 50 years of age. If congenital vesicoureteral junction abnormalities are the cause, the problem occurs in younger children or young adults.

Etiology

Reflux can be caused by congenital malformations and by infectious processes in which edema and fixation of the intramural ureter and urethra interfere with normal flow. Neuromuscular malfunctions may contribute to reflux, as can bladder neck obstruction, which builds up intravesical pressure until it finally overwhelms the resistance of the ureteral sphincters.

Risk Factors

Risk factors for reflux include any disorder that causes obstruction. Chronic UTIs increase the risk of scarring and, therefore, obstruction. Bladder neck contracture after prostatectomy (see Chap. 75) is another risk factor, as is BPH itself. There is no primary prevention, but those clients with obstructive disorders should be closely checked for reflux.

Pathophysiology

If there is urethral obstruction, the main result is an ever present residual urine that often leads to the development of UTIs. The continual presence of urine can also change detrusor tone, thereby increasing the bladder's capacity and raising the threshold required to initiate the micturition reflex.

Renal damage and infection are the two primary problems resulting from vesicoureteral reflux. Because the capacity of the renal pelvis is only 5 ml, any larger amounts of urine can cause renal parenchymal changes, whether they result from ureteral obstruction or reflux. The increased hydrostatic pressure leads to renal cortical atrophy and calicectasis (dilation of the renal calix). The destruction of the kidney tissue, often asymptomatic and undetected, can proceed to end-stage renal disease. The kidneys are usually protected from ascending infections by the vesicoureteral sphincters. However, with reflux, any pathogens in the bladder are carried through the ureters to the kidney. This problem leads to repeated pyelonephritis (kidney infection), which eventually causes chronic renal failure with or without increased hydrostatic pressure.

Clinical Manifestations

The major symptoms exhibited by those clients are symptoms of obstruction and retention. The bladder will be distended if the obstruction is in the bladder neck but not if the obstruction is in the vesicoureteral junction or higher. If the obstruction is higher, then the client may exhibit signs and symptoms of renal failure.

DIAGNOSTIC ASSESSMENT

The major diagnostic studies are cystoscopy to look for signs of obstruction, ureteroscopy to look at the vesicoureteral junction, and IVP to look at the entire collecting system. Blood studies such as blood urea nitrogen and creatinine determinations are done to assess renal function.

Medical Management

There are few medical treatments for urinary reflux; the primary treatment is surgical.

DIETARY MANAGEMENT

There is no specific dietary treatment for urinary reflux. If the kidneys are damaged, then the client would be on a low-protein diet.

Surgical Management

The presence of renal damage, from the reflux, usually calls for surgical intervention. Surgery is also indicated for obstruction at the ureteropelvic junction, for intractable infection, and if the problem is not resolved by maturation. Because the most common causes of reflux are ureteral defects, surgical procedures that focus on correcting reflux involve the ureter (e.g., reimplantation of the ureter).

Postoperatively, a urethral or suprapubic catheter keeps the bladder empty to reduce tension on the suture line. A ureteral catheter will also be inserted into each ureter involved in the surgical procedure. This tiny, semirigid catheter is inserted into the ureter with its tip frequently placed in the renal pelvis. The distal end extends through the bladder and out through the urethra or through an abdominal incision. A ureteral catheter (1) splints the ureter to facilitate healing, (2) prevents obstruction from edema after surgery or other trauma in the area, and (3) drains urine.

Complications

The major complications to monitor for are problems associated with the ureteral catheters postoperatively. They can clog or become dislodged prematurely. Ureteral catheters are rarely irrigated by the nurse.

Nursing Management

The nurse should carefully assess clients who are at high risk for obstruction for any signs or symptoms of urinary reflux. The client who is being diagnosed for urinary reflux will require support during this diagnostic process.

Preoperative preparation for ureteral surgery is similar to that required by any client requiring surgery (see Chap. 19).

Postoperatively, the nurse must closely monitor the output of the ureteral catheter. Because the renal pelvis holds only 5 ml, ureteral catheters must be kept patent. Never clamp them! Any unexpected reduction in urine flow requires prompt intervention.

Several conditions can interfere with the flow of urine through these catheters. The catheters are easily plugged with mucous shreds, blood clots, and chemical sediment. Also, ureteral peristalsis occasionally pushes the catheters out of the ureter into the bladder.

Monitor the output from these catheters closely. Each catheter, ureteral and urethral, should drain into its own collection bag so the source of the reduced flow will be noticed immediately. Measure and record the output of each catheter every hour for the first 24 hours and then every 4 to 8 hours until they are removed. Most of the urine will drain from the ureteral catheters for the first 48 to 72 hours postoperatively. As the inflammation decreases, urine flows around ureteral catheters and is drained by the urethral or suprapubic catheters.

If catheter irrigation is ordered by the physician, use strict aseptic technique. A maximum of 5 ml of irrigating solution, usually normal saline, should be allowed to flow in by gravity, or irrigated with *very* gentle force. Never irrigate this catheter with use of force. If patency cannot be established, notify the physician immediately.

Take special care not to dislodge the catheter accidentally. If the catheter is not sutured in place, secure it carefully to the skin with tape.

Assess the color of the urine frequently. Expect that the color will progress from bright red to clear yellow over a matter of days. If the urine does not clear, further investigation may be necessary.

Modification of Plan of Care for the Elderly

There are no specific modifications for the older client, although men with BPH are in the higher risk group.

Post-hospital Care

DISCHARGE TEACHING

Discharge teaching is dependent on a variety of factors: (1) the cause of the reflux, (2) the treatment done, and (3) the amount of renal damage that occurred.

If reflux is caused by BPH, the probable treatment would be prostatectomy and the discharge instructions would be based on the exact type of surgery done (see Chap. 75). If the cause is a problem with the vesicoureteral junction, then the teaching will possibly include information about catheter care at home, because these clients have a catheter in place longer.

If there is permanent renal damage, then the teaching will be similar to that given to a client with chronic renal failure (see Chap. 50).

HOME HEALTH CARE NEEDS

The major home health care need would center around care of a urethral or suprapubic catheter.

FOLLOW-UP CARE

The client with renal involvement should have renal function closely monitored, at regular intervals, for about 1 year so that any changes could be detected early.

BLADDER NEOPLASMS

Definition

Most bladder cancers are papillomatous growths within the bladder lumen, although these growths may infiltrate the bladder wall.

Incidence

Bladder cancer is the most frequent neoplasm of the urinary tract. It accounts for approximately 3 per cent of all deaths due to cancer. It occurs most frequently in the fifth to seventh decades. Also, it appears in men two to three times more often than in women, although the incidence in women is rising. This cancer is now the fifth most common cancer in men and the tenth most common cancer in women. It affects Caucasians twice as often as African Americans. It is more common in people living in the northern states as opposed to those living in the southern states.

Etiology

The disease process has several possible causes. There seems to be a strong correlation between cigarette smoking and the incidence of bladder cancer. Industrial exposure to certain substances or conditions also may cause bladder cancer. These include aniline dyes, aromatic amines like benzidine and naphthylamine, leather finishings, metal machinery, and processing petroleum products. Attempts to connect coffee consumption and bladder cancer have produced contradictory findings. Another controversy relates artificial sweeteners to the incidence of bladder cancer, although recent studies find no significant increase in bladder cancer from these.

Risk Factors

The major risk factor for bladder cancer is exposure to cigarette smoke. The best method of preventing bladder cancer is to avoid cigarette smoke, through either smoking or second-hand smoke.

Pelvic radiation, the use of cyclophosphamide (Cytoxan), chronic cystitis, bladder calculus disease, schistosomiasis, and a large phenacetin intake are all predisposing factors in the development of bladder cancer. Many of these are not amenable to primary prevention, but clients who are exposed to these factors should be monitored closely for the development of bladder cancer.

Pathophysiology

Cigarette smoking, either active or passively receiving second-hand smoke, may result in carcinogenic metabolites produced by abnormal tryptophan metabolism.

Most bladder cancers start as papillomas that undergo malignant changes. Nodular tumors occur less frequently but may also invade the bladder wall. Cellular proliferation is chiefly in the transitional epithelium (90 per cent), although squamous cell (6 per cent) or adenocarcinoma (2 per cent) may occur.

Staging of the tumor indicates the depth of penetration into the bladder wall and its degree of metastasis. Staging must be done before selection of the treatment mode. For clinical staging, the physician needs to review at least the laboratory results from an excretory urogram, cystoscopy, biopsy, and bimanual examination under anesthesia. To check for specific areas of metastasis as well as for staging, chest radiography, lymphangiography, isotope bone scans, computed tomography, and liver function analysis are needed. Figure 49-7 illustrates the usual staging schema.

- Stage 0 ($T_0N_0M_0$) tumor is limited to the mucosa.
- Stage A ($T_1N_0M_0$) tumor indicates invasion no farther than the submucosa.
- Stage B_1 ($T_2N_0M_0$) tumor extends not more than halfway through the muscle layer.
- Stage B_2 ($T_{3a}N_0M_0$) tumor penetrates more deeply into the muscle layer but not into the fat.
- Stage C ($T_{3b}N_0M_0$) tumor has infiltrated beyond the muscle layer but is not metastatic, nor is it invading adjacent structures.
- Stage D_1 ($T_{4a}N_{1-3}M_0$) tumor metastasizes to the pelvic lymph nodes.
- Stage D_2 ($T_{4a}N_4M_1$) tumor metastasizes beyond the pelvis.

Common sites for metastasis include liver, bones, and lungs. As the tumor progresses, it extends into the rectum, vaginal and soft tissue, and retroperitoneal structures. The prognostic "dividing line" lies between B_1 and B_2; tumors staged C or D on the scale have a much poorer prognosis. Superficial tumors have a good chance of being eradicated or stabilized, although recurrence is frequent. Less than 25 per cent of clients with deeply invasive tumors have a 5-year survival rate; aggressive adenocarcinoma results in an average survival rate of 21 months.

Because the incidence of recurrence is high, it is crucial to do follow-up examinations with cystoscopy. In a study of 114 clients, the interval between the original intervention and the recurrence of tumor ranged from 3 months to 27 years. Nineteen per cent involved a new tumor of a higher grade, and 22 per cent of the tumors were of a more advanced stage. Most recurrences of superficial tumors represent lesions that can be controlled by transurethral resection.

Clinical Manifestations

Painless hematuria is most frequently the first sign of bladder cancer, and it occurs in 75 per cent of all cases. Unfortunately, the bleeding is initially intermittent, which often causes a delay in seeking health care diagnostic services. As the disease progresses, the client may experience frequent bladder irritability with dysuria. Finally, gross hematuria, an obstruction, or development of a fistula may force the client to seek help.

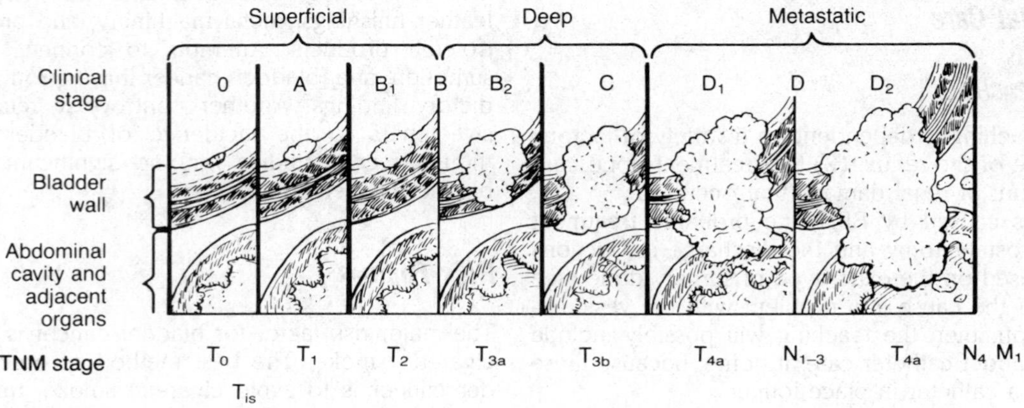

▲ *Figure 49-7*

The Jewett-Marshall clinical staging of bladder cancer. Diagram shows degree of tumor infiltration at each stage and compares it with the TNM system.

DIAGNOSTIC ASSESSMENT

The most basic test for bladder cancer is urinalysis. The presence of blood in the urine, especially if no other cause is apparent, warrants further tests. Cystoscopy should be done to visualize the tumor directly and to biopsy the lesion for cytologic study. Flow cytometry can be done to examine the DNA content of the urine cells. Cytology on a total voided urine specimen, obtained in the late morning and sent immediately to the laboratory, is done to check for the presence of malignant cells. Cytology can also be done on specimens obtained during cystoscopy. The specimen is obtained when the bladder is irrigated with a solution of Ringer's lactate.

Another examination is the IVP, which evaluates not only the bladder but also the ureters and kidneys. Computed tomography, magnetic resonance imaging, and ultrasonography may also be done to assess the bladder and surrounding structures, such as the rectum or uterus, possible sites of spread. A tumor marker, the carcinoembryonic antigen level, can also be evaluated.

Medical Management

Several forms of intervention are used in the medical management of bladder cancer, including chemotherapy and radiation therapy. Radiation therapy is more accepted for advanced disease, although it is used on early tumors outside the United States and is being studied for such use in the United States. Bladder cancers are poorly radiosensitive and therefore require high doses of radiation.

Intracavitary radiation applies radiation to the bladder malignancy while the adjacent tissues are protected. Radium seeds are inserted through a cystoscope or through a suprapubic opening in the bladder and placed directly in the tumor. Otherwise, radiation therapy may begin by the insertion of an indwelling catheter, with its balloon filled with isotopes, or the planting of seeds in the uterus or vagina. Save the urine from clients undergoing this intervention and send it to the radioisotopes laboratory for monitoring. Learn your health care facility's policies about isolation of the client, with precautions to be taken. In general, clients with implants are in a private room with limited visiting rights (see Chap. 22 for more information).

External supervoltage radiation, rather unsuccessful by itself, is effective when used in combination with surgery or chemotherapy. It may be used preoperatively to inactivate tumor cells that might disseminate during surgery and to control micrometastasis. Hyperbaric radiation therapy increases the oxygen tension of the tumor cells and therefore radiosensitivity. Palliative radiation may be used to relieve pain, bowel obstruction, and leg edema secondary to venous or lymphatic obstruction or to control bladder hemorrhage.

Several interventions are now being tried to treat bladder cancer. One such intervention is the use of hematoporphyrin derivative, which selectively goes to malignant cells, making them more photosensitive. Phototherapy or laser therapy is then used to destroy tumor cells.

The client receiving radiation therapy is at an increased risk for developing complications. The most frequent complications include severe cystitis and proctitis causing dysuria, frequency, urgency, nocturia, and diarrhea. Delayed adverse effects, such as ileitis, colitis, persistent cystitis, and bladder ulceration and hemorrhage, may occur as late as 6 to 12 months after radiation.

Radiation therapy also increases the risk of fistula formation. A fistula is an abnormal passage between two organs or between an organ and the skin. This allows intercommunication of secretions and other substances. After radiation to the bladder, a vesicovaginal fistula (in women) or a colovesical fistula (in men) may develop.

A fistula is suspected when urine leaves the body from an unnatural site such as the vagina, when fecal material or air appears in the urine, or when the client suffers from recurrent UTIs. Diagnosis is confirmed by IVP, cystoscopy, or sigmoidoscopy. To further delineate the path of a fistula, a dye such as Congo red or indigo carmine is instilled into the urinary tract, and all outlets are identified. UTI is also common with a fistula.

Before surgical repair of the fistula is undertaken, the client must maintain a continuous flow of urine from the kidney through temporary urinary diversion, either externally or with catheters. Surgical repairs often require multiple stages. The primary goal is to excise the fistula and reestablish tissue integrity.

Postoperatively, urinary diversion is maintained until the surgical site is well healed. If catheters are in place, irrigate only after consulting the physician.

The major side effects of chemotherapy include hemorrhagic cystitis and bladder irritation. Local application of formalin may control bladder hemorrhaging that results from the cancer or the treatments.

PHARMACOLOGIC MANAGEMENT

Pharmacologic agents can be administered preoperatively, postoperatively, or instead of surgery. Vitamin A analogs are being investigated for "chemoprevention" capabilities during the preneoplasia period. Antineoplastic chemotherapy is administered both topically and systemically. Intravesical instillation of an alkylating chemotherapeutic agent is the most common method; it provides concentrated topical treatment with relatively little systemic absorption. Thio-TEPA, mitomycin C, doxorubicin (Adriamycin), and cyclophosphamide (Cytoxan) are all used for this purpose.

More recently, bacille Calmette-Guérin (BCG) has been used as an intravesical agent. It is now considered more effective than the older agents and is being used more commonly than even thio-TEPA, especially in carcinoma in situ and stage A tumors. Usually the medication is injected into the bladder through a urethral catheter, the catheter is clamped or removed, and the client is asked to retain the fluid for 2 hours, and possibly to change position every 2 hours from side to side and supine to prone. The client then voids (or the catheter is unclamped) and is then instructed to drink two glasses of water to help flush the bladder. These treatments are typically repeated weekly for 4 to 8 weeks and then monthly for varying periods.

Systemic agents include cisplatin (Platinol), doxorubicin (Adriamycin), methotrexate, cyclophosphamide (Cytoxan), and pyridoxine. These agents have proved effective in prolonging life, even for metastatic disease.

DIETARY MANAGEMENT

There is no particular diet modification associated with treatment of bladder cancer. If the client develops radiation proctitis, a low-residue diet is ordered.

Surgical Management

Surgical therapy is commonly used to treat bladder cancer. Surgical intervention ranges from local resection and fulguration of the tumor to total cystectomy, which also requires diversion of normal urinary flow.

The simplest procedure, done for very early superficial tumors for cure or sometimes for inoperable tumors for palliation, is the transurethral resection (TUR) of the tumor and fulguration (destruction of tissue by electrical current through electrodes placed in direct contact with the growth).

A segmental or partial cystectomy may be done in some instances. Up to half of the bladder can be removed. During the initial postoperative period, bladder capacity is markedly reduced. The postoperative bladder may be able to hold no more than 60 ml. However, over several months, bladder tissue regenerates, increasing its capacity from 200 to 400 ml.

When the client is determined to have potentially curable disease that is too advanced for TUR or intravesical chemotherapy, the treatment of choice is total cystectomy or radical cystectomy and urinary diversion. Total cystectomy entails removal of the bladder and urethra in women and the bladder, urethra, prostate, and seminal vesicles in men. Radical cystectomy also involves the dissection of the pelvic lymph nodes and, in women, may include the removal of the uterus, fallopian tubes, and ovaries. This procedure is necessary when the tumor is invasive and involves the trigone, or whenever the malignancy cannot be treated adequately by less radical methods.

When the bladder and urethra are removed, permanent urinary diversion becomes required. Several alternatives for this are possible. The entire surgery may be done in one step with urinary diversion and cystectomy performed at the same time. The surgery may also be done in two stages, with urinary diversion performed during the first operation and cystectomy done several weeks later. Radiation therapy may be given between treatments.

Urinary diversion is essential after total or radical cystectomy and removal of the urethra. In addition, it may help to establish adequate urinary drainage in clients with meningomyelocele, exstrophy of the bladder, neurogenic bladder, mechanical obstruction to the outflow of urine, severe interstitial or hemorrhagic cystitis, or trauma to the lower urinary tract interfering with normal function.

Ureters may be implanted into the colon so urine passes through the rectum, or the ureters may simply empty through an opening in the skin. Openings into the kidney are established to drain urine directly from the renal pelvis into an external collection system. Figure 49–8 illustrates the variety of urinary diversion methods used.

Ureterosigmoidostomy and ureteroileosigmoidostomy are two outdated methods of diversion resulting in the excretion of urine through the rectum, mixed with feces. This procedure is not done anymore because of the severe problems of chronic pyelonephritis and hyperchloremic acidosis associated with it. Other surgeries can provide continence without the complications.

Cutaneous ureterostomy attaches the ureter to the surface of the abdomen where urine flows directly into a drainage appliance without an intermediary conduit. There are several variations of this procedure.

- A single or bilateral ureterostomy brings the distal end of the ureter out through the abdominal wall, creating one or two stomas as appropriate.
- A transureteroureterostomy produces only one stoma, because one ureter is connected to the other ureter.
- A double-barreled ureterostomy forms two stomas in very close proximity as both ureters are brought to the surface together.
- A loop ureterostomy is usually a temporary diversion that brings the midsection of the ureters to the skin surface for drainage. The rest of the urinary tract is left intact, allowing normal urinary functioning to be reestablished later. For clients with ureterostomies, infection, obstruction to urine flow, and skin irritation are potential problems.
- A vesicostomy produces a hole in the abdomen directly over the bladder. After suturing the bladder to the abdominal wall, the surgeon forms a stoma from the bladder wall. Through this stoma, the bladder can be emptied.

Nephrostomy is insertion of catheters into the renal pelvis by surgical incision or a percutaneous puncture procedure. In the surgical approach, a balloon- or mushroom-tipped catheter is connected to an external drainage system. In percutaneous nephrostomy, a trocar is inserted under fluoroscopy by direct puncture into the renal pelvis or calix. Then a flexible small-gauge needle is used to instill contrast material to verify proper location. By use of angiographic wire as a guide, the nephrostomy tube is placed and connected to a closed drainage system. The entire procedure is done under local anesthesia. It is important to stabilize the tube to prevent dislodgement. Figure 49–9 shows a percutaneous nephrostomy tube in place and a suggested method for stabilization.

If the nephrostomy tube is used to divert urine flow while the ureters are repaired, it may be temporary. It is more often permanent, especially if the ureters are removed as part of a cystectomy. Because of the high

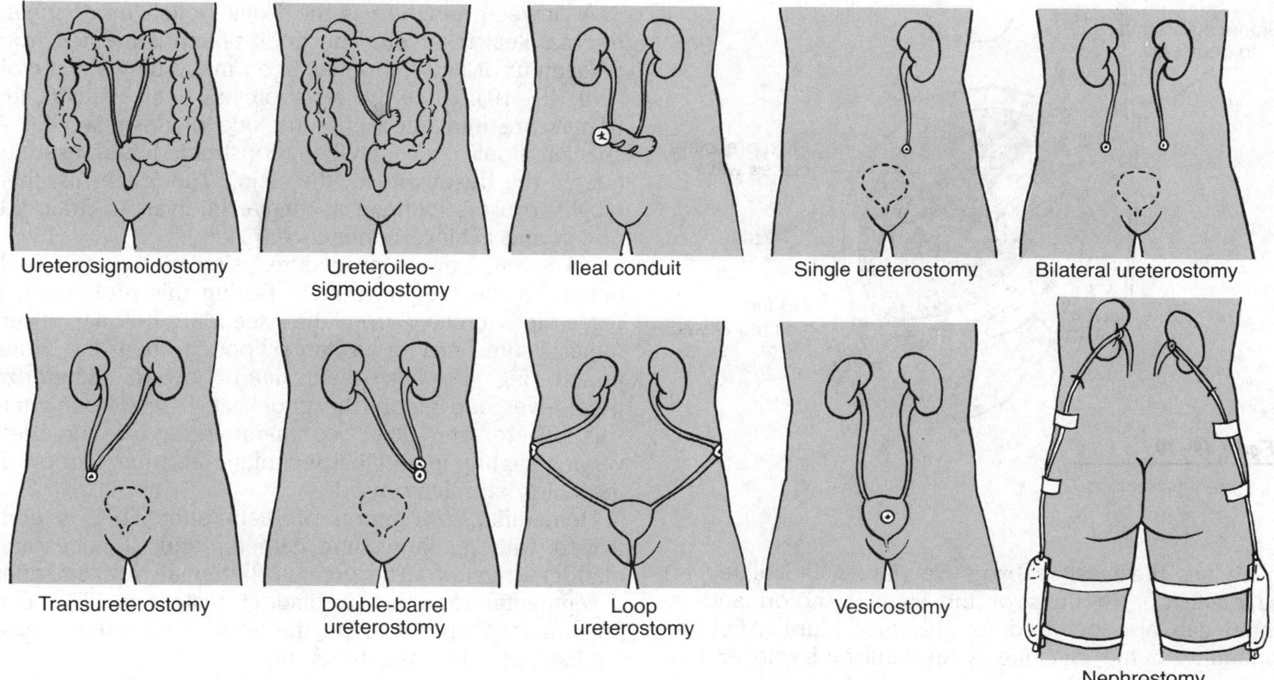

▲ *Figure 49–8*

Surgical alternatives for urinary diversion.

risk of infection and calculus formation, nephrostomy is a last resort and considered only a palliative measure. Other complications include erosion of the collection system by the catheter, hemorrhage, mucosal edema, obstruction of the catheter, and perforation of the calix during catheter insertion.

An ileal conduit, also called ureteroileostomy, ileal bladder, or Bricker's procedure, is the most common urinary diversion alternative now available. Using a segment of the intestine as a conduit, this procedure constructs a system so urine is emptied through an opening in the skin. Usually, a portion of the terminal ileum,

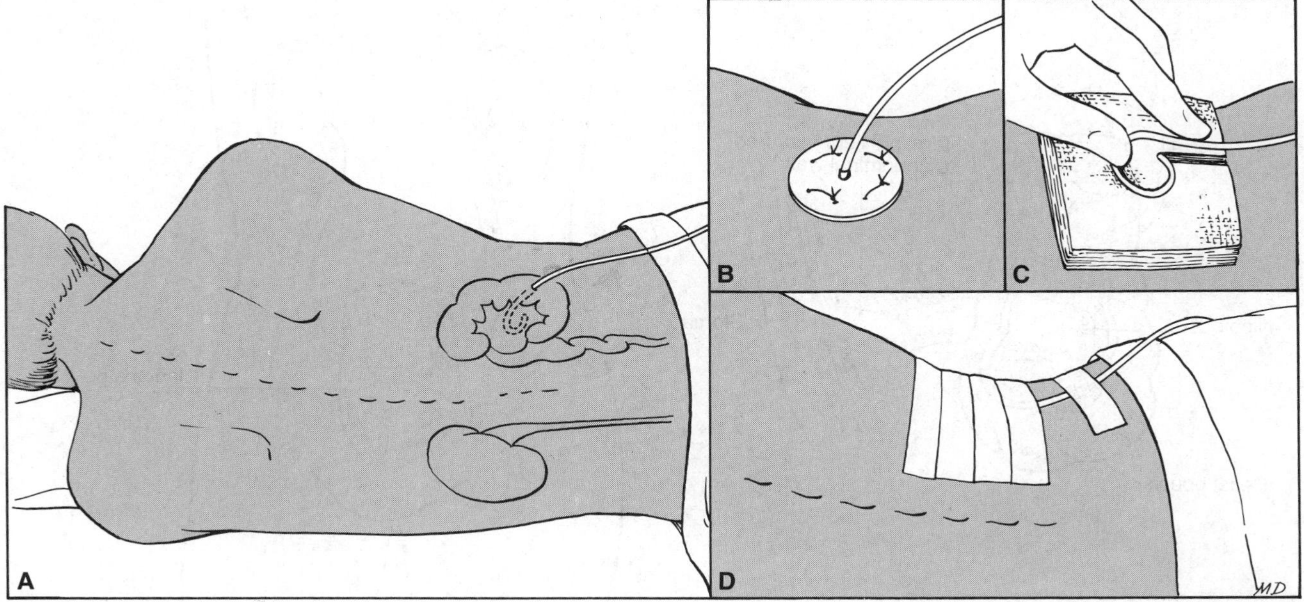

▲ *Figure 49–9*

Percutaneous nephrostomy tube and suggested method for stabilization. *A*, Insertion point in kidney. *B*, Securing nephrostomy tube to skin with sutured disc. *C*, Snip 4 × 4 with sterile scissors, cover disc with 4 × 4 as shown, and loop tubing. *D*, Cover entire 4 × 4 with tape. (Adapted from Cain, L., and Bigongiari, L., [1982]. The percutaneous nephrostomy tube. *American Journal of Nursing, 82*:296.)

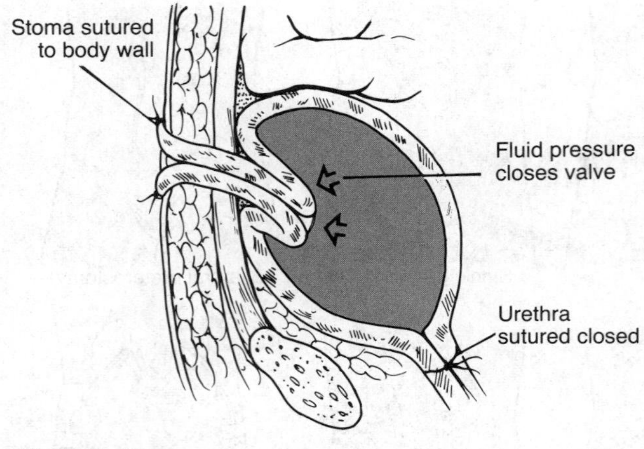

▲ *Figure 49–10*

A continent vesicostomy.

which has the least reabsorptive power, is isolated for the diversion. Portions of the sigmoid colon and jejunum can also be used for this procedure. After the continuity of the intestine is reestablished with end-to-end anastomosis, the proximal end of the segment is closed. The distal end is brought out through a hole created in the abdominal wall and sutured to the skin to form a stoma. The ureters are then implanted into the ileal segment. The urine flows into the conduit and is continually propelled out through the stoma by peristalsis. Because the ileal segment is not a reservoir, there is minimal absorption of electrolytes. This avoids the imbalances that occur when the rectum serves as a reservoir. An ileal conduit requires the client to wear an appliance for collecting urine.

A newer procedure is the Kock pouch or continent internal ileal reservoir. The Kock pouch is created from a segment of ileum that has been made into a reservoir (Fig. 49–10). Once the reservoir has been created, the ureters are implanted into the side of the reservoir. A special nipple valve is then constructed and used to attach the reservoir to the skin. The client is then taught to use a catheter at regular intervals to drain the pouch and achieve continence.

An even newer procedure, similar to the Kock pouch, is the Indiana pouch. During this procedure, a reservoir is created from the ascending colon and terminal ileum, making a larger pouch than the Kock pouch (Fig. 49–11). Clients learn how to catheterize themselves and empty the pouch at 4- to 6-hour intervals. There are other continent reservoir surgeries, varying slightly in surgical technique and the portion of the colon and ileum used.

Hematuria, a common problem after TUR, is controlled with an indwelling catheter and, if necessary, bladder irrigation. The greatest potential problem after a segmental resection is bladder distention. This can put too much pressure on the area of resection, causing leakage and possibly rupture.

A radical cystectomy can cause several complications. It is a very invasive surgery, lasting hours, that leaves the client at risk for most of the usual postoperative complications including shock, hemorrhage, and thrombophlebitis. The pelvic lymph node dissection can predispose to the development of lower extremity lymphedema. Male clients who have undergone a radical cystectomy and radical pelvic node dissection may be impotent postoperatively; however, newer nerve-sparing procedures have lessened the risk of this occurring. Men will have a "dry" orgasm, however, be-

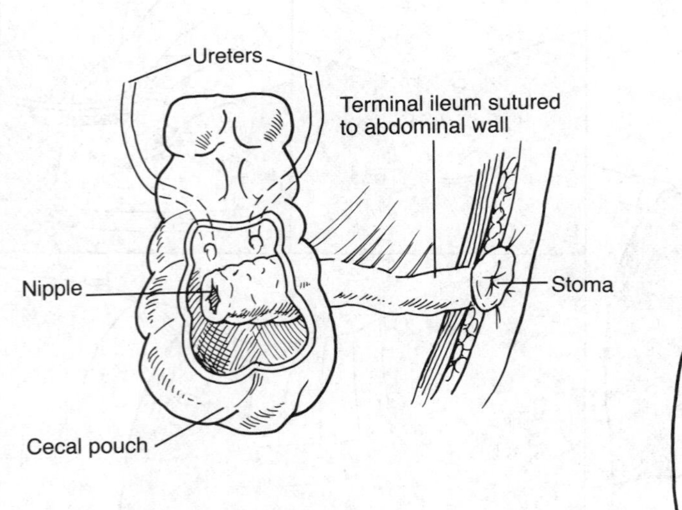

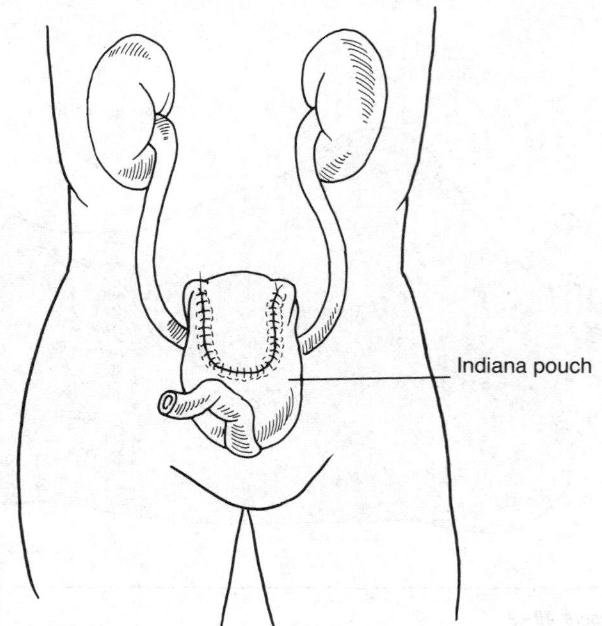

▲ *Figure 49–11*

Indiana pouch procedure.

cause the prostate and seminal vesicles have been removed.

The most common complication of the ileal conduit is the late development of obstruction at the ureteroileal anastomosis. Other complications include pyelonephritis, leakage at the anastomosis site, stenosis anywhere along the system, hydronephrosis, calculi, peristomal hernia, uremia, skin irritation, ulceration, and stomal defects.

The complications of a Kock pouch or an Indiana pouch include incontinence, difficult catheterization, urinary reflux and possible pyelonephritis, obstruction, bacteriuria, electrolyte imbalances, or absorptive problems.

Nursing Management

ASSESSMENT

The nurse should begin the assessment of the client being evaluated for bladder cancer with a careful history, looking especially for exposure to known risk factors.

The nurse should also question the client about changes in the urine or in urination, noting changes in color, frequency, and amounts of urine. The presence of hematuria should always be investigated further.

NURSING INTERVENTION

Nursing Diagnosis: Injury, High Risk for R/T radiation therapy and chemotherapy.

Planning: Expected Outcomes. The client will not develop problems related to radiation therapy or chemotherapy, as evidenced by absence of hemorrhagic cystitis.

Implementation. Intervention for the side effects of radiation therapy includes administering antispasmodics, increasing the client's fluid intake, and administering urinary tract antiseptics for the cystitis. The client with proctitis requires a low-residue diet and agents to decrease intestinal motility. Complete information on nursing care for clients receiving radiation therapy is covered in Chapter 22.

Nursing care for the client receiving chemotherapy is covered in Chapter 22. If the client has intravesical chemotherapy, the nurse should remember to treat the urine as a biohazard, the same as any other chemotherapy that needs to be disposed of properly.

Nursing Diagnosis: Urinary Elimination, Altered (Dysuria) R/T presence of tumors.

Planning: Expected Outcomes. The client will have tumors diagnosed early to eliminate the dysuria.

Implementation. Nursing care after TUR is covered in detail in Chapter 75. The client will have some hematuria and, until the bleeding ceases, an indwelling urethral catheter. Sometimes the catheter will be attached to a continuous or intermittent closed bladder irrigation system to prevent blood clots. Nursing intervention is similar to that after a cystoscopy or TUR of the prostate. This includes adequate intake of fluids, analgesics, and antispasmodics as needed.

Nursing care for the client who has had segmental resection centers on maintaining constant urinary drainage so the bladder does not become distended, straining the suture line. The client usually has both a urethral and a suprapubic catheter. The suprapubic catheter is usually left in for 2 weeks, until complete healing has occurred, so the client will be discharged with the catheter in place.

Nursing Diagnosis: Knowledge Deficit R/T diagnostic tests, surgery, and care of urinary diversion.

Planning: Expected Outcomes. The client will understand the diagnostic tests, surgery, and care of the urinary diversion, as evidenced by client's statements and demonstration of ability to care for his or her own diversion.

Implementation. Preoperative preparation of clients undergoing diversionary surgery includes (1) giving teaching guidelines concerning urinary diversion and (2) encouraging acceptance of the fact that diversion results in the elimination of urine through the skin, rectum, or specially constructed stoma and not through the urethral meatus as was once "normal."

In addition to general physical and emotional preparation, the client's bowel may need the following special attention: a nonresidue diet for several days, sterilization of the bowel with neomycin, and bowel cleansing with cathartics or enemas.

If the surgeon plans to construct a stoma, the site is selected during the preoperative period. An enterostomal therapist should be involved in the care at this point and throughout the care of this client. The main criterion for stomal placement is that the site will allow the faceplate of the drainage appliance to bind securely to the abdominal surface. This means that the surgeon must avoid the umbilicus, rib margins, pubis, and iliac crests. Placing the stoma directly on the client's waistline will cause excessive pressure by clothing. The client is observed in the supine, standing, and sitting positions during the selection process. Usually the stoma is created in the right or left lower quadrant of the abdomen.

Skin irritation or breakdown is a constant threat to the client who has undergone urinary diversion. Advise the client to prevent urine from contacting the skin. This can be achieved in part by using a well-fitted and properly attached appliance (Fig. 49–12). The opening in the adhesive backing of the temporary pouch or faceplate of the permanent appliance should be not more than 3 mm larger than the stoma. The faceplate opening will need to be remeasured after the edema in the stoma recedes. Each time the pouch is changed, the skin around the stoma should be cleaned with soap and water and thoroughly dried. Any adhesive material

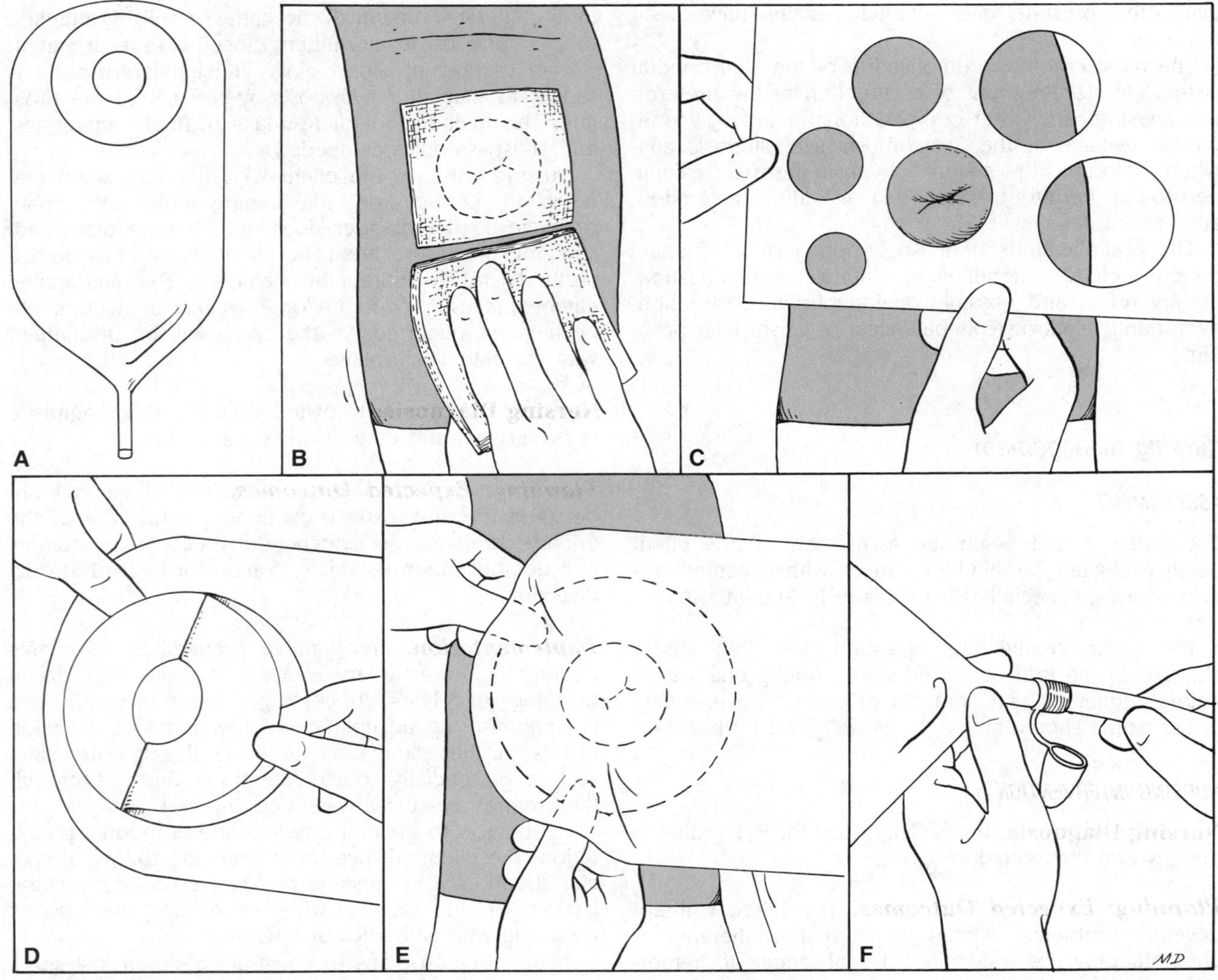

▲ *Figure 49–12*

Applying a disposable ostomy pouch. *A*, Gather supplies: ostomy pouch, ostomy belt, skin barrier, stoma template, gauze pads, pouch clip or rubber band, safety pin, and clean gloves. Clamp or rubber band end of pouch to prevent leakage during procedure. Make sure that lighting is adequate and that client is comfortable and understands procedure. Wash hands and don clean examining gloves. *B*, Gently remove old pouch, using warm water or adhesive solvent around seal if necessary. Place gauze pad over stoma to prevent leakage as you gently cleanse peristomal area with moist gauze. *C*, Measure stoma with stoma template. Trace shape onto skin barrier and adhesive, using template. Cut openings no more than 3 mm larger than stoma. *D*, Remove backing from adhesive surface of disposable ostomy pouch. *E*, Center pouch opening over stoma with pouch drain pointing to floor. (If client ambulates frequently, pouch drain should point to client's feet.) Make sure seal is complete. *F*, Connect drainage tubing to ostomy pouch if appropriate. Secure tubing (with rubber band around tubing, pin rubber band to sheets if client is immobile).

adhering to the skin must be removed with adhesive remover. If crystals are present on the skin, wash with a diluted vinegar solution to help remove them. A gauze pad or tampon should be placed over the stoma during cleansing to prevent urine from flowing out over the skin. Remove this pad or tampon just as the appliance is reapplied. The appliance should be changed early in the morning, because urine production is slowest at this time.

Because urine is not as corrosive to the skin as feces is, a skin barrier is not always used. However, some authorities suggest that a skin barrier be applied prophylactically. If a barrier is used, its stoma opening is cut just large enough to fit over the stoma and applied next to the skin before attaching the pouch or faceplate. A skin bond cement or adhesive disc may help the faceplate stick more securely to the skin. A non–water-soluble adhesive spray will allow the client to go swimming.

Once the skin is properly prepared, the nurse or individual can complete application of the appliance. With a temporary pouch, the paper is removed from the adhesive backing, and the opening in the back is placed over the stoma. Affix the adhesive portion firmly to the skin, avoiding creases and wrinkles. The temporary pouch may attach to a continuous, closed drainage system.

For a permanent appliance, stretch the pouch onto the faceplate so that it will lie smoothly. Carefully center the faceplate over the stoma and adhere it to the skin. For added security, nonallergic adhesive tape strips may be placed around the edges of the temporary pouch or the faceplate. A belt may hold the faceplate in place, especially if the client engages in strenuous activities. For added security, this belt may be worn continuously. If a belt is used, caution the client against excessive tightness, which may lead to pressure sores under the faceplate. Whatever type of pouch is used, direct the opening at the bottom toward the floor to ensure adequate drainage.

A permanent pouch usually has a valve in the bottom that can be opened and closed, allowing the urine to collect for intermittent emptying. Alternatively, the pouch may be drained by gravity into a bedside bag (especially at night) or a leg bag. The self-contained pouch drainage system allows the client to resume most, if not all, former activities with very little or no change in style of dress. However, caution the client to empty the pouch frequently; the weight of accumulating urine may pull the faceplate away from the skin and cause leakage. Advise the client also to check the seal often if heavily perspiring.

Odor is a common problem with urinary stomas. Noxious odors result mostly from poor hygiene, alkaline urine, normal breakdown of urine (ammonia), and the ingestion of certain foods, such as asparagus. Although permanent appliances are rarely used today, to control odors in them, wash reusable appliances thoroughly with soap and lukewarm water. The pouch can also be soaked in dilute white vinegar or in a commercial deodorant product for 20 to 30 minutes. Rinse the pouch and allow it to dry.

For all appliances, deodorant tablets are available that can be placed in the pouch while it is being worn. Ingestion of methionine can alleviate the smell of ammonia, and acidifying the urine reduces odor. Because diluted urine is less odiferous, adequate fluid intake is most helpful in preventing odor.

Care for the client with a Kock or Indiana pouch is similar to that of any client with a urinary diversion, except there is no pouch. The client will have a Medena tube in place to drain the urine continuously until the pouch has healed. The catheter may be irrigated with normal saline to wash out any clots or mucus that might plug it. The Medena catheter is removed 3 to 4 weeks after the surgery, and the client is taught the self-catheterization procedure. At the beginning, the client is taught to insert the catheter every 2 to 3 hours to drain the pouch. Later, the interval can be every 4 to 6 hours during the day and once during the night.

Nursing Diagnosis: Self-Esteem Disturbance and Body Image Disturbance R/T urinary diversion.

Planning: Expected Outcomes. The client will have a normal self-concept, body image, and self-esteem after the urinary diversion, as evidenced by the client's return to normal life.

Implementation. Whatever diversion alternative is selected, assume that the client and significant others will need a great deal of emotional support. Changing the normal route of urine flow and the client's usual micturition pattern will change the client's self-image, including alterations in emotional, psychosocial, and perceptual reactions. Preoperative counseling should fully explain the expected anatomic and physiologic alterations, including their possible effect on the client. Counseling should also present ways to maintain the client's current life style. Community associations and their resources, such as the United Ostomy Association and the American Cancer Society, are a tremendous help to the client undergoing diversion. Remember that most clients experience denial as a defense mechanism both pre- and postoperatively. Thus, the nurse must share hope and faith when guiding the client and significant others through their initial unwillingness to accept the procedure. You may need to restrict teaching content to essentials and frequently repeat instructions before learning actually takes place. Postoperatively, the client and significant others may need help to look at the stoma and to accept it as part of the total self.

Nursing Diagnosis: Injury, High Risk for R/T postoperative complications such as hemorrhage, paralytic ileus, stomal ischemia, and blocking of ureteral catheters.

Planning: Expected Outcomes. The client will not develop postoperative injury, as evidenced by vital signs within preoperative norms, presence of active bowel sounds within 3 to 4 days postoperatively, pink stoma, and at least 30 to 60 ml urine output via ureteral catheters.

Implementation. Postoperative nursing management of the client includes routine monitoring of the vital signs, inspection of the incision, and other postoperative intervention as described in Chapter 19. The client often has a nasogastric tube in place, because postoperative ileus is a common complication. If the client has nephrostomy tubes, they are connected to a bedside drainage system. Keep tubing patent to prevent obstruction to the free flow of urine. Also keep the drainage system closed to help prevent pyelonephritis. If the client has a stoma, there will be a temporary, clear plastic pouch over the stoma that connects to a gravity drainage system. Sometimes ureteral catheters are used to splint the ureters while they heal. These catheters, usually removed before the client is discharged, may extend through the stoma but are ordinarily visible just inside the stomal opening.

For all postoperative clients after diversion, nursing intervention includes the following actions:

- Measure urine output every hour for the first 24 hours, and afterward at least every 8 hours.
- Check the ostomy bag for leaks and the skin under it

for irritation every 4 hours initially and then every 8 hours.

- Inspect the stoma every hour for the first 24 hours after surgery. This will give you a baseline from which you can quickly detect deviations. Then, if there are no problems, extend intervals to every 4 hours and then every 8 hours.
- Note the stoma's size, shape, and color. An edematous stoma is expected in the immediate postoperative period. However, other changes may indicate complications, warranting action from the physician. A dusky or cyanotic color of the stoma may denote an insufficient blood supply and the onset of necrosis. This is an emergency! The reduced blood supply may result from (1) the surgical technique, (2) an appliance faceplate that is too small or improperly centered, or (3) peristomal protective materials that have been poorly applied. Other complications with the stoma include prolapse (protrusion from the skin) or retraction into the abdomen beneath the skin.
- Watch for signs of peritonitis, because leakage at the site of the anastomosis or ureteral separation from the conduit causes urine to seep into the peritoneal cavity.
- Observe for bleeding. Although bleeding from the stoma may indicate a surgical defect, it is also common for the intestinal mucosa, which is very fragile, to bleed during a change of appliance or because of a poorly fitted collection pouch.

Stenosis of the stoma may occur from scarring during stomal maturation. If the opening on the faceplate is too large, epithelial hyperplasia, or thickening of the peristomal skin, may contract the stoma. Clients with urinary diversion are also prone to uric acid and calcium stone disease. The onset of urinary stone development usually occurs at least 2 years postoperatively and sometimes as long as 5 to 10 years later. UTI is a perpetual threat because of the exposure of the urinary tract. Obstruction anywhere in the urinary tract will interfere with normal urine flow.

Nursing Diagnosis: Skin Integrity, High Risk for Impaired R/T irritation of peristomal skin.

Planning: Expected Outcomes. The client will not develop an altered skin integrity or irritation of peristomal skin, as evidenced by intact, clear skin.

Implementation. Intervention for any skin irritation must begin promptly. Check the pH of the urine; strongly alkaline urine irritates the skin and facilitates crystal formation. If urine cultures identify UTI, it must be treated. The appliance should be checked carefully to find any leakage and to determine whether the skin is sensitive to anything used in the process of application. Skin irritation may also result from changing the pouch too frequently. A general recommendation is that the pouch be left in place as long as it is not leaking. During changes of the appliance, leave the skin open to the air as much as possible. When the appliance is reattached, dust the skin with Stomahesive powder and apply a pouch with a Stomahesive skin barrier. Karaya cannot be used with urinary pouches because urine corrodes the karaya.

Skin irritation around the stoma is often caused by a yeast infection. Nystatin creams or powders are used to treat this. Nystatin powder is applied directly over the irritated skin area and then sealed to the skin with a liquid skin barrier.

Nursing Diagnosis: Sexuality Patterns, Altered R/T potential postoperative impotence in men after radical cystectomy.

Planning: Expected Outcomes. The client will accept alternative methods of sexual expression as evidenced by client's statements.

Interventions. Male clients have a high risk of impotence after a radical cystectomy related to the extent of the resection. It is important for them to receive counseling both before and after the surgery so they can begin to adjust to any alterations. Chapter 75 discusses alterations in male sexuality in detail.

EVALUATION

To evaluate the care that has been given, the nurse formulates outcome criteria. If the goals were not met, alterations in the plan and interventions will be needed. The nurse must continually evaluate the outcomes and modify the interventions as needed.

Modification of Plan of Care for the Elderly

The major modification for older clients with urinary diversion centers around possible difficulties they may have with self-care of the appliance. Changing the appliance requires some degree of dexterity, and older clients are more likely to have arthritis and other disabilities that limit their ability to manipulate the pouches. They may require assistance or modification of teaching so they can retain some independence.

Post-hospital Care

Long-term nursing intervention aims to maintain a functional urinary system and prevent complications. It takes time for the client and significant others to adjust to the client's body. Even though counseling may have been excellent during the preoperative period, the reality of the diversion usually produces further anxiety, depression, and anger. The client may need help at first to look at or even talk about the stoma. As soon as possible, the client must begin to help care for the stoma, peristomal skin, and drainage system, gradually assuming more responsibility until achieving independence.

DISCHARGE TEACHING

Clients who have undergone urinary diversion need the enterostomal therapist's and the nurse's help and encouragement to regain their independence and accept their new body image. A well-balanced teaching plan includes both the client and significant others. To implement the teaching plan, the nurse must

- Encourage clients to take an active role in their care as soon as possible.
- Create an environment as similar as possible to that of the client's home.
- Help the client organize the equipment and procedures necessary for stomal care.
- Teach the client how to remove and reapply the appliance, empty the pouch, and attach it to the night drainage system.
- Discuss adaptations the client may need to make while traveling.
- If necessary, help the client select new clothing that will not constrict the drainage pouch.
- Emphasize how important it is to maintain a daily fluid intake of at least 2000 ml.
- Teach the client how to select the proper foods and fluids.
- Give clear, written instructions regarding when to contact the physician (e.g., changes in color or quantity of urine output, cloudy or foul-smelling urine, or stomal color changes).

The client with a suprapubic catheter or Medena tube will have to be taught to care for it before discharge. This client will come home with a urinary pouch on and will continue to wear it until the surgically created pouch completely heals.

HOME HEALTH CARE NEEDS

The client with a new urinary diversion should be followed at home by a visiting nurse to ensure that the client is correctly caring for the diversion. The client must also be told where to obtain supplies needed to care for the diversion.

FOLLOW-UP CARE

The client with bladder cancer should be followed and assessed for recurrence of the cancer. The client should also continue to be seen by an enterostomal therapist, especially at the postoperative office visit, to be sure that no problems have arisen concerning the ostomy.

URINARY BLADDER CALCULI

Definition

Urinary calculi (urolithiasis) are stones within the urinary system. Stones are primarily formed in the kidney, although some originate in the bladder. This section discusses only bladder stones; nephrolithiasis is discussed in Chapter 50.

Incidence

Primary bladder calculi are rare. Kidney stones may pass into the bladder and linger. Renal lithiasis is a common problem. Some regions of the country have a higher frequency of stone formation, such as the southern states and the Great Lakes region. It is more common in men than in women and occurs more frequently in young adults and early middle adulthood. Once a client has had calculi, they tend to recur at a rate of 50 per cent in 5 to 10 years.

Etiology

Infection, presence of a foreign body, failure to empty the bladder normally, and obstruction within the urinary tract all contribute to the formation of bladder calculi. The two primary causative factors are urinary stasis and supersaturation of urine with poorly soluble crystalloids, such as calcium crystals, which precipitate easily in the urine. Hypercalcemia predisposes to calculi formation by the increased calcium excreted in the urine.

Risk Factors

Risk factors for stone formation in the bladder include those things that cause stasis, retention, or supersaturation of the urine. These include stressors such as immobility that increases stasis, dehydration that leads to supersaturation, and an increase in calcium or other ion in the urine. Other major risk factors include having had urinary calculi previously, bladder outlet obstruction, neurogenic bladder, and prolonged indwelling catheterization.

These risk factors have primary preventions that can be implemented. Frequent turning of immobilized clients, a high fluid intake, and decreased calcium in the diet in susceptible individuals help prevent stones. These will also help decrease the recurrence of stones.

Some stones are composed of uric acid. The prime risk factor for these stones is an alteration in purine metabolism as seen with gout. Controlling the production and excretion of uric acid can help prevent these stones.

Pathophysiology

The exact mechanism of stone formation has not been clearly defined. A primary factor in stone formation is the supersaturation of the urine with elements such as calcium, phosphate, and oxalate. Certain factors contribute to the ease of stone formation. These factors include the pH of the urine, the amount of solute in the urine, and the amount of solution or urine. Problems with purine metabolism predispose to the formation of uric acid stones.

Prolonged immobility leads to urinary stasis and, because of calcium mobilization from the bones, an increase in serum and urine calcium. If the fluid intake is also inadequate, then the calcium saturating the urine is more likely to precipitate out and form stones.

The pH of the urine also contributes to stone formation or stone dissolution. Uric acid and cystine stones are more likely to precipitate in acid urine; calcium phosphate and struvite stones are more common in alkaline urine. Oxalate stones are not affected by urine pH.

Clinical Manifestations

Calculi range in size from almost undetectable to several centimeters in diameter. Stones formed in the kidney may continue to grow in the bladder. As long as these stones remain in the bladder, the client will probably be asymptomatic, because pain is associated with stones that migrate. However, some people do experience cystitis symptoms. A very large stone lodged against the bladder neck during micturition may cause a heavy feeling in the suprapubic region, a decreased bladder capacity, and an intermittent urinary stream. The stone may partially or totally obstruct urine or cause mucosal trauma if it enters the urethra.

DIAGNOSTIC ASSESSMENT

The major diagnostic examination for radiopaque stones is a simple radiograph, a flat plate of the abdomen. Uric acid stones are not radiopaque (cannot be seen on x-ray film); however, an elevated serum uric acid, with symptoms of stones, may be diagnostic of these stones.

When the stones are passed, they are analyzed for their components. It is important to identify the exact stone composition so exact preventive measures can be implemented.

Medical Management

If urinary stones are suspected, the nurse must strain all urine through a urine strainer or at least four layers of gauze pads. After straining, inspect the filter or pads carefully for stones; if any are found, send them to the laboratory for stone analysis. During the period that the urine is being filtered, encourage the client to drink 3000 to 4000 ml of fluid per day (unless contraindicated). This helps wash out the stones and hinders their formation by diluting the urine. The type of fluid is dependent on the type of stone; if it is calcium, acid-ash fluids should be taken to help the calcium remain in solution.

Sometimes just waiting for a time will allow the stones to pass naturally from the bladder. However, if this does not occur, or if a cystogram shows that the calculus is too large to pass safely through the urethra, more invasive treatment is necessary.

PHARMACOLOGIC MANAGEMENT

There are no particular medications used to treat calcium stones. If the client has uric acid stones, medications to lower uric acid such as allopurinol (Zyloprim) should be given. If the client is in pain, narcotics and antispasmodics are used.

DIETARY MANAGEMENT

Once the components of the stone have been identified, diet modification will be used to help prevent recurrence. A low-calcium, low-oxalate diet is used for calcium or oxalate stones, and a low-purine diet for uric acid stones.

Surgical Management

Sound waves may be applied externally to break up stones in the kidney or ureter (see Fig. 50–9). Also, the physician may remove small bladder stones transurethrally or with a cystoscope. Large stones may be broken up with an instrument called a lithotrite (stone crusher). This procedure is called litholapaxy, and it is followed by complete irrigation of the bladder to wash out stones. In lithotripsy, an electrohydraulic lithotrite delivers an electrical charge to fragment a stone.

If the stone cannot be removed transurethrally, a suprapubic approach may be used. In a procedure called cystolithotomy, the surgeon makes a suprapubic incision into the bladder and removes the stones.

Possible complications after litholapaxy and lithotripsy include hemorrhage, urinary retention, infection, and possible stone recurrence.

Nursing Management

When a client is admitted with a diagnosis of bladder calculi, the major nursing responsibilities center around maintaining adequate urine output. The nurse should force fluids up to 4000 ml a day, unless otherwise contraindicated, so that good output is ensured. All urine must be strained to be sure that the stone is recovered and sent for analysis. If the stone does not pass, the nurse should prepare the client for a more invasive procedure.

Postoperatively, after litholapaxy, the nurse must monitor for signs of hemorrhage, urinary retention, infection, and stone recurrence. Maintain the client on a high fluid intake and, if prescribed, administer intermittent bladder irrigations to wash out possible stone fragments. The nurse should continue to strain all urine.

Nursing care after cystolithotomy is similar to the care of a client after suprapubic prostatectomy (see Chap. 75).

Modification of Plan of Care for the Elderly

There are no specific modifications for the older client except the increased risk of complications of surgery associated with aging (see Chap. 19).

Post-hospital Care

DISCHARGE TEACHING

The client must be taught methods for avoiding recurrence or for at least detecting the stones early if they recur. This includes teaching the client to increase fluid intake; void every 2 hours; maintain an acidic urine pH (unless the stones are uric acid); change diet to low-calcium, low-phosphate for calcium stones or low-purine for uric acid stones; and take medications to improve excretion of uric acid for uric acid stones. The client should also be taught to recognize any signs of recurrence.

HOME HEALTH CARE NEEDS

The client does not usually require any specific home health care after the stone is passed or removed.

FOLLOW-UP CARE

The client should be followed at intervals for signs of recurrent calculi. Follow-up urinalysis and blood measures for the presence of the stone-causing agents are done at intervals.

NEUROGENIC BLADDER DYSFUNCTION

Definition

The term "neurogenic bladder" refers to several bladder dysfunctions, all of which are caused by lesions of the central or peripheral nervous systems. Their manifestations depend on the site of the lesion.

There are five major types of neurogenic bladder dysfunction (Fig. 49-13): (1) uninhibited, (2) sensory paralytic (detrusor muscle hyperreflexic), (3) motor paralytic (detrusor muscle areflexic), (4) autonomous, and (5) reflex.

Neurogenic bladder dysfunctions may also be classified according to the level of the lesion within the central nervous system. Dysfunctions related to lesions in the upper motor neuron occur above the sacral segments of the spinal cord; lesions in or below the sacral vertebrae produce lower motor neuron bladders. Upper motor neuron bladders are spastic or hyperreflexic; lower motor neuron bladders are areflexic or atonic.

Incidence

The incidence of neurogenic bladder dysfunctions is dependent on the incidence of the various neurologic injuries or disorders that cause these problems. With certain disorders, 100 per cent of clients will develop a neurogenic bladder (such as with transection of the cord); with other neurologic disorders, fewer clients will be affected (such as with multiple sclerosis).

Etiology

The uninhibited neurogenic bladder produces "infant-like" or uninhibited voiding. The urge to void causes urine excretion. This type is caused primarily by lesions in the corticoregulatory tracts (e.g., cerebrovascular accidents, multiple sclerosis).

The sensory paralytic bladder results from an interruption in the lateral spinal tracts (e.g., tabes dorsalis, diabetic neuropathy, and pernicious anemia). Because of the sensory loss, the client cannot perceive bladder filling. This lack of perception leads to chronic retention with overflow incontinence.

A motor paralytic bladder is the most uncommon type and is caused by lesions in the motor outflow from sacral vertebrae 2 to 4 (S2 to S4). Disease processes that cause this dysfunction include poliomyelitis, tumor, trauma, and infection. This dysfunction may be temporary if it is caused by a bacterial or viral infection. Although there is full sensation of bladder filling, even to the point of pain, the client is unable to initiate micturition.

The individual with an autonomous neurogenic bladder can neither perceive bladder fullness nor initiate or maintain urination without some type of "assistance" (such as applying external pressure on the abdomen). Retention and incontinence are common problems. This type occurs after destruction of all nerve connections between the bladder and the central nervous system at S2, S3, or S4 (e.g., trauma, inflammatory processes, spinal anesthesia, or malignancy).

Finally, transection of the spinal cord above the sacral segments causes a reflex neurogenic bladder. There is no sensation, and the bladder contracts reflexively but does not empty completely. A client's neurogenic bladder may involve a combination of one or more nervous system dysfunctions.

Risk Factors

Risk factors for neurogenic bladder disorders include tumors, neurologic disorders, and trauma to the nervous system. Accidents are the most preventable cause of this problem; tumors and many neurologic diseases are not preventable.

Pathophysiology

Lesions at the lower motor neuron level of the spinal cord often directly interfere with the reflex arc and lead to inappropriate interpretation of efferent and afferent impulses. When the bladder fills, the message is transmitted through afferent fibers to the brain cortex. The injury, however, keeps these impulses from being correctly interpreted, leading to no impulse for micturition. A flaccid bladder with urinary retention is the result.

With upper motor neuron lesions, impulses are not transmitted to or from the lower spinal areas to the cortex. When the client's bladder distends, no sensation is transmitted. Because the lower cord is intact,

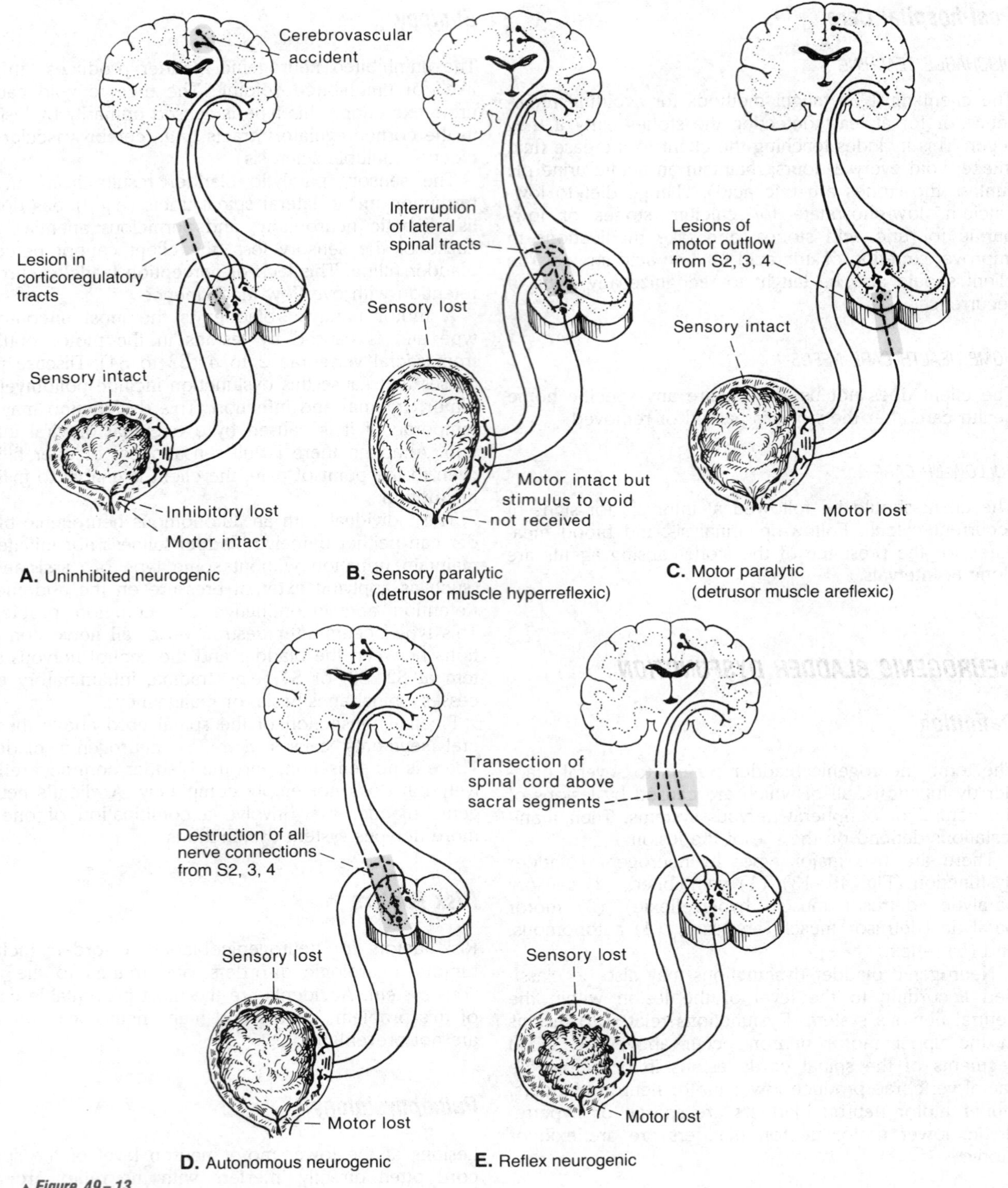

▲ *Figure 49–13*

Types of neurogenic bladder dysfunction.

however, activity of the reflex arc can occur, and the client will have reflex incontinence of urine.

When the damage is to the cortical area itself, such as with a stroke or trauma, the client cannot correctly interpret the impulses that are being transmitted.

The client with a dysfunctional bladder is more likely than normal to develop serious UTIs, skin breakdown associated with incontinence, and even renal disease due to chronic overdistention of the bladder.

Clinical Manifestations

The major clinical manifestation of neurogenic bladder dysfunctions is either retention or incontinence. The client may or may not feel a need to void or may not even feel a sense of bladder distention. The diagnosis is often made from the type of neurologic dysfunction that has occurred.

DIAGNOSTIC ASSESSMENT

Urodynamic studies including an electromyogram may be done to help determine the extent of neurologic involvement in the retention or incontinence.

Medical Management

If possible, some form of bladder training is attempted for the client with neurogenic bladder dysfunction. This includes a bladder training program with or without intermittent catheterization, pharmacologic therapy, and sometimes surgical intervention.

PHARMACOLOGIC MANAGEMENT

A number of medications are used to treat neurogenic bladder dysfunction (see Tables 49-1 and 49-3). Antispasmodics and anticholinergics (e.g., dicyclomine, propantheline, and flavoxate) are given to relieve uninhibited or reflex bladder contractions. Phenoxybenzamine and other alpha-adrenergic blocking agents may be used. Bethanechol chloride may help stimulate an atonic bladder. Other pharmacologic agents, described in the discussion of incontinence, may be similarly useful.

DIETARY MANAGEMENT

There are no particular nutritional needs for clients with neurogenic bladder dysfunction; however, they should be encouraged to maintain a high fluid intake of at least 3000 ml a day. They also should be encouraged to drink fluids that promote an acidic urine, which helps prevent UTIs in these clients.

Autonomic dysreflexia or hyperreflexia is a serious, potentially life-threatening complication that can affect spinal cord-injured clients during a bladder training program or if their urinary system becomes obstructed. This condition results from excessive autonomic response to normal stimuli and affects primarily clients with upper motor neuron lesions. The most frequent cause is bladder distention, although autonomic dysreflexia can be triggered by visceral distention or stimulation of pain receptors in the skin. Its most common manifestations are hypertension, bradycardia, throbbing headache, flushing, diaphoresis above the level of the lesion, blurred vision, nasal congestion, nausea, and pilomotor spasm ("goose bumps"). If left untreated, this problem can lead to retinal hemorrhage, seizures, or stroke. Teach the client to recognize its earliest symptoms and summon help immediately because this is a medical emergency.

Surgical Management

If the conservative measures are ineffective in treating the neurogenic bladder, surgical intervention may be necessary. External sphincterotomy or incision of the bladder neck may restore normal bladder emptying. Interrupting innervation to the bladder reflex can aid an uninhibited bladder. Injection of alcohol into the subarachnoid space or rhizotomy (cutting) of the sacral nerves increases bladder capacity by inhibiting reflex bladder contractions, without interfering with normal sphincter function. Sometimes the physician will do a temporary sacral nerve block before surgery to evaluate the potential candidate. Also, electrodes may be implanted in the thoracic or cervical levels of the spinal epidural space and then attached to a percutaneous stimulator. As soon as the client learns to regulate the electrical stimulation properly, the device can be used to interfere with the reflex bladder contractions. Finally, only if all else fails, urinary diversion may be performed to provide the client with a more manageable urinary system.

Surgery is not always successful in alleviating the problems associated with neurogenic bladder dysfunction. Some clients cannot be helped surgically; therefore, learning other methods of bladder control is important.

Nursing Management

Neurogenic bladders are difficult to control, so you will need to teach many clients with this problem how to stimulate the micturition reflex and maintain urination. Assist the client by providing external pressure on the abdomen, which helps contract the detrusor muscle. Have the client lean forward or try pushing on the abdomen with the hand or arm. Have the client breathe deeply to force the diaphragm downward. In addition, wearing a corset or girdle provides an extra source of external pressure.

Another method to help the client learn to empty the bladder is the Credé maneuver. The Credé maneuver involves placing the fingers over the bladder and pressing down slowly. Pressure is exerted downward toward the symphysis pubis as though "milking" the urine out of the urinary system. The nurse or client should use caution when performing this technique. If the client suffers from sphincter dyssynergia (failure of muscular coordination) or if the sphincter does not readily relax, the Credé maneuver can lead to sphincter damage. This maneuver also could result in ureteral reflux if there is any obstruction of outflow.

The client can use several other methods to initiate and maintain micturition. Locate trigger points on the body (e.g., lower abdomen, inner thighs, and pubic area) and explain how to stimulate them by stroking, pinching, or applying ice. Stretching the anal sphincter also relaxes the reflexes of the external urethral sphincter because they are both innervated by the pudendal nerve. The client leans forward while sitting on the toilet and inserts two gloved fingers into the anus.

The fingers are then either widened apart or pulled posteriorly. The male must be careful to avoid touching the glans penis, which stimulates the bulbocavernosus reflex, contracting the external sphincter.

The nurse should always be prepared for the development of autonomic dysreflexia. If the client suddenly develops symptoms of severe hypertension (sometimes >300/180), flushing, and a pounding headache, the nurse must act immediately. Nursing interventions would involve removing the triggering stimuli, for example, reestablishing urine flow or removing fecal impaction if necessary. Removal of a fecal impaction should be done only after a topical anesthetic has been inserted into the rectum for avoiding further stimulation. In addition, a catheter may be necessary, or if one is already in place, patency of the system must be restored by irrigating or removing kinks and obstructions in the system. Monitor vital signs every 5 minutes and raise the head of the bed to semi-Fowler's position. Medications, such as diazoxide (Hyperstat), phenoxybenzamine hydrochloride (Dibenzyline), guanethidine sulfate (Ismelin), propantheline bromide (Pro-Banthine), phentolamine mesylate (Regitine), and mecamylamine hydrochloride (Iversine), relieve both acute symptoms and the chronic recurrence of episodes. Intrathecal administration of tetracaine hydrochloride may block nerve conduction.

For the treatment of long- or short-term bladder atony, an intermittent catheterization program is an alternative to long-term indwelling catheterization. This program consists of inserting a straight urethral catheter into the bladder at specified intervals, draining the urine, and removing the catheter. The catheter may be inserted by the client (self-catheterization), by a significant other, or by anyone properly trained. Encourage clients with bladder atony to learn self-catheterization as soon as possible because it increases independence and mobility.

Sterile catheterization technique is necessary in health care facilities because of the high risk for nosocomial infections. However, authorities recommend that clean, rather than sterile, technique be used for catheterization outside health care facilities. Studies show no increase in the rate of UTIs in comparing clean with sterile technique. Clean technique is also easier and less expensive for the client. For reducing the risk of bacteriuria, urinary antiseptics and acidification or bladder irrigations with antibiotics and antiseptics are given with each catheterization.

The main procedural differences between clean and sterile technique are

- Gloves are not worn for clean technique. Thus, the client must wash hands thoroughly before starting.
- A clean rather than sterile catheter is used.
- Females may chose not to use lubricant because the urethra is short and because they are less susceptible to traumatic urethritis; they may, however, use it.

The catheter should be washed thoroughly after use with soap and water and stored in a plastic sandwich bag or other clean container. Depending on the type of catheter, it may be periodically sterilized by boiling.

During self-catheterization, the client may sit or stand. When the female stands, she should keep one foot on the floor while placing the other on a chair or toilet seat to help her identify the meatus. The female may use a mirror while learning but should not become dependent on it, because she may find herself in situations without one.

Timing is the key success factor in intermittent catheterization programs. Catheterization must be carried out at specified intervals throughout the 24-hour period. A client who is incapable of adhering to this schedule is not an appropriate candidate for the program. The interval between catheterizations is set according to the degree of continence. The average interval for adults is every 4 hours, but the client usually has to start at intervals of 2 to 3 hours.

There are various opinions concerning the amount of fluid intake allowed. Some programs allow fluid as desired, whereas others restrict fluid intake to varying degrees. This aspect of the program requires systematic investigation. Clinicians generally recommend that the client drink small amounts of fluid at specified times (e.g., 250 ml or less within 2 hours for an adult). Ingestion of large amounts of fluid within a short period can cause bladder distention and reflux.

Two main parameters indicate success of an intermittent catheterization program: a catheter-free bladder and absence of bacteriuria. These results may be due to several factors, including intermittent bladder distention, which stimulates the normal micturition reflex, and reactivation of the bladder's normal antibacterial properties. Other advantages include increased independence, better hygiene, reduced incidence of complications arising from a retention catheter, decreased cost, and ease of sexual relations.

Intermittent catheterization is not a panacea, however. The program requires that the client assume a great deal of personal responsibility. Some clients are not sufficiently motivated to fulfill the responsibilities involved in self-catheterization. Also, problems can occur when the client is away from home, for instance, at a movie, in a restaurant, or without access to facilities in which the catheterization can be easily performed, such as on a plane. Poor technique can cause UTI, urethral trauma, and stricture. Bladder calculi may result from pubic hairs inadvertently pushed into the bladder by the catheter, where they become the nidus for stones. Also, some people develop a silent hydronephrosis secondary to obstruction, infection, or reflux due to abnormally high resting bladder pressures. This condition is discovered only with an IVP and monitoring of renal function, both of which should be done frequently. Silent hydronephrosis can be reversed by inserting an indwelling catheter and lowering the bladder pressure.

Modification of Plan of Care for the Elderly

Older clients are more likely to have other problems that may interfere with their ability to use the self-catheterization program to control bladder dysfunction.

They may still be able to use this method if they have a significant other who can help with the catheterization process. Be careful, however, not to force the older client into a dependent state if this is inappropriate.

Post-hospital Care

DISCHARGE TEACHING

The focus of discharge teaching is self-care. The nurse must teach the client and significant others a bladder training program and, if appropriate, self-catheterization. The nurse needs to assess the client's ability to perform self-care procedures while the client is still in the hospital, if possible. Written materials and even diagrams can be given to the client to reinforce the teaching.

HOME HEALTH CARE NEEDS

The client needs to be assessed in the home setting to ensure that the client is able to function there as well as in the hospital. A visiting nurse may be needed to complete the client's education of self-catheterization or bladder training.

FOLLOW-UP CARE

The client should have urinary function monitored at regular intervals, including renal function tests and regular IVPs. The client should also be taught to call the physician at the first sign of UTI or other urinary problem.

BLADDER TRAUMA

Definition

Bladder trauma is defined as a blunt or penetrating injury to the bladder that may or may not cause bladder rupture.

Incidence

Bladder trauma is often related to automobile accidents, when the seat belt compresses the bladder; it is a fairly common problem.

Etiology

A bladder distended by urine can rupture with a direct blow to the abdomen. This injury commonly occurs from wearing a seat belt in an automobile accident. The bladder may also be punctured by bullets, knives, bony splinters from a fractured pelvis, or internal instruments such as a catheter, sound, or cystoscope.

Risk Factors

Accidents are the greatest risk factor for bladder trauma and, when possible, should be prevented. In seat belt trauma, a distended bladder is more likely to rupture.

Pathophysiology

When the bladder ruptures, whatever the cause, urine spills into the peritoneal cavity and continues to leak while the bladder is not intact. Urine leaking into the peritoneal cavity causes peritonitis or pelvic cellulitis to develop.

Clinical Manifestations

Bladder injuries usually produce a pain low in the abdomen or pain referred to the shoulder and hematuria. If the client has a history of an injury or blow to the abdomen, this should arouse suspicion of bladder injury. The client may also demonstrate difficulty voiding (e.g., small amounts of bloody urine or inability to void at all).

DIAGNOSTIC ASSESSMENT

Diagnostic tests to assess bladder trauma include cystography and a voiding cystourethrogram. This allows assessment of both the intactness of the bladder and the bladder's ability to empty.

Medical Management

The first treatment for suspected bladder injury is insertion of a Foley or suprapubic catheter to monitor for hematuria or a complete lack of urine and to divert urine away from the site of injury. Any injury, other than a simple contusion or very small perforation, will require surgical repair. If blood is coming from the meatus, urethral disruption may be present. In this case, the client should not be catheterized until it is determined whether the urethra is disrupted.

Surgical Management

Bladder injuries usually require surgical interventions. After a urethral or suprapubic catheter has been inserted, surgical repair of the damaged bladder wall is done. The extravasated urine in the perivesical space should be drained. If the pelvis is fractured, this is repaired before the bladder to prevent further injury.

The major complication after bladder repair occurs if urinary drainage is not maintained. Healing will be delayed, and fistulas or leakage may develop.

Nursing Management

Assessment of the client at high risk for bladder injury is very important. The nurse should closely monitor the client's urine output for both amount and the presence of hematuria. The nurse should report any anuria to the physician immediately.

Postoperatively, the nurse must maintain urinary drainage to prevent tension on the sutures in the bladder. The nurse may also have to change dressings around a Penrose drain left in to allow any urine remaining in the pelvis to drain.

Modification of Plan of Care for the Elderly

There are no specific modifications for the aged client, only the modifications associated with surgery covered in Chapter 19.

Post-hospital Care

DISCHARGE TEACHING

Because the client may be discharged with an indwelling or suprapubic catheter, it is important the client and significant others be taught how to care for this catheter.

HOME HEALTH CARE NEEDS

The client's self-care abilities should be assessed for the possible need for assistance at home. If the client or significant others are unable to care for the catheter, a visiting nurse must be arranged.

FOLLOW-UP CARE

The client will need to be seen by the physician after discharge for assessment of healing and to have the catheter removed. A suprapubic catheter allows the client to begin to void normally before the catheter is removed. If the client has a urethral catheter, this will have to be removed before the client can begin to void normally. If clients do not void within 8 hours of removal of the catheter, they will have to have the catheter reinserted.

CONGENITAL ANOMALIES OF THE BLADDER

Exstrophy of the bladder is a serious anomaly that develops when the symphysis pubis fails to close in utero. In this condition, the lower anterior abdominal wall and anterior bladder wall are absent. The open bladder protrudes through the abdominal surface. Urinary diversion after surgical removal of the bladder is usually done at an early age. The diversion may require revision as the child grows, and children who had the diversion in the past can have it revised to a continent diversion today. Urinary diversions are discussed earlier in the chapter.

▼ URETHRAL DISORDERS

URETHRITIS

Urethritis is inflammation of the urethra. It is a common problem associated with venereal disease (see Chap. 77 for incidence) and may be seen with cystitis. The most common causes of urethritis in men are gonorrhea and chlamydial infection. In women, it is often caused by feminine hygiene sprays, perfumed toilet paper and sanitary napkins, spermicidal jellies, UTIs, and changes in the vaginal mucosal lining.

Any irritant in contact with the urethra has the potential of causing urethritis. In men, prevention of gonorrhea is the primary way to prevent urethritis. In women, avoidance of perfumed toilet paper and sanitary napkins and of feminine hygiene sprays helps prevent the development of urethritis. If the woman uses spermicidal jelly, she should be aware of the risk of developing urethritis. Sexual intercourse itself has not been shown to cause urethritis.

With exposure to the irritant, the mucosal lining of the urethra becomes highly inflamed. The mucosa becomes swollen and painful, and pus may be produced. The presence of pus cells is referred to as pyuria. The lining is red and irritated, and the lips of the meatus may be swollen.

As with cystitis, assessment reveals burning on urination, frequency, and nocturia. In women, a history reveals exposure to the causative agents. The client may also complain of very low abdominal or perineal pain or discomfort. Pus may be present in the urine (pyuria) even without the presence of bacteria in the urine. Male clients frequently exhibit a discharge, but not females.

Culture and sensitivity testing of the urine may be negative. If the cause is venereal disease, then tests for this are positive. The diagnosis is often made on the basis of the client's history and symptoms.

Management of urethritis includes removing its cause and, if it is caused by microorganisms, administering systemic and topical antibiotics. Sitz baths, especially with baking soda in the water, and high fluid intake are also helpful. The client should be told to avoid sexual intercourse until the symptoms subside. Although sexual intercourse has not been shown to cause urethritis, the use of lubricants with intercourse seems to decrease irritation in women who have had frequent attacks. Refer to Table 49-1 for common medications. The physician may also prescribe topical estrogens.

This problem is usually not treated surgically. If strictures occur, then the urethra is dilated with sounds. If there is scarring at the meatus, a meatotomy may be done.

URETHRAL TUMORS

The most common urethral tumors are condylomas in the male and caruncles. Caruncles are common in women aged 40 to 65 years and are thought to result from chronic irritation such as urethritis. Malignant tumors are uncommon in both sexes but occur more frequently in women than in men. On histologic examination, the tumors found most often in men are squamous cell and transitional cell carcinomas; neoplasms in the female are usually adenocarcinomas or squamous cell carcinomas. The structure of the urethral wall and the degree of lymph drainage mean localized metastasis is fairly common, primarily to the inguinal and lymph nodes. In women, infiltration may involve the vulva and vagina. Further metastasis is usually to the lung, liver, bone, and brain.

Whether the tumor is benign or malignant, its manifestations are similar. Assessment reveals bleeding, urinary obstruction, dysuria, palpable urethral mass, urethral discharge, perineal pain, and urinary incontinence. Diagnosis is made by cystoscopy and biopsy of the tumor.

The surgical treatment for benign or superficial malignant tumors is transurethral fulguration or excision, although total or subtotal urethrectomy may be necessary for larger lesions. Other modes of intervention that are successful include podophyllum cream and thio-TEPA and BCG instillations. The tumors do recur.

As with all cancers, recommended intervention for malignant urethral tumors depends on the degree of neoplastic invasion. Surgery and irradiation are the acceptable choices. Surgery usually involves radical procedures. Partial of total urethrectomy may be performed; often, permanent urinary diversion is required. However, research is continuing on the use of silicone rubber tubing to replace urethras. In addition, men may face partial or total penectomy, whereas women may need anterior pelvic exenteration and vulvectomy with a urinary diversion. Radical excision of the pelvic lymph nodes is sometimes necessary.

URETHRAL TRAUMA

The urethra, as well as the bladder, may be injured in pelvic fractures. Falling astride an object, such as the bar on a boy's bike, with sudden force to the groin may cause urethral contusion and laceration. Injury may occur during medical or surgical interventions or be self-inflicted. Penetrating wounds also cause urethral damage.

Urethral damage is indicated if the client is unable to partially or totally pass urine through the urethra. Even if the client can pass some urine through the urethra, voiding will cause urinary extravasation. Extravasation results in increased swelling of the scrotum or inguinal areas, which can result in sepsis and necrosis. Bleeding may occur at the external meatus, and blood may also extravasate into the surrounding tissues, giving the area an ecchymotic appearance. The two most common complications of urethral trauma are the (1) development of urethral strictures and (2) risk of impotence in men. Impotence occurs because the cavernous tissue of the penis, blood vessels, or nerves supplying this area are damaged.

Proper management of urethral injuries is controversial. Clinicians generally agree that urinary drainage must first be established with either a urethral or suprapubic catheter; some physicians suggest an immediate primary surgical repair of the urethra, whereas others prefer to wait 2 to 3 weeks to see if the urethra will heal itself without surgery. During any waiting period, the client must be monitored for signs of developing sepsis and continuing extravasation of urine.

CONGENITAL ANOMALIES OF THE URETHRA

Urethral anomalies are not common. Those that do occur include absence or atresia of the urethra, urethral stricture, fistulas, and misplacement of the meatus. Misplacement of the meatus (hypospadias and epispadias) is discussed in Chapter 75.

▼ URETERAL DISORDERS

URETERITIS

Ureteritis is an inflammation of the ureter commonly associated with pyelonephritis (see Chap. 50). Once the kidney infection is cured, ureteral inflammation usually subsides. Unfortunately, chronic pyelonephritis causes the ureter to become fibrotic and inhibited by strictures.

URETERAL CALCULI

Calculi have been discussed in this chapter and in Chapter 50. When small stones form in the kidneys, they often move into the ureters. This can lead to ureteral colic, a syndrome of gastrointestinal and GU symptoms and severe pain. The stones irritate the mucosal lining of the ureter and cause a ureterointestinal reflex that irritates the surrounding intestine. If the right ureter is affected, the symptoms may mimic appendicitis. The client will complain of distention, constipation, and right lower quadrant pain. If the left ureter is affected, the symptoms range from nausea and vomiting to diarrhea. The pain is left-sided, usually left lower quadrant.

The incidence, etiology, risk factors, and pathophysiology of calculi in the ureters are the same as for bladder calculi discussed earlier. Treatment is essentially the same as for bladder calculi with a basket extraction through cystoscopy and the use of electrohydraulic lithotripsy. A newer type of laser therapy is being used to disintegrate the stone so the fragments are allowed to pass. The surgery to remove a stone is called ureterolithotomy. This surgery requires the placement of ureteral catheters and a Penrose drain. The care of both is discussed earlier in this chapter.

URETERAL NEOPLASMS

Tumors that arise primarily in the ureter are rare. Ureteral neoplasms usually extend from renal or bladder neoplasms or from tumors originating in the bowel, uterus, or ovary. Those primary neoplasms that do occur usually first appear as a papillary transitional cell or squamous cell carcinoma. These tumors are most frequently found in the lower third of the ureter. In men, ureteral cancer occurs predominantly in the sixth and seventh decades of life. This form of cancer rarely affects women.

In later stages of ureteral cancer, there is extension outside the ureter to adjacent structures and regional lymph nodes or distant metastasis. Common sites for metastasis include the lungs and liver.

Usually, the first sign of ureteral malignancy is gross hematuria. The tumor normally develops painlessly until obstruction occurs. At this point, the client may experience flank pain. Diagnosis is made through urine cytology, IVP, cystoscopy, ultrasonography, and computed tomography.

Treatment for ureteral cancer almost exclusively involves surgical excision and resection, although radiation may also be used in advanced cases with local extension. When the lesion is located in the middle or proximal third of the ureter, the surgical procedure usually involves nephroureterectomy, which removes the kidney, ureter, and attached segment of the bladder on the affected side. However, if the tumor is in the distal third of the ureter and noninvasive, a more conservative surgery may be used. In this case, just the distal portion of ureter is resected with ureteral reimplantation. Silicone rubber, Teflon, polytetrafluorourethane, and bovine carotid heterograft are used to replace the resected ureter, thereby facilitating reimplantation in the bladder. Pre- and postoperative intervention is similar to that for clients undergoing nephrectomy, ureteral reimplantation, or segmental resection of the bladder.

If the decision is made not to perform any of these procedures, some palliative measure may be needed to prevent or alleviate ureteral obstruction. Urinary diversion may be performed, as described previously, or a ureteral stent catheter may be placed into the ureter during cystoscopy to maintain its patency. The older catheter, a flanged, winged stent (Gibbon's stent), or the newer double J stent are made to prevent migration up the ureter or dislodgement by ureteral peristaltic waves or gravity.

URETERAL TRAUMA

The ureters are located deep within the abdomen and are protected by the spine and surrounding musculature, so ureteral injury from trauma is not common. Most accidental injury to the ureters occurs during surgery. Perforation or tearing may occur during manipulation of intraureteric catheters or other instruments. The ureters may be occluded by ligating sutures or a misplaced clamp or may be transected during pelvic surgery; many surgeons insert ureteral stents before pelvic procedures in order to more easily identify the ureters and prevent transection. Gunshot and stab wounds may also traumatize the ureters; although uncommon, blunt trauma or rapid deceleration such as in a car accident can tear these structures.

Direct visualization of the injury may first indicate its presence, especially if it occurred as a complication of surgery. However, trauma is frequently not discovered until signs and symptoms develop. Hematuria may be present, but the most common indications are anuria, kidney pain, or symptoms of extravasation of urine. As the urine seeps out into the tissues, pain may develop in the lower abdomen and flank. As extravasation continues, there may be sepsis, paralytic ileus, a palpable intraperitoneal mass, and the appearance of urine in an external wound. An IVP and cystoscopy are the most definitive means of diagnosis.

Surgical intervention primarily involves repair of the defect, preferably with end-to-end anastomosis. However, more radical procedures such as cutaneous ureterostomy, transureteroureterostomy, and reimplantation may be necessary. The surgeon may use prosthetic ureteral implants. A nephrectomy is performed if obstruction or sepsis has caused severe renal damage. Significant extravasation of urine may require the surgeon to open the abdomen and drain the urine. However, some physicians feel that such urine will be reabsorbed without sequelae as long as it is sterile. It is essential to treat sepsis aggressively.

CONGENITAL ANOMALIES OF THE URETERS

The ureter that follows an abnormal course or has an abnormal distal opening is the most common congenital ureteral anomaly. For example, a retrocaval ureter hooks around the vena cava before it returns to the proper side of the pelvis and enters the bladder appropriately. In women, the ureters may open directly into the urethra or vagina, rather than opening into the bladder. Also, ureteral openings into the bladder may connect to abnormal portions of its wall. During micturition, this anomaly often results in a backflow of urine. Treating these problems may require reimplanting the distal ends of the ureters or replacing the ureters.

Other deviations include duplicate ureters, abnormal dilation of the ureters, and congenital ureteropelvic obstruction.

Duplicate ureters, arising from the same renal pelvis, occur in several variations:

- The ureters on one side may unite at some point along the way.
- Both may open in the normal portion of the trigone.
- Both may open into the urethra or vagina.

Surgical intervention is usually not necessary unless complications develop such as obstruction, infection, and inadequate renal function. Incontinence is also a major reason for surgical intervention when the ureters open into the urethra or vagina.

Abnormal dilation of the ureter (ureterocele or megaureter) is characterized by dilation and pouching of the ureteric wall just adjacent to the vesicoureteral junction. It causes problems because of its refluxing or obstructive effects. Although it may be asymptomatic, the defect can result in flank pain due to backflow pressure on the kidney. This condition predisposes the client to recurrent UTIs.

Congenital ureteropelvic obstruction occurs at the junction of the renal pelvis and the ureter. This anomaly is usually bilateral. A mild obstruction may never cause symptoms of a urinary tract disorder. As long as the kidney produces urine at a rate below 6 ml/min, the ureter can generally handle the flow. However, urine production above this rate causes urine to back up into the kidney, which results in hydronephrosis. Assessment reveals nausea, vomiting, and abdominal or flank pain in response to fluid overload, diuretic therapy, or uncontrolled diabetes mellitus. If the condition is symptomatic, treatment is surgical reimplantation of the ureters.

Summary

Urinary system disorders can be extremely problematic for clients, and the nurse can play a major role in the prevention and treatment of these disorders. Many of the disorders of the urinary system are chronic or lead to chronic problems. Some of the problems can drastically alter the client's self-concept and lifestyle. These problems can range from incontinence to urinary diversions. Clients experiencing these problems require a great deal of support from the nurse so that the client can adapt to the changes in his or her life. Problems also can be life threatening, and the nurse must help ensure that the client receives prompt treatment.

Bibliography

1. Abraham, P., & Smith, C. (1984). Medical evaluation and management of calcium nephrolithiasis. *Medical Clinics of North America, 68,* 281.
2. Acute dysuria in women (1984). *American Family Physician, 29,* 291, June 1984.
3. Adams, M. C., et al. (1992). Conversion of an ileal conduit to a continent catheterizable stoma. *Journal of Urology, 147*(1), 126-128.
4. Ahlering, T. E., et al. (1991). A comparative study of the ileal conduit, Kock pouch and modified Indiana pouch. *Acta Urology Belgium, 59*(2), 303-313.
5. Akaza, H., et al. (1984). Bladder cancer induced by noncarcinogenic substances. *Journal of Urology, 131,* 152.
6. A little-known staph in UTI. *Emergency Medicine 16,* 58, October 15, 1984.
7. Amendola, M., et al. (1983). Bladder calculi complicating intermittent clean catheterization. *American Journal of Radiology, 141,* 751.
8. A new look at cystitis in women (1984). *Patient Care, 18,* 16.
9. Arthur, R. R., et al. (1986). Association of BK viruria with hemorrhagic cystitis in recipients of bone marrow transplants. *New England Journal of Medicine, 315,* 230.
10. Artificial sphincter (1984). *American Family Physician, 30,* 283.
11. Avoiding a voiding problem (1983). *Transition, 1,* 55.
12. Babaian, R. J., & Smith, D. B. (1991). Effect of ileal conduit on patients' activities following radical cystectomy. *Urology, 37*(1), 33-35.
13. Bagley, D., et al. (1985). *Urologic endoscopy: A manual and atlas.* Boston: Little, Brown & Co.
14. Bell, D., & Frentz, G. (1983). Urinary tract infections in the elderly. *Geriatrics, 38,* 42.
15. Bennett, J., et al. (1984). 10-year experience with adenocarcinoma of the bladder. *Journal of Urology, 131,* 262.
16. Bernstein, I. T., et al. (1991). Bricker's ileal conduit urinary diversion with a simple non-refluxing uretero ileal anastomosis. *Scandanavian Journal of Urology and Nephrology, 25*(1), 29-33.
17. Blaivas, J. G. (1990). Diagnostic evaluation of urinary incontinence. *Urology, 36*(Suppl 4), 11-20.
18. Bradshaw, T. (1983). Making male catheterization easier for both of you. *RN, 46,* 43.
19. Branner, G., & Bush, W. (1984). Ultrasonic destruction of kidney stones. *Western Journal of Medicine, 140,* 227.
20. Brodeff, A. (1984). Alleviating stubborn UTI in women. *Patient Care, 18,* 176.
21. Burgers, J. K., et al. (1990). Improved technique for creation of ileal conduit stoma. *Journal of Urology, 44*(5), 1188-1191.
22. Burns, P. B., & Swanson, G. M. (1991). Risk of urinary bladder cancer among blacks and whites: The role of cigarette use and occupation. *Cancer Causes and Control, 2*(6), 371-379.
23. Burns, P., et al.: Kegel's exercises with biofeedback therapy for treatment of stress incontinence. *Nurse Practitioner 10,* 28.
24. Cass, A. (1983). Genitourinary trauma. *Postgraduate Medicine, 74,* 99.
25. Choi, B. C., & Nethercott, J. R. (1991). A proportionate mortality study on risk of bladder cancer among rubber workers. *Cancer Detection and Prevention, 15*(5), 403-406.
26. Chyou, P. H., et al. (1992). A prospective study of the attributable risk of cancer due to cigarette smoking. *American Journal of Public Health, 82*(1), 37-40.
27. Costello, A. J., & Bowsher, W. G. (1992). Radiotherapy as a treatment for bladder cancer. *Australia and New Zealand Journal of Surgery, 62*(1), 81-83.
28. Diokno, A., et al. (1983). Fate of patients started on clean intermittent self-catheterization therapy 10 years ago. *Journal of Urology, 129,* 1120.
29. Drach, G. W. (Ed.) (1986). New perspectives on management of upper and lower urinary tract infection. *Urology, 27*(Suppl 2), 2-30.
30. Droller, M. (1984). Immunotherapy in genitourinary neoplasia. *Urology Clinics of North America, 11,* 643.
31. Dugan, J. (1984). Winning the battle against incontinence. *Nursing, 84, 14,* 59.
32. Engram, B. (1983). Ten easy ways to improve your urologic nursing care. *Nursing 83, 13,* 49.
33. Eure, G. R., et al. (1992). Bacillus Calmette-Guérin therapy for high risk stage T1 superficial bladder cancer. *Journal of Urology, 147*(2), 376-379.
34. Faro, S. (1992). New considerations in treatment of urinary tract infections in adults. *Urology, 39*(1), 1-11.
35. Felsen, D., et al. (1991). Inflammatory mediators and interstitial cystitis. *Seminars in Urology, 9*(2), 102-107.
36. Frentz, G., & Lang, E. (1983). Bladder injury. *Emergency Medicine, 15,* 111.
37. Frentz, G., et al. (1983). Urethral trauma. *Emergency Medicine, 15,* 63.
38. Ghoneim, M. A., et al. (1992). Further experience with the urethral Kock pouch. *Journal of Urology, 147*(2), 361-365.
39. Gleeson, M. J., & Griffith, D. P. (1990). Urinary diversion. *British Journal of Urology, 66*(2), 113-122.
40. Hanno, P. M., & Wein, A. J. (1991). Conservative therapy of interstitial cystitis. *Seminars in Urology, 9*(2), 143-147.
41. Harris, R. (1984). Acute urinary tract infections and subsequent problems. *Clinical Obstetrics and Gynecology, 27,* 874.
42. Harwood, A. (1983). Urologic emergencies. *Emergency Medicine, 15,* 112.
43. Hermann, G. G., et al. (1992). Recombinant interleukin-2 and lymphokine-activated killer cell treatment of advanced bladder cancer: Clinical results and immunological effects. *Cancer Research, 52*(3), 726-733.
44. Herzog, A. R., & Fultz, N. H. (1990). Epidemiology of urinary incontinence: Prevalence, incidence, and correlates in community populations. *Urology, 36*(Suppl 4), 2-10.
45. Hooton, T. M., et al. (1991). Single-dose and three-day regimens of ofloxacin versus trimethoprim-sulfamethoxazole for acute cystitis in women. *Antimicrobial Agents and Chemotherapy, 35*(7), 1479-1483.
46. Jeter, K., Faller, N., & Norton, C. (1990). *Nursing for continence.* Philadelphia: W.B. Saunders.

47. Jolleys, J. V. (1991). Factors associated with regular episodes of dysuria among women in one rural general practice. *British Journal of General Practice, 41*(347), 241-243.
48. Krebs, M., et al. (1984). Prevention of urinary tract infection during intermittent catheterization. *Journal of Urology, 131,* 82.
49. Krieger, J. N. (1990). Urinary tract infections in women: Causes, classification, and differential diagnosis. *Urology, 35*(Suppl 1), 4-7.
50. Loening, S. (1984). Chemotherapy as an adjuvant to cystectomy and for advanced urothelial cancer. *Urologic Clinics of North America, 11,* 699.
51. London, R. (1984). Diverticulum of the urinary bladder. *American Family Physician, 30,* 151.
52. Marchant, D. (1983). Urinary incompetence in the female. *Hospital Medicine, 19,* 49.
53. Matsuura, T., et al. (1991). Assessment of the long-term results of ileocecal conduit urinary diversion. *Urology International, 46*(2), 154-158.
54. Mizutani, Y., et al. (1992). Effects of bacille Calmette-Guérin on cytotoxic activities of peripheral blood lymphocytes against human T24 lined and freshly isolated autologous urinary bladder transitional carcinoma cells in patients with urinary bladder cancer. *Cancer, 69*(2), 537-545.
55. Mohr, J. (1984). Overcoming stress incontinence: a twofold approach. *Transition, 2,* 38.
56. Morrison, A. (1984). Advances in the etiology of urothelial cancer. *Urologic Clinics of North America, 11,* 557.
57. Nomhold, P. (1984). Sex and the Foley catheter. *Nursing 84, 14,* 98.
58. Nordstrom, G. M., & Nyman, C. R. (1991). Living with a urostomy: A follow up with special regard to the peristomal-skin complications, psychosocial and sexual life. *Scandanavian Journal of Urology and Nephrology (Suppl), 138,* 247-251.
59. Nurse, D. E., et al. (1991). Problems in the surgical treatment of interstitial cystitis. *British Journal of Urology, 68*(2), 153-154.
60. Oliver, J. R., et al. (1991). Correction of incontinent ileocolic urostomy with Kock's nipple valve. *Gynecology Oncology, 43*(2), 178-181.
61. Pow-Sang, J. M., et al. (1992). Conversion from external appliance wearing or internal urinary diversion to a continent urinary reservoir (Florida pouch I and II): Surgical technique, indications and complications. *Journal of Urology, 147*(2), 356-360.
62. Ronald, A. (1984). Current concepts in the management of urinary tract infections in adults. *Medical Clinics of North America, 68,* 335.
63. Rottkamp, B. (1985). A holistic approach to identifying factors associated with an altered pattern of urinary elimination in stroke patients. *Journal of Neurosurgical Nursing, 17,* 37.
64. Rubin, R. (1984). Infections of the urinary tract. *Scientific American Medicine, 7,* 1.
65. Samodai, L., et al. (1991). The efficacy of intravesical BCG in the treatment of patients with high risk superficial bladder cancer. *International Urology and Nephrology, 23*(6), 559-567.
66. Sander, S., & Beisland, H. (1984). Application of laser beam technology in the treatment of bladder tumors. *Progress in Clinical and Biological Research, 162B,* 365.
67. Scott, D., et al. (1984). Stress-coping response to genitourinary carcinoma. *Nursing Research, 33,* 325.
68. Seidman, A. D., & Scher, H. I. (1991). The evolving role of chemotherapy for muscle infiltrating bladder cancer. *Seminars in Oncology, 18*(6), 585-595.
69. Skinner, D., et al. (1984). Techniques of creation of a continent internal ileal reservoir (Kock pouch) for urinary diversion. *Urologic Clinics of North America, 11,* 741.
70. Slate, W. (1982). *Disorders of the female urethra and urinary incontinence.* Baltimore: Williams & Wilkins.
71. Smith, C. (1984). When should the stone patient be evaluated: Early evaluation of single stone formers. *Medical Clinics of North America, 68,* 455.
72. Smith, P., & Hetherington, J. (1984). Hydrostatic bladder distention for bladder cancer. *Progress in Clinical and Biological Research, 162B,* 309.
73. Snowden, D., & Phillips, R. (1984). Coffee consumption and risk of fatal cancers. *American Journal of Public Health, 74,* 820.
74. Sobota, A. (1984). Inhibition of bacterial adherence by cranberry juice: Potential use for the treatment of urinary tract infections. *Journal of Urology, 131,* 1013.
75. Soloway, M. (1984). Intravesical and systemic chemotherapy in the management of superficial bladder cancer. *Urologic Clinics of North America, 11,* 623.
76. Spinelli, J. J., et al. (1991). Mortality and cancer incidence in aluminum reduction plant workers. *Journal of Occupational Medicine, 33*(11), 1150-1155.
77. Staff (1986). What is interstitial cystitis and what can be done about it? *American Journal of Nursing, 86*(1), 13-14.
78. Stanton, S. (1984). *Clinical gynecologic urology.* St. Louis: C.V. Mosby.
79. Stone, A. R., et al. (1991). Role of the immune system in interstitial cystitis. *Seminars in Urology, 9*(2), 108-114.
80. Utz, D., & Farrow, G.: Carcinoma in situ of the urinary tract. *Urologic Clinics of North America, 11,* 735.
81. van den Broek, P., et al. (1985). Bladder irrigation with povidone-iodine in prevention of urinary-tract infections associated with intermittent urethral catheterization. *Lancet, 1,* 563.
82. van der Werf-Messing, B. H. P. (1984). Carcinoma of the urinary bladder treated by interstitial radiotherapy. *Urologic Clinics of North America, 11,* 659.
83. Walsh, P. C., et al. (Eds.) (1986). *Campbell's Urology* (5th ed.). Philadelphia: W.B. Saunders.
84. Webster, D. (September, 1990). Comparing patients' and nurses' views of interstitial cystitis: A pilot study. *Urologic Nursing,* 10-13.
85. Wishnow, K. I., et al. (1992). Stage B (P2/3A/N0) transitional cell carcinoma of bladder highly curable by radical cystectomy. *Urology, 39*(1), 12-16.

Chapter 50

Nursing Care of Clients with Renal Disorders

By producing urine, the kidneys regulate the body's fluid, electrolyte, and acid-base balances while removing toxic substances from the blood. The kidneys play a significant role in erythropoietin and prostaglandin synthesis, in insulin degradation, and in the renin-angiotensin-aldosterone system.

This chapter identifies the common disease processes and injuries that interfere with normal renal function. Although the effects of extrarenal influences on the kidneys are briefly described, the primary purpose of this chapter is to discuss specific renal pathologic processes. Because of the potential seriousness of any renal problem, the client and significant others will have physical as well as psychosocial needs. Nurses should know about both aspects and be constantly aware of the need for appropriate intervention.

RENAL DISORDERS ASSOCIATED WITH EXTRARENAL CONDITIONS AND NEPHROTOXINS

Many conditions primarily located in other parts of the body affect the kidneys. Examples of these include sepsis, hypertension, and diabetes mellitus. Description of the renal implications of these conditions is brief here. For further discussion, see Chapters 14, 20, 44, and 61.

EXTRARENAL CONDITIONS

Diabetes Mellitus

One of the most common extrarenal diseases affecting the kidney is diabetes mellitus. Diabetic nephropathy, a progressive process, frequently leads to renal failure. Approximately 30 per cent of clients with end-stage renal disease have diabetes mellitus. Researchers estimate that 25 to 50 per cent of clients with insulin-dependent diabetes mellitus (IDDM or type I) will develop end-stage renal disease within 10 to 20 years of beginning insulin therapy. Renal disease can also develop in the non-insulin-dependent diabetic. The incidence of proteinuria is about 25 per cent after 20 years of diabetes.[16]

Several pathologic changes lead to renal failure in clients with diabetes mellitus. The most frequent is a characteristic intercapillary glomerulosclerosis, or scarring of the capillary loops. Progressive microangiopathy, nephrosclerosis, affects the afferent and efferent arterioles and eventually causes scarring of the glomerulus, tubules, and interstitium. Pyelonephritis, kidney infection, may cause scarring and subsequent ischemia in the renal parenchyma. It may also lead to renal papillary necrosis and sloughing of the papillae. Neurogenic bladder dysfunction may contribute to renal failure. The high incidence of urinary tract infection or the increased pressure in the kidney caused by the back-up of urine may be the cause.

Initially, the sclerotic, or hardening, process of glomerulosclerosis increases renal vascular resistance, contributing to systemic hypertension. This does not cause renal insufficiency. Indeed, the glomerular filtration rate (GFR) may increase as much as 20 to 50 per cent above the GFR of normal nondiabetics during this early or "silent" phase. It is now recognized that microalbuminemia (measurable by assay) occurs quite some time before clinical proteinuria. If diagnosed, this may be a much earlier harbinger of eventual renal failure. As more nephrons are destroyed, available functioning renal tissue decreases, and the client begins to demonstrate clinical proteinuria (a key sign), hypertension, edema, and manifestations of renal failure.

The kidney metabolizes 30 to 40 per cent of insulin, so as renal function diminishes, the degradation of insulin also decreases, which results in a lower insulin requirement for the client. Renal failure may be initially identified when the client is undergoing evaluation for recurrent insulin reactions. Researchers hope the sclerotic process can be slowed by (1) carefully controlling hypertension, (2) appropriately adjusting insulin therapy, and (3) restricting dietary protein. However, the client inevitably develops renal failure within 5 to 10 years after the appearance of significant proteinuria, regardless of diabetic control.

Hypertension

Because the kidneys receive such a large share of the cardiac output, renal function can affect or be affected by alterations within the cardiovascular system. The flow of blood determines the GFR, which directly affects renal function. Hypertension is one condition that can either cause or be affected by renal disese. For example, renovascular hypertension results from renal artery stenosis or renal infarction, a condition that activates the renin-angiotensin-aldosterone system and increases systemic blood pressure. Renal hypertension arising from parenchymal renal disease (e.g., glomerulonephritis, polycystic disease, pyelonephritis) usually results from the kidney's decreasing ability to excrete salt and water. Other causes include increased renin release due to increased glomerular perfusion and inadequacy of renal vasodilatory substances such as occurs with analgesic nephropathy. Whereas renovascular hypertension accounts for up to 15 per cent of all systemic hypertension, in renal failure clients, 80 to 85 per cent of hypertension is a result of excess salt and water retention.[16]

On the other hand, sustained systemic high blood pressure adversely affects the kidneys. Researchers estimate that microscopically evident nephrosclerosis is present in clients with uncontrolled hypertension for more than 5 years, although all other renal diagnostic tests may be normal. This kidney damage is the direct result of degenerative changes in the arterioles and interlobular arteries caused by increased blood pressure. There is a direct correlation between the duration and degree of elevated blood pressure and the severity of renal vascular disease. However, progression of the disease frequently can be halted or slowed by bringing the hypertension under control. This means that client teaching is vital to controlling the hypertension and preventing renal failure.

Hypotension

Cardiovascular shock, or hypotension, also affects renal function. Renal vasoconstriction reduces renal blood flow. However, because of the autoregulation capabilities of the kidneys (see Chap. 47), GFR remains at a functional level until the advanced stages of systemic shock, at which time acute renal failure develops. Restoring the systemic blood pressure usually reverses the renal vasoconstriction, and kidney function returns, generally within 2 to 8 weeks. A period of polyuria may follow the correction of hypovolemia, although the mechanisms for this are unclear. Before renal function returns to normal, another oliguric period may occur, followed by a "mobilization phase" that shifts sequestered fluid into the intravascular space. This may cause some hypertension until the kidneys can remove the extra fluid. Careful assessment of the client's fluid status and meticulous fluid management are crucial during these recovery phases.

Cardiovascular Disease

Cardiac disease influences kidney function primarily through its effect on the cardiac output and circulating blood volume. The hemodynamic and hormonal changes of cardiac disease may decrease the kidneys' ability to excrete sodium and water. This, in turn, increases intravascular congestion and edema and establishes a pathologic cycle.

Hemodynamic changes also occur with normal aging. Blood flow to the kidneys decreases by up to 50 per cent by 70 years of age, and GFR decreases by up to 40 to 50 per cent. Renal function deteriorates as glomeruli become sclerotic and atrophy.

Peripheral Vascular Disease

Thromboembolic disease can affect the renal circulation and cause infarction of the tissue supplied by the affected blood vessel. The interstitial hypertonicity and low oxygen pressure found in the renal medulla seem to favor sickling of red blood cells in the kidney's juxtamedullary region in clients with sickle cell disease. These cell masses cause gross hematuria as venules rupture; papillary necrosis; renal infarction; concentrating disturbances due to interference with the "countercurrent mechanism"; nephrotic syndrome; pyelonephritis; and, finally, renal failure. The kidney is the organ most affected in disseminated intravascular coagulation, in which diffuse clotting consumes clotting factors and causes hemorrhage in affected areas throughout the body.

Sepsis

Extrarenal sepsis may affect kidney function either through its effect on the systemic circulation or through its stimulation of the immune system. Renal reactions to septic shock are similar to those described under Hypotension. Immunologic injury leading to glomerulonephritis is described later. Occasionally, pathogens may break away from extrarenal foci of infection and travel to the kidney to establish additional sites.

Pregnancy

Pregnancy has a definite influence on kidney function. Collecting system dilation and kidney enlargement begin during the first trimester of pregnancy and may persist 9 to 12 weeks after delivery. Renal blood flow and GFR increase by 30 to 50 per cent during pregnancy, contributing to increased creatinine clearance and decreased uric acid excretion. These normal changes must be taken into account when laboratory findings are interpreted in pregnant women. Pregnancy also increases the likelihood of proteinuria (usually transient), polyuria, and nocturia. These disorders are possibly caused by external bladder compression and alterations in antidiuretic hormone metabolism.[32]

Many other extrarenal disease processes influence kidney function. These include neoplastic disease, connective tissue disorders, and metabolic disturbances.

NEPHROTOXINS

Nephrotoxins are substances that have specific, destructive effects on renal cells. They can cause five types of renal injury: (1) acute tubular necrosis, (2) defects in the tubular transport system, (3) interstitial nephritis, (4) vasculitis, and (5) nephrotic syndrome.

Nephrotoxic substances found in the environment include heavy metals, such as mercurial compounds, lead, cadmium, bismuth, arsenic, copper, and phosphorus; carbon tetrachloride; ethylene glycol; trichloroethylene; carbon monoxide; and chlorinated hydrocarbons. Exposure to many of these substances occurs in industrial locations. Other environmental nephrotoxins include snake venom and certain mushrooms. Their most frequent renal result is acute tubular necrosis. Some also cause tubular transport defects and nephrotic syndrome. Box 50-1 shows some of the common nephrotoxic agents.

All five types of kidney damage may result from nephrotoxic reactions to medications (see Box 50-1). The two most common medications causing renal damage are antibiotics and certain analgesics. Because the kidneys are the major route of excretion for many antibiotics, renal tissue is directly exposed to these compounds. The longer the exposure, the higher the risk of renal toxic effects. Pre-existing renal disease, decreased renal blood flow, electrolyte imbalances, and concurrent use of other nephrotoxic medications enhance a medication's nephrotoxic effect. High-risk antibiotics include cephalosporins, sulfonamides, polymyxins, aminoglycosides, and amphotericin B. Careful monitoring of renal function tests identifies early

Box 50-1. Nephrotoxins

Antibiotics

Aminoglycosides
Tetracyclines
Amphotericin B
Cephalosporins
Sulfonamides (Co-trimoxazole)
Bacitracin
Polymyxin
Colistin

Heavy Metals

Lead
Mercury
Arsenic
Copper
Gold
Lithium

Poisons

Mushrooms
Insecticides
Herbicides
Snake bites

Anesthetics

Contrast Dyes

Organic Solvents

Glycols
Gasoline
Kerosene
Turpentine
Tetrachloroethylene

Other Drugs

Heroin
Dextran
Mannitol
Interleukin-2
Cisplatin
Amphetamines

nephrotoxic reactions so causative medications can be discontinued or the dose decreased. Besides using these medications as briefly as possible, maintaining a high fluid intake and carefully maintaining only a therapeutic blood level may prevent nephrotoxic effects. A high urine output keeps the medication dilute within the kidney and helps prevent any crystallization of the compound.

The risk of renal damage from excessive use of certain analgesics has received more attention in recent years. Salicylates, acetaminophen, phenacetin, and nonsteroidal anti-inflammatory drugs are the most common causative agents. Short-term overdose or long-term consistent use of these medications may cause acute tubular necrosis or chronic renal failure. Researchers estimate that between 5 and 10 per cent of all clients with end-stage renal disease have analgesic nephropathy.[60]

Anesthesia reduces the kidney's vasoconstrictive ability, which helps protect it against systemic blood pressure drops; thus, the kidney is made more vulnerable to the effects of shock. In addition, certain anesthetics, particularly methoxyflurane, have a direct nephrotoxic effect. Administering this general anesthetic can cause acute tubular necrosis and has been associated with fatal acute renal failure. Halothane may also adversely affect renal function. Higher serum concentrations of sodium thiopental have been found in clients with renal disease than in clients with normal kidney function who receive an equal dose.

Other common medications that may have nephrotoxic effects include aggressive use of diuretics that cause hypovolemia, probenecid, phenytoin, low-molecular-weight dextran, rifampin, phenindione, lithium, and gold therapy. Nurses must know the possible adverse effects of any medication a client takes so proper assessments and intervention are initiated.

Radioiodinated contrast agents used in radiographic and computed tomographic (CT) studies have been associated with acute tubular necrosis. Risk factors include being over 60 years old; pre-existing renal insufficiency, especially diabetic nephropathy; dehydration; low cardiac output with pre-existing renal disease; proteinuria; hypoalbuminemia; multiple myeloma; and multiple contrast studies within a 24-hour period. Using nondye studies whenever possible and keeping the client well hydrated throughout the test reduce the incidence of acute renal failure. Baseline renal function tests before the contrast study should be available to compare with post-test findings. Monitor urine output carefully for several hours after the study is completed.

▼ ACQUIRED DISORDERS

PYELONEPHRITIS

Definition

Pyelonephritis is an inflammation of the renal pelvis caused by a bacterial infection.

Incidence

Clients with insulin-dependent diabetes have an increased tendency to develop pyelonephritis. Clients with chronic renal calculi and those who are pregnant also have a greater tendency to develop pyelonephritis. Clients who have had acute pyelonephritis are likely to have a recurrence within several weeks of the initial attack.

Etiology

Sometimes an infection may be a primary disease, as happens with calculus, malignancy, hydronephrosis, or trauma that has reduced host resistance. However, most kidney infections appear to be extensions of infectious processes located elsewhere; the bladder is the most common site. Chapter 49 discusses the etiology and pathogenesis of infections in the lower urinary tract. The bacteria spread to the kidney primarily by traveling up (ascending) the ureter to the kidney. Blood and lymphatic circulation also provide channels for the organisms. Ureteral reflux, which allows infected urine back into the ureter, and obstruction, which causes urine to back into the ureter and allows organisms to multiply, are the most common causes of ascending urinary tract infections.

There are two main types of pyelonephritis: acute and chronic. They differ, primarily, in their clinical picture and long-term effects.

Acute Pyelonephritis. Acute pyelonephritis often occurs after bacterial contamination of the urethra or after instrumentation such as catheterization or cystoscopy.

Chronic Pyelonephritis. Chronic pyelonephritis is more likely to occur after chronic obstruction with reflux or chronic disorders. It is a slowly progressive disease usually associated with recurrent acute attacks, although there may be no history of acute pyelonephritis.

Risk Factors

Pregnant clients and clients with a history of diabetes, hypertension, chronic renal calculi, chronic cystitis, and new developments or changes in seizure activity are at an increased risk of developing pyelonephritis. The presence of structural abnormalities of the urinary tract, the presence of foreign bodies such as stones or tubes, and mechanical drainage also increase the risk.

Prevention is best accomplished through early detection, complete treatment, and diligent follow-up of the problem.

Pathophysiology

Pyelonephritis occurs when bacteria enter the renal pelvis, causing an inflammatory response and an increase in white blood cells. The inflammation leads to edema and swelling of the involved tissue, beginning at the papillae and sometimes spreading to the cortex.

As the infection is treated and the inflammation recedes, fibrosis and scar tissue may develop. The calices become blunted with scarring in the interstitial tissues. If the infections recur, more and more scar tissue is developed; fibrosis and altered tubular reabsorption and secretion lead to decreased renal function.

Acute Pyelonephritis. Acute pyelonephritis is associated with the development of renal abscesses, perinephric abscesses, emphysematous pyelonephritis, and chronic pyelonephritis that can lead to renal failure.

The course of acute pyelonephritis is usually short. However, it often recurs, either as a relapse of a previous infection not eradicated or as a new infection; 20 per cent of these recurrences take place within 2 weeks of completion of therapy.[64] A client must be treated adequately for preventing the development of chronic pyelonephritis. The infection may also progress to bacteremia.

Chronic Pyelonephritis. This disease is characterized by a combination of caliceal abnormalities and overlying cortical scarring. The kidney becomes contracted, and the number of functioning nephrons decreases as they are replaced by scar tissue. Renal failure may ensue, although the development of uremia is less frequent than is commonly thought.[2]

Clinical Manifestations

Acute Pyelonephritis. Acute pyelonephritis is characterized by enlarged kidneys, focal parenchymal abscess formation, and accumulation of polymorphonuclear lymphocytes around and within the renal tubules. It may cause minimal symptoms or may be asymptomatic. Typically, however, the client seems in acute distress and appears toxic.

Assessment reveals high fever, chills, nausea, flank pain on the affected side, headache, muscular pain, and general prostration. The pain often radiates down the ureter or toward the epigastrium and may be colicky if the infection is complicated by calculi or sloughed renal papillae. Percussion or deep palpation over the costovertebral angle elicits marked tenderness. Frequently the client has experienced dysuria, frequency, urgency, and other signs of cystitis for several days. The urine may be cloudy or bloody, is foul-smelling, and demonstrates a marked increase in white cell casts and white blood cells.

Chronic Pyelonephritis. This disease has no specific symptoms of its own. Thus, it is frequently diagnosed incidentally when the client is being evaluated for hypertension or its complications. Hypertension itself is the most frequent manifestation of the disease.

DIAGNOSTIC ASSESSMENT

Acute Pyelonephritis. Urine culture and sensitivity studies are the primary diagnostic tests with a physical examination. Studies may be done for calculi, especially with recurrent infections, because calculi may seed and cause reinfection, particularly with *Proteus*. X-ray studies such as of the kidney, ureter, and bladder (KUB) and intravenous pyelography (IVP) are also done. A cystourethrogram is often done, especially after an initial episode of pyelonephritis, to look for underlying defects, particularly any cause of reflux. Magnetic resonance imaging or CT scan may also be used to evaluate the kidney size or the presence of other problems.

Chronic Pyelonephritis. Abnormal laboratory studies may show azotemia, pyuria, anemia, acidosis, and proteinuria. They may also demonstrate a poor concentrating ability.

Medical Management

Acute Pyelonephritis. Intervention aims at (1) eliminating the pathogenic organisms with appropriate antibiotics as identified by urine culture and sensitivity study and (2) removing any component contributing to decreased host resistance. If calculi are found during the work-up for the cause of recurrent infection, appropriate treatment is instituted.

Chronic Pyelonephritis. Medical management focuses on preventing further renal damage. If bacteria are found, appropriate antibiotics are given, as in acute pyelonephritis. Above all, hypertension must be controlled. Additional intervention depends on the degree of renal failure that has already occurred.

PHARMACOLOGIC MANAGEMENT

Antibiotics, specific to the bacteria present, are given to treat pyelonephritis (see Table 49-1). Although they may be administered orally or by use of the single large-dose method described in Chapter 49, the usual method involves parenteral antibiotics for 3 to 5 days until the client has been afebrile for 24 to 48 hours; oral administration follows for 2 to 4 weeks. The client must understand that prolonged antibiotic therapy suppresses recurrent infections, so completing therapy is of vital importance.

Additional pharmacologic therapy may be needed to correct any predisposing factors.

DIETARY MANAGEMENT

Nutrition is not used to treat pyelonephritis directly, unless renal failure has occurred. The causes, however, may require dietary alterations. For example, if the cause is related to calculi, the dietary management discussed in Chapter 49 would be appropriate. If the client suffers from recurrent urinary tract infections, then the acid-ash diet discussed in Chapter 49 would be appropriate.

Surgical Management

Surgery is done only to correct any underlying defects that might have caused the pyelonephritis, such as obstruction, reflux, or calculus.

Nursing Management

ASSESSMENT

Assessment of the client with pyelonephritis begins with a thorough history and physical examination, with close attention paid to the presence of risk factors, hypertension, and costovertebral angle (CVA) tenderness. The nurse should look for the presence of the signs and symptoms of pyelonephritis.

NURSING INTERVENTION

Nursing Diagnosis: Fluid Volume Deficit, High Risk R/T fever, nausea, vomiting, and possible diarrhea.

Planning: Expected Outcomes. The client will not develop fluid volume deficit, as evidenced by balanced intake and output, maintenance of adequate hydration, and no signs of dehydration.

Implementation. The nurse should prepare the client for the diagnostic tests and probable antibiotic therapy. Clients with severe nausea and vomiting may require intravenous fluids. Overhydration may dilute antimicrobials, diminishing the effectiveness of these drugs. Refer to Chapter 49 for specific information on the nursing care of the client with cystitis.

Nursing Diagnosis: Pain R/T abdominal pain, headache, muscular pain, fever, and nausea.

Planning: Expected Outcomes. The client will have no pain or have pain controlled, as evidenced by client's statement.

Implementation. Medications can be given to control the pain caused by calculi that may have precipitated the problem. The CVA tenderness should decrease as the antibiotics control the infection. Medication for nausea can be given as needed with antipyretics for high fevers. The urinary symptoms subside quickly once antibiotic therapy is begun.

Nursing Diagnosis: Urinary Elimination, Altered R/T dysuria, pyuria, and frequency.

Planning: Expected Outcomes. The client will return to normal urinary elimination, as evidenced by the absence of dysuria, pyuria, and frequency.

Implementation. Adequate treatment of the infection quickly reverses the dysuria, pyuria, and frequency. Urinary analgesics described in Chapter 49 can also help the client with these problems.

Nursing Diagnosis: Knowledge Deficit R/T prevention of recurrent infections.

Planning: Expected Outcomes. The client will understand how to prevent recurrent infections, as evidenced by client's statements and no recurrence of infection.

Implementation. The preventive measures for acute and chronic pyelonephritis are similar to those for cystitis (see Chap. 49). It is important to prevent permanent renal damage.

EVALUATION

The nurse will evaluate whether the expected outcomes have been met. If they were not, the plan and interventions will be altered to better meet the client's needs.

Modification of Plan of Care for the Elderly

The major difference for older clients is that their kidneys may be less able to recover from a severe infection. Antibiotic therapy should be monitored closely, because the older adult's sensitivity and response to the medication may vary. Older adults may also have altered blood levels of antibiotics because perfusion changes with age.

Post-hospital Care

DISCHARGE TEACHING

When the acute infection subsides, instruct the client to continue to follow-up care. This includes completing the full course of antibiotic therapy and repeating urine cultures. Also teach ways of preventing further infections anywhere in the urinary tract (see Chap. 49).

HOME HEALTH CARE NEEDS

No specific home health care is needed unless the client develops renal failure. This is discussed later in this chapter.

FOLLOW-UP CARE

It is vital for the client to return for follow-up urine cultures and possibly for other diagnostic tests if the cause of the pyelonephritis is not clear. The client needs to understand the importance of follow-up cultures because bacteriuria may be present but asymptomatic. The client must also be told to report any signs of recurrence immediately so retreatment can be initiated.

ACUTE GLOMERULONEPHRITIS

Definition

Glomerulonephritis is a term that encompasses a variety of diseases, most of which are caused by an immunologic reaction that, in turn, results in proliferative and inflammatory changes within the glomerular structure.

Two forms of glomerulonephritis are included in the category of acute glomerulonephritis: postinfectious glomerulonephritis and infectious glomerulonephritis. Of the two, postinfectious glomerulonephritis, also called acute poststreptococcal glomerulonephritis, is the most common.

Incidence

Although the exact incidence of acute glomerulonephritis is unknown, it is twice as common in men as in women.

Etiology

Box 50-2 is a classification system based on etiology.

Classically, the causative factor is a beta-hemolytic streptococcal infection elsewhere in the body, although other organisms may be responsible. Typically, it occurs about 21 days after a respiratory or skin infection.

Postinfectious glomerulonephritis is primarily a disease of children, 95 per cent of whom recover fully. It does, however, sometimes occur in adults. Approximately 30 per cent of adults with this disease progress to chronic renal failure.[77]

Box 50-2. Classification of Glomerulonephritis Based on Etiology

- Glomerulonephritis, primary
  - Acute glomerulonephritis
    - Postinfectious glomerulonephritis
    - Infectious glomerulonephritis
  - Membranoproliferative glomerulonephritis
  - Rapidly progressive glomerulonephritis
  - Idiopathic membranous glomerulonephritis
  - IgA nephropathy
  - Chronic glomerulonephritis
  - Lipoid nephrosis
  - Focal glomerular sclerosis
- Glomerulonephritis, secondary to systemic disease
  - Goodpasture's syndrome
  - Hemolytic-uremic syndrome
  - Henoch-Schönlein syndrome
  - Polyarteritis
  - Progressive systemic sclerosis
  - Systemic lupus erythematosus
  - Wegener's granulomatosis

Infectious glomerulonephritis is also associated with bacterial, viral, or parasitic infections elsewhere in the body. It differs from postinfectious glomerulonephritis in that it occurs during or within a few days of the original infectious process.

Risk Factors

There are no specific risk factors for this disorder because it is actually an immunologic disorder that occurs in response to either endogenous (those already in the body) or exogenous (those associated with infections) antigens.

Pathophysiology

Glomerulonephritis is an immunologic disorder that results in inflammatory and proliferative changes within the glomerulus. Because the primary function of the glomerulus is to filter blood, most cases of glomerulonephritis result from trapping of circulating antigen-antibody complexes within the glomerulus. This causes inflammatory damage and impedes glomerular function, reducing the glomerular membrane's capacity for selective permeability. The source of the antigens may be either exogenous (e.g., poststreptococcal infection) or endogenous (e.g., systemic lupus erythematosus). Evidence also indicates that some antigen-antibody complexes may form in situ within the kidney.

In addition to this immune complex nephritis, glomerulonephritis may also be produced by the fixing of antibodies to the glomerular basement membrane. An example of this is Goodpasture's syndrome, which involves pulmonary hemorrhage and glomerulonephritis.

The primary pathologic process of glomerulonephritis, lipoid nephrosis, and focal glomerular sclerosis is proliferation and inflammation. However, lipoid nephrosis and focal glomerular sclerosis are characterized by degeneration.

Acute glomerulonephritis can become a fulminant process, proceeding quickly to uremia or to chronic glomerulonephritis. However, most clients start to recover within 14 days. Most clinical signs return to normal within several weeks, although the hematuria and proteinuria may be present for longer periods. If complete recovery does not occur within 2 years, it probably will not occur at all. Some use the term "subacute glomerulonephritis" to designate disease that lasts more than 6 to 8 weeks. Although most of the signs and symptoms of the acute disease have disappeared, the client is still very susceptible to exacerbation of glomerulonephritis. The term "latent glomerulonephritis" refers to an asymptomatic condition characterized by the presence of significant albumin and cast levels in the urine for more than 1 year after the acute onset. These findings indicate continued but slow parenchymal changes.

Clinical Manifestations

The development of acute glomerulonephritis may be insidious or sudden. Classic symptoms of sudden onset include hematuria with red cell casts and proteinuria. Fever, chills, weakness, pallor, anorexia, nausea, and vomiting may be present. Generalized edema, particularly facial and periorbital swelling, is a typical finding. The client may have ascites, pleural effusion, and congestive heart failure.

The client frequently has headache and moderate to severe hypertension. Visual acuity may be reduced owing to retinal edema. Abdominal or flank pain, probably caused by kidney edema and distention of the renal capsule, may be present. Oliguria, and even anuria, may be present for several days; the longer this persists, the more irreversible the kidney damage.

In contrast, the disease may be so mild that the client reports vague weakness, anorexia, and lethargy.

DIAGNOSTIC ASSESSMENT

Diagnosis is usually based on the presence of an underlying infection and an elevated antistreptolysin O titer. The disease, however, may even be discovered on the basis of a routine urinalysis.

Examining the urine usually provides the information necessary for a definitive diagnosis of acute glomerulonephritis. Gross hematuria and proteinuria are the cardinal findings. The urine, which may be scanty in amount, is typically dark, smoky or cola-colored, or red or brown in hue. The proteinuria produces a persistent and excessive foam. There is a low pH and a specific gravity in the mid- to high-normal range due to the kidneys' decreased ability to concentrate.

There are other studies that assist in the diagnosis. Serum urea nitrogen and creatinine levels will be elevated, and creatinine clearance rates will be down. C-reactive proteins and antistreptolysin O titer are usually elevated, and serum complement level is low. Hematocrit and hemoglobin studies indicate anemia.

Medical Management

Medical intervention aims to eliminate antigens, to alter the client's immune balance, and to inhibit or alleviate the inflammation for prevention of further renal damage and improvement of kidney function.

Plasmapheresis may be used in some research protocols for certain types of glomerulonephritis, including rapidly progressive glomerulonephritis. This intervention is used in conjunction with immunosuppressive therapy. This technique is designed to remove the specific circulating antibody or mediators of the inflammatory response. Large volumes of the client's plasma are cyclically removed and replaced with fresh frozen plasma by use of a continuous-flow blood cell separator.

PHARMACOLOGIC MANAGEMENT

Antibiotic therapy (e.g., penicillin for streptococcal organisms) is used to treat the predisposing infections. Volume overload and hypertension are treated with diuretics, antihypertensives, and restriction of dietary sodium and water. Corticosteroids and immunosuppressive agents (e.g., azathioprine and cyclophosphamide) may be used.

DIETARY MANAGEMENT

A low-sodium diet is used to treat the hypertension and fluid overload. If renal failure develops, then protein and other nutrients and electrolytes will be limited.

Complications

Common complications are congestive heart failure with pulmonary edema, and increased intracranial pressure. Renal failure may develop. Appropriate monitoring, including vital signs, intake and output, and weights, is essential. Recognizing complications early facilitates prompt medical intervention.

Surgical Management

Surgery is not used to treat glomerulonephritis. If the kidney is abscessed or completely destroyed, a nephrectomy may be performed.

Nursing Management

ASSESSMENT

A comprehensive history should be taken from the client with suspected glomerulonephritis about recent upper respiratory tract or skin infections or a history of glomerulonephritis. The client should also be questioned about systemic disorders that might be present, such as lupus. Any recent invasive procedures should also be noted.

Physical examination may reveal ascites, pleural effusion, and signs of congestive heart failure with pulmonary edema. The urine should be closely examined for color, amount, and presence of any abnormal substances. The vital signs should be closely checked, especially the blood pressure.

NURSING INTERVENTION

Nursing Diagnosis: Nutrition, Altered: less than required R/T anorexia and altered renal function.

Planning: Expected Outcomes. The client will maintain adequate nutritional intake, as evidenced by no weight loss, absence of a negative nitrogen balance, and normal electrolytes.

Implementation. It is important to protect the kidneys while they are recovering their function. The diet prescribed by the physician is generally high-calorie and low-protein. This diet avoids protein catabolism and allows the kidney to rest because it handles fewer protein molecules and metabolites. The degree to which protein is restricted depends on the amount excreted in the urine and the client's individual requirements. Sodium is also restricted, depending on the amount of edema present. Anorexia, nausea, and vomiting may interfere with adequate intake, requiring creative intervention on the part of the nurse. A dietician can help plan the client's diet around these restrictions.

Nursing Diagnosis: Fluid Volume Excess R/T reduced urine output.

Planning: Expected Outcomes. The client will maintain balanced intake and output, as evidenced by no signs of edema or fluid overload.

Implementation. Appropriate fluid balance is important. Careful monitoring of daily weights and intake and output helps determine the progress of the edema and thus provides an estimate of renal function. Daily measuring of edematous parts (e.g., legs and abdomen) also provides useful, objective data. The client's allowable fluid intake is based on the results of these measurements. Fluid intake is usually restricted. Thirst may be relieved by sucking on hard candies or lemon slices or by using ice chips rather than a glass of water. Assist the client to "plan" fluid distribution during the day (e.g., with meals).

Nursing Diagnosis: Activity Intolerance R/T fatigue.

Planning: Expected Outcomes. The client will obtain an adequate balance of rest and activity, as evidenced by absence of complaints of fatigue.

Implementation. Rest is essential—both physical and emotional. As mentioned, there is a direct correlation between activity and the amount of hematuria and proteinuria. Exercise also increases catabolic activity. The allowable amount of activity depends on the results of serial urinalyses. Bed rest followed by a period of very limited activity may continue for several weeks to months. Therefore, the client may need assistance in arranging personal matters, such as family, home, job, finances, and community responsibilities. Encourage the client to talk about any fears or concerns and, if necessary, help the client deal with the emotional reactions expected during a long-term illness with a questionable prognosis. Only after handling these problems will the client be able to rest emotionally. Appropriate diversionary activities may help the client cope with prolonged physical immobility.

Nursing Diagnosis: Skin Integrity, High Risk for Impaired R/T edema.

Planning: Expected Outcomes. The client will not develop skin breakdown, as evidenced by continued intact skin.

Implementation. Edema interferes with cellular nutrition, which makes the client more susceptible to skin breakdown. Therefore, take precautions to prevent this complication. Interventions include good hygiene, massage, and position changes as well as the use of other prophylactic measures, such as mattress devices. Use research-based tools to assess the client's risk of breakdown.

Nursing Diagnosis: Infection, High Risk for R/T altered immune response secondary to treatment.

Planning: Expected Outcomes. The client will not develop an infection, as evidenced by normal temperature.

Implementation. Glomerulonephritis markedly diminishes a client's natural defenses to infection, especially to streptococcal organisms. Moreover, immunosuppressives and corticosteroids further reduce host resistance. Although isolation is not necessary, take care to protect the client from others with obvious infectious processes. General supportive measures help boost the client's defense mechanisms. Too, you should teach the client appropriate ways to avoid infections.

EVALUATION

The nurse must evaluate client outcomes based on the established plan of care. If these goals were not achieved, the plan and interventions must be revised to meet the client's needs.

Modification of Plan of Care for the Elderly

The older client is at greater risk for renal damage because of the pre-existing effects of age on the kidneys. The older client is also more likely to have concurrent chronic diseases that may have affected the kidneys. Treatment is the same, however.

Post-hospital Care

DISCHARGE TEACHING

The client's learning needs will depend on the amount of renal damage done by the disease. If it is minimal, the client will need to be told to avoid infections and avoid any stressors on the kidneys.

If the client develops renal failure, teaching will have to be much more involved. If the client develops renal failure and requires dialysis, a great deal of teaching will be necessary. This information is covered later in this chapter.

HOME HEALTH CARE NEEDS

The level of home health care follow-up correlates with the degree of renal damage.

FOLLOW-UP CARE

The client's renal function will be assessed at frequent intervals for monitoring the status of the kidneys.

CHRONIC GLOMERULONEPHRITIS

Chronic glomerulonephritis is a heterogeneous category of diseases with varying causes. All the previously described forms of glomerulonephritis can progress to a chronic state. Sometimes, glomerulonephritis is first seen as a chronic process.

As the glomeruli and tubules are destroyed by the pathologic process, the kidneys shrink and become severely contracted. Fibrous and scar tissue replaces functioning renal tissue. Sclerosis of renal blood vessels also occurs. The destruction rates vary.

The disease has a very insidious onset. In fact, many years may pass before findings of renal insufficiency or renal failure appear. Common symptoms include malaise, weight loss, edema, increasing irritability and mental cloudiness, metallic taste in the mouth, polyuria and nocturia due to the kidney's inability to concentrate urine, headache, dizziness, and digestive disturbances. As the disease progresses, these symptoms intensify, and the client may experience respiratory difficulty and angina.

The cardinal symptom of this disease is hypertension. It is not uncommon for the client to experience complications such as nosebleed, signs of arteriosclerosis, cardiomegaly, and hemorrhage into the kidneys, lungs, retina, or cerebrum. Edema increases as heart failure becomes more severe and the serum albumin decreases. Examination of the eyegrounds shows vascular changes and edema of the discs. Urinalysis shows a fixed specific gravity, small amounts of proteinuria except during exacerbation, casts, white blood cells, renal tubular cells, and consistent hematuria. Anemia tends to be severe.

Chronic glomerulonephritis progresses over an extended period, often as long as 30 years. When it progresses to end-stage renal failure, dialytic therapy must be instituted or the client will die.

Medical treatment involves dialysis, transplant, and control of the accompanying symptoms. Chemotherapy with anti-inflammatory agents and anticoagulants may be used. Controlling edema and hypertension with diet and decreased fluid intake is imperative.

Nursing interventions focus on the need for consistent monitoring, symptomatic relief, education of the client about the disease and its management, and helping the client and significant others cope with a long-term illness.

TUBULOINTERSTITIAL DISEASES (INTERSTITIAL NEPHRITIS)

Traditionally, the term "interstitial nephritis" has been used to designate a category of renal disease characterized by the presence of inflammatory cells in the spaces between the renal tubules. However, not all disease processes included in this classification are inflammatory. Therefore, the term "tubulointerstitial disease" is being advocated as the label for this category of renal disorders.

Classification

Tubulointerstitial diseases are commonly classified as either acute or chronic.

ACUTE TUBULOINTERSTITIAL DISEASE

The acute form usually represents an allergic reaction and has a rapid onset. Assessment findings typically are the result of tubular injury. Symptoms often include fever, skin rash, eosinophilia, oliguric renal failure, and occasionally gross hematuria. The disease may progress along any of three courses: complete recovery, rapid progression to renal failure and death, or movement to the chronic form. Although corticosteroids are frequently used, their value is unclear. Treatment is similar to that for acute renal failure.

CHRONIC TUBULOINTERSTITIAL DISEASE

In chronic tubulointerstitial disease, there is progressive interstitial fibrosis and usually chronic inflammatory cell infiltration with tubular atrophy. In the terminal stages, the altered renal vasculature and renal structure make the disease indistinguishable from chronic pyelonephritis.

Pathophysiology

The morphologic findings for tubulointerstitial disease include interstitial edema, cellular infiltration of the interstitium, tubular cellular atrophy and flattening, and interstitial fibrosis. As the disease progresses, renal involvement extends beyond the tubules to progressive fibrosis of Bowman's capsule with secondary involvement of the glomeruli.

Potential causes of this pathologic process are many: acute pyelonephritis; septicemia; analgesic abuse, especially with phenacetin, aspirin, and acetaminophen; immunologic mechanisms, e.g., renal allograft, systemic lupus erythematosus, and Sjögren's syndrome; heavy metal toxicity; drug toxicity; hypercalcemia; and hypocalcemia.

Additionally, several medication hypersensitivities may contribute, e.g., rifampin, penicillin and its analogs, sulfonamides, cephalosporins, allopurinol, captopril, cimetidine, azathioprine, phenytoin, thiazide, lithium, nonsteroidal anti-inflammatory agents, and possibly furosemide.

Clinical Manifestations

An early sign of tubulointerstitial disease is a sudden, unexplained decrease in renal function that may be mild to severe. Specifically, there is an inability to concentrate urine, salt-wasting, and poor acidification of the urine leading to metabolic acidosis. Finding a variety of urine sediment abnormalities is common, too. Because they are not effectively reabsorbed in the tubules, glucose, uric acid, phosphates, amino acids, and bicarbonate will appear in the urine. Severe bicarbinaturia is an indicator of renal tubular acidosis. Proteinuria is less severe than with other renal disease. Systemic hypertension is a common finding.

MEMBRANOPROLIFERATIVE GLOMERULONEPHRITIS

As with acute glomerulonephritis, membranoproliferative glomerulonephritis is most common in children and young adults. Although it may be preceded by a streptococcal infection, more frequently the antigen is not identified. Its indications generally are nephrotic syndrome, microscopic or gross hematuria, and proteinuria. Although remissions may occur, they tend to be short-lived; the general course of the disease is a gradual progressive chronic renal failure.

Medical treatment so far has been disappointing. Renal transplants have been performed, but the disease almost always recurs. Chronic renal dialysis therapy is necessary. Nursing interventions are a combination of those for acute and chronic glomerulonephritis.

RAPIDLY PROGRESSIVE GLOMERULONEPHRITIS

Rapidly progressive glomerulonephritis is a fulminant variation of the disease. Its stimulus may be a streptococcus, staphylococcus, pneumococcus, virus, or collagen disease—or something thus far unidentified. More frequent among men, it strikes at any age but has a peak incidence between the ages of 40 and 60 years. It often begins insidiously and, without effective intervention, relentlessly progresses to renal failure and death within a period of weeks to months.

Initial symptoms include hematuria, edema, hypertension, nausea, vomiting, abdominal pain, diarrhea, proteinuria, oliguria or anuria, and acidosis. On morphologic examination, this condition is a diffuse proliferative inflammation that encircles the glomerulus, encroaches on Bowman's capsule, and apparently compresses the glomerular tufts.

Intravenous methylprednisone has been successful in treating some clients. Immunosuppression and anticoagulant therapy have also been used with inconsistent results. Nursing interventions are similar to those for other forms of glomerulonephritis.

IDIOPATHIC MEMBRANOUS GLOMERULONEPHRITIS

Idiopathic membranous glomerulonephritis is primarily a disorder of adults; peak onset is between the ages of 40 and 70 years. Immunologic challenge is less frequent than with other types, and the antigen source may not be known. Most clients present with asymptomatic proteinuria or nephrotic syndrome, and at least half of them have impaired renal function when the disease is first identified through renal biopsy. The prognosis for these clients is mixed: approximately 25 per cent experience spontaneous remission, 25 per cent have a persistent nephrotic syndrome, 25 per cent have persistent proteinuria, and 25 per cent progress to renal failure despite all treatment. Later stages of this disease become indistinguishable from chronic glomerulonephritis.

IgA NEPHROPATHY

IgA nephropathy, also called Berger's disease, was first described in 1968. It is a focal proliferative process occurring most frequently in children and young adults. There is still much to learn about this disease. Originally, it was believed to be relatively benign because of its seemingly nonprogressive nature. However, evidence suggests it may be chronic; approximately 25 per cent of clients demonstrate deteriorating renal function. The effectiveness of various treatments is still being studied.

LIPOID NEPHROSIS

Lipoid nephrosis, also called minimal change glomerulonephritis, is similar to the forms of glomerulonephritis described previously except that instead of proliferative and inflammatory changes, its pathologic change is degenerative. Although it can occur at any age, it is primarily a childhood disease and is the most common cause of nephrotic syndrome in children.

Its main morphologic finding is marked lipid accumulation in the proximal tubules and large numbers of fat bodies excreted in the urine. Overall, this disease has a good prognosis, especially when corticosteroids are given. There is, however, a tendency for spontaneous remission and repeated relapses. More information can be found in any pediatric nursing text.

FOCAL GLOMERULAR SCLEROSIS

Some authorities believe that focal glomerular sclerosis is a form of lipoid nephrosis, whereas others consider it a separate entity. Although it is primarily a disease of young children, its incidence in adults peaks between the ages of 30 and 50 years.

Histopathologic features include segmental or glial sclerosis. Initial clinical presentation shows nephrotic syndrome or persistent proteinuria. Adults commonly demonstrate hypertension and renal insufficiency.

The prognosis of this disease is poor, although the rate of deterioration varies widely. Complete remissions are rare. Steroids and immunosuppressive agents have been used but with disappointing results. Renal transplants have been successful temporarily, but the original disease almost invariably recurs. Therefore, the client may require chronic renal dialysis therapy.

NEPHROTIC SYNDROME

Definition

The nephrotic syndrome is a set of clinical symptoms arising from protein-wasting secondary to diffuse glomerular damage.

Incidence

Because of the multiple causes of this syndrome, it is a frequent sequela of both renal disorders and systemic diseases such as diabetes and lupus.

Etiology and Risk Factors

The causes of nephrotic syndrome are numerous; the most common is glomerulonephritis or some systemic disorder such as diabetes mellitus, lupus erythematosus, amyloidosis, hepatitis B, syphilis, carcinoma, leukemia, infectious disease, and preeclampsia. Other predisposing factors include allergic reactions; medication and drug reactions, e.g., penicillamine, anticonvulsants, probenecid, captopril, gold salts, heroin, and nonsteroidal anti-inflammatory medications; renal vein thrombosis; sickle cell disease; and congestive heart failure.

Pathophysiology

The pathophysiologic mechanism of this disorder is the abnormal permeability of the glomerular basement membrane to protein molecules, particularly albumin. These proteins are excessively filtered into the tubules and excreted into the urine. The resultant hypoalbuminemia alters the oncotic pressure within the vascular tree, and fluid moves into the interstitial spaces, initiating the development of edema. This stimulates plasma renin activity and augments aldosterone production so the kidney retains sodium and water, thus adding to the accumulation of extracellular fluid.

Potential complications include the effects of extracellular fluid accumulation and the progressive development of renal failure. The client may also experience severe hypovolemia, thromboembolism, secondary aldosteronism, abnormal thyroid function, and increased susceptibility to infections. Osteomalacia may also occur.

Clinical Manifestations

On the basis of this pathophysiologic mechanism, the clinical picture of nephrotic syndrome presents a classic constellation: proteinuria, hypoalbuminemia, and edema. Hyperlipidemia is usually found and is thought to result from increased hepatic lipoprotein synthesis in response to decreased serum albumin. Depending on the degree of renal failure, some level of normocytic anemia is common. Edema is usually the client's chief problem. Although its onset may be insidious, it becomes massive, and complications of the swelling may be seen. The skin frequently has a characteristic waxy pallor due to the edema rather than to the anemia. Other symptoms include anorexia, malaise, irritability, and amenorrhea or abnormal menses. The amount of proteinuria may account for losses of 4 to 30 g daily. Serum albumin concentrations may drop as low as 1 to 2.5 g/100 ml. The urine typically contains granular and epithelial cell casts and fat bodies. Some hematuria may be present.

DIAGNOSTIC ASSESSMENT

The urinalysis is the main diagnostic test; high amounts of protein are found in the urine.

Medical Management

The primary aim of medical treatment is to heal the leaking glomerular basement membrane and to stop loss of protein in the urine. The cycle of edema would then be broken. Much of the intervention concentrates on decreasing the client's edema.

Unless the client is hyponatremic, fluids are not usually restricted. The client's fluid balance should, however, be carefully monitored via daily weights, girth measurements, and intake and output determinations. These data are important because weight loss may represent true tissue loss from protein rather than from lost fluid.

PHARMACOLOGIC MANAGEMENT

Steroids are successful with some clients, depending on the cause of their disease. Cytotoxic agents such as cyclophosphamide and chlorambucil, indomethacin, anticoagulants, and antiplatelet agents may be used.

Loop diuretics, such as furosemide, are typically included in the medication regimen. Plasma volume expanders, such as salt-poor albumin, plasma, and dextran, may be administered to raise the oncotic pressure within the vascular tree. This pulls fluid from the extracellular spaces, making it available for kidney filtration. Diuresis in elderly clients must be handled with particular caution because of their reduced capability to tolerate sudden shifts in intravascular volume.

There is a significant incidence of renal vein thrombosis among clients with nephrotic syndrome. Because of this, some clients are placed on long-term anticoagulation. The client needs to know how to monitor for possible hemorrhage and should be encouraged to carry identification describing medications being taken.

DIETARY MANAGEMENT

Although some physicians recommend a diet containing a normal level of protein with good biologic value, others prescribe a diet of high biologic value protein with adequate carbohydrate and calorie intake. A daily protein intake of 1 to 1.5 g/kg daily with over 35 kcal/kg/day for prevention of further protein breakdown is generally recommended.[16]

Because the kidneys have a reduced capacity to excrete sodium, a mild sodium restriction is usually instituted. The level and duration of salt restriction are controversial issues. Because the client must take in the necessary protein and calories, the diet needs to be as palatable as possible.

Nursing Management

Nursing interventions are designed to help the client maintain health, manage the edema, cope with long-term illness, and learn about the disease and its treatment.

In addition to helping the client comply with the medication regimen, nursing interventions assist the client to achieve and maintain maximal health. Much of this is accomplished through presenting learning materials to the client and significant others. For example, teach the client that the amount of exercise allowed is based, at least in part, on the severity of the edema. Bed rest is imposed only during severe edema, and as the fluid level moves toward normal, the client is allowed more activity.

Because edema interferes with cellular nutrition, skin care is vital. During acute stages, the client and significant others may need help dealing with the accompanying malaise, anorexia, and depression. Also assess signs and symptoms of electrolyte imbalance associated with aggressive diuresis required for the client with central edema.

HYDRONEPHROSIS

Hydronephrosis is the distention of the renal pelvis and calices by an obstruction of normal urine flow. Urine production continues, and the urine is trapped proximal to the obstruction. The cause of the occlusion may include calculus, tumor, scar tissue, or a kink in the ureter.

Whatever the cause, the accumulating urine exerts pressure on the renal pelvis wall. At low to moderate pressures, the kidney may dilate with no obvious loss of function. Over time, sustained or intermittent high pressure causes irreversible nephron destruction. In addition to the pressure-related problems, pyelonephritis is always a risk because of urinary stasis.

Medical treatment aims to relieve the obstruction permanently and prevent infection. After the obstruction is relieved, postobstructive diuresis occurs, possibly leading to fluid and electrolyte imbalances including dehydration. Removal of the obstruction results in a sudden release of the pressure on the renal parenchyma caused by the trapped urine, which leads to the diuresis. The kidney will gradually begin to concentrate urine appropriately. Diuresis can, however, lead to fluid depletion if it continues.

Potential fluid volume deficit related to increased urine output is the most important nursing problem. Because of the dangers involved in postobstruction diuresis, it is crucial to monitor the client closely after an obstruction is released. Make frequent assessments, including hourly outputs; daily weights; vital signs every 30 minutes for the first 4 hours and then every 2 hours; urine for specific gravity, albumin, and glucose; and edema. Make periodic serum electrolyte and glucose determinations as well. Consider the expected presence of severe fatigue caused by urinary losses and the need for frequent observations. Fluid management during this period is crucial; hourly fluid replacement is based on the previous hour's output.

UREMIC SYNDROME

Uremia literally means "urine in the blood." This term and the term "uremic syndrome" describe a set of symptoms that result from loss of renal function. This loss may be sudden or may develop over a long period. It may be self-limiting or irreversible. Sudden loss of kidney function, such as occurs in damage from trauma, shock, toxins, or acute glomerulonephritis, brings on uremia rapidly and usually causes a severe deterioration of the client's condition. Gradual loss of kidney function over an extended period may occur with glomerulonephritis, hypertension, chronic pyelonephritis, and other diseases.

Because the kidneys perform a wide variety of functions, the effects of uremia occur not only within the kidneys themselves but also within other organ systems. Because of the time factor, chronic renal failure produces more degenerative changes in the body than does acute uremia. However, both types have many of the same consequences, and unless the process can be halted, coma, convulsions, and death result.

ACUTE RENAL FAILURE

Definition

Acute renal failure (ARF) refers to the abrupt loss of kidney function. Over a period of hours to a few days, the GFR falls, accompanied by concomitant rise in serum creatinine and urea nitrogen. A healthy adult eating a normal diet needs a minimum daily urine output of approximately 400 ml to excrete the body's waste products through the kidneys. An amount lower than this indicates a decreased GFR. Oliguria refers to daily outputs of urine between 100 and 400 ml; anuria refers to outputs less than 100 ml.

Incidence

The incidence of ARF will depend on the underlying cause. The most common causes of ARF are hypotension and prerenal hypovolemia.

Etiology

The numerous causes of ARF can be categorized into three major areas: prerenal, renal, and postrenal (Fig. 50-1).

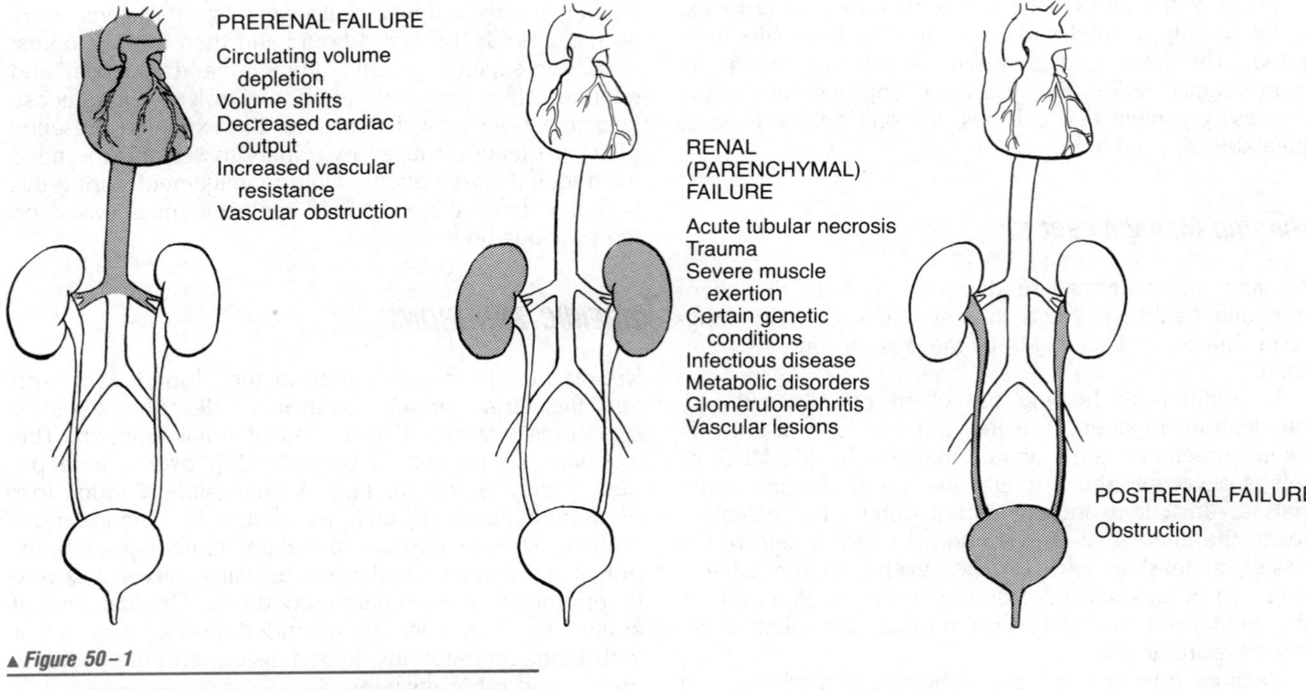

▲ *Figure 50-1*

Causes of acute renal failure: prerenal, renal, and postrenal.

PRERENAL CAUSES

Prerenal causes interfere with renal perfusion. The kidneys depend on an adequate delivery of blood to be filtered by the glomeruli. Therefore, a reduced renal blood flow obviously decreases the GFR. Conditions that contribute to decreased renal blood flow include (1) circulatory volume depletion, such as may occur with diarrhea, vomiting, hemorrhage, excessive use of diuretics, burns, renal salt-wasting conditions, and glycosuria; (2) volume shifts, e.g., "third space" sequestration of fluid, vasodilation, and gram-negative sepsis; (3) decreased cardiac output, such as during cardiac pump failure, pericardial tamponade, and acute pulmonary embolism; (4) increased vascular resistance, e.g., anesthesia and hepatorenal syndrome; and (5) vascular obstruction, e.g., bilateral renal artery occlusion or dissecting aneurysm.

RENAL CAUSES

Renal causes refer to parenchymal changes from disease or nephrotoxic substances. Acute tubular necrosis is the most frequent renal cause of ARF, accounting for approximately 75 per cent of cases.[50] This destruction of the tubular epithelial cells is the result of impaired renal perfusion or direct damage from nephrotoxins. In addition to the nephrotoxins described previously, acute tubular necrosis may also be caused by the presence of heme pigments, such as myoglobin and hemoglobin, which are liberated from damaged muscle tissue. This release may result from trauma (rhabdomyolysis) such as surgery, crush injury, and electric shock or from nontraumatic conditions such as severe muscle exertion, genetic conditions (e.g., diabetes mellitus and malignant hyperthermia), infectious disease, and metabolic conditions (e.g., hypokalemia, phosphatemia, and heatstroke).[68]

Additional renal causes of ARF include glomerulonephritis; microvascular and large vascular lesions, as in hemolytic-uremic syndrome; thrombosis; vasculitis; scleroderma; trauma; atherosclerosis; tumor invasion; and cortical necrosis, which is caused by prolonged vasospasm of the cortical blood vessels.

POSTRENAL CAUSES

Postrenal causes leading to ARF arise from obstruction in the urinary tract, anywhere from the tubules to the urethral meatus. Common sources of obstruction include prostatic hypertrophy, calculi, invading tumors, surgical accidents, and retroperitoneal fibrosis. Obstruction caused by retroperitoneal fibrosis is difficult to identify unless it is bilateral. This is because the unobstructed kidney continues to function normally, and if the affected kidney is only partially obstructed, it may even become polyuric as it loses its ability to concentrate.

In managing the client with ARF, it is important to determine whether the disorder originates in the prerenal, renal, or postrenal area before intervention begins. Appropriate interventions require determining the origin of the disorder.

Risk Factors

This condition may be preventable with close monitoring by the nurse of the client at risk. Because hypotension and hypovolemia are two causes with the highest mortality rate, early diagnosis and reversal of these problems can save the client's life. The nurse must carefully monitor the vital signs and urine output of clients at risk for the development of ARF.

Nephrotoxic agents are another risk factor for this condition. The nurse should always be aware of the action and potential side and toxic effects of any medication administered to the client.

Pathophysiology

The pathogenesis of ARF is not clear. One hypothesis is that the damaged tubules cannot conserve sodium normally, which leads to renin-angiotensin-aldosterone system activation. This redistributes the renal vascular supply by increasing the tone of both the afferent and efferent arterioles. The resulting ischemia may cause an increase in vasopressin, cellular swelling, inhibition of prostaglandin synthesis, and further stimulation of the renin-angiotensin system. The reduced blood flow decreases glomerular pressure, GFR, and tubular flow; thus, oliguria occurs.

There is also a theory that cellular and protein debris within the tubule obstructs the lumen, which raises the intratubular pressure. This increasing oncotic pressure opposes filtration pressure until glomerular filtration stops. A biochemical theory claims that decreased renal blood flow leads to decreased oxygen delivery to the proximal tubules; this causes reduction in cellular adenosine triphosphate, which increases cytosolic and mitochondrial calcium concentrations. The result of this process is cell death and tubular necrosis. Vasomotor nephropathy, causing spasms of peritubular capillaries, may result in tubular damage. Other possible pathogenic mechanisms include leakage of filtered urine through damaged tubules back into the peritubular capillaries and chemical or morphologic changes in the basement membrane of the glomerular capillary, which decreases nephron filtration. The reversibility of this is dependent on the level of destruction of the basement membrane.[34]

The mortality rate for ARF may be as high as 50 per cent; the highest mortality rates occur when the failure is caused by trauma or surgery. The lowest mortality rate is for ARF caused by nephrotoxic substances (discussed earlier). When obstruction or glomerulonephritis is the cause, the mortality rate is low.

The clinical course of ARF is marked by several phases. The onset, or initiating, phase covers the period from the precipitating event to the development of renal symptoms. Symptoms may begin immediately or a week after the precipitating event. The oliguric-anuric or nonoliguric phase lasts 1 to 8 weeks. The longer the persistence, the poorer the prognosis. Dialytic therapy may be required during the oliguric-anuric phase.

A gradual or abrupt return to glomerular filtration and leveling of the blood urea nitrogen (BUN) signals the diuretic phase. Urine output may be 1000 to 2000 ml/day, which may lead to dehydration; 25 per cent of the deaths from acute renal failure occur during this phase. The recovery phase lasts 3 to 12 months. During this time, the client often returns to a prerenal failure activity level. In actuality, mild tubular abnormalities, including glycosuria and decreased concentrating ability, may continue for years, and the client will continually be at risk for fluid and electrolyte imbalance, especially during times of stress.

The effects of ARF are widespread. The major consequences include (1) fluid and electrolyte imbalances (fluid overload or depletion, hyperkalemia, hyponatremia, hypocalcemia, and hypermagnesemia); (2) acidosis; (3) increased susceptibility to secondary infections; (4) anemia; (5) platelet dysfunction; (6) gastrointestinal complications (anorexia, nausea, vomiting, diarrhea or constipation, and stomatitis); (7) increased incidence of pericarditis; and (8) uremic encephalopathy characterized by apathy, defective recent memory, episodic obtundation, dysarthria, tremors, convulsions, and coma. Wound healing is impaired. Other symptoms are usually a result of these sequelae.

Clinical Manifestations

The most common overall sign of ARF is alteration in the expected urine output. Usually this is oliguria or anuria, but polyuric ARF accounts for 30 per cent of the cases.[31]

There are two varieties of ARF: nonoliguric and oliguric.

Nonoliguric Renal Failure. Although nonoliguric, or polyuric, ARF is being recognized more often, whether it is an entity in and of itself or a phase of oliguric ARF remains controversial. Clients with nonoliguric renal failure may excrete as much as 2 L/day, and this needs to be recognized as a possible sign of ARF. The urine produced is dilute and nearly isomolar, indicating that not all nephrons have stopped filtering. Hypertension and tachypnea, with signs of fluid overload, are frequently found. However, the client may also demonstrate signs of extracellular fluid depletion, such as dry mucous membranes, poor skin turgor, and orthostatic hypotension. Nonoliguric renal failure is usually associated with less morbidity and mortality than is the oliguric form, probably because of the lesser degree and shorter duration of azotemia.

Oliguric Renal Failure. In oliguric ARF, urine production usually falls below 400 ml/day. However, remember that the aging kidney normally loses its concentrating ability, and the renal function becomes more susceptible to insult. Therefore, the older client may have developed oliguria at urine volumes of 600 to 700 ml/day.[51]

The clinical manifestations of oliguric ARF depend on the causation. In prerenal failure, assessment findings are quite diverse, depending on the underlying condition. The client will frequently have a history of a precipitating event, such as hemorrhage or cardiac insult. The urine has a high specific gravity and osmolarity, and there is little or no proteinuria. Urine sediment is usually normal, although it may contain a few hyaline and granular casts. There is very little urinary sodium excretion. The BUN : creatinine ratio is significantly elevated, reaching levels of 10 : 1 to 40 : 1.

Systemic signs of intrinsic renal failure may include edema, weight gain, hemoptysis from elevated left ventricular end-diastolic pressure, weakness from anemia, and hypertension. The urine has a fixed specific gravity, a high sodium concentration, and definite proteinuria. In the case of glomerulonephritis, there will be hematuria and red blood cell and hemoglobin casts. Acute tubular necrosis will cause "muddy-brown" granular casts. If there has been significant tissue damage, elevated levels of serum creatinine, phosphokinase, and potassium can be expected.

Urine produced in postrenal failure may have fixed specific gravity and elevated sodium concentration with little or no proteinuria. Urine sediment is generally normal. The most definitive signs are those indicating obstruction, as described with calculi and neoplasms. Wide fluctuations between anuria and polyuria may indicate intermittent urinary tract obstruction.

DIAGNOSTIC ASSESSMENT

Urinalysis, urine specific gravity and sodium levels, and serum creatinine and urea nitrogen are common diagnostic tests for ARF. The amount of urine in relation to intake is also important in formulating the diagnosis. To measure the exact amount of urine output or obtaining a specimen for culture and sensitivity, the client may need to be straight catheterized.

Medical Management

The medical management of ARF is largely based on preventing and treating its effects. As with any disease process, prevention is the primary intervention. Attaining and maintaining adequate hydration and diuresis in high-risk clients is crucial, as is the prevention of contributing factors. Once ARF has developed, prompt recognition and action facilitate restoration of optimal renal function. Correction of the underlying condition may be all that is necessary in ARF due to prerenal disorders. Postrenal causes must be rectified. In the meantime, the sequelae of ARF require specific intervention.

Treatment for ARF usually takes place in an intensive care unit. Much of the care revolves around physiologic monitoring and interventions that center primarily on maintenance of fluid and electrolyte balance and nutrition.

Dialysis is frequently required for treatment of ARF. Indications for dialysis include significant volume overload, uncontrolled hyperkalemia or acidosis, progressive uremia as evidenced by rising BUN and creatinine concentrations, altered central nervous system function, and pericarditis. Dialysis is discussed later in this chapter.

Secondary infections are a significant cause of death in clients with ARF. The client must be monitored carefully for infectious processes; if these occur, they should be treated aggressively. Indwelling urethral catheters are avoided because of their great potential for introducing infection.

Pericarditis occurs in as many as 18 per cent of clients with renal failure. Assessment findings include pleuritic pain that may be relieved by an upright position, pericardial friction rub, tachycardia, and fever. Treatment is usually begun with steroids or nonsteroidal anti-inflammatory agents. Pericardiocentesis and pericardiectomy may be necessary if cardiac function is compromised.

Other problems call for symptomatic relief. There is a rise in the number of seizures and a decrease in the seizure threshold secondary to the rising BUN. These seizures may be relieved by intravenous phenytoin or phenobarbital. Anemia is treated by transfusions or the use of recombinant erythropoietin. Erythropoietin is the hormone produced by the kidney to stimulate red cell production. Erythropoietin is used in chronic renal failure, although its use in ARF has not been studied extensively. Bleeding tendencies may be minimized by correcting vitamin K deficiencies as well as by lowering the serum BUN level, because BUN interferes with platelet aggregation.

PHARMACOLOGIC MANAGEMENT

Fluid replacement must be done very carefully for the avoidance of fluid overload. Fluid replacement volumes are usually calculated on the basis of some fraction of the previous day's urine output plus an amount (e.g., 400 ml) to account for the usual insensible loss that occurs during a 24-hour period. Losses from other sources, such as vomiting and diarrhea, are added to the daily allotment. Unless the client is on total parenteral nutrition, some physicians use a daily weight loss of 0.2 to 0.5 kg/day as a measure of the success of the fluid replacement program. This represents usual daily weight loss from catabolism and loss of lean body mass.

Diuretic therapy may be used, although it remains controversial. Furosemide and mannitol are the pharmacologic agents most frequently used, and they must be administered cautiously. It is important to replace fluids as needed to maintain adequate blood flow and perfusion to the kidneys. These diuretics may affect the outcome of nonoliguric ARF, which generally has a better prognosis than does anuric or oliguric renal failure.

Electrolyte replacement is based primarily on urine and serum electrolyte concentrations. Hyperkalemia is probably the most dangerous imbalance because of its contribution to cardiac arrhythmias and arrest. In addition to the kidney's inability to excrete potassium, this electrolyte is released in greater quantities from the body cells when acidosis is present and is further increased by rapid tissue catabolism. Electrocardiographic monitors are frequently used. Cation-exchange resins may be administered orally or rectally to facilitate excretion of potassium through the gastrointestinal tract. Sorbitol, an osmotic cathartic, is given with cation-exchange resins to induce a diarrhea to eliminate the potassium ions that were exchanged for sodium ions in the resins. Potassium-containing foods and medications should be avoided. The administration of 50 per cent glucose and regular insulin, with sodium bicarbonate if necessary or calcium gluconate intravenously, can temporarily prevent cardiac arrest in an emergency by moving potassium into the cells and temporarily reducing serum potassium levels.

Hyponatremia is usually an effect of dilution rather than a true lack of sodium. Therefore, intervention is actually a factor of proper fluid replacement (i.e., fluid restriction and self-correction). Hyperphosphatemia is treated with decreased dietary intake and phosphate binders. Antacids containing magnesium should be avoided. Physostigmine may be used for hypermagnesemia, and intravenous magnesium sulfate for hypomagnesemia.

Metabolic acidosis usually results from the accumulation of acid waste products. Sodium bicarbonate, sodium lactate, or sodium acetate may be used on a short-term basis to correct this condition. Dialysis is usually used for severe acidosis.

DIETARY MANAGEMENT

Proper nutrition is crucial. A high-calorie, low-protein diet is usually prescribed. It may also be low in sodium and potassium. The protein must be of high biologic value (complete), containing the essential amino acids to reduce the nitrogenous waste products. Adequate carbohydrate intake reverses the process of gluconeogenesis. During the acute phases, intake should be 135 to 150 nonprotein kcal for each 6.25 g of protein ingested; this ratio is considered adequate for prevention of protein catabolism.[50] Low-potassium liquid supplements may also be used. If oral intake is not sufficient to meet requirements, tube feedings or total parenteral nutrition, including intralipids, may be instituted.

Nursing Management

ASSESSMENT

The nurse should assess the client for the presence of risk factors for the development of ARF. The nurse must carefully monitor the client for the development of ARF. Because hypovolemia is a common cause, the nurse must assess the client closely for this problem. The most important assessment the nurse can make, therefore, is fluid balance.

Once the client has been diagnosed with ARF, the nurse must carefully assess the client for the development of complications such as pleural effusion, pericarditis, acidosis, and uremia.

NURSING INTERVENTION

Nursing Diagnosis: Fluid Volume Deficit R/T hypovolemia, followed by Fluid Volume Excess R/T inability of kidneys to produce urine secondary to ARF.

Planning: Expected Outcomes. The client will not develop fluid volume deficit and ARF; if ARF does occur, the client will not develop fluid volume excess or will have it managed with dialysis, as evidenced by return to balanced intake and output.

Implementation. Careful monitoring of fluid balance indicators is crucial to the management of ARF. Accurate intake and output measurements guide the fluid replacement regimen. It is important to compare these values, looking for 24- to 48-hour trends. Vital signs, including postural blood pressures, apical pulses, skin turgor, and mucous membranes, are checked approximately every 4 hours depending on the severity of the illness. Daily weights are carefully obtained. Internal blood pressure measurements may be done. Urine specific gravity, usually an indication of fluid balance, may be negated by intrinsic renal disease. Heart sounds, lung sounds, and mental status may indicate the presence of fluid imbalances.

Once the physician has determined the client's fluid allotment, the nurse must be sure the regimen is followed. This means carefully monitoring fluid intake to make certain that the prescribed amount is taken. Many times, this amount represents a fluid restriction for the client, which causes a problem with thirst. The nurse helps the client stay within the prescribed restriction with careful oral hygiene, judicious use of ice chips, lip ointments, and appropriate diversionary activities. Placing the allotted water in a spray bottle may help to spread out the amount taken. Fluid from nutrition must be taken into account. To conserve fluids for the client, the nurse can administer medications with meals, if possible.

Nursing Diagnosis: Nutrition, Altered: Less than Body Requirements R/T anorexia secondary to renal failure or dietary restrictions.

Planning: Expected Outcomes. The client will maintain adequate nutrition, as evidenced by sufficient intake to prevent protein catabolism.

Implementation. The client frequently experiences anorexia, nausea, and stomatitis accompanying renal failure. That combined with the general unpalatability of the diet makes adequate nutrition a challenge for the nurse and client. Working with the client to plan a diet that is most acceptable is important. The therapeutic dietician is a good resource. Provide a pleasant environment at mealtime. Food prepared in an attractive manner and presented in small amounts may help. Medications to alleviate the discomfort of nausea and stomatitis are useful. Parenteral nutrition may be instituted if the client's nutritional status cannot be maintained with oral intake.

Nursing Diagnosis: Skin Integrity, High Risk for Impaired R/T poor cellular nutrition.

Planning: Expected Outcomes. The client will not develop impaired skin integrity, as evidenced by intact skin.

Implementation. The poor systemic nutrition and edema accompanying renal failure may cause skin breakdown. Meticulous skin care, frequent turning, and special mattresses are very important. Range-of-motion exercises facilitate movement and increase circulation.

Nursing Diagnosis: Infection, High Risk for R/T lowered resistance.

Planning: Expected Outcomes. The client will not develop infection, as evidenced by normal vital signs and white blood cell count.

Implementation. The client with ARF is compromised and very susceptible to secondary infections, which represent a stress that the kidneys cannot handle. Urethral catheters are avoided if possible. If they must be used, provide meticulous catheter care. Nursing intervention must be designed to prevent infection in the usual high-risk sites (e.g., respiratory tract, wounds, central catheters, and mouth). The nurse must also be alert to early signs of infection so aggressive medical treatment may be instituted.

Nursing Diagnosis: Anxiety R/T unknown outcome of disease process.

Planning: Expected Outcomes. The client will not exhibit signs of anxiety, as evidenced by calmness and ability to focus on disease and its outcomes (within the limits of altered mental status related to elevated BUN).

Implementation. Because the client's physical needs are so obvious, it is easy to forget that the client, as well as significant others, will be anxious and frightened. Give frequent, careful explanations and remain cognizant of the need for emotional and psychosocial support. Be aware that the client may be mechanically ventilated and not able to articulate feelings and fears.

EVALUATION

The evaluations of outcomes of client goals must be done continually. If the goals have not been met, the nurse must revise the interventions to meet those needs.

Modification of Plan of Care for the Elderly

The major difference with older clients is their increased risk for developing ARF because of their cardiovascular instability. The older adult has more difficulty maintaining a homeostatic fluid balance. There is also a greater likelihood that older clients have some pre-existing renal damage, especially men related to benign prostatic hypertrophy and the obstruction it causes.

Post-hospital Care

DISCHARGE TEACHING

The client and significant others will require a great deal of teaching about renal function, the signs and symptoms of renal failure, and the need for possibly ongoing treatment. The client and significant others will have to understand what signs and symptoms might indicate further renal damage or that the client has developed chronic renal failure.

HOME HEALTH CARE NEEDS

Most care for ARF takes place in the intensive care unit. Once the client begins to recover, transfer will be made to a general floor, and the client will eventually be discharged. The significant others caring for the client will have to be able to monitor progress by measuring the client's weight, intake and output, and dietary modifications. They may require some visiting nurse follow-up.

FOLLOW-UP CARE

The client will need to be closely followed by a nephrologist at frequent intervals for at least a year after ARF is reversed so that deterioration of renal function can be monitored.

CHRONIC RENAL FAILURE

Definition

Chronic, or irreversible, renal failure (CRF) is a progressive reduction of functioning renal tissue such that the remaining kidney mass can no longer maintain the body's internal environment. It can develop insidiously over many years or can occur as a result of a bout of ARF from which the client fails to recover.

Incidence

As the life expectancy increases and medical science is able to prolong life, the incidence of CRF has been increasing.

Hypertension and diabetes are the most common causes of CRF, accounting for over 60 per cent of the clients seen on dialysis. Men and women are equally affected by the problem; the incidence is highest among middle-aged clients.

Etiology

The causes of CRF are numerous. Throughout this section, various injuries and disease processes that may potentially end in renal failure have been discussed. Chronic glomerulonephritis, acute renal failure, polycystic kidney disease, obstruction, repeated bouts of pyelonephritis, and nephrotoxins are examples of causes. Systemic diseases such as diabetes mellitus, hypertension, lupus erythematosus, polyarteritis, sickle cell disease, and amyloidosis may produce renal failure.

The most common causes of CRF are diabetic and hypertensive nephropathy, glomerulonephritis, chronic pyelonephritis, and then other disorders.

Risk Factors

Clients with a variety of renal and systemic diseases are at risk for CRF. These include diseases such as glomerulonephritis, obstructions, ARF, hypertension, diabetes mellitus, and lupus.

In order to decrease the risk that these diseases will lead to CRF, the client should be closely followed and receive adequate treatment to control or slow the progress of these problems before they progress to end-stage renal failure. Some conditions, such as lupus and diabetes, however, can progress to failure despite close treatment.

Pathophysiology

The pathogenesis of CRF portrays deterioration and destruction of nephrons with progressive loss of renal function. As the total GFR falls and clearance is reduced, the serum urea nitrogen and creatinine clearance levels rise. Remaining functioning nephrons hypertrophy as they are required to filter a larger load of solutes. One of the consequences of this is that the kidneys lose their ability to concentrate urine adequately. In an attempt to continue excreting the solutes, a large volume of dilute urine is passed, which makes the client susceptible to fluid depletion. The tubules gradually lose their ability to reabsorb electrolytes. Occasionally, this can result in "salt-wasting," in which the urine contains very large amounts of sodium, which leads to more polyuria.

As renal damage advances and the number of functioning nephrons declines, the total GFR decreases further. Thus, the body becomes unable to rid itself of water, salt, and other waste products through the kidneys. When the GFR is less than 10 to 20 ml/min, clinical uremia is evident. The body becomes increasingly toxic.

The result of CRF is uremia and death, treatment with dialysis, or transplantation. The introduction of Medicare funding to pay for dialysis in 1973 opened the option of dialysis to clients suffering from CRF (see Ethical Issues in Nursing).

Clinical Manifestations

Because of the wide diversity of contributing elements and disease processes, the early stages of renal failure are varied. However, as the destruction of nephrons progresses to its end stage, the manifestations become very similar and are classified as uremic syndrome.

The projected clinical course of irreversible renal disease is as follows:

- Normal functioning.
- Reduced renal reserve, in which the BUN may be high-normal, but there are no clinical symptoms. Normal functioning is evident as long as the client is not exposed to unusual physiologic or psychosocial stress.
- Renal insufficiency demonstrates a more advanced pathologic process with mild azotemia when the client is on a general diet. Impaired urine concentration with nocturia and mild anemia are common findings. Renal function is easily impaired by stress.
- Renal failure causes severe azotemia, acidosis, impaired urine dilution, severe anemia, and a number of electrolyte imbalances, such as hypernatremia, hyperkalemia, and hyperphosphatemia.
- Finally, end-stage renal disease is characterized by two groups of clinical symptoms: deranged excretory and regulatory mechanisms; and a distinctive grouping of gastrointestinal, cardiovascular, neuromuscular, hematologic, integumentary, skeletal, and hormonal symptoms.

The clinical manifestations of CRF—with its retention of nitrogenous waste products; changes in fluid, electrolyte, and acid-base balances; and loss of normal kidney functions—are present throughout the body. No organ system is spared. Renal alterations (described previously) include the kidney's inability to concentrate urine and regulate electrolyte excretion. Polyuria progresses to anuria, and the client loses normal diurnal patterns of voiding. In addition, all normal functions of the kidney become curtailed and are eventually lost. This includes regulation of acid-base balance, regulation of blood pressure, synthesis of 1,25 dihydroxycholecalciferol, biogenesis of erythropoietin, degradation of insulin, and synthesis of prostaglandins. Refer to Chapter 47 for more information about these functions.

Electrolyte Imbalances. Although many clients maintain a normal serum sodium level, electrolyte balances may be upset by impaired excretion and utilization. The salt-wasting properties of some failing kidneys, in addition to vomiting and diarrhea, may cause hyponatremia. Apparent hyponatremia may be a dilutional effect of water retention. Late in the disease, the problem becomes hypernatremia, and the salt and water retention often contribute to hypertension and congestive heart failure.

Because the kidneys are very efficient potassium excretors, potassium levels usually remain within normal limits until late in the disease. However, hyperkalemia then becomes a challenging problem. Catabolism, potassium-containing medications, trauma, blood transfusions, and acidosis contribute to potassium excess.

Hypocalcemia occurs as a result of decreased conversion of 25-hydroxycholecalciferol to 1,25-dihydroxycholecalciferol and a reduced intestinal absorption of calcium. At the same time, phosphate is not excreted, which causes hyperphosphatemia. This combination stimulates the parathyroid glands to secrete parathyroid hormone in an attempt to facilitate phosphate excretion and raise the serum calcium level by the resorption of calcium from bone. Osteomalacia, osteitis fibrosa, and osteosclerosis are commonly seen in CRF clients as a result of these metabolic alterations in calcium, phosphorus, parathyroid hormone, and vitamin D. Some clients may develop hypercalcemia because of persistent secretion of parathyroid hormone.

Mildly elevated serum magnesium levels are found early in the disease. However, these do not usually reach a dangerous level unless the client is receiving magnesium-containing laxatives or antacids.

Metabolic Changes. In advancing renal failure, BUN and serum creatinine rise as waste products of protein metabolism accumulate in the blood. The proteinuria accompanying renal disease and inadequate dietary intake of proteins often cause hypoproteinemia, which decreases the intravascular oncotic pressure. Serum uric acid is often high but is not commonly associated with signs of gout.

Carbohydrate intolerance results from impaired insulin production and metabolism. Four mechanisms are responsible: peripheral insulin antagonism, impaired insulin secretion, prolonged insulin half-life directly related to kidney malfunction, and abnormalities in circulating insulin. Therefore, special care is needed in adjusting insulin doses for clients with diabetes mellitus complicated by renal failure. Results of glucose tolerance tests must be carefully interpreted.

Elevated triglycerides is almost a universal finding. This type IV hyperlipidemia is thought to be caused by increased production of lipids by the liver in response to the elevated blood glucose and insulin levels. At the same time, there seems to be reduced assimilation of lipids in the peripheral tissues, possibly because of the blockage of lipoprotein lipase activity.

Metabolic acidosis occurs because of the kidney's inability to excrete hydrogen ions as a result of decreased reabsorption of sodium bicarbonate and decreased formation of dihydrogen phosphate and ammonia. This condition accentuates hyperkalemia and the reabsorption of calcium from the bones.

Pericarditis is usually related to accumulation of uremic toxins and is rarely due to infection. Symptoms include pericardial pain (often relieved by an upright position), tachycardia, pleural friction rub, and fever. The condition may progress to pericardial effusion and cardiac tamponade, a life-threatening complication.

Hematologic Changes. The primary hematologic effect of renal failure is anemia, usually normochromic and normocytic. Frequently, it is the fatigue, weakness, and cold intolerance accompanying the anemia that initiate the evaluation leading to a diagnosis of renal failure. The mild anemia found in the early stages is usually due to reduced erythropoiesis. Later, hemolysis, gastrointestinal losses, and clotting abnormalities may add to the severity of the condition. Occasionally, the client will be iron- or folate-depleted from nutritional deficiencies. Bleeding tendencies become apparent as the disease progresses. Platelet abnormalities are the primary defect responsible for bleeding in the uremic client. The accumulation of uremic toxins interferes with platelet adhesiveness.

Gastrointestinal Changes. The entire gastrointestinal system is affected. Transient anorexia, nausea, and vomiting are almost universal. Clients often experience a constant, bitter, metallic, or salty taste, and their breath commonly smells fetid, fishy, or ammoniacal. Stomatitis, parotitis, and gingivitis are common problems due to poor oral hygiene and the formation of ammonia from salivary urea. Accumulations of gastrin (due to increased secretion abnormalities of gastric acid physiology) may be a major cause of ulcer disease. Esophagitis, gastritis, colitis, gastrointestinal bleeding, and diarrhea may be found. Serum amylase levels may be increased, although they may not indicate actual pancreatitis.

Constipation is a common problem. It is often the result of phosphate-binding agents; restriction of fluids and high-fiber foods, many of which are potassium- and phosphorus-rich; and decreased activity. Constipation provides a particular challenge, because the usual interventions for prevention and treatment are contraindicated in the client with renal failure.

Immunologic Changes. Impairment of the immunologic system makes the client very susceptible to infection. Several factors are involved, including depression of humoral antibody formation, suppression of delayed hypersensitivity, and decreased chemotactic function of the leukocytes. Immunosuppression is an important part of the medical management of CRF. Immunosuppression after transplantation is discussed later in this chapter.

Changes in Medication Metabolism. Finally, renal failure has a serious effect on medication metabolism. The uremic client is at very high risk for medication toxicity owing to the effect of renal changes on the pharmacokinetics (absorption, distribution, metabolism, and excretion) of otherwise therapeutic medications. There are three main causes of this toxicity: (1) a high plasma level of the medication due to low serum albumin, decreased binding sites, impaired renal excretion, or impaired hepatic metabolism of the medication; (2) increased sensitivity to the medication due to uremia-induced changes in the target organ; and (3) a metabolic load because of the administration of the medication, e.g., hypoalbuminemia means less protein available for binding. There are various tables and formulas that help guide dosage decisions. Remember that medication dosages must be altered and that the usual dosage ranges in the medication literature are not safe for the client with CRF. Assess the client carefully for toxic reactions.

Cardiovascular Changes. At least 50 to 65 per cent of deaths occurring during chronic renal failure result from cardiovascular complications.[44] The most frequent clinical manifestation is hypertension produced through (1) the mechanisms of volume overload; (2) stimulation of the renin-angiotensin system; (3) sympathetically mediated vasoconstriction, e.g., increased levels of dopamine beta-hydroxylase; and (4) the absence of prostaglandins. Any of the many systemic complications of prolonged high blood pressure may be found.

The effects of volume overload on the heart are seen, including left ventricular hypertrophy and congestive heart failure. Heart failure may also result from anemia, arteriovenous shunt, complications of coronary artery disease, electrolyte imbalance, acidosis, myocardial calcification, and thiamine depletion. Arrhythmias may be caused by hyperkalemia, acidosis, hypermagnesemia, and decreased coronary perfusion.

Atherosclerosis is accelerated because of (1) abnormal carbohydrate and lipid metabolism; (2) impaired fibrinolysis, which leads to the development of microemboli; and (3) hyperparathyroidism. Arterial calcifications have been identified, the ankles being the most common early location. Other sites include the abdominal aorta, feet, pelvis, hands, and wrists. These vascular calcifications also occur within the heart itself, particularly at the mitral valve.

Respiratory Changes. Some of the respiratory effects, such as pulmonary edema, can be attributed to fluid overload. Pleuritis is a frequent finding, especially when pericarditis develops. A characteristic condition called uremic lung is a type of pneumonitis that responds well to fluid removal. Acidosis causes a compensatory increase in respiratory rate as the lungs try to eliminate excess hydrogen ions.

Musculoskeletal Changes. The musculoskeletal system is affected fairly early in the disease process, and bone reabsorption found on x-ray examination may be the first sign of renal failure in some clients. The most prevalent problem, affecting up to 90 per cent of clients with CRF, is renal osteodystrophy. This condition develops insidiously and takes several forms: osteomalacia, osteitis fibrosis, osteoporosis, or osteosclerosis. The development of this manifestation results from interrelationships between the kidney-bone-parathyroid and calcium-phosphate–vitamin D connections. As the GFR decreases, phosphate excretion decreases, and calcium elimination increases. The abnormal levels of calcium and phosphate stimulate the release of parathyroid hormone, which mobilizes calcium from the bones and facilitates phosphate excretion.

As the renal failure progresses, the kidney no longer converts vitamin D to its active form, 1,25-dihydroxycholecalciferol. The lack of this substance interferes with calcium absorption from the intestine and paradoxically facilitates phosphate retention. Thus, mineralization of the bone with calcium and phosphate is impaired. Demineralization of the bone frees more calcium and phosphorus into the blood. As the disease progresses even further, the parathyroid gland may become unresponsive to the normal feedback system and continue to produce parathyroid hormone, causing acceleration of renal osteodystrophy. A partial parathyroidectomy is the treatment of choice when hypercalcemia and high plasma levels of parathyroid hormone cannot be controlled with medication.

In addition to bone demineralization, this process also leads to calcification deposits in the subcutaneous, vascular, and visceral tissues throughout the body. In the advanced stages of this process, joint pain is severe. The client may also report diffuse and generalized bone and muscle pain. Bone deformities and frequent fractures are common. In children, bones fail to calcify, causing growth retardation. Tissue calcifications may be lethal if they develop in vital tissues, such as cerebral, coronary, or pulmonary vessels.

Some clients complain of muscle cramps. These may be due to osmolarity changes of the body fluids.

Integumentary Changes. Integumentary problems are particularly uncomfortable for some clients with CRF. Severe and intractable pruritus may be due to secondary hyperparathyroidism and calcium deposits in the skin. The skin is also often very dry because of atrophy of the sweat glands. Pruritus can lead to excoriated skin because of continued scratching.

Several color changes are found in renal failure. The bleeding tendencies often result in increased bruising, petechiae, and purpura. These do not usually cause problems themselves, but their presence may be alarming to the client. The pallor of anemia is evident. The cause of retained urochrome pigments, making the skin orange-green or gray in color, is not clear.

Hair is brittle and tends to fall out, and nails are thin and brittle. Characteristic red bands that develop on the nails are called Muercke's lines. Another nail pattern that has been observed is a "half-and-half" nail with the proximal half normally white and the distal portion brown.

Neurologic Changes. Although dialysis has reduced the incidence of neurologic changes, some clients experience these problems early in the disease process. Peripheral neuropathy causes many symptoms such as burning feet, inability to find a comfortable position for the legs and feet ("restless leg syndrome"), gait changes, footdrop, and paraplegia. These symptoms move up the extremities and may extend to include the upper extremities. Initially, it is primarily a problem of the sensory system, but if left untreated, it may progress to the motor system. Nerve conduction becomes slower, and deep tendon reflexes and vibratory sense are diminished.

Central nervous system involvement is demonstrated through forgetfulness, inability to concentrate, short attention span, impaired reasoning ability and judgment, increased nervous irritability, nystagmus, twitching, dysarthria, seizures, central nervous system depression, and coma. Involvement of the cranial nerves may alter any of the senses. Hearing threshold levels show a definite high-frequency deficit early in the disease, and hearing progressively deteriorates. Uremic amaurosis is a very sudden onset of bilateral blindness, which seems to reverse itself in hours to days. Eyes often contain calcium salts, which give them an irritated appearance.

Reproductive Changes. Reproductive system changes can be very alarming. Women often experience menstrual irregularities, particularly amenorrhea, and infertility. However, there have been women with CRF who have conceived and successfully carried their pregnancies to term. Men frequently report impotence resulting from both physiologic and psychosocial causes. They may also experience testicular atrophy, oligospermia, and reduced sperm motility. Both sexes report decreased libido, which may be due to both physiologic and psychosocial factors.

Endocrine Changes. CRF also affects the endocrine system. The effect on insulin utilization has been discussed earlier, as has parathyroid function. Pituitary hormones, such as growth hormone and prolactin, may be increased in some people. The levels of luteinizing hormone and follicle-stimulating hormone vary greatly from client to client. Thyroid-stimulating hormone is usually at a normal level, but it may demonstrate a blunted response to thyrotropin-releasing hormone; this results in the common finding of hypothyroidism.

Psychosocial Changes. Psychosocial changes occur, probably as the result of both the physiologic alterations and the extreme stress placed on the client by the presence of a chronic, life-threatening disease. Behavior changes are greatly influenced by the client's personality. Expected alterations include marked personality changes, labile emotions, increased demand on others, withdrawal, depression, agitation, delusions, and psychosis.

DIAGNOSTIC ASSESSMENT

Many laboratory tests are performed, including serum sodium, potassium, urea nitrogen, creatinine, phosphorus, creatinine clearance, calcium, and pH levels; urinalysis and urine creatinine clearance; and complete blood count. The normal ratio of BUN to creatinine is 20 : 1. This ratio remains the same as both the creatinine and BUN rise.

A KUB is usually done first to determine whether there is a problem with the structure of the renal system. An IVP and CT scan can be done to assess renal structure and function. Renal angiography may also be done to assess the blood supply to and through the kidneys.

Medical Management

Conservative intervention does not cure the disease but may retard its progress. Eventually, most clients will require renal replacement therapy. However, even successful dialysis and transplant do not preclude the potential for death from complications of renal failure or its treatment.

After the correction of contributing factors, control of blood pressure and fluid and dietary adjustments are the mainstays of conservative intervention for the client with CRF. The five goals of medical management are to (1) preserve renal function, (2) delay the need for dialysis or transplant as long as feasible, (3) improve body chemistries, (4) alleviate extrarenal manifestations as much as possible, and (5) provide an optimal quality of life for the client and significant others.

Pruritus can be very aggravating. Many interventions have been tried, including topical emollients and lotions, antihistamines, intravenous lidocaine, and ultraviolet B light, but relief has been inconsistent and often temporary. Subtotal parathyroidectomy has helped some, but there have been reports of recurrence. Dialysis seems to relieve the symptoms effectively for many clients.

Neurologic manifestations require safety measures to protect the client from injury. Anticonvulsants and sedatives may be used. Phenothiazines are potentiated by uremia and should be avoided. Reduction in mental function, related to the rising BUN, requires more patience in explaining and reexplaining things to the client.

DIALYSIS

There are two types of dialysis: peritoneal dialysis and hemodialysis. Each may be used to relieve symptoms of renal failure temporarily until the client regains kidney function or to sustain life in the client with irreversible kidney disease. In the latter case, the dialysis must continue for the rest of the client's life unless a successful kidney transplantation is done. Dialysis is also used to control uremia and to physically prepare the client to receive a transplanted kidney. Dialysis is frequently necessary to keep the client alive until a suitable donor kidney is found. If the transplanted kidney does not immediately function adequately, dialysis may help prevent uremia until the kidney functions sufficiently.

Dialysis is usually accomplished through both ultrafiltration and diffusion. Ultrafiltration refers to the removal of fluid from the blood by the use of either osmotic or hydrostatic pressure to produce the necessary gradient. Diffusion is the passage of particles (ions) from an area of high concentration to an area of low concentration. Both processes occur across a semipermeable membrane, one with pores large enough to allow certain particles to pass through but too small to allow the passage of larger particles. When the two solutions are separated by a semipermeable membrane, solute particles will move toward the solution with lesser concentration. Simultaneously, water will move toward the solution in which the solute concentration is greater.

When dialysis is used as a substitute for kidney function, the semipermeable membrane used is either the peritoneal membrane (for peritoneal dialysis) or an artificial membrane (for hemodialysis). This membrane must have pores large enough to allow the passage of electrolytes, urea, and creatinine but too small to allow passage of blood cells and other protein molecules. The blood and a specially prepared electrolyte solution called dialysate are placed in compartments on opposite sides of the membrane.

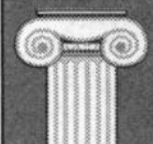

ETHICAL ISSUES IN NURSING

Do Clients with Renal Failure Have an Unconditional Right to Dialysis?

Renal dialysis is by far one of the most significant medical breakthroughs of modern time. It is so common now that the significance of such technology is often overlooked. In the United States, most dialysis clients receive government subsidies for their treatment. It has become a standard that clients with renal failure receive dialysis without personal financial consequence. Dialysis in and of itself does not automatically cause an ethical dilemma. The dilemma arises, however, when dialysis, funding, and client rights are combined.

Do clients with renal failure have an unconditional right to dialysis? From a humanitarian standpoint, financial constraints should not cloud the right to health care of any kind. But from a utility standpoint, is this approach realistic, given the cost of dialysis and the relative few who benefit as opposed to the health of the population at large?

Clients with renal failure are faced with many systemic problems. In addition to such physical and emotional problems, the cost of their treatment over their lifetime can be exorbitant. These clients do have a right to care, but perhaps limits should be set regarding the kind of technologic care that is rendered.

Is the use of all available technology a right of all clients under all conditions? There is no one answer to this question. This question is posed to make all health care workers think about what the right to health care means to them. Do all clients with renal failure have an unconditional right to dialysis treatments?

Goals of Dialysis Therapy. The four basic goals of dialysis therapy are to

- remove the end products of protein metabolism, such as urea and creatinine, from the blood
- maintain a safe concentration of serum electrolytes
- correct acidosis and replenish the blood's bicarbonate buffer system
- remove excess fluid from the blood.

Remember that solute particles and water can move freely across the membrane in either direction between the blood and the dialysate. With this in mind, note that if the client's blood has a higher concentration of urea, creatinine, and certain electrolytes than does the prepared dialysate solution, these particles will move into the dialysate solution, thus lowering the level in the blood. Likewise, if the blood is deficient in a substance such as bicarbonate, a higher concentration of this substance in the dialysate will cause it to move into the blood, raising the blood level. Excess fluid can be removed from the blood by increasing the particle concentration of the dialysate with a component such as dextrose. This increased particle concentration will cause water to move into the dialysate while at the same time the dextrose moves into the blood. The tendency is always toward an equalization of concentration of the two solutions.

Peritoneal Dialysis. Peritoneal dialysis involves repeated cycles of instilling dialysate into the peritoneal cavity, allowing time for substance exchange, and then removing the dialysate. The procedure is useful for both ARF and CRF and for fluid and electrolyte imbalances. It has been used for overdoses of drugs and toxins, but because its clearance is much slower than that with hemodialysis, it may not be satisfactory for this purpose. One of the primary advantages of peritoneal dialysis is its relative ease, which allows it to be used in community health care facilities without all the sophisticated equipment needed for hemodialysis. It can be easily managed at home and often provides the client more independence and mobility than hemodialysis does.

Peritoneal dialysis may be used for clients with severe cardiovascular disease, especially those whose problems would be worsened by the rapid changes in urea, glucose, electrolytes, and fluid volume that occur during hemodialysis. Some physicians prescribe peritoneal dialysis for their diabetic patients for reducing the risk of retinal hemorrhage from the heparin used during dialysis treatment. Peritoneal dialysis is the dialytic treatment of choice for children.

Contraindications to peritoneal dialysis include hypercatabolism, in which peritoneal dialysis is unable to adequately clear uremic toxins, and poor condition of the peritoneal membrane due to adhesions and scarring. Certain other conditions may be relative contraindications to peritoneal dialysis; these include obesity, history of ruptured diverticuli, abdominal disease, respiratory disease, recurrent episodes of peritonitis, abdominal malignancies, severe vascular disease, and extensive abdominal surgery with drains or tubes that may increase risk of infection.

Types of Peritoneal Dialysis. There are three types of peritoneal dialysis: intermittent, continuous ambulatory, and continuous cycle.

Continuous Ambulatory Peritoneal Dialysis (CAPD). In CAPD, the dialysate is instilled into the abdomen and left in place for 4 to 8 hours. The empty dialysate bag is folded up and carried in a pouch or pocket until it is time to drain the dialysate. The bag is later unfolded and placed lower than the insertion site so the fluid drains by gravity flow. When full, the bag is changed, and new dialysate is instilled into the abdomen as the process continues. In CAPD, there are usually four dialysis cycles every 24 hours, including an 8-hour dwell overnight. There are two major advantages to this procedure: (1) because there is no need for machinery, electricity, or a water source, the client can go about almost any desired activity during dialysis; and (2) because the continuous exchange process closely resembles normal renal function, the body more easily maintains homeostasis, and there are fewer dietary and fluid restrictions. For diabetic management, insulin can be added to the dialysate.

Continuous Cycle Peritoneal Dialysis (CCPD). CCPD is similar to CAPD in that it is a continuous dialysis process but different in that it requires a peritoneal cycling machine. In this procedure, there are usually three cycles done at night and one cycle with an 8-hour dwell done in the morning. The advantage of this procedure is that the peritoneal catheter is opened only for the on and off procedures, which reduces the risk of infection.

Intermittent Peritoneal Dialysis (IPD). IPD is not a continuous dialysis procedure like CAPD and CCPD. Dialysis is performed for 10 to 14 hours, three to four times a week, with use of the same peritoneal cycling machine as in CCPD. Hospitalized patients may be dialyzed up to 24 to 48 hours at a time if they are catabolic and require additional dialysis time. There are variations in scheduling IPD, such as nightly tidal peritoneal dialysis, in which treatment is performed for 8 to 12 hours each night with no daytime dwells.

Dialysis Procedure. The dialysate is usually allowed to run into the peritoneal cavity by gravity flow. The dialysate is warmed to prevent chilling of the client and to dilate the peritoneal blood vessels, thus facilitating substance exchange. Two liters are usually instilled in adults, although smaller amounts may be needed at first until the client adjusts. Care must be taken to prevent air from entering the peritoneal cavity throughout the entire procedure.

"Dwell time" is the period during which the dialysate is left in the cavity. In IPD, equilibrium between the dialysate and the body fluids usually occurs within 15 to 30 minutes, with the maximum exchange happening within the first 5 minutes. Therefore, the solution is typically left in place 30 to 45 minutes for manual dialysis or 10 to 20 minutes when an automatic cycler is used. The fluid is then allowed to run out through the catheter by gravity. In CAPD and CCPD procedures, the dwell time is prolonged to 4 to 8 hours with a solution that allows continuous exchange and better clearance of certain elements.

The number of dialysis cycles depends on the normalization of body fluids and blood chemistries, as indicated by laboratory studies. Peritoneal clearance is influenced by several factors, including the size of the membrane area, blood flow to the peritoneum, and alterations in the permeability of the peritoneal membrane.

Preparation. Before catheter insertion, the client must be fully prepared. The client needs to know exactly what will happen and what to do during the dialysis process, and what kind of results can be expected from the treatment. Informed consent must be obtained. Baseline weight, vital signs, and blood chemistries provide important data for later comparison. Mild sedation may be provided. The bladder and bowel should be emptied. The abdomen is shaved and prepped. If dialysis is to begin immediately, the equipment needs to be entirely ready with the dialysate warmed to 37° C (98.6° F) in order to optimize clearance of uremic metabolites; all tubing is flushed to prevent air from entering the cavity.

Catheter Insertion. Catheter insertion may be performed in the operating room or at the bedside under local anesthesia. The preferred insertion site is 3 to 5 cm below the umbilicus, an area that is relatively avascular and has less fascial resistance. For the placement of an acute rigid stylet catheter, an incision is made, and a stylet or large bore needle is inserted through the incision. Fluid is infused to expand the peritoneal cavity, and the catheter is inserted with the tip in the pelvic gutter.

There are several types of soft catheter that are inserted for acute or chronic peritonal dialysis. These are generally inserted in the operating room under local anesthesia. The clients are medicated before the procedure to relax them and reduce discomfort. The catheters are tunneled under the skin before they enter the peritoneal cavity to stabilize the catheter and reduce the risk of infection.

Figure 50-2 illustrates three types of peritoneal catheters. The Tenckhoff catheter has two Dacron felt cuffs bonded to the catheter. Over a period of 1 to 2 weeks, there is an ingrowth of fibroblasts and blood vessels into the cuffs, which fix the catheter in place and provide an effective barrier against dialysate leakage and bacterial invasion. Notice in Figure 50-2 that a subcutaneous tunnel is created for the catheter to further reduce direct bacterial invasion into the peritoneum. The other catheters illustrated also have cuffs that provide stable placement.

Complications of Peritoneal Dialysis. Although peritoneal dialysis is considered a safe procedure, there are a number of complications that can be attributed to it.

Peritonitis. Peritonitis is the major concern. Manifestations include fever, rebound tenderness, nausea, malaise, and a cloudy dialysate output. If peritonitis develops, appropriate antibiotics are added to the dialysate; in addition, systemic antibiotics may be used. Bacteria may enter the peritoneal cavity through contaminated dialysis fluid, a contaminated catheter lumen, or the catheter insertion site.

Laboratory tests routinely used to diagnose peritonitis include white blood cell counts with differential, culture and sensitivity, and Gram stain of the peritoneal fluid. Peritonitis is diagnosed when the dialysate white blood cell count is greater than 100/mm³ and neutrophils are greater than 50 per cent. Routine cultures may not grow the causative organism, but a Gram stain will be positive in 9 to 40 per cent of the samples.

Catheter-Related Complications. Catheter problems include displacement and plugging. Obstruction may be due to malposition, adherence of the catheter tip to the omentum, or infection. Constipation can reduce catheter flow, possibly because peristalsis facilitates outflow. A bisacodyl suppository may be used prophylactically even if the client is not constipated. Fluid leakage

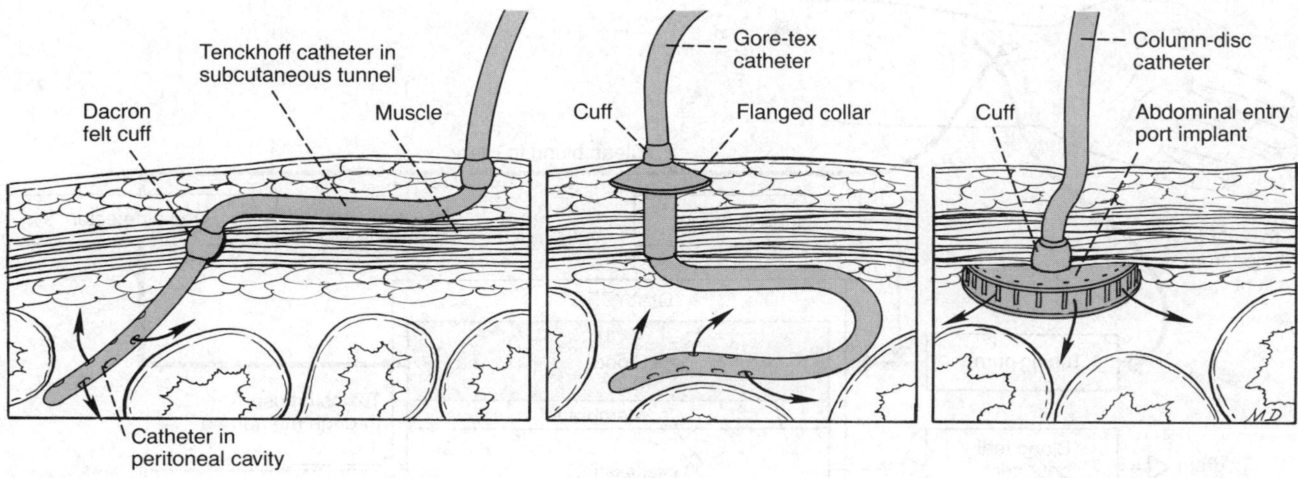

▲ **Figure 50-2**

Three types of peritoneal dialysis catheters. Tenckhoff catheter has two Dacron felt cuffs that hold catheter in place and prevent dialysate leakage and bacterial invasion; subcutaneous tunnel also helps prevent infection. Gore-tex catheter has Dacron cuff above a flanged collar. Column-disc catheter has cuff and large abdominal entry port implant.

may indicate improper catheter function, incomplete healing of the insertion site, or excessive instillation. Especially in the early stages, it is sometimes necessary to use small-volume instillations. Bloody effluent is usually insignificant and will disappear spontaneously. However, it may indicate bowel perforation, which is most likely to occur in cachectic clients or where there are abdominal adhesions. Fecal material returned in the dialysate or massive diarrhea after instillation may also signal perforation. Bladder perforation can also occur if the bladder has not been emptied before catheter insertion.

Dialysis-Related Complications. Pain during dialysis may result from rapid instillation, incorrect dialysate pH or temperature, dialysate accumulation under the diaphragm, or excessive suction during outflow. Some pain is expected in the early stages but should disappear after 1 to 2 weeks. Low back pain may develop with continuous dialysis procedures because of the abdominal weight affecting posture; appropriate exercises help relieve this problem. Hernia formation may occur. Systemic cardiovascular and neurologic effects are usually the result of fluid and electrolyte imbalances. Especially during small-volume exchanges, a significant amount of the dialysate fluid may be absorbed by the body. Hypoalbuminemia leading to hypovolemia often occurs because the peritoneal membrane allows the passage of albumin, as much as 100 g/day if the client is infected. This is especially a problem if dietary intake of protein is poor, the client is infected, or dialysis treatment is used for several consecutive days. Hyperglycemia may occur in diabetic clients as a result of absorption of glucose from the dialysate and electrolyte changes. These clients require extra insulin. Respiratory difficulties may occur during dwell time because of pressure on the diaphragm.

Hemodialysis. Hemodialysis is used for clients with acute or irreversible renal failure and fluid and electrolyte imbalances. It is usually the treatment of choice when toxic agents, such as barbiturate overdose, need to be removed from the body quickly.

Historical Overview. The first development of an "artificial kidney" was in 1943 in the Netherlands. In 1960, Scribner reported the first successful treatment of clients with CRF. In the early years, although the technology was available, the exorbitant cost and the lack of equipment required that a stringent selection process be followed in choosing clients who would be allowed to have hemodialysis. Clients were screened as to their motivation, intelligence, emotional stability, and rehabilitative potential. In essence, it had to be decided who among the many potential candidates would best be able to cope with the program and who would make the biggest contribution to society.

In 1972, an amendment to the Social Security Act ensured that anyone with CRF would be able to have any lifesaving treatment needed. In 1973, Medicare took over the financial responsibility for many clients on hemodialysis. Thus, the availability of this treatment mode for clients with irreversible renal failure has become more prevalent. Generally self-selection is the only criterion used now. As a result, the population receiving hemodialysis now represents a wide cross section in terms of age, rehabilitative potential, and socioeconomic status. This is a costly program. In 1991, over 130,000 clients were on chronic dialysis in the United States, and more than 7000 kidney transplants had been performed.

Dialysis Procedure. The procedure for hemodialysis involves diverting toxin-laden blood from the client into a dialyzer and then returning the clean blood to the

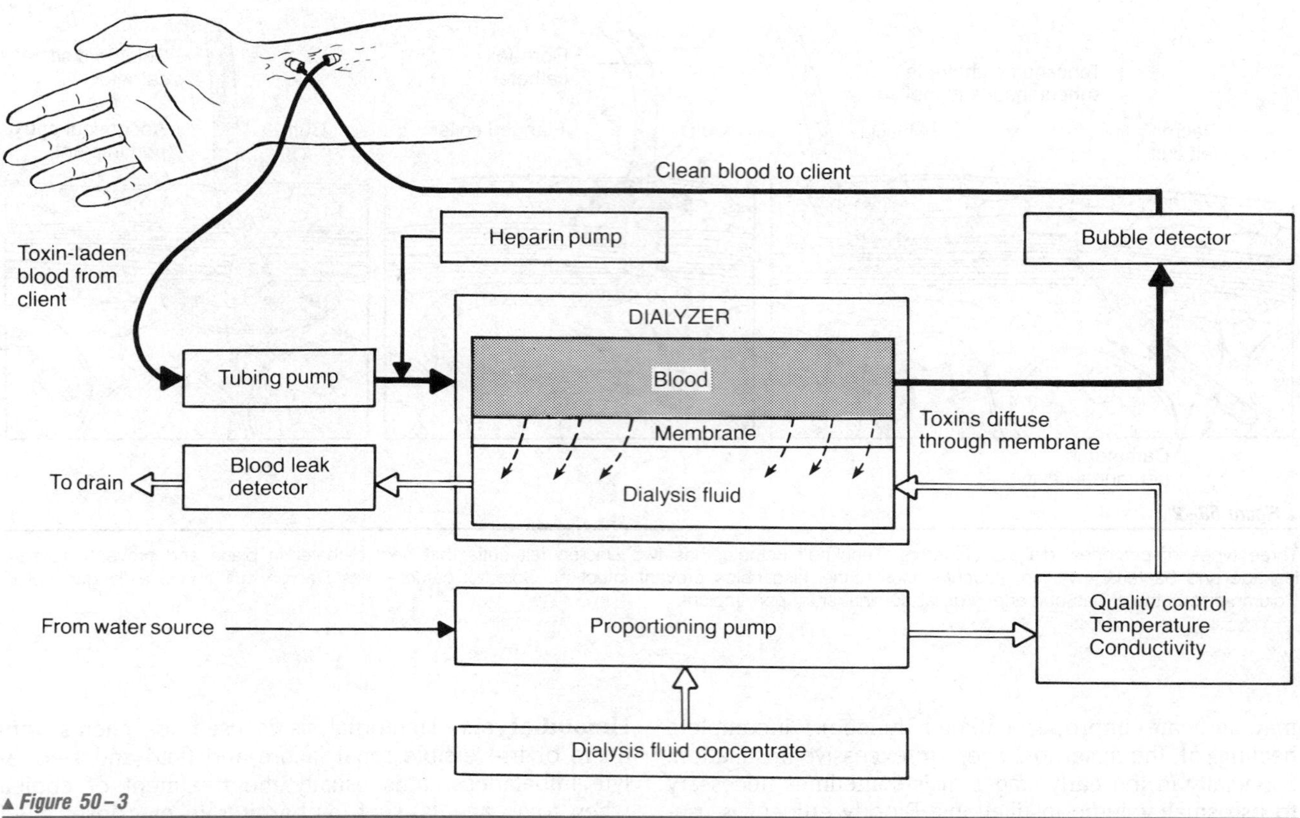

▲ *Figure 50–3*

Typical hemodialysis system. Toxin-laden blood from client diffuses across membrane within dialyzer into dialysis fluid. Clean blood is returned to client.

client. Figure 50–3 schematically illustrates a typical hemodialysis system. While the blood is within the dialyzer, the dialysis fluid is delivered by a mechanical proportioning pump to flow on the other side of the membrane. Toxins diffuse across the membrane from the blood to the dialysate. Strict asepsis must be maintained throughout the procedure.

One of the vital aspects of hemodialysis is the establishment and maintenance of adequate blood access. Without it, hemodialysis cannot be done. The major routes of access are external arteriovenous shunts and subclavian catheters for acute dialysis and internal arteriovenous fistulas and grafts for chronic dialysis.

The external arteriovenous shunt (Fig. 50–4) requires the surgical placement of two cannulas into the forearm or leg. The two Silastic cannulas are connected together to form a U shape. Blood flows from the client's artery through the shunt into the vein.

When the client is to be connected to the hemodialyzer, a tube leading to the membrane compartment is connected to the arterial cannula. Blood then fills the membrane compartment and flows back to the client by way of a tube connected to the venous cannula. When the dialysis is completed, the arterial cannula is clamped. Once the blood in the membrane compartment has been returned to the body, the venous can-

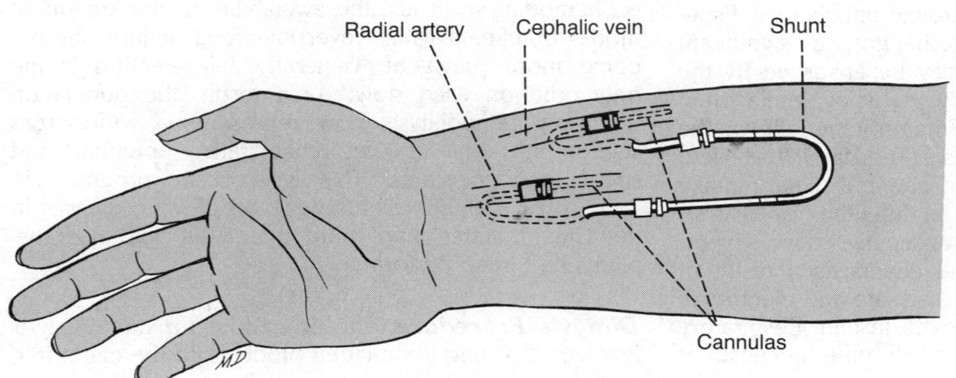

▲ *Figure 50–4*

External arteriovenous shunt provides access to blood for hemodialysis. Arterial cannula is connected to dialyzer, and blood returns through venous cannula. When not connected to hemodialyzer, arterial cannula is connected to venous cannula with a U-shaped shunt and secured carefully to skin.

nula is clamped, and the ends of the two cannulas are reattached to form their U. This access can be created quickly and so is particularly suited to situations in which dialysis must be started immediately. Infection at the site of insertion and clotting are frequent complications that often necessitate moving the cannula sites. Other problems that occur with shunts are accidental dislodgement, hemorrhage, and skin erosion.

The internal arteriovenous fistula is the access of choice for chronic dialysis clients. The fistula is created through a surgical procedure in which an artery in the arm is anastomosed to a vein in an end-to-side, side-to-side, side-to-end, or end-to-end fashion (Fig. 50–5*A*). This creates an opening or fistula between a large artery and a large vein. The flow of arterial blood into the venous system causes the veins to become engorged (Fig. 50–5*B*). These fistulas require 2 to 6 weeks to mature before they can be used, which makes this approach inappropriate for immediate hemodialysis. Peritoneal dialysis or external arteriovenous shunts may be used while the fistula is maturing.

The internal arteriovenous graft is used primarily for chronic dialysis. This access uses an artificial graft made of Gore-Tex or a bovine carotid artery to create an artificial vein for blood flow. The graft is used in clients who do not have adequate blood vessels for surgical creation of a fistula. One end of the artificial graft is anastomosed to an artery, tunneled under the skin, and anastomosed to a vein. The graft can be used 2 weeks after insertion. Complications include clotting, aneurysms, and infection.

Once the access is placed and ready for use, two 15- or 16-gauge needles are placed in the vein at each dialysis treatment (Fig. 50–5*C*). A pump pulls arterial blood out of the vein by way of the fistula and into the hemodialyzer. Blood returns to the client by a tube connected to the other needle. Another method of accessing the fistula is with single-needle dialysis. This device means that only one puncture is required each time, but there may be significant recirculation of dialyzed blood, meaning that clearance rates are decreased. Internal arteriovenous accesses may cause hand swelling or ischemia ("steal syndrome"), carpal tunnel syndrome, hemorrhage, thrombosis, and aneurysms.

Besides the arm, the lower leg is the most common site used for venous access. Figure 50–6 shows two alternative sites, the subclavian area and the thigh.

Subclavian and femoral catheters can be inserted at the bedside for use as a vascular access. Subclavian catheters may be used as a temporary or permanent access for hemodialysis. Permanent catheters are surgically placed in the operating room and have Dacron cuffs that are implanted under the skin to anchor the catheter in place. Femoral catheters are always a temporary source of blood flow and must be replaced frequently to prevent infection.

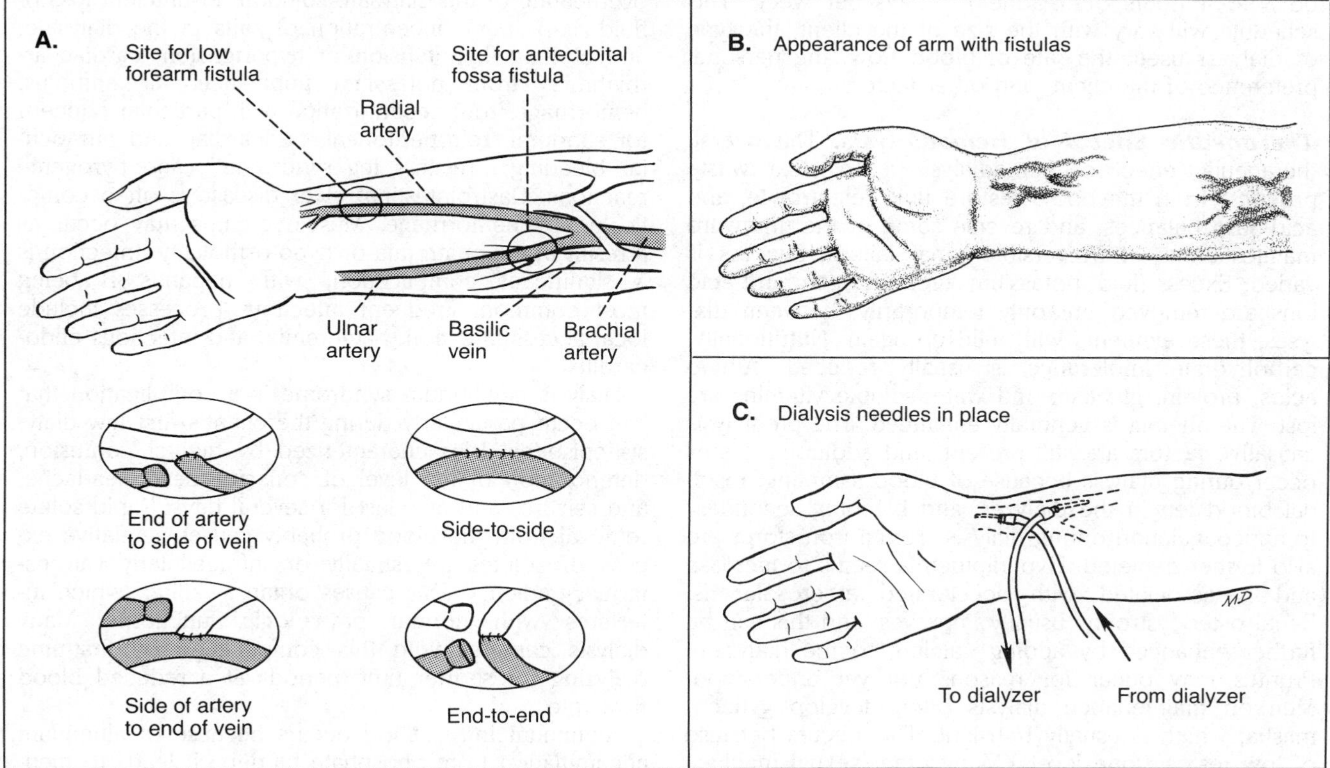

▲ **Figure 50–5**

Internal arteriovenous fistula. Surgical creation of an arteriovenous anastomosis provides easy access to blood for hemodialysis. This method reduces risk of infection and makes external shunts unnecessary except during hemodialysis. The internal fistula must be created 2 to 6 weeks before it can be used. Note that in this illustration, arteries, not veins, are toned.

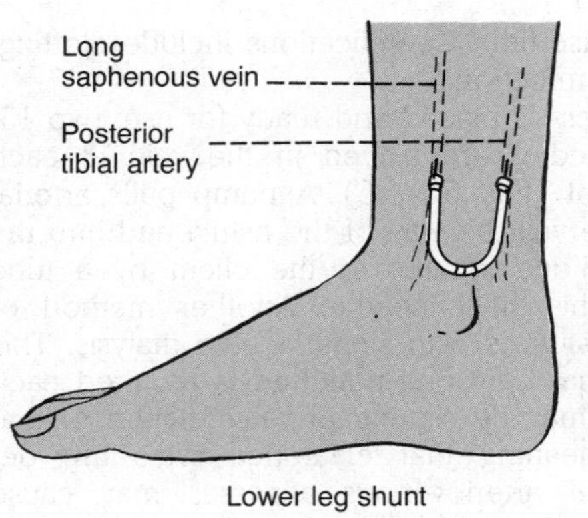

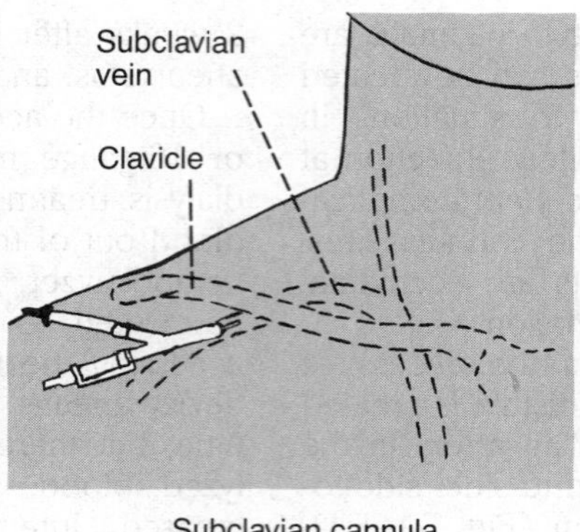

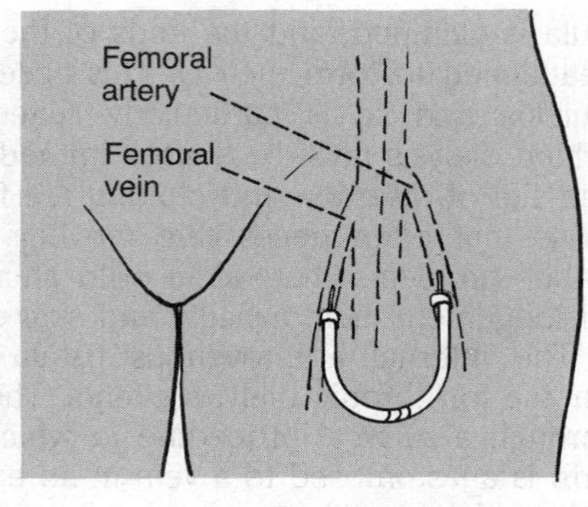

▲ Figure 50–6

Alternative access areas for hemodialysis: ankle, clavicle, and thigh.

Dialyzers. There are several types of dialyzers available. These include flat plate and hollow fiber mold. Choice of a particular system is mostly a matter of preference. The dialysate solution is altered to fit the client's need.

Hemodialysis Schedules. Hemodialysis as a treatment for irreversible renal failure must be continued intermittently for the client's lifetime, unless a successful kidney transplant is done. A typical schedule would be 3 to 4 hours of treatment 3 days per week. This schedule will vary with the size of the client, the type of dialyzer used, the rate of blood flow, the personal preference of the client, and other factors.

Therapeutic Effects of Hemodialysis. The overall therapeutic effect of hemodialysis is to clear waste products from the body; restore fluid, electrolyte, and acid-base balances; and reverse some of the untoward manifestations of irreversible renal failure. Success is varied. Excess fluid, potassium, urea nitrogen, and acid ions are removed but only temporarily; between dialyses, these elements will build up again. Nutritionally, carbohydrate intolerance is usually reduced. Amino acids, protein, glucose, and water-soluble vitamins are lost. The anemia is generally enhanced. The predialysis causative factors are still present, and additional losses occur during dialysis because of blood sampling, residual blood left in the dialyzer, and bleeding secondary to anticoagulation during dialysis. Serum iron stores are also further depleted. Hyperlipidemia seems to increase and is associated with accelerated atherosclerosis. Renal osteodystrophy usually improves, and this can be further enhanced by adding calcium to the dialysate. Pruritus may occur for reasons not yet understood. Men on maintenance dialysis often develop gynecomastia, which is usually transient. This occurs because of low testosterone levels. Many other sexual manifestations of uremia are reversed after a period of adaptation.

The usual effect of hemodialysis on serum concentration of medications is increased clearance. This is therapeutic in the case of overdose. Dosage schedules are altered to prevent dialysis loss of medications as much as possible. Supplemental doses may be necessary in order to maintain therapeutic levels of certain pharmacologics.

Complications of Long-Term Hemodialysis. In addition to therapeutic effects, there are a number of complications involved with chronic hemodialysis. These include technical problems, such as blood leaks, overheating of the dialysate solution, insufficient loss of fluid, improper concentration of salts in the dialysate, and clotting; hypotension or hypertension; cardiac arrhythmias from potassium imbalance; air embolus; hemorrhage from heparinization with particular concern for subdural, retroperitoneal, pericardial, and intraocular bleeding; "restless leg syndrome"; and pyrogenic reactions. Gastrointestinal ulcer disease is often complicated by hemorrhage. Muscle cramps may occur as a result of hyponatremia or hypo-osmolality. Infection is a significant complication, with hepatitis B being most common. Frequent infectious processes include local access infection, bacteremia, and infectious endocarditis.

Dialysis equilibrium syndrome is a complication that can occur particularly during the client's first few dialysis episodes. It is characterized by mental confusion, deterioration of the level of consciousness, headache, and seizures and may last for several days. Rapid solute removal from the blood probably causes a relative excess of solutes interstitially or intracellularly (an osmotic gradient). This causes organ swelling, which interferes with normal physiologic function.[48] Many dialysis centers avoid this complication by first-time dialyzing for shorter time periods at a reduced blood flow rate.

Aluminum intoxication occurs because of aluminum accumulation from phosphate binders. It leads to mental cloudiness, dementia, and infiltration of the bone with aluminum leading to significant pain. Aluminum chelating agents may be administered so that aluminum is freed up and dialyzed from the body.

PHARMACOLOGIC MANAGEMENT

Diuretics may be used early to stimulate excretion of water by the kidneys. The appearance of edema indicates fluid overload, but some physicians prefer to have a little end-of-the-day edema so it is more evident that fluid depletion is not a danger. Thirst is not a reliable indicator; if thirst were used as a guide, fluid overload would be inevitable. As the failure progresses, it usually becomes necessary to restrict fluid intake. Although authorities differ in their exact amounts, daily fluid allowances may be 400 to 1000 ml plus measured output.

Vitamin supplements for water-soluble vitamins (e.g., folic acid, pyridoxine, ascorbic acid) are usually given because low-protein diets are typically deficient in these. Water-soluble vitamins may need to be replaced in clients on dialysis therapy. Vitamin A supplements should be avoided unless total parenteral nutrition is to be used exclusively for several weeks. Vitamin D supplements may be necessary. Work is being done to determine the efficacy of replacing trace elements, such as iron and zinc.

Acidosis contributes to many of the undesirable effects of CRF. Sodium bicarbonate may be used to correct this imbalance. Shohl's solution, a mixture of sodium citrate and citric acid, may be administered, although it may also promote stomatitis.

Iron sulfate and folic acid are used only if the anemia is caused by a deficiency of the respective factor. Parenteral iron is frequently given rather than the oral form. Androgens may be administered if the kidneys are in place, but their effect is questionable. Transfusions may be used if the client is symptomatic.

The primary treatment for anemia in CRF clients is erythropoietin, a hormone produced in the kidney to stimulate red blood cell production. Erythropoietin has been produced by recombinant DNA and is available for intravenous administration. With adequate iron stores, anemia can be corrected in most clients within 3 to 4 months.

Much of the treatment for renal osteodystrophy involves dietary and medication regulation of calcium, phosphorus, and acidosis, as directed. The parathyroidism must also be brought under control. Vitamin D in its active form may be used, although it must be administered with care because of its severe side effects from metastatic calcifications. Calciferol helps promote bone mineralization by increasing the intestinal absorption of calcium and decreasing circulating parathyroid hormone and alkaline phosphatase. Some advocate subtotal parathyroidectomy if all other methods fail.

Fluid and sodium regulation are the major interventions for congestive heart failure. Other cardiovascular manifestations are managed much the same as for those clients without CRF, but diuretics are not used except in the very early stages of conservative management. Hypertension must be aggressively controlled with stronger medications. Antihypertensive drugs are administered as necessary in relation to renal function and nephrotic response. Pericarditis may be managed with nonsteroidal anti-inflammatory agents but may require pericardial aspiration or pericardiectomy. Tamponade (fluid in the pericardium) necessitates pericardial drainage. Some work is being done with local steroid instillation through an indwelling pericardial catheter. If conservative methods are unsuccessful, cardiac surgery to achieve revascularization or to replace a diseased valve may be performed.

DIETARY MANAGEMENT

Dietary adjustment is dictated by many components of CRF, including accumulation of nitrogenous waste products, impaired excretion of electrolytes, vitamin deficiencies, and continued catabolism. The wasting syndrome is a major problem. The client with renal failure constantly loses body weight, muscle mass, and adipose tissue.

Specific adjustments of the dietary elements often depend on the results of blood chemistries. Although there is some debate concerning whether and how to restrict proteins, studies are now indicating that maintaining a daily intake of high biologic value protein below 50 g may slow the progression of renal failure. Generally, recommendations range from no restriction other than avoiding high-protein fad diets to restrictions of 1 g/kg/day. This protein must be of high biologic value so the essential amino acids can be used more efficiently with less nitrogenous waste. This restriction of proteins also limits accumulation of acid, potassium, and phosphate.

It is also important to provide adequate nonprotein calories to prevent or reduce catabolism. One recommendation is 40 to 50 kcal/kg/day of carbohydrates and fats. As the renal disease progresses, the client's ability and willingness to take in adequate nutrition diminishes, and the challenge becomes not only to maintain appropriate intake of nonprotein calories but to satisfy protein needs as well. In these instances, elemental diets, enteral feedings, or total parenteral nutrition may be used instead of or in addition to regular food intake.

Dietary electrolytes may be encouraged or restricted. The regulation of sodium is a delicate matter. At times the kidneys are salt-wasters, and sodium must be encouraged to replace that which is lost. More frequently, however, the kidneys retain sodium and dietary intake. Some feel there should be a moderate restriction with careful monitoring of urinary sodium excretion as a guideline. Serial monitoring of data indicating fluid status also gives important information about sodium needs. Many regimens are used.

Potassium is frequently restricted. Clients must be reminded not to use salt substitutes because they contain potassium chloride. When *hyperkalemia* becomes evident, restriction of potassium in food and fluids is instituted. In an emergency situation, when the serum potassium is above 7.0, intravenous glucose ($D_{50}W$), insulin, and calcium gluconate or oral or rectal sodium polystyrene sulfonate (Kayexalate), a cation-exchange resin, may be given. Dissolving the resin in gingerale helps to (1) prevent it from sticking to the teeth and (2) mask its gritty texture. Sorbitol is usually given with the resin to avoid constipation and counteract the sodium retention that can occur. Dialysis is also effective in removing potassium from the blood.

If serum calcium levels are low, adequate calcium intake is important. Dietary sources may be supplemented with calcium carbonate, calcium lactate, or calcium gluconate. Supplements are definitely needed for clients receiving dialysis therapy. However, if serum calcium levels are high, dietary restriction may be recommended. Phosphorus is restricted. In addition, phosphate-binding gels such as aluminum hydroxide, aluminum carbonate, and calcium carbonate may be used to further reduce phosphorus levels. These agents must be administered cautiously in clients who have had a parathyroidectomy for secondary hyperparathyroidism, because aluminum deposition on bony surfaces is enhanced. Aluminum intoxication also leads to encephalopathy and osteomalacia. Finally, a mild magnesium restriction may be imposed.

Surgical Management

Renal transplantation is the surgical implantation of a human kidney from one client to another. This procedure is performed as an intervention for irreversible kidney failure.

The first successful kidney transplant was performed in the early 1950s, and transplantation has been accepted as a viable alternative for the treatment of end-stage renal disease. A successful transplant prolongs life and markedly improves the quality of life. The client is freed from the restrictions of dialysis and from the reversible manifestations of uremia. However, the procedure is certainly not without risk. In addition to the surgical risks, the immunosuppressive medications that must be taken for the life of the kidney have some potentially serious complications that are discussed later in this chapter.

Over the years, both recipient and graft survival rates have greatly improved. One-year graft survival rates are 85 to 90 per cent in living related donor transplants and 75 to 80 per cent with cadaver kidneys.

The primary limiting factor in the number of transplants done is the availability of kidneys. The Uniform Anatomical Gift Act allows clients to give permission before their own death for the use of their organs for transplantation after their death (requires family consent at the time of potential donation). In 1992, Required Request legislation was passed, which mandates that hospitals ask family members of dying clients who may be suitable organ donors if they would consider donation. There are also regional and national networks known as Organ Procurement and Transplant Networks (OPTN) and the United Network of Organ Sharing (UNOS) that have been organized to coordinate the recovery and distribution of organs and tissue for transplantation. Despite these efforts to increase donation, the loss of potentially suitable organs is still very high owing primarily to lack of awareness and acceptance by health care professionals, families, and the community as a whole. Solution of this problem will require extensive professional and public education about donation and perhaps more legislation enabling organ donation.

Selection of a transplant recipient is based on careful evaluation of the client's medical, immunologic, psychosocial, and social statuses. The decision is usually made by the client, significant others, and physician working together. Recipient selection is usually from the group less than 70 years of age who have an estimated life expectancy of 2 years or more and in whom the transplant will improve the quality of life.[62] Important psychosocial concerns include the client's (1) feelings about transplant, (2) understanding and acceptance of the risks and chances of graft survival, and (3) family and social obligations.

Although there are few absolute contraindications to transplantation, some physical conditions markedly increase the risk for the client, primarily because long-term immunosuppressive medications are necessary to avoid graft rejection. Infection and active malignancy are the only absolute contraindications to transplantation. Clients with liver disease, psychological disorders, advanced atherosclerosis, hypertension, respiratory disease, and gastrointestinal bleeding need particular consideration.

SELECTION OF CADAVER DONOR

Because of the higher graft survival rates, the most desirable source of kidneys for transplant is living related donors who match the client closely. Willing family members are screened for ABO blood group, tissue type, human leukocyte antigen (HLA) suitability, and mixed lymphocyte culture stimulation index. The donors are carefully screened and must be in excellent health. Living related donors are also carefully assessed for emotional well being and complete understanding of the donation process and outcome. However, the location of enough suitable living related donors for clients needing transplants is essentially impossible. Therefore, most kidneys for transplantation are cadaver organs.

Potential cadaver renal donors must meet the criteria for brain death and the following criteria: under 60 years of age, normal renal function, no malignant disease outside the central nervous system, no generalized infection, no significant hypertension, no abdominal or renal trauma, negative hepatitis B antigen and human immunodeficiency virus (HIV) antibody, and continuous ventilation and heart beat until the kidneys are surgically removed from the body. Warm ischemic time is the time elapsed between cessation of perfusion and cooling of the kidney plus the time required for anastomosis of the renal artery to the recipient's iliac artery. Maximum allowable warm ischemic time for a usable kidney is 30 to 60 minutes. The kidney can be cooled and the maximum time for transplantation increased to 24 to 48 hours. Once a potential donor has demonstrated cerebral death, it is crucial to restore intravascular volume, wean from vasopressors, and establish diuresis.

TRANSPORTATION OF KIDNEY

Once permission has been obtained to remove a suitable cadaver kidney, the major problem becomes one of preserving the kidney during transportation to the recipient so that maximal renal function is maintained. Preservation times also allow adequate time for (1) tissue typing and (2) preparation of the recipient for surgery. Commonly used methods for preservation include simple cold storage, in which the kidney is flushed with a chilled electrolyte solution, and hypothermic pulsatile perfusion. If properly preserved, kidneys can now be kept for 72 hours before implantation, although most kidneys are transplanted within 48 hours.

If the potential donor is a living relative, careful physical and psychosocial assessment is necessary. After histocompatibility has been established, probably the main criterion is that the donor have two properly functioning kidneys, because continued life after the unilateral nephrectomy depends on adequate renal function in the remaining kidney. Full evaluation of the entire urinary tract is done. The donor also receives a complete examination to rule out any systemic disease that may render the donor unsuitable. Potential family donors must be psychologically evaluated as to their real desire to donate a kidney and their ability to make a lifelong adjustment to voluntarily losing a kidney. Frequently, evaluation of the donor is done by a team different from that caring for the recipient to avoid conflict of interest. Discussions with the donor should be held in strictest confidence; if the donor decides not to donate, the medical team frequently cites a physical contraindication to help ensure continued acceptance of the potential donor by the family.

Personal and family relationships are very important factors in the decision to accept a potential donor. A variety of motivations have been reported, including strong altruistic drives, hopes to restore previously destroyed family ties, and religious beliefs. Tremendous pressure may be brought to bear on the potential donor by the recipient and the rest of the family.

If the potential donor is a minor, special legal precautions must be taken during the evaluation period. To neutralize conflict of interest, the court usually assigns guardians ad litem for the child. The final decision is made by these people and the court. The use of small children is controversial; strong opinions are found on both sides of the issue.

The kidney is surgically placed extraperitoneally in the iliac fossa. The renal artery is anastomosed to the recipient's hypogastric artery and the renal vein to the recipient's iliac vein. Figure 50-7 illustrates this position.

Usually the kidney begins to function immediately. Sometimes adequate functioning is delayed a few days. Hemodialysis may be performed until good function is established.

COMPLICATIONS

Graft Rejection. Except for identical twin donor and recipient, the major postoperative complication is graft rejection. This is an immunologic attack against the foreign donor organ that the body has recognized as foreign tissue. The reaction is stimulated by foreign histocompatibility antigens (see Chap. 24). There are three main types of clinical rejection: hyperacute, acute, and chronic. Hyperacute rejection (rare now)

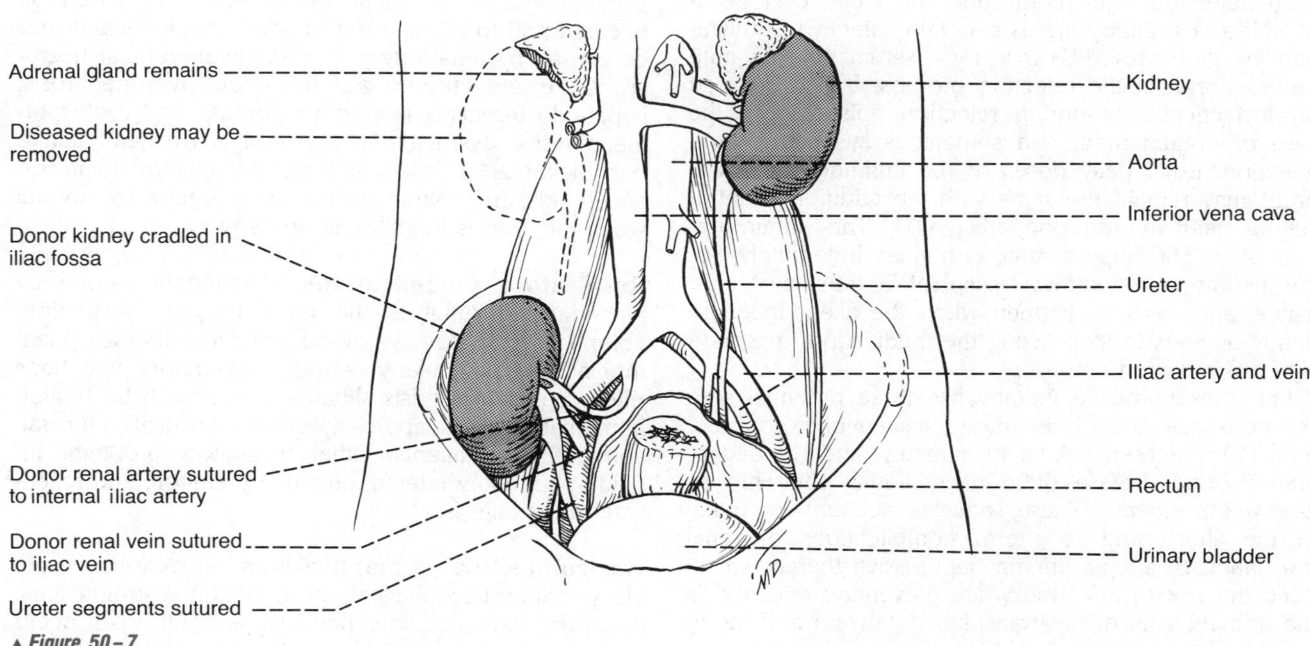

▲ *Figure 50-7*

Transplanted kidney placement.

occurs any time from the moment of revascularization of the kidney to 48 hours postoperatively. It appears to be caused by circulating cytotoxic antibodies in a presensitized client or transmitted staphylococcus alpha toxin or streptococcal infection. The result is destruction of the kidney, and the intervention is immediate donor nephrectomy to avoid the development of disseminated intravascular coagulopathy and microangiopathic hemolytic anemia.

Acute rejection usually occurs within 6 weeks after transplant; 3 months is the most common time, but rejection can occur as late as 2 years after transplantation. A cell-mediated process, it produces interstitial edema and vasculitis within the kidney. Clinical signs of this reaction include fever, malaise, elevated white blood cell count, acute hypertension, graft tenderness, and signs of deteriorating renal function. Treatment is usually initiated with high-dose steroids. If steroids are ineffective, treatment is instituted with a monoclonal antibody called OKT_3 or polyclonal antibodies ATG/ALG/ALS (discussed in detail in Chap. 24).

Chronic rejection occurs slowly over a period of months to years. It mimics CRF, although it is mediated differently in relation to the immunologic process and is resistant to therapy.

The signs of transplant rejection include fever, graft tenderness, anemia, and malaise. Urography, renal scan, ultrasonography, and CT scan are among the diagnostic tools used, mainly to rule out other causes of the symptoms.

Antirejection therapy revolves around the use of immunosuppressive drugs, which block the body's normal immune responses. A combination of azathioprine, cyclosporine, and prednisone is used most frequently for maintenance.

Cyclophosphamide is sometimes used in place of azathioprine. The use of monoclonal antibodies for acute rejection, with prednisone and either cyclophosphamide or azathioprine, is generally effective. Antilymphocyte globulin (ALG) is a horse serum that has antibodies useful in the rejection process. It can be used prophylactically or during rejection episodes. In the case of documented, and sometimes suspected, graft rejection, usual daily doses of the immunosuppressive drugs may remain the same with the addition of intravenous methylprednisone/OKT_3/ATG. The administration of immunosuppressants continues indefinitely, for the lifetime of the kidney transplant. Sudden discontinuance, such as may happen when the client independently decides to stop taking the medication, triggers a vigorous rejection episode.

Immunosuppressive therapy has three potential serious consequences: (1) increased susceptibility to infection, (2) increased risk of malignancy, and (3) degenerative bone disease often necessitating total hip or knee replacements. These sequelae account for many of the short- and long-term complications of renal transplant. Balancing immunosuppressive therapy to reduce the risk of infection while preventing rejection is the primary goal of posttransplant follow-up and monitoring.

Infection. Mortality rates for infectious disease in renal transplant clients have decreased dramatically over the past 6 to 8 years. However, infection remains a potential problem and represents the most serious life-threatening complication in the early transplant period. Urinary tract infections, pneumonia, and sepsis are most commonly seen. Causative agents include bacteria (especially in the early postoperative period), viruses, and fungi. Viral and fungal complications include herpes and, more commonly, cytomegalovirus infection, which can occur in more than 50 per cent of clients who receive transplants. Immunosuppressive drugs can mask early signs of infection, so by the time infections are recognized, they may be well advanced. Sometimes immunosuppressive therapy is reduced for a short time while the infection is brought under control.

Urinary Tract Complications. There are several complications that may occur within the urinary tract. Although rare, spontaneous rupture of the kidney may occur, usually within 14 days of the transplant. It is probably caused by rejection or ischemic damage or by some intrinsic renal disease. Leaking of urine from the ureteral-bladder anastomosis causes the development of a urinoma, which eventually puts pressure on the kidney and ureter, reducing renal function. Fistula formation includes caliceal-cutaneous, ureteral, and vesical. Long-term uremia and steroid therapy may be predisposing factors. Surgical repair may be undertaken as well as tapered alternate-day steroid therapy. Other urinary tract complications include ureteral, bladder, or pelvic leaks; obstruction; reflux; and lymphoceles. A ureteral catheter is used early in the postoperative period to decompress the bladder and monitor urine output.

Cardiovascular Complications. Cardiovascular complications may be local or systemic. Hypertension occurs in 50 to 60 per cent of adult recipients and may be caused by renal artery stenosis, acute tubular necrosis, acute and chronic graft rejection, hydronephrosis, hyperaldosteronism, large-dose steroids, and cyclosporine. Cardiac dysrhythmias and congestive heart failure may occur as a result of fluid and electrolyte imbalances. Plasma erythropoietin titers return to normal when the graft is functioning properly.

Respiratory Complications. Pneumonia caused by bacteria and fungi is the most frequent respiratory complication. Cytomegalovirus and *Pneumocystis* pneumonias are particularly serious. Respiratory infections often represent a crisis situation and should be treated immediately with appropriate antimicrobial, antiviral, and antifungal agents. Other respiratory problems include pulmonary edema, pulmonary emboli, and reactivated tuberculosis.

Gastrointestinal Complications. Infections, especially oral and esophageal, are common gastrointestinal sequelae. Noninfectious hepatitis and cirrhosis occur and may be associated with the use of hepatotoxic medications such as azathioprine. Peptic ulcer disease is a particularly problematic consequence in the presence of prednisone. Impaired gastric metabolism and increased secretion due to stress-induced epinephrine release enhance the development of ulcers. Elevated histamine levels, hyperparathyroidism, and hypercalcemia may also contribute. Histamine-receptor antagonist and antacid therapy are always instituted after transplant. Pancreatitis may also occur, although its pathogenesis is not entirely clear.

Integumentary Complications. Skin carcinomas are particularly common. Other dermatologic sequelae include infection, purpura, acne, and alopecia. Wound healing may be slowed because of poor nutritional status, low serum albumin, and steroid therapy.

Miscellaneous Complications. Other systems are also affected by posttransplant complications. Steroid-induced diabetes mellitus may develop. Musculoskeletal sequelae include osteoporosis and myopathy. Aseptic bone necrosis is primarily due to corticosteroid therapy. The reproductive problems described in CRF frequently disappear after transplantation. The incidence of gynecologic malignancies is higher than in the general population, with cervical cancer dominating. Successful pregnancies have been completed after transplant. Steroid-induced cataracts, glaucoma, and retinitis secondary to cytomegalovirus infection may occur.

Death. The overall mortality rate 2 years posttransplant is about 10 per cent.[38] This represents a dramatic decrease in the past two decades, when deaths 2 years posttransplant were nearly 40 to 50 per cent. In particular, the decreased death rate due to infection in the first 2 years after transplant has been dramatic. Advances in immunosuppressive therapy and the treatment of infectious diseases have contributed to the overall improvement. Cardiovascular deaths remain the leading cause of death in the late transplant period. Myocardial infarction, stroke, and congestive heart failure are the primary causes of death.

Nursing Management

ASSESSMENT

When the client is suspected of having CRF, the nurse must take a complete history, paying close attention to the presence of risk factors. It is important to question clients about past and present medications, diet and weight changes, energy levels and the presence of unexplained fatigue, and the pattern of urinary elimination.

The nurse will assess the client for the presence of the multiple effects of CRF on all body systems, such as the presence of cardiovascular or respiratory abnormalities, neurologic changes, gastrointestinal problems, or skin changes.

The nurse will also assess the client's understanding of CRF, the diagnostic tests that will be done, and the possible treatment regimens. The client's level of anxiety and ability to cope with this chronic disease should be assessed. The nurse should also involve the family in the assessment to determine their ability to cope with the client's disease and treatments.

When the client has been diagnosed with CRF and is being treated with peritoneal dialysis, the nurse must assess the client's and significant others' understanding of the treatment regimen. The client and significant others, the nephrologist, and the nephrology nurse discuss the use of peritoneal dialysis and decide which type most meets the client's needs. The client's understanding of the treatment is also important to assess, as is the client's ability to cope with the treatment regimen. The family's ability to cope and their ability to support the client is also vital to assess.

Once the client has begun peritoneal dialysis, the priority assessment for the nurse is the presence of an infection. The insertion site should be carefully inspected for redness or other signs of infection. The nurse should also carefully assess the effluent after it is drained for the presence of cloudiness, fibrin streaks, or blood. The vital signs and weight are monitored closely.

If the client is undergoing hemodialysis, the priority assessment becomes the patency of the venous access site. It is vital that this site be assessed for possible occlusion or, if it is an external site, for the presence of infection. The client's understanding of the access site and care of it should be noted.

If the client is to receive a renal transplant, the client's understanding of the procedure and follow-up regimen must be assessed. The client's ability to cope with a complex medication regimen after the transplant must also be assessed.

NURSING INTERVENTION

Nursing Diagnosis: Fluid Volume Deficit or Fluid Volume Excess R/T impaired renal function.

Planning: Expected Outcomes. The client will not develop a fluid volume deficit or excess, as evidenced by no signs of edema or dehydration.

Implementation. Fluid volume deficits or overloads are a cardinal problem caused by CRF. The current fluid status must be known and fluid intake carefully regulated, depending on this information. Monitor fluid status by observing daily weight, orthostatic blood pressure, skin turgor, and mucous membrane moistness and by meticulous intake and output comparisons. Give learning guidelines to clients being followed on an ambulatory basis concerning (1) how to weigh themselves and (2) how to interpret the relationship of daily weight loss or gain to their need for sodium and water. Help clients understand that vomiting, diarrhea, and working or playing in a hot environment may cause excessive fluid loss and must be prevented or controlled. Teach clients how to take their blood pressure.

Once the fluid allowance for the day has been determined, help the client follow the recommendation. The assistance needed usually concerns restricting fluid intake. Offer suggestions about reducing thirst and moistening dry mucous membranes with lip balms, frequent oral hygiene, ice chips, or spray bottles. Spread out fluid intake over a longer period of time. If intravenous fluids are used, carefully attend to them to ensure proper administration rates.

Nursing Diagnosis: Nutrition, Altered: Less than Body Requirements R/T anorexia, nausea, and dietary restrictions secondary to renal failure.

Planning: Expected Outcomes. The client will maintain adequate nutrition, as evidenced by maintenance of weight without loss of muscle mass.

Implementation. Dietary management is vital in the conservative management of CRF. Anorexia results from many of the manifestations of irreversible renal failure, emotional depression, and a frequently unpalatable diet. Thus, a major nursing challenge is helping the client take in adequate nutrition while minimizing uremic toxicity. This problem grows as the disease progresses and clients tend to develop an aversion to meat and other sources of protein. To help stimulate the client's appetite, take measures to relieve nausea and vomiting, stomatitis, and other gastrointestinal manifestations. Diet counseling is essential for compliance, and the nurse should arrange for dietary consultation if appropriate. The client needs to know how to translate the dietary regimen into a palatable, understandable food program. The nurse may help the client select and prepare foods and learn where to obtain special foods if necessary. Exercise may also improve appetite.

Nursing Diagnosis: Constipation R/T medications, fluid and dietary restrictions, and decreased activity level.

Planning: Expected Outcomes. The client will not develop constipation, as evidenced by client having a bowel movement at least every other day.

Implementation. Constipation is almost a universal problem for clients with CRF. Fluid restrictions, inability to eat most high-fiber foods, and activity intolerance reduce the ability to use customary measures for preventing constipation. In addition, phosphate-binding agents contribute to this problem. Bran, which is not rich in potassium or phosphorus, can be used. Stool softeners are often administered on a regular basis, although care must be taken with those agents containing significant calcium and sodium. If necessary, bulk laxatives (e.g., psyllium hydrophilic mucilloid) may be given. It is important that the recommended amount of fluid be taken with the powder, and this amount must be subtracted from the day's fluid allotment. Stimulant and lubricant laxatives should be used only if necessary, especially compounds containing magnesium or phosphorus. If none of these measures is effective, small-volume, gentle stimulant enemas may be used sparingly, but large-volume enemas must be avoided because of possible fluid and saline absorption. Renal failure clients are at risk for the development of diverticular disease.

Nursing Diagnosis: Activity Intolerance R/T anemia and altered renal function.

Planning: Expected Outcomes. The client will have a balance of rest and activity, as evidenced by absence of fatigue or complications related to immobility.

Implementation. Rest is important to any client whose body is under a great deal of stress. Encourage frequent naps. Insomnia is frequently a problem, and the nurse may need to make suggestions about how to solve this problem (e.g., presleep quiet time and establishing a presleep routine). Hypnotics and sedatives must be used very cautiously because they may alter mentation. The client also needs to establish and maintain an appropriate exercise program. Strenuous exercise, however, is discouraged because it increases catabolism.

Nursing Diagnosis: Skin Integrity, High Risk for R/T edema, dryness of skin, and pruritus.

Planning: Expected Outcomes. The client will not develop impaired skin integrity, as evidenced by intact skin.

Implementation. Dry skin is a common problem. Moisturizing oils in the bath water or applied directly to the skin help correct this problem. Whereas the use of soaps may need to be curtailed, keep the skin clean, because the client is susceptible to secondary infection. If edema is present, avoid sustained pressure on the area. The potential for skin breakdown is particularly acute in the diabetic patient. Observe for poor circulation and areas of breakdown or infection.

Nursing Diagnosis: Family Coping, High Risk for Impaired R/T chronic illness and uncertain future of client.

Planning: Expected Outcomes. The family will cope with the client's chronic illness and uncertain future, as evidenced by acceptance of client's problems and ability to support client.

Implementation. Clients with CRF face an uncertain future, one that promises continued deterioration, but with an unknown course and timetable. In addition, the disease itself produces behavioral manifestations that contribute to the client's susceptibility to stress. Clients are often required to make important decisions about the choice of treatment modes at a time when they do not feel well. The client and significant others have many questions about such things as family, job or school, dependency, and sex life. The client often suffers from a reduced self-esteem. The nurse needs to encourage the client and significant others to discuss feelings and concerns, using therapeutic communication techniques. To develop an individualized nursing care plan, the nurse also needs to assess how the client handled change and stress before onset of the illness.

Nursing Diagnosis: Knowledge Deficit R/T disease process and its treatment.

Planning: Expected Outcomes. The client will understand disease process and treatment regimen, as evidenced by client's ability to describe disease and treatment and to participate in treatment regimen.

Implementation. Teaching is a crucial part of the nursing management plan. Most of the time, the client will be followed on an ambulatory basis and will be responsible for following the recommended treatment regimen. The client and significant others must know about normal renal function and how the disease has altered it, the details of the management protocol and how to follow it, a number of self-assessment skills as described earlier, and when to seek professional consultation about possible complications.

Although clients with renal disease need to learn about their disorder, they may not always be ready to learn. Anxiety itself interferes with learning. In addition, the disease retards normal mental functioning; memory deficits and a short attention span may require simple presentations and frequent repeating of information. Retained learning must be continually evaluated.

Significant others may be especially frustrated during teaching sessions by the client's inability to grasp the concepts being presented. The client often seems out of touch with reality. Significant others need reassurance that this is an effect of the disease itself and that the client will become more capable of learning, especially after institution of dialysis.

With the exception of insertion and removal of the peritoneal catheter, peritoneal dialysis is primarily a nursing intervention. The nurse monitors the client, plans care, and, in many instances, teaches the client how to do the procedure independently.

Nursing Diagnosis: Fluid Volume Excess or Fluid Volume Deficit R/T fluid shifts between blood and dialysate.

Planning: Expected Outcomes. The client will not develop fluid volume excess or deficit, as evidenced by absence of disequilibrium syndrome.

Implementation. Throughout the process, carefully monitor the client's vital signs, including postural blood pressure, pulse, weight, and intake and output. Fingersticks for blood glucose are done. Watch for the development of hypovolemia and the retention of dialysate. The amount of desired fluid loss will be determined by the dialysis physician. If fluid cannot be drained during dialysis, check the system for kinks or other obstructions. Report fluid accumulations exceeding the limits set in the dialysis orders to the physician.

Nursing Diagnosis: Infection, High Risk for R/T presence of indwelling peritoneal catheter and instillation of dialysate.

Planning: Expected Outcomes. The client will not develop an infection, as evidenced by normal white blood cell count, absence of fever, and clear dialysate.

Implementation. Because peritonitis is the main complication of peritoneal dialysis, aseptic technique must be used throughout the procedure. Masks are worn by the nurse and client anytime the peritoneal dialysis circuit is opened. Gloves are worn by anyone touching the catheter during all connections and disconnection procedures. The catheter will be soaked before and after these procedures in a povidone-iodine solution. Dressing changes will be ordered per specific unit protocol. Be sure dressings are kept dry at all times.

Nursing Diagnosis: Pain, High Risk for R/T instillation of dialysate.

Planning: Expected Outcomes. The client will have pain controlled, as evidenced by client's statement.

Implementation. If discomfort is present, it can be relieved in several ways, including slowing the rate of flow, elevating the head, massaging the abdomen, or having the client move around. Analgesics may be necessary. If eating makes the client uncomfortable, serve small meals frequently and also try to coordinate the meals with drainage periods.

Nursing Diagnosis: Breathing Pattern, Ineffective R/T pressure of dialysate.

Planning: Expected Outcomes. The client will have an effective breathing pattern, as evidenced by absence of shortness of breath.

Implementation. Because of pressure on the diaphragm by the dialysate, its full excursion may be reduced. The immobilized client may be at risk for the development of respiratory problems. Encourage the client to cough and deep breathe regularly. The client also needs to be alert for early signs of compromised respiratory function.

Nursing Diagnosis: Knowledge Deficit R/T peritoneal dialysis and its impact.

Planning: Expected Outcomes. The client will understand peritoneal dialysis and its impact, as evidenced by client discussion.

Implementation. The client and significant others may have significant levels of anxiety and many concerns about peritoneal dialysis and its impact on their lives. Therapeutic communication by the nurse helps them cope with these concerns. If the client will be having long-term dialysis, the client and significant others may have a prolonged relationship with the nurse, and the nurse should be constantly working to establish and maintain a supportive, therapeutic rapport with them. If the client is immobilized during the day for treatment, the nurse may need to help the client develop appropriate diversionary activities.

The client and significant others need to know about peritoneal dialysis and how to work with its ramifications. Because so many clients continue this treatment mode in their homes, this knowledge needs to be complete and detailed. They require a complete training program so they can handle the entire dialysis process independently.

Most of the care required by the client during and after hemodialysis falls within the realm of nursing. Providing this care requires specialized training.

Continuous monitoring during dialysis provides vital information about the progress of the treatment and allows early diagnosis of potential complications. There should be a well-organized plan for observing and recording vital signs, dialysate composition and temperature, functioning of the entire dialysis system, blood flow, and clotting times. The nurse should also be alert to early signs of potential complications as listed earlier. The nurse often serves as case manager and coordinates the services provided by the nephrology team that includes the physician, nurses, social worker, and dietician.

Nursing Diagnosis: Injury, High Risk R/T trauma to hemodialysis venous access site.

Planning: Expected Outcomes. The client will not suffer injury to venous access site, as evidenced by continued patency of site.

Implementation. Careful attention to the access site is important to its life expectancy. Care of the access site is designed to prevent infection and clotting. A dressing is used to protect cannulas and subclavian catheters from infection. The access must also be protected from trauma that could cause clotting, bleeding, or physical disruption of the access. Blood pressure measurement should not be taken on, or blood drawn from, the limb containing the access. Between dialysis periods, the skin over the fistula or graft requires only routine care with soap and water.

Nursing Diagnosis: Knowledge Deficit R/T nutritional needs during dialysis.

Planning: Expected Outcomes. The client will understand nutritional needs during dialysis and possible home dialysis program, as evidenced by discussion with client.

Implementation. Providing adequate nutrition is often easier during dialysis and for a time afterward. Dialysis usually relieves many of the gastrointestinal problems that frequently interfere with adequate intake. Food and fluid restrictions are usually liberalized just before dialysis but are reimposed afterward. As a result, sodium and water are metabolized and ready to be dialyzed during actual dialysis.

Dietary noncompliance remains a major problem during maintenance dialysis, and it may require all the nurse's knowledge and creativity to help the client follow the recommended regimen.

Nursing Diagnosis: Individual Coping, Ineffective R/T effects of long-term hemodialysis.

Planning: Expected Outcomes. The client will cope effectively with effects of long-term hemodialysis, as evidenced by client's ability to look at alternatives and discuss plans.

Implementation. Much of the care required by clients on chronic hemodialysis and significant others revolves around psychosocial aspects of dialysis. Clients on maintenance dialysis often have ambivalent feelings. On one hand, they realize that hemodialysis is their tie with life. Yet, the many restrictions and lifestyle changes imposed on them make continuation of the program extremely difficult. Clients often report that they feel in limbo between the worlds of life and death.

The process of adaptation to a loss is a part of adjustment. It is not uncommon for clients to feel quite grateful and optimistic at the start of their dialysis treatments. Usually they have felt ill for some time, and they view the intervention as a route to survival and a hope for feeling well again. It takes a few days or weeks for them to fully realize the permanent place of dialysis in their lives. Depression during this period is expected. The suicide rate among clients on dialysis has been estimated at 100 times that of the general population.

Three of the most common psychosocial problems are change in body image, dependency-independency conflict, and daily facing potential death. The client's own feelings of weakness and illness plus the presence of the arteriovenous fistula and dialysis equipment are constant reminders that the client is no longer a "whole person." These clients often play one of three roles: (1) professional patient, in which all of life revolves around the dialysis; (2) rebel, in which the client acts noncompliant or mischievous; or (3) adult, in which the client uses appropriate coping skills and is able to focus outward. Relationships with relatives and friends, job, and community roles and responsibilities will probably be altered. Changes in sexuality emphasize the problem even further. The client's normal need for independence is continually threatened by dependence on the dialysis equipment and care providers. This is especially true of adolescents and young adults. Other emotional problems that have been identified include the need for identity, safety, control of the environment, love, esteem, and communication. The stress on marital relationships and significant others is extreme.

Assistance for the client and significant others must begin before dialysis is started. They need to fully understand the intervention and its implications. Encourage them to discuss their feelings. It is often difficult for clients to voice concerns about continuing dialysis because of its significance. These feelings are often, albeit subconsciously, supported by the nurses; it is sometimes difficult for care providers to accept a client's decision to stop treatment and choose ultimate death instead. The nurses, who often become a kind of "family" to the client, must provide a continued, unified, supportive approach and be ready to accept the whole gamut of reactions to dialysis by the client and significant others. It is helpful to know the client's usual patterns of response to stress. If clients have sound psychosocial coping mechanisms and help from those around them, they usually accommodate themselves to the situation and plan their lives realistically. Clients who handle stress poorly or who have little support from others may never make an adequate adjustment. Active participation by clients in their care is a valuable tool in helping to meet several of the needs identified here.

Nursing Diagnosis: Family Coping, Ineffective R/T chronic treatment and possible home dialysis program.

Planning: Expected Outcomes. The client will cope with chronic treatment, as evidenced by family's ability to work with client and offer support.

Implementation. The number of clients availing themselves of home dialysis is about 15 per cent of all clients receiving dialytic therapy. The cost of this type of program is less than in-center dialysis, and usually the client's quality of life is improved. Home dialysis offers the client more access to significant others and greater feelings of independence and control. However, this type of treatment also produces stress on personal relationships, especially to the person who becomes the "dialyzer helper." Some spouses have voiced concern about the lack of free time and increased responsibility; others see it as an opportunity to give something back to their spouse or loved ones. Some states have funding available to pay for a non–family member to serve as dialysis helper. In some instances, this may reduce tension and improve the quality of life for the family.

Clients for home dialysis programs must be selected carefully. Criteria might include stability of relationships, psychosocial stability, financial support, and lack of severe physical complications. A successful program requires care providers who are advocates of home dialysis, a good training program, and the provision of good support services (e.g., nursing, medical, and social services; provision of supplies; equipment maintenance; dietary counseling; home visits; and retraining as necessary).

Nursing Diagnosis: Knowledge Deficit R/T renal transplant and therapeutic regimen.

Planning: Expected Outcomes. The client will understand the transplant and therapeutic regimen, as evidenced by discussion with client.

Implementation. The donor and recipient must be prepared for postsurgical psychological reactions. Strong emotional ties often develop between the donor and recipient during the evaluation period, and the donor frequently feels responsible for the success or failure of the graft postoperatively. Graft rejection is usually devastating to these clients. Also, the need to protect the remaining kidney may give rise to later feelings of anger. Postoperative traumatic reactions by the donor are less likely in clients who have good inner resources, flexible defense mechanisms, and good mental health. Another source of postoperative stress for the donor is the fact that families tend to pay more attention to the recipient because of the continued possibility of graft rejection. The donor often feels abandoned. However, strong, long-lasting, positive effects include identification of a source of inner strength, a more positive self-image, and a general "sense of feeling good" about saving someone's life.

The donor may be assured that the remaining kidney will assume adequate total renal functioning. The renal blood flow and GFR of the remaining kidney have been reported to increase to 70 to 80 per cent of the preoperative levels of both kidneys together. Within 2 to 6 years, the 24-hour creatinine clearance levels often recover 85 to 87 per cent. This increased function is probably facilitated by tubular hypertrophy and hyperplasia.

Preoperative preparation of both the living donor and the recipient includes all aspects of general preoperative care as outlined in Chapter 19. In addition, there are several concerns unique to the recipient. Adequate conservative management and dialysis should have placed the client in as close to a nontoxic state as is feasible. All infections must be eradicated, gastrointestinal ulcers treated, and any lower urinary tract malfunctions corrected. Sometimes, when the bladder is unable to receive urine from the transplanted kidney, a urinary diversion procedure, such as ileal conduit, may be done before the transplant itself. Immunosuppressive therapy may be started at least 24 hours before surgery.

Bilateral nephrectomy may be performed before the transplantation procedure if any of the following conditions are present: persistent or active bacterial pyelonephritis, infected stone disease, uncontrolled renin-mediated hypertension, infected polycystic kidneys, selected rapidly progressive glomerulonephritis, or renal malignancy. The decision to do a nephrectomy can be safely delayed until the posttransplant period when surgeons may determine it necessary because of recurrent urinary tract infection.

Nursing Diagnosis: Infection, High Risk R/T immunosuppressive therapy.

Planning: Expected Outcomes. The client will not develop an infection, as evidenced by absence of fever and no signs of infection (may be masked by steroids).

Implementation. Much of nursing management is aimed at prevention, early recognition, and treatment of complications plus measures to facilitate maximal renal function and help the client attain an optimal quality of life. Immediate postoperative care of both the donor and recipient encompasses the care required by anyone having surgery, as described in Chapter 19. Care of the donor resembles that of anyone having a nephrectomy. The additional care required by the recipient is partially suggested by the potential complications. The nurse must be constantly aware of the signs and symptoms of these sequelae. Handwashing and universal precautions are measures taken to protect the client from potential sources of infection within the environment.

Because of the high incidence and seriousness of pneumonia to the client with a renal transplant, preventive respiratory treatment is essential. Coughing and deep-breathing exercises are started immediately. These exercises are painful, and the nurse can use analgesics judiciously and put external pressure over the incision to help the client cough and breathe more effectively.

Wound care must be done with use of the strictest aseptic technique because the client does not have much resistance to bacterial invasion. Delayed wound healing makes the client susceptible to dehiscence longer than usual. If the client has a fistula or graft for hemodialysis, it will be left in place in case dialysis is needed postoperatively.

Oral hygiene is important because of the high incidence of stomatitis and bacterial and fungal infections. Antifungal mouthwashes may be used. Oral fluids are usually instituted after 12 to 24 hours.

Collaborative Problem: Injury, high risk for R/T postoperative complications.

Planning: Expected Outcomes. The client will not develop postoperative complications, as evidenced by vital signs within preoperative range, return of normal bowel function, and return of urinary function.

Implementation. Maintain circulatory function. Frequently monitor blood pressure, pulse, respiration, central venous pressure, weight, and hourly or half-hourly intake and output. For monitoring renal function and maintaining electrolyte balance, serial laboratory determinations of hemoglobin, hematocrit, BUN, creatinine, electrolytes, white blood cell count, and platelets will be followed closely. Postoperatively, manage intravenous fluids carefully; the amount of fluid infused is frequently based on the previous hour's output. A high urine output is usually desired.

Bowel function should be carefully assessed before oral intake is allowed. As bowel peristalsis returns, the diet will be advanced. Unless the client is demonstrating rejection or hypertension, there may be no dietary restrictions. As soon as the client begins taking oral food and fluids, antacid therapy is begun.

Nursing Diagnosis: Body Image Disturbance R/T medications and the presence of a transplanted kidney.

Planning: Expected Outcomes. The client will not develop a disturbance in body image, as evidenced by client's statements about self and willingness to be with others.

Implementation. Psychosocially, the client must be helped to incorporate a new kidney as a part of the whole being. Education and counseling need to be provided to the client to enhance changes in lifestyle that will promote good health-seeking behavior and compliance with transplant medications. If the graft fails, expected reactions include anger, hostility, guilt, and a helplessness/hopelessness syndrome. Relatives and friends may mirror these feelings. Role changes, so well established during the chronic illness period, may be difficult, such as the family member who no longer feels needed as the "care giver." Likewise, the client may have difficulty giving up the sick role.

Economic concerns also need to be addressed. Immunosuppressive medications, particularly cyclosporine, are very costly. Currently, Medicare covers payment of these drugs for 365 days after the client is discharged from transplant admission. After that time, other sources of funding need to be explored to ensure compliance with medications.

EVALUATION

The nurse must evaluate whether the established goals have been met. If they were not, the nurse must alter the plan and interventions to ensure that the client's needs are met.

Modification of Plan of Care for the Elderly

One of the major modifications for an older client will be the possible limits of options available for treatment. Renal transplant is not routinely done on elderly clients. Clients over age 60 years are evaluated on an individual basis; clients as old as 75 years have been successfully transplanted. The types of dialysis will be evaluated on the basis of the presence of other chronic disorders the client may have that would limit the ability to comply with any treatment.

Older clients may have had multiple abdominal surgeries with the development of adhesions that will limit the usefulness of peritoneal dialysis. They are more likely to have pre-existing cardiovascular problems that may limit the usefulness of many venous access sites.

Post-hospital Care

DISCHARGE TEACHING

Clients with CRF have a wide variety of learning needs. They and their significant others must understand the disease, its outcome, and the treatment regimen. Diet teaching is important with all the possible treatment regimens and medications that the client will need for the rest of life.

A good teaching program is essential for clients with chronic peritoneal or hemodialysis or transplants and their significant others. Give carefully constructed guidelines concerning

- medications—purpose, dosage, administration, side effects, and toxic effects
- manifestations of infection, venous access blockage, or graft rejection
- how to avoid infections and how to manage them when they occur
- the dietary regimen and its preparation
- information about the transplant that must be given to dentists and other physicians
- the importance of an exercise program to help maintain body function and to maintain muscle mass despite steroid therapy.

HOME HEALTH CARE NEEDS

If clients are on home dialysis, they will need more assistance at home with both the set-up and the maintenance of their dialysis.

Help the client arrange activities and lifestyle to avoid highly stressful situations. Additionally, the client may need job retraining. In essence, the client and significant others require your knowledge and assistance in adjusting to a lifelong chronic illness, often with complex, continuous therapy.

FOLLOW-UP CARE

Long-term care usually continues throughout the client's lifetime. Clients need continued physical and psychosocial support. The importance of complying with recommended medical management regimens and follow-up evaluation schedules must be emphasized and periodically reinforced.

RENAL CALCULI

Definition

Although calculi can form anywhere in the urinary tract, the most frequent site is in the kidney. These stones may travel down the urinary tract with or without resultant damage, may lodge anywhere along the tract, or may stay within the kidney.

Incidence

Researchers estimate that approximately 12 per cent of the male population will develop a renal stone by the age of 70 years. The incidence rate of males in the United States is 123.6 per 100,000 per year.[16] Also, more than 200,000 Americans each year are admitted to hospitals because of nephrolithiasis (kidney stones). Many more people pass urinary stones without even knowing it, and others are treated on an ambulatory basis in emergency rooms and clinics.

Etiology

A number of etiologic factors influence renal stone formation. The presence of precipitators in the urine includes protein matrix and bacteria or inflammation elements. Increased solute concentration occurs because of fluid depletion or an increased solute load. This increased concentration predisposes to the precipitation of crystals, such as calcium, uric acid, and phosphate. Urinary pH influences the solubility of certain crystals, with some crystal types precipitating readily in acid urine and some in alkaline urine. Abnormal pH levels occur in (1) renal tubular acidosis, with the administration of carbonic anhydrase inhibitors, (2) in the presence of urea-splitting organisms, and (3) in severe, chronic diarrhea.

Not only does the deficiency of inhibitors predispose the client to develop renal stones, but there may be "anti-inhibitors" in the urine, such as aluminum, iron, and silicone. Drinking water and magnesium trisilicate are common sources of silicone. Certain medications may induce stone formation through various modes. Commonly used medications with this potential side effect include acetazolamide, absorbable alkali (e.g., calcium carbonate and sodium bicarbonate), and aluminum hydroxide. Massive doses of vitamin C increase urinary oxalate concentration. Anything that results in urinary stasis predisposes a client toward stone formation, because the crystals in unmoving urine precipitate more readily. Common conditions include urinary tract obstruction and immobilization.

Development of urinary lithiasis is probably the result not of any single factor but of multiple phenomena. One of the questions still unanswered is why some clients form stones whereas others do not. This problem is particularly important with recurrent "stoneformers."

Risk Factors

Risk factors for stone formation include anything that causes either stasis or supersaturation of the urine. This includes stressors such as immobility, which increases stasis; dehydration, which leads to supersaturation; and an increase in calcium or other ion in the urine. Another major risk factor is having had urinary calculi previously.

These risk factors have primary preventions that can be implemented. Frequent turning of immobilized clients, a high fluid intake, and decreased calcium in the diet in susceptible individuals help prevent stones. These will also help decrease the recurrence of stones.

The prime risk factor for uric acid stones is an alteration in purine metabolism as seen with gout. Controlling the production and excretion of uric acid can help prevent these.

Pathophysiology

Regardless of the specific type of calculus, the process of stone formation is one of crystallization. Current theory identifies three factors that may be involved in this process: urine saturation, inhibitor deficiency, and the production of matrix. Generally, crystal growth involves nucleation, in which crystallites are formed from supersaturated urine. Growth proceeds by aggregation to form larger particles. One of these particles may travel down the urinary tract until it is trapped at some narrow point where it becomes the nidus for stone formation. Substances such as citrate, pyrophosphate, magnesium, and glycosaminoglycans have been identified that chelate stone constituents so that they are not available for stone formation. These are called inhibitors; when present in adequate amounts, they interfere with crystal aggregation. Also, a fibrous matrix of urinary organic matter (mostly mucoproteins) may form in the kidney or bladder, producing a substance into which crystallites are deposited and trapped. This, then, becomes the nidus for a stone.[1] The excessive production of this mucoprotein may, in part, account for the family history of renal stones among those clients with calculi.

Renal calculi may be of one crystalline type only or a combination of types. Approximately 80 per cent of all urinary tract stones contain calcium, usually as calcium phosphate or calcium oxalate. Calcium stones may range from very small particles, often called sand or gravel, to giant staghorn calculi, which may fill the entire renal pelvis and extend up into the calices (Fig. 50-8). They have a peak onset in the third decade and primarily afflict men.

Hypercalciuria, or an increased solute load of calcium in the urine, is caused by three main components: (1) a high rate of bone reabsorption, which liberates calcium (hyperparathyroidism; Paget's disease; immobility; osteolysis caused by malignant tumors of the breast, lung, and prostate; Cushing's disease); (2) gut absorption of abnormally large amounts of calcium (milk-alkali syndrome, sarcoidosis, excessive intake of vitamin D); and (3) impaired renal tubular absorption of filtered calcium (renal tubular acidosis). About 35 per cent of all clients who form calcium stones do not have high serum levels of calcium and have no apparent cause for their hypercalciuria. This condition is called idiopathic hypercalciuria.

There are two variants of hypercalciuria. In one, the primary abnormality is increased intestinal absorption of calcium or increased bone reabsorption. The resulting higher serum calcium level triggers increased renal filtration of calcium and parathyroid hormone suppression. This in turn decreases tubular reabsorption, thereby increasing the concentration of calcium in the urine. The other abnormality involves "renal leak" of calcium caused by a tubular defect. The resulting mild hypocalcemia stimulates parathyroid hormone production, which increases intestinal absorption of calcium. This cycle then fits into the previous one, causing an increased solute load of calcium. Clients with this problem are often called "calcium-wasters."

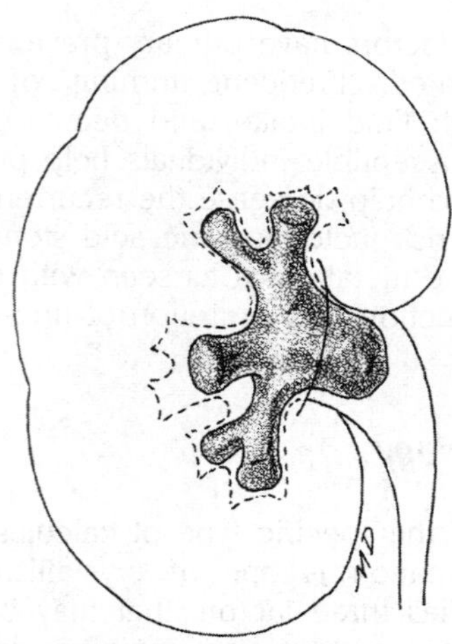

▲ **Figure 50-8**

Staghorn calculus.

The second most frequent crystal to cause stones is oxalate, which is relatively insoluble in urine. Its solubility is only slightly affected by changes in urinary pH. The mechanism for oxalate availability is unclear but may be closely related to diet. The disease is most common in areas where cereals are a major dietary component and least common in dairy farming regions. Some conditions in which the incidence of oxalate stone increases may be related to hyperabsorption of oxalate (e.g., inflammatory bowel disease); postileal resection or small bowel bypass surgery; overdose of ascorbic acid, which metabolizes to oxalate; familial oxaluria; and methoxyflurane anesthetic. There is also some thought that a concurrent fat malabsorption causes calcium binding, which frees oxalate for absorption.

Struvite stones, also called triple phosphate, are composed of calcium, magnesium, and ammonium phosphate. Their cause is certain bacteria, usually *Proteus,* which contain the enzyme urease. This enzyme splits urea into two ammonia molecules, which raise the urine pH. Phosphate precipitates in alkaline urine. This action is responsible for the label "urea-splitter" given to these organisms. The stones formed in this manner are staghorn calculi (see Fig. 50-8). Abscess formation is common, sometimes the result of erosion into the perinephric space. These stones are particularly difficult to eliminate because the hard stone forms around a nucleus of bacteria, protecting them from antibiotic therapy. Any small fragment left after surgical removal of the stone begins the cycle again.

Uric acid stones are caused by increased urate excretion, fluid depletion, and a low urinary pH. Hyperuricuria is the result of either increased uric acid production or the administration of uricosuric agents. Approximately 25 per cent of clients with primary gout and about 50 per cent of individuals with secondary gout develop uric acid stones. A high dietary intake of purine-rich foods may predispose susceptible clients to uric acid stone formation. Also, treating neoplastic disease with agents that cause rapid cell destruction may increase the urine's uric acid concentration. Moreover, a link between hyperuricuria and calcium stone formation may exist. It seems uric acid crystals absorb some of the crystal inhibitors normally found in urine.

Cystinuria is the result of a congenital metabolic error inherited as an autosomal recessive disorder. Cystine stones typically appear during childhood and adolescence; development in adults is very rare.

Xanthine stones also occur as the result of a rare hereditary condition in which there is a xanthine oxidase deficiency. This crystal precipitates readily in acid urine.

Despite the type of stone that forms, the potential damage is essentially the same: pain, obstruction, and tissue trauma with secondary hemorrhage and infection.

Clinical Manifestations

The most characteristic symptom of renal or ureteral calculi is a sharp, severe pain with a sudden onset. Depending on the site of the stone, this pain may be called either renal colic or ureteral colic. Renal colic originates deep in the lumbar region and radiates around the side and down toward the testicle in the male and the bladder in the female. Ureteral colic radiates toward the genitalia and thigh. When the pain is severe, the client will usually exhibit nausea, vomiting, pallor, and diaphoresis and be quite anxious. Urinary frequency may occur. The pain lasts for minutes to days and can be somewhat resistant to narcotic intervention. Pain may be intermittent, which usually means that the stone has moved. Physicians hypothesize that the ureter dilates just proximal to the calculus, which allows urine to pass, relieving the ureteral distention. Then, as the stone moves and sets up a new obstruction site, the pain returns. The pain subsides when the stone reaches the bladder.

Pain caused by renal stones is not always severe and colicky in nature. In fact, it may be a dull, aching, or heavy feeling. This is particularly true during the early stages of hydronephrosis. Sometimes, there may be no sensation, and the first clue the client has is when a "clink" sounds against the toilet when the stone passes.

DIAGNOSTIC ASSESSMENT

The major diagnostic test is a KUB or flat plate of the abdomen to visualize the stone. An IVP is also done to determine if any obstruction is present and, if it is, how severe it is.

Medical Management

MECHANICAL INTERVENTION

If it is decided that the stone will not pass before complications occur, mechanical intervention may be used. Depending on the position of the calculus, cystoscopy may be done. Additionally, one or two ureteral catheters may be inserted past the stone. From this point, several different interventions are appropriate. The catheters may be left in place for 24 hours. Their presence drains the urine trapped proximal to the stones and dilates the ureter, which may prompt spontaneous movement of the calculus. Otherwise, the catheters may mechanically guide the stones downward as they are removed. A continuous chemical irrigation may be established to dissolve the stone. Finally, an attempt may be made to manipulate or to dislodge the stone. A variety of special catheters with loops and expanding baskets may be inserted through the cystoscope and used to snare the stone. The postprocedure care of these clients is the same as that following cystoscopy (see Chap. 48). Chapter 49 describes the care of a client with indwelling catheters.

A noninvasive mechanical procedure for breaking up stones so they can pass spontaneously or be removed by other methods is extracorporeal lithotripsy. Figure 50-9 shows how this procedure works. The client is placed in a specially designed tub with the trunk submerged in water. Then, an underwater electrode generates shock waves via a reflector that fragments kidney stone. The client is strapped to a frame and may be sedated during the procedure, because it usually lasts for 30 to 40 minutes and immobility is essential. After the procedure, the client may experience some renal colic that needs spasmolytics. Early ambulation and adequate diuresis are important to fully "wash out" the stone fragments.

Another aspect of intervention is preventing stone recurrence. Although many people with a urinary stone will never have another, researchers estimate that 25 to 30 per cent of them will develop recurrent lithiasis. The recurrence rate is reportedly as high as 60 per cent. The ability to predict who will and who will not have a recurrence is still unreliable. Stone recurrence usually happens within a 2- to 3-year period, but many occur as long as 20 years later. As the number of recurrences increases, the interval between stones tends to become shorter. Thus, prevention is a lifelong program.

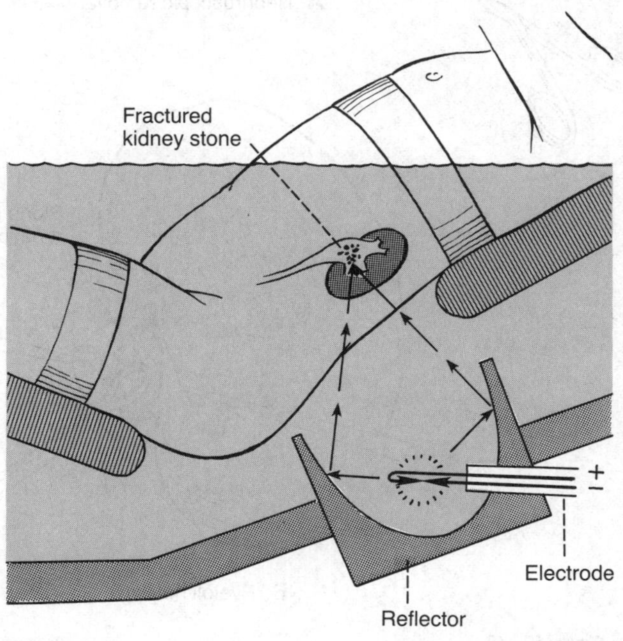

▲ *Figure 50-9*

Extracorporeal lithotripsy. Electrically generated shock waves fracture kidney stones.

Two objectives are essential to the total preventive regimen. First, any underlying contributing problem must be corrected (e.g., metabolic and anatomic). Parathyroidectomy may be performed in the case of intractable hypercalcemia. Second, infection must be avoided or aggressively treated for all stone types because it places additional stress on the kidneys.

PHARMACOLOGIC MANAGEMENT

There are no particular medications used to treat calcium stones. If the client has uric acid stones, medications to lower uric acid such as allopurinol (Zyloprim) should be given. The client is treated with narcotics and antispasmodics.

DIETARY MANAGEMENT

Once the components of the stone have been identified, diet modification will be used to help prevent recurrence. A low-calcium, low-oxalate diet is used to prevent calcium or oxalate stone recurrence, and a low-purine diet is used to prevent uric acid stone recurrence.

Surgical Management

Percutaneous lithotripsy is an invasive procedure in which tubes are inserted in the area of stone formation. Contrast dye is injected, and forceps are used to remove the stones. If the stones are too large to remove with forceps, ultrasonic waves can be used to break up the stones for easier removal.[16]

Surgical intervention may be performed through a percutaneous approach or by open procedures. The development of advanced fiberoptic equipment has made the percutaneous route the most common. Because the incision is so small, surgical risk is minimal, and the client recuperates quickly. If the client has a significant infection, antibiotics probably will be given for at least 1 day before the procedure. Small, free-lying stones may simply be retrieved by use of a nephroscope. In this instance, a needle is inserted through the skin into the kidney. The tract into the kidney is dilated, and the nephroscope is inserted through the tract. Figure 50-10*A* shows a nephroscope in place. The stone may be removed by alligator forceps or a stone basket. Irrigation to flush the stone out of its resting place may be done.

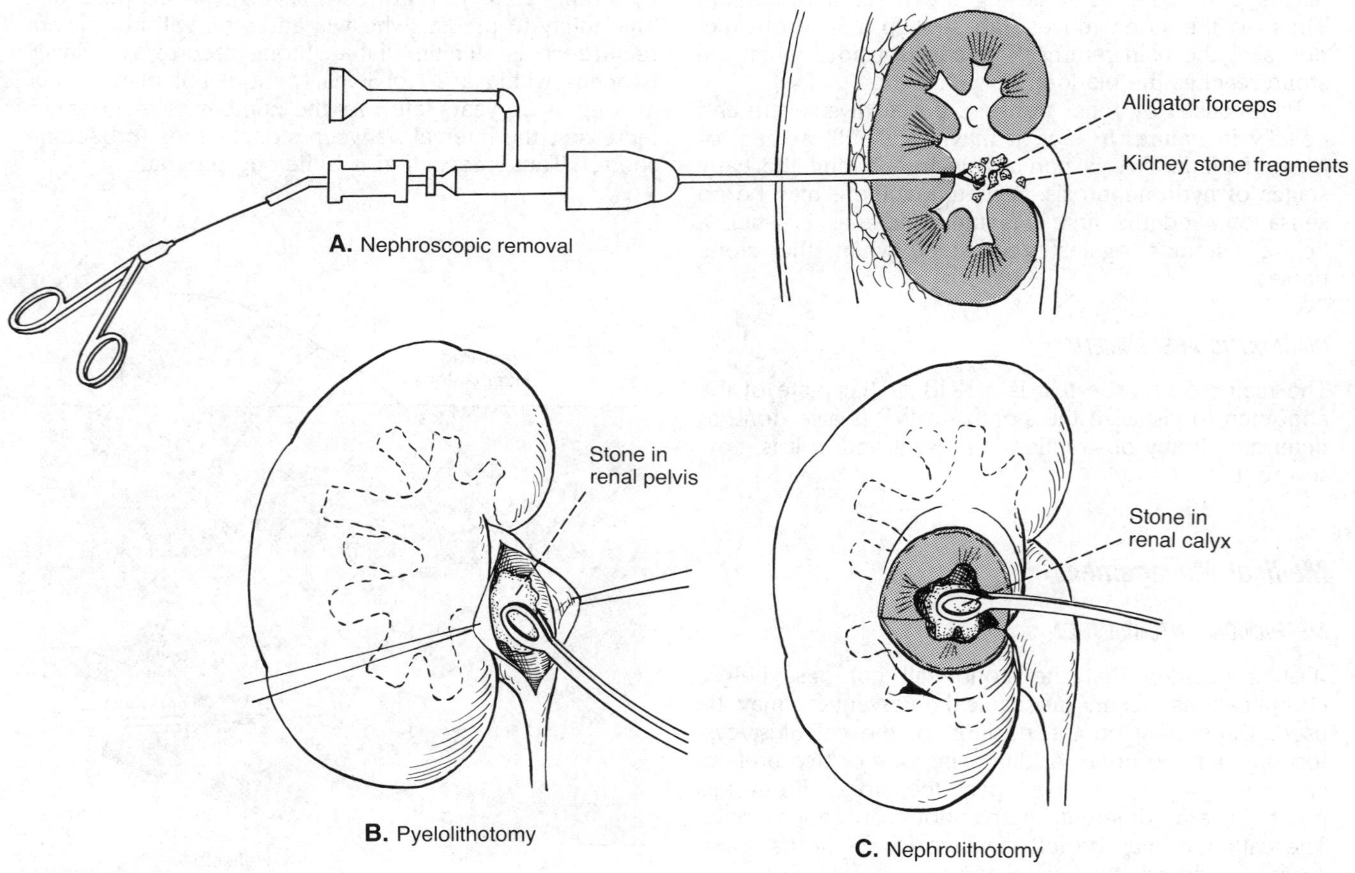

▲ **Figure 50-10**

Surgical techniques for removal of kidney stones.

If the stone is too large, one of several methods may be used to break it up into smaller fragments (litholapaxy). A punch lithoclast helps to fragment the stone. An ultrasound nephroscope may be inserted into the kidney and subharmonic sound waves used to shatter the stone. Electrohydraulic lithotripsy involves inserting an electric probe through the nephroscope to produce shock waves to the stone. Chemolysis may also help break up the stone, especially with uric acid, struvite, and cystine stones. Two nephrostomy tubes are placed, one to keep the chemical solution flowing freely around the stone and the other to provide effective drainage to prevent hydrostatic pressure in the kidney. Sodium bicarbonate, organic acids, and chelating solutions are the most common.[73]

After the procedure, a nephrostomy tube remains in place for 1 to 5 days. The client may be sent home with the nephrostomy tube. A nephrotomogram is then done to determine whether all stone fragments were removed. If the kidney is clear, the tube will be removed and a bulky dressing placed over the site. Be certain that a high fluid intake is maintained during the post-procedure period to flush out any fragments. Recommended daily amounts are 3000 to 4000 ml. Monitor for, or teach the client to monitor for, complications such as infection, hemorrhage, and extravasation of fluid into the retroperitoneal cavity.

If these procedures do not successfully remove the stone, an open surgical procedure may be required. A stone lodged in the ureter will require a ureterolithotomy, which involves incision into the affected ureter. The approach may be through a lower abdominal or flank incision. The stone is removed, any strictures are repaired, and the incision is closed. The stone is removed from the renal pelvis by a pyelolithotomy, and from the renal calix by a nephrolithotomy. Figure 50–10*B* and *C* illustrates these two procedures.

If constricted or tortuous ureters cause recurrent calculi, one of two procedures may be used to correct the problem. An ileal ureter, using a segment of the ileum between the renal collecting system and the bladder, may be constructed. This creates a wide-bore passage that replaces the original ureter. A renal autotransplant may also be performed. Here the kidney is transplanted to the ipsilateral or contralateral pelvis. A flap of bladder tissue is raised, formed into a large-caliber tube, and anastomosed to the renal pelvis. The bladder wall is then sutured to reestablish its continuity. These procedures are used very selectively.[59]

The physician may decide that a partial or total nephrectomy is necessary because of extensive kidney damage, overwhelming renal infection, or severe ureteropelvic junction obstruction or, in the case of abnormal renal parenchyma, to prevent stone recurrence. This procedure is used much less now than in the past and is usually considered a "last resort" intervention.

Possible complications after litholapaxy include hemorrhage, urinary retention, infection, and possible stone recurrence.

Nursing Management

ASSESSMENT

As with any disease, the history the client gives is very important in identifying the problem. Full information about the onset of symptoms and the pattern of pain is vital. Family history of calculi is suggestive. Evaluate recent dietary habits. For instance, a large intake of purines may be significant, and drinking large amounts of fruit juices or tea facilitates oxalate precipitation. The client should be asked about recent medications and the presence of any contributing factors, such as urinary tract infection, immobility, or gout.

Physical findings primarily center on two things: the urine and x-ray studies. Be certain to strain all urine being voided through several layers of gauze or through a commercial urine strainer. Carefully examine all debris in the bedpan or urinal. Save any stone material so the stone's composition can be analyzed as a basis for treatment and to show how much has passed through the urinary tract. Also, monitor urine for hematuria. A routine urinalysis gives important information about the pH, the specific gravity, and the presence of red blood cells, white blood cells, crystals, and casts. Collect 24-hour urine specimens, if necessary, to determine the daily output of possible causative crystals. A urine culture will help identify urinary tract infection. Blood levels of constituent elements, such as calcium, phosphorus, and uric acid, may be determined. Stones containing calcium and cystine are radiopaque and will show up on a KUB x-ray film. IVP and retrograde pyelography are an important part of the evaluation process.

NURSING INTERVENTION

Nursing Diagnosis: Pain R/T irritation from stone movement.

Planning: Expected Outcomes. The client will have pain relieved or controlled, as evidenced by client's statement.

Implementation. Controlling the client's pain is a primary objective of nursing intervention. Large doses of narcotics and possibly antispasmodics are given to control the client's pain because the client cannot force fluids and ambulate if the pain is too severe.

Nursing Diagnosis: Injury, High Risk for R/T possible obstruction.

Planning: Expected Outcomes. The client will not suffer an injury from an obstruction, as evidenced by normal output.

Implementation. All urine must be strained. Whenever the client voids, the urine is strained through a strainer or a gauze pad so any stones or sediment can be saved and sent for analysis. The stone analysis will help determine what measures are needed to prevent recurrence.

Nursing Diagnosis: Injury, High Risk for R/T postoperative complications.

Planning: Expected Outcomes. The client will not develop injury, as evidenced by absence of hemorrhage, vital signs within preoperative limits, and normal white blood cell count and temperature.

Implementation. If the client had surgery to remove the stone, then postoperative nursing interventions will depend on the incision's location and the type of drainage tubes present. With a flank incision, care is similar to that needed after nephrectomy. The client with an abdominal incision, however, requires the same care as anyone having major abdominal surgery (see Chap. 19).

The nurse needs to know that the incision probably will drain large amounts of urine for days to weeks after surgery. Intervention includes frequent dressing change around the Penrose drain and protection of the skin against the urinary drainage. A nephrostomy tube may be left in place attached to a drainage bag. Care should be taken to ensure a free flow of urine. Sterile technique is always used to prevent infection.

Nursing Diagnosis: Knowledge Deficit R/T fluid requirements, dietary restrictions, and medications.

Planning: Expected Outcomes. The client will understand fluid requirements, dietary restrictions, and medications, as evidenced by discussion with client.

Implementation. The nurse has a major role in helping the client develop and maintain an effective, individual regimen to prevent recurrence. The nurse should help the client establish health habits that prevent renal stone recurrence, teach about the disease and its implications, and provide support during the follow-up period. The three main components of a preventive regimen are fluids, diet, and medications.

The client's fluid intake should be high enough to ensure 2500 to 3000 ml or more of urine output per day. This will require at least 3000 to 4000 ml of fluid daily; more will be needed under certain situations (e.g., hot weather, fever, diarrhea). The increased urine volume resulting from this high fluid intake decreases the concentration of solutes and alleviates urinary stasis. The kind of fluid the client drinks depends on dietary restrictions. At least half of the fluid should be water, which usually has a low calcium content. The fluid intake needs to be as consistent as possible throughout the 24-hour period. Clients are usually advised to drink one glass every hour during the day and two large glasses just before going to bed. This will usually mean that they will need to void about midway through the night, when they can drink another glass of water. These clients will probably need help adjusting their lifestyles to accommodate the need for frequent bathroom breaks.

There is some controversy regarding dietary restrictions because of the uncertain therapeutic effectiveness of and problems in long-term compliance with this regimen.

For planning recommended dietary restrictions, the results of a stone analysis are essential. Some stone constituents require specific diet adjustments in order to avoid stone formation. Hypercalciuria may be controlled by limiting excessive calcium intake. Clients with oxalate stones should avoid high-oxalate foods: tea, instant coffee, cola drinks, beer, rhubarb, beans, asparagus, spinach, cabbage, chocolate, citrus fruits, apples, grapes, cranberries, peanuts, and peanut butter. Megadoses of vitamin C increase oxalate excretion in the urine.

If the stone is composed of uric acid, the client should be on a low-purine diet. This limits foods such as aged cheeses, wine, and organ meats.

Medications may also be used to reduce the incidence of recurrent calculi. Teach the client about these agents and the need for long-term administration. Medications frequently used to control calcium stone formation may include phosphates, thiazide diuretics, and allopurinol. Phosphates reduce urinary calcium and increase the excretion of pyrophosphate, which is responsible for inhibiting crystal formation. Methylene blue may decrease calcium oxalate crystal formation. Clients with these conditions should also avoid calcium-containing antacids.

Cholestyramine, an anion-exchange resin, binds oxalate and promotes its excretion by the intestine. It does have the potential side effect of severe vitamin K deficiency. Because pyridoxine (vitamin B_6) deficiency increases crystal excretion, B_6 may be given to clients who have oxalate stones. Magnesium oxide also decreases oxalate excretion, and isocarboxazid apparently blocks the metabolism of oxalate. Allopurinol, a xanthine oxidase inhibitor, may be used to prevent oxalate and uric acid stone formation. Uricosuric agents should be avoided; they increase uric acid excretion in the urine, thus increasing the solute concentration.

One of the most frequent components of the medication regimen for triple phosphate or struvite stones is long-term antibiotics as an attempt to control the infection. Acidification of the urine, administration of phosphate-binding gels, and dietary restrictions of phosphate are also used. Cystine stone-formers are treated with D-penicillamine or mercaptopropionylglycine, which transform L-cystine into a water-soluble disulfide derivative. Clients treated with these medications usually need supplemental vitamin B_6.

Adjusting the urinary pH as a means to control precipitation of crystals is a possible treatment. An acidic urine, with a pH below 6, is used to prevent possible calcium and triple phosphate or struvite stones. Chapter 49 describes methods for acidifying the urine. Additionally, methionine or ammonium salts may be used. Uric acid and xanthine stones are inhibited in alkaline urine; alkalinization of the urine is usually accomplished with sodium bicarbonate, citrate, or acetazolamide.

EVALUATION

The nurse should evaluate whether the established goals have been met for this client. If the goals were not met, the nurse must alter the plan of care and interventions so that the client's needs are met.

Modification of Plan of Care for the Elderly

There are no specific modifications for the older client except the increased risk of complications of surgery associated with aging (see Chap. 19).

Post-hospital Care

DISCHARGE TEACHING

The client must be taught methods to avoid recurrence or to at least detect the stones early if they recur. This includes teaching the client to increase fluid intake; void every 2 hours; maintain an acidic urine pH (unless the stones are uric acid); change diet to low-calcium, low-phosphate with calcium stones or low-purine with uric acid stones; and take medications to improve excretion of uric acid with uric acid stones. The client should also be taught to recognize any signs of recurrence.

HOME HEALTH CARE NEEDS

The client does not usually require any specific home health care after the stone is passed or removed.

FOLLOW-UP CARE

The client should be followed at intervals for signs of recurrent calculi. Follow-up urinalysis and blood measures for the presence of the stone-causing agents are done at intervals.

RENAL CANCER

Definition

Benign kidney tumors are rare. Classifications include lymphangioma, lipoma, medullary fibroma, adenoma, leiomyoma, and oncocytoma. When large tumors occur, it is relatively impossible to distinguish them from malignant tumor by x-ray examination. If other diagnostic tests are also inconclusive, nephrectomy may be done.

Incidence

At least 85 per cent of all renal tumors are malignant. There are approximately 5000 to 7000 deaths yearly as a result of adult kidney cancer. The figure represents 1 to 3 per cent of all malignancies. The tumors are most frequently found between the ages of 50 and 70 years. They affect men more frequently than women.

Etiology

The exact cause of renal tumors is unknown. There have been some links established between kidney cancer and tobacco, lead, cadmium, and phosphates. A genetic link has also been postulated.

Pathophysiology

Renal cell carcinoma, or adenocarcinoma, is the most frequent type of tumor; it accounts for 90 per cent of all kidney neoplasms. Tumor growth begins in the renal cortex and usually continues for some time before it produces symptoms. It can grow very large and tends to compress adjacent renal parenchyma rather than infiltrate it. The tumor, usually avascular, tends to surround blood vessels and stenose them. The lungs and mediastinum are the most frequent metastatic sites for this tumor. Liver, bone, skin, spleen, renal vein, and brain are other common sites.

Other types of renal cancer include nephroblastoma, sarcoma, and epithelial tumors within the renal pelvis. Nephroblastoma, or Wilms' tumor, is primarily a childhood disease, although it occasionally occurs in adults. The prognosis for adults is worse than for children, with some sources reporting only a 25 per cent survival rate.[65] For further discussion of this type of tumor, refer to a pediatric nursing text. Sarcoma is infrequent, typically arising in the renal capsule. Most tumors of the renal pelvis are primarily urolithelial in origin and include three different tissue types: transitional cell, squamous cell, and adenocarcinoma.

Staging of the tumor helps delineate the appropriate treatment to be used. Figure 50–11 illustrates the typical staging system for renal carcinoma.

Spontaneous regression of renal adenocarcinoma reportedly occurs in fewer than 1 per cent of all cases. Most of these regressions developed after nephrectomy and involved metastatic areas. However, authorities consider these episodes as more evidence the disease has a definite immunologic or hormonal link.

The prognosis partially depends on the stage at time of treatment. Five-year survival rates for stage I are about 65 per cent, for stage II about 40 per cent; 10-year rates drop to 40 per cent and 35 per cent. Five-year survivals are rare for stages III and IV.

Clinical Manifestations

Symptoms of renal malignancies vary, and tumor growth may advance significantly before the disease is discovered. It is not uncommon for the client to demonstrate signs and symptoms not apparently related to renal disease. Frequently, a palpable abdominal mass found during a routine physical examination arouses the first suspicion. The average time between the onset

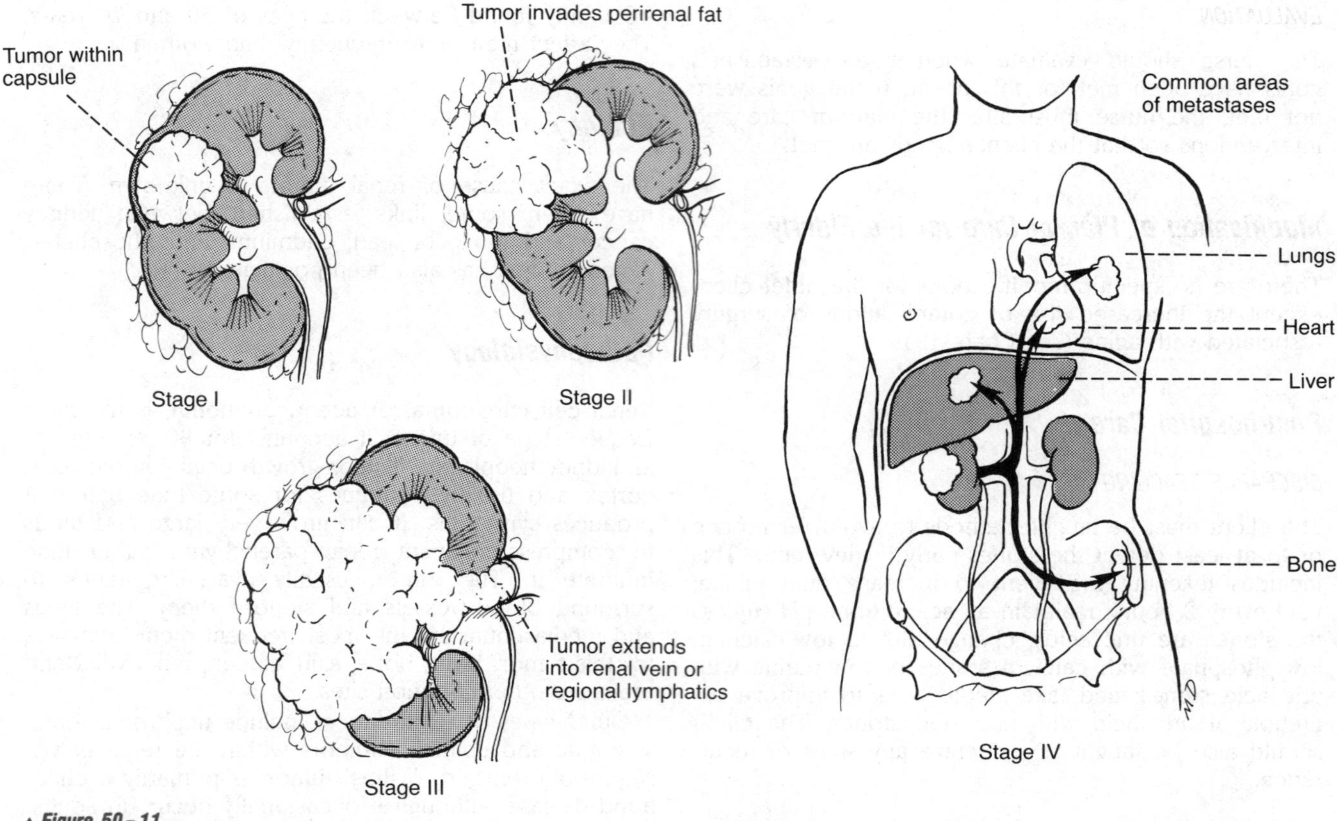

▲ *Figure 50–11*

Staging system for renal carcinoma. Stage I tumor is confined within renal capsule; stage II tumor extends beyond renal capsule, with invasion of local perinephric fat, but no metastasis; stage III tumor extends into renal vein or involves local lymphatics; and stage IV tumor has metastasized to other parts of the body.

of hematuria and the onset of pain is 9 months, and 14 months between the initial pain and diagnosis. Many times, extrarenal manifestations are found before a diagnosis of renal cancer is confirmed. As many as 35 per cent of all clients have metastasis when the final diagnosis of a renal neoplasm is made.

The common triad of symptoms includes hematuria, flank pain, and a palpable abdominal or flank mass. The hematuria is usually gross and intermittent, which helps explain the client's delay in seeking medical advice. The clinical picture also contains a combination of the following frequent assessment findings: fever, weight loss and cachexia, fatigue, hypertension, amyloidosis, thrombophlebitis, anemia, erythrocytosis, hypercalcemia, abnormal serum liver profile, and an elevated sedimentation rate. Less frequent findings include peripheral neuropathy, inferior vena cava obstruction, priapism, and varicocele. Hydronephrosis may occur if the tumor obstructs the ureteropelvic junction. The incidence of pulmonary embolus as a presenting manifestation may be more frequent than has been previously thought because of the high rate of vena cava and renal vein involvement. Plasma erythropoietin, renin, and chorionic gonadotropin levels are elevated, and prostaglandin production increases in renal cell carcinoma.

DIAGNOSTIC ASSESSMENT

Several diagnostic tests help confirm a diagnosis of renal cancer. IVP is probably the most helpful in identifying a space-occupying lesion. Ultrasonography helps differentiate between a cyst and a solid mass. Other noninvasive procedures include CT scan, nephrotomography, and radioisotope studies. Arteriography evaluates the renal vascular system. Renal biopsy, usually done percutaneously, provides definitive data about the lesion.

Medical Management

Radiation therapy may be used in adjunction with chemotherapy and surgery. Irradiation is most useful in preoperative preparation of the tumor. It is sometimes also used postoperatively to (1) destroy residual or recurrent tumor cells, (2) treat lymphatic involvement, and (3) treat metastatic sites, such as the bones, palliatively.

PHARMACOLOGIC MANAGEMENT

Clinical investigation continues to search for an effective chemotherapeutic regimen. Medroxyprogesterone and testosterone have been used as hormonal therapy, but their effectiveness has been short-lived. Vinblastine seems the most effective single agent, with response rates of 25 per cent. Attempts with combination regimens seem to raise toxic effects without improving response rates. Many agents are being studied, but renal cancer cells seem insensitive to chemotherapeutic or hormonal agents, possibly because of their slow growth rate.

Immunotherapy seems to have some promise in treating renal cancer. Stimulants to the immune system have shown some positive results as long as the tumor is not too large and the immunodepression is not too severe. Natural and recombinant leukocyte interferon both show some response in treatment as well. Interleukin-2 has been approved by the Food and Drug Administration for expanded clinical trials in renal cancer.

Surgical Management

The conventional and principal intervention for renal cancer is nephrectomy. Radiation and chemotherapy may be part of the medical regimen but are usually adjuncts to surgical kidney removal. For renal cell carcinoma, the surgical procedure of choice is generally radical nephrectomy, including removal of the kidney, the adrenal gland, and perinephric fat with the retroperitoneal lymphatics. Lymphadenectomy remains controversial. When the tumor is located in the renal pelvis, a nephroureterectomy is usually performed because of a tendency for transitional cell cancer to "seed" down the ureter into the bladder. With nephroureterectomy, a cuff of the adjacent bladder is removed. Even in advanced cases, when prognosis is poor, nephrectomy may be done to relieve pain and for hematuria. If the neoplastic disease is bilateral, or if there is a solitary functioning kidney, a partial nephrectomy may be done on at least one kidney, leaving enough renal tissue to support life without long-term dialysis. If partial nephrectomy is not possible in either instance, the entire kidney will be removed and the client placed on dialysis. These clients may be candidates for renal transplant, but they are usually maintained on dialysis for about a year in order to observe for recurrence of the disease.

Preoperative intervention may help shrink the tumor, making it easier to resect during surgery. Irradiation helps reduce the size of the tumor, although slowly. Renal artery embolization of the affected kidney may be done to infarct the tumor and reduce its vascularity, thereby reducing the risk of hemorrhage. This is usually done by placing one of several things into the renal artery to occlude it: absorbable gelatin sponge, metal coil, barium, subcutaneous fat, isobutyl-2-cyanoacrylate, absolute ethanol, and temporary balloons. This procedure may also be performed to control hemorrhage in an inoperable kidney. In addition, some researchers believe embolization may stimulate an immune response against the dying cancer cells.[10]

Preoperative preparation of the client having renal surgery includes general guidelines as described in Chapter 19. Increase fluid intake if indicated to ensure adequate excretion of waste products before surgery. Give emotional support because the client may be anxious, not only about the surgery but about the prospects for adequate postoperative urinary function. If the remaining kidney functions adequately, the client can be assured this kidney will fully meet the body's elimination needs. (See the discussion about renal transplantation for more information about this.)

Nursing Management

Nursing management of the client with renal cancer must include general aspects of care for any neoplastic disease (see Chaps. 21 and 22). Most specific to the client with kidney cancer is the care required after nephrectomy and nephroureterectomy.

Postoperative care is similar to that for laparotomy. One of the biggest challenges is reestablishing effective breathing patterns. Deep breathing and coughing are very difficult because the incision is so close to the diaphragm. Liberal use of narcotics (including the use of patient-controlled analgesia) to relieve pain and external mechanical support to the chest and abdomen with pillows or hands helps the client to do deep-breathing and coughing exercises more effectively. Incentive spirometers provide immediate feedback regarding the effectiveness of the deep breathing. Surgically induced or spontaneous pneumothorax does occur occasionally after nephrectomy, so be prepared for this possibility by assessing for sudden shortness of breath and loss of breath sounds on the affected side.

Careful monitoring of urine output is essential. Measure output hourly to identify renal failure as early as possible. Meticulous catheter care is necessary to prevent postoperative urinary tract infection.

The incision used for nephrectomy is extensive and causes significant discomfort. Muscular pain may develop as a result of the prolonged position maintained during surgery. This pain may be relieved by analgesics (including the use of patient-controlled analgesia), proper positioning, massage, and heat.

Paralytic ileus is a common problem. Interventions include carefully assessing the client's gastrointestinal status postoperatively, beginning oral intake only after adequate bowel function has been established, and early exercise (i.e., ambulation).

The skin impairment depends on the size and location of the surgical incision and the number and type of drains present. Wound care is routine; dressing changes are performed as needed for the amount of drainage.

To help reduce feelings of anxiety, continue to keep the client and significant others informed about the progress made. All should be encouraged to express their concerns and to talk with one another. The need for this support will continue throughout the follow-up period.

Post-hospital Care

The major follow-up depends on the stage of cancer and the need for further treatment.

RENAL CANDIDIASIS

Bacteria cause most instances of pyelonephritis. However, the incidence of renal candidiasis is increasing. Primary renal candidiasis is most common in women with diabetes mellitus. Manifestations of this disease include obstruction secondary to bezoar (tangled hyphae or clumps of yeast cells) in the ureter; progressive oliguria, sometimes alternating with episodic diuresis; ureteral colic; passing tissue- or stonelike material; pyuria; and progressive renal failure. Diagnosis is based on the presence of fungi in several properly collected urine cultures; the presence of serum *Candida* precipitins; and selected radiologic findings, such as hydronephrosis, caliceal erosion, and the presence of filling defects called fungus balls. Amphotericin B and flucytosine are the keys to medical management, although these medications present problems of dosage and nephrotoxicity. Surgery to remove obstruction or nephrectomy may be needed for severe disease.

RENAL ABSCESS

A renal abscess (or renal carbuncle), a localized infection within the cortex of the kidney, usually forms when smaller infectious foci or microabscesses combine in the renal parenchyma. It is usually secondary to urinary tract infection with enterobacteriaceae, often complicated by renal calculi and obstruction. Other organisms, coming from extrarenal sites, may also cause this infectious process. For example, the client will frequently give a history of recent cutaneous furuncles.

Clients with renal abscess typically have high fever and moderate to severe pain. This pain is usually constant and is felt in either the upper quadrant of the abdomen or in the costovertebral area; it sometimes resembles renal colic. Unlike pyelonephritis, the urine is usually sterile, because the abscess does not reach into the urinary collecting system. Other symptoms of this infectious process include weakness, anorexia, weight loss, night sweats, and leukocytosis.

Medical and nursing interventions for renal abscess resemble those for acute pyelonephritis. Aggressive antibiotic therapy is usually successful. A needle aspiration of the abscess may be done for culture and sensitivity study on the contents. This helps pinpoint the appropriate antimicrobial to be used. Surgical incision and drainage of the abscess sometimes is necessary. If so, nursing intervention expands to include postoperative care of the incision. A drain will be left in place for some time.

PERINEPHRIC ABSCESS

A perinephric abscess involves the fatty tissue surrounding the kidney. It may be an extension of a renal infectious process (most common) or may have spread hematogenously from an extrarenal infection. The abscess may spread in several directions, extending to the peritoneal cavity, chest, or skin.

Assessment findings are the same as with a renal abscess—fever, tenderness, flank or loin pain, and other signs of sepsis—with the possible addition of swelling over the site.

Medical and nursing interventions are almost identical to those for renal abscess. Appropriate antibiotics are administered, and symptomatic interventions are undertaken. Because of the nature of a perinephric abscess, incising and draining are needed more frequently than with renal abscess. After this surgical procedure, there may be profuse drainage from the wound; frequent dressing changes and nursing intervention are required to prevent or treat skin excoriation.

RENAL TRAUMA

Serious kidney injury is relatively rare because of the protection afforded by the rib cage, the back's heavy muscles, and the tough capsule surrounding the kidney. Traffic accidents and falls wherein the client lands on the abdomen, flank, or back are the most common cause of injury, usually resulting in blunt trauma. Kidney lacerations are also associated with fractures of the spine and ribs as well as penetrating injuries from bullets and knives.

Assessment

The type of injury the client has suffered gives the first real key to identifying renal trauma. There frequently are multiple serious injuries, and renal trauma may not be immediately apparent. Hematuria (gross or microscopic) is a cardinal sign and is found in approximately 80 per cent of cases. Remember, however, that serious renal injury can occur without hemorrhage, so clear urine should not negate a possible diagnosis. Other findings include shock, flank pain, and the development of a palpable mass in the affected flank area or over the eleventh or twelfth rib. Paralytic ileus may also occur. Grey Turner's sign refers to bruises over the flank and lower back secondary to retroperitoneal hemorrhage. A KUB, IVP, retrograde pyelography, renal scan, ultrasonography, CT scan, and renal arteriography all help confirm the kind and amount of kidney injury.

Classification

Figure 50-12 illustrates the five categories of traumatic injury that can occur to the kidney: contusion with

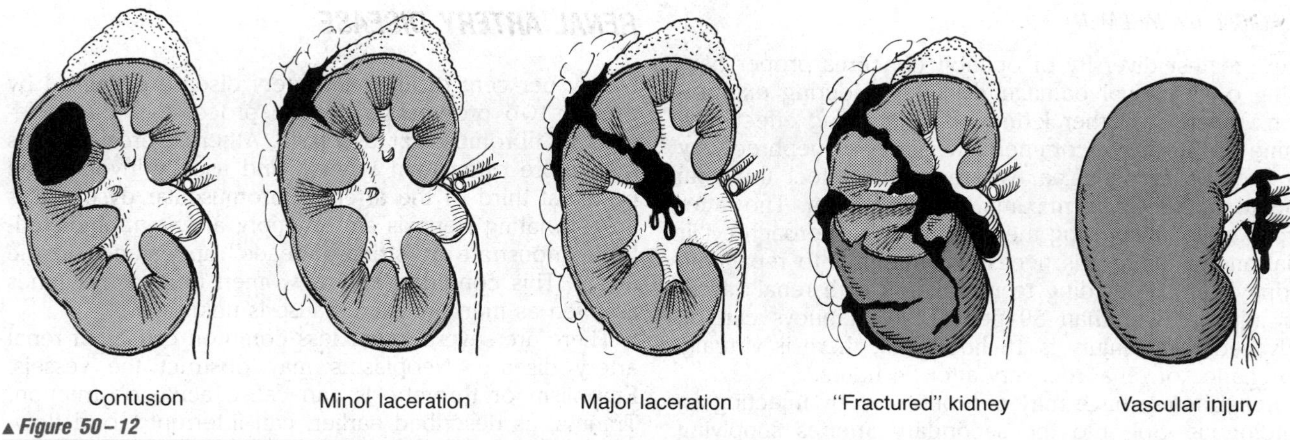

▲ **Figure 50–12**

Categories of renal trauma: contusion (intrarenal hemorrhage); minor laceration (subcapsular hemorrhage); major laceration (hemorrhage into renal pelvis); fractured kidney (shattered rupture); and vascular (pedicle) injury (damaging renal blood supply).

intrarenal hemorrhage, minor laceration (rupture with subcapsular hemorrhage), major laceration (rupture into the renal pelvis), "fractured" kidney (shattered rupture), and vascular (pedicle) injury. A contusion involves development of a hematoma that remains confined within the renal parenchyma. Rupture of the kidney may cause hemorrhage between the capsular wall; bleeding may or may not reach into the renal pelvis. A shattered or "fractured" kidney results in hemorrhage throughout the renal tissue. The pedicle holds the renal artery and other vital circulatory and nervous system connections for the kidney. Injury to the pedicle may well jeopardize the life of the kidney. A pedicle injury may occur with or without intrarenal hemorrhage.

Complications

In addition to the immediate problems of hemorrhage and loss of functioning renal tissue, kidney trauma makes the client highly susceptible to a number of other problems. Even in closed injuries, there is a high risk for sepsis leading to the development of kidney and perinephric abscesses. Secondary hemorrhage is not uncommon. Other complications include hypertension due to fibrosis and ischemic kidney; renal artery thrombosis; arteriovenous aneurysms; fistula formation due to extravasation of urine; and the development of urinomas and pseudocysts.

Management

Intervention for renal trauma is controversial and centers on whether to pursue a conservative or a surgical path. Most physicians agree that kidney contusion calls for conservative treatment. Other minor injuries, such as small subcapsular hematomas and minor lacerations without extravasation, may also be better followed conservatively. Major injuries, such as renal fracture, parenchymal injury with major arterial occlusion, avulsion injuries or tears in the renal artery or vein, and parenchymal lacerations with extending perirenal hematomas or urinary extravasation, may require surgical exploration. Possible indicators for exploration include continued moderate to severe hemorrhage and continued urine extravasation. Urine extravasation itself is not definite grounds for surgery, because sterile urine usually resolves or encapsulates spontaneously. However, it sometimes produces severe tissue reaction and causes fistula formation. The pocket of extrarenal urine may also become obstructive.

CONSERVATIVE MANAGEMENT

Conservative treatment, which primarily involves waiting and watching, is possible because the retroperitoneal space allows tamponade. In the absence of other injuries, a client with microscopic hematuria and normal IVP may be followed on an ambulatory basis with careful instructions about activity restrictions and the need for adequate hydration. If there is gross hematuria, the client is placed on bed rest until the urine clears. Serial observations of the urine, hematocrit, and vital signs are made to watch the progress of the hemorrhage. Sequential urine specimens may be collected to compare current and previous urine color and turbidity. Even if replacement fluids are not needed, a prophylactic intravenous line may be established, and a type and crossmatch for blood may be done. If a hematoma is present or the IVP demonstrates extravasation of the urine, the client may receive antibiotics to prevent sepsis. The physician prescribes blood transfusions if the hematocrit is low. After the urine is cleared, the client will be allowed to be more active. After discharge from the health care facility, the client needs follow-up blood pressure checks and IVPs to rule out the development of secondary hypertension and anatomic derangement of the renal system.

SURGICAL MANAGEMENT

The greatest diversity of opinion concerns proper handling of the renal damage discovered during exploration. When the other kidney is functioning effectively, some physicians recommend free use of nephrectomy to avoid later sequelae, whereas others feel the goal should be salvaging maximal renal function. The latter group advocates giving the conservative approach a fair trial and, if surgery is necessary, attempts to repair the kidney before deciding to remove it. With renal vascular injury, fewer than 50 per cent of kidneys can be salvaged if the injury is 18 hours old; there is virtually no chance of renal recovery after 24 hours.

Renal hemorrhage may be controlled by injecting an autologous clot into the secondary arteries supplying the bleeding site. Blood is drawn from the client and allowed to clot. The clot is then injected angiographically. Normal endothelium has a strong clot-lysing effect, so the clot disappears after a period of several hours from the normal adjacent vasculature and affects only the damaged portion.

If a kidney repair is attempted rather than nephrectomy, the surgical procedure aims to debride devitalized tissue, achieve hemostasis, establish a watertight seal of the collecting system, approximate the renal parenchymal edges, and drain the renal fossa. Two surgical techniques increase the successful outcome of repair attempts. Extracorporeal or bench surgery allows the kidney to be removed from the body in order to better visualize and manipulate the organ during the repair process; the kidney returns to the body by autotransplantation. During the time outside the body, the kidney is maintained either by hypothermia or by a perfusate mechanically pulsed through it. The slush technique, involving immersing the kidney in iced saline slush, decreases the metabolism and oxygen requirement of the renal tissue, allowing longer intraoperative ischemic times. This does cause some systemic hypothermia, but not significantly. Pedicle vascular injury may also be repaired. If these techniques fail, nephrectomy is necessary. Postoperative nursing diagnoses and interventions are as described previously.

Nursing interventions during conservative treatment center on monitoring urinary elimination patterns and helping the client to cope and to comply with the medical regimen. Anxiety is common and requires supportive intervention on the part of the nurse. Imposed activity restrictions may result in problems with bowel elimination and adequate fluid intake, circulation, and respiratory function. The client being followed on an ambulatory basis needs an appropriate teaching plan covering health maintenance activities and the need for a follow-up program.

▼ Renal Vascular Abnormalities

The kidneys depend on adequate blood circulation to nourish tissues and to provide blood for filtration so they can perform their intended functions. Anything that interferes with the normal circulatory flow significantly reduces renal capabilities.

RENAL ARTERY DISEASE

Ninety per cent of all renal artery disease is caused by one or two progressive disease processes: atherosclerosis or fibromuscular dysplasia. Atherosclerosis affects men more often than women and usually involves the proximal third of the artery. Fibromuscular dysplasia is an alternating stenosis and dilation; arteriographic studies demonstrate a "string-of-beads" appearance in the artery. This condition affects women four to five times as often as men; its exact cause is unknown.

There are several other less common causes of renal artery disease. Neoplasms may obstruct the vessels. Embolism or thrombosis can cause acute obstruction. Trauma, as described earlier, can interrupt blood flow. The renal artery may be purposely occluded to produce a "medical nephrectomy" or total renal infarction; this may be done preoperatively in the case of renal adenocarcinoma or to control proteinuria or hypertension. Shredded Gelfoam may be used, or a liquid substance that polymerizes instantly when it contacts blood may be injected into the renal artery. A dissecting aneurysm in the renal artery may also interrupt renal circulation.

The end result of any of these conditions, if severe enough, is reduced renal blood flow. This, in turn, causes renal parenchymal ischemia and, finally, renal atrophy. The role of renal artery disease in renovascular hypertension is also well documented, and it alone may indicate treatment of the condition.

Because of the kidney's compensatory mechanisms, the gradual development of renal artery stenosis from atherosclerosis and neoplasms may give rise to very few symptoms, at least until the resulting hypertension and decreasing renal function become evident. However, acute obstruction makes itself known relatively quickly. Symptoms of this sudden episode include flank pain over the affected kidney or abdominal pain and fever. Atrial arrhythmias are a frequent finding, although because they often alternate with periods of normal sinus rhythm this symptom can be missed. Urinalysis may be normal, and blood chemistries may show an elevated aspartate aminotransferase and lactic dehydrogenase. An IVP will demonstrate a nonfunctioning kidney, and a renal scan will show no arterial blood flow.

RENAL TUBERCULOSIS

Tuberculosis of the kidney, which affects men more frequently than women, occurs when the causative organism, *Mycobacterium tuberculosis*, reaches the kidney via the bloodstream from another source in the body, usually the lungs. Once the organism arrives at the kidney, it may become dormant for many years. By the time it again becomes active, the original infection is often well healed. Frequently, the primary tubercular site was asymptomatic, which makes it difficult to identify renal tuberculosis on the basis of history.

The clinical course of renal tuberculosis is generally very slow, and clinical signs and symptoms often do not become evident until the later stages of the disease. Early disease involves the renal cortex or medulla. Tissue destruction extends in all directions, eventually eroding into a calix at the tip of the papilla and progressing to rupture into the renal pelvis. Once the infection reaches the pelvis, it spreads along the mucosa. This allows the causative organisms full access to the rest of the kidney and permits them to move down the urinary tract where they can infect any of the urinary organs. If untreated, this destructive process will continue to form large, caseating masses, which coalesce to destroy kidney tissue. X-ray examination at this time will show the kidneys to have a "moth-eaten" appearance.

Organisms reaching the lower urinary tract usually result in fibrosis and stricture formation and destruction of the ureterovesical valve. If these processes stenose the ureter, thus reducing the exit for pus and urine from the infected kidney, renal destruction will accelerate. Descending tubercle bacilli may also lodge in the male reproductive organs, causing reduced function.

When renal tuberculosis becomes evident, assessment findings are often nonspecific. Renal symptoms may be preceded by general malaise, weight loss, low-grade fever, and night sweats, but these are not as frequent as with pulmonary tuberculosis. Symptoms of cystitis, as described in Chapter 49, are often the presenting indications. Flank pain may be present, and hematuria and pyuria are common. Males frequently have signs and symptoms of epididymitis. A culture of *Mycobacterium tuberculosis* grown from the urine helps confirm a definitive diagnosis of renal tuberculosis. The specimens for culture are collected on at least three successive mornings. Because tubercle bacilli shed intermittently, three to 12 negative cultures are needed to exclude the diagnosis of active renal tuberculosis absolutely.

Chemotherapy with antitubercular agents has reduced the need for surgical intervention. Multiple therapy that typically combines several medications (rifampin, ethambutol, isoniazid and pyridoxine, streptomycin, cycloserine, and sodium para-aminosalicylate) is the most common intervention. Because tubercle bacilli divide slowly, the medications are usually given in a single daily dose. However, if side effects develop, the day's dose may be divided. See Chapter 39 for further information on antitubercular medications.

Surgical intervention includes total or partial nephrectomy or cutaneous ureterostomy. Permanent urinary diversion may be necessary if strictures are severe or bladder damage is irreparable. Indications for surgery include persistent infection that does not respond to chemotherapy, intractable pain, hemorrhage, uncontrollable hypertension, renal malignancy, and progressive strictures.

If surgery is needed, preoperative and postoperative nursing interventions will be similar to those for any client having major surgery (see Chap. 19).

During the acute phase, nursing interventions involve assisting with diagnostic procedures, protecting against the spread of the causative organisms, providing symptomatic relief for the client, and assisting the client with the medication regimen. Because tuberculosis arouses a great deal of fear and a feeling of social isolation, expect your nursing diagnoses to include fear and anxiety for the client as well as for the significant others. Help these clients to discuss and work through their feelings. Listen to their concerns and help them seek additional counseling if necessary.

Renal tuberculosis is a prolonged illness that requires long-term care and support. Because the client is usually followed on an ambulatory basis, instruction in self-care frequently is the primary nursing intervention. One of the biggest problems with clients recovering from renal tuberculosis is continued compliance with the prescribed medical and nursing regimens, especially when the client begins to feel better. Help the client understand the need for continuous medication therapy and continuing follow-up examinations. The client must also understand the importance of maintaining general good health, such as proper nutrition, adequate rest, and good hygiene. During recovery, give the client positive feedback for adhering to the regimens, if appropriate. If not, use problem-solving techniques to help the client reestablish compliance with the regimens.

In response to reduced renal circulation, collateral circulation helps preserve the kidney if sufficient development takes place before the total obstruction. Collateral circulation, in addition to a marked reduction in filtration, renal work, and oxygen requirements, allows the kidney to tolerate ischemic periods for up to several weeks. In acute total occlusion, a normal kidney can remain viable for approximately 2 hours before infarction and tissue necrosis begin.[58]

Treatment of the ischemic kidney usually involves surgical revascularization. Arterial endarterectomy may be done with follow-up anticoagulant or antiplatelet therapy. Percutaneous transluminal renal angioplasty is a procedure in which the vessel is reamed out with use of a balloon catheter. If the vessel cannot be recanalized, a renal artery resection with end-to-end anastomosis or an aortorenal bypass graft procedure may be performed.

In the postoperative period after an aortorenal bypass graft procedure, the client may experience an initial exacerbation of hypertension. The cause of this development is unclear, but researchers believe it is related to systemic vasoconstriction secondary to general anesthesia and intraoperative hypothermia, severe pain, or transient renin secretion caused by the clamping of the aorta and manipulation of the kidney. This episode usually lasts no more than 48 hours, but it can be significant and may require medical intervention. Nurses must monitor the blood pressure frequently.

RENAL VEIN DISEASE

The primary process involving the renal vein is thrombosis. Obstruction in venous drainage increases interstitial pressure, which reduces renal function. Assessment findings of this condition include severe lumbar pain, renal enlargement, proteinuria, and hematuria. If the obstruction is bilateral, oliguria and azotemia will occur. Contributing factors include diabetic nephropathy, chronic glomerulonephritis, renal amyloidosis, collagen vascular disease, hypercoagulable states, pregnancy, use of oral contraceptives, and nephrotic syndrome.

Kidney survival depends, in large part, on the degree of collateral circulation development before the vessel was totally occluded. Embolectomy or ligation of the renal veins may be done, and anticoagulants may be prescribed. Intravenous streptokinase is used to lyse the occluding clot. If enough renal damage has occurred, nephrectomy is an option.

▼ CONGENITAL DISORDERS

Renal congenital anomalies usually refer to the number, position, form or size, and structure of the kidneys. There may be an abnormal blood supply, although malformations that significantly affect renal function are rare. Anomalies of the ureteropelvic junction usually obstruct at that point and result in hydronephrosis. Typically, this situation is diagnosed and treated during childhood.

▼ Congenital Anomalies Involving Kidney Number and Position

Renal agenesis indicates the absence of one or both kidneys. Having only one kidney presents no difficulty if it functions adequately. A client can live normally with one properly functioning kidney, as kidney donors aptly demonstrate. Bilateral agenesis, on the other hand, is fatal. In unilateral agenesis, the functioning kidney is at high risk for additional anomalies.

Supernumerary kidneys, the presence of more than two kidneys, is usually asymptomatic and is found during IVP. The extra ureter enters either the ipsilateral ureter or the bladder.

Ectopic, or malpositioned, kidneys are usually found in the pelvis, although thoracic kidneys have been documented. Problems associated with this anomaly include respiratory difficulties, pain from pressure on nerves or surrounding structures, and difficulty in childbirth. Occasionally one kidney may be across the midline so that both kidneys are on the same side. This condition usually remains undiscovered until infection or obstruction requires x-ray examination.

▼ Congenital Anomalies Involving Kidney Form and Size

Anomalies of kidney form and size include aplasia, hypoplasia, dysplasia, and horseshoe kidney. Aplastic kidneys are small and contracted and contain no functioning renal tissue. Renal hypoplasia produces miniature kidneys with some functioning tissue. Although clinically this condition may be completely asymptomatic, it may be the origin of hypertension and recurrent urinary tract infection.

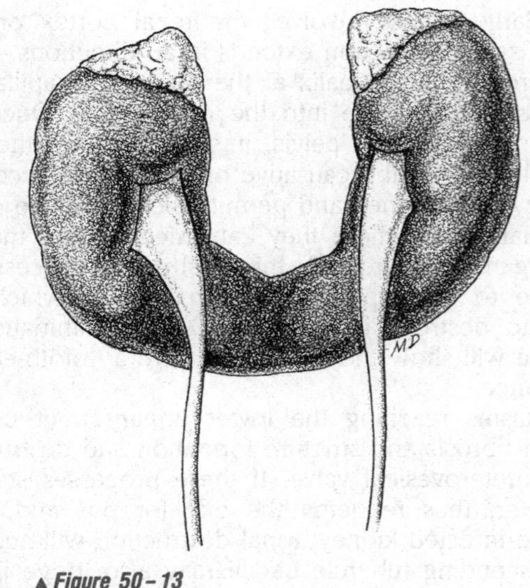

▲ Figure 50–13
Horseshoe kidney.

Horseshoe kidney results when two kidneys are joined into a single organ whose shape somewhat resembles a horseshoe (Fig. 50–13). The kidneys are connected, usually at the lower poles, by an isthmus of tissue. Because the developmental error interferes with normal ascent and medial rotation, the kidney is usually located in the lower lumbar region with its pelvis facing anteriorly. Although horseshoe kidney may be asymptomatic, it carries with it a predisposition to hydronephrosis and infection secondary to ureteropelvic junction obstruction and calculus formation.

▼ Congenital Anomalies Involving Cystic Disease

A congenitally abnormal kidney structure usually denotes the presence and progression of cysts within the renal tissue. This disorder ranges from a simple, solitary cyst to almost complete replacement of the functioning renal structures by cystic tissue. A simple renal cyst commonly originates superficially within the renal parenchyma. It is slow-growing and usually produces no symptoms until adulthood, when it may cause a heaviness and pain in the abdomen and may become a palpable mass. Diagnosis may be complicated because renal cysts closely resemble malignant tumors; differentiation between the two is vital. As long as a simple renal cyst remains asymptomatic, intervention usually is unnecessary. If needed, the cyst may be aspirated with a needle, or a partial nephrectomy to surgically remove the cyst may be performed.

POLYCYSTIC KIDNEYS

Polycystic disease of the kidney is a hereditary disorder in which grapelike cysts containing serous fluid, blood, or urine replace normal kidney tissue (Fig. 50-14). The condition may strike during childhood or adulthood. In infancy, the disease usually results in death within days, although in milder forms the disease will not appear until childhood. Infantile polycystic kidney disease is an autosomal recessive trait, requiring both parents to carry the gene. It is a very rare disorder that affects both kidneys and often the liver.[16] Adult polycystic disease has an incidence rate of 1 per 250 to 1 per 5000 and accounts for about 10 per cent of the clients receiving dialysis or transplantation. It is inherited as an autosomal dominant trait. It usually appears after 40 years of age, although it may begin as early as age 20 years or as late as age 80 years.

Adult polycystic disease displays diverse manifestations. The most common manifestations are dull, aching lumbar or flank pain, which may be colicky in nature, and hematuria. Other common urinary tract findings are proteinuria, palpable kidney masses, pyuria, calculi, and uremia. Early in the disease, the ability to concentrate urine decreases. Hypertension with resultant cardiac enlargement and heart failure are classic findings. Polycystic liver disease occurs in approximately one third of the cases, and cystic lesions are sometimes found in the thyroid, lung, pancreas, spleen, ovary, testis, epididymis, uterus, and bladder. Cerebral aneurysms occur in about 2 per cent of clients with polycystic kidney disease.[46]

The kidney can become so enlarged that it causes severe pressure on other organs, with production of additional extrarenal symptoms. The ultimate result of this disease is renal failure. As the disease slowly progresses, renal nephrons are destroyed, renal function deteriorates, and uremia ultimately results. The mean duration of polycystic kidney disease from the onset of symptoms to the development of uremia varies a great deal and may be 15 to 30 years or more. It is impossible to predict who of those carrying the gene will go on to develop end-stage renal disease.[16]

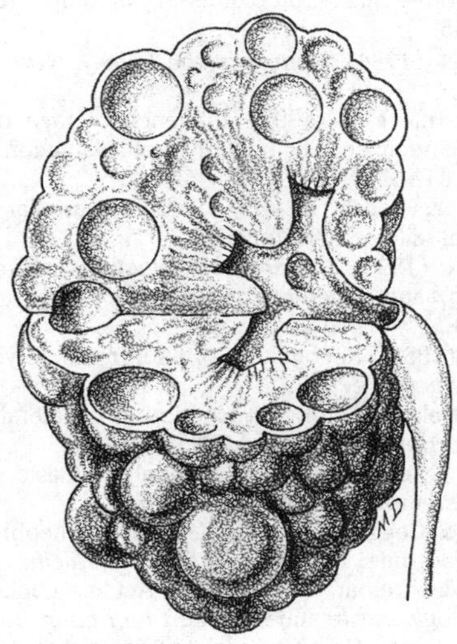

▲ **Figure 50-14**

Polycystic kidney disease.

There is no known way to arrest the progress of the destructive cysts, so conservative medical treatment deals with preserving kidney function. Urinary tract infection is the most common complication because of the distorted renal architecture, and chronic infection may occur because of the development of resistant bacteria. Aggressively controlling hypertension is essential.

Unlike clients with increasing creatinine clearance rates caused by other kidney diseases, those with polycystic kidney disease seem to waste rather than retain sodium. Thus, they need an increased sodium and water intake. Percutaneous cyst puncture may bring palliative relief of obstruction or aid in draining an abscess. Once end-stage renal disease develops, hemodialysis or renal transplantation may be used. Nursing interventions for clients with renal failure are discussed earlier.

Genetic counseling is advisable because of the hereditary nature of the disease. This is particularly recommended if the disease is diagnosed during the childbearing years. However, because the disease typically appears after the childbearing period, the likelihood of transmitting the disease to another generation is greatly increased. Therefore, counseling the extended family is essential once the disease has been identified.

ADULT-ONSET MEDULLARY CYSTIC DISEASE

This condition, sometimes called uremic sponge kidney or medullary polycystic disease, is also an autosomal dominant disorder. It is similar to polycystic disease in all aspects except that it progresses to uremia very rapidly after its onset in the second or third decade of life. Prognosis is poor, although hemodialysis and renal transplantation may be successful interventions.

MEDULLARY SPONGE KIDNEY

Medullary sponge kidney is a cystic disorder that produces spaces at the apex of the renal pyramids. Onset peaks during adolescence or between the ages of 30 and 40 years. Infection, calculi, pain, and hematuria are potential complications. However, renal function usually remains adequate unless the client develops uncontrolled infection or calculi.

▼ Other Hereditary Renal Disorders

Other hereditary renal disorders include chronic nephritis, congenital nephrotic syndrome, distal renal tubular acidosis, idiopathic hypercalciuria, and nephrotic diabetes insipidus. Many of these conditions are fatal during childhood, but some persist into adulthood and are discussed in the appropriate units of this text.

Summary

Renal disorders are highly complex diseases. The nurse must have a clear understanding of the structure and function of the renal system in order to care for clients with these conditions. Treatments for renal disease may require the client to undergo many lifestyle changes, and the teaching provided by the nurse can influence the success of the client's adaptation. Clients requiring renal transplantation may be critically ill and need complex nursing interventions, whereas those undergoing dialysis require more long-term management. It is important for the nurse to be able to work with clients whatever treatments they are receiving.

Bibliography

1. Abraham, P., & Smith, C. (1984). Medical evaluation and management of calcium nephrolithiasis. *Medical Clinics of North America, 68,* 281.
2. Adler, S. (1980). An approach to diagnosis and treatment of pyelonephritis. *Consultant, 20,* 207.
3. Almond, P. S., et al. (1992) Renal transplant function after ten years of cyclosporine. *Transplantation, 53*(2), 316–23.
4. Andress, D., et al. (1985). Effect of parathyroidectomy on bone aluminum accumulation in chronic renal failure. *New England Journal of Medicine, 312,* 468.
5. Andreucci, V. (1984). *Acute renal failure: Pathophysiology, prevention.* Boston: Martinus Nijhoff Publishing.
6. Baer, C. L., & Lancaster, L. E. (1992). Acute renal failure. *Critical Care Nursing Quarterly, 14*(4), 1–21.
7. Barry, J., (1983). Procurement and preservation of cadaver kidneys. *Urologic Clinics of North America, 10,* 205.
8. Bellomo, R., et al. (1991). Continuous arteriovenous haemodiafiltration in the critically ill: Influence on major nutrient balances. *Intensive Care Medicine, 17*(7), 399–402.
9. Berger, B., & Vincenti, F. (1984). Diabetic nephropathy: managing complications and using current therapy. *Consultant, 24,* 81.
10. Biggers, R. (1983). Renal carcinoma. *Hospital Medicine, 19,* 38.
11. Binkley, L. (1984). Keeping up with peritoneal dialysis. *American Journal of Nursing, 84,* 729.
12. Blaivas, J. G. (1990). Diagnostic evaluation of urinary incontinence. *Urology, 36*(Suppl 4), 11–20.
13. Branner, G., & Bush, W. (1984). Ultrasonic destruction of kidney stones. *Western Journal of Medicine, 140,* 227.
14. Braun, W. (1983). Histocompatibility testing in clinical renal transplantation. *Urologic Clinics of North America, 10,* 231.
15. Brenner, B. (1983). *Acute renal failure.* Philadelphia: W. B. Saunders.
16. Brenner, B. M., & Rector, F. C. (Eds.) (1990). *The kidney (4th ed.).* Philadelphia: W. B. Saunders.
17. Cecka, J. M., et al. (1992). Analyses of the UNOS Scientific Renal Transplant Registry at three years—early events affecting transplant success. *Transplantation, 53*(1), 59–64.
18. Cogan, M., & Garovoy, M. (1985). *Introduction to dialysis.* New York: Churchill-Livingstone.
19. Cohen, A., & Rosenstein, E. (1985). A nephropathy associated with disseminated tuberculosis. *Archives of Internal Medicine, 145,* 554.
20. Comty, C., & Collins, A. (1984). Dialytic therapy in the management of chronic renal failure. *Medical Clinics of North America, 68,* 399.
21. Cummings, N., & Klahr, S. (1985). *Chronic renal disease: Causes, complications, and treatment.* New York: Plenum Medical Book Co.
22. Dolleris, P. M. (1992). Diuretic and vasopressor usage in acute renal failure: A synopsis. *Critical Care Nursing Quarterly, 14*(4), 28–31.
23. Drach, G. W. (Ed.) (1986). New perspectives on management of upper and lower urinary tract infection. *Urology, 27*(Suppl 2), 2–30.
24. Dunn, M. (1984). Clinical effects of prostaglandins in renal disease. *Hospital Practice, 19,* 99.
25. Epstein, M. (1985). Aging and the kidney: clinical implications. *American Family Physician, 31,* 123.
26. Evans, R., et al. (1985). The quality of life of patients with end-stage renal disease. *New England Journal of Medicine, 312,* 553.
27. Ferrans, C., & Powers, M. (1985). The employment potential of hemodialysis patients. *Nursing Research, 34,* 273.
28. Fouque, D., et al. (1992). Controlled low protein diets in chronic renal insufficiency: A meta-analysis. *British Medical Journal, 304*(6821), 216–220.
29. Gjertson, D. W., & Terasaki, P. I. (1992). The large center variation in half-lives of kidney transplants. *Transplantation, 53*(2), 357–367.
30. Gleeson, M. J., & Griffith, D. P. (1990). Urinary diversion. *British Journal of Urology, 66*(2), 113–122.
31. Goldstein, M. (1982). The varieties of renal failure. *Emergency Medicine, 14,* 32.
32. Harris, J., et al. (1978). The kidney and pregnancy. *American Family Physician, 18,* 97.
33. Harter, H., & Goldberg, A. (1985). Endurance exercise training: an effective therapeutic modality for hemodialysis patients. *Medical Clinics of North America, 69,* 159.
34. Harter, H., & Martin, K. (1982). Acute renal failure: Classification evaluation and clinical consequences. *Postgraduate Medicine, 72,* 175.
35. Henrich, W., & Campbell, W. (1983). The systemic β-adrenergic pathway to renin secretion relationships with the renal prostaglandin system. *Endocrinology, 113,* 2247.
36. Herzog, A. R., & Fultz, N. H. (1990). Epidemiology of urinary incontinence: Prevalence, incidence, and correlates in community populations. *Urology, 36*(Suppl 4), 2–10.
37. Higashihara, E., et al. (1992). Clinical aspects of polycystic kidney disease. *Journal of Urology, 147*(2), 329–332.
38. Hill, M. N., et al. (1991). Changes in causes of death after renal transplantation, 1966 to 1987. *American Journal of Kidney Disease, 17*(5), 512–518.
39. Hirsch, D. (1985). Limited-protein diet: A means of delaying the progression of chronic renal disease? *Canadian Medical Association Journal, 132,* 913.
40. Hou, S. (1985). Pregnancy in women with chronic renal failure. *New England Journal of Medicine, 312,* 836.
41. Hricik, D. E., et al. (1992). Withdrawal of steroids after renal transplantation—clinical predictors of outcome. *Transplantation, 53*(1), 41–45.
42. Javadpour, N. (1984). *Cancer of the kidney.* New York: Thieme-Stratton.
43. Kerman, R. H., et al. (1992). Influence of race on crossmatch outcome and recipient eligibility for transplantation. *Transplantation, 53*(1), 64–67.
44. Kotler, M., & Segal, B. (1984). Cardiovascular problems in chronic renal failure. *Geriatrics, 39,* 69.
45. Krieger, J. N. (1990). Urinary tract infections in women: Causes, classification, and differential diagnosis. *Urology, 35*(Suppl 1), 4–7.
46. Kutcher, R. (1981). Recognition of adult renal polycystic disease. *Hospital Medicine, 17,* 37.
47. Liu, P. L., et al. (1992). Renal function in unilateral nephrectomy subjects. *Journal of Urology, 147*(2), 337–339.
48. MacKenzie, T., et al. (1985). Hemodialysis: Basic principles and practice. *Postgraduate Medicine, 77,* 95.
49. Maffey, R., & Coggins, C. (1985). Glomerulonephritis and acute nephrotic syndrome. *Scientific American Medicine, 8,* 1.
50. Mars, D., & Treloar, D. (1984). Acute tubular necrosis—pathophysiology and treatment. *Heart and Lung, 13,* 194.
51. Mitchell, J. (1980). Chronic renal failure in the elderly: What to look for when it starts. *Geriatrics, 35,* 28.
52. Moore, J., & Maher, J. (1984). Management of chronic renal failure. *American Family Physician, 30,* 204.

53. Morris, P. (1984). *Kidney transplantation: Principles and practice.* New York: Grune & Stratton.
54. Murphy, L., & Cole, M. (1983). Renal disease: nutritional implications. *Nursing Clinics of North America, 18,* 57.
55. Navarro, M., et al. (1991). Anemia of chronic renal failure: Treatment with erythropoietin. *Childhood Nephrology and Urology, 11*(3), 146-151.
56. Nicolaisen, G., et al. (1985). Renal trauma; re-evaluation of the indications for radiographic assessment. *Journal of Urology, 133,* 183.
57. Nolph, K. (1985). *Peritoneal dialysis.* Boston: Martinus Nijhoff Publishers.
58. Novick, A., et al. (1984). Revascularization to preserve renal function in patients with atherosclerotic renovascular disease. *Urologic Clinics of North America, 11,* 447.
59. Olsson, C. (1983). Ileal ureter and renal autotransplantation. *Urologic Clinics of North America, 10,* 685.
60. OTC analgesic abuse (1983). *American Family Physician, 27,* 196.
61. Pirsch, J. D., et al. (1992). The effect of donor age, recipient age, and HLA match on immunologic graft survival in cadaver renal transplant recipients. *Transplantation, 53*(1), 55-59.
62. Rao, K. (1984). Status of renal transplantation: A clinical perspective. *Medical Clinics of North America, 68,* 427.
63. Rehan, A. (1985). Hemodialysis emergencies. *Emergency Medicine, 17,* 138.
64. Ronald, A. (1984). Current concepts in the management of urinary tract infections in adults. *Medical Clinics of North America, 68,* 335.
65. Roth, D., et al. (1984). Nephroblastoma in adults. *Journal of Urology, 132,* 108.
66. Rubenstein, E. (Ed.) (1984). Evaluation of renal morphology. *Scientific American Medicine, 7,* 1.
67. Sanai, T., et al. (1991). Effect of different doses of aluminum hydroxide on renal deterioration and nutritional state in experimental chronic renal failure. *Mineral and Electrolyte Metabolism, 17*(3): 160-165.
68. Schulze, V. (1982). Rhabdomyolysis as a cause of acute renal failure. *Postgraduate Medicine, 72,* 145.
69. Sheinfeld, J., et al. (1985). Selective pre-transplant nephrectomy: Indications and perioperative management. *Journal of Urology, 133,* 379.
70. Shelter, M. (1984). Renal arteriogram and cystourethrogram. *RN, 47,* 89.
71. Sinnek, K., et al. (1984). Chronic renal failure: effect of hemodialysis on gastric hormones. *American Journal of Surgery, 148,* 732.
72. Slatopoisky, E., et al. (1986). Calcium carbonate as a phosphate binder in patients with chronic renal failure undergoing dialysis. *New England Journal of Medicine, 315,* 157.
73. Smith, A., & Lee, W. (1983). Percutaneous stone removal procedures including irrigation. *Urologic Clinics of North America, 10,* 719.
74. Smith, C. (1984). When should the stone patient be evaluated: Early evaluation of single stone formers. *Medical Clinics of North America, 68,* 455.
75. Smollens, P. (1984). Acute renal failure. *Hospital Medicine, 20,* 95.
76. Staff (1986). What is interstitial cystitis and what can be done about it? *American Journal of Nursing, 86*(1), 13-14.
77. Stark, J. (1982). Acute poststreptococcal glomerulonephritis. *Nursing 82, 12,* 114.
78. Stein, J. H. (1992). Acute renal failure: Lessons from pathophysiology. *Western Journal of Medicine, 156*(2), 176-182.
79. Stone, L. (1984). Percutaneous nephrolithotripsy. *AORN Journal, 39,* 773.
80. Trimarco, B., et al. (1985). Role of prostaglandins in the renal handling of a salt load in essential hypertension. *American Journal of Cardiology, 55,* 116.
81. Walsh, P. C., et al. (1986). Campbell's Urology (vol. 3, 5th ed.). Philadelphia: W. B. Saunders.
82. Watson, A., & Whelton, P. (1985). Acute renal failure: Key components of evaluation and therapy. *Consultant, 25,* 25.
83. Watson, A., et al. (1985). Nephrotic syndrome: An orderly approach can guide successful management. *Consultant, 25,* 59.
84. Webster, D. (1990). Comparing patients' and nurses' views of interstitial cystitis: A pilot study. *Urologic Nursing, 11,* 10-13.

Gastrointestinal Disorders

Unit 12

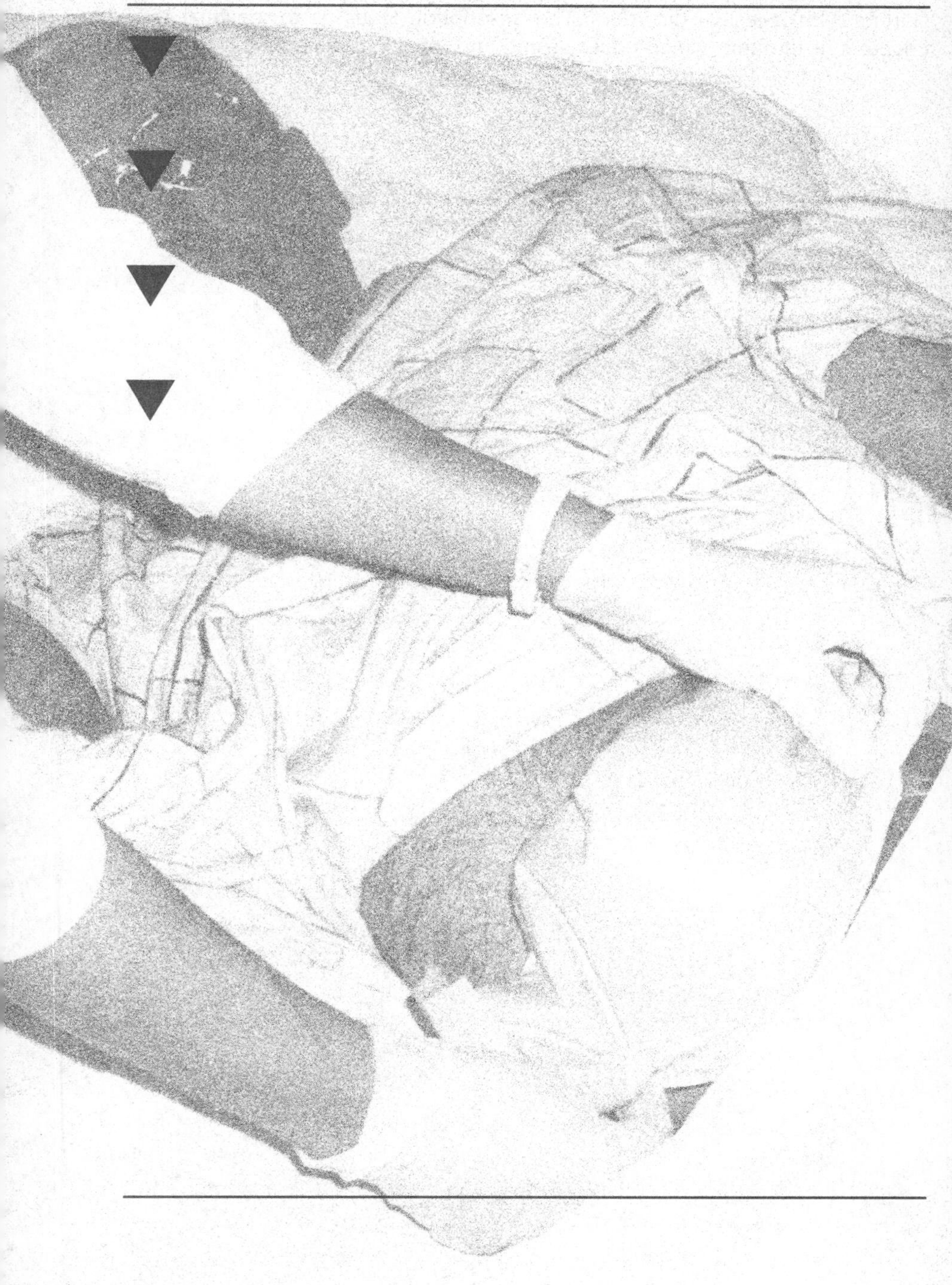

A functional gastrointestinal (GI) tract is necessary for health and, in most cases, for life itself. However, the GI system is subject to many disorders that can interfere with normal ingestion, absorption of nutrients, and the normal elimination of waste products produced by these processes.

This unit focuses on the nursing care of clients with GI disorders. It consists of five chapters. Chapter 51 discusses GI structure and function. Chapter 52 provides a basis for a thorough assessment of the GI tract. The major components of this chapter are the health history, the physical assessment of the GI tract, and an explanation of diagnostic tests used to assess GI function. Chapter 53 begins a description of GI tract disorders, starting with ingestive disorders. The description leads us to the final two chapters in the unit, which cover gastric and intestinal disorders.

Chapter 51

Structure and Function of the Gastrointestinal System

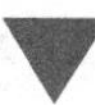

The gastrointestinal (GI) tract, also called the digestive tract or alimentary canal, is a hollow muscular tube that extends from the mouth to the anus (Fig. 51-1). Its principal function is to provide the body with fluid, nutrients, and electrolytes.

Normally, the GI tract is the source of intake for the body. Raw materials taken in through the mouth are metabolized for energy, tissue building, and so forth. The GI tract also disposes of the wastes from this digestive process.

ACTIVITIES OF THE TRACT

The four major activities of the GI tract are (1) secretion of electrolytes, hormones, and enzymes to be used in breakdown of the ingested materials; (2) movement of ingested products; (3) digestion of food and fluids; and (4) absorption of end products into the bloodstream.

Secretions

There are two general types of secretions in the GI tract: (1) mucous secretions, which are produced throughout the entire length of the tract; and (2) digestive secretions, which are produced in the mouth, stomach, duodenum, and jejunum. Mucous secretions protect and lubricate the walls of the tract. Digestive secretions (enzymes and electrolytes) break down ingested food so that it can be absorbed.

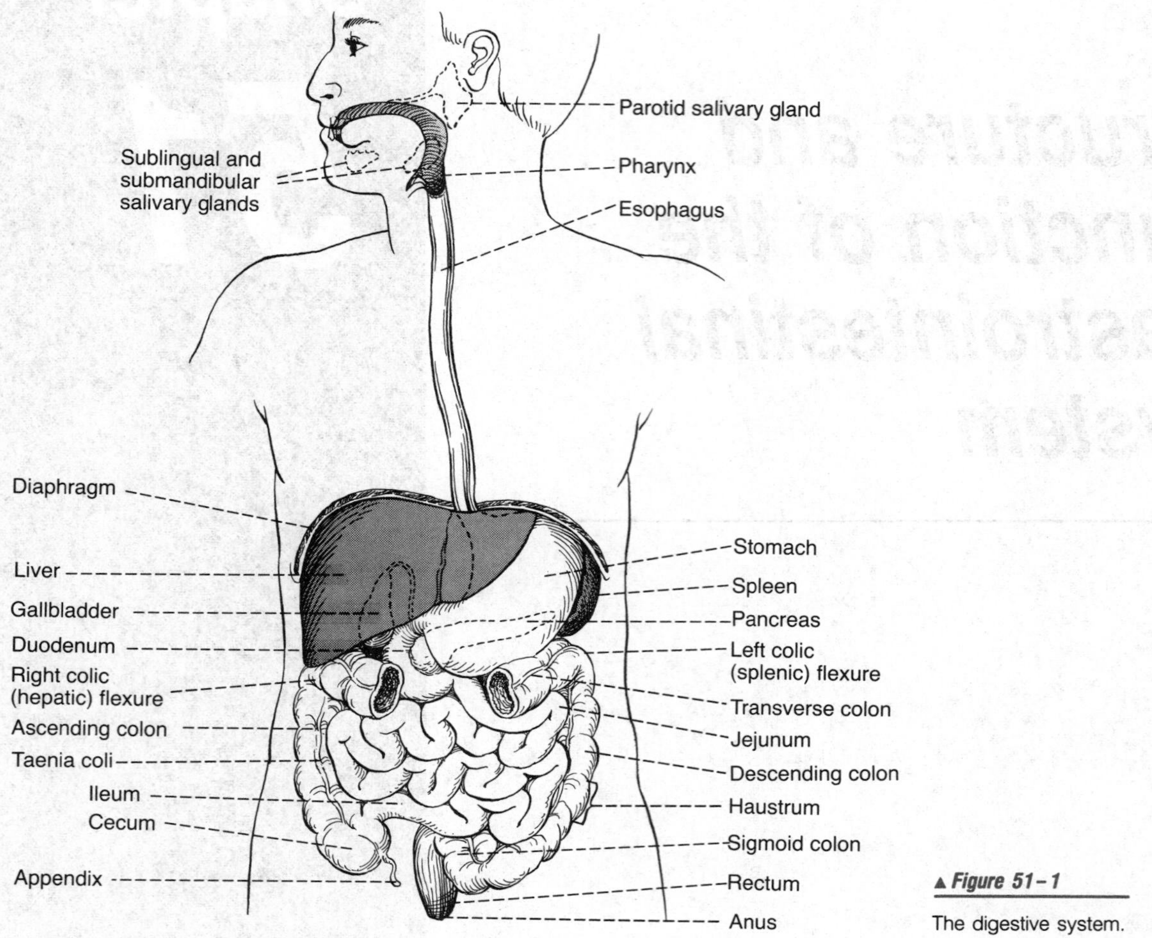

▲ *Figure 51-1*

The digestive system.

Motility

There are two types of movements in the GI tract, mixing and propulsive; both are produced by rhythmic contractions of the smooth muscle fibers that lie in the walls of the stomach and gut. These fibers vary somewhat from one segment of the tract to another. However, they usually consist of an outer longitudinal layer, an inner circular layer, and a thin layer in the deeper portion of the mucosa. See Figure 51-2 for a typical cross section of the gut.

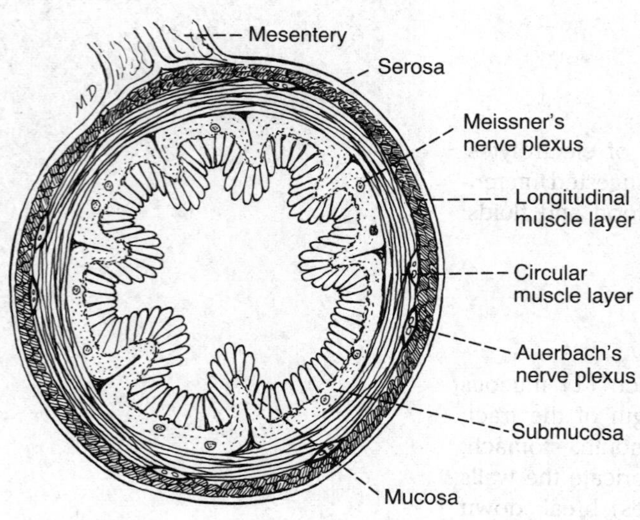

▲ *Figure 51-2*

Typical cross section of the GI tract.

Mixing movements, sometimes called segmentation contractions, are rhythmic contractions between individual segments of bowel that alternate with contractions occurring at the midpoint of each segment. Peristalsis is a wave of muscle contraction in the bowel wall that pushes the bolus of food ahead of it (Fig. 51-3). This type of movement occurs in all smooth muscle tubes of the body and can go in either direction from the point of stimulation. In the bowel, the waves usually move toward the anus.

Digestion and Absorption

During digestion, food is broken down into chemical compounds small and simple enough to be absorbed into the bloodstream by diffusion or active transport. The digestive process begins in the mouth.

THE MOUTH

Structure

The mouth (also called the oral or buccal cavity) is formed by the cheeks, the hard palate (anterior portion

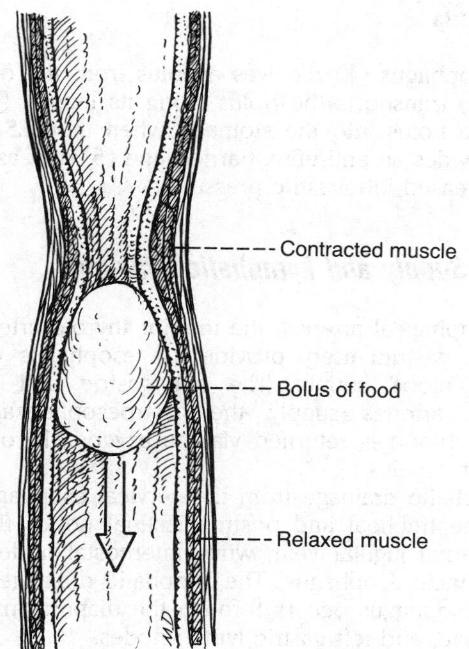

▲ *Figure 51-3*

Peristalsis moves food through the GI tract by pushing bolus ahead of a wave of muscle contraction.

of the roof of the mouth), the soft palate (posterior portion of the roof of the mouth), and the tongue. The lips are folds of flesh that surround the opening of the mouth.

Chewing and Its Functions

Chewing begins digestion by preparing food for swallowing. It is controlled by reflex activity via the fifth cranial nerve. Chewing is stimulated by the presence of food in the mouth.

The functions of chewing are

- To break food products into smaller portions
- To break down any fibrous coverings in order to allow digestive enzymes access to the food particles
- To prevent trauma to the mucous lining of the esophagus by making the food smoother

To preserve chewing capabilities, a person must maintain dental health. An individual exerts pressures ranging from 25 to 275 pounds during the chewing process, depending on the nature of the food and the teeth involved. Dentures are not as effective for chewing as natural teeth, and poorly chewed foods are not readily digested.

Saliva and Its Functions

Saliva is secreted by the sublingual and submandibular glands under the tongue and by the parotid glands near the ears, opposite the second molars.

Saliva lubricates and softens the food mass and dissolves the most soluble components of food, thus stimulating the taste buds. Saliva contains the enzyme ptyalin (amylase), which breaks down starches to maltose. The action of ptyalin continues in the fundus of the stomach, where food is mixed with gastric secretions.

Swallowing (Deglutition)

Food in the mouth, called a bolus, is swallowed in three phases: (1) the oral phase, (2) the involuntary pharyngeal phase, and (3) the esophageal phase.

The time it takes for the bolus to reach the stomach depends on the consistency of the bolus and the individual's body position. Fluids tend to arrive ahead of the peristaltic wave, and the more solid masses may arrive after it. The bolus travels faster when the individual is in a vertical position. Esophageal transport requires the coordination of peristalsis with relaxation of the lower esophageal sphincter (Fig. 51-4).

THE ESOPHAGUS

Structure

The esophagus, a hollow muscular tube, lies posterior to the trachea and larynx at the level of the sixth cervical vertebra. It extends vertically through the mediastinum and diaphragm to the level of the 11th thoracic vertebra. The esophagus connects the hypopharynx with the stomach and serves as a passage for food from mouth to stomach.

The esophageal wall consists of four layers: (1) mucosa, (2) submucosa, (3) muscularis, and (4) serosa. These four basic layers compose the entire GI tract, although slight modifications occur in different regions.

In the upper esophagus, the muscle is striated but acts like smooth muscle, contracting and relaxing as the bolus travels through the tube. The body of the esophagus is composed of smooth muscle that serves to propel food toward the stomach. The areolar layer connects the muscular and mucous layers and contains the blood and lymph vessels. The mucous layer in the proximal half of the esophagus contains glands that secrete mucus to lubricate the bolus. Mucus also protects the esophageal mucous membrane from trauma resulting from passage of partially chewed food products.

The body of the esophagus is composed of cervical and thoracic segments. At the proximal end is the upper esophageal sphincter (UES). The distal segment is composed of the ampulla and vestibule and includes the lower esophageal sphincter (LES). The LES is not a distinctive sphincter but a zone of increased pressure that provides a physiologic barrier to protect the esophageal mucosa from the effects of gastric reflux (the return or backflow of gastric secretions).

The pressure and competence of the LES is normally increased by gastrin and parasympathetic drugs. Substances such as secretin, cholecystokinin (CCK), anticholinergics, cigarettes, fatty foods, and alcohol decrease LES pressure.

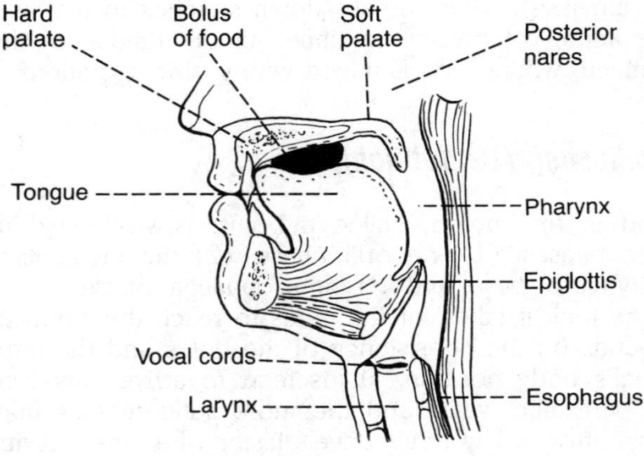

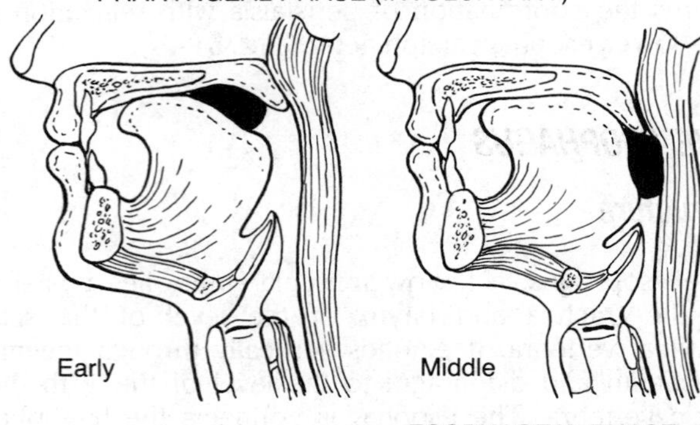

Late

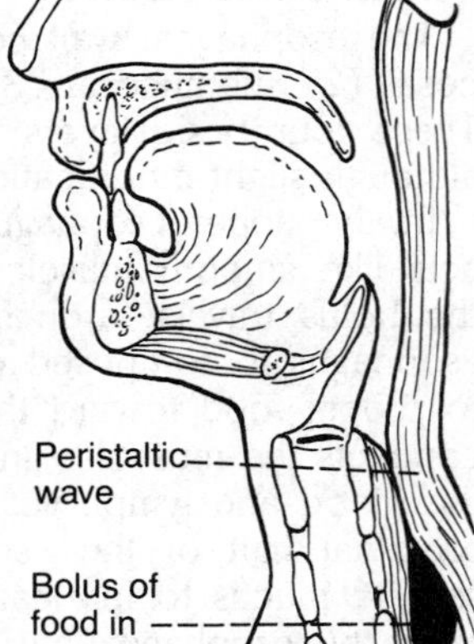

▲ **Figure 51-4**

Swallowing occurs in three phases: (1) Voluntary or oral phase. Tongue presses food against hard palate, forcing it toward pharynx. (2) Involuntary, pharyngeal phase. Early: wave of peristalsis forces bolus between tonsillar pillars. Middle: soft palate draws upward to close posterior nares, and respirations cease momentarily. Late: vocal cords approximate and larynx pulls upward, covering airway and stretching esophagus open. (3) Involuntary, esophageal phase. Relaxation of upper esophageal (hypopharyngeal) sphincter allows peristaltic wave to move bolus down esophagus.

Decreased sphincter pressure can cause gastric reflux, resulting in epigastric pain and indigestion. On the other hand, increased pressure can be manifested as dysphagia (difficulty swallowing).

Functions

The esophagus (1) receives a bolus from the oropharynx, (2) transports the bolus along its length, (3) propels the bolus into the stomach when the LES opens, (4) provides an antireflux barrier, and (5) acts as a vent for increased intragastric pressure.

Blood Supply and Lymphatic Drainage

The esophageal arteries, the inferior thyroid artery, and the left gastric artery provide the esophagus with its arterial blood supply. The left gastric and inferior phrenic arteries supply the gastroesophageal area. Venous blood is returned via the azygos, thyroid, and left gastric veins.

Lymphatic drainage from the cervical esophagus and from the tracheal and postmediastinal nodes flows to the internal jugular vein, while intercostal nodes drain the thoracic esophagus. The lymphatic drainage of the lower esophagus occurs through the diaphragmatic, intracardiac, and left gastric lymph nodes.

Innervation

Both the sympathetic and parasympathetic fibers of the autonomic nervous system provide innervation to the esophagus. The sympathetic fibers emanate from cervical and thoracic ganglia and from preganglionic fibers of the greater and lesser splanchnic nerves. Parasympathetic innervation from the vagus nerve extends along the anterior and posterior esophageal walls. Both sympathetic and parasympathetic stimuli are received by the LES.

Motor Activity

Peristaltic waves are an involuntary reflex of the glossopharyngeal nerves stimulated by the act of swallowing. Secondary stimulation of peristalsis occurs with dilatation of the lower half of the esophagus and is probably reflex in origin.

THE STOMACH

Structure

The stomach is located in the upper portion of the abdomen, to the left of the midline. The lower esophageal, or cardiac, sphincter divides the esophagus and stomach, which, on contraction, closes the stomach off from the esophagus. The stomach has a capacity of approximately 1500 ml and has three anatomic divisions (Fig. 51-5):

1. The fundus, which lies above and to the left of the cardiac sphincter.
2. The body or central area.
3. The lower area, called the antrum or pyloric region.

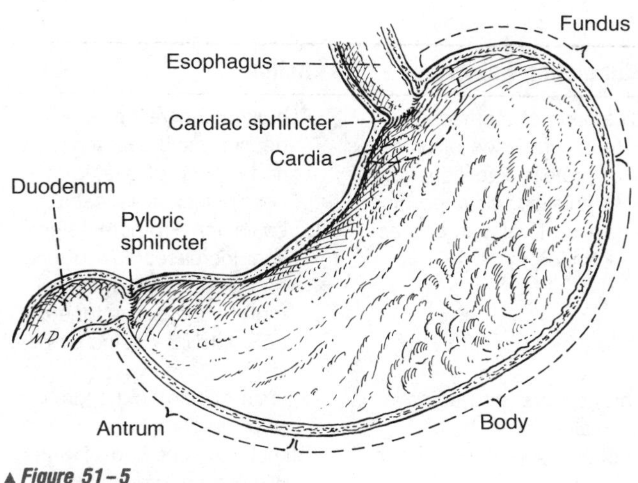

▲ **Figure 51-5**

Anatomy of the stomach.

The outlet from the distal end of the stomach and the duodenum is called the pyloric sphincter. It permits the flow of chyme from the stomach.

The stomach wall has four layers: (1) serosa, (2) muscularis, (3) submucosa, and (4) mucosa. The serosal outer layer is the visceral peritoneum. The muscular layers (tunica muscularis) produce peristaltic activity of the stomach as it churns food during digestion. The submucosa (or tela submucosa) connects the muscular and mucous layers of the stomach wall and contains the blood, lymph channels, and nerve plexus.

The epithelial lining of the stomach contains many microscopic glands:

- Cardiac glands secrete mucus.
- Peptic (chief) cells secrete mucus and pepsinogen. Pepsinogen is converted to pepsin, a proteolytic enzyme.
- Parietal (oxyntic) cells secrete hydrochloric acid and water. The parietal cells are stimulated by gastrin to produce hydrochloric acid, which helps digestion of protein. These cells also produce the intrinsic factor that allows vitamin B_{12} to be absorbed.
- Neck cells secrete mucus.
- Pyloric glands secrete gastrin and mucus.

Functions

The functions of the stomach include storage, mixing, liquefaction of the bolus of food into chyme, and control of passage of food into the duodenum. The first stage of protein breakdown occurs in the stomach. The major portion of the mechanical breakdown of food occurs in the antrum (Fig. 51-5). At the distal end of the stomach, the pyloric sphincter permits the flow of chyme from the stomach into the duodenum. Digestion of starches, which begins in the mouth by the action of ptyalin, continues in the stomach. Digestion can last for as long as 30 minutes, or until the mixing function of the stomach allows its acid contents to inactivate the ptyalin. Digestion of fats in the stomach is minimal. Small quantities of water, alcohol, glucose, and some drugs may be absorbed through the gastric mucosa. Most organisms are destroyed by the acidic gastric juice.

Blood Supply

The stomach's arterial blood supply is from the celiac artery, which branches off the lesser and greater curvatures. Gastric arteries, from the splenic artery, supply the fundus. The portal vein provides the venous drainage of the stomach. The right and left gastroepiploic veins drain the greater curvature, while the right gastric and coronary veins drain the lesser curvatures. Lymph nodes of the stomach arise in the submucosa and drain into the thoracic duct.

Innervation

The stomach is innervated by both the sympathetic and parasympathetic systems. The vagus nerve supplies parasympathetic innervation. When stimulated, the vagus nerve causes (1) increased gastric secretion of acid, gastrin, and pepsin; and (2) increased gastric motor activity.

The greater splanchnic nerves and the celiac ganglia supply the sympathetic innervation. The sympathetic nerves inhibit gastric secretion and motility. They are stimulated by muscle contraction, distention, and inflammation.

Auerbach's plexus (motor function) and Meissner's plexus (sensory function) lie within the gastric wall. These nerve plexuses provide intrinsic innervation for the stomach. Both begin in the esophageal wall and extend the length of the gut. Auerbach's plexus lies between the longitudinal and circular muscle layers; Meissner's plexus is in the submucosa.

Stimulation of Auerbach's plexus generates gastric motility, increasing the intensity and rate of contractions and the release of gastrin from the antrum. Meissner's plexus functions with Auerbach's plexus to coordinate the motor and secretory activity of the gastric mucosa.

Secretion

The stomach secretes 1500 to 3000 ml of gastric juice per day. Its major secretions are hydrochloric acid, pepsin, and mucus. Gastric juice contains mucin, intrinsic factor, lipase, pepsinogen, and protein. Gastric acid secretion is directly stimulated by distention of the stomach and the presence of protein. Gastric acid secretion is also stimulated by vagal activity, acetylcholine, histamine, and the hormone gastrin (Table 51-1). Gastrin is released when the stomach becomes distended with food.

Hydrochloric acid and pepsin provide the corrosive power of gastric secretions. Pepsin is the most active factor in the digestive process of the stomach, acting to break down proteins to polypeptides, proteases, and

TABLE 51–1. Digestive Hormones

Hormone	Source	Stimulating Factors	Action
Gastrin	C cells of gastric antrum; duodenal mucosa	Distention of stomach by food, presence of products of protein digestion, vagal stimulation, elevated blood levels of calcium and epinephrine	Stimulates secretion of HCl, pepsin, pancreatic enzyme, and growth of gastric mucosa. Relaxes ileocecal sphincter. Promotes digestion. Increases flow of bile and gastric and intestinal motility. Increases tone of LES. Inhibits gastric emptying
Enterogastrone	Duodenal mucosa	Fats, sugars, and acids in small intestine	Inhibits gastric acid secretion and motility
Secretin	Duodenal mucosa	Fats and sugars in small intestine	Stimulates secretion of watery alkaline pancreatic fluid; augments CCK; decreases gastric acid secretion; stimulates secretion of pancreatic digestive enzymes and bile from liver; stimulates pepsinogen release
Cholecystokinin (CCK)	Duodenal and jejunal mucosa	Products of fat digestion in duodenum	Augments secretin in stimulating secretion of alkaline pancreatic juice and digestive enzymes; stimulates gallbladder contraction; inhibits gastric emptying; stimulates pepsin secretion; stimulates motility of small bowel
Gastric inhibitory peptide (GIP)	Duodenal and jejunal mucosa	Presence of glucose, fat, and amino acid in duodenum	Inhibits gastric acid and pepsin secretion and gut motility; stimulates secretion of intestinal juice and insulin
Vasoactive intestinal peptide (VIP) (structurally related to secretin)	Intestinal mucosa, central nervous system, genitourinary system	None known	Stimulates insulin release, pancreatic enzyme secretion, and intestinal secretion of electrolytes and water; inhibits gastric acid secretion; dilates peripheral blood vessels and lowers blood pressure
Motilin	Small intestine, especially duodenum and upper jejunum	None known	Diminishes speed of gastric emptying and stimulates gastric acid secretion and pepsin; stimulates bicarbonate secretion of pancreas
Somatostatin	Hypothalamus and pineal gland, stomach, intestine (duodenum), Auerbach's plexus, pancreas	Secretin, CCK, glucagon; acid in duodenum	Inhibits secretion of gastrin, VIP, GIP, secretin, and motilin; inhibits gastric duodenal, gallbladder motility, and intestinal motility, and intestinal Na^+ and Cl^- absorption
			Inhibits gastric acid, pancreatic enzyme, and bicarbonate secretion, and intestinal motility

peptones (Table 51-2). Peptic activity is greatest at pH levels less than 3.5. Pepsin is stimulated by food, whereas mucus has a neutralizing effect, which protects the stomach mucosa.

The three phases of gastric secretion are cephalic, gastric, and intestinal.

- The cephalic (nervous) phase of digestion is dependent on stimulation of gastric secretions by receptors in the brain that are mediated by the vagus nerve. This phase is stimulated by hunger and by the odors, sight, smell, thought, and discussion of food. The cephalic phase results in secretion of acid, pepsin, and mucus.
- The gastric (hormonal) phase of secretion occurs when the bolus of food reaches the antrum. This phase consists of three mechanisms. When the food enters the stomach, the long vagovagal reflex, local enteric reflexes, and gastrin mechanisms are excited. These mechanisms lead to the secretion of gastric juice. This phase continues for several hours, until the acidity of the gastric contents reaches 1.5 or less.
- The intestinal phase includes both nervous and hormonal mechanisms. This phase is stimulated by food entering the duodenum, resulting in the secretion of a small amount of gastrin by the intestine. This process, in turn, stimulates gastric secretion of pepsin and mucus. The duodenal pH then decreases, resulting in the release of secretin, which inhibits gastric secretion and slows gastric emptying.

INHIBITION OF GASTRIC SECRETIONS

Gastric secretions are decreased by (1) vagal stimulation, (2) increased osmolality of food, (3) fat, (4) enterogastrone, (5) alterations in blood flow, and (6) inflammation, such as gastritis. Decreased gastric secretion also results from a duodenal acid pH of 1.5 or less and an antrum pH of 3.0, both of which block the release of gastrin.

In addition, hormonal mechanisms in the small bowel may inhibit gastric secretion. The presence of acid, fat, and protein breakdown products, or any irritating factor, in the duodenum causes the release of secretin and CCK. These substances are especially important for control of pancreatic secretion, and CCK promotes emptying of the gallbladder. The release of these substances inhibits gastric secretion of the parietal cells and the stomach's motor activity. Also, they decrease gastric emptying, inhibit peptic digestion, and facilitate pancreatic enzyme activity. Stimulation of the duodenum—by distention, or the presence of acid, hypotonic or hypertonic substances, carbohydrates, fats, or protein products—causes the enterogastric vagus reflex arc to slow gastric motility and secretions. Digestive hormones and enzymes are listed in Tables 51-1 and 51-2.

Motor Activity

The stomach empties slowly, accommodating itself to the ability of the duodenum to receive and act on the contents. Tonic contraction of the stomach musculature causes the pressure within it to remain almost constant, whether it is empty or full. Mixing of chyme and emptying of the stomach occur by means of slow, mild, rhythmic peristaltic waves that begin about every 30 seconds at the fundus and continue over the antrum to

TABLE 51-2. Digestive Enzymes

Enzyme	Source	Action and Products
Carbohydrates		
Pytalin (salivary amylase)	Parotid and submaxillary glands	Break starch into maltose and limit dextrins (polysaccharides into disaccharides)†
Pancreatic amylase (more potent than ptyalin)	Pancreas	Break starch into maltose and limit dextrins (polysaccharides into disaccharides)†
Maltase*	Intestinal mucosa	Breaks maltose into glucose
Dextrinase	Intestinal mucosa	Breaks alpha limit dextrins into glucose†
Lactase*	Intestinal mucosa	Breaks lactose into galactose and glucose
Sucrase*	Intestinal mucosa	Breaks sucrose into glucose and fructose
Proteins		
Pepsin I, II, III	Chief cells of gastric mucosa	Breaks dietary proteins into polypeptides of various sizes
Enterokinase	Duodenal mucosa	Activates trypsin
Trypsin	Pancreas	Splits polypeptide chains
Peptidases* (several)	Intestinal glands	Splits polypeptides into amino acids
Fats		
Gastric lipase (tributyrase)	Gastric mucosa	Digests butter fat
Pancreatic lipase	Pancreas	Splits emulsified fats into monoglycerides
Intestinal lipase*	Intestines	Splits neutral fats into glycerol and fatty acids

* Secreted mainly in brush border of epithelial cells; digests food substances on outside surfaces of microvilli before or during absorption through epithelium.

† Small polymers present when starch is broken down.

the pylorus. The rugae of the stomach walls also contribute to the mixing of chyme.

As chyme is ready to be discharged through the pyloric sphincter into the duodenum, pressure builds up within the pylorus. The pyloric sphincter opens, allowing chyme to pass through. The sphincter then closes to prevent backflow. This process is repeated until all the food in the stomach is emptied into the duodenum. The pressure and rate of emptying are affected by viscosity, volume, physical state, osmotic activity, acidity of the food, and receptivity of the small bowel, as well as by exercise, drugs, emotions, pain, position, and other chemical and mechanical factors. The enterogastric reflex and enterogastrone (the hormone secreted by the small bowel) both act to inhibit the emptying of the stomach.

The greater the acidity and caloric density, and the more the osmolarity varies from that of body fluids, the more slowly the stomach empties. Fats move more slowly than any other dietary constituents.

THE SMALL INTESTINE

Structure

The small intestine is about 22 ft long and about 1 inch in diameter. It is divided into three segments:

1. The duodenum, which begins at the pyloric valve of the stomach and extends about 25 cm (10 inches) until it joins the jejunum.
2. The jejunum, 2.5 m (8 ft) long, which is the middle section of the small intestine and extends to the ileum.
3. The ileum, 3.6 m (12 ft) long, which is the terminal section. The ileum joins the colon at the ileocecal valve. This valve controls the flow into the large intestine and prevents reflux into the small intestine.

Four coats cover the small intestine: (1) the outer serous layer (tunica serosa), (2) muscular layer (tunica muscularis), (3) submucous layer (tela submucosa), and (4) inner mucous layer (tunica mucosa) (Fig. 51-6).

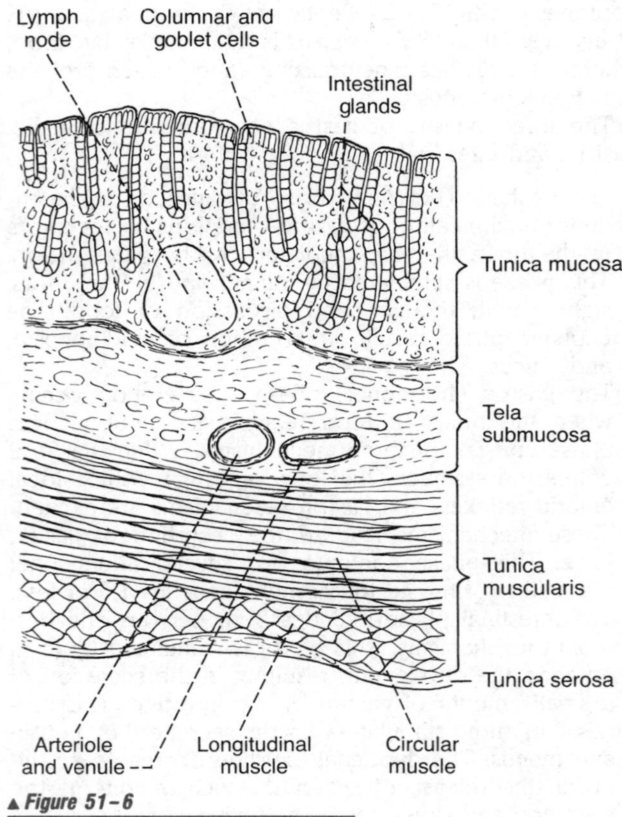

▲ **Figure 51-6**

Cross section of wall of small intestine.

The tunica serosa of the small intestine constitutes the peritoneum. This serous membrane lines the walls of the abdominal and pelvic cavities. The tunica muscularis is subdivided into the outer longitudinal and inner circular muscle layers. The tela submucosa contains blood vessels, lymphatics, Meissner's nerve plexus, and Brunner's glands (in the duodenum), which secrete mucus. Glands in the tunica mucosa also secrete mucus. The mucous and submucous layers are arranged in folds that provide a surface for secretion, digestion, and absorption.

The circular folds of the mucosa and submucosa are large and permanent. The villi, small, finger-like projections, are in continuous motion, stirring the intestinal contents. The villi are composed of columnar cells under which lie blood capillaries and a lymph channel called a lacteal. Digested food is absorbed from the villi. Fats are absorbed from the lacteals. The microvilli are microscopic processes on the surface of the epithelial cells. Together, these structures increase the surface area of the small intestine 600-fold, enlarging its total surface area to equal approximately 250 m^2, the size of a tennis court! This area is also known as the brush border.

Solitary and aggregated lymph nodes (Peyer's patches) are present in the small intestinal mucosa. Solitary nodes are small and connect directly with lymph vessels in deeper tissues. The aggregated lymph nodes occur mainly in the ileum.

Functions

The small intestine (1) completes digestion of foods, (2) absorbs the products of digestion, and (3) secretes hormones that help control the secretion of bile, pancreatic juice, and intestinal secretions. The residues are then moved on into the large intestine.

Blood Supply

Except in the duodenum, arterial blood supply to the small intestine is derived from the superior mesenteric artery. Arterial blood from the hepatic artery supplies the duodenum. Venous drainage is via the superior mesenteric vein, which unites with the inferior mesenteric, splenic, and gastric veins and then empties into the portal system.

Innervation

Stimulation of the sympathetic system inhibits the motility of the small intestine. Stimulation of the parasympathetic system increases intestinal tone and motility. The nerve supply to the small intestine passes through Auerbach's plexus within the intestinal wall. As within the other sections of the GI tract, the sensory fibers of the sympathetic system carry pain, whereas those of the parasympathetic system regulate intestinal activity.

Secretion

Hormonal secretion in the small intestine helps control bile, pancreatic juice, and intestinal secretions. The duodenal (Brunner's) glands are stimulated by glucagon and duodenal mucosa. These glands produce and release mucus not only in response to intestinal hormones but also in the presence of chyme and vagal stimulation. Sympathetic stimulation inhibits the secretion of mucus by Brunner's glands, which may explain the high incidence of peptic ulcers in this area of the GI tract. The goblet cells of the intestinal mucosa also secrete mucus.

The crypts of Lieberkühn are small pits that line the entire surface of the small intestine. These cells secrete about 2 liters per day of clear, yellowish, almost pure extracellular fluid with a slightly alkaline pH of 7.5 to 8.0. This fluid is absorbed rapidly by the villi. The epithelial cells of the mucosa covering the villi contain digestive enzymes. The enzymes found in the small intestine include (1) enterokinase, which activates trypsin; (2) maltase, lactase, and sucrase, which change disaccharides into simple sugars; and (3) nuclease, which facilitates hydrolysis of nuclein and nucleic acids. Other enzymes that hydrolyze peptides also are present.

In addition to the secretions from the small intestine, the pancreas secretes enzymes, bicarbonate, and water into the duodenum, which acts on chyme to digest substrates. Pancreatic secretion depends on the action of two duodenal hormones, secretin and CCK.

Secretin stimulates secretion of watery alkaline pancreatic fluid and also augments CCK. CCK stimulates bile secretion from the gallbladder. The gallbladder serves as a reservoir for bile after its manufacture in and secretion from the liver. Bile secretion from the liver is stimulated by vagal stimulation, secretin, increased liver blood flow, and high levels of bile salts in the blood. Bile aids fat digestion (see Chap. 56).

Flora

The small intestine flora are predominantly gram-positive lactobacilli, streptococci, and staphylococci. *Aerobacter aerogenes, Bacteroides, Candida albicans, Escherichia coli, Proteus, Pseudomonas,* and *Streptococcus faecalis* are also found. Bile acids and gastric acid may inhibit bacterial proliferation in the intestine.

Absorption

During the process of digestion and the preparation of end products for absorption, the following transformations occur in the small intestine:

- Carbohydrates are changed to monosaccharides and a few disaccharides. Carbohydrate digestion takes place primarily in the jejunum.
- Proteins are changed to amino acids and a minute quantity of dipeptides.
- Fats are changed to fatty acids, monoglycerides, diglycerides, and a few triglycerides.

The end products of digestion are absorbed along with water and electrolytes by diffusion and by active transport. Carbohydrates and proteins are absorbed by active transport along with sodium in a mutually dependent relationship in which neither material is transported without the other. Fatty acids are absorbed by diffusion, whereas most of the electrolytes are absorbed actively. Water diffuses by osmosis as a result of these other transport systems. Diffusion, active transport, and osmosis are discussed in Chapter 14.

Absorption of up to 8 liters of fluid daily occurs in the small intestine. Glucose, water-soluble vitamins, protein, and fat are absorbed primarily in the jejunum. The ileum acts mainly as a reserve to absorb these substances, and it is also the site of bile salt absorption. The duodenum and ileum share the function of active sodium transport. Vitamin B_{12} absorption takes place in the ileum, provided the stomach has secreted intrinsic factor and calcium ions are present. Iron absorption occurs in the duodenum and jejunum.

Digestion and absorption in the small bowel are very efficient. The chyme obtained from the terminal ileum contains no digestible carbohydrates, very few lipids, and only 15 to 17 per cent nitrogen-containing substances, most of which are bacterial or desquamated epithelial cells and the remains of digestive secretions. Generally, only 500 to 1000 ml of fluid passes into the large intestine.

Motor Activity

The motility of the small intestine is a result of the autorhythmicity of the smooth muscle, the intrinsic nerve impulses, and the hormonal effects of intestinal secretions. The chyme normally moves forward at an average rate of about 1 to 2 cm per minute, and remains in the small intestine for 3 to 10 hours.

As in other parts of the GI tract, the principal movements of the small intestine are (1) peristalsis and (2) mixing (or segmental) contractions. Although movements are divided into two categories, each type of contraction results in both mixing and propulsive activity.

Peristalsis or propulsive activity waves propel the chyme through the tract. Rhythmic segmental peristaltic waves are circular contractions that occur in the jejunum, resulting in mixing and absorption.

Peristalsis occurs by reflex as a result of mucosal stretching of the longitudinal and circular muscle layers when the chyme enters a segment of the intestine. Serotonin, produced by the intestinal glands, and acetylcholine cause contraction of the longitudinal muscle. Contraction of the circular muscle occurs through Meissner's plexus, and motor stimulation through Auerbach's plexus. This activity results in emptying of the intestinal segment.

A peristaltic rush is a powerful peristaltic wave that begins in the duodenum and passes to the ileocecal valve in a few minutes. Its purpose is to relieve the intestine of an irritating substance. A peristaltic rush can be caused by any intense chemical or mechanical irritation or by extreme distention.

Mixing movements consist of the alternate contraction of circular muscle fibers. They bring the chyme into close contact with (1) the glands and secretions involved with digestion and (2) the villi for absorption.

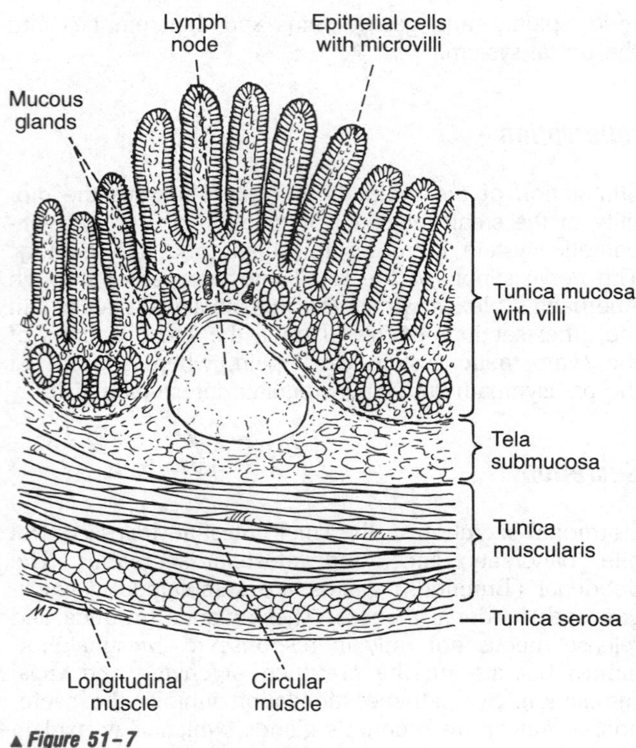

▲ *Figure 51-7*

Cross section of wall of large intestine.

THE LARGE INTESTINE

Structure

The large intestine, extending from the ileocecal valve to the anus, is approximately 5 to 6 ft long and 2 inches in diameter. It is divided into three segments: (1) cecum, (2) colon, and (3) rectum. Note in Figure 51-1 that these parts are not separated by valves or sphincters.

An outer serous layer (tunica serosa) covers the large intestine (Fig. 51-7). The muscular layer (tunica muscularis) is divided into an outer layer of longitudinal muscles and an inner layer of circular muscles. The longitudinal muscles are broken up into bands called taeniae coli. These bands run the length of the large intestine but are shorter than the intestine, causing the colon to pucker, thereby forming sacs or pouches called haustra. The submucous areolar layer (tela submucosa) contains arteries, veins, and lymphatic vessels, and it secretes mucus. This layer connects the muscular layer to the inner mucous layer.

The Cecum. The cecum comprises the first 2 to 3 inches of the large intestine. It connects with the ileum at the ileocecal valve. Relaxation of the cecum allows ileal contents to enter the cecum. The distal end of the cecum forms a blind pouch to which is attached the vermiform appendix. The appendix is located in the lower right quadrant of the abdomen (see Fig. 51-1).

The Colon. The colon is divided into four sections: (1) ascending, (2) transverse, (3) descending, and (4) sigmoid colon. The ascending colon lies just above the ileocecal valve. It continues up the right side of the abdomen to the lower border of the liver, where the section known as the hepatic flexure bends to the left. Extending horizontally from the liver across the abdomen is the transverse portion of the colon. At the spleen, the splenic flexure bends downward. Extending from the spleen down the left side of the abdomen is the descending colon. The S-shaped turn, the sigmoid colon, lies within the pelvis.

Anatomically the colon is larger in diameter than the small bowel and does not contain villi. The only significant secretion is mucus.

The major functions of the colon are to (1) absorb the remaining water, urea, and electrolytes (sodium and chloride); (2) secrete mucus in the proximal half, and (3) store the feces in the distal half until defecation.

Rectum and Anus. The final segments of the large intestine, the rectum and the anus, extend from the sigmoid colon to the anus. Two sphincter muscles (internal and external) control the opening of the anus.

The distal portion of the rectal walls form longitudinal folds, called rectal or anal columns. These folds terminate about $\frac{1}{2}$ inch from the anus and are connected to each other by transverse folds of tissue called valves. Pockets formed by the valves are called sinuses or crypts. Because the external portion of the anal opening is lined with skin that changes at this point to mucosa, this area is sometimes designated as the mucocutaneous border.

The venous drainage and nerve supply also change at this point. Above this line, venous drainage is into the portal system. Below this line, drainage is into the vena cava. The autonomic nervous system supplies innervation above the line, and the somatic nervous system supplies innervation below it.

The anal canal is about 1 inch long. At the level of the crypts lies the dentate or pectinate line. This important landmark divides the (1) squamous epithelium (below) and columnar epithelium (above), and (2) somatic nerve supply (below) and autonomic supply (above). The line also marks the division between internal and external hemorrhoids. Lymphatic drainage below the pectinate line goes largely to the inguinal nodes, while lymphatic drainage above this line goes to the pararectal and lateral pelvic (obturator) plexuses.

Functions

The major functions of the large intestine are to

- Complete absorption of water, chloride, and sodium;
- Reduce the volume of chyme;
- Manufacture vitamins, including some B vitamins and K;
- Form feces;
- Expel feces from the body.

Blood Supply

The cecum and colon receive their arterial blood supply from branches of the superior and inferior mesenteric arteries. The rectum and anal canal receive arterial blood from the superior, middle, and inferior rectal arteries. The superior and inferior mesenteric veins carry venous blood from the large intestine to the hepatic portal vein and then to the liver.

Innervation

The intramural nerve plexuses that lie within the layers of the bowel wall are responsible for nervous stimulation of the large intestine. Recall that these are known as Auerbach's and Meissner's plexuses. These nerves maintain the continuous tone of the bowel and also stimulate movements.

The plexuses are stimulated by the parasympathetic nervous system and, in general, cause an increase in tone of the gut, a decrease in tone of the sphincters, and an increase in frequency, volume, and velocity of contractions. The cranial division of the parasympathetic nervous system mediates impulses via the vagus nerve from the esophagus to the proximal colon. The distance from the midcolon to the anus is controlled by the sacral division of the parasympathetic nervous system.

Sympathetic innervation comes via nerve fibers that leave the spinal cord between T8 and L3. The nerve impulses then pass through ganglia, such as the celiac and mesenteric, and spread to all parts of the gut. In general, they reduce peristaltic activity and increase the tone of sphincters. Sympathetic effects on the bowel are minimal; this is known because denervation has only short-term effects.

Motor Activity

As food passes through the ileocecal valve, it accumulates in the proximal haustrum of the ascending colon. When the haustrum is completely distended, the walls contract and squeeze the contents into the next haustrum. This process continues, thereby moving the food through the colon. This movement is called haustral churning.

Mass peristalsis involves slow, forceful waves that occur when the bowel is evacuated. Mass peristalsis occurs two or three times a day and is stimulated by the gastrocolic reflex. Distention of a segment of the bowel or any irritation of the bowel mucosa may initiate a peristaltic wave.

Secretion

The mucosa of the large bowel contains the crypts of Lieberkühn. Secretion consists of water, mucus, potassium, and bicarbonate, resulting in alkaline secretions. Mucus is the major secretory product. It lubricates, allows passage of the fecal residue, protects the mucosa from injury, and binds fecal particles into a formed mass.

Mucus production is stimulated by the parasympathetic nervous system and is increased by bacterial, mechanical, or chemical colonic irritation. Its alkalinity helps to counteract the effects of acid formation from the bacterial action.

Flora

The alkaline reaction of the large intestine permits the growth of organisms whose main functions are to putrefy and break down remaining proteins and indigestible residue. These organisms include *E. coli, A. aerogenes, Clostridium perfringens,* and *Lactobacillus.*

Intestinal bacteria convert urea to ammonium salts and ammonia. Bacterial action in the large bowel causes the formation of gases, which provide bulk and help propel the feces. This action also synthesizes nutritional factors such as vitamin K, thiamine, riboflavin, vitamin B_{12}, folic acid, biotin, and nicotinic acid.

Absorption

Absorption of sodium, chloride, and water occurs in the large bowel and reduces the volume of chyme from 500 ml in the cecum to 100 ml of fluid in the feces. The colon is capable of absorbing 90 per cent of the sodium and water it receives.

Feces

Feces are three-fourths water and one-fourth solid matter. The solid matter includes food residues, digestive enzymes, dead cells, bile pigments, salts, and mucus.

Thirty per cent of the fecal mass consists of bacteria, and another 30 per cent is fat. The outer surface of feces is usually basic, and the inner part is acidic. The nature of the diet does not change the stool's content except for the amount of cellulose.

Substances that absorb water or prevent the movement of water form a soft bulky mass of fecal material and stimulate colonic movement. The feces are expelled through the act of defecation.

Defecation

The defecation reflex is stimulated by distention of the rectum, which occurs when feces and gas are propelled into the rectum from the descending colon. As the pressure within the rectum rises and the internal and external sphincters relax, distention sets the defecation reflex in motion.

Voluntary suppression of defecation is achieved by contracting the striated muscles of the pelvic floor and external sphincter. On the other hand, if an individual elects to defecate on stimulation of the reflex, performance of the Valsalva maneuver will augment the pressure within the colon by increasing intra-abdominal pressure. Specifically, the person increases the pressure by contracting the abdominal muscles and exhaling against a closed glottis. This strain causes cardiovascular alterations. There is a slight bradycardia at the beginning of the maneuver, which changes to tachycardia during the Valsalva maneuver and then back to bradycardia. Intrathoracic pressure increases, thus inhibiting blood return to the heart. Blood pools in the extremities, thereby reducing cardiac filling and output. This cardiovascular effect sometimes makes a person feel lightheaded. In extreme cases, some people feel faint. When the urge to defecate is voluntarily suppressed, the rectum relaxes and the desire to defecate disappears.

EFFECTS OF AGING ON THE GASTROINTESTINAL TRACT

Physiologic changes in the GI tract are known to occur with aging. In the mouth, teeth may loosen from the loss of supporting gums and bone. Circulation in the gums is reduced, and aging teeth darken and may become uneven and fracture. Decreased output of the salivary glands leads to dryness of mucous membranes and increased susceptibility to breakdown. This decrease can cause difficulty swallowing and decreased stimulation of taste buds.

Changes also occur in the ability to digest and absorb food due to a decrease in the secretions of digestive enzymes and bile. In the stomach, atrophy of gastric mucosa leads to a decreased secretion of hydrochloric acid. A decrease in hydrochloric acid causes a decrease in the absorption of iron and vitamin B_{12}, and leads to a proliferation of bacteria. This decrease in iron and vitamin B_{12} leads to the development of anemia. An increase in the bacteria in the gut can lead to diarrhea and infection. With a decrease in bile secretion, absorption of fats and fat-soluble vitamins (A, D, E, and K) becomes impaired. This decreased absorption of fat can lead to weight loss, and the decrease in the fat-soluble vitamins can lead to a variety of problems such as altered calcium metabolism and bleeding from the decrease of vitamin K (needed to synthesize prothrombin).

In the large intestine, peristalsis decreases and nerve impulses are dulled. In addition, muscular tone of the intestinal wall and abdominal muscle strength are decreased. These changes can result in a decreased sensation to defecate and an increased incidence of constipation.

Summary

A thorough knowledge of the structure and function of the GI system helps the nurse provide knowledgeable care to clients with disorders in these areas. In order to provide effective interventions, the nurse must understand the normal physiology of this system and the digestive organs.

Bibliography

1. Barkin, J., & Rogers, A. (Eds.) (1989). *Difficult decisions in digestive diseases*. Chicago: Year Book Medical Publishers.
2. Bayless, T. M. (1989). *Current therapy in gastroenterology and liver disease* (vol. 3, 3rd ed.). St. Louis: C. V. Mosby.
3. Beck, J. E. (Ed.) (1985). *Bockus gastroenterology* (4th ed.). Philadelphia: W. B. Saunders.
4. Berne, R., & Levy, M. (Eds.) (1988). *Physiology* (2nd ed.). St. Louis: C. V. Mosby.
5. Bickel, H. (Ed.) (1983). *Digestion and absorption of nutrients*. Ft. Lee, NJ: J. K. Burgess.
6. Bongiovanni, G. L. (Ed.) (1988). *Essentials of clinical gastroenterology* (2nd ed.). New York: McGraw-Hill.
7. Braunwald, E., et al. (Eds.) (1987). *Harrison's principles of internal medicine* (11th ed.). New York: McGraw-Hill.
8. Cheli, R., et al. (1988). *Gastric protection*. New York: Raven Press.
9. Cheli, R. (1986). *Gastric secretion: A physiologic and pharmacologic approach*. New York: Raven Press.
10. Gitnick, G. (Ed.) (1988). *Handbook of gastrointestinal emergencies* (2nd ed.). New York: Elsevier Science Publishing.
11. Gitnick, G., et al. (Eds.) (1988). *Principles and practice of gastroenterology and hepatology*. New York: Elsevier Science Publishing.
12. Given, B. A., & Simmons, S. J. (1984). *Gastroenterology in clinical nursing* (4th ed.). St. Louis: C. V. Mosby.
13. Granger, D. N., et al. (1985). *Clinical gastrointestinal physiology*. Philadelphia: W. B. Saunders.
14. Groth, K. (1988). Age-related changes in the gastrointestinal tract. *Geriatric Nursing, 9*(5), 278–280.
15. Guyton, A. C. (1991). *Textbook of medical physiology* (8th ed.). Philadelphia: W. B. Saunders.
16. Hamilton, H., & Rose, M. B. (1985). *Gastrointestinal disorders*. Springhouse, PA: Springhouse Corporation.
17. Hayworth, M. F., & Jones, A. L. (1988). *Immunology of the gastrointestinal tract and liver*. New York: Raven Press.
18. Helleman, J. & Vantrappen, G. (1984). *Gastrointestinal tract disorders in the elderly*. New York: Churchill Livingstone.
19. Johnson, L. R., et al. (1987). *Physiology of the gastrointestinal tract* (2nd ed.). New York: Raven Press.
20. Kirsner, J. B., & Shorter, R. G. (Eds.) (1988). *Diseases of the colon, rectum, and anal canal*. Baltimore: Williams & Wilkins.

21. Matteson, M. A. (1988). Age-related changes in the gastrointestinal system. In M. A. Matteson & E. S. McConnell (Eds.), *Gerontologic nursing: Concepts and practice* (pp. 265–278). Philadelphia: W. B. Saunders.
22. Sabiston, D. C., Jr. (1991). *Textbook of surgery: The biologic basis of modern surgical practice* (14th ed.). Philadelphia: W. B. Saunders.
23. Schroeder, S. A., et al. (1988). *Current medical diagnosis and treatment.* Norwalk, CT: Appleton & Lange.
24. Sernka, T., & Jacobson, E. (1983). *Gastrointestinal physiology: The essentials.* (2nd ed.). Baltimore: Williams & Wilkins.
25. Shaffer, E., & Thomson, A. B. R. (1989). *Modern concepts of gastroenterology.* New York: Plenum Publishing Corporation.
26. Sleisenger, M. H., & Fordtran, J. S. (Eds.). (1989). *Gastrointestinal disease: Pathophysiology, diagnosis, and management* (4th ed.). Philadelphia: W. B. Saunders.
27. Snape, W. J., Jr. (Ed.). (1989). *Pathogenesis of functional bowel disease.* New York: Plenum Publishing Corporation.
28. Thomson, J. C., et al. (1987). *Gastrointestinal endocrinology.* New York: McGraw-Hill.
29. Wyngaarden, J. B., & Smith, L. H. (Eds.). (1988). *Cecil textbook of medicine* (18th ed.). Philadelphia: W. B. Saunders.

Chapter

52

Assessment of Clients with Gastrointestinal Disorders

Assessment of the gastrointestinal (GI) tract involves a detailed health history as well as a comprehensive physical examination of the client's oral cavity and abdomen.

HISTORY

DEMOGRAPHIC DATA

A review of demographic data about the client, such as age, sex, and religion, are helpful when assessing the GI tract. Many GI disorders are associated with age and sex. For example, some GI cancers occur more frequently in the elderly and more frequently in males, whereas others are more common in women. Ulcerative colitis occurs more frequently in young and middle-aged adults and in clients of Jewish descent.

Personal and Family History

To continue the history, the nurse should note the client's general health status as well as previous GI disorders and surgery. The nurse should question whether the client currently has or previously has had a change in bowel habits, GI bleeding, jaundice, ulcers, colitis, or unexplained weight loss. Any medications taken routinely such as aspirin, vitamin supplements, laxatives, enemas, or antacids may be important. For example, large doses of aspirin can contribute to ulcer disease. Long-term use of laxatives or enemas could cause bowel dependency.

A family history of many GI disorders may influence a client's risk level. The nurse should ask the client whether any family member has had ulcers, colitis, or GI cancer. Many of these diseases have a higher incidence within families. For example, ulcerative colitis and Crohn's disease tend to occur in families, and duodenal ulcers occur more frequently in clients with blood group O, suggesting a genetic cause.

DIET HISTORY

When assessing GI tract function, a diet history is an essential component of the health history. The client's dietary practices and nutritional status are often factors in GI disorders. These practices are influenced by the client's cultural and religious background, individual preferences, and his or her physical and mental well-being. The client should describe the usual foods and fluids that are typically consumed. The nurse can then evaluate, often with the assistance of a clinical dietician, the quality of the foods ingested and the client's understanding of a balanced diet.

The nurse should explore the relationship between food intake and GI symptoms. The nurse should assess the client's usual and current appetite. Other symptoms, such as nausea and vomiting and difficulty swallowing, should be noted.

CHIEF COMPLAINT

A thorough assessment of the client's current health problem is necessary and often a key component of the health history. Many GI symptoms are vague and have baffling causes, so the nurse must explore each symptom in detail. Begin by asking the client why he or she is seeking health care. Ask the client the following questions about the chief complaint and present illness when conducting a symptom analysis.

Onset. When was the problem first noted? Was the onset gradual or sudden? What was the client doing when the problem was first noticed?

Duration. How long does the problem last? Does it occur occasionally, or is it persistent? Is there a pattern to the problem? If the problem is pain, note whether the pain is continuous or intermittent.

Quality and Characteristics. Ask the client to describe the problem. If the problem is diarrhea, ask the client to describe the stool's appearance.

Severity. Ask the client to describe, on a scale of 1 to 10, how bad the problem is. Does it interfere with his or her ability to perform usual daily activities?

Location. Where does the client feel the problem occurs? Does the pain spread to other areas of the body? What happens to the client when the symptoms occur?

Precipitating Factors. Is there anything that seems to bring on the problem? Does anything make it worse or better? When does it occur? Is it related to eating, drinking, or activity?

Relieving Factors. Is there anything the client can do to relieve the problem? Has he or she tried medications, position changes, or anything else for relief?

Associated Symptoms. Are there any other symptoms that bother the client when the problem is present? Does the client lose appetite, get nauseated, vomit, or have diarrhea?

Common GI symptoms include nausea, vomiting, stomach pain (gastritis), abdominal pain, diarrhea, constipation, abdominal distention, flatulence, dysphagia, heartburn, and indigestion (dyspepsia). The client may also report symptoms such as dry mouth, halitosis, sore mouth, difficulty chewing or swallowing, food intolerance, vomiting of blood (hematemesis), belching, bloody stool (melena), abdominal cramping, anal pruritus or burning, or rectal bleeding. Symptoms associated with the hepatic, biliary, and pancreatic systems may also occur and be reported as GI disturbances (see Chap. 57).

While conducting the health history interview, the nurse notes the client's general health status. A *diet history* and *nutritional assessment* as well as assessment of the client's *elimination patterns* are important data for both baseline information and for future comparisons. Ask the client what foods are usually consumed on a daily basis. Note whether there are differences in the diet on weekends and holidays. Determine whether the client is knowledgeable about basic human nutrition and whether the client's diet is nutritionally sound. Specifically inquire about snacks, intake of sugar, salt, fiber, and fluids. Many GI problems are a result of dietary habits; for example, inadequate fiber intake is a factor in constipation, diverticular disease, and colorectal cancer. See Chapter 11 for a discussion of diet history and nutritional assessment. Note whether the client reports a *change* in elimination patterns (see Chap. 11).

PAST MEDICAL HISTORY

The nurse collects data about previous hospitalizations, major illnesses, surgeries, use of medications, and allergies as part of the past medical history.

Major Illnesses and Hospitalizations

The nurse asks the client about past problems with the GI system. Has the client been hospitalized or treated for peptic ulcer, anemia, hiatal hernia, jaundice, gallbladder disease, colitis, cancer, or a change in bowel habits? Has the client ever had surgery of the oral cavity, throat, stomach, abdomen, or rectal area? If so, determine dates and outcomes of the procedures. Ask whether the client has had diagnostic tests involving the GI system, such as a barium swallow, upper GI studies, or x-ray studies of the lower GI tract.

Medications

Obtain detailed information about prescribed and over-the-counter medications, both currently used and previously taken. Does the client take antacids? If so, determine the type and the frequency taken. Over-the-counter preparations for indigestion often contain sodium bicarbonate (baking soda), which is readily absorbed and may lead to metabolic alkalosis if ingested in sufficient quantities. Also, ask about the use of aspirin and aspirin compounds, which may contribute to gastritis and gastric bleeding. Does the client take a vitamin or mineral supplement? Does the client take laxatives or use enemas to aid elimination? Long-term use of laxatives and enemas can cause dependence.

Allergies

The nurse inquires about allergies to foods, taking care to distinguish between actual allergic response and client dislikes of certain foods. If the client reports food allergies, determine what GI symptoms result, such as cramping, flatulence, diarrhea, or other symptoms such as hives or dyspnea.

FAMILY HISTORY

A family history of certain GI problems may influence a client's current and past health problems. The nurse asks the client if any family members have had cancer, ulcers, or colitis. Many of these diseases have a higher incidence within families, for example, ulcerative colitis and Crohn's disease. Duodenal ulcers also occur more frequently in clients with blood group O, suggesting a genetic cause.

Other disorders to inquire about include jaundice, alcoholism, hepatitis, cancer of the colon, intestinal polyps, obesity, peptic ulcers, and irritable bowel syndrome.

PSYCHOSOCIAL HISTORY AND LIFESTYLE

Sociologic and psychological factors as well as the physical environment can affect health.

Occupation

Ask the client about his or her occupation. Are there factors present that are toxic if ingested or absorbed such as arsenic, mercury, or carbon tetrachloride? Does the client travel as part of his or her job requirements, which can lead to exposure to unfamiliar foods, pathogens, or parasites?

Habits

Certain habits have a known effect on the GI system. Alcohol can cause gastritis and eventual hepatic damage if it is used excessively. Nicotine irritates the GI mucosa and is linked to oral and esophageal cancers.

Ask the client whether there are aspects of the work or home environments that are stress provoking, such as in interpersonal relationships, job security, or financial concerns. Can the client relate his or her GI symptoms to stressful situations, such as epigastric pain, nausea, diarrhea, or peptic ulcers?

REVIEW OF SYSTEMS

The nurse questions the client about other areas related to the GI system. Inquire about the condition of the oral cavity, such as the presence of dental caries, number and condition of teeth, condition of the gingivae, use of dentures and their fit, problems of the oral cavity (e.g., lesions, odor, excess salivation or dryness, sore tongue). Does the client have difficulty chewing or swallowing? Any change in appetite or weight? If pain is reported with eating, is it related to specific foods or associated events? Has the client had a change in bowel habits or stool characteristics? Are there problems with hemorrhoids? Specifically, ask about problems of the hepatic and biliary systems such as jaundice, pruritus, ascites, dark-colored urine, pale stools, or bleeding problems.

Detailed questions for the review of systems (ROS) are found in Chapter 11, Table 11-5.

▼ PHYSICAL EXAMINATION

ASSESSING THE ORAL CAVITY

Begin the GI physical assessment with the oral cavity. Assessment of the oral cavity involves inspection and palpation. The nurse puts on gloves, faces the client, and begins by inspecting the lips. The lips are inspected for abnormal color, lesions, nodules, and symmetry.

Good illumination and instrumentation are essential in performing an oral cavity assessment (Fig. 52-1). A headlight provides direct illumination and a head mirror provides indirect lighting of the mouth, both allowing the examiner's hands to be free to handle the equipment. A penlight may also be used.

After applying gloves, the examiner asks the client to remove any dentures or partial appliances in order to better visualize all areas of the mouth. The oral assessment begins at the left side of the client's mouth and continues in a clockwise fashion. The oral mucosa is inspected for redness, pallor, swelling, ulcers, or leukoplakia. The gums are inspected for redness, pallor, recession, ulcers, and bleeding. Examine the teeth for evidence of dental caries, and dentures and missing or broken teeth. The tongue is inspected for color, ulcers, abnormal coatings, swelling, or a deviation to one

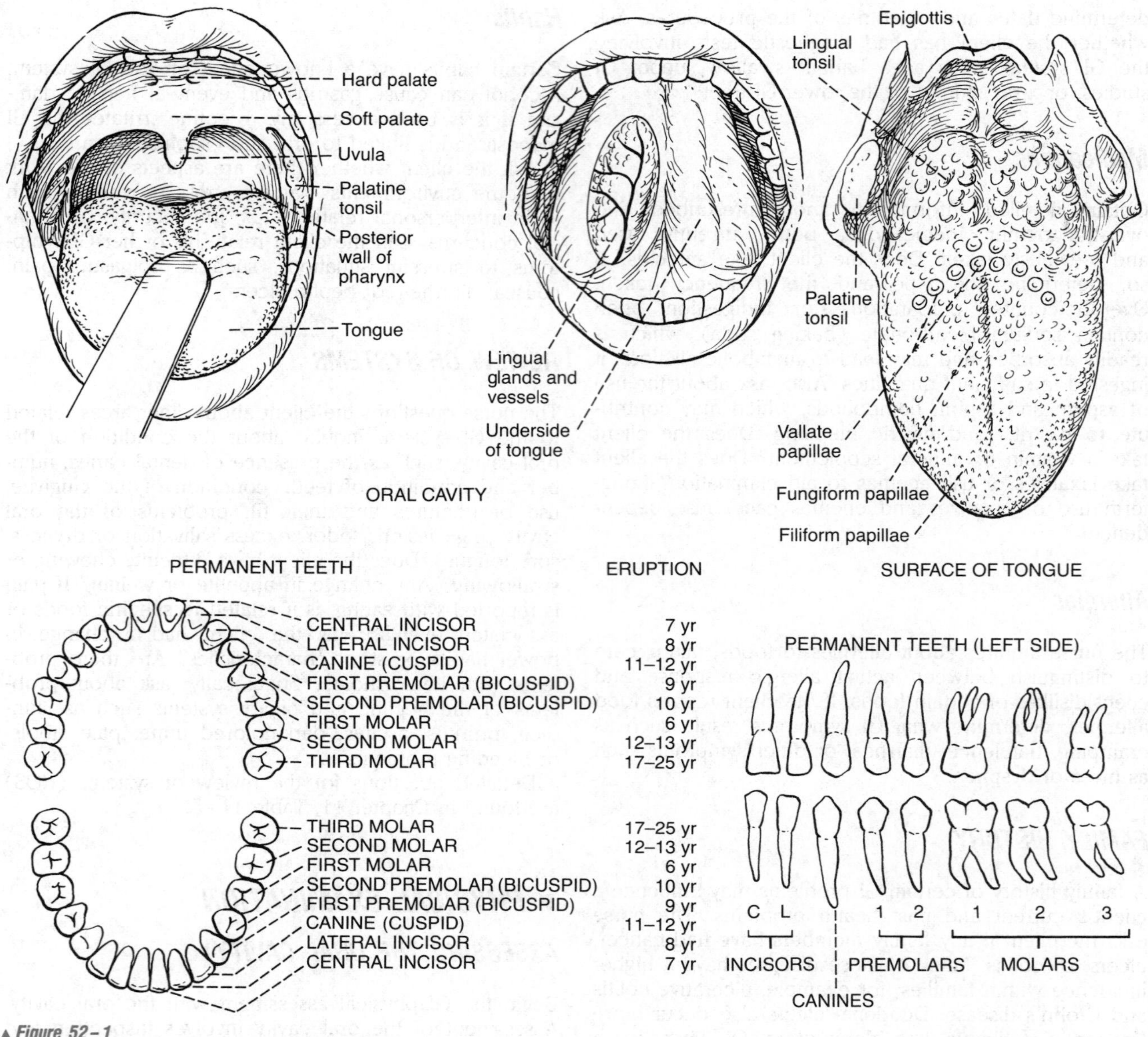

▲ *Figure 52–1*

Assessing the oral cavity: terminology and normal findings.

side. Using the tongue blade or gauze as a retractor, the examiner moves the tongue to inspect the mucous membranes. The client is instructed to protrude the tongue and move it from side to side and upward and downward. This allows the examiner to observe the tongue for voluntary or involuntary movement. Abnormal tongue movement may be due to infiltration of muscle or nerve by tumor or nerve entrapment. While depressing the tongue, the examiner asks the client to say "ah." Examine the pharynx for any tonsil abnormalities, lesions, ulcers, uvular deviations, and any unusual mouth odor. The lips, gingiva, buccal mucosa, and tongue are palpated, and the area is checked for any masses, swellings, or tenderness (Fig. 52–1).

ASSESSING THE ABDOMEN

To assess the client's abdomen, have the client in a supine position with the arms at the side. Bending the knees slightly helps to relax the abdominal muscles. The nurse begins in the right upper quadrant and proceeds in a clockwise manner (Fig. 52–2). When assessing the abdomen, the nurse proceeds in the following sequence: inspection, auscultation, percussion, and palpation. This sequence varies from other body systems because, in the GI system, auscultation is performed in the abdomen before percussion and palpation. This is because percussion and palpation can increase intestinal activity and, therefore, alter bowel sounds. The nurse must be knowledgeable about the

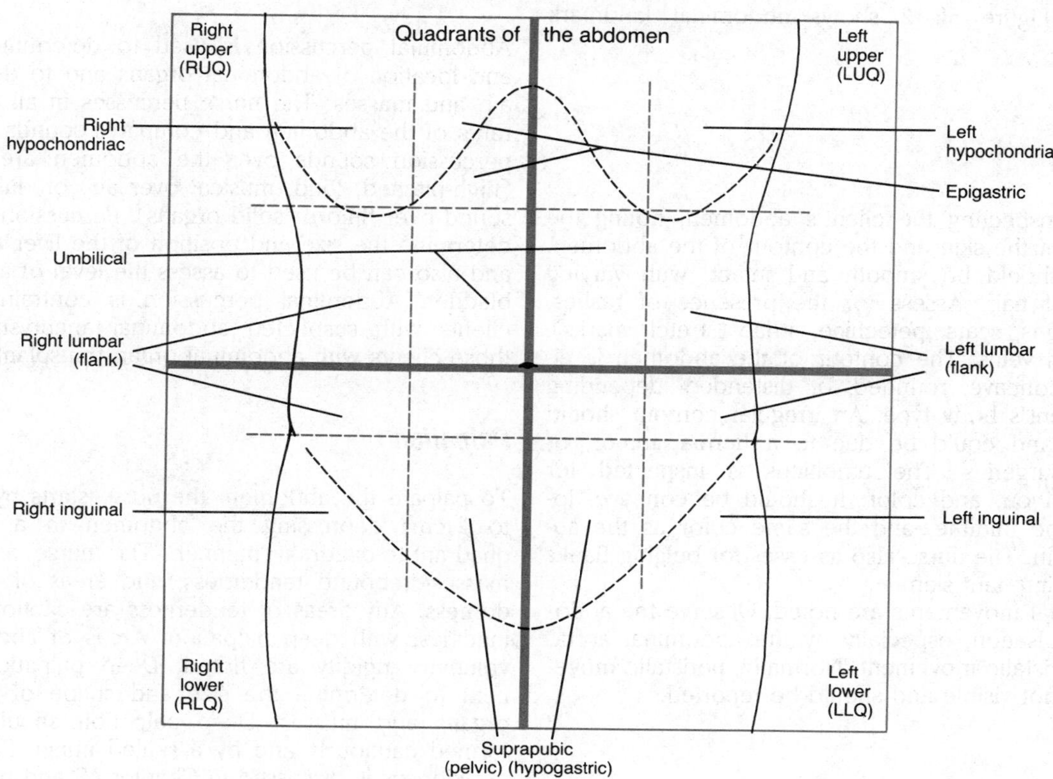

QUADRANTS OF THE ABDOMEN AND THEIR UNDERLYING ORGANS*

Right Upper Quadrant (RUQ)
- Adrenal gland (right)
- Colon (hepatic flexure and portions of ascending and transverse)
- Duodenum
- Kidney (portion of right)
- Liver (right lobe)
- Gallbladder
- Pancreas (head)
- Pylorus

Left Upper Quadrant (LUQ)
- Adrenal gland (left)
- Colon (splenic flexure and portions of transverse and descending)
- Kidney (portion of left)
- Liver (left lobe)
- Pancreas (body)
- Spleen
- Stomach

Right Lower Quadrant (RLQ)
- Appendix
- Bladder (if distended)
- Cecum
- Colon (portion of ascending)
- Kidney (lower pole of right)
- Ovary (right)
- Salpinx (uterine tube; right)
- Spermatic cord (right)
- Ureter (right)
- Uterus (if enlarged)

Left Lower Quadrant (LLQ)
- Bladder (if distended)
- Colon (sigmoid and portion of descending)
- Kidney (lower pole of left)
- Ovary (left)
- Salpinx (uterine tube; left)
- Spermatic cord (left)
- Ureter (left)
- Uterus (if enlarged)

* Small intestine loops in all quadrants.

ANATOMIC REGIONS OF THE ABDOMEN AND THEIR UNDERLYING ORGANS

Right hypochondriac
- Right lobe of liver
- Gallbladder
- Portion of duodenum
- Hepatic flexure of colon
- Portion of right kidney
- Adrenal gland (right)

Epigastric
- Pyloric end of stomach
- Duodenum
- Pancreas
- Portion of liver

Left hypochondriac
- Stomach
- Spleen
- Tail of pancreas
- Splenic flexure of colon
- Upper pole of left kidney
- Adrenal gland (left)

Right lumbar
- Ascending colon
- Lower half of right kidney
- Portion of duodenum and jejunum

Umbilical
- Omentum
- Mesentery
- Lower duodenum
- Jejunum and ileum

Left lumbar
- Descending colon
- Lower half of left kidney
- Portions of jejunum and ileum

Right inguinal
- Cecum
- Appendix
- Ileum (lower end)
- Right ureter
- Right spermatic cord
- Right ovary

Suprapubic
- Ileum
- Bladder
- Uterus (in pregnancy)

Left inguinal
- Sigmoid colon
- Left ureter
- Left spermatic cord
- Left ovary

▲ **Figure 52–2**

Quadrants and anatomic regions of the abdomen and their underlying organs.

underlying structures of the abdomen for accurate assessment. Figure 52–2 shows abdominal landmark mapping.

Inspection

Begin by inspecting the client's abdomen, noting the condition of the skin and the contour of the abdomen. The skin should be smooth and intact, with varying amounts of hair. Assess for the presence of rashes, discolorations, scars, petechiae, striae (stretch marks), and dilated veins. The contour of the abdomen is either flat, concave, rounded, or distended, depending on the client's body type. An irregular contour should be noted and could be due to a hernia, tumor, or previous surgeries. The umbilicus is inspected for shape, position, and color. It should be concave, located at the midline, and the same color as the abdominal skin. The nurse also assesses for bulging flanks and glistening, taut skin.

Abdominal movements are noted. Observe the abdomen for pulsation, especially by the abdominal aorta, and for peristaltic movement. Normally, peristaltic movements are not visible and should be reported.

Auscultation

Auscultation of the abdomen begins by listening with the diaphragm of the stethoscope and provides information on bowel and vascular sounds. The stethoscope is lightly pressed on the abdominal wall in all four quadrants. As air and fluid move through the GI tract, soft clicks and gurgles can be heard every 5 to 15 seconds. The frequency and character of bowel sounds should be noted with a normal frequency rate of 5 to 35 bowel sounds per minute. Bowel sounds may be irregular. Rapid, high-pitched, loud bowel sounds are hyperactive and may occur normally in a hungry client or in a client with gastroenteritis. Hypoactive bowel sounds occur at a rate of one every minute or longer, and can be seen in clients with a paralytic ileus or after bowel surgery. To determine the absence of bowel sounds, the nurse must listen in each quadrant for at least 5 minutes. Make sure the bladder is empty because a full bladder can interfere with sounds.

The nurse next uses the bell of the stethoscope to auscultate vascular sounds. Three abnormal sounds should be listened for: a bruit, venous hum, or friction rub. The nurse listens over the aorta, renal arteries, and iliac arteries. No bruits should be auscultated. A bruit heard over the aorta could indicate the presence of an aneurysm. A continuous venous hum heard in the periumbilical area can indicate engorged liver circulation. Listen for a friction rub, which sounds like two pieces of leather rubbing together, over the liver and spleen. If the sound is heard, it can indicate a hepatic tumor or splenic infarct.

Percussion

Abdominal percussion is used to determine the size and location of abdominal organs and to detect fluid, air, and masses. The nurse percusses in all four quadrants of the abdomen and compares sounds. Normally, percussion sounds over the abdomen are tympanic (high-pitched, loud, musical over air) or dull (thudlike sound over fluid or solid organs). Percussion is used to determine the size and position of the liver and spleen and also can be used to assess the level of a distended bladder. Abdominal percussion is contraindicated in clients with suspected abdominal aneurysms and in those clients with abdominal organ transplants.

Palpation

To palpate the abdomen, the nurse starts by lightly (1 to 2 cm) depressing the abdomen in a systematic quadrant-to-quadrant manner. The nurse assesses for masses, rebound tenderness, and areas of direct tenderness. Any areas of tenderness are cautiously examined last with deep palpation. Areas of abdominal involuntary rigidity are noted. Deep palpation is used next to determine the size and shape of abdominal organs and masses. Deep palpation should be performed cautiously and by a skilled nurse. Palpation of the kidneys is discussed in Chapter 48 and palpation of the liver and spleen in Chapter 57. Further discussion of palpation techniques is in Chapter 12.

▼ DIAGNOSTIC TESTS

Diagnostic measures are performed to locate the nature and level of the problem associated with diseases of the GI tract. The general methods of diagnosis include (1) laboratory tests (Table 52–1), (2) radiographic tests, (3) endoscopy, (4) gastric analysis, (5) cytologic studies, and (6) magnetic resonance imaging. Hematologic studies and electrolyte determinations reveal the general status of the person but do not give specific information about GI disorders.

LABORATORY TESTS

Carcinoembryonic Antigen

Carcinoembryonic antigen (CEA) is a glycoprotein normally produced during the first or second trimester of fetal life. Normally, production is halted before birth. Increased CEA levels in clients other than neonates may indicate the presence of colorectal or other cancer. This test is not useful as a screening tool because increased CEA levels are also seen in cirrhosis, hepatic disease, and alcoholic pancreatitis and in clients who smoke heavily. The test is used to assist in preoperative staging of colorectal cancer, monitor the

TABLE 52-1. Normal Findings and Significance of Abnormal Findings in Common Laboratory Tests Used to Assess GI Function

Test	Normal Findings	Significance of Abnormal Findings
Complete Blood Count		
Red blood cells	4.2 to 5.4 million/mm³ (women) 4.5 to 6.2 million/mm³ (men)	Decreased values indicate possible anemia or hemorrhage
Hemoglobin	12 to 16 g/dl (women) 14 to 18 g/dl (men)	Increased values indicate possible hemoconcentration, caused by dehydration
Hematocrit	38% to 46% (women) 42% to 54% (men)	
Electrolytes		
Potassium	3.5 to 5.0 mg/L	Decreased values indicate possible GI suction, diarrhea, vomiting, intestinal fistulas
Calcium	8.0 to 10.5 mg/dl	Decreased values indicate possible malabsorption
Sodium	135 to 145 mg/L	Decreased values indicate possible malabsorption and diarrhea
D-Xylose	Blood levels peak (25 to 40 mg/dl) 2 hours after ingestion 80 to 95% excreted in 5 hours	Decreased values indicate possible malabsorption
CEA	Less than 5 ng/ml (nonsmokers)	Increased values indicate possible colorectal cancer and inflammatory bowel disease
Fecal Analysis		
Stool for occult blood	Negative	Presence indicates possible peptic ulcer, cancer of the colon, ulcerative colitis
Stool for ova and parasites	Negative	Presence indicates infection
Stool cultures	No unusual growth	Presence of pathogens may indicate shigella, salmonella, *Staphylococcus aureus,* or *Bacillus cereus*
Stool for lipids	2 to 5 g/24 h (normal diet)	Increased values indicate possible malabsorption syndrome and Crohn's disease

effectiveness of cancer therapy, and test for recurrence of colorectal and other cancers. It is referred to, therefore, as a tumor marker. CEA levels usually return to normal within 6 weeks of successful treatment. A continued elevation suggests residual or recurrent tumor. Normally, serum CEA values are less than 5 ng/ml in nonsmokers.

Client Preparation. These laboratory tests require a venipuncture. In these tests, as well as in all diagnostic tests, the nurse should explain the purpose and procedure to the client, and evaluate the client's understanding. There is no follow-up care for this procedure.

D-Xylose Absorption Test

Measurement of blood and urine levels of absorbed D-xylose helps evaluate the absorption qualities of the small intestine and aids in the diagnosis of malabsorption. D-Xylose is a monosaccharide absorbed in the small intestine.

Client Preparation. The client receives nothing by mouth 10 to 12 hours before the test. Before the administration of D-xylose, a blood sample and a first-voided morning urine specimen are collected.

Procedure. D-Xylose is given orally in water. All urine is then collected for a specified time, and blood is drawn 2 hours after D-xylose is given. The client is instructed to remain in bed during the test because activity affects the test results.

Fecal Analysis

Stool examinations that may aid in the diagnosis of GI tract disorders include stool for occult blood, stool for ova and parasites, stool cultures, and stool for lipids.

STOOL FOR OCCULT BLOOD

Stool can be examined for occult blood to detect GI bleeding and aid in the early diagnosis of colorectal cancer. The guaiac or orthotoluidine test is commonly used.

Client Preparation. If the orthotoluidine test is used, the client may be instructed to eat a high-fiber diet for

48 to 72 hours before the collection of the stool specimen. Red meats, poultry, fish, turnips, and horseradish should be avoided. The following medications should be withheld for 48 hours before the test: iron preparations, bromides, rauwolfia derivatives, steroids, indomethacin, and colchicine. Other tests for occult blood do not require dietary restrictions.

Procedure. The nurse or the client usually collects a total of three stool specimens (over 3 successive days). A wooden applicator is used to apply the stool to one side of guaiac paper. After applying the required solution, color is immediately noted. A positive result, which is blue coloration, should be reported. There is no follow-up care for this procedure.

STOOL FOR OVA AND PARASITES

Stool for ova and parasites is collected to detect intestinal infections caused by parasites and their ova (eggs).

Client Preparation. The client should be instructed to avoid drugs such as castor oil, mineral oil, or antidiarrheal compounds, all of which may alter the feces. The client should be informed that the test usually requires three stool specimens, one taken every other day or every third day.

Procedure. The nurse should collect the stool and send it immediately to the laboratory. The nurse should wear gloves when obtaining the specimen. Fresh warm stool is required. If it cannot be examined within 30 minutes, the nurse should place the specimen in a preservative per hospital protocol. There is no follow-up care for this procedure.

STOOL CULTURES

Stool cultures are performed to identify pathogenic organisms in the GI tract. If a stool culture shows no pathogens, detection of viruses can be performed by immunoassay or electron microscopy, which may help in the diagnosis of nonbacterial gastroenteritis.

Client Preparation. The nurse should report if the client is or has been taking any antibiotics recently.

Procedure. Stool should be collected using sterile technique and a sterile stool container. The stool may be collected for 3 consecutive days. There is no follow-up care.

STOOL FOR LIPIDS

Stool can also be examined for lipids. Normally, dietary lipids are almost completely absorbed in the small intestine. Excessive secretion of fecal fats (steatorrhea) may occur in various digestive and absorptive disorders.

Client Preparation. The client should be instructed to eat a high-fat diet and refrain from alcohol for 3 days before the test and during the collection period. The client should avoid drugs that interfere with the test such as mineral oil, neomycin, and potassium chloride.

Procedure. The nurse should collect a 72-hour stool specimen, storing it on ice. There is no follow-up care.

RADIOGRAPHIC TESTS

Flat Plate of the Abdomen

A flat plate of the abdomen is an x-ray study performed to visualize abdominal organs. This test can reveal abnormalities such as tumors, obstructions, abnormal gas collectives, and strictures.

Client Preparation. For this procedure, the client should be dressed in a hospital gown without any belts or jewelry. There is no follow-up for this procedure.

Upper Gastrointestinal Series (Barium Swallow)

An upper GI series permits radiologic visualization of the esophagus, stomach, duodenum, and jejunum. It can aid in the detection of strictures, ulcers, tumors, polyps, hiatal hernias, and motility problems.

Client Preparation. The client is not allowed to have food or fluids for 6 to 8 hours before the test. The nurse should instruct the client about the procedure and about the barium preparation.

Procedure. The client drinks a radiopaque contrast medium (barium) while standing in front of a fluoroscopy tube. The client may be asked to move to other positions, such as lying on the x-ray table.

Follow-up Care. A laxative is usually ordered to help expel the barium and prevent a fecal impaction. The nurse should assess the abdomen for distention and bowel sounds. The nurse should also observe the stool to determine whether the barium has been completely eliminated. Initially, the client's stool is white in color but it should return to its normal brown color within 72 hours. Constipation with a distended abdomen may indicate a barium impaction.

Lower Gastrointestinal Series (Barium Enema)

A lower GI series is performed to visualize the position, movements, and filling of the colon. This test can aid in the detection of tumors, diverticuli, stenosis, obstructions, inflammation, ulcerative colitis, and polyps.

Client Preparation. In this procedure, adequate bowel preparation is essential and varies among institutions. A typical preparation for most adults includes placing the client on a low-residue or clear liquid diet for 2 days prior to the test. The client usually receives a potent laxative and an oral liquid preparation for cleansing the bowel the day before the test. The client receives nothing by mouth after midnight. The morning of the examination, a suppository or a cleansing enema may be administered. If ultrasounds, abdominal scans, or colonoscopy are also indicated, they should be performed first because the barium will interfere with these tests.

Procedure. During a lower GI series, a radiopaque contrast medium (barium) is instilled rectally and radiographs are taken with or without fluoroscopy. Air contrast studies can also be used for more detail. The procedure is often uncomfortable and can be very tiring, especially for the elderly.

Follow-up Care. A laxative or cleansing enema is often given after the test to empty the large bowel and prevent barium impaction. Stools are white for 24 to 72 hours following the examination. The client should increase the intake of liquids to prevent a fecal impaction. The client should report any pain, bloating, absence of stool, or bleeding.

Computed Tomography

Tomography uses a beam of radiation to detect density differences in tissue. The computerized data are visualized as cross sections of the body. Computer tomography (CT) is used mainly to identify masses such as neoplasms, cysts, focal inflammatory lesions, and abscesses of the liver, pancreas, and pelvic areas. CT aids in evaluation of local tumor spread, especially if barium studies suggest the presence of tumor growth beyond the bowel wall (Fig. 52-3). Although CT has the advantage of providing a three-dimensional image, other diagnostic procedures are more valuable for most disorders of the gut. To distinguish normal bowel from abnormal intraperitoneal masses, dilute oral barium or other contrast media may be administered.

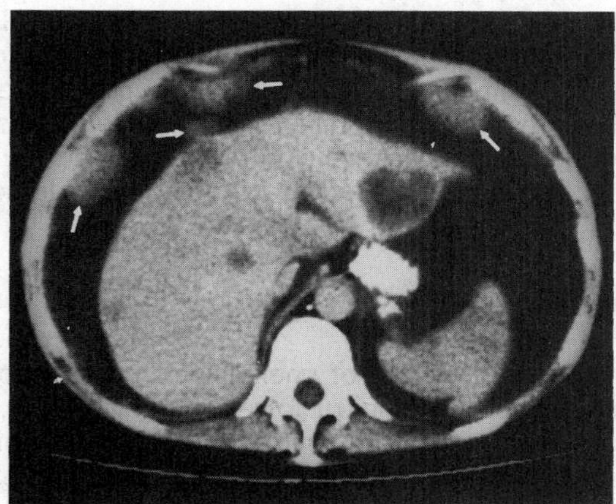

▲ *Figure 52-3*

CT of metastatic colon cancer. Scan of the upper abdomen shows ascites, peritoneal implants *(arrows)*, and hepatic metastases. The metastatic lesion in the left lobe of the liver has undergone partial necrosis. Its central necrotic cavity has a low density similar to that of the ascitic fluid. A thick, irregular margin of solid tumor tissue surrounds the cavity. (From Berk, J. E., et al. (1985). *Bockus' gastroenterology* (4th ed.). Philadelphia: W. B. Saunders.)

Client Preparation. The client usually receives nothing by mouth after midnight before the test. The client should be taught about this painless procedure. If contrast is to be used, the client should be asked about an allergy to iodine.

Procedure. A radiation detector is used to visualize three-dimensional images of abdominal structures. This test may require the administration of a contrast material. The client will have to lie still and hold his or her breath when asked. No follow-up care is needed.

ENDOSCOPY

Endoscopy is the direct visualization of the GI system by means of a lighted, flexible tube. It is more accurate than radiologic examination because the physician can directly observe sources of bleeding and surface lesions and determine the status of healing tissues.

Upper Gastrointestinal Endoscopy

Upper GI tract endoscopy includes esophagoscopy, gastrostomy, and esophagogastroduodenoscopy (EGD) (see Plate 11). These procedures are useful for examining clients with acute or chronic GI bleeding, pernicious anemia, esophageal injury, dysphagia, substernal pain, and epigastric discomfort. Upper GI endoscopy should not be performed on clients with severe cardiovascular disease.

Client Preparation. To prevent aspiration of the stomach contents into the lungs, the client receives nothing by mouth for 8 hours before the procedure. The client may receive an anticholinergic medication to decrease oropharyngeal secretions and to prevent reflex bradycardia. Sedatives, narcotics, or tranquilizers such as diazepam (Valium) or meperidine (Demerol) also may be given before the procedure to help relax the client. The client's dentures and any removable bridges should be removed prior to the procedure to prevent dislodgement. The client's oral cavity also should be carefully assessed for the presence of infection or any lesions.

A local anesthetic is sprayed on the posterior pharynx to ease the discomfort and prevent gagging when the tube is inserted. This anesthetic often tastes unpleasant and makes the tongue feel swollen. The client should not swallow saliva after the throat has been anesthetized. Saliva can drain from the side of the mouth. The musculature of the tract tends to react with spasms and gagging if premedication is not used.

Endoscopic procedures require a signed consent. Provide complete preprocedure teaching because learning about the endoscopy enhances the client's cooperation. Tell the client not to drive a motor vehicle for at least 12 hours after the test if sedation was used during the procedure.

Procedure. After being medicated, a flexible, fiberoptic endoscopy tube is passed orally into the esophagus, stomach, and pylorus and duodenum. Some endoscopes are equipped with a camera to enable the physician to obtain color photographs. Other endoscopic tubes have equipment for performing a biopsy or securing cells for cytologic examination if cancer is suspected. Single polyps are sometimes removed via an endoscope.

Follow-up Care. Vital signs are checked frequently as ordered. The client is also placed on one side to prevent aspiration while the sedation and local anesthesia wear off. The client receives nothing by mouth until the gag reflex returns (2 to 4 hours). Many endoscopic procedures are performed on an outpatient basis. The physician may order anesthetic throat lozenges or normal saline gargles for throat irritation or hoarseness.

Assess the client after an endoscopy for signs of perforation, which include bleeding, fever, and dysphagia. The client with cervical perforation has crepitus (crackling) in the neck from the leakage. Neck and throat pain, aggravated by swallowing or moving, may also occur. Midesophageal perforation can result in referred substernal or epigastric pain. Also, assess for cyanosis, pleural effusion, and back pain. Distal esophageal perforation may result in shoulder pain, dyspnea, or symptoms similar to those of perforated ulcer.

Lower Gastrointestinal Endoscopy (Colon Endoscopy)

Direct visualization of the bowel through a proctoscope, sigmoidoscope, or colonoscope is called colon endoscopy. This procedure is used when a client has a history of constipation, diarrhea, or lower GI bleeding. Colonic endoscopy is useful in diagnosing cancer, strictures, polyps, and ulcerative or inflammatory bowel lesions. Colon endoscopy is contraindicated in patients with inflammatory bowel disease, toxic megacolon, or strictures. This procedure sometimes is complicated by rectal bleeding and, rarely, bowel perforation.

Proctosigmoidoscopy

Proctosigmoidoscopy is the endoscopic examination of the distal sigmoid colon, the rectum, and the anal canal. This test helps diagnose malignant and benign neoplasms, and detect hemorrhoids, polyps, fissures, fistulas, and abscesses within the anal canal and rectum. Health professionals recommend this procedure for clients over 40 years of age on an annual or biennial basis because this examination helps diagnose malignancy at an early stage.

Client Preparation. To prepare the client for proctosigmoidoscopy, clearly explain the preparation for the procedure, the position for examination (knee chest or left lateral), and the discomfort that may accompany passage of the scopes. For example, because the rectum is sensitive to temperature changes, the examining instrument will feel cool. Explain that the instrument will be advanced slowly.

When the entire colon is to be examined, the client usually (1) receives a clear liquid diet 24 hours before the test, (2) takes a cathartic the night before the procedure, and (3) receives a cleansing enema the morning of the test to cleanse the bowel. If bleeding or severe diarrhea is present, examination may be carried out without bowel preparation. To promote visualization, the client is placed in an inverted position (knee chest) that allows the sigmoid colon to straighten. A left lateral Sims' position is suitable for clients who are aged, weak, or very ill.

Procedure. A rigid proctoscope and a sigmoidoscope (rigid or flexible) are used to examine the bowel. Flexible fiberscopes decrease the possibility of perforation and permit examination above the rectosigmoid junction. The procedure involves three separate steps:

1. A digital examination, during which the examiner dilates the anal sphincter in order to detect an obstruction that might make the rest of the examination difficult.
2. Sigmoidoscopy, during which a 25- to 30-cm (10- to 12-inch) sigmoidoscope is inserted into the anus to visualize the distal sigmoid colon and rectum. A flexible sigmoidoscope also makes it possible to visualize the descending colon. The examiner may obtain specimens from suspicious-looking areas of the colon.
3. Proctoscopy, during which a 7-cm ($2\frac{3}{4}$-inch) rigid proctoscope is inserted into the anus. This procedure helps the physician visualize the lower rectum and anal canal.

Follow-up Care. The client is observed for signs of perforation, such as bleeding, pain, and fever. Label and send any specimens obtained during the test to the laboratory immediately. Following the procedure, let the client rest for a few minutes in the supine position before standing up to avoid postural hypotension and fainting. For discomfort, a sitz bath may be ordered.

Colonoscopy

If a client has a history of unexplained constipation or diarrhea, rectal bleeding, or lower abdominal pain, and if results from a barium enema and proctosigmoidoscopy are inconclusive, the physician may perform a colonoscopy. Colonoscopy provides visualization of the lining of the large intestine through a flexible endoscope, which is inserted rectally.

Procedure. For colonoscopy, the client is usually sedated and placed on the left side with the knees flexed. Once the lubricated colonoscope is inserted into the anus, a small amount of air is instilled to help the physician visualize the bowel lumen. When the colonoscope reaches the sigmoid junction, the client may be moved to the supine position, making it easier to advance the colonoscope past the splenic flexure. During the test, encourage the client to relax. Monitor vital signs throughout the procedure, watching for a vasovagal response leading to hypotension and bradycardia.

Follow-up Care. The nurse monitors vital signs as ordered. The nurse should assess for signs of perforation, such as abdominal pain, bleeding, or fever.

EXFOLIATIVE CYTOLOGY

Exfoliative cytology, developed by George Papanicolaou, is the study of cells that have sloughed off from a tissue. This procedure is used to distinguish between benign and malignant lesions. Malignant cells, which exfoliate more readily than normal cells, are collected by lavage and sent to the laboratory for analysis. Cells of the esophagus, stomach, small intestine, and colon can be examined.

Client Preparation. A written consent is obtained. The client is placed on a liquid diet. For colon studies, laxatives and enemas are administered. The nurse should explain the procedure to the client.

Procedure. In this procedure, cells are obtained from saline lavage through a nasogastric tube, from a proctoscope, or during an endoscopy.

Follow-up Care. The client is allowed to rest and resume an appropriate diet.

GASTRIC ANALYSIS

Gastric analysis is performed to measure secretions of hydrochloric acid and pepsin in the stomach. It can aid in the diagnosis of duodenal ulcer, Zollinger-Ellison syndrome, gastric carcinoma, and pernicious anemia. There are two tests performed in gastric analysis: (1) the basal cell secretion test and (2) the gastric acid stimulation test.

Client Preparation. The client receives nothing by mouth 12 hours before the test. A nasogastric tube is inserted, and any contents left in the stomach are removed. The client should avoid taking drugs that interfere with gastric acid levels (e.g., cholinergics, antacids).

Procedure. The client's nasogastric tube is attached to suction, and stomach contents are collected every 15 minutes for 1 hour. The nurse must properly label the specimens with the time and volume. If the basal secretion test suggests abnormal gastric secretion, a gastric acid stimulation test is usually performed immediately.

The gastric acid stimulation test measures the amount of gastric acid for 1 hour after subcutaneous injection of a drug that stimulates gastric acid secretion (pentagastrin, beta zole [Histalog]). If abnormal results occur, usually radiographic studies or endoscopy are performed to determine the cause.

A markedly increased level of gastric secretion may indicate Zollinger-Ellison syndrome, whereas moderately increased levels indicate a duodenal ulcer. Decreased levels of gastric secretion could indicate gastric ulcer or carcinoma.

Follow-up Care. If the nasogastric tube is left in place, it should be clamped or attached to low intermittent suction if ordered.

Bernstein Test

This test is performed to determine whether or not the client's symptoms of chest pain are related to acid perfusion of the esophageal mucosa.

Client Preparation. The client should receive nothing by mouth the night before the test. The nurse should prepare the client for insertion of a nasogastric tube.

Procedure. A nasogastric tube is inserted, and gastric contents are aspirated. Alternatively, 0.9 per cent NaCl (normal saline) and 0.1 per cent HCl are instilled into the lower esophagus. If the client experiences no pain, the test is considered negative. If pain occurs, 0.9 per cent NaCl is administered until the pain ceases. To ensure that the pain is caused by acid perfusion, the 0.1 percent HCl is readministered. After the test, the nasogastric tube is withdrawn.

Follow-up Care. After the procedure, the client may receive an antacid.

ULTRASONOGRAPHY

Ultrasonography is a noninvasive diagnostic procedure during which sound waves are passed into the body in order to produce an image or photograph of an organ or tissue on an oscilloscope.

Diagnosticians use ultrasonography on the GI system to identify pathophysiologic processes in the pancreas, liver, gallbladder, spleen, and retroperitoneal tissue. Ultrasound can identify fluid, masses (e.g., tumors), adipose tissue, and hematoma. Diagnosis of an abdominal abscess can be made with ultrasonography. Ultrasound enhances the physical examination because palpable masses and areas of tenderness can be correlated with anatomic structures while the person is on the examining table. Gas in the abdomen may interfere with ultrasound waves.

Client Preparation. The client may be required to have nothing by mouth 8 to 12 hours before the procedure to reduce bowel gas. Reassure the client that the test is painless and safe.

Follow-up Care. There are no specific precautions or observations related to ultrasound.

MAGNETIC RESONANCE IMAGING

Magnetic resonance imaging (MRI) is a noninvasive test that can be used in addition to other GI diagnostic tests. An MRI produces cross-sectional images of soft tissue and blood vessels by using magnetic fields. The test is used to study blood flow and identify tumors, infections, and other decreased tissue. The test is contraindicated in clients with pacemakers, aneurysm clips, or orthopedic screws because of the magnetic field.

Client Preparation. The client may not receive anything by mouth for 6 hours before the procedure. The client should be instructed that the test requires that the client lay still during the procedure, which can take from 60 to 90 minutes. All jewelry and metal should be removed.

Procedure. The client lies on a narrow table that slides into a magnetic body scanner. A strong magnetic field is created around the client, which allows the image of tissue to be produced. The client will hear a clanging noise during the procedure. There is no follow-up care.

Summary

Once the nurse has a thorough knowledge of the structure and function of the GI system, the nurse must understand the diagnostic assessment of these organs. Systematic assessment of the client with possible disorders in the GI system can lead to prompt diagnosis and treatment. The nurse can facilitate this diagnostic process by adequately preparing the client for the diagnostic procedures and by assisting with or actually collecting assessment data.

Bibliography

1. Barkin, J., & Rogers, A. (Eds.). (1989). *Difficult decisions in digestive diseases.* Chicago: Year Book Medical Publishers.
2. Bayless, T. M. (1989). *Current therapy in gastroenterology and liver disease* (Vol. 3, 3rd ed.). St. Louis: C. V. Mosby.
3. Beck, J. E. (Ed.). (1985). *Bockus gastroenterology* (4th ed.). Philadelphia: W. B. Saunders.
4. Beck, M. L. (1989). Percutaneous endoscopic gastrostomy. *American Journal of Nursing, 89,* 76.
5. Berne, R., & Levy, M. (Eds.). (1988). *Physiology* (2nd ed.). St. Louis: C. V. Mosby.
6. Bongiovanni, G. L. (Ed.). (1988). *Essentials of clinical gastroenterology* (2nd ed.). New York: McGraw-Hill Book Co.
7. Braunwald, E., et al. (Eds.). (1987). *Harrison's principles of internal medicine* (11th ed.). New York: McGraw-Hill Book Co.
8. Cheli, R., et al. (1988). *Gastric protection.* New York: Raven Press.
9. Clinical highlights: Blood in the stool. (1983). *Hospital Medicine, 19,* 249.
10. Cotran, R. S., et al. (1989). *Robbins' Pathologic Basis of Disease* (4th ed.). Philadelphia, W. B. Saunders Company.
11. Dent, T. L., et al. (1985). *Surgical endoscopy.* Chicago: Year Book Medical Publishers.
12. Dunphy, J. E., & Way, L. W. (1983) *Current Surgical Diagnosis and Treatment* (6th ed.). Los Altos, CA: Lange Medical Publications.
13. Fishbach, F. (1988). *A manual of laboratory diagnostic tests* (3rd ed.). Philadelphia: J. B. Lippincott.
14. Gale, M. E., & Robbins, A. H. (1983). CT scans of the abdomen: Indications and basic interpretation. *Hospital Medicine, 19,* 10.
15. Gitnick, G., et al. (Eds.). (1988). *Principles and practice of gastroenterology and hepatology.* New York: Elsevier Science Publishing Co.
16. Given, B. A., & Simmons, S. J. (1984). *Gastroenterology in clinical nursing* (4th ed.). St. Louis: C. V. Mosby.
17. Granger, D. N., et al. (1985). *Clinical gastrointestinal physiology.* Philadelphia: W. B. Saunders.
18. Gryska, P., et al. (1987). Screening asymptomatic patients at high risk for colon cancer with full colonoscopy. *Diseases of the Colon and Rectum, 30,* 18–20.
19. Guyton, A. C. (1991). *Textbook of medical physiology* (8th ed.). Philadelphia: W. B. Saunders.
20. Hamilton, H., & Rose, M. B. (1985). *Gastrointestinal disorders.* Springhouse, PA: Springhouse Corp.
21. Hayworth, M. F., & Jones, A. L. (1988). *Immunology of the gastrointestinal tract and liver.* New York: Raven Press.
22. Hochman, R. B. (1982). X-ray clues to esophageal disorders. *Hospital Medicine, 18,* 33.
23. Jarvis, C. (1992). *Physical examination and health assessment.* Philadelphia: W. B. Saunders Company.
24. Johnson, R. A., et al. (1982). Flexible sigmoidoscopy. *Journal of Family Practice, 14,* 757.
25. Johnson, L. R., et al. (1987). *Physiology of the gastrointestinal tract* (2nd ed.). New York: Raven Press.
26. Kirsner, J. B. (1985). The stomach. In W. A. Sodeman, & T. M. Sodeman (Eds.), *Pathologic physiology: mechanisms of disease* (7th ed.). Philadelphia: W. B. Saunders Co.
27. Kirsner, J. B., & Shorter, R. G. (Eds.). (1988). *Diseases of the colon, rectum, and anal canal.* Baltimore: Williams & Wilkins.
28. Miller, H., et al. (1982). *New diagnostic techniques.* New York: Grune & Stratton.
29. Sabiston, D. C., Jr. (1991). *Textbook of surgery: The biologic basis of modern surgical practice* (14th ed.). Philadelphia: W. B. Saunders.
30. Schroeder, S. A., et al. (1988). *Current medical diagnosis treatment.* Norwalk, CT: Appleton & Lange.
31. Sernka, T., & Jacobson, E. (1983). *Gastrointestinal physiology: The essentials* (2nd ed.). Baltimore: Williams & Wilkins.
32. Shaffer, E., & Thomson, A. B. R. (1989). *Modern concepts of gastroenterology.* New York: Plenum Publishing Corp.
33. Shiau, Y. (1987). Clinical and laboratory approaches to evaluate diarrheal disorders. *Critical Reviews in Clinical Laboratory Science, 25,* 43–63.
34. Sleisenger, M. H., & Fordtran, J. S. (Eds.). (1989). *Gastrointestinal disease: Pathophysiology, diagnosis, and management* (4th ed.). Philadelphia: W. B. Saunders.
35. Snape, W. J., Jr. (Ed.). (1989). *Pathogenesis of functional bowel disease.* New York: Plenum Publishing Corp.
36. Swartz, M. H. (1989). *Textbook of physical diagnosis.* Philadelphia: W. B. Saunders.
37. Thomson, J. C., et al. (1987). *Gastrointestinal endocrinology.* New York: McGraw-Hill Book Co.
38. Urosevich, P. R. (Ed.). (1983). *Performing GI procedures.* Springhouse, PA: Intermed Communication.
39. Warden, M. J., et al. (1987). Role of colonoscopy and flexible sigmoidoscopy in screening for colorectal cancer. *Diseases of the Colon and Rectum, 30,* 52–54.
40. Waye, J. D. (1987). Expanding uses of therapeutic endoscopy. *Hospital Practice, 22,* 143.
41. Winawer, S. J., et al. (1982). Current status of fecal occult blood testing in screening for colorectal cancer. *Ca—A Cancer Journal for Clinicians, 32,* 100.
42. Wyngaarden, J. B., & Smith, L. H. (Eds.). (1988). *Cecil textbook of medicine* (18th ed.). Philadelphia: W. B. Saunders.

Chapter 53

Nursing Care of Clients with Ingestive Disorders

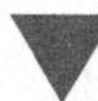

People depend on their mouths for the ingestion of food and fluids, the pleasures of taste, and the ability to communicate verbally. Nevertheless, the oral cavity is subject to many disorders, such as tooth decay, periodontal disease, and tumors, that sometimes destroy vital oral structures. Disorders of the oral cavity threaten the client's general health (especially nutrition and fluid and electrolyte balance), communication, and lifestyle. Assessment, preventive care, and early intervention help clients maintain optimal oral health.

DENTAL DISORDERS

A person must have healthy teeth and gums for good general health. Health care professionals (nurses, dentists, dental physicians) strive to preserve healthy gums and natural teeth for as long as possible for these reasons:

A person's natural teeth are almost always more functional in masticating food than a dental prosthesis,
Effective mastication of food helps promote efficient digestion, and
Efficient digestion of food results in healthy gastrointestinal function and good general health.

The most frequent sources of tooth loss are dental decay and periodontal disease. Plaque is the major cause of both caries (decay) and periodontal disease.

DENTAL PLAQUE

Definition

Dental plaque is a soft mass of proliferating bacteria with a scattering of leukocytes, macrophages, and epithelial cells in a sticky polysaccharide-protein matrix that adheres to the teeth. Plaque is transparent and colorless, and escapes detection unless it (1) absorbs pigment from within the oral cavity or (2) is stained in the dental office by a disclosing solution. It can be removed only by mechanical cleansing.

Pathophysiology

Food contributes to plaque formation. Bacterial enzymes liquify food debris after a meal and use some of the carbohydrates, along with saliva, to form plaque. The polysaccharide dextran, the major component of the intercellular matrix, envelopes the plaque bacteria and attaches them to each other and to the tooth surface. The sticky organic film begins to collect on the teeth within hours of eating or brushing. Carbohydrates contribute to plaque formation because they supply energy for the biosynthesis of macromolecules and the proliferation of bacteria.

DENTAL CARIES

Definition

A dental caries (tooth decay) is an erosive process that can cause progressive demineralization and destruction of the outer enamel of the tooth. If the condition is not treated, eventual damage to the pulp can occur.

Incidence

It has been estimated that 90 to 99 per cent of the population in the United States have experienced dental disorders. Many Americans fail to act to maintain healthy teeth.

Etiology

Dental decay has many causes. Basically, decay depends on (1) the resistance of the tooth enamel, (2) the nature of the plaque (including its bacterial population), and (3) the diet ingested. Of these factors, dental plaque is probably the most important.

Risk Factors

One of the major risk factors for dental caries is poor dental care. Many people do not follow simple dental hygiene measures such as daily brushing and regular visits to the dentist. Prevention includes daily brushing and flossing; dental visits with cleaning; in children, the application of fluoride; and maintaining a healthy diet.

Pathophysiology

Many dentists accept the theory that dental decay occurs when the acids produced by bacteria in the plaque begin to decalcify the inorganic tooth enamel when pH falls below 5.6. The plaque itself initially offers some protection against the acid because of its buffering qualities. For decay to progress, both acid-producing cariogenic bacteria and carbohydrates must be present in the mouth. Any carbohydrate in the mouth will stimulate bacterial acid production, but sucrose seems to stimulate the most acid. The longer carbohydrates remain in the mouth after ingestion, the longer it takes for the pH to return to normal levels. Therefore, increased frequency of food ingestion (particularly sticky substances such as caramels or honey) causes the acid level in the mouth to elevate for longer periods of time, increasing the risk of cavity production.

Clinical Manifestations

The major symptom of dental caries is pain in the affected tooth, especially when the tooth comes in contact with heat, cold, or certain foods.

Diagnostic Assessment

The dentist diagnoses caries through direct examination of the teeth and through x-ray studies.

Medical Management

The best treatment for dental caries is prevention. Encourage clients in your care to perform regular brushing and flossing, eat a diet low in simple carbohydrates, use fluoride, and schedule regular visits to the dentist for examination, cleaning, and treatment of dental caries.

Increasing the resistance of the enamel also helps prevent caries. The resistance of the enamel increases with the ingestion of fluoridated water during tooth formation and the continued use of fluoride throughout life. The daily use of fluoride rinses produces a more acid-resistant structure, enhances tooth mineralization, and interferes with bacterial growth. In addition, the dentist may apply topical fluoride to the teeth, especially in children.

Surgical Management

Treatment of dental caries may include (1) drilling out cavities and filling them with material to restore the tooth, (2) removal of the entire tooth (extraction) if the cavity cannot be filled, and (3) preservation of the tooth by root canal therapy (pulpectomy), followed by proper restoration.

Any number of teeth can be removed because of disease. Teeth are usually replaced with some type of dental prosthesis (crowns, dentures, or by dental implants). If only one tooth or a few teeth are being removed, the procedure is usually performed with local anesthesia, removing several teeth or having a full-mouth extraction may require sedation or general anesthesia.

In root canal therapy, the entire pulp of the tooth is removed. The canal space within the roots are then filled aseptically and sealed to prevent infection. Subsequent restoration of the tooth is essential to retain the tooth in a normal functional relation with the rest of the dentition.

In a pulpectomy or root canal, the entire pulp of the tooth is removed. The cavity of the tooth is then aseptically filled and sealed to prevent infection. The tooth remains rooted in the gingiva and can still be used by the client.

PERIODONTAL DISEASE

Definition

Periodontal disease is defined as a spectrum of disorders of the gums ranging from gingivitis, in its least destructive form, to periodontitis, in its worst form.

Incidence

This is a very common problem and probably affects more than 90 per cent of the population to some degree. It is equally divided among men and women.

Etiology

Plaque accumulating on the teeth is the major cause of both caries and periodontal disease. Once plaque has hardened to form calculus, it can be removed only by dental professionals with specialized instruments.

Risk Factors

The major risk factor for caries and periodontal disease is poor dental hygiene. The best way to prevent these problems is by preventing the accumulation of plaque. This is best accomplished through proper brushing, flossing, and regular dental check-ups. Fluoridation also helps strengthen enamel. A high intake of sugar can weaken enamel.

Pathophysiology

Plaque formation and subsequent bacterial colonization results in gingival inflammation (gingivitis) if the plaque is not removed by proper brushing and flossing. Pockets of inflammation form (Fig. 53–1) and gradually deepen. Eventually, inflammation causes destruction of the underlying tissues and separation of the gingiva from the tooth. In periodontitis, the inflammation extends from the gums into the alveolar bone and periodontal ligament, destroying supporting structures for the teeth (Fig. 53–2). As a result, the teeth loosen and may require extraction.

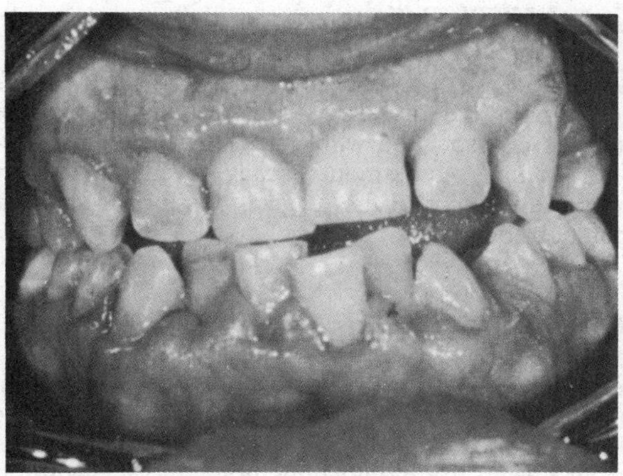

▲ *Figure 53–1*

Gingivitis with erythema and inflammatory enlargement of gingiva. (From Shklar, G. [1984]. The oral cavity, jaws, and salivary glands. In S. L. Robbins, et al. [Eds.], *Pathologic basis of disease* [3rd ed.]. Philadelphia: W. B. Saunders Co., p. 773.)

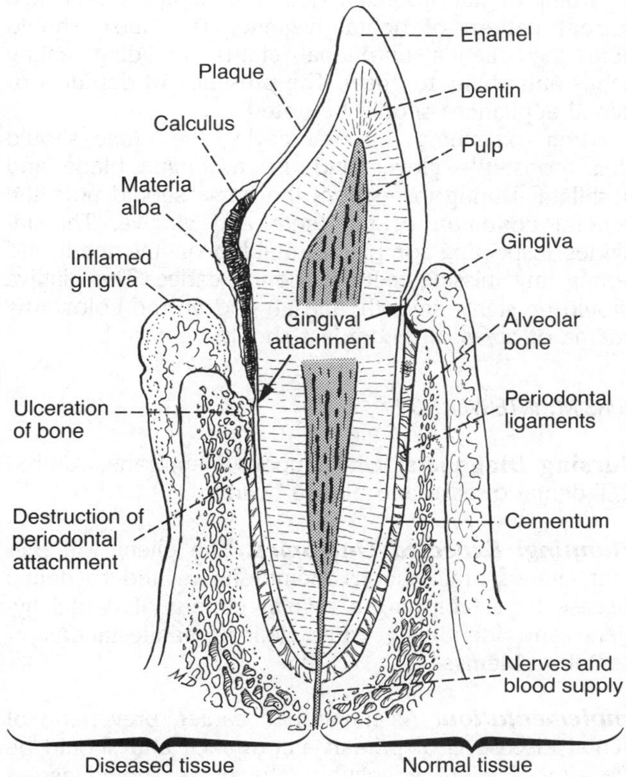

▲ *Figure 53–2*

Periodontal disease. A tooth with normal tissues on right side, periodontal disease on left side. Note destruction of alveolar bone and periodontal fibers that normally hold tooth in place.

Clinical Manifestations

The early form of periodontal disease is gingivitis. The late form of the disease is periodontitis or pyorrhea. Gingivitis is associated with gums that bleed from even minor trauma. Assessment usually reveals some alterations in the color of the gingiva, possibly swelling and ulceration, but rarely pain.

Medical Management

Prevention is the most effective method for controlling periodontal disease. Plaque removal remains the best defense against gingivitis and, thus, periodontal disease. Simply rinsing the mouth does not remove plaque, because plaque cannot be removed without friction. Friction dislodges both plaque and other debris. Plaque can be decreased by thorough cleansing, decreasing the frequency of meals, and reducing the ingestion of between-meal snacks, especially sticky, adherent ones. Good oral hygiene is based on tooth brushing, the use of dental floss, interdental cleaners, and water irrigation.

Nursing Management

ASSESSMENT

The nurse should obtain a dental history from the client regarding dental problems, dental visits, and the client's current pattern of dental hygiene. The nurse should note the client's nutritional status including eating habits and ability to chew. The presence of dentures or dental appliances should be noted.

When examining the oral cavity, the nurse should wear nonsterile gloves and use a tongue blade and flashlight. During inspection, the nurse should note the general condition of the teeth and gingiva. This includes inspecting for plaque buildup on the teeth and noting any missing teeth or dental caries. The gingiva should be shiny, smooth, and an uneven red color. Any edema or areas of tenderness should be noted.

NURSING INTERVENTION

Nursing Diagnosis: Oral Mucous Membrane, Altered R/T dental disease and plaque buildup.

Planning: Expected Outcomes. The client will prevent altered oral mucous membrane related to dental disease by establishing a regular pattern of dental hygiene and identifying early clinical manifestations of dental problems.

Implementation. As mentioned earlier, prevention of dental disease is of primary importance and should be the aim of client education. The nurse should assess the client's current dental hygiene practices, making sure the client brushes, rinses, and flosses properly. The nurse should also assess the client's diet, especially for refined and hidden sugars. The use of fluoride, both in rinses and added to water supply, can also be helpful, barring any medical restrictions. The nurse should also teach the client about the importance of undergoing regular dental examinations every 6 months and the importance of early detection of minor irritations and infections.

Collaborative Problem. High risk for injury R/T hemorrhage after oral surgery.

Planning: Expected Outcomes. Injury will be prevented after oral surgery, as evidenced by absence of bleeding.

Implementation. Postoperative care for a tooth extraction includes assessing the oral cavity for bleeding and monitoring vital signs (if the client stays in an inpatient facility or recovery area). A gauze pad is usually placed over the extraction site, and the client is instructed to bite down gently on the pad to maintain pressure. Ice also may be applied to the site to decrease the blood flow and edema. Small amounts of bleeding may be normal, but the nurse should notify the physician if bleeding occurs for longer than 1 hour.

The client usually requires analgesics to control pain. The client should be instructed to eat soft foods and avoid hot or cold foods for several days. The client also should gently rinse the mouth with normal saline, but should avoid brushing any remaining teeth for one day.

EVALUATION

The nurse must evaluate client outcomes based on the established plan of care. If these goals were not achieved, the plan and interventions must be revised to meet the client's needs.

Modifications of Plan of Care for the Elderly

Remember, there are changes that occur in the oral cavity of the elderly client. The oral mucosa is more susceptible to injury because of atrophy of the mucosa and a decrease in salivation. The teeth of the elderly are more prone to caries, and many clients have lost some or all of their teeth. There also may be a decrease in oral motor functions (chewing and swallowing). There is often an inability to perform normal hygiene practices resulting from a decrease in manual dexterity and strength.

The goal of dental care in the elderly is to retain permanent teeth as long as possible. Tooth loss is not a normal part of aging and is usually the result of periodontal disease or dental caries.

Post-hospital Care

DISCHARGE TEACHING

To prepare the client for discharge, the nurse should provide oral and written instructions on dental hygiene, signs and symptoms of complications, and instructions on a balanced diet. If the client has new dentures, the client should be able to demonstrate proper care of them.

DENTAL EMERGENCIES

A client who fractures a tooth must see a dentist immediately. Entry of bacteria into the canal of the tooth and the resulting infection may cause a dental abscess. An avulsed tooth is a tooth torn from the mouth by trauma. If it is found, reimplantation of the tooth should be attempted as soon as possible. It should be placed in a cool normal saline solution and reimplanted by the dentist or oral surgeon after the wound has been irrigated. Once the tooth has been reimplanted, wires or splints are used to stabilize it in place. Root canal therapy is required in cases of avulsion. Teeth that are imbedded into the gum should be left alone but followed by a dentist. They usually return to normal position within 1 month.

Emergencies such as deep lacerations of the gums and fractures of the jaw must be treated by an oral surgeon. These lacerations bleed freely, because of the mouth's excellent blood supply. Application of local pressure to the site provides the best first-aid intervention. In any wound of this nature, prevent aspiration by carefully removing debris from the mouth. Either gently irrigate the mouth or allow the client to rinse the mouth.

Post-extraction hemorrhage can be (1) primary, occurring within an hour or two of the extraction and usually caused by dislodging of the clot, or (2) secondary, probably caused by infection in the socket or a loose clot. Application of local pressure provides emergency intervention for both types of hemorrhage. Additional treatments include (1) applying a sterile gauze pad over the extraction site and (2) asking the client to bite down on the gauze to produce hemostasis. Sometimes biting down on a moistened tea bag is a successful home remedy. The pressure helps stop bleeding and the tannic acid in the tea helps promote hemostasis. If bleeding continues, the client should always return to the dentist.

▼ ORAL DISORDERS

▼ Stomatitis

Stomatitis is an inflammation of the oral cavity. It may be of infectious origin or a symptom of a systemic condition. It may be caused by mechanical or chemical trauma. Jagged teeth, cheek biting, and mouth breathing may result in mechanical trauma. Certain foods and drinks and sensitivity to mouthwashes or dentifrices may produce chemical trauma.

The inflammatory sloughing of tissue allows organisms to multiply; thus, stomatitis may lead to infection by viruses, bacteria, yeasts, or fungus.

Stomatitis is classified as primary or secondary depending on the cause. Primary stomatitis includes aphthous stomatitis, herpes simplex, and Vincent's angina. Secondary stomatitis is caused when the client's resistance is lowered and an opportunistic infection results. Secondary stomatitis can be caused by a local or systemic disorder. Systemic disorders that can affect the oral mucous membranes include allergies, bone marrow disorders, nutritional disorders, or disorders resulting from immunosuppressive therapy or immunodeficiency.

APHTHOUS STOMATITIS (CANKER SORE)

Definition

Canker sores are recurrent, small, ulcerated lesions of the soft tissues of the mouth, including the lips, tongue, and inside the cheeks.

Incidence

Canker sores can appear in all age groups, although young adults are more frequently affected. The incidence is also higher in females than in males.

Etiology

Although the etiology is unknown, possible causes include emotional stress, trauma, vitamin deficiency, food and drug allergies, endocrine imbalances, and viral infections.

Risk Factors

High stress is one of the major risk factors along with viral infections like colds. Prevention is almost impossible because the exact etiology is unknown.

Pathophysiology

These lesions start as small, reddened areas that undergo central necrosis and ulceration. The lesions are not infective but are simply inflammatory, and they heal within several weeks without treatment.

Clinical Manifestations

Assessment usually reveals a well-circumscribed erythematous macule that undergoes necrosis (Fig. 53–3). Necrosis results in a well-defined pseudomembranous ulcer with an erythematous border. Lesions, although painful, are not contagious and heal spontaneously within 1 to 2 weeks.

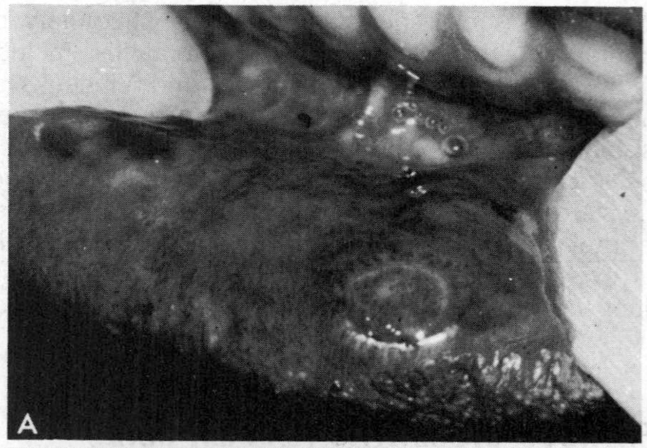

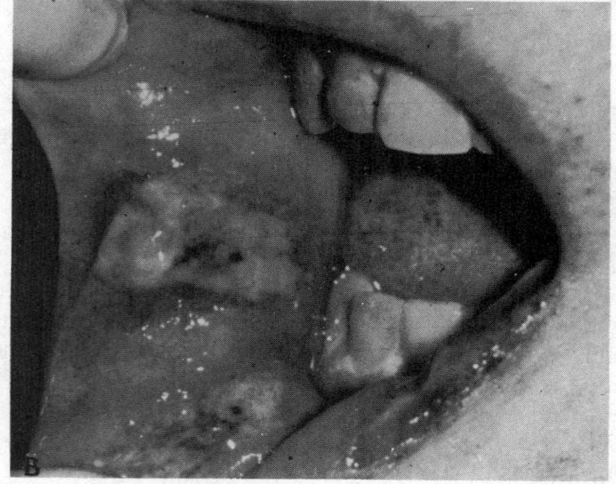

▲ **Figure 53-3**

Aphthous stomatitis. *A*, Discrete round ulcer. *B*, Large necrotic lesions. (From Shklar, G. [1984]. The oral cavity, jaws, and salivary glands. In S. L. Robbins, et al. [Eds.], *Pathologic Basis of Disease* (3rd ed.), Philadelphia: W. B. Saunders Co., p. 778.)

Medical Management

Medical treatment with topical or systemic steroids may shorten the healing time. In addition, to suppress the recurrence of sores, suggest that clients prone to allergic reactions should avoid tomatoes, chocolate, eggs, shellfish, milk products, nuts, and citrus fruits. Some dentists report that the routine administration of systemic steroids may also prevent recurrence.

HERPES SIMPLEX

Definition

Herpes simplex is a form of inflammation and ulceration caused by a viral infection.

Incidence

By the age of 5 years, 90 per cent of the population has had an infection, usually asymptomatic, of primary herpes simplex. Secondary herpes is often seen in clients receiving immunosuppressants and in those with human immunodeficiency virus (HIV), or acquired immunodeficiency syndrome (AIDS).

Etiology

Stomatitis caused by the *herpes simplex virus* (HSV) can occur as a primary or secondary infection. Primary HSV infection occurs as a result of the initial exposure to the virus and is often asymptomatic. Secondary HSV infection takes the form of *herpes labialis* (fever blister, cold sore). The current theory is that respiratory infections, sunlight, a fever, or emotional stress can reactivate the virus. Clients vary greatly in their susceptibility to secondary herpes simplex.

Risk Factors

Age is one of the risk factors for primary herpes, because it is most common in children. Immunosuppression is the highest risk factor for secondary herpes. There are no preventive measures for either of these factors other than early detection and appropriate treatment once they develop.

Pathophysiology

When the client is first infected with the primary herpes virus, lesions appear in the oral cavity. These vesicals, which appear throughout the oral cavity, rupture to form ulcerated areas that resemble canker sores and heal within several weeks. The client's tongue appears heavily coated with a characteristic white coating. The infection may produce symptoms of generalized infection in the client.

Secondary herpes is a recurrent infection that appears to lie dormant after the primary herpes infection. Any infection, especially upper respiratory infections, fever, or even sunlight can reactivate the virus.

Clinical Manifestations

Assessment reveals clear, vesicular lesions, most often appearing at the mucocutaneous junction of the lips and face. The lesions are contagious, last about 1 week, and heal without scarring (Plate 12). Later in the course of the infection, the tongue may appear coated, and the client may complain of a foul breath odor.

Medical Management

PHARMACOLOGIC MANAGEMENT

General pain may be treated with analgesics. Unless the ulcer is secondarily infected, antimicrobial treatment does not affect the progress of the ulcer. Local ointments and anesthetics may soothe lesions. Clients who are immunocompromised are started on intravenous acyclovir (Zovirax). Clients with competent immune systems also may be given acyclovir but in oral or topical forms.

VINCENT'S ANGINA (NECROTIZING ULCERATIVE GINGIVITIS, TRENCH MOUTH)

Definition

Vincent's angina is an acute bacterial infection of the gingiva.

Incidence

Vincent's angina occurs in adults, and the incidence increases with age. This is probably related to the increased susceptibility to infections and changes in the oral cavity that occur with aging.

Etiology

This acute inflammatory gum disease is caused by resident flora in the mouth, fusiform bacteria, and spirochetes. Precipitating factors include poor oral hygiene, nutritional deficiencies, lack of rest and sleep, local tissue damage, and debilitative diseases such as infectious mononucleosis, nonspecific viral infections, bacterial infections, blood dyscrasias, and diabetes mellitus. This condition is not contagious.

Risk Factors

The above-mentioned precipitating factors are the major risk factors associated with this condition. Poor hygiene, nutritional deficiencies, and lack of rest and sleep are all avoidable.

Pathophysiology

When systemic disease lowers one's resistance, susceptibility to one's own flora increases. The disease has a sudden onset and causes erythema and ulceration of the gingiva. The disease affects the entire oropharynx. Once the tonsils are removed, this disorder rarely recurs.

Clinical Manifestations

Assessment reveals ulcers covered with a pseudomembrane. A smear from ulcer exudate identifies the causative organisms. Clients with Vincent's angina often have an elevated white blood cell count (WBC). The client may complain of a foul taste, pain, a choking sensation, fever, thick secretions, anorexia, and occasionally, lymphadenopathy.

Medical Management

Medical management consists of removing the devitalized tissue and correcting the underlying cause with rest, improved oral hygiene, a bland diet, and vitamins. Pain medications and peroxide mouthwashes promote comfort.

▼ Other Oral Disorders

CANDIDIASIS (MONILIASIS)

Definition

Candidiasis (thrush) is caused by the organism *Candida albicans* that is part of the normal flora of the oral cavity.

Incidence

Candidiasis of the oral cavity is commonly seen in clients who are immunosuppressed, such as those receiving chemotherapy or clients with HIV infection or AIDS. There is also a higher incidence in clients with diabetes mellitus and those who are pregnant, under stress, on high doses of or prolonged antibiotic therapy, or on prolonged periods of tube feeding.

Etiology

When the client becomes immunosuppressed or has a decrease in some of the normal oral flora, an overgrowth of the normal flora *Candida* can occur.

Risk Factors

The major risk factors are immunosuppression and the prolonged use of antibiotics that disrupts the normal flora. Clients with either risk factor should be monitored closely, and often, prophylactic treatment is started for these high-risk clients.

Pathophysiology

Candidiasis is a secondary infection resulting from either an immunodeficiency or prolonged use of antibiotics. When the normal flora is disrupted, an overgrowth of the *Candida* organism may occur.

Clinical Manifestations

Assessment reveals white patches on the tongue, palate, and buccal mucosa (Plate 13). These lesions adhere firmly to the tissues and are difficult to remove. The lesions are often referred to as milk curds because of their appearance. Clients will often describe the lesions as dry and hot. Clients who have recurrent candidiasis infections should be examined for a possible systemic cause.

Nursing Management

ASSESSMENT

The nurse should assess whether the client has pain, tenderness, bleeding in any part of the oral cavity, or any febrile episodes. The client should be questioned about a history of previous infection elsewhere in the body and the use of any medications such as antibiotics. The client also should be questioned about a history of treatment with radiation or chemotherapy, because both can affect the oral mucosa.

In order to perform the oral assessment, the nurse should have a tongue blade and good lighting. The nurse should inspect the oral cavity noting any areas of inflammation and whether vesicular eruptions, ulcers, white patches, or erythematous gingivae exist. The client should be examined by a dentist to rule out infection of dental origin.

NURSING INTERVENTION

Nursing Diagnosis: Pain R/T altered oral mucous membrane and ulcerations.

Planning: Expected Outcomes. The client will not have pain or will have pain controlled, as evidenced by the client verbalizing pain relief and the ability to maintain normal nutrition.

Implementation. The nurse must assess for oral pain and administer analgesics, such as aspirin or acetaminophen, as ordered. Topical agents and topical swishes often provide pain relief. A change in diet to liquid or pureed foods often eases the discomfort of eating. The client should avoid spicy foods, citrus juice, and hot liquids.

Clients with painful lesions cannot tolerate commercial mouthwashes because of the high alcohol concentration in these products. A solution of warm water, half-strength hydrogen peroxide, or mouthwash formulas specific to many institutions are better tolerated and may promote healing.

Collaborative Problem. High risk for infection R/T altered oral mucous membrane, ulcerations, and decreased resistance.

Planning: Expected Outcomes. Infection will not develop or will be controlled, as evidenced by healing of lesions, absence of fever or elevated WBC, and no evidence of secondary infection.

Implementation. If painful oral lesions are present, the nurse may suggest modifications in the client's oral hygiene regimen. Gauze pads may replace toothbrushes, and oral rinses may be needed to cleanse the area of debris and promote healing. Oral pharyngeal cultures should be taken if infection is suspected. Antibiotics and antifungal agents may be used when positive cultures are found. Antifungal agents are frequently given as oral liquids to swish and swallow.

EVALUATION

The nurse must evaluate client outcomes based on the established plan of care. If these goals were not achieved, the plan and interventions must be revised to meet the client's needs.

Post-hospital Care

DISCHARGE TEACHING

On discharge, the client should be given oral and written instructions regarding a dental hygiene regimen, diet, medications, and signs and symptoms of complications. The client should demonstrate to the nurse proper techniques of dental hygiene.

HOME HEALTH CARE NEEDS

Minimal home health care preparation is required unless the client requires alternate feeding routes. If the client is receiving tube feedings, referral to a home health care agency may be appropriate.

FOLLOW-UP CARE

The client should be followed by a physician or a dentist, or both, to assess for recurrence.

▼ TUMORS OF THE ORAL CAVITY

▼ Benign Tumors of the Oral Cavity

The most common benign tumors of the mouth are fibromas, lipomas, neurofibromas, and hemangiomas. As with benign tumors in other parts of the body, oral tumors cause problems primarily by occupying space and causing pressure. Benign tumors are usually excised if they cause functional or cosmetic problems.

▼ Premalignant Tumors of the Oral Cavity

LEUKOPLAKIA

Definition

Leukoplakia is a potentially precancerous, yellow-white or gray-white lesion. It may occur in any region of the mouth. The size and shape of lesions vary, but they are

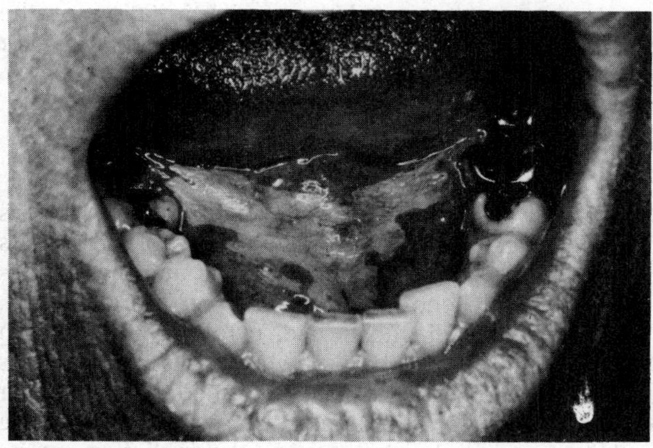

▲ Figure 53-4

Leukoplakia of floor of mouth. This lesion, which was symptomatic, had been present for 4 years and was related to cigarette smoking. (From Silverman, S., Jr. [1985]. Oral medicine. In J. B. Wyngaarden & L. H. Smith, Jr. [Eds.], *Cecil Textbook of Medicine* [17th ed.]. Philadelphia: W. B. Saunders Co., p. 666.)

usually elevated with a roughened or leathery surface and have clearly defined borders (Fig. 53-4).

Incidence

Leukoplakia is a common disorder of the oral mucous membranes, usually seen in the fifth decade of life. Men are twice as affected as women; however, the incidence in women is increasing.

Etiology

Leukoplakia results from chronic irritation of the mucosa by physical, thermal, or chemical factors. It also sometimes arises from systemic factors, such as poor nutrition or syphilis.

ERYTHROPLAKIA

Definition

Erythroplakia is a red, velvety-appearing patch that is often indicative of early squamous cell carcinoma.

Incidence

Erythroplakia occurs most frequently in the sixth and seventh decade of life, with men and women equally affected.

▼ Malignant Tumors of the Oral Cavity

Cancers of the oral cavity account for less than 5 per cent of total cases of body malignancies. Cancers in this area most frequently are seen in the fifth and sixth decades of life, affecting men more frequently than women. Cancers of the oral cavity are most often associated with alcohol consumption and tobacco use. With the increase of tobacco use in the younger age groups, especially the use of smokeless tobacco, and by women, the age and sex ratios are changing.

BASAL CELL CARCINOMA

Definition

Basal cell carcinoma of the oral cavity occurs primarily in the lips. It starts as a small scab that develops into an ulcer with a characteristic pearly border.

Incidence

Cancer of the mouth accounts for about 4 per cent of all cancers. Basal cell carcinoma is the second most common oral cancer.

Etiology

Basal cell carcinoma primarily occurs as a result of excessive exposure to sunlight. It tends to occur more commonly in fair-skinned individuals who are exposed to sunlight.

SQUAMOUS CELL CARCINOMA

Definition

Squamous cell carcinoma is a malignant growth arising from tiny flat squamous cells that line mucous membranes.

Incidence

Squamous cell carcinoma is the leading type of oral cancer. Most tumors occur in clients older than 45 years of age. Common sites of squamous cell carcinoma include the lower lip and the tongue. Approximately 95 per cent of cancers found on the tongue are squamous cell carcinomas. The tongue represents 1 to 1.5 per cent of all malignancies in the United States.

Etiology

The primary cause of squamous cell carcinoma is chronic irritation of the mucous lining of the mouth and oral cavity. The overuse of alcohol and tobacco are the primary causes of oral irritation. In combination, tobacco and alcohol are extremely destructive to the oral mucosa.

Risk Factors

There are a number of risk factors associated with squamous cell carcinoma of the oral cavity. Tobacco and alcohol are the primary risk factors, and primary prevention is simple if excessive use of these substances is avoided. Other risk factors include poor oral hygiene with bacterial irritation; physical trauma, as from jagged teeth or improperly fitting dentures; chemical and thermal trauma from tobacco, alcohol, oral tobaccos and snuff, or hot or spicy foods or drinks; malnutrition; syphilis or cirrhosis of the liver; and a family history of oral cancer.

Most of these risk factors are amenable to primary prevention such as use in moderation, good oral hygiene, and adequate nutrition.

Pathophysiology

Squamous cell carcinoma develops from tiny cells that line the oral cavity. It can occur on the lips, buccal mucosa, tongue, floor of the mouth, and tonsils (Fig. 53-5). Squamous cell carcinoma is usually well differentiated and has a less than 10 per cent metastasis rate. Cells metastasize by direct infiltration of local lymph nodes and can extend into the buccal fat and even to the mandible.

Clinical Manifestations

Symptoms of squamous cell carcinoma may include the presence of a sore or lesion in the oral cavity. Red-appearing (erythroplakia) squamous cell carcinomas may not be well delineated and often bleed easily. Because squamous cell carcinomas usually grow slowly, they may be large before symptoms are detected.

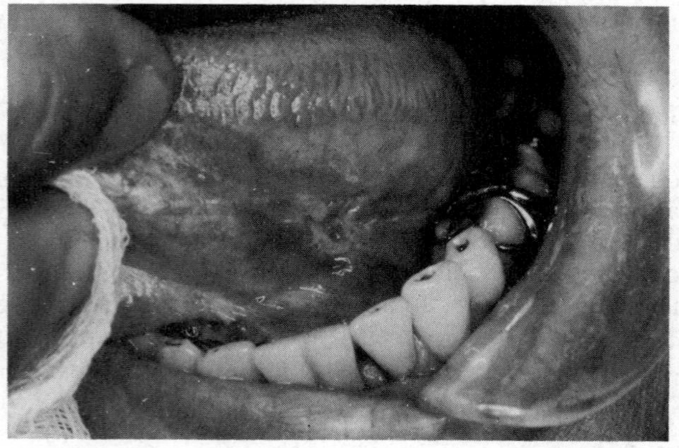

▲ **Figure 53-5**

Oral squamous carcinoma. This early cancer at the junction of the tongue and mouth floor was noticed 3 weeks earlier. It was at first mistaken for a traumatic ulcer. (From Silverman, S., Jr. [1985]. Oral medicine. In J. B. Wyngaarden, & L. H. Smith, Jr. [Eds.], *Cecil Textbook of Medicine* [17th ed.]. Philadelphia: W. B. Saunders Co., p. 667.)

Other symptoms can include a mild irritation of the tongue, sore throat, trouble with wearing dentures, or pain in the tongue or ear.

Diagnostic Assessment

Only biopsy of lesions positively confirms a diagnosis of oral cancer. Cytologic examination of suspicious mucosa, while valuable in screening, unfortunately is not used widely enough to reduce the mortality rate. To be a valuable diagnostic aid, cytologic examination must be followed by biopsy when questionable cells are found. Biopsies may be performed with local or general anesthesia. To diagnose carcinoma at the base of the tongue, a laryngoscopic examination must be performed.

Medical Management

The survival rate for clients with oral cancer depends on the site and staging of the tumor (Table 53-1). Cancer of the lip has one of the highest cure rates of oral cancers. Squamous cell carcinoma of the tongue has the poorest prognosis because of the tongue's extensive vascular and lymphatic supply. Management of oral cancers includes radiation therapy, chemotherapy, and surgery, and again depends on the site and staging of the tumor.

Treatment of oral cancers with radiation can be given by external beam or interstitial radiation therapy. The external beam passes through the skin or mucous membrane to the tumor. Interstitial radiation involves implanting radioactive seeds into the tissue for a specific period of time. Because interstitial radiation affects local tissue, it is used for small lesions that have not infiltrated the surrounding tissue. The client with interstitial radiation is hospitalized and placed on radiation precautions while the materials are active (see Chap. 22).

PHARMACOLOGIC MANAGEMENT

The effectiveness of chemotherapy for the treatment of oral cancers remains to be determined. Several chemotherapeutic agents are used to treat clients with head and neck cancers (Box 53-1).

Surgical Management

Surgical management of oral cancers can range from local excision of small tumors to extensive surgery for invasive tumors. Small tumors can be treated in outpatient facilities by local excision, radiation, or laser therapy. Small tumors of the floor of the mouth can be locally excised with or without removing a portion of the mandible. Small tumors in the anterior floor of the mouth can be excised and the area reconstructed with the use of a split-thickness skin graft. A thin layer of skin, usually from the anterior thigh, can line the surgi-

TABLE 53-1. TNM Staging of Cancers of the Lip and Oral Cavity

Primary Tumor (T)

TX	Primary tumor cannot be assessed
T0	No evidence of primary tumor
Tis	Carcinoma in situ
T1	Tumor 2 cm or less in greatest dimension
T2	Tumor more than 2 cm but not more than 4 cm in greatest dimension
T3	Tumor more than 4 cm in greatest dimension
T4 (lip)	Tumor invades adjacent structures (e.g., through cortial bone, tongue, skin of neck)
T4 (oral cavity)	Tumor invades adjacent structures (e.g., through cortical bone, into deep [extrinsic] muscle of tongue, maxillary sinus, skin)

Regional Lymph Nodes (N)

NX	Regional lymph nodes cannot be assessed
N0	No regional lymph node metastasis
N1	Metastasis in a single ipsilateral lymph node, 3 cm or less in greatest dimension
N2	Metastasis in a single ipsilateral lymph node, more than 3 cm but not more than 6 cm in greatest dimension; or in multiple ipsilateral lymph nodes, none more than 6 cm in greatest imension; or in bilateral or contralateral lymph nodes, none more than 6 cm in greatest dimension
N2a	Metastasis in a single ipsilateral lymph node more than 3 cm but not more than 6 cm in greatest dimension
N2b	Metastasis in multiple ipsilateral lymph nodes, none more than 6 cm in greatest dimension
N2c	Metastasis in bilateral or contralateral lymph nodes, none more than 6 cm in greatest dimension
N3	Metastasis in a lymph node more than 6 cm in greatest dimension

Distant Metastasis (M)

MX	Presence of distant metastasis cannot be assessed
M0	No distant metastasis
M1	Distant metastasis

Stage Grouping

Stage 0	Tis	N0	M0
Stage I	T1	N0	M0
Stage II	T2	N0	M0
Stage III	T3	N0	M0
	T1	N1	M0
	T2	N1	M0
	T3	N1	M0
Stage IV	T4	N0, N1	M0
	Any T	N2, N3	M0
	Any T	Any N	M1

cal site, allowing the client to maintain good mobility and function of the tongue. Xeroform gauze is usually placed over the skin graft and sutured into place. This can restrict the tongue, causing aspiration of secretions. Because of this packing and as a result of postoperative edema, a tracheostomy tube is usually placed until edema subsides and the oral airway is patent. The client receives nothing by mouth for 7 to 10 days after surgery to allow for healing. A feeding tube (nasogastric, gastrostomy, or percutaneous endoscopic gastrostomy [PEG]; see Chap. 54) is used to provide nutrition until the client can resume oral feedings.

Invasive tumors require extensive surgical excision and usually involve removal of associated lymph nodes. Depending on the location, procedures may include a glossectomy (removal of the tongue), mandibulectomy (removal of the mandible), or hemiglossectomy (removal of part of the tongue). A radical neck dissection is an extensive procedure that involves removal of all tissue under the skin, from the jaw down to the clavicle, and from the anterior border of the trapezius muscle to the midline. To remove the cervical lymph nodes in this procedure, the sternocleidomastoid muscle, the spinal accessory nerve, and the jugular vein have to be removed. A modified radical neck dissection involves removal of the lymph nodes only and is preferred when the disease is confined to mobile lymph nodes. (see surgical management of cancer of the larynx). The commando procedure is a very extensive oral operation in which part of the mandible is excised along with the oral lesion. This procedure is often combined with a radical neck dissection.

Nursing Management

ASSESSMENT

The nurse should carefully question the client about his or her symptoms. A common finding is that of a painful ulcer. The client should also be assessed for difficulty in swallowing, white or red patches on the oral mucosa, bleeding in the mouth, lumps in the neck, pain referred to the ear, foul odor, and hoarseness. The nurse should question the client concerning the use of

Box 53-1. Chemotherapeutic Agent Used in the Treatment of Head and Neck Cancers

- Bleomycin
- Cisplatin
- Cyclophosphamide
- Doxorubicin (Adriamycin)
- 5-Fluorouracil
- Hydroxyurea
- Methotrexate
- Vincristine

alcohol and tobacco, oral hygiene habits, and exposure to the sun. The nurse must also assess the rehabilitative needs of the client. Surgery can result in disfigurement and alterations in speech, and can cause the client to experience depression related to a change in body image.

NURSING INTERVENTION

Nursing Diagnosis: Knowledge Deficit R/T prevention of oral lesions and treatment of lesions should they occur.

Planning: Expected Outcomes. Client will understand and comply with measures to maintain oral mucosa, as evidenced by statements of understanding of substances and activities to avoid, no evidence of lesions, and verbalization of understanding of treatment regimen, including surgery.

Implementation. The nurse should teach the client about the disease itself and treatment protocols. Because irritation is related to the development of leukoplakia, instruct the client to eliminate tobacco, very hot drinks, and spicy foods. If dentures fit poorly, the client needs to consult with a dentist immediately for new ones. Give the client with poor nutrition guidelines for improving the diet. Supply pamphlets outlining the basic nutrients for good health, and refer the client to a dietician as needed.

Again, the best intervention for oral cancers is prevention. Advise clients to

- Avoid chemical, physical, and thermal oral trauma;
- Perform careful, frequent oral hygiene, preferably three times daily;
- See a dentist if they have ill-fitting dentures; and
- See a physician for any mouth lesion that does not heal in 2 to 3 weeks.

If the client is receiving radiation or chemotherapy, the nurse should instruct the client about possible side effects of these forms of treatment. The nurse should provide the client with comfort measures to minimize the side effects, such as using antiemetics to prevent nausea and vomiting.

If the client is scheduled for a surgical resection, the nurse should ensure that the client understands the procedure to be performed and all implications (such as a temporary or permanent tracheostomy). The client should receive adequate support before surgery to help the client cope with a possibly radically altered appearance. Instructions regarding postoperative procedures will depend on the extent of the surgical resection. Clients should be instructed on the need for frequent vital signs, intravenous activity, the availability of analgesics for pain, and oxygen therapy after surgery. The purpose and care involved with a feeding tube also should be explained.

Nursing Diagnosis: Nutrition, Altered: Less than Body Requirements R/T oral pain and difficulty eating and swallowing.

Planning: Expected Outcomes. The client will maintain weight or show weight gain before surgery, as evidenced by an increase in intake, weight remaining stable, or weight gain of 1 pound/week preoperatively.

Implementation. The location, size, and pain associated with a tumor often interferes with the client's ability to eat. Small, frequent feedings often promote intake. Administering an analgesic 30 to 45 minutes prior to a meal often decreases pain associated with eating. The nurse should provide oral care before and after meals to remove oral odors and debris.

Unfortunately, treatments such as radiation alter salivation and taste perception. Xerostomia (dryness of the mouth) usually improves with the use of pilocarpine and artificial saliva. Suggest that the client chew sugarless gum or suck on sugarless candy drops to increase moisture. The client should perform frequent oral rinses with cool water to reduce dryness.

Nursing Diagnosis: Injury, High Risk for R/T surgical procedure, including hemorrhage, ineffective airway clearance, and possible wound infection.

Planning: Expected Outcomes. The client will not develop injury, as evidenced by absence of excessive bleeding, maintenance of a patent airway, and wound healing without signs of infection.

Implementation. The extent of nursing care required by the client after surgery depends on the extent of the procedure. After local excisions, the nurse teaches the client how to perform hygiene gently. If a dressing and packing are in place, the nurse monitors the amount of drainage. After the dressing and packing are removed, the client should rinse the oral cavity with a mild half-strength form of hydrogen peroxide and water or saline solution every 4 hours to remove debris and promote healing.

With more extensive surgery, the suture lines must be protected from trauma. Oral hygiene and oral suctioning are usually not implemented until healing has begun and the physician decides this type of cleaning can be performed.

Hemorrhage can occur at any time, from the first few days after surgery to several days after surgery. Hemorrhage can be massive because of the large vessels that supply the mouth and oral area. Should bleeding occur, apply local pressure on the site until the physician can be notified. Surgical repair may be required. If an extensive resection was performed requiring skin grafts, the nurse should monitor the site every shift for drainage and for signs of infection.

The most critical postoperative intervention is to maintain a patent airway. If the surgical procedure has been extensive, there is usually a tracheostomy in place, which helps prevent respiratory difficulty arising from edema of the oral and pharyngeal structures. Clients at risk for ineffective airway clearance should be in semi to high Fowler's position after surgery to promote venous lymphatic drainage. The client may have a dusky appearance about the face from venous congestion. Pulse oximeter readings also should be used to determine whether or not the client is sufficiently oxygenated.

For the client with a tracheostomy, some blood-tinged mucus is normal in tracheal secretions for the first 48 hours after surgery. Bright red bleeding from the tracheostomy tube or site is a sign of hemorrhage.

Nursing Diagnosis: Nutrition, Altered: Less than Body Requirements R/T altered oral mucosa and surgical procedure.

Planning: Expected Outcomes. The client will maintain or gain weight after surgery, as evidenced by a stabilization of weight and possibly a 1 pound/week weight gain.

Implementation. Immediately after surgery, the nurse should monitor intravenous hydration. Bowel sounds should be assessed every shift. The return of bowel sounds is often an indication to begin tube feedings. Before each tube feeding, the nurse should properly assess the client for proper tube placement (see Chap. 54). Nutritional supplements may be administered by pump or bolus feedings.

Once the edema has subsided, adequate healing has occurred, and the tracheostomy tube has been removed, the client may be restarted on oral feedings. The client should be cautioned about a decrease in sensation in the oral cavity after surgery. Swallowing should be carefully assessed before the client begins to eat, and the client should be taught to avoid putting food directly on the surgical resection site. After meals, the client should always perform good oral hygiene.

Nursing Diagnosis: Impaired Verbal Communication R/T presence of tracheostomy.

Planning: Expected Outcomes. Client will be able to communicate using alternate forms of communication, as evidenced by ability to continue communication with staff and significant others.

Implementation. The nurse should help clients who cannot communicate verbally to express their needs, concerns, and feelings. The nurse should assess the client's literacy and then provide paper for the client to write on as a substitute for talking or provide the client with a picture board to use for communicating any needs. The nurse should check on the client frequently to reduce any anxiety and loneliness. The nurse also should place the call light within easy reach and respond to the light in person promptly.

The client should be allowed to communicate by gestures or written notes if this approach puts the client at ease. Most important, the nurse's manner should communicate acceptance, compassion, and caring. It is common to treat clients who cannot talk as though they cannot hear or understand. Be alert to any tendency to treat these clients as though they were mentally incompetent or deaf. The nurse should help the client avoid social isolation by taking the client for walks and meeting others. Friendly social encounters and physical activity can help alleviate depression in this client.

EVALUATION

The nurse must evaluate client outcomes based on the established plan of care. If these goals were not achieved, the plan and interventions must be revised to meet the client's needs.

Post-hospital Care

DISCHARGE TEACHING

On discharge, the nurse should supply the client and family with complete instructions regarding diet, medications, signs and symptoms of complications, and any treatments such as wound or tracheostomy care.

HOME CARE NEEDS

Clients who have undergone extensive surgery may need a referral to a home health care agency for possible assistance with respiratory support (home oxygen), nutritional support, and wound care.

FOLLOW-UP CARE

The client will need to be seen by the physician after discharge to ensure complete healing of any extensive surgical wounds. If the client has a tracheostomy, it may be permanent or may be closed at a later date.

▼ DISORDERS OF THE SALIVARY GLANDS

INFLAMMATION

Parotitis, also known as surgical mumps, involves inflammation of the parotid glands. It is the most common inflammatory condition affecting the salivary glands. Inflammation probably results from inactivity of the gland caused by certain medications, such as diuretics, and lack of oral intake, such as that seen in postoperative clients. As secretions of the salivary glands diminish, oral bacteria have an opportunity to invade the gland and multiply. Interventions involve

- Administering frequent oral hygiene to keep the bacterial count of the mouth low,
- Keeping the client well hydrated, and

▸ Suggesting that the client use sugarless hard candies or chew sugarless gum to stimulate secretions of the glands.

CALCULI

Stones, or calculi, form in the salivary glands when the glands are inactive and the client has a metabolic condition favoring the precipitation of salts. A focus or nidus is necessary for stimulating salt precipitation. Assessment reveals that irritation from the stones causes local inflammation, swelling, and pain when the gland is stimulated to secrete, as during chewing. Intervention requires local excision. Stones occur most commonly in the submaxillary glands, probably because of (1) the longer length of the duct and (2) production of viscous alkaline secretions.

TUMORS

Most tumors in the salivary glands are benign. The most frequently seen malignant tumor is adenocarcinoma. Both types of tumors are characterized by enlargement. Pain occurs when expansion within the capsule of the gland creates pressure on sensory nerves. The treatment of choice for both benign and malignant tumors is usually surgical excision. If the tumor has recurred or is highly malignant, radiation therapy may be used.

▼ DISORDERS OF THE ESOPHAGUS

The esophagus is a muscular tube that begins at the base of the pharynx and ends below the diaphragm. Its primary purpose is to transport a bolus of food from the mouth to the stomach while preventing reflux of gastric contents. The most common symptom of esophageal disease is dysphagia. Other symptoms include regurgitation, pain (which is probably linked with spasm), and heartburn.

DYSPHAGIA

Dysphagia, or difficulty with swallowing, can be caused by any esophageal disorder. Specific causes include neuromotor malfunction, such as cerebrovascular accident (CVA), the most common cause of dysphagia; mechanical obstruction, such as tumors of the larynx; cardiovascular abnormalities, such as aneurysms; and neurologic diseases, such as multiple sclerosis.

Mechanical Obstruction

Mechanical obstructions causing dysphagia include congenital defects (see Foster's *Family-Centered Nursing Care of Children*), carcinoma, and acquired conditions such as hiatal hernia. When an obstruction narrows the esophageal lumen, clients first experience dysphagia only with solid foods. Later, dysphagia becomes associated with semisolid foods and liquids. Finally, these clients are unable to swallow their own saliva. Obstructive disorders, particularly esophageal carcinoma, may be accompanied by weight loss and cachexia.

Cardiovascular Abnormalities

Dysphagia also may result from cardiovascular abnormalities, particularly in the elderly. Specific conditions that cause vascular dysphagia include an enlarged heart, an aortic aneurysm, and calcification of the descending aorta. Figure 53-6 demonstrates the relationship of the heart and great arteries to the esophagus.

Neurologic Diseases

Dysphagia also may be caused by certain neurologic diseases such as CVA, multiple sclerosis, poliomyelitis, and amyotrophic lateral sclerosis.

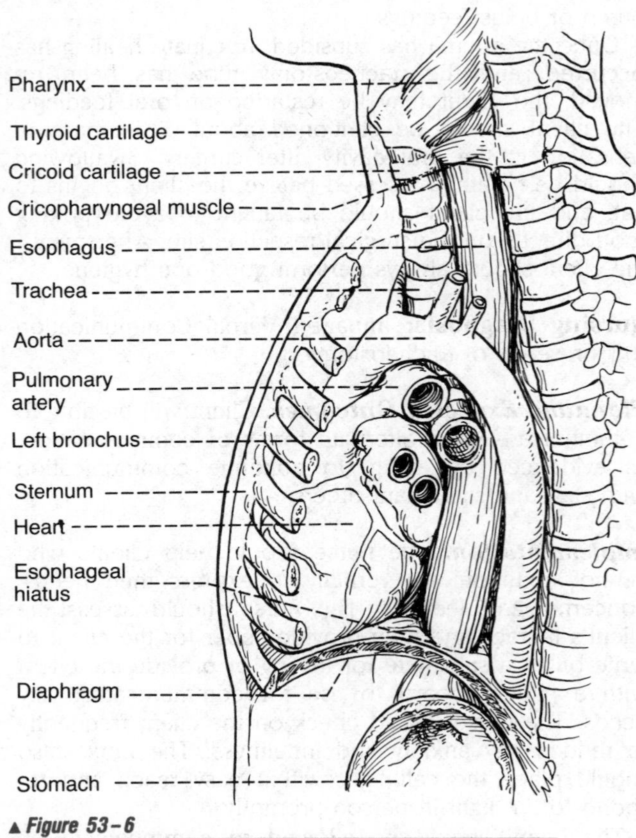

▲ **Figure 53-6**

Relationship of the heart and great arteries to the esophagus.

Other Causes

Dysphagia can be experienced after swallowing if food gets caught in the esophagus. Relief may be obtained by drinking liquids to force the impacted bolus through the narrow segment, or retching may dislodge the food.

REGURGITATION

Regurgitation is the ejection of small amounts of chyme or gastric juice from the mouth without antecedent nausea. It is usually caused by an incompetent lower esophageal sphincter (LES). Regurgitation occurring immediately after swallowing results from structural or motor abnormality in the LES. Factors contributing to regurgitation include abnormal motor activity, increased abdominal pressure, and sphincter abnormality. Regurgitation occurs with pylorospasm, lesions proximal to the cardia, achalasia, hiatal hernia, reflux esophagitis, and esophageal ulcer or malignancy. Stooping or lying down facilitates the flow of gastric contents into the esophagus, thus exacerbating regurgitation.

PAIN

Pain, which sometimes is constant and may occur only with swallowing, suggests diffuse esophageal spasm. Pain may result from alterations of the mucosa due to reflux disease, radiation, or viral infection. Pain that affects the esophageal mucosa and occurs with swallowing is called odynophagia. The client usually describes the pain as sharp, constricting, sticking, crushing, stabbing, or knifelike. Odynophagia is usually severe, quite distressing, and often associated with a deep and long-lasting pain. The pain, located substernally, may radiate to the neck, back, upper thorax, and shoulder. Pain may occur throughout the day and can be confused with angina. Odynophagia can be triggered by a cold, or carbonated beverage or solid food passing through the esophagus. The most common cause is the reflux of gastric contents into the esophagus.

HEARTBURN

Heartburn (pyrosis, indigestion, or dyspepsia) is another common manifestation of esophageal disease. Generally, it is a painful sensation of warmth and burning in the lower retrosternal midline. Clients may use the term "heartburn" to describe very different sensations. Therefore, find out exactly what this term means to the client experiencing the symptom. Heartburn usually means substernal, midline burning, which tends to radiate, generally in waves, upward to the neck because of abnormalities of the LES. Clients often describe this discomfort as cramping or knotting. Heartburn is often experienced with postural changes such as bending, stooping, or lifting, as well as when someone gulps food or liquids or ingests alcohol. Symptoms often are relieved by standing. Heartburn also arises in the presence of refluxed gastric or duodenal contents. Disorders most commonly associated with heartburn are reflux esophagitis, hiatal hernia, achalasia, and gastric stasis. Heartburn is common in clients with pyloric or duodenal ulcers and LES disorders.

There are many pathologic conditions of the esophagus. Achalasia, diffuse spasm, gastroesophageal reflux disease, hiatal hernia, diverticula, and esophageal neoplasms are discussed in the following section.

ACHALASIA

Definition

Achalasia is a disorder characterized by progressively increasing dysphagia, with the client eventually having great difficulty swallowing and expressing the feeling that "something is stuck in the throat."

Incidence

Achalasia commonly occurs in the third to fourth decades of life and appears with equal incidence in men and in women.

Etiology

Achalasia is a chronic, progressive disease that is considered idiopathic in origin. Occasionally, the client can relate the onset to an episode of acute dysphagia, but usually achalasia has an obscure onset and is only noticed when the dysphagia becomes severe.

Risk Factors

Because achalasia is an idiopathic condition, there are no identified risk factors. It is believed there may be a familial incidence of achalasia.

Pathophysiology

Achalasia is characterized by impaired motility of the lower two thirds of the esophagus. The LES fails to relax normally with swallowing.[22] Inadequate functioning occurs because (1) nerve impulses are unable to pass through the esophagus or (2) sympathetic receptors are absent from the LES. There also may be degeneration of the ganglion cells or impairment of impulses from Auerbach's plexus (see Chap. 51). Impaired propulsion and a constricted LES result in accumulation of food and fluid within the lower esophagus. When hydrostatic pressure exceeds the force of resistance of the LES, the contents pass into the stomach.

Complications

Complications of achalasia include esophagitis with resultant ulceration. Aspiration of regurgitated esophageal contents may result in atelectasis and other pulmonary problems.

Clinical Manifestations

The initial symptom of achalasia is dysphagia. Food and fluid do not pass through the region of the LES. In the early stages of achalasia, the client also may have substernal pain due to spasms of the esophagus or may be unable to belch. The client may regurgitate undigested food eaten many hours earlier as well as large amounts of mucus that have been stimulated by esophageal irritation. As achalasia progresses, symptoms increase in frequency and severity. Upper respiratory infections, emotional disturbances, overeating, and pregnancy may aggravate the problem.

Diagnostic Assessment

Diagnostic tests used to determine the presence of achalasia include the barium swallow, endoscopy, and manometry. The barium swallow is considered positive for achalasia if it reveals nonpropulsive waves and esophageal dilation. Also, barium may be retained. Endoscopy helps determine the status of the LES, dilation, and the presence of food. Manometry (measurement of pressure in the esophagus) confirms the diagnosis.

Medical Management

Treatment of achalasia is aimed at relieving symptoms.

PHARMACOLOGIC MANAGEMENT

Medications have been investigated that relax the LES or lower esophageal pressures, such as anticholinergic drugs, gastrointestinal hormones, and calcium channel blockers. Pain is controlled with non-narcotic and narcotic analgesics.

DIETARY MANAGEMENT

Changes in diet can often ease the pressure and reflux in the client with achalasia. Small, frequent feedings ease the passage of food, and semisoft, warm foods are better tolerated than cold, hard foods. The client should avoid hot, spicy, and iced foods as well as alcohol and tobacco. All foods should be chewed thoroughly to add saliva to the mixture, providing lubrication and allowing the bolus to pass more easily from the esophagus to the stomach. The client should experiment with different positions to reduce pressure while eating. To prevent nocturnal reflux of food, the client should sleep with the head of the bed elevated.

Surgical Management

Surgical management of achalasia can involve dilating the esophageal sphincter (esophageal dilation) or enlarging the sphincter (esophagomyotomy). Esophageal dilation or bougienage forcefully dilates the lower esophagus and sphincter (Fig. 53-7). It is used to help correct not only achalasia but esophageal spasms and strictures. Vigorous dilatation has a 75% success rate. This procedure is performed with a local anesthesia under radiologic guidance.

A more complex procedure, esophagomyotomy (Heller's procedure) may have to be performed. In this procedure, the surgeon enlarges the vestibule by incising the circular muscle fibers down to the mucosa (Fig. 53-8). Complications of esophagomyotomy include reflux esophagitis and re-stenosis. If a client cannot swallow for long periods, a gastrostomy tube may be inserted. There are two methods to insert a gastrostomy tube. The first involves making an incision in the wall of the abdomen and suturing the tube to the gastric wall. The second method is called a PEG. Under local anesthesia, the physician inserts a cannula into the stomach through an abdominal incision. A suture is threaded through the cannula. A second physician uses an endoscope to pull the suture through the client's mouth. The PEG tube is attached and advanced down the esophagus, through the abdominal incision, where it is secured internally and externally by crossbars (Fig. 53-9).

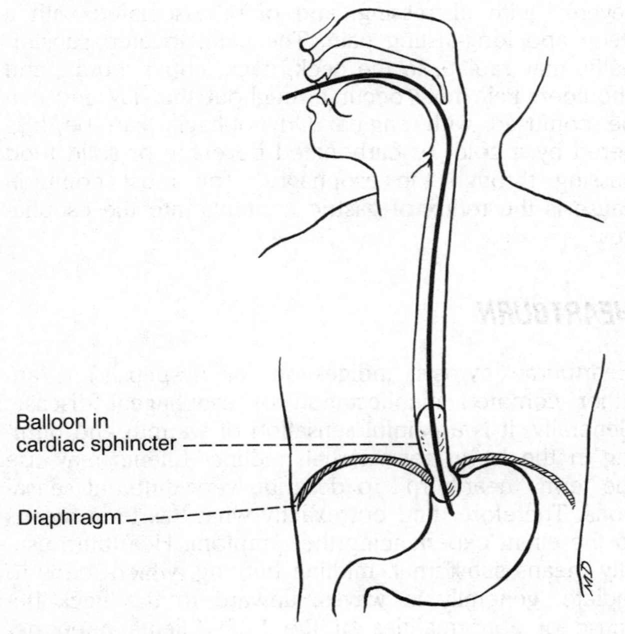

▲ **Figure 53-7**

Bougienage relieves dysphagia by dilating the lower esophageal sphincter.

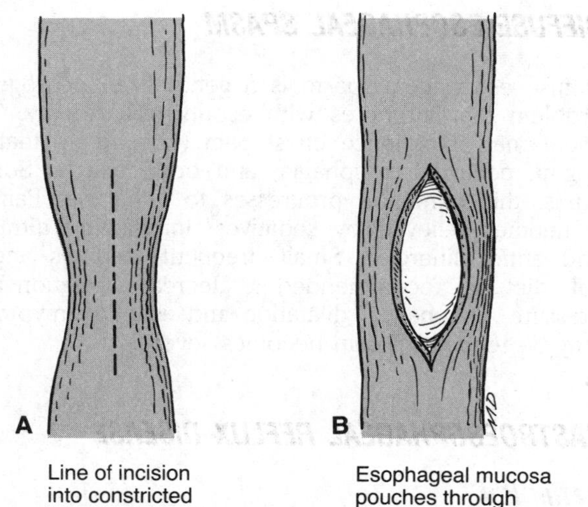

▲ **Figure 53–8**

Esophagomyotomy (Heller's procedure) is the surgical procedure of choice when a segment of esophagus narrows and causes functional obstruction.

Nursing Management

ASSESSMENT

The nurse needs to obtain a history noting the symptoms the client is experiencing. The onset and duration of symptoms with factors that aggravate symptoms should be assessed. The nurse should note any methods the client uses for relief.

Respiratory symptoms also should be assessed because the respiratory tract can be affected with reflux or regurgitation. The nurse should assess the client's nutritional status, noting any weight changes and the effects of esophageal symptoms on dietary habits and the client's respiratory status.

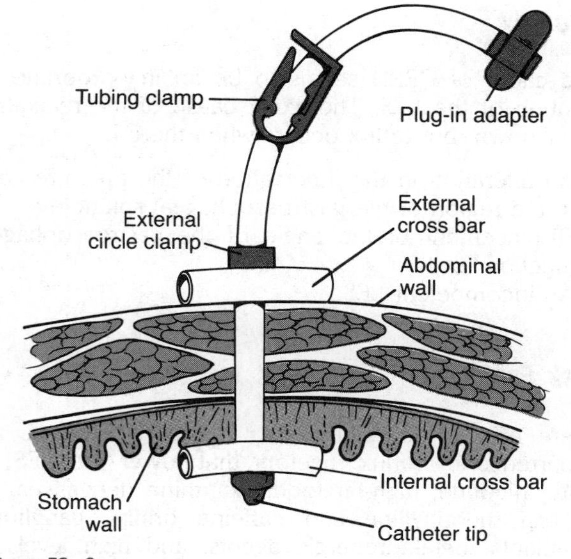

▲ **Figure 53–9**

Abdomen with PEG.

NURSING INTERVENTION

Nursing Diagnosis: Nutrition, Altered: Less than Body Requirements R/T dysphagia.

Planning: Expected Outcomes. The client will maintain an adequate nutritional intake, as evidenced by maintenance of ideal body weight or gaining back any weight lost at a rate of 1 pound/week.

Implementation. The nurse should consult with the client concerning dietary habits and assess the client's intake of nutrients daily. A baseline weight should be obtained, and the client should be weighed daily. The nurse should teach the client about changes in dietary habits that may relieve symptoms.

Nursing Diagnosis: Pain, Acute and Chronic, R/T episodes of gastric reflux.

Planning: Expected Outcomes. The client will experience a decrease in pain or absence of pain, as evidenced by the client verbalizing a decrease in or absence of pain and the client's ability to maintain oral intake.

Implementation. As stated, pain can be decreased or relieved through the use of medications, dietary changes, and repositioning the client. The nurse should assess the client every shift to determine whether or not the use of medications, changes in diet, and positioning were effective in controlling or relieving pain.

Nursing Diagnosis: Knowledge Deficit R/T preoperative preparation.

Planning: Expected Outcomes. The client will understand and be adequately prepared for surgery, as evidenced by client questions and statements of understanding.

Implementation. Clients undergoing esophageal dilatation should be told that they will be awake during the procedure. A local anesthetic will be sprayed on the throat, and the client may receive an analgesic or tranquilizer. The client should take long slow breaths during the passage of the bougies. As the bag is inflated, the client may feel a brief feeling of discomfort. Esophageal dilatation is often performed on an outpatient basis.

Esophagomyotomy is a more complex procedure. The client will require a general anesthetic and remain hospitalized for several days. The nurse should instruct the client undergoing an esophageal procedure about all usual preoperative procedures, such as taking nothing by mouth after midnight, intravenous fluids, and preoperative medications. The nurse should also discuss pain control, chest tubes, drains, surgical dressings, and the presence of a nasogastric or gastric tube.

Collaborative Problem. High risk for injury R/T surgical procedure and presence of chest tubes.

Planning: Expected Outcomes. Injury will be prevented, as evidenced by absence of hemorrhage, no signs of perforation, normal temperature, and absence of signs of problems associated with the chest tubes such as respiratory distress.

Implementation. After the performance of esophageal dilatation, the nurse should monitor the client for signs of perforation, such as elevated temperature, chest or shoulder pain, and subcutaneous emphysema. If any of these manifestations are noted, the nurse should notify the physician immediately. The client will require an x-ray study to determine whether or not air is in the mediastinum, indicating perforation.

After an esophagomyotomy, the client will have a thoracotomy incision and chest tubes in place. The nurse will need to maintain chest tube drainage, the nasogastric or gastric drainage system, and manage the client's pain. (See Chap. 37 for care of the client with chest tubes.)

EVALUATION

The nurse must evaluate client outcomes based on the established plan of care. If these goals were not achieved, the plan and interventions must be revised to meet the client's needs.

Modification of Plan of Care for the Elderly

In older adults, an attempt is made to treat the client with more local measures (pain medications, positioning, and dietary modification) and, possibly, esophageal dilatation.

Post-hospital Care

DISCHARGE TEACHING

The client should receive written and oral instructions regarding diet, medications, and symptoms of respiratory complications related to esophageal reflux and aspiration.

Clients who have undergone an esophagomyotomy should be instructed to sleep with the head of the bed elevated and recognize signs and symptoms of respiratory complications. The client should be instructed about signs and symptoms of infection and esophageal perforation, and instructed to notify the physician if any of these problems occur.

HOME HEALTH CARE NEEDS

A home health care agency should be consulted to assist the client with any home health care needs related to medications, wound care, and diet, and to provide an ongoing evaluation of the client's condition. A referral to a social worker also might be needed to assist the client with financial assistance, counseling, and specialized equipment.

DIFFUSE ESOPHAGEAL SPASM

Diffuse esophageal spasm is a generalized neurogenic problem that interferes with esophageal motility. The client may experience chest pain (resembling that of angina pectoris), dysphagia, and odynophagia. Sometimes, this condition progresses to achalasia. Pain is sometimes relieved by sedatives, long-acting nitrates, and anticholinergics. Small, frequent feedings and a soft diet are recommended to decrease irritation and pressure. Esophageal dilatation and esophagomyotomy may be required if pain becomes severe.

GASTROESOPHAGEAL REFLUX DISEASE

Definition

Esophageal reflux is defined as the backward flow of gastric contents into the esophagus. Gastroesophageal reflux disease (GERD) is a term used to describe a syndrome resulting from esophageal reflux. Reflux exposes the esophageal mucosa to the gastric contents and gradually breaks down the esophageal mucosa. This condition is sometimes referred to as reflux esophagitis. This reflux is often associated with a sliding hiatal hernia. However, reflux causing complications can occur without a hiatal hernia, and clients with a hiatal hernia may not have symptoms of reflux.

Incidence

GERD can occur in any age group. It is estimated that 10 per cent of the population has daily symptoms from GERD and as much as one third of the population has monthly symptoms.[13] Symptoms are often overlooked and attributed to stress.

Etiology

The cause of GERD seems to be an inappropriate relaxation of the LES. The exact cause of the relaxation is unknown, but reflux occurs when there is

- An alteration in the innervation of the pressure zone in the region of the gastroesophageal sphincter;
- Displacement of the angle of the gastroesophageal junction; and
- An incompetent LES.

Risk Factors

There are several factors that seem to increase the occurrence of reflux. Factors that lower the LES include nicotine; high-fat foods; xanthine derivatives, including theophylline and caffeine drinks; ganglionic stimulants; beta-adrenergic agents; and high levels of estrogen and progesterone.

Avoiding some of the agents is possible, such as

caffeinated drinks, smoking, and high-fat foods. If specific medications are implicated, the client can be warned about the occurrence of GERD and counseled on methods to relieve the irritation.

Pathophysiology

Normally, a high-pressure zone exists in the region of the gastroesophageal sphincter. High-pressure prevents reflux but permits the passage of food and liquids. When there is an alteration in this region, reflux occurs.

Reflux esophagitis also may occur with gastric or duodenal ulcer, after esophageal or gastric surgery, after prolonged vomiting, or after prolonged gastrointestinal intubation. The reflux most often consists of hydrochloric acid or gastric and duodenal contents containing bile acid and pancreatic juice. Frequent or prolonged reflux results in inflammation of the esophageal mucosa (esophagitis). The degree of reflux esophagitis present depends on the (1) frequency of the reflux, (2) contents of the gastric reflux, (3) buffering ability of the saliva and mucus secretion, and (4) rate of gastric emptying.

Clinical Manifestations

Clients with GERD may experience a sudden or gradual onset of symptoms. The client may complain of heartburn, odynophagia, dysphagia, acid regurgitation, water brash (the release of salty secretions in the mouth), or eructation. Pain in GERD is typically referred to as a burning sensation that moves up and down. If the condition is severe, the pain may radiate to the back, neck, or jaw. Pain usually occurs after meals and is relieved with antacids or fluids. Discomfort sometimes accompanies activities that increase intra-abdominal pressure, such as lifting or straining. The client may state that discomfort occurs when lying supine or when the stomach is distended. Discomfort may be relieved by standing and walking. Dysphagia resulting from edema, spasm, or a narrowed lumen is intermittent and worse at the beginning of meals. Responses to pain-relieving measures (e.g., nitroglycerin) help to differentiate between esophagitis and problems of cardiac origin (e.g., angina pectoris).

Diagnostic Assessment

Diagnosis rests on the demonstration of reflux. Barium swallow, esophageal manometry, esophagoscopy, esophageal biopsy, cytologic examination, analysis of gastric secretions, and acid perfusion tests confirm the diagnosis of GERD (see Chap. 51).

Medical Management

PHARMACOLOGIC MANAGEMENT

Drug therapy for GERD usually starts with antacid therapy. Antacid therapy often provides prompt relief. Typically, the client takes 30 ml of antacid 1 hour before and 2 to 3 hours after each meal. Clients typically tolerate combination products such as Mylanta or Maalox. Gaviscon is another excellent antacid because of its foaming action.

If symptoms are severe or persist, the client may be prescribed histamine receptor antagonists such as ranitidine (Zantac) or famotidine (Pepcid). Bethanechol (Urecholine) may be added for clients with severe symptoms because it has been found to increase LES pressure and prevent reflux. Because bethanechol is a cholinergic drug, it is usually given with antacids and a histamine receptor antagonist because it can increase the secretion of gastric acid. It should be taken before meals.

Metoclopramide (Reglan) may be prescribed because it increases LES pressure by stimulating the smooth muscle of the gastrointestinal tract and increasing the rate of gastric emptying. It is taken before meals.

Anticholinergic drugs, calcium channel blockers, and theophylline should be avoided because they appear to decrease LES pressure or delay gastric emptying.

DIETARY MANAGEMENT

In mild cases of GERD, diet changes may be sufficient to relieve symptoms. The prescribed regimen of therapy should include having the client

- Restrict the diet to small, frequent feedings (4 to 6/day);
- Drink adequate fluids at meals to assist food passage;
- Eat slowly and chew thoroughly to add saliva to the food;
- Avoid extremely hot or cold foods as well as spices, fats, alcohol, coffee, chocolate, and citrus juices;
- Avoid eating and drinking for 3 hours before retiring to prevent the common problem of nocturnal reflux;
- Elevate the head of the bed 6 to 8 inches to prevent nocturnal reflux;
- Lose weight if overweight to decrease the gastroesophageal pressure gradient; and
- Avoid tobacco, salicylates or phenylbutazone, which may aggravate esophagitis.

Surgical Management

Surgery is used with clients who do not respond to medical management. Any one of three different procedures may be used. They are the Nissen fundoplication, Hill's operation, or Belsey's repair. The Nissen fundoplication is most frequently used and involves a gastric wraparound (Fig. 53-10). An abdominal approach is usually used and the fundus is wrapped 360° around the lower esophagus. An increase in pressure or volume in the stomach closes the cardia and blocks reflux into the esophagus. The surgery creates a valve-like substitute sphincter with inherent contractibility.

The Hill operation narrows the esophageal opening and anchors the stomach and distal esophagus to the

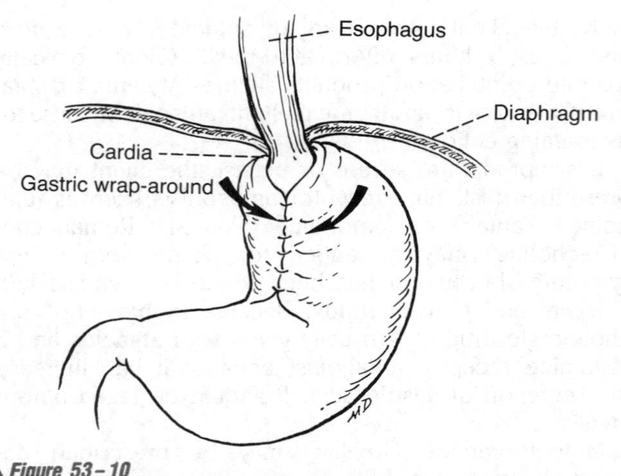

▲ **Figure 53–10**

Nissen fundoplication for hiatus hernia. The gastric fundus is wrapped around the distal esophagus and sutured to itself.

median arcuate ligament (posterior gastropexy). This procedure reinforces the sphincter and re-creates the gastroesophageal valve. In the Hill procedure, there is a partial wraparound (180° of the stomach around the esophagus using an abdominal approach).

The Belsey (Mark IV) repair consists of plicating the anterior and lateral aspects of the stomach onto the distal esophagus. This creates the esophagogastric angle without opening the esophagus. This creates the esophagogastric angle without opening the diaphragm. This procedure has a 280° esophageal wraparound and a thoracic approach.

Clients undergoing a surgical procedure are encouraged to follow the antireflux medical regimen, because the recurrence rate is significant.

Clients with severe reflux may have an Angelchik prosthesis inserted. In this procedure, a laparotomy is performed and a synthetic C-shaped silicone prosthesis is tied around the distal esophagus (Fig. 53–11). The

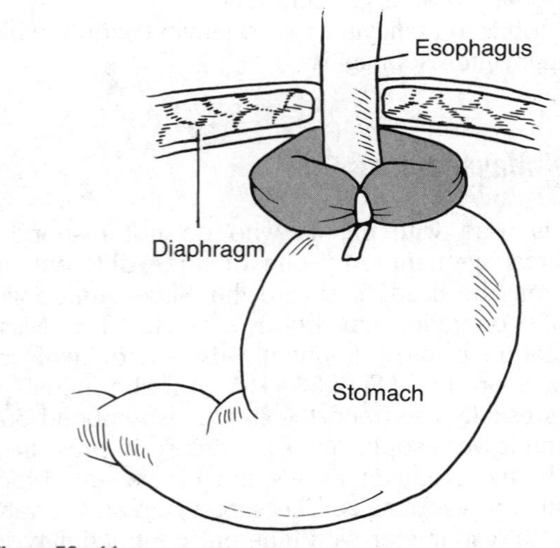

▲ **Figure 53–11**

Angelchik antireflux prosthesis.

prosthesis anchors the LES in the abdomen and reinforces sphincter pressure. The success of this procedure is variable, depending on the severity of the problem. Clients with severe reflux may find this procedure unsuccessful.

Nursing Management

ASSESSMENT

The nurse should identify what symptoms the client has been experiencing. The nurse should note when symptoms started, their frequency and severity, and the relationship of symptoms to food and various food products. The nurse also should assist in maintaining the clients general appearance and nutritional status.

NURSING INTERVENTION

Nursing Diagnosis: Pain R/T irritation of the esophagus caused by gastric reflux.

Planning: Expected Outcomes. The client's pain will decrease or be absent, as evidenced by the client verbalizing that the pain is decreased or absent.

Implementation. The nurse should teach the client about the prescribed diet regimen and evaluate both the client's understanding and the effectiveness of the treatment. The nurse should administer medications ordered for the pain and document the effectiveness of the medications.

Collaborative Problem. High risk for injury R/T surgical procedure and presence of chest tubes.

Planning: Expected Outcomes. Injury will be prevented, as evidenced by absence of hemorrhage, no signs of infection, normal temperature, and absence of signs of problems associated with the chest tubes such as respiratory distress.

Implementation. Preoperative care is basically the same as for other surgeries. Preoperative procedures such as laboratory tests, preoperative medications, and taking nothing by mouth before surgery should be taught. The nurse should teach the client the importance of coughing and deep breathing after surgery to prevent respiratory complications. If a thoracic approach is used, the client should be instructed on the purpose and care associated with chest tubes. Clients may have a nasogastric tube in place after surgery to prevent stomach distention. The client should be taught the purpose and care associated with a nasogastric tube.

If a thoracic approach was used, the client will have a chest tube (see Chap. 37 for the care of the client with a chest tube). Postoperative breathing can be painful, so the client must cough and deep breathe to avoid respiratory complications. With an abdominal incision, there is a greater chance of a wound infection.

The nurse needs to assess the wound drainage for signs of infection.

The client will have a nasogastric tube, and tube patency should be maintained to avoid stomach distention. Fluids are usually resumed after 24 hours and the diet is progressively advanced as tolerated as peristalsis returns. Small, frequent meals should be provided to avoid overloading the stomach.

After fundoplication, the client could experience gas-bloat syndrome. This condition occurs if the wrap of the fundus is too tight, causing bloating and the inability to eructate. Clients should avoid carbonated beverages, drinking with a straw, and gas-producing foods. Ambulation can assist peristalsis in removing air from the gastrointestinal tract. The condition is usually temporary. Clients should be instructed to report dysphagia, epigastric fullness, bloating, or excessive rumbling to their physician.

EVALUATION

The nurse must evaluate client outcomes based on the established plan of care. If these goals were not achieved, the plan and interventions must be revised to meet the client's needs.

Post-hospital Care

DISCHARGE TEACHING

The client should be able to

- List substances that cause recurrence of condition and that should be avoided (alcohol, aspirin, chocolate, and caffeine);
- Discuss a diet that meets nutritional requirements and will not interfere with the function of the LES, including the restriction of food and fluid before bedtime;
- Describe the dosage, action, and side effects of prescribed medications such as antacids and list over-the-counter medications to avoid; and
- State the proper position for sleeping, with the head of the bed elevated.

FOLLOW-UP CARE

The client should know what symptoms to watch for that indicate the need for immediate follow-up care, including the recurrence of symptoms, especially nausea and vomiting, hematemesis, or symptoms of obstruction.

HIATAL HERNIA

Definition

A hiatal hernia, also referred to as a diaphragmatic hernia, is a condition in which the cardiac sphincter becomes enlarged, allowing the stomach to pass into the thoracic cavity. There are two types of hernias, sliding hernias (type I), and rolling or paraesophageal hernias (type II). In a sliding hernia, the upper stomach and the gastroesophageal junction are displaced upward into the thorax (Fig. 53–12*A*). Sliding hernias account for approximately 90 per cent of the total cases of esophageal hiatal hernias.

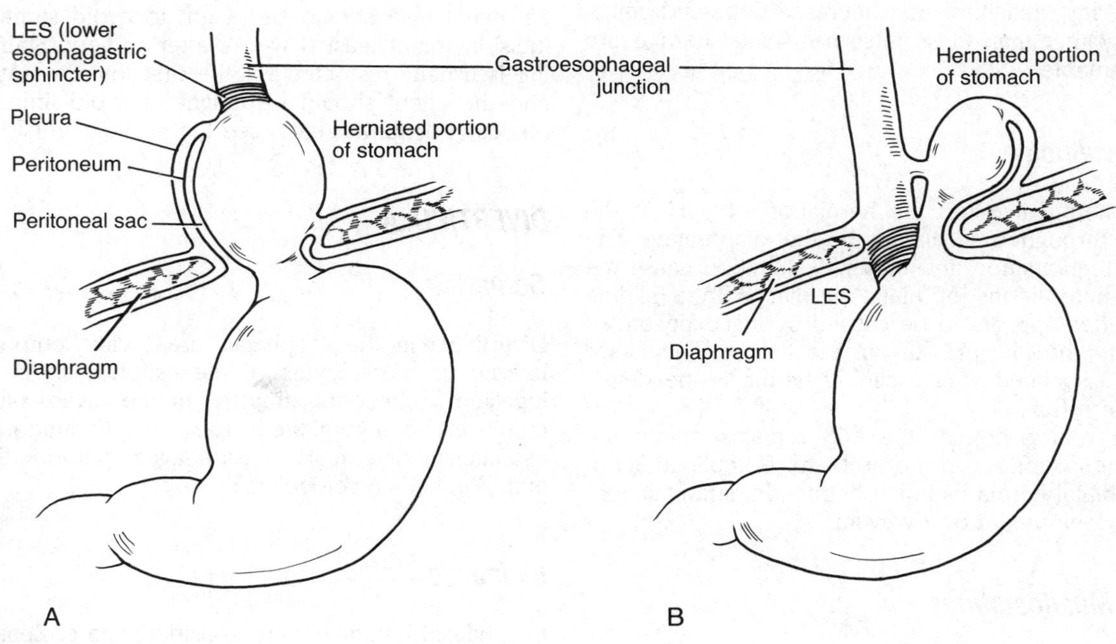

▲ **Figure 53–12**

A, Sliding and, *B*, rolling hiatal hernias.

With a rolling hernia, the gastroesophageal junction stays below the diaphragm, but all or part of the stomach pushes through into the thorax (Fig. 53–12*B*).

Incidence

The incidence of hiatal hernia is estimated as 5 per 1000 in the general population and may be as high as 60 per cent in clients over 60 years of age.[29a] Women tend to be more affected than men, and the incidence increases significantly with age. Sliding hiatal hernias may be noted in infants, but they usually do not produce symptoms until the person reaches middle age. Rolling hiatal hernias are rarely noted in infants.

Etiology

Hiatal hernias are related to muscle weakness in the esophageal hiatus, which loosens the esophageal supports and allows the lower portion of the stomach to rise into the thorax. As with other hernias, the muscle weakness is caused by a variety of conditions, such as aging, congenital muscle weakness, trauma, surgery, or anything that increases intra-abdominal pressure.

Risk Factors

Risk factors for the development of hiatal hernias are any factors that lead to both weakness of the diaphragmatic muscle and increases intra-abdominal pressure. The pressure may be increased by conditions such as obesity, pregnancy, or ascites.

Primary prevention of the hiatal hernia can be accomplished, or at least delayed, by losing weight and avoiding any activities that increase intra-abdominal pressure. Other than these measures, hiatal hernias are not preventable.

Pathophysiology

A hiatal hernia involves the herniation of part of the stomach through a weakness in the diaphragm. The resulting regurgitation and motor dysfunction cause the major manifestations of hiatal hernia. With a sliding hernia, reflux appears to be caused by the exposure of the LES to the low pressure in the thorax. The major problem associated with a sliding hernia is the development of reflux.

With a rolling hernia, the LES remains below the diaphragm so reflux is not a problem. Complications of a rolling hiatal hernia include obstruction, strangulation, and the development of a volvulus.

Clinical Manifestations

Manifestations of hiatal hernia vary in kind and severity. In sliding hiatal hernias, clients may have heartburn 30 to 60 minutes after meals. In addition, reflux may result in substernal pain.

The client with a rolling hiatal hernia does not have symptoms of reflux. The client may complain of a feeling of fullness after eating or have difficulty breathing. Some clients experience chest pain similar to that of anginal pain. Pain is usually worse when the client assumes a recumbent position.

Medical Management

The medical management for the client with a hiatal hernia is the same as that for the client with GERD.

DIAGNOSTIC ASSESSMENT

Hiatal hernias are diagnosed by a barium swallow, with fluoroscopy, showing the position of the stomach in relation to the diaphragm.

Nursing Management

The nursing care of the client with a hiatal hernia is the same as that for a client with GERD. As with GERD, the most common nursing diagnosis is pain related to irritation of the esophagus caused by gastric reflux.

Post-hospital Care

DISCHARGE TEACHING

The client should be taught the appropriate diet modifications, drug therapy, and positioning. The postsurgical client also should be taught to avoid straining the incision for at least 6 weeks after surgery. Stair climbing is usually restricted for the first few days at home, and the client should be taught to avoid lifting heavy objects. For further care, see the section on GERD.

DIVERTICULA

Definition

Diverticula in the esophagus are saclike outpouchings in one or more layers of the esophagus. As food is ingested, it becomes trapped in the diverticulum and can later be regurgitated. The most common type of esophageal diverticula is esophageal pulsion diverticulum (Zenker's diverticulum).

Incidence

Esophageal diverticula are considered rare. Zenker's diverticulum occurs three times more frequently in men than women.

Etiology

The cause of esophageal weakness could be a congenital defect, esophageal trauma, scar tissue, or inflammation.

Risk Factors

There are two categories of diverticula—(1) traction and (2) pulsion. In traction diverticula, the esophageal mucosa has pulled outward from the esophagus. Traction diverticula are most commonly found in the middle esophagus. In pulsion diverticula, the esophageal mucosa has pushed outward through a defect in the esophageal musculature. Pulsion diverticula are most commonly found in the upper esophagus.

Clinical Manifestations

Initially, the client usually complains of difficulty swallowing. Other symptoms may include belching, regurgitation of undigested food, halitosis, and a sour taste in the mouth. Coughing also may occur because of irritation of the trachea from regurgitated food.

Diagnostic Assessment

A barium swallow is performed to locate diverticulum. Endoscopy is usually contraindicated because the diverticulum may be perforated by the endoscope.

Medical Management

Medical management of symptoms from a diverticulum is achieved through dietary management and positioning. Small frequent feedings of semisoft foods often facilitate passage of food. The client should note what foods relieve or exacerbate the symptoms.

To prevent reflux of food, the client should have the head of the bed raised for 2 hours after meals. Nocturnal reflux can often be prevented by sleeping with the head of the bed elevated. The client also should avoid constrictive clothes and vigorous exercise after eating.

Surgical Management

When symptoms become severe, surgery may be indicated. A cervical approach is used for Zenker's diverticulum, whereas a thoracic approach is used for diverticulum located lower in the esophagus. In both procedures, the diverticulum is excised and the esophageal mucosa is reanastamosed.

Nursing Management

ASSESSMENT

The nurse should obtain a history from the client, noting symptoms. The nurse should note the onset and duration of symptoms, and whether or not they occur at mealtimes or at night. The nurse also should assess the client's respiratory status because regurgitation can cause respiratory complications.

NURSING INTERVENTION

Nursing Diagnosis: Pain R/T dysphagia.

Planning: Expected Outcomes. The client will have a decrease in pain or an absence of pain, as evidenced by the client verbalizing that the pain is decreased or absent, and by the client's ability to maintain oral intake.

Implementation. The nurse should teach the client about the necessary changes in diet and how positioning can control symptoms. The nurse should encourage the client to try various foods and various positions to evaluate which are most effective.

Collaborative Problem. High risk for injury R/T surgical procedure and possible chest tubes.

Planning: Expected Outcomes. Injury will be prevented, as evidenced by absence of hemorrhage, no signs of infection, normal temperature, and absence of signs of problems associated with the chest tubes such as respiratory distress.

Implementation. The nurse should discuss the normal preoperative routines. The client should be told they will not be permitted to take anything by mouth after surgery and will have a nasogastric tube. If a thoracic approach is used, the preoperative and postoperative nursing care is similar to that for clients having thoracic surgery and chest tubes (see Chap. 37 for the care of the client after a thoracotomy and with chest tubes).

After surgery, the client's nasogastric tube will be attached to low suction. The nurse should assess the amount and color of the drainage during each shift. The nurse should check for continued bloody nasogastric drainage as well as for signs of external bleeding. The nurse should not irrigate or reposition the nasogastric tube unless it is specifically ordered by the physician.

The client will receive intravenous fluids until tube feedings are begun. Once fluids and supplemental feedings are begun, the nurse should record the client's response. The nurse should assess the client for signs of esophageal perforation, such as chest pain, elevated temperature, and subcutaneous emphysema.

The nurse should assess the client's pain and administer analgesics as ordered. After surgery, the head of the bed should be elevated 30 degrees to decrease edema. Frequent practice of oral hygiene increases the client's comfort.

EVALUATION

The nurse must evaluate client outcomes based on the established plan of care. If these goals are not achieved, the plan and interventions must be revised to meet the client's needs.

Modification of Plan of Care for the Elderly

Older adults are treated more conservatively, using diet and positioning rather than surgery. Surgery may entail too much risk for the older client.

Post-hospital Care

DISCHARGE TEACHING

The client who had surgery may be discharged with a nasogastric or a gastrostomy tube in place to allow for esophageal healing. The client should have written and verbal instructions about tube feedings, diet, and positioning.

HOME HEALTH CARE NEEDS

A visiting nurse should see the client at home to ensure that the tube feedings are being tolerated well.

FOLLOW-UP CARE

The client who has had surgery will need to be seen at intervals until the feeding tube can be removed.

ESOPHAGEAL NEOPLASMS

Definition

Cancer of the esophagus takes the form of either squamous cell carcinoma or adenocarcinoma of the esophageal mucosa.

Incidence

In the United States, the incidence of squamous cell cancer of the esophagus is 4 per 100,000 males. The incidence is twice as high in men as in women, and it is higher in black, Japanese, and Chinese males than in white males. In Northern China, the incidence among males is very high (130 per 100,000). Adenocarcinoma of the esophagus occurs less often than squamous cell cancer and develops primarily in the distal esophagus.

Etiology

The cause of esophageal neoplasms is unknown, but researchers are studying environmental differences between locations with a low and a high incidence. In the Western world, evidence points to heavy smoking, nutritional deficiencies, and habitual ingestion of alcohol, hot foods, and hot drinks as underlying etiologic factors.

In other parts of the world, contaminants in the soil and food, high levels of nitrosamines, smoking opium, and nutritional deficiencies (especially fruits and vegetables) have been linked to the condition. Chronic irritation from other esophageal problems such as achalasia, hiatal hernia, and stricture play a minor role in the development of esophageal cancer.

Risk Factors

The major risk factors are long-term use of alcohol and tobacco combined with poor nutrition. The presence of achalasia, hiatal hernia, reflux, stricture, or poor oral hygiene increases the risk of developing esophageal cancer.

These are very preventable causes. Prevention particularly should be targeted toward the black male population in this country, because their risk is so much higher.

Pathophysiology

Malignant tumors of the esophagus begins as slow-growing benign tissue changes. The majority of cancers are squamous epidermoid tumors that are commonly found in the middle or upper third of the esophagus. Esophageal tumors expand locally and very rapidly, and early spread to the lymph nodes is common. Because the esophagus has no serosal layer to limit its extension, it spreads rapidly. The rich lymphatic supply to the mucosa provides an excellent means for the tumor to metastasize widely. The tumors are typically intraluminal, ulcerating lesions that both encircle the esophageal wall and extend upward and downward.

The disease is progressive and almost always fatal. As it progresses, most clients experience some pulmonary complications because of the formation of tracheal-esophageal fistulas that result in aspiration. If the condition is untreated, total esophageal obstruction is the inevitable outcome of the disease. Infiltration into blood vessels may predispose the client to hemorrhage.

Clinical Manifestations

Typically the first symptoms are dysphagia or odynophagia. Unfortunately, these manifestations are usually not apparent until the tumor involves the whole circumference of the esophagus. By the time the client becomes aware of a swallowing problem and seeks medical care, the tumor frequently has invaded the deeper layers of the esophagus and, sometimes, adjacent structures such as the bronchus.

At first, dysphagia is usually mild and intermittent, occurring only after ingestion of solid food (especially meat). Soon, dysphagia becomes constant, and signs of esophageal obstruction appear. These signs include an increase in salivation and mucus in the throat, nocturnal aspiration, regurgitation, and inability to swallow even liquids.

Diagnostic Assessment

The diagnosis is confirmed by barium swallow, endoscopy, cytologic examination, and direct biopsy. Computerized tomography (CT) scans provide an excellent definition of the size of the primary lesion and the extent of nodal involvement.

Medical Management

Treatment of esophageal cancer depends on the location, size of the tumor, metastases, and the condition of the client. If the cancer is found in an early stage, the treatment is directed toward cure; however, it is usually detected in the late stages, whereby treatment becomes palliative and aimed specifically at allowing the client to continue eating.

Radiation therapy is often used alone or in conjunction with surgery, either before or after surgery. Radiation provides palliation by reducing the tumor size and slowing tumor growth. High-dose radiation therapy may cause stenosis of the esophagus, so radiation treatments are usually administered over a 6-to-8-week period to minimize this effect.

PHARMACOLOGIC MANAGEMENT

Chemotherapy, combining several drugs, provides symptomatic relief. Chemotherapy combined with radiation and surgery is being studied.

DIETARY MANAGEMENT

Maintaining nutrition is a major goal for the client with esophageal cancer. In the beginning of the disease process, the client may be able to tolerate small, frequent feedings of soft or semisoft foods. As the disease progresses, feeding tubes may be needed. If necessary, a feeding gastrostomy or jejunostomy may be created. Short-term hyperalimentation may be used to improve the client's nutritional status before surgery. Proper positioning after meals is necessary in the client with frequent regurgitation, as well as in the client with a prosthesis. The head of the bed should always be elevated 30 degrees.

Surgical Management

Esophageal dilatation may be necessary throughout the course of the disease to treat strictures and tumor obstruction. The treatment should be performed by the physician as often as needed to relieve dysphagia.

In advanced disease, a prosthesis may be inserted to bypass the tumor or to prevent aspiration in clients who develop fistulas. The prosthesis can maintain esophageal patency but can perforate the esophagus as the tumor size increases or become dislodged.

Surgery may be performed for cure or palliation, depending on the extent of the disease. There are three surgical procedures that can be performed. An esophagectomy is the removal of all or part of the esophagus. The resected esophagus is replaced with a Dacron graft. The esophagogastrostomy involves resecting the lower portion of the esophagus and anastomosing the remainder to the stomach, brought up into the thorax. The third procedure, esophagoenterostomy (also known as a colon interposition), involves resecting the esophagus and replacing it with a segment of the descending colon.

Nursing Management

ASSESSMENT

The nurse needs to obtain data concerning the client's nutritional status. Most clients complain of dysphagia that is both persistent and progressive. The client initially may have difficulty swallowing solid foods and then progressively have difficulty swallowing soft foods and liquids.

A careful assessment of dysphagia is important. Other symptoms such as odynophagia, regurgitation, chronic cough, increased secretions, and hoarseness (due to involvement of the larynx) also are important to assess.

NURSING INTERVENTION

Nursing Diagnosis: Nutrition, Altered: Less than Body Requirements R/T client's inability to swallow.

Planning: Expected Outcomes. The client will maintain an adequate nutritional status, as evidenced by maintenance of stable body weight or slowed weight loss.

Implementation. The nurse must monitor the client's nutritional status throughout treatment. Daily weights, intake and output, and calories are carefully monitored. In the beginning, the nurse should teach the client about diet changes that can make eating easier.

As the disease progresses, the nurse may have to provide tube feedings. The nurse must assess skin integrity around the feeding tube for impairment of skin integrity due to leakage of gastric juices. The skin around the opening should be washed with a gentle soap and thoroughly dried twice daily or as needed. Protective ointments such as zinc oxide or Karaya may be applied to the skin for further protection.

Nursing Diagnosis: Swallowing, Impaired, High Risk for R/T esophageal obstruction from tumor.

Planning: Expected Outcomes. The client will not suffer from impaired swallowing, as evidenced by absence of choking and maintenance of patent airway.

Implementation. Many problems arise when the client is unable to swallow. The client can easily choke on saliva and mucous secretions, and must spit frequently or drool. Constant wiping of saliva from the lips can cause irritation, cracking of the skin, and open lesions. Because it is impractical to collect this quantity of secretions in tissues, the client should carry a receptacle to receive the saliva. To prevent oral lesions and infections, and to provide comfort, the nurse should administer or assist with frequent oral care.

Nursing Diagnosis: Individual Coping, Ineffective, High Risk for R/T changes in body image and potentially terminal prognosis.

Planning: Expected Outcomes. The client will effectively cope with the alterations in body image and potentially terminal prognosis, as evidenced by client's maintenance of activities and continued social interaction by the client.

Implementation. In addition to meeting the client's physical needs, the nurse must provide emotional support. The gastrostomy tube may cause an alteration in body image and increased dependency. The drooling or need to spit constantly also may cause the client a great deal of emotional distress.

The poor prognosis of esophageal cancer necessitates psychologic support and interventions aimed at helping the client and significant others prepare for the client's peaceful death.

Collaborative Problem. High risk for injury R/T surgical procedure.

Planning: Expected Outcomes. Injury will be prevented, as evidenced by absence of atelectasis, fever, wound infection, or problems associated with the chest tubes.

Implementation. Before surgery, clients usually require 2 to 3 weeks of nutritional support. Often, this support includes tube feedings or hyperalimentation. The client's weight and fluid and electrolyte status are monitored. The nurse should provide extensive instruction on postoperative respiratory care, including turning, coughing and deep breathing, and chest physiotherapy. The client should be taught about all incisions, wound drainage tubes, feeding tubes, and chest tubes that may be present after surgery. Oral care should be performed four times a day to help prevent infection postoperatively. If an esophagoenterostomy is performed, a complete bowel preparation is performed before surgery.

After surgery, respiratory care is a high priority. The client may be placed on a ventilator (see Chap. 37 for care of a client receiving mechanical ventilation) in a critical care unit. Otherwise, the client must turn, cough, and deep breathe every hour. The nurse must carefully assess the client's respiratory status and report any signs of atelectasis or pneumonia, and supplemental oxygen is administered. Pain medication must be administered frequently, and the nurse should assist the client in splinting the incision while coughing. The client is placed in a semi-Fowler's position to prevent reflux. The nurse should continually monitor the chest tube drainage for amount, color, and patency.

The nurse must assess the client's fluid and electrolyte status. The drainage from the nasogastric, gastric, and all drainage tubes should be monitored at least every shift. The client will not be permitted to take anything by mouth for 4 to 5 days until peristalsis returns. During the first 24 hours after surgery, nasogastric or gastric drainage is bloody but should then change to a greenish yellow color. If bloody drainage continues, it could indicate bleeding at the suture line and should be reported.

Leakage at the site of anastomosis may appear about 5 to 7 days after surgery. The nurse must assess the client for early symptoms of shock as well as signs of fever, fluid accumulation at the wound site, and any signs of inflammation. The nurse should check all dressings for signs of bleeding, drainage, or separation of the suture lines.

The client should be started on small sips of water. If this intake is tolerated, the quantity is slowly increased. The nurse must supervise the client, making sure the client stays in an upright position, and monitor for signs of leakage at the anastomosis site. If this is tolerated, the client gradually progresses to pureed and semisolid foods. The client must be taught the importance of small, frequent feedings and always sitting upright with meals and for 1 hour after meals to prevent overdistention of the stomach and reflux.

EVALUATION

The nurse must evaluate client outcomes based on the established plan of care. If these goals were not achieved, the plan and interventions must be revised to meet the client's needs.

Post-hospital Care

DISCHARGE TEACHING

The client and family should be given written and oral instructions concerning wound healing, nutritional support, respiratory care, and medications. The client should be taught about possible wound and respiratory complications, and symptoms that should be reported immediately.

HOME CARE NEEDS

The nurse should make appropriate referrals to community agencies. Most clients need a significant amount of assistance at home. The family should be given information about services offered from the American Cancer Society and local hospice care.

VASCULAR DISORDERS

The principal vascular disorder of the esophagus is varices. Because esophageal varices result from portal hypertension, this condition is discussed with liver disorders in Chapter 58.

TRAUMA

Major traumatic conditions of the esophagus include chemical burns, presence of foreign bodies, and injuries from external forces, such as endoscopic equipment. Chemical burns occur from the ingestion of acids or alkalis and sometimes from highly spiced foods. Thermal burns can result from drinking extremely hot liquids. Foreign bodies are most apt to lodge in the natural narrow spots of the esophagus. Trauma can cause esophageal perforation with resultant contamination of the mediastinum and stricture formation as healing occurs.

Treatment for esophageal strictures involves dilatation of the esophagus or surgical excision of the diseased portion, and reanastamosis or interposition of a piece of gut from the stomach or colon (see the section on esophageal neoplasms).

Summary

Disorders of the mouth and esophagus range from fairly simple problems, such as dental caries, to complex and potentially lethal problems, such as cancer of the esophagus. Disorders throughout this oral esophageal area, no matter how small, however, can interfere with the client's nutritional intake. The nurse must always remember this fact when assessing and caring for clients with these disorders.

Bibliography

1. Adams, G., Haselow, R. (1983). Oral and pharyngeal cancer: early diagnosis for optimal treatment (Part I). *Hospital Medicine, 19,* 173.
2. Adams, G., Haselow, R. (1983). Oral and pharyngeal cancer: Early diagnosis for optimal treatment (Part II). *Hospital Medicine, 19,* 241.
3. American Cancer Society. (1992). *Cancer facts and figures.* New York: Author.
4. Auld, E. M. (1988). Oral health. *Geriatric Nursing, 9,* 340-341.
5. Baird, S. B., et al. (1991). *Cancer nursing: A comprehensive textbook.* Philadelphia: W. B. Saunders.
6. Barkin, J., & Rogers, A. (Eds.) (1989). *Difficult decisions in digestive diseases.* Chicago: Year Book Medical Publishers.
7. Beahrs, O. H., et al. (Eds.) (1988). *Manual for staging cancer* (3rd ed.). Philadelphia: J. B. Lippincott.
8. Beck, J. E. (Ed.). (1985). *Bockus gastroenterology* (4th ed.). Philadelphia: W. B. Saunders.
9. Blaney, G. M. (1986). Mouth care—basic and essential. *Geriatric Nursing, 7,* 242-243.
10. Bongiovanni, G. L. (Ed.) (1988). *Essentials of clinical gastroenterology* (2nd ed.). New York: McGraw-Hill.
11. Braunwald, E., et al. (Eds.) (1987). *Harrison's principles of internal medicine* (11th ed.). New York: McGraw-Hill.
12. Cameron, J. L. (Ed.) (1989). *Current surgical therapy.* Philadelphia: B. C. Decker.
13. Castell, D. O. (1986). Medical therapy for reflux esophagitis: 1986 and beyond. *Annals of Internal Medicine, 104,* 112-114.
14. Cohen, D. J., & Starling, J. R. (1986). Surgery for reflux esophagitis. *AORN Journal, 43,* 858-864.
15. Cumming, C. W., & Schuller, D. (1986). *Otolaryngology—head and neck surgery* (vol. 1). St. Louis: C. V. Mosby.
16. Davis, J. H., et al. (Eds.) (1990). *Clinical surgery.* St. Louis: Mosby-Year Book.
17. Dental dye pinpoints cavities (1985). *Gallagher Medical Report, 3,* 1.
18. Dreizen, S. (1984). Systemic significance of glossitis. *Postgraduate Medicine, 75,* 207.

18a. Foster, R. L., et al. (Eds.) (1989). *Family-centered nursing care of children.* Philadelphia: W. B. Saunders.

19. Frank-Stromberg, M. (1989). The epidemiology and primary prevention of gastric and esophageal cancer. *Cancer Nursing 12*(2), 53-64.
20. Gitnick, G. (Ed.) (1988). *Handbook of gastrointestinal emergencies* (2nd ed.). New York: Elsevier Science Publishing.
21. Gitnick, G., et al. (Eds.) (1988). *Principles and practice of gastroenterology and hepatology.* New York: Elsevier Science Publishing.
22. Given, B. A., & Simmons, S. J. (1984). *Gastroenterology in clinical nursing* (4th ed.). St. Louis: C. V. Mosby.
23. Groenwald, S. L., et al. (Eds.) (1991). *Cancer nursing: Principles and practice* (2nd ed.). Boston: Jones and Bartlett.
24. Guyton, A. C. (1991). *Textbook of medical physiology* (8th ed.). Philadelphia: W. B. Saunders.
25. Hamilton, H., & Rose, M. B. (1985). *Gastrointestinal disorders.* Springhouse, PA: Springhouse Corporation.
26. Hayworth, M. F., & Jones, A. L. (1988). *Immunology of the gastrointestinal tract and liver.* New York: Raven Press.
27. Johnson, L. R., et al. (1987). *Physiology of the gastrointestinal tract* (2nd ed.). New York: Raven Press.
28. Lynch, D. (1984). Ulcerations of the tongue. *Postgraduate Medicine, 75,* 207.
29. Newland, J. R. (1984). Benign lingual lesions of intrinsic origin: Differential diagnosis. *Postgraduate Medicine, 75,* 152.

29a. Payne, W. S., & Ellis, F. H., Jr. (1984). Esophagus and diaphragmatic hernias. In S. I. Schwartz, et al. (Eds.), *Principles of surgery* (4th ed, pp. 1063-1112). New York: McGraw-Hill.

30. Peterson, D. E., et al. (Eds.) (1986). *Head and neck management of the cancer patient.* New York: Martinus Nijhoff.
31. Sabiston, D. C., Jr. (1991). *Textbook of surgery: The biologic basis of modern surgical practice* (14th ed.). Philadelphia: W. B. Saunders.
32. Schroeder, S. A., et al. (1988). *Current medical diagnosis treatment.* Norwalk, CT: Appleton & Lange.
33. Schweiger, J. L., et al. (1980). Oral assessment: How to do it. *American Journal of Nursing, 80,* 654.
34. Shaffer, E., & Thomson, A. B. R. (1989). *Modern concepts of gastroenterology.* New York: Plenum Publishing Corporation.
35. Shklar, G. (1984). The oral cavity, jaws, and salivary glands. In S. L. Robbins, et al. (Eds.), *Pathologic basis of disease* (3rd ed.). Philadelphia: W. B. Saunders.
36. Sleisenger, M. H., & Fordtran, J. S. (Eds.). (1989). *Gastrointestinal disease: Pathophysiology, diagnosis, and management* (4th ed.). Philadelphia: W. B. Saunders.
37. Spechler, S. J., & Goyal, R. K. (1986). Barrett's esophagus. *New England Journal of Medicine, 315,* 362.
38. Thomson, J. C., et al. (1987). *Gastrointestinal endocrinology.* New York: McGraw-Hill.
39. Widmann, F. (1987). *Goodall's clinical interpretation of laboratory tests* (10th ed.). Philadelphia: F. A. Davis.
40. Wyngaarden, J. B., & Smith, L. H. (Eds.) (1988). *Cecil textbook of medicine* (18th ed.). Philadelphia: W. B. Saunders.
41. Zinner, S. H., et al. (1988). *Assessing the risk of herpes in immunocompromised patients.* (Monograph No. 729). Research Triangle Park, NC: Burroughs Welcome.

Chapter 54

Nursing Care of Clients with Gastric Disorders

Digestion, which starts in the mouth, continues in the stomach. Protein breakdown and the secretion of gastric juices begin this next phase of digestion. Recall from Chapter 51 that the chief functions of the stomach are (1) to mix and liquefy the bolus of food into chyme and (2) to regulate the flow of gastric contents into the upper intestine. The rate of gastric emptying depends on the volume of food ingested, the size of the particles, the amount of acid production, and the nature of the ingested food. Very little absorption takes place within the stomach. However, the stomach does absorb alcohol, small quantities of water, glucose, and some medications such as acetylsalicylic acid.

GENERALIZED CLINICAL MANIFESTATIONS

Manifestations of gastric dysfunction are caused by (1) excessive gastric secretions that feed on stomach mucosa, (2) excessive motility, or (3) retention of gastric contents. The most prominent symptoms are pain, acid eructation, anorexia, belching, nausea, vomiting, hemorrhaging, and diarrhea.

Pain, the most characteristic symptom, usually results from chemical irritation of nerve endings. Nerve irritation develops when acid comes into contact with the eroded stomach mucosa. It also results from stretching and contracting of the stomach, caused in turn by increased motility and increased smooth muscle tension, as is found in an obstruction.

Anorexia, a loss of appetite, is often experienced by clients with malignancy or various other disorders. Hunger is normally caused by a number of stimuli, including contraction of the empty stomach. When the stomach empties slowly or there is gastric stasis because of a gastric disorder, anorexia can result.

Nausea is a result of conditions that increase tension on the walls of the stomach, duodenum, or lower end of the esophagus. Unpleasant stimuli or distention, gastritis, and carcinoma of the stomach can produce nausea. Vomiting may follow nausea or occur without it. Recall from Chapter 51 that vomiting is caused by stimulation of the emetic center. Vomiting is stimulated by

- the chemoreceptor trigger zone (CTZ) in the fourth ventricle. The CTZ is stimulated by various drugs and body toxins. Conversely, medications of the phenothiazine derivative groups, such as chlorpromazine and prochlorperazine, depress vomiting caused by chemoreceptor stimulation.
- nerve impulses, which can be excited by (1) direct mechanical stimuli, as in increased intracranial pressure, (2) chemical stimuli from blood-borne metabolites or toxic substances, and (3) sympathetic and parasympathetic afferent nerve impulses through the vagus, glossopharyngeal, vestibular, and splanchnic nerves. The most sensitive receptors are located in the proximal duodenum.
- unpleasant odors, subjects, and sights that stimulate higher center impulses
- distention of stomach or duodenum
- decreased gastric motility
- pain, because the pain centers are close to the vomiting centers in the medulla
- increased intracranial pressure

Bleeding results from local trauma or irritations that cause erosion or ulceration of the gastrointestinal mucosa. The disorders involved include stomach neoplasms, gastric ulcer, gastritis, anastomotic (marginal) ulcers, and duodenal ulcers. Duodenitis can also cause bleeding. Although bleeding may arise from numerous causes, up to three quarters of all cases of upper gastrointestinal tract bleeding result from esophagogastric varices (venous), hemorrhagic gastritis (capillary), or peptic ulcer. Ulcers account for 80 per cent of all upper gastrointestinal tract hemorrhage.[10]

Diarrhea can be caused by increased peristalsis resulting from an increased gastrocolic reflex or from the effort of the stomach and intestines to eliminate a local irritant.

Belching and *flatulence* result predominantly from swallowed air. It is easy to swallow air during eating and drinking, especially for nervous clients who ingest food rapidly. Frequently, clients attempt to belch to relieve a vague feeling of distress in the stomach caused by swallowed air. Attempting to belch with the mouth closed sometimes adds more air to the stomach than it removes.

Dyspepsia (indigestion) can be caused by such factors as strong emotions, gastrointestinal tract disease, eating too rapidly, inadequate chewing, gas-forming foods (e.g., beans and cabbage), or food allergy.

NUTRITIONAL SUPPORT

Nutritional support is commonly required for clients with gastrointestinal problems. Two types of nutritional support commonly used are enteral nutrition and parenteral nutrition.

Enteral Nutrition

Enteral nutrition is nutrients (containing needed fats, carbohydrates, and proteins) that the client takes in via the gastrointestinal tract system. This nutrition can be supplemental to the general diet or can replace oral intake totally. In the case of clients with gastric and many gastrointestinal tract disorders, this nutrition is often given through intestinal tubes, rather than simply orally.

All kinds of intestinal tubes exist for the administration of enteral feedings in clients who are unable to take them orally. There are nasogastric, gastric, duodenal, and jejunal tubes. Tube feedings are administered either as a bolus feeding or by continuous infusion. The feeding can be administered by bolus push, gravity drainage, or infusion pump. The choice of the type of infusion and method of delivery will depend on the disease and the client's ability to tolerate the feedings.

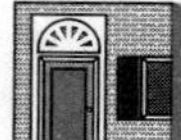

BRIDGE TO HOME HEALTH CARE

Nasogastric Feedings

Knowing how to maintain patency of the nasogastric tube facilitates the transition from hospital to home care. Consistently flushing the tube after each feeding with water followed by cola enhances the longevity of the tube. Teach the patient and family to secure the tube firmly to the nose or to either side of the face or position of comfort. Always determine whether the tube has remained in place prior to starting any infusion.

Referral to a home care agency provides the family with an important resource. They can contact agency staff if the nasogastric tube is accidentally removed or if other difficulties occur, such as cramping, nausea, diarrhea, or displacement.

Management of the nasogastric feeding tube varies with the type of infusion: continuous with a pump, bolus, or by gravity. There are numerous commercial feedings available to meet the individual's nutritional needs; the doctor and dietician are responsible for assessing those needs. However, the client may tolerate one better than the other.

Positioning at a 45-degree angle or greater helps the client tolerate the feedings. Changing the rate and frequency of infusion may decrease or eliminate nausea, diarrhea, or abdominal cramping.

Successful nasogastric tube feedings begin in the hospital and can continue at home with cooperation of the client and his or her family, home care nurse, and physician.

Commercially prepared tube feedings contain nutrients. The physician, usually in consultation with the nutritionist, will determine the appropriate solution for each client. Many health care facilities mix their own tube feedings, which can then be tailored to suit the client.

Problems associated with tube feedings include a variety of fluid and electrolyte disturbances. The client's fluid and electrolyte status is monitored closely, and the make-up of the feeding is altered to accommodate any disturbances. Diarrhea is also a common but controllable problem associated with these feedings. Usually decreasing the concentration of the feeding or slowing the rate of administration controls the problem.

When the client is receiving tube feedings via a nasogastric or gastrostomy tube, an important nursing function is to check tube placement at regular intervals, especially before bolus feedings, to prevent aspiration (see Bridge to Home Health Care). Tube placement can be assessed by either aspirating tube contents for the presence of gastric contents or injecting air with a syringe while listening over the stomach for the movement of the air. This client should also be carefully positioned for preventing aspiration. When the feedings are administered, the client should be in semi- or high-Fowler's position, on the right side.

Another important nursing intervention is to check for residual after the feedings. Either at regular intervals or usually 1 hour after bolus feedings, the nurse aspirates the tube to assess the amount of feeding left in the stomach. If the residual is high, then problems may exist at the gastric outlet.

Parenteral Nutrition (Total Parenteral Nutrition or Hyperalimentation)

Two types of solution are administered when the client receives hyperalimentation, amino acid-dextrose solutions and fat emulsions. The amino acid-dextrose solution can contain additives such as electrolytes, sodium, potassium, chloride, calcium, magnesium, phosphate, and trace elements (zinc, copper, chromium, and manganese).

Many clients with gastrointestinal tract disorders are unable to ingest, digest, or absorb sufficient nutrients to maintain themselves in a state of anabolism or positive nitrogen balance. These clients include those who

- have debilitating diseases such as malabsorption of the bowel
- are unable to eat adequate amounts of nutrients
- have gastric cancer or cancer cachexia
- are undergoing chemotherapy or radiotherapy
- have anorexia nervosa
- have excessive metabolic needs (e.g., extensive burns or draining wounds)

Total parenteral nutrition (TPN) may also be used to rest the gastrointestinal tract when there is a fistula or inflammatory bowel disease or after an intestinal obstruction is removed. TPN is most commonly administered through an indwelling subclavian catheter inserted by the supraclavicular, intraclavicular, antecubital fossa, or internal jugular route into the superior vena cava (Fig. 54-1). A Hickman or Broviac catheter or subcutaneous port can also be used. TPN is usually administered in a large vein because solutions used for TPN are hypertonic. Most fat emulsions, however, are isotonic.

Complications that may occur during or after insertion of the catheter are due to (1) accidental perforation of the pleura leading to pneumothorax or hemothorax, (2) injury to the brachial plexus or the artery, (3) air embolism, or (4) subclavian venous thrombosis. Other major complications of TPN therapy are infection, hyperglycemia, hypoglycemia, and other electrolyte imbalances.

Clients receiving TPN are very susceptible to infection, especially *Candida* septicemia. Concentrated glucose solutions provide a good medium for bacterial growth. Contamination of the catheter, solution, insertion site, tubing, or filters can lead to infection. Therefore, exercise stringent surgical asepsis in hanging TPN solutions, assisting with line insertion, or changing solutions or dressings.

A filter is commonly used in the intravenous tubing to trap bacteria and particles. The solution and administration equipment must be changed every 24 hours. Dressing changes are done every 48 to 72 hours on the basis of hospital policy, except right after the catheter placement (then dressings are usually changed every 24 hours for the first 10 days). Povidone-iodine (Betadine) or an antibiotic ointment is often applied to the catheter insertion site with each dressing change, and an occlusive dressing is applied. Unused solution is always discarded.

When the rate of glucose infusion is faster than the rate of glucose metabolism, hyperglycemia results. If hyperglycemia persists, the renal threshold for glucose

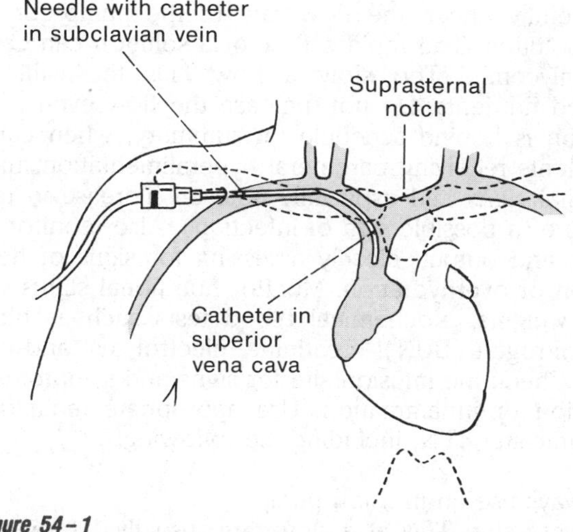

▲ **Figure 54-1**

Insertion of catheter into superior vena cava via right subclavian vein. Once in place, this catheter may be used for TPN administration.

reabsorption is exceeded, and osmotic diuresis with subsequent dehydration and electrolyte depletion occurs. An infusion pump is always used to avoid this complication. Mechanical infusion pumps provide greater accuracy in administration of solutions and help prevent wide fluctuations in rate. Check the infusion rate every hour.

Blood sugar is usually monitored every 6 hours. Even with steady rates, the client's blood sugar may be elevated because of the high levels of glucose being administered. The physician will often order a varying amount of regular insulin to be given, which is based on the client's blood sugar levels.

One of the body's major responses to high blood glucose levels, such as those found in clients receiving TPN, is increased insulin output from the pancreas. When a hypertonic glucose infusion is abruptly interrupted, insulin levels remain high while glucose levels decline, which results in rebound hypoglycemia. Kinking of the tubing or catheter by position changes, occlusion of the catheter, failure of the mechanical pump, or allowing the infusion bottle to run dry can cause cessation of solution flow and subsequent hypoglycemia.

Venous thrombosis is another possible complication. It is characterized by neck vein distention (unilateral); unilateral edema of the arm, neck, or face; and shoulder pain. If this is suspected, notify the physician immediately.

Maintain strict aseptic technique during the insertion of the catheter, with dressing changes, and in changing bottles, filters, and intravenous tubing. Clinicians have developed rigid guidelines for accomplishing these duties, and they must be carefully followed. Procedures may vary in detail. To change the dressing, wear a mask and sterile gloves; apply an antiseptic solution, such as povidone-iodine, and an antibiotic ointment to the insertion site. After application of a dry, sterile dressing or transparent dressing, use tape to form an occlusive dressing that is impervious to air and small amounts of moisture.

Carefully check the flow rate of the pump for the TPN solution. Too rapid a flow of a solution can cause hyperglycemia. Too slow a flow fails to instill the needed nutrients. Do not increase the flow even if the infusion is behind schedule. In summary, when caring for clients receiving parenteral hyperalimentation, monitor vital signs and especially note an increase in temperature (a possible sign of infection). Also monitor the intake and output, closely assessing for signs of dehydration or overhydration. Monitor nutritional status with daily weights, biochemical blood tests such as blood urea nitrogen (BUN), creatinine, electrolytes, and minerals. Check the infusion site for signs and symptoms of infection or inflammation. Use appropriate techniques to administer TPN, including the following:

- ▶ Always use an infusion pump.
- ▶ Always start TPN at a slow rate (usually 1 L over 24 hours). In some institutions, 10 per cent dextrose is given first. The rate is then advanced over 1 to 2 days until the rate desired to meet the client's nutritional requirements is met.
- ▶ Do not abruptly discontinue TPN. If TPN stops or the next bottle is unavailable, administer a 10 per cent dextrose solution until the correct fluid can be obtained.

▼ EATING DISORDERS

Over the past several decades, eating disorders have become of increasing concern to nurses and other health care professionals. Anorexia nervosa and bulimia are now recognized as potentially life-threatening problems. Clients suffering from these disorders are frequently seen by medical-surgical nurses. The nurse must understand these disorders to help clients recover.

ANOREXIA NERVOSA

Definition

Anorexia nervosa is a loss of at least 15 to 25 per cent of ideal body weight due to voluntary restriction of food intake. Clients with anorexia nervosa (usually young women) experience (1) severe weight loss, (2) related physiologic changes associated with starvation, including cessation of menses, and (3) a complex of distorted mental perceptions such as alterations in body image, weight phobia, and obsessive self-starvation associated with the fear of being fat.

Incidence

The incidence of anorexia nervosa is increasing; the high-risk group is American girls between the ages of 12 and 18 years (estimated 1 of 20).[11] It most commonly occurs in females from the middle and upper class in the Western culture. Males account for approximately 5 to 10 per cent of the population with anorexia nervosa. There is an increased incidence of anorexia nervosa in participants of sports or professions that require low body weight, such as gymnasts, wrestlers, and ballet dancers.

Etiology

The cause of anorexia nervosa is not fully understood. It appears to be the result of many factors interacting in a vulnerable client. The importance of each factor to a client can vary.

Risk Factors

Young women with low self-esteem seem to be the highest risk group because they see thinness as a way to improve their self-confidence. The culture in this country that seems to worship the thin model encourages young girls to try to match this appearance.

Education by the nurse can help prevent this problem. Education should center around the avoidance of fad diets, proper nutrition, and ways to build self-confidence safely. The other important factor is to recognize the disorder early in high-risk young women.

Pathophysiology

The obvious pathologic changes associated with anorexia nervosa are physiologic, but the real disorder is psychological. The pathophysiologic changes include changes associated with the effects of starvation.

Untreated, this disorder can be fatal when life-threatening fluid and electrolyte imbalances occur because of the limited intake.

Clinical Manifestations

Clients usually seek medical attention when weight loss is apparent. The client is usually under the age of 25 years. Other symptoms, probably due to the state of starvation, include amenorrhea, cachexia, constipation, fine hair over the body, dry and sandpaper-like skin, bradycardia, periods of hyperactivity, hypothermia, and hypotension. The blood pressure may be as low as 60/40. To induce weight loss, anorexics often subsist on fewer than 600 calories/day, or if they eat more, they vomit. Eventually, severe dieting causes extreme wasting and cachexia. The facial puffiness, due to parotid hypertrophy, contrasts with the wasting of the rest of the body (Fig. 54-2).

Clients usually deny the existence of any problem, except a feeling of being fat. They seem to enjoy losing weight as evidence they are achieving their goals. They often exhibit bizarre rituals associated with food, including hoarding food or handling it in ritualistic ways (such as lining up peas and then eating them one at a time).

DIAGNOSTIC ASSESSMENT

Clients often suffer from profound anemia diagnosed by a complete blood count. Electrolyte abnormalities such as hypokalemia, hypochloremic metabolic acidosis, metabolic alkalosis, or hypoglycemia may be present. If the client is dehydrated, the BUN may be elevated. Often serum cholesterol levels are elevated, although the reason for this is not fully understood. Other diagnostic tests may include a chest radiograph and electrocardiogram. Often, psychological testing is done by a psychiatrist as part of the diagnostic process.

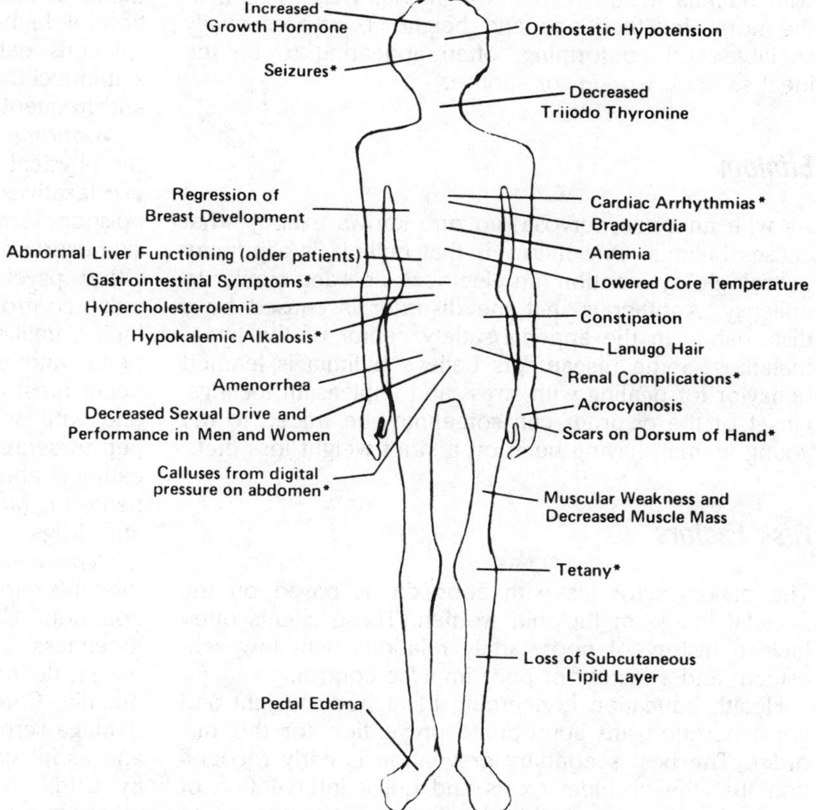

▲ *Figure 54-2*

Physical signs of anorexia nervosa. The signs found in patients with bulimic complications are starred (*); those primarily due to starvation are without an asterisk. (From Andersen, A. E. [1985]. *Practical comprehensive treatment of anorexia nervosa and bulimia.* Baltimore: The Johns Hopkins University Press.)

Medical Management

Nutritional rehabilitation and improvement of self-image are necessary for the client with anorexia. Intervention must first focus on improving the state of nutrition so the client can undertake psychotherapy for the underlying problem. Eating is the preferred method of achieving weight gain, but sometimes the client refuses to comply. In this case, the physician may institute tube feedings. In addition, the client may receive a combined program of psychotherapy and behavior modification. Intervention normally involves the client's significant others.

BULIMIA NERVOSA

Definition

Bulimia, also known as compulsive eating with self-induced vomiting, is another nutritional disorder. Bulimia can overlap with anorexia nervosa, that is, anorexic clients may have bulimia episodes.

Incidence

Bulimia is a common problem, especially among young women during late adolescence and young adulthood. Clients are typically normal weight and from middle- to upper-class socioeconomic background. Most clients with bulimia maintain their weight but weigh less than the norm for their age and height. They are usually sociable and conforming, often appearing to be the ideal student, worker, or spouse.

Etiology

As with anorexia nervosa, no one knows exactly what causes bulimia. One theory is that bulimia is a primary neurologic dysfunction, an electrical disorder, similar to epilepsy. Another is that the disorder is caused by a disturbance in the appetite/satiety center of the hypothalamus. Some researchers believe bulimia is learned behavior for dealing with stress and unpleasant feelings. Onset of the disorder can sometimes be traced to the young woman having been on a strict weight loss diet.

Risk Factors

The major factor, as with anorexia, is based on the societal image of the thin woman. These clients often have a history of poor family relations with low self-esteem and a history of poor impulse control.

Health education concerning ideal body weight and good nutrition are appropriate prevention for this disorder. The best secondary prevention is early recognition that the problem exists and quick intervention of mental health care providers to help the client come to terms with the behavior.

Pathophysiology

Clients often binge after some psychological-emotional factor such as depression, anxiety, anger, or even boredom. Bulimics ingest tremendous amounts of food during these binges without extremes of hunger as the trigger. They may feel some hunger as a trigger; however, the intake of food is out of proportion to the hunger being felt.

Bulimics often do experience weight gains on low-calorie diets and may have a history of being overweight. When they restrict their intake, they may have difficulty losing weight. They find that a large intake of food followed by purging controls their weight.

Clients are aware that the eating pattern is abnormal and they fear they will lose complete control and be unable to stop eating at all. Other types of excessive behavior may be exhibited, such as alcohol or drug abuse or sexual promiscuity. The client has poor impulse control resulting in overindulgence in many aspects of life.

Clinical Manifestations

Assessment reveals a history of repeated binge-eating episodes (rapid consumption of a large amount of food in 2 hours or less), with an awareness of abnormality and a fear of being unable to stop eating. Eating binges are followed by a depressed mood and self-deprecating thoughts. Manifestations of bulimia include consumption of high-calorie and easily ingested foods, inconspicuous eating, abdominal pain, excessive sleeping, self-induced vomiting, repeated attempts to lose weight, and frequent weight fluctuations of 10 pounds or more.

Vomiting, the primary method of purging, decreases the physical pain of abdominal distention. Some clients use laxatives or severely restrictive diets after a bulimia episode. Amphetamines, diuretics, fasting, and excessive exercise may also be used to avoid gaining weight. Other psychological symptoms include impaired impulse control, fear of obesity, and low self-esteem. Bulimics, unlike clients with anorexia, report a strong appetite and usually binge several times a day. Binges occur most often in the late afternoon and evening and end with self-induced vomiting. Binges normally happen in secret. Clients with bulimia are aware that their eating is abnormal and may express concern about this behavior. Many clients with bulimia also abuse alcohol and drugs.

Depression, marked by feelings of gloom, suicidal thoughts, irritability, and impaired concentration, is common. Clients with long-term bulimia also report loneliness, boredom, and anger. Except for frequent weight fluctuations, there are no known clinical signs of bulimia. Chronic vomiting, however, can lead to tooth damage (erosion of the enamel), irritation of the throat and esophagus, swelling of the salivary glands (caused by acidic reflux and constant stimulation), fluid and electrolyte imbalances, and occasionally fistulas of the upper gastrointestinal tract. Laxative abuse may further aggravate fluid and electrolyte imbalance and may cause rectal bleeding.

Medical Management

Intervention for bulimia includes pharmacotherapy, aversion therapy, and psychotherapy; sometimes a monoamine oxidase inhibitor medication (tranylcypromine sulfate) may be ordered to decrease the client's urge to binge. The most widely used modes of treatment are individual psychotherapy and self-help groups. Intervention for bulimia has two goals: (1) to interrupt the binge/purge cycle by helping the client gain control of eating habits and (2) to change attitudes toward food, eating, body size, and self. Family therapy is also recommended to improve family interactions. Clients are encouraged to strengthen and explore relationships with family members.

OBESITY

Definition

Obesity is defined as weight 20 per cent or greater than the desirable weight for adults of a given sex and height.

Etiology

Obesity is usually caused by a caloric intake that exceeds the energy expenditure. A number of metabolic abnormalities are present in obese clients but are probably the result of obesity rather than the cause. When food intake equals metabolic needs, weight remains fairly constant throughout life. A weight gain sometimes accompanies aging because the client does not adjust food intake to lowered metabolism and diminished activity.

Complications

Atherosclerosis and its associated ischemic heart disease are caused by the altered metabolism of obesity. Hypertension and left ventricular hypertrophy occur because blood must be pumped through an enlarged vascular bed. Diabetes mellitus is four times more common in the obese client. Also, recent studies indicate a link between obesity and breast, endometrial, and ovarian cancer.

Medical Management

Activity increases both the energy output and the caloric deficit of a client after a weight loss diet. Thus, it is an excellent intervention. Any obese client on a calorie-restricted program should also have a planned, gradually increasing exercise program to help weight loss and muscle tone.

Most clients need the support and encouragement of others who understand the extreme difficulty of losing weight. The best intervention for obesity is appetite reeducation, in which the client learns to eat and be satisfied with nutritious, well-balanced foods that are low in calories. Support groups such as TOPS (Take Off Pounds Sensibly), a nonprofit organization, and Weight Watchers help some clients. Overeater Anonymous Groups use the Alcoholics Anonymous approach. Most of these groups teach nutrition as well as weight loss dieting. Because weight tends to be self-sustaining, vigilance and continued support are needed to maintain weight losses. No approach will work, however, unless the client is motivated to lose weight.

Obesity is controlled with dietary changes. A weight loss diet must provide fewer calories than the client's energy expenditure while consistently supplying the nutrients necessary for health. Extreme obesity is sometimes treated with fasting, or complete abstinence from food. Fasting can be tolerated for repeated periods of 10 to 15 days if the client is under medical supervision and fluids and vitamins are provided. An average weight loss of 1 lb/day results from fasting. Complications include postural hypotension, anemia, cardiac irregularities, decreased uric acid excretion, and hyperuricemia that is reversed when the fast ends but may then result in uric acid neuropathy and fluid retention. Because of those possible complications, the fasting client should be hospitalized.

Surgical Management

Clients who do not respond to dietary methods of weight loss may require surgical procedures to lose weight. There are a number of surgical procedures that can help the obese client. Many surgical approaches are designed to reduce the ability of the body to ingest or absorb ingested nutrients.

Food intake can be reduced by jaw wiring. Subcutaneous fat can be excised in a procedure called lipectomy. Both have advantages and disadvantages and do not always cause permanent weight reduction.

There are more permanent surgical approaches to weight loss. One approach, used in the past, involved severing the jejunum 14 inches from its beginning and anastomosing this end to the terminal ileum 4 inches above the ileocecal valve. This left the client with 18 inches of small bowel. This jejunal bypass surgical technique has been abandoned because of complications, especially hepatic failure.

The surgical procedure currently done is the gastroplasty or gastric stapling. The gastric stapling or gastroplasty involves stapling the top part of the stomach, with creation of a small pouch to receive ingested food. A small opening left in the line of staples allows food to enter the rest of the stomach slowly. Depending on the size of the pouch created, the client can eat only about 30 ml of food every 5 minutes until satisfied. Before surgery, the client should receive psychiatric evaluation and begin participation in a support group. Because these clients are high surgical risks, an extensive preoperative assessment should be conducted. Postoperatively, special care must be taken with the nasogastric tube for preventing disruption of the suture line. Pulmonary complications often occur with gastric stapling.

Nursing Management of Eating Disorders

ASSESSMENT

A thorough history is necessary to differentiate the type of eating disorder from other illnesses. The nurse should carefully collect demographic data such as age and sex and get a thorough past medical history. The nurse should note the client's weight history, including the onset of the weight loss or weight gain and the reason for the change in weight. Information about the client's attitude and behavior related to food and weight are important. The client should describe his or her typical pattern of eating and be asked about the use of any appetite-suppressing medication, laxatives, and self-induced vomiting. Exercise patterns can also be important. A sexual history including a menstrual history should be taken; it should be noted whether amenorrhea is present.

NURSING INTERVENTION

Nursing Diagnosis: Nutrition, Altered: Less than Body Requirements R/T inadequate food intake (anorexia nervosa).

Planning: Expected Outcomes. The client will maintain body weight within normal limits for client, as evidenced by steady weight gain of 2 to 4 lb/week until ideal weight is reached.

Implementation. When caring for a client with anorexia nervosa, the nurse should help the client select foods from all four food groups. The client is usually allowed to refuse a specific number of foods, such as two or three, so some sense of control is felt. The client must eat only those foods provided by the dietary department and must eat all the meal. Someone should remain with the client, talking, for at least 1 hour after meals so the client is supported and purging is prevented. Maintain an accurate calorie count on the client. The diet should allow the client to gain 2 to 4 lb/week. Weigh the client at regular intervals.

The nurse can help prevent the development of anorexia nervosa through education. By helping the public learn about the disease and its causes and manifestations, the nurse can help prevent its development. The nurse can teach all clients a healthy, well-balanced diet. The nurse should speak out against fad diets and rapid weight loss approaches. If the client is overweight and seeking to lose weight, the nurse should refer the client to a dietician and discourage fad diets.

Nursing Diagnosis: Nutrition, Altered: More than Body Requirements R/T increased food intake (bulimia nervosa, obesity).

Planning: Expected Outcomes. The client will maintain body weight within normal limits for client, as evidenced by steady weight loss of 2 lb/week until ideal weight is reached.

Implementation. The nurse must teach the client how to select a healthy diet with portions that are the correct size. Clients should be encouraged to eat slowly and to develop a regular exercise pattern. Exercise is important especially in bulimics and the obese for it allows increased calorie intake.

The nurse needs to help the client approach food, eating, and self-image in a new way. The nurse needs to help the client learn to eat a balanced diet from the four basic food groups. The nurse can help the client learn to choose proper foods in the right portions. The nurse can help provide supervision and emotional support for the client to overcome stressful periods and break the cycle of binge/purge.

Collaborative Problem. Cardiac Output, High Risk for decreased R/T alterations in rhythm caused by hypokalemia (anorexia nervosa and bulimia).

Planning: Expected Outcomes. The client will maintain normal cardiac output, as evidenced by absence of cardiac dysrhythmias and adequate tissue perfusion.

Implementation. Monitor the client's serum potassium at regular intervals. If the potassium is low, administer potassium supplements as ordered. If the potassium is at a dangerous level, intravenous replacement may be required. The client's potassium should return to normal once the diet is normalized and the condition controlled.

Nursing Diagnosis: Body Image Disturbance R/T misconception of body size or negative feedings (all disorders).

Planning: Expected Outcomes. The client will develop a more normal image of self, as evidenced by client's statements concerning self and by client's ability to overcome eating disorder.

Implementation. The nurse needs to recognize that clients suffering from eating disorders often have low self-esteem. These clients see the regulation of food and exercise of self-control in eating patterns and amounts as ways to prove themselves successful. It is important that the client's significant others help the client find other areas of self-regard unrelated to food.

EVALUATION

The nurse must evaluate whether the client has been able to achieve the goals. If the goals were not achieved, the nurse must revise the plan and interventions to meet the client's needs.

Post-hospital Care

A client whose behavior indicates a motivation to comply with treatment regimens may be discharged home. Clients with anorexia nervosa or bulimia nervosa must have inpatient or outpatient therapy before discharge. If the client does not follow the treatment regimen, referral to a facility specializing in eating disorders may be necessary.

▼ INFLAMMATORY AND NEOPLASTIC DISORDERS

ACUTE GASTRITIS

Definition

Gastritis is inflammation of the gastric mucosa. Gastritis is classified as either acute or chronic.

Incidence

The incidence of gastritis is highest in the fifth and sixth decades of life; men are more frequently affected than are women. There is greater incidence in clients who are heavy drinkers and smokers.

Etiology

The acute form of gastritis may present with nausea and vomiting, epigastric discomfort or eructation, hemorrhage, malaise, and anorexia. It usually stems from the ingestion of a corrosive, erosive, or infectious substance. Aspirin and other nonsteroidal anti-inflammatories, digitalis, chemotherapeutics, steroids, acute alcoholism, and food poisoning (typically due to *Staphylococcus* organisms) are common causes. In addition, food substances that can precipitate acute gastritis include excessive amounts of tea, coffee, mustard, paprika, cloves, and pepper. Foods with a rough texture or those eaten at an extremely high temperature can also damage the stomach mucosa. Ingestion of corrosive agents such as lye or drain cleaner also causes acute gastritis.

Disorders linked with acute gastritis include uremia, shock, central nervous system lesions, hepatic cirrhosis, portal hypertension, and prolonged emotional tension.[27] Acute gastritis is usually of short duration unless the gastric mucosa has suffered extensive damage.

Risk Factors

Ingestion of gastric irritants is a major risk factor. These include aspirin, alcohol, caffeine, and other irritants listed in the preceding section. The primary preventive measure is to avoid these agents if possible. Other measures include the use of enteric-coated aspirin to avoid irritation or medications such as the histamine (H_2)-receptor antagonists to decrease gastric acidity.

Gastritis may also occur secondary to a variety of diseases such as cirrhosis, shock, and uremia, or it may follow treatments such as chemotherapy and radiation therapy. If the client is at high risk because of the presence of one of these disorders or treatments, then the best prevention is early detection and treatment.

Pathophysiology

The mucosal lining of the stomach normally protects it from the action of the gastric acid. This mucosal barrier is composed of prostaglandins. If this barrier is penetrated, gastritis will occur, with resultant injury to the mucosa. When hydrochloric acid comes into contact with the mucosa, injury to small vessels occurs with edema, hemorrhage, and possible ulcer formation. The damage associated with acute gastritis is usually limited.

Clinical Manifestations

Assessment typically reveals epigastric discomfort, abdominal tenderness, cramping, eructation, severe nausea and vomiting, and sometimes hematemesis. Sometimes gastrointestinal bleeding is the only symptom. When contaminated food is the cause of gastritis, the client usually develops diarrhea within 5 hours of ingestion of the offending substance.

DIAGNOSTIC ASSESSMENT

Diagnosis is based on a detailed history of food intake, medications taken, and any disorders related to gastritis. Also, the physician may perform a gastroscopic examination with a biopsy.

Medical Management

Intervention involves removing the cause or treating the condition symptomatically. Vomiting frequently responds to medications of the phenothiazine group; pain responds to antacids or H_2 antagonists such as aluminum-magnesium combinations (Maalox) or ranitidine hydrochloride (Zantac). Initially, foods and fluids are withheld until nausea and vomiting subside. Once the client can tolerate foods, the diet includes decaffeinated tea, gelatin, toast, and simple, bland substances. The client should avoid spicy foods, caffeine, and large, heavy meals. In the continued absence of nausea, vomiting, and bloating, the client can slowly return to a normal diet.

CHRONIC GASTRITIS

Definition

This condition appears in three different forms:

- *Superficial gastritis,* which causes a reddened, edematous mucosa with hemorrhages and small erosions.
- *Atrophic gastritis,* which occurs in all layers of the stomach, develops frequently in association with gastric ulcer and gastric cancer, and is invariably present in pernicious anemia. It is characterized by a decreased number of parietal and chief cells.
- *Hypertrophic gastritis,* which produces a dull and nodular mucosa with irregular, thickened, or nodular rugae. Hemorrhages occur frequently.

Etiology

Peptic ulcer disease or gastric surgery may lead to chronic gastritis. Other risk factors are similar to those for acute gastritis, such as alcohol, smoking, and certain medications. Chronic gastritis is associated with atrophy of the gastrin glands. After gastric resection with a gastrojejunostomy, bile and bile acids may reflux into the remaining stomach, causing the condition.

Risk Factors

The risk factors for chronic gastritis are similar to those for acute gastritis. *Helicobacter pylori* infection can lead to chronic atrophic gastritis, which predisposes to the development of gastric cancer. Age is also a risk factor; chronic gastritis is more common in older adults.

Pathophysiology

The initial pathophysiologic changes associated with chronic gastritis are the same as with acute gastritis. After being thickened and erythematous, the lining of the stomach becomes thin and atrophic. Continued deterioration and atrophy lead to loss of function of the parietal cells. When the acid secretion decreases, the source of the intrinsic factor is lost, which results in the inability to absorb vitamin B_{12}; this leads to the development of pernicious anemia.

Chronic gastritis usually heals without scarring but can cause hemorrhage and ulcer formation. The atrophic changes eventually result in minimal amount of acid being secreted into the stomach. This achlorhydria is a major risk factor for the development of gastric cancer.

Clinical Manifestations

Symptoms are vague and may be absent (because the problem is not an increase in hydrochloric acid). Assessment may reveal anorexia, a feeling of fullness, dyspepsia, belching, vague epigastric pain, nausea and vomiting, and intolerance of spicy or fatty foods.

Medical Management

Intervention begins once the physician rules out cancer as a causative factor. Discomfort may lessen with a bland diet, small frequent meals, antacids, anticholinergics, sedatives, and avoidance of foods that cause symptoms. Sometimes the physician prescribes corticosteroids in the hope of inducing some parietal cell regeneration. Administer vitamin B_{12} if the client has pernicious anemia.

Surgical Management

If conservative measures have not controlled bleeding, surgery may be necessary. Partial gastrectomy, pyloroplasty, vagotomy, or total gastrectomy may be indicated with severe erosive gastritis. These procedures are discussed in the section on peptic ulcer disease.

Nursing Management of Acute and Chronic Gastritis

ASSESSMENT

When assessing the client with gastritis, the nurse should carefully focus on risk factors. The client's diet, patterns of eating, use of prescription and over-the-counter drugs, and lifestyle, including the use of alcohol and cigarettes, are assessed.

NURSING INTERVENTION

Nursing Diagnosis: Pain R/T irritation of the gastric mucosa.

Planning: Expected Outcomes. The client will experience relief of discomfort by removing irritating agents, as evidenced by client's statement of pain relief.

Implementation. The nurse should focus on teaching the client about the causes of gastritis and foods that may aggravate the disease. The nurse should help the client assess factors that increase symptoms, such as stress or fatigue, and assist the client with techniques to reduce the discomfort.

Gaviscon, an antacid that produces a soothing foam, is the best antacid for this problem. H_2-receptor antagonists also may produce relief of the pain.

Nursing Diagnosis: Nutrition, Altered: Less than Body Requirements R/T decreased appetite, nausea and vomiting, and pain.

Planning: Expected Outcomes. The client will experience improved nutritional intake by eating a balanced diet, as evidenced by weight gain or cessation of weight loss.

Implementation. If the nausea and vomiting are severe, the client may be given nothing by mouth until these problems decrease in severity. Once the pain and nausea associated with gastritis have subsided, the client is usually willing to follow a prescribed, well-balanced diet. The nurse can help the client identify foods and beverages that stimulate the development of gastritis and encourage the client to avoid these agents.

EVALUATION

The nurse must always evaluate the degree to which the goals have been achieved. If they were not completely achieved, the nurse must reexamine the nursing care plan and revise goals and interventions as needed.

Post-hospital Care

DISCHARGE TEACHING

The nurse should provide oral and written instructions about untoward signs and symptoms, diet therapy, and prescribed medications.

FOLLOW-UP CARE

The client with chronic gastritis should be seen by the physician at regular intervals and tested for the development of gastric cancer. This is particularly important for the client diagnosed with *H. pylori* infection and atrophic gastritis because these are closely related to gastric cancer.

PEPTIC ULCER DISEASE

Definition

Peptic ulceration is a break in continuity of esophageal, gastric, or duodenal mucosa. It may occur in any part of the gastrointestinal tract that comes into contact with gastric juices (hydrochloric acid and pepsin). The ulcer may be found in the esophagus, stomach, duodenum, or (after gastroenterostomy) jejunum.

Incidence

The incidence of peptic ulcer disease occurs in approximately 10 per cent of the population. Gastric ulcers are more likely to occur during the fifth and sixth decades of life; duodenal ulcers more commonly occur during the fourth and fifth decades for men. For women, the occurrence is about 10 years later in life. Men are more likely to develop both gastric and duodenal ulcers.

Etiology

Peptic ulceration depends on the defensive resistance of the mucosa relative to the aggressive force of secretory activity. The defensive resistance of the mucosa depends on (1) mucosal integrity and regeneration, (2) the presence of a protective mucous barrier, (3) adequate blood flow to the mucosa, (4) the ability of the duodenal inhibitory mechanism to regulate secretion, and (5) possibly the presence of adequate gastromucosal prostaglandins. The aggressive factors relate to the volume of hydrochloric acid and biliary acid. Ulceration occurs when aggressive factors exceed the defensive ones. The aggressive nature of the gastric juice may be the result of hypersecretion of gastric juices, increased stimulation of the vagus, decreased inhibition of gastric secretions, increased capacity or number of the parietal cells to secrete acid, or increased response of the parietal cells to stimulation.[27] Certain medications increase the risk of ulcer formation (see Acute Gastritis), as do a variety of medical conditions including Crohn's disease, Zollinger-Ellison syndrome, and hepatic and biliary disease.

Risk Factors

Smoking is a major risk factor associated with peptic ulcer disease, as are ulcerogenic agents such as steroids, aspirin, caffeine, and alcohol. Stress has also been shown to increase the risk, especially of duodenal ulcers, because they are more likely to be associated with an increase in acid secretion. The presence of Crohn's disease, Zollinger-Ellison syndrome, and hepatic and biliary disease also increases the risk of ulcer formation.

Prevention of peptic ulcers is geared toward the avoidance of ulcerogenic agents and the cessation of smoking. Stress management may also be helpful in lowering the risk of ulcers.

Pathophysiology

Endocrine hormones such as adrenocorticotropic hormone (ACTH) and cortisone may affect mucosal cell secretion by changing (1) the structure of the mucosa or (2) the amount or type of mucus produced. Adrenocorticosteroids may increase the susceptibility of the mucosa, or they may reduce the rate of renewal of mucosal cells and the formation of granulation tissue. Emotional stress can cause an increase in gastric secretion, blood supply, and gastric motility by way of thalamus stimulation to the vagal nerves. Hormonal influence takes place via the hypothalamus through the pituitary adrenal route. When clients undergo stress reactions, the sympathetic nervous system causes the blood vessels in the duodenum to constrict, which makes the mucosa more vulnerable to trauma from gastric acid and pepsin secretion. Upon activation of the adrenal cortex, mucus production decreases, and gastric secretion increases. Together, these factors result in an increased vulnerability of the client to ulceration. Stress reactions thus cause an upset in the aggressive-defensive balance. Prolonged stress from burns, severe trauma, and so forth can produce "stress ulcers," or stress erosive gastritis, within the gastrointestinal tract.

Certain medications may contribute to gastroduodenal ulceration by altering gastric secretion, producing localized damage to mucosa, interfering with the reparative process, or delaying the healing process. Anti-inflammatory agents such as indomethacin decrease mucosal resistance and should be used with caution. Reserpine and caffeine stimulate acid production. Caffeine stimulates acid/pepsin secretions, vascular stasis, and mucosal anoxia; phenylbutazone (Butazolidin) impairs cell metabolism. Chemotherapeutic agents or antimetabolites damage both normal and neoplastic cells of the gastroduodenal mucosa. Alcohol stimulates acid production, and aspirin ingestion is frequently related to local mucosal damage and suppressed mucus secretion.

Zollinger-Ellison syndrome is a condition characterized by abnormal secretion of gastrin by a rare islet cell tumor in the pancreas. Pathophysiologic changes associated with this syndrome include hypergastrinemia and diarrhea secondary to fat malabsorption from decreased duodenum-inactivating pancreatic lipase or from acid-induced injury of the villi. Besides gastric secretion, there is hyperplasia of the gastric mucosa induced by the trophic effects of gastrin. Treatment of the Zollinger-Ellison syndrome is aimed at suppression of acid secretion.

Duodenal ulcers may result from increased gastric acid secretion, increased motility, and increased gastric emptying time. Sometimes, clients with normal gastric acid secretion develop duodenal ulcers. This is related to a very rapid gastric emptying; the gastric acid irritates the duodenal mucosa.

Treated ulcers usually heal without difficulty. However, untreated ulcers or those not responding to treatment can result in perforation, hemorrhage, or obstruction, conditions that may require surgical treatment. Some ulcers recur after healing, particularly if the risk factors associated with their development are not modified.

Critically ill clients are susceptible to stress ulcers. Gastric mucosal changes due to stress develop within 72 hours in 78 per cent of clients with greater than 35 per cent burns. Stress ulcers manifest with superficial gastric erosions, often accompanied by painless massive gastric hemorrhage. The client characteristically has multiple lesions, usually small and superficial, that do not extend through the muscularis mucosa. These lesions may give the appearance of "oozing blood." The mechanism causing stress ulcerations is unknown but probably involves ischemia. In the presence of acid, ischemia can produce erosive gastritis and ulcerations. Increased hydrogen ion back-diffusion and decreased mucosal perfusion may also contribute to stress ulcer formation. Low gastric pH (high acidity) is necessary for stress ulcer development.

Researchers continue to seek the precise mechanism by which stress ulcers occur. Few symptoms accompany stress ulcer. These ulcerations are typically painless unless perforation occurs, but fortunately this is rare. Upper gastrointestinal tract hemorrhage is the major sign of stress ulcer. About 10 per cent of clients experience dyspepsia before hemorrhage, but typically there are no warning symptoms. Once stress ulcers cause profound hemorrhage, the mortality rate rises to about 50 per cent.

Table 54–1 distinguishes the types of peptic ulcers.

DUODENAL ULCERS

Duodenal ulcers, which have a higher incidence than gastric ulcers, usually occur within 1.5 cm of the pylorus. They are usually characterized by high gastric acid secretion, although, as mentioned, some are associated with normal gastric secretion associated with rapid emptying of the stomach. Hypersecretion of acid is attributed to a greater mass of parietal cells. Stimuli for acid secretion include protein-rich meals, calcium, and vagal stimulation. Clients with duodenal ulcers experience low pH levels in the duodenum for longer periods. They are sensitive to gastrin and secrete excess gastrin. Finally, clients with duodenal ulcers have more rapid gastric emptying. Combined with hypersecretion of acid, rapid emptying of food from the stomach reduces the buffering effect of a food and results in a large acid load in the duodenum. Within the duodenum, inhibitory mechanisms and pancreatic secretion may be insufficient to control the acid load.

GASTRIC ULCERS

Gastric ulcers, which tend to heal within a few weeks, form within 1 inch of the pylorus of the stomach in an area of gastritis. Gastric ulcers are probably caused by a break in the "mucosal barrier." The barrier, which differs from the layer of glycoprotein mucus that overlies the gastric epithelium, normally allows hydrochloric acid to be secreted into the stomach without injury to the epithelial cells. An incompetent pylorus may decrease mucus production, the usual gastric defense. The reflux of bile acids through an incompetent pylorus into the stomach may break the mucosal inflammation. Decreased blood flow to the gastric mucosa may also alter the defensive barrier. Decreased blood flow may make the duodenum more susceptible to gastric acid and pepsin trauma. The recurrence rate in gastric ulcer is lower than in duodenal ulcer.

STRESS (STRESS-EROSIVE GASTRITIS) AND DRUG-INDUCED ULCERS

Besides peptic and gastric ulcers, acute gastric erosion, frequently called stress ulcers or stress-erosive gastritis, can occur after an acute medical crisis. Six major assaults that give rise to gastroduodenal ulcerations are

- severe trauma or major illness
- severe burns (sometimes called Curling's ulcers)
- head injury or intracranial disease (frequently called Cushing's ulcers)

TABLE 54-1. Classification of Peptic Ulcers

Assessment Data	Duodenal Ulcers	Gastric Ulcers
Location of ulcer	1/4 to 1 inch from pylorus	Junction of fundus and pylorus, some in antrum
Acid secretion	Increased	Normal to decreased
Serum pepsinogen I	Increased	Normal
Serum gastrin		
Fasting	Normal	Elevated
Postprandial	Elevated	
Blood group	Most frequently type O	No difference
Age of onset	25 to 50 years	Peaks 45 to 54 years
Gender predominance	Men to women, 4:1	Men to women, 2:1
Associated gastritis	None	Common and increased
Pain	Occurs on empty stomach, 2 to 3 hr after meals or in middle of night; relieved by food and antacids	Variable pain pattern; may be made worse by food; antacids ineffective
Nutritional status	Usually well nourished	Probably malnourished
Malignancy potential	Rare, no increase in incidence	Occurs in approximately 10% of clients
Bleeding pattern	Melena more common than hematemesis	Hematemesis more common than melena
Recurrence	May occur as marginal ulcers after surgery	Recurrence unlikely after surgery

- drug ingestion (e.g., aspirin and alcohol) that acts on the gastric mucosa
- shock
- sepsis

Clinical Manifestations

PAIN

The principal symptom experienced by the client with ulcers is an aching, burning, cramplike, gnawing pain. The pain has a definite relationship to eating. With gastric ulcers, food may cause the pain, and vomiting may relieve it. Clients with duodenal ulcers have pain on an empty stomach, and discomfort may be relieved by the ingestion of food or antacids. Clients usually describe the pain as circumscribed in an area 2 to 10 cm in diameter, between the xiphoid cartilage and the umbilicus. Gastric ulcer pain often occurs in the upper epigastrium, with localization to the left of the midline, whereas duodenal pain is in the right epigastrium. Ulcer pain also varies with the site, size, or penetration of the ulcer or the amount of surrounding fibrotic tissue.

In duodenal ulcers, steady pain near the midline of the back between the sixth and tenth thoracic vertebrae with radiation to the right upper quadrant may indicate perforation of the posterior duodenal wall. Fullness or hunger may also be present. Distention of the duodenal bulb produces epigastric pain, which may radiate to the back and thorax. Hydrochloric acid secretion may produce edema and inflammation, with resultant pain, or may activate motor changes, with increased spasm, intragastric pressure, and increased motility, also with resultant pain. In addition, ulcer pain tends to occur within distinct periods (periodicity).

The pain in both gastric and duodenal ulcers tends to recur daily for a while; it and all symptoms then disappear for months or years, to be followed eventually by another episode of pain.

NAUSEA AND VOMITING

Clients with duodenal ulcer usually have a normal appetite unless pyloric obstruction is present. Carcinoma, gastric ulcers, or gastritis may be associated with anorexia, weight loss, and dysphagia. Vomiting occurs more often with gastric ulcer than with uncomplicated duodenal ulcer. It also occurs more frequently when the ulcer is in the pylorus or antrum. Vomiting usually results from gastric stasis or pyloric obstruction. The client with a gastric ulcer or pyloric obstruction typically vomits undigested food. Severe retching and vomiting may suggest an esophageal tear.

BLEEDING

Clients with ulcers often bleed when the ulcer erodes through a blood vessel. Bleeding may occur as massive hemorrhage or may be occult from slow oozing. Approximately 25 per cent of clients with gastric ulcers may experience bleeding.

DIAGNOSTIC ASSESSMENT

Ulcers are diagnosed on the basis of symptoms, x-ray evidence, and endoscopy. The history and physical examination do not yield much significant data in an uncomplicated peptic ulcer. A complete blood count with decreased hematocrit and hemoglobin values may indicate bleeding. Stool for occult blood might also be positive, if bleeding is present.

The major diagnostic tests are an upper gastrointestinal tract series and esophagogastroduodenoscopy (EGD). The EGD has several advantages. It allows the physician to take tissue specimens and treat the ulcer with either multipolar electrocoagulation (MPEC) or heater-probe therapy (see Medical Management).

Medical Management

The primary objective of intervention for peptic ulcer is to provide stomach rest. This may include such approaches as neutralizing or buffering hydrochloric acid, inhibiting acid secretion, and decreasing the activity of pepsin and hydrochloric acid. Specific measures include medications, physical and emotional rest, dietary management, and stress reduction.

Response to the therapeutic program will vary with the client's perception of his or her health status and the degree to which lifestyle influences the ulcer disease. If intervention succeeds, the client will (1) experience a decrease in pain with eventual elimination of all ulcer pain and related symptoms; (2) eat a nutritionally sound diet and report an increased tolerance to food; (3) comply with the medication schedule; and (4) identify stressors and develop ways of dealing with or modifying them.

PHARMACOLOGIC MANAGEMENT

Medications are prescribed for clients with peptic ulcer for three major reasons: (1) to reduce secretions (hyposecretory drugs), (2) to neutralize acid (antacids), and (3) to protect the mucosal barrier (mucosal barrier fortifiers) (Table 54-2).

Hyposecretory Agents. Hyposecretory agents, which cause a reduction in acid secretions, include the anticholinergics, prostaglandin analogs, H_2-receptor antagonists, anticholinergics, and antacids.

H_2-Receptor Antagonists. H_2-receptor antagonists block histamine-stimulated gastric secretions (basal and stimulated) and are thus effective in the management of ulcer disease.

Ranitidine hydrochloride (Zantac), one of the typical agents of the H_2-receptor antagonists, blocks the action of H_2-receptors and appears to inhibit gastrin release. It inhibits pepsin secretion and reduces the volume of gastric secretion. Maximal doses reduce food-stimulation secretion of acid by 75 to 85 per cent in 3 hours. This medication appears to be effective in healing both gastric and duodenal ulcers. Ranitidine and famotidine (Pepcid) cause fewer complications than does the older agent cimetidine (Tagamet).

The client generally takes H_2-receptor antagonists every 6 hours for short-term management until the ulcer heals and symptoms subside, then once a day at bedtime. Although H_2 blockers are much more effective than are anticholinergic drugs acting alone, their effect is potentiated by anticholinergics. H_2-receptor antagonists do not appear to affect the rate of pepsin secretion or of gastric motility. The ulcer may recur after these medications have been discontinued, although rebound hyperacidity does not occur when they are stopped.

Prostaglandin Analogs. Prostaglandins are local tissue hormones that are formed from essential fatty acids. These hormones seem to be present in various forms in almost every tissue of the body. Two prostaglandins, E_1 and E_2 (PGE_1 and PGE_2), inhibit the secretion of gastric acid. Misoprostol (Cytotec) is a drug in this category.

Anticholinergics. Excessive hydrochloric acid secretion and gastric motility can be partially prevented by decreasing vagal stimulation. Anticholinergics, as well as rest and sedation, accomplish this by blocking the action of acetylcholine on smooth muscles. This blockage decreases gastric motility and inhibits gastric secretions. Anticholinergics also delay gastric emptying time, thus prolonging the effect of foods and antacids. Reduced motility and consequent slowed gastric emptying cause a feeling of fullness. No proof exists that anticholinergics increase the rate of ulcer healing. However, they may enhance pain relief by relieving gastric distress caused by gastric spasm and hyperperistalsis.

Anticholinergics are best given 1 hour after meals, when food-stimulated acid is at its peak. Their effects last 4 to 5 hours. Do not give anticholinergics to clients who are bleeding, because the stomach may become distended. These agents are also contraindicated in clients who have pyloric obstruction, glaucoma, urinary retention, or achalasia. Dicyclomine hydrochloride (Bentyl) is a common anticholinergic used for clients with ulcers.

Unfortunately, anticholinergics suppress basal secretion more effectively than they suppress secretion in response to food. Also, to achieve sufficient suppression of secretion, the client must receive a large dose, which causes intolerable side effects: dryness of mouth, blurred vision, constipation, and sometimes urinary retention due to bladder atony. For these reasons and because the H_2-receptor antagonists work better, anticholinergics are not used as frequently as they once were.

Antacids. The ideal antacid decreases acidity, is effective for a prolonged period, is pleasant to take orally, is not constipating or cathartic in nature, and is not absorbed—thereby eliminating systemic effects.

Calcium carbonate is a potent antacid but is constipating and triggers gastrin release, causing a rebound acid secretion. Magnesium carbonate and magnesium oxide are also potent antacids but are laxatives. They are sometimes prescribed to counteract the constipating effects of calcium carbonate. Frequently, the client takes these antacids alternately or balances dosages of each to produce a stool of the desired consistency.

Aluminum hydroxide, aluminum phosphate, and aluminum carbonate are less effective because they only partially neutralize the acid. Sodium bicarbonate, a potent antacid, has a very brief effect and is absorbed systemically. Antacids that combine the effects of mag-

TABLE 54–2. Medications Commonly Used to Treat Peptic Ulcers

Medication	Action	Side Effects	Nursing Implications
Hyposecretory Agents			
Histamine (H_2)–Receptor Antagonists			
Cimetidine (Tagamet)	Same action as Zantac	Fever, rash, headache, dizziness, somnolence, confusion (especially in elderly), hypotension, diarrhea, neutropenia, gynecomastia, and impotence	Monitor mental status of elderly; do not take antacids within 1 h of Tagamet; take with meals and at bedtime; interacts with theophylline, phenytoin, warfarin, and beta blockers; continue treatment for at least 8 weeks to ensure healing.
Ranitidine hydrochloride (Zantac)	Inhibits gastric acid secretion by blocking H_2 receptors on parietal cells	All side effects rare including nausea, constipation, bradycardia, increased liver enzymes, and headache	Give antacids at least 1 hr before or 2 hr after Zantac; can be given in single bedtime dose; use cautiously in clients with liver or renal disorders; absorption not affected by food; interacts minimally with other drugs
Famotidine (Pepcid)	Same action as Zantac	Headache, diarrhea, constipation, nausea, flatulence, increased blood urea nitrogen and creatinine, and rash	Should not be taken longer than 8 weeks without physician's specific order; may be given with antacids; can be given in single bedtime dose; has no significant drug interactions
Nizatidine (Axid)	Same action as Zantac	Diarrhea, rash bronchospasms, somnolence, joint pain, and sweating	Give as single bedtime dose or, if given twice a day, one dose at bedtime; assess for excessive drowsiness; monitor and record stools; do not give antacids within 1 h of Axid; must be taken 4 to 8 weeks for ulcer healing; notify physician if somnolence or rash develops
Prostaglandin Analogs			
Misoprostol (Cytotec)	Suppresses secretion of gastric acid and stimulates production of cytoprotective mucus	Diarrhea, nausea, abdominal discomfort, headache, and dizziness	Cannot be used in pregnancy because it stimulates uterine contractions; use for treatment in peptic ulcer disease currently under investigation; considered equivalent to cimetidine in ability to heal duodenal ulcers; useful in treating gastric ulcers also; recommended for clients on long-term aspirin or nonsteroidal anti-inflammatory drug therapy

Table continued on following page

TABLE 54-2. Medications Commonly Used to Treat Peptic Ulcers Continued

Medication	Action	Side Effects	Nursing Implications
Anticholinergics			
Dicyclomine hydrochloride (Bentyl)	Muscarinic antagonist; inhibits secretion of gastric acid in large doses	Headache, palpitations, dizziness, constipation, paralytic ileus, urinary hesitancy and retention, and dry mouth	Do not use in clients with obstructive uropathy, gastrointestinal obstruction, ulcerative colitis, unstable cardiovascular status, or toxic megacolon; use carefully in clients with narrow angle glaucoma, hyperthyroidism, hiatal hernia, congestive heart failure, hepatic or renal disease; give 1/2 hour before meals and at bedtime; monitor vital signs and urine output; report blurred vision; maintain good fluid intake
Antacids			
Aluminum hydroxide (Amphogel)	Buffers and neutralizes acid in gastrointestinal tract	Constipation, anorexia, intestinal obstruction, and hypophosphatemia	Give 1 to 2 hr after meals and at bedtime; do not give within 1 to 2 hr of H_2-receptor antagonists, enteric-coated drugs, or tetracycline; monitor and treat constipation; shake suspension well before use; follow tablets with water; contains salt, so contraindicated in large doses or long-term use with clients on sodium-restricted diets; used in clients with renal failure
Magnesium oxide (Mag-Ox)	Increases gastric pH to reduce pepsin activity; strengthens gastric mucosal barrier and esophageal sphincter tone	Diarrhea, nausea, and hypermagnesemia	Do not use in clients with renal disease; monitor for development of symptoms of hypermagnesemia; alter with aluminum or combination product if diarrhea occurs; do not give within 1 to 2 hr of H_2-receptor antagonists, tetracycline, or enteric-coated tablets
Aluminum-magnesium combinations (Riopan, Maalox, Mylanta, Gelusil)	Increases gastric pH to reduce pepsin activity; strengthens gastric mucosal barrier and esophageal sphincter tone	Mild constipation or diarrhea	Do not use in clients with renal disease; monitor bowel movements and signs of hypermagnesemia; Riopan low in sodium; do not give within 1 to 2 hr of H_2-receptor antagonists, tetracycline, or enteric-coated tablets
Calcium carbonate (Tums, Titralac)	Increases gastric pH to reduce pepsin activity; strengthens gastric muco-	Constipation, gastric distention, rebound hyperacidity, hypercalcemia, and	Do not use in clients with renal disease; do not give with milk; monitor for

TABLE 54–2. Medications Commonly Used to Treat Peptic Ulcers Continued

Medication	Action	Side Effects	Nursing Implications
	sal barrier and esophageal sphincter tone	hypophosphatemia	symptoms of hypercalcemia and constipation; do not give within 1 to 2 hr of H_2-receptor antagonists, tetracycline, or enteric-coated tablets
Mucosal Barrier Fortifiers			
Sucralfate (Carafate)	In presence of mild acid condition, forms viscid and sticky gel and adheres to ulcer surface, forming a protective barrier	Dizziness, constipation, sleepiness, nausea, and gastric discomfort	Best on an empty stomach, 1 hr before meals and at bedtime; monitor for constipation; pain and ulcer symptoms may subside, urge client to take entire prescribed regimen; drug minimally absorbed, so few adverse reactions

nesium and either aluminum or calcium are on the market, such as Maalox and Mylanta.

Antacids are ordered to buffer gastric acid. They do not influence healing or prevent recurrence. They do, however, prevent the formation of pepsin, the protein-digesting enzyme. Antacids may also reduce the pyloroduodenal tone. For treatment of active peptic ulcer disease, sufficient antacid must be used to neutralize the hourly production of acid. Raising gastric pH from 1.3 to 2.3 produces 90 per cent neutralization of gastric acid.

Generally, the goal of antacid therapy is to maintain a gastric pH of 3.0 to 3.5. For optimal effect, the client should take antacids about 1 hour after meals or feedings, at bedtime, and during periods of "rebound."

Some clinicians recommend that the antacid be mixed with water to ensure that it enters the stomach and does not simply coat the esophagus. Clients with esophageal reflux or hiatal hernia should take alginic acid, an additive present in Gaviscon. Alginic acid forms a viscous solution that floats to the top of the gastric contents and protects the esophageal mucosa. Table 54–3 summarizes what to watch for with antacids.

Mucosal Barrier Fortifiers. Mucosal barrier fortifiers are effective in (1) preventing hydrogen ion back-diffusion into the mucosa and (2) stimulating mucus production, which results in accelerated gastric ulcer healing.

Sucralfate is a sulfonated disaccharide that forms complexes with proteins at the base of a peptic ulcer. These complexes form a protective coat that prevents further digestive action of both acid and pepsin. Sucralfate does not inhibit acid secretion and has minimal acid-neutralizing ability. Instruct the client to take the recommended dosage of sucralfate 1 hour before each meal and at bedtime, but not within 30 minutes of antacids, as needed for pain.

DIETARY MANAGEMENT

In uncomplicated ulcer disease, few physicians favor strict dietary changes. There is little evidence that diet treatment promotes or accelerates healing. Foods known to increase gastric acidity or cause discomfort should be avoided, such as coffee, alcohol, and milk.

COMPLICATIONS

Hemorrhage. Hemorrhage varies from minimal, manifested by occult blood in the stool (melena), to massive, in which the client vomits bright red blood (hem-

TABLE 54–3. Precautions for Antacid Administration

Giving Antacids With	May Result In
Amphetamines or quinidine	Delayed drug elimination
Chlorpromazine and other phenothiazines	Decreased absorption with magnesium-aluminum
Diazepam (Valium)	Increased absorption rate
Dicumarol	Increased absorption with magnesium hydroxide
Digoxin (Lanoxin)	Decreased absorption (some antacids)
Enteric-coated tablets	Increased tablet dissolution and absorption rate
Iron salts	Decreased iron absorption: magnesium trisilicate or carbonates
Propranolol (Inderal)	Decreased drug absorption (aluminum hydroxide)
Tetracycline	Decreased absorption (especially with calcium, magnesium, and aluminum)

Adapted from Rosenberg, J. M., & Kirschenbaum, H. L. (1982). What to watch for with antacids. *Nursing Research, 31,* 54.

atemesis). The usual symptom of gastrointestinal tract bleeding is either the vomiting of coffee ground–colored material or the passing of tarry stools. Acid digestion of blood in the stomach results in a granular dark emesis, whereas digestion in the duodenum or below may result in a black stool. Hemorrhage tends to occur more often with gastric ulcers, especially among the elderly.

Although the onset of hemorrhage may be associated with fatigue, nervous tension, upper respiratory tract infection, dietary indiscretion, alcoholism, or irritating drugs, there may be no known precipitating factor. Bleeding may manifest as either hematemesis or melena. Melena may occur with gastric ulcers but is more common with duodenal ulcers. Hematemesis usually indicates bleeding proximal to the ligament of Treitz at the duodenal level.

Symptoms depend on the severity of the hemorrhage. In mild bleeding (less than 500 ml), the client may experience only slight weakness and diaphoresis. Severe blood loss of more than 1 L per 24 hours may cause manifestations of shock, such as hypotension, weak thready pulse, chills, palpitations, and perspiration.

Intervention for massive bleeding aims to treat hypovolemic shock, prevent dehydration and electrolyte imbalance, and stop the bleeding. The client, who should be fasting, receives intravenous fluids until the bleeding subsides. The nurse or physician may insert a nasogastric tube in the presence or absence of blood in the stomach to assess the rate of bleeding, to prevent gastric dilation, and to administer cool saline lavage for gastric cooling. Gastric cooling, although controversial, may curtail hemorrhage through its vasoconstrictive effect. Iced saline is not used because it may lead to more mucosal damage by decreasing perfusion to the gastric mucosa and may cause a vagal response, decreasing systemic perfusion.

Arterial administration of vasopressin (via an infusion pump) can also successfully control acute hemorrhage. Vasopressin has few complications if given intravenously for less than 36 hours to control the bleeding.

Another approach to the control of bleeding is selective arterial embolization via angiography. The emboli may consist of autologous blood clots with or without an absorbable gelatin sponge. A modified clot may be made with a mixture of the client's own blood, aminocaproic acid, and platelets. The client must remain on absolute bed rest for several days after bleeding has subsided. Rest decreases blood pressure and gastrointestinal tract activity. When bleeding stops, the client is allowed bathroom privileges. If the individual requires narcotics, administer them with caution. Morphine sulfate can cause nausea and vomiting. However, it may calm the client who is extremely restless and apprehensive.

During the first few days of hemorrhaging, gastric pH should be maintained between 5.5 and 7.0. To accomplish this, administer ranitidine intravenously every 4 hours for 4 days as prescribed. Monitor gastric pH at least each shift. Anticholinergics are not recommended for treatment of gastric hemorrhage. Administer antacids for 1 week to complement the ranitidine, but remember to give them 1 hour before or 2 hours after the ranitidine so the antacids do not interfere with its absorption. The client may require antacids every 30 minutes after starting intake of food or fluids. Antacids increase pH by direct hydrogen ion buffering.

If bleeding continues beyond 48 hours, recurs, or is associated with perforation or obstruction, surgery may be indicated. Increased surgical risk is associated with prolonged bleeding, multiple transfusions, debilitation, electrolyte imbalances, and increased age. Surgical procedures include partial gastric resection, excision of the ulcer, or vagotomy and pyloroplasty. Vagotomy and pyloroplasty with ligation of the eroded vessel may also be performed.

Blood volume depletion presents a major problem for the client who has severely hemorrhaged. For those who have suffered a massive upper gastrointestinal tract hemorrhage, a primary objective of intervention is to replace blood volume. Restlessness and tachycardia are the earliest symptoms of hypovolemia. The client will also have a greatly decreased urine output, which should be monitored via a Foley catheter.

Two endoscopic procedures have been found to be safe and effective in treating bleeding ulcers: multipolar electrocoagulation (MPEC) and heater-probe therapy. In MPEC, a bipolar electric current cauterizes the bleeding lesion; in heater-probe therapy, direct heat cauterizes the lesion. Both procedures stop bleeding.

Perforation. Perforation is usually a surgical emergency. When the ulcer perforates, gastroduodenal contents empty through the anterior wall of the stomach into the peritoneal cavity, resulting in chemical peritonitis, bacterial septicemia, and hypovolemic shock. Peristalsis diminishes, and paralytic ileus develops.

Perforation occurs most frequently with duodenal ulcers. Perforation develops when an ulcer erodes through the tunica muscularis. The client experiences sudden, sharp, severe pain beginning in the midepigastrium. As peritonitis develops, the pain spreads over the entire abdomen, which then becomes tender, hard, and rigid. (See discussion of peritonitis in Chap. 55.)

The degree of pain depends on the amount and type of contents spilled. Characteristically, the pain causes the client to bend over or draw the knees up to the abdomen in an effort to decrease the tension on the abdominal muscles. If the perforation occurs on the posterior gastric wall, however, it may erode through to adjacent organs and become sealed, causing few symptoms. Manifestations of pancreatitis usually develop when a perforation erodes into the pancreas.

If perforation occurs, the client needs immediate replacement of fluid, blood, and electrolytes and administration of antibiotics. Nasogastric suction should be instituted to drain gastric secretions and thus prevent further peritoneal spillage. A small perforation that closes immediately by adhering to the adjacent tissues usually causes only a small loss of gastric contents. In this instance, the client may recover without surgery. When surgery is necessary, the surgeon (1) evacuates the escaped gastric contents, (2) cleanses the peritoneal cavity by flushing it out with normal saline or an antibiotic, and (3) closes the perforation by patching it with a bit of omentum. Vagotomy and hemigastrectomy or vagotomy and pyloroplasty can provide definitive control of both ulcer and its complications.

After surgery, administer antibiotics to combat peritonitis. The nasogastric tube remains in the stomach until peristalsis returns. Postoperative complications include subphrenic abscess, hemorrhage, duodenal or gastric fistula, atelectasis, or pneumonia.

Obstruction. Long-standing ulcer disease causes scarring from repeated ulcerations and healing. Scarring at the pylorus frequently causes pyloric obstruction manifested most often by pain at night when the stomach cannot be emptied by peristalsis. Pyloric obstruction can also lead to vomiting. Surgery, a pyloroplasty, is usually required to correct the problem.

Surgical Management

Surgery of the stomach is performed to (1) reduce its acid-secreting ability, (2) remove a malignant or potentially malignant lesion, (3) treat a surgical emergency that develops as a complication of peptic ulcer disease, or (4) treat clients who do not respond to medical intervention. Most chronic, recurring ulcers are eventually treated surgically. Surgery for prevention of ulcer recurrence is performed to (1) facilitate enterogastric regurgitation of mucous secretions, bile, and pancreatic juice; (2) decrease the secretory capacity of the stomach by removing the parietal cells; (3) remove stimuli for hydrochloric acid secretion by cutting the vagus nerve; and (4) eliminate the gastrin hormone mechanisms by antrectomy.

If the physician suspects cancer in a gastric lesion, surgery is generally indicated. When an ulcer does not respond to intensive medical therapy and a definite diagnosis cannot be made by radiographic and endoscopic examination, surgery is performed to remove the lesion and make certain it is not malignant.

Emergencies such as acute obstruction, perforation, and acute intractable hemorrhage are usually treated by surgical intervention immediately. Hemorrhage sometimes responds to medical management, but when medical approaches (such as cooling, vasoconstriction, and neutralization of the acid) do not stop the bleeding, emergency surgery is required to save the client's life.

The surgical approaches for reducing acidity of the stomach are (1) severing nerves that stimulate the acid-secreting cells and (2) removing the acid-secreting portions of the stomach.

VAGOTOMY

Vagotomy is performed to eliminate the acid-secreting stimulus to gastric cells. There are three types of vagotomy: (1) truncal, (2) selective, and (3) proximal (Fig. 54-3*A*). Truncal vagotomy involves completely cutting each vagus nerve. In selective vagotomy, the surgeon partially severs the nerves to preserve the hepatic and celiac branches. Proximal vagotomy also involves partial cutting, but in this instance, only the parietal cell mass is denervated; innervation of both the antrum and the pyloric sphincter is preserved. Cutting the vagal nerve fibers selectively avoids the problems of impaired

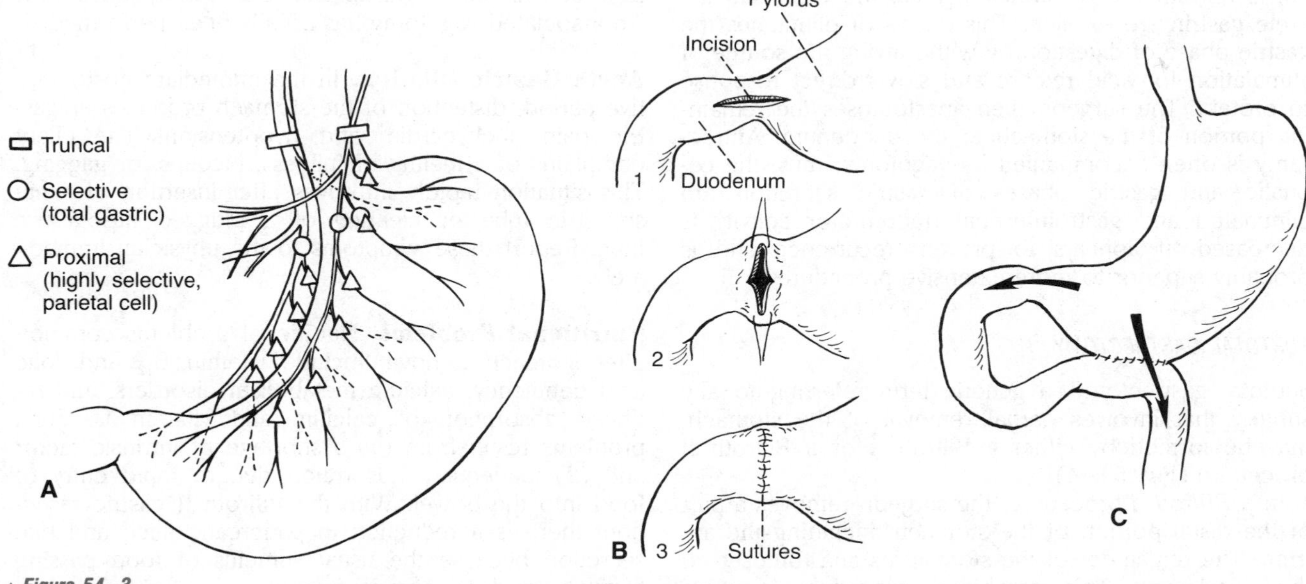

▲ *Figure 54-3*

Vagotomy and drainage. *A*, Sites at which the three types of vagotomy are performed. *B*, Pyloroplasty provides a larger opening from stomach to duodenum to enhance emptying after vagotomy. *C*, Gastroenterostomy, another associated surgical procedure, creates a passage between the body of the stomach and the jejunum.

emptying and diarrhea that follow the truncal vagotomy. It also eliminates the necessity for a drainage anastomosis to offset the gastric stasis. In addition, proximal vagotomy reduces acid secretion and preserves the function of the antrum.

VAGOTOMY WITH PYLOROPLASTY

Vagotomy with pyloroplasty involves cutting the right and left vagus nerves and widening the existing exit of the stomach at the pylorus. This procedure prevents stasis and enhances emptying, thereby preventing belching, weight loss, and feelings of fullness (Fig. 54–3*B*).

GASTROENTEROSTOMY

A simple gastroenterostomy (Fig. 54–3*C*) permits regurgitation of alkaline duodenal contents, thereby neutralizing gastric acid. In this procedure, a drain is made in the bottom of the stomach and sewn to an opening made in the jejunum. Because this neutralization interferes with the inhibition of gastrin release, a net increase in acid secretion may result. If the gastroenterostomy drains the stomach, it reduces motor activity in the pyloroduodenal area. Drainage also diverts acid away from the ulcerative area, which facilitates healing. A gastroenterostomy does not reduce the secretory capacity of the parietal cell mass, and the gastrin mechanism continues to function. Gastroenterostomy should be combined with vagotomy to reduce vagal influences.

ANTRECTOMY

Antrectomy is performed to reduce the acid-secreting portions of the stomach. The procedure removes the entire antrum of the stomach; thus, the cells that secrete gastrin are excised. This delays or eliminates the gastric phase of digestion by withdrawing the source of stimulation for acid release and slows direct response to protein. The surgeon then anastomoses the remaining portion of the stomach to the duodenum. Antrectomy is often accompanied by vagotomy; thus, the cephalic and gastric phases of gastric secretion are eliminated and gastrointestinal tract motor activity is decreased. It appears to prevent recurrence and is probably superior to more extensive procedures.

SUBTOTAL GASTRECTOMY

Subtotal gastrectomy, a generic term referring to any surgery that involves partial removal of the stomach, may be formed by either a Billroth I or a Billroth II procedure (Fig. 54–4).

In a *Billroth I* procedure, the surgeon removes a part of the distal portion of the stomach, including the antrum. The remainder of the stomach is anastomosed to the duodenum. This combined procedure is more properly called gastroduodenostomy. It decreases the incidence of dumping syndrome that often occurs after a Billroth II procedure.

A *Billroth II* resection involves reanastomosis of the proximal remnant of the stomach to the proximal jejunum. Note that pancreatic secretions and bile continue to be secreted into the duodenum even after gastrectomy. Because these secretions are necessary for digestion, a route to the intestine must be preserved for them. Surgeons prefer the Billroth II technique for treatment of duodenal ulcer because recurrent ulceration develops less frequently with this procedure.

TOTAL GASTRECTOMY

Total resection of the stomach is the principal intervention for extensive gastric cancer. This surgery involves removal of the stomach, with anastomosis of the esophagus to the jejunum, an esophagojejunostomy (Fig. 54–5). To perform total gastrectomy, the surgeon enters the chest; thus, the client returns to the recovery room with chest tubes.

COMPLICATIONS

Marginal Ulcers. A marginal ulcer can develop where gastric acids contact the operative site, either at the site of the anastomosis or in the jejunum. This ulceration may cause scarring and obstruction of the passages. Hemorrhage and perforation can also occur.

Hemorrhage. The reported incidence of hemorrhage after gastric surgery is 1 to 3 per cent. It is usually caused by a splenic injury or slippage of a ligature. Assess the client postoperatively for signs and symptoms of bleeding and intraperitoneal hemorrhage.

Alkaline Reflux Gastritis. Alkaline reflux gastritis due to duodenal contents occurs after gastric surgery in which the pylorus has been bypassed or removed. It also occurs after pyloroplasty and gastrojejunostomy. An associated vagotomy has usually been performed.

Acute Gastric Dilation. In the immediate postoperative period, distention of the stomach produces epigastric pain, tachycardia, and hypotension. The client complains of a feeling of fullness, hiccups, or gagging. This situation rapidly improves after insertion of a nasogastric tube or clearing of a plugged nasogastric tube. Report these symptoms to the physician immediately.

Nutritional Problems. Nutritional problems common after stomach removal include vitamin B_{12} and folic acid deficiency, calcium metabolism disorders, and reduced absorption of calcium and vitamin D. Such problems result from (1) a shortage of intrinsic factor and (2) inadequate absorption due to rapid entry of food into the bowel. With the Billroth II gastric resection, there is a reduction in pancreatic juice and bile secretion because the usual stimulus of food passing through the duodenum is missing.

Dumping Syndrome. This postprandial problem occurs after gastric resection because ingested food

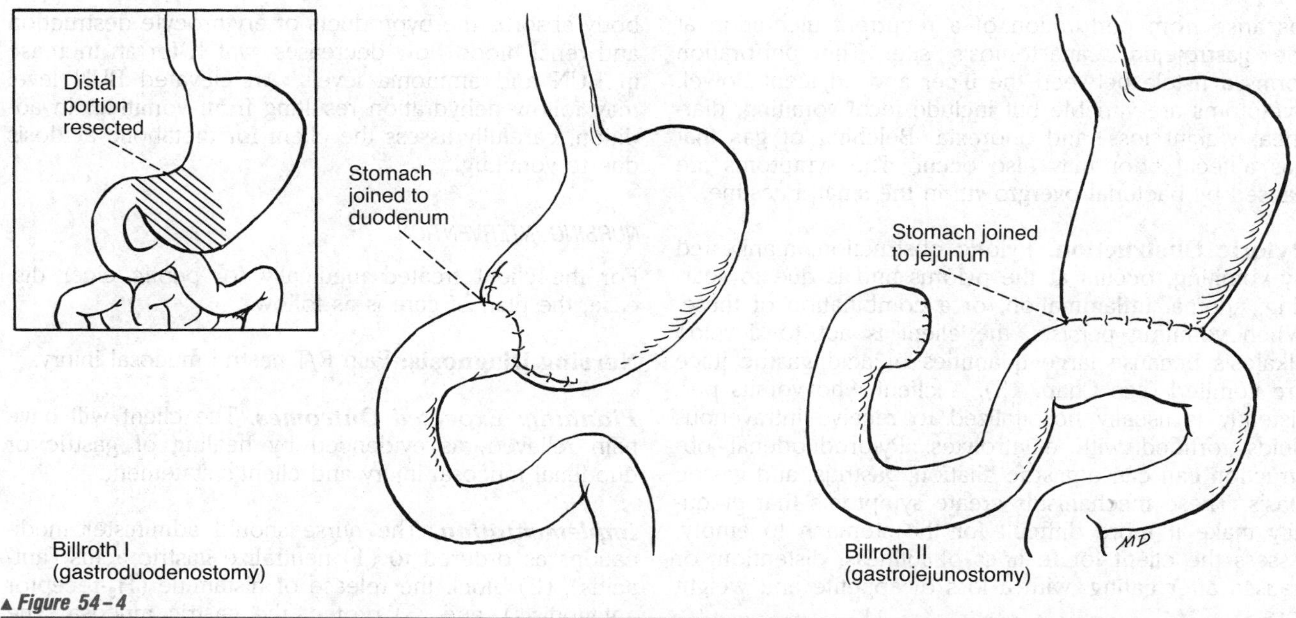

▲ **Figure 54-4**

Subtotal gastrectomy removes acid-secreting portions of the stomach. After removing the distal stomach *(inset),* a surgeon sutures the remaining portion of the stomach to the duodenum (Billroth I procedure) or to the proximal jejunum (Billroth II procedure).

rapidly enters the jejunum without proper mixing and without the normal duodenal digestive processing. It usually subsides in 6 to 12 months. Early manifestations, which occur 5 to 30 minutes after eating, involve the vasomotor disturbances of vertigo, tachycardia, syncope, sweating, pallor, palpitation, diarrhea, and

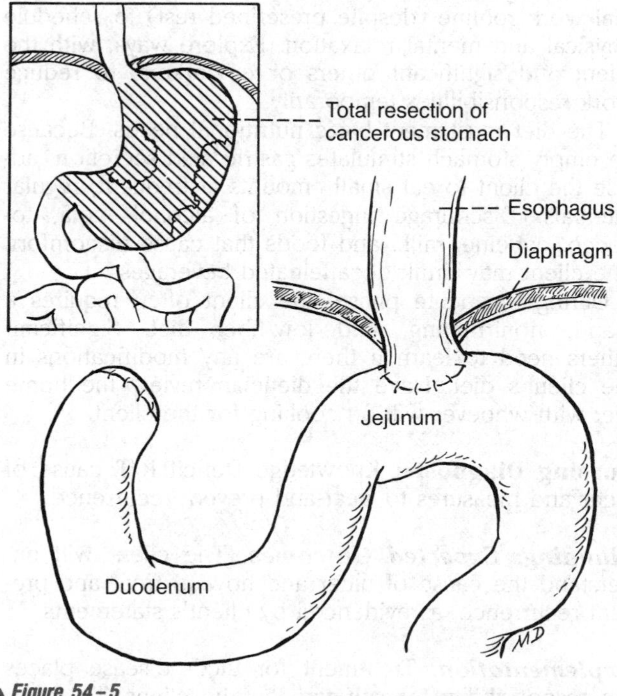

▲ **Figure 54-5**

Total gastrectomy *(inset)* with anastomosis of esophagus to jejunum (esophagojejunostomy) is the principal intervention for extensive gastric cancer.

nausea with the desire to lie down. The client's blood pressure and pulse may either rise or fall. Dumping syndrome is most common after the Billroth II procedure. Intestinal manifestations of dumping include epigastric fullness, distention, discomfort, abdominal cramping, nausea (with only occasional vomiting), and borborygmi (rumbling in the bowel). The client may experience tenesmus (a desire to defecate). Pain is not present.

Early manifestations are probably due to rapid movement of extracellular fluids into the bowel to convert the rapidly entering hypertonic bolus into an isotonic mixture. This rapid fluid shift decreases the circulating blood volume. A jejunum distended with food and fluid increases intestinal peristalsis and motility.

Late manifestations, which occur 2 to 3 hours after eating, are a result of (1) the rapid entry of high-carbohydrate food into the jejunum, (2) a rise in blood sugar, and (3) excessive insulin.

Management of dumping syndrome involves decreasing the amount of food taken at one time and maintaining a high-protein, high-fat, low-carbohydrate, dry diet. Gastric emptying can be delayed by (1) eating in a recumbent or semirecumbent position, (2) lying down after meals, (3) increasing the fat content in the diet, and (4) not taking fluids 1 hour before, with, or 2 hours after meals.

The client may also take sedatives and antispasmodics to delay gastric emptying. When symptoms persist, surgical intervention may include (1) reducing the size of the gastroenterostomy or (2) converting a Billroth II resection to a Billroth I by inserting a short segment of jejunum between the duodenal stump and the stomach.

Gastrojejunocolic Fistula. This postoperative complication follows recurrent peptic ulcer disease. The fistulas arise from perforation of a recurrent ulceration at the gastrojejunal anastomosis site. The perforation forms a fistula between the ulcer and adjacent bowel. Symptoms are variable but include fecal vomiting, diarrhea, weight loss, and anorexia. Belching of gas that has a fecal odor may also occur. The symptoms are caused by bacterial overgrowth in the small intestine.

Pyloric Obstruction. Pyloric obstruction, manifested by vomiting, occurs at the pylorus and is due to scarring, edema, inflammation, or a combination of these. When vomiting persists, the client is apt to develop alkalosis because large quantities of acid gastric juice are vomited (see Chap. 15). A client who vomits persistently is usually hospitalized to receive intravenous fluids fortified with electrolytes. Pyloroduodenal obstruction can cause gastric dilation, gastritis, and gastric stasis. These mechanisms create symptoms that gradually make it more difficult for the stomach to empty. Assess the client for feelings of fullness, distention, or nausea after eating, with a loss of appetite and weight loss.

Management of obstruction focuses on restoring fluid and electrolytes and decompressing the dilated stomach; if necessary, surgical intervention is instituted.

Nursing Management

ASSESSMENT

Nursing assessment involves gathering both psychosocial and pathophysiologic data concerning the client. To assess psychosocial aspects involving ulcer disease, ask the client about

- Familial incidence of ulcer
- Ingestion of medications causing gastric irritation
- Cigarette smoking
- Alcohol intake
- Stressors
- Coping patterns

Questions about lifestyle, occupation, work, and leisure can yield valuable information. Physical assessment includes accurately observing and immediately reporting to the physician symptoms that help pinpoint the diagnosis or that might indicate the presence of a complication. Symptoms include pain, vomiting, and occasionally bleeding and changes in appetite. Always obtain a complete history of previous ulcer attacks, including frequency, duration, manifestations, and response to intervention.

Assessment also involves describing the bleeding, including hematemesis and melena; note is made of such factors as the color, amount, consistency, and frequency. Bright red blood usually signifies new bleeding, whereas dark red blood indicates old bleeding. In severe bleeding, always maintain an accurate and up-to-date record of the client's hemoglobin, hematocrit, red blood cell count, and fluid intake and output.

Because of shock, the client may experience a decreased renal blood flow, which causes a decrease in renal excretion and glomerular filtration rate. As the body absorbs the byproducts of erythrocyte destruction and renal blood flow decreases, watch for an increase in BUN and ammonia levels. An elevated BUN level may follow dehydration resulting from vomiting. In addition, carefully assess the client for metabolic acidosis due to vomiting.

NURSING INTERVENTION

For the client treated medically for peptic ulcer disease, the plan of care is as follows.

Nursing Diagnosis: Pain R/T gastric mucosal injury.

Planning: Expected Outcomes. The client will have pain relieved, as evidenced by healing of gastric or duodenal mucosal injury and client's statement.

Implementation. The nurse should administer medications as ordered to (1) neutralize gastric acids (antacids), (2) block the release of histamine (H_2-receptor antagonists), and (3) protect the gastric mucosa. The nurse must assess the effectiveness of the medication on the client's pain and notify the physician if the pain is not relieved by these medications.

Avoidance of strenuous physical activity decreases gastric secretions and peristalsis. Thus, a primary nursing goal is to promote recovery by helping the client achieve rest, both physically and mentally. Be alert for factors that interfere with the client's rest. Arrange the environment to encourage relaxation. If certain visitors or telephone calls agitate the client, discourage these visits or calls until the client improves.

Encourage clients who attempt to carry on their normal work routine (despite prescribed rest) to schedule physical and mental relaxation. Explore ways, with the client and significant others or coworkers, to reduce work responsibilities temporarily.

The diet must meet basic nutritional needs. Because an empty stomach stimulates gastric acid secretion, advise the client to eat small amounts at frequent, regular intervals. Discourage ingestion of alcohol, cola, tobacco, caffeine, milk, and foods that cause discomfort. The client may drink decaffeinated beverages.

During the acute phase, the client often requires a bland, nonirritating, and low-fiber diet. Significant others need to learn if there are any modifications in the client's diet. Have the dietician review the home diet with whoever will be cooking for the client.

Nursing Diagnosis: Knowledge Deficit R/T cause of ulcer and measures to treat and prevent recurrence.

Planning: Expected Outcomes. The client will understand the cause of ulcer and how to treat and prevent recurrence, as evidenced by client's statements.

Implementation. Treatment for ulcer disease places the responsibility for self-care on the client. To maintain good self-care, the client must understand the pathophysiologic process underlying ulcer development and the rationale underlying intervention.

The nurse can help the client to (1) understand the pathogenesis of the ulcer and the significance of the pain; (2) realize that healing takes place rapidly when the irritating effect is removed; (3) understand what caused the condition to develop and what must be done to lessen the stimulation; (4) discover which substances cause pain by stimulating secretion of gastric juices, and eliminate them from the diet until the ulcer heals; (5) understand the importance of continuing the medical regimen, although pain is gone, until healing is completed; and (6) recognize that once maintenance therapy stops, the ulcer recurrence rate is over 50 per cent.

The nurse should instruct the client to use acetaminophen instead of aspirin preparations, when these are needed. Teach the client to examine the labels of all nonprescription medications, particularly cold remedies, for aspirin (acetylsalicylic acid), other salicylates, nonsteroidal anti-inflammatories such as ibuprofen and phenylbutazone, adrenocorticosteroids, and ACTH. These medications are ulcerogenic (cause ulcers), particularly when combined. If any of these medications must be taken, advise the client to check with the physician first, eat between meals, and use H_2-receptor antagonists or antacids.

Helping clients with ulcers cope with psychosocial problems is a vital part of intervention. Take time to learn about their stressors. Discussing coping and relaxation techniques may enable clients to better deal with their problems.

Collaborative Problem. Injury, high risk for R/T complication (e.g., hemorrhage, perforation, obstruction).

Planning: Expected Outcomes. The client will not suffer any injury, as evidenced by the absence of hemorrhage, perforation, or obstruction.

Implementation. The nurse must monitor for the development of complications of ulcers including hemorrhage, perforation, or obstruction. The nurse should monitor vital signs closely for the development of symptoms of shock that might occur if bleeding is present. Document and report the occurrence of melena or hematemesis. If hemorrhage occurs, treat immediately to stop hemorrhage and prevent shock (see Chap. 20).

Monitor the client for the development of perforation. Assess the abdomen for pain, tenderness, or rigidity. Report suspected perforation to the physician immediately and prepare the client for possible surgery. The client should also be monitored for the development of gastric obstruction. If the client vomits, the nurse should record the frequency and consistency (digested or undigested food or hematemesis) of the vomitus. If pyloric obstruction is present, the client will require a nasogastric tube and intravenous fluids until the problem is corrected surgically.

For the client undergoing surgery for peptic ulcer disease, the plan of care is as follows.

Nursing Diagnosis: Knowledge Deficit R/T preoperative preparation, postoperative care, diet, and long-term prevention of recurrence.

Planning: Expected Outcomes. The client will understand preoperative preparation, postoperative care, diet, and long-term prevention of recurrence, as evidenced by client's statements and no recurrence of ulcer disease.

Implementation. Surgical intervention for gastric and duodenal conditions may be either a planned procedure or an emergency. When emergency surgery is required (e.g., for acute obstruction, perforation, or hemorrhage), the client is very ill and usually frightened. Provide calm, efficient, knowledgeable care and explain what is being done. Note and respond to the client's nonverbal behavior. Help significant others provide the client with empathy and emotional support.

When cancer is suspected, the client may want to talk about fears and concerns. Listen to the client carefully, respond to cues, and offer support and understanding. The client may wish to attend to personal matters before surgery (e.g., check a will, see a minister).

When elective surgery is done, the client will probably have an extensive series of preoperative examinations, such as a gastrointestinal tract series, endoscopy, and perhaps acid-secretion studies (see Chap. 52). These may be done on an outpatient basis.

Preoperative teaching should include an explanation of what surgery generally involves. Explain that the client will have (1) either a nasogastric tube or possibly a gastrostomy tube and suction and (2) intravenous infusion in the hand or arm for fluids until the surgical site heals. Thoroughly demonstrate and discuss the importance of deep-breathing exercises. Warn clients that the high abdominal incision makes deep breathing very uncomfortable. The high incision also increases the risk of respiratory complications.

Postoperatively, some clients need help to reduce the number of stressors in their lives. Strategies for altering lifestyle may be an important part of the rehabilitation and recovery plan. When complications such as dumping syndrome occur, the client may feel disappointed. Many clients expect a rapid recovery and may be unprepared when complications do develop. Most clients can learn to control symptoms and lead a fairly normal life.

Collaborative Problem. Injury, high risk for R/T postoperative complications (immediate and delayed).

Planning: Expected Outcomes. The client will not suffer injury related to postoperative complications (immediate and delayed), as evidenced by decreasing bloody drainage from nasogastric tube, absence of abdominal distention, and normal breath sounds.

Implementation. Nursing care after gastric surgery is the same as postoperative care for any client recovering from major abdominal surgery. In addition to general postoperative care, the nurse should

- check the drainage from the nasogastric tube
- ensure that the tube is attached to suction, as ordered
- assess the operative site for excessive drainage; too much fluid in the remaining gastric stump could cause increased pressure and injury
- note the color and consistency of drainage from the operative site and report bleeding or hemorrhaging

Immediate complications after gastric surgery include gastric dilation, obstruction, hemorrhage, and disruption of the suture line. Also, observe for general surgical complications such as shock, hemorrhage, pulmonary problems, thrombosis, evisceration, and infection. Nausea and vomiting should not occur if the nasogastric tube is patent. Carefully measure and document intake (oral and intravenous) and output (urine, suction, and wound drainage).

The client will return from surgery with a nasogastric or gastrostomy tube for preventing the retention of gastric secretions. The nurse should carefully assess for abdominal distention. The nasogastric or gastrostomy tube should not be repositioned after gastric surgery and should be irrigated gently, *only* if specifically ordered.

The color of the drainage in the nasogastric tube may be bright during the early hours after surgery but should become dark red by the end of 24 hours.

Keep the client comfortable with liberal administration of pain medications. This helps the client to cooperate more fully during deep-breathing and coughing exercises. Give fluids by intravenous infusion as ordered until edema and swelling have diminished enough to allow fluids to pass the operative area (seen as a decrease in the gastric tube output).

Nursing Diagnosis: Nutrition, Altered: Less than Body Requirements R/T decreased nutrient absorption secondary to dumping syndrome.

Planning: Expected Outcomes. The client will maintain adequate nutrition, as evidenced by client's ability to maintain weight at normal level and no evidence of dumping syndrome.

Implementation. When healing has occurred, begin oral intake by giving the client clear water, usually 30 ml at a time. Aspirate the tube an hour or so later to see if the fluid has been retained. When gastrointestinal function has returned (e.g., active bowel sound, passing flatus) and the client tolerates clear water, the nasogastric tube is usually removed and the diet progressed. Next, progress to soft foods and eventually to a regular diet of five or six small meals a day. The diet should not begin too early or progress too rapidly. The client may experience discomfort, at first, if too much food is taken at one time.

Clients need to know that convalescence after gastric surgery tends to be slow. It may be 3 months before clients regain strength and even partial ability to eat in a more normal manner. It may take a year or so before they can eat three normal meals a day. Observe the client postoperatively for persistent gastric disturbances.

EVALUATION

The nurse must evaluate the degree to which the goals and outcomes have been achieved. If the client's goals have not been met, the plan and interventions must be revised so they can be met.

Post-hospital Care

DISCHARGE TEACHING

Preparation for going home must be gradual, so start your teaching program early during the client's stay in the health care facility. The client should have verbal and written instructions on medications and treatments.

FOLLOW-UP CARE

The client who has had gastric resection should be seen at intervals to be assessed for the development of pernicious anemia.

GASTRIC CANCER

Definition

Gastric cancer refers to the malignant neoplasms found in the stomach, usually adenocarcinoma, although they may be malignant lymphomas.

Incidence

For unknown reasons, the incidence of stomach cancer in the United States has diminished steadily during the last four decades. Despite the reduced incidence, this is the sixth most common cause of death from cancer in the United States. The incidence of gastric cancer in the United States has decreased from 25 to 4 per 100,000 during the past 40 years.[4]

Although little is known of the cause, it is known that stomach cancer is twice as common in men as in women, more common in American whites, and more frequent in clients who have pernicious anemia. It often develops in conjunction with atrophic gastritis and affects individuals who (1) have a low socioeconomic status, (2) live in an urban area, (3) eat smoked fish, or (4) are exposed to background radiation or trace metals in the soil. Worldwide mortality rates vary greatly, possibly owing to differences in diet, genetics, and soil composition. The presence of *H. pylori* in the stomach increases the incidence of gastric cancer.

Etiology

Although there are no specific etiologic factors associated with gastric cancer, several factors do seem associated with the development of the disease. These include chronic atrophic gastritis, achlorhydria, and pernicious anemia. The changes in the mucosa may lead to an increase in the absorption of carcinogens from the diet, such as pickled foods, salted fish, and nitrates. Smoking also appears to be associated with an increased incidence of gastric cancer. There may also be a genetic factor because it does seem to run in families.

Risk Factors

Metal craftsmen, coal miners, bakers, and those working in dusty, smoky, and sulfur dioxide–containing environments are at greater risk. Wood or tobacco smoke, nitrite food preservatives, and overheated fat products may predispose clients to stomach cancer.

Avoidance of the carcinogenic agents is important, especially in clients with other risk factors such as chronic gastritis, *H. pylori* infection, and pernicious anemia. Cessation of smoking is a good primary preventive measure.

Pathophysiology

Gastric cancer most often arises from the mucous lining of the stomach. The majority of these cancers occur in the lesser curvature of the stomach in the pyloric and antral regions.

Most carcinomas of the stomach develop in its lower half. Prognosis is best for stomach cancer involving polypoid lesions, poor for ulcerating cancers, and poorest for infiltrating forms. Stomach cancer spreads by (1) direct extension into the pancreas, (2) the lymphatics, or (3) hematogenous infiltration of the liver, lungs, and bones. The particular route depends on the location and type of tumor. Some penetrate, some ulcerate, and some spread along the tissue planes (Table 54–4).

The disease is resectable in early stages before it has invaded the wall of the stomach. The 5-year survival rate is about 90 per cent for local disease; this rate drops to less than 10 per cent for stage III disease. In advanced gastric cancers, the survival rate is almost zero. Lesions higher in the stomach, especially around the cardia, have a poor prognosis because of the usual lateness of diagnosis.

Clinical Manifestations

Because the symptoms occur late, stomach cancer is seldom diagnosed in an early stage. Furthermore, unless hemorrhage or perforation occurs, manifestations are vague and indefinite. The presence of a palpable mass, ascites, or bone pain from metastasis may be the first symptom. Symptoms vary, depending on the location of the tumor in the stomach. If the neoplasm grows near the cardia, the client may experience dysphagia from early involvement of the esophagus. If the neoplasm is near the pylorus, symptoms may occur from obstruction.

Assessment reveals weight loss, a vague indigestion, anorexia, or a feeling of fullness or mild discomfort so insidious that the client does not recognize it as abnormal or seek medical assistance. Discomfort may be brought on or relieved by food. Anemia from blood loss commonly occurs, and occult blood may be present in the stool. The presence of lactic acid and a high lactate dehydrogenase level in the gastric juice suggests carcinoma.

TABLE 54–4. TNM Classification for Gastric Carcinoma

Primary Tumor (T)	
T_x	Primary tumor cannot be assessed
T_0	No evidence of primary tumor
T_{is}	Carcinoma in situ: intraepithelial tumor without invasion of lamina propria
T_1	Tumor invades lamina propria or submucosa
T_2	Tumor invades muscularis propria or subserosa
T_3	Tumor penetrates serosa (visceral peritoneum) without invasion of adjacent structures
T_4	Tumor invades adjacent structures
Lymph Node (N)	
N_x	Regional lymph node(s) cannot be assessed
N_0	No regional lymph node metastasis
N_1	Metastasis in perigastric lymph node(s) within 3 cm of edge of primary tumor
N_2	Metastasis in perigastric lymph node(s) more than 3 cm from edge of primary tumor, or in lymph nodes along left gastric, common hepatic, splenic, or celiac arteries
Distant Metastasis (M)	
M_x	Presence of distant metastasis cannot be assessed
M_0	No distant metastasis
M_1	Distant metastasis
Stage Grouping	
0	$T_{is}N_0M_0$
IA	$T_1N_0M_0$
IB	$T_1N_1M_0$
	$T_2N_0M_0$
II	$T_1N_2M_0$
	$T_2N_1M_0$
	$T_3N_0M_0$
IIIA	$T_2N_2M_0$
	$T_3N_1M_0$
	$T_4N_0M_0$
IIIB	$T_3N_2M_0$
	$T_4N_1M_0$
IV	$T_4N_2M_0$
	Any T, any N, M_1

DIAGNOSTIC ASSESSMENT

Upper gastrointestinal tract x-ray examination and gastroscopy diagnose gastric cancer. Gastroscopy allows the lesion to be viewed directly. Cytologic brushing and biopsy can be used to diagnose cancer cells.

Medical Management

There is little effective medical treatment for gastric carcinoma. Clients may receive chemotherapy and radiation therapy, but the primary treatment for this condition is surgical resection.

At present, best results are achieved with multiple drug combinations. Those giving the best results are fluorouracil (5-FU), mitomycin C, and doxorubicin (Adriamycin). The combination of radiation and chemotherapy after surgery may be done.

TPN (hyperalimentation) is a method for providing nutrition to the client intravenously, thus bypassing the gastrointestinal tract.

Surgical Management

Surgery is the only intervention that effectively treats stomach cancer. Unfortunately, because the diagnosis is usually late, surgery is more often palliative than curative. Gastrectomy, either partial or complete, depending on tumor location, is the usual procedure. Ideally, the surgeon removes all local growth and the associated lymph nodes. When an extensive tumor makes resection impractical or impossible and the pylorus is obstructed, the surgeon may perform a palliative gastroenterostomy (surgical creation of a passage between the stomach and small intestine). Chemotherapy and, less often, radiation may be used with surgery.

Nursing Management

ASSESSMENT

As mentioned, the symptoms associated with gastric cancer are usually vague. Clients may present with symptoms similar to ulcer disease, but often symptoms are not present until the tumor is advanced. The nurse should note on the client's history any risk or predisposing factors to the development of gastric carcinoma. These include a history of chronic gastritis, pernicious anemia, gastric surgery, or smoking. The nurse should also note in the client history if the client ingests large amounts of nitrates, smoked fish, salty foods, or pickled foods.

NURSING INTERVENTION

Nursing Diagnosis: Pain, Acute R/T gastric erosion; and Pain, Postoperative R/T high surgical incision.

Planning: Expected Outcomes. The client will have pain controlled or experience a reduction in pain, as evidenced by client's statements.

Implementation. It is very important that the client receive pain relief. Pain that is not controlled can interfere with sleep and eating and contribute to overall physical and mental deterioration. See Chapter 16 for a detailed explanation of pain control.

Nursing Diagnosis: Nutrition, Altered: Less than Body Requirements R/T decreased appetite, pain, possible gastric obstruction, and nausea and vomiting.

Planning: Expected Outcomes. The client will maintain nutritional intake to meet metabolic requirements, as evidenced by maintenance of normal body weight.

Implementation. Nutritional therapy is a very important aspect of management of the client with gastric cancer. TPN or jejunostomy tube feedings may be used postoperatively (or for inoperable clients) to maintain the nutritional status.

Nursing Diagnosis: Fear R/T knowledge deficit, treatment, and life-threatening illness.

Planning: Expected Outcomes. The client will have fear reduced or controlled, as evidenced by client's ability to understand and discuss disease and treatment options.

Implementation. The client needs an explanation of the disease and all treatment options. The nurse needs to reinforce information to the client as needed. The client also needs to have preoperative teaching concerning operative procedures (nothing by mouth; holding area; intravenous infusions). Information will help decrease the client's fear.

Postoperative complications include hemorrhage, obstruction, anemia, nutritional deficiency, dumping syndrome, duodenal stump leakage, gastric dilation, and delayed gastric emptying.

EVALUATION

The nurse must evaluate the degree to which the goals and outcomes have been achieved. If the client's goals have not been met, the plan and interventions must be revised so they can be met.

Post-hospital Care

DISCHARGE TEACHING

The client should have verbal and written instructions regarding medications, treatments, and follow-up care.

HOME HEALTH CARE NEEDS

A home health care referral can assist the client with emotional support and treatments and provide an ongoing assessment of the client's condition. The nurse might also refer the client to a dietician, clergyman, and hospice team. Various community support groups are also available, such as I Can Cope.

FOLLOW-UP CARE

The client will be followed for signs of recurrence if the treatment was successful. If the treatment was unsuccessful, palliative care will be needed.

▼ CONGENITAL DISORDERS

ESOPHAGEAL ATRESIA WITH TRACHEOESOPHAGEAL FISTULA

Atresia of the esophagus with a fistula from the lower pouch and a blind upper pouch (type III) is described as the "classic picture" of the disease. There are six types of esophageal atresia that can be present; the largest percentage are type III. There are a wide variety and combination of approaches in treatment, depending on the type and condition of the infant. Ligation of the fistula usually takes place immediately. The esophagus is repaired at the same time if the infant's condition allows. If there is too wide a gap between the proximal and distal pouches in esophageal atresia without fistula or if a leak occurs in the anastomosis, a reconstruction of the esophagus (colon transposition, colon transport, esophageal replacement) is performed.

The prognosis for complete recovery depends on many factors. The most common complication is stricture at the anastomosis site. Regularly scheduled dilation with Tucker dilators is necessary if stricture is present.

Summary

Gastric disorders are common; unless treated promptly and completely, they can continue to cause problems throughout the client's life. The nurse must often help clients learn a new way of eating to obtain and maintain health. This is a difficult task; however, unless the client modifies behavior, especially eating behaviors, many of the gastric disorders simply recur. The focus of nursing interventions will be education and modifications of the client's behavior to a healthier pattern.

Bibliography

1. Achkar, E. (1985). Peptic ulcer disease: Current management in the elderly. *Geriatrics, 40*(9), 77-83.
2. Akridge, K. (1989). Anorexia nervosa. *Journal of Obstetric, Gynecologic, and Neonatal Nursing, 18,* 25-30.
3. American Cancer Society (1986). Gastric cancer. *CA: A cancer journal for clinicians, 36.*
4. American Cancer Society (1987). *Cancer facts and figures.* New York: Author.

4a. American Cancer Society (1992). *Cancer facts and figures.* New York: Author.

5. Andersen, A. E. (1985). *Practical and comprehensive treatment of anorexia nervosa and bulimia.* Baltimore: The Johns Hopkins University Press.
6. Baird, S. B., et al. (1991). *Cancer nursing: A comprehensive textbook.* Philadelphia: W. B. Saunders.
7. Bardhan, K. D. (1986). Gastric ulcer: Sparing patients from surgery. *Geriatric Medicine, 40*(5), 41-44.
8. Barkin, J., & Rogers, A. (Eds.) (1989). *Difficult decisions in digestive diseases.* Chicago: Year Book Medical Publishers.
9. Beahrs, O. H., et al. (Eds). (1988). *Manual for staging cancer* (3rd ed.) Philadelphia: J. B. Lippincott.
10. Beck, J. E. (Ed.) (1985). *Bockus gastroenterology* (4th ed.). Philadelphia: W. B. Saunders.
11. Botoman, V. A., & Black, H. R. (1984). Weight loss: Guide to evaluating patients. *Consultant, 24,* 258.
12. Bowers, W. A. (1987). Medical complications of anorexia nervosa and bulimia: Implications for rehabilitation counselors. *Journal of Rehabilitation, 53,* 55-58.
13. Broadwell, D. C., & Jackson, B. S. (Eds.) (1982). *Principles of ostomy care.* St. Louis: C. V. Mosby.
14. Brooks, F. P., et al. (1985). *Peptic ulcer disease: Contemporary issues in gastroenterology.* New York: Churchill Livingstone.
15. Burns, R. A., & Davis, W. S. (1985). Recurrent aphthous stomatitis. *American Family Physician, 32,* 99.
16. Cheli, R., et al. (1987). *Gastritis: A critical review.* New York: Springer-Verlag.
17. Cohen, E. L. (1984). Epiglottitis in the adult. *Postgraduate Medicine, 75,* 309.
18. Correa, P. (1991). Is gastric carcinoma an infectious disease? *New England Journal of Medicine, 325*(16), 1170-1171.
19. Cotran, R. S., et al. (1989). *Robbins pathologic basis of disease.* Philadelphia: W. B. Saunders.
20. Cushman, K. E. (1986). Symptom management: A comprehensive approach to increasing nutritional status in the cancer patient. *Seminars in Oncology Nursing, 2*(1), 30-35.
21. De Fazio, F. (1985). To control painless worry. *American Health, 4,* 16.
22. Douglas, H. O. (1986). Current management of gastric cancer: Analysis of recent advances. *Current Concepts in Oncology, 8*(3), 3-8.
23. Farinati, F., et al. (1988). Gastric ulcer and stomach aging: Pathophysiology and clinical implications. *Gerontology, 34,* 297-303.
24. Frank-Stromberg, M. (1989). The epidemiology and primary prevention of gastric and esophageal cancer. *Cancer Nursing 12*(2), 53-64.
25. Garner, D. M., & Garfinkel, P. E. (Eds.) (1985). *Handbook of psychotherapy for anorexia nervosa and bulimia.* New York: Guilford.
26. Gitnick, G. L. (Ed.) (1983). *Gastroenterology.* New York: John Wiley & Sons.
27. Given, B., & Simmons, S. (1984). *Gastroenterology in clinical nursing* (4th ed.). St. Louis: C. V. Mosby.
28. Grabinar, J. (1987). Upper GI pain: Causes, clues, and action. *Geriatric Medicine, 47*(8), 67-70.
29. Groenwald, S. L., et al. (1991). *Cancer nursing: Principles and practice* (2nd ed.). Boston: Jones and Bartlett.
30. Guyton, A. C. (1991). *Textbook of medical physiology* (8th ed.). Philadelphia: W. B. Saunders.
31. Gwirtsman, H. E., et al. (1983). Neuroendocrine abnormalities in bulimia. *American Journal of Psychiatry, 140,* 559.
32. Hamilton, H., & Rose, M. B. (1985). *Gastrointestinal disorders.* Springhouse, PA: Springhouse Corporation.
33. Johnson, C., & Connors, M. E. (1987). *The etiology and treatment of bulimia nervosa: A biopsychosocial perspective.* New York: Basic Books.
34. Kandel, G. (1990). Management of nonvariceal upper GI hemorrhage. *Hospital Practice, 25,* 167-184.
35. Karb, V. (1988). GI drugs: Histamine antagonists, sucralfate and metoclopramide. *Journal of Neuroscience Nursing, 20,* 202.
36. Katz, K., & Hollander, D. (1988). Outpatient management of duodenal ulcer disease. *Hospital Medicine, 24,* 95-103.
37. Kirsner, J. B. (1985). The stomach. In W. A. Sodeman, Jr., & T. M. Sodeman (Eds.), *Pathologic physiology: Mechanisms of disease* (7th ed.). Philadelphia: W. B. Saunders.
38. Konopad, E., & Noseworthy, T. (1988). Stress ulceration: A serious complication in critically ill patients. *Heart and Lung, 17,* 339-348.
39. Kopeski, L. M. (1989). Diabetes and bulimia: A deadly duo. *American Journal of Nursing, 89,* 482-485.
40. Levinson, M. (1989). Gastric stress ulcer. *Hospital Practice, 24,* 59-67.
41. Marble, D., & Ward, J. (1989). Managing NSAID-induced peptic ulcer. *Drug Therapy, 19,* 34-45.

42. Marks, R. G. (1984). Anorexia and bulimia: Eating habits that can kill. *RN, 14,* 44.
43. Martin, L. F., et al. (1985). Bleeding from stress gastritis. Has prophylactic pH control make a difference? *American Surgeon, 51,* 189-193.
44. Mickley, D. W. (1988). Eating disorders. *Hospital Practice, 23,* 58-62.
45. Miles, M. W. (1988). Bulimia nervosa and gender identity: Symbols of a culture. *Holistic Nursing Practice, 3,* 55-56.
46. Nelis, G. F., & Misiewicz, J. J. (1985). *Peptic ulcer disease: Basic and clinical aspects.* Boston: Martinus Nijhoff.
47. Nonsurgical alternative to NG tube (1983). *Nursing Life, 3,* 10.
48. Parrsonett, J., et al. (1991). *Helicobacter pylori* infection and the risk of gastric carcinoma. *New England Journal of Medicine, 325*(16), 1127-1136.
49. Pattern of binge/purge (1984). *American Journal of Nursing, 84,* 33.
50. Peterson, W. L. (1985). Gastrointestinal hemorrhage. In J. B. Wyngaarden & L. H. Smith, Jr. (Eds.), *Cecil textbook of medicine* (18th ed). Philadelphia: W. B. Saunders.
51. Potts, N. L. (1984). Eating disorders—the secret. *American Journal of Nursing, 84,* 32.
52. Preece, P. E., et al. (1986). *Cancer of the stomach.* New York: Grune & Stratton.
53. Present, D., et al. (1980). Treatment of Crohn's disease with 6-mercaptopurine. *New England Journal of Medicine, 302,* 981.
54. Price, S., & Wilson, L. (1982). *Pathophysiology: Clinical concepts of disease processes* (2nd ed.). New York: McGraw-Hill.
55. Pries, J. M. (1982). Coping with reflux esophagitis in the aged. *Geriatrics, 37,* 57.
56. Provenzale, J. (1983). Anorexia nervosa: Thinness as illness. *Postgraduate Medicine, 74,* 83.
57. Rodman, M. J., & Smith, D. W. (1985). *Pharmacology and drug therapy in nursing* (3rd ed.). Philadelphia: J. B. Lippincott.
58. Roth, G. (1986). *Breaking free from compulsive eating.* New York: Signet.
59. Sabiston, D. C., Jr. (1991). *Textbook of surgery: The biologic basis of modern surgical practice* (14th ed.). Philadelphia: W. B. Saunders.
60. Sanger, E., & Cassino, T. (1984). Eating disorders: Avoiding the power struggle. *American Journal of Nursing, 84,* 31.
61. Schroeder, S. A., et al. (1988). *Current medical diagnosis treatment.* Norwalk, CT: Appleton & Lange.
62. Sernka, T., & Jacobson, E. (1983). *Gastrointestinal physiology: The essentials* (2nd ed.). Baltimore: Williams & Wilkins.
63. Siler, W. (1985). Pathogenic factors in erosive gastritis. *American Journal of Medicine, 29,* 45-48.
64. Skinner, S. M. (1985). Gastric lavage. *Nursing '85, 12,* 56M-56O.
65. Sleisenger, M. H., & Fordtran, J. S. (1989). *Gastrointestinal disease* (4th ed.). Philadelphia: W. B. Saunders.
66. Spiro, H. M. (1983). *Clinical gastroenterology* (3rd ed.). New York: Macmillan Publishing.
67. Strange, J. M. (1983). An expert's guide to tubes and drains. *RN, 46,* 35.
68. Strickland, R. G. (1983). Acute and chronic gastritis. *Hospital Medicine, 19,* 148.
69. Symmonds, R. E. (1983). Surgery for morbid obesity. *Postgraduate Medicine, 74,* 183.
70. Theophylline-induced gastroesophageal reflux (1983). *Nurses' Drug Alert, 4,* 30.
71. U.S. Department of Health and Human Services (1988). *Cancer of the stomach.* (NIH Publication No. 88-2978). Bethesda: National Cancer Institute.
72. Viste, A., et al. (1988). Postoperative complications and mortality after surgery for gastric cancer. *Annals of Surgery, 207,* 7-13.
73. Walsh, B. T. (1988). *Eating behavior in eating disorders.* Washington, DC: American Psychiatric Press.
74. Wang, J. (1988). Stomach cancer. *Seminars in Oncology Nursing, 4,* 258.
75. White, J. H. (1984). Bulimia, utilizing individual and family therapy. *Journal of Psychosocial Nursing, 22,* 22.
76. Wyngaarden, J. B., et al. (1992). *Cecil Textbook of Medicine* (19th ed.). Philadelphia: W. B. Saunders Company.

Chapter 55

Nursing Care of Clients with Intestinal Disorders

GENERALIZED CLINICAL MANIFESTATIONS

Manifestations of intestinal disorders vary according to which function (motility, digestion, or absorption) is disturbed and the cause of this disturbance. The major manifestations of dysfunction are hemorrhage, pain, tenderness, distention, vomiting, malabsorption, constipation, diarrhea, abdominal masses, or abnormal fecal contents.

Hemorrhage

Bleeding may be caused by trauma, ulceration, inflammation, or a growth that erodes through a blood vessel (Fig. 55-1). The usual manifestation is blood in the stool (melena) rather than in the emesis (hematemesis). The amount of bleeding varies from a minute quantity that is invisible except by testing (occult blood) to large quantities that cause the stools to be bright red to tarry black. Because color comes from the digestive processes acting on the blood, the examiner can use the amount of color change to determine the level of the bowel in which bleeding occurs. The rapidity with which the chyme passes through the bowel also affects stool color passed in a certain period and what color changes occur. For instance, slow bleeding from the duodenum may not increase peristalsis and may produce a tarry stool. If the rate of bleeding or of peristalsis increases, subsequent stools may become brighter in color.

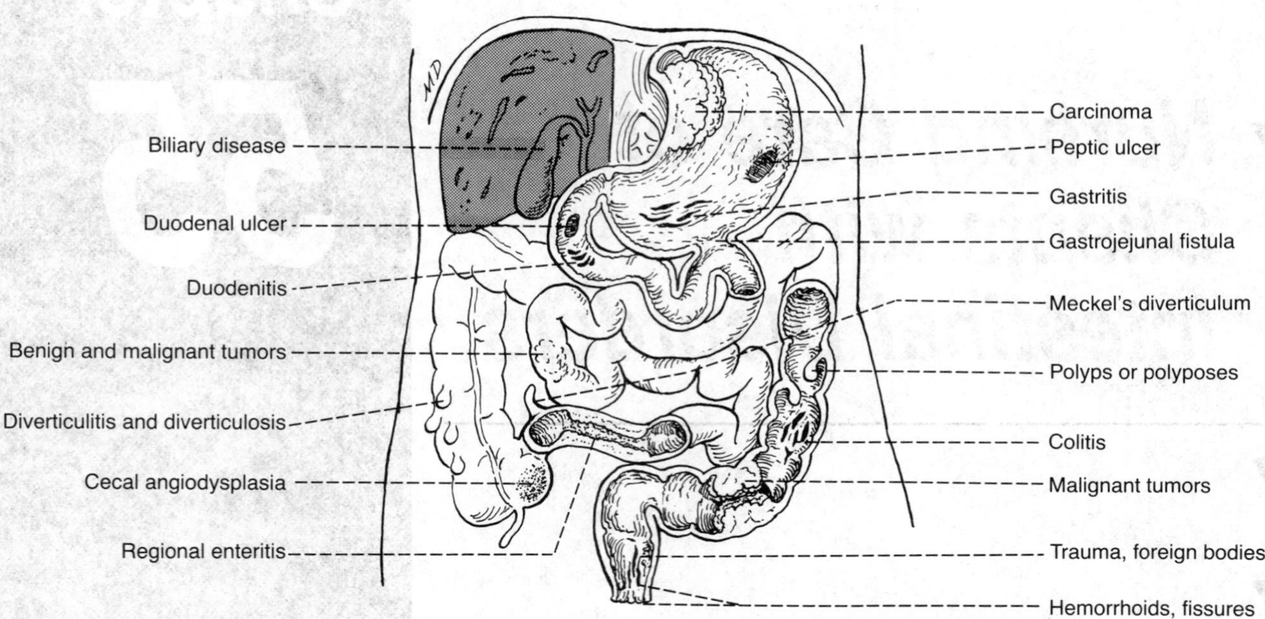

▲ *Figure 55–1*

Causes of GI bleeding.

Pain

Pain results from stimulation of nerve endings in the muscular or submucosal layers of bowel wall and from increased tension when the bowel is distended. Discomfort occurs in various places, including the involved portion of the bowel, another previously diseased area, or a nearby somatic portion of the body (referred pain). Previous surgical procedures also influence the location at which pain is felt.

Obstruction of blood supply to the intestine also can cause pain. Acute or partial occlusion of the mesenteric artery causes intermittent pain during digestion because of the increased need for blood at that time. This is sometimes called intestinal angina. Occlusion can occur in the major artery or one of the smaller branches.

Nausea and Vomiting

In intestinal disorders, nausea results from distention of the duodenum. If vomiting occurs and is fecal in nature, it originates from the bowel and is usually due to a high small intestinal obstruction.

Malabsorption

Malabsorption is a defect in the mechanism by which food is absorbed by the small intestinal mucosa. In the intestinal phase of absorption, the intestinal villi secrete enzymes that stimulate intestinal motility and facilitate absorption. The active transport mechanism moves absorbed nutrients from the lumen of the small bowel to the intestinal submucosa and from the submucosa to the body's tissues by way of the circulatory or lymphatic system. Abnormalities may result from (1) loss of ileal function; (2) decreased production of pancreatic enzyme, especially inadequate secretion of lipase; (3) inflammation of the intestinal mucosa; or (4) any surgical loss of absorptive mucosa, such as gastric, small bowel, or colon resection.

Diarrhea

Rapid propulsion of intestinal contents through the small bowel usually results in diarrhea.

Constipation

Constipation, a very common symptom, can be caused by inadequate fluid or bulk, mechanical blockage of the passage of intestinal contents (by a tumor), or slow peristalsis.

Abnormalities in Fecal Content

The presence of fats or other abnormal constituents normally absorbed from the stool indicates malabsorption. Other fecal abnormalities that may aid in diagnosis are bacteria, parasites, pus, blood, and abnormal quantities of mucus from the colon.

GASTROINTESTINAL INTUBATION

Gastric and intestinal tubes are inserted for several purposes: decompression, lavage, gastric analysis, and tube feedings. Decompression relieves the pressure caused by gastrointestinal (GI) contents and gases that remain in the stomach or bowel because of some obstruction. Long intestinal tubes are sometimes used to dilate or release an obstruction. Postoperative, decompression removes secretions that cannot pass through the GI tract because of edema and decreased gastric motility. Intubation helps prevent vomiting, distention, and obstruction.

Lavage is the irrigation or washing out of an organ. Gastric lavage washes out the stomach. It is used most frequently as an emergency treatment in poisoning. Lavage is also used for exfoliative cytology.

Tube feeding or *enteral nutrition* is a method of giving clients fluids and nutrients via a tube when oral intake is inadequate or impossible.

Types of Tubes

Two types of tubes are used for decompression. Short nasogastric tubes are used for the stomach, and long tubes for the rest of the GI tract (Table 55-1).

SHORT TUBES

These include the Levin and Salem sump tubes. Short tubes are long enough to extend into the stomach but not into the bowel. These tubes are attached to intermittent suction.

Levin Tube. The Levin tube is an older, single-lumen tube used to remove fluid or gas or to obtain a specimen of gastric contents.

Salem Sump Tube. This is a double-lumen tube used to empty and decompress the stomach. The "pigtail" lumen on the Salem vents the tube and protects gastric mucosa from being sucked against the tube.

LONG TUBES

The long tubes extend into the small bowel, sometimes for its entire length. They are between 6 and 10 feet long, and are used to prevent gas and fluid accumulation in the intestine, which is usually due to intestinal obstruction. The more common long tubes are the Miller-Abbott, Cantor, and Harris tubes.

Miller-Abbott Tube. This is a double-lumen, 3 meter (10 foot) tube. One lumen is used to introduce mercury or to inflate the balloon at the end of the tube, and the other is used for aspiration. Markings on the tube indicate how far the tube has been passed.

Cantor Tube. This tube is used for aspirating intestinal contents and has only one lumen. It is 3 meters (10 feet) long, and larger than the others. It has 4 to 5 ml of mercury in a bag at the end, which is wrapped about the tube before insertion. For intestinal intubation, the tube is threaded through the nose into the stomach and then through the pylorus, where peristaltic activity of the bowel carries it to the desired intestinal area.

Harris Tube. This is a single-lumen, mercury-weighted tube, 180 cm (6 feet) long. It has a metal tip that is introduced into the nostril after being lubricated. The weight of the mercury carries the bag by gravity. This tube is used for suction and irrigation.

Sometimes, it is difficult to get intestinal tubes to pass through the pylorus. The client is instructed to lie on the right side. Once the tube has passed into the duodenum, it is advanced, as ordered, an additional 4.8 to 9.6 cm (2 to 4 inches) every hour or half-hour. Once the tube has reached the desired location, it is taped securely to prevent further advancement.

Insertion of Tubes

Gastrointestinal tubes are generally inserted through the nose into the stomach or small intestine; rarely, they are inserted through the mouth. Explain each step of the intubation procedure at the client's level of understanding. Assist the client to obtain a high Fowler's position, because this makes intubation easier. Measure the distance on the tube from the tip of the nose to the ear lobe, plus the distance from the ear lobe to the tip of the xiphoid process (called the NEX measurement). Mark this distance on the tubing with adhesive.

After measuring the tube, lubricate it and gently insert it through the nares and posterior nasal pharynx and into the oropharynx. Once the tube is in the oropharynx, instruct the client to swallow. This measure is important because the sphincter at the proximal end of

TABLE 55-1. Gastric and Intestinal Tubes

	Length	Size (French)	Lumen	Other Characteristics
Short Tubes				
Levin type (plastic or rubber)	125 cm (50″)	12, 16, 18	Single	
Salem sump	120 cm (48″)	12, 14, 16, 18	Double	Sump-type suction
Long Tubes				
Cantor	300 cm (10′)	16	Single	Mercury weighted
Harris	180 cm (6′)	14, 16	Single	Mercury weighted
Miller-Abbott	300 cm (10′)	12, 14, 16, 18	Double	Mercury weighted

the esophagus remains closed except during swallowing. The larynx rises during swallowing, stretching the cricopharyngeal muscle and causing it to relax, thus reducing resistance to the tube. Swallowing also enables the tube to enter the esophagus rather than the trachea. After the tube passes the sphincter, advance it into the stomach.

To verify placement, perform at least two of the following activities: (1) aspirate gastric contents, (2) instill air into the tube with a syringe and listen with a stethoscope for air passing into the stomach (preferred method), (3) measure the pH of the aspirant, or (4) check the x-ray study of the tube with radiopaque lines. After confirming placement, secure the tube to the nose with hypoallergenic tape. (This procedure is used for short tubes only; long tubes need to be able to advance).

Suction

When suction is applied to a GI tube to remove accumulated gas and fluid, it is important to ensure that the GI mucosa is not traumatized. Excessive negative pressure causes the mucosa to be sucked into the openings on the tube, impairing the effectiveness of the suction and injuring the mucosa. Intermittent suction is commonly used to avoid this problem. Since mucus tends to plug the openings of these tubes, irrigate the openings as ordered to maintain or check their patency.

Nursing Management

It is very important to maintain the clients comfort while the tube is in place. Some helpful nursing interventions include the following:

- Gently clean and lubricate the external nares. They may become sore from crusted secretions around the tube.
- Tape the tube in a manner that prevents irritation to the nares.
- Administer frequent oral hygiene to remove debris, increase comfort, maintain a healthy oral cavity, and stimulate saliva secretion. The client's mouth is usually dry because the absence of chewing prevents the normal stimulus to salivary secretions and because mouth breathing results from the presence of the tube.
- If possible, let the client chew gum or suck on sour candies or ice chips to help stimulate salivation.
- Brush the client's teeth or assist the client to do so.
- Request an order for anesthetic mouth rinses or lozenges because clients frequently suffer sore throats from the presence of the tube.

Placement of the tube in the throat may result in cricoid chondritis (irritation of the cricoid cartilage of the larynx) and laryngeal injuries. Presenting symptoms include localized odynophagia, pain radiating to the ears, sore throat, stridor, bloody sputum, and mild hoarseness. Assess for these potential complications and report your findings immediately. The physician may order anesthetic lozenges or gargles to relieve the symptoms.

Frequently assess the material aspirated via the tube for color, odor, and quantity. Report any changes to the physician. You may need to send samples of these secretions to the laboratory for analysis. Measure contents of the suction bottles to maintain an accurate record of GI losses. Metabolic alkalosis may result from a major loss of water and electrolytes.

Remember that the irrigating solution instilled into a GI tube is counted as intake. Keep accurate records of how much is instilled and how much is aspirated from the tube during irrigations. Normal saline is often the irrigating solution of choice because water, a hypotonic solution, increases electrolyte loss through osmotic action if the tube is irrigated often.

ENTERAL FEEDINGS

It is a challenge to provide both short- and long-term nourishment for clients with a wide variety of GI and nonintestinal disorders such as coma. Instilling essential nutrients and calories directly into the stomach or intestine by way of a GI tube (tube feeding) is one method of providing nourishment.

GI feedings have a number of advantages over parenteral nutrition. There are many physiologic benefits associated with enteral feedings. They help to maintain GI structure (villi height and number) and the mucosal barrier. They also help to maintain GI motility that discourages bacterial overgrowth.

There are potential problems associated with enteral feedings, such as tube obstruction; aspiration; diarrhea; distention; constipation; hyperglycemia; hyperosmolar, hyperglycemic, nonketotic dehydration (HHNK); tube feeding syndrome; hypercapnia; and electrolyte abnormalities.

Routes and Formulas

Routes for tube feeding vary according to the client's condition. Feedings can be given via nasoenteric or nasogastric (NG) tubes. A physician sometimes performs surgery to place an esophagostomy, gastrostomy, percutaneous gastrostomy (PEG), jejunostomy, or needle catheter jejunostomy tube. Commonly, a feeding ostomy is created for clients requiring prolonged therapy.

The physician or dietician prescribes the amount, frequency, and kind of tube feeding. Many commercially prepared enteral feeding formulas are available. They differ in osmolality, digestibility, caloric density, lactose content, viscosity, fat content, and expense.

Formula selection is made on an individual basis and is dependent on factors such as the client's ability to digest and absorb nutrients, concurrent health problems, and anatomic site of the tube. For example, when administering jejunal feedings, which bypass the normal gastric and duodenal digestive processes, it may be more desirable to use a defined or elemental formula whose nutrients are in their simplest forms (e.g., proteins in the form of dipeptides or amino acids rather than intact protein) so absorption is enhanced.

Methods of Administration

CONTINUOUS FEEDING METHOD

The continuous feeding method is the method of choice for the critically ill and for clients fed via the small intestine. Continuous-drip feeding helps to minimize cramping, nausea, and diarrhea.

INTERMITTENT FEEDING METHOD

With the intermittent feeding method, the feeding is given periodically, using an administration set and adjusting the drip rate to the client's tolerance. For example, a scheduled feeding of 400 ml is given over 30 minutes four to six times a day. Intermittent feedings are often the preferred method for clients on home tube-feeding regimens because they can be free of the feeding apparatus for part of the day and are able to engage in regular activities between feedings.

BOLUS FEEDING METHOD

For many years, the bolus method was the common procedure for tube feeding, and although theoretically obsolete, it is still occasionally practiced. To administer bolus feedings, pour a prescribed amount of room temperature formula (usually 250 to 400 ml) slowly into the barrel of an Asepto syringe or funnel that is attached to the end of the GI tube (Murphy drip). The formula flows by gravity into the stomach or small intestine. This method is likely to cause nausea, vomiting, aspiration, diarrhea, or cramping because large amounts of formula are given over a short period of time. The continuous and intermittent feeding methods are preferable.

Volumetric or peristaltic pumps are often employed to maintain a constant flow rate. Tubes smaller than 10 Fr require a pump designed specifically for enteral feeding to keep them patent.

Nursing Management

ASSESSMENT

When administering tube feedings, review the (1) type of formula; (2) time, frequency, and amount of feeding; and (3) specific indications for the client. Most clients need an acclimatization period to adjust to tube feeding, generally starting at a low rate and gradually increasing until the client is receiving the desired amount of formula.

NURSING INTERVENTION

Collaborative Problem. Potential complication respiratory–atelectasis pneumonia R/T aspiration of tube feeding.

Planning: Expected Outcomes. The nurse will prevent aspiration.

Implementation. The client should be sitting upright or have the head of the bed elevated 30 degrees. During the feedings, monitor for signs of intolerance, which include cramping, diarrhea, nausea, vomiting, aspiration, glycosuria, and diaphoresis.

Before each tube feeding, explain the procedure to the client and significant others. Always check the placement of the tube. Gently aspirate gastric contents with a syringe, and measure the pH of the gastric contents. Remember antacids and gastric acid inhibitors can alter the pH. X-ray confirmation is the most reliable way to ensure proper placement, but this method is impractical in most situations and is used almost exclusively to confirm initial tube placement. Injecting air into small bore tubes is not always an accurate way to determine placement, because small-bore tubes can lodge in the bronchus without causing respiratory distress.

Check gastric residuals by aspirating stomach contents before each feeding, or every 4 to 8 hours. A residual greater than 50 percent of the previous hour's intake indicates delayed gastric emptying. Notify the physician before giving additional formula. Reinstall the residual feeding to prevent excessive fluid and electrolyte losses unless the residual appears abnormal, e.g., contains coffee ground–like material that is usually old blood. If this problem occurs, notify the physician.

To administer tube feedings, pour the formula into the bag attached to the feeding administration set. Connect the administration tubing to the feeding tube, and start the feeding by releasing the clamp on the tubing or turning on the pump. Assess the client's reaction to the feeding. If abdominal cramps develop, you may need to decrease the infusion rate. If the cramps continue, stop the infusion and notify the physician.

After the meal, the client should remain in a sitting position or with the head of the bed elevated to 30 degrees and turned on the right side for at least 30 minutes to encourage gastric emptying and discourage regurgitation and aspiration. Make sure the client is comfortable and place the call light within easy reach. Chart the time of the meal, amount of formula and water given, amount of residual, and the client's response to the feeding. Return to check on the client in 20 minutes, or sooner as needed.

The feeding tube should be flushed with 20 to 30 ml of water before and after intermittent feedings, every 4 hours during continuous feedings, and before and after any medications are administered via the feeding tube. If an obstruction occurs, try flushing the tube with water, cola, cranberry juice, meat tenderizer, or pancreatic enzymes. Before the last two items are used, be sure the tube is not in the lungs, because these agents could cause severe trauma to lung tissue.

In order to minimize bacterial contamination, the feeding set should be changed every 24 hours.

Nursing management of the client receiving enteral feeding involves the same principles as does caring for someone with a nasal or oral tube. Possible complications include (1) vomiting and aspiration if the stomach is overfilled; (2) plugging of the tube; (3) dislocation of the tube into trachea or lungs, thereby causing aspiration of anything passed through the tube; (4) development of ulcerations and dried secretions in the nares; and (5) tracheoesophageal fistula, which is a breakdown of the anterior esophageal wall, resulting from prolonged contact between the nasogastric tube and a tracheostomy tube, if present. With the development of soft, small bore tubes, this last complication has become very rare. Suspect tracheoesophageal fistula when gastric contents appear in tracheal excretion. If it is not apparent, food coloring can be added to the feeding so when the lungs are suctioned, the coloring would be apparent. Notify the physician, because this condition requires immediate intervention.

Nursing Diagnosis: Fluid Volume Deficit, High Risk for R/T excess fluid loss or inadequate intake.

Planning: Expected Outcomes. The client will not develop a fluid volume deficit, as evidenced by absence of signs of dehydration, no diarrhea, and adequate intake of fluids.

Implementation. The client must be assessed for dehydration. Clients receiving tube feedings may lose fluids from excessive diarrhea, excessive protein intake, or osmotic diuresis. They also may not take in enough water. If the client continues to have problems with diarrhea, slow the rate of infusion or change to a more defined formula.

The nurse should carefully monitor for changes in skin turgor, vital signs, intake and output, mucous membrane moisture, level of consciousness, fever, and disorientation. The client's electrolyte and BUN levels must be measured at regular intervals. Daily weights also should be obtained. Monitor for osmotic diuresis from high glucose load, especially if the infusion rate is increased. Keeping the formula at a constant infusion rate also can help ensure intake, as does routinely irrigating the tube with at least 30 ml of water every 4 hours. If sufficient water is not given, it will be taken from the tissues.

Nursing Diagnosis: Constipation R/T immobility and possible dehydration.

Planning: Expected Outcomes. The client will not be constipated, as evidenced by the client having at least one bowel movement every other day with soft formed stool.

Implementation. The client's hydration status must be assessed to determine if dehydration is a possible cause of the constipation. Increasing the water intake may be a simple solution to this problem. The client should be encouraged to ambulate as much as possible to lessen the effect of immobility on bowel function.

If the constipation continues, a stool softener may need to be ordered. The formula of the feeding also could be changed to a fiber-enriched formula to improve defecation. Sometimes simply allowing the client to use the toilet or a bedside commode can improve defecation.

The tube feedings should be discontinued if the client develops severe nausea, vomiting, increased abdominal girth, or epigastric and left upper quadrant pain, or if there is a large residual volume after feeding. It is important to stop the feedings because the client could vomit and aspirate.

Nursing Diagnosis: Diarrhea R/T enteral feedings.

Planning: Expected Outcomes. The client will not exhibit diarrhea, as evidenced by the client having at least one bowel movement every other day with soft, formed stool.

Implementation. The nurse should monitor the client for the presence of diarrhea. Possible causes of diarrhea include bacterial contamination of the formula, lactose intolerance, osmotic action caused by hyperosmolar fluids, fecal impaction, concurrent drug therapy (especially antibiotics or elixirs containing sorbitol), and low serum albumin. The nurse should carefully assess the bowel sounds for hyperactivity and notify the physician if they are found.

The perianal skin should be carefully cleaned after each bowel movement and a skin barrier applied to prevent skin excoriation. If the diarrhea continues, the nurse must carefully monitor the client for signs of fluid and electrolyte imbalances.

Nursing Diagnosis: Knowledge Deficit R/T tube feeding regimen for home feeding.

Planning: Expected Outcomes. The client will understand how to self-administer tube feedings at home, as evidenced by the client's ability to demonstrate correct procedures and through the client's ability to explain possible problems and solutions.

Implementation. Some clients who require long-term enteral feeding are candidates for home enteral feeding programs. The nurse or dietician assesses the client's home environment and lifestyle before planning the program. Significant others should be included in teaching efforts. It is easy for the client to use prepared formulas rather than preparing them himself. The use of prepared formulas also ensures that the client will receive all the required nutrients. When chewing is important to the client's mental state, allow the client to chew food and spit it out.

Intermittent nocturnal feedings are the method of choice for home feedings so the client can be free of the equipment for at least part of the day.

Be sure that the client and significant others are taught proper storage of the formula, care of the administration apparatus, maintenance of tube patency, what complications to monitor for, and when to notify the physician.

EVALUATION

The nurse must evaluate client outcomes based on the established plan of care. If these goals were not achieved, the plan and interventions must be revised to meet the client's needs.

▼ DISORDERS OF THE LARGE AND SMALL BOWEL

▼ Inflammatory Disorders

Inflammation can occur in any portion of the bowel and can be caused by (1) organisms, (2) toxins produced by organisms, (3) infiltration of the bowel wall by granulomatous processes, (4) injury from radiation, or (5) medications. All types of organisms, from viruses to large parasites, can cause inflammation.

VIRAL AND BACTERIAL INFECTIONS: GASTROENTERITIS AND DYSENTERY

Definition

Gastroenteritis is an inflammation of the stomach and intestinal tract that primarily affects the small bowel. It is associated with abdominal cramps, diarrhea, vomiting, and fever.

Dysenteries are inflammatory conditions affecting the colon. They are exhibited by severe bloody diarrhea and abdominal cramping.

Incidence

Viral gastroenteritis occurs throughout the world and is common. It often occurs in epidemic outbreaks.

Dysenteries caused by *E. coli* and *Shigella* also occur worldwide. *Shigella* occurs more frequently in children under 10 years of age and in homosexual populations.

Infection with *Clostridium difficile*, also known as pseudomembranous colitis, is a bacterial dysentery commonly seen in clients who have been receiving large doses of antibiotics or who have taken antibiotics for a long period of time. The condition is becoming increasingly common in the hospitalized population.

Another cause of dysentery is *Salmonella*, which is also referred to as food poisoning. *Salmonella* is associated with ingestion of contaminated eggs or poultry, or other food composed of these contaminated products.

Etiology

The cause of gastroenteritis is usually a virus or bacteria. The virus varies and is often referred to as the 'flu.' In staphylococcal food poisoning, the bacteria produce a toxin when infected foods are allowed to remain warm for a time before being eaten.

Amebic and bacterial organisms such as *Entamoeba histolytica*, *Shigella bacilli*, *Escherichia coli*, or *Salmonella* cause most dysenteries. The organisms are transmitted by ingestion of contaminated foods and drinking water. Infected individuals carry these organisms in the large bowel. Cholera also causes dysentery-like symptoms. *Clostridium difficile*, another common cause of dysentery, occurs when the normal flora of the bowel is depressed by antibiotics.

Risk Factors

Viral gastroenteritis is often associated with crowds and frequently occurs more in the fall and winter months. Yearly, different vaccines are available for viral enteritis, based on the likely viral source for that given year.

The risk factors for gastroenteritis caused by food poisoning are improper handling and storage of foods, or food handling by infected individuals. Proper food handling and storage are the best method to prevent food poisoning.

The risk factors for dysentery include (1) overcrowding, (2) poor sanitary conditions, and (3) food remaining at a temperature high enough for organisms to incubate and colonize easily. Preventive measures for dysentery revolve around cleanliness and proper sanitation.

The major risk factor for gastroenteritis caused by *Clostridium difficile* is the use of antibiotics, either for long periods or in high doses. Careful prescription of antibiotics and frequent assessment of clients for continued need of these drugs can help prevent this dysentery. It is, however, not a completely preventable problem, because some clients require these medications for long periods and in high doses.

Pathophysiology

If *Staphylococcus* organisms multiply sufficiently, they can cause a violent gastroenteritis to develop in 2 to 4 hours. Bacterial or viral food poisoning usually develops within 16 hours after ingestion of contaminated food. Gastroenteritis temporarily disables people, but the condition is of short duration and usually is not serious, except in infants, the very elderly, and weakened or debilitated individuals. These clients are at risk for life-threatening fluid and electrolyte imbalances.

Diarrhea associated with dysentery is caused, in part, by the inflammatory action of the organisms on the lining of the bowel. The organisms can invade and actually destroy the mucosal lining of the bowel, leading to fluid leaking into the bowel.

Endotoxins produced by the infective organisms stimulate the mucosal cells lining the bowel, leading to further diarrhea. These mucosal cells increase secretion of water and electrolytes into the intestinal lumen. The active secretion of chloride and bicarbonate ions in the small bowel leads to the inhibition of sodium reabsorption. In order to balance the excess sodium, large amounts of protein-rich fluids are secreted into the bowel, overwhelming the large bowel's ability to reabsorb the fluid.

Dysentery can prove fatal in the debilitated, aged, and very young persons. Early detection and intervention with fluids and electrolytes are critical to prevent death or disability.

Clinical Manifestations

Assessment reveals possible vomiting, profuse diarrhea, and resultant severe fluid and electrolyte loss. Varying amounts of blood may be present in the stool, and the client may experience a mild-to-severe temperature elevation, depending on the causative organism.

Management

Management of gastroenteritis includes resting the GI tract and replacing fluids. Rest with nothing by mouth until the vomiting has stopped is the best intervention. If the client has fluid depletion, an intravenous agent such as 0.45 per cent NaCl (hypotonic) is administered. A potassium supplement may be ordered if the client's serum potassium level is low.

The client is started on small amounts of clear liquids, as tolerated. The client may be given Gatorade or other electrolyte replacement beverage. The diet is advanced after 24 hours, as tolerated. In gastroenteritis, the infecting agents need to be eliminated, so drugs that decrease intestinal motility are not administered.

If the infecting organism is *Shigellosa*, an anti-infective agent such as sulfamethoxazole with trimethoprim (Bactrim, Septra) is administered. In the case of prolonged diarrhea in which the stool is leukocyte positive, antibiotics are given.

Antidiarrheals and antispasmodics may be given, but their use is controversial. Because many of these medications slow intestinal motility, they may actually increase the severity of the infection because these drugs keep the infection in contact with the bowel longer. The nonsystemic antidiarrheals, such as kaolin and pectin (Kaopectate) or bismuth subsalicylate (Pepto-Bismol), coat the intestinal mucosa, decrease intestinal secretions, and decrease the diarrhea. To be effective, these agents must be given frequently (every 30 minutes) in doses of 30 to 60 ml.

PROTOZOAL INFECTIONS: AMEBIASIS AND GIARDIASIS

Amebiasis produces diarrhea when a protozoan (*E. histolytica*) invades the lining of the colon. Symptoms include rectal inflammation and blood, pus, and amoebae in the stool. Metronidazole (Flagyl) is the drug of choice to treat this condition.

Giardiasis, a diarrheal illness, is caused by the protozoan, *Giardia lamblia*. It generally spreads through the water system or spoiled food. Symptoms begin several weeks after exposure. Onset is abrupt with symptoms of nausea, vomiting, excessive foul flatulence, and malabsorption, which causes weight loss. The vast majority of clients, however, are asymptomatic. Organisms infect the small intestinal mucosa and submucosa and are found in the stool. The medication of choice to treat this is tinidazole (Fasigyn). Other agents that may be used include metronidazole (Flagyl), quinacrine (Atabrine), and furazolidone (Furoxone). At present there is no chemoprophylactic agent that is effective in curing giardiasis.

PARASITIC INFESTATIONS

The intestinal tract may be infested with any of several species of parasitic worms, including *Ascaris* (roundworms), *Enterobius* (pinworms), *Trichinella spiralis* (which causes trichinosis), and various species of tapeworms. These parasites are found worldwide and, often, in the poorer regions of the United States. Worm infestations can cause serious and even fatal disease if the parasites are not eradicated from the intestinal tract. Worms also may cause urinary tract infections or pruritus ani. Fortunately, most of these parasites are susceptible to medications such as mebendazole and pyrantel pamoate. Piperazine and quinacrine hydrochloride also may be used, but they produce more side effects. Treatment for all household members may reduce reinfection.

Schistosomiasis is caused by a blood fluke (a parasitic worm). It is prevalent worldwide. The cercariae of the parasite penetrate the skin, migrate to the liver via the lungs, and remain in intrahepatic portal venules while the worm matures. The mature worm, which does not multiply within humans, then moves into its final habitat. Depending on the species involved, the worm may settle in the veins of the large bowel, small bowel, or bladder, where it lays eggs. These eggs, which form pseudotubercles, are commonly found in the liver and veins of the abdomen and lungs but have been identified in every system of the body, including the nervous system. Some eggs are excreted in the urine or feces. Without adequate sewage disposal, the eggs may be deposited in water that contains a susceptible snail, thus continuing the cycle.

In humans, schistosomiasis may have no symptoms. It may be mild or severe, depending on the species of worm involved and the number present. The prognosis is usually good, although there is an increase in the incidence of bladder cancer in clients with this parasite. Schistosomes do not multiply within the body, but a large number may be present owing to repeated infections. Their lifespan is probably about 3 to 5 years but may be as much as 30 years. Thousands of worms have been removed from a single client.

Schistosomiasis begins with dermatitis at the site of penetration, followed by a fever in 20 to 60 days, and later, by symptoms from the extrusion of eggs. Laboratory studies must examine the eggs or worms and identify the species before pharmacologic treatment can begin. Medications of choice include oxamniquine, metrifonate, praziquantel, and niridazole.

Nursing Management of Intestinal Infections and Infestations

ASSESSMENT

Most clients present with an acute onset of diarrhea. Carefully note a description of the diarrhea, including onset, number of stools, color, consistency, and accompanying symptoms such as nausea and vomiting. The nurse should ask the client about recent foreign travel, eating habits, and antibiotic use.

The nurse should assess the abdomen. Examination may reveal hyperactive bowel sounds, distention, and tenderness. Dehydration may be present depending on the amount of fluids lost. Metabolic alkalosis from bicarbonate loss is also a potential problem.

NURSING INTERVENTION

Nursing Diagnosis: Diarrhea R/T intestinal hypermotility.

Planning: Expected Outcomes. The client will have cessation of diarrhea, as evidenced by a decrease in the number of stools and the solid consistency of feces.

Implementation. The nurse must carefully examine all stool for blood and mucus, and must accurately record intake and output. The nurse must examine the anal area for irritation. After cleaning the area, a moisture barrier (e.g., petroleum jelly, zinc oxide) can be applied.

The nurse administers medications to treat the specific cause of the diarrhea, such as antibiotics and antiparasitics. Antidiarrheals also may be ordered if the diarrhea is uncontrollable.

Nursing Diagnosis: Fluid Volume Deficit, High Risk for R/T GI fluid and electrolyte losses.

Planning: Expected Outcomes. The client will have return of normal fluid and electrolyte balance, as evidenced by normal serum electrolytes and balanced intake and output.

Implementation. If the client shows signs of fluid and electrolyte imbalance, intravenous fluids may have to be started until oral fluids are tolerated. Clear liquids with electrolytes are then started in small amounts until the client can tolerate the diet advanced to include toast and saltines. If this diet is tolerated, the diet is usually advanced to a bland diet, then a general diet as tolerated.

EVALUATION

The nurse must evaluate client outcomes based on the established plan of care. If these goals were not achieved, the plan and interventions must be revised to meet the client's needs.

Post-hospital Care of Clients with Intestinal Infections and Infestations

The nurse gives written and oral instructions regarding diet and rest. The client should be given instructions to report any continued problems. Home health care needs are usually minimal unless the client is unable to prepare meals or obtain rest. The client must be reminded to wash his or her hands well and to maintain absolute cleanliness if other family members are sharing the bathroom.

APPENDICITIS

Definition

Appendicitis is an inflammation of the vermiform appendix that develops most commonly in adolescents and young adults.

Incidence

Appendicitis can occur at any age, but is rare in clients younger than 2 years of age and reaches a peak incidence in clients between the ages of 20 and 30 years old. It is not common in older adults, but when it does occur in this age group, rupture is more common.

Etiology

Appendicitis can be caused by (1) a fecalith (a fecal calculus or stone) that occludes the lumen of the appendix, (2) kinking of the appendix, (3) swelling of the bowel wall, (4) fibrous conditions in the bowel wall, and (5) external occlusion of the bowel by adhesions.

Risk Factors

There are no particular risk factors for appendicitis. It is not preventable, so early detection of the condition is important.

Pathophysiology

When the appendix becomes obstructed, the intraluminal pressure increases, leading to decreased venous drainage, thrombosis, edema, and bacterial invasion of the bowel wall. With continued obstruction, perforation will result.

After the initial obstruction, the appendix becomes increasingly hyperemic, warm, and covered with exudate progressing to gangrene and perforation.

Clinical Manifestations

The classic manifestations begin with acute abdominal pain, which comes in waves. At first, the pain may be perceived merely as discomfort that makes the client feel that passing flatus or having a bowel movement will bring relief. Unfortunately, many clients take a laxative during this period, which may lead to rupture of the appendix and peritonitis. The pain typically starts in the epigastrium or periumbilical region. It then shifts to the right lower quadrant as the inflammatory process spreads to involve the serosal layers of the bowel, thereby bringing the inflammatory process into contact with the peritoneum. The pain becomes steady rather than intermittent, and the client often guards the area by lying still and drawing the legs up to relieve tension on the abdominal muscles. Assessment also may reveal vomiting that begins after the pain starts, loss of appetite, low-grade fever, coated tongue, and bad breath.

DIAGNOSTIC ASSESSMENT

Mild leukocytosis is usually present, with the white blood cell count between 10,000 and 15,000. Physical findings confirm the diagnosis. Pain at McBurney's point, which lies midway between the right anterior superior iliac crest and the umbilicus, may be diagnostic.

Medical Management

There is no medical treatment as such for appendicitis. Until surgery can be performed, intravenous fluids and antibiotics are administered.

Surgical Management

Surgical intervention involves removing the appendix (i.e., appendectomy) within 24 to 48 hours of onset of the symptoms. When the operation is performed in time, the mortality rate is less than 0.5 per cent. Delay usually causes rupture of the organ and resultant peritonitis. Surgery is frequently delayed, however, because the diagnosis is difficult to make and clients often seek medical aid belatedly. Older clients may have very few symptoms and do not seek aid until after perforation has occurred.

Diagnosis also can be difficult in very young children. Numerous diseases, including mesenteric adenitis, ovarian cyst, cholelithiasis, renal or ureteral calculi, diverticulitis, and Meckel's diverticulum, mimic appendicitis. The client may require antibiotics and surgical drainage if perforation occurs.

Nursing Management

The client is usually admitted with severe abdominal pain. The nurse should carefully assess the pain, especially to determine its location. The client also should be assessed for the presence of peritonitis (see section on Peritonitis). Carefully assess the client's vital signs, fluid and electrolyte status, and laboratory data. The client with appendicitis should fast in preparation for surgery.

NURSING INTERVENTION

Nursing Diagnosis: Pain, Acute R/T inflammation.

Planning: Expected Outcomes. The client will understand why pain medication is held preoperatively and have pain controlled postoperatively, as evidenced by client verbalization.

Implementation. The client will have pain medication withheld until the diagnosis is confirmed. Sometimes, pain medication will not be given until the client is actually ready for surgery. The nurse should never give an enema or a laxative, or apply heat to the abdomen of the client with appendicitis, because these actions could lead to perforation.

An abrupt change in the character of the pain preoperatively could indicate perforation. Postoperatively, pain control, as outlined in Chapters 16 and 19, should be practiced.

Nursing Diagnosis: Fluid Volume Deficit, High Risk for R/T vomiting.

Planning: Expected Outcomes. The client will have fluid and electrolyte balance maintained, as evidenced by balanced intake and output and electrolytes within normal limits.

Implementation. As soon as the client is admitted, intravenous fluids are started to maintain fluid balance, with electrolytes added as needed. If the client is vomiting, a nasogastric tube is inserted. Intake and output should be carefully measured and discrepancies reported to the physician.

Nursing Diagnosis: High Risk for Infection R/T rupture of appendix.

Planning: Expected Outcomes. The client will not develop an infection or will have rupture diagnosed early, as evidenced by removal of appendix before rupture or prompt treatment.

Implementation. The client's vital signs must be checked regularly, monitoring closely for an increase in temperature and a change in pulse and blood pressure that may signify a ruptured appendix. The client's pain also should be closely monitored. If the pain becomes generalized throughout the abdomen and the abdomen becomes rigid and boardlike, rupture may have occurred.

If a rupture of the appendix is suspected, the symptoms should be reported to the physician immediately so the client can be prepared for surgery. Preoperative antibiotics are usually administered to decrease the infection.

After surgery, the nurse will monitor vital signs, urine output, level unconsciousness, and intravenous therapy, and assess the client's respiratory status and the surgical wound. The client may have a drain, and if the appendix ruptured, packing may be present. The nurse must assess the dressings, provide wound care, reposition the client, and adequately manage the client's pain.

EVALUATION

The nurse must evaluate client outcomes based on the established plan of care. If these goals were not achieved, the plan and interventions must be revised to meet the client's needs.

Modification of Plan of Care for the Elderly

Although the incidence of appendicitis is low in older adults, if it does occur in this age group, rupture is more likely.

Post-hospital Care

DISCHARGE TEACHING

The client with uncomplicated appendicitis should resume normal activity in 2 to 4 weeks. Discharge teaching and post-hospital care for the client with a routine appendectomy are the same as for any client after surgery.

If the client had a ruptured appendix with an infected wound, the client will have to be taught the proper way to care for the wound. Wound care usually includes irrigation of the wound with sterile saline and application of a sterile dressing, at least, several times a day.

HOME HEALTH CARE NEEDS

The nurse should assess the client's ability to function at home and to care for the wound. A home health care referral may be needed to assist the client with physical needs.

FOLLOW-UP CARE

The client with a ruptured appendix may have to return for surgery after the abscess has walled off. The client with an infected wound will have to be seen at intervals to ensure that the wound is healing properly.

PERITONITIS

Definition

Peritonitis is the inflammation of the peritoneal membrane. The peritoneum is a semipermeable two-layered sac filled with approximately 1500 ml of fluid that covers all the organs in the abdominal cavity. Because it is well supplied with somatic nerves, stimulation of the parietal peritoneum that lines the abdominal and pelvic cavities causes sharp, well-localized pain. The visceral peritoneum is relatively insensitive.

Incidence

The incidence of peritonitis caused by perforation or rupture of abdominal viscus is hard to determine. Data usually relate to the underlying cause.

Etiology

Peritonitis can be primary or secondary, or acute or chronic. The major sources of inflammation are from the gastrointestinal tract, from the external environment, and through the bloodstream. The peritoneum is able to produce an inflammatory reaction and wall off a localized process to combat an infection, if (1) the stimulus is not too massive or (2) the source of infection does not continue. For instance, a perforation (e.g., of a gastric ulcer) that continues to drain contaminants into the peritoneal cavity will overcome the ability of the peritoneum to localize and combat the inflammatory process.

Specific causes of peritonitis are listed in Box 55-1.

Normal bacterial flora of the intestine become a source of infection when they enter the sterile peritoneal cavity. The most common organism is *E. coli*, although *streptococci*, *staphylococci*, and *pneumococci* also may be involved.

Risk Factors

There are no specific risk factors for peritonitis, because the condition is a result of another problem. The major preventive measure to consider with this disorder is early diagnosis of clients at risk for developing the condition secondary to one of its many causes. Early diagnosis and the initiation of early treatment help to prevent spread of the infection.

Pathophysiology

Peritonitis creates severe systemic effects. Circulatory alterations, fluid shifts, and respiratory problems can cause critical fluid and electrolyte imbalances. The circulatory system undergoes great stress from several

Box 55–1. Causes of Peritonitis

Gangrenous cholecystitis
Ruptured gallbladder
Perforated carcinoma of the stomach
Perforated gastric or duodenal ulcer
Ruptured spleen
Acute pancreatitis
Penetrating wound of the GI tract
Ulcerative colitis
Gangrenous obstruction of the small bowel due to (1) adhesions, (2) carcinoma, (3) volvulus, or intussusception
Perforation of Meckel's diverticulum
Mesenteric thrombosis
Perforation of a diverticulum
Regional ileitis
Appendicitis with perforation
Ruptured retroperitoneal abscess
Strangulated hernia
Puerperal infection
Salpingitis
Septic abortion
Ruptured bladder
Iatrogenic perforation

sources. The inflammatory response shunts extra blood to the inflamed area of the bowel to combat the infection. Peristaltic activity of the bowel ceases. Fluids and air are retained within its lumen, raising pressure and increasing fluid secretion into the bowel. Thus, the circulating blood volume diminishes.

The inflammatory process increases oxygen requirements at a time when the client's ability to ventilate has been reduced. The client has difficulty ventilating because of abdominal pain and increased abdominal pressure, which elevates the diaphragm.

Clinical Manifestations

Manifestations of peritonitis vary depending on the cause. Pain may be either localized or generalized. Well-localized pain that causes rigidity of abdominal muscles and pain that increases with any pressure or motion of the abdomen is characteristic of peritonitis. Also, the client usually experiences nausea, vomiting, and possibly a low-grade fever. Assessment reveals (1) absence of bowel sounds and (2) shallow respirations because the client is trying to avoid the pain caused by body movement.

DIAGNOSTIC ASSESSMENT

The client with peritonitis commonly has an elevated white blood cell (WBC) count (20,000/mm^3) with a high neutrophil count. Abdominal x-rays studies are performed, which may show dilation and edema of the intestines, or free air or fluid in the abdominal cavity. If the client is vomiting, signs of altered fluid and electrolyte balance also may be present.

Medical Management

If peritonitis is advanced and surgery is contraindicated because of shock and circulatory failure, oral fluids are prohibited and intravenous fluids are necessary for replacement of electrolyte and protein losses. Usually, a long intestinal tube is inserted through the nose into the intestine to reduce pressure within the bowel. Once the infection has become walled off and the client's condition improves, surgical drainage and repair can be attempted.

The other major treatment for peritonitis is intravenous antibiotic therapy with potent broad-spectrum agents.

Surgical Management

Surgery may be performed to prevent peritonitis, such as with an appendectomy for an inflamed appendix or a colon resection for inflamed diverticuli. If the perforation is not prevented, then the major surgical intervention is incision and drainage of the abscess once it is walled off.

Nursing Management

ASSESSMENT

The nurse must obtain a thorough history including specific information about the client's pain. The nurse should assess the abdomen, noting the presence of bowel sounds. The abdomen should be palpated, noting if the abdomen is firm, distended, or rigid. Areas of tenderness should be noted. The nurse also should assess for the presence of rebound tenderness. The client probably has a high fever, indicating peritonitis.

NURSING INTERVENTION

Nursing Diagnosis: Injury and Infection, High Risk for R/T possible perforation and ischemia.

Planning: Expected Outcomes. The client will not develop an infection or complications of peritonitis, or will have infection and complications adequately treated, as evidenced by normal vital signs, no sign of inflammation, absence of shock, renal failure, adult respiratory distress syndrome (ARDS), or sepsis.

Implementation. Clients with peritonitis are acutely ill. They are started on broad-spectrum antibiotics immediately on admission to the hospital.

Surgery is usually performed to repair the perforated organs as soon as clients are stable enough to withstand the stress of surgery. During surgery, any leakage can be cultured so specific antibiotic therapy can be implemented. The peritoneal cavity is usually thoroughly irrigated with an antibiotic solution during surgery to decrease the bacterial count. The wound is often packed open, or at least with drains, so infection can be treated.

Postoperatively, the nurse must carefully monitor clients for the development of postoperative complications such as ARDS, sepsis, and shock. The vital signs should be closely monitored and any signs of sepsis, such as a drop or increase in temperature or drop in blood pressure, reported immediately.

Nursing Diagnosis: Fluid Volume Deficit, High Risk for R/T vomiting.

Planning: Expected Outcomes. The client will maintain normal fluid volume, as evidenced by adequate output, good skin turgor, and moist mucous membranes.

Implementation. Intravenous fluids are administered along with antibiotic therapy. In the client with peritonitis, the nurse must maintain the NG tube (see Gastrointestinal Intubation). The nurse also must monitor the client's fluid balance by assessing vital signs, urine output, skin turgor, intravenous fluid replacement, weight, and mucous membrane integrity.

Evaluation. The nurse must evaluate client outcomes based on the established plan. If these goals were not achieved, the plan and interventions must be revised to meet the client's needs.

Post-hospital Care

The client should be provided with verbal or written instructions regarding wound care, medications, and activity restrictions.

INFLAMMATORY BOWEL DISEASE

Inflammatory bowel disease (IBD) includes two chronic inflammatory disorders: (1) Crohn's disease (regional enteritis) and (2) ulcerative colitis. Both diseases are characterized by periods of exacerbation and remission. These chronic, recurrent diseases predominantly affect younger people. Treatment is symptomatic and responses are often unpredictable. Frequently, clients with IBD require surgery, which may be followed by recurrence. Because of the similarities between Crohn's disease and ulcerative colitis, we compare and contrast these two conditions throughout the following discussion of IBD (Table 55–2).

Definition

Crohn's Disease. Crohn's disease (regional enteritis) is a chronic relapsing disease that may develop discontinuously in any segment of the alimentary tract. The most common location is the terminal ileum. Crohn's disease more characteristically involves the entire thickness of the bowel wall (transmural) but particularly the submucosa. The mortality rate is not high, but recurrences and complications can result in disability.

Ulcerative Colitis. In contrast to Crohn's disease, which is transmural and segmental, ulcerative colitis is a disease that spans the entire length of the colon and involves only the mucosa and submucosa. The disease usually starts in the rectum and distal colon, and spreads upward beyond the rectosigmoid valve to involve most of the sigmoid and descending colon.

Ulcerative colitis causes inflammation, thickening, congestion, edema, and minute lacerations that ooze blood and eventually develop into abscesses. The edema may lead to extreme friability of the mucosa, so bleeding occurs from any minor trauma.

Incidence

Crohn's Disease. Crohn's disease is more common in whites and among Jewish people. There is an increased incidence within families. It occurs at all ages but more often in the third decade of life. Both sexes are affected equally.

Ulcerative Colitis. Ulcerative colitis is more common than Crohn's disease. It occurs at all ages, but has a higher incidence among young adults, women, and Jewish people. It has demonstrated a familial tendency.

Etiology

Crohn's Disease. The cause of Crohn's disease is unclear, although the literature suggests there is some genetic or hereditary basis. The disease is also considered autoimmune in nature.

Ulcerative Colitis. Several theories have attempted to explain the cause of ulcerative colitis. One theory is that the disease is of bacterial origin, because many clients have a history of bacterial infection before the onset of the condition. Researchers have also suspected an allergic reaction as a basis of the disease. Others believe that ulcerative colitis may be due to an altered immunity, because colon antibodies have been found. Still others suggest that destructive enzymes and a lack of protective substances in the bowel wall cause the inflammatory process. An emotional disturbance can precipitate an exacerbation or prolong an attack of the disorder, but it is not the primary cause.

Risk Factors

Crohn's Disease. The only risk factors identified for Crohn's disease are genetic ones. There are no preventive measures that can be taken.

Ulcerative Colitis. There are no preventable risk factors associated with ulcerative colitis. Once the client has the disease, controlling stress can help keep the disease in remission.

TABLE 55–2. Differentiation Between Crohn's Disease and Ulcerative Colitis

Characteristic	Regional Enteritis (Crohn's Disease)	Ulcerative Colitis
General Description		
Age at onset	Young	Young to middle
Pathology and Anatomy		
Depth of involvement	Transmural (all layers of submucosa)	Mucosa and submucosa
Rectal involvement	50%	95%
Right colon involvement	Frequent	Occasional
Small bowel involvement	Involved, ileum narrow	Usually normal
Distribution of disease	Segmental	Continuous
Inflammatory mass	Chronic and extensive	Rare (crypt abscess)
Cobblestone-like mucosa and granuloma	Common	Absent
Mesentery lymph involvement	Edema and hyperplasia	Not involved
Toxic megacolon	Occasional	Occasional
Steatorrhea	Frequent	Absent
Malignancy results	Rare	After 10 years
Fibrous stricture	Common	Absent
Clinical		
Course of disease	Slowly progressive	Remissions and relapses
Rectal bleeding	Occasional	Common (90–100%)
Abdominal pain	Colicky (45%)	Predefecation (60–70%)
Hematochezia	Unusual or absent	Almost always present
Diarrhea	Present (65–85%)	Early and frequent (80–95%)
Vomiting	Present (35%)	Present (15%)
Nutritional deficit	Common	Common
Weight loss	Present (60–70%)	Present (20–50%)
Fever	Present (35%)	Present (10%)
Anal abscess	Common (75%)	Occasional (10%)
Fistula and anorectal fissure fistula	Common (80%)	Rare (10–20%)
Systemic Manifestations		
Arthritis	20%	Uncommon (10%)
Peripheral sacroilitis	18%	18–20%
Hepatobiliary involvement	Uncommon	15% cholestatic dysfunction 19–38% fatty liver 30–50% pericholangitis
Skin: erythema nodosum, pyoderma gangrenosum	Common	Present (5–10%)
Nephrolithiasis	Occasional	Rare

Pathophysiology

Crohn's Disease. Lesions typically develop in several separated segments of bowel. They are grossly visible and their color is dramatically different from that of normal tissue. Examination of the bowel tissue by oscopy reveals edematous, heavy, reddish purple areas. Granular spots also may be present. Enlarged lymph nodes appear in the submucosa, and Peyer's patches are seen in the intestinal mucous membrane. These areas undergo small superficial ulceration with granulomas and fissures. Fissures may completely penetrate the bowel wall, leading to fistulas and abscesses. Collections of lymphocytes throughout the mucosa, submucosa, and serosa are the only microscopic features of Crohn's disease. The small bowel wall becomes congested and thickened, and the lumen narrows. The mucosa has an erythematous, cobblestone-like appearance. In later stages of the disease, the intestinal wall becomes permanently fibrosed, thickened, and narrowed.

Small bowel–related complications of Crohn's disease include malabsorption, kidney stones, gallstones, and hydronephrosis. Anorectal problems include internal fistulas and abscesses. Nephrolithiasis, hydronephrosis, and growth retardation are other complications. Fissure in ano is the most common lesion and is directly related to the severity of the diarrhea, which produces ulceration of the perianal skin. Pain commonly accompanies defecation. Perianal abscess may appear during the active phase of IBD. Pain is aggravated by walking, sitting, and defecation.

Assessment may reveal an area of induration, swelling, and redness. Internal fistulas characterize Crohn's disease of the ileum and right colon. Rectovaginal fistulas may occur in women. Incontinence is common owing to breakdown in the relatively thin rectovaginal septum. Fistulas into the bladder precipitate recurrent urinary infections and, in some instances, even fecaluria. Treatment may include either drainage to control infection or excision.

Arthritis is a transient, acute, painful swelling present in 20 per cent of clients with Crohn's disease. It may be polyarticular or monarticular. It most commonly affects the knees, ankles, and wrists. The client seldom suffers permanent limitation of motion.

Toxic megacolon is an extreme dilatation of a segment of the diseased colon (often the transverse) that results in complete obstruction. Toxic megacolon usually occurs during an acute exacerbation and may follow hypokalemia, a barium enema, or the use of anticholinergics, narcotics, corticosteroids, or antibiotics. Bacterial overgrowth contributes to the development of toxic megacolon.

Assessment reveals paralytic ileus, dehydration, fever, tachycardia, lethargy, leukocytosis, decreased serum protein and albumin levels, anxiety, and prostration. In addition, perforation and peritonitis may complicate toxic megacolon.

Ulcerative Colitis. The appearance of the colon depends on the stage, activity, and severity of the disease. The most characteristic lesion of ulcerative colitis is an inflammatory infiltrate called crypt abscess. This abscess consists of polymorphonuclear leukocytes, lymphocytes, red cells, and cellular debris appearing at the base of the glandular crypts. The crypt abscess secretions result in purulent discharge. The abscesses may become necrotic and may ulcerate.

Infections secondary to ulcerative colitis produce further inflammatory reactions in the mucosa and submucosa. When the inflammatory lesions heal, scarring and fibrosis, with narrowing, thickening, and shortening of the colon and loss of haustral folds, may follow.

Cancer of the colon is more common among clients with ulcerative colitis than among the general population. The incidence is greatly increased among those who develop ulcerative colitis before the age of 16 and those who have had the condition for more than 20 years.

Complications of ulcerative colitis vary with its severity and location. Ankylosing spondylitis and clubbing of the fingers are found in a few clients. Anemia and nutritional deficiency may occur, causing dry skin that lacks turgor. In addition, assessment reveals erythema, pustules, abscesses, and neurodermatitis.

Toxic megacolon is an extreme dilatation of a segment of the diseased colon (often the transverse) that results in complete obstruction. Toxic megacolon usually occurs during an acute exacerbation, and it may follow hypokalemia, a barium enema, or the use of anticholinergics, narcotics, corticosteroids, or antibiotics. Bacterial overgrowth contributes to this complication.

Assessment reveals paralytic ileus, dehydration, fever, tachycardia, lethargy, leukocytosis, decreased serum protein and albumin levels, anxiety, and prostration. In addition, perforation and peritonitis may complicate toxic megacolon.

Clinical Manifestations

Crohn's Disease. Crohn's disease may have acute manifestations, but the condition is usually slow and unaggressive. The client may be treated for mild and intermittent symptoms months before the diagnosis of Crohn's disease is made.

Assessment typically reveals abdominal pain, diarrhea, and weight loss due to nutritional deficits. The pain is usually intermittent. Terminal ileum involvement produces pain in the periumbilical region. The client experiences jejunal pain in the upper and left midabdomen. Pain of the ileum is intermittent and is felt in the lower right quadrant. A constant aching, soreness, or tenderness usually indicates advanced disease. The client may experience relief of discomfort after passing stool or flatus.

Diarrhea is usually less severe than that associated with ulcerative colitis. Stool consistency is typically soft or semi-liquid. Malabsorption, associated with steatorrhea, may develop. If so, stools may be foul-smelling and fatty. Urgency to expel stools may awaken the person at night. In contrast to ulcerative colitis, the client rarely passes gross blood.

Passage of blood indicates ulceration. The client with severe steatorrhea, diarrhea, or long-standing enteritis may have associated nutritional deficits, weight loss, anorexia, pain, anemia, debility, fatigue, and metabolic disturbances. Nutritional deficits arise from (1) a reduction in the intestinal absorptive surface; (2) impaired absorption of fat, vitamin B_{12}, folic acid, iron, calcium, and vitamins A,C,D,E and K; and (3) malabsorption of protein and carbohydrates. Alterations in bile salt and vitamin metabolism may result from surgery or mucosal defects. Metabolic requirements increase because of the inflammatory process and infection, decreased food intake, and nutrients lost in the feces owing to rapid GI transit time. Electrolytes lost from diarrhea include sodium, potassium, chloride, the trace elements (magnesium, zinc, copper), and minerals.

Nitrogen excretion remains normal if there is no loss of protein from the inflammatory exudate. The consequence of malnutrition may include

- Loss of immunocompetence,
- Decreased resistance to infection,
- Diminished wound healing,
- Diminished pancreatic enzyme output,
- Impaired healing (fistula and surgical wounds),
- Decreased iron-binding capacity resulting from chronic infection or blood loss,

Temperature elevation may occur with (1) acute inflammation; (2) associated fistulas, abscesses, or sinus tracts, or (3) rheumatoid manifestations. Sudden, severe, right lower quadrant pain, leukocytosis, and tenderness accompany the elevated temperature. Nausea and vomiting are rare unless there is a small bowel obstruction.

Additional acute inflammatory symptoms include pain in the lower right quadrant, cramping, tenderness, flatulence, nausea, and diarrhea. Borborygmus and increased peristalsis also may develop. Pain sometimes mimics acute appendicitis or bowel perforation, and symptoms may be confused with those of ulcerative colitis. If anal disease occurs, fissures, fistulas, skin tags, ulcers, and strictures may be present.

The client may experience periods of remission interrupted by exacerbations of active Crohn's disease. Because exacerbations often follow dietary indiscretions, emotional upsets, or illness, inquire into the client's life events at the time of the exacerbation.

Ulcerative Colitis. The predominant symptom of ulcerative colitis is rectal bleeding. Clients often experience diarrhea, possibly 20 or more stools per day. The severity and frequency of diarrhea depends on the extent of involved colon. Severe diarrhea can cause a loss of 500 to 17,000 ml of water in 24 hours. Liquid stools occur with tenesmus and may contain blood, mucus, and pus. A sense of urgency and cramping abdominal pain may occur with the diarrhea. The client typically experiences colicky pain in the lower left quadrant.

Nausea, vomiting, anorexia, weight loss, and decreased serum potassium may occur with severe disease. In addition, the client loses plasma proteins, prothrombin, and fluids. The development of anemia depends on the degree of blood loss, severity of the illness, and dietary iron intake.

When the disease is acute, the client develops fever. Severe diarrhea or vomiting may cause metabolic acidosis. Physical findings include tenderness in the lower left quadrant, guarding, and (in severe ulcerative colitis) abdominal distention. Following remissions, ulcerative colitis may recur after bouts of emotional stress, dietary indiscretion, or the ingestion of irritants such as laxatives or antibiotics. Physical exertion, respiratory infections and overfatigue also may cause an attack. As in Crohn's disease, it is important to inquire into the client's life events prior to recurrences.

DIAGNOSTIC ASSESSMENT

Crohn's disease and ulcerative colitis produce similar symptoms. Clients with both disorders suffer from abdominal pain, fever, diarrhea, fluid imbalances, and weight loss. Remissions are followed by exacerbations of acute disease. Although bleeding is more common in ulcerative colitis, clients with severe Crohn's disease often experience bloody diarrhea.

Physical assessment may reveal certain characteristic manifestations. The general appearance of clients with IBD varies from reasonably healthy to wasted, drawn, and malnourished, with varying degrees of pallor. Some clients have a fever and tachycardia. They usually report a steady and progressive weight loss. Inspection reveals a flat or concave shape of the abdomen, with visible peristaltic activity. Palpation of the abdomen reveals tenderness over the area of inflamed bowel. Increased bowel sounds are heard on auscultation. The rectal sphincter is found to be tight, the rectum empty, and the anal area irritated. Hemorrhoids and, in Crohn's disease, perianal abscess, fistula, or ulcers may be apparent.

Decreased levels of hematocrit and hemoglobin are usually noted. A barium enema study with air contrast is often performed to differentiate between ulcerative colitis and Crohn's disease. The client with suspected IBD routinely undergoes colonoscopy. Biopsy and cytologic studies also help distinguish between carcinoma, ulcerative colitis, and Crohn's disease.

Medical Management

Medical treatment, which primarily aims to control the symptoms, is similar for ulcerative colitis and for Crohn's disease. Because the inflammatory process in Crohn's disease involves deeper layers of the bowel wall and is more chronic, healing may occur more slowly than in ulcerative colitis. Thus, anti-inflammatory therapy, including steroids, is required for longer periods in Crohn's disease than in ulcerative colitis.

Fluids, electrolytes, and blood are replaced as needed to maintain the client's homeostasis. Physical activity should be kept to a minimum during the acute attack to decrease intestinal motility. The client with mild attacks may work but needs extra rest. The client with fever, toxemia, frequent bowel movements, bleeding, or pain sometimes requires bed rest. Failure of the inflamed colonic mucosa to reabsorb water and electrolytes, bile salts, and lactose interferes with control of diarrhea. The extent of large bowel involved in the disease influences the severity of diarrhea. The client should keep a record of the number of stools, their consistency and color, and the presence of blood.

PHARMACOLOGIC MANAGEMENT

Antidiarrheal preparations may provide symptomatic benefit (Table 55–3). Loperamide (Imodium) is superior to diphenoxylate (Lomotil) in controlling diarrhea of Crohn's disease, with fewer side effects. Opiates for diarrhea control may cause distention and megacolon. Hydrophilic mucilloids, such as psyllium or methylcellulose, may improve the consistency of stools and rectal continence. Antispasmodic medications such as belladonna extract, propantheline bromide, glycopyrrolate, or dicyclomine hydrochloride may reduce postprandial pain and diarrhea.

Diarrhea associated with IBD may be treated successfully by antimicrobial agents such as sulfasalazine. The specific action is unknown, but the medication is retained by the connective tissue of the intestinal mucosa. Side effects include headache, malaise, dizziness, aching, epigastric distress, lethargy, depression, nausea, and vomiting. In an attempt to control diarrhea, tincture of opium and paregoric are sometimes given. Bowel rest and parenteral hyperalimentation may result

TABLE 55-3. Drugs Used in the Treatment of Diarrhea

Drug	Daily Dosage	Nursing Intervention
Diphenoxylate hydrochloride with atropine sulfate (Lomotil)	5 mg, four times daily (altered doses for elderly are not specifically established)	1. Assess number of stools and consistency throughout treatment 2. Assess fluid and electrolyte balance 3. Assess for dry mouth, tachycardia, rash, and urinary retention 4. May be administered with food if GI irritation occurs 5. Assess for abdominal distention, pain, and fever
Loperamide hydrochloride (Imodium)	4 mg initially, then 2 mg after each loose stool. Maximum dose 16 mg daily	1. Assess number of stools 2. Assess for drowsiness, dry mouth, N/V, constipation 3. Assess for abdominal distention, pain, and fever
Opium preparations (opium tincture, paregoric)	Paregoric: 5 to 10 ml, one to four times daily Tincture: 0.6 ml, four times a day	1. Assess for N/V 2. Dilute opium tincture in 15 to 30 ml of liquid 3. Assess for abdominal distention, pain, and fever

N/V, nausea/vomiting

in restored immunocompetence, greater resistance to infection, correction of nutritional deficiencies, and relief of edema and bowel inflammation.

Clients who fail to respond to general supportive measures may require anti-inflammatory medications. Adrenal steroids and corticotropin may be used with other therapy to reduce the body's response to inflammation. Steroids do not cure IBD, but by reducing inflammation, they may modify its course. The systemic effects of IBD also respond to steroids.

Antacids or histamine receptor antagonists should be given during steroid therapy to prevent gastric ulceration. Steroids decrease adrenal function and may impair resistance, causing defective healing of abscesses and fistulas. Remember that steroids may mask the symptoms of infection. They are not recommended for clients suffering from dehydration, potential perforation, or severe fluid and electrolyte imbalance. Steroids may be given intravenously, intramuscularly, rectally, or orally. Oral forms include hydrocortisone, prednisolone, and prednisone. Hydrocortisone also can be administered rectally as an enema or suppository. Corticosteroids interfere with intestinal absorption of calcium.

6-Mercaptopurine, an immunosuppressive agent, is used when other treatment modalities fail and can be effective against chronic, unrelenting Crohn's disease and many of its complications. The medication should be used during the chronic phase. To be effective, therefore, the client must receive steroids or ACTH beforehand.

During acute exacerbations, the client is given anticholinergic medications to relieve abdominal cramps and help control diarrhea. Anticholinergics, antidiarrheal agents, and antispasmodics allow the colon to rest and decrease the gastrocolic reflex. Anticholinergics may decrease muscle spasm and discomfort but have little effect on diarrhea. Withhold these medications if there are signs of obstruction. Treatment with these agents may cause further iatrogenic problems.

Medications commonly used to prevent or control infections include the sulfonamides and antibiotics. If antibiotic therapy is effective, you will note a decrease in temperature, number of stools, and bleeding. Antibiotics may be given to control secondary bowel inflammation and infection. Sulfasalazine is the most commonly prescribed sulfonamide for management of both ulcerative colitis and Crohn's disease. Sulfasalazine can interfere with folate absorption and use.

DIETARY MANAGEMENT

Total parenteral nutrition is indicated for the client who (1) fails to respond to medical intervention, (2) is being prepared for surgery, or (3) has had an intestinal resection. This feeding method provides bowel rest by removing all stimulation of secretion and by decreasing fecal bulk. Weight gain, positive nitrogen balance, and a temporary remission of symptoms can occur. Total parental nutrition appears to be more useful in Crohn's disease than in ulcerative colitis. When oral food and fluids are resumed, they should be chemically and mechanically nonirritating and high in calories, protein, and minerals. Exclude foods such as cocoa, chocolate, citrus juices, cold or carbonated drinks, nuts, seeds, popcorn, and alcohol.

Elemental diets provide nutritionally balanced meals. They are residue free, low in fat, and digested mainly in the upper jejunum. Unfortunately, many of the enteral formulas are not very palatable, and client compliance often is low.

Anemia and vitamin B_{12} deficiencies should be corrected nutritionally. Folate deficiency, which may be due to therapeutic use of sulfasalazine, may be prevented by increasing dietary intake of folate, giving sulfasalazine between meals, or supplementing the intervention regimen with folic acid.

A diet high in protein and calories is given in an attempt to restore normal nutritional levels but is not always well tolerated. Eating tends to increase diarrhea and anorexia, and nausea and vomiting are often present.

Complications

Nutritional deficiencies are the most common complications of IBD. These deficits derive from (1) decreased intake, (2) increased nutritional requirements, (3) increased losses, and (4) side effects of certain medications. Diarrhea causes fluid and electrolyte losses with resultant muscle wasting and edema. Malabsorption due to bacterial overgrowth or mucosal involvement of the bowel may cause further problems. Deficiencies of all the fat-soluble vitamins A, D, E, and K, and folate may develop. Vitamin K deficiency causes bleeding tendencies. Clients usually limit their dietary intake to control pain and diarrhea.

Therapeutic interventions such as special diets, antibiotic agents, and anti-inflammatory medications also may cause anorexia or stomatitis. Specific nutritional and metabolic problems caused by IBD include diminished absorption of vitamin B_{12} and trace metals including zinc, calcium, and magnesium and decreased reabsorption of bile salts.

Extraintestinal manifestations occur frequently in clients with IBD and complicate its management. Manifestations involve the joints (most common symptom), skin, eyes, and mouth. The major skin manifestations are erythema nodosum and pyoderma gangrenosum. Local tissue involvement can cause rectal complications, such as anal fissures, and bowel complications, such as local abscesses, perforation, and stenosis from healing lesions. Infrequent nonspecific manifestations include osteoporosis, liver disease, peptic ulceration, and amyloidosis.

Surgical Management

Surgery is commonly used to treat ulcerative colitis, but not Crohn's disease, except to treat complications. When medical management fails and the condition provides intractable, surgical intervention is usually indicated for ulcerative colitis. Surgery may be indicated in both conditions for complications such as perforation, hemorrhage, obstruction, toxic megacolon, abscess, fistula, and intractability.

Possible procedures that may be performed to treat ulcerative colitis include a total proctocolectomy with a permanent ileostomy, and restorative procedures such as an ileorectal anastomosis, an ileoanal reservoir, and a Kock pouch.

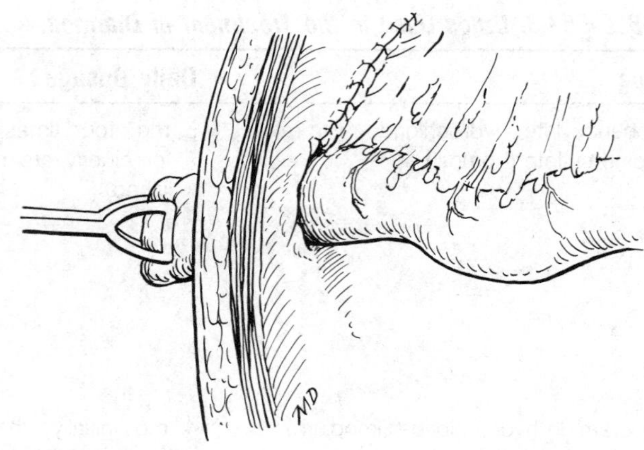

▲ Figure 55-2

Ileum being drawn through abdominal wall to form ileostomy stoma.

In a total proctocolectomy, the colon and rectum are removed and the anus closed. The terminal ileum is brought out through the abdominal wall and a permanent ileostomy formed (Fig. 55-2).

Ileorectal anastomosis is another possible form of surgical management. The colon is resected, leaving a rectal stump. The terminal ileum is then anastomosed to this stump (Fig. 55-3). The client will have diarrhea postoperatively; however, in time, the stool usually becomes more solid.

Ileorectal anastomosis, an early alternative to the total proctocolectomy, has several problems, however. The remaining rectum is often still affected by the disease, and further treatment, even eventual resection, is often required. There is also a significant incidence of rectal cancer among clients who have had this surgery. The newer procedures have essentially eliminated the

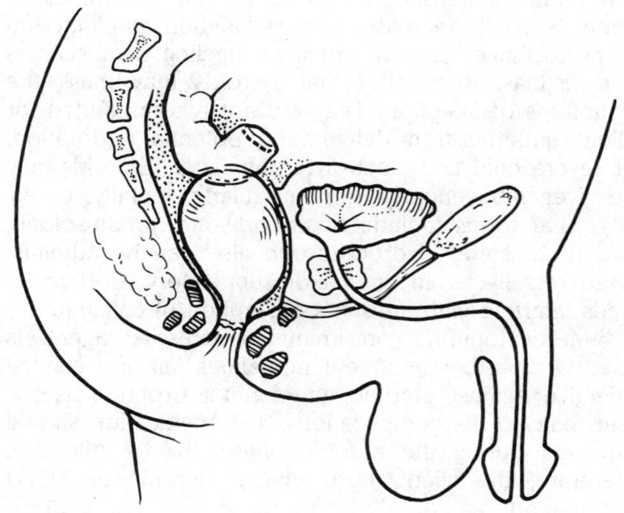

▲ Figure 55-3

Ileorectal anastomosis following subtotal colectomy. This operation eliminates proctectomy with its attendant complications but does not provide definitive treatment for ulcerative colitis.

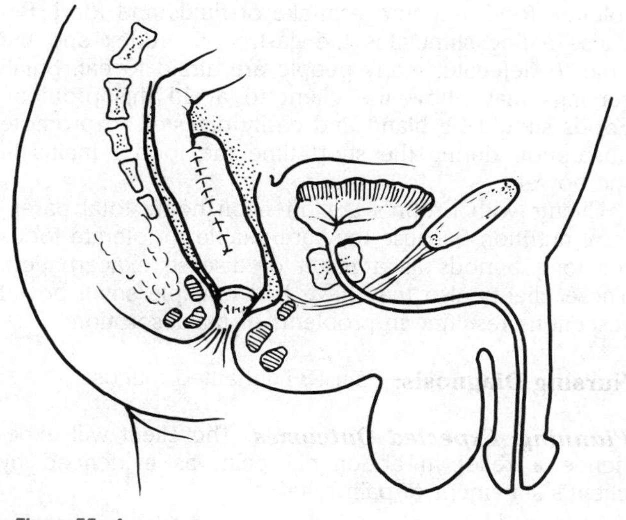

▲ *Figure 55-4*

Ileal "J" pouch-anal anastomosis. The two-loop ileal pouch is simple to construct, provides adequate storage capacity, and is evacuated spontaneously and fully.

need for this procedure because safer, more effective options are available.

The ileoanal reservoir (also known as a J pouch) prevents the need for an ostomy and preserves the rectal sphincter muscle. The rectal mucosa is excised and the colon removed. An ileoanal reservoir is then created in the anal canal, and a temporary loop ileostomy is formed. After healing has taken place, the ileostomy is reversed and stool drains into the reservoir (Fig. 55-4).

A continent ileostomy, or a Kock pouch, is a procedure in which reservoir or pouch is constructed from a loop of ileum. This allows stool to be stored intra-abdominally until it is drained by the client from a nipple valve made from an intussuscepted portion of ileum (Fig. 55-5). The client has a flat stoma on the right side of the abdomen.

This continent ileostomy, or Kock pouch, has advantages because the client (1) does not need to wear an external pouch, (2) has minimal skin problems, and (3) usually has no leakage of stool or flatus. The client drains the pouch several times per day using a catheter, usually when a feeling of fullness occurs.

After the formation of the Kock pouch, suture line leakage with local or generalized peritonitis (the most frequent complication with the reservoir) occurs in the early postoperative period. Other complications, including fistula formation, sliding of the valve, and obstruction with food residue, may occur later in the recovery period.

In Crohn's disease, surgery is used only to treat the complications, because even when the diseased portion is removed, there is a 50 per cent incidence of recurrence. The physician may prescribe antibiotics to control infection. During surgical resection for Crohn's disease, attempts are made to preserve as much of the small intestine as possible. Two thirds of the small intestine may be removed with no ill effects if the remaining portion is normal. However, resection of the distal ileum results in the client's inability to absorb

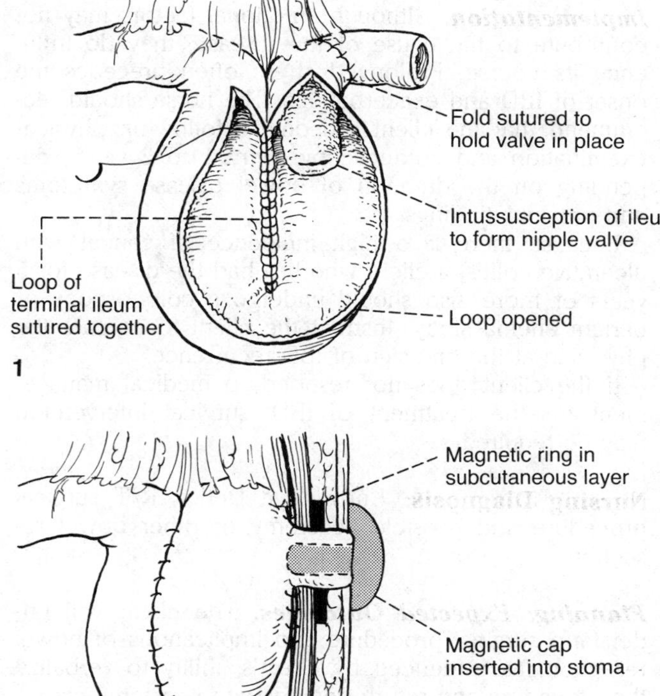

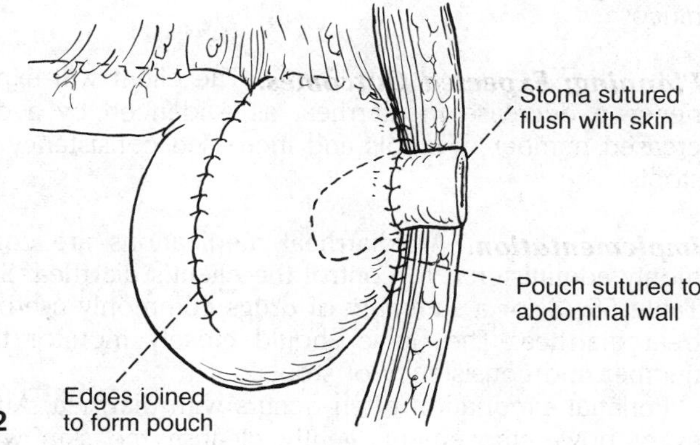

▲ *Figure 55-5*

Continent ileostomy (Kock pouch) with Maclet ring device. *1*, Loop of terminal ileum is sutured together and cut open. Using forceps, surgeon intussuscepts distal ileum to form nipple valve. *2*, Free edges sutured together to form reservoir; stoma sutured flush with skin, and pouch sutured to abdominal wall. *3*, Magnetic ring is implanted in subcutaneous layer and stoma closed with magnetic cap.

vitamin B_{12}, and removal of more than 6 to 8 feet results in impaired absorption of glucose, fat, and protein. If the colon is diseased, an ileotransverse colectomy (right colon and ileum), segmental colectomy, or total colectomy may be performed. A total colectomy with ileorectal anastomosis may be the surgery of choice.

Complications

For 1 to 3 weeks after extensive small bowel resection, the client may be unable to tolerate oral intake and may have further losses in body protein or lean body mass. Total parenteral alimentation is given until oral intake can be resumed. Diarrhea usually occurs during the first 6 weeks after surgery. Anemia (from iron deficiency, steatorrhea, or decreased protein absorption) also may ensue. Paralytic ileus is another possible complication.[30]

Nursing Management

ASSESSMENT

The nurse should assess the client's bowel elimination pattern, noting the number of stools, color, and consistency, as well as the presence of blood or steatorrhea. The nurse also should assess the abdomen noting bowel sounds, and the location of pain.

NURSING INTERVENTION

Nursing Diagnosis: Diarrhea R/T inflamed intestinal mucosa.

Planning: Expected Outcomes. The client will experience a decrease in diarrhea, as evidenced by a decreased number of stools and increased consistency of stools.

Implementation. Antidiarrheal medications are commonly administered to control the client's diarrhea. See Table 55–3 for a summary of drugs commonly used to treat diarrhea. The nurse should closely monitor the number and consistency of stools.

Perianal excoriation often occurs with diarrhea. After every bowel movement, gently cleanse the skin with warm water, and apply a protective moisture barrier product.

Nursing Diagnosis: Altered Nutrition: Less than Body Requirements R/T diarrhea and malabsorption.

Planning: Expected Outcomes. The client will increase nutritional uptake to meet metabolic requirements, as evidenced by weight stabilization and, possibly, weight gain.

Implementation. The nurse also must monitor the client's nutritional intake. The type of diet ordered depends on the condition of the client. If the client can tolerate food, encourage intake of fluids and food. Because eating stimulates the gastrocolic reflex and the urge to defecate, many people are afraid to eat. Small servings may allow the client to avoid this problem. Foods should be bland and easily digested to promote absorption during the short time the food remains in the bowel.

Clients with Crohn's are often on home total parenteral nutrition because they are unable to tolerate foods for long periods as a result of disease exacerbation. These clients also may have had multiple small bowel resections resulting in problems of malabsorption.

Nursing Diagnosis: Pain R/T inflamed mucosa.

Planning: Expected Outcomes. The client will experience a relief in abdominal pain, as evidenced by client's statement of pain relief.

Implementation. The nurse must assess the client's pain and give pain medications as ordered. The nurse should note any changes in the client's complaints of pain, because they may indicate the development of complications. Narcotics are generally used sparingly so they do not mask symptoms.

Nursing Diagnosis: Ineffective Individual Coping, High Risk for R/T stress of disease and exacerbations R/T stress.

Planning: Expected Outcomes. The client will cope effectively with the disease, as evidenced by fewer exacerbations and client's improved coping style.

Implementation. Although emotional factors may not contribute to the cause of the disease, they do influence its course. Prolonged stress often precedes the onset of IBD and exacerbations. The nurse should recommend that the client schedule a follow-up physical examination and colonoscopy every 1 to 2 years, depending on the duration of bowel disease symptoms and previous findings.

Because there is a high incidence of cancer with ulcerative colitis, a client who has had the disease for 5 years or more also should undergo a colonoscopy or barium enema study. Instruct the client to contact the physician at the first sign of IBD recurrence.

If the client does not respond to medical management for the treatment of IBD, surgical intervention may be required.

Nursing Diagnosis: Knowledge Deficit R/T surgical procedure and possible ileostomy or other bowel resection.

Planning: Expected Outcomes. The client will understand surgical procedure and implications of bowel resection, as evidenced by client's ability to verbalize the procedure and return demonstrate ileostomy care.

Implementation. If the client is scheduled for an ileostomy, then ostomy surgery, a procedure that may provoke a life crisis, must be fully explained to the client. In some instances, a preoperative visit from a member of an ostomy association may be helpful. An enterostomal therapist should assist with the preoperative preparation. Before surgery, the site of the ileostomy is selected, consideration being given to the location of the disease, body contours, convenience, and the type of clothing the client wears. If an ostomy pouch is indicated, the client may wear the pouch for 1 to 2 days before surgery to ensure comfort with the site selected. In order to provide assistance and support, the nurse must assess the client's body image and feelings about loss of a major body part.

If the client is not having an ileoproctectomy, but one of the continence-sparing surgeries, extensive teaching is still required. The client needs to understand the type of bowel resection to be performed and the implications of this surgery. Some procedures may require a temporary ileostomy (ileoanal reservoir), whereas others will require some altered elimination by the client (Kock pouch).

Nursing Diagnosis: Injury, High Risk for R/T postoperative complications such as stomal cyanosis, distention, intestinal obstruction, and fluid and electrolyte imbalances.

Planning: Expected Outcomes. The client will not suffer injury, as evidenced by minimal distention, rapid return of normal peristalsis, and absence of fluid and electrolyte imbalance.

Implementation. The nurse must monitor the stoma after surgery. The nurse should ensure there is no pressure on the stoma that could interfere with circulation. The color of the stoma should be assessed at frequent intervals. If the color becomes pale, dusky, or cyanotic, the nurse should immediately notify the physician. If the blood supply to the stoma is compromised, the stoma may require surgical revision.

A nasogastric, gastrostomy, or jejunostomy tube will be in place for several days after surgery to remove gases and fluids that would increase intestinal distention and put pressure on the suture line. The drainage must be accurately noted. The passage of flatus indicates return of peristalsis. As bowel sounds return, clamp the tube as prescribed and give the client ice chips and water. When the client has tolerated this for a minimum of 24 hours, the tube is usually removed and clear liquids given.

Although most ileostomies are uneventful postoperatively, several complications can occur. The most common is an intestinal obstruction that may be caused by lumen obstruction, adhesions, food, or stomal edema. Early signs include anorexia, abdominal cramps, no ileostomy drainage, or a foul, brown, watery discharge in the pouch, or visible peristalsis. Other early postoperative complications include hemorrhage, hypoxia, and fluid and electrolyte imbalance. If there are severe or prolonged problems with absorption, an elemental diet or parenteral nutrition may be necessary.

Nursing Diagnosis: Ineffective Individual Coping R/T disturbance of body image and self-concept secondary to ostomy.

Planning: Expected Outcomes. The client will experience a positive body image and self-concept, as evidenced by the client's statements and ability to care for his or her own ostomy without embarrassment.

Implementation. A few days after surgery, the client needs to begin to confront the stoma and to begin integrating its function and appearance into his or her body image. The nurse must help the client look at and touch the stoma as soon as possible. The nurse should always use proper terms for the stoma and equipment.

Clothing can be a concern for the client with an ostomy, and clothing options need to be discussed with the client. The client should be discouraged from wearing a tight waistband that might rub on the stoma. The client should be encouraged to try on various outfits to ensure that the stoma and pouch are invisible. A visit with another client with an ostomy often helps the client realize that the ostomy is easily hidden beneath the clothing.

Encourage the client to verbalize feelings about the stoma and its appearance. The client may be very accepting of the stoma because the illness (ulcerative colitis) is now gone and the client's life may be more normal and productive than it had been with the disease. Young men and unmarried women may express the greatest concern about body image. It is also important to find out how family or significant others now view the client. Again, this might be a positive response, because the client may have been chronically ill prior to the surgery and now seems much healthier.

The client needs to be aware of the nearest ostomy supply center so equipment will be easy to obtain. Clients may want to join the local ostomy association for emotional support. This organization often helps clients regain lost self-esteem and improves their self-concept and body image. The successful rehabilitation of others helps clients believe that they, too, can return to a normal lifestyle.

Nursing Diagnosis: Knowledge Deficit R/T ileostomy care, care following ileorectal anastomosis, care of an ileoanal reservoir, or care of a continent ileostomy.

Planning: Expected Outcomes. The client will understand proper care of (1) an ileostomy, (2) an ileorectal anastomosis, (3) ileoanal reservoir, or (4) a continent ileostomy, as evidenced by (1) ability to apply own appliance correctly, without leakage, and to empty pouch appropriately, (2) absence of perianal breakdown, (3) absence of fecal leakage, or (4) ability to empty reservoir correctly and absence of leakage.

Implementation

Ileostomy. The client must soon begin to master the skills needed to provide self-care. Initially, the client can simply observe the care of the stoma. Stoma care is the area of greatest concern to the client with an ileostomy. Begin by telling the client what the stoma looks like; that it extends 1 to 2 cm beyond the abdominal wall and is very red and swollen at first. Assure the client that permanent changes in stoma size usually occur within the first 3 to 4 months after surgery when the swelling subsides, with the stoma shrinking to a slightly smaller permanent size.

When changing the pouch, the client should learn to check the size and color of the stoma and the odor of the drainage. Also, check the stoma for signs of irritation or cyanosis.

When the ileostomy begins to function, the output is minimal. As the client takes in more food, the drainage becomes thicker in consistency and has a weak odor. The discharge is irritating to the skin because of the alkaline contents of the effluent. Because an ileostomy drains continuously, a pouch must be worn and the stoma must be covered with gauze when the pouch is being changed.

The pouch should be cut to fit about 1⁄16 to 1⁄8 inch larger than the stoma. If the pouch does not fit well, severe skin irritation can occur. Skin irritation can vary from redness to weeping dermatitis or ulceration. Irritation also can result from adhesives or frequent removal of the appliance. The skin should be washed and rinsed thoroughly between changes.

If skin irritation does occur, the nurse should first check the fit of the pouch. The best initial treatment for this problem would be to reapply the ostomy appliance (one with a karaya or hydrocolloid skin barrier), ensuring a proper fit and seal. The skin barrier of the appliance is usually sufficient to protect and heal the skin. If this method does not work, other barriers must be used. A wide variety of skin care products are available. If the problems continue, an enterostomal therapist should be consulted for further assistance.

Skin infection also can occur. *Candida* is the most common cause. The peristomal skin takes on a rashlike appearance. An antifungal powder such as nystatin should be applied directly to the affected skin area. The barrier can then be applied over the powder.

The frequency with which the ileal pouch needs to be emptied varies with each client. It should be emptied when the pouch is approximately 1⁄3 to 1⁄2 full. The client should be taught to empty the pouch during times of low output, usually before meals, at bedtime, and on arising in the morning.

When changing the pouch, all equipment should be ready before the old one is removed. Remove the old pouch carefully. A piece of gauze may be held over the stoma until the new pouch is attached. Encourage the client to inspect and touch the stoma at this time. Remind the client with a new ileostomy to take ostomy supplies along when traveling. The client may want to keep supplies handy in a shaving or cosmetic case instead of a suitcase.

Many different types of pouches are available (Fig. 55-6). Clients should try to find the best pouch for their needs. Small ileostomy drainage pouches are available for small adults and children. Foods such as eggs, fish, onions, cabbage, or greens cause stool odor; therefore, deodorizing solutions and tablets may be placed in the pouch. Spinach, parsley, yogurt, and buttermilk decrease drainage odor.

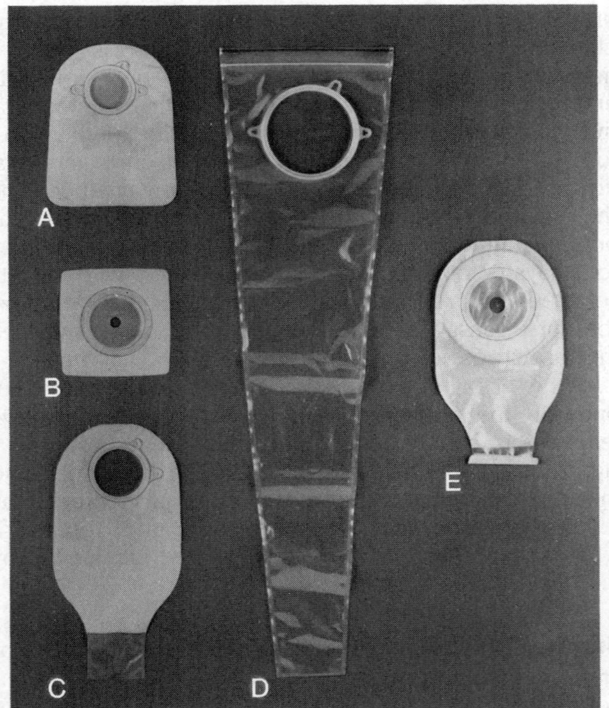

▲ **Figure 55-6**

Colostomy and ileostomy pouches. *A*, Closed two-piece colostomy pouch. *B*, Skin barrier (second piece of two-piece pouches). *C*, Two-piece drainable colostomy and ileostomy pouch (transparent or flesh colored). *D*, Colostomy irrigation sleeve. *E*, One-piece drainable colostomy and ileostomy pouch with clamp.

The client also needs special instructions regarding prescription and over-the-counter medications. Enteric-coated tablets, such as iron preparations, vitamins, and hormones, multilayer tablets, time-release capsules, and gelatin capsules may not be absorbed in the small intestine. The client should note if any medications are obvious in the pouch drainage. The physician will need to prescribe different medications or different forms of the medication.

The client who has had an ileostomy needs to pay close attention to fluid intake. It is very easy for this client to become dehydrated. The approximate output from an ileostomy is 1200 to 1500 ml per day. The client must monitor this output for any increase that could lead to severe fluid and electrolyte balance.

A low residue diet that is high in protein, carbohydrates, and calories is recommended after the surgery. Supplemental vitamins A, D, E, K, and B_{12} may be needed. Berries, whole-grain cereals, and raw fruits and vegetables can cause problems for clients with an ileostomy. Omit any foods that cause discomfort or diarrhea. Ingested foods will pass through the ileostomy within 4 to 6 hours. It is not advisable to eat a large meal close to bedtime.

Ileostomy clients must learn to chew their food well because the shortened bowel transit time means that poorly chewed food will be passed undigested. High-fiber and high-cellulose foods may absorb excessive moisture, leading to swelling and possibly constipation or even obstruction. Foods that should be avoided or limited include popcorn, peanuts, tough fibrous meats, skinned vegetables, rice, bran, and coconuts.

These clients often find, however, that their postoperative diet is less restrictive than the diet they followed with the disease. Their diet was often very restricted preoperatively because so many foods increased the diarrhea and other symptoms. These clients often gain weight after surgery, sometimes to the point that they must begin to restrict their caloric intake.

Some clients with ileostomies tend to develop calcium oxalate, uric acid, or urinary calculi. Uric acid stones tend to form when urine volume is low and the urine is persistently acidic. Ingestion of sodium bicarbonate or potassium citrate will alkalinize the urine. Allopurinol may be used if uric acid levels remain elevated. Fluid intake should be at least 1500 ml per day.

Ileorectal Anastomosis. The client with an ileorectal anastomosis does not have to learn about stoma or pouch care. The major goal of teaching centers around the importance of defecating before the rectum becomes overly distended. Most clients find that they have 4 to 5 stools per day once their bodies have adjusted to the surgical alteration.

The feces in these clients is often described as pasty in consistency, and appears to contain fewer electrolytes than the drainage from a traditional ileostomy. It may take up to 1 year for the client's altered bowel to adapt.

Clients having the ileoanal anastomosis must understand the importance of follow-up meetings with the physician. They must understand that the remaining mucosa can become diseased with ulcerative colitis or Crohn's disease, requiring further resection and possibly formation of an ileostomy. They also need to know that they are at an increased risk for the development of rectal cancer. These clients have to receive regular proctoscopic examinations following their surgery.

The client should learn to avoid foods that may have caused diarrhea in the past. It is best to try new foods one at a time so the effect can be determined. The diet is usually not limited; however, it should include adequate fluids to avoid dehydration.

Ileoanal Reservoir. The client with the ileoanal reservoir also has no need to learn about stoma or pouch care. The client will learn to respond to the sensation to defecate so spillage does not occur. After the bowel adapts to the surgical alteration, the stool becomes more formed and many clients will have only 2 to 4 stools per day. The client should maintain an adequate fluid intake.

Continent Ileostomy, or Kock Pouch. During the surgical formation of the Kock pouch, an evacuation catheter is inserted. A skin barrier and special gauze dressing are then applied. These hold the catheter in an upright position to avoid stress on a healing nipple valve. It is imperative to avoid distention of the ileostomy reservoir in the early postoperative period because of the pressure it would cause on the suture line. Thus, it is emptied every 2 hours for about 2 weeks.

Carefully observe for the start of ileal drainage, which usually starts 3 to 4 days postoperatively. About 2 weeks after surgery, the catheter is removed from the pouch. The marked catheter may then be used to drain the pouch. The intervals between drainings are gradually increased each week until the ileostomy is emptied two to four times per day but not at night.

To empty the reservoir, the client should sit up. The catheter is lubricated with a water-soluble lubricant and inserted into the stoma through the valve. Contents are allowed to drain by gravity through the catheter into the toilet, with complete drainage occurring in 3 to 5 minutes. A small gauze dressing is then applied over the stoma. The equipment is cleaned with mild soap and rinsed, and can be carried in a plastic case.

The reservoir volume continues to increase to a maximum of around 600 ml in 6 months. The client needs an oral intake of at least eight 8-oz glasses of fluid per day. No long-term restrictions are placed on physical activities. Tell the client to wear Medic Alert identification bracelet and carry a brief description of the pouch and drainage procedure in case of emergency.

The client needs to learn about dietary restrictions associated with a continent ileostomy. Foods that could cause a blockage of the valve and the stoma need to be avoided. These include foods such as mushrooms and nuts. All foods need to be chewed thoroughly so partly digested food will not occlude the stoma.

Nursing Diagnosis: Sexual Dysfunction R/T concern about ileostomy.

Planning: Expected Outcomes. The client will not develop a sexual dysfunction, as evidenced by client's ability to return to preillness sexual functioning and role.

Implementation. The ileostomy may cause concern about sexual activity and pregnancy. The nurse should encourage the client to express any such concerns and to discuss them with the sexual partner. Impotency is uncommon, and psychological reasons should be explored if it does occur. Pregnancy and normal vaginal delivery are possible. The United Ostomy Association has a wide variety of booklets available for individuals with an ostomy. Topics include "Sex, Pregnancy and the Female Ostomate," "Sex, Courtship and the Single Ostomate," "Sex and the Male Ostomate," and "Insight into the Emotional Aspects of Ileostomies and Colostomies." The American Cancer Society also has resources available.

The client and sexual partner should be encouraged to discuss sexuality and to verbalize any fears. Clients can be taught activities to lessen the intrusiveness of the pouch such as emptying it before intercourse, wearing a soft flannel pouch cover, and being open to using different positions for intercourse. If there are problems, a sexual therapist should be consulted for further information and assistance.

EVALUATION

The nurse must evaluate client outcomes based on the established plan of care. If these goals were not achieved, the plan and interventions must be revised to meet the client's needs.

Modification of Plan of Care for the Elderly

Crohn's disease and ulcerative colitis occur less often in the older age groups. The treatment, however, when it does occur in this age group is the same as for the younger client.

If the aged client has an ileostomy or other diversion, teaching may take a little longer, but most older clients can learn to care for themselves without difficulty. If the client has an ileostomy, issues such as eyesight and dexterity are important. Sometimes the older client cannot manipulate the clamp used to close the pouch. If the client is unable to manipulate the equipment, a family member may have to assume that responsibility. Carefully assess the older client's ability to care for self and the appliance.

Post-hospital Care

DISCHARGE TEACHING

Clients with IBD should be referred to the Crohn's and Colitis Foundations of America for support groups and information. The client with an ileostomy should be encouraged to join the ileostomy association associated with the American Cancer Society.

Postoperative care and care of the stoma or diversion should be reinforced before the client is discharged.

HOME HEALTH CARE NEEDS

The client will need to know where to purchase the necessary equipment to care for an ileostomy. If the client was experiencing difficulty with self care, a visiting nurse should probably see the client at home to follow-up on learning needs (see Bridge to Home Health Care).

FOLLOW-UP CARE

The client will need to be seen by the physician at regular intervals if the disease is being controlled medically. If the client had surgical resection, the client will be seen after the surgery to ensure that healing has occurred. If the client has Crohn's disease, the client will need to be followed for disease recurrence. The client may need a follow-up visit to an enterostomal therapist to ensure that the appliance fits well and that the client does not have any problems with stoma care.

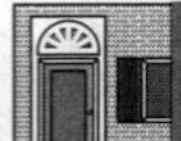

BRIDGE TO HOME HEALTH CARE

The Client with an Ostomy

In bridging the ostomy client from hospital to home care, it is vital to provide information on where to purchase supplies for the ostomy. Written instructions should be given, including the brand name, order number, size of pouch, skin barrier, and pouch deodorants, as well as the name, address, and phone number of a local medical supply facility. Ostomy supplies are very expensive; therefore, an issue of the *Ostomy Quarterly*, which lists mail order companies that sell equipment at a discount, is appreciated by clients. Talking with other ostomates at a local United Ostomy Association meeting may help to find several money-saving ideas. United Ostomy Association's phone number is 213-413-5510. *The Ostomy Book* by Barbara Dorr Mullen and Kerry Anne McGinn is an excellent publication written especially for clients and their families.

▼ Neoplastic Disorders

BENIGN TUMORS

Various kinds of benign tumors are found in the bowel. Polyps are the most commonly found benign tumor of the large bowel. A polyp is a lesion that projects into the lumen of the bowel. Some polyps have stems (pedunculated), whereas others do not (sessile). Polyps are usually benign lesions, but some types are precursors of cancer (i.e., premalignant tumors). Polyps are dangerous in two ways: (1) they can mask the presence of a malignant tumor and (2) they may serve as the focus for bowel obstruction or intussusception. Benign bowel tumors produce manifestations similar to those of malignant tumors. Some benign tumors bleed profusely and cause abdominal discomfort. Bleeding benign tumors are usually removed surgically.

CANCER OF THE SMALL BOWEL

Only about 1 per cent of all GI cancers involve tumors of the small bowel. The average age of onset is 53 to 58 years. Most tumors are in the ileum, with the remainder almost equally divided between the duodenum and jejunum. Symptoms are vague and nonspecific, and include weight loss, pain, anemia, nausea, vomiting, obstruction, palpable mass, and hemorrhage. Surgery is the only intervention that offers hope of cure. Unfortunately, even with early diagnosis and bowel resection, only about 20 per cent of clients survive for 5 years. With late diagnosis, the 5-year survival rate decreases to about 5 per cent.

COLON CANCER

Definition

Cancers of the colon are usually adenocarcinomas.

Incidence

In both sexes, colonic and rectal cancer is the second most frequent cause of death from cancer in the United States. It ranks just behind lung cancer as cause of cancer deaths in the United States. It occurs with the same frequency in men and women. Most tumors are found in the distal portion of the large bowel, from the sigmoid colon to the anus. In recent years, the incidence of carcinoma of the right colon has increased, whereas that of the rectosigmoid area has decreased.

Even though early diagnosis reduces mortality, many clients still do not take advantage of screening techniques. Survival following diagnosis of colon cancer correlates with the stage of tumor invasion (Box 55–2).

Etiology

The cause of colon cancer is not definitely known. There are identifiable predisposing factors, however. It does seem to be related to low-residue, high-fat diets and highly refined foods. There also seems to be a familial tendency for colon cancer. The risk of cancer increases with chronic ulcerative colitis, granulomas, and familial polyposis.

Epidemiologic students indicate that diet may be a major factor in the development of cancer of the large bowel. Studies on bulk in stool and the rate of transit of fecal matter have so far given mixed results. Some researchers propose that metabolic and bacterial end products are carcinogenic and that constipation allows a longer contact with the bowel wall, thus increasing the probability of cancer developing.

Risk Factors

There are a number of known risk factors for colon cancer. These include

Family history of colon cancer;
Previous colon cancer;
Over age 40;
Ulcerative colitis;
High-fat, low-residue diet that is high in refined foods;
Familial polyposis;
Adenomatous polyps; and
Living in highly industrialized, urban societies.

Many of these risk factors have no primary prevention, so early detection is more important. Early detection includes yearly digital rectal examinations for adults over 40, proctoscopic examination after age 50, and stool guaiac following the rectal examinations. Reducing the amount of fats and refined foods and increasing the amount of fiber in the diet may help reduce the risk of colon cancer.

Box 55–2. TNM Classification of Colorectal Cancer

Primary Tumor (T)

TX Primary tumor cannot be assessed
T0 No evidence of primary tumor
Tis Carcinoma in situ
T1 Tumor invades submucosa
T2 Tumor invades muscularis propria
T3 Tumor invades through muscularis propria into subserosa, or into nonperitonealized pericolic or perirectal tissues
T4 Tumor perforates visceral peritoneum, or directly invades other organs or structures

Lymph Node (N)

NX Regional lymph nodes cannot be assessed
N0 No regional lymph node metastasis
N1 Metastasis in 1 to 3 pericolic or perirectal lymph nodes
N2 Metastasis in 4 or more pericolic or perirectal lymph nodes
N3 Metastasis in any lymph node along course of a major vascular trunk

Distant Metastasis (M)

MX Presence of distant metastasis cannot be assessed
M0 No distant metastasis
M1 Distant metastasis

Stage Grouping

0	Tis	N0	M0
I(A)	T1	N0	M0
	T2	N0	M0
II(B)	T3	N0	M0
	T4	N0	M0
III(C)	Any T	N1	M0
	Any T	N2	M0
	Any T	N3	M0
IV(D)	Any T	Any N	M1

Pathophysiology

The majority of malignant tumors (at least 50 per cent) occur in the rectal area; another 20 to 30 per cent are found in the sigmoid and descending colons. The remainder are found in the transverse and ascending colons, with twice as many found in the ascending colon as in the transverse colon.

Cancers of the colon almost always develop from adenomatous polyps. As this tumor becomes malignant, it increases in size within the lumen and begins to invade the bowel wall.

Colon cancer is staged using Duke's classification, with Duke's A having an 80 to 90 per cent 5-year survival rate; Duke's B, about a 60 per cent 5-year survival rate; Duke's C, a 25 to 40 per cent 5-year survival rate; and Duke's D, less than a 5% 5-year survival rate.

Malignant bowel tumors spread by (1) direct extension to a nearby organ, as to the stomach from the transverse colon; (2) lymphatic and hematogenic channels, usually to the liver; and (3) seeding or implanting of cells into the peritoneal cavity.

The urinary bladder, ureters, and reproductive organs are frequently involved by direct extension. Also, the formation of a fistula between the bladder and the bowel or between the bowel and vagina is not uncommon. Blood-borne metastasis extends most frequently to the liver but also may involve the lungs, kidneys, and bones.

Clinical Manifestations

Symptoms of colon cancer include rectal bleeding, changed bowel habits, intestinal obstruction, abdominal pain, weight loss, anorexia, nausea and vomiting, anemia, and palpable mass (Fig. 55-7). In general, tumors in the small bowel and right colon are more likely to cause abdominal pain, nausea, and vomiting. Because the large intestine distends, there are fewer early symptoms. Tumors in the left colon and rectum are more likely to cause passage of blood or mucus, an alteration in bowel habits, and a feeling that the bowel is not empty after defecation. Bleeding is the symptom that often alerts the client to seek health care. When the tumor occludes the bowel, obstructive symptoms result.

Symptoms of carcinoma vary according to the area in which the tumor is found and the type of tumor involved. Tumors in the right colon are unlikely to cause obstruction because of its large lumen and the liquid quality of the feces. At this location, lesions often ulcerate, resulting in anemia. Anorexia, weight loss, weakness, and debility may be present at the time of diagnosis.

Lesions of the ascending and transverse colon often present with progressive obstruction. Tumors in the descending colon and rectum frequently cause obstructive symptoms but not weight loss, anemia, or dyspepsia. Most clients also report a change in bowel habits.

DIAGNOSTIC ASSESSMENT

One third of malignant tumors of the distal colon and rectum can be felt with the examining finger. This makes digital rectal examination one of the more important diagnostic methods. A stool guaiac test is done to test for GI bleeding. Carcinoembryonic antigen (CEA) may be elevated in colon cancer and aids in determining the progress of the disease. X-ray studies of the colon may show either a filling defect or a stricture. Ultrasound and CT help establish tumor size and metastasis. A sigmoidoscopy can identify more than one half of the tumors. Flexible fiberoptic scopes permit better visualization into the right colon, extend the diagnostic capabilities of the procedure, and allow biopsy (see Chap. 51).

Early diagnosis improves the survival rate. American Cancer Society guidelines for early detection include routine annual digital rectal examination beginning at age 40, an annual stool guaiac test at age 50, and a sigmoidoscopy every 3 to 5 years, after two negative sigmoidoscopy examinations performed 1 year apart, after age 50. It is vital to explain to clients the necessity for early detection and the importance of reporting symptoms such as rectal bleeding and a change in bowel habits to their physician.

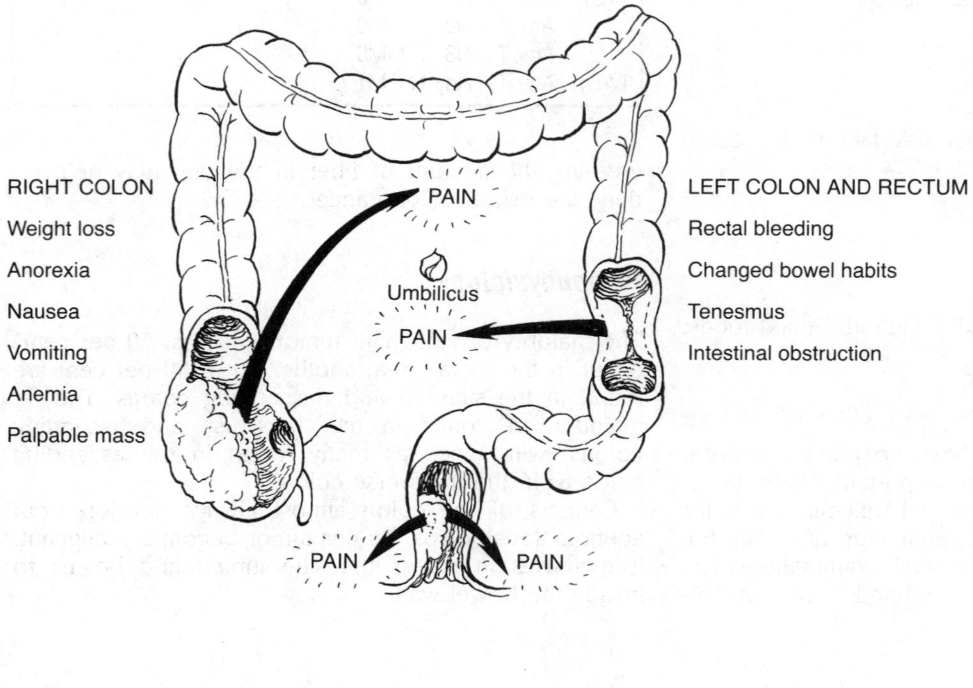

▲ *Figure 55-7*

Symptoms of carcinoma in colon. Pain usually radiates toward umbilicus or perianal area.

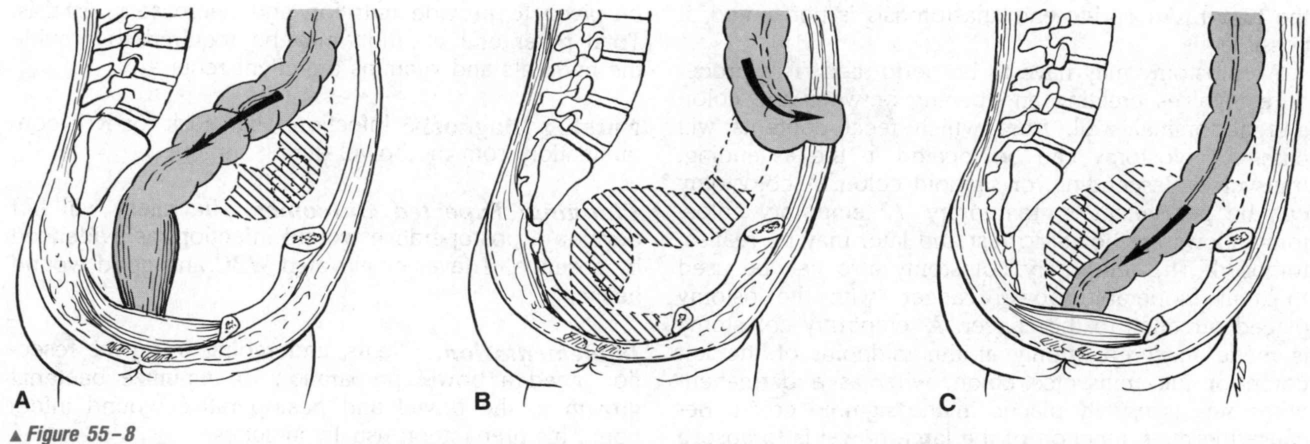

▲ Figure 55-8

Resecting malignant tumors in rectosigmoid segment of bowel. *A*, Anterior resection with primary anastomosis is used for cancer at any point in bowel except terminal rectum. Associated lymph nodes are resected. *B*, Abdominoperineal (anteroposterior) resection with formation of permanent colostomy (Miles operation) for cancer involving the anus and terminal portion of the rectum. *C*, Proctosigmoidectomy with "pull-through" and preservation of external sphincter muscles is appropriate when tumor is in proximal rectum and unlikely to metastasize further.

Medical Management

The primary treatment for colon cancer is surgery; however, medical treatment is used as an adjunct to improve survival in tumors that cannot be completely removed. Radiation therapy is often given before surgery in the hope that the malignant cells will not metastasize, and to reduce the size of the tumor and thus make it more resectable.

Local interventions at the tumor site after surgery include the implantation of isotopes into the tumor area and electrocoagulation. Interstitial implant includes radium, cesium, or cobalt. Iridium has been used in the rectum.

Chemotherapy has had limited success, although 5-fluorouracil has produced some positive results. Recently, research has been conducted to improve this picture by using combinations of medications. Levamisol is the newest agent to be given with 5-fluorouracil. This combination has improved survival in Duke's C tumors. Leucovorin also may be given with 5-fluorouracil, with or without levamisol to increase its effects. Chemotherapy may be used to reduce metastasis and control symptoms of metastasis. In clients with liver metastasis, intrahepatic arterial chemotherapy may be administered.

Surgical Management

Intervention depends on the type of tumor, its location and stage, and on the client's general condition (see Box 55-2). A variety of surgical procedures are performed to treat colorectal cancer (Figs. 55-8 and 55-9). All procedures entail colon resection. The tumor is removed with several inches of colon on either side of

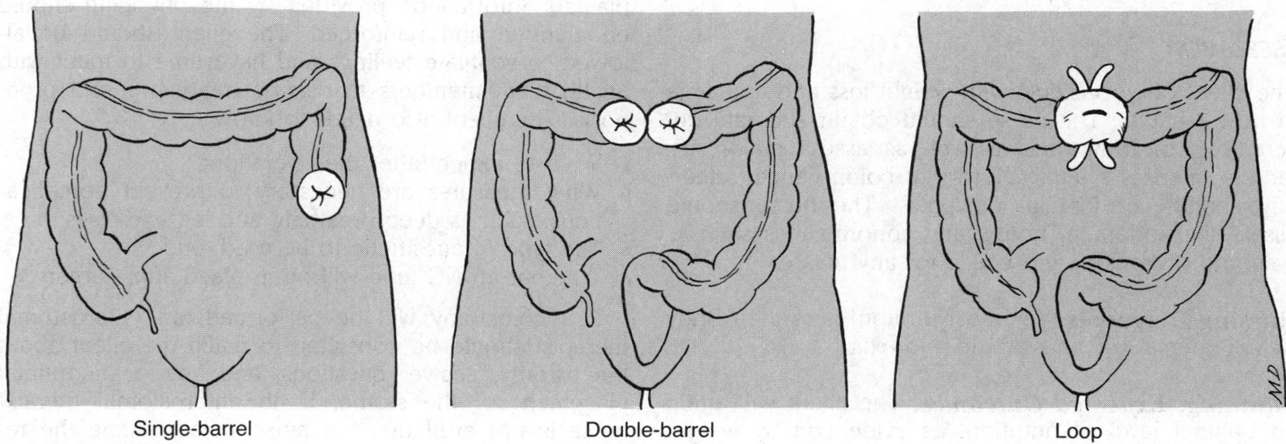

▲ Figure 55-9

Types of colostomies. Single-barrel colostomies are usually permanent. Double-barrel colostomies are usually temporary, and stomas may be adjacent or several inches apart. Loop colostomies are temporary and formed by bringing a loop of colon through the abdominal wall and supporting it with a plastic brace.

the tumor. An end-to-end anastomosis is performed, if possible.

A colostomy may have to be performed. This procedure involves creating an opening between the colon and abdominal wall, from which fecal contents will pass. A colostomy can be located in the ascending, transverse, descending, or sigmoid colon. A colostomy can be permanent or temporary. A temporary colostomy allows the bowel to rest and later may be reanastomosed. The temporary colostomy also can be used to treat inoperable bowel cancer, with the ostomy placed proximal to the cancer. A temporary colostomy is made most commonly at the midpoint of the left colon or the transverse colon, whereas a permanent colostomy is usually placed in the sigmoid colon. Because the main function of the large bowel is to absorb water, the colostomy is easier to manage nearer the sigmoid colon than in the transverse or right colon because the stool is formed.

A colostomy may also be single- or double-barreled. When only one loop of bowel is opened onto the abdominal surface, it is called an end colostomy; the client has only one stoma. A double-barreled colostomy is one in which both loops, distal and proximal, are open on the abdominal wall. An end colostomy is permanent if the bowel distal to it has been resected. A double-barreled colostomy may be closed later depending on the disease present. A double-barreled colostomy can be two separate stomas, a loop with one stoma with two openings, or one stoma and a Hartmann's pouch (distal bowel closed off and placed left intra-abdominal).

Rectal tumors may require an abdominal-perineal resection, with the formation of a permanent or end colostomy. The affected colon and entire rectum is excised and the anus closed. Newer surgical techniques allow low sigmoid tumors to be removed while leaving the rectal sphincter intact. This allows for normal bowel elimination to be maintained.

Nursing Management

ASSESSMENT

The client often presents with weight loss and a change in bowel habits. The nurse should obtain accurate descriptions of symptoms as well as assess major risk factors, such as a family history of colon cancer, ulcerative colitis, or familial polyposis. The nurse should assess the abdomen, noting any abnormalities such as pain and distention, and check for any masses.

Nursing Diagnosis: Altered Nutrition: Less than Body Requirements R/T nausea and anorexia.

Planning: Expected Outcomes. The client will attain an optimal level of nutrition, as evidenced by weight regain (or absence of weight loss), and normal serum electrolytes and protein levels.

Implementation. Preoperatively, a diet high in calories, protein, and carbohydrates but low in residue may be given to provide nutrition and decrease peristalsis. Total parenteral nutrition may be required to provide the nutrients and vitamins the client requires.

Nursing Diagnosis: Infection, High Risk for R/T contamination from the bowel during surgery.

Planning: Expected Outcomes. The client will not develop a postoperative wound infection, as evidenced by absence of fever or elevated WBC and good wound healing.

Implementation. Clients undergoing a bowel resection need a bowel preparation to minimize bacterial growth in the bowel and postoperative wound infection. This preparation usually includes

- A low-residue or liquid diet to reduce the fecal contents of the bowel;
- Administration of cathartics orally such as polyethylene glycol-electrolyte solution (Go-LYTELY) or other agent, which is usually started at least 24 hours preoperatively;
- Administration of antibiotics, such as sulfonamides and possibly neomycin and cephalexin; usually by mouth, for 24 to 48 hours preoperatively;
- Administration of enemas to cleanse the bowel (the inside of the bowel lumen should be as clean and bacteria free as possible); and
- Blood transfusions to correct severe anemia.

Nursing Diagnosis: Anxiety R/T impending surgery and diagnosis of cancer.

Planning: Expected Outcomes. The client will have a decrease in anxiety, as evidenced by the client's ability to understand preoperative teaching and respond appropriately.

Implementation. The nurse should identify the client's level of anxiety and provide supportive efforts. Clients should have all treatments and procedures fully explained. Information provided by the physician should be clarified and reinforced. The client should be allowed to ventilate feelings and have time to meet with health team members to discuss treatments and prognosis. The client also needs to know

- What to expect after the operation;
- What measures are necessary to prevent complications, such as deep breathing and leg exercises;
- The type of anesthetic to be used; and
- Whether an NG tube will be in place after surgery.

If a colostomy will be performed, an enterostomal therapist should be consulted to teach the client about the ostomy, answer questions, and advise an optimal placement of the stoma. If an enterostomal therapy nurse is not available, the nurse must assume the responsibility for teaching the client about the stoma. The client may be concerned with sexual dysfunction after surgery. The physician should explain this risk to the client, and the nurse should provide support to the client.

Nursing Diagnosis: Injury, High Risk for R/T postoperative complications, including infection, hemorrhage, wound disruption, thrombophlebitis, and abnormal stomal function.

Planning: Expected Outcomes. The client will not develop an injury, as evidenced by absence of signs of infection, no bleeding, and no evidence of wound disruption, thrombophlebitis, stomal ischemia, or bowel spillage.

Implementation. Immediate postoperative interventions are the same as those used for any major abdominal surgery. Additionally, if a colostomy was created, the nurse should monitor colostomy output and use special care to keep fecal contents from the colostomy (which contain bacteria) away from the surgical incision.

When creating a temporary loop colostomy, the surgeon brings a loop of bowel out through a wound that is separate from the surgical incision. To keep the loop from slipping back into the abdominal cavity, the surgeon places a rod or bridge beneath it. Two or three days postoperatively the surgeon opens the bowel, usually with a cautery. Because there are no sensory nerve endings in the bowel wall, this procedure is essentially painless, except for some cramping. The surgeon usually indicates which is the proximal loop and which is the distal loop.

The nurse should assess for the return of peristalsis. Indications include (1) passage of flatus and (2) return of bowel sounds, which can be heard with a stethoscope. The client may remain on gastric suction until peristalsis returns. It usually takes several days before the client can receive food and fluids and, as the client tolerates food, slowly advance to a regular diet.

Abdominal cramps commonly occur after surgery, as does distention of the bowel. Distention is uncomfortable and may cause pressure on suture lines. The insertion of a rectal tube for 20 to 30 minutes per physician order will help if the rectum contains gas.

Postoperatively, if an abdominal-perineal resection with creation of an end colostomy was performed, the nurse must assess not only the abdominal wound but a large draining perineal wound. Drains are often left in the incision and may be attached to a suction device such as a Hemovac. When suction is not used, you may need to change the client's dressing. The nurse should assess the character, volume, and odor of the drainage. Should the drainage in any way suggest a developing infection, the nurse should take a culture of the wound to identify the organism.

In the immediate postoperative period, sump drainage is often placed in the perineal wound. The sump tube is attached to suction, allowing the wound to heal from its deepest portion without forming an abscess. If a Penrose drain is used, rectal dressings will need to be changed frequently because the large, deep wound drains profusely. It will take several weeks to months for the wound to heal completely because of its size. The client should be prepared to wear a rectal dressing throughout the healing period.

The perineal wound can be very painful, and the client should receive sufficient pain medication to control the pain. Once the packing is removed, the wound is irrigated and the client should take a sitz bath 3 to 4 times a day. The client will find a side-lying position much more comfortable.

The client's stoma must be assessed closely for the presence of stomal ischemia. The stoma should be very red and moist. If it becomes dark or dusky, the nurse must immediately report this to the surgeon. Clients may have a colostomy pouch over the stoma. Be sure that this pouch is not applying any pressure to the stoma, interfering with its blood supply. When you change the pouch or empty it, prevent contamination of the surgical wound by fecal discharges. Monitor the return of bowel function by observing the type and quantity of discharges from the stoma.

The high lithotomy position associated with the abdominal-perineal resection is associated with an increased risk of the development of postoperative phlebitis. In order to prevent this problem from developing, the client will often receive subcutaneous injections of heparin, usually 5000 units every 12 hours both before and after surgery. Sequential pressure stockings or thigh high antiemboli hose also must be worn. The client also needs to perform leg exercises both before and after surgery. The nurse should monitor the client for the development of symptoms of thrombophlebitis, such as redness, swelling, or the presence of Homans' sign.

Nursing Diagnosis: Ineffective Individual Coping, High Risk for R/T disturbance in self-concept.

Planning: Expected Outcomes. The client will adjust to changes in body image, as evidenced by the client's ability to identify and use effective coping methods in dealing with disease and losses experienced.

Implementation. The nurse must provide emotional support while the client begins the process of adjusting to the colostomy. It is also important to provide extensive teaching regarding how to care for the colostomy.

A client's reactions to a new colostomy may range from apparently easy acceptance to total withdrawal from social contacts. How well clients adjust depends partly on their attitude toward excretory functions, previous knowledge about colostomies, and general ability to adjust to stressful situations.

Some clients refuse to look at the stoma and find it very difficult to accept its presence, whereas others begin to participate in stoma care almost immediately. The nurse's reactions and manner toward the client and the care required can affect the client's adjustment. For some clients, the colostomy represents a "cure"; whereas for others, it is merely palliation, as for those with extensive cancer.

Watson[113] has compared the phases of adjustment to an "ostomy" with the psychological phases experienced by a person in any crisis. The stages are (1) shock, (2) defensive retreat, (3) acknowledgment, and (4) adaptation. Watson points out that during the first two stages, clients need a great deal of support, a realistic appraisal of their situation, and encouragement to participate in their own care. Clients must reach the acknowledgment phase before they are able to achieve any real rehabilitative gains. Once clients begin to care for their stoma with a degree of success, they are moving toward the final or adaptive level.

The client's significant others also must adjust to the colostomy. Nurses help significant others by listening to their reactions and interpreting the client's problems to them.

Continuing sexual relationships are one major concern for clients with colostomies and their significant others. There is no physical reason the client cannot enjoy normal sexual relationships, although a small number of men become impotent after a radical perineal dissection. If this complication occurs, the physician may recommend a urology consultation to discuss treatment options for impotence. Psychological barriers may cause problems. With love, patience, understanding, and good hygienic practices, there should be no problem. However, it may take several months after surgery before a couple manage to reestablish a satisfactory sexual relationship.

Nursing Diagnosis: Knowledge Deficit R/T end colostomy care, irrigation, and possible complications associated with colostomies.

Planning: Expected Outcomes. The client will understand care of the end colostomy, as evidenced by the client's ability to apply the pouch; care for peristomal skin; irrigate colostomy, if applicable; and prevent or treat any associated problems.

Implementation. Carefully assess the client's physical condition and emotional and mental attitude toward the colostomy before attempting to teach ostomy self-care. Pace the teaching to the client's level of acceptance of the colostomy and ability to manage it.

The client should be taught how to apply the pouch to the stoma correctly. The client first should be taught to examine the stoma. A healthy stoma is red and slightly raised. The skin around the stoma should be clear, without evidence of irritation. The skin around the stoma should be cleaned well with a mild soap and water and dried well before the new pouch is applied. The skin should be treated with a skin barrier and the new pouch applied, cut about 1/16 to 1/8 inch larger than the stoma. The pouch should be changed about every 4 to 5 days or more often if leakage occurs. If it is changed after the bowel has evacuated, there will be less risk of spillage during the change.

The client also should be taught how to empty the pouch when it is about one-half full. The client should be shown how to clean out the pouch when emptying it. The client should demonstrate the ability to empty and change the pouch independently before discharge. See the section on ileostomy care for further information.

The client must regularly cleanse the skin around the stoma to prevent irritation. Excoriation due to the constant presence of moisture can usually be prevented or healed with a light dusting of karaya or other powder. Too much powder will prevent the pouch from sticking, however.

Clients with end colostomies can be taught to regulate the colostomy through regular irrigation. Clients who are physically, mentally, and emotionally capable should be encouraged to attempt irrigation and regulation, especially clients who had regular bowel habits before surgery and no other bowel disease. Although clients do not have to irrigate their colostomies, all clients who are able should be given the option of learning this technique. Some clients, in spite of irrigation, may never gain regularity. If they have not become regulated within 6 months, they probably will not.

Irrigation is taught in much the same way the nurse would teach clients to self-administer an enema. See the Client Education Guide. The best time for irrigation is when the client formerly had a daily bowel movement, because the bowel is already 'trained' to evacuate at this time.

Clients find that by irrigating the bowel daily or every other day, the bowel evacuates after the irrigation and then does not empty until it is irrigated again.

If there is difficulty inserting the catheter, let a little solution flow in and rotate the catheter. If it will not go in, teach the client to apply gloves or a finger cot, lubricate the finger, and gently pass it into the stoma. This method will often dislodge any feces that may be near the stoma. If the client cannot pass a catheter and no obstruction is felt digitally, the client should notify the physician.

If cramping occurs, stop the solution temporarily, take a few deep breaths, and restart the solution slowly.

Never use more than 1000 ml, irrigate more than once a day, or irrigate if diarrhea is present.

If there is no return after irrigation, the client should ambulate, gently massage the abdomen, and try drink-

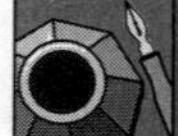

CLIENT EDUCATION GUIDE

Colostomy Irrigation

1. Assemble all the irrigation equipment and pouch, skin care products, and new colostomy pouch.
2. Remove and discard the old pouch.
3. Clean the peristomal skin.
4. Apply the irrigating sleeve and close off the distal end or place it into the toilet.
5. Using 500 to 1000 ml of warm tap water, suspend the solution container about 18 inches above the stoma, clear the air from the irrigation tubing, insert the lubricated catheter (water-soluble lubricant) 2 to 4 inches into the stoma (NEVER FORCE THE CATHETER), and allow the solution to flow gently into the colon.
6. Once all solution has been instilled, either allow the majority of the stool to pass into the toilet and then close off the pouch for another 30 to 45 minutes or simply close off the end of the pouch until the bowel evacuates.
7. Once the bowel has emptied, simply remove the sleeve, clean the stoma, and cover it with a small pouch or a gauze pad.

ing some warm water. If there is still no return, apply a pouch and try the irrigation again the next day. If there is no return, call the physician.

Diarrhea is a serious problem for clients with colostomies. Medications to slow the motility of the bowel should be prescribed by the physician. Two problems can result from diarrhea: (1) excoriation of skin from digestive juices that have not been reabsorbed and (2) electrolyte imbalance when the condition persists. Encourage the client to drink water, broth, and plain tea; no solid food should be ingested until bowel motility returns to normal.

When hard stools are present, the client has difficulty evacuating the bowel and irrigating the colostomy. Fecal impactions also can occur. Sometimes the physician prescribes a stool softener such as dioctyl sodium sulfosuccinate (Colace). The client also needs to reevaluate the diet and increase the amount of fruit, vegetables, fiber, and water if constipation persists.

Flatus is an embarrassing problem because client may have no control over its passage and no sensations to indicate when it is about to pass. The noise of the passage of gas can make clients avoid social situations. Clients can be taught how to muffle the passage of gas from their colostomies. Women may hold their purses or arms over the colostomy and men may hold their folded jackets or hats over the stoma to disguise the noise. Odor-proof pouches and those with charcoal filter discs are commonly available, but the most satisfactory way to control flatus is by proper diet. Because every client is different, clients have to learn by trial and error which foods cause gas. In general, nuts, cabbage, sauerkraut, broccoli, corn, cauliflower, and legumes are gas-forming foods. Swallowing air by eating too rapidly, chewing gum, or drinking carbonated beverages also cause intestinal gas.

Strictures of the stoma may occur after some surgeries because the rectus muscles of the abdominal wall tend to close over the artificial opening made through them. Some clients, especially those who do not irrigate, may be taught to dilate their stoma with a gloved, lubricated finger. This is usually not a problem in clients who irrigate because the irrigation nipple dilates the stoma.

EVALUATION

The nurse must evaluate client outcomes based on the established plan of care. If these goals were not achieved, the plan and interventions must be revised to meet the client's needs.

Post-hospital Care

Clients need support and knowledgeable advice as they learn to live with their colostomies. The enterostomal therapy nurse can help the client learn to manage and accept the ostomy, and to achieve a smooth transition from the health care facility to the home. Some cities have established ostomy rehabilitation clinics to help clients, and most large communities have an ostomy association that has contact with the American Cancer Society. These support groups are helpful because clients can share their ostomy concerns with others who have similar problems.

DISCHARGE TEACHING

After major bowel surgery, advise clients that it may be several weeks before they regain their strength. Also, tell them that when segments have been removed from the bowel, bowel habits may alter until the body adjusts to the situation. The nurse may need to teach the client and significant others how to change dressings at home, because wounds may not be healed totally by the time the client is discharged. In general, teaching should include

- How to change dressings correctly,
- Dietary or activity restrictions that the client must follow,
- Signs and symptoms of intestinal obstruction and perforation, and
- How to care for a colostomy, if applicable

HOME HEALTH CARE NEEDS

A home health care referral can add to the client's peace of mind, identify problems that might not otherwise be known, and ensure necessary follow-up care.

FOLLOW-UP CARE

Clients having problems with the colostomy should see an enterostomal therapy nurse. The client with an abdominal or perineal resection will need follow-up from the surgeon to ensure the perineal wound is healing properly.

▼ Other Disorders of the Large and Small Bowel

HERNIATIONS

Definition

A hernia is the abnormal protrusion of an organ, tissue, or part of an organ through the structure that normally contains it. Hernias most frequently occur in the abdominal cavity as a result of a congenital or acquired weakness of abdominal musculature.

Incidence

Hernias can occur at any age and in either sex. Indirect inguinal hernias are the most common type and typically occur in men. Direct hernias are found more commonly in older adults. Incisional or ventral hernias occur most often in clients who had poor wound healing after surgery. Obese or pregnant clients are more likely to develop umbilical hernias.

Etiology

Two factors must be present for a hernia to occur: (1) a defect in the integrity of the muscular wall and (2) increased intra-abdominal pressure.

Risk Factors

Congenital muscle weakness is one risk factor combined with the factors that increase intra-abdominal pressure. The muscle weakness cannot be prevented, but exercises can be performed to strengthen weak muscles. Because obesity is one cause of increased intra-abdominal pressure, it can be prevented by weight control. Avoiding heavy lifting and straining also reduces intra-abdominal pressure. Early diagnosis is important to prevent incarceration and strangulation.

Pathophysiology

Defects in the muscular wall may be congenital owing to weakened tissue or a wide space at the inguinal ligament, or may be caused by trauma. Intra-abdominal pressure most commonly increases as a result of pregnancy or obesity. Heavy lifting also causes increased pressure, as do coughing and traumatic injuries from blunt pressure. When two of these factors coexist, with some tissue weakness, the person may develop a hernia. Increased pressure without a weakness is not likely to cause a hernia. Weakness, in addition to being present from birth, is acquired as part of the aging process. As clients age, muscular tissues become infiltrated and are replaced by adipose and connective tissues.

When the contents of the hernia sac can be replaced into the abdominal cavity by manipulation, the hernia is said to be reducible. Irreducible and incarcerated are terms that refer to a hernia that cannot be reduced or replaced by manipulation. When pressure from the hernia ring (the ring of muscular tissue through which the bowel protrudes) cuts off the blood supply to the herniated segment of bowel, the bowel becomes strangulated. Incarcerated hernias usually become strangulated. This situation is a surgical emergency because unless the bowel is released, it soon becomes gangrenous owing to a lack of blood supply.

Hernias may penetrate through any defect in the abdominal wall, through the diaphragm, or through some internal structure within the abdominal cavity (Fig. 55–10). For this discussion, only the more common types of hernias are covered. The most common hernias are the inguinal (both indirect and direct), femoral, umbilical, and incisional. (Hiatal hernia was discussed in Chap. 53.)

INDIRECT INGUINAL HERNIA

This herniation occurs through the inguinal ring and follows the spermatic cord through the inguinal canal. It is more common in males than in females because of the space allowed for the testicles to descend. There is a high incidence of these hernias among infants and young persons. The incidence increases again among clients in their 50s, and then the incidence gradually decreases. These hernias can become extremely large and often descend into the scrotum.

DIRECT INGUINAL HERNIA

This hernia passes through the abdominal wall in an area of muscular weakness, not through a canal as do indirect inguinal and femoral hernias. It is more common in the elderly. Direct inguinal hernias gradually develop in an area that is weak because of congenital deficiency in the number of fibers it contains.

FEMORAL HERNIA

A femoral hernia occurs through the femoral ring and is more common in females than in males. It begins as a plug of fat in the femoral canal that enlarges and gradually pulls the peritoneum, and almost inevitably

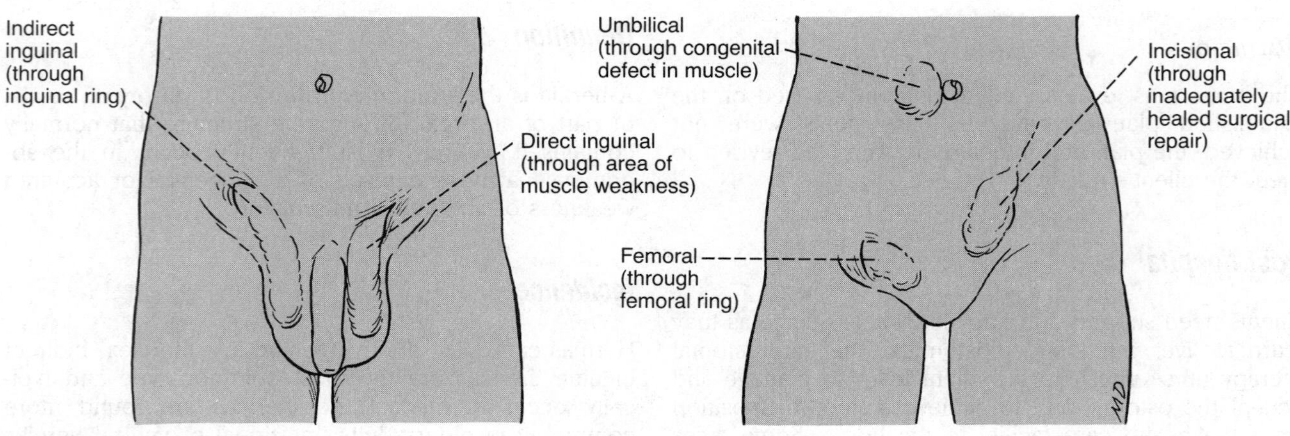

▲ **Figure 55–10**

Common types of herniation.

the urinary bladder, into the sac. There is a high incidence of incarceration and strangulation with this type of hernia.

UMBILICAL HERNIA

Umbilical herniation in the adult is more common in women and is due to increased abdominal pressure. It usually occurs in obese clients and in multiparous women.

INCISIONAL OR VENTRAL HERNIA

This type of hernia occurs at the site of a previous surgical incision that has healed inadequately because of postoperative problems such as infection, inadequate nutrition, extreme distention, or obesity.

Medical Management

Hernias that are not strangulated or incarcerated can be mechanically reduced. A truss also can be used to keep the hernia reduced. A truss is a firm pad held in place by a belt. The pad is placed over the hernia after it has been reduced and left in place to prevent the hernia from recurring. The client is taught to apply the truss daily before arising. The client should carefully inspect the skin under the truss for any sign of breakdown.

Surgical Management

A hernia repair is performed using a small incision directly over the weakened area. The intestine is then returned to the perineal cavity, the hernia sac excised, and the muscle closed tightly over the area. Hernias in the inguinal region are usually repaired under a spinal or local anesthetic. Many hernia repairs are now performed as outpatient procedures.

Some repairs are difficult because there is insufficient muscle mass to keep the intestines in place. In this case, mesh grafts are used to reinforce the area of herniation. Clients with difficult repairs are usually hospitalized for 1 to 2 days to receive prophylactic antibiotics.

Nursing Management

The nurse should make certain the client voids after surgery, because urinary retention is a common problem, especially in male clients. Return the client to a general diet as soon as the client tolerates food. When general anesthesia is used, postoperative progress is slower. Assure the client that during the immediate postoperative period the hernia will not recur. Some clients hesitate to become active because of this fear. Obese patients progress slower, heal more slowly, and may need more encouragement to participate in postoperative activities.

Following an inguinal hernia repair, an ice pack is usually applied to the incisional area to control pain and decrease swelling. In male clients, the scrotal area should be carefully assessed for swelling. An ice pack also can be applied to the scrotal area. To decrease scrotal swelling, the scrotum should be elevated and a scrotal support worn when the client is up.

The client should be told not to engage in heavy lifting from 4 to 6 weeks after surgery.

DIVERTICULAR DISEASE

Definition

Diverticular disease is the term used to describe diverticulosis and diverticulitis. Diverticulosis refers to the presence of noninflamed outpouchings of the intestine. Diverticulitis is inflammation of a diverticulum. A diverticulum is a blind outpouching or herniation of intestinal mucosa through the muscular coat of the large intestine, usually the sigmoid colon.

Incidence

Diverticular disease is common in men and women over 45 years of age and in the obese. It is present in approximately one third of the population over age 60 years. It is more common in the United States, the United Kingdom, Australia, and France.

Etiology

Lower-fiber diets have been implicated in the development of diverticula, because these diets decrease the bulk in the stool and predispose the person to the development of constipation. In the presence of muscle weakness in the bowel, this increase in intraluminal pressure can lead to the formation of diverticula.

The causes of diverticulosis include atrophy or weakness of the bowel muscle, increased intraluminal pressure, obesity, and chronic constipation.

Diverticulitis occurs when undigested food blocks the diverticulum, leading to a decrease in the blood supply to the area and predisposing the bowel to invasion of bacteria into the diverticulum.

Risk Factors

The highest risk factor for the development of diverticulum is chronic constipation. A low-fiber diet is one of the leading causes of chronic constipation. The major risk factor for the development of diverticulitis is the ingestion of indigestible roughage, such as corn, popcorn, and tomatoes or cucumbers with seeds, in clients with diverticulosis because these foods can block the opening of the diverticulum and trigger inflammation.

The best way to prevent diverticulosis is to maintain adequate bowel habits by consuming a high-fiber diet that helps prevent constipation. Once the condition has developed, avoiding indigestible bulk may help prevent inflammation of the diverticula.

Pathophysiology

Diverticula have narrow, flasklike necks, which communicate with the bowel lumen. Weak points in the bowel muscularis exist where branches of the blood vessels penetrate the colonic wall. These weak points create areas for bowel protrusion when there is increased intraluminal pressure.

Diverticula frequently develop in the sigmoid colon because of the high pressures in this area required to move the stool into the rectum.

Diverticulitis may be acute or chronic. If the diverticulum is not infected (diverticulosis), these lesions cause few problems. However, when fecaliths do not liquefy and drain from the diverticulum, they may become trapped and cause irritation and inflammation (diverticulitis).

The inflamed area becomes congested with blood and may bleed. Diverticulitis can lead to perforation when the trapped mass in the diverticula erodes the bowel wall. Chronic diverticulitis can result in increased scarring and, eventually, narrowing of the bowel lumen, potentially leading to obstruction.

Clinical Manifestations

Symptoms produced by diverticulitis depend on the extent of the inflammation and the site of occurrence. Discomfort includes episodic, dull, or steady left-quadrant or midabdominal pain. Assessment also reveals alteration in bowel habits (constipation, diarrhea, or both), increased flatus, anorexia, and low-grade fever. The inflammatory process usually subsides within several weeks. If the infection penetrates the pelvic floor or retroperitoneal tissues, abscesses may result. Extension of the inflammation to adjacent organs can lead to fistulas of the bladder or vagina and peritonitis. Repeated inflammation can result in narrowing of the bowel and obstruction.

Rectal bleeding occurs in about 15 per cent of clients. Stools also may contain mucus. Urinary frequency can occur if the inflammation is in the proximity of the bladder. Straining, coughing, or lifting causes an increase in intra-abdominal pressure and symptoms. The clinician may palpate a tender mass on digital and rectal examinations.

Medical Management

Asymptomatic diverticular disease requires no specific therapy other than modification of the client's diet. Mild disease can be treated by (1) adherence to a high-fiber diet and (2) prevention of constipation with bran and bulk laxatives (hydrophilic colloids). Advise clients to notify the physician of any change in bowel movement pattern (constipation or diarrhea) or character (presence of mucus or blood), or if fever, abdominal pain, or urinary symptoms develop.

Diverticulitis may be treated conservatively with medical intervention by allowing the colon to rest. Clients with acute diverticulitis are not permitted anything by mouth, may have an NG tube, and receive parenteral fluids until pain, inflammation, and temperature decreases. When the acute episode begins to subside, they can ingest oral liquids and, later, a progressively more inclusive diet.

Intervention also aims to control inflammation. Administer prescribed antibiotics and advise the client to (1) avoid activities that increase intra-abdominal pressure, such as bending, lifting, stooping, coughing, or vomiting; (2) drink at least eight glasses of water every day, and (3) reduce weight if client is obese.

Surgical Management

Surgery is indicated for clients who develop complications, such as hemorrhage, obstruction, abscesses, or perforation. Surgical procedures usually include ligation and removal of the sac or resection of involved bowel if there are complications. With abscess or obstruction, the surgeon performs a colon resection with a temporary colostomy, which is left in place until the client's condition improves. For some clients, the temporary colostomy alone allows the bowel to rest and heal. For further information on the care of these clients see the section on colon resections.

MECKEL'S DIVERTICULUM

Meckel's diverticulum is an outpouching of the bowel, a vestige of embryonic development found on the ileum within 10 cm of the cecum. The pouch may be lined with gastric mucosa or may contain pancreatic tissue. The gastric mucosal lining sometimes ulcerates and bleeds or perforates. In addition, the diverticulum may become inflamed and mimic appendicitis. Meckel's diverticulum is sometimes attached to the umbilicus by a fibrous band and may be the focus around which the bowel twists, causing obstruction. Treatment involves surgical excision of the diverticulum.

OBSTRUCTION

Definition

Partial or complete impairment of the forward flow of intestinal contents is known as an intestinal obstruction. Most obstructions occur in the small bowel, especially in the ileum, the narrowest segment. Obstructions of the small intestine are a common surgical emergency. Obstruction produces nausea, vomiting, dehydration, and severe pain. Intestinal obstruction has a high mortality rate if it is not diagnosed and treated within 24 hours.[30]

Incidence

The incidence of obstruction depends on its cause.

Etiology

Obstruction of the small intestine may be caused by narrowing of the intestinal lumen due to inflammation, neoplasms, adhesions, hernia, volvulus, intussusception, food blockage, or compression from outside the intestine. Paralytic ileus, vascular problems such as mesenteric embolus or thrombus, or hypokalemia from diuretics or antihypertensive agents also may result in small bowel obstructions. Infections of the abdomen and sometimes of the thoracic cavity, such as lobar pneumonia, peritonitis, or pancreatitis, frequently produce an ileus of infectious origin.

Cancer accounts for approximately 80 per cent of obstructions of the large intestine, with most occurring in the sigmoid colon. Other causes include diverticulitis and ulcerative colitis. For instance, factors causing intestinal obstructions may be (1) mechanical, (2) neurogenic, and (3) vascular.

Risk Factors

MECHANICAL FACTORS

Adhesions. Adhesions are probably the most common cause of obstruction in the small and large intestines combined. Adhesions form after abdominal surgery, and for unknown reasons some clients develop massive adhesions. Irritants that remain in the abdomen following surgical procedures enhance the formation of adhesions. These fibrous bands of scar tissue can become looped over a portion of the bowel. These loops can then become either (1) the focus around which the bowel can twist (volvulus) (Fig. 55-11) or (2) the band that mechanically obstructs the bowel by external pressure. The presence of multiple adhesions increases the risk of obstruction.

Hernia. An incarcerated hernia may or may not cause obstruction, depending on the size of the hernia ring. However, the potential for obstruction is always present in any hernia. A strangulated hernia is always obstructed, because the bowel cannot function when its own blood supply is cut off.

Volvulus. Volvulus is a twisting of the bowel that frequently occurs about a stationary focus (e.g., tumor or Meckel's diverticulum) in the abdominal cavity (see Fig. 55-11). It can cause infarction of the bowel and can occur in either the large or small bowel. Volvulus can sometimes be corrected without surgical intervention. Successful decompression of the bowel with a long

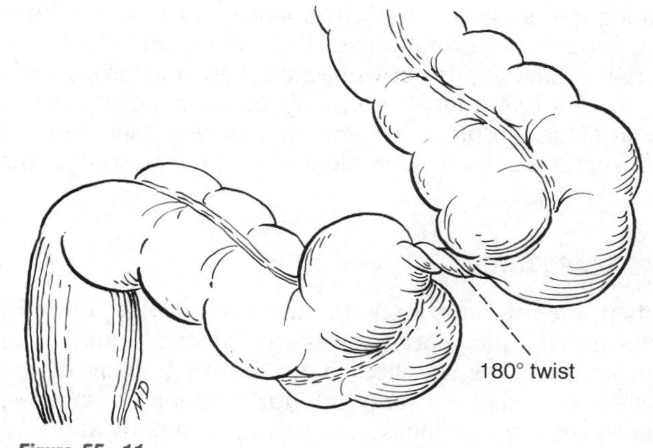

▲ *Figure 55-11*

Volvulus. Intestine twists at least 180 degrees, causing obstruction and ischemia.

tube releases pressure against the proximal end of the loop, thus allowing a small bowel volvulus to relax.

Intussusception. Intussusception, that sometimes complicates IBD, is a telescoping of the bowel on itself (Fig. 55-12). The condition is often associated with tumor of the large bowel. Peristaltic action telescopes the proximal bowel into the bowel distal to it. Intramural lesions often cause intussusception.

Tumors. In the large bowel, tumors are the chief cause of obstruction. The process develops slowly and, because of the large lumen of the bowel, may become advanced before a fecal mass lodges at the constricted site and precipitates an acute obstructive process. In the small bowel, obstructive symptoms are frequently the first sign of a tumor. Even though the lumen of the small bowel is smaller, manifestations still do not occur early in the process because the intestinal contents are liquid.

NEUROGENIC FACTORS

An adynamic (or functional) obstruction, sometimes called a "paralytic ileus," is caused by a lack of peristaltic activity. Paralytic ileus commonly occurs after

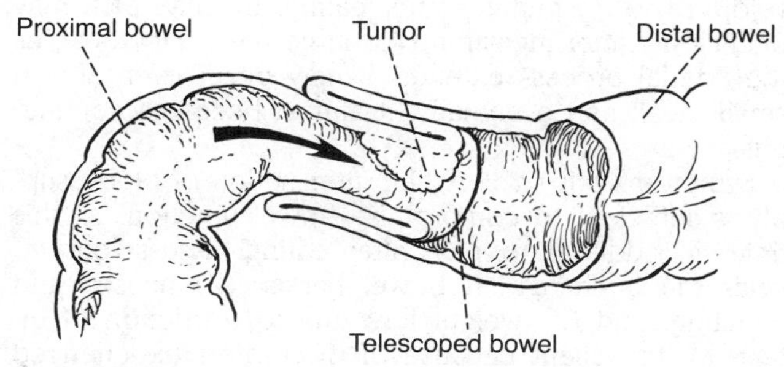

▲ *Figure 55-12*

Intussusception. Portion of bowel telescopes into adjacent (usually distal) bowel.

abdominal surgery. The bowel ceases to function for a few hours to several days. Procedures in which the surgeon handles the bowel extensively and procedures in the retroperitoneal area may cause a postoperative neurogenic problem. Treatment involves aspiration of the secretions by gastric suction until the bowel begins to function.

VASCULAR FACTORS

When the blood supply to any part of the body is interrupted, the part ceases to function and pain occurs. Blood is supplied to the bowel by way of the celiac and superior and inferior mesenteric arteries. These vessels have anastomotic intercommunications at the head of the pancreas and along the transverse bowel. Obstruction of blood flow can arise as a result of (1) complete occlusion (mesenteric infarction) or (2) partial occlusion (abdominal angina).

Complete Occlusion (Mesenteric Infarction). Any occlusion of arterial blood supply to the bowel, as in mesenteric thrombosis, effectively stops bowel function. The usual cause is an embolus. The extent of the resulting symptoms is determined by (1) the size of the vessel that is occluded, (2) the length of bowel that is without a supply of blood, and (3) the rapidity with which the occlusion occurs.

An acute occlusion, at its onset, causes intense abdominal pain, usually without any signs of advanced intestinal obstruction. This is because the pain results from ischemic tissue rather than from obstruction. As the process advances, fever, leukocytosis, shock, and other symptoms of bowel gangrene develop. Acute mesenteric obstruction constitutes a surgical emergency and carries a high mortality rate (approximately 75 per cent).

Surgical intervention must be initiated early. Sometimes, an embolectomy can restore circulation. The surgeon also must resect necrotic segments of the bowel.

Partial Occlusion (Abdominal Angina). This condition usually results from atherosclerosis of the mesenteric arteries. It is a common although often asymptomatic problem. It is found in 33 per cent of routine autopsies. Because there is an increased need for oxygenation during the digestive process, pain may develop 15 to 30 minutes after eating. Initially, pain may occur only after ingestion of a large meal. However, as the arterial process extends, it may occur even after a small meal, and eventually, it almost becomes continuous.

Symptoms arise only when interruption of blood supply is sufficient to compromise bowel function. At this time, in addition to pain after eating, assessment reveals (1) a change in bowel habits, (2) nausea and vomiting, and (3) weight loss due to restriction of intake by the client because of discomfort experienced when eating. Vascular or bypass grafts can sometimes improve the blood supply to the affected portion of the bowel.

Pathophysiology

Normally, 7 to 8 liters of electrolyte-rich fluid are secreted by the bowel, and most of it is reabsorbed. When the bowel is obstructed, this fluid is partially retained within the bowel and partially eliminated by vomiting, causing severe reduction in circulating blood volume, resulting in hypotension, hypovolemic shock, and diminished renal and cerebral blood flow. Because fluid is lost but blood cells are not, the hematocrit and hemoglobin increase, thus increasing the potential for vascular occlusive disorders such as coronary, cerebral, and mesenteric thrombosis.

For instance, with the onset of an instruction, fluids and air collect proximal to the site of the problem, causing distention. Manifestations occur sooner and are more intense in a small bowel blockage because the small bowel is narrower and normally more active. The large volume of secretions from the small bowel adds to the distention. The only significant secretion from the large bowel is mucus.

Distention causes a temporary increase in peristalsis as the bowel attempts to force the material through the obstructed area. Within a few hours, the increased peristalsis ends and the bowel becomes flaccid, thus decreasing pressure within the lumen and slowing the process caused by the obstruction. Increased pressure within the bowel reduces its absorptive ability, which increases the fluid retention still further. Soon the intraluminal pressure reduces venous return, which increases venous pressure, congestion, and vessel fragility. This process, in turn, raises the capillary permeability and allows plasma to extravasate into the bowel lumen and into the peritoneal cavity. The bowel wall becomes permeable to bacteria, and bowel organisms enter the peritoneal cavity. Increasing pressure in the bowel wall soon slows arterial blood flow, causing necrosis and, in some cases, toxemia and peritonitis.

Strangulation of the bowel results in decreased arterial blood supply. Necrosis and perforation may force intestinal contents into the peritoneal cavity, causing peritonitis. Bacteria proliferate in the strangulated bowel and may form an endotoxin. When the endotoxin is released into the peritoneal cavity or systemic circulation, there is rapid circulatory collapse with endotoxic shock, accounting for the high mortality rate associated with this condition. These complications are especially likely to occur in elderly persons, who tend to have atherosclerotic narrowing of these vessels, making thrombosis more likely.

Clinical Manifestations

Manifestations of intestinal obstruction depend on (1) the level and length of bowel involved, (2) the degree to which the obstruction interferes with blood supply, (3) the completeness of the obstruction, and (4) the type of lesion producing the obstruction.

Intestinal obstruction affects the bowel at local and systemic levels. Local changes in the bowel wall include congestion, fragility, decreased circulation, and increased pressure. Increased pressure leads to reverse peristalsis, producing vomiting that helps prevent overdistention of the bowel. These local effects result from (1) loss of fluids, electrolytes, and plasma; (2) bacterial proliferation; and (3) perforation. Systemic effects include decreased extracellular fluid and circulating blood volume, toxemia, and peritonitis.

The client with small bowel obstruction typically experiences abdominal pain in rhythmically recurring waves. The pain results from distention and the small intestine's peristaltic efforts to push its contents past the obstruction. Small intestine pain is felt in the upper and midabdomen, whereas colonic pain is experienced in the lower abdomen. Soon after the small intestine becomes distended, the nurse can see the peristaltic waves and hear accompanying high-pitched tinkling sounds. The client usually becomes nauseated and vomits, which brings some relief from the pain, provided the obstruction is high or proximal to the ileum.

If the obstruction lies below the ileum, vomiting fails to empty the bowel completely, allowing the accumulation of fluids, residue, and gases. As the muscles become atonic, loops of the small bowel dilate, compounding the problem of distention. Eventually, severe distention may raise the diaphragm, thereby inhibiting respirations. Hypoxia (due to inadequate respirations and decreased circulating blood volume and hypotension) often develops. Vomiting is more severe if the obstruction is located high in the small bowel. At first, vomitus is composed of semidigested food and chyme and, later, becomes watery and contains bile. Finally, the client vomits dark fecal material owing to bacterial growth in the fluid that has stagnated in the obstructed bowel.

When the colon is obstructed, the competent ileocecal valve prevents regurgitation and the pressure within the lumen increases, resulting in distention. In some cases, the cecum may perforate. Obstruction of the colon results in altered bowel habits, lower abdominal pain, a desire to defecate, distention, and borborygmi. Vomiting is not a common symptom because of the competent ileocecal valve. In the presence of an incompetent ileocecal valve, distention progresses to the small intestine. Vomiting that accompanies large intestine obstruction is a very late symptom, and occurs only secondarily to a distended small intestine.

Clients with vomiting may experience severe fluid and electrolyte imbalances. They lose not only water but also sodium, chloride, potassium, and bicarbonate. The result is an acute extracellular volume deficit (dehydration), which, in turn, decreases the circulating blood volume. Hydrogen ion imbalances frequently occur in intestinal obstructions, with metabolic acidosis being the most common problem.

DIAGNOSTIC ASSESSMENT

Specific diagnostic tests include flat plate x-ray studies, which will show gas shadows; barium or radiopaque x-ray studies; and complete blood studies. Increased hemoglobin and hematocrit values may indicate dehydration. Leukocytosis may point to a strangulated bowel. A decrease in sodium, potassium, and chloride levels and a rise in the nonprotein nitrogen and BUN levels may indicate small bowel obstruction.[30]

Medical Management

The major treatment for an intestinal obstruction is the insertion of an intestinal tube (see the section on intestinal tubes). Often, an intestinal tube both decompresses the bowel and breaks up the obstruction.

In adynamic ileus, the best intervention is rest and prevention of distention by gastric suction. Medications are not effective in stimulating bowel activity. The bowel will respond when it completely recovers from the effects of obstruction.

Surgical Management

If intestinal intubation does not relieve the obstruction, surgery is the only remaining option. The major objective in treating bowel obstruction is to relieve the cause and thus eliminate the problem. However, the cause is not always immediately obvious. Diagnosis of the cause of the acute abdominal condition may be difficult and must frequently be made during surgery. The nurse needs to document specific observations to aid the physician in the diagnosis.

In the majority of vascular and mechanically caused obstructions, surgical excision of the cause is the only intervention. Surgery relieves the obstruction and removes any ischemic bowel. Relieving the obstruction should reestablish bowel patency. The type of surgery depends on the location and type of obstruction. The surgeon may reform bowel resection, colostomy, or a bypass procedure.

Nursing Management

ASSESSMENT

The nurse should obtain a complete history of the onset of symptoms, eating patterns, food tolerance, vomiting episodes, stools (number per day and appearance), and distention.

During physical assessment, note the following:

- Abdominal distention,
- The quality of bowel sounds,
- The presence and extent of dehydration, and
- Muscle guarding or signs of abdominal pain.

A lack of bowel sounds indicates peritoneal irritation or adynamic ileus. Usually, in the case of bowel obstruction, auscultation reveals high-pitched peristaltic rushes with high, metallic tinkling sounds.

NURSING INTERVENTION

Nursing Diagnosis: Fluid Volume Deficit R/T vomiting, decreased intestinal reabsorption of fluid, and decreased intestinal secretions.

Planning: Expected Outcome. The client will maintain fluid balance, as evidenced by balanced intake and output, no signs of dehydration, and blood pressure within the client's normal range.

Implementation. The nurse must maintain good fluid balance in the client with an obstruction by carefully replacing fluids and electrolytes. The nurse administers parenteral fluids with sodium chloride, bicarbonate, and potassium added as ordered.

Maintain an intestinal tube attached to suction to relieve the vomiting and distention (see the section on care of a client with intestinal tubes). If the obstruction is not mechanical, an intestinal tube can achieve decompression. If the obstruction is due to adhesions, hernia, or tumors, the tube stops at the point of obstruction and keeps the bowel decompressed above the obstruction.

Note the progress of an intestinal tube, the amount and type of drainage, and relief of distention and nausea. Assess and measure emesis and drainage from the intestinal tube. Document color, odor, consistency, and volume. Inform the physician about blood levels of sodium, potassium, and bicarbonate, and the pH of the blood, all reflecting fluid and electrolyte balance.

Nursing Diagnosis: Altered Gastrointestinal Tissue Perfusion, High Risk for R/T intestinal obstruction.

Planning: Expected Outcomes. The client will not develop an alteration in tissue perfusion to the bowel, as evidenced by the return of normal peristalsis and usual bowel elimination.

Implementation. The client will have the intestinal tube inserted to help relieve the obstruction. The nurse must recognize and immediately report to the physician symptoms such as emesis, increasing distention and pain, and temperature elevation, all of which are signs of bowel strangulation.

If the blood supply becomes impaired, the client will require emergency surgery. The nurse must prepare the client for this procedure. Antibiotics are often given before surgery. The nurse must be careful about administering narcotics, because these medications may mask symptoms of increasing obstruction or impaired blood flow.

The client with a bowel obstruction with impaired tissue perfusion requires an emergency bowel resection. (See the section on care of a client after a bowel resection with or without a colostomy.)

EVALUATION

The nurse must evaluate client outcomes based on the established plan of care. If these goals were not achieved, the plan and interventions must be revised to meet the client's needs.

Post-hospital Care

DISCHARGE TEACHING

The learning needs of the client depend on the resolution of the obstruction. If the obstruction was relieved without surgery, the client needs to learn ways to prevent recurrence and maintain bowel elimination. The client needs to maintain an adequate nutritional intake so lost weight can be regained.

If the client had surgery, the learning needs vary based on the surgical procedure performed. The client with a temporary colostomy needs to learn to care for the colostomy. Without a colostomy, the client's learning needs are the same as for any client after a bowel resection.

FOLLOW-UP CARE

The client needs to be seen at intervals after the obstruction is relieved to ensure that it has not recurred. The client's nutritional status also should be monitored to ensure that adequate nutrition is maintained.

IRRITABLE BOWEL SYNDROME

Definition

Irritable bowel syndrome (IBS) is a functional disorder of motility in the small and large intestines. It develops without organic disease or anatomic abnormality. Other descriptive names for this condition are spastic colon, irritable colon, nervous indigestion, functional dyspepsia, pylorospasm, spastic colitis, intestinal neuroses, and laxative or cathartic 'colitis.'

Incidence

IBS is the most common gastrointestinal disorder in Western society, accounting for 50 per cent of subspecialty referrals. It is more common in women than men and occurs during middle age.[122]

Etiology

Several factors appear to be involved in the pathogenesis of IBS:

- Prediverticular disease characterized by increased width of the sigmoid circular muscles, increased segmentation, and nonpropulsive intraluminal pressures;
- Psychological stress;
- A low-residue diet; and
- Lactose intolerance.

Risk Factors

Risk factors associated with IBS include diets high in rich foods such as creams and fats. Other foods such as fresh fruits also seem to trigger the diarrhea. Gas-producing foods such as carbonated beverages and beans cause severe bloating. Alcohol and smoking, both gastric stimulants, increase gastric stimulation, and increase the diarrhea.

Stress is another factor that increases the incidence of IBS. Alterations in sleep and rest may precipitate the problem.

Prevention primarily centers around diet modification. A well-balanced diet that avoids the problematic foods is best. Once the client has identified that a certain food is stimulating the condition, that food should be avoided. Stress reduction is also helpful in preventing attacks of the disease.

Pathophysiology

IBS appears to be a disorder of GI motility; this motility may be altered by any number of factors, including diet and emotions. The alteration in the motility can cause diarrhea, constipation, or alternating diarrhea and constipation. The structure of the bowel mucosa is not altered, although the disease continues whenever the client is exposed to the causative agents. The causative agents vary among clients; however, most clients can clearly identify their agents.

Clinical Manifestations

The client with IBS is usually found to have some combination of the following symptoms: abdominal pain, altered bowel function, constipation or diarrhea, hypersecretion of colonic mucus, dyspeptic symptoms (flatulence, nausea, anorexia), and some degree of anxiety or depression. Symptoms vary in intensity. Roughage, fruits, alcohol, and fatigue aggravate or precipitate symptoms.

Emotional disturbances affect the autonomic nervous system (ANS) and its innervation of the bowel. Disturbances of ANS function probably alter motor activity and transit time. Symptoms may mimic various organic and systemic diseases. Pain may be steady or intermittent, and there may be a dull deep discomfort with sharp cramps in the morning or after eating. The typical pattern consists of lower left quadrant abdominal pain, constipation, and diarrhea. There may be tenderness over the sigmoid area.

Diarrhea tends to be the major problem but not usually at night. Nocturnal diarrhea tends to be associated with organic disease of the bowel. Examination of the stool reveals mucus but not blood. Eating may aggravate pain and defecation, and passing flatus or stool may provide temporary relief. Spastic contractions sometimes occur with stools that are small, dry, hard, and pellet-like. Other symptoms include abdominal disturbances such as nausea, distention, dyspepsia, eructation (belching), and borborygmus due to aerophagia and decreased gas motility. Anorexia, foul breath, sour stomach, flatulence, and cramps also may be present. Associated behavioral disturbances are anxiety, tension, nervousness, depression, sleep disturbances, weakness, or difficulty concentrating.

DIAGNOSTIC ASSESSMENT

Because there are no confirmatory diagnostic tests or histologic features for IBS, diagnosis generally is made by excluding other diseases. Diagnostic techniques, therefore, must eliminate the possibility that the client has organic GI disease.

Clients over age 50 suspected of having IBS must be carefully evaluated to rule out malignancy or other diverticular disease. When functional bowel disease develops, the client usually gives a history of nervousness and emotional disturbances. The client also may be conscious of the bowel and frequently use cathartics and enemas. Palpation may demonstrate abdominal tenderness, particularly along the course of the colon.

Sigmoidoscopy or colonoscopy may reveal spasm and mucus in the colonic lumen. A barium enema is usually performed. A complete blood count and stool examination is needed to rule out the presence of occult blood, ova, parasites, and pathogenic bacteria.

Medical Management

Treatment is palliative and supportive. Advise the client to limit responsibilities, seek rest, and adopt measures to decrease stress. The client can control symptoms through diet, medication, and regular physical activity. The client must continue with routine follow-up assessment and care.

PHARMACOLOGIC MANAGEMENT

Sedative and antispasmodic medications may help the client feel more relaxed. Taking vegetable mucilages such as psyllium hydrophilic mucilloid (Metamucil) can increase stool bulk.

DIETARY MANAGEMENT

Increased fiber in the diet helps control IBS through the production of bulkier stools and reduction of tension in the walls of the sigmoid colon. Fiber helps manage both constipation and diarrhea. In constipation, the softer, bulkier, and heavier stools produced by dietary fiber tend to decrease transit time. In diarrhea, the fiber diet helps absorb water, giving form to the stool and increasing transit time.

Sources of fiber include unprocessed Miller's bran, packaged bran cereals, whole wheat, and fresh vegetables. Clients should drink six to eight glasses of water daily, because increased water helps regulate stool consistency and frequency. If diarrhea is a problem, the client needs to avoid foods that may cause diarrhea, such as cold drinks, and drink liquids between meals rather than at mealtime.

Nursing Management

The nurse should reinforce the physician's explanation of the nature of the disorder, the intervention plan, and the prognosis. Make it clear to the client that the bowel responds to stress, foods, and medications. Stress the importance of regular hours, nourishing meals, and adequate sleep, exercise, and recreation. The nurse should help the client reestablish a regular bowel routine.

The nurse should reinforce diet teaching to the client. Advise the client with diarrhea to (1) limit foods that are normally gas producing or irritating; (2) avoid caffeinated beverages, alcohol, and foods containing nondigestible carbohydrates, such as beans; and (3) exclude milk and milk products.

ACQUIRED MEGACOLON

Acquired megacolon is a dilation of the colon above an area of obstruction. It may be secondary to any cause of severe constipation or obstruction (functional cause, rectal disease). In acquired megacolon, clients usually are incontinent of stool. Acquired megacolon usually occurs in the very young or very old. The treatment for acquired megacolon involves a retraining of bowel habits, behavior modification, removing impactions by using enemas or laxatives, and relief of any obstructions.

▼ DISORDERS OF THE ANORECTAL AREA

The major function of the rectum is to store feces until evacuation. When feces enter the rectum, peristalsis occurs. Many disorders in the rectal area result from constipation or failure to empty the rectum when peristalsis occurs.

At the mucocutaneous border of the anal canal, the mucous membrane changes to skin that has cutaneous somatic nerve endings. Because of this anatomic structure, lesions of the external anal canal are very painful. The two most common symptoms are bleeding and pain. Drainage of mucus and fecal matter and irritation of the skin from organisms can cause intense itching.

Hemorrhoids and skin tags may protrude from the anal opening, and there may be drainage of pus from abscesses. Bright red blood per rectum usually indicates a lesion of the left colon or anorectal region. Blood on the toilet paper alone usually indicates perianal disease, whereas blood on the surface of a formed stool may suggest a polyp or carcinoma of the left colon or rectum. Blood mixed with the stool suggests inflammatory bowel disease or carcinoma of the proximal colon. Blood in the toilet bowl after the passage of formed stool suggests hemorrhoidal bleeding. All rectal bleeding must be evaluated by a physician.

Hemorrhoids are the most common source of bright red blood in the stool. Carcinoma is the most serious source. Clinical features of rectal carcinoma often mimic those of hemorrhoids (sense of incomplete evacuation, stool caliber changes, and tenesmus). Carcinoma is suspected if there has been a change in bowel habits, loss of weight, or both.

HEMORRHOIDS

Definition

Hemorrhoids are perianal varicose veins. Hemorrhoids may be internal or external (Fig. 55–13). Internal hemorrhoids are varicosities of the superior hemorrhoidal plexus occurring above the mucocutaneous border (pectinate line) and are covered by mucous membrane and are innervated by the autonomic nervous system.

External hemorrhoids are dilatations of the inferior hemorrhoidal plexus that lie below the mucocutaneous junction and are covered by anal skin. As these vessels dilate, they stretch the overlying mucous membrane and skin and eventually protrude down the anal canal. This bulging plexus may be traumatized or pushed outside the anus by the passage of hard stool. Anal fissures are sometimes mistaken for hemorrhoids.

Incidence

Hemorrhoids are a common disorder, affecting both men and women of any age, but the incidence is increased in clients between 20 to 50 years of age. Enlargement of hemorrhoids is caused by increased intra-abdominal pressure. Pregnancy, congestive heart failure, prolonged sitting or standing, and cirrhosis with portal hypertension also increase the incidence of hemorrhoids.

Etiology

Both internal and external hemorrhoids may result from: (a) the many anastomoses between the plexuses and (b) the lack of valves in the veins of the superior hemorrhoidal plexus, which leads into the portal vein. Internal hemorrhoids are frequently caused by portal hypertension. Several causes contribute to acute enlargement of hemorrhoids, including constipation, diarrhea, and prolonged straining. Congestive heart failure also can cause hemorrhoids.

Risk Factors

Any condition that increases the constipation, intra-abdominal pressure, and hemorrhoidal venous pressure increases the risk of the development of hemorrhoids. Prevention of constipation through increased roughage in the diet is an excellent measure to decrease the risk of hemorrhoid development.

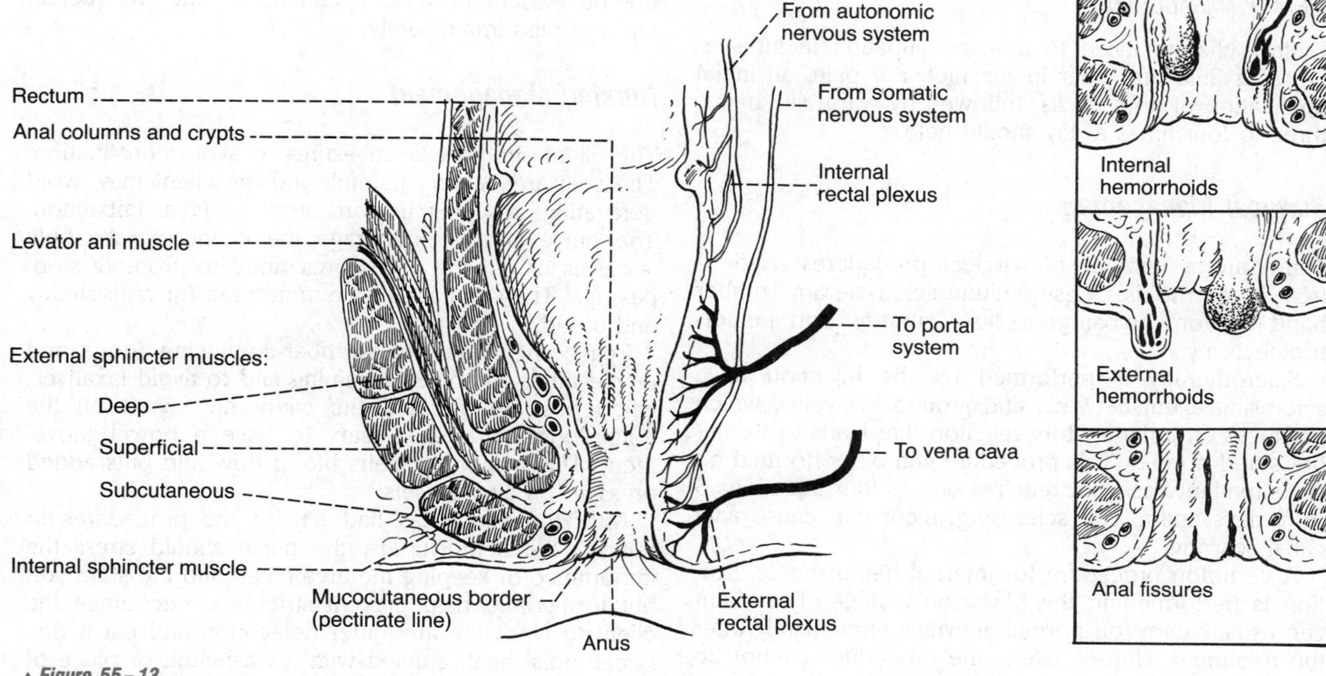

▲ *Figure 55–13*

Structure of the anus and common disorders: internal hemorrhoids, external hemorrhoids, anal fissures.

Pathophysiology

Straining during a bowel movement increases intra-abdominal and hemorrhoidal venous pressures, leading to distention of the hemorrhoidal veins. When the rectal ampulla is filled with formed stool, venous obstruction is believed to occur. As a result of the repeated and prolonged increase in this pressure and the obstruction, permanent dilation of the hemorrhoidal veins occurs. As a result of the distention, thrombosis and bleeding also may occur.

Clinical Manifestations

The major symptom of external hemorrhoids is an enlarged mass at the anus. Internal hemorrhoids are characterized by bleeding and prolapse. Other symptoms include rectal itching and constipation. Pain may be present if there is associated thrombosis. The blood is bright red and may be seen in the stool or on the toilet tissue. A prolapse may occur in severe cases after exercise or after prolonged standing. Hemorrhoids may prolapse during defecation and spontaneously return, or the client may need to replace them manually. In some clients, hemorrhoids are prolapsed at all times.

DIAGNOSTIC ASSESSMENT

External hemorrhoids are diagnosed by visual examination; internal hemorrhoids are diagnosed through history, digital palpation, and proctoscopy. Asking the client to strain during assessment causes the veins to enlarge, thus aiding diagnosis.

Complications

Primary complications of hemorrhoids are bleeding, thrombosis, and hemorrhoidal strangulation. Severe bleeding from prolonged trauma to the vein during defecation can cause iron deficiency anemia. Blood oozes or may even spurt out following a bowel movement. Thrombosis within the hemorrhoids can occur at any time and is manifested by intense pain. Strangulated hemorrhoids, prolapsed hemorrhoids in which blood supply is cut off by the anal sphincter, can result in thrombosis when blood within the hemorrhoid clots. Assessment reveals a severe pain, extreme edema, and inflammation. Application of cold packs and elevation of the buttocks may allow the prolapsed hemorrhoid to reduce itself spontaneously.

Medical Management

Medical therapy is used only for small, uncomplicated hemorrhoids with mild symptoms. Treatment involves (1) reducing pressure by treating the constipation and (2) relieving pain with heat application and astringent lotions. No other intervention is required.

PHARMACOLOGIC MANAGEMENT

Constipation unrelieved by diet may require use of a stool softener (Colace) or a hydrophilic psyllium preparation. Use of a topical anesthetic or steroid preparation such as lidocaine (Xylocaine) or steroid creams also reduces pain or itching.

DIETARY MANAGEMENT

Dietary changes used to treat constipation include increasing fluid and fiber in the diet. For pain, an initial application of cold packs, followed by warm sitz baths, three to four times a day should help.

Surgical Management

There are a number of surgical procedures used to treat hemorrhoids. These include sclerotherapy, rubber band ligation, cryosurgery, laser surgery, and hemorrhoidectomy.

Sclerotherapy is performed by the injection of a sclerosing agent between and around the veins, which produces an inflammatory reaction that leads to thrombosis and fibrosis. This procedure can be performed on an outpatient basis but requires one to four injections 5 to 7 days apart. The sclerosing agent can cause anal canal scarring.

A common procedure for internal hemorrhoids, ligation is performed in the physician's office. The client can usually carry on normal activities immediately after the treatment. Unfortunately, the procedure cannot be used for external hemorrhoids and may be only temporarily effective. The surgeon inserts a ligator, a small, double-lumen cylinder with a small rubber band on the inner layer, through an anoscope. The hemorrhoid is then grasped with forceps and pulled through the ligator. The rubber band is placed around the neck of the hemorrhoid. Although bleeding can occur, the most common problem is some pain during ligation. The client takes a bulk laxative after the procedure to avoid local trauma from a hard fecal mass. In 8 to 10 days, the rubber band cuts through the neck of tissue, and the tissue sloughs.

Cryosurgery, freezing of the hemorrhoids, is performed less commonly today. It is also an outpatient procedure. The freezing of the tissue leads to necrosis and sloughing of the hemorrhoids. The problems associated with this procedure are the prolonged periods of drainage, amount of foul drainage, the presence of large residual skin tags, and possibly, incomplete destruction of the hemorrhoids.

Laser removal is the newest procedure. This also is performed on an outpatient basis. The hemorrhoid is burned off with the laser. There is minimal bleeding, although the procedure causes some pain.

With a hemorrhoidectomy, the vein is excised and the area is either left open to heal by granulation or sutured closed. The open method is very painful but has a high rate of success. The sutured method, although far less painful, is more likely to cause infection and result in poor healing.

Complications

Complications include infection, stricture formation as the lesion heals, and hemorrhage. Hemorrhage may occur immediately after surgery or about 10 days later as a result of sloughing of tissue. Also, bleeding may not be evident because it can occur into the rectum and not pass immediately.

Nursing Management

The client should take measures to avoid constipation. The anal area is very painful, and the client may avoid defecating, resulting in hard stool or fecal impaction. The nurse should encourage the client to take bulk laxatives or mineral oil as prescribed to promote stool passage. The stool should be monitored for consistency and blood.

Teach the client to eat fiber-containing foods and ample fluids to prevent straining and to avoid laxatives, when possible. Remind the client not to sit on the toilet longer than necessary to have a bowel movement. This position impairs blood flow and puts added pressure on anal vessels.

After the client has had any of the procedures to remove the hemorrhoids, the nurse should stress the importance of keeping the area clean and the stool soft but formed, to help prevent strictures. Encourage the client to wash the area after defecation and pat it dry. Local moist heat, applied with a washcloth or piece of cotton to the anal opening for a few minutes, is soothing and cleansing, and promotes healing. Never apply heat in the immediate postoperative period because of the increased risk of hemorrhage. Most physicians prescribe sitz baths three or four times a day or as the client desires, beginning 12 hours after surgery.

Postoperative complications requiring nursing assessment include hemorrhage and urinary retention. The proximity of the bladder and tenderness in the area sometimes makes urination difficult. Reestablishment of bowel habits is another potential postoperative problem. The client may need instruction on the relationship of proper diet and adequate fluid intake to bowel regularity, the physiology of defecation, and the importance of establishing a regular bowel routine.

After a hemorrhoidectomy, the client should take a warm sitz bath after each bowel movement or three to four times per day to relieve discomfort and spasm and to promote healing. Perianal irritation may be relieved with zinc oxide ointment. The most convenient perianal dressing is a sanitary napkin, although if there is no drainage, the client requires no dressing. The stools can be regulated by increasing dietary fiber intake, with the goal of one soft stool daily.

Postoperative pain can be controlled with parenteral and then oral analgesics. Warn the client to avoid vigorous perianal wiping during the immediate postoperative period. The client is usually given a stool softener and mineral oil to soften and lubricate the first stool. Warn clients that fainting can occur, through pain and vagal stimulation, during the first postoperative bowel movement.

PILONIDAL CYST

A pilonidal cyst occurs at the base of the sacrum, usually contains hair, and becomes infected, forming an abscess and then a sinus tract. It is most common in young adults, especially males. It may result from hairs that penetrate the skin and cause sinus tracts to form. Constant irritation (e.g., from clothing) can cause hairs to become embedded and then infected.

Acute pain and swelling result, followed by a discharge. Treatment involves surgical excision of the abscess. Healing is slow, and if the infectious process is not completely removed, the condition may recur. The client also may receive antibiotics.

RECTAL FISSURE (FISSURE-IN-ANO)

A rectal fissure is an ulceration or tear of the lining of the anal canal, usually on the posterior wall. An acute fissure occurs as a result of excessive tissue stretching and possibly from passage of a hard or large stool through the area. The skin tear is very tender and tends to reopen at subsequent periods of defecation.

Chronic fissures are usually secondary to cryptitis (infectious material retained in the anal crypts). Sharp pain accompanies defecation, followed by burning. Severe muscle spasm of the sphincter usually accompanies chronic conditions. The client may try to avoid defecation, which aggravates the condition.

If the acute lesion does not heal with local dilatations, cleansing, and control of constipation, the tract can be excised surgically. A chronic fissure usually does not heal spontaneously and requires surgery.

The nurse should advise the client to (1) keep the stool soft with Metamucil, mineral oil, or Colace as prescribed; (2) have a bowel movement daily; and (3) clean the area after defecation, preferably with warm water. Sitz baths aid healing and may relieve pain. Suppositories with a local anesthetic may help constipation.

RECTAL FISTULA (FISTULA-IN-ANO)

A fistula is a sinus tract that develops between two body cavities or between a body cavity and the external environment. A rectal fistula is a tract that leads from the anal canal to the skin outside the anus, or from an abscess to either the anal canal or the perianal area. It usually is preceded by an abscess. A fistula may heal over temporarily and then open and drain periodically.

This is a chronic condition for which surgery is the only cure. The surgeon excises the tract and cleans the area, leaving it open to heal by granulation. It may heal very slowly and be very painful. Advise the client to keep the area clean, especially after a bowel movement.

RECTAL ABSCESS

Rectal abscesses form in several locations; Figure 55–14 illustrates the common ones. Most abscesses begin as cryptitis, with the formation of cysts that extend through the tubular ducts into the submucosal spaces. They also may originate from abrasions of the local tissues, with the entry of a virulent organism.

Treatment involves draining the abscess and surgical excision of any associated fistulas. It may take two stages of surgery to accomplish the needed resection.

TUMORS OF THE RECTUM

Carcinoma and melanoma both can occur at the anus but are rare, constituting less than 5 per cent of rectal cancers. They spread by local extension into the perirectal spaces and then to the inguinal nodes. Surgical

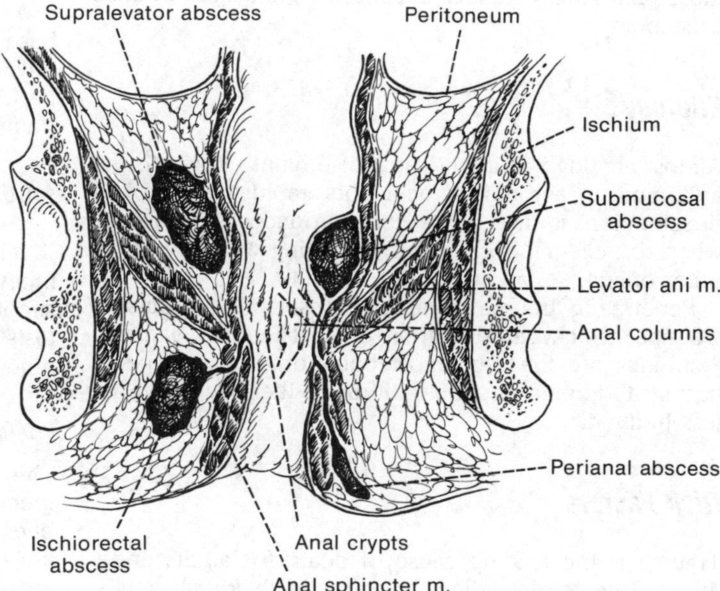

▲ Figure 55–14

Abscesses of the anorectal area.

intervention involves excision of the anus with an abdominoperineal resection. Preoperative irradiation and chemotherapy are other modes of intervention for anal cancer. Regional intra-arterial infusion of 5-fluorouracil as palliative therapy can relieve pain and improve the quality of life for the client with rectal cancer.

Cancer of the anal canal or lower rectum can coexist with other rectal conditions, and the client may falsely attribute bleeding to a hemorrhoid instead of carcinoma. Anal cancers are more common in African Americans and usually occur in clients with pre-existing anal and perianal problems such as a fistula. Bleeding, pain, and tenesmus are characteristic symptoms. The client is usually aware of a lump near the anus that has bled and gradually becomes more and more painful, particularly during or just after a bowel movement. Many cancers are not diagnosed until they are large, and by then, the prognosis is poor. A physician should investigate every case of rectal bleeding, even though it may be attributable to hemorrhoids or some other local rectal condition.

▼ ABDOMINAL TRAUMA

BLUNT OR PENETRATING TRAUMA OF THE ABDOMEN

Definition

Blunt or penetrating trauma to the abdomen refers to the accidental or intentional trauma causing internal injuries.

Incidence

Most blunt abdominal trauma is caused by the automobile steering wheel or pedestrian accidents, whereas most penetrating trauma is caused by gunshot wounds or stabbings.

Etiology

Almost any kind of injury can cause blunt trauma to the abdomen. In automobile accidents, rapid, uncontrolled deceleration is the force that produces the trauma when the client's body hits the steering wheel or some other object.

Penetrating trauma commonly results from gunshot wounds, which cause a great deal of internal damage. Stabbings are the next most common cause of penetrating abdominal wounds, although these wounds are less traumatic.

Risk Factors

Trauma is the leading cause of death for adults under 40 and the third leading cause of death for all adults. Although not all of these cases of trauma are abdominal trauma, abdominal injuries are common with motor vehicle accidents.

One method of prevention is wearing seat belts, which could decrease abdominal trauma in case of accidents.

Pathophysiology

Blunt trauma to the abdomen can cause shearing, crushing, or compressing forces that can cause rupture of bowel and other abdominal structures.

Gunshot wounds have the potential of damaging every structure in the abdomen. The gunshots may perforate the stomach or bowel, causing peritonitis and sepsis.

Stab wounds produce less trauma to internal abdominal structures because the abdominal organs have more time to shift out of the way of the penetrating instrument.

Clinical Manifestations

Assessment of the client first involves obtaining a thorough history of the accident so the degree of blunt trauma can be estimated. For penetrating trauma, careful assessment of the position of entry and possibly exit wounds is vital.

The client may show signs of an acute abdomen with either type of trauma. With both injuries, either internal or external hemorrhage may occur. If the bowel is ruptured, signs and symptoms of peritonitis are present. All abdominal drainage is closely assessed for the presence of bowel contents.

DIAGNOSTIC ASSESSMENT

Abdominal lavage is commonly used to assess the presence of bleeding in all abdominal wounds. This involves performing paracentesis following the instillation of a crystalloid solution into the peritoneal cavity.

A CT scan of the abdomen is now considered the base assessment of intra-abdominal injury. Angiography, intravenous pyelography, and other studies may be performed to assess different organs and the degree of trauma suffered.

Medical Management

If minimal blunt trauma was sustained without severe injury to any abdominal organs, then the client may simply be observed for problems once the diagnostic tests have been conducted. Penetrating trauma always requires some type of surgical intervention.

PHARMACOLOGIC MANAGEMENT

The client's pain is treated conservatively until the degree of trauma has been determined. If the bowel has been ruptured, large doses of intravenous antibiotics are given to control infection. If hemorrhage and shock are present, intravenous fluids, colloids, and vasopressors may be used.

DIETARY MANAGEMENT

The client receives nothing by mouth until the abdomen has been assessed and found to be intact.

COMPLICATIONS

The major complications of trauma are hemorrhage, shock, peritonitis, and sepsis.

Surgical Management

The treatment of choice for abdominal trauma with injury to the abdominal contents is an exploratory laparotomy. Depending on the exact injury found, the surgery may be as simple as a closure of tears or as complex as a bowel resection and even a temporary colostomy.

Nursing Management

Careful assessment of the client's injury is vital. The nurse must often prepare the client for immediate emergency surgery. The nurse must prepare the client as quickly as possible, knowing that postoperatively, much more teaching and support will be required.

Post-hospital Care

If the client developed peritonitis or had an ostomy performed, the client may need follow-up care from a visiting nurse. This care can involve the administration of antibiotics at home, further ostomy teaching, or wound care for an open draining wound.

DISCHARGE TEACHING

The client may need teaching regarding home health care that may include ostomy care and extensive wound care. The client or significant others may have to learn to change dressings and to care for an open, draining wound.

FOLLOW-UP CARE

Usually, once the injuries and repair have had sufficient time to heal and the infection has been adequately treated, the client will return to the hospital to have the ostomy closed and the bowel returned to normal.

▼ CONGENITAL DISORDERS

HIRSCHSPRUNG'S DISEASE

Definition

Hirschsprung's disease, also called congenital megacolon, is a colonic dilation that results from a functional obstruction of the rectum.

Incidence

This disorder predominantly affects male newborns and is present in about 1 in 5000 live births. It is often associated with congenital defects including Down syndrome and genitourinary abnormalities.

Etiology

The functional obstruction associated with Hirschsprung's disease is due to a congenital absence of intramural neural plexus (aganglionosis). Affected bowel is unable to transmit normal peristaltic waves, resulting in a hypertrophied and dilated portion of intestine proximal to this area.

Pathophysiology

Hirschsprung's disease is characterized by a congenital absence of autonomic ganglion cells from the intramural plexus of the colon. The ganglion are absent from the anorectal junction, the rectum, and sometimes from parts of the sigmoid colon.

Complications of Hirschsprung's disease include fluid and electrolyte imbalances and possible perforation of the distended bowel.

Clinical Manifestations

Children with Hirschsprung's disease have intestinal obstruction and meconium ileus present in the first few days of life. Later in life, clients present with severe constipation and recurrent fecal impactions. Children with only a small segment of bowel involved may not demonstrate symptoms until after surgery.

DIAGNOSTIC ASSESSMENT

In Hirschsprung's disease, digital examination shows the rectum to be empty. A barium enema study also confirms the absence of stool and usually shows a narrowed distal segment of bowel. A definitive diagnosis of Hirschsprung's is made from a full-thickness biopsy.

Surgical Management

In Hirschsprung's disease, if obstruction is present, often a temporary colostomy is necessary. In some cases, a regular program of enemas can provide decompression. A number of surgical procedures can be performed. Each of the major operations consists of dissecting the dilated bowel along with the portion of aganglionic bowel and then anastomosis. Later, most children do achieve bowel control, but it is seldom completely normal. Anal dilatation may be required.

Bibliography

1. Abrams, J. S. (1984). *Abdominal stomas: Indications, operative techniques, and patient care.* Boston: John Wright PSG.
2. Alterescu, K. V. (1987). Colostomy. *Nursing Clinics of North America, 22,* 281-290.
3. Alterescu, V. A. (1985). The ostomy: What do you teach the patient? *American Journal of Nursing, 85,* 1250-1253.
4. American Cancer Society. (1991). *1992 Cancer facts and figures.* New York: Author.
5. Bartlett, J. G. (1991). *1991 Pocketbook of infectious disease therapy.* Baltimore: Williams & Wilkins.
6. Bates-Jensen, B. (1989). Psychological response to illness: Exploring two reactions to ostomy surgery. *Ostomy/Wound Management, 23,* 24-30.
7. Bongiovanni, G. L. (1988). *Essentials of clinical gastroenterology* (2nd ed.) New York: McGraw-Hill.
8. Bragg, V. (1989). Continent intestinal reservoir: Ileostomy option. *Ostomy/Wound Management, 23,* 32-41.
9. Braun, J., et al. (1991). Anal sphincter function after intersphincteric resection and stapled ileal pouch-anal anastomosis. *Diseases of the Colon and Rectum, 34*(1), 8-16.
10. Braunwald, E., et al. (Eds.). (1987). *Harrison's principles of internal medicine.* New York: McGraw-Hill.
11. Broadwell, D. (1987). Peristomal skin integrity. *Nursing Clinics of North America, 22,* 321-332.
12. Broadwell, D., & Jackson, B. S. (1982). *Principles of ostomy care.* St. Louis: C. V. Mosby.
13. Celestin, L. R. (1987). *A colour atlas of the surgery and management of intestinal stomas.* Chicago: Year Book Medical Publishers.
14. Cohen, L. Z., et al. (Eds.). (1985). *Gastrointestinal disorders.* Springhouse, PA: Springhouse Corp.
15. Collins, S. M. (1988). The irritable bowel syndrome. *Canadian Medical Association Journal, 138,* 309-316.
16. Dobkin, K. A., & Broadwell, D. (1986). Nursing considerations for the patient undergoing colostomy surgery. *Seminars in Oncology Nursing 2,* 249-255.
17. Doughty, D. B. (1986). Colorectal cancer: Etiology and pathophysiology. *Seminars in Oncology Nursing, 2,* 235-241.
18. Dozois, R. R. (Ed.). (1985). *Alternatives to conventional ileostomy.* Chicago: Year Book Medical Publishers.
19. Dozois, R. R., et al. (1988). Newer operations for ulcerative colitis and Crohn's disease. *Surgical Clinics of North America, 68,* 1339-1352.
20. Dunphy, J. E., & Way, L. W. (1983). *Current surgical diagnosis and treatments* (6th ed.). Los Altos, CA: Lange Medical Publications.
21. Dworken, H. (1982). *Gastroenterology: Pathophysiology and clinical applications.* Boston: Butterworth Publications.
22. Edwards, J., & Krause, S. (1987). Helping the emergency colostomy patient through reality shock. *Nursing '87, 17*(7), 63-64.
23. Erickson, P. (1987). Ostomies: The art of pouching. *Nursing Clinics of North America, 22,* 311-320.
24. Frank, M. S., et al. (1983). Pharmacotherapy of inflammatory bowel disease, Part 2: metronidazole. *Postgraduate Medicine, 74,* 155.
25. Freely, J., et al. (1981). Reduction of liver blood flow and propranolol metabolism by cimetidine. *New England Journal of Medicine, 304,* 692.
26. Gale, M. E., & Robbins, A. H. (1983). CT scans of the abdomen: indications and basic interpretation. *Hospital Medicine, 19,* 10.
27. Gerver, L. (1983). Antidiarrheals: ensuring their safe use. *Nursing 83, 13,* 17.
28. Gilman, C. J. (1984). Improving survival in patients with rectal cancer. *American Family Physician, 29,* 165.
29. Gitnick, G. L. (Ed.). (1983). *Gastroenterology.* New York: John Wiley & Sons.
30. Given, B., & Simmons, S. (1984). *Gastroenterology in clinical nursing* (4th ed.). St. Louis: C. V. Mosby Co.
31. Goldner, F. (1981). Office management of diverticulosis. *Hospital Medicine, 17,* 83.
32. Goldstein, F. (1980). Inflammatory bowel disease—better prospects. *Consultant, 20,* 68.
33. Gramse, C. A. (1983). Diverticular disease. *Nursing 83, 13,* 56.
34. Grant, A., & Skyring, R. (1981). *Clinical diagnosis of gastrointestinal disease.* Oxford: Blackwell Scientific Publications.
35. Greenberger, N. (1981). *Gastrointestinal disorders: A pathophysiologic approach.* (2nd ed.). Chicago: Year Book Medical Publishers.
36. Greer, J. (1980). Hemorrhoids. In B. Eiseman (Ed), *Prognosis of surgical disease.* Philadelphia: W. B. Saunders.
37. Grunberg, K. J. (1986). Sexual rehabilitation of the cancer patient undergoing ostomy surgery. *Journal of Enterostomal Therapy, 13,* 148-152.
38. Guyton, A. C. (1991). *Textbook of medical physiology* (8th ed.). Philadelphia: W. B. Saunders.
39. Hallgren, T., et al. (1990). The stapled ileal pouch—anal anastomosis: A randomized study. *Scandinavian Journal of Gastroenterology, 25*(11), 1161-1168.
40. Halsted, C. H., et al. (1981). Sulfasalazine inhibits the absorption of folates in ulcerative colitis. *New England Journal of Medicine, 305,* 1513.
41. Hardy, T. G., et al. (1980). Management of inflammatory bowel disease: an effective and concise approach. *Diseases of the Colon and Rectum, 23,* 244.
42. Hassey, K. M. (1987). Radiation therapy for rectal cancer and the implications for nursing. *Cancer Nursing, 10,* 311-318.
43. Hendrix, T. R. (1981). Management of inflammatory bowel disease. *Hospital Medicine, 17,* 40.
44. Hocking, M. P., & Vogel, M. P. (1991). Woodward's postgastrectomy syndromes (2nd ed.). Philadelphia: W. B. Saunders.
45. Hollander, D., & Pelot, D. (1983). Diseases of the small intestine. In G. L. Gitnick (Ed.), *Gastroenterology.* New York: John Wiley & Sons.
46. Horowitz, I., & Talansky, A. (1980). Clinical differentiation of inflammatory bowel disease. *Hospital Medicine, 16,* 20.
47. Howell, D. A., & Almy, T. P. (1981). Current medical management of diverticular disease. *Consultant, 21,* 160.
48. International Association of Enterostomal Therapy. (1989). *Standards of care: Patient with colostomy.* Irvine, CA: Author.
49. Joachim, G., et al. (1987). Inflammatory bowel disease: Effects on life-style. *Journal of Advanced Nursing, 12,* 483-487.
50. Johnson, R. A., et al. (1982). Flexible sigmoidoscopy. *Journal of Family Practice, 14,* 757.
51. Kallman, H. (1983). Constipation in the elderly. *American Family Physician, 27,* 179.
52. Keighley, M. (1981). Prevention of infection in colo-rectal surgery. In J. M. Watts, et al. (Eds.), *Infection in surgery.* London: Churchill Livingstone.
53. Kelman, G., & Minkler, P. (1989). An investigation of quality of life and self-esteem among individuals with ostomies. *Journal of Enterostomal Therapy, 16,* 4-11.
54. Khan, A. H. (1984). Colorectal carcinoma: Risk factors, screening, early detection. *Geriatrics, 39,* 42.
55. Kies, M. (1982). Fluorouracil for colorectal cancer. *Journal of the American Medical Association, 247,* 2826.
56. Kirsner, J. B. (1985). The stomach. In W. A. Sodeman, Jr., & T. M. Sodeman (Eds.), *Pathologic physiology: mechanisms of disease,* (7th ed.). Philadelphia: W. B. Saunders.
57. Kirsner, J. B. (1980). Observations on the medical treatment of inflammatory bowel disease. *Journal of the American Medical Association, 243,* 557.
58. Kirsner, J. B., & Shorter, R. G. (1982). Recent developments in "nonspecific" inflammatory bowel disease, Part 1. *New England Journal of Medicine, 306,* 775.
59. Kirsner, J. B., & Shorter, R. G.: (1982). Recent developments in "nonspecific" inflammatory bowel disease, Part 2. *New England Journal of Medicine, 306,* 837.
60. Kirsner, J. B., & Shorter, R. G. (Eds). (1988). *Inflammatory bowel disease* (3rd ed.). Philadelphia: Lea & Febiger.
61. Korelitz, B. I. (1982). What is considered good medical care in Crohn's disease? In B. I. Korelitz (Ed.), *Inflammatory bowel disease: experience and controversy.* Boston: John Wright PSG.
62. Korelitz, B. I. (1983). Pharmacotherapy of inflammatory bowel disease. *Postgraduate Medicine, 74,* 165.
63. LaMont, J. T. (1982). Recommendations for inflammatory bowel disease. *Geriatrics, 37,* 93.
64. Lamphier, T. A. (1981). Small-bowel obstruction: Think of it early. *Consultant, 21,* 165.

65. Leibach, J. R., & Cerda, J. J.: (1981). Office management of hemorrhoids. *Hospital Medicine, 17,* 17.
66. Libbus, M. K. (1983). Enterobiasis. *Nurse Practitioner, 8,* 17.
67. Marion, A. W., et al. (1983). Anorectal surgery—hemorrhoids. *Diseases of the Colon and Rectum, 23,* 211.
68. Messner, R. L., et al. (1986). Early detection: The priority of colorectal cancer. *Cancer Nursing, 9*(1), 8-14.
69. Michael, R. M. (Ed.). (1981). Methyldopa colitis. *Nurses' Drug Alert, 5,* 73.
70. Moertel, C., & Thynne, G. (Eds.) (1982). *Cancer medicine* (2nd ed.). Philadelphia: Lea & Febiger.
71. Myer, S. A. (1984). Overview of inflammatory bowel disease. *Nursing Clinics of North America, 19*(1), 3-10.
72. Neilan, B. A. Colorectal cancer. *Clinical Geriatric Medicine, 3,* 625-635.
73. Neufeldt, J. (1987). Helping the inflammatory bowel disease patient cope with the unpredictable. *Nursing '87, 17*(8), 47-49.
74. Nortridge, J. A. (1982). Helpful hints for assessing the ostomate. *Nursing 82, 12,* 72.
75. Nuccio, M. A., & Sparks, C. (1983). Intestinal parasites: Diagnostic and treatment guidelines. *Nurse Practitioner, 8,* 47.
76. Palmer, E. D. (1982). Identifying irritable bowel syndrome. *Hospital Medicine, 18,* 116.
77. Porter, J. A., et al. (1989). Complications of colostomy. *Diseases of the Colon and Rectum, 32,* 299-303.
78. Present, D., et al. (1980). Treatment of Crohn's disease with 6-mercaptopurine. *New England Journal of Medicine, 302,* 981.
79. Price, S. A., & Wilson, L. M. (1986). *Pathophysiology: Clinical concepts of disease processes* (3rd ed.). New York: McGraw-Hill.
80. Rainer, W. (1986). *Stoma therapy: An atlas and guide for intestinal stomas.* New York: Thieme.
81. Rakel, R. E. (Ed.). (1990). *Conn's current therapy 1990.* Philadelphia: W. B. Saunders.
82. Rankin, G. B. (1981). Crohn's disease: Its recognition and complications. *Primary Care, 8,* 309.
83. Rawls, D., & Dyck, W. (1984). Previewing new drugs, reviewing current therapy. *Consultant, 24,* 85.
84. Rideout, B. W. (1987). The patient with an ileostomy: Nursing management and patient education. *Nursing Clinics of North America, 22*(2), 253-262.
85. Robbins, R. D. (1982). The role of hyperalimentation in the treatment of Crohn's disease. In B. I. Korelitz (Ed.), *Inflammatory bowel disease: experience and controversy.* Boston: John Wright PSG.
86. Robbins, S. L., et al. (1984). *Pathologic basis of disease* (3rd ed.). Philadelphia: J. B. Lippincott.
87. Rodman, M. J., & Smith, D. W.: *Pharmacology and drug therapy in nursing,* (3rd ed.). Philadelphia: J. B. Lippincott.
88. Rogers, A. I. (1981). (3rd ed.). Diagnosis: rectal bleeding. *Hospital Medicine, 17,* 55.
89. Sabiston, Jr., D. C. (1991). *Textbook of surgery: The biological basis of modern surgical practice* (14th ed.). Philadelphia: W. B. Saunders.
90. Schartz, S. I., et al. (1984). *Principles of surgery,* (4th ed.). New York: McGraw-Hill.
91. Schrock, T. R. (1983). Large intestine. In L. W. Way (Ed.), *Current Surgical Diagnosis & Treatment* (6th ed.) Los Altos, CA: Lange Medical Publications.
92. Schroeder, S. A., et al. (1989). *Current medical diagnosis and treatment.* Norwalk, CT: Appleton & Lange.
93. Segal, H. L., (1981). Clues to cancer of the digestive system. *Consultant, 21,* 101.
94. Sernka, T., & Jacobson, E. (1983). *Gastrointestinal physiology: The essentials,* (2nd ed.). Baltimore: Williams & Wilkins.
95. Sherlock, P. (1983). Cancer surveillance in inflammatory bowel disease. *Postgraduate Medicine, 74,* 191.
96. Shinehouse, P. M. (Ed.). (1987). *Gastrointestinal problems.* Springhouse, PA: Springhouse Publishing.
97. Shipes, E. (1987). Psychosocial issues: The person with an ostomy. *Nursing Clinics of North America, 22,* 291-302.
98. Silverstein, F. E., & Rubin, C. E. (1980). Gastrointestinal endoscopy. In K. J. Isselbacher, et al. (Eds.), *Harrison's principles of internal medicine,* (9th ed.). New York: McGraw-Hill.
99. Simmons, M. (1984). Using the nursing process in treating inflammatory bowel disease. *Nursing Clinics of North America, 19,* 11.
100. Singleton, J. W. (1980). Medical therapy of inflammatory bowel disease. *Medical Clinics of North America, 64,* 1117.
101. Sircus, W., & Smith, A. (1980). *Scientific foundations of gastroenterology.* Philadelphia: W. B. Saunders.
102. Smith, L. (1983). Symptomatic internal hemorrhoids: what are your options? *Postgraduate Medicine, 73,* 323.
103. Sleisenger, M. H., & Fordtran, J. S. (Eds.). (1989). *Gastrointestinal disease: Pathophysiology, diagnosis, and management* (4th ed.). Philadelphia: W. B. Saunders.
104. Smith, L. E. (1989). Surgical therapy in ulcerative colitis. *Gastroenterology Clinics of North America, 18*(1), 99-110.
105. Sparks, S. M., & Taylor, C. M. (1991). *Nursing diagnosis reference manual.* Springhouse, PA: Springhouse Publishing.
106. Stratton, J. W., & Mackeigan, J. M. (1982). Treating constipation. *American Family Physician, 25,* 139.
107. Thorbjarnarson, B. (1983). Intussusception: current concepts. *Hospital Medicine, 19,* 13.
108. Tilson, M. D. (1980). Pathophysiology and treatment of short bowel syndrome. *Surgical Clinics of North America, 60,* 1273.
109. Tollison, J. W., & Griffin, J. W. (1980). High-fiber diet and colorectal disease. *American Family Physician, 22,* 121.
110. Trainor, M. A. (1982). Acceptance of ostomy and the visitor role in a self-help group for ostomy patients. *Nursing Research, 31,* 102.
111. Urosevich, P. R. (Ed.) (1983). *Performing GI procedures.* Springhouse, PA: Intermed Communication.
112. U. S. Department of Health and Human Services (1981). *Cancer of the colon and rectum.* Washington, DC: National Cancer Institute, DHHS.
113. Watson, P. G. (1985). Meeting the needs of patients undergoing ostomy surgery. *Journal of Enterostomal Therapy, 12,* 121-124.
114. Watts, R. C. (1985). The ostomy: How is it created? *American Journal of Nursing, 85,* 1242-1243.
115. Way, L. W. (1988). *Current surgical diagnosis and treatment.* Norwalk, CT: Appleton & Lange.
116. Weiss, B. D. (1983). Traveler's diarrhea: Update 1983. *American Family Physician, 27,* 193.
117. Whitehead, W. E., et al. (1980). Irritable bowel syndrome: Physiological and psychological differences between diarrhea-predominant and constipation-predominant patients. *Digestive Diseases and Sciences 25,* 404.
118. Wicks, L. J. (1986). Treatment modalities for colorectal cancer. *Seminars in Oncology Nursing, 2,* 242-248.
119. Williams, S. (1989). *Nutrition and diet therapy* (6th ed.). St. Louis: C. V. Mosby.
120. Wilson, C. (1984). The diagnostic work-up for the patient with inflammatory bowel disease. *Nursing Clinics of North America, 19*(1), 51-60.
121. Witt, M. E., et al. (1987). Adjuvant radiotherapy to the colorectum: Nursing implications. *Oncology Nursing Forum, 14*(3), 17-21.
122. Wyngaarden, J., & Smith, L. (1988). *Cecil textbook of medicine,* (17th ed.). Philadelphia: W. B. Saunders.

Unit 13

Liver, Biliary Tract, and Exocrine Pancreatic Disorders

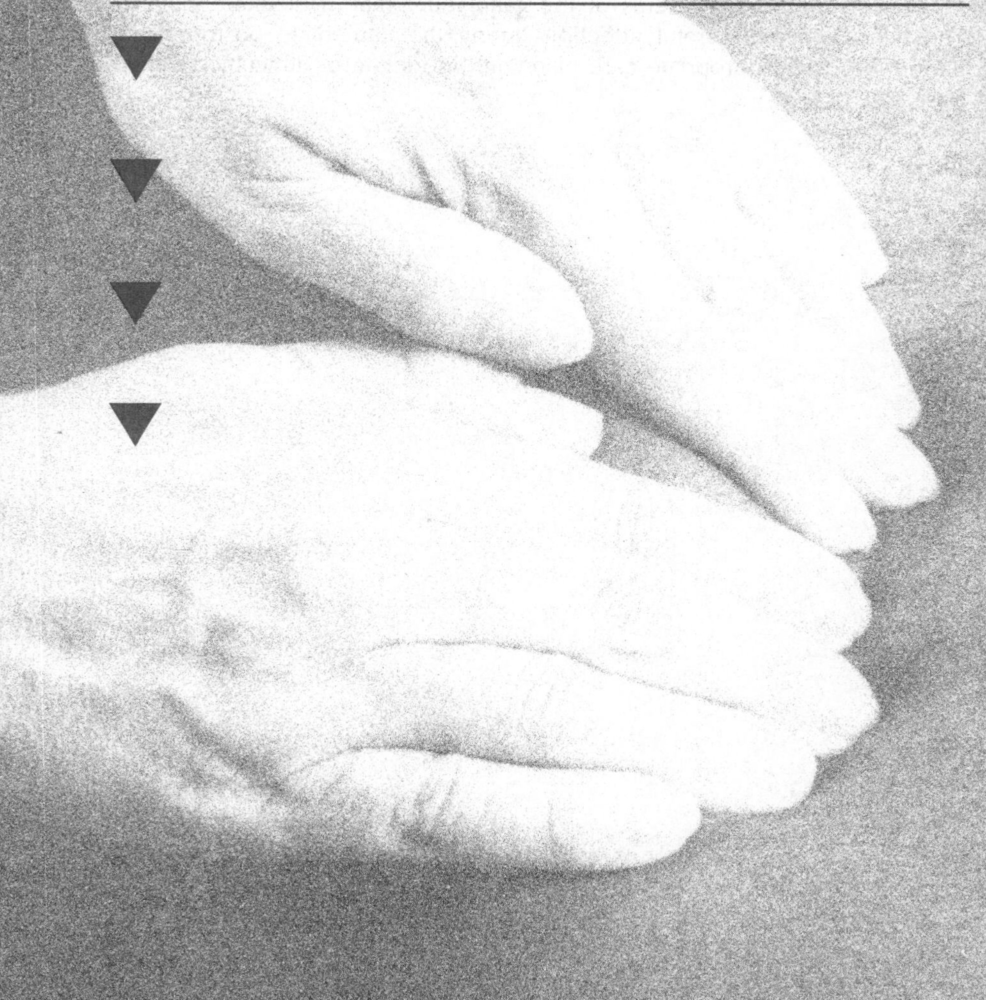

The liver, biliary tract, and exocrine pancreas are located together in the upper abdominal cavity, where they facilitate digestion and metabolism. The liver, in addition, detoxifies chemicals, destroys bacteria in the blood, synthesizes blood-clotting factors, and assists in regulation of blood volume. This unit explores the coordinated and independent functions of the liver, biliary tract, and exocrine pancreas. Assessment of this system is also covered. It identifies disorders related to one or common to all, and discusses current medical treatment and nursing management.

Chronic, progressive disorders of the liver, biliary tract, and exocrine pancreas alter the client's lifestyle and require long-term assessment and management. Severe hepatic and pancreatic damage demands intensive, complex nursing interventions. When these disorders are due to drug or alcohol dependence, the lifestyle of the client may be in conflict with traditional cultural values. In these situations, the nurse must care for the client and meet the client's needs without allowing preconceived ideas to influence the care.

Acute, episodic problems of the gallbladder may necessitate surgery. The client requires careful attention during the immediate postoperative period but, with appropriate care planning, no long-term difficulties should arise.

Chapter 56

Structure and Function of the Liver, Biliary System, and Exocrine Pancreas

STRUCTURE OF THE LIVER

The liver is the largest organ in the body, representing 2 per cent of body weight. It lies in the upper right quadrant of the abdomen, just below the diaphragm. The rib cage encloses the liver except for the lower margin (Fig. 56-1). The lungs extend over the liver's upper portion. The lower portion of the liver provides a roof for the stomach and intestines. A peritoneal covering blankets most of the liver and also the adjacent gallbladder (Fig. 56-2).

Note in Figure 56-2 that the liver divides at the falciform ligament into two major lobes, right and left. These two lobes, in turn, divide into superior and inferior portions of the posterior, anterior, medial, and lateral segments.

The hepatic artery supplies the liver with about one third of its blood, while the portal vein supplies the other two thirds. The hepatic artery carries oxygenated blood; the portal vein carries deoxygenated blood. The superior and inferior mesenteric veins and the splenic vein, which receive blood from the pancreas, spleen, stomach, intestines, and gallbladder, join to form the portal vein. The portal vein carries nutrients, metabolites, and toxins from the digestive organs to the liver for processing, detoxification, or assimilation. Agents such as prothrombin and fibrinogen (both vital to clotting) are added to the blood within the liver. The vasculature of the liver has been called the antechamber of the heart because it takes in all the gastrointestinal and splenic blood via the portal vein and returns it to the right side of the heart by way of the hepatic veins. Hence, any process

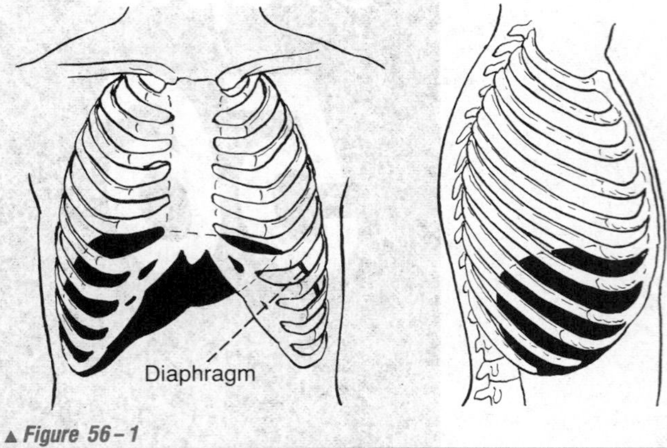

▲ *Figure 56-1*

The liver, shown here from an anterior and right lateral view, is located just below the diaphragm.

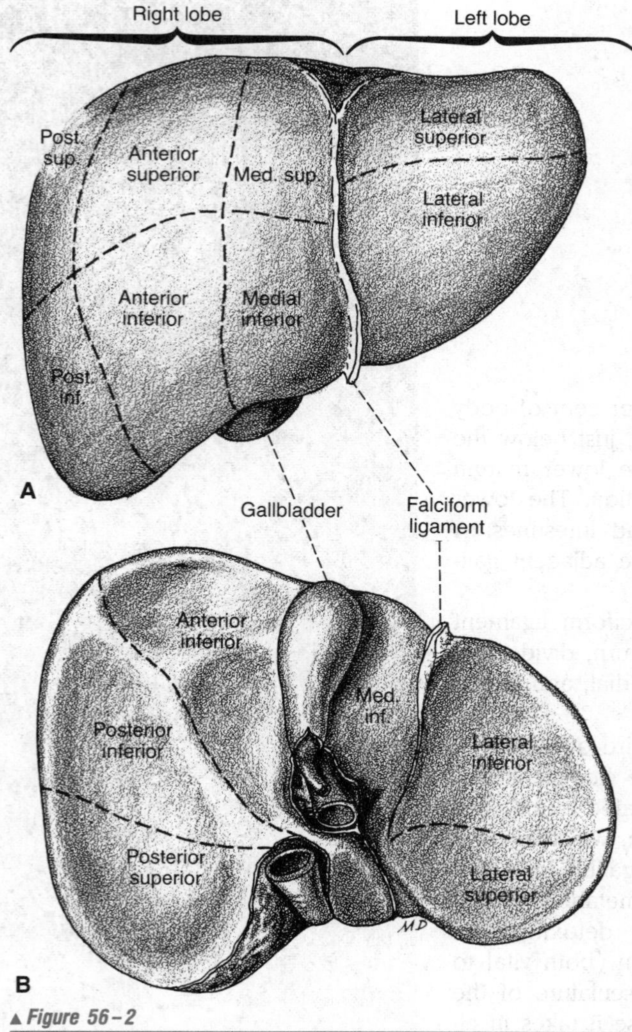

▲ *Figure 56-2*

Segments of right and left lobes of the liver. *A*, Anterior view. *B*, Inferior view.

impeding blood flow through the right atrium of the heart causes liver engorgement. Similarly, any process impeding blood flow through the liver causes engorgement of vessels draining the digestive organs.

Examine the hepatic portal system in Figure 56-3. In general, a portal circulation system is one in which blood from one or more organs circulates through another organ before returning to the heart.

The functional unit of the liver is the liver lobule, with the hepatocyte being the major cell. In the liver lobule, these cells are arranged hublike around a central vein. One side of the polyhedral hepatocyte faces the hepatic sinusoids, the capillary system of the liver. The other side faces the bile canaliculi. Incoming blood from the portal vein and the hepatic artery enters the sinusoids. As this blood passes through the liver lobules, many substances are exchanged between the blood and the hepatocytes. Lymphatic ducts drain waste products. Bile is formed in the hepatocytes, is secreted into the bile canaliculi, and then travels through bile ductules to the gallbladder. Endothelial and Kupffer's cells form the walls of the sinusoids. Kupffer's cells are an important part of the mononuclear phagocyte system (formerly called the reticuloendothelial system). The blood then courses into the central vein, the hepatic veins, and the inferior vena cava. The basic structure of a liver lobule is illustrated in Figure 56-4.

STRUCTURE OF THE BILIARY TRACT

The gallbladder (Fig. 56-5) is a small, pear-shaped sac that can hold approximately 100 to 150 ml of bile. It receives its arterial blood supply from the cystic artery, which branches off the right hepatic artery. Venous blood is drained via the cystic veins. The celiac plexus, the vagus nerve, and the right phrenic nerve supply the gallbladder's innervation.

Bile is transported from the liver through the right and left hepatic ducts. The gallbladder serves as a reservoir for bile produced in the liver. Bile is necessary for the digestion of dietary fat. The gallbladder concentrates the bile, releases it into the cystic duct, which empties into the common bile duct, and finally into the small intestine (specifically the duodenum) (Fig. 56-6). When there is fat present in the intestine, a valve at the confluence of the common bile duct and the duodenum, called the sphincter of Oddi, opens to allow bile to flow into the intestinal tract. When there is no fat present, the sphincter remains closed and bile backs up into the gallbladder, where it is stored.

STRUCTURE OF THE PANCREAS

The pancreas is a large, many-lobed gland that structurally resembles the salivary glands. It is located posterior to the greater curvature of the stomach. The head of the pancreas lies in the concavity of the duodenum, and its tail rests against the spleen (Fig. 56-6). The liver lies above the pancreas, and the stomach

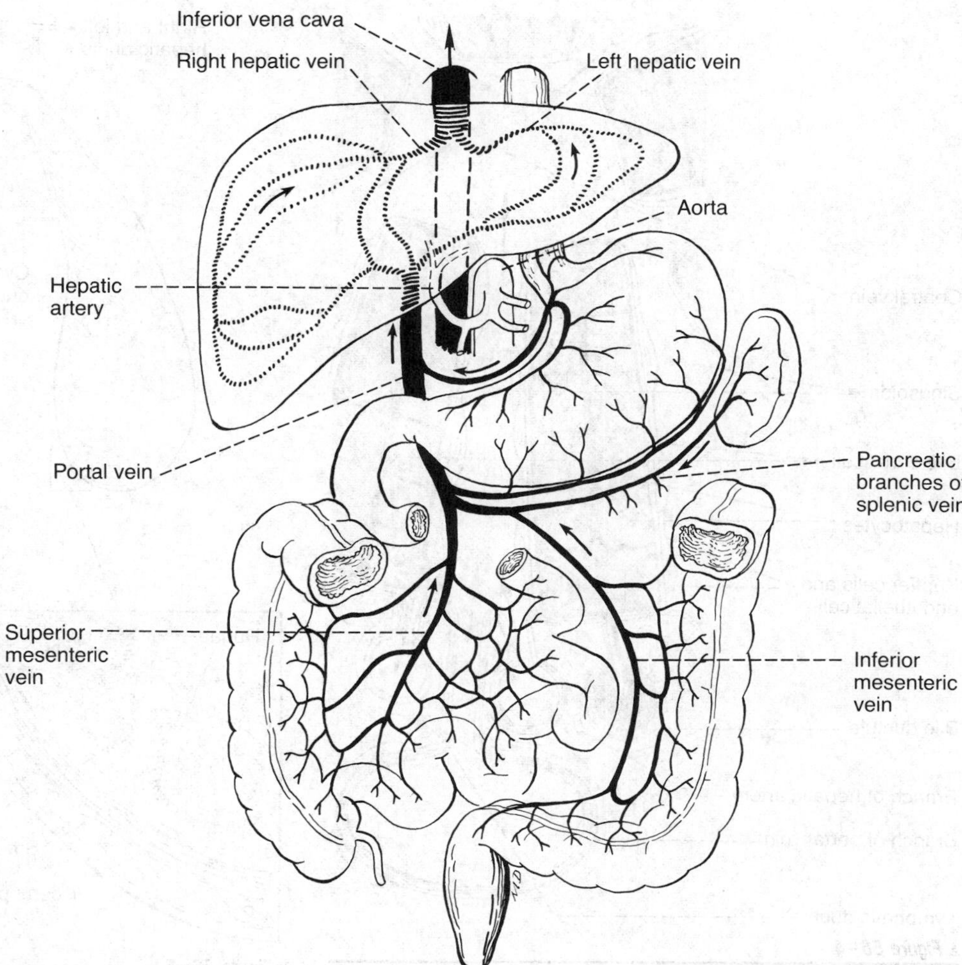

▲ *Figure 56-3*

Hepatic portal system supplies the liver with blood from the digestive organs.

passes close to the anterior surface. Major blood vessels, namely the aorta, inferior vena cava, and hepatic artery, are located very near the head of the pancreas and, thus, greatly complicate extensive surgery in this area.

The pancreas functions as (1) an endocrine gland, secreting insulin and glucagon directly into the bloodstream; and (2) an exocrine gland, secreting multiple digestive enzymes into a system of ducts. These ducts flow into the duct of Wirsung and empty into the duodenum. The site where the duct of Wirsung joins the common bile duct and enters the duodenum is referred to as the ampulla of Vater (Fig. 56-6). The sphincter of Oddi controls the release of both pancreatic juices and bile into the duodenum. The exocrine function of the pancreas is discussed in this unit. Endocrine function and disorders are discussed in Chapter 60.

METABOLIC FUNCTIONS OF THE LIVER, BILIARY TRACT, AND PANCREAS

The liver, biliary system, and exocrine pancreas produce, detoxify, and store many substances in the body. The substances produced aid in the digestion, assimilation, and use of nutrients by the body.

Liver Functions

BILE PRODUCTION

The liver normally produces and secretes between 600 and 1200 ml of bile each day. The basic components of bile are water, bile salts, bilirubin, cholesterol, fatty acids, lecithin, sodium, potassium, calcium, chloride, and bicarbonate ion. Water is the most abundant component of bile, followed by bile salts. Because bile is concentrated in the gallbladder, this water and a large portion of the electrolytes (not calcium ions) are reabsorbed by the gallbladder mucosa.

Bile salts are produced by the liver in a quantity of about 0.5 g a day. The precursor of these bile salts is cholesterol, supplied either by the diet or synthesized by the liver through fat metabolism. Bile salts function in two ways. First, they function an emulsifying or detergent function, decreasing the surface tension of fat particles in the food, allowing the agitation of the intestine to break the fat globules into a much smaller

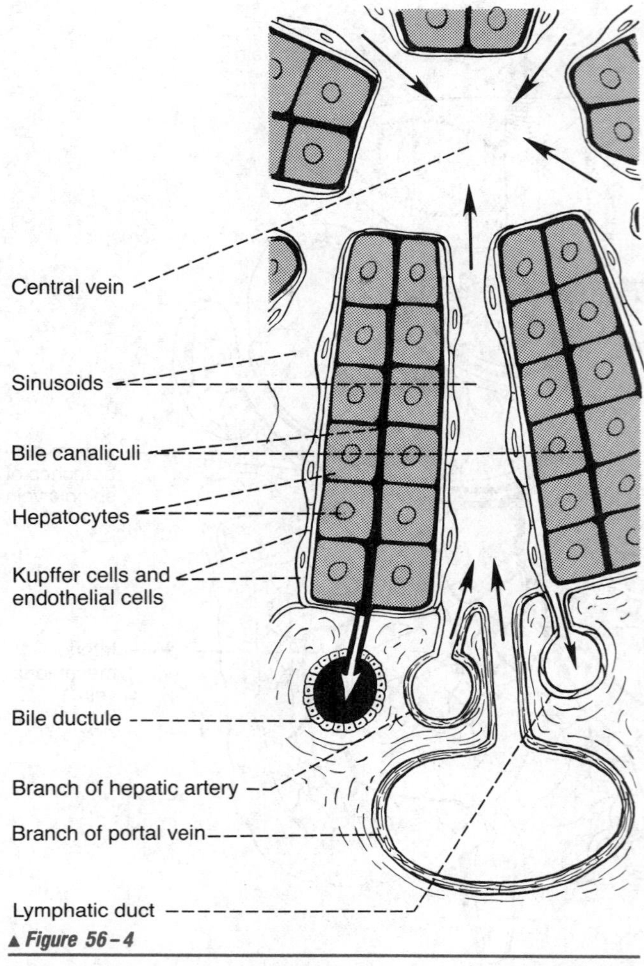

▲ *Figure 56–4*

Diagram of a liver lobule. As blood from the portal vein and hepatic artery flows through the sinusoids toward the central vein, substances are exchanged between the blood and the hepatocytes. Lymphatic ducts drain the waste products. Bile produced in the hepatocytes is secreted into the bile canaliculi and travels through the bile ductules to the gallbladder.

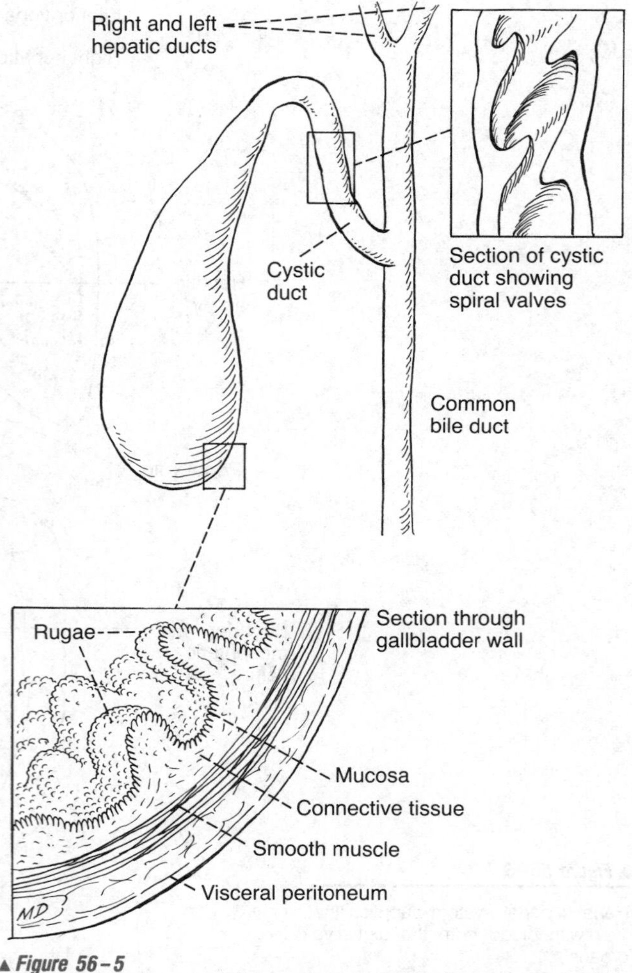

▲ *Figure 56–5*

The gallbladder stores bile until needed to digest fat in the duodenum. Insets show a longitudinal section of spiral valves in the cystic duct and a section of the gallbladder wall.

size. Second, they help in the absorption of fatty acids, monoglycerides, cholesterol, and other lipids from the intestine.

The next most abundant component of bile is bilirubin. Bilirubin, an orange-yellow or greenish yellow pigment in the bile, is the product of hemoglobin breakdown (Fig. 56–7). Cholesterol, a precursor of bile acid, may precipitate unless enough bile salts are present to keep it in suspension.

Biliverdin is the first pigment to be formed during bile production. This greenish pigment is soon reduced to unconjugated bilirubin and released into the plasma. Lecithin is a fatty substance and a phospholipid, that is, a substance containing phosphorus, fatty acids, and a nitrogen base.

Cholesterol is a bile precursor supplied either through the diet or synthesized by the liver. It is highly insoluble in water and may precipitate unless enough bile salts are present to keep it in suspension. When the balance of cholesterol, lecithin, and bile salts is disturbed, cholesterol or other components may precipitate and form gallstones.

The liver continuously secretes bile, which is then stored in the gallbladder until it is needed in the duodenum for digestion. The gallbladder can hold only 20 to 60 ml of bile at a time; however, up to 450 ml is produced in about 12 hours. The gallbladder can manage this amount because water, sodium, chloride, and most small electrolytes are reabsorbed by the gallbladder mucosa. This process concentrates the bile from 5 to 20 times.

The gallbladder continues to store the bile until fatty foods enter the small intestine and stimulate the release of cholecystokinin. Cholecystokinin stimulates contractions of the gallbladder wall, and this process combined with simultaneous relaxation of the sphincter of Oddi allows the bile to flow into the duodenum and mix with the food. The gallbladder is also stimulated by cholinergic nerve fibers that also stimulate intestinal motility and secretion in other parts of the gastrointestinal tract. The gallbladder empties poorly in the absence of fatty foods but empties completely within 1 hour after a meal with adequate fat. Reabsorption of bile salts is almost total, and recycling occurs as they return to the liver.

The sphincter of Oddi must relax completely if adequate emptying is to occur. There are three mechanisms that help this occur: (1) cholecystokinin has a weak relaxant effect on the sphincter; (2) rhythmic contractions of the gallbladder wall transmit peristaltic waves down the common bile duct to the sphincter, leading to partial relaxations; and (3) relaxation phases of intestinal peristaltic waves cause the greatest relaxation of the sphincter and the intestinal wall.

CARBOHYDRATE METABOLISM

The major functions of the liver in relation to glucose metabolism are (1) *glycogenesis,* the conversion of glucose to glycogen, (2) *glycogenolysis,* the breakdown of glycogen to glucose, (3) storage of glycogen, (4) conversion of galactose and fructose to glucose, and (5) *gluconeogenesis,* the conversion of amino acids to glucose.

When glucose is not needed, the body stores it as glycogen. Later, if glucose is needed, the liver can break down glycogen to release glucose. If the blood sugar drops precipitously, gluconeogenesis occurs, which maintains a normal blood glucose.

LIPID (FAT) METABOLISM

The major functions of the liver in relation to fat metabolism are (1) oxidation of fatty acids for energy, (2) formation of most lipoproteins, (3) synthesis of cholesterol and phospholipids, and (4) synthesis of fat from proteins and carbohydrates.

The liver provides energy from fats by splitting them into glycerol and fatty acids, followed by the oxidation of the fatty acids, leading to the release of tremendous amounts of energy. The liver is responsible for a major part of the metabolism of fats.

Most of the cholesterol synthesized in the liver is converted into bile salts, whereas the remainder is transported in the lipoproteins throughout the body. Phospholipids are also synthesized in the liver and transported in lipoproteins. The cholesterol and phospholipids help form cell membranes and intracellular structures and are involved in cellular function.

PROTEIN METABOLISM

Although carbohydrate and fat metabolism are important, human survival depends on the liver's role in protein metabolism. The primary functions of the liver in relation to protein metabolism are (1) deamination of amino acids, (2) formation of urea for the removal of ammonia from the body, (3) formation of plasma proteins, and (4) biotransformation of substances, hormones, drugs, and other chemicals.

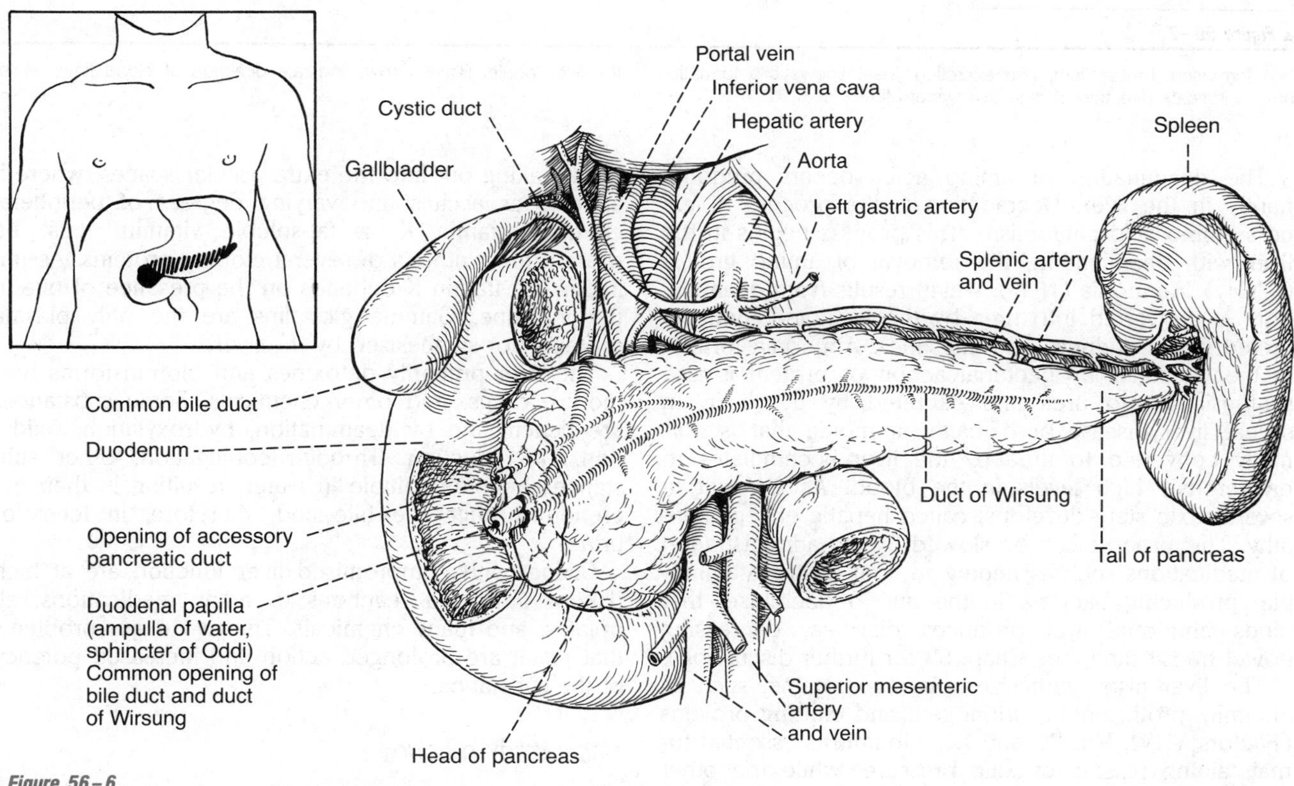

▲ Figure 56-6

Pancreas and adjacent organs. Inset shows anatomic location of pancreas behind stomach.

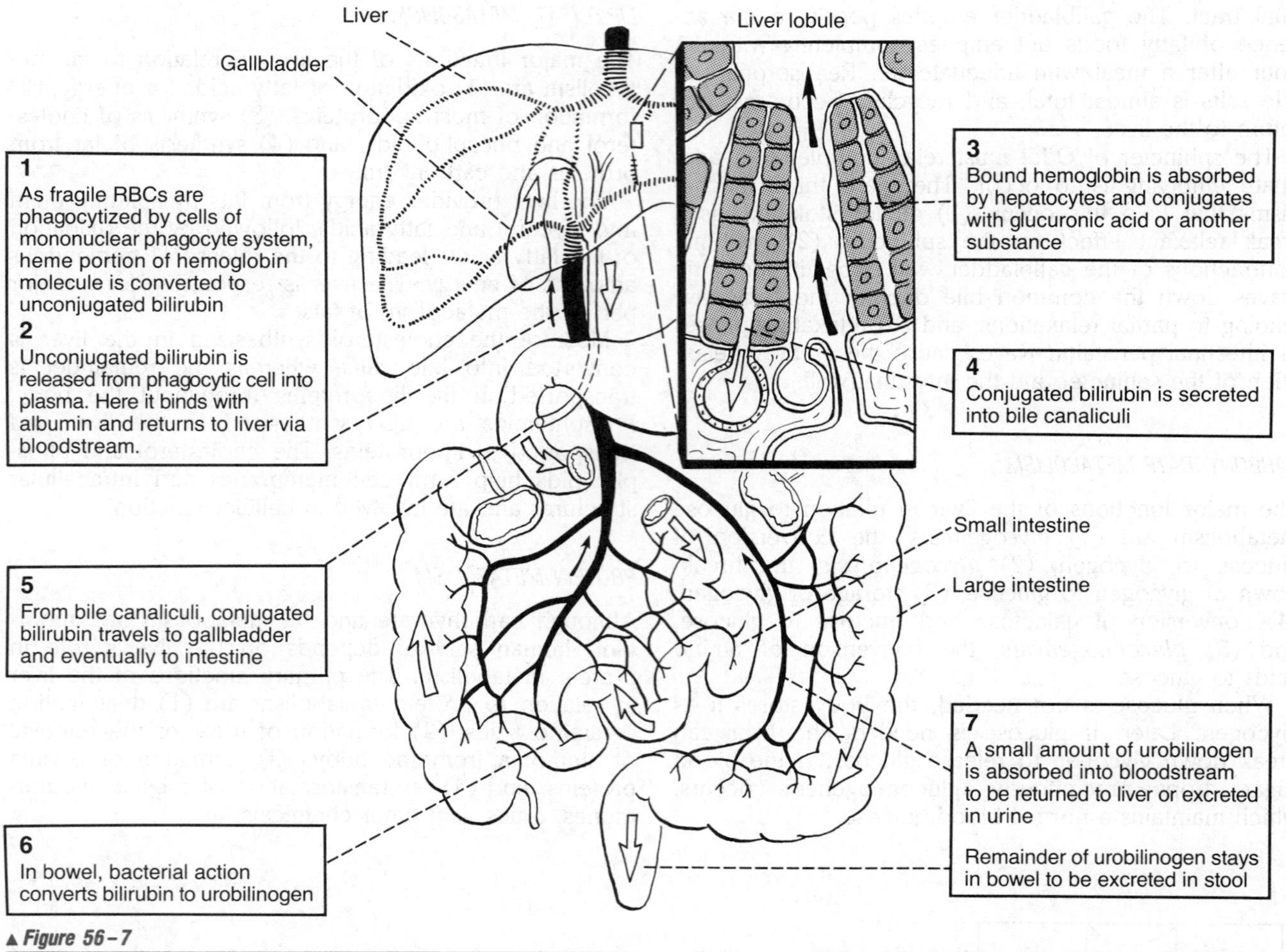

Liver
Gallbladder
Liver lobule
1
As fragile RBCs are phagocytized by cells of mononuclear phagocyte system, heme portion of hemoglobin molecule is converted to unconjugated bilirubin
2
Unconjugated bilirubin is released from phagocytic cell into plasma. Here it binds with albumin and returns to liver via bloodstream.
3
Bound hemoglobin is absorbed by hepatocytes and conjugates with glucuronic acid or another substance
4
Conjugated bilirubin is secreted into bile canaliculi
Small intestine
Large intestine
5
From bile canaliculi, conjugated bilirubin travels to gallbladder and eventually to intestine
7
A small amount of urobilinogen is absorbed into bloodstream to be returned to liver or excreted in urine
Remainder of urobilinogen stays in bowel to be excreted in stool
6
In bowel, bacterial action converts bilirubin to urobilinogen

▲ ***Figure 56-7***

Bile formation, metabolism, and excretion. Inset shows bile formation in the liver lobule. Black arrows indicate direction of blood flow; white arrows indicate direction of digestive system flow.

The deamination of amino acids occurs predominantly in the liver. Degradation is the process of excess amino acid catabolism. This process begins in the liver with deamination, the removal of amino groups ($-NH_2$). Ammonia (NH_3), which results from deamination, is converted into urea by the liver and then excreted by the kidneys and intestines. Ammonia formed in the intestines by bacterial action or protein is also synthesized into urea and excreted by the liver. In severe liver disease or damage, ammonia that is normally converted to urea by the liver accumulates to dangerously high levels in the blood. As a result, a severe toxic state develops, called hepatic encephalopathy. This process can be slowed by the administration of medications such as neomycin, that destroys ammonia, producing bacteria in the gut, or lactulose, that binds ammonia and produces diarrhea, decreasing bowel transit time (see Chap. 58 for further discussion).

The liver also synthesizes plasma proteins, such as albumin, prothrombin, fibrinogen, and clotting proteins (Factors V, VI, VII, IX, and X). Albumin is essential for maintaining plasma oncotic pressure, while the other proteins contribute to blood clotting (see Chap. 45). Plasma oncotic pressure prevents intravascular fluid from leaking out into the extravascular spaces, where it appears as ascites and varying degrees of peripheral edema. Vitamin K, a fat-soluble vitamin, must be present for synthesis of several clotting proteins. Assimilation of vitamin K depends on the presence of bile in the intestine. Gamma globulins are the only plasma proteins not synthesized by the liver.

The liver primarily detoxifies and biotransforms hormones, drugs, and other chemicals. Some substances are deactivated by deamination, hydroxylation, oxidation, or reduction. Through conjugation, other substances become soluble in water, resulting in their excretion through the bile and, therefore, in feces or urine.

Clients with compromised liver function are at high risk of untoward reactions to many medications, all opiates, and many chemicals. The two major problems that result are prolonged action and increased potency of the substance.

CIRCULATORY FUNCTION

The liver processes more than 1000 ml of blood a minute circulating through its sinusoids from the portal vein, and more than 350 ml of blood a minute from the hepatic artery. More than one fourth of the resting cardiac output, therefore, is found in the liver at any given time.

Because of its size and sinusoid passages, the liver is a reservoir for storing large quantities of blood. When major systemic blood loss occurs, the liver provides an emergency blood supply of about 500 ml, or up to 1 liter if the pressure in the right atrium is high.

Blockage within the portal venous system, often caused by cirrhosis, leads to increased pressures within the system, called portal hypertension. The result is an increase in pressure in the venous system draining into the liver, with subsequent distention and a decrease in the flow of blood from the liver to the heart (see Chap. 58 for further discussion).

The blood flowing through the intestine picks up bacteria, which then flows into the liver. Kupffer's cells, the phagocytic macrophages that line the hepatic sinuses, serve as filters that remove bacteria and other debris from the blood as it enters the liver from the portal vein. By engulfing foreign particles, Kupffer's cells render many potential toxins and pathogens harmless. Less than 1 per cent of the bacteria entering the portal system from the intestine pass on to the systemic circulation.

Biliary Tract Functions

The bile ducts and gallbladder function as a collecting and concentrating system and as a reservoir for bile (Fig. 56-7). Following surgical removal of the gallbladder, the bile ducts act as reservoirs and body processes proceed normally, but the ability to excrete large quantities of bile after the ingestion of a fatty meal is lost. The function of the gallbladder was described in detail previously in this chapter.

Exocrine Pancreatic Functions

The pancreas normally produces 1200 to 3000 ml of pancreatic juice daily. Pancreatic juice is a clear alkaline solution carrying three major types of digestive enzymes.

- Pancreatic amylase splits carbohydrates to dextrins and maltose.
- Pancreatic lipase hydrolyzes fat to yield glycerol and fatty acids.
- Pancreatic trypsin is one of a group of enzymes, including chymotrypsin and carboxypolypeptidase, that split proteins.

Trypsin is activated in the intestine, and, in turn, activates other proteolytic enzymes. The pancreas stores a special trypsin inhibitor to prevent autodigestion of pancreatic tissue. A dysfunction of the inhibitor may cause pancreatitis. The pancreatic juices, therefore, digest all three major types of food: proteins, carbohydrates, and fats. These enzymes are all secreted by the acini of the pancreatic glands. These juices also contain large quantities of bicarbonate ions that neutralize the acid chyme from the stomach present in the duodenum. The bicarbonate ions and water are secreted in large amounts mainly by the ductules and ducts leading from the acini. The amount of bicarbonate ion secreted here leads to amounts four to five times higher than that in the plasma.

Pancreatic secretion is stimulated by four basic factors: (1) acetylcholine, from the parasympathetic vagus nerve endings as well as other cholinergic nerves in the enteric nervous system; (2) gastrin, large quantities of which are secreted during the gastric phase of digestion; (3) cholecystokinin, secreted by the duodenum and upper jejunal mucosa when food enters the small intestine; and (4) secretin, secreted by the duodenal and jejunal mucosa when highly acidic food enters the small intestine.

The first three, acetylcholine, gastrin, and cholecystokinin all stimulate the acinar cells more than the ductal cells. This causes large amounts of digestive juices to be secreted, but with little fluid with these enzymes. These enzymes remain stored in the pancreas until they are washed into the duodenum by fluid secretion. Secretin, however, stimulates large amounts of bicarbonate ion to be secreted to neutralize the acidic foods, but causes minimal secretion of the enzymes.

There are three phases of pancreatic secretion. The first is the cephalic phase. During this phase, the release of acetylcholine is stimulated by the same impulses that cause secretion in the stomach. The acetylcholine causes moderate amounts of pancreatic enzymes to be secreted, but little actually flows into the duodenum because there is little water and electrolytes being secreted.

The gastric phase is characterized by further nervous stimulation of enzyme secretion. Also, the large amount of gastrin formed in the stomach stimulates more enzyme secretion. Because there is still little fluid, the enzymes remain in the gland.

During the intestinal phase, chyme enters the intestine, stimulating secretin and drastically increasing the amount of fluid in the pancreatic juice. Cholecystokinin also causes more enzymes to be secreted at the same time.

Secretin stimulates the production of copious amounts of bicarbonate ions without the stimulation of the acinar cells and, therefore, the enzymes. Secretin is released when the pH in the duodenum is less than 4.5, increasing even more if the pH is below 3.0. This immediately results in large amounts of sodium bicarbonate in pancreatic juices being secreted and entering the duodenum. The acid from the stomach is immediately neutralized, stopping all peptic activity. This is a protective mechanism since the mucosa of the small bowel cannot tolerate the acidic pH of the gastric secretions.

Pancreatic enzymes work best in a neutral or slightly alkaline environment. The bicarbonate has a pH of about 8.0, raising the pH of the solution so the pancreatic enzymes function efficiently.

The presence of food in the small intestine stimulates the secretion of cholecystokinin. Cholecystokinin stimulates the secretion of large amounts of pancreatic enzymes by the acinar cells.

PHYSIOLOGIC CHANGES ASSOCIATED WITH AGING

With aging, liver, biliary system, and exocrine pancreatic functions all begin to deteriorate. In the liver, there is a decrease in the number and size of hepatic cells, leading to a decrease in both liver weight and mass. Fibrotic tissue also increases, leading to a decrease in protein synthesis, liver enzymes, and cholesterol synthesis.

The decrease in enzyme activity diminishes the liver's ability to detoxify drugs, increasing the risk of toxic levels of a variety of medications in the elderly.

The pancreas is also affected by the process of aging. There is calcification of the pancreatic vessels, and the size of the ducts change through distention and dilation. These changes lead to a decrease in the production of lipase, resulting in a decrease in fat absorption and digestion. The older client also may experience a decreased absorption of fat-soluble vitamins and an increase of fat excreted through the feces (steatorrhea).

Summary

A thorough knowledge of the structure and function of the liver, biliary tract, and exocrine pancreas will help the nurse provide knowledgeable care to clients with disorders in these areas. In order to provide effective interventions, the nurse must understand the normal physiology of these organs.

Bibliography

1. Arias, I. M., et al. (1988). *The liver: Biology and pathobiology.* New York: Raven Press.
2. Bayless, T. M. (1989). *Current therapy in gastroenterology and liver disease, vol. 3, (3rd ed.).* St. Louis: The C. V. Mosby.
3. Beck, J. E. (Ed.) (1985). *Bockus gastroenterology* (4th ed.). Philadelphia: W. B. Saunders.
4. Bongiovanni, G. L. (Ed.) (1988). *Essentials of clinical gastroenterology* (2nd ed.). New York: McGraw-Hill Book Co.
5. Braunwald, E., et al. (Eds.) (1987). *Harrison's principles of internal medicine* (11th ed.). New York: McGraw-Hill Book Co.
6. Gitnick, G. (Ed.) (1988). *Handbook of gastrointestinal emergencies* (2nd ed.). New York: Elsevier Science Publishing Co.
7. Gitnick, G. (Ed.) (1989). *Modern concepts of acute and chronic hepatitis.* New York: Plenum Publishing Corp.
8. Gitnick, G., et al. (Eds.) (1988). *Principles and practice of gastroenterology and hepatology.* New York: Elsevier Science Publishing Co.
9. Go, V. L. W., et al. (1986). *The exocrine pancreas: Biology, pathobiology, and disease.* New York: Raven Press.
10. Guyton, A. C. (1991). *Textbook of medical physiology* (8th ed.). Philadelphia: W. B. Saunders.
11. Hayworth, M. F., & Jones, A. L. (1988). *Immunology of the gastrointestinal tract and liver.* New York: Raven Press.
12. Johnson, L. R., et al. (1987). *Physiology of the gastrointestinal tract* (2nd ed.). New York: Raven Press.
13. Schiff, L., & Schiff, E. R. (1987). *Diseases of the liver* (3rd ed.). Philadelphia: J. B. Lippincott.
14. Seeff, L. B., & Lewis, J. H. (Eds.) (1989). *Current perspectives in hepatology.* New York: Plenum Publishing Corp.
15. Setchell, K. D. R., et al. (1988). *The bile acids.* New York: Plenum Publishing Corp.
16. Shaffer, E., & Thomson, A. B. R. (1989). *Modern concepts of gastroenterology.* New York: Plenum Publishing Corp.
17. Sherlock, S. (1985). *Diseases of the liver and biliary system.* Oxford: Blackwell Scientific.
18. Sleisenger, M. H., & Fordtran, J. S. (Eds.) (1989). *Gastrointestinal disease: Pathophysiology, diagnosis, and management* (4th ed.). Philadelphia: W. B. Saunders.
19. Soloway, R. D. (Ed.) (1983). *Chronic active liver disease.* New York: Churchill Livingstone.
20. Thomson, J. C., et al. (1987). *Gastrointestinal endocrinology.* New York: McGraw-Hill Book Co.
21. Wyngaardern, J. B., & Smith, L. H. (Eds.) (1988). *Cecil textbook of medicine* (18th ed.). Philadelphia: W. B. Saunders.
22. Zakim, D., & Bayer, T. D. (Eds.) (1990). *Textbook of liver disease* (2nd ed.). Philadelphia: W. B. Saunders.

Chapter 57

Assessment of Clients with Hepatic, Biliary Tract, and Exocrine Pancreatic Disorders

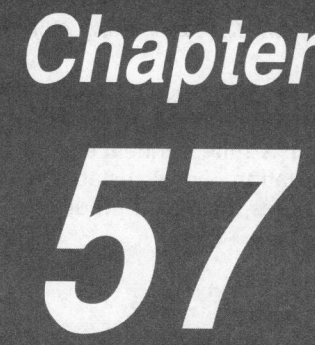

Assessment of the liver, biliary tract, and exocrine pancreas may reveal inflammation, fibrosis, lithiasis, or neoplasms. Underlying causative factors may include poor dietary habits, substance abuse, or environmental problems. Bacteriologic, biochemical, radiographic, and surgical diagnostic procedures provide only partial assessment data. For thorough assessment, analyze the client's presenting symptoms, nutritional status, lifestyle, activities of daily living, and health history.

HISTORY

In assessment of clients with hepatic, biliary, and exocrine pancreatic disturbances, a thorough history includes an account of (1) the present illness and presenting symptoms, (2) recent skin or mucous membrane disruption, and (3) psychosocial history and lifestyle patterns, including environmental and occupational history.

During collection of historical data, help the client recall experiences and onset of symptoms by placing them in a time sequence. Linking events and disease manifestation helps establish the diagnosis and, in some cases, can even predict the course of the disease.

Chief Complaint

Thorough investigation of the client's chief complaint is necessary for accurate assessment. Similar to gastrointestinal symptoms, the symptoms of the hepatic, biliary and pancreatic systems may be vague and have puzzling causes. Each reported symptom is explored by the nurse during the symptom analysis (see Chap. 11).

Common symptoms related to the hepatic, biliary, and pancreatic systems include problems associated with the gastrointestinal, neurologic, genitorurinary, integumentary, or cardiovascular systems. The nurse asks the client about the following symptoms:

Gastrointestinal

- Abdominal pain? Inquire about the site, type, and frequency of pain. Right upper quadrant discomfort suggests gastrointestinal organ dysfunction. The distress may or may not be colicky in nature.
- Nausea?
- Vomiting?
- Anorexia?
- Chronic indigestion? This may be a sign of cholecystitis.
- Fatty food intolerance? This also may be diagnostic of cholecystitis.
- Disturbed bowel pattern? Constipation or diarrhea?
- Melena (blood in the stool)?
- Clay-colored stools?
- Steatorrhea (bulky, foul, fatty stools)?

Neurologic

- Mild depression?
- A clouded sensorium?
- Irritability?
- Drowsiness? Dramatic neurologic symptoms can signal the development of hepatic encephalopathy.

Genitourinary

- Dark yellow or tea-colored urine?

Integument

- Jaundiced skin?

Cardiovascular

- Nose bleeds or bruises easily?
- Hemorrhoids?
- Ascites (fluid accumulation in peritoneal cavity)?
- Edema of limbs?

In addition, the client may have yellow sclerae, fever, intolerance to alcohol, intolerance to medications of any kind, extreme fatigue, and weight loss.

Past Medical History

MAJOR ILLNESSES AND HOSPITALIZATIONS

The client is asked to describe past problems with jaundice, hepatitis, abdominal pain, gallbladder disease, anemia, or changes in bowel elimination such as diarrhea, clay-colored stools, and melena. Has the client ever been hospitalized for any of these problems or ever had surgery of the liver or gallbladder? Ask the client to recall if diagnostic procedures such as a gallbladder x-ray study, liver biopsy, or ultrasound examination of the gallbladder have ever been performed. Has the client ever received a transfusion of blood or blood products?

Recent Skin or Membrane Disruption. Blood tests, transfusions of blood products, dental procedures, ear piercing, tattooing, and any intravenous injection with a potentially contaminated needle are important to assess. Note any unexplained puncture holes. Such breaks in the skin may be the route of entry for hepatitis virus (types B or C) or other pathogens.

MEDICATIONS

Specifically inquire about medications the client is taking currently or previously, including over-the-counter drugs. Many drugs and chemicals are potentially hepatotoxic such as alcohol, gold compounds, mercury, phosphorus, anabolic steroids, acetaminophen, isoniazid, halothane, sulfonamides, arsenic, thiazide diuretics, and anti-cancer drugs such as methotrexate. Other medications to ask about are oral contraceptives, anesthetic agents, and antipsychotic drugs, which may cause liver damage.

Family History

The nurse asks the client if any family members have had cancer (especially of the bowel or liver), jaundice, hepatitis, alcoholism, obesity, or gallbladder disease. Incidence of these problems in family members increase the client's risk status for their occurrence.

Psychosocial History and Lifestyle

Assessment of the client's psychosocial history and lifestyle patterns provide data about his or her physical and psychologic status. Include questions about the client's occupation, environment, and habits.

OCCUPATIONAL AND ENVIRONMENTAL FACTORS

Ask about the client's occupation and work environment. Are there factors present that are known to cause liver damage? For example heavy metals, such as mercury and lead, and chemicals, such as carbon tetrachloride, are known hepatotoxins. Does the client engage in activities that increase the risk of exposure to substances causing hepatitis or pancreatitis? Ask about the following:

- Any close contact with hazardous waste or polluted water
- Travel in hepatitis or pancreatitis endemic areas
- Eating raw or steamed shellfish from polluted water
- Contact with hepatitis-infected animals or people
- Ingestion of mushrooms that were not purchased in a store

HABITS

The nurse asks the client about eating patterns, and use of alcohol and other recreational substances, such as use of illicit drugs.

Eating patterns are important. Investigate

- Food preferences
- Daily consumption of proteins, carbohydrates, fats, and sodium
- Changes in eating patterns, including onset of changes
- Meal preparation—by whom, style of preparation
- Recent development of food intolerances

Carefully explore the client's use of alcohol and other mind-altering substances. Pay attention to alcohol use patterns, because alcoholism often accompanies liver and pancreatic disease, such as fatty infiltration of the liver.

The nurse is alert to whether the client provides confusing or conflicting data. Does the client alter behavior in any way as the assessment proceeds? For example, does the client become angry, silent, or tearful? If significant others are present, do they corroborate the client's story? The client who does not acknowledge a substance abuse problem may not provide reliable information regarding usage. The client who takes illicit drugs may be unwilling to describe drug use patterns. If the client's history is suspected to be unreliable, significant others are asked to provide additional information. (See Chap. 79 for a discussion of alcoholism and other drug use.)

Review of Systems (ROS)

During the ROS, the nurse includes questions about the gastrointestinal system, mental status, genitourinary system, integument, and cardiovascular system (see discussion under "Chief Complaint"). Specifically inquire about jaundice, pruritus (itching), abdominal swelling (edema or ascites), dark-colored urine, clay-colored stools, bleeding tendencies (purpura), spider angioma (spider nevi or telangiectasia), fatigue, and weight loss. Detailed questions for the ROS are found in Chapter 11, Table 11-5.

PHYSICAL EXAMINATION

Physical assessment for liver, biliary, or pancreatic dysfunction involves careful exploration of the entire body.

Begin by assessing the client's general appearance and health status. Is there yellowing of the client's sclerae and integument? (See section on jaundice.) Does the client appear acutely or chronically ill? Is there a tense facial expression or fidgety movement indicating discomfort or pain?

Assess the client's nutritional status. Weigh the client and determine the amount of subcutaneous fat and muscular development. (Nutritional assessment is discussed in Chapter 12.) Obesity may accompany gallbladder disease. Malnutrition may exist in clients with a substance abuse history or cirrhosis. Ascites may account for recent rapid onset of weight gain with accompanying loss of muscle mass.

Next, assess the abdomen. Prior to examination, ask the client to point to any painful area and examine that section last. As stated earlier, hepatic and biliary pain is often located in the right upper quadrant. Pain that is dull and difficult to localize or describe may arise from an organ (viscera). Somatic pain is sharp, bright, easy to localize, and arises from nerve endings in the peritoneum.

Inspect the abdomen for ascites (fluid-filled abdomen) and prominent venous collateral networks common to cirrhosis. Characteristics of ascites include a distended abdomen with tight and glistening skin, bulging flanks, and prominent abdominal veins.

Palpate and percuss the abdomen, especially the liver and spleen. Perform light palpation initially to assess for muscle guarding or tenderness. Observe the client for facial grimaces, tensing, or other indications of discomfort. Next, perform deep palpation to evaluate tenderness, indicating possible inflammation. Light and deep palpation are discussed in Chapter 12. Because the peritoneum is often involved, evaluate for localized peritoneal irritation. Press the abdomen firmly at a point away from any tender area and then quickly remove the examining hand. Severe pain accompanies this maneuver when inflammation is present, indicating rebound tenderness.

Liver size is assessed by percussing the span of the liver at the right midclavicular line (RMCL) and the midsternal line (MSL). The nurse begins by percussing in the RMCL either superior or inferior to the estimated borders of the liver. Superiorly, the nurse begins at the third intercostal space (ICS) over lung resonance and percusses down the thorax until the sound changes to dull. This level is marked on the skin with a pen. Inferiorly, the nurse starts over a tympanic area and percusses upward until the sound changes to dull. This, too, is marked with the pen. At the MSL, the nurse percusses upward from above the umbilicus from tympany to dull and marks the change with the pen. Superiorly, the nurse percusses down the sternum until the percussion note changes. This, too, is marked. The distance between each set of marks is measured. At the RMCL, the liver span ranges from 6 to 12 cm ($2\frac{1}{2}$ to 5 in) and at the MSL, it ranges from 4 to 8 cm ($1\frac{1}{2}$ to 3 in). The lower border of the liver at the RMCL is usually at the right costal margin and the upper border is between the fifth and seventh ICSs. Liver size varies with body size. Measurements larger than the norms indicated liver enlargement. The client is asked to take a deep breath and hold it while the nurse percusses the lower liver border in the RMCL again. Deep inspiration causes the liver to descend lower into the abdomen from pressure of the diaphragm. The distance of liver descent is marked and measured and ranges from 2 to 3 cm (about 1 in). The nurse uses the marked level of liver descent as a guide for later palpation of the liver.

Spleen size may be determined by percussion, particularly if the spleen is enlarged. The spleen is located by percussion as a small area of dullness just posterior to the left midaxillary line (LMAL) between the sixth and tenth ribs. It normally has a span of approximately 7 cm (2½ to 3 in). If the spleen enlarges, the area of dullness shifts inferiorly below the tenth rib and anteriorly toward or beyond the left anterior axillary line (LAAL).

Percussion also is used to assess the presence of ascites in the abdomen by observing for a fluid wave. The client is supine. Two nurses are needed to perform this assessment maneuver. One nurse places the edges of his or her hands on the client's abdominal midline to stabilize the abdominal wall. The second nurse places one hand on one side of the client's abdomen while briskly tapping the opposite side of the abdomen with the other hand. The second nurse feels for the movement of a fluid wave against the palpating hand opposite to the side percussed.

Liver palpation is performed with the nurse standing at the client's right side. One of two bimanual techniques may be used. The nurse places the left hand under the client's right posterior thorax over the eleventh and twelfth ribs and pushes the thorax upward. The right hand is placed below the right costal margin at the previously marked level of liver descent as determined by percussion. The fingers point upward toward the costal margin. The nurse then gently pushes up and in as the client takes a deep breath using the abdominal muscles. As the client inhales, the nurse feels for the liver's edge to slip over the fingertips as it descends. If felt, the liver's edge is firm, sharp, smooth, and regular. The nurse palpates at several points medially and laterally to assess the edge along its inferior border. In the second technique, the nurse places the right hand below the right costal margin as described. The left hand is superimposed on the right hand. The remainder of the maneuver is performed as described earlier. The liver is difficult to palpate in clients who are obese, tense, or have taut abdominal muscles from being physically fit. Abnormal findings include the liver feeling hard, nodular, and tender. If extreme ascites is present, the liver edge will be nonpalpable.

Spleen palpation is performed in a manner similar to that for the liver, except it is on the left side of the abdomen below the costal margin. If percussion has shown that the spleen is enlarged, the nurse does not usually palpate it because of the possibility of rupture. The client is asked to turn onto the right side, allowing gravity to bring the spleen forward and down, closer to the abdominal wall. The nurse places the left hand behind the client's left posterior rib cage and pushes forward while palpating with the right hand. The spleen is normally nonpalpable. Congestion from portal hypertension results in enlargement of the spleen. This is a common finding in cirrhosis.

Blunt percussion (fist percussion) is performed to determine organ tenderness over the liver. This maneuver is performed after all other abdominal assessment techniques are completed to avoid producing discomfort should organ tenderness exist. When assessing for *liver tenderness*, the nurse uses *only* indirect fist percussion over the costal margin at the RMCL to avoid trauma to the liver. This is also known as the "liver tap." For comparison, indirect fist percussion is also performed over the left costal margin at the MCL. The nurse informs the client what is going to be done to avoid the reaction of surprise that may be misinterpreted as tenderness. The client's reaction to the blows is noted.

In addition to assessment of the abdomen, observe for systemic signs suggestive of hepatic, biliary, or pancreatic dysfunction. Such signs include jaundice, purpura, hair loss, weight loss, gynecomastia, spider angiomas, and reddened palms (palmar erythema).

While taking the history and performing physical assessment, continue assessment of the client's mental and neurologic status. Informally observe the client's verbal and nonverbal behavior. Notice facial expressions at rest and while talking. Try to assess the client's mood. Is there evidence of anxiety, depression, apathy, anger, exhaustion, or hostility? If possible, directly question the client regarding sensorium. Note the presence of confusion, disorientation, or lethargy. Question the client's use of alcohol or other drugs. Since handwriting deteriorates with diminishing liver function, record a handwriting sample for subsequent comparison, should the client develop progressive hepatocellular damage (see also Chap. 58).

DIAGNOSTIC TESTS

A client with dysfunction of the liver, biliary tract, or pancreas frequently requires multiple diagnostic measures. No single laboratory test, radiographic study, or surgical procedure yields sufficient data to confirm a diagnosis or establish the degree of malfunction. Afford the individual a sense of self-worth and understanding during repeated diagnostic procedures. This helps gain the person's cooperation and also reduces the fatigue and anxiety that frequently accompany these experiences.

Laboratory Studies

Familiarize yourself with common laboratory tests of liver, biliary, and pancreatic function. Refer to Table 57-1 for a summary of these tests.

Ultrasonography

Ultrasonography uses high-frequency sound waves to examine the interior of the body. In abdominal ultraso-

TABLE 57–1. Laboratory Tests of Liver, Biliary, and Pancreatic Function

Measurement	Normal Value*	Procedure	Interpretation
Biliary Excretion			
Serum bilirubin Direct (conjugated) Indirect (unconjugated) Total	 0.1 to 0.3 mg/100 ml 0.2 to 0.8 mg/100 ml 0.1 to 1.0 mg/100 ml	Blood drawn without special preparation; protect sample from ultraviolet light	Direct bilirubin increased with impaired biliary excretion, causing conjugated fraction to accumulate in plasma Indirect bilirubin increased with excessive erythrocyte hemolysis Total bilirubin measures direct and indirect levels together
Urine bilirubin	0	Urine collection (urine appears smoky or tea-colored); protect from light	Urine bilirubin measures conjugated bilirubin only; increased with impaired bile excretion
Urine urobilinogen	0 to 4 mg/24 hr or 0.1 to 1.0 Ehrlich unit	24-hr or 2-hr afternoon collection placed in brown refrigerated bottle with sodium carbonate	Urine urobilinogen decreased with impaired bile excretion; increased with erythrocyte hemolysis
Fecal urobilinogen	40 to 280 mg/24 hr	Entire stool to laboratory	Fecal urobilinogen decreased with impaired bile excretion; increased in erythrocyte hemolysis
Serum cholesterol	150 to 250 mg/100 ml	Blood drawn after low-cholesterol diet for 12 h	Cholesterol elevated when excretion blocked by bile duct obstruction, but reduced when severe liver damage reduces ability to synthesize it
Carbohydrate Metabolism			
Serum amylase Serum pancreatic isoamylase Urine amylase	80 to 150 Somogyi U/100 ml or 56 to 190 IU/liter (depends on test used)	Blood drawn without special preparation 2-, 12-, or 24-h urine collection with no preservative unless specified	Pancreatic digestive enzyme released with breakdown of acinar cells; serum levels increase 2 to 3 hr after pain onset with pancreatitis and return to normal in 24 to 48 hr; elevations not directly correlated with severity; amylase test measures both pancreatic and salivary amylase; pancreatic isoamylase is a more specific test; urinary levels elevated longer with pancreatitis
Protein Metabolism			
Total protein	6 to 8 gm/100 ml	Blood drawn without special preparation	Less plasma protein synthesized in liver damage (albumin, alpha and beta globulins); gamma globulins produced by plasma cells, not liver
Serum albumin	3.5 to 5.5 gm/100 ml		
Serum globulin Include alpha$_1$, alpha$_2$, beta, gamma	2.5 to 3.5 gm/100 ml		
A/G ratio (albumin/globulin)	1.5/1 to 2.5/1	Same as above	A decrease in the ratio may indicate chronic liver disease
Blood ammonia	<75 μg/100 ml	Blood drawn without special preparation	Reduced synthesis of urea from body ammonia in severe hepatocellular damage produces elevated blood ammonia
Methemalbumin	Absent	Fluid from peritoneal or pleural tap analyzed	Product of hemoglobin digestion elevated when blood released into body fluids, as in hemorrhagic pancreatitis
Fat Metabolism			
Serum lipase	0 to 1.5 U	Blood drawn from fasting person	Pancreatic digestive enzyme released with breakdown of acinar cells

Table continued on following page

TABLE 57–1. Laboratory Tests of Liver, Biliary, and Pancreatic Function Continued

Measurement	Normal Value*	Procedure	Interpretation
Metabolism of Foreign Substances			
Bromsulphalein (BSP) excretion	<5% retention in 1 hr	Control blood taken after fasting for 12 h, BSP given, blood drawn at intervals	Dye retained with diminished hepatocellular ability to remove it from blood and excrete it; infrequently used
Serum Enzymes†			
Aspartate aminotransferase (AST) (formerly SGOT)	5 to 40 U/ml	Blood drawn without special preparation	Serum aspartate aminotransferase, alanine aminotransferase, and lactic dehydrogenase released from damaged liver, heart, kidney, and muscle cells; levels not directly correlated with degree of damage; elevations above 400 U accompany acute hepatocellular alteration
Alanine aminotransferase (ALT) (formerly SGPT)	5 to 35 U/ml		
Lactate dehydrogenase (LDH)	Varies with units used		
Alkaline phosphatase (ALP)	Varies with method and age of person	Blood drawn without special preparation	Increase in biliary obstruction; produced by cells lining the biliary tract; this enzyme is also found in bone, intestine, and placenta
Serum 5′-nucleotidase	0.3 to 3.2 Bodansky units	Blood drawn without special preparation	Enzyme located mainly in liver and confirmation of liver disease occurs if ALP and this both elevated
Serum gamma glutamyl transpeptidase (GGTP)	<65 IU/liter	Blood drawn without special preparation	Enzyme located in liver and kidney; elevation of GGTP and ALP significant indication of liver disorders
Hepatitis Antigens and Antibodies	Negative for antigens Positive or negative for antibodies, depending on history	Blood drawn without special preparation	Antigens indicate hepatitis; antibodies indicate past or present hepatitis or immunization (hepatitis B)
Hemostatic Function			
Prothrombin time (PT)	12 to 15 sec	Blood drawn without special preparation	Assesses function of extrinsic pathway in clotting process (factors I, II, V, VII, X) PT prolonged with (1) decreased synthesis due to liver cell damage or (2) decreased vitamin K absorption due to bile duct obstruction Vitamin K necessary for liver to synthesize prothrombin (factor II)
Platelets	150,000 to 400,000/mm³	Blood drawn without special preparation	May fall when spleen is enlarged in portal hypertension
Exocrine Pancreatic Function		Oral bentiromide given after overnight fast; urine is collected for 6 h	Pancreatic chymotrypsin splits bentiromide; para-aminobenzoic acid (PABA), a breakdown product, is excreted in urine; less PABA is excreted with pancreatic insufficiency
Antigens Associated with Cancer			
Alpha-fetoprotein (AFP)	<10 ng/mg	Blood drawn without special preparation	AFP is synthesized by fetus but not by healthy adult; AFP level >1000 ng/ml usually indicates hepatocellular carcinoma

* Normal values may differ significantly between laboratories.

† Trends in elevation are of particular importance in predicting the rapidity with which the liver is failing. If levels rise, fall, then rise again, liver failure may be occurring.

nography, the examiner passes a transducer over the abdomen. The technique proceeds rapidly and requires little or no preparation. Depending on the area to be examined, the individual may or may not fast prior to the procedure. Ultrasonography is noninvasive and generally accurate. Because it does not involve x-rays, it is safe for pregnant women. It lacks the ionizing radiation or other untoward side effects of radiologic procedures using contrast media. (A discussion of radiologic techniques follows.) Because of the low risk involved, the health practitioner may recommend ultrasonography as the initial diagnostic study.

Ultrasonographic examination provides valuable diagnostic information for liver, pancreatic, and biliary tract conditions. It is a valuable diagnostic tool for presence of tumors as well as patency of vessels.

Radiologic Studies

Many of the procedures used to diagnose disorders of the liver, pancreas, and biliary tract involve the use of x-rays. Plain x-ray films of the abdomen may show diaphragm elevation due to hepatic enlargement or calcification in the abdominal organs. Upper or lower gastrointestinal series using barium contrast medium also provide important information about the accessory organs of digestion, that is, the liver, gallbladder, and pancreas.

Radiologic studies using iodinated contrast media permit visualization of tubes or vessels. Before all of these procedures, question the person about known hypersensitivity to iodine or seafood.

ORAL CHOLECYSTOGRAPHY (GALLBLADDER SERIES)

This is an x-ray test for gallbladder or cystic duct disease. Oral cholecystography has been the standard examination for gallstone detection for almost 50 years. Although still clinically useful, it does predispose the client undergoing study to greater risks than does the similarly accurate cholecystosonography.

The evening before the examination, the client ingests a radiopaque dye determined by the fat content of the evening meal. If the client has a regular or low-fat dinner, the client may receive sodium ipodate (Oragrafin). After a high-fat dinner, the client must be given iopanoic acid (Telepaque). These dyes contain iodine. Carefully observe the client for allergic reactions even when the health history reveals no known allergies to iodine or seafood. Possible hypersensitive reactions include nausea and vomiting, diarrhea, abdominal pain, rash, and anaphylaxis.

Conjugation of the dye occurs in the liver. Be aware that these dyes are potentially toxic to the liver and kidneys. This is especially true in clients with preexisting hepatic or renal failure.

Following excretion of the opaque medium into the bile, the gallbladder concentrates the contrast medium.

During the test, radiography permits visualization of the gallbladder. When contraction of the gallbladder is desirable, the client consumes a high-fat meal during the procedure. Following an oral cholecystogram, some people experience burning on urination due to the presence of the dye in the urine. Forcing fluids decreases this problem.

Poor or no visualization of the gallbladder indicates gallbladder disease, presumably because biliary obstruction prevents passage of the dye. Occasionally, stones can be visualized as shadows within the opaque medium. The test results are accurate only when gastrointestinal and liver function allow absorption and conjugation of the dye.

CHOLANGIOGRAPHY

A cholangiogram or cholangiopancreatogram allows visualization of the bile ducts. Following administration of an organic iodine dye called iodipamide meglumine (Cholografin), x-ray filming begins.

Again, assess for iodine allergies. Possible allergic reactions include dyspnea, tachycardia, sweating, nausea, vomiting, and chills.

Also, to prevent renal damage, instruct the client to drink ample amounts of fluid following administration of the dye.

There are four types of cholangiograms.

1. Intravenous cholangiography is used for common bile duct visualization. The radiopaque dye burns intensely upon injection.
2. Percutaneous cholangiography involves injecting the dye directly into the ductal system, directly through the skin via a long, slender needle.
3. Retrograde cholangiography involves passage of an endoscope through the mouth into the duodenum. After location of the ampulla of Vater, the examiner passes a catheter into the common bile duct and, possibly, the pancreatic duct. Dye is injected through the catheter into the duct.
4. T-tube cholangiography involves injecting dye into the preexisting bile drainage tube.

In all four types of cholangiography, failure of the opaque dye to pass through the bile ducts provides evidence of duct obstruction.

ANGIOGRAPHY

This x-ray procedure allows visualization of the visceral vessels in order to identify abnormalities of vascular structure and function, observe masses, and note sites of bleeding. Angiography is helpful in the study of the pancreas, spleen, and portal system. Recall that it is also employed in diagnosing disorders of the kidneys, lower extremities, and gastrointestinal tract. To inject the contrast media, the examiner usually introduces a needle into the femoral artery. Next, the needle is exchanged for a catheter, which is then passed into the celiac artery or one of its branches (superior mesenteric or hepatic). After contrast media injection, rapid sequence filming is done.

Following angiography, assess the needle insertion site for signs of bleeding, because with liver conditions clients often have concurrent clotting disorders.

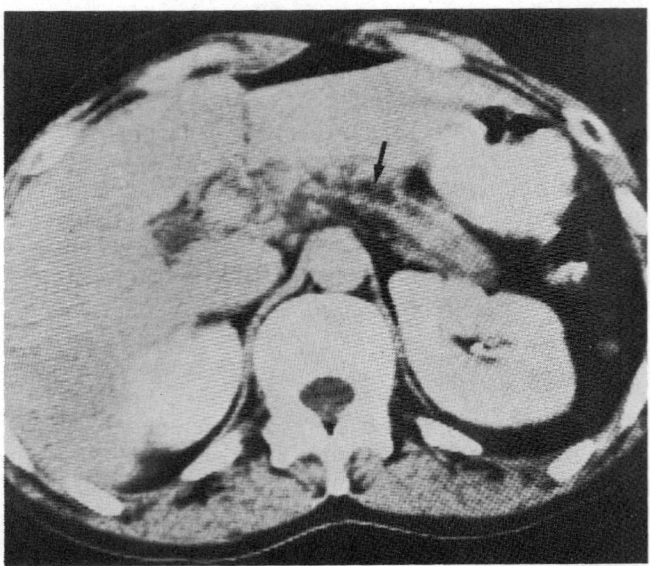

▲ **Figure 57-1**

CT scan of chronic pancreatitis. There is pancreatic atrophy and a dilated pancreatic duct *(arrow)* but no evidence of pancreatic calcification. (From Moss, A. A., et al. [1983]. *Computed tomography of the body.* Philadelphia: W. B. Saunders.)

COMPUTED TOMOGRAPHY

Computed tomography (CT) is another radiologic technique used to diagnose and evaluate liver, biliary tract, and gallbladder disease. A CT scan is performed by rotating a finely focused x-ray beam around the client. A computer then assembles data from the detector and provides an image. The constructed image yields a cross-sectional view (Fig. 57-1). Contrast media, when used, enhance the picture. Very dense structures, such as bone, appear white; less dense matter is gray; air is black.

Radionuclide Scanning

Radionuclide scanning, or scintigraphy, involves the intravenous infusion of gamma-emitting isotopes. Following infusion, a scintillation detector passes over the abdomen. This procedure investigates biliary duct patency and indicates whether a tumor or abscess is present in the liver, gallbladder, or pancreas. Useful isotopes include colloidal gold (^{198}Au), gallium (^{67}Ga), technetium (^{99}Tc), and selenium (^{75}Se). ^{67}Ga accumulates in inflamed tissue. ^{99}Tc evaluates liver and biliary tract function. ^{75}Se is useful in identifying pancreatic abnormalities.

Paracentesis

The purpose of paracentesis, or peritoneal tap, is to extract fluid accumulations in the peritoneum (ascites) to relieve intra-abdominal tension, which can impair the client's respiratory status, or to obtain the fluid to send for culture. The nurse actively participates in this procedure, which usually takes place at the bedside. Beforehand, instruct the client regarding the purpose of the procedure and the steps involved, and obtain written permission. Ask the client to void immediately prior to the procedure to decrease the risk of bladder puncture. Have the client sit upright on the edge of the bed, with feet resting on a stool and back well supported. Following cleansing of the skin and infiltration with a local anesthetic, the physician, using sterile technique, inserts a long aspirating needle with a syringe to collect a fluid specimen. To drain ascitic fluid (if desired), the physician inserts a trocar aseptically through a small stab wound below the umbilicus. This allows fluid (usually several liters) to drain slowly through a catheter into a collection bottle.

The major complication of paracentesis is *hypovolemia* and shock secondary to fluid drainage from the peritoneum, and the resulting fluid shift from intravascular to interstitial space as well as the sudden change in intra-abdominal pressure on the vessels. This fluid shift is exacerbated by hypoalbuminemia.

Assess vital signs and peripheral circulation every few minutes during and immediately following paracentesis. Observe for hypovolemic shock: pallor, tachycardia, decreased blood pressure, and oliguria and dyspnea.

Hepatic encephalopathy due to reduced tissue perfusion is another complication arising from drainage of ascitic fluid. Because of the high protein concentration of ascitic fluid, the physician may prescribe albumin infusions for 24 hours following paracentesis to compensate for protein losses. Potassium depletion may occur following multiple paracentesis procedures. Infection, peritonitis, and bleeding due to vessel trauma occasionally complicate paracentesis.

Carefully assess for abdominal pain following paracentesis. Monitoring the site for persistent leakage of ascites is also important.

Peritoneoscopy

Insertion of a peritoneoscope through an abdominal stab wound permits direct visualization of the liver and peritoneum. Visualization of structural changes aids in the diagnosis of cirrhosis and cancer. During peritoneoscopy, the examiner may take photographs and perform a biopsy.

Peritoneoscopy is relatively safe and simple. Contraindications include infections of the abdominal cavity, clotting disorders, or intestinal obstruction. In addition, the person must be able to cooperate throughout the procedure. Obesity and ascites interfere with test results.

To prepare an individual for peritoneoscopy:

- Check that written consent has been obtained.
- Check the laboratory record to make certain the person has normal or adequate clotting factors. If not, inform the physician.

- Check the client and health care record for contraindications to pre-procedural medications.
- Inquire as to whether the client is sensitive to local anesthetics.
- Prepare the skin, and administer pre-procedural medication when appropriate.
- Instruct the client to take nothing by mouth and to empty the bowel and bladder just before the procedure begins.
- Provide adequate teaching before and during the actual procedure.
- Explain that it may be difficult to breathe when air is placed into the abdominal cavity.
- Instruct the client to elevate the abdominal wall by holding the breath to protect major organs during needle insertion.

When peritoneoscopy includes liver biopsy, 24 hours of bed rest follow the procedure. If biopsy is not performed, the person resumes activity following recovery from effects of medication. Complications are uncommon and more often occur secondary to biopsy.

Possible post-peritoneoscopy complications are pneumothorax, subcutaneous emphysema, air embolism, bile peritonitis, perforation of a hollow organ, and shoulder or abdominal pain.

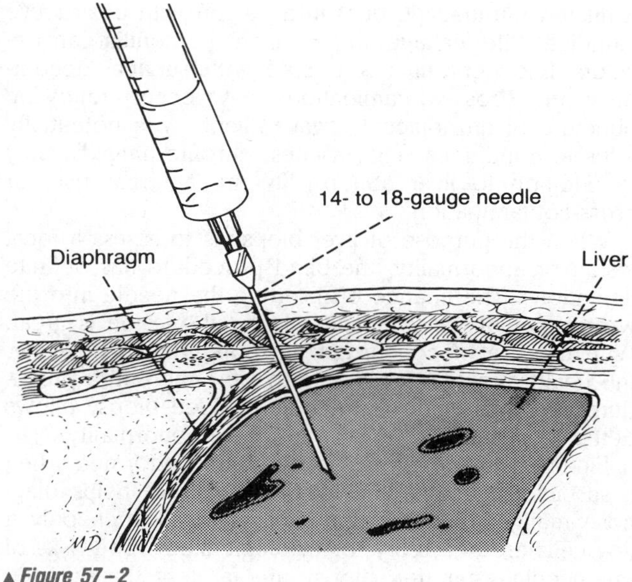

▲ *Figure 57–2*

Percutaneous liver biopsy requires cooperation. The individual must be able to lie quietly and hold his or her breath after exhaling.

Biopsy

Biopsy is the single most valuable diagnostic study to the physician. It involves the removal of a sample of living tissue for analysis. Biopsies may be open or closed procedures. An open biopsy necessitates a general anesthetic and a major abdominal incision. A client may have an open biopsy at the time of a concurrent operative procedure. An advantage of the open biopsy is that the surgeon can observe the entire liver, identify grossly altered tissue, and remove the biopsy specimen for study.

A closed biopsy or percutaneous liver biopsy is a simpler procedure than open biopsy. It involves aspiration of a core of tissue via needle for histologic study. The conventional percutaneous liver biopsy is a blind procedure (Menghini's technique). The primary limitation of Menghini's technique is that the surgeon is unable to see where the needle is going. Nevertheless, this procedure may be appropriate for determining the cause of general hepatic disease (diffuse parenchymal involvement).

Contraindications to percutaneous liver biopsy are severe thrombocytopenia, local infection of lung base, prolonged prothrombin time, peritonitis, massive ascites, an uncooperative client, and extrahepatic obstructive jaundice, especially with an enlarged gallbladder. The client with cancer or amyloidosis has an increased risk of post-procedure hemorrhage. Also, if the client is unable to remain still and cooperate during the procedure, the surgeon could accidentally puncture an organ.

To prepare for percutaneous liver biopsy, the client fasts for at least 6 hours before the test. The procedure is usually performed at the bedside using a local anesthetic. Place the client either in the supine position or in a lateral position with the upper arm elevated. Less frequently, you may ask the person to assume a prone position. During insertion of the needle, have the client exhale and then hold the breath on expiration for 5 to 10 seconds to avoid puncturing of the diaphragm (Fig. 57–2).

Following percutaneous liver biopsy, perform the following nursing assessments and interventions:

- Monitor vital signs for the first 8 to 12 hours.
- Carefully assess for tachycardia and decreasing blood pressure, which may indicate hemorrhage.
- Observe for pain in the right upper quadrant of the abdomen due to a subcapsular accumulation of blood or bile, or at the right shoulder as a result of blood on the undersurface of the diaphragm.
- Maintain the client on bed rest for 24 hours following the procedure. The right side-lying position for the first 1 to 2 hours decreases the risk of hemorrhage and bile leakage.
- Administer post-procedure medications on an individual basis, depending on the person's physical status.
- Give vitamin K if prescribed.
- Assess respiratory status for signs of dyspnea.

Inherent risks following biopsy include hemorrhage and puncture of adjacent organs or structures. Hemorrhage, the most serious complication, may result from penetration of the arterial tree or a distended vein radicle. Hemorrhage may occur during the first 24 hours after the biopsy procedure. The risk of hemorrhage is increased if vascular channels are distended or if the individual breathes during needle insertion into the liver. Puncture of a lung can cause pneumothorax. A large biopsy needle (14- to 18-gauge) can penetrate a dilated intrahepatic duct in a person with obstructive jaundice. Bile leakage and resultant peritonitis can develop. Bile peritonitis is treated with surgical decompression. Cross-contamination may occur following puncture of an adjacent organ. Clients with potentially effusive conditions (e.g., ascites, chronic lung disease) in addition to liver abnormality are at great risk for cross-contamination.

When the purpose of liver biopsy is to assess a focal lesion or abnormality, the blind procedure has definite limitations. The chance of inserting the needle into the wrong part of the liver and missing the lesion is great. With the use of concurrent ultrasonography, however, the health practitioner is able to view the entire procedure and thus guide the needle. Guided biopsy allows better localization of a focal lesion or abnormality.

Fine-needle aspiration biopsy, often performed when a suspicious area of the liver is localized, helps diagnose malignancy. This approach is ideal when only a few cells are necessary for cytologic study. The risks of fine-needle aspiration biopsy are far less than guided regular biopsy, since the tissue sample is much smaller. Also, this procedure greatly reduces any risk of tumor metastasis along the needle track.

There are few contraindications to the guided regular or fine-needle aspiration biopsy procedures. People with impaired coagulation associated with liver disease, however, may not be appropriate candidates for the closed procedure. When biopsy is indicated for these clients, a new "plugged" biopsy procedure[28a] minimizes the risk of hemorrhage. This procedure allows injection of absorbable gelatin material on withdrawal of the biopsy needle. The gelatin material applies pressure to the bleeding site and closes the potential track. The client must be able to hold his or her breath for a period of up to 15 seconds.

Portal Pressure Measurements

Measurements of portal pressure and flow help to (1) diagnose portal hypertension, (2) indicate the severity of portal hypertension, and (3) guide decisions as to appropriate intervention, which may include surgery. Also, the indirect calculation of sinusoid pressure helps determine the location of an obstruction in the liver and thus identify the underlying disorder.

Portal pressure measurements are minor surgical procedures that are performed in the operating room or a special studies laboratory. Often, the surgeon concurrently injects contrast media. These measures require standard preoperative and postoperative care, with special postoperative assessment of the incision site for hematoma formation.

The major portal pressure measurements are

- Wedged hepatic vein pressure (WHVP). In this procedure, portal pressure is obtained indirectly by percutaneous hepatic vein catheterization. The examiner uses either an arm vein or a femoral vein.
- Umbilical vein catheterization. This procedure allows the direct measurement of portal pressure.
- Splenic pulp manometry. During manometry, the examiner places a needle between two of the lower ribs, inserting a manometer into the spleen.

Instruct the person to hold his or her breath during needle insertion and passage. Carefully observe for bleeding or pneumothorax afterward.

Analysis of Duodenal or Biliary Drainage

Duodenal and biliary drainage analysis assists in the diagnosis of cholelithiasis when the cholecystogram is inconclusive. Also, these procedures provide an alternative for clients allergic to iodine who cannot undergo cholecystography or cholangiography.

To prepare for the test, instruct the client to fast for 8 hours before the study. The study involves insertion of a single-lumen nasogastric tube into the stomach. Stomach contents are aspirated and the tube slowly advanced until the aspirate changes to clear, golden, and alkaline. At this point, the tube is in the duodenum, and clear golden bile (sometimes called "A" bile) is collected.[9]

The next step is to increase the flow of bile into the duodenum. Instillation of magnesium sulfate into the tube, or intravenous administration of secretin (sometimes followed by pancreozymin), stimulates bile flow. After administering these bile flow stimulants, it should be possible to aspirate 30 to 60 ml of concentrated bile from the duodenum, sometimes known as "B" bile. Bile can also be collected through an endoscope.

Collected fluid is sent to the laboratory to be analyzed for volume and bicarbonate, enzyme, and bile content. Disproportions in the bile and pancreatic juice fractions indicate obstruction in the bile or pancreatic duct. The presence of cholesterol crystals indicates lithiasis.

Summary

Once the nurse has a thorough knowledge of the structure and function of the liver, biliary tract, and exocrine pancreas, the nurse must examine the diagnostic assessment of these organs. Systematic assessment of the client with possible disorders in the liver, biliary tract, and exocrine pancreas can lead to prompt diagnosis and treatment. The nurse can facilitate this diagnostic process by adequately preparing the client for the diagnostic procedures and by assisting with or actually collecting assessment data.

Bibliography

1. Arias, I. M., et al. (1988). *The liver: Biology and pathobiology.* New York: Raven Press.
2. Axon, A. T. (1989). Endoscopic retrograde cholangiopancreatography in chronic pancreatitis: Cambridge classification. *Radiologic Clinics of North America, 27*(1), 39–50.
3. Balthazar, E. J. (1989). CT diagnosis and staging of acute pancreatitis. *Radiologic Clinics of North America, 27*(1), 19–37.
4. Bayless, T. M. (1989). *Current therapy in gastroenterology and liver disease* (vol. 3, 3rd ed.). St. Louis: The C. V. Mosby Co.

5. Berne, R., & Levy, M. (Eds). (1988). *Physiology* (2nd ed.). St. Louis: The C. V. Mosby Co.
6. Bongiovanni, G. L. (Ed.) (1988). *Essentials of clinical gastroenterology* (2nd ed.). New York: McGraw-Hill Book Co.
7. Braunwald, E., et al. (Eds.) (1987). *Harrison's principles of internal medicine* (11th ed.). New York: McGraw-Hill Book Co.
8. Clouse, M. E. (1989). Current diagnostic imaging modalities of the liver. *Surgical Clinics of North America, 69*(2), 193–234.
9. DaCunha, J. P., et al. (1985). *Nurse's clinical library, gastrointestinal disorders*. Springhouse, PA: Springhouse Corporation.
10. Early test for liver cancer. (1984). *Science Digest, 92,* 40.
11. Ebersol, P., & Hess, P. (1989). *Toward healthy aging: Human needs and nursing response* (3rd ed.). St. Louis: The C. V. Mosby Co.
12. Foster, P., et al. (1984). Prospective comparison of three noninvasive tests for pancreatic disease. *British Medical Journal 289,* 13.
13. Gallbladder disease induced by parenteral nutrition (1985). *American Family Physician, 31,* 310.
14. Gillinsky, N. H. (1987). The role of pancreatic function testing in the 1980's. *South African Medical Journal, 71*(4), 235–238.
15. Gitnick, G., et al (Eds.) (1988). *Principles and practice of gastroenterology and hepatology*. New York: Elsevier Science Publishing Co.
16. Go, V. L. W., et al. (1986). *The exocrine pancreas: Biology, pathobiology, and disease*. New York: Raven Press.
17. Granger, D. N., et al. (1985). *Clinical gastrointestinal physiology*. Philadelphia: W. B. Saunders.
18. Guyton, A. C. (1991). *Textbook of medical physiology* (8th ed.). Philadelphia: W. B. Saunders.
19. Haynes, J., et al. (1982). Hereditary pancreatitis. *American Family Physician 25,* 153.
20. Hayworth, M. F., & Jones, A. L. (1988). *Immunology of the gastrointestinal tract and liver*. New York: Raven Press.
21. Heiss, F., et al. (1984). Common bile duct calculi: nonsurgical therapy. *Postgraduate Medicine, 75,* 109.
22. Heiss, F., et al. (1984). Common bile duct calculi: surgical therapy. *Postgraduate Medicine, 75,* 88.
23. Holland, P., & Hussain, I. (1989). Biliary lithotripsy: Nonsurgical treatment of gallstones. *Society of Gastrointestinal Assistants Journal, 3,* 158–162.
24. Jeffery, R. B. (1989). Sonography in acute pancreatitis. *Radiologic Clinics of North America, 27*(1), 5–17.
25. Johnson, L. R., et al. (1987). *Physiology of the gastrointestinal tract* (2nd ed.). New York: Raven Press.
26. Kosel, K., et al. (1982). Total pancreatectomy and islet cell autotransplantation. *American Journal of Nursing, 82,* 568.
27. Kozarek, R. A., & Sanowski, R. A. (1981). Endoscopic papillotomy. *American Family Physician, 23,* 111.
28. Levitt, M. D. (1985). Pancreatitis. In J. B. Wyngaarden, & L. H. Smith, Jr. (Eds.), *Cecil textbook of medicine* (17th ed.). Philadelphia: W. B. Saunders.
28a. Liver biopsy (1985). *American Family Physician, 31*(4), 238.
29. Liver biopsy with a view (1984). *Emergency Medicine, 16,* 127.
30. Maddrey, W. C. (1984). Axioms on chronic hepatitis. *Hospital Medicine, 13,* 6.
31. Marta, M. R. (1987). Endoscopic retrograde cholangeopancreatography: Its role in diagnosis and treatment. *Focus on Critical Care, 14*(5), 62–63.
32. Mosley, J. W., et al. (1990). Non-A, non-B hepatitis and antibody to hepatitis C virus. *JAMA, 263,* 77–78.
33. Pancreatitis from mercaptopurine: Nurses' drug alert. (1985). *American Journal of Nursing, 9,* 68.
34. Rakel, R. E. (1990). *Conn's current therapy*. Philadelphia: W. B. Saunders.
35. Rifkin, M. D., et al. (1984). Detection of liver and gallbladder calcification. *American Family Physician, 29,* 247.
36. Sabiston, D. C., Jr. (1991). *Textbook of surgery: The biologic basis of modern surgical practice* (14th ed.). Philadelphia: W. B. Saunders.
37. Schiff, L., & Schiff, E. R. (1987). *Diseases of the liver (3rd ed.).* Philadelphia: J. B. Lippincott.
38. Schroeder, S. A., et al. (1988). *Current medical diagnosis and treatment*. Norwalk, CT: Appleton & Lange.
39. Seeff, L. B., & Lewis, J. H. (Eds.) (1989). *Current perspectives in hepatology*. New York: Plenum Publishing Corp.
40. Septimus, E. J. (1984). Seroprevalence of hepatitis B markers in health-care workers at a teaching medical center at two community hospitals. *Advances in Therapy, 1,* 215.
41. Sleisenger, M. H., & Fordtran, J. S. (Eds.) (1989). *Gastrointestinal disease: Pathophysiology, diagnosis, and management* (4th ed.). Philadelphia: W. B. Saunders.
42. Swenson, S. A. (1984). Diagnosis: hepatic neoplasms. *Hospital Medicine, 20,* 190.
43. Toskes, P. P. (1983). Bentiromide as a test of exocrine pancreatic function in adult patients with exocrine insufficiency. *Gastroenterology, 85,* 565.
44. Van Landingham, S., & Roberts, J. (1984). Pancreatic pseudocyst. *Hospital Medicine, 20,* 71.
45. VanSonneberg, E., et al. (1989). Imaging and interventional radiology for pancreatitis and its complications. *Radiologic Clinics of North America, 27*(1), 65–72.
46. Widmann, F. (1987). *Goodall's clinical interpretation of laboratory tests* (10th ed.). Philadelphia: F. A. Davis.
47. Witkin, G. B., et al. (1987). Choosing liver function tests. *Emergency Medicine, 19*(20), 22–46.
48. Wyngaarden, J. B., & Smith, L. H. (Eds.) (1988). *Cecil textbook of medicine* (18th ed.). Philadelphia: W. B. Saunders.
49. Yatto, R., & Siegel, J. (1984). Cholestasis: an alternative to surgery in older patients. *Geriatrics, 39,* 113.
50. Zakim, D., & Boyer, T. D. (Eds.) (1990). *Textbook of liver disease* (2nd ed.). Philadelphia: W. B. Saunders.

Chapter 58

Nursing Care of Clients with Hepatic Disorders

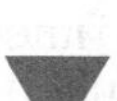

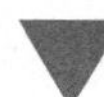

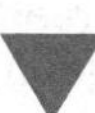

HEPATIC DISORDERS

Jaundice

Definition

Jaundice, or icterus, is the yellow pigmentation of the sclerae, skin, and deeper tissues due to excessive accumulation of bile pigments in the blood. Bilirubin (bile pigment), a product of red blood cell breakdown, is deposited in the skin and excreted in the urine when present in the blood in excessive amounts (hyperbilirubinemia). This characteristic makes jaundice a valuable indicator for a variety of disorders involving either hemolysis or biliary obstruction. When there is an obstruction blocking the flow of bile into the intestine, jaundiced individuals may have clay-colored stools due to the lack of bilirubin and its metabolites in the intestine. For a description of normal bilirubin metabolism, see Figure 56-7.

Etiology

Jaundice can be classified according to the location of the pathologic change. Jaundice may occur because of a problem (1) in the blood before reaching the liver (prehepatic jaundice), (2) within the liver itself (hepatic jaundice), or (3) after the bilirubin leaves the liver (post-hepatic or obstructive jaundice). The pathologic causes underlying these three types of jaundice are outlined briefly here and in more detail in Table 58-1.

PREHEPATIC JAUNDICE

Prehepatic jaundice results from excessive red blood cell destruction. It may be due to transfusion reactions, hemolytic anemia, severe burns, or defective albumin binding. The liver normally compensates for the increased unconjugated bilirubin it receives by increasing its rate of bilirubin conjugation. The excess can then be excreted in the urine and feces. Prehepatic jaundice disappears once the rate of hemolysis slows.

HEPATIC JAUNDICE

Hepatic jaundice is due to defective uptake, conjugation, or transport of bilirubin within the liver. Liver cell dysfunction or necrosis caused by hepatitis, for example, or defective bile transport in the bile canal and small bile duct can cause hyperbilirubinemia. Stagnation of bile in the hepatic cells or in the intrahepatic or extrahepatic bile ducts is called cholestasis. Unknown channels absorb the pooled bile components into the bloodstream. Although "obstructive jaundice" usually refers to posthepatic jaundice, an obstruction within the liver can make this term appropriate for hepatic jaundice as well.

POSTHEPATIC (OBSTRUCTIVE) JAUNDICE

Posthepatic (obstructive) jaundice results from impaired bilirubin transport and excretion in the biliary system. In this case, the problem arises from obstruction of an extrahepatic bile duct, for example, occlusion of the common duct by gallstones.

Clinical Manifestations

Manifestations of jaundice include yellow sclera, yellowish-orange skin, clay-colored feces, tea-colored urine, pruritus, fatigue, and anorexia.

Diagnostic Assessment

Table 58-1 presents the laboratory diagnostic tests that are used to identify the underlying cause and type of jaundice. The following are diagnostic tests consistent with jaundice:

- Increased levels of direct (conjugated) serum bilirubin (>0.4 mg/100 ml) because bilirubin returns to the plasma when it cannot be excreted
- Increased indirect (unconjugated) serum bilirubin values (>0.8 mg/100 ml)
- Absence of bilirubin in the urine (unconjugated bilirubin is water soluble)
- Increased urine urobilinogen (>4 mg/24 h)
- Reduced fecal urobilinogen (<40 mg/24 h) because it does not reach the intestine
- Increased alkaline phosphatase and cholesterol serum levels because they cannot be excreted into the bile as normal
- In extreme cases of fulminant liver failure, unusually low cholesterol level, indicating the liver's inability to synthesize it at all
- Increased serum bile salts with consequent deposition in the skin, causing pruritus
- Prolonged prothrombin time (>40 seconds) owing to reduced absorption of fat-soluble vitamin K

Medical Management

Treatment for jaundice aims to resolve the underlying disease. See Chapter 46 for a discussion of interventions in hemolytic anemia (prehepatic anemia). Time and rest compose the primary treatment for resolution of jaundice in hepatitis. Treatments for hepatic jaundice are discussed later. Treatments for posthepatic jaundice include dissolution therapy or surgical removal of the obstruction.

Surgical Management

Surgical exploration of the common bile duct (choledochostomy) enables the diagnostician to differentiate between choledocholithiasis (stone in the common bile duct) and tumor. If carcinoma (usually of the pancreas head) is discovered during exploration, the surgeon may perform a palliative anastomosis of the gallbladder to the jejunum to bypass the common bile duct (see Chap. 59).

Nursing Management

ASSESSMENT

The client should be closely observed for the development of jaundice. Often, the first symptom the client notices is a change in taste, manifesting as a distaste for a food or drink the client liked, such as coffee. The sclera should be checked daily for the development of the yellow coloration. Pruritus is another early sign of developing jaundice.

NURSING INTERVENTION

Nursing Diagnosis: Skin Integrity, Impaired R/T pruritus.

Planning: Expected Outcomes. The client will have itching controlled, as evidenced by client's statements of relief, decreased dryness of skin, and a decrease in scratching by the client.

Implementation. Pruritus is probably caused by an accumulation of bile salts in the skin, resulting from

TABLE 58-1. Types of Jaundice (Icterus)

			Laboratory Tests									
			Conjugated (Direct) Bilirubin	Unconjugated (Indirect) Bilirubin	Total Bilirubin	Urine Bilirubin	Urine Urobilinogen	Fecal Urobilinogen	Aspartate Aminotransferase (SGOT*)	Alanine Aminotransferase (SGPT†)	Partial Thromboplastin Time	Prothrombin Time
	Causes	**Assessment**	0.1–0.3 mg/100 ml	0.2–0.8 mg/100 ml	0.1–1.0 mg/100 ml	0	0–4 mg/day	40–280 mg/day	5–40 U/ml	5–35 U/ml	30–40‡ sec	12–15 sec
Prehepatic jaundice	Excessive hemolysis due to transfusion reactions, hemolytic disease of newborn, severe burns, bacterial toxins, venoms, hypotonic parenteral solutions, etc. Defective albumin binding.	Liver function usually normal; compensates for ↑ bilirubin by ↑ metabolism of bilirubin.	normal	↑	↑	none	↑	↑	normal	normal	normal	normal
Hepatic jaundice	Liver's inability to conjugate or transport bilirubin to canaliculi for excretion due to hepatitis, liver congestion, cirrhosis, metastatic cancer, prolonged use of medications metabolized by liver, etc.	Liver may be enlarged. Abdomen may be tender. May have bruising or bleeding due to vitamin K malabsorption.§	↑	normal or slight ↑	↑	↑	↑↓	↓	↑	↑	prolonged	prolonged
Posthepatic jaundice (obstructive)	Blocked flow of bile into duodenum due to inflammation, scar tissue, stones, or tumors in liver, biliary, or pancreatic system.	↑ Level of unconjugated bilirubin if liver cell function is diminished. May have bruising or bleeding due to vitamin K malabsorption (bile is necessary for vitamin K absorption).§ Abdomen may be tender. Stools are clay-colored (bile gives stool its dark color). Urine is brown or foamy (conjugated bilirubin is excreted in urine).	↑	normal or ↑	↑	↑	↓	absent or ↓	normal or ↑	normal or ↑	prolonged	prolonged

* Serum glutamic-oxaloacetic transaminase.
† Serum glutamic-pyruvic transaminase.
‡ Normal values will vary among laboratories.
§ Parenteral vitamin K will improve prothrombin time only if jaundice is due to posthepatic cause.
Adapted from Gannon, R. B., & Pickett, K. (1983). Jaundice. *American Journal of Nursing 83*, 404.

obstructed biliary excretion. Some clients experience only mild itching. Others suffer such extreme itching that they may tear at their skin or scratch in their sleep.

Oral cholestyramine resin provides some relief by binding bile salts in the intestine so they can be excreted. Antihistamines also may relieve the itching. Phenobarbital has been effective in some cases because of its ability to enhance bile flow.

Nursing Diagnosis: Self-Esteem Disturbance R/T yellowing of skin and sclerae.

Planning: Expected Outcomes. The client will cope with self-esteem disturbance, as evidenced by the client's not isolating him- or herself and being able to discuss feelings associated with jaundice.

Implementation. A highly visible sign of illness, jaundice may have a considerable emotional impact and may impair body image. Jaundice and its manifestations can dominate the client's feelings and require ongoing emotional support and information to reduce unfounded fears.

Nursing Diagnosis: Knowledge Deficit R/T cause of jaundice.

Planning: Expected Outcomes. The client will understand the cause of jaundice, as evidenced by the client's statements and ability to redefine illness.

Implementation. Clients often wonder why they are jaundiced, how long the condition will last, and how to cope with the problem. The nurse should take the time to explain the condition in a manner appropriate to the client's knowledge base and desire to learn about the illness.

Jaundice usually begins to disappear within 4 to 6 weeks. The return of normal stool and urine colors are an indication of resolution.

EVALUATION

The nurse must evaluate client outcomes on the basis of the established plan of care. If these goals were not achieved, the plan and interventions must be revised to meet the client's needs.

▼ Hepatitis

Simply stated, hepatitis is inflammation of the liver. This inflammation may be caused by a virus, bacteria, or toxic substance. Jaundice usually develops, and the liver is tender. Other systemic manifestations depend on the causative agent and the degree of organ disruption.

There are several different types of hepatitis. These include viral, toxic, chronic, and alcoholic hepatitis.

VIRAL HEPATITIS

Definition

There are four major types of identified viral hepatitis: hepatitis A, hepatitis B, hepatitis C, and delta hepatitis. Although the symptoms are similar, each of these conditions is caused by a different virus and differs in incubation period, mode of transmission, and severity (Table 58–2). Other types of hepatitis have also been identified recently.

Previously, when a client had a viral hepatitis that was unidentified, the condition was termed non-A or non-B hepatitis. Now that hepatitis C has been identified, all unidentified strains of hepatitis are referred to as non-A, non-B, non-C hepatitis. Little is known currently about hepatitis C.

There has recently been a fourth hepatitis virus identified, delta hepatitis. This is usually found with hepatitis B.

Incidence

Hepatitis occurs worldwide.

Hepatitis A. Hepatitis A is endemic in some areas of the world, especially areas with poor sanitation. Epidemics do occur in countries with good sanitation, however.

Hepatitis B. Hepatitis B is found worldwide, even in remote areas. Its incidence increases in areas of high population density and poor hygiene.

Hepatitis C. The incidence of hepatitis C is not fully known. Because it is now possible to screen blood for the hepatitis B antigen before transfusion, most post-transfusion hepatitis is probably caused by hepatitis C or by a newly identified strain of hepatitis.

Delta Hepatitis. The incidence of delta hepatitis is not known; however, it is always found with hepatitis B.

Etiology

Agents that may cause viral hepatitis include hepatitis A virus, hepatitis B virus, Epstein-Barr virus (infectious mononucleosis virus), cytomegalovirus, rubella, herpes simplex, varicella, retrovirus, yellow fever virus, coxsackievirus, adenovirus, or Marburg virus.

Hepatitis A. Hepatitis A, also known as short incubation hepatitis, infectious hepatitis, and MS_1 hepatitis, is caused by an RNA virus of the enterovirus family.

Causes of epidemics include infected water, milk, or food, especially raw shellfish from contaminated waters. In the general population, those under 15 years of age are at the most risk.

TABLE 58-2. Comparison of Four Types of Viral Hepatitis

Factor	Hepatitis A	Hepatitis B	Hepatitis C	Delta Hepatitis
Incidence	Endemic in areas of poor sanitation Common in fall and early winter	Worldwide, especially in drug addicts and clients and others exposed to blood and blood products Occurs all year	Posttransfusion Those working around blood and blood products Occurs all year	Found in conjunction with hepatitis B
Incubation period	15-45 days	28-180 days	7-8 weeks	Same as hepatitis B
Risk factors	Close personal contact Handling feces-contaminated wastes	Health care workers in contact with blood and blood products Hemodialysis and post-transfusion clients Homosexually active males and drug abusers	Same as for hepatitis B	Same as hepatitis B
Mode of transmission	Infected feces, fecal-oral route May be airborne if copious secretions Shellfish from contaminated water Also parenteral	Parenteral Sexual contact Fecal-oral route	Contact with blood and body fluids	Co-infects with hepatitis B, close personal contact
Severity	Usually not fatal	More serious; may be fatal	Not known	Increased mortality with hepatitis B
Diagnostic tests	IgM positive in acute infection IgG positive after infection	HB_sAg, HB_cAg, and HB_eAg positive	Not identified	HD Ag positive
Vaccine	Vaccine under development	Hepatitis B vaccine	None	None

Note. HB_sAg, hepatitis B surface antigen; HB_cAg, hepatitis B core antigen; HB_eAg, hepatitis B e antigen.

Hepatitis B. The major sources of this infection are carriers and clients with the acute process. Contact with the serum of an infected client is the major mode of transmission. The virus also may be transmitted by other body fluids, such as saliva and semen. Hepatitis B virus can survive on environmental surfaces for at least a week.

Hepatitis C. Hepatitis C is transmitted parenterally through the blood, by personal contact, and possibly by the fecal-oral route. In contrast to hepatitis A, but similar to hepatitis B, hepatitis C may be spread by carriers.

Delta Hepatitis. Delta hepatitis is transmitted only through blood contact, so it is seen most commonly in clients exposed to blood and blood products, such as drug-addicted and hemophiliac individuals.

Risk Factors

Hepatitis A. Hepatitis A spreads from person to person by close contact or by the handling of feces-contaminated articles. Because the infected client's feces contain the virus before the onset of manifestations, the remaining household members are at risk.

People who work with animals imported from areas where hepatitis A is endemic are at increased risk, as are individuals who eat raw or steamed shellfish.

This problem also may spread in an institution such as a day care center, prison, or facility for developmentally disabled people.

Hepatitis B. Health care workers are at high risk for hepatitis B because of their close contact with the blood of carriers. Clients who have multiple blood transfusions or dialysis are also vulnerable to this infection. Other high-risk populations are homosexually active males, morticians, persons who undergo tattooing, and parenteral drug abusers.

Hepatitis C. Because hepatitis C is also parenterally transmitted, the risk factors are similar to those for hepatitis B.

Delta Hepatitis. The risk factors for delta hepatitis are the same as for hepatitis B.

To a great extent, viral hepatitis can be prevented by proper controls within the home, community, and health care facility setting.

PREVENTION

Hepatitis A

Personal Hygiene. Because transmission of hepatitis A and possibly C is by the fecal-oral route, good personal hygiene is important. Food handlers must wash their hands thoroughly. In some facilities, the disease is present because residents are unable to care for themselves properly. Care providers must supervise handwashing by ambulatory residents. Personnel in day care centers need to wash their hands carefully after changing diapers.

Water Supply. Treatment of municipal water supplies prevents transmission of hepatitis A virus. Private water supplies can be sources of contamination and need to be under government or some other type of control. Polluted fishing waters pose a threat. Shellfish that come from these waters can be a major source of hepatitis A.

Restaurants. Local health authorities need to monitor eating establishments. Serologic screening of food handlers for hepatitis A reduces its transmission. Because the disease can be transmitted via food, a client with active hepatitis A should not work in food services.

Animal Care. Isolating newly imported animals for a 2-month period reduces the incidence of hepatitis A among people who handle them. If isolation is impossible, these individuals need to wear protective clothing and use good handwashing technique. If the risk of contamination is high, some physicians prescribe prophylactic standard immunoglobulin.

Passive Immunization. Again, physicians may prescribe standard immunoglobulin. Adverse effects of intramuscular injection include pain, tenderness, and at times hematoma formation. Immune globulin is helpful prophylaxis both before and after exposure. Immune globulin (gamma globulin, Gammar) is administered intramuscularly after exposure but not after the development of clinical symptoms. Clients who live in or visit areas of high risk for hepatitis A can be protected for about 2 months by immune serum. The earlier in the incubation period that the prophylactic immune serum is given, the greater the protection.

Hepatitis B

Control of Blood, Blood Products, and Skin-Piercing Instruments. Remember that hepatitis B is transmitted by the serum of the infected client. Therefore, blood, blood products, and instruments that pierce the skin and contact the vascular system are all potential sources of contamination. Some donor-related precautions that decrease the incidence of hepatitis B are (1) screening of donors' blood for hepatitis B virus surface antigen (HB_sAg), (2) use of volunteer rather than paid donors, (3) registration of carriers, and (4) sharing of accurate records between institutions. It is possible to reduce the transfusion recipient's exposure to hepatitis B by using blood products only when necessary, using only the necessary amount of blood or blood products, cross-checking laboratory data to reduce errors of reported results, and encouraging clients who are having elective surgery to donate their own blood (autologous transfusions).

Many health care facilities use disposable equipment, especially needles and syringes, to reduce hepatitis transmission. Nondisposable equipment must be sterilized to prevent virus transmission. All health care workers, of course, follow the Centers for Disease Control universal precautions.

Personal Hygiene. Good personal hygiene by clients with hepatitis B or hepatitis B carriers also reduces transmission. Such clients should not share razors, toothbrushes, wash cloths, cigarettes, or other personal items with others.

Passive Immunization. Standard immunoglobulin may contain antibodies against hepatitis B. However, another preparation called specific *hepatitis B* immunoglobulin contains much higher levels of antibody. The vaccine is usually given in three doses. The second and third doses are given 1 month and 6 months after the initial dose. Physicians may prescribe hepatitis B immunoglobulin for postexposure prophylaxis when there has been percutaneous exposure to blood that contains HB_sAg.

Active Immunization. Hepatitis B vaccine may provide active immunization before exposure to hepatitis B virus. The injection is best given into the deltoid muscle. Authorities recommend this killed virus vaccine for persons in the high-risk categories for hepatitis B. It may be used in conjunction with specific hepatitis B immunoglobulin after documented exposure to hepatitis B.

Hepatitis C. Recall that transmission of hepatitis C is similar to that of hepatitis B. Therefore, many of the same measures are probably useful in its prevention. Physicians sometimes prescribe standard immunoglobulin for postexposure passive immunization to hepatitis C. However, this intervention has not yet been well documented and needs further research. As with hepatitis A, there is no vaccine for active immunization against hepatitis C.

Delta Hepatitis. Because delta hepatitis must coexist with hepatitis B, the hepatitis B vaccine can help prevent delta hepatitis also. The precautions that help prevent hepatitis B also are useful in preventing delta hepatitis.

Table 58-3 summarizes the immunizations for hepatitis A, hepatitis B, hepatitis C, and delta hepatitis.

TABLE 58–3. Immunizations for Hepatitis A, B, C, and Delta Hepatitis

Immunization Type	Hepatitis Type: A	B	C	Delta
Active	Vaccine under development	Hepatitis B vaccine (killed virus) Before exposure	No vaccine	No vaccine
Passive	Standard immunoglobin Before and after exposure	Specific hepatitis B immunoglobin (preferred) Standard immunoglobin After exposure	Standard immunoglobin (of questionable value) After exposure	Standard immunoglobin (of questionable value) After exposure

Pathophysiology

The physical manifestations of viral hepatitis reflect liver cell damage. Hepatocytes are damaged by the body's immune response to the virus, which alters cellular function. The degree of functional impairment depends on the amount of hepatocellular damage. The endoplasmic reticulum (responsible for protein and steroid synthesis, glucuronide conjugation, and detoxification) is the first organelle to undergo change. Liver functions that depend on these processes are altered, with the degree of impairment depending on the amount of damage to the endoplastic reticulum. Kupffer's cells increase in size and number. Vascular and ductule tissues undergo inflammatory changes. The hepatocytes generally heal in 3 to 4 months.

HEPATITIS A

Antibodies to hepatitis A are of two types. The IgM antibody develops soon after infection and remains in the body for 6 to 8 weeks; it is, therefore, an indicator of current infection. The IgG antibody against hepatitis A develops several weeks after infection and persists for years, providing immunity against the disease; it is, therefore, an indicator of past infection.

Clients who are otherwise healthy usually recover from hepatitis A without major sequelae. Although hepatitis A has a low mortality rate, fulminant hepatitis A may result. The fulminant form resembles acute liver failure. It causes severe illness and even death.

HEPATITIS B

The hepatitis B virus is a DNA virus that has an inner core and a surface envelope. The body forms antibodies to hepatitis B virus core antigen (HB_cAg) and surface antigen (HB_sAg). The presence of HB_sAg in the blood denotes (1) a previous or resolving infection with hepatitis B; (2) a continuing, chronic infection; or (3) immunization with immunoglobulin or hepatitis B vaccine.

HEPATITIS C

Little specific information is available about hepatitis C. Neither a specific antigen nor antibody has been found.

DELTA HEPATITIS

Delta hepatitis is a defective RNA virus, requiring the helper function of hepatitis B. An antigen, HD Ag, and an antibody, anti-HD, have been identified.

Typically clients with viral hepatitis completely recover from the illness in 3 to 16 weeks. Mortality from hepatitis A is low, except for the fulminant form. Clients with hepatitis B tend to develop more complications. One in ten clients develops chronic active hepatitis as a result of hepatitis B, often leading to destruction of the liver. Cirrhosis may follow a severe case of hepatitis B or chronic active hepatitis. Primary hepatocellular carcinoma is a potential complication of chronic hepatitis.

Clinical Manifestations

Clients with viral hepatitis all experience liver inflammation and other sequelae that are similar. Hepatitis B and delta hepatitis are usually the most severe, although they may be asymptomatic in some clients. The onset of manifestations varies according to the incubation period and the degree of infectivity.

Symptoms of viral hepatitis are systemic and vary from client to client. Symptoms might include jaundice, lethargy, irritability, myalgia, arthralgia, anorexia, nausea, vomiting, abdominal pain, diarrhea or constipation, fever, and other flulike symptoms. Pruritus (itching) is typically mild and transient and may be more intense at its onset and termination. Jaundice is first seen in the sclera of the eyes and mucous membranes. Anicteric (without jaundice) hepatitis may or may not precede jaundice. Children with hepatitis are usually anicteric. Adults often note the appearance of darker urine and clay-colored stools a few days before clinical jaundice develops. The other symptoms often abate when jaundice appears, but they also may worsen.

If irritability and drowsiness become severe, the nurse assesses for the possibility of hepatic encephalopathy. Deterioration of handwriting is an early sign of hepatic encephalopathy; thus, clients should be asked to write their name each shift and their writing should be observed closely for changes. Asterixis, an abnormal muscle tremor sometimes called liver flap, may accompany encephalopathy. This sign is easily elicited by applying a blood pressure cuff and noting if the flapping is present when the cuff is released. Mild depression is not uncommon, owing to (1) the nature of the illness (weakness, jaundice, itching, and nausea), (2) its length and cost, (3) confinement, and (4) forgetfulness and the inability to concentrate on completion of activities of daily living (ADLs).

Anemia may occur because of the decreased lifespan of erythrocytes. Erythrocyte destruction results from liver enzyme alterations. A transient hyperglycemia sometimes develops, and a client with diabetes may need to increase insulin dosage at this time. The liver is larger than normal with hepatitis and tender on palpation. Some people develop spider angiomata, palmar erythema, and gynecomastia, which disappear during the recovery period. A small percentage (5 to 15 per cent) of clients experience splenomegaly or enlargement of the posterior cervical lymph nodes. Occasionally, hepatitis B is accompanied by arthralgias, rash, vasculitis, or glomerulonephritis.

Major assessment findings and their pathophysiologic bases are summarized in Table 58-4.

Occasionally, the person develops cholestatic viral hepatitis syndrome. This uncommon disease process resembles mechanical obstruction. It is thus difficult to differentiate cholestatic viral hepatitis from biliary tract obstruction due to gallstones, strictures, and tumors. The cause and pathophysiology of this hepatitis variant are unclear. Cholestatic viral hepatitis syndrome causes jaundice, itching, and the typical flulike and gastrointestinal problems of hepatitis, but the symptoms often last longer and are more severe. The serum bilirubin reaches levels of 10 to 15 mg/100 ml. Diagnostic studies reveal elevations of serum lipoproteins, globulins, cholesterol, and alkaline phosphatase. Rarely does the liver progressively enlarge.

Other clients may manifest fulminant viral hepatitis. This life-threatening form resembles acute liver failure with manifestations of encephalopathy (increased excitability, insomnia, somnolence, and impaired mentation). The liver rapidly decreases in size. Other problems include gastrointestinal bleeding, disseminated intravascular coagulation, fever with leukocytosis and neutrophilia, hepatorenal problems of oliguria and azotemia, edema and ascites, hypotension, respiratory failure, hypoglycemia, bacterial infection of respiratory and/or urinary tract, and thrombocytopenia and coagulopathy. The prognosis is poor, and death may occur before jaundice appears. A liver transplant may be performed to save the client's life.

TABLE 58-4. Hepatitis Assessment Data

Assessment Data	Pathophysiologic Bases
Jaundice, clay-colored stools (no pigment); ↑ serum bilirubin; darkened urine (bilirubin and urobilin)	Impaired excretion of conjugated bilirubin Urobilin in blood excreted through kidneys instead of bowel
Pruritus	Bile salt accumulation in skin
Abdominal pain in right upper quadrant	Stretching of Glisson's capsule (surrounding liver) due to inflammation
Fever	Release of pyrogens in inflammatory process
Fatigue and weakness	Reduced energy metabolism by liver
Anorexia, nausea, vomiting	Changes in stomach or bowel
Bleeding tendencies	Reduced prothrombin synthesis by injured hepatic cells Reduced fat-soluble vitamin K absorption due to reduced bile in intestine
Anemia	Decreased red blood cell life due to liver enzyme alterations, hemorrhage

HEPATITIS A

The fecal-oral route is the major path of transmission, although parenteral transmission does occur rarely. Hepatitis A has an incubation period of about 15 to 45 days. The client with hepatitis A excretes the virus in the stool throughout the preicteric (prejaundice) stage and is probably free of the virus within 7 to 9 days after jaundice develops.

The client with the primary infection can transmit the virus to others before precautions can be started. Secondary infections tend to occur in household members about every 20 to 30 days.

HEPATITIS B

Hepatitis B has an incubation period of 28 to 180 days.

HEPATITIS C

The incubation period for hepatitis C is usually 7 to 8 weeks, although longer incubations have been observed. This can probably be accounted for by the existence of more unidentified strains.

DELTA HEPATITIS

The incubation period for delta hepatitis is the same as for hepatitis B.

DIAGNOSTIC ASSESSMENT

The serologic markers of viral hepatitis are presented in Table 58-5. Presence of HB_sAg in the blood usually indicates that the individual is infectious. HB_sAg is sometimes called the Australian antigen. Another antigen, HB_eAg, is often associated with the progression from acute hepatitis to chronic hepatitis and indicates a highly infectious state.

The serum aminotransferases first elevate and then begin to fall as the bilirubin starts to increase. Levels that rise, peak, drop, and then rise again indicate se-

TABLE 58–5. Serologic Markers of Viral Hepatitis

	Marker Results				
	Hepatitis A Antibody				
Hepatitis Type	***IgM***	***IgG***	***HB_sAg***	***HB_sAb***	***HB_cAb***
Hepatitis A					
Acute	+	−	−	−	−
Immune	−	+	−	−	−
Hepatitis B					
Acute	−	−	+	−	+
Immune	−	−	−	+	+ or −
Chronic	−	−	+	+ or −	+ or −
Hepatitis C	Serologic markers in development				

Note. HB_sAg, hepatitis B surface antigen; HB_sAb, hepatitis B surface antibody; HB_cAb, hepatitis B core antibody.

vere liver damage and a poor prognosis. Jaundice occurs as bilirubin rises above 2.5 mg/100 ml. Bilirubin that rises above 20 mg/100 ml and remains elevated for a long period may indicate severe liver necrosis, which has a poor prognosis. Mild prolongation of the prothrombin time sometimes occurs. The gamma globulin fraction and alkaline phosphatase elevate in some clients. If hepatitis B is responsible, detection of HB_sAg is possible even before the level of aspartate aminotransferase (formerly serum glutamic-oxaloacetic transaminase) rises.

Medical Management

Five important interventions for clients with viral hepatitis are (1) rest, (2) proper diet, (3) emotional support, (4) relief of pruritus, and (5) correction of knowledge deficits regarding the disease.

PHARMACOLOGIC MANAGEMENT

If given early, standard immunoglobulin (proteins capable of acting as antibodies and formerly termed immune serum globulin) can prevent hepatitis A or decrease the severity of symptoms. The hepatitis A virus does not remain in the blood long; therefore, there is no healthy carrier state for hepatitis A, as there is for hepatitis B.

Few medications are available for treating viral hepatitis. Antibiotics are not prescribed. Immunoglobulin, although not used to treat viral hepatitis, does provide prophylactic assistance for family members. Antiemetics decrease nausea and vomiting, but phenothiazines should not be used because they are biotransformed in the liver and therefore potentially toxic.

The corticosteroids are not necessary in uncomplicated cases of acute viral hepatitis, and authorities question their use in several cases. Corticosteroids may decrease the serum aminotransferase and bilirubin levels. However, they have no affect on liver necrosis or regeneration.

Estrogens can raise serum bilirubin levels. Therefore, clinicians need to evaluate the use of oral contraceptives during acute viral hepatitis.

The administration of cholestyramine or ursidiol can relieve the pruritus associated with severe cholestatic liver disease. This medication acts by bonding bile salts in the intestine.

All in all, clinicians administer very few medications to clients with hepatitis. Medications such as chlorpromazine, aspirin, acetaminophen, and a variety of sedatives are given as infrequently as possible because they all have the potential to damage an already damaged liver.

DIETARY MANAGEMENT

A diet high in carbohydrates and calories with moderate amounts of fat and protein is recommended. Meals should be given in small portions and given four to six times daily. The client's food preferences should be accommodated.

Nursing Management

ASSESSMENT

The nurse always begins by questioning the client about possible exposure to risk factors to assess the type of hepatitis present. The presence of common symptoms, especially jaundice, is assessed, as are signs of progression of the disease, such as hepatic encephalopathy (see section on hepatic encephalopathy). Liver function studies are monitored to assess the progression of the disease.

NURSING INTERVENTION

Nursing Diagnosis: Activity Intolerance R/T extreme fatigue.

Planning: Expected Outcomes. The client will maintain adequate rest to conserve energy, as evidenced by compliance with activity restrictions and a gradual increase in activity to pre-illness level.

Implementation. Fatigue associated with hepatitis may interfere with ADLs. Most clients experience the greatest fatigue during the anicteric phase and begin to feel stronger during the icteric phase. Fatigue may persist, however, even after the jaundice clears. During the period of severe fatigue, the client should be advised to rest in bed. Most clients who feel capable of being up and around can do so without any harm, if they rest after meals and do not engage in any activity to the point of being overly tired. Because prolonged bed rest itself can lead to weakness, a reasonable activity level is more conducive to recovery than enforced bed rest.

ADLs such as bathroom privileges, personal hygiene, and feeding should be encouraged unless they cause excessive fatigue. The client should be advised to plan rest periods while jaundiced, especially after meals. Clients who engage in excessive activity too early in the recovery phase sometimes experience a relapse, possibly leading to liver failure.

Nursing Diagnosis: Physical Mobility, Impaired R/T prolonged bed rest.

Planning: Expected Outcomes. The client will regain mobility and not suffer from the complications of immobility, as evidenced by increasing mobility and the absence of complications.

Implementation. In very severe cases of hepatitis, the client may need to remain in bed for a prolonged period. In this case, the nurse needs to intervene to prevent the complications of prolonged immobility, e.g., pressure sores, contractures, anorexia, and depression. For detailed information on preventing problems due to immobility, see Chapter 66.

Nursing Diagnosis: Nutrition, Altered: Less Than Body Requirements R/T anorexia, nausea, bile stasis, and altered absorption and metabolism.

Planning: Expected Outcomes. The client will maintain an intake of the required calories to maintain weight, as evidenced by no weight loss and possible weight gain.

Implementation. To help the client meet the nutritional requirements associated with hepatitis, the nurse should

- Provide a nutritious breakfast. Anorexia usually worsens during the day, so breakfast may be the best tolerated meal.
- Encourage the client to avoid heavy, greasy food, which can induce nausea.
- Devise a dietary plan for a diet high in protein (75 to 100 g) and carbohydrates (300 to 400 g) and moderate in fat (60 to 100 g). This diet is optimum to allow recovery of injured liver cells. The amounts of protein and fat are decreased only if there is a problem with their digestion and metabolism. If the client has no problem with protein metabolism, a normal intake is helpful for tissue repair. However, clients with very severe hepatitis who are in danger of developing hepatic encephalopathy require a diet low in protein (due to the buildup of ammonia in the blood). Alterations in fat metabolism differ according to the degree of interruption in bile production and excretion.
- Suggest multiple small meals. This allows the client with anorexia to ingest a diet of 2500 to 3000 calories more comfortably. Also, candy, juice, sweetened tea, and carbonated drinks can supply calories when nausea is a problem.
- Remind the client to avoid alcohol, because it is an extremely hepatotoxic agent.
- Tell the client that vitamin supplements are not generally necessary in uncomplicated hepatitis, provided the diet is adequate in nutrition. Vitamin K supplements as ordered may be administered if the prothrombin time is longer than normal.

Clients who develop severe nausea and vomiting may obtain relief from antiemetics. However, before these medications are administered, their effect on liver functions should be reviewed. Phenothiazines such as chlorpromazine (Compazine) are usually contraindicated. Clients who are unable to tolerate any oral intake may require intravenous nutrition.

Nursing Diagnosis: Anxiety R/T uncertainty of the effects of hepatitis.

Planning: Expected Outcomes. The client will have a decrease in anxiety, as evidenced by the ability to discuss his or her feelings about disease.

Implementation. Clients with hepatitis should be encouraged to express their feelings concerning (1) their illness, (2) the duration and cost of the illness, (3) alterations in home life and in finances (especially for the parent of young children and/or the sole breadwinner), (4) the effect of the illness on future health problems, and (5) the possibility of death if they are very ill. The nurse should suggest psychosocial and financial counseling for the client who is disturbed by the illness. Teaching and subsequent understanding will greatly decrease anxiety.

Nursing Diagnosis: Tissue Integrity, Impaired R/T pruritus.

Planning: Expected Outcomes. The client will have pruritus relieved, as evidenced by the client's statements of comfort and the absence of scratching.

Implementation. Clients with severe jaundice may suffer pruritus. See section on jaundice for a discussion of nursing interventions for itching.

Nursing Diagnosis: Knowledge Deficit R/T the disease and its course.

Planning: Expected Outcomes. The client will understand the disease and its treatment, as evidenced by the client's ability to state the causes of the disease and rationales for treatment.

Implementation. Teaching for the client with hepatitis varies with the causative agent. In addition to teaching how to prevent recurrence and spread, the nurse instructs the client to return to former activity levels slowly in order to avoid a relapse. Instructions concerning the diet need to be clear.

EVALUATION

The nurse must evaluate client outcomes on the basis of the established plan of care. If these goals were not achieved, the plan and interventions must be revised to meet the client's needs.

Modification of Plan of Care for the Elderly

Older clients are at higher risk for liver damage because they are more likely to have already had some changes in the liver. They are at greater risk for developing complications.

Post-hospital Care

DISCHARGE TEACHING

One of the primary areas covered is teaching the client and significant others to avoid reinfection or possible spread of the infection to other family members. The client is also taught to avoid alcohol and medications such as aspirin or sedatives due to their hepatotoxicity.

The client must understand the need for adequate rest so the liver can heal on its own. The client needs to be active enough to prevent complications of immobility but not so active as to risk relapse. The client also should be encouraged to maintain an adequate intake of nutrients to promote healing.

The client and significant others should be taught to avoid sexual activity until there is no longer a chance of disease transmission. They should check with their physician before resuming sexual relations.

HOME HEALTH CARE NEEDS

The client may need help at home after discharge because limits on activity will still have to be maintained. The client may need help with housework or shopping.

FOLLOW-UP CARE

The client needs to be seen at regular intervals after discharge to ensure that the liver is healing and no further damage has occurred.

TOXIC HEPATITIS

Toxic hepatitis occurs after exposure to hepatotoxins. These substances cause liver alterations by initiating either drug-induced hepatitis or drug-induced cholestasis. Either of these responses may be dose related and predictable or idiosyncratic and unpredictable, depending on the chemical nature of the hepatotoxin or the genetic make-up of the individual. Idiosyncratic hepatotoxicity is often due to hypersensitivity (immune response). Some substances cause liver damage because they are converted to toxic metabolites. Table 58-6 lists some hepatotoxic agents. Liver necrosis occurs within 2 or 3 days after acute exposure to a dose-related hepatotoxin. However, several weeks may pass before manifestations of idiosyncratic reactions appear. Clients with either process develop abnormal reactions to liver function tests.

Clients who are repeatedly exposed to some hepatotoxins in minimal amounts but over long periods of time may develop cirrhosis. Individuals experiencing a hypersensitivity reaction may demonstrate eosinophilia, fever, arthralgia, and sometimes xanthomatosis (an excessive accumulation of lipids brought about by faulty lipid metabolism).

TABLE 58-6. Substances Known To Be Hepatotoxic

	Type of Liver Alteration	
	Hepatitis	**Cholestasis**
Dose-related	acetaminophen *Amanita phalloides* (mushroom) aspirin benzene carbon tetrachloride chloroform methotrexate tetracyclines	oxymetholone
Idiosyncratic	alpha-methyldopa sulfasalazine halothane isoniazid nitrofurantoin phenytoin quinidine	allopurinol anabolic steroids carbamazepine chlordiazepoxide chlorpromazine chlorpropamide diazepam erythromycin estolate flurazepam oral contraceptives

Nursing intervention consists of removal of the causative agent, rest, alleviation of side effects (e.g., cholestyramine for pruritus), high-calorie diet with fats if tolerated, high-protein diet if there is no evidence of impending hepatic encephalopathy, and steroids for hypersensitivity reactions.

Renal failure sometimes appears as a complication of toxic hepatitis. Assessment and interventions for renal failure are discussed in Chapter 50.

CHRONIC HEPATITIS

Chronic hepatitis exists when liver inflammation continues beyond a period of 3 to 6 months. This disease process may manifest as chronic persistent hepatitis (CPH) or chronic active hepatitis (CAH). CPH is usually benign and seldom progressive. CAH is more serious and differential diagnosis is of utmost importance. Definitive diagnosis and decisions regarding appropriate intervention depend on liver biopsy findings. Figure 58-1 compares biopsy findings in CPH and CAH.

Chronic Persistent Hepatitis

CPH may follow acute hepatitis and may represent a protracted course of the acute illness. Initially, about two thirds of clients with chronic persistent hepatitis have symptoms of acute viral hepatitis. Recurrent epi-

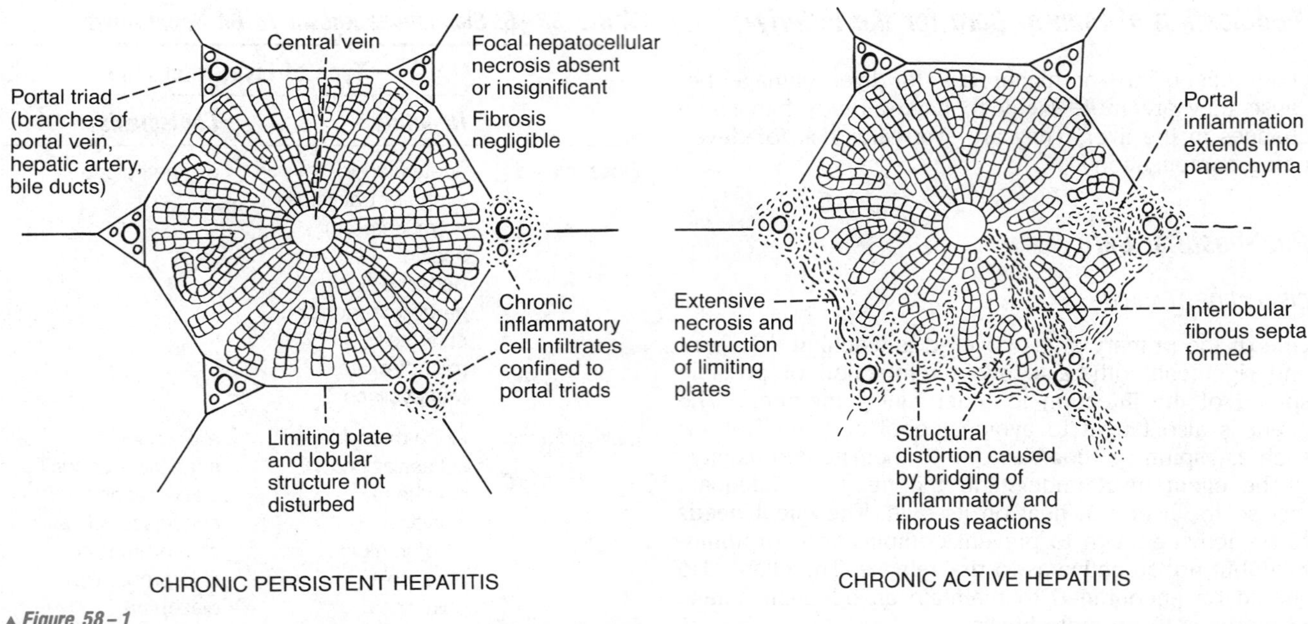

▲ *Figure 58–1*

Comparison of biopsy findings in chronic persistent hepatitis and chronic active hepatitis. Inflammation is confined to portal triads in chronic persistent hepatitis but extends into parenchyma in chronic active hepatitis.

sodes are not acute in nature, and extrahepatic involvement seldom occurs. Fibrotic liver and cirrhosis develop rarely, but clients with CPH generally have an excellent prognosis. Figure 58–2 illustrates common manifestations of CPH.

Chronic Active Hepatitis

CAH causes a more severe illness. It leads to hepatic inflammation, hepatic necrosis, and progressive fibrosis. Cirrhosis usually occurs with this variant. In addition to the manifestations of chronic liver disease, seroimmunologic alterations and extrahepatic abnormalities characterize chronic active hepatitis.

In most instances, CAH results from an idiopathic cause or from the hepatitis B virus. Idiopathic CAH occurs more frequently in females (Fig. 58–3), whereas hepatitis B CAH occurs more commonly in males. The pathogenesis in hepatitis B CAH may be an

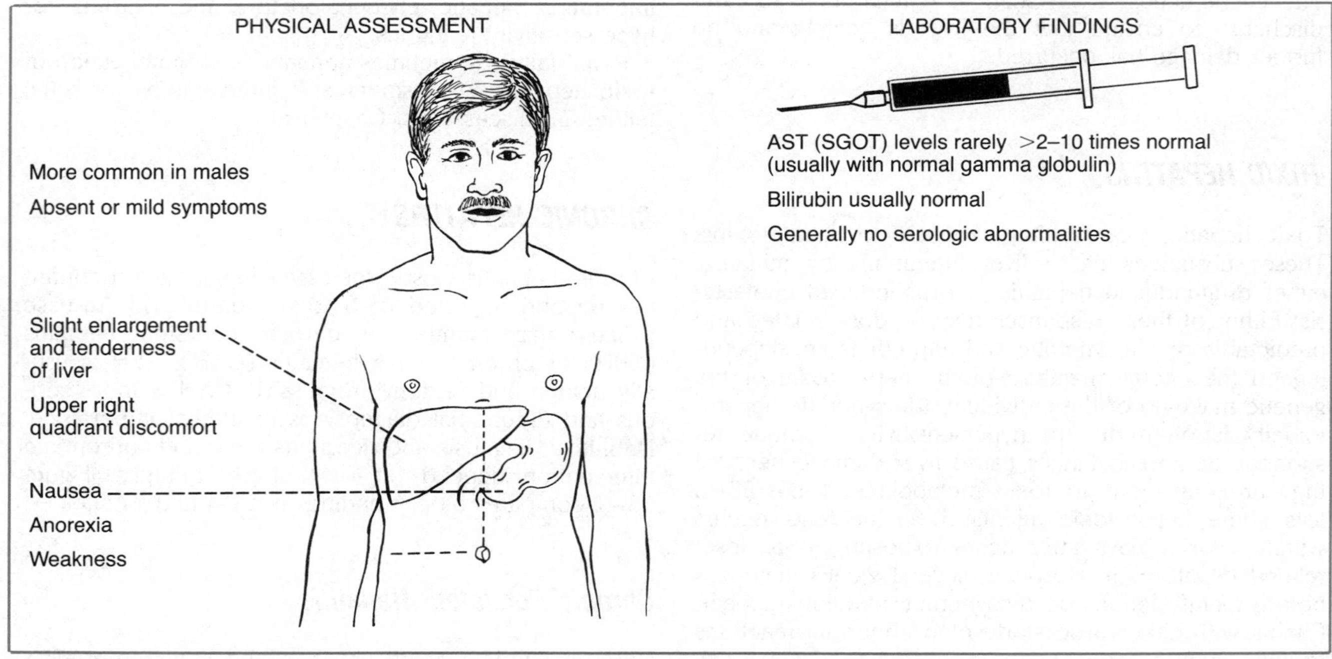

▲ *Figure 58–2*

Chronic persistent hepatitis: common assessment findings. AST, aspartate amino transferase; SGOT, serum glutamic-oxaloacetic transaminase.

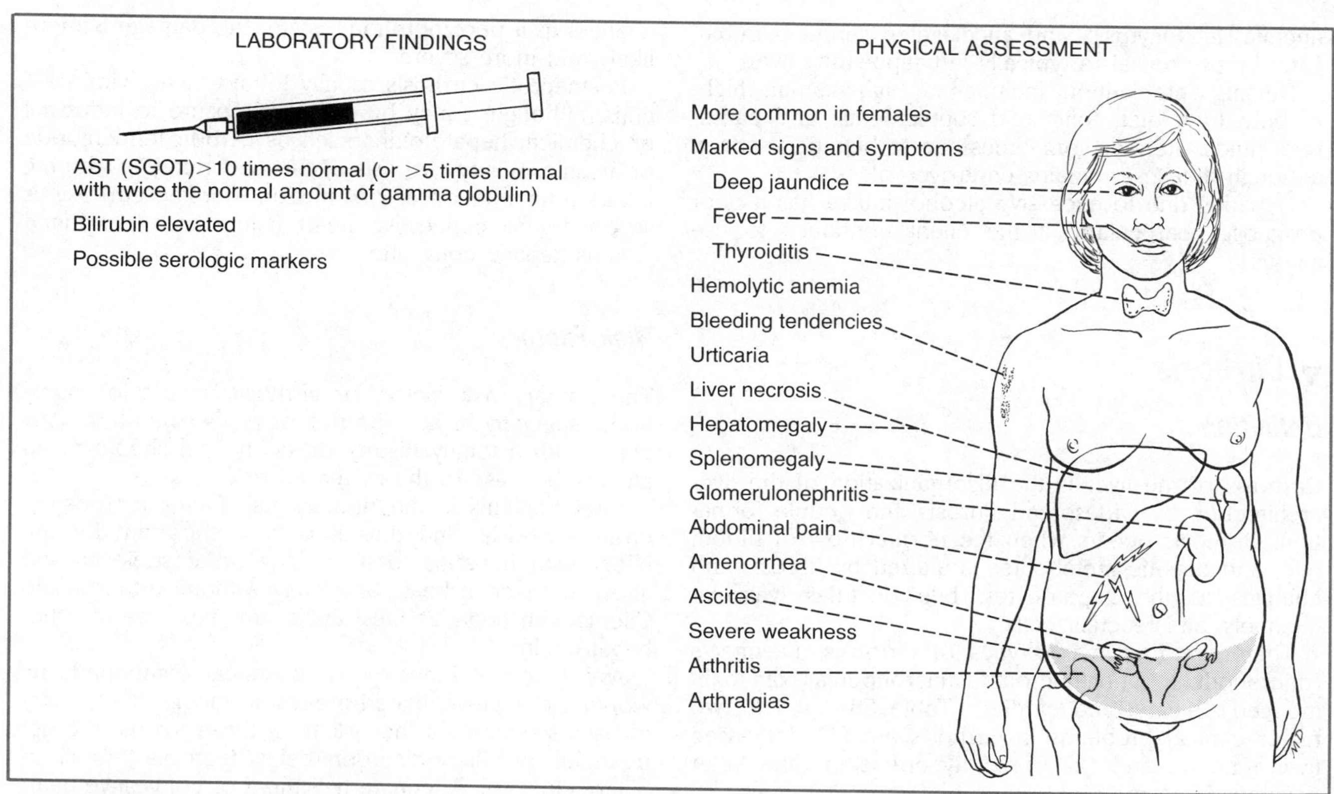

▲ *Figure 58-3*

Chronic active hepatitis (idiopathic): common assessment findings. AST, aspartate aminotransferase; SGOT, serum glutamic-oxaloacetic transaminase.

autoimmune response to HB_sAg. Cytomegalovirus infection during an immunosuppressed state is another viral cause. CAH may also follow acute hepatitis C, post-transfusion hepatitis, or delta hepatitis. When CAH presents in adolescents, it may arise from Wilson's disease, a hereditary disorder. In addition, alphamethyldopa, dantrolene, nitrofurantoin, and isoniazid cause inflammatory changes consistent with CAH. Discontinuing the medication usually resolves the inflammatory process.

The onset of CAH is slow. Some clients report the symptoms of acute viral hepatitis, cirrhosis, or extrahepatic problems. Clients go to the acute care setting primarily for liver biopsy and the identification of extrahepatic sequelae, e.g., thyroiditis, hemolytic anemia, amenorrhea, arthritis, urticaria, or glomerulonephritis.

Nursing intervention involves medications and supportive management. As stated, it is important to discontinue medications that may be causing inflammatory changes. The physician may prescribe steroids for a period of 3 to 5 years. Clients who cannot tolerate large doses of steroids may benefit from azathioprine and smaller steroid doses. Clinicians generally do not recommend steroid therapy for asymptomatic CAH, especially in elderly clients. In addition to pharmacologic intervention, bed rest is encouraged during the active phase of the disease. The client usually remains at home to convalesce. There may be periods of remission, but liver necrosis continues.

With steroid therapy, fatigue and anorexia resolve in a few days or weeks. Laboratory values return to normal within weeks or months. The physician reduces the dose of steroids in small increments to prevent a relapse and allow the adrenal glands time to resume normal secretion.

Untreated CAH has a high mortality rate. Death results from hepatic failure, bleeding varices, hepatic encephalopathy, or primary hepatocellular carcinoma.

Liver transplantation is a consideration for those individuals with end-stage liver disease that can no longer be medically managed.

ALCOHOLIC HEPATITIS

Alcoholic hepatitis is either an acute or a chronic inflammation of the liver. It is caused by parenchymal necrosis resulting from heavy alcohol ingestion. Although sometimes reversible, this condition is the most frequent cause of cirrhosis. This fact is important because cirrhosis of the liver is a common cause of death among adults in the United States.

Clinical manifestations of alcoholic hepatitis usually develop following a recent bout of heavy drinking. Assessment reveals anorexia, nausea, abdominal pain, splenomegaly, hepatomegaly, jaundice, ascites, fever, and encephalopathy. Laboratory studies typically show anemia, leukocytosis, and an elevated serum bilirubin. Liver biopsy reveals a typically fatty-appearing liver.

Nursing intervention includes a high-vitamin, high-carbohydrate diet; folic acid supplements; and parenteral fluids. Steroids sometimes have a beneficial effect, although their use remains controversial.

Hepatitis due to excessive alcohol intake has a poor prognosis, particularly if the client continues to use alcohol.

▼ Cirrhosis

Definition

Cirrhosis of the liver is the disorganization of the liver architecture by widespread fibrosis and nodule formation. Cirrhosis occurs when the normal flow of blood, bile, and hepatic metabolites is altered by fibrosis and changes in the hepatocytes, bile ductules, vascular channels, and reticular cells.

There are four major types of cirrhosis: Laennec's (micronodular), postnecrotic (macronodular or toxin induced), biliary, and cardiac (Table 58-7). The two major clinical problems in cirrhosis are (1) decreased liver function and (2) portal hypertension. The latter develops in severe cirrhosis.

Incidence

Only 10 to 15 per cent of clients with chronic alcoholism develop cirrhosis; however, more than 65 per cent of all cases of cirrhosis are related to alcohol. Laennec's cirrhosis is therefore the most common type. Men are more likely than women to develop Laënnec's cirrhosis. Cirrhosis is the fourth leading cause of death in clients between 35 and 54 years of age. It is the ninth leading cause of death overall in the United States and may occur at any age.

Worldwide, postnecrotic cirrhosis is the most common type of cirrhosis. It is also more common in women. Mortality is higher from all types of cirrhosis in men and non-whites.

Etiology

The exact causes of cirrhosis have not been clearly identified. Genetic predisposition with a familial tendency, as well as a hypersensitivity to alcohol is seen in alcoholic cirrhosis.

Laennec's or micronodular cirrhosis is most commonly found in clients who chronically abuse alcohol. However, it is also found in nondrinkers. The quantity of alcohol that causes the diffuse scarring of micronodular cirrhosis varies from client to client.

Any chemical or organism that causes liver destruction and irregular patchy regeneration predisposes a client to cirrhosis. In Laennec's cirrhosis, it is the hepatotoxic nature of alcohol that causes the damage. If the client is in a poor nutritional state, the damage is more likely and more severe.

Postnecrotic cirrhosis usually follows acute viral hepatitis, although it may be due to exposure to industrial or chemical hepatotoxins such as carbon tetrachloride or arsenic. Biliary cirrhosis occurs secondary to chronic biliary inflammation or obstruction. Cardiac cirrhosis is secondary to congestive heart failure with prolonged venous hepatic congestion.

Risk Factors

The primary risk factor for cirrhosis is alcohol ingestion, especially in the absence of proper nutrition. Any client with a family history of alcoholism should avoid alcohol because of the increased risk.

Viral hepatitis is the primary risk factor for postnecrotic cirrhosis, and thus it is very important for the client with hepatitis to avoid any other stressors and allow the liver to heal completely without further insult. Clients with hepatitis must avoid any exposure to other hepatotoxins.

Avoidance of industrial or chemical compounds by working in well-ventilated areas and taking other safety measures decreases the risk from these toxins. Prompt treatment of biliary disorders helps decrease the risk of biliary cirrhosis. Adequate treatment of congestive heart failure can help prevent cardiac cirrhosis.

Pathophysiology

Cirrhosis is the final stage in many types of liver insults. The cirrhotic liver usually has a nodular consistency, with bands of fibrosis (scar tissue) and small areas of regenerating tissue. There is extensive destruction of hepatocytes. This alteration in the architecture of the liver alters the flow in the vascular system and lymphatic bile duct channels. Periodic exacerbations are marked by bile stasis, precipitating jaundice.

Portal hypertension develops in severe cirrhosis. Recall that the portal vein receives blood from the intestines and spleen. Thus, an increase of pressure in the portal vein causes (1) a reverse flow of blood and enlargement of the esophageal, umbilical, and superior rectus veins, which may result in bleeding varices; (2) ascites (fluid accumulation in the peritoneum); and (3) incomplete clearing of metabolic wastes, leading to hepatic encephalopathy.

Continuation of the process from unknown causes or from alcohol abuse usually results in death from hepatic encephalopathy, bacterial infection (Gram negative), peritonitis (bacterial), hepatoma (liver tumor), or complications of portal hypertension.

Clinical Manifestations

Table 58-8 identifies the clinical manifestations of advanced cirrhosis and their pathophysiologic bases. Figure 58-4 illustrates the characteristics of severe cirrho-

TABLE 58-7. Comparison of Macronodular, Biliary, and Cardiac Cirrhosis

Definition	Etiology	Pathology	Assessment Data	Diagnosis and Prognosis	Intervention
Macronodular cirrhosis (postnecrotic)					
Most common worldwide form Massive loss of liver cells, with irregular patterns of regenerating cells	Post-acute viral (types B and C) hepatitis Post-intoxication with industrial chemicals Some infections and metabolic disorders	Liver small and nodular	Similar to Laennec's except less muscle wasting and more jaundice	Needle biopsy of liver establishes pathologic process Within 5 years 75% die of complications ↑ Serum aminotransferases ↑ Gamma globulins	Treat complications as needed
Biliary cirrhosis					
Bile flow is decreased with concurrent cell damage to hepatocytes around bile ductules	*Primary* Chronic stasis of bile in intrahepatic ducts Cause unknown Autoimmune process implicated *Secondary* Obstruction of bile ducts outside of liver	Early-stage biopsy reveals inflammatory process with necrosis of cells and ducts Hepatocytes are lost and scar tissue remains End stage similar to postnecrotic	Generalized pruritus Dark urine Pale stools Jaundice Impaired bile flow Steatorrhea ↓ absorption of fat-soluble vitamins Elevated serum lipids ↑ Cholesterol deposits in subcutaneous tissues Signs of portal hypertension	Elevated serum bilirubin levels Early: 3-10 mg/100 ml Late: >50 mg/100 ml High elevations of alkaline phosphatase ↑ Gamma globulins ↑ Blood lipids Presence of lipoprotein X ↑ Serum bile salts Hypoprothrombinemia ↑ Antimitochondrial antibody in primary cases ↑ Serum copper in primary cases	*Primary* Treatment is symptomatic, e.g.: High-calorie diet; lower intake of fats by 30-40 gm/day if problems develop Cholestyramine for pruritus Supplement of fat-soluble vitamins *Secondary* Treatment to relieve mechanical obstruction
Cardiac cirrhosis					
Chronic liver disease associated with severe right-sided long-term congestive heart failure (fairly rare)	Atrioventricular valve disease Prolonged constrictive pericarditis Decompensated cor pulmonale	*Early* Dark-colored liver enlarged by blood and edema fluid *Late* Liver capsule thickens and nodular scarring occurs	Slight jaundice, enlarged liver, and ascites in person with severe cardiac impairment over 10-year span RUQ pain during acute congestion Cachexia Fluid retention Circulatory problems	↑ Conjugated bilirubin in serum ↑ Bromosulphalein ↓ Albumin in serum ↑ Serum aminotransferases ↑ Alkaline phosphatase Liver biopsy	Cause of chronic congestive failure is treated if possible

RUQ, right upper quadrant.

sis. Manifestations of cirrhosis diminish if the process is arrested at an early stage.

Cirrhosis is a disease that initially progresses slowly. Thus people with cirrhosis often discover they have the condition when they are seeking health care for other problems. In the early stages of cirrhosis, assessment findings include hepatomegaly (enlarged liver), vascular changes, and abnormal laboratory tests. Palpation reveals a firm (scarred), lumpy (nodular), usually enlarged liver (although the liver becomes hard and shrunken in late cirrhosis).

In advanced cirrhosis, assessment reveals severe

TABLE 58–8. Advanced Cirrhosis Assessment Data

Assessment Data	Pathophysiologic Bases
Emaciation, ascites	Malnutrition, portal hypertension, hypoalbuminemia, and hyperaldosteronism
Splenomegaly	Portal hypertension
Lower leg edema	Hypoalbuminemia, hyperaldosteronism, and pressure of massive ascites obstructing venous return from legs
Prominent abdominal wall veins (caput medusae)	Collateral vessels bypass scarred liver to carry portal blood to superior vena cava; portal hypertension causes dilation
Internal hemorrhoids	Superior rectal veins dilate with pressure of portal hypertension
Palmar erythema, spider nevi, altered hair distribution; amenorrhea, atrophy of testicles, gynecomastia	Probably decreased hormone metabolism in liver, resulting in manifestations of estrogen excess
Bleeding tendency, especially gastrointestinal	Hypoprothrombinemia, thrombocytopenia; portal hypertension and esophageal varices; peptic ulcers common in alcoholism
Anemia	Gastrointestinal blood losses; erythrocyte destruction in enlarged spleen; folic acid deficiency due to inadequate diet
Renal failure	Rapidly failing hepatic function; occasionally precipitated by volume depletion; hepatorenal syndrome
Infections	Leukopenia due to enlarged, overactive spleen; bacteria in portal blood bypass liver, so not removed by Kupffer cells
Encephalopathy	Ammonia, no longer removed by liver, accumulates to levels toxic to brain
Initial or recurrent symptoms of hepatitis (jaundice)	Chronic viral, toxic, or alcoholic hepatitis progressing to cirrhosis may have inflammatory exacerbations
Esophageal varices	Collateral veins in esophagus bypass scarred liver to carry portal blood to superior vena cava; portal hypertension causes dilation

complications such as ascites, gastrointestinal bleeding from varices, or encephalopathy. Splenomegaly (enlarged spleen) indicates severe portal hypertension. Anemia, leukopenia, or thrombocytopenia may result from splenomegaly.

DIAGNOSTIC ASSESSMENT

Laboratory results reveal impaired hepatocellular function: elevated liver serum enzymes (aspartate aminotransferase, alanine aminotransferase, and lactate dehydrogenase), reduced BSP dye excretion, hypoalbuminemia, and elevated prothrombin time. Liver biopsy provides definitive diagnosis and its follow-up sequelae.

Medical Management

Three goals guide the medical management of a client with cirrhosis:

- Maximization of liver function. Although cirrhosis is a progressive, degenerative disorder, steps are taken to minimize trauma risk and maximize regeneration, thereby slowing the course of the disease and prolonging life. A nutritious diet and adequate rest are important. In postnecrotic or posthepatic cirrhosis, the physician may prescribe corticosteroids to reduce manifestations of cirrhosis and improve liver function.
- Prevention of infection. This goal is accomplished by adequate rest, diet, and environmental control. Before the discovery of antibiotics, infection was the major cause of mortality in clients with cirrhosis.
- Control of disabling complications. Ascites, bleeding esophageal varices, and hepatic encephalopathy are discussed in depth later in this chapter. They are the most feared complications of cirrhosis. Renal failure (hepatorenal syndrome) and infection also are deadly.

Management of the client with postnecrotic (macronodular), biliary, and cardiac cirrhosis is essentially the same as that of the clients with Laennec's cirrhosis.

PHARMACOLOGIC MANAGEMENT

Corticosteroids may be used for postnecrotic cirrhosis. The B vitamins and fat-soluble vitamins (vitamins A, D, E, and K) are commonly given to clients with Laennec's cirrhosis. Other medications may be used to treat the complications, such as diuretics for ascites (discussed later in this chapter).

DIETARY MANAGEMENT

A nutritious diet is recommended for cirrhosis. The diet should be high in protein (as long as the blood ammonia levels are normal) and calories. Fat intake need not be restricted.

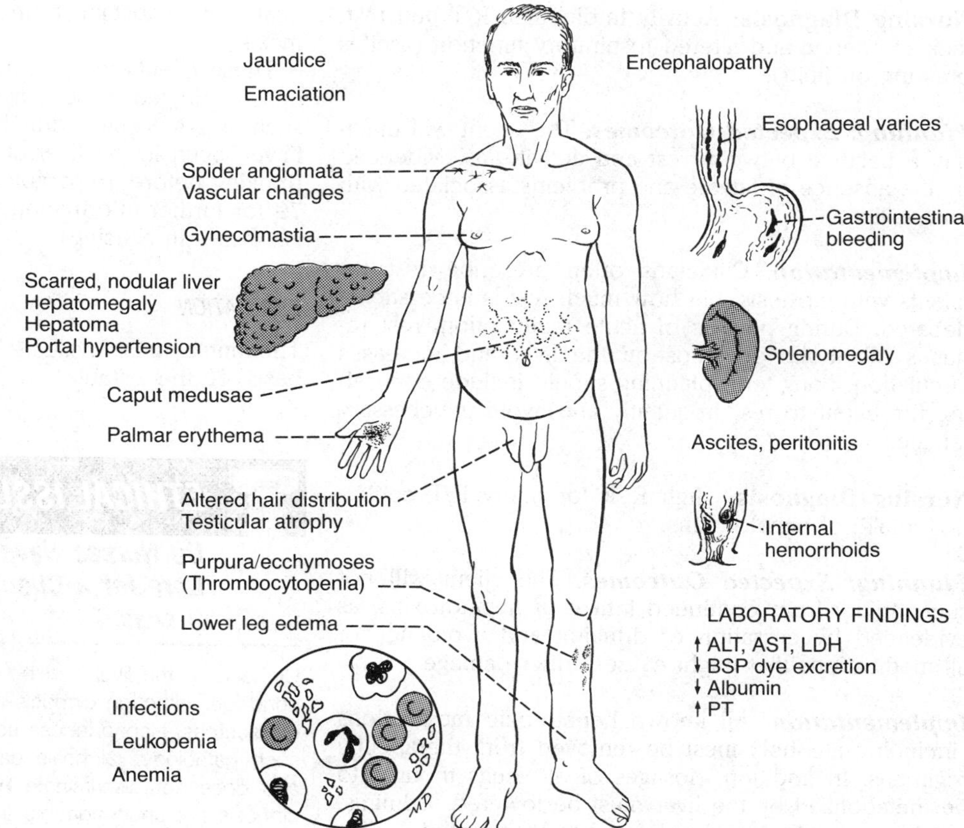

▲ ***Figure 58-4***

Liver cirrhosis: common assessment findings. ALT, alanine aminotransferase; AST, aspartate aminotransferase; LDH, lactate dehydrogenase; BSP, sulfobromophthalein (Bromsulphalein); PT, prothrombin time

Surgical Management

Surgery is not used to treat cirrhosis, although it is used to treat some of the complications.

Nursing Management

ASSESSMENT

Because the symptoms of cirrhosis are sometimes vague and nonspecific, the client may not be aware of the disease's early symptoms. The nurse closely assesses the client for the presence of any of the early symptoms, such as hepatomegaly, and carefully checks the laboratory data for any indication that cirrhosis is present.

As the disease progresses, the nurse should assess for symptoms of complications of cirrhosis, such as ascites, portal hypertension, or hepatic encephalopathy. These are discussed later.

When a client with cirrhosis is hospitalized, the nurse uses laboratory data and the client's physical and psychosocial assessment data to guide care planning.

NURSING INTERVENTION

Nursing Diagnosis: Nutrition, Altered: Less Than Body Requirements R/T anorexia, impaired liver function, decreased absorption of fat-soluble vitamins, and diarrhea.

Planning: Expected Outcomes. The client will take in adequate nutrition, as evidenced by no weight loss and no signs of malnutrition.

Implementation. The diet should provide ample protein to rebuild tissue, but not enough protein to precipitate hepatic encephalopathy. The diet should supply sufficient carbohydrates to maintain weight and spare protein. Fat restriction is not necessary. Total daily calories should range between 2000 and 3000. The client is placed on daily weight, intake and output, and calorie counts to assess fluid and nutritional balance. The laboratory and nutritional panels are closely monitored for signs of improvement or further deterioration.

If the client has ascites or edema, sodium and possible fluids should be restricted in the diet. Small frequent meals will make it easier for clients with anorexia to ingest enough food. Adequate rest and a stable environmental temperature should be ensured to allow optimal use of calories.

The physician usually prescribes a maintenance multivitamin preparation and administers therapeutic levels of vitamins in severe malnutrition. Also, vitamins A, D, E, and K are supplied if fat absorption is present. The client with severe malabsorption may require intravenous vitamins with calcium gluconate supplementation.

Nursing Diagnosis: Activity Intolerance R/T bed rest, lack of energy, and altered respiratory function (ascites pressing on fluid).

Planning: Expected Outcomes. The client will maintain a balance between rest and activity, as evidenced by the absence of fatigue and problems associated with immobility.

Implementation. Clinicians often prescribe rest for clients with cirrhosis, but how much rest is necessary is debated. During periods of acute malfunction, rest reduces metabolic demands on the liver and increases circulation. Long-term planning should include counseling the client to rest frequently and avoid unnecessary fatigue.

Nursing Diagnosis: High Risk for Injury R/T continued intake of hepatotoxins.

Planning: Expected Outcomes. The client will not suffer injury from continued intake of hepatotoxins, as evidenced by cessation of drinking and avoidance of all medications that might cause further damage.

Implementation. All known hepatotoxic medications (including alcohol) must be removed from therapeutic regimens. In addition, dosages of all drugs thought to be metabolized by the liver must be lowered. Administration of sedatives and opiates is to be avoided.

Collaborative Problem. High Risk for Hemorrhage R/T bleeding tendencies.

Planning: Expected Outcomes. Hemorrhage will be prevented, as evidenced by absence of bleeding, normal vital signs, and urine output of at least 30 ml/h.

Implementation. The nurse monitors the client for bleeding gums, purpura, melena, hematuria, and hematemesis. The nurse protects the client from physical injury due to falls or abrasions and gives injections to the client only when absolutely necessary, using only small-gauge needles. The nurse should be sure to apply gentle pressure after an injection.

The nurse teaches the client to avoid vigorous nose blowing and straining with bowel movements. Sometimes stool softeners may be ordered. The nurse advises the client to use a soft toothbrush and refrain from flossing until the bleeding has improved.

Nursing Diagnosis: Knowledge Deficit R/T disease and long-term treatment.

Planning: Expected Outcomes. The client will understand the disease and the implications of long-term management, as evidenced by the client's statements.

Implementation. The client and significant others are provided with information in preparation for care at home. Clients with cirrhosis live longer if they get adequate rest, abstain from alcohol, and eat nutritious meals.

Those clients with a history of alcohol abuse should be encouraged to seek assistance from support groups such as AA to stop drinking. Even if cirrhotic changes have begun in the liver, it is vital for the client to stop drinking before irreparable damage occurs. See Chapter 79 for further information on alcoholism (also see Ethical Issues in Nursing).

EVALUATION

The nurse must evaluate the client outcomes on the basis of the established plan of care. If these goals

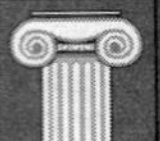

ETHICAL ISSUES IN NURSING

Do Nurses Have an Obligation to Care for a Client with a Lifestyle Disease?

Cirrhosis of the liver can be a very serious and often deadly condition. Although cirrhosis may be caused by several different sources, alcohol abuse accounts for a large percentage of such pathology. Cirrhosis can affect both men and women and does not discriminate by age. The end stages of liver cirrhosis are uncomfortable for the client as well as for those who care for him or her.

Health care workers who are not specialized in substance abuse often care for those persons who have abused alcohol or other pharmacologic substances. These clients appear in all nursing care settings, e.g., medical-surgical, intensive care, obstetric-gynecologic, and home health care. Because many nurses have not had formal training in the care of substance abusers, it is easy to misunderstand these clients. Caring for a person who has destroyed his or her liver through years of alcohol abuse is difficult, knowing that the problems were purely self-induced. When care givers see these clients and their families go through such an emotional experience all because the clients could not control their alcohol consumption, it is easy to judge the clients harshly. For example, if the client becomes demanding, requiring more nursing time, it is easy to think unkindly of him or her, figuring that, after all, had the client not abused him- or herself, the client would not be in this situation.

It is difficult not to prejudge persons with conditions brought about by their own substance abuse. Health care providers, although they may not approve of such abuse, have a responsibility to assist in the care of those who are in need. In the case of the alcoholic client with liver cirrhosis, the nurse can refer the client and/or family to a substance abuse center or other such services. Nurses who have the potential for caring for substance abusers on an ongoing basis should receive special training in the care of such persons. It is natural to feel that those who abuse anything should more or less receive whatever comes from such activity; however, health care workers must look beyond the abusive personality and treat the person holistically.

were not achieved, the plan and interventions must be revised to meet the client's needs.

Modification of Plan of Care for the Elderly

There are no particular modifications for the older client, other than the possibility that the liver has been damaged previously.

Post-hospital Care

DISCHARGE TEACHING

Discharge teaching first addresses the need for the client to avoid the ingestion of hepatotoxins, especially alcohol. Other medications that should be avoided are also specified to the client. The client should be encouraged to seek help (for example, from AA) with alcohol abstinence.

The client and significant others are taught the need for a nutritious diet. The diet should be rich in vitamins with high enough calories and protein (unless encephalopathy is present, in which case protein is limited). A list of foods to be included in the diet is given to the client and family. If the client is experiencing edema, the client will probably be on a low-sodium diet, possibly with fluid restrictions. If the client is on a thiazide diuretic, the diet should be high in potassium.

The significant others and the client are taught signs of progressive liver failure. The family should know what symptoms they need to report to the physician and when to seek immediate assistance, such as when bleeding from varices or a decrease in the level of consciousness occurs.

HOME HEALTH CARE NEEDS

The home health care needs vary greatly among clients with cirrhosis. Those with milder disease may not need any assistance at home, whereas clients with encephalopathy may need extensive home care.

FOLLOW-UP CARE

The client is seen at regular intervals to follow the progress of the disease. Periodic blood tests are performed to assess liver damage.

▼ Complications of Cirrhosis

PORTAL HYPERTENSION

Definition

Portal hypertension occurs when there is a persistent increase in the pressure in the portal venous system as a result of increased resistance or obstruction of the blood flow through the portal venous system.

Incidence/Etiology

Most cases of portal hypertension in the United States relate to cirrhosis. The portal vein is likely to be obstructed by a thrombus; a tumor is the next most common cause. Table 58-9 identifies factors that may cause portal hypertension.

Pathophysiology

Recall that the normal flow to and from the liver depends on proper functioning of the portal vein (70 per cent of inflow), the hepatic artery (30 per cent of inflow), and the hepatic veins (outflow). Disease processes that damage or alter the flow of blood through the liver or its major vessels are responsible for the development of portal hypertension (Table 58-9). The amount of liver dysfunction varies with the initial process, the length of the process, and individual differences.

Normal portal pressure is 5 to 10 mm Hg. Portal hypertension exists when the pressures rise above 25 mm Hg and collaterals form as a result of poor blood flow through major venous channels. The spleen

TABLE 58-9. Factors in the Pathogenesis of Portal Hypertension

Increased vascular resistance
Intrahepatic
Cirrhosis
Infiltrations (e.g., tumors, sarcoidosis)
Polycystic disease
Schistosomiasis
Noncirrhotic portal fibrosis (hepatic phlebosclerosis)
Portal vein
Thrombosis
Tumor
Infection (pyelophlebitis)
Hepatic veins
Thrombosis (Budd-Chiari syndrome)
Veno-occlusive disease
Sustained high splanchnic inflow
Splenomegaly
Diffuse atrioventricular shunts(?)
Major atrioventricular fistulas
Inadequate decompression via venous collaterals
Esophageal
Retroperitoneal
Periumbilical
Hemorrhoidal

From LaMont, J. T., & Isselbacher, K. J. (1977). Cirrhosis. *In* G. W. Thorn, et al. (Eds.), *Harrison's principles of internal medicine* (8th ed., p. 1611) New York: McGraw-Hill.

and other organs that empty into the portal system also begin to undergo the effects of congestion. Eventually, clinical manifestations arise.

Clinical Manifestations

In clients with portal hypertension, assessment reveals slightly tortuous epigastric vessels that branch off the area of the umbilicus and lead toward the sternum and ribs *(caput medusae);* an enlarged, palpable spleen; internal hemorrhoids; bruits, which may be heard over the upper abdomen; and ascites, which typically appears when there is concurrent liver disease.

DIAGNOSTIC ASSESSMENT

Direct measurement of portal pressure is possible only during laparotomy. The diagnosis of portal hypertension often relies on indirect measurements of portal pressure—liver scans, splenoportography, abdominal angiography, liver biopsy, and other laboratory data (see Chap. 57). Radiography and endoscopy procedures may be used to differentiate variceal hemorrhage from other types of gastrointestinal bleeding.

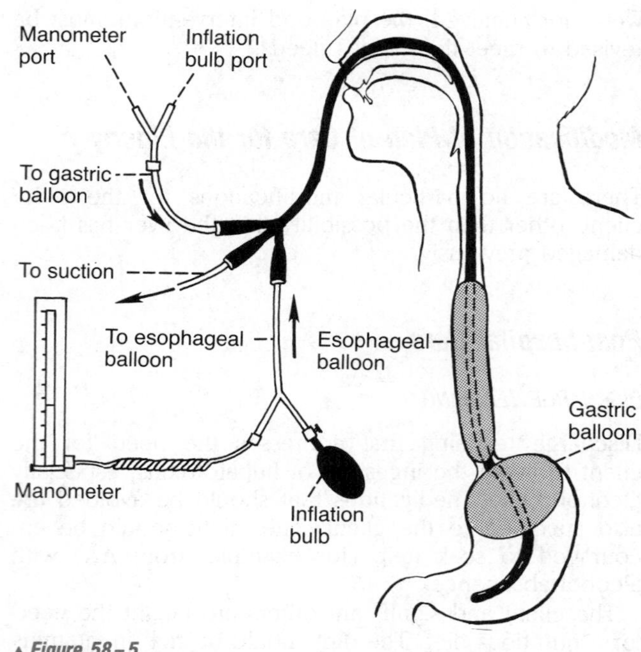

▲ Figure 58-5

A Sengstaken-Blakemore tube may be used to control ruptured esophageal varices, a potential complication of portal hypertension.

Complications

Hemorrhage constitutes the major life-threatening complication of portal hypertension. As portal pressure rises, the superior rectal veins, abdominal wall veins, and esophagogastric veins dilate and distend. These swollen, dilated veins are called varices. Various factors can contribute to the rupturing of varices: portal pressure, increased intrathoracic pressure (coughing and straining at stools), irritation by food or alcohol, and erosion by gastric juices (Fig. 58-5). Veins of the stomach and esophagus are most subject to rupture.

Another mechanism that leads to hemorrhage involves the spleen. The splenic vein merges with the superior mesenteric vein to form the portal vein. When pressure increases in the portal system, damage to the spleen occurs. Damage to the spleen is not proportional to the increase in portal pressure. As the spleen enlarges, it tends to destroy blood cells, and especially platelets, which then increases the risk of hemorrhage and anemia.

Hepatic encephalopathy is an extremely dangerous complication of portal hypertension. This problem usually arises following a period of bleeding into the gastrointestinal tract. Digestion of this blood takes place in the intestines. Because blood is a protein substance, this process increases ammonia in the gut and bloodstream. In turn, the excessive ammonia disturbs brain function. Hepatic encephalopathy is discussed later in this chapter.

Medical Management

Nonsurgical approaches to treat varices include the administration of propranolol and sclerotherapy. To perform sclerotherapy, the physician passes an endoscope into the esophagus and injects a sclerosing agent (e.g., morrhuate sodium) that flows into the varices. The sclerosing agent initially causes inflammation of the vein wall and then fibrosis. The physician may give repeated injections over a period of weeks until the varices are no longer prominent.

Death often follows rupture of esophageal varices. To stop hemorrhage, health practitioners perform emergency measures: administration of vasopressin, balloon tamponade, injection sclerotherapy, direct ligation of the bleeding varices, transhepatic embolization of the left gastric vein, or even urgent portocaval shunt surgery. Cold saline lavage is probably ineffective, but is done while waiting to transport the client to surgery or the gastrointestinal laboratory. Fluids, especially volume expanders and blood products, are administered to maintain volume. Vital signs should be closely monitored throughout this period. This is a very critical time for nursing intervention and can be a very stressful time for the client, family, and the nurse.

Applying pressure to ruptured varices via balloon tamponade may stop the hemorrhage. For this intervention, the clinician inserts a Sengstaken-Blakemore or Minnesota tube into the stomach and inflates the esophageal and gastric balloons (Fig. 58-5). The pressure of the balloon against the varices may stop the bleeding. It is important to release this pressure periodically to prevent tissue necrosis. The esophageal balloon is not left inflated for more than 24 hours. Also, it is important to remove secretions and saliva that accumulate above the balloon to prevent aspiration. The Minnesota tube actually has a fourth port for aspiration of secretions above the esophageal balloon.

PHARMACOLOGIC MANAGEMENT

Propranolol (Inderal) reduces portal pressure. Administered on a long-term basis, it appears to decrease the risk of bleeding from esophageal varices. Propranolol is a beta-blocker, and therefore it reduces the heart rate and masks the early manifestation of hypoglycemia should it occur.

Administration of vasopressin (Pitressin) achieves temporary lowering of portal pressure. These agents reduce portal blood flow by constricting afferent arterioles. Direct infusion of vasopressin into the superior mesenteric artery is most effective. Sometimes vasopressin is administered intravenously. Systemic side effects include hyponatremia, myocardial ischemia, and stimulation of uterine and gastrointestinal contraction (cramping and diarrhea).

Surgical Management

There are several surgical approaches that reduce the danger of hemorrhage from varices caused by portal hypertension. Surgical approaches include a variety of portosystemic shunt procedures to reduce portal pressure.

Surgical creation of a portosystemic shunt reduces portal hypertension by sending portal blood directly into the inferior vena cava, bypassing the liver (Fig. 58-6). Such a procedure decreases portal hypertension and thus the risk of rupturing esophageal varices. This process increases the incidence of hepatic encephalopathy, however, because the shunted blood is not cleared of toxic substances. For this reason, clinicians usually reserve portosystemic shunt procedures for clients who have had one or more episodes of bleeding varices.

Figure 58-6 illustrates some of the many portacaval shunt procedures possible. The goal of these procedures is threefold:

1. To reduce portal blood flow enough to prevent variceal hemorrhage.
2. To preserve enough blood inflow to the liver to prevent hepatic encephalopathy and hepatic failure.
3. To increase client comfort (this is a palliative procedure).

Achievement of these goals requires a delicate balance between the reduction of expendable blood flow and the preservation of essential blood flow.

Nursing Management

ASSESSMENT

The major assessment for the nurse to make is the presence of hemorrhage. The other important assess-

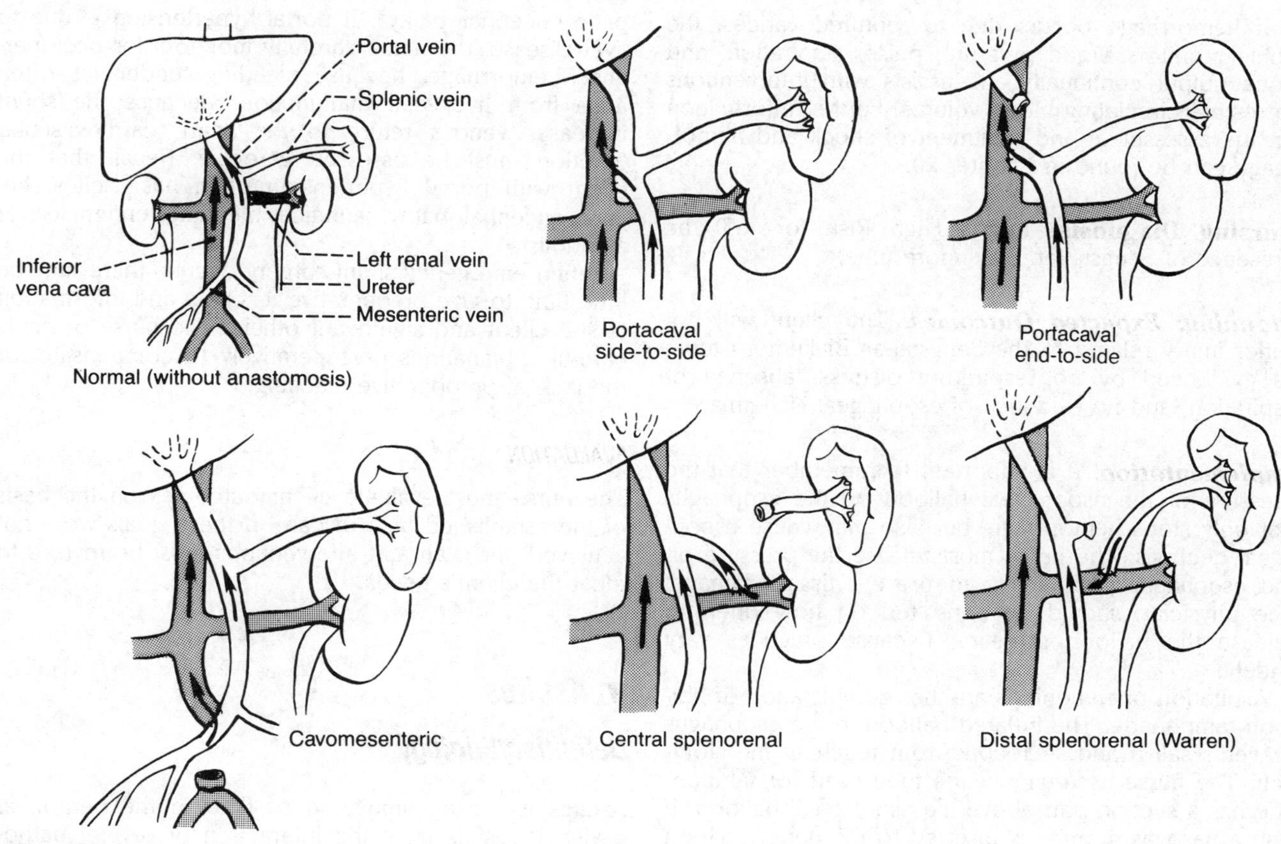

▲ *Figure 58-6*

Some types of portacaval shunt procedures used to reduce portal hypertension.

ments are the client's condition after any interventions to treat the hemorrhage, such as the functioning of the Sengstaken-Blakemore tube. The client's vital signs are continuously assessed for any significant changes.

NURSING INTERVENTION

Collaborative Problem. Decreased cardiac output R/T blood volume loss secondary to rupture of esophageal varices and resultant hemorrhage.

Planning: Expected Outcomes. An adequate cardiac output will be maintained as evidenced by the return of vital signs to normal and no further bleeding.

Implementation. The client can learn activities to help decrease the risk of rupture of esophageal varices. The nurse should teach the client to

- Avoid straining maneuvers that increase intra-abdominal or intrathoracic pressure.
- Avoid rough foods that may traumatize the esophagus or spicy foods that may irritate the esophageal mucosa.
- Develop an emergency plan if the client has severe esophageal varices that may rupture. Included in this plan should be a list of all emergency telephone numbers. The plan should be discussed with both the client and significant others.

If hemorrhage occurs due to ruptured varices, the nurse monitors blood pressure, pulse, respiration, and urine output continually and assists with interventions to restore circulating blood volume. Further information on the assessment and treatment of shock and hemorrhage can be found in Chapter 20.

Nursing Diagnosis: Injury, High Risk for R/T the presence of Sengstaken-Blakemore tube.

Planning: Expected Outcomes. The client will not suffer injury related to the Sengstaken-Blakemore tube, as evidenced by no respiratory distress, absence of aspiration, and no evidence of esophageal ischemia.

Implementation. It is important to remember that the pressure of the esophageal balloon on the esophagus not only stops hemorrhage, but also may cause esophageal necrosis. The nurse must release the pressure on the esophagus periodically to prevent tissue damage. The physician should be consulted on how often to release the balloon pressure, because practices vary widely.

Aspiration pneumonia is another complication of balloon tamponade. The inflated balloon in the esophagus prevents saliva and secretions from reaching the stomach. The nurse ascertains if the tube used for tamponade has a suction port above the esophageal balloon. If not, a nasogastric tube is inserted to the upper balloon level or suctioning performed frequently to remove accumulating fluid.

Tubes inserted through the nose may cause erosion of the nares, especially if traction is applied to the tamponade (practices differ). To prevent this complication, the nurse cleans and lubricates the external nares. Padding is provided if necessary.

The last complication of balloon tamponade is airway obstruction. This occurs when the gastric balloon deflates or breaks and the traction on the tube pulls the esophageal balloon up into the oropharynx. Scissors should be kept at the bedside in case this emergency arises. The nurse cuts the tube and pulls it out to restore airway patency. To prevent this complication, the nurse may label each port of the tube to prevent accidental deflation of the gastric balloon.

Nursing Diagnosis: Thought Processes, Altered, high risk for R/T development of hepatic encephalopathy secondary to shunt procedure.

Planning: Expected Outcomes. Hepatic encephalopathy will be prevented or will be diagnosed early, after the shunt surgery, as evidenced by no decreased level of consciousness and no increase in blood ammonia level.

Implementation. If the client with portal hypertension undergoes portosystemic shunt surgery, the nurse provides postoperative care as described in Chapter 19. In addition, the client is assessed for hepatic encephalopathy (see the section on clinical manifestations of hepatic encephalopathy). If portal hypertension is due to liver disease, the nurse carefully monitors for postoperative hemorrhage, because bleeding tendencies often arise from liver cell malfunction. Because the shunt increases venous return to the heart, cardiovascular function must be assessed carefully. Recall that the client with portal hypertension often has ascites, hepatic encephalopathy, jaundice, bleeding tendencies, or alcoholism.

When emergency shunt surgery occurs, there may be little time to give preoperative teaching and information to the client and significant others. The nurse presents careful explanations postoperatively to compensate for the lack of preoperative teaching.

EVALUATION

The nurse must evaluate client outcomes on the basis of the established plan of care. If these goals were not achieved, the plan and interventions must be revised to meet the client's needs.

▼ Ascites

Definition/Etiology

Ascites is the accumulation of fluid in the peritoneal cavity. It results from the interaction of several pathophysiologic changes. Portal hypertension, lowered plasma colloidal osmotic pressure, and sodium retention all contribute to this condition. Disease processes that lead to these events include cirrhosis of the liver, right-sided heart failure, tuberculous peritonitis, cancer, and complications of pancreatitis.

Pathophysiology

Any process that blocks the flow of blood through the liver sinusoids to the hepatic veins and vena cava causes an increase in hydrostatic pressure in the portal venous system. Most commonly, this problem develops in cirrhosis of the liver or right-sided heart failure. As portal pressure increases, plasma leaks directly from the liver capsule and the congested portal vein into the peritoneal cavity. Congestion of lymph channels occurs, leading to the leakage of more plasma into the peritoneal cavity. Loss of plasma proteins into ascitic fluid from the portal system reduces oncotic pressure in the vascular compartment. Reduction in oncotic pressure limits the vascular system's ability to hold onto or collect water.

In addition, hepatocellular damage reduces the liver's ability to synthesize normal amounts of albumin. Decreased albumin synthesis leads to hypoalbuminemia, which is exacerbated by leakage of protein into the peritoneal cavity. The circulating blood volume decreases from the loss of colloid osmotic pressure. The secretion of aldosterone increases to stimulate the kidneys to retain sodium and water. As a result of hepatocellular damage, the liver is unable to inactivate the hormone aldosterone. Thus, sodium and water retention continues. More fluid is held, and the volume of ascites grows.

In summary, the three mechanisms that underlie ascites formation are

- Portal hypertension resulting in increased plasma and lymphatic hydrostatic pressures,
- Hypoalbuminemia resulting in decreased colloid osmotic pressure, and
- Hyperaldosteronism resulting in renal sodium and water retention.

Clinical Manifestations

Ascitic fluid typically produces abdominal distention, bulging flanks, and a protruding (downward) umbilicus. Figure 58-7 depicts a client with ascites before therapy. Although large accumulations of ascitic fluid are obvious, small or moderate amounts may be more difficult to diagnose.

DIAGNOSTIC ASSESSMENT

Diagnostic tests to confirm the presence of ascites include paracentesis, abdominal x-ray studies, ultrasonography, and computed tomographic scan. These tests may locate fluid in the peritoneal cavity. A paracentesis provides samples of fluid for analysis. Findings help determine the source of the ascites, such as the finding of malignant cells.

Medical Management

The goal of intervention for ascites is to correct fluid and electrolyte imbalances by improving renal sodium excretion and restricting sodium and water intake. This involves discontinuing medications that inhibit prostaglandin synthesis (e.g., aspirin and indomethacin) and thus impair renal sodium excretion.

The use of repeated paracenteses for removal of ascitic fluid has fallen into disfavor. Repeated removal of fluid, protein, and electrolytes from the body causes severe disturbances of homeostasis.

PHARMACOLOGIC MANAGEMENT

Diuretics, especially spironolactone, are useful in decreasing fluid retention. In addition, the physician may prescribe intravenous administration of albumin.

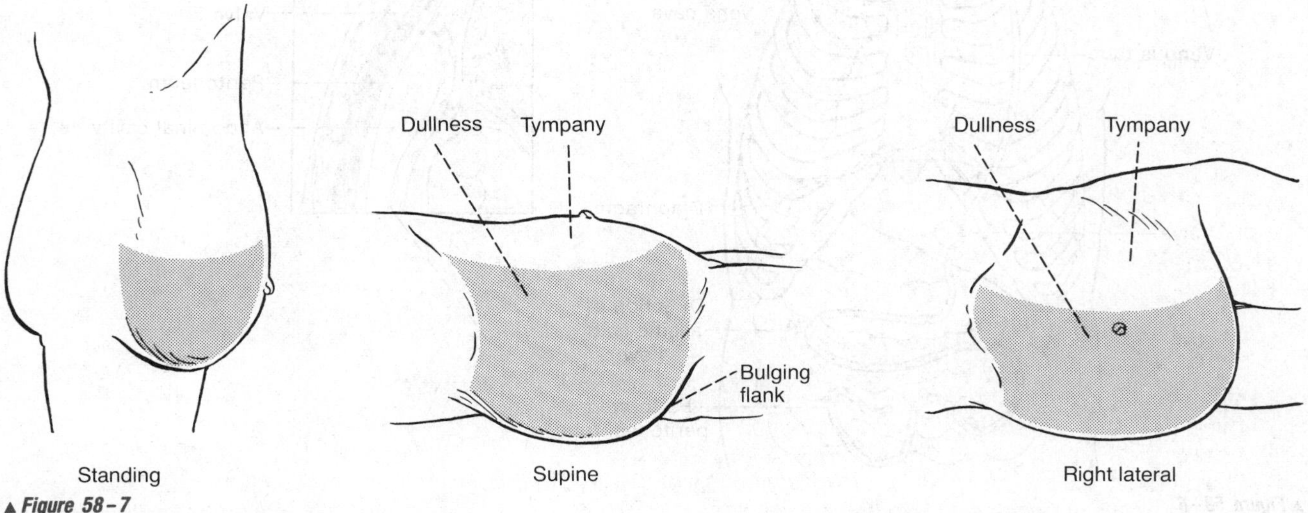

▲ **Figure 58-7**

Assessing fluid levels in ascites.

DIETARY MANAGEMENT

The diet is a low-sodium diet with restriction of fluids. Protein intake is moderate unless the client has signs of hepatic encephalopathy.

Surgical Management

The client with refractory and disabling chronic ascites may obtain relief from the insertion of a peritoneovenous shunt (e.g., LeVeen or Denver shunt). As Figure 58-8 shows, a properly functioning shunt moves fluid from the peritoneal (abdominal) cavity into the venous blood of the superior vena cava. Resolution of ascites may be dramatic after implantation of a peritoneovenous shunt.

Complications of shunt implantation include infection, disseminated intravascular coagulation, congestive heart failure, and shunt clotting.

Nursing Management

ASSESSMENT

Some simple assessments that can be performed at the bedside are as follows:

- Percuss the abdomen. If the client has ascites, the sound will be dull.
- Turn the client laterally and percuss the abdomen (Fig. 58-7). Because ascitic fluid flows to the lowest point in the abdomen, it will move downward when the client turns. This causes a shift in the area where dullness is heard.
- Tap the abdomen to elicit a fluid wave.

The amount of distress that the ascites is causing also should be assessed. The nurse assesses whether the fluid is interfering with sleeping, eating, and breathing.

NURSING INTERVENTION

Collaborative Problem. Fluid volume excess in third space combined with fluid volume deficit in intravascular space R/T fluid shifts secondary to portal hypertension, hypoalbuminemia, and hyperaldosteronism.

Planning: Expected Outcomes. A normal balance of fluid between the intracellular and extracellular spaces will be maintained, as evidenced by absence of hypovolemia, normal serum albumin, decreased abdominal girth, and normal blood pressure.

Implementation. The client is on a fluid restriction that must be strictly followed. To better space the fluids, the nurse may give medications with meals, if possible, so these fluids can be used for the medications. The abdominal girth should be measured daily and sometimes twice a day, and daily weights should be taken. Aspirin should be avoided because it stimulates prostaglandin secretion.

The client is monitored closely after a paracentesis. The nurse checks vital signs frequently to ensure that the client tolerated the procedure well and checks the dressing carefully to ensure that excessive amounts of fluid are not lost.

Nursing Diagnosis: Breathing Pattern, Ineffective R/T increased intra-abdominal pressure on diaphragm.

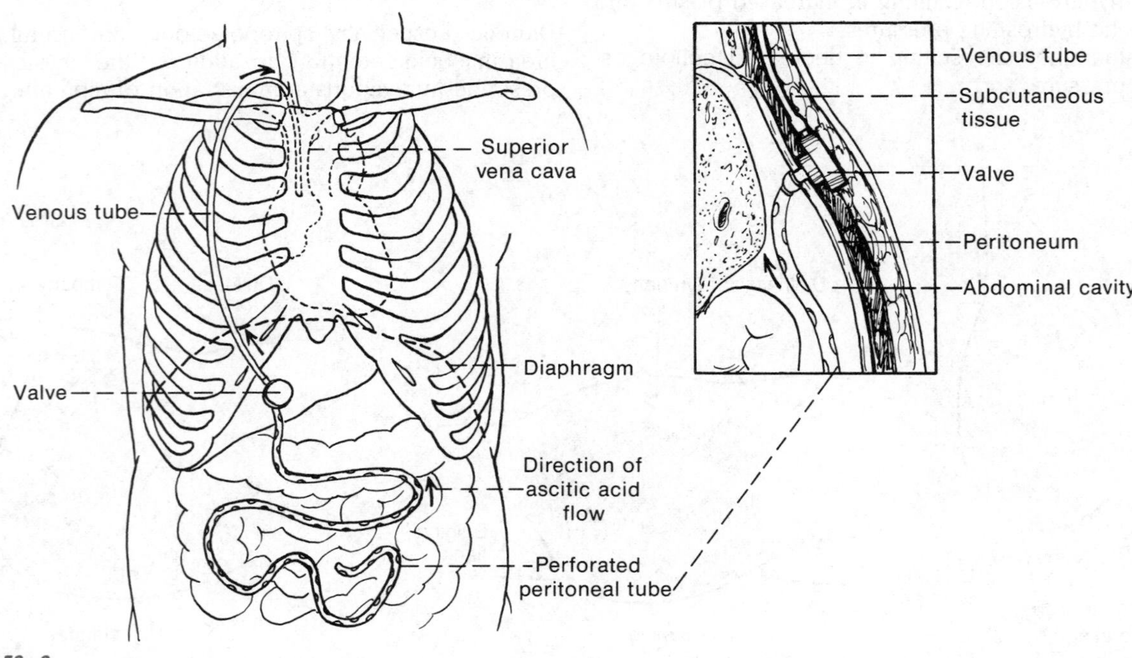

▲ *Figure 58-8*

LeVeen peritoneovenous shunt for chronic ascites moves fluid from the peritoneal (abdominal) cavity into the superior vena cava.

Planning: Expected Outcomes. The client will not suffer from an ineffective breathing pattern, as evidenced by the absence of shortness of breath and the presence of normal respiratory excursion.

Implementation. The nurse positions the client in high Fowler's position to facilitate breathing and monitors the client's respiratory status for the development of atelectasis or pneumonia. The client is asked to cough and take a deep breath hourly to maintain adequate respiratory function. The client may need to use an incentive spirometer or receive ultrasonic treatments if the cough is ineffective.

Nursing Diagnosis: Skin Integrity, High Risk for or Actual Impaired R/T immobility, edema, and pressure from the abdomen.

Planning: Expected Outcomes. The client will not develop impaired skin integrity, as evidenced by intact skin.

Implementation. The nurse turns the client frequently, providing adequate support for the distended abdomen. If the client is on bed rest, a specialty mattress is used to prevent skin breakdown. The client's skin is carefully inspected daily and lotions and creams used if necessary.

Nursing Diagnosis: Knowledge Deficit R/T ascites, treatment, and self-care following discharge.

Planning: Expected Outcomes. The client will understand ascites, its treatment, and self-care following discharge, as evidenced by the client's statements and compliance with the treatment regimen and abstention from alcohol.

Implementation. The nurse discusses the causes of ascites with the client, making sure that the client understands ways to slow the recurrence. The nurse ensures that the client understands the need for dietary modifications, fluid restrictions, and home health care needs. The client must be helped to understand that all alcohol intake must be stopped. Refer the client to AA for assistance with abstinence if necessary.

EVALUATION

The nurse must evaluate client outcomes on the basis of the established plan of care. If these goals were not achieved, the plan and interventions must be revised to meet the client's needs.

▼ Hepatic Encephalopathy

Definition/Etiology

Hepatic encephalopathy encompasses a spectrum of central nervous system (CNS) disturbances. These disturbances may appear in conjunction with severe liver injury, liver failure, or portal shunt. The etiology of this disorder is the liver's inability to metabolize ammonia to form urea that is then excreted. Ammonia is a CNS depressant. Changes during the initial stages of hepatic encephalopathy include reduced mental alertness, confusion, and restlessness. Loss of consciousness, seizures, and irreversible coma occur in the terminal stage.

Pathophysiology

Hepatic encephalopathy is characterized by elevations of ammonia levels in the blood and cerebrospinal fluid. Ammonia is produced when protein is broken down in the gastrointestinal tract by bacteria; in the liver; and, in lesser amounts, by gastric juices and peripheral tissue metabolism. The kidneys are another source of ammonia in the presence of hypokalemia.

Normally, the liver converts ammonia into glutamine, which is stored in the liver and later converted to urea and excreted through the kidneys. Blood ammonia rises when the liver cells are unable to perform this conversion. Failure of the liver to perform this important function may be due to liver cell damage and necrosis. It also may result from shunting blood from the portal system directly into systemic venous circulation (bypassing the liver). In either case, as blood ammonia levels rise, many unusual compounds begin to form. Some of these (e.g., octopamine) apparently act as false neurotransmitters in the CNS. Ammonia also is a CNS toxin, with glial and nerve cells greatly affected, leading to altered CNS metabolism and function.

Any process that increases protein in the intestine, such as increased dietary protein or gastrointestinal bleeding, causes elevated blood ammonia levels and possibly signs of hepatic encephalopathy in clients with hepatocellular failure or portal shunt.

Although intervention usually alleviates hepatic encephalopathy, the client may succumb to circulatory or respiratory complications, infection, or delirium and convulsions. Mortality is high among clients who progress into coma with hepatic failure. Health practitioners often use dramatic measures to reduce toxic levels of ammonia in the blood. Such measures include peritoneal dialysis and exchange transfusions, which involve removal and replacement of approximately 80 per cent of the client's blood. A liver transplant may be performed for cases of fulminant liver failure.

Clinical Manifestations

Manifestation of hepatic encephalopathy progresses from mild mental confusion to deep coma. Hepatic encephalopathy impairs memory, attention, concentration, and rate of response. Sleep pattern reversal often occurs, with the client awake at night and sleepy during the day. The nurse evaluates handwriting and speech for significant changes. Asterixis (liver flap) may be present. Some clients with hepatic encephalopathy develop hyperventilation with respiratory alkalosis. The presence of methylmercaptan causes a characteristic odor on the breath called fetor hepaticus.

As the client's condition deteriorates, characteristic delta waves appear on the electroencephalogram. As the syndrome progresses, the client's level of consciousness slowly diminishes, and confusion becomes more severe. However, the level of CNS depression commonly fluctuates.

Coma may eventually ensue, deepening until there is no pain response and the reflexes, including corneal, are completely absent. Table 58-10 lists the stages of hepatic encephalopathy.

DIAGNOSTIC ASSESSMENT

Laboratory results show elevated blood ammonia and cerebrospinal fluid glutamine. Although findings help to confirm the diagnosis of encephalopathy, they are not specific to this entity.

The nurse monitors serum ammonia levels, electrolytes, blood gases, and hepatic function tests (bilirubin, albumin, prothrombin, and enzymes) throughout the course of this syndrome. These clinical findings help determine the degree of imbalance and the extent of hepatic injury and malfunction (see Chap. 57).

Medical Management

The goals of intervention for clients with hepatic encephalopathy are (1) control or reduce further degenerative processes, (2) correct present metabolic imbalances, and (3) preserve remaining physiologic functioning.

TABLE 58-10. Stages of Hepatic Encephalopathy

Stage 1
Fatigue
Restlessness
Irritability
Decreased intellectual performance
Decreased attention span
Diminished short-term memory
Personality changes
Sleep pattern reversal

Stage 2
Deteriorated handwriting
Asterixis
Drowsiness
Confusion
Lethargy
Fetor hepaticus

Stage 3
Severe confusion
Unable to follow commands
Deep somnolence, but arousable

Stage 4
Coma
Unresponsive to painful stimuli
Possible decorticate or decerebrate posturing

Five principles guide intervention in hepatic encephalopathy:

1. Reduce protein in the intestine. Reducing dietary protein serves to reduce protein in the intestine. If no other precipitating factors are present, this alone may eliminate symptoms.
2. Prevent gastrointestinal bleeding, or, if it occurs, quickly remove the blood from the gastrointestinal tract with lactulose enemas.
3. Reduce bacterial production of ammonia. Neomycin and lactulose are useful pharmacologic agents for this purpose.
4. Eliminate fluid and electrolyte imbalances, hypoxia, infection, and sedation.
5. Maintain safety and function in the unconscious client. The immobile client who lacks reflexes is vulnerable to numerous complications.

PHARMACOLOGIC MANAGEMENT

Neomycin and lactulose are given to reduce the bacteria in the intestinal tract. Because neomycin is not absorbed into the circulation, it exerts a powerful effect on the intestinal bacteria responsible for ammonia production. Undesirable side effects result from the depletion of intestinal flora (e.g., diarrhea and vitamin K deficiency). Since neomycin is ototoxic and nephrotoxic, avoid its use in clients with renal insufficiency.

DIETARY MANAGEMENT

Protein might be totally eliminated from the diet, with an intake of fruit juices and intravenous fluids, although this radical restriction leads to catabolism of the client's own protein stores. The usual protein restriction is 20 to 40 g/day. The client with chronic hepatic encephalopathy may need to adjust to a long-term, low-protein diet (50 to 60 g/day), which can be difficult.

Nursing Management

ASSESSMENT

When working with a client susceptible to hepatic encephalopathy, the nurse uses interviewing and assessment techniques to evaluate psychophysiologic status. For example, has the client's normally neat handwriting become sloppy and difficult to read? Is speech slow and slurred? The nurse observes for personality changes with labile feeling states and elicits flapping tremor (asterixis or liver flap) by asking the client to dorsiflex the hand with the rest of the arm resting on the bed. The hand cannot be held steady.

The nurse, who is with the client over time, is often the best person to assess a change in level of mental functioning. Early detection of a depressed or confused level of consciousness greatly improves the client's chances of recovery. To make nursing progress notes relevant, the nurse should describe behavior vividly and objectively ("States pigeons are pecking at his bedclothes") rather than offer interpretations that may have a different meaning for each reader ("Seems more confused"). As the client progresses into coma, the nurse makes ongoing neurologic checks to determine the level of consciousness. See Unit 6 for neurologic assessment of comatose clients.

NURSING INTERVENTION

Nursing Diagnosis: Knowledge Deficit R/T reduction in protein in the diet and long-term pharmacologic intervention with neomycin.

Planning: Expected Outcomes. The client will understand and comply with the reduction in protein in the diet and long-term pharmacologic intervention with neomycin, as evidenced by the client's following a low-protein diet and stating reasons why neomycin should be taken.

Implementation. It is important that the client understand the importance of the protein-reduced diet in order to have the motivation to remain on this diet.

In addition to ensuring a low-protein diet, the nurse assesses for signs of gastrointestinal bleeding, checking for bright blood in the stool or for black, tarry stools. Bleeding results in protein accumulation in the gastrointestinal tract, which exacerbates hepatic encephalopathy. To reverse the progression of symptoms, constipation must be prevented. Cathartics and enemas hasten the exit of protein material from the intestine.

Nursing Diagnosis: Diarrhea R/T laxative action of lactulose.

Planning: Expected Outcomes. The client will have diarrhea controlled, as evidenced by a decrease in the number of diarrheal stools.

Implementation. Intervention for severe hepatic encephalopathy commonly combines neomycin therapy with protein restriction and bowel cleansing. The physician may prescribe maintenance doses of neomycin and a low-protein diet for clients with chronic hepatic encephalopathy. Lactulose is a combination of galactose and fructose that passes through the intestine unchanged. The physician may prescribe lactulose to decrease ammonia by trapping ammonium ions in the bowel. The appropriate lactulose dosage causes two to three soft stool evacuations daily. Diarrhea may be a side effect. The physician may reduce the dosage to prevent further electrolyte imbalance.

Nursing Diagnosis: Fluid Volume Deficit R/T bleeding, decreased intake, and ascites.

Planning: Expected Outcomes. The client will maintain a balanced fluid volume, as evidenced by normal blood pressure, absence of edema, absence of ascites, and balanced intake and output.

Implementation. Hypovolemia often precipitates hepatic encephalopathy by reducing hepatocellular perfusion. Fluid balance must be achieved, maintained, and monitored to prevent further hepatic injury, reduced renal perfusion. Intravenous fluids are delivered evenly over time. Vital signs and central venous pressure are monitored frequently. If necessary, urine output is measured hourly.

Electrolyte and acid-base disturbances may precipitate hepatic encephalopathy or develop during its course. Laboratory tests indicate what replacement therapy is necessary.

Collaborative Problem. High risk for injury R/T loss of protective mechanisms secondary to hepatic coma.

Planning: Expected Outcomes. Injury or complications of immobility will be prevented or will be diagnosed early, as evidenced by absence of corneal abrasions or problems related to immobility.

Implementation. Hypoxemia may precipitate hepatic encephalopathy by damaging the hepatic cell. To prevent and treat hypoxemia, the nurse attends to respiratory interventions (e.g., maintaining a patent airway).

Concurrent infection, with protein accumulating from tissue catabolism, requires rapid intervention. The client is particularly vulnerable to nosocomial infections. Nurses should wash their hands thoroughly and take other measures to prevent cross-contamination.

The nurse must be alert to possible harmful accumulations of ammonia due to diuretic therapy. Hypokalemia from the use of diuretics contributes to hepatic encephalopathy by increasing ammonia production in the kidney.

Finally, depressants may precipitate coma. Their use should be avoided. If agitation occurs in early encephalopathy, agents that are excreted partially through the kidney instead of the liver (e.g., phenobarbital) are administered. Phenobarbital should be administered with caution! The nurse should know which narcotics, tranquilizers, and sedatives are biotransformed by the liver. They are often contraindicated in clients with decreased hepatic function.

The immobile client who lacks reflexes is vulnerable to numerous complications. Preventing complications requires intensive nursing intervention. Pneumonia and skin breakdown may be prevented by turning the client frequently and promoting lung aeration.

Physiologic agitation may appear as the body accumulates metabolic substances. Therefore, the client should be protected from self-injury, i.e., by lowering the bed and padding the side rails. See Unit 6 for further discussion of the comatose client and the client with neurologic disturbances.

EVALUATION

The nurse must evaluate client outcomes on the basis of the established plan of care. If these goals were not achieved, the plan and interventions must be revised to meet the client's needs.

Post-hospital Care

DISCHARGE TEACHING

The discharge teaching for the client with cirrhosis who has experienced complications is extensive. The family or significant others need to know how to decrease the incidence of complications from cirrhosis. The nurse reviews the potential complications and how to prevent or treat them with the care givers. All medications, along with scheduled times of administration and intended, side, and adverse effects, are reviewed.

HOME HEALTH CARE NEEDS

The client's home may need to be altered to adjust for limitations in mobility. Safety precautions should be taken to help prevent any injury to the client. The client's bedroom should be set up near the bathroom facilities when the client is receiving diuretics.

FOLLOW-UP CARE

The client's status needs to be followed closely. The client's care givers need to be aware of any changes that would require immediate medical attention. Diagnostic testing at regular intervals is continued to monitor the status of the liver.

▼ Fatty Liver

Lipid infiltration is one of the more common metabolic diseases of the liver. These infiltrations cause liver enlargement and increased firmness and may result in decreased function. Liver biopsy establishes a definite diagnosis. Studies reveal that triglyceride is the major lipid, but small amounts of cholesterol and phospholipid also may have infiltrated the liver.

Major causes of lipid infiltrations include chronic alcoholism, protein malnutrition in early life, diabetes mellitus, obesity, Cushing's syndrome (natural or induced), jejunoileal bypass, prolonged intravenous hyperalimentation, chronic illnesses that interfere with normal cell nutrition, some hepatotoxins (carbon tetrachloride and DDT), and Reye's syndrome in children.

Clients with moderate to severe lipid infiltration are frequently asymptomatic. However, clients with massive infiltration experience anorexia, abdominal pain, and sometimes jaundice. Laboratory studies demonstrate BSP (Bromsulphalein) retention and elevated serum alkaline phosphatase and bilirubin levels.

Recovery begins after the source of the problem is removed and metabolic balance and adequate nutrition are restored. Residual damage, if it occurs, usually follows persistent fatty infiltration and chronic alcoholism. Fat embolization may occur and can cause death.

Nursing intervention for clients with fatty infiltration of the liver includes (1) preparing the client for diagnostic procedures, (2) giving emotional support by allowing verbalization of concerns and fears, (3) giving supportive physical care, and (4) designing teaching guidelines that promote proper diet and prevent a recurrence.

▼ Liver Neoplasms

Tumors of the liver are either primary or metastatic in origin. Primary liver tumors may arise from hepatocytes, connective tissue, blood vessels, or bile ducts. These tumors are either benign or malignant (Figure 58–9). Figure 58–10 presents a classification of the primary liver neoplasms.

Metastatic malignant tumors arise from the gastrointestinal tract (particularly the colon), the breasts, and the lungs.

PRIMARY LIVER NEOPLASMS

Adenomas

Adenomas are benign hepatic cell tumors. The incidence of this type of tumor is increasing. Researchers

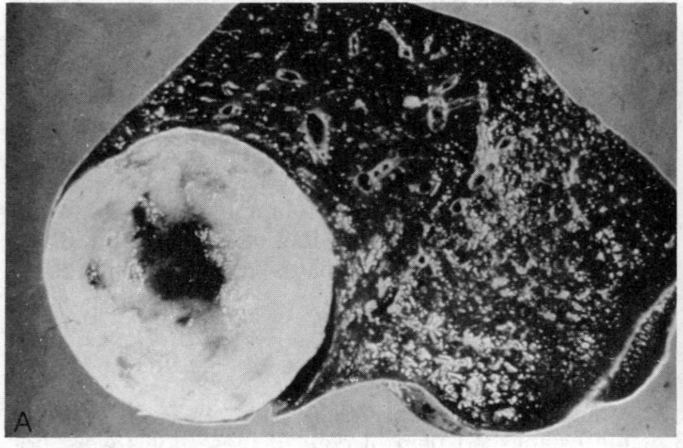

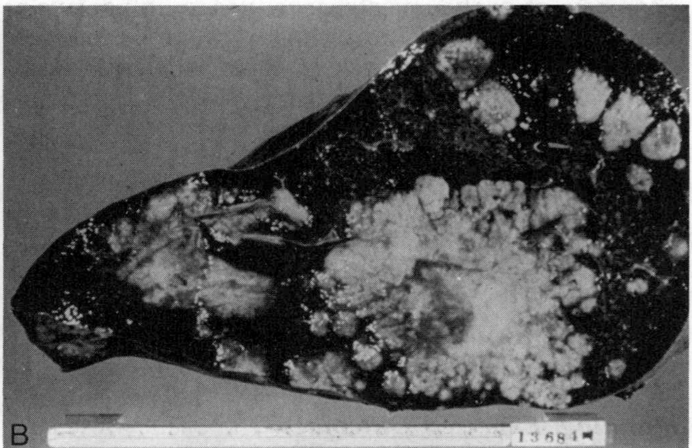

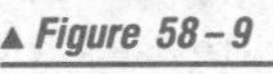
▲ Figure 58–9

Benign liver tumor *(A)* and metastatic malignant liver tumor *(B)*.

postulate that there is an association between some adenomas and either oral contraceptives used by women or androgens used by men.

Although these tumors are classified as benign, they are nevertheless dangerous because of their vascularity. A benign adenoma may rupture, with consequent hemorrhage. Hepatic arteriography is a valuable early diagnostic test for this condition. Liver biopsy is helpful but poses a danger due to the problem of possible hemorrhage. Other liver function tests usually reveal normal findings.

Intervention for benign adenomas depends on its cause. Simply discontinuing oral contraceptives or androgens when a tumor appears to be hormone dependent may correct the condition. Otherwise, treatment may include surgical excision of the involved liver segment. If acute hemorrhage precipitates surgery, the surgeon may perform a hepatic lobectomy.

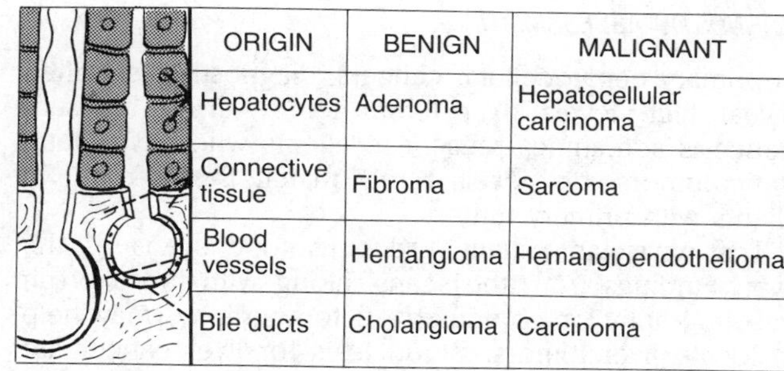

ORIGIN	BENIGN	MALIGNANT
Hepatocytes	Adenoma	Hepatocellular carcinoma
Connective tissue	Fibroma	Sarcoma
Blood vessels	Hemangioma	Hemangioendothelioma
Bile ducts	Cholangioma	Carcinoma

▲ *Figure 58-10*

Classification of primary liver neoplasms.

Primary Hepatocellular Carcinoma

Primary hepatocellular carcinoma (malignant hepatoma) occurs more frequently in men. Etiologic factors that may contribute to hepatoma are hepatitis B, chronic liver disease, hemochromatosis, certain mycotoxins (aflatoxins), anabolic steroid use, polyvinylchloride, nitrosamines, and long-term androgen therapy.

Primary hepatocellular carcinoma is the main cause of death from cancer in many areas of the world, including sub-Saharan Africa and parts of Asia.

Benign hepatic tumors have an excellent prognosis if they can be removed surgically before they rupture and cause death from hemorrhage.

Following the diagnosis of liver cancer and if intervention fails to terminate the tumor process, the individual usually dies of hepatic failure within 4 to 6 months.

METASTATIC TUMORS

Definition/Incidence

Metastatic tumors of the liver are tumors that began elsewhere in the body and have spread to the liver. The liver is one of the common sites of metastasis for all cancers. In the United States, metastatic tumors of the liver are more common than primary liver tumors.

Etiology/Risk Factors

The liver is a common site of metastatic tumors because of a variety of anatomic factors. Melanomas and tumors from the gastrointestinal tract, lung, and breast lead to liver metastasis more frequently than do tumors of the prostate, skin, or thyroid.

Pathophysiology

The liver is a common site of metastasis because of the liver's high rate of blood flow, size, and portal drainage from the major abdominal organs. Metastatic tumors spread to the liver by (1) direct extension from adjacent organs (stomach and gallbladder), (2) the hepatic arterial system, and (3) the portal venous system. Also, as a result of cell migration, the surface of the liver may become seeded with metastatic cells.

Unfortunately, these metastatic tumors may be far advanced before clinical manifestations or laboratory findings indicate their presence. For this reason, this condition usually carries a poor prognosis. Interventions with radiotherapy and chemotherapy may be only palliative.

Clinical Manifestations

Clients with primary (benign and malignant) and secondary (metastatic) tumors often present with similar signs and symptoms. Early indicators of liver neoplasm are usually vague. The client may report minor temperature elevation and gastrointestinal symptoms. Common manifestations include right upper quadrant distress and tenderness, abdominal distention, diarrhea or constipation, and nausea. Diagnostic studies and physical examination may reveal the following: hepatomegaly, liver mass, friction rub or bruit over the liver, positive angiography, hypoproteinemia, blood-tinged ascites, decreased liver function, elevated alkaline phosphatase, and reversal of albumin/globulin ratio.

Some clients also may develop metabolic derangement such as polycythemia, blood sugar disorders, and high levels of calcium. Other clients may present with high leukocytosis and anemia. Jaundice occurs more often when the bile ducts are the primary site or the tumor mass obstructs a major outflow duct. Still other manifestations may be present, but they vary according to the concurrent pathologic condition. At times, the tumor process causes elevation of the diaphragm and some respiratory problems.

Although neoplasms of the liver create numerous clinical manifestations, many of these manifestations may not occur until the tumors have grown quite large. Malignant tumor cells may have replaced as much as 90 per cent of normal liver tissue before liver insufficiency becomes clinically evident.

DIAGNOSTIC ASSESSMENT

In primary hepatocellular cancers, diagnostic tests often reveal high levels of α-fetoprotein (AFP). This substance is sometimes present in clients who have metastatic tumors, but levels rarely match those found in clients with primary tumors.

The physician usually orders isotope scans of the liver. Findings from the scans, along with those of ultrasonography or computerized tomography, may help to locate liver tumors. Blood tests for liver cancer are under development.

Liver biopsy is very helpful in diagnosis. The route of access may be percutaneous, direct via laparotomy, or through a peritoneoscope. Each method has its limitations. Percutaneous procedures may cause seeding of tumor cells along the exit pathway. Laparotomy requires anesthesia and therefore may be too dangerous. Peritoneoscopy may be impossible if there are extensive adhesions. Because all of these biopsy procedures require membrane puncture, the nurse must be sure the client has an acceptable prothrombin time.

Medical Management

Dearterialization of the liver by hepatic artery ligation or occlusion decreases oxygen supply to the liver. As a result, tumor cells undergo a reduction in number and activity. Although the portal vein carries a sufficient oxygen supply to nourish the hepatocytes, the client should be observed carefully for signs of liver failure. The physician may prescribe a combination of chemotherapy and dearterialization.

Irradiation of liver tumors may provide temporary relief. Percutaneous biliary drainage or the internal placement of a biliary drain helps increase the passage of bile into the duodenum and decrease jaundice and discomfort.

Post-intervention, it is important to monitor the AFP levels in clients with primary liver tumors to assess their progress.

PHARMACOLOGIC MANAGEMENT

Regional perfusion of the liver via the hepatic artery helps relieve pain and/or slow tumor growth. During surgery, the surgeon may implant a chemotherapy infusion pump. Such pumps, filled percutaneously, deliver medication continuously into the hepatic artery. In metastatic growths, the physician may prescribe systemic chemotherapy to reduce tumor size and pain.

Surgical Management

For tumors that are small and confined to one liver segment or lobe, the surgeon may perform resection of the segment or lobe if the client is able to withstand the stress of surgery.

Nursing Management

Nursing diagnoses and interventions for clients with liver neoplasms vary according to the amount of liver dysfunction. The nurse should plan to assess the client for metabolic malfunctions, bleeding problems, ascites, edema, inability to biotransform endogenous and exogenous (drug) wastes, hypoproteinemia, jaundice, and endocrine complications.

The nurse takes time to prepare the client in the diagnostic stage for the various procedures and assesses carefully for post-procedure complications. See Chapters 21 and 22 for detailed discussion of nursing care for clients with malignant tumors.

▼ Liver Transplant

Liver transplant is now considered a feasible form of intervention for a variety of end-stage liver diseases. The following are some of the most common:

- Primary biliary cirrhosis (adult)
- Hepatitis—chronic or fulminant (usually adult)
- Sclerosing cholangitis (adult)
- Biliary atresia (pediatrics)
- Alpha-1 antitrypsin deficiency (usually pediatric)
- Confined hepatic malignancy (adult or pediatric)
- Wilson's disease
- Budd-Chiari syndrome (hepatic vein obstruction)

There are two general approaches to liver transplant: (1) *orthotopic* (the diseased liver is removed during transplant) and (2) *heterotopic* (the diseased liver is left in during transplant). Orthotopic transplant is by far the more common of the two.

As with other forms of transplant, immunosuppressive therapy (cyclosporine and newer experimental medications) prevents the rejection of the transplanted liver. Matching proper organ size and blood and tissue type is the most crucial factor in finding suitable donors.

The appropriate candidate for liver transplant is younger than 55 and not suffering from life-threatening complications such as bleeding varices, advanced cardiac disease or severe hypertension, advanced catabolism, active alcoholism, or metastatic malignancy. The client must be stable psychologically and should have good support systems for the complex postoperative course.

Surgery can last anywhere from 6 to 20 hours. The surgery involves anastomosis of veins, arteries, and biliary ducts. Postoperative complications include infection, rejection, hemorrhage, atelectasis, and acute renal failure. Rejection most commonly occurs between the 4th and 10th postoperative days. Symptoms of acute rejection include fever, tachycardia, right upper quadrant or flank pain, and increasing jaundice. Steroids are used to attempt to stop the rejection; otherwise, rapid deterioration of liver function occurs.

The nurse must closely monitor the client during the postoperative period. Table 58–11 lists the postopera-

TABLE 58–11. Postoperative Liver Transplant Nursing Assessment, Interventions, and Rationales

Assessment/Intervention	Rationales
Observe for signs of respiratory compromise.	Client may be on ventilator for 24 to 48 hours postoperatively. Incision under diaphragm limits excursion due to pain and edema. May have chest tube in place.
Monitor fluid and electrolyte status.	Client is somewhat fluid overloaded from receiving extensive volumes of blood products administered during the long surgical procedure. This overload could lead to pulmonary edema and congestive heart failure.
Monitor for signs of bleeding.	Coagulopathy and thrombocytopenia may persist into the early postoperative period. The transplant procedure itself consists of several vascular anastomoses that may be source of hemorrhage.
Monitor blood pressure, pulse, central venous pressure, and pulmonary artery pressures.	Correlation of these factors can help diagnose early changes in the cardiac and circulatory status.
Follow immunosuppressive protocols.	The amount of immunosuppressant varies for each client. Maintaining proper levels of immunosuppressive drugs helps prevent rejection.
Monitor wound drains and bile drains for patency.	Obstruction of wound drains causes increased intra-abdominal pressure from accumulation of ascites and blood. Obstruction of bile flow can cause damage to the liver and the biliary system.
Keep the client and significant others informed of changes and requirements.	The level of acuity may be alarming to both the client and significant others; in addition, the client is likely to have difficulty expressing concerns because of grogginess and the presence of an endotracheal tube.
Teach the client and significant others about the procedures required postoperatively.	Both the client and significant others require education about procedures such as cholangiogram, liver biopsy, and abdominal ultrasound. Much of the teaching is done preoperatively unless the client required an emergency transplant as a result of fulminant liver failure.

tive nursing assessments and interventions and explains the rationale for each. The other major nursing function is teaching the client and significant others about long-term care (Table 58–12).

▼ Liver Abscess

Liver abscess usually develops after one of the following three conditions:

- *Bacterial cholangitis,* which results from obstruction of the bile ducts by stone or stricture
- *Portal vein bacteremia,* which may develop following bowel inflammation or organ perforation
- *Amebiasis* (infestation with amebae from tropical or subtropical areas)

Other predisposing factors are diabetes mellitus, infected hepatic cysts, metastatic liver tumors with secondary infection, and diverticulitis.

The client commonly reports right-sided abdominal and tight shoulder pain. Assessment also reveals liver enlargement, tenderness, nausea, vomiting, weight loss, fever, and diaphoresis. At times, the client may develop a right pleural effusion. The liver's proximity to the base of the right lung contributes to this process.

Liver scans are extremely valuable in diagnosis. Other useful diagnostic measures include ultrasound, computerized tomography, or arteriography. Laboratory data reflect slight to marked elevations of aminotransferase, alkaline phosphatase, and bilirubin. High levels indicate the presence of concurrent obstruction. A positive blood culture occurs in some cases.

Intervention for hepatic abscess consists of (1) percutaneous drainage of the abscess with antimicrobial therapy, (2) surgical drainage of large abscesses with postoperative antimicrobial therapy, or (3) antimicrobial therapy without drainage for a few months. Any concurrent problem disposing the client to abscess requires attention as well. These clients are very ill. Early diagnosis and intervention reduce mortality from liver abscess to about 10 per cent.

Abscesses due to amebic infestation *(Entamoeba histolytica)* are similar to other liver abscesses. The major difference in intervention is that physicians prescribe metronidazole (Flagyl) or chloroquine phosphate (Aralen) instead of broad-spectrum antibiotics. It is important to dispose of feces carefully and wash hands to prevent transmission of this organism.

When caring for the client with liver abscess, the nurse assesses vital signs regularly. High temperature and rapid pulse may indicate the presence of general sepsis, a likely complication. Movement, coughing, and deep breathing should be encouraged to prevent or limit pulmonary complications related to hepatic ab-

TABLE 58-12. Client Education Post-Liver Transplant

Areas of Teaching	Required Content
Medication management	Explain to client why each medication is important, as well as when to take each and what to do if medication is forgotten and not taken on time.
Dietary management	Although most clients do not go home with dietary restrictions, some clients may require a low-sodium diet. All clients need a nutritious diet to help with healing.
Signs of infection	Explain what to do when fever, cough, malaise, nausea/vomiting, headache, or other untoward symptoms are present. Include the importance of avoiding self-medication with over-the-counter drugs and when to call the physician.
Signs of rejection	The client should be told to report any changes in liver function, such as jaundice, to the physician. The client needs to know that any changes in liver function tests may indicate rejection.
Activity and exercises	The client should resume activities slowly. Although there are very few limitations on normal physical activities, more vigorous ones may require the physician's permission.

scess. The client's fluid intake is increased and skin care is provided in the event of hyperpyrexia.

The nurse helps the client's significant others accept the seriousness of the condition and provides a supportive environment that allows close associates to express fears and concerns.

▼ Hemochromatosis

Hemochromatosis is a disorder of iron metabolism. It is, however, often associated with portal hypertension and it causes hepatomegaly. Thus, we include it with liver disorders.

This process, which is relatively uncommon, affects men more often than women. Primary hemochromatosis, a recessive inherited metabolic defect, causes increased iron absorption from the gastrointestinal tract. Secondary hemochromatosis is caused by alcoholism, excessive dietary intake of iron, or conditions that require repeated blood transfusions (e.g., chronic anemias).

Total body iron in most clients ranges from 2 to 5 g. Clients with hemochromatosis often have levels of 20 g or higher. The excess iron travels to parenchymal cells, where it is deposited as ferritin or hemosiderin. The liver and pancreas are most at risk. The heart, spleen, kidney, and skin undergo less damage. As these organs become fibrotic, loss of function occurs. As a result, the more common problems associated with hemochromatosis include diabetes, enlarged liver, cirrhosis, cardiac disease, increased skin pigmentation, and arthritis.

Diagnosis depends on the presence of (1) elevated plasma iron levels (above 150 μg/ml), (2) greater than 60 per cent saturation of iron-binding protein (transferrin), and (3) signs of specific organ dysfunction. Liver biopsy provides the most definitive method for establishing a diagnosis.

Intervention involves phlebotomy on a biweekly or weekly basis over a 1- or 2-year period (2 ml of blood = 1 mg of Fe). Once the excess iron has been removed from the body, two or three maintenance phlebotomies per year keep body iron normal. If diagnosis of hemochromatosis occurs before cirrhosis develops, phlebotomy will reverse or prevent all the manifestations except arthropathy and hepatocellular carcinoma. Desferrioxamine mesylate, a chelating agent, also facilitates the removal of iron from the body.

When severe tissue damage with marked clinical symptoms occurs prior to diagnosis, the prognosis extends from 1 to 8 years. The health practitioner manages the liver disease, cardiac disease, and diabetes as necessary. Death usually follows cardiac failure, cirrhosis, hepatocellular carcinoma, hematemesis, or pneumonia.

▼ Amyloidosis

Amyloid is a proteinaceous substance that can infiltrate the liver and other organs. Accumulation of amyloid deposits causes tissues to cease functioning.

Clinicians may classify amyloidosis according to the type of protein that forms the amyloid deposits. The most common form of amyloidosis (primary amyloidosis) involves deposit of light-chain amyloid formed from immunoglobins. This abnormal protein material causes the most damage to tissues of cardiac, smooth muscle, skin, kidney, and liver origin. However, light-chain amyloid can accumulate in every organ except the central nervous system.

Amyloidosis due to deposition of protein A is associated with chronic inflammation in conditions such as tuberculosis, rheumatoid arthritis, ankylosing spondylitis, osteomyelitis, and bronchiectasis. Tissues most disturbed by this type of amyloidosis include those of the spleen, kidney, and liver.

Amyloidosis becomes a problem when it begins to interfere with organ function. Although many organs may be afflicted, the liver receives the greatest damage. Assessment reveals that hepatomegaly is the most noticeable effect of this pathologic process. Liver function remains relatively unaffected. Clinical jaundice rarely appears.

Liver biopsy provides excellent diagnostic data, but there is a high incidence of postbiopsy hemorrhage or liver rupture. Bleeding probably results from amyloid infiltration of the walls of small blood vessels. Clinicians find that gingival, skin, or rectal biopsy provides sufficient diagnostic data.

The physician may prescribe chemotherapy to treat light-chain amyloidosis and provide symptomatic relief. When kidney, heart, or gastrointestinal tract involvement occurs, the afflicted person usually experiences progressive deterioration. Assessment and interventions are designed for the specific organs involved. Death typically follows cardiac failure.

Intervention for amyloidosis associated with chronic inflammation consists of removing the primary cause and administering antimicrobial therapy to relieve chronic infection.

▼ LIVER INJURIES

Liver injury usually results from a penetrating injury or blunt trauma. Either may lead to laceration and hemorrhage.

Penetrating injuries are usually knife or missile wounds (gunshot). A knife wound generally is superficial and leaves a sharp clear edge, while missile wounds cause perforations through the liver tissue, i.e., entrance and exit points. The higher the velocity of the missile, the greater the damage. Often, a close-range missile injury is fatal because of the large amount of damage.

Blunt trauma (e.g., from a steering wheel or a fall) can have various effects, from small hematomas that remain under the liver capsule to large, starlike lacerations from severe impact forces. Intervention for hemorrhage constitutes the major immediate problem after injury. The nurse monitors victims of trauma carefully for the falling blood pressure and tachycardia that may indicate hemorrhage. The problem is more difficult when the liver's blood vessels or bile ducts receive damage as well. Later complications include bile peritonitis and abscess formation.

Intervention for liver injuries consists of hemorrhage control, débridement, and drainage. It may be necessary to remove liver lobes, but more often the major goal is to control hemorrhage. When a damaged blood supply causes sloughing of a hepatic segment, hemorrhage follows as a late problem.

Common postoperative problems include pulmonary infections and abscess formation. Clients are assessed postoperatively for manifestations of infection, e.g., fever, chills, difficulty breathing, and so forth. Interventions to prevent pneumonia are performed. For information on preventing postoperative complications, review Chapter 19.

▼ CONGENITAL CONDITIONS IN WHICH CLIENT SURVIVAL INTO ADULTHOOD IS EXPECTED

Three of the more common diseases of the liver in which survival into adulthood is expected are Wilson's disease, Caroli's syndrome, and congenital hepatic fibrosis.

WILSON'S DISEASE

Wilson's disease leads to an accumulation of copper in the tissue of the liver, brain, and kidney. The primary signs of this disorder are abnormal liver functions and neurologic changes. Hepatic symptoms may occur from early childhood to adulthood. This disease is usually chronic in nature, but also may be acute. The acute form is often fatal unless a transplant can be performed. One of the hallmarks of this disease is the presence of Kayser-Fleischer rings around the iris of the eye. These rings are caused by copper deposits. Copper deposits also can be seen on liver biopsy. Penicillamine is the drug of choice as an anti-copper agent.

CAROLI'S SYNDROME

Caroli's syndrome is characterized by dilated bile ducts and cyst formations. The condition may be localized or widespread. It usually presents soon after birth but may not be diagnosed until early adulthood. Fever and bacterial cholangitis are usually two manifestations that lead to diagnosis. Other symptoms may include right upper quadrant pain and jaundice, both of which may be caused by obstruction of the biliary tract by a cyst(s) or stone(s). Treatment consists of antibiotics, external biliary drainage, or even transplant.

CONGENITAL HEPATIC FIBROSIS

Congenital hepatic fibrosis is characterized by portal hypertension caused by portal fibrosis. It usually presents as an upper gastrointestinal bleeding from gastric or esophageal varices. Treatment ranges from blood transfusions and sclerotherapy to portacaval shunting (see Fig. 58-6).

Summary

Hepatic disorders are complex and difficult for all involved. The nurse needs to have a thorough understanding of the liver and its functions to care for these clients. Many hepatic disorders are the result of the client's lifestyle, further complicating an already difficult problem. The nurse must therefore consider both the physiologic and psychosocial problems associated with many hepatic disorders. Helping the client make appropriate lifestyle changes is an important nursing function.

Bibliography

1. American Cancer Society. (1992). *Cancer facts and figures*. New York: Author.
2. Anderson, F. D. (1986). Portal-systemic encephalopathy in the chronic alcoholic. *Critical Care Quarterly, 8*(4), 40-50.

3. Arias, I. M., et al. (1988). *The liver: Biology and pathobiology.* New York: Raven Press.
4. Bayless, T. M. (1989). *Current therapy in gastroenterology and liver disease* (Vol. 3, 3rd ed.). St. Louis: C. V. Mosby.
5. Beasley, R. P., & Hwang, H. Y. (1984). Hepatocellular carcinoma and hepatitis B virus. *Seminars in Liver Disease, 4,* 113–121.
6. Braunwald, E., et al. (Eds.). (1987). *Harrison's principles of internal medicine* (11th ed.). New York: McGraw-Hill.
7. Cerilli, J. G. (Ed.). (1988). *Organ transplantation and replacement.* Philadelphia: J. B. Lippincott.
8. Clouse, M. E. (1989). Current diagnostic imaging modalities of the liver. *Surgical Clinics of North America, 69*(2), 193–234.
9. Colonna, J. O., et al. (1988). The quality of survival after liver transplantation. *Transplantation Proceedings, 20*(Suppl. 1), 594–597.
10. Ebersol, P., & Hess, P. (1989). *Toward healthy aging: Human needs and nursing response* (3rd ed.). St. Louis: C. V. Mosby.
11. Epskin, M. (1985). Renal complications of liver disease. *Clinical Symposia, 37*(5), 3–33.
12. Gitnick, G. (Ed.). (1988). *Handbook of gastrointestinal emergencies* (2nd ed.). New York: Elsevier Science.
13. Gitnick, G. (Ed.). (1989). *Modern concepts of acute and chronic hepatitis.* New York: Plenum.
14. Gitnick, G., et al. (Eds.). (1988). *Principles and practice of gastroenterology and hepatology.* New York: Elsevier Science.
15. Gregory, D. H. (1984). Hepatitis B vaccine. *Postgraduate Medicine, 75,* 199.
16. Gregory, P. B. (1984). Cirrhosis of the liver. *Scientific American Medicine, 7,* 1.
17. Gregory, P. B. (1984). Chronic hepatitis. *Scientific American Medicine, 7,* 1.
18. Grimson, A. E. S., et al. (1986). A randomized trial of vasopressin and vasopressin plus nitroglycerin in the treatment of acute variceal hemorrhage. *Hepatology, 6,* 410–413.
19. Guyton, A. C. (1991). *Textbook of medical physiology* (8th ed.). Philadelphia: W. B. Saunders Company.
20. Hayworth, M. F., & Jones, A. L. (1988). *Immunology of the gastrointestinal tract and liver.* New York: Raven Press.
21. Keith, J. S. (1985). Hepatic failure: Etiologies, manifestations and management. *Critical Care Nurse, 5*(1), 60–86.
22. Keown, P. A., et al. (1987). Cyclosporine: A double-edged sword. *Hospital Practice, 22*(5), 207–220.
23. Klopp, A. (1984). Shunting malignant ascites. *American Journal of Nursing, 84,* 212.
24. Kolts, B., and Spindel, E. (1984). Chronic active hepatitis. *American Family Physician, 29,* 228.
25. Kusne, S., et al. (1988). Infections after liver transplantation: An analysis of 101 consecutive cases. *Medicine, 67,* 132–143.
26. Lightdale, C. J. (1984). Liver cancer: Making optimal use of current diagnostic aids. *Consultant, 24,* 271.
27. Maddeux, M. S. (1989). The pharmacology and complications of immunosuppressive therapy. *Problems of General Surgery, 6*(2), 85–96.
28. Maddrey, W. C. (1984). Axioms on chronic hepatitis. *Hospital Medicine, 13,* 6.
29. Maloney, J. P. (1986). Surgical interventions in the alcoholic patient with portal hypertension. *Critical Care Quarterly, 8*(4), 63–73.
30. Mifliori, R., & Simmons, R. L. (1988). Infection prophylaxis after organ transplantation. *Transplantation Proceedings, 20*(3), 395–399.
31. Miller, H. D. (1988). Liver transplantation: Postoperative ICU care. *Critical Care Nurse, 8*(6), 19–31.
32. Mosley, J. W., et al. (1990). Non-A, non-B hepatitis and antibody to hepatitis C virus. *Journal of the American Medical Association, 263,* 77–78.
33. Newell, J. (1984). Portal systemic encephalopathy. *Nurse Practitioner, 9,* 26.
34. Oberfield, R. A., et al. (1989). Liver cancer. *Ca: A Journal for Clinicians, 39,* 206–218.
35. Quinless, F. W. (1985). Severe liver dysfunction. *Focus on Critical Care, 12*(1), 24–32.
36. Rakel, R. E. (1990). *Conn's current therapy.* Philadelphia: W. B. Saunders Company.
37. Ricci, J. A. (1987). Alcohol induced upper GI hemorrhage: Case studies and management. *Critical Care Nurse, 7*(1), 56–65.
38. Rollins, B. J. (1986). Hepatic veno-occlusive disease. *American Journal of Medicine, 81,* 297–306.
39. Sabiston, D. C., Jr. (1991). *Textbook of surgery: The biologic basis of modern surgical practice* (14th ed.). Philadelphia: W. B. Saunders Company.
40. Schade, R. R. (1987). The changing indicators for liver transplantation. *Transplantation Proceedings, 19*(Suppl. 3), 2–6.
41. Schiff, L., & Schiff, E. R. (1987). *Diseases of the liver* (3rd ed.). Philadelphia: J. B. Lippincott.
42. Schindler, M. S., & Eastwood, G. L. (1987). Delta hepatitis: A deadly corollary to hepatitis B. *Journal of Critical Illness, 2,* 91–100.
43. Schroeder, S. A., et al. (1988). *Current medical diagnosis treatment.* Norwalk, CT: Appleton & Lange.
44. Schumann, D. (1983). Correction of ascites with peritoneovenous shunting: A study of clinical management. *Heart and Lung, 12,* 248.
45. Sebesin, S. M., et al. (1987). Status of liver transplantation. *Annals of Surgery, 200,* 524–534.
46. Seeff, L. B., & Lewis, J. H. (Eds.). (1989). *Current perspectives in hepatology.* New York: Plenum.
47. Septimus, E. J. (1984). Seroprevalence of hepatitis B markers in healthcare workers at a teaching medical center at two community hospitals. *Advances in Therapy, 1,* 215.
48. Sherlock, S. (1985). *Diseases of the liver and biliary system.* Oxford: Blackwell Scientific.
49. Smith, S. L. (1985). Liver transplantation: Implications for critical care nursing. *Heart and Lung, 14,* 617–627.
50. Soloway, R. D. (Ed.). (1983). *Chronic active liver disease.* New York: Churchill Livingstone.
51. Swenson, S. A. (1984). Diagnosis: hepatic neoplasms. *Hospital Medicine, 20,* 190.
52. Van Ness, M. M., & Hall, L. W. (1986). A treatable form of liver disease. *Consultant, 26,* 143.
53. Vargo, R. L., & Rudy, E. B. (1989). Infection as a complication of liver transplant. *Critical Care Nurse, 9*(4), 52–62.
54. Vyas, G. N., et al. (1984). *Viral hepatitis and liver disease.* Orlando: Grune & Stratton.
55. When hepatitis B comes back with a vengeance. (1986). *Emergency Medicine, 18,* 207.
55a. Werzberger, A., et al. (1992). A controlled trial of a formalin-inactivated hepatitis A vaccine in healthy children. *New England Journal of Medicine, 327*(7), 453–457.
56. Williams, B. A. H., et al. (1991). *Organ transplantation: A manual for nurses.* New York: Springer.
57. Wyngaarden, J. B., & Smith, L. H. (Eds.). (1988). *Cecil textbook of medicine* (18th ed.). Philadelphia: W. B. Saunders Company.
58. Zakim, D., & Bayer, T. D. (Eds.). (1990). *Textbook of liver disease* (2nd ed.). Philadelphia: W. B. Saunders Company.

Nursing Care of Clients with Biliary and Exocrine Pancreatic Disorders

BILIARY DISORDERS

CHOLELITHIASIS (GALLSTONES)

Definition

The biliary system is composed of the gallbladder, bile ducts, and the cystic duct. The cystic duct (from the gallbladder) joins with the hepatic duct (from the liver) to form the common bile duct (see Fig. 56–5). Recall from Chapter 56 that the function of the biliary system is to transport bile (secreted by the liver) from the gallbladder (where it is stored) into the duodenum.

Disorders of the gallbladder and ducts are extremely common. Within the United States alone, biliary tract disorders account for more than a half million hospitalizations annually. Disorders include gallstones, inflammatory conditions, infections, tumors, and congenital malformations.

The two most common conditions are cholelithiasis (presence of gallstones) and associated cholecystitis (inflammation of the gallbladder). Approximately 98 per cent of clients who present with symptomatic gallbladder disease have gallstones. Malignancies and congenital anomalies of the biliary system are relatively uncommon.

Before we discuss biliary tract disorders, note the list of terms that are used in association with these conditions, presented in Table 59-1.

Incidence

It is estimated that 20 million people in the United States have gallstones, and that 475,000 cholecystectomies are performed every year. Studies show that the incidence of gallstones increases with age, as do the risks associated with cholelithiasis. Women account for nearly 70 per cent of those treated for gallstones, although studies have suggested that the mortality rate is higher in men. Twice as many white Americans are affected than black Americans. The prevalence of this disease is much the same in Europe and Australia. Most of our present knowledge of cholesterol gallstones comes from the study of Pima Indian women is Southwestern United States, in whom the occurrence is 75 per cent between the ages of 25 and 34 years old. Pigment stones are dominant in Asians and in black Americans.

Etiology

The etiology of gallstone disease is not well understood. Based on various theories, there are four possible explanations of stone formation.

First, bile may undergo a change in composition. Studies of clients with cholesterol gallstones indicate that their bile is supersaturated with cholesterol but deficient in bile salts. The cholesterol saturation of bile seems to increase with age. Changes in bile composition, however, do not completely explain why gallstones form.

Second, gallbladder stasis may lead to bile stasis. Bile stasis may (1) change bile composition, (2) supersaturate bile with cholesterol, and (3) precipitate some bile constituents. Gallbladder stasis may result from decreased contractility of the gallbladder and spasm of the sphincter of Oddi. Total parenteral nutrition (TPN) without oral intake for longer than 1 month is associated with gallbladder sludge formation and cholelithiasis. Delayed emptying of the gallbladder may correlate with hormonal factors. This may explain why gallstones seem to be associated with pregnancy.

Third, infection may predispose a person to stone formation. Inflammatory debris can form a nidus (point of origin) for stone growth. The related tissue injury may alter the composition of bile by increasing the reabsorption of bile salts and lecithin. Particular organisms may also play a part in stone formation by altering the composition of bile. For example, *Escherichia coli* increases the amount of bilirubin available for pigment stones and *Streptococcus faecalis* reduces bile salts.

Finally, genetics also seems to play some role in stone formation, as evidenced by the prevalence in the Pima and Chippewa Indians.

TABLE 59-1. Biliary Tract Terminology

Term	Definition
Chole-	Pertaining to bile
Cholang-	Pertaining to bile ducts
Cholangiography	X-ray study of bile ducts
Cholangitis	Inflammation of bile duct
Cholecyst-	Pertaining to gallbladder
Cholecystectomy	Removal of gallbladder
Cholecystitis	Inflammation of gallbladder
Cholecystography	X-ray study of gallbladder
Cholecystostomy	Incision & drainage of gallbladder
Choledocho-	Pertaining to common bile duct
Choledocholithiasis	Stones in common bile duct
Choledochostomy	Exploration of common bile duct
Cholelith-	Gallstones
Cholelithiasis	Presence of gallstones
Cholescintography	Radionuclide imaging of biliary system

Risk Factors

Conditions that predispose clients to gallstone formation include

- Diabetes mellitus;
- Multiple pregnancies;
- Vagotomy, a surgery that results in decreased gallbladder motility;
- Ileal disease or resection, which results in bile salt depletion;
- Long-term parenteral nutrition, which results in decreased gallbladder motility;
- Cirrhosis of the liver;
- Chronic hemolytic disorders, which result in increased bile pigments;
- Obesity;
- Exogenous estrogen administration;
- Pancreatitis;
- Caloric restriction with certain diets;
- Chlofilerate therapy (for treating hyperlipidemia);
- Cholestyramine therapy

Although obesity is a preventable risk factor, most of the risk factors are not. Maintaining a low-fat diet and weight reduction helps prevent gallstone formation. Clients with these conditions should be aware of their increased risk.

Pathophysiology

Gallstones are generally divided into the following three groups: (1) cholesterol stones, (2) pigment stones, or (3) mixed stones. The incidence of a pure stone formation is rare, so stones are generally classified by the predominant constitution.

Cholesterol stones are the most common; the incidence of cholesterol stones increases with age and is prevalent in women. The stones are usually smooth and are whitish yellow to tan in color. *Pigment stones* are present in about 30 per cent of the clients with cholelithiasis in the United States. In these clients, the bile contains an excess of unconjugated bilirubin. Pigment stones are subdivided into black (associated with hemolysis and cirrhosis) and earthy calcium bilirubinate stones (associated with infection in the biliary system). *Mixed stones* may be a combination of cholesterol and pigment stones or either of these stones with some other substance. Calcium carbonate, phosphates, bile salts, and palmitates constitute the more common minor constituents of stones. Exactly why or how stones form is as yet unclear. We do know that most gallstones are formed in the gallbladder but may also form in the common duct or hepatic ducts of the liver. We do not know, however, the actual incidence because some stones do not cause symptoms and pass through the ducts into the bowel unnoticed.

The pathologic findings are best interpreted from the clinical manifestations of the disease, which may be acute or chronic. Once a client becomes symptomatic, treatment and follow up are essential to prevent progression to a more severe, and sometimes fatal, complication of gallbladder disease. Approximately one third of these complications are due to free perforation, which occurs when a gangrenous area becomes necrotic and bile breaks into the peritoneal cavity. Peritonitis with systemic distribution of pepsin has a mortality rate of approximately 20 per cent. Pericholecystic abscess accounts for 50 per cent of the complications and is the least severe, with a mortality rate of approximately 15 per cent. Abscess formation occurs while the perforation is walled off by omentum or adjacent organs such as the colon, stomach, or duodenum.

Much less frequently (approximately 15 per cent of clients), a fistula occurs when the gallbladder becomes attached to a portion of the gastrointestinal (GI) tract and perforates it. The duodenum is the most common site, followed by the colon. Occasionally, a stone is discharged into the small intestine. If the stone is large enough, it can obstruct the narrow terminal ileum, causing gallstone ileus.

Clinical Manifestations

Manifestations of biliary system disorders are similar to those of a number of other conditions. Box 59–1 lists some of the more common diseases that must be differentiated from acute and chronic cholecystitis.

Fewer than half of the clients with gallstones report any distress because gallstones cause no symptoms unless complications develop. The primary symptom is pain or biliary colic. This pain usually follows the temporary obstruction of the gallbladder outlet. Characteristically, the pain starts in the upper midline area. It may radiate around to the back and right shoulder blade, although some clients complain that it passes straight through to the back and substernal areas.

The client is often restless, changing positions frequently to relieve the pain's intensity. Pain may persist for only a few hours or several days and the interval between attacks is variable.

Box 59–1. Disorders with Symptoms Similar to Those of Chronic and Acute Cholecystitis

Chronic Cholecystitis

Angina pectoris
Chronic pancreatitis
Esophagitis
Hiatal hernia
Peptic ulcer
Pyelonephritis
Spastic colitis

Acute Cholecystitis

Acute appendicitis
Acute hepatitis
Acute myocardial infarction
Acute pancreatitis
Acute pyelonephritis
Intercostal neuritis
Intestinal obstruction
Perforated ulcer
Pleurisy
Renal calculus
Right lower lobe pneumonia

Jaundice only appears when common duct obstruction is present. If the stone is blocking the cystic duct, the person may develop signs of acute cholecystitis (see the section on acute cholecystitis). If the stone lodges in the common duct, gallstones may be complicated by cholangitis (inflammation of the bile ducts) and pancreatitis.

Nausea and vomiting may occur, and occasionally, self-induced vomiting alleviates the symptoms. Assessment may further reveal a history of flatulence, bloating, dyspepsia, belching, an intolerance to fatty foods, and vague upper abdominal sensations. Often, clients who have these problems still have them after cholecystectomy.

Assessment of these clients becomes important in light of the fact that symptoms of biliary colic and coronary artery disease are remarkably similar. Considering the prevalence of both these problems, accurate diagnosis is essential.

Many times, the diagnosis is made based on the symptoms alone. Physical findings are present only during an attack with pain, with pain being the cardinal symptom. The right upper quadrant or epigastric area is tender to palpation with voluntary muscle guarding, but signs of peritonitis are absent. The gallbladder is not palpable, and the temperature is normal.

DIAGNOSTIC ASSESSMENT

Blood tests are unremarkable. Jaundice is not present unless there is common duct obstruction. Diagnosis of cholelithiasis may involve abdominal ultrasonography, computerized axial tomography, cholescintography, cholangiography, cholecystography, or rarely, biliary drainage examination.

Current tends, however, point to the use of endoscopic retrograde cholangiopancreatography (ERCP) and endoscopic retrograde catheterization of the gallbladder (ERCG) in diagnoses. Refer to Chapter 57 for a discussion of these procedures. Biliary ultrasonography (cholecystosonography) may be the initial study because it is accurate, safe, does not use radiation, and can be performed without preparation.

Medical Management

For clients with symptomatic cholelithiasis, treatment is dictated by the severity of symptoms. An oral analgesic may be prescribed, and the client may be instructed to avoid those foods that precipitated the attack. It may mean hospitalization and (1) administration of parenteral analgesics for the discomfort of biliary colic (nitroglycerin may reduce colic as well); (2) insertion of a nasogastric tube for the symptomatic relief of vomiting or for those who have probable pancreatitis; (3) maintenance of fluid and electrolyte balance with intravenous fluids; and (4) monitoring for progression of abdominal complications, which may include bile duct obstruction, cholangitis, pancreatitis, acute calculous cholecystitis, and subsequent sepsis and death.

Retrograde endoscopy for stone removal is an important nonsurgical alternative. To remove a gallstone from the common bile duct, the physician passes an endoscope orally into the duodenum, then passes a wire snare into the common bile duct through the ampulla of Vater, securing and removing the obstructing stone. The physician may elect to enlarge the ampulla of Vater by endoscopic papillotomy to allow passage of stones. If stones remain in the common bile duct after cholecystectomy and a T-tube is still in place, the physician may pass a stone-retrieving basket or other device through the T-tube tract to remove the stone.

Because the gallbladder is left in place in all interventions except cholecystectomy and laparoscopic cholecystectomy, the recurrence of stones is likely. Investigation continues on long-term prevention of the recurrence of gallstones.

Another important nonsurgical intervention is the use of oral administration of dissolution agents for cholesterol gallstones. The use of chenodeoxycholic acid is not widely used because of its tendency to produce dose-related diarrhea. However, ursodeoxycholic acid (ursodiol) has become widely used because it is effective and produces no side effects. Both drugs act by reducing the amount of cholesterol in bile; however each drug uses a different mechanism. Oral chenodeoxycholic acid is contraindicated in clients with liver disease and, subsequently, in women of childbearing years because of its hepatotoxic effects on the developing fetus. There is evidence that these two drugs, administered together, produce a slightly better effect than when they are used individually, and interestingly, diarrhea does not occur when the two drugs are combined.

Surgical Management

Whether or not to operate on a client with asymptomatic cholelithiasis (silent gallstones) is another area for debate. When is prophylactic gallbladder removal appropriate? The potential for serious complications (e.g., acute cholecystitis; choledocholithiasis, sepsis) can pose a significant risk. Elderly persons and people with insulin-dependent diabetes have a high incidence of gallstones. Because such people are at high risk during acute biliary attacks and emergency procedures, surgeons recommend that they undergo elective cholecystectomy to avoid later emergency surgery.

CHOLECYSTECTOMY

Cholecystectomy consists of excising the gallbladder from the posterior liver wall and ligating the cystic duct, vein, and artery. The surgeon usually approaches the gallbladder through a right subcostal incision (Fig. 59-1). Common duct exploration may also occur through this incision site, if necessary. When stones are suspected in the common duct, an operative cholangiography may be performed (if it had not been ordered, preoperatively). Also, the surgeon may dilate the common duct if it is not already dilated as a result of a pathologic process. This facilitates stone removal. The surgeon passes a fine instrument into the ducts to collect the stones, either whole or after crushing them.

Following exploration of the common duct, the surgeon usually inserts a T-tube to ensure adequate bile drainage during duct healing. The T-tube also provides a route for postoperative cholangiography or stone dissolution, when appropriate.

Following cholecystectomy the client should be monitored for the usual postoperative complications; such as hemorrhage, pneumonia, thrombophlebitis, uri-

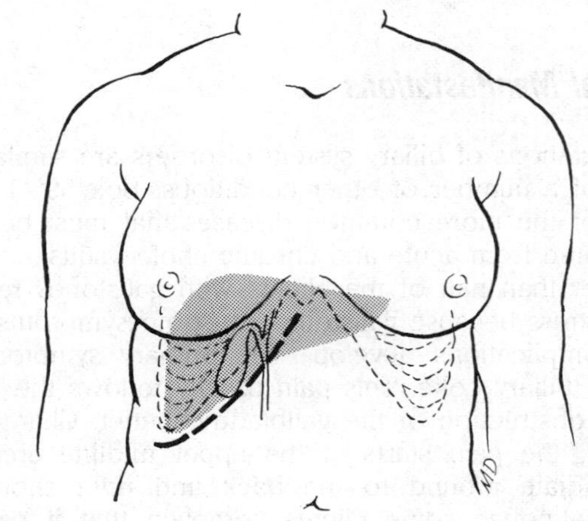

▲ Figure 59-1

Right subcostal incision.

nary retention, and ileus. The risk of bile leakage into the abdominal cavity is more specific for surgeries involving the gallbladder. With hemorrhage and bile leakage, the client feels severe pain and tenderness in the right upper quadrant, abdominal girth increases, bile or blood may leak from the wound, blood pressure drops, and tachycardia develops.

Cholecystectomy is the most common surgical intervention for gallstones. However, changes in medical care reimbursement have initiated the innovation of laparoscopic cholecystectomy. In its infancy, certain criteria are used to determine which clients are good candidates for the procedure. Clients are usually admitted for a 23-hour stay.

Using general anesthesia, carbon dioxide is used to create pneumoperitoneum through a needle inserted near the umbilicus. Also, near the umbilicus, an endoscope is inserted through a small incision to view the gallbladder and determine the feasibility of success by this procedure. Three other small incisions are created, one for grasping the gallbladder, one for suction and irrigation, and another for dissection instruments and applying clips.

Risks from this procedure include hemorrhage, bile duct injury, and injury to other organs. However, the advantages of small scars and a short hospital stay have influenced the increased use of this procedure. Although the possible postoperative complications are the same as with traditional cholecystectomy, the client who undergoes this procedure is at lesser risk because they are ambulatory sooner and usually require only oral analgesia.

EXTRACORPOREAL SHOCK WAVE LITHOTRIPSY

Extracorporeal shock wave lithotripsy may be used in a selected group of clients. These clients should have symptomatic cholelithiases with fewer than four stones, each less than 3 cm in diameter. Contraindications for the procedure are the presence of common duct stones, recent acute cholecystitis, cholangitis, and pancreatitis.

Minor complications may include ecchymosis over the area of entry of the shock waves, gross hematuria through microscopic hematuria because of the close proximity of the right kidney, and biliary pain when large fragments pass through the cystic duct.

PERCUTANEOUS CHOLECYSTOLITHOTOMY

With a percutaneous cholecystolithotomy, surgeons extract stones using cystoscopes, stone baskets, and instruments designed for nephrolithotomy. Stones too large to extract manually can be fragmented using a lithotriptor or laser fiber. General anesthesia is not necessary for this procedure.

Research is currently taking place in the use of percutaneous insertion of a contact dissolution agent. With this procedure, a catheter is inserted into the gallbladder percutaneously and methyl tert-butyl ether (MTBE) is instilled directly into the gallbladder to dissolve cholesterol gallstones. When small amounts are infused and withdrawn four to six times per minute, stones dissolve in 1 to 3 days. Results from early treatments have been excellent.

Nursing Management

ASSESSMENT

If the client is being admitted for evaluation and treatment of symptoms, the nurse's assessment should focus on collecting subjective and objective data, and noting the client's response to ordered therapeutics (i.e., analgesics). The client's symptoms should be carefully assessed to help determine the diagnosis. The client's knowledge of the diagnostic process also should be assessed.

The client should be closely monitored for symptoms of obstruction from the gallstones. Vital signs should be checked at regular intervals to note inflammation associated with the stones.

Generally, surgical management for cholelithiasis is elective and is not performed in an emergency situation, unless obstruction has occurred. Consequently, the client is typically knowledgeable about the procedure and the rationale for it. The client should be assessed, however, concerning knowledge of preoperative and postoperative care.

NURSING INTERVENTION

Nursing Diagnosis: Pain R/T biliary spasms.

Planning: Expected Outcomes. The client will demonstrate an absence or a decrease in pain, as evidenced by client verbalizing that pain is absent or decreased and is resting quietly.

Implementation. The nurse should administer pain medications as ordered and document and report effectiveness of the medication. Meperidine (Demerol) is the drug most frequently ordered. Morphine is contraindicated because it may increase spasm of the sphincter of Oddi. Nitroglycerin may be ordered sublingually to relax smooth muscle and, thereby, decrease colic.

Other comfort measures may be helpful. Providing a quiet environment and using relaxation techniques such as a backrub or positioning may promote rest and enhance the effects of the analgesics given.

Nursing Diagnosis: Fluid Volume Deficit, High Risk for R/T vomiting and nasogastric suctioning.

Planning: Expected Outcomes. The client will maintain adequate hydration, as evidenced by normal skin turgor, moist oral mucous membranes, and urinary output equal to or greater than 30 ml/hr.

Implementation. If the client continues vomiting, obtain an order for a nasogastric tube with a suction attachment to relieve distention and vomiting. Suction also removes the gastric juices that stimulate cholecystokinin, which, in turn, causes painful contractions of the gallbladder.

The nurse should administer intravenous fluids as ordered. Assess and document intake and output, communicating discrepancies to the physician. Assess the client for signs of dehydration, such as dry mucous membranes, poor skin turgor, and urinary output less than 30 ml/hr. For a detailed discussion of fluid and electrolyte imbalances and nasogastric suction, see Chapters 14 and 54.

Nursing Diagnosis: Knowledge Deficit R/T treatment modalities and diagnostic procedures.

Planning: Expected Outcomes. The client will indicate understanding of therapeutics and diagnostics, as evidenced by verbalizing understanding and anxiety decreased.

Implementation. The client who is in acute pain may have a short attention span. Give explanations that are simple and direct when the client is the most comfortable, if possible. Providing too much information when the client is in acute distress will only frustrate the client, and little will be understood or retained. Also, assessing the client's and significant other's level of understanding and learning needs is helpful in giving them the information that is most pertinent to them. Provide simple and concise written information or films as well as verbal instruction if appropriate.

Nursing Diagnosis: Injury, High Risk for R/T medication during retrograde endoscopy for stone removal.

Planning: Expected Outcomes. The client will remain free from injury following retrograde endoscopy, as evidenced by passage of stones and no further occurrence.

Implementation. Clients who undergo retrograde endoscopic papillotomy or stone removal will have a local anesthetic sprayed on the back of their throats. This intervention facilitates the passing of the endoscope. After the endoscopic papillotomy, carefully check for the return of the gag reflex below allowing oral intake. If these clients receive sedation, raise the side rails on the bed for their protection and keep the call light within reach.

Nursing Diagnosis: Knowledge Deficit R/T oral dissolution agents.

Planning: Expected Outcomes. The client will indicate an understanding of treatment, as evidenced by his or her ability to verbalize indications for drugs and side effects and will be able to verbalize dosage and administration instructions.

Implementation. After assessing the level of understanding and learning needs, teach the client about the purpose of the oral dissolution therapy, expected responses, and possible untoward reactions. Because the medication must be taken over a long period of time, help the client devise ways to remember to take the medication daily. For example, a pillbox divided into the days of the week clearly indicates whether or not the client has missed a medication dose.

Nursing Diagnosis: Preoperative Knowledge Deficit R/T surgery and recovery.

Planning: Expected Outcomes. The client will indicate understanding, as evidenced by ability to verbalize information regarding the surgical procedure; ability to demonstrate accurate coughing, deep breathing, and leg exercises; and ability to verbalize information given regarding immediate postoperative course.

Implementation. The nurse should reinforce information given to the client regarding the surgical procedure. Determine the level of understanding and the learning needs of the client and significant other. Material should be provided that can be read or viewed at the client's own pace, if available. Verbal instruction and demonstration is necessary to ensure the client can perform postoperative exercises (turning, coughing, deep breathing, and wound splinting) accurately as well as understand their importance.

The client also needs to have some knowledge of what to expect postoperatively (e.g., intravenous fluids; T-tube placement and drainage, if applicable; and pain control and activity). Studies have shown that preoperative teaching alone significantly decreases the risk of developing postoperative complications.

Nursing Diagnosis: Anxiety R/T the procedure and unknown outcome.

Planning: Expected Outcomes. The client will express and demonstrate feelings of comfort and show decreasing signs of anxiety, as evidenced by calmly discussing apprehension, verbalizing that anxiety is decreasing, and ventilating feelings regarding the surgical procedure and diagnosis.

Implementation. Assess the client's level of anxiety by listening and observing. Reassure and acknowledge that the unknown is frightening. Thoroughly explain those things that may frighten the client, such as diagnostic or preparatory procedures. Allow significant others to stay with the client as appropriate.

Collaborative Problem. High risk for injury R/T postoperative complications of hemorrhage, infection, fluid and electrolyte imbalance, pulmonary changes (atelectasis, pneumonia), urine retention, ileus, decreased GI motility.

Planning: Expected Outcomes. The client will receive appropriate assessments and interventions for early detection and prevention of injury from postoperative complications, as evidenced by stable vital signs; normal pulmonary function; normal GI function; laboratory values within normal limits; normal urinary function, which returns within 6 to 8 hours postoperatively; an intact incision that does not exhibit redness, odor, or purulent drainage; and no signs of thrombus or embolus.

Implementation. Take routine postoperative vital signs and assess for signs and symptoms of shock, such as cyanosis, diaphoresis, cold clammy skin, decreased blood pressure, and increased pulse. As vital signs are checked, the nurse should check dressings and drain tubes at the same time for unusual amounts of bleeding or drainage. If any of the above mentioned symptoms or changes occur, vital signs should be checked frequently and the doctor should be notified.

The client should change position at least every 2 hours. While the client is awake for turning, help him or her to cough and deep breath. Some hospitals use devices such as incentive inspirometry to encourage lung expansion and spontaneous coughing. When using these devices, it is helpful to demonstrate their use prior to surgery.

Lungs should be auscultated for rales, rhonchi, and diminished breath sounds every 4 hours for the first 24 hours and every 8 hours thereafter. If the client had a cholecystectomy, it will be even more difficult to take deep breaths and cough because of the location of the incision. Extra care should be taken to ensure that the client is kept comfortable enough that normal respiration is possible. Many physicians and nurses believe that smaller doses of narcotics given more frequently are beneficial. Splinting the incision helps as well.

Measure intake and output every 4 hours or more frequently, if ordered. Assess amounts for discrepancies. It is not unusual for new postoperative clients to be behind on fluids for the first few hours, so you would not expect the output to equal the intake initially. However, you should assess the client for edema along with the lung sounds every 4 hours as another assurance that the client is tolerating the fluids that are being infused.

Unless the client is otherwise compromised (i.e., acutely ill at the time of surgery or has a history of other health problems such as heart disease or diabetes), laboratory work will probably not be ordered until the following day. These values should be monitored for indications of fluid and electrolyte imbalance (see Chap. 14).

Generally, the client voids within 6 to 8 hours after surgery. If he or she does not, the bladder should be assessed for distention. It is normal for even the otherwise healthy client not to be able to void because of pain, discomfort, and position and not to feel the need to void because of the effects of anesthesia and narcotics. The physician may order the client to be catheterized to empty the bladder initially. Also, the client may need an indwelling foley until he or she is able to ambulate.

Occasionally, following surgery on the gallbladder, the client will return with a nasogastric tube to suction. This should be checked frequently to ensure that it is patent and that placement is good for adequate drainage. A plugged or displaced tube causes distention, nausea, and vomiting, which, in turn, decreases comfort and may place undue stress on the surgical site. Bowel sounds should be auscultated every 8 hours to note when bowel activity returns and that it is returning normally. Depending on the surgery, the client may or may not be allowed oral intake before bowel sounds return.

For the more involved surgical procedure such as a cholecystectomy, clients are usually not allowed a normal diet until they have begun to pass flatus. After the client is allowed to have fluids or food, the nurse should continue to assess the client for abdominal distention and normal bowel sounds to ensure that the intake is being tolerated. Early activity also helps the return of intestinal motility, so the client should be encouraged to begin progression of regular activities as soon as possible.

Many physicians order antiembolism stockings or some sort of sequential compression device to help prevent pooling of blood in the lower extremities and, thus, the development of thrombosis. However, the benefit of regular leg exercises should not be overlooked as a beneficial preventative measure. Even when the client is able to ambulate, leg exercises should continue. The nurse must also assess the lower extremities at least every 8 hours for redness, swelling, pain, and whether Homan's sign is present.

If the dressings are to be changed by the nurse, the incision should be checked simultaneously for redness, swelling, drainage characteristics and amounts, and odor. If drains are present such as a T-tube, the drainage should be observed for its characteristics and amount, also. The client's temperature must be checked at least every 4 hours or more frequently, if necessary. Care must be taken to keep the dressing and incision clean and dry because moisture enhances bacterial growth. Subjective complaints of increased pain may be the first sign that an infectious process is taking place. This is why it is important for the nurse to document the location, type, and amount of pain routinely so that comparison can be made and a significant change in condition will be noted immediately. Many times it is the nurse's assessment that alerts the physician and facilitates the diagnosis of infection.

Nursing Diagnosis: Pain R/T surgical procedure and incision.

Planning: Expected Outcomes. The client will verbalize feelings of comfort and rests quietly, as evidenced by verbalizing pain relief, blood pressure and heart rate within normal limits, and ability to tolerate postoperative exercises and activities.

Implementation. The nurse should assess and document the level, location, and type of pain, as well as the client's response to pain medication. The nurse may need to intervene and obtain new medication orders if the medication is ineffective as ordered. It may be necessary to administer medication to coincide with activity to keep the client active. Nonpharmacologic comfort measures are helpful as well. Providing a quiet environment (even limiting visitors, if necessary), changing the client's position, and rubbing the client's back are all important in relaxing the client and enhancing the effects of the pain medication. Be sure to assist the client in splinting the incision and to instruct the client on the best way to get out of bed and lie down.

Nursing Diagnosis: Oral Mucous Membranes, Altered R/T NPO status, intubation, and nasogastric suctioning.

Planning: Expected Outcomes. The client will maintain normal oral mucosa, as evidenced by intact, moist oral cavity and verbalizing decreased or absence of discomfort.

Implementation. Oral care should be offered at least every 2 hours while he or she is taking nothing by mouth. This may consist of rinsing the mouth with water, using mouthwash, swabbing with a moist swab, or assisting the client to brush his or her teeth. The oral mucous membranes should be assessed at least every 8 hours for their integrity, color, and moistness. While the client is taking nothing by mouth, it may be helpful to place a wet washcloth over the lips to humidify the air as he or she breathes. Offering ice chips or sips of liquid as soon as allowed will provide much relief also.

Nursing Diagnosis: Knowledge Deficit R/T home health care needs.

Planning: Expected Outcomes. The client will accurately verbalize and demonstrate home health care needs and skills, as evidenced by ability to verbalize signs and symptoms of infection; demonstrate wound care; state medications, their purpose, side effects, and administration instructions; and state activity and dietary restrictions.

Implementation. The nurse should begin to teach the client about home health care as soon after surgery as possible to assess the client's learning potential and teaching needs. Instruction should include wound care and dressing changes with return demonstration, as well as how to assess for signs and symptoms of infection.

Be sure the client is knowledgeable about what signs and symptoms should be reported to the physician and how to contact the physician. The client should be instructed to report jaundice, dark-colored urine, pale-colored stools, and pruritus. If the client is discharged with a drain or T-tube in place, he or she should know the purpose of the tube, how to secure it, how to empty it, what amounts of drainage can be expected, and abnormal characteristics of drainage.

Explain and reinforce activity and dietary restrictions thoroughly. Instruct and then question the client as to what medications they are discharged with, what adverse effects are possible, and what the dosage and frequencies are.

EVALUATION

The client will be evaluated based on the expected outcomes. If the outcomes are not achieved, the plan and implementations should be revised.

Modification of Plan of Care for the Elderly

Gallstones in the elderly may not cause pain, fever, or jaundice. Mental confusion, shakiness, and an elevated alkaline phosphatase may be the only manifestations of gallstones in the elderly. Nonsurgical decompression techniques may be preferred in high-risk elderly clients.

When the older client has a cholecystectomy, he or she is at greater risk for injury related to anesthesia, pain medications, and sometimes, the response to the trauma of surgery. Postoperative care should be modified to prevent this injury. Especially in the immediate postoperative period, the side rails should be up, the bed in low position, and the call light within easy reach.

Depending on the older client's response to anesthesia and pain medication, frequent reorientation to the environment and circumstances may be necessary. Remind the older client how to summon help and why it is important that he or she does not get up alone. Be sure that all intravenous lines and drain tubes are secure to prevent the client from inadvertently disconnecting or dislodging them.

In particular, older adults have a tendency to become confused following surgery (especially at night), so the nurse must be alert to this possibility and may need to take precautions, such as use of soft wrist or vest restraints or a device such as a bed-check machine, which is placed under the client and sounds an alarm if it senses weight is no longer on it.

Post-hospital Care

DISCHARGE TEACHING

The client treated medically may be sent home with oral analgesics or other medications for comfort as well as an oral dissolution agent. Be sure the client and significant other is able to relate all necessary information to the nurse before discharge. Diet instructions may be necessary if ingestion of food precipitated the attack (i.e., if a fatty food caused the biliary colic, the client should receive information on a low-fat diet).

Also, the client should be given information on what to do should another attack occur. The client has probably been encouraged by the physician to consider elective cholecystectomy or other surgical intervention before the gallbladder disease progresses further. Written material on gallbladder disease should be provided at this time to aid in understanding and decision making.

ACUTE CHOLECYSTITIS

Definition

Acute cholecystitis refers to acute inflammation of the gallbladder wall.

Incidence

There is an increased incidence of cholecystitis in clients who are overweight, especially those with sedentary lifestyles. Certain ethnic groups, including Chinese, Jews, and Italians, also have a higher rate of the disease.

Etiology

The exact etiology of cholecystitis is unknown. Gallstones are a major cause of acute cholecystitis along with anything that affects normal gallbladder function or affects the blood supply to the organ. Anatomic abnormalities such as kinking or twisting of the bile ducts can lead to acute disease.

Risk Factors

The major preventable risk factors are sedentary lifestyle and obesity. If the client increases his or her level of activity and maintains a low-fat diet, the risk of cholecystitis can be reduced.

Pathophysiology

Acute calculous cholecystitis is a common complication of cholelithiasis. In fact, calculous cholecystitis accounts for 95 per cent of all cases. It appears to be caused by obstruction of the cystic duct, which, in turn, causes distention of the gallbladder. Subsequently, (1) venous and lymphatic drainage is impaired, (2) proliferation of bacteria occurs, (3) localized cellular irritation and/or infiltration takes place, and (4) areas of ischemia may develop. The inflamed gallbladder wall is edematous and thickened, and may have areas of gangrene or necrosis. Empyema is a term used to describe the gallbladder that contains pus, which is the equivalent of an intra-abdominal abscess and may be associated with severe sepsis. Recurrent episodes of acute cholecystitis cause fibrosis of the wall of the gallbladder.

Complications of untreated acute cholecystitis are usually associated with septic complications. Others are consequences of ischemia and gangrene: perforation, pericholecystic abscess, and fistula.

Acalculous cholecystitis (cholecystitis without stones) is far less common than cholecystitis due to gallstones. It apparently can be triggered by (1) multiple blood transfusions, (2) gram-negative bacterial sepsis, or (3) tissue damage after burns, trauma, or extensive surgery. Other possible contributing factors include hyperalimentation, prolonged fasting, hypotension, anesthesia, narcotic analgesics, and mechanical ventilation with positive end-expiratory pressure. Clients with diabetes mellitus and systemic arteritis are also prone to this condition.

Clinical Manifestations

Inflammation of the gallbladder may be an acute or a chronic process. The most common and reliable finding on physical examination is tenderness in the right upper quadrant, epigastrium, or both. Although clients with chronic and acute cholecystitis may complain of the same type of pain, the distinguishing factor is the severity and persistence of the pain. Chronic cholecystitis rarely lasts more than a few hours, whereas acute cholecystitis may last several days.

Pain in acute cholecystitis may be located in the epigastric, subscapular, or right upper quadrant areas. Sometimes, the pain is referred to the right scapula. The pain usually starts suddenly, steadily increases, and reaches a peak in about 30 minutes. During examination of the abdomen, extreme tenderness often causes the client to guard the upper right quadrant. When palpating the right subcostal area, ask the client to take a deep breath. If the client experiences extreme tenderness and stops breathing on inspiration, you have elicited Murphy's sign. About 75 per cent of clients with acute cholecystitis have experienced biliary colic episodes in the past.

In addition to pain, assessment of people with acute cholecystitis reveals the following problems:

- Nausea and vomiting occur in 60 to 70 per cent of the clients.
- Approximately 80 per cent of all clients have an elevated temperature but this may be absent in the elderly, immunocompromised clients, and those on steroidal therapy.
- Mild jaundice occurs in only 10 per cent of the cases.

See Table 59–2 for a summary of assessment data for cholecystitis and cholelithiasis.

Biliary calculi and focal gallbladder tenderness are the most reliable indicators of acute cholecystitis, particularly if other assessment data support this diagnosis.

DIAGNOSTIC ASSESSMENT

Diagnostic examinations for acute cholecystitis include the following:

- Biliary ultrasonography is often the initial diagnostic procedure. Sonographic findings consistent with acute cholecystitis include (1) cholelithiasis, (2) focal tenderness over the gallbladder (sonographic Murphy's sign), (3) thickening of the gallbladder wall (greater than 3 mm), and (4) distention of the gallbladder lumen (greater than 5 cm).

TABLE 59-2. Cholecystitis and Cholelithiasis: Assessment Data

Assessment Data	Pathophysiologic Basis
Abdominal pain, most commonly right upper quadrant or epigastric; often radiates to back	In cholelithiasis, ductal spasm when a stone moves from gallbladder into ducts may cause waves of pain (biliary colic)
	In cholecystitis, pain may be steady (because of inflammation) and increases in severity with peritoneal extension
Nausea and vomiting	Distention of bile ducts initiates impulses to vomiting center
Fat intolerance	Contraction of inflamed gallbladder to release bile to digest fat often precipitates pain
Fever and leukocytosis	Response to inflammation
Jaundice	In cholelithiasis, obstruction to common bile duct causes increased serum bilirubin
	In cholecystitis, edema sometimes obstructs the duct enough to increase bilirubin levels

- Aminotransferase, alkaline phosphatase, and bromosulfa phthalein parameters may be slightly abnormal.
- An abdominal x-ray study occasionally reveals the enlarged gallbladder. In 15 per cent of cases, the gallstones contain enough calcium to be visible on film.
- Radionuclide imaging (cholescintography) can provide additional information (when the diagnosis is clinically obscure) by pinpointing cystic duct obstruction. Confirmation is based on nonvisualization of the gallbladder.
- The white blood cell count is elevated in 85 per cent of clients, with the exception of the elderly or those on steroidal therapy.

Refer to Chapter 57 for a discussion of other diagnostic techniques.

Medical Management

Clients suspected of having acute cholecystitis should be hospitalized, and initial management should include administration of antibiotics effective against organisms found in the bile in approximately 80 per cent of the clients. These organisms include both gram-positive and gram-negative aerobes and anaerobes: *Escherichia coli, Klebsiella aerogenes, Streptococcus faecalis, Clostridium welchii, Proteus* species, *Enterobacter* species, and anaerobic streptococci.

Further medical management is the same as for symptomatic cholelithiasis (see the section on cholelithiasis).

Surgical Management

Once the diagnosis of acute cholecystitis is made, the decision for early or delayed cholecystectomy depends on the risk factors. Delayed surgery is usually the correct decision in those clients who have unstable angina, significant carotid artery disease, congestive heart failure, cirrhosis, and other conditions that would increase their risk.

Cholecystectomy for acute cholecystitis is more difficult than elective surgery because of the distended gallbladder. Usually, the gallbladder must be decompressed first to allow complete visualization of all surrounding structures and avoid injury to the extrahepatic bile ducts.

Cholecystotomy is usually performed only when cholecystectomy is too dangerous given all the risk factors. Although the procedure relieves the obstruction, the cure depends on the ability of the client's defense to resolve the inflammatory process. The treatment of the complications of cholecystotomy is usually cholecystectomy.

Nursing Management

Assessment of these clients becomes extremely important because several other disease entities may produce the same symptoms (see Table 59-1). The nurse collects subjective and objective data and notes the client's response to ordered therapeutics. The nursing care plan is the same as for medical management of cholelithiasis except that it is certain these clients will receive a course of antibiotics. Also, the client should be observed for the development of complications. For more information on nursing management, see the section on nursing management for surgical intervention in cholelithiasis.

ACUTE ACALCULOUS CHOLECYSTITIS

Acute acalculous (absence of stones) cholecystitis accounts for approximately 4 to 8 per cent of all cases of acute cholecystitis. Although it has not been proved, this condition is estimated to be increasing. It has a tendency to occur after or in association with other conditions, especially major trauma, burns, or surgery. Other preceding conditions include multiple transfusions, childbirth, bacterial sepsis, and debilitating diseases such as sarcoidosis, polyarteritis nodosa, and lupus erythematosus. However, no apparent precipitating factor is present in as many as 50 per cent of the clients.

The pathologic process does not differ from that of the calculous type except that the incidence of gangrene and perforation is higher. It is conjectural whether this is an inherent feature of the disease or the result of delayed diagnosis.

Recognition of the disease may be delayed when the client cannot communicate well because of concomitant disease, post-traumatic, or postoperative states. The symptoms are the same as acute calculous cholecystitis — pain in the right upper quadrant, epigastrium, or both, and vomiting. However, although pain is the cardinal symptom in the calculous type, it may be obscured or absent in acalculous cholecystitis because of narcotic administration, decreased level of consciousness, or abdominal pain from an incision or other disease process. Significant physical findings are the same as those of acute calculous cholecystitis and the same diagnostic procedures are used.

The standard treatment is emergency cholecystectomy because of the increased risk of gangrene and perforation.

CHRONIC CHOLECYSTITIS

Chronic cholecystitis sometimes arises as a sequela to acute cholecystitis. Typically, however, it develops independently of acute cholecystitis. In addition, it is almost always associated with gallstones. Chronic cholecystitis principally affects middle-aged and older obese women. The female-to-male ratio is 3 : 1.

Assessment data for chronic cholecystitis are similar to those of acute cholecystitis with certain exceptions. In chronic states, (1) the pain is less severe, (2) the temperature is not as high, and (3) the leukocyte count is lower. Vague symptoms of dyspepsia, fat intolerance, heartburn, and flatulence accompany chronic cholecystitis. The client has usually experienced these manifestations for a long time as well as repeated attacks (mild or severe) of acute cholecystitis. Eventually fibrous tissues begin to replace the normal muscle and mucosal tissues of the gallbladder. As a consequence, the gallbladder loses its ability to concentrate bile.

Diagnosis of chronic cholecystitis largely depends on ultrasonography. Other diagnostic procedures provide supplementary information. Diagnostic findings include (1) cholelithiasis, (2) gallbladder wall thickening (greater than 3 mm), and (3) delayed visualization or nonvisualization of the gallbladder on radionuclide scanning. Scarring from chronic inflammation may partially or completely obstruct the cystic duct and, thus, account for this delay in visualization or nonvisualization.

It may be difficult to differentiate chronic cholecystitis from other disorders. Conditions that mimic the manifestations of cholecystitis (acute and chronic) appear in Table 59-1. The diagnostic process serves to rule out these conditions.

Conservative interventions include (1) a low-fat diet; (2) weight reduction; and (3) administration of anticholinergics, sedatives, and antacids. When medical intervention is ineffective, cholecystectomy may be the treatment of choice. About 90 per cent of clients obtain relief of symptoms after cholecystectomy. Ninety-five per cent of removed gallbladders contain stones.

CHOLEDOCHOLITHIASIS AND CHOLANGITIS

Definition

Choledocholithiasis is defined as stones in the common duct. Common bile duct calculi can arise from the gallbladder or hepatic ducts. Thus, common duct stones can occur in the absence of a gallbladder and are termed primary common duct stones. Cholangitis is inflammation of the bile duct.

Incidence

Common duct stones are found in 8 to 16 per cent of clients with cholelithiasis. The incidence increases with age to approximately 25 per cent in clients over 60 years of age. Frequently, inflammation or bacteria are present, and cholangitis may develop.

Etiology

The etiology is essentially the same as for cholelithiasis. This condition is sometimes combined with a narrowing of the papilla, trapping stones.

Risk Factors

The risk factor for choledocholithiasis is that a small stone passes from the gallbladder and lodges in the common bile duct.

Pathophysiology

The pathophysiology is essentially the same as for cholelithiasis.

Clinical Manifestations

Common duct calculi may be asymptomatic or cause biliary colic, bile duct obstruction, cholangitis, or pancreatitis. Early symptoms of choledocholithiasis are not easily distinguished from gallbladder colic or acute cholecystitis. Pain may be mild or severe and cannot be differentiated from gallbladder pain. Jaundice is intermittent if obstruction is intermittent but may be progressive if the stone becomes impacted.

Chills and fever, slight abdominal discomfort, and mild elevation of serum bilirubin are signs of cholangitis. The white blood cell count is normal except when cholangitis is present. It is characteristic, however, to see elevation of serum bilirubin and alkaline phosphatase. Serum amylase should always be measured to determine whether or not pancreatitis is present.

Infrequently, symptoms of cholangitis are accompanied by shock and confusion, coma, or other central nervous system symptoms. This signals the presence of acute toxic cholangitis, a condition in which infected bile or pus is under pressure within the duct system. Emergency decompression of the duct system is necessary to prevent death.

DIAGNOSTIC ASSESSMENT

To determine the diagnosis, ultrasonography may be performed but is not reliable in the detection of common duct stones, although it can detect common duct dilation. Endoscopic retrograde cholangiography is indicated for those clients who have bile duct obstruction (as indicated by persistent jaundice) or bile duct dilatation on ultrasonography. It allows visualization and endoscopic sphincterotomy when indicated.

Medical Management

Medical management involves antibiotic therapy when cholangitis is present.

Surgical Management

Surgical management in some form is usually necessary for symptomatic choledocholithiasis. Common duct stones in a client who has previously had a cholecystectomy is best treated by endoscopic sphincterotomy. The success rate is approximately 90 per cent. Extracorporeal shock wave lithotripsy is used when stones are too large to extract via the endoscopic approach. Success can be achieved in 70 to 85 per cent of these complicated cases. Most common duct stones are found and removed at the time of cholecystectomy.

Choledochostomy consists of opening the common duct surgically, removing stones, and inserting a T-tube for drainage. Choledochostomy may be performed in conjunction with cholecystectomy. If not, a cholecystectomy may be necessary at a later date.

Surgical traumas or the presence of stones may result in ductal edema following choledochostomy. Inserting a T-tube prevents bile from spilling into the peritoneal cavity and maintains patency of the duct (Fig. 59-2). T-tubes may be attached to continuous gravity drainage or to collapsible bags in the dressing site.

Avoid tension on long tubing and obstruction by kinking. Carefully measure drainage from the T-tube. The T-tube usually drains 300 to 500 ml in the first 24 hours. This amount decreases to less than 200 ml after

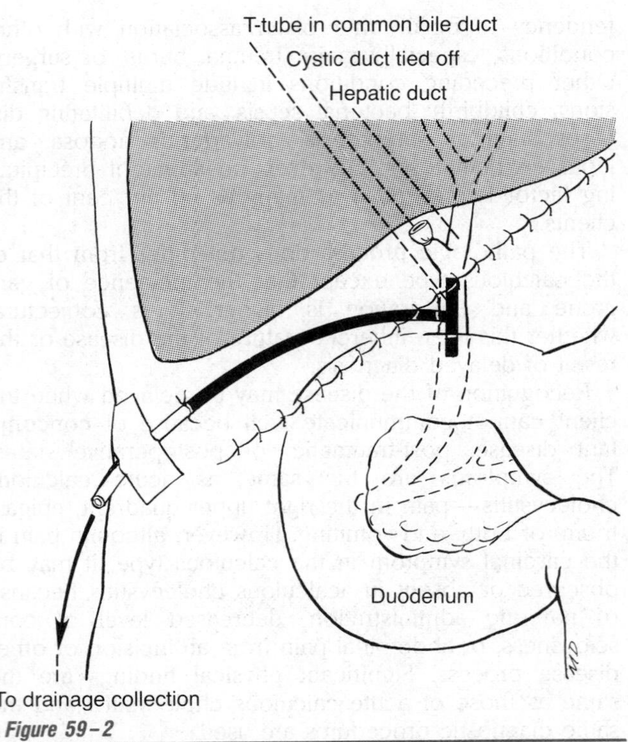

▲ *Figure 59-2*

T-tube placement. The surgeon ties off the cystic duct and sutures the T-tube into the common bile duct, with the short arms of the T-tube toward the hepatic duct and duodenum. The long arm of the T-tube exits the body near the incision site. Skin suture and tape secure placement.

3 to 4 days. Record the volume and color of the drainage. To prevent excessive loss of bile, place the drainage bag for the T-tube at the level of the abdomen rather than hanging the bag below the bed. At this height, bile flows into the bag only when pressure is high in the biliary tree.

Excessive T-tube drainage may indicate obstruction. Occasionally, it signals development of a biliary fistula. Excessive bile losses may necessitate recycling the client's bile drainage. You may return the bile through a nasogastric tube or orally in a medium such as fruit juice.

Thick bile or bile containing blood clots may cause lack of drainage or inadequate amounts of drainage from the T-tube. Without intervention, bile may begin to leak from the choledochotomy site instead of through the T-tube. To prevent this problem, the physician may decide to irrigate the tube with sterile saline.

On rare occasions, tube dislodgement causes failure of the T-tube to drain. The tube may dislodge from the common duct when the client moves from a supine to a sitting position. This complication may result from excessive tension during T-tube insertion in surgery.

After a few days, you will probably clamp the T-tube during meals to aid fat digestion. The tube remains in place for about 10 days. When T-tube cholangiogram indicates absence of obstruction, the surgeon may decide to remove the T-tube. If a retained stone is discovered, the client may go home with the T-tube in place. The surgeon may remove the stone through the T-tube tract with a catheter at a later time.

Nursing Management

Nursing management is the same as for the client with cholelithiasis.

SCLEROSING CHOLANGITIS

Sclerosing cholangitis is an inflammatory disease of the bile ducts that causes fibrosis and thickening of their walls and multiple short, concentric strictures. The disease is progressive and gradually causes cirrhosis, portal hypertension, and death from hepatic failure. It may also predispose the client to the development of cholangiocarcinoma. Some cases are associated with inflammatory bowel disease, 70 per cent of which are ulcerative colitis.

The cause has been linked to altered immunity, toxins, and infectious agents. Approximately two thirds of cases occur in clients under the age of 45, and the male-to-female ratio is 3:2.

Usually, the clients present with fatigue, anorexia, weight loss, jaundice, and pruritus. They sometimes complain of vague upper abdominal pain. The diagnosis is usually made by endoscopic retrograde cholangiography, clinical findings, and liver biopsy.

Medical management consists of corticosteroids and long-term antibiotic therapy when cholangitis is a recurrent problem. Immunosuppressants, bile acid–binding agents, colchicine, and penicillamine have been used. However, these agents do not alter the slow progressive course of the disease. Urodeoxycholic acid (Ursodiol), which improves primary biliary cirrhosis, is now being evaluated in the treatment of sclerosing cholangitis.

The success of surgical intervention is limited by the progressive nature of the disease and the recurrent cholangitis. Surgery is generally limited to procedures to open the ducts. Cholecystectomy should not be performed unless there is definite evidence of cholecystitis or cholelithiasis. Although surgical therapy may be lifesaving in some circumstances, it has to be considered palliative in the overall context of the disease. The most definitive management of these clients is liver transplantation.

CARCINOMA OF THE GALLBLADDER

Although cancer of the gallbladder is the most common malignant lesion of the biliary tract, it only accounts for 5 per cent of all cancers at the time of autopsy. Of all clients who develop this malignancy, 91 per cent are over the age of 50 and the incidence in women is three to four times that of men. However, the incidence of bile duct cancer is predominant in men. American Indians, Hispanics, Inuit, northeastern Europeans, Israelis, and Japanese immigrants to the United States are at greatest risk of developing cancer of the gallbladder. At least 70 per cent of these clients have gallstones. Adenocarcinoma accounts for 82 per cent of all cases.

The clinical presentation differs depending on the stage of the disease. There is no distinct pattern because the symptoms are dependent on the site of the lesion, its extent, and the presence or absence of preexisting biliary symptoms. However, pain occurs in 66 per cent, weight loss in 59 per cent, jaundice in 51 per cent, anorexia in 40 per cent, and a right upper quadrant mass in 40 per cent of clients.

The prognosis of cancer of the gallbladder is poor. About 88 per cent die within the first year, and only about 4 per cent are alive within 5 years. The long-term survivors are generally those in whom the diagnosis of cancer had not been made prior to cholecystectomy and was determined by pathology.

At this point, treatment modalities and their effectiveness are widely debated. Treatment varies from radical resection, to palliative relief of duct obstruction, to chemotherapy or radiation.

CONGENITAL ANOMALIES

Congenital anomalies of the gallbladder are very rare. Absence of the gallbladder seems to have a genetic link because several family members may be affected. Clients with no gallbladder may be asymptomatic, and the condition is discovered only at the time of autopsy or other surgical procedure.

Double and triple gallbladders are also rare, the latter being more so. Double gallbladders may share a common cystic duct and be completely separated, or they may be divided by a septum. An ectopic location of the gallbladder is another rare occurrence.

▼ DISORDERS OF THE EXOCRINE PANCREAS

A client with a pancreatic disorder may have problems with both digestion and glucose use. Disorders of the pancreas fall into four groups: (1) inflammatory, (2) neoplastic, (3) traumatic, and (4) genetic. Box 59–2 lists pancreatic disorders under each category. The following sections include a discussion of exocrine illness. See Chapter 60 for coverage of hormonal disorders. Measures used to diagnose disorders of the pancreas include various laboratory and radiographic studies.

ACUTE PANCREATITIS

Definition

Acute pancreatitis is an inflammation of the pancreas that may result in autodigestion of the pancreas by its own enzymes.

Box 59–2. Classification of Pancreatic Disease

Inflammatory

Acute pancreatitis
Relapsing acute pancreatitis
  In acute and relapsing acute pancreatitis, function and morphologic restoration may occur as causes (e.g., alcohol, gallstones) are eliminated
Relapsing chronic pancreatitis
  Chronic pancreatitis with acute exacerbations
Chronic pancreatitis
  Permanent structural and functional damage has occurred; may be related to nutritional, metabolic, or endocrine factors.

Neoplastic

Parenchymal origin (acinar cells)
  Adenoma
  Acinar cell adenocarcinoma
Ductal origin
  Cystadenoma
  Adenocarcinoma
Islet cell origin
  Insulinoma
  Gastrin-producing tumor
  Vasoactive intestinal peptide (VIP)–producing tumor
  Glucagonoma
  Other tumors derived from amine precursor uptake and decarboxylation (APUD) cells

Traumatic

Nonpenetrating or blunt trauma
Penetrating injuries

Genetic

Cystic fibrosis
Hereditary and familial pancreatitis

Reprinted with permission from Arvanitakis, C., & Cooke, A. R. (1978). Diagnostic tests and exocrine pancreatic function and disease. *Progress in Gastroenterology, 74,* 932. Copyright 1978 by American Gastroenterological Association.

Incidence

Pancreatitis, or inflammation of the pancreas, may be acute or chronic. Acute pancreatitis is a fairly common but potentially lethal inflammatory process that results in varying degrees of pancreatic edema, fat necrosis, and hemorrhage. Typically, the manifestations of acute pancreatitis disappear once causative factors are eliminated. Nine out of ten clients experience the disease with mild to moderate symptoms and improve with supportive care. Conversely, in one out of ten clients, the condition evolves into a severe life-threatening form of acute pancreatitis. Studies have revealed that the late complication of multisystem organ failure and pancreatic abscess contributed to most of the deaths. Pulmonary edema and congestion are also contributory factors to the mortality rate.

Etiology

In 90 per cent of the cases of acute pancreatitis, the cause is related to excessive alcohol intake or biliary tract disease. Alcohol abuse is the major cause of acute pancreatitis in urban areas of the United States. In other areas of the United States, Asia, and Europe, gallstone-associated pancreatitis is predominant. Although the exact mechanism of alcohol-related injury is unknown, the association is undeniable. Several theories exist regarding the effect of alcohol on the pancreas, but research continues. In gallstone-related pancreatitis, it is believed that gallstones migrating through the ampulla of Vater cause diversion of bile into the pancreatic duct and subsequent bile-induced pancreatic parenchymal injury.

Other causes include

- Hyperlipidemia, which may occur secondary to nephritis, castration, or exogenous estrogen administration, or it may occur as hereditary hyperlipidemia;
- Hypercalcemia arising as a result of hyperparathyroidism;
- Familial cases with no definite mechanism defined;
- Pancreatic trauma, such as penetrating or blunt external trauma, intraoperative manipulation, or ampullar manipulation and pancreatic ductal overdistention during ERCP;
- Pancreatic ischemia during episodes of hypotensive shock, cardiopulmonary bypass, visceral atheroembolism, or vasculitis;
- Drugs that have been linked to acute pancreatitis. Although azathioprine and estrogens have been directly linked with disease, many other drugs are felt to have a probable association;
- Other general causes, such as pancreatic duct obstruction, duodenal obstruction, viral infection, scorpion venom, and idiopathic causes.

Risk Factors

Alcohol abuse is a high-risk factor for the development of pancreatitis. Avoidance of alcohol is the best way to decrease the risk of the disease. The other major risk factor is cholecystitis and cholelithiasis.

Pathophysiology

The precise mechanism causing pancreatic damage remains unclear. The pathologic changes occurring in the pancreas may be due to premature activation of proteolytic and lipolytic pancreatic enzymes. These enzymes are normally activated in the duodenum. Note in Table 59–3 that the pancreas normally releases pro-

TABLE 59-3. Pancreatic Enzymes

Enzyme	Catalyzes the Hydrolysis of:
Amylase	Carbohydrates into maltose and dextrins
Lipase	Fats into glycerol and fatty acids
Proteases:	Proteins into peptides and amino acids
Trypsinogen Chymotrypsinogen Procarboxypeptidase Proaminopeptidase	Proteases are secreted in an inactive form, otherwise they would destroy pancreatic tissue. Once in the intestine, enterokinase acts on trypsinogen, converting it to trypsin. Trypsin then acts on the other proteases to convert them to active enzymes

Box 59-3. Ranson's Early Prognostic Signs of Acute Pancreatitis

At Admission

Age over 55 years
WBC > 16,000 cells/mm^3
Blood glucose > 200 mg/dl
Serum lactate dehydrogenase > 350 IU/L
SCOT > 250 U/dl

During Initial 48 hours

Hematocrit falls > 10 per cent points
BUN elevation > 5 mg/dl
Serum calcium falls to < 8 mg/dl
Arterial PO_2 < 60 mm Hg
Base deficit > 4 mEq/L
Estimated fluid sequestration > 6 L

Data from Ranson, J. H. C., et al. (1974). Prognostic signs and the role of operative management in acute pancreatitis. *Surg Gynecol Obstet, 139*:69.

tease in an inactive form. Once in the intestine, the action of intestinal enterokinase converts pancreatic trypsinogen (one of the proteases) into trypsin. In pancreatitis, however, the activation of the proteases and lipases occurs prior to secretion into the intestine. This causes tissue damage in the pancreas.

Exactly how the enzymes become active in the pancreas is unknown, but they may be triggered by reflux of bile from the duodenum into the pancreatic duct or by pancreatic duct obstruction. The net effect of this enzymatic activation is autodigestion of the pancreas. Once pancreatic inflammation begins, a vicious circle continues the process of further tissue damage and enzyme activation. As the process becomes chronic, destruction of pancreatic parenchyma occurs.

The clinical course of up to 90 per cent of clients with acute pancreatitis follows a self-limited pattern. However, in 10 to 15 per cent of clients, a severe form of illness develops that requires a lengthy hospitalization, complications, and significant rates morbidity and mortality. These clients present a major medical challenge by requiring an intensive care setting, hemodynamic monitoring, and frequent laboratory and radiographic evaluation.

One way to predict the severity of attack and overall prognosis is to use the predictive criteria identified by Ranson in 1974 (Box 59-3). Clients with two or less prognostic signs essentially have no mortality and generally require supportive care. Clients with three or four signs have a mortality rate of approximately 15 per cent. If five or six prognostic signs are present, intensive care is required and the mortality rate reaches 50 per cent. Clients with seven or more of these prognostic signs have an even higher mortality rate and truly test the limits of modern medicine.

Clinical Manifestations

Symptoms in clients presenting with acute pancreatitis can vary from mild nonspecific abdominal pain to profound shock with coma and ultimate death. The predominant clinical feature is abdominal pain, which normally begins in the midepigastrium and achieves maximal intensity several hours into the illness. In most clients, the pain has a penetrating quality, which radiates to the back. In clients with alcohol-associated pancreatitis, the pain often begins 12 to 48 hours after an episode of inebriation. However, those with gallstone-associated pancreatitis typically experience pain after a large meal. Nausea and vomiting frequently accompany the pain.

Physical examination typically reveals fever, tachycardia, epigastric tenderness, and abdominal distention. Severe hemorrhagic pancreatitis may produce two distinctive signs: Turner's sign (bluish discoloration of the left flank) and Cullen's sign (bluish discoloration of the periumbilical area). These signs, which occur in less than 3 per cent of the cases, are the result of blood-stained retroperitoneal fluid. Jaundice may be seen in clients with gallstone-associated pancreatitis but otherwise is uncommon in the initial phase of the disease.

Clients with severe pancreatitis may exhibit severe circulatory complications such as hypotension, hypovolemia, hypoperfusion, and obtundation. As many as one third of the clients have evidence of left pleural effusion or left hemidiaphragmatic elevation.

Other clinical findings include subcutaneous fat necrosis and cerebral abnormalities such as belligerence, confusion, psychosis, and coma. It is speculated that the cerebral abnormalities are caused by hyperosmolality, hypoperfusion, and hypoxia, cerebral fat embolism, or disseminated intravascular coagulopathy. Transient hyperglycemia is found in 50 per cent of the clients, probably as a result of damage to the islets. Hypocalcemia occurs in up to 30 per cent (Table 59-4).

TABLE 59-4. Acute Pancreatitis: Assessment Data

Assessment Data	Pathophysiologic Basis
Extreme epigastric or umbilical pain, extending into back and flank	Edematous distention of pancreatic capsule; local peritonitis due to enzyme release into peritoneum; ductal spasm, or pancreatic autodigestion stimulated by increased enzyme secretion while eating
Persistent vomiting	Pain stimulates vomiting center; intestinal peristalsis reduced because of localized peritonitis
Abdominal distention, fever	Paralytic ileus of small bowel loop due to localized peritonitis
Shock and cardiac dysfunction	Release of pyrogens by tissue breakdown Hypovolemia caused by the loss of fluid into the retroperitoneal space and decreased preload into the heart, the release of kinins that cause peripheral vasodilation and increased vascular permeability and toxemia
Hypocalcemia, usually mild, although tetany is possible	Calcium may be deposited in areas of fat necrosis; undigested intestinal fat traps calcium in feces
Impaired glucose tolerance	Some degree of islet involvement
Jaundice	Common bile duct obstruction by pancreatic edema
Pleural effusion	Spread of inflammation into surrounding tissues

DIAGNOSTIC ASSESSMENT

Serum amylase is the most widely used test in the diagnosis of pancreatitis; however, the absence of hyperamylasemia does not exclude the diagnosis. The absence of hyperamylasemia may reflect extensive pancreatic necrosis or the failure of a chronically diseased gland. In most cases, hyperamylasemia is seen within 24 hours of the onset of symptoms and resolves within 7 days. If hyperamylasemia persists, it may indicate the development of complications.

The measurement of urinary amylase has been indicated as a sensitive index of the disease. Urinary amylase elevations persist for a longer period of time. Again, however, hyperamylasuria is not a true indicator of acute pancreatitis.

Some support the use of amylase-creatinine clearance ratio in the diagnosis. Unfortunately, acute pancreatitis may occur with a normal amylase-creatinine clearance ratio.

The elevation of serum lipase is a more accurate indicator of acute pancreatitis because lipase is solely of pancreatic origin. Also, the duration of hyperlipasemia often exceeds that of hyperamylasemia. However, hyperlipasemia may be seen in perforated peptic ulcer, acute cholecystitis, and intestinal ischemia.

Serum lipase is one of the most specific for acute pancreatitis. Serum lipase may be seen in clients with hereditary hyperlipidemia-associated pancreatitis or in alcohol-induced pancreatitis.

Additionally, a white blood cell count above 10,000 cells/mm^3 is common; also, hyperglycemia, mild azotemia, abnormal liver function tests, and hypocalcemia may be present.

Chest film findings are supportive but not specific for acute pancreatitis. They include left basilar atelectasis, elevated left hemidiaphragm, and left pleural effusion. These findings reflect the presence of a significant peridiaphragmatic retroperitoneal inflammatory process occurring in the region of the pancreas.

Abdominal films may reveal nonspecific abnormalities; presence of air in the duodenal loop indicating duodenal ileus; sentinel loop sign, representing a dilated proximal jejunal loop; colon cutoff sign, which is distention of the transverse colon, gallstones, or pancreatic calcifications.

Although no findings on upper GI series are specific for acute pancreatitis, the studies may reveal widening of the duodenal loop and anterior displacement of the stomach.

Ultrasound can be used to detect pancreatic edema and acute peripancreatic fluid collections but may be limited by the presence of air and fluid-filled loops of bowel.

Nearly all acute pancreatitis clients have some abnormality on CT scan. Pancreatic changes include parenchymal enlargement, edema, or necrosis. A CT scan is also helpful in identifying other structural changes that develop such as pancreatic pseudocyst, abscess, or phlegmon. A magnetic resonance imaging (MRI) study reveals the same information as computed tomography (CT).

Although endoscopic retrograde pancreatography has no role in the standard diagnostic evaluation of the majority of clients with acute pancreatitis, it has proved helpful in some clients with recurrent pancreatitis by identifying correctable abnormalities such as duct abnormalities.

Medical Management

Acute pancreatitis is commonly associated with massive fluid isolation. Fluids can accumulate in the bowel secondary to ileus or in the peripancreatic region because of edema. Fluids also can be lost in the form of emesis. Therefore, an essential first step in the management of these clients is replacing lost body fluids, correcting hypovolemia, and restoring electrolyte balance. Normally, the success of fluid and electrolyte restoration is monitored by assessing the client's response by checking his or her heart rate, blood pressure, and urinary output. In clients with preexisting cardiac, pulmonary, or renal disease, or in clients with severe pancreatitis, invasive monitoring, including urinary catheterization, central venous pressure monitoring, or monitoring cardiac output and filling via a Swan-Ganz catheter, is indicated.

Those with severe hemorrhagic pancreatitis may require blood transfusions or transfusion of clotting factors to correct abnormal coagulation problems.

Often, a variety of electrolyte abnormalities are encountered. Clients with severe and persistent vomiting may require saline solutions containing potassium chloride. Serum calcium may be depressed secondary to hypoalbuminemia. Mild hyperglycemia is usually corrected with fluid volume replacement, but marked hyperglycemia or glycosuria requires careful insulin administration.

Respiratory complications may require supportive measures such as oxygen administration and physical therapy, or the lesser supportive measures such as endotracheal intubation and positive pressure ventilation.

Treatment may involve attempts to suppress pancreatic exocrine function. Therapy to decrease these enzymes may include nasogastric suction, or administration of histamine H_2-receptor antagonists, antacids, anticholinergics, glucagon, calcitonin, somatostatin, and proglumide.

It may be necessary to perform peritoneal dialysis to rid the peritoneum of potentially toxic compounds commonly found in exudate from acute pancreatitis. A-histamine, vasoactive kinins, elastase, prostaglandins, phospholipase A, trypsin, and chymotrypsin may mediate adverse systemic effects, such as hypotension, pulmonary failure, hepatic failure, and altered vascular permeability. This mode of therapy is usually reserved for those clients who show early clinical deterioration in spite of maximal intensive care support.

PHARMACOLOGIC MANAGEMENT

Pain is usually treated with administration of narcotic analgesics, with meperidine being the drug of choice. Morphine is contraindicated because it potentially may cause spasm of the sphincter of Oddi, which could then potentiate ongoing pancreatic parenchymal injury.

Antibiotics, in theory, are not necessary in most mild to moderate cases. However, prophylactic antibiotics may be ordered, particularly in the more severe cases of pancreatitis.

DIETARY MANAGEMENT

Oral intake is prohibited initially but generally can be resumed once abdominal pain and tenderness have improved. Caution must be taken because premature return to oral intake has been associated with the development of pancreatic abscess and reactivation of pancreatic inflammation. Clients with severe cases may need to be supported nutritionally by the parenteral route. Administration of carbohydrate- and amino acid-based solution along with lipids as a source of calories may be necessary.

Surgical Management

Operative intervention is indicated in four specific circumstances: (1) uncertainty of diagnosis, (2) treatment of pancreatic sepsis, (3) correction of associated biliary tract disease, and (4) progressive clinical deterioration despite optimal supportive care.

When caring for clients following pancreatic surgery, the nurse should (1) have a clear idea of the surgical procedure performed, its purpose, steps, and dangers; (2) be aware of the location and purpose of each drain inserted during surgery—if there are multiple drains, especially external drains, assess each one for proper function; (3) continually assess tubes or drains that are in place for decompression; and (4) if a T-tube or internal stent becomes nonfunctional, bring it to the surgeon's attention immediately to prevent leakage at the internal insertion site. Leakage may lead to peritonitis or fistula formation.

Following pancreatic excision, find out how much pancreatic tissue was removed. When there is a decrease in endocrine tissue, control of blood sugar with insulin and diet becomes necessary. Exocrine loss does not pose immediate postoperative problems but will necessitate lifelong enzyme replacement when the client returns to oral food ingestion.

COMPLICATIONS

It has been previously discussed how difficult it may be to diagnose acute pancreatitis and to exclude other potentially fatal diagnoses. When such a condition exists, exploratory laparotomy is indicated to eliminate processes such as perforated viscus or acute mesenteric ischemia. Then if uncomplicated acute pancreatitis is present, no manipulation is needed and the surgery is terminated. In presumed gallstone-associated pancreatitis, cholecystectomy and intraoperative cholangiography are favored. In clients with severe hemorrhagic pancreatitis with necrosis, débridement of necrotic tissue is performed and retroperitoneal drainage is established.

Treatment of pancreatic abscess combines antibiotic therapy and surgical drainage. Operative débridement is necessary to remove the thick, debris-filled, pastelike collections of infected necrotic material.

Correction of Associated Biliary Tract Disease. Formerly, biliary tract surgery for gallstone-associated pancreatitis was deferred for up to 8 weeks. However, up to 50 per cent of clients awaiting elective surgery had a recurrence of pancreatitis. Now, most surgeons proceed with surgery as soon as the initial symptoms of pancreatitis resolve.

When clients with severe pancreatitis do not respond to medical management, operative intervention may be indicated to débride necrosis, or again to exclude other possible diagnoses as causative factors.

Nursing Management

ASSESSMENT

Until a confirmed diagnosis is made, nursing should concentrate on treating the symptoms and preparing clients for diagnostic procedures. Assessing and documenting subjective and objective data may assist in making the diagnosis. Also, much of the nurse's role in these instances is teaching the client and significant others regarding procedures and their rationale. Keep in mind that the degree of nursing intervention is directly related to the severity of illness and client's overall condition.

NURSING INTERVENTION

Nursing Diagnosis: Pain R/T inflammation of the pancreas and surrounding tissue, biliary tract disease, obstruction of pancreatic ducts, and interruption of the blood supply.

Planning: Expected Outcomes. Client will demonstrate absence or decrease in pain, as evidenced by verbalizing that pain is absent or decreased and resting quietly.

Implementation. The nurse should assess the location, severity, and character of the pain as well as the onset, duration, and precipitating or relieving factors. This assessment should be documented, and significant changes should be reported. Evaluate the client's response to pain and therapies used to decrease discomfort.

Not allowing the client to take anything by mouth not only rests the GI tract but also decreases pancreatic stimulation. Keep in mind that even ice chips can stimulate enzymes and increase pain. Nasogastric suctioning helps decrease distention and, thereby, promote comfort. Check the system frequently to ensure that the nasogastric suction is functioning properly to avoid pooling and stimulation of enzyme secretion.

Be sure to administer pain medications in a timely manner. Remember that opiate narcotics may stimulate spasm of the ducts and increase pain. Demerol is usually the drug of choice. Other drugs may be ordered (such as anticholinergics) to quiet the pancreas and decrease enzyme secretion.

Again, remember that nonpharmacologic measures are often helpful in decreasing pain, relaxing the client, and enhancing the effects of narcotics. Positioning (side-lying, knee-chest position with a pillow pressed against the abdomen or a sitting position with the trunk flexed may be helpful), back rubs, relaxation techniques, and providing a quiet environment all help promote comfort and rest.

Nursing Diagnosis: Anxiety and Fear R/T change in health status, change in environment, and fear of pain returning.

Planning: Expected Outcomes. The client will express and demonstrate decreasing signs of anxiety, as evidenced by calmly discussing apprehensions, verbalizing that anxiety and fear is decreasing, and displaying behavior associated with relaxation (e.g., rests quietly).

Implementation. Assess the client's level of anxiety by listening and observing. Reassure and acknowledge that the unknown is frightening. Explain procedures that may be frightening to the client. Remember that clients in pain or acute anxiety may have a shortened attention span, so instruction should be simple and direct. Allow significant others to remain with the client as appropriate for added reassurance and comfort.

Collaborative Problem: Fluid Volume Deficit and Electrolyte Imbalance R/T vomiting, nasogastric suctioning, NPO status, shifting of body fluids, fever, and diaphoresis.

Planning: Expected Outcomes. The client will receive appropriate assessments and interventions for early detection or prevention of fluid and electrolyte imbalance.

Implementation. Monitor vital signs for changes in pulse and blood pressure (fluid volume changes) and respirations (acid-base imbalance). If the client is in the intensive care setting, hemodynamic monitoring should be assessed for changes in fluid status (see Chap. 14), and heart monitor rhythm changes may be a first indication of electrolyte imbalance (see Chap. 14). The nurse should check laboratory values as they are ordered for significant changes and observe for physical symptoms indicating hyperglycemia, hypocalcemia, and hypokalemia. The nurse should monitor the client's response to fluid administration and blood products by checking for edema, lung sounds, skin turgor, mucus membranes, and monitoring the intake and output. Significant changes should be reported promptly because these clients are at increased risk.

Nursing Diagnosis: Breathing Pattern, Ineffective R/T abdominal distention or ascites, pain, or respiratory complications.

Planning: Expected Outcomes. The client will maintain an effective breathing pattern, as evidenced by a respiratory rate within normal limits, relaxed respiratory effort, absence of cyanosis, and clear lungs.

Implementation. The nurse should assess the client's respirations for rate and effort. Assessments should include lung auscultation for decreased lung sounds (potential for atelectasis), rales or rhonchi (potential for pneumonia and pleural effusion), and cyanosis. Many times, these clients are on bed rest, which precludes the need for prophylactic nursing interventions of pulmonary hygiene (e.g., turning, coughing, deep breathing, and incentive spirometry). Keeping the client comfortable with the administration of pain medications enhances full inspiration and normal breathing patterns. Positioning, such as placing the client in semi-Fowler's or a side-lying position, may facilitate normal respirations.

Nursing Diagnosis: Nutrition, Altered: Less than Body Requirements R/T nausea and vomiting, NPO status, and nasogastric suctioning.

Planning: Expected Outcomes. The client will maintain adequate nutritional status, as evidenced by maintaining normal body weight, keeping blood sugar within normal limits, and finding no evidence of muscle wasting.

Implementation. Again, depending on the severity of illness, these clients may take nothing by mouth for an extended length of time. When extended fasting is necessary, nutrition is provided through hyperalimentation and lipids (see Chap. 54). Nursing assessment should include the overall nutritional status of the client by checking daily weights, tissue integrity, and the presence of adequate body fat and muscle mass.

You will recall in earlier discussion, acute pancreatitis clients are allowed to have an oral diet when all abdominal pain and tenderness have resolved. However, if oral intake is resumed too soon, reexacerbation of symptoms may occur. Therefore, the nurse should monitor the client's response to oral intake carefully and begin intake slowly with liquids and progress to a normal diet. It may be necessary to administer antispasmodics, anticholinergics, and antacids to reduce gastric and pancreatic secretions. Also, if the pancreas has been severely damaged, it may be necessary to give replacement pancreatic enzymes to replace enzyme deficit and aid in digestion. The nurse then must monitor the effects of these drugs.

Nursing Diagnosis: Knowledge Deficit R/T causes of pancreatitis, treatment, possible complications, and home health care.

Planning: Expected Outcomes. The client and significant other will accurately verbalize home health care needs, as evidenced by being able to verbalize an understanding of diet; list medications, including indications, dosage, frequency, and side effects; and list signs and symptoms of recurrence.

Implementation. The nurse should begin preparing clients for discharge by assessing their level of understanding and learning needs. Discuss the medication regimen, including the medication's purpose, dosage, frequency, and possible side effects. The client may require an insulin supplement because of pancreatic damage. Teaching should begin as soon as possible to ensure that the client and significant other are fully prepared to deal with glucose monitoring, diet, and insulin administration (see Chap. 61 for Diabetic Teaching). Instruct the client about dietary restrictions, such as restricting alcohol, tea, coffee, spicy foods, and heavy meals that stimulate pancreatic secretions and attacks of pancreatitis. Clients should understand the benefit of eating small, frequent meals that include high-protein, low fat, and moderate to high carbohydrate foods. Ensure that the client is aware of which symptoms may indicate that pancreatitis is recurring and understands the importance of reporting these symptoms immediately. These symptoms include steatorrhea (fatty-looking stools); severe back or epigastric pain; persistent gastritis, nausea, and vomiting; weight loss; elevated temperature; and symptoms of hyperglycemia.

Nursing Diagnosis: Injury, High Risk for R/T malfunction of pancreatic drains or loss of endocrine and exocrine function secondary to removal of the pancreas.

Planning: Expected Outcomes. The client will not experience injury, as evidenced by proper draining of pancreatic drains, and no symptoms of hypoglycemia or digestive disorders related to absence of exocrine enzymes.

Implementation. The nurse should assess for placement of drains, the location of the drains (internal or external), and proper function and patency of the drains. If the drains do not appear to be functioning, the physician should be notified immediately.

The nurse should assess the functional ability of remaining pancreatic tissue following excision of pancreas, determining both endocrine and exocrine functioning for long-term implications. If the client has lost all endocrine function, he or she will require insulin (see Chap. 61). Continue to monitor the client for signs of hypoglycemia.

With the loss of exocrine function, replacement of pancreatic enzyme function with medications such as pancrelipase (Pancrease) will be necessary. When the client begins to eat, the nurse should watch for the development of diarrhea and steatorrhea, which indicates that insufficient pancreatic enzymes are present.

Nursing Diagnosis: Knowledge Deficit R/T care, postoperative nutritional needs, diabetic care, and pancreatic enzyme replacement.

Planning: Expected Outcomes. The client will understand discharge instructions, as evidenced by the ability to describe and demonstrate appropriate wound care, diet, proper diabetic care, and correct administration and side effects of medication regimen.

Implementation. Assess the knowledge of the client and significant others before providing appropriate learning guidelines prior to discharge. Provide instructions for wound care. The client will require alterations in his or her diet to reflect the new status as a diabetic. Provide teaching guidelines regarding nutritional needs and appropriate low-fat, diabetic diet (see Chap. 61).

Provide the client with important information concerning diabetes, including information about hyperglycemia (polyuria, polydipsia, and polyphagia) and information about hypoglycemia. See Chapter 61 for further information on diabetic teaching.

Provide the client with information about pharmacologic therapy (pancreatic enzymes), including the medication action, side effects, and when to notify the physician.

Nursing Diagnosis: Individual Coping, Ineffective R/T alcohol abuse.

Planning: Expected Outcomes. The client will learn to cope with life more effectively, as evidenced by admitting alcohol is a problem, seeking help with alcohol abstinence, and seeking long-term support to develop more effective coping strategies.

Implementation. The client must be encouraged to face the problem that alcohol ingestion is causing. Spend time with the client and encourage verbalization of problem. Facilitate counseling for alcohol abuse by recommending groups such as Alcoholics Anonymous to the client and supporting the client's decision to join such a program. Discuss supportive services available as necessary with the client and significant others.

The nurse also can help the client by working with significant others so they better understand the problems with alcohol and can better help the client.

EVALUATION

The client will be evaluated based on the expected outcomes. If the outcomes are not achieved, the plan and the interventions should be revised.

Modification of Plan of Care for the Elderly

The older client may be less able to survive the life-threatening effects of pancreatitis. Treatment is the same, although surgery may not be performed unless the condition becomes life threatening.

Post-hospital Care

DISCHARGE TEACHING

The client with loss of pancreatic endocrine function requires extensive teaching regarding diabetes and diabetic care (see Chap. 61).

All clients require teaching on good nutrition to maintain adequate output. The client will need to understand and follow a nutritious, low-fat diet.

Avoidance of alcohol is another area of postoperative teaching for these clients. The client needs to understand the problems that alcohol is creating and the need to stop drinking before irreversible damage is done.

HOME HEALTH CARE NEEDS

The client should probably be seen by a visiting nurse after discharge to assess the client's ability to follow the postoperative regimen.

FOLLOW-UP CARE

The client will need to be seen at regular intervals to ensure that the postoperative regimen is being followed. The client's ability to abstain from alcohol should be carefully assessed and further counseling provided.

CHRONIC PANCREATITIS

Chronic pancreatitis is a progressive, inflammatory, destructive disease of the pancreas. The incidence of chronic pancreatitis in the United States is about four cases per 100,000 population. Chronic pancreatitis involves progressive fibrosis and degeneration of the pancreas.

Characteristically, the pancreas is progressively destroyed by repeated flare-ups of usually mild attacks of pancreatitis. After repeated attacks of acute pancreatitis, this inflammatory process results in scarring and calcification of pancreatic tissue and the damage is irreversible, affecting both endocrine and exocrine pancreatic functions. Within the United States (and other industrial countries), chronic alcoholism is the most frequent cause of chronic calcifying pancreatitis. Protein malnutrition is a cause of this disease in some other parts of the world. Other causes include hyperparathyroidism, congenital anomalies, and pancreatic trauma.

In chronic pancreatitis, as in acute pancreatitis, dull pain alternates with severe pain, vomiting, fever, and jaundice. When sitting in bed with knees flexed and pressing a pillow to the abdomen, the client may experience some pain relief. The client generally experiences more pain when lying supine.

Because food may aggravate the pain, the client usually decreases food intake, resulting in weight loss. Reduction in digestive enzyme secretion eventually causes malnutrition and contributes to this weight loss.

Eventually, because of involvement of the islet tissue, the client develops hyperglycemia with manifestations of diabetes. Insulin-dependent diabetes mellitus occurs in up to one third of clients.

The client also suffers from (1) abdominal distention with flatus and cramps and (2) frequent passage of foul fatty stools (steatorrhea). Thus, the clinical group of symptoms that serves as a classic presentation of chronic pancreatitis is abdominal pain, weight loss, diabetes, and steatorrhea.

Additionally, many clients present with a history of narcotic analgesic abuse in an effort to control pain.

Pain or digestive disturbance may motivate a person with chronic pancreatitis to seek help.

Because of a reduced amount of functioning tissue in chronic pancreatitis, pancreatic enzyme analysis may be normal. Blood studies may reveal a mild leukocytosis. X-ray studies may show reduced bowel motility, calcifications, and adhesions. Both ultrasonography and the more expensive CT study provide useful diagnostic data. Angiography indicates vascular changes. Cholangiography and cholecystography show biliary alterations, which may be either a cause or a consequence of the pancreatic disorder.

Pancreatitis frequently reveals bloody fluid that is high in amylase and methemalbumin from hemoglobin digestion. Other studies may be in order, especially when the diagnosis is obscure.

The three areas that are treated medically are (1) control of pain, (2) treatment of endocrine insufficiency, and (3) treatment of exocrine insufficiency.

The control of pain can be a major problem and is generally the sole indication for surgical intervention. For alcohol-related pancreatitis, total abstinence from alcohol is imperative and sometimes successful in itself in pain relief. Control of diet may decrease painful stimulation of pancreatitis enzyme secretion. Attempts to control pain pharmacologically should begin with non-narcotic analgesics and progress to narcotic analgesics, if needed.

Exogenous insulin therapy may be necessary because of destruction of islet tissue. Exocrine insufficiency is treated with exogenous pancreatic enzyme therapy. This therapy may include lipase, trypsin, or histamine H_2-receptor antagonists.

The three major goals of surgical intervention for chronic pancreatitis are to (1) correct the primary tract disease (ampullar procedure), (2) relieve ductal obstruction (ductal drainage), and (3) relieve pain (ablative procedure). Several surgical approaches are available. Major operations are summarized in Figure 59-3.

The prognosis in chronic pancreatitis is good if acute attacks decrease in frequency. Replacement therapy for chronic fat indigestion permits a fairly normal life. If the client continues to drink alcohol, the prognosis is poor. Repeated attacks eventually cause death from shock or renal failure.

PANCREATIC PSEUDOCYST

Pancreatic pseudocysts are localized collections of pancreatic secretions (high concentrations of amylase, lipase, and trypsin) in a cystic structure usually adjacent to the pancreas rather than within the parenchyma. These pseudocysts account for up to 75 per cent of all cystic lesions of the pancreas. Pancreatic pseudocysts develop in up to 10 per cent of clients after an attack of acute alcoholic pancreatitis, but they may be associated with acute pancreatitis of other causes, chronic pancreatitis, trauma, and pancreatic neoplasm.

The most common clinical picture of a client with pancreatic pseudocyst involves abdominal pain, early satiety, nausea, and vomiting. Less common symptoms include pruritus, jaundice, sepsis, and hemorrhage. Essentially, diagnosis of pseudocyst is made through the same assessment as that used with pancreatitis.

Treatment is based on the presence or absence of symptoms, the client's age, and size of the cyst. In about 25 per cent of the cases, the pseudocyst resolves spontaneously. Clients with this condition are followed with frequent ultrasound study to determine whether or not the cyst is decreasing in size. However, persistent symptoms or pseudocyst-related complications require operative intervention.

Surgical procedures range from internal drainage of the pseudocyst (cystojejunostomy, cystogastrostomy, and cystoduodenostomy), pancreatic resection, distal pancreatectomy, and least frequent, percutaneous or endoscopic drainage.

PANCREATIC CANCER

There are approximately 28,000 cases of cancer of the pancreas in the United States each year. It is the fifth most common cause of cancer death, exceeded only by lung, colorectal, breast, and prostate cancer. Ninety per cent of pancreatic cancer clients die within the first year after diagnosis. Cancer of the pancreas is more common in blacks than in whites, smokers than nonsmokers, and males than females.

It appears to be linked to diabetes mellitus, use of alcohol, history of previous pancreatitis, and the ingestion of a high-fat diet.

Duct cell adenocarcinoma accounts for over 90 per cent of malignant pancreatic exocrine tumors. The most common site of origin is the pancreatic head. Less common types of pancreatic exocrine cancer include cystadenocarcinoma and acinar cell carcinoma.

Periampullary adenocarcinomas originate in the region of the ampulla of Vater. Clients typically present with jaundice, weight loss, and abdominal pain. The majority of clients are managed operatively by either resection or palliative therapy.

Carcinomas of the tail and body of the pancreas represent up to 30 per cent of pancreatic carcinomas. Clients usually present with significant weight loss and abdominal pain. Because of their location, these tumors generally grow to a large size before symptoms occur and the diagnosis is made. Therefore, the resectability rate is low (less than 7 per cent), and the prognosis is poor (5 to 6 month mean survival).

Cystadenocarcinoma of the pancreas is most frequently seen in women between the ages of 40 and 60 and accounts for less than 2 per cent of all pancreatic exocrine neoplasms.

Acinar cell carcinoma of the pancreas is very rare, has no sexual predominance, and is given surgical treatment as that used for ductal adenocarcinoma.

PANCREATIC TRAUMA

The pancreas is injured in less than 2 per cent of clients with abdominal trauma. Two thirds of pan-

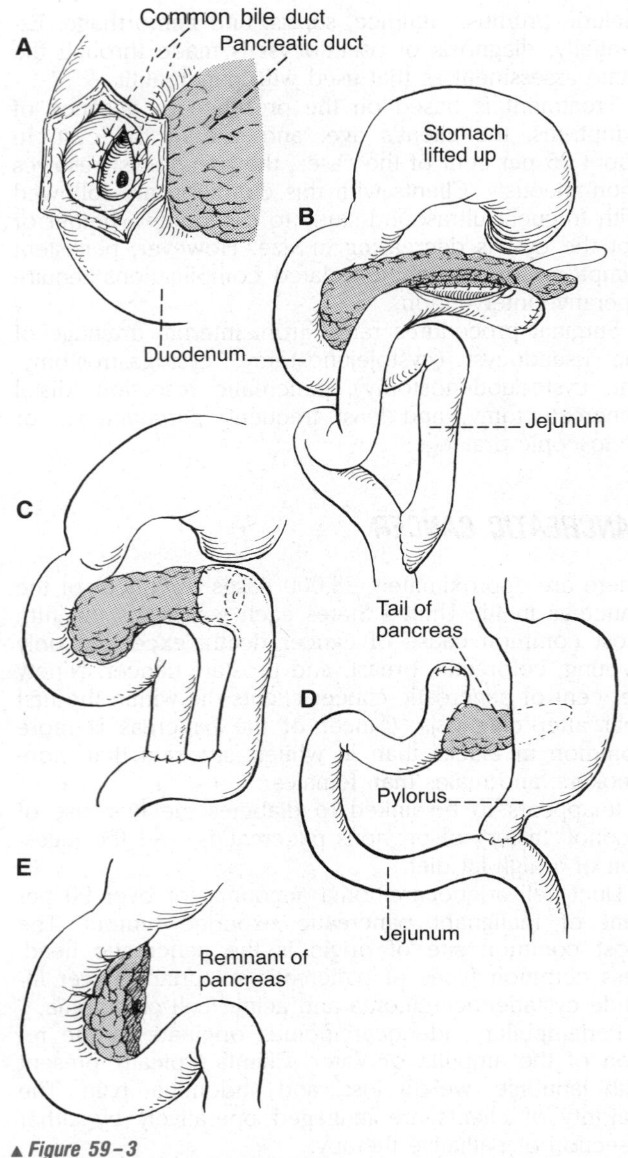

A. **Sphincteroplasty (ampullary)**
Indicated for stenosis of sphincter of Oddi with dilatation of pancreatic duct. This procedure has limited application in pancreatitis and frequency is decreasing.

B. **Side-to side pancreaticojejunostomy (ductal drainage)**
Indicated when gross dilatation of pancreatic ducts is associated with septa and calculi. The most successful with rates of 60-90 percent.

C. **Caudal pancreaticojejunostomy (ductal drainage)**
Indicated to the uncommon cases of isolated proximal pancreatic ductal stenosis not involving the ampulla.

D. **Pancreaticoduodenal resection (ablative) (with preservation of pylorus)**
Indicated when major changes are confined to head of pancreas. Preservation of pylorus avoids usual gastric resection sequelae.

E. **Subtotal pancreatectomy (ablative)**
Indicated when other operations fail and when ducts are unsuitable for decompression. Because metabolic sequelae are significant, this procedure is declining in popularity.

▲ *Figure 59–3*

Operations for chronic pancreatitis.

creatic injuries are associated with penetrating abdominal trauma, and the rest are due to blunt trauma. Clients with penetrating abdominal trauma show signs of hemorrhage, progressive peritonitis, and hypovolemia.

The presentation of blunt pancreatic trauma is varied. The majority of clients with blunt trauma have injuries to surrounding organs and vascular structures, and pancreatic trauma is discovered on treatment of these other injuries. In clients without injury to other areas, the only findings may be mild epigastric pain and tenderness; progressive deterioration will yield the diagnosis of pancreatic injury.

Treatment involves surgery to control hemorrhage, debride nonviable tissue, preserve viable tissue, and provide drainage of pancreatic secretions.

CYSTIC FIBROSIS

Cystic fibrosis (CF) is a hereditary, chronic disease characterized by abnormal secretions of the exocrine glands. It is genetically transmitted as an autosomal recessive trait. Approximately 4 to 5 per cent of the population are carriers, and the incidence in the United States is about 1 in every 1600 to 2000 white births.

Pancreatic exocrine function is affected by decreased lipase released into the bowel. This results in malabsorption of lipids and causes blockage of the pancreatic ducts with thick mucus. Pancreatic degeneration, fibrosis, and atrophy of tissues follow, with eventual development of fatty infiltration and loss of function. The intestines have thick, viscous mucus, which may cause a thick mass within the bowel. The lack of pancreatic enzymes causes steatorrhea.

Pulmonary complications are the most physically visible. These clients have obvious respiratory compromise, with frequent bronchopneumonia and chronic bronchitis.

Recent improvements in the management of infants and children with CF have led to a greater number of adults with CF. Typically, these clients have a small stature and appear somewhat emaciated. They are barrel-chested and have clubbed fingers.

Because the digestive problems encountered with CF are generally managed with diet and oral administration of pancreatic enzymes and fat-soluble vitamins, these clients are hospitalized for treatment of respiratory compilations rather than for intestinal problems. The current trend is to hospitalize the client routinely for thorough pulmonary hygiene with a full course of intravenous antibiotics (with emphasis on antifungals) and respiratory therapy.

Nursing diagnoses that may apply to people with CF include

- Ineffective Airway Clearance R/T thick, viscous, mucous secretions from the submucosal glands of the respiratory tract
- Altered Nutrition: Less than Body Requirements R/T lack of pancreatic enzymes
- Knowledge Deficit R/T dietary management of CF

Interventions for clients with CF include

- Prophylactic pulmonary support—expectorants, postural drainage, antibiotics, and exercise;
- Administration of pancreatic enzymes;
- Dietary management—high-protein, high-calorie, high-salt, and low-fat diet
- Replacement of fat-soluble vitamins.

Summary

Biliary and exocrine pancreatic disorders are common but are extremely complex and diverse. The nurse needs a thorough understanding of the biliary and pancreatic anatomy and physiology to understand these disorders. Some of these conditions are treated without further difficulty, such as cholecystitis, whereas others can become chronic and lead to a wide variety of other problems, such as pancreatitis. Teaching is vital to the care of these clients, so the nurse must understand these conditions so appropriate teaching plans can be initiated.

Bibliography

1. Addison, N. V., & Finan, P. J. (1988). Urgent and early cholecystectomy for acute gallbladder disease. *British Journal of Surgery, 75,* 141.
2. Akiyama, H., et al. (1990). Percutaneous treatments for biliary diseases. *Radiology, 176,* 25.
3. Bates, D. M., & Girvin, G. W. (1987). Biliary tract disease. Is there a difference in men? *American Journal of Surgery, 153,* 532.
4. Birkenfeld, S., et al. (1988). Choledochoduodenostomy for benign and malignant biliary diseases. *Surgery, 53,* 658.
5. Biorsch, G., et al. (1988). Clinical evaluation, ultrasound, cholescintography, and endoscopic retrograde cholangiography in cholestasis: A prospective comparative study. *Journal of Clinical Gerontology, 10,* 185.
6. Bova, J. G. (1985). Cholecystitis: Diagnostic benefits of current radiologic techniques. *Consultant, 25,* 216.
7. Calhoun, R., & Willbanks, O. (1987). Coexistence of gallbladder disease and morbid obesity. *American Journal of Surgery, 154,* 655.
8. Carey, W. D. (1984). Biliary cirrhosis: Two causes with similar effects but different treatment. *Consultant, 24,* 89.
9. Cappell, M. S. (1991). Hepatobiliary manifestations of the acquired immune deficiency syndrome. *American Journal of Gastroenterology, 86,* 1.
10. Cotton, P. B. (1990). Critical appraisal of therapeutic endoscopy in biliary tract disease. *Annual Review of Medicine, 41,* 211.
11. DaCunha, J. P., et al. (1985). *Nurse's clinical library, gastrointestinal disorders.* Springhouse, PA: Springhouse Corporation.
12. Diehl, A. K., et al. (1987). Coronary risk factors and clinical gallbladder disease: An approach to the prevention of gallstones? *American Journal of Public Health, 77,* 841.
13. Fisher, R. L. (1989). Hepatobiliary abnormalities associated with total parenteral nutrition. *Gastroenterology Clinics of North America, 18,* 645.
14. Fitzgerald, E. J., & Toi, A. (1987). Pitfalls in the ultrasonographic diagnosis of gallbladder diseases. *Postgraduate Medical Journal, 63,* 525.
15. Gallbladder disease induced by parenteral nutrition (1985). *American Family Physician, 31,* 310.
16. Gilliland, T. M., & Trcyerso, L. W. (1990). Cholecystectomy provides long-term symptom relief in patients with acalculous gallbladders. *American Journal of Surgery, 159,* 489.
17. Groer, M. W., & Skekleton, M. E. (1989). *Basic pathophysiology: A holistic approach.* St. Louis: C. V. Mosby.
18. Gutman, H., et al. (1988). Changing trends in surgery for benign gallbladder disease. *American Journal of Gastroenterology, 83,* 545.
19. Guyton, A. C. (1991). *Textbook of medical physiology* (8th ed.). Philadelphia: W.B. Saunders.
20. Haynes, J., et al. (1982). Hereditary pancreatitis. *American Family Physician, 25,* 153.
21. Heiss, F., et al. (1984). Common bile duct calculi: Nonsurgical therapy. *Postgraduate Medicine, 75,* 109.
22. Heiss, F., et al. (1984). Common bile duct calculi: Surgical therapy. *Postgraduate Medicine, 75,* 88.
23. Isaksson, G., & Ihse, I. (1983). Pain reduction by an oral pancreatic enzyme preparation in chronic pancreatitis. *Digestive Diseases and Sciences, 28,* 97.
24. Jurf, J. B., et al. (1990). Cholecystectomy made easier. *American Journal of Nursing,*
25. Jurkovich, G. I., et al. (1988). Cholecystectomy. Expected outcome in primary and secondary biliary disorders. *American Surgeon, 54,* 40.
26. Klar, E., et al. (1990). Pancreatic ischemia in experimental acute pancreatitis: Mechanism, significance, and therapy. *British Journal of Surgery, 11,* 1205.
27. Kosel, K., et al. (1982). Total pancreatectomy and islet cell autotransplantation. *American Journal of Nursing, 82,* 568.
28. Kozarek, R. A., & Sanowski, R. A. (1981). Endoscopic papillotomy. *American Family Physician, 23,* 111.
29. Kulhman, J. E., et al. (1989). Complications of endoscopic retrograde sphincterotomy: Computed tomographic evaluation. *Gastrointestinal Radiology, 14,* 127.
30. Lee, S. P. (1990). Pathogenesis of biliary sludge. *Hematology, 12,* 2005.
31. Levitt, M. D. (1992) *In* J. B. Wyngaarden, et al. (Eds.), Pancreatitis. *Cecil textbook of medicine* (19th ed.). Philadelphia: W. B. Saunders.
32. McCance, K. L., & Huether, S. E. (1990). *Pathophysiology. The biologic basis for disease in adults and children.* St. Louis: The C. V. Mosby Company.

33. Miller, F. J., & Rose, S. C. (1990). Intervention for gallbladder disease. *Cardiovascular and Interventional Radiology, 13,* 264.
34. Miyake, H., et al. (1989). Prognosis and prognostic factors in chronic pancreatitis. *Digestive Diseases and Sciences, 34,* 449.
35. Montori, A., & Masoni, L. (1988). Impact of biliary tract endoscopy on benign and malignant diseases. *Surgical Endoscopy, 2,* 159.
36. Ohara, N., & Schaefer, J. (1990). Clinical significance of biliary sludge. *Journal of Clinical Gastroenterology, 12,* 291.
37. Pancreatitis from mercaptopurine: nurses drug alert, (1985). *American Journal of Nursing, 9,* 68.
38. Pettiti, D. B., & Sidney, S. (1988). Obesity and cholecystectomy among women: Implications for prevention. *American Journal of Preventive Medicine, 4,* 327.
39. Pigott, J. P., & Williams, G. B. (1988). Cholecystectomy in the elderly. *American Journal of Surgery, 155,* 408.
40. Reber, H. A. (1990). The cause and management of the pain of chronic pancreatitis. *Gastroenterology Clinics of North America, 19,* 895.
41. Ritchie, A. C. (1990). *Boyd's textbook of pathology.* Philadelphia: Lea and Febiger.
42. Sabiston, D. C. Jr. (1991). *Textbook of surgery. The biological basics of modern surgical practice.* Philadelphia: W. B. Saunders Company.
43. Sugawa, C., & Wiencek, R. G. Jr. (1988). Endoscopic retrograde sphincterotomy in the treatment of biliary tract disease. *American Surgeon, 54,* 412.
44. Urban, M. H. (1989). Endoscopic retrograde cholangiopancreatography. A diagnostic outpatient procedure. *AORN Journal, 50,* 572.
45. van Heerden, J. A., et al. (1991). Early experience with percutaneous cholecystolithotomy. *Mayo Clinic Procedures, 66,* 1005.
46. Vogelzang, R. L., & Nemcek, A. A. Jr. (1988). Percutaneous cholecystostomy: Diagnostic and therapeutic efficacy. *Radiology, 168,* 29.

Unit 14

Metabolic Disorders

The endocrine system often is considered one of the most complex systems within the human body. It is only in recent times that endocrine function has been understood and well defined. Prior to that time, the study of glands and hormones was considered to be more in the realm of ritual and magic than science and medicine. Endocrine disorders were not regarded as treatable physiologic problems. With the advent of endocrinology and the increased understanding of the system, nurses have found themselves deeply involved in the care of clients with endocrine disorders.

The nurse has a major role in the care of clients with endocrine disorders. The nurse is involved in assessment of these disorders as well as the care of clients during treatment. Many of these disorders require minimal hospital care, only during initial diagnosis and when severe complications occur. These clients remain at home, only seeking health care at periodic intervals. After extensive instruction, these disorders are usually controlled by the clients themselves.

Chapter 60 covers the structure and function of the endocrine system as well as assessment of the system and all potential disorders. The remainder of this unit discusses the specific disorders of the pituitary gland, endocrine pancreas, thyroid, parathyroid glands, adrenal glands, and gonads.

Chapter 60

Structure and Function; Assessment of Clients with Metabolic Disorders

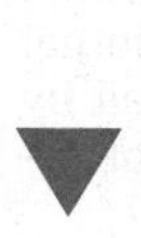

STRUCTURE AND FUNCTION OF THE ENDOCRINE SYSTEM

The endocrine system, in conjunction with the nervous system, controls and integrates body function. These two systems operate together to maintain homeostasis. Closely related in their functions, they are indistinguishable from one another in certain characteristics. For example, the adrenal medulla and the posterior pituitary glands are of neural origin. If they are destroyed or removed, the functions of these glands are partially taken over by the nervous system.

Although the communicative and integrative roles of the endocrine and nervous systems are similar, the precise ways in which each system functions differ. The nervous system sends its messages along nerve fibers, and these neural responses are swift and selective. Also, neural effects usually are rapid in onset and of short duration. In contrast, the endocrine system sends its messages in the form of hormones via the bloodstream. Hormonal effects have a slower onset than neural effects but a longer duration of action. The actions of the endocrine system may be localized to one area, or generalized to all the cells of the body.

STRUCTURE

There are two type of glands: (1) exocrine and (2) endocrine. Exocrine glands release their secretions into ducts on body surfaces, such as the skin or internal organs like the lining of the intestinal tract. Exocrine glands include the liver, pancreas (an exocrine and endocrine gland), the breast, and lacrimal glands for tears. In contrast, endocrine glands release their secretions directly into the blood (Fig. 60–1). Endocrine glands include the

islets of Langerhans in the pancreas,
gonads (ovaries and testes),
adrenal, pituitary, thyroid and parathyroid glands, and thymus.

The endocrine glands are shown in Figure 60–2.

HORMONES AND THEIR FUNCTIONS

The word hormone is derived from the Greek term hormon, which means to set in motion, arouse, or excite. Hormones set into motion various processes that govern life. The endocrine system has five general functions:

1. Differentiation of the reproductive and central nervous systems in the developing fetus.
2. Stimulation of sequential growth.
3. Coordination of the reproductive systems.
4. Maintenance of optimal internal environment.
5. Initiation of corrective and adaptive responses when emergency situations occur.

The disorders that occur when the endocrine system is not functioning properly affect growth, reproduction, and adaptation to stress.

Classification

In terms of their chemical structure, hormones are classified as water soluble or lipid soluble. Water-soluble hormones include polypeptides (e.g., insulin, glucogon, ACTH, gastrin) and catecholamines (e.g., dopamine, norepinephrine, epinephrine). Lipid-soluble hormones include steroids (e.g., estrogen, progesterone, testosterone, glucocorticoids, aldosterone) and thyronines (e.g., thyroxine). Water-soluble hormones act via a second messenger system, whereas steroid hormones are freely permeable to the cell membrane.

Characteristics

Although each hormone is unique in its own structure and function, all hormones have the following characteristics.

Hormones are secreted in one of three patterns. *Diurnal* secretion is a pattern that rises and falls within a 24-hour period. Cortisol is as example of a diurnal hormone. Cortisol levels rise in the morning and fall by evening. *Pulsatile and cyclic* patterns of hormonal se-

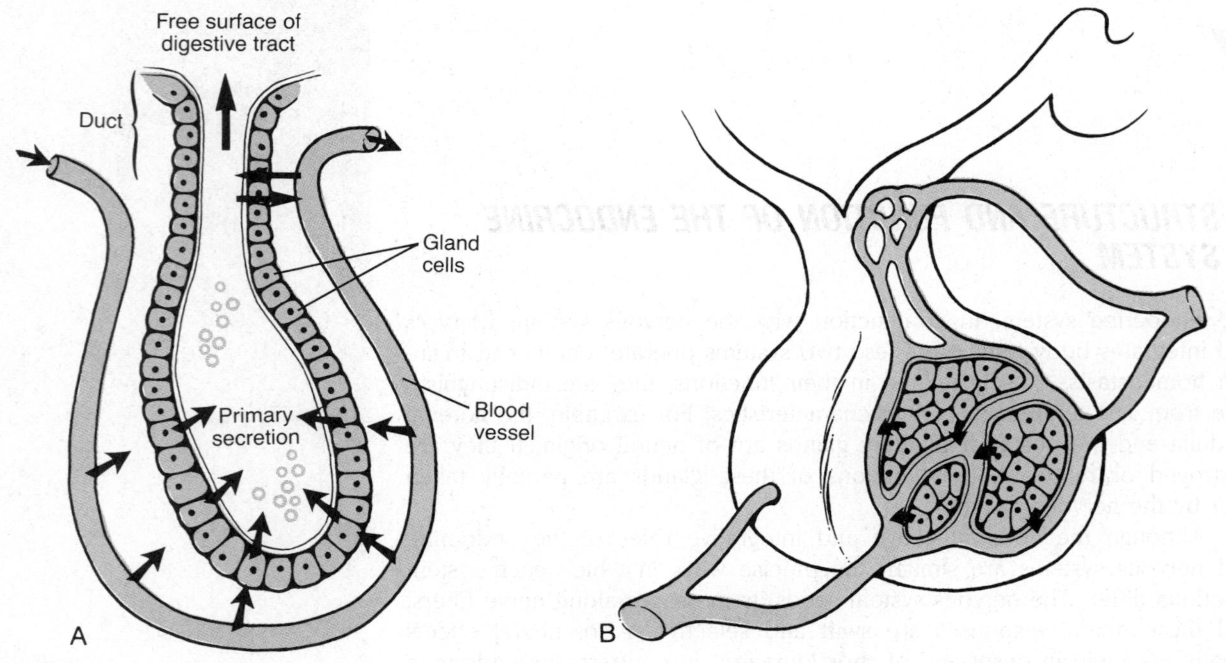

▲ *Figure 60–1*

Differences between endocrine and exocrine gland function. *A*, Exocrine secretions pass through a duct to reach their final destination, which are free surfaces of the body (e.g., internal surfaces such as the lining of the gastrointestinal tract, or external surfaces such as the skin). *B*, Endocrine glands, on the other hand, are generally ductless. Hormones are released from the cells of the gland into the interstitial fluid, from which they may pass into the blood to circulate throughout the body.

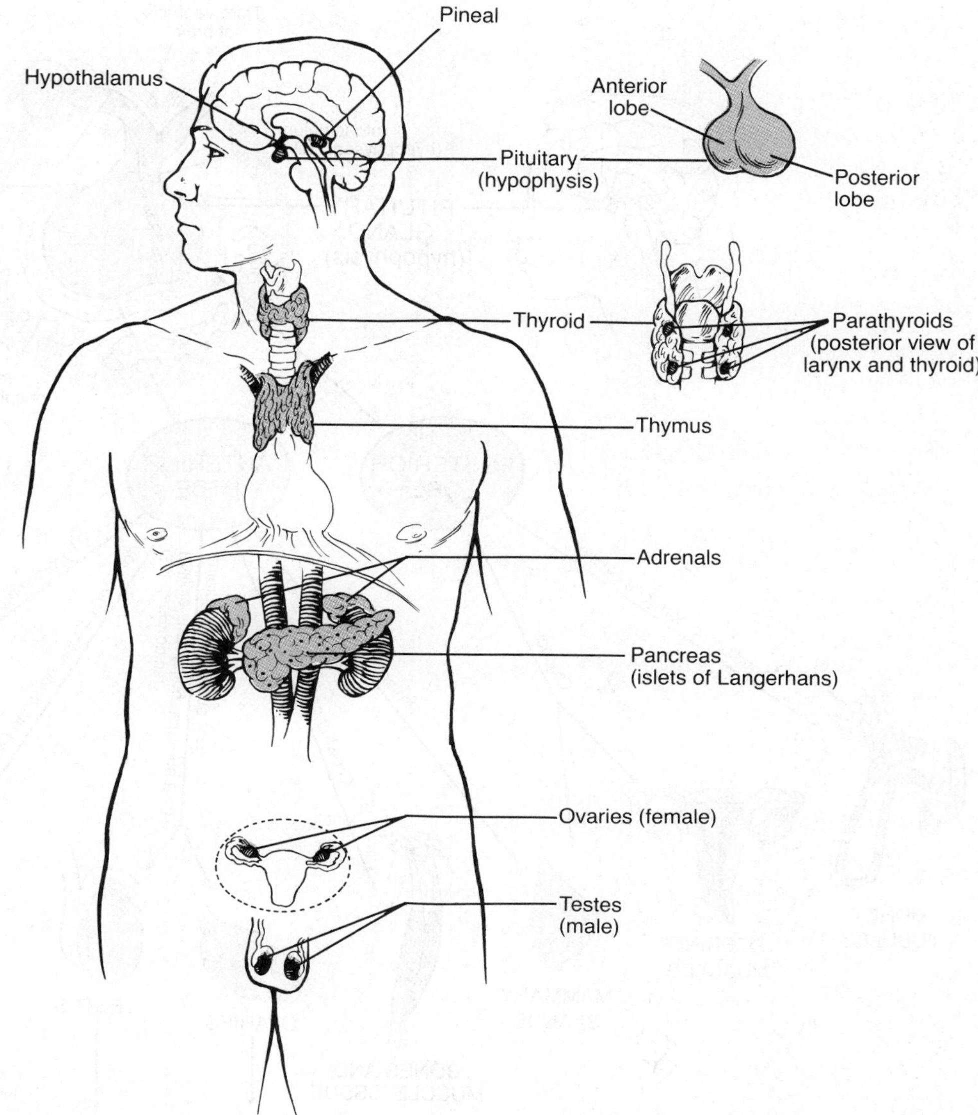

▲ **Figure 60-2**

Organs of the endocrine system.

cretion rise and fall along another time frame, such as monthly. Estrogen is a cyclic hormone with peaks and troughs (low points) to produce a menstrual cycle. The third type of hormonal secretion is *variable* and depends on levels of other substrates. Parathyroid hormone is secreted in response to serum calcium levels.

Hormones operate within a feedback system. Feedback loops can be positive or negative and allow the body to be maintained in an optimum environment.

Hormones control the rate of cellular activity. They do not initiate biochemical changes.

Hormones affect only cells that contain appropriate receptors, which initiate a specific function.

Hormones have independent and interdependent functions. The release of hormones from one gland often triggers the release of hormones from other glands.

Hormones are constantly deactivated by the liver or other cellular mechanisms and are excreted by the kidney.

Regulation

ROLE OF THE HYPOTHALAMUS AND PITUITARY GLANDS

The two major endocrine glands are the hypothalamus and the pituitary glands. Endocrine activity is controlled directly or indirectly by the hypothalamus, which links the nervous system to the endocrine system. In response to input from other areas of the brain and from other hormones in the blood, neurons in the hypothalamus secrete several releasing and inhibiting hormones. These hormones act on specific cells in the pituitary gland that regulate the production and secretion of pituitary hormones. The hypothalamus and pituitary gland are connected by a stalk of tissue called the infundibulum (Fig. 60-3).

The hormones secreted from each endocrine gland and the action of the hormones are listed in Table 60-1. Note that each of the hormones affects organs and tissues that are far removed from the location of its

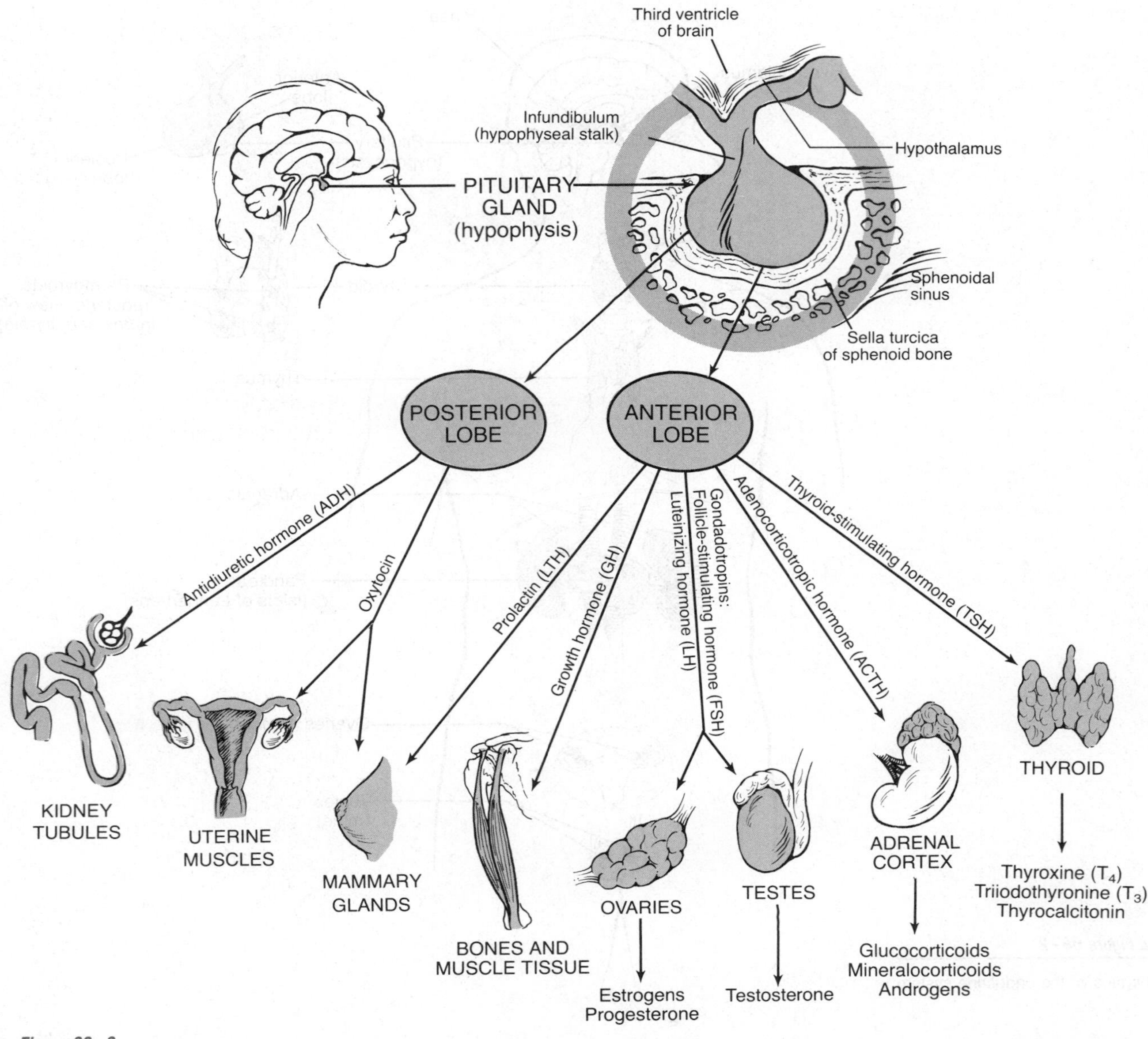

▲ *Figure 60–3*

The pituitary gland is suspended from the hypothalamus by the infundibulum. Shown here are hormones released by the pituitary gland and the target tissues they act on.

parent gland. For example, oxytocin, which is released from the posterior lobe of the pituitary gland, causes uterine contractions. The pituitary hormones that govern the secretion of hormones from other glands are called tropic hormones. Glands influenced by the hormones are called target glands (Fig. 60–3).

The prostaglandins are a form of hormone, but their action is different from the other hormones. Rather than exerting a response in tissues far from their synthesizing tissues, prostaglandins appear to exert their effect in the tissue that synthesizes them. Prostaglandins inhibit gastric secretion, relax smooth muscle in the airway, increase urine flow, increase or decrease blood pressure, and stimulate uterine contraction.

FEEDBACK SYSTEMS

Blood levels of hormones are also controlled by *negative feedback*. Once a hormone level is sufficient to produce its intended effect, further elevations in the hormone level are prevented by negative feedback. Rising levels of hormone negate the initial change that triggered the hormone release. For example, an increased secretion of adrenocorticotropic hormone (ACTH) from the anterior pituitary gland stimulates a rise in the release of cortisol from the adrenal cortex, causing a decrease in the release of more ACTH. Blood levels of substances other than hormones can also trigger hormone release and are controlled through a

TABLE 60-1. Endocrine Structure, Function, and Assessment

Gland	Hormone	Action of Hormone and Target Gland
Pituitary		
Anterior lobe	Growth hormone (GH)	Stimulates growth of body tissues and bones
	Prolactin	Stimulates mammary tissue growth and lactation
	Thyrotropic hormone (TSH)	Stimulates thyroid gland
	Gonadotropic hormones (LH and FSH)	Affect growth, maturity, and functioning of primary and secondary sex organs
	Adrenocorticotropic hormone (ACTH)	Stimulates steroid production by the adrenal cortex
	Melanocyte-stimulating hormone (MSH)	May stimulate adrenal cortex; may affect pigmentation
Posterior lobe	Antidiuretic hormone (ADH, vasopressin)	Promotes reabsorption of water by the distal tubules and collecting ducts of the kidney, thus decreasing urine output
	Oxytocin	Stimulates ejection of milk from mammary alveoli into the ducts; stimulates uterine contractions; may possibly be involved in the transport of sperm in the reproductive tract of the female
Thyroid	Thyroxine (T_4) Triiodothyronine (T_3)	Increases metabolic activity of almost all cells; stimulates most aspects of fat, protein, and carbohydrate metabolism
	Thyrocalcitonin	Lowers serum calcium and elevates phosphate levels; opposite effect from that of PTH
Parathyroid	Parathormone (PTH)	Increases calcium levels and decreases phosphate levels; increases resorption of bone
Adrenal		
Cortex	Hormones divided into three main groups:	
	Glucocorticoids (primarily cortisol)	Promotes carbohydrate, protein, and fat catabolism; increases tissue responsiveness to other hormones
	Mineralocorticoids (Aldosterone)	Tend to increase sodium retention and potassium excretion
	Androgens (male hormones)	Govern certain secondary sex characteristics
		All corticoids are important for defense against stress or injury
Medulla	Epinephrine (Adrenalin) (80%) Norepinephrine (20%)	Elevates blood pressure; converts glycogen to glucose when needed by muscles for energy; increases heart rate; increases cardiac contractility; dilates bronchioles
Ovaries	Estrogens and progesterone	Stimulate development of secondary sex characteristics; effect repair of the endometrium after menstruation
Testes	Testosterone	Essential for normal functioning of male reproductive organs; stimulates development of male secondary sex characteristics
Pancreas		
Islets of Langerhans	Insulin	Promotes metabolism of carbohydrates, protein, and fat, thus decreasing blood glucose levels
	Glucagon	Mobilizes glycogen stores, thus raising blood glucose levels
	Somatostatin	Decreases secretion of insulin, glucagon, growth hormone, and several gastrointestinal hormones (gastrin, secretin)

feedback system. The release of insulin from the islets of Langerhans in the pancreas is driven by blood glucose levels. A feedback system is shown in Figure 60-4.

ACTIVATION OF TARGET CELLS

Once the hormone reaches the target cell, it can influence how the cell functions in one of two methods: (1) through the use of intracellular mediators or (2) by activating the genes within the cell (Fig. 60-5). One intracellular mediator is cyclic AMP, which is bound to the inner surface of the cell membrane. When the hormone attaches to the cell, the action of the cell is altered in some way. For example, when the pancreatic hormone glucagon binds to liver cells, elevated levels of cyclic AMP promote the breakdown of glycogen to glucose. When hormones activate cells by interacting with genes, the gene synthesizes m-RNA and ultimately proteins (i.e., enzymes, steroids). These substances affect cellular reactions and processes.

THE EFFECTS OF AGING ON THE ENDOCRINE SYSTEM

The interaction of the endocrine system with the aging process has generated much study, but most data are inconclusive. The endocrine system has never been implicated as the cause of aging. There are changes in the endocrine glands and target organs that occur as a result of aging, however.

There may be a loss of self-regulation, leading to autoimmune or immunodeficiency disorders such as diabetes.

Theories of programmed change examine the genetic control of cell function. These theories suggest that cells are programmed to function only for a given time. The changes in the reproductive system, such as menopause, are an example of this theory.

As a result of changes with aging and disease, the target organs may lose their ability to respond to hormones. In addition, the hypothalamus and pituitary may be altered by changed levels of neurotransmitters.

Theories of stress and adaptation suggest that body structures wear out in time and are no longer able to adapt to stressors. This theory may help explain the inability of the elderly to respond to illness and stress.

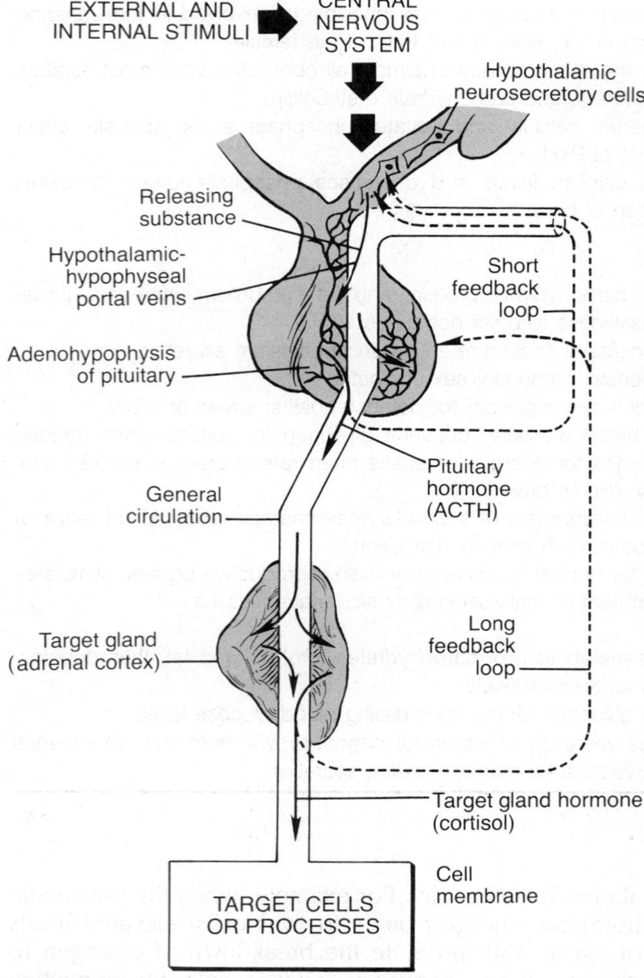

▲ *Figure 60–4*

Regulation of hormone secretion by negative feedback. When the calcium level in the blood falls below normal, the parathyroid glands are stimulated to release more parathyroid hormone. This hormone acts to increase the calcium level in the blood, thus restoring homeostasis. If the calcium level exceeds normal, the parathyroid glands are inhibited and slow their release of hormone. This diagram has been simplified. Calcitonin, a hormone secreted by the thyroid gland, works antagonistically to parathyroid hormone and is important in lowering blood calcium concentration.

THE ENDOCRINE GLANDS

Pituitary Structure and Function

The pituitary gland lies securely cradled within a small recess in the sphenoid bone called the sella turcica (Fig. 60–3). About 70 per cent of the gland is the anterior lobe, or adenohypophysis. The posterior lobe, or neurohypophysis, comprises the rest.

Three basic cell types compose the adenohypophysis: (1) eosinophils, (2) basophils, and (3) chromophobes. The adenohypophysis synthesizes and releases six hormones (Table 60–1): growth hormone (GH), ACTH, thyroid-stimulating hormone (TSH), prolactin (PRL), follicle-stimulating hormone (FSH), and luteinizing hormone (LH). Of these hormones, only GH and PRL act directly on the body's nonendocrine target tissues. The other four hormones stimulate the target glands governed by the pituitary (thyroid, adrenal cortex, testes, and ovaries), thereby indirectly influencing body structure and function (e.g., growth, intellectual and sexual development, and metabolism).

Target glands depend on stimulation from the anterior pituitary hormones to synthesize target gland hormones. If stimulation is excessive, the target gland becomes overactive; for example, too much ACTH from the pituitary stimulates the adrenal cortex to produce excessive amounts of cortisol, thereby causing hypertrophy and Cushing's disease. Conversely, inadequate pituitary production of a hormone causes the target gland to become hypoactive; for example, insufficient production of ACTH can cause secondary adrenocortical insufficiency.

The posterior lobe of the pituitary is called the neurohypophysis because it is of neural (rather than glandular) origin. An extension of the hypothalamus, the posterior lobe stores and releases antidiuretic hormone (ADH) and oxytocin (a hormone that stimulates uterine and mammary gland contractions).

The production and release of anterior pituitary hormones is regulated by hypothalamic hormones. Note in Figure 60–3 that the hypothalamus lies above the pituitary gland and is connected to it by the hypophyseal (pituitary) stalk.

The hypothalamus continuously monitors information regarding the internal and external milieu via the central nervous system. These messages are transmitted to the pituitary gland by hypothalamic peptide hormones called releasing hormones. They travel within the portal blood that flows from the hypothalamus to the anterior pituitary, causing the release of hormones from the anterior pituitary gland.

The hypothalamus communicates with the posterior pituitary gland by way of nerve fibers in the hypophy-

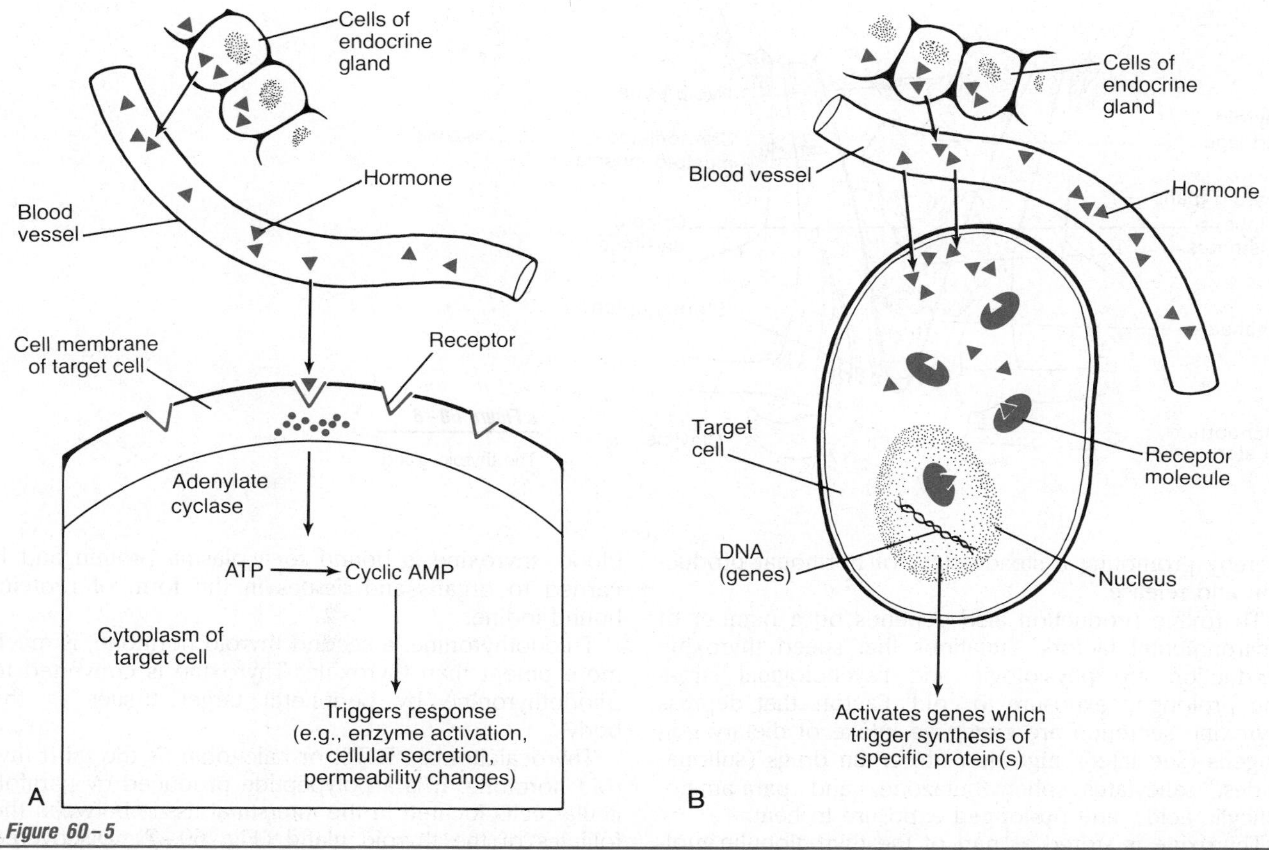

▲ *Figure 60–5*

There are two mechanisms by which a hormone influences cellular function. *A*, Intracellular mediators, especially cyclic AMP, trigger various cellular responses, such as the production of an enzyme. *B*, Genes can also be activated by hormones (e.g., steroids). Genes then produce messenger RNA, which triggers the production of proteins, such as enzymes.

seal stalk. Synthesis of the two posterior pituitary hormones occurs within the hypothalamus. The hormones then are transmitted to the posterior pituitary, where they are stored and released.

Thyroid and Parathyroid Structure and Function

THYROID

The thyroid gland is located in the neck, just below the cricoid cartilage. It is shaped somewhat like the letter H. The right and left lateral lobes lie on either side of the trachea. The lobes are connected by a thin mass of tissue called the isthmus, which stretches over the surface of the trachea (Fig. 60–6). Each of the two lobes is composed of irregularly shaped lobules. These lobules, in turn, consist of a multitude of tiny sacs called follicles (Fig. 60–7) filled with a jelly-like, iodine-containing substance called colloid. The main component of colloid is thyroglobulin—the storage form of the hormone thyroxine.

Thyroxine is one of the three hormones secreted by the thyroid gland; triiodothyronine and thyrocalcitonin are the other two. The major role of thyroxine is to regulate body metabolism. Thyroxine also aids in

- Regulating growth and development (both physical and mental);
- Carbohydrate, fat, and protein metabolism;
- Reproduction; and
- Resistance to infection.

Thyroxine ensures that oxygen consumption and heat production keep pace with the body's needs and activities. Too much thyroxine causes a dangerous increase in metabolism and a high rate of oxygen consumption. Conversely, too little results in a sluggish metabolism, a slowing of physical and mental function in the adult, and retardation of growth and development in the child.

Thyroxine production depends on (1) ingestion of sufficient protein and iodine and (2) the release of a vital anterior pituitary hormone called thyroid-stimulating hormone (TSH), thyrotropin, or thyrotropic hormone. TSH, as the name implies, stimulates the thyroid gland to produce thyroxine. TSH release is controlled by a negative feedback system: low serum levels of thyroxine stimulate increased secretion of TSH, and high serum levels of thyroxine inhibit TSH secretion,

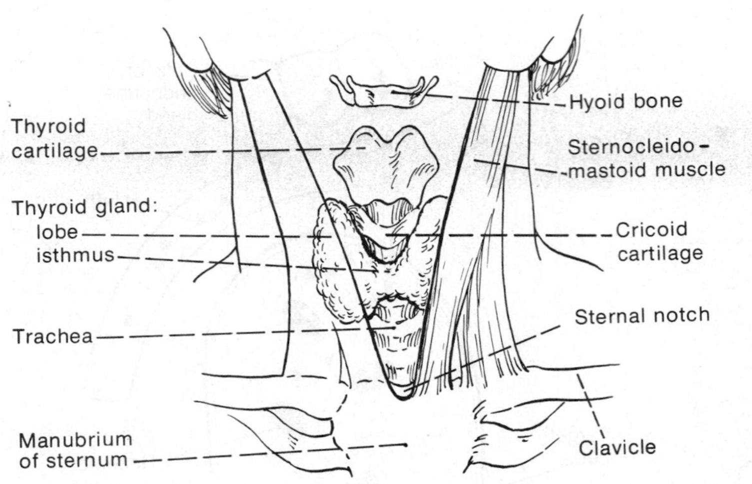

▲ *Figure 60–6*

The thyroid gland.

thereby promoting a steady state of hormonal production and release.

Thyroxine production also depends on a number of environmental factors. Situations that speed thyroxine production are physiologic and psychological stress and prolonged exposure to cold. Factors that depress thyroxine secretion are excessive intake of dietary goitrogens (see later), ingestion of certain drugs (sulfonamides, salicylates, phenylbutazone, and para-aminosalicylic acid), and prolonged exposure to heat.

Thyroxine is stored as part of the thyroglobulin molecule in the thyroid follicles. Whenever the body's circulating thyroxine levels drop too low, thyroxine is released from thyroglobulin into the blood. Within the blood, thyroxine is bound to a plasma protein and is carried to organs and tissues in the form of protein-bound iodine.

Triiodothyronine, a second thyroid hormone, is much more potent than thyroxine. Thyroxine is converted to triiodothyronine by peripheral target tissues in the body.

Thyrocalcitonin (TCT), or calcitonin, is the third thyroid hormone. It is a polypeptide produced by parafollicular cells located in the interstitial tissue between the follicles of the thyroid gland (Fig. 60–7). Discovered during the 1960s, calcitonin is capable of lowering both plasma calcium and phosphate. Calcitonin acts in a manner opposite to that of parathormone. Its effect on maintaining calcium balance is minor compared with that of parathormone.

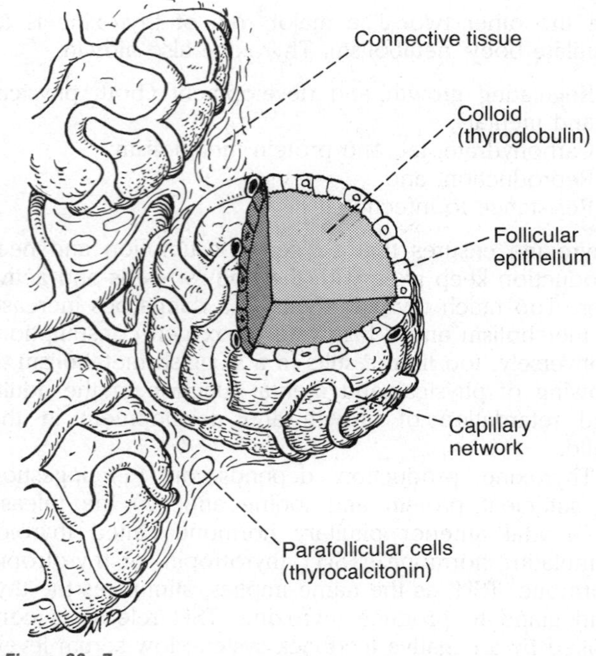

▲ *Figure 60–7*

Microscopic view of the thyroid gland.

PARATHYROID

The parathyroid glands are four small glands near to, attached to, or embedded in the thyroid gland. The hormone secreted by the parathyroid gland is a polypeptide substance called parathormone (PTH). The functions of PTH are to

- Control calcium and phosphate metabolism (see Chap. 14);
- Increase resorption of bone, thereby maintaining normal serum calcium levels; and
- Maintain an inverse relationship between serum calcium and phosphate levels, thereby fostering normal excitability of nerves and muscles.

The regulation of PTH release depends on a feedback relationship between the level of serum calcium and the level of PTH in the blood. Note that, when serum calcium is elevated, PTH secretion decreases, resulting in decreased mobilization of calcium ions from bone and lowering of serum calcium. Conversely, when serum calcium levels are low, PTH secretion increases, resulting in increased mobilization of calcium from bone and an increase in serum calcium levels.

Adrenal Structure and Function

The adrenal glands are small vital endocrine structures that lie next to each kidney (Fig. 60-8). Each adrenal gland is composed of an inner core, the medulla, and an outer shell, the cortex. Both contribute to survival and well being, but only the cortex is essential for life.

ADRENAL MEDULLA

The adrenal medulla is a part of the sympathetic nervous system. It releases two potent hormones, epinephrine and norepinephrine. These hormones prepare an individual to meet and deal with threat and danger. During stressful situations, epinephrine acts (1) on the liver to convert glycogen into glucose, and (2) on the heart to increase cardiac output. It is the release of epinephrine that produces the cold sweat, pounding heart, deep rapid breathing, and a wide-eyed blank expression experienced in times of emergency. Norepinephrine produces extensive vascular constriction and marked rise in blood pressure (BP) (Table 60-1).

Overactivity of the adrenal medulla is usually caused by a catecholamine-producing tumor called a pheochromocytoma. This tumor is usually (but not always)

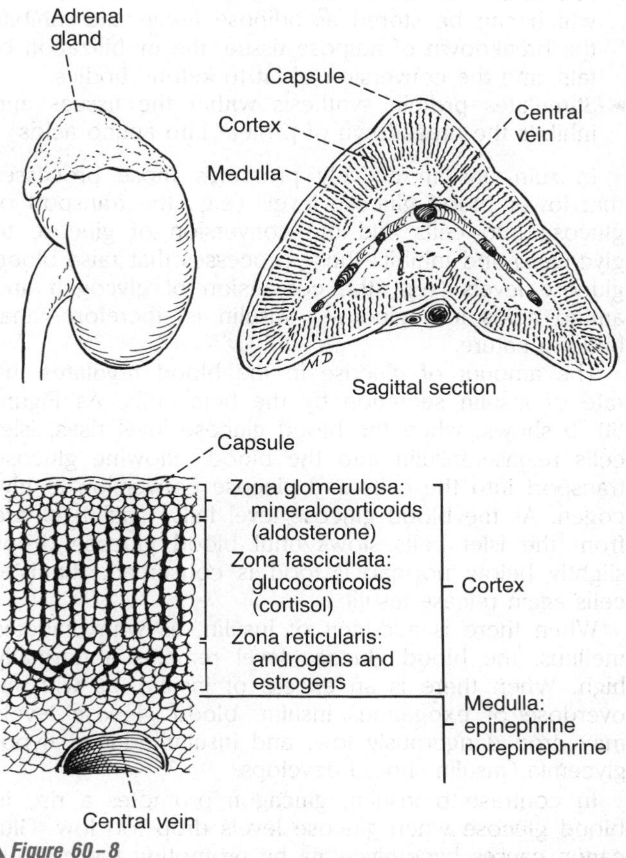

▲ *Figure 60-8*

The adrenal glands top the kidneys. A cortex surrounds the inner medulla and central vein. The cortex and medulla secrete specific hormones.

found in the adrenal gland. Pheochromocytomas produce hypertension, hypermetabolism, and hyperglycemia. Surgical removal of the tumor is usually curative.

ADRENAL CORTEX

The adrenal cortex is essential for survival. Loss of the adrenocortical hormones leads to death. The adrenal cortex synthesizes three classes of steroid hormones: (1) mineralocorticoids, (2) glucocorticoids, and (3) androgens. All of them are synthesized from cholesterol. As Boyd helpfully reminds us:

> For persons with a desire to memorize things easily, the 3 functions [of the hormones of the adrenal cortex] may be represented by the letter S, as salt, sugar and sex. For the others, these categories are the mineralocorticoids, the glucocorticoids, and the androgenic hormones.[5]

Mineralocorticoids. The mineralocorticoids (primarily aldosterone in humans) are produced in the zona glomerulosa of the adrenal cortex (Fig. 60-8). They regulate electrolyte balance by promoting sodium retention and potassium excretion. These physiologic activities, in turn, help sustain normal BP and cardiac output. Mineralocorticoid deficiency (Addison's disease) leads to hypotension, hyperkalemia, decreased cardiac output, and (in acute cases) shock. Mineralocorticoid excess results in hypertension and hypokalemia.

Glucocorticoids. The glucocorticoids are produced in the zona fasciculata (Fig. 60-8). Cortisol is the major glucocorticoid in humans. Cortisol has the following effects on the body.

Glucose Metabolism. Amino acids, lactate, and pyruvate are converted in the liver to glucose (gluconeogenesis), which raises the blood glucose level.

Protein Metabolism. Tissue catabolism increases. Amino acids are transported into the extracellular fluid and to the liver, where they are converted to glucose. Tissue wasting is the result.

Fluid and Electrolyte Balance. Sodium retention and potassium excretion increase. Excessive glucocorticoid secretion results in hypervolemia and hypertension due to sodium and water retention. Note the similarity between these effects of the glucocorticoids and those of the mineralocorticoids.

Inflammation and Immunity. The glucocorticoids suppress the inflammatory response to tissue injury and the protective immune response to invasion by infectious agents. Recall from Chapter 3 that Selye called the glucocorticoids anti-inflammatory corticoids. He believed that the principal action of glucocorticoids was to suppress inflammation in response to stress. In some cases, suppressing inflammation can be beneficial. For example, persons with arthritis (joint inflammation) obtain pain relief with cortisone injections. On the other hand, excessive glucocorticoids impede healing, decrease antibody formation, lower the number of circulating eosinophils and lymphocytes, and lower resistance to infection.

Stressors. Insufficient production of glucocorticoids (as noted in Addison's disease) decreases resistance to stress. Such individuals can die in shock following relatively minor trauma unless they quickly receive an injection of glucocorticoid (hydrocortisone).

Sex Hormones. The adrenal cortex secretes small amounts of sex steroids from the zona reticularis (Fig. 60–8). Normally, the adrenals secrete few androgens and estrogens compared with the large amounts of sex hormones secreted by the gonads. Excess production of sex hormones by the adrenal gland, however, does cause symptoms. For example, excessive release of androgens causes virilism, whereas excessive release of estrogens (e.g. from an adrenal carcinoma) causes gynecomastia and sodium and water retention.

The Pancreas

The pancreas, a large fish-shaped organ that lies behind the stomach, is both an exocrine and an endocrine gland. The exocrine role of the pancreas is carried out by cells within the tubular and acinar units of the gland. These cells secrete hormones and digestive enzymes that catalyze the digestion of proteins, carbohydrates, and fats.

ENDOCRINE FUNCTION OF THE PANCREAS

The endocrine functions of the pancreas are carried out by the islets of Langerhans. The islets, containing alpha, beta, and delta cells, are scattered throughout the pancreatic tissues. The islet cells are arranged in cords and are separated by a rich blood supply of capillaries. Insulin and glucagon, two hormones secreted by the islets, play a vital role in the control of carbohydrate metabolism. Insulin, synthesized by the beta cells, also helps control fat and protein metabolism. Insulin is a powerful hypoglycemic agent; insulin lowers blood sugar levels by promoting the passage of glucose into the cells. Conversely, glucagon, synthesized by alpha cells, is a hyperglycemic agent. It raises blood sugar by promoting the conversion of glycogen (the principal storage form of carbohydrate in mammals) to glucose within the liver. Somatostatin and gastrin are synthesized by the delta cells. Gastrin is used in the metabolism of foods, and somatostatin decreases the secretion of insulin, glucagon, growth hormone, gastrin, and secretin. Research is currently being conducted to explore the clinical usefulness of somatostatin.

HORMONAL FACTORS REGULATING CARBOHYDRATE METABOLISM

The hormones that regulate carbohydrate metabolism include the following: (1) insulin, (2) glucagon, (3) adrenocorticotropic hormone (ACTH), (3) corticosteroids, (4) epinephrine, and (5) thyroid hormone.

Insulin and Glucagon

Insulin and glucagon are the two principal hormones controlling carbohydrate metabolism. Both hormones are small proteins. Insulin, the hypoglycemic factor, also helps regulate fat and protein metabolism. More specifically, it

- Stimulates the active transport of glucose into muscle and adipose tissue cells. For glucose to cross the cell membrane, insulin must connect with a receptor on the cell membrane. Some clients with diabetes mellitus have enough insulin but too few receptor sites, which thus reduces glucose transport into the cell. Others have inadequate insulin production from the pancreas. When insulin levels are inadequate, or insulin is unable to connect with a receptor, glucose remains outside the cells, raising the serum glucose levels above normal.
- Regulates the rate at which carbohydrates are used by cells for energy.
- Promotes the conversion of glucose to glycogen for storage and inhibits the conversion of glycogen to glucose.
- Promotes the conversion of fatty acids into fat, which can be stored as adipose tissue and inhibits the breakdown of adipose tissue, the mobilization of fats, and the conversion of fat to ketone bodies.
- Stimulates protein synthesis within the tissues and inhibits the breakdown of protein into amino acids.

In sum, insulin actively promotes those processes that lower blood glucose levels (e.g., the transport of glucose into cells and the conversion of glucose to glycogen) and inhibits those processes that raise blood glucose levels (e.g., the conversion of glycogen and amino acids into glucose). Insulin is, therefore, anabolic in nature.

The amount of glucose in the blood regulates the rate of insulin secretion by the beta cells. As Figure 60–9 shows, when the blood glucose level rises, islet cells release insulin into the blood, allowing glucose transport into the cells and glucose conversion to glycogen. As the blood glucose level falls, insulin release from the islet cells slows until blood glucose drops slightly below normal. If food is consumed, the islet cells again release insulin.

When there is a deficit of insulin, as with diabetes mellitus, the blood glucose level remains abnormally high. When there is an excess of insulin, as with an overdose of exogenous insulin, blood glucose levels may drop dangerously low, and insulin-induced hypoglycemia (insulin shock) develops.

In contrast to insulin, glucagon promotes a rise in blood glucose when glucose levels drop too low. Glucagon causes hyperglycemia by promoting the conversion of liver glycogen to glucose. Clients with diabetes mellitus often experience abnormalities in the secretion of both insulin and glucagon. Diseases involving only

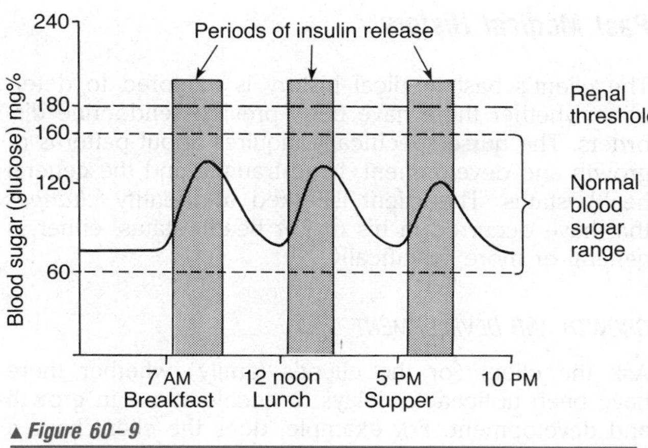

▲ **Figure 60-9**

Insulin release and its effect on blood glucose levels following meals.

the alpha cells (glucagon secretion—either excess or deficiency) are rare.

What factors are necessary for the synthesis and release of insulin and glucagon? These essential hormones depend on the following three requirements:

- A healthy pancreas with functioning alpha and beta cells.
- A diet adequate in protein. Both insulin and glucagon are protein substances.
- Normal potassium (K^+) levels. Insulin affects potassium mostly by inhibiting its leaving the cell.

When insulin or glucagon secretion is deficient, the person may receive the missing hormone by exogenous means. When injected, glucagon reverses hypoglycemia caused by excessive insulin. The person cannot take either of these hormones orally because they are inactivated within the gastrointestinal tract by proteolytic enzymes.

Other Hormonal Factors

Although insulin and glucagon play the predominant roles in carbohydrate regulation, the following hormones also influence blood glucose levels:

- Adrenocorticotropic hormone (ACTH) and the glucocorticoids of the adrenal cortex raise the serum glucose by increasing the formation of new glucose by the liver (gluconeogenesis) and decreasing the use of glucose in peripheral tissues. ACTH and the glucocorticoids also promote lipolysis and protein catabolism.
- Epinephrine, also released during stress, stimulates a rise in blood glucose by promoting the conversion of glycogen to glucose. Thyroid hormone stimulates almost all aspects of protein, fat, and carbohydrate metabolism.

Ovaries and Testes

The structure and function of the reproductive organs are described in Chapter 73.

▼ ASSESSMENT OF THE ENDOCRINE SYSTEM

Assessment of the endocrine system is often difficult because of the variety of symptoms that may occur. Each body system is affected by hormones; thus, clinical signs and subjective symptoms may be specific or nonspecific. Additionally, symptoms may be related to causes other than endocrine disorders. Thorough health history interviewing and physical examination assist in the diagnostic process.

HISTORY

Throughout the history interview, the nurse gathers information about the client's present condition and previous medical history. The history begins with the biographic data and proceeds to the chief complaint, including a symptom analysis (see Chap. 11). Additional subjective data are collected about the client's past medical history, family history, psychosocial history and lifestyle, and a review of systems (ROS).

Biographic Data

The nurse notes the client's age, because the endocrine system is affected by the aging process. Fewer hormones may be produced, or their effect on the target organs is decreased. For example, the incidence of diabetes mellitus increases with age.

Chief Complaint

The client's presenting symptoms may be specific or nonspecific. Common nonspecific symptoms include fatigue and depression, often accompanied by altered alertness, decreased energy, sleep pattern disturbances, weight changes, altered mood and affect, changes in the condition of the skin and hair, altered general appearance, and sexual dysfunction. Some symptoms are specific for certain endocrine disorders, as the following examples illustrate.

- *Mental status changes*. The client may report increased nervousness, lability of mood, mental confusion, and depression. Extreme alterations in consciousness such as coma may occur in uncontrolled diabetes mellitus.
- *Changes in vital signs*. Body temperature and pulse rate may be elevated due to hyperthyroidism. Kussmaul's respirations (deep rapid breathing) are a classic sign of diabetic ketoacidosis. Tumors of the adrenal glands, causing increased secretion of epinephrine (e.g., pheochromocytoma), can result in hypertension. Insufficient ADH from the pituitary gland can cause dehydration, whereas oversecretion can cause excessive retention of body water.
- *Palpitations*. Increased heart rate with sweating and flushing can occur in hyperthyroidism and also in pheochromocytoma.

- *Tremors.* Uncontrolled tremors can be a possible indication of hyperthyroidism.
- *Fatigue.* May signify emotional stress and/or pathophysiologic changes.
- *Weakness.* Weakness may be generalized or localized. Localized weakness often indicates a neurologic problem, which can be a complication of an endocrine disorder.
- *Appetite changes.* The client may report polyphagia (excessive hunger) associated with diabetes mellitus or anorexia (lack of appetite).
- *Weight changes.* Eating more but losing weight may indicate diabetes mellitus or hyperthyroidism. Clients with hypothyroidism may gain weight.
- *Polydipsia and polyuria.* Abnormal thirst plus passage of large amounts of urine may indicate diabetes mellitus.
- *Changes in bowel status.* Frequent loose stools are a sign of hyperthyroidism, while constipation can indicate hypothyroidism.
- *Abnormalities involving the sexual organs and libido.* Menstrual cycle irregularities (including amenorrhea), loss of libido, loss or premature development of secondary sexual characteristics, impotence, and infertility are sexual changes characteristic of endocrine disorders.
- *Untoward changes in appearance.* Acromegaly produces enlargement of the hands and feet and a coarsening of the facial features.
- *Adrenocortical hyperfunction (Cushing's syndrome).* Adrenocortical hyperfunction is manifested in moon facies, thin extremities, and truncal obesity.
- *Growth abnormalities.* Growth may be delayed, stunted (dwarfism), excessive (gigantism), or inappropriate (acromegaly).
- *Skin and tissue changes.* Hyperpigmentation occurs in chronic adrenocortical insufficiency (Addison's disease). Areas of hypopigmentation (vitiligo) may indicate other endocrine disorders. Delayed tissue healing and susceptibility to infection are associated with diabetes mellitus. Hard, nonpitting edema occurs in adult hypothyroidism (myxedema).
- *Hair.* Excessive hair (hirsutism) in women may indicate ovarian or adrenocortical disorders. Axillary and pubic hair loss may indicate a pituitary disorder. Hair feels soft and silky in hyperthyroidism and coarse, dry, and brittle in hypothyroidism.
- *Eyes.* Exophthalmos (bulging eyes) is an important characteristic of hyperthyroidism. A pituitary tumor may cause partial or total loss of vision. Diabetes may cause temporary blurred vision or permanent blindness.
- *Bone and joint problems.* Clients with hyperparathyroidism often develop bone pain, cysts, and fractures. Cushing's syndrome produces a rapid breakdown of bone.
- *Renal colic and stones.* Renal problems such as stone development may follow the bone disorders found in hyperparathyroidism.
- *Tetany, paresthesias, and muscle cramps.* These manifestations may develop in clients with insufficient PTH.

Past Medical History

The client's past medical history is explored to determine whether there have been previous endocrine disorders. The nurse specifically inquires about patterns of growth and development, head trauma, and the general health status. The client is asked to identify *changes* that have occurred in his or her health status, either in general or more specifically.

GROWTH AND DEVELOPMENT

Ask the client (or the client's family) whether there have been noticeable delays or accelerations in growth and development. For example, does the client have a history of being small or large for his or her chronologic age and ethnic background? The nurse also asks about family members' growth patterns so that valid comparisons are made.

The client is asked about changes in body size that may have occurred since physical maturation. Have there been changes in the size of the hands, feet, or head circumference? For example, has the client had to get shoes in a larger size? gloves? rings? hats? Similarly, ask the client about changes in secondary sex characteristics. For example, has there been increased amounts of facial hair (women) or decreased amounts (in men, thus less need for shaving)? For both men and women, the nurse asks whether there have been changes in pubic or axillary hair such as the amount and its distribution. Does the female client have problems with menstruation, infertility, or pregnancy?

MAJOR ILLNESSES AND HOSPITALIZATIONS

Ask the client to identify whether there is a history of head trauma such as a forceful blow. Trauma can lead to hypopituitarism. Has the client been hospitalized for surgery to the head or neck? Is there a history of chemotherapy or radiation therapy to the head or neck? Disorders to ask about include primary brain tumors, metastatic tumors, meningitis, brain infarctions, diabetes mellitus, diabetes insipidus, hypertension, and goiter.

MEDICATIONS

All medications, past and current, are included for identification. The nurse specifically asks about use of hormones and steroids, including name, dose, and duration of use. Does the client have a history of using anabolic steroids?

FAMILY HISTORY

When assessing a client with an endocrine disorder, inquire into the family history. A number of endocrine disorders are inherited or at least associated with a familial trend.

The nurse asks whether there are family members who have or have had problems similar to those of the client. Disorders to inquire about include growth and development problems, obesity, goiter, hypothyroidism or hyperthyroidism, hypertension, low blood pressure (hypotension), diabetes mellitus, diabetes insipidus, autoimmune diseases (Addison's disease), and problems with the adrenal gland (e.g., pheochromocytoma).

Psychosocial History and Lifestyle

The nurse inquires about the client's stress tolerance and coping patterns. Stressors can be either physiologic (illness) or emotional. Ask about job-related stressors such as amount of time spent on the job both in the work setting and at home. Are there strained interpersonal relationships among workers and/or management that contribute to increased stress levels? Are there opportunities for the client to retreat from the workplace and engage in recreational activities? Also ask about the home environment and family interpersonal relationships and obligations. What are the client's support systems? Does the client verbalize that current coping strategies are effective? If possible, the nurse asks family members to corroborate or help identify behavior changes.

The nurse considers other aspects of lifestyle and coping and asks the client about habits such as smoking, exercise, diet, and sleep patterns. Ask the client to describe the usual patterns as well as changes that may have occurred (see Chap. 11).

Review of Systems

A careful ROS is important if an endocrine problem is suspected. All body systems are reviewed because endocrine disorders can affect the entire body with multisystem effects. Detailed questions for the ROS are found in Chapter 11, Table 11-5.

PHYSICAL EXAMINATION

Physical examination of the endocrine system is integrated throughout the interaction with the client beginning with the history interview. As the client responds to questions, the nurse observes the client's level of consciousness (orientation, alertness), memory, affect, and speech patterns. Signs of anxiety or nervousness are noted. All body systems are examined as the nurse assesses in a systematic manner from head-to-toe (see Chap. 12).

General Appearance. Observe the client's state of dress, growth and development, level of consciousness, orientation, body size. Measure height and weight and compare to published norms. Observe extremities for proportion to rest of body.

Vital signs. Measure and assess vital signs. The temperature will be elevated in hyperthyroidism or may be low normal or below normal in hypothyroidism. Observe respirations for change in rate and rhythm. Blood pressure changes include hypotension, hypertension, widening pulse pressure, and orthostatic changes along with pulse changes.

Integument. Observe hair texture and distribution over body surfaces. Note brittleness or alopecia. Inspect skin for color, pigmentation, striae, ecchymosis. Palpate skin for texture, thickness, moisture, diaphoresis. Inspect and palpate nails for color, texture, brittleness, ridges, peeling.

Head. Inspect head contour and shape. Note symmetry of facial features. Observe skin color for erythema or rash over cheeks. Observe the client's facial expression for anxiety.

Eyes. Inspect and palpate eyebrows, noting hair distribution. Observe eye position, symmetry, shape, and lid lag. Assess visual acuity, Extraocular movements (EOMs), and visual fields. Inspect for lens opacity, eye edema.

Nose. Inspect mucosa for swelling and color. Listen for noisy breathing.

Mouth. Note size and shape of jaw. Inspect oral mucosa color and condition of teeth (mottling). Note malocclusion. Observe tongue size and activity for fasciculations.

Neck. Listen to the client's voice for hoarseness or huskiness. Note speech clarity, pitch and volume. Ask the client to swallow and observe for difficulty swallowing or pain; repeat this maneuver with the neck hyperextended. Inspect the neck for symmetry, alignment, thickness or bulging over the thyroid gland, and midline position of the trachea. Note presence of hyperpigmentation. Observe for forceful pulsations over the carotid arteries. The thyroid gland is palpated unless it is noticeably enlarged (vigorous palpation can stimulate release of thyroid hormone, which increases the risk of precipitating a thyroid crisis in a client with thyroid hyperplasia). If the thyroid gland is enlarged, the nurse auscultates the lobes for *bruits*.

Palpation of the thyroid gland is performed by either one of two techniques (Fig. 60-10). In the anterior approach, the nurse gently runs a finger down the anterior neck, locating the thyroid and cricoid cartilages and the isthmus of the thyroid gland. The isthmus feels soft and compressible compared with the firmer cartilage ring just superior to it. The nurse asks the client to swallow while the isthmus is palpated. It should rise in the neck and should not be enlarged. To palpate the lobes of the thyroid gland, the nurse flexes the client's head toward the side of the lobe being palpated to relax the neck muscles. The nurse's right hand gently displaces the client's thyroid toward his or her right while the head is flexed toward the right. The nurse's left fingers palpate the right lobe while the client swallows and the gland rises in the neck. This procedure is

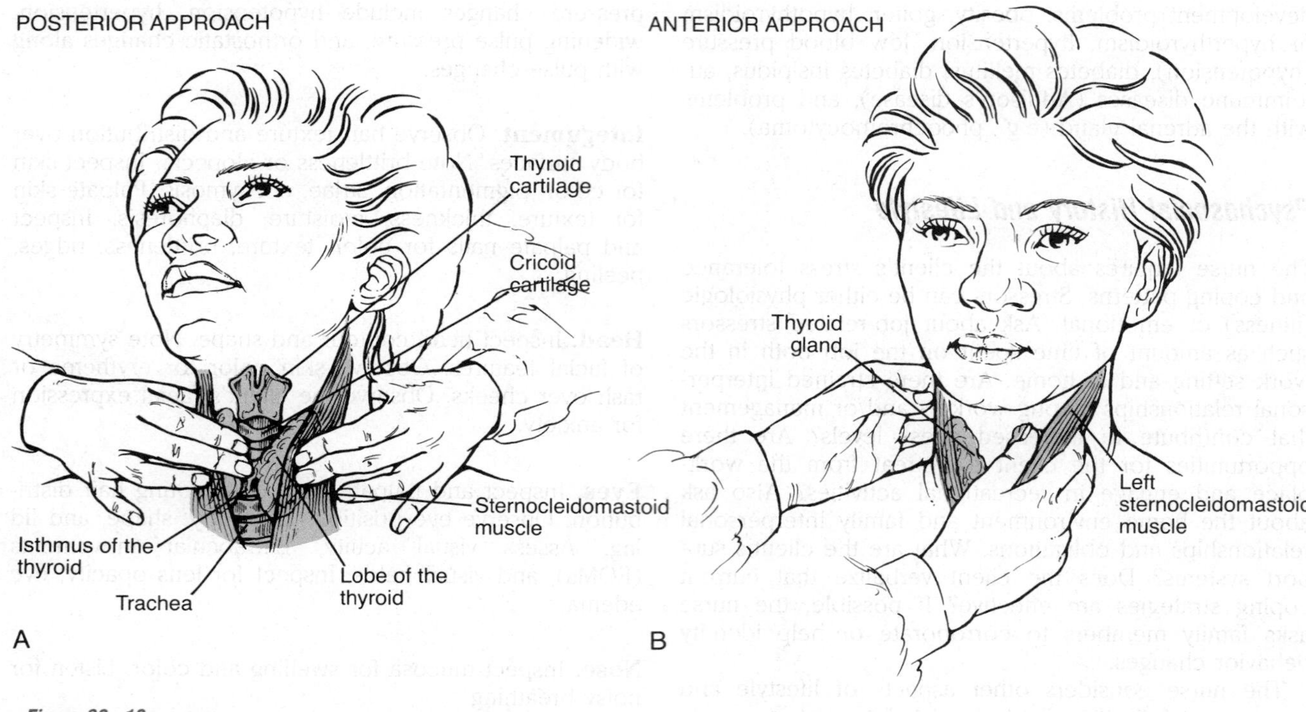

▲ *Figure 60–10*

Palpation of the thyroid. *A*, Posterior approach for thyroid palpation. The examiner stands behind the client. The client is asked to lower the chin to relax the neck muscles and turn the head slightly to the right. To examine the right lobe of the thyroid, the examiner uses the finger of the left hand to displace the trachea slightly to the right. This moves the thyroid laterally. The lobes can then be palpated by the fingers of the right hand. Projection of the thyroid can be assisted by having the client drink water.

B, Anterior approach to thyroid palpation. The examiner stands in front of the client. To examine the right lobe of the thyroid, the examiner uses the fingers of the left hand to displace the trachea slightly to the right. With the fingers of the left hand, the thyroid is palpated. The client is asked to swallow and flex the head slightly and turn. Thyroid enlargement can also be assessed for by palpating deep on each side of the sternocleidomastoid muscle.

repeated for palpating the client's left lobe by having the client flex the head toward his or her left, displacing the thyroid to the client's left with the left hand and feeling with the right fingers. The thyroid gland is normally nonpalpable. If it is palpable, the nurse notes the texture of the gland because it is usually smooth and firm, without lumps, roughness, hardness, asymmetry, or tenderness. In the posterior approach, the nurse stands behind the client and reaches both hands around the neck to locate the isthmus with the fingers. The rest of the procedure is similar to that of the anterior approach.

Extremities. Examine the arms and legs for size, shape, symmetry, and their proportion to the trunk. The distance from the symphasis pubis to the heel is usually about half of a body's total height. Note peripheral edema. Palpate and rate peripheral pulse amplitude (see Chap. 12). Assess deep tendon reflexes and observe their relaxation time (see Chap. 28).

Upper Extremities. Ask the client to extend the hands with palms down; observe for fine tremors. Inspect for thenar wasting, Dupuytren's contracture, and nail clubbing (see Chap. 36). Assess grip strength and muscle strength of the fingers and arms (see Chap. 65).

Lower Extremities. Note the color and distribution of hair. Assess the size of the feet in proportion to the rest of the client's body. Inspect for corns and calluses. Separate the toes and observe for deformities and skin changes such as thickening, fissures, or nail thickening. Palpate and rate pedal pulses. Assess leg muscles for weakness (see Chap. 65.).

Thorax. Inspect for gynecomastia in males. Auscultate for extra heart sounds, such as a systolic murmur (see Chap. 41).

Abdomen. Note areas of hyperpigmentation such as in scars or striae. Observe the client for signs of pain when lightly palpating.

Genitalia. Observe the pattern of pubic hair distribution, particularly in female clients. A diamond-shaped (male) pattern is indicative of a masculinizing tumor. Note the size of the testes and the clitoris for comparison to expected norms.

The remainder of endocrine assessment is with diagnostic studies, as the only endocrine glands accessible to physical examination are the thyroid and gonads. Assessment of the gonads is discussed in Chapter 73.

DIAGNOSTIC TESTS

Tests of the endocrine system involve several general types of clinical evaluations. Blood levels of the various hormones are obtained through radioimmunoassay (RIA) and enzyme immunoassay (EIA). RIA is a technique in which antibodies to the hormone and radioactively tagged hormones are placed in a test tube with untagged hormone. The two types of hormones compete for sites on the antibodies. If most of the radiotagged hormone is bound to the antibody, there is a decreased amount of client hormone. EIA is performed like the RIA, except that enzymes are used instead of radioisotopes. This method allows hormones, such as thyroid hormone, to be tested in small amounts.

The client may have anxiety over the test and its possible results. Many clients with endocrine disorders have been misdiagnosed for years due to the discrete symptoms of the disorders. After the diagnosis is made, the client and family will need help to cope with the diagnosis and need for ongoing care.

Pituitary Function

The structure of the pituitary gland can be assessed with skull x-ray study, computed tomography (CT), or magnetic resonance imaging (MRI). Tumors of the pituitary may be visualized with these studies.

Hormonal disorders due to malfunctioning of the pituitary can lead to a wide variety of clinical manifestations, depending on which hormone is involved. Growth hormone and antidiuretic hormone are discussed here.

Growth hormone (GH) is secreted in a diurnal pattern, and the level of growth hormone can be assayed. It is usually drawn in the morning to determine basal levels; usual levels are 3 μg/ml. Growth hormone can be stimulated with (1) levodopa (500 mg orally), (2) insulin (0.1 units/kg intravenously), or (3) bromocriptine (5 mg orally). Following the stimulus, blood is drawn at intervals up to 120 minutes. GH levels usually peak 60 minutes after the stimuli.

An absence of antidiuretic hormone leads to diabetes insipidus. To diagnose diabetes insipidus, the client is given a water deprivation test. Water is withheld for 4 to 18 hours, and during this time, the client's vital signs, urine output, and urine specific gravity are assessed hourly. Hypovolemic shock can develop from dehydration. A client without diabetes insipidus decreases urine output and increases urine osmolarity. The client with diabetes insipidus is not able to respond and continues to produce high volumes of dilute urine (low osmolarity).

Thyroid Function

A number of tests are available to assess thyroid function. A brief overview of the purposes of each of these diagnostic tests follows, as well as a discussion of factors that interfere with testing. The most important tests are outlined in Table 60–2.

Serum Thyroxine (T_4) and Triiodothyronine (T_3). Radioimmunoassay can now measure serum concentrations of T_4 and T_3. T_4 is transported in the blood largely bound to thyroid-binding globulin; conditions that affect thyroid-binding globulin levels will alter the serum T_4 concentration. For example, pregnancy and oral contraceptives both increase serum T_4. Phenytoin (Dilantin) may alter these values in euthyroid people, causing T_3 and T_4 readings to be low.

T_3 Resin Uptake. T_3 (like T_4) circulates in the bloodstream attached to plasma proteins and to erythrocytes. However, T_3 tends to bind far more readily to plasma proteins than to erythrocytes. T_3 binds to erythrocytes only when plasma protein binding sites are limited.

If thyroid function is low or if serum protein levels are high, resin uptake of T_3 is depressed. On the other hand, if thyroid function is increased above normal or serum protein levels are low, resin uptake of T_3 is elevated. When compared with serum T_4 or T_3 levels, this test can detect abnormal plasma thyroid-binding globulin levels.

Radioiodine (^{131}I) Uptake and Excretion Test. The body cannot distinguish between radioactive or "tagged" iodine and nonradioactive iodine. Consequently, the thyroid takes up radioactive iodine and processes it exactly as it does regular iodine. Furthermore, radioiodine is excreted in the urine just as is ordinary iodine. Thus, a scintillation scanner can measure the amount of radioactive iodine in the thyroid after administration of a radioiodine preparation. The laboratory may measure the person's urine output of radioactive iodine following the test.

Many factors can distort findings. Question the person about the following medications, procedures, and activities to ensure more accurate test results. Be certain to inform the physician if the person answers "yes" to any of the following questions:

- Have you taken any iodine-containing medications within the last 30 days? Any estrogens that can cause a false elevation?
- Have you undergone x-ray studies of the gallbladder, ureters, bronchi, fallopian tubes, or heart within the last 10 years?
- Within the last 2 weeks, have you eaten principally seafoods? (Seafood is so rich in iodine that ^{131}I uptake could show a falsely low reading.)

Thyrotropin-Releasing Hormone Stimulation Test. Thyrotropin-releasing hormone (TRH) is released from the hypothalamus, and it normally stimulates release of TSH from the pituitary. During the TRH stimulation test, people with thyroid disorders are given TRH intravenously. If TSH levels rise, the pituitary is functioning normally. TSH levels do not rise (1) in hyperthyroidism or (2) if the pituitary cells that secrete TSH are diseased.

Serum Cholesterol. Serum cholesterol is not a specific test of thyroid function, because its levels are

TABLE 60–2. Thyroid Function Tests

Test	Preparation	Procedure	Normal Findings	Significance of Abnormal Findings
Serum thyroxine (T_4) or triiodothyronine (T_3)	No food or water restrictions. Question person concerning medications recently taken	Sample of venous blood drawn and sent to laboratory	4.5–11.5 μg/100 ml of serum (adults)	Low concentration of thyroxine or triiodothyronine indicates hypothyroidism. Excessive concentrations of thyroid hormones indicates hyperthyroidism
Serum thyroid-stimulating hormone (TSH)	No restrictions	Sample of venous blood drawn and sent to laboratory	1 to 10 μ units/ml	Elevated levels indicate primary hypothyroidism
Radioiodine uptake test (^{131}I uptake)	No food or water restrictions. Reassure person that doses of radioiodine used for tests are extremely small and not harmful. Notify physician of recent ingestion of seafood and iodine-containing medication or recent x-ray studies	Person receives tracer dose of ^{131}I. 24-h urine specimen is started at time of drug administration. After 24 h, scintillation counter is placed over thyroid gland to measure exact amount of radioactivity emitting from gland. 24-h urine specimen is labeled and sent to lab for analysis	15 to 35 per cent uptake. Urine excretion: 40 to 80 per cent ^{131}I within first 24 h	(1) *Uptake results:* early high peak in ^{131}I uptake indicates hyperthyroidism. Persistent low ^{131}I uptake indicates hypothyroidism. (2) *Urine excretion:* excretion less than 40 per cent indicates hyperthyroidism. Excretion greater than 80 per cent indicates hypothyroidism
Triiodothyronine (T_3) resin uptake	No food and water restrictions. No special preparation	Blood sample drawn from person and sent to laboratory for incubation with T_3 and resin particles	Standardized in each lab	Depression of resin uptake of T_3 may indicate hypothyroidism. Elevation of resin uptake of T_3 may indicate hyperthyroidism.
Thyrotropin-releasing hormone (TRH) stimulation test	No restrictions	Person receives TRH IV. Serum TSH is measured in serum drawn before and 30 min after TRH injection	Increase in TSH	No rise in TSH in pituitary disease (secondary hypothyroidism) or hyperthyroidism

influenced by many factors in addition to thyroid hormone levels. Nevertheless, the serum cholesterol level tends to be relatively elevated in primary hypothyroidism, which may explain why this condition is accompanied by a marked tendency toward atherosclerosis. Persons with hyperthyroidism usually have a relatively low serum cholesterol level.

Serologic Tests. Many thyroid disorders are presumed to have an autoimmune basis, such as Hashimoto's thyroiditis, some types of myxedema, and Graves' disease (a form of hyperthyroidism). Consequently, serologic tests may be performed to determine if the person's blood contains any antithyroid antibodies.

Basal Metabolic Rate. The basal metabolic rate (BMR) is estimated by measuring the amount of oxygen consumed by the body under basal conditions during a given time, that is, while the person is in a state of complete mental and physical relaxation. Factors that can alter test results include inadequate rest before the examination, anxiety and emotional stress, a noisy environment, and previous ingestion of medications that effect metabolism. The BMR, once the major test of thyroid function, has been largely replaced by newer, more sophisticated diagnostic techniques.

Achilles Tendon Reflex Recording. The Achilles tendon reflex test measures the amplitude and duration of the ankle jerk with a special instrument, which is used to tap the strong tendon at the back of the heel. People with hyperthyroidism tend to experience a more rapid tendon reflex. Individuals who have underactive thyroid glands, have diabetes mellitus, or are pregnant have a slower reflex and a prolonged relaxation time.

Adrenal Function

Adrenal function tests are divided into medullary and cortical types. Adrenal hormones include cortisol, aldosterone, and adrenocorticotropic hormone (ACTH). Medullary hormones include the catecholamines.

Cortisol is secreted in a diurnal pattern, and levels are assessed at 8:00 AM and 8:00 PM. A cortisone suppression test is the suppression of the pituitary ACTH with dexamethasone. Normally after administration of dexamethasone, 24-hour levels of ketosteroid in the urine drop 50 per cent. Dexamethasone can also be given at midnight, and then serum cortisol assessed at 8:00 AM. In clients with increased adrenocortical stimulation, there will not be a decrease in ketosteroid production in urine or serum levels of cortisol.

Plasma levels of aldosterone, angiotensin II, renin can be measured at any time. Plasma levels of aldosterone can be increased by giving potassium, restricting sodium, or having the client assume an upright position. Plasma levels of aldosterone can be decreased by infusing saline.

Serum levels of ACTH can be assessed after the infusion of synthetic ACTH. Urine levels of ketosteroid would be expected to rise to 25 mg/24 hr; plasma levels of cortisol should rise to 10 to 40 μg/100 ml. Urine levels of ketosteroid can be measured with 24-hour urine specimens. These substances are metabolites of the hormones produced by the adrenal cortex. A preservative is required for the collection bottle, and if the client has an indwelling catheter, the bag is placed on ice.

The adrenal cortex can be assessed for tumors by x-ray study CT, and MRI scans.

The function of the adrenal medulla can be assessed through urine levels of catecholamines and their metabolites (vanillylmandelic acid [VMA]). A 24-hour urine sample is collected and assayed. The medulla can be suppressed with the administration of ganglionic blocking agents. These agents normally decrease the urine levels of catecholamines. In clients with pheochromocytoma, a tumor of the adrenal medulla, there is a negligible effect. An old test, which involved manipulation of blood pressure, is seldom performed today to assess for pheochromocytoma.

Pancreatic Function

Diagnostic assessment of pancreatic function is discussed in Chapters 56 and 61.

ABNORMALITIES OF THE ENDOCRINE SYSTEM: AN OVERVIEW

Classification of Endocrine Disorders

Primary Hyperfunction of Endocrine Glands. Major causes include benign tumors and hyperfunctional states that are not linked with tumor growth and autoimmune conditions. Malignant hormone-secreting tumors occur but are uncommon.

Primary Hypofunction of Endocrine Glands. Causes include infection, congenital absence of the gland, and tumor growths that destroy the glands. In addition, there is evidence that certain hypofunctional disorders of the thyroid, parathyroid, pancreas, and adrenal glands may be autoimmune in nature.

Secondary Failure of Endocrine Glands. Hypofunction of the gonads, thyroid, and adrenal cortex may develop secondary to pituitary insufficiency.

Secondary Hyperfunction of Endocrine Glands. The endocrine glands may be stimulated to overproduce a hormone due to pituitary overstimulation. Cushing's disease is overproduction of ACTH due to excess stimulation by the pituitary.

Functional Disorders. Endocrine disease develops secondary to pituitary disorders and as a consequence of nonendocrine disease. For example, hyperparathyroidism may complicate renal failure, and hyperaldosteronism may develop secondary to cirrhosis of the liver.

Failure of the Target Cell to Respond to a Hormone. For example, the bones may fail (for unknown reasons) to grow linearly despite the administration of human growth hormone.

Production of an Abnormal or Unusual Hormone by an Endocrine Gland. These congenital disorders are classified as inborn errors of metabolism. An example is congenital adrenal hyperplasia.

Production of a Hormone by a Nonendocrine Organ. Ectopic secretion of hormones by nonendocrine tumors is a fairly common cause of glandular hyperfunction. Tumors most frequently linked with ectopic syndromes are cancers of the lungs, thymus, and pancreas.

Iatrogenic Endocrine Disease. Causes include (1) prescribed administration of hormones either for hormonal replacement therapy or as a pharmacologic method for controlling inflammation, obesity, infertility, and so forth; (2) surgical removal of a gland; and (3) destruction of a gland by irradiation.

Altered Degradation of the Hormone. Degradation of the hormone may be altered by antibodies before they reach the target cell.

Failure of the Feedback System. Failure of the feedback system may fail to recognize the need for a particular hormone, or the feedback system may respond inappropriately.

Summary

The endocrine system works in unison with the nervous system to maintain homeostasis. There are two types of glands: Endocrine, which release hormones into the blood, and exocrine, which release hormones into ducts. Endocrine glands include the pancreas, gonads, adrenal, thyroid, parathyroid, and thymus glands. Assessment of the client includes the usual history and physical examination. Blood levels of the various hormones can be determined.

Bibliography

1. Bates, B. (1991). *A guide to physical examination* (5th ed.). Philadelphia: J.B. Lippincott.
2. Corbett, J. (1991). *Laboratory tests and diagnostic procedures with nursing diagnoses* (3rd ed.). Norwalk, CT: Appleton and Lange.
3. Jarvis, C. (1992). *Physical examination and health assessment.* Philadelphia: W.B. Saunders.
4. McCance, K., & Huether, S. (1990). *Pathophysiology.* St. Louis: C.V. Mosby.
5. Price, S., & Wilson, L. (1992). *Pathophysiology* (4th ed.). St. Louis: C.V. Mosby.
6. Sheldon, H. (1988). *Boyd's introduction to the study of disease* (10th ed.). Philadelphia: Lea & Febiger.
7. Solomon, E., et al. (1990). *Human anatomy and physiology* (2nd ed.). Philadelphia: W.B. Saunders College Books.
8. Spence, A., & Mason, E. (1987). *Human anatomy and physiology* (3rd ed.). Menlo Park: CA: Benjamin Cummings Co.
9. Wilson, J., & Foster, D. (1992). *Williams textbook of endocrinology* (8th ed.). Philadelphia: W.B. Saunders.

Chapter

61

Nursing Care of Clients with Endocrine Disorders of the Pancreas

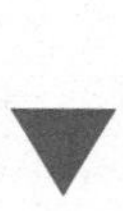

DIABETES MELLITUS

Definition

Diabetes mellitus is a metabolic disorder characterized by glucose intolerance. It is a systemic disease caused by an imbalance between insulin supply and insulin demand. Insulin is produced by the pancreas and normally maintains the balance between high and low blood glucose levels. In diabetes mellitus, either there is not enough insulin or the insulin that is produced is ineffective, resulting in high blood glucose levels. Diabetes mellitus also causes disturbances of protein and fat metabolism. These abnormalities are associated with micro- and macrovascular and neuropathic changes.

There are two main types of diabetes mellitus: insulin-dependent (IDDM) and non–insulin-dependent (NIDDM) (Table 61–1).

TABLE 61-1. Types of Diabetes Mellitus

Factors	IDDM (Type I)	NIDDM (Type II)
Synonyms	Juvenile diabetes, labile or brittle diabetes	Adult or maturity-onset diabetes, or mild diabetes
Age of onset	Usually occurs before 30 years of age but may occur at any age	Usually occurs in clients over 35 years of age, but can occur in children
Type of onset	Usually abrupt	Insidious
Endogenous insulin production	Little or none	Below normal, normal, or above normal
Incidence	10%	85-90%
Ketosis	May occur	Unlikely to occur
Insulin injections	Required	Necessary for only 20-30% of clients
Body weight at onset	Ideal body weight or thin	80% of clients are obese
Management	Diet, exercise, and insulin	Diet, exercise, oral hypoglycemic agent and/or insulin

IDDM, insulin-dependent diabetes mellitus; NIDDM, non-insulin-dependent diabetes mellitus.

Incidence

Approximately 12 million Americans have diabetes, and about 6 million of these clients do not know it. Approximately 600,000 new cases of diabetes are reported in the United States each year. Twice as many blacks between the ages of 45 and 65 years have diabetes than do white Americans, and Hispanics are three times as likely to develop diabetes mellitus. Native Americans have the highest rate of NIDDM in the world. Nearly one third of clients with diabetes mellitus are over the age of 60 years.

Most clients in the United States (85 to 90 per cent) who develop diabetes mellitus are non-insulin-dependent (NIDDM or type II). Approximately 10 per cent are insulin-dependent (IDDM or type I), and about 2 per cent of diabetes is secondary to other causes (i.e., medications, receptor problems, genetic disease, hormonal changes). Gestational diabetes develops in about 2 to 5 per cent of all pregnancies.

In 1987, the cost of care for clients with diabetes mellitus was $20.4 billion. This figure includes hospital and nursing home care, laboratory tests, physician fees, pharmacy supplies, and workdays lost from premature deaths and disability.

Diabetes with its complications is the third leading cause of death by disease in the United States; 100,000 clients will die from diabetes mellitus and its complications this year. Even when diabetes does not kill, it can produce major permanent disabilities. Diabetes mellitus is

- the leading cause of new blindness in adults
- the leading cause of new cases of renal failure (one fourth of all clients requiring dialysis have diabetes)
- responsible for 50 to 70 per cent of all nontraumatic amputations in the United States
- responsible for an increased risk of coronary artery disease and strokes. Clients with diabetes are twice as likely to have coronary artery disease and three times as likely to suffer a stroke.

Over the previous decades, the incidence of diabetes in the United States has steadily increased. Diabetes mellitus is becoming more frequent for a number of reasons: (1) life expectancy is longer today; this increases the population of older clients, who are more susceptible to diabetes; (2) obesity, which predisposes clients to diabetes, has increased in the general population; and (3) treatment with insulin has lowered the mortality rate among clients with IDDM; as a result, clients with diabetes marry and have children who are predisposed to the development of diabetes.

Etiology

INSULIN-DEPENDENT DIABETES MELLITUS

Both genetic and environmental factors seem to precipitate IDDM. There are currently three areas of ongoing research investigating the cause of IDDM. Because the highest incidence of new cases of IDDM occurs during the winter months, it is believed that environmental factors have a role in the development of diabetes. In clients who are predisposed to the development of diabetes, certain viruses, such as coxsackie B (and, rarely, mumps and rubella), are an etiologic factor. These viruses attack the islet cells of the pancreas, which renders them useless for producing insulin.

It appears also that there is some autoimmune response in the development of IDDM. Apparently, some trigger causes the body to develop islet cell antibodies and anti-insulin antibodies. These antibodies attack the beta cells of the pancreas (where insulin is produced) and also the insulin molecules themselves. Circulatory islet cell antibodies are found in approximately 85 per cent of all newly diagnosed IDDM clients.

Heredity is also believed to have a role in the development of IDDM. Siblings of clients with diabetes have 10 times the risk of developing diabetes over the general population. Certain HLA antigens (DR3 and DR4) on specific chromosomes appear to predispose clients to the development of IDDM.

NON-INSULIN-DEPENDENT DIABETES MELLITUS

Viruses and HLA antigens do not appear to have a role in the development of NIDDM. Heredity, however, does have a major role. Research also indicates that obesity is one of the most important determinants for the development of NIDDM. Approximately 80 per cent of all clients with NIDDM are obese (20 per cent over ideal body weight). Overweight clients require more insulin for metabolizing the food they eat. Hyperglycemia develops when the pancreas cannot secrete enough insulin to match the body's needs or when the number of insulin receptor sites is decreased or altered (as often occurs with obesity). Increasing age may be a risk because the pancreas becomes more sluggish with age in clients who are already predisposed to diabetes.

Risk Factors

Clients with a family history of diabetes are at far greater risk for developing diabetes, especially NIDDM. Primary prevention of NIDDM centers on maintaining as ideal a body weight as possible. Secondary prevention is the initiation of weight reduction measures and exercise programs by dieticians, nurses, and exercise physiologists or physical therapists.

Because diabetes cannot always be prevented, health agencies strive to diagnose diabetes in its early stages, often before clients are aware of the symptoms. Screening is a form of secondary prevention.

The nurse should suspect diabetes in anyone who (1) is obese; (2) suffers from excessive thirst, hunger, urination, and weight loss; (3) has given birth to a baby over 9 lb; (4) has a family history of diabetes; or (5) is over the age of 40 years. Anyone who is found to have an elevated blood glucose level during screening should be referred to a physician for more conclusive tests.

Primary prevention of IDDM is aimed at identifying the specific environmental factors responsible for initiating the development of IDDM. Not all clients with the genetic predisposition to diabetes develop IDDM, so obviously some environmental triggers are also responsible. Secondary prevention with immunosuppressive agents, such as cyclosporine, has been proposed to prevent beta cell destruction. However, because immunosuppression has such severe side effects, long-term use, especially in children, is unrealistic.

Tertiary prevention, the prevention of complications in known diabetes, is discussed throughout the chapter.

Pathophysiology

IDDM is associated with inflammation of the islets of the pancreas. This process, called insulitis, appears to be an autoimmune response. Infection with coxsackievirus B has been shown to be the likely trigger of the autoimmune response, although other etiologic factors may also exist, such as inherited susceptibility. After infection with the virus, the beta cells inappropriately express an antigen. The antigens on the beta cells are recognized and destroyed by circulating T cells. The process of cellular destruction is marked by the appearance of islet cell antibodies. Islet cell antibodies occur in up to 85 per cent of newly diagnosed insulin-dependent diabetics. In addition to the destruction of beta cells, alpha cells (which produce glucagon) are also destroyed. Therefore, there is a lack of insulin and a relative excess of glucagon.

Sometimes the pancreas will attempt to produce near-normal or normal levels of insulin during a "honeymoon phase," usually noted after initial diagnosis. This phase may last 6 months or longer, but eventually, in true diabetes, the client will develop signs of hyperglycemia again.

NIDDM is due to a refractoriness to insulin in the cell membrane receptor. The development of this form of diabetes is consistent with all the pathophysiologic changes seen in long-term obesity, with one exception. In obesity, insulin resistance is compensated by increased insulin production. In diabetes, the pancreas cannot compensate for problems in the receptors by increasing insulin production. Some newer theories suggest that over time, the high levels of circulating insulin that occur with obesity "insulinize" the cells, making them more resistant to the action of insulin. Research is being conducted to study a problem called "postreceptor deficits" in which the glucose enters the cell but still cannot produce energy. It is seen in non-insulin-dependent types of diabetes.

METABOLIC EFFECTS OF DIABETES

Without insulin, three major metabolic problems occur: decreased utilization of glucose, increased fat mobilization, and increased protein utilization.

Decreased Utilization of Glucose. In diabetes, cells that require insulin as a carrier for glucose can take in only about 25 per cent of the glucose they require for fuel. Nerve tissues, erythrocytes, and the cells of the intestines, liver, and kidney tubules do not require insulin for glucose transport. The skeletal and cardiac muscles and adipose tissues rely on insulin for glucose transport. Glucose remains in the blood, and blood glucose levels rise (hyperglycemia). The glucose level continues to rise because the liver cannot store glucose as glycogen without insulin.

In an attempt to restore balance and normal levels of glucose, the kidney excretes the excess glucose. Sugar appears in the urine (glucosuria). Glucose excreted in the urine acts as an osmotic diuretic and causes excretion of increased amounts of water. This process results in fluid volume deficit.

Increased Fat Mobilization. Fortunately, the body can rely on fat stores for energy when glucose is not available. Unfortunately, the process of fat metabolism leads to the formation of breakdown products called ketones. Ketones accumulate in the blood and are excreted through the kidneys and lungs. Ketone levels can be measured in the blood and urine and can serve as an indicator of diabetes. Ketones interfere with acid-base balance by producing hydrogen ions. The pH can fall, and the client can develop metabolic acidosis. (Metabolic acidosis is discussed later.) In addition, when ketones are excreted, sodium is also eliminated, which results in sodium depletion and further acidosis. When ketones are excreted, they also increase osmotic pressure and cause increased fluids to be lost.

When fats are used for a primary source of energy, the body lipid level can rise to five times normal. This elevated level can lead to atherosclerosis.

Increased Protein Utilization. Lack of insulin also causes protein wasting. Normally, proteins are constantly being broken down and rebuilt. Without insulin to stimulate protein synthesis, the balance is altered, and there is increased catabolism. Amino acids are converted to glucose in the liver, which further compounds the elevated glucose levels. Untreated, the diabetic appears thin and emaciated.

The pathophysiologic process of diabetes continues and leads to many acute and chronic complications. They are discussed later in this chapter.

Clinical Manifestations

CARDINAL SIGNS OF DIABETES

The excretion of glucose and ketones leads to increased urine output and thirst. Extra food is eaten but cannot be metabolized, which leads to hunger, and the client loses weight. These processes result in the four cardinal signs of diabetes: *polyuria, polydipsia, polyphagia, and weight loss* (Table 61-2).

The client with IDDM usually presents with the cardinal signs and symptoms and sometimes already has complications such as ketoacidosis (discussed later in this chapter).

Clients with NIDDM may also develop the cardinal signs and symptoms; however, because many of these clients are elderly, they may not recognize the abnormal thirst or frequent urination as abnormal for their age. More commonly, they may only experience visual blurring, neuropathic complications (such as pain in the feet), or infections. NIDDM is commonly diagnosed while the client is hospitalized for another problem.

DIAGNOSTIC ASSESSMENT

Blood Glucose (Blood Sugar). A blood sample for determination of glucose level may be drawn at any time and requires no preparation of the client. The results should be within normal limits for both nondiabetics and diabetics in good control. Elevated blood glucose levels may occur after meals, after stressful events, if the sample was drawn from above an intravenous site, or in clients with diabetes.

Elevated blood sugar levels (hyperglycemia) warrant investigation if the client is not a known diabetic. Conditions that cause hyperglycemia include glucocorticoid imbalances such as Cushing's syndrome, increased epinephrine levels such as after trauma, excess growth hormone secretion, and pregnancy. Fluctuations in blood glucose over 24 hours are shown in Figure 61-1.

Hypoglycemia also warrants investigation in the nondiabetic. Conditions that may lead to hypoglycemia include tumors of the pancreas, a lack of cortisone with Addison's disease, extensive liver disease, and pituitary disorders.

Fasting Blood Sugar. For fasting blood sugar tests, the client may not eat for 4 hours, but water intake may continue. If the client has a dextrose intravenous solution infusing, the results of the test will not be accurate. If the client is a known diabetic, food and insulin are withheld until after the specimen is drawn. Average normal values for adults are 70 to 110 mg/100

TABLE 61-2. Cardinal Signs of Diabetes

Clinical Manifestations	Pathophysiologic Bases
Polyuria (frequent urination)	Water not reabsorbed from renal tubules because of osmotic activity of glucose in the tubules
Polydipsia (excessive thirst)	Polyuria causes severe dehydration, which causes thirst
Polyphagia (excessive hunger)	Tissue breakdown and wasting cause a state of starvation that compels the client to eat excessive amounts of food
Weight loss (primarily insulin-dependent diabetes)	Glucose not available to cells; thus, the body breaks down fat and protein stores for energy

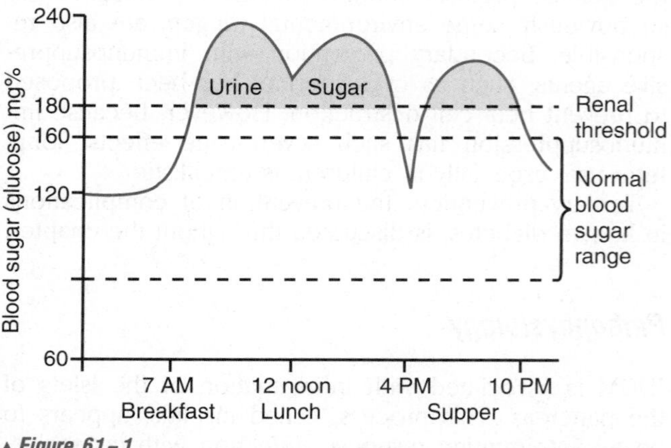

▲ *Figure 61-1*

Blood glucose levels throughout the day in a client with uncontrolled diabetes mellitus. Sugar appears in the urine when blood glucose exceeds 180 mg/100 ml (renal threshold). (Adapted from Kozak, G. P. [1982]. *Clinical diabetes mellitus*. Philadelphia: W. B. Saunders.)

ml but vary with laboratories. As a general rule, in an adult, a fasting blood sugar level over 140 mg for two to three times indicates diabetes.

Postprandial Blood Sugar. These blood glucose levels are tested after meals. Sometimes the client is given a standard amount of glucose, but most commonly the sample is drawn after a standard meal. The purpose of the meal is to determine how well the carbohydrates are digested. After 2 hours, the blood sugar level should return to normal. Nurses accurately record the meal eaten and ascertain that the sample was drawn 2 hours after eating.

Blood Glucose Finger Sticks. In the past, most diabetics were monitored by self-testing of urine for glucose and ketones and occasional venipuncture samples. Urine samples of glucose were largely inaccurate, even though fresh urine was used. The invention of self-monitoring devices for blood sugar has revolutionized diabetes care. These new machines use reagent strips and a photometer and have a digital readout of blood sugar values. There are two major drawbacks to this method: the need to stick oneself; and the cost of the monitor, strips, lancets, and wipes. The cost is commonly $1000 to $2150 a year, but it is worth the improved control.

Blood glucose monitoring tests must be performed with extreme care and accuracy. The Joint Commission on Accreditation of Hospitals and other regulating bodies dictate the procedure and frequency for quality control of meters. Most devices have some type of control process for determining accuracy of the machine. Manufacturers' instructions must be followed exactly because test results are used to adjust insulin or oral hypoglycemic dosages, exercise regimens, and dietary management. The devices are technique-dependent, and because treatment is based on results, accuracy is a major concern. Clients can check their machine by drawing a sample for a laboratory analysis, doing a self-stick at the same time, and comparing results.

Self-monitoring of blood glucose is recommended for all clients with IDDM, clients with NIDDM who require glucose, pregnant women, clients who have an insulin pump, and clients who have widely fluctuating blood glucose levels.

Glycosylated Hemoglobin. Glucose normally attaches itself to the hemoglobin molecule on a red blood cell. Once attached, it cannot dissociate. Therefore, the higher the blood glucose levels have been, the higher are the glycosylated hemoglobin results. Glycosylated hemoglobin is the average of blood glucose control over the previous 3 months.

Glycosylated hemoglobin can be sampled at any time during the day, in contrast to a fasting blood sugar specimen, which is drawn before breakfast. This advantage allows the test to be done during a client's initial visit to a physician in order to obtain a more accurate assessment of the client's compliance with the prescribed plan of care, evaluate a client with wide fluctuations in blood glucose levels, or manage blood glucose levels during pregnancy.

Glycosylated Albumin (Fructosamine). Glycosylated albumin (fructosamine) is a measure of blood glucose control over the previous 7 to 10 days. This test may be used in conditions in which close control of blood glucose is desirable.

Connecting Peptide. Connecting peptide (C-peptide) attaches two chains of insulin molecules. C-peptide tests measure the level of endogenous insulin production. If the C-peptide level is normal, it can mean that the client is not producing enough or any insulin.

Glucose Tolerance Test. The oral glucose tolerance test is considered one of the best methods of diagnosing diabetes. However, because there are so many factors that render the test invalid, many hospitalized clients are diagnosed by fasting blood sugar levels. Bed rest, infection, trauma, medications, and stress can alter the test results.

The client needs to be on a normal diet for several days before the test is done. The test is usually done in the morning so that the client is in a fasting state. At the start of the test, a blood sample for fasting blood glucose level and a urine sample for glycosuria are taken. The client is then given 100 g of glucose to drink. Blood and urine samples are taken at 1-, 2-, and 3-hour intervals afterward. The client cannot eat after the glucose ingestion but can drink water to stimulate urine production.

The results of the samples are plotted on a graph to see how long it takes blood glucose to return to normal levels. Diabetics either take longer to return to normal or never return to normal. In a client below the age of 55 years, the blood sugar should return to normal in 2 hours, with a peak of 120 to 160 mg. In clients over 55 years, the peak may be as high as 200 mg, and normal values may not return for over 3 hours.

Urine Ketone Levels. Urine levels of ketones (acetone, acetoacetic acid, and beta-hydroxybutyric acid) can be tested by dip-strips or tablets. The color change on the strip on in the test tube indicates the amount of ketone present. The presence of ketones indicates that the body is using fat as a major source of energy. Fats are used when glucose is not available, such as in diabetes, in periods of starvation, or with use of rapid weight loss diets, especially those high in protein.

Criteria for diagnosis of diabetes are listed in Box 61–1.

Medical Management

To date, there is no cure for diabetes. Consequently, the overall goal of care for clients with diabetes is control or regulation of blood sugar rather than cure. When diabetes is successfully regulated, the client avoids the complications of hyper- and hypoglycemia,

Box 61-1. Criteria for Diagnosis of Diabetes Mellitus

Diabetes Mellitus (Adult)

- Elevation of plasma glucose (≥200 mg/100 ml) and classic symptoms of diabetes, including polydipsia, polyuria, polyphagia (extreme hunger), and weight loss
- Fasting plasma glucose > 140 mg/100 ml on two occasions or oral glucose tolerance test (OGTT) values > 200 mg/100 ml at 2 hours and at one intervening point between 0 and 2 hours

Impaired Glucose Tolerance

Fasting blood glucose < 140 mg/100 ml and 2-hour blood sugar level ≥ 140 and <200 mg/100 ml with one intervening blood sugar level ≥ 200 mg/100 ml after a 75-g glucose load

Gestational Diabetes Mellitus

Diagnosis is confirmed when two or more of the following blood sugar levels are met or exceeded when a 100-g glucose load is used rather than 75 g

Fasting blood sugar ≥ 105 mg/100 ml
1-hour ≥ 190 mg/100 ml
2-hour ≥ 165 mg/100 ml
3-hour ≥ 145 mg/100 ml

with minimal disruption to a normal lifestyle (Nursing Research). Unfortunately, clients with diabetes may develop complications despite their own vigorous efforts to carefully control their disease.

Diabetes control depends on the proper interaction of three factors: (1) food, (2) insulin or oral medication to lower blood glucose, and (3) exercise.

The intervention planned for the treatment of diabetes must be individualized. It needs to be based on the client's age, lifestyle, nutritional needs, maturation, activity level, occupation, and ability to independently perform the skills required by the treatment plan (i.e., monitoring of blood sugar levels, insulin injection).

CRITERIA FOR GOOD CONTROL OF DIABETES

Diabetes is generally considered under control when the following conditions are met:

- The client is of optimal weight and enjoys good health.
- Glycosylated hemoglobin is in normal range (normal values vary between laboratories).
- Fasting blood glucose level is under 140 mg/100 ml.
- Blood glucose level is no higher than 180 mg/100 ml 1 to 2 hours after meals.

DIETARY MANAGEMENT

Dietary management is discussed first, because diet is considered the cornerstone of diabetic management. The balanced nutritional plan for clients with diabetes has a twofold purpose: (1) to discourage the ingestion of foods with high sugar and fat content and (2) to correct or avoid obesity. Table 61-3 outlines the contrasting strategies clinicians use for regulating the diet of clients who are either obese but not insulin-dependent or not obese but insulin-dependent.

Some of the nutritional goals for clients with diabetes are to (1) achieve normoglycemia, as possible, (2) maintain lipids within a normal range (cholesterol, low-density lipoproteins, high-density lipoproteins, triglycerides), (3) prevent wide swings in the blood glucose levels, (4) have normal growth and development in children and adolescents, and (5) meet individualized weight loss goals (usually 1 to 2 lb per week as appropriate). It is now known that hyperglycemia and hyperlipidemia promote the complications of diabetes. Therefore, the emphasis for clients with diabetes is on controlling concentrated sweets and fat intake.

The current recommendations for the distribution of calories are

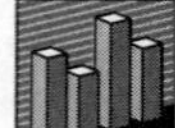

NURSING RESEARCH

A client's health beliefs can influence the performance of behaviors that affect health; these factors are addressed in a health belief model. The purpose of this research study was to determine whether selected health beliefs of clients with diabetes can be modified with education and treatment and the extent to which these beliefs are related to adherence to treatment plans and blood glucose levels.

Baseline health beliefs were measured in 119 clients, 66 per cent had NIDDM, 50 per cent were female, and the mean duration of the disorder was 10.1 years. A 14-point health belief scale was designed by the researchers. The tool focused on several perceptions: severity of diabetes, susceptibility to complications, cost of treatment, benefits of treatment, and ability to follow recommendations by the health care team. In addition, the client's locus on control, compliance and glycosated hemoglobin levels was measured.

All clients were assessed prior to beginning diabetes education. The education methods were directed at various perceptions. For example, the client with a low perception of severity was taught about the seriousness of diabetes and so on.

The pre-education and post-education health belief scores, and glycosated hemoglobin were correlated. Modest but statistically significant increases occurred in perceptions of severity, benefits of treatment, and ability to carry out recommendations. Glycosated hemoglobin levels dropped significantly but did not correlate with health beliefs or compliance.

Certain health beliefs can be modified with education. The long-term effect of this program needs to be studied.

▼▼▼

Woodridge, K. L., et al. (1992). The relationship between health beliefs, adherence and metabolic control of diabetes. *The Diabetes Educator, 18* (6), 495-500.

TABLE 61–3. Comparison of Dietary Intervention for Insulin-Dependent and Non–Insulin-Dependent Diabetes

Intervention	Insulin-Dependent (nonobese client)	Non–Insulin-Dependent (obese client)
Calories	No special caloric restrictions	Restrict calories; weight loss often decreases blood sugar level to within normal limits
Size and frequency of meals	Routine (e.g., 3 meals/day) with regular and appropriate snacks	Optional, but total calories/day should provide for 0.5–1 kg (1–2 lb) weight loss/week
Hypoglycemia	Prevent by increasing calories during increased exercise or stress; intervene with foods high in simple sugars (orange juice, hard candy)	Prevent by regular, reasonable diet; provide strategies for regulating meal plans
Exercise	Exercise planned with appropriate insulin and glucose adjustments	Exercise usually needed to promote weight loss

- 55 to 60 per cent carbohydrates
- 30 per cent fats
- 12 to 20 per cent proteins

The current recommendations from the American Dietetic Association and the American Diabetes Association call for less fat in the meal plan than was previously allowed because of the known increased risk for myocardial infarctions, strokes, and other blood vessel diseases in clients with diabetes.

Carbohydrates should be mostly complex, including foods high in soluble fiber such as corn, oats, peas, apples, potatoes, broccoli, carrots, and dried beans. In addition to being filling, these foods lower glucose and cholesterol levels and insulin requirements. Fats should be primarily polyunsaturated or monounsaturated. Proteins should come from low-fat sources too.

Recent research has indicated that clients with diabetes may not have to eliminate all simple sugars from their diets. Concentrated sweets should be avoided, but 5 per cent of the diet can be sucrose as long as it is eaten at intervals and with other foods.

Overweight NIDDM clients should stay on a weight loss diet. Weight reduction slows the release of glucose into the bloodstream and increases the number of insulin receptor cells, with lessening of the defects that might impair normal use of glucose. Blood sugar levels begin to improve with as little as a 5- to 10-lb weight loss. An example of food exchanges by number of calories for a sample day is shown in Figure 61–2, and carbohydrate exchanges are in Box 61–2.

PHARMACOLOGIC MANAGEMENT

Oral Hypoglycemic Agents. Some clients with NIDDM may require oral hypoglycemic agents for lowering blood glucose levels. Oral hypoglycemic agents are *not* insulin. They lower the blood sugar in part by stimulating the pancreatic beta cells to release insulin. They also appear to make target tissues more sensitive to the effects of insulin by increasing the number of receptor sites and by enhancing insulin's action at the postreceptor sites. Some of them also work to decrease glucose production (gluconeogenesis) in the liver.

The two classifications of oral hypoglycemic agents are the sulfonylureas (Table 61–4) and the biguanides. The biguanides have been banned in the United States since 1977 because of the increased risk of lactic acidosis. One that is currently approved in several other countries, metformin, may soon be available in the United States, however.

The average candidate for the oral hypoglycemic agents (1) is over the age of 40 years, (2) has no history of ketosis, (3) is not pregnant, (4) is on less than 40 units of insulin per day, and (5) has mild to moderate symptoms of hyperglycemia.

Box 61–2. Carbohydrate Food Exchange List

Carbohydrate Replacement

Fruit exchange = 15 g carbohydrate
Bread/starch exchange = 15 g carbohydrate
Milk exchange = 12 g carbohydrate

The following contain approximately 15 g carbohydrate

½ c applesauce
½ banana
15 grapes
¾ c mandarin oranges
⅓ c pineapple
⅛ c peaches, pears, cherries
¾ c dry cereal (except Bran)
½ c Bran cereal, Shredded Wheat
½ c corn, peas, potato, lima beans
1 slice bread
3 c popcorn
3 graham cracker squares
½ c diet pudding, custard
½ c pasta
⅓ c rice
6 saltine crackers
½ c sherbet (½ of container)
½ c vanilla ice cream
6 vanilla wafers
1 c milk
1 c *plain* yogurt
½ c apple, orange, pineapple, grapefruit juices
⅓ c regular cranberry, grape, prune juices

		NUMBER OF FOOD EXCHANGES												
	CALORIES	800	1000	1200	1400	1500	1600	1800	2000	2200	2400	2500	3000	3400
Breakfast	Meat			1	1	1	1	1	1	1	1	1	2	2
	Bread/starch	1	1	1	1	2	2	2	2	2	2	2	3	3
	Fruit	1	1	1	1	1	1	1	1	1	2	2	2	2
	Fat				1	1	1	1	1	1	1	2	2	2
	Skim milk		1	1	1	1	1	1	1	1	1	1	1	1
AM snack	Bread/starch				1	1	1	1	1	1	1	1	2	2
	Fruit								1	1	1	1	1	2
	Skim milk													
Lunch	Meat	2	2	2	2	2	2	3	3	3	3	3	4	5
	Vegetable	1	1	1	1	1	1	1	1	1	1	1	1	1
	Bread/starch	1	1	1	2	2	2	2	2	3	3	3	3	3
	Fruit	1	1	1	1	1	1	1	1	1	1	2	2	2
	Fat		1	1	1	1	1	1	1	1	1	1	1	1
	Skim milk										1	1	1	1
PM snack	Bread/starch			1	1	1	1	1	1	1	1	1	2	2
	Fruit						1	1	1	1	1	1	1	2
	Skim milk													
Dinner	Meat	2	2	2	2	2	2	2	3	3	3	3	4	5
	Vegetable	1	1	1	1	1	1	1	1	1	1	1	1	1
	Bread/starch	1	1	1	1	1	2	2	2	3	3	3	3	3
	Fruit	1	1	1	1	1	1	1	1	1	1	2	2	2
	Fat		1	1	1	1	1	1	1	1	1	1	1	1
	Skim milk									1	1		1	1
Bedtime snack	Meat							1	1	1	2	2	2	2
	Bread/starch		1	1	1	1	1	2	2	2	2	2	2	2
	Fruit						1	1	1	1	1			2
	Fat								1	1	1	1		
	Skim milk	1/2	1/2	1	1	1	1	1						1

▲ *Figure 61–2*

Sample diabetic food exchanges.

Oral hypoglycemic agents are contraindicated in clients with IDDM, pregnant or breastfeeding women, surgery clients, and those with allergies to sulfa.

Side effects of the oral hypoglycemic agents include (1) hypoglycemia, especially in the elderly; (2) skin rashes in about 2 per cent of all clients; (3) gastrointestinal disturbances in about 5 per cent of all cases; and (4) a disulfiram-like effect in about 35 per cent of all clients taking chlorpropamide. These symptoms include a severe flushing, nausea, and vomiting. Chlorpropamide also has a long half-life (up to 36 hours) and should be discontinued 24 to 48 hours before surgery because of its potential for causing hypoglycemia during surgery. As a result of its long half-life, it should also be used with caution in the elderly. The syndrome of inappropriate antidiuretic hormone occurs in 4 per cent of clients who receive chlorpropamide.

Glipizide should be administered about one half hour before a meal because its absorption is retarded by food. Both glipizide and glyburide have fewer side effects and less drug interaction with other medications than do the other oral hypoglycemic agents.

Insulin Therapy. All clients with IDDM must inject insulin daily. Some clients with NIDDM may *require* insulin if diet, exercise, and oral hypoglycemic agents are ineffective. Some medications such as prednisone may elevate blood glucose levels and necessitate insulin injections.

Insulin lowers blood sugar by (1) promoting the

TABLE 61-4. Oral Hypoglycemic Agents

Agent	Starting Dose	Maximal Dose	Duration of Action	Frequency	Metabolism
First-generation					
Tolbutamide (Orinase)	0.5 g	2.0-3.0 g	6-12 hr	1-3/day	By liver to inactive product
Tolazamide (Tolinase)	100 mg	1.0 g	12-24 hr	1-2/day	By liver to active and inactive products requiring renal route
Acetohexamide (Dymelor)	250 mg	1.5 g	12-18 hr	1-2/day	Same as tolazamide
Chlorpropamide (Diabinase)	100-250 mg	0.5 g	60 hr	1/day	Approximately 70% by liver to less active products but renal route imperative
Second-generation					
Glyburide (Diabeta; Micronase)	2.5-5.0 mg	20 mg*	16-24 hr	1-2/day	By liver to mostly inert products
Glipizide (Glucotrol)	2.5-5.0 mg	40 mg*	12-24 hr	1-2/day	By liver to inert products

* Lower levels of glyburide and glipizide have been effective in reducing blood glucose by 25 per cent at 15 mg/day.

transport of glucose into the cells and (2) inhibiting the conversion of glycogen and amino acids to glucose. There are several different types of insulin. They are grouped according to speed of action in the body: (1) rapid-acting, (2) intermediate-acting, and (3) long-acting. Table 61-5 compares and contrasts these insulins. Whereas all types of insulin have the same basic action (i.e., the reduction of blood sugar), they differ in onset, peak, and duration of hypoglycemic effect and thus in the time period in which an insulin reaction is likely to occur.

If blood sugar is difficult to control, two different insulins can be mixed and administered as a single injection. For example, NPH (neutral protamine Hagedorn) and regular insulin can be mixed to provide for both the immediate and daylong insulin needs. Lente, Semilente, and Ultralente insulins may be mixed with each other. When regular insulin is mixed with Lente or Ultralente, the zinc in the intermediate- and long-acting insulin can cause prolonged actions of the regular insulin.

The absorption and duration of insulin varies by anatomic site. Insulin injected into the abdomen is absorbed fastest, and as a consequence, the duration is shortest. Moving the injection site to the arm, leg, or buttocks progressively slows absorption and lengthens duration.[1] See Figure 61-3 for insulin regimens.

Insulin Sources. There are three sources of insulin: beef, pork, and "human." If the source is not specified

TABLE 61-5. Types of Insulin

Action	Preparation	Appearance	Action in Hours: *Onset*	*Peak*	*Duration*
Short	Insulin injection				
	Regular insulin	Clear	½-1	2-4	6-8
	Insulin, zinc suspension				
	Semilente insulin	Cloudy	½-1	2-8	8-16
Intermediate	Isophane insulin suspension				
	NPH insulin	Cloudy	1-2	6-12	18-26
	Insulin, zinc suspension				
	Lente insulin	Cloudy	1-3	6-12	18-26
Long	Protamine zinc insulin suspension (seldom used)				
	Protamine zinc insulin	Cloudy	4-6	18-24	28-36
	Extended insulin zinc suspension				
	Ultralente insulin	Cloudy	4-6	14-24	36
Premixed	70% NPH, 30% regular	Cloudy	½	2-12	18-24

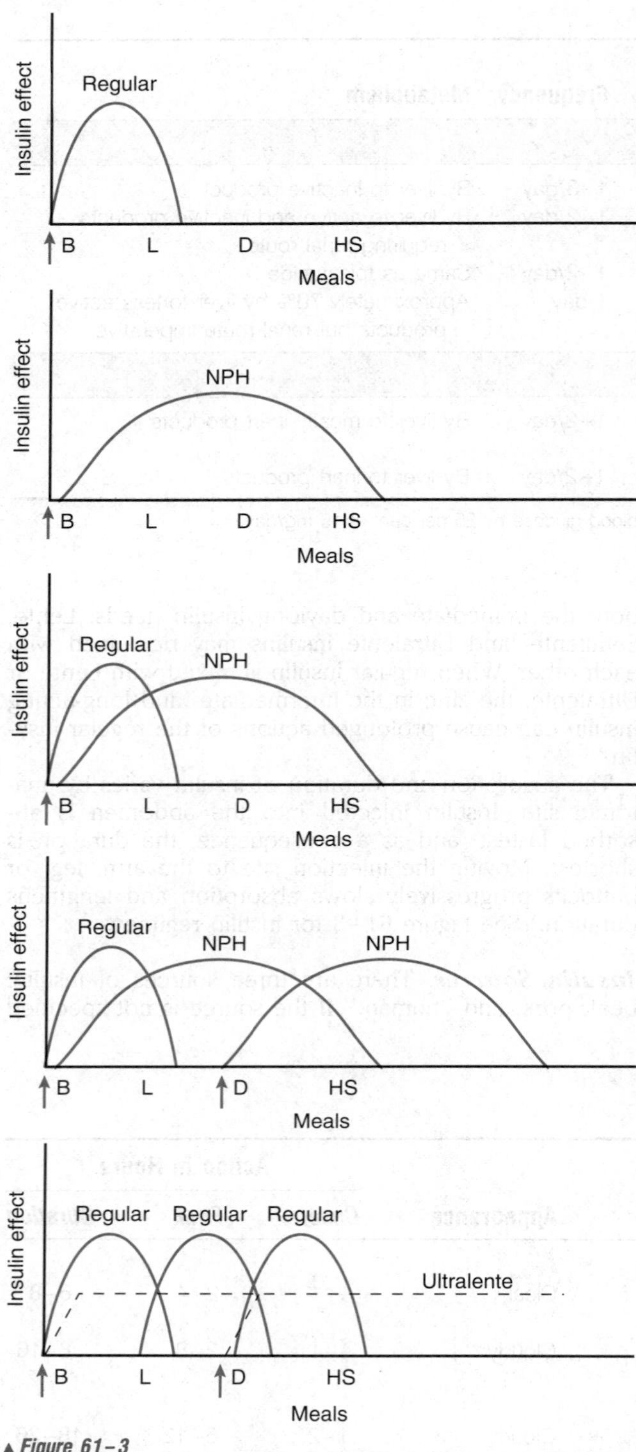

▲ **Figure 61-3**

There are a variety of insulin regimens, of which these are only a few. Some clients require only one injection a day, whereas others may require split mixed doses (i.e., NPH or Ultralente and regular insulin) or several doses of the same insulin (i.e., NPH). Insulin regimens must be individualized for each client. (B, breakfast; L, lunch; D, dinner; HS, bedtime.)

on the bottle, the bottle contains a mixture of beef and pork. Pork insulin differs chemically from human insulin at one amino acid in the molecule. Beef insulin differs from human at three amino acids. Human insulin is produced commercially by recombinant DNA technology. Human insulin is also produced by chemically modifying porcine insulin. Human insulin may have a shorter duration and onset of action than beef/pork insulin. The peak may also be affected in intensity. Human insulin dosages may need to be reduced, therefore, if a client changes from animal-source insulin to human insulin.

Insulin Dosage. Insulin dosage varies greatly. Two major considerations determine insulin dosage.

Requirements of the Client. The insulin requirement usually increases when a client (1) is seriously ill, (2) develops an infection, (3) undergoes surgery, (4) suffers trauma, or (5) is going through puberty.

Client's Response to Insulin Injections. Because clients with diabetes vary widely in their response to insulin, the process of regulating insulin dosage may require several weeks. The starting dose of insulin is usually determined to be between 0.5 and 1 unit/kg body weight/day. Clients will optimally monitor their blood sugar at home, and physicians will regulate insulin on the basis of blood glucose level, diet, exercise, and other factors such as stress. Many clients are now initiated on insulin therapy as outpatients because metabolic demands with hospitalization may be quite different from when the client is at home.

Insulin Pumps. Small portable pumps for the continuous administration of regular insulin are now sometimes used. The small pump, worn externally, injects insulin subcutaneously into the abdomen through an indwelling needle site that is usually rotated daily. Insulin is normally infused at a low, "basal" rate (i.e., a rate that matches the client's basal metabolic needs), with additional infusion of larger amounts (boluses) of insulin before meals.

Insulin pumps often improve blood glucose control by means of continuous subcutaneous insulin infusion. However, they do not have a built-in feedback mechanism for monitoring blood glucose levels. To benefit from an insulin pump, the client must comply with dietary requirements and usually must deliver the correct premeal bolus of insulin. Clients must also monitor their blood glucose levels four to six times a day and make decisions regarding dosages by use of problem-solving skills (Fig. 61-4).

These pumps store insulin either in syringes or in a disposable reservoir. Only regular insulin is used with the pump. Disposable or rechargeable batteries power the pumps. Some of the newer pumps are no larger than a credit card.

Complications arising from use of insulin pumps include

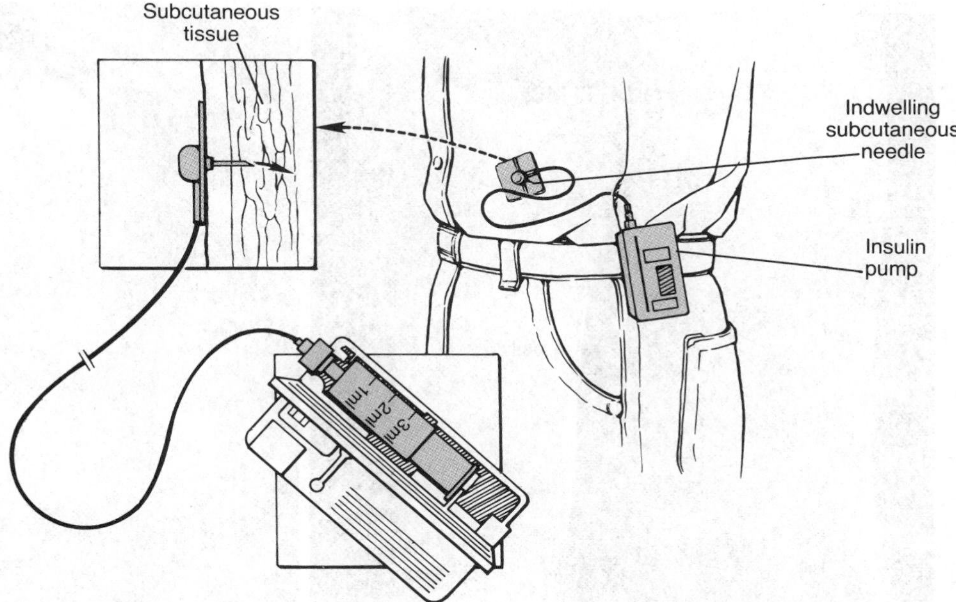

▲ **Figure 61-4**

Insulin pump is worn externally with an indwelling subcutaneous needle usually placed in the abdomen.

- local infection at the injection site
- hypoglycemia due to error in calculating insulin dosage or to pump malfunction
- diabetic ketoacidosis due to injection of insufficient insulin for meeting regular or increased metabolic needs

For initiation of insulin pump therapy, the client must be carefully supervised in either an inpatient or outpatient setting. During this time, the clinician adjusts the pump for basal and bolus doses before meals according to the client's usual diet and exercise regimen and previous insulin requirements. Researchers are currently trying to produce an implantable pump that will not only administer insulin but also monitor blood sugar levels much as a normal pancreas does.

Some clinicians and clients may decide to use an intensive insulin therapy program (IIT) rather than insulin pump therapy. In IIT, the client must be willing to monitor blood glucose levels four to six times a day and take three to five insulin injections a day. Throughout the initiating period of the pump or IIT, assess the client's knowledge concerning (1) the meal plan, (2) monitoring techniques, (3) management goals, and (4) symptoms of and intervention for hyperglycemia and hypoglycemia. The client also needs to be made aware of the extra financial and emotional burdens. The family and significant others need to be involved in the teaching process. Finally, the client needs to know there are no guarantees currently that either protocol will definitely prevent long-term complications. A 10-year study called the Diabetes Control and Complications Trial, which ended in 1992, should help define whether good control of diabetes does indeed prevent long-term complications.

Complications of Insulin Therapy. Insulin therapy may be complicated by one or more of the following conditions: hypoglycemia; tissue hypertrophy, atrophy, or both at the site of injection; erratic insulin action; insulin allergy; and insulin resistance.

Hypoglycemia. Clients usually experience symptoms of hypoglycemia (such as altered consciousness, tachycardia, or increased perspiration) when the blood glucose level drops to 60 mg/100 ml or less. In diabetes, an overdose of insulin, late or skipped meals, or overzealous exercise may cause hypoglycemic reactions. Hypoglycemia is discussed later in this chapter.

Tissue Hypertrophy or Atrophy. Tissue hypertrophy involves thickening of the subcutaneous tissues at injection sites (Fig. 61-5*A*). Tissue atrophy, in contrast, involves a loss of subcutaneous fat at the injection site. A hypertrophied area may feel lumpy and hard or spongy and soft. Tissue changes due to atrophy may be slight, causing only a dimpling of the tissues, or they may be extensive, causing large "craters" (Fig. 61-5*B*).

Erratic Insulin Action. Some clients respond erratically to insulin (i.e., with periods of hypoglycemia followed by periods of hyperglycemia). Box 61-3 lists the important causes of erratic insulin action.

Insulin Allergy. Clients who develop allergies during insulin therapy are usually sensitive to the insulin itself. Most insulin manufactured today, however, is extremely pure. Clients who do exhibit allergies to beef insulin can be switched to human insulin, which is identical to the body's own insulin.

Insulin Resistance. The client who is insulin-resistant requires more than 200 units of insulin per day. Insulin resistance may be caused by specific insulin antagonists

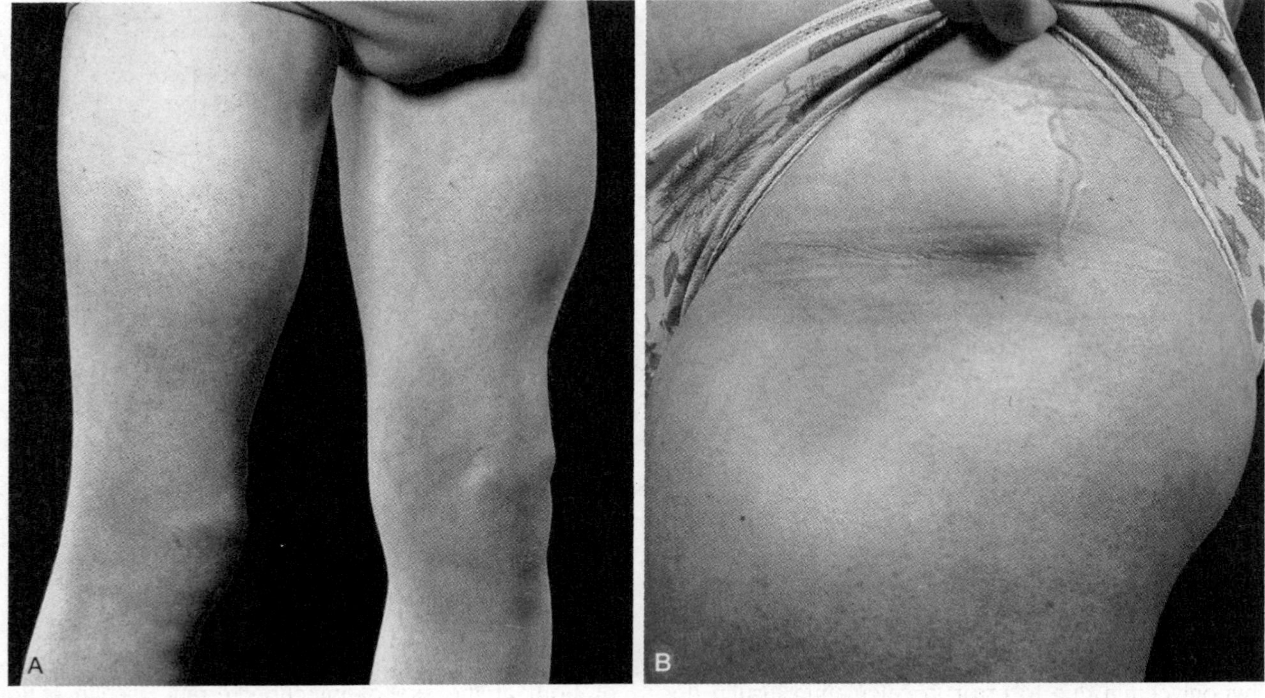

▲ *Figure 61–5*

A, Lipohypertrophy at insulin injection sites. This is a consequence of the lipogenic effect of insulin. *B*, Lipoatrophy at insulin injection sites. This is caused by high circulating levels of insulin antibody. (From Besser, G., et al. [1988]. *Clinical diabetes: An illustrated text.* London: Gower Medical Publishing.)

within the blood or by circulating antibodies that link to insulin, making it unavailable to the target tissue.

To treat insulin resistance, the clinician may first attempt to give the client human insulin. If human insulin fails, the clinician must then order as high a dosage of insulin as is needed to control the client's diabetes. Consequently, dosages may range from as low as 80 units/day to as high as thousands of units per day. There are special preparations of U-500 insulin available for those clients who require high insulin dosages. Some clients (up to 75 per cent) respond to prednisone 60 to 100 mg/day.

Box 61–3. Causes of Erratic Insulin Action

- Dietary (overeating, irregular meals, omission of snacks, and so forth)
- Insulin technique errors
  - Inaccurate measurement (visual problems)
  - Failure to rotate injection sites
  - Injecting insulin at sites of lipodystrophy
  - Inadequate mixing
  - Frozen or outdated insulin
  - Improper dosage adjustment
- Psychological errors
  - Deliberate omission or overdosage of insulin
  - Inaccurate blood or urine tests
  - Feigned insulin reactions
  - Marital or parental tensions
- Chronic overdosage of insulin (Somogyi effect)
- Intermittent use of hyper- or hypoglycemic drugs (aspirin, phenylbutazone, steroids, birth control pills, alcohol, beer, cough syrups, thiazides, nicotinic acid, etc.)
- Irregular exercise or rest periods

SOMOGYI EFFECT

The Somogyi effect (also known as rebound hyperglycemia) is a rapid decrease in the blood glucose that generates the release of counterregulatory hormones (epinephrine, cortisol, glucagon). Glucose is then released from muscle and liver cells, which causes a rapid rise in blood glucose. The hypoglycemia may be caused by (1) autonomic neuropathy, which results in no early warning signs of hypoglycemia; (2) inappropriate timing of insulin; the client's insulin may be peaking at 2:00 to 3:00 AM when blood glucose levels may be lower because of decreased metabolism; (3) exercise without adequate caloric intake; or (4) excessive insulin treatment, in which the client has consistently high glucose in the morning. Checking the glucose around 3:00 AM should help in differentiating the cause.

DAWN PHENOMENON

The dawn phenomenon is an early morning (5:00 to 6:00 AM) increase in the blood glucose levels that is usually associated with the release of growth hormone.

Monitoring the blood glucose at 3:00 AM should help to differentiate whether the hyperglycemia is related to the release of nocturnal growth hormone. If the 3:00 AM blood glucose level is normal and the 8:00 AM blood sugar is elevated, chances are the cause is the dawn phenomenon. To correct this, the clinician may change the time the evening insulin is given. For example, intermediate insulin may be given at 10:00 PM, which would peak around the same time as the release of growth hormone.

"HONEYMOON" PHASE

Shortly after a client with IDDM is newly diagnosed, the few remaining islet cells can "kick in," resulting in an apparent disappearance of symptoms. Warn clients and their families that the honeymoon phase happens and that diabetes does not go away. This phase can last up to 6 months or longer. The client may need very little or no insulin during this time. A C-peptide level can be obtained to determine whether the client is making insulin. The client and family will usually know when this phase is over, however, because the blood glucose rises without any other change in activity, diet, and so forth.

EXERCISE

A program of planned exercise can greatly benefit the client with diabetes. Exercise (1) lowers the blood sugar by increasing carbohydrate metabolism, (2) facilitates weight reduction and proper weight maintenance, (3) increases high-density lipoproteins and decreases triglycerides, (4) decreases blood pressure, and (5) decreases stress and tension.

There are three components to fitness: flexibility, muscle strength, and cardiovascular endurance. Aerobic exercises use large muscles in repetitive motion, improve circulation, and strengthen the heart and lungs. These exercises also help lower blood glucose. Examples of aerobic exercise include jogging, bicycling, swimming, skiing, dancing, and walking.

Goals of Exercise. The goals of planned exercise are as follows.

- Exercise to 60 to 75 per cent of the maximal heart rate for the client's age. This is determined by subtracting present age from 220 and multiplying by 60 to 75 per cent. Thus, a client 20 years old could exercise to a heart rate of 120 to 150 beats per minute, but a client 60 years old could exercise only to a heart rate of 96 to 120 beats per minute.
- Exercise for a period of 20 to 45 minutes at the desired heart rate.
- Exercise a minimum of three times a week.

Clients with diabetes must consult their clinician before starting an exercise program. Many clients with diabetes may not be able to exercise intensely to a calculated heart rate because of pre-existing heart conditions, age, or joint problems. The client should be helped to choose an exercise and set reasonable goals, because any increase in activity level is beneficial. Walking is usually well tolerated. Using an exercycle or swimming is possible when foot problems exist. Clients with diabetes must start any new activity at a well-tolerated intensity level and duration, gradually (over a period of weeks or months) increasing the activity until they reach their exercise goals. They should have warm-up and cool-down periods before and after the exercise. It is best to exercise at the same time of day, when possible. Because regular exercise is so important, have the client plan an alternative activity in case environmental or other factors make the usual exercise difficult. Unplanned exercise can be dangerous for clients taking insulin or oral hypoglycemic agents. During periods of exercise, the muscles are stimulated to take up glucose. Therefore, blood glucose levels can abruptly fall. Clients with blood sugar levels at or near 300 mg/100 ml should *not* exercise because vigorous activity can also raise the blood sugar level by releasing stored glycogen.

Surgical Management

PANCREAS TRANSPLANTS

Some clients with IDDM are now receiving pancreas transplants. The first pancreas transplant was completed in 1963. Today, most pancreas transplants are done in clients who have IDDM and who have had a kidney transplant. This is usually because the antirejection medications (i.e., cyclosporine) have such severe side effects, which include hyperglycemia and nephrotoxicity. The client's own pancreas is left intact (98 per cent of its function is exocrine), and the new pancreas is usually anastomosed to the iliac artery and vein, where insulin can enter the systemic pathway. The exocrine secretions of the new pancreas drain into the bladder and are not absorbed. The client survival rate is 98 per cent after transplant; the pancreas remains functional in 60 per cent of clients.[22] Research is being conducted on the use of transplanted pancreatic islets rather than the entire pancreas.[23]

Nursing Management

ASSESSMENT

The assessment of the client with diabetes depends on the situation under which the condition was diagnosed. Some clients are admitted with the classic symptoms of IDDM that has advanced all the way to ketoacidosis. Clients with NIDDM are frequently diagnosed during the treatment of hypertension, visual changes, or urinary tract, vaginal, or skin infection.

All clients with diabetes need (1) assessment of their health history, including family history, diet, and educational level; (2) a complete physical examination focused on the common acute and chronic manifestations of diabetes (discussed later in the chapter); (3) laboratory findings for diagnostic assessment; (4) a complete evaluation of home life, daily schedule, and lifestyle; and (5) consideration of health beliefs (see Nursing Research).

Clients with newly diagnosed diabetes need extensive education for self-management. Long-term diabetics also need to have their management of diabetes reviewed. Many times, the nurse can discover some errors in their self-care or introduce them to newer technologies.

As in all chronic disorders, the client's physical condition, age, and basic personality must be considered when interventions are planned. For example, a client with IDDM may rebel if the diet and activities are too strictly controlled. Rebellion, in turn, may result in a self-destructive refusal to comply with any restrictions on diet or activity. Another client may ritualize the diabetic regimen to the point that it totally dominates life. An anxious client may worry so much about diabetes that the accumulated stress actually raises the blood sugar!

Always investigate the client's habits and attitudes toward the illness before deciding on a plan of intervention and teaching. Tailor the plan as much as possible to the client's personality and lifestyle.

NURSING INTERVENTION

Nursing Diagnosis: Health Maintenance, Altered R/T lack of knowledge about diabetes mellitus.

Planning: Expected Outcomes. The client will relate the basic pathophysiologic mechanism of diabetes mellitus; explain the need for insulin, exercise, and diet in the treatment; and list the clinical manifestations of acute and chronic complications.

Implementation. The nurse or diabetes educator explains the basic pathophysiologic mechanism of diabetes to the client and family. Sometimes the information is given through classes or by videotape. The client should also be given some form of written information for reinforcement of the material. If the client is newly diagnosed with diabetes, ample time must be given for questions. In addition, the nurse monitors for possible denial or anger about the diagnosis as part of a coping response. These coping responses are accepted and discussed with the client.

If the client has had diabetes for a while, the nurse assesses for the need for refresher material. The client is asked whether he or she wishes to review material on diabetes and is asked to relate some basic pathophysiology. If the nurse notices a deficiency, the client is encouraged to review the disease once again.

Nursing Diagnosis: Health Maintenance, Altered R/T blood and urine testing.

Planning: Expected Outcomes. The client will state personal goals for urine ketone and blood glucose testing parameters; demonstrate correct techniques for blood glucose tests (including timing of tests); demonstrate correct technique for urine ketone test (including timing of test); test blood glucose at regular times, including when ill and when traveling; prick the side of the finger, because there are less nerve endings there and more blood is available; test urine for ketones when glucose is high (over 250 mg/100 ml) or when ill; keep a record of all tests performed and bring this record to regular, scheduled follow-up visits; and store testing materials away from heat, light, and moisture.

Implementation. All clients with newly diagnosed diabetes mellitus require teaching about urine and blood glucose monitoring. Even clients with diabetes who are admitted for other reasons may require review or update of information for self-care.

Newer, easier, and more accurate blood glucose meters are constantly being made available. Only the basics are covered in this discussion, so the nurse must keep up-to-date on each meter's advantages and disadvantages.

There are many different kinds of meters available today. Each client needs to be evaluated so that the proper meter is obtained. The client's ability to calibrate the meter and visually interpret the digital reading needs to be considered. Some meters can be connected to a computer, which can convert the client's blood glucose results into bar graphs or other printouts. There are glucose meters available for the visually impaired, which give audio commands to use the device and announce the blood sugar.

In addition to demonstrating the techniques of blood glucose self-monitoring, discuss the normal blood sugar range, goals for good control (individualized for each client), when to test, how to record test results, and what to do for abnormal results. Consult a diabetes educator for assistance in helping the client choose an optimal meter.

Some clients visually read blood glucose strips when they are not able or willing to purchase a meter. Make sure the client is not colorblind, or these results will be inaccurate. Compare the client's results with a blood glucose meter to check for accuracy.

Remember that with some meters and strips there is a 15 per cent difference between capillary blood and venous blood glucose levels. The capillary blood reading will be lower. When insulin is being adjusted, make sure this difference is accounted for. As long as there is a consistent source of blood, no adjustment will be required.

Both health care agencies and clients need to verify the accuracy of their blood glucose determinations. The Joint Commission on Accreditation of Hospitals and other regulating bodies dictate the procedure and frequency for quality control of meters used in health care agencies. Many glucose meters are technique-dependent. Because treatment is based on results, correct methods of use must be ensured. Clients can (1) perform a self-test, (2) simultaneously send a blood specimen to the laboratory, and (3) compare results. Manufacturers of meters also provide quality control testing solutions, which clients should be instructed to use routinely (i.e., weekly). Quality control of glucose monitors is a constantly changing area; nurses and clients must keep updated.

Urine testing for sugar is rarely done now. Urine, however, can be tested for ketones (beta-hydroxybutyric acid, acetoacetic acid, and acetone). These substances appear in the urine of (1) clients who are fasting, (2) clients with IDDM who are insulin-deficient, and (3) clients with IDDM or NIDDM who have a secondary illness.

Ketones result from fat metabolism and therefore are present when someone is fasting. In a client with diabetes, however, the presence of ketones may indicate a serious illness, diabetes ketoacidosis. Ketoacidosis is discussed further in the acute complications section of this chapter.

Nursing Diagnosis: Health Maintenance, Altered R/T lack of knowledge about dietary management of diabetes.

Planning: Expected Outcomes. The client will state the relationship of dietary management to blood sugar control; choose foods that meet the caloric needs and offer a well-balanced diet; recognize the times when it is necessary to substitute a food to maintain blood sugar; discuss with the health care team difficulties seen in compliance with plans for diet; maintain blood sugar within preset parameters; and maintain weight within preset parameters.

Implementation. A balanced nutritional plan is important for all clients whether they have diabetes or not. Emphasize to the client and family that they are not eating a diabetic diet but rather a balanced meal plan.

A registered dietician (preferably a certified diabetes educator) should always be consulted for initial evaluation and teaching of any client with a new diagnosis of diabetes. Each client should receive an individualized meal plan based on ethnic, religious, and cultural background; eating, cooking, and work habits; and food preferences.

Ideally, the nurse and dietician working together will develop teaching goals for the nutritional plan. All clients need to know the basics, which will include the following.

- Avoid adding sugar to coffee, cereal, and so forth.
- Avoid foods sweetened with sugar or honey (e.g., jellies, jams, cakes, ice cream).
- Check blood sugar levels regularly.
- Keep periodic appointments with health care providers for evaluation of blood glucose control.
- Be consistent regarding amount, distribution, and timing of nutrients.
- Increase amount of carbohydrate in the meal before sustained exercise.
- Limit intake of saturated fat and cholesterol.

Some clients will need or want more specific information about the exchange diet and how to measure or weigh foods until the portion size can be accurately estimated. Again, the dietician should instruct the client and significant others on this. The nurse can reinforce and answer questions as appropriate.

Practical examples that can be used in food preparation to help decrease the fat and caloric content are listed in the Client Education Guide.

The client with diabetes who requires strict dietary control and insulin or oral hypoglycemic agents should be advised as follows.

- Eat all of the food prescribed; if a meal cannot be finished, always compensate for the uneaten portion of food by eating a comparable amount of calories and nutrients as a snack later in the day.
- Eat meals and snacks at regular times; if a meal is delayed, drink a glass of milk or eat a cracker while waiting in order to avoid an insulin reaction.
- Never skip a meal, but take the carbohydrate portion of the meal in the form of soup, regular soda, or juice when there is loss of appetite.
- Take precautions to avoid hypoglycemic reactions during periods of prolonged or unusual exercise by increasing caloric intake as needed.

Remember that the obese client with NIDDM may not require insulin or oral hypoglycemic agents if adequate weight control is maintained. Sometimes the fact that insulin can be avoided is enough of an impetus for clients to lose weight if they know they may be able to avoid insulin injections.

Remember, too, that the client with NIDDM is usually over 40 years of age and has a lifelong history of eating habits. The nurse should set goals with this in mind. If the client normally eats three eggs and four pieces of bacon for breakfast, the nurse will need to set realistic goals that may include having the client eat only one egg per day and two pieces of bacon. Then the goal of no bacon and three eggs per week can be gradually obtained. Many clients also associate food with love, memories of childhood, religious rituals, ethnic holidays, and special personal occasions such as birthdays, weddings, and the like. Collaborate with the dietician,

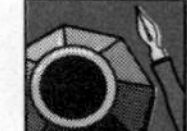

CLIENT EDUCATION GUIDE

Food Preparation Techniques

- Use only water-packed fruits and artificially sweetened gelatin desserts, beverages, and so forth.
- Oils and margarines that are liquid at room temperature are better than those that are hard (i.e., shortening).
- Include foods high in fiber such as whole grains, vegetables, legumes, and fresh fruits.
- When dining out, order standard foods (e.g., broiled fish, baked potato); avoid casseroles, gravies, fried foods, and sweetened desserts.
- Avoid alcohol if possible. Limit alcohol to 2 ounces or less daily taken with meals or snacks. Alcohol should never be drunk on an empty stomach because of its ability to cause hypoglycemia if the client takes insulin or oral hypoglycemic agents. Use water or nonsweetened mixes if desired.
- Use noncaloric sweeteners and fat substitutes.

client, and family to allow certain foods to be eaten at certain times. For example, for a birthday, angel food cake without icing might be an alternative to cake with frosting.

The nurse can evaluate whether the client's needs were met by (1) evaluating blood sugar results, (2) evaluating client's weight loss or gain, and (3) evaluating lipid levels.

It is important to work with the client, significant others, and dietician to arrange a meal plan that is practical and relevant for each client.

Nursing Diagnosis: Health Maintenance, Altered R/T insulin injections.

Planning: Expected Outcomes. The client will state that insulin lowers blood sugar; state the type or types of insulin prescribed and the onset, peak, and duration of each; take injections at regular times, 30 to 60 minutes before meals, every day, even when ill; wash hands before preparing insulin injection; demonstrate proper mixing of insulin; withdraw prescribed dosage, using sterile technique; when on two types of insulin, withdraw the prescribed dosage of each insulin into one syringe without contaminating either bottle (regular insulin is drawn up first); demonstrate the correct technique of insulin injection; rotate injections according to a definite plan; store at least one extra bottle of insulin in the refrigerator and not use insulin past the expiration date; purchase insulin syringes before all of current supply has been used; wear a Medic-Alert bracelet or necklace, or carry an identification card; state symptoms and treatment of hypoglycemia; and always carry something for treatment of hypoglycemia.

Implementation

Insulin Administration. Administered correctly, insulin acts as a lifesaving medication for the insulin-dependent client. Administered incorrectly, insulin may cause complications ranging from tissue damage to lethal hypoglycemia (insulin shock). To administer insulin properly, the client must be familiar with information about insulin concentrations, syringes, storage, preparation for injection, site selection and rotation, and techniques for self-injection.

Insulin Concentrations. Insulin is prescribed in units. Thus, pharmaceutical companies prepare types of insulin (NPH, regular, Lente) in 10-ml glass vials that contain 100 units/ml. U-100 insulin contains 100 units of insulin per milliliter. Some clients requiring very large doses of insulin (i.e., over 150 units/day) may require U-500 insulin. Insulin is available only in glass vials because it adheres to plastic.

Insulin Syringes. U-100 syringes are available for the administration of insulin. At home, clients can reuse syringes up to four times. In order to reuse a syringe, after injecting, expel any remaining insulin in the syringe and recap the needle. The entire syringe is then refrigerated.

Insulin Storage. Insulin should never be frozen or kept at temperatures over 80° F. Insulin may be kept at room temperature for 1 month. If it is not used in 1 month, it should be refrigerated; there is some deterioration of insulin potency when it is not refrigerated. Clients should be instructed never to leave their insulin in a car or in the baggage compartment of an airplane because of possible temperature alterations.

Preparation and Injection of Insulin. The client needs to learn to draw up insulin into a syringe and obtain an accurate dose. The client should be taught how to maintain sterility while working with the syringe, how to recap the needle safely, and how to dispose of used syringes. If the client has lost vision, visiting nurses can prepare the syringes for the client in advance.

If clients must mix two insulins in the same syringe, the regular insulin should be drawn up first. Then it can be given immediately or within 24 hours.

Site Selection and Rotation. At the present time, insulin cannot be taken orally because it is destroyed by the stomach enzymes. Some diabetic clients need insulin injections throughout life. Over time, the repeated use of an injection site can result in either atrophy or hypertrophy of the tissues. These abnormal tissue changes may cause decreased absorption of the injected insulin with consequent loss of control. For prevention of tissue changes, choose the injection site carefully and rotate sites systematically. The sites for injections should be (1) easily accessible (use thighs, upper arms, abdomen, and lower back; Fig. 61–6), (2) relatively insensitive to pain (avoid the midline of the body where there are numerous nerve endings), and (3) relatively normal in appearance and to touch.

Insulin absorption varies from site to site. For avoidance of dramatic changes in daily insulin absorption, instruct the client to give injections in one site, about an inch apart, until the whole area has been used, then change to another site. Instruct the client to avoid sites above muscles that will be exercised heavily that day, because exercise increases the rate of absorption. The client who is on two injections daily may use one site for the morning insulin and another site for the evening insulin. Some clinicians instruct their clients to use only the abdomen because of its more even absorption. Emphasize to the diabetic client the importance of adhering to a definite injection plan for avoiding tissue damage.

Techniques for Self-Injection. The majority of clients who take insulin learn to give their own injections. It is primarily the nurse's responsibility to instruct clients with diabetes in the technique of preparing insulin and giving injections to themselves. The amount of teaching needed depends on the client's familiarity with insulin and the injection equipment. Teaching guidelines for clients with IDDM are discussed later in this chapter.

Equipment that the client must purchase for home use includes (1) insulin of the type prescribed, (2) absorbent cotton, (3) approved syringes with needles,

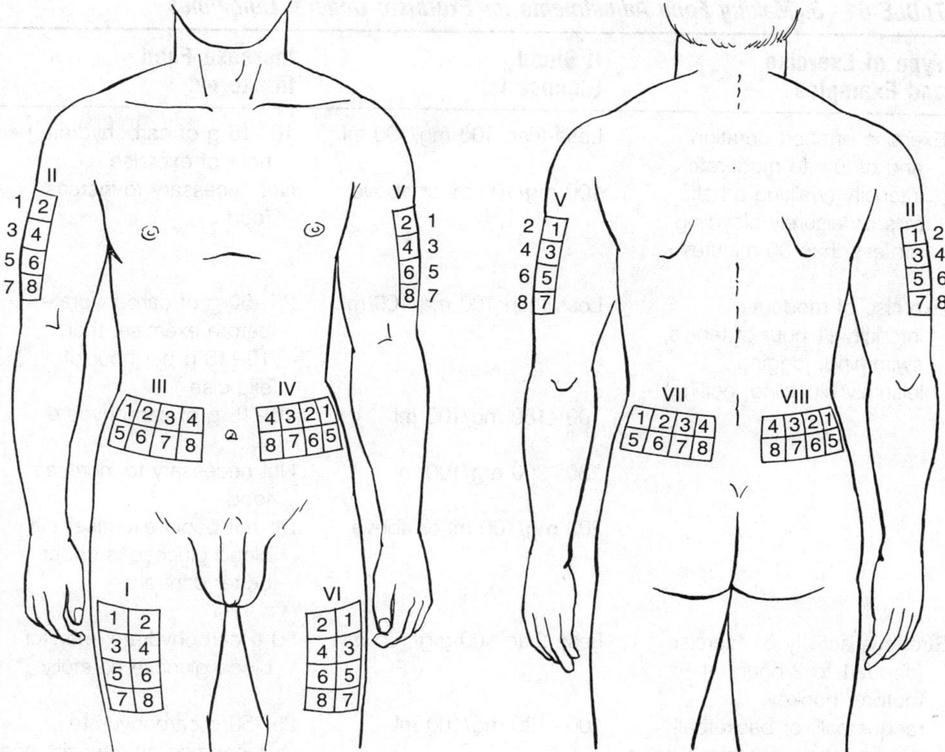

▲ ***Figure 61–6***

Insulin injection sites. To avoid overuse of injection sites and dramatic changes in daily insulin absorption, use an approved method of site rotation. One method is to begin with site I (right thigh), give injections consecutively at points 1 to 8, then move to site II (right arm) (e.g., a client on one injection daily would inject insulin into the right thigh for 8 days, then into the right arm for 8 days).

and (4) 70 per cent ethyl or 91 per cent isopropyl alcohol.

Although the prospect of daily injections for life is far from pleasant, the client's attitude toward this intervention may be largely influenced by the nurse. A matter-of-fact attitude helps the client understand and accept responsibility for self-care. Schedule a teaching/learning session for self-injection techniques. Some clients find it difficult to inject the needle into their own skin. For these clients, the nurse might select the site and inject the needle. Then, as the first step in self-injection, have the client push in the plunger and remove the needle. As the client gains confidence, self-injecting will seem less traumatic.

Use of Oral Hypoglycemic Agents. Warn clients not to ingest a large number of aspirin (i.e., over 12 to 14) when taking the sulfonylureas because aspirin tends to increase the hypoglycemic effect of these agents.

Also, instruct clients taking oral hypoglycemic agents to notify the physician at once should they develop an infection or febrile illness. When ill, clients have a greater need for insulin. Consequently, they may need temporary insulin injections until they recover.

Nursing Diagnosis: Health Maintenance, Altered R/T exercise.

Planning: Expected Outcomes. The client will follow a normal activity schedule so that diet and insulin dosage are in balance with the regular activity level while interventions are being planned; eat additional food if exercising more than usual (generally, the equivalent of a bedtime snack is adequate for preventing hypoglycemia); monitor glucose levels before and after activities; relate that the effects of exercise can be felt up to 12 to 24 hours later, including hypoglycemia; and recognize that time and practice will be needed to learn how much energy is expended in various activities and be able to regulate the diet accordingly. The client will state that insulin is injected in sites away from the exercising lines of the body; for example, insulin should not be injected in the thighs shortly before riding a bike. The client should exercise with someone else who is familiar with the symptoms of hypoglycemia and its treatment. The client should state that if a hypoglycemic reaction is experienced (even a mild one) after eating a snack, more food is needed before that particular activity. If, on the other hand, blood glucose is elevated, more food than necessary has been eaten for that activity.

Implementation. The insulin-dependent client must regulate activity so that the rate of energy expenditure balances the amount and type of insulin and food intake. Because glucose can enter the cell without insulin during exercise, the client needs a lighter diet or more insulin when exercising less than usual. If exercising more than usual, the client needs either to eat more food or to lower the insulin dosage. Any variation in one factor necessitates adjustment of the other two factors. Encourage the non–insulin-dependent client to

TABLE 61-6. Making Food Adjustments for Exercise: General Guidelines

Type of Exercise and Examples	If Blood Glucose Is:	Increase Food Intake by:	Suggestions of Food to Use
Exercise of short duration and of low to moderate intensity (walking a half mile or leisurely bicycling for less than 30 minutes)	Less than 100 mg/100 ml	10-15 g of carbohydrate per hour of exercise	1 fruit or 1 starch/bread exchange
	100 mg/100 ml or above	Not necessary to increase food	
Exercise of moderate intensity (1 hour of tennis, swimming, jogging, leisurely bicycling, golfing)	Less than 100 mg/100 ml	25-50 g of carbohydrate before exercise, then 10-15 g per hour of exercise	½ meat sandwich with a milk or fruit exchange
	100-180 mg/100 ml	10-15 g of carbohydate	1 fruit or 1 starch/bread exchange
	180-300 mg/100 ml	Not necessary to increase food	
	300 mg/100 ml or above	Do not begin exercise until blood glucose is under better control	
Strenous activity or exercise (about 1 to 2 hours of football, hockey, racquetball, or basketball games; strenuous bicycling or swimming; shoveling heavy snow)	Less than 100 mg/100 ml	50 g carbohydrate; monitor blood glucose carefully	1 meat sandwich (2 slices of bread) with a milk and fruit exchange
	100-180 mg/100 ml	25-50 g carbohydrate, depending on intensity and duration	½ meat sandwich with a milk or fruit exchange
	180-300 mg/100 ml	10-15 g carbohydrate	1 fruit or starch/bread exchange
	300 mg/100 ml or above	Do not begin exercise until blood glucose is under better control	

From Franz, M. J., & Norstrom, J. (1990). *Diabetes actively staying healthy (DASH): Your game plan for diabetes and exercise.* Minneapolis: International Diabetes Center.

exercise in order to foster weight loss, improve blood glucose control, and burn excess calories.

Table 61-6 describes various exercises (including their intensity and duration) and corresponding suggested dietary adjustments.

EVALUATION

The degree of expected outcome attainment (stable blood glucose levels) is evaluated on an ongoing basis. A few days are required for many of the teaching goals for the newly diagnosed diabetic to be accomplished.

Modification of Plan of Care for the Elderly

A client with diabetes over the age of 65 years who has had diabetes mellitus for a period of time will probably experience some complications. The normal changes of aging will only compound these problems and make self-care more difficult. Some elderly clients may lack the dexterity or the ability to monitor their blood glucose levels or inject their own insulin. They may need to have a family member or significant other do this.

Clients who are elderly and are newly diagnosed with diabetes mellitus may find it very difficult to change or alter their lifelong eating habits. If they are not used to a regular exercise program, this may also be difficult to implement because of cardiovascular concerns or other disorders (such as arthritis).

The quality of life is essential. Optimal blood sugar levels may not be possible for some in this group. It is important to remember, however, that some clients *will* be able to perform the skills necessary for good blood sugar control. Discuss with the client and family what is their optimal blood sugar control.

Post-hospital Care

DISCHARGE TEACHING

Before discharge, the client and family must have a full understanding of diabetes and its management with blood glucose monitoring, insulin injections, and exercise. Because diabetes is a chronic disorder, the client needs time to adapt as well as to learn about the many changes occurring. Discussions should be held about the potential compliance with any regimen. The client should be encouraged to anticipate a usual day at work, school, or home and taught how and when insulin would be given, how blood glucose would be monitored, and what type of foods would be eaten.

FOLLOW-UP CARE

Diabetic clients need ongoing care for monitoring their self-care ability. Glycosylated hemoglobin levels are usually checked, as is the client's log of daily glucose levels and insulin. Female clients will need to increase their insulin during menses.

The chronic changes that occur from diabetes are also assessed on an ongoing basis. The client's vision, kidney function, degree of neuropathy, hypertension, and condition of the skin are assessed.

If the client is elderly or dibilitated, visiting nurses may be an excellent asset for the client. A referral to the visiting nurses should be started before discharge (see Bridge to Home Health Care).

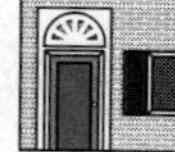

BRIDGE TO HOME HEALTH CARE

The Diabetic Client

Normal foot care activities can be a real difficulty for the diabetic client. These clients may have diminished vision and difficulty reaching their feet because of their diabetes or other chronic diseases. Peripheral vascular complications, other circulatory problems, and the decrease of sensation and lack of healing in extremities can combine to make even routine foot care a hazard. These hazards have been noted among the home visit and health maintenance population, especially when the clients are elderly.

The home health care nurse completes an initial assessment and evaluates the client's mobility, gait, hygiene, hydration, color, temperature, edema, pain, and sensation. Circulation is checked by palpating pedal pulses and blanch/return time of nail beds. The nails are evaluated for thickness and discoloration due to possible fungal infection. The nurse needs to ask, "Who has been cutting your nails?" When the nurse plans to trim toenails for a diabetic client, check for physician's orders.

Toenails are easiest to cut after they are soaked in warm, soapy water or just after bathing. It is important to be able to see both sides of the cutting instrument before you cut, and then to protect your eyes from "flying" toenail pieces. Cut the nail to follow the curve of the toe: not so straight across that edges are created that cause pressure on adjacent toes, and not so rounded or short that tissue is left unprotected. File the nail with an emery board to smooth the edges and prevent clothing snags and nail damage. If nails have not been cut for an extended time, do not try to remove too much of the nail. Use a manicure stick to gently push the cuticle back under the nail. Tell the client that you will trim a portion of the nail today; ask the client to soak the feet daily, and return in 2 weeks for further trimming. If the nails are so thick that they cannot be cut with a nipper or clipper, refer the client to a podiatrist.

▼ ACUTE COMPLICATIONS OF DIABETES MELLITUS

HYPERGLYCEMIA AND DIABETIC KETOACIDOSIS

Definition

Hyperglycemia is an elevated blood glucose level over 120 mg/100 ml. Hyperglycemia results when glucose cannot be transported to the cells because of a lack of insulin. Without available carbohydrates for cellular fuel, the liver converts its glycogen stores back to glucose (glycogenolysis) and increases the biosynthesis of glucose (gluconeogenesis). Unfortunately, however, these responses aggravate the situation by raising the blood sugar even higher.

In IDDM, as the need for cellular fuel grows more critical, the body begins to draw on its fat and protein stores for energy. Excessive amounts of fatty acids are mobilized from adipose tissue cells and transported to the liver. The liver, in turn, accelerates the rate at which it produces ketone bodies (ketogenesis) for catabolism by other body tissues, particularly muscle. As fat metabolism increases, the liver may produce too many ketone bodies. Ketone bodies accumulate in the blood (ketosis) and are excreted into the urine (ketonuria). Metabolic acidosis develops from the acidic (pH lowering) effect of the ketones acetoacetate and beta-hydroxybutyrate. This condition is called diabetic ketoacidosis. Severe acidosis may cause the diabetic client to lose consciousness, a condition often called diabetic coma.

Incidence

Diabetic ketoacidosis is a fairly common complication of diabetes and a common cause of hospital admission.

Etiology

Diabetic ketoacidosis is primarily a complication of IDDM, although non–insulin-dependent clients can also develop ketoacidosis during periods of extreme stress. Causes of diabetic ketoacidosis commonly include (1) taking too little insulin; (2) omitting doses of insulin; (3) failing to meet an increased need for insulin due to surgery, trauma, pregnancy, stress, puberty, or infections; and (4) developing insulin resistance owing to insulin antibodies.

Risk Factors and Prevention

Primary prevention of diabetic ketoacidosis is through client education. Clients with diabetes should learn to

- Take insulin as discussed.
- Monitor blood glucose frequently (at least before each meal and at bedtime).
- Monitor urine ketones when blood glucose levels rise (above 250 mg/100 ml).

- Schedule regular appointments with the physician for regular review of blood glucose results, weight gain or losses, and general health and well-being.
- Recognize signs and symptoms of infection (a major cause of diabetic ketoacidosis). The first sign of an infection in a foot or leg—or upper respiratory, urinary tract, or vaginal infection—should be reported immediately to the physician. Other stressors, such as family or emotional problems, can also precipitate diabetic ketoacidosis.

Call the physician if any of the following develops:

Anorexia, nausea, vomiting, or diarrhea
Ketonuria persisting for more than 8 hours
A febrile illness or infection
Any sign or symptom of acidosis

Emphasize to the client that the greatest weapons against diabetic ketoacidosis are (1) regular, daily self-monitoring of blood glucose; (2) adherence to the diabetes management program; and (3) early recognition of and intervention for mild ketosis.

Pathophysiology

In diabetic ketoacidosis, there is a relative or absolute lack of insulin. Insulin may be present, but there is not a sufficient amount for the increased need for glucose due to the stressors present (i.e., infections).

When the body lacks insulin and cannot use carbohydrates for energy, it resorts to fats and proteins. Ketosis and metabolic acidosis represent the final stages in the body's struggle for fuel. Figure 61-7 summarizes the pathophysiologic mechanism involved. The process of catabolyzing fats for fuel gives rise to four pathologic events: (1) incomplete lipid metabolism, (2) dehydration, (3) metabolic acidosis, and (4) electrolyte and acid-base imbalances.

INCOMPLETE LIPID METABOLISM

Normal fat metabolism is discussed first. The three ketone bodies (beta-hydroxybutyrate, acetoacetate, and acetone) are the intermediate products of fat metabolism. In normal metabolism, ketone bodies are used by cells for energy as needed, buffered by the body's buffer systems, oxidized, and finally excreted as carbon dioxide and water.

In the client with diabetes lacking sufficient insulin, however, fat metabolism (and thus the production of ketone bodies) accelerates. As ketone production speeds, the body's capacity to oxidize the ketones is exceeded, and these intermediate products of fat metabolism are excreted in the urine. Once the number of ketone bodies overwhelms the kidney's capacity to excrete them, they accumulate in the blood.

Meanwhile, to defend itself against the rising ketosis, the body uses its three lines of defense against acidosis. The first line of defense is immediate buffering. Hydrogen ions produced from synthesis of acetoacetate react with bicarbonate to form carbonic acid, which is converted by carbonic anhydrase to carbon dioxide and water. The lungs excrete the carbon dioxide, and the kidneys excrete acetoacetate in the urine. The phosphate buffer system buffers other ketone bodies.

Within minutes, the respiratory system (the second line of defense) becomes activated, and some acetone as well as carbon dioxide is exhaled. As a result, respirations increase in depth and rate (Kussmaul's respirations), and the breath has a "fruity" or acetone odor.

The renal system (the third line of defense) can excrete between 30 and 100 g of ketone bodies every day to control ketoacidosis, but the kidney requires over 24 hours to become fully functional. Also, the ammonia mechanism is activated, which removes excess hydrogen.

In uncontrolled ketoacidosis, the rising tide of ketone bodies eventually overwhelms the body's defenses against hydrogen excess. With its buffer, respiratory, and renal defense systems depleted, the body finally succumbs to its acid overload, and diabetic coma can ensue.

DEHYDRATION

Clients with ketoacidosis lose fluids from several sources. They excrete large amounts of urine in an attempt to eliminate excessive glucose and ketone bodies. Second, acidosis can cause severe nausea and vomiting, with resultant further losses of fluid and electrolytes (notably sodium and chloride). Finally, water is lost in the breath as the body attempts to rid itself of excessive acetone and carbon dioxide. Typically, clients in diabetic coma lose an amount of water equivalent to 15 per cent of body weight and approximately 40 g of sodium. Severe dehydration resulting from these fluid losses may be followed by hypovolemic shock and lactic acidosis.

LACTIC ACIDOSIS

When water losses are critical, blood volume falls, which results in hemoconcentration. Hemoconcentration in turn impedes blood circulation, causing a severe, generalized tissue anoxia accompanied by the production of large amounts of lactic acid. The rise in lactic acid within the blood adds more hydrogen to the body's already overwhelming acid load.

ELECTROLYTE IMBALANCE

As the pH of the blood decreases (acidosis), the accumulating hydrogen moves from the extracellular fluid to the intracellular fluid. Hydrogen moving into the cells promotes the movement of potassium out of the cells into the extracellular fluid, which results in severe intracellular potassium depletion. Initially, the intracellular potassium loss may go unrecognized because serum potassium levels are often normal or elevated. As the resulting osmotic diuresis continues, however, much potassium is excreted in the urine. If the client becomes severely dehydrated, hemoconcentration and ol-

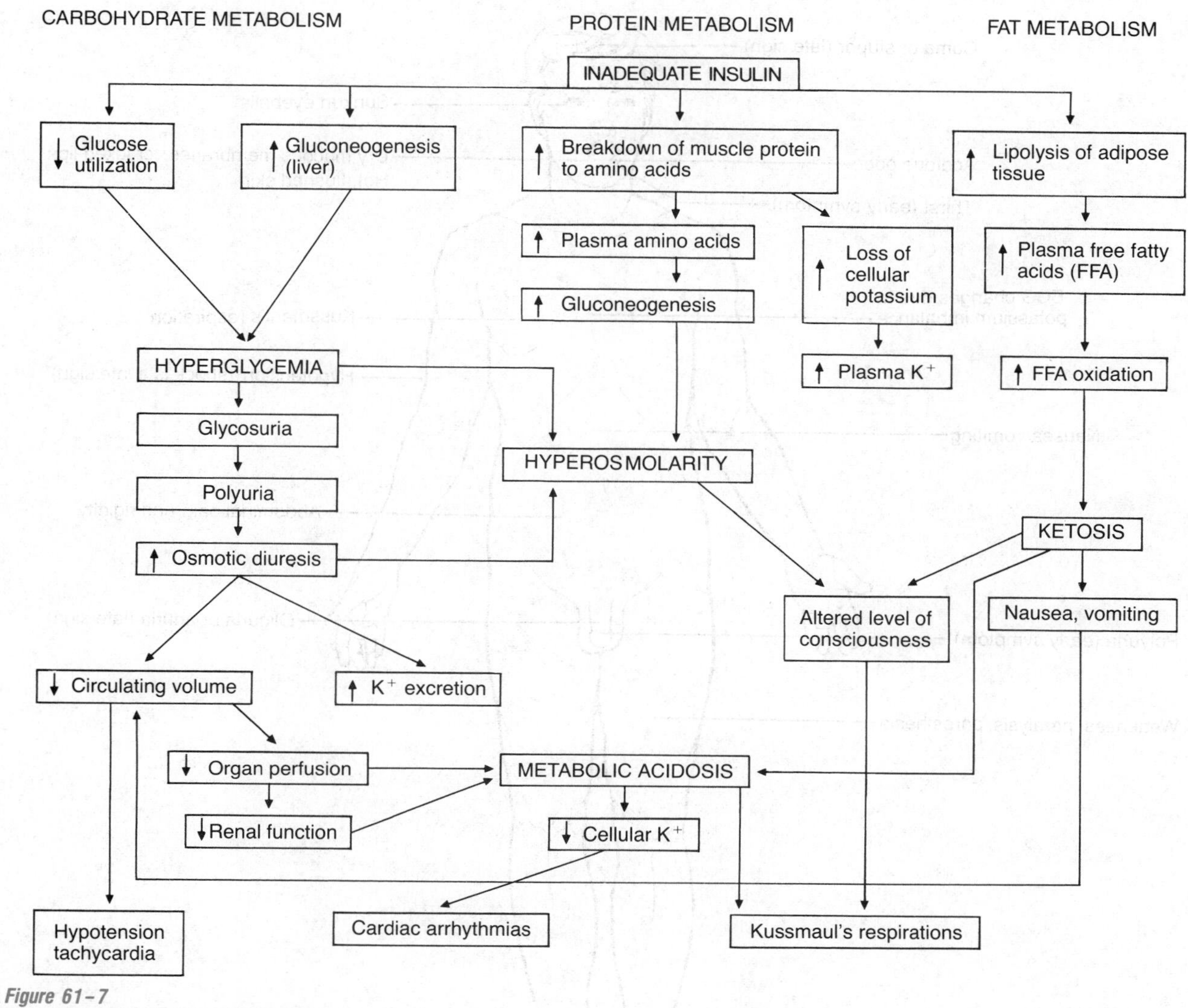

▲ *Figure 61–7*

Pathophysiology of diabetic ketoacidosis.

iguria may cause the serum potassium levels to rise still higher.

In addition to potassium losses, the client in metabolic acidosis loses excessive amounts of sodium, phosphate, chloride, and bicarbonate in the urine and vomitus.

Clinical Manifestations

Clinical manifestations of the client in diabetic ketoacidosis are presented in Figure 61–8.

Collaborative Management

Dehydration resulting in hypovolemic shock, acute tubular necrosis, and uremia are major causes of death in untreated diabetic ketoacidosis. Diabetic ketoacidosis is an emergency. Rapid medical care and nursing intervention are essential.

Management goals in diabetic ketoacidosis are to (1) correct fluid and electrolyte imbalances, (2) restore normal circulating blood volume, (3) shift from a state of fat catabolism to a state of carbohydrate catabolism by providing insulin, and (4) identify and correct those factors that precipitated the ketoacidosis.

Intravenous infusions of isotonic saline (0.9 per cent sodium chloride) are started immediately. Usually, the client receives 1000 ml of isotonic solution intravenously during the first hour, followed by 2000 to 8000 ml more of solution over the next 24 hours. Clients with compromised cardiovascular function may require slower intravenous fluid replacement.

Hemodynamic readings, vital signs (including blood pressure, pulse, and respirations), and level of consciousness need to be assessed frequently (every 1 to 2 hours initially). The development of rhonchi or rales may indicate overhydration. Dehydration and hemoconcentration can lead to thrombus formation. Unilateral leg edema or shortness of breath or other signs of

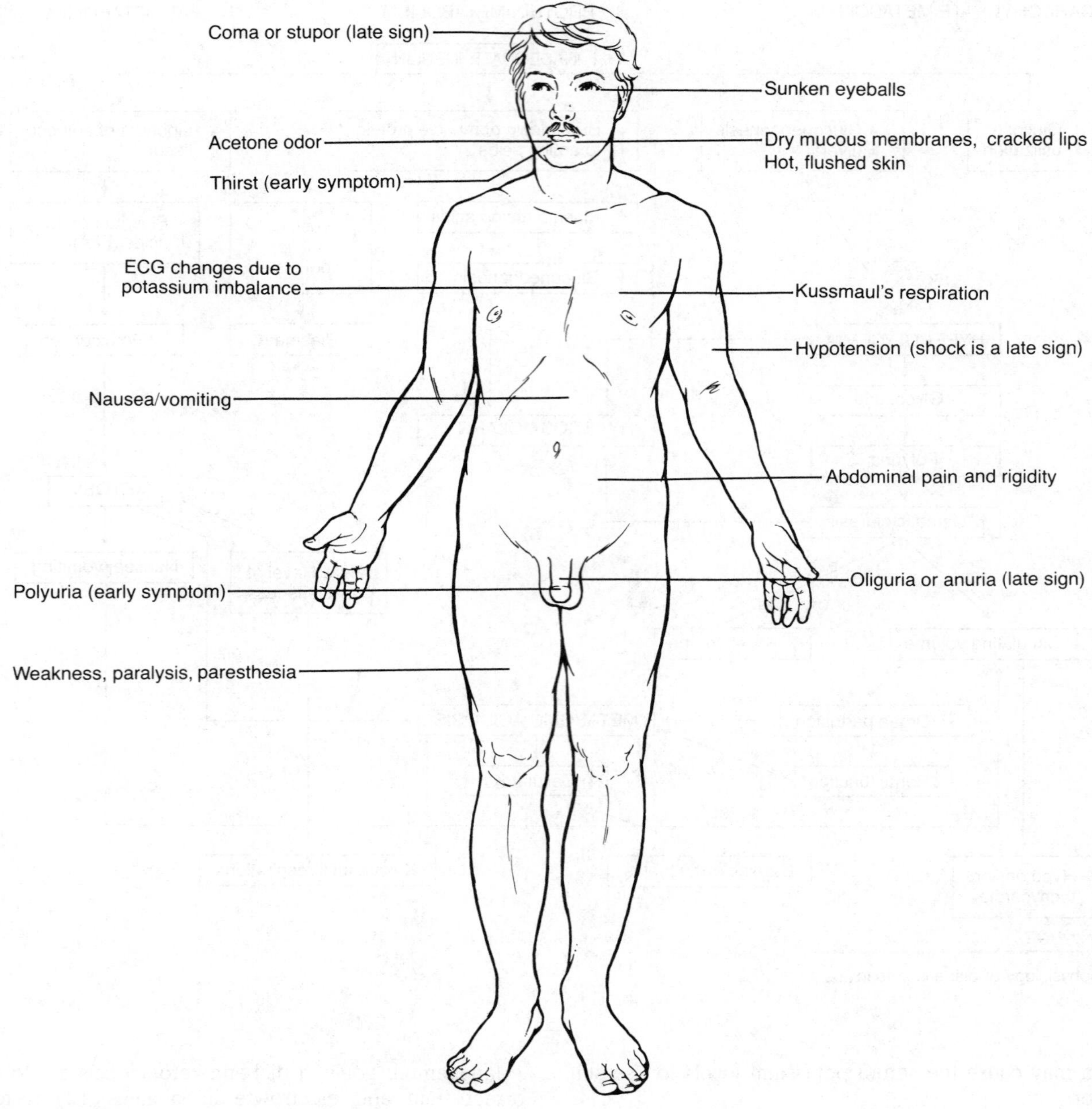

▲ *Figure 61-8*

Clinical manifestations of diabetic ketoacidosis.

a pulmonary embolus or a deep vein thrombus need to be reported immediately.

A nasogastric tube may be necessary if the client is comatose or is vomiting and is likely to aspirate. The client's mouth may be dry because of the nasogastric tube and dehydration. Frequent oral care is important.

Assess weight, skin turgor, and hematocrit for the client in diabetic ketoacidosis. When the client is sufficiently hydrated, skin turgor improves, weight increases, and the hematocrit drops to normal levels.

Bowel sounds should be assessed frequently for changes. Once the client can tolerate fluids, fluid intake is encouraged. Drinking broth is beneficial because it contains needed sodium chloride. Intake and output are recorded accurately. Most clients require a urinary catheter. Because clients with diabetes are more prone to infection, aseptic catheter care is essential.

REVERSING SHOCK

If the client is in circulatory collapse, the physician may order blood, albumin, or other plasma volume expanders, such as dextran, to be administered alternately with normal saline solutions. Also, the client may receive combinations of colloids and saline solution that raise the serum levels of both sodium chloride and plasma protein.

RESTORING POTASSIUM BALANCE

Potassium leaves the cells in untreated ketoacidosis, and transient hyperkalemia develops. However, once intervention begins, the client may develop dangerous hypokalemia with weakness, extreme dyspnea, and even cardiac arrest. Hypokalemia occurs because potassium reenters the cells (along with glucose) with insulin administration, and potassium is excreted in the urine with rehydration and renal function restoration. General agreement exists on the following points of assessment and intervention.

- Frequently assess and measure urine output. Do not administer potassium to a client with low urine output; dangerous hyperkalemia may develop. Notify the physician promptly if the urine output falls dramatically or is less than 30 ml/hr.
- Assess the client continuously for signs of hyperkalemia (bradycardia, cardiac arrest, weakness, flaccid paralysis, oliguria) or hypokalemia (weakness, flaccid paralysis, paralytic ileus, cardiac arrest). Hyperkalemia may be present during the first 4 hours of intervention. Hypokalemia usually develops 4 to 24 hours after the initial intervention.
- Carefully monitor the client's electrocardiogram. Flattening or inversion of the T wave and prolonged QT intervals indicate hypokalemia. Peaking of T waves, loss of P wave, and a disrupted QRS complex indicate hyperkalemia (see Chap. 14).
- Plan to begin potassium administration 2 hours or more after the client's admission to the health care facility and after adequate urine output is ensured.
- When the client has recovered sufficiently to resume eating and drinking, give foods and liquids high in potassium such as orange juice or bananas.

Sodium chloride and phosphate levels also need to be closely monitored. Sodium is replaced as described in the preceding. Phosphate levels can vary the same as potassium does and can be replaced intravenously. Sometimes the physician will alternate potassium chloride with potassium phosphate in the intravenous fluid.

CORRECTING pH

Clinicians usually administer sodium bicarbonate only to clients with a pH of 7.1 or below. Such replacement therapy partially corrects the metabolic acidosis. As the client's condition improves, normal body mechanisms restore the blood pH to normal (see also Chap. 15).

Low-dosage insulin therapy (5 to 10 units/hr) will be ordered for the client in diabetic ketoacidosis. The client in ketoacidosis may receive an initial bolus of regular insulin (0.3 to 0.4 units/kg) in the emergency room. Before starting an infusion of insulin, ask whether the client has already received insulin that day. Insulin should never be given subcutaneously to someone in diabetic ketoacidosis because the subcutaneous tissues are dehydrated and poorly perfused with blood from dehydration and hypovolemic shock. Insulin can be given intramuscularly, but blood glucose levels are much easier to control if it is given intravenously through an infusion pump.

Blood glucose levels need to be monitored every 1 to 2 hours initially, preferably with a blood glucose meter. Rapid blood sugar results allow the nurse to adjust the insulin infusion rapidly and correctly. Dextrose is usually added to the intravenous solution when the blood sugar reaches 250 mg/100 ml for preventing hypoglycemia.

PREVENTING CEREBRAL EDEMA

Although it is an uncommon complication, cerebral edema may develop in some clients with diabetic ketoacidosis. The exact cause is unknown, but it occurs more frequently in children. The mortality rate with cerebral edema exceeds 50 per cent. The client's level of consciousness and other neurologic signs (i.e., severe headache) must be closely assessed for prevention of this catastrophic event. Normally, clients with ketoacidosis become more responsive and alert as the intervention program progresses. If the client's neurologic status deteriorates, notify the physician promptly. Management of cerebral edema precipitated by diabetic ketoacidosis differs little from management of cerebral edema resulting from other problems. Steroids, mannitol, and furosemide (Lasix), are commonly used (see Chap. 29).

Some clients in diabetic ketoacidosis can have their blood sugar levels controlled by a glucose controller. The client is connected to this machine, and it acts like an artificial pancreas. It administers insulin or glucose on the basis of the client's blood sugar levels.

When diabetic ketoacidosis is resolved, regular or intermediate-acting insulin should be administered subcutaneously a half hour before the infusion is discontinued because the intravenous regular insulin has a very short half-life.

Post-Hospital Care

DISCHARGE TEACHING

Prior to discharge, the nurse reviews the situation(s) leading to DKA and institutes teaching of risk factor reduction. See earlier discussion of primary risk reduction.

HYPERGLYCEMIC, HYPEROSMOLAR, NONKETOTIC COMA

Overview

Hyperglycemic, hyperosmolar, nonketotic coma (HHNK) is another acute complication of diabetes. It is a variant of diabetic ketoacidosis. HHNK is characterized by extreme hyperglycemia (800 to 2000 mg/100 ml), mild or undetectable ketonuria, and the absence of acidosis. HHNK is most commonly seen in older aged clients with NIDDM.

The precipitating factors of HHNK may be the same as those precipitating diabetic ketoacidosis, such as infections, medications (i.e., thiazide diuretics, steroids, and phenytoin), or stress. For some clients, HHNK is their first indication of having diabetes. Total parenteral nutrition (hyperalimentation) and dialysis may also precipitate HHNK if the client receives solutions containing large amounts of glucose.

The major difference between HHNK and diabetic ketoacidosis is the lack of ketonuria with HHNK. Because there is some residual ability to secrete insulin in NIDDM, the mobilization of fats for energy is avoided.

When there is an absence of adequate insulin, blood becomes concentrated with glucose. Glucose is too large to pass into cells; therefore, osmosis of water occurs from the interstitial spaces and cells to dilute the glucose in the blood. Osmotic diuresis occurs. Eventually, the cells become dehydrated.

The client's fluid intake can initially balance the loss of fluid and glucose through the urine. The imbalance gradually becomes more severe as the client cannot match intake to output. In time, the client becomes obtunded and unable to respond to thirst. At this point, the process is self-perpetuating.

Clinical manifestations of HHNK are polyphagia, polydipsia, polyuria, glucosuria, dehydration, abdominal discomfort, hyperpyrexia, hyperventilation, changes in sensorium and coma, hypotension, and shock. Lactic acidosis can develop.

Management

HHNK is treated with vigorous fluid replacement. A common intervention is to infuse 2 L of hypotonic saline solution (0.45 per cent) over a 2-hour period. As in diabetic ketoacidosis, potassium, sodium, chloride, and phosphates are administered intravenously. Insulin is given via an infusion pump but usually at lower dosages because the client is producing some insulin. Dextrose is added to the intravenous fluid when the blood sugar reaches around 250 mg/100 ml for preventing hypoglycemia. Because many clients in HHNK are elderly and have other cardiovascular or renal disorders, fluid volume and electrolyte changes must be carefully assessed.

As the population ages, an increasing number of clients will experience HHNK, and nurses need to be alert for its signs and symptoms. Before discharge, the nurse reviews the causes of HHNK with the client and family, including insulin injection and blood glucose testing techniques. The nurse helps the client understand how serious these acute complications are and how to prevent them in the future.

HYPOGLYCEMIA (INSULIN REACTION)

Overview

Hypoglycemia is defined as a blood glucose level less than 60 mg/100 ml. Most clients who take insulin experience a hypoglycemic reaction at some time. Hypoglycemic reactions result from (1) an overdose of insulin or, less commonly, a sulfonylurea; (2) omitting a meal or eating less food than usual; (3) overexertion without additional carbohydrate compensation; (4) nutritional and fluid imbalances due to nausea and vomiting; and (5) alcohol intake.

Low blood glucose levels trigger an adrenergic response that stimulates the liver to convert glycogen (stored glucose) into glucose. In addition, the reticular activating system is stimulated to a state of wakefulness and alertness. When the liver's supply of glycogen is exhausted and glucose is not replaced, brain damage can occur.

Untreated prolonged hypoglycemia can result in coma. When the brain is deprived of glucose, brain cells are destroyed, which can cause permanent brain damage; memory loss, decreased learning ability, and even paralysis can result.[4] Brain damage develops when the brain is deprived of needed glucose after a drastic drop in blood sugar. In this respect, hypoglycemic shock is more dangerous than diabetic ketoacidosis. Some medications, such as propranolol and sulfamethoxazole, can mask the symptoms of hypoglycemia, and clients may not know they are having a reaction.

The time period during which the client is most likely to experience an insulin reaction depends on (1) the type of insulin given, (2) the client's response to that type of insulin, and (3) the timing of the insulin injection. When insulins are given in the morning, short-acting preparations tend to produce reactions before lunch; intermediate-acting insulins, 2 or 3 hours before dinner; and long-acting insulins, between 2:00 AM and breakfast. NPH or Lente insulin injected before dinner (5:00 PM) can cause hypoglycemia around 2:00 AM when the normal blood glucose level is lowest because of the decrease in metabolism.

Early clinical manifestations of an insulin reaction (hypoglycemia) include headache, weakness, irritability, lack of muscular coordination, and apprehension. Because epinephrine is released when the blood glucose drops abnormally low, the client usually becomes diaphoretic. In addition, these clients may behave as if they are drunk or psychotic. Some clients may become combative, and others may stare at the wall and become unresponsive to verbal commands.

Clinical manifestations of hypoglycemia at night may include bizarre nightmares, restlessness, diaphoresis, sleeplessness, or confusion. These symptoms can be misinterpreted as "sundown syndrome" in the elderly. If the client exhibits these symptoms or complains of a headache when arising, check blood glucose levels the next morning around 3:00 AM.

Management

Management of hypoglycemia depends on the severity of the reaction. For reversal of mild hypoglycemia, instruct the client to drink a glass of orange juice or to eat hard candy. This should be followed by a small snack of carbohydrate and protein such as half a sandwich or graham crackers and milk. A blood glucose test (with a glucose meter) should be performed as soon as the symptoms are recognized for determining the blood glucose level. If a meter is not available, it is safer to assume and treat hypoglycemia. Retest the blood glucose in 15 to 30 minutes and treat again if the blood is not over 100 mg/100 ml. Continue testing until the blood sugar goes above 100 mg/100 ml. Some clients who have had high blood sugar levels (over 250 mg/100 ml) for a long period of time may experience signs and symptoms of hypoglycemia even if their blood sugar level is 110 to 120 mg/100 ml. They have become accustomed to high glucose levels and perceive normal blood sugar levels as too low.

As an alternative to orange juice or candy, some clients purchase glucose tablets or a glucose gel. Clients who are tempted to go off their diet by candy may prefer commercial products such as the gel.

Never force an unconscious or semiconscious client to drink liquids because fluid may be aspirated into the lungs. The unconscious client with severe hypoglycemia needs glucagon or intravenous glucose immediately. Family members of clients with diabetes can administer glucagon at home in the event of a serious hypoglycemic reaction. Glucagon, administered intramuscularly or subcutaneously, may eliminate the need for emergency department intervention. The pharmacy dispenses glucagon in the form of a powder with the diluent in a separate vial. Instruct the family how and when to mix and inject glucagon and that the client may experience nausea or vomiting upon awakening.

The client who experiences severe hypoglycemia in the hospital usually receives 20 to 50 ml of 50 per cent glucose by intravenous push. Once the client fully regains consciousness, orange juice is given, followed by a longer-acting carbohydrate and protein snack.

Because insulin reactions are so common, newly diagnosed diabetic clients must understand (1) why reactions occur, (2) when reactions are most likely to occur, (3) early clinical manifestations of hypoglycemia, (4) the danger of severe or repeated reactions, (5) the importance of early intervention, and (6) how to prevent insulin reactions. Whenever a client is begun on insulin or an oral hypoglycemic agent, teaching must include clinical manifestations and management of hypoglycemia.

Once a client develops and then fully recovers from an episode of hypoglycemia, the nurse needs to thoroughly reassess the intervention program. In some cases, insulin reactions develop because the client carelessly prepares insulin dosages, fails to eat, or exercises excessively. Talk to the client who is careless about the dangers of repeated insulin reactions. Stress the importance of conscientious adherence to the therapeutic program.

In other cases, hypoglycemia develops because the prescribed insulin dosage is too large or the client's dietary intake is too small. Instruct the client to record the time and probable cause of any hypoglycemic episodes on the blood test record. The health care team can then evaluate the record together, making appropriate changes. Teach the client with IDDM to adjust diet and insulin by monitoring results. Finally, be certain that the client with diabetes obtains a diabetic identification tag or bracelet and an identification card from the clinician or the local diabetes association. Sometimes, clients who are suffering an insulin reaction behave as if they are intoxicated or mentally disturbed. By carrying proper identification, the client can avoid being arrested at a time when emergency care is desperately needed. Table 61-7 compares the data and interventions for diabetic ketoacidosis, HHNK, and hypoglycemia.

As with many chronic disorders, the client needs to develop a positive self-concept and a feeling of control. Help the client and significant others understand the complications associated with diabetes. Equally important, the nurse should assist the client to develop and maintain interventions that meet emotional and social needs as well as physical ones.

HYPERFUNCTION OF THE ISLETS OF LANGERHANS (HYPERINSULINISM)

Overview

Hyperinsulinism is excessive secretion of insulin by the pancreas. It is either organic or functional in origin. Organic hyperinsulinism is usually caused either by hyperplasia (overgrowth) of the islets or by an adenoma of the pancreas that secretes excessive amounts of insulin.

Functional hyperinsulinism develops with far greater frequency than does the organic form. In this case, the exact cause of insulin hypersecretion remains unknown. However, functional hyperinsulinism frequently strikes tense, anxious clients who also have various manifestations of autonomic nervous dysfunction (e.g., neurocirculatory asthenia and excessive diaphoresis). Second, this disorder may be a forerunner of diabetes mellitus. Finally, functional hyperinsulinism sometimes follows gastrectomy. After removal of the stomach, ingested carbohydrates pass directly into the small bowel (the "dumping syndrome") and are absorbed. The sudden, resultant hyperglycemia causes excessive insulin release, with symptoms of hypoglycemia appearing 1 to 2 hours later (see Chap. 53).

Because oversecretion of insulin causes an abnormally low blood glucose level, manifestations of hyperinsulinism are identical to those of hypoglycemia previously discussed (e.g., hunger, weakness, tremor, sweating, personality changes). The client and family are taught the usual clinical manifestations of, intervention for, and preventive measures for hypoglycemia. Repeated or prolonged attacks may ultimately result in progressive and irreversible neuropathy, retinal hemorrhages, cerebrovascular accidents, permanent personality changes, and intellectual damage.

Management

The goals of intervention in functional hyperinsulinism are to control and to prevent the symptoms of hypo-

TABLE 61-7. Acute Complications of Diabetes

	Diabetic Ketoacidosis (DKA)	**Hyperglycemic, Hyperosmolar, Nonketotic Coma (HHNK)**	**Hypoglycemia**
Type of diabetes	Insulin-dependent	Non-insulin-dependent, nondiabetic client	Insulin-dependent or non-insulin-dependent
Clinical manifestations	History of warm and dry skin, nausea, vomiting, flushed appearance, dry mucous membranes, soft eyeballs, Kussmaul's respirations or tachypnea, abdominal pain, alterations in level of consciousness, hypotension, tachycardia, acetone breath Polyuria (early) Oliguria/anuria (late)	Same as DKA except Kussmaul's respirations and acetone breath usually not present Alterations in level of consciousness Nausea and vomiting not present	Cool and moist skin or diaphoresis, pallor Tachycardia, thready pulse Nausea, loss of appetite, hunger, malaise Visual disturbances, headache Alterations in level of consciousness: memory loss, confusion, hallucinations, generalized or focal seizures, status epilepticus, primitive movements (sucking, smacking lips, picking or grasping, Babinski's reflex) may be present
Precipitating factor	Undiagnosed diabetes Skipping insulin dose Puberty Infection Cardiovascular disorder Other physical or emotional stress such as pregnancy or surgery	Undiagnosed diabetes Infection or other stress Medications: Dilantin, thiazide diuretics, mannitol steroids Dialysis Hyperalimentation Acute pancreatitis Central nervous system disorders Major burns rehydrated with high volumes of glucose	Delay or omission of meal Insulin overdosage Excessive exercise
Onset of symptoms	Slow (hours to days)	Slow (hours to days)	Rapid (minutes to hours)
Laboratory findings			
Blood glucose	300-1500 mg/100 ml	600-3000 mg/100 ml	60 mg/100 ml or less
Serum sodium	Normal or decreased	Elevated	Normal
Serum potassium	Normal or elevated at first, then decreased	Same as DKA	Normal
Blood urea nitrogen	Elevated	Elevated	Normal
Serum ketones	Elevated	Normal	Normal
White blood cells	Elevated	Elevated	Normal or elevated
Hematocrit	Elevated	Elevated	Normal
Urine glucose	Elevated	Elevated	Normal
Urine ketones	Elevated	Normal	Normal
Arterial blood gas	Metabolic acidosis with compensatory respiratory alkalosis	Normal (metabolic acidosis of shock is profound and prolonged)	Normal or slight respiratory acidosis
pH	Less than 7.3	Usually normal or slightly decreased	
Osmolarity	300-350 mg/100 ml	Usually over 350/100 ml	
Intervention	Insulin IV fluids such as normal saline, possibly half normal saline Potassium when urine output is adequate Sodium bicarbonate if pH is less than 7.0	Insulin IV fluids such as half normal or 0.45% normal saline Potassium when urine output is adequate	Candy, glucose gel or tablets, orange juice if awake 50% dextrose IV push, 5-10% D/W IV drip, or glucagon if unconscious Follow with a complex carbohydrate and protein (e.g., cheese and crackers)

D/W, dextrose in water; IV, intravenous.

glycemia. Interventions include psychological counseling, diet, medications, and follow-up care.

Emergency intervention for acute hypoglycemic attacks is the same as that for an insulin reaction, that is, immediate administration of a simple carbohydrate in any quickly digested form (orange juice). However, for permanently alleviating organic hyperinsulinism, surgery is required. The operation involves either removing the insulin-secreting tumor or resecting hyperplastic pancreatic tissue. In a few cases, partial or total pancreatectomy becomes necessary.

Clients who are anxious may find relief by learning to relax more fully and more frequently. The help of a psychiatrist may be needed in extreme cases. Sedation may help the anxious client relax. Anticholinergic medications may help control the "dumping syndrome."

In the past, some physicians have advised a high-protein, low-carbohydrate diet. Most authorities now recommend a diet of normal composition but with no large meals or concentrated sweets. Six small meals rather than three large meals may also be helpful. The client should ingest carbohydrates of the slowly assimilated variety (e.g., starches and vegetables).

Advise clients with functional hyperinsulinism to schedule periodic physical examinations so they can be assessed for the signs of overt diabetes mellitus.

▼ CHRONIC COMPLICATIONS OF DIABETES MELLITUS

Before the discovery of insulin, complications in clients with diabetes had little significance because the life expectancy of a client with IDDM was short. Today, most diabetic clients can expect to live much longer. Unfortunately, the long-term complications of diabetes are relentless. They can be divided into those resulting from disorders of the microcirculation (neuropathy, retinopathy, and nephropathy) and of the macrocirculation (peripheral vascular lesions, coronary artery disease, stroke, hypertension, and infection). They are summarized in Table 61–8.

The increased glucose levels in the diabetic create an imbalance of substances used for making the matrix between cells. Enzyme systems normally convert glucose to other sugars such as sorbitol and fructose to lower blood sugar. Sorbitol and fructose, as well as glucose, accumulate in the basement membrane of the cell and between the cells. Intracellular accumulations of sorbitol cause intracellular edema and affect function.

The microcirculation is affected by extracellular accumulation of glucose, sorbitol, and fructose. The thickened basement membrane increases the distance that nutrients and waste products must travel to and from the cell. As a result, the cells receive inadequate oxygen and nutrition and cannot rid themselves of waste. Most of the long-term complications of diabetes mellitus are related to the cell's inability to receive nutrition and rid itself of waste because of the thickened membrane. Unfortunately, the process starts as early as 2 years after the onset of diabetes.

The widespread effects of microangiopathy can be disastrous. The eyes and kidneys are the organs most seriously affected. Vascular degeneration within the retina can cause microaneurysms, retinal hemorrhages, and eventual blindness. Small vessel changes within the kidney eventually result in intercapillary glomerulosclerosis and renal failure.

NEUROPATHY

Neuropathy is the most common chronic complication of diabetes. Even though nerve fibers do not have their own blood supply, they depend on the diffusion of nutrients and oxygen across the membrane. When axons and dendrites are not nourished, their transmission of impulses slows. In addition, sorbitol accumulates in nerve tissue, further diminishing both sensory and motor function. Clients with diabetes may develop both temporary and permanent neurologic problems during the course of their illness. Identified causes of diabetic neuropathy include vascular insufficiency, chronic elevations in blood glucose levels, hypertension, cigarette smoking, and increasing age. Clients may present with mononeuropathy or polyneuropathy and may have sensory or motor impairment, depending on which nerves are involved.

Peripheral Nerve Degeneration

This common form of diabetic neuropathy tends to develop in stages. During its earliest stage, the affected client usually suffers from temporary episodes of pain and tingling in the extremities (particularly the feet). Later, the pain may grow more nagging and constant. Discomfort becomes particularly troublesome at night. Finally, in the months or years after development of diabetes, the client may experience a painless neuropathy characterized by an inability to perceive pain. Painless neuropathy is a dangerous condition. Clients may be totally unaware of injury, particularly of the lower extremities.

Atherosclerosis results in reduced blood supply to the feet, which causes intermittent claudication, cold feet, paresthesias, infections, delayed healing of foot lesions, ulceration, and gangrene of the extremities. Clients with diabetes are five times more likely than is the general population to develop gangrene. Lesions of the extremities may become so severe that the client faces amputation of the toes, foot, or leg. For decreasing the risk of foot infections, clients with diabetes are taught the principles of good foot care. (See Client Education Guide.)

POLYNEUROPATHY

Polyneuropathy is damage to a variety of nerves with resultant weakness, pain, various paresthesias, sensory loss, and decreased or absent reflexes. Amyopathy is

TABLE 61–8. Long-term Complications of Diabetes

Complication	Clinical Manifestations	Prevention	Intervention
Vascular Changes			
Macroangiopathy (atherosclerosis)		Control blood sugar levels	
Coronary artery disease	Angina pain	Control hypertension Diet low in cholesterol and saturated fat	Medical management Surgical intervention when necessary
Cerebrovascular disease	Fainting episodes Paralysis		
Peripheral vascular disease	Intermittent claudication	Avoid cigarette smoking Regular exercise program Daily foot inspection and foot care aimed at prevention and early intervention	
Microangiopathy			
Retinopathy	Advanced stages lead to blindness	Regular eye examinations every 6 months to 1 year Control hypertension Control blood sugar levels	Photocoagulation Vitrectomy
Nephropathy	Fluid accumulation Fatigue Increased incidence of hypoglycemia	Prompt, vigorous treatment of urinary tract and kidney infections Low-protein diet	Hemodialysis Peritoneal dialysis Renal transplantation Decrease insulin dose
Neuropathy			
Peripheral neuropathy	Numbness, tingling, or pain in extremities	Daily foot inspection and foot care aimed at prevention and early intervention	Tricyclic antidepressants Pentoxifylline (Trental) Capsaicin
Autonomic neuropathy	Nausea, vomiting, and abdominal discomfort from delayed emptying of gastric contents	Maintain blood sugar near normal levels	Metoclopramide 3 or 4 times a day before meals
	Diarrhea or constipation		
	Urinary retention or incontinence		Bladder training using Credé's and other techniques
	Decreased sweating		Metoclopramide Self-catheterization 9-Fluorohydrocortisone Support stockings Metoclopramide
	Fainting episodes		
	Male impotence		Implantation of penile prosthesis if desired
	Vaginal dryness in the female		Lubrication jelly during intercourse
	Silent myocardial infarction		Medical or surgical intervention

wasted muscle mass and decreased response to infection due to nerve damage leading to weakness in the pelvic girdle and legs.

Autonomic Neuropathy

Autonomic neuropathy causes a variety of problems seen in the autonomic nervous system. Gastroparesis is slowed digestion. Clients experience bloating and feelings of fullness. Because digestion is slowed, dietary regulation of blood glucose is also impaired. Gastroparesis may be diagnosed when the client is having increasing problems with self-regulation. Other clinical manifestations of autonomic nerve damage include diarrhea or constipation, urinary incontinence or retention, decreased sweating, orthostatic hypotension, and impotence in men. Also, clients with diabetes depend

TABLE 61–8. Long-term Complications of Diabetes Continued

Complication	Clinical Manifestations	Prevention	Intervention
Cranial neuropathy	Diplopia Pain in the orbit of the eye Ptosis	Regular eye examinations Control blood sugar	Control blood sugar

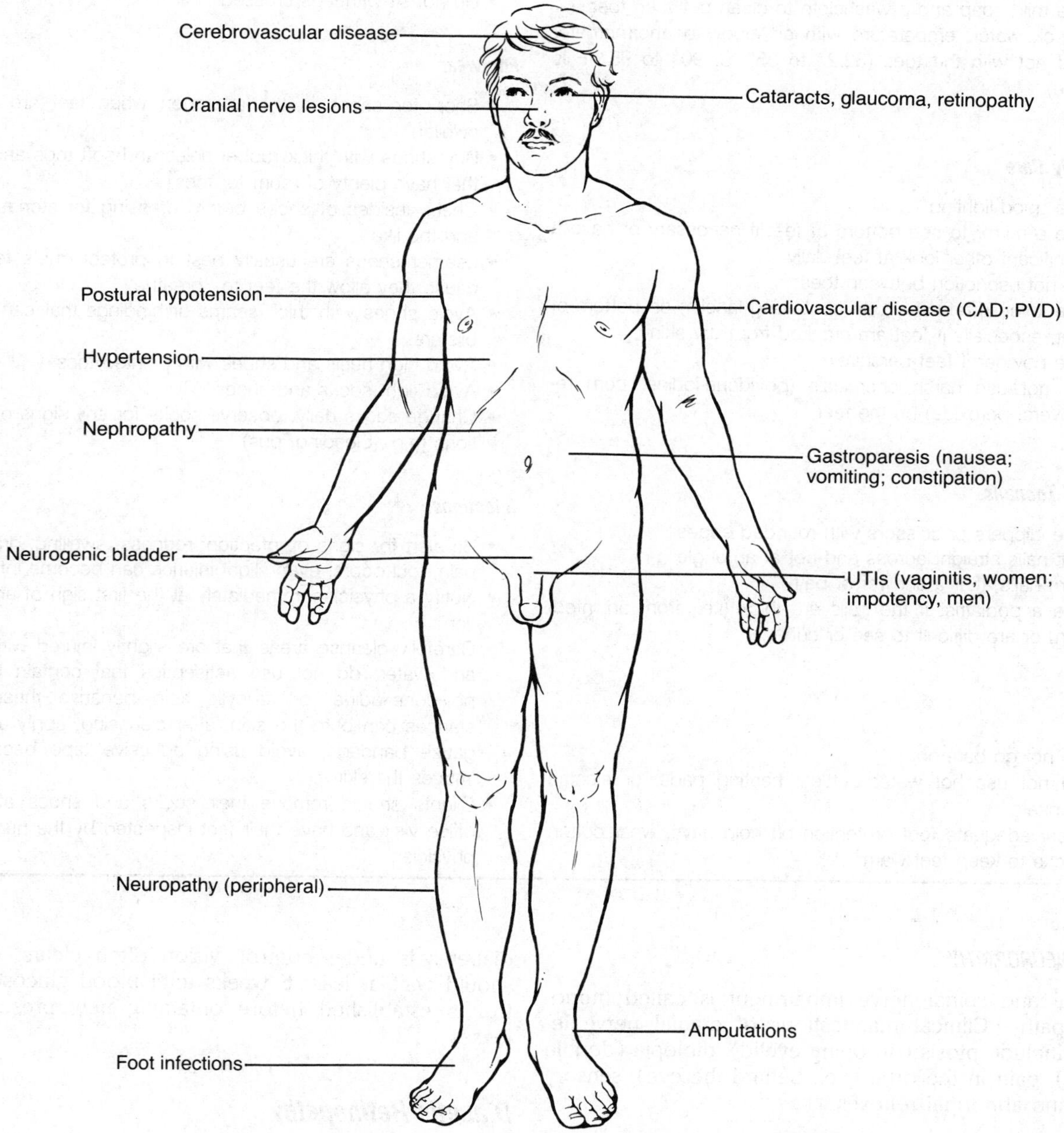

on an intact autonomic nervous system to signal development of hypoglycemia. Clients with damaged autonomic nerves may find it difficult to recognize when they are becoming hypoglycemic. Be sure to alert clients to this problem when teaching the management of hypoglycemia.

Some clients with autonomic neuropathy may also have "silent myocardial infarctions" without angina. The first symptom may be shortness of breath due to congestive heart failure. Clients may also experience no increase in heart rate with stress or exercise because of the decrease in nerve innervation to the heart.

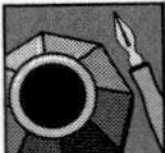

CLIENT EDUCATION GUIDE

Foot and Skin Care

- Do not soak feet unless otherwise directed to do so
- Use mild soap and a washcloth to clean between toes
- Check water temperature with an elbow or thermometer and not with the toes (32.2° to 35° C, 90° to 95° F is safe)

For Daily Care

- Use good lighting
- Use a mirror to see bottom of feet if necessary or have a significant other look at feet daily
- Do not use lotion between toes
- Use lotion (preferably one containing lanolin) on bottom of feet, especially if feet are cracked from dry skin
- Use powder if feet perspire
- Do not use harsh chemicals (povidone-iodine, corn removers, peroxide) on the feet

Care of Toenails

- Use clippers or scissors with rounded edges
- Cut nails straight across and not at an angle
- Trim nails after a shower or bath
- See a podiatrist if the nails are thick (i.e., from an infection) or are difficult to see or cut

Safety

- Do not go barefoot
- Do not use hot water bottles, heating pads, or electric blankets
- Wear adequate foot protection on cold days; wear cotton socks to keep feet warm
- Turn lights on in dark hallways and rooms
- Do not sit with legs crossed

Footwear

- Shop for shoes in the afternoon when feet are a little swollen
- Buy shoes with thick rubber soles and soft tops and ones that have plenty of room for toes
- Check insides of shoes before dressing for stones, pins, and the like
- Leather shoes are usually best to protect one's feet because they allow the feet to "breathe"
- Avoid shoes with thick seams or bindings that can cause blisters
- Avoid high heels and shoes with pointed toes
- Avoid tight socks and shoes
- Change socks daily; observe socks for any signs of infections (e.g., bleeding, pus)

Infections

- Be alert for signs of infection: redness, swelling, drainage, pain, foul odors; even slight injuries can become infected
- Notify a physician immediately at the first sign of an infection
- Carefully cleanse areas that are slightly injured with soap and water; do not use antiseptics that contain phenol, povidone-iodine, or salicylic acid because these substances can burn the skin; after cleansing, apply a sterile gauze bandage; avoid using adhesive tape because it irritates the skin
- Clients should remove their socks and shoes at every office visit and have their feet inspected by the nurse and physician

MONONEUROPATHY

Cranial and spinal nerve impairment is called mononeuropathy. Clinical manifestions of cranial nerve lesions include ptosis (drooping eyelid), diplopia (double vision), pain in the orbit (i.e., behind the eye), sensory loss, and abnormal reflexes.

OCULAR DISORDERS

Diabetes is the leading cause of new cases of blindness in adults in the United States today. The most common eye complications include blurred vision, diabetic retinopathy, and cataracts.

Blurred Vision

Blurred vision usually results from an abnormally elevated blood sugar level. Consequently, once the client's diabetes is under control, vision often clears. Clients should wait at least 6 weeks until blood glucose control is established before obtaining new prescription lenses.

Diabetic Retinopathy

Diabetic retinopathy is a major cause of blindness among clients with diabetes. Diabetes may be severely complicated by microangiopathy or vascular degeneration of the small vessels supplying the eyes and kidneys (see Fig. 33-16). The retina, which is the most essential structure of the eye, has the highest rate of oxygen consumption of any tissue in the body. Consequently, if the retina is deprived of oxygen-carrying blood from the destruction of its capillaries, tissue anoxia swiftly develops. Background retinopathy is the early phase of retinopathy. Microaneurysms (outpouching) develop and allow fluid to leak. Vision is not usually affected in this stage. In proliferative retinopathy, the weakened, damaged vessels may rupture, causing retinal hemorrhage and exudates. Hemorrhage is followed by the growth of new capillaries into the vitreous, called neovascularization, and by retinal scar tissue formation. Contraction of this scar tissue can result in retinal detachment.

Although many clients develop some degree of retinopathy, most do not suffer visual impairment. Whether a client develops retinopathy is related in part to the length of time the client had diabetes. Sixty to 70 per cent of clients who have had diabetes more than 15 years develop retinopathy. When retinopathy does occur, it tends to develop slowly and insidiously. Direct ophthalmoscopic observation of vascular changes within the retina and fluorescein angiography confirm the diagnosis.

Unfortunately, to date there is no cure for this condition. Diabetic retinopathy may progress to permanent blindness, either partial or total. The progression of diabetic retinopathy can sometimes be slowed by maintaining good blood glucose control. Hypertension, if present, must also be controlled.

The most common intervention for diabetic retinopathy is photocoagulation, a procedure that destroys retinal tissue or blood vessels. The physician performs photocoagulation with a laser beam or xenon arc. Another intervention involves the actual removal of vitreous hemorrhages, which thereby minimizes tension on the retina by a procedure called vitrectomy (see Chap. 33).

Clients should have their eyes checked, preferably by an ophthalmologist, every 6 to 12 months. Many clients with retinopathy have no signs or symptoms, so routine examination by a qualified professional is essential.

Cataracts

A cataract is an opacity of the lens. Fortunately, surgical removal of the cataracts or use of glasses or implanted lenses helps restore vision in the majority of clients.

Clients who are visually impaired may continue to give their own insulin injections by using syringe magnifiers or other available devices. In some cases, the nurse may need to plan for a family member or home health care nurse to draw up the insulin for the client. Self-monitoring of blood glucose may be done with a special device that announces the result or with the help of another person. The Association for the Blind provides training that enables many visually impaired clients to maintain independence in daily living. Strenuous exercise increases intraocular pressures in the eye, as does heavy lifting, so warn the client with severe retinopathy against these activities.

KIDNEY DISEASE

Pyelonephritis

Clients with diabetes are susceptible to kidney infections, particularly recurrent pyelonephritis. Females are most susceptible to renal and bladder infections. Approximately one half of all women who have diabetes for 10 or more years have developed at least one kidney or bladder infection during that time. Fortunately, sulfonamides, antibiotics, and the urinary antiseptics successfully treat the majority of renal infections.

Diabetic Nephropathy

A second and far more devastating form of kidney disease is diabetic nephropathy. A consequence of microangiopathy, nephropathy involves damage and eventual obliteration of the capillaries that supply the glomerulus of the kidney. Damage of the glomerular capillaries in turn leads to a complex of pathologic changes and symptoms (intercapillary glomerulosclerosis, nephrosis, gross albuminuria, and hypertension). Some clients now check their microalbumin levels at home. This test can detect very small quantities of urinary albumin, which can indicate very early renal disease. With worsening of the nephrosis, chronic renal failure ensues. Unless the client can be maintained with hemodialysis or receives a renal transplant, uremia eventually causes death (see Chap. 49).

Clients with nephropathy monitor their blood sugar levels and blood pressure at home. They are taught to eat a low-protein diet and avoid nephrotoxic drugs (like gentamicin). If the client must have a contrast dye for radiographic study, mannitol may be ordered, but the client must drink fluids after the test to clear the dye from the kidneys.

Like diabetic retinopathy, diabetic nephropathy cannot be cured. However, prompt and adequate intervention for renal and bladder infections can prevent these causes of renal failure. Control of hypertension and efforts to normalize the blood glucose can contribute to a delay in the development of nephropathy or a decrease in its progression.

INFECTIONS

Clients with diabetes are susceptible to infections of many types. Infections, once they occur, are difficult to treat. Infected areas heal slowly because the damaged vascular system cannot carry sufficient oxygen, white blood cells, nutrients, and antibodies to the injured site. Infections increase the need for insulin and the possibility of ketoacidosis. Areas of the skin particularly subject to local infection by yeast organisms include the neck, axillae, and groin. In addition, obese women may develop raw, infected areas under their breasts.

Teach clients to prevent severe foot problems by instructing them to visually and manually inspect their feet for blisters, sores, cuts, and ingrown nails. Emphasize to older clients that their ability to perceive pain may be diminishing and that they must rely on their senses of touch and sight to protect themselves from injury. Also point out that even trivial injuries (particularly of the feet) require immediate intervention for preventing the development of severe complications.

▼ SPECIAL SITUATIONS IN THE CARE OF DIABETICS

SURGICAL CARE OF CLIENTS WITH DIABETES MELLITUS

Undergoing surgery is a stressful experience for anyone, but for the client with diabetes, surgery imposes several additional stressors. Surgery interrupts the client's usual therapeutic regimen; the diet must be temporarily changed, and the dosage of insulin or oral hypoglycemic agent readjusted; the stress of surgery raises serum glucose levels; the client is prone to infection; and the surgical incision itself becomes a new portal of entry for infectious agents. Furthermore, postoperative healing in these clients may be slow owing to vascular disease.

To offset these problems, clients with diabetes require special intervention, both preoperatively and postoperatively. Specific interventions vary, depending on whether the client has IDDM or NIDDM and whether the surgery is elective or emergent.

Preoperative and Intraoperative Management

The goal of preoperative care for clients with diabetes is thorough regulation of blood glucose levels before surgery. Clients with IDDM will need to be closely monitored for several days or even weeks before elective surgery in order to stabilize their condition and thereby decrease surgical risk. Sometimes, a poorly controlled insulin-dependent client requires emergency surgery. In this situation, the surgeon must make the critical decision between operating on a hypo- or hyperglycemic client and postponing an emergency operation until the diabetes is controlled. In either case, the client will need constant monitoring of vital signs, frequent laboratory and bedside glucose meter studies, and vigilant nursing intervention.

In contrast to clients who have IDDM, clients with well-controlled NIDDM usually undergo surgery with only slightly more risk than the general population. Typically, preoperative preparation for clients with diabetes includes

- preoperative laboratory tests, including (1) fasting and preprandial blood glucose levels; (2) glycosylated hemoglobin; (3) electrolytes, blood urea nitrogen, and creatinine; (4) complete blood count; (5) electrocardiogram and cardiac enzymes; and (6) chest radiograph
- early morning scheduling of the surgery so that the client's diet and insulin regimen undergo as little disruption as possible
- omission of food, water, and oral hypoglycemic agents on the morning of surgery. One long-acting hypoglycemic agent, chlorpropamide, should be discontinued 1 to 2 days before surgery because of its long half-life.
- beginning an intravenous infusion of insulin for those clients who are insulin-dependent or insulin-requiring. Glucose (5 per cent) is usually also administered to prevent the possibility of hypoglycemia. If the surgery is relatively minor (i.e., cataract removal), the surgeon may order a 5 per cent dextrose solution infusion begun and one half the usual intermediate-acting insulin administered. The anesthesiologist in the operating room can monitor blood glucose levels.
- a blood glucose determination performed and reported to the physician within 1 hour before the operation for ensuring that the client (NPO since midnight) will not develop hypoglycemia while in surgery

Once the client arrives in surgery, management again depends on the severity of the diabetes and the extent of the surgery. Regular insulin, based on the client's blood glucose levels according to a sliding scale or an insulin protocol, can be given intravenously. Subcutaneous insulin should not be given intraoperatively because its absorption is affected by body temperature, circulatory blood volumes, and certain types of anesthetics.

Postoperative Management

After surgery, the goals of postoperative management are to stabilize the client's vital signs, correct fluid and electrolyte imbalances, reestablish control of the diabetes, prevent wound infection, and promote wound healing. The following are important postoperative interventions:

- Administer prescribed intravenous infusions and regular insulin until the client is able to take oral nourishment.
- Once the client is able to tolerate fluids, offer fluids that contain calories for prevention of hypoglycemia. Once the client can eat, an American Diabetes Association diet, which consists of three meals a day with between-meal snacks, should be provided. Discuss the client's caloric level with a registered dietician so that enough calories for postoperative wound healing are being provided.
- Obtain blood sugar level four to six times daily.
- Resume the client's prescribed preoperative insulin type (e.g., NPH, Lente) and dosage once blood glucose control is reestablished.
- Observe for signs of hypoglycemia after surgery. These may include a decrease in the blood pressure or an increase in the heart rate in a client who is still unresponsive from anesthesia.
- Avoid catheterization if at all possible for help in preventing bladder infections.
- Change wound dressings with meticulous sterile technique for prevention of wound infection.
- Observe for signs of skin breakdown and treat, especially if peripheral vascular disease or neuropathy is present.
- Assess the client's wound and incision frequently for signs of infection. Be alert for abnormal amounts of drainage or foul-smelling drainage.

TRAVEL

All clients with diabetes face special challenges when they travel. They may travel across different time zones, and chances are their mealtimes will be altered. Discuss with the client how to accommodate diabetes when traveling. Most airlines now offer special meals that are well balanced. Insulin should never be packed in the luggage; it should be carried on board.

SICK DAY GUIDELINES

Clients should be taught never to skip their insulin or oral hypoglycemic agent when they are experiencing an acute illness. They should monitor their blood glucose four to six times per day when they are nauseated or febrile. They should have a plan of care for illness before they actually are ill. Some clients who normally do not take insulin may need it during an illness, and other clients who normally do not take a fast-acting insulin may need that. If the client cannot follow the normal meal plan, fluids such as orange juice, gelatin, or broth should be taken. Work out an appropriate plan with the dietician.

FORMAL DIABETES INSTRUCTION

Learning to live with diabetes requires that the client (1) grasp unfamiliar factual material (e.g., the nature of diabetes and insulin), (2) learn to perform certain diagnostic procedures (e.g., blood testing), and (3) permanently change certain behavior patterns such as eating habits and recreational activities (see Ethical Issues in Nursing). Like any student, the client with diabetes needs scheduled classes, planned instruction, appropriate reading materials, demonstrations of new procedures (e.g., blood tests and insulin preparation), and the opportunity to perform these procedures with supervision.

Instruct clients with diabetes either individually or in groups, depending on the policy of the individual health care facility and the number of staff members available for teaching. Group instruction offers the advantage of bringing clients with diabetes together to discuss common problems and share feelings.

Next, the nurse needs to plan the client's course of instruction. Many hospitals and outpatient clinics employ certified diabetes educators who can help the nurse implement teaching; refer to the institution's standardized teaching program for ensuring that all important points are discussed and reinforced by the nurse and the diabetes educator. Integrate teaching throughout the day. For example, basic foot care can be taught while helping clients with their bath. Include a checklist and have spaces for recording the date when instruction has taken place as well as the dates for retesting to measure how well the client has learned the material. Information for establishing quality diabetes programs can be obtained from the American Association of Diabetes Educators and the American Diabetes Association. Lists of names for cookbooks and free diabetes client education information can also be obtained from them.

The client may not learn everything while hospitalized. Some clients will need continual training in an outpatient setting. Sometimes the nurse can only provide the basic information that clients will need to know for preventing acute problems. The outpatient classes or instructions can provide them with more detailed information on sick day guidelines, exercise, and the like. Do not overwhelm the client by giving all the information in 1 to 2 days. Prioritize teaching!

Remember that clients will go through the phases of the grief stages (fear, denial, anger, bargaining, depression, and acceptance) when learning they have diabetes. Listen and observe for cues about what the client and significant others are saying and doing. If they are denying they have diabetes, they probably will not listen to discussion about the complications of diabetes or how to draw up insulin. Help them deal with their denial and their feelings and move on from there.

Diabetes affects the whole family, not just the client. Include the client's significant other as much as possible in discussions. Utilize the interdisciplinary team to

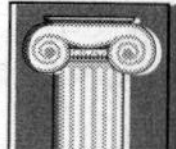

ETHICAL ISSUES IN NURSING

How Do Nurses Teach Compliance to Diabetic Clients?

With proper care, those with diabetes have a very good chance of living their lives to the fullest with few complications. However, there are complications that may arise no matter how meticulous a client is regarding the diabetic treatment plan. Even so, the best defense against long-term complications is to follow one's prescribed diabetic treatment plan closely.

Diabetic clients are seen in all different health care settings. They may be seen in an office setting for high blood pressure or at a clinic for an eye examination. In other words, nurses will see clients with diabetes for reasons other than primarily their diabetes. Many times, these other reasons are adversely affected by diabetes (as in hypertension, glaucoma, and weight gain). It is important that nurses in all settings speak to their diabetic clients about their disease (no matter what the presenting problem is). Because diabetes requires daily behavioral restrictions, predominantly dietary, diabetic clients may need more reinforcement than other clients do. If a nurse sees a client with high blood pressure who is also a diabetic, the nurse can take an opportunity to do some teaching. Noncompliance among diabetics is high most probably because the disease touches on so many aspects of their lives.

Diabetic education is important not only for the new-onset diabetic but also for the long-term diabetic. Health care providers should take advantage of every opportunity to assess their diabetic client's level of understanding and feelings about the disease. It is through this education that diabetic clients are given their best defense against the complications of their disease.

provide a balanced approach to diabetes teaching/support. The social worker, nurse, dietician, and physician are all valuable members of the diabetes teaching team. Work out a plan of care that involves them also.

A poor self-image may result in a client's wondering if insulin injections, blood glucose monitoring, and dietary restrictions are worth the effort. The client's and family's attitude can affect their compliance with and adherence to the diabetes regimen. Counseling may be necessary for obtaining good diabetes control.

Summary

Diabetes mellitus is a chronic disease characterized by abnormalities in carbohydrate, fat, and protein metabolism. There are two major categories of diabetes: insulin-dependent and non-insulin-dependent. Diet, exercise, and insulin replacement are the main forms of treatment. Acute complications include hyperglycemia with diabetic ketoacidosis and hypoglycemia. Chronic complications are relentless and are due to impaired circulation in small and large vessels. Because diabetes is chronic, nursing management focuses on teaching the client and family how to manage the disorder on a day-to-day basis and how to assess for the complications.

Bibliography

1. Albisser, A. M., & Sperlich, M. (1992). Adjusting insulins. *The Diabetes Educator, 18* (3), 211-219.
2. American Diabetes Association, American Dietetic Association (1988). *Nutrition guide for professionals: Diabetes education and meal planning.* Alexandria, VA: American Diabetes Association.
3. Besser, G. M., et al. (1988). *Clinical diabetes: An illustrated text.* New York: Gower Medical Publishing.
4. Bischoff, L. C., Warzak, W. J., MaGuire, K. B. et al. (1992). Acute and chronic effects of hypoglycemia on cognitive and psychomotor performance. *Nebraska Medical Journal, 77* (9), 253-263.
5. Broadstone, V. L., et al. (1987). Diabetic peripheral neuropathy. Part I. Sensorimotor neuropathy. *The Diabetes Educator, 13* (1), 30-35.
6. Campbell, K. (1990). Insulin update. *The Diabetes Educator, 16* (1), 60-61.
7. Davidson, M. (1986). *Diabetes mellitus: Diagnosis and treatment* (2nd ed.). New York: John Wiley and Sons.
8. Dunning, D. (1989). Diabetes now: safe travel tips for the diabetic. *RN, 52* (4), 51-55.
9. Frantz, M., & Norstrom, J. (1990). *Diabetes actively staying healthy (DASH): Your game plan for diabetes and exercise.* Minneapolis: International Diabetes Center.
10. Galloway, J., et al. (1988). *Diabetes mellitus.* Indianapolis: Eli Lilly & Co.
11. Gavin, J. F. (1988). Diabetes and exercise. *American Journal of Nursing, 88* (2), 178-180.
12. Guthrie, D. (1988). *Diabetes education: A core curriculum for health professionals.* Chicago: American Association of Diabetes Educators.
13. Hernandez, C. G. (1989). The pathophysiology of diabetes mellitus: an update. *The Diabetes Educator,* 15 (2), 162-170.
14. Holler, H., & Pastors, J. (1991). Nutrition guidelines and meal planning: a step-by-step teaching process. *Diabetes Spectrum, 4* (2), 58-61, 104-107.
15. Kopeski, L. M. (1989). Diabetes and bulimia: a deadly duo. *American Journal of Nursing, 89* (4), 482-485.
16. Kozak, G. (1982). *Clinical diabetes mellitus.* Philadelphia: W.B. Saunders.
17. Kroll, L., & Beaver, R. (1989). *Joslin diabetes manual* (12th ed.). Philadelphia: Lea and Febiger.
18. Levin, M. E. (1986). Pathophysiology of diabetic foot lesions. In J.K. Davidson, *Clinical diabetes mellitus: A problem-oriented approach* (pp. 383-396). New York: Thieme.
19. Ley, B., & Goldman, D. (1991). Sick day management: preparing for the expected. *Diabetes Spectrum, 4* (3), 173-176.
20. Nathan, D. (1988). Modern management of insulin-dependent diabetes mellitus. *Medical Clinics of North America, 72* (6), 1365-1378.
21. National Diabetes Data Group (1979). Classification and diagnosis of diabetes mellitus and the categories of glucose intolerance. *Diabetes, 28* (12), 1039-1057.
22. Nettles, A. T. (1992). Pancreas transplantation: A University of Minnesota perspective. *The Diabetes Educator, 18* (3), 232-238.
23. Pyzdrowski, K. L., Kendall, D. M., Halter, J. B. et al. (1992). Preserved insulin secretion and insulin independence in recipients of islet autografts. *The New England Journal of Medicine, 327* (4), 220-226.
24. Reynolds, C. (1985). Management of the diabetic surgical patient. *Postgraduate Medicine, 77*(1), 265-279.
25. Robertson, C. (1989). Coping with chronic complications...diabetes. *RN, 52* (9), September, 34-43.
26. Saltiel-Berzin, R. (1992). Managing the surgical patient who has diabetes. *Nursing, 22* (4), 34-42.
27. Saudek, C., et al. (1990). Implanted insulin pumps: a status report. *Practical Diabetology,* 18-20.
28. Schneider, S. (1986). Exercise and physical training in the treatment of diabetes mellitus. *Comprehensive Therapy, 12* (1), 49-56.
29. Skillman, T. G. (1978). Diabetic ketoacidosis. *Heart and Lung, 7* (4), 594-602.
30. Steil, C. F., & Deakins, D. (1990). Today's insulins: what you and your patient need to know. *Nursing, 20* (8), 34-40.

Chapter 62

Nursing Care of Clients with Thyroid and Parathyroid Disorders

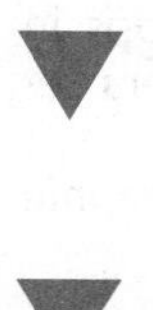

THYROID DISORDERS

There are many terms to describe normal and abnormal states of thyroid function. Euthyroid signifies normal thyroid function and secretion.

Thyroid abnormalities are basically of three types: (1) enlargement of the thyroid (goiter), (2) hyperfunction (hyperthyroidism), and (3) hypofunction (hypothyroidism). The last two conditions represent disorders of thyroid hormone secretion.

Enlargement of the thyroid gland may or may not be associated with abnormalities of hormone secretion. An enlarged thyroid may result from (1) lack of iodine, (2) inflammation, or (3) benign or malignant tumors. Enlargement may also appear in hyperthyroidism, especially Graves' disease.

Hyperthyroidism is characterized by overactivity of the thyroid gland, hypersecretion of thyroid hormone, and increased body metabolism and heat production. Clients suffering from severe hyperthyroidism may become overactive to the point of mania and psychosis. Conversely, hypothyroidism is characterized by underactivity of the thyroid, hyposecretion of thyroid hormone, and decreased body metabolism and heat production. In its most extreme form, myxedema coma, body metabolism slows almost to the point of death.

Both hyperthyroidism and hypothyroidism adversely affect cardiac function. Sustained tachycardia in hyperthyroidism and sustained bradycardia with cardiac enlargement in hypothyroidism result in cardiac failure.

Because the thyroid hormone acts on nearly all body tissues, excessive or deficient secretion of this hormone affects various body systems. The hypometabolic, hypoactive state associated with a deficiency of thyroxine (T_4) or triiodothyronine (T_3) is called hypothyroidism. The hypermetabolic, overactive state associated with an excess of T_4 or T_3 is called hyperthyroidism. Both conditions affect the general rate of metabolism, the cardiovascular system, the muscular system, the nervous system, the gastrointestinal system, and other endocrine glands.

Hyperthyroidism often produces an effect opposite to that of hypothyroidism. Therefore, interventions for these two conditions can also be sharply contrasted. The goal of care in hypothyroidism is to increase the client's metabolism by correcting the thyroid hormone deficiency. Thus, the major intervention is thyroid hormone administration. Conversely, the goal of care in hyperthyroidism is to slow the client's racing metabolic state by correcting the thyroid hormone excess.

HYPOTHYROIDISM

Definition

Hypothyroidism refers to a deficiency of thyroid hormone in the adult resulting in slowed body metabolism due to decreased oxygen consumption by the tissues and pronounced personality changes. The term hypothyroidism is not synonymous with myxedema.

Myxedema is a complication of hypothyroidism characterized by a generalized hypometabolic state. Myxedema coma is a life-threatening situation in which all body systems are severely compromised by the hypometabolic state.

Incidence

Hypothyroidism affects women more than men (about 4:1). Although hypothyroidism may be congenital and therefore present at birth, the highest incidence is between 30 and 60 years of age. More than 95 per cent of all clients with hypothyroidism have the primary form of the disease. Central hypothyroidism resulting from pituitary or hypothalamic disease accounts for fewer than 10 per cent of the cases of hypothyroidism. Myxedema is most commonly identified in postmenopausal, hypothyroid women in their 60s.

Etiology

There are several types of hypothyroidism: (1) primary, (2) secondary, and (3) tertiary.

Primary hypothyroidism may be caused by (1) congenital defects of the thyroid (cretinism), (2) defective hormone synthesis, (3) iodine deficiency (prenatal and postnatal), (4) antithyroid drugs, (5) surgery or radioactive therapy for hyperthyroidism, and (6) following chronic inflammatory diseases such as Hashimoto's disease, amyloidosis, and sarcoidosis.

Secondary hypothyroidism develops when there is insufficient stimulation of the normal thyroid gland; consequently, thyroid-stimulating hormone (TSH) levels are increased. This may start as a malfunction of the pituitary or hypothalamus. It may also be caused by peripheral resistance to thyroid hormone.

Tertiary or central hypothyroidism can develop if the hypothalamus fails to produce thyroid-releasing hormone (TRH) and subsequently does not stimulate the pituitary to secrete TSH. This may be due to a tumor or other destructive lesion in the hypothalamic region.

There are two major forms of simple goiter: endemic and sporadic. Endemic goiter is principally caused by nutritional iodine deficiency. It tends to occur in "goiter belts," geographic areas characterized by soil and water deficient in iodine. Major "goiter belts" within the United States are the Midwest, Northwest, and Great Lakes region. Endemic goiter typically occurs in the winter and fall and is twice as prevalent in women as in men. Also, because the need for thyroid hormone is particularly great during growth spurts, pregnancy, and lactation, goiter commonly develops in adolescents, pregnant women, and nursing mothers residing in iodine-deficient regions.

Sporadic goiter is not restricted to any geographic area. Major causes include

- genetic defects resulting in faulty iodine metabolism
- ingestion of large amounts of nutritional goitrogens (goiter-producing agents that inhibit T_4 production), such as rutabagas, cabbage, soybeans, peanuts, peaches, peas, strawberries, spinach, and radishes, all of which contain goitrogenic glycosides
- ingestion of medicinal goitrogens, e.g., thioureas (propylthiouracil), thiocarbamides (aminothiazole, tolbutamide), and iodine in large doses. Some people take iodine-containing solutions as a tonic.

Risk Factors

Endemic goiter occurs in clients living in areas that are iodine-deficient in the soil and water. The use of iodized salt and food additives has almost eliminated this problem in this country.

Congenital hypothyroidism cannot be prevented, so secondary prevention with early diagnosis is vital if retardation is to be prevented by early intervention.

Pathophysiology

The thyroid gland needs iodine to synthesize and secrete its hormone. If a client's diet lacks sufficient amounts of iodine or if the production of thyroid hormone is suppressed for any other reason, the thyroid enlarges in an attempt to compensate for hormonal deficiency. Under these circumstances, goiter is essentially an adaptation to a deficiency of thyroid hormone. Enlargement of the gland occurs in response to in-

TABLE 62–1. *Signs and Symptoms of Hypothyroidism and Hyperthyroidism*

System	Hypothyroidism	Hyperthyroidism
Cardiovascular	↓HR + ↓SV: ↓CO Myocardial O_2 demand ↓ ↑Peripheral vascular resistance Possible hypertension Hyperlipidemia Hypercholesterolemia Distant heart sounds	↑HR + ↑SV: ↑CO ↑O_2 consumption Systolic BP ↑ 10–15 mm Hg Diastolic BP ↑ 10–15 mm Hg Palpitations Rapid, bounding pulse Possible congestive heart failure, edema
Hematologic	Normocytic, normochromic anemia Macrocytic anemia (pernicious) Easy bruising	No specific changes
Respiratory	Reduced hypoxic drive Hypercapnic ventilatory drive Respiratory muscle weakness Possible CO_2 retention on ABGs Dyspnea	↑Respiratory rate and depth Shortness of breath
Renal	Fluid retention ↓Urinary output ↑Total body water Dilutional hyponatremia ↓Production of erythropoietin	Fluid retention ↓Output
Gastrointestinal	↓Peristalsis Anorexia Possible weight gain Constipation ↓Protein metabolism ↑Serum lipids Delayed glucose uptake ↓Glucose absorption	↑Peristalsis ↑Appetite Weight loss Diarrhea ↑Use of adipose and protein stores ↓Serum lipids ↑Gastrointestinal secretions Vomiting, abdominal pain
Musculoskeletal	Transient pain Muscle cramps and stiffness Slow movements ↑Bone density ↓Bone formation and resorption	Negative nitrogen balance Malnutrition Fatigue Muscle weakness Proximal muscle wasting Incoordination due to tremors
Integumentary	Dry, coarse, scaly skin Hair that falls out Thick, brittle nails Expressionless face Periorbital edema Thick, puffy skin: face and pretibial areas Cold intolerance	Profuse sweating Moist skin Flushed, warm skin Hair: fine, soft, straight, possible hair loss Heat intolerance
Endocrine	Normal to enlarged thyroid	Thyroid usually enlarged Bruit over thyroid
Neurologic	↓DTRs Muscle sluggishness Fatigue, somnolence Slow, deliberate speech Apathy, depression, paranoia Impaired short-term memory Lethargy	↑DTRs Fine tremors Nervousness, restlessness Emotional instability: anxiety, worry, paranoia
Reproductive	Females: menorrhagia, anovulation, irregular menses, decreased libido Males: decreased libido, impotence	Females: amenorrhea, irregular menses, ↓fertility, ↑tendency for spontaneous abortion Males: impotence, decreased libido ↓Sexual development prepuberty
Other	Myxedema	Exophthalmos

ABGs, arterial blood gas analyses; BP, blood pressure; CO, cardiac output; CO_2, carbon dioxide; DTRs, deep tendon reflexes; HR, heart rate; O_2, oxygen; SV, venous oxygen.

creased pituitary secretion of TSH. TSH stimulates the thyroid to secrete more T_4 when blood T_4 levels are low. Eventually, the gland may become so large that it compresses structures in the neck and chest, causing respiratory symptoms and dysphagia.

Decreased levels of thyroid hormone lead to an overall slowing of the basal metabolic rate. This slowing of all body processes leads to achlorhydria, decreased gastrointestinal tract motility, bradycardia, slowed neurologic functioning, and a decrease in heat production.

The most important changes caused by the decreased levels of thyroid hormone are those affecting lipid metabolism. There is a resultant increase in serum cholesterol and triglyceride levels and an increase in arteriosclerosis and coronary heart disease in clients suffering from hypothyroidism.

The thyroid hormones also play a role in the production of red blood cells, so clients with hypothyroidism also show signs of anemia, with possible vitamin B_{12} and folate deficiency.

The myxedema, a mucinous edema, is caused by an accumulation of hydrophilic proteoglycans in the interstitial spaces. The reason for this problem remains unclear.

Clinical Manifestations

The symptoms of hypothyroidism depend on whether it is mild or complicated with myxedema or by myxedema coma. Clients with mild hypothyroidism (the most common form) may be asymptomatic or may experience vague symptoms so ordinary as to escape detection. For example, clients may experience mild sensitivity to cold, lethargy, dry skin or hair, forgetfulness, depression, and some weight gain. On the other hand, clients with the more rare and severe coma develop a multitude of striking symptoms. They slow drastically in both physical and mental reactions and appear abnormally fatigued and apathetic (Table 62-1).

Myxedema is characterized by a dry, waxy type of swelling with abnormal deposits of mucin in the skin and other tissues. The edema is of the nonpitting type and is common in the pretibial and facial areas.

Myxedema coma is characterized by a drastic decrease in the metabolic rate, hypoventilation leading to respiratory acidosis, hypothermia, and hypotension. Myxedema coma may be brought on by stress such as surgery, infection, or noncompliance with thyroid treatment.

Typically, clients with goiter seek medical advice when the goiter grows large enough to distort the appearance of the neck (Fig. 62-1). They may also experience respiratory distress and difficulty swallowing if the goiter is very large. The client with simple goiter rarely has symptoms until the gland enlarges enough to produce normal amounts of T_4.

The client's physical appearance also changes (Fig. 62-2). Often, obesity develops, features become coarse, hair becomes dry and sparse, and the skin feels dry, flaky, and inelastic. In addition, clients with hypothyroidism suffer an intolerance to cold because of a decreased metabolic rate. The client's ability to sweat also diminishes. Constipation and fecal impaction due

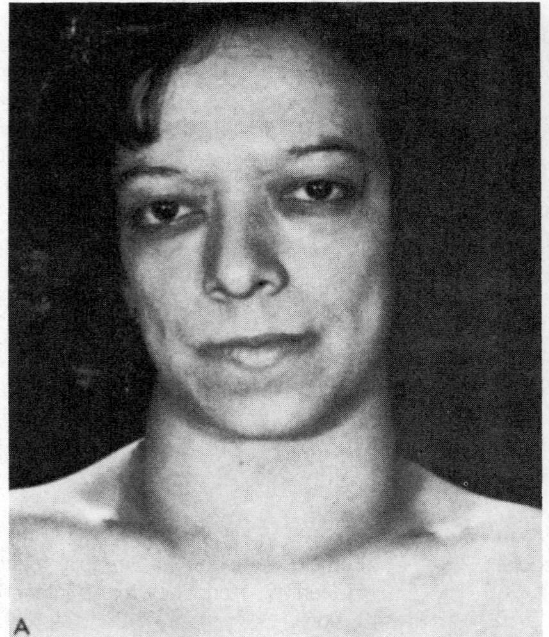

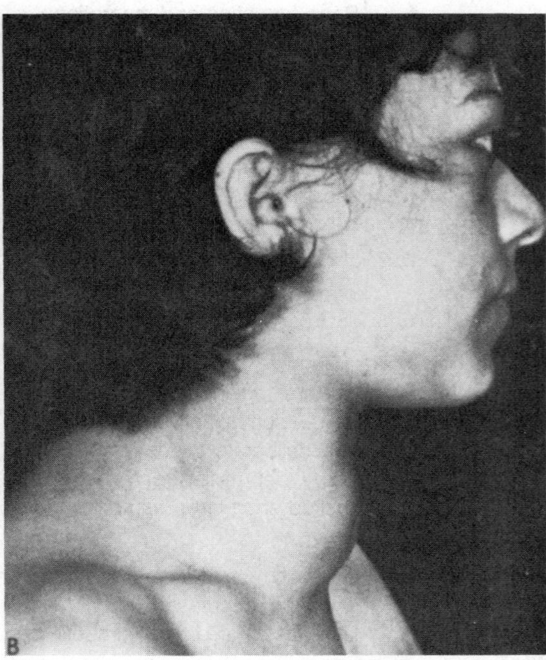

▲ ***Figure 62-1***

Massive thyroid enlargement due to diffuse toxic goiter. *A*, Front view. *B*, Side view. (From Wilson, J. D., & Foster, D. W. [1992]. *Williams textbook of endocrinology* [8th ed.]. Philadelphia: W. B. Saunders.)

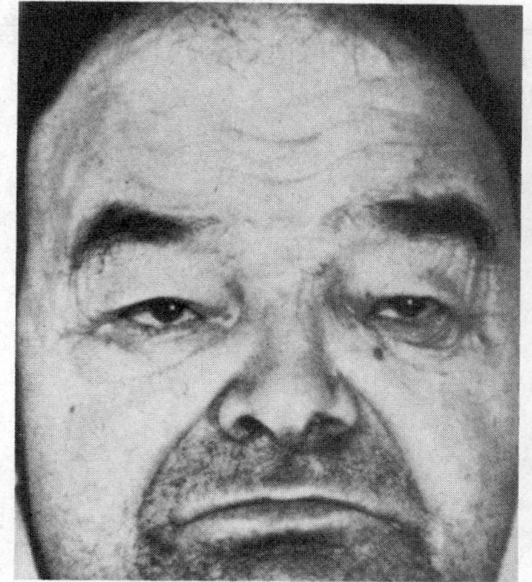
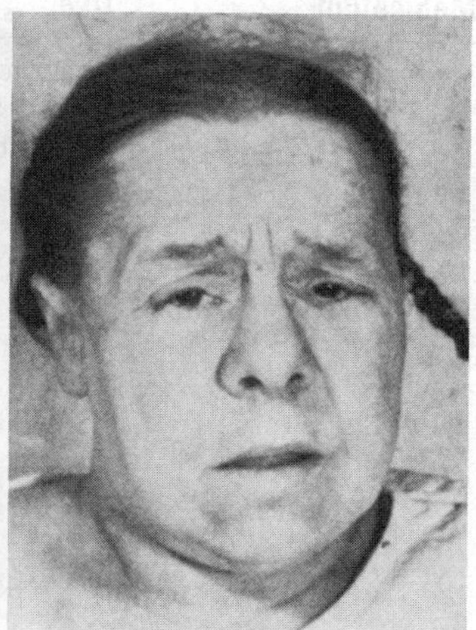

▲ *Figure 62-2*

Typical facial appearance of myxedematous clients. (From Wilson, J. D., & Foster, D. W. [1992]. *Williams textbook of endocrinology* [8th ed.]. Philadelphia: W. B. Saunders.)

to slowed peristaltic action and lack of normal physical activity constitute serious problems. Also, there is increased susceptibility to infection. When myxedema develops, the client looks puffy and edematous owing to infiltration of fluid into the interstitial tissues.

The major complication of hypothyroidism is myxedema coma. This is an extremely rare condition. Unrecognized and undiagnosed hypothyroidism may progress to myxedema coma.

DIAGNOSTIC ASSESSMENT

Diagnostic tests for hypothyroidism confirm the clinical picture of hypometabolism and depressed thyroid activity (Table 62-2). Serum TSH level is elevated in hypothyroidism as an attempt to compensate for low levels of T_3 and T_4. Radioactive iodide uptake (RAIU) is decreased in hypothyroidism. A tracer dose of ^{131}I is given, and a thyroid scan is done 24 hours later to determine the uptake of ^{131}I.

Clients with myxedema may also have hypercholesterolemia, hyperlipidemia, and proteinemia as a result of T_4 changes on the synthesis, mobilization, and degradation of serum lipids. Elevated lipid levels may be a contributing factor to the later development of cardiac problems. Dilutional hyponatremia may develop as a result of the marked impairment of water excretion related to decreased delivery of sodium and volume to the distal renal tubules as a result of decreased renal blood flow. Elevated creatine phosphokinase, aspartate aminotransferase, and lactate dehydrogenase may also develop secondary to altered metabolism.

Diagnosis of simple goiter is confirmed by history and laboratory tests. The client is often euthyroid; the symptoms and diagnostic signs of hypothyroidism are seldom present because the gland enlarges enough to produce normal amounts of T_4.

TABLE 62-2. Diagnostic Tests for Hypothyroidism and Hyperthyroidism

Test	Results in Hypothyroidism	Results in Hyperthyroidism
TRH	Increased	Decreased
TSH	Increased	Decreased
Serum T_4	Normal-low	Increased
Serum T_3	Normal-low	Increased
F, T_4	Decreased	High normal-increased
F, T_3	(not used)	Increased

F, free; TRH, thyroid-releasing hormone; TSH, thyroid-stimulating hormone; T_4, thyroxine; T_3, triiodothyronine.

Medical Management

PHARMACOLOGIC MANAGEMENT

Hypothyroidism. The goals of treatment for hypothyroidism are to correct thyroid hormone deficiency, reverse symptoms, and prevent further cardiac and arterial damage.

For hypothyroidism to be reversed permanently, the client usually needs to take thyroid hormone preparation throughout life. Available thyroid medications include sodium levothyroxine (Synthroid), liothyronine sodium (Cytomel), and desiccated thyroid, converted in the body to both T_4 and T_3 (Table 62-3). Sodium levothyroxine is the principal form of replacement therapy. Dosages vary with age, the severity of the hypothyroidism, general medical condition (particularly cardiovascular disorders), and client response to medical treatment.

Clients with cardiac complications must be started on small doses of thyroid hormone. Large doses could precipitate heart failure or myocardial infarction by increasing body metabolism, myocardial oxygen requirements, and consequently the workload of the heart.

Once clients have responded to thyroid hormone therapy, they are placed on a lifetime maintenance dose of T_4 daily. Clients are also told to stop all pharmacologic goitrogens such as sulfonamides, salicylates, lithium.

The drug of choice for thyroid replacement is sodium levothyroxine (Synthroid) (see Table 62-3). Desiccated thyroid and sodium liothyronine (Cytomel),

TABLE 62-3. Medications Used to Treat Thyroid Disorders

Medication	Use	Usual Daily Dosage	Side Effects	Nursing Implications
Propylthiouracil (PTU)	Antithyroid medication used to treat hyperthyroidism	100 mg PO tid	Nausea, vomiting, diarrhea, loss of taste, skin changes, headache, dizziness, drowsiness, lymphadenopathy, hypersensitivity, agranulocytosis, hypothyroidism	Use carefully in combination with any drug that causes agranulocytosis; monitor blood counts; should not be used in the last trimester of pregnancy or during lactation; report any symptoms of infection; give every 8 hr around the clock; urge continued compliance because response is slow
Methimazole (Tapazole)	Antithyroid medication used to treat hyperthyroidism	5–20 mg PO tid	Agranulocytosis, headache, drowsiness, diarrhea, nausea and vomiting, jaundice, urticaria, arthralgia, lymphadenopathy	Use carefully in pregnancy; monitor thyroid function closely; check CBC periodically; watch for signs of hypothyroidism, colds, other infections; stop drug if rash or lymphadenopathy occurs; give with meals to decrease gastrointestinal effects; store in light-resistant containers
Saturated solution of potassium iodide (SSKI)	Antithyroid medication that blocks thyroid hormone production and release; used to treat hyperthyroidism	0.1–0.3 ml tid for 10–14 days before thyroidectomy	Diarrhea, nausea and vomiting, stomach pain, hypothyroidism, hypersensitivity, iodine poisoning, irregular heart beat, productive cough	Use with caution in clients with tuberculosis, hyperkalemia, acute bronchitis, impaired renal function, or cardiac disease; safety not established in pregnancy, lactation, or childhood; give after meals with fruit juice; monitor potassium level; avoid sudden withdrawal; keep in light-protected bottle; avoid use of over-the-counter drugs containing iodine; restrict iodine-rich foods and iodized salts; ensure preoperative compliance
Radioactive iodine (^{131}I)	Antithyroid medication that destroys thyroid tissue; used to	4–10 millicuries PO for hyperthyroidism, 50–150 millicuries	Feeling of fullness in neck, metallic taste, hypothyroidism,	Contraindicated in pregnancy and lactation for hyper-

TABLE 62–3. Medications Used to Treat Thyroid Disorders Continued

Medication	Use	Usual Daily Dosage	Side Effects	Nursing Implications
	treat hyperthyroidism; may be used to treat thyroid cancer	for thyroid cancer	possible increased risk of leukemia later in life	thyroidism; stop all antithyroid medications 1 week before ^{131}I administration; monitor thyroid function closely; give on empty stomach; institute radiation precautions on body secretions for 3 days after ingestion; teach client to avoid close, prolonged contact with children for a week, should also sleep alone for a week; client should not resume antithyroid medications for 6 weeks
Levothroxine sodium (Synthroid)	Thyroid replacement medication T_4 used to treat hypothyroidism	0.2–0.5 mg IV for myxedema coma; initially 0.25–0.1 mg PO daily increased until response to 0.1–0.4 mg PO daily for hypothyroidism	Rare hyperthyroidism, tremors, hunger, palpitations, headache, nervousness, tachycardia, insomnia, heat intolerance, weight loss	Use with caution in clients with acute MIs, hypertension, renal insufficiency, or diabetes and in elderly or pregnant clients; give a single dose in AM; watch for adverse effects early in treatment; do not use to treat depression or obesity; stress need for lifetime replacement; toxicity may last for weeks with overdosage; monitor for improvement of symptoms
Liothyronine sodium (Cytomel)	Thyroid replacement medication T_3 used to treat hypothyroidism	For myxedema, 5 μg daily increased to 50–100 μg daily maintenance dose; for thyroid hormone replacement, use 5 μg daily increasing to 12.5–25 μg PO daily	Signs of hyperthyroidism, diarrhea, abdominal cramps, vomiting, tachycardia, weight loss, heat intolerance	Use with caution in clients with acute MIs, hypertension, renal insufficiency, or diabetes and in elderly or pregnant clients; give a single dose in AM; watch for adverse effects early in treatment; smaller doses required for older clients; monitor pulse, blood pressure, and thyroid function

CBC, complete blood count; IV, intravenously; MIs, myocardial infarctions; PO, orally; tid, three times daily.

once commonly used in replacement therapy, are now used infrequently because of problems with fluctuating plasma levels and side effects. Dosage is based on the age of the client. Children and the elderly receive smaller doses.

Simple Goiter. The goals for treatment of simple goiter are to halt further enlargement of the thyroid gland and to promote regression of the gland.

When enlargement is a compensatory reaction to iodine deficiency and consequent suppression of T_4 secretion, the client can be treated with preparations of iodine and thyroid hormone. Iodine is administered in the form of either strong iodine solution (Lugol's solution) or saturated solution of potassium iodide (SSKI drops). Iodine actually decreases the size and vascularity of the enlarged gland. However, the availability of iodized salt and thyroid hormones has made this replacement therapy with iodine obsolete in the United States.

Myxedema Coma. The goal of treatment for myxedema coma is to reverse the condition to save the client's life. Supportive measures are begun immediately, such as maintaining a patent airway, giving oxygen, and replacing fluids intravenously. The client is kept warm, and vital signs are closely monitored until the client begins to recover from the coma.

Sodium levothyroxine is given intravenously with glucose and corticosteroids. When administering thyroid hormone to a client with myxedema heart disease, assess the client carefully for anginal pain, dyspnea, or orthopnea.

DIETARY MANAGEMENT

If the hypothyroidism and goiter are due to iodine deficiency, the client should be on a diet higher in iodine. This is accomplished simply by switching to iodized salt. Dietary goitrogens such as turnips, soybeans, rutabagas, and to a lesser degree, seafood, green leafy vegetables, carrots, and peanuts should also be avoided.

Surgical Management

Surgery is done for goiter that is very large, not responding to treatment, or putting too much pressure on other structures in the neck. Surgery is discussed in detail under Hyperthyroidism (see later).

Nursing Management

ASSESSMENT

The nurse should carefully assess the client for the presence of signs and symptoms of hypothyroidism. Obtain a careful history; look for the signs and symptoms that reflect a decrease in metabolic functions such as weight gain, excessive sleeping, and generalized fatigue.

The nurse should also take a thorough diet history, looking particularly at the intake of iodine. The clients should also be questioned regarding the intake of goitrogenic substances and residence in a "goiter belt."

The nurse should question the client about other medical conditions that might be present, such as a previous history of hyperthyroidism treated with surgery or radioactive iodine, both of which predispose to hypothyroidism. The nurse should also question the client about the use of medications that may lead to hypothyroidism; lithium, aminoglutethimide, sodium or potassium perchlorate, or cobalt can decrease thyroid metabolism.

The client should also be observed for the physical signs of hypothyroidism, such as periorbital and facial edema, a blank facial expression, a thick tongue, and generalized slowing of all muscle movement.

NURSING INTERVENTION

Nursing Diagnosis: Nutrition, Altered: More than Body Requirements R/T slowed metabolic rate.

Planning: Expected Outcomes. The client will return to normal weight, as evidenced by a loss of at least 2 lb/week.

Implementation. When thyroid medication is begun, the client's activity level and decreased edema often lead to significant initial weight loss without alteration of the diet. Typically, however, the appetite also increases as the medication begins to work. It is important, therefore, to provide a low-calorie diet until the weight stabilizes at the ideal body weight.

Nursing Diagnosis: Activity Intolerance R/T weakness and apathy secondary to decreased metabolic rate.

Planning: Expected Outcomes. The client will develop increased tolerance to activity, as evidenced by a return to pre-illness activity levels.

Implementation. Once thyroid hormone replacement is begun, the client returns to a level of physical and mental activity that should gradually improve with the hormone therapy.

Nursing Diagnosis: Constipation R/T decreased peristalsis secondary to slowed metabolic rate and activity intolerance.

Planning: Expected Outcomes. The client will return to a normal pre-illness bowel pattern, as evidenced by a bowel movement at least every other day.

Implementation. The nurse needs to implement measures to prevent constipation and fecal impaction. As the hypothyroidism reverses and cardiac status improves, encourage more activity. Advise the client to drink six to eight glasses of water every day and to eat foods high in fiber such as fresh fruits, vegetables, and grains. If this is ineffective, a stool softener or cathartic may be indicated.

Nursing Diagnosis: Skin Integrity, High Risk for Impaired R/T edema and dryness secondary to infiltration of fluid into interstitial spaces.

Planning: Expected Outcomes. The client will have all skin remain intact, as evidenced by absence of injury and resolution of edema.

Implementation. The nurse must monitor the sacrum coccyx, elbows, scapula, and other pressure points for signs of redness or tissue breakdown. The nurse must remember that edematous tissues are more prone to decubitus ulcer formation. The client should be placed on a strict turning schedule and on a pressure reduction mattress.

Nursing Diagnosis: Hypothermia R/T slowed metabolic rate.

Planning: Expected Outcomes. The client will not develop hypothermia, as evidenced by a normal body temperature.

Implementation. Provide the client with a comfortable, warm environment. Remember that hypothyroidism sharply increases sensitivity to cold. If necessary, supply extra clothing and warm blankets.

Nursing Diagnosis: Social Isolation R/T lethargy, weakness, apathy, and changes in appearance.

Planning: Expected Outcomes. The client will return to a pre-illness level of social interaction, as evidenced by increasing interaction with others and statements of acceptance of reversibility of appearance changes.

Implementation. The nurse must reassure the client and significant others that the client's appearance and energy level will gradually improve with thyroid hormone therapy.

Ongoing assessment of the client undergoing treatment for goiter is necessary because further enlargement or growth of nodules within the tissues may indicate thyroid cancer.

Collaborative Problem: Injury, high risk for R/T hypersensitivity to anesthetics, sedatives, and narcotics secondary to decreased metabolic rate.

Planning: Expected Outcomes. The nurse will prevent injury to the client, as evidenced by normal responses to anesthesics, sedatives, and narcotics by the client.

Implementation. The client should not receive sedatives unless it is absolutely necessary. If a sedative or narcotic must be given, administer no more than one half to one third the usual dose and then assess the client carefully for signs of respiratory depression or a decreased level of consciousness.

Collaborative Problem: Decreased cardiac output, high risk for R/T sustained bradycardia, edema, and decreased urine output.

Planning: Expected Outcomes. The client will have a normal cardiac output maintained, as evidenced by normal heart rate, evidence of normal perfusion, absence of edema, and urine output of at least 30 ml/hr.

Implementation. As the client takes the hormone replacement, the edema and puffiness will start to lessen. The nurse should continue to monitor intake and output, which becomes more balanced. Urine output should significantly increase during thyroid therapy. The client's daily weight will be monitored.

To help prevent further strain on the already overburdened heart, always help the client to turn so the client is not straining and placing an extra burden on the heart. If any new cardiac symptoms occur, notify the physician immediately. Do not give thyroid hormone until the physician has reappraised the client's condition.

When administering thyroid preparations, assess the client carefully for symptoms of thyrotoxicosis (i.e., tachycardia, increased appetite, diarrhea, sweating, agitation, tremor, palpitations, shortness of breath). If any of these symptoms develop during thyroid therapy, notify the physician at once so the dosage can be reduced.

Nursing Diagnosis: Knowledge Deficit R/T pharmacologic regimen, nutrition, and follow-up care.

Planning: Expected Outcomes. The client will understand the pharmacologic regimen, nutrition, and follow-up required for control of the condition, as evidenced by client's statements and compliance with therapeutic regimen.

Implementation. Once clients are mentally alert, evaluate their knowledge level regarding the disorder and the importance of taking thyroid hormone daily for life. Develop and implement a teaching plan based on each client's needs. Also, provide a written list of the symptoms of thyroid deficiency or excess. Instruct the client and significant others to phone the physician if those symptoms develop.

Endemic goiter can be prevented by the use of iodized salt. Adults require at least 50 μg of iodine per day. However, an adequate iodine intake guaranteed to prevent goiter is 200 to 300 μg/day. Iodized salt, used in the United States since 1924, contains 1 part iodine for every 100,000 parts of salt. Thus, the average person, who ingests approximately 6.2 g of salt a day, is also taking 474 μg of iodine daily if the salt is iodized.

Many clients do not understand the need for iodized salt as a goiter preventive. Some believe that any additive to food or water is harmful and therefore do not use iodized salt. These two problems, plus the fact that many modern foods are processed with cheaper noniodized salt, contribute to the potential for development of simple goiter. Nurses need to educate the public regarding the importance of iodized salt.

EVALUATION

The nurse must evaluate client outcomes on the basis of the established plan of care. If these goals have not been achieved, the plan and interventions must be revised to meet the client's needs.

Modification of Plan of Care for the Elderly

Subclinical hypothyroidism is the combination of elevated TSH levels and normal T_3 and T_4 levels without symptoms. Subclinical hypothyroidism occurs in up to 15 per cent of postmenopausal women.

The most common causes of subclinical hypothyroidism are listed in order of frequency: autoimmune thyroiditis, Hashimoto's thyroiditis, previous thyroid surgery or radioactive treatment, and noncompliance with prescribed T_4 replacements.

Medical treatment is not indicated for those clients who are without symptoms. Those clients with generalized complaints of hypothyroidism may benefit from small doses of T_4, which thus proves that their condition was symptomatic rather than subclinical. Remember, a principal hazard in giving T_4 to an elderly client is the development of ischemic heart disease as evidenced by angina. Client response to therapy and serum levels must be observed closely.

The difficulty in diagnosing hypothyroidism in the elderly is that the symptoms are usually vague and generic to other disease processes. Hypothyroidism must be considered in the differential diagnosis of a variety of conditions affecting the elderly client.

Post-hospital Care

DISCHARGE TEACHING

The discharge teaching centers around the need to understand and follow the medication regimen, symptoms of hyperthyroidism and hypothyroidism, diet, and when to seek medical attention. Teach the client about the need for iodized salt. The client should also be taught to eat a high-fiber diet for preventing constipation.

FOLLOW-UP CARE

The client needs to have thyroid hormone levels checked at intervals until these levels are stabilized and then at regular intervals to be sure the client is maintaining normal levels.

HYPERTHYROIDISM

Definition

Hyperthyroidism is defined as excessive secretion of thyroid hormone; thyrotoxicosis refers to the clinical manifestations that occur when the body tissues are stimulated by this increased thyroid hormone.

Incidence

Hyperthyroidism is a highly preventable endocrine disorder. Like most thyroid conditions, it is predominantly a disorder of women. It affects women four times as often as it does men, especially young women between the ages of 20 and 40 years.

Etiology

Hyperthyroidism may be due to the overfunctioning of the entire gland or, less commonly, may be caused by single or multiple functioning adenomas of thyroid cancer. Also, overtreatment of myxedema with thyroid hormone may result in hyperthyroidism. The most common form of hyperthyroidism is Graves' disease (toxic, diffuse goiter), which has three principal hallmarks: (1) hyperthyroidism, (2) thyroid gland enlargement (goiter), and (3) exophthalmos (abnormal protrusion of the eyes). Graves' disease is likely to be an autoimmune disorder. About 60 to 80 per cent of clients with Graves' disease have circulating autoantibodies that react against thyroglobulin. Also, thyroid-stimulating immunoglobulins (TSI) are present in the serum of 95 per cent of hyperthyroid clients. Evidently, TSI are autoantibodies that react against a component of the thyroid cell membranes, stimulating enlargement of the thyroid gland and secretion of excess thyroid hormone. TSI apparently are not involved in the development of exophthalmos. Also, the severity of the hyperthyroidism cannot be determined by TSI levels in the serum.

Risk Factors

Because the disorder is probably autoimmune in nature, there are no known risk factors or preventive measures.

Pathophysiology

Hyperthyroidism is characterized by loss of the normal regulatory controls of thyroid hormone secretion. Because the action of thyroid hormone on the body is stimulatory, hypermetabolism results, with increased sympathetic nervous system activity.

The excessive amounts of thyroid hormone stimulate the cardiac system and increase the number of beta-adrenergic receptors. This leads to tachycardia and increased cardiac output, stroke volume, adrenergic responsiveness, and peripheral blood flow.

Metabolism increases greatly, leading to a negative nitrogen balance, lipid depletion, and a resultant state of nutritional deficiency.

Hyperthyroidism also results in the alteration of secretion and metabolism of hypothalamic, pituitary, and gonadal hormones. If hyperthyroidism occurs before puberty, sexual development is delayed in both sexes, but after puberty it results in decreased libido in men and women. After puberty, women will also exhibit menstrual irregularities and decreased fertility.

Clinical Manifestations

Because hyperthyroidism is caused by an excess secretion of thyroid hormone, the clinical picture of Graves' disease is in many ways opposite to that of myxedema. Assessment reveals a client who appears extremely agitated and irritable, with a hand tremor at rest. Despite a ravenous appetite, weight loss occurs as a result of the quickened metabolism. Because of the high levels of circulating thyroid hormone, the client's body processes literally "speed up." Manifestations include loose bowel movements, heat intolerance, profuse diaphoresis, tachycardia, and incoordination due to tremor. Also, the skin becomes warm and smooth because of accelerated circulation to the tissues. The hair appears thin and soft (see Table 62-1).

Moreover, the client's emotions are adversely affected by the turbulent activity within the body. Moods may be cyclic, ranging from mild euphoria to extreme hyperactivity or delirium. The excessive hyperactivity in turn leads to extreme fatigue and depression, again followed by episodes of overactivity, and so forth. As a result of the client's chaotic emotional state, interpersonal relationships may deteriorate, further accentuating the emotional disturbance.

Goiter, the second characteristic of Graves' disease, is due to hyperplasia and hypertrophy of the thyroid cells. The gland may enlarge up to three to four times its normal size. Cellular overgrowth results in the release of excessive amounts of thyroid hormone into the blood.

Exophthalmos is the third major manifestation of Graves' disease. The client who suffers from exophthalmos has protruding eyes and a fixed stare due to the accumulation of fluid in the fat pads and muscles that lie behind the eyeballs. Because the eyes are surrounded by unyielding bone, edema forces them forward out of their sockets, producing the typical facies of exophthalmos (Fig. 62-3). In severe cases, clients may be unable to close their eyelids and must have their lids taped shut to protect the eyes. Without intervention, severe exophthalmos can progress to corneal ulceration or infection and loss of vision. In some cases, exophthalmos is not reversed by intervention.

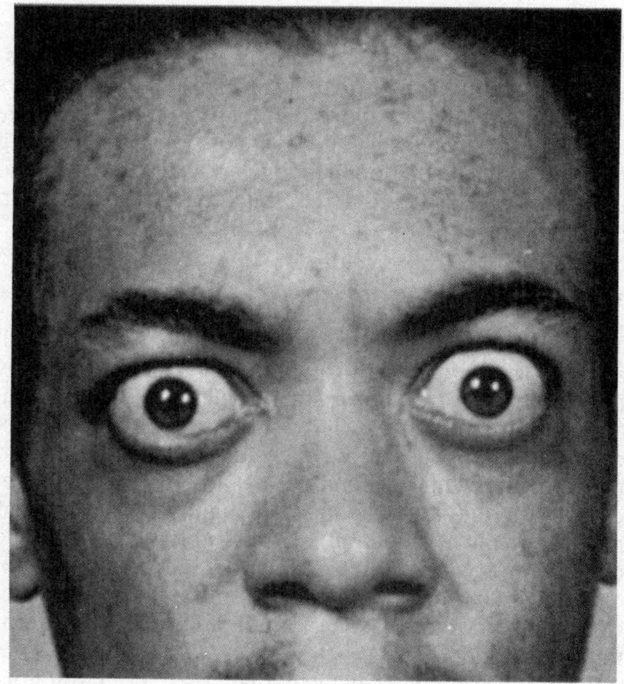

▲ *Figure 62-3*

Extreme exophthalmos in hyperthyroidism. Because the eyes are surrounded by unyielding bone, fluid accumulation in the fat pads and muscles behind the eyeballs causes protruding eyes and a fixed stare in the client with exophthalmos. Without intervention, the client with severe exophthalmos may be unable to close the eyelids and may develop corneal ulceration or infection. Eventually, this can result in total loss of vision. (From Delp, M. H., & Manning, R. T. [1981]. *Major's physical diagnosis* [9th ed.]. Philadelphia: W. B. Saunders.)

DIAGNOSTIC ASSESSMENT

Graves' disease is diagnosed on the basis of (1) the client's often striking physical appearance (enlarged neck, protruding eyes, agitated expression); (2) the symptoms of agitation, restlessness, and weight loss; and (3) laboratory findings. The serum thyroid hormone levels are usually all elevated, although they occasionally may be within the normal range (so-called euthyroid Graves' disease). Serum cholesterol levels are usually depressed. Refer to Table 62-2 for usual laboratory findings.

Complications

The three major complications of Graves' disease are (1) exophthalmos, (2) heart disease, and (3) thyroid storm (thyroid crisis, thyrotoxicosis).

EXOPHTHALMOS

Unlike the manifestations of goiter and hyperthyroidism, exophthalmos does not necessarily regress with therapy. Diuretics may alleviate some of the periorbital edema. Glucocorticoids such as prednisone are given in large doses to reduce inflammation of the periorbital tissues. Unfortunately, steroids produce many undesirable side effects, including acute psychoses. Estrogen therapy is occasionally of value in postmenopausal women. Methylcellulose eye drops, 1/4 per cent four times daily, help reduce eye irritation. Radiation therapy to the retro-orbital tissues may help in severe cases. Surgical decompression of the orbits may be performed when all other measures fail to correct the exophthalmos. This procedure may save the client's vision when eye changes are severe.

A number of general nursing interventions also help to reduce eye discomfort and prevent corneal ulceration and infection. Instruct clients with exophthalmos to wear dark glasses. Warn them to avoid getting dust or dirt in their eyes. When they cannot close their eyelids easily or at all, have them wear a sleeping mask (available in drug stores) or lightly tape the eyes shut with nonallergic tape. Elevate the head of the bed at night and have the client restrict salt intake to relieve edema.

HEART DISEASE

Heart disease, the second complication of Graves' disease, poses a serious threat. Tachycardia almost always accompanies thyrotoxicosis, and atrial fibrillation may also appear. Congestive heart failure is found among older clients with long-standing thyrotoxicosis. The treatment of these cardiac complications is discussed in detail in Unit 9.

THYROID STORM (THYROTOXICOSIS)

Thyroid storm (thyrotoxicosis) is a sometimes fatal, acute episode of thyroid overactivity characterized by high fever, severe tachycardia, delirium, dehydration, and extreme irritability. It was once a commonly occurring crisis but seldom develops today, thanks to modern intervention techniques. Factors that may precipitate thyroid storm include undiagnosed or untreated hyperthyroidism, infection, thyroid ablation, metabolic catastrophes, surgery, trauma, labor and delivery, myocardial infarction, pulmonary embolus, medication overdosage, or inadequate preparation of clients for thyroid surgery.

Thyroid storm is a clinical diagnosis; no laboratory tests serve to differentiate hyperthyroidism from thyroid storm in general.

Because it is an emergency, thyroid storm requires heroic intervention for control. The high fever is treated with hypothermic blankets; dehydration is reversed with intravenous fluids. Treatment of thyroid storm involves suppressing hormonal release, inhibiting hormonal synthesis, blocking conversion of T_4 to the more active T_3, and inhibiting the effects of thyroid hormone on body tissues as well as treating the precipitating cause, if known. Blockade of thyroid hormone release is usually achieved by the administration of iodides such as SSKI given orally. Sodium iodide may be given intravenously. Glucocorticoid dexamethasone and propylthiouracil are also commonly used oral drugs. Beta-blockers are given to decrease the effects of sympathetic nervous system stimulation and for treating tachycardia.

Medical Management

PHARMACOLOGIC MANAGEMENT

The goals of care for clients with Graves' disease are to curtail the excessive secretion of thyroid hormone and to prevent and treat complications. Choice of intervention is based on (1) age, (2) goiter size, and (3) whether other health problems exist.

The three major forms of therapy are (1) antithyroid medication, (2) radioiodine, and (3) surgery.

Antithyroid Medication Therapy. This intervention is recommended for clients under 18 years of age and for pregnant women. The major medications used to control hyperthyroidism include the thioureas, propylthiouracil, and methimazole (see Table 62-3). Adrenergic blocking agents may also be administered as adjunctive therapy.

Propylthiouracil is the most commonly used antithyroid medication. It corrects hyperthyroidism by impairing thyroid hormone synthesis. With the usual dosage regimen, propylthiouracil ameliorates Graves' disease within 4 to 8 weeks. However, several months may pass before symptoms completely abate. Once euthyroid, the client is given a maintenance dose of propylthiouracil, usually three times daily. Propylthiouracil, although an ideal medication in many ways, causes significant side effects in about 9 per cent of clients using it.

The most serious toxic effect is agranulocytosis (see Chap. 24). A white blood cell (WBC) count should be obtained before initial administration of the medication. Instruct clients to report a sore throat, fever, or rash immediately to their physician so that further WBC tests can be performed and their condition evaluated. Less severe adverse reactions include mild allergies (rash and pruritus). Rarely, the client develops hepatitis or drug fever.

Methimazole (Tapazole) acts to block the action of thyroid hormone in the body. Unfortunately, methimazole also produces agranulocytosis in a small percentage of people.

Iodine therapy is prescribed for two reasons: (1) to reduce the vascularity of the thyroid gland before subtotal or total thyroidectomy and (2) to treat "thyroid storm" (see earlier). Iodine preparations temporarily act to prevent release of thyroid hormone into the circulation by increasing the amount of thyroid hormone stored within the gland. However, the stored thyroid hormone is eventually released back into the circulation, once again producing hyperthyroidism. For this reason, iodine preparations are usually given only for a 10- to 14-day period before surgery. If iodine is given for a longer period or if it is given alone (i.e., not in combination with propylthiouracil), the thyroid gland may "escape" before thyroidectomy. "Escape of the thyroid" means that the iodine is no longer capable of maintaining thyroid hormone storage. As a result, thyroid hormone floods the circulation, and hyperthyroidism returns in a more severe form than before.

The iodine medication of choice is SSKI. Lugol's solution is also used but is more expensive than SSKI and tends to inactivate antithyroid preparations within the bowel.

Adrenergic blocking agents are sometimes given as adjunctive therapy to control the activity of the sympathetic nervous system. There is now evidence that these agents are of great benefit to the "hyperthyroid heart," which has an increased sensitivity to catecholamines and an increased number of beta-adrenergic receptor sites. Therefore, these agents help lessen distressing symptoms such as palpitations and tachycardia. Tremor and nervousness may also be alleviated by adrenergic blocking agents. These medications include propranolol and reserpine.

Radioiodine Therapy. Therapy with ^{131}I is principally prescribed for middle-aged and elderly clients. This intervention offers many advantages: it is economical, is simple to administer, and can be prescribed on an outpatient basis. Radiotherapy is contraindicated for pregnant women and is rarely used for children.

The rationale behind ^{131}I therapy for Graves' disease is simple. The thyroid gland is unable to distinguish between regular iodine atoms and radioiodine atoms. Consequently, when the client receives a dose of ^{131}I, the thyroid gland picks up the radioiodine and concentrates it just as it would regular iodine. As a result, the cells that concentrate ^{131}I to make T_4 are destroyed by the local irradiation. Thus, thyroid hormone secretion diminishes, and the signs of hyperthyroidism and goiter disappear. However, because radioiodine destroys thyroid cells, one of the major possible complications of ^{131}I therapy is myxedema. Therefore, assess for symptoms of hypothyroidism after ^{131}I therapy.

^{131}I is administered orally dissolved in water. Dosage is determined both by the size of the gland and by the thyroid's uptake of a tracer dose of radioiodine. After receiving the radioiodine, the client may go home unless the dosage is extremely large. In the latter case, the client must be placed in isolation for several days to prevent radioactive contamination. The symptoms of hyperthyroidism usually subside within 6 to 12 weeks after ^{131}I administration. Sometimes, resistant clients require a second or (in rare cases) third dose of radioiodine. Once they become euthyroid, clients still need regular medical check-ups, because hypothyroidism may develop several years after radiotherapy. Clients who become hypothyroid require lifelong hormone replacement with thyroid preparations.

DIETARY MANAGEMENT

The client with hyperthyroidism needs a high-calorie, high-protein diet to compensate for the hypermetabolic state of the body. A diet of 4000 to 5000 calories with high protein levels may be necessary to prevent the negative nitrogen balance and weight loss that occurs.

Surgical Management

Surgery for hyperthyroidism has been performed since the early 1880s. Ideally, those selected are young and free from any condition that makes them poor operative risks (e.g., diabetes, heart disease, renal disease, drug allergies).

A thyroidectomy (removal of the thyroid gland) may be total or partial. Total thyroidectomy is performed to remove thyroid cancer. Clients who undergo this operation must take thyroid hormone on a permanent basis. Subtotal thyroidectomy is performed to correct hyperthyroidism and extreme cases of simple goiter. Approximately five sixths of the gland is removed, but because one sixth of the functioning gland is left intact, hormonal replacements may not be necessary.

Preoperative preparation for a subtotal thyroidectomy is extremely important. The client must be euthyroid before the operation, if possible. If the client is not euthyroid, the risk of thyroid storm occurring postoperatively is greatly increased. Therefore, preoperative care for clients with Graves' disease includes administration of (1) antithyroid drugs to suppress secretion of thyroid hormone and (2) iodine preparations to reduce the size and vascularity of the organ, thereby diminishing the chance of hemorrhage. Clients should be adequately rested, at optimal weight, and in good health before entering the operating room. Adequate preoperative preparation may take as long as 2 to 3 months.

Surgical treatment is effective in most people with Graves' disease. A small percentage remain hyperthyroid, and some develop hypothyroidism. Rarely, vocal cord paralysis or hypoparathyroidism may develop as a result of nerve damage or inadvertent removal of parathyroid gland tissue, respectively.

Nursing Management

ASSESSMENT

The nurse should begin the assessment by obtaining a complete client history. By asking questions concerning weight, appetite, activity, heat intolerance, and bowel activity, the nurse can assess for the presence of typical signs and symptoms of hyperthyroidism.

The nurse should assess the client for all the typical clinical manifestations associated with Graves' disease. Symptoms of the hypermetabolic state may be obvious with apparent weight loss, and exophthalmos may be readily apparent. The client should also be questioned regarding visual difficulties, fatigue, weakness, tremors, or insomnia.

The nurse should also question significant others about mood alterations experienced by the client. Mood swings, irritability, decreased attention span, and manic behavior may be experienced by the client with hyperthyroidism. Although the client may not be aware of some of the mood changes, the significant others can usually notice the change.

NURSING INTERVENTION

Nursing Diagnosis: Nutrition, Altered: Less than Body Requirements R/T accelerated metabolic rate.

Planning: Expected Outcomes. The client's weight loss will stop, as evidenced by client's ability to take in sufficient calories to return to ideal body weight.

Implementation. Provide the client with a well-balanced, high-calorie diet. Clients with Graves' disease are usually extremely hungry because of the increased metabolism. Six full meals a day may be needed to satisfy their appetite. However, they may lose weight rapidly despite unusually large meals. Also, they usually are in a state of negative nitrogen balance. Therefore, encourage them to eat foods that are nutritious and contain ample amounts of protein, carbohydrates, fats, and minerals. Discourage eating of foods that increase peristalsis and thus result in diarrhea (e.g., highly seasoned, bulky, or fibrous foods). Clients should be weighed daily, and weight losses of more than 2 kg (4.4 lb) should be reported. If they continue to appear malnourished despite an ample diet, supplemental vitamins, particularly vitamin B complex, may be needed.

Nursing Diagnosis: Activity Intolerance R/T exhaustion secondary to accelerated metabolic rate.

Planning: Expected Outcomes. The client will be able to engage in normal level of activity, as evidenced by client's ability to maintain a proper balance of rest and activity to prevent exhaustion.

Implementation. Provide the client with an environment that is restful both mentally and physically. It is a challenge to help hyperthyroid clients relax. Assign these clients to a private room to promote rest and to prevent them from disturbing others through hyperactivity and restlessness.

Collaborative Problem. Injury, high risk for: corneal ulcerations, infection, and possible blindness R/T inability to close eyelids secondary to exophthalmos.

Planning: Expected Outcomes. The nurse will prevent corneal ulceration, infection, or blindness, as evidenced by no further development of exophthalmos.

Implementation. The treatment should be started as soon as possible once the diagnosis is made so exophthalmos can be avoided, because the condition is irreversible. The client should use artificial tears and eye patches as needed to prevent irritation if the exophthalmos has already occurred.

Nursing Diagnosis: Hyperthermia R/T accelerated metabolic rate.

Planning: Expected Outcomes. The client will not exhibit hyperthermia, as evidenced by return to normal body temperature.

Implementation. Provide the client with a cool environment. Remember that clients with Graves' disease suffer from heat intolerance. Use only a lightweight sheet for the top cover, and give them light loose pajamas. If the client is diaphoretic, the nurse may need to change the bedsheets and clothes frequently.

Nursing Diagnosis: Social Interaction, Impaired R/T extreme agitation, hyperactivity, and mood swings.

Planning: Expected Outcomes. The client will not suffer from impaired social interaction, as evidenced by client's ability to interact without difficulty without agitation, hyperactivity, or mood swings.

Implementation. Explain to significant others that any bizarre, difficult behavior is likely to be temporary and should steadily improve with intervention. Maintain a quiet, understanding manner when caring for clients with Graves' disease. Accept their irritation and emotional outbursts as normal expressions of the disease.

Incorporate occupational therapy into care planning. The occupational therapist may be able to provide clients with simple activities designed to distract them from focusing on the disorder (e.g., putting together a puzzle with large pieces, molding clay, watching television). For a very restless client, discuss with the physician the need for a sedative (such as Valium) or possibly one of the adrenergic blocking agents.

Collaborative Problem: High risk for injury R/T preoperative preparation, euthyroid state, and surgical procedure.

Planning: Expected Outcomes. The client will not suffer injury, as evidenced by client's statements of understanding of preoperative preparation; euthyroid state preoperatively; and absence of hemorrhage, respiratory distress, loss of voice, hypocalcemia, tetany, or thyroid storm.

Implementation. Clients must be carefully prepared for a thyroidectomy for avoidance of complications (such as thyroid storm, hemorrhage). Outcomes of successful preparation of clients for thyroid surgery include

- The client is euthyroid before entering the operating room. Tests of thyroid function must be within normal limits.
- Signs of thyrotoxicosis are greatly diminished or absent. The client appears rested and relaxed.
- Weight and nutritional status are normal, and any weight losses suffered earlier have been regained.
- Cardiac problems are under control, pulse rate is normal, and electrocardiographic tracings taken preoperatively show no dangerous arrhythmias.

For help in meeting these outcomes, the client undergoing a thyroidectomy is treated with antithyroid drugs, iodine preparations, bed rest, a nutritious diet, and supplemental vitamins. Thorough preparation may take months. However, once good health has been restored, the client can undergo surgery with confidence that the operation will be successful and the symptoms alleviated.

The immediate goals of postoperative care after a thyroidectomy are to (1) maintain airway patency, (2) decrease the strain in the suture line, (3) relieve discomfort from the sore throat and tracheal irritation, (4) prevent pooling of respiratory secretions, and (5) prevent or relieve the complications of thyroidectomy.

Typical postoperative orders, their rationale, and important associated nursing interventions are outlined in Table 62–4. Assemble the equipment at the bedside before the client returns from surgery (e.g., blood pressure cuff and stethoscope, additional pillows, oxygen, suction equipment, intubation supplies, and a tracheostomy set). Ampules of calcium gluconate should also be on hand in the medicine room or on the emergency cart.

Major complications after a thyroidectomy may include

- respiratory obstruction due to edema of the glottis, bilateral laryngeal nerve damage, or tracheal compression from hemorrhage

TABLE 62-4. Postoperative Orders, Rationale, and Associated Nursing Interventions After Thyroidectomy

Postoperative Order	Rationale	Associated Nursing Interventions
Vital signs every 15 min until stable; then every 30 min for next 12 h	After thyroidectomy, hemorrhage and respiratory obstruction may develop. Elevated pulse and hypotension indicate hemorrhage and shock. Dyspnea, stridulous respirations, and retraction of neck tissues indicate respiratory obstruction.	Check dressing after checking vital signs. Observe for bleeding at front, sides, and back of neck. Examine back of client's neck and shoulders for bleeding because blood tends to drain posteriorly. Check dressing for tightness; uncomfortable tautness may indicate bleeding into tissues. Loosen dressing and call surgeon immediately.
Semi-Fowler's position when conscious unless client is hypotensive; support head and neck with pillows and sandbags; ambulate second day as tolerated	Immobilization of head and neck is essential to prevent flexion and hyperextension of neck with resultant strain on suture line. Semi-Fowler's position is used for comfort.	Place sandbags on either side of client's head for immobilization and maintenance of good alignment. Warn client not to extend or hyperextend neck; reassure client that sandbags will prevent moving head too much. Gently rub back of client's neck to relieve tension. Support client's head and neck when moving or changing position.
Fluids by mouth as tolerated; if nausea or vomiting, notify surgeon; soft diet on afternoon of second day	Give intravenous fluids if nauseated or vomiting. Otherwise, start oral fluids as soon as client is fully conscious.	Maintain intake and output record for 2 or 3 days. Assess for difficulty swallowing. Normally this problem lasts for only 1 or 2 days postoperatively. Weigh client once a full diet is started; weight lost during early postoperative period should be regained.
Meperidine (Demerol) or morphine sulfate, every 3–4 hr as needed for pain in throat area	Demerol and morphine sulfate are both used during early postoperative period to relieve pain and promote rest.	Do not give narcotics if respirations below 12/min or if respiratory congestion; consult physician for further orders.
Cough and deep breathe every half hour; suction mouth and trachea if necessary	Pooling of mucous secretions in trachea, bronchi, and lungs will cause respiratory obstruction with resultant atelectasis and pneumonia. Secretions must be raised to prevent respiratory complications.	Instruct client to cough and deep breathe as taught during preoperative period. If client cannot raise secretions, gently suction mouth and trachea. Do not oversedate clients with profuse respiratory secretions; give narcotics judiciously.
Tracheostomy set, endotracheal tube, laryngoscope, and oxygen on hand in room	Acute respiratory obstruction due to hemorrhage, edema of glottis, laryngeal nerve damage, or tetany is an emergency. Equipment for establishing an airway and administering oxygen must be available for immediate use.	Continuously assess for signs of airway obstruction, e.g., increasing restlessness, tachycardia, apprehension, cyanosis, stridulous respirations, and retraction of neck tissues. Report any of these signs to surgeon immediately.
Continuous mist inhalation until chest clear	Humidification of air promotes easier breathing and helps to liquefy mucous secretions.	Keep doors closed so that moist air is retained in room.
Rectal temperature every 4 hr for 24 hr, then orally	One of the first signs of thyroid storm is an elevated temperature.	Carefully assess for signs of thyroid storm: elevated temperature, extreme restlessness, agitation, and tachycardia. Report any elevation over 37.7° C (100° F) rectally or 37.2° C (99° F) orally.

- hemorrhage
- weakness and hoarseness of the voice due to trauma or damage of one laryngeal nerve
- hypocalcemia and tetany resulting from accidental removal of one or more parathyroid glands
- thyroid storm

Temporary hoarseness and voice weakness may occur if there has been unilateral injury to the recurrent laryngeal nerve during surgery. To assess the client's voice, ask "What is your name?" as soon as full recovery from anesthesia occurs. Have the client speak every 30 to 60 minutes thereafter, and carefully note any voice changes. If hoarseness or voice weakness is present, reassure the client the problem will probably subside in a few days. Discourage unnecessary talking to minimize hoarseness.

Muscular twitching and hyperirritability of the nervous system may indicate hypocalcemic tetany. Hypocalcemia can develop after thyroidectomy if the parathyroid glands are accidentally removed during surgery. Symptoms may develop 1 to 7 days after surgery. If the client develops numbness and tingling around the mouth, fingertips or toes, muscle spasms, or twitching, call the physician immediately. Make sure calcium gluconate ampules are available.

Nursing Diagnosis: Knowledge Deficit R/T medications, eye care, and possible complications.

Planning: Expected Outcomes. The client will understand eye care and possible complications, as evidenced by client's statements and ability to comply with medication regimen.

Implementation. Once the immediate postoperative period and its dangers have passed, turn your attention to teaching. Several important areas should be included in your teaching. First, teach the client how to support the weight of the head and neck when sitting up in bed. Show clients how to place their hands at the back of the head when flexing the neck or moving. Usually, they are able to perform this maneuver by the first postoperative day. Second, as the wound heals (around the second to fourth postoperative day), instruct the client in range-of-motion exercises for prevention of contractures. With the surgeon's permission, teach clients to flex the head forward and laterally, to hyperextend the neck, and to turn the head from side to side. Have them perform these exercises several times every day. Third, if a total thyroidectomy has been performed, give instruction concerning self-administration of thyroid medications, as outlined previously under Hypothyroidism.

EVALUATION

The nurse must evaluate client outcomes on the basis of the established plan of care. If these goals have not been achieved, the plan and interventions must be revised to meet the client's needs.

Modification of Plan of Care for the Elderly

Hyperthyroidism in the elderly accounts for 10 to 15 per cent of all thyrotoxic clients. Some clients present with typical symptoms of hyperthyroidism, especially when the diagnosis is Graves' disease. However, hyperthyroidism in the elderly is also notorious for presenting with atypical or minimal symptoms. It is often overlooked because the symptoms and signs are not the usual ones. The symptoms are frequently attributed to aging. Weight loss, lack of eye findings, and normal-sized thyroid glands are frequently found on assessment. Many clients actually appear apathetic instead of hyperactive. Cardiovascular abnormalities such as congestive heart failure, atrial arrhythmias (usually digoxin resistant), and various degrees of heart block are much more common in the elderly. A relative lack of tachycardia has been documented; approximately 40 per cent of elderly clients have heart rates less than 100.

The diagnosis of hyperthyroidism is established by appropriate laboratory tests. It is usual to find an elevated T_4 and a suppressed TSH. Therapy for hyperthyroidism in the elderly is radioactive iodine.

Post-hospital Care

DISCHARGE TEACHING

Teach the client the medication regimen and the need for lifelong replacement therapy. Make an appointment for the clinic or physician's office after discharge. Emphasize that the client who has had a thyroidectomy must see a physician at least twice yearly for averting possible complications (e.g., hypothyroidism, hypoparathyroidism, or recurrent hyperthyroidism).

HOME HEALTH CARE NEEDS

The nurse should teach the client how to care for the incision once it has healed with the use of lanolin cream to soften the wound. This will help to lessen the scar.

FOLLOW-UP CARE

As stated previously, the client needs to have the levels of thyroid hormone measured at regular intervals until the replacement medication is adjusted to a maintenance dose. The client should then see the physician twice a year for check-ups.

THYROIDITIS

Definition

Thyroiditis simply means inflammation of the thyroid gland. It appears in three basic forms: (1) acute suppurative, (2) subacute granulomatous and lymphocytic, and (3) chronic (Hashimoto's disease).

Incidence

Acute and subacute thyroiditis are uncommon disorders. Acute thyroiditis is more common in women, usually between the ages of 20 and 40 years, although it does occur in both children and the elderly; 80 per cent of the cases of subacute granulomatous thyroiditis are in women between the ages of 40 and 50 years. There also appears to be a genetic predisposition for the subacute disease. Chronic thyroiditis is more common in women than in men and most commonly occurs in the third to fifth decade of life.

Etiology

Acute suppurative thyroiditis is an uncommon inflammatory disease usually caused by bacterial invasion of the thyroid gland. *Streptococcus pyogenes, Staphylococcus aureus,* and *Pneumococcus pneumoniae* are the most common etiologic agents.

Subacute granulomatous thyroiditis is a self-limiting inflammatory condition. No etiologic agent has yet been identified, although it may be viral in origin and frequently follows a respiratory infection. Recently, autoimmune abnormalities have been described. There also appears to be a genetic predisposition to the development of both subacute granulomatous and lymphocytic thyroiditis.

Chronic thyroiditis (Hashimoto's thyroiditis), a long-term inflammatory disorder, is the most common form of thyroiditis. Like Graves' disease, chronic thyroiditis has an autoimmune basis. Genetic predisposition also plays a role in its causation.

Pathophysiology

The inflammation associated with the autoimmune thyroiditis results in enlargement of the gland or goiter. In subacute thyroiditis, hyperthyroidism occurs; in chronic thyroiditis, the client remains euthyroid or in some cases hypothyroid if the gland is destroyed by the autoimmune process. Occasionally in chronic thyroiditis, the client may appear hyperthyroid because of the leakage of previously produced thyroid hormone from damaged cells. There are immune antibodies found in diagnostic tests in subacute lymphocytic thyroiditis.

Clinical Manifestations

Symptoms of acute thyroiditis include abrupt onset of unilateral anterior neck pain, with possible radiation to the ear or mandible on the affected side. Fever, diaphoresis, and other symptoms of bacterial toxicity may also be present.

Subacute granulomatous thyroiditis is usually painful, whereas subacute lymphocytic thyroiditis is usually painless. Assessment data may include characteristic anterior, unilateral neck pain that may occur with an abrupt onset. Radiation to the ear on the ipsilateral side may occur. Symptoms like viral infection may be present that consist of myalgia, low-grade fever, lassitude, and sore throat.

Subacute lymphocytic thyroiditis is characterized by occasional hyperthyroidism and a painless goiter. The goiter is very firm, diffuse, and mildly enlarged.

Symptoms of chronic thyroiditis include painless, asymmetric enlargement of the gland, which in turn causes pressure on the surrounding structures and can lead to dysphagia and respiratory distress. Most clients are euthyroid; about 20 per cent are hypothyroid, and less than 5 per cent are hyperthyroid.

DIAGNOSTIC ASSESSMENT

Clients with acute thyroiditis are typically euthyroid by laboratory tests.

For subacute granulomatous thyroiditis, laboratory findings reveal hyperthyroidism in approximately 50 per cent of the clients. With subacute lymphocytic thyroiditis, laboratory diagnosis includes decreased RAIU, elevated T_3 and T_4, and frequently positive thyroid antibodies.

In chronic thyroiditis, immune antibodies are usually positive. The other thyroid function tests may be normal, increased, or decreased.

Medical Management

The course of Hashimoto's thyroiditis varies. Some clients experience spontaneous remission, whereas others remain stable for years. In approximately one third of the cases, hypothyroidism develops owing to gradual atrophy of the gland. Intervention is directed toward reducing the size of the gland and correcting any thyroid function abnormalities.

Acute thyroiditis usually responds to parenteral antibiotic therapy.

Treatment for subacute granulomatous thyroiditis includes salicylates, nonsteroidal anti-inflammatory agents, and oral glucocorticoids such as prednisone.

The treatment goal for subacute lymphocytic thyroiditis is to provide relief of symptoms from the hyperthyroidism with beta-adrenergic blocking agents. Antithyroid medications are not indicated.

Surgical Management

Acute thyroiditis that does not respond to medical treatment may require incision and drainage of the affected gland.

Nursing Management

Nursing care for clients with thyroiditis is usually supportive until the diagnosis is made. The care then, as with other thyroid disorders, revolves around helping the client learn correct medication administration. If surgery is necessary, then care is the same as discussed earlier.

Post-hospital Care

DISCHARGE TEACHING

As with other clients with thyroid disorders, discharge teaching is centered on making sure that clients understand their medication and how to take it.

FOLLOW-UP CARE

Clients should have their thyroid functions measured at regular intervals after discharge for monitoring the development of hyperthyroidism or hypothyroidism and for testing the effectiveness of medication.

THYROID CANCER

Definition

There are four distinctive histologic types of thyroid cancer: papillary, follicular, medullary, and anaplastic. Benign adenomas and malignant thyroid tumors constitute the third cause of thyroid enlargement (hypothyroidism and hyperthyroidism constitute the first two causes). Like other benign tumors, most thyroid adenomas are usually well encapsulated and consequently do not spread out or extend into other tissues.

Incidence

Malignant tumors of the thyroid are rare. They account for approximately three to four new cases per 100,000 population per year in the United States. Thyroid cancer accounts for approximately 0.2 per cent of cancer deaths; it develops mainly in women between the ages of 40 and 60 years. Females are affected 2.5 : 1.

Etiology

Benign adenomas are usually not dangerous, although they rarely grow large enough to cause respiratory symptoms by pressing against the trachea. Occasionally, however, malignant transformation occurs, and the benign nodules become cancerous. Also, malignant transformation of benign nodules can apparently follow prolonged stimulation of the thyroid gland by the pituitary hormone TSH.

Risk Factors

Thyroid carcinoma occurs more frequently among clients who have received large doses of radiation to the head and neck. Prevention centers around avoiding radiation to the area, shielding the thyroid area if possible if radiation is done, and closely following clients who had radiation to that area.

Pathophysiology

There are four major types of thyroid cancer: (1) papillary adenocarcinoma, (2) follicular adenocarcinoma, (3) medullary carcinoma, and (4) anaplastic carcinoma. The incidence, characteristics, intervention, and prognosis of each of these thyroid cancers are compared in Table 62 – 5.

Clinical Manifestations

The major manifestation of thyroid cancer is the appearance of a hard, painless nodule in an enlarged thyroid gland. The nodule itself is typically solitary, rapidly enlarging, and "cold" (i.e., it does not take up radioactive iodine) as opposed to benign adenomas, which may take up radioactive iodine. Also, if the tumor has already metastasized, the client's lymph nodes are sometimes palpable. In long-standing cases, the client may suffer from respiratory difficulty and dysphagia, again due to the enlarged thyroid's pressing against neck structures.

DIAGNOSTIC ASSESSMENT

Thyroid cancer is diagnosed by fine-needle aspiration and biopsy.

Medical Management

Chemotherapy, ^{131}I, or external radiation may also be used for metastasis. These have been discussed previously.

Surgical Management

Treatment usually includes removal of all or part of the thyroid. Neck resection may be done for metastases to the neck. Thyroid surgery is covered earlier in this chapter.

As with a thyroidectomy for noncancerous lesions, the major complications postoperatively are respiratory distress, recurrent laryngeal damage, hemorrhage, and hypoparathyroidism.

Nursing Management

Nursing care for the client with thyroid cancer is similar to the care of any client undergoing a thyroidectomy. The client will also need the support and teaching a

TABLE 62–5. Types of Thyroid Cancer: Incidence, Characteristics, Intervention, and Prognosis

Type	Incidence	Characteristics	Intervention	Prognosis
Papillary adenocarcinoma	Comprises 60% of thyroid cancers Mainly affects clients in 40s	Slow-growing firm tumor Palpable nodule Spreads to regional nodes in approximately 50% of cases Radiation-related thyroid cancer with 10- to 20-year latency period	Total or near-total thyroidectomy Others recommend lobectomy and isthmectomy	Excellent if cancer restricted to thyroid gland Surgery usually curative
Follicular adenocarcinoma	Comprises 15% of thyroid cancers Mainly affects clients in 50s	Slow-growing nodule with about 15% metastasis to regional nodes at diagnosis Associated with radiation, iodine deficiency, endemic goiter	Total thyroidectomy	Good but inferior to that of papillary adenocarcinoma
Medullary carcinoma	Comprises 5–10% of thyroid cancers Mainly affects clients 40–50s	Tumor is hereditary and familial Tends to secrete adrenocorticotropic hormone, serotonin Metastases to surrounding structures at diagnosis in 50%	Total thyroidectomy Radical neck resection if metastasis	Poor; mean survival = 6.6 years
Anaplastic carcinoma	Comprises 5–15% of thyroid cancers Mainly affects clients 60–70s	Highly malignant Grows rapidly Local and widespread metastasis within 1 year	Combination of thyroidectomy, external radiation therapy, chemotherapy, and tracheostomy as needed	Grave; mean survival = 6.2 months; 5-year survival = 7.1%

cancer client requires. If the client is to undergo chemotherapy, then additional teaching is needed.

Post-hospital Care

DISCHARGE TEACHING

If the client has total thyroidectomy, replacement of the thyroid hormone is necessary. Discharge teaching is centered on making sure the client understands the medication and how to take it.

HOME HEALTH CARE NEEDS

There are no special home health care needs other than the needs of a client after thyroidectomy or the home health care needs for a client on chemotherapy or radiation therapy.

FOLLOW-UP CARE

The client should be checked at regular intervals for recurrence and also should have thyroid function monitored.

▼ PARATHYROID DISORDERS

HYPERPARATHYROIDISM

Definition

Hyperparathyroidism is a disorder caused by overactivity of one or more of the parathyroid glands. Hyperparathyroidism is classified as primary, secondary, or tertiary.

Incidence

Hyperparathyroidism usually occurs in clients over the age of 60 years and affects women 2:1 in a population of 1000. It is not age-related in the renal client.

Etiology

Primary hyperparathyroidism develops when the normal regulatory relationship between serum calcium levels and parathyroid hormone (PTH) secretion is interrupted. This occurs when either an adenoma or hyperplasia of the gland exists without an identifying injury.

Secondary hyperparathyroidism occurs when the glands are hyperplastic from malfunction of another organ system. This is usually the result of renal failure but may also occur with osteogenesis imperfecta, Paget's disease, multiple myeloma, and carcinoma with bone metastasis.

Tertiary hyperparathyroidism occurs when PTH production is irrepressible (autonomous) in clients with normal or low serum calcium levels.

Risk Factors

The risk factors vary on the basis of whether it is primary, secondary, or tertiary. In the presence of other disorders, the best secondary prevention is early detection in those clients who are at high risk. Screening of the serum calcium level is important in these clients so interventions can be taken early.

Pathophysiology

The normal function of PTH is to increase bone resorption, thereby maintaining the proper balance of calcium and phosphorus ions within the blood (see Chap. 56). Excessive circulating PTH leads to bone damage, hypercalcemia, and kidney damage.

BONE DAMAGE

Oversecretion of PTH causes excessive osteoclast growth and activity within the bones. Osteoclasts are large multinuclear cells that are active in promoting resorption of bone. When bone resorption is increased, calcium is released from the bones into the blood, causing hypercalcemia. Thus, the bones suffer demineralization as a result of calcium loss. In time, the bones may become so fragile that they cause pathologic bone changes including kyphosis of the dorsal spine and compression fractures of the vertebral bodies. Also, as the uncontrolled osteoclast proliferation continues, the skeleton may develop cystic lesions. If this condition is not corrected, the client eventually may develop a severe bone disease called *osteitis fibrosa cystica* (von Recklinghausen's disease of bone).

HYPERCALCEMIA

An increased serum calcium level is the consequence of bone resorption due to excessive PTH secretion. Hypercalcemia eventually results in hypercalciuria (excessive calcium in the urine). Also, because of the high serum calcium levels, excess calcium may precipitate as calcium phosphate in the kidneys, lungs, muscles, heart, and eyes. Hypercalcemia can stimulate hypergastrinemia, abdominal pain, and peptic ulcer disease. Pancreatitis is also influenced by high serum calcium levels.

KIDNEY DAMAGE

Excessive PTH levels cause hyperphosphaturia. As serum calcium continues to rise in hyperparathyroidism, excessive amounts of both phosphorus and calcium are excreted and lost from the body. Large amounts of both calcium and phosphate are being excreted by the renal system, so calcium phosphate may be deposited within the renal tubules, causing a kidney condition called *nephrocalcinosis*. Calcium salts are quite insoluble in urine. Thus, kidney stones composed of calcium phosphate may be found in the urine of clients with primary hyperparathyroidism.

If hyperparathyroidism is surgically treated early in its course, the chance of total recovery is good. Bone pain may disappear within 3 days after removal of parathyroid tissue, and bone lesions may heal completely. Unfortunately, serious renal disease may not be reversible by parathyroid surgery.

Clinical Manifestations

Some clients with hyperparathyroidism may be entirely asymptomatic. Others suffer from a myriad of symptoms arising from the skeletal disease, renal involvement, gastrointestinal tract disorders, and neurologic abnormalities (Table 62–6).

Manifestations of bone disease range from backache, joint pain, and bone pain to pathologic fractures of the spine, ribs, and long bones. In long-standing cases, assessment reveals deformity and bending of the bones.

TABLE 62–6. Characteristics of Hyperparathyroidism and Hypoparathyroidism

Hyperparathyroidism	Hypoparathyroidism
Increased bone resorption	Decreased bone resorption
Elevated serum calcium levels	Depressed serum calcium levels
Depressed serum phosphate levels	Elevated serum phosphate levels
Hypercalciuria and hyperphosphaturia	Hypocalciuria and hypophosphaturia
Decreased neuromuscular irritability	Increased neuromuscular activity, which may progress to tetany

Symptoms of renal involvement include (1) polyuria and polydipsia; (2) the appearance of sand, gravel, or stones within the urine; (3) azotemia; and (4) hypertension due to renal damage. Without intervention, renal insufficiency may progress to fatal renal hypertension and uremia.

Hypercalcemia mainly produces gastrointestinal tract manifestations (e.g., thirst, nausea, anorexia, constipation, ileus, and abdominal pain). Often, clients have a history of peptic ulcer or gastrointestinal tract bleeding. Assessment may also reveal psychiatric symptoms. Listlessness, depression, and paranoia are sometimes associated with high levels of serum calcium. Finally, calcium may form calcification within the eyes, impairing vision.

The major complications of hyperparathyroidism are the symptoms associated with hypercalcemia and those associated with treatment such as dehydration, hypocalcemia, and gastrointestinal tract symptoms.

DIAGNOSTIC ASSESSMENT

The diagnosis of hyperparathyroidism mainly rests on laboratory and x-ray findings. Serum calcium is elevated, whereas serum phosphate is depressed; urine calcium and phosphorus are both high. In addition, alkaline phosphatase is elevated among the 25 per cent of affected clients who have associated bone disease. Also, clients with skeletal damage have the following characteristic x-ray findings: diffuse demineralization of bones, bone cysts, subperiosteal bone resorption, and loss of the lamina dura surrounding the teeth (Table 62-7).

Medical Management

The treatment of hyperparathyroidism includes (1) lowering severely elevated calcium levels, (2) increasing urinary calcium excretion with diuretics, and (3) long-term management of hypercalcemia with drugs to increase bone resorption of calcium.

PHARMACOLOGIC MANAGEMENT

Serum calcium levels are lowered by hydration and calciuresis. Hydration may be achieved with a normal saline infusion. Normal saline is the fluid of choice because it both expands the volume and acts in the kidney to inhibit the resorption of calcium. Furosemide (Lasix), a loop diuretic, may also be used to promote calciuresis. Thiazide diuretics are not used since they promote calcium retention in the kidneys.

Drugs that inhibit bone resorption include mithramycin (Mithracin), gallium nitrate (Ganite), phosphates, and calcitonin. Mithramycin is a cancer chemotherapeutic agent that is very effective in lowering serum calcium levels. The hypocalcemic effect is seen after 24 hours and lasts for about 1 to 2 weeks. The dose is about one tenth that used for cancer treatment, so the adverse effects are proportionally lower.

A newer drug, gallium nitrate, is now being used more often because it has even fewer side effects. Glucocorticoids may be used to reduce hypercalcemia by decreasing gastrointestinal absorption of calcium. Etidronate (Didronel) or calcitonin may be used to decrease the release of calcium by bones. Drugs used to treat hypercalcemia are summarized in Table 62-8.

DIETARY MANAGEMENT

The client with hypercalcemia should be on a low-calcium, low-vitamin D diet.

Surgical Management

Definitive treatment of hyperparathyroidism is surgical removal of the gland or glands causing hypersecretion of PTH. Usually, only the diseased parathyroid glands are resected. However, if all four glands are hyperplastic, three and one-half glands are removed. Fortunately, one half of a parathyroid gland is usually sufficient to maintain normal levels of circulating PTH.

Autotransplantation of the parathyroid glands is a useful modality for the management of clients with certain forms of hyperparathyroidism. After partial parathyroidectomy, it is possible to transplant the remaining healthy parathyroid tissue to a safer location, such as the brachioradialis muscle of the forearm. Reexploration of the neck in the future may cause laryngeal nerve damage and influence complications from the original surgery. Transplants take some time to come to full effect. Clients must be supplemented with calcium and vitamin D for prevention of hypoparathyroidism and hypocalcemia until the transplant matures.

The complications after parathyroidectomy are similar to those after thyroidectomy. Hypocalcemia is a potentially life-threatening complication even if some parathyroid glands are left untouched because edema decreases their function. The client can also develop respiratory distress related to either hemorrhage or recurrent laryngeal nerve damage.

Nursing Management

ASSESSMENT

There are no obvious signs or symptoms of hyperparathyroidism and the resultant hypercalcemia. The nurse should elicit a good history from the client to see if any of the risk factors for developing the condition exist.

The client may exhibit some psychosocial changes that the nurse could assess, such as lethargy, drowsiness, memory loss, or emotional lability, all signs of hypercalcemia.

NURSING INTERVENTION

Nursing Diagnosis: Injury, High Risk for R/T demineralization of bones resulting in pathologic fractures.

TABLE 62-7. Diagnostic Test of Parathyroid Function: Purpose, Procedure, Normal Range, and Interpretation of Abnormal Findings

Test	Purpose	Procedure	Normal Range	Interpretation of Abnormal Findings	Remarks
Total serum calcium	Measures amount of ionized and non-ionized calcium in serum	Venous blood to laboratory	4.8–5.2 mEq/L or 8–11 mg/100 ml	Elevated in hyperparathyroidism; depressed in hypoparathyroidism, tetany, rickets, nephrosis, and osteomalacia	Normally 50% of total serum calcium is ionized; amount of ionized calcium available decreases in alkalosis
Qualitative urinary calcium (Sulkowitch test)	Measures roughly amount of calcium in urine; used as quick method for diagnosing if tetany is due to hypoparathyroidism	Collect urine specimen and send to laboratory	Fine white precipitate should form when Sulkowitch reagent is added to urine specimen	Absence or decreased density of precipitate indicates low serum calcium and hypoparathyroidism	Medications that elevate serum calcium levels include vitamin D, parathyroid injection, and dihydrotachysterol
Quantitative urinary calcium (calcium deprivation test)	Measures exact amount of calcium in 24-hr urine specimen	Collect 24-hr urine specimen and send to laboratory	75–175 mg calcium per 24 hr	Elevated in hyperparathyroidism; depressed in hypoparathyroidism	Foods high in calcium include milk, cheese, molasses, turnip greens, and dandelion greens
Serum phosphorus	Measures amount of inorganic phosphorus in serum	Venous blood to laboratory	1.3–1.75 mEq/L (2.5–4.5 mg/100 ml) in adults	Elevated in hypoparathyroidism, uremia, and alkalosis; depressed in hyperparathyroidism, rickets, and osteomalacia	There is an inverse relationship between serum calcium and serum phosphorus
Serum alkaline phosphatase	Measures amount of alkaline phosphatase in serum; aids in diagnosing bone and liver disorders	Venous blood to laboratory	2.0–5.0 Bodansky units	Elevated in hyperparathyroidism, osteomalacia, rickets, healing fractures, and pregnancy and after ingestion of large amounts of vitamin D	Alkaline phosphatase is an enzyme normally present in small amounts in serum; some medications causing false elevations of alkaline phosphatase levels include allopurinol, some androgens, colchicine, erythromycin, methyldopa, some oral contraceptives, procainamide, and tolbutamide
PTH (parathyroid hormone) radioimmunoassay test	Measures level of PTH in serum	Venous blood to laboratory	Depends on serum calcium concentration	High concentrations indicate hyperparathyroidism	When evaluated in conjunction with serum calcium levels, this is the most specific test for hyperparathyroidism

TABLE 62-8. Drugs Used to Treat Hypercalcemia

Medication	Dosage	Side Effects	Nursing Implications
Furosemide (Lasix)	Up to 100 mg IV	Volume depletion and dehydration, orthostatic hypotension, hypokalemia, hypochloremic alkalosis, hyperuricemia, dilutional hyponatremia, hypocalcemia, hypomagnesemia	Monitor intake and output carefully; monitor blood pressure and pulse; give with 0.9% sodium chloride; monitor serum electrolytes; watch calcium level closely
Mithramycin (Mithracin)	25 μg IV daily for 1 to 4 days	Thrombocytopenia, bleeding tendencies, nausea and vomiting, facial flushing, diarrhea; increased BUN and creatinine; decreased serum calcium, potassium, and phosphorus; anorexia	Therapeutic effect in hypercalcemia may not be seen for 24 to 48 hr and may last 3 to 15 days; monitor serum electrolytes, liver enzymes, and BUN and creatinine; monitor platelet count and watch for bleeding; watch for sudden drop in serum calcium; check closely for signs of hypocalcemia; give antiemetics before administration to reduce nausea
Etidronate disodium (Didronel)	5 mg/kg PO daily as single dose 2 hr before meals, up to dose of 20 mg/kg	Diarrhea, nausea, bone pain, increased risk of fractures, elevated serum phosphate	Do not administer with food or antacids; monitor serum phosphate; tell client that onset of therapeutic effect may take several months; do not give for more than 6 months continuously, stop, then restart after 3 months; monitor renal function
Gallium nitrate (Ganite)	100–200 mg/m² daily for 5 consecutive days	Increased BUN and creatinine, hypocalcemia, decreased serum bicarbonate, transient hypophosphatemia, anemia, hypotension, nausea and vomiting	Administer IV with 0.9% sodium chloride; monitor serum calcium, bicarbonate, and phosphate; check blood pressure at intervals; monitor renal function; check for signs of anemia
Calcitonin (Calcimar)	0.5–1 mg SC daily or 2 to 3 times a week	Nausea and vomiting, urinary frequency, flushing of face and hands, hypocalcemia	Administer at bedtime to decrease nausea and vomiting; monitor for signs of hypocalcemia; treatment may last for 6 months; monitor serum phosphate; warn client about transient facial flushing

BUN, blood urea nitrogen; IV, intravenously; PO, orally, SC, subcutaneously.

Planning: Expected Outcomes. The client will not suffer injury, as evidenced by absence of pathologic fractures or hypercalcemia.

Implementation. Protect the client from accidents. If bone involvement exists, the client may develop pathologic fractures from even small bumps or minor falls. Keep the client's bed in low position and use side rails. If the client is weak or has joint or skeletal disease, assist in ambulation.

Nursing Diagnosis: Urinary Elimination, Altered R/T renal involvement secondary to hypercalcemia and hyperphosphaturia.

Planning: Expected Outcomes. The client will return to a normal urinary output, as evidenced by no development of stones and urine output of 30 to 60 ml/hr.

Implementation. The client should take in at least 3000 ml of fluid a day. Dehydration is dangerous for clients with hyperparathyroidism because it both increases the serum calcium level and promotes the formation of renal stones. Cranberry and prune juice may help make the urine more acidic. High urinary acidity helps prevent renal stone formation, because calcium is more soluble in an acidic urine than in an alkaline urine.

If the client has a kidney stone, strain all urine to detect gravel and stones. Save any specimens of abnormal urine for the physician to examine and for laboratory analysis. Also, observe the urine for blood and assess the client for renal colic (see Chaps. 49 and 50).

Nursing Diagnosis: Nutrition, Altered: Less than Body Requirements R/T anorexia and nausea.

Planning: Expected Outcomes. The client will have an adequate intake, as evidenced by absence of nausea and return to or maintenance of ideal body weight.

Implementation. Encourage a low-calcium diet to correct hypercalcemia. Explain to the client that the omission of milk and milk products from the menu may help alleviate some of the distressing gastrointestinal symptoms. The client who suffers from peptic ulcers will need to take antacids or histamine-receptor antagonists.

Nursing Diagnosis: Constipation R/T adverse effects of hypercalcemia on the gastrointestinal tract.

Planning: Expected Outcomes. The client will maintain a normal bowel pattern, as evidenced by a bowel movement daily.

Implementation. The nurse must work to prevent constipation and fecal impaction resulting from hypercalcemia. Help the client to be as active as possible, depending on the extent of bone disease. If constipation continues despite these measures, obtain an order for a stool softener or laxative.

Collaborative Problem: High risk for injury R/T preoperative drug sensitivities and postoperative complications.

Planning: Expected Outcomes. The client will not suffer injury, as evidenced by no medication reactions preoperatively and the absence of respiratory distress, hemorrhage, and hypocalcemia after surgery.

Implementation. If the client is on digitalis, administer this medication with extreme caution. Clients with hypercalcemia are hypersensitive to digitalis and may quickly develop toxic symptoms.

During the postoperative period, new problems arise, some of which are the reverse of those found preoperatively. During the immediate postoperative period, nursing care is similar to that after thyroidectomy, that is, assess the client carefully for hemorrhage, airway obstruction, injury to the recurrent laryngeal nerve, and tetany. Also watch for signs of hormonal imbalance.

Mild tetany due to the drop in serum calcium is expected after the removal of the parathyroid tissue. Typically, the uncomfortable tingling of the hands and around the mouth that follows parathyroid resection usually disappears without problem. This mild tetany is usually temporary; however, if it persists or is severe, calcium gluconate is administered intravenously to relieve symptoms.

Clients with bone disease require additional therapy after surgery. Removal of the parathyroid glands reduces bone resorption, and because bone rebuilding proceeds at a rapid rate, the client can develop the "hungry bones" syndrome. This is characterized by hypocalcemia and severe tetany resulting from the rapid utilization of calcium by the bones. For preventing low serum calcium levels due to bone recalcification, instruct these clients to eat foods high in calcium. Tetany is treated with injections of calcium gluconate. For maintaining adequate calcium levels, oral calcium preparations are usually given for months until the skeletal tissues have been rebuilt. Finally, clients are usually encouraged to ambulate as soon as possible after surgery, because weight-bearing speeds the recalcification process.

EVALUATION

The nurse must evaluate client outcomes on the basis of the established plan of care. If these goals have not been achieved, the plan and interventions must be revised to meet the client's needs.

Modification of Plan of Care for the Elderly

Hyperparathyroidism in the elderly is an overlooked disease. It is estimated that 1 per 1000 men and 2 per 1000 women over the age of 60 years experience hyperparathyroidism. This disease often goes undiagnosed in the elderly because symptoms in the early stages are subtle and attributed to old age, depression, or anxiety. The symptoms only intensify as the level of serum calcium continues to rise and other physiologic and functional changes occur. Laboratory diagnosis is made the same as for a client younger than 60 years old, but treatment may be complicated by medical problems and medication.

Post-hospital Care

DISCHARGE TEACHING

Clients and significant others need to understand discharge medications that may be needed for continued control of the hypercalcemia. The client and significant others should also be taught about any dietary restrictions of calcium or phosphorus.

HOME HEALTH CARE NEEDS

If the client suffered from severe osteoporosis or pathologic fractures, some assistance may be required at home. The client may need a visiting nurse to help assess the current home situation and make recommendations on how it could be made safer. The home will need to be cleared of articles such as throw rugs that might increase the client's risk of falling. The client may also need assistive devices such as a railing in the bathroom, a bedside commode, or a walker.

FOLLOW-UP CARE

The client will need to have calcium levels measured at intervals to be sure that they remain within the normal range.

HYPOPARATHYROIDISM

Definition

Hyposecretion of the parathyroid glands produces a syndrome opposite that of hyperparathyroidism. Thus, serum calcium levels are abnormally low, serum phosphate levels are abnormally high, and pronounced neuromuscular irritability (tetany) may develop.

Incidence

Idiopathic hypoparathyroidism strikes children nine times as often as adults and affects twice as many women as men.

Etiology

The causes of hypoparathyroidism are either iatrogenic or idiopathic. Iatrogenic causes of hypoparathyroidism include (1) accidental removal of the parathyroid glands during thyroidectomy, (2) infarction of the parathyroid glands resulting from an inadequate blood supply to the glands during surgery, and (3) strangulation of one or more of the glands by postoperative scar tissue.

Idiopathic hypoparathyroidism, like Graves' disease and Hashimoto's thyroiditis, may be an autoimmune disorder with a genetic basis. This type of hypoparathyroidism is far less common than the iatrogenic form.

Risk Factors

The major risk factor for hypoparathyroidism is thyroid or parathyroid surgery. The only preventive measure is early detection through close monitoring of clients who have had these procedures.

Pathophysiology

PTH normally acts to increase bone resorption, which in turn maintains proper serum calcium levels. The hormone also regulates phosphate clearance by the renal tubules, thereby maintaining the correct inverse balance between serum calcium and serum phosphate. Consequently, when parathyroid secretion is reduced, bone resorption slows, serum calcium levels fall, and severe neuromuscular irritability develops. Somewhat paradoxically, calcifications form in various organs (e.g., the eyes and basal ganglia). Also, without sufficient PTH, fewer phosphorus ions are secreted by the distal tubules of the kidney, renal excretion of phosphate decreases, and serum phosphate levels rise.

The client may fully recover from the effects of hypoparathyroidism if the condition is diagnosed early, before the advent of serious complications. Unfortunately, cataracts and brain calcifications, once formed, are irreversible.

Clinical Manifestations

The symptoms of hypoparathyroidism are mainly caused by low serum calcium levels. They are always more severe in clients who have an elevated serum pH (alkalosis) from any cause (e.g., ingesting antacids, hyperventilation). Symptoms worsen because when the pH of the blood rises, the amount of ionized calcium drops, although total serum calcium remains the same. With less ionized calcium available to the body, the symptoms resulting from hypocalcemia become more severe until the alkalosis is corrected.

Acute Hypoparathyroidism. This condition is caused by accidental damage to parathyroid tissues during thyroidectomy. It is characterized by greatly increased neuromuscular irritability, which results in tetany. Clients with tetany experience painful muscle spasms, irritability, grimacing, tingling of fingers, laryngospasm, and arrhythmias. Assessment also reveals Chvostek's and Trousseau's signs. In some cases, tetany is so severe that a tracheostomy is required to correct acute respiratory obstruction secondary to laryngospasm.

Chronic Hypoparathyroidism. This condition is usually idiopathic. It causes lethargy; thin, patchy hair; brittle nails; dry, scaly skin; and personality changes. Ectopic calcifications may appear in the eyes and basal ganglia. Thus, the client may develop cataracts and permanent brain damage accompanied by psychosis or convulsions. In addition, severe persistent hypocalcemia adversely affects the heart, causing arrhythmias and eventual cardiac failure.

DIAGNOSTIC ASSESSMENT

The diagnosis of hypoparathyroidism is based on

- presence of Chvostek's sign (spasms of facial muscles after a tap on the side of the face, signifying hyperirritability of the facial nerve)
- presence of Trousseau's sign (carpal spasms of the fingers and hand after application of a blood pressure cuff to the arm)
- numbness and tingling around the mouth and fingertips
- laboratory findings of low serum calcium, high serum phosphate, and low or absent urinary calcium
- x-ray studies showing calcification of the basal ganglia
- eye examinations that may reveal the early development of cataracts due to the formation of calcifications within the lens of the eye

Complications

If treatment is not begun rapidly in acute hypoparathyroidism, death can result from the respiratory obstruction secondary to the tetany and laryngospasms.

In chronic hypoparathyroidism, the complications are calcifications in the eye and basal ganglia that can occur if the treatment is delayed.

Medical Management

Acute hypoparathyroidism (with its major manifestation of acute tetany) is a *life-threatening* disorder. The three goals of emergency care are to (1) elevate serum calcium levels as rapidly as possible, (2) prevent or treat convulsions, and (3) control laryngeal spasm and consequent respiratory obstruction.

The goal of intervention for clients with chronic hypoparathyroidism is to restore the serum calcium level to normal concentrations. This is done more gradually than with acute hypoparathyroidism.

PHARMACOLOGIC MANAGEMENT

For acute hypoparathyroidism, to elevate the serum calcium levels quickly, the physician will prescribe 10 per cent calcium gluconate solution in an intravenous infusion. While administering the calcium gluconate, instruct the client to inhale carbon dioxide by breathing into a paper bag. This causes a mild metabolic acidosis, which serves to elevate the amount of ionized calcium in the blood.

Once the condition has stabilized and the dangers of tetany have passed, the client is given oral calcium salts and vitamin D to maintain normal serum calcium levels.

For chronic hypoparathyroidism, the client is given oral calcium salts (either calcium gluconate, calcium lactate, or calcium chloride) and vitamin D. Commercially available forms of vitamin D include calciferol (vitamin D_2), dihydroxycholecalciferol, and dihydrotachysterol (Hytakerol). Although calciferol is a more reliable and less expensive drug than dihydrotachysterol or dihydroxycholecalciferol, all three forms of vitamin D are effective in correcting hypocalcemia. They are all obtainable as either tablets or oily liquids.

DIETARY MANAGEMENT

The client with hypoparathyroidism should be on a diet high in calcium but low in phosphorus.

Surgical Management

Surgery is not done to treat hypoparathyroidism. It is often the cause of this disorder.

Nursing Management

ASSESSMENT

The nurse should carefully assess the client at risk for acute hypoparathyroidism, such as the postthyroidectomy client, for the development of hypocalcemia. The nurse should question the client for any sign of numbness and tingling around the mouth or in the fingertips or toes. The nurse should also check for a positive finding of Chvostek's or Trousseau's sign. It is also important to assess for any sign of respiratory distress secondary to laryngospasm.

In the client with chronic hypoparathyroidism, the nurse should assess the client for the presence of the obvious physical changes such as dry skin and hair. The nurse should also assess for the presence of a Parkinson's-like syndrome or the presence of cataracts. The nurse should also assess the teeth because pits may encircle the teeth, indicating enamel hypoplasia.

NURSING INTERVENTION

Collaborative Problem: Injury, high risk for R/T severe tetany secondary to decreased serum calcium levels.

Planning: Expected Outcomes. The client will not suffer any injury, as evidenced by calcium levels returning to normal range and by normal respiratory rate and blood gases within normal limits.

Implementation. When caring for clients with severe hypoparathyroidism, always be ready for the client with tetany to suffer laryngeal spasm and respiratory obstruction. Always have an endotracheal tube, laryngoscope, and tracheostomy set available when caring for clients with acute tetany.

When a client is at risk for sudden hypocalcemia, such as after thyroidectomy, an ampule of intravenous calcium gluconate is usually kept at the client's bedside for immediate use if necessary.

Nursing Diagnosis: Knowledge Deficit R/T diet and medication regimen.

Planning: Expected Outcomes. The client will understand the diet and medication, as evidenced by client's statements and ability to follow diet and medication regimen.

Implementation. Teaching is the priority for the client with chronic hypoparathyroidism because this client will require lifelong medication and dietary modification.

When teaching the client about take-home medications, make sure the client knows that all forms of the vitamin D, except dihydroxycholecalciferol, are slowly assimilated by the body. Warn the client that it may take a week or longer, therefore, for the symptoms to improve.

EVALUATION

The nurse must evaluate client outcomes on the basis of the established plan of care. If these goals have not been achieved, the plan and interventions must be revised to meet the client's needs.

Post-hospital Care

DISCHARGE TEACHING

Teach the client about a diet high in calcium but low in phosphorus. Remind the client to omit cheese and milk products from the diet, because these foods have a high phosphorus content.

Tell the client that calcium supplements may be obtained in either tablet or solution form, depending on the client's preference. Oral calcium administration is usually discontinued once the client responds successfully to the vitamin D preparations.

FOLLOW-UP CARE

Emphasize the importance of lifelong medical care for the client with chronic hypoparathyroidism. Instruct the client to have the serum calcium level checked by a physician at least three times a year, every year. Normal blood serum calcium levels must be maintained to prevent complications. If hypercalcemia or hypocalcemia develops, the physician will need to adjust the treatment regimen to correct the imbalance.

Summary

The nurse must make careful assessments of clients with thyroid or parathyroid disorders. These disorders can be controlled and the symptoms reversed if they are diagnosed in a timely manner and prompt and proper treatment is begun. The nurse is an important resource for these clients with all the education they require. The nurse is also responsible for the close monitoring the client requires after surgery on either the thyroid or parathyroid gland. The client is particularly vulnerable during this postoperative period, and high-level nursing surveillance and intervention can mean the client recovers successfully.

Bibliography

1. Auwerx, J., et al. (1984). Altered parathyroid set point to calcium in familial hypocalciuric hypercalcaemia. *Acta Endocrinologica, 106,* 215.
2. Aviolo, L. V. (1987). Primary hyperthyroidism recognition and management. *Hospital Practice, 22*(9), 69–74.
3. Bagdade, J. D. (1987). *The yearbook of endocrinology.* Chicago: Year Book.
4. Beck-Peccoz, P., et al. (1985). Decreased receptor binding of biologically inactive thyrotropin in central hypothyroidism. *New England Journal of Medicine, 312,* 1085.
5. Besser, G. M., & Cudworth, A. G. (Eds.) (1987). *Clinical endocrinology. An illustrated text.* Philadelphia: J. B. Lippincott.
6. Bondeson, A. G., et al. (1984). Chronic parathyroiditis associated with parathyroid hyperplasia and hyperparathyroidism. *American Journal of Surgical Pathology, 8,* 211.
7. Bouma, D. J., et al. (1982). Follow-up comparison of short-term versus 1-year antithyroid drug therapy for the thyrotoxicosis of Graves' disease. *Journal of Clinical Endocrinology and Metabolism, 55,* 1138.
8. Brunt, L. M., & Wells, S. A. (1987). Advances in the diagnoses and treatment of medullary thyroid carcinoma. *Surgical Clinics of North America, 67,* 263–279.
9. Bybee, D. E. (1987). Saving lives in thyroid crisis. *Emergency Medicine, 19*(16), 20–30.
10. Canonica, G. W., et al. (1983). Why thyroid is major site of thyroid autoantibody synthesis in autoimmune thyroid disease. *Lancet, 1,* 1163.
11. Cross, A. J., et al. (1983). Dopamine D_1 receptors in human parathyroid gland in vitro and in vivo studies. *Life Sciences, 22,* 743.
12. DeGroot, L. J. (Ed.) (1984). *The thyroid and its diseases.* New York: John Wiley and Sons.
13. DeGroot, L. J. (Ed.) (1989). *Endocrinology* (2nd ed.). Philadelphia: W. B. Saunders.
14. DeRubertis, F. R. (1985). Hypocalcemia: etiology and management. *Hospital Medicine, 21,* 3.
15. DuFour, D. R., et al. (1983). Factors related to parathyroid weight in normal persons. *Archives of Pathology and Laboratory Medicine, 107,* 167.
16. Felig, P., Baster, J. D., & Broadhaus, A. (Eds.) (1987). *Endocrinology and metabolism.* New York: McGraw-Hill.
17. Gever, L.N. (1985). Understanding and teaching thyroid hormone therapy. *Nursing 84, 8,* 30.
18. Goltzman, D., et al. (1984). Discordant disappearance of bioactive and immunoreactive parathyroid hormone after parathyroidectomy. *Journal of Clinical Endocrinology and Metabolism, 58,* 70.
19. Greenspan, F. S., & Forsham, P. H. (1986). *Basic and clinical endocrinology.* (2nd ed.). Los Altos, CA: Lange Medical.
20. Halbert, S. P., et al. (1983). A rapid standardized enzyme immunoassay for autoantibodies to thyroglobulin. *Clinica Chimica Acta, 127,* 69.
21. Harada, T., et al. (1987). Current treatment of Graves' disease. *Surgical Clinics of North America, 67,* 299–314.
22. Haslett, C., et al. (1983). Rheumatic heart disease and thyroid status. *Scottish Medical Journal, 28,* 17.
23. Hennemann, G. (Ed.). *Thyroid hormone metabolism.* New York: Marcel Dekker.
24. Ingbar, S. H., & Braveman, L. E. (1986). *Werners' the thyroid* (5th ed.). Philadelphia: J. B. Lippincott.
25. Johnson, D. (1983). Pathophysiology of thyroid storm: Nursing implication. *Critical Care Nurse, 8,* 80.
26. Kawamura, S., et al. (1983). Serum thyroglobulin changes in patients with Graves' disease treated with long-term antithyroid drug therapy. *Journal of Clinical Endocrinology and Metabolism, 56,* 507.
27. Lazarus, J. H., & Hall, R. (Eds.) (1988). *Hypothyroidism and goitre.* Philadelphia: Bailliere Tindall.

28. Lennquist, S. (1987). The thyroid nodule: diagnoses and surgical treatment. *Surgical Clinics of North America, 67,* 213-232.
29. Lever, E. G., et al. (1983). Coexisting thyroid and parathyroid disease—are they related? *Surgery, 94,* 893.
30. Levey, G. S., & Levey, B. A. (1985). Cardiovascular effects of thyroid disease. *Hospital Medicine, 21,* 147.
31. Lyerly, H. K. (1991). Hyperthyroidism. In D. C. Sabiston, Jr. (Ed.), *Textbook of surgery: The biological basis of modern surgical practice* (14th ed, pp. 568-579). Philadelphia: W. B. Saunders.
32. Martin, C. R. (1985). *Endocrine physiology.* New York: Oxford University Press.
33. Mazzaferri, E. L. (Ed.) (1986). *Textbook of endocrinology* (3rd ed.). New York: Elsevier Science.
34. Mazzaferri, E. L., et al. (1988). Solitary thyroid nodule: diagnoses and management. *Medical Clinics of North America, 72,* 1177-1211.
35. McConnell, E. A. (1985). Assessing the thyroid. *Nursing 85, 15*(5), 60.
36. McGraw, D. A., et al. (1982). Parathyroid function in persistent hyperparathyroidism in relationship to gland size. *Kidney International, 22,* 662.
37. McMillan, J. Y. (1988). Preventing myxedema coma in the hypothyroid patient. *Dimensions in Critical Care Nursing, 7,* 136-145.
38. Metz, R. M., & Laeson, E. B. (Eds) (1985). *Blue book of endocrinology.* Philadelphia: W.B. Saunders.
39. Molzahn, A. E. (1984). Parathyroid hormone as a uremic toxin. *Journal of Nephrological Nursing, 1,* 13.
40. O'Neil, J. (1987). Thyroid crisis. *Nursing 87, 17*(11), 335-338.
41. Powell, B. L., et al. (1984). Thyroid cancer. *American Family Physician, 30,* 185.
42. Roher, H. D., & Goretzki, P. E. (1987). Management of goiter and thyroid nodules in an area of endemic goiter. *Surgical Clinics of North America, 67,* 233-249.
43. Saffos, R. O., et al. (1984). The normal parathyroid and borderline with early hyperplasia: a light microscopic study. *Histopathology, 8,* 407.
44. Sawin, C. T. (1988). Hypothyroidism. *Medical Clinics of North America, 69,* 989-1003.
45. Sherwood, L. M. (1988). Diagnosis and management of primary hyperparathyroidism. *Hospital Practice, 23*(3), 9-10.
46. Shoemaker, W. C., et al (Eds.) (1989). *Textbook of critical care* (2nd ed.). Philadelphia: W. B. Saunders.
47. Solomon, B. (1984). Endocrinology: a future challenge for critical nurses. *Dimensions of Critical Care Nursing, 3,* 68.
48. Stiges-Serra, A., & Caralps-Riera, D. (1987). Hyperparathyroidism associated with renal disease. *Surgical Clinics of North America, 67,* 359-377.
49. Takagi, H., et al. (1983). Polymorphism of parathyroid glands in patients with chronic renal failure and secondary hyperparathyroidism. *Endocrinologica Japonica, 30,* 463.
50. Vander Velden, P. C., et al. (1984). Histamine and parathyroid activity. *Hormone and Metabolic Research, 16,* 269.
51. Van Middlesworth, L. (1989). Effects of radiation on the thyroid gland. *Advances in Internal Medicine, 34,* 265-284.
52. Wells, S. A., & Ashley, S. W. (1991). The parathyroid glands. In D. C. Sabiston, Jr. (Ed.), *Textbook of surgery: The biological basis of modern surgical practice* (14th ed, pp. 598-615). Philadelphia: W. B. Saunders.
53. When hypercalcemia won't calm down (1986). *Emergency Medicine, 18,* 103.
54. Wiener, J. D. (1983). Relative ineffectiveness of exogenous triiodothyronine as a thyroid suppressive agent. *Journal of Endocrinological Investigation, 6,* 69.
55. Wilson, J., & Foster, D. (Eds.) (1992). *Williams textbook of endocrinology* (8th ed.). Philadelphia: W. B. Saunders.
56. Wyngaarden, J. B., & Smith, L. H. (Eds.) (1988). *Cecil textbook of medicine* (18th ed.). Philadelphia: W. B. Saunders.

Chapter 63

Nursing Care of Clients with Adrenal, Pituitary, and Gonadal Disorders

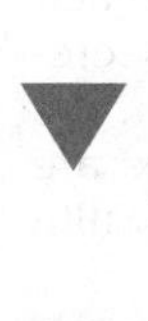

ADRENOCORTICAL DISORDERS

Glandular hypofunction and hyperfunction characterize the major disorders of the adrenal cortex. Underactivity of the adrenal cortex results in a deficiency of glucocorticoids, mineralocorticoids, and adrenal androgens. Overactivity results in excessive production of glucocorticoids, mineralocorticoids, and androgens or estrogens.

Adrenal Insufficiency

Hypofunction of the adrenal cortex can originate from a disorder within the adrenal gland itself (primary adrenal insufficiency), or it may be due to hypofunction of the pituitary-hypothalamic unit (secondary adrenal insufficiency). Adrenocortical insufficiency can be either chronic or acute.

CHRONIC PRIMARY ADRENAL INSUFFICIENCY (ADDISON'S DISEASE)

Definition

Addison's disease is a condition that occurs as a result of a disorder within the adrenal gland. Primary adrenal insufficiency, or Addison's disease, was named for Thomas Addison, who first described this condition more than 100 years ago.

Incidence

Addison's disease strikes only 4 of 100,000 persons. Adrenal insufficiency affects all age groups and both sexes.

Etiology

At one time, most cases of Addison's disease were a complication of tuberculosis. Today, 70 per cent are considered idiopathic in origin. Since one-half to two-thirds of clients with idiopathic Addison's disease have circulating autoantibodies that react specifically against adrenal tissue, this condition may have an autoimmune basis. In addition, a few cases of Addison's disease are caused by neoplasm, amyloidosis, or systemic fungal infections.

Risk Factors

The major risk factors for Addison's disease are the diseases listed under the section on etiology. There are no known risk factors for the idiopathic disease.

Pathophysiology

Adrenocortical hypofunction results in decreased levels of both mineralocorticoids (aldosterone), glucocorticoids (cortisol), and androgens.

Aldosterone deficiency causes numerous fluid and electrolyte imbalances. Aldosterone normally promotes conservation of sodium (Na^+) (and consequently water) and excretion of potassium (K^+). A deficiency of aldosterone causes increased sodium excretion, which results in the following chain of events: (1) water excretion increases, (2) extracellular volume becomes depleted (dehydration), (3) hypotension develops, (4) cardiac output decreases, and (5) the heart becomes smaller as a result of its diminished workload. Eventually, hypotension becomes severe and cardiovascular activity weakens, leading to circulatory collapse, shock, and death. Although the body excretes excess sodium, it retains excess potassium. Potassium levels of more than 7 mEq/L result in arrhythmias and, possibly, cardiac arrest.

Glucocorticoid deficiency causes widespread metabolic disturbances. Remember that the glucocorticoids promote gluconeogenesis and have an "anti-insulin" effect. Consequently, when glucocorticoids become deficient, gluconeogenesis decreases, with resultant hypoglycemia and liver glycogen deficiency. The client grows weak, exhausted, and suffers from anorexia, weight loss, nausea, and vomiting. Emotional disturbances can develop, ranging from mild neurotic symptoms to severe depression. In addition, glucocorticoid deficiency diminishes resistance to stress. Surgery, pregnancy, injury, infection, or salt loss due to profuse diaphoresis can cause an addisonian crisis (acute adrenal insufficiency). Finally, cortisol deficiency results in a failure to inhibit anterior pituitary secretion of adrenocorticotropic hormone (ACTH) (Fig. 63-1).

Melanocyte-stimulating hormone (MSH) stimulates the epidermal melanocytes, which manufacture melanin, a dark pigment. Increased ACTH secretion leads to increased pigmentation of the skin and mucous membranes. Thus, clients with Addison's disease have increased levels of ACTH and a bronzed, or tanned, appearance.

Androgen deficiency fails to produce symptoms in men with Addison's disease because the testes supply adequate amounts of sex hormones. However, women depend on the adrenal cortex for an adequate secretion of androgens.

The hormones secreted by the adrenal cortex are essential to life. Untreated Addison's disease is ultimately fatal.

Clinical Manifestations

The onset of Addison's disease is usually insidious. The client experiences mild fatigue, languor, irritability, weight loss, nausea, vomiting, and postural hypotension weeks or months before diagnosis of the disease. As the disorder progresses, symptoms intensify. In the 19th century, Addison vividly described the manifestations of this debilitating and potentially fatal condition:

> The patient, in most of the cases I have seen, has been observed gradually to fall off in general health; he becomes languid and weak, indisposed to either bodily or mental exertion; the appetite is impaired or entirely lost; . . . the pulse small and feeble . . . excessively soft and compressible; the body wastes . . . slight pain or uneasiness is from time to time referred to the region of the stomach, and there is occasionally actual vomiting . . . it is by no means uncommon for the patient to manifest indications of disturbed cerebral circulation. . . . We have discovered a most remarkable, and, so far as I know, characteristic discoloration taking place in the skin—sufficiently marked indeed as generally to have attracted the attention of the patient himself, or of the patient's friends. . . . It may be said to present a dingy or smoky appearance, or various tints of shades of deep amber or chestnut brown. . . . The body wastes . . . the pulse becomes smaller and weaker, and . . . the patient at length gradually sinks and expires.

For those receiving appropriate intervention, the prognosis is now excellent.

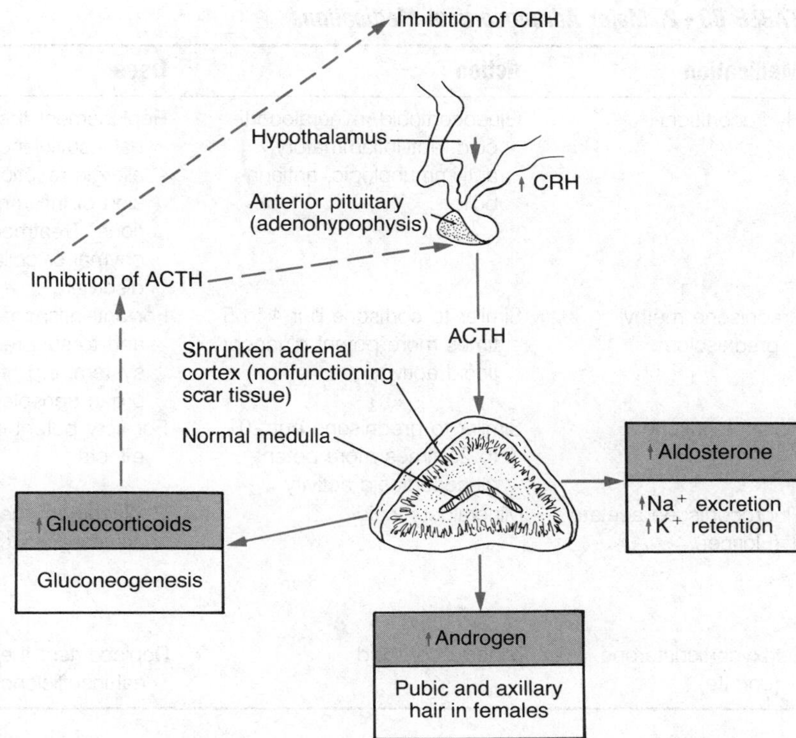

▲ *Figure 63-1*

Effects of Addison's disease. Dashed arrows show feedback mechanisms.

DIAGNOSTIC ASSESSMENT

Diagnosis of Addison's disease depends primarily on blood and urine hormonal assays. Diagnostic tests of adrenalcortical function include

- *ACTH stimulation test:* This is the most reliable screening test for Addison's disease. The procedure follows: Baseline plasma cortisol is drawn (Time '0'). Plasma cortisol response to ACTH is then measured by administering 250 μg synthetic ACTH intravenously; 45 minutes later, a blood sample is drawn. The cortisol concentration should be greater than 20 μg/dl.
- *Plasma ACTH:* Failing the screening test, plasma ACTH will accurately categorize clients with primary (high) and secondary (normal or low) adrenal insufficiency.
- *Serum electrolytes:* The serum sodium is usually decreased, while potassium and calcium are usually increased (Table 63-1).

Medical Management

PHARMACOLOGIC MANAGEMENT

Addison's disease was once fatal within months. Today, with the manufacture of synthetic corticosteroids, clients with Addison's disease can live normal, active lives provided they receive adequate glucocorticoid replacement (Table 63-2). Clients should be carefully assessed for signs of hypercortisolism that can result from excessive long-term cortisol therapy.

Table 63-1. Routine Laboratory Findings Suggesting Addison's Disease

Blood chemistry	Low serum Na^+ (<130 mEq/L)
	High serum K^+ (>5 mEq/L)
	Ratio of serum Na^+:K^+ (<30:1)
	Low fasting blood glucose level (<50 mg/100 ml)
	Decrease in CO_2 combining power (<28 mEq/L)
	Elevated BUN (>20 mg/100 ml)
Hematology	Relative lymphocytosis
	Increased eosinophils

Data from Bethune, J. E. (1989). The diagnosis and treatment of adrenal insufficiency. In L. DeGroot (Ed.), *Endocrinology and metabolism* (2nd ed.). Philadelphia: W. B. Saunders.

Fludrocortisone acetate (Florinef) also should be taken daily, 100 μg by mouth, as mineralocorticoid replacement therapy.

Nursing Management

ASSESSMENT

The client's vital signs should be monitored closely while the disease is being diagnosed. Check the pulse carefully, at least every 4 hours. Report drops in blood pressure below the baseline.

TABLE 63–2. Major Adrenocortical Medications

Medication	Action	Uses	Side Effects
Hydrocortisone	Glucocorticoid, mineralocorticoid, anti-inflammatory, anti-immunologic, antianabolic	Replacement therapy for adrenal insufficiency. Control of allergic reactions. Suppression of inflammatory reactions. Treatment of mesenchymal or collagen disorders	Overdosage produces Cushing's syndrome
Prednisone methylprednisolone	Similar to cortisone but 4 to 5 times more potent glucocorticoid activity	For anti-inflammatory action and to suppress immune system, e.g., following organ transplants	Similar to cortisone but less mineralocorticoid activity
Dexamethasone	Similar to prednisone but 20 to 25 times more potent glucocorticoid activity	For very potent glucocorticoid effects	Similar to prednisone
Fludrocortisone acetate (Florinef)	Mineralocorticoid	Replacement therapy for adrenal insufficiency	Mineralocorticoid effects: hypertension, edema due to sodium retention, muscle weakness, and arrhythmias due to hypokalemia
Deoxycorticosterone (cortate)	Mineralocorticoid	Replacement therapy for adrenal insufficiency	Mineralocorticoid effects: same as for Florinef

Assess for signs and symptoms of increased physical vitality and emotional well-being. Assess bony prominences to avoid pressure sores in immobilized clients. With therapy, listlessness and exhaustion should gradually lessen and disappear.

Monitor for exposure to cold and infections. Immediately inform the physician if signs of infection develop, such as a sore throat or burning on urination. Remember, the client with Addison's disease cannot tolerate stress. Infection imposes additional stress on the body, and cortisol levels need to be higher during infectious illnesses.

Carefully assess for signs of sodium and potassium imbalance (see Chap. 10). If steroid replacement therapy is inadequate, sodium loss and potassium retention continue uncorrected. If steroid dosage is too high, excessive amounts of sodium and water are retained and potassium excretion is high.

NURSING INTERVENTION

Nursing Diagnosis: Knowledge Deficit R/T self-administration of steroid medications.

Planning: Expected Outcomes. The client will understand how to take steroids correctly, as evidenced by the client's statements and compliance with therapeutic regimen.

Implementation. Provide the client and significant others with written instructions for self-administration of steroids. This information should include the

- Actions of prescribed hormones (hydrocortisone, fludrocortisone)
- Importance of taking the medications daily, without fail, exactly as prescribed.
- Principles of self-administration of oral medications (e.g., check the label on the bottle before taking the medication, document when medications are taken and their side effects.)
- Signs of over- and underdosage.
- Importance of hydrocortisone self-injection when unable to tolerate oral medication (due to nausea/vomiting) and during times of acute stress (auto accident, trauma) because the body is unable to compensate for its need for additional glucocorticoid coverage.
- Need for an intramuscular self-injection kit to be available at all times.
- Client's and significant others' ability to demonstrate ability to prepare medication, draw up medication into syringe, and perform injections (normal saline) prior to discharge.
- Need for a Medic Alert bracelet worn to indicate the diagnosis and/or need for cortisol replacement.
- Need for the client to contact health care provider if questions arise after discharge from medical center. Emphasize to clients who take glucocorticoids they must call the physician to get a dosage increase when experiencing stressful situations, e.g., emotional upheavals, dental extractions, minor surgery, or upper respiratory infections. In addition, temporary mineralocorticoid dosage increases may be indicated if the client experiences profuse diaphoresis, for any reason (strenuous physical exertion, heat spells, fever). The general rule of thumb is to double the dosage for up to 1 week, depending on the symptoms, and then resume the normal dosage. Clients should be encouraged to consult their physician for dose adjustment. The medication will need

to be administered intramuscularly when nausea and vomiting prevent oral administration.

Finally, clients must be reminded to adhere to semiannual appointments with their physician, even when they are in good health and the process of self-medication is proceeding smoothly. As in diabetes mellitus, the control of Addison's disease is a lifelong responsibility.

Nursing Diagnosis: Injury, High Risk for R/T acute adrenal insufficiency secondary to addisonian crisis (adrenal crisis).

Planning: Expected Outcomes. The client will not suffer injury, as evidenced by the absence of hypotension, shock, or other signs of acute adrenal insufficiency.

Implementation. The nurse should closely monitor for signs and symptoms of addisonian crisis, including (1) sudden profound weakness; (2) severe abdominal, back, and leg pain; (3) hyperpyrexia followed by hypothermia; (4) peripheral vascular collapse; (5) coma; and (6) renal shutdown and death.

The development of an adrenal crisis constitutes a medical emergency that must be treated rapidly and vigorously. The three major goals of intervention are to (1) reverse shock, (2) restore blood circulation (the client usually suffers from a deficit of at least 20 per cent of ECF volume), and (3) replenish the body with essential steroids.

Immediately on admission, a rapid infusion of 1000 ml of normal saline is administered with water-soluble glucocorticoid (hydrocortisone phosphate or hydrocortisone sodium succinate) added. The dosage of the prescribed glucocorticoid is gradually reduced. It is administered intramuscularly or intravenously every 6 hours during the first day of crisis and every 8 hours of the second day, and is gradually reduced thereafter.

Plasma, oxygen, and vasopressor medications may be indicated. Antibiotic therapy is appropriate if an infection triggered the crisis. Throughout the emergency period, the nurse must monitor blood pressure, administer intravenous infusion and medications, monitor hourly urine output and report oliguria (a sign of shock), minimize exposure to emotional and physical stress, and observe for symptoms of glucocorticoid overdose and overhydration, such as generalized edema due to fluid retention, hypertension, flaccid paralysis resulting from hypokalemia, psychoses, and loss of consciousness.

With rapid, efficient intervention, addisonian crisis usually passes by 12 hours. The client's condition stabilizes, and the convalescent period begins. When the client is able to tolerate food and fluids by mouth, steroid replacement can be administered orally.

After the immediate crisis is past, the nurse needs to help the client prevent further development of adrenal insufficiency. Identification bracelets and emergency kits should be obtained for all clients with Addison's disease prior to their discharge from the hospital. Clients should be instructed to carry these items at all times. The client's name and diagnosis should appear on the identification bracelet, and a wallet card should state the client receives daily hydrocortisone, and that the medication must be administered by injection in any emergency.

Dexamethasone can be kept in a prepared syringe in an emergency kit with sterile alcohol wipes for cleaning the injection site. The kit also should contain written information on the client's diagnosis, medication prescription, dosage schedules, and emergency phone numbers, including the physician's name and phone number.

EVALUATION

The nurse must evaluate client outcomes based on the established plan of care. If these goals were not achieved, the plan and interventions must be revised to meet the client's needs.

Modification of Plan of Care for the Elderly

When older clients suffer from Addison's disease, the symptoms are often more pronounced because their adrenal function may already be decreased from the aging process. The elderly also may be more sensitive to the side effects of steroid therapy such as osteoporosis, hypertension, diabetes, and so on because these problems may already exist in the client.

Post-hospital Care

DISCHARGE TEACHING

The client has significant teaching needs prior to discharge. The client must understand the proper self-administration of steroids, implications of the side effects, and what to do if problems arise. The discharge teaching these clients receive will directly affect their ability for self-care.

FOLLOW-UP CARE

The client must be seen at regular intervals so the effects of the medication can be assessed. The client also must be aware of the need to seek medical attention in case of severe stress or illness so the dosage of steroids can be altered by the physician.

SECONDARY ADRENAL INSUFFICIENCY

Definition

Secondary adrenal insufficiency is defined as that caused by other conditions outside the adrenals.

Etiology

Causes of adrenocortical insufficiency include

- Bilateral adrenalectomy
- Hemorrhagic infarction and necrosis of the adrenal glands. Adrenal apoplexy can develop as a complication of meningococcal septicemia or anticoagulant therapy.
- Hypopituitarism resulting in decreased secretion of ACTH by the pituitary gland, causing decreased secretion of cortisol and androgens by the adrenal gland (secondary adrenal insufficiency) (see Fig. 63-2, which illustrates the hypothalamic-pituitary-adrenal axis).
- Suppression of hypothalamic-pituitary secretion of ACTH due to hypercortisolism caused by either (1) exogenous administration of corticosteroids, or by (2) oversecretion of corticosteroids by an adrenal tumor. In both cases, the adrenal glands atrophy and become filled with lipids. Because the circulating levels of corticosteroids remain high, these clients do not develop symptoms of adrenocortical insufficiency unless steroid therapy is discontinued suddenly or the tumor is resected. Fortunately, if corticosteroid drug therapy is terminated by gradually reducing the dosage each day, adrenal gland function usually returns to normal.

Nursing Management

Assessment reveals that clients with secondary adrenal insufficiency experience cortisol deficiency. Aldosterone continues to be secreted in sufficient amounts.

Treatment involves administering glucocorticoids, as in Addison's disease. Mineralocorticoid replacement is unnecessary. Client teaching should include instruction regarding the need to wear an emergency identification bracelet and carry an emergency kit for hydrocortisone injection in case an adrenal crisis occurs.

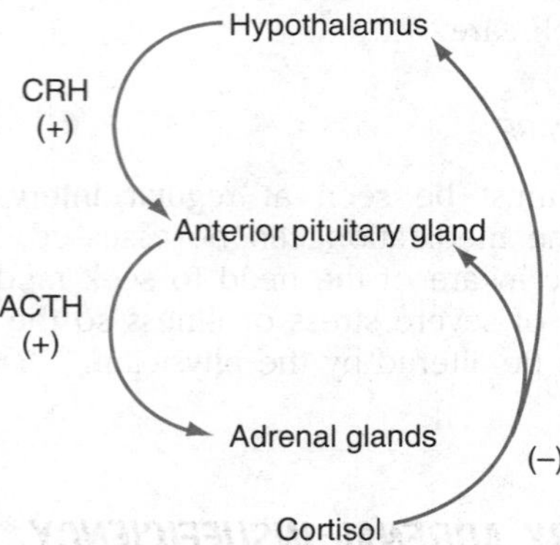

▲ *Figure 63-2*

The hypothalamic-pituitary-adrenal (HPA) axis, demonstrating stimulation and feedback between the hypothalamus, anterior pituitary, and adrenal glands.

▼ Adrenocortical Hyperfunction

Hyperfunction of the adrenal cortex can result in excessive production of glucocorticoids, mineralocorticoids, and androgens. The three major conditions of adrenocortical hyperfunction are

1. Cushing's syndrome (glucocorticoid excess),
2. Conn's syndrome or aldosteronism (aldosterone excess), and
3. Congenital adrenal hyperplasia (adrenogenital syndrome, androgen excess)

HYPERCORTISOLISM (CUSHING'S SYNDROME)

Definition

Cushing's syndrome was first described by Harvey Cushing in 1932. It results from overactivity of the adrenal gland, with consequent hypersecretion of glucocorticoids.

Incidence

Cushing's syndrome is a relatively rare condition. It occurs mainly in women, and the average age of onset is 20 to 40 years of age. It can, however, be seen up to age 60 years.

Etiology

The hypersecretion of cortisol can be caused by the following factors:

- A cortisol-secreting adrenal tumor. Adrenal tumors are responsible for approximately 30 per cent of cases of Cushing's syndrome. Most (85 per cent) are benign, but 15 per cent are malignant.
- Adrenal hyperplasia is caused by overproduction of ACTH. The two sources of excessive ACTH secretion are

  1. Pituitary hypersecretion and pituitary tumors cause approximately 70 per cent of cases of Cushing's syndrome. These usually benign tumors are either small basophil adenomas or large chromophobe adenomas. Pituitary hypersecretion of ACTH resulting in glucocorticoid excess is called Cushing's disease.
  2. Ectopic secretion of ACTH (ectopic ACTH syndrome). ACTH-secreting tumors located outside the pituitary gland constitute a rare cause of Cushing's syndrome. The bronchial carcinoid tumor is frequently linked with ectopic ACTH syndrome.

Additionally, iatrogenic Cushing's syndrome, another form of the disorder, results from exogenous administration of synthetic glucocorticoids in supraphysiologic amounts.

Risk Factors

One of the major risk factors for increased levels of cortisol is the administration of exogenous steroids. Whenever steroids are administered, a degree of excess is present. Placing the client on the lowest amount of steroids possible can help to control this problem.

Other risk factors are outlined in the section on etiology. These factors are related to hyperplasia of the adrenal gland, either as a primary disorder or secondary to excessive amounts of ACTH. In the latter case, control of the primary disease decreases the adrenal hyperplasia. There are no particular preventive measures.

Pathophysiology

When Cushing's syndrome develops, the normal function of the glucocorticoids (see Chap. 60) becomes exaggerated and the classic picture of the syndrome emerges (Fig. 63–3). This exaggerated physiologic action of glucocorticoids appears as

- Persistent hyperglycemia ("steroid diabetes").
- Protein tissue wasting, which results in

  Weakness due to muscle wasting
  Capillary fragility, resulting in ecchymosis
  Osteoporosis due to bone matrix wasting. Osteoporosis can become so severe that even mild trauma can cause fractures. Compression fractures can develop in the osteoporotic spine, leading to kyphosis and loss of height.

- Potassium depletion, leading to hypokalemia, arrhythmias, muscle weakness, and renal disorders.
- Sodium and water retention, which causes edema and hypertension.
- Hypertension, which eventually predisposes the individual to left ventricular hypertrophy, congestive heart failure, and cerebral vascular accidents.
- Abnormal fat distribution (in conjunction with edema), results in a moon-shaped face, a dorsocervical fat pad on the neck (buffalo hump), and truncal obesity with slender limbs. Also, pink and purple striae appear on the breasts, axillary areas, abdomen, and legs due to thinning of skin. Striking changes occur in appearance following both development and cure of Cushing's syndrome. Old photographs can be useful in recognizing changes over time.
- Increased susceptibility to infection and lowered resistance to stress increase vulnerability to microorganisms of all types. Due to suppression of the inflammatory response, people with Cushing's syndrome can show few signs of infection. The client also demonstrates poor wound healing.
- Possible increased production of androgens can cause virilism in women. Manifestations of virilism include acne, thinning of scalp hair, and hirsutism (abnormal growth and distribution of hair).
- Mental changes include memory loss, poor concentration and cognition, euphoria, and depression. Some clients develop "steroid psychosis." Depression can predispose the client to suicidal thoughts.

Clinical Manifestations

Figure 63–3 demonstrates the clinical picture of a client with hyperadrenalism. The pathophysiology of the disease also provides a clear picture of the client with this hyperplasia.

DIAGNOSTIC ASSESSMENT

Although there is a classic "Cushingoid" appearance to clients with hypercortisolism, it is important to perform diagnostic studies to confirm the diagnosis.

Laboratory tests for Cushing's syndrome reflect hyperglycemia, fluid and electrolyte disturbances, and immunosuppressive responses that characterize excessive glucocorticoid secretion. Thus, in Cushing's syndrome, glucose tolerance decreases and glucosuria appears. The white blood cell count often rises above 10,000/mm^3, but the total eosinophil count can drop below 50 cells/mm^3. Also, lymphocytes can fall below 20 per cent. Both urinary 17-hydroxysteroids (HS) and blood cortisol rise to high levels.

Normally, plasma cortisol follows a diurnal pattern, rising in the early morning (10 to 25 μg/dl), then gradually falling to less than 10 μg/dl in the evening, and approaching undetectable levels near midnight. Clients with Cushing's syndrome have elevated plasma cortisol levels throughout the day and can demonstrate a loss of diurnal variation.

Urinary free cortisol (UFC) measurement is used as a screening test to identify elevated urinary excretion of free cortisol. Clients with Cushing's syndrome will have UFC levels above 100 μg/day.

The overnight dexamethasone suppression test is often used in the differential diagnosis of Cushing's syndrome. It can be performed on an outpatient basis.

Day 1: Administer dexamethasone, 1 mg PO at 11 PM
Day 2: Draw plasma cortisol level at 8 AM

The normal range is below 5 μg/dl. Severe stress or depression can cause false-positive results (i.e., plasma cortisol greater than 5 μg/dl despite otherwise normal endocrine function). If dexamethasone fails to suppress the hypothalamic-pituitary-adrenal (HPA) (see Fig. 63–2) axis and the morning cortisol level is greater than 5 μg/dl, an abnormality of feedback is suggested that is compatible with Cushing's syndrome.

The standard dexamethasone suppression test (performed over 6 consecutive days) differentiates Cushing's disease (caused by pituitary oversecretion of ACTH) from other causes of Cushing's syndrome.

Days 1 to 6: Collect 24 h urine for UFC.
Days 1 to 2: Baseline.
Days 3 to 4: Low-dose dexamethasone test; 0.5 mg PO q 6 h

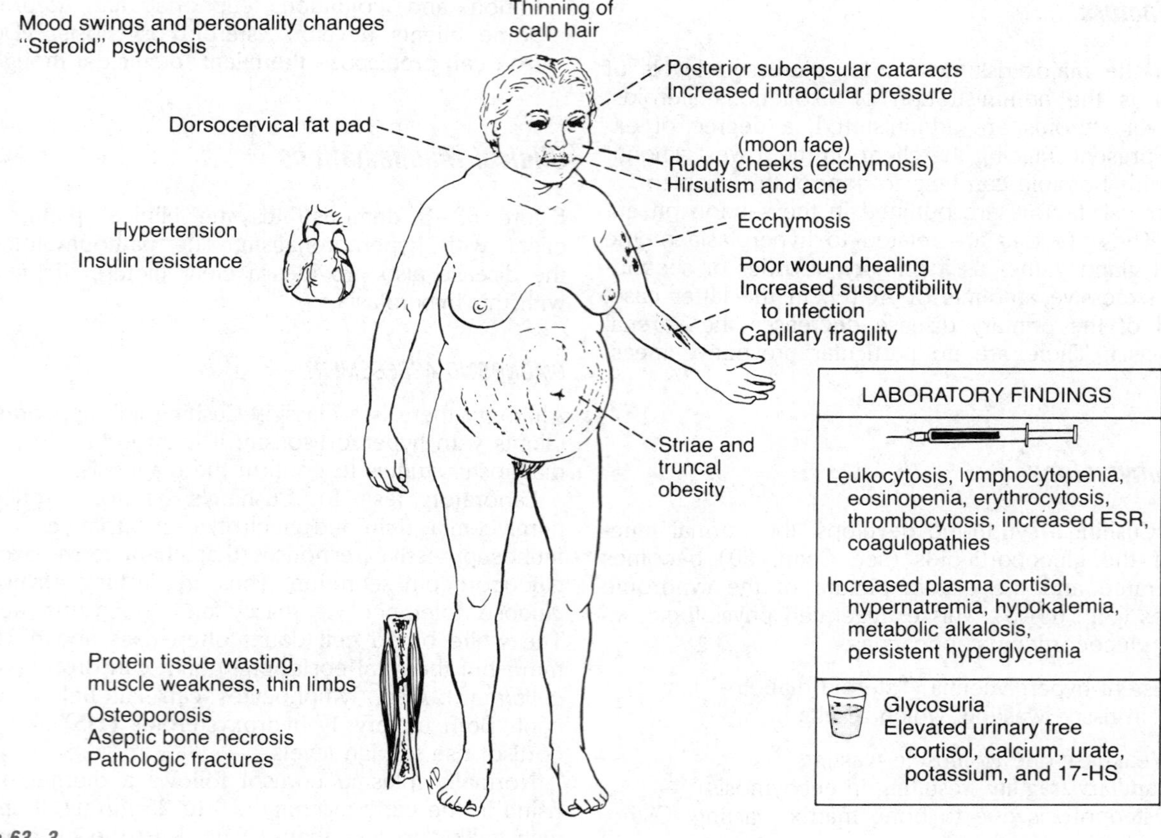

▲ *Figure 63–3*

Assessment data for Cushing's syndrome. Inset refers to laboratory findings.

Days 5 to 6: High-dose dexamethasone test; 2 mg PO q 6 h

The results show that suppression is interpreted as a fall in basal 17-HS of more than 50 per cent. This is compatible with Cushing's disease and ectopic ACTH secretion.

Dexamethasone suppresses pituitary secretion of ACTH. Thus, by the second day of dexamethasone administration, levels of urinary 17-HS should be less than 2 mg in normal subjects. In the client with Cushing's disease (a pituitary disorder), levels of 17-HS drop due to a pathologic disruption in the HPA axis. ACTH-secreting pituitary adenomas are relatively resistant to dexamethasone. Cushing's syndrome and an ectopic ACTH-secreting tumor, on the other hand, usually do not respond to dexamethasone (i.e., levels of 17-HS do not decrease).

The plasma ACTH test demonstrates that low ACTH levels point toward an adrenal tumor as the cause of hypercortisolism. The overproduction of cortisol from the adrenal tumor provides negative feedback to the pituitary gland, which responds by decreasing ACTH release. The high cortisol level also provides feedback to the hypothalamus, which decreases release of cortisol-releasing hormone (CRH).

The presence of an ectopic ACTH-producing tumor usually yields a normal or elevated ACTH level. ACTH production from the tumor is independent of pituitary production of ACTH, and so despite negative feedback to the hypothalamic-pituitary unit, ACTH levels will remain high.

The inferior petrosal sinus sampling test (IPSS) is a radiologic test used to isolate the source of ACTH secretion (whether it is within the pituitary gland or not, and if so, where within the gland). The left and right petrosal sinuses carry blood from the pituitary gland to the jugular veins. Catheters are threaded into the inferior petrosal sinus via the femoral veins. By sampling ACTH levels drawn from the right and left petrosal sinuses, the side of the pituitary gland producing ACTH can be identified. If ACTH levels from the petrosal sinuses are greater than that from a peripheral site (the arm), a pituitary tumor is identified as the source of hypercortisolism. If central ACTH levels (petrosal) and peripheral ACTH levels (arm) are equivalent, an ectopic ACTH-secreting tumor is likely. The development of this test has allowed neurosurgeons to perform a hemi-hypophysectomy and remove only the half of the pituitary gland that contains the microadenoma. Prior to the availability of IPSS, the entire gland usually had to be removed due to the difficulty in localizing these "invisible" tumors.

An adrenal CT scan is performed to seek an adrenal mass in the right or left adrenal gland. Contrast dye is used, when possible, to enhance the clarity of the scan.

Medical Management

Although surgery is the usual treatment for primary adrenal hyperplasia, other palliative treatments are available (Table 63-3). Radiation therapy can be used to treat primary pituitary tumors and other ACTH-secreting adenomas. Radiation can be either internally or externally applied to the pituitary gland for tumors. Internally, the radiation is applied through a transphenoidal implant. Radiation must be used with care because of the proximity of the optic nerve. Radiation is not always effective in even palliative treatment of tumors and may destroy normal tissue. For ACTH-secreting adenomas such as lung tumors, palliation is possible. See Chapter 22 for a discussion of care of the client undergoing radiation therapy.

PHARMACOLOGIC MANAGEMENT

Medications that interfere with ACTH production or adrenal hormone synthesis are available. Mitotane (Lysodren) is a cytotoxic antihormonal agent that inhibits corticosteroid synthesis without destroying cortical cells. Aminogluthethamide (Cytadren) and trilostane (Modrastane) are other cytotoxic agents that block the synthesis of glucocorticoids and adrenal steroids.

Cyproheptadine (Periactin) is used less commonly to treat hypersecretion due to pituitary abnormalities resulting in increased ACTH levels. This agent appears to interfere with the ACTH production, thereby decreasing the effect on the adrenals.

Surgical Management

The resection of most pituitary tumors causing Cushing's syndrome is performed via transsphenoidal hypophysectomy. Occasionally, large or anatomically complex tumors are excised via a transfrontal approach. (See the section on hypophysectomy).

For Cushing's syndrome due to adrenal tumor (or possibly ectopic ACTH-secreting tumor), an adrenalectomy can be performed to remove the gland containing the tumor. In cases of ectopic ACTH-secreting tumors, the tumor can be difficult to localize. If no source is found, a bilateral adrenalectomy can be performed to interrupt the production of cortisol in response to ACTH produced by the tumor, or the client can be treated with antiglucocorticoids while continuing to search for the tumor.

Nursing Management

ASSESSMENT

The nurse begins by collecting a careful history from the client with potential Cushing's syndrome. The client

TABLE 63-3. Therapies Prescribed for Cushing's Syndrome, Cushing's Disease, and Ectopic ACTH Syndrome

Condition	Responsible Lesion	Therapies	Remarks
Cushing's syndrome	Adrenal tumor (benign or malignant)	Adrenalectomy (surgical excision)	Adrenalectomy for a benign unilateral tumor; usually curative Bilateral adrenalectomy must be followed by lifelong administration of corticosteroids
	Adrenal carcinoma with widespread metastases	Surgery and chemotherapy: o,p'-DDD	Chemotherapy largely unsuccessful
Cushing's disease	Pituitary tumor (or unidentified lesion) that secretes excessive amounts of ACTH	Microsurgical resection of pituitary adenoma	Pituitary surgery is successful in 95 per cent of cases
		Irradiation of pituitary gland	Irradiation successful in 75 per cent of cases; therapeutic effects not apparent for months following initiation of therapy
		Total bilateral adrenalectomy (corrects adrenal hyperplasia due to excessive ACTH stimulation)	Total bilateral adrenalectomy must be followed by lifelong replacement therapy with a glucocorticoid and mineralocorticoid
Ectopic ACTH syndrome	Extra-adrenal malignant tumor	Surgical removal of ectopic malignant tumor; chemotherapy used to control hypercorticism and promote remission in individuals with inoperable cancer	Surgery rarely successful because metastasis usually occurs before diagnosis; chemotherapy purely palliative

may well exhibit the characteristic clinical manifestations identified previously.

The client will require support during the diagnostic phase of the disease. There is often a great deal of uncertainty at this point about the cause of the disorder. The client will require thorough explanations as to why these tests must be performed before treatment can be started.

During the preoperative phase, the client with Cushing's syndrome requires expert nursing assessment and care. The crucial problems of hypertension, edema, possible heart disease, diabetes mellitus, increased susceptibility to infection, decreased resistance to stress, and emotional lability must all be assessed and then brought under control prior to surgical treatment.

NURSING INTERVENTION

Collaborative Problem. High risk for infection R/T lowered resistance to stress and compromised immune response.

Planning: Expected Outcomes. Infection will not develop or will be detected early, as evidenced by absence of leukocytosis, fever, or other signs of infections.

Implementation. Protect clients from exposure to infectious organisms. Isolate them from health care personnel and significant others with contagious disorders. Employ careful handwashing technique before contact with client.

Because glucocorticoids suppress immune and inflammatory reactions, clients with Cushing's syndrome may experience only mild symptoms, even in the presence of a severe infection. A slight elevation in body temperature may indicate the presence of a severe infection.

Collaborative Problem. High risk for injury: fractures, hypertension, or diabetes R/T osteoporosis, sodium and water retention, or the presence of an insulin antagonist.

Planning: Expected Outcomes. Injury will not occur, as evidenced by absence of fracture, hypertension, or hyperglycemia.

Implementation. The nurse must protect the client against falls and accidents. Clients with Cushing's syndrome have osteoporosis and tend to develop fractures even with mild trauma. Keep the bed in the lowest position, and raise side rails for protection. Assist clients with ambulation to avoid falls.

Monitor vital signs at frequent intervals. Assess the client carefully for signs of severe hypertension, e.g., elevated blood pressure (BP), headache, failing vision, irritability, and dyspnea. Check for postural hypotension (encourage position change slowly to avoid injury from sudden drop in BP).

Obtain daily weight in a consistent manner. If sodium intake is reduced, edema and weight should diminish. Test urine for glucose and acetone daily or perform daily blood glucose levels via finger stick. Positive results may indicate the development of diabetes mellitus (steroid diabetes) due to the insulin antagonist action of the excessive cortisol.

Nursing Diagnosis: Activity Intolerance R/T fatigue and muscle weakness from protein wasting, persistent hyperglycemia (and possible diabetes mellitus), and potassium depletion.

Planning: Expected Outcomes. Client will not experience activity intolerance, as evidenced by client's ability to balance rest and activity.

Implementation. The nurse must promote mental and physical rest for the client with Cushing's syndrome. It is important to minimize stress and confusion so the client can achieve maximal periods of rest.

Nursing Diagnosis: Skin Integrity, Impaired, High Risk for R/T tissue catabolism (thinning of skin), decreased connective tissue, and edema secondary to sodium and water retention.

Planning: Expected Outcomes. Client will not develop impaired skin integrity, as evidenced by intact skin.

Implementation. The client's skin should be meticulously monitored for the presence of breakdown. The client is extremely prone to breakdown from the tissue catabolism. Avoid the use of tape or other irritants that may result in skin tearing or excoriation.

Nursing Diagnosis: Thought Processes, Altered (Memory Loss, Cognitive Impairment, Mood Swings, Euphoria, Depression) R/T increased levels of glucocorticoids and ACTH.

Planning: Expected Outcomes. Client will not suffer from altered thought process, as evidenced by decrease in symptoms of memory loss, cognitive impairment, or mood swings or will have symptoms minimized.

Implementation. The nurse must anticipate clients' mood swings. Clients can become easily upset by changes in their appearance caused by the disease process. They also can become alarmed by the bizarre feelings and emotions they experience. Reassurance should be given, explaining that appearance and moods should gradually return to normal after the disorder is treated (see Fig. 63–3) unless the treatment requires the client to receive steroid replacement. If clients have to receive steroid therapy, they will continue to experience some of side effects.

Nursing Diagnosis: Knowledge Deficit R/T the disease, surgery, and proper diet.

Planning: Expected Outcomes. Client will understand the disease, planned surgery, and proper diet, as evidenced by client's statements of understanding and client's ability to choose correct diet.

Implementation. It is important for clients to understand their condition and the proposed treatment. Clients should be given the opportunity to ask questions about the treatment and should be assessed for their understanding of it.

Encourage a diet low in calories, carbohydrates, and sodium but with ample protein and potassium content. Such a diet promotes weight loss, reduction of edema and hypertension, control of hypokalemia, and rebuilding of wasted tissue. The client with diabetes mellitus or gastric ulcers requires a special diet (see Chaps. 61 and 54, respectively).

Collaborative Problem. High risk for injury R/T surgical procedure.

Planning: Expected Outcomes. Injury will not occur or will be detected early, as evidenced by absence of shock, hemorrhage, infection, or addisonian crisis.

Implementation. On the morning of surgery, administer a glucocorticoid preparation (intramuscular [IM] or intravenous [IV]) as prescribed. A water-soluble cortisol preparation (diluted in an IV infusion) may be given throughout the surgical procedure. Cortisol protects the client from the development of acute adrenal insufficiency during adrenalectomy. Even if the surgeon plans to remove only one adrenal gland, temporary glucocorticoid support may be needed until the remaining adrenal gland begins to secrete sufficient amounts of cortisol. Because of the excessive secretion of cortisol by the tumorous gland, the healthy gland can atrophy and require time to readjust.

During the immediate postoperative phase, major goals are to (1) prevent shock, (2) prevent infection, (3) sustain adequate cortisol levels, and (4) control pain and incisional discomfort.

Observe for signs of shock due to hemorrhage (hypotension, and rapid, weak pulse). The nurse should document vital signs every 15 minutes, measure urine and record hourly output, observing for oliguria, a sign of shock and renal shutdown. Administer IV fluids, pressor amines, and corticosteroids as prescribed.

Remember that the signs of addisonian crisis resemble shock. The client should be closely assessed for the development of this complication, and IV cortisol should be administered in high doses until the symptoms subside. The client will continue to require increased amounts of steroids until the remaining adrenal returns to a normal level of functioning and the stress associated with the treatment subsides.

Encourage clients in coughing, turning, and deep breathing to prevent respiratory infections. Employ meticulous sterile technique with wound care to prevent infection. Ileus is less common because the flank approach is usually used.

Nursing Diagnosis: Knowledge Deficit R/T self-administration of replacement hormones.

Planning: Expected Outcomes. Client will understand self-administration of replacement hormones, as evidenced by the client's ability to repeat and comply with instructions and that the client does not develop addisonian crisis or adrenal insufficiency.

Implementation. Following bilateral adrenalectomy, lifelong glucocorticoid replacement is essential. If only one adrenal gland has been removed, daily cortisol replacement continues until the remaining gland functions normally (usually 6 to 12 months later). Prior to discharge, the client, family, and significant others need instruction on self-administration of replacement hormones (hydrocortisone). The client and significant others should successfully demonstrate the self-injection technique before discharge from the hospital.

EVALUATION

The nurse must evaluate client outcomes based on the established plan of care. If these goals were not achieved, the plan and interventions must be revised to meet the client's needs.

Modification of Plan of Care for the Elderly

Elderly clients may exhibit excessive symptoms from Cushing's syndrome because these clients may already exhibit many of the characteristic manifestations, such as osteoporosis, hypertension, and diabetes. The client also is more prone to the side effects of steroid replacement therapy.

Post-hospital Care

DISCHARGE TEACHING

The discharge teaching is the same as for the client with Addison's disease (see the section on Addison's disease).

FOLLOW-UP CARE

Follow-up care is the same as for the client with Addison's disease because the client will require steroid replacement (see the section on Addison's disease).

PRIMARY HYPERALDOSTERONISM (CONN'S SYNDROME)

Definition

Aldosterone is the most powerful of the mineralocorticoids. Its primary role is to conserve sodium, and it also promotes potassium excretion.

Incidence

The exact incidence of Conn's syndrome is unknown. It strikes females twice as often as males and appears most frequently in middle-aged clients.

Etiology

Hypersecretion of aldosterone due to an adrenal lesion results in primary hyperaldosteronism. In contrast, secondary hyperaldosteronism arises as a consequence of edematous disorders (cardiac failure, cirrhosis of the liver with ascites, and nephrotic syndrome). It also develops in clients with hypertension due to destructive renal artery disease.

The major cause of primary hyperaldosteronism is a benign, aldosterone-secreting tumor called an aldosteronoma. Although sometimes the diagnostician finds multiple tumors, the causative factor in 90 per cent of clients is a single adenoma. Rarely, Conn's syndrome develops as a consequence of adrenocortical carcinoma.

Risk Factors

There are no particular risk factors for primary hyperaldosteronism. The risks for secondary hyperaldosteronism include chronic heart failure, cirrhosis with ascites, nephrotic syndrome, and hypertension due to destructive renal artery disease. The preventive measures, therefore, are successful treatment and control of the causative disease process. The more successfully these factors are controlled, the less secondary hyperaldosteronism will be present.

Pathophysiology

Aldosterone affects the tubular reabsorption of sodium and water, and the excretion of potassium and hydrogen ions in the renal tubular epithelial cells (Fig. 63-4). This leads to the development of hypernatremia, hypervolemia, hypokalemia, and metabolic alkalosis. With the hypervolemia and hypernatremia, the blood pressure increases, often to very high levels, and renin production is suppressed. The hypertension can lead to cerebral infarcts and to renal damage.

Secondary hyperaldosteronism is due to the continuous secretion of aldosterone secondary to the high levels of angiotensin II, resulting, in turn, from high plasma renin activity. The decreased renal perfusion due to a variety of causes is the underlying mechanism.

Clinical Manifestations

Clients with primary hyperaldosteronism experience hypertension, hypernatremia, and hypokalemia. Without intervention, they can develop all the complications of chronic hypertension, such as visual disturbances, heart failure, renal damage, and cerebrovascular accident.

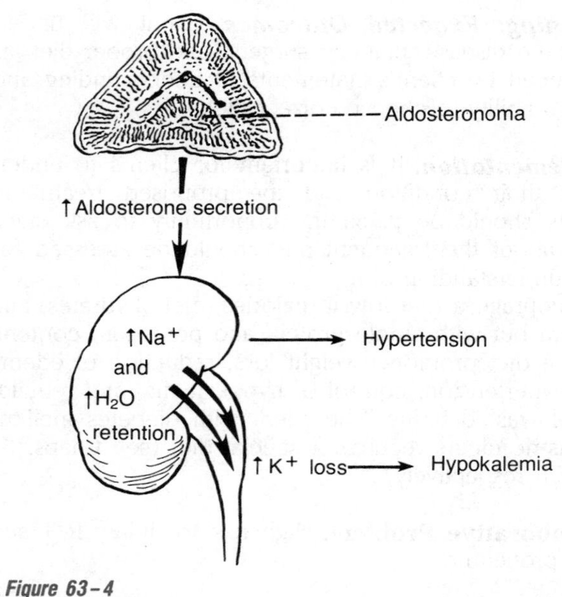

▲ *Figure 63-4*

Effects of primary aldosteronism. Excessive aldosterone secretion causes increased Na^+ and water retention and increased excretion of K^+.

Hypokalemia results from excessive urinary excretion of K^+ (see Chaps. 14 and 15). This problem, in turn, causes muscle weakness, paralysis, or cardiac arrhythmias, because K^+ loss reduces normal neuromuscular irritability. In addition, excessive excretion of K^+ results in polyuria. The large urinary output leads to polydipsia (excessive thirst). Finally, hypokalemia leads to metabolic alkalosis from (1) shifting of H^+ into the cells in exchange for K^+ and (2) exchange of H^+ within the tubular cells for Na^+ from the tubular urine. Metabolic alkalosis causes a decrease in ionized calcium levels, which can result in tetany and respirator suppression (see Chaps. 14 and 15).

Despite sodium retention, clients with hyperaldosteronism rarely develop overt edema. Although extracellular increases moderately, excessive water is normally excreted in the urine with potassium ions. Over time, the kidneys tend to adjust physiologically to excessive secretion of aldosterone, so water excretion reaches an equilibrium with sodium intake. The ability of the kidneys to eventually "escape" from the sodium- and water-retaining action of aldosterone is sometimes called the escape phenomenon.[56]

DIAGNOSTIC ASSESSMENT

Diagnosis of primary hyperaldosteronism is based on low serum potassium, alkalosis, and elevated urinary or plasma aldosterone with low plasma renin levels. Additionally, radiographic studies can reveal cardiac hypertrophy resulting from chronic hypertension. Radionuclide scanning techniques using radiolabeled iodocholesterol allow visualization of the tumors.

Medical Management

The three goals of intervention for clients with primary hyperaldosteronism are to (1) reverse hypertension, (2) correct hypokalemia, and (3) prevent kidney damage. In two thirds of the cases, removal of the aldosterone-secreting tumor completely resolves the hypertension. Most clients have normal BP readings by the third postoperative month.

Unfortunately, the renal complications resulting from long-term hypertension tend to be progressive. Therefore, clients with primary hyperaldosteronism need to be diagnosed and treated early in the course of the disease.

PHARMACOLOGIC MANAGEMENT

If clients cannot be treated surgically, they are often given spironolactone (Aldactone) to increase sodium excretion and to treat the hypertension and hypokalemia. The client's potassium level should be carefully monitored for the development of hyperkalemia, especially if the client has been receiving potassium supplements or has been on a high-potassium diet.

Surgical Management

Surgery is the treatment of choice for primary hyperaldosteronism. A unilateral or bilateral adrenalectomy must be performed. Clients undergoing a unilateral adrenalectomy may need temporary replacement of glucocorticoids, while those requiring bilateral adrenalectomies will need permanent replacement (see the section on Addison's disease). Clients usually receive glucocorticoids preoperatively to prevent any adrenal hypofunction.

Nursing Management

The nurse must help prepare the client for the diagnostic assessment so the diagnosis of hyperaldosteronism can be achieved rapidly and treatment performed before permanent damage occurs. The nurse should administer prescribed medications and closely monitor the client for hypertension or renal damage. The preoperative and postoperative management is the same as that described previously under Cushing's syndrome (see the section on Cushing's syndrome).

CONGENITAL ADRENAL HYPERPLASIA

Congenital adrenal hyperplasia (CAH) is a rare condition characterized by virilism. It results from excessive secretion of androgens by the adrenal cortex. CAH results from an inherited enzyme deficiency, which, in turn, leads to a number of pathologic consequences (Fig. 63-5). Without the missing enzyme, the body cannot synthesize adequate amounts of cortisol. Cortisol, by means of negative feedback, normally inhibits ACTH secretion from the anterior pituitary gland (see Fig. 63-2).

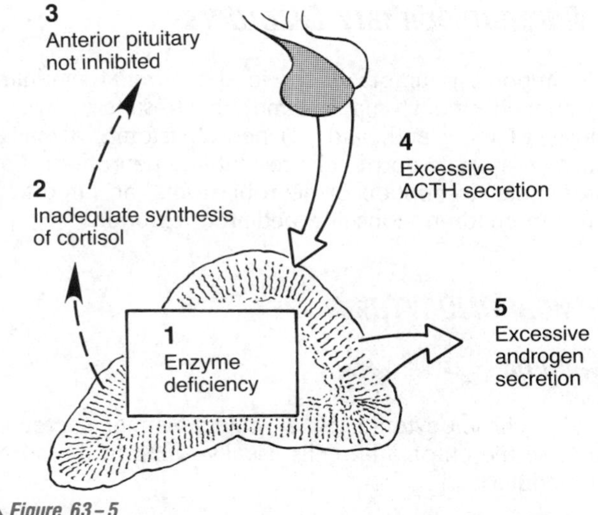

▲ *Figure 63-5*

Congenital adrenal hyperplasia (CAH). Enzyme deficiency ultimately leads to excessive androgen secretion.

Without the inhibitory effects of cortisol, the pituitary gland continues to secrete ACTH and blood levels rise. Excessive stimulation of ACTH results in hyperplasia of the adrenal glands and hypersecretion of sex steroids. Finally, excessive production of androgenic steroids causes virilization.

The symptoms of CAH differ, depending on the age, sex, and particular enzyme deficiency of the client. A female infant can be born with pseudohermaphroditism, or masculinization of the female external genitalia. Older girls and women can develop hirsutism, clitoral enlargement, balding, breast tissue atrophy, and a masculine physique. Virilizing changes in boys and men are less obvious. CAH is primarily congenital, but it occasionally occurs in adulthood.

Other manifestations of CAH (depending on the specific enzyme deficiency) can include salt wasting accompanied by hypotension and dehydration, or excessive salt and water retention accompanied by hypertension. In addition, many clients suffer from disturbances of self-image and sexual dysfunction because of their abnormal appearance and development.

Diagnostic findings that confirm CAH include an elevated 17-hydroxyprogesterone or other key steroid intermediate that can be suppressed by glucocorticoid administration.

Treatment for CAH involves the administration of cortisol preparations to (1) correct the cortisol deficiency and (2) inhibit ACTH production by the anterior pituitary gland. This, in turn, reverses adrenal hypertrophy and overproduction of androgenic steroids.

In addition, client education should include instruction on the need to wear an emergency identification bracelet and carry an emergency hydrocortisone replacement kit.

If an adrenal tumor is causing masculinization, it must be removed surgically.

▼ Adrenomedullary Disorders

Two important tumors occur in the adrenal medulla: (1) pheochromocytoma, a tumor that results in hyperactivity of the gland, and (2) neuroblastoma, a malignant tumor made up of cells resembling neuroblast. For a complete description of neuroblastoma, an important tumor in children, consult a pediatric textbook.

PHEOCHROMOCYTOMA

Definition

A pheochromocytoma is a catecholamine-secreting tumor of the chromaffin cells usually found in the adrenal medulla.

Incidence

Pheochromocytomas are rare, causing about 0.1 per cent of the cases of hypertension. The condition is slightly more common in women than in men. Although the disease can occur at any age, it is most common in middle age and rarely occurs after age 60 years.

Etiology

The exact cause of pheochromocytomas is unknown. In some cases, pheochromocytomas appear to have a hereditary basis. They often occur in association with neuroectodermal diseases and with medullary cancer of the thyroid gland.

Risk Factors

Pregnancy and stress can precipitate and amplify the manifestations of pheochromocytoma.

Pathophysiology

The pheochromocytoma, usually less than 200 g, is composed of chromaffin cells, so named because they stain a dark color with chromium salts. In 80 to 90 per cent of cases, pheochromocytomas arise within the adrenal medulla. Occasionally, however, they develop from the chromaffin tissues, forming the sympathetic paraganglia.

Pheochromocytomas are typically benign; less than 10 per cent are malignant. Because of the excessive amounts of epinephrine and norepinephrine they secrete, they can produce severe symptoms and even death (Table 63-4). Without early intervention, the client is at risk for cerebral hemorrhage and cardiac failure. Fortunately, if pheochromocytomas are discovered early in their development, they can usually be eliminated by surgical removal.

TABLE 63-4. Comparative Effects of Epinephrine and Norepinephrine

Epinephrine	Norepinephrine
Cardiovascular System	
Constricts superficial blood vessels; in small doses, dilates muscle, brain, and coronary vessels, thus shunting blood supply to organs; essential for "fight or flight"	Constricts all blood vessels (especially peripheral), causing increased peripheral resistance
Raises blood pressure	Raises blood pressure greatly
Increases cardiac output	Decreases cardiac output because of increased peripheral resistance
Increases pulse dramatically	Increases pulse moderately
Constricts spleen, shunting stored red blood cells into general circulation	
Increases coagulability of blood	
Respiratory System	
Increases rate and depth of respirations	
Dilates bronchi	
Nervous System	
Stimulates central nervous system, increasing alertness and producing a feeling of fright, excitation, and impending doom	
Dilates pupils	Dilates pupils
Inhibits gastrointestinal tract	Inhibits gastrointestinal tract
Metabolism	
Increases nonesterified fatty acid level of blood	Increases nonesterified fatty acid level of blood
Promotes conversion of glycogen to glucose	
Increases body metabolism	Increases body metabolism slightly

Data from Campese, V. M., & DeQuattro, V. (1989). Functional components of the sympathetic nervous system: Regulation of organ systems. In L. DeGroot (Ed.), *Endocrinology and metabolism* (2nd ed.). Philadelphia: W. B. Saunders.

Clinical Manifestations

The client with pheochromocytoma can experience symptoms similar to diabetes mellitus (elevated blood glucose and glucosuria), essential hypertension (elevated BP, headaches), hyperthyroidism (increased metabolic rate, diaphoresis, agitation, rapid pulse, emotional outbursts) and psychoneurosis (emotional instability).

Hypertension is the principal manifestation of pheochromocytoma, and can be persistent, fluctuating, intermittent, or paroxysmal in nature. Typically, the client has episodes of high blood pressure accompanied by pounding headaches. Other manifestations of sympathetic overactivity include sweating, apprehension, palpitations, nausea, and vomiting. The excessive release of catecholamine also results in excessive conversion of glycogen into glucose in the liver. Consequently, hyperglycemia and glucosuria occur during attacks. Such manifestations can develop spontaneously or be precipitated by emotional stress, physical exertion, or change in body position.

Acute attacks can be associated with profuse diaphoresis, dilated pupils, and cold extremities. Severe hypertension can precipitate a cerebral vascular accident or sudden blindness.

DIAGNOSTIC ASSESSMENT

Because pheochromocytoma is curable, early and accurate diagnosis is essential. Current methods of diagnosis include the following:

1. History and physical examination. The client may describe symptomatic attacks over weeks, months, or even years. The BP may change with exertion or emotional upset. In long-standing cases, complications of hypertension (e.g., visual disturbances), symptoms of heart disease (dyspnea, edema), and manifestations of kidney damage (albuminuria, proteinuria, and increased blood urea nitrogen) can exist.
2. Chemical tests. Two hormonal assay tests are useful in diagnosing pheochromocytoma:
   (a) Assay of the urinary catecholamines and their metabolites (metanephrines and vanillylmandelic acid [VMA]). Assays of catecholamines are performed on single-voided urine specimens, 2- to 4-hour specimens, and 24-hour urine specimens. The normal range of urinary catecholamines is up to 14 μg/100 ml of urine, with higher levels occurring in pheochromocytoma.
   (b) Determinations of plasma catecholamine concentrations. Assays of urinary VMA levels are performed on 24-hour urine specimens only. Advise clients to avoid tea, chocolate, vanilla, and all fruits for at least 2 days before urine collection begins. Also, remind them not to take any medications for 2 to 3 days before the test. Normally, the amount of VMA is less than 7 mg per 24 hours. Urinary VMA rises in clients with pheochromocytoma.

   The laboratory also performs a direct assay of catecholamines in the blood. The normal range of catecholamines in the blood is epinephrine, 0.02 to 0.2 μg/L, and norepinephrine, 0.1 to 0.5 μg/L.
3. X-ray imaging. Various radiographic techniques can help confirm and identify adrenomedullary tumor location, such as CT scan and magnetic resonance imaging (MRI).
4. Miscellaneous nonspecific laboratory tests. In the presence of pheochromocytoma, the basal metabolic rate increases, blood sugar rises abnormally, and glycosuria can occur.

Medical Management

PHARMACOLOGIC MANAGEMENT

Alpha-adrenergic blocking agents such as phentolamine (Regitine) can be used in an IV bolus or IV drip for hypertensive crisis. Oral phenoxybenzamine (Dibenzyline) is used preoperatively to control the blood pressure prior to definitive treatment, surgical removal of the affected gland.

Surgical Management

The primary treatment for a pheochromocytoma is surgical removal of one or both adrenal glands, depending on whether the tumor is unilateral or bilateral. The procedure is the same as that described for treatment of Cushing's syndrome.

Surgical removal can cure the client, provided the growth is discovered before cardiovascular damage becomes permanent. The operation, however, is not without danger. There are two serious hazards. First, excessive discharge of pressor hormones during induction of anesthesia or manipulation of the tumor can cause extreme rises in BP and cardiac arrhythmias. Second, following resection of the tumor, BP can fall precipitously.

Nursing Management

ASSESSMENT

It is important to assess and control the client's blood pressure preoperatively. The client must be closely monitored for the development of stressful episodes before treatment has begun. It is also important to assess the client's neurologic status in case the client has a stroke from the extremely elevated blood pressure.

NURSING INTERVENTION

Collaborative Problem. High risk for injury R/T excessive release of epinephrine and norepinephrine preoperatively.

Planning: Expected Outcomes. Injury will not occur or will be detected early, as evidenced by the absence of hypertensive episodes and cardiovascular or cerebral damage.

Implementation. During the preoperative phase, the goal of treatment is to prevent attacks of acute paroxysmal hypertension, thereby decreasing the risk of further damage to the cardiovascular system. Important nursing interventions include (1) promoting rest and relief from stress; (2) administering prescribed sedatives; (3) providing a high vitamin, mineral, and caloric diet; (4) prohibiting beverages with caffeine such as coffee and tea; and (5) monitoring vital signs. In most cases, the physician will prescribe an alpha-adrenergic blocking agent such as phenoxybenzamine.

Collaborative Problem. High risk for injury R/T postoperative hypotension, hemorrhage, and shock.

Planning: Expected Outcomes. Injury will not occur or will be detected early, as evidenced by normotensive state and the absence of hemorrhage, shock, or addisonian crisis.

Implementation. The first 24 to 48 hours after surgery is a critical period demanding vigilant nursing assessment and intervention. During the immediate postoperative period, nursing interventions include observation for signs of shock and hemorrhage.

Following removal of the tumor, profound shock can develop as catecholamine levels drop. Hypotension can persist for 24 to 48 hours. Hemorrhage can occur due to the high vascularity of the adrenal glands. To prevent postoperative shock

- Give IV fluids as prescribed, such as blood, plasma, dextran, or glucose in water to maintain blood volume.
- Administer IV pressors as prescribed at a rate sufficient to maintain BP within a safe range. Check BP as often as is necessary to titrate the medication.
- Carefully measure hourly urinary output. If the client voids less than 30 ml per hour, notify the physician. Oliguria can signify impending shock and consequent renal shutdown.
- Assess the client for signs of hemorrhage. Check the dressing every half hour for bloody drainage. If the client is bleeding internally, an abdominal hematoma can develop, resulting in paralytic ileus. Symptoms of paralytic ileus include abdominal pain, distention, severe nausea, vomiting, and diminished or absent bowel sounds.
- If cortical tissue was resected during surgery, assess the client closely for signs of adrenal insufficiency (see the section on addisonian crisis). If both adrenal glands have been removed, the client must receive cortisol replacement for life.

Nursing Diagnosis: Pain R/T surgery, headache, and other manifestations of pheochromocytoma.

Planning: Expected Outcomes. Client will not suffer pain, as evidenced by client's statements, normotensive state, and absence of evidence of painful expression.

Implementation. When administering medication for incisional pain, monitor BP frequently. Remember that narcotics, particularly meperidine, produce hypotension as a side effect; however, withholding pain medication also can lead to hypotension and severe pain. It is important to control the pain so the client's level of stress will decrease.

Nursing Diagnosis: Knowledge Deficit R/T self-administration of corticosteroids.

Planning: Expected Outcomes. Client will understand self-administration of steroids, as evidenced by client's ability to explain administration and client's compliance with medication regimen.

Implementation. Once the critical postoperative period is over, most clients pass through an uneventful convalescence. Clients who will be self-administering corticosteroids need instruction concerning the administration and side effects (see the section on Addison's disease).

EVALUATION

The nurse must evaluate client outcomes based on the established plan of care. If these goals were not achieved, the plan and interventions must be revised to meet the client's needs.

Modification of Plan of Care for the Elderly

The elderly client is more likely to suffer damage related to any hypertensive episodes associated with the pheochromocytoma because their cardiovascular and cerebrovascular systems are likely to be weaker and prone to damage from the elevated pressure.

Post-hospital Care

DISCHARGE TEACHING

The discharge teaching for the client on steroids is the same as that for the client with Addison's disease (see the section on Addison's disease).

FOLLOW-UP CARE

The follow-up care is the same as for the client with Addison's disease if the client requires steroid replacement (see the section on Addison's disease).

▼ ANTERIOR PITUITARY DISORDERS

Disorders of the pituitary gland occur most frequently in the anterior lobe (Table 63–5 and see Fig. 60–2). Major causes of pituitary disease include (1) functioning tumors, (2) nonfunctioning tumors, (3) pituitary infarction, (4) genetic disorders, and (5) trauma. The three principal pathologic consequences of pituitary disorders are (1) hyperpituitarism, (2) hypopituitarism, and (3) local compression of brain tissue by expanding tumor masses.

HYPERPITUITARISM

General Information

Hyperpituitarism is defined as oversecretion of one or more of the hormones secreted by the pituitary gland. It is primarily caused by a hormone-secreting pituitary

TABLE 63-5. Pituitary Hormones

Name	Releasing Factor	Target Cells	Response	Increased Level	Decreased Level
Anterior Pituitary					
GH	GHRH	Bone, muscle	Stimulates growth; promotes active transport of amino acids into cell and influences lipid, CHO, and CA^{2+} metabolism	Child: gigantism (before epiphyseal closure); child grows very tall. Adult: acromegaly (after epiphyseal closure); bones increase in thickness; increase in soft tissue growth.	Child: dwarfism. Adult: lethargy, increased weight, loss of reproductive function, premature aging.
ACTH	CRH	Adrenal cortex	Stimulates adrenal gland secretion of mineralocorticoids and glucocorticoids	Cushing's disease: increased amounts of cortisol and aldosterone	Addison's disease: decreased cortisol and aldosterone, increased MSH
TSH	TRH	Thyroid	Stimulates thyroid to increase secretion of thyroxine (controls rate of most chemical reactions in body)	Goiter; increased BMR; decreased weight; increased cardiac output, HR, and BP; increased cerebration; fine muscle tremors	Reduced thyroid activity; decreased BMR; increased weight; decreased cardiac output, HR, and BP; decreased cerebration; somnolence
Prolactin		Breast	Stimulates breast to lactate	Amenorrhea	Too little milk
FSH	LHRH	Ovaries, testes	Stimulates growth of ovaries and sperm		Late puberty
LH	LHRH	Ovaries, testes	Growth of follicles and increased secretion of estrogen and progesterone; increased testosterone secretion in the male	Excess testosterone, menstrual cycle disturbance	Amenorrhea; diminished progesterone and testosterone
Posterior Pituitary					
Oxytocin	Labor, sucking	Uterus, breasts	Stimulates uterus to contract at childbirth; stimulates lactation	Precipitate childbirth, excess milk	Prolonged childbirth, diminished milk
ADH (vasopressin)	Dehydration	Arterioles, distal renal tubule	Vasoconstriction of arterioles to increase arterial pressure; increased water reabsorption in distal tubules, stimulates smooth muscle of GI tract	Increased BP, decreased urinary output, edema	Diabetes insipidus, dilute urine, increased urinary volume

Adapted from Davis, J., and Mason, C.: *Neurologic Critical Care.* New York: Van Nostrand Reinhold Co., 1979. BMR, basal metabolism rate; CRH, cortisol releasing hormone.

tumor, typically a benign adenoma. Syndromes associated with hyperpituitarism are Cushing's syndrome, acromegaly, amenorrhea, galactorrhea, hyperthyroidism, and rarely, hypergonadism in the male.

The diagnosis of hyperpituitarism involves radiologic and laboratory testing. Measurement of plasma levels of hormones such as growth hormone (GH), ACTH, follicle-stimulating hormone (FSH), and luteinizing hormone (LH) usually establishes the diagnosis of pituitary hormone hypersecretion. CT scan and MRI can allow visualization of pituitary tumors.

Pituitary tumors produce both systemic effects and local manifestations. Systemic effects include (1) excessive or abnormal growth patterns due to overproduction of GH, (2) abnormal milk secretion (galactorrhea), and (3) overstimulation of one or more of the target glands, resulting in the release of excessive thyroid, sex, or adrenocortical hormones.

Locally, pituitary tumors produce symptoms because the bony cranium that houses the tumor cannot expand to accommodate a growing mass. Local manifestations include visual field abnormalities, resulting from pressure on the optic chiasma; headaches; and somnolence.

GIGANTISM AND ACROMEGALY

Definition

Gigantism and acromegaly are both disturbances of growth that arise from an oversecretion of GH. Gigantism, an overgrowth of the long bones, develops in children before the age when the epiphyses of the bones close. Clients suffering gigantism may grow to 9 defeet tall.

Acromegaly is a disease of adults and develops after closure of the epiphyses of the long bones. As implied by its name, acromegaly (*"akron"* is the Greek word for "extremity") is marked by increases in bone thickness and hypertrophy of the soft tissues.

Incidence

There is a low incidence of gigantism and acromegaly. The acidophilic, GH-producing tumors that cause acromegaly, however, are the second most common type of hyperpituitarism.

Etiology

Gigantism and acromegaly result from GH-secreting adenomas of the anterior pituitary gland.

Risk Factors

There are no identified risk factors for the development of a GH-producing tumor. Also, there is no familial tendency for development of these tumors.

Pathophysiology

Acidophilic, GH-producing tumors are characterized by an excessive secretion of GH. The increased amounts of GH lead to rapid growth in all body tissues. This increased growth leads to giantism, if it occurs before closure of the epiphysis, and acromegaly, if it occurs after epiphyseal closure.

Clients with giantism also often develop hyperglycemia with degeneration of the beta cells of the islets of Langerhans in the pancreas. About 10 per cent of the clients go on to develop full-blown diabetes mellitus.

As the tumor continues to grow, the size often results in destruction of the entire pituitary gland, leading to hypopituitarism. The size of the tumor also can result in pressure on the optic nerve, which crosses directly above the pituitary gland, leading to blindness.

Prognosis depends on the age at which the client develops an oversecretion of GH and seeks health intervention. Many of the somatic changes are irreversible, and the longer the client is in a hypopituitary state, the higher the mortality rate. Thus, the earlier the diagnosis, the more likely the client is to benefit from treatment.

Clinical Manifestations

Clients with acromegaly have a characteristic appearance. Note in Figure 63-6 the coarsening of the facial features, the prognathism (protrusion of the jaw), and the broad hands with spadelike fingers that characterize the disease. In addition, clients with acromegaly develop local manifestations such as headache, diplopia, blindness, and lethargy, due to compression of brain tissue by the tumor. In advanced cases, clients can suffer from associated hormonal disturbances such as diabetes mellitus, goiter, Cushing's disease, changes in libido, and menstrual disorders.

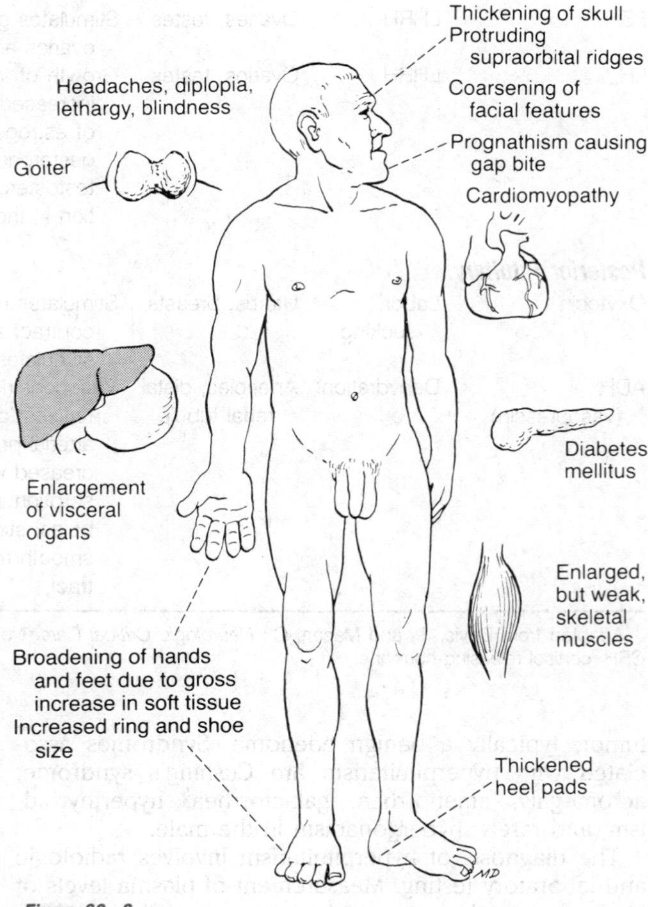

▲ **Figure 63-6**
Assessment data for acromegaly.

Medical Management

Treatment for pituitary tumors can be accomplished through irradiation of the pituitary gland to destroy the tumor. This is usually performed through a radiation implant via the transsphenoidal approach.

PHARMACOLOGIC MANAGEMENT

Bromocriptine (Parlodel) can reduce the levels of growth hormone and decrease tumor size. This agent can be used if the levels of growth hormone remain high after surgery or until the effects of radiation occur.

Surgical Management

The treatment of choice for both gigantism and acromegaly is a surgical hypophysectomy. Partial or complete removal of the pituitary gland occurs during surgical resection of pituitary tumors.

Surgeons prefer the transsphenoidal route for clients with tumors remaining within the sella turcica, or tumors with only moderate suprasellar extension. This approach avoids disturbing the cranium and avoids scarring. Access to the pituitary gland is obtained through an incision made in the upper gum line. Preoperatively, the client's sinuses are cleansed and antibiotic nasal spray is used.

The surgeon, when performing a transsphenoidal hypophysectomy, takes muscle or fat from the thigh and places it in the tumor cavity. The nasal cavities are then packed with vaseline gauze, and a mustache dressing is applied under the nose. Following surgery, the need for cortisone replacement may be permanent.

Nursing Management

ASSESSMENT

Most clients are frightened by the prospect of undergoing surgical removal of the pituitary gland. Provide the client and significant others with emotional support and comfort throughout the preoperative period. The initial symptoms are vague; therefore, clients have often seen many physicians in the past and have had multiple examinations and tests seeking a diagnosis. The client and family might be fearful, skeptical, or relieved at the final diagnosis of a pituitary tumor. The nurse's assessment should include the client's (1) reaction to the diagnosis, (2) expectations of surgery, (3) educational needs related to diagnosis and treatment plan, and (4) available support network following discharge.

The nurse's physical assessment of the client includes baseline vital signs and weight as well as neurologic assessment. These findings are essential to establish a baseline for postoperative comparison. To perform the neurologic assessment, check

- Pupil equality and reactivity to light;
- Handgrip for strength, equality, and ability to release on command;
- Level of consciousness;
- Orientation to time, place, person, and situation;
- Appropriate response to stimuli; and
- Visual acuity and visual fields.

NURSING INTERVENTION

Nursing Diagnosis: Knowledge Deficit R/T surgery and possible outcomes.

Planning: Expected Outcomes. The client will understand the planned surgery and possible outcomes, as evidenced by client's statements, questions, and ability to describe the procedure and outcomes.

Implementation. The client should have the surgery explained in detail, along with potential outcomes of surgical treatment. Use drawings of the brain to explain the transsphenoidal approach. Prepare the client for the presence of an indwelling urinary catheter, IV lines, and any other lines or monitors that may be needed after surgery. Tell the client vital signs will be closely monitored following surgery.

Preoperative preparation also includes coaching the client in deep-breathing exercises and assisting in keeping records of intake and output. **Warn clients to avoid coughing, sneezing, or blowing their nose after surgery.**

Collaborative Problem. High risk for injury R/T postoperative complications.

Planning: Expected Outcomes. Injury will not occur from surgery, as evidenced by the absence of addisonian crisis, balanced output, no signs of increased intracranial pressure, normal temperature, and absence of symptoms of cerebrospinal fluid leakage or meningitis.

Implementation. Prior to surgery, the client usually receives an injection of or intravenous cortisol. Glucocorticoids help the client to tolerate the stress of an operation that can result in loss of adrenocortical function.

Treatment following transfrontal hypophysectomy resembles that for any craniotomy (see Chap. 30). Immediately after surgery, assess for signs of cerebral edema and rising intracranial pressure (elevated BP, widened pulse pressure, low pulse rate, pupil changes, altered respiratory pattern).

The pituitary no longer produces tropic hormones; therefore, watch for signs of target gland deficiencies, such as adrenal insufficiency and hypothyroidism. In addition, diabetes insipidus can occur temporarily due to antidiuretic hormone (ADH) deficiency. Maintain strict documentation of intake and output. Notify the physician if urine output is greater than 200 ml/h with a specific gravity of less than 1.005.

Assess the client carefully for signs of meningitis, a potential complication of surgery. Report any temperature elevation, severe headache, irritability, or nuchal rigidity.

The client who has undergone transsphenoidal hypophysectomy requires frequent oral hygiene using a gauze sponge, and the lips should be lubricated with petroleum jelly. The client should not brush the teeth for 2 weeks after surgery.

The nasal packing is usually removed in 2 to 5 days. After its removal, observe the client for rhinorrhea, which can indicate a cerebrospinal fluid (CSF) leak. Have the client report frequent postnasal drainage. Collect any serous drainage and test it for the presence of cerebrospinal fluid (see Chap. 28) or send it to the laboratory for analysis. It is possible for the muscle or fat graft to dislodge, causing a CSF leak. Instruct the client to avoid sneezing, coughing, and bending over from the waist to avoid disrupting the graft.

Nursing Diagnosis: Knowledge Deficit R/T self-administration of pituitary replacement hormones.

Planning: Expected Outcomes. The client will understand the self-administration of medication, as evidenced by the client's statements, ability to comply with postoperative medication regimen, and absence of symptoms of hypopituitarism.

Implementation. As stated earlier, people who have undergone complete hypophysectomy must take cortisone replacements for the rest of their lives. Instruct these clients to avoid gastric irritation by taking cortisone with milk, food, or an antacid. Advise clients to notify the physician if they develop frequent gastritis, tarry stools, or frank blood in the stools.

Some clients also may require thyroid or sex hormone replacement. In addition, some will need vasopressin replacement to treat diabetes insipidus. Diabetes insipidus is usually transient following surgery but can persist, indicating the need for chronic hormone replacement.

EVALUATION

The nurse must evaluate client outcomes based on the established plan of care. If these goals were not achieved, the plan and interventions must be revised to meet the client's needs.

Post-hospital Care

DISCHARGE TEACHING

Client teaching must include self-administration of hormones, side effects, and signs of overdosage or underdosage of prescribed hormones.

HOME HEALTH CARE NEEDS

If the client has suffered from arthritic changes, assess the client's home so any obstacles can be removed and the client can be fitted with any necessary assistive care devices.

FOLLOW-UP CARE

Because the client is on many hormones, imbalances can develop as a result of the hypophysectomy. It is important, therefore, to stress the importance of maintaining follow-up appointments. Advise clients to obtain a physical check-up at least every 6 months and whenever symptoms of imbalance appear.

CUSHING'S DISEASE

Recall that Cushing's disease is one form of Cushing's syndrome. It results from oversecretion of ACTH by a pituitary tumor, which, in turn, results in oversecretion of adrenocortical hormones. See Figure 63–2, which illustrates the H-P-A axis.

SEXUAL DISTURBANCES

Excess secretion of gonadotrophic hormones (LH, FSH) from pituitary tumors can produce sexual precocity in children. Excess prolactin secretion can cause amenorrhea or galactorrhea (excessive flow of milk) in women. Physicians consider surgical removal to be the treatment of choice for radiologically apparent tumors.

Clients with increased prolactin secretion and no radiologic or neurologic evidence of a pituitary tumor often respond to bromocriptine, an ergot-like compound. Clients with prolactinomas can be successfully treated with bromocriptine. Bromocriptine, a dopamine agonist, inhibits prolactin secretion. Surgery is no longer the treatment of choice in most of these cases.

HYPOPITUITARISM

Definition

In contrast to hyperpituitarism, hypopituitarism is a deficiency of one or more of the hormones produced by the anterior lobe of the pituitary. When both the anterior and posterior lobes fail to secrete hormones, the condition is called panhypopituitarism.

Incidence

Hypopituitarism and panhypopituitarism are rare disorders.

Etiology/Pathophysiology

The five most important causes of hypopituitarism and the pathophysiology associated with each are discussed below.

HYPOPHYSECTOMY

This procedure (removal or destruction of pituitary) is sometimes performed as a palliative measure for clients with diabetic retinopathy or breast cancer. This procedure results in an absolute absence of all pituitary hormones and the need for their replacement.

NONSECRETING PITUITARY TUMORS

There are two types of nonsecreting pituitary tumors that cause hypopituitarism: nonfunctioning chromophobe adenoma and craniopharyngioma. As these tumors expand, they eventually compress and obliterate pituitary tissue, thereby diminishing the secretion of pituitary hormones.

DECREASED GROWTH HORMONE

When children are born with a deficiency of GH, they become dwarfed in stature unless they are given injections of human growth hormone (HGH). Clients with GH deficiency are normally proportioned and have normal intelligence.

POSTPARTUM PITUITARY NECROSIS

Hypopituitarism can develop after postpartum hemorrhage and circulatory collapse. The fall in BP following the baby's delivery evidently causes necrosis of the gland due to anoxia. This leads to an absence of all hormones.

FUNCTIONAL DISORDERS

Functional hypopituitarism develops whenever the pituitary gland fails to receive adequate nourishment and dies. Causes include starvation and systemic diseases such as anorexia nervosa, severe anemia, and gastrointestinal tract disorders.

Clinical Manifestations

The pituitary has enormous functional reserve; therefore, manifestations of hypopituitarism usually do not appear until 75 per cent of the pituitary has been obliterated by tumors or thromboses. Symptoms depend on the age of onset as well as the hormones that are deficient.

Specific disorders resulting from pituitary hyposecretion include

- Short stature. Severely stunted growth results from either: (1) congenital lack of GH or (2) the development of space-occupying intracranial tumors, meningitis, or brain injury during early childhood.
- Secondary adrenocortical insufficiency. Adrenal insufficiency can follow diminished synthesis of ACTH by the pituitary gland, which, in turn, causes diminished secretion of adrenocortical hormones by the adrenal cortex (see Fig. 63-2).
- Hypothyroidism. Because the synthesis of thyroid hormone depends on thyroid-stimulating hormone (TSH), therapeutic ablation or pathologic destruction of the pituitary gland causes hypothyroidism unless the client receives thyroid hormone (see Chap. 62).
- Sexual and reproductive disorders. Deficiencies of the gonadotropins (LH and FSH) can produce sterility, diminished sexual drive, and decreased secondary sex characteristics. Decreased FSH and LH lead to infertility and amenorrhea, diminished spermatogenesis, and testicular atrophy.

DIAGNOSTIC ASSESSMENT

Diagnosis of GH deficiency rests on the inability of stimulating agents such as L-dopa, arginine, and insulin to increase plasma GH levels.

Measurement of ACTH levels can be performed to diagnose secondary adrenal insufficiency. Cortisol levels are low in both primary and secondary hypothyroidism; however, when it is a primary deficiency, ACTH levels are high. In the client with secondary hypopituitarism, the ACTH levels are low.

Low serum thyroid hormone levels, together with low serum TSH levels, establish the diagnosis of hypothyroidism.

Sexual and reproductive disorders are diagnosed by low levels of sex steroids and low levels of plasma FSH and LH.

Medical Management

Treatment for hypopituitarism involves (1) removal, if possible, of the causative factor (e.g., tumors) and (2) permanent replacement of the hormones secreted by the target organs.

PHARMACOLOGIC MANAGEMENT

Injections of HGH successfully treat GH deficiency. Previously, HGH was scarce and available for only a few clients, but HGH produced by recombinant DNA technology is now available.

Medications prescribed to replace hormones include (1) corticosteroids for correction of secondary adrenocortical insufficiency, (2) thyroid hormone for treatment of myxedema, and (3) sex hormones to correct hypogonadism.

Nursing Management

Assessment of the client with hypopituitarism revolves around assessment of the various target organs that are dependent on pituitary secretions. See the discussion of specific disorders for further information.

Nursing interventions also are directed at the problems from the deficiency at the target organ. See the appropriate sections for specific interventions.

POSTERIOR LOBE (NEUROHYPOPHYSEAL) DISORDERS

Unlike the adenohypophysis, disease rarely destroys the neurohypophysis. Even if the posterior lobe becomes damaged or is surgically destroyed with the anterior lobe, hormonal deficiencies usually do not develop. This is because the hypothalamus continues to synthesize oxytocin and ADH. On the other hand, if the hypothalamus suffers damage, deficiencies of oxytocin and ADH develop even if the neurohypophysis is healthy and intact.

The major disorder of the posterior lobe is ADH deficiency (diabetes insipidus) (Fig. 63-7). Excessive ADH causes the syndrome of inappropriate ADH secretion (SIADH), which can occur with lung cancer, head injuries, cranial surgery, pituitary tumors, encephalitis, poliomyelitis, and myxedema.

Researchers have not documented oxytocin imbalances. For further information on oxytocin, consult an obstetric textbook.

DIABETES INSIPIDUS

Definition

Diabetes insipidus is a deficiency of ADH resulting in a physiologic imbalance of water.

Incidence

Diabetes insipidus is a rare disorder.

Etiology

Diabetes insipidus results from a deficiency of ADH. Causes of ADH deficiency (diabetes insipidus) are categorized as follows:

- Central or neurogenic diabetes insipidus due to (1) abnormalities in the hypothalamus and pituitary gland from familial or idiopathic causes (primary diabetes insipidus), (2) destruction of the gland by tumors in the hypothalamic-pituitary region, trauma, infectious processes, vascular accidents, or metastatic tumors from the breast or lung (secondary diabetes insipidus), and (3) medications such as phenytoin (Dilantin), alcohol, and lithium carbonate, can interfere with the synthesis or release of ADH in some clients.
- "Nephrogenic" diabetes insipidus. Owing to an inherited defect, the kidney tubules cannot respond to ADH.

Risk Factors

Risk factors include head injuries, infections, and other factors that lead to destruction of the gland. Certain medications also may lead to the development of diabetes insipidus. Prevention is mainly related to identification of risk factors and early detection.

Pathophysiology

The major functions of ADH are to (1) promote water reabsorption by the kidney and (2) control the osmotic pressure of the extracellular fluid. Thus, when ADH production decreases excessively, the kidney tubules fail to reabsorb water, and consequently, the client excretes large amounts of dilute urine. As in diabetes mellitus, clients with diabetes insipidus excrete excessive amounts of urine. Urine in diabetes mellitus contains large amounts of glucose, whereas urine in diabetes insipidus is highly dilute and contains no glucose.

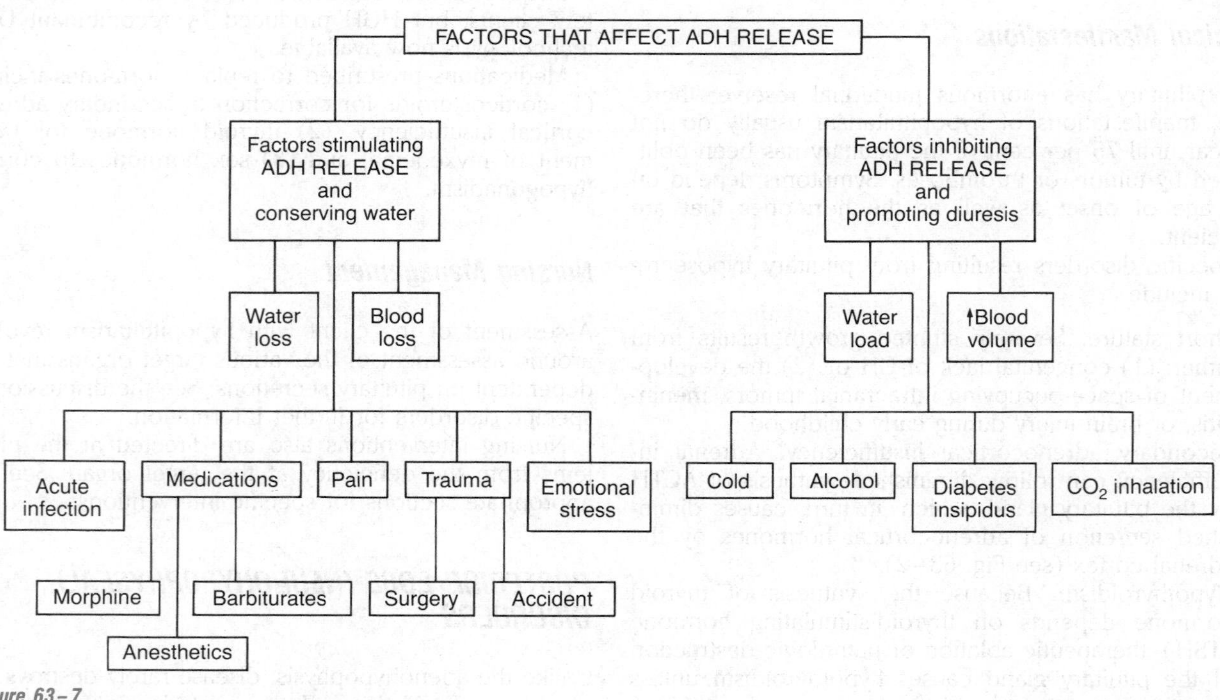

▲ Figure 63-7

Factors that stimulate and inhibit the release of ADH.

Clinical Manifestations

Diabetes insipidus can arise slowly, or can appear suddenly following injury or infectious disease. Its two major manifestations are polyuria and polydipsia. The thirst mechanism in some clients with diabetes insipidus, however, may not be intact. The client can drink and excrete 5 to 10 liters of fluid per day! The urine is very dilute, with a specific gravity of 1.001 to 1.005 (normal specific gravity is 1.001 – 1.030). The client must drink fluid almost continuously to avoid severe dehydration and hypovolemic shock.

DIAGNOSTIC ASSESSMENT

Diabetes insipidus can be diagnosed by a water deprivation test. Instruct the client not to drink water, to concentrate the urine. Test results are positive for diabetes insipidus if the urine remains dilute. Clients with nephrogenic diabetes insipidus do not respond to ADH injection.

Medical Management

PHARMACOLOGIC MANAGEMENT

Clients with diabetes insipidus often benefit from administration of the benzothiadiazine diuretics, either alone or in combination with sulfonylurea chlorpropamide.

In addition, injection of vasopressin (aqueous Pitressin) can control the symptoms of diabetes insipidus. Pitressin typically alleviates polyuria, and usually polydipsia, for 24 to 72 hours. The synthetic polypeptide desmopressin acetate (DDAVP) can be insufflated through the nose in the morning and at bedtime. This medication has largely replaced vasopressin tannate for long-term treatment of clients with severe diabetes insipidus.

After administering vasopressin, clients need to be assessed for signs and symptoms of water intoxication, which can lead to fluid overload, cerebral edema, and seizures (see Chap. 14).

Surgical Management

Surgical resection of the tumor can cure clients with diabetes insipidus secondary to a tumor.

Nursing Management

Assessment of the client with suspected diabetes insipidus should center around monitoring of the client's intake and output. The client should be asked about the presence of excessive thirst or urination. The client's fluid and electrolyte balance must be closely monitored. The client also should be assessed for exposure to risk factors.

The nursing interventions center around maintaining adequate hydration, electrolyte balance, and preventing complications. The nurse should not only administer the ordered vasopressin or synthetic ADH but also should assess the effectiveness of the medication. The client also must learn self-administration of either the injections or the nasal spray.

If the client undergoes surgical resection of a tumor of the pituitary, provide nursing care for the hypophysectomy client (see the section on hypophysectomy).

SYNDROME OF INAPPROPRIATE ANTIDIURETIC HORMONE (SIADH)

Definition

SIADH is a disorder associated with excessive amounts of ADH, resulting in a water imbalance.

Incidence

SIADH is one of the most common causes of hyponatremia, although the exact incidence of SIADH itself is not known.

Etiology

There are a wide variety of causes of SIADH, including the stress of surgery and many disorders and medications.

Risk Factors

Treatment of diabetes insipidus with vasopressin can lead to SIADH if excessive amounts are administered. Care must be taken when vasopressin is administered so this complication does not occur.

A variety of malignancies are risk factors for SIADH. It is important to monitor the high-risk client for sudden fluid retention or weight gain.

Pathophysiology

SIADH is the opposite of diabetes insipidus. Instead of large fluid losses, clients with SIADH may have water intoxication due to fluid retention. Factors that affect ADH secretion are summarized in Figure 63 – 7.

Under normal circumstances, ADH regulates serum osmolality. When serum osmolality falls, a feedback mechanism causes inhibition of ADH. This, in turn, promotes increased water excretion by the kidneys to raise serum osmolality to normal. When this feedback mechanism fails and ADH levels are sustained, fluid retention results. Ultimately, serum sodium falls, resulting in hyponatremia and water intoxication.

Clinical Manifestations

Central nervous system dysfunction, characterized by alterations in level of consciousness, seizures, and coma, can become evident when serum sodium falls to 120 mEq/L or less.

Hyponatremia can result in diminished gastrointestinal function, and this problem is further complicated by the need for fluid restriction.

DIAGNOSTIC ASSESSMENT

Diagnosis rests on the presence of hyponatremia with a normal or expanded plasma volume.

Medical Management

Treatment for SIADH includes fluid restriction, very careful replacement of sodium chloride, administration of diuretics and demeclocycline (a tetracycline that increases free-water clearance), and correction of the cause, if possible.

The physician also can prescribe cathartics or low-volume, hyperosmolar fluid enemas. In general, administration of tap water or saline enemas should be avoided because the fluid can be absorbed from the bowel and contribute to water intoxication.

Treatment is the same as for any client with dilutional hyponatremia (see Chap. 14).

Nursing Management

ASSESSMENT

The client with suspected SIADH should have fluid status and electrolytes closely monitored. The client's cardiovascular status also should be assessed regularly so any alterations are immediately noted.

The client's weight should be recorded, and any gain of more than 2 pounds should be reported to the physician. The client's neurologic status should be monitored so any alterations related to the hyponatremia are immediately diagnosed and treatment can be started.

NURSING INTERVENTION

Nursing Diagnosis: Injury, High Risk for R/T to the danger of cerebral edema, water intoxication, and CNS dysfunction.

Planning: Expected Outcomes. The client will not suffer injury, as evidenced by absence of signs of increased intracranial pressure, hypertension, altered level of consciousness, or seizures.

Implementation. Nursing care for clients with SIADH includes accurate assessment of fluid balance, daily weights, and careful and frequent assessment of neurologic status.

Position the client so the person's head is flat or raised no more than 5 degrees, unless contraindicated. This position helps prevent possible development or worsening of cerebral edema. It also avoids stimulation of receptors in the atrium of the heart that are sensitive to volume changes and that can increase ADH secretion. See Chapter 29 for further information on cerebral edema.

The nurse should perform frequent neurologic checks and notify the physician if any significant changes occur. Continue to monitor the client's mental status by assessing the client's orientation to person, place, and time.

See Chapter 14 for information on the nursing care associated with dilutional hyponatremia.

Nursing Diagnosis: Fluid Volume Excess R/T excessive secretion of ADH secondary to SIADH.

Planning: Expected Outcomes. The client will not develop fluid volume excess or will have the excess resolved without injury, as evidenced by return to normal blood pressure, absence of edema, and balanced intake and output.

Implementation. Clients with SIADH will have significant fluid restrictions, often as low as 500 to 600 ml/24 h. The intake and output and daily weights must be closely monitored. A continued imbalance of intake and output, with intake higher than output, should be immediately reported. If the client's weight increases by 2 pounds or more in a 24-hour period, it may represent fluid retention. The client also will be maintained on a very low sodium intake and diuretics administered.

Once the client has begun to recover, the output should increase significantly, becoming greater than the intake until balance is restored. The client's weight should begin to decrease gradually.

EVALUATION

The nurse must evaluate client outcomes based on the established plan of care. If these goals were not achieved, the plan and interventions must be revised to meet the client's needs.

Post-hospital Care

DISCHARGE TEACHING

If the client's SIADH has not been resolved, the client and significant others will have to understand the continued need for sodium and fluid restrictions. The client also should learn to weigh daily and to report any excessive gain (2 pounds or more a day). Clients should be taught to avoid the use of aspirin or nonsteroidal anti-inflammatory agents because these drugs can increase the hyponatremia.

HOME HEALTH CARE NEEDS

The client should have access to a scale so his or her weight can be monitored regularly.

FOLLOW-UP CARE

The client with chronic SIADH will need to be followed closely by the physician on a regular basis. The client should be reminded of the need to notify the physician whenever changes in his or her condition occur.

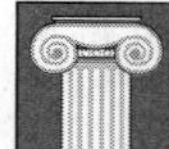

ETHICAL ISSUES IN NURSING

What Is a Nurse's Role in Influencing Parental Gender Selection for Hermaphrodite Babies?

The birth of a baby is usually a much anticipated and happy event. A healthy "perfect" little baby is the usual expected outcome of labor and delivery. When a baby is born that is less than perfect, the event becomes a very somber and concerned one, especially when the outcome was not expected, that is, detected through ultrasound or other prenatal testing. For many pregnant women, prenatal care was never sought, so complications may go undetected up until the time of birth.

There are occasions, although rare, when a complication arises in which a baby is born with both male and female genitalia (hermaphroditism). In such cases, the parents have to decide which gender they wish to assign to the child. Several factors may influence their decision, such as what predominant physical genitalia is present and chromosomal data. The gender decision does not need to be made right away, but should be made as soon as possible so surgical procedures and other therapies may begin. The parents also need to begin to identify with their baby as a person of a certain gender. This process is a very emotional and stressful one.

How can the nursing staff assist in fulfilling the needs of these parents? What happens when the parents decide on a gender that perhaps goes against the recommendations of the medical staff? Perhaps the parents want to have the child brought up as a male because they have two female children already, but the medical recommendation is that the child be raised as a female?

This issue, although rare, does happen, and the nursing staff is closely related to the situation. The parents may ask questions of the staff such as "What would you do in our situation?" or seek advice regarding similar issues. Nursing staff do have an obligation to care for the parents of such babies as well as the babies themselves. Referrals for counseling, social work and other related services would be of benefit for such families. Even though parents may make decisions that the health care team may not agree with, nurses can help the parents have the opportunity to receive all available information through appropriate teaching and referrals. By doing this, the staff establishes a setting in which a truly informed decision may be made.

▼ GONADAL DISORDERS

TESTICULAR DYSFUNCTION

Testicular dysfunction can be primary, as a disorder of testicular function, or secondary, as a disorder of hypothalamic-pituitary function. Primary testis dysfunction can involve the seminiferous tubules (germ cells or Sertoli's cells), Leydig's cells, or both. Germ cell abnormalities cause infertility by disrupting spermatogenesis.

Secondary sexual development and virilization are normal because testosterone production is not interrupted. When Leydig cell function is impaired, testosterone production falls, and virilization is impaired.

Causes of primary hypogonadism include genetic defects (see Ethical Issues in Nursing), malnutrition, trauma, infection, renal failure, radiation, chemotherapy, and environmental toxins (e.g., lead, alcohol). The cause, however, is usually unknown. Klinefelter's syndrome (XXY) is an example of a genetic disorder causing primary testicular failure.

Secondary testicular dysfunction is frequently referred to as hypogonadotropic hypogonadism and results from the inadequate secretion of gonadotropins. This complication leads to infertility and hypoandrogenism. The extent of LH and FSH deficiency and the age of onset determine clinical manifestations. Prepubertal hypogonadism leads to eunuchoidal body proportions, small testes, and a lack of virilization.

Examples of secondary hypogonadism include hypothalamic or pituitary tumors, trauma, degenerative lesions, and radiation. Kallmann's syndrome, a deficiency of GnRH production by the hypothalamus, is an example of congenital secondary testicular dysfunction.

Clients with Kallmann's syndrome fail to mature normally due to gonadotropin deficiency. Midline defects such as cleft lip or palate, color blindness, anosmia, and ataxia are common findings in these clients.

Summary

Adrenal, pituitary, and gonadal disorders are not common, but are extremely complex and diverse. The nurse needs a thorough understanding of the adrenal, pituitary, and gonadal anatomy and physiology to understand these disorders. Most of these conditions are acute and affect many body systems, such as hypopituitarism, whereas others can become chronic and lead to a wide variety of other problems, such as Addison's disease. Teaching is vital to the care of these clients, so the nurse must understand these conditions so appropriate teaching plans can be initiated.

Bibliography

1. Anderson, L. D., et al. (1986). Endocrine and metabolic systems. In J. Thompson, et al. (Eds.), *Clinical nursing.* (pp. 823–942). St. Louis: C. V. Mosby.
2. Baxter, J. D. (1988). Principles of Endocrinology. In J. B. Wyngaarden & L. H. Smith (Eds.), *Cecil textbook of medicine* (pp. 1252–1267). Philadelphia: W. B. Saunders.

3. Becker, K. L. (1990). General principles of endocrinology. In K. Becker (Ed.), *Principles and practice in endocrinology and metabolism* (pp. 2-80). Philadelphia: J. B. Lippincott.
4. Berkow, R. (Ed.) (1982). *Merck manual.* Rahway, NJ: Merck Sharp & Dohme Research Laboratories (14th ed.).
5. Boyd, W., & Sheldon, H. (1984). *An introduction to the study of disease* (9th ed.). Philadelphia: Lea & Febiger.
6. Boyd, A. E., III, et al. (1986). Disorders of the hypothalamus and anterior pituitary. In P. Kohler (Ed.), *Clinical endocrinology* (pp. 11-52). New York: Wiley.
7. Campese, V. M., & DeQuattro, V. (1989). Functional components of the sympathetic nervous system: Regulation of organ systems. In L. DeGroot (Ed.), *Endocrinology and metabolism* (2nd ed., pp. 1738-1756). Philadelphia: W. B. Saunders.
8. Christy, N. P. (1975). Disease of the endocrine system: General considerations. In P. B. Beeson & W. McDermott (Eds.), *Cecil-Loeb textbook of medicine* (pp. 1662-1667). Philadelphia: W. B. Saunders.
9. DeQuattro, V., et al. (1989). Pheochromocytoma: Diagnosis and therapy. In L. DeGroot (Ed.), Endocrinology (2nd ed., pp. 1780-1797). Philadelphia: W. B. Saunders.
10. Drass, J. A., et al. (in press). Endocrine and Metabolic Systems. In J. Thompson, et al. (Eds.), *Mosby's manual of clinical nursing* (pp. 876-967). St. Louis: C. V. Mosby.
11. Frohman, L. A. (1988). Neuroendocrine regulation and its disorders. In J. B. Wyngaarden & L. H. Smith (Eds.). *Cecil textbook of medicine* (pp. 1280-1289). Philadelphia: W. B. Saunders.
12. Guthrie, D. W., et al. (1983). The disease process of diabetes mellitus: definition, characteristics, trends, and developments. *Nursing Clinics of North America, 18*,617.
13. Haffner, S. M., et al. (1986). Hyperinsulinemia in a population at high risk for non-insulin-dependent diabetes mellitus. *New England Journal of Medicine, 315*(4), 220-224.
14. Harris, R. B., et al. (1984). Comprehensive nursing care of the patient with pheochromocytoma. *Heart and Lung, 13*,82.
15. Imperato-McGinley, J. (1988). Disorders of sexual differentiation. In J. B. Wyngaarden & L. H. Smith (Eds.), *Cecil textbook of medicine* (pp. 1390-1404). Philadelphia: W. B. Saunders.
16. Larsen, P. R. (1988). The thyroid. In J. B. Wyngaarden & L. H. Smith (Eds.), *Cecil textbook of medicine* (pp. 1315-1331). Philadelphia: W. B. Saunders.
17. Levey, G. S., & Levey, B. A. (1985). Cardiovascular effects of thyroid disease. *Hospital Medicine, 21,* 147.
18. Liddle, G. W. (1982). Adrenal cortex. In P. B. Beeson et al. (Eds.), *Cecil textbook of medicine* (16th ed.). Philadelphia: W. B. Saunders.
19. Matsumoto, A. M., (1985). The testis. In J. B. Wyngaarden & L. H. Smith (Eds.), *Cecil textbook of medicine* (18th ed., pp. 1404-1421). Philadelphia: W. B. Saunders.
20. Loriaux, D. L. (1990). The adrenal glands. In K. Becker (Ed.), *Principles and practice in endocrinology and metabolism* (pp. 92-246). Philadelphia: J. B. Lippincott.
21. Loriaux, D. L., & Cutler, J. B. Jr. (1986). Diseases of the adrenal glands. In P. Kohler (Ed.), *Clinical endocrinology* (pp. 167-238). New York: Wiley.
22. McConnell, E. A. (1985). Assessing the thyroid. *Nursing 85, 15,* 60.
23. Meikle, A. W. (1989). Secretion and metabolism of the corticosteroids and adrenal function and testing. In L. DeGroot (Ed.), *Endocrinology* (2nd ed., pp. 1610-1632). Philadelphia: W. B. Saunders.
24. Moses, A. M., & Streeten, D. H. P. (1986). Disorders of the hypothalamic-neurohypophyseal system. In P. Kohler (Ed.) *Clinical endocrinology* (pp. 53-72). New York: Wiley.
25. Nelson, D. H. Cushing's syndrome. In L. DeGroot (Ed.), *Endocrinology* (2nd ed., 1989, pp. 1660-1675). Philadelphia: W. B. Saunders.
26. Propst, C. L. (1983). Nursing care of a patient undergoing transsphenoidal hypophysectomy. *Journal of Neurosurgical Nursing, 15,* 332.
27. Rebar, R. W. (1988). The ovaries. In J. B. Wyngaarden & L. H. Smith (Eds.), *Cecil textbook of medicine* (18th ed., pp. 1425-1446). Philadelphia: W. B. Saunders.
28. Reichlin, S. (1985). Neuroendocrinology. In J. D. Wilson & D. W. Foster (Eds.), *Williams textbook of endocrinology* (7th ed., pp. 492-567). Philadelphia: W. B. Saunders.
29. Robertson, G. L. (1990). The endocrine brain and pituitary gland. In K. Becker (Ed.), *Principles and practice in endocrinology and metabolism* (pp. 92-246). Philadelphia: J. B. Lippincott.
30. Solomon, B. (1984). Endocrinology: A future challenge for critical nurses. *Dimensions of Critical Care Nursing, 3*,68.
31. Treadwell, P. (1984). Nursing care study: Adrenalectomy. *Nursing Mirror, 157,* 48.
32. Tyrell, J. B., & Baxter, J. D. (1988). Disorders of the adrenal cortex. In J. B. Wyngaarden & L. H. Smith (Eds.), *Cecil textbook of medicine* (pp. 1340-1360). Philadelphia: W. B. Saunders.
33. Volner, J. S. (1983). Endocrine dysfunction associated with pituitary adenomas and pituitary surgery. *Journal of Neurosurgical Nursing, 15,* 325.

Musculoskeletal Disorders

Unit 15

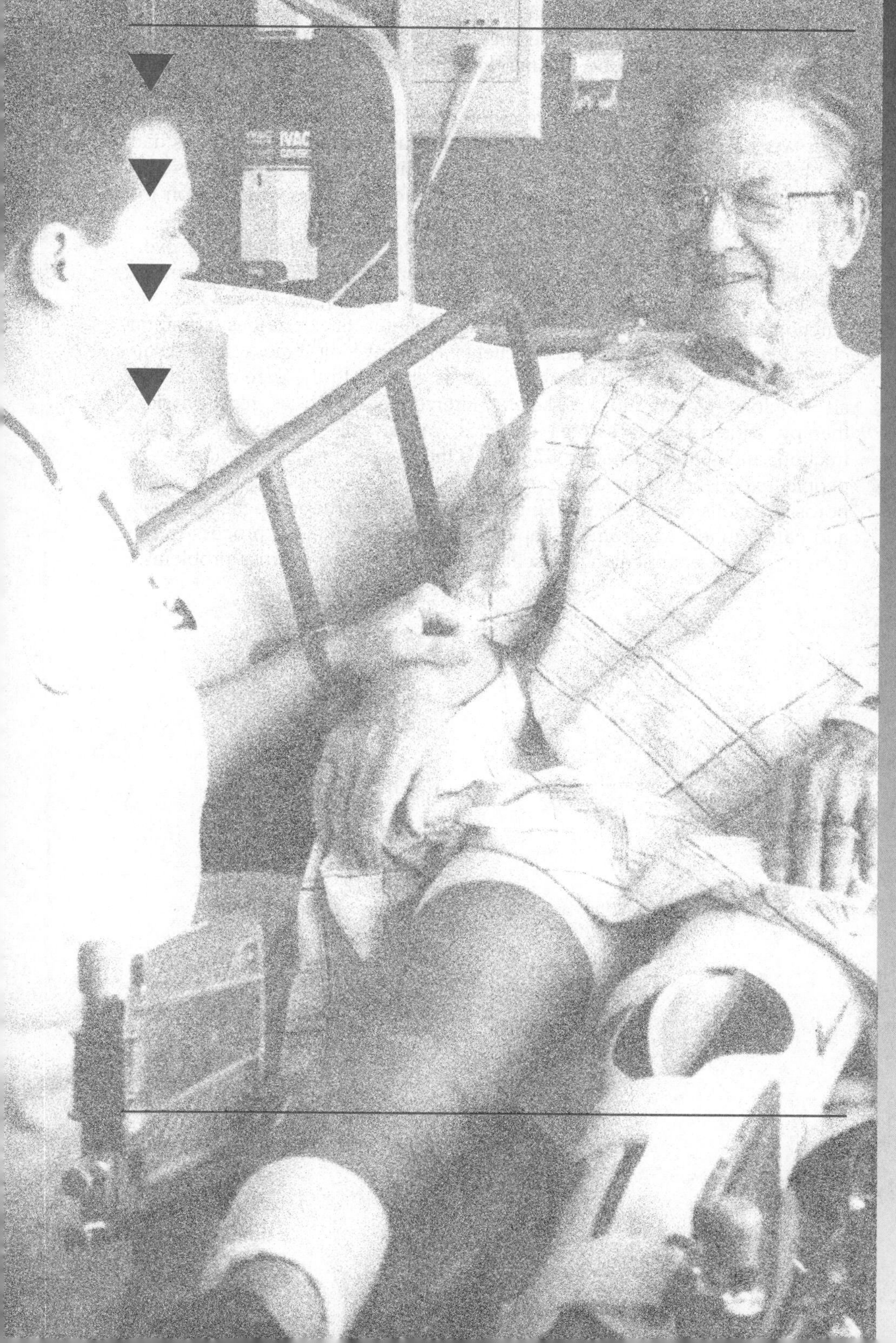

The need to move and maintain a desirable position is a basic human need. Physiologically, the musculoskeletal system enables movement and position changes. The bony skeleton provides support and movable parts. Musculature facilitates movement. Psychosocially, our emotions, thoughts, and relationships with others affect movements we make and positions we assume. These movements are nonverbal gestures.

Movement serves two general purposes. First, movement is necessary to perform normal activities of daily living. Second, movement in itself is a source of pleasure. There is increasing interest in performing activities that contribute to physical fitness. This is partly because such activities promote physical health and also because they are pleasurable. People who enjoy exercise programs describe feelings of well being or a "high" that comes from regular physical activity.

Musculoskeletal disorders are among the oldest known diseases. Fractures were apparently a common injury, and the treatment of fractures had reached a sophisticated level by the time of Hippocrates. Arthritis was also common at the time of the Roman empire and presumably the reason for extensive bathing pools throughout the Roman empire.

This unit consists of five chapters. Chapter 64 presents a brief overview of musculoskeletal structure and function. Chapter 65 discusses nursing and medical assessment and intervention relating to musculoskeletal function and musculoskeletal problems. Chapter 66 describes common clinical problems experienced by clients who have musculoskeletal disorders. In this chapter, the nursing process is applied to the care of individuals requiring typical musculoskeletal intervention, such as rest, physical therapy, assistive devices (e.g., crutches, canes, walkers, supports), casts, traction, and surgery. Chapter 67 applies the nursing process to the care of people experiencing metabolic musculoskeletal disorders, such as osteoporosis, Paget's disease, bone tumor, osteomyelitis, osteomalacia, scoliosis, and carpal tunnel syndrome. Chapter 68 applies the nursing process to the care of people experiencing musculoskeletal injury and overuse problems.

Chapter 64

Structure and Function of the Musculoskeletal System

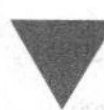

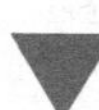

The musculoskeletal system is composed of various connective tissues, bone, muscle, cartilage, tendon, and ligament. The joint, an articulation of two or more bones, represents the functional unit of the system.

STRUCTURE OF THE SKELETAL SYSTEM

The body contains 206 bones, which are divided into two major categories: the axial and appendicular skeletons. The axial skeleton consists of 80 bones, which include the skull, vertebral column, and thorax. The appendicular skeleton has 126 bones and consists of the bones in the legs, arms, shoulder, and pelvis (Fig. 64–1).

Bones vary greatly in size and shape, but regardless of their shape, bones have the same general structure. The outer surface cover of the bone is called the periosteum. The outer layer of periosteum contains blood vessels and nerves. Some of the vessels and nerves reach the inner portions of the bone through Volkmann's canals. The inner layer of periosteum is attached to the bone by collagenous fibers, called Sharpey's fibers, that penetrate the bone. The outer portion of bone (the cortex) is dense and hard. The cortex is a group of bony layers packed closely together. The cortex is also called compact bone. Compact bone is highly

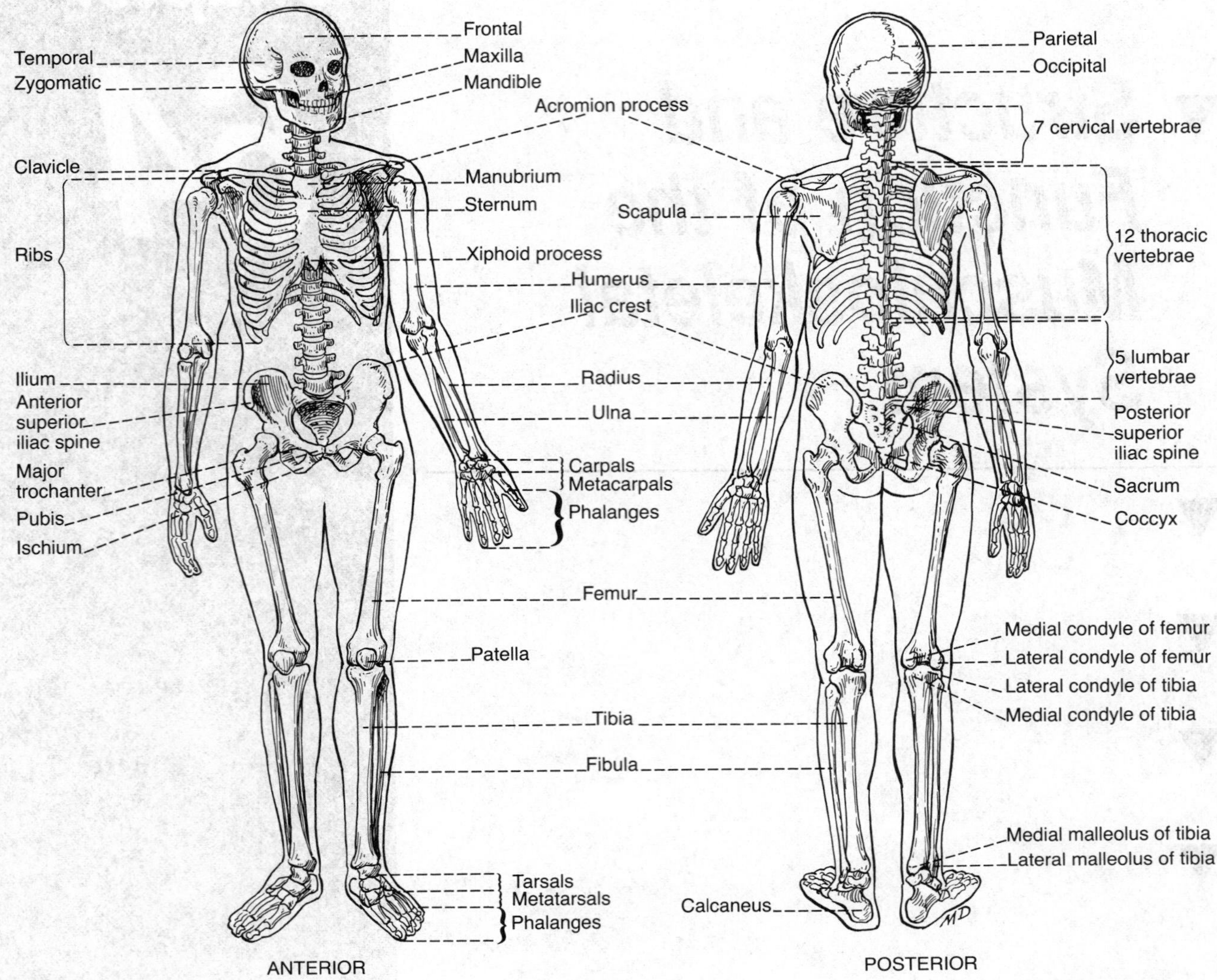

▲ *Figure 64–1*

Human skeleton.

organized, solid, and extremely strong. Compact bone is organized into structural units, called haversian systems. Each haversian system is made up of a central canal called the haversian canal; concentric layers of bone matrix called lamellae; tiny spaces between the lamellae called lacunae, which contain osteocytes; and small channels called canaliculi (Fig. 64–2). Each haversian system looks like a separate cylinder, and together, they look like concentric rings. The large haversian canal runs through the center of long bones and contains blood vessels and nerves. The blood vessels transport nutrients to the bone, and wastes away from the bone.

The middle portion of bone lacks a haversian system and, instead, is filled with trabeculae (beams) of bone, which are weak individually but together form a strong bracing system. The trabeculation looks spongy, and thus, this portion is called spongy bone. The trabeculae are filled with marrow for the formation of blood cells. The pattern of the bracing can vary between bones, and it is determined by the stress placed on the bone. The internal blood supply is connected to the periosteum through channels, called Volkmann's canals.

Mature bone is rigid connective tissue, and like other tissues, it is a living organ. Bone contains three types of cells: (1) osteoblasts, (2) osteocytes, and (3) osteoclasts. Osteoblasts are bone-forming cells; they lay down new bone. Osteocytes are osteoblasts that are found in the bone matrix. Osteoclasts are cells that resorb (remove) damaged or old bone cells during periods of growth or repair. Bone cells allow bone to grow, repair itself and change shape. Even mature bone constantly changes, with new cells being formed and old cells being destroyed. The bone cells are surrounded by extracellular elements of tissue, called the bone matrix. The matrix contains collagen, fibers, proteins, carbohydrate-protein complexes, minerals, and ground substance. Ground substance is a gelatinous material that acts as a medium for the diffusion of nutrients, oxygen, and metabolic wastes between bone cells and blood vessels.

Bone Classification According to Shape

Long Bones. Long bones (e.g., humerus, radius) consist of epiphysis, articular cartilage, diaphysis, periosteum, and medullary cavity. The epiphysis (end of long bones) is composed of cancellous bone. It is the location of muscle attachment and increases joint stability. Articular cartilage covers long bone ends and provides smooth surfaces for joint movement. The diaphysis (composed of compact bone) is the main shaft of a long bone. It provides structural support. The metaphysis is the flared part of a long bone between the epiphysis and diaphysis. It is the growth area during bone development. In adults, the metaphysis joins to the epiphysis. In children, it is a cartilaginous area that actively produces bone to create longitudinal growth. The periosteum is fibrous connective tissue that covers bone. The medullary cavity (marrow) is in the center of the diaphysis (Fig. 64-2*A*).

Short Bones. Short bones (e.g., carpals, tarsals) consist of cancellous bone covered by a thin layer of compact tissue.

Flat Bones. Flat bones consist of cancellous bone encased in two flat plates of compact bone. Examples are the ribs, skull, scapula, and portions of pelvic girdle. Flat bones protect soft body parts or provide large surfaces for muscle attachments.

Irregular Bones. Irregular bones are of differing shapes, such as vertebrae, ear ossicles, mandible. Irregular bones are similar to other bones in structure and composition.

Sesamoid Bones. Sesamoid bones are small, rounded bones adjacent to joints and encased in tendon and fascial tissue, such as patella (knee cap). Sesamoid bones increase the leverage of muscles.

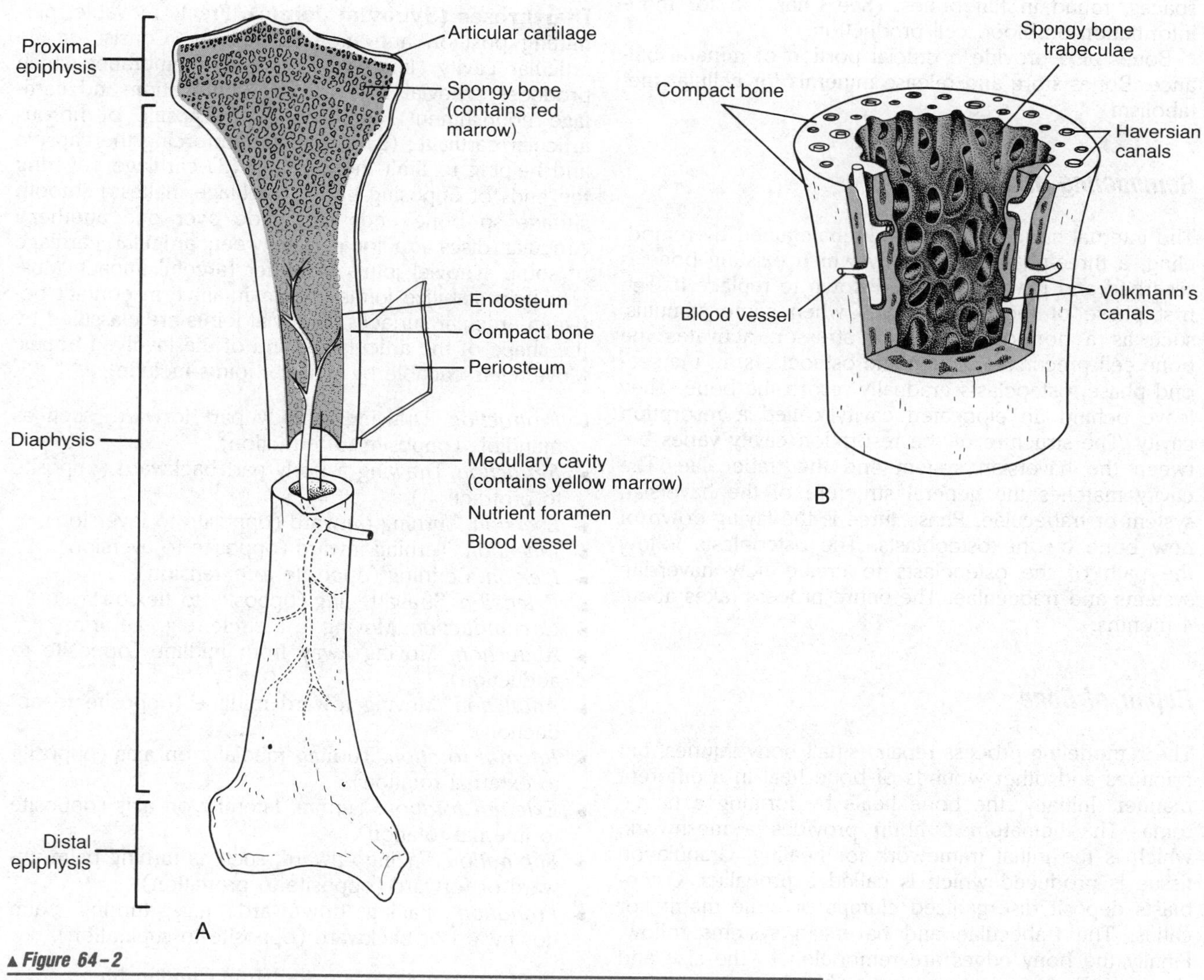

▲ *Figure 64-2*

Osseous tissue. *A*, Macroscopic appearance of a long bone; *B*, haversian system of compact bone.

FUNCTION OF THE SKELETAL SYSTEM

Bones give form to the body, support various tissues and organs and permit movement by providing attachments for tendons and ligaments. The skull and rib cage, for example, provide support for the brain, special senses and lungs. Movement of the body is permitted by the articulation of joints and their attached muscles.

Bone protects the hematopoietic system, which manufactures blood cells. The marrow cavities within various bones serve as sites for blood cell formation. In adults, blood cells form in marrow cavities in the skull, vertebrae, ribs, sternum, shoulder, and pelvis. There are two types of bone marrow: yellow and red. The yellow marrow is found in the shafts of long bones and extends into the haversian systems. Yellow marrow is connective tissue composed of fat cells. Yellow marrow does not produce blood cells, except during times of increased blood cell need. Red marrow has the hematopoietic function (manufactures red and white blood cells). Red marrow is located in the cancellous bone spaces, found in flat bones. (See Chap. 45 for more information on blood cell production.)

Bones also provide a crucial portion of mineral balance. Bones store and release minerals for cellular metabolism.

Remodeling of Bone

The internal structure of bone is maintained by remodeling, a three-phase process by which existing bone is resorbed and new bone is laid down to replace it. The first phase of the cycle begins when some stimulus, such as a hormone, drug, or stressor, activates the bone cell precursors to become osteoclasts. In the second phase, osteoclasts gradually resorb the bone. They leave behind an elongated cavity called a resorption cavity. The structure of the resorption cavity varies between the haversian system and the trabeculae. The cavity matches the general structure of the haversian system or trabeculae. Phase three is the laying down of new bone by the osteoblasts. The osteoblasts follow the path of the osteoclasts to create new haversian systems and trabeculae. The entire process takes about 4 months.

Repair of Bone

The remodeling process repairs small bony injuries, but fractures and other wounds of bone heal in a different manner. Initially, the bone heals by forming a hematoma. The hematoma's fibrin provides a meshwork, which is the initial framework for healing. Granulation tissue is produced which is called a procallus. Osteoblasts deposit disorganized clumps of bone matrix, or callus. The trabeculae and haversian systems follow. Finally the bony edges are remodeled to the size and shape of the bone before it was injured.

STRUCTURE AND FUNCTION OF THE ARTICULAR SYSTEM

Articulations (joints) are places of union between two or more bones. Movement does not always occur at joints.

Groups of Joints

Categorization is according to degree of movement.

Synarthroses. No movement, such as skull suture joints and temporary cartilage connection between the epiphysis and diaphysis of long bone (replaced by bone during maturation).

Amphiarthroses. Slight movement, such as pubic symphysis and connection of ligaments where radius articulates with ulna.

Diarthroses (Synovial Joints). Freely movable, permitting position and motion changes. Consist of (1) articular cavity (lined with synovial membrane, which produces synovial fluid for joint lubrication and cartilage nourishment) enclosed by a capsule of fibrous articular cartilage; (2) ligaments reinforcing the capsule and helping to limit motion; and (3) cartilage covering the ends of opposing bones (cartilage makes a smooth surface so bone ends can glide over one another). Articular discs are located between articular cartilage of some synovial joints to buffer forceful impact. Muscles help stabilize joints and maintain firm contact between articular surfaces. Synovial joints are classified by the shape of the articulating end of the involved bones. Movements capable by synovial joints include

- *Protraction.* Drawing a body part forward, such as mandible (opposite to retraction).
- *Retraction.* Drawing a body part backward (opposite to protraction).
- *Eversion.* Turning outward (opposite to inversion).
- *Inversion.* Turning inward (opposite to eversion).
- *Flexion.* Bending (opposite to extension).
- *Extension.* Straightening (opposite to flexion).
- *Circumduction.* Moving in a circle, e.g., an arm.
- *Abduction.* Moving away from midline (opposite to adduction).
- *Adduction.* Moving toward midline (opposite to abduction).
- *Internal rotation.* Turning medially on axis (opposite to external rotation).
- *External rotation.* Turning laterally on axis (opposite to internal rotation).
- *Supination.* Facing upward, such as turning palm upward or forward (opposite to pronation).
- *Pronation.* Facing downward, e.g., turning palm downward or backward (opposite to supination).

Various joint motions are shown in Chapter 65.

STRUCTURE AND FUNCTION OF THE MUSCULAR SYSTEM

Muscles make up 40 to 50 per cent of body weight (Fig. 64-3). Muscles produce movement by contraction.

Types of Muscle

Striated (Skeletal) Muscle. This type is voluntary muscle of the skeletal system. It is composed of muscle and connective tissue. Muscle fibers are arranged in bundles (fasciculi) held together by connective tissue. Groups of bundles are similarly bound together. Tendons (i.e., bands of strong inelastic fibrous tissue) attach muscle to bone. The entire muscle is encased in a tough muscle sheath of connective tissue that contains blood and lymph vessels and nerve fibers. Nerve fibers (each may supply over 100 individual muscle cells) carry impulse-messages to muscles. Endings of motor nerve fibers are called motor end plates or myoneural junctions. A continuous flow of stimuli maintains muscle tone, i.e., keeps muscles partially contracted, in a state of readiness for movement. To generate heat and power, muscle cells require large amounts of oxygen (O_2) and glucose. Muscles thus have a rich vascular (blood) supply. An oxygen debt develops during exercise if O_2 cannot be delivered to muscles in concentrations great enough to metabolize accumulations of lactic acid. Following exercise, increased O_2 consumption is necessary to relieve oxygen debt.

Cardiac Muscle (myocardium). This type is involuntary muscle that occurs only in the heart. Striated crosswise and longitudinally.

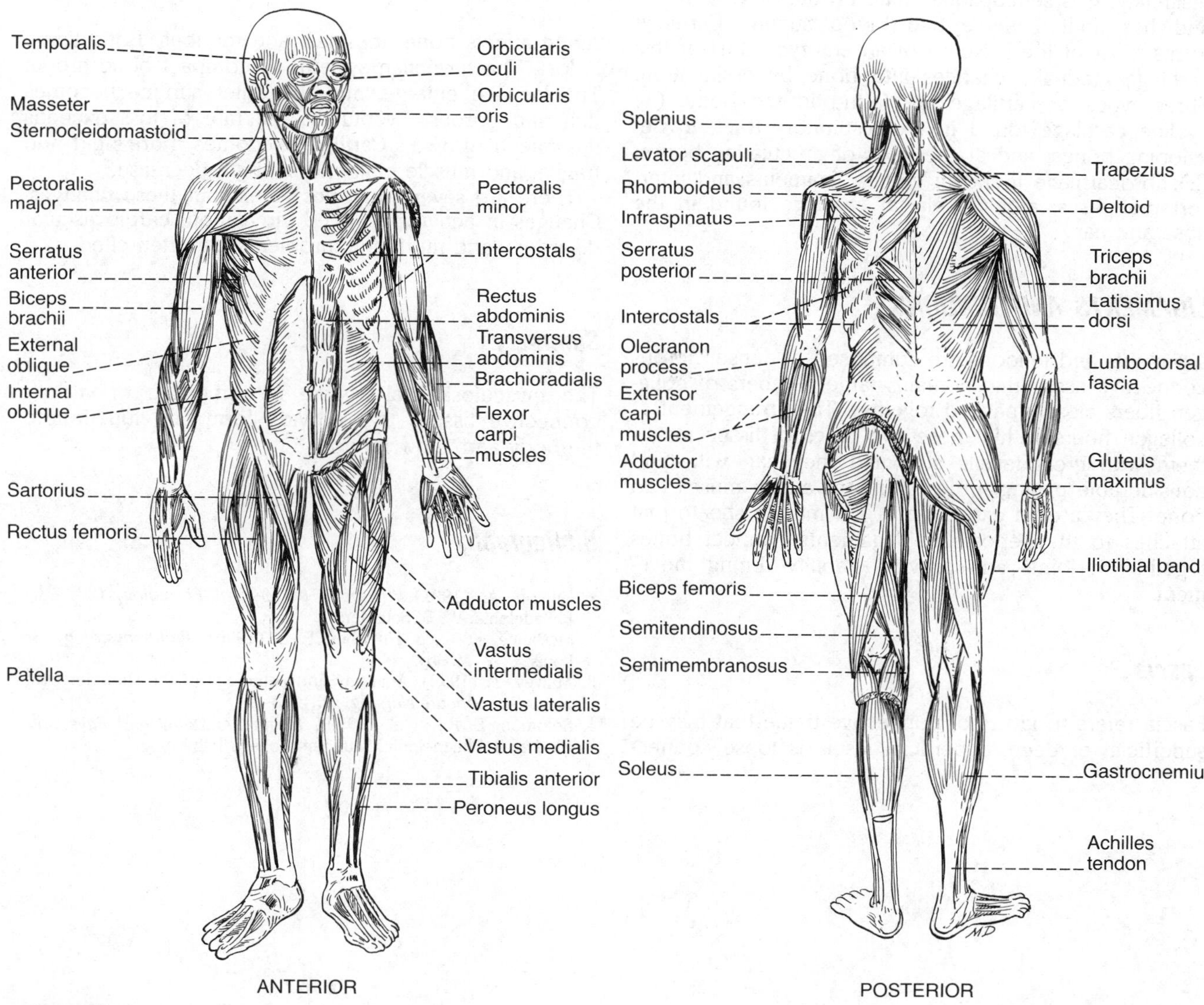

▲ **Figure 64-3**

Principal muscle groups.

Smooth Muscle. This type is involuntary, nonstriated muscle present in hollow structures, such as the digestive tract, blood vessels, urinary bladder, and other areas, including the eye. The muscle is controlled by the autonomic nervous system.

Individual Skeletal Muscles. Skeletal muscles are named according to (1) action, such as flexor, extensor; (2) shape, such as quadrilateral, pennate; (3) origin, that is, stationary attachment of muscle to skeleton; (4) insertion, that is, movable attachment of the muscle; (5) number of divisions; (6) location; or (7) direction of fibers, that is, transverse.

CARTILAGE

Cartilage is one type of dense connective tissue prevalent throughout the musculoskeletal system. It can resist forces of tension and compression with considerable resiliency. It is semiopaque (bluish-white or gray color) and has limited nerve and blood supply. Cartilage forms most of the skeleton of an embryo. Most of this cartilage gradually changes into bone by ossification. Three types of cartilage are found in the body: (1) hyaline cartilage found in the respiratory tract, in developing bones, and at the ends of articulating bones; (2) fibrocartilage found in certain ligaments and intervertebral discs; and (3) elastin cartilage found in the nose and ear.

LIGAMENTS AND TENDONS

Ligaments and tendons are composed of dense, fibrous connective tissue that contains large numbers of collagen fibers closely packed together. The arrangement of collagen fibers within these two types of tissue instills them with great tensile strength. They can withstand considerable pulling forces. Tendons attach muscles to bone. They are an extension of the muscle sheath that attaches to the periosteum. Ligaments connect bones together at joints and provide stability during movement.

Fascia

Fascia refers to layers of connective tissue that may be superficial or deep. Superficial fascia is loose connective tissue immediately under the skin. Deep fascia is dense, fibrous connective tissue found surrounding muscle, between muscles, and binding bundles of nerves and blood vessels together.

Bursa

A bursa is a small sac of connective tissue lined with synovial membrane that produces synovial fluid. Bursae are commonly located at joints to prevent friction and relieve pressure where one body part moves on another. Examples of bursae are between the (1) patella and skin, (2) olecranon process and skin, and (3) head of the humerus and acromion process.

EFFECTS OF AGING ON THE MUSCULOSKELETAL SYSTEM

Aging affects bone, muscles, and tendons. Bone tissue is lost. The haversian systems in compact bone erode. The lacunae enlarge, and the outer surface becomes thin and porous. Eventually, the rate of loss exceeds the rate of growth. Cartilage becomes more rigid and fragile, and muscle bulk and strength decrease.[2]

There are several theories to explain these changes. Changes in activity, reduced circulation, cardiovascular disorders, and nutritional problems are often cited.

Summary

The musculoskeletal system is composed of various connective tissues that provide form and function to the body and allow motion.

Bibliography

1. Guyton, A. (1991). *Textbook of Medical Physiology* (8th ed.). Philadelphia: W. B. Saunders.
2. McCance, K. L., & Huerther, S. E. (1990). *Pathophysiology*. St. Louis: C. V. Mosby.
3. Mulvey, T. (1988). Anatomy and pathology of the shoulder complex. *Orthopaedic Nursing, 7*(3), 23–28.
4. Solomon, E. P., et al. (1990). *Human Anatomy and Physiology* (2nd ed.). Philadelphia: Saunders College Publishing.

Chapter 65

Assessment of Clients with Musculoskeletal Disorders

Assessment of the musculoskeletal system includes the client's history, physical examination, and diagnostic studies. The health history provides direction for further musculoskeletal system assessment. For example, the musculoskeletal physical examination can be either general (as in a screening examination) or local (for a specific problem or injury). Similarly, diagnostic tests can be either general or specific.

HISTORY

The musculoskeletal history includes the client's biographic data, chief complaint (including symptom analysis), past medical history, family history, psychosocial history and lifestyle data, and review of systems. Information is collected to help determine the nature and extent of current disorders. If the client's chief complaint is related to trauma, the history interview is brief and focused on the cause of injury or it may be deferred, depending on the extent of the injury. Once the client's condition is stable, a more complete history is obtained.

Biographic Data

Personal information helps the nurse know the client as an individual. This enables personalized care planning. For example, knowing where the client lives and the kind of transportation used helps the nurse understand the energy expenditure the client needs to keep an appointment. Identifying and getting to know significant others is essential in planning care. The client's age and sex may suggest possible causes for musculoskeletal symptoms. For example, 85 per cent of people over age 70 have some osteoarthritis; osteoporosis occurs most often in postmenopausal women; Reiter's syndrome is most common in men between the ages of 20 and 40; and osteogenic sarcoma is rare after age 40. Carpal tunnel syndrome occurs more often in women than in men.

Chief Complaint

The client is asked to describe the reason for seeking health care. Common symptoms related to the musculoskeletal system include pain, tenderness, muscle tightness, muscle weakness, joint stiffness, cramps, muscle spasms, swelling, redness, deformity, reduced movement or joint range of motion (ROM), sensory changes, and other abnormal sensations. Activities of daily living (ADLs) may be affected. The nurse asks the client and significant others to relate their perceptions of the problem and its cause. Their answers often provide not only information about areas for further assessment but also clues about personal fears and concerns.

The nurse conducts a symptom analysis for each symptom the client reports (see Chap. 11). Examples of assessment questions for typical musculoskeletal symptoms follow.

PAIN

"Point to the pain's exact location." Poorly localized pain is usually associated with blood vessels, joints, fascia, or periosteum. "Describe the pain. Is it an ache, sharp pain, throbbing?" Throbbing pain is usually bone related and aches are often muscular. Sharp pain is associated with fractures and bone infection. "Does anything make the pain worse? Temperature changes? Movement? Lifting or carrying something heavy?" Pain associated with movement is typical of joint problems. Degenerative hip conditions produce pain during weight-bearing and during and after walking. Degenerative knee problems produce pain during and after walking. Vertebral disc herniation produces pain on bending or lifting and tends to radiate down one leg or the other. Pain associated with osteoarthritis is worse in cold, damp weather. "Is pain worse at any particular time of day? Does the pain wake you up or prevent you from sleeping at night?" Inflammation of bursae or tendons is worse at night. Degenerative joint pain is often worse at the end of a day. "Is pain relieved with rest?" Most musculoskeletal pain is helped by rest. "What medications help relieve the pain?" Pain from inflammation is usually helped by aspirin or nonsteroidal anti-inflammatory drugs. Narcotics are usually required for traumatic injury. "Have you had any recent injuries?" Sometimes a client does not relate a fall or other injury with current symptoms. Is the pain associated with chills, fever, rash, or sore throat? Joint pain occurring 10 to 14 days after sore throat may be from rheumatic fever.

JOINT STIFFNESS

"Point to which joints are stiff. Are your joints always stiff? How long does the stiffness last?" Some conditions, such as ankylosing spondylitis, have remissions and exacerbations. "What time of day is the stiffness worst?" With degenerative joint disease, stiffness is often most severe in the morning after inactivity in bed. "What relieves the stiffness? Temperature changes? Exercise?" Coldness and lack of use generally increase joint stiffness. Heat may reduce muscle spasm. Heat to a recently injured joint may increase stiffness by increasing bleeding into and swelling of the joint. "Does the joint lock? Can you hear or feel bones rubbing together?" Bone malalignment within a joint causes locking (joint cannot move). Crepitus (sound of bone ends rubbing together) indicates fractures or joint destruction. "Do you have pain or weakness in muscles with certain movements?" Weakness in muscles may be due to various neuromuscular disorders. "If weakness is present, does it impair usual activities?"

SWELLING

"How long have you had the swelling? Do you also have pain?" Swelling and pain often accompany bone and muscle injury. With degenerative joint disease, swelling often does not develop for some time, maybe weeks, after pain is present or it may not develop at all. "Is movement limited by the swelling?" Limited movement is associated with soft tissue damage and swelling within a joint. "Does rest give relief? Does elevating the part give relief?" Elevation reduces swelling in acute injuries. "Have you had a cast on this body part recently?" Removing a cast can precipitate temporary swelling. A casted extremity may have muscle atrophy. "Has the area been hot or red?" Redness and heat indicate inflammation, infection, or recent injury; not usually present with degenerative conditions.

DEFORMITY AND IMMOBILITY

"Has the deformity developed suddenly or gradually?" A gradually developing mass may indicate a tumor. "Is movement limited? Is movement limitation always present? Is it worse after activity? Does any particular body position make it worse or better?" Immobility from degenerative joint disease varies with the severity of the condition. "How does the deformity affect your daily activities? Do you use any supportive equipment such as crutches, a walker, or bandages?" Use of such aids indicates the severity of the disability.

SENSORY CHANGES

"Do you have a history of back pain or injury? If yes, where is the pain located? Does the pain travel, for example, down the back of the leg? Do you have problems walking? Do you have any loss of feeling anywhere? Any tingling or burning sensation? Is loss of feeling associated with any pain?" Pressure on nerves or blood vessels can occur from swelling, tumors, or fractures, causing sensation loss. Sensory changes may be associated with pain in an arm or hand.

Past Medical History

The nurse asks the client about a number of past health problems because there are many diseases that can affect the musculoskeletal system. Both childhood and adult-onset disorders are explored because of the possible long-term effects.

Previous trauma, accidents, or surgery involving bones or joints is carefully assessed. The client may have sustained fractures, dislocations, strains, or sprains. Previous accidents leading to bony fracture may predispose the client to degenerative changes.

CHILDHOOD AND INFECTIOUS DISEASES

Some health conditions affect the musculoskeletal system either directly or indirectly. For example, diabetes may predispose the client to degenerative joint disease. Blood dyscrasias, such as hemophilia, may cause bleeding in joints that produces pain, swelling, tenderness, and deformity. Psoriasis may precede psoriatic arthritis. Trauma producing cartilage damage may precipitate degenerative changes in a relatively young person. Ask about a history of tuberculosis, poliomyelitis, inflammatory and/or degenerative arthritis, scurvy, rickets, osteomyelitis, soft tissue infection, fungus infection of bones or joints, and neuromuscular disorders. Ask about infections which can be a source of secondary bacterial infection, such as ears, tonsils, sinuses, genitourinary system, or pelvic inflammatory disease. Seek detailed information about any of these conditions, if present.

IMMUNIZATIONS

Document the date of the client's last immunizations, especially tetanus and polio. Specifically, inquire whether the client has had a tuberculin skin test, the date, and the results. Some clients may report a history of positive reaction to the PPD test but do not have active tuberculosis. Inoculation with the bacille Calmette-Guérin (BCG) vaccine usually results in the client having a positive PPD test result from that time on.

MAJOR ILLNESSES AND HOSPITALIZATIONS

In addition to diseases such as diabetes mellitus, tuberculosis, poliomyelitis, and arthritis, ask the client about hospitalizations related to musculoskeletal disorders, including trauma. If the client or significant others cannot remember details, ask for permission to obtain the medical records. Ask about past or present minor and major injuries, including the circumstances of the injury, diagnosis of injury, treatment received, duration of treatment, and any current problems resulting from the injury.

Musculoskeletal injury includes fractures, sprains, strains, and joint dislocations. Some injuries are minor and are treated on an ambulatory basis, whereas others are major and require prolonged hospitalization, surgery, or rest and immobilization. Ask whether the client has any residual impairment from the injury such as a need to use assistive devices, such as a cane, crutches, or walker. Also inquire whether there has been a need to change or adjust ADLs because of lingering limitations.

MEDICATIONS

Question the client carefully about past and present prescription and over-the-counter medications. Ask the reasons for taking each medication, its dose, frequency, how long it was taken, and any observed side effects. Ask specifically about medication used for musculoskeletal problems, such as muscle relaxants, salicylates, nonsteroidal anti-inflammatory drugs (NSAIDs), and steroids. Some medications affect the musculoskeletal system. For example, corticosteroids can precipitate necrosis of the head of the femur, leading to septic arthritis, and can also precipitate muscle weakness. High doses of anticoagulants can produce hemarthrosis (blood in joints); anticonvulsants may cause osteomalacia; phenothiazines may produce gait disturbances; potassium-depleting diuretics may produce cramps and muscle weakness; and amphetamines and caffeine cause generalized, increased motor activity. For the postmenopausal woman, inquire about use of hormonal replacement therapy with estrogen, which has been shown to modify the effects of osteoporosis.

FAMILY HISTORY

Genetically related family history is important to identify musculoskeletal problems that have a familial predisposition, such as arthritis, ankylosing spondylitis, gout, Heberden's nodes in osteoarthritis, muscular dystrophy, and scoliosis. Thirty per cent of people with psoriatic arthritis have a family history of psoriasis.

PSYCHOSOCIAL HISTORY AND LIFESTYLE

The integrity of the musculoskeletal system allows people to function effortlessly. Yet there are many factors that can disrupt that integrity. The nurse inquires about the client's daily activities and habits. When assessing clients with chronic illnesses and degenerative processes, the nurse asks if the disorder has affected the client's interactions with others or friends and the client's view of himself/herself. Crippling illnesses often curtail social activity and decrease self-esteem.

DAILY ACTIVITIES

Are there any everyday activities that the client finds difficult or impossible, such as opening containers, pouring liquids, cutting up food; dressing; using zippers; fastening or unfastening buttons, snaps, or hooks; grooming; combing hair; applying makeup; running a bath and testing water temperature; washing the hair; shaving; writing; getting out of the house; climbing stairs; or getting in and out of chairs or cars? Ask if there is anything in everyday life the client wants to do that symptoms prevent.

Occupation. Ask whether a lot of heavy lifting or strenuous activity is typical. This can cause muscle strain, degenerative vertebral disc problems, and other trauma. Low back pain can arise from jobs involving a lot of driving. Habitually carrying heavy objects, such as a mail bag, shoulder bag, attaché case, or other equipment, causes musculoskeletal problems by placing uneven pressure on the spinal column.

Habits. The client's habits and lifestyle can increase the risk of developing musculoskeletal disorders. Similarly, musculoskeletal impairment affects the ability to perform ADLs. Document details of the client's typical recreational activities and exercise pattern. Lack of exercise produces poor muscle tone, which leads to muscle strain. Sporadic exercise in poorly toned muscles causes muscle injury and spasm. In addition, the lack of warm-up increases the likelihood of injury. Fractures and other trauma can arise from contact sports, such as football and hockey. Achilles tendon damage can arise from improperly landing on the heels while jogging. Pain in arm joints can arise from racket sports such as tennis and squash, which require a strong grasp, wrist extension, and forearm rotation. Ask about typical footwear. High-heeled shoes can shorten the Achilles tendons and pitch the center of gravity forward, leading to lordosis.

Try to ascertain the client's attention to safety. Ask about safety practices at work and at home. Does the client use the recommended equipment for recreational activities, such as correct shoes? Does the client wear safety goggles when using power tools or scraping paint? There is a high incidence of accidental injury among people who pay little attention to safety practices.

Dietary history is important to provide clues to musculoskeletal problems. For example, obesity stresses weight-bearing joints and predisposes the client to ligamentous instability, particularly of the lower back. Poor calcium intake can precipitate fractures due to bone decalcification. Ask the client to list foods eaten on a typical day. Dietary history forms help with dietary assessment and teaching. Adequate dietary intake of vitamins A and D, calcium, and protein is important for musculoskeletal health. Ask about recent major weight changes. Excessive weight gain can place stress on the musculoskeletal system.

Review of Systems

The nurse asks the client about problems such as muscle pain, spasm or tenderness; joint pain, stiffness, pain, swelling, or redness; weakness; limited movement; clumsiness; crepitus; backache; and changes in joints or bones. Each reported problem is investigated with a symptom analysis, as well as an inquiry about the effect the problem has had on the client's ability to perform ADLs.

Assessment findings from other body systems sometimes indicate musculoskeletal problems. For example, (1) pain or burning when urinating is associated with Reiter's syndrome; (2) cardiovascular symptoms such as tachycardia and hypertension may accompany gout; (3) chronic diarrhea may occur when arthritis is associated with colitis or other gastrointestinal problems; (4) conjunctivitis may indicate Reiter's syndrome, and nongranulomatous uveitis may occur with ankylosing spondylitis; (5) skin changes may indicate musculoskeletal problems, e.g., dry skin over thumb and first two fingers with carpal tunnel syndrome; (6) cramping leg pain upon activity may signal intermittent claudication; (7) generalized muscle cramping may result from electrolyte imbalances; and (8) joint pain associated with recent chills, fever, or sore throat may be due to rheumatic fever.

Detailed questions for the review of systems (ROS) are found in Chapter 11, Table 11–5.

PHYSICAL EXAMINATION

Like other body system assessments, assessment of the musculoskeletal system proceeds in a systematic manner to avoid missing hidden problems. Use an examining room big enough for the client to move around. Natural lighting is best to assess skin color changes and swelling. Artificial light distorts some assessment findings. During musculoskeletal assessment, have the client sit, stand, and walk (unless any position is contraindicated by the client's condition).

The *musculoskeletal assessment* includes inspection and palpation of *muscle masses* for symmetry, involuntary movements, tenderness, tone, and strength; *joints* for symmetry, crepitus, tenderness or pain, and ROM; and *bones* for deformity. The nurse also tests the muscle stretch or deep tendon reflexes (DTRs) using a percussion hammer.

General Musculoskeletal Examination

Using inspection and palpation, examine each body part. First examine the body at rest. Then assess ROM and muscle strength (see discussion below).

First have the client sit on the edge of the examining table. Look at the client's general appearance and body build. Examine the head, neck, shoulders, and upper extremities.

Then have the client stand, and examine the chest, back, and ilium. Observe posture; body build; body contours; body alignment; and the cervical, thoracic, and lumbar spine. Also observe the relationships of various body parts to each other, e.g., relationship of feet to legs, legs to hips, and hips to pelvis. Ask the

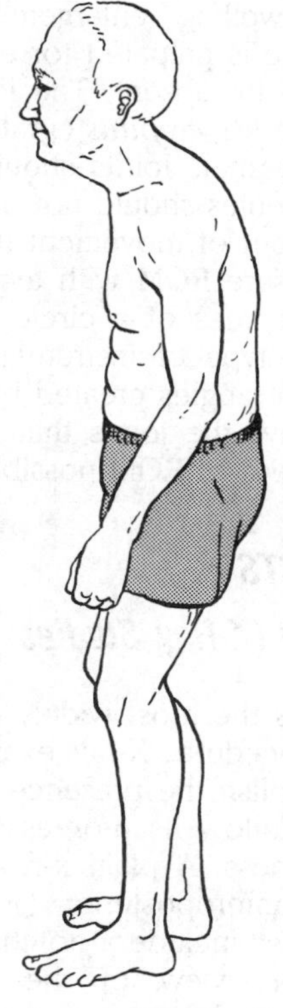

▲ Figure 65-1

When doing a musculoskeletal assessment, have the client stand and walk, if possible. Observe stance, joint mobility, and posture. If this man were assessed only while reclining, his posture, curvature of the spine, and limited range of motion may not have been observed.

client to walk and observe gait, body mobility, joint motion (Fig. 65-1). While observing movement and gait, watch for gait patterns associated with specific disorders (see Chapter 28), objective evidence of discomfort, indications of joint stiffness or muscle weakness, lack of coordination, or deformities. Observe the client's stance and note any spinal deformities (Fig. 65-2), such as (1) kyphosis, i.e., abnormally increased roundness of the thoracic curve (Fig. 65-2A); (2) scoliosis, that is, an obvious lateral deformity of the spine (Fig. 65-2B; or (3) lordosis, i.e., abnormal increase in the lumbar curve (Fig. 65-2C). Other observable abnormalities include genu varum, that is, "bowed" legs (Fig. 65-2D), and genu valgum, that is, "knock-knees" (Fig. 65-2E). The terms "varus(-um)" and "valgus(-um)" refer to the direction in which the apex of a deformity lies in relationship to the midline. In other words, with a varus deformity the apex of the deformity points away from the midline. With a valgus deformity it points toward the midline. These terms are used to describe the direction of a deformity in any body region.

Last, have the client lie supine and examine the hips, knees, ankles, and feet.

MUSCLES

The nurse compares each muscle group with its contralateral side. Muscles should be free of *fasciculations* (fine muscle twitches) and smooth, without bulges or lumps. Palpate muscle groups gently, from a proximal to distal direction, feeling the *muscle tone* (i.e., the state of tension in a muscle at rest, which is felt as firmness). Muscles should feel firm, smooth, and bilaterally equal in size and be nontender. A slight increase in mass or *hypertrophy* on the dominant side is normal, whereas *atrophy,* or decreased muscle size, on either side is abnormal. If muscle groups are noticeably asymmetric in size, use a tape measure to assess limb circumference. Differences of 1 cm or less are considered within normal variation.

Assess *muscle strength* while putting the client's joints through active ROM. If detailed assessment of muscle strength is necessary, each major muscle group can be assessed separately. Follow the guidelines in Table 65-1. (Note the sternocleidomastoid and trapezius muscles are tested as part of the head and neck (i.e., cranial nerve) examination and are omitted from the table.) Test muscle strength by asking the client to repeat ROM while resistance is applied. Note the strength the client uses against the resistance. If there is

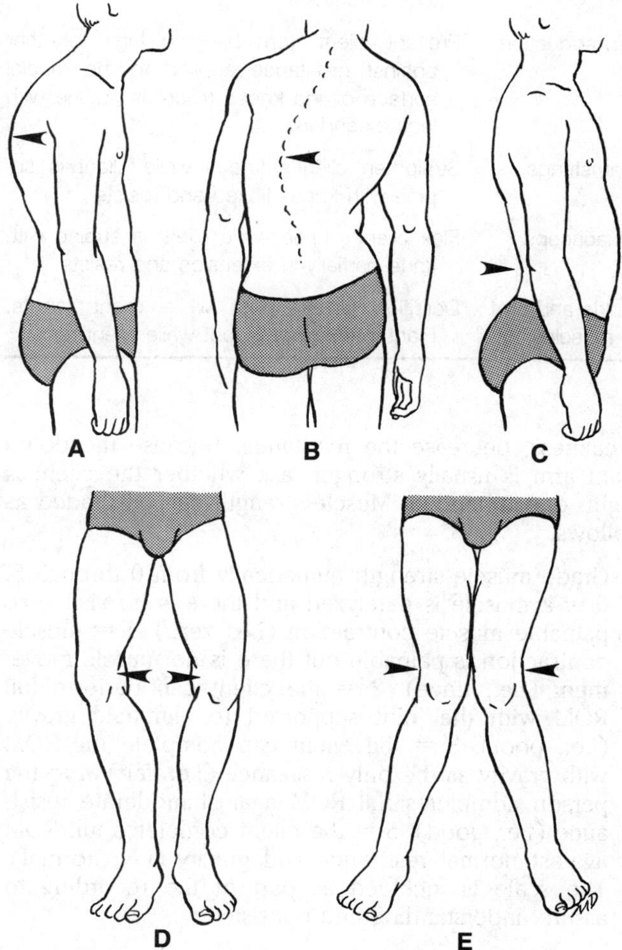

▲ Figure 65-2

Musculoskeletal deformities observable during assessment. *A,* Kyphosis. *B,* Scoliosis. *C,* Lordosis. *D,* Genu varum. *E,* Genu valgum. Black arrowheads indicate the deformities.

TABLE 65-1. Assessing Muscle Strength

Muscle Group	Technique
Deltoid	Push down client's arm while it is held up and client resists
Biceps	Hold client's arm in extension while it is fully extended and client flexes arm
Triceps	Keep client's arm in flexion while it is flexed and client extends arm
Wrist and finger muscles	Push client's fingers together while client spreads them and resists
Grip strength	Try to pull crossed index and middle fingers out from the client's grasp
Hip muscles	Hold down client's leg while it is fully extended and client lifts it off the table (client is supine)
Hip abduction	Prevent client from spreading legs apart against resistance applied to the lateral surface of the knees (client is supine with legs extended)
Hip adduction	Prevent client from bringing legs together against resistance applied to the medial surface of the knees (client is supine with legs extended)
Hamstrings	Straighten client's knees while client is supine with knees flexed and resists
Quadriceps	Flex client's knee while client is supine with knee partially in extension and resists
Ankle and foot muscles	Dorsiflex client's foot while client resists. Plantar flex client's foot while client resists

weakness, decrease the resistance. Because the dominant arm is usually stronger, ask whether the client is right- or left-handed. Muscle strength can be graded as follows.

- Grade muscle strength numerically from 0 through 5. 0 = a muscle is paralyzed and there is no visible or palpable muscle contraction (i.e., zero). 1 = muscle contraction is palpable but there is no muscle movement (i.e., trace). 2 = the client can perform full ROM with the joint supported to eliminate gravity (i.e., poor). 3 = the client can complete full ROM with gravity as the only resistance (i.e., fair). 4 = the person completes full ROM against moderate resistance (i.e., good). 5 = the client completes full ROM against normal resistance and gravity (i.e., normal). The scale is included as part of the recording to assure understanding and consistency.

JOINTS AND BONES

The nurse inspects the joints and bones and compares findings bilaterally. They should be symmetric and without redness, swelling, enlargement, or deformity. Each joint and bone is palpated for edema and tenderness, which should be absent. The joints also are palpated as they move for *crepitus* (grating sound or feeling), which is abnormal. Joints should feel smooth as they move, and nodules should not be present. ROM is the maximum amount of movement that a healthy joint is capable of. Measure ROM with a goniometer, which is based on the degrees of a circle (Fig. 65-3). This flexible, protractor type of instrument is placed on a joint to measure the angles created by joint movement. Figure 65-4 displays the joints that are assessed, and the types and degrees of ROM possible.

DIAGNOSTIC TESTS

Roentgenography (X-Ray Studies, Radiography)

Roentgenography is the most widely used musculoskeletal diagnostic procedure. X-ray examinations are important to (1) establish the presence of a musculoskeletal problem, (2) follow its progress, and (3) evaluate treatment effectiveness. A plain x-ray film is common, usually from an anteroposterior (AP) and/or lateral view. Common views include a notch (posterior or less commonly anterior) view of the knee in flexion, oblique (45-degree angle) view, and a sunrise or patella view of the underside of the patella. The client is asked to remove any radiopaque objects that could appear on the x-ray film, such as jewelry. No additional preparation is needed except possibly analgesics for some clients. If possible, the client may be asked to move into various positions so that x-ray films may be taken from the most useful angles. This may be difficult or painful. X-ray tables are very hard. Analgesia and other pain-relieving interventions may be needed after x-ray.

Studies Using Contrast. Other specialized radiographic procedures allow more precise visualization. An arthrogram is a radiographic examination of soft tissue

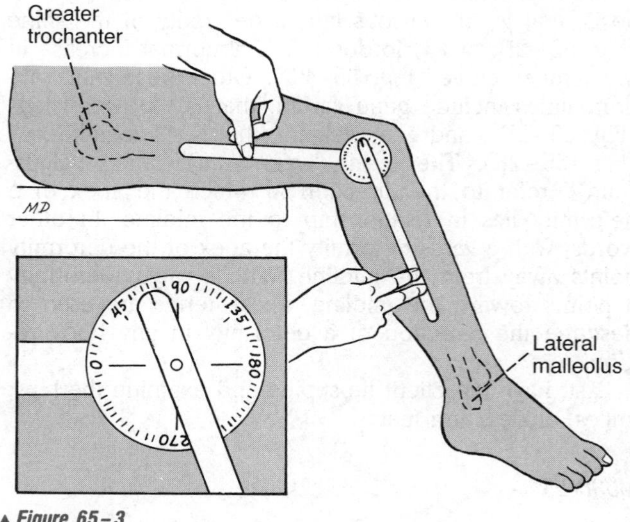

▲ *Figure 65-3*

Use of goniometer to measure joint range of motion.

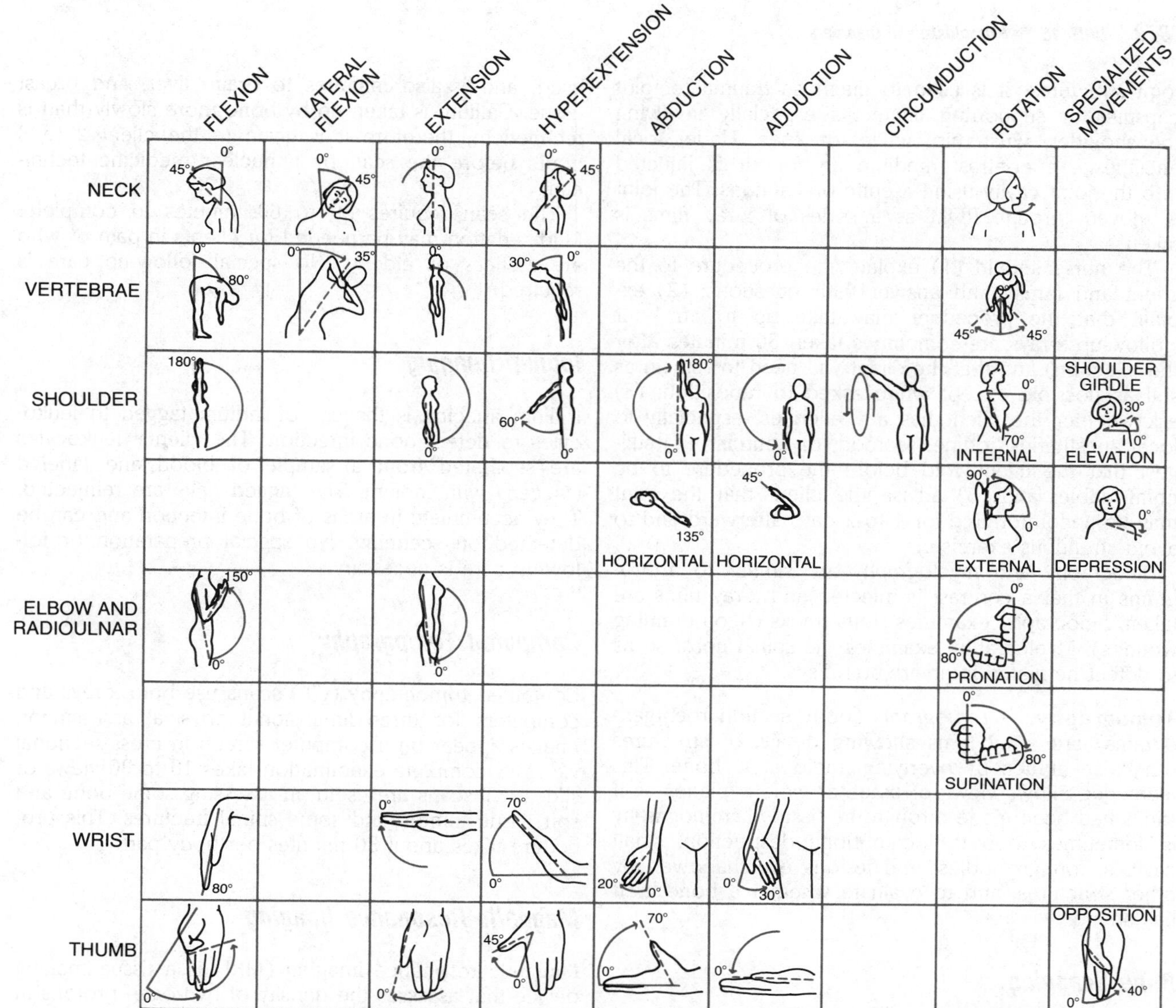

	FLEXION	LATERAL FLEXION	EXTENSION	HYPEREXTENSION	ABDUCTION	ADDUCTION	CIRCUMDUCTION	ROTATION	SPECIALIZED MOVEMENTS
NECK	0° 45°	0° 45°	0°	0° 45°					
VERTEBRAE	0° 80°	0° 35°		30° 0°				45° 45°	
SHOULDER	180° 0°		0°	60°	180° 0°	0°		0° 70° INTERNAL	SHOULDER GIRDLE 30° 10° 0° ELEVATION
					45° 135° HORIZONTAL	45° HORIZONTAL		90° 70° 0° EXTERNAL	0° DEPRESSION
ELBOW AND RADIOULNAR	150° 0°		0°					0° 80° PRONATION	
								0° 80° SUPINATION	
WRIST	80°		0°	70° 0°	20° 0°	0° 30°			
THUMB	0°		0°	45° 0°	70° 0°	0°			OPPOSITION 0° 40°
FINGERS	90° 0°				45° 0° 45°				
HIP	120° 0°		0°	30° 0°	45° 0°			45° INTERNAL	PELVIC GIRDLE 10° 0° ELEVATION
								0° EXTERNAL	0° 10° DEPRESSION
KNEE	135° 0°								
ANKLE	20° 0° DORSI-		0°	0° PLANTAR FLEXION					15° 0° EVERSION; 35° 0° INVERSION
TOES	0° 45°		0°	70° 40° 0°	20° 0° 0° 10°	0°			RIB CAGE ELEVATION 25° 0°; DEPRESSION 25° 0°

▲ ***Figure 65–4***

Joint range of motion (ROM). All joints are at 0 degrees when in anatomic position. ROM begins at 0 degrees, as shown by solid lines. Attainment of the average normal ROM is shown by dotted lines and the number of degrees in the angle formed by the two lines. Shoulder flexion and abduction to 180 degrees include scapular motions. Hip flexion to 120 degrees is with the knee flexed.

joint structures. It is used to diagnose trauma to joint capsules or supporting ligaments especially involving the shoulder, wrist, hip, ankle, or knee. Under local anesthesia, a contrast medium and/or air is injected into the joint cavity using aseptic precautions. The joint is moved through ROM as a series of x-ray films is taken.

The nurse should (1) explain the procedure to the client and family and answer their questions; (2) explain that the procedure may take up to an hour (follow-up x-rays are sometimes taken 30 minutes after the injection) and that the client will need to remain as still as possible except when asked to reposition; (3) ask whether the client has any allergies, especially to local anesthetics, iodine, seafood, or contrast; (4) suggest that the client void before the procedure to be comfortable; and (5) advise the client that the joint may be uncomfortable for 1 to 2 days afterward and to avoid strenuous exercise.

Sinography and myelography are similar to arthrograms in that a contrast is injected and x-ray films are taken. Sinography examines sinus tracks (deep draining wounds). Myelography examines the spinal cord, so as to detect herniated intervertebral discs.

Tomography. *Tomograms* (body section roentgenograms) are x-ray films showing details of structures otherwise hidden by overlying, radiopaque bone. This technique allows views of tissue at various planes as if slices had been made through the tissue. Laminography is sometimes used to locate bone destruction, small cavities, foreign bodies, and lesions overshadowed by other structures, and to evaluate whether a bone graft has united.

Bone Scanning

Radioisotopes that are taken up by bone are injected intravenously (usually technetium ^{99m}Tc). This substance migrates to bone. The whole body is usually scanned, although only an extremity may be scanned if a stress fracture is suspected (i.e., pinhole scan). Bone scanning is used to detect malignancies, osteomyelitis, osteoporosis, and some fractures (especially pathologic fractures). The isotope collects in these areas, indicating abnormal bone metabolism. The isotope does not collect in poorly perfused bone. The nurse (1) explains the procedure to the client and family and answers their questions; the procedure takes about 1 hour, during which the client lies supine; (2) reassures the client that the procedure is not painful and there are no harmful effects from the isotopes; and (3) suggests that the client urinate before the procedure for comfort.

After the scan, no special precautions are required. There is minimal radioactivity in the isotope and therefore no hazard to the nurse. The isotope is excreted in urine and feces.

Gallium Scan

Gallium scans are similar to bone scans, but the test is more specific to bone disorders. Gallium is the isotope used, and it also migrates to brain, liver, and breast tissue. Gallium is taken up by bone more slowly than is technetium, therefore it is given to the client 2 to 3 hours before the scan by a nuclear medicine technician.

The scan requires 30 to 60 minutes to complete. Mild sedation may be needed for clients in pain or who are restless or elderly. No special follow-up care is required.

Indium Imaging

Indium imaging is the use of indium tagged to leukocytes to detect bone infection. The clients' leukocytes are separated from a sample of blood and labeled (tagged) with indium. The tagged cells are reinjected. They accumulate in areas of bone infection and can be detected on scanning. No special preparation or follow-up care is necessary.

Computed Tomography

Computed tomography (CT) scans use both x-rays and computers for three-dimensional physical assessment. Images appear on a computer screen in cross-sectional views. A complete examination takes 10 to 30 views or slides. CT scans are useful in assessing some bone and soft tissue tumors and some spinal fractures. This procedure takes about 30 minutes per body part.

Magnetic Resonance Imaging

Magnetic resonance imaging (MRI) is a tissue-imaging device that assesses the density of hydrogen protons in the body. Because bone marrow and soft tissue are high in hydrogen, MRI facilitates the early diagnosis of many conditions, such as knee problems, degenerative bone disease and tumors. The client is slid inside a horizontal cylinder (a giant solenoid) and exposed to a magnetic field that is roughly 15,000 times greater than the earth's natural magnetic field. Radio waves knock protons out of their polarized alignment. When the radio waves are shut off, the protons swing back into alignment, releasing a measurable amount of energy. This process allows MRI to make rapid, detailed, and efficient pictures of body tissue. The nurse (1) explains the procedure to the person and significant others and answers their questions (they may be anxious about the new procedure; if possible, show them the equipment); (2) reassures the person that no discomfort is experienced with this procedure; (3) explains that the procedure takes about 15 to 20 minutes per body part; and (4) suggests that the person urinate before the procedure for comfort.

Biopsy

A biopsy is the removal and histologic examination of tissue for diagnostic purposes. Disorders such as infection and cancer of the bone and atrophy and inflammation of the muscle are detected. Bone or muscle may be biopsied during surgery or through a needle or bore not requiring a surgical incision. The latter are called aspiration, punch, or needle biopsies. Sometimes aspiration biopsy with radiographic control is performed, such as into the spine. Bone biopsies are taken in the radiology department or an operating room under sterile conditions to prevent osteomyelitis. Local anesthesia is used. Bone or muscle biopsies take about 30 minutes.

Following the biopsy the nurse monitors the site for bleeding, swelling, and hematoma development. Because dressings usually surround the biopsy site, assessment is performed through analysis of the client's pain. Mild to moderate discomfort is usual; more severe levels of pain may signal complications. The biopsy site is elevated for 24 hours to reduce edema. Vital signs are monitored every 4 hours for 24 hours. A mild analgesic is usually required. Ongoing assessments of the site for signs of infection are performed by the nurse or client when discharged.

Arthroscopy

Arthroscopy is common and a very useful diagnostic tool. An arthroscope is a small fiberoptic instrument that allows endoscopic examination of various joints, including the hip, knee, shoulder, elbow, and wrist, without making a large incision into the joint. Diagnoses made via arthroscopy are 98 per cent accurate. Arthroscopy can be used for assessment and/or treatment. For example, biopsies can be taken, articular cartilage abnormalities can be assessed, or loose bodies can be removed and cartilage trimmed. Arthroscopy is usually an outpatient procedure performed under local anesthesia. The client is usually home and back to work sooner than if an arthrotomy (opening the joint) were performed. Arthroscopy is contraindicated in clients whose joint flexion is less than 50 per cent (e.g., in fibrous ankylosis) or if skin or wound infection is present at the site. Complications are rare but include infection, hemarthrosis (blood in the joint), swelling, synovial rupture, joint injury, or thrombophlebitis (Fig. 65-5).

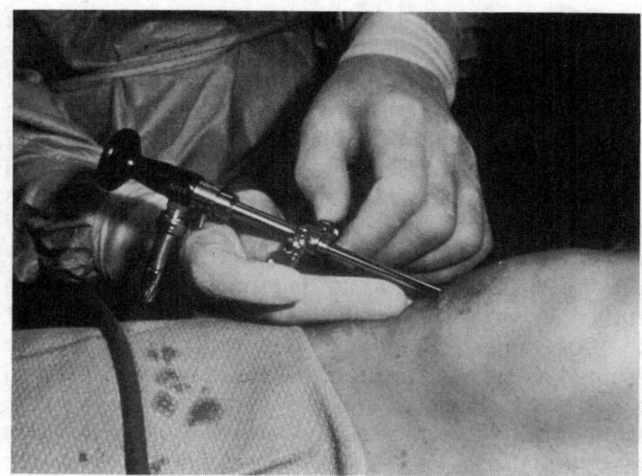

▲ *Figure 65-5*

An arthroscope inserted into the knee joint.

NURSING MANAGEMENT

The nurse explains the procedure to the client and family and answers their questions.

TABLE 65-2. Synovial Fluid Analysis

Tests	Measurement and Norms
Mucin clot test	The addition of 5 per cent acetic acid to normal joint fluid results in a thick ropy clot that will not fragment when shaken. Fluid from an acutely inflamed joint results in a stringy loose clot
Viscosity	After taking normal synovial fluid between the thumb and index finger, a string of fluid 1 to 2 inches long will develop as the thumb and index finger are separated. Inflamed joints produce synovial fluid that is watery
Color, clarity, amount	Normal joint fluid varies from yellow to straw, is clear, and is present in the joint in only minute quantities. Inflamed joints produce increased fluid that is turbid and gray in color
White blood cells	Normal synovial fluid has a low concentration, with predominately mononuclear cells. WBC greater than 2000 per mm^3 occurs in osteoarthritis; WBC greater than 100,000 with sepsis and polymyalgia rheumatica
Glucose	Blood and synovial fluid glucose levels need to be determined simultaneously in the fasting patient. If the joint fluid glucose level is less than 50 per cent of that of the blood, pyogenic infection should be suspected. However, greater differentials can occur with RA
Crystal studies	Presence of crystals in the synovial fluid indicates gout or pseudogout
Rheumatoid factor	RF may be found in synovial fluid before becoming evident in the blood. However, RF in synovial fluid is nonspecific, and cannot be relied on to provide meaningful support for a diagnosis of RA

RA, Rheumatoid arthritis; RF, rheumatoid factor; WBC, white blood cell.
From Schoen, D. (1988) Assessment for arthritis. *Orthopaedic Nursing*, 7(2), 31-39.

Instruct the client to fast from midnight the night before. Be sure the client and family know where the procedure will be performed and by whom and that appropriate consent forms are understood and signed. If a local anesthetic will be used, tell the client that there may be mild discomfort as it is administered and a thumping sensation may be felt as the arthroscope is inserted. Teach the client to watch for indications of post-procedure infection, such as temperature elevation, local inflammation at the incision site, and to report this promptly. Ensure necessary pain relief after the procedure. Tell the client a normal diet may be resumed as soon as desired. Advise that unless surgical excision is performed and the surgeon gives specific instructions, walking is usually permitted after sensation has returned, but excessive exercise should be avoided for a few days.

Arthrocentesis

Arthrocentesis is a method of aspirating synovial fluid, blood, or pus via a needle inserted into the joint cavity. It is used to diagnose rheumatoid arthritis and other inflammatory conditions or to remove fluid to relieve pain. The procedure is done under local anesthesia with aseptic precautions. Medication may be instilled into the joint if necessary, such as to alleviate inflammation. Apply a compression bandage following arthrocentesis and rest the joint for 8 to 24 hours. Results of synovial fluid analysis are summarized in Table 65-2.

Electromyography

Electromyography (EMG) is used to assess lower motor neuron lesions. It measures the electrical potential associated with skeletal muscle contractions. Needles are inserted into muscles. Recordings of muscular electrical activity are then traced on an audiotransmitter, on an oscilloscope, and on recording paper. EMG helps diagnose neuromuscular conditions.

Nurses (1) explain the procedure to the client and family; (2) teach that needle insertion is uncomfortable; and (3) instruct the person not to take any stimulants or sedatives for 24 hours before the procedure.

Bone Mineral Content

Methods used to measure bone density are performed to diagnose osteoporosis, because the condition is not evident on x-ray study until 30 to 50 per cent of the bone mass is lost. One method of measuring bone mass is the use of single photon absorptiometry. This technique measures the amount of radioisotopes absorbed by the bone. Radioisotope is passed beneath a bone, usually the forearm, and the amount is read from above the arm by a detector. The test takes about 10 minutes. There are several other techniques that can detect osteoporosis in other sites, such as the spine and hips. No preparation is required; the client may require teaching about osteoporosis once the findings are known.

TABLE 65-3. Common Laboratory Studies Used in Diagnosing Musculoskeletal Conditions

Test/Normal Value	Significance of Results
Erythrocyte sedimentation rate (ESR) Normal: Westergren's method: men, 0-15 mm/h women, 0-20 mm/h Wintrobe's method: men, 0-9 mm/h women, 0-15 mm/h	Elevations common in arthritic conditions, infection, inflammation, cancer, cell or tissue destruction
Tests of Mineral Metabolism	
Calcium 8.0-10.5 mg/dl or 4.5-5.5 mEq/L	Decreased levels found in osteomalacia, osteoporosis Increased levels found in bone tumors, Paget's disease, healing fractures
Alkaline phosphatase 30-90 IU/L	Elevations found in bone cancer, osteoporosis, osteomalacia, Paget's disease
Phosphorus 2.5-4.0 mg/dl	Increased levels found in healing fractures, osteolytic metastatic tumor diseases
Muscle Enzymes	
Aldolase A 1.3-8.2 U/dl	Elevations in muscular dystrophy, dermatomyositis
Aspartate aminotransferase 10-50 mU/ml	Found in skeletal muscle, but primarily heart and renal cells
Creatine phosphokinase 15-150 IU/L	Increased levels found in traumatic injuries, progressive muscular dystrophy, polymyositis
Lactate dehydrogenase (LDH_4, LDH_5) 60-150 IU/L	Elevations in skeletal muscle necrosis, extensive cancer, progressive muscular dystrophy

Laboratory Tests

Table 65-3 lists the most common laboratory tests for clients with musculoskeletal disorders. Chapter 26 includes laboratory tests specific for rheumatic problems.

Summary

The musculoskeletal system assessment begins with a complete history including symptom analysis. Diagnostic studies commonly include x-ray study, and in recent years, arthroscopy has been performed to diagnose and treat joint disorders in one procedure.

Bibliography

1. Bryan, V. (1990). Troubleshooting arthroscopic equipment. *Orthopaedic Nursing, 9* (1), 18–25.
2. Jarvis, C. (1992). Physical Examination and Health Assessment. Philadelphia, W. B. Saunders.
3. Pavlik, M. (1991). Measuring bone mineral content. *Orthopaedic Nursing, 10* (2), 39–42.
4. Peters, V., & Ferkel, R. (1989). Arthroscopic surgery of the ankle. *Orthopaedic Nursing, 8* (5), 12–19.
5. Schoen, D. (1988). Assessment for arthritis. *Orthopaedic Nursing, 7* (2), 31–39.
6. Swartz, M. (1989). *Textbook of Physical Diagnosis*. Philadelphia: W. B. Saunders.
7. Zubay, R. (1988). Understanding magnetic resonance imaging from a nursing perspective. *Orthopaedic Nursing, 7* (6), 17–23.

Chapter 66

Common Musculoskeletal Interventions

Orthopaedic interventions are some of the oldest recorded areas of medical practice. The nurse treating the client with musculoskeletal disorders is challenged to deal with traditional methods and to stay current with change. Casts often appear awkward and daunting, and some would feel traction is barbaric, but both methods play an important part in immobilizing and aligning fractures.

No matter what form of treatment the client undergoes, the nurse can have a direct impact on the outcome for the client. Clients with musculoskeletal disorders suffer problems related to immobility and have common nursing diagnoses of impaired physical mobility, diversional activity, self-care deficit, and knowledge deficit. This chapter discusses the common interventions for clients with musculoskeletal impairments—some very old, some very new. All interventions challenge the nurse to plan care that promotes independence and a return to self-care.

REST

Rest is an essential intervention for many clients with musculoskeletal problems. Following trauma or for clients with rheumatic disorders, rest promotes healing and minimizes inflammation, swelling, and pain. Rest is sometimes achieved by immobilizing affected joints with splints or casts. Splints prevent joint deformities and minimize pain by relieving muscle spasms.

Unfortunately, however, bone, joint, and muscle deconditioning occurs. The bone demineralization that occurs with immobility appears to be secondary to decreased stress on bones. Decreased range of motion (ROM) results from an increased density of connective tissue around the joint. Muscle mass is also decreased by immobility. This deconditioning process is normal during prolonged immobilization. Use of physical therapy and nursing interventions are essential to avoid the problems associated with deconditioning.

Box 66-1. Purposes of Traction

- Reduce fractures and/or dislocations and maintain alignment.
- Decrease muscle spasms and relieve pain.
- Correct, lessen, or prevent deformities.
- Promote rest of a decreased or injured part.
- Promote exercise.

▼ TRACTION

Therapeutic traction (pull) is accomplished by exerting a pull (on the head, body, or limbs) in two directions, that is, pull of traction and pull of countertraction. Traction often is produced by weights. Countertraction may be produced with either (1) the person's body weight or (2) other weights. The traction and countertraction must be equal in order to be therapeutic.

When using traction, it is important to (1) support and stretch the extremity in a direction that properly aligns bone fragments (traction is exerted on the distal fragment to align it with the proximal fragment), (2) not overstretch the limb (overstretching excessively distracts bone fragments), and (3) maintain stretching forces that are constant in amount and direction until bone union occurs. Weights used to treat fractures with traction may be gradually reduced by the physician as the injured bone heals.

When traction is properly applied in bed, the person is centered in the bed and the affected part is held aligned by a constant two-way pull. When applied to a long bone, the direction of traction is in line with the bone's long axis. When applied to the head or pelvis, the pull is in line with the person's spinal column. The bed is usually elevated or tilted under the part in traction; for example, the foot of the bed may be elevated when traction is applied to lower extremities. If the bed is not properly tilted, countertraction from the client's body weight is inadequate. Then the person tends to slide in the direction of the traction force. This defeats the purpose of the traction apparatus, and effective traction is not achieved on the injured part. With some types of traction, countertraction is applied with ropes, pulleys, and weights pulling in a direction opposite to that of the traction. The purposes of traction are listed in Box 66-1.

METHODS OF APPLYING TRACTION

Traction may be applied (1) manually, by pulling on the body part with the hands; (2) mechanically, by exerting a pull on the body part with ropes and pulleys; (3) with devices inserted in casts (plaster traction); or (4) with braces (e.g., hyperextension braces).

Major disadvantages of most types of traction are that prolonged hospitalization and bed rest are necessary. Advantages of traction include (1) a greater potential for exercising joints and muscles than is possible with casts and (2) elimination of the need for surgery and its risks.

TRACTION TECHNIQUES

Continuous versus Intermittent Traction

Traction may be continuous (constant pull) or intermittent (pull periodically relieved by lifting the weights). Continuous traction typically is used to treat some fractures or dislocations. Intermittent traction may be used to treat arthritis (e.g., to reduce flexion contractures) or low back disorders (e.g., to reduce pain and muscle spasm). Always assume that traction is continuous unless the physician specifically states it should be intermittent. Prescriptions for intermittent traction state the precise length of time traction is to be applied.

Running versus Suspension Traction

Running traction (straight traction) exerts a direct pull on the affected part without a hammock or splint to provide balanced support. It pulls in one plane and may be unilateral or bilateral. Running traction may be applied to the skin (skin traction) or skeleton (skeletal traction). Buck's extension (see the section on skin traction) is an example.

Suspension traction (balanced traction) exerts a pull on the affected part and also supports the extremity in a hammock or splint held in place by balanced weights attached to an overhead bar (Fig. 66-1*E*). Countertraction is supplied by a system of ropes, pulleys, and weights. With suspension traction, the pull remains the same even when the person moves because countertraction takes up any slack caused by the movement. Thus, suspension traction allows more movement and activity than does running traction. This makes it easier to care for the client and improves the client's comfort and well being. Also, by increasing circulation to the affected part and by decreasing prolonged pressure on weight-bearing areas, suspension traction reduces possible complications.

Suspension traction may be either skeletal or skin and may use any type of splint or hammock. Examples of suspension traction are Russell's traction (Fig. 66-1*B*) and a Thomas splint with a Pearson attachment. The traction must be continuous to be effective.

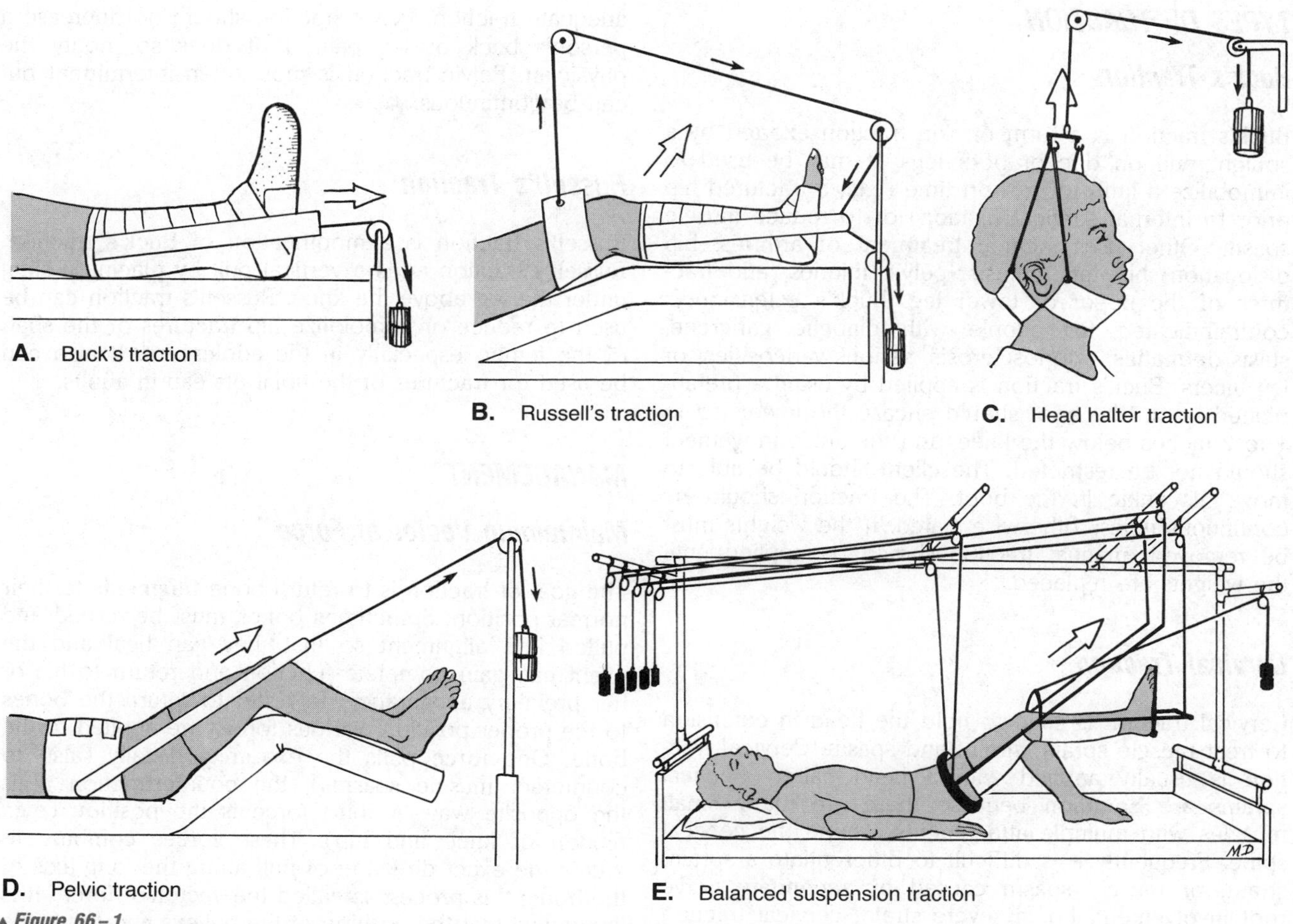

▲ *Figure 66–1*

Some common types of traction used in treating musculoskeletal problems. Solid arrows show pull on cables; open arrows show traction pull on body.

Skin Traction

Skin traction applies traction to the underlying skeletal system and other structures, such as muscles. It may be applied by (1) using commercially prepared adhesive backed materials or (2) encircling a body part with a halter, corset, or sling. A halter may be used to apply traction to the head, and a corset or sling may be used to apply traction to the pelvis. An anklet or bandage may be used with a splint to apply temporary traction to the ankle. Countertraction is provided by the person's weight when the bed is tilted down toward the head.

Skeletal Traction

Skeletal traction is accomplished by surgically inserting metal wires (Kirschner wires) or pins (Steinmann pins) through bones or by anchoring metal tongs (Crutchfield, Barton, or Vinke tongs) in the skull. The traction apparatus is then attached to the metal insertion. Skeletal traction applied to the skull is discussed in Chapter 32. Kirschner wires and Steinmann pins are round stainless steel rods typically inserted (with a drill) perpendicular to and completely through bones. A traction bow is attached to the wire or pin and the traction force is applied to the bow (also called spreader, stirrups, or calipers). The insertion site of pins, wires, or tongs determines the location where traction force is applied.

Wires and pins are not inserted through joints. They are inserted so that they only penetrate skin, subcutaneous tissue, and bone. Joints, muscles, tendons, arteries, and nerves are avoided. Wires and pins should not pass through a fracture hematoma. Also, they are not inserted through skin that is infected, is abraded, or has a rash. Inserting skeletal pins or wires is a sterile procedure performed under local or general anesthesia. Since the skin is opened for the placement of wires and pins, bone infection (osteomyelitis) is a potential complication.

In the past, skeletal traction was used until bone healing took place. Now, its most common use is to reduce unstable fractures of long bones until the client is able to undergo more definitive surgical treatment, such as insertion of intramedullary nails and various plates.

TYPES OF TRACTION

Buck's Traction

Buck's traction is a form of skin traction exerted by a straight pull on one or both legs. It may be used to immobilize a limb for a short time (e.g., a fractured hip prior to internal surgical fixation) or to reduce muscle spasm. Other uses include treatment of arthritis, hip dislocation, hip tuberculosis, pelvic injuries, and fractures of the upper or lower leg. Buck's extension is contraindicated for people with diabetic gangrene, stasis dermatitis, arteriosclerosis, serious varicosities, or leg ulcers. Buck's traction is applied by using a prefabricated boot. The boot should encase the lower leg to 1 to 2 inches below the knee, and the ankle movement should not be restricted. The client should be able to move his ankle in the boot. The traction should be continuous unless otherwise stated. If the weights must be removed, manual traction should be applied until the weights are replaced.

Cervical Traction

Cervical traction is used to hold the head in extension to treat muscle sprain, strain, and spasm. Cervical traction is usually applied with a head halter. Cervical sprains are common because there are many small muscles with multiple attachments around the cervical spine. Frequently it is difficult to differentiate a sprain, strain, or muscle spasm caused by secondary nerve root involvement. For a severe strain, cervical traction of 4 to 6 pounds may be used for several days.

Cervical traction can also be skeletal traction, as used with skull tongs or a halo apparatus. These types of traction are used to stabilize fractures or dislocations of the cervical or upper thoracic spine. The tongs or pins are inserted aseptically using general or local anesthesia. The skull tongs (Gardener-Wells, Crutchfield, or Vinke) are a running traction with weight attached to the tongs and the client is used as countertraction. The halo apparatus consists of a head piece with four pins, two anterior and two posterior. The head piece attaches to a body jacket. The purpose of halo traction is immobilization.

Pelvic Traction

Pelvic traction is accomplished with a belt applied just above and encircling the iliac crests. The belt attaches to a spreader bar and pulley system. Traction is applied to the lumbar spine. Some physicians order pillows beneath the legs; others want the foot of the bed elevated. If the backrest is excessively elevated, the client slides down in bed, creating a shearing force on the sacrum. This is undesirable. The most desirable position is the William's position (hips and knees each flexed 30 degrees). An overhead trapeze helps the person lift up off the bed. A snug-fitting pelvic belt ensures adequate traction. Pelvic traction should not increase a person's back or leg pain. If it does so, notify the physician. Pelvic traction is most often intermittent but can be continuous.

Russell's Traction

Russell's traction is a modification of Buck's traction. Russell's traction adds a vertical pull by placing a sling under the leg above the knee. Russell's traction can be used to reduce or immobilize hip fractures or the shaft of the femur, especially in the adolescent. It also can be used for fractures of the tibial plateau in adults.

MANAGEMENT

Maintaining Vector of Force

The goal of traction is to return bone fragments to their normal position. Sometimes bones must be turned and pulled into alignment so that they can heal and the client can gain complete function and return to his or her preinjury appearance. In order to return the bones to the proper position, various forces are applied to the bone. One force pulls the extremity distally (also to counteract muscle spasms), the countertraction pulls the opposite way. A third force is the position (e.g., flexion of knee and hip). These forces combine to create the exact direction of pull along the long axis of the bone; this process is called the vector of force. It is imperative that the position of the pulleys and the angle of splints not be adjusted without physician direction.

Preventing Complications

Short-term problems with traction are related to immobility (e.g., pneumonia, pressure ulcers) and malalignment of bony fragments. Nurses reduce or prevent the complications of immobility. Physicians monitor the progress of bony alignment by follow-up x-ray studies.

Long-term complications include osteomyelitis (see Chap. 67) and erosion/slipping of the pin due to excess weight. If the pin moves, it can be reinserted if needed.

Removing Traction

When skeletal traction is to be removed, prepare the skin around the pin site according to the physician's instructions. A physician removes a wire by (1) depressing the skin around the wire end, (2) cutting the wire beneath the skin surface, and then (3) pulling the wire through from the opposite side. Cutting one end of the pin prevents the bone from exposure to the contaminated end of the pin. Cover skin insertion and exit incisions with small sterile dressings. Clients will often be placed in a cast to allow complete bone healing.

Nursing Management

When planning nursing intervention for people in traction, it is important to know (1) the nature of the injury, (2) the purpose of the traction, (3) how the traction device accomplishes its purpose, (4) permitted movements and positions, (5) potential complications associated with traction, and (6) appropriate intervention to prevent complications.

If possible, prepare the client physically and psychosocially before using traction. Because of their formidable appearance, some traction set-ups look like implements of torture rather than like helpful therapeutic devices! Explain to the client and family the purposes of traction and reasons why specific body positions must be maintained for long periods of time. Make sure they understand contraindicated movements or positions. Explain that moving into contraindicated positions defeats the purpose of traction and disrupts healing. Explain that traction helps tight muscles to relax and that the client will probably feel more comfortable after a few hours. The physician tells the client how long traction is likely to be maintained.

Neurovascular assessment is essential when applying skeletal traction. Before a pin is inserted, establish neurovascular baseline measurements for later comparison between preinsertion and postinsertion assessment. Neurovascular assessment includes color, warmth, movement, sensation, pedal pulses, and capillary refill.

Periodically assess a skeletal traction apparatus. Sometimes the sharp ends of the wires or pins extend beyond the bow. If so, place corks or adhesive tape over these protruding ends to prevent injury to people or damage to clothing. Frequently inspect skin around pin sites for signs of infection, such as odor, redness, drainage. Some physicians cover these stab wounds with sterile dressings and do not want dressings disturbed unless there is evidence of infection. Others prescribe for dressings to be changed daily and for pin sites to be cleaned with antiseptic solution, followed by application of antibiotic ointment. Assess wrapped extremities for indications of constriction. Swelling is most likely to occur 24 to 48 hours after injury.

Much nursing intervention is directed at preventing complications from (1) prolonged immobility and (2) the traction equipment itself. (see Nursing Care Plan).

Cover the affected limb (or limbs) without interfering with the traction, such as wrapping the limb in a lightweight blanket. Do not allow coverings to press on the footplate of leg traction. Also, be sure ropes and pulleys remain free. Change linen by proceeding from the top to the bottom of the bed. Do not jerk the client by catching linens in traction equipment.

Once muscle spasms have subsided, about 48 to 72 hours after the application of traction, the client should have only mild discomfort when still. Pain may be reported with movement; adequate analgesia should be used preventively.

A client confined in traction, especially if it continues for some time, may experience a diversional activity deficit. This problem can occur because of inadequate environmental stimulation or lack of variation. It is particularly common in young adults and elderly clients. Appropriate nursing intervention focuses on preventing sensory deprivation. Plan varied activities of interest to the person to fill each day, such as radio, television, reading, and writing. Be sure a telephone is convenient to maintain contact with significant others. Sit with, talk with, and touch the client as appropriate. Place the client's bed beside a window, keep the door open as possible, and visit frequently.

Provide normal aids to orientation, such as accurate clock, current calendar and publications, clean glasses, and hearing aids, if worn by the client. Prism glasses may help a person read more easily while lying flat. Have the radio and television clearly tuned, but do not leave them on continuously if the person cannot control them independently. Continuous noise can increase confusion.

Some clients in traction are not able to perform many usual self-care activities independently. Other clients can do a lot themselves, provided necessary equipment and supplies are placed within easy reach. Be aware of which activities a client can and cannot perform, such as washing the feet. The client can also have control of care by being included in scheduling of procedures such as bath or linen changes.

Use a fracture bedpan (small, flat bedpan with a tapering slope from front to back) for a person in traction. For enemas, use a large bedpan, however. Some women prefer a kidney basin for urination. If the client can use a trapeze, position and remove a bedpan while the person raises the hips off the mattress.

Immediately following traction removal a client is often weak and unsteady. If a limb was immobilized, it may have some muscle atrophy. Orthostatic hypotension may occur if the client has been bedridden for several days or more. To combat this problem, help the client very gradually resume a sitting (and later standing) position. Elevate the head of the bed a little bit at a time to combat orthostatic hypotension. Raising the bed to a full sitting position may require several days. Have adequate help and provide careful physical support when a client first sits on the edge of the bed or gets out of bed. Safety precautions are imperative to prevent falls until the nurse is sure the client has secure balance, self-support, and strength.

Prepare client for a lack of proprioceptor response (awareness of body position, movement, and posture) following traction removal. Explain that the client may feel faint or weak, and that joints may be stiff or unstable. Weakened limbs may require temporary support at their joints, and crutches may be needed for a while.

▼ CASTS

Casts are temporary devices of plaster or fiber glass that immobilizes a body part, usually an extremity. However, clients can wear casts over the torso also. The purposes for a cast include (1) immobilization; (2)

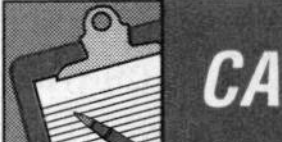

CARE PLAN

The Client in Skeletal Traction

Nursing Diagnosis/ Collaborative Problem	Planning: Expected Outcomes	Implementation: Nursing Interventions	Rationales
At risk for Impaired Skin Integrity R/T inability to change position secondary to skeletal traction	Client will retain intact skin, as evidenced by • no reddened areas • no abrasions	Assess pressure points (sacrum, heels under ropes and bones) every shift	Common pressure points for clients in supine position
		Provide skin care every shift by lifting client	Clients in traction cannot turn
		Apply therapeutic mattress to bed	Some mattresses (Geomatt) reduce surface pressure. Eggcrate mattresses improve comfort
Impaired Physical Mobility R/T confinement in traction	Client will not experience complications of immobility, as evidenced by • maintaining preinjury ROM in joints • not developing thrombophlebitis • having a bowel movement every other day • maintaining clear lung sounds	Place all joints (except those immediately proximal and distal to fracture) through ROM q shift	ROM assists to maintain muscle tone.
		Assess lung sounds q shift	Immobility and use of analgesia may cause hypoventilation and atelectasis
		Teach client to deep breathe and cough q shift	Deep breathing and coughing hyperventilate and clear secretions
		Assess for clinical manifestations of thrombophlebitis: unilateral leg edema or pain Do not rely on Homans' sign as an indicator	The presence of Homans' sign is not an accurate indicator of thrombophlebitis; other signs are assessed
		Monitor bowel movement	Constipation is a side effect of immobility
		• Encourage fluids and food containing fiber	Fiber and fluids assist to add bulk and soften bowel movement, making its passage easier
		• Administer laxatives prn	Laxative irritates or stimulates the colon
High Risk for Injury R/T traction	Client will sustain no injury while in traction	Ensure that weights hang freely from pulleys	If weights rest on the bed or floor, the traction is not effective
		Ensure that knots in the rope do not catch in the pulleys	Traction is not effective when knots catch in pulleys
		Add and remove weights slowly with physician's order	Slow, steady pull reduces muscle spasms
		Pin site care per agency policy	Reduce risk of infection
		Adjust the position of the bed	

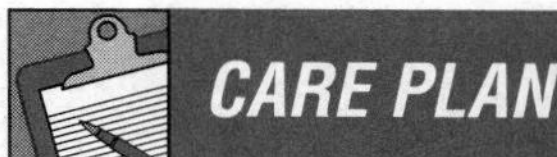

CARE PLAN

The Client in Skeletal Traction Continued

Nursing Diagnosis/ Collaborative Problem	Planning: Expected Outcomes	Implementation: Nursing Interventions	Rationales
Potential for compartment syndrome and neurovascular compromise	Nurse will monitor for symptoms and signs of compartment syndrome q shift	Monitor color, warmth, movement, and sensation of extremity distal to traction q shift Assess pedal (radial) pulse q shift Monitor reports of degree of pain and relief by analgesia	Signs and symptoms of compartment syndrome include pallor, pulselessness, cool extremities, inability to move, loss of or change in sensation, and pain that is not relieved with usual analgesia

prevention or correction of deformity; (3) maintenance, support, and protection to realign bone; and (4) promotion of healing, which allows early weight bearing for ambulation. The types of casts are described in Box 66-2, and shown in Figure 66-2.

Box 66-2. Types of Casts

Name of the Cast	Description
Short arm	Used to treat stable metacarpal, carpal, distal radius, or humerus fractures, or wrist sprains. Cast extends from the palm and thumb to mid-arm. May include a thumb spica for thumb fractures, or may be a hanging cast for humerus fractures.
Short leg	Used to treat fractures of the tibia, fibula, and ankle. Cast extends from the foot to below the knee. May be weight-bearing or non-weight-bearing.
Long leg	Used to treat unstable fractures of the femur, tibia, and/or fibula. Cast extends from foot to hip and holds the knee in flexion if fracture is unstable, to prevent weight-bearing. If weight-bearing is permitted, a cylinder cast is used.
Cast brace	Used to treat a stable distal femur fracture. Cast consists of two parts, above and below the knee, with a hinge at the knee to allow ROM.
Hip spica	Used to treat fractures of the hip and to immobilize the hip(s). Cast extends from mid-trunk to foot or feet, hips abducted with an abductor bar. Opening made in cast for elimination of urine and feces. Fairly uncommon today.

APPLYING A CAST

Cast Materials

Plaster of Paris (anhydrous calcium sulfate) is a chalky white powder made by removing water from gypsum. Plaster of Paris bandages are individual rolls of precut crinoline impregnated with plaster. They are available in various sizes. The body part to be casted determines the amount of plaster used; for example, a short leg walking cast uses four to five rolls, whereas a short wrist cast takes about two rolls.

Synthetic casting materials are made of fabric impregnated with high-density thermoplastic resin or fiber glass. These materials provide strong, lightweight casts that set in about 20 minutes. Unlike plaster of Paris, synthetic casts maintain their shape and firmness even if they become wet. However, if a synthetic cast becomes wet, it must be thoroughly dried to prevent skin maceration. If there is no incision under the cast, a synthetic cast can be dried with a cast dryer or hair blow dryer on a low setting.

Procedure

A cast may be applied in a physician's office, a clinic, an emergency room, or at a hospital bedside. In a hospital, the client is usually taken to an equipped cast room for cast application. Explain the procedure to the client and family. If a fracture is to be reduced before a cast is applied, the client is usually given an anesthetic. Cast application must be performed quickly. It is helpful to have a nurse present to concentrate on the client's needs. The procedure for skin preparation and casting is the same whatever body part is being casted and whether a plaster or synthetic cast is being applied. Skin preparation includes thoroughly cleaning the skin. Closely examine the skin while preparing it. Document lesions, unremovable dirt, and foreign particles.

After skin is prepared, it may be covered with stockinette or padding. Make sure these coverings fit

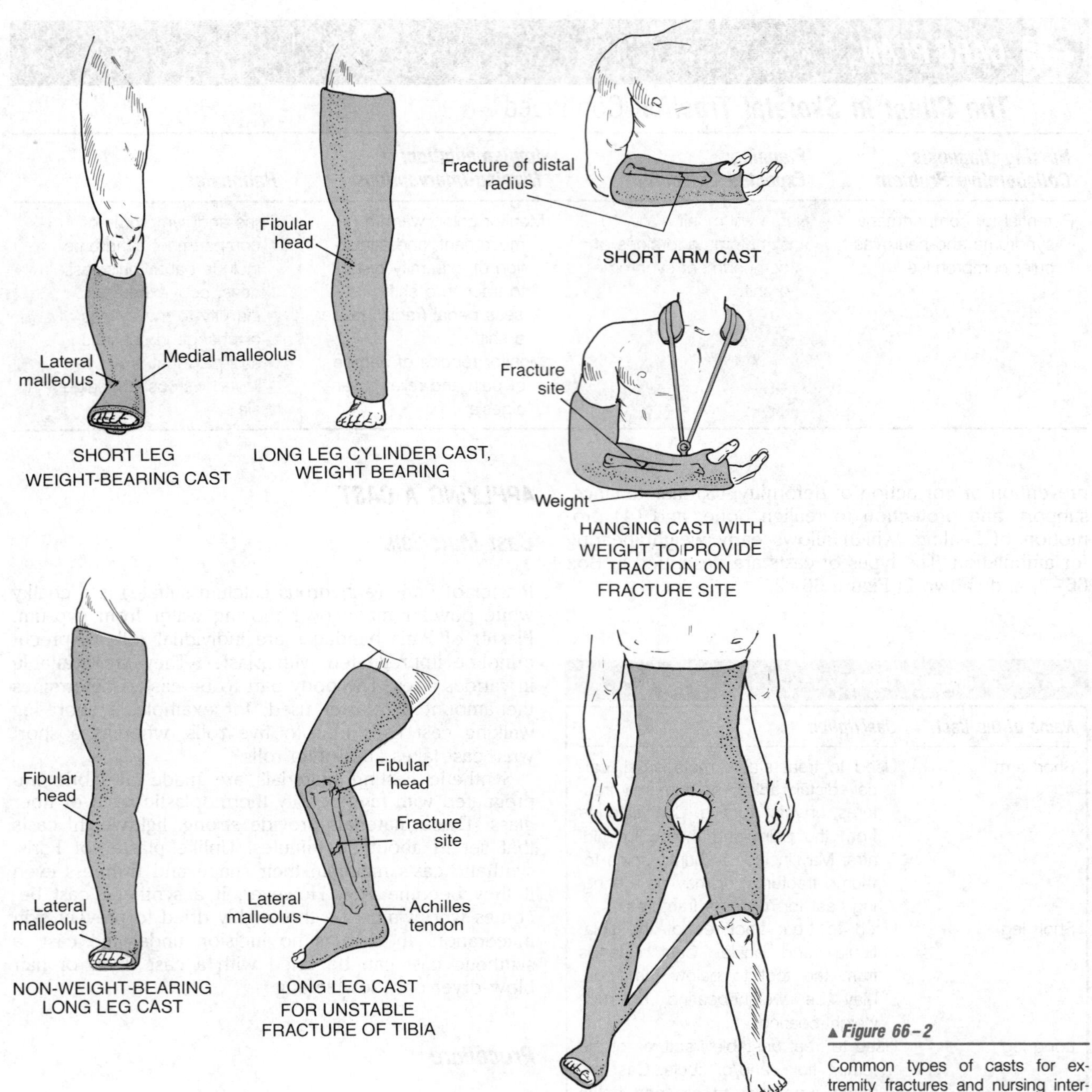

▲ *Figure 66-2*

Common types of casts for extremity fractures and nursing interventions.

smoothly, without wrinkles. Wrinkles or uneven surface can abrade skin and lead to skin breakdown. Stockinette is a soft knit material, available in rolls of various widths in a bias-cut (for circumferential wrapping) or tubular form without seams (to completely encircle a body part). Always cut tubular stockinette longer than the expected finished cast length, so that the excess portions can be pulled. Whether fiber glass or plaster of Paris is used, the area to be casted should be covered with a stockinette and then padding. When using the fiber glass material, the padding should be of a synthetic material. The padding may be applied more heavily over a bony prominence, but use caution because too much padding can cause pressure. When padding is applied, make sure it is smooth and even so that it does not become the cause of pressure sores.

Plaster-filled bandages are submerged in a bucket of clean water one at a time, the excess water is removed, and the bandage is applied to encircle the body part. Plaster bandages are applied wetter than are synthetic bandages. If a large plaster cast is being applied, the water in the cast bucket should be changed because sediment accumulates (see later). Use of clean dipping water speeds up cast setting.

During cast application, an assistant may support the extremity. Always support the extremity from underneath in the palms of the hands in such a way that pressure is not applied to any one area. Do not press finger tips into the cast or rest the cast on a hard or sharp surface. Doing so would cause flattening or indentations in the cast that could result in pressure problems.

Never empty plaster-laden water into an ordinary sink because plaster sediment will solidify and plug the plumbing. If a sink with a plaster trap is not available, wait for sediment to settle into the bottom of the plastic-lined bucket, then drain off the water from the top. Scrape the plaster sediment off the bottom of the pan and dispose of it into the garbage.

As soon as the casting procedure is complete, the client's skin is cleaned of excess casting material. An x-ray may be performed to verify correct bone alignment.

Drying Casts

Synthetic casts are dry to touch in a few minutes, but take about 20 minutes to set completely. Synthetic casts dry with a thermal reaction and may feel hot. Also, the surface is sticky and should be handled only while wearing gloves. Plaster casts set rapidly but take several hours to dry completely (large casts may take several days). The water from a newly applied cast (green cast) eventually evaporates, leaving a mature cast of full strength. Factors influencing the drying time of a plaster cast include (1) the amount of water to be evaporated from the cast; (2) the thickness of the cast, such as the number of layers of plaster bandages; and (3) the surrounding environment, such as humidity, temperature, and air circulation.

Promote the circulation of warm, dry air around a damp cast to enhance moisture evaporation and speed the drying process. Warn a person being casted that heat (both plaster of Paris and fiber glass generate heat) is created during the cast's early setting (hardening) stages. The sensation of heat under a cast can be frightening if it is not understood. Allow the heat generated in a newly applied cast to dissipate into circulating air. During the green period (while the cast is still damp), a casted person may feel cold and chill easily. Provide adequate covering while also allowing air to circulate around the cast. If the client has a large cast, avoid excessive chilling by covering some parts of the cast for a brief time and rotating the exposed portions.

Unless contraindicated, turn a person in a green cast periodically to expose more of the casted area to air. Occasionally, a cast dryer or a hair dryer may be used to facilitate drying. However, never place a dryer too close to a cast or focus it on one spot. Rapid drying can burn skin under a cast or crack the cast. Never use a dryer over a recently operated area without a physician's order because the heat can cause bleeding. A wet plaster of Paris cast is musty smelling, is dull on percussion, is gray in appearance, and feels cold to the touch. A dry plaster cast is odorless, is resonant when percussed, is white in appearance, and feels similar to the room temperature. Wet, or green, fiber glass casts appear a creamy color and feel hot to touch. The surface also is sticky. The surface should not be touched without gloves until the cast is "dry" (about 20 minutes). A fiber glass cast should be placed as you would a plaster cast. Do not place a fiber glass casted area over drainage containing pads, such as bluepads, because paper and plastics will adhere and become a permanent part of the cast.

Place new casts on plastic-protected pillows to protect them from pressure and flattening while drying. Once completely dry, a cast can be placed on a hard surface if the person wishes (e.g., a casted arm may rest on a table), but it is usually more comfortable to rest the casted area on pillows.

WINDOWING AND BIVALVING A CAST

Cutting windows in casts and bivalving casts are two techniques commonly used to relieve or prevent excessive pressure in casted body areas, or to provide access to or visualization of certain body parts. Windows may be cut (in dried casts) (1) to prevent uncomfortable abdominal distention (e.g., in a body cast or hip spica); (2) to assess a radial pulse (e.g., to check circulation in a casted arm); (3) to inspect areas of discomfort or areas of suspected tissue damage; and (4) to remove drains or care for wounds.

Bivalving a cast means splitting it along both sides (1) to allow tissue swelling, (2) so half of it can be removed to facilitate care and the taking of x-ray films, (3) so the cast can be removed and reapplied while a person is learning to adjust to being without a cast, or (4) to make a half-cast for use as an intermittent splint (e.g., to prevent deformities). Once a cast is bivalved, either half can be removed easily without disturbing alignment. When reapplying a bivalved cast, the client's extremity should be handled carefully with care not to pinch skin between the two cast halves. When both halves of the cast are properly fitted, secure them with a wrap.

COMPLICATIONS

Although casts are protective and therapeutic, they can also cause serious complications, such as swelling of the casted part, or vascular or nerve damage sustained during injury or treatment, such as from surgery, fracture reduction, or vascular emboli or thrombi. The cast, because it is inflexible and meant to restrict movement, can cause pressure and constriction of the casted limb. Complications can arise from impaired blood flow or innervation, which may head to paralysis, paresis or paraesthesia, or anesthesia. In extreme cases, amputation may be necessary. Careful assessment is essential

TABLE 66-1. Clinical Manifestations of Complications from Cast Use

1. Impaired blood flow producing soft tissue ischemia, e.g., due to pressure in casted extremity. Clinical manifestations may include
   - ▶ Pulselessness: slow nail bed capillary refill, as evidenced by refill greater than 3 seconds;
   - ▶ Skin pallor, blanching, cyanosis, or coolness;
   - ▶ Pain, swelling, painful edema peripheral to cast;
   - ▶ Paresthesias (tingling, prickling), heightened sensitivity, numbness; hypesthesia (diminished sensitivity to touch); anesthesia (numbness); and
   - ▶ Motor paralysis of previously functioning muscles
2. Nerve damage from pressure where a nerve passes over a bony prominence. Clinical manifestations may include
   - ▶ Increasing, persistent, localized pain;
   - ▶ Hypesthesia (diminished sensitivity); anesthesia (numbness); paresthesias (tingling, prickling, heightened sensitivity, numbness);
   - ▶ Feelings of deep pressure; and
   - ▶ Motor weakness or paralysis not previously present
3. Infection, tissue necrosis, e.g., due to skin breakdown. Clinical manifestations may include
   - ▶ Musty, unpleasant odor over cast and/or at ends of cast
   - ▶ Drainage through cast or cast opening
   - ▶ Sudden unexplained body temperature elevation
   - ▶ "Hot spot" felt on cast over lesion
4. Compartment syndrome, which compromises circulation, viability, and function of tissues within the compartment. Clinical manifestations may include
   - ▶ A dramatic increase in pain, that is no longer controlled by analgesia
   - ▶ Loss of movement
   - ▶ Loss of sensation
   - ▶ Pain with passive motion
   - ▶ Pulselessness
5. Cast syndrome occurs with body casts and may be fatal if untreated. Possible assessment findings include
   - ▶ Prolonged nausea; repeated vomiting
   - ▶ Abdominal distention; vague abdominal pain

to prevent serious complications. Clinical manifestations of complications are found in Table 66-1. These complications are discussed in Chapter 67, in the section on complications of fractures.

Nursing Management

ASSESSMENT

Thorough assessment and prompt intervention are essential to prevent cast-related complications. Establish an assessment pattern and always make observations sequentially. For example, in a casted extremity, assess (1) color, (2) movement of distal fingers or toes, (3) warmth, (4) sensation, (5) swelling, and (6) pulses distal to cast (abbreviated CMWS). Another helpful way of remembering some significant assessment findings with cast-related complications is the 6 Ps mnemonic: pain, pallor, paralysis, pulselessness, paresthesia, and poikilothermia (skin cold to the touch). Document and report any abnormalities.

Feel skin temperature in areas distal to the cast, such as the hand, foot, fingers, and toes. Compare skin temperature on a casted extremity with the opposite extremity. Arterial insufficiency causes abnormal coolness in exposed fingers and toes. Feel the surface of the cast by placing the palm of your hand on the cast and moving it over the cast's entire surface. "Hot spots" (areas that feel warmer than other areas) may indicate tissue necrosis or infection under the cast. "Wet spots" may indicate a need for drying or drainage beneath the cast.

When assessing peripheral pulses, compare casted and uncasted limbs. Peripheral pulses are absent with impaired arterial blood flow. Assess the radial pulse at the wrist of a casted arm and the dorsalis pedis pulse on the dorsum of the foot of a casted leg. Occasionally, the client's cast covers the dorsum of the foot and pulses cannot be palpated. In this situation, the nurse must rely on other assessment parameters.

Assess a person's awareness of pinpricks and light touch in areas distal to a cast. Hypesthesia or anesthesia indicates serious damage to a limb. Assess for indications of peroneal nerve damage in a casted leg and median, ulnar, or radial nerve damage in a casted arm (see Box 66-3 and Fig. 66-3). When assessing for sensory losses, review the client's history to determine whether such losses were present before cast application.

Assess skin color distal to the cast. Look for indications of circulatory impairment, such as pallor, blanch-

Box 66-3. Nursing Assessment of Lower Extremity Nerve Function

Deep Peroneal Nerve

- ▶ Runs through anterior compartment of lower leg.
- ▶ Innervates toe extensors.
- ▶ Supplies sensation to web between first and second toes.

Superficial Peroneal Nerve

- ▶ Runs through lateral compartment of leg.
- ▶ Autonomous zone at base of third, fourth, and fifth toes.
- ▶ Supplies sensation to dorsolateral aspect of foot.

Tibial Nerve

- ▶ Runs through posterior compartment of leg.
- ▶ Supplies sensation to base of toes and sole of foot.

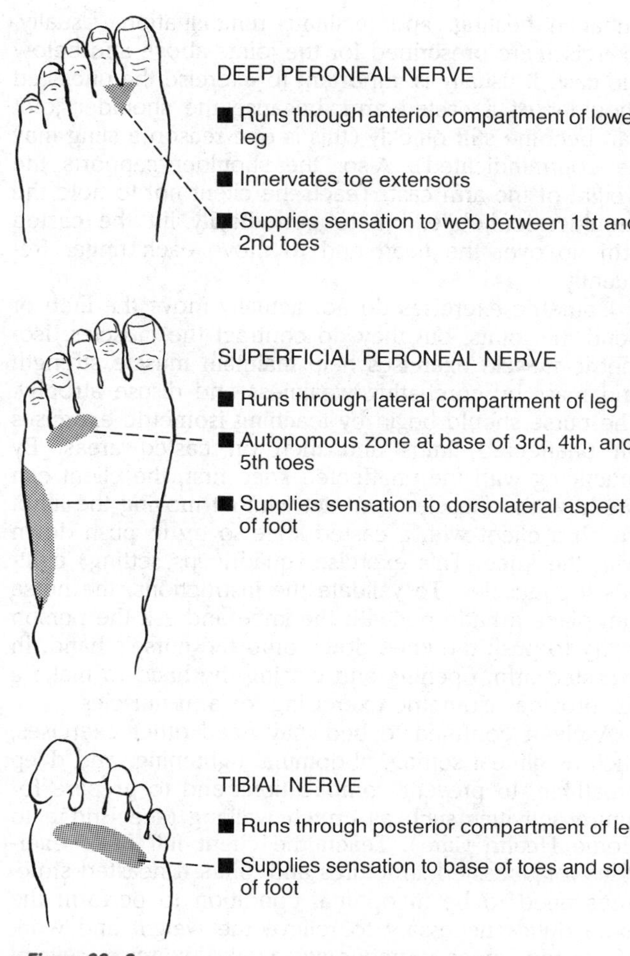
DEEP PERONEAL NERVE
■ Runs through anterior compartment of lower leg
■ Innervates toe extensors
■ Supplies sensation to web between 1st and 2nd toes
SUPERFICIAL PERONEAL NERVE
■ Runs through lateral compartment of leg
■ Autonomous zone at base of 3rd, 4th, and 5th toes
■ Supplies sensation to dorsolateral aspect of foot
TIBIAL NERVE
■ Runs through posterior compartment of leg
■ Supplies sensation to base of toes and sole of foot

▲ ***Figure 66-3***

Nursing assessment of lower extremity nerve function.

ing, and cyanosis. Cyanosis results from impaired venous return, such as that due to soft tissue constriction. Cyanosis may be a late indication of impaired circulation. Pallor or blanching may indicate arterial insufficiency.

A blanching test assesses circulation by observing nailbed capillary refill time. Compare capillary refill time in the casted limb with that on the unaffected side. However, this is not a conclusive test since nailbed capillary refill can remain fairly normal even though a limb is pulseless.

Ask the client to move fingers or toes on the casted limb. Movement should be easy and painless, unless the person's injury restricts motion. Motion paralysis of fingers or toes may be due to primary nerve damage, or the person may be unable to move because of pain. Painful motion usually indicates excessive swelling. A person can wiggle the toes by active flexion, and they will return to neutral position by passive recoil. This indicates complete loss of extensor power. Document these findings and notify the physician. Moving the fingers or toes (even very gently) of an ischemic limb is extremely painful. Motor paralysis is a late symptom of ischemia.

Assess skin around cast edges for skin damage or swelling. Injury to an extremity and subsequent treatment (e.g., reduction, surgery) usually produce swelling, which progresses for the first 12 to 24 hours after injury or surgery. Swelling may be the greatest for the first 24 to 48 hours. Although mild swelling of exposed fingers and toes is not unusual, moderate or severe swelling associated with pain and discoloration is abnormal. When a casted part swells markedly, structures within the cast are constricted and severe complications result. Swelling may obstruct blood flow.

Assess the cast surface for indications of wound drainage (stains) or bleeding. Closely inspect areas of the cast that cover wounds (e.g., surgical incisions or accidental wounds) and all pressure points (for indications of damage to underlying skin). When an area of drainage or bleeding becomes visible, document the time, date its appearance, and describe the observation. Drainage on the surface of fiber glass casts may not appear at the area of the wound or incision. Because of the make up of the cast, the drainage may not wick outward but may wick to the dependent area if the cast is flat, or the drainage may be found posterior and superior if the limb is elevated. The drainage may even seep out of the cast at the posterior and superior aspect of the elevated cast or the distal end of a dependent cast. Continued assessment is, of course, necessary.

Smell for odors indicative of tissue necrosis and infection. A cast often develops a sour smell after being worn a while, from perspiration and normal sloughing of outer skin layers. However, pathologic tissue necrosis emits an easily detectable, musty, strong, offensive odor. If the odor of mildew is present, especially with a fiber glass cast, the cast may have become wet at one time and not thoroughly dried. If this event has occurred, the physician should be notified and the cast will probably be removed.

INTERVENTION

Intervention to prevent or relieve excessive swelling typically includes (1) full-length elevation of the cast higher than the person's heart, (2) exercising the fingers or toes to stimulate circulation, and (3) placing ice bags around the cast. Pressure caused by swelling must be relieved by cutting the cast before irreversible damage occurs. Pressure (without swelling) by the edge of a cast against skin may be relieved by a position change or loosely padding the uncomfortable area.

Positioning. Because a cast is heavy and inflexible, a client wearing a cast can easily lose his or her balance and fall. Safety straps should be used to secure a casted client being transported and to assist with transfer procedures, such as to a cart. Safety straps may be required to make sure that a green cast is handled properly. Footdrop may develop in a casted leg. The foot should be splinted or supported at a 90-degree flexion in the ankle. Protect the toes of a casted foot from the pressure of bedclothing; stockings may provide warmth.

A casted extremity should be elevated to minimize swelling and promote drainage. This procedure is especially important for the first 24 to 48 hours. Elevating a casted part stimulates circulation and reduces swelling (and thus pressure within the cast). Elevate casted extremities on rubber or plastic-protected pillows. A casted arm may be placed in a sling or arm immobilizer when the person is ambulatory. Support the entire arm, including the elbow, wrist, and hand (wristdrop leads to neurovascular complications), and keep the fingers higher than the elbow (to minimize swelling). If a sling or immobilization is not used, the person should be encouraged to exercise the uncasted joints such as the shoulder or elbow to prevent complications of disuse. Use a pillow to elevate the arm while sitting if this position is more comfortable.

Expose the buttocks of a person in a hip spica or body cast to prevent soiled or damp clothing during urination and to provide adequate skin care. Position the client carefully and comfortably on a fracture bedpan designed for use by clients wearing body casts or hip spica casts. Slightly raise the head of the bed to facilitate elimination and to prevent body excrement from running up under the cast. Raising head and shoulders slightly to use a bedpan is usually allowed unless the client is in shock, is hemorrhaging, or has a spinal injury. Damp, soiled casts become odorous and may mold or break. Dampness also causes skin irritation and may increase the risk of infection if an open wound is present.

Frequent position changes are essential to prevent complications of immobility. A client with a cast often needs help to turn in bed. If possible, give the client turning instructions and encourage practice before the cast is applied. The nurse should always have adequate help to move and position a casted person; that is, to turn a person with a heavy cast, at least one other staff member should help the nurse and one person should always be on each side of the bed. Three or four people may be needed to turn a person in a body or hip spica cast. Wet casts are particularly heavy. Good body mechanics should be used to prevent injury to the client or the nurse.

People in casts can often bear weight as soon as the cast is dry. Synthetic casts can be walked on immediately after application. Plaster casts require 36 to 48 hours before bearing weight. Weak, aged, and debilitated clients often find the weight of a cast difficult to deal with and may tire rapidly when ambulating for the first few times. Observe them closely to prevent excessive fatigue and accidents. Pain may be experienced the first few times that a casted leg is lowered to a dependent position. Prepare the client for this pain. Explain that pain is not unusual and that it occurs as blood rushes into the leg. Initially, the nurse can assist the client to lower the leg for brief periods and gradually lengthen the time of dependence. Once the client's leg becomes accustomed to the increased blood, pain subsides.

Exercises. The nurse should instruct the client in exercises to stimulate circulation, increase venous return, enhance healing, and facilitate rehabilitation. Usually, exercises are prescribed for the joints above and below the cast. It usually is important to exercise the uncasted shoulder of a casted arm, because the shoulder joint can become stiff quickly (this is one reason a sling may be contraindicated). Also, the shoulder supports the weight of the arm cast. Teach the client not to hold the shoulder immobile, but to periodically lift the casted arm up over the head and to move each finger frequently.

Isometric exercises do not actually move the limb or bend the joints, but they do contract the muscles. Isometric muscle exercises help maintain muscle strength and mass by combating weakness and disuse atrophy. The nurse should begin by teaching isometric exercises on unaffected limbs and then on casted areas. By practicing with the unaffected knee first, the client can see how the muscles contract without moving the limb. Teach a client with a casted knee to try to push down with the knee. This exercise (quadriceps setting) tightens leg muscles. To validate the instructions, the nurse can place a hand beneath the knee and ask the person to try to push the knee down onto the nurse's hand. In a casted arm, opening and closing the hand to make a fist provides isometric exercising for arm muscles.

A client confined to bed may need other exercises, such as gluteal setting, abdominal tightening, and deep breathing, to prevent complications and to prepare for future activities such as crutch walking (see Bridge to Home Health Care). Teach the client full ROM exercises for uncasted structures and joints. Uncasted structures need to be in optimal condition to perform the extra duties necessary to relieve the weight and work of casted areas. Encourage active exercise several times a day. Self-care activity provides significant indirect exercise.

Nutrition. Increased dietary fiber helps people with reduced mobility maintain normal bowel elimination. A person in a body cast or hip spica cast may need to avoid gas-forming foods to prevent abdominal distention. A general, well-balanced diet promotes wound healing.

DISCHARGE TEACHING

The nurse should teach the client and significant others about skin care and how to prevent skin damage, as discussed later. Skin care includes assessing the client's skin condition, washing and drying the skin, applying emollient lotions, and turning frequently. Skin areas subjected to irritation or pressure can rapidly develop into pressure sores. All exposed skin areas and all pressure areas, that is, the back of the head, ears, elbows, iliac crests, sacrum, and heels, should be inspected frequently, especially around the edges of the cast. Look for friction rubs, swelling, irritation, or discoloration, such as redness, blanching, cyanosis. Notify the physician of any indications of skin problems including irritation or pressure.

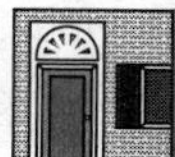

BRIDGE TO HOME HEALTH CARE

Clients with Casts and Braces

Bridging hospital to home care for persons with casts and braces involves teaching, monitoring, case management, ingenuity, and encouragement. A client with a brace or ankle-foot orthosis needs to know who to contact if the fit of the device changes. In extremity braces, all straps should be comfortably tight without leaving marks on the skin. With leg braces, the bars parallel the shape of the leg but generally do not touch the leg. If a short leg brace has a T-strap on the lateral side of the shoe, it goes against the ankle and the cinch strap goes around the medial upright. This prevents ankle inversion. Any strap that is too tight can cause swelling distal to that strap. Sometimes a washcloth under a strap can provide needed padding. Use a magic marker to label "top front" of a body jacket or Jewett brace. A rolled washcloth can also be used to relieve a pressure area in a body jacket.

A cast should not be too tight nor too loose. Watch fingers or toes for discoloration or swelling. These digits should be wiggled as much as possible to help maintain circulation. Initially, keep the casted extremity elevated on pillows, rolled blankets, or even balloons. If swelling is severe, the extremity may need to be suspended from a vertical pole such as an IV pole or coat rack. An elastic wrap, strips of a sheet, or a towel can be used to keep the extremity in place.

To relieve discomfort caused by a cast, a doubled ziplock bag of ice, or even a jar of ice, can be placed on or next to the cast. Never insert anything under a cast because of the potential to injure skin or damage the padding. Itching can sometimes be relieved by dribbling alcohol down the skin inside the cast.

A cast will create inconvenience and frustration with usual personal hygiene routines. Wrap the cast in a plastic bag and secure all open edges with tape in order to keep the cast dry during a bath or shower. A commercial shower chair or a lawn chair can also be used. Care should be taken that the tub surface is not scratched, as that can lead to rusting. Be sure to provide a nonslip surface. If only a tub is available, water can be poured over the client with a pan or pitcher. A foot stool may be necessary to prop up a casted leg while using the toilet.

Persons with casts and braces face challenges with dressing. Reacher sticks or other assistive devices may be needed. For relatively short-term needs, seams of some garments may need to be opened, cuts made, and larger sizes borrowed or purchased from a thrift store. If there is to be long-term brace use, zippers can be placed in the inner seams of pant legs to allow braces to be worn under clothing or even just to facilitate easier dressing. Consulting with a physical or occupational therapist who could provide further suggestions may be of benefit.

Never insert any object beneath a cast or scratch the skin under a cast. Notify the physician if an object is caught beneath a cast. Often, itching under a cast is extremely uncomfortable (especially in hot weather), and the client is tempted to slip some object under the cast to scratch. Explain that this practice is dangerous and should not be done because (1) skin may be broken and infection may develop; (2) scratching wrinkles the padded surface under the cast and this may cause skin breakdown; and (3) the scratcher object may become caught under the cast and cause pressure and skin breakdown. Also, tell the client not to pull stockinette or padding out from under the cast. Explain that these materials are there to protect the skin. Itching beneath the cast can be reduced by blowing cool air or sprinkling powder into the cast. Powder cannot be used when open wounds are present.

While giving skin care, inspect the condition of the cast and check its fit. Excessively loose casts usually need replacing. Sometimes casts are somewhat loose in the morning but fit more securely later in the day, such as after a casted leg has been dependent during ambulation. Notify the physician of deteriorated, cracked, molded, soft, or broken cast areas or loose bracing bars. The physician may reinforce weakened or soiled cast areas.

Follow-up Care

Cast changes are often necessary when a cast no longer fits because of weight changes or muscle atrophy. Sometimes, cast changes are necessary for additional treatment or so the area can be inspected. During cast changes, assess and care for the client's skin.

Cast Removal. The length of time a client wears a cast varies with the type and extent of injury, disease, or surgery and the rate of healing. A cast is usually removed with an electric cast cutter, which resembles a small electric saw with a circular blade. Because of its appearance and noise, a cast cutter is often frightening. Show the client the cast cutter before using it and explain that it cannot cut skin because the blade does not whirl around and cut like a saw. Rather, it breaks the cast by oscillating or vibrating rapidly back and forth sideways. When a cast cutter is used, the client may feel sensations of heat, vibrations, or pressure. Very rarely, a client suffers a burn from the cast cutter blades. A cast spreader may also be used to spread open a cut cast so that underlying padding material can be cut. Equipment used to remove casts is shown in Figure 66-4.

Skin under a casted area often becomes very sensitive and is mottled and covered with yellow-brown scales or crusts of dead skin, oil, and exudate. Muscles under a cast may appear atrophied, and the extremity feels stiff and weak from inactivity. New aches and pains may appear with movement following cast removal, and muscles and tissues are subjected to new stresses and strains. The client's balance is altered, because removing a cast removes weight. The client needs to be prepared.

Gentle soaking and washing for a few days after a cast is removed returns skin to its normal appearance. Many clients want to vigorously scrub the skin, but this

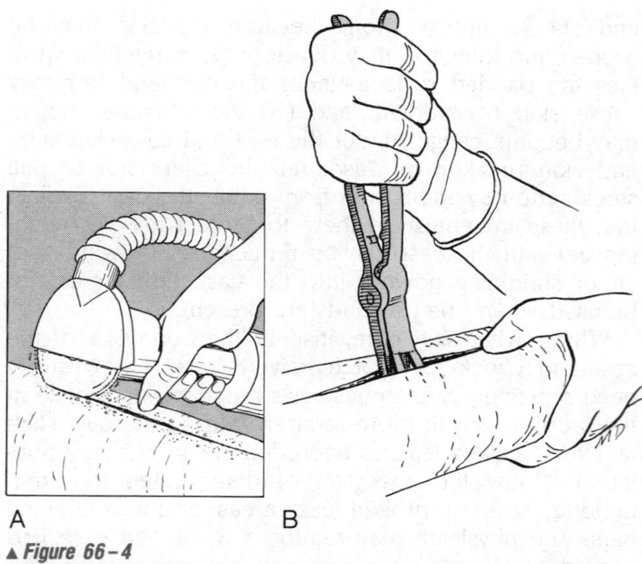

▲ *Figure 66-4*

A, A cast saw ("cast cutter") with its oscillating blade "vibrates" plaster and synthetic cast material apart with precision speed. The vibrating motion prevents the client's skin from being cut. *B*, A cast spreader is a useful tool in aiding cast removal. It is used to open a cast so padding material can be cut.

often causes irritation. After a gentle washing, dry the skin and lubricate it with cocoa butter, lanolin, or another emollient to promote softening. Because newly uncasted skin is sensitive and can burn easily, advise the person to prevent overexposure to the sun.

Following cast removal, swelling may develop for a while when the involved limb is dependent. Elevate the limb when sitting or lying down. Swelling decreases with increased activity and improved muscle tone and circulation. Sometimes the physician recommends elastic bandages or stockings during ambulation to minimize swelling. Encourage ambulation because intermittent weight bearing acts as an effective venous pump.

Rehabilitation. Rehabilitation instructions are given by the physician according to the client's condition. A physical therapist often participates in rehabilitative care following cast removal. For example, a physical therapist may teach and supervise graded active exercises (to stimulate circulation and increase muscle strength) and joint ROM, and perform other prescribed activities such as whirlpool baths to force joints and muscles during recovery (by passive stretching exercises, resistive exercises, or forced movements). Placing excessive demands on stiff, weakened limbs may further impair motion by increasing fibrosis and excessively engorging the area with blood.

External Fixation

An external fixator may be used as an alternative to either a cast or traction. Some common external fixators are the Hoffmann, Anderson, Haynes, or Struder devices. External fixators can be used on arms, legs, and occasionally, fingers or the pelvis. These devices are made of aluminum, titanium, or nylon. An external fixator is a device consisting of pins that are placed in bone and attached to a rigid external frame. The open pin sites and wound need ongoing assessment and wound care. Usually, the client is ambulatory with a non-weight-bearing gait.

▼ MUSCULOSKELETAL SURGERY

Musculoskeletal Surgical Procedures

Musculoskeletal procedures may reconstruct, replace, or remove diseased or injured structures or correct deformities. They may be performed on bone (e.g., bone grafting, osteotomy, total hip and knee replacements, arthrodesis) or soft tissues (e.g., tendon transfer, lateral release, tenotomy, and rotator cuff repair). Common musculoskeletal surgical procedures include arthroscopy, arthroplasty, arthrodesis, osteotomy, tenotomy, and bone grafting.

ARTHROSCOPY

Arthroscopy (see Chap. 65) is used for two purposes, diagnosis and treatment.

Diagnosis is the main purpose. Athroscopy is also the surgery type of choice for

- Excising tears of the meniscus,
- Removing foreign bodies and adhesions,
- Biopsy of synovial disorder or partial synovectomy, and
- Patellar shavings (smoothing knee cartilage) due to arthritis or chondromalacia.

Clients undergoing arthroscopy usually have the procedure performed on an outpatient basis. The wounds are usually covered by an elastic bandage. The bandage may be removed within 3 days, and the client returns to normal activity within 3 weeks. Home instructions to the client should include signs and symptoms of infection.

ARTHROPLASTY

Arthroplasty is used to reestablish movement of diseased or painful joints. Common arthroplasties are total hip, knee, shoulder, elbow replacements, or wrist replacements. (See Chap. 26).

ARTHRODESIS

Arthrodesis produces artificial ankylosis or fusion that leaves a joint permanently immobile, repairing a joint by fusing joint surfaces. Advancements in total joint replacements (hip, knee, shoulder, elbow) have made this procedure uncommon. Arthrodesis is a procedure that is used as a last resort.

OSTEOTOMY

Osteotomy is a surgical procedure used to realign the bone by removing a wedge from it. The most common disorders behind osteotomies are varus and valgus deformities of the knee due to osteoarthritis. Varus deformities refer to alateral angulation, and valgus refers to a medial deformity. The tibia or femur is wedged so as to realign the knee. The purpose of the surgery is to maintain joint function but also to stabilize the joint and relieve pain. Usually, the client is in the hospital for 3 to 5 days for pain management and gait training.

TENOTOMY

Tenotomy, cutting a tendon, is often used to release contracture related to spasticity such as that which occurs with cerebrovascular accident (CVA) or cerebral palsy.

BONE GRAFTING

Bone grafting is transplanting pieces of cancellous or compact bone to new locations. Grafts may be (1) autogenous (obtained from the person having the transplant), (2) homogeneous (obtained from another human being), or (3) heterogeneous (obtained from an animal or synthetic material).

Nursing Management

PREOPERATIVE MANAGEMENT

Musculoskeletal surgical procedures are often elective, allowing time to prepare clients physically and psychosocially. Provision of preoperative and postoperative physical and psychosocial support is essential. Before musculoskeletal surgery, some clients have had long, tiring, and painful periods of illness, such as in clients requiring joint replacement for arthritis. They often have mixed feelings of hope and dread. They hope surgery will reduce pain and increase mobility, but they also fear that it will increase their suffering and disability.

Preoperative intervention to prevent possible postoperative infection is essential. Bone is more susceptible to infection than soft tissue. Bone infection (osteomyelitis) is difficult to treat and can lead to permanent disability, such as chronic infection or joint stiffness. Bone union will not occur if infection is present. Specific skin preparation for musculoskeletal surgery varies, but the underlying principles are the same. Skin preparation is performed meticulously in a nontraumatic manner. In surgery, open traumatic wounds such as compound fractures are cleaned carefully, because they may be contaminated. Preparation is performed under aseptic conditions and usually by the surgeon.

POSTOPERATIVE MANAGEMENT

Prolonged immobilization is usually necessary for bone healing. As with any type of surgery, postoperative intervention focuses on preventing complications from (1) the surgical procedure, (2) a presurgical pathologic process, and (3) the necessary immobilization. Careful assessment and prompt intervention are essential. Possible postoperative complications include shock (see Chap. 20), thrombophlebitis (see Chap. 44), pulmonary embolism (see Chap. 39), and fat embolism (see Chap. 68), and compartment syndrome (see Chap. 67).

General care includes assessment of dressings and drainage. Check dressings frequently and document drainage. Using aseptic technique, reinforce saturated dressings to minimize the introduction of infection by capillary action. Document casts stained from blood seepage or serous or purulent drainage, including the dimensions of stained areas, such as "a circle of bloody drainage about 1 inch in diameter." Compare measurements with previous measurements to assess whether or not drainage has stabilized or is increasing. Report unusual drainage.

Position, turn, and exercise the client postoperatively according to physician's instructions. Frequently, assess the person's posture and position to ensure that healing is occurring in correct alignment and to prevent other complications. Operated extremities are usually elevated postoperatively to prevent or minimize swelling. Support limbs along their entire length (e.g., do not place a pillow just under the heel or knee).

Following surgery, clients with joint disease should use movement to prevent the joints from becoming stiff and immobile. Early ambulation is desirable but sometimes cannot be started until adequate bone healing has occurred. Soft tissues heal more quickly than does bone. Thus, while a skin incision may be healed, the underlying bone may not be. Convalescence may be prolonged after bone injury or bone surgery, especially when weight-bearing structures are involved. Follow physician's instructions about whether weight may be placed on an affected limb while the client is standing or walking. The nurse should have adequate help when assisting a person to move or get out of bed. The person probably fears falling or being injured.

Postoperative rehabilitation may include occupational therapy, prosthetics, bracing, and physical therapy (e.g., gait training, muscle reeducation, exercise, heat application, massage). It is important to keep the person mobilized and participating in safe self-care activities.

After discharge from a health care facility, contact continues with the physician and other health care professionals, as necessary. Community health nurses may make home visits. Before discharge, learning/teaching sessions are essential to make the client and family aware of indicated and contraindicated activities. They also need information about indications of complications.

POSTOPERATIVE REHABILITATION

Therapeutic exercises have many benefits, including maintaining or restoring adequate joint activity, preventing muscular atrophy and other deformities, building or maintaining muscular bulk and strength, maintaining or improving joint ROM, building endurance, and stimulating circulation. Exercises include (1) active or passive joint ROM exercises to preserve joint motion; (2) quadriceps setting exercises to stabilize the knees; (3) gluteal and abdominal muscle tightening to improve trunk stability; (4) lifting exercises to increase biceps strength.

Exercises such as resistive, isometric, and ROM can be performed with the client on bed rest. The client can be instructed on how to do the appropriate exercises. A sign demonstrating the appropriate exercise or list of exercises can be posted at the bedside and the client instructed on the frequency for each exercise. By posting the exercises, the client can take an active part in the plan of care. When the care plan includes exercise, the physical therapist also becomes involved. Physical therapy has as its goals (1) maintaining or improving joint ROM, dexterity, and strength; (2) reducing or relieving pain and swelling; (3) relieving muscle spasms; (4) preventing complications associated with inactivity; and (5) teaching self-care and ambulation techniques.

Physical therapy and nursing work as a team. Often, the physical therapist sees the client once or twice a day to teach exercises or gait training. The nurse, in turn, takes on the responsibility to reinforce these instructions. A care plan can be written with input from the physical therapist or to compliment a program set up by the physical therapist for the client.

▼ ASSISTIVE DEVICES

CRUTCHES

Two important points about crutch fitting and crutch use are

- *Crutches must be of correct length.* If they are too long, they cause excessive pressure and rubbing in the axilla. Excessive axillary pressure can cause nerve damage (to branches of the brachial plexus) and arm paralysis (crutch palsy or crutch paralysis). Arm paralysis may be evidenced by numbness or wrist drop. If the client is unable to make a fist, he or she may be experiencing wristdrop. Crutches that are too short can slip, and the person may fall.
- *People using crutches are prone to accidents.* Never walk on crutches in stocking feet, slippers, or high-heeled shoes. Prevent accidents by (1) teaching people proper crutchwalking (Client Education Guide), (2) pointing out possible hazards, and (3) teaching environmental safety consciousness, such as keeping floors litter free and dry and opening doors carefully.

CANES

The cane needs to be long enough for the person to extend the elbow and bear weight on the hand grasping the cane. For safety, a cane needs a soft, pure rubber suction tip and a curved handle with a comfortable hand grip.

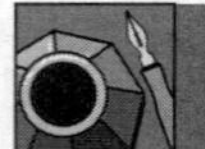

CLIENT EDUCATION GUIDE

Crutch Walking, Gaits

Gaits	
Two Point	Some weight-bearing is permitted bilaterally. The right leg and left crutch move simultaneously, then the left leg and right crutch simultaneously.
Three Point	No weight-bearing or partial weight should be allowed on the affected leg. Both crutches and the affected leg move in unison, while the body weight is supported on the unaffected leg. (The affected leg may be used for balance if partial weight is allowed).
Four Point	Weight-bearing is permitted on both legs. Crutches and feet are moved alternately. Left crutch, right foot, right crutch, left foot.
Swing Through	No weight-bearing should be allowed on the affected legs. Both crutches move forward, and both legs swing through between the crutches, while the weight is borne by the crutches.
Stairs	*Up*—lead with the unaffected leg; the crutches and affected leg move together. *Down*—The crutches and the affected leg lead.
Walkers	Lift the walker and place it ahead, walk up to the walker. Do not slide the walker. Do not use the walker as a base to come to standing.
Cane	The cane is used on the side opposite of the affected leg. The cane and affected leg move in unison, while weight is borne on the unaffected leg.

WALKERS

Walkers of different kinds are available. Some people find it helpful to use walkers before trying crutches. Walkers provide better support and stability than crutches (Fig. 66-5). Walkers are useful for the older client and clients who have trouble with balance. The walker should be adjusted so the elbow is slightly bent (30 degrees or less). Exercises to prepare for using a walker include resistance exercises to strengthen triceps muscles (may be performed in bed). Some walkers have underarm supports similar to those used on crutches.

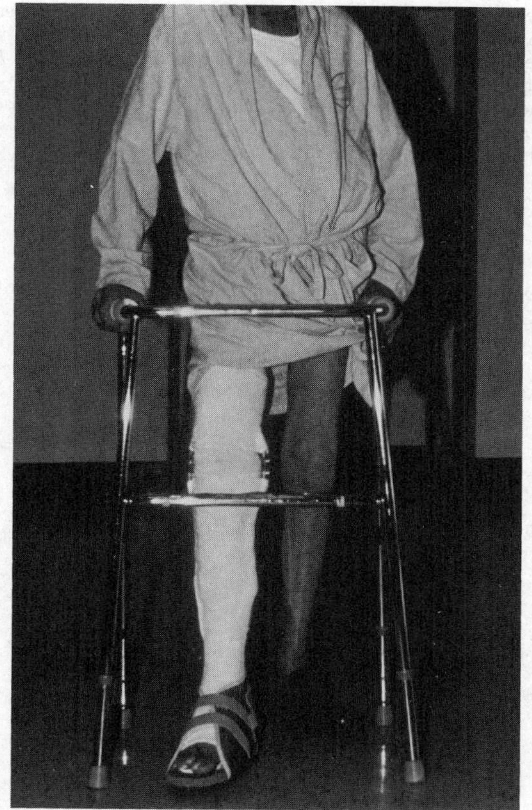

▲ **Figure 66-5**

Older individuals often feel secure ambulating with the aid of a walker. They sometimes have difficulty maneuvering two crutches and find a walker is secure and helps in getting up out of a chair.

SUPPORTS

Various supports such as braces or straps may be part of the treatment for musculoskeletal disorders. Braces and supports can be used to the back, neck and any joint of the arms and legs. Braces and supports are a common sight in the treatment of musculoskeletal complications, in which the goal is support yet early mobility. Braces or supports to joints are often hinged and can be adjusted to allow controlled ROM during the healing process. An orthotist or occupational therapist makes individualized heavy-duty braces that require precise fitting. Often, a person's appearance and body image are altered by a brace. This factor may be difficult to adjust to.

Supports need careful fitting, application, and maintenance. Teach the client and family to assess the skin frequently for indications of skin damage. Use a mirror to examine areas that cannot otherwise be seen. If a person has impaired sensation, visual skin inspection is even more important. In a health care facility, nurses may initially assess the client's skin. Adjustments may be needed to fit the appliance properly.

Teach the client and family how the support works and the reasons for wearing it. Informed and involved clients are more likely to comply with treatment. If used incorrectly, supports may be detrimental to the client's condition. If supports do not fit comfortably and correctly, clients may become discouraged and not wear them, and the condition may worsen.

Summary

Orthopedic interventions are some of the oldest medical treatments. Despite their longevity, they are not without risk. The client in traction must be assessed for correct anatomic bone alignment and the complications of immobility. Clients in casts are usually discharged, so the main focus of nursing is education for self-care. Following orthopedic surgery, the client is observed for common postoperative complications and is rehabilitated with walkers, crutches, cane, or braces for ambulation and support.

Bibliography

1. Amadio, P., Jr., & Cummings, D. M. (1986). Nonsteroidal antiinflammatory agents: An update. *American Family Physician, 34*(10), 147.
2. Berg, E. E. (1990). Progress in orthopaedic surgery: The 1980's in review. *Orthopaedic Nursing, 9*(5), 29-31.
3. Bevy, J. (1986). The adolescent in a spica cast. *Orthopaedic Nursing, 5*(3), 22-23.
4. Browner, C. M., et al. (1987). Haloimmobilization brace care; an innovative approach. *Journal of Neuroscience Nursing, 19*(1), 24-29.
5. Christopher, M. A. (1986, July). Home care for the elderly: In three-part harmony. *Nursing 86, 16,* 50.
6. Consensus Conference (1986, August). Prevention of venous thrombosis and pulmonary embolism. *Journal of the American Medical Association, 256,* 744.
7. Dutka, M. (1986). Elbow and wrist arthroscopy: Perioperative nursing care. *Orthopaedic Nursing, 5*(4), 29-34.
8. Evaris, McCollister, C. (1990). *Surgery of the musculoskeletal system* (2nd ed., Vol. 3). Churchill Livingstone.
9. Foster, C. (1986, July). Central circulatory adaptations to exercise training in health and disease. *Clinics in Sports Medicine, 5,* 589.
10. Frontera, W. R., & Adams, R. P. (1986). Endurance exercise: Normal physiology and limitations imposed by pathological processes. *Physician and Sports Medicine, 14*(8), 94.
11. Funk, J. R., et al. (1990). Tibial osteotomy. *Orthopaedic Nursing, 9*(2), 29-34.
12. Griffin, M. (1986). In the mind's eye. *American Journal of Nursing, 86*(7), 804.
13. Krupp, M. A., et al. (1985). *Current medical diagnosis and treatment.* Los Altos, CA: Lange Medical.
14. Lane, P. L. (1990). Crutchwalking. *Orthopaedic Nursing, 9*(5), 31-37.
15. Lorig, K. (1985, July). Osteoporosis. *Healthline, 4,* 9.
16. MacArthur, B. J. (1986). Arthroscopy of the shoulder. *Orthopaedic Nursing, 5*(4), 26-28.
17. Meloche, A. T. (1987). Disorders of the knee: Genu valgum and chondromalacia patellae. *Orthopaedic Nursing, 6*(3), 41-45.
18. Morris, L., et al. (1988). Nursing the patient in traction. *RN, 51*(1), 26-31.
19. Morris, L, et al. (1988). Special care for skeletal traction. *RN, 51*(2), 24-29.
20. Muhlenkamp, A., & Joyner, J. (1986). Arthritis patients' self-reported affective states and their caregivers' perceptions. *Nursing Research, 35*(1), 24.
21. Newschwander, D. E., et al. (1989). Limb lengthening and the Ilizarov external fixator. *Orthopaedic Nursing, 8*(3), 15-21.

22. Olson, B. (1990). Self-care needs of patients in the halo brace. *Orthopaedic Nursing, 9*(1), 27–33.
23. Osbourne, L. J., et al. (1987). Traction: A review with nursing diagnosis and interventions. *Orthopaedic Nursing, 6*(4), 14–18.
24. Pellins, T. A., et al. (1986). *NAON core curriculum for orthopaedic nursing* (1st ed.). Pitman, NJ: Anthony J. Jannetti.
25. Peters, V. J., et al. (1989). Arthroscopy surgery of the ankle. *Orthopaedic Nursing, 8*(5), 12–18.
26. Shepard, R. J. (1986, July). Physical training for the elderly. *Clinics in Sports Medicine, 5,* 515.
27. Stevenson, C. K. (1985, June). Take no chances with fat embolism. *Nursing 85, 15,* 58.
28. Steywood Jones, I. (1990). Making sense of . . . traction. *Nursing Times, 86*(23), 39–41.
29. Tucker, L. E. (1985, July). Back pain due to visceral disease. *Hospital Medicine, 21,* 125.
30. Zimmer (1980). *The traction handbook.* Warsaw, IN.

Chapter

67

Nursing Care of Clients with Musculoskeletal Disorders

METABOLIC BONE DISEASE

Metabolic bone disease may result from an inappropriate function of the parathyroid gland, vitamin deficiency, estrogen deficiency, and malabsorption syndrome. Osteoporosis, osteomalacia, and Paget's disease can cause severe deformity, significant restriction of activity, lost income, and increased health care costs.

OSTEOPENIA

Osteopenia is a condition that is common to all metabolic bone diseases characterized by a reduction in bone mass greater than expected for age, race, or sex. The causes of osteopenia include a decrease in bone formation, inadequate bone mineralization, or excessive bone deossification. Osteopenia is not a diagnosis but a term to describe an apparent lack of bone on radiographic studies.

OSTEOPOROSIS

Definition

Osteoporosis literally means porous bones. Bones that were once strong become fragile. Osteoporosis is a common age-related metabolic bone disease in which there is severe general reduction in the skeletal bone mass and an increased susceptibility to fractures, especially in the wrist, hip, and vertebral column. Bone resorption occurs faster than bone formation.

Osteoporosis can be classified into primary and secondary forms. Primary or type I postmenopausal osteoporosis is the most common and cannot be associated with an underlying medical condition. Secondary or type II osteoporosis results from an associated underlying condition, such as hyperparathyroidism, or an iatrogenic cause, such as long-term corticosteroid or heparin administration.

Primary osteoporosis can be divided into two subgroups. The first or type I postmenopausal osteoporosis occurs in women between the ages of 51 and 75 years of age. The bone loss is primarily in the cancellous bone trabecular network, resulting in fractures of the vertebrae or distal radius (Colles' fracture). Type II senile osteoporosis occurs in those individuals older than 70 years of age, affecting women twice as often as men. This results in equal trabecular and cortical bone loss with fractures of the hip and vertebrae being most common.

Incidence

In the United States alone, osteoporosis affects 25 million individuals and is responsible for more than 1.3 million fractures each year, most of which occur after age 65. More than 250,000 osteoporosis related hip fractures occur annually and these happen three times more often in women than men. The American health care system spends in excess of $10 billion to pay for the acute costs associated with these fractures as well as the medical, long-term, and social costs of osteoporosis. Among individuals with hip fractures, 50 per cent will need some help with activities of daily living and 15 to 25 per cent require placement in a long-term care institution. The mortality rate for elders with hip fractures is higher than 50 per cent.

One third of American women over age 50 will eventually have a compression or vertebral fracture of the spine. Osteoporosis occurs in about one fourth of all elderly people with the incidence of the disease greater in men than women (at least 5 : 1) with white women being affected more often than black women. Research reveals that black women have 10 per cent more bone mass than Caucasian women.

Etiology and Risk Factors

The exact etiology of osteoporosis is unknown; however several risk factors increase the risk that osteoporosis will occur (Box 67-1).

Box 67-1. Risk Factors for Osteoporosis

- Advanced Age
- Hereditary tendencies including blonde or red hair, freckles, and fair skin
- Northern European background
- Female
- Caucasian
- Postmenopausal
- Thin, small framed body
- Inactive or bedridden
- Calcium deficient diet
- Vitamin D deficiency
- Heavy cigarette smoking
- Heavy caffeine intake
- Alcohol consumption to excess
- Long-term corticosteroid use
- Long-term heparin use
- Long-acting psychotropic drugs
- Use of antacids
- Use of laxatives
- Cushing's disease
- Parkinson's disease
- Dementia
- Bilateral oophorectomy
- Endocrine disorders
- Type II diabetes
- Scoliosis
- Rheumatoid arthritis with no disability
- High-protein diet
- Anorexia and bulimia with resultant amenorrhea
- Excessive exercise

Women are at a high risk for early bone loss related to menopause. In postmenopausal women, estrogen production and bone calcium storage decrease. Estrogen appears to protect against bone loss. Accelerated bone loss also occurs with women who have early or surgically induced menopause, amenorrhea as a result of prolactin-producing pituitary tumors or anorexia nervosa, or in those who undertake intense long-distance running associated with undernourishment. These situations are all accompanied by estrogen deficiency, which is likely to be a major determinant of accelerated bone loss. Bone loss also occurs when estrogen therapy is withdrawn.

The susceptibility to fracture may be, in part, hereditary. The presence of the so-called "dowager hump" or collapse and wedging of vertebra in a mother may indicate a risk for her daughters.

Other hereditary factors include Northern European traits, such as blonde or red hair, the presence of freckles, and fair skin. Petite, thin women, especially those who do not exercise are at greater risk because they have less bone to lose than larger, big-boned women. Similarly, small-framed, thin men are more at risk than men with larger frames and more body weight.

PREVENTION

Once the clinical expression of osteoporosis has occurred, treatment is less than satisfactory. Therefore, it is important to identify those individuals at risk early, in order to initiate therapy when it will have maximum efficacy. Strategies for preventing osteoporosis are most efficient when started early in life.

Adequate calcium intake requires consuming more dairy products, which provide about 75 per cent of the calcium in the average diet. Most authorities recommend that women consume 1000 to 1200 mg of calcium per day before menopause.

National surveys of dietary intake have shown that many Americans are not consuming enough calcium. In fact, many women and adolescent girls actually consume less than half of what is recommended for growth and maintenance of bone. The United States Recommended Daily Allowances (USRDAs) are labeling standards. The USRDA for calcium is 1000 mg per day and for vitamin D, it is 400 international units. Foods rich in calcium include milk, dairy products, and leafy green vegetables (see Chap. 14).

Some individuals have difficulty digesting milk due to a lack of the enzyme lactase, which breaks down the milk sugar lactose. Acidophilus milk, yogurt, and hard cheeses may be tolerated because of the way they are processed.

Vitamin D plays a major role in both calcium absorption and its incorporation into bone. Vitamin D is the key that allows calcium to leave the intestine and enter the bloodstream. Vitamin D is formed naturally in the body after exposure to sunlight. Vitamin D supplements may be necessary for the institutionalized or homebound individual.

Common therapeutic modalities may include the administration of vitamin D, calcium, calcitonin (available in parenteral form), estrogen preparations, (available as a transdermal patch), and sodium fluoride.

Sodium fluoride is an experimental therapy that significantly increases trabecular bone mass, although clinical trials suggest it may also increase the rate of hip fracture. The hormone calcitonin is naturally secreted by the thyroid in response to increased amounts of serum calcium. With aging, the calcitonin level decreases and is less effective in inhibiting bone resorption, so bone mass is lost. Calcitonin therapy must be given parenterally each day for 12 to 18 months, at which time bone resorption either stabilizes or slightly increases bone mass.

Calcium supplements vary (Table 67–1) and may be absorbed differently, as well as being contraindicated in individuals with a history of renal stones, granulomatous conditions, or hypercalemic conditions. Excessive serum calcium can cause damage to the urinary system; therefore, calcium supplements should be prescribed by a physician or nurse practitioner. A lumbosacral brace for vertebral fractures, surgical repair of fractures when indicated, and pain management are key interventions.

Individuals who exercise regularly generally have a higher peak bone mass because bone responds to exercise by becoming stronger. Weight-bearing exercise, such as walking, jogging, or stair climbing, is recommended over non-weight-bearing exercise such as cycling or swimming. However it is important to note that some type of physical activity is better than none. The 1984 National Institutes of Health (NIH) Consensus Development Conference on Osteoporosis recommends participation in activities such as walking, tennis, hiking, and ballroom dancing.

Pathophysiology

Throughout the lifespan, new bone is formed (osteoblastic activity) while old bone is resorbed (osteoclastic activity.) Two major theories have been proposed regarding the development of osteoporosis. The most popular theory suggests an increase in osteoclastic activity causing bone resorption or thinning. The second theory suggests that osteoporosis may result from decreased osteoblastic activity perhaps from less efficient or short-lived bone-forming cells.

Bone mass or density peaks between 30 and 35 years of age. After the peak years, calcium stored in the spongy bone (cancellous mass) leaves the tissue. Bone trabeculae are decreased in numbers and width, while marrow spaces are widened, and the bone mass decreases as calcium leaves the compact bone (cortical mass).

With osteoporosis, the supporting skeletal structures are weak, so even minimal stress can cause fractures. Spinal fractures occurring with osteoporosis are usually "compression fractures" and are very painful. They occur when one or more vertebrae simply collapse from carrying the weight of the upright body.

Clinical Manifestations

Clinical manifestations may reveal shortened stature, difficulty in bending over, marked kyphosis of the thoracic spine (dowager's hump), or impaired breathing due to deformities of the spine and rib cage (Fig. 67–1).

Back pain and fractures are the most characteristic presenting symptoms. Vertebral compression fractures (often multiple and most commonly T12 to L2), proximal femur fractures (femoral neck and intertrochanteric), distal radius fractures, and pelvic fractures are the most common fracture types. The loss of height secondary to multiple fractures is characteristic of individuals with osteoporosis. Bone loss can occur in the jaw bone, which, along with oral health problems, may lead to tooth loss or improperly fitting dentures. This complication may lead to changes in the appearance of the individual's face. These changes in addition to the shortened stature and kyphosis associated with osteoporosis may have a profound negative impact on the individual's self-esteem.

At present, there is no way in which an individual can tell if he or she has low bone mass from a family or personal history. Medical tests are available that

TABLE 67–1. Calcium Supplement Types

Form of Calcium	Per Cent of Elemental Calcium	Dietary Characteristics	Cautions	Side Effects	Considerations
Calcium carbonate	40	Take 1 hour after meals and at bedtime	Do not take with milk or food high in vitamin D	Constipation, gastric distention, flatulence, acid-rebound nausea, hypercalcemia, hypophosphatemia, milk alkali syndrome	Avoid if too little or no stomach acid secretions
Calcium lactate	13	Milk and yogurt are main source Powder form = 650 mg/level tsp	Contains lactose	Less constipating; same as above	Avoid if lactose-intolerant; symptoms are: gas, bloating, cramps or diarrhea
Calcium gluconate	9	Sweet		Less constipating; same as above	Must be taken frequently because of low concentration
Chelated calcium					Calcium anchored to a protein or yeast, amino acid not absorbed any better than standard calcium
Calcium levulinate	13	Bitter salty taste			
Calcium chloride	27	Used to pickle foods		Irritates stomach	Tends to irritate stomach
Calcium orate	10				
Bone meal	31		May contain lead	Same as above	Not well absorbed
Dolomite	22		Same as above		

Calcium Supplement Types

Brand	Milligrams/Pill	Source of Calcium
Alka-2 antacid (chewable)	200 mg	calcium carbonate
Calcet	153 mg	calcium gluconate, lactate, carbonate
Calcium lactate—Arco	83 mg	calcium lactate
Chelated calcium—Arco	150 mg	calcium, amino acid chelate
Caltrate 600 (chewable)	600 mg	calcium carbonate
Chooz antacid gum (chewable)	200 mg	calcium carbonate
Dical D capsules (133 IU vitamin D added)	117 mg	dibasic calcium phosphate
Dical D wafers (chewable, 200 IU vitamin D added)	232 mg	dibasic calcium phosphate
Os-Cal 250 (125 IU vitamin D added)	250 mg	calcium carbonate
Os-Cal 500 (high potency)	500 mg	calcium carbonate
Tums antacid (chewable)	200 mg	calcium carbonate
Tums E-X (chewable)	300 mg	calcium carbonate

Prepared by Barbara M. Schultz, RN, BSN, C, a patient care and education coordinator at the Veterans Administration Domiciliary, White City, Oregon.

From Urrows, S. T., et al. (1991). Profiles in osteoporosis. *American Journal of Nursing, 91*(2), p. 36.

measure bone mass in various sites in the body. These tests, called absorptiometry or densitometry, are safe and painless. Dual-Energy X-ray Absorptiometry (DXA) provides a measurement of the amount of bone tissue in the hip and spine. This technique is now widely used because of the shortened examination time (about 5 minutes), slightly lower radiation levels than previous scans and increased precision measurements. With information obtained from bone mass measurements, family history, and risk factor assessment, the individual's likelihood to fracture can be predicted.

There are no definitive laboratory tests that confirm a diagnosis of primary osteoporosis. A battery of tests is performed to rule out secondary osteoporosis or other metabolic bone diseases. These tests include serum calcium, phosphorus, and alkaline phosphatase, which

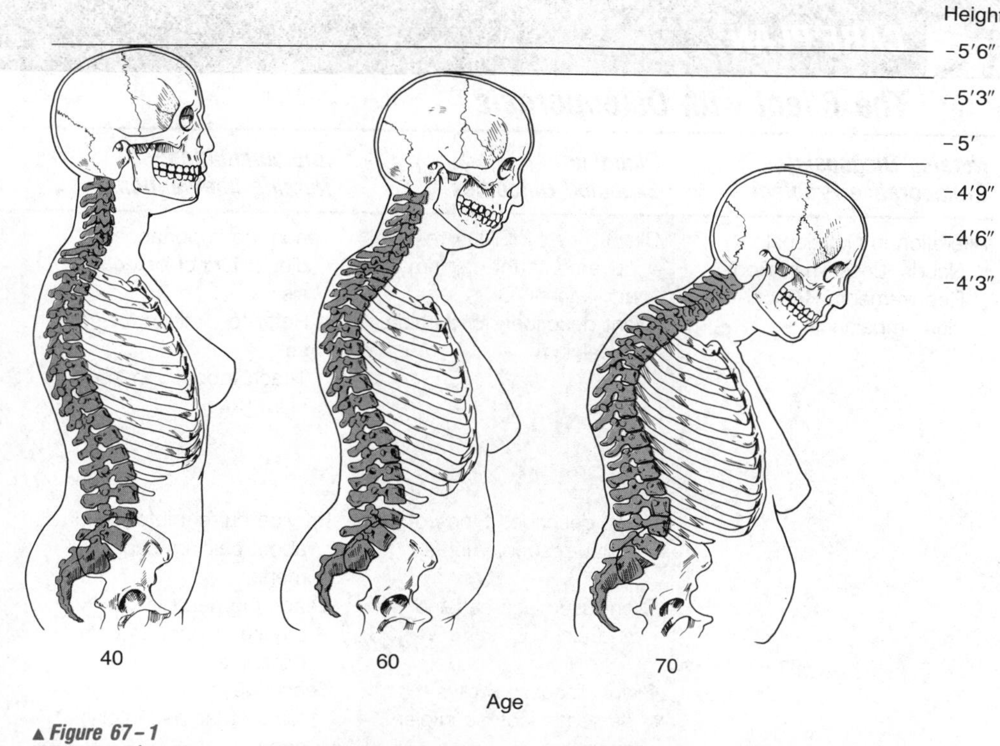

▲ *Figure 67–1*

Osteoporotic changes. Normal spine at age 40, and osteoporotic changes at ages 60 and 70. These changes can cause a loss of height and can result in the deformity called dowager's hump in the upper thoracic spine.

are normal in this condition. Serum osteocalcin is elevated. Urinary calcium is initially high, then returns to normal.

Bone biopsy may be performed when diagnosis by noninvasive measures is considered unreliable or when there has not been a positive response to therapy.

Medical Management

Intervention in the care of the client with osteoporosis focuses on the symptoms expressed.

Important goals are adequate nutrition, strengthening exercises, mobility in a hazard-free environment, and pain management. Fracture is usually the first symptom that causes an individual to seek medical intervention; therefore, the plan should include further fracture prevention techniques.

Many of the nonsurgical management interventions are given for the treatment of the disease, as well as for the prevention of osteoporosis. These include diet and drug therapy used to slow bone resorption and promote new bone growth.

Nursing Management

Nursing management for the client with osteoporosis is shown in the Nursing Care Plan.

Post-hospital Care

DISCHARGE TEACHING

The teaching plan for the client with osteoporosis includes fall prevention, an exercise program, diet management, and drug therapy.

The client who has developed a fracture can be discharged home, to an extended care facility for intensive rehabilitation, or to a permanent residence, if support systems are not in place.

The first priority is to assess the home environment for potential safety hazards. Evaluation of the home setting is performed by reviewing the admission assessment, discussions with the client, and consultation with a specialist in social services. For the client who has sustained a fall and fractured a bone, discussion about fall prevention strategies is imperative.

Alterations to the home and a referral for a home safety evaluation by a visiting nurse may be helpful. Handrails in the bathroom, removal of scatter rugs, and increased lighting are some of the modifications that may be necessary.

PAGET'S DISEASE (OSTEITIS DEFORMANS)

Overview

Paget's disease is defined as a disorder of bone architecture characterized by an initial phase of increased

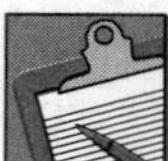

CARE PLAN

The Client with Osteoporosis

Nursing Diagnosis/ Collaborative Problem	Planning: Expected Outcomes	Implementation: Nursing Interventions	Rationales
Alteration in Nutritional Needs: Less Than Body Requirements R/T calcium imbalance	Client meets USRDA requirements for calcium and vitamin D Client describes foods high in calcium	Teach the importance of diet in further osteoporosis Refer to dietitian for consult Teach foods high in calcium	Dietary calcium is needed to maintain serum calcium levels, to maintain bone mass Foods high in calcium include plain yogurt, dairy products, seafood, sardines, green vegetables, calcium fortified orange juice, and cereals
	Client describes types of calcium supplements	Provide current information about calcium supplements	
	Client uses less caffeine and alcohol	Teach the need to decrease alcohol and caffeine intake	Excessive alcohol and caffeine use increase bone resorption
	Client discusses ways to decrease lactose intolerance	Teach ways to avoid symptoms of lactose intolerance	Lactose intolerance is caused by the inability to break down milk sugar lactose. Use of acidophilus milk, as well as commercially prepared lactase, decreases the symptoms of lactose intolerance
Impaired Physical Activity R/T osteoporosis	Client complies with physical mobility plan to level of independent ADLs	Consult with physical therapy to develop exercise program Weight-bearing exercises Strengthening exercises Discuss benefits of walking at least ½ mile three times a week Teach the importance of exercise in prevention of osteoporosis	Weight-bearing exercises increase bone formation. Strengthening exercises increase muscle tone and circulation. NIH Consensus on Osteoporosis 1984 recommends walking, tennis, hiking, and ballroom dancing
	Client uses assistive devices to perform independent ADLs	Assist with ADLs, allowing client to remain independent	Pain may limit client's ability to perform ADLs
		Evaluate need for assistive devices for ADLs and home use	Devices may be needed for independent ADLs
	Client identifies and avoids potential hazards, thereby avoiding falls and fractures resulting from minimal injury	Establish a hazard-free hospital environment Provide adequate lighting Adjust bed to lowest position with side rails up, when client is in bed Place necessary articles within client's reach including call light, water pitcher, telephone and eyeglasses Keep client area free of spills and clutter	Establishment of a hazard-free environment will reduce the risk from falls or minimal injury

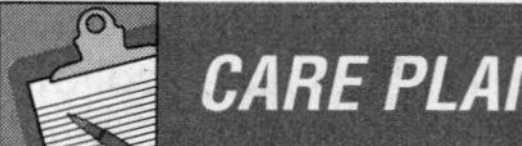

CARE PLAN

The Client with Osteoporosis Continued

Nursing Diagnosis/ Collaborative Problem	Planning: Expected Outcomes	Implementation: Nursing Interventions	Rationales
Pain R/T fracture (vertebral, Colles' wrist, hip)	Client experiences pain reduction or relief so client may be independent	Assess pain medication needs	Client may not be receiving adequate medication due to inadequate dosing, the need for around the clock administration, or iatrogenic causes. Therefore plan medication schedule with client
	Client uses alternative measures to reduce or alleviate pain	Teach alternative modalities for pain relief	Alternative modalities have been found effective in reducing pain. Include comfort measures such as positioning, warm compresses, application of assistive devices, distraction, imagery, biofeedback, and hypnosis

rate of bone tissue breakdown by osteoclasts, followed by excessive abnormal bone formation by osteoblasts. The diseased bone is structurally weak and prone to fractures. Paget's disease most frequently produces painful deformities of the femur, tibia, lower spine, pelvis, and cranium.

The exact cause of Paget's disease is unknown. One theory suggests that perhaps a slow virus with a long latent period causes Paget's disease. Although no definite hereditary pattern has been established, a familial clustering has been reported.

Paget's disease occurs worldwide, but it appears to afflict those of northwestern European extraction in North America. It is seen less frequently in Africa, Asia, and Scandinavia. In the United States, 2.5 million people over the age of 40 are affected, and is more common in males than females.

Many individuals are diagnosed because they have experienced some sort of trauma, and their radiographic studies demonstrate the characteristic changes of the disease. Ten to twenty per cent of individuals with the disease are asymptomatic. Before clinical manifestations occur, radiographic studies show increased bone expansion and density. After symptoms have developed, the bone shows a characteristic mosaic appearance (Fig. 67-2). A bone scan may be useful when radiographs are unreliable, and to determine whether a lesion in pagetoid bone is active or inactive. Computed tomography scans and magnetic resonance imaging improve visualization of bone and are diagnostically useful.

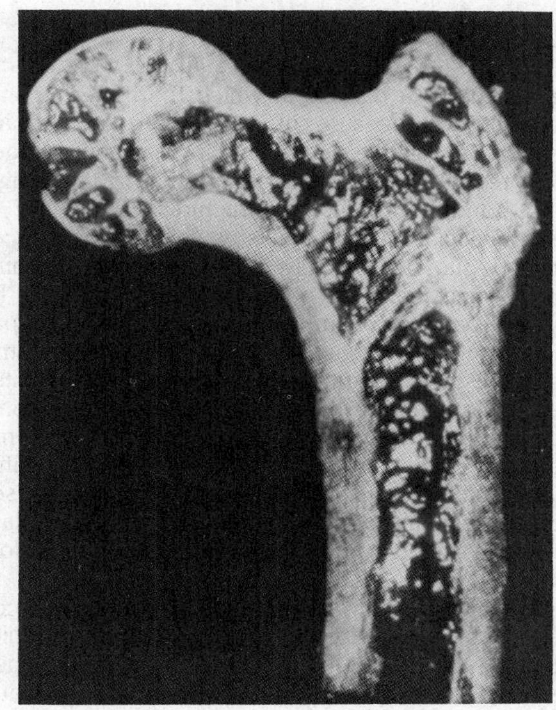

▲ **Figure 67-2**

Example of pagetoid bone, demonstrating the characteristic mosaic pattern on radiographic study. (From Merkow, R. L., & Lane, J. M. [1990]. Paget's disease of bone. *Orthopaedic Clinics of North America, 21*[1], 173.)

In symptomatic Paget's disease, the most common presenting complaints include one or more of the following: bone pain, skeletal deformity (barrel shaped chest or bowing of tibia/femur, or kyphosis), changes in skin temperature, pathologic fractures through diseased bone and symptoms related to nerve compression. Diseased bone pressing on the cranial nerves may result in vertigo, hearing loss with tinnitus, and blindness. Rheumatoid arthritis, ankylosing spondylitis, gout, and calcific periarthritis are commonly associated with Paget's disease.

An increase in hydroxyproline during a 24-hour urine collection indicates osteoclastic activity. A normal or increased serum calcium, anemia, and increased alkaline phosphatase are indicative of the disease process.

Management

The primary indication for treatment is pain. Analgesics such as aspirin, indomethacin, or ibuprofen may decrease bone pain. Further orthopedic treatment may be indicated for severe disabling arthritis, severe bowing deformities of the femur or tibia, and pathologic fractures. Calcitonin and etidronate, both of which retard bone resorption, may be administered, especially in painful pseudofracture. The cytotoxic antibiotic mithramycin (Mithracin) may be used to decrease serum calcium, urinary hydroxyproline, and serum alkaline phosphatase.

OSTEOMALACIA

Overview

Osteomalacia is a disease in which the bone becomes abnormally soft because of a disturbed calcium and phosphorous balance secondary to a vitamin D deficiency, resulting in marked deformities of the weight-bearing bones and pathologic fractures.

Osteomalacia mainly affects women, and it is endemic in Asia. Occasionally, the disease can be found in strict vegetarians or postgastrectomy patients. Primary hypoparathyroidism, renal tubular disorders, pancreatic insufficiency, hepatobiliary disease, and small intestine disease contribute to the incidence of osteomalacia. Women who have had multiple frequent pregnancies and who have breastfed their children may have a higher incidence of the disease as well as individuals on long-term anticonvulsants, tranquilizers, sedatives, muscle relaxants, or antidiuretics. Osteomalacia is similar to rickets, which occurs in children; therefore, the condition is called adult rickets.

Osteomalacia is always due to an inadequate concentration of calcium or phosphorus in the body fluids. Inadequate calcium or vitamin D in the diet may cause a decrease in the absorption of calcium from the intestine. Increased urinary excretion of calcium or the loss of calcium or phosphorous during pregnancy and lactation may cause osteomalacia.

Osteomalacia is characterized by widespread decalcification and softening of bones, especially in the spine, pelvis, and lower extremities. Bones become bent and flattened as they soften. In the spine, scoliotic and kyphotic deformities are present. Coxa vara deformity of the femoral neck due to pressure on the femoral neck is common.

Serum calcium and phosphorus levels are reduced, and the alkaline phosphatase level is moderately elevated. Urinary calcium and creatinine excretion levels are low.

Radiographic studies indicate generalized demineralization with trabecular bone loss. Pseudofractures (milkman's fractures) and cyst formation are common. Compression fractures, and bowing and bending deformities of the long bones are often present. Biopsy may assist in diagnosis.

Management

Intervention for osteomalacia includes vitamin D administered daily until signs of healing take place when a daily low maintenance dose is continued. Adequate intake of calcium and phosphorous as well as protein should be ensured. Supplemental calcium in the form of lactate or gluconate is administered.

▼ OTHER MUSCULOSKELETAL DISORDERS

SCOLIOSIS

Overview

Scoliosis is defined as a lateral curvature of the spine when viewing from the posteroanterior view. The spine would normally appear straight in this plane. Adult scoliosis is a spinal curvature existing after skeletal maturity. A curve may present in any area of the spine—cervical, thoracic, thorocolumbar, and lumbar. There is usually a second compensatory curve in the opposite direction. The most common curve pattern is a right thoracic, which produces a rib prominence.

The prevalence of scoliosis in the general population ranges from 2 to 4 per cent. If the individual has a positive family history for scoliosis, the risk for the occurrence of scoliosis is greater. Many adults with scoliosis have been diagnosed as children; have been observed for spinal curve progression; and have undergone exercise regimens, bracing, casting, and even some surgical intervention. Other individuals with scoliosis have never been formally diagnosed, and the curve has progressed, causing cardiopulmonary problems, resulting in the seeking out of medical care.

Adult scoliosis occurs in individuals aged 40 years or older. Most cases are idiopathic and are defined as a structural spinal curvature of unknown etiology, which arises during adolescence and persists into adulthood. Curves of less than 40 degrees, without symptoms, generally remain stable and do not require intervention. A progressive curve (more than 65 degrees) in the thoracic spine may be responsible for shortness of breath and fatigue. Other symptoms may include back pain, progressive spinal curvature accompanied by decreased height, cardiopulmonary failure, and cosmetic deformity. Evaluating the character, severity, and specific location of back pain helps determine whether or not the pain is caused by scoliosis. A progressive curve in the lumbar spine may be responsible for low back fatigue and pain. Back pain associated with scoliosis is usually located at the apex of the curve on either the convexity or the concavity. Early degenerative changes include spinal stenosis. If nerve root entrapment occurs, surgery is indicated.

Diagnosis is based on radiographic findings of a curvature of greater than 10 degrees, combined with structural changes in the spine, including vertebral rotation. Functional scoliosis occurs as a result of leg-length discrepancy or posture.

Management

Surgical procedures for adults include the application of spinal instrumentation either through an anterior or posterior approach. These include the Cotrel-Dubousset system, Harrington rod system, Harrington rods with spinous process wiring (Drummond or Wisconsin technique), Luque rods with sublaminar wires, Dwyer and Zielke procedures, as well as the creation of bone-grafted fusions (Fig. 67–3). The type of instrumentation used is based on the discretion of the surgeon. Other considerations include diagnosis, magnitude of the curve, flexibility of the curve, inherent strength of the bone, and the individual's ability to wear postoperative immobilization.

Nursing management focuses on education of the client about postoperative care, pain control, providing adequate fluid replacement, and progressive ambulation.[20]

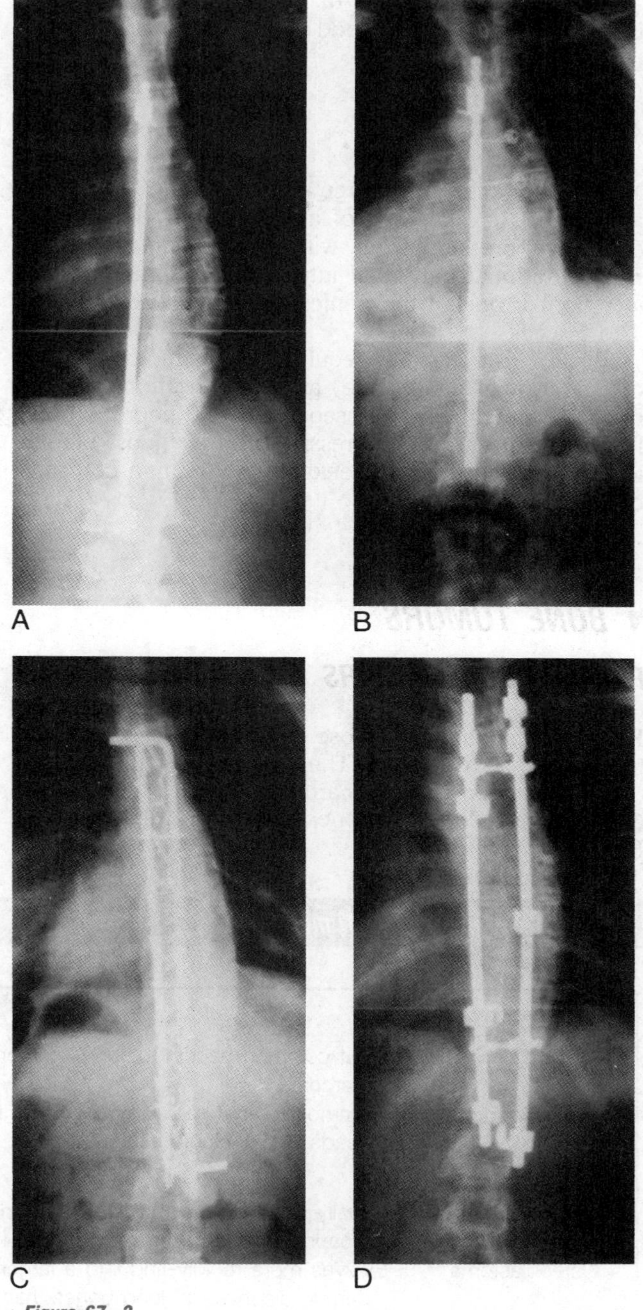

▲ **Figure 67–3**

Examples of surgical instrumentation used to correct scoliosis. Thoracic scoliosis with *(A)* Harrington rod instrumentation, *(B)* Harrington rod with spinous process wiring, *(C)* Luque instrumentation, and *(D)* Cotrel-Dubousset instrumentation. (From Rodts, M. F. [1987]. Surgical intervention for adult scoliosis. *Orthopaedic Nursing,* 6[6], 12.)

OSTEOMYELITIS

Overview

Osteomyelitis is a term used to describe any infection of the bone. Acute osteomyelitis responds to a 4- to 6-week course of intravenous antibiotics, whereas chronic osteomyelitis persists longer than 4 weeks and involves sequestered (necrotic bone that has separated from living tissue) areas of infection.

Osteomyelitis is generally bacterial in origin but may also be caused by viral or fungal infections. *Staphylococcus aureus* in the most common organism but *Eschericha coli, Klebsiella, Proteus, Pseudomonas,* and *Salmonella* may also cause osteomyelitis. These organisms may be directly introduced into the bone, or they may be spread from adjacent soft tissue infection or travel through the blood to the infected site. The causative bacterial agent is able to multiply readily in bone because bone has a slow circulatory system.

Clinical manifestations of osteomyelitis include fever, usually above 101° F (38° C); localized pain or tenderness; erythema (redness); heat; and swelling around the affected bone.

Early diagnosis is important to prevent progression of the infection. Symptoms are based on the area affected. Diagnostic tests include radionuclide bone scans, gallium scans, indium scans, computed tomography and magnetic resonance imaging. In acute osteomyelitis, radiographic changes are usually not visible till 2 to 3 weeks after onset. Laboratory findings include an elevated white blood count (WBC), an elevated erythrocyte sedimentation rate (ESR), and if bacteremia is present, a positive blood culture for the organism causing the infection.

Management

Needle aspiration or a percutaneous needle biopsy may assist with the diagnosis of acute osteomyelitis as well as relieve pressure from within the bone. Treatment requires administration of intravenous or intramuscular injection of one of the penicillin type of antibiotics for 4 to 6 weeks.

Chronic osteomyelitis requires sequestrectomy (surgical removal of dead bone) and saucerization (removal of scar or infected tissue, sequestra, and necrotic bone, leaving a saucer-like depression). Intravenous antibiotics are used for 4 to 6 weeks, followed by a course of oral antibiotics.

▼ BONE TUMORS

PRIMARY BONE TUMORS

Primary bone tumors (those originating in bone) may be benign or malignant. The two major types include (1) chondrogenic (from cartilage) and (2) osteogenic (from bone). Primary bone tumors are described in Box 67-2.

Management

The treatment of primary bone lesions is radical surgery, combined with radiation or chemotherapy. Radiation and chemotherapy are described in Chapter 22.

SURGICAL MANAGEMENT

The customary treatment of bone and soft tissue sarcomas has been amputation. Over the past 2 decades, much progress has been made in understanding the tumor, chemotherapy, and radiation therapy, thereby enabling salvage of the limb. Research has shown that clients have the same disease-free survival rate with limb-sparing operations as those who have amputations.[25]

Before surgery, the client undergoes chemotherapy and radiation therapy to decrease the tumor size and treat small metastases. During surgery, the tumor and a margin of normal bone are removed. The defect created by tumor removal is filled in with bone allograft. Bone grafts are usually from cadaveric donors. The recipients of bone allografts do not require immunosuppressive treatment because the bone is frozen after harvesting. Freezing diminishes the immune response of the bone tissue. The risk of contracting human immunodeficiency virus is well over 1 in 1,000,000.[40] The bone graft is secured with metallic pastes and screws.

NURSING MANAGEMENT

Prior to surgery, the health care team discusses the options with the client and family (many clients are

Box 67-2. Primary Bone Tumors

Classification/Name	Description
Benign chondrogenic	
Osteochondroma	Most common benign tumor. Commonly found in the femur and tibia; about 10 per cent develop into sarcoma
Endochondroma	Common to mature hyaline cartilage in hands, feet, ribs, spine, sternum, or long bones. Frequently leads to pathologic fractures.
Benign osteogenic	
Osteoid, Osteomas	Usually small tumors with clearly outlined area of reactive bone. Common to the proximal femur, tibia, scaphoid bone of the wrist, talus, or calcaneus of the foot. Causes pain at night.
Osteoblastoma	Evolves more rapidly and into a larger tumor than an osteoid osteoma. Found in the vertebrae, distal femur, diaphysis of long bones, hands, and feet.
Giant cell tumor	Aggressive and extensive lesion. Has a tendency to recur and metastasize to the lung. Commonly found in the distal femur, tibia, distal radius, sacrum, proximal humerus, and proximal fibula. Produces pain, edema, and limitation in movement.
Malignant osteogenic	
Osteosarcoma	Most common malignant bone tumor. Occurs in the metaphysis of lone bones, at the sites of the most rapid bone growth. Common to the distal femur, proximal tibia, and proximal humerus. Can be induced by ionizing radiation, and may follow therapeutic radiation. Causes pain, swelling, and pathologic fracture. Serum alkaline phosphatase is markedly elevated. Prognosis improving with combination therapies, reaching 65 per cent survival.
Ewing's sarcoma	Common to young adults and found in the pelvis and lower extremities. Metastasizes quickly to the lungs and other bones. Clinical manifestations include pain, edema, low grade fever, leukocytosis, and anemia. Improving prognosis with aggressive therapy, 65 per cent survival rate.
Chondrosarcoma	Common to the pelvis, ribs, proximal femur, and proximal humerus.
Fibrosarcoma	Common to the femur and tibia.

adolescents or young adults). Autologous blood donations prior to surgery are not permitted for tumor resection; therefore, the family may wish to donate blood.

Following surgery, the limb is immobilized and elevated. Pain is usually severe and controlled with narcotic analgesics through epidural or patient-controlled analgesia modes. Postoperative anemia may require transfusion. Complications of the surgery typify other orthopedic surgeries: infection, deep vein thrombosis, and nonunion of the bone grafts. Ambulation is begun the day after surgery, and the client is taught to walk with crutches.[34, 40]

METASTATIC BONE TUMORS

Skeletal metastases are the most common form of malignant bone tumors, and virtually every malignant tumor can metastasize to bone. Evidence suggests that distant metastases seem to develop from tumor seed cells that travel through the lymphatic system, blood vessels, and other surrounding tissues. Primary lesions of the prostate, the breast, the kidney, the thyroid, and the lung most commonly seek to metastasize to bone. The femur, the pelvis, the ribs, and the vertebrae are the most commonly affected bone sites. Pathologic fractures are common, especially in the acetabulum and proximal femur. Serum levels of alkaline phosphatase and calcium and sedimentation rate may be elevated.

Pain may occur before changes are detectable on radiographic studies. Diagnosis may be made through radiographic studies, incisional biopsy, or frozen section. Many bone tumors produce typical patterns on radiographic studies. Whenever malignant lesions are suspected, anteroposterior, and lateral chest films and computerized tomograms of the chest are taken to detect pulmonary metastases. A scintigraphy (bone scan) is performed to locate additional osseous lesions. Computerized tomography and magnetic resonance imaging are used to detect soft tissue involvement and the location of tumor and neurovascular structures.

▼ DISORDERS OF THE HAND

CARPAL TUNNEL SYNDROME

Carpal tunnel syndrome is a frequently seen painful disorder caused by pressure on the median nerve at the wrist. The exact cause is unknown and is often seen in those with recent fractures, arthritis, lipomas, ganglion, or congenital anomaly. This condition may develop in people with histories of strenuous or repetitive use of the hands.

Early clinical manifestations include burning or tingling pain in the thumb, index, and middle fingers. Aching pain may radiate to the upper extremity and, occasionally, to the shoulder, neck, and chest. Pain may be episodic or constant and exacerbated at night and by movement. The physical examination reveals the presence of Tinel's sign (tingling or shocklike pain) elicited by light percussion over the median nerve, at the wrist. Phalen's sign (hand tingling with acute wrist flexion) may also be present.

Treatment ranges from nonsteroidal anti-inflammatory agents, splints, and steroid injections, to surgical release. The client is advised to limit the specific motion that aggravates carpal tunnel syndrome.

DUPUYTREN'S CONTRACTURE

Dupuytren's contracture is a flexion deformity that most often affects the ring finger at the proximal joint. The exact cause is unknown, but the disorder may be inherited, and may also be seen with gout, arthritis, diabetes, epilepsy, and with alcoholism. The condition most often occurs bilaterally, but when only one side is affected, the right hand is involved twice as frequently as the left. It is seen most often in the late fifth and early sixth decades of life.

Initial assessment findings may reveal a bulky proliferation of tissue and contracting band palpated on the palmar crease opposite the ring or affected finger. Treatment includes finger-stretching exercises and surgical resection of the thickened palmar fascia.

GANGLION

A ganglion is the most common benign soft tissue mass in the hand consisting of a round cyst-like lesion overlying or adjacent to the wrist joint or tendon. The synovium surrounding the tendon degenerates, allowing the tendon sheath to buckle and weaken. The onset may be gradual or sudden, and it may be posttraumatic. Clinical manifestations include localized pain and a freely moveable mass. Symptoms are exacerbated by dorsiflexion of the wrist. Treatment includes the aspiration of the ganglion followed by an injection of corticosteroid into the joint. Nonsteroidal anti-inflammatory agents (NSAIDs) are prescribed. Surgical excision may be necessary if symptoms persist and range of motion is impaired. Ganglion formation may recur in some instances.

▼ DISORDERS OF THE FOOT

HALLUX VALGUS

The hallux valgus (bunion) deformity is the most common disorder of the foot. Although the terms hallux valgus and bunion are frequently used synonymously, they actually refer to separate elements of the same disorder. It is defined as a painful swelling of the bursa when the great toe deviates laterally at the metatarsophalangeal (MTP) joint. The problem may be congenital, or may be acquired by wearing shoes that are too short or too narrow. Females are affected more frequently than males.

Initial assessment findings include a painful valgus deformity of the great toe and callus formation on the bottom of the feet. Weight-bearing radiographic studies of both feet are performed.

Treatment includes suggesting the use of open-toed shoes made with soft leather or sneakers. Metatarsal pads relieve some of the pressure from weight-bearing. Intra-articular corticosteroid injections are given for acute bursitis, and analgesics are administered for pain. Simple bunionectomy involves osteotomy (bone resection) of the first metatarsal, removing the bony overgrowth and bursa. Kirschner wires are inserted vertically through the toes and remain in place for 3 weeks postoperatively. Corks are placed on the tips of the wires for protection.

HAMMER TOE

Hammer toe deformity is a flexion contracture of the proximal interphalangeal joint with extension or slight hyperextension of the distal interphalangeal joint. Hammer toe deformity often accompanies hallux valgus deformity.

Clinical manifestations may include a family history of hammer toe, rheumatoid arthritis, and clawfeet. Shoes may fit incorrectly, and there is often pain upon walking, with alterations in stride length. Corns may be present on the dorsum of the toe.

Treatment includes the use of pads to cushion the foot from the shoe, removal of corns, and passive stretching exercises. Surgical intervention involves osteotomy of the toe and resection of the proximal phalanx. In the very young child, surgery may consist of

TABLE 67–2. Clinical Features of Major Muscular Dystrophy Types

Clinical Features	Duchenne MD	Clinical Features	Limb Girdle MD
Incidence:	most common	Incidence:	not infrequent
Age at onset:	generally before age 3	Age at onset:	usually by second decade
Inheritance:	sex-linked recessive gene, autosomal less than 10 per cent	Inheritance:	usually autosomal recessive, may occur as autosomal dominant
Pattern of muscle involvement:	onset: selected symmetric weakness of proximal pelvic muscles. 3 to 5 years later shoulder girdle muscles become involved	Pattern of muscle involvement:	proximal shoulder and pelvic girdle
Late muscle involvement:	all muscles, including facial oculopharyngeal and respiratory	Late muscle involvement:	periphery; brachioradialis, hand and calf
Pseudohypertrophy:	calf muscles	Pseudohypertrophy:	occurs in less than one-third of cases
Contractural deformities:	common	Contractural deformities:	late, milder than Duchenne MD
Scoliosis/kyphoscoliosis:	common, late	Scoliosis/kyphoscoliosis:	mild, late
Heart involvement:	yes	Heart involvement:	very rare
IQ:	decreased	IQ:	normal
Course:	steadily progressive	Course:	much variation between patients, but is slowly progressive

Clinical Features	Becker MD
Incidence:	less common
Age at onset:	majority between ages 5–15
Inheritance:	sex-linked recessive gene
Pattern of muscle involvement:	similar to Duchenne MD
Late muscle involvement:	face is spared
Pseudohypertrophy:	calf muscles
Contractural deformities:	less common
Scoliosis/kyphoscoliosis:	not severe
Heart involvement:	late, uncommon
IQ:	normal
Course:	slowly progressive

Modified from Doleysh, N., et al. (1991). Neuromuscular disorders. In S. W. Salmond, et al. (Eds), *Core curriculum for orthopaedic nursing* (2nd ed., p. 301). Pitman, NJ: National Association of Orthopaedic Nurses.

transplanting the flexor tendons to the extensor sides of the toes.

MORTON'S NEUROMA (PLANTAR NEUROMA)

Morton's neuroma, also known as a plantar neuroma or plantar digital neuritis, is the thickening of a nerve or the formation of a small tumor, secondary to pressure, in the area around the lateral branch of the medial plantar nerve. Pain is described as a severe, burning sensation, usually occurring in the web space between the third and fourth toes. Treatment is the surgical excision of the neuroma. Palliative measures may include steroid injection and insertion of a metatarsal arch to relieve pressure.

▼ MUSCULAR DISORDERS

MUSCULAR DYSTROPHY

Muscular dystrophy (MD) is a progressive, hereditary, degenerative disease of skeletal muscle. There are many forms of muscular dystrophy (Table 67-2), each with its own distinct characteristics and causes. All are progressive.

Three theories have evolved regarding the pathophysiology of muscular dystrophy. The membrane theory, which states that the cell membrane has been genetically altered, compromising the integrity of the cell and making it vulnerable to degeneration, is the most popular hypothesis. The neurogenic theory suggests a disturbance in the nerve-muscle interaction. The vascular theory proposes that a lack of blood flow causes muscle and tissue degeneration.

Diagnosis of muscular dystrophy is often difficult, because the clinical manifestations are varied and similar to other muscular disorders such as myasthenia gravis or polymyositis. Muscle weakness is characteristic of all types. Elevated enzyme levels of creatine phosphokinase (CPK), abnormal muscle biopsy results, and an abnormal electromyogram (EMG) are found with muscular dystrophy.

Treatment includes corrective surgery for scoliosis or flexion contractures, long-leg braces, spinal braces, and exercise programs, including breathing exercises for respiratory decompensation. The prognosis for muscular dystrophy depends on the type and severity of the disease.

Summary

The focus of this chapter was on musculoskeletal disorders. These disorders include metabolic bone diseases, such as osteoporosis. Osteoporosis is a common disorder that results from loss of bone mineralization. Bone tumors were also discussed. They can be benign or malignant primary lesions or metastatic tumors. Bone salvaging procedures are becoming more common in the management of these tumors.

Bibliography

1. Aloia, J. F. (1989). *Osteoporosis: A guide to prevention and treatment*. Champaign, Illinois: Leisure Press.
2. Barden, R. M., & Sinkora, G. L. (1991). Bone stimulators for fusions and fractures. *Nursing Clinics of North America, 26*(1), 89-103.
3. Bender, L. H. (1991). Osteogenesis imperfecta. *Orthopaedic Nursing*, 10(4), 23-31.
4. Boden, S. D., & Kaplan, F. S. (1990). Calcium homeostasis. *Orthopaedic Clinics of North America, 21*(1) 31-42.
5. Bridwell, K. H. (1988). Cotrel-Dubousset instrumentation. *Orthopaedic Nursing, 7*(1), 11-16.
6. Brosnan, H. (1991). Nursing management of the adolescent with idiopathic scoliosis. *Nursing Clinics of North America, 26*(1), 17-31.
7. Carrasco, C. H., & Murray, J. A. (1989). Giant cell tumors. *Orthopaedic Clinics of North America, 20*(3), 395-405.
8. Doheny, M. O., & Sedlak, C. A. (1987). Body image considerations for the adult scoliosis patient having spinal fusion surgery. *Orthopaedic Nursing, 6*(6), 18-22.
9. Doleysh, N., et al. (1991). Neuromuscular disorders. In S. W. Salmond, et al. (Eds.), *Core curriculum for orthopaedic nursing* (2nd ed., pp. 299-303). Pitman, New Jersey: National Association of Orthopaedic Nurses.
10. Einhorn, T. A., et al. (1990). Nutrition and bone. *Orthopaedic Clinics of North America, 21*(1), 43-50.
11. Fueyo, L. (1991). Hand. In S. W. Salmond, et al. (Eds.), *Core curriculum for orthopaedic nursing* (2nd ed, pp. 239-250). Pitman, New Jersey: National Association of Orthopaedic Nurses.
12. Gagliardi, B. A. (1991). The impact of Duchenne muscular dystrophy on families. *Orthopaedic Nursing, 10*(5), 41-48.
13. Gertner, J. M., & Root, L. (1990). Osteogenesis imperfecta. *Orthopaedic Clinics of North America, 21*(1), 151-162.
14. Gitelis, S. & Schajowicz, F. (1989). Osteoid osteoma and osteoblastoma. *Orthopaedic Clinics of North America, 20*(3), 313-325.
15. Haberman, E. T., & Lopez, R. A. (1989). Metastatic disease of bone and treatment of pathological fractures. *Orthopaedic Clinics of North America, 20*(3), 468-486.
16. Hahn, T. J. (1988). Metabolic bone disease. In W. Kelley, et al. (Eds.), *Textbook of rheumatology* (3rd ed., pp. 1714-1748). Philadelphia: W. B. Saunders.
17. Hansel, M. J. (1988). Fractures and the healing process. *Orthopaedic Nursing, 7*(1), 43-48.
18. Hay, E. K. (1991). That old hip: The osteoporosis process. *Nursing Clinics of North America, 26*(1), 43-51.
19. Ignatavicius, D. D. (1991). Interventions for clients with musculoskeletal disorders. In D. D. Ignatavicius & M. V. Bayne (Eds.), *Medical-surgical nursing: A nursing process approach.* (pp. 733-777). Philadelphia: W. B. Saunders.
20. Jacobs-Zacny, J. M., & Horn, M. J. (1988). Nursing care of the adolescents having posterior spinal fusion with Cotrel-Dubousset instrumentation. *Orthopaedic Nursing, 7*(1), 17-22.
21. Kaiser, J. M., and Piasecki, P. A. (1991). Tumors. In S. W. Salmond, et al. (Eds.), *Core curriculum for orthopaedic nursing* (2nd ed, pp. 407-425), Pitman, New Jersey: National Association of Orthopaedic Nurses.
22. Kanis, J. A. (1990). Editorial: Osteoporosis and osteopenia. *Journal of Bone and Mineral Research, 5*(3), 209-211.
23. Klein, M. J., et al. (1989). Osteosarcoma: Clinical and pathological considerations. *Orthopaedic Clinics of North America,* 20(3), 327-345.
24. Lamphier, P. C. (1985). Primary bone tumors. *Orthopaedic Nursing, 4*(5), 17-23.
25. Limb-sparing treatment of adult soft tissue sarcoma and osteosarcoma. Consensus Conference. (1985). *Journal of the American Medical Association,* 254, 1791-1794.
26. Lindsay, R. (1989). Osteoporosis: An updated approach to prevention and management. *Geriatrics, 44*(1), 45-52.
27. Lisanti, P., & Tompkins, J. S. (1991). Pain. In S. W. Salmond, et al. (Eds.), *Core curriculum for orthopaedic nursing* (2nd ed, pp. 95-107). Pitman, New Jersey: National Association of Orthopaedic Nurses.

28. Liscum, B. (1992). Osteoporosis: The silent disease. *Orthopaedic Nursing, 11*(4), 21-25.
29. Maier, T., & Pietrocarlo, T. (1991). The foot and footwear. *Nursing Clinics of North America, 26*(1), 223-231.
30. Martin, M. E. (1989). Oral antibiotics for the treatment of patients with chronic osteomyelitis. *Orthopaedic Nursing, 8*(3), 35-38.
31. Merkow, R. L., & Lane, J. M. (1990). Paget's disease of bone. *Orthopaedic Clinics of North America, 21*(1) 171-189.
32. Mitchell, N. R., et al. (1991). Infection. In S. W. Salmond, et al. (Eds.), *Core curriculum for orthopaedic nursing* (2nd ed, 251-263). Pitman, New Jersey: National Association of Orthopaedic Nurses.
33. Mooney, N. E. (1991). Pain management in the orthopaedic patient. *Nursing Clinics of North America, 26*(1), 81-84.
34. McCaffery, M., Beebe, A. (1989). *Pain: Clinical manual for nursing practice*. St. Louis, C. V. Mosby.
35. Mosher, C. M. (1991). The Papineau bone graft: A limb salvage technique. *Orthopaedic Nursing, 10*(3), 27-32.
36. National Osteoporosis Foundation. (1991). *Boning up on osteoporosis: A guide to prevention and treatment*. University of Connecticut Health Center. Farmington, Connecticut.
37. Nestle Information Services. (1991). Osteoporosis: The silent thief. *Worldwide, 3*(2), 1-8.
38. Parker, B. C. (1988). Rehabilitative aspects of nerve injuries of the hand. *Orthopaedic Nursing, 7*(1), 29-34.
39. Pavlik, M. (1991). Measuring bone mineral content. *Orthopaedic Nursing, 10*(2), 39-43.
40. Piasecki, P. A. (1991). The nursing role in limb salvage surgery. *Nursing Clinics of North America, 26*(1), 33-41.
41. Prior, J. C., et al. (1990). Spinal bone loss and ovulatory disturbances. *New England Journal of Medicine, 323*(18), 1221-1271.
42. Rodts, M. F., (1987). Surgical intervention for adult scoliosis. *Orthopaedic Nursing, 6*(6), 11-17.
43. Rodts, M. F., & Ruda, S. C. (1991). Spine. In S. W. Salmond, et al. (Eds.), *Core curriculum for orthopaedic nursing* (2nd ed, pp. 357-361). Pitman, New Jersey: National Association of Orthopaedic Nurses.
44. Sauers, K. F. (1991). Self-concept. In S. W. Salmond, et al. (Eds.), *Core curriculum for orthopaedic nursing* (2nd ed, pp. 109-115). Pitman, New Jersey: National Association of Orthopaedic Nurses.
45. Tomaski, A. M., & Dobert, J. H. (1991). Metabolic bone disease. In S. W. Salmond, et al. (Eds.), *Core curriculum for orthopaedic nursing* (2nd ed, pp. 265-279). Pitman, New Jersey: National Association of Orthopaedic Nurses.
46. Urrows, S. T., et al. (1991). Profiles in osteoporosis. *American Journal of Nursing, 91*(12), 32-37.
47. Weinerman, S. A., & Bockman, R. S. (1990). Medical therapy of osteoporosis. *Orthopaedic Clinics of North America, 21*(1) 109-119.
48. Zwolski, K., et al. (1991). Miscellaneous disorders. In S. W. Salmond, et al. (Eds.), *Core curriculum for orthopaedic nursing* (2nd ed, pp. 430-433). Pitman, New Jersey: National Association of Orthopaedic Nurses.

Chapter 68

Nursing Care of Clients with Musculoskeletal Trauma or Overuse

MUSCULOSKELETAL INJURIES

Fractures

Definition

A fracture is a disruption of normal bone continuity that occurs when more stress is placed on a bone than it is able to absorb. Surrounding soft tissue injury often also occurs. Although some fractures are life threatening (because of associated hemorrhage and shock), most are not.

Classification

FRACTURE PATTERN

There are more than 150 different types of fractures classified in various ways. Some of the more common types are described later (Fig. 68-1). The following terms help establish generally the pattern of a fracture:

- *Closed (simple) fracture.* An uncomplicated fracture with intact skin over the fracture site, that is, bone does not protrude through the skin (Fig. 68-1*A*).

- *Open (compound) fracture.* A break in the skin is present over the fracture site. The wound communicates from the skin (externally) to the fractured bone (internally). Because of this communication with the external environment, an open fracture is always potentially infected (Fig. 68-1*B*). Open fractures are further divided into grades of severity.

Grade I: skin puncture with minimal tissue damage.
Grade II: as in grade I, with skin and muscle contusion.
Grade III: a wound larger than 6 to 8 cm with damage to blood vessels, nerves, muscles, and skin.

- *Complete fracture.* Fracture line extends through the entire bone substance, that is, the periosteum is disrupted on both sides of the bone (Fig. 68-1*C*).
- *Incomplete (partial) fracture.* Fracture line extends part way through the bone, that is, bone continuity is not completely disrupted. This type of fracture is also called a willow, green-stick, or hickory-stick fracture (Fig. 68-1*D*).
- *Displaced fracture.* Bone fragments are separated at the fracture line (Fig. 68-1*E*).
- *Comminuted fracture.* More than one fracture line, and bone fragments are crushed or broken into several pieces (Fig. 68-1*F*).
- *Impacted fracture ("telescoped fracture"), or compression fracture.* One bone fragment is forcibly driven into another adjacent bone fragment (Fig. 68-1*G* and I).
- *Pathologic fracture.* The fracture occurs as a result of underlying bone disorders such as osteoporosis or tumor. Usually occurs with minimal trauma (Fig. 68-1*H*).
- *Greenstick fracture.* Fracture in which one side of the bone is broken and the other side is bent (Fig. 68-1*J*).

The above-mentioned terms describing fractures may be used in combination to provide more complete description, such as a client may have a "closed, complete fracture that is displaced."

When a fracture of an extremity divides a bone into two fragments, the fragments are referred to as the proximal (uncontrollable) fragment and the distal (controllable) fragment. The proximal fragment is the section of bone nearer the body. This fragment cannot be manipulated or moved when the fractured bones are being set (i.e., therapeutically correctly aligned) because of its muscle attachments and location. The distal fragment (farther away from the body) can be manipulated or moved to realign it with the proximal fragment.

Summarized in the next section are some terms used to describe the direction of fracture line in relation to the affected bone's longitudinal axis.

- *Linear fracture.* Fracture line runs parallel to the bone's long axis.
- *Oblique fracture.* Fracture line is at an oblique angle (about a 45-degree angle) to the shaft (axis) of the bone (Fig. 68-1*A* and *B*).
- *Longitudinal fracture.* Fracture line extends longitudinally (Fig. 68-1*D*).
- *Transverse fracture.* Fracture line is straight across the bone, that is, right angle to the bone's axis (Fig. 68-1*C*).
- *Spiral fracture.* Fracture line forms a spiral encircling the bone (Fig. 68-1*E*).
- *Stellate.* Central fracture point with several fissures radiating outward.

FRACTURE LOCATION

In long bones fractures are described as being proximal, distal, or midshaft, based on their location on the bone. Other terms include angulation fracture, avulsion fracture, blowout fracture (results from blow that fractures the floor of the orbit of the eye), compression fracture (Fig. 68-1*I*), and a fatigue or march fracture (fracture of metatarsals due to long marches).

Some fractures are named for the physician who first described them. Two common examples are

- *Colles' fracture.* A common fracture in which the distal radius is fractured within 1 inch of articular surface.
- *Pott's fracture.* Occurs at the medial malleolus of the tibia and fibula, and often is associated with rupture of the internal lateral ligament or chipping off of a piece of the medial malleolus, or both. The tibiofibular articulation is seriously disrupted.

Fractures involving or close to joints are described as

- *Articular fracture* (joint fracture). Fracture involving a joint surface.
- *Extracapsular fracture.* Fracture near a joint but not entering the joint capsule.
- *Intracapsular fracture.* Fracture within a joint capsule.
- *Epiphyseal fracture.* Fracture involving ossification center at the extremity of long bones. These fractures may result in alterations in bone growth.

Fractures are also classified according to their causes. For example, a stress fracture may occur in a bone that is subjected to prolonged, unaccustomed muscular action. Pathologic fractures occur in diseased bones (Fig. 67-1*H*), such as bones with osteoporosis.

FRACTURE DISPLACEMENT

Displacement of the fracture ends and fragments of bone depend on the causative force and degree of spasm in surrounding muscles. Displacement may occur sideways, at an angle (angulated), as an override, rotated, or offset.

Incidence

The incidence of fractures varies with the site of the fracture. Rib fractures are the most common bone frac-

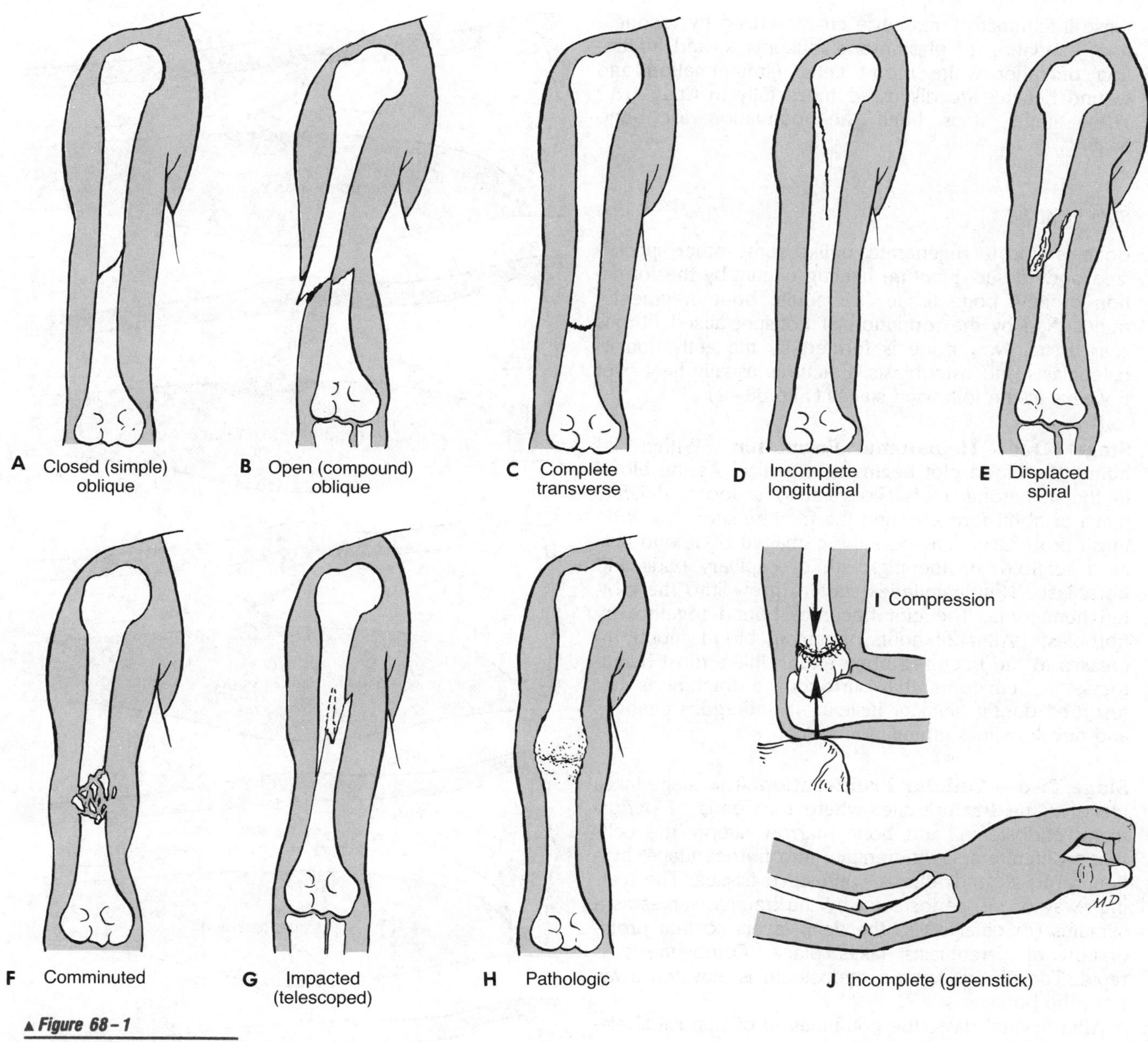

▲ *Figure 68-1*

Common types of fractures.

ture in adults. Femoral fractures are most common in young and middle-aged adults. The elderly client often fractures the hip and wrist.

Etiology

The most common cause of fracture is direct trauma to the bone. Motor vehicle accidents and falls are the primary mechanism of injury. In addition, primary bone disease such as osteoporosis or metastatic bone cancer can weaken the bony structure and lead to fracture.

The amount of trauma required to fracture a bone can vary. Fractures occur from direct or indirect force, and are affected by biologic and behavioral factors. Direct force is the result of a moving object contacting the bone. Indirect force can be caused by contracting muscles exerting a powerful pulling force on the bone.

Pathophysiology

When a bone is broken, the periosteum and blood vessels in the cortex, marrow, and surrounding soft tissues are disrupted. Bleeding occurs from the damaged ends of the bone and from nearby soft tissues (muscles). A hematoma forms in the medullary canal, between the fractured ends of the bone and beneath the periosteum. Bone tissue immediately adjacent to the fracture dies. This necrotic tissue stimulates an intense inflammatory response characterized by vasodilation, exudation of plasma and leukocytes, and infiltration of other white blood cells. (Inflammation and wound healing are discussed more fully in Chap. 18.) These initial steps build the foundation for bone healing.

BONE HEALING

Bone is able to regenerate, unlike some other specialized body tissue. Fracture healing occurs by the formation of new bone tissue (to reunite bone fragments) rather than by the formation of nonspecialized fibrous scar tissue. New bone is formed by the activation of osteoclasts and osteoblasts. Fractures usually heal over 6 weeks in the following stages (Fig. 68-2).

Stage One—Hematoma Formation. Within 24 hours, the blood clot begins to organize. As the blood in the hematoma clots (coagulates), a loose, delicate mesh of fibrin forms around the fracture site. This fibrin mesh protectively encloses the damaged bone and acts as a scaffold for the ingrowth of capillary buds and fibroblasts. New capillaries start to grow into the clotted hematoma. The clot becomes bound together by fibroblasts. After 24 hours, the main blood supply increases to the fractured bone ends. Unlike most hematomas, a hematoma that surrounds a fracture is not resorbed during healing. Instead, it undergoes changes and develops into granulation tissue.

Stage Two—Cellular Proliferation. This stage takes place at the fracture site, where torn ends of periosteum, endosteum, and bone marrow supply the cells that proliferate and differentiate into fibrocartilage, hyaline cartilage, and fibrous connective tissues. The tearing away of the periosteum, by the trauma, serves as a stimulus (or catalyst) to the deep layers so that proliferation of osteoblasts takes place. Osteogenesis is rapid. The fibrous layer a periosteum is elevated away from the bone.

After several days, the combination of periosteal elevation and the granulation tissue forms a collar around the end of each fragment. The collars eventually advance, unite, and form a bridge across the fracture site.[7]

Stage Three—Procallus Formation. Six to ten days after injury, the granulation tissue changes and a provisional callus (procallus) forms. Newly formed cartilage and bone matrix (derived in part from the undamaged periosteum and endosteum of adjacent bone margins) disperse through the soft tissue callus. They increase in number until a provisional callus is established. This provisional callus is a large, loosely woven mass of bone and cartilage that is considerably wider than the normal bone's diameter. It secures the bone fragments but does not provide strength. A provisional callus extends some distance beyond the fracture line, serving as a temporary splint. In an uncomplicated fracture, the provisional callus usually reaches its maximal size about

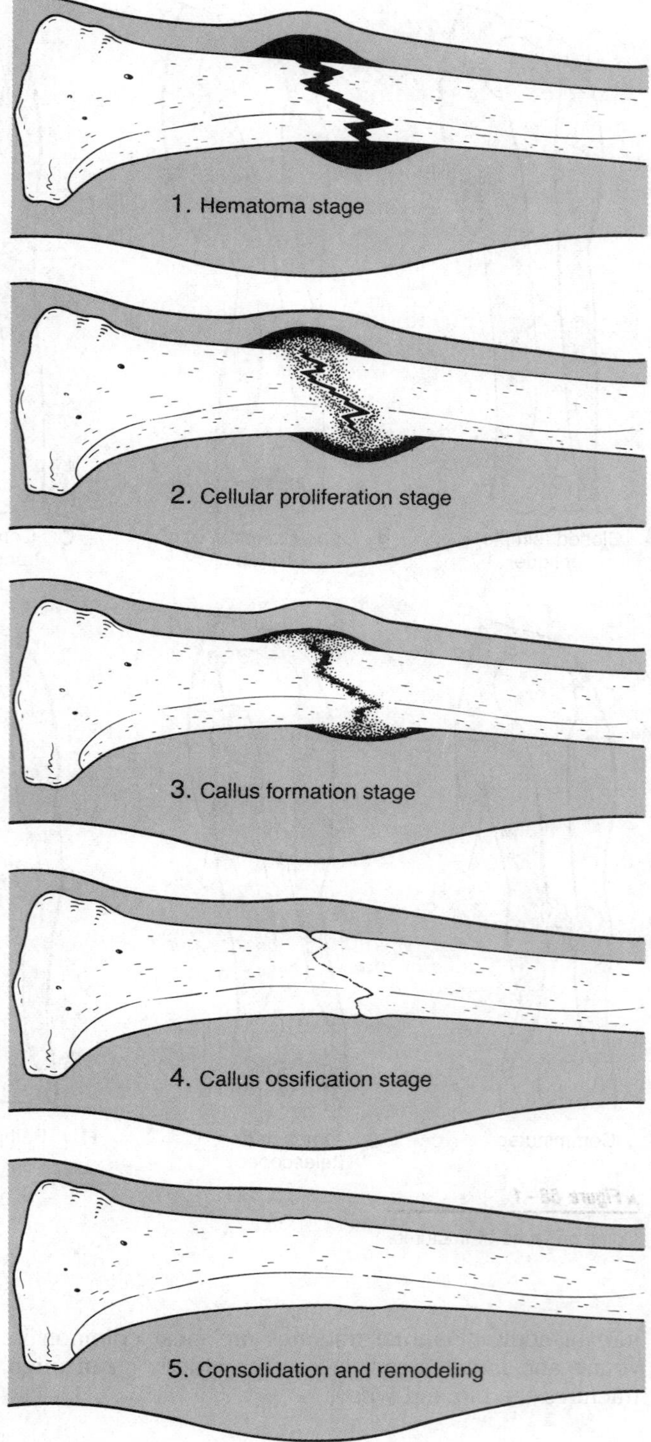

▲ **Figure 68-2**

Stages of fracture healing. Possible complications during hematoma stage include prevention of coagulation and loss of hematoma through (a) open fracture, (b) débridement, or (c) action of fibrinolytic synovial fluid. Possible complications during cellular proliferation stage include interruption of vascular network by (a) motion or infection; (b) a hostile environment because of an inadequate blood supply; (c) unbridgeable gaps between bone ends; or (d) devitalization of periosteal, intramedullary, or extraosseous mesenchymal tissues from which red cells originate. A possible complication during the callus formation stage is that the collagen matrix may be rendered nonossifiable by hypercortisonism or scurvy.

14 to 21 days after the injury. This mass is subsequently remodeled (see later).

Stage Four — Ossification. A permanent callus of true, rigid bone eventually forms by the deposition of calcium salts, which knits the fractured bone ends together. Ossification first forms an external callus (between the periosteum and cortex), next an internal callus (medullary plug), and finally an intermediate callus (between the cortical fragments). During the third to tenth weeks of healing, the callus converts into bone. This formation of bone firmly binds together the fractured ends and completes healing.

Stage Five — Consolidation and Remodeling. At the same time that true bone is forming, the callus is remodeled by osteoblastic and osteoclastic activity. In effect, excess bone is chiseled away and absorbed from the callus. This remodeling process is governed by the stresses imposed on it by muscles and weight bearing. Remodeling occurs according to Wolff's law, which basically states that a bone's structure is determined by its function, that is, the stresses and strains placed on it.

Healing Time. Healing time varies with the type of fracture and type of bone. Spongy bone heals more rapidly than compact bone because of the rich blood supply. Impacted fractures require several weeks to heal, whereas displaced fractures may require months to years for complete healing.

Different bones also heal over different time frames. The bones of the arm may heal in 3 months whereas the tibia and femur require 6 months or longer. The more surface area the fracture fragments have, the more rapidly they heal. For example spiral fractures heal more rapidly than transverse fractures.

Most function returns in 6 months after bony union takes place, but complete function may not be regained for a year or more. In a year, a simple fracture will resume an almost normal appearance if aligned correctly. A fracture that has healed in excellent position may still have some reduced joint motion.

Conditions that Modify Healing. Because healing of fractures is a continuous sequential process, any interruption in the process may result in delayed healing. Bone healing may be delayed by inadequate mobilization of the fragments, decreased blood supply, interposition of soft tissues into the fracture site, or infection.

When a bone is completely transsected, immobilization is necessary to rigidly hold the fracture fragments in place. Inadequate immobilization allows movement of the fragments, which opens the hematoma and actually reverses the healing processes.

During the time of healing, adequate blood supply to the bone is critical. If both ends of the fracture have blood supply, the fracture will heal (as long as no other complications develop). Decreased blood supply may occur from swelling of soft tissues at the fracture site or traumatic severance of the major vessels feeding the bone.

If one fragment has lost its blood supply and, therefore, is dead, the living fragment must unite with the dead fragment. Bony union will be slow and often requires rigid immobilization. If both fragments are dead, revascularization is required.

When bony fragments are distant from each other and separated by soft tissue, the soft tissue seals off the bone surface. When the surface is covered, a hematoma is not able to form and the formation of granulation tissue is inhibited. This leads to poor union of the fracture site.

Infection is a likely complication in open fractures. The open area is a rich culture medium for bacteria to infect tissues and bone itself. If osteomyelitis (bone infection) does develop, the healing process is retarded because the infection destroys newly forming bone and interrupts blood supply.

Clinical Manifestations

Many factors affect the clinical manifestations a fracture may produce, such as site, severity, type of fracture, and amount of damage to other structures. Some fractures produce few clinical manifestations and would not be detected if x-ray films were not taken to assess the injury. Various combinations may be present:

- *Deformity*. Strong muscle pull may cause bone fragments to override; therefore alignment and contour changes occur, such as (1) angulation, rotation, limb shortening; (2) bone depression; or (3) altered curves in the injured site especially when compared with the opposite site.
- *Swelling*. Edema may appear rapidly from localization of serous fluid at the fracture site and extravasation of blood into adjacent tissues.
- *Bruising (ecchymosis)*. From subcutaneous bleeding.
- *Muscle spasm*. Involuntary muscle contraction near the fracture.
- *Tenderness*. Over fracture site due to underlying injuries.
- *Pain*. Immediate severe pain at the time of injury. Following injury, pain may result from muscle spasm, overriding of the fractured ends of the bone, or damage to adjacent structures.
- *Impaired sensation (numbness)*. May occur from nerve damage or nerve entrapment from edema, bleeding, or bony fragments.
- *Loss of normal function*. May result from instability of the fractured bone, pain, or muscle spasm. Paralysis may be caused by nerve damage.
- *Abnormal mobility*. Movement of a part that is normally immobile, due to instability when long bones are fractured.
- *Crepitus*. Grating sensations or sounds felt or heard if the injured part is moved. Crepitus results from broken bone ends rubbing together.
- *Hypovolemic Shock*. May result from blood loss or other injuries.

DIAGNOSTIC ASSESSMENT

Radiology or fluoroscopy is used to confirm the diagnosis of a fracture by showing the location of the fracture and the direction of fracture line (Fig. 68-3). Findings vary according to site and type of fracture. X-ray films of fractured bones are taken in two planes and include the joint above and the joint below the fracture (to identify dislocations or subluxations). Anteroposterior (AP) and lateral views are commonly taken (1) before reduction, (2) after reduction, and (3) periodically during the healing process.

Complications

Possible early complications of fractures include arterial damage, compartment syndrome, fat embolism, infection, shock, and Volkmann's ischemic contracture.

Arterial Damage. Arterial damage may consist of contused, thrombosed, lacerated, severed, or spastic arteries. Arteries may be constricted by bandages or casts that are too tight. Indications of arterial damage include variable or absent pulse, swelling, pallor or patch cyanosis distal to the fracture, continuing blood loss, pain, a large fracture hematoma, poor capillary return, poorly filled veins in a cold extremity, and paralysis or anesthesia distal to the fracture (in the absence of known neurologic injury). Promptly report and document assessment findings indicating arterial complications. Emergency intervention may include splitting or removing tight encircling casts or bandages, elevating or changing the position of the injured part, reducing fractures or dislocations, or surgery.

Compartment Syndrome. Compartment syndrome is a serious complication of fractures. Compartments are made up of muscles, bones, nerves, and blood vessels wrapped by a fibrous membrane. A compartment, therefore, is a closed space. Following trauma, edema or bleeding can occur within the compartment. Because a compartment is a closed space, the edema or bleeding exerts pressure on the pliable muscles, nerves, and vessels. Compartment syndrome can also develop if external pressure is applied, such as from a cast or tight dressing.

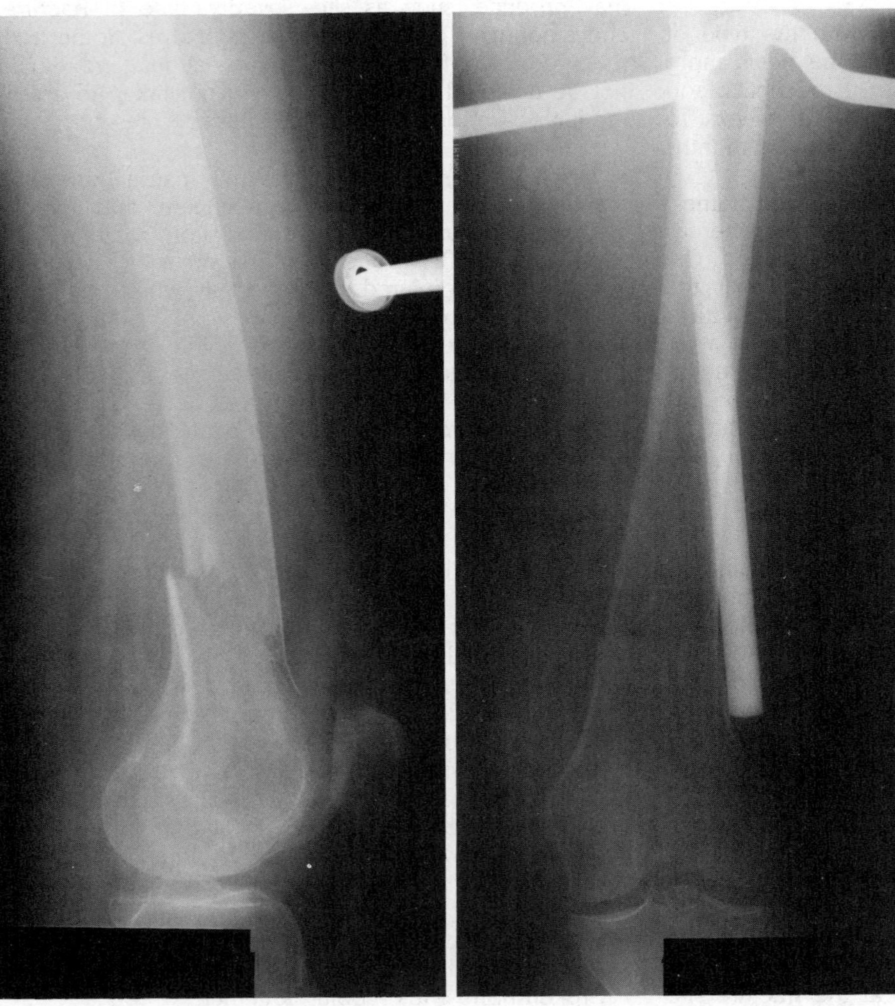

▲ *Figure 68-3*

Fracture of the supracondylar femur *(A)*, reduction of the fracture with traction *(B)*. The fracture was eventually pinned.

Clinical manifestations of compartment syndrome are ischemic pain that is not controllable with narcotic analgesics, pain with elevation due to decreased arterial inflow, and pain when the area is touched or moved. In addition to the pain, the client will have weak active movement, paresthesias (needles-and-pins sensation), diminished or absent pulses, coolness, or pallor. Nursing assessment is described in Figure 66-3.

Compartment syndrome is managed by removing the cause of the compression. The cast or dressing is loosened or removed. If it is due to edema or bleeding, a fasciotomy (incision into the fascia) is performed. Sometimes the incision is left open until the swelling decreases. If it is left untreated, compartment syndrome leads to a functionless extremity or requires amputation.

Fat Embolism. Fat embolism is a relatively uncommon but potentially life-threatening complication of long-bone and pelvis fractures. Fat embolism syndrome (FES) occurs 24 to 48 hours after injury. The etiology of FES includes direct damage to the lung, soft tissue injury, hypotension, and aspiration of blood or gastric contents. The pathophysiology of FES is similar to that of adult respiratory syndrome. Two theories exist to explain the problem: (1) the mechanical and (2) biochemical theories. The mechanical theory states that trauma causes disruption of the fragile veins and fat cells in the bone marrow at the fracture site. Fat globules enter the circulation, aided by the increased interstitial pressure at the hematoma on the fracture site. The biochemical theory proposes that there is a stress-related release of catecholamines following trauma. The catecholamines mobilize lipids from adipose tissue and cause of chylomicron emulsion stability. The chylomicrons coalesce into large droplets, which embolize to the lung.

Once fat droplets enter the circulation, the fat is too large to pass through pulmonary circulation. They lodge in the capillaries and break down into fatty acids. Free fatty acids are toxic to lung parenchyma, capillary endothelium, and surfactant. The result is pulmonary hypertension.

The nurse must have a high index of suspicion for FES. The classic picture of the client with FES includes altered mental status, tachypnea, tachycardia, hypoxemia, petechiae, and fever. Many times, it is difficult to distinguish FES from pulmonary embolism. The distinguishing features are listed in Table 68-1.

Infection. Infection following a fracture may result from contamination of open fractures, or it can be introduced at the time of surgery. Compound fractures may be complicated by tetanus or gas gangrene.

Pseudomonas is another common infectious agent. Any infection can lead to delayed union or osteomyelitis.

Gas gangrene infections may develop in deep, grossly contaminated wounds. Gas gangrene is caused by anaerobic bacteria (various species of *Clostridia*). These organisms produce a characteristic cellulitis in which gas is present under the skin. *Assessment reveals* (1) a precipitous drop in hemoglobin, (2) temperature elevation, (3) rapid pulse, (4) pain, (5) sudden local puffiness (with discoloration of tissues), and (6) thin, watery, extremely foul-smelling exudate. Crepitation may be felt, on palpation of the skin, due to the presence of gas bubbles in muscles and subcutaneous tissue. Treatment of gas gangrene involves opening the wound widely to admit air and permit drainage. Generous, multiple incisions are made through the skin and fascia. Sutures and any gangrenous material are removed and the wound is irrigated. Anti-infective agents are administered. If massive gangrene develops, amputation is necessary.

Shock. Most musculoskeletal injuries are not life threatening. However, some are because of shock resulting from blood loss and increased capillary permeability, leading to decreased oxygenation.

Volkmann's Ischemic Contracture. This serious and potentially crippling condition of the hand or forearm arises from a complication of a fracture around the elbow joint or forearm bones. It begins as a compartment syndrome that compromises arterial and venous circulation. If it is not relieved, pressure causes prolonged ischemia and muscle is gradually replaced by fibrous tissue that traps tendons and nerves. The typical end result is a permanent, stiff, clawlike deformity of the arm and hand. Often, anesthesia and paralysis are also present. Volkmann's ischemic contracture most commonly arises after a supracondylar fracture of the humerus. It may also occur following other fractures of the elbow joint and forearm, crushing injuries of the forearm, excessive use of forearm muscles, and from tight bandages or casts. To avoid permanent deformity, compartment syndromes must be recognized and treated early.

LONG-TERM COMPLICATIONS

Delayed Union. Delayed union is the failure of a fracture to consolidate within the time usually required for union. Delayed union is usually due to a retardation of the healing process from the previously discussed factors such as decreased blood supply. Delayed union usually is correctable with additional time and the application of weight bearing to the fracture site.

Nonunion. Nonunion is the failure of a fracture site to consolidate and produce a complete, firm, and stable union after 6 to 9 months. Nonunion is characterized by excessive motion in the fracture site that leads to a false joint or *pseudoarthrosis*. The risk factors to nonunion are the same as presented earlier. Nonunion is commonly treated with bone grafts (Fig. 68-4).

Malunion. Malunion is the healing of a fracture site with an increased degree of angulation or deformity. Malunion seen early in fracture healing can be corrected with adjustment of traction or reimmobliza-

TABLE 68–1. Comparison of Characteristics for Pulmonary Embolism and Fat Embolism Syndrome

Characteristics	Pulmonary Embolism	Fat Embolism Syndrome
Pathophysiology and etiology	Local venous trauma	Fat globulin release from long bone or multiple fractures
	Venous stasis	
	Hypercoagulability	Stress-related release of catecholamines that mobilize lipids from adipose tissues
Risk factors	Immobility	Hypovolemia/shock
	Age > 40	Delayed immobilization or surgery
	History of heart disease, especially myocardial infarction or congestive heart failure	Multiple traumatic injuries
		Joint replacement
	Prior history of DVT or pulmonary embolus	
	Surgery/trauma to hip, pelvis, or knee	
	Obesity	
Clinical manifestations*	Dyspnea	Dyspnea
	Chest pain	
	Apprehension/anxiety	Restless, agitated, confused, stuporous
	Cough/hemoptysis	
	Tachypnea	Tachypnea > 30/min
	Localized rales	Diffuse rales (late)
	Tachycardia	Tachycardia > 140/min
	Low-grade fever	Fever > 103° F
	Thrombophlebitis	Petechial skin rash
Diagnostic assessment	ABGs ($P_{O_2} < 80$ mm Hg)	Hypoxemia ($P_{O_2} < 60$ mm Hg)
	Chest radiograph	Chest radiograph
	Electrocardiogram	Electrocardiogram
	Lung scan	Laboratory
	Pulmonary angiography	Thrombocytopenia
		↓ Hemoglobin
		Fat in urine and blood
		Increased sedimentation rate
		Increased levels of fibrin split products
Prevention	Early ambulation	Immobilize fractures
	Leg elevation	Adequate hydration
	Elastic stockings	O_2
	Leg exercises	Corticosteroids
	Intermittent pneumatic compression	
	Medications	
	Anticoagulants	
	Antiplatelet agents	
Management	Anticoagulation	O_2
	Surgical intervention	Fluid replacement
	IVC interruption	Mechanical ventilation with PEEP
	Embolectomy	Corticosteroids
		Maintain adequate hemoglobin

* Occur within 48 to 72 hours in venous thromboembolism. Occur within 24 to 48 hours in fat embolism.
ABGs, arterial blood gases; DVT, deep vein thrombosis; IVC, inferior vena caval; PEEP, positive end expiratory pressure.
Modified from Slye, D. (1991). Orthopedic complications. *Nursing Clinics of North America, 26*(1), 113–132.

tion. Malunion after healing is usually treated with surgery.

Medical Management

Primary goals of treatment of a fracture are to return an injured limb to maximal function, prevent complications, and obtain the best possible cosmetic result.

The physician may need to manipulate a fracture to restore peripheral pulses distal to the fracture and to reduce normal compression or stretching of nerves. With a displaced fracture, there may be damage to large blood vessels and a hematoma may develop in the soft tissues. Blood loss may be considerable. Massive hemorrhage accompanying a fracture is a surgical emergency. Vital signs are closely monitored, and the client is kept NPO in case surgery is needed.

Fracture reduction restores the injured bone to normal anatomic alignment, position, and length and brings the fractured fragments into close approximation with one another. Fracture reduction is usually painful and requires anesthesia.

Fortunately, not all fractures require reduction. For example, undisplaced fractures do not need reduction because the bone fragments are already correctly aligned. Splinting is used with such fractures to prevent future displacement. A few fractures, such as distal phalanges, cannot be adequately splinted and are treated by resting the part until healing occurs.

Fractures may be reduced in three basic ways used singly or in combination.

Traction. (See Chap. 66.) With reduction traction, considerable pull is exerted on the distal fragment of a fracture to align it with the less manageable proximal fragment. The amount of traction needed to achieve alignment is usually intense and is applied for just a short time. Once a fracture has been reduced, the amount of weight applied through the traction set-up is the smallest amount required to maintain proper alignment and apposition of bone fragments.

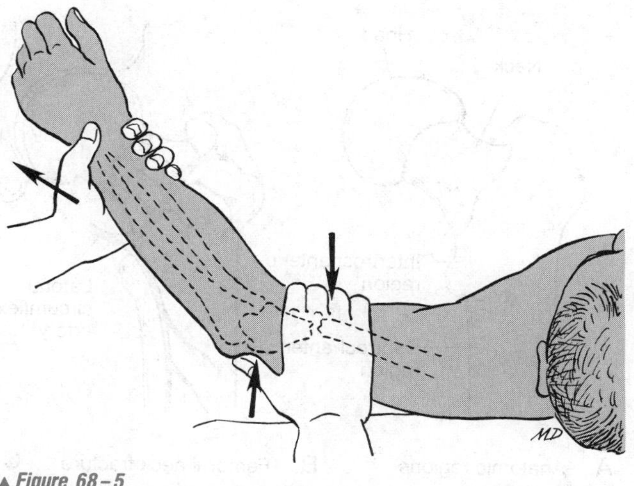

▲ Figure 68-5

Closed (manipulative) reduction to realign a supracondylar fracture.

Closed Reduction (Manipulation). A physician performs closed reduction by manually applying traction to lock the ends of a fragment together and restore normal bone alignment (Fig. 68-5). A surgical incision is not needed. Three basic maneuvers used for manipulation are (1) traction and countertraction, (2) angulation, and (3) rotation. Manipulation requires skill and tactile sensitivity to reverse the causal force of the fracture. Following a closed reduction, x-ray films are taken and a cast is usually applied.

Open Reduction. An incision is made, and the fracture is aligned during surgery under direct vision. At the time of surgery, various internal fixation devices may be applied to the fractured bone to maintain alignment (e.g., screws, plates, pins, wires, nails), or rods may be placed through bone fragments, fixed to the sides of the bone, or inserted directly into the bone's medullary cavity. For some fractures, open reduction is the treatment of choice, such as for compound fractures that are comminuted, accompanied by serious neurovascular injuries, or fractures with widely separated fragments, or soft tissue interposed between bone fragments. Open reduction is usually needed for fractures of the femur and fractured joints. Although internal fixation devices initially help immobilize a fracture and prevent deformity, they are not a substitute for bone healing. If proper bone healing does not occur, the metallic internal fixation devices succumb to stress, loosen, or break.

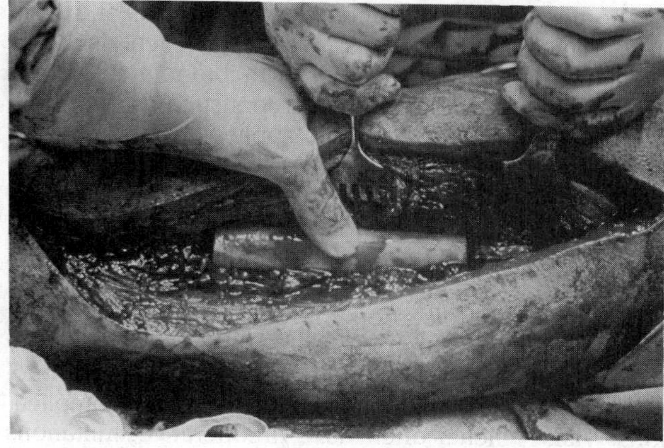

▲ Figure 68-4

Bone grafting is sometimes used to correct fracture nonunion. Available bones are stored in a "bone bank" under refrigeration until required for a recipient.

▼ Management of Specific Fractures

HIP FRACTURES

Definition

Hip fractures are generally divided into three types: (1) femoral neck, (2) intertrochanteric, and (3) subtrochanteric (Fig. 68-6). Fractures of the femoral neck and intertrochanteric regions constitute 97 per cent of hip fractures.[14]

Incidence

Hip fractures are the leading traumatic injury in the elderly, and with degenerative arthritis increasing in frequency with age, hip surgery is a very common orthopedic procedure. In 1980, 267,000 hip fractures were reported in the United States; 90 per cent of these fractures occurred in clients over 65 years of age. This figure is expected to rise to 500,000 per year by the early 1990's.[14]

Etiology

Hip fractures result from two major changes seen with aging. The most significant loss in the aged is the loss

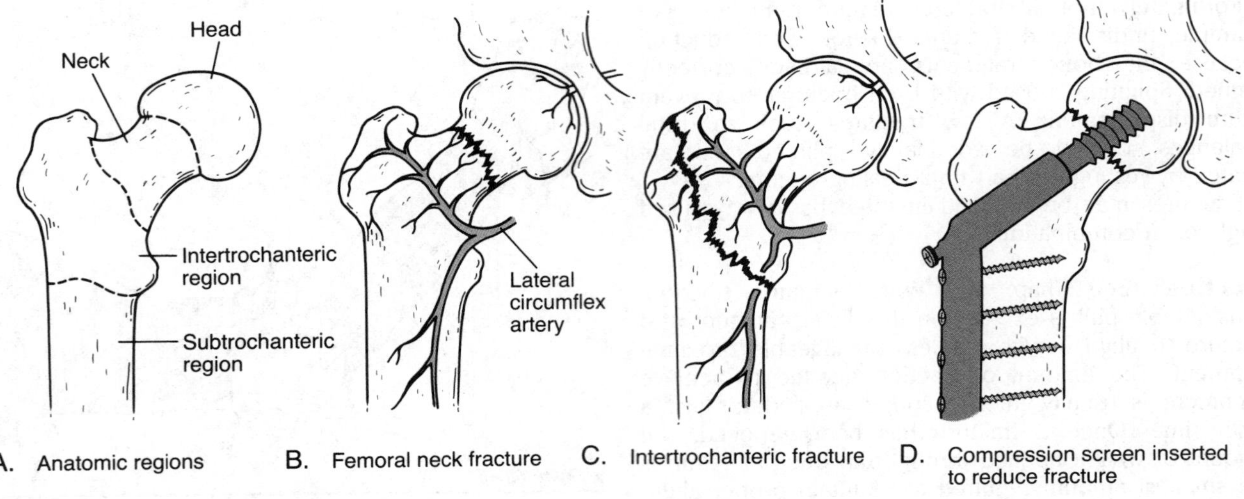

▲ Figure 68-6

A, Normal proximal end of femur. *B*, Intracapsular fracture of proximal end of femur. Note blood supply. *C*, Extracapsular intertrochanteric fracture. Note effect of fracture on blood supply. *D*, Femoral neck fracture with compression screw inserted for reduction.

of postural stability, leading to an increased incidence of falls. The amount of bone mass has been shown to be equal in clients who fall and age-matched controls. This leads to the conclusion that falling is the more significant etiology.

Decreased bone mass does contribute to hip fractures, however. Bone mass decreases linearly with age. The combination of decreased bone mass and tendency toward falls explains why the incidence of hip fracture doubles every 5 years after the age of 50.

Pathophysiology

The pathophysiology of fracture injury was discussed earlier in this chapter.

Femoral neck fractures are often called the unsolved fracture because there is a significant failure rate after primary fixation.[14] For the most part, complications are due to the anatomic features of the proximal femur. The femoral neck and head lie entirely within the joint capsule and, therefore, have no periosteum. Secondly, the arterial supply to the femoral head is usually disrupted by fracture fragments. These facts often lead to nonunion and avascular necrosis (tissue death due to a lack of blood supply) of the femoral head.

Intertrochanteric fractures are usually comminuted and more osteoporotic, leading to difficulty with good anatomic reduction of the fragments and fixation. Because this section of bone has a periosteum and the vascular supply is not affected, avascular necrosis and nonunion are uncommon complications.

Clinical Manifestations

The client or family reports a history of a fall. Even accidents that seem relatively minor, such as slipping out of a chair onto the floor, can produce hip fracture in the aged. Objective findings include a shortened, externally rotated hip and sometimes deformity along the lateral side of the hip. There may also be ecchymosis and tissue trauma from the fall. Other sites of tissue trauma may also be present, such as forehead or hand lacerations.

DIAGNOSTIC ASSESSMENT

Hip fracture is confirmed by x-ray study. Other diagnostic tests may be used to assess the client's readiness for surgery and anesthesia. A complete blood count, electrolyte levels, urinalysis, chest x-ray study, and electrocardiogram are the most common tests.

Medical Management

Treatment plans vary depending on the type of fracture, other injuries sustained during the fall, and concurrent medical conditions. While the client is being stabilized for surgery, perhaps with blood transfusions or correction of underlying disorders such as heart failure, skin traction is commonly applied to the leg (e.g., Buck's traction [see Chap. 66]). Traction assists to realign the fractures and reduce muscle spasms in the extremity. In general, the client is taken for surgical repair quickly, because placing an elderly person at bed rest increases the risks of immobility.

The number of disorders the client has (concomitant illnesses) increases the risk of morbidity and mortality with hip fracture. Nursing home residents with hip fractures are at increased risk of perioperative complications. These clients often have preoperative limitations in mobility and can seldom return to any form of ambulation. Because of the limited progress clients can make and their surgical risk, sometimes hip fractures in these clients are not surgically repaired.

SURGICAL MANAGEMENT

The primary goal of surgery is to provide a solid union of fracture sites to allow for early weight bearing and functional recovery.

Femoral Neck Fractures. Four surgical procedures are common to repair femoral neck fractures: (1) a Knowles pin; (2) a Jewett nail (Fig. 68-7*A*); (3) a sliding nail or compression screw (Fig. 68-7*B*); and (4) hemiarthroplasty or total hip arthroplasty. Following fixation with a Knowles pin, full weight bearing is not allowed because the pin does not pull the fracture fragments together (a process called compression). The Jewett nail also does not provide compression of the fragments, but it is a stronger device and the client can usually bear weight after surgery. The compression screw is the most commonly used device and has an advantage of drawing the fracture fragments together. The alignment of the fractures increases healing and allows for weight bearing. A hemiarthroplasty, with replacement of the femoral component of the hip with a noncemented metallic prosthesis, can be performed. This procedure allows the client to have full weight bearing. But when the hip prosthesis is used, there is a risk of postoperative dislocation. Because of the problems with nonunion after hip fracture, a complete hip replacement can also be performed. Total hip arthroplasty is discussed in Chapter 26.

Intertrochanteric Fractures. The most widely used device for repair of intertrochanteric fractures is the sliding nail or compression screw. Following surgery, clients cannot bear weight. These clients also have a poorer functional outcome and higher mortality than clients with fractures of the femoral neck.

Postoperative Complications. There are several complications that can result from both the surgery and the postoperative immobility; three will be discussed here. They include deep vein thrombosis, pressure ulcers, and delirium.

Deep Vein Thrombosis. The incidence of deep vein thrombosis in clients not receiving prophylaxis is reported to be 40 to 60 per cent following hip surgery. Because approximately 20 per cent of clients with deep vein thrombosis develop pulmonary embolus, the prevention of thrombosis is essential. Measures to decrease the risk of deep vein thrombosis include the use of aspirin, heparin, warfarin, low molecular weight dextran, and external pneumatic compression devices. Antiembolism stockings are also commonly used.

Pressure Ulcers. Pressure ulcers occur in 20 to 70 per cent of clients following hip fracture. It should be recognized that significant pressure has often been applied to the skin before the client is admitted to the nursing unit, from lying on a hard floor or hard surfaces in ambulances and emergency departments and x-ray departments. Prevention of ongoing ischemia is critical and can be accomplished by decreasing the risk of pressure through the use of eggcrate mattresses, excellent skin care, early ambulation, and elevation of the heels from the bed with rolled towels. Identification of high-risk clients can be made through the use of

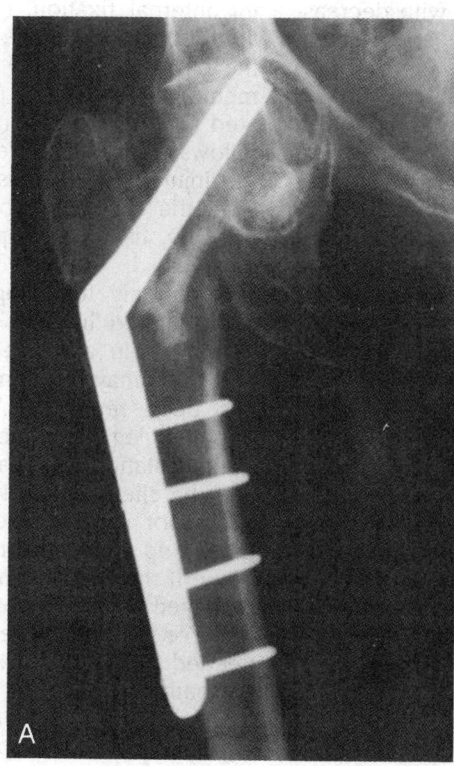

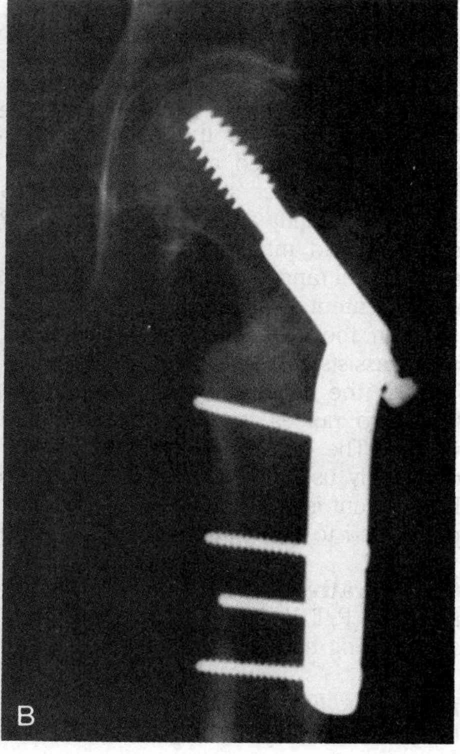

▲ *Figure 68-7*

A, A single piece Jewett nail fixation of an intertrochanteric fracture. With medial displacement of the fracture fragments, the rigid nail has penetrated the femoral head, causing pain and limitation of motion of the hip. *B*, Femoral neck fracture repaired using a Richards compression screw. The screw is driven into the femoral head and is locked in place by a set screw on its lateral end. (From Ochs, M. [1990]. Surgical management of the hip in the elderly patient. *Clinics in Geriatric Medicine, 6* [3], 571-587.)

assessment tools such as the Braden tool, presented in Chapter 18.

Delirium. Postoperative confusion usually occurs in response to systemic stressors rather than the result of central nervous system disorders. Medications, infection, impaction, and hypoxemia are common causes of delirium.

Rehabilitation. Physical therapists teach the client how to ambulate, and most clients are moved to a chair the day after surgery. Eventual recovery of clients after the repair of hip fractures is influenced by premorbid dementia, preoperative immobility, presence of intertrochanteric fracture, and advanced age.[1] Several large series report that of clients surviving 1 year after a fracture, only 50 per cent achieve prefracture functional status.[14]

Nursing Management

ASSESSMENT

On admission, the client is usually weighed before being placed in bed. A complete assessment is performed, including the assessment of abrasions or other injuries from the fall.

Nursing Diagnosis: Physical Mobility, Impaired R/T prescribed limitations in movement and pain.

Planning: Expected Outcomes. The client will maintain adequate strength to regain physical mobility once able to ambulate, as evidenced by performing exercises while bedridden, transferring to the chair with decreasing need for assistance once ambulatory, and walking with a walker safely.

Implementation. The client is encouraged to perform various exercises for the upper and lower extremities. A trapeze is placed above the bed to facilitate upper arm and shoulder strength. Exercises such as quadriceps setting, gluteal setting, and leg movements up and down in bed maintain some muscle strength. Passive and active range of motion exercises should also be implemented.

When the client is allowed to be in the chair, the nurse assists the client to the edge of the bed while keeping the legs abducted. The client is assisted by at least two nurses to stand and then balance with the walker. The degree of weight bearing that the client can safely use must be reinforced as the client stands. If the client is unable to stand, a complete lift is usually performed to assist the client to the chair.

Collaborative Problem. High risk for dislocation of the hip R/T inappropriate stress on the joint and surrounding tissues.

Planning: Expected Outcomes. The nurse will monitor the client for clinical manifestations of hip dislocation and position the client to decrease the risk of dislocation.

Implementation. Handle the operated leg gently following hip surgery. Before moving the client, explain what is going to happen and how the client can help. An overbed trapeze helps with moving. Teach the client how to use the trapeze. Avoid extremes of position following hip surgery. Keep the leg abducted, i.e., out to the side, at all times. Never adduct the leg past the body's midline (e.g., over the other leg), or the head of the femur (or prosthesis) may dislocate out of the acetabulum. Place a pillow or A-frame between the client's legs to help maintain abduction and to remind the client not to cross the legs.

Avoid acute flexion of the operated hip. This can be caused by excessive elevation of the head of the bed. Check the physician's instructions about how high the head of the bed can be safely elevated. Some can have the head of the bed raised 35 to 40 degrees. If the head of the bed can be somewhat elevated, instruct the client not to lean farther forward, because this practice further flexes the hip and may cause dislocation.

Prevent external rotation of the leg on the operated side by placing a trochanter roll beside the external aspect of the thigh. Without this intervention, the operated leg may tend to lie slightly externally rotated when the person is supine.

Turn the client only with the physician's order following hip surgery. Commonly after hip surgery the client can be turned to the unoperated side. Following hip pinning, some people are permitted to turn to either side. However, after other types of hip surgery, such as total hip replacement, turning is not permitted for several days. When helping a client to turn following internal fixation, (1) avoid adduction of the operated leg and excessive movement, (2) prevent strain on the hip, and (3) keep the leg and hip in proper alignment. If the client is permitted to turn onto the operated side, roll the client gently toward you after placing pillows between the legs. The bed acts as a splint for the injured leg. If it is not permitted to turn to either side, the client may be able to lift straight up off the bed by using a trapeze for back care and linen changes.

Commonly following an anterior surgical approach, the operated limb is positioned so it is internally rotated and in a neutral or an abducted position. The individual may be permitted to sit up unless the capsule has been removed. With a posterior approach the operated leg is positioned in slight abduction and external rotation (a change from "typical" positioning) and the client lies fairly flat.

Do not position the bed too low when a client is getting up after hip surgery. Less hip strain and bending occur if the bed is somewhat elevated. Be sure the bed is locked so it will not move while the client is getting up. For the same reasons, elevated toilet seats are needed following hip surgery once the client can go to the bathroom.

Usually when a client first gets up in a chair following hip surgery, the operated leg is kept extended, well supported, and elevated. Once the operated leg may be lowered, the client should sit with hips even with knees. Tell the client not to cross the legs but to keep both feet on the floor. Crossing the legs adducts the operated leg and can dislocate the hip. The first few times the leg is lowered, assess for swelling and discoloration.

Collaborative Problem. High risk for compartment syndrome R/T leg edema and bleeding

Planning: Expected Outcomes. The nurse will monitor the client for clinical manifestations of compartment syndrome

Implementation. The nurse monitors the color, capillary refill, warmth, movement, sensation, pedal pulses, and ability to dorsiplantar flex the operative leg using the nonoperative leg as a control. Clinical manifestations of compartment syndrome include pallor, pulselessness, paresthesias, pain, and paralysis of the leg. These findings must be reported to the physician immediately. Compartment syndrome was discussed earlier.

Nursing Diagnoses: Pain R/T trauma and surgical repair of a fractured hip

Planning: Expected Outcomes. The client will experience improved comfort, as evidenced by less facial grimacing and guarding with movement, ability to transfer to the chair or ambulate without reports of pain, and using a decreasing amount of narcotics for pain relief.

Implementation. Most surgical and traumatic pain is managed with narcotic analgesics until the pain subsides somewhat. Usually within 3 to 4 days, less potent narcotics and non-narcotic analgesics are used for pain relief.

The treatment of clients with discomfort from lying in one position (supine) can be decreased by placing a small folded bath towel beneath the lumbar spine and by moving the legs slightly in bed.

Epidural Analgesia. Some clients are being pain managed with epidural narcotics. Epidural narcotics relieve most or all of the pain but carry some significant side effects. If the client is receiving epidural narcotics, the nurse must closely monitor the client for respiratory depression, hypotension, loss of motion and sensation in the legs, and infection at the catheter site. Before ambulating a client with an epidural infusion, the nurse closely assesses for sensation by asking about numbness and by touching the client's legs with an alcohol wipe. The ability to lift the legs from the bed is also assessed. Once the client is moved to the chair, the blood pressure measurement should be reassessed to detect orthostatic hypotension. Clients with epidural anesthetics have decreased venous return due to the lack of muscle activity in the legs. They can very quickly develop orthostasis and faint.

Nursing Diagnosis: Constipation, High Risk for R/T side effects of narcotics and immobility

Planning: Expected Outcomes. The client will decrease risk of constipation by consuming high-fiber and bulk foods, adequate fluids, and having a bowel movement every 2 to 3 days.

Implementation. The nurse determines the client's usual defecation pattern and monitors for the return of bowel sounds after surgery. Once the client is eating, foods with fiber such as bran and prunes should be encouraged. Some clients find that hot fluids such as coffee stimulate the bowels. Bowel programs should be instituted in the morning after breakfast because the gastrocolic reflex is strongest at that time. Docusate sodium (Colace) and other stool softeners are commonly prescribed. In addition, the client may require suppositories or enemas to maintain a normal bowel movement schedule. When possible, the client should be placed on a bedside commode to facilitate moving the bowels.

EVALUATION

The degree of expected outcome attainment is assessed frequently, usually daily. Some of the expected outcomes for mobility may require extended periods of time to accomplish, depending on the status of the client before surgery.

Post-hospital Care

DISCHARGE TEACHING

Since many of the clients with fractured hips are covered by Medicare, their hospital stay is very short and only a portion of rehabilitation can be accomplished. Finding a location for ongoing rehabilitation is a collaborative effort among all members of the health care team, the client, and family.

Many clients benefit from transfer to an extended care facility, where they can complete their rehabilitation. Ochs[14] questions whether the clients see as much benefit when transferred to a community nursing home where little rehabilitation is offered. Many clients remain as nursing home residents after a year because rehabilitation was incomplete and the client cannot maintain self-care.

FOLLOW-UP CARE

At the time of dismissal, most clients cannot walk more than a few feet and transfer from bed to chair or wheelchair. In addition to ongoing rehabilitation, these clients need complete care to provide food, hygiene, and other needs for daily living. If the client is sent home, the nurse and social worker ascertain that the client's family can safely move the client and that other activities of daily living are provided for the client.

FRACTURES OF THE FEMUR SHAFT

Fermoral shaft fracture most often results from severe violence and occurs in young or middle-aged people. Fractures of the proximal femur are more common in the elderly. A fractured femur shaft commonly causes marked displacement and deformity, and extensive soft tissue damage with swelling. It is essential that the leg be protectively immobilized during transportation, such as with an air splint or Thomas splint. Blood loss at the time of injury is often considerable and the client often develops shock. If the fracture is relatively simple and the client is in good general condition with no skin damage, treatment by open reduction and internal fixation (ORIF) by intramedullary rod insertion may be used (Fig. 68-8). This allows immediate ambulation (with guarded weight bearing).

Fractures of the distal end of the femur may be reduced by continuous skeletal traction and manipulation, or internal fixation with rods, nails and plates, or screws. A complication of these fractures is tearing or compression of the sciatic nerve or popliteal artery. Care of the client in skeletal traction is discussed in Chapter 66.

FRACTURES OF THE PELVIS

Pelvic fractures occur in nearly 30 per cent of all multiple trauma injuries. Pelvic fractures are associated with injuries to the major arteries, lower urinary tract, uterus, testes, bowel and rectum, abdominal wall, and spine and spinal cord. Pelvic fractures can result in hemorrhage (the pelvis can hold as much as 4 liters of blood), and usual clinical manifestations include hypotension, pain with pressure applied to the pelvis, and bleeding into the peritoneum or urinary tract.

Management of pelvic fractures depends on the severity of the fracture. Unstable, weight-bearing pelvic fractures are treated with external fixation devices and through open reduction with internal fixation. Less severe fractures of non-weight-bearing portions can be successfully treated with bed rest and traction.

Nursing management centers around maintaining adequate circulation to the skin because the client in traction can seldom turn. Low air loss beds (e.g., Kinair) are beneficial. In addition, the client needs adequate pain control, assessment of neurovascular status, and assessment for complications such as thrombophlebitis and fat embolism.

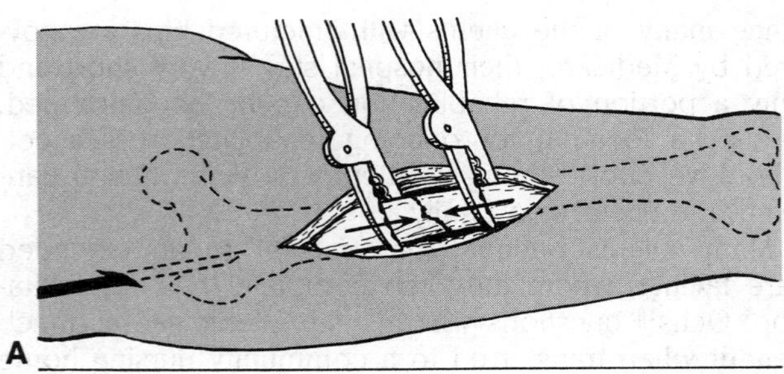

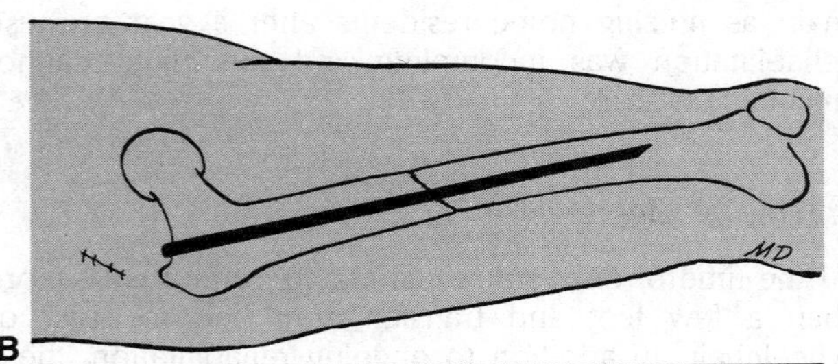

▲ *Figure 68-8*

Open reduction and internal fixation of a fractured shaft of femur. *A*, Fractured bone ends are realigned by open reduction. Intramedullary nail is inserted through the proximal end of femur. *B*, Fractured bone ends secured in correct position with intramedullary nail.

FRACTURES OF THE TIBIA AND FIBULA

Fractures of the lower leg, tibia, and fibula are most commonly casted after reduction if necessary. Complex fractures may require traction or external fixation. Open fractures of the distal third of the leg are often slow to heal in many people owing to diminished blood supply from artherosclerosis.

FRACTURES OF THE FOOT

Minimally displaced fractures of the foot are treated with open walking shoes, casts, or braces to reduce direct contact with the fracture site and splint the area. In fractures with significant displacement, open reduction and casting may be necessary. A Pott's fracture occurs at the medial malleous of the tibia and fibula. Pott's fracture can occur from supination and eversion, pronation and abduction, or pronation and eversion. The mechanism of injury can produce a variety of fracture patterns. Open and closed reduction may be needed.

FRACTURES OF THE UPPER EXTREMITY

Humerus. Fractures of the proximal humerus are common in the elderly. The fracture may be impacted or displaced. Impacted fractures are usually immobilized with a sling. Displaced fractures are treated by surgical open reduction and fixation with pins. Fractures of the dominant arm in elderly clients often make them dependent and immobile. There is also an increased risk of falling because balance is reduced due to the loss of the use of the arm.

Fractures of the shaft of the humerus are usually managed with traction via a hanging arm cast or splint. Sometimes, the fracture is surgically reduced and repaired with intermedullary rods or plates and screws (ORIF). Nonunion is a common complication of humeral shaft fractures, and bone grafting may be required.

Fractures of the condyles of the humerus usually occur from a direct blow. These fractures can result in damage to the brachial or median nerves. The fracture is treated with ORIF, although skeletal traction and casts can be used.

Radius and Ulna. Colles' fracture is a fracture of the distal radius resulting from a fall on an outstretched hand. It is most common in women. The distal radius has a large percentage of cancellous bone, the type that is most commonly affected by osteoporosis. These fractures can be treated by ORIF, splints, casts, or external fixation, depending on their severity.

The radius and ulna usually fracture together. The fracture may be treated with ORIF or casted. Closed reduction with casting is the most common form of treatment.

Olecranon. Fractures of the olecranon are common and usually result from a fall onto the elbow. Treatment includes closed reduction and long arm casting. Healing is slow and so is rehabilitation of range of motion in the elbow once the cast is removed. Six weeks to two months is the usual length of time the cast is left on, and several months may be required for full return of function.

Wrist and Hand. The most common bone fractured in the hand is the carpal scaphoid, and this injury most often occurs in young men. A fracture of one or more of the bones in the wrist and hand can occur. Closed reduction and casting is the usual treatment. Casts are usually worn for 6 to 12 weeks.

Fractures of the metacarpals and phalanges are seldom displaced. They are immobilized with splints for 10 days for phalangeal fractures, and 3 to 4 weeks for fractures of the metacarpals.

Nursing Management

The nurse assess the client's radial and ulnar arteries as well as color, warmth, movement, sensation, and capillary refill in the fingers. The client's arm should be elevated on two pillows. During the night, the client needs frequent assessment to be certain the arm does not become dependent. The arm can quickly swell and occlude arterial and nerve supply to the hand. Cast care should be taught to the client and family (see Chap. 66).

▼ Sport Injuries

OVERUSE SYNDROMES

Overuse syndromes are common sport-related problems. They begin insidiously, and although uncomfortable, they do not completely stop a person's activity. Thus, the person may continue to exercise. However, continuing exercise sets up a cycle that worsens the overuse syndrome (Ethical Issues in Nursing). Overuse syndromes relate to specific athletic activities, such as excessive running. Gradually an overload of stress produces microtrauma, causing inflammation and pain. Stopping the activity that is producing the syndrome usually corrects the problem. Intervention consists of resting the injured part, ice applications, and performing supervised, gradual rehabilitative exercises of the part before returning to athletic activity. Runners may be difficult to treat. They are often compulsive about their sport, resist resting from it, and therefore, tend not to comply with treatment.

People at greatest risk for overexercising and overuse injury are (1) competitive athletes; (2) first-time athletes; (3) "born again" athletes, that is, individuals who were once very active and begin exercising again after a decade or so of sedentary living; and (4) people recovering from injury. Some authorities suggest that exercising 5 days a week is beneficial and relatively safe, while exercising 6 or 7 days a week greatly increases the risk of injury including overuse injury. Anatomic variants, that is, bone malalignment, also increase risk for overuse injury.

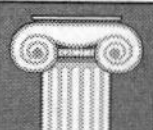

ETHICAL ISSUES IN NURSING

Should People Be Encouraged To Continue in a Sporting Event When They Are Injured?

Sports-related injuries are often a result of musculoskeletal overuse. The weekend athlete may experience muscle strain, but the week of inactivity allows the strain to heal. Members of organized sports teams may sustain more severe injuries than the weekend athlete because they may not be allowed a period of inactivity to rest their strains and sprains. Athletes may even be encouraged to continue playing with injuries, thus making the injuries worse. Steroid injections have been used on athletes with sports injuries to allow the athletes to continue playing, and in doing so, may cause the player irreversible damage to the injured areas.

Should people be encouraged to continue in a sporting event when they are injured? The reasonable answer is, of course, no; however, there is a fair amount of pressure placed on a team member to continue, especially in college and professional sports in which performance is measured in wins and losses. The emphasis is placed on the end, or outcome, of the sporting event rather than on the means, or people involved in the process. In classic teleological theory, the best outcome is winning the event, without consideration of who gets hurt in the process.

Considerations for nursing practice related to such injuries might include the use of a deontological theory. This theory would argue that the means do not justify the end. That is, to continue to play on an injury in order to win is not the right thing to do. This theory makes good health sense, because as clients should not be encouraged to participate in activities that would cause further injury.

Overuse syndromes may be prevented by avoiding factors that precipitate overuse injury, such as

- *Training errors* such as progressing too fast, lack of conditioning
- *Improper technique,* such as arm problems from poor tennis technique
- *Improper equipment,* such as incorrect shoes for the sport
- *Unsafe environmental factors,* such as a slippery surface

Overuse syndromes can be grouped into four categories according to severity. In general, intervention depends on severity more than on the specific type of injury (Table 68-2).

Some common overuse syndromes of the leg follow:

- *Patellar tendinitis* ("jumper's knee") is caused by repetitive stress on the patellar tendon during jumping. The person experiences tenderness at the insertion of the patellar tendon on the tibia.
- *Plantar fasciitis* produces heel pain during or immediately after exercise and often on arising in the morning. It is caused by repetitive stress on the long plantar ligament that attaches to the plantar (sole) surface of the calcaneus (heel bone) with its fibers fanning out and attaching to the forefoot.
- *Chondromalacia* is a painful patella caused by repeated quadriceps contractions with the knee semiflexed, e.g., during running, mountain climbing, skiing. Symptoms are usually diffuse aching, worsened by climbing stairs or hills, and weakness of the vastus medialis. Chondromalacia is more common in women athletes than in men.
- *Stress fractures* are partial or complete fractures of bone that are due to recurrent submaximal trauma. They are common in but not confined to the lower limbs. Early stress fractures are difficult to identify on x-ray examination. Clinical manifestations include localized swelling and point tenderness across a bone. Most stress fractures are "hairline fractures" of the bone, and therefore, it takes several weeks for new bone to be seen. Most stress fractures are preventable with proper preconditioning and preseason training.

Stretching is extremely important before exercise requiring joint flexibility. Flexibility is determined mainly by muscles and much less by capsules and tendons. Stretching exercises affect muscles and are, therefore, important in increasing general flexibility. Stretching exercises also help maintain and increase range of motion (ROM) around a joint. They do not increase endurance or strength. Stretching exercises should be static, i.e., should hold muscles in a stretched position for a few moments rather than repeatedly stretching and relaxing them. Static stretching (1) reduces the danger of overstretching or tissue damage, (2) causes less muscle soreness than a bouncing or ballistic stretch, and (3) relieves muscle soreness when it does occur. Box 68-1 summarizes some ways of preventing injuries in fitness programs.

▼ Strains

Overview

Strain is trauma to the body of a muscle or attachment of a tendon caused by overstretching, misuse, or overextension. Strains usually arise from twisting or

TABLE 68-2. Grades of Overuse Injuries

	Grade I	Grade II	Grade III	Grade IV
Assessment				
History	Hurts after, not during, activity	Hurts after and sometimes during activity	Hurts during and after activity	Hurts all the time
Physical examination	Generalized tenderness over area	Generalized tenderness over area	More localized tenderness	Localized tenderness
X-rays	Negative	Negative	Usually negative	May be positive
Bone scan	Negative	Negative	May be positive	Usually positive
Type of Tissue Injured	Soft tissue	Soft tissue	Soft, hard, or bony tissue	Hard or bony tissue
Management	Ice Treat underlying problem	Ice Correct underlying problem Anti-inflammatory medication, e.g., aspirin Decrease exercise 25 to 33 per cent	Ice Correct underlying problem Anti-inflammatory medication, e.g., aspirin, NSAIDs; possibly prednisone Decrease exercise 50 to 75 per cent	Ice Correct underlying problem Anti-inflammatory medication, e.g., aspirin, NSAIDs; possibly prednisone Stop exercising altogether

Adapted from The athlete's leg (1985). *Emergency Medicine,* 17,83.

Box 68–1. Preventing Injuries in Fitness Programs

Lack of fitness is one of the main causes of sport injury.

Warm-up and Stretching Exercises

Always warm up and stretch before strenuous exercises. Warm up means to begin and finish exercises gradually. Stretching exercises increase muscle flexibility.

Pacing

Build up an exercise program gradually. It takes at least 6 to 8 weeks to get into strong condition. Add small, gradual increments of exercise. Proceed gradually and do not overdo. Tired muscles are prone to injury.

Intensity

When preparing for a specific event, plan training programs accordingly, that is, a marathon demands a more intense training program than does a shorter race.

Capacity Level

Exercise to the capacity of physiologic limits.

Strength

Build strength gradually to gain greater endurance, speed, and power.

Motivation

Success in an exercise program depends on individual motivation.

Relaxation

Relaxation exercises relieve fatigue and tension.

Routine

Regular exercise is more valuable and less likely to lead to injury than bursts of activity followed by long periods of inactivity.

wrenching movements. They may be acute (e.g., occur during unaccustomed vigorous exercise) or chronic (e.g., develop after repetitive muscle overuse). Strains may occur in any age group and in any body part that contains muscles and tendons.

There are three classifications of strains.

First-Degree Strain. This condition is identified by the gradual onset of muscle spasms, discomfort, and loss of range of motion. No edema or ecchymosis is present. It involves pulling of the musculotendinous unit.

Second-Degree Strain. This condition is identified by extreme muscle spasms, pain, and edema develop immediately after injury. The area remains tender after acute symptoms subside. Ecchymosis develops within a few hours. This type of strain involves tearing or straining of the musculotendinous unit.

Third-Degree Strain. This condition is identified by severe muscle spasms, point tenderness, and edema at the rim of injury. There is a sensation of sudden tearing, or a snapping or burning sensation. There is very limited range of motion due to spasms. This degree of injury usually represents a complete rupture of the musculotendinous unit.

Management

X-ray examination is required to rule out the possibility of fracture. Ecchymosis develops later.

Acute strains require rest, and possibly splinting. Elevate the injured part. Ice pack applications for the first 24 to 48 hours after injury reduce swelling. Heat may then be prescribed for comfort, to encourage reabsorption of blood and fluid, and to promote healing. Surgical repair may be necessary if rupture is present at the tendon-bone interface. During healing (4 to 6 weeks) movement of the injured part should be minimal. Activity should never be such that it produces symptoms, such as swelling or pain. After mature scar tissue has formed, the part can be gradually and progressively exercised. Avoid overactivity during rehabilitation.

▼ Sprains

A sprain is a ligament injury resulting from overstress causing damage to ligament fibers or their attachment. They commonly result from sudden injury or forced hyperextension. Sprains may be mild (grade 1), moderate (grade 2), or severe (grade 3). A mild sprain tears a few ligament fibers, but there is no loss of function and the ligament is not weakened. Therefore, protection of the ligament is not vital. A moderate sprain tears a portion of a ligament, producing some loss of function. Protection is vital to prevent further tearing. A severe sprain completely tears a ligament either from its attachment or within the ligament body itself. Complete rupture often requires surgical repair. Approximation of the ligament ends is important to ensure strength and stability of the ligament (Fig. 68–9).

Upper extremity sprains often result from overstressing a joint during sports activity, while attempting to break a fall, or while bracing during a motor vehicle accident. Ankle sprains are often the result of missteps, motor vehicle accidents, or sports injuries. Cervical sprains most often result from whiplash injuries.

On physical examination, the severity of a sprain may not be apparent. With severe sprains the person may say the joint feels loose or like "something coming apart." The person may describe what feels like a snap,

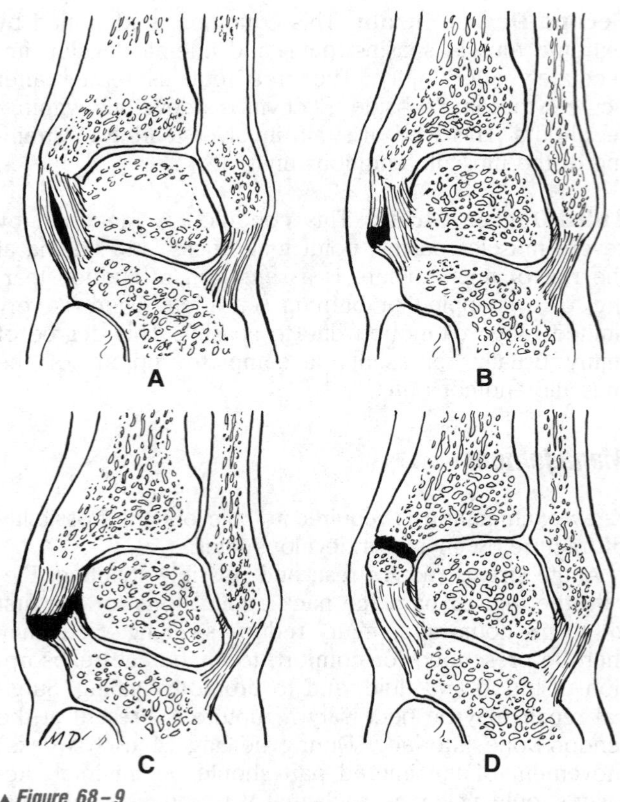

▲ *Figure 68-9*

Various types of sprain. (This figure shows the ankle.) *A*, Mild (grade 1) sprain. There is a small hematoma in a localized ligament area. A few fibers are separated. *B*, Moderate (grade 2) sprain. More severe fiber tearing than in *A*. No more than half the fibers are torn. *C*, Severe (grade 3) sprain. Tearing is completely through the ligament. *D*, Sprain fracture. Ligament is completely torn off, and a fragment of bone is torn off also.

pop, or tearing. This usually indicates severe injury. The amount of swelling also indicates severity. Diffuse swelling (grade 1 sprains) results from microscopic ligament tearing, whereas severe swelling (grade 3 sprains) comes from bleeding into the tissues. Ecchymosis does not necessarily indicate either the severity or site of the injury. For example, gravity causes bruising in a part of the foot distal to a sprained ankle.

Following a sprain injury, tenderness to palpation develops, which is well localized at first and later becomes more diffuse. Other assessment findings include swelling, severe pain, discoloration, decreased motion (limited joint motion and function), and disability. Disability may not be very severe initially but may be extensive after 2 to 3 hours. X-ray study may show soft tissue swelling but no evidence of bone or joint injury.

Immediate intervention includes elevating the injured joint and applying ice. The joint may be immobilized by splinting, casting, or taping. Immobilization may continue from 3 to 4 weeks. Casting helps approximate the ligament ends and alleviates pain. A mature scar forms in connective fibrous tissue in 4 to 6 weeks. Following complete healing the person needs a carefully planned exercise program.

▼ Dislocations and Subluxations

Dislocation and subluxation are both displacements of a joint from its normal position. Dislocation is the separation of both articulating surfaces. Subluxation occurs when the articulating surfaces lose partial contact. These injuries usually occur from direct or indirect pressure to the joint. For example, trying to break a fall down the stairs by holding on to a railing would dislocate the shoulder. A displaced bone may impede blood supply, tear ligaments, rupture blood vessels, damage nerves, and rupture muscle attachments. Dislocations and subluxations disrupt a joint by tearing the capsule and ligaments. They are often accompanied by a fracture of the joint surface.

Dislocations and subluxations may or may not produce visible deformity. Dislocation may alter the length of an affected extremity. Localized joint pain and loss of function may occur. A dislocation differs from a fracture in that it partially immobilizes a joint. (A fracture site typically has abnormal free movement.) X-ray films show the abnormality, that is, complete or partial separation of the articulating surfaces. Some dislocations reduce themselves, leaving a sprain. Others require therapeutic reduction. Before treatment, assess and document the neurovascular status of parts distal to the injury. Once diagnosis is confirmed by x-ray examination, the dislocation or subluxation is reduced.

Prompt intervention is essential to prevent complications, that is, ischemia or aseptic necrosis (resulting from impaired blood supply to parts distal to the dislocation), and impaired nourishment of the articulating cartilage in the injured joint. Reduction is usually performed without surgery (closed reduction). Occasionally, surgery (open reduction) is required, that is, for some knee injuries that completely rupture ligaments. Closed manipulation is performed under general anesthesia. The physician pulls on the joint with a gradual steady pull and moves the bone back into correct alignment.

Following reduction of a dislocation or subluxation, the joint is immobilized by a splint or cast. Immobilization may be needed for 3 to 6 weeks. Encourage prescribed active exercise of adjacent nonimmobilized joints. After immobilization is removed, encourage active motion of the injured part, that is, voluntary muscle contraction. Passive stretching can be harmful.

▼ Low Back Pain

Low back pain occurs in the low lumbar, lumbosacral, or sacroiliac areas. It often relates to degenerative processes and musculotendinous strain caused by stress from the human upright posture. The lumbar area is the most easily injured part of the back and is the most common site of back pain. Back pain can also occur from (1) a ruptured vertebral disc or herniation of the nucleus pulposus; (2) back or pelvic fractures, tumors, or infection (e.g., osteomyelitis); (3) inflammation such as ankylosing spondylitis; (4) congenital back deformities; (5) muscle spasm associated with strain or sprain; or (6) back strain from stretched abdominal muscles due to obesity or pregnancy.

Much low back pain can be prevented by proper posture, strong abdominal and leg muscles, using proper lifting techniques, and keeping oneself in good physical condition. Education can help people considerably with low back pain problems. Back schools are often offered through health care facilities. They aim at teaching people with chronic (and sometimes acute) back pain proper body mechanics, exercises, and other noninvasive practices to manage their pain (see Client Education Guide).

Pain

Back pain may be relieved by bed rest, local heat, local ice, analgesia (e.g., aspirin), and muscle relaxants. Traction is occasionally needed to relieve muscle spasm but bed rest is usually sufficient. After the acute pain is relieved, a lumbosacral corset and muscle-strengthening exercises may be prescribed to strengthen back support structures. Narcotic analgesics should be avoided.

SPECIFIC BACK PAIN PROBLEMS

- *Degenerative changes* (osteoarthritis). Osteoarthritis in intervertebral discs and posterior articulating facets often occurs along with spinal stenosis. These conditions occur mainly in middle-aged people. Assessment findings include early morning stiffness and pain made worse by sitting or standing. Walking usually brings some relief. Spinal stenosis is relieved most by lying down. Sciatic radiation may occur. Symptoms are increased by fatigue, obesity, and muscle tension.
- *Osteoporosis*. Osteoporosis is the most common disorder causing low back pain (see also Chap. 67).
- *Spondylolysis and spondylolisthesis*. The breaking down of a vertebra (spondylolysis) or the forward slipping of a vertebra (spondylolisthesis) often results from stress fractures. Frequently, they involve the fifth lumbar vertebra. These conditions may be asymptomatic or cause low back pain with or without sciatic radiation. Acute symptoms are relieved by bed rest and analgesics.
- *Compression fractures*. Compression vertebral fractures may be caused by minimal trauma. Cancer or osteoporosis is considered as the cause of repeated fractures due to only minimal trauma. Stable fractures respond to bed rest and analgesics.
- *Scoliosis*. Degenerative changes develop more rapidly in people with scoliosis than in those without such deformities. Uncorrected scoliosis in adults can cause back pain, which can be helped by surgical intervention.

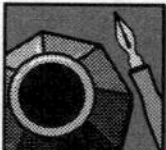

CLIENT EDUCATION GUIDE

Techniques for Managing Chronic Back Pain

Walking, Standing, and Sitting

Maintain erect posture.
Avoid prolonged standing or sitting. Change position frequently.
Avoid cramped, uncomfortable, or tense positions.
Walk, stand, and sit as tall as possible. When walking, hold head erect, chin tucked in slightly, and hold stomach in. The abdominal muscles help support the lower back.
When sitting, use a footstool to keep knees level with hips. Keep both feet on the floor. Keep your back against the chair back (do not slouch). Use a rolled towel as needed to support the lower back.
Stand with lower back as flat as possible. (Avoid "hollow" of the back.) Tuck hips in by tightening abdominal muscles.
Avoid excessive hip and knee extension.
When standing for some time, place one foot on a small stool to relieve lumbar lordosis. Lean body slightly forward and place hands in front of body.
Avoid bending, lifting, twisting at waist level.
Do not wear high-heeled shoes.
Squat with a straight lower back.
Alternate activity with periods of rest.

Exercising

Begin a fitness program with the approval of a physician.
Start a fitness program slowly.
Use a program that provides general fitness as well as a specific back-conditioning exercise.
In each session, begin exercises gradually (warm up) and at the end slow down gradually (cool down). Do not start and end exercises abruptly.
Avoid exercises that hyperextend the back, e.g., straight leg sit-ups or back bends.
Avoid exercises that have caused you back pain previously. While standing straight, place your hands on your hips and bend over backwards. Hold for 30 to 60 seconds. While sitting, bend at the waist and place your head on your knees. Hold for 2 to 5 minutes. While lying flat on the floor, place your legs on a chair and hold for up to 15 minutes.

▼ Anterior Cruciate Ligament Injury

The ligaments of the knee stabilize the joint and control into motion. The anterior cruciate ligament (ACL) is the strongest and least compliant ligament with the knee. It functions primarily to prevent anterior displacement of the tibia on the femur as well as to control the rotary stability of the knee joint.

The ACL is susceptible to injury and is the most frequently completely torn ligament of the knee. Two basic mechanisms of injury exist. In the first type of injury, an excessive valgus force is applied to the knee. This type of force damages the medial collateral ligament (MCL) and the ACL. Clipping in football is a common cause of this type of injury. The second type of injury to the ACL occurs with hyperextension while the leg is internally rotated. This mechanism causes isolated ACL rupture and more subtle symptoms. This type of injury commonly occurs while skiing, and during basketball or gymnastics.

At the time of injury, there is a snapping sensation and, at times, a popping noise. Within hours, the knee becomes tense, swollen, stiff, and painful. If it is not treated, the knee will give way, leading to falls. The knee loses support during lateral pivots. The Lachman test results are positive, showing an anterior shift of the lateral tibial plateau. The Lachman test is one of the most sensitive tests used to assess ACL damage. The examiner holds the distal end of the femur and it is displaced posteriorly while the examiner attempts to pull the tibia forward. When the ACL has been damaged, the tibia will travel forward. The drawer test for ACL damage is not as reliable because the femur is held in a neutral position. False-negative results occur frequently using the drawer test.

ACL tears can be repaired within several weeks of injury and still allow the return of function and stability. Various devices, including autograft and artifical ligament materials, have been used for reconstruction. Reconstruction after the surgery requires an effective balance between mobilization and immobilization. Some clients are treated with continuous passive motion machines (CPM). They are placed in the recovery room and provide support to the limb as well as put the knee through preset degrees of passive range of motion. The CPM is used at least 3 hours a day or until full ROM is achieved.

When the CPM is not used, the limb is placed in long leg limb brace set at 40 degrees flexion for 1 week. The client is taught to do isometric quadriceps setting, bent knee leg raises, and foot exercises. Over the course of the next 4 to 6 weeks, progressive ROM is added to the brace.

A newer form of reconstruction is through artificial grafts to reconstruct the ACL. These clients can undergo rapid rehabilitation, obtaining full range of motion in 3 to 4 days most of the time.

Summary

Musculoskeletal trauma may range from simple strains and sprains to very complex open, compound fractures that are life threatening. The nurse's role in the care of these clients is primarily to reduce the complications of immobility and teach the client how to prevent further injury.

Bibliography

1. Barangan, J. (1990). Factors that influence recovery from hip fracture during hospitalization. *Orthopaedic Nursing 9*(5), 19-29.
2. Bullock, B., & Rosendahl, P. (1984). *Pathophysiology*. Boston: Little, Brown and Company.
3. Folcik, M. (1991). Meniscal injuries. *Nursing Clinics of North America, 26*(1), 181-198.
4. Folcik, M. (1988). Winter sports injuries. *Orthopaedic Nursing, 7*(6), 25-28.
5. Funk, J., MacBrair, B., & Peterson, A. (1990). Tibial osteotomy. *Orthopaedic Nursing, 9*(2), 29-36.
6. Gross, R. (1991). Initial assessment and management of a patient with a gunshot wound to the femur. *Orthopaedic Nursing, 10*(6), 9-13.
7. Hansell, M. (1988). Fractures and the healing process. *Orthopaedic Nursing, 7*(1), 43-50.
8. Herron, D., & Nance, J. (1990). Emergency department nursing management of patients with orthopedic fractures from motor vehicle accidents. *Nursing Clinics of North America 25*(1), 71-84.
9. Johnson, L. (1989). Operative management of unstable pelvic fractures. *Orthopaedic Nursing, 8*(4), 21-26.
10. Martin, M. (1989). Oral antibiotics for treatment of patients with chronic osteomyelitis. *Orthopaedic Nursing, 8*(3), 35-40.
11. Mims, B. (1989). Fat embolism syndrome: A variant of ARDS. *Orthopaedic Nursing, 8*(3), 22-27.
12. Mooney, N. (1991). Pain management in the orthopedic patient. *Nursing Clinics of North America 26*(1), 73-88.
13. Nelson, L., Taylor, F., Adams, M. & Parker, D. (1990). Improving pain management for hip fractured elderly. *Orthopaedic Nursing, 9*(3), 79-83.
14. Ochs, M. (1990). Surgical management of the hip in the elderly patient. *Clinics in Geriatric Medicine, 6*(3), 571-585.
15. Peters, V., & Ferkel, R. (1989). Arthroscopic surgery of the ankle. *Orthopaedic Nursing, 8*(5), 12-20.
16. Reinhard, S. (1988). Case managing community services for hip fractured elders. *Orthopaedic Nursing, 7*(5), 42-49.
17. Rothenberg, J. (1991). Innovations in treating anterior cruciate ligament injury. *Orthopaedic Nursing, 10*(2), 17-26.
18. Shea, K., & Folcik, M. (1989). Water sports injuries. *Orthopaedic Nursing, 8*(6), 11-17.
19. Slye, D. (1991). Orthopedic complications: Compartment syndrome, fat embolism syndrome and venous thromboembolism. *Nursing Clinics of North America, 26*(1), 113-132.
20. Smrcina, C. (1991). Stress fractures in athletes. *Nursing Clinics of North America, 26*(1), 159-166.
21. Smrcina, C. (1988). Case study: Shoulder injury. *Orthopaedic Nursing, 7*(3), 57.
22. Wittington, C., & Carlson, C. (1991). Anterior cruciate ligament injuries: Evaluation, arthroscopic reconstruction and rehabilitation. *Nursing Clinics of North America, 26*(1) 149-158.

Unit 16

Integumentary Disorders

Skin, the largest and most visible organ of the body, plays a critical role in a client's physical and mental health. Nurses in both outpatient and inpatient practice settings have a unique opportunity to affect a client's dermatologic care significantly. Nurses have more prolonged contact with the skin than do most other health care professionals. Despite being the largest organ of the body, many rarely take skin as seriously as other organ systems such as the heart or the lung. Clients must appreciate the important role that the skin plays and should recognize that some skin conditions are indeed life-threatening. Forecasts indicate that in the year 2000, as many as 1 in 75 Americans will be afflicted by malignant melanoma, a life-threatening, often fatal skin cancer; and burn injury continues despite many advances in fireproofing homes and clothes.

Skin is integral to self-image and self-esteem. Each client's unique appearance is established through the skin. The skin was once thought to reflect the "normal aging process" and how that aging process affected the genetic skin types our parents gave to each of us. We now know it more likely reveals the cumulative amount of sun exposure that each client has gotten over a lifetime. It is hoped that with education, untanned skin will once again be viewed as attractive and healthy. Likewise, cosmetic surgery should not be considered surgery for vanity, but surgery to improve self-esteem.

Today's society has a long-standing prejudice about imperfect skin that needs to be dispelled. Historically, skin diseases have been perceived as divine punishment for being spiritually and physically "unclean." Subtle punishment for skin diseases still exists basically because of ignorance about the skin condition. For example, a woman with atopic dermatitis may sit isolated and shunned in a waiting room because others view her scratching and eczematous lesions as contagious. A waitress is encouraged to work in the back of the kitchen so that customers will not notice the healed burn scars on her hands and body. Vitiligo, loss of pigment in the skin, is sometimes incorrectly labeled "white leprosy," and the list goes on. Clients experiencing visible chronic skin problems often experience withdrawal from social situations, altered interpersonal relationships, and increased social isolation. When these clients seek professional care for skin problems, psychosocial as well as physical concerns need to be met.

The intent of the following chapters is to provide information that will promote optimal nursing care and outcomes for clients experiencing skin disorders, trauma, and surgery. The bibliography in each chapter provides information in greater depth.

Chapter 69

▼ Structure and Function; Assessment of Clients with Integumentary Disorders

▼ STRUCTURE AND FUNCTION OF THE SKIN

STRUCTURE

Skin is the largest body organ and comprises 15 to 20 per cent of body weight. If stretched out flat, adult skin surface would be about 6 by 3 feet. Skin has three layers—(1) epidermal (epidermis), (2) dermal (dermis), and (3) subcutaneous (subcutaneous fat) (Fig. 69-1)—as well as epidermal appendages (i.e., eccrine glands, apocrine glands, sebaceous glands, hair follicles, and nails).

Epidermis

The epidermis is the thin, stratified outer skin layer in direct contact with the external environment. The thickness of the epidermis ranges from 0.04 mm on the eyelids to 1.6 mm on the palms and soles. The epidermis consists of five layers and four cell types. Dermasomes, which are points of intercellular attachment that are critical for cell-to-cell adhesion, are also found in the epidermis (Fig. 69-2).

KERATINOCYTES

Keratinocytes are the principal cells of the epidermis. All five layers of epidermis consist of keratinocytes. Each layer of cells gradually differentiates into the next. The name of each layer, from inner to outermost, reflects evolving differentiation: (1) stratum germinativum (basal cell layer),

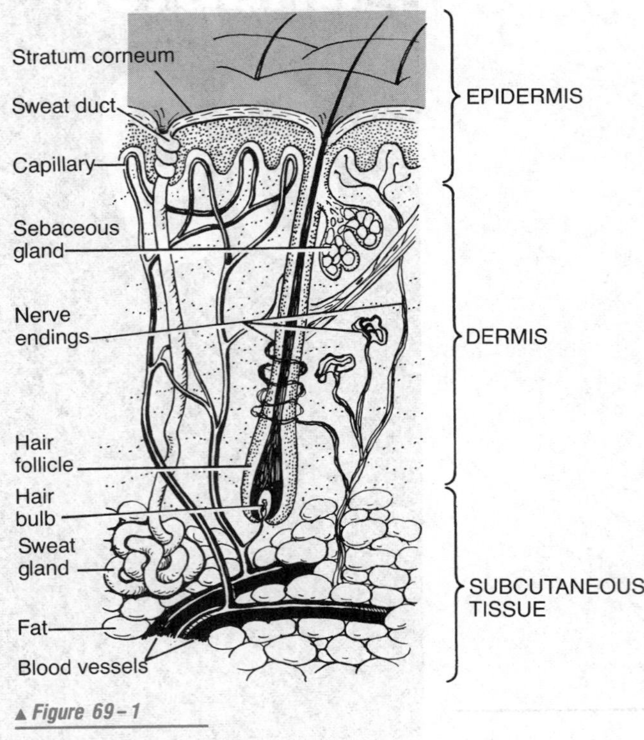

▲ Figure 69–1

Overall skin structure.

(2) stratum malpighii (prickle cells), (3) stratum granulosum (nucleated granular cells), (4) stratum lucidum (thin transparent layer), and (5) stratum corneum (the horny layer of dead keratinized cells). Keratinocytes produce keratin in a complex process as the cells begin in the basal cell layer, constantly change, and move upward through the epidermis. The entire process of differentiation from basal cell layer to horny cell layer requires 3 to 4 weeks. Thus, the epidermis constantly regenerates itself, providing a tough keratinized barrier.

MELANOCYTES

Melanocytes are epidermal pigment-producing cells that are intermittently found wedged between basal cells. Melanocytes produce melanosomes (pigment granules) that contain melanin (skin pigment). Skin color is produced by four pigments: (1) exogenously formed carotenoids (yellow), (2) melanin (brown), (3) oxygenated hemoglobin in capillaries (red), and (4) reduced hemoglobin in venules (blue). Melanin has the greatest role in skin color and is produced in the epidermis and in corresponding layers of hair follicle. Melanin is not produced in the dermis; however, it can be deposited in the dermis from the epidermis through various processes such as inflammation. Skin color differences result from the size and quantity of melanosomes as well as from the rate of melanin production. In blacks, there is an increase in the size and number of melanosomes—not melanocytes—as well as increased melanin production. The melanosomes in blacks are large, discrete, and dispersed. In whites, the melanosomes are small and aggregated and produce less melanin. Sun exposure initially increases the size and functional activity of both melanocytes and melanosomes. With chronic sun exposure, there is an increase in concentration of melanocytes as well as in the size and functional activity.

MERKEL CELLS

Merkel cells are in the basal layer but can usually be located only by electron microscopy. They are thought to be touch receptors on palms, soles, and oral and genital epithelium but are very scarce. A rare but highly malignant tumor called Merkel cell carcinoma derives from these cells.

LANGERHANS CELLS

Langerhans cells are scattered among the keratinocytes located primarily in the epidermis; however, they can

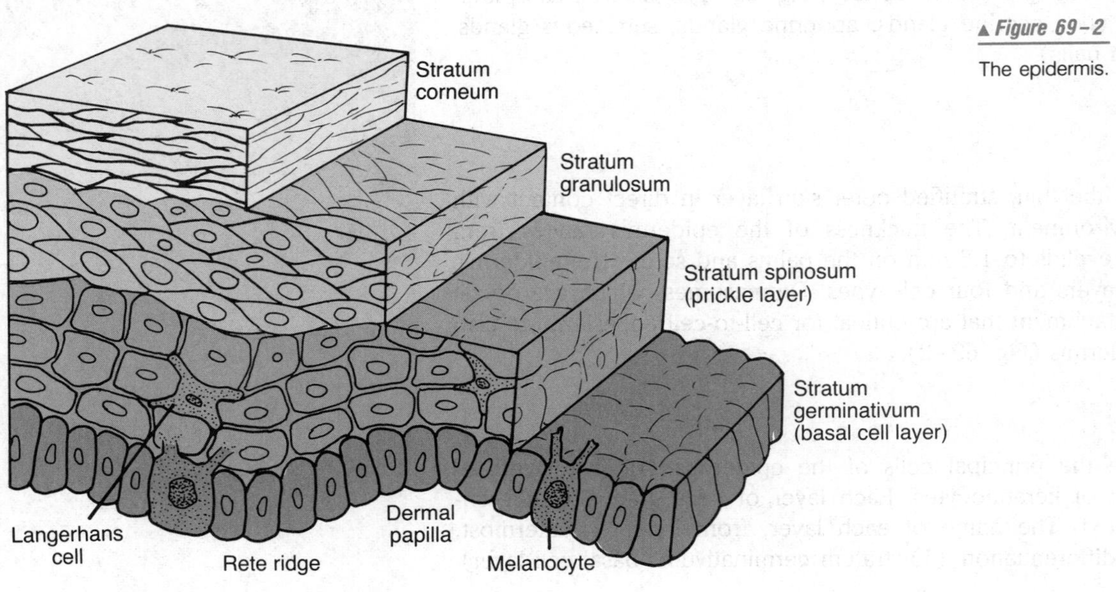

▲ Figure 69–2

The epidermis.

be seen in the dermis. These cells originate in the bone marrow and migrate to the epidermis. Langerhans cells play a role in the cell-mediated immune reactions of the skin.

Epidermal Appendages

Epidermal appendages are downgrowths of epidermis into the dermis and consist of (1) eccrine glands, (2) apocrine units, (3) sebaceous glands, (4) hair, and (5) nails.

ECCRINE GLANDS

Eccrine glands are sweat-producing glands that play an important role in thermoregulation; they are found throughout the skin except on the vermilion border of the lip, nail bed, glans penis, and labia minora. They are more numerous on the palms, soles, forehead, and axillae. Eccrine glands consist of two types of cells: (1) large, pale cells and (2) small, dark-staining cells. Sweat has the same composition as plasma in a less concentrated form. The main stimulus for eccrine gland secretion is heat. However, exercise and emotional stress also stimulate sweat production via cholinergic innervation. These glands exit the body independently of the hair shaft.

APOCRINE GLANDS

The function of the apocrine glands, which occur primarily in the axillae, breast areolae, anogenital area, ear canals, and eyelids, is not known. It is theorized that these glands may be evolutionary remnants in humans and serve lower order animals in sexual arousal. Mediated by adrenergic innervation, they secrete a milky substance that becomes odoriferous when altered by skin surface bacteria. These glands do not function until puberty and require a high output of sex hormone for activity.

SEBACEOUS GLANDS

Sebaceous glands are found throughout the skin except on the palms and soles. They are most abundant on the face, scalp, upper back, and chest. Sebaceous glands are associated with hair follicles that open onto the skin surface, where sebum is released. Sebum is a mixture of sebaceous gland-produced lipids and epidermal cell-derived lipids. Androgen is responsible for sebaceous gland development. In utero androgen causes the neonatal acne. Sebum production is higher in men.

HAIR AND HAIR FOLLICLES

Hair is a nonviable protein end product found on all skin surfaces except the palms and soles; it serves primarily as an ornament for humans. Each hair follicle functions as an independent unit and goes through intermittent stages of development. It develops from the mitotic activity of the hair bulb. Hair in different regions of the body spends different fractions of time in phases of growth. Scalp hair grows for 3 to 10 years, involutes in a 2-to-3 week period, and rests for 3 to 4 months. In a typical adult scalp, 85 to 90 per cent of hairs are in an anagen (growth) phase. The remainder are in a telogen (rest) phase. About 75 to 100 hairs are lost each day. As a rule, the growing phase of hair on the eyebrows, trunk, and extremities does not exceed 6 months. Its resting phase is 3 to 4 months. Hair shape depends on what it looks like on cross section. Straight hair has a round cross section, curlier hair has an oval or ribbonlike cross section. Curved follicles also affect the curliness of hair. Melanocytes in the bulb determine hair color. Hair follicles usually occur with sebaceous glands, and together they form a pilosebaceous unit.

NAILS

Nails are horny scales of epidermis (see Fig. 69-1). A nail matrix is the source of specialized, nonkeratinized cells that differentiate into keratinized cells, which make up the nail protein. The matrix for nail formation is located in the proximal nail bed. It grows forward from the nailfold to cover the nail bed. Fingernails grow about 0.1 mm/day. Their complete reproduction takes 100 to 150 days. Toenails grow one third as fast as fingernails do. A damaged nail matrix, which may result from trauma or aggressive manicuring, produces a distorted nail. Nails are also sensitive to physiologic changes (i.e., they grow more slowly in cold weather and during periods of illness). Nails and hair consist of keratinized and, therefore, "dead" cells. The ingestion of gelatin has not been shown to increase nail growth or strength.

Dermis

The dermis, a dense layer of tissue beneath the epidermis, gives the skin most of its substance and structure. It varies from 1 to 4 mm in thickness and is thickest over the back. The dermis contains fibroblasts, macrophages, mast cells, and lymphocytes that promote wound healing. The skin's lymphatic, vascular, and nerve supplies, which maintain equilibrium in the skin, are in the dermis.

The dermis is divided into two parts: (1) papillary dermis and (2) reticular dermis. The papillary dermis, which contains increased amounts of collagen, blood vessels, sweat glands, and elastin, is in contact with the epidermis. The reticular dermis also has collagen but with increased amounts of mature elastic tissue.

The epidermis and dermis meet at the dermoepidermal junction. This area contains wavelike projections from the dermis called papillae. They correspond to reciprocal structures in the epidermis. The subepidermal basement membrane zone is a semipermeable filter that permits fluid exchange of components, such as nutrients, metabolites, and waste products.

Apart from sight and hearing, the major human sensory apparatus is in the skin. Sensory fibers responsible

Table 69-1. Skin Structure and Function

Structure	Normal Function	Effects of Abnormalities	Clinical Correlation
Epidermis			
Stratum corneum	Protection (from trauma, microbes)	Scaling (with excess)	Psoriasis
	Barrier (prevents fluid, electrolyte, and chemical loss)	Reduced barrier (with loss)	Burns, ulcers
Keratinocytes (squamous cells)	Synthesis of keratin, 14-day migration through epidermis	Impaired barrier function	Ichthyosis
		Malignant transformation	Squamous cell epithelioma
Melanocytes	Melanosome production	Increased pigmentation after inflammation	Suntan
	Melanin (protection from sunburn, ultraviolet carcinogenesis)	Malignant transformation	Malignant melanoma
	Determine skin color	Decreased or absent pigmentation	Albinism, vitiligo
Langerhans cells	Antigen presentation	Allergic contact dermatitis	Poison ivy
		Hyperplastic states	Histiocytosis X
Basal cells	Epidermal reproduction (average of 457 hr between cell divisions), producing one basal cell and one squamous cell	Accelerated production	Psoriasis
		Malignant transformation	Basal cell epithelioma
Epidermal Appendages			
Eccrine unit	Thermoregulation by perspiration	Fluid/electrolyte shifts (up to 6 L/hr)	Heat stroke, arrhythmia
		Reduced heat dissipation (when absent)	Anhidrosis
Apocrine unit	Production of apocrine sweat (no known significance)	Staining of clothing, odor	Chromhidrosis
Hair follicle	Protection, adornment	Disturbance of anagen:telogen ratio	Alopecia, hirsutism, postpregnancy hair thinning
Nails	Protection and mechanical assistance	Subungual thickness	Psoriasis
		Separation of nailplate from nail	Fungal infections

for pain, touch, and temperature form a complex network in the dermis. There are four primary types of sensation: pain, touch, cold, and warmth. Pain may be caused by physical, chemical, or mechanical stimulation. Touch stimuli are received by hair follicles and the intervening skin. Itching arises from terminal nerve endings close to the skin surface; itching does not occur when the epidermis is absent. Temperature sense probably occurs through free sensory nerve endings in the epidermis.

Subcutaneous Fat

The subcutaneous layer is a specialized layer of connective tissue. It is sometimes called the adipose layer because of its fat content. This layer is absent in some places such as the eyelids, scrotum, areola, and tibia. Age, heredity, and many other factors influence the thickness of the subcutaneous layer. Subcutaneous fat is generally thickest on the back and buttocks, giving shape and contour over bone. The primary functions of this layer are the insulation from extremes of hot and cold, as a cushion to trauma, and as a source of energy and hormone metabolism.

FUNCTION

The skin is a morphologically complex structure that serves several functions essential to life. The skin differs anatomically and physiologically in different areas of the body. Primary functions of the skin include protection, homeostasis, thermoregulation, and sensory perception. Table 69-1 summarizes major skin structures and functions.

Protection

The skin protects the body against many forms of trauma, including mechanical, thermal, chemical, and

Table 69–1. Skin Structure and Function Continued

Structure	Normal Function	Effects of Abnormalities	Clinical Correlation
Epidermal Appendages			
Sebaceous glands	Production of sebum (lipid mixture)	With overproduction; obstruction of sebum flow	"Oily" skin Acne
Dermis			
Collagen, reticulum, elastin	Major skin proteins; contribute to skin texture	Abnormal molecular structure Altered structure	Ehlers-Danlos syndrome Wrinkles, saggy skin
Fibroblasts	Collagen synthesis; provide vital structural skin strength and wound healing	Excessive collagen formation Synthesis failure	Scurvy Fragile skin
Macrophages	Phagocytosis of foreign substances and microbes; initiation of inflammation and repair	Defects in function, delayed wound healing	Job's syndrome
Mast cells	Provide histamine for vasodilation and chemotactic factors for inflammatory responses	Release vasoactive molecular mediators after allergic stimulus	Urticaria
Lymphatic glands	Removal of microbes and excess interstitial fluids	Inadequate drainage	Chronic edema
Blood vessels	Provide metabolic skin requirements, thermoregulation	Ischemia and necrosis, altered cutaneous blood flow	Diabetic peripheral vascular disease, arterial and venous ulcers, erythroderma with possible hypothermia, heart failure, heart attack
Nerve fibers	Perception of heat/cold, pain, itching	Reduced threshold for itching	Atopic dermatitis, pruritus
Subcutaneous Adipose Tissue			
	Energy storage and balance, trauma absorption	Abnormal structure, fat atrophy	Lipoma, obesity

radiant. The intact tough epidermal layer is a mechanical barrier. Bacteria, foreign matter, other organisms, and chemicals penetrate it with difficulty. The oily and slightly acid secretions of its sebaceous glands protect the body further by limiting the growth of many organisms. The thickened skin of the palms and soles provides additional covering to absorb the constant trauma to these areas.

Homeostasis

Skin forms a barrier that prevents excessive loss of water and electrolytes from the internal environment and also prevents the subcutaneous tissues from drying out. The effectiveness of this impermeable membrane is readily recognized when one observes the extreme loss of fluids that occurs with damage to the skin, such as with burns and other injuries. Insensible loss of water and electrolytes occurs only through pores in this effective barrier.

Thermoregulation

The skin, under normal conditions, adjusts metabolic heat production to heat loss in order to maintain the thermal balance of the body and the internal temperature of the body, which is approximately 37° C (98.6° F). The rate of heat loss depends primarily on the surface temperature of the skin, which is in turn a function of the skin's blood flow.

The vascular supply to the skin, much more extensive than is needed for tissue nourishment, is regulated by central and local neural and hormonal processes.

Sensory Reception

The primary function of the receptors in the skin is to sense temperature (hot and cold), pain, light touch, and pressure. Different nerve endings are responsible for responding to each different stimuli, and they have varying concentrations over the body. For example, fingertips are more densely innervated than is the skin on the back.

EFFECTS OF AGING ON THE INTEGUMENTARY SYSTEM

The skin undergoes numerous changes that one can see and feel throughout the lifespan. Many of these changes are natural, unchangeable, and harmless. Other changes may be bothersome or painful and often are treated in a variety of ways until there is acceptable resolution or acceptance of the condition. Other skin changes may go unnoticed and not be bothersome because they are slowly growing, such as senile keratosis.

Adolescence

During puberty, hormone secretion stimulates the maturation of hair follicles, sebaceous glands, and apocrine and eccrine units in certain body areas. Hair follicles on the face (males), pubic region, and axilla activate to produce coarse terminal hairs. Folliculitis (hair follicle infection) may occur on the thighs and buttocks. Sebaceous glands on the face, chest, and upper back become functional, and mild acne (inflammation of a pilosebaceous follicle) may occur. As the apocrine glands increase sweat production, perspiration and body odor become noticeable for the first time. These normal changes bother some teenagers. Skin irritation (excessive dryness) may result from the excessive application of commercial skin products such as astringents or other products marketed for "oily" skin.

Pigmented nevi, which may be flat or papular lesions, are other noticeable changes that occur during adolescence. The most common nevi are junctional, dermal, and compound nevi. These lesions are benign cluster melanocyte-like cells. The tendency to freckle is genetically inherited. These small, brown, macular lesions appear on sun-exposed areas and are promoted by sun exposure.

New nevi can appear after adolescence. Pigmented lesions that appear much later in life are called lentigo or senile lentigo. At any age, raised, pigmented lesions that bleed or change in color or size should be assessed by a physician. Such a lesion may simply be an irritated nevus requiring minor care or may have early malignant changes, for example, malignant melanoma (see Chap. 70 for discussion of malignant melanoma).

Adulthood

Temporary hormonal changes account for some of the adult skin changes. Pregnancy and birth control pills may change hormonal status and thus skin structures that are hormonally linked. Temporary changes in hair growth patterns and a temporary thinning of hair after pregnancy are common. Melasma is a condition of blotchy hyperpigmentation on the cheeks and forehead, the pathogenesis of which is unknown. Many etiologic factors have been implicated, such as pregnancy, oral contraceptives, and genetics. Melasma disappears after pregnancy, discontinuance of oral contraceptives, or correction of hormonal abnormalities. Hormonal and genetic changes also produce a recognizable male pattern baldness (alopecia). Family history reveals a balding tendency that passes to subsequent generations. Excessive facial body hair in women can be an androgen-related problem.

Hereditary and environmental factors play a major role in many of the skin changes that occur in adults. Actinic keratosis (slightly raised, red, scaly papules), sebaceous cysts (enclosed cyst in the dermis), and acrochordon or "skin tags" (small flesh-colored papules) commonly occur singly or in combination. Some lesions (i.e., seborrheic keratosis and acrochordon) may be removed for cosmetic reasons, if desired. Actinic keratosis and sebaceous cysts need assessment and may be removed (Chap. 70): actinic keratoses because of their premalignant status, and sebaceous cysts because of their infectious potential.

Older Adulthood

The skin of older clients reflects the cumulative influence of the environment, decreased circulation, and diminished function of a variety of skin structures. As the stratum corneum becomes thinner, the skin reacts more readily to minor changes in humidity, temperature, and other irritants. Wrinkles appear as the collagen becomes weakened and there is decreased subcutaneous fat. Wrinkling is also caused by excessive sun exposure, effects of gravity, and cigarette smoking. Epidermal thinning makes the skin more transparent in the elderly. Small, bright red domes (cherry angiomas) are created by dilated blood vessels that form loops; these are harmless and often occur on the trunk. Seborrheic keratoses are raised black or brown spots or wartlike growths that look as though they have been pasted on the skin surface. These are common and also an inherited trait; they are not contagious or precancerous but are easily removed if cosmetically bothersome. Hair and nail growth is decreased, and nails become brittle. Loss of pigment causes gray hair.

Lentigines (liver spots)—various-sized black or brown, flat lesions—are common. These macules may appear anywhere and have nothing to do with the liver. Those on the dorsum of the hand or the face are probably promoted by prolonged sun exposure. The skin may also have a leathery or coarse appearance from excessive exposure to ultraviolet light. Because there is no known treatment for these lesions, protection from ultraviolet light is the only preventive measure (see later discussion).

▼ ASSESSMENT OF THE INTEGUMENTARY SYSTEM

A thorough health history assists in diagnosis of integumentary disorders, such as occupationally related contact dermatitis, or in revealing psychosocial aspects of disease processes. Many medications can cause skin changes as a result of side effects. The physical examination can confirm integumentary disorders as well as reveal disorders that the client may have omitted during the history.

HISTORY

The history includes asking questions about the chief complaint, past medical history, medications, allergies, family history, psychosocial history and lifestyle including occupational and travel history, and a review of systems.

Chief Complaint

The most common problems related to the integument are itching (pruritus), dryness, rashes, lesions, ecchymoses, lumps, and masses. The nurse asks about changes in the skin, hair, and nails that may be related to the chief complaint. Sample questions that attempt to elicit pertinent information related to the presenting dermatologic problem are listed in Table 69-2. Ask only one question at a time. Remember to pause after each question to give the client time to answer. A symptom analysis is completed, which includes definition of the problem, onset, location, duration, evolution of the lesion or eruption, aggravating and relieving factors, medical intervention, self-treatment, and compliance/treatment factors.

Past Medical History

Various systemic diseases have cutaneous manifestations. It is important to find out whether the client has other systemic illness relevant to the skin, that is, immunologic, endocrine, collagen, vascular, renal, or hepatic conditions. Information on recent exposure to infectious or childhood diseases is helpful, as is knowing the immunization status. Previous trauma and surgical intervention may give the explanation for unusual lesions or location. History of past allergic reactions to foods or medications is important for avoiding inadvertent reaction through readministration.

Medications. Prescription as well as over-the-counter medications that the client is currently taking or has recently finished should be noted. Sensitivity to antibiotics or other drugs in the form of a drug rash may not occur until the end of a routine course of the drug. Photosensitizing drugs (i.e., phenothiazides, tetracyclines, diuretics, sulfonamides) may cause a sunburn-like rash in areas of sun exposure. Topical preparations may include many preservatives or active ingredients that are known sensitizers. The most commonly encountered are neomycin, ethyl aminobenzoate (Benzocaine), and diphenhydramine hydrochloride (Benadryl).

Table 69-2. Dermatologic Assessment History: Sample Questions

Information Needed	Questions
Chief complaint	"Please tell me what brings you here today."
Definition of problem (onset, location)	"Tell me more about the problem. Where did it start? Have you noticed this problem before?"
Duration	"When did it start? Does it come and go? Has it changed? Has it become better or worse?"
Accompanying symptoms	"Did you have any feelings—such as fatigue, nausea, skin tightness, skin burning—before this problem started? Does it itch?"
Evolution of lesion or eruption	"How does it feel now? Are you experiencing any discomfort? Do you feel tenderness, tightness? Does clothing irritate your skin? Do you have any problems sleeping? Does it limit any of your activities? Has it interfered with your normal daily routine?"
Aggravating factors/relieving factors	"Have you noticed whether the problem worsens after any of these activities: eating particular foods? using cosmetics? using soaps? wearing clothing? Do changes in temperature or climate affect the problem? does it worsen or improve with changes in season? Are you more comfortable when warm or when cool?"
Medical intervention	"Did you see a physician about this? Were you told what the problem was? Was any treatment recommended? Did it help?"
Self-treatment	"What have you tried to do on your own to get relief? What did you use? What over-the-counter or home remedies have you tried? What do you do yourself that helps the problem?"
Compliance/treatment failure	"How often were you able to apply or take prescribed medication? Were you able to complete prescribed treatment? How did you use the medication? (e.g., How did you apply it? How did you take it? For how long? Why did you stop?)"

Allergies. The nurse asks the client about allergies to medications and foods (see previous discussion under Medications). Are there certain foods that, when ingested, cause itching, burning, or eruption of skin rashes? Foods high in citric acid and chocolate are common culprits. Fresh fruits that have been treated with pesticides or preservatives may also be problematic, as may prepared foods containing preservatives.

PSYCHOSOCIAL HISTORY AND LIFESTYLE

Psychosocial factors influencing the dermatologic disorders often play a large role, particularly in long-term and chronic processes. Skin disease can greatly affect lifestyle and self-image. Cultural and familial influences on how to care for a particular disorder may conflict with prescribed therapies. Misconceptions about skin problems (i.e., acne lesions can be scrubbed away) need to be determined and corrected. Visually or physically disabling chronic skin diseases have been associated with chronic unemployment, poor mental health, and even suicide.

Socioeconomic factors cannot be ignored. Compliance with outlined therapies and return for follow-up care are influenced by social expectations or financial ability to pay for medications or treatments. When recommending desired therapies or medications, the nurse considers the impact on the client's day-to-day routine, as well as what type of prescription insurance plan the client may or may not have. Many topical therapies, whether covered by insurance or not, are expensive, and expense is a factor that impacts compliance.

Habits. The nurse inquires about the client's habits. Determine the frequency of hygiene practices, what products are used (e.g., soaps, lotions, abrasives), and whether cosmetics are used. Record products used, including brand names. Review the client's diet history for intake of sufficient nutrients, such as water; protein; vitamins A, D, E, and C; and dietary fat. Also ask about exercise and sleep patterns, which affect circulation, nourishment, and repair of the skin. Does the client engage in recreational activities that incur prolonged exposure to the sun, unusual cold, or other conditions that may damage the integument?

Occupational and Travel History. Occupational history is significant because a large number of skin problems are caused or worsened by exposure to irritants and chemicals in the home and work environment. It is important to understand what the client comes in contact with and to what extent. This could explain situations such as the chronic reflaring of hand eczema whenever the client uses certain glues and glazes during a hobby project, or the total body rash secondary to chemical mists penetrating nonprotective gear at the work site.

Travel history can be helpful. This is especially true if the travel included hiking or exposure to any variety of outdoor wonders that have resulted in dermatologic disorders such as poison ivy, sumac, and oak or Lyme disease.

Family History

A family history helps determine genetic predisposition to skin disorders as well as predisposition to parasitic or other conditions based on the family's lifestyle and living environment. Many dermatologic disorders or systemic disorders with a dermatologic presentation are passed on genetically to other family members. Genetically transmitted dermatologic conditions include alopecia (loss of patches of hair), ichthyosis, atopic dermatitis, and psoriasis. Systemic diseases with dermatologic manifestations include diabetes mellitus, blood dyscrasia, and collagen vascular diseases (lupus erythematosus). Other diseases, such as scabies, are likely to be passed on to family members because of close and frequent exposure.

Review of Systems

A complete history of skin changes is important. The nurse specifically asks about past problems with unusual itching, dryness, lesions, rashes, lumps, ecchymoses, and masses. Has the client had problems with moles or other lesions, especially if they have undergone changes in size, shape, or color? A more complete list of questions for the review of systems appears in Chapter 11, Table 11-5.

PHYSICAL EXAMINATION

Examination of the skin is done as thoroughly as the examination of any other body organ. It cannot be done properly in the hall or at a quick glance, which is often asked of the dermatologist or the nurse. Inspection, palpation, and olfaction are used to assess hair, nails, and skin. Effective assessment requires knowledge, awareness, and practice in describing skin of individuals of all ages and different lifestyles and in recognizing normal and abnormal skin changes.

Terminology

The terms used in dermatology have frequently been referred to as a foreign language and have been known to inhibit health care providers from using the correct terminology for skin disease. The problem relates to inability to correctly identify extremely large numbers of similarly appearing, troublesomely named diseases. Use of standard terminology is important and often leads to differential diagnosis. The intent of this section is to clarify some of the commonly used dermatology terminology and to assist the nurse in recognizing and describing skin disorders. Table 69-3 is a glossary of commonly used dermatologic terms.

Types of Lesions

Examination and diagnosis of skin disorders are dependent on identifying skin lesions or changes. Two major

Table 69-3. Glossary of Dermatologic Terms

Actinic	Pertaining to ultraviolet light (UVL)
Amelanotic	Without pigment
Circinate (pronounced *sir-sin-ate*)	Circular
Circumscribed	Limited to a certain area by sharply defined border
Coalesce	To merge one with another
Comedo	Plug in a skin duct containing keratin (blackhead)
Cytotoxic	Toxic to cells
Dermatome	Area of skin supplied by a single dorsal nerve root
Dermatophyte	Fungus that enters the skin's surface causing infection
Desquamation	Scaling, peeling of epidermis
Discoid	Coinlike
Eczematous	General term for disease process characterized by blisters, weeping, crusting, and inflammation
Erythema	Redness
Exacerbation	Worsening of disease state
Exfoliative	Shedding of skin in fairly large quantities
Folliculitis	Hair follicle inflammation
Guttate	Small, water drop-sized lesions, usually widespread
Hives	Spontaneously occurring wheals
Hyperkeratosis	Thickening of stratum corneum, usually from repeated pressure or friction
Hyperpigmentation	Increased or excessive skin pigmentation (melanin) causing an area of skin to be darker than surrounding areas
Hypopigmentation	Decreased pigmentation
Indurated	Hard (tissue)
Intertrigo	Irritation of body areas with opposing skinfolds that are subject to friction
Lesion	Detectable change from normal skin structure
Maceration	Tissue softening or disintegration from excessive moisture
Milia	Small, white papules
Mosaic	Resembling inlaid material
Perioral	Around the mouth
Periungual	Under the nailplate
Pigmentation	Degree of skin or mucous membrane color
Plantar	Pertaining to sole of the foot
Polymorphic	Existing in many forms
Pruritus	Itching
Punctate	Pinpoint or dot-shaped
Sclerosis	Hardening or induration of skin
Sebum	Lipid excretion produced by sebaceous glands
Tautness	Degree of skin tightness
Texture	Tactile or visual skin characteristics, e.g., coarseness, dryness
Ultraviolet light (UVL)	Electromagnetic radiation from the sun (wavelengths 4-400 nm)
Urticaria	Wheals (hives)
Verruca	Lesion characterized by surface roughness, e.g., wart
Wheal	Lesion found in hives

types of lesions are distinguished: *primary* and *secondary* lesions.

The primary lesion is the first lesion to appear on the skin and has a visually recognizable structure. Figure 69-3 pictures and describes 10 primary lesions: macule, papule, plaque, nodule, tumor, wheal, vesicle, bulla, cyst, and pustule.

When changes occur in the primary lesion, it becomes a secondary lesion. These changes may be brought about by the client or the client's environment and often occur in the epidermal layer. These changes may result from many factors including scratching, rubbing, medication, natural disease progression, or processes of involution and healing. Figure 69-4 pictures and describes the following secondary lesions: scale, crust, erosion, ulcer, scar, lichenification, excoriation, fissure, and atrophy.

Examination Environment

A well-lit, private room with moderate temperature and neutral, white, or cream-colored walls is best for assessment. Excessive warmth can produce changes in skin color (e.g., redness) by causing vasodilation. Colored walls can affect normal skin hue (color). Ask the

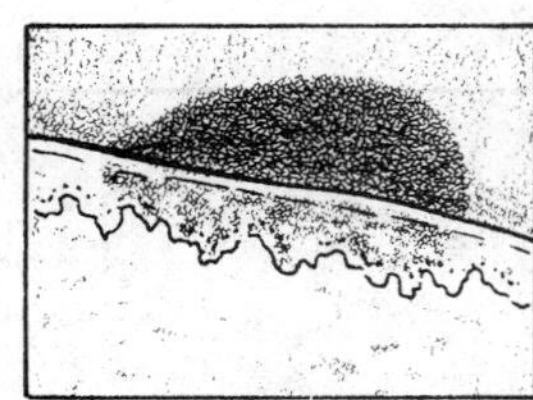

MACULE: Skin color change without elevation, i.e., flat (e.g., freckles or petechia). Described as a "patch" if greater than 1 cm (e.g., vitiligo).

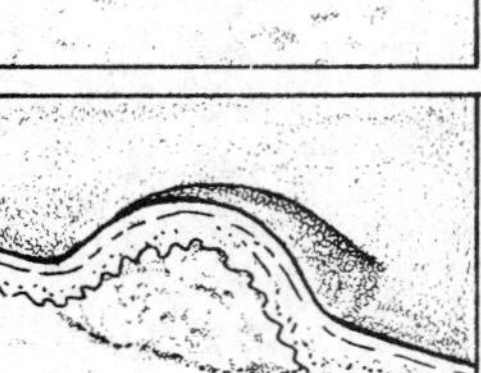

PAPULE: Elevated, solid lesion of less than 1 cm, varying in color (e.g., warts or elevated nevus).

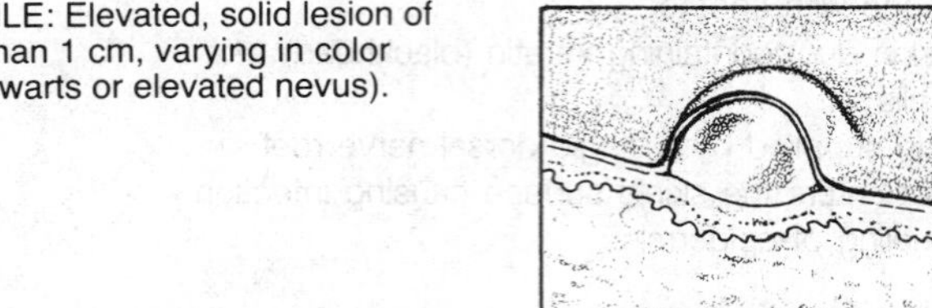

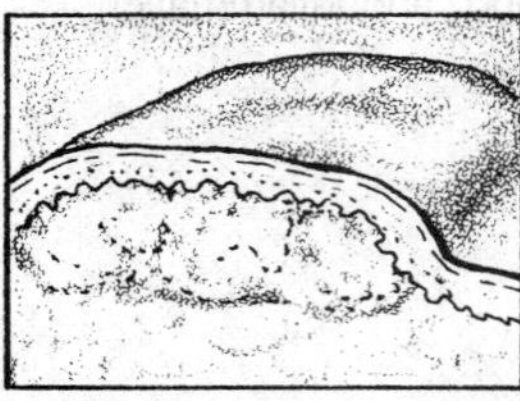

PLAQUE: Raised, flat lesion formed from merging papules or nodules.

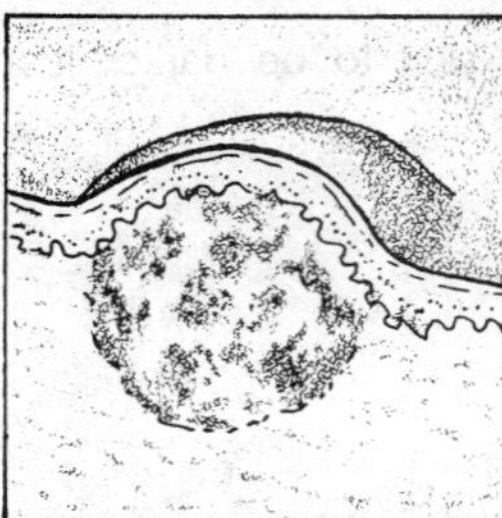

NODULE: Larger than a papule. Raised solid lesion extending deeper into the dermis.

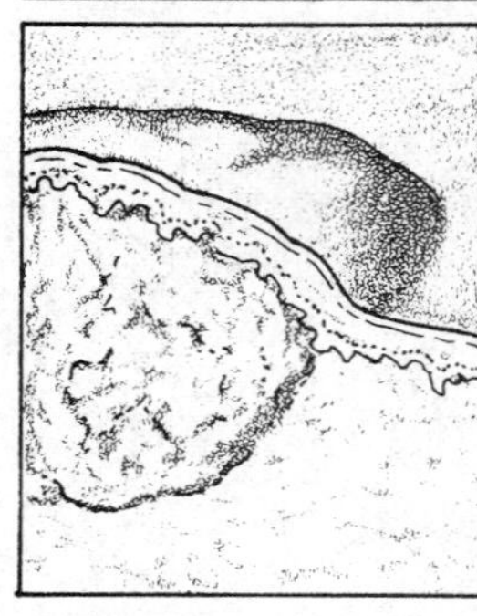

TUMOR: Larger than a nodule. Elevated firm lesion that may or may not be easily demarcated.

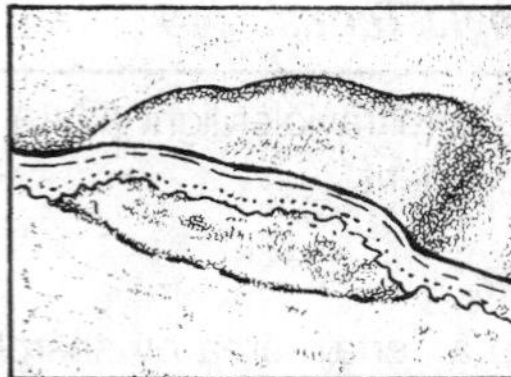

WHEAL (hive): Fleeting skin elevation that is irregularly shaped because of edema (e.g., mosquito bite or urticaria).

VESICLE (blister): Elevated, sharply defined lesion containing serous fluid. Usually less than 1 cm (e.g., blister, chickenpox, or herpes simplex).

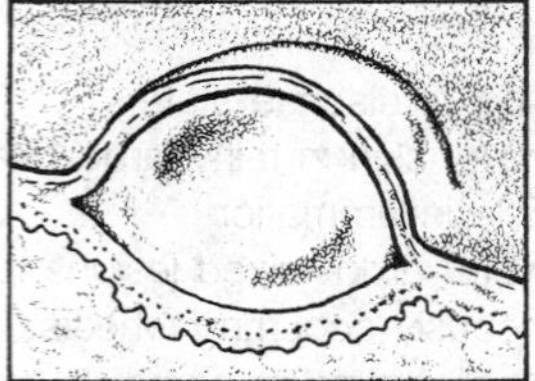

BULLA (plural, *bullae*): Large, elevated, fluid-filled lesion greater than 1 cm (e.g., second-degree burn).

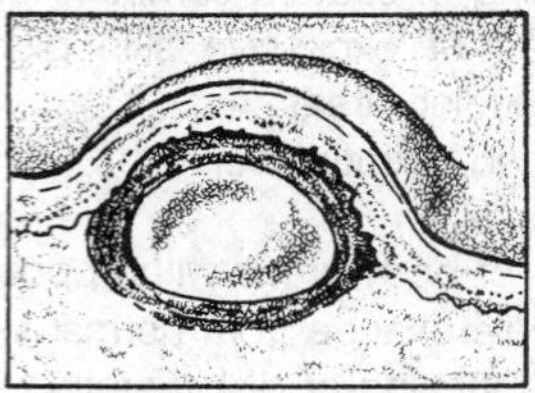

CYST: Elevated, thick-walled lesion containing fluid or semisolid matter.

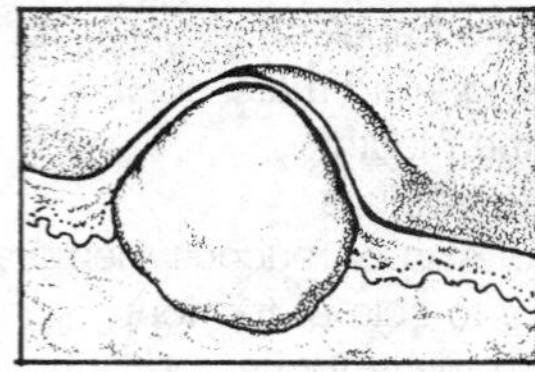

PUSTULE: Elevated lesion less than 1 cm containing purulent material. Lesions larger than 1 cm are described as boils, abscesses, or furuncles (e.g., acne, or impetigo).

▲ *Figure 69–3*

Primary lesions: visually recognizable structural changes in the skin that have specific characteristics.

client to undress for a complete examination; provide a gown. Tell the client that all skin surfaces will be examined. Avoid unnecessary exposure as the examination proceeds.

Depth of Examination

Examination is systematic and as complete as appropriate. A total body skin examination includes hair, scalp, nails, mucous membranes, and the skin. Begin at the head and proceed to the toes. General changes can alter total body skin color (i.e., jaundice, cyanosis, pallor), thickness, turgor, temperature, and vascularity (i.e., purpura, petechiae). General findings such as these can suggest systemic disease and may require complete physical examination and appropriate work-up. The diagnosis of skin disease is accomplished by careful observation and work-up of individual lesions. This discussion is limited to assessment of hair, scalp, nails, and skin lesions.

Although the nurse may examine the client's integument over the complete body surface at one time, this usually is not done in the screening examination. Rather, integument assessment is integrated throughout the physical examination as each body region is examined. However, for the purpose of discussion, assessment of the integument is presented here as a separate body system. Significant or abnormal findings are commonly reported as part of each regional assessment rather than separately.

Assessment of Hair, Scalp, and Nails

HAIR AND SCALP

Hair distribution patterns are examined for symmetry and distribution according to age and sexual development. Fine hair covers much of the body and is of the same color as scalp hair. Increased distribution occurs normally in the axillae and pubic areas. Excess body hair is known as *hirsutism.*

The hair and scalp are inspected under good light. If the nurse suspects lesions or infestation with lice, gloves are worn. The hair is inspected and palpated for distribution, thickness, texture, lubrication, and signs of infestation or infection. Natural hair color varies greatly (the nurse asks the client if hair dye is used because it alters texture). Hair should be resilient and distributed evenly over the scalp. Individual hair shaft diameter can range from thin and fine to thick and coarse; the shape of hair fibers can be straight, curly, or wavy. Texture and lubrication are affected by the type of hair care products used (e.g., harsh shampoo, curling irons, or hair dryers) as well as by a protein-deficient diet or health problems such as febrile illness, all of which tend to leave hair dry and brittle. Hair loss or thinning *(alopecia)* can result from genetic predisposition to baldness or a health problem such as recent chemotherapy.

The *scalp* is inspected and palpated for lesions, excoriation (from scratching), lumps, or bruises, which should be absent. Hair shafts are examined for the presence of nits, which are the eggs of the human head louse *(Pediculus capitis)* and appear as particles of oval dandruff. The areas behind the ears and along the

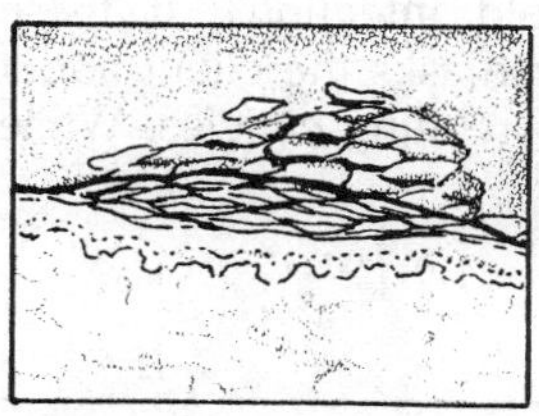
SCALE: Dried fragments of sloughed epidermal cells, irregular in shape and size and white, tan, yellow, or silver in color (e.g., dandruff, dry skin, or psoriasis).

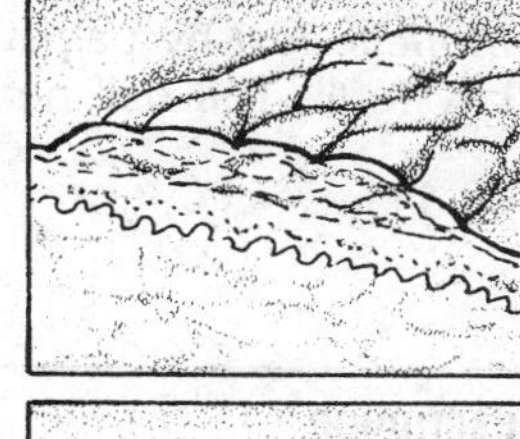
LICHENIFICATION: Epidermal thickening resulting in elevated plaque with accentuated skin markings. Usually results from repeated injury through rubbing or scratching (e.g., chronic atopic dermatitis).

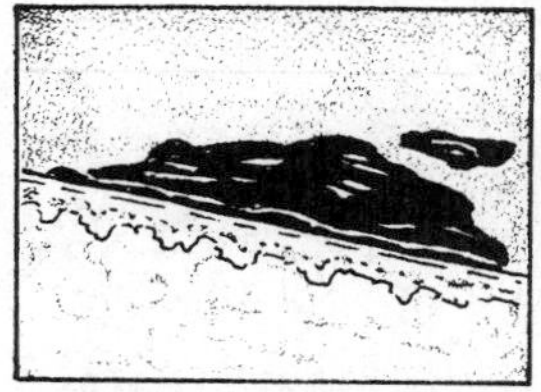
CRUST: Dried serum, sebum, blood, or pus on skin surface producing a temporary barrier to the environment (e.g. impetigo).

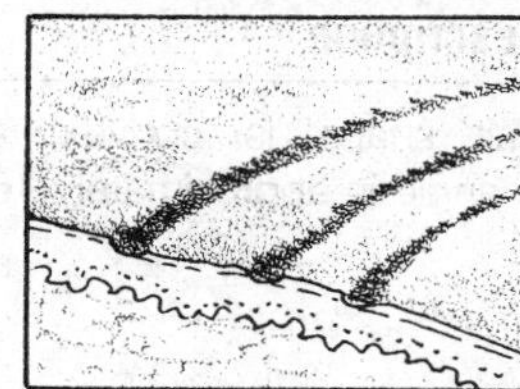
EXCORIATION: Superficial, linear abrasion of epidermis. Visible sign of itching caused by rubbing or scratching (e.g., atopic dermatitis).

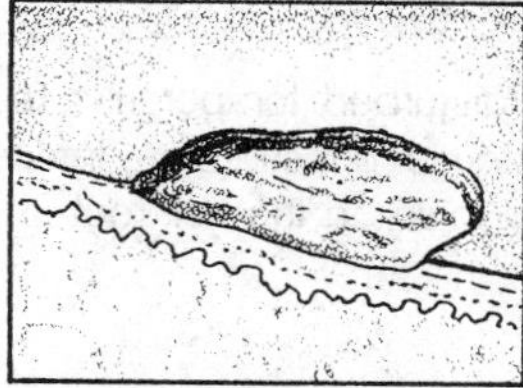
EROSION: A moist, demarcated, depressed area due to loss of partial- or full-thickness epidermis. Basal layer of epidermis remains intact (e.g., ruptured chickenpox vesicle).

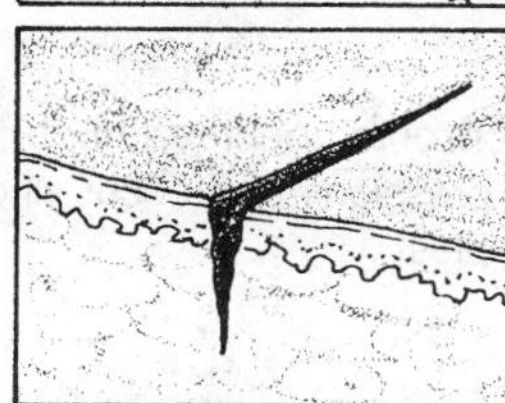
FISSURE: Deep linear split through epidermis into dermis (e.g., tinea pedis).

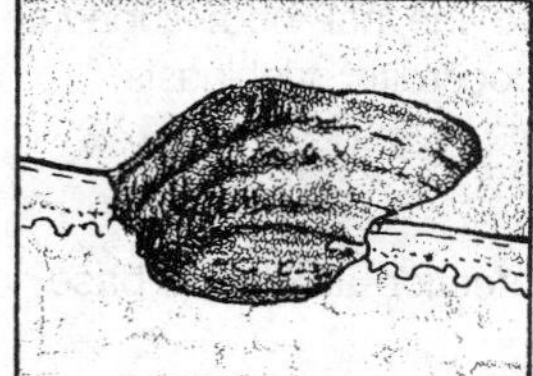
ULCER: Irregularly shaped, exudative, depressed lesion in which entire epidermis and upper layer of dermis are lost. Results from trauma and tissue destruction (e.g., stasis ulcer).

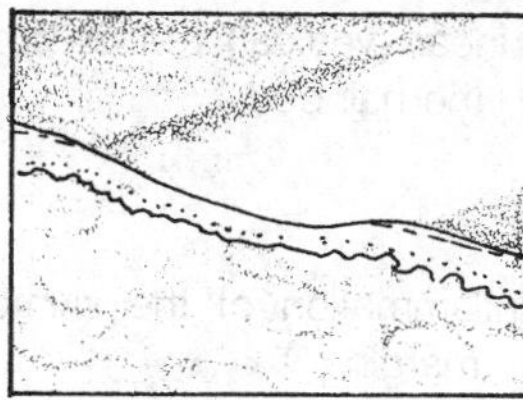
ATROPHY: Wasting of epidermis in which skin appears thin and transparent, or of dermis in which there is a depressed area (e.g., arterial insufficiency).

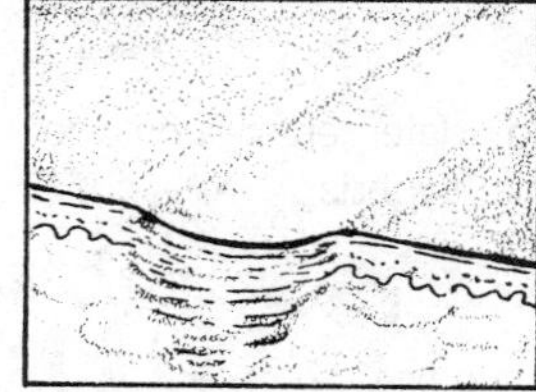
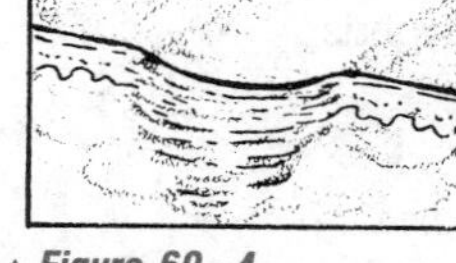
SCAR: Mark left on skin after healing. Replacement of destroyed tissue by fibrous tissue.

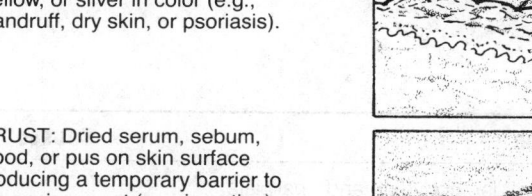

▲ **Figure 69–4**

Secondary lesions: primary lesions that have changed owing to the natural progression of the lesion or to physical change (i.e., scratching, irritation, or secondary infection).

back of the neck are often where adult lice bite the scalp, which results in pustular lesions. It is difficult to see adult lice on the scalp; they are very small (1 to 2 mm) with gray-white bodies.

If lesions are seen, the nurse describes them and asks the client about recent trauma or injury to the head. If the client has not already provided information during the health history interview, the nurse conducts a symptom analysis.

NAILS

Inspect the client's nails for color, shape, texture, integrity, and thickness (Table 69-4). The nails reflect the client's overall health, indicating nutrition and respiratory status. The nailplate is usually transparent and colorless and, when viewed from the side, has a convex *shape*. The vascular bed underlying the nailplate gives the nail its color. In Caucasian clients, the *color* is pink, whereas it is darker in dark-skinned clients. A deficiency in hemoglobin is seen in the nail bed as pallor, and decreased arterial circulation appears as cyanosis. The nurse performs a *blanche test* by palpating the nail beds to assess capillary refill. The nail bed is pressed firmly for 5 seconds, then quickly released while the rate of color return to the nail bed is observed. Color return should be immediate within 3 to 5 seconds. When palpated, the nail bed feels firm with no softness (i.e., bogginess) or tenderness.

Texture is smooth; healthy nails are of uniform thickness with no signs of dryness, softness, brittleness, splitting, peeling, ridges, or pitting. The *angle* formed between the nailplate and posterior nailfold is approximately 160 degrees without separation. Changes in nail shape and nail bed angle can indicate health problems. Clubbing of the nails is an increase of more than 160 degrees in the angle between the nailplate and nail base. The nail base of a clubbed nail is spongy and soft on palpation. These changes result from hypoxia (diminished tissue oxygenation). Nail clubbing commonly occurs in clients with congenital heart defects or chronic lung disease.

The tissue surrounding the nail should appear intact without signs of inflammation, jagged edges (hangnail), or dryness. Inferior or lateral nailfold inflammation is a sign of paronychia (i.e., nailfold infection). If these abnormalities are noted, the nurse asks the client about nail care habits such as biting or cutting cuticles. While

Table 69-4. Assessing the Nails

Assessment Finding	Description	Causes
Normal nail (About 160 degrees)	Nail shape is convex, and nailplate angle is approximately 160 degrees	
Beau's line (Beau's line)	Horizontal depression in nailplate; depressions can occur singly or in multiples	Nail growth is disturbed temporarily; related to systemic illness (e.g., infection) or direct injury to the nail root
Splinter hemorrhages	Linear (vertical) red or brown streaks in the nail bed	Minor trauma to the nail bed; subacute bacterial endocarditis; trichinosis
Paronychia	Inflammation of the skinfold at the nail margin	Trauma; skin infection at the nail base
Spoon shape	Nail shape is concave as the nail curves upward from the nail bed	Use of strong detergents; iron deficiency anemia; syphilis
Clubbing	Increased angle between nailplate and nail base	Long-standing hypoxia

examining the fingers and toes, the nurse may note common abnormalities such as calluses or corns. A *callus* is a flat, painless thickening of a circumscribed area of skin. Calluses usually occur on the hands and feet. A *corn* is a horny induration and thickening of the skin caused by friction and pressure.

Assessment of Skin

COLOR

Overall skin color is assessed during the health history interview. A more thorough assessment is conducted as the nurse proceeds through the remainder of the physical examination. The nurse observes the client's face and visible skin surfaces for color tones, which should be congruent with the client's stated race. Abnormal findings include pallor (paleness), flushing or a ruddy complexion, cyanosis (blue cast), jaundice (yellow cast), and areas of irregular pigmentation. There is normal variation from one region of the body to another, particularly in those areas protected from the sun and exposure by clothing, which will be lighter. Overall color should be uniform. Skin tone may range over a variety of colors including light ivory to deep brown or blue-black, yellow to olive, or light pink to dark, ruddy pink.

Areas that are less pigmented reveal abnormal findings more readily than do heavier pigmented surfaces. For example, *pallor* is best seen in the buccal (mouth) mucosa, especially in clients with dark skin. *Cyanosis* is evident more readily in less pigmented areas such as the nail beds, lips, and palms. *Jaundice* sharply contrasts with the white of the sclera, especially in dark-skinned clients who have more carotene deposits. Jaundice is best assessed in dark-skinned clients by inspecting color changes in the hard palate.

Local areas of color change are examined closely by the nurse. *Hyperpigmentation* describes areas of increased pigmentation; *hypopigmentation* describes areas of decreased pigmentation. Skin color also results from the circulation supply; an increased blood supply may indicate the redness of inflammation *(rubor)*, whereas extreme pallor may be a result of anemia or impeded arterial circulation to the area.

MOISTURE

Moisture refers to the skin's hydration level for both wetness and oiliness. Overall skin moisture is dry but not excessively so and often reflects ambient temperature and humidity levels. Moistness usually occurs in intertriginous areas such as the axillae and groin. Skin that feels overly moist and cool (i.e., clammy) is abnormal.

TEMPERATURE

Temperature is assessed with the dorsum of the hand. The skin should feel uniformly warm, because it reflects circulation. Areas of hypothermia or hyperthermia are compared with the same area on the opposite side.

TEXTURE

The nurse palpates texture by stroking the skin lightly with the fingertips. The skin should feel smooth, soft, and resilient. There should be no areas of lumps or unusual thickening or thinning (atrophy).

TURGOR

Turgor is the skin's elasticity and is measured by the time it takes for the skin and underlying tissue to return to its original contour after being pinched up. The skin over the forearm is lightly pinched between the nurse's thumb and index finger, then released. If the skin remains elevated (i.e., tented) more than 3 seconds, turgor is decreased. Normal turgor is a return to baseline contour within 3 seconds when the skin is mobile and elastic. Turgor decreases with age as the skin loses elasticity.

EDEMA

The nurse palpates for edema, particularly if areas of taut, shiny skin are noted on inspection. Edema is the collection of fluid in underlying tissues that separate the skin's surface from pigmented and vascular layers, which results in a blanched appearance. It is an abnormal finding. Edematous areas are palpated for consistency, temperature, shape (i.e., extent), tenderness, and mobility. The nurse presses a finger firmly against the edematous area for 5 seconds to assess for *pitting edema,* that is, a residual indentation left by the finger's pressure when the fluid is displaced from the underlying tissue. The depth of pitting is expressed in millimeters or centimeters. Because of a variation in rating scales, it is more accurate for the nurse to state the depth of pitting rather than to rate it. Areas examined by the nurse for edema include over the sacrum (especially in bed-ridden clients), the feet, ankles, and over the tibia on the shins.

TENDERNESS

Tenderness is an abnormal finding and is elicited as the nurse palpates. There should be no areas of tenderness in a healthy, uninjured client.

ODOR

The skin should be free of pungent odors. Odors, when noted, are usually present in the axillae and skinfolds or open wounds and are related to the presence of bacteria on the skin, inadequate hygiene, or infection.

LESIONS

Inspect the skin for detectable lesions. It is important to assess and describe the findings about any lesions in an orderly fashion: location, distribution, size; arrangement; color; configuration; secondary changes; and presence of drainage. Skin lesions are also palpated to determine the characteristics of contour (e.g., flat, raised, or depressed), size, consistency (e.g., firm, soft), mobility, and tenderness. Lesions can be mobile or immobile (fixed to underlying tissue).

Location, Distribution, and Size. Location is described in reference to anatomic landmarks. The nurse measures lesions for size, because this helps to classify their type (e.g., macule, papule). If there are multiple lesions, the distribution pattern could be helpful in determining the diagnosis. Extent of the presence of the lesions is noted. Lesions can be localized (confined to a specific area), regional, or generalized (present over a large surface). Compare sides bilaterally to determine if lesions are symmetric or asymmetric. Another commonly noted distribution is in sun-exposed areas. Certain diseases have a classic lesion distribution, such as herpes zoster (following along a nerve root dermatome). Table 69-5 gives other descriptions of common distributions. Figure 69-5 depicts the common locations of common skin disorders found during physical examination.

Arrangement. The arrangement refers to the pattern of nearby lesions. Two of the typical patterns include "linear" and "satellite," which can also be helpful in confirming diagnosis. Linear lesions are found in a straight line (i.e., scabies). Satellite lesions are the small peripheral lesions around a central larger lesion (i.e., diaper candidiasis).

Table 69-5. Terminology for Skin Lesion Configuration and Distribution

Configuration*	Description
Annular	Ring-shaped
Iris	Concentric rings, "bull's eyes"
Gyrate	Spiral-shaped
Linear	Forming a line
Nummular	Coinlike
Polymorphous	Occurring in several forms
Punctate	Marked by points or dots
Serpiginous	Snakelike
Distribution†	
Solitary	Single lesion
Satellite	Single lesion occurring in close proximity to but separate from a large group of lesions
Grouped	Clustered
Confluent	Merged together
Diffuse	Widely distributed
Discrete	Separate from other lesions
Generalized	Diffusely distributed
Localized	Limited, clearly defined
Symmetric	Bilaterally distributed
Asymmetric	Unilaterally distributed
Zosteriform	Bandlike distribution of lesions along a dermatome

* Position of lesions relative to other lesions.
† Grouping, or pattern, of lesions over entire skin surface.

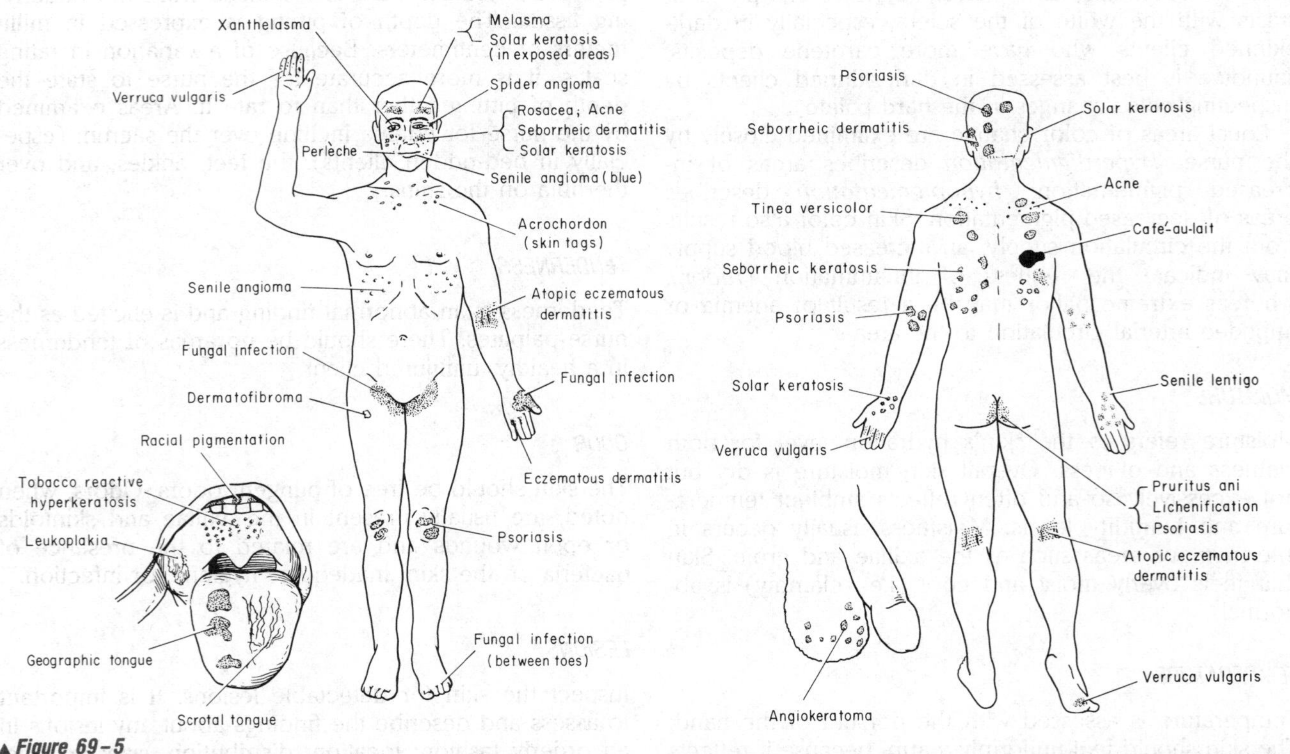

▲ **Figure 69-5**

Common disorders encountered during physical examination of the skin. (From Fitzpatrick, T. B., Eisen, A. Z., Wolff, K., et al. [1987]. *Dermatology in general medicine* [3rd ed.]. New York: McGraw-Hill.)

Color. Skin lesions can assume a wide variety of colors; they may be flesh-colored, brown, red, yellow, tan, or blue. Color can be influenced by many factors, including the client's normal skin color, which often makes it hard to accurately describe. Slight color changes can best be assessed in areas having the least amount of natural pigmentation and those with superficial capillary beds (i.e., buccal membrane of the mouth, mucosa, lips, nail beds, ocular conjunctiva, palms, and soles). These areas are especially important in assessing darkly pigmented skin.

Configuration. Configuration refers to the shape or the outline of the lesion. Most lesions are circular. The term nummular is used for a circular lesion when it is the diameter of a large coin (i.e., nummular eczema). Annular describes lesions found with an active ring-shaped border and some central clearing (i.e., granuloma annulare). Table 69-5 gives the description of other configurations that may be found during assessment.

DIAGNOSTIC TESTS

Before a diagnostic skin procedure (or treatment), the nurse should perform an assessment and document findings. Nursing intervention for diagnostic procedures includes explaining the procedure to the client and significant others, allowing them to ask questions and express concerns. Teach them appropriate wound care and indications of possible side effects and complications that should be reported, such as prolonged bleeding or infection (indicated by swelling, redness, increased discomfort, temperature elevation). Provide instructions (preferably written) for follow-up care as well as follow-up appointment and telephone number. Documentation of diagnostic procedures (exactly what was done and by whom) and the specific location of the lesion must be completed by appropriate personnel.

KOH Examination and Fungal Culture

Fungal infection of skin, hair, or nails may be confirmed by microscopic identification and culture of scrapings from the area. Any scaly dermatitis may be scraped for this test. Typical sites are the scalp, intertriginous areas (between the toes, axillae, groin, under or between the breasts, abdominal folds), and the nailfold. Fine scales from the edge of the site are gently scraped with a #15 scalpel blade or the edge of a glass slide onto a second glass slide. A drop of 10 to 20 per cent potassium hydroxide (KOH) is added to the scale, and a coverslip is placed over the specimen. Gentle pressure is applied to the coverslip to flatten the scales. The slide may be gently heated to dissolve the keratin or the cells more quickly. The scrapings are examined under the microscope. For a culture, scrapings from a suspicious lesion are obtained and implanted onto the appropriate culture medium. For a nail culture, an altered, dystrophic nail is snipped and implanted into the medium. Debris from the nail's subungual area is less suitable for culturing.

Tzanck's Smear

Tzanck's smear is the microscopic assessment of fluids and cells from vesicles or bullae. The presence of multinucleated giant cells establishes a diagnosis of viral infection, such as herpes simplex or herpes zoster. After gentle cleaning of an intact, recently evolved vesicle, the blister's top is removed and its base is scraped with a scalpel or small curet. The debris is smeared onto a slide, which is properly identified and sent for cytologic assessment.

Scabies Scraping

The test for scabies is most accurate when a papule that has not been scratched is chosen. The most difficult part of this procedure is finding the proper lesion from which to take the specimen, and it often requires several areas being prepped. When visible, a linear burrow is sampled in order to look for the mite or its eggs or feces. The best method is to shave off the top of the lesion with a #15 scalpel blade. The shavings are placed on a microscope slide, covered with immersion oil and a coverslip, and examined under low power on the microscope. Local anesthesia is not necessary, and fine bleeding should be expected. There will be some discomfort when the lesion is opened.

Wood's Light Examination

Wood's light examination is assessment with a high-pressure mercury lamp that transmits long-wave ultraviolet light (UVA; 360 nm); it has several diagnostic uses. For example, it (1) detects superficial fungal and bacterial skin infections, (2) delineates pigmentary disorders by highlighting the degree of contrast between lesions and normal skin color, and (3) accentuates the contrast between hypopigmented and totally amelanotic areas. Wood's light ("black light") examination is done in a darkened room. The procedure is painless.

Patch Testing

Patch testing is done to attempt to identify substances that produce allergic skin responses. This testing is very time-consuming; it requires individuals skilled in correctly placing the test as well as a skilled evaluator to read and interpret the results. Patch testing is often done to differentiate between an *irritant* contact dermatitis and an *allergic* contact dermatitis. Small amounts of various substances or allergens are applied to the skin on aluminum discs placed on a special tape. The client and significant others need to understand that whereas potential allergic substances (allergens) can produce inflammatory skin reactions, compounds of low concentration are used to prevent possible excessive irritation. Patch testing should not be performed if acute dermatitis is present. The potential allergen could worsen the dermatitis. The tape must be worn for 48 hours without disturbing the patches, and interpretations are made at 48, 72, and 96 hours and sometimes at 1 week. An eczematous response at the test site with erythema, papules, or small vesicles indicates a positive reaction and confirms an allergic contact sensitivity to the substance on the disc.

Biopsy

Skin biopsy is the removal of a skin tissue specimen for histologic (cellular microscopic) assessment. There are three types: shave, dermal punch, and surgical excision. In all three procedures, local anesthesia is used, and small-gauge needles (26- to 30-gauge) are recommended to limit trauma to the skin. Clean or sterile technique as appropriate should be used in dealing with the biopsy site. The specimen is placed in formalin solution, properly identified, and sent for pathologic assessment.

SHAVE BIOPSY

This procedure is performed to obtain tissue for analysis from possibly malignant epidermal growths, except potential melanoma (Fig. 69-6*A*). After skin cleansing and infiltration of local anesthesia, tissue is removed with a lateral motion by use of a scalpel with a #15 blade. Alternatively, a specimen can be obtained by snipping with curved tissue scissors or a special instrument called a keratome, which shaves off the top layer of skin. Tissue removed includes the epidermis and upper portions of the dermal layers. Hemostasis of the biopsy site is obtained by applying pressure, by using ferric subsulfate (Monsel's solution) or aluminum chloride solution, or by electrodesiccation (cautery).

PUNCH BIOPSY

A dermal punch biopsy uses a circular instrument with a sharp cutting edge to remove a specimen of skin that includes epidermal, dermal, and subcutaneous tissue. This method is used for biopsy of a well-developed, mature lesion (Fig. 69-6*B*). An appropriate size of punch biopsy is chosen (from 2 to 6 mm). The skin site is cleaned, and a local anesthetic is injected. Skin surrounding the lesion is stretched taut and the punch pressed firmly downward into the skin site. The instrument is rotated back-and-forth in a cutting motion that frees the lesion from surrounding tissue. The specimen is then gently grasped with a tissue forceps or needle, and its base is severed with scissors or a scalpel blade. Depending on the size of the biopsy, hemostasis can be achieved with pressure or application of ferric subsulfate (Monsel's solution) or aluminum chloride solution. The oval defect may be closed with a 4-0 or 5-0 silk or nylon suture to produce a linear scar. Sutures are removed after about 7 to 14 days (with facial biopsies, 3 to 5 days).

SURGICAL EXCISION BIOPSY

This biopsy is used (1) when it is necessary to excise a lesion totally (e.g., when full skin thickness is needed), (2) when a lesion's borders are indistinct from

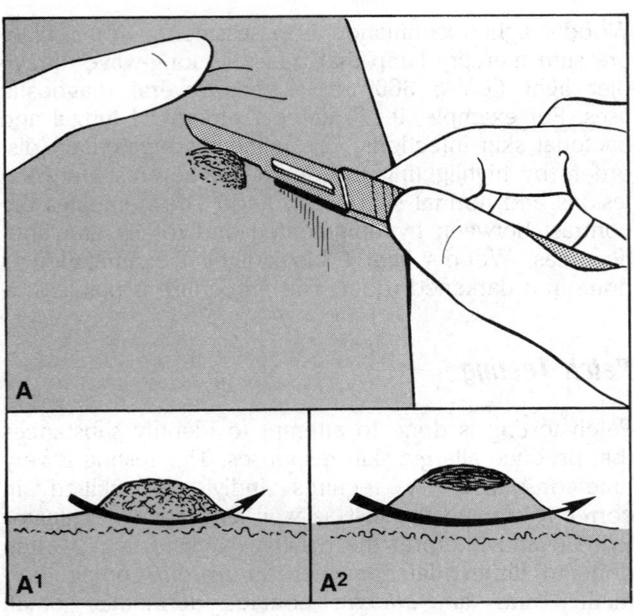

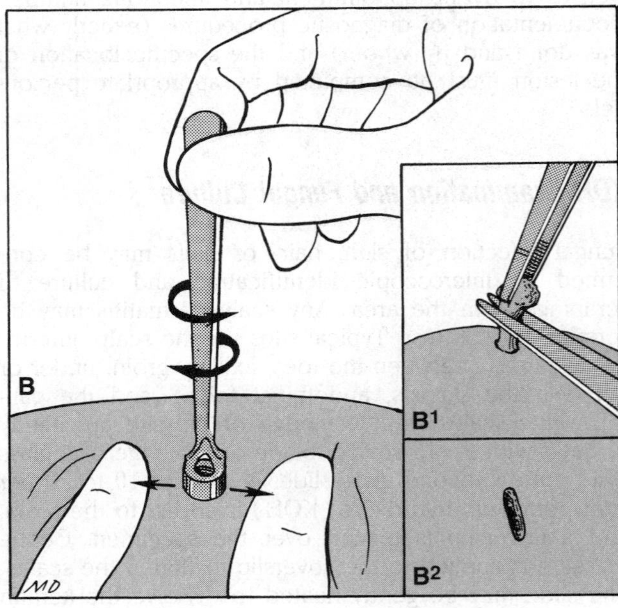

▲ Figure 69-6

Skin biopsies. *A*, Shave biopsy. A tissue specimen is obtained by use of a scalpel (#15 blade) in a horizontal-lateral motion. *B*, Punch biopsy. A tissue specimen is obtained with the instrument pressed down firmly on the skin. The specimen is freed from surrounding tissue by a rotary back-and-forth cutting motion; the specimen base is severed with tissue scissors.

surrounding skin, or (3) when there is a recurrent or aggressive cancer, such as malignant melanoma. The site is cleaned, the excisional lines are marked with a gentian violet pen, and local anesthetic is administered. The lesion is excised with a scalpel by a variety of surgical techniques; a commonly used one is an elliptical incision. Hemostasis is achieved with pressure and ligation (suturing closed) of superficial vessels. The incision is closed with sutures. The suture site is rinsed with saline-dampened gauze. A pressure dressing of sterile nonadhering gauze is applied and taped in place.

Nursing Management

Depending on the size of the excision, the nurse should instruct the client to avoid the use of aspirin and products containing aspirin for 48 hours before the biopsy to avoid a prolonged postprocedure bleeding time. If the client uses anticoagulants (e.g., heparin or coumadin), notify the physician. If the client has a history of cardiac valve replacement, the nurse should be sure prophylactic antibiotics are prescribed. The client should eat a light meal before the procedure to avoid syncope (fainting episodes).

Following the procedure, the nurse covers all biopsy sites with an antibiotic ointment and a clean or sterile dry dressing and pressure dressings when appropriate. Remind the client that follow-up assessment is necessary and plan a follow-up appointment for suture removal. Tell the client how biopsy results will be reported.

Summary

Even though the skin is the largest organ in the body, it is often taken for granted. During the course of a lifetime, gallons of caustic chemicals contact the skin, yet the skin repairs itself quickly. When disorders do occur, the nurse is often the first health care provider to recognize them. Thorough assessment is important for accurate diagnosis and proper care.

Bibliography

Arnold, H. L., Odom, R. B., & James, W. D. (1990). *Andrew's diseases of the skin*. Philadelphia: W. B. Saunders.

Burrage, R., et al. (1991). Physical assessment. An overview with sections on the skin, eye, ear, nose and neck. In W. Chenitz, et al. (Eds.), *Clinical gerontological nursing*. Philadelphia: W. B. Saunders.

Caughman, S., et al. (1989). Cutaneous signs of internal cancer. *Patient Care, 23*(2), 28-41.

Chapel, T., et al. (1988). Cutaneous signs of infection. *Patient Care, 22*(13), 185-197.

Dellasega, C., & Burgunder, C. (1991). Perioperative nursing care for the elderly surgical patient. *Today's OR Nurse, 13*(6), 12-17.

Fitzpatrick, T. B., and Eisen, T. B. (1992). *Dermatology in general medicine*. Hightstown, NJ: McGraw-Hill.

Jarvis, C. (1992). *Physical examination and health assessment*. Philadelphia: W. B. Saunders.

Jaubovic, H., & Ackerman, A. (1985). Structure and function of the skin. In S. Moeohella & H. Hurley (Eds.), *Dermatology* (2nd ed., vol. 1) Philadelphia: W. B. Saunders.

Kreisberg, S., et al. (1989). Skin signs of endocrine disease. *Patient Care, 23*(6), 73-86.

Pogue, S. (1992). Nursing assessment of the elderly for dermatologic procedures. *Dermatology Nursing, 4*(1), 15-23.

Rudy, S. (1991). From conception to birth: the development of the skin and nursing implications. *Dermatology Nursing, 3*(6), 381-392.

Chapter 70

Nursing Care of Clients with Integumentary Disorders

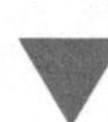
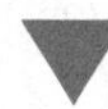
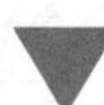

GENERAL PRINCIPLES OF DERMATOLOGIC NURSING

Many effective treatments are available for skin problems. Some are specific to certain conditions. Some treatments are directed at skin cellular metabolism; these include (1) altering skin temperature, (2) reducing or increasing blood flow, (3) adapting delivery of oxygen to and from skin tissue, (4) altering inflammatory responses, and (5) adapting absorption of toxins and mediators. Dermatologic intervention includes (1) topical medications, (2) soaks and wet wraps, (3) protective dressings, (4) skin lubricants, and (5) ultraviolet light (UVL) therapy.

TOPICAL MEDICATIONS

Pharmacologic Therapy

Topical therapy can be used to (1) restore hydration, (2) alleviate symptoms, (3) reduce inflammation, (4) protect the skin, (5) reduce scale and callus, (6) cleanse and debride, and (7) eradicate causative organisms. Topical medications are chosen both for the action of the active ingredients (which are delivered directly to the skin surface) and for the vehicle (base in which the medication is suspended). Topical medications have many different actions and cover a large spectrum of drug categories, including antibacterial, antifungal, and antipruritic (Table 70-1).

TABLE 70-1. Dermatologic Medications

Category	Example	Action	Nursing Intervention
Acne products	Benzoyl peroxide (Benzagel, Benzamycin, Desquam, PanOxyl, Xerac)	Keratolytic Bacteriostatic Decreases production of irritant-free fatty acids in follicle	Applied once or twice a day after washing area Observe for dryness or redness
	Tretinoin (Retin-A)	Vitamin A acid Decreases cohesiveness of epithelial cells, increasing cell mitosis and turnover; an irritant causing desquamation	Applied once daily at bedtime, 20 minutes after washing area Instruct client to expect some redness and peeling within a week, lasting 3 to 4 weeks Flare-up of acne may occur in first 2 to 4 weeks before improvement Clearing of acne requires 2 to 3 months Avoid excessive sun exposure, and use sunscreen daily Keep agent away from eyes
Antibacterials	Bacitracin ointment Polysporin ointment	Alter chemistry of microorganism's structure: denature proteins, increase cell wall permeability, and interfere with metabolism	Clean skin of adherent crust and debris before application Apply ointments frequently (2 to 3 times daily), as prescribed
Antibiotics	*Topical* Erythromycin (T-Stat, Erycette, Benzamycin) Clindamycin (Cleocin-T) Mupirocin (Bactroban)	Suppressive effects on inflammatory response; effective on papular and pustular lesions	Apply as prescribed Observe for redness, itching, or burning
Antifungals	*Topical* Nystatin (Mycostatin) Clotrimazole (Lotrimin) Oxiconazole (Oxistat) Naftifine (Naftin)	Alter cell wall permeability	A 2- to 3-week course of twice daily application is necessary for adequate treatment Overapplication can irritate sensitive, damaged skin
Antimetabolites	5-Fluorouracil (Efudex, Fluoroplex)	Interfere with DNA synthesis Inhibit thymidylate synthetase activity Effective in treating large areas of sun-damaged skin having premalignant or malignant lesions, e.g., basal cell epithelioma	Apply medication with gloved hand, avoiding mucous membranes and eyes Describe to the client expected response to the medication, e.g., a brisk inflammatory response with burning and itching Advise client to avoid sun exposure, which can increase the intensity of reaction to medication
Antiparasitics	Permethrin (Nix) Lindane (Kwell) Permethrin (Elimite)	Unknown	Avoid getting in eyes Observe for signs of reinfestation

TABLE 70–1. Dermatologic Medications Continued

Category	Example	Action	Nursing Intervention
			Observe for side effects (e.g., rash, redness, itching, burning, tingling) Full course of therapy needs to be completed Wash clothing in hot water or dry-clean Seal clothing that cannot be washed or dry-cleaned in plastic for 30–35 days All sexual contacts must also be treated
Antipruritics	*Lotions/Pastes* Phenol (0.5–2%) Menthol (0.1–2%) Camphor (1–3%) Calamine lotion Baths/cornstarch Oatmeal Aveeno	Antihistamine effect, blocking histamine and serotonin effects Cool and soothe skin	Apply frequently to reduce discomfort, unless medication contains an anesthetic ingredient (e.g., lidocaine); avoid the eyes If it contains anesthetic ingredient, apply as prescribed (2 to 4 times daily)
	Wet Dressings Potassium permanganate (1 : 4000–1 : 16,000) Aluminum acetate Burow's solution (1 : 10–1 : 40) Boric acid (1 tablespoon in 1 L of water) Normal saline (2 teaspoons salt in 1 L of water) Magnesium sulfate (8 teaspoons in 1 L of water) Silver nitrate 0.25%	Cool and soothe Some germicidal activity	Assess for contact sensitivity Use caution when entering and exiting tub; most solutions are slippery Protect linens from stains with wet dressings
Antiseptics	Chlorhexidine gluconate (Hibiclens)	Effective against staphylococci, streptococci, and gram-positive bacteria	Use for irrigating and cleansing wounds, but not for packing, because it may cause dermatitis
	Acetic acid (0.25%) solution	Effective against *Pseudomonas*	Protect healthy skin with a layer of petrolatum, because it excoriates the skin
	Hydrogen peroxide (3%)	Breaks up necrotic tissues	Use to irrigate and clean necrotic tissues from wounds Inhibits tissue formation, so avoid use in healing wounds
Corticosteroids	Hydrocortisone (Hytone) Alclometasone (Aclovate) Triamcinolone (Kenalog) Fluocinolone (Synalar) Mometasone (Elocon) Halcinonide (Halog) Betamethasone (Diprosone) Diflorasone (Psorcon) Clobetasol (Temovate)	Reduce blood flow by vasoconstrictive effects Antimitotic effect; slow epidermal cell production Reduce erythema and itching by anti-inflammatory action *Note:* Potent corticosteroids should be avoided in treating face, neck, and intertriginous sites because	Apply in even amounts Monitor length of prescribed topical administration to avoid long-term side effects Use care in clients with systemic bacterial, fungal, or viral infections May be applied to hydrated skin or with occlusive dressings to increase

Table continued on following page

TABLE 70–1. Dermatologic Medications Continued

Category	Example	Action	Nursing Intervention
		increased side effects may occur	penetration
Dressings	Duoderm Tegasorb Opsite Zinc oxide in Unna's boot	Physical protectants	Physical skin protectants should be used according to manufacturer's direction
Emollients/protectants	Vaseline Aquaphor ointment Eucerin cream Moisturel cream Neutrogena emulsion	Emollients provide a temporary barrier, protecting and softening skin Protectants cover skin and alleviate irritation	Apply evenly and smoothly; most useful when applied immediately after bathing Reapplication is required to provide protection when product has been absorbed or has worn off
Keratolytics	Salicylic acid (Duofilm, Duoplant, Occlusal, Ionil shampoo, T/Sal shampoo, Meted shampoo, Keralyt gel) Lactic Acid (Duofilm, LactiCare lotion)	Soften keratin and loosen cornified epithelium of the stratum corneum Debride excessive scale Used in varying concentrations to treat conditions ranging from dry, ichthyotic scalps or skin to warts	Apply only to involved area; can produce irritation and erythema in normal skin If prescribed for scale debridement, discontinue as soon as scale disappears If erythema and irritation occur, seek physician's approval to reduce frequency of use
Sunscreens	PABA PABA esters Cinnamates Salicylates Anthranilates Benzophenone	Provide protection through absorption, reflection, and scattering of ultraviolet radiation	Apply liberally 30 minutes to 1 hour before sun exposure Reapply after swimming or sweating or with prolonged ultraviolet exposure
Tars	*Coal Tar Products* Psorigel T-Derm Estar gel	Keratolytic Keratoplastic Photosensitizing Antipruritic	May be applied locally to specific lesions or widely to skin Do not apply to face or intertriginous sites Explain drug's photosensitizing properties to client

Topical Vehicles

Examples of various topical vehicles (Table 70–2) include ointments, creams, gels, aerosols, lotions, powders, and pastes. Ointments are more occlusive and therefore provide better delivery of the medication by preventing water loss from the skin. However, in some cases, especially periods of excessive heat or humidity, this occlusion may result in increased itching or skin infection; in these situations, creams may be better tolerated. Although creams spread more easily, they are less occlusive and may produce increased drying in some clients. Sprays and lotions are available for use on the scalp or other hairy areas. The various ingredients used to formulate the different bases may be irritating to individual clients, and care must be taken in recommending any product.

Both the active ingredient and the vehicle must be appropriate for the condition being treated. For acute dermatosis (i.e., weeping, blistering lesions), an aqueous (water-based) compound provides a drying effect. An ointment-based greasy vehicle has the opposite effect; it promotes lubrication and occlusion and helps treat the dryness and scaling caused by chronic dermatosis. Differences in skin permeability also influence the effectiveness of topical medications. For example, absorption increases in inflamed skin. Depending on the medication and the specific condition, topical medication may be specifically applied to localized lesions or to larger skin surfaces. When increased absorption of the medication is needed, topical medication may be prescribed for application under an occlusive dressing (Table 70–3). Ointments, creams, and gels have greatly increased absorption if they are applied to skin that is wet.

Topical Corticosteroids

Corticosteroids are the most commonly used topical medication. A large selection of topical steroids, ranging from very low potency to extremely high potency, is available today. Clients should be informed of what strength topical steroid they are given and the potential side effects. The lowest potency corticosteroid that is effective should be used. Rebound (exacerbation or worsening) of the condition can occur if treatment is stopped abruptly.

Clients must clearly understand how, when, and where to use topical steroids. Properly applying the medication evenly and sparingly one or two times daily to the affected areas can eliminate many potential problems. It is rarely helpful to apply the topical corticosteroid more than twice per day. This increases the

TABLE 70–2. Topical Medication Vehicles

Category	Example	Action	Use	Nursing Implications
Powders	Talc, cornstarch	Absorbs fluid	Intertriginous dermatitis	Dry surface before applying to prevent caking; reapply often
Lotions				
Suspension-based	Calamine lotion	Leaves a thin film of powder as water evaporates	Pruritus	Shake lotions well before applying Observe for overdrying of skin Apply in long, even strokes along direction of hair growth
Solutions	Salicylic acid	Leaves a film of powder as alcohol base evaporates	Warts	Shake well before applying; observe for skin overdrying and dry, tight skin for alcohol Apply as above
Aerosols	Triamcinolone acetonide aerosol	Leaves a thin film after alcohol evaporates	Pruritus, when direct application is painful	Shake well before applying; prevent inhalation by turning client's face to the side
Gels	Fluocinonide gel	Promotes drying of the skin	Eczema Pruritic rash	Observe for skin drying; avoid application to open skin areas (it burns)
Creams	Hydrocortisone cream	Leaves medication on skin after evaporation	Pruritus	Apply in thin layer along direction of hair growth Use during daytime Need to be reapplied often because perspiration or drainage may remove them
Ointments				
Water-in-oil	Eucerin	Lubricates skin	Dermatitis	Removable with soap and water
Absorbent	Aquaphor	Lubricates skin	Severe dermatitis	Difficult to remove; may feel greasy
Water-repellent	Petrolatum	Promotes absorption of water and medication	Severe dermatitis	Retains heat, difficult to remove; observe for maceration; avoid use in hair-bearing areas

TABLE 70-3. Occlusive Dressings

Purpose/Desired Effect	Nursing Implications
Produces airtight barrier, usually with plastic film Enhances absorption of topically applied medication (e.g., corticosteroids, keratolytics) by preventing evaporation Increases stratum corneum rehydration Softens hyperkeratotic areas by moisture retention	Clean skin site of debris and "old" medication before applying prescribed topical medication Apply topical medication while skin is still damp Apply plastic film (Saran wrap) snugly Use plastic bags for feet, polyethylene gloves for hands, plastic shower caps for scalp Press air out; seal borders with paper tape Leave dressing intact for 2-12 hours (as prescribed); then remove and gently clean the site Observe and document complications, e.g., maceration, oozing, signs of secondary fungal or bacterial infection, and folliculitis When occlusive dressings are used in conjunction with topical corticosteroids, frequent, prolonged use can result in permanent skin changes; these include striae, nonhealing ulcerations, telangiectasias, erythema, and skin atrophy

chance of side effects, makes the therapy more costly, and does not increase effectiveness. As the skin disorder improves, the frequency of use may be changed or a less potent topical corticosteroid prescribed. When the skin disease disappears or comes under good control, a tar preparation, moisturizer, or other topical preparation may be substituted.

SOAKS AND WET WRAPS

Soaks can be done in a variety of ways and serve several purposes. A wet environment softens dry epidermis and aids in removal of crusts. Removal of cellular skin debris promotes healing and improves absorption of topical medication. The risk of infection is decreased by the removal of necrotic tissue and occlusive crusts. Cooling also results from the gradual evaporation of water and acts as an anti-inflammatory, thus reducing itching.

Soaks can be accomplished by either soaking the affected area or bathing for 15 to 20 minutes in warm — not hot — tap water. The agent added to the soaks is the least important aspect of this therapy. Addition of substances such as colloidal oatmeal (Aveeno) or starch to the bath water is soothing to a certain population of clients but does nothing to increase water absorption. Tar preparations (Balnetar, T/Derm) have an anti-inflammatory effect and can be helpful in some eczematous and psoriatic conditions. Aluminum acetate (Burow's solution, Domeboro) and povidone-iodine (Betadine) are also effective antibacterial substances but additionally have drying effects. Bath oils are not recommended because they give the client a false sense of lubrication and make the bathtub very slippery. Clients leaving the bath should remove excess water by gently patting with a soft towel. They should immediately apply the recommended occlusive substance. Immediate application of the occlusive substance to the damp skin is the most important detail, because if the skin is not occluded within 3 to 5 minutes, evaporation will begin to occur.

Wet wraps used immediately after soaking and occlusion can optimize hydration and topical therapy; this also promotes cooling of the skin. Wet wraps and occlusion can be done in a variety of ways. The location and severity of lesions often determine the choices. Total-body wet wraps can be accomplished by putting on wet pajamas or wet long underwear followed by dry pajamas or a dry or plastic sweatsuit. The hands and feet can be covered by wet tube socks or wet cotton gloves followed by dry tube socks. Any extremity or the trunk can be covered by wet Kerlix and occluded with Ace bandages or by pieces of tube socks, wet followed by dry. The face can be wrapped with two layers of wet Kerlix followed by two layers of dry Kerlix held in place with Spandex netting or other tubular dressings; holes are cut out for eyes, nose, and mouth. If the dressing becomes dry, it should be rewetted before removal because debridement by wet-to-dry method produces tissue damage and pain. Gentle débridement usually still occurs if dressings are removed when damp.

PROTECTIVE DRESSINGS

Dressings and bandages allow control of the affected skin's environment and remain important in the treatment of wounds, ulcers, and recalcitrant dermatitis. Protection is the primary function of the dressings. Dressings limit the exposure of injured skin to dirt, mechanical trauma, and irritants. Ulcers and denuded skin heal more quickly when kept damp by an occlusive or semiocclusive dressing because regenerating epithelium migrates more easily across a moist surface. These wounds are less painful when kept damp, and enhanced absorption of topical medications will occur. Occlusive or semiocclusive dressings range from adhesive strips, nonstick gauze (Telfa), and petrolatum-impregnated gauze to dressings such as Duoderm and Opsite. Snug dressings such as elastic wraps over the lower legs effectively reduce edema and decrease healing time in stasis ulcers.

Finally, Unna's boot, a dressing designed to be removed only by medical personnel at a later visit, can be extremely useful for treatment of stasis ulcers that have venous insufficiency or when there is a concern about client compliance, scratching (neurodermatitis), or even self-injury. Unna's boot is a fixed, protective dressing that stimulates granulation tissue and restores epithelial growth. Dressings impregnated with zinc oxide paste, glycerin, and gelatin harden into a castlike dressing after application. Thus, the skin is protected from mechanical injury, and venous return is promoted. With use of warm water, the damaged skin surface is gently irrigated for removal of previous medication and debris. The damaged skin area is then measured and assessed. Prescribed topical agents (i.e., antibiotic ointments) may be applied. Next, starting at the dorsum of the foot, the dressing is applied. It is wrapped obliquely over the heel and up the calf. The greatest pressure is applied at the ankle and the lower third of the leg. The boot is completed just below the popliteal space. A layer of tube gauze is applied over the dressing. For additional support, an Ace bandage is secured appropriately with tape. Unna's boot is removed weekly for assessing damaged skin and cleaning normal skin.

Ideally, the area of damaged skin decreases, granulation tissue forms, and signs of chronic inflammation are reduced. Treatment continues for weeks until improvement occurs. It is important to explain to the client and family to keep the dressing dry and intact, and that Unna's boot needs to be removed if there is excessive drainage or localized pain (signs of infection). Routine follow-up is very important.

SKIN LUBRICANTS

Agents to hydrate the skin play an important therapy in many xerotic, pruritic, and inflammatory skin disorders. Measures to prevent skin dryness include elimination of drying compounds, which may include soaps and solvents, and use of emollients such as humectants, occlusive agents, and keratin-softening agents.

Skin is dry not because it lacks oil but because it lacks water. The primary means of correcting dryness is to add water to the skin and then apply a hydrophobic occlusive substance to retain the absorbed water. To seal in the water, the use of occlusives such as white petrolatum (Vaseline), Aquaphor ointment, or Crisco is very effective.

Frequent use of emollients should be encouraged. Clients often prefer cosmetically elegant products because they are formulated into lotions that can be poured from bottles and rubbed into the skin without leaving a greasy residue. Although the chemicals in these lotions provide benefit, the water loss continues. There are many moisturizers available in the form of lotions and creams. Lotions and creams may be irritating and drying because of an evaporative effect of the water and multiple ingredients used as preservatives, solubilizers, and fragrances. Lotions contain more water than creams do and thus evaporate more quickly.

If emollient products are not successful, it may be necessary to try more potent agents. Humectants are substances such as urea (Aquacare/HP 10 percent, Carmol 20 per cent) that attract and hold water, which results in transepidermal water migration. The alpha-hydroxy acids such as lactic acid (LactiCare) or ammonium lactate (LacHydrin) may be tried; these hold moisture and decrease the rough scale that creates the sensation of dryness. Also popular with clients are additives such as aloe, vitamin E, jojoba, elastin, and collagen. No scientific evidence has shown that these have special, intrinsic properties beyond their minimal lubricating effects.

ULTRAVIOLET LIGHT THERAPY

Artificially reproduced forms of UVL are used therapeutically with topical or systemic photosensitizing drugs to cause desquamation (shedding or peeling of epidermis). UVL also temporarily suppresses mitosis of the basal cell layer by inhibiting DNA mitosis. Ultraviolet A (UVA) and ultraviolet B (UVB) are used to treat diseases responsive to UVL, such as psoriasis, vitiligo, cutaneous T-cell lymphoma, uremic pruritus, chronic eczematous eruptions, and, more rarely, acne vulgaris. Currently, three treatment modalities involve UVL: (1) Goeckerman and modified Goeckerman regimen, and (2) photochemotherapy or PUVA (psoralen plus UVA).

Every client must have a complete history and physical examination before initiation of any UVL therapy for assessment of multiple factors. Record highlights of the client's history; take care to include complete medication history because the client could be taking one or more of the many photosensitizing drugs (i.e., thiazide diuretics, tetracyclines). Clients should also be asked specifically about previous herpes simplex infections because these can be stimulated by UVL. Pretreatment assessment includes identifying solar-induced skin malignancies, cataracts, or lupus erythematosus. Clients with a history of basal cell or squamous cell epitheliomas are at risk for developing additional neoplastic changes with this treatment. Thus, potential benefit is weighed against potential risk. A complete ophthalmologic examination is important before treatment is started and yearly thereafter during long-term treatment. A history of cataract formation is a potential contraindication to PUVA therapy. Anyone showing early cataract changes needs extra photoprotective measures (e.g., the complete occlusion of goggles or PUVA glasses) and more frequent ophthalmologic assessments (every 3 to 6 months). The skin changes of clients with lupus erythematosus are aggravated by sun exposure, so photochemotherapy is contraindicated. Before therapy is initiated, an antinuclear antibody test (ANA titer) should rule out this condition.

Be aware that because treatments to the face and genitalia increase risk for cumulative effect of UVL, minimal exposure is indicated. Periodic assessments must be done throughout the course of therapy for signs of actinic damage (e.g., severe wrinkling, "tissue paper" transparency) or cutaneous malignancy. Posttherapy clients must be observed for potential side effects including dry skin, pruritus, and potential delayed (36 to 48 hours after exposure) phototoxic reaction (such as erythema, vesicles, and pain).

Goeckerman Regimen

The most common type of phototherapy is the Goeckerman regimen and variants of it. This method uses the photosensitizing, keratoplastic, and antipruritic properties of topical tar preparations in conjunction with UVL in UVB wavelengths. It is often used to treat psoriasis vulgaris and atopic dermatitis. The procedure includes a therapeutic tar emulsion bath followed by an application of topical tar medication (e.g., crude coal tar in petrolatum). Several hours later, a specific dose of UVL is administered to the skin surface. If the client's condition is severe, hospitalization or daily care in an ambulatory or day care setting may be necessary for this treatment. Outpatient phototherapy combined with treatment baths and tar applications at home can be helpful for less severe involvement.

Photochemotherapy

Photochemotherapy or PUVA combines oral or topical 8-methoxypsoralen with UVA. PUVA is used to treat severe, unresponsive forms of psoriaris, atopic dermatitis, and cutaneous T-cell lymphoma and for cosmetic therapy in clients with alopecia areata or vitiligo. The potent systemic photosensitizing medications increase skin sensitivity to long-wave UVL (UVA). In conjunction with exposure to artificially reproduced forms of UVA (PUVA therapy), these medications induce repigmentation (melanin production) in vitiligo and have an antimitotic effect in psoriasis and cutaneous T-cell lymphoma. Dosage is determined by body weight. The medication in taken orally with food to minimize nausea 1½ to 2 hours before UVL irradiation. Topical medication is used to treat localized sites or in clients in whom systemic administration is contraindicated (such as clients with liver or renal disease).

Clients taking these photosensitizing medications must protect the skin from ambient UVL irradiation before and for 8 hours after taking the medication. The client should (1) wear protective clothing, such as long sleeves, (2) apply sunscreen to exposed skin, (3) minimize natural skin exposure, and (4) wear dark green or brown plastic sunglasses that are capable of screening both UVA and UVB to protect the eyes for 48 hours after taking the medication.

PSYCHOSOCIAL ASPECTS OF SKIN DISORDERS

Anger, frustration, and anxiety are commonly experienced by clients with skin disorders, which often exacerbates the condition. Clients with underlying skin disease are more likely to respond to stress, frustration, embarrassment, or any emotionally upsetting event with itching and scratching. Excitability and arousal of the central nervous system from an emotional upset can intensify the vasomotor and sweat responses in the skin and lead to the itch-scratch cycle (see Pruritus). In some instances, scratching is used as an expression of anger, because typically it will get an immediate response from those nearby. The added dimension of family hostility, rejection, and guilt can damage the family structure.

Learning about the acute or chronic nature of the given disorder, the exacerbating factors, and the management measures that can control it is important for both the client and family members. Maintaining a healthy outlook is important. Counseling and other psychosocial intervention is often very helpful for dealing with the frustrations of skin disease. It is especially helpful to adolescents and young adults, who may consider the lesions disfiguring or unattractive.

The client education needs of those affected by skin disease are vast. Health care providers need to consistently provide information that includes detailed skin care plans, general disease information, and availability of client-oriented support organizations as well as updates on hopeful research results. Most clients will forget or confuse the important skin care recommendations without written instructions. Clearly outlining the skin care recommendations to the client in both a verbal and written manner is essential for good outcomes (Client Education Guides). Nurses play the major role in providing this important aspect of care. Adequate time and client teaching materials are needed to provide education in an effective manner. Nurses should be resourceful in obtaining or writing educational materials and instruction sheets. Client education pamphlets are available through a variety of sources, including the many dermatologically oriented client support groups, professional dermatology agencies such as the Dermatology Nurses' Association, and the American Academy of Dermatology.

▼ COMMON SKIN DISORDERS

PRURITUS

Overview

Pruritus (itching) is one of the most common manifestations of skin problems; it is a symptom, not a disease. Pruritus has been defined as an unpleasant skin sensation producing a strong desire to scratch, localized to or generalized over a body area. It can lead to damage if scratching injures the skin's protective barrier, possibly with resultant infection and scarring. Relieving this symptom, especially for chronically ill clients, is a nursing challenge because of its common occurrence and the major effect it may have on a client's quality of life.

Pruritus can be a secondary symptom of conditions ranging from dry skin to carcinoma. Systemic diseases that can cause generalized and severe pruritus include chickenpox, severe liver disease, diabetes mellitus, uremia due to chronic renal failure, drug hypersensitivities,

CLIENT EDUCATION GUIDE

Skin Self-examination

What You Will Need: a bright light; a full-length mirror; a hand mirror; two chairs or stools; a blow dryer; body maps; a pencil. Examine your face, especially the nose, lips, mouth, and ears—front and back. Use one or both mirrors to get a clear view. Thoroughly inspect your scalp, using a blow dryer and mirror to expose each section to view. Get a friend or family member to help, if you can. Check your hands carefully: palms and backs, between the fingers and under the fingernails. Continue up the wrists to examine both front and back of your forearms. Standing in front of the full-length mirror, begin at the elbows and scan all sides of your upper arms. Do not forget the underarms. Next focus on the neck, chest, and torso. Women should lift breasts to view the underside. With your back to the full-length mirror, use the hand mirror to inspect the back of your neck, shoulders, upper back, and any part of the back of your upper arms you could not view previously. Still using both mirrors, scan your lower back, buttocks, and backs of both legs. Sit down; prop each leg in turn on the other stool or chair. Use the hand mirror to examine the genitals. Check front and sides of both legs, thigh to shin; ankles, tops of feet, between toes, and under toenails. Examine soles of feet and heels.

From The Skin Cancer Foundation (1992). *Skin cancer: If you can spot it, you can stop it.* New York: The Skin Cancer Foundation.

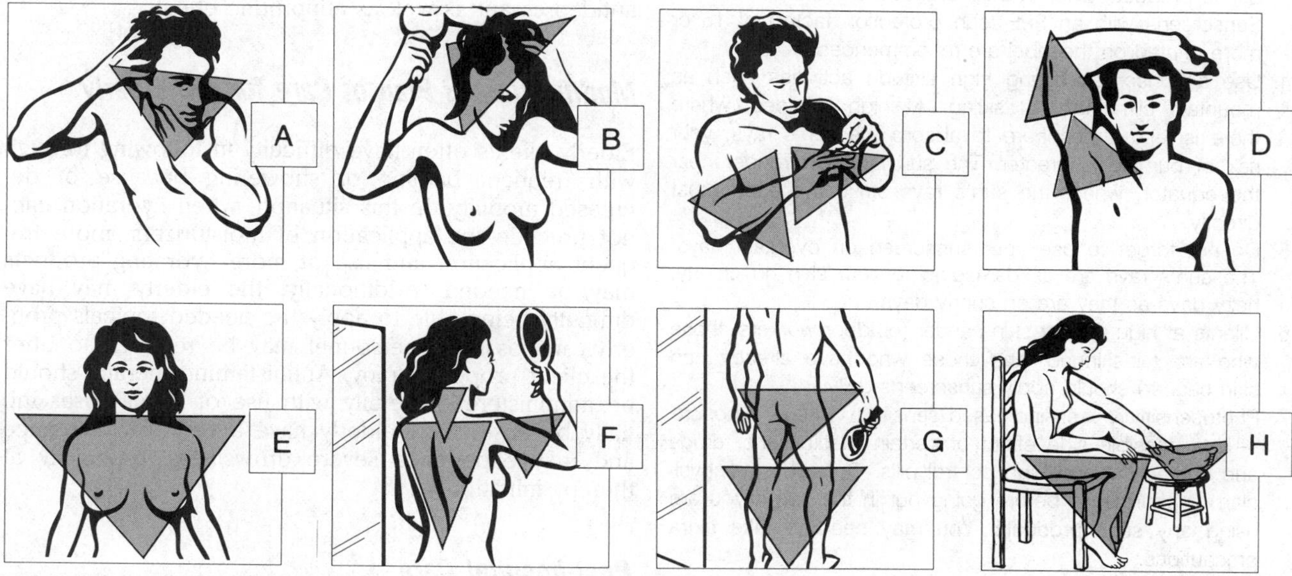

intestinal parasites, and neoplastic conditions (i.e., leukemia and lymphoma).

Stimulation of itching can be initiated by almost any chemical or physical substance, especially if skin is damaged. Once the itch sensation is established, the client has an almost uncontrollable urge to scratch. Scratching leads to further skin damage and increased inflammation. Pruritus therefore increases, and so does the urge to scratch. Thus, the *itch-scratch-itch cycle* develops. In order to minimize skin trauma caused by scratching, fingernails should be kept short.

The client will usually volunteer subjective reports of the degree and location of itching. Listen carefully to the client's description of the severity and location of pruritus and (2) seek information about how pruritus interferes with activities of daily living. Objective signs include excoriations or other secondary skin changes such as lichenification. Document all assessment findings.

Management

Appropriate management of the itching requires a complete assessment that attempts to discover the underlying cause and knowledge of appropriate therapeutic modalities for treatment.

Dry skin may either be the source of or contribute to pruritus, and it is often helpful to employ good hydration (see Xerotic Eczema) in addition to any other topical therapy. One bath or shower per day for 15 to 20 minutes with warm water and a mild soap should be immediately followed by the application of an emollient, with or without other topical medications, to prevent evaporation of water from the hydrated epidermis. Other topical medications often added to emollients to help alleviate itching include menthol (0.25 to 0.5 per cent), camphor (0.25 to 0.50 per cent), urea (10 to 20 per cent), and lactic acid (12 per cent). Camphor and menthol produce a cooling effect. Topically applied

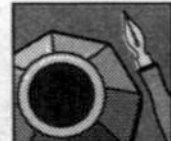

CLIENT EDUCATION GUIDE

Simple Guidelines to Help Protect You from the Damaging Rays of the Sun

1. Minimize sun exposure during the hours of 10 AM to 2 PM (11 AM to 3 PM daylight saving time), when the sun is strongest. Try to plan your outdoor activities for the early morning or late afternoon.
2. Wear a hat, long-sleeved shirt, and long pants when out in the sun. Choose tightly woven materials for greater protection from the sun's rays.
3. Apply a sunscreen before every exposure to the sun and reapply frequently and liberally, at least every 2 hours, as long as you stay in the sun. The sunscreen should always be reapplied after swimming or perspiring heavily, because products differ in their degrees of water resistance. Sunscreens with an SPF (sun protection factor) of 15 or more printed on the label are recommended.
4. Use a sunscreen during high altitude activities such as mountain climbing and skiing. At high altitudes, where there is less atmosphere to absorb the sun's rays, your risk of burning is greater. The sun is also stronger near the equator, where the sun's rays strike the earth most directly.
5. Do not forget to use your sunscreen on overcast days. The sun's rays are as damaging to your skin on cloudy, hazy days as they are on sunny days.
6. Clients at high risk for skin cancer (outdoor workers, those who are fair-skinned, and those who have already had skin cancer) should apply sunscreens daily.
7. Photosensitivity—an increased sensitivity to sun exposure—is a possible side effect of certain medications, drugs and cosmetics, and birth control pills. Consult your physician or pharmacist before going out in the sun if you are using any such products. You may need to take extra precautions.
8. If you develop an allergic reaction to your sunscreen, change sunscreens. One of the many products on the market today should be right for you.
9. Beware of reflective surfaces! Sand, snow, concrete, and water can reflect more than half the sun's rays onto your skin. Sitting in the shade does not guarantee protection from sunburn.
10. Avoid tanning parlors. The ultraviolet light emitted by tanning booths causes sunburn and premature aging and increases your risk of developing skin cancer.
11. Keep young infants out of the sun. Begin using sunscreens on children at 6 months of age, and then allow sun exposure with moderation.
12. Teach children sun protection early. Sun damage occurs with each unprotected sun exposure and accumulates over the course of a lifetime.

From The Skin Cancer Foundation, New York.

antihistamines and anesthetics are relatively ineffective and are best avoided because they can be potent allergic sensitizers. This is especially true if these products are used on inflamed skin. Use of topical corticosteroids should be reserved for the treatment of a specific steroid-responsive dermatosis. Long-term application of topical steroids, especially on skin not affected with an eczematous condition, may result in thinning of the skin, striae, telangiectasias, and easy bruising.

Systemic antihistamines may be prescribed. They are most helpful in disorders in which histamine is the principal mediator but may be of benefit through sedative or even placebo effect. A trial of H_1-blocker antihistamine (hydroxyzine, diphenhydramine, chlorpheniramine) is appropriate either on a regular schedule or as indicated for itching. Tricyclic antidepressants (doxepin hydrochloride, amitriptyline hydrochloride) have a high binding capacity for histamine H_1-receptors and may be helpful for clients who would benefit from their antidepressant as well as antipruritic effect.

Modification of Plan of Care for the Elderly

Elderly clients often have difficulty in following through with frequent bathing or showering because of decreased mobility. In this situation, when hydration cannot precede the application of moisturizers, more frequent application and use of more hydrating products may be needed. Additionally, the elderly may have difficulty being able to apply the needed topicals properly, and assistive personnel may be required to offer the client proper therapy. Antihistamine therapy should be administered carefully with use of small doses initially because many elderly have a very low tolerance and may experience severe drowsiness, especially at therapy initiation.

Post-hospital Care

DISCHARGE TEACHING

Home health care instructions are very important and always most helpful when given in written format (see Bridge to Home Health Care). While providing instruction, it is very important to remember that things that irritate some clients do not irritate others. See section on implementation under alteration in comfort in the care plan on atopic dermatitis.

▼ Eczematous Disorders

Eczema is not a specific disease. Dermatitis and eczema are terms that may be used interchangeably to describe a group of disorders with a characteristic appearance. A few examples of eczema or dermatitis (and abbreviated definitions) include allergic contact dermatitis (eruptions from allergy to poison ivy, sumac, or oak or proven allergen); irritant dermatitis (eruption

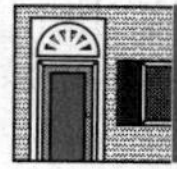

BRIDGE TO HOME HEALTH CARE

Skin Care

Minor skin problems are not the focus of client care during hospitalization for major illnesses. When the client returns home to convalesce, minor problems often surface as the primary complaint during recovery. The home health care nurse needs to perform assessment on the initial home visit and be very alert to problems not identified on the referral. Frequently, the nurse discovers edema, redness, abrasions, tears, or minor skin wounds on the first home visit.

Assessment of the skin system can provide a clue to underlying disease and the body's defense against the present illness. Poor skin turgor will alert the nurse to focus on nutrition and hydration as important needs for client recovery.

Assessment for skin intactness will alert the nurse to focus on health of the skin. Extremely dry skin not only is a discomfort to the client but may deteriorate further. The nurse should evaluate the client's need for assistance with personal care and determine whether skin care instruction is appropriate or skin care by a home health care aide is needed. Thorough assessment helps the nurse determine the frequency of home health care aide visits required for ensuring good skin care.

from direct contact with cosmetics, chemicals, dyes, or detergents); nummular eczema (appearance of coin-shaped, oozing, crusting patches); seborrheic dermatitis (yellowish-pink scaling of scalp, face, and trunk); stasis dermatitis (eruption resulting from peripheral venous disorders); and atopic dermatitis (characteristic distribution of eczema in clients with a family history of an allergic disorder). Eczema/dermatitis has three primary stages; eczema may manifest in any one of the three stages, or the three stages may coexist.

Acute dermatitis is characterized by extensive erosions with serous exudate or by intensely pruritic, erythematous papules and vesicles on a background of erythema. *Subacute dermatitis* is characterized by erythematous, excoriated, scaling papules or plaques that are either grouped or scattered over erythematous skin. Often, the scaling is so fine and diffuse that the skin acquires a silvery sheen. *Chronic dermatitis* is characterized by thickened skin and increased skin marking secondary to rubbing and scratching (lichenification); excoriated papules, fibrotic papules, and nodules (prurigo nodularis); and postinflammatory hyper- and hypopigmentation.

ATOPIC DERMATITIS

Definition

Atopic dermatitis is a common, chronic, relapsing, pruritic type of eczema. The word "atopic" refers to a group of three associated allergic disorders: asthma, allergic rhinitis (hay fever), and atopic dermatitis.

Incidence

According to several studies, 75 to 80 per cent of clients with atopic dermatitis have a personal or family history of allergic disorders. Atopic dermatitis is a common disorder affecting 0.5 to 1 per cent of the people in all parts of the world.

Etiology and Risk Factors

The exact cause of atopic dermatitis is unknown. Xerosis is usually worse during periods of low humidity; winter in northern latitudes may aggravate pruritus.

Pathophysiology

Compared with normal skin, the dry skin of atopic dermatitis has a reduced water-binding capacity, a higher transepidermal water loss, and a decreased water content. Although the underlying biochemical abnormality for xerosis in atopic dermatitis is unknown, clinically noninflamed, nonichthyotic skin in atopic dermatitis contains a mild inflammatory infiltrate and epidermal edema (spongiosis). Whether these pathologic findings cause the dry skin or are a result of the dry skin is unknown. Water loss leads to further drying and cracking of the skin, which leads to more itching. Rubbing and scratching of itchy skin are responsible for many of the clinical changes seen in the skin.

Clinical Manifestations

Atopic dermatitis begins in many clients during infancy. This form of dermatitis is called acute dermatitis, and the child has a red, oozing, crusting rash. As the child grows, the skin tends to show the chronic form of dermatitis with thickened dry texture, brownish-gray color, and scale. The rash tends to become localized to the large folds of the extremities as the client becomes older. It is found mainly on elbow bends, backs of knees, neck, sides of the face, eyelids, and the backs of hands and feet. Hand and foot dermatitis becomes a significant problem in some clients.

Pruritus is the major symptom of atopic dermatitis and causes the greatest morbidity. The urge to scratch may be mild and self-limiting, or it may be intense, leading to severely excoriated lesions, infection, and scarring.

Complications

Clients with atopic dermatitis have a tendency to develop viral, bacterial, and fungal skin infections. It is not clear whether these cutaneous infections arise secondary to a disruption of normal barrier function or reduced local immunity. The most common viral infection is herpes simplex, which tends to spread locally or become generalized. Honey-colored crusting, extensive serous weeping, folliculitis, pyoderma, and furunculosis indicate bacterial infection usually secondary to *Staphylococcus aureus* in clients with atopic dermatitis. Clients with atopic dermatitis are heavily colonized with *S. aureus*. Superficial fungal infections may also appear more frequently in atopic clients.

Medical Management

The goal of therapy is to break the inflammatory cycles that cause excess drying and cracking as well as the itching and scratching. Primary prevention begins with daily skin care that hydrates and lubricates the skin. The health care team's understanding of each client's disease pattern and the discovery and reduction of exacerbating factors are crucial to effective management of this chronic disorder. Other factors that must be considered include irritants, allergens, physical environment, and emotional stresses.

Hydration is the key to management but is often difficult to achieve. Soaks followed by application of occlusive substances is usually prescribed (see Soaks and Wet Wraps).

Aeroallergens may be inciting factors in this disorder. Clients should avoid exposure to allergens to which there is a positive test finding and for which a high degree of suspicion exists that dermatitis is precipitated by them. Stringent restrictions on clients are unjustified. It is important to attempt to identify and eliminate triggers that cause the atopic dermatitis to flare. Many of these triggering factors are the same irritants that contribute to generalized pruritus (see Pruritus).

PHARMACOLOGIC MANAGEMENT

Occlusives, moisturizers, topical corticosteroids, and tar preparations can all be used topically in various combinations to control atopic dermatitis. Topical steroids are a very important component of therapy in treating eczema (see topical corticosteroids). All of these preparations will be best absorbed into hydrated skin or by using wet wraps and occlusion. Topicals containing chemicals or drugs that would cause skin eruptions themselves are avoided.

Systemic medications may include antibiotics and antihistamines. The use of a systemic corticosteroid is rarely warranted in atopic dermatitis. Some clients or parents view the systemic use of steroids as a "quick cure" and find them much easier to use than hydration and topical therapy; however, they should be avoided in this chronic non-life-threatening disorder. Although there may be dramatic improvement with their use, the rebound after their discontinuation is equally dramatic. The side effects of long-term systemic steroid use are both unpleasant and dangerous.

When a short-term course of oral steroid therapy is given, it is important to taper the dosage as it is discontinued. Intensified skin care should also be instituted during the taper to suppress flaring of the dermatitis.

Recent research has suggested a variety of new therapeutic approaches. There are promising results with the use of the new immune response modifiers thymopentin and interferon-gamma for therapy of severe atopic dermatitis as well as with etretinate and other experimental modalities. Clients with severe, recalcitrant disease should be updated of research advances and encouraged to participate in trials when possible for preventing a sense of hopelessness.

DIETARY MANAGEMENT

Dietary management of atopic dermatitis has continued to be a controversial subject. The significance of food allergies is not known in the causation of atopic dermatitis or what percentage of atopic dermatitis clients have food allergies. The most common allergens that appear to be important are eggs, cow's milk, soy, wheat, nuts, and fish. Known allergens are avoided. Care must be taken to avoid inadvertent malnutrition when any type of restrictive diet is used.

Nursing Management

The client with atopic dermatitis should be assessed for present hygienic habits (e.g., does the client bathe with soap and hot water?), present medication regimen, exposure to known allergens, environmental exposure, and history of skin eruptions.

Nursing management of the client with atopic dermatitis is presented in the nursing care plan.

Modification of Plan of Care for the Elderly

Dermatitis is a common skin disorder in the elderly. It may be caused by hypoproteinemia, venous insufficiency, allergens, irritants, or underlying malignancy such as leukemia or lymphoma. Because the elderly client often takes multiple medications, dermatitis from drug-drug interaction is considered. The fragility of the skin as a result of the flattened epidermal-dermal junction and loss of dermis should be considered in planning any form of treatment. Most aged clients do not need a daily bath and should avoid hot water for bathing as well as soap. Tepid water and nondrying bath agents should be used.

Post-hospital Care

DISCHARGE TEACHING

If dermatitis is due to an allergen, the client should be advised to avoid the allergen. However, this advice must be given within reason. For example, if the client is found to be allergic to cat dander and the cat is the client's only companion, the client may not be required to dispose of the cat, but perhaps the places the cat goes in the home can be restricted. Air conditioning can help reduce aeroallergen exposure at home or in the workplace. Food allergens can be avoided only if the client reads the labels on prepackaged food or prepares all food from scratch. Clients will need to be taught about medication regimens as well as techniques for self-care.

XEROTIC ECZEMA (DRY SKIN)

Xerotic (dry) skin is dehydrated, erythematous, scaling, and finely cracked. Xerosis occurs in patches and may involve any skin surface. It is common in elderly clients. If xerosis is severe, the skin is tight, itchy, and painful. In low humidity, which is especially prevalent in artificially heated rooms in wintertime, excessive water is lost from the stratum corneum. Water loss causes xerotic chapping. The problem is accentuated by use of drying skin cleansers, soaps, disinfectants, and solvents and infrequent use of moisturizers.

Environmental factors play a large role, especially those that increase water loss in the skin. Any factors that decrease the relative humidity exacerbate this condition, such as cold or dry winter air, especially in artificially heated rooms.

The treatment of xerotic skin consists primarily of correcting dryness and avoidance of irritating factors. Teaching the client correct daily skin care is essential in treating this condition. See earlier discussion.

STASIS DERMATITIS

Overview

Stasis dermatitis is the development of areas of very dry skin and sometimes shallow ulcers on the lower legs primarily due to venous insufficiency. The process of dermatitis begins with edema of the leg due to slowed venous return. The client commonly has a history of varicose veins or deep vein thrombosis. As the venous stasis continues, the tissue becomes hypoxic from inadequate blood supply. As the blood pools, hemoglobin is released from the red blood cell and deposited in the tissues. This poorly nourished tissue begins to necrose. The clinical manifestations include itching, a feeling of heaviness in the legs, brown-stained skin, and open shallow lesions (Fig. 70-1). The lesions are very slow to heal because of the lack of oxygenated blood.

Management

The legs need improved venous return. This can be accomplished with leg elevation and support hose. Clients should be instructed to raise the legs during the day, especially if they are employed at a job in which they stand still in one area for long periods of time (e.g., cashier). Stasis ulcers are treated with wet-to-dry dressings for debridement of the area, Unna's boots, and skin grafts.

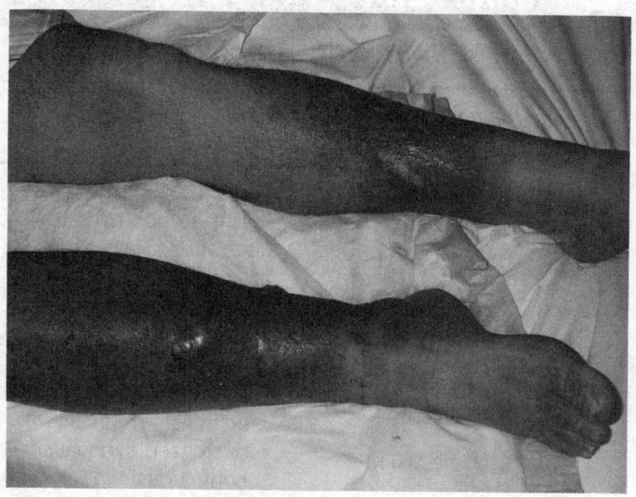

▲ **Figure 70-1**

Stasis dermatitis and cellulitis. This client has stasis dermatitis in the left leg and blisters from cellulitis in the right leg.

CONTACT DERMATITIS

Contact dermatitis is an inflammatory response of the skin to chemical or physical allergens. *Irritant contact dermatitis* is due to exposure to a chemical or physical irritant. Clinical manifestations range from mild erythema to vesicles to ulceration (Fig. 70-2). *Allergic*

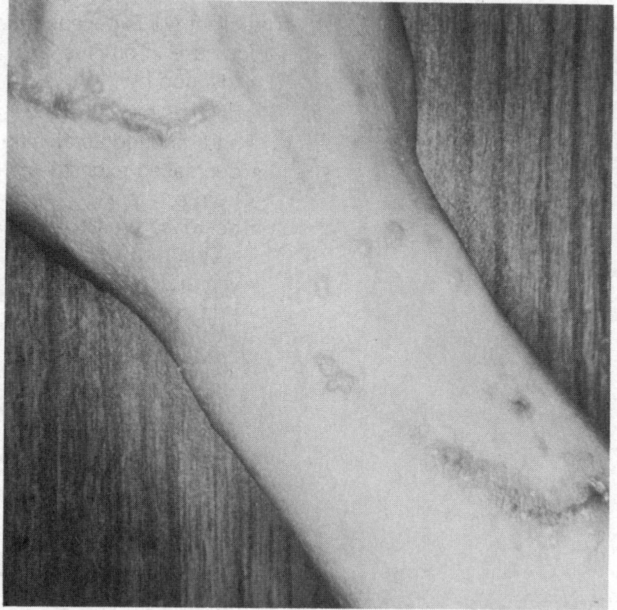

▲ **Figure 70-2**

Contact dermatitis of the hand from poison ivy exposure.

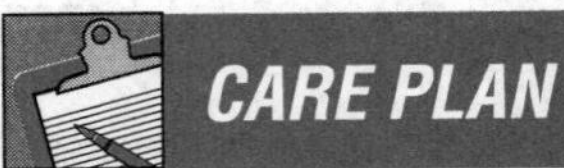

CARE PLAN

The Client with Atopic Dermatitis

Nursing Diagnosis/ Collaborative Problem	Planning: Expected Outcomes	Implementation: Nursing Interventions	Rationales
Skin Integrity, Impaired R/T cutaneous dryness	The client will maintain skin that has good hydration and reduced inflammation, as evidenced by • verbalizing increased skin comfort • decreased flaking and scaling • decreased redness • decreased excoriations from scratching • healing of previous areas of breakdown	Bathe at least once every day for 15 to 20 minutes. Immediately upon leaving the bath, apply an appropriate emollient or prescribed topical. Bathe more often when signs and symptoms increase.	Soaking saturates the stratum corneum. Application of an occlusive moisturizer 2 to 4 minutes after the bath is critical for preventing evaporation of water from the hydrated epidermis.
		Use warm water—not hot.	Hot water causes vasodilation, which increases pruritus.
		Use superfatted soaps (i.e., Dove or Basis) or soaps for sensitive skin (i.e., Neutrogena, Moisturel, Aveeno, Oilatum, Purpose). Avoid bubble baths.	The use of drying soap may compound the problem. Superfatted soaps are less alkaline and less drying to the skin.
		Apply occlusive topical emollient or prescribed topical preparation 2 to 3 times per day.	Ointments and creams seal in water and thereby hydrate the skin. The particular emollient selected depends mostly on client preference and whether the ingredients in the base are irritants.
Alteration in comfort, R/T pruritus	The client will experience a decrease in pruritus, as evidenced by • decrease in observed and reported scratching • decreased excoriations from scratching • decreased restlessness during sleep • verbalizing increased skin comfort	Explain the itching symptom as it relates to cause (i.e., dryness of the skin) and the principles of the selected therapy (i.e., hydration) and the itch-scratch-itch cycle.	Understanding the physiologic or psychological process and principles of itching and its treatment increases cooperation
		Wash all new clothes before wearing for removal of formaldehyde and other chemicals, and avoid use of fabric softeners.	Pruritus is often precipitated by irritant or allergic effects of certain chemicals or components of fabric softeners.
		Change to a milder detergent and add a second rinse cycle to ensure removal of soap.	Residual laundry detergent in clothing may be irritating. The actual laundry soap that is used is not the key, but rather that all soap is rinsed out so that an irritant effect is avoided.
		Wear open-weave, loose-fitting, cotton-blend clothing. Avoid over-dressing, rough or wool fabrics, and tightly woven fabrics.	Light cotton-blend clothing allows air circulation and minimizes perspiration, which intensifies itching.

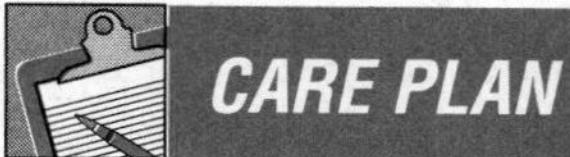

The Client with Atopic Dermatitis Continued

Nursing Diagnosis/ Collaborative Problem	Planning: Expected Outcomes	Implementation: Nursing Interventions	Rationales
		Work and sleep in comfortable surroundings with a fairly constant temperature (68–75°) and humidity level (45–55 per cent). Air conditioning in the home, particularly the bedroom, may be beneficial.	Extremes of temperature cause pruritus frequently secondary to vasodilation and increased cutaneous blood flow. In addition to providing a cooler environment, air conditioning will decrease aeroallergen exposure.
		Keep fingernails very short, smooth, and clean.	Trimmed nails prevent damage and infection to the skin.
		Appropriate use of antihistamines may reduce itching to some degree.	Histamine is the most commonly known itch mediator. The sedating antihistamines also provides relief.
		Use sunscreen on a regular basis.	Sunburn may cause flare of dermatitis.
		Immediately after swimming, take a shower or bath, washing with a mild soap from head to toe, and then apply an appropriate moisturizer.	Residual chlorine or bromine on the skin after swimming in a pool may be irritating.
Infection, High Risk for R/T • skin excoriation • decreased resistance to cutaneous viral, fungal, and staphylococcal organisms	The client will be free of infectious lesions, as evidenced by absence of pustules, exudate, or crusting	Explain to client the signs of infection and be sure the client understands that presence of these signs indicates need for medical intervention.	Infections are a potentially serious complication of disorders of open skin.
			Leftover medications may be outdated and may be inappropriate treatment.
		Ensure that the client understands the importance of not self-treating with leftover medication at home.	Medications can become contaminated and lead to infection or lose their potency.
		Emphasize that it is important to take the antibiotic on schedule and the entire course.	To completely eradicate the infectious organism.
Body Image Disturbance R/T • skin lesions • response of significant others to appearance	The client will exhibit a positive self-concept, as evidenced by • engaging in social activities • expressing feelings of importance, self-worth • enjoying interpersonal interactions	Encourage client to teach others that eczema is not contagious unless severely infected.	Eczema can be mistaken for impetigo or as an indication of uncleanliness, causing social isolation.
		Encourage client and significant others to share feelings with each other regarding the client's appearance and the chronic nature of eczema.	Unidentified fears and concerns may hinder interpersonal relationships.
		Reinforce client's sense of identity and personal competence. Encourage self-management of eczema and understanding that controlling scratching will greatly reduce lesions.	Allowing client to determine need for various treatment modalities, such as when to initiate wet wraps or minor alterations in topical therapy, promotes positive self-concept.

contact dermatitis is a delayed hypersensitivity reaction from contact with an allergen. This response is due to action of the T lymphocyte. Clinical manifestations begin at the site of exposure with itching, stinging, erythema, and edema but then extend to more distant sites.

Management of contact dermatitis begins by determining the causative agent. Determining the agent usually begins by interviewing the client for recent exposure to chemicals, metals, and the like. Patch testing is done to determine the specific agent, if necessary. Pain and itching may be controlled with topical medications or wet dressings. Antihistamines and steroids may be required.

INTERTRIGO

Overview

Intertrigo is superficial inflammatory dermatitis that occurs when two skin surfaces rub, which prevents adequate ventilation. Friction, heat, and moisture cause erythema and maceration, itching, and burning. Erosions and fissures with erythema and secondary bacterial or *Candida albicans* infection may form. Intertrigo is common in hot, humid weather in neck creases, axillae, antecubital fossae, perineal and finger and toe webs, abdominal skinfolds, and beneath the breast, particularly in obese clients.

Management

The treatment for intertrigo is to eliminate maceration by promoting drying and to aerate the body skinfolds. For mobile clients, it is important to review environmental changes that promote drying of the body folds, such as light clothing or periodic removal of clothing to dry off. Care recommendations are very dependent on the degree of involvement and the overall condition of the skin. If the skin is still intact, recommendations include washing the area gently with tap water twice daily, rinsing, and drying the area, followed by liberal application of a talc-containing powder or a cellulose-containing powder (i.e., Zeasorb) for extra absorption. Never use cornstarch because it encourages *C. albicans* overgrowth. If inflammation is present, low-potency topical corticosteroids in nonocclusive vehicles (i.e., hydrocortisone 1 or 2½ per cent cream or lotion) or combination steroid-antibiotic (Vytone 1 per cent) preparations may initially be helpful, but long-term use should be avoided. Apply cool, wet soaks with tap water or Burow's solution three to four times daily for removal of exudate if secondary infection is present. In the event of fissuring, use of an antiseptic drying dye preparation (i.e., Castaderm) to these areas once daily is effective but messy and may sting on application. Applying folded gauze or clean cotton handkerchiefs in skinfolds promotes healing by keeping skin surfaces apart.

PSORIASIS VULGARIS

Overview

Psoriasis vulgaris is a chronic, recurrent, erythematous, inflammatory disorder involving keratin synthesis. Pruritus can be severe. Psoriasis occurs in both sexes, usually commencing in early adulthood. The term "vulgaris" means common.

The cause of psoriasis vulgaris is unknown. However, alterations in cyclic nucleotides, and possible immunologic abnormalities have been noted. Genetic predisposition is also possible.

Rapidly proliferating epidermal cells form small, scaly patches of skin that develop into erythematous, dry, scaling patches of various sizes. The course of psoriasis vulgaris is prolonged and unpredictable. Anxiety and stress often precede flare-ups. Exacerbations and remissions are common. It usually recurs at intervals and lasts for increasingly longer periods. Spontaneous clearing is uncommon. Psoriatics have greater than normal colonization of *Staphylococcus* on plaques. Psoriatics who are human immunodeficiency virus (HIV)-positive are at high risk for infection from self-inoculation.

Psoriatic patches are covered with silvery white scales. The eruptions (usually symmetric) commonly occur on the scalp, elbows, knees, and sacral regions (Fig. 70-3). Lesions may develop at the site of a previous injury, which is known as Koebner's phenomenon. A generalized eruption may occur with severe psoriasis vulgaris. A rare form of psoriasis (pustular psoriasis) produces generalized, sterile cutaneous pustules. Severe systemic involvement can be fatal. About 15 to 20 per cent of clients with psoriasis have psoriatic arthritis, which primarily affects the distal joints and may be deforming. Nail dystrophies and pitting occur in approximately 30 to 50 per cent of clients.

Medical Management

Mild psoriasis may be treated locally with natural sunlight or topical therapy, including tar preparations and topical corticosteroids (see Topical Corticosteroids) or intralesional corticosteroids. Injecting small, diluted amounts of corticosteroids (e.g., triamcinolone acetonide) into or just below a lesion gives a high drug concentration to a localized site. Potential localized side effects include atrophy, hypopigmentation, infection, and, rarely, ulceration. Keratolytic agents (e.g., salicylic acid) may remove scale and allow greater penetration of topical agents.

Anthralin is an effective topical therapy for psoriasis with widespread discrete lesions consisting primarily of thick plaques. There are varying methods of application of this topical. With all methods, it is important to apply medication only to the affected lesions, avoiding contact with normal surrounding skin. The client should wash hands immediately after application, leave medication on for the prescribed period of time, then re-

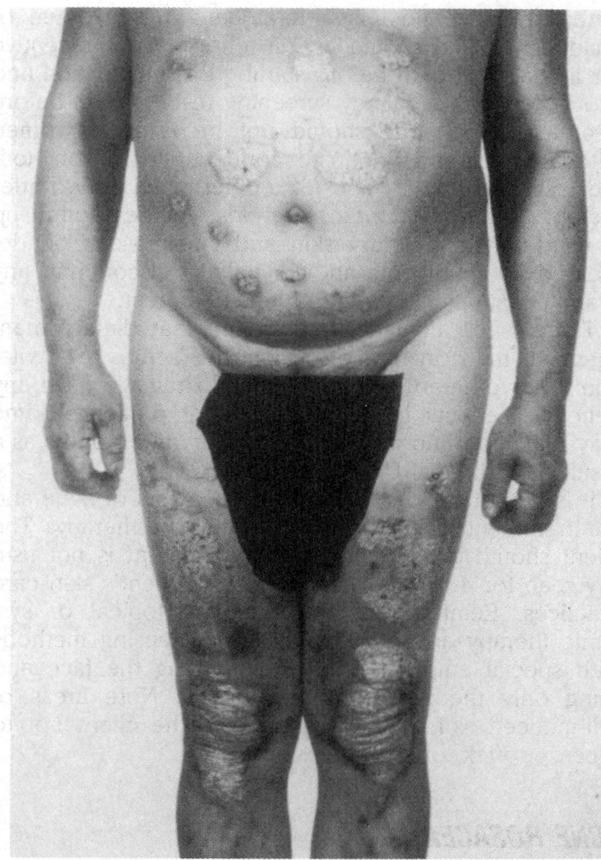

▲ *Figure 70-3*

Psoriasis vulgaris. (From Grizzard, D. [1991]. Understanding the pathophysiology of psoriasis: A nursing perspective. *Dermatology Nursing,* 3[5], 305-311.)

move it by showering or bathing. Anthralin products have the potential to stain fabric, hair, skin, nails, furniture, and bathroom fixtures. For avoidance of excessive staining, it is recommended that medication be carefully applied and that as much medication as possible be removed with tissue or previously stained towel before bathing.

Scalp care with psoriasis consists of removing scales and treating inflammation. Tar shampoos with keratolytic agents, followed by topical corticosteroid lotions, are useful. It is often necessary to use steroids under occlusion (under dressings) for percutaneous absorption to be enhanced. There is no consistently effective treatment of psoriatic involvement of the nails. Usually, the scalp and nails improve with remission of psoriasis on the body surface.

Widespread involvement may require whole-body irradiation with UVL (see earlier).

Systemic treatment is sometimes prescribed for widespread psoriasis. The vitamin A derivative etretinate (Tegison) has been shown to be useful in pustular and erythrodermic psoriasis but not as useful in chronic plaque-type psoriasis. The mode of action may involve the correction of abnormal polyamine metabolism or leukocyte migration. The side effects of etretinate are similar to those of the oral retinoid isotretinoin (see Acne Vulgaris). Because of the teratogenicity of the drug and the extremely long half-life, its use in women of childbearing age is unwarranted.

Antimetabolites (e.g., methotrexate) in small doses are useful for inhibiting DNA synthesis. Methotrexate is a folic acid antagonist used to treat psoriasis that is unresponsive to all topical therapies; it is reserved for the most severe cases. Methotrexate is potentially toxic to the renal, hepatic, and hematopoietic systems. Thus, baseline assessment (e.g., blood chemistry, complete blood count, and liver biopsy) is important before this medication is started. During treatment, periodic assessments are needed, including repeat liver biopsy. If any serious side effects develop, such as bone marrow depression (decreased white blood cell count and platelet count) or gastrointestinal tract bleeding, treatment is discontinued. For limiting potential liver damage, the client is advised not to consume alcohol throughout therapy. Because methotrexate may cause chromosomal abnormalities, effective birth control methods are important both for women and men before and during treatment. Nausea, the most common side effect, can be limited by taking methotrexate with food or taking prophylactic antiemetics.

Nursing Management

Although the physician orders the medical regimen for the client, the nurse and the physician collaborate in the ongoing assessment of the client's response to treatment and the development of new lesions.

The nurse's role in client care centers on teaching the client about the UVL light treatments and medications. In addition, the nurse should assist the client in coping with an altered self-concept. The appearance of skin lesions may make the client feel "dirty" or untouchable. In addition, the smell of the tar preparations and the stain may add to the psychological reaction. The client is also at high risk for secondary infection in the open lesions. The client should be taught to keep the creams or ointments on and keep the areas clean and dry.

In order to keep psoriasis in remission, the client needs to control the causative factors. Adequate rest, nutrition, and exercise promote health. Stress should be minimized, and illness and infection treated early.

ACNE VULGARIS

Overview

Acne is a common, self-limiting, multifactorial disorder. One of four clients affected has enough significant disease to seek professional treatment. Potential facial disfigurement is a major concern. Acne requires active treatment for control until it spontaneously resolves. The three types of acne lesions are comedones, pustules, and cysts; all involve the hair follicles and large sebaceous glands (pilosebaceous units) on the face, neck, and upper trunk. A comedone (most common lesion) is a hair follicle filled with debris. It is either a blackhead (an open follicle) or a small, flesh-colored papule (with a closed follicular orifice). Erythematous papules and pustules occur at the inflammatory stage of closed comedones. Cysts (actually deep nodules) may produce scarring (deep triangular pits).

Acne is initiated by androgenic hormones that activate sebaceous glands. Sebum production increases, which encourages colonization by anaerobic diphtheroids *(Corynebacterium acnes).* The irritant effect of bacterial byproducts and excessive follicle keratinization block follicle patency. There is no scientific evidence that factors such as chocolate, nuts, or fatty foods affect acne. However, exacerbations coinciding with the menstrual cycle result from hormonal activity. Heat, humidity, and excessive perspiration also have a role in increased acne.

Management

Treatment depends on the severity of acne. To prevent scarring, it is important to suppress inflammation. See Table 70-1 regarding further discussion of the following acne medications. Benzoyl peroxide (Desquam, Benzagel, Persa-Gel, Panoxyl) 5 per cent and 10 per cent has a potent antimicrobial effect. It will reduce the size and number of comedones present and may inhibit sebum secretion. Topical antibiotics (Cleocin T, T-Stat, Benzamycin) are also used. Tretinoin (Retin-A) has been found to be one of the most effective comedolytic agents, used alone or in combination with benzoyl peroxide. The irritant effects sometimes limit its usefulness. Clients should receive written instructions regarding use of tretinoin.

Failure of response to topicals indicates needed evaluation for addition of oral antibiotics (tetracycline or erythromycin). Tetracycline or erythromycin administered over an extended period (e.g., several months) suppresses *C. acnes* and decreases inflammation. Long-term systemic antibiotics can cause monilial vaginitis and gastrointestinal symptoms, and clients should be informed how to monitor for these and what interventions to take. Improvement may not be apparent for 4 to 6 weeks.

Hormone therapy may be indicated for severe cystic acne. Medication containing estrogens suppresses sebaceous gland activity. Estrogenic therapy requires treatment through a minimum of three to four menstrual cycles.

In severe cystic acne resistant to standard management, isotretinoin (Accutane) is used to inhibit inflammation. Dosage is determined by body weight and is taken in divided, daily doses for several months. The drug has many side effects and requires frequent follow-up visits and laboratory evaluations. Adverse effects include elevated triglycerides, skin dryness, cheilitis (lip inflammation), and eye discomfort (i.e., dryness, burning). Isotretinoin is a teratogen; thus, women of childbearing age should use an effective contraceptive for at least 1 month before starting this medication and should have a pregnancy screening test 2 weeks before treatment. This drug should not be used in women without strict and adequate contraception throughout the course of therapy and for a determined period after therapy. Reinforce the fact that close medical follow-up is needed and that dry skin and cheilitis can be decreased by emollients and lip balms. Discontinue any vitamin A supplements during this treatment.

There is no convincing evidence that dietary management, mild drying agents, abrasive scrubs, oral vitamin A, cryotherapy, or incision and drainage have any beneficial effects in the management of acne. Some may notice an improvement in the summer months as a result of additional UVL exposure.

It is important to explain the mechanism of acne and the treatment plan and to set goals of therapy. The client should understand that improvement is not usually seen for 4 to 8 weeks. Assess the client's skin care practices. Reinforce compliance with topical or systemic therapy and appropriate skin cleansing methods with special emphasis on not scrubbing the face and using only the agreed upon topicals. Note areas of self-induced skin damage and teach the client not to squeeze, prick, or pick at lesions.

ACNE ROSACEA

This chronic, inflammatory eruption, characterized by erythema, papules, pustules, and telangiectasis, occurs on the face, especially the nose. Unlike in acne vulgaris, comedones are generally not seen. Acne rosacea has an insidious onset, usually between ages 30 and 50 years, and affects women more frequently than men. It is more common in fair-skinned clients with a history of easy facial flushing. Precipitating factors that appear to make the flushing worse include tea, coffee, alcohol (wine), caffeine-containing products, sunlight, extremes of hot and cold, spicy foods, and emotional stress. Sebaceous hyperplasia of the nose (rhinophyma) is often associated with years of chronic acne rosacea resulting in a "W. C. Fields nose." This results from chronic inflammation and increased connective tissues and may be mistaken for an indication of excessive alcohol consumption. Ocular changes such as eyelid inflammation and conjunctivitis may occur.

Avoidance of the stimuli that trigger acne rosacea may be sufficient for mild disorders. Clients should be instructed to avoid factors that provoke their facial vasodilation, such as caffeine, excessive sunlight, alcohol (especially wine), temperature extremes, hot liquids, and spicy foods. Systemic antibiotics usually are necessary. Remind the client that improvement with systemic antibiotics will be gradual. Antibiotics are given in small, usually tapered doses for long periods. Relapse is common in clients who discontinue therapy. Topical therapy with nonfluorinated topical corticosteroid cream can be used to reduce inflammation.

▼ Bullous Disorders

PEMPHIGUS

Pemphigus is a chronic disorder that results in the development of blisters (called bullae). It is fairly uncommon in the general population but has an increased incidence in the Jewish and Mediterranean peoples. There are several types of pemphigus: pemphigus vulgaris, pemphigus foliaceous, and pemphigus erythematosus. This discussion focuses on pemphigus vulgaris, the most common type.

Pemphigus is an autoimmune disease caused by circulating IgG autoantibodies. These autoantibodies react with the intracellular cement or the substance that holds epidermal cells together. The reaction causes intraepidermal blister (bulla) formation and acantholysis (loss of cohesion between epidermal cells).

Clinical manifestations include flaccid bullae that rupture easily, emitting a foul-smelling drainage and leaving crusted, denuded skin. The lesions are common on the face, back, chest, groin, and umbilicus. Even slight pressure on an intact blister causes it to spread to adjacent skin, which is called Nikolsky's sign.

Management includes large doses of steroids and immunosuppressives. Plasmapheresis has had some success with pemphigus. If the client has a large portion of denuded skin, the management is similar to that for a burn client. The client is at increased risk for infection, fluid and electrolyte imbalance, and stress response complications (i.e., stress ulcers, body system failure). In addition, nursing management focuses on self-concept and pain management. Potassium permanganate baths may be used to reduce the risk of infection, control the odor of the drainage, and ease the pain.

▼ Infectious Disorders

Several organisms lead to skin infections. Common skin infections are described in Table 70-4. A few will be discussed in detail in the text.

ERYSIPELAS AND CELLULITIS

Overview

Erysipelas is an acute, superficial, rapidly spreading inflammation of the dermis and lymphatics. The usual causative agent is beta-hemolytic streptococcus group A. The organism enters tissue via an abrasion or wound. Fever and leukocytosis (elevated white blood cell count) are present. The skin is elevated beginning with a small, bright red area. The involved area spreads peripherally to become a plaque with sharp, indurated borders. Lesions are most common on the face and extremities. Recurrence in the same area is common, possibly because of underlying lymphatic obstruction.

Cellulitis is a suppurative inflammation of the dermis and subcutaneous tissues without sharp, indurated borders that spreads widely through tissue spaces (see Fig. 70-1). The skin is erythematous, edematous, tender, and sometimes nodular. *Streptococcus pyogenes* is the usual cause of this infection; however, other pathogens may be responsible. Lymphangitis may occur; if cellulitis is untreated, gangrene, metastatic abscesses, and sepsis result.

Clients at increased risk for erysipelas and cellulitis include the elderly and clients with lowered resistance from diabetes, malnutrition, steroid therapy, and the presence of wounds or ulcers. Other predisposing factors include the presence of edema or other cutaneous inflammation or wounds (e.g., tinea, eczema, burns, trauma). There is a tendency for recurrence, especially at sites of lymphatic obstruction.

Management

Erysipelas and cellulitis are treated by systemic antibiotics; penicillin is the antibiotic of choice. Before antibiotics are administered, a culture and sensitivity test of the wound should be taken, although it is usually difficult to yield an organism on culture. Soaks may reduce edema and inflammation. The enzymes that facilitate a rapid spread of infection also seem to produce other significant manifestations such as high fever, tachycardia, confusion, and hypotension; appropriate interventions should be taken if these occur. Monitor the client's temperature and administer prescribed antipyretic medication. Prevent cross-contamination by teaching the client careful handwashing and careful disposal of linen, clothing, dressings, and so forth. Universal precautions should be used as appropriate.

HERPES ZOSTER

Overview

Herpes zoster (Fig. 70-4) or shingles is an infection caused by the same virus that causes varicella (chickenpox). Although herpes zoster is much less communicable than is varicella, clients who have not had varicella may develop it after exposure to a client with herpes zoster. An increased incidence of herpes zoster occurs in clients with lymphoma, leukemia, and acquired immunodeficiency syndrome (AIDS), probably because of their decreased immunologic response. Diagnostic tests are often not necessary because of the specific characteristics of herpes zoster. A Tzanck smear will demonstrate multinucleated giant cells (see Chap. 69).

In herpes zoster, clusters of grouped vesicles appear unilaterally along cranial or spinal nerve dermatomes after 1 to 2 days of pain, itching, and hyperesthesia.

TABLE 70–4. Common Skin Infections

Name	Organism	Clinical Manifestations	Management
Parasitic			
Scabies	*Sarcoptes scabiei*	Multiple straight or wavy thread-like lines beneath the skin, itching	Application of a scabicide with retreatment of the residual eggs in 1 week. All clothing and linen should be washed and dried in hot cycles or dry cleaned
Lice	*Pediculus humanis/ Phthirus pubis*	Intense itching, scratch marks may be evident	Application of pediculicides. For head lice, the shampoo should be worked into dry hair until it is saturated. A fine-toothed comb should be used to remove the dead lice and nits. Brushes and combs should be washed in the pediculicide also. For body lice, a pediculicide lotion is applied to involved body areas. Clothing should be washed and dried in hot cycles or dry cleaned. Family members or close contacts should be treated, too
Bacterial			
Impetigo	Streptococcus A	Pruritic vesicle or pustule that breaks and leaves a thick honey-colored crust	Antibiotics until cultured include erythromycin or dicloxacillin. Use of mupirocin being studied. Teach control of contagiousness; infection is contagious as long as skin lesions are present. Thorough hand washing, separate laundry for client's linens, separate washing of client's dishes
Folliculitis, furuncles, carbuncles	*Staphylococcus aureus*	White pustules on forehead, chest, upper back, neck, thighs, groin, and axillae. Furuncles are deeper inflamed nodules. Carbuncles are interconnected furuncles. Often rupture expelling purulent, foul smelling thick drainage	Localized folliculitis is treated with warm compresses, gentle washing and topical antibiotics. Furuncles are treated as folliculitis and are incised and drained (I&D) to avoid rupture. Carbuncles are treated with systemic antibiotics and I & D. Teach men to use disposable razors. Reduce spread of infection by careful handwashing and separate laundry of linens
Fungal			
Candidiasis	*Candida albicans*	Appearance depends on location. In the mouth, it is called thrush, and appears as white plaques with an underlying red base with fissures on corners of the mouth. Skin lesions are pruritic, red, and moist with eroded scales. Skin lesions are common to the axilla, gluteal, perianal, and interdigital folds. Vaginal thrush causes intense itching and a cheesy drainage	Eliminate or control the predisposing factors such as antibiotics (which alter the flora), malnutrition, diabetes, immunosuppression, pregnancy, or use of birth control pills. Use topical antifungal powders and creams. Keep the skin dry, keep the environment cool
Tinea (several locations) Tinea corposis (ringworm) Tinea capitiis (on scalp) Tinea cruris (jock itch) Tinea pedis (athlete's foot)	Variety of dermatophytes	Tinea capitus presents as patchy hair loss, inflammation, scales, and folliculitis. Tinea corposis appears as round red macules and papules with scales. They have advancing borders and healing centers. Tinea cruris appears as red lesions with raised borders. Tinea pedis causes scaling, maceration, pain, and vesicles.	Infection is controlled with antifungal solutions and creams. Acute lesions may require wet dressings, keratolytic agents, or both to remove the scales. Client is taught to reduce risk by thoroughly drying after a bath or shower, wearing absorbent underwear and socks, applying talc to intertriginous areas, and wearing open shoes during warm weather

TABLE 70–4. Common Skin Infections Continued

Name	Organism	Clinical Manifestations	Management
Viral			
Herpes simplex	Herpes simplex virus	Vesicles preceded by sensation of itching or burning. Clear exudate from vesicles, followed by crusting. Common to the nose, lips, cheeks, ears, and genitalia.	No cure available today. Treatment includes pain relief and topical anesthetics. Acyclovir, an antiviral drug, may decrease viral shedding and hasten healing. Avoiding the sun or using sunscreens reduces recurrent lesions on the lips. Reduce contagiousness by frequent handwashing, not picking at lesions, avoiding intercourse and kissing while lesions are active, and not sharing lipsticks. Try to identify (and avoid or control) personal triggers for lesions
Warts	Human papilloma virus	Rough, flesh, or gray-colored skin protrusion	Numerous therapies, some over-the-counter. May require electrodesication or cryosurgery. Intralesional injections of cytotoxic drugs may also be used

Because they follow nerve pathways, the lesions do not cross the body's midline; however, the nerves of both sides may be involved. Herpes zoster lesions evolve into crusts on the skin and ulcers on the superficial mucous membrane (Fig. 70–4).

The eruption clears in about 2 weeks unless the period between the pain and the eruption is longer than 2 days. In the latter situation, a prolonged convalescence may be expected. Residual pain, postherpetic neuralgia, and itching are the major problems with herpes zoster. The pain may be constant or intermittent and vary from light burning to a deep visceral sensation. The duration of the pain can be weeks or months to years. Unfortunately, in the elderly, the pain generally lasts months to years. Another potential complication is trigeminal herpes zoster involving the facial and acoustic nerves; ophthalmic involvement requires close medical attention for avoidance of ocular complications.

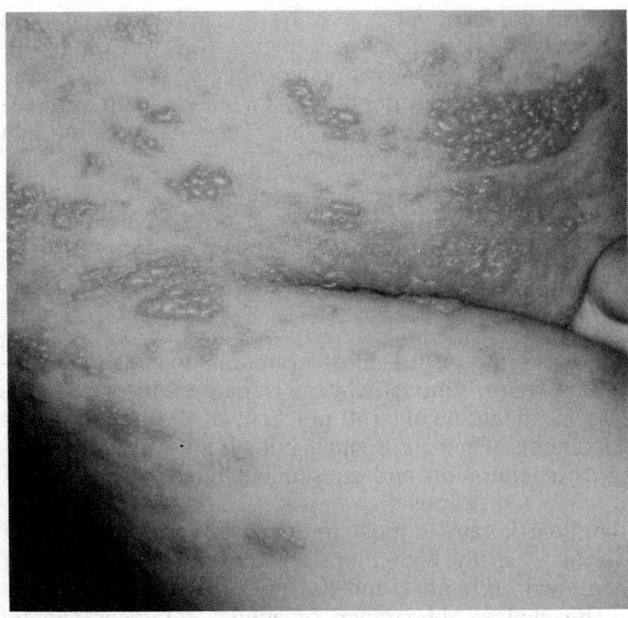

▲ **Figure 70–4**

Herpes zoster of the groin.

Management

Treatment for herpes zoster is acyclovir (Zovirax) given in large dose orally or smaller dose intravenously five times daily. Acyclovir, when started early in the course of the disease, reduces acute pain as well as accelerates healing. The role of acyclovir in preventing postherpetic neuralgia remains unclear. Use of systemic corticosteroids appears to decrease the incidence of postherpetic neuralgia in clients over the age of 50 years. Analgesics and sedatives are prescribed for pain relief.

Topical therapy is primarily symptomatic: applications of cool compresses, use of cooling antipruritic preparations (see Table 70–1), and measures to prevent secondary infection. If pain is present, the client's normal pain tolerance and current pain level must be assessed. Systemic analgesics are usually required, and occasionally narcotics; however, in chronic pain, these may be addictive alternatives. Assess the effectiveness and side effects of prescribed analgesics. Because postherpetic neuralgia can last a long time, the client and significant others need continued intervention and support. Chronic pain management may include use of tricyclic antidepressants, phenothiazines, and other local physical modalities.

▼ Nail Disorders

Disorders of the nail can be indicators of several dermatologic processes, such as an infection of the nail (e.g., paronychia), a fungal infection of the nail (e.g., onychomycosis), a dermatologic disease with prominent nail changes (e.g., psoriasis), or pigmentary abnormalities of the nail (e.g., melanoma).

Unguis incarnatus (ingrown nail) is the most frequent nail condition caused by improper nail trimming and by wearing tight or ill-fitting shoes. It primarily involves the great toes. A painful, warm inflammatory reaction results from excessive lateral growth of the nail into the nailfold. The nail acts as a foreign body, promoting granulation tissue. Decrease inflammation with warm soaks for 20 minutes several times a day. If the problem is minor, lifting the lateral portion of the nail by inserting a cotton wick prevents contact with the nailfold. Sometimes, the involved segment of the nailfold needs to be excised.

Paronychia or infection around the nail is characterized by red, shiny skin often associated with painful swelling. These infections frequently result from trauma, picking at the nail, or disorders such as dermatitis. Often these become secondarily infected with bacteria or fungus, which later involve the nail. As with ingrown toenail, warm soaks three or more times a day may reduce pressure and pain; however, incision and drainage of inflamed sites is frequently required. Appropriate cultures of the purulent material and the nail should be obtained. Onychomycosis is the term applied to any fungal infection of the nail, whether it is due to dermatophytes or candidiasis. Prescribed topical or systemic antibiotic or antifungal therapy with emphasis on the need for compliance is important for good outcome.

Clients should understand the importance of reducing trauma and irritation to involved nails by (1) trimming nails straight across to reduce further separation; (2) avoiding overmanicuring or self-induced trauma; (3) limiting chemical irritants such as soaps, cleansers, and nail products; and (4) keeping the nails dry.

▼ CANCER OF THE SKIN

▼ Precursors to Cancer

Precursors to cancer of the skin include recurrent skin trauma and various skin lesions. In order to understand the role of prevention of skin cancer, they are discussed here.

SUNBURN

Overview

Sunburn is an acute inflammatory skin response which occurs as a reaction to excessive exposure to sunlight. Dermatopathologic changes include the production of epidermal cells that have cytoplasmic and nuclear changes. These changes are cumulative over the lifespan and lead to an increased incidence of skin cancer.

A first-degree sunburn produces mild, tender erythema followed by desquamation (peeling), which heals without scarring. Second-degree sunburn causes more extreme erythema and edema, and blistering results from damage to the epidermal cells. Deep sunburns are uncommon unless they are induced by artificial sources such as tanning lamps or booths. Deep sunburn produces burns resembling a pathophysiologic response (see Chap. 71).

Management

Prevention is obviously the best therapy for sunburn. Client teaching emphasizing sun protection should never be omitted when caring for the sunburned client (see Client Education Box).

Treating sunburn involves decreasing inflammation and rehydrating the damaged skin. For localized, first-degree sunburn, apply cool tap water soaks for 20 minutes or until the skin is cool. This limits skin destruction, prevents edema, and potentially reduces blisters. Tepid tap water baths are indicated for large sunburned areas. After a bath or soak, apply water-based emollients, preferably refrigerated for an additional cooling effect. Emollients should also be applied throughout the day to soothe and relieve dryness. Lotions or foams containing camphor or menthol (e.g., Sarna) can also be beneficial.

For second-degree sunburn, apply continuous cool, normal saline soaks or soaking baths to reduce oozing and edema. Aspirate very large blisters, and apply sterile dressings. Avoid debridement unless there is evidence of secondary bacterial infection. Silver sulfadiazine may be prescribed. Avoid use of over-the-counter remedies containing local anesthetics (Benzocaine, Nupercaine, or Xylocaine) because they are rarely effective and have the potential of contact sensitivity.

Prostaglandin inhibitors (aspirin, indomethacin) may be used to reduce the erythema and inflammation. Topical corticosteroids may be prescribed to be used sparingly in nonocclusive vehicles (i.e., cream or lotion) for their vasoconstrictive effects. Systemic corticosteroids are prescribed only for clients with very extensive, painful burns, but their use has declined in favor of prostaglandin inhibitors.

ACTINIC KERATOSIS

Overview

Actinic keratosis, the most common epithelial precancerous lesion among whites, is caused by sun exposure. It affects nearly 100 per cent of the elderly white population. There is a small but definite risk of malignant degeneration and subsequent metastatic potential in neglected lesions.

Actinic keratosis most frequently occurs in areas of chronic, usually high-intensity sun exposure, including face, neck, forearms, and dorsum of the hand.

The clinical appearance of actinic keratoses can be quite varied. The typical lesion is an irregularly shaped, flat, slightly erythematous macule or papule with indistinct borders and an overlying hard keratotic scale or horn. In some cases, the erythema or horn may be absent. This scale can be periodically shed or peeled off, but then it regrows. The lesion varies in size from pinhead to several centimeters and is often more easily palpated than observed. Single lesions may be seen, but more often they appear in groups on a background of sun-damaged skin. It is often difficult to distinguish a large or hypertrophic actinic keratosis from a squamous cell carcinoma without histologic diagnosis.

Management

Topical application of 5-fluorouracil (5-FU, Efudex), a topical antimetabolite, is presently one of the best approaches to treatment of widespread actinic damage with multiple lesions. The advantage of 5-FU is that large areas of widespread disease can be treated at the same time. Use of 5-FU not only removes the majority of premalignant and superficial malignant lesions that can be seen but also will uncover and destroy clinically undetectable lesions of this type. However, the major disadvantage is the therapeutic inflammatory response that often accompanies successful treatment. This response sequence is erythema usually followed by vesiculation, erosion, ulcerations, necrosis, and epithelialization.

The medication should be applied with a gloved hand, carefully avoiding eyes, nose, mouth, and scrotum. A porous gauze dressing may be applied over the medication for cosmetic reasons without increase in reaction. However, occlusive dressing should be avoided because of increased inflammatory response. Medication should be continued until the inflammatory response reaches the erosion, necrosis, and ulceration stage, at which time the medication should be stopped. The usual duration of therapy is 2 to 4 weeks; the client may experience extreme discomfort requiring pain medication by this point. At the time 5-FU is stopped, topical corticosteroid creams may be applied to decrease inflammation and provide the client with additional pain relief. Complete healing of the lesions may not be evident for 1 to 2 months after cessation of therapy.

SURGICAL MANAGEMENT

Cryotherapy. Liquid nitrogen is usually applied with a cotton applicator or spraying device and requires no local anesthetic (Fig. 70-5*A*). The client does note a small amount of discomfort at the time of freezing, which may linger afterward. Application of a warm, damp washcloth intermittently to the site may bring the client relief. Freezing frequently results in inflammation with blister formation, and blister care should be re-

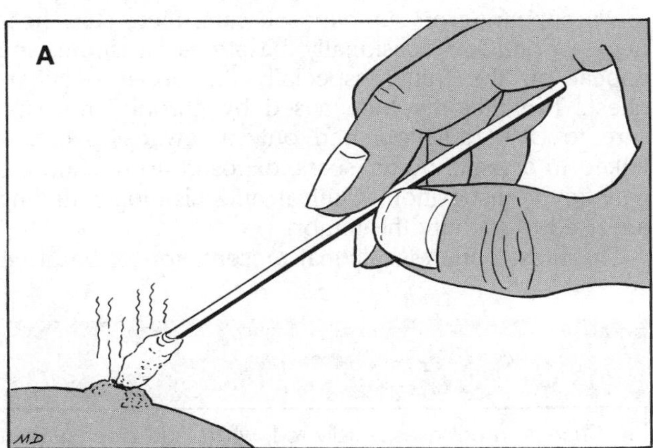

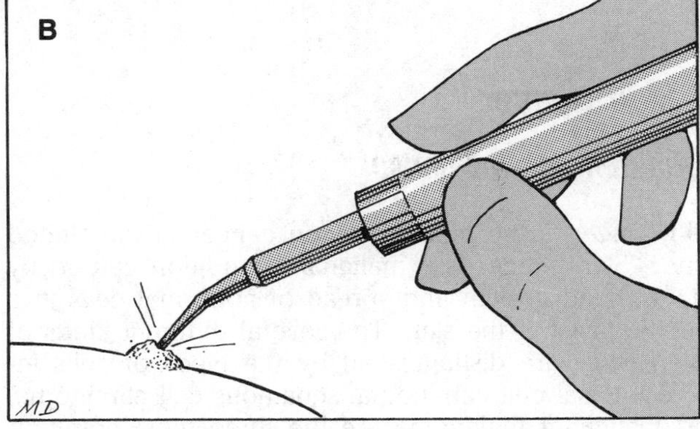

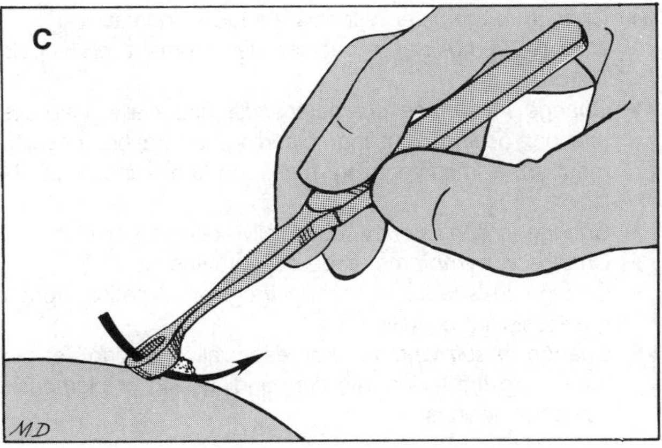

▲ **Figure 70-5**

Methods for destroying skin lesions. *A*, Cryotherapy. Liquid nitrogen is applied with a saturated cotton-tipped applicator directly to the lesion or sprayed on. This causes tissue destruction by freezing. *B*, Electrodesiccation. Tissue is destroyed by heat from an electrical current; note gloved hand. *C*, Curettage. A curet (cutting instrument) removes tissue by scraping or scooping; note gloved hand.

viewed with the client. Care must be taken to avoid overfreezing the site, which may result in scarring. Cryotherapy is cost-effective, is easy to perform, and has minimal side effects.

Electrodesiccation and Curettage. Electrodesiccation produces superficial destruction through bursts of electrical current and is usually done under local anesthesia (Fig. 70-5*B*). The tissue is destroyed by mechanical disruption of cells and heat. The tissue is removed by scraping or scooping with a loop-shaped instrument called a curet (Fig. 70-5*C*). This method does provide tissue for histologic diagnosis if needed. The wounds usually heal quickly with adequate wound care. Wound care should emphasize keeping the wound site moist with some nonsensitizing topical antibiotic ointment such as bacitracin.

Shave or Excisional Biopsy. Shave or excisional biopsy is indicated on lesions that are large or hypertrophic or have other characteristics of a cutaneous malignancy (induration, erythema, erosion). It is often difficult to distinguish a large or hypertrophic actinic keratosis from a squamous cell carcinoma without histologic diagnosis. Biopsy should also be done on lesions that persist after adequate treatment with 5-FU. Local anesthesia is given for a biopsy and allows electrodesiccation to be done painlessly after biopsy. Excisional biopsy requires primary closure of the site and may be a more extensive procedure than the lesion will warrant; however, it ensures removal of the entire growth.

▼ Skin Cancer

Definition and Incidence

Skin cancer is the most common cancer in the United States. Skin cancer is a malignant condition caused by uncontrolled growth and spread of abnormal cells in a specific layer of the skin. The several different kinds of skin cancer are distinguished by the types of cells involved. Basal cell carcinoma, squamous cell carcinoma, and malignant melanoma are the three most common types of skin cancer. More than 90 per cent of all skin cancers fall into the first two classifications. Both basal cell carcinoma and squamous cell carcinoma are slow-growing tumors that have a cure rate of 95 per cent or greater with early treatment.

Etiology and Risk Factors

The cause of skin cancer is well known. Prolonged or intermittent exposure to UVL radiation from the sun, especially when it results in sunburn and blistering, plays a key role in the induction of skin cancer, especially malignant melanoma. The majority of all nonmelanoma skin cancers occur on parts of the body unprotected by clothing (face, neck, forearms, and backs of hands) and in clients who have received considerable exposure to sunlight. All clients are at risk for skin cancer regardless of skin tone and hair color; however, some clients are at much greater risk than others are. In general, clients with red, blond, or light-brown hair with light complexions or freckles, many of Celtic or Scandinavian origin, are most susceptible; blacks and Asians are least susceptible.

Danger signals in moles are presented in Box 70-1. Suspicious lesions should be examined by a physician.

The history of a client's pattern of reaction to acute sun exposure is correlated with the client's tendency to get actinic keratosis and skin cancer. Those who never tan and always burn after 1 to 2 hours of midday summer sun are most susceptible. Those who burn once or twice at the beginning of summer and then tan are somewhat less susceptible. Those who never burn and always tan are the least susceptible. The most severely affected clients usually have a history of long-term occupational (farmers, construction workers, surveyors, sailors) or recreational (swimmers, skiers, surfers, sunbathers) sun exposure.

Clinical Manifestations

BASAL CELL CARCINOMA

Basal cell carcinoma, the most common form of skin cancer, is a malignant epithelial tumor of the skin that arises from the basal cells contained in the epidermis.

The tumor is usually painless and slow-growing, generally appearing on sun-exposed skin, face, ears, head, neck, or hands. Occasionally, basal cell carcinoma may appear on the trunk, especially the upper back and chest. The majority are caused by chronic overexposure to UVL radiation, and only a few cases can be linked to arsenic, burns, scars, exposure to radiation, or genetic predisposition. Clinical and histologic findings are used to identify the tumor.

The most common clinical presentation of basal cell

Box 70-1. Danger Signals Suggestive of Malignant Transformation in Pigmented Nevi

- *Change in color,* especially red, white, and blue; sudden darkening; mottled shades of brown or black
- *Change in diameter,* especially sudden increase
- *Change in outline,* especially development of irregular margins
- *Change in surface characteristics,* especially scaliness, erosion, oozing, crusting, bleeding, ulceration, development of a mushrooming mass on the surface of the lesion
- *Change in consistency,* especially softening or friability
- *Change in symptoms,* especially pruritus
- *Change in shape,* especially irregular elevation from a previously flat condition
- *Change in surrounding skin,* especially "leaking" of pigment from the lesion into surrounding skin or pigmented "satellite" lesions

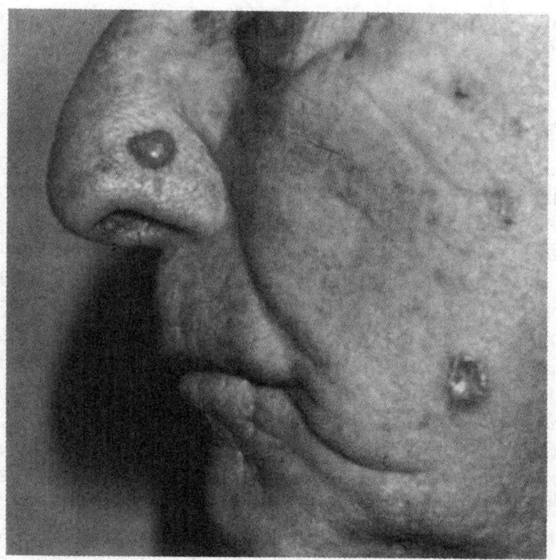

▲ *Figure 70-6*

Two forms of basal cell carcinoma. (From Black, J. [1991]. Reconstructive surgery in the elderly. *Plastic Surgical Nursing, 11*[4], 151–167.)

carcinoma is the nodular lesion (Fig. 70-6). This is a dome-shaped papule with a well-defined border containing a classic "pearly" texture. Basal cell carcinoma has this flesh-colored "pearly" or shiny appearance because it does not keratinize. Telangiectatic vessels frequently overlie the lesion. As the lesion enlarges, the center may flatten or ulcerate; however, the border will still be raised and give a "rolled" appearance (Color Plate 14).

Basal cell carcinomas almost never metastasize. They can, however, be locally destructive and invasive through tissue. This is particularly true on the face, where a lesion can invade deep structures with resultant loss of an eye, ear, or nose. If untreated, the tumor can invade through bone and brain. However, if the tumor is identified and treated early, local excision or even nonexcisional destruction is usually curative.

Clients who have had one basal cell carcinoma are at greater risk for developing others. Recurrences of previously treated basal cell carcinomas are also possible but more unusual. The possible recurrence generally occurs within the first 2 years after removal or therapy.

SQUAMOUS CELL CARCINOMA

Squamous cell carcinoma is the second most common skin cancer in whites. It is a tumor of the epidermal keratinocytes and rarely occurs in dark-skinned clients. It is found on areas often exposed to the sun, typically the rim of the ear, the face, the lips and mouth, and the dorsa of the hands. Squamous cell carcinoma is more difficult to characterize than is basal cell carcinoma. These tumors are poorly marginated; the edge often blends into surrounding sun-damaged skin. Squamous cell carcinoma may present as an ulcer, flat red area, cutaneous horn, indurated plaque, or hyperkeratotic papule or nodule (Fig. 70-7). Often they present as a red- to skin-colored papule surmounted by varying amounts of scale. These lesions grow more rapidly than does a basal cell carcinoma (Color Plate 15). These tumors are potentially dangerous because they may infiltrate surrounding structures, metastasize to lymph nodes, and be subsequently fatal.

MALIGNANT MELANOMA

Malignant melanoma is a cancer of melanocytes; it is the deadliest form of skin cancer. The incidence and death rate from melanoma are rising worldwide. In countries populated with fair-skinned whites, the incidence of melanoma and mortality have risen by 7 to 15 per cent per year, more than doubling over the past

▲ *Figure 70-7*

Squamous cell carcinoma of the lip. (From Black, J. [1991]. Reconstructive surgery in the elderly. *Plastic Surgical Nursing, 11*[4], 151–167.)

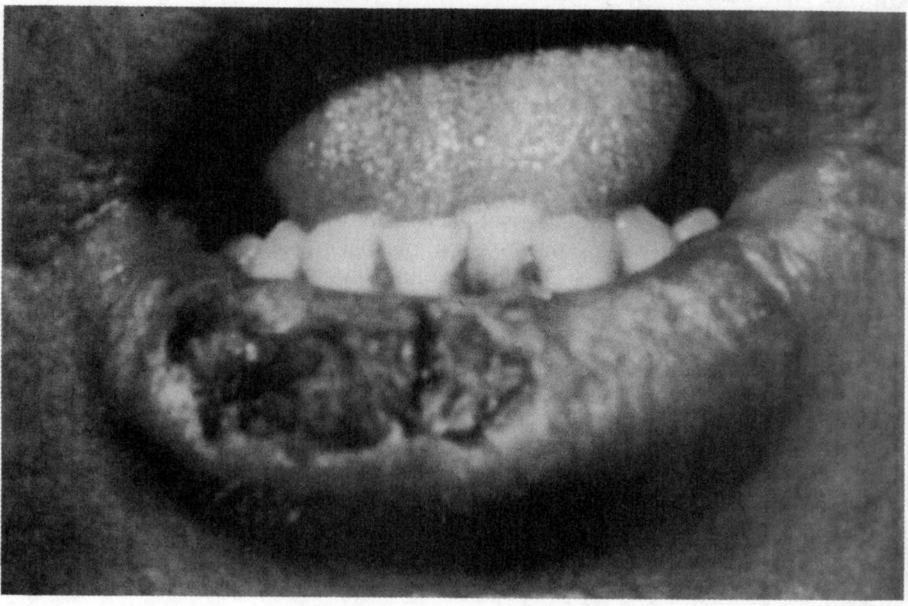

decade. Whites have 10 times the incidence that blacks do.

UVL continues to be one of the most important causes of malignant melanoma. However, melanoma can appear anywhere on the body, not just on sun-exposed areas. The majority of malignant melanoma appears to be associated with the intensity rather than the duration of sunlight exposure, in contrast to basal cell and squamous cell carcinomas. Melanoma tends to be observed more often in whites who move to sunny climates, or in professionals who take short vacations with intense sun exposure, than in clients who suffer from chronic sun exposure. The suspicion of melanoma is based on history as well as clinical appearance (Color Plate 16). The tumor can metastasize, usually to the brain, lungs, bones, liver, and skin, and is ultimately fatal. The prognosis of melanoma has become more predictable. Clinically, metastatic melanoma is universally fatal. Prognosis and mortality of melanoma that is not clinically metastatic at presentation depend critically on the depth of the lesion at the time of excision. The more superficial or "thin" the tumor, the better the prognosis.

Medical Management

Medical management begins by having a high index of suspicion for any type of skin cancer but specifically melanoma. The need for early detection cannot be overstressed in dealing with malignant melanoma. Any indication, whether it is a high-risk client or a suspicious lesion, is adequate reason for referral.

Surgical Management

Treatment of any and all skin cancer requires removal of the lesion. The tumor removed needs to have a specified margin free of tumor (differs depending on type of skin cancer) to guarantee full removal of the skin cancer.

A special surgery technique primarily used for the removal of skin malignancies such as basal cell and squamous cell carcinoma is Mohs surgery. Mohs surgery is also indicated for primary lesions in areas where preservation of normal skin is necessary (e.g., eyelids, pinna, nasolabial folds). The technique is based on a series of excisions. Careful microscopic tissue assessment "maps" the presence or absence of malignant cells within each specimen. The procedure may be lengthy. After all tumor tissue is removed, the wound is closed with sutures or with a flap (see Chap. 72) or allowed to close by secondary intention.

Basal cell and squamous cell carcinoma can also be excised and the area closed primarily or with a skin flap. The advantage of this technique is that it requires much less time, and the scar is controllable as a fine line. The tumor is completely excised with adequate margins of tumor-free tissue. If there is doubt about the adequacy of margins, the specimen is sent for pathologic diagnosis (frozen section). Surgery can be combined with Mohs technique.

MELANOMA

The treatment for malignant melanoma is wide local excision. There is no role at present for chemotherapy or radiation therapy as the initial treatment.

Surgical excision begins with a biopsy for determining the stage of the cancer. Biopsies are performed whenever the client cannot be assured that a lesion is benign. Excisional biopsy is the removal of the lesion and a narrow margin of normal-appearing tissue. This tissue is examined, and the melanoma is staged (Fig. 70–8).

Surgeons differ on their timing for the definitive surgery. Some surgeons excise the lesion after frozen-section examination while the client is still on the operating bed. Other surgeons wait for the results of permanent-section pathologic diagnosis and then proceed with definitive treatment. The final excision is usually completed within 1 week of biopsy. Nurses should be aware that although there is theoretic risk of tumor spread during biopsy, there is no convincing evidence that waiting 1 to even 6 weeks after biopsy jeopardizes the outcome. In fact, sometimes the delay allows the client time to prepare for surgery, both physically and psychologically.

Wide excision of the tumor with a 1- to 3-cm margin of normal-appearing skin is the treatment. The margin is based on the type of melanoma. The area is closed in surgery, either primarily (skin edges sewn together) or with grafts of flaps.

Advanced Metastatic Melanoma. Most clients with metastatic melanoma live less than 1 year.[3] There is no cure today for metastatic melanoma, but some therapies will improve the quality of life. A treatment plan is arranged on the basis of several factors: site of the tumor, number of metastases, rate of tumor growth, previous treatments, response to treatment, age of the client, general health of the client, and desires of the client.

Some treatments include surgery to remove metastatic lesions, radiation therapy, chemotherapy, and local hyperthermia. Of course, the client can opt for no further treatment. Immunotherapy and hormonal therapy are currently investigational.

▼ Cutaneous T-Cell Lymphoma (Mycosis Fungoides)

Overview

Cutaneous T-cell lymphoma (CTCL), also known as mycosis fungoides or Sézary syndrome, is a malignant disease involving the T helper cells. Malignant T cells in the blood migrate to the skin, where they have an

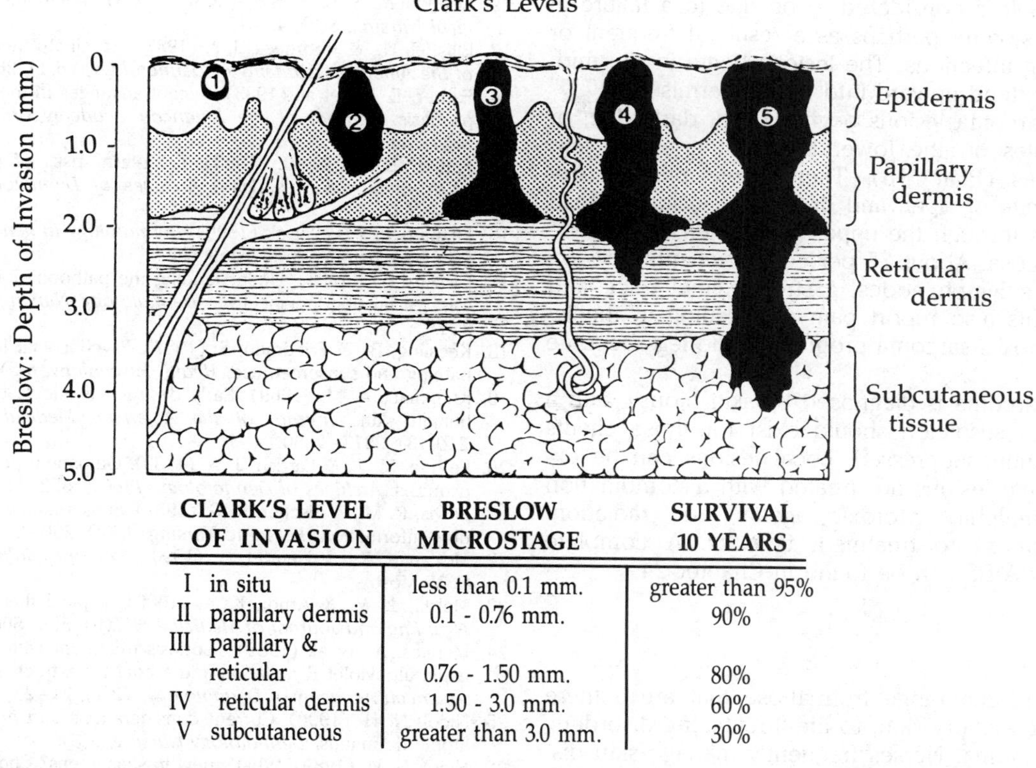

CLARK'S LEVEL OF INVASION	BRESLOW MICROSTAGE	SURVIVAL 10 YEARS
I in situ	less than 0.1 mm.	greater than 95%
II papillary dermis	0.1 - 0.76 mm.	90%
III papillary & reticular	0.76 - 1.50 mm.	80%
IV reticular dermis	1.50 - 3.0 mm.	60%
V subcutaneous	greater than 3.0 mm.	30%

▲ *Figure 70–8*

The combination of Clark's level of invasion and Breslow's depth of invasion allows prediction of 10-year survival in melanoma. (From Eisenbaum, S. L., & Black, J. M. [1988]. Melanoma. *Plastic Surgical Nursing, 8*[2], 42–47.)

affinity for the epidermis. The malignant cells continue to grow and change, eventually moving into the dermis. The cause is not known. This disease has exacerbations and remissions but is invariably fatal. Median life span after tissue biopsy is 5 years. Virtually every organ, especially the liver, spleen, and lungs, may be involved. There seems to be a correlation between high exposure to environmental toxins and this disease.

CTCL is an extremely difficult disorder to diagnose and is often misdiagnosed. In its early stages, CTCL can clinically mimic eczematous processes. The initial erythematous papules resemble eczematous conditions, including psoriasis and seborrheic dermatitis. The original eruptions of CTCL may be either transitory or prolonged and sometimes are pruritic. Clinical manifestations' include eversion of the eyelids and hyperkeratosis of the palms and soles, often with fissuring. Finally, the plaques form tumors that ultimately ulcerate. Tumors can also develop spontaneously in previously unaffected areas, and eventual visceral or organ involvement ensues. Clients often feel desperate by the time diagnosis is confirmed, which adds to the psychological difficulties.

Management

Control of pruritus is essential at all stages and is accomplished by rehydration of the skin, various dry skin therapies (see xerotic eczema), topical corticosteroids, and UVB therapy (see Ultraviolet Light Therapy). Prevention of secondary infections is important. Nitrogen mustard administered topically acts as a cytotoxin. It is applied daily and is often initial treatment. Photophoresis, a treatment involving the removal of small amounts of blood that is irradiated and then returned to the body, is used frequently in more advanced stages. Total-body electron beam therapy with or without adjuvant chemotherapy is a favorably aggressive approach often used. Unfortunately, even if these therapies succeed in clearing the skin, the disorder is still fatal because of systemic involvement.

▼ Kaposi's Sarcoma

Kaposi's sarcoma is a vascular malignancy that presents as a skin disorder. It has a long history. Kaposi's sarcoma used to be a skin disease common in 50- to 60-year-old men of Jewish or Mediterranean descent. It was seen less frequently in clients who were African black, homosexual, or immunosuppressed (e.g., renal transplant clients). Recently, Kaposi's sarcoma has been seen in many clients with AIDS.

The cause of Kaposi's sarcoma is not known, although the human immunodeficiency virus and cytomegalovirus have been suggested as the cofactors in its development. It is considered to be due to a failure in the immune system, perhaps as a result of frequent or overwhelming infections. The lesions begin in the middermis and extend upward into the epidermis.

Kaposi's sarcoma lesions begin as red, dark blue, or purple macules on the lower legs that coalesce into larger plaques (Plate 16). These large plaques frequently ulcerate or open and drain. The lesions spread by metastasis through the upper body, then to the face and oral mucosa. About 75 per cent of clients develop lesions of the lymph nodes, gastrointestinal tract, and lungs.[16] Clients also report pain and itching in the lesions; as Kaposi's sarcoma progresses, the legs become edematous.

Kaposi's sarcoma is diagnosed by skin biopsy, and a high index of suspicion should exist for those clients who are immunosuppressed. Local lesions can be excised. Systemic lesions are treated with a combination of interferon-alpha, cytotoxic agents, and radiation. General response to treatment is poor. A complete discussion of AIDS can be found in Chapter 24.

Summary

Skin disorders can range from those that are a mere nuisance, such as dry skin, to life-threatening disorders, such as melanoma. Nurses frequently manage skin disorders independently; therefore, a thorough knowledge of the use of topical medications and therapies is critical. Because much of skin care is provided by the client or family, the nurse must use excellent teaching skill to convey needed self-care information.

Bibliography

1. Abel, E. A., et al. (1986). Drugs in exacerbation of psoriasis. *Journal of the American Academy of Dermatology, 15*(11), 1007-1022.
2. Arndt, K. W. (1989). *Manual of dermatological therapeutics* (4th ed.). Boston: Little, Brown.
3. Balch, C.M., & Milton, C.W. (1985). *Cutaneous melanoma.* Philadelphia: W. B. Saunders.
4. Carter, D. M. (1987). Basal cell carcinoma. In T. B. Fitzpatrick, et al. (Eds.), *Dermatology in general medicine* (pp. 759-765). New York: McGraw-Hill.
5. Clark, R. A. F., & Adinoff, A. D. (1989). Aeroallergen contact can exacerbate atopic dermatitis: patch tests as a diagnostic tool. *Journal of the American Academy of Dermatology, 2*(4), 863-869.
6. Clark, R. A. F., et al. (1990). Atopic dermatitis. In M. Sams & P. Lynch (Eds.), *Principles and practice of dermatology* (pp. 365-380). Philadelphia: W. B. Saunders.
7. Clark, R. A. F., et al. (1990). Current concepts in the management of the patient with atopic dermatitis. *Modern Medicine, 58*(3), 78-94.
8. Cunliffe, W. J. (1987). Evolution of a strategy for the treatment of acne. *Journal of the American Academy of Dermatology, 16*(3), 591-599.
9. Dicken, C. H. (1984). Retinoids: a review. *Journal of the American Academy of Dermatology, 11*(10), 541-552.
10. Dunn, M. L., et al. (1988). Treatment options for psoriasis. *American Journal of Nursing, 88*(8), 1082-1087.
11. du Vivier, A., & McKee, P. H. (1986). Malignant tumors of the skin. In A. du Vivier (Ed.), *Atlas of clinical dermatology* (pp. 7.2-7.36). Philadelphia: W. B. Saunders.
12. Eisenbaum, S. L., & Black, J. M. (1988). Melanoma. *Plastic Surgical Nursing, 8*(2), 42-47.
13. Ellis, C. N., & Voorhees, J. J. (1987). Etretinate therapy. *Journal of the American Academy of Dermatology, 16*(1), 267-291.
14. Farber, E. M., et al. (1983). Recent advances in the treatment of psoriasis. *Journal of the American Academy of Dermatology, 8*(3), 311-321.
15. Farber, E. M., et al. (1983). Long-term risks of psoralen and UV-A therapy for psoriasis. *Archives of Dermatology, 119*(5), 426-431.
16. Fitzpatrick, T. B., et al. (1990). *Dermatology in general medicine* (4th ed.). New York: McGraw-Hill.
17. Glizzard, D. (1991). Understanding the pathophysiology of psoriasis. A nursing perspective. *Dermatology Nursing, 3*(5), 305-314.
18. Keesling, B., & Friedman, S. (1987). Psychosocial factors in sunbathing and sunscreen use. *Health Psychology, 6*(5), 477-493.
19. Klingman, A. M. (1969). Early destructive effects of sunlight on human skin. *Journal of the American Medical Association, 210*(13), 2377-2390.
20. LeVine, M. J., & Parrish, J. A. (1980). Outpatient phototherapy of psoriasis. *Archives of Dermatology, 116*(5), 552-554.
21. Lewis, R. M., & Fischer, R. G. (1987). Sunscreen agents, pediatric drug information. *Pediatric Nursing, 13*(4), 200-201.
22. McCance, K., & Heurter, S. (1990). *Pathophysiology.* St. Louis: C. V. Mosby.
23. Melski, J. W., & Arndt, K. A. (1980). Topical therapy for acne. *New England Journal of Medicine, 302*(9), 503-506.
24. Menkes, A., et al. (1985). Psoriasis treatment with suberythemogenic ultraviolet B radiation and a coal tar extract. *Journal of the American Academy of Dermatology, 12*(1), 21-25.
25. Nicol, N. H. (1990). Current considerations and management of atopic dermatitis. *Dermatology Nursing, 2*(3), 129-138.
26. Nicol, N. H. (1989). What's new in sunscreens? Choices, choices, choices. *Pediatric Nursing, 15*(4), 417-418.
27. Nicol, N. H. (1989). Actinic keratosis: preventable and treatable like other precancerous and cancerous skin lesions. *Plastic Surgical Nursing, 9*(2), 49-55.
28. Nicol, N. H. (1989). Early detection and prevention of skin cancer. *Dermatology Nursing, 1*(1), 11-20.
29. Nicol, N. H. (1987). Atopic dermatitis: the (wet) wrap-up. *American Journal of Nursing, 87*(12), 1560-1564.
30. Nicol, N. H., & Clark, R. A. F. (1988). Therapy of atopic dermatitis. In E. Farmer & T. Provost (Eds.), *Current therapy in dermatology—2.* Philadelphia: B. C. Decker.
31. Pathak, M. A., et al. (1987). Preventive treatment of sunburn, dermatoheliosis and skin cancer with sunprotective agents. In T. B. Fitzpatrick, et al. (Eds.), *Dermatology in general medicine* (pp. 1507-1522). New York: McGraw Hill.
32. Provan, A., & Phillips, T. (1991). An overview of moist wound dressings: the under cover story. *Dermatology Nursing, 3*(6), 393-400.
33. Rosen, T., et al. (1983). *The nurse's atlas of dermatology.* Boston: Little, Brown.
34. Salasche, S. J. (1988). Actinic keratosis and keratoacanthoma. In E. Farmer & T. Provost (Eds.), *Current therapy in dermatology—2* (pp. 74-76). Philadelphia: B. C. Decker.
35. Sams, V. M., & Lynch, P. J. (1990). *Principles and practice of dermatology.* New York: Churchill Livingstone.
36. Schwartz, R. A., & Stoll, H. L. (1987). Epithelial precancerous lesions. In T. B. Fitzpatrick, et al. (Eds.), *Dermatology in general medicine* (pp. 733-743). New York: McGraw-Hill.
37. Scotto, J., & Fears, T. R. (1987). The association of solar ultraviolet and skin melanoma incidence among caucasians in the United States. *Cancer Investigation, 5*(4), 275-283.
38. Shelk, J. (1991). Phototherapy: a nursing overview. *Dermatology Nursing, 3*(6), 401-410.
39. Smith, D. P., & Nicol, N. H. (1991). Controlling pruritus. In D. P. Smith (Ed.), *Comprehensive child and family nursing skills: Assessment and intervention* (pp. 503-510). St. Louis: C. V. Mosby.
40. Stern, R. S., et al. (1984). Isotretinoin and pregnancy. *Journal of the American Academy of Dermatology, 10*(5), 851-854.
41. Stern, R. S., et al. (1986). Risk reduction for nonmelanoma skin

cancer with childhood sunscreen use. *Archives of Dermatology, 122*(5), 537–544.

42. Stern, R. S., et al. (1984). Topical versus systemic agent treatment for papulopustular acne. *Archives of Dermatology, 120*(12), 1571–1578.
43. Stoll, H. L., & Schwartz, R. A. (1987). Squamous cell carcinoma. In T. B. Fitzpatrick, et al. (Eds.), *Dermatology in general medicine* (pp. 746–758). New York: McGraw-Hill.
44. Vickers, C. F. H. (1980). The natural history of atopic eczema. *Acta Dermato-Venereologica (Stockh), 92* (Suppl.), 113.
45. Werner, Y. (1986). The water content of the stratum corneum in patients with atopic dermatitis. *Acta Dermato-Venereologica (Stockh), 66,* 282–284.
46. Wilkner, N. E., & Weston, W. L. (1988). Skin neoplasms. In R. W. Schrier (Ed.), *Medicine: Diagnosis and treatment* (pp. 513–530). Boston: Little, Brown.

Chapter 71

Nursing Care of Clients with Burn Injury

Definition

Injuries that result from direct contact or exposure to any thermal, chemical, electrical, or radiation source are termed burns. Burn injuries occur when energy from a heat source is transferred to the tissues of the body. The depth of injury is a function of temperature and the duration of exposure.

Incidence

Burn care has improved in recent decades, resulting in a lower mortality rate for victims of burn injuries.[26] Dedicated burn centers have been established with multidisciplinary burn team members who work together to care for the burn client and family. Advances in prehospital and inpatient care have contributed to survival. However, despite these advances, many people are still injured and die each year from burns. In the United States, two million people seek medical attention every year for injuries caused by burns; of these, 70,000 are hospitalized with severe injuries. Burn injuries are the third leading cause of accidental death in all age groups. Males tend to be injured more frequently than females, except in the elderly (older than 70 years).[25]

Etiology

Burn injuries are categorized according to their mechanism of injury.

THERMAL BURNS

Thermal burns are caused by exposure to or contact with flame, hot liquids, semiliquids (steam), semisolids (tar), or hot objects. Specific examples of thermal burns are those sustained in residential fires, explosive automobile accidents, scald injuries, clothing ignition, and ignition of poorly stored flammable liquids.

CHEMICAL BURNS

Chemical burns are caused by tissue contact with strong acids, alkalis, or organic compounds. The concentration of the chemical, duration of contact, and the amount of tissue exposed determine the extent of a chemical injury. Chemical burns can result from contact with certain household cleaning agents and various chemicals used in industry, agriculture, and the military. More than 25,000 products capable of causing chemical injuries have been identified.[20]

ELECTRICAL BURNS

Electrical burns are caused by heat that is generated by the electrical energy as it passes through the body.[36] The extent of the injury is influenced by the duration of contact, voltage level, and the pathway the electrical current takes as it passes through the body. Electrical injuries can result from contact with exposed or faulty electrical wiring or high-voltage power lines. Individuals struck by lightning also sustain an electrical injury.

RADIATION BURNS

Radiation burns are the least common type of burn injury and are caused by exposure to a radioactive source. These types of injuries have been associated with the use of ionizing radiation in industry or from therapeutic radiation sources in medicine. A sunburn from prolonged exposure to ultraviolet rays is also considered to be a type of radiation burn.

Risk Factors

Data collected from the National Burn Information Exchange reveals that 75 per cent of all burn injuries result from the actions of the victim, with many of these injuries occurring in the home environment. The client over age 70 is at a high risk for burn injury. This section will address risk factors in the adult; the reader is referred to a pediatric text for specific information on burns in children.

Contact with scalding liquids in either the kitchen or bathroom is often cited as a common mechanism of injury.[13, 25, 80] Overturned coffee pots and cooking pans spilling hot liquid and grease, overheated foods, liquids cooked in microwave ovens, and hot tap water have been identified as specific causes.[24, 57] Efforts to reduce the incidence of scald injuries have included the recommendations of the Consumer Products Safety Commission and Underwriters Laboratory that the maximum temperature on the thermostats of hot water heaters be lowered and a warning label identifying the potential for injury be applied to the water heater.[4] Antiscald devices have also been developed that, when installed at the faucet or shower head, shut off the flow of water when the temperature rises above a predetermined temperature, typically 43.3° C.

Clothing ignition during routine meal preparation has also been cited, particularly in the elderly population.[47, 71, 79] Although this is a well-documented problem, no flammability standards exist for adult clothing manufacturers, as they do for children's sleepwear manufacturers.

Public education for primary prevention of burn injuries has included the following recommendations:[24, 56, 79]

- Turning pot handles toward the back of the stove
- Purchasing a stove with controls on the front or side to reduce the likelihood of clothing ignition as one reaches across the hot elements
- Placing a screen around any heating appliance to function as a barrier
- Adjusting the thermostat setting on water heaters to produce a temperature of 130° F (54.5° C) or lower

Residential fires are another common cause of burn injuries. Chimneys, vent flues, fixed heating units, fireplaces, central-heating systems, wood-burning stoves, ignition of wood-shingled roofs, cigarettes, and human error have all been implicated. Cigarette-related ignition of furniture and mattresses is the single leading cause of fire deaths.[1] Preventive efforts have included the following recommendations:[1, 56, 74]

- Routine cleaning and checking of heating units and chimneys
- Careful attention to the installation and use of fuels for wood-burning stoves
- Treatment of wood-shingled roofs with a fire-retardant coating
- Installation of residential sprinkler systems
- Use of a fire-safe cigarette
- Presence of an operable smoke detector and fire extinguisher

Of primary importance in reducing injuries from residential fires is the presence of an operable smoke detector and fire extinguisher. It has been estimated that the risk of dying in a residential fire is reduced 50 per cent when an operable smoke detector is in place.[29] Some suggest that insurance carriers should refuse to issue hazard insurance for residential properties if smoke detectors and fire extinguishers are not on the premises.[74]

Pathophysiology

CUTANEOUS BURNS

The pathophysiologic changes that occur immediately following a cutaneous burn injury depend on the extent or size of the burn. For smaller burns, the body's response to injury is localized to the injured area. However, with more extensive burns, i.e., 25 per cent of the total body surface area (TBSA) or greater, the body's response to injury is systemic and proportional to the extent of the injury. Extensive burn injuries affect all major systems of the body.

Cardiovascular System. Immediately following a burn injury, vasoactive substances (catecholamines, histamine, serotonin, leukotrienes, and prostaglandins) are released from the injured tissue. These substances initiate changes that cause an increase in capillary permeability, allowing plasma to seep into surrounding tissues. Direct heat injury to vessels further increases capillary permeability. Direct injury to cell membranes permits sodium entry and potassium exit from the cell. Overall, this creates an osmotic gradient leading to increases in intracellular and interstitial fluid and further depletes intravascular fluid volumes.[59] Extensive burns result in generalized body edema in both burned and nonburned tissues[22] and a decrease in circulating intravascular blood volume. Heart rate increases in response to the catecholamine release and to the relative hypovolemia, yet initial cardiac output falls.[8] Hematocrit levels are elevated, demonstrating hemoconcentration from the loss of intravascular fluid. In addition, evaporative fluid losses through the burn wound are 4 to 20 times greater than normal[82] and remain elevated until complete wound closure is obtained. The result is a decrease in organ perfusion. If the intravascular space is not replenished with intravenous fluids, hypovolemic (burn) shock and ultimately death for the victim of an extensive burn may result.

At approximately 18 to 36 hours post-burn, the capillary permeability decreases,[60] but it does not normalize until 2 to 3 weeks following the injury.[8] Cardiac output returns to normal and then increases to meet the hypermetabolic needs of the body at approximately 24 hours post-burn. This change in cardiac output occurs even before circulating intravascular volume levels are restored to normal.[8] The initial rise in hematocrit falls to below normal by the third or fourth day post-burn due to red blood cell loss and damage at the time of injury. The body begins to reabsorb the edema fluid and diureses the excess fluid over the ensuing days and weeks (Fig. 71–1).

Renal and Gastrointestinal Systems. The body responds initially by shunting blood from the kidneys and decreasing glomerular filtration rate, causing oliguria. Blood flow to the mesenteric bed is also diminished, leading to the development of intestinal ileus and gastrointestinal dysfunction in clients with burns greater than 25 per cent of TBSA.[68]

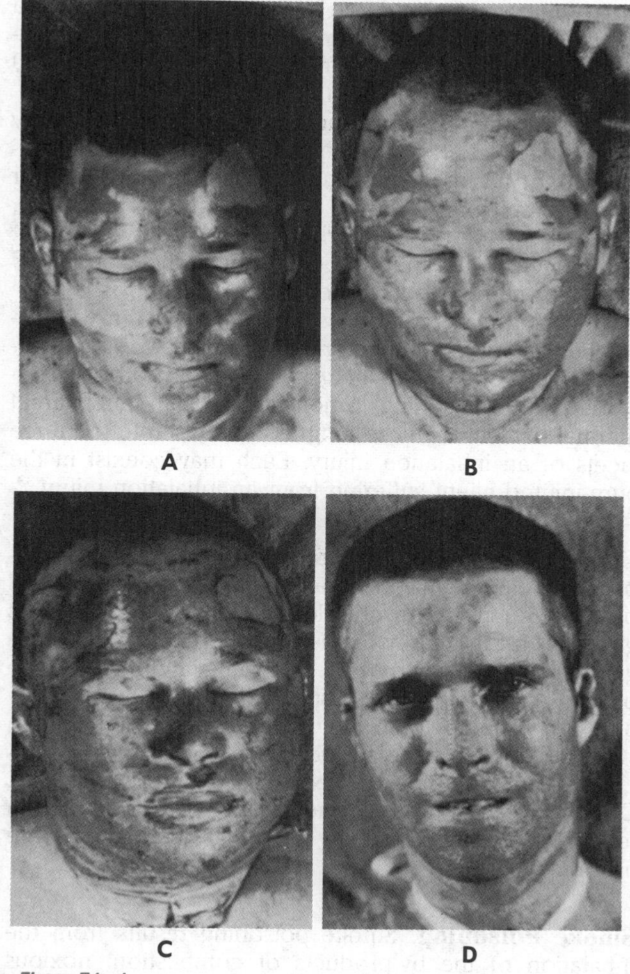

▲ *Figure 71–1*

Facial edema at various times following a burn injury to the face and neck. Edema worsens over the first 24 to 48 hours following a burn. *A*, 3 hours after burn. *B*, 8 hours after burn. *C*, 24 hours after burn, when the edema has typically maximized. *D*, Complete healing after 40 days. (From Artz, C. P., et al. [1979]. *Burns—a team approach.* Philadelphia: W. B. Saunders Company.)

Immune System. Immune system function is depressed. Depression of lymphocyte activity, a decrease in immunoglobulin production, suppression of complement activity, and an alteration in neutrophil and macrophage functioning are evident following extensive burn injuries.[6, 31, 45, 64] Together, these changes result in some degree of immunosuppression, increasing the risk of infection and life-threatening sepsis.

Respiratory System. The client may exhibit modest pulmonary artery hypertension, resulting in a decrease in arterial oxygen tension levels and lung compliance even when the client sustains no inhalation injury.[21]

SMOKE INHALATION

The inhalation of smoke and resulting pulmonary injury are often associated with flame injuries, particularly if the victim was trapped in an enclosed, smoke-filled space (e.g., a residential fire). The incidence of inhalation injuries has been estimated to be as great as 30 per cent for persons injured in a fire.[63]

Clinical manifestations suggestive of inhalation injury include facial burns, erythema or swelling of the oropharynx or nasopharynx, singed nasal hairs, agitation or anxiety, tachypnea, flaring nostrils, stridor, wheezing, dyspnea, hoarse voice, carbonaceous (sooty) sputum, and cough. Fiberoptic bronchoscopy and xenon-133 lung scan can be used to confirm the diagnosis.[2, 19, 65]

The pulmonary pathophysiology that occurs with inhalation injury is multifactorial and relates to the severity and type of smoke or gases inhaled. Carbon monoxide (CO) poisoning, smoke poisoning, and direct thermal or heat injury to lung tissue constitute the three facets of an inhalation injury. Each may coexist in the burn-injured client suffering from an inhalation injury.[33]

Carbon Monoxide Poisoning. CO is a common by-product released when organic substances (e.g., wood or coal) burn. It is a colorless, odorless, and tasteless gas that has an affinity for hemoglobin that is 200 times greater than that of oxygen. With inhalation of CO, the oxygen molecules are displaced and CO reversibly binds to hemoglobin to form carboxyhemoglobin (COHb). Tissue hypoxia occurs from an overall decrease in the blood's oxygen-delivering capability. COHb levels are easily monitored via blood serum levels in the clinical setting. Associated symptoms are listed in Table 71-1.

Smoke Poisoning. Smoke poisoning results from the inhalation of the by-products of combustion: noxious chemicals and particulate matter. The pulmonary response includes a localized inflammatory reaction, a decrease in bronchial ciliary action, and a decrease in alveolar surfactant. Mucosal edema in the smaller airways occurs, leading to audible wheezing on auscultation. After several hours, sloughing of the tracheobronchial epithelium may occur and hemorrhagic tracheobronchitis may develop. If the disease process continues, adult respiratory distress syndrome may follow.

Direct Thermal (Heat) Injury. Thermal burns to the lower airways of the pulmonary system are rare due to the protective reflex closure of the glottis and the ability of the respiratory tract to exchange heat effectively.[62] However, thermal burns to the lower airways can occur with the inhalation of live steam or explosive gases or with aspiration of scalding liquids. Thermal burns to the upper airways (mouth, nasopharynx, pharynx, and larynx) are more common and generally appear erythematous and edematous with mucosal blisters or ulcerations. The mucosal edema can lead to upper airway obstruction, particularly during the first 24 to 48 hours post-burn. Therefore, all clients with head and neck burns should be suspect for developing an airway obstruction and immediately considered for endotracheal intubation.

TABLE 71-1. Clinical Manifestations of Carbon Monoxide (CO) Poisoning

CO Level (%)	Clinical Manifestations
5-10	Impaired visual acuity
11-20	Flushing, headache
21-30	Nausea, impaired dexterity
31-40	Vomiting, dizziness, syncope
41-50	Tachypnea, tachycardia
>50	Coma, death

Adapted from Cioffi, W. G., & Rue, L. W. (1991). Diagnosis and treatment of inhalation injuries. *Critical Care Clinics of North America, 3*(2), 195.

Classification of Burn Severity

The severity of a burn injury is assessed with respect to the risk of mortality and the risk of cosmetic or functional disability.[3] Factors that influence injury severity include:

- Burn depth (Fig. 71-2)
- Burn size (percentage of TBSA)
- Burn location
- Age
- General health
- Mechanism of injury

BURN DEPTH

Burn depth can be divided into four categories based on the elements of the skin that are damaged: (1) superficial, (2) partial thickness, (3) full thickness, and (4) fourth degree. Most burn wounds that require medical intervention are a combination of partial- and full-thickness burns. A partial-thickness burn is shown in color plate 17. A full-thickness burn is shown in color plates 18 and 19. The appearance, sensation, and course of these burns are compared in Table 71-2.

BURN SIZE

The size of a burn is determined by one of two techniques: (1) the rule of nines or (2) the Lund and Browder method. Burn size is expressed as a percentage of TBSA. The accuracy of the calculation varies with the method and the experience of the individual making the determination.[11, 30]

The rule of nines was introduced in the late 1940s as a quick assessment tool for estimating burn size.[53] The basis of this rule is that the body is divided into anatomical sections, each of which represents 9 per cent or a multiple of 9 per cent of the TBSA (Fig. 71-3). This method is easy, requiring no diagrams to determine the percentage of TBSA injured. Therefore, it has been used in emergency departments where the initial triage occurs.

The Lund and Browder method modifies the percentages for body segments according to age and provides a more accurate estimate of burn size. It uses a diagram of the body, divided into sections with the

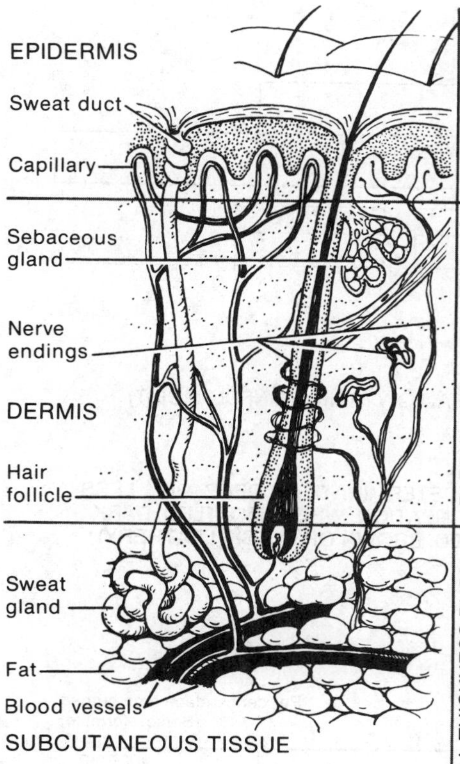

EPIDERMIS
Sweat duct
Capillary
Sebaceous gland
Nerve endings
DERMIS
Hair follicle
Sweat gland
Fat
Blood vessels
SUBCUTANEOUS TISSUE

	APPEARANCE	SENSATION	COURSE
SUPERFICIAL BURN	Mild to severe erythema; skin blanches with pressure	Painful Hyperesthetic Tingling Pain eased by cooling	Discomfort lasts about 48 hours Desquamation in 3–7days
PARTIAL-THICKNESS BURN	Large thick-walled blisters covering extensive area (vesiculation) Edema; mottled red base; broken epidermis; wet, shiny, weeping surface	Painful Sensitive to cold air	Superficial partial-thickness burn heals in 14–21 days Deep partial-thickness burn requires 21–28 days for healing Healing rate varies with burn depth and presence or absence of infection
FULL-THICKNESS BURN	Variable, e.g., deep red, black, white, brown Dry surface Edema Fat exposed Tissue disrupted	Little pain Insensate	Full-thickness dead skin suppurates and liquefies after 2–3 weeks Spontaneous healing impossible Requires removal of eschar and subsequent split- or full-thickness skin grafting Hypertrophic scarring and wound contractures likely to develop without preventive measures

▲ ***Figure 71-2***

Burn injury classification according to the depth of injury.

TABLE 71-2. American Burn Association Severity Classification for Burn Injuries

Major Burn Injury

- 25% total body surface area (TBSA) burn in adult
- 20% in children < 10 years
- 20% in adults > 40 years
- Burns involving the face, eyes, ears, hands, feet, and perineum likely to result in functional or cosmetic impairment or disability
- High-voltage electric burn injury
- All burn injuries with concomitant inhalation injury or major trauma

Moderate Burn Injury

- 15-25% TBSA in adult
- 10-20% in children < 10 years
- 10-20% in adults > 40 years
- <10% TBSA full-thickness burn without cosmetic or functional risk to burn involving the face, eyes, ears, hands, feet, perineum

Minor Burn Injury

- <15% TBSA in adults
- <10% TBSA in children < 10 years
- <10% TBSA in adults > 40 years
- No risk of cosmetic or functional impairment or disability

From American Burn Association. (1984). Guidelines for service standards and severity classification in the treatment of burn injury. *Bulletin of the American College of Surgeons, 69*(10), 24-28.

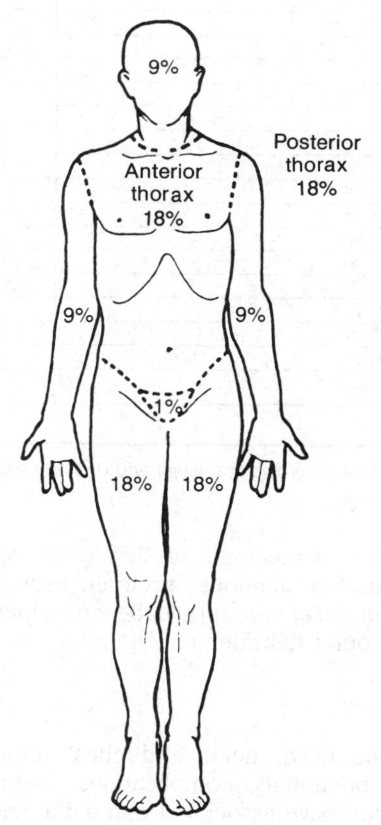

▲ ***Figure 71-3***

The "rule of nines" provides a quick method for estimating the extent of a burn injury.

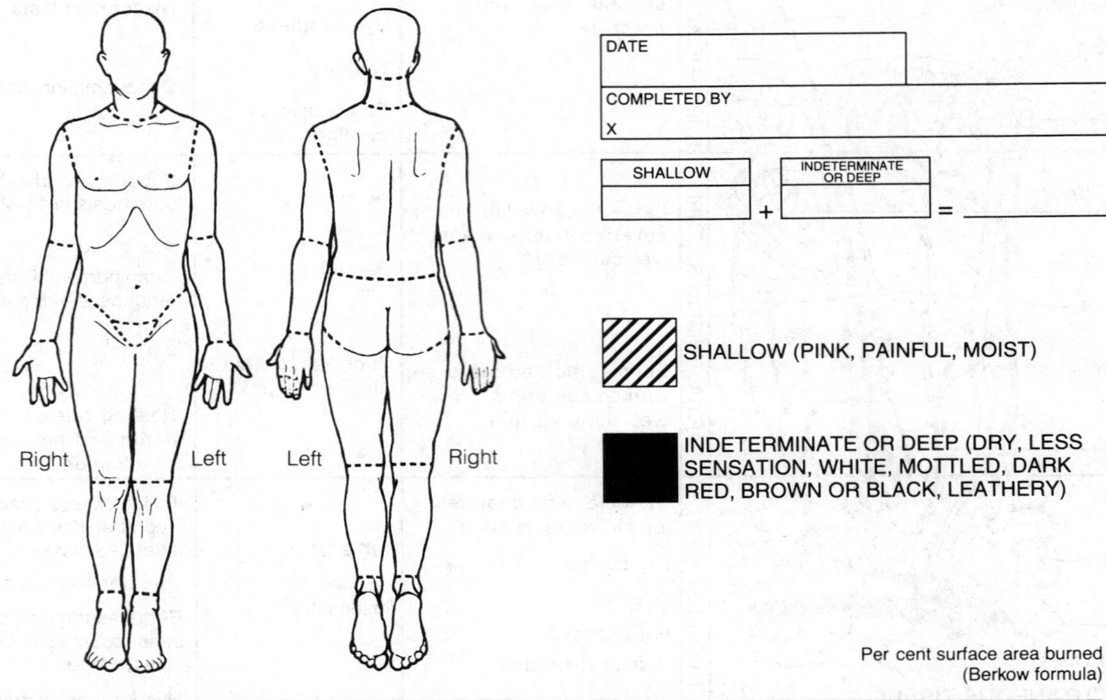

Per cent surface area burned (Berkow formula)

AREA	1 YEAR	1 to 4 YEARS	5 to 9 YEARS	10 to 14 YEARS	Y 15 YEARS	ADULT	SHALLOW	INDETER-MINATE OR DEEP
Head	19	17	13	11	9	7		
Neck	2	2	2	2	2	2		
Ant. Trunk	13	13	13	13	13	13		
Post.Trunk	13	13	13	13	13	13		
R. Buttock	2½	2½	2½	2½	2½	2½		
L. Buttock	2½	2½	2½	2½	2½	2½		
Genitalia	1	1	1	1	1	1		
R. U. Arm	4	4	4	4	4	4		
L. U. Arm	4	4	4	4	4	4		
R. L. Arm	3	3	3	3	3	3		
L. L. Arm	3	3	3	3	3	3		
R. Hand	2½	2½	2½	2½	2½	2½		
L. Hand	2½	2½	2½	2½	2½	2½		
R. Thigh	5½	6½	8	8½	9	9½		
L. Thigh	5½	6½	8	8½	9	9½		
R. Leg	5	5	5½	6	6½	7		
L. Leg	5	5	5½	6	6½	7		
R. Foot	3½	3½	3½	3½	3½	3½		
L. Foot	3½	3½	3½	3½	3½	3½		
TOTAL								

▲ ***Figure 71–4***

A sample chart for recording the extent and depth of a burn injury using the Lund and Browder formula.

representative percentage of TBSA for ages greater than 1 year. For the most accurate estimate of burn size, the burn diagram should be confirmed following the initial wound débridement.[54]

BURN LOCATION

Burns of the head, neck, and chest frequently have associated pulmonary complications. Burns involving the face often have associated corneal abrasions. Burns of the ears are prone to auricular chondritis and are susceptible to infection and further loss of tissue. Burns of the hands and joints often require intense physical and occupational therapy and have implications for loss of work time and/or permanent physical and vocational disability. Burns involving the perineal area are prone to autocontamination by urine and feces. Circumferential burns of extremities may produce a tourniquet-like effect and lead to vascular compromise. Circumferential thorax burns may lead to inadequate chest wall expansion and pulmonary insufficiency.

AGE

The client's age affects the severity and outcome of the burn. Mortality rates are higher for children less than 4 years of age, particularly in the 0- to 1-year age group and for clients over 65.[13,15,45,53,71]

High mortality and morbidity statistics in the elderly burn client result from the combination of functional impairments (slower reaction time, impaired judgement, and decreased mobility), living alone, and environmental hazards.[13] Compounding this vulnerability to burn injury is the thinning of the skin and atrophy of skin appendages. Situations such as bathing and cooking may lead to a burn.[71, 80]

GENERAL HEALTH

Debilitating cardiac, pulmonary, endocrine, and renal disease—specifically, diabetes, cardiopulmonary insufficiency, alcoholism, and renal failure—have been observed to influence the client's response to injury and treatment.[47, 68] The mortality rate for clients with preexisting cardiac disorders is 3.5 to 4 times higher than for burn clients without cardiac disorders.[33] Alcoholic clients with burns had a threefold increase in mortality rate over that of the nonalcoholic client with burns. In addition, those alcoholic clients who survived their burn injury had longer hospital stays.[41] Obese clients are also at increased risk of cardiopulmonary complications.[81]

MECHANISM OF INJURY

The mechanism of injury is another factor used to determine the severity of injury. In general, any burn associated with inhalation injury requires special consideration.

In electrical burns, heat is generated as the electricity travels through the body, resulting in internal tissue damage. Cutaneous burn injuries may be negligible but muscle and soft tissue damage may be extensive, particularly in high-voltage electrical injuries. The voltage, type of current (direct or alternating), contact site, and duration of contact are important considerations because they may affect morbidity. Alternating current is more dangerous than direct current. It is often associated with cardiopulmonary arrests, ventricular fibrillation, tetanic muscle contractions, and long bone or vertebral compression fractures.[68] In addition, victims of electrical injuries may have fallen from the point of electrical contact and sustained associated injuries. In chemical burns, systemic toxicity from cutaneous absorption may occur.

The American Burn Association has published a severity classification schedule for burn injuries (Table 71-2). These guidelines are intended to assist the clinician in determining injury severity for the burn client. This classification schedule separates injuries into major, moderate, or minor burn injuries. Clients with major burns are usually transferred to a specialized burn care facility after local emergency treatment has been provided. Clients with moderate burns can usually be treated on an inpatient basis at the receiving hospital. Clients with minor burns usually receive initial care in the emergency department and are then discharged for follow-up care on an outpatient basis.[3]

Management

The multiple organ system response that occurs following a burn injury necessitates an interdisciplinary approach. The nurse is responsible for developing a plan of care that is based on assessment data reflecting the physical and psychosocial needs of the client and family or significant other.[9]

Nursing diagnoses, related goals, and treatments are presented in the Nursing Care Plan, and the phase(s) of recovery in which they are most applicable are specified. The clinical course of the burn client can be divided into three phases: the emergent and resuscitation phase, the acute phase, and the rehabilitation phase.[16, 67]

THE EMERGENT PHASE

The emergent phase begins at the time of injury and concludes with the restoration of capillary permeability, usually at 48 to 72 hours following the injury. The primary goal during the emergent phase of recovery is to prevent hypovolemic (burn) shock and to preserve vital organ functioning. Pre-hospital care, emergency department management, and the resuscitation period are included within this phase and are discussed separately.

Pre-hospital Care. Pre-hospital care of the burn victim begins at the scene of the accident and concludes when institutional emergency medical care is obtained (Box 71-1). Pre-hospital care should begin with removing the victim from the source of the burn and/or

Box 71-1. Guidelines for Pre-Hospital Care of Burn Victims

1. Remove the victim from the source of the burn:
   - Extinguish burning clothes,
   - Remove saturated clothing (chemical or scald burns),
   - Cool the tar burn,
   - Copiously irrigate a chemical burn,
   - Turn off electricity or remove the electrical source using dry, nonconductive object.
2. Assess the ABCs:
   - Establish airway,
   - Ensure adequate breathing (100% oxygen via non-rebreather face mask for suspected inhalation injury),
   - Assess circulation.
3. Assess for associated trauma.
4. Conserve body heat.
5. Consider need for intravenous fluid administration.
6. Transport.

Data from Trunkey, D. D. (1983). Transporting the critically burned patient. In T. L. Wachtel, et al. (Eds.): *Current Topics in Burn Care.* Rockville, MD: Aspen Publications.

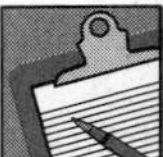

CARE PLAN

The Burn-Injured Adult Client

Nursing Diagnosis/ Collaborative Problem	Planning: Expected Outcomes	Implemention: Nursing Interventions	Rationales
(E) Fluid Volume Deficit R/T increased capillary leak and large fluid shift from intravascular to interstitial space	Client will have improved fluid balance, as evidenced by urine output of 30–50 ml/h, clear sensorium, pulse rate < 120 bpm without dysrhythmias, and blood pressure within expected range for age and medical history (pain control achieved).	Assess for hypovolemia q 1 hour × 36 hours. Obtain admission weight. Weigh client daily. Monitor and document hourly intake and output. Administer intravenous (IV) fluid and electrolyte replacement per physician's order. Monitor serum electrolytes and hematocrits.	Fluid shifts lead to hypovolemia. Weight is an accurate index of fluid balance. Urine output is a measure of effectiveness of fluid resuscitation. IV fluids are used to restore fluid volume. Hyperkalemia and elevated hematocrit are common findings.
Collaborative Problem (E) Potential for paralytic ileus R/T stress from injury	The nurse will monitor for normoactive bowel sounds, absence of abdominal distention, flatus production, and normal bowel movements.	Assess need for placement of nasogastric (NG) tube. Assess bowel function: • Auscultate bowel sounds q 4 hours. • Observe for abdominal distention. • Monitor gastric output and amount, color, and presence of blood and pH.	Ileus is common in burns >20–25% BSA. Bowel sounds indicate peristalsis is present. Abdominal distention indicates ileus. Gastric output may require fluid replacement. Gastric ulcers are common following major burns.
Collaborative Problem (E) Potential for renal failure R/T presence of hemachromagens in the urine due to deep burn and/or crush injury	The nurse will monitor for visible urinary hemachromagens and adequate urine output of 75–100 ml/h.	Monitor and document hourly urine output and urine color. Ensure patency of urinary catheter. Administer IV fluids per physician's order. Send urine samples for urine myoglobin/hemoglobin levels per physician's order.	Urine is red or dark brown when hemachromagens are present. Catheter can become plugged with hemachromagens. Hemachromagens are flushed from the body. Provides quantitative information on risk of renal failure.
(E, A) Impaired Gas Exchange R/T carbon monoxide poisoning, smoke poisoning, and heat damage to lungs	Client will have improved gas exchange, as evidenced by unlabored respirations of 16–24/min, $PaO_2 > 90$ mm Hg, $PaCO_2$ 35–45 mm Hg, $SaO_2 > 95\%$, and clear bilateral breath sounds.	Assess for signs of respiratory distress as evidenced by restlessness, confusion, labored breathing, tachypnea, dyspnea, diminished and/or adventitious breath sounds, tachycardia, decrease in PaO_2 and SaO_2 levels, cyanosis.	Impaired gas exchange can lead to respiratory distress from hypoxemia.

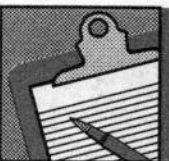

CARE PLAN

The Burn-Injured Adult Client Continued

Nursing Diagnosis/ Collaborative Problem	Planning: Expected Outcomes	Implemention: Nursing Interventions	Rationales
		Monitor arterial blood gas and carboxyhemoglobin levels per physician's order.	Provides data on effectiveness of respiration/oxygenation.
		Monitor SaO_2 levels continuously.	Provides noninvasive oxygenation data.
		Administer oxygen therapy as prescribed.	Reduces hypoxemia
		Instruct client on the use of incentive spirometer.	Encourages deep breathing.
		Elevate head of bed (HOB)	Facilitates lung expansion.
		Monitor need for endotracheal intubation.	Intubation may be required to maintain oxygenation.
(E, A) Ineffective Airway Clearance R/T tracheal edema, airway epidermal sloughing, and depressed pulmonary ciliary action from inhalation injury	Client will have effective airway clearance, as evidenced by clear bilateral breath sounds, clear to white pulmonary secretions, effective mobilization of pulmonary secretions, and unlabored respirations of 16–24/min.	Have client turn, cough, and deep breathe q 1–2 hours × 24 hours, then q 2–4 hours while awake.	Facilitates clearance of upper airways.
		Place oral suction device within client's reach for independent use.	Encourages removal of oral secretions and expectorated sputum.
		Perform endo- or nasotracheal suction prn, and monitor and document character of sputum.	Removes secretions from upper airway. Sputum color, consistency, odor, and amount may indicate infection.
(E, A) Altered Peripheral Tissue Perfusion R/T from constricting circumferential burns	Client will have adequate peripheral perfusion, as evidenced by pulses present by palpation or Doppler, capillary refill of unburned skin < 2 seconds, absence of numbness or tingling, and absence of increased pain with active range-of-motion (ROM) exercises.	Remove all constricting jewelry and clothing.	May compromise circulation as edema ensues.
		Limit use of constricting blood pressure cuffs in affected extremity.	May reduce arterial inflow and venous return.
		Monitor arterial pulses by palpation or ultrasonic flow detector (Doppler) hourly × 72 hours	Pulses will diminish with circulation impairments.
		Assess capillary refill of unburned skin on affected extremity	Capillary refill will be prolonged with impaired circulation.
		Assess pain level with active ROM exercises	Ischemic tissues cause pain.
		Elevate affected extremities above the level of the heart.	Reduces dependent edema formation.
		Encourage active ROM exercises.	Promotes venous return and reduces muscle atrophy.
		Anticipate and prepare client for escharotomy	Escharotomy is used to restore circulation to compromised tissues.

Care Plan continued on following page

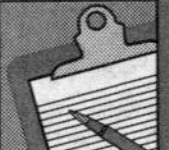

CARE PLAN

The Burn-Injured Adult Client Continued

Nursing Diagnosis/ Collaborative Problem	Planning: Expected Outcomes	Implemention: Nursing Interventions	Rationales
		Post-Escharotomy care: Assess adequacy of circulation: • Check pulses • Note color, movement, and sensation of affected extremity	These data indicate adequacy of perfusion.
		Control post-escharotomy bleeding with pressure, electrocautery, or suturing of bleeding vessels.	Viable tissue beneath eschar bleeds.
(E, A) Hypothermia R/T epithelial tissue loss and fluctuating ambient air temperatures	Client will remain normothermic, as evidenced by core body temperature between 99.6° and 101.0° F.	Monitor client's rectal or core temperature as indicated (hourly during the emergent phase and post-surgery).	Hypothermia may follow loss of skin as a thermal regulator and with some anesthetics.
		Limit the amount of body surface area exposed during wound care.	Exposure leads to hypothermia. Heat is lost in open wounds and after hydrotherapy by evaporation.
		Limit hydrotherapy treatment sessions to 30 minutes or less with water temperature 98° - 102.0° F.	
		Use external heat shields/radiant heat lamps.	External source of heat.
		Keep procedure rooms and surgical suites warm.	
		If air-fluidized therapy bed is in use, monitor and maintain appropriate bed temperature and consider reducing the flow of fluidization if hypothermia develops.	Heat is lost due to convection.
Collaborative Problem (E, A) High Risk for Stress Ulcers R/T neurohormonal stress response from the burn injury	The nurse will monitor for gastrointestinal bleeding and will maintain gastric pH > 5.	Monitor and document gastric pH values and heme content q 2 hours while NG tube is in place.	Acidic gastric secretions may lead to bleeding.
		Administer antacids and/or H_2 receptor antagonists per physician's order.	Reduces gastric acid content.
		Monitor stools for occult blood.	Stress ulcers cause bleeding, which may be excreted in stools.
(A) Altered Nutrition: Less Than Body Requirements R/T	Client will have adequate nutrition, as evidenced	Obtain accurate pre-burn weight.	Caloric needs are based on pre-burn weight.

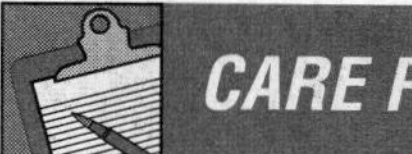

CARE PLAN

The Burn-Injured Adult Client Continued

Nursing Diagnosis/ Collaborative Problem	Planning: Expected Outcomes	Implemention: Nursing Interventions	Rationales
increased metabolic needs for wound healing	by maintaining 85–90% of pre-burn weight.	Consult dietician.	Dieticians perform nutritional assessments.
		Assess eating habits/patterns, food preferences, food allergies within 72 hours of admission.	Establishes a baseline.
		Record caloric intake (calorie counts).	Quantitative data on caloric intake.
		Weigh client daily to follow weight trends (exception: if operative procedure limits movement).	Weight should be stable if caloric needs are being met.
		Provide oral hygiene each shift and prn.	Prevents stomatitis, enhances appetite.
		Provide an aesthetically pleasing environment.	Conducive to eating.
		Schedule treatments to provide for uninterrupted meal times.	Interruptions may decrease calorie intake.
		Allow a period of rest prior to meal time if the client has endured a painful procedure or treatment.	Pain decreases appetite.
		Provide aids and devices for eating utensils.	Facilitates self care.
		Encourage family/SO to bring favorite foods from home.	Client may be willing to eat familiar foods. Foods must be nutritionally sound.
		Provide nutritious supplements between meals.	Caloric needs are often too high to be eaten in three meals.
		Provide positive reinforcement for eating.	Anorexic clients may believe there is no benefit to eating.
		Consider other methods to meet caloric needs, such as tube feeding, total parenteral nutrition	Oral feeding may not provide adequate calories for healing.
(E, A) High Risk for Infection R/T loss of skin barrier, impaired immune response, presence of invasive catheters (indwelling urinary catheter and intravenous catheters), and invasive procedures (venous and arterial blood sampling and bronchoscopy)	Client will have no burn wound microbial invasion, as evidenced by (quantitative wound cultures < 100,000 organisms); core body temperature will maintain 99.6°–101.0° F; will have no swelling, redness, or purulence at invasive line insertion sites; and will have negative	Administer tetanus prophylaxis prn.	Anaerobic environment beneath eschar may allow tetanus organism to grow.
		Maintain infection control techniques.	Prevent cross contamination.
		Instruct family/SO on infection control measures.	Promote compliance.
		Enforce strict handwashing.	Minimize incidence of cross-contamination.
		Assess for clinical signs of infection: discoloration of	Burn wound is open and client is immunocompro-

Care Plan continued on following page

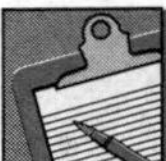

CARE PLAN

The Burn-Injured Adult Client Continued

Nursing Diagnosis/ Collaborative Problem	Planning: Outcomes	Implementation: Nursing Interventions	Rationales
	blood, urine, and sputum cultures.	wounds or drainage, odor, delayed healing; headache, chills, anorexia, nausea; change in vital signs; hyperglycemia and glycosuria; paralytic ileus, confusion, restlessness, hallucinations.	mised; therefore, local wound infection or systemic infection is a risk.
		Before reapplying topical cream, cleanse and rinse the burn wound.	To remove wound debris that would prevent cream from adhering to the wound.
		Debride wound of loose, nonviable tissue.	These tissues are a medium for bacterial growth.
		Shave or cut body hair in and around wound margins (exception: eyebrows and eyelashes).	Hair is contaminated and prevents cream adherence.
		Apply topical therapy (antimicrobial agent or temporary wound covering).	Provides wound coverage.
		Assess for signs of infection at catheter insertion site twice a day.	
(E, A, R) Pain R/T burn injury, exposed nerve endings, treatments, and anxiety	Client will have more comfort as evidenced by verbalizing relief or control of pain/discomfort and identifying factors that contribute to pain/discomfort.	Assess client's response to pain with wound care, physical therapy, and at rest (background pain).	Establishes a baseline.
		Medicate prior to painful procedures: 45 minutes for oral, 30 minutes for intramuscular, 5–10 minutes for IV. Do NOT administer intramuscular medications to clients with major burns during the emergent phase.	Adequate time allowed for onset of analgesia. Intramuscular injections are not given because of erratic and diminished circulation impairing absorption.
		Explore relaxation technique, music therapy, guided imagery, distraction, and hypnosis.	Nonpharmocologic analgesics.
		Explain all procedures to the client and allow time for preparation.	To reduce anxiety.
		Talk to the client while providing care and performing procedures.	Promotes client's trust.
		Assess for the need of anxiolytic medications.	Anxiety decreases pain threshold.
		Document the client's response to prescribed medications and nonpharmocologic treatments.	Evaluate effectiveness of interventions.

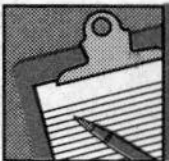

CARE PLAN

The Burn-Injured Adult Client Continued

Nursing Diagnosis/ Collaborative Problem	Planning: Expected Outcomes	Implementation: Nursing Interventions	Rationales
(A, R) Self-Care Deficit (Grooming, Bathing, Eating, Elimination) R/T functional deficits resulting from the burn injury, pain, dressings, splints, and enforced immobility	Client will have less self-care deficit and will demonstrate increased participation in self-care.	Assess the client's ability to provide self-care.	Provides a baseline.
		Consult with occupational therapy regarding the need for assistive devices.	Promotes self-care.
		Encourage client to participate in self-care tasks.	Helps to motivate client and overcome fear and dependency.
		Ensure that the client has adequate time to accomplish tasks.	Helps establish self control.
		Provide positive reinforcement when tasks are accomplished.	Promotes independence and motivation.
(E, A, R) Impaired Physical Mobility R/T edema, pain, dressings, splints, surgical procedures, and wound contractures	Client will have improved physical mobility, as evidenced by returning to maximum activities of daily living with minimal disability and disfigurement.	Assess ROM and muscle strength in burned areas prone to develop contractures for q day and prn.	Determine baseline.
		Maintain burned areas in position of physiologic function within limits imposed by associated injuries, grafting, other therapeutic devices (see Table 71–6 for positioning recommendations).	Prevent/reduce contracture development.
		Explain rationale for activities and positioning to client and family. Reinforce prn.	Improves compliance.
		Consult physical and occupational therapy for an individualized rehabilitation schedule. Adjust schedule as needed.	Will provide needed devices and teaching for ambulation and ROM.
		Wrap burned legs and/or unburned legs with donor sites with Ace wraps (figure 8 technique) before placing in any dependent position. As healing progresses, other elasticated support bandages can be worn.	Decrease capillary venous stasis, which impairs graft healing.
		Encourage active ROM q 2–4 hours while awake unless contraindicated because of a recent grafting procedure.	Control post-resuscitation edema and prevent muscle atrophy, tendon adherence, joint stiffness, and capsular shortening.

Care Plan continued on following page

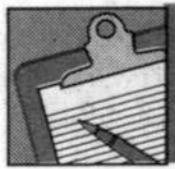

CARE PLAN

The Burn-Injured Adult Client Continued

Nursing Diagnosis/ Collaborative Problem	*Planning: Expected Outcomes*	*Implementation: Nursing Interventions*	*Rationales*
		Ambulate client to chair or walking (unless contraindicated by a recent grafting procedure or other injuries).	Ambulation promotes muscle strength and cardiopulmonary reserve. After grafting, clients remain on bed rest.
		Provide passive exercise and stretching if client is unable to actively participate (ie., comatose or paralyzed).	Passive ROM maintains joint motion and muscle tone.
(A, R) High Risk for Self-Esteem Disturbance R/T threatened or actual change in body image, physical loss, and loss of role responsibilities	Client will develop improved self-esteem as evidenced by making social contact with others outside of immediate family, developing effective coping mechanisms through the stages of recovery, and verbalizing feelings about self-concept.	Determine previous coping style.	Determine baseline, previous coping styles will be tried by client.
		Provide an atmosphere of acceptance.	
		Explain projected appearance of burns and grafts during different phases of wound healing.	Provides information; may reduce misconceptions.
		Allow client to progress at own pace through stages of denial, grief, and acceptance of injury and recovery.	Clients progress at varying rates depending on the degree of injury, perception of injury, support systems, and previous coping styles.
		Assess need for limit setting for maladaptive behavior. Consult with burn team members to establish limits and treatment plan. Explain and assist family/SO to maintain same limits.	Maladaptive behavior is harmful and is usually controlled by setting limits for all to follow.
		Promote client's self-confidence:	
		• Ensure continuity of care providers.	Promotes trust.
		• Discuss all activities and procedures prior to initiation.	Reduces anxiety.
		• Support client's role in care and treatment.	Motivates client; reduces fear.
		• Keep client informed of progress.	
		• Provide honest, positive reinforcement.	Do not provide false hope of functional return if there is irreparable damage.
		• Help family/SO to interact with client.	Family may be fearful and require guidance.
		Encourage interaction with others outside immediate family day passes.	Facilitates societal reintegration.
		Help prepare client for so-	Provides rehearsal of

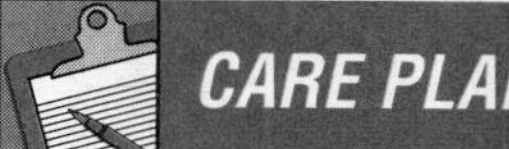

CARE PLAN

The Burn-Injured Adult Client Continued

Nursing Diagnosis/ Collaborative Problem	Planning: Expected Outcomes	Implementation: Nursing Interventions	Rationales
		cial interactions after discharge by discussing potential situations and how client might deal with them.	events and reduces anxiety.
		Make home health care nurse or physical therapist referral as indicated.	To assess client's adjustment at home, ability to continue with needed therapy, further teaching, and care requirements.
(E, A, R) High Risk for Ineffective Family Coping R/T the emergent and critical nature of the injury and separation from family/friends	Family will have improved coping strategies, as evidenced by verbalizing goals of treatment regimen; emotional stressors, concerns, and behaviors; and understanding and knowledge of available support services.	Prior to family's/SO's initial visit:	
		• Communicate extent of burn and changes in client's appearance;	Preparation to reduce degree of fright.
		• Provide family/SO with information that meets their basic needs.	Common needs of family members.
		• Provide brief, simple explanations of procedures and equipment.	Simple explanations more readily retained.
		Determine how the client and family/SO have coped with past stress.	Provides a baseline.
		Assist client with dealing with stress by providing coping strategies such as diversion and relaxation techniques.	Provides client with new strategies.
		Allow for uninterrupted visitation during visiting hours if possible.	Assists client to cope.
		Provide family/SO with daily updates regarding changes in client's condition.	Maintains realistic perception of client's progress.
		Consult with psychologist, psychiatrist, social worker, or psychiatric clinical nurse specialist prn.	These professionals may assist client to improve coping strategies.
		Encourage family/SO attendance at support group meetings for family members.	Provides support and helps to dispel misconceptions.
		For impending client transfer, provide family/SO with support services to assist with their travel.	To reduce anxiety during transition.

Note. E, emergent phase; A, acute phase; R, rehabilitation phase. Data from Dyer, C., & Roberts, D. (1990). Thermal trauma. *Nursing Clinics of North America, 25(1)*,101–115; Burgess, M. C. (1991). Initial management of a patient with extensive burn injury. *Critical Care Nursing Clinics of North America, 3(2)*,175–177; Duncan, D. J., & Driscoll, D. M. (1991). Burn wound management. *Critical Care Nursing Clinics of North America, 3(2)*,202–204; Carlson, D. E., & Jordan, B. S. (1991). Implementing nutritional therapy in the thermally injured patient. *Critical Care Nursing Clinics of North America, 3(2)*,229–231.

eliminating the source of the heat. This action requires some consideration of the mechanism of injury so as to avoid further injury to the victim and/or injury to the rescuer.

Emergency Department Management. The care in the emergency department is a continuation of that administered at the scene. If little or inadequate assessment and/or treatment has been done, pre-hospital care is provided in the emergency department. Treatment of the burn wound (debridement and dressings) should not take precedence over the evaluation and treatment of any associated life-threatening problems.[82]

Minor Burns. Care of the client with minor burn injuries is frequently provided on an ambulatory or outpatient basis. In making the decision whether to discharge a client, consideration of (1) the client's ability to follow instructions and provide self-care and (2) the home environment is important. Discharging a client to "home" who has no home and who lives on the street can lead to a poor recovery and outcome.

Emergency department care of minor burn wounds includes (1) pain management, (2) tetanus prophylaxis, (3) initial wound care, and (4) teaching.

Pain management is often achieved with small doses of morphine or meperidine in the emergency department.[67] Oral analgesic agents are prescribed for outpatient use.

The current protocol for tetanus prophylaxis is the same for clients with minor burns as for clients with any other type of injury. Clients who have been previously immunized against tetanus but not within the past 5 years should receive a tetanus toxoid booster. For clients not immunized, tetanus human immune globulin and the first of a series of active immunizations with tetanus toxoid should be administered.[70, 85]

Wound care for minor burns consists of cleansing; debridement of loose, nonviable tissue; removal of any damaging agents (chemicals, tar, etc.); and application of topical antimicrobial creams or ointments and a sterile dressing. It is during this time that the nurse has a major responsibility for teaching home wound care and the clinical manifestations of infection that would necessitate the client's return to medical care. Other teaching needs include the need to perform active range-of-motion (ROM) exercises to maintain normal joint function and to decrease edema formation and possibility of scar formation, although it is minimal to nonexistent with minor, superficial burn wounds. The need for any follow-up evaluations or treatments should be confirmed with the client at this time.

Major Burns. For clients with extensive burn wounds, the emergency department management includes

- Reevaluation of airway, breathing, and circulation (ABCs) and associated trauma,
- Initiation of fluid resuscitation,
- Placement of indwelling urinary catheter,
- Placement of nasogastric tube,
- Vital signs/baseline laboratory studies,
- Pain management,
- Tetanus prophylaxis,
- Data collection, and
- Wound care.

With the exception of chemical burns, the burn wound should not take precedence over other life-threatening trauma or complications. The adequacy of the airway, breathing, and circulation should be reestablished and a re-evaluation for any associated trauma performed. The oropharynx is inspected for evidence of erythema, blisters, or ulcerations, and the need for endotracheal intubation considered. If inhalation injury is suspected, administration of 100 per cent oxygen via a tight fitting non-rebreather face mask continues until carboxyhemoglobin levels fall below 15 per cent.[65] Hyperbaric oxygen may also be used (see Chapter 18).

For adults with burn injuries affecting more than 15 per cent of TBSA, intravenous fluid resuscitation is generally required. Peripheral intravenous access through nonburned skin, proximal to any extremity burns, is preferred. For those clients with extensive burns or limited peripheral intravenous access sites, cannulation of a central vein (subclavian, internal or external jugular, or femoral) by a physician may be necessary. The per cent of burn injury is determined and fluid resuscitation begun. Table 71–3 outlines the fluid resuscitation formulas currently used.

Resuscitation. The resuscitation period begins with initiation of fluid resuscitation measures and concludes when capillary integrity returns to near-normal levels and the large fluid shifts have decreased.

Fluid resuscitation is initiated to minimize the deleterious effects of fluid shifts. The goal of fluid resuscitation is to maintain vital organ perfusion while avoiding the complications of inadequate or excessive therapy.[65] Several formulas used to calculate fluid requirements are listed in Table 71–3. In the calculation of fluid infusion rates, the time of injury, and not the time the fluid resuscitation was initiated, serves as time zero.

Although each formula is different, generally the first 24 hours post-burn dictates the infusion of a balanced salt solution. The exact amount of fluid is based on the client's weight and the extent of injury. Other factors to be considered include the presence of an inhalation injury, a delay in initiation of resuscitation, or deep tissue damage. These factors tend to increase the amount of intravenous fluid required for adequate resuscitation above the calculated amount. With the exception of the Evans and Brooke formula, colloid-containing solutions are not given during this period due to the changes in capillary permeability that allow leakage of protein-rich fluid into the interstitial space, increasing edema formation. During the second 24 hours post-burn, colloid-containing solutions are administered, along with 5 per cent dextrose and water in varying amounts.

It is important to remember that all resuscitation formulas serve only as guides and should be adjusted according to the client's physiologic response. Successful or adequate fluid resuscitation in the adult is sig-

TABLE 71-3. Fluid Resuscitation Formulas Used in Burn Care

	First 24 Hours			Second 24 Hours		
Formula Name	**Electrolyte-Containing Solution**	**Colloid-Containing Solution**	**Dextrose in Water**	**Electrolyte-Containing Solution**	**Colloid-Containing Solution**	**Dextrose in Water**
Evans	Normal saline 1 ml/kg/% burn	1 ml/kg/% burn	2000 ml	½ of first 24-hour requirement	½ of first 24-hour requirement	2000 ml
Brooke	Lactated Ringer's 1.5 ml/kg/% burn	0.5 ml/kg/% burn	2000 ml	½–¾ of first 24-hour requirement	½–¾ of first 24-hour requirement	2000 ml
Modified Brooke	Lactated Ringer's 2 ml/kg/% burn	None	None	None	0.3–0.5 ml/kg/% burn	Titrate to maintain urine output
Parkland	Lactated Ringer's 4 ml/kg/% burn	None	None	None	0.3–0.5 ml/kg/% burn	Titrate to maintain urine output
Hypertonic Saline Solution	Fluid containing 250 mEq of sodium/L to maintain hourly urine output of 70 ml in adults	None	None	Same solution to maintain hourly urine output of 30 ml in adults	None	None

Adapted from Rue, L. W., & Cioffi, W. G., Jr. (1991). Resuscitation of thermally injured patients. *Critical Care Nursing Clinics of North America, 3*(2), 185; and Wachtel, T. L., & Fortune, J. B. (1983). Fluid resuscitation for burn shock. In T. L. Wachtel et al. (Eds.), *Current topics in burn care* (p. 44). Rockville, MD: Aspen Publishers, Inc.

naled by stable vital signs, adequate urine output, palpable peripheral pulses and clear sensorium (see the Care Plan).

An indwelling urethral catheter should be placed to measure hourly urine production. Urine output is the most readily available and reliable indicator for determining the adequacy of fluid resuscitation.[65, 68]

Circumferential burns of the extremities and of the thorax may compromise circulation and respiration, respectively. These complications are more likely to occur during resuscitation, when fluid shifts into the interstitial tissues are at their peak. With circumferential burns of the extremities, elevating the extremity above the level of the heart helps reduce dependent edema; however, circulatory compromise may still occur. Frequent assessment of distal extremity perfusion is necessary.

An escharotomy is the appropriate treatment for circulatory compromise due to circumferential burns. The physician makes a lengthwise incision through eschar, relieving the constriction to circulation (Fig. 71-5). It is generally performed at the bedside and without anesthesia because the eschar does not bleed and there is no pain. Viable tissue beneath the burn may bleed though. The wound with an escharotomy can be dressed in the usual fashion. If adequate tissue perfusion does not return, a fasciotomy may be necessary. This procedure, in which the fascia is incised, is performed in the operating room under anesthesia.

Likewise, escharotomy can be performed on thorax burns to improve ventilation. Following these escharotomies, the nurse monitors for improvement of ventilation.

Many centers advocate the placement of a nasogastric tube for clients with burns of 20 to 25 per cent or more of TBSA to prevent emesis and reduce the risk of aspiration.[67, 68] Gastrointestinal dysfunction results from the intestinal ileus that develops almost universally in these clients during the early post-burn period. All oral fluids should be restricted at this time.

Vital signs provide baseline information as well as additional data for determining the adequacy of resus-

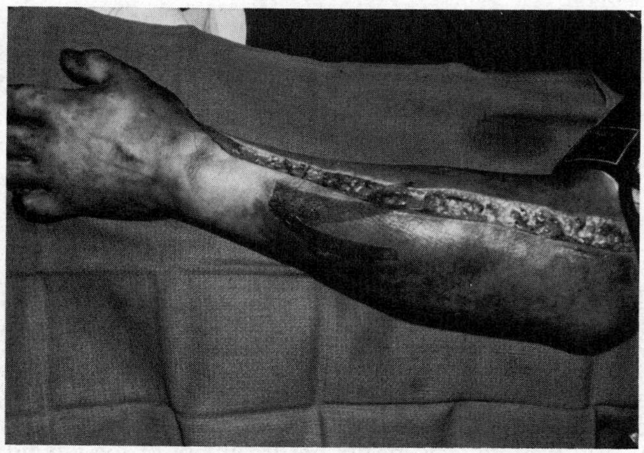

▲ *Figure 71-5*

Escharotomy. Incision is made through the constricting burn eschar to permit expansion of the underlying subcutaneous tissues as edema forms. (Courtesy of the University of Washington Burn Center at Harborview Medical Center, Seattle, WA.)

citation. Baseline laboratory studies should include blood glucose, blood urea nitrogen, creatinine, serum electrolytes, and hematocrit levels. Arterial blood gas and COHb levels should also be obtained, particularly if an inhalation injury is suspected. A chest x-ray study should be obtained for all clients with extensive burns or inhalation injury. Other laboratory tests as well as x-ray studies to rule out fractures or associated trauma need to be obtained on an as-needed basis. Depending on the circumstances of the injury, an alcohol and/or drug screen may be indicated. Continuous electrocardiographic monitoring should be initiated on all clients with major burn injuries, particularly those suffering from a high-voltage electric injury,[68] or with a history of cardiac ischemia or dysrhythmia.

Pain management is achieved through the administration of intravenous narcotic agents, typically morphine. The intramuscular or subcutaneous routes are not used because absorption from the soft tissues is unreliable during this period when hypovolemia and large fluid shifts are occurring. The oral route for pain medication administration is not used due to the likelihood of gastrointestinal dysfunction.

Tetanus prophylaxis for a client with a major burn is the same as for one with a minor burn (see earlier discussion).[82, 98]

Data collection is an important responsibility of the emergency room team. The client, individuals at the scene, and the emergency medical technicians should be questioned regarding the accident.[16] Useful information includes the time of injury, the level of consciousness at the scene, whether the injury occurred in an enclosed or open space, the presence of associated trauma, and the mechanism of injury. If the victim has suffered a chemical burn, knowledge of the offending agent, its concentration, duration of exposure, and whether irrigation was initiated at the scene is useful. For victims of electrical injuries, knowledge of the source, type of current, and the current voltage is useful in determining the extent of injury. Information concerning the client's past medical history as well as general health should be obtained. Specifically, information regarding any cardiac, pulmonary, endocrine, or renal disease should be obtained because it may have implications for treatment. Known allergies should also be identified as well as the client's current medication regime.

Wound care in the emergency department consists of covering the wound with a clean, dry sheet and blankets to maintain body heat. Clients with burns of the head and face should be positioned with their head elevated and all burned extremities elevated on pillows above the level of the heart. These measures help decrease dependent edema formation. For small burns, application of a cool, sterile compress aids in pain control. Unless transport time to the receiving medical facility is prolonged, no further treatment of the wound is generally necessary.

Consideration of transferral to a specialized burn care facility is appropriate for all clients with major burn injuries. Prompt contact with the receiving burn center is important to facilitate a smooth transfer.

THE ACUTE PHASE

The acute phase of recovery following a major burn begins when the patient is hemodynamically stable, capillary permeability is restored, and diuresis has begun. This is generally considered to be at 48 to 72 hours after the time of injury.[67] Many of the same principles of care outlined for the emergent phase apply to the acute phase; however, more emphasis is placed on restorative therapies. The acute phase continues until wound closure is achieved.

Medical management of the client during the acute phase focuses on

- Infection control,
- Wound care,
- Wound closure,
- Nutritional support,
- Pain management, and
- Physical therapy.

Infection Control. Sources of infection for the burn-injured client include autocontamination from (1) the oropharynx, (2) fecal flora, and (3) unburned skin and cross-contamination from (4) staff, (5) visitors, and (6) the air.[68] Specific infection control practices and isolation techniques exist for all burn centers.[49] These practices differ and include the use of gloves, caps, masks, shoe covers, scrub clothes, and plastic aprons. Strict handwashing is stressed to reduce the incidence of cross-contamination between clients. Staff and visitors are generally prevented from client contact if they suffer from any skin, gastrointestinal, or respiratory tract infections.

Wound Care. Care of the burn wound is ultimately aimed at promoting wound healing. Daily wound care involves cleansing, débridement, and dressing of the burn wound.[78]

Hydrotherapy. The wound is cleansed by the use of hydrotherapy.[77] This is accomplished by immersion (Fig. 71–6, *A* & *B*), showering, or spraying (Fig. 71–6*B*). A hydrotherapy session of 30 minutes or less is optimal for clients with acute burns.[78] Longer time periods may increase sodium loss (water is hypotonic) through the burn wound, heat loss, and pain and stress. During hydrotherapy, the wounds are gently washed using a variety of solutions: dilute sodium hypochlorite,[28, 42] dilute povidone-iodine,[18, 34, 38] and dilute chlorohexidine.[19, 85] Care should be taken to minimize bleeding and to maintain body temperature during this procedure. To prevent cross-contamination between clients, single-use, plastic hydrotherapy tub liners are available. Clients excluded from hydrotherapy are generally those who are hemodynamically unstable and those with new grafts.[18] If hydrotherapy is not used, wounds are washed and rinsed while in bed prior to the application of antimicrobial agents.

Débridement. Burn wound débridement involves the removal of the eschar. This serves to promote wound healing by preventing bacterial proliferation in and

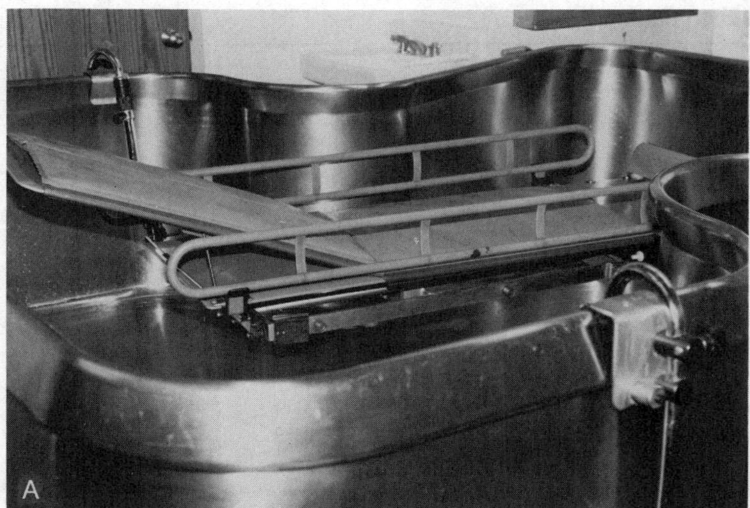

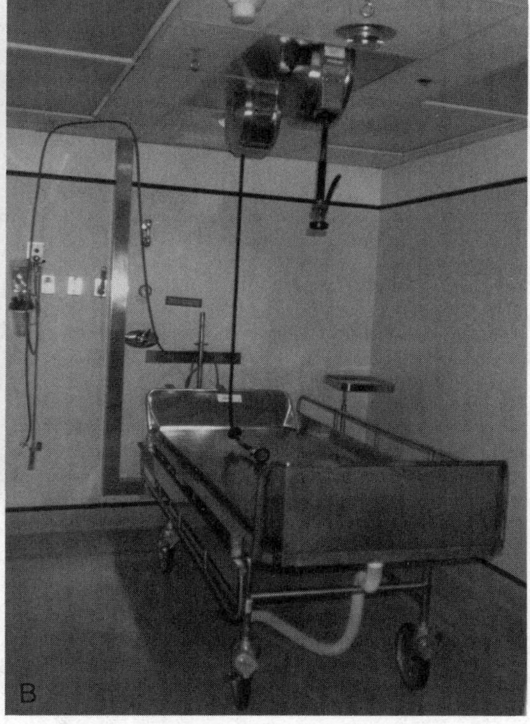

▲ *Figure 71–6*

A, Hubbard tank used for immersion hydrotherapy treatment of burn wounds. (Courtesy of the Burn Center at the Washington Hospital Center, Washington, DC.) *B*, Spray table used for hydrotherapy treatments of burn wounds. The long, flexible hose allows for ease in washing of the wounds. (Courtesy of the University of Washington Burn Center at Harborview Medical Center, Seattle, WA.)

under the eschar.[28] Débridement of the burn wound is accomplished through mechanical, enzymatic, or surgical means.

Mechanical Débridement. Mechanical débridement can be accomplished with the careful use of scissors and forceps to lift and trim away loose eschar. Dressing changes are another effective means of mechanical débridement. This is accomplished by the use of wet-to-dry and wet-to-wet dressings. Mechanical débridement of the burn wound can be extremely painful; therefore, effective pain management is paramount.

Enzymatic Débridement. Enzymatic débridement involves the application of commercially prepared proteolytic and fibrinolytic topical enzymes. These products selectively digest necrotic tissue, facilitating eschar removal. They require a moist environment to be effective and are applied directly to the burn wound. Pain and bleeding are major problems with this treatment and should be assessed continuously throughout treatment. Enzymatic débridement agents are contraindicated for wounds communicating with major body cavities, exposed nerves, or nervous tissue and in fungating neoplastic ulcers.[12]

Surgical Débridement. Surgical débridement of the burn wound involves excision of devitalized tissue. Two techniques are currently used: tangential excision and fascial excision.[32] In tangential excision, very thin layers of eschar are sequentially shaved until viable tissue is reached. Fascial excision involves removing the burn tissue and underlying fat down to fascia. This technique is frequently used for very deep burns.

Use of Specialized Wound Coverings. Deep partial- or full-thickness burn wounds are treated initially with topical antimicrobial agents. These agents are applied once or twice daily following cleansing, débridement, and inspection of the wound. The nurse assesses for eschar separation, the state of the granulation tissue or the presence of reepithelialization, and signs of infection.[27] The most commonly used topical antimicrobial agents are listed in Table 71–4. Although no one agent is universally used, many burn centers choose silver sulfadiazine cream as the initial topical treatment for burn wounds.

Open Versus Closed Methods. Burn wounds are treated using either an open or closed dressing technique. For the open method, the antimicrobial cream is applied and then left open to the air without gauze dressings. The agent is reapplied as needed, although formal reapplication occurs every 12 hours due to the agent's duration of activity. The advantages of this method include increased visualization of the wound, easier mobility and joint ROM, and simplicity in wound care. The disadvantages include an increased chance of hypothermia from exposure and the psychological difficulty for the client of continuously viewing the wound.[10]

In the closed method of wound care, gauze dressings of various types are used. Dressings are prepared by applying a 1/16 inch thick layer of cream prior to hydrotherapy (Fig. 71–7). When applied, the gauze is carefully wrapped from the distal portion of the extremity proximally, to ensure that circulation is not compromised. No two burn surfaces should be allowed to touch, because this could promote webbing of

TABLE 71–4. Topical Antimicrobial Agents Used in Burn Care

Agent	Antimicrobial Spectrum	Application	Side Effects	Nursing Considerations
Water-based creams				
1% Silver sulfadiazine	Broad spectrum, including some fungi and yeast	2 times daily, 1/16-inch thickness Gauze dressing not required	Transient leukopenia typically appearing after 2 or 3 days of treatment Macular rash	
Mafenide acetate	Broad spectrum, little antifungal activity	2 times daily, 1/16-inch thickness Gauze dressing not required	Hyperchloremic metabolic acidosis from bicarbonate diuresis due to the inhibition of carbonic anhydrase Pain/burning sensation on application to superficial burns Maculopapular rash	Assess for side effects. Assess adequacy of pain management. If pain and discomfort continue, consider other topical treatments Use cautiously in clients with acute renal failure.
Solutions				
5% Mafenide acetate	Broad spectrum	Gauze dressing required and moistened with solution for application to the wound	Pain on application Pruritus Skin rash Fungal colonization	Remains investigational and requires informed consent. Assess for side effects. Assess adequacy of pain management.
0.5% Silver nitrate	Broad spectrum, including *Candida* species	Multiple layers of gauze dressing required and moistened with solution for application to the wound	Hyponatremia Hypochloremia Hypokalemia Hypocalcemia	Check serum electrolytes daily. Penetrates eschar poorly. Rewet dressings every 2 hours to avoid wound desiccation. Protect the environment. Stains everything a blackish-brown color.

digits, contracture development, and poor cosmetic outcome. The advantages of the closed method technique are decreases in evaporative fluid and heat loss from the wound surface. In addition, gauze dressings may aid in debridement. The disadvantages of the use of gauze dressings are mobility limitations and a potential decrease in effective ROM exercises. Wound assessment is also limited to the times when dressing changes are performed.

Wound Closure

Temporary Wound Coverings. Temporary wound coverings are frequently used as a kind of wound "dressing." Table 71–5 outlines the most common biologic, biosynthetic, and synthetic wound coverings available today. These products are temporary wound coverings, each having specific indications. The character of the wound (depth of injury, amount of exudate, location of the wound on the body, and phase of recovery) and treatment goals are considered when choosing the most appropriate wound covering.

Autografting is the surgical removal of a thin layer of the client's own unburned skin (Fig. 71–8) and application of it to the excised burn wound. This procedure occurs in the operating room while the client receives anesthesia. Skin grafts can be applied in either a sheet (sheet graft) or meshed form (meshed graft) and are referred to as split-thickness skin grafts. A sheet graft is applied to the excised wound bed without alteration in its integrity. Sheet grafts are often used to graft facial burns. In contrast, a meshed graft contains many little slits, called interstices, that allow for expansion of the

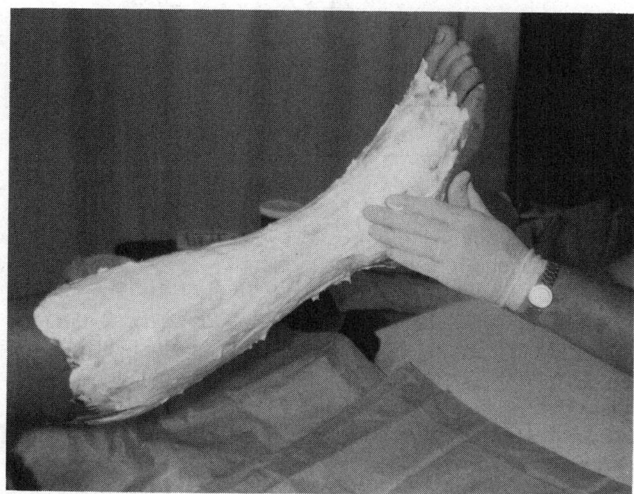

▲ Figure 71-7

Silver sulfadiazine, a common antimicrobial cream used in burn care, is applied to the burn wound using a sterile, gloved hand. (Courtesy of the University of Washington Burn Center at Harborview Medical Center, Seattle, WA.)

donor skin. Meshing permits coverage of larger areas or irregularly shaped wounds and allows for drainage from a bleeding wound bed. When healed, the meshed pattern of the skin graft remains visible. When a thicker layer of skin is removed, consisting of the epidermis and a portion of the dermis, this is considered a full-thickness skin graft. For all autografts, the area of the body where the skin was removed is referred to as the donor site.

In addition to routine postoperative nursing care, care of the client following autografting includes:

- Assessment of bleeding from the graft site
- Proper positioning and immobilization of the graft site
- Donor site care
- Care of specialized autografts (e.g., cultured epithelial autografts)

Assessment of Bleeding. Bleeding beneath an autograft may prevent successful adherence of the graft to the excised wound and ultimately result in some degree of graft loss, particularly beneath sheet grafts.

Small amounts of blood or serum beneath sheet grafts can be removed by gently rolling (use sterile cotton swab) the fluid from the center of the graft to the periphery where it can be absorbed with a sterile gauze pad. For large accumulations, aspiration of the blood/serum using a small-gauge needle and syringe has been found to be effective.

Positioning and Immobilization. Autografts are immobilized following surgery, generally 3 to 7 days. This period of immobilization allows the autograft time to adhere and attach to the wound bed. Immobilization can be accomplished in a variety of ways. Proper positioning, splinting, traction, and limb restraints have been used to prevent unwanted movement and shearing of grafts. The nurse also implements various actions to reduce the hazards of immobility.

Donor Site Care. Various types of dressings are used to cover donor sites, depending on the size, location, and condition of adjacent skin or tissue. Nursing care depends on the type of dressing used. For example, a fine-mesh gauze dressing is allowed to dry, often assisted by radiant heat lamps. Once new epithelium forms beneath it, the gauze can be gently lifted and trimmed away. Removal of the gauze prior to this time will reinjure the donor site. Donor sites treated with synthetic, semipermeable polyurethane films are often dressed with a compression bandage. This dressing, applied in the operating room, is left in place for several days to promote adherence of the polyurethane film to the donor site and reduce fluid accumulation. When the compression dressing is removed, the polyurethane film is left intact until new epithelium forms beneath it. Donor sites dressed with a specialized nylon fabric are often stapled, sutured, or taped in place. A compression dressing is applied in the operating room and left in place for at least 48 hours after surgery. At this time, the compression dressing can be removed and the donor site left open to the air. Staples and sutures should be removed by the third to fifth day after surgery. The nylon fabric remains adhered to the donor site and is peeled away once reepithelialization occurs beneath it (typically 10 to 14 days).

Despite the differences in nursing care, the donor site wound requires the same meticulous care as other partial-thickness wounds in order for healing to occur and infection to be prevented. If the donor site becomes infected, the dressing should be gently removed or soaked off. The wound can then be thoroughly cleaned and an antimicrobial agent applied. Once the donor site has healed, lubricating lotions can be applied to soften the area and reduce itching. Donor sites can be reused once complete healing has occurred.

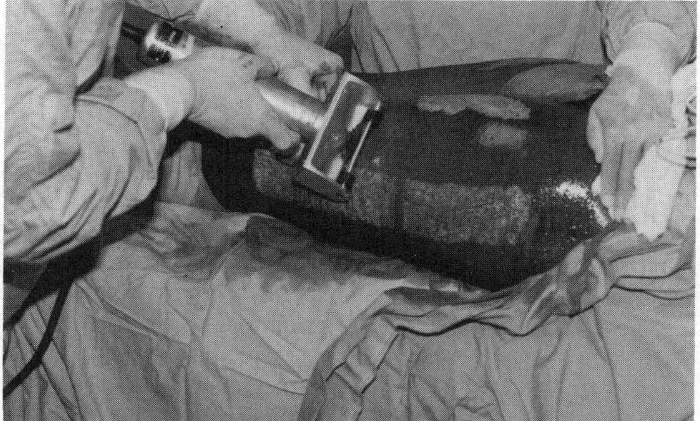

▲ Figure 71-8

The harvesting of donor skin from the anterior-lateral portion of the client's thigh. (Courtesy of the Burn Center at the Washington Hospital Center, Washington, DC.)

TABLE 71-5. Temporary Wound Coverings Used in Burn Care

Category/Examples	Description	Indications	Nursing Considerations
Biologic			
Amnion	Amniotic membranes collected from human placentas	To protect partial-thickness burns To protect granulation tissue prior to autograft application	Cover dressing is changed every 48 hours with amnion.
Allograft homograft	Donated human cadaver skin harvested within 24 hours after death	To debride exudative wounds To cover excised wounds and test for receptivity prior to autograft application To cover and protect meshed autografts	Observe for wound exudate and signs of infection that may be indicative of a wound infection beneath the allograft/xenograft.
Xenograft heterograft	Porcine skin is harvested after slaughter, then cryopreserved or lyophilized for storage	To promote healing of clean, superficial partial-thickness wounds	Xenograft over granulation tissue is changed every 2-5 days. For superficial wounds, ensure that the wound is clean and well rinsed. Apply xenograft with slight overlapping of edges to allow for shrinkage. Trim away xenograft when skin beneath it has healed.
Biosynthetic Biobrane (Winthrop Pharmaceuticals, New York City)	Nylon fabric bonded to a silicone rubber membrane containing collagenous porcine peptides	Donor site dressing Protective cover over meshed autografts To promote healing of clean superficial partial-thickness wounds	Secure to the surrounding intact skin by staples, skin closure strips, tape, or sutures and then wrap with a gauze dressing. This outer dressing can be removed by 48 hours to check for adherence of the Biobrane. Once adherence has occurred, the tape, sutures, and staples can be removed. The Biobrane can then be left exposed to the air. New and healing donor sites of the legs require support during ambulation. The figure 8 Ace wrapping technique is recommended to minimize trauma to newly formed capillaries. Assess for infection beneath the fabric and at wound periphery.
Integra (Marion-Merrell Dow, Inc., Kansas City, KS)	Bilaminate substitute composed of collagen (dermal analog) and a Silastic covering (epidermal analog) The dermal analog is allowed to incorporate into the wound, becoming permanent.	For application to excised wounds	The silastic portion is removed after several days, providing a wound bed for placement of a very thin split-thickness skin graft. Assess for infection. Protect the grafted site from mechanical shearing forces.

Nutritional Support. Maintenance of adequate nutrition during the acute phase is essential in promoting wound healing and in preventing infection. Basal metabolic rates may be 40 to 100 per cent higher than normal levels, depending on the extent of the burn.[37] This response is thought to be the result of a reset in the hypothalamic-adrenal axis, leading to an increase in heat production.[14] Metabolic rates decrease as wound coverage is achieved. In addition, glucose metabolism is altered following a burn injury, resulting in hyperglycemia. Low levels of insulin during the emergent phase, inhibition of insulin activity by increased levels of circulating catecholamines, and increased gluconeogenesis during the acute phase have all been implicated in causing hyperglycemia in the burn client.

Aggressive nutritional support is required to meet the increased energy requirements necessary to promote healing and prevent the untoward effects of catabolism.

Formulas are used to estimate energy requirements by factoring several different indices: weight, sex, age, extent of burn, and activity or injury.

$$(25 \text{ kcal} \times \text{body weight (kg)}) + (40 \text{ kcal} \times \% \text{ TBSA burn}) = \text{kcal/day}$$

Aggressive nutritional support is generally indicated for the burn client with any one of the following: 30 per cent or greater TBSA burn, a clinical course requiring multiple operations, the need for mechanical ventilatory support, a compromised mental status, and a poor preburn nutritional state.[17]

Methods for delivering nutritional support include oral diet, enteral tube feedings, peripheral parenteral nutrition, total parenteral nutrition, and a combination of these modalities. The preferred route is by oral or enteral feedings; however, the decision of how to best meet the nutritional needs should be individualized for all clients. Typically, parenteral nutrition is reserved for clients with a prolonged ileus or clients who fail to meet their nutritional needs by the enteral route.

Pain Management. Physiologic factors that have an impact on pain include the depth of injury, extent, and stage of wound healing. Typically, partial-thickness burns and newly harvested donor sites are exquisitely painful due to stimulation of exposed nerve endings. In contrast, full-thickness burns are insensate because the superficial nerve endings have been destroyed. However, nerve endings located at the wound's periphery can be extremely sensitive. Psychological factors that influence the perception of pain include anxiety, fear, and the client's ability to cope. Social factors include past experiences with pain, personality, family background, circumstances surrounding the injury, and separation from family and home. It is important to remember that the perception of pain and response to painful stimuli are individual and that the treatment plan should be individualized as well.

The most common approach to pain control is the use of pharmocologic agents.[43] Morphine, codeine, and meperidine are the most commonly used narcotic analgesics to control the pain associated with burn injuries and treatment.[66] Other pharmocologic modalities used include patient-controlled analgesia, inhalation analgesics such as nitrous oxide, pain cocktails, and narcotic agonist-antagonist agents.[58] Nonsteroidal anti-inflammatory agents are also prescribed for the treatment of mild to moderate pain.[43]

Nonpharmocologic modalities used to treat burn-related pain include hypnosis, guided imagery, art and play therapy, relaxation technique, distraction, biofeedback, and music therapy.[43, 58] These modalities have been found to be effective in decreasing anxiety and thereby decreasing the perception of pain[51] and are often used as adjuncts to the pharmocologic treatment of burn pain.

Physical Therapy. Maintenance of optimal physical functioning in the client with a burn injury is a challenge for the entire burn team. Nurses work closely with occupational and physical therapists to identify the rehabilitative needs of burn clients. An individualized program of splinting, positioning, exercise, ambulation, activities of daily living, and pressure therapy should be implemented early in the acute phase of recovery to maximize functional recovery and cosmetic outcome.

Wound contracture and hypertrophic scarring are two major problems for the burn client.[83] Wound contractures are typically more severe with extensive burns. Areas seemingly predisposed to contracture are the hands, head, neck, and axilla.[46]

Measures used to prevent and treat wound contractures include therapeutic positioning, ROM exercises, splinting, and client/family education.[39, 83]

Therapeutic Positioning. Table 71–6 lists corrective and therapeutic techniques for positioning clients with specific areas of burn injury during periods of inactivity or immobilization. Allowing the burn client to assume a position of comfort most often contributes to contracture formation. Therefore, proper positioning should be maintained for the burn client while both in and out of bed. These techniques position the affected area opposite to the anticipated contracture or deformity. (Fig. 71–9).

Exercise. Active ROM exercises are prescribed early in the acute phase of recovery to reduce edema and maintain strength and joint function. In addition, activities of daily living can be effective in maintaining function and ROM. Ambulation also maintains strength and ROM of the lower extremities and should be initiated as soon as the client is physiologically stable. Passive ROM and stretching exercises should be included as part of the daily treatment plan if the client is unable to perform active ROM exercises.[83]

Splinting. Splints are used to maintain proper joint positioning and prevent or correct contractures. Two types of splints are frequently used: static and dynamic. A static splint immobilizes the joint. Static splints do not replace exercise and are frequently applied for periods of immobilization, during sleeping hours, and in the uncooperative client who cannot maintain proper

TABLE 71-6. Therapeutic Positioning for the Burn-Injured Client

Burned Area	Therapeutic Position	Positioning Techniques
Neck		
Anterior	Extension	No pillow Small towel roll beneath cervical spine to promote neck extension
Circumferential	Neutral toward extension	No pillow
Posterior or Assymetrical	Neutral	No pillow
Shoulder/axilla	Arm abduction to 90–110°	Splinting Arms positioned away from the body and supported on arm troughs
Elbow	Arm extension	Elbow splint Elbows positioned in extension with slight bend at the elbow (no greater than 10° elbow flexion) Arms supported on arm troughs with the forearm in slight pronation
Hand		
Wrist	Wrist extension	Hand splint
Metacarpal Interphalangeal Joints (MCP)	MCP flexion at 90°	Hand splint
Proximal and distal interphalangeal joints (PIP/DIP)	PIP/DIP extension	Hand splint
Thumb	Thumb abduction	Hand splint with thumb abduction
Web spaces	Finger abduction	Web spacers of gauze, foam, or thermoplastics to decrease webbing formation
Hip	Hip extension	Supine with the head of bed flat and legs extended Trochanter roll to maintain neutral hip rotation (toes should be pointing toward the ceiling) Prone positioning
Knee	Knee extension	Supine with knees extended (toes should be pointing toward the ceiling) Prone positioning with feet extended over the end of the mattress Sitting in chair with legs extended and elevated Knee splint
Ankle	Neutral	Padded footboard Ankle positioning devices (avoid ankle inversion and eversion positions)

positioning.[83] In contrast, dynamic splints exercise the affected joint. Care must be taken to ensure that all splints fit properly and do not apply pressure that could lead to further tissue or nerve damage.

Education. Client and family education regarding correct positioning and the need for continued exercise is very important. Written guides and handouts on positioning, splinting, and exercise routines can facilitate learning and cooperation.[39]

Control of Scarring. Hypertrophic scarring results from an overabundant deposition of collagen in the healed burn wound. The severity of hypertrophic scarring depends on several factors: burn depth, race, age, and type of autograft.[42] The nonoperative method for minimizing hypertrophic scarring is pressure therapy (Fig. 71-10).[83]

Several products are commercially available that provide continuous pressure over the healing burn wound. During the early stages of wound healing, elastic wraps and bandages can be used to apply continuous pressure to the healing skin while it is still fragile and vulnerable to mechanical shearing. Ultimately, custom-fit antiburn scar support garments can be ordered and worn 23 hours a day until the burn scar tissue has matured (typically 18 months to 2 years post-burn).

Surgical options for the treatment of wound contractures and hypertrophic scarring include (1) split-thickness and full-thickness skin grafts, (2) skin flaps, (3) Z-plasties, and (4) tissue expansion. These surgical options are discussed in Chapter 72.

THE REHABILITATION PHASE

The rehabilitation phase of recovery represents the final phase of burn care (see Bridge to Home Health Care). Although this phase overlaps the acute care phase and lasts well beyond the acute inpatient hospitalization, the goals and principles of physical rehabilitation are similar to those previously described. Ultimately, a burn rehabilitation program is designed for the client to gain independence through achievement of maximal functional recovery. Measures to promote wound healing,

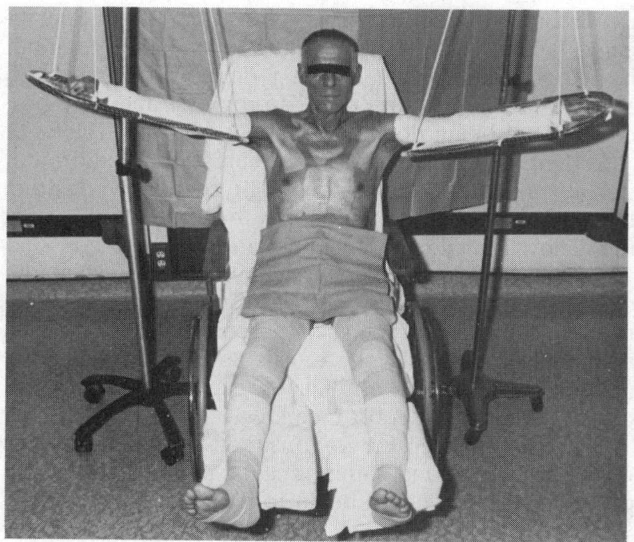

▲ Figure 71–9

Example of therapeutic positioning for a client with extremity burns. Note that the client's arms are abducted and his legs are wrapped with Ace wrap bandages in a figure 8 pattern to reduce dependent edema formation and provide pressure therapy support.

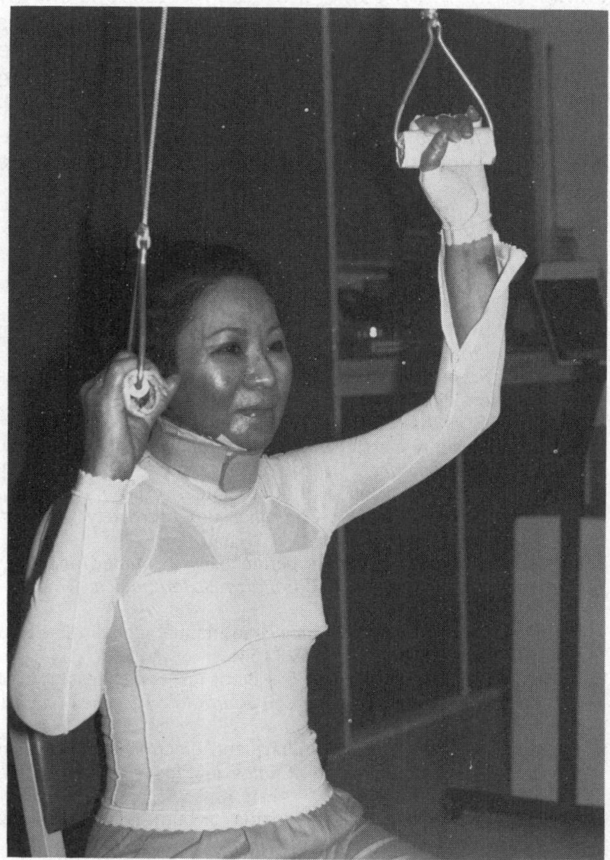

▲ Figure 71–10

Client wearing custom-fit antiscar support garment. When worn 23 hours a day, this garment is effective in providing pressure therapy over healing burn wounds. Pressure therapy helps to minimize the development of hypertrophic scarring.

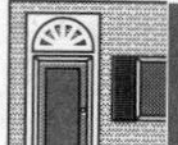

BRIDGE TO HOME HEALTH CARE

Rehabilitation of the Burn Client

As adults recover at home from the trauma of a burn, they face two specific challenges. The first is physical healing; the second is the emotional trauma. Clients with extensive burns may require many months or years of complex, expensive reconstructive surgery. Members of the home health care team must be sensitive to the physical, emotional, and sexual needs of the client and the client's family. It is the responsibility of the home health care nurse to ask questions and encourage the client and family to formulate theirs. Does the home need to be modified before the client is dismissed from the hospital? Is special equipment needed? What changes can be expected in the next month? The next year? Will future surgery be scheduled? What benefits and difficulties can be expected as a result of surgery? What preparation will the client and family need?

The client who has been severely burned often requires physical therapy at home or on an outpatient basis. A high-calorie, high-protein diet may be prescribed to facilitate healing. Skin care is another concern. The client with burns requires a supply of lotion or oil to apply to the new skin and scabbed areas. While healing, these areas feel tight and dry, which can lead to itching and pain. Eucerine cream, Nivea oil (not cream), Keri lotion, or any lanolin-rich lotion may be applied and covered with a dressing of loose gauze or loose cotton underclothing. This covering protects and absorbs some of the excess oil and at the same time prevents excess drying. This oil should not replace antibiotic creams but can be used in addition on the surrounding healed areas.

The client with severe burns experiences emotional trauma. The client's independence, lifestyle, education, career, and future goals are disrupted or permanently changed. Memories about the accident/injury, nightmares, a sense of loss, and self-esteem problems are not resolved at the time of hospital discharge. Instead, new challenges face clients as they leave the security and acceptance of the hospital environment. Burns can produce very visible and disfiguring effects. Clients and their families require anticipatory guidance and encouragement as they cope with curious glances, stares, and questions. Role playing may be an effective technique to use with clients and their families. The home health care nurse can help families anticipate and discuss such emotions as frustration, anger, and depression and develop strategies to resolve them in constructive ways.

prevent or minimize deformities and hypertrophic scarring, increase strength and function, and provide emotional support and education are part of the ongoing rehabilitation process.[83]

Special Considerations

PSYCHOSOCIAL CONSIDERATIONS

Psychological rehabilitation is equally as important as physical in the overall recovery process. A myriad of psychological and emotional responses to burn injuries have been identified, ranging from fear to psychosis.[27] A victim's response is influenced by age, personality, cultural and ethnic background, extent and location of injury, and the resulting impact on body image. In addition, separation from family and friends and the change in the client's normal role and responsibilities affect the reaction to burn trauma.

Nursing care should focus on maximizing the client's psychosocial recovery through appropriate interventions (see care plan and Ethical Issues in Nursing).

Four stages of psychosocial responses following burn trauma have been characterized by Lee: (1) impact, (2) retreat or withdrawal, (3) acknowledgment, and (4) the reconstructive period.[48]

The period of impact occurs immediately post-injury and is characterized by shock, disbelief, and feelings of being overwhelmed. The client and family may be aware of what is happening but may be coping with the situation poorly. Studies indicate that the families of critically ill patients have a need for assurance, proximity to their ill family member, and information. Specifically, families want to know how their family member is being treated, what is being done for him or her, specific facts about the client's progress, and why procedures are being done.[52]

Retreat is characterized by repression, withdrawal, denial, and suppression. Although seemingly destructive, these coping strategies may be protective in that they allow the client to maintain an intact psyche.

The third phase, acknowledgment, begins when the client accepts the injury and resultant change in body image. Mourning of actual or perceived losses may be apparent. During this phase, clients may benefit from meeting with other burn-injured clients in one-to-one contact or group support meetings.

The final phase, the reconstructive period, begins when the client and family accept the limitations imposed by the injury and begin to plan for the future.

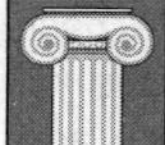

ETHICAL ISSUES IN NURSING

Should Severely Burned Clients Be Allowed to Refuse Treatment?

People who have sustained severe burns are perhaps the most fragile of all clients. The road to recovery is a long and hard process, and full recovery may never occur. In the most severe cases, the treatments for these clients may take months and induce intense pain. Even though months of whirlpool and débridement treatments may be required with the client put through severe pain with each treatment, death may be the end result. Even if death does not occur, return to a "normal" life may never happen.

Should the severely burned client be allowed to die without any medical intervention save pain management? Should there be a set of criteria that a client must meet to determine what treatment options are offered to him or her? These criteria, of course, would be based on the client's best interests, respect for the client's dignity as a person, and the availability of resources. Should clients be allowed to refuse treatments, even if their chance of survival is good, simply because they believe the potential quality of their life will be too low?

Currently there are national statistics based on age, depth of the burns, degree of inhalation damage, and the like that assist care givers in the burn unit in calculating the potential survival rate of a given burn client. The survival rate does assist in the recommended treatment options, but clients may still choose death over treatment. When in such a physical and mental state, are clients competent to make such a final decision regarding their own survival? There are, undoubtedly, many challenges facing both clients and care givers in the burn unit setting. Each case should be individually evaluated, and care givers should always be sensitive to the client and the client's family members. There are many uncomfortable ethical questions regarding the care of burn clients and the answers are no less comfortable, if the questions are answered at all.

Summary

Nursing care of the burn-injured client is both complex and challenging. The psychological and physical trauma sustained following a burn injury can be devastating for both victim and the family or significant other. As a key member of the burn team, the nurse is responsible for an individualized plan of care that reflects the client's total condition as he or she progresses through the different phases of recovery. Priority issues and care will change as the client moves from the critical emergent phase onto and ultimately through the rehabilitative period. Therein lies the challenge to the burn care nurse.

Bibliography

1. Achauer, B. M., & McGuire, A. (1989). Fire safe cigarettes—an update. *Journal of Burn Care & Rehabilitation 10*(2), 173–174.
2. Agee, R. N., et al. (1976). Use of 133-xenon in early diagnosis of inhalation injury. *Journal of Trauma, 16*(3), 218–224.
3. American Burn Association. (1984). Guidelines for service standards and severity classification in the treatment of burn injury. *Bulletin of the American College of Surgeons, 69*(10), 24–28.
4. American National Standards Committee. (1981). *Standard Z21.10.1.* Washington, DC: Consumer Product Safety Commission.
5. Arturson, G. (1961). Capillary permeability in burned and nonburned areas in dogs. *Acta Chirurgica Scandinavica, 274,* 55–135.
6. Arturson, G., et al. (1969). Changes in immunoglobulin levels in severely burned patients. *Lancet, 1,*546.
7. Ayoub, C., & Pfeifer, D. (1979). Burns as a manifestation of child abuse and neglect. *American Journal of Diseases of Children, 133*(9), 910–914.
8. Baxter, C. R. (1974). Fluid volume and electrolyte changes in the early post-burned period. *Clinics in Plastic Surgery, 1*(4), 693–709.
9. Bayley, E. W., et al. (1990). Standards for burn nursing practice. *Journal of Burn Care & Rehabilitation 10*(4), 362–374.
10. Bayley, E. W. (1990). Wound healing in the patient with burns. *Nursing Clinics of North America, 25*(1), 205–222.
11. Berry, C. C., et al. (1982). Differences in burn size estimates between community hospitals and a burn center. *Journal of Burn Care & Rehabilitation 3*(3), 176–177.
12. Boots Pharmaceuticals, Inc. (1991). *Travase ointment—*

indications and usage (Product Monograph). Lincolnshire, Ill: Author.
13. Brodzka W., et al. (1985). Burns: Causes and risk factors. *Archives of Physical Medicine and Rehabilitation, 66*(11), 746-752.
14. Burdge, J. J., et al. (1986). Nutritional and metabolic consequences of thermal injury. *Clinics in Plastic Surgery, 13*(1), 49-55.
15. Burdge, J. J., et al. (1988). Surgical treatment of burns in elderly patients. *Journal of Trauma, 28*(2), 214-217.
16. Burgess, M. (1991). Initial management of a patient with extensive burn injury. *Critical Care Nursing Clinics of North America, 3*(2), 165-179.
17. Carlson, D. E., & Jordan, B. S. (1991). Implementing nutritional therapy in the thermally injured patient. *Critical Care Nursing Clinics of North America, 3*(2), 221-235.
18. Carrougher, G., & Marvin, J. (1989). Mechanical debridement: Views from University of Washington Burn Center at Harborview, Seattle, Washington [Editorial]. *Journal of Burn Care & Rehabilitation, 10*(3), 271-272.
19. Cioffi, W. G., & Rue, L. W. (1991). Diagnosis and treatment of inhalation injuries. *Critical Care Nursing Clinics of North America, 3*(2), 191-198.
20. Curreri, P. W. (1979). Chemical burns. In C. P. Artz, et al. (Eds.), *Burns: A team approach*, (pp. 363-369). Philadelphia: W. B. Saunders Company.
21. Demling, R. H. (1987). Fluid replacement in burned patients. *Surgical Clinics of North America, 67*(1), 15-30.
22. Demling, R. H., et al. (1984). Role of thermal injury-induced hypoproteinemia on edema formation in burned and nonburned tissue. *Surgery, 95*(2), 136-144.
23. Dyer, C., & Roberts, D. (1990). Thermal trauma. *Nursing Clinics of North America, 25*(1), 85-117.
24. Feldman, K. W., et al. (1978). Tap water scald burns in children. *Pediatrics, 62*(1), 1-7.
25. Feller, I., et al. (1982). Burn epidemiology: Focus on youngsters and the aged. *Journal of Burn Care & Rehabilitation, 3*(5), 285-288, 336.
26. Feller, I., et al. (1980). Improvements in burn care, 1965 to 1979. *Journal of the American Medical Association, 244*(18), 2074-2078.
27. Freeman, J. W. (1984). Nursing care of the patient with a burn injury. *Critical Care Nurse, 4*(6), 52-68.
28. Gordon, M. K. (1987). Burn wound care: Silver sulfadiazine application. [editorial]. *Journal of Burn Care & Rehabilitation, 8*(5), 429.
29. Hall, J. R., Jr. (1985). A decade of detectors: Measuring the effect. *Fire Journal, 79*, 37-43.
30. Hammond, J., & Ward, C. G. (1987). Transfers from emergency room to burn center: Errors in burn size estimate. *Journal of Trauma, 27*(10), 1161-1165.
31. Heideman, M., et al. (1978). Complement activation and hematologic hemodynamic and respiratory reactions early after soft tissue injury. *Journal of Trauma, 18*(10), 696-700.
32. Heimbach, D. M. (1987). Early excision and grafting. *Surgical Clinics of North America, 67*(1), 93-107.
33. Heimbach, D. M. (1983). Smoke inhalation: Current concepts (pp. 31-38). In T. L. Wachtel, et al. (Eds.), *Current topics in burn care*. Rockville, MD: Aspen Publications.
34. Helvig, B., & Curry, V. (1989). Mechanical debridement: Views from Shriners Hospitals for Crippled Children, Burn Unit, Galveston, Texas [Editorial]. *Journal of Burn Care & Rehabilitation, 10*(3), 272-273.
35. Herndon, D. N., et al. (1988). Inhalation injury in burned patients: effects and treatment. *Burns, 14*(5), 349-356.
36. Hunt, J. L., et al. (1976). The pathophysiology of acute electric injuries. *Journal of Trauma, 16*(5);355-340.
37. Ireton, C. S., et al. (1986). Evaluation of energy expenditures in burn patients. *Journal of the American Dietetic Association, 86*(3), 331-333.
38. Jarvis, R., & Weireter, L. J. (1989). Mechanical debridement: Views from Sentara Norfolk General Hospital, Norfolk, Virginia [Editorial]. *Journal of Burn Care & Rehabilitation 10*(3), 273.
39. Johnson, C. L., & Cain, V. J. (1985). The rehab guide. *American Journal of Nursing, 85*(1), 48-50.
40. Jones, C. A., et al. (1979). Nursing care of the burned child. In W. C. Bailey (Ed.), *Pediatric burns*. Chicago: Year Book Medical Publishers.
41. Jones, J. D., et al. (1989). Alcohol use and burn injury. *Journal of Burn Care & Rehabilitation, 12*(2), 148-152.
42. Ketchum, L. D., et al. (1974). Hypertrophic scars and keloids. *Plastic and Reconstructive Surgery, 53*(2), 140-154.
43. Kibbee, E. (1984). Burn pain management. *Critical Care Quarterly, 7*(3), 54-62.
44. Knaysi, G. A., et al. (1968). The rule of nines: Its history and accuracy. *Plastic and Reconstructive Surgery, 41*(6), 560-563.
45. Kohn, J., & Cort, D. F. (1969). Immunoglobulins in burned patients. *Lancet, 1*, 836.
46. Kraemer, M. D., et al. (1988). Burn contractures: incidence, predisposing factors, and results of surgical therapy. *Journal of Burn Care & Rehabilitation, 9*(3), 261-265.
47. Kravitz, M., et al. (1985). Thermal injury in the elderly: Incidence and cause. *Journal of Burn Care & Rehabilitation, 6*(6), 487-489.
48. Lee, J., (1970). Emotional reactions to trauma. *Nursing Clinics of North America, 5*(4), 577-587.
49. Lee, J. L., et al. (1985). Survey of isolation techniques [Abstract]. *Proceedings of the American Burn Association, 17*, 82.
50. Lenoski, E. F., & Hunter, K. A. (1977). Specific patterns of inflicted burn injuries. *Journal of Trauma, 17*(11), 842-846.
51. Leonard, L. G., et al. (1982). Chemical burns: Effect of prompt first aid. *Journal of Trauma, 22*(5), 420-423.
52. Leske, J. S. (1991). Overview of family needs after critical illness: From assessment to intervention. *AACN Clinical Issues in Critical Care Nursing, 2*(2), 220-226.
53. Linn, B. S. (1980). Age differences in the severity and outcome of burns. *Journal of the American Geriatrics Society, 28*(3), 118-123.
54. Lund, C. C., & Browder, N. C. (1944). The estimation of areas of burn. *Surgery, Gynecology and Obstetrics 79*(4), 352-358.
55. McLoughlin, E., & McGuire, A. (1990). The causes, cost, and prevention of childhood burn injuries. *American Journal of Diseases of Children, 144*(6), 677-683.
56. Maley, M. P. (1987). Children should be seen—not hurt. *Journal of Burn Care & Rehabilitation, 8*(2), 135-136.
57. Maley, M. P. (1989). Scald burns associated with tap water. *Journal of Burn Care & Rehabilitation, 10*(2), 172-173.
58. Marvin, J. (1987). Pain management in the burn patient: Excerpts from a symposium on pain management at Harborview Hospital, Seattle, Washington, July 23, 1986. *Journal of Burn Care & Rehabilitation, 8*(4), 307-318.
59. Monafo, W. W., Jr. (1971). The treatment of burns: Principles and practices. St. Louis, MO: Warren H. Green.
60. Moncrief, J. A. (1979). Replacement therapy. In C. P. Artz, et al. (Eds.), *Burns: A team approach* (pp. 169-192). Philadelphia: W. B. Saunders Company.
61. Moncrief, J. A. (1979). The Body's Response to Heat. In C. P. Artz, et al. (Eds.), *Burns: A team approach* (pp. 23-44). Philadelphia: W. B. Saunders Company.
62. Moritz, A. R., et al. (1945). The effects of inhaled heat on the air passages and lung: An experimental investigation. *American Journal of Pathology, 21*(2), 311-332.
63. Moylan, J. A., & Chan, C. (1978). Inhalation injury—an increasing problem. *Annals of Surgery, 188*(1), 34-37.
64. Munster, A. M., et al. (1970). The effect of thermal injury on serum immunoglobulins. *Annals of Surgery, 172*(6), 965-969.
65. Nebraska Burn Institute. (1990). Advanced burn life support manual. Lincoln, NE: Author.
66. Perry, S. (1982). Management of pain during debridement: A survey of US. burn units. *Pain, 13*, 267-280.
67. Philbin, P., & Marvin, J. A. (1982). Management of the pediatric patient with a major burn. *Journal of Burn Care & Rehabilitation, 3*(2), 118-125.
68. Pruitt, B. A., Jr., & Goodwin, C. W., Jr. (1990). Burn injury. In E. E. Moore, et al. (Eds.), *Early care of the injured patient*, (pp. 286-306). Philadelphia: Dekker.
69. Purdue, G. F., et al. (1990). Obesity: A risk factor in the burn patient. *Journal of Burn Care & Rehabilitation, 11*(1), 32-34.
70. Robson, M. C., & Kucan, J. O. (1983). The burn wound. In T. L.

Wachtel, et al. (Eds.), *Current topics in burn care.* (pp. 55-63). Rockville, MD: Aspen Publications.

71. Rossignol, A. M., et al. (1985). Consumer products and hospitalized burn injuries among elderly Massachusetts residents. *Journal of the American Geriatrics Society, 33*(11), 768-772.
72. Rue, L. W., & Cioffi, W. G., Jr. (1991). Resuscitation of thermally injured patients. *Critical Care Nursing Clinics of North America, 3*(2), 181-189.
73. Sadowski, D. A. (1987). Burn wound care: silver sulfadiazine application: Feature protocol from Shriners Burns Institute, Cincinnati. *Journal of Burn Care & Rehabilitation* 8(5), 429-431.
74. Silverstein, P., & Lack, B. (1987). Fire prevention in the United States—are the home fires still burning? Surgical Clinics of North America 67(1), 1-14.
75. Slater, H., & Gaisford, J. C. (1981). Burns in the older patient. J Am Geriatri 29(2), 74-76.
76. Stratta, R. J., et al. (1983). The management of tar and asphalt injuries. *American Journal of Surgery* 146(6); 766.
77. F. A. Davis Company. (1989). *Taber's cyclopedic medical dictionary* (16th ed.). Philadelphia: Author.
78. Thomson, P. D., et al. (1990). A survey of burn hydrotherapy in the United States. *Journal of Burn Care & Rehabilitation, 11*(2), 151-155.
79. Trunkey, D. D. (1983). Transporting the critically burned patient. In T. L. Wachtel, et al. (Eds.), *Current topics in burn care.* (pp. 11-14). Rockville, MD: Aspen Publications.
80. Turner, D. G., et al. (1989). Cooking-related burn injuries in the elderly: Preventing the "granny gown" burn. *Journal of Burn Care & Rehabilitation, 10*(4), 356-359.
81. Van Rijin, O. J. L., et al. (1989). The etiology of burns in developed countries: review of the literature. *Burns, 15*(4), 217-221.
82. Wachtel, T. L., et al. (1983). Initial management of major burns. In T. L. Wachtel, et al. (Eds.): *Current topics in burn care.* (pp. 25-30) Rockville, MD: Aspen Publications.
83. Wachtel, T. L., & Fortune, J. B. (1983). Fluid resuscitation for burn shock. In T. L. Wachtel, et al. (Eds.), *Current topics in burn care.* (pp. 41-53). Rockville, MD: Aspen Publications.
84. Ward, R. S. (1991). The rehabilitation of burn patients. *Critical Reviews in Physical and Rehabilitation Medicine, 2*(3), 121-138.
85. Warden, G. D. (1987). Outpatient care of thermal injuries. *Surgical Clinics of North America, 67*(1), 147-157.
86. Williamson, J. (1989). Actual burn nutrition care practices—a national survey (part II). *Journal of Burn Care & Rehabilitation, 10*(2), 185-194.
87. Wolfort, K. D., et al. (1970). Surgical management of cutaneous lye burns. *Surgery, Gynecology and Obstetrics, 131,* 873-876.

Chapter 72

Nursing Care of Clients Having Plastic Surgery

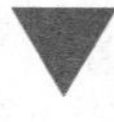

PLASTIC SURGERY

Definition

Plastic surgery is the surgical subspecialty concentrating on the restoration of function and form to body structures damaged by trauma, the aging process, disease processes such as skin cancer, and congenital defects. Plastic surgeons repair defects in skin and underlying tissue, sometimes including the skeletal framework. Plastic surgeons and nurses approach the plastic surgery client as a whole being. They intervene as a team to help the client deal with the psychosocial impact of deformity on body image as well as the physical aspects of surgery.

AESTHETIC AND RECONSTRUCTIVE SURGERY

Plastic surgery can be divided into two major areas: (1) aesthetic (cosmetic) surgery and (2) reconstructive surgery.

Aesthetic plastic surgery alters the appearance of any physical feature that is already within "normal" range. Thus, it is elective and typically not covered by insurance. People seek aesthetic plastic surgery for many reasons, e.g., to look younger, maintain a job, or improve self-image. People often have high expectations of aesthetic plastic surgery and may be dissatisfied with anything but "perfect" results (see Ethical Issues in Nursing).

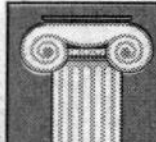

ETHICAL ISSUES IN NURSING

Should a Psychological Profile of the Client Be Required Before Cosmetic Surgery Is Performed?

Plastic surgery procedures may be performed for various reasons, including cosmetics, reconstruction, traumatic repair, hand surgery, scar revision, and skin grafting. When most people think of plastic surgery, they think of procedures such as "face lifts," "nose jobs," and breast implants—in other words, procedures that are done for purely cosmetic purposes. Although there is a market for purely cosmetic procedures, a large percentage of plastic surgeries are reconstructive in nature.

Should people who wish to have plastic surgery for reasons that are not medically indicated be required to undergo a psychological profile prior to surgery? Should plastic surgeons have set psychological criteria that a client must meet to qualify for a cosmetic procedure? The purpose of such psychological assessments would be to help the person truly understand why he or she desires a cosmetic procedure. Some clients who have a desire to improve their physical person may not be satisfied with the results of a certain surgery and seek out additional cosmetic procedures, never being totally satisfied with the end products. This desire for physical perfection that is never really satisfied could stem from deeper psychological feelings. Because some clients are not dealing with such psychological barriers, they will never really be happy with the physical changes that cosmetic surgery provides.

Psychological profiles may assist those who work in plastic surgery to better understand the needs of those clients seeking cosmetic surgery. Such profiles may also help those who care for clients who have had cosmetic surgery. However, is the plastic surgery team obligated to help all their cosmetic surgery patients understand all of the psychological reasons that they desire such surgeries? Perhaps such an in-depth psychological assessment is not needed. However, if they do not assess basic psychological reasons for cosmetic surgery, the providers may not be acting beneficently. In a free-market system such as exists in the United States, the consumer is always right; should this hold true for consumers who elect to have cosmetic procedures for the "wrong" reasons?

Reconstructive surgery attempts to restore an abnormal body part to normal. The abnormality may be due to injured tissue, disease, or missing tissues, or may be causing other medical problems. People undergoing reconstructive surgery are typically motivated to try to gain increased function of body parts and improve their appearance. Although they may hope that plastic surgery will make them "normal," they usually know this may be unrealistic.

Initial reconstructive procedures focus on saving a person's life. For example, following a burn injury, skin grafting may be performed to reduce fluid and heat loss and the risk of infection. Later, additional reconstructive surgery is performed to restore physical function, and finally to improve the person's appearance. Reconstructive plastic surgery is used to repair or reconstruct traumatic injuries, congenital defects, and acquired deformities such as cancer.

Incidence

The "incidence" of plastic surgery procedures is not recorded. They are becoming quite common though. Technology and plastic surgery techniques have improved rapidly in recent times. Plastic surgery is able to address successfully many problems (e.g., amputated digits, breast reconstruction following mastectomy, and unsightly birthmarks) that were not repairable just a few years ago.

Etiology

There are many disorders that may be corrected or improved through plastic surgery. Disorders range from life threatening (e.g., burns) to disorders within the realm of normal but unacceptable to the client. It is a normal desire to want to physically resemble one's peers reasonably closely, e.g., to have acceptably "normal" facial features. The desire to be attractive or beautiful is a desire present in people of all cultures, but the perception of what is attractive varies.

Adorning the body with paints or scars dates from ancient times to the present (e.g., lipstick, nail polish, tattoos). Some people decorate the body by wearing objects in their noses, ear lobes, or lips. Western society pressures people to continue to look young (perhaps by exercise) and combat the normal physical changes of aging (perhaps by plastic surgery). For many years, people were limited to highlighting their positive features with make-up and clothing. Plastic surgery can correct their negative features.

BODY IMAGE

A significant portion of any deformity rests in the client's perception of it. Perceptions develop in part from body image. Body image describes an individual's perception of his or her body—how the *person* thinks he or she looks, rather than an objective assessment of the person's characteristics. Body image is a factor in determining an individual's self-image, self-concept, and self-esteem. Individuals with a positive body image display more confidence and interact more easily with others. Body image changes continually, depending on individual expectations and feedback from others.

An individual with a physical deformity, real or perceived, can have a severely damaged body image. Even the usual processes of aging can be detrimental to body image. People's perception that they look like they're "getting old" can impair their level of confidence, affect their behavior, and interfere with their interactions in society. Body image is an important factor in the nursing assessment of the client having plastic surgery.

Prevention

Primary prevention of disorders requiring plastic surgery is directed at reducing congenital disorders through prenatal care and genetic counseling. Plastic surgery is also used in the treatment of malignancies; therefore, primary prevention focuses on cancer detection and treatment. Conditions requiring aesthetic surgery generally are not preventable.

Clinical Manifestations

Most clients with conditions requiring plastic surgery have some degree of deformity. The deformity can be *actual,* that is, objectively measured by others, such as a missing breast or deviated septum. Deformity can also be *perceived,* that is, the client is aware of the deformity, but it may not be noticeable to others. Fine facial wrinkling indicative of aging is an example.

DIAGNOSTIC ASSESSMENT

All clients must be assessed for their physical readiness for surgery. Prior to a major operation, a complete blood cell count is taken, electrolyte levels are assessed, and a chest x-ray study and electrocardiogram (for clients over 40) are performed. Other diagnostic assessments vary with specific procedures.

Medical Management

In this section, basic principles and practices in plastic surgery are discussed. Specific techniques are discussed later in the chapter.

RECONSTRUCTIVE LADDER

One of the greatest challenges in plastic surgery is reconstructing deformities. The reconstructive ladder is a guide to plan reconstruction. The following questions are asked:

- *What tissue is missing?* Does the client have bone, muscle, subcutaneous tissue, or skin missing? If only skin is missing (e.g., burns), skin grafts are used for reconstruction. People with large pressure sores may be missing muscle, subcutaneous tissue, and skin, and a rotation flap containing all these tissues may be used to repair the defect. Facial trauma may cause loss of bone as well as other tissues and vascularized bone may be used in reconstruction.
- *Where is tissue available?* Some small defects have adequate tissue for repair nearby. This is ideal, since the tissue can be lifted from its base and rotated into the defect. Nearby tissue has the same color, thickness, and hair-bearing tendencies, contributing to a more natural appearance. If the tissue needed is not nearby, it may be moved from its location and attached to the defect by microscopic anastomosis (i.e., suturing small vessels and nerves with the aid of a microscope). Reconstruction with this technique is called free flap reconstruction.
- *What deficit might result from moving donor tissue?* Obviously, a person does not want a larger defect in the donor site than the area being reconstructed! For example, a toe is often used to reconstruct a missing finger, but it is unlikely a person would give up a finger to rebuild a toe.
- *What is the simplest method to achieve the desired results?* The simplest method to close any wound is simple suturing. More complex methods are used if adequate tissue is not available for primary closure or if a greater defect would result from simple suturing. For example, a defect on the cheek could be closed by suturing, but as it healed it would pull the eyelid down into ectropion. Another method of closing a wound is to use a flap of tissue and rotate it onto the wound, maintaining the flap's own blood supply. Skin grafting is the third choice for reconstruction. The most complex form of wound closure is the free flap of skin, subcutaneous tissue, and possibly muscle or bone. Blood vessels nourishing a flap are attached to the wound vessels using an operating microscope.

MINIMAL SCARRING

Skin Lines. Plastic surgeons strive for minimal postoperative scarring. The quality of scarring is affected by many variables. The client's age, general health, skin type, and healing ability are important. Surgical technique and the quality of wound care also affect the healing process.

Every individual has normal lines and skinfolds (Fig. 72-1). Incisions made perpendicular to these lines result in more obvious scars. Incisions made parallel to the lines heal camouflaged by natural skinfolds. Incisions can also be hidden in the scalp or by the eyebrow or concealed by clothing. A long incision parallel to these lines is less visible than a shorter incision placed at right angles. No amount of care in suturing can ensure an aesthetic scar if the incision is positioned at right angles or obliquely to the lines of minimal tension. Skinfolds and wrinkles become more pronounced with age, further obscuring incision lines.

Elliptical Incision. When excising a lesion, the surgeon designs the incision lines longer than the lesion (Fig. 72-2). The resulting defect is elliptical, and the skin edges can be approximated easily. When the defect is round, tissues bunch up at the ends of the incision, resulting in "dog ears." [21]

Suturing Techniques. To heal with minimal scarring, the edges of the skin incision must be approximated precisely without undue tension. The suture lifts up the skin edges while it approximates them. Each suture puncture represents a miniature wound, and scar tissue forms at the site of each puncture. Suture lines must be kept clean, or stitch abscesses will develop and increase scarring. Sutures removed within 7 days leave no discernible suture marks or tracks. Unfortunately,

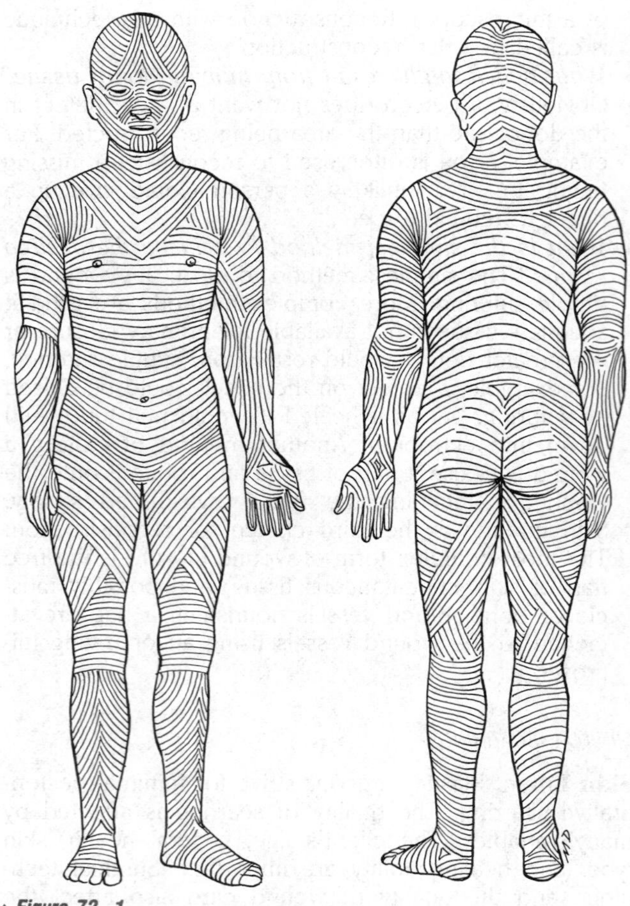

▲ Figure 72-1

Langer's lines. These lines are important in surgery. To minimize scar formation, the surgeon makes incisions parallel to these lines rather than at right angles to them. Langer's lines are natural cleavage lines formed by the skin's fibrous tissue. See the lines in the palms of your hands.

the skin on some areas of the body (e.g., the back) is tough and slower to heal and requires that sutures remain for a longer period of time. It is difficult to achieve fine scarring in these areas.

SURGICAL MODALITIES

Flaps and Grafts. Raw or exposed tissue left to its own heals slowly by secondary intention. Skin coverage is managed by approximating skin edges, covering the area with a graft, or transferring a flap. Most plastic surgery procedures are based on the transfer of tissue, either locally or to distant areas of the body.

A graft is tissue (e.g., skin, bone, nerve, or vessel) that is harvested without a blood supply from a donor site. It is transferred to a recipient site, where it develops a new blood supply. For the tissue to remain viable, or take, there must be a healthy vascular supply at the recipient site. The graft is anchored in position, and the area is immobilized until a new blood supply to the graft is established. Skin grafts always result in scars.

Skin grafts are used extensively to resurface exposed surfaces. The grafts vary in thickness from very thin split-thickness skin grafts (STSGs), which contain epidermis and a very thin layer of dermis, to full-thickness grafts (FTSGs), which contain epidermis and all of the dermis. Thinner grafts are more likely to contract during healing, but are also more likely to develop adequate blood supply. FTSGs are used in areas where contraction would limit function, such as on the hand or over joints. FTSGs leave a full-thickness defect in the donor site that must be closed, either primarily or with an STSG or a flap.

A flap is tissue that is elevated with its blood supply intact. Local flaps are rotated or advanced to reconstruct an adjacent defect (Fig. 72-3). Free flaps are harvested from one area of the body to reconstruct a defect in a distant area. The donor tissue (skin, muscle, bone, or a combination of these) (Table 72-1) is detached from its blood supply at the donor site and reattached by microvascular anastomosis to arteries and veins at the recipient site.

Microvascular Surgery. The development of microvascular techniques has made it possible to reconstruct defects that were previously untreatable. For example,

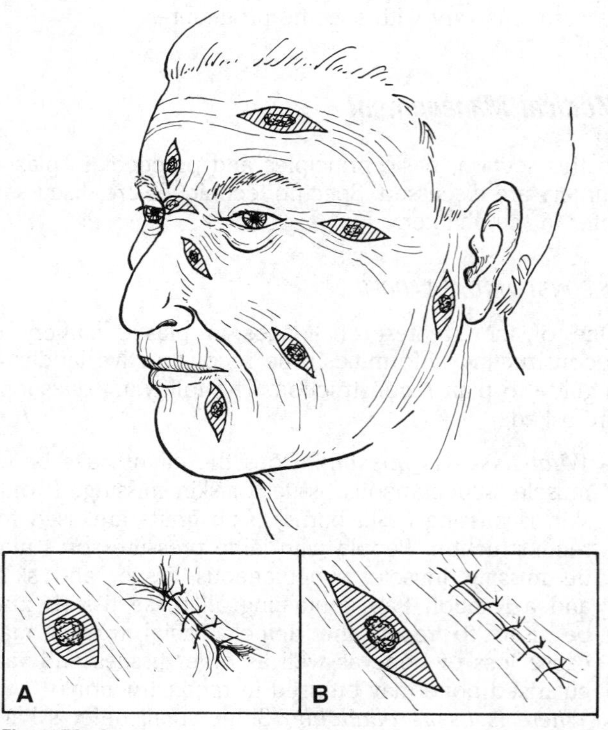

▲ Figure 72-2

Examples of elliptical excisions around skin lesions. Note that the incisions are placed along normal skin lines so the scars are hidden. Shaded area shows area of tissue removed with each lesion. *A*, If the ellipse is too short, puckers or "dog ears" form at the ends of the incision. This creates an unsightly scar. *B*, Correct length of elliptical incision for minimal scarring. (Redrawn from Grabb, W., & Smith, J. [1979]. *Plastic surgery* [3rd ed.]. Boston: Little, Brown.)

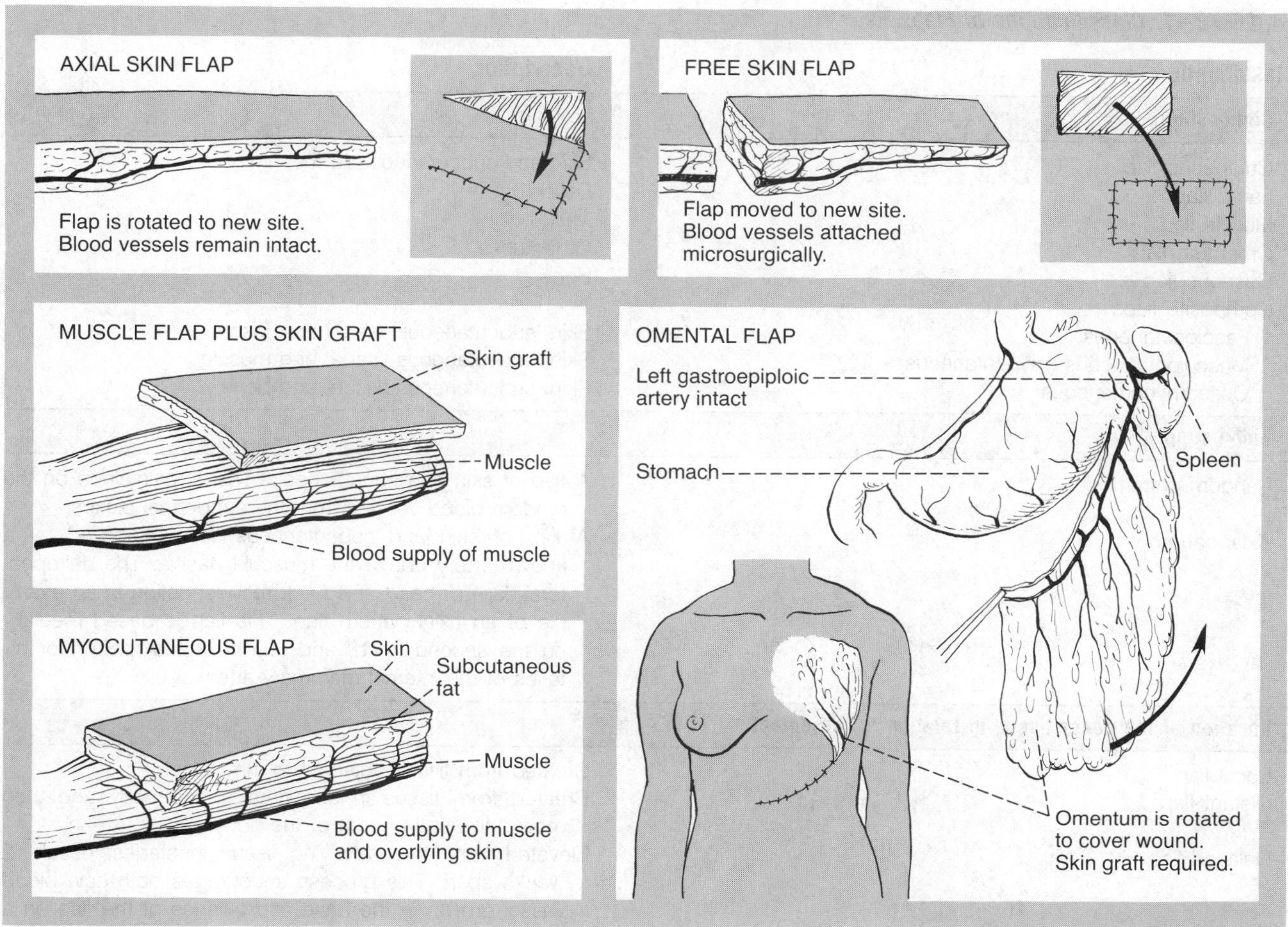

▲ *Figure 72–3*

Common flaps.

tissue from the forearm can be used in facial reconstruction. In some cases, sophisticated microvascular procedures have replaced less effective reconstructive approaches. Cumbersome metal implants were once used for mandibular reconstruction. Vascularized iliac bone, fashioned in the shape of a mandible, can now be transferred to reconstruct the jaw. The iliac bone and tissue with an intact blood supply are much more resistant to infection.

Adequate blood flow may be difficult to maintain in the anastomosed vessels in free flap, owing to vasospasm and edema. When the flap becomes engorged with blood, a leech may be used to remove the excess blood. A sterile leech is applied by the surgeon. The leech injects an anticoagulant into the wound and removes blood. The therapy is usually effective in 30 minutes. Because of the anticoagulant in the wound, blood flow usually remains adequate after the leech is removed.

Implants. Implant material can be used to augment or replace tissue in all parts of the body. Polymers such as medical-grade silicone rubber are used most frequently in plastic surgical procedures. Silicone prostheses can be very soft (breast prostheses), flexible (finger and toe joints), or rigid (bones and joints). Stainless steel; Vitallium; and titanium plates, screws, and wire are used to approximate, replace, and stabilize bone fragments (Fig. 72–4). Injectable collagen can be used to fill out skin depressions and fine wrinkles.

Facial structures (including the nose, chin, ears, orbital floor, and malar complex), breasts, bones and joints, and genitalia are often augmented or reconstructed with implant material. Material for implants must be biocompatible and not rejected by body tissues. It must not cause severe foreign body reaction or infection. Implants must be noncarcinogenic, nontoxic, nonallergenic, and sterile when implanted.

In 1991, the use of implants for breast augmentation was placed under strict regulations. The long-term risks of their use are being studied. The nurse caring for clients with breast implants must remain up to date by reading the scientific literature.

Skin Expansion. Skin expansion is a technique used to increase the amount of local tissue available to re-

TABLE 72-1. Classifications of Flaps

Classification	Description
Composition	
Cutaneous flap	Skin and subcutaneous tissue
Facial flap	Fascia
Muscle flap	Muscle
Omentum flap	Omentum
Osseous flap	Bone
Composite flaps	
Fasciocutaneous	Skin, subcutaneous tissue, and fascia
Musculocutaneous (myocutaneous)	Skin, subcutaneous tissue, and muscle
Osseomyocutaneous	Skin, subcutaneous tissue, and bone
Blood supply	
Random pattern	A flap of skin and subcutaneous tissue maintained on the random blood vessels from the subdermal plexus.
Axial pattern	A flap of skin and subcutaneous tissue supplied by a known artery above the muscular fascia. The deltopectoral flap for head and neck reconstruction is an example of an axial pattern flap. This flap is based medially on the second, third, and fourth anterior perforator arteries of the internal mammary artery.
Location of the donor tissue in relation to the defect	
Local flap	Created from tissue adjacent to the defect.
Distant flap	Created from tissue in one area of the body and then moved to another area of the body.
Delayed flap	Elevated from the underlying tissue in stages, usually 2 weeks apart. This process encourages both new blood vessel growth in the base and reliance of the flap on a more central vessel. When the blood vessels in the base have developed adequate blood supply to support the flap, it is transposed.
Free flap	Completely detached from donor site. Blood vessels are reattached at recipient site.
Method used to mobilize donor tissue	
Advancement flap	Moved directly forward to cover a defect rather than rotated.
Island flap	Has an intact donor blood vessel transferred to a new site, usually through a skin tunnel. The transrectus abdominal myocutaneous flap is an example of an island flap. The donor tissue is located in the abdomen and transferred beneath the abdomen to the chest wall.
Pedicle flap	An old term used to describe flaps based on a long stalk or pedicle that contained blood vessels and nerves. The flap is very mobile, depending on its length.
Transpositional flap (rotational flap)	Turned at an angle to the donor site. The defect created by the flap is usually closed with a skin graft.
Function	
Innervated flap	Contains a known nerve or branch of a nerve within the pedicle. Flaps for coverage of finger defects use innervated tissue.
Noninnervated flap	Contains a random supply of nerves. Eventually obtains sensation through lateral ingrowth of nerves.

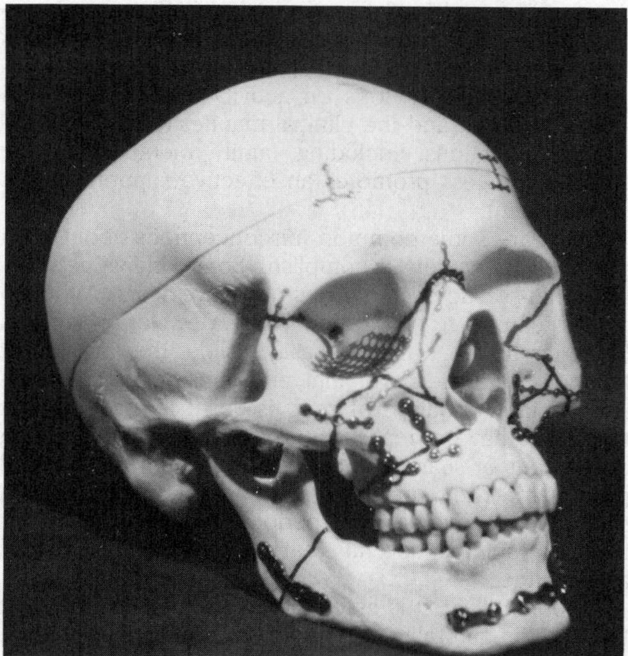

▲ *Figure 72-4*

Titanium plates and screws.

construct a defect. An inflatable silicone balloon is placed under the skin or muscle flap adjacent to a defect. The expander is inflated sequentially over several weeks or months, to stretch the overlying tissue. When there is sufficient tissue to resurface the adjacent defect, the balloon is removed, and the flap is contoured (shaped) and advanced to cover the defect.

Liposuction. Liposuction or suction-assisted lipectomy is a technique used (1) to aspirate fatty tissue from areas resistant to diet and exercise (lipodystrophy), (2) to contour flaps, and (3) to remove lipomas (benign fatty tumors). It is also used adjunctively with other plastic surgery procedures to create better contour and enhance the aesthetic result.

A blunt, hollow cannula is inserted through a very small incision (Fig. 72-5). The cannula, attached to a powerful suction machine, is passed back and forth through the subcutaneous tissue, sucking adipose tissue and creating a series of tunnels. The blunt tip pushes aside nerves and blood vessels. Precise surgical technique avoids ridges and dimpling on the surface as fatty tissue is suctioned away. Complications of liposuction include hematoma, skin necrosis, infection, and undesirable scars or skin dimpling.

Many clients expect the results of liposuction to be immediate. Usually up to 6 months is required for final results to be apparent after edema subsides and subcutaneous tissue heals.

Lasers. The laser (acronym for *l*ight *a*mplification by *s*timulated *e*mission of *r*adiation) is a coagulating, vaporizing, and cutting tool used frequently in plastic surgery. A precise beam of laser light is directed onto tissue. The light is converted into heat energy that is absorbed by the cells. Cells heat up, lose their moisture, and are destroyed.

The advantages of laser surgery include precision and accuracy of cell destruction, with reduced bleeding and swelling, and sometimes less postoperative pain. Operating time may be longer, but tissue damage is less, and the postoperative infection rate is lower.

There are different colors and wavelengths of laser light. Each is absorbed differently, depending on cell pigment and water content. The CO_2 laser is primarily a cutting and vaporizing tool. Its energy is absorbed by the water in cells, and therefore it penetrates tissue only superficially. The CO_2 laser is used primarily to excise or vaporize lesions such as warts, keloids, and vascular lesions. Argon, copper vapor, and pulsed dye laser energy are preferentially absorbed by hemoglobin and are used primarily for coagulating. These types of lasers are used to treat birthmarks (e.g., port-wine stain), superficial vascular lesions, and pigmented lesions.

Craniofacial Surgery. Craniofacial surgery is an approach for reconstructing facial bones through an incision on the top of the skull. The skin and muscles over the forehead and face are lifted off the bones and muscles. Once the face is free of its soft tissue drape, bones are rearranged to correct congenital or acquired deformities. Bone grafts from the ribs, iliac crest, or skull may provide bone for reconstruction. Adults likely to undergo craniofacial surgery are those with facial fractures and facial skeletal tumors.

Serious risks accompany craniofacial surgery, i.e., death from increased intracranial pressure, blindness, brain damage, and infections such as meningitis and osteomyelitis of the skull.

Postoperative care focuses on managing intracranial pressure, airway patency, and postoperative edema. The length of hospitalization varies with the underlying etiology.

CLIENT SELECTION PROCESS

The success of a plastic surgery procedure is determined by the degree to which it meets the client's

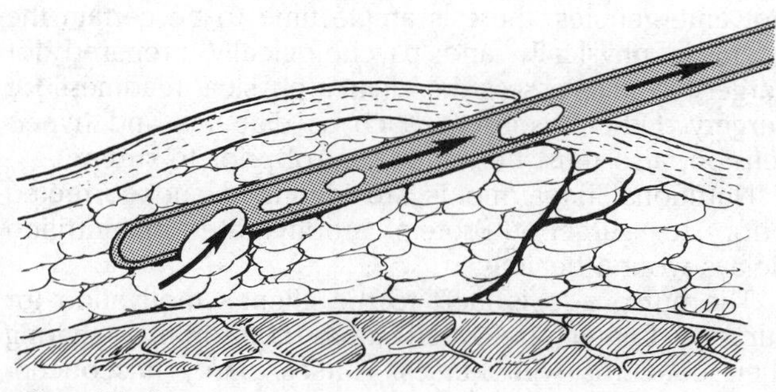

▲ *Figure 72-5*

Suction-assisted lipectomy. To prevent extracting subdermal fat, the surgeon directs the opening of the suction cannula toward the muscle fascia.

expectations. A surgical procedure may produce excellent clinical results, but the client will not consider it a success unless it achieves a specific appearance or level of function. Therefore, it is essential that the surgeon and nurse understand what the client expects and that the client have a realistic view of what can and cannot be accomplished by surgery.

Because most procedures affect appearance, clients make a considerable emotional commitment when they elect to have plastic surgery. There is no ideal candidate for plastic surgery, but there are characteristics that indicate an individual would be at risk for achieving an unsatisfactory result. In addition to good physical health, the client must be psychologically healthy. Assessing the client's motivation is essential. Plastic surgery does not cure an individual's underlying emotional problems or alleviate major stress. An external change does not make a happy, well-adjusted person out of an individual who is unhappy, poorly adjusted, or excessively stressed. Clients who expect plastic surgery to do so are poor candidates for plastic surgery. Nurses help identify appropriate candidates for surgery.

DOCUMENTATION THROUGH CLINICAL PHOTOGRAPHY

Photographs are used extensively in plastic surgery. It is essential to document the client's condition prior to any surgical intervention. Once changes have been made in appearance, it is very difficult to remember the details of the original situation. Photographic documentation provides an accurate record.

In office settings, nurses commonly photograph the client before and after surgery. By protecting the client's privacy and explaining the importance of photographic documentation, the nurse can make a photo session much less uncomfortable and embarrassing. The client must give written permission for photographs to be taken, especially if they are to be used for teaching purposes in addition to documentation for the medical record.

Nursing Management

PREOPERATIVE

Because the majority of plastic surgery procedures are not emergencies, there is ample time to be certain the client is physically and psychologically prepared for surgery. Nurses assess the client's physical readiness for surgery. Other disorders, such as diabetes and hypertension, also must be under control prior to surgery.

Nutritional impairments are identified and corrected prior to surgery. Protein-carbohydrate malnutrition delays wound healing.

The nurse also is alert to the client's motivation for surgery. Clients are often more comfortable sharing their concerns with nurses. Nurses clarify misconceptions about the surgery and/or results. Serious unrealistic expectations are conveyed to the surgeon.

Preoperative teaching includes helping the client develop realistic postoperative expectations. The client must understand how the surgery will affect usual routines. Thorough planning ensures minimum disruption in routines. Preoperative teaching must include information about restrictions on activity, the location and extent of scars, and the clinical manifestations of possible complications. Including family members in the teaching process promotes an effective support system for the client.

There are some common misconceptions about what plastic surgery can accomplish. Some individuals believe that plastic surgery does not leave scars. Although some scars can be hidden from view or placed in locations that not are not easily visible, the nurse must help clients understand that any incision in tissue results in the formation of scar tissue. It is essential that the client have a realistic expectation of the location and extent of scarring that will result from the surgical procedure. The nurse must remind the patient that a scar matures over a long period of time. Some scars take as long as several years to achieve their final appearance.

Preoperatively, it is essential to reinforce the fact that the body is naturally asymmetric. Left and right breasts, ears, eyes are not identical in size, shape, or position. Most of these discrepancies are seldom noticed, but plastic surgery clients have a heightened sensitivity to all aspects of appearance. In preparing the client for realistic postoperative expectations, the surgeon and nurse must reinforce the fact that perfect symmetry is not a realistic expectation.

Survival of tissue that has been manipulated during surgery depends on promoting adequate blood flow. The nurse teaches the client to avoid anything that inhibits blood flow to the tissue. Aspirin and aspirin-containing compounds interfere with platelet agglutination and can promote bleeding and hematoma formation. Nicotine is a potent vasoconstrictor and can interfere with tissue perfusion. Smoking can result in flap necrosis and the loss of a significant amount of tissue. The client is also taught to elevate the surgical site.

POSTOPERATIVE ASSESSMENT

The surgical site is inspected every 2 hours if no dressing is present. Dressings put on by the surgeon are not removed to make assessments. The nurse assesses and documents pain, pressure, bleeding, skin color, temperature, sensation, presence of blisters (discussed shortly), presence or absence of edema or seroma (accumulation of serosanguineous drainage), and blanching time.

Any indications of complications at the surgical site are reported to the surgeon, including cool, pale, or cyanotic skin; increased (prolonged) blanching time as compared with preoperative findings; and changes in sensation, e.g., tingling. Abnormal pain, pallor, or cyanosis in transferred skin is immediately reported to the surgeon.

Assess the surgical site for venous stasis and edema. Either can seriously impair tissue perfusion. Venous stasis increases local tissue hypoxia because metabolic tissue waste is not removed promptly. Local tissue hypoxia can cause tissue necrosis. Prolonged blanching time is an early assessment finding that indicates venous stasis. Venous engorgement makes the flap appear blue. Any sign of decreased vascularity (change in color or temperature, size, or tightness) must be reported immediately. Tissue oxygenation monitors may also be used.

Blisters (small blebs of serum) indicate reduced circulation and impaired tissue viability. The nurse documents and reports to the surgeon the presence of blisters. Sometimes, blisters under a skin graft need to be drained. When prescribed, this is accomplished by inserting a small (25-gauge), sterile needle into the blister and letting the fluid run out onto a sterile dressing. A standing p.r.n. order may be given for this intervention. Large accumulations may require surgical removal.

The amount of pain is assessed. Donor sites commonly are more painful than recipient sites.

The client's ability to cope with a temporary or permanent, perceived or actual, disfigurement is also assessed. The nurse assesses the client's coping mechanisms. Some coping mechanisms may be effective; others may be ineffective. Men may have more difficulty expressing their feelings about their appearance than women. The nurse listens to the client, alert for positive and negative statements about the self. The degree of anxiety and fear is noted. The nurse assesses the client's willingness or unwillingness to touch or look at involved body areas, and the client's comfortableness in being near other people.

NURSING INTERVENTION

Nursing Diagnosis: Tissue Perfusion, Altered Peripheral, High Risk for R/T tissue transfer.

Planning: Expected Outcomes. The client will have adequate peripheral tissue perfusion, as evidenced by usual color of skin, no pallor or cyanosis, warm and dry skin, blanching in 3 to 5 seconds, no edema or blebs, intact incisions, and controllable pain.

Implementation

Postoperative Flaps. Many plastic surgery procedures involve flaps. Failure of all or part of a flap can result in significant tissue loss. Flap failure is a devastating experience, physically and emotionally. Not only does the defect remain unrepaired, but the tissue used for the reconstruction is also sacrificed. The client's emotions are also devastated.

Protecting the blood supply to a flap is a primary nursing responsibility. Nursing interventions are designed to avoid factors that can jeopardize blood flow. Tension on the flap can stretch or kink the feeding blood vessels, reducing the flow of blood to the tissues. A blood clot can restrict blood flow. The first sign of compromised blood flow is pallor.

The nurse positions the client so that he or she is comfortable and the flap is relaxed and elevated. Gravity promotes edema and venous congestion, both of which impede blood flow. Interventions to increase venous return include elevating the involved body part and applying elastic stockings or wraps as prescribed.

A hematoma under a flap can be a severe complication. It can place pressure on vessels and inhibit blood flow. Hematomas can also precipitate an infection and release toxic substances. Increasing swelling and a feeling of tightness and pressure are danger signs. Hematomas can be removed if recognized early. Continued evaluation ensures that any factors inhibiting vascularity are reported and addressed immediately.

When an engorged flap is going to be treated with leeches, the nurse answers questions about the plan with the client. The client may express fear, disgust, or apprehension about the use of leeches.

Implants. Postoperatively, assessment and intervention focus on preventing displacement of the implant, ensuring adequate blood flow to the operative site, and preventing infection. Implants themselves are not painful, but the surgical procedure causes mild to moderate pain. Infection is a serious complication that could result in having to remove the implant. Excellent wound care is imperative. The nurse must teach the client to recognize the clinical manifestations of infection so that treatment can be initiated quickly. Pain that is unrelieved with analgesics must be investigated. Changes in temperature and local changes such as drainage, increasing edema, hyperemia, and increasing skin temperature may indicate a developing infection or implant rejection.

The process of skin expansion involves an extended period of time, commitment, and significant, although temporary, disfigurement. It is essential that the client be motivated, well prepared for the experience, and compliant. The client must be able to make additional trips to the doctor's office where the expander will be inflated under sterile conditions. Each expander has an injection site into which a sterile needle is inserted percutaneously. Saline is injected slowly until the tissue is very tight over the expander. Sometimes a small amount of saline needs to be withdrawn to reduce discomfort. The tightness may be uncomfortable for several hours but subsides as the tissue begins to expand.

The nurse teaches the client to keep the incision and the injection site clean and dry to prevent infection. It is important that the client understand that pressure on the expander compromises blood flow and could cause tissue breakdown. Infection is a serious complication and may require that the expander be removed altogether. If the incision line dehises, exposing the expander, it does not usually result in aborting the treatment. Fluid can be removed from the expander to relieve the tension. When the incision has healed sufficiently, expansion can begin again.

In most cases, the patient can camouflage the expander with clothing. So that no pressure is placed on the expander, the clothing must be loose. The client should sleep in a position that protects the expander from pressure. Those clients with expanders in exposed areas like the neck or scalp must be able to cope with

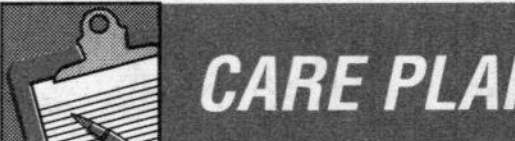

CARE PLAN

The Client Having Plastic Surgery

Nursing Diagnosis/ Collaborative Problem	Planning: Expected Outcomes	Implementation: Nursing Interventions	Rationales
High Risk for Body Image Disturbance in Self-Concept R/T perceived or actual disfigurement	The client will have improved self image with incorporation of changed body part into body image as evidenced by: • Effective coping and appropriate use of defense mechanisms • Verbalizes feelings comfortably and appropriately • Expresses satisfaction with changed body image • Able to openly verbalize feelings • Makes positive statements about self • Normal level of anxiety and normal fears • No indications of depression • Comfortably looking at self in mirror and/or touching deformed body area, healed surgical site, or other scars • Able to be with others comfortably	Continue to assess apparent self-concept, coping methods, defense mechanisms, degree of anxiety, and fears frequently	Continued assessment provides data about degree of self-concept
		Assist client to explore and express feelings	Allowing the client to express feelings assists client to work through feelings
		Be sensitive to client's feelings and needs	Sensitivity is imperative to facilitate open communication
		Acknowledge client's feelings	Using phrases such as "I know how you feel" builds barriers to communication. "You are angry" or "you seem depressed" identify the feeling
		Present reality	Building false hope is detrimental. Reality need not be brutal, however. Healing is unpredictable, questions should be referred to the surgeon.
		Demonstrate appropriate feelings of value and positive regard toward client	Nurse must believe and respect client to facilitate feelings of self-worth
		Provide necessary physical care if client is de-	Do not force the client to view or touch self

the temporary physical inconvenience and insult to body image.

Nurses are instrumental in assisting the client to disguise the deformity caused by the expander. For example, when one breast is being expanded prior to reconstruction, the other breast will not match in size or shape. The nurse assists the client in padding the other breast to a size equal to the expanded breast to reduce obvious asymmetry.

Liposuction. Because moderate to large quantities of tissue and fluid can be removed during liposuction, the nurse must assess the client for signs of hypovolemia and electrolyte imbalance (syncope, dizziness, and abnormal blood values). If drains are used, assessing the quantity and quality of drainage is important.

Compression dressings or elastic compression garments may be used to help collapse the tunnels and prevent fluid collection (hematoma and seroma), maintain the desired body contour, and promote healing. Dressings usually remain in place for at least 24 hours. Nurses must ensure that dressings remain smooth and uniform or contour irregularities can result. Sometimes the client wears a compression garment for several weeks postoperatively to promote good healing.

Following liposuction, clients rest for several hours. They may gradually resume normal activity except for strenuous exercise. It may be 4 to 6 weeks before the client attains the preoperative level of exercise. Resuming activity too rapidly may result in soreness and swelling. Bruising is common following liposuction and may take weeks to disappear completely.

The nurse reinforces that results may not be apparent for 6 months following surgery. This period of time is required for complete resolution of edema and reconnection of soft tissues.

Laser Surgery. Laser energy generates intense heat and clients experience a burning sensation. The tissue reaction can be similar to a first-degree burn with blistering.

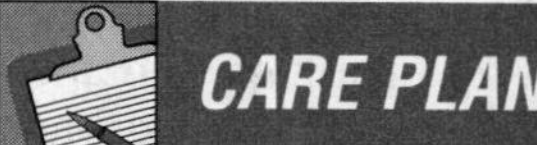

CARE PLAN

The Client Having Plastic Surgery Continued

Nursing Diagnosis/ Collaborative Problem	Planning: Expected Outcomes	Implementation: Nursing Interventions	Rationales
		pressed. (Depressed clients may be unable to meet these needs, since they lack energy or desire to do so.)	
		Gently assist client to look at and touch deformity or healed surgical site. (Help incorporate it into client's self-concept and body image.)	Desensitization begins in safe environments and proceeds to new situations. Client is prepared for stares and remarks
		Encourage client to begin meeting in public to begin desensitization to reactions of others, such as by taking walks in halls.	
		Assist client, as necessary, to be with others, walking in halls.	
		Discuss reaction of others to client. Support grief reactions.	
		Prepare visitors and family members before seeing client if facial deformity is present	Allows family members time to prepare and control reactions
		Look for vocal expression or hand gestures if facially disfigured	Facial expression may be limited in clients with extensive facial scars or skin grafting

Ointment applied to the affected area for 2 to 4 weeks keeps the tissue moist until healing is complete. It is also essential that the area treated with laser energy be protected from sun exposure for several weeks.

Laser treatment to remove large pigmented lesions may require many operations. A single application may address only a small portion of the lesion, and the results are appreciated slowly as the site heals. Clients must be prepared for the length of time required and the inconvenience of multiple procedures.

Craniofacial Surgery. Postoperative care following craniofacial surgery includes elevating the head of the bed to reduce edema. The head can and should be turned while being supported behind the coronal incision line. Care must be taken that no pressure is placed on areas of bone grafts. The client can lie supine or on the nonoperative side but not directly on the operated side of the head or cheek, because pressure on the bony grafts may dislodge them. Neck flexion is permitted. Frequent neurologic assessment is important for increasing intracranial (Chap. 29) and intraocular pressure. Diplopia (double vision) is usually due to edema, is temporary, and may be helped with alternating eye patches. Relatively mild doses of analgesics or narcotics may control discomfort. However, the donor sites for rib or iliac bone grafts are often very painful. Analgesics that contain aspirin are avoided because they increase risk of bleeding.

Care of the client with Body Image Disturbance, High Risk for R/T perceived or actual disfigurement is discussed in the care plan.

EVALUATION

The degree of expected outcome attainment is evaluated prior to discharge from the postanesthesia area, hospital room, or office setting. Because the clinical manifestations of impaired tissue perfusion may develop hours after surgery, the client needs thorough education in order to detect reportable problems.

Modification of Plan of Care for the Elderly

Many elderly clients have both aesthetic and reconstructive surgery. The nurse ascertains that the client understands the surgical plans, often by using education forms with large print. Many elderly clients routinely take anticoagulants and therefore tend to bleed more easily. Pressure dressings may be required for a longer period of time. Finally, some clients may resist not being independent with driving and self-care. Safety issues must be discussed. For example, the side effects of anesthetics and narcotics as well as facial edema and dressings prohibit driving after facial surgery.

Post-hospital Care

DISCHARGE TEACHING

Discharge teaching depends on the specific operation and surgeon's preferences. Client teaching and general discharge teaching have been discussed.

▼ FACIAL REJUVENATING SURGERY

In childhood, skin is very elastic and is supported at maximum distension by the adipose tissue (sometimes called "baby fat"). During aging, the skin loses elasticity and the subcutaneous fat diminishes and changes in character. Skinfolds and wrinkles become increasingly noticeable. The tissues around the eyes and jowls sag, producing a drooping, weary or worried expression.

The rate of skin changes varies among individuals. Weight loss, sun exposure, and genetic tendencies affect the speed and character of the changes. There is no ideal time to have surgery. Some people elect to have surgery very early to prolong a youthful appearance. Others wait until the effects of the aging process are pronounced. The client's physical and psychosocial health and support system determine the appropriateness of surgery.

Rhytidectomy

Rhytidectomy, also called a face lift, removes the larger skin wrinkles and folds from the face and neck. Physical signs of aging occur throughout the body but are most obvious to others on the face. Rhytidectomy may restore a more youthful appearance to the face (maybe 5 to 10 years younger), e.g., by removing wrinkles from the forehead and along the eyes and mouth (Fig. 72-6).

Rhytidectomy is usually performed on a day surgery basis under general or local anesthesia with intravenous sedation. Incisions are made along the ear and out into the hair-bearing scalp (Fig. 72-7). Through the incisions, excess facial skin is undermined and pulled back toward the ear. Upon completion of the operation, facial compression dressings are applied.

The most common complications of a face lift are hematoma, hair and skin loss, and nerve injury. Hematomas are caused by small bleeding points that start bleeding again after the wound is closed. Large hematomas can cause tissue necrosis and must be surgically removed. Hematoma formation occurs most often in individuals who smoke. Hair loss is presumably due to altered circulation to hair follicles. The hair usually regrows. Skin loss occasionally develops behind the ear, and may be due to swelling or hematoma. Such a wound is allowed to heal by secondary intention and does not result in a very large scar. Nerve damage causing facial paralysis is a rare but devastating complication of facial surgery. Occasionally, facial paralysis is due to nerve compression by a suture. When facial paralysis is observed, immediate surgical exploration to correct the problem (e.g., release a suture) and prevent permanent damage is necessary.

Preoperatively, prior to rhytidectomy, the person thoroughly shampoos the hair and washes the face well. Men carefully shave.

Postoperatively, the client is assessed for hematoma development, e.g., increasing facial asymmetry associated with pain or tightness on one side of the face. The nurse reports these findings immediately to the surgeon and makes certain the client understands the importance of also doing so at home. Large hematomas are removed surgically, because of potential skin necrosis due to pressure from the hematoma on blood vessels nourishing the skin. The nurse also assesses blood pressure and reports elevations, because this increases the risk of bleeding. Use antiemetics to reduce nausea and vomiting. Vomiting increases blood pressure and the risk of bleeding.

Teach the client to keep the head of the bed elevated for 1 week to minimize edema and rest the face for 1 week to achieve fine, unnoticeable scars (minimize talking and chewing, i.e., take a soft diet). The surgeon usually removes dressings the morning after rhytidectomy. The face may then be gently washed, and creams and cosmetics applied. However, the suture line should not be touched with soap, water, creams, or cosmetics until healing is complete. Washing the hair is usually postponed for 48 hours. Dandruff shampoo is avoided.

Blepharoplasty

Blepharoplasty is the surgical removal of excessive tissue from the upper or lower eyelid. If eyelid tissue obstructs vision, blepharoplasty is classified as reconstructive. The aging process causes a loss of elasticity and relaxation of eyelid skin. Excessive eyelid tissue occurring in young and middle-aged people may be inherited, be an allergic reaction, or result from cardiovascular or thyroid disease. Complete medical assess-

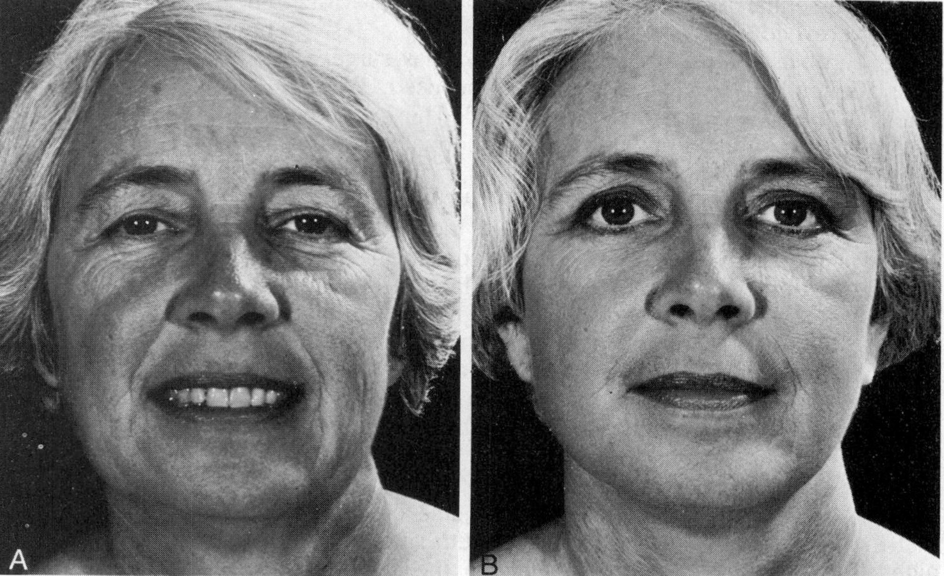

▲ *Figure 72–6*

Before *(A)* and after *(B)* a face lift (rhytidectomy) and blepharoplasty. (From Baptist, G. (1985). Perioperative nursing roles for the aesthetic surgical patient. *Plastic Surgical Nursing* 5(3), 86–93.)

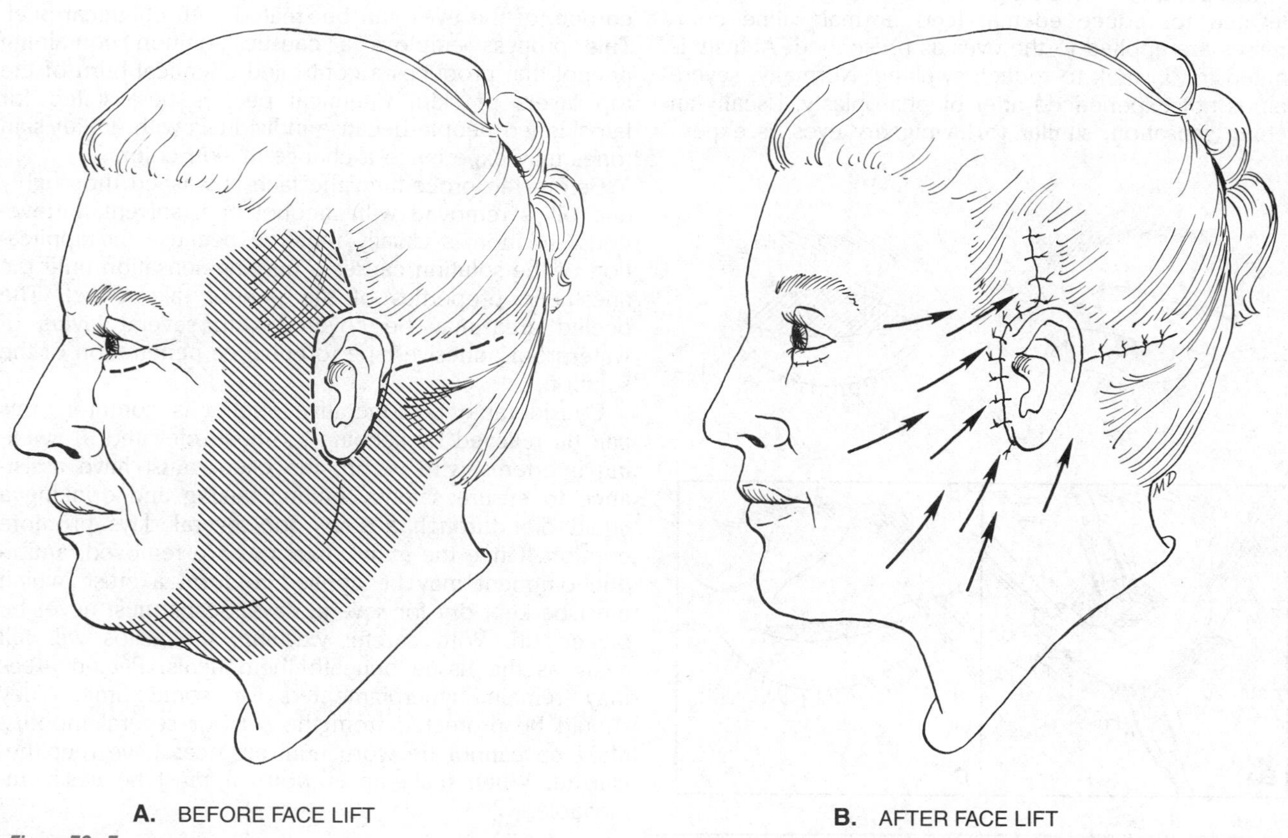

▲ *Figure 72–7*

Face lift (rhytidectomy) and blepharoplasty. Face lifts remove large wrinkles and folds of skin from the face and neck. *A*, Shaded area shows amount of tissue removed. The incision lines for the face lift go around the ear and into the hair-bearing scalp. Other incisions may also be used for face lifts. Note also the incision line beneath the eyelid for the blepharoplasty (to remove excess eyelid tissue). *B*, The postoperative near-final result, with tightened facial skin and neck folds.

ment is essential to rule out these physical causes of excessive eyelid skin.

Blepharoplasty is usually performed on a day surgery basis. General or local anesthesia can be used. Wide elliptical incisions are made on the eyelid. The excised wedge of excess tissue is lifted off and herniated fat is removed (Fig. 72-8).

A lower-lid blepharoplasty incision is placed one eighth of an inch below the edge of the eyelid. It begins at the tear duct and extends to the laugh lines on the eye's outer border. Extending the incision to the side of the eye prevents buckling of the tissues during healing. Sutures are removed on the third or fourth postoperative day. Rapid, uneventful recovery is typical. Blepharoplasty can be performed alone or with rhytidectomy (face lift). Complications from blepharoplasty are rare.

Because blepharoplasty clients are not hospitalized, preoperative nursing care is brief. The nurse confirms that the person has taken nothing by mouth since midnight. The presence of food or liquid in the stomach may necessitate postponing the operation. Preoperative near and distant vision is assessed in each eye by asking the person to read from a book as well as from something in the distance with the eye not being examined covered. These baseline data are critical to assess postoperative visual changes.

Postoperatively following blepharoplasty, the head is elevated to reduce edema. Iced normal saline compresses are applied to the eyes as prescribed. Activity is limited for 1 week to reduce swelling. Normally, severe pain is not experienced after blepharoplasty. Usually an itching sensation, similar to having dry eyes, is experienced owing to slight corneal swelling. This can be prevented with cold wet dressings.

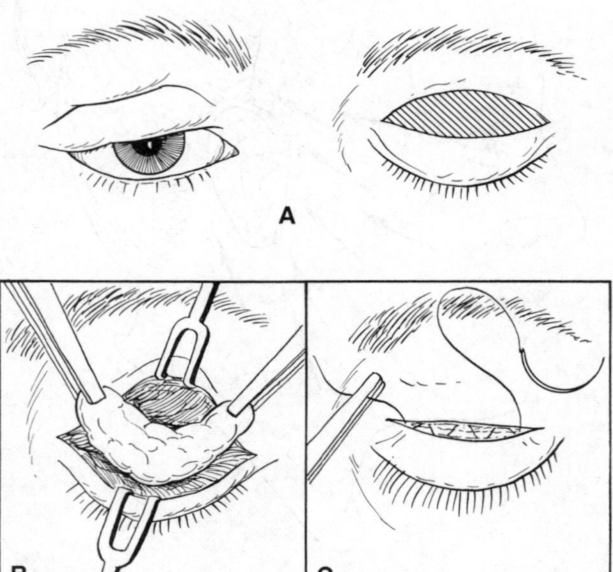

▲ Figure 72-8

Blepharoplasty. An elliptical incision is made in the eyelid and through it excess tissue and fat are removed. *A*, The amount of tissue to be removed *(shaded area)* and the incision lines. *B*, The removal of herniated fat from beneath the skin and the muscles. *C*, Closure of the wound.

Postoperatively, the nurse teaches the client the following:

1. Report changing vision or eye pain not relieved by prescribed analgesia immediately to the surgeon.
2. Apply cold compresses to the eyes as prescribed (typically for 24 to 48 hours after surgery). At home, clean wash cloths soaked in ice water work well. The cloths should be damp and changed frequently.
3. Sleep on the back with the head elevated for the first 48 hours. Lying on one side causes facial edema on that side, increasing tension on the suture lines.
4. Avoid bending over from the waist for 48 hours.
5. Avoid vigorous activity for 1 month.
6. Bruising and swelling are common around the eyes. Hence, the client may want to wear sunglasses. The nurse shows the client how to apply and remove the eyeglasses carefully to avoid bumping the incisions.

Adjunctive Procedures

CHEMICAL PEEL

Rhytidectomy does not remove all the wrinkles of the face. The fine lines around the mouth and at the corners of the eyes can be treated with chemical peel. This process employs a caustic solution containing phenol that produces a controlled chemical burn of the top layers of skin. Chemical peel is best suited for fair-skinned people because individuals with darker skin tones may experience a change in skin color.

Before the procedure, the face is washed thoroughly and oil is removed with alcohol or a solvent. Intravenous sedation is usually required because the application of the solution causes a burning sensation until the anesthetic properties of the phenol take effect. The peeled area may be covered with several layers of waterproof adhesive tape to enhance penetration of the solution.

Considerable postoperative edema is common; this can be relieved by keeping the head elevated. If swelling interferes with vision, the client must have assistance to ensure safety. Limiting talking and drinking a liquid diet through a straw for several days promote comfort. Once the initial dressings are removed, antibiotic ointment may be applied to form a crust, which must be kept dry for several days. Scabs must never be picked off. With careful washing, the scabs will fall away as the tissue beneath them heals. Peeled areas may remain hyperpigmented for some time. They should be protected from the sun for several months. Make-up cannot be worn until all areas have reepithelialized. When make-up is worn, it must be easily removable.

TRICHLORACETIC ACID PEEL

Trichloracetic acid is a form of chemical peel. The chemical is brushed on the skin until the skin frosts.

DERMABRASION

Dermabrasion is a process of sanding away the surface layers of skin on cheeks and forehead to remove pitting and surface blemishes, leaving a smoother skin surface. The healing process and nursing care following dermabrasion are similar to those following a chemical peel.

COLLAGEN INJECTION

Collagen is sometimes injected to fill in small wrinkles or depressed blemishes in the skin.

The client's reaction to collagen is tested before treatment because some individuals experience induration (hard, raised area) and swelling at the injection site. Clients with autoimmune disorders are not candidates for collagen injection.

Following collagen injections, the face should not be washed and face cream or make-up cannot be applied for 3 to 4 hours. Normal skin care can then continue. Exposure to strong sunlight, alcohol consumption, and excessive exercise can cause mild swelling and should be avoided as prescribed, e.g., for a week.

▼ OTHER ELECTIVE FACIAL SURGERY

RHINOPLASTY

Rhinoplasty is the surgical correction of external nose deformities. Rhinoplasty is frequently performed as day surgery, under local anesthesia and sedation or general anesthesia. Incisions are made inside the nose. Procedures are individualized and may include reshaping the bony dorsum of the nose, the tip of the nose, and/or cartilage along the nares (nostrils). The nasal bones may be fractured to achieve a desirable result. Following surgery, the inside of the nose is packed and an external splint applied.

Preoperative nursing care focuses on teaching the client to breath through the mouth after surgery and not to touch the nose. Postoperatively, assess for bleeding. While the person is sleepy from the anesthetic, excessive swallowing may be the only sign of bleeding. Examine the back of the throat with a flashlight to look for blood. Some bleeding is normal down the back of the throat and on the nasal packs and dressings. The nurse promptly reports excessive bleeding to the surgeon. The head of the bed is kept elevated to control postoperative edema. Nasal packing can be very uncomfortable. Pain management is important and can usually be achieved with oral analgesics, e.g., codeine or acetaminophen. Aspirin is avoided for 1 week before and 3 weeks after surgery.

In preparation for discharge, client education typically includes the following:

1. Sleep with the head of the bed elevated for 1 week.
2. Do not remove the external splints or nasal packing.
3. Do not blow the nose. Sneeze only with the mouth open.
4. Remain on a soft diet for 2 days.
5. Avoid decongestant nasal sprays because they are vasoconstrictors and they decrease the blood supply needed for healing.
6. After nasal packs and external splints are removed, the nose will remain swollen and bruised for a while. Wait 3 months before judging the final results of the surgery.

▼ BREAST SURGERY

POSTMASTECTOMY BREAST RECONSTRUCTION

Mastectomy for breast cancer or other breast disease not only disfigures but also causes emotional trauma (Chapter 78). For many women planning to have a mastectomy, the knowledge that breast reconstruction is possible reduces some of their anxiety. It is important that the client realize that the cosmetic results will not match the opposite breast. The reconstructed breast does not feel like a normal breast but it has distinct advantages over external prostheses in feel and appearance in clothes.

Breast reconstruction can be performed immediately after mastectomy (during the same operation) or many years later. The timing of the reconstruction varies with the woman's preference and the surgeon's opinion. Disadvantages to immediate reconstruction are an increased risk of poor tissue perfusion and hematoma owing to the just-completed mastectomy. There is also concern that a woman might deny the seriousness of the cancer (possibly reducing motivation for follow-up treatment with radiation therapy) if the breast is reconstructed immediately. On the positive side, breast reconstruction does not reduce the effectiveness of radiation therapy, and it may provide psychologic strength for the woman to undergo radiation and chemotherapy.

Breast reconstruction is usually a collaborative effort among the general surgeon, the plastic surgeon, and the oncologist. A variety of reconstructive approaches are available and depend on the situation.

- Inserting a tissue expander. A tissue expander is inserted under the chest tissues and expanded slowly, by adding fluid via percutaneous injection. After a few weeks, when the chest tissue has expanded, the expander is removed and an implant inserted.
- Rotating the latissimus dorsi muscle. This large flat muscle is in the back. The muscle and skin can be lifted up from the back, tunneled through the axilla, and formed into a breast mound on the chest. An implant is then inserted. The incision is positioned so that it can be hidden under the brassiere. Functional loss of strength and shoulder abduction and loss of ability to pull occur following latissimus dorsi breast reconstruction.
- The transrectus abdominal musculocutaneous flap (TRAM) flap is breast reconstruction using abdominal muscle and skin. This form of reconstruction

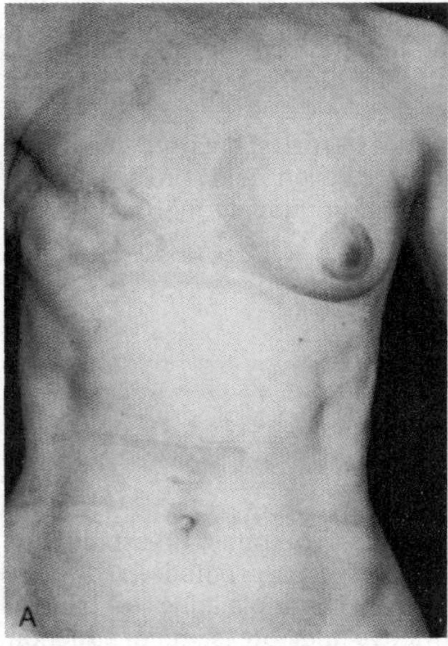

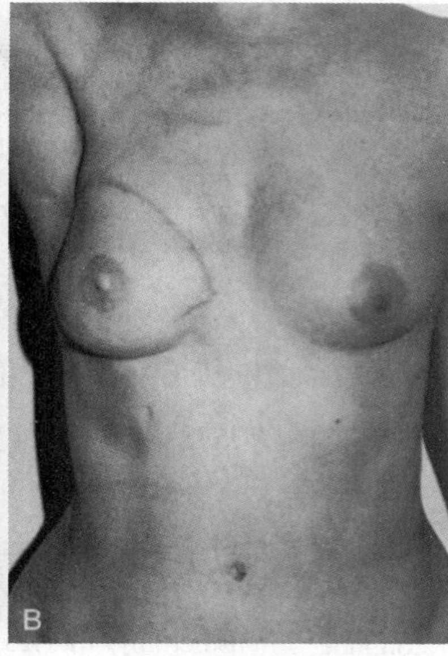

▲ **Figure 72-9**

Preoperative (*A*) and postoperative (*B*) transverse rectus abdominus myocutaneous reconstruction. (From Lerberg, L., & Prin, J. [1991]. TRAM breast reconstruction. *Plastic Surgical Nursing,* 11[2], 58-61.)

does not usually require a prosthesis. The tissue can be rotated to the chest wall with the blood vessels intact, or the blood vessels can be reattached as a free flap through microsurgery. The donor site in the abdomen is closed as a modified abdominoplasty (Fig. 72-9). Although the contour of the abdomen is improved (flattened), the scar is usually visible.

To undergo a TRAM flap, the patient must have sufficient redundant abdominal tissue. Previous abdominal surgery and smoking can be contraindications if the blood supply to the TRAM is impaired.

▶ Free flaps, including flaps from the gluteal area and TRAM, have also been used for reconstruction.

The breast reconstruction techniques just discussed rebuild the breast mound. Some women elect to have the nipple-areola also replaced. In order to achieve symmetry, nipple reconstruction may be delayed for several months following breast reconstruction. During the healing process, the contour of the reconstructed breast may change slightly as the incisions heal and edema subsides. Nipples can be reconstructed from a variety of grafts, tattooing, or a combination of graft and tattooing (Fig. 72-10).

The nipple-areola area can be reconstructed by taking tissue from the contralateral nipple, labial tissue or a local flap from breast skin. A projectile nipple is created from ear cartilage. An areola can also be tatooed or grafted on the breast mound.

Nursing Management

Preoperative nursing care includes reinforcing the surgeon's discussion and teaching the woman about the planned procedure and postoperative care. If surgery is being performed for known or suspected cancer, the nurse facilitates the expression of feelings, e.g., powerlessness, disbelief, anger, fear, or depression.

In addition to providing the postoperative nursing care required by any person having surgery (Chap. 19), after reconstructive breast surgery the nurse assesses the flap or breast area, color, temperature, and capillary refill. The nipple-areola complex is also assessed if possible. Dressings are usually cone-shaped, with the nipple-areola complex open for assessment. A dusky, deep-red, purple, or black-edged areola indicates circulation impairment. The nurse documents assessment findings and immediately reports any that indicate possible complications to the surgeon.

Pain management varies with type of surgery. Epidural analgesia has been used in breast reconstruction. When epidural analgesia is used, the nurse assesses the respiratory rate, degree of pain relief, presence of numbness or paralysis in lower extremities every 2 hours. Caution must be used to protect the client from falling when ambulating.

A woman with a recent subpectoral implant needs to

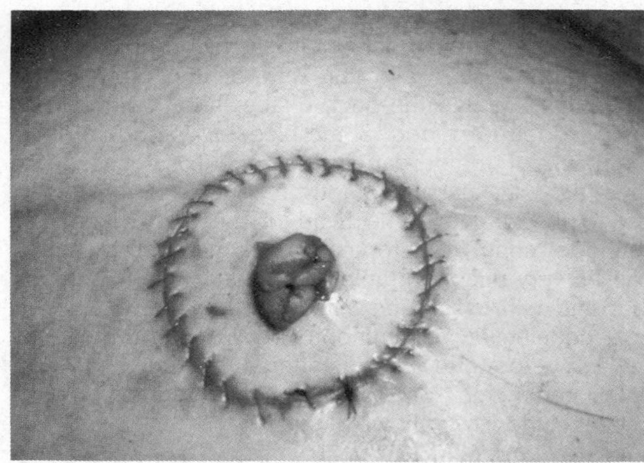

▲ **Figure 72-10**

Nipple-areolar reconstruction. (From Hutcheson, H. A. [1989]. Nipple and areolar reconstruction. *Plastic Surgical Nursing,* 9[3], 105-110.)

know that initially the implant feels very firm and is higher on the chest than a normal breast. Over time the muscle stretches, allowing the implant to drop and soften. Women with subpectoral implants do not wear bras, because the implant needs to move into the pocket created in the chest wall. Women having other types of surgery may or may not return from the operating room wearing a bra to support the breasts. A front-closing support bra, without wires, is preferred. Wearing a bra also helps some women feel more normal, encouraging a return to wellness.

Psychosocial readjustment to breast reconstruction, including incorporation of the reconstructed breast into the woman's body image, usually occurs 3 to 4 months after surgery. Following augmentation, most women incorporate a breast implant into their body image within 60 days. They often report increased self-confidence, increased feelings of equality and self-worth, and improved sexual relationships.

OTHER BREAST SURGERY

Reduction Mammoplasty

Reduction mammoplasty surgically reduces the size of large pendulous breasts. Women usually seek such surgery to reduce the physical and psychosocial discomforts of large breasts, e.g., back pain, bra strap indentations in the shoulders, inability to wear normal clothing styles, intertriginous dermatitis (skin breakdown under large breasts) from skin folds resting on each other, and being the subject of jokes or uncomfortable comments about breast size. These procedures may also be performed for men with gynecomastia (breast enlargement).

Many breast reduction techniques exist. Excess breast tissue is removed through incisions under the breast, and the nipple is (Fig. 72–11). The nipple is transposed on a pedicle of tissue or grafted onto the newly formed breast. A possible complication is loss of blood supply to the nipple-areola complex.

Subcutaneous Mastectomy

Some women develop premalignant lesions, have a high risk of breast cancer, have had cancer in one breast, or have multiple suspicious breast nodules. These women may elect to undergo prophylactic mastectomy (a mastectomy done to prevent cancer) on one or both breasts. One alternative to simple prophylactic mastectomy is subcutaneous mastectomy, during which almost all breast tissue is removed. An implant is inserted immediately, or tissue expanders may be used. This operation reduces the risk of cancer later develop-

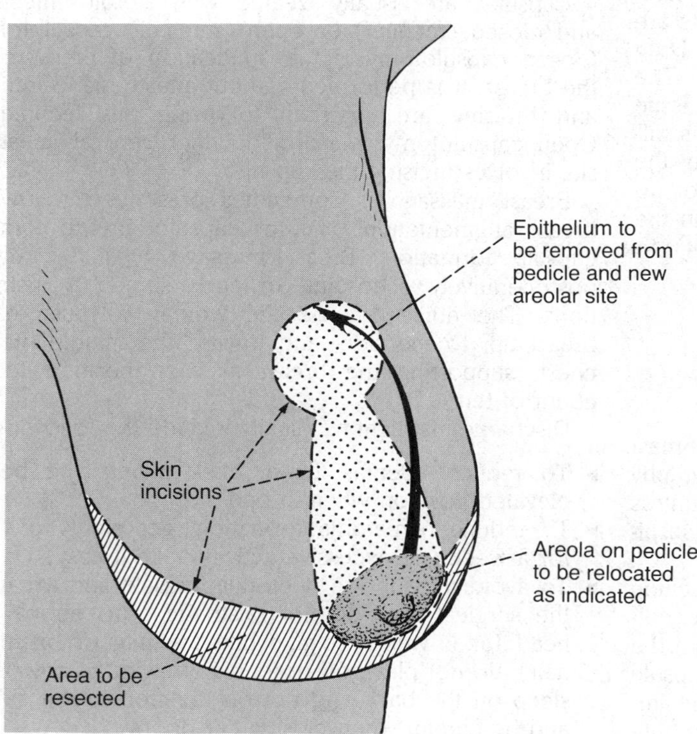

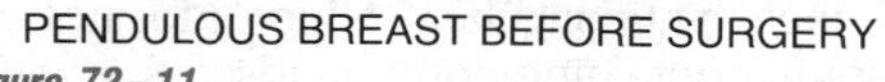
PENDULOUS BREAST BEFORE SURGERY

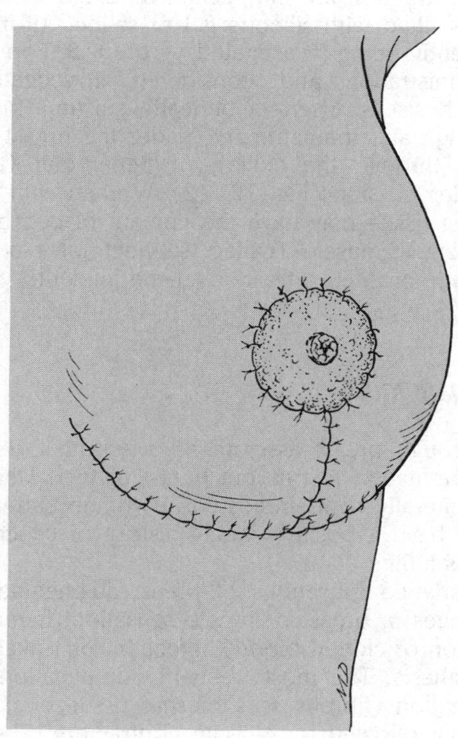
SAME BREAST AFTER RECONTOURING

▲ *Figure 72–11*

Reduction mammoplasty. Breast size is surgically reduced. Excess breast tissue is removed through incision lines as shown, and breast shape is recontoured. Nipple is relocated (e.g., moved higher) on a pedicle of tissue. The pedicle supplies the nipple with blood until new blood vessels form.

ing in the operated breast. However, a few women develop tumors in the remaining bit of breast tissue within the nipple.

Mastopexy

Mastopexy is the correction of mammary ptosis (drooping) to achieve an improved breast contour and position. Mastopexy may be performed with subcutaneous mastectomy or on normal breasts to improve contour and is part of a reduction mammoplasty.

BREAST AUGMENTATION

Overview

Breast augmentation materials used in the past to enlarge breasts have included fatty tissue tumors (lipomas) and paraffin and silicone injections. There are potential problems with all augmentation materials. Lipomas are resorbed into body tissue. Silicone injections have significant complications, including breast nodules, emboli, and death. Silicone is no longer used in injectable form for breast augmentation or breast reconstruction.

Current prostheses used for breast augmentation or reconstruction are thin, seamless, silicone rubber envelopes filled with silicone gel or saline. All implants are currently being investigated by the U.S. Food and Drug Administration and considered investigational. The prosthesis is inserted beneath existing breast tissue through an inframammary (under the breast), transaxillary (through the axilla), or periareolar (around the nipple) incision (Fig. 72-12). Women with little or no breast tissue may have the implant placed beneath the pectoralis muscle (called subpectoral placement) to provide protective tissue over the implant.

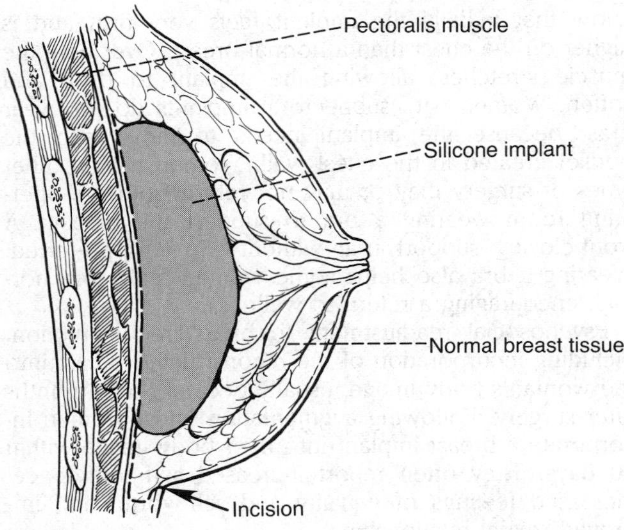

▲ Figure 72-12

Augmentation mammoplasty is achieved by inserting a saline filled implant beneath normal breast tissue (shown here) or beneath the pectoralis muscle. An inframammary approach is illustrated. Before beginning the retromammary dissection, the surgeon creates a subcutaneous flap. The incision is represented by a dashed line.

Management

Thorough breast assessment is essential before breast augmentation to rule out breast cancer. Mammography is generally contraindicated in women under 35, unless they have a positive family history of cancer or suspicious lumps.

Early complications of breast augmentation include changes in breast or nipple sensation, hematoma (collection of clotted blood), infection, or leakage from the prosthesis. The most frequent complication is capsule formation (fibrous sacs of scar tissue enclose the implant) followed by capsule contracture. These complications cause excessive breast firmness and distortion of the breast into a hard round ball. Possible causes of capsular contracture include infection, seroma (a collection of serosanguineous fluid) or hematoma formation, or impurities in the implant. Probably the basic problem is that scar tissue forms around the prosthesis to wall it off because it is a foreign substance.

Capsules are usually treated with steroid injection and closed (manual) or open (surgical) capsulotomy. Closed capsulotomy is the application of pressure to the breast. It is performed without anesthesia. Soreness and bruising are common following this technique. Open capsulotomy, performed under general anesthesia, involves incising the capsule.

Breast massage is sometimes prescribed following breast augmentation or after capsulotomy to reduce capsule formation. Breast massage typically begins postoperatively according to each surgeon's instructions. The nurse teaches the woman to push each breast up, to the side, and toward the middle of the chest, supporting the breast in each position for a count of ten.

Discharge instructions usually include the following:

- To reduce edema, for a week maintain a head-elevated position when in bed.
- To reduce hematoma formation, get plenty of rest for a week (no excessive activity; take it easy).
- To avoid moving the pectoralis muscle and irritating the surgical site, do not raise the arms above the head for 3 weeks (e.g., while washing or brushing hair), do not play golf or tennis or swim for 6 weeks, sleep on the back and not on the stomach or sides, and be careful when closing car doors.
- Because of their anticoagulant effect, do not use aspirin or aspirin-containing compounds.
- Notify the physician if bleeding or a fever over 37.6° C (99.6° F) develops.

▼ BODY CONTOURING SURGERY (LIPECTOMY)

Overview

Body contouring surgical procedures (lipectomy) remove excess skin folds or subcutaneous fat from various body parts, including the abdomen, thighs, arms, and buttocks. Suction lipectomy was discussed earlier.

Abdominoplasty is the removal of excess abdominal skin and fat and the repair and tightening of stretched abdominal muscles. An incision is made across the lower abdomen, and the skin and subcutaneous tissues are lifted off the muscles and fascia to the costal margin. The excess skin and fatty tissue are excised and recontoured. The umbilical stalk is detached and reattached once the overlying skin is in its proper position.

During abdominoplasty, the surgeon repairs diastasis (lateral separation of the rectus abdominis muscles, a benign condition occurring during pregnancy) and/or umbilical hernias when present. Indications for abdominoplasty include abdominal skin flaccidity (e.g., after multiple pregnancies and following major weight loss) and marked striae from pregnancy. An indwelling urinary catheter and surgical drains are inserted and compression stockings are applied in surgery.

Generally, obesity is best treated by diet and exercise before any body contouring surgery is performed. The exception is some people who may become highly motivated to follow a weight-reducing diet after such surgery. Careful preoperative assessment is necessary to try to identify such individuals. Individuals who have experienced major weight loss may develop excess loose skin and subcutaneous tissue over the abdomen, thighs, and arms. This tissue may hang in large folds and is greater in older people who have lost skin elasticity. Removing excess tissue usually requires more than one operation. The surgery is lengthy and there is risk of major blood loss. As much as 10 lb of redundant tissue has been surgically removed during one of these operations.

Nursing Management

Preoperative nursing care includes teaching the client having abdominoplasty that drains and a urinary catheter will be in place, a blood transfusion may be required, and an intravenous infusion is continued until a diet is tolerated. Also, the person (1) needs to lie in a contouring position (i.e., mid-Fowler's position with knees bent; see inset) when in bed postoperatively to decrease tension on the suture lines and (2) needs to walk "hunched over" until the abdominal skin relaxes, as swelling decreases. The client is taught postoperative pain management techniques. Abdominoplasty is an abdominal operation and therefore is uncomfortable. Adequate analgesia and other pain-relieving measures are essential.

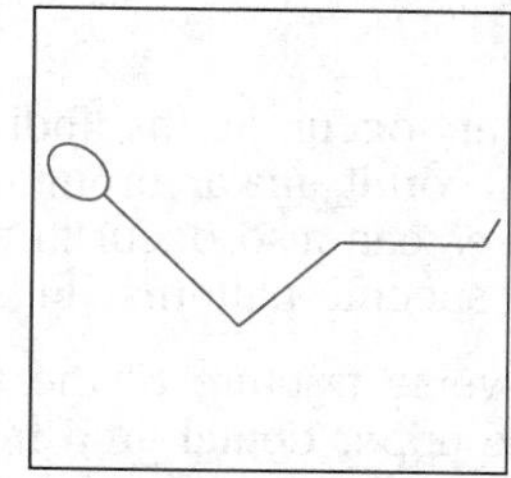

Postoperative care is based on principles of flap care and wound healing. It is essential that the blood supply to tissue be preserved.

▼ TRAUMATIC INJURY REPAIR

FACIAL INJURIES

Injuries to the face are a common result of automobile accidents and physical violence. Although they may be serious, facial injuries are seldom fatal. Proper management helps to avoid sensory impairment and permanent disability and can minimize disfigurement.

Lacerations

Facial lacerations can range from very small (.50 cm) that can be repaired under local anesthesia to extensive lacerations with soft tissue injury requiring repair under general anesthesia. Prior to closure, wounds are cleansed of debris and devitalized tissue.

Facial lacerations and facial soft tissue injuries are usually distressing to the injured person and family. Although it is important to remain optimistic about the outcome and reduce anxiety, it is also essential to provide accurate information. Teaching includes the fact that whenever there is an injury a scar forms. Scar revision can also be performed later.

Excellent wound care, including cleansing and applying prescribed topical antibiotics, promotes the healing of facial abrasions and lacerations. A person who is NPO and has dried blood in the mouth needs frequent oral care. If the person's mouth has sutures, the mouth is simply rinsed with saline. Oral care *must* be performed, however. With severe facial trauma, soft toothbrushes suffice for oral care. Waterpiks may further damage such injuries and are usually contraindicated. The nurse takes measures to prevent aspiration during oral care.

The nurse teaches the person and family to keep facial incision lines clean by applying a prescribed topical antibiotic. Skin incisions must not get wet (e.g., when showering), because moisture allows bacteria to enter the wound along the sutures. Infected incisions tend to produce more scar tissue. (Wound care is also discussed in Chap. 18.)

Facial Fractures

Facial fractures can occur in the individual bones of the face: the nasal, orbit, malar prominence, mandible, or maxilla. Fractures can also occur in patterns. Le Fort fractures occur in specific patterns (Fig. 72-13):

- Le Fort I: transverse fracture of the alveolar process separating the upper dental arch from the maxilla
- Le Fort II: fracture of the midface, maxilla, and orbits
- Le Fort III: fracture of the orbits that leads to craniofacial dissociation

The client with facial fractures has often been involved in an auto accident, an assault, or a sports injury. Pain, improper bite (malocclusion), swelling, bruising, diplopia (double vision), facial asymmetry, enophthalmos (sunken eye), or exophthalmos (bulging eye) are other clinical manifestations of facial fractures. Diagnostic assessment includes x-ray studies. Life-threatening problems such as airway obstruction, hemorrhage, or cervical spine injury that may accompany facial trauma must be managed immediately. Repair of facial fractures can be delayed for up to 3 weeks and still achieve good results.

Like all fractures, facial fractures must be reduced, stabilized, and immobilized to ensure proper healing. Methods vary according to the location of the fractures. Nasal fractures are reduced, splinted, or stabilized with nasal packing and immobilized with an external nasal splint that usually remains for at least 1 week.

Fractures of the mandible and maxilla and Le Fort fractures can be reduced and stabilized with intermaxillary fixation (wiring the upper and lower jaws together in occlusion) using arch bars. The jaws usually remain wired from 4 to 6 weeks. When small plates and screws are used to stabilize bone fragments, intermaxillary fixation may not be necessary.

Blowout fractures of the orbit can involve trapping of orbital structures between bone fragments, which may result in diplopia or enophthalmos. The integrity of the orbital floor is reestablished surgically and stabilized with wire or small plates and screws. Implant material or bone graft might be used to complete the reconstruction. Malar (cheekbone) fractures may produce facial asymmetry. These fractures may also be stabilized with wire or small plates with screws. Malar implants may be necessary to reestablish facial symmetry.

Nursing Management

The nurse assesses airway patency and breath sounds every 2 hours or more often if bleeding is present. Suction equipment is present at the bedside. The client is taught to breath through the nose. Trying to open the mouth may dislocate the fracture. When the client has intermaxillary wiring, wire cutters should be with the client at all times. If airway problems develop that cannot be managed with suction, the wires should be cut. The nurse and client need to be informed which wires should be cut. There are usually two wires on each side of the mouth and they are the only wires present that attach the top and bottom teeth.

Facial edema and ecchymosis may be present. The head of the bed is elevated. Liquid tears may be needed if the client has reduced blinking.

The nurse assesses the client for diplopia and blurry vision. When these disorders are present, the nurse assists the client's ambulation to prevent injury.

The client remains on a liquified diet until the wires

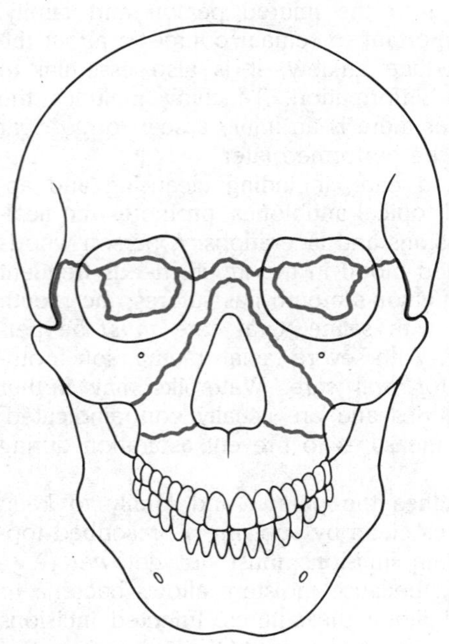

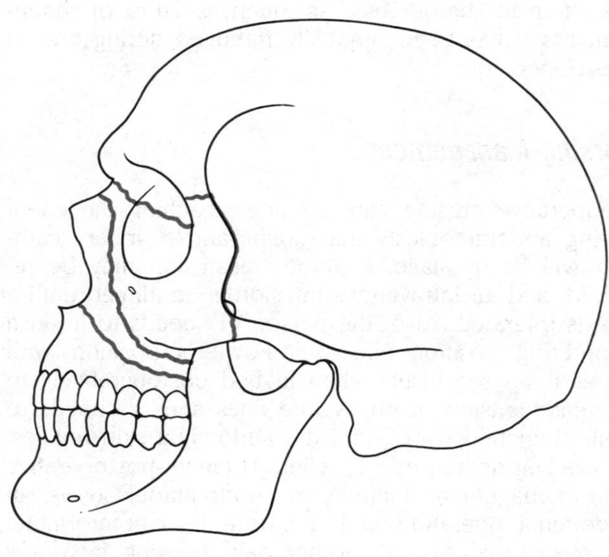

▲ Figure 72-13

Le Fort fractures.

are removed. Without adequate nutrition, clients can lose 10 to 20 lb during convalescence. The client is taught how to blenderize food and maintain adequate balances of carbohydrates, fat, protein, and calories. Milkshakes can be made with a wide variety of foods. High-calorie food supplements can augment the regular diet, and liquid multivitamins may be useful. Alcoholic and carbonated beverages can cause nausea and fizz and foam in the back of the throat, leading to airway problems and are to be avoided.

The nurse assesses the client for clear rhinorrhea or otorrhea. Rhinorrhea or otorrhea may indicate leaking cerebrospinal fluid (CSF), which must be reported to the physician. With CSF leakage, there is the potential for developing meningitis. To assess for rhinorrhea or otorrhea, the nurse observes bed linens because CSF dries in concentric, halo-like rings and does not crust.

Initially, the nurse and client must establish a means of communication. Although talking is possible through clenched teeth, hand signals or writing may be most effective initially. Trying to open the mouth may dislocate the fracture. Clients initially require reassurance that they will not choke or suffocate.

Oral hygiene aids in healing of oral wounds, prevents infection and destruction of teeth and gums, increases comfort, and enhances self-esteem. Rinsing the mouth with water or a mouthwash followed by a waterpik on low pressure removes particles from the front of the mouth while the tissues are still tender. Once the initial swelling and tenderness subside, the teeth must be brushed and the mouth rinsed following every meal and at bedtime. Pieces of paraffin wax can be placed on the open ends of the wires if they irritate buccal surfaces.

Prior to discharge, the client and family need to be taught about the wires and diet and oral care. Once the incisions have healed, the client can resume normal activities. However, while the jaws are wired, the client must carry a wire cutter and know which wires to cut. A well-balanced blenderized diet and oral care should be continued.

TRAUMATIC AMPUTATIONS

Immediate care of a person following a traumatic amputation, like that of any other injured person, focuses on life-saving activities (see Chap. 80). Hemorrhage is controlled with direct pressure on the bleeding points. Tourniquets and cautery are not used. They may damage surrounding tissue and prevent replant. All amputated parts, including small pieces of tissue, are sent to the health care facility with the injured person. As soon as possible (1) these parts are rinsed with sterile normal saline, (2) the parts are wrapped in sterile wet gauze, (3) the parts are sealed in a watertight bag, and (4) the bag is placed in ice. Cooling the amputated part reduces metabolism, increasing the time the part can survive without blood. For example, an amputated finger can survive for 18 hours if effectively cooled. Although the part is rinsed with normal saline, it is never stored or left in normal saline or on dry ice or frozen, because this causes extensive cellular damage.

Replantation surgery is performed under regional block or general anesthesia. An operating microscope guides the surgical reattachment of arteries, veins, tendons, and nerves. With severe injuries, such an operation may take 12 to 18 hours. Following surgery, incisions are dressed, the extremity is immobilized with casts or splints, and the entire extremity is elevated.

Following replantation, a person requires careful, frequent nursing assessment (every 15 minutes) and documentation of the replanted part's color, temperature, and capillary refill. A reimplanted part may have blocked arterial or venous blood flow, which, if not immediately corrected surgically, will cause the part to die. Toes and fingertips are usually left uncovered for assessment. Doppler assessments help assess pulses in the part. Temperature probes are often placed on the extremity. The surgeon usually states the ideal temperature range for replantations. A temperature decrease of 2° C or more in an hour or a decline to 32° C (89.6° F) demands immediate attention and is promptly reported to the surgeon. Aspirin is usually prescribed to reduce blood-clotting tendencies. A temperature at 34° to 36°C (93.2° to 96.5° F) is considered excellent for a replanted finger. Owing to lengthy anesthesia (18 to 24 hours), nursing care also focuses on monitoring recovery from anesthesia.

An active rehabilitation program usually begins 2 weeks after injury and continues for months. Joint motion initially may be restricted by pins through joints and by bulky dressings. Because peripheral nerves take a long time to regenerate, protective sensation may be absent for months. The person must be careful to avoid injuring the part. Rehabilitation is accomplished through prescribed active and passive range-of-motion exercises several times each day.

Psychosocial adjustment following replantation varies with each person. Grieving over the loss of appearance and function of the extremity (the replant never achieves normal complete function and appearance) is a normal reaction that requires support. Praise and encouragement during rehabilitation are very helpful.

The nurse teaches the person to avoid activities and substances that cause vasoconstriction (which precipitates necrosis) for 2 weeks after surgery, e.g., tobacco, nicotine, cocaine, and/or amphetamines. Air conditioning is harmful. The client is taught to avoid cold and chilling, e.g., by wearing extra clothing and having the car prewarmed before entering to prevent vasoconstriction.

A final indication of the success of replantation is return of sensory-motor nerve function in the reimplanted part.

Summary

Effective nursing care makes a significant difference in postoperative outcomes for plastic surgery clients. Nursing care includes interventions to maintain both physiological and psychological homeostais. Successful plastic surgery procedures require a significant degree of client compliance with treatment protocols. With shortened hospital stays and an increased number of outpatient procedures, effective client teaching is imperative to ensure that the client has realistic expectations of surgery and meets postoperative responsibilities.

Bibliography

1. American Society of Plastic and Reconstructive Surgical Nurses. (1989). *Core curriculum for plastic and reconstructive surgical nursing.* Pitman, NJ: Author.
2. Apfelberg, D. (1986). The role of lasers in current plastic surgical practice. *Plastic Surgical Nursing, 6*(1), 10-15.
3. Baptist, G. (1987). Abdominoplasty: Surgical technique and nursing care. *Plastic Surgical Nursing, 7*(2), 41-46.
4. Belger, D. (1989). A care plan for the patient having hand surgery. *Plastic Surgical Nursing, 9*(3), 126-128.
5. Black, J. (1990). Complications following blepharoplasty. *Plastic Surgical Nursing, 10*(4), 151-155.
6. Black, J. (1991). Reconstructive surgery in the elderly. *Plastic Surgical Nursing, 11*(4), 151-162, 167.
7. Black, J., & Mangan, M. (1991). Body contouring and weight loss surgery for obesity. *Nursing Clinics of North America, 26*(3), 777-788.
8. Chick, K., et al. (1989). Nursing care of adults having craniofacial surgery. *Plastic Surgical Nursing, 9*(1), 16-19.
9. Cohen, T., et al. (1992). *Wound healing: Biochemical and clinical aspects.* Philadelphia: W. B. Saunders Company.
10. Daniel, R., & Farkas, L. (1988). Rhinoplasty, Image and reality. *Clinics in Plastic Surgery, 15*(1), 1-10.
11. Dillerud, E. (1990). Abdominoplasty combined with suction lipoplasty: A study of complications, revisions and risk factors in 487 cases. *Annals Plastic Surgery, 25*(5), 333-343.
12. Fisher, J., et al. (1988). Surgical alternatives in subcutaneous mastectomy reconstruction. *Clinics in Plastic Surgery, 15*(4), 667-676.
13. Frioch, S., et al. (1990). Ambulatory surgery. A study of patient's and helpers' experiences. *AORN Journal, 52*(5), 1000-1009.
14. Furnas, H., & Rosen, J. (1991). Monitoring in microvascular surgery. *Annals of Plastic Surgery, 26*(3), 265-272.
15. Georgiade, N., et al. (1987). *Essentials of plastic, maxillofacial and reconstructive surgery.* Baltimore: Williams & Wilkins.
16. Gilboa, D., et al. (1990). Emotional and psychosocial adjustment of women to breast reconstruction and detection of subgroup(s) at risk for psychological morbidity. *Annals of Plastic Surgery, 25*(5), 397-401.
17. Goodman, T. (1988). Flaps and grafts in plastic surgery. *AORN Journal, 48*(4), 678-690.
18. Goodman, T. (1987). Tissue expansion: A new modality reconstructive surgery. *AORN Journal, 46*(2), 198-216.
19. Goodman, T., & White, S. (1988). Microvascular reconstruction. *AORN Journal, 48*(4), 666-676.
20. Hinojosa, R. (1991). Breast reconstruction through tissue expansion. *Plastic Surgical Nursing, 11*(2), 52-57.
21. Hopwood, M., & Kay, J. (1986). Anesthetic considerations in prolonged reconstructive surgeries. *Plastic Surgical Nursing, 6*(2), 52-54.
22. Hutcheson, H. (1987). Breast reconstruction using abdominal tissue: A nursing diagnoses approach. *Plastic Surgical Nursing, 7*(1), 11-16.
23. Hutcheson, H. (1991). Epidural analgesia in the postoperative patient: A nursing perspective. *Plastic Surgical Nursing, 11*(1), 6-10, 27.
24. Hutcheson, H., & Bostwick, J. (1989). Nipple and areola reconstruction. *Plastic Surgical Nursing, 9*(3), 105-109, 119.
25. Hutcheson, H., & Hartrampf, C. (1986). Breast reconstruction using abdominal tissue. *Plastic Surgical Nursing, 6*(3), 97-104.
26. Hutcheson, H., et al. (1991). Breast reconstruction using the inferior gluteus free flap. *Plastic Surgical Nursing, 11*(2), 65-71.
27. Keene, A. (1991). Perioperative assessment and nursing implications for the elderly. *Plastic Surgical Nursing, 11*(4), 143-150.
28. Kroll, S., et al. (1990). Long-term survival after chest-wall reconstruction with musculocutaneous flaps. *Plastic and Reconstructive Surgery, 86*(4), 697-701.
29. Lawson, E. (1986). Psychological aspects of the lipoplasty patient. *Plastic Surgical Nursing, 6*(3), 108-112.
30. Lerberg, L., & Prin, J. (1991). TRAM breast reconstruction. *Plastic Surgical Nursing, 11*(2), 58-61.
31. Mangan, M. (1986). Patient education with tissue exanders. *Plastic Surgical Nursing, 6*(2), 76-78.
32. McCain, L. (1992). Making a difference in the breast implant issue. *Plastic Surgical Nursing, 12*(1), 28-30.
33. McCarthy, J. (1991). *Plastic surgery.* Philadelphia: W. B. Saunders Company.
34. Meland, N., & Weimar, R. (1991). Microsurgical reconstruction: Experience with free fascia flaps. *Annals of Plastic Surgery, 27*(1), 1-8.
35. Napoleon, A., & Lewis, C. (1990). Psychological considerations in the elderly cosmetic surgery candidate. *Annals of Plastic Surgery, 24*(2), 165-169.
36. O'Hara, M. (1991). Beauty and the beast: Nursing care of the patient undergoing leech therapy. *Plastic Surgical Nursing, 11*(3), 101-104.
37. Roeder, J., & White, S. (1990). Tissue expansion for the treatment of keloids. *Plastic Surgical Nursing, 10*(3), 114-117, 125.
38. Rubayi, S., et al. (1990). Myocutaneous flaps: Surgical treatment of severe pressure ulcers. *AORN Journal, 52*(1), 40-56.
39. Russell, B., & Russell, R. (1990). The role of the plastic surgery nurse collagen specialist. *Plastic Surgical Nursing, 10*(2), 51-60.
40. Salisbury, C., & Kaye, B. (1987). Complications following rhytidectomy. *Plastic Surgical Nursing, 7*(3), 76-83.
41. Salzarulo, M. (1986). Nursing aspects of microvascular surgery. *Plastic Surgical Nursing, 6*(2), 56-60.
42. Smith, J., & Aston, S. (1992). *Grabb and Smith's plastic surgery.* Boston: Little, Brown.
43. Solomon, M., & Granick, M. (1990). Plastic surgery in the elderly. *Clinics in Geriatric Medicine, 6*(3), 633-657.
44. Steuer, K. (1991). Facial fractures. *AORN Journal, 54*(4), 773-795.
45. Teimourian, K. (1989). Complications associated with suction lipectomy. *Clinics in Plastic Surgery, 16*(2), 385-394.
46. Vander Kam, V., & Achauer, B. (1990). Lasers in plastic surgery: Applications and nursing interventions. *Plastic Surgical Nursing, 10*(3), 107-111, 125.
47. Walsh, K. (1991). Breast reconstruction using the latissimus dorsi flap. *Plastic Surgical Nursing, 11*(2), 43-51.
48. Watson, D., & James, D. (1990). Intravenous conscious sedation. *AORN Journal, 51*(6), 1512-1523.
49. Wengle, H. (1986). The psychology of cosmetic surgery: A critical overview of the literature 1960-1982. *Annals of Plastic Surgery, 16*(5), 435-443.
50. Westlake, C. (1991). Commitment to function: Microsurgical flaps. *Plastic Surgical Nursing, 11*(3), 95-100.
51. Williams, L. (1991). Mastopexy. *Plastic Surgical Nursing, 11*(3), 130-132.
52. Williams, L., & Peters, C. (1989). Blepharoplasty. *Plastic Surgical Nursing, 9*(1), 28-30.
53. Williams, L., & Peters, C. (1989). Rhinoplasty. *Plastic Surgical Nursing, 9*(2), 82-85.
54. Williams, L., & Peters, C. (1990). Reduction mammaplasty. *Plastic Surgical Nursing, 10*(2), 84-87.
55. Williams, L., & Peters, C. (1989). Rhytidectomy. *Plastic Surgical Nursing, 9*(4), 163-165.

Unit 17

Reproductive Disorders

Clients experiencing disorders of sexual structure and function are often reluctant to tell anyone about their problems because of shyness, embarrassment, and fear that private, sexual aspects of their lives will need to be discussed. They may fear being asked to disclose more about themselves than they want. Thus, unless symptoms become acute, clients experiencing reproductive and sexual disorders often put off seeking the help of health professionals.

When helping clients with reproductive and sexually related problems, remember to consider the client's psychosocial as well as physical needs. Emotional and social factors are often involved with physical problems. Be especially caring and supportive of clients who are seeking help for disorders that involve the genitalia. These clients are likely to be embarrassed and threatened by this invasion of what is probably a very private part of their lives. Allow clients to be involved in decision making and keep them informed about what is happening to them. This helps them maintain a sense of control and reduces the sense of powerlessness. Competent management of the technical aspects of care and scrupulous attention to asepsis, combined with preparation and instruction about assessment procedures and intervention, give the client added reassurance in these awkward circumstances.

Health professionals are often required to discuss reproduction and sexuality with clients. If they cannot do this openly, comfortably, and nonjudgementally, they should not try to do so. It is better to make an appropriate referral to someone who can. Health professionals who are uncomfortable talking about reproduction and sexuality need to find ways to clarify their own feelings and attitudes about sexuality and thus increase their professional competency. Nurses are not in the business of judging other people's sexual behavior. The nurse's purpose is to help others to achieve life satisfactions in ways that are comfortable and desirable to each.

This unit covers normal female and male reproduction and reproductive disorders. Sexually transmitted diseases and breast disorders also are covered in this unit.

Chapter 73

Structure and Function of the Female and Male Reproductive Systems

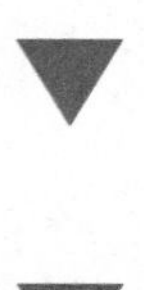

STRUCTURE AND FUNCTION OF THE FEMALE REPRODUCTIVE SYSTEM

Gonads

The gonads are the sex glands of the female (ovaries) and male (testes). The primary function is to form the cells of human reproduction. The ovaries produce ova; the testes produce spermatozoa.

Gonadal development begins during the fifth week of fetal life. Gonadal differentiation occurs in the seventh and eighth weeks of gestation with the development of the testes in the male and the ovaries in the female. In the male, the wolffian ducts develop into the epididymis, vas deferens, and seminal vesicles. The müllerian ducts regress. In the female, the wolffian ducts regress and the müllerian ducts develop into fallopian tubes, uterus, and upper vagina. The external genitalia, the glans penis, and scrotum, are complete in the male by 14 weeks of gestation. The clitoris, labia majora, and labia minora are complete in the female by 11 weeks of gestation.

▼ Female Reproductive Structure

The female reproductive organs (also called female genitalia, female genitals, or female organs of generation) consist of (1) externally (collectively termed the vulva or pudendum), the mons pubis (veneris), labia majora, labia minora, clitoris, fourchette, fossa navicularis, vestibule, vestibular bulb, Skene's ducts (glands), Bartholin's glands, vaginal opening (introitus), and possibly, hymen and (2) internally, two ovaries, two fallopian tubes, the uterus, and the vagina (Fig. 73-1).

EXTERNAL FEMALE GENITAL STRUCTURE

The external female genital structures play a role in sexual stimulation and as a barrier to protect the body from foreign materials.

Mons Pubis (Veneris)

This rounded pad of flesh lies over the symphysis pubis. It is covered with hair following puberty.

Labia Majora

These two elongated folds of tissue are separated by a cleft. Within the cleft, the vagina and urethra open. The labia majora connect anteriorly and posteriorly with commissures (the posterior one is not clearly defined).

Labia Minora

These are two small, thin, elongated folds of tissue. They lie one on each side, between the labia majora and vaginal opening, just inside and enclosing the vagina's vestibule. The labia minora each divide anteriorly, before uniting. They form the clitoris' hoodlike prepuce and enclose the clitoris.

Clitoris

This small, elongated, highly sensitive erectile structure is located under the anterior labial commissure. It is partly hidden by the anterior portion of the labia minora. Usually covered by a prepuce, the clitoris is homologous to the male penis.

Fourchette

Located at the vagina's posterior commissure, this tense band of mucous membrane connects the posterior end of the labia minora.

Fossa Navicularis

This cul-de-sac, located anterior to the fourchette, separates the fourchette from the hymen. Following rupture of the hymen or parturition (childbirth), the fossa navicularis disappears.

Vestibule

The vagina's vestibule is an almond-shaped space between the labia minora. The clitoris is at the vestibule's anterior angle, and the fourchette is its posterior boundary. The vestibule's covering mucous membranes are delicate and pink. The four major structures opening into the vestibule are the (1) urethra, (2) vagina (posteriorly), and (3 and 4) two secretory ducts of Bartholin's glands (laterally). The perineum is posterior to the vestibule, between it and the anal region.

Vestibular Bulbs

These two sacculated collections of veins (homologous to the male corpus spongiosum) lie on either side of the vagina.

Skene's Ducts (Glands, Tubules)

The openings of these two glands lie on either side of the urethra's floor, just inside the urethral opening.

Bartholin's Glands (Vulvovaginal Glands)

These two small mucous glands (homologous to the male bulbourethral glands) lie on either lateral wall of the vagina's vestibule. They are at the base of the labia majora, close to the vaginal opening. During sexual excitement, Bartholin's glands apparently secrete large amounts of mucus, lubricating the vagina for sexual activity.

Vaginal Opening (Introitus)

The vagina is discussed later. The hymen, a fold of mucous membrane that may or may not be present, partially covers the opening to the vagina. The hymen may be ruptured in various ways, for example, during exercise, sexual activity, surgery, vaginal examination, and insertion of menstrual tampons. In the past, the presence or absence of a hymen was used as proof of a woman's virginity or sexual activity. This unfortunate practice, based on chauvinism and inaccurate folklore, has caused many women to bear serious consequences. Pregnancy has been known to occur even with an undisturbed hymen. A ruptured or absent hymen does not necessarily indicate the loss of virginity.

Perineum

The female perineum (perineal body) refers to the external area between the vulva and the anus. It is lo-

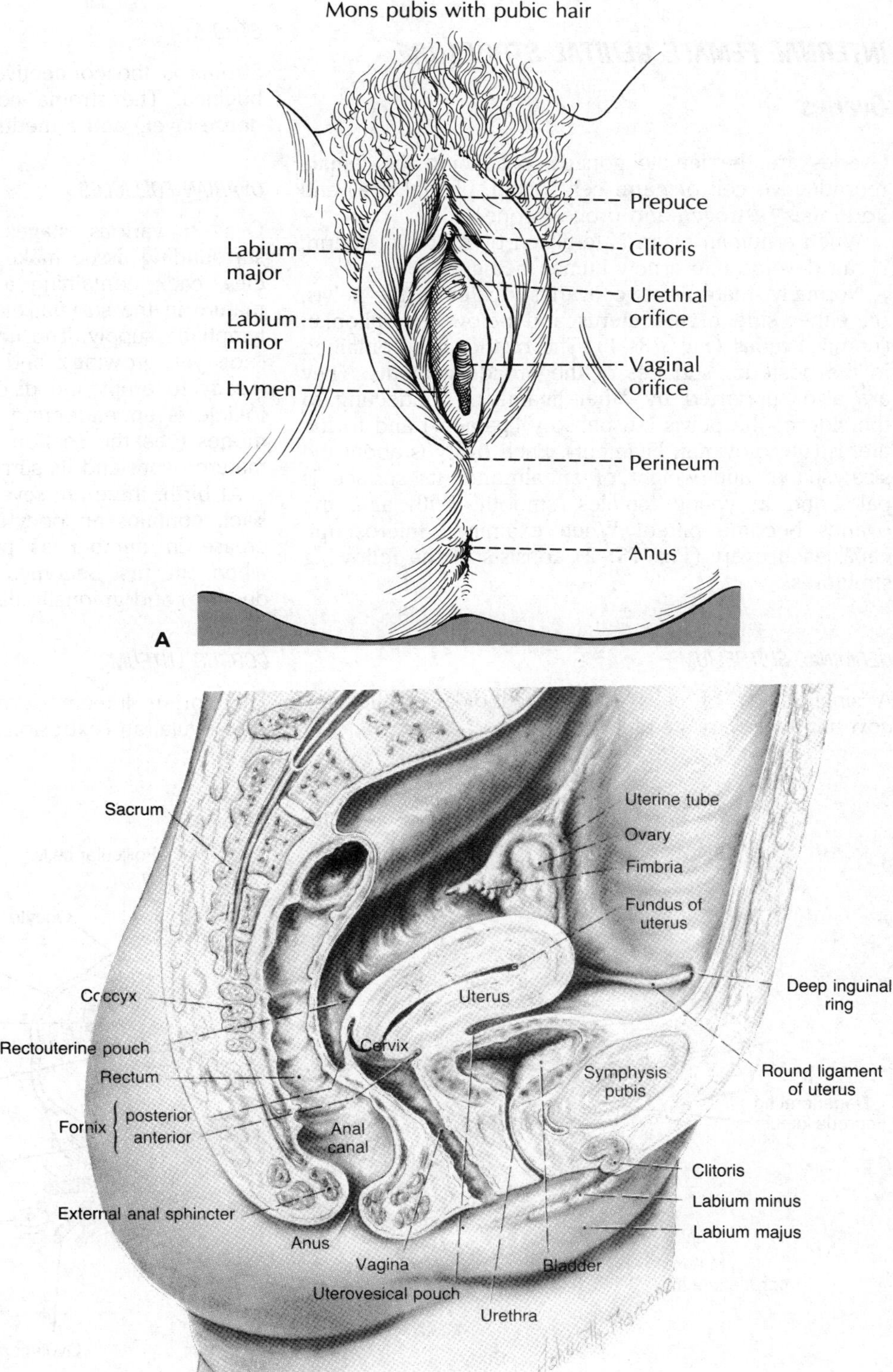

▲ Figure 73-1

A, Anatomic landmarks of external female genitalia. *B*, Midsagittal section of the female pelvis. (*B* from Jacob, S. W., et al. [1982]. *Structure and function in man* [5th ed., p. 602]. Philadelphia: W. B. Saunders.)

cated between the thighs, below the pelvic diaphragm and in front of the rectum and anus.

INTERNAL FEMALE GENITAL STRUCTURE

Ovaries

Ovaries are the female gonads, producing the female reproductive cell or germ cell (ovum, pleural ova) and hormones (estrogen and progesterone).

When a human ovum is fertilized by a human sperm, it can develop into a new human being.

Normally, there are two ovaries located in the pelvis, on either side of the uterus and below the fallopian (uterine) tubes (Fig. 73-1). The ovaries are contained in the posterior surfaces of the broad ligaments. They are also supported by other ligaments connecting to the side of the pelvis (suspensory ligament) and to the uterus (utero-ovarian ligament). Each ovary is about the size, shape, and weight of an almond. Its surface is pale, and in young females, smooth. With age, the ovaries become pitted. When examined microscopically, each ovary (Fig. 73-2) consists of the following structures.

GERMINAL EPITHELIUM

A single layer of cells (simple, cuboidal epithelium) covering the ovary's surface.

TUNICA ALBUGINEA

The tunica albuginea is a capsule of dense, collagenous connective tissue beneath the germinal epithelium.

STROMA

Stroma is the connective tissue beneath the tunica albuginea. The stroma consists of a cortex (an outer, dense layer) and a medulla (an inner, loose layer).

OVARIAN FOLLICLES

Ova in various stages of development with their surrounding tissue make up the ovarian follicles. Follicles, each containing a developing ovum, grow and mature in the stroma, close to an abundant blood and lymphatic supply. The cortex contains primary follicles (not yet growing) and mature or graafian follicles (ready to erupt and discharge mature ova). A mature follicle is an endocrine gland secreting estrogen hormones (see the section on estrogen). It consists of a mature ovum and its surrounding tissues.

At birth, there are several hundred thousand follicles. Each contains an oocyte (end-stage ovum). They decrease in number as puberty approaches (the time when one first becomes functionally capable of reproduction) and gradually disappear around menopause.

CORPUS LUTEUM

The corpus luteum develops from a graafian follicle after ovulation (extrusion of a mature ovum). This glan-

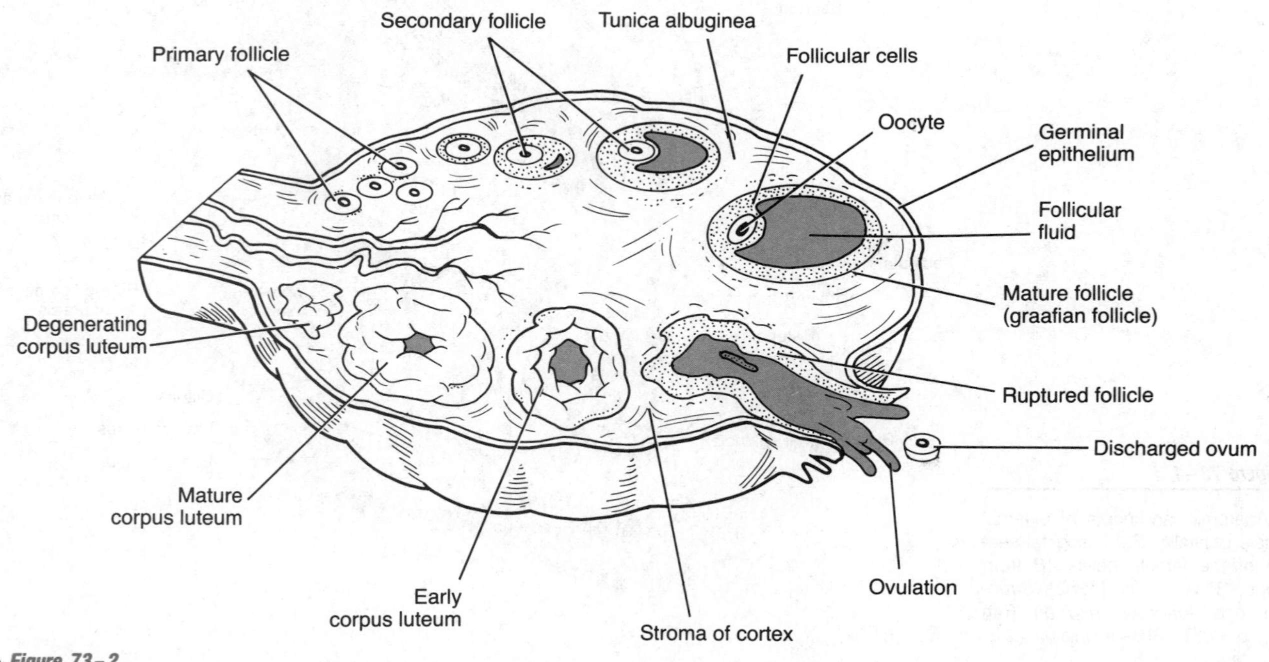

▲ **Figure 73-2**

Histology of the ovary. Diagram of parts of an ovary in sectional view. Arrows indicate the sequence of developmental stages that occur as part of the ovarian cycle. (From Tortora, G. J. [1983]. *Principles of human anatomy* [3rd ed., p. 641]. New York: Harper & Row.)

dular body produces the progesterone and estrogen hormones (see sections on estrogen and progesterone).

Fallopian Tubes

Two fallopian tubes connect the uterus to the ovaries and are the usual site of fertilization. They convey either the fertilized or the unfertilized ovum to the uterus. Each fallopian tube is about 4 inches long. Although thin, the walls of the tubes have a serosal covering, a muscular layer, and a mucous lining. The mucous lining contains hairlike cilia that undulate, sweeping the ovum (along with muscular contractions) toward the uterus.

Supported by ligaments, each fallopian tube has four subdivisions: (1) the fibrinated end, nearest to the ovary, with small, finger-like projections that cup over the ovary like a funnel; (2) the ampulla, the widest, longest part of the tube (where fertilization usually occurs); (3) the isthmus, a narrow, short, wavy portion of the tube adjacent to the uterus; and (4) the straight intramural (interstitial) portion, passing through the uterine wall.

Uterus

The hollow, thick-walled, muscular organ (1 to 2 inches thick) looks like an inverted pear. The organ is about 2 inches long, 2 inches at the widest portion, 1 inch wide at the narrowest point, that is, the cervix. The uterus is located in the pelvic cavity slightly below and between the fallopian tubes, almost at a right angle to the vagina (the passageway between the cervix and the vulva).

The normal uterus is movable in all directions. However, it maintains a normal position in the body cavity through the action of various ligaments and the pelvic floor. The right and left margins of the uterus are anchored by a pair of broad ligaments. A pair of uterosacral ligaments, on each side of the rectum, connect the uterus to the sacrum. The main ligaments that maintain the position of the uterus are the cardinal (lateral cervical) ligaments. If these ligaments are weak, the uterus is likely to drop into the vagina, that is, prolapse. The cardinal ligaments run between the pelvic wall and the cervix and vagina. Round ligaments extend from the external genitalia to the uterus, just below the fallopian tubes.

The uterus is divided into three anatomic areas: (1) fundus, (2) corpus, and (3) cervix. The fundus (dome) is the area between the insertion of the two fallopian tubes. The corpus (body) of the uterus is the largest portion, separated from the cervix by a slight constriction (isthmus). The cervix (neck) attaches to and projects into the vagina for a short distance. The cervical opening into the vagina is termed the external os. Its opening into the uterus is called the internal os or isthmus. Contents of the cervical canal include glands producing a mucin secretion. The cervix normally extends backward and downward. Usually, it forms almost a right angle with the vagina (angle of anteversion).

The body of the uterus is usually bent forward (anteflexion) over the urinary bladder. It is separated from the bladder by the uterovesical pouch. The rectum is behind the uterus. The posterior wall of the uterus is separated from the sigmoid colon above and behind the rectouterine pouch (cul-de-sac of Douglas). This cavity, an extension of the peritoneal cavity, usually contains coils of ileum.

The uterus has three functional layers: (1) parametrium, the thin peritoneal and fascial covering of the uterus; (2) myometrium (bulk of the uterus), a muscular layer composed of three layers, mainly of involuntary muscles; and (3) endometrium, the mucous membrane lining the inner surface of the uterus. The superior two thirds of the endometrium responds cyclically to hormones. Menstrual flow results from shedding of the endometrial lining when the ovum is not fertilized. A fertilized ovum implants in the endometrium.

Vagina

This musculomembranous canal connects the uterus, through the cervical opening, with the external genitalia. The vagina has three layers: (1) epithelium, (2) fibrous connective tissue, and (3) muscular layer. The vagina's upper third attaches to the cervix. At the level of attachment, there is a shallow space in front called the anterior fornix. Also, there are two lateral fornices and a deep posterior fornix.

The mucosa of the inner surface of the vaginal wall folds over in small ridges extending laterally upward. This rugal pattern adds to the vagina's elasticity, making it very distensible. The rectum is posterior to its lower two thirds.

The vagina's smooth rugal pattern and elasticity diminish with age during the menopausal and postmenopausal years. The vagina can easily become infected from urethral or rectal secretions, and vice versa.

PELVIC BLOOD SUPPLY, INNERVATION, AND LYMPHATIC DRAINAGE

Blood Supply

The most important blood supply to the external genitalia comes from the internal iliac (hypogastric) artery, a division of the common iliac artery. This artery branches to supply the pelvic floor, pelvic walls, and pelvic viscera. Two branches of this artery are the (1) uterine artery and (2) vaginal artery. The former provides a rich vascular bed to the uterus, and the latter to the vaginal walls. The ovarian artery (that arises at the level of the renal artery) supplies blood to the ovaries, fallopian tubes, and body of the uterus. Venous drainage roughly parallels the arterial supply.

Innervation

Both the sympathetic and parasympathetic autonomic nervous systems innervate pelvic structures. The uterine myometrium is innervated only by the sympathetic nerve fibers. The perineum is principally supplied by the pudendal nerve.

Lymphatic Drainage

The pelvic lymphatics consist of a rich network of superficial and deep systems that roughly parallel the blood supply. There is an intermingling of the pelvic lymphatics and blood vessels. This is significant to the potential spread of cancer.

BREAST STRUCTURE AND FUNCTION

Breasts have an important role in our culture. Sexuality and femininity are associated with breasts. Because breasts are visible, their size and shape are often viewed as a measure of one's sexuality, femininity, and attractiveness. The physiologic function of female breasts to feed infants is equally important.

A breast (mammary duct) is a modified sebaceous gland and a skin appendage (Fig. 73–3). The female breast extends vertically from the second to sixth rib and horizontally from the sternum to the midaxillary line. It lies entirely within the anterior chest wall's superficial fascia. The largest part of the breast rests on fascia of the pectoralis major and the remainder on fascia of the serratus anterior. An average nonlactating breast weighs between 150 and 250 g, and a lactating breast weighs 400 to 500 g.

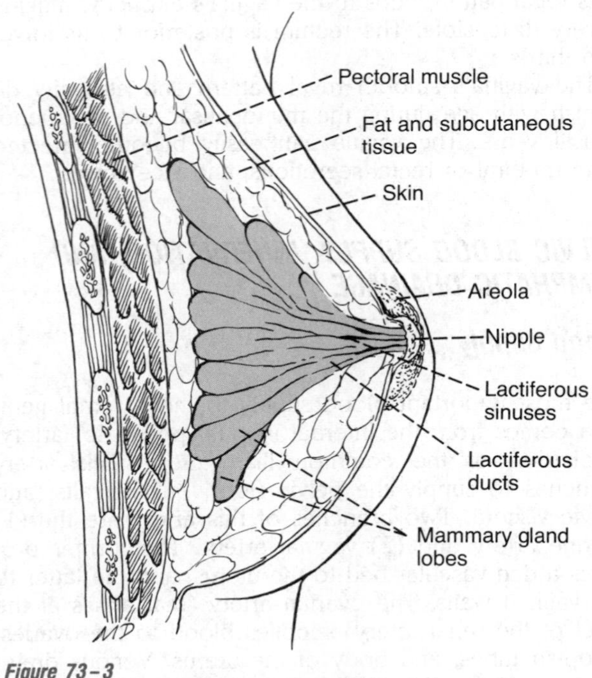

▲ **Figure 73–3**

The structure of the female breast.

The parenchyma of a breast consists of ductular, lobular, and acinar epithelial structures. The stroma of a breast is made of fibrous and fatty tissue. The central and upper portions are mostly glandular and the periphery is mostly fatty. A breast consists of 12 to 20 lobes subdivided into lobules. These, in turn, are made up of acini. Breast lobes are arranged like the spokes of a wheel around the nipple. Each lobe is drained by a duct, 12 to 20 of which open on the nipple. Each duct opens independently on the surface of the nipple and has a dilated ampulla just before its opening. The largest amount of a breast's glandular tissue is located in its upper lateral quadrant. A projection of breast tissue extends from this quadrant into the axilla, i.e., the tail of Spence. Because the upper quadrant and the tail of Spence contain the largest amount of breast tissue, this is the area where the majority of tumors occur (see Fig. 78–1).

A breast is fixed to the overlying skin and underlying pectoral fascia with fibrous bands (Cooper's ligaments). A fascial cleft on the breast's undersurface permits breast mobility. The nipple is located at the fourth intercostal space. Its base is surrounded by a circular pigmented area called the areola. The administration of estrogen increases pigmentation of the areola at any age. The areolar epithelium contains some small hairs and sebaceous glands, sweat glands, and accessory mammary glands. The sebaceous glands (Montgomery's glands) enlarge during pregnancy and lactation to lubricate the nipple.

The two main sources of a breast's blood supply are the lateral mammary artery and the lateral thoracic artery. These arteries form an extensive network of anastomoses. The main veins follow the arterial pattern. Lymphatic pathways, in general, follow the pathways of the veins. There are three types of lymphatic drainage of the breast: (1) cutaneous or superficial lymphatic drainage from the skin, (2) areolar lymphatic drainage from the areola and nipple, and (3) glandular lymphatic drainage from deep glandular tissue (Fig. 73–4). The radical mastectomy, sometimes used to treat breast cancer, is based on lymphatic drainage pathways. In less radical surgery, axillary dissection determines the number of lymph nodes involved. This involvement is the best indictor of prognosis. Nerve supply is derived from the anterior and lateral branches of the fourth to sixth intercostal nerves.

Three types of physiologic changes affect the breast, i.e., those related to (1) growth and development, (2) the menstrual cycle, and (3) pregnancy and lactation.

The hormones estrogen and progesterone act synergistically with pituitary growth hormones prolactin and corticotropin to produce breast development and function. Estrogen is responsible for the growth of the breast and periductal stroma. Progesterone promotes the development of lobular and acinar structures. During the normal menstrual cycle, the cyclic secretion of these hormones is responsible for female breast structure. After menopause, the ovaries stop producing es-

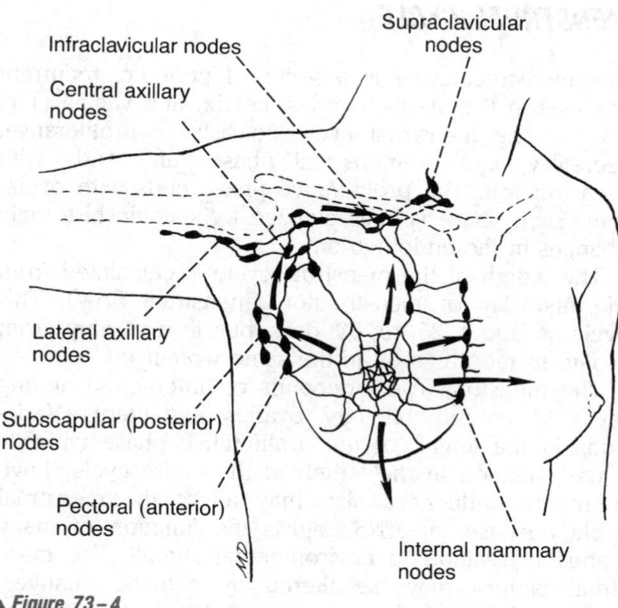

▲ *Figure 73–4*

Routes of lymphatic drainage from the breast. These routes are very important routes of spread of breast cancer.

trogen and progesterone. Estrogen is then produced by the adrenals through stimulation from the anterior pituitary. During this life stage, there is a continuous involution of the breast with loss of the glandular elements and tissue atrophy.

During pregnancy, estrogen, progesterone, and pituitary hormones increase, increasing breast vascularity and the permeability and dilation of breast lymphatics. When pregnancy ends, prolactin initiates lactation. Prolactin and corticoptropin help maintain lactation. The "letting down" (flow) of milk is a complex response involving a mother's subjective response and the mechanical stimulation of suckling. Suckling releases the pituitary hormone oxytocin into the bloodstream. This causes the mammary acini to contract and release milk into the duct system.

The male breast is similar to that of a preadolescent girl. It has a few ducts surrounded by connective tissue. Estrogen can cause a man's breast to enlarge (gynecomastia; see Chap. 78) due to growth of ducts and supporting tissue. Accumulation of fat in obese men can also make the breasts appear large.

▼ Female Reproductive Function

FEMALE SEXUAL DIFFERENTIATION

The female reproductive system develops between week 5 and 18 of gestation. Wolffian ducts regress and müllerian ducts develop into fallopian tubes, uterus, and upper vagina. The ovary secretes estradiol and progesterone. These sex steroids affect the growth, differentiation, and function of the female reproductive system.

FEMALE HORMONES

The ovaries manufacture hormones that (1) stimulate sexual desire; (2) interact with the hypothalamic-pituitary unit and the uterus for ovarian changes (follicular development, ovulation, corpus luteum formation), pregnancy (implantation of a fertilized ovum), or menstruation; and (3) have additional effects elsewhere in the body.

Estrogens

Estrogens (female sex hormones) produce cyclic changes in the uterine endothelium and vaginal epithelium. Estrogens are steroids secreted in both sexes by the adrenal cortex and, in women, by the ovary (main source) and placenta. Natural estrogens include estradiol, estrone, and estriol. When administered therapeutically, estrogens are usually given orally as a conjugate or as diethylstilbestrol (DES), a synthetic estrogenic substance.

Estrogens may be used therapeutically as a replacement hormone during menopause. They are administered, often alternating with progesterone, in the lowest effective dose (see the section on menopause).

The effects of hormones on menstruation are discussed later. The main effects of estrogenic stimulation on the body occurs at puberty, and include breast growth (fatty tissue deposition, pigmentation), fat deposition in the vulva, pubic and axillary hair growth, bony pelvis growth and broadening, vaginal epithelial changes, and general growth.

Estrogens also influence (1) positive nitrogen balance maintenance; (2) calcium and phosphorus metabolism and calcium retention in bones; (3) sodium chloride retention and, hence, sodium and water balance; (4) control of blood proteins and lipids; (5) the vascular and skeletal systems; and (6) thyroid function, insulin production, and adrenal function. It is not known precisely how these systems interact. Thus, it is controversial whether or not estrogen replacement should be given during menopause. Osteoporosis (increased bone porosity) is associated with estrogen deficiency in adult women.

Progesterone

Progesterone is a steroid hormone with varied functions. For example, it helps prepare the endometrium to receive and implant the fertilized ovum. After implantation, progesterone promotes development of the placenta (a spongy structure in the uterus that provides nourishment for a developing fetus) and the mammary glands.

Progesterone is used therapeutically to treat threatened abortion and menstrual problems, for example, dysmenorrhea, amenorrhea. It is obtained from the placenta and the corpus luteum.

Progesterone plays a minor role in sodium and water balance. It also influences nitrogen balance, breast function, and body temperature during the menstrual cycle.

MENARCHE

Menarche, the beginning of menstrual life, is an important developmental milestone in a woman's life. The event is biologic, psychological, and social. A young woman experiencing menarche needs to understand what is happening to her. Psychosocial support and knowledge of how to take care of herself are essential.

Menarche is preceded by characteristic body changes occurring between ages 9 and 16. Breast development varies but takes about 4 to 5 years. The average age for menarche in the United States is now 12.8 years.

Dramatic changes in body image occur. Girls appear to act differently after menarche, and they see themselves differently. The body image is reorganized toward greater sexual maturity and feminine differentiation.

Many factors affect the age at which menarche occurs. Genetic factors are significant. Hence, a late-maturing girl is likely to have a late-maturing mother or father. Undernourished young women are likely to experience delayed menarche. Menarche occurs later in girls who exercise extensively, such as athletes or dancers. Menarche may be delayed by several conditions, such as diabetes mellitus, congenital heart disease, and ulcerative colitis. Menarche can occur earlier than average with other conditions, such as hypothyroidism, central nervous system (CNS) tumors, and head trauma. Girls start to menstruate after their growth spurt has peaked and usually grow only 2 to 3 inches more after the onset of menstruation.

Ideally, girls should be taught about menarche as pubertal changes begin to occur. Girls who feel adequately prepared both physically and psychosocially for menarche have a more positive initial experience with menstruation. Information about menstrual physiology, menstrual hygiene, and the personal experience is useful. Having appropriate sanitary products ready for use when menarche does occur is also helpful. The girl's mother or significant female is critical in providing information and support. Some women need preparation for fulfilling this role. Sex education also should be included in the preparation for menarche. Information should be provided about reproduction, and sexually active teenagers require contraceptive counseling.

Early menstrual cycles are often irregular and anovulatory (menstrual flow is not preceded by ovulation, production, and discharge of an ovum). Although regular menstrual cycles may not occur for several years, any individual cycle may be ovulatory and, thus, potentially fertile.

MENSTRUAL CYCLE

The menstrual cycle is a series of periodic, recurrent changes in the uterus, ovaries, cervix, and vagina (Fig. 73-5). The menstrual cycle consists of proliferative, secretory, and premenstrual phases and ends with menstruation. The proliferative phase ends with ovulation. Each phase is characterized by specific histologic changes in the endometrium.

The length of the menstrual cycle is calculated from the first day of menstruation (menstrual flow). This cycle is about 25 to 32 days but it may vary from month to month (even in the same woman).

The menstrual cycle depends on interaction among the CNS, anterior pituitary, ovaries, and uterus. Variations in the length of the proliferative phase typically cause variation in the length of the entire cycle. Environmental influences also may affect the menstrual cycle because the CNS adjusts the function of many glands in relation to environmental stimuli. The menstrual pattern may be altered by climatic changes, emotionally traumatic experiences, stress, or acute or chronic illness.

Proliferative Phase

The proliferative phase of the menstrual cycle depends on the ration of follicle-stimulating hormone (FSH) to luteinizing hormone (LH).

In the ovary, after menstrual flow has begun, primary follicles (containing oocytes, i.e., primitive ova) and follicular cells begin to develop under the influence of FSH from the anterior pituitary gland (Fig. 73-5). The thecal (stromal) cells surrounding ova produce estrogens. The level of estrogen produced by these cells begins to rise, which signals the pituitary to inhibit FSH production and to stimulate secretion of LH. Then, acting together, the two pituitary hormones stimulate further estrogen production. Estrogens, in turn, further inhibit FSH release from the anterior pituitary. The LH hormone becomes dominant, stimulating further maturation of the follicle.

About 2 days before ovulation, one follicle (now called a graafian follicle) reaches full maturity. The remaining primary follicles degenerate, that is, follicle atresia takes place. The graafian follicle migrates to the ovary's cortex, where it ruptures through the ovary's wall (ovulation).

Meanwhile, in the uterus, related changes are occurring primarily in response to estrogen from the developing follicle. At the end of a menstrual flow, the uterine endometrium (containing surface epithelium, glands, connective tissue, spaces, and blood vessels) is very thin. Much of it has sloughed off during menstrual flow. Estrogen begins creating a new endometrial surface layer and restoring the uterine epithelium. It stimulates growth of glands and stroma. The epithelium becomes thicker and more vascular. Endometrial proliferation peaks about 2 days before ovulation.

The cervix also undergoes changes. The most impor-

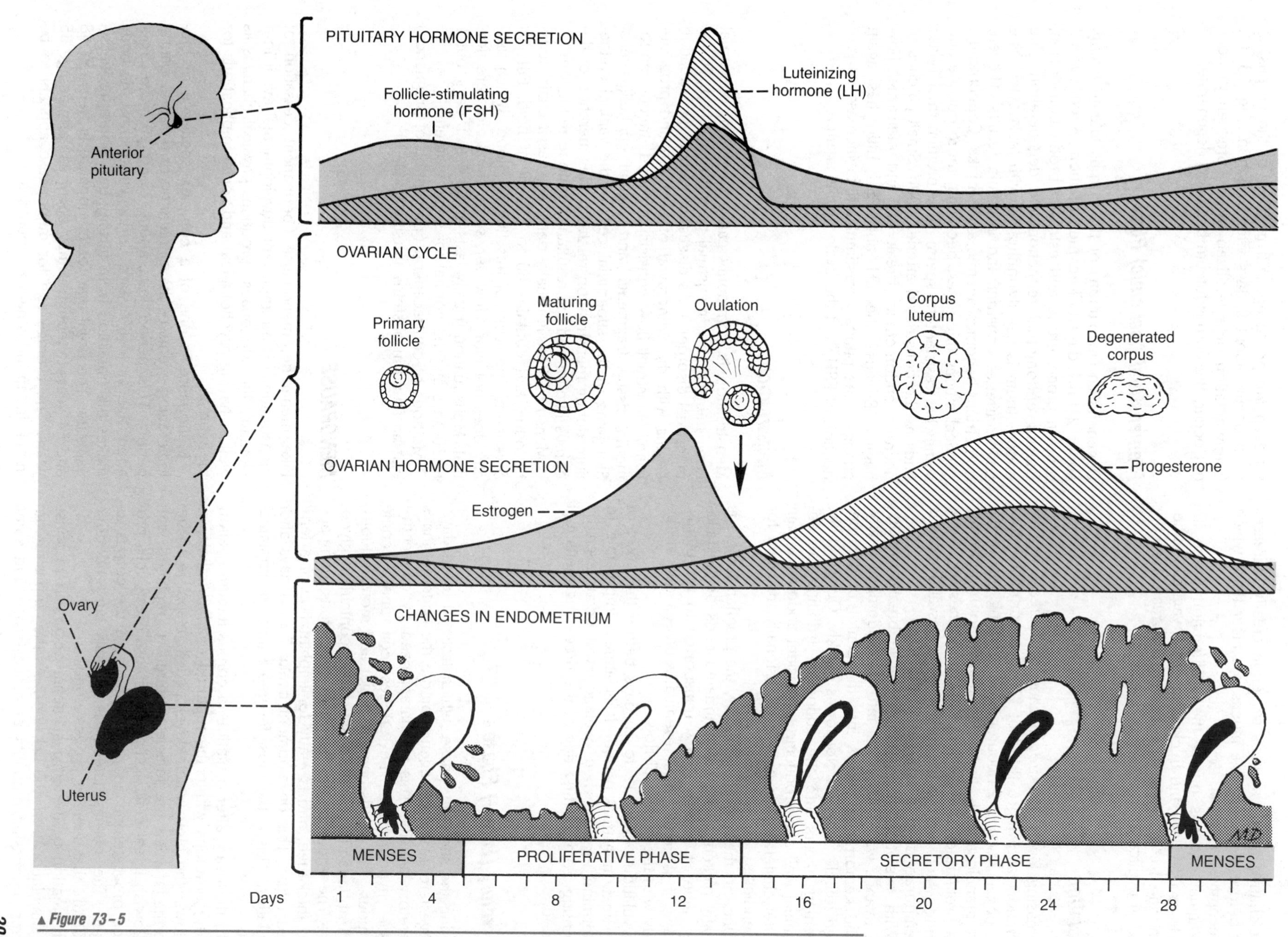

▲ ***Figure 73–5***

Menstrual (uterine) cycle. Note hormonal control of the menstrual cycle and the effects on ovaries *(center)* and endometrium *(below).*

tant change is that mucous secretion greatly increases just before ovulation. The mucus is a clear fluid, which is receptive to sperm.

Vaginal changes during the proliferation phase include proliferation and thickening of the vaginal epithelium due to estrogen. This change is greatest at the time of ovulation.

Ovulation

Increasing levels of estrogen cause a decrease in FSH secretion, allowing a flood of LH to occur. This process occurs over a 24-hour period, causing the thecal and granulosa cells lining the follicle to hypertrophy and proliferate. The LH flood also produces ovulation, during which the ovarian follicle collapses and there is a temporary drop in estrogen production.

With ovulation, the graafian follicle breaks through the ovary's wall and passes into the abdominal cavity. Some hemorrhage occurs into the center of the ruptured follicle, where a clot forms quickly. Occasionally, bleeding occurs into the abdomen, irritating the abdominal wall and producing a transient abdominal pain (mittelschmerz). This pain is occasionally mistaken for appendicitis.

Once in the abdominal cavity, the graafian follicle is usually picked up by the fimbriated ends of the fallopian tube. It is then slowly transported to the uterus. Unless it is fertilized, it eventually passes out of the body with the menstrual flow.

Ovulation occurs 12 to 15 days before the onset of the next menstrual period. It is almost impossible to determine exactly when ovulation will occur even by counting from the first day of the preceding menstrual period.

Secretory (Luteal) Phase

During the secretory phase, which lasts 10 to 14 days, progesterone and estrogen promote the endometrium's secretory activity. This is characterized by connective tissue hypertrophy. The arteries coil and become tortuous. The glands become larger and more tortuous, and abundantly secrete a substance containing glycogen. The endometrium becomes edematous, compact, and thickened, and is ready for implantation of a fertilized ovum. This development peaks 7 to 8 days after ovulation. This is the most favorable time for implantation.

In the ovary after ovulation, a corpus luteum (yellow body) develops within the ruptured ovarian follicle, as follows: the clot, which developed in response to hemorrhage when the follicle ruptured, is replaced with yellowish luteal cells containing lipids. These cells produce progesterone and eventually form the corpus luteum. The corpus luteum is actually an endocrine structure that secretes progesterone.

Formation of the corpus luteum occurs in response to stimulation from the LH flood. As the corpus luteum forms, increasing amounts of progesterone and some estrogen are produced. Full maturity of the corpus luteum occurs about 9 days after ovulation (Fig. 73–6). If implantation of a fertilized ovum (pregnancy) does not occur, the corpus luteum begins to degenerate.

Premenstrual (Ischemic) Phase

Degeneration (involution) of the corpus luteum occurs about 2 to 4 days before menstruation. A concurrent drop in progesterone and estrogen production occurs, causing endometrial retraction and degeneration. The endometrium is heavily infiltrated with leukocytes. The coiled arteries constrict and ischemia results. The endometrium becomes anemic and shrinks. Concurrently, cervical mucus decreases, becoming more opaque and somewhat resistant to sperm. The premenstrual phase ends as the constricted arteries open. Small patches of necrotic endometrium break off, and menstrual flow begins. Because the LH and FSH ratio has again changed, the pituitary is stimulated to increase its production of FSH, and the cycle begins again.

Menstruation

Menstruation is commonly called a period, menstrual flow, menses, or a menstrual period (see Chap. 76 for menstrual disorders). As discussed earlier, menstruation begins with the withdrawal of estrogen and progesterone. Menstrual flow consists of blood, mucus, endometrial tissue fragments, and vaginal epithelial cells. Sloughing of the superficial cells of the vaginal epithelium during menstruation relates to degeneration of the corpus luteum and the resultant hormone reduction.

Menstrual flow is usually dark red, has a characteristic odor, and contains 60 to 150 ml of fluid. Fifty to seventy-five per cent of this fluid is blood, which usually does not clot. However, some small clots are normal. Menstruation usually lasts about 4 to 5 days, but 1 to 10 days may be normal for some women.

Methods of contraception (prevention of pregnancy) can be found in obstetric nursing texts.

MENOPAUSE

Like menarche, menopause (permanent cessation of menstruation) is an important developmental event in a woman's life. Menopause produces physical changes as well as having psychological and social implications for the woman.

Menopause is one of a complex sequence of biologic aging events of the climacteric or perimenopausal period. This period lasts about 15 to 20 years from about age 40 to 60 years, during which time the body makes the transition from fertility to a nonreproductive capacity. The usual age for menopause is between 48 and 54 years, although it may occur as early as age 35 years. The average age for menopause appears to be increasing in industrialized countries.

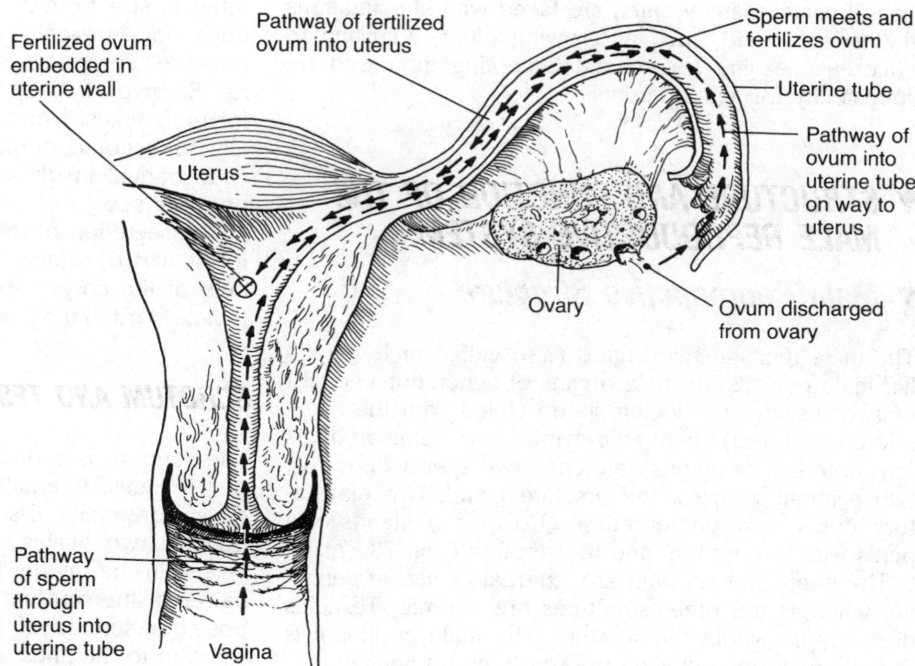

▲ *Figure 73-6*

Pathways of sperm and ovum in the female reproductive organs. (Modified from Miller, B. F., & Keane, C. B. [1992]. *Encyclopedia & dictionary of medicine, nursing, & allied health* [5th ed., p. 1085]. Philadelphia: W. B. Saunders.)

The pattern of menstrual cessation varies. It may be abrupt but more often occurs over 1 to 2 years. Periodic menstrual flow gradually occurs less frequently, becoming irregular and less in amount. Anovulatory cycles are common during this time, and occasional episodes of profuse bleeding may be interspersed with episodes of scant bleeding. Menopause is said to have occurred when there have been no menstrual periods for 12 consecutive months. Any spontaneous uterine bleeding after this time is abnormal and requires investigation. Unplanned pregnancy may occur during the premenopausal period. Advise sexually active women to use contraception for at least 6 months after menses have ceased.

Causes of Menopause

The cause of menopause is not known. However, certain predictable physiologic changes and experiences occur. Premenopausal ovaries contain abundant germinal structures in various stages of development. During the climacteric, a gradual decrease in the number of maturing ovarian follicles and a parallel decline in the production of ovarian estrogen occur. Over time, as the ovaries become unresponsive to pituitary hormones, and toward the end of the climacteric, the ovaries atrophy. Other changes associated with the menopause, such as hot flashes and vaginal atrophy, are related to decreased estrogen production.

Most women experience menopause without difficulty. The menopausal woman of today is younger looking, active, and has more positive attitudes about menopause than in the past.[1] The stereotype of the typical menopausal woman, who is miserable with a diffuse range of symptoms for which she seeks medical assistance, has been disproved. Research shows that menopause itself does not cause poorer health or greater use of health care.[13] The perimenopause marks the beginning of the healthy aging process in women. However, some women do become distressed enough to require professional assistance.

Menstrual variation such as irregular menses, skipped periods, and occasional scanty or moderately heavy menses may happen a year or two before menopause occurs. Usually, these variations do not require any intervention.

Although further study is needed about psychosexual changes associated with the perimenopausal period, it is likely that any changes that occur are the result of a complex interaction among anatomic, physiologic, psychological, and social factors. Vaginal lubrication may be decreased in the perimenopausal years, and this dryness may cause discomfort or bleeding with intercourse. Estrogen replacement therapy can usually relieve this discomfort. Some studies have reported lessened interest in sexual activity among menopausal women, but other authors claim freedom from pregnancy allows women to relax and enjoy intercourse more.

Menopause is not a disease. Most women pass through menopause with minimal or no problems. With increased life expectancy, the typical woman can spend over a third of her life in the postmenopausal years. This can be a time to set new goals and gain a new lease on life. Nurses can help counter some misconceptions and negative connotations often associated with menopause by stressing the normal and positive aspects of the experience. The nurse should help to clarify misconceptions about menopause and differentiate menopausal physiologic manifestations from midlife developmental changes. During the menopausal years, many women are faced with life situations that affect mood, such as growing older, adjusting to children's leaving home, and accepting increased responsibility for aging parents.

▼ STRUCTURE AND FUNCTION OF THE MALE REPRODUCTIVE SYSTEM

▼ Male Reproductive Structure

The male reproductive organs (also called male genitalia, male genitals, or male organs of generation) consist of two testicles producing sperm (filled with the seminiferous tubules), two epididymis, two seminal ducts (vas deferens or ductus deferens), two spermatic cords, two seminal vesicles, the prostate gland, two ejaculatory ducts, two bulbourethral (Cowper's) glands, the penis with the urethra, and the scrotum (Fig. 73-7).

The penis and scrotum are external or visible genitalia, whereas the other structures are internal. Testicles normally lie within the scrotum. The male perineum is the external area between the scrotum and anus.

PENIS AND RELATED STRUCTURES

The penis is both a sexual organ (organ of copulation) and an organ for urination. This cylindric, pendulous structure suspends from its attachment to the pubic arch. The skin of the penis is dark, hairless, thin, and loose (permitting considerable distention).

Structurally, the penis consists mainly of erectile tissue, covered by skin, and is arranged into 3 columns. Two columns of erectile tissue *(corpus cavernosum)* form two lateral columns. The median column *(corpus spongiosum)* contains the urethra, which forms a pathway for eliminating urine and semen. Each corpus is enclosed in a fascial sheath *(tunica albuginea)*. All are surrounded by a thick fibrous envelope *(Buck's fascia)*. The portion of the penis between its end or head and its attachment to the pubic bone is the shaft.

In males, the urethra's external opening (meatus or orifice) is in the glans (glans penis), that is, the cone-shaped end or head of the penis. The glans is the distal portion of the corpus spongiosum. The expanded proximal portion of the glans is the corona, and its junction and the corpus cavernosa is the coronal sulcus. A flap of movable skin (foreskin or prepuce) covers the glans.

Smegma is a cheesy, thick, odoriferous secretion of sebaceous glands occurring under this hood of skin. (In females, smegma occurs around the clitoris, under the labia minora.)

Usually, the penis is flaccid. However, with varied stimuli (physical stimulation, sexual excitement) it becomes firm and erect. An erection occurs as the corpus cavernosum fills with blood. The tissue becomes congested (hyperemic) with an unusual amount of blood. Following orgasm (climax of sexual excitement) and ejaculation (expulsion of semen), the erection leaves as hyperemia subsides. An erect penis may differ in size from a flaccid penis. Penis size, however, does not physically influence either partner's sexual pleasure. The penis is homologous to the female clitoris. Embryos initially have all the necessary structures for both sexes. Normally, sexual organs develop gradually to become predominantly either female or male, with gradual involution of the sexual structures of the opposite sex.

The secretion of the bulbourethral (Cowper's) glands forms part of semen. These two small glands above the bulb of the corpus spongiosum are homologous to the female Bartholin's glands.

SCROTUM AND TESTES

The scrotum is a double pouch hanging from the root of the penis. Internally, beneath the scrotal skin, muscular contractile tissue *(tunica dartos)* separates the pouch's two halves. Externally, the scrotal skin is bisected in the middle by a *raphe* (ridge) where the two halves of the scrotum join. The raphe extends from the posterior surface of the penile shaft under the entire scrotum to the anus.

Each half of the scrotum contains (1) a testicle with its epididymis and (2) part of a spermatic cord. The spermatic cord is held together by spermatic fascia. Each cord is made up of nerves, testicular vessels (spermatic artery, vein, lymph vessels), and the vas deferens. The vas deferens (ductus deferens, seminal duct) is the testicle's excretory duct. It is the continuation of the epididymis and is a tube of musculature about 45.7 cm (18 inches) long. The vas deferens conveys sperm from the testicle to the prostatic urethra, that is, from the epididymis to the ejaculatory duct. The ejaculatory duct then conveys semen into the urethra.

The scrotum's left side hangs lower than the right because the left spermatic cord suspends the testicles and extends from them into the inguinal ring. The cord goes through the inguinal canal, and the vas deferens continues into the abdominal cavity. It passes behind the bladder, anterior to the rectum, to join the duct of the seminal vesicle, becoming the ejaculatory duct. The spermatic cord is movable for protection from trauma and facilitates optimal spermatogenesis, that is, mature, functional sperm formation.

Testicles are the male gonads. They produce the male hormone (testosterone) and the male reproductive cells (sperm).

Testicles (testes) are smooth, solid, oval structures about 4.0 cm long and 2 to 2.5 cm wide. An inelastic, dense, fibrous *tunica albuginea* encloses each testicle.

The epididymis is a small, oblong body resting on and beside each testicle's posterior surface. Each epididymis consists of a convoluted tube 3.9 7 to 6.1 m (13 to 20 feet) long. A testicle's upper end is capped by the head of an epididymis. The body of an epididymis attaches to a testicle's posterior surface. At the lower end of a testicle, the tail of an epididymis becomes continuous with the vas deferens that join other vessels to form the spermatic cord. The head of an epididymis contains 12 to 20 testicular efferent ducts.

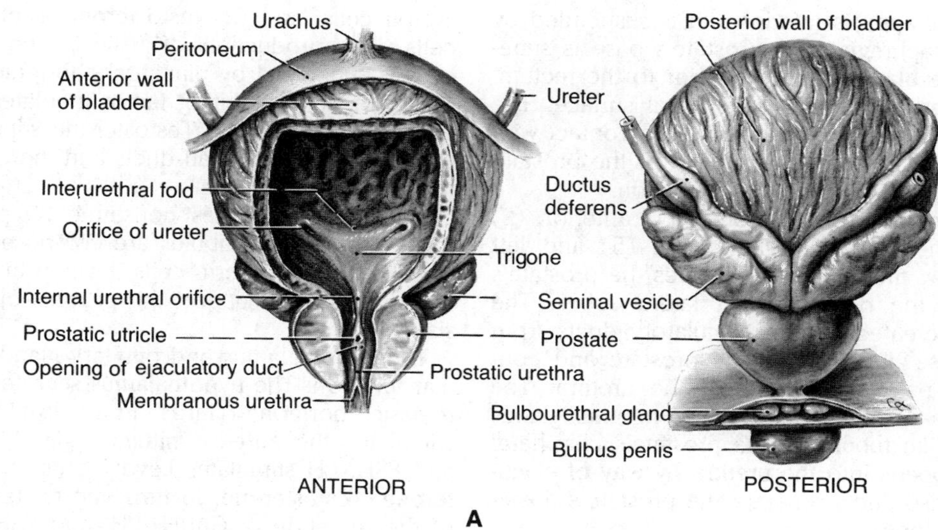

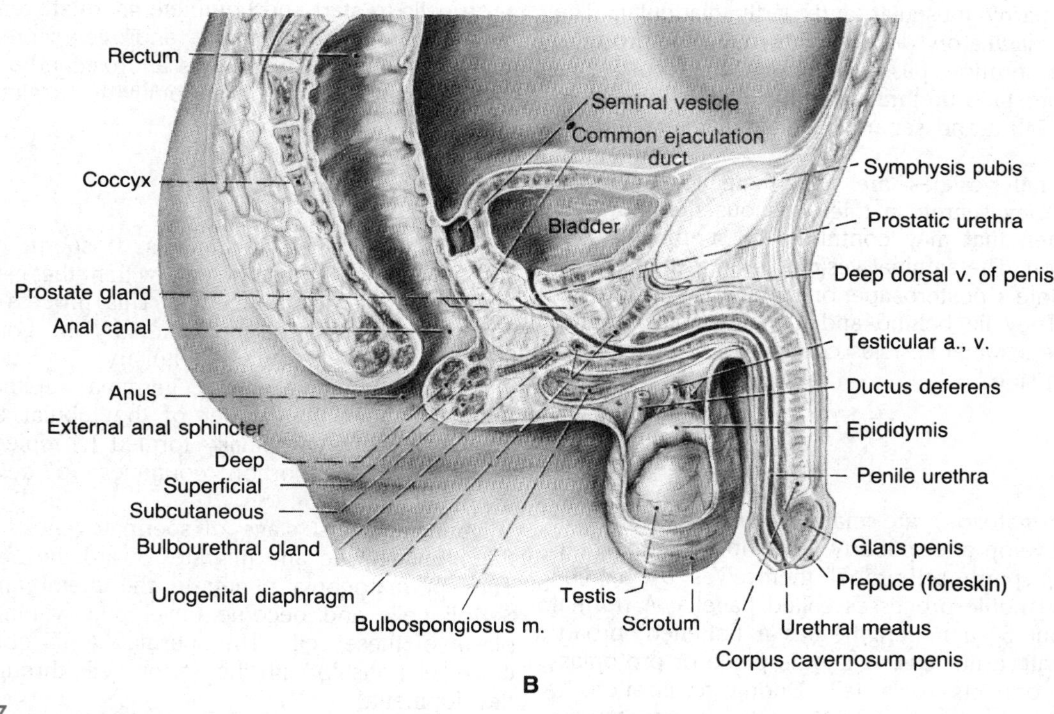

▲ *Figure 73-7*

A, Internal and external aspects of the male urinary bladder and related structures. *B*, Midsagittal section of the male pelvis and external genitalia. (From Jacob, S. W., et al. [1982]. *Structure and function in man* [5th ed., pp. 536, 597]. Philadelphia: W. B. Saunders.)

Many lobules, separated by septa, divide a testicle. These lobules lead to straight ducts that join a plexus from which efferent ducts lead to the epididymis. Each lobule contains 1 to 3 seminiferous tubules. Each testicle has 600 to 1200 seminiferous tubules. Their combined length is almost a mile! Sperm (spermatozoa) are produced within these tubules. Between the seminiferous tubules are interstitial cells called the *cells of Leydig*, the source of testosterone, the male hormone.

PROSTATE AND RELATED STRUCTURES

The prostate gland surrounds the neck of the male urinary bladder and urethra. In childhood, the prostate is small, but with puberty, it grows to the size of a walnut. The adult prostate gland (see Fig. 73-7) lies like a flattened cone in the pelvis, about 2 cm posterior to the symphysis pubis. A normal adult male's prostate weighs 15 to 20 g and is 4 to 6 cm long. The prostate is inverted, so its apex is inferior and is suspended by the urogenital diaphragm. The prostate's base is superior and is at the bladder neck, anterior to the rectum. The bladder overlies the prostate's basal surface. The posterior surface of the prostate is in close contact with the rectal wall. This is the only surface of the prostate available for direct examination by palpation.

The prostate consists of five lobes: (1) anterior, (2) posterior, (3) median, (4) right lateral, (5) and left lateral. A shallow, median furrow divides the prostate's lower part into the right and left lateral lobes. The middle lobe is created by the ejaculatory ducts from either side. These ducts pierce the prostate and converge with the prostatic portion of the urethra. The prostate consists of (1) periurethral or internal glands and (2) follicle-like tubules in the prostate's peripheral portion, which opens into the urethra by way of ejaculatory ducts. These ducts separate the prostate's posterior and median lobes.

A firm fibrous capsule, containing smooth muscle fibers in its inner layer, encloses the prostate. The prostate is partly muscular and partly glandular. The urethra and ejaculatory ducts pass through the prostate. The urethral portion passing through the prostate is called the prostatic urethra. Prostatic muscle fibers encircle the urethra and separate the prostate's glandular tissue.

The seminal vesicles are two 5-cm long, saclike structures. They secrete a thick, viscous fluid forming part of semen that may contribute to sperm nutrition and activation. The seminal vesicles are closely applied to the prostate's posterosuperior surface (as in the vas deferens). They lie behind and closely parallel to the bladder. The seminal vesicles connect to the vas deferens on each side.

SPERM

Sperm (spermatozoa) are mature male sex or germ cells that develop after puberty. Resembling tadpoles in appearance, sperm self-propel themselves by hairlike tails, that is, motile processes called flagella. A normal sperm (about 51 μ in length) has a flattened, broad, oval head with a nucleus. A middle piece or protoplasmic neck connects to a tail. During fertilization, a sperm's head pierces an ovum (female reproductive or germ cell). The sperm's tail is lost when fusion of two cells occurs. Sperm are produced in seminiferous tubules of the testicles. Sperm develop in great quantities from spermatids (spermoblasts) and are stored in the vas deferens.

▼ Male Reproductive Function

MALE SEXUAL DEVELOPMENT

Development of the male genitalia requires two hormones: (1) müllerian duct inhibiting factor, secreted by Sertoli cells, and (2) testosterone, secreted by Leydig cells. The production of testosterone by the Leydig cells is supported by placental chorionic gonadotropin. Müllerian duct inhibiting factor mediates the involution of the müllerian duct. Testosterone supports the differentiation of the wolffian ducts and the differentiation of male external genitalia.

Seminiferous tubules constitute 90 per cent of the mature testis. The tubules are composed of germ cells and Sertoli cells. Germ cells develop into spermatozoa, and Sertoli cells support the process of spermatogenesis.

The hypothalamus and pituitary gland regulate testicular function. The hypothalamus secretes gonadotropin-releasing hormone (GnRH) in a pulsatile fashion. GnRH stimulates the anterior pituitary gland to produce LH and FSH. LH stimulates Leydig cells to produce testosterone. Testosterone, in turn, modulates the regulation of the secretion of GnRH, LH, and FSH through negative feedback to the hypothalamus and pituitary gland. FSH and testosterone stimulate the Sertoli cells and germ cells to start and complete spermatogenesis.

Testosterone is the primary androgen secreted by the testis. The testis also secretes androstenedione and estradiol. Estradiol may be important for skeletal maturation in the male.

SPERMATOGENESIS

Spermatogenesis is the process of sperm production and development that occurs within the seminiferous tubules during active sex life. This process begins at puberty as a result of stimulation by the gonadotropic hormones from the anterior pituitary.

Spermatogonia are the germinal epithelial cells found in the outer border of the tubular epithelium. These cells are continually formed to replenish themselves, while a portion continues to develop into sperm.

During the first stage of spermatogenesis, the spermatogonia divide and migrate toward the *Sertoli cells.* The spermatogonia penetrate the membranes of the Sertoli cells and become enveloped within the cytoplasm of these cells. The spermatogonia continue this close relationship with the Sertoli cells throughout their development.

During the 24 days when it is in contact with Sertoli cells, the spermatogonia changes and enlarges to form a primary spermatocyte. After this development, the spermatocyte splits into two secondary spermatocytes, each with only 23 chromosomes. After 2 to 3 days, the spermatocytes undergo a second division to form four spermatids, each with 23 chromosomes, half the original number. This means that the sperm that eventually fertilizes the female ovum contains half the genetic material, while the ovum contains the other half.

The period of spermatogenesis from germinal cell to sperm takes about 74 days. During this time, the spermatocytes lose some cytoplasm, the chromatin material of the head reorganizes to form a compact head, and the remaining cytoplasm and cell membranes collect at one end of the cell to form the tail of the sperm.

Hormonal Stimulation

Testosterone is essential for the growth and division of the germinal cells that form the sperm. Luteinizing hormone stimulates the Leydig cells to secrete testosterone. Follicle-stimulating hormone stimulates the Sertoli cells promoting spermatogenesis. Estrogens are formed from testosterone when the Sertoli cells are stimulated by FSH. This estrogen appears to be essential in spermatogenesis. Growth hormone promotes early division of the spermatogonia.

Maturation in the Epididymis

After the sperm are formed in the seminiferous tubules, they spend several days passing through the epididymis. After the sperm have spent about 24 hours in the epididymis, they become motile. The sperm also become capable of fertilization, a process called maturation.

Sperm are stored in small amounts in the epididymis but are mainly stored in the vas deferens and the ampulla of the vas deferens. With low levels of sexual activity, the sperm can be stored there up to a month, maintaining their motility and fertility. When sexual activity is frequent, sperm may be stored only a few days.

PROSTATIC FLUID

The prostate produces prostatic secretion, an opalescent, thin, slightly alkaline fluid that forms part of the semen. Prostatic secretion aids the passage of sperm and helps keep them alive, supplying them with emergency food, if needed. Prostatic secretion is manufactured in a network of branching glands embedded in muscle within the prostate. This muscle contracts during ejaculation, and prostatic secretions are ejected through the ejaculatory ducts into the urethra.

SEMEN

Semen (seminal fluid or ejaculate) is a viscid, thick, opalescent secretion discharged by males at the climax of sexual excitement or orgasm. It contains sperm and other secretions. About 10 per cent of the semen is composed of sperm and fluid from the vas deferens, with about 60 per cent of the semen made up of fluid from the seminal vesicles. The remaining 30 per cent of semen is composed of prostatic fluid and small amounts of mucus from the bulbourethral glands.

With sexual climax, the fluid and sperm are ejaculated through the urethra. Semen is slightly alkaline, with a pH of about 7.5. The prostatic fluid contains a clotting enzyme, which causes the fibrinogen of the seminal vesicle fluid to form a weak coagulum that holds the semen near the uterine cervix. The coagulum dissolves in about 15 to 30 minutes at which time the sperm becomes highly motile. The sperm can live within the vagina for 24 to 48 hours after ejaculation (see Fig. 73-6).

Summary

A thorough knowledge of the structure and function of the female and male reproductive systems is important if the nurse is to provide safe, effective care for clients with problems associated with the reproductive system. The nurse must be sensitive to the delicate nature of problems associated with this system, because many disorders affect sexuality.

Bibliography

1. Avis, N. E., & McKinley, S. M. (1991). A longitudinal analysis of women's attitudes toward the menopause: Results from the Massachusetts Women's Health Study. *Matures, 13,* 65-79.
2. Bobak, I. M., et al. (1989). *Maternity and gynecologic care* (4th ed.). St. Louis: C. V. Mosby.
3. Cooke, B. A., & Sharpe, R. M. (1988). *The molecular and cellular endocrinology of the testis.* New York: Raven Press.
4. DeGroot, L. J., et al. (Eds.) (1989). *Endocrinology* (2nd ed.). Philadelphia: W. B. Saunders.
5. Diczfalusy, E., & Bygedman, M. (1987). *Fertility regulation today and tomorrow.* New York: Raven Press.
6. Droegmueller, W., et al. (1987). *Comprehensive gynecology.* St. Louis: C. V. Mosby.
7. Gruhn, J. G., & Kazer, R. R. (1989). *Hormonal regulation of the menstrual cycle.* New York: Plenum Publishing Co.
8. Guyton, A. C. (1991). *Textbook of medical physiology* (8th ed.). Philadelphia: W. B. Saunders.
9. Jones, H. W., et al. (Eds.) (1988). *Novak's textbook of gynecology* (11th ed.). Baltimore: Williams & Wilkins.
10. Knobil, E. (1988). *The physiology of reproduction.* New York: Raven Press.
11. Leung, P. C. K., et al. (Eds.) (1987). *Endocrinology and physiology of reproduction.* New York: Plenum Publishing Co.
12. Manhesh, V. B., et al. (Eds.) *Regulation of ovarian and testicular function.* New York: Plenum Publishing Co.
13. McKinley, J. B., et al. (1987). Health status and utilization behavior associated with the menopause. *American Journal of Epidemiology, 125*(1), 110-121.
14. Negro-Vilar, A., et al. (Eds.) (1988). *Andrology and human reproduction.* New York: Raven Press.
15. Newton, M., & Newton, E. R. (1988). *Complications of gynecology and obstetric management.* Philadelphia: W. B. Saunders.
16. Soules, M. R. (1989). *Problems in reproductive endocrinology and infertility.* New York: Elsevier Science Publishing Co.
17. Wynn, T. M., & Jollie, W. (Eds.) (1989). *The biology of the uterus* (2nd ed.). New York: Plenum Publishing Co.
18. Yen, S. S. C., & Jaffe, R. (1986). *Reproductive endocrinology: Physiology, pathophysiology, and clinical management* (2nd ed.). Philadelphia: W. B. Saunders.

Chapter

74

Assessment of Clients with Reproductive Disorders

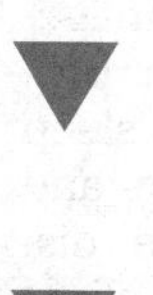

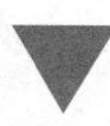

ASSESSING WOMEN EXPERIENCING GYNECOLOGIC CONDITIONS

In recent years, there has been an increased emphasis on women's health concerns and on the importance of health promotion activities for women. Because many women receive most, if not all, of their primary health care with reproductive needs, a broader concept of gynecologic care is needed. Nurses participating in this area of health care must focus not only on the gynecologic condition but also on the woman's total health maintenance needs. A thorough assessment includes the usual health history and physical examination as well as a review of the woman's lifestyle, health habits, self-perception, body image, and developmental stage with consideration of cultural, religious, socioeconomic, and educational factors. These factors influence the woman's health and health-seeking behaviors. A nonjudgmental attitude and respect for the woman's values will allow the nurse to provide more effective care. The woman's cultural or ethnic background, socioeconomic status, or sexual preference should not limit her access to or quality of health care.

Psychosocial Impact of Gynecologic Problems

For many women, the genital organs and reproductive capacity have symbolic significance. Thus, problems in this area can affect her sexuality and sense of femininity. Gynecologic problems may be associated with changes in a woman's self-concept, body image, personal identity, and role performance. Reproductive capabilities and the experience of sexuality and sexual activities may be affected. There may be psychosocial consequences for some women experiencing gynecologic disorders. For this reason, psychological assessment is especially important. A woman's outward reaction to gynecologic problems does not necessarily correlate with either her inner experience or the seriousness of the condition.

Sensitivity is vital in interviewing a woman. The nurse does not press for information that the client appears hesitant to reveal. Remember that the woman herself may not understand her own responses. Empathetic listening is supportive, often lessening the stress the woman experiences.

Fear may be expressed because of a suspicion the woman holds of unhealthy changes in the genitals or of unwanted pregnancy. There may be anxiety and embarrassment in the anticipation of a pelvic examination. Women may consider the pelvic examination unpleasant despite the insignificant risk of injury or physical pain. Other feelings that may be expressed include humiliation, guilt, or anger. In the event of deep, powerful feelings, women may avoid seeking gynecologic care. It has been suggested that intrusive gynecologic procedures may evoke memories or strong reactions in women who have experienced childhood sexual abuse or sexual assault.[8] The opportunity to express and discuss feelings with a nurse skilled in therapeutic communication may help these women cope more effectively and follow through with appropriate care. Such therapeutic conversations can provide opportunities for clarifying a woman's misconceptions about her diagnosis, proposed treatment, or preventive care. Many women have never received accurate information about reproductive problems.

▼ Approach to Gynecologic Care

Women have the right to be informed and to participate actively in decisions about their health. A supportive, respectful attitude on the part of the nurse promotes the woman's participation in her care and cooperation. The nurse also is alert for sexist attitudes in the health care system, which may lead to women's health complaints being ignored or unnecessary prescriptions being written. The nurse can act as an advocate for the woman, positively influencing her perception of health care and the importance of health maintenance. Common misconceptions include

- surgical removal of the uterus means that menopause will begin
- an extensive hysterectomy (without vaginectomy) ends sexual activity (an extensive hysterectomy removes the top of the vagina, the uterus, and the paracervical and paravaginal tissues; a vaginectomy removes one third to one half of the vagina)
- removing reproductive organs makes a woman less womanly
- removing one ovary produces sterility
- a suspicious Pap test always means cancer

Providing privacy and creating an environment that is conducive to the expression of feelings allow a woman to discuss her concerns openly. It is important to assess the woman's understanding of health care information and to elicit her perception of her needs and problems. The nurse may need to repeat information, especially if the woman is anxious or stressed, for example, when information is received during a pelvic examination. Nurses can provide a sensitive, humane orientation to gynecologic health care. Through teaching and counseling, nurses provide valuable impetus to health maintenance for women.

The annual gynecologic examination provides opportunity for the nurse to discuss health maintenance activities with women. For example, a health visit for a Pap smear is a good time to teach breast self-examination and to talk about risk factors associated with gynecologic cancer. It also is a good time to provide information about developmental changes such as adolescence, menarche, or menopause and about menstrual hygiene and menstrual symptom management. Information on the ways the woman can promote her health through diet, exercise, adequate sleep and rest, stress management, cessation of smoking, and general risk factor identification also should be discussed. If appropriate, the nurse provides the client with information about protection against sexually transmitted diseases (STDs).

▼ Gynecologic Assessment

After establishing rapport with the woman, the nurse performs a comprehensive gynecologic nursing assessment appropriate to the situation. (For review of a comprehensive history and psychosocial assessment, see Chap. 11). Physical examination discussion follows in this chapter. This information is a basis for nursing intervention.

HISTORY

The health history for the gynecologic system includes data related to the breast as well as genitoreproductive systems. The nurse also inquires about other general information as it relates to the reproductive system.

Chief Complaint

The client is asked to describe her problem in her own words. These data alert the nurse to the possible nature of the client's problem as well as to the level of the client's understanding of the problem. This information provides direction for the nurse during the remainder of the health history interview. The nurse asks the client to relate the history of the problem, including a symptom analysis (see Chap. 11).

Past Medical History

The past medical health history has many components significant to the reproductive system. These include childhood and infectious diseases, immunizations, major illnesses and hospitalizations, medications, allergies, gynecologic history, family history, psychosocial history, and review of systems.

CHILDHOOD AND INFECTIOUS ILLNESSES

The most common childhood infectious illness to affect a woman of childbearing age is rubella. The nurse specifically asks if the client has had rubella or has been immunized against it. The woman who is contemplating pregnancy should have a rubella titer analysis for determining whether immunity exists. Maternal rubella during the first trimester increases the risk to the fetus for congenital disorders. If the titer is negative (i.e., immunity is lacking), the woman is encouraged to receive an immunization. A woman who is already pregnant should not be immunized. If a woman elects to be immunized, the nurse advises the client not to become pregnant for at least 3 months after the immunization.

MAJOR ILLNESSES AND HOSPITALIZATIONS

The nurse asks the client about major illnesses such as diabetes, hypertension, thrombophlebitis, angina, anemia, thyroid disorders, cholecystitis, hepatitis, and migraine headaches. Diabetes is associated with increased morbidity and mortality in women who are pregnant or who take oral contraceptives. Pregnancy and oral contraceptive use also is linked with higher morbidity and mortality rates in women with a history of cardiovascular diseases such as angina, hypertension, and thrombophlebitis. Anemia can result from menstrual disorders such as dysfunctional uterine bleeding, or it can be aggravated even by normal menstruation. Endometrial implants (endometriosis) can cause painful menstruation and fertility problems so that the woman who wishes to become pregnant may need treatment with medication and surgery for the implants to be reduced or removed. Hypothyroidism and hyperthyroidism affect the menstrual cycle, as can other endocrine disorders. Renal and urinary tract disorders can interfere with sexual function.

Women with a history of migraine headaches or seizure disorders should avoid oral contraceptives because of an associated increased risk of occurrence with their use. Cholecystitis may be aggravated by oral contraceptives; hepatitis and other liver disorders are a contraindication for taking estrogen because of its route of metabolization. The progesterones in oral contraceptives thicken respiratory secretions, which complicates the treatment of women with asthma or chronic obstructive respiratory disorders.

The nurse asks the client about surgery involving the reproductive system. Specific surgical procedures include dilation and curettage, tubal ligation, cryosurgery, cystocele and rectocele repair, hysterectomy, oophorectomy, and salpingectomy. Inquire about interruptions to pregnancies, such as planned or spontaneous abortion.

MEDICATIONS

A complete medication history is obtained for prescription, over-the-counter, and recreational drugs. Diuretics are often prescribed for women who are subject to premenstrual edema. There also are many over-the-counter preparations for premenstrual "bloating." The significance of oral contraceptives has already been discussed. Use of other hormones should also be determined, such as thyroid preparations. Recreational drugs including amphetamines, barbiturates, marijuana, and other hallucinogens can affect sexual behavior and physiologic function of the reproductive system.

ALLERGIES

The nurse asks the client specifically about allergies to penicillin, sulfonamides, and latex or rubber. Genitourinary disorders such as vaginitis and urinary tract infections are often treated with penicillin and sulfa compounds. Latex and rubber are used in contraceptive devices such as diaphragms and some condoms; allergy eliminates their use for contraception.

GYNECOLOGIC HISTORY

The gynecologic history includes the following. For the menopausal or elderly woman or the woman who has had a hysterectomy, the nurse asks only the appropriate questions.

Breast History. Ask the client about breast pain or tenderness and its occurrence in relationship to the menstrual cycle. Many women experience breast tenderness before menses onset. Also inquire whether the woman has had or currently has breast lumps or masses. If a lump is present, ask the woman to describe its location, onset, and size and whether it is painful. Determine if the lump has changed shape, size, consistency, or amount of tenderness since it was first noticed and if the lump changes during the menstrual cycle. Ask the woman the date of her last menstrual period in order to better evaluate a breast lump. The breasts become more firm and cystic during the luteal phase so that the best time to perform breast palpation is 7 to 10 days after menses onset.

The nurse also asks about discharge from the nipple. Nipple discharge is abnormal in women who are not pregnant or lactating. If discharge is present, determine color, consistency, amount, and odor.

Inquire about the practice of breast self-examination on a monthly basis. Ask not only about frequency of performance but also about technique to determine if the woman could benefit from a review of the procedure and supervised practice. Note whether the woman includes the axillary nodes as part of her self-examination. Last, ask if there is a history of breast cancer in blood-related female relatives, such as mother, sister, maternal aunts, or maternal grandmother. Incidence of breast cancer in these relatives increases a woman's risk of breast cancer occurrence.

Menstrual History. Determine the woman's age at menarche. Ask the woman to specify the first day of bleeding of her last menstrual period and that of her previous last menstrual period. How long were these menstrual periods? Were they regular? If not, what deviations occurred? How heavy was the flow? (Ask the number of pads used.) Document the woman's usual duration of menses, amount and type of flow, interval between menses, and any dysmenorrhea, premenstrual symptoms, or menopausal symptoms.

Contraceptive History. Document the woman's current contraceptive method (if any), her satisfaction with the method, duration of use, any contraceptive problems, and any desire to change methods. Ask about previous contraceptive methods, problems encountered, and reason for discontinuation. Ask if she wants any contraceptive information. For women at risk for pregnancy (those of reproductive age, not sterilized, and heterosexually active), determine whether they wish to become pregnant.

Sexual History. After careful psychosocial and environmental preparation, the nurse obtains a sexual history using a direct approach and terms the woman understands. The purpose of a sexual history is to identify sexual problems and give the woman an opportunity to ask questions or express concerns. Begin with general questions about whether the woman is satisfied and comfortable with her current sexual activity. A nonjudgmental approach is essential. Follow up on any concerns or issues she raises (Table 74-1). See also Chapters 7 and 11 for further information on sexuality assessment.

Obstetric History. If the woman is in her childbearing years, ask if she thinks she may be pregnant. (Pregnancy may contraindicate mammography or other radiologic studies.) If the woman has been pregnant, obtain information about each pregnancy, including the delivery and postpartum period. Document details of any difficulties or complications (physical or psychosocial). Record any spontaneous abortions or voluntarily interrupted pregnancies. If the woman has never been pregnant or has no living children, ask whether children were or are desired. If the woman has relinquished a child for adoption, explore her feelings about it. See also Chapter 11 for detailed questions to assess the obstetric history.

Past Gynecologic/Genitourinary History. Ask about previous problems with genitourinary infections and vaginitis. Determine whether the woman has had a previous pelvic infection. If so, what was the treatment prescribed? Ask whether the woman has previously had an STD and about problems or complications resulting from the disease. Determine whether the woman experiences urinary incontinence and the circumstances when incontinence occurs. See also Chapter 48 for assessment of urinary incontinence.

Reproductive Health Practices. The nurse seeks information about menstrual, sexual, and gynecologic hygiene. Ask about the frequency of gynecologic examinations and whether the woman performs monthly breast self-examination as necessary. Determine whether the woman protects herself against STD, if appropriate. See also Chapter 11 for discussion of health risk management.

Family History

There are a number of diseases with a familial tendency that can affect the reproductive system. In addition to breast cancer, the nurse asks about other types of cancer, especially of the reproductive organs. Also inquire about diabetes mellitus, hypertension, cerebrovascular accidents (stroke), angina, myocardial infarction, anemia, and endocrine disorders including hypo- and hyperthyroidism.

For women who were born between 1940 and 1975, ask if their mothers had a history of taking diethylstilbestrol (DES) during pregnancy. In utero exposure to DES is associated with increased incidence of cervical adenosis and adenocarcinoma of the cervix and vagina in these women.

Psychosocial History and Lifestyle

There are many factors in the psychosocial history that can have an effect on reproductive function. The nurse assesses the following areas.

OCCUPATIONAL AND ENVIRONMENTAL FACTORS

Many toxic substances are known to affect or suspected of affecting sexual function and reproductive ability adversely. Ask about exposure to chemicals and environmental pollutants.

HABITS

The nurse assesses the client's use of caffeine, alcohol, and cigarette smoking. These substances as well as numerous other drugs can be harmful to a developing fetus (see Ethical Issues in Nursing). Cigarette smoking has been linked to increased morbidity in women who also take oral contraceptives. Women who consume a high-fat diet have increased incidence of breast cancer.

Other aspects of psychosocial assessment of the reproductive system have been discussed earlier. The nurse must remain sensitive to the client and her expressed and unexpressed fears and concerns.

Review of Systems

Before the physical examination, the nurse reviews the physical health history, proceeding from head to toe.

TABLE 74-1. Sexual Health Assessment

Sexual health assessment may include consideration of the client's current

- Knowledge about sexuality
- Attitudes about sexuality and toward sexual partner(s)
- Level of comfort and feelings of adequacy regarding own sexuality
- Concerns about sexuality of significant others
- Perception of own sex role and that of sexual partner(s)
- Sexual self-concept as a female or male
- Fears and anxiety about intimacy and other aspects of sexuality
- Self-perception of own body (body image)
- Ability to function sexually, e.g., to obtain an erection and control ejaculation, to please sexual partner, to achieve pain-free orgasm, to reproduce, to obtain adequate contraception, to obtain sufficient vaginal lubrication, to give and receive effective sexual stimulation and pleasure
- Typical sexual patterns and activities, e.g., partner choice (female, male, spouse, extramarital, multiple, single, same partner, different partners), frequency of sexual activity, type of sexual activity (vaginal, anal, oral, masturbation), partner satisfaction, self-satisfaction
- Level of interest in sexual activity (sex drive)
- Level of satisfaction regarding current sexual opportunity and activity
- Physical health problems affecting sexuality, e.g., menstrual problems, pregnancy, medication, surgery (colostomy, surgical amputation, recent heart surgery or brain surgery), paralysis, illness (hypertension, diabetes, recent myocardial infarction, "stroke"), injury (recent spinal cord injury, recent head injury, burns, traumatic amputations), sexually transmitted disease, genitourinary problems

Sexual History

There is no single approach to taking a sexual health history. Information obtained may relate to historical (past) information about the following:

Both Females and Males

- Pregnancies (information about unplanned pregnancies)
- Fertility management
- Genitourinary problems
- Sexually transmitted disease
- Sexual abuse, e.g., incest, rape, pedophilia, battering
- Relationship-partner history, e.g., number of sexual partners, sexual orientation (bisexual, homosexual, heterosexual)
- First experience of sexual activity
- Early sexual development and influences
- Adolescent sexual experiences
- Sexual techniques used, e.g., masturbation, intercourse (oral, vaginal, anal)
- Role models for sexuality, e.g., peers, parents, guardians, famous people, advertising models
- Spiritual-philosophical models influencing the client's sexuality

Females

History specific to menstruation, abortion, pregnancy

Males

History specific to impotence, noctural emissions

Areas of particular concern to the reproductive system for women include the cardiovascular system (hypertension, angina, myocardial infarction, and thrombophlebitis if oral contraceptives are taken concurrently), endocrine disorders such as hypo- and hyperthyroidism and disorders of the pituitary gland, liver disorders, and cholecystitis. In addition, the nurse asks about problems involving the urinary tract and reproductive system such as urinary tract infection, urine incontinence, vaginitis, and any bleeding disorders associated with menstruation (e.g., amenorrhea, dysmenorrhea, breakthrough bleeding, menorrhagia, post-coital bleeding). Detailed questions for the review of systems are found in Chapter 11, Table 11-5.

PHYSICAL EXAMINATION

A standard gynecologic examination includes the following physical assessment and laboratory data:

- vital signs (temperature, pulse, respiration, blood pressure)
- height
- weight

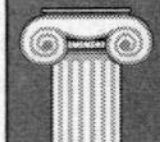

ETHICAL ISSUES IN NURSING

Should Pregnant Women Who Engage in Substance Abuse Be Held Liable for Damage to the Fetus?

The rights of procreation are continually challenged as technology allows more and more reproductive options. Much controversy exists around reproductive issues such as abortion, in vitro fertilization, surrogate motherhood, sperm banks, and genetic selection (to name a few). There is, however, controversy surrounding the right to reproduce that does not involve any modern technology. This controversy surrounds the responsibilities of the mother to her unborn baby.

Pregnant women who engage in substance abuse often are directly responsible for physical and mental handicaps that their babies are born with. These babies, who might otherwise have been healthy, will live their lives with disabilities that could have been prevented had their mothers not abused drugs or alcohol. Should such women be legally prosecuted for the harm they have inflicted on their children? Although a woman has a right to do with her own body what she wants, abusing toxic substances does not simply affect her body alone. Should a woman who gives birth to a baby addicted to cocaine and perhaps disabled for life be ordered by the courts not to ever procreate again? Is court-ordered sterilization ever ethically justified? Society has an obligation to help care for its members who are physically and mentally handicapped. Does society also have a responsibility to see that its members (however potential they might be) are not treated in such ways that intentional physical and mental handicaps result in order not to overburden the society? (Intentional means that had substance abuse not occurred, perhaps the handicaps might not have either.)

Nurses who care for babies and children who are handicapped from maternal substance abuse may develop negative feelings for the parents of such babies and children. It is hard to see the innocent suffer, no matter what the cause. It is very important that care givers in these situations express their concerns and emotions in an arena in which it is safe to do so, for instance, in team care conferences or informal sessions with a peer or social worker.

- complete blood count
- urinalysis
- pelvic examination and Pap smear
- physical assessment of heart, lungs, breasts and axillae, thyroid, and abdomen

Refer to Chapter 41 for heart assessment, Chapter 36 for lung assessment, Chapter 60 for thyroid assessment, and Chapter 52 for assessment of the abdomen. Physical examination of the breasts and axillae and the reproductive organs follows. Unusual or abnormal findings during the gynecologic history or physical examination require obtaining additional data. (See Chap. 12 for details of general physical assessment techniques.)

Breast and Axilla Examination

The breast and axilla examination is an important part of the annual gynecologic examination. Good lighting is essential. Some examiners complete this portion of the examination before assessing the anterior lungs and heart. Because the breasts are sensitive and closely associated with sexuality, other nurses delay examining them until there has been more "hands on" interaction with the client during the lungs and heart assessments and sequence this portion of the physical examination to follow the heart. Others integrate the assessments so that the client is sitting for those portions of the heart, breast, and axillae examination before being assisted to a supine position for the remaining portions. Any of these sequencing patterns is acceptable as long as the nurse is thorough and the client can tolerate the position changes. The nurse instructs the client in this procedure while performing it. See Chapter 78 for further information in breast self-examination.

The nurse asks the client when the last menstrual period began. Breasts are usually tender the week before menses onset and the least tender the week after. If the client reports that one breast is tender, the nurse begins palpation with the opposite breast. Thorough examination requires the client to have both breasts exposed for bilateral comparison.

INSPECTION

The nurse begins inspecting the breasts while the client is seated. Inspection is done while the client sits quietly (1) with arms at the sides, (2) with the hands raised over the head, and (3) with the hands pressed firmly on the hips or pressed together to tighten the pectoral muscles; women who have large or pendulous breasts are also examined while leaning forward at the waist, facing forward, and with the breasts hanging down (Fig. 74-1). The breasts are inspected for symmetry, size, shape, contour, skin characteristics including vascular pattern, and nipple and areolae characteristics in all positions.

The breasts are symmetric, although it is not unusual for one breast to be slightly larger than the other. They should point laterally and hang evenly between the third and fourth ribs with the nipples approximately level with the fourth intercostal space when the client sits with arms at the sides. With aging and loss of tissue elasticity, the breasts hang lower. Contour is even without signs of dimpling (retraction), masses, or surface flattening, which are abnormal. Skin color is the same as that of the abdomen. *Striae* (i.e., stretch marks from rapid skin stretching) may be present; recent striae are reddened, but they become paler with time. If venous patterns are noticeable, they should be symmetric. There should be no local areas of hyperpigmentation or edema.

The client is asked to raise the arms over the head while the nurse examines the lateral and under surfaces of each breast. The contraction of the pectoral muscles will emphasize any signs of retraction or skin flattening.

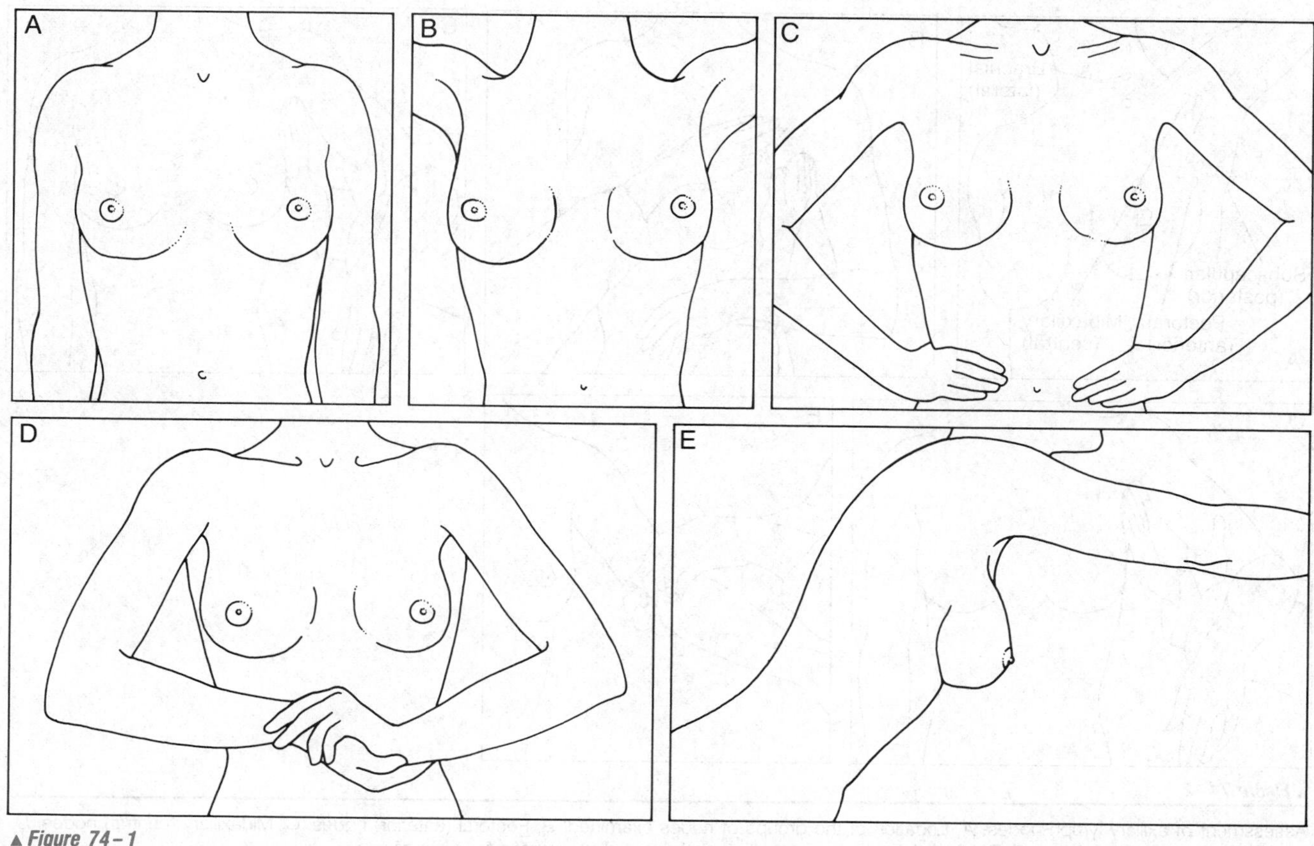

▲ Figure 74–1

Positions for breast examination. *A*, Arms at sides. *B*, Hands raised over head. For tightening pectoral muscles, the examiner asks the client to press hands firmly on hips *(C)* or to press hands together *(D)*. *E*, Breasts may also be examined with the woman leaning forward at the waist, allowing the breasts to hang down.

Areas of redness or excoriation may be noted in women with large breasts from brassiere rubbing. The breasts should elevate evenly so that the areolae remain at the same level. The client is then asked to put hands on hips and press inward firmly while the nurse repeats inspection for masses, retraction, or skin flattening.

The *areolae and nipples* are inspected for size, shape and contour, symmetry, surface characteristics, and masses or lesions. *Areolae* are pink in Caucasians and darker in dark-skinned clients. Slight asymmetry is common, but the nipples should point in symmetric directions. The shape is round or oval. Masses or lesions are abnormal. There may be prominence of *Montgomery's tubercles* around the nipple, which is normal. The *nipples* are round, equal in size, of the same color, soft, and smooth. If one or both nipples are inverted, the nurse asks whether this is a recent occurrence or has been present for a while and for how long. Recent nipple inversion is abnormal, and the client is referred to the physician for follow-up. There should be no rashes, crusts, cracks, or discharge unless the client is in the later stages of pregnancy, when *colostrum* (a yellowish fluid) may leak from the nipples.

The *axillae* are inspected for rashes, masses, and areas of unusual pigmentation, which should be absent. Axillary hair is present unless the client removes it by shaving or with a depilatory.

PALPATION

Palpation of axillae and breasts is done while the client is seated, although breast palpation is facilitated with the client supine. Clients with large and pendulous breasts, with a history of breast masses or cancer, or who are at increased risk for breast cancer should have their breasts palpated in both positions.

Palpation of the axillae includes examination of five sets of *lymph nodes,* which are illustrated in Figure 74–2. The client is encouraged to relax the arm, which assists in relaxing the muscles and eases palpation. The nurse begins by palpating the edge of the pectoralis major muscle along the anterior axillary line, using a bimanual technique if necessary, to examine the pectoral (anterior) nodes. Then the nurse reaches high up into the axilla at the midaxillary line to palpate the midaxillary (central) nodes against the ribs and serratus anterior. The subscapular (posterior) nodes are palpated along the posterior axillary fold along the anter-

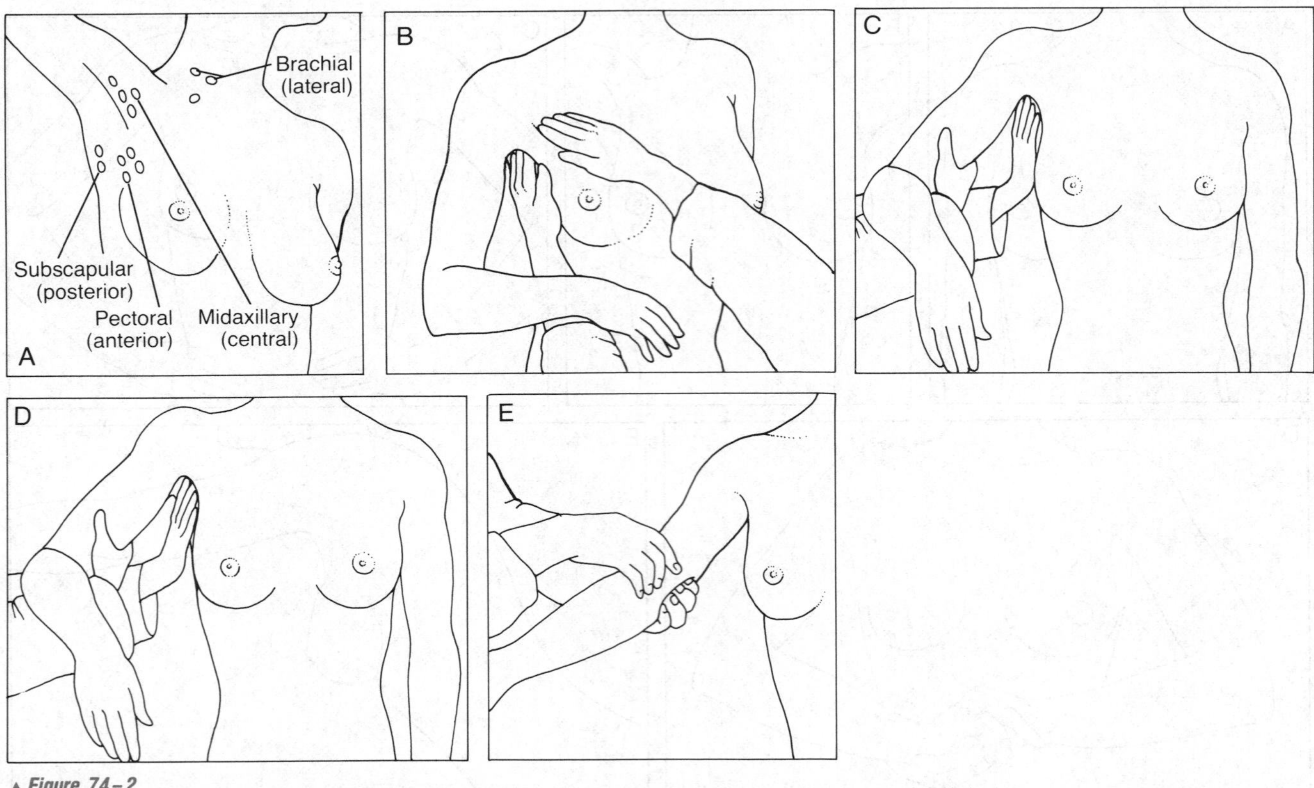

▲ Figure 74-2

Assessment of axillary lymph nodes. *A*, Location of the groups of nodes examined. *B*, Pectoral (anterior) nodes. *C*, Midaxillary (central) nodes. *D*, Subscapular (posterior) nodes. *E*, Brachial (lateral) nodes. Axillary nodes are also palpated for male clients.

ior edge of the latissimus dorsi. The brachial (lateral) nodes are palpated along the upper inner arm along the humerus. Last, the infraclavicular area is palpated (the supraclavicular nodes, which receive lymphatic drainage from the breasts, were examined with the neck nodes). All nodes should be nonpalpable, although the detection of one or two small, nontender, mobile central nodes is often normal. Abnormal findings include firm, fixed nodes that may or may not be tender. If nodes are palpated, the nurse notes the number of nodes felt, location, size, shape, mobility, tenderness, and consistency.

Breast palpation is conducted systematically so that all breast tissue, including the *tail of Spence* in the upper outer quadrant, is examined. Any one of several approaches may be used as long as the nurse palpates each portion of the breasts, areolae, and nipples. The breast and areola may be palpated in concentric circles, in a wheel-and-spokes pattern, or back and forth from the superior to inferior aspects. When the client is sitting, the nurse may prefer to use a bimanual technique, especially if the breasts are large. When supine, the client has a small folded towel under the shoulder to enhance breast flattening against the chest wall, and the arm is placed behind the head.

The nurse slides the fingers along the tissue using a rotary motion to press the breast against the chest wall. The fingers remain in contact with the skin surface. The nurse will feel a firm, curved ridge along the inferior breast, which is the *inframammary ridge*. Breast consistency varies from firm and elastic in young women to stringy and nodular in older women. If the client reports a mass, the nurse begins palpation with the unaffected breast so that there is a basis for comparison. The nurse pays particular attention to the upper outer quadrant and tail of Spence, where most of the glandular tissue is located and 50 per cent of breast lesions are found. There should be no masses or local areas of increased warmth. If a lump or mass is felt, its characteristics are noted, including exact location (and the position the client is in for the palpation) with the areola for a reference point, size, shape, contour, consistency, mobility, tenderness, and discreteness. The breast can be visualized as having four quadrants plus the tail; the location of lesions can be diagrammed in the written record.

The *areola and nipple* are palpated gently. The nipple is compressed between the thumb and index finger in an attempt to express any discharge, which should be absent. Erection and wrinkling of the nipple with manipulation is normal.

Breast Self-Examination

Breast self-examination (BSE) is a technique that all women can use to assess their own breasts. The American Cancer Society recommends that all women over the age of 20 years perform monthly BSE.[1a] Teaching the skills of BSE can be life-saving and is one of nursing's most important activities. With regular BSE, malignancy may be discovered early and effectively treated. Regular monthly BSE is an essential health maintenance activity.

Women familiar with their own normal breast characteristics can easily notice the development of abnormalities early. Nurses have many opportunities to encourage and educate men and women about this important health maintenance procedure. Individualized instruction in BSE that guides the client in self-examination produces more thorough BSE performance than films, pamphlets, or posters. As with any teaching procedure, it is desirable to allow a return demonstration and time for discussion and questions.

The nurse emphasizes that the breasts easily lend themselves to self-examination by palpation and inspection in a mirror. Sexual partners may help perform breast examinations.

Techniques of BSE for a woman are described in Figure 74-3. As part of BSE instruction, teach about the risk factors of breast cancer (see Chap. 78). Each woman should be aware of her own risk factors. Emphasize the importance of obtaining professional consultation as soon as breast abnormalities are noted. It is important not to delay. Mention the following statistics: (1) 80 per cent of breast lumps are not cancer;[1b] (2) women who were taught and practiced BSE had tumors more amenable to treatment at diagnosis than women with breast cancer who did not perform BSE;[22a] (3) one study showed that after 5 years, 75 per cent of those women who perform BSE are alive compared with only 57 per cent of those who did not.[10a] BSE definitely contributes to the early detection and improved survival of clients with breast cancer.

Factors Affecting BSE Practice. All women should do monthly BSE. However, studies have shown that only 37 per cent,[4a] 27 per cent to 51 per cent,[22c] 54 per cent,[26a] or 47 per cent[28a] comply. Women who are highly motivated, are concerned about their susceptibility, perceive social support for doing BSE, and are able to identify more benefits than barriers to BSE report greater frequency.[3a] Some of the barriers identified are never having been taught,[10d] lack of confidence in abilities,[10c] perception of low risk,[22c] belief it is unnecessary after menopause, forgetfulness, embarrassment, cultural or religious taboos regarding touching oneself, and fear of finding something. In the past, finding a cancerous lump meant losing a breast.[10c] Now, cancer can be diagnosed at an earlier stage, and small, localized breast cancer can be treated with lumpectomy and radiation therapy and possibly chemotherapy and hormonal therapy.

IMAGING TECHNIQUES

Various techniques have been tried in an effort to identify early-stage breast cancer in women accurately and safely when assessment indicates breast lesions. Such techniques are also important to find an effective method to screen women without clinically apparent findings. At present, only mammography has been shown to be useful for widespread use. Ineffective techniques include ultrasonography, light scanning, and thermography. Computed axial tomography (CT) scanning and magnetic resonance imaging (MRI) are being investigated.

Mammography. A mammogram is a soft tissue radiologic breast examination. Two common methods to obtain mammograms are (1) film/screen mammography (Fig. 74-4), and (2) xeromammography (Fig. 74-5). The first method uses a roentgen (x-ray) film. The second method is a radiographic process in which an aluminum plate with an electrically charged selenium layer is exposed to x-rays and an electrostatic image is transferred to plastic-coated paper. Whether film/screen mammographic or xeromammographic units are used, it is important that the equipment be designed and used exclusively for mammograms. Each technique has its own strengths and limitations. Both provide mammograms at acceptably low radiation doses.[25a]

With mammography, it is possible to identify some breast cancers before they reach a size that could be detected by palpation. The Breast Cancer Demonstration Project (BCDP) included 280,000 participants who were followed mammographically for at least 5 years.[30a] This project showed that mammography alone was responsible for discovering disease in 41.6 per cent of the cancers detected—impressively high in the diagnosis of small cancers.

Current indications for mammography include[10b] (1) to assess breasts when a diagnosis of potentially curable cancer has been made, and as follow-up on the noninvolved breast every 1 to 3 years after treatment, (2) to assess questionable breast masses or other abnormal physical findings to help determine whether or where a biopsy should be performed, (3) to search for undetected breast cancer when assessing a woman with metastatic cancer if the original site is unknown, and (4) to screen women according to the American Cancer Society guidelines. The ACS recommends a baseline mammogram for all women between the ages of 35 and 40 years and mammography screening of asymptomatic women aged 40 to 49 years at intervals of 1 to 2 years and annually over age 50 years. A woman who is at high risk for breast cancer should follow the recommendations of her physician.

It is not uncommon for the nurse to be asked, "Should I have a mammogram?" The nurse must be able to answer this important question. Women need to know not only the risk factors associated with the development of breast cancer (see Chap. 78) but also the risks and benefits of procedures used for breast cancer screening and detection. Some common questions and possible answers about mammography include:

- *How often should I have a mammogram?* Use the ACS guidelines for the age and risk group.
- *Cost?* Prices vary. Inquire at the facility where the mammogram will be performed. Tell the client it is worthwhile to compare prices.
- *Time involved?* About 15 to 30 minutes to complete the procedure. Results are usually available within 7 to 21 days, depending on the facility.

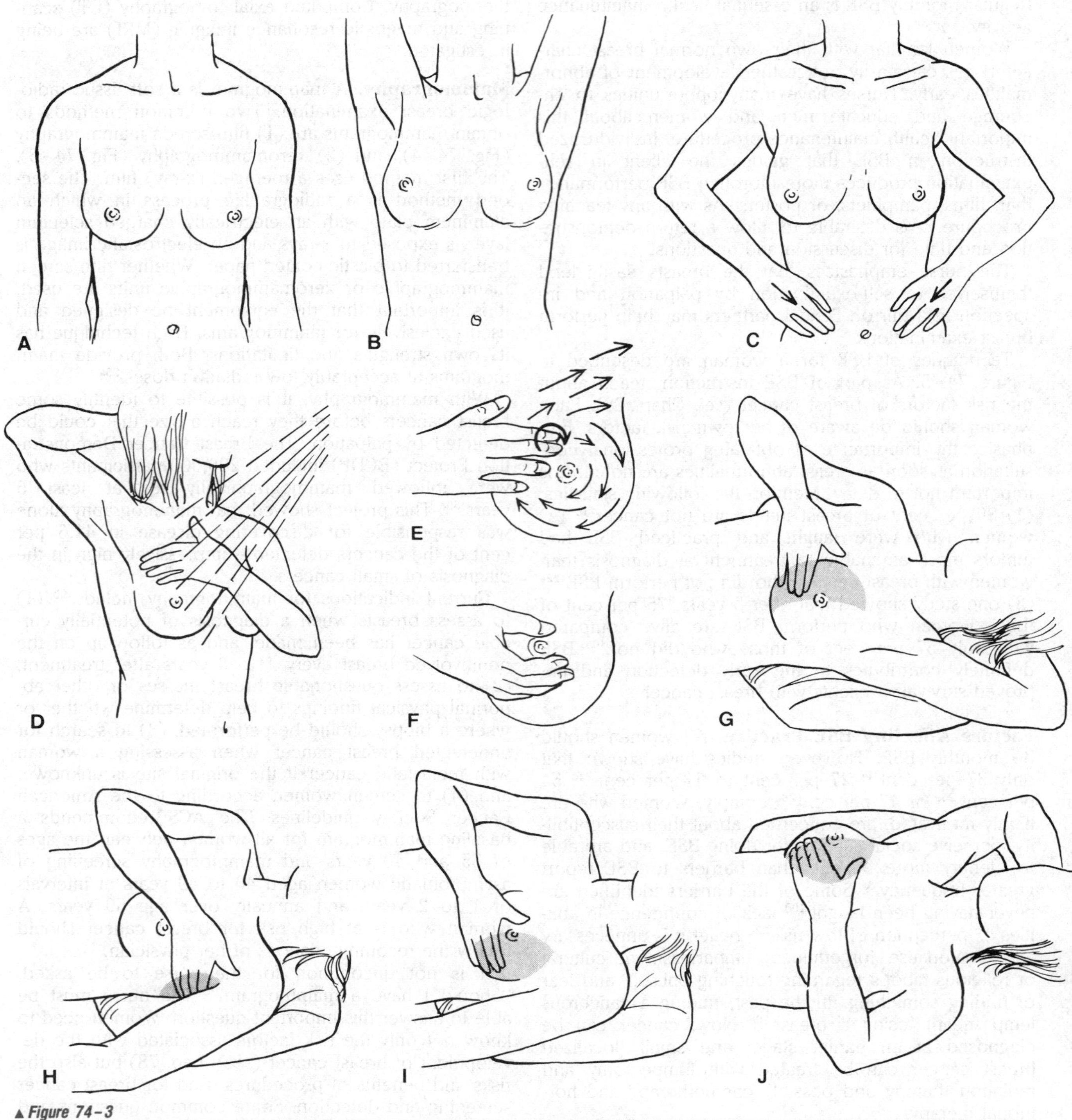

▲ **Figure 74–3**

Self-examination of female breasts and axillae. Accomplished by observation and palpation. Various positions are assumed for *observation* while standing in front of a mirror. *A*, Arms relaxed at sides. Next, lean forward. *B*, Raise arms high overhead. Press arms behind head. *C*, Rest palms on hips and firmly press inward to flex chest muscles. *D*, In shower, examine breast contours. *E*, Method of palpating breast. With fingers flat, gently press in small circular motions around an imaginary clock face, i.e., begin at 12 o'clock. Move an inch at a time toward nipple. *F*, As a final step, squeeze nipple gently between thumb and index finger. Palpation of breast is accomplished while lying down. *G*, Position to examine inner breast. *H*, Position to examine axilla. *I*, Position to examine outer breast. *J*, Entire process is repeated for opposite breast and axilla. (See text for discussion of technique and observations.)

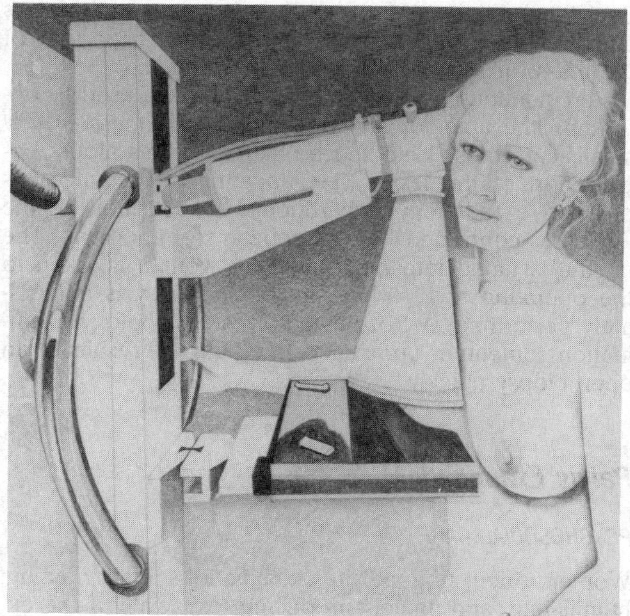

▲ Figure 74-4

Mammography, a technique for x-raying the breast, is the most reliable mechanical method for detecting a breast cancer before it can be felt. It is also used to help diagnose breast cancer in women with symptoms. (From U.S. Dept. of Health and Human Services: *The breast cancer digest*. Bethesda, MD: NIH Publication No. 84-1691, 1984.)

- *Is there pain?* Some discomfort may be experienced through use of a balloon attachment with the pressure needed to flatten the breast (done to decrease radiation exposure).
- *Where is it available?* At most health care facilities. Make sure the facility has a dedicated machine certified by the American College of Radiology.
- *Is there a risk in the exposure to the radiation?* The long-term effects of yearly mammography are being studied, although it is thought to be harmless. Both film/screen and xeromammography use the smallest dose possible.

Ductograms and pneumocystograms are specialized techniques done in conjunction with a mammogram. In a ductogram, a radiocontrast dye is injected through the areolar orifice of the duct. This is done to determine whether there is a filling defect, duct ectasia, or obstruction.

After aspiration of a nonpalpable cyst under mammographic guidance, a pneumocystogram is done by injecting air into the cyst and then performing another mammogram. The air fills the cyst cavity. The pneumocystogram helps visualize the walls of the cyst.

Ultrasonography. Ultrasound of the breast involves scanning with an automated whole breast scanner and a hand-held real-time sector scanner, very useful in determining the consistency of breast masses. It differentiates cystic (fluid-filled) from solid lesions. It cannot differentiate benign from solid cancerous lesions. Ultrasound is useful in confirming the fluid consistency of cystic-appearing lesions seen on a mammogram. It is also useful in guiding fine needle aspiration of cysts and other breast masses. Ultrasonography is painless and does not involve a radiation risk.

Transillumination. Light-scanning and diaphanography are other names for transillumination. Infrared or visible light is transmitted through the breast. Transillumination is based on the concept that there is preferential absorption of light by malignancies. This technique is currently not in use because it has limited resolution and is not sensitive enough to be effective.

Thermography. Thermography measures the infrared energy produced by metabolic activity in tissue. The increased vascularity of a tumor is recorded by heat-sensitive film. Thermography is no longer used in detecting breast lesions because it is not sensitive or ef-

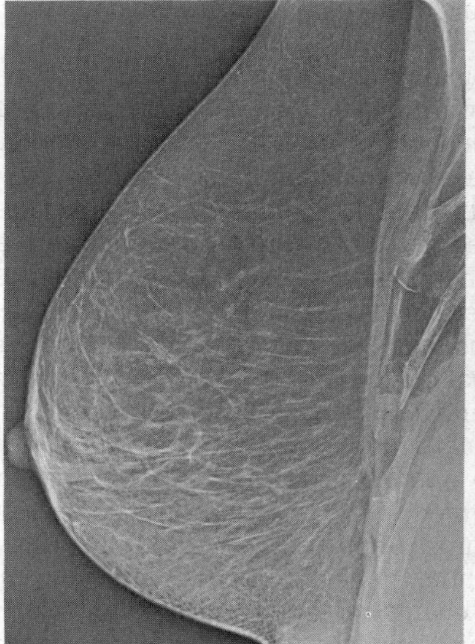

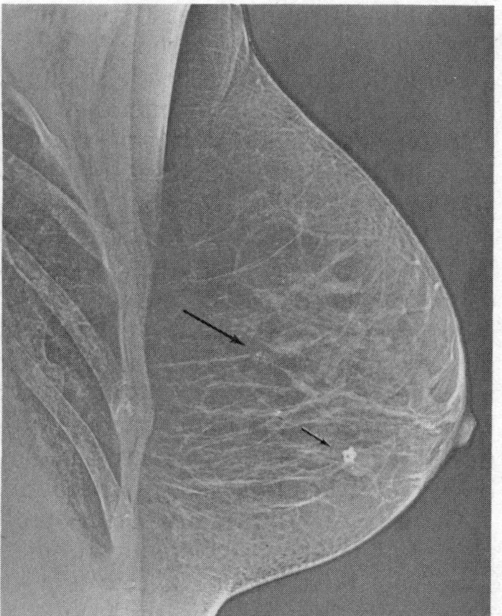

▲ Figure 74-5

Xeromammography, performed prior to a planned biopsy of a palpable mass that proved to be benign *(small arrow)*, revealed the presence of an otherwise occult cancerous lesion *(large arrow)*. (From Lippman, M. E.: *Diagnosis and management of breast cancer*. Philadelphia: W. B. Saunders Co., 1987.)

fective enough to identify occult (hidden) lesions deep in the breast.

Computed Axial Tomography Scanning. CT scanning provides cross-sectional images of the breast, mediastinum, axilla, supraclavicular area, and tissue adjacent to the chest wall. CT scanning may be useful in staging breast cancer, but it is currently not in use for routine screening and the diagnosis of breast cancer.

Magnetic Resonance Imaging. MRI is done with the client within a large magnet that provides a uniform static magnetic field around the client. The electric signals of the tissue are measured and used to construct an image of the breast. It has not been proved effective in screening for breast lesions.

LABORATORY STUDIES

No laboratory tests can screen for breast cancer. Some progress has been made in identifying biologic tumor markers for breast cancer that detect metastatic disease. Elevations in carcinoembryonic antigen (CEA), alkaline phosphatase, ferritin, and 2-glutamyltranspeptidase seem to be associated with the recurrence of breast cancer. Other possible tumor markers that have been studied include C-reactive protein, acid glycoprotein, sialyl transferase, urinary hydroxyproline/creatinine ratio, and gross cystic disease fluid protein.

BIOPSY

Biopsy is essential to diagnose breast cancer. No treatment should be undertaken without an unequivocal histologic diagnosis of cancer. Core needle biopsy is a simple procedure that is useful during an office visit to confirm and expedite the diagnosis of a clinically obviously malignant breast mass. A small core of tissue is obtained with a special needle, e.g., Vim-Silverman needle, and a histologic diagnosis is made.

Fine needle aspiration (FNA) is a slightly different procedure in which a needle and syringe are used to aspirate cells from a breast mass or fluid from a cyst. The cells are fixed on a slide (as in a Pap smear), and a cytologic diagnosis is made. Mammography is useful in guiding the needle for the FNA examination of nonpalpable lesions. FNA cytologic examination is useful for confirming the diagnosis of clinical and mammographic findings of a fibroadenoma, fibrocystic condition, inframammary lymph nodes, fat necrosis, subareolar papillomatosis, chronic subareolar abscess, and cancer. If the cytologic interpretation is that the specimen is acellular or has only blood and adipose cells present, then a biopsy or further evaluation is needed to rule out breast cancer. Both FNA and core needle biopsy take only a small amount of cells and tissue from a lesion. False-negative results are possible, so an open biopsy may still need to be performed.

Open biopsy, the biopsy procedure most often used, is performed in an operating room under general or local anesthesia. About 35 per cent of clients requiring an open biopsy for a breast lesion have a malignancy. Excisional biopsy removes the entire mass that was palpated. Incisional biopsy removes only a portion of the mass for histologic assessment.

Percutaneous needle localization may be used to determine the area for an open biopsy if a mass is very small, e.g., those detected by mammograms alone. Localization of the lesion (i.e., locating it accurately) is done in a radiology department. The position of the lesion is confirmed with a repeat mammogram. The needle is taped into place and the woman is taken to the operating room where an open biopsy is immediately performed. A frozen section is a pathology examination sometimes performed to obtain the results of an open biopsy quickly.

Pelvic Examination

PSYCHOSOCIAL CARE

Women often find pelvic examinations embarrassing, humiliating, and anxiety-producing, especially if the examination is incorrectly performed in rough or hurried ways. Insensitive professional treatment causes damage to women, producing fear, humiliation, submission, and low self-esteem. Memories of an uncomfortable or otherwise unpleasant pelvic examination may make women avoid such examinations. Thus, gynecologic health care may not be obtained.

The nurse must put a woman at ease before and during pelvic examination. The nurse makes the client more comfortable by being nonjudgmental, relaxed, and competent. All actions are explained before the nurse proceeds. Quick movements are avoided because they may cause the client to tense muscles, which results in greater discomfort. Client comfort is enhanced when the nurse is gentle, provides privacy, keeps the woman warm, warms hands and instruments, uses lubricant to ease insertion during invasive maneuvers, and cleans the perineum after the examination. Scrupulously protect the woman's dignity, and communicate comfortably with her before, during, and after the examination. With use of a mirror during the examination, show the woman her anatomy, if she desires, to ease the teaching/learning process.

When a pelvic examination is an experience in which a woman participates and retains a sense of power and self-control as well as an educational experience, it is usually less dreaded. Encourage the woman to ask questions and express concerns, feelings, and wishes. Some women are afraid the examiner can detect their personal sexual secrets from a pelvic examination. The nurse makes an effort to provide these clients with a sense of control about self-disclosure so they do not feel the nurse is prying or can "read their past."

The nurse remains professional and avoids actions or remarks that may be misconstrued by the client as being demeaning or sexually provocative (e.g., using firm touch instead of gentle stroking). The nurse is prepared by knowing that a client may become sexually stimulated and alters the sequence of the examination, if necessary, but continues in a professional manner. Some agencies dictate that a male examiner be accompanied by a woman assistant when examining a woman.

PREEXAMINATION PREPARATION

Instruct a woman not to douche, have intercourse, or use any vaginal products for 2 to 3 days before a pelvic examination. Just before the examination, ask the woman to empty her bladder and bowels to make the examination more comfortable and accurate. If necessary, collect a urine specimen at this time. Ask the woman to remove enough clothing to allow examination of the abdomen and perineal structures. If a breast examination is planned, have the woman disrobe completely and put on a gown. The nurse asks the woman about previous experiences with pelvic examinations and acknowledges any feelings she may have. If this is the client's first examination, explain the procedure fully and show her how the speculum works. All women should be told what examinations will be performed. Telling the woman when she will be touched can help her avoid tensing up, which produces unnecessary discomfort.

PELVIC EXAMINATION EQUIPMENT

The following equipment is used during a pelvic examination:

- vaginal speculum (appropriate size)
- materials for obtaining smears and cultures for cytologic study, such as Papanicolaou (Pap) smear, including sterile cotton-tipped swabs, vaginal spatulas (wooden or plastic) or cytology brush, glass slides and glass cover slides, cytology fixative, and culture plates for gonorrhea screening
- good light source
- water-soluble lubricant
- examination gloves (appropriate size)

Long forceps and cotton balls may be used after smears and cultures have been obtained or to clean the cervix or vaginal areas so that any suspicious areas may be examined more easily. Have biopsy equipment available in case the examination reveals that such procedures are necessary.

EXAMINATION POSITION (see Chap. 12, Table 12-1)

The client is assisted in assuming a dorsal recumbent or lithotomy position and kept draped until the nurse is ready to proceed. In a lithotomy position, the woman's buttocks need to be flush with the end of the table. The client does not have to put her feet into stirrups if only the external genitalia are examined. The nurse assists the client to flex and abduct her hips and knees while arms are at the sides or crossed over the chest. Adjust the height and distance of the stirrups from the examination table to match the woman's height. Being in a lithotomy position with one's perineum exposed is uncomfortable and embarrassing. Do not keep a woman exposed any longer than necessary. The client's head may be elevated on a small pillow. Clients who have lower back pain or hip deformity may be unable to assume this position; an alternative position is necessary, such as Sims' (see Table 12-1), or an assistant may be needed to help the client abduct one or both legs. There must be an adjustable light source. The nurse wears nonsterile, disposable examining gloves.

PELVIC EXAMINATION TECHNIQUE

The nurse, with special preparation, may perform the complete pelvic examination. Two persons should be present during a pelvic examination, and one should be a woman. While the examiner is performing the examination, the second person offers the woman emotional support, gives aid during the examination, and protects the examiner against accusations of sexual abuse.

The nurse assesses secondary sexual characteristics (e.g., pubic hair distribution, developmental stage of external genitalia) during the examination of genitalia and rectum because these areas are uncovered at this time. The nurse must be familiar with the normal characteristics of the external genitalia and rectum for clinical competency when assessing skin integrity, administering vaginal and rectal medications or enemas, inserting urinary drainage catheters, and assessing changes during labor. A pelvic examination consists of four parts done in the following order.

External Genitalia Assessment. The nurse inspects the external genitalia and perineum (Fig. 74-6). Before touching the client's perineum, the nurse places one hand on the client's thigh to avoid startling her. The *mons pubis* is a mound of tissue superior to the labia. In adults, it is usually covered by *pubic hair* distributed as an inverse triangle over the mons, anterior perineum, and medial aspects of the upper thighs. The hair is inspected for nits and the skin for parasites, irritation, inflammation, edema, and lesions. There is no offensive odor present. Discharge, if present, is minimal and clear.

Perineal skin is slightly darker than that of the rest of the body. The *labia majora* are symmetric, rounded, and full. If the client has had a previous vaginal delivery, the labia majora gape slightly and the *labia minora* are evident. After menopause, the labia majora slowly atrophy. They are free of edema, inflammation, or lesions. The labia minora are thinner than the labia majora, and one side may be larger than the other. The nurse gently separates the labia majora and labia minora to inspect the vulva and remaining external structures. The nurse places the thumb and index finger of the nondominant hand inside the labia minora and retracts the tissues laterally. A firm hold is needed to avoid unnecessary manipulation of sensitive tissues.

The nurse inspects the clitoris, urethral meatus, hymen (if present), and vaginal orifice (introitus); presence is noted of discharge, inflammation, edema, or lesions, which should be absent. The *clitoris* is approximately 1 cm wide and 2 cm long and of the same color as the rest of the vulva. It can be the site of

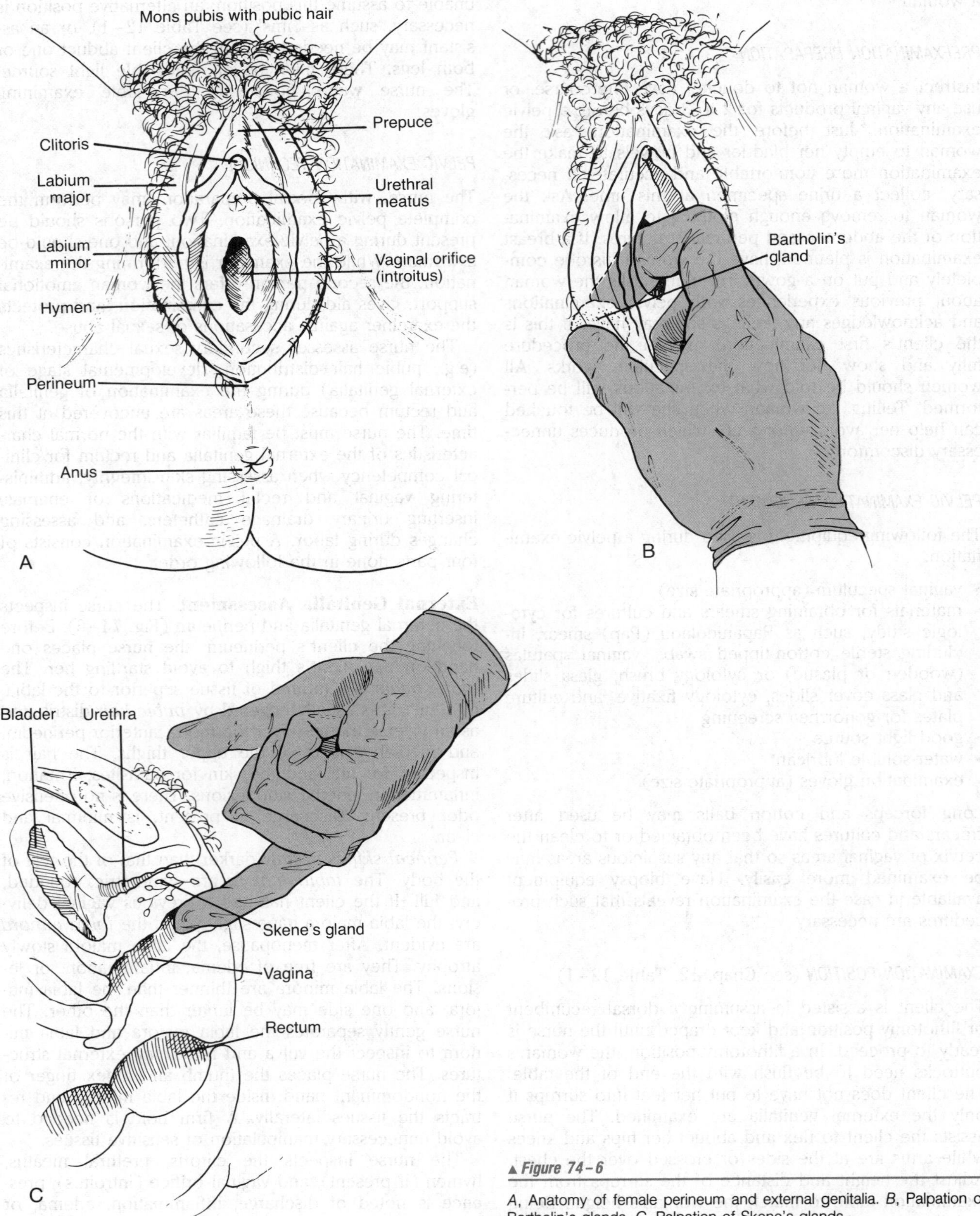

▲ *Figure 74–6*

A, Anatomy of female perineum and external genitalia. *B*, Palpation of Bartholin's glands. *C*, Palpation of Skene's glands.

syphilitic chancres in young women, and the site of dry, scaly, nodular lesions that are malignant in older women. When examining the *introitus,* the nurse also inspects the *hymen,* which is just inside the introitus. The hymen may be prominent and restrict the vaginal opening in a virgin, or it may be mostly absent in a sexually active client. *Bartholin's glands* are found near the posterior of the introitus and normally are not visualized or palpable. If inflammation and edema are present near the posterior introitus, the nurse palpates each gland between thumb and index finger. The index finger is inserted into the introitus and rotated laterally and posteriorly (Fig. 74-6*B*). The gland is palpated against the thumb at the posterior aspect of the labia majora. The maneuver is repeated for the other side.

The *urethral meatus* is between the clitoris and introitus and can be difficult to locate, particularly in women who have had a vaginal delivery. It is a small slit just above the vaginal opening and the same color as surrounding tissues. In women who have had several vaginal deliveries, the opening may be located just inside the vaginal orifice. The meatus is free of discharge, inflammation, or swelling. If these are present, the nurse palpates *Skene's glands* (paraurethral glands), which are at both sides of the urethral meatus (Fig. 74-6*C*). They usually are not visualized or palpable. The nurse inserts a gloved index finger palm-up into the introitus and approximately 1 inch (2.5 cm) into the vagina. The nurse then presses gently upward to palpate the glands and notes their characteristics. The index finger is drawn along the vaginal wall as it is removed from the vagina so that any discharge is "milked" from the glands into the urethra and out the meatus. If discharge is present, the nurse collects a specimen for culture and changes gloves before proceeding further with the examination.

In the final portion of the physical examination of external female genitalia, the nurse assesses the integrity of the *pelvic floor musculature.* The nurse inserts the index and middle fingers into the vagina and asks the client to contract her pelvic floor muscles as if trying to stop the flow of urine. In a nulliparous client, the muscles will constrict around the nurse's fingers with more tone than will those of a client who has had a vaginal delivery. Next the client is asked to bear down as if straining to void. The nurse feels for bulging of the vaginal walls that presses down against the introitus. If the anterior wall of the vagina bulges, the client probably has a *cystocele* (prolapse of the urinary bladder). A posterior vaginal wall bulge is often a result of a *rectocele* (rectal wall prolapse). Both of these are common in multiparous or obese clients.

Vaginal Speculum Examination. Wearing gloves, the examiner inserts a prewarmed vaginal speculum gently into the vagina (Fig. 74-7) *without* lubricants (lubricants interfere with the accuracy of the various cytologic examinations, such as the Pap smear). Vaginal speculum insertion is easier and more comfortable for the woman if the speculum is warmed in warm water. If lubricant is used, it is water-soluble. The nurse places the index and middle fingers of the nondominant hand in the vaginal orifice and gently pulls posteriorly. Ask the client to bear down while looking for a cystocele or rectocele. Place the end of the speculum blades, which are in a closed position, into the vaginal orifice. Gently move the speculum inward, opening the blades to observe the vaginal walls and cervix. Offer the woman a mirror if she wishes to see her cervix.

Vaginal *mucous membranes* are moist and pink, without discharge. If a discharge is present, it should be thin and white to clear in color. Abnormal findings include dry or inflamed mucosa; discharge that may be thick, curdy, yellow, green, odorous, or profuse; ulcers; lesions; masses; and bulges of the vaginal wall (e.g., rectocele, cystocele).

The *cervical os* is usually round but may be irregularly shaped after pregnancy. It is pink and smooth; a discharge is usually present, which varies from thin and clear to thick, white, and stringy, depending on the phase of the menstrual cycle. Abnormal findings include unusual color of the mucosa, abnormal consistency of discharge, ulcerations, growths, masses, nodules, inflammation, and bleeding. If abnormal discharge is present, a culture is obtained.

Before the speculum is removed from the vagina, a Pap smear and culture, if indicated, are obtained. The speculum blades are left slightly open as they are withdrawn for visualizing the vaginal walls.

Bimanual Examination. One or two fingers of the dominant hand are lubricated and inserted gently into the vagina, and the other hand is placed on the lower abdomen (Fig. 74-8). The pelvic contents are palpated between the fingers in the vagina and the hand on the abdomen. The *cervix* is located and assessed. The size, shape, surface characteristics, consistency, position, mobility, and tenderness of the *uterine body* and *fundus* are assessed. Last, each of the *adnexal areas* (left and right) is palpated. Normal *ovaries* may or may not be palpated, and normal *fallopian tubes* are not palpable. Postmenopausal ovaries should not be palpable.

A normal cervix can be gently moved sideways without pain. The cervix should feel smooth and firm, located deep in the vagina on the anterior wall. It usually points away from the fundus of the uterus, posteriorly. Abnormal findings include tenderness or pain with palpation, immobility, and an abnormal position.

The uterus is typically in an anterior position and retroverted in some women. It is normally firm, smooth, mobile, and nontender and is approximately 7.5 cm (3 inches) in length. Abnormal findings include prolapse into the vagina, feeling hard or soft, being fixed in position, irregular contour, enlargement, or tenderness.

A normal ovary is 4 to 6 cm in diameter and feels smooth, firm, and oval. Slight tenderness on palpation is normal, but uncomfortable tenderness or pain or masses are not.

Rectovaginal Examination. With insertion of one finger into the rectum (Fig. 74-9), the rectal tissues can be assessed for abnormalities, for example, hemor-

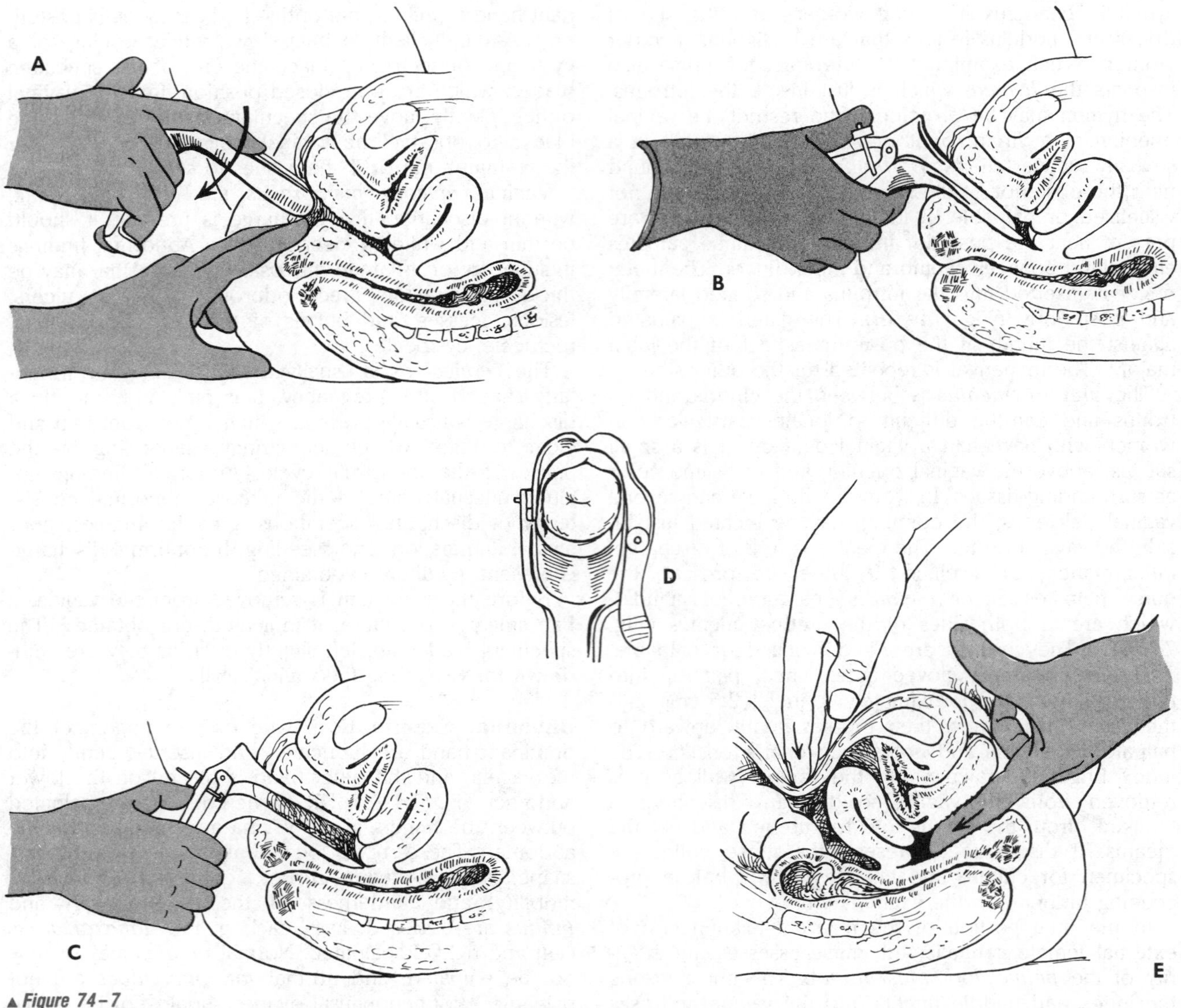

▲ *Figure 74–7*

Pelvic examination and insertion of the vaginal speculum. *A*, The speculum blades are turned obliquely, and any pressure is directed downward onto the perineum. *B*, After full insertion, the blades are rotated to a horizontal position. *C*, Squeezing the speculum handles opens the blades. *D*, A full view of the cervix and cervical os. *E*, The bimanual examination. The abdominal hand presses the pelvic organs toward the intravaginal hand to be palpated.

rhoids. Rectal examination also confirms uterine position. If the uterus is retroverted, the body and fundus are palpated. The adnexal areas are reassessed, and the rectovaginal septum and cul-de-sac are palpated. Normal pelvic organs can be palpated through the posterior cul-de-sac. Abnormal masses or normal ovaries are often felt in the cul-de-sac. If there has been blood in the vagina, a stool specimen may be tested for occult blood.

The nurse asks the client to bear down, then places the pad of the gloved middle finger over the anus. Gentle pressure is applied until the sphincter begins to relax. The tip of the finger is inserted into the rectum while the index finger is inserted into the vagina. If the uterus is retroverted, it may be felt through the rectovaginal wall. The rectovaginal wall is firm, smooth, and resilient. The cervix feels smooth, round, firm, and movable without tenderness. The nurse may mistake the cervix or a vaginal tampon (if one is left in place) for a rectal mass.

If a stool specimen is needed for occult blood, it is obtained at this time. When the examination is completed, the nurse assists the client to sit up and offers tissues or wipes for perineal hygiene.

If well performed, a vaginal examination in women who have no pathologic conditions usually causes no or minimal discomfort. Some discomfort may occur during palpation of the ovaries during the bimanual and rectal examination. Acknowledge this, and help the woman relax by asking her to bear down during rectal examination and to breathe deeply through her mouth during ovary palpation. After the examination is com-

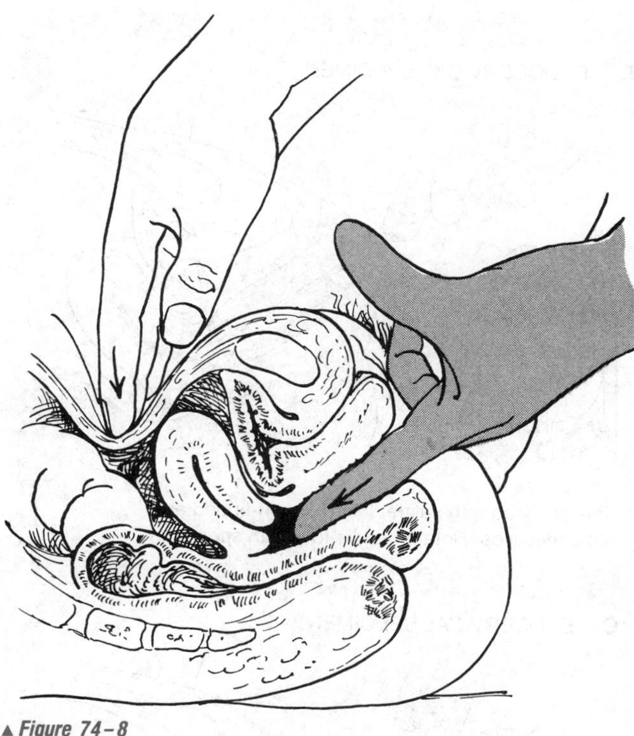

▲ Figure 74–8

Bimanual examination. The abdominal hand presses the pelvic organs toward the intravaginal hand to be palpated.

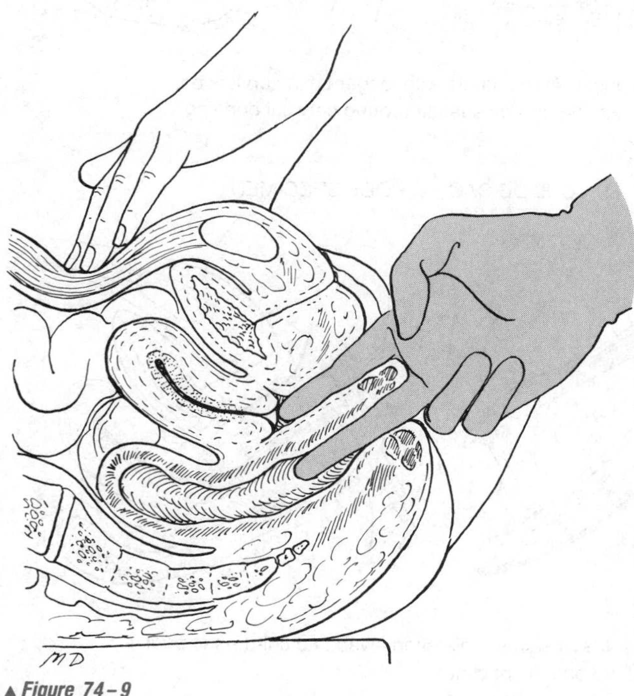

▲ Figure 74–9

Rectovaginal examination. The examiner combines bimanual and rectal examination by inserting the index finger in the woman's vagina and the middle finger in the rectum.

pleted, give instructions and conduct appropriate health teaching.

Sometimes abnormal cervical or vaginal tissue, a suspicious mass, or other problem is found during a pelvic examination. Perhaps colposcopy or biopsy of the abnormal tissue will be performed. Further examination under anesthesia may be necessary for exploration of a suspicious mass or unexplained tenderness. A pelvic examination is conducted before various other gynecologic tests (e.g., colposcopy, microscopic cervical examination, hysterosalpingogram, tubal patency) and before surgeries (such as laparoscopy or laparotomy).

DIAGNOSTIC TESTS

A complete blood count (CBC), urinalysis, and Pap smear are part of the annual gynecologic examination.

Cytology

Cytology is the examination of the structure, function, and formation of any cells (Fig. 74–10). In a gynecologic context, cytology refers to a Papanicolaou (Pap) smear. The Pap smear or test identifies preinvasive and invasive cervical cancer.

Papanicolaou Smear

A Pap test is based on the fact that cells (normal and abnormal) are shed from the lining of the uterus and cervix and pass into both cervical and vaginal secretions. When a cytologic smear is made of these secretions and examined under a microscope, early cellular changes may be detected before disease becomes clinically apparent. The Pap test is up to 95 per cent accurate in diagnosing early cervical carcinoma, when correct sampling and handling techniques are used. It is much less accurate (about 40 per cent) in detecting endometrial carcinoma.

Smears for the Pap test consist of a small amount of secretions taken from (1) the vaginal pool, located in the posterior fornix, and (2) the endocervix and ectocervix. These secretions are smeared separately on clean and dry slides, or they may be placed on one slide divided into sections. The slides are marked with C for cervix and V for vaginal pool. Immediately after the smears are made on the slides, they are fixed, by use of either a commercial spray or fixative solution. It is important to fix the secretions before they dry. Cells in the specimen may be distorted if they dry, which makes accurate reading difficult or impossible. Lubricant is not used on the vaginal speculum for the same reason.

Obtaining a Pap smear is usually painless. The American Cancer Society[1] currently recommends that women who are or have been sexually active, or have reached age 18 years, should have annual Pap tests and pelvic examinations. After a woman has had three or more consecutive satisfactory normal annual exami-

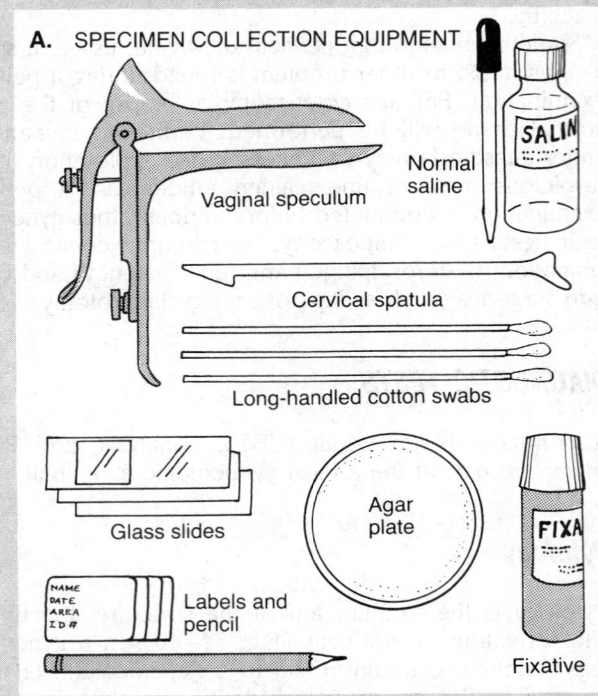

B. ENDOCERVICAL SPECIMEN

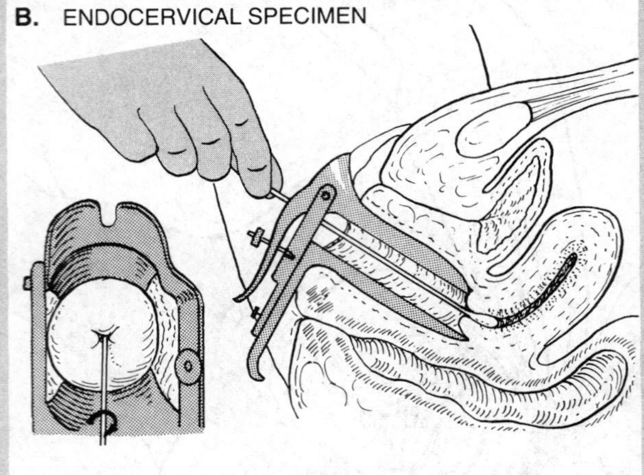

Moisten swab with saline. Insert cotton-tipped end into cervical os. Rotate handle to obtain specimen.

C. EXOCERVICAL SPECIMEN

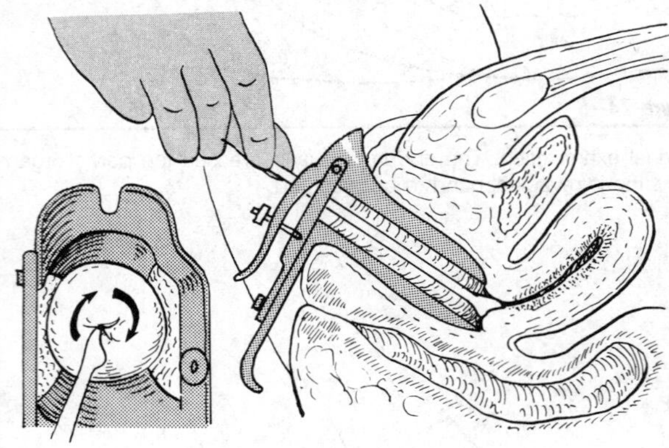

Insert Ayre spatula with longer tip in cervical os. Rotate end of spatula around cervical opening.

D. CUL-DE-SAC POOL SPECIMEN

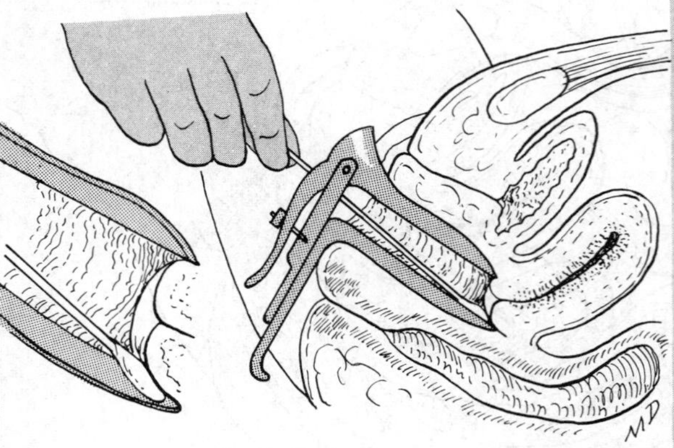

Insert saline-moistened swab into cul-de-sac pool to obtain specimen.

E. SLIDE PREPARATION

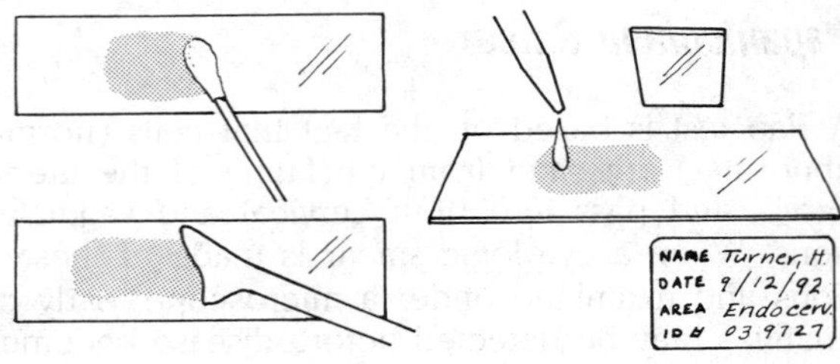

Smear specimen evenly on glass slide. Add drop of saline and cover with cover glass. Label with name, date, area of sample, identification number.

F. GONOCOCCAL CULTURE

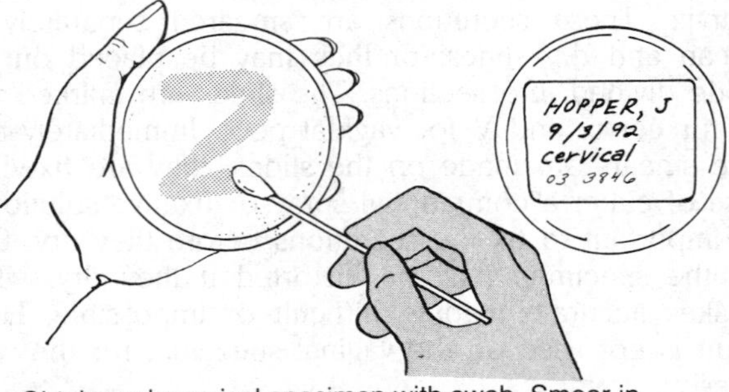

Obtain endocervical specimen with swab. Smear in Z-pattern on agar plate. Spray with fixative. Cover and label as above.

▲ *Figure 74–10*

Cervical cytology specimen collection.

nations, the Pap test may be performed less frequently at the discretion of her physician. Many physicians, however, continue to recommend annual examinations. For women at high risk, an endometrial tissue sample should be taken at menopause. The Pap test should be continued after menopause. Vaginal smears are obtained for Pap smear in women who have had a hysterectomy (see Chap. 76).

Be sure the woman knows when and where she can get the results of her Pap test. In the past, a numerical classification system ranging from class I (no abnormal or atypical cells present) to class V (probable malignancy) was used to report findings. Descriptive reports are currently preferred because they are more useful in clinical decision making. Such reports either classify findings as normal or describe more fully the cellular changes seen. Specific infections may also be identified, and hormonal assessment may be done. A Pap test may be used to follow some abnormalities, and women may be taught to get their own specimens.

A suspicious Pap smear does not necessarily mean that the woman has a malignancy. There is about a 5 per cent false-positive or false-negative rate for the Pap test, and this rate may be much higher if the specimen was incorrectly collected or handled. However, having an abnormal Pap smear can be a frightening experience. Careful interpretation of cytologic findings to a woman is very important. She needs ample opportunity to ask questions, to discuss concerns and feelings, and to participate in follow-up care planning.

If the woman's cervix appears abnormal to the naked eye during the examination, then colposcopy may be done during the examination, if it is available (see section on colposcopy). If the results of the Pap smear show a vaginal infection is present, the woman may be treated for the vaginitis and the Pap test repeated later. If the results of the Pap test show dysplasia or abnormal tissue, then treatment will vary according to the extent of the lesion, the grade of the dysplasia, and the preference of the woman and her physician. For more information on cervical cancer, see Chapter 76.

Wet Smear

The wet smear is used to detect vaginal infection with *Candida albicans, Trichomonas vaginalis,* or organisms that cause bacterial infections. A copious specimen of discharge from the vaginal vault is obtained with a cotton-tipped swab and placed in about 1 ml of warm normal saline (to separate the cells), mixed to produce a suspension, and then placed on a glass slide for microscopic examination.

Cervical Culture

A cervical culture may be done to detect infection with *Neisseria gonorrhoeae* or *Chlamydia trachomatis.* A cotton-tipped swab is rotated in the endocervical canal for obtaining a specimen and then rolled in a Z pattern onto a culture medium. The culture medium should be at room temperature before inoculation with the specimen.

Endometrial Smear

An endometrial smear is made in a manner similar to a Pap smear (Fig. 74-11). An endometrial smear is obtained by swabbing the uterine lining to get cells and secretions for examination. This test differs from a Pap test in that the cervix must be dilated under sterile conditions to get the specimen. The procedure is usually done during the first 12 hours after the onset of menses, because the cervix is easier to enter at this time. Cervical dilation may cause cramping, which is usually relieved by analgesics and heat application to the lower abdomen.

The American Cancer Society[1] recommends that women at high risk for developing endometrial cancer have an endometrial tissue smear performed at menopause. Subsequent smears are recommended by calculating the client's risk.

Endometrial Biopsy

A sample of endometrial tissue can be obtained for histologic study on an outpatient basis through the technique of endometrial biopsy. Endometrial tissue may be analyzed for menstrual disturbances, infertility, or endometrial cancer. The biopsy is performed after bimanual examination of the uterus. Because the biopsy may cause cramping, the woman may receive a paracervical block to relieve the discomfort. After dilating the cervix, the physician passes a sounding instrument into the uterus to measure the depth of the uterine cavity. Then the physician inserts a cutting or aspirating instrument into the uterus and removes a small amount of tissue from the fundus for examination. Again, if cramping persists after the procedure, administer analgesics as ordered or apply heat to the lower abdomen.

Colposcopy

Colposcopy involves using a magnifying instrument (colposcope) to examine the cervical epithelium, vagina, and vulva (Fig. 74-12). A colposcope is a stereoscopic binocular microscope, usually used with a magnification power of 15. Colposcopy is indicated for all women with Pap smears showing dysplasia and may be used to examine any suspicious lesion in the lower genital tract. In this office/clinic procedure, the woman is placed in lithotomy position and her cervix is exposed with a vaginal speculum. A solution of 3 per cent acetic acid (common household vinegar) is applied to remove mucus and debris and to dehydrate the cells slightly on the cervix. The cervix and upper vagina are then inspected with the colposcope. Epithelial abnormalities can be detected as well as specific lesions. Biopsy is usually performed at the time of colposcopy if a suspicious lesion is present and can easily

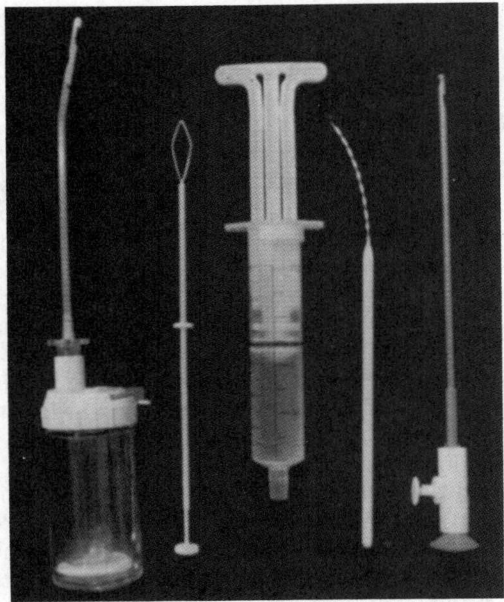

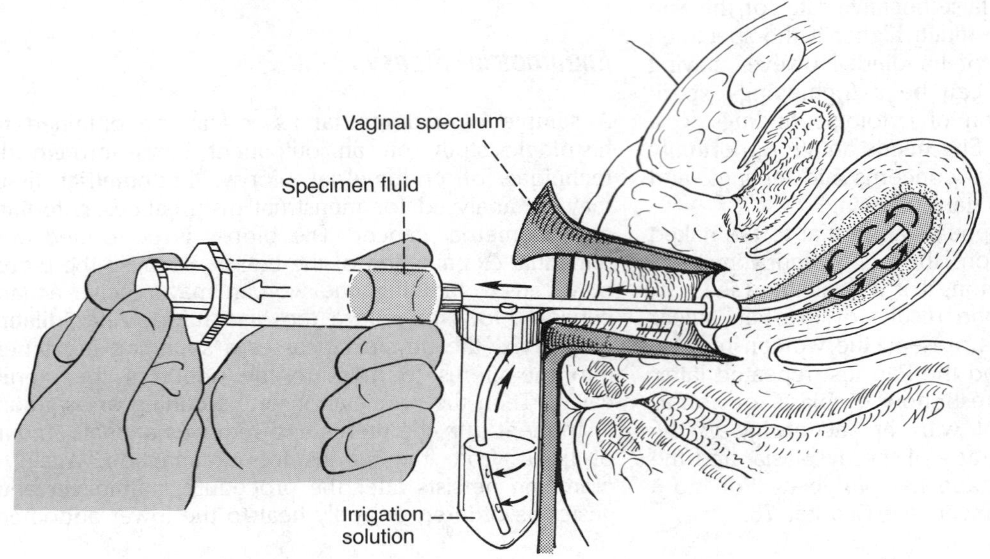

▲ Figure 74-11

A, Endometrial sampling devices for uterine cancer screening. *Left to right:* Vakutage, Accurette, syringe for Karman cannula, Mi-Mark helix, and Karman cannula. *B*, Gravlee Jet Washer performing endometrial uterine lavage with sterile normal saline under negative pressure. Cells loosened by the "washing" are obtained for cytopathologic examination. Arrows indicate the flow of the irrigating solution and collection of the specimen. Fluid does not enter the fallopian tubes. A rubber plug at the cervical os helps create an airtight, negative pressure within the uterus. Arrows within the uterus show circulation of fluids within the uterus. (From Boone, M. I., et al. [1984]. Uterine cancer screening by the family physician. *American Family Physician, 30:*157.)

be done in the office or clinic without the use of anesthesia.

Use of colposcopy increases the diagnostic accuracy and reduces the need for biopsy. The procedure is safe and painless and can be done on pregnant women. Explain to the woman that the procedure is like a pelvic examination and that when the speculum is in place, a large microscope will be used to look at the cervix. The scope is not inserted into the vagina.

Cervical Biopsy

Biopsies of suspicious cervical lesions identified with the naked eye or with colposcopic magnification are usually performed in the outpatient setting with the use of little or no anesthesia. A solution of 3 percent acetic acid can be applied to the cervix to identify areas suspicious for dysplasia, metaplasia, or malignancy. These areas undergo a color change and appear white.

In an unusual situation, when colposcopy cannot identify an abnormal lesion on the cervix or vagina, Schiller's test may be performed. Schiller's iodine solution is applied to the vagina and cervix. Normal tissue takes up the stain and appears a homogeneous mahogany-brown color. Usually, abnormal tissue does not take stain as well and may appear light yellow instead. This is a positive finding and can indicate areas that need to be biopsied. A biopsy may be done when a cervical lesion is first noted or delayed until about 1 week after the menstrual period (when the cervix is least vascular). Multiple biopsies are usually obtained at specific sites with biopsy forceps (Fig. 74-13). Hemostasis is achieved with topical application of silver ni-

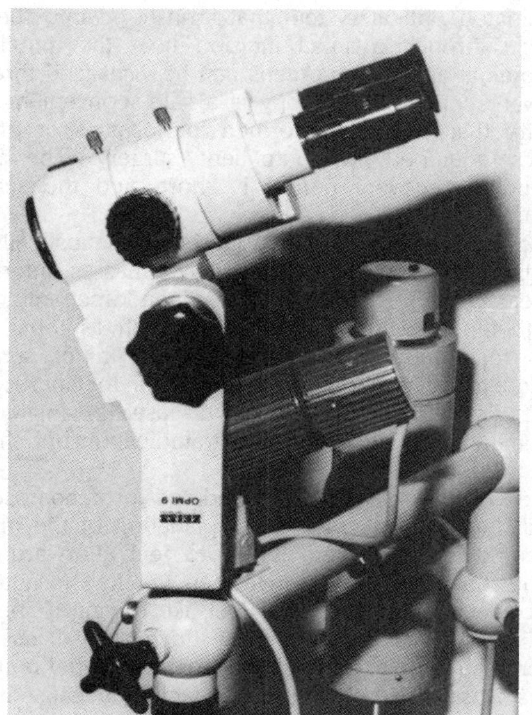

▲ **Figure 74-12**

A colposcope, used to evaluate clients with an abnormal Papanicolaou smear and a grossly normal cervix. (From Hacker, N. F., & Moore, J. G. [1992]. *Essentials of obstetrics and gynecology* [2nd ed.]. Philadelphia: W. B. Saunders.)

trate or Monsel's solution. The biopsies are usually somewhat painful. For ruling out disease in the endocervical canal, endocervical curettage may be performed.

Allow the woman to rest for a short time before going home. Instruct her to avoid activity for the next 24 hours. Although she may note a small amount of blood-tinged vaginal discharge, any excessive bleeding should be reported to the physician immediately. Advise her to abstain from vaginal sexual activity, avoid tampons, and avoid douching for several days to achieve hemostasis, lessen trauma, and promote healing.

Cold Knife Conization

Today, colposcopy, biopsy, and endocervical curettage have largely replaced conization, but there are some circumstances in which it is indicated. When the lesion is in the endocervix or when the Pap smear suggests invasive carcinoma, conization may be done. The goal of conization is to excise the cervical lesion entirely by cutting out a cone-shaped section of tissue with an adequate surgical margin. Conization is usually performed in an outpatient room under general or spinal anesthesia. After excision of the conization specimen, curettage of the remaining endocervical canal is usually performed. The carbon dioxide laser can be used in place of cold knife cone biopsy. Laser conization is carried out the same way as the cold knife procedure is. Postoperative care is similar to that after dilation and curettage. Vaginal packing may be used to control bleeding for 24 to 48 hours. Immediate complications include intraoperative or postoperative hemorrhage. Tell the woman that some vaginal discharge (often blood-tinged) usually occurs after 3 to 5 days and that her next two to three menstrual periods may be prolonged, heavier than usual, and possibly preceded by a dark-brown premenstrual discharge. Bleeding can occur about 1 week after surgery when the absorbable suture placed in the surgical bed reabsorbs. Complications are rare after conization but include infection, incompetent cervix, or cervical stenosis.

Culdoscopy

Culdoscopy allows visualization of structures in the cul-de-sac through a culdoscope, a lighted hollow tubelike instrument. This allows the physician to inspect this area and thus avoid exploratory surgery when faced with puzzling diagnostic problems that may or may not require surgical intervention. Laparoscopy has replaced culdoscopy in most settings because it provides superior visualization of the entire pelvis, especially the cul-de-sac, and permits a more complete visualization of the abdominal cavity. *Culdocentesis* is similar to culdoscopy except that a needle is inserted through the posterior fornix into the cul-de-sac to facilitate drainage. The cul-de-sac may be aspirated for assessing various gynecologic conditions such as ectopic pregnancy or ovarian malignancy.

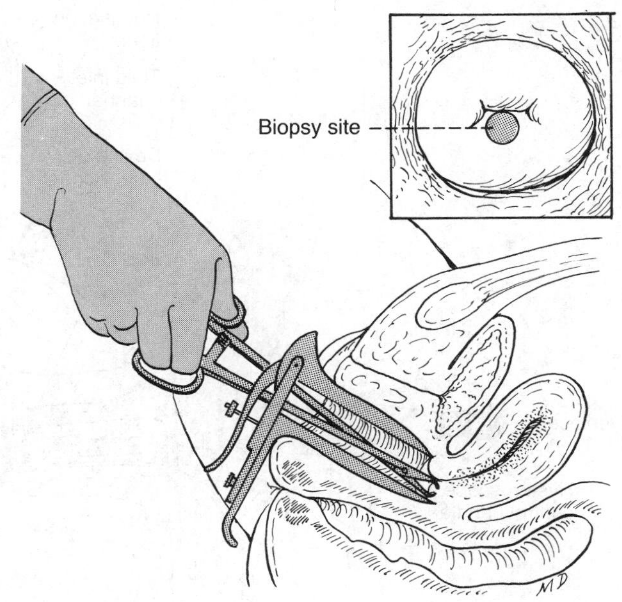

▲ **Figure 74-13**

Cervical biopsy.

Hysteroscopy

In this technique, the intrauterine cavity is directly viewed through an endoscope called a hysteroscope (Fig. 74-14). Hysteroscopes have a fiberoptic lighting system and employ 5 per cent glucose in water, highly viscous dextran solutions, or carbon dioxide as the uterine-distending medium. The hysteroscope is passed into the uterus via the vagina. The uterine cavity is distended and may be rinsed to clear away blood and secretory debris that would obstruct vision. In addition to direct visualization of the uterine cavity, directed biopsies and resections of endometrial abnormalities can be done. The hysteroscope can also be used to deliver a laser beam into the uterus for therapeutic procedures. Hysteroscopy may be used for (1) ruling out organic causes in abnormal uterine or postmenopausal bleeding, (2) suspected leiomyomas or polyps, (3) removal of intrauterine device with missing string, (4) infertility evaluation, and (5) surgical techniques for uterine abnormalities. Hysteroscopy is contraindicated if the woman (1) has acute pelvic inflammatory disease, recurrent chronic upper genital tract infection, or recent uterine perforation; (2) has or is suspected of having cervical malignancy; or (3) is pregnant. Complications include bleeding, uterine perforation, infection, and perhaps bowel injuries.

Laparoscopy

A laparoscope is a commonly used diagnostic and therapeutic tool (Fig. 74-15). It is a telescope with an illuminated optical system that is inserted into the abdomen through a small incision near the umbilicus. Abdominal and pelvic organs can be visualized through a laparoscope. Laparoscopy is a safe, convenient procedure that can be performed in hospitals or office/clinics equipped for outpatient surgery. The post-procedure recovery period is short, and the scar is small.

Laparoscopy may be performed (1) diagnostically for conditions such as pelvic pain, pelvic masses, infertility, suspected ectopic pregnancy, and endometriosis; and (2) therapeutically for procedures such as tubal ligations for contraceptive purposes and minor surgical procedures. The main contraindication to laparoscopy is serious cardiac or pulmonary disease. Previous lower abdominal surgery is not a contraindication but should be considered.

Preoperatively, a woman scheduled for a laparoscopy should be given a complete explanation of the procedure and how she can expect to feel afterward. She should have someone drive her to the hospital or clinic, because she may not feel like driving if she has local anesthesia and should not drive at all if she has general anesthesia. She will be more comfortable if she wears loose-fitting clothes to the facility, because it will be easier to prepare to go home after the procedure. Typically, women having laparoscopy in a same-day surgical setting can go home 2 to 4 hours after the procedure.

The woman is usually instructed to have nothing by mouth past midnight on the day the laparoscopy is scheduled. Depending on the physician's preference, a cathartic or enema and a partial perineal shave might

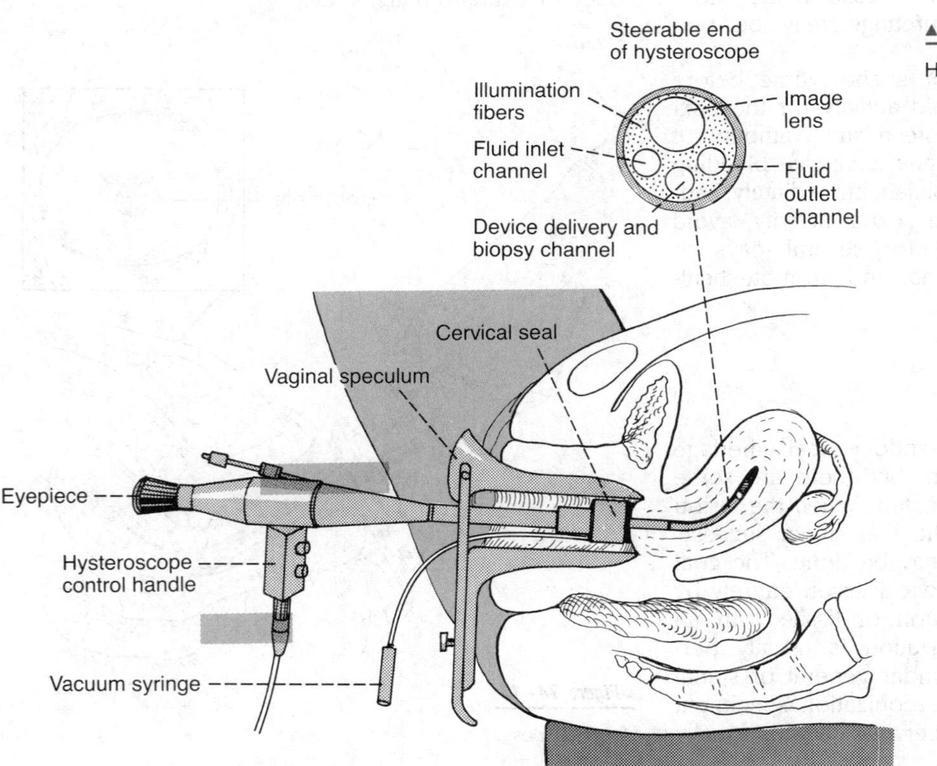

▲ *Figure 74-14*

Hysteroscopy.

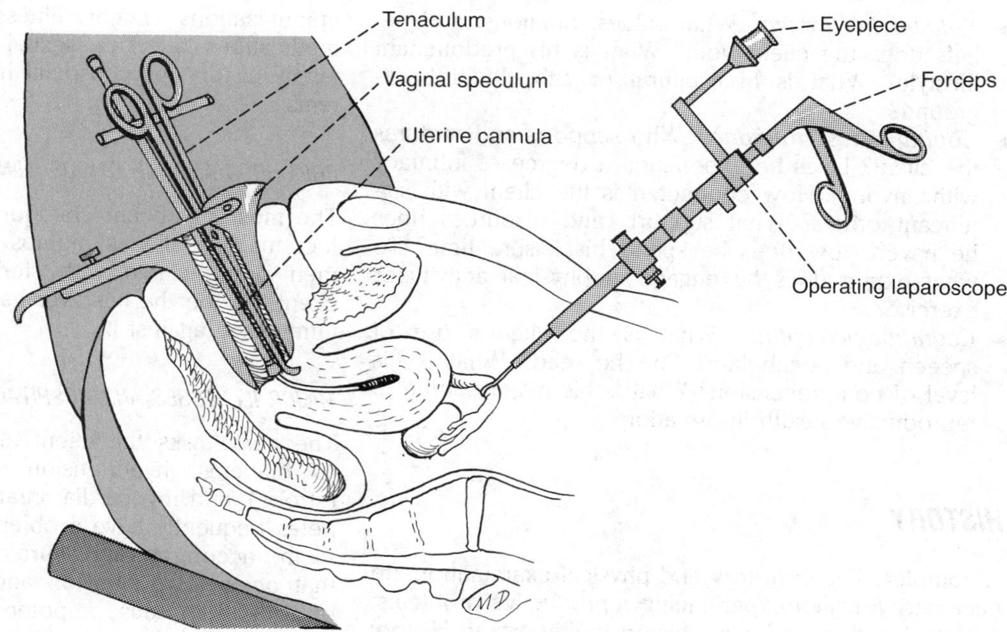

▲ Figure 74-15

Laparoscopy.

be required (usually they are not). Abdominal skin preparation (scrubbing and shaving) is done in the operating room.

Postoperatively, take vital signs every 15 minutes for the first hour, or until the client is stable. If local anesthesia has been used, the woman can have fluids and a light snack as soon as she wants. After general anesthesia, the woman may have fluids and a light snack as soon as she is fully awake and has no nausea. Explain to the client that she may experience mild to moderate transient shoulder pain or a feeling of "bloatedness" as a result of the carbon dioxide or nitrous oxide used to distend the abdomen during the procedure (separating the organs and allowing better visualization). The discomfort usually lasts only a few hours and may be relieved by comfortable positioning or mild analgesics. The woman also may experience mild incisional pain or abdominal cramping for the first few hours or days after the procedure, which is usually relieved by rest. If the woman had general anesthesia, she might have a sore throat from intubation or a sore chest from insufflation. These symptoms usually disappear within 48 hours. Teach her to keep the incision clean and dry. After it heals, the scar will be barely noticeable. Sexual intercourse can be resumed within a week or less.

▼ ASSESSING MEN WITH REPRODUCTIVE/URINARY TRACT DISORDERS

Male reproductive problems are common disorders experienced by men of all ages. Assessing men's reproductive/urinary tract disorders requires expertise on the part of the nurse. This expertise is required in both the history and psychosocial assessment, as well as physical examination skills. The nurse must display sensitivity and tact when working with these clients because men are often uncomfortable discussing issues associated with these disorders.

PSYCHOSOCIAL ASSESSMENT

An overview of assessment areas pertinent to males with reproductive disturbances is presented here. When taking a nursing history for such men, consider the following factors. The nurse will probably not be able to obtain detailed information in each of these areas, but the outline will signal areas that will help understand each man and his significant others as individuals and avoid stereotypic and possibly judgmental nursing care.

- *Self-concept.* How has the client's health affected how he feels about himself? How do his partner and significant others feel about him? What is his posture, dress, grooming? What is his emotional response? What is his mood or feeling tone?
- *Role-relationships.* Who are the important people to this client? Who accompanied him to the health care facility? Who does he say is his most significant other? How was the client's health affected? How is he able to carry out his various social roles (e.g., partner, husband, friend, father, worker)? How has his health affected his economic situation and his partner/significant others?
- *Communication.* How does the client communicate both verbally and nonverbally with (1) the nurse, (2) his significant others? Does he maintain eye contact? Does he use gestures or touch? How does he speak (e.g., volume, tone, vocabulary, repetition)?

- *Value-belief system.* What values, opinions, and beliefs does the client hold? What is his predominant lifestyle? What is his cultural or subcultural background?
- *Coping, stress tolerance.* Who supports and nurtures the client? Does he experience a degree of intimacy with anyone? How connected is the client with significant others? What supports and resources does he have? How does he spend his leisure time? To what extent does he engage in physical activity or exercise?
- *Cognitive-perceptual.* What is the client's use of speech and vocabulary? Can he read? What is his level of comprehension? What is his major source of reproductive health information?

HISTORY

A complete health history and physical examination are necessary for men experiencing reproductive problems. A sexual and reproductive history is important. History taking provides an opportunity to (1) give men permission to express sensitive concerns, (2) identify myths and misinformation held by the client, (3) give health information, (4) offer referrals, and (5) facilitate further communication. Those aspects of history taking that address major risk factors pertinent to men's reproductive health are discussed here.

Chief Complaint

The client may present with problems related to the genitourinary, reproductive, or sexual systems. Areas in a chief complaint may include

- systemic disturbances, such as weight loss, fever, and malaise
- voiding disturbances, such as frequency, polyuria, oliguria, nocturia, pyuria, enuresis, dysuria, urgency, or incontinence
- disturbances in the character of urine, such as hematuria, pyuria
- gastrointestinal disturbances, such as nausea, vomiting, anorexia, abdominal discomfort, constipation, or diarrhea
- reproductive disturbances, infertility, history of STDs, genital lesions, or genital discharge in self and partner; genital trauma
- sexual functioning, whether sexually active or celibate; changes in sexual desire; changes in erectile ability; decreased ejaculatory ability; gynecomastia; effects of symptoms, disability, chronic disease, trauma, surgery, or treatment on sexual functioning

For each reported symptom the client reports, the nurse conducts a symptom analysis (see Chap. 11).

Past Medical History

Significant past medical history for the male reproductive system includes childhood and infectious diseases, immunizations, major illnesses and hospitalizations, medications, allergies, sexual and reproductive history, family history, psychosocial history, and review of systems.

CHILDHOOD AND INFECTIOUS ILLNESSES

The most significant childhood infectious illness to affect male fertility is mumps. Its occurrence in young men is associated with sterility. The nurse asks the client whether he has ever had the mumps or has been immunized against it.

MAJOR ILLNESSES AND HOSPITALIZATIONS

The nurse asks the client about major illnesses such as diabetes, hypertension, cerebrovascular accident (stroke), and myocardial infarction. Men who have diabetes frequently have problems with impotency related to the accompanying neurologic and vascular changes that occur. Hypertension and its serious complication of stroke can cause impotence because of physiologic or psychological factors. Impotence may also occur in men who have had myocardial infarctions because of a fear of precipitating another heart attack as a result of sexual excitement and activity. The nurse is alert to the man's concerns and fears and remains nonjudgmental, offering the support of counseling and referral to peer groups established for this purpose. Renal and urinary tract disorders can interfere with sexual functioning because of the close physiologic and anatomic relationships. Endocrine disorders can also interfere with sexual performance.

The nurse asks the client about surgery involving the reproductive system. Specific surgical procedures include herniorrhaphy, vasectomy, prostatectomy, varicocelectomy, and testicular torsion repair.

MEDICATIONS

Obtain a complete medication history for prescription, over-the-counter, and recreational drugs. Some medications prescribed for hypertension may cause impotence (e.g., methyldopa, clonidine, guanethidine, and hydralazine). Tranquilizers can interfere with sexual performance. Recreational drugs that alter behavior can also affect physiologic reproductive function, for example, marijuana and other hallucinogenics.

ALLERGIES

Ask the client specifically about allergies to penicillin and sulfonamides and to rubber or latex. Male genitourinary disorders are often treated with these antibiotics, and latex and rubber are ingredients found in condoms as well as in the gloves used by the examiner during the rectal examination.

SEXUAL AND REPRODUCTIVE HISTORY

The sexual and reproductive history for a man includes the following. See also Chapters 7 and 11 for further information on sexuality assessment.

Breast History. Data should be collected about the breast and axilla for both men and women. The nurse asks the client about breast pain or tenderness, masses, lumps, and nipple discharge. If any of these symptoms is present, a symptom analysis is performed (see Chap. 11). Ask whether the man or his sexual partner has noticed any changes in breast tissue, such as enlargement (*gynecomastia*). Gynecomastia can occur in obese or elderly men. Ask whether the client performs breast self-examination, similar to that done by a woman. Breast self-examination should be performed on a regular, monthly basis following the same guidelines as those for a woman. If the client does not perform breast self-examination, offer to teach him the technique.

Contraceptive History. Document the man's current contraceptive method (if any), his satisfaction with the method, effect of contraception on sexual function, and any desire to change methods. Has the man used contraceptive methods previously, and if so, were there problems leading to their discontinuation?

Sexual History. The nurse inquires about the client's patterns of sexual relationships. Can the man relate the total number of sexual partners he has had and the frequency of sexual activity? Multiple partners and contacts increase the client's risk of STD as well as human immunodeficiency virus (HIV) infection. Does the man use condoms during sexual intercourse? Does the client engage in homosexual or bisexual relationships, both of which increase the risk of HIV infection?

Does the client have any sexual concerns, such as an inability to attain or maintain an erection? If so, the nurse asks whether this is a problem that occurs frequently or occasionally. Is the client able to discuss sexual concerns with his partner? Have he and his partner developed ways to cope with or adjust to disturbances in sexual function? If sexual dysfunction exists, does the client wish a referral or consultation with a sexual counselor?

Throughout the interview, the nurse asks questions directly. Instead of beginning questions with "why" (which puts the client on the spot to justify his behavior), the nurse phrases questions in such a way that it is assumed the client has performed in this way. This interview technique helps preserve the client's dignity and self-esteem instead of making him feel guilt or shame.

Past Genitourinary History. Ask about past problems with genitourinary infections, such as prostatitis. Determine whether the client has had a previous pelvic examination. Are there problems with urine incontinence or dribbling, hesitancy, weak urine stream, or other symptoms? Also see Chapter 48 for assessment of the urinary system.

Reproductive Health Practices. The nurse inquires about sexual and reproductive hygiene. How often does the man perform self-examinations of the breast and testes? Does he protect himself against STDs? See also Chapter 11 for discussion of health risk management.

Family History

Ask if there is a family history of infertility, diabetes, hypertension, cerebrovascular accidents (stroke), or endocrine disorders. Like women whose mothers took DES during pregnancy, men exposed to DES in utero are at increased risk for congenital anomalies including structural defects of the genitourinary system and decreased semen levels.

Psychosocial History and Lifestyle

In addition to those areas previously discussed under psychosocial assessment, the nurse assesses the following areas.

OCCUPATIONAL AND ENVIRONMENTAL FACTORS

Determine the type of work and recreational activities of the client for identifying risk of exposure to chemicals, pesticides, heat, heavy metals, hormones, and radiation. These materials can directly affect the number and integrity of sperm and germal tissue.

HABITS

Assess the client's use of caffeine, alcohol, smoking tobacco, and marijuana. These substances may affect the sperm count, contribute to impotence, or decrease the libido. The use of recreational drugs is discussed previously.

Review of Systems

When conducting the review of systems, ask specifically about diabetes, hypertension, stroke, myocardial infarction, angina, endocrine disorders, renal disorders, and urinary tract problems. Detailed questions for the review of systems are found in Chapter 11, Table 11-5.

PHYSICAL EXAMINATION

Skillful history taking can help establish a therapeutic relationship that facilitates successful physical examination. Many men find physical examination for problems of the reproductive system stressful and embarrassing. Genitals are viewed by many as private and even unclean.

Nurses can make a reproductive and sexual physical examination more comfortable for the man by sharing normal findings while proceeding. Explain each step carefully. Ways of increasing the client's comfort during examination include maintaining eye contact, proceeding in an unhurried manner, and involving the client in self-examination.

Sometimes a man will have an erection during an examination. This possibility is lessened by a kind yet professional manner and a firm yet gentle touch. If the man does have an erection, explain that this is normal and does not have any sexual connotation.

Physical examination for reproductive problems focuses on findings that may be associated with reproductive or sexual problems. These may be

- inflammatory (e.g., enlarged, tender, movable, or fixed lymph nodes in the inguinal regions)
- endocrinologic and genetic (e.g., general body appearance for indications of conditions such as Cushing's syndrome or acromegaly; hair distribution; gynecomastia)
- neurologic (e.g., gross neurologic examination of the lower extremities)
- vascular (e.g., status of femoral and pedal pulses)
- traumatic (e.g., hernia)

The nurse follows an orderly approach for the physical examination and teaches the client how to do similar self-examinations regularly. The male breast and axilla are included here as part of the examination of the reproductive system.

Breast Examination

It is important that the nurse examine the breasts of male clients. Although the incidence of breast cancer in men is low, it does occur because men have glandular tissue beneath each nipple. Likewise, the axillary nodes are examined for men.

Inspect and palpate the breasts and axillae while the man is sitting, following the same guidelines as discussed for the female breast examination. The male breast is flat and symmetric without nodules, edema, or ulceration. Enlargement (gynecomastia) may occur in obese or elderly men. Unilateral enlargement that persists past puberty is abnormal. Palpation reveals a small, flat disc of glandular tissue under the areola. There should be no masses or discharge present. Axillary nodes should be nonpalpable (see Fig. 74–2).

Male Genitalia

The nurse ensures that the client's urinary bladder is empty. The client may be supine or lying on his side with legs spread slightly for the first portion of the genitalia examination but will be asked to stand when the nurse assesses for inguinal herniation. An alternative position is to have the client stand for the entire examination of the genitalia while the nurse is seated on a stool. Because the male urethra is the common conduit for both urine and semen, examination of the male reproductive tract also includes assessment of the urinary system. The nurse wears nonsterile, disposable examining gloves.

The nurse inspects the external genitalia and perineum (Fig. 74–16), observing the *pubic hair and skin.* The nurse must be familiar with normal growth and development of the male genitalia. Observe the client's general appearance and body build. Notice hair distribution. Pubic hair distribution is triangular with hair covering the symphysis pubis, base of the penis, and inner aspects of the thighs. Hair distribution may also spread toward the umbilicus in a diamond pattern. Hair is inspected for nits and the skin for parasites, rashes, excoriation, and lesions. Masses, lesions, edema, and offensive odors should be absent. *Scrotal skin* is darker than other skin surfaces, loose, and wrinkled.

The *penis* includes the penile shaft, prepuce (foreskin), glans, and urethral meatus (Fig. 74–17). The nurse inspects and palpates these structures for lesions, nodules, swelling, inflammation, atrophy, and discharge. *Penile skin* in the unerect penis is wrinkled. The *foreskin,* if present, covers the glans. The foreskin is absent in a circumcised client. The nurse instructs the client to retract the foreskin to expose the *glans,* which is easily accomplished. The nurse may note a small amount of cheesy, thick, white, odoriferous *smegma* between the glans and the foreskin, which is normal. If other discharge is noted, the nurse obtains a specimen for culture. The area between the glans and foreskin is a common site for venereal lesions. It is normally free of lesions; if any are present, the nurse palpates them for tenderness, size, shape, and consistency.

Next, the nurse inspects the *urethral meatus,* which is located at the tip of the penis and looks like a slit. Malposition of the meatus on either the underside of the penile shaft *(hypospadias)* or upper side *(epispadias)* is usually a congenital condition. The meatus is pink and without ulcers, scars, inflammation, or discharge. The nurse gently compresses the glans between thumb and index finger to open the meatus and inspects for discharge. If the client reports a urethral discharge, the nurse asks the client to compress the penis from base to tip between his thumb and fingers in an attempt to express a discharge. If one is expressed, the nurse obtains a specimen for culture or microscopic examination.

The *penile shaft* is gently palpated between the thumb and first two fingers. It is smooth and semifirm, and the skin moves easily over underlying structures. The penis is free of nodules, thickened or hard areas, and tenderness.

The *scrotum* is inspected and palpated for symmetry, size, shape, and swelling. The scrotum has a right and left half, each containing a testis, epididymis, and vas deferens. The left testis usually hangs lower than the right. Scrotal size varies with ambient temperature; cold results in contraction, and warmth in relaxation. The nurse asks the client to hold the penis to one side and then the other and to lift the scrotum up while she inspects. The skin is loose, without tenseness. The *testes* are oval, approximately 2 cm by 4 cm (4/5 inch by 1 3/5 inches). On palpation, they are smooth, firm, and rubbery without nodules, masses, or tenderness. Elderly clients have smaller, less firm testes. In younger, adolescent males, the nurse notes that both testes are present in the scrotum. Testes may temporarily migrate as a result of being touched during examination or

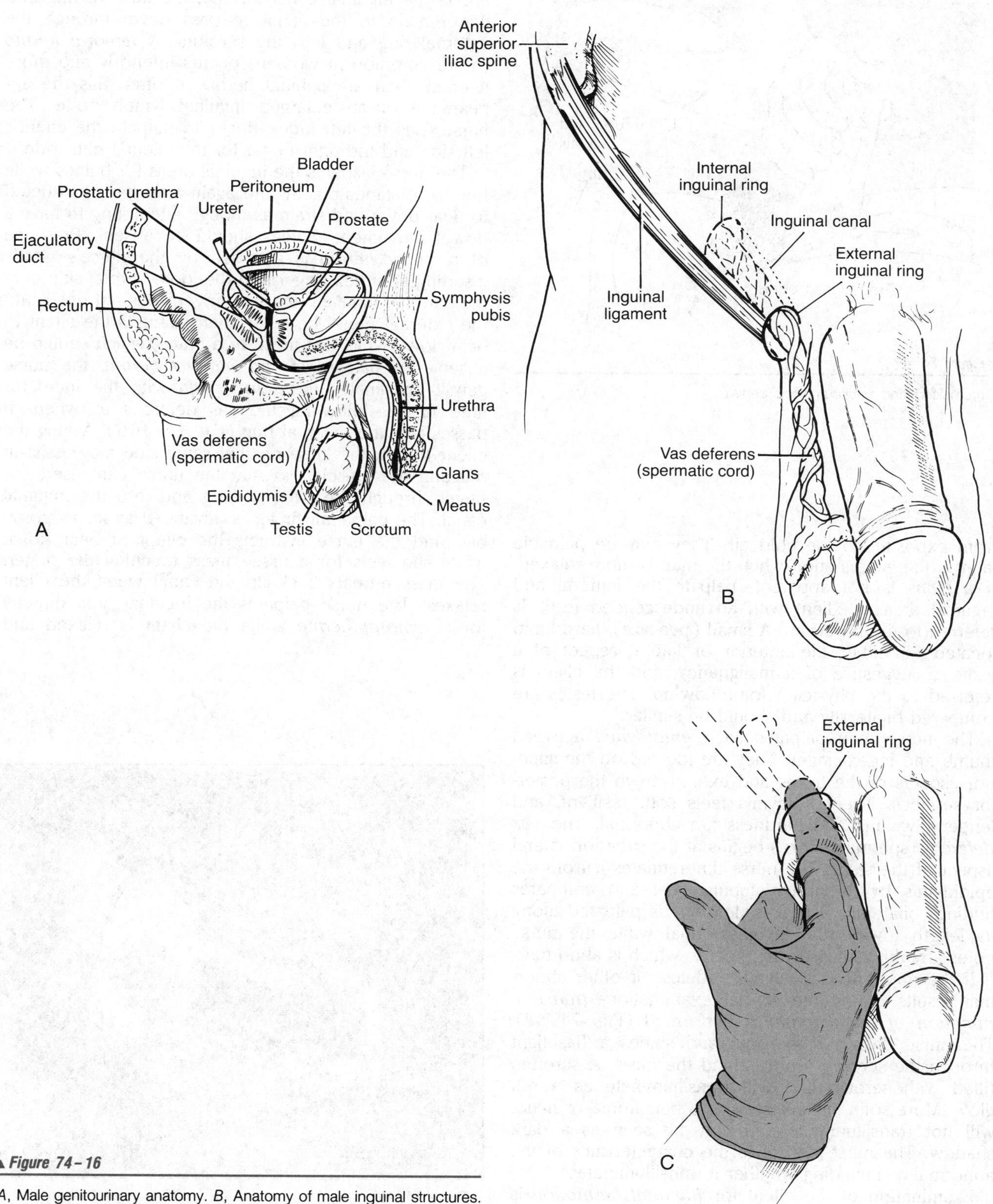

▲ *Figure 74–16*

A, Male genitourinary anatomy. *B*, Anatomy of male inguinal structures. *C*, Palpation for detecting an indirect hernia.

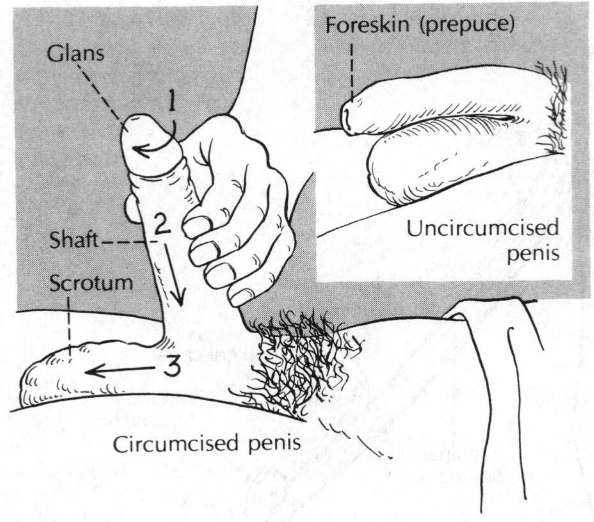

▲ *Figure 74–17*

Circumcised and uncircumcised penis.

from exposure to the cold air. They may be palpable later in the examination when the man is more relaxed. If a testis is not apparent, palpate the femoral and inguinal area. A client with an undescended testis is referred to the physician. A small (pea-size), hard lump located on either the anterior or lateral aspect of a testis is suggestive of a malignancy, and the client is referred to the physician for follow-up. The testes are compared bilaterally and should be similar.

The nurse then palpates each *epididymis* between thumb and index finger. They are located on the superior aspects of the testes and extend down the posterior surfaces. The epididymis feels soft, resilient, and tender. Swelling and hardness are abnormal. The *vas deferens* (spermatic cord) begins at the superior, lateral aspect of the testis. The nurse differentiates it from the epididymis by its firmer, tubular feel and compares findings bilaterally. The vas deferens is palpated along its length toward the inguinal canal while the nurse notes any thickening or asymmetry, which is abnormal.

If the nurse finds swelling, nodules, or other abnormal results during the scrotal examination, *transillumination of the scrotum* is performed (Fig. 74–18). The nurse darkens the room and shines a flashlight through the scrotum from behind the mass. A scrotum filled with serous fluid will transilluminate as a red glow. More solid lesions, such as a hematoma or mass, will not transilluminate and may be seen as a dark shadow. The nurse describes the characteristics of the abnormality, including whether it transilluminates.

Examination of the client for *inguinal herniation* is best performed while the client stands. A *hernia* is a prolapse or protrusion of a loop of intestine through the inguinal wall or canal. A *direct inguinal hernia* enters the inguinal canal behind the external ring because of a weakened abdominal wall; it does not pass through the inguinal canal. An *indirect inguinal hernia* enters the inguinal canal through the internal ring and can remain in the canal or pass down through the external ring and into the scrotum. A *femoral hernia* (more common in women) occurs inferiorly and more laterally than an inguinal hernia; it often has the appearance of an enlarged inguinal lymph node. The nurse uses the left index finger to palpate the client's left side and the right finger for the client's right side.

The nurse inspects the inguinal areas for bulges while the client stands quietly and again after he is instructed to bear down and strain as though attempting to have a bowel movement. Bulges should be absent. Presence of a *direct hernia* is assessed by the nurse's gently inserting an index finger into the loose scrotal skin over the external inguinal ring; the finger does not enter into the external ring. The nurse then instructs the client to bear down while she feels for a bulge, which should be absent. To palpate for an *indirect hernia,* the nurse gently invaginates the scrotal skin with the index or little finger, following the vas deferens to where it passes into the external ring (Fig. 74–16*C*). Asking the client to flex the knee on that same side may assist in relaxing the muscles so that the nurse can insert the finger through the external ring and into the inguinal canal. The palpating finger is advanced as far as possible, and the nurse instructs the client to bear down while she feels for a tissue mass touching the finger. The mass retreats back up the canal when the client relaxes. The nurse palpates the inguinal area directly for a *femoral hernia* while the client is relaxed and

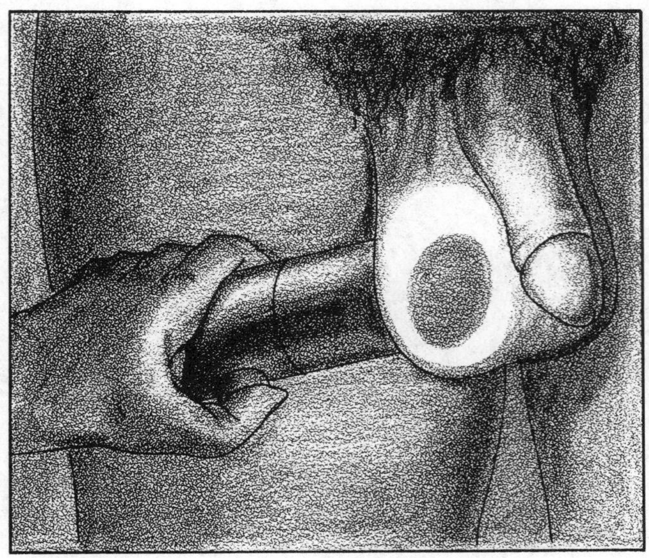

▲ *Figure 74–18*

Transillumination of the scrotum. In a darkened room, place a strong, lighted flashlight next to the scrotum as shown. Light normally passes through the scrotum (transillumination), but this does not occur with testicular tumor. A hydrocele will shine red.

again after he is instructed to bear down. A palpable mass should be absent.

After examination of the anterior male genitalia, the nurse assesses the rectum and prostate gland. A rectal-prostatic examination should be performed during physical examination annually for men over 40 years of age. This assesses (1) for evidence of STD; (2) the prostate gland for alterations in size, consistency, and evidence of tumors; and (3) for acute and chronic infection. Impress on the man the importance of regular rectal-prostatic examination as the best way to detect prostatic cancer early enough for effective treatment.

Just before rectal-prostatic examination, ask the client to empty his bladder. Collect a urine specimen at this time if one is needed. Explain that this makes the examination more comfortable and more accurate. Also explain that it is normal to experience sensations of having to urinate or defecate during the examination.

Two possible positions for the client during rectal examinations are (1) knee-chest position with buttocks elevated or (2) bending over from the hip with elbows placed either on the knees or on the examining table. (See discussion of examination positions in Chap. 12, Table 12-1.)

The nurse wears a glove on the examining hand and applies water-soluble lubricant to the examining finger. To perform the examination, place a hand on the client's hip to stabilize his position and to reassure him. Observe the perineum and perianal areas for lesions, hemorrhoids, inflammation, or discoloration. Ask the client to "bear down," explaining that this helps relax the anus and makes it easier to insert the examining finger. Insert the ball of the finger toward the anterior wall of the rectum. The normal prostate is located 2 to 5 cm beyond the anal sphincter along the anterior wall of the rectum. It is normally about 4 cm long and 5 cm wide (Fig. 74-19*A* and *B*). The prostate is shaped like a doughnut around the neck of the urethra (Fig. 74-19*C*). The posterior and lateral lobes only can be felt through the rectal wall (Fig. 74-19*D* and *E*). The lateral lobes should be symmetric. A normal prostate should feel smooth, rubbery, and firm, rather like the base of the thumb. Benign prostatic hypertrophy feels larger than normal, with a firmer consistency like that of the chin. Tenderness and bogginess (like the cheek of the face) may indicate acute or chronic prostatitis. Carcinoma feels "stony hard" or like a "hard nodule," that is, a circumscribed area of induration. Any induration is abnormal. The seminal vesicles (superior and lateral to the prostate) are normally nonpalpable.

Prostatic massage may be indicated even when the client is asymptomatic, in order to diagnose prostatitis. Roll the pad of the index finger across the prostate, starting laterally and superiorly and moving toward the midline of the prostate (Fig. 74-19*F*). Then, strip (or "milk") the area of the seminal vesicles, starting laterally and superiorly, toward the midline (Fig. 74-19*G*). Send resultant meatal secretions for microscopic examination. Large numbers of pus cells suggest prostatitis. Acid-fast organisms may be identified by staining. Cultures may be needed to identify organisms such as gonococci, chlamydiae, or tubercle bacilli. If a culture is required, the glans of the penis must be cleaned and the bladder emptied to clean the urethra before prostatic massage. Collect meatal secretions in sterile culture media.

Anus and Rectum

This portion of the physical examination is a potential source of embarrassment and discomfort to the client. The nurse manipulates tissues slowly to avoid causing unnecessary discomfort and uses a professional, matter-of-fact manner. Some agencies limit the extent of rectal examination performed by nurses without advanced preparation and skills to inspection of the anus. However, the nurse must be familiar with rectal structures and assessment findings when performing a digital assessment for fecal impaction or administering rectal medications. (See Chapter 52 for further information on GI assessment.)

The position for rectal examination depends on the circumstances of the examination. When the rectal examination is conducted as part of the screening physical examination, a female client is examined in the lithotomy position immediately after examination of the genitalia. The examiner uses a bimanual approach with index finger in the vagina and second finger in the rectum. If only the anus and rectum are to be examined, the client is assisted in assuming Sims' position (Table 12-1) or dorsal recumbent position. Male clients are examined in Sims' position if only the anus and rectum are being examined. If the rectal examination is performed as part of the screening examination, the client stands and leans across the examining table (Table 12-1). This position is often used to facilitate palpation of the prostate gland. Alternative positions are discussed in Table 12-1. Clients are draped for preventing unnecessary and embarrassing exposure. For all clients, the nurse wears disposable examining gloves and uses water-soluble lubricant. A specimen of stool is usually obtained for occult blood (guaiac) testing at the time of the examination.

INSPECTION

The nurse uses the nondominant hand to spread the buttocks apart in order to visualize the perianal area. *Perianal skin* is darker than the skin of the surrounding buttocks and should be intact. The *anal area* has coarse skin and is moist without hair. The anus is closed without sign of *rectal prolapse* (i.e., protrusion of rectal mucous membrane through the anus). The perianal area is without fissures (cracks), excoriation, rash, inflammation, ulceration, abscess, lumps, fistula openings, or *hemorrhoids*. Hemorrhoids are dilated veins seen as skin protrusions that are reddened. The nurse then instructs the client to bear down as if having a bowel movement while she inspects for abnormalities such as rectal prolapse, internal hemorrhoids, polyps, and rectal fissures. The increased intra-abdominal pres-

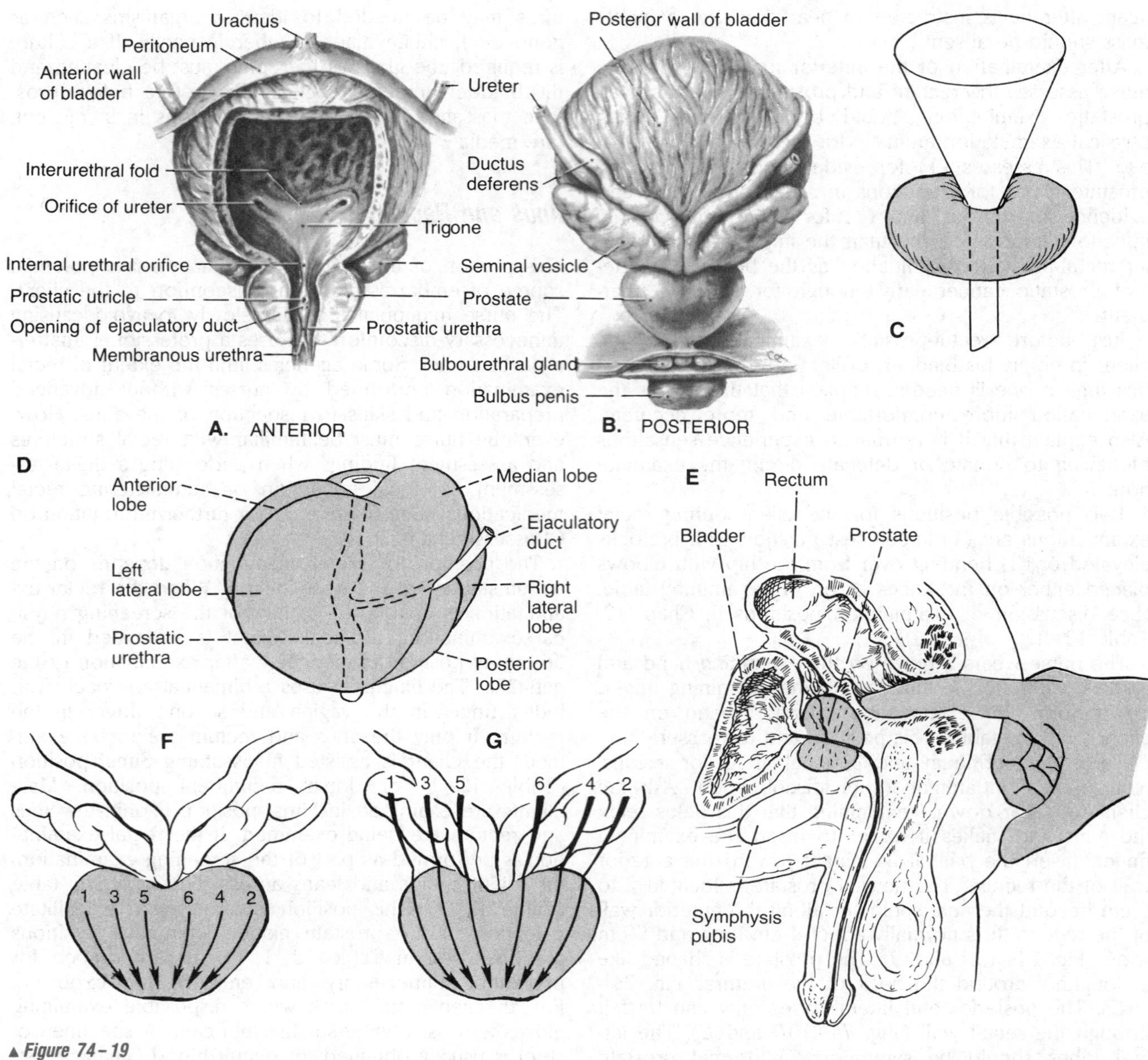

▲ *Figure 74–19*

Rectal-prostatic assessment. *A* and *B*, Anterior and posterior views of the prostate gland. *C*, Diagrammatic representation of the anatomic position of the prostate gland. It lies around the urethra rather like a doughnut around the outlet of a funnel. *D*, Posterior and lateral lobes of the prostate. *E*, Rectal examination. Insert a gloved index finger into the anus while the client is "bearing down." Palpate all surfaces. *F*, Prostate massage. Roll the pad of the index finger across the prostate, starting laterally and superiorly and moving toward the midline of the prostate. *G*, Seminal vesicles and prostate massage. Use the same technique as for prostate massage, but extend the finger higher over the area of the seminal vesicles. (*A* and *B* from Jacob, S. W., & Francone, C. A. [1989]. *Elements of anatomy and physiology* [2nd ed.]. Philadelphia: W. B. Saunders.)

sure may cause abnormalities to become more prominent.

PALPATION

The nurse lubricates the index finger of the dominant hand and places it over the client's anus. The client is instructed to bear down, and as the anal sphincter relaxes, the nurse inserts the index finger slowly and gently into the anal canal, pointing the finger toward the umbilicus. It is normal for the client to feel like having a bowel movement. If insertion is difficult or the nurse meets with resistance or rectal bleeding, the examination is stopped.

The *anal canal* extends toward the umbilicus approximately 3 cm (1 inch), where it joins the rectum at the anorectal junction. While the nurse's finger is in the anal canal, the client is instructed to tighten the anal muscles around the finger. The nurse assesses the *anal sphincter tone,* which is normally strong. The nurse then rotates her finger around the *anal wall* to assess for nodules, masses, or tenderness, which should be absent. The index finger is advanced slowly to the *anorectal junction,* where the rectum widens and turns posteriorly along the coccyx and sacrum. The nurse continues to palpate around the *rectal wall* and along the curve of the *coccyx,* which is mobile. The nurse advances the index finger to its fullest extent, approximately 6 to 10 cm (2 to 4 inches) into the rectum, palpating for tenderness or masses. The rectal mucosa is smooth and nontender. If an abnormality is palpated, the nurse describes the location (e.g., left lateral wall 1 cm proximal to internal anal sphincter) and characteristics. Once the nurse has inserted the index finger fully, she instructs the client to bear down again while she feels for a mass descending from above against the palpating finger; this should be absent.

In the *female client,* the nurse palpates the *cervix* of the uterus through the *rectovaginal wall* along the anterior rectum (Fig. 74-20*A*). The rectovaginal wall is firm, smooth, and resilient. The cervix feels round, smooth, firm, and movable without tenderness. The nurse may mistake the cervix or a vaginal tampon for a rectal mass.

In the *male client,* the nurse palpates the *prostate gland* through the anterior rectal wall (Fig. 74-20*B*). It is felt as a rounded, heart-shaped structure approximately 2.5 to 4 cm (1 to 1 1/2 inches) in diameter with discrete borders. The nurse feels for the *median sulcus* (groove), which separates the posterior prostate gland into two lateral lobes. The gland is firm, rubbery, nontender, and movable. Enlargement, bogginess, nodules, hardness, or tenderness is abnormal.

As the nurse withdraws her finger from the client's rectum, she observes for the presence of *stool* on the glove. Feces, if present, is normally brown. Mucus or blood and black, tarry, light tan or gray stool is abnormal. The nurse tests a sample of the stool for *occult blood,* which should be negative. If presence of STD is suspected, the nurse also obtains a rectal culture. The nurse wipes the perianal area and informs the client that the physical examination is completed.

DIAGNOSTIC TESTS

Various diagnostic tests may be used to assess male reproductive disturbances. Men and their significant others are often anxious about diagnostic tests. Reduce anxiety by giving careful explanations before and during the tests. It is much less frightening if a client knows what to expect and is included in the process.

Learn the specific preparation necessary for each test. Sometimes sedation or pain relief is required. Informed consent authorization may be necessary. Physiologic preparations may be required (e.g., fasting, enema). During the test, keep the client informed about what is happening. Help him maintain specific positions as required. Observe the client carefully during and after the test for adverse reactions, such as pain, excessive anxiety, pallor, or nausea.

Cystoscopy

A cystoscope is indispensable in both assessment and treatment of urologic problems. It is a metal instrument with optical systems providing a magnified illuminated image of the bladder. Flexible cystoscopes are also available and make the procedure much more comfortable for the client. Some indications for cystoscopy are (1) to determine the source of urinary bleeding, (2) to determine the cause of unexplained urinary symptoms, (3) to determine the source of pyuria, (4) to catheter-

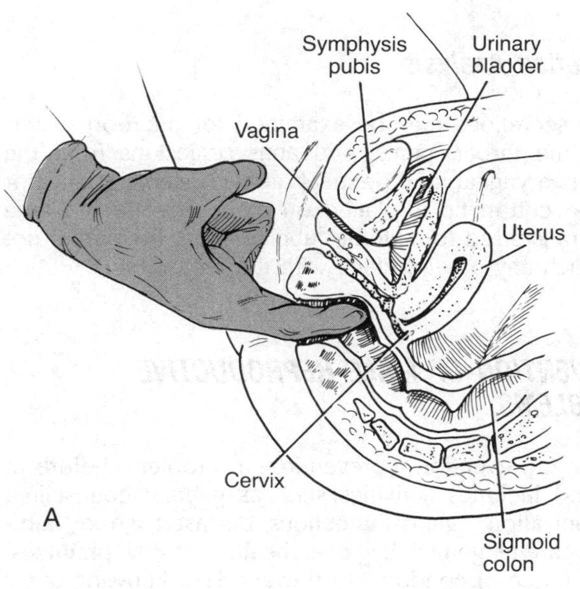

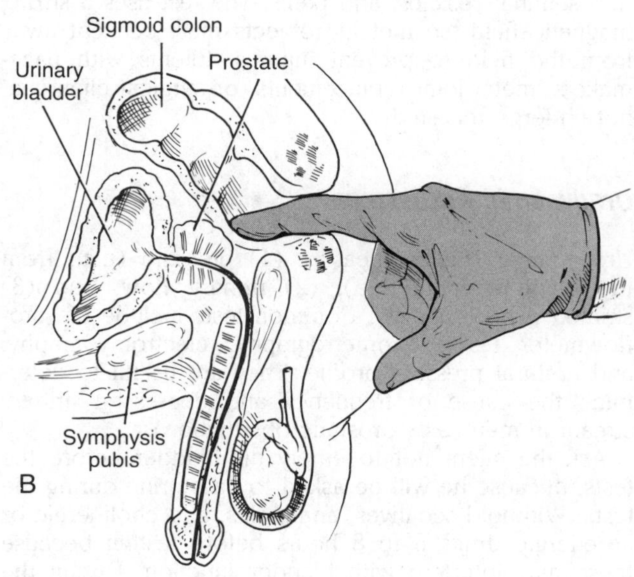

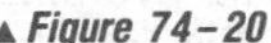
▲ **Figure 74-20**

Palpation of the rectum: *A,* female; *B,* male.

ize the ureters to localize the infection and subsequent treatment, (5) to obtain biopsy specimens, and (6) for follow-up examinations. A cystoscopy may be done in a urologist's office or (if the client is quite symptomatic) in an operating room before surgery. Inspection of the bladder interior includes looking for trabeculation, diverticula, and bladder neck contracture and checking the size and contours of the prostatic lobes.

Computed Tomography

Computed tomographic scans are used in the clinical staging of testicular tumors and prostatic cancer. The client lies on an x-ray table, which moves him into various positions while scans are taken at various planes. If an injectable contrast medium is used, ask the client about any history of allergies. The procedure takes about 30 minutes.

Ultrasonography

Ultrasonic waves (sound waves too high in frequency for the human ear to hear) are "bounced off" tissue surfaces and produce an electronic image of body structures that can differentiate masses. This technique is used to visualize an enlarged prostate or scrotum. This procedure is done transrectally to help detect prostate lesions.

Magnetic Resonance Imaging

Magnetic resonance images are reflections of hydrogen densities in body tissues induced by a strong magnetic field. This method provides very clear images of soft tissues. Magnetic resonance imaging may be used to visualize pelvic structures, including the prostate, bladder, seminal vesicles, and penis. The test uses a strong magnetic field, so metallic objects must be kept away from the field to prevent injuries. Clients with pacemakers, metal joint replacements, or surgical clips cannot undergo this study.

Urodynamic Assessment

Urodynamic studies measure (1) pressure (e.g., from the bladder or urethra), (2) urinary flow, and (3) striated muscle activity. Common tests include the uroflowmeter test, cystometrography, electromyography, and urethral pressure profile. They are useful to determine the cause of frequency and decreased urinary stream in men (e.g., prostatic obstruction).

Ask the client not to empty his bladder before the tests, because he will be asked to pass urine during the tests. Withhold sedatives, analgesics, and cholinergic or adrenergic drugs 6 to 8 hours before testing because these may interfere with bladder function. During the tests, the client is asked to void into a funnel or commode connected to a uroflowmeter, which measures voiding patterns (i.e., rate, time, volume, effort needed to initiate stream, strength and continuity of stream). During cystometrography, a urethral or suprapubic catheter is inserted and residual urine measured. Then, 30 ml of saline solution at room temperature is introduced into the bladder, followed by 30 ml of fluid at 110° to 115° F. The client is asked to describe sensations as the bladder fills (e.g., need to void, nausea, flushing, discomfort, temperature). The bladder is drained, the catheter is connected to a cystometer, and normal saline or carbon dioxide is slowly introduced into the bladder. A transducer connected to the catheter records pressure changes in the bladder. The client is asked to report when he first feels the need to void, and then when he feels an urgent need to void. He voids when the bladder reaches its full capacity.

An electromyogram assesses sphincter activity during voiding. A needle electrode is inserted through the perineum into the external sphincter. Normally, sphincter activity ceases during voiding and resumes when the man stops voiding. The urethral pressure profile involves slowly withdrawing a catheter through the urethra. A transducer connected to the catheter measures the pressure as it is withdrawn.

All these tests may be quite uncomfortable and embarrassing for the client. Document intake and output for 24 hours after the test. Document and report any hematuria.

Scans

Scans may be used to assess testicular abnormalities (e.g., torsion, epididymitis, abscess, tumors, hydroceles, varicoceles, and spermatoceles). A radioactive substance is administered intravenously, and several scans are taken. Before a scan is taken, ask the client if he has any history of allergies.

Secretion Analysis

Body secretions may be examined for microorganisms from the throat, penis, and anus or lesions from the oral, pharyngeal, and perineal areas. A sterile applicator with a cotton tip is placed on or in the affected area and transferred to a sterile tube or slide. Be careful not to touch any other surface with the applicator.

PREVENTION OF MALE REPRODUCTIVE PROBLEMS

Primary prevention (preventing a problem before it occurs) includes activities such as genetic counseling; immunization against infectious diseases; good nutrition; careful genital hygiene; healthy sexual practices, such as use of condoms to prevent STD; knowing one's partner; avoiding multiple sex partners; and avoiding sex (oral or genital) with a person who has genital lesions.

Secondary prevention (detecting and treating a problem before symptoms occur) includes activities such as screening (e.g., assessing large numbers of "healthy" people for hypertension) and self-examination (see following).

Tertiary prevention (correcting a problem and preventing further deterioration) is provided by most health professionals who provide care for clients experiencing acute and chronic diseases.

Self-Examination

Self-examination of the perineal and genital areas, including the penis, scrotum, and testes, is important. The nurse takes every opportunity to talk with men about this part of self-directed health care. Teach self-examination to all males past puberty. Such secondary prevention practices can be taught anywhere, including all health care settings, schools and colleges, and workplace clinics. Self-examination can identify potential problems early when treatment is likely to be more successful; for example, testicular self-examination can detect testicular cancer while it is treatable.

Most men are used to touching their own genitals when urinating, bathing, or masturbating, but it may take a while for them to get used to touching their genitals for health assessment. It takes practice for a man to feel confident in doing self-examinations. After a time, however, he becomes familiar with his own genital anatomy and can identify abnormal changes. Explain the procedure carefully and provide opportunities to ask questions and express concerns. Whenever possible, give the client literature to take home (the American Cancer Society publishes a useful pamphlet on testicular self-examination).

When teaching genital self-examination to men, include the following.

- Develop a habit of doing self-examination once a month. Connect it in your mind with some other monthly event (e.g., paying bills, receiving the first pay check of the month).
- Use a mirror to check inaccessible places (e.g., buttocks, perianal area, scrotum).
- Look for any changes from normal, such as swelling, lumps, tenderness, lesions, discoloration, asymmetry, or discharge.
- The best time to do a testicular self-examination is after a shower when you are warm, the scrotum is relaxed, and the testicles are easier to examine. When the testicles are cold, the scrotum pulls close to the body, making the testicles hard to feel. The left testicle is usually lower than the right because of a longer cord.
- The technique for testicular self-examination is as follows: hold the scrotum in the palms of your hands and examine each testicle with thumb and fingers of both hands. Index and middle fingers should be on the underside of each testicle and thumbs on the top. Roll the testicles between your thumb and fingers (Fig. 74-21).

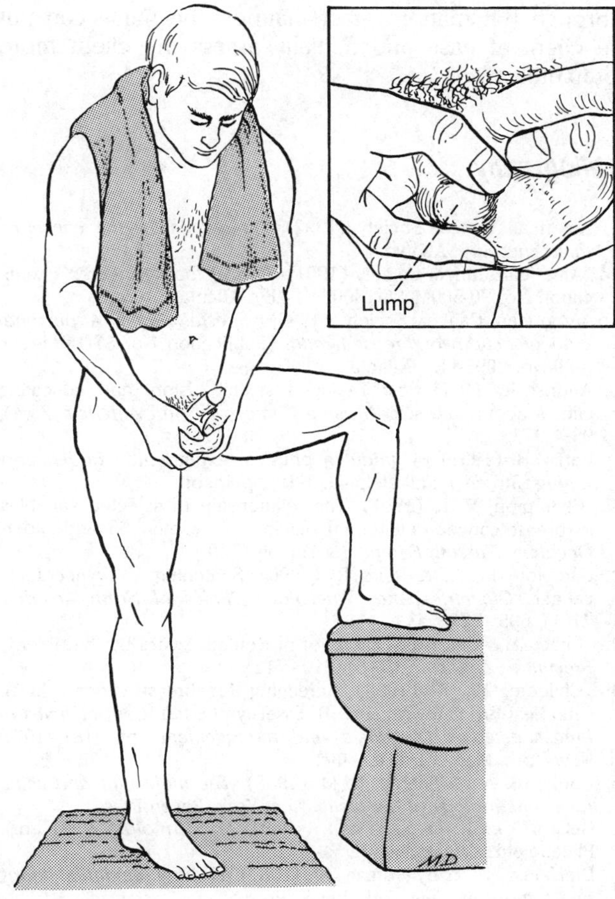

▲ *Figure 74-21*

Testicular self-examination. See text for details of procedure.

- A normal testicle is shaped like an egg and is about 4 cm (1 5/8 inches) long. It feels firm but not hard (rather like an ear lobe), even rubbery, and quite smooth with no lumps.
- Examine the epididymis (a storage tube found on the side, behind the testicles). Each epididymis should feel soft and may be spongy.
- Examine the spermatic cords, which ascend from the epididymis behind the testicles. They are normally firm, smooth, tubular structures.
- Do not hesitate to seek professional assessment and advice about anything unusual you find. It is better to learn that everything is all right than to wait too long.

Summary

It is very important for the nurse to understand the proper assessment of the male and female reproductive systems. The nurse must be aware not only of the physiology of this system but also of the psychological implications associated with any reproductive disorders. The nurse must exhibit a concerned, caring attitude when assessing clients with reproductive disorders because disorders within this system are so laden with psychosocial overtones. By assessing the client in a thorough but matter-of-fact manner, the nurse can put the client at ease and actually assess the client more completely.

Bibliography

1. American Cancer Society (1992). *Guidelines for the cancer-related check-up.* Atlanta.

1a. American Cancer Society (1991). *Cancer facts & figures.* (Publication No. 90-500M-NO. 5008.91-LE). Atlanta.

1b. American Cancer Society (1989). *Special touch: A personal plan of action for breast health.* (Publication No. 87-1MM-Rev. 9/89-No. 2095-LE). Atlanta.

2. Andrist, L. C. (1988). Taking a sexual history and educating clients about safe sex. *Nursing Clinics of North America, 23*(4), 959-973.

3. Bates, B. (1991). *A guide to physical examination and history taking* (5th ed.). Philadelphia: J. B. Lippincott.

3a. Champion, V. L. (1991). The relationship of selected variables to breast cancer detection behaviors in women 35 and older. *Oncology Nursing Forum, 18*(4), 733-739.

4. Campion, M. J., & Reid, R. (1990). Screening for gynecologic cancer. *Obstetrics and Gynecology Clinics of North America, 17*(4), 695-727.

4a. Chao, A., et al. (1987). Use of preventative care by the elderly. *Preventive Medicine, 16*(5), 710-712.

4b. Chilcote, W. A. (1988). Screening for breast cancer. In S. Grundfest-Broniatowski & C. B. Esselstyn (Eds.), *Controversies in breast disease: Diagnosis and management* (pp. 181-197). New York: Marcel Dekker, Inc.

5. Cooke, B. A., & Sharpe, R. M. (1988). *The molecular and cellular endocrinology of the testis.* New York: Raven Press.

6. DeGroot, L. J., et al. (Eds.). (1989). *Endocrinology* (2nd ed.). Philadelphia: W. B. Saunders.

7. Diczfalusy, E., & Bygedman, M. (1987). *Fertility regulation today and tomorrow.* New York: Raven Press.

8. Droegmueller, W., et al. (1987). *Comprehensive gynecology.* St. Louis: C. V. Mosby.

9. Dugan, K. A. (1985). Diagnostic laparoscopy under local anesthesia for evaluation of infertility. *Journal of Obstetric, Gynecologic, and Neonatal Nursing, 14,* 363-366.

10. Fogel, C. I., & Lauver, D. (1990). *Sexual health promotion.* Philadelphia: W. B. Saunders.

10a. Foster, R. S., & Costanza, M. C. (1984). Breast self-examination practices and breast cancer survival. *Cancer, 53*(4), 999.

10b. Frankl, G. (1988). Screening and detection of breast cancer. In M. E. Lippman, et al. (Eds.), *Diagnosis and management of breast cancer* (pp. 10-21). Philadelphia: W. B. Saunders Co.

10c. Glenn, B. L., & Moore, L. A. (1990). Relationship of self-concept, health locus of control, and perceived cancer treatment options to the practice of breast self-examination. *Cancer Nursing, 13*(6), 361-365.

10d. Gonzalez, J. T. (1990). Factors relating to frequency of breast self-examination among low income Mexican American women: Implications for nursing practice. *Cancer Nursing, 13*(3), 134-142.

10e. Gray, M. E. (1990). Factors related to practice of breast self-examination in rural women. *Cancer Nursing, 13*(2) 100-107.

11. Grimes, J., & Burns, E. (1987). *Health assessment in nursing practice* (2nd ed.). Boston: Jones & Bartlett.

12. Gruhn, J. G., & Kazer, R. R. (1989). *Hormonal regulation of the menstrual cycle.* New York: Plenum.

12a. Habegger, D., & Ellerhorst-Ryan, J. M. (1988). Needle localization for nonpalpable breast lesions. *Oncology Nursing Forum, 15*(2), 192-194.

13. Hacker, N. F., & Moore, J. G. (1992). *Essentials of obstetrics and gynecology* (2nd ed.). Philadelphia: W. B. Saunders.

14. Helderman, G., et al. (1990). Comparing two sampling techniques for endocervical cell recovery on Papanicolaou smears. *Nurse Practitioner, 15*(11), 30-32.

14a. Helvie, M. A., et al. (1990). Radiographic guided fine needle aspiration of non-palpable breast lesions. *Radiology, 174*(3141), 657-661.

15. Jarvis, C. (1992). *Physical examination and health assessment.* Philadelphia: W. B. Saunders.

16. Jones, H. W., et al. (Eds.). (1988). *Novak's textbook of gynecology* (11th ed.). Baltimore: Williams and Wilkins.

17. Kaunitz, A. M., & Grimes, D. A. (1988). The woman over 50: endometrial sampling in older women. *Contemporary Obstetrics and Gynecology, 31*(Suppl.), 85.

18. Kisslo, J., et al. (1988). *Doppler color flow imaging.* New York: Churchill Livingstone.

19. Knobil, E. (1988). *The physiology of reproduction.* New York: Raven Press.

19a. Lashley, M. E. (1987). Predictors of breast self-examination practice among elderly women. *Advances in Nursing Sciences, 9*(4), 25-34.

20. Lee, P., et al. (1988). Accuracy of Papanicolaou smears: art or science? *Journal of Reproductive Medicine, 33,* 795-798.

21. Leung, P. C. K., et al. (Eds.). (1987). *Endocrinology and physiology of reproduction.* New York: Plenum.

22. Manhesh, V. B., et al. (Eds.). *Regulation of ovarian and testicular function.* New York: Plenum.

22a. Mant, D., et al. (1987). Breast self-examination and breast cancer stage at diagnosis. *British Journal of Cancer, 55*(2), 207-211.

22b. Masood, S., et al. (1989). The potential value of mammographically guided fine-needle aspiration biopsy of nonpalpable breast lesions. *American Surgeon, 55*(4), 226-231.

22c. McMillan, S. C. (1990). Nurses' compliance with American Cancer Society guidelines for cancer prevention and detection. *Oncology Nursing Forum, 17*(5), 721-736.

23. Morrison-Beedy, D., & Robbins, L. (1989). Sexual assessment and the aging female. *Nurse Practitioner, 14*(12), 35-45.

23a. National Cancer Institute (1988). *Breast exams: What you should know.* (NIH Publication No. 90-2000). Washington, D.C.

24. Nelson, J. H., et al. (1984). *Dysplasia, carcinoma in situ, and early invasive cervical carcinoma.* New York: American Cancer Society.

25. Newton, M., & Newton, E. R. (1988). *Complications of gynecology and obstetric management.* Philadelphia: W. B. Saunders.

25a. Pennes, D. R., & Adler, D. D. (1988). Mammography: Changing roles and concepts. In J. K. Harness, et al. (Eds.), *Breast cancer: Collaborative management* (pp. 79-95). Chelsea, MI: Lewis Publishers, Inc.

26. Pleatman, M. A., & Cardona, R. R. (1990). Detection of breast cancer. *Obstetrics and Gynecology Clinics of North America, 17*(4), 729-740.

26a. Philip, J., et al. (1986). Clinical measures to assess the practice and efficiency of breast self-examination. *Cancer, 58*(4), 973-977.

27. Primrose, R. B. (1984). Taking the tension out of pelvic exams. *American Journal of Nursing, 84,* 72-74.

28. Quilligan, E. J., & Zuspan, F. P. (1990). *Current Therapy in Obstetrics and Gynecology* (3rd ed.). Philadelphia: W. B. Saunders.

28a. Richardson, J. L., et al. (1987). Frequency and adequacy of breast cancer screening among elderly Hispanic women. *Preventive Medicine, 16*(6), 761-774.

29. Saite, A. (1989). Cervical cytology in general practice. *New Zealand Nursing Journal, 82*(1), 18-19.

30. Seidel, H. M., et al. (1987). *Mosby's guide to physical examination.* St. Louis: C. V. Mosby.

30a. Seidman, H., et al. (1987). Survival experience in the breast cancer detection demonstration project. *CA—A Cancer Journal for Clinicians, 37*(5), 258-291.

31. Smith, D. B. (1989). Discussing sexuality. *Oncology Nursing Forum, 16*(1), 106.

32. Soules, M. R. (1989). *Problems in reproductive endocrinology and infertility.* New York: Elsevier.

33. Swartz, M. H. (1989). *Textbook of physical diagnosis.* Philadelphia: W. B. Saunders.

34. Szydlo, V. L. (1988). Approaching a male adolescent about a pelvic exam. *American Journal of Nursing, 88,* 1052-1056.

35. Wynn, T. M., & Jollie, W. (Eds.). (1989). *The biology of the uterus* (2nd ed.). New York: Plenum.

36. Yen, S. S. C., & Jaffe, R. (1991). *Reproductive endocrinology: Physiology, pathophysiology, and clinical management* (3rd ed.). Philadelphia: W. B. Saunders.

Chapter 75

Nursing Care of Men With Reproductive and Urinary Disorders

Today, men are showing more interest in being actively involved in health maintenance. This is evident in (1) the increasing interest by men in fitness, (2) men's increased attainment of lifestyle factors related to fitness (such as stopping smoking), and (3) men's increased participation in childbirth and parenting. As men learn to express their interest in general health maintenance, nurses can extend these interests to reproductive and urinary health maintenance.

PSYCHOSOCIAL FACTORS INFLUENCING REPRODUCTIVE HEALTH

When caring for men experiencing sexual, reproductive, or urinary problems, the nurse needs to plan sensitive care to meet the psychosocial and physical needs of men undergoing very personal procedures. Remember, the urinary system and reproductive system are the same, so any problem in the urinary system may be seen as a threat to the man's reproductive system and sexuality. Men are often reluctant to ask for help because they see any problem as a potential threat to their sexuality and embarrassing.

There are many stereotypes concerning men's reluctance to complain or seek health care. Some are true, because men are less likely than women to seek health care and some men do complain less. What is important for the nurse to remember, however, is that urinary or reproductive problems and sexual preference are very personal, and the client may be very hesitant to talk about these problems (see Ethical Issues in Nursing).

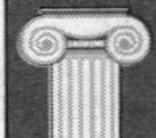

ETHICAL ISSUES IN NURSING

Should a Client's Sexual Lifestyle Influence His Nursing Care?

Personal attitudes toward sexuality help make us who we are. Our sexuality is an important part of how we identify with ourselves as well as others. Attitudes toward others who may not view sexuality in the same way influence our relationship with those people.

Homosexuality, especially among men, is a subject that produces various responses. Recently, AIDS has caused a negative reaction toward gay males because at first the HIV virus was seen primarily in homosexual men. Although this virus now is seen in heterosexual as well as homosexual populations, a negative association with homosexuals remains.

Health care providers take care of many kinds of people who are certain to have different attitudes about sexuality. Nurses may or may not be aware of the sexuality of their clients. Those who care for homosexual men need to confront their own feelings about providing such care, which may reflect social discomfort or the fear of contracting the HIV virus. Although this fear is a reality for many health care professionals, all clients should be treated equally and with respect and dignity. Also, the use of universal precautions may alleviate some of the apprehensions associated with the HIV virus. The sexuality of clients is just as private as the sexuality of caregivers, and the respect shown toward one's own private lifestyle should be shown equally to others, no matter what personal attitudes are held.

Because men may be reluctant to ask for help, skillful therapeutic interaction is essential to help them express their concerns. The nurse should be very sensitive and give the client permission to talk about his problem. The nurse should be sensitive to the client's discomfort and attempt to put the client at ease. Statements such as "Many men are concerned about how this problem will affect their sex lives," "It is common to worry about how your partner might feel about this problem," and "What are some of your concerns?" may help the client begin to talk about his concerns.

Giving men permission to express their feelings and health-related concerns draws them and their significant others into the process of health care. Teaching men reproductive and urinary health maintenance and self-care contributes to their overall health.

PHYSICAL FACTORS AFFECTING MALE REPRODUCTION

Some men find reproductive assessment difficult and need considerable support. Some men simply refuse to participate, perhaps fearing abnormal results. Masturbation is necessary to obtain a semen sample, and some men find this difficult for personal, cultural, or religious reasons. Many men may not know what chemicals they have been exposed to at their work place. In the United States, not all states have right-to-know laws that require employers to inform workers (1) of any use of toxic agents, (2) of possible harmful effects from toxic agents that are used, and (3) how to avoid exposure to these toxic agents.

Assessment of reproductive problems in men includes (1) careful reproductive history-taking of men at risk and their partners, including exposure to hazards from occupations, hobbies, and environment; (2) sexual history of men at risk and their partners; (3) semen analysis; and (4) hormonal studies, e.g., radioimmunoassay for follicle-stimulating hormone (FSH), luteinizing hormone (LH), and testosterone.

Environmental and Occupational Agents

The effects of a variety of chemical agents on the male reproductive system are well documented. In 1977, the toxicity of the pesticide dibromochloropropane (DBCP) was dramatically linked to adverse testicular effects in workers in a California plant manufacturing the chemical.[35] The workers suspected the problem when they realized as a group they had conceived few children. Interesting findings were made: (1) low sperm counts correlating with the length of time men had worked in the plant and (2) higher than normal levels of FSH and LH. Some men's sperm counts improved after they were no longer exposed to the pesticide. DBCP has also been found in community water supplies in California and Arizona. It has since been banned for agricultural use in the United States except use on Hawaiian pineapples (little residue having been found on pineapples).[34]

Other agents associated with adverse reproductive effects in men include (1) anesthetic gases used in operating rooms and dentists' offices; (2) carbon disulfide from rubber vulcanization; (3) estrogen during manufacturing; (4) the pesticides ethylene dibromide and chlordecone (Kepone); (5) inorganic lead from smelters, painting, and printing; (6) inorganic mercury from manufacturing and dental work; (7) microwaves leaking from machines; (8) neurotoxins from the manufacture of polyurethane foam; (9) ionizing radiation from x-rays and gamma-emitting radioisotopes; (10) uoulene diamine from chemical manufacturing; and (11) waste water treatment at petroleum refineries.[34]

Reproductive effects of chemical exposure vary, including abnormal sperm counts, loss of motility, impotence, spontaneous abortion, birth defects, and decreased libido (sex drive).[34]

Pharmacologic Agents

Whenever a man is taking any drug, the possibility of sexual or reproductive health effects should be considered during nursing assessment. When planning nursing care, always review the specific use and action of drugs being taken by clients. Asking a man the simple question "Have there been any changes in your sexual activity? Why?," because part of nursing history can reveal problems that may be corrected by medication changes.

Some drugs may actually enhance sexual and reproductive functioning, such as clomiphene citrate (Clomid), which increases the sperm count. Other drugs depress sexual and reproductive functioning, such as phenytoin (Dilantin), which decreases spermatogenesis. The effects of some drugs are variable, enhancing functioning in one man and depressing it in another. Drugs that delay ejaculation (alcohol, cocaine, and amphetamines) may improve sexual functioning in a man who ejaculates prematurely. However, overuse of such drugs may lead to other problems, such as erectile dysfunction.

Many drugs (prescription, over-the-counter, and recreational) are known to have sexual and reproductive effects in males. Others may not have been identified yet.

Major sexual and reproductive effects of drugs on men include (1) decreased desire for sex (libido), (2) decreased erectile ability (impotence), (3) decreased ejaculatory ability, (4) decreased sperm quality, and (5) gynecomastia. The following drugs may have one or more of such effects:

- Antihypertensives may cause impotence. These drugs include (1) diuretics, such as spironolactone (Aldactone) and chlorthalidone (Hygroton); (2) metoprolol (Lopressor); and (3) others, such as methyldopa (Aldomet), clonidine (Catapres).
- Antipsychotics, such as chlorpromazine (Thorazine) and thioridazine (Mellaril) may lead to impaired ejaculation and priapism (prolonged, persistent erection without ejaculation).
- Tricyclic antidepressants, such as amitriptyline (Elavil) and imipramine (Tofranil), may lead to a decrease in libido.
- Monamine oxidase inhibitor (MAO) antidepressants, such as phenelzine (Nardil) and tranylcypromine (Parnate), may lead to a decrease in libido.
- Hormones, such as, progestins, antiandrogens, and androgens, may lead to almost any of the above-mentioned problems, including impotence and gynecomastia.
- Sedative-hypnotics and tranquilizers, such as diazepam (Valium), chlordiazepoxide (Librium), barbiturates such as secobarbital (Seconal) and pentobarbital (Nembutal), methaqualone (Quaalude), and ethyl alcohol, may lead to a decrease in libido.
- Stimulants, such as amphetamines (Obestrol-10) and cocaine, may lead to impotence and changes in libido.
- Chemotherapeutic agents, such as chlorambucil (Leukeran) and cyclophosphamide (Cytoxan), may lead to decreased sperm quality.
- Opiates, such as morphine, heroin, and methadone (Dolophine), may lead to impotence.
- Recreational drugs, such as marijuana, lysergic acid diethylamide (LSD), phencyclidine piperidine (PCP), and tobacco may lead to decreased libido and impotence.

Many other drugs also have been found to affect sexual or reproductive functioning in males, including digoxin (Lanoxin), griseofulvin (Fulvicin), and cimetidine (Tagamet), which may cause gynecomastia; disopyramide phosphate (Norpace), disulfiram (Antabuse), and trimethoprim-sulfamethoxazole (Bactrim-Septra) may cause impotence; and metronidazole (Flagyl) may cause a decrease in libido.

Systemic Conditions

Sexual dysfunction and other reproductive problems may be associated with medical or surgical conditions, such as diabetes mellitus, renal disease, prostate surgery, and spinal injury. It is important to assess a man's previous level of sexual functioning. Nurses must be aware of the wide range of normal sexual and reproductive function in order to reassure clients about their normalcy. What may be normal for one man may be considered abnormal by another and, therefore, a cause for concern.

INFERTILITY

In 1982, one out of every eight couples in the United States were considered infertile (i.e., unprotected intercourse did not result in a pregnancy over a 12-month period). Requests for infertility services are increasing rapidly, now numbering in the millions.

Male infertility is extensive, occurring in 5 to 10 per cent of married men. Ten to 15 per cent of marriages are childless, and another 10 to 15 per cent have fewer children than they would like. In 30 to 50 per cent of such marriages, it is the man who is infertile. However, the two partners are best treated together. Minimal fertility in one partner can be offset by strong fertility in the other. On the other hand, if both are minimally fertile, infertility is more likely.

An awareness of these statistics alerts health care professionals to clients who may have concerns about infertility but who have difficulty expressing them.

Etiology

Causes of male infertility include

- *Pre-testicular:* endocrinopathy and sexual dysfunction, such as excessive ejaculation frequency;
- *Testicular:* varicocele (varicose testicular vein), failure of testicle to produce sperm, such as due to effects of drugs, environmental factors, development of chromosomal abnormalities, mumps orchitis, and spinal cord injury;
- *Post-testicular:* ejaculatory dysfunction, obstruction, such as from trauma, infection, and surgery;
- *Genitourinary:* infection; and
- *Immunologic:* sperm antibodies in one or both partners.

Diagnostic Assessment

Both the man and his partner may need help and support to express concerns and fears about infertility. Failure to conceive may make severe demands on the couple, threatening their individual self-concepts, sex roles, relationship, and sexual interaction. Guilt and blame about previous sexual activity, sexually transmitted diseases (STDs), or abortion may come between them. Fear and anxiety may be lessened by the taking involved a nursing history. This also provides the nurse with the opportunity to give support, respond to questions, and explain diagnostic and treatment procedures.

Assessment of male infertility includes obtaining a detailed history (sexual, medical, and reproductive) and a thorough physical examination. Semen analysis includes (1) gross examination, noting volume, viscosity, and color; and (2) pH, concentration, motility, morphology, and sperm agglutination. Other, more specific tests of sperm function include the fructose concentration and the Sims-Huhner test to assess the penetration of cervical mucus by sperm. Additional tests are performed for azoospermia (absence of sperm in the semen) or oligozoospermia (less than normal number of sperm in the semen). Other studies include tests for sperm antibodies in serum and chromosome karotyping to detect genetic abnormalities.

Endocrinologic studies assess FSH, LH, prolactin, and serum testosterone levels, all of which can help to identify endocrinologic causes of the infertility. For example, if FSH levels are high, there is probably arrested spermatogenesis. If FSH is normal, azoospermia or oligozoospermia is probably due to obstruction in the post-testicle ducts, which may be corrected by microsurgery. A testicular biopsy provides further information about spermatogenesis.

A genitourinary source of infertility can be assessed through a urinalysis, urine culture, serum creatinine, and an examination of prostatic secretions.

Medical Management

Thorough and complete infertility assessment is expensive and is often ineffective. It is more effective to prevent infertility from developing. Clients who either want to conceive at present or may want to conceive in the future can try to prevent infertility by

- Avoiding excessive intake of alcohol;
- Avoiding tobacco, marijuana, and other recreational drugs;
- Decreasing exposure to occupational and environmental hazards, including toxic substances and radiation;
- Keeping the scrotum cool, e.g., avoiding excessive heat, hot baths, and tight clothing;
- Avoiding transmission of sexually transmitted organism by limiting the number of sexual partners and using condoms, diaphragms, contraceptive foam, and other spermicides, especially with new partners (STDs, particularly gonorrhea and those caused by *Chlamydia trachomatis,* may account for up to 30 per cent of cases of infertility in populations at high risk);
- Developing effective means of stress reduction; and
- Eating a well-balanced nutritious diet.

Treatment for pre-testicular causes of male infertility varies. No treatment is available for primary testicular failure or hypogonadism. Testosterone may be prescribed to correct low testosterone levels. Hyperprolactinemia may be treated by surgical removal of a pituitary tumor or by administration of bromocriptine (Parlodel).

Treatment for male sexual dysfunction is discussed in the section on Erectile Dysfunction. For oligozoospermia caused by excessive frequency of ejaculation, the couple may be recommended to have intercourse only once every 36 hours during the woman's periovulatory period, because it takes 24 hours for a normal sperm count to be generated after ejaculation.

Treatment of testicular causes of male infertility also varies. Reduced spermatogenesis from testicular atrophy due to infection may be treated by (1) avoiding factors that depress spermatogenesis, such as drugs, heat, alcohol, marijuana; (2) keeping the testes cool by avoiding hot baths and tight clothing, or using a commercially prepared, water-dampened scrotal cooling device (keeping the testes cool seems to improve the sperm count); and (3) good nutrition. Medication, such as human chorionic gonadotropin (hCG) testosterone (Depo-Testosterone), is sometimes prescribed, with varying degrees of success. Varicocele is treated surgically.

Treatment for post-testicular causes of male infertility involves correcting ejaculatory abnormalities and obstruction. Ejaculatory abnormalities may be corrected by the split-ejaculate technique. The first half of the ejaculate contains more sperm than the second half. This first half may be used for artificial insemination or deposited in the vagina during intercourse, followed by withdrawal of the penis. Absence of ejaculation or retrograde (backward) ejaculation may be treated with drugs such as ephedrine, imipramine, or antihistamines. Artificial insemination may be done using sperm from urine obtained by centrifuge. Obstructive infertility is treated by surgery.

Appropriate antimicrobial drugs are used to treat genitourinary infections. Immunologic causes of male infertility may be treated with steroids and artificial insemination of sperm that have been washed to remove antibodies contained in the sperm.

Referral for counseling or support groups, or both, for infertile couples may be appropriate. A nationally known support group in the United States is RESOLVE, Department P, Box 474, Belmont, MA 02178.

ERECTILE DYSFUNCTION

Erectile dysfunction (impotence) was once thought to be entirely psychogenic in origin. We now know there are physiologic causes in about half the cases. The number is even higher in men over 50 years of age.

Psychogenic Dysfunction

Indications of psychogenic erectile dysfunction include

- Normal and sustained erection during foreplay, but loss of erection at the moment of intromission (penetration);
- Normal erection with some sexual partners but not with others;
- Normal erection with masturbation but not with partners;
- Sudden onset of total impotence in a man under age 40; and
- Alternating periods of normal function and total impotence.

ASSESSMENT

Assessment begins with carefully gathering the client's sexual and medical history and physical assessment. Physiologic causes must be eliminated. It is not true that nothing is physically wrong with a man if he can achieve a partial erection. Men with diabetic, vasculogenic, neurogenic, or endocrine pathologic conditions and men using certain drugs (see the section on Infertility) may be able to achieve some erectile activity, especially in the morning. Therefore, all medical possibilities, including drug use, are assessed and documented before an erectile problem is considered psychogenic.

Physical examination includes complete blood count; urinalysis; examination of prostatic secretions; liver function studies; thyroid function tests; assessment for diabetes mellitus; and serum creatine, serum testosterone, LH, and prolactin tests.

Psychometric testing, including the Minnesota Multiphasic Personality Inventory, Derogatis Sexual Function Inventory, or the Walker Sex Form, may be used to assess psychologic functioning.

MEDICAL MANAGEMENT

Treatment for erectile dysfunction of psychogenic causes includes various psychotherapeutic approaches. The best and most well-known approach is that developed by Masters and Johnson in the 1960s, which uses behavioral modification techniques.

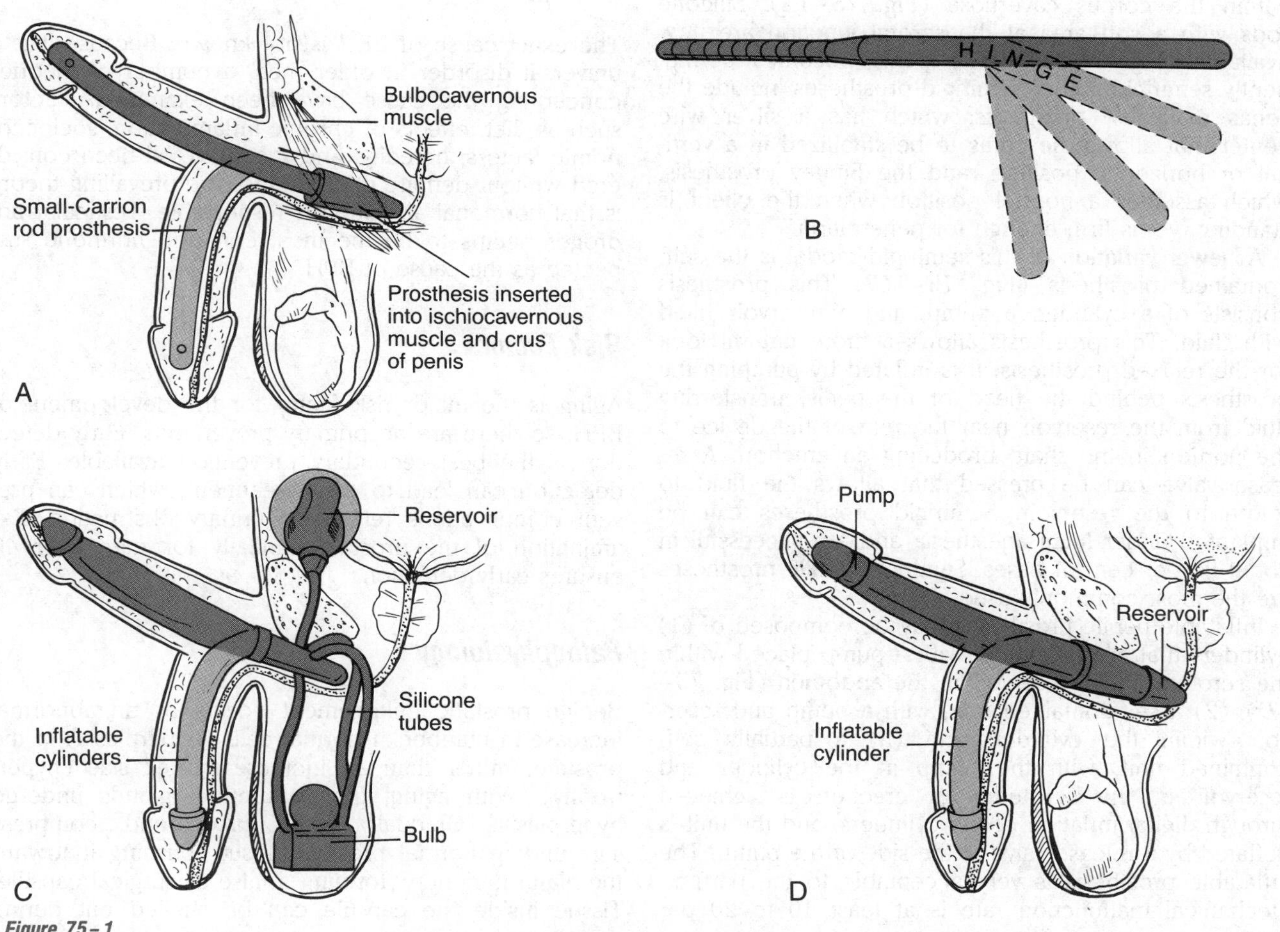

▲ **Figure 75-1**

Penile prostheses. *A*, Small-Carrion prosthesis consisting of plastic rods. *B*, Flexrod semirigid penile implant. *C*, Inflatable penile prosthesis. *D*, Self-contained penile prosthesis.

Physiologic Dysfunction

ASSESSMENT

As stated previously, there are many tests that can be performed to identify physiologic causes of erectile dysfunction.

MEDICAL MANAGEMENT

Treatment for physiologic erectile dysfunction includes medical treatment, such as discontinuing or modifying the drugs that affect sexual functioning or treating endocrine abnormalities.

SURGICAL MANAGEMENT

Surgical treatment includes the use of penile prostheses, intracavernosal injections (using papaverine or prostin), and penile revascularization. Various penile prostheses are available. There are basically three types: (1) semirigid, (2) self-contained, and (3) inflatable. There are also vacuum erection devices that have been in use the last several years.

The original semirigid penile prosthesis (Small-Carrion) consists of a pair of plastic rods inserted within the corpus cavernosa (Fig. 75-1*A*). Silicone rods with a soft area at the scrotal junction are now available (Fig. 75-1*B*). The penis becomes permanently semirigid. Other semirigid prostheses include the Jonas malleable prosthesis, which has a silver wire center that allows the penis to be stabilized in a vertical or horizontal position, and the Finney prosthesis, which assumes a normal position when the client is standing, yet is firm enough for penetration.

A newer variation of this semirigid model is the self-contained prosthesis (Fig. 75-1*C*). This prosthesis consists of a cylinder, a pump, and a reservoir filled with fluid. This prosthesis allows a more natural look for the relaxed prosthesis. It is inflated by pumping the prosthesis behind the head of the penis, transferring fluid from the reservoir near the rear of the device to the portion in the shaft, producing an erection. A release valve can be pressed that allows the fluid to return to the reservoir. Semirigid prostheses can be implanted under local anesthesia and are successful in about 95 per cent of cases. Semirigid penile prostheses are the most commonly used.

Inflatable penile prostheses may be composed of (1) cylinders that are inflatable, with a pump placed within the scrotum and a reservoir in the abdomen (Fig. 75-1*D*), (2) a self-contained unit, with a pump and reservoir within the cylinder; and (3) a partially self-contained unit, with the pump in the cylinder and reservoir in the scrotum. An erection is achieved through digital inflation of the cylinders, and the unit is deflated by a release valve at the side of the pump. The inflatable prosthesis is very acceptable to the partner. Mechanical malfunction rate is at least 10 to 20 per cent.

Penile revascularization may be used to correct vasculogenic erectile dysfunction. This surgical approach is still in its infancy. Currently, microsurgical techniques are being tried to revascularize the dorsal or central penile arteries.

▼ PROSTATE DISORDERS

BENIGN PROSTATIC HYPERTROPHY

Definition

With aging, the prostatic tissue undergoes benign hypertrophy and hyperplasia. Benign prostatic hypertrophy (BPH) is one of the most common disorders affecting men. The prostate is the urologic organ most frequently affected by benign and malignant neoplasms.

Incidence

It is estimated that by age 50, 50 per cent of men have some degree of BPH; the incidence increases to more than 75 per cent in men over age 80. It is more common in white men.

Etiology

The exact cause of BPH is not known. Because it is a universal disorder in older men, a number of theories concerning the cause have been examined. Factors such as diet, effects of chronic inflammation, socioeconomic factors, heredity, and race have all been considered without definite conclusions. The prevailing theory is that hormonal alteration is responsible. Testicular androgen seems to be the most common hormone suspected as the cause of BPH.

Risk Factors

Aging is the major risk factor for the development of BPH, so there are no primary preventions. Early detection is the best secondary prevention available. Early detection can lead to early treatment, which can prevent complications related to urinary obstruction. Examination of the prostate annually for men over 40 ensures early detection.

Pathophysiology

Benign prostatic enlargement occurs by an abnormal increase in number of normal cells (hyperplasia) in the prostate, rather than an increase in cell size (hypertrophy). With aging, the periurethral glands undergo hyperplasia. Gradually, they grow and compress surrounding normal prostatic tissue, pushing it toward the gland periphery, forming a false or surgical capsule. Tissue inside the capsule can be shelled out during surgery.

Potential complications of prostatic enlargement (Fig. 75-2) include (1) impeded urinary outflow and

(2) urinary reflux (backward flow) because of decompensation of the ureterovesical junction. Decompensation results from long-term elevated bladder pressure. Thickening, trabeculation (fibromuscular bands), and bladder wall diverticula may occur. Bladder diverticula may retain urine, causing infection and calculi development. Fishhooking of the ureters entering the bladder is common (i.e., ureters looping downward like a fishhook as they enter the bladder). The ureters may be compressed and obstructed by the thickened bladder wall, causing hydroureter (ureter abnormally distended with urine). A similar situation (hydronephrosis) may develop in the kidneys, because urine flow is obstructed in the ureters and urine backs up. In this situation, the pelvis and renal calyces distend with urine and the renal parenchyma atrophies. Ultimately, prolonged urinary obstruction or reflux can cause renal insufficiency (Fig. 75-2).

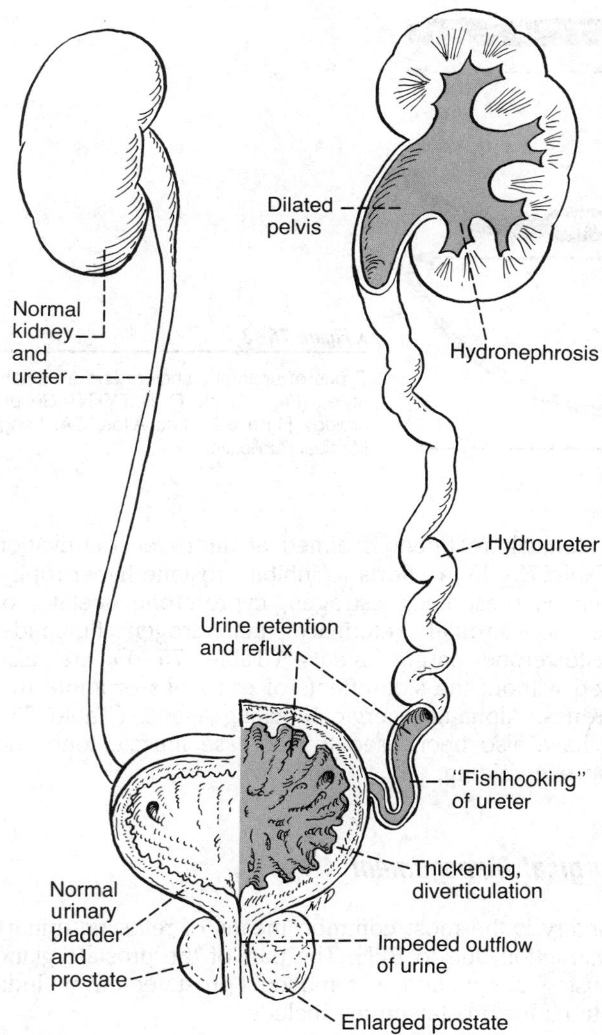

▲ *Figure 75-2*

Complications of benign prostatic hypertrophy. Left side of illustration shows normal kidney, ureter, bladder, and prostate. Right side shows potential complications.

Clinical Manifestations

BPH usually develops slowly and may persist for a long time in a silent state without creating a major problem. As the man becomes older, he may assume that increasing frequency of urination is part of aging. Reduction in both the size and force of urinary stream is abnormal and should be assessed.

With developing BPH, the urinary stream first lacks force, then becomes weak and dribbling. The man feels unable to empty his bladder, and either strains to urinate or urinates more frequently. There may be blood in the urine (a symptom more common in benign hypertrophy than in cancer).

As the prostate enlarges, there is a danger of complete urinary obstruction and retention. Retention may be precipitated by (1) the man becoming chilled, (2) drinking alcoholic beverages, (3) an infection, (4) delay in voiding, and (5) bed rest. Some medications may also provoke retention, such as decongestants, anticholinergics, and antidepressants. Obstruction can be a painful emergency requiring catheterization. If retention is long-standing and large amounts of urine are removed, observe the person carefully for signs of shock. Figure 75-3 shows various types of urethral catheters.

DIAGNOSTIC ASSESSMENT

BPH is assessed by (1) a general physical examination, including rectal examination; (2) laboratory examination of blood, urine, and renal function; (3) x-ray examination including intravenous pyelogram and cystography, and (4) instrumental examination, including catheterization and cystoscopy.

The client should be asked about the size and force of the urinary stream. A uroflow test may be performed. Straight catheterization after voiding assesses the amount of residual urine. Other studies used to assess obstruction include (1) urethral pressure profile and (2) electromyelography (EMG) of the sphincter muscles.

Rectal examination and prostatic massage for a sample of prostatic secretion can be performed. The secretion can be examined under the microscope for pus cells, which may indicate infection. Urine, obtained before prostatic massage, may be normal in asymptomatic men, or it may show infection by the presence of red or white blood cells and an alkaline pH.

The enlarged prostate may cause urinary back pressure, leading to renal damage. Assessing for indication of renal problems is, therefore, important, and renal function studies must be included in the assessment.

Medical Management

Some men find their symptoms considerably relieved by conservative interventions. The client can learn some techniques that will decrease his symptoms and possible complications. Explain to the man that if his bladder is distended rapidly, it can increase his symptoms and precipitate acute retention; the hypertrophic

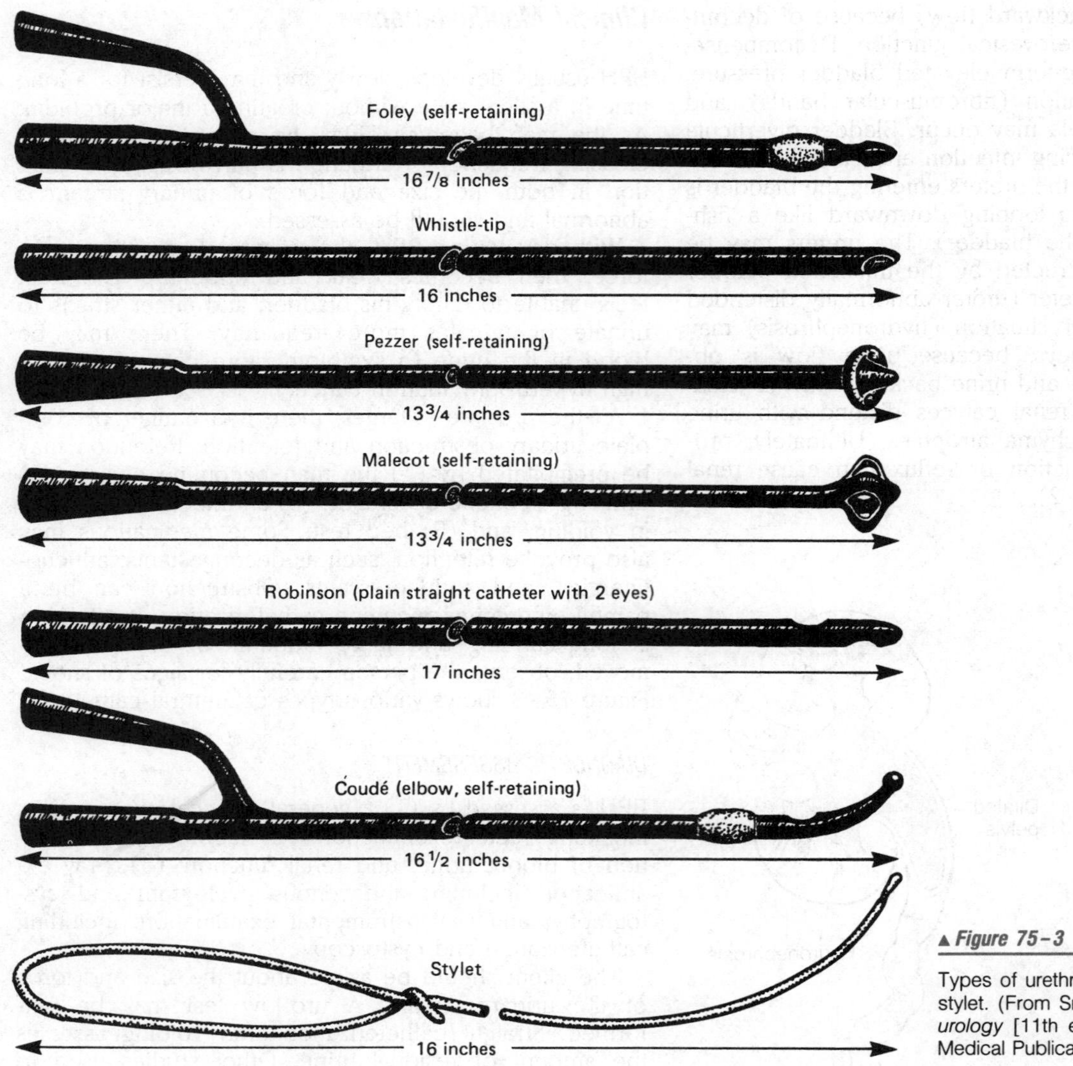

▲ *Figure 75-3*

Types of urethral catheters and a catheter stylet. (From Smith, D. R. [1984]. *General urology* [11th ed.]. Los Altos, CA: Lange Medical Publications.)

muscle of the bladder can lose its tone if distended quickly. Advise the client to (1) void whenever the urge to do so is felt and not put it off, (2) avoid taking large quantities of fluid over a short period, and (3) avoid alcohol, because its diuretic effect, with the volume of fluid, increases bladder distention. Alcohol intake is the most common precipitating factor for acute urinary retention.

Prostatic massage, sexual intercourse, and hot sitz baths may relieve symptoms by releasing a small amount of prostatic fluid, which reduces the edema. Urinary frequency is then decreased, and stream flow is increased.

Mild or asymptomatic BPH may be associated with prostatitis, which causes increased prostatic swelling and worsening of symptoms. Antibiotics may relieve acute symptoms and possibly delay surgery. Sympathomimetic drugs such as phenylpropanolamine and phenylephrine, found in common cold and cough remedies, worsen BPH. Warn the client not to take any of these medications.

Medical treatment is aimed at androgen deprivation (Table 75-1) in efforts to inhibit prostatic hypertrophy, such as prescribing estrogen, cyproterone acetate, or the nonsteroidal veterinary antiandrogen flutamide. Testosterone-sparing agents (Table 75-1) are also used without the side effects of estrogens or antitestosterones. Alpha-adrenergic blocking agents (Table 75-1) have also been used to decrease muscle tone and improve voiding.

Surgical Management

Surgery is the most common means of relieving urinary obstruction due to BPH. The part of the prostate gland causing obstruction is removed (prostatectomy). Indications for prostatectomy include

- Upper urinary tract dilatation (hydroureter, hydronephrosis) and impaired renal function;
- Severe discomfort and inconvenience for the person;

TABLE 75-1. Selected Medications Used to Treat Benign Prostatic Hypertrophy

Medication	Action
Testosterone-Ablating Agents	
▶ diethylstilbestrol (DES) ▶ flutamide (Eulexin) ▶ gonadotropin-releasing hormone analogs (GnRH) ◆ nafarelin acetate (Synarel) ◆ buserelin (Suprefact-investigational) ◆ leuprolide (Lupron) ◆ goserelin acetate (Zoladex) ▶ cyproterone acetate (Androcur)	Testosterone-ablating agents decrease the amount of circulating testosterone levels, leading to suppression of prostatic tissue growth. Estrogens inhibit prostatic growth by suppressing release of luteinizing hormone-releasing agent, leading to a decrease in testosterone. Flutamide is an antiandrogen that competes with testosterone for androgen receptor sites. GnRH inhibits the release of pituitary gonadotropin, preventing testosterone biosynthesis. Cyproterone is a synthetic antiandrogen that acts as an androgen-receptor inhibitor.
Testosterone-Sparing Agents	
▶ finasteride (Proscar)	A 5-α reductase inhibitor that blocks dihydrotestosterone without suppressing circulating testosterone. Decreases prostatic tissue without affecting potency or libido.
Alpha-adrenergic Blocking Agents	
▶ phenoxybenzamine (Dibenzyline) ▶ terazosin (Hytrin) ▶ prozasin (Minipress)	There is abundant autonomic innervation of the bladder neck and prostatic smooth muscle. Prostatic obstruction is due in part to the neurogenic tone of the bladder neck and prostatic smooth muscle. These agents block the alpha receptors, improving urination by decreasing outlet obstruction.

- Total urinary obstruction;
- Vesical (urinary bladder) calculus, indicative of long-standing obstruction associated with BPH and infection;
- Long-standing urinary obstruction that impairs renal function;
- Severe and prolonged hematuria (recurrent bleeding);
- Chronic urinary retention; and
- Recurrent urinary tract infections.

Enlarged prostate tissue may be removed by various approaches (Fig. 75-4). These approaches include (1) transurethral resection, (2) suprapubic prostatectomy, (3) retropubic prostatectomy, and (4) perineal prostatectomy. The method used depends on the size of the prostate and the general health of the person. The term prostatectomy is really a misnomer. The procedure is actually an adenectomy of new tissue growth, and the true prostate and fibrous capsule are not removed. The entire prostatectomy is removed only during a radical prostatectomy, which is used only for some prostatic cancers.

Transurethral Resection. Transurethral resection of the prostate (TURPs) is the most widely used of all prostatic surgical techniques. TURPs is especially suitable for men with relatively small prostatic enlargements, or who are poor surgical risks. No incision is made. Repeated TURPs may be needed because of postoperative urethral strictures, bladder neck scarring, and prostatic tissue regrowth.

TURPs is performed by inserting a resectoscope through the urethra (Fig. 75-4*A*). Two types of resectoscopes may be used; (1) hot-loop resectoscope, which has a movable loop of wire that cuts tissue with a high-frequency current; or (2) a cold-punch resectoscope (rarely used), which punches out tissue, piece by piece, with a circular knife blade. In both cases, the surgeon is able to visualize the inside of the bladder by inserting a telescope through the resectoscope. Bleeding is controlled by cauterization. Irrigating fluid can be passed into and out of the area through the resectoscope, and debris falls back into the bladder and is then washed out. Closed-system, sterile gravity irrigation is used with a solution of isotonic irrigation fluid. Water is never used, because during surgery the client absorbs about 900 ml of irrigating fluid through the tissues and veins at the operative site. Water could precipitate hemolysis and acute renal failure. Surgery must be completed within about 60 to 90 minutes to avoid excessive blood loss and absorption of irrigating fluid. Monitoring fluid and electrolyte balance and renal function before, during, and after surgery is important. Fluid absorption (water intoxication or dilutional hyponatremia) during surgery can produce hypervolemia. Postoperative assessment includes observing for hypertension, bradycardia, weakness, and seizures.

Suprapubic Prostatectomy. This surgical approach is through a lower abdominal incision (Fig. 75-4*B*). Indications for this procedure include (1) a prostate too large to be resected transurethrally; (2) bladder abnormality (e.g., diverticula or calculi); (3) the presence of large, pedunculated middle lobe or lateral prostatic lobes; or (4) a need to explore the abdomen.

An incision is made into the bladder, and the en-

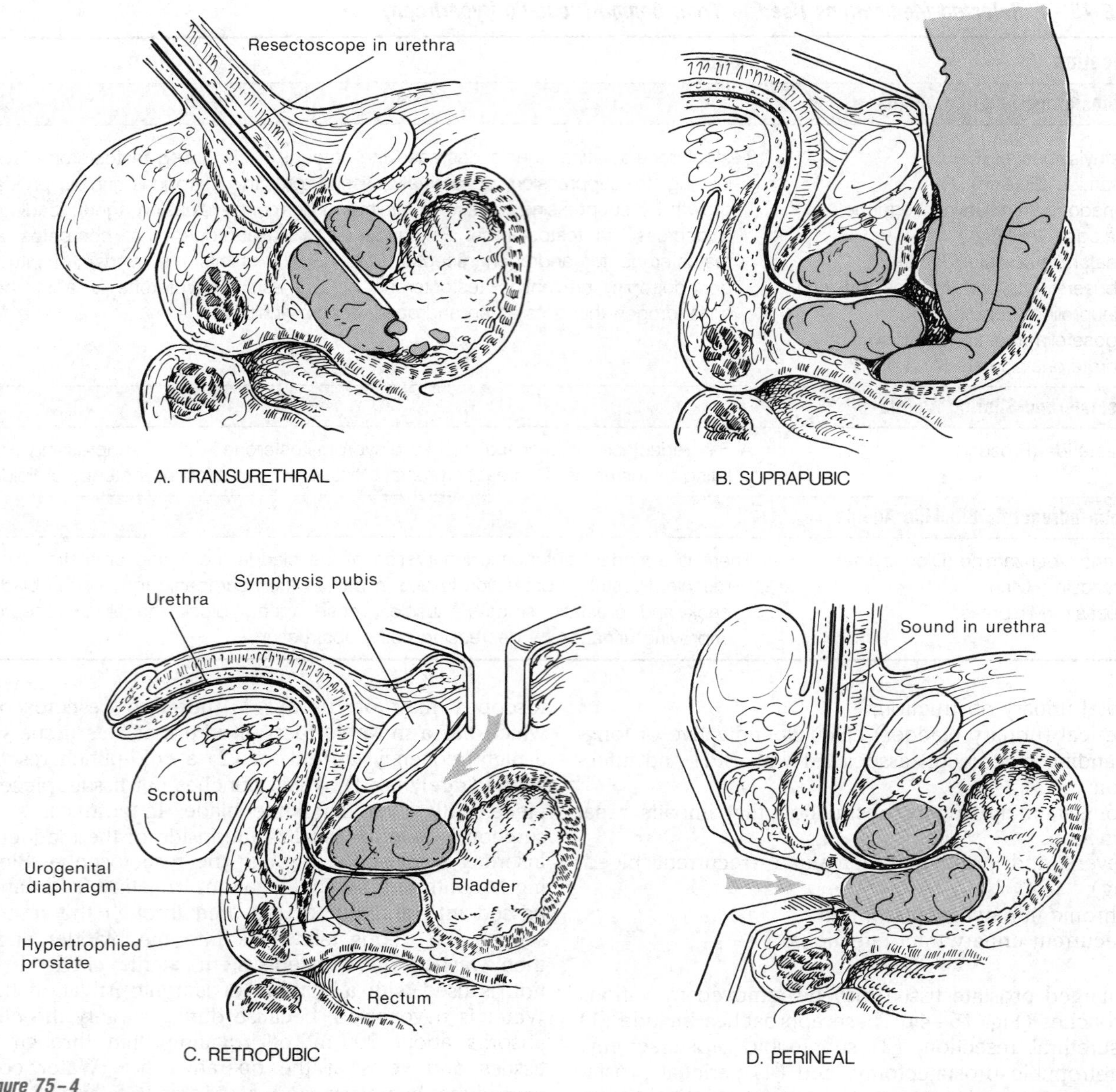

▲ *Figure 75–4*

Surgical approaches to the prostate. *A*, Transurethral resection prostatectomy (TURP) is a closed method of treatment, i.e., no incision is made and the hyperplastic prostate tissue is removed through a resectoscope (like a cystoscope) inserted through the penis. *B*, Suprapubic (transvesical) prostatectomy is an open method of treatment in which the hyperplastic prostatic tissue is enucleated through the anterior walls of the abdomen and bladder. *C*, Retropubic (extravesical) prostatectomy is an open method in which a low abdominal incision is made between the pubic arch and the bladder. *D*, Perineal prostatectomy is an open method involving an incision between the anus and the scrotum.

larged tissue is enucleated by blunt dissection. Both suprapubic and urethral catheters are inserted. An advantage of suprapubic prostatectomy is that bladder abnormalities can be treated concurrently, because an incision is made into the urinary bladder. Thorough exploration and complete tissue removal are facilitated. Disadvantages include (1) difficulty in obtaining hemostasis (therefore, assess for shock and hemorrhage); (2) bladder spasms; (3) urinary leakage into an abdominal wound around the suprapubic catheter; and (4) relatively prolonged and uncomfortable convalescence. Incontinence sometimes occurs. A small number of men experience erectile dysfunction after this procedure.

Retropubic Prostatectomy. Retropubic prostatectomy is the most recently developed open method (Fig, 75–4*C*). A low abdominal incision facilitates approaching the prostate without entering the bladder. Indications for use are (1) when the prostate is too large to be removed transurethrally and (2) presence of severe urethral stricture. Advantages include direct visualization of the prostate and direct hemostasis in the prostatic fossa. A disadvantage is that any associated pathologic condition in the bladder cannot be treated, because the bladder is not entered. Also, osteitis pubis (pubic bone inflammation) may occur. A suprapubic catheter may be inserted to control bleeding, or constant bladder irrigation may be used. Infrequent complications include incontinence and erectile dysfunction (impotence). Postoperative urinary leakage may occur for a few days after the catheter is removed.

Perineal Prostatectomy. An incision is made into the perineum, between the anus and the scrotum (Fig. 75–4*D*). The perineal prostatectomy is performed to treat prostatic cancer. Because of possible postoperative erectile dysfunction, it is not performed to treat BPH.

A subtotal prostatectomy may be performed when enlarged glands are filled with calculi or when abscesses fail to respond to treatment. In a subtotal prostatectomy, the entire gland and capsule are removed, but the seminal vesicles and sections of the vas deferens are left in place. A major disadvantage is that the procedure is carried out in a lithotomy position, which is contraindicated for people with arthritis or cardiopulmonary disease. Complications include (1) a stronger likelihood of erectile dysfunction than with other procedures, (2) rectourethral fistula, (3) urinary tract infections, (4) epididymitis, and (5) urinary retention.

Other Procedures. There are other newer surgical procedures used to treat BPH. These include the transurethral incision of the prostate (TUIP), balloon dilation of the prostate, microwave/hyperthermia of the prostate, transurethral laser incision of the prostate (TULIP), and the insertion of prostatic stents.

The TUIP is an option for men with small prostates causing outlet obstruction. This procedure has fewer postoperative complications and can be performed under local anesthesia for high-risk clients. Greater client satisfaction has also been reported with this procedure, with many clients reporting no change in ejaculation, making this an excellent procedure for younger men with small glands.

Transurethral balloon dilation of the prostate (TUDP) is another new procedure that has become increasingly popular. The concept of dilating the prostate is not new because sounds, bougies, and metal dilators have been used, but the balloon is new. The procedure is actually not surgical, but it is invasive. It involves the insertion of a small catheter into the urethra, with the positioning of a balloon within the prostatic urethra and inflating it to apply pressure to the enlarged gland, causing it to dilate. The balloon is carefully placed inside the prostatic urethra in a variety of ways. Care is taken to ensure that the balloon does not migrate downward, damaging the sphincter, or upward into the bladder, negating the effect. The balloon is inflated to a diameter of a 75 to 90 French catheter and left in place for 15 minutes. The client has a urethral catheter overnight.

This surgical procedure can be performed under local anesthesia, and there is no associated blood loss, making it appropriate for many high-risk clients. The hospital stay is short, and there are few postoperative complications. There are two major concerns with this procedure. First, because no tissue is removed, prostatic cancer could be missed. The other concern is the length of time this procedure will be effective. Because it is such a recent innovation, clients have not been followed long enough to determine whether or not recurrence of the obstruction is common.

Microwave hyperthermia is one of the newest procedures being performed. Microwave hyperthermia is delivered via a rectal probe over a period of 4 to 10 treatments. Each treatment lasts about 60 minutes and is performed without anesthesia on an outpatient basis. The treatment has shown some promising results to date, although the ultimate efficacy has not been shown.

TULIP is the newest treatment. It is similar to the TUIP, but a laser is used to make the incision. So far, few results are available, but those data that are available look promising. The procedure results in minimal blood loss, no irrigation, and the client does not need a catheter after surgery.

The remaining new treatment is the insertion of a prostatic stent. This procedure is used for clients who are extremely poor operative risks. This hollow tube can be inserted through an endoscope into the prostatic urethra, where it holds the urethra open mechanically. It is safer than an indwelling urethral catheter because there is no risk of infection. The stent can be left in place for 4 to 6 weeks without problems. If left in place longer than this, epithelial cells will grow over the stent.

The most common early complication is postoperative bleeding. Other complications include (1) retrograde ejaculation (semen passing into the bladder instead of out through the penis) because of bladder neck surgical trauma, (2) urethral stricture, (3) bladder neck constriction, (4) urinary incontinence, and (5) epididymitis.

There is no treatment for retrograde ejaculation. The condition should be explained to the client so they are not frightened by this. The condition will result in sterility because the sperm are ejaculated into the bladder.

Urethral stricture can be treated postoperatively with dilation with urethral sounds. If the stricture is severe, a urethroplasty can be performed. Bladder neck contractures, if severe, also can be treated with surgical reconstruction.

Urinary incontinence is usually caused by trauma to the urinary sphincter. The client can decrease the symptoms by performing perineal exercises to improve muscle control. Kegel exercises are described in Chapter 49.

Epididymitis is a preventable complication if a vasectomy is performed at the same time as the prostatectomy. Tying the vas deferens prevents retrograde bacterial infection or inflammation of the epididymis. If the prostate is removed in its entirety, or is almost completely removed, the client will be sterile anyway.

Other possible complications are urinary tract infection, obstruction, accidental displacement of the catheter, incontinence, impotence, and recurrence of symptoms.

Nursing Management

ASSESSMENT

Men often have only a vague understanding about what an enlarged prostate is and may be afraid of the tests and their results. Carefully explain each part of the assessment process. Show the client and significant others a picture of the reproductive organs and prostate, and explain the effects of enlargement on urine excretion.

The client should be asked to describe all urinary symptoms, including the pattern of urination, presence of urgency, frequency, decreased or altered urinary stream, hesitancy, or nocturia. The nurse should question the client about the presence of hematuria.

The ability of the client to empty his bladder also must be assessed. The client's bladder should be palpated for distention. If the client is unable to void, the need for a urethral catheter should be assessed.

Careful preoperative assessment in both physical and psychosocial areas is important. The client's knowledge about the surgery and its outcomes should be assessed. Because so many types of treatment are possible, the client may not understand the implications of the treatment he will be receiving.

NURSING INTERVENTION

Collaborative Problem. Altered urinary elimination: frequency, urgency, hesitancy, change in stream, incontinence; retention, or nocturia R/T urethral obstruction.

Planning: Expected Outcomes. The client will not develop symptoms of BPH, as evidenced by absence of frequency, urgency, hesitancy, change in stream, incontinence, retention, or nocturia.

Implementation. The man may have preoperative urinary difficulties, such as obstruction, urinary retention, and diminished renal function. These problems may require early admission to the health care facility for treatment. An indwelling catheter may be inserted, or drainage may be achieved by cystostomy. Assess the client carefully for signs of shock due to post-obstructive diuresis.

Never force a urinary catheter. If it cannot be inserted with gentle pressure, contact a urologist. Emergency catheterization for complete bladder obstruction requires a urologist's skills and possibly special instruments, such as insertion of a stylet (thin wire) into the catheter lumen, metal catheters, or other firm, specially angled catheters (coudé).

Nursing Diagnosis: Fear and Anxiety R/T hospitalization, urinary problems, and treatments.

Planning: Expected Outcomes. The client will have fear and anxiety controlled, as evidenced by client's statements of understanding, ability to ask questions, and ability to rest quietly.

Implementation. Fear and anxiety may be lessened by taking a nursing history and giving appropriate explanations. Respond to the concerns of the client and significant others with empathetic listening, accurate information, and ongoing support. Restating the explanations given by the surgeon and anesthetist when securing informed consent may be necessary, because stressed clients frequently forget what they have been told.

Informed consent requires that the man understand the risks (e.g., possible sexual dysfunction, including erectile dysfunction, retrograde ejaculation, infertility) and short- and long-term benefits (e.g., relief of urinary symptoms and arrested reduction in renal function).

Nursing Diagnosis: High Risk for Fluid Volume Deficit R/T urinary symptoms and self-imposed fluid restriction.

Planning: Expected Outcomes. The client will not develop fluid volume deficit, as evidenced by intake of at least 2 liters of fluid a day.

Implementation. It is important to improve the client's nutritional status preoperatively, especially fluid balance. Many clients limit their fluid intake to combat the symptoms of frequency and urgency they experience as a result of the prostatic enlargement. Clients increase their risk of urinary tract infection and even renal or cardiovascular dysfunction with this limited intake. The client should maintain, unless otherwise contraindicated, an intake of at least 2500 to 3000 ml/day to correct dehydration and azotemia (nitrogen waste products in the blood).

Nursing Diagnosis: High Risk for Self-Esteem disturbance R/T threats to sexuality from disease and treatment.

Planning: Expected Outcomes. The client will not develop a disturbance in self-concept as evidenced by client's willingness to discuss sexual issues.

Implementation. Most men undergoing prostatectomy are over age 50. The aging process compounds the psychosocial threat involved in intimate surgery. Such men may experience disturbing changes in self-concept, including body image, self-esteem, role performance, and personal identity. Sexual concerns may be a part of these changes.

It is usually helpful if the man and significant others can talk about these concerns with a supportive person. They need reassurance that their concerns (including fears of being unable to perform sexually) are common to men who undergo major surgery. Recommendations for any restrictions on sexual intercourse and alternative sexual activity are best given in collaboration with the physician. Men who leave health care facilities with incontinence, weakness, pain, and indwelling catheters may have additional concerns and self-doubts.

Significant others also need support following prostatectomy. They may not understand what is happening and may be concerned about potential or actual changes in their relationship.

Collaborative Problem. High risk for fluid volume deficit R/T postoperative hemorrhage.

Planning: Expected Outcomes. The client will not develop fluid volume deficit, as evidenced by absence of hemorrhage and maintenance of at least 30 ml of urine output every hour.

Implementation. Carry out the nursing assessment described in Chapter 19 to identify hemorrhage. In addition, observe the wound drains, wound packing, and catheter drainage for excessive bleeding. Wound drains may be in place after perineal, retropubic, or suprapubic prostatectomies. A suprapubic urinary catheter positioned directly into the bladder through the abdominal wall is in place after suprapubic prostatectomies. Sometimes, the balloon of the indwelling catheter (Foley type) is inflated with 30 ml or more of fluid, up to 100 ml (rather than the usual 5 ml) to promote hemostasis at the operative site.

Some hematuria (blood in the urine) is usual for several days after surgery. However, frank bleeding, arterial or venous, may occur during the first day after surgery. Arterial bleeding is bright red, has numerous clots, and is viscous. Blood pressure may fall, and emergency surgical intervention may become necessary. Venous bleeding in the prostatic area may be controlled by increasing the pressure (adding fluid) in the ballooned end of the urethral catheter and pulling the catheter tightly so the balloon moves into the prostatic fossa, then taping the catheter to the thigh (called applying traction). Traction is left in place for 24 hours or more and released by the physician when the bleeding has stopped. The physician also can remove fluid slowly from the balloon as the bleeding decreases.

Overdistention of the bladder must be avoided because it can precipitate secondary hemorrhage by placing undue strain on freshly coagulated blood vessels.

Nursing Diagnosis: Pain R/T surgery and bladder spasms.

Planning: Expected Outcomes. The client will have pain relieved or controlled, as evidenced by client's report.

Implementation. Pain control following surgery is discussed in Chapter 19. Additional pain can occur after prostatectomy if urinary drainage tubes become obstructed. The best intervention is to prevent catheters from becoming blocked. If a man experiences pain after a prostatectomy, first assess the drainage apparatus for patency. Relief of obstruction often alleviates pain without the need for analgesics. Clots are often the cause of the obstruction.

Bladder spasms also may occur because of bladder overdistention or irritation from an indwelling catheter balloon. Antispasmodic medications, such as belladonna and opium (B & O) suppositories or propantheline bromide (Pro-Banthine), may be prescribed prophylactically to help prevent bladder spasms, especially in clients who require traction. They may cause complications, however (clients with severe cardiac disease or glaucoma should not receive these agents). Antispasmodic drugs can cause constipation, and straining at stool can precipitate bleeding from the operative site, so stool softeners, such as docusate sodium (Colace) often are given.

Collaborative Problem. High Risk for Injury R/T presence of urinary catheters, irrigation, or suprapubic drains.

Planning: Expected Outcomes. The client will not develop an injury such as infection, catheter obstruction, water intoxication, or injury due to the catheter, as evidenced by absence of fever; normal white blood cell count; adequate wound healing; adequate catheter drainage; hyponatremia, hypertension, or other signs of water intoxication; excessive bleeding or trauma from the catheter; urinary retention after catheter removal; or fistula formation.

Implementation. Indwelling catheters (urethral or suprapubic) are generally used to facilitate urinary drainage after all types of prostatectomies (Fig. 75-4). Various types of catheter irrigation systems may be used with these catheters. Closed irrigation, referred to as a constant bladder irrigation (CBI) (Fig. 75-5), permits either constant or intermittent irrigation without the hazard of breaking aseptic technique. Isotonic irrigating fluid is used for intermittent irrigation, incorporating small amounts (usually 60 to 100 ml); for continuous irrigation, enough to maintain outflow of clear or slightly pink urine. The fluid must be isotonic, because water could lead to a depletion of electrolytes or water intoxication (see Chap. 14).

Frequently assess drainage from the catheter. Because the client usually receives intravenous fluid postoperatively, urinary catheters should be draining. Keep accurate records of intake and output, accounting for the amount instilled with the irrigation.

While a urinary catheter is in place, it must be kept patent (open, clear, and unobstructed). Urinary flow may become obstructed in various ways, such as with, blood clots, prostatic chips, mucous plugs, kinked tubing, tube displacement. The nurse should frequently assess catheter patency to make sure it is draining.

The catheter may become blocked by clots or sediment, leading to complications, such as infections, bladder distention, and painful bladder spasms. Some bladder spasms occur with bladder distention, whereas others are a response to irritation from the catheter balloon (from excessive fluid in the balloon to prevent bleeding).

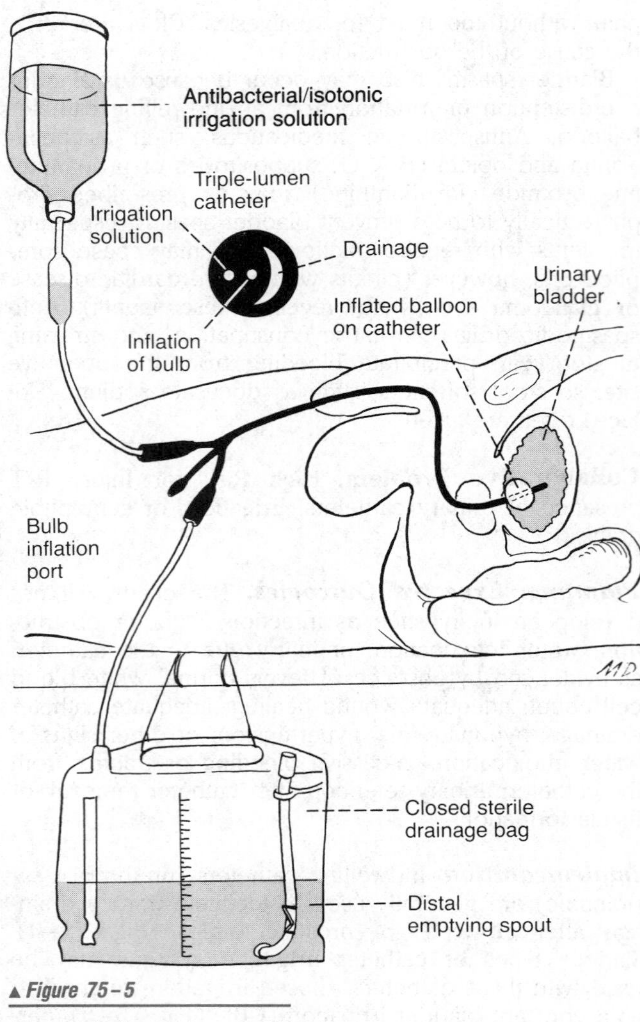

▲ *Figure 75-5*

Closed irrigation system, or CBI.

It is important to prevent bladder overdistention, such as during irrigation or as a result of urinary obstruction. Bladder overdistention can cause hemorrhage by placing undue strain on freshly coagulated blood vessels. The nurse should assess the client for bladder overdistention by shutting off continuous irrigation and palpating the lower abdomen. If overdistention is present, catheter irrigation may clear clots or plugs and restore urinary drainage.

If there is resistance to the introduction of irrigating fluid into the catheter, or if there is no return of irrigating fluid through the tubing, **do not force the fluid.** If this occurs, contact the surgeon immediately. If a catheter cannot be cleared, it may have to be removed and a new one inserted. This procedure is usually performed by the surgeon.

The client may be confused immediately after surgery and may accidentally pull out the catheter. Tell the client repeatedly that he has a tube in his bladder through his penis or abdomen (whichever it is), and remind him not to touch it. A displaced or removed urinary catheter following prostatic surgery is painful and disrupts recovery. If the client does pull the catheter out, contact the surgeon for reinsertion.

The nurse should observe the client carefully for local or systemic indications of infection. Handle catheters, drainage apparatus, and urine collection carefully to avoid introducing microorganisms into the urinary tract. Aseptic technique is especially important after a perineal prostatectomy because of a high possibility of infection in a wound so close to the anal area. Meticulous aseptic technique is also necessary around the area of insertion of a suprapubic catheter.

The surgeon may make the initial dressing change and delegate subsequent wound care to the nurses. The man may be taught to change his own dressing. When a perineal incision is present, a double-tailed T-binder may be used to secure dressings. Cross the tails over the incisional area, and position one tail on each side of the scrotum. Then, pull the tails up to the waistband and tie them securely. Prevent wound trauma after perineal surgery by avoiding the use of enemas, rectal tubes, or rectal thermometers. Clean the wound thoroughly after each bowel movement.

The length of time urethral catheters are left inserted varies according to surgeon preference, the client's recovery, and the type of surgery. After perineal prostatectomy, a urethral catheter may be left in place for 12 to 14 days to allow for healing of the resected bladder neck and urethra. Following a simple TUR, it may be removed after 2 to 3 days if the urine remains clear. Sometimes the catheter is removed early if it is causing problems, such as bladder spasms.

After a urethral catheter is removed (and after a TUR), the nurse should monitor the client closely for signs of urinary retention and urethral strictures. Indications of urinary retention include inability to pass urine and bladder overdistention. Indications of urethral stricture include a small urinary stream, dysuria, and straining to urinate. The nurse should talk to the client and significant others about the importance of urinating when the client first feels a desire to do so. Holding the urine may increase the possibility of retention.

Temporary urinary frequency or incontinence may occur after the catheter is removed. The nurse must be understanding of the man's feelings and keep him dry without embarrassing him. Keep reminding him and his significant others these problems are temporary, but they may take some time to resolve. Urinary control usually returns quickly in young men, whereas in older men, a period of dribbling for up to 3 months is not unusual. Perineal exercises may reduce this problem (see the section on Knowledge Deficit). Additional surgery is sometimes required for persistent incontinence.

Wound drains are usually removed earlier than suprapubic drains. The suprapubic drain is left in place until urinary function has returned. Once the client is voiding well, the suprapubic drain can be removed. If it is removed before the client has returned to a normal voiding, the wound may not heal properly, leading to fistula formation.

Nursing Diagnosis: Knowledge Deficit R/T postoperative exercises and return of urinary function.

Planning: Expected Outcomes. The client will understand postoperative exercises and return of urinary function, as evidenced by client's statements.

Implementation. Throughout the postoperative period, explain each procedure and expectation, such as not to strain at stool, to the client and encourage his participation. Specific teaching opportunities for the client and significant others are appropriate and include the following categories.

Catheters, Wound Drains, Urinary Drainage, and Irrigation. Provide information about related procedures. Answer questions patiently. Tell the client and significant others that it is important not to touch the equipment, pull out the tubes, or obstruct the drainage. Help the man learn ways of turning and getting out of bed without pulling on the catheter or kinking the drainage tubing. Remind the client not to lie on the tubing. Show the client and significant others how to make sure the tubing always remains above the level of the drainage bag, because if the tubing falls at or below the drainage bag the flow of urine may be impeded and actually pass back into the bladder.

Common Sensations. Common sensations experienced by clients after a prostatectomy are that (1) the ureteral catheter may cause bladder spasms and a sensation of needing to pass urine, and (2) following removal of a catheter, dribbling of urine and a sense of urgency may occur.

Urinary and Wound Drainage. Urinary and wound drainage, such as bloody urine, is not unusual early in the postoperative period.

Permission to Tell Nurses of Concerns or Discomforts. Many men find it difficult to admit to discomfort or pain, such as from bladder spasms. Ask them frequently about this problem, and remind them of the importance of letting you know (see Chap. 16).

Self-Help Activities. Self-help activities include drinking increased amounts of fluids while a catheter is in place, performing bed exercises, incorporating early ambulation, and measuring fluid intake and urinary output. Prolonged sitting increases intra-abdominal pressure and may precipitate bleeding. Therefore, the man should avoid sitting except during meals. After he leaves the health care facility, driving an automobile or taking prolonged automobile rides should be avoided until at least 2 weeks after surgery, when the risk of bleeding lessens. Strenuous exercise is also contraindicated.

Advise the client not to strain during defecation for at least 6 weeks after surgery, because this can lead to bleeding from the operative site. Docusate sodium (Colace), prune juice, and milk of magnesia are usually satisfactory bowel stimulants during this time.

Perineal Exercises. Perineal exercises help the client regain urinary sphincter control. From the second or third postoperative day, teach the client to breathe normally while contracting abdominal, gluteal, and perineal muscles 12 to 25 times/h. A good way to describe this action is "Contract your muscles as if you have to pass urine urgently and there is no place to relieve yourself."

Another helpful exercise is to squeeze the rectal sphincter tensely while relaxing other body muscles. Teach the man to place his hands on his abdomen to assess abdominal tension. The abdomen should not be tense and a Valsalva maneuver should not occur when the exercise is performed correctly. During these exercises, it may help the man concentrate if he says aloud words such as relax and squeeze. Encourage the man to establish a planned schedule of exercising during waking hours and continue this routine until complete urinary control is achieved.

Advice on Leaving the Health Care Facility. The client is usually discharged 2 to 3 days after a TUR and up to 10 days after a radical perineal prostatectomy. Be sure he knows when and where to contact his surgeon next, and how to get in touch with health care professionals if he has concerns before that time. Tell the client to be sure to report to his surgeon any bleeding, infection, or obstructed urine flow. However, give him support and permission to discuss any concern with a health care professional.

Advise the client to avoid strenuous activity for 4 to 6 weeks (e.g., mowing the lawn, lifting more than 20 pounds). He will probably need extra rest while at the same time maintaining a balance of activity with ambulation. He may drive a car when given permission, usually after his first visit to the physician.

Advise the client to continue a high daily intake of nonalcoholic fluids to minimize clot formation. If he is discharged home with an indwelling catheter, provide him and his significant others with appropriate information (see Bridge to Home Health Care).

Nursing Diagnosis: High risk for Sexual Dysfunction R/T removal of prostate, retrograde ejaculation, and sterility.

Planning: Expected Outcomes. The client will not develop sexual dysfunction, as evidenced by client statements and the client's ability to discuss fears and concerns with staff.

Implementation. Retrograde ejaculation consists of the ejaculation of semen into the bladder rather than through the urethra. The man experiences erection and orgasm, but normal ejaculation does not occur. Retrograde ejaculation may occur after a prostatectomy because when the prostatic capsule contracts, the semen passes more easily into the bladder rather than through the urethra. Semen passes into the bladder and mixes with the urine, producing cloudy urine. Advise the man to observe his urine for cloudiness and tell his physician if it occurs.

Erectile dysfunction (impotence) is a rare complication of prostatectomy and is more likely to occur after

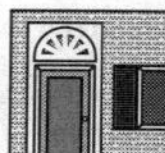

BRIDGE TO HOME HEALTH CARE

Catheter Insertion in the Home Setting

When inserting a catheter in the home setting, there is rarely the convenience of a hospital bed. Often, the lighting is not ideal. Although supplies may be sent home from the hospital with the client, obtaining the supplies is usually the responsibility of the home health care nurse.

For the female client who is obese or arthritic, try a posterior approach by having her turn on her side facing away from you. If you are using swabs to cleanse the meatal area, insert the last swab slightly into the vagina to identify the vaginal opening. A sterile Q-tip can also be used. Also, if you do insert the catheter in the vagina by mistake, leave it there and it will mark the opening so that you will not reinsert it into the same place. If there is no immediate urine return, one method of verifying placement is to slightly insert your fingertip into the vagina and feel for the catheter.

Male catheters are frequently inserted by the female home health care nurse. You may want to make a shared visit with an experienced home health care nurse for the first time or two to give yourself a little more confidence. If you are having difficulty inserting the catheter in a male client, remove the catheter and insert 3 to 5 ml of K-Y gel directly into the meatus by using a sterile syringe without the needle. If you know the catheter change is going to be difficult, instill the K-Y gel first. Then, when you meet resistance, use steady, easy pressure and rotate the catheter slowly until it finally slips through the constricture.

Most urologists use lidocaine (Xylocaine) gel for inserting male catheters, so you may request an order from the physician for Xylocaine gel. Insert it just like the K-Y gel, and wait a few minutes before inserting the catheter. This will relieve some of the pain and help the client relax.

Remember, if the client has had a catheter inserted for a long time, you may not get an immediate urine return. Have the person drink a glass of water and wait 15 to 30 minutes. Because it may be some time before the home health nurse returns, it is especially important that the client has been instructed to drink adequate fluids, observe the color and amount of urine, and report changes to the nurse or physician.

a perineal prostatectomy than the other types. If this problem occurs, it is important to reinforce the man's masculine image. This is mainly achieved through supportive caring of significant others. Nurses may be able to help significant others understand what is happening so they can provide the necessary support.

Referral for sexual counseling may be helpful. The man needs to know that he can still please a partner and that sometimes lovemaking techniques other than intercourse may even be necessary. The couple may need information about alternatives to intercourse such as cuddling, stroking, or manual or oral stimulation to orgasm. Talking about options may enhance communications between the man and his partner. A penile implant may be considered (see the section on Erectile Dysfunction).

EVALUATION

The nurse must evaluate client outcomes based on the established plan of care. If these goals were not achieved, the plan and interventions must be revised to meet the client's needs.

Post-hospital Care

DISCHARGE TEACHING

As stated previously, the client should be taught about potential urinary incontinence and the exercises that should decrease it. They are also taught about any further need for treatment with some therapies, such as recurrence years after a TUR.

Clients should be taught to maintain a high fluid intake (2000 to 3000 ml/day) to ensure a good urine output. Clients who had undergone TUR or balloon dilation also must be taught about the possibility of recurrence, because prostatic tissue that is left can continue to hypertrophy.

HOME HEALTH CARE NEEDS

There are no specific home health care needs for this client. The only equipment the client may have is a catheter, which should be removed within several weeks of surgery.

FOLLOW-UP CARE

The client should be encouraged to discuss any sexual problems that occur after the surgery. If necessary, sexual counseling may be required.

The client should be seen after surgery to be checked for the development of urethral strictures or bladder neck contractures. Clients may need urethral dilation following surgery.

If the entire gland was not removed, clients should continue yearly check-ups for the development of prostate cancer.

PROSTATE CANCER

Incidence

Prostate cancer is the most common cancer among men and the third leading cause of death among men in the United States.[7] Most clients with clinically detectable prostate cancer are over age 50; therefore, the man's risk of prostatic cancer increases with each decade after age 50. Young men, however, seem to have more aggressive disease and are more likely to have metastasis at time of diagnosis.

Black men have a higher incidence than white men in this country, whereas Japanese-Americans have the lowest incidence.

Etiology

The cause of prostatic cancer is unknown, but epidemiologic studies suggest several associated factors.

GENETIC TENDENCY

The condition tends to occur more in certain families. In the United States, black men are at greater risk than white men (it is not clear whether this is due to genetic or environmental factors, e.g., income and exposure to occupational hazards, which tend to place blacks at higher risk than whites).

HORMONAL FACTORS

Although exact mechanisms and factors are not known, the incidence of prostatic cancer is higher in men (1) who had a late puberty, (2) who have high frequency of sexual experience, (3) with a history of multiple sexual partners, and (4) with higher fertility. Because the risk of prostatic cancer increases with age, it may be associated with the hormonal shifts associated with aging, such as lower amounts of androsterone and higher serum levels of estrogen and estradiol.

DIET

Differences in mortality rates from prostatic cancer between Asians and Caucasians have been associated with dietary differences. Japanese men have low rates of prostatic cancer, yet those who migrate to the United States experience increasing rates, which suggests dietary habits as factors. High fat consumption (typical of American diets) can alter cholesterol and steroid metabolism, which may increase the risk of cancer. Green and yellow vegetables (typical of Japanese diets) could have a protective effect against prostatic cancer.

CHEMICAL CARCINOGENS

Occupational and environmental hazard exposure to carcinogens may increase the risk of prostatic cancer. There is a higher incidence in urban areas, which suggests air pollution may be a factor. Occupations linked to higher rates of prostatic cancer include (1) employment in fertilizer, textile, and rubber industries; and (2) work with batteries containing cadmium.

VIRUSES

The observation by electron microscopy of virus particles in carcinomatous prostatic tissue suggests that viruses may be associated with the disease. Gonorrhea is also associated with an increased incidence of prostatic cancer, although it is assumed that people with gonorrhea are exposed to a virus concurrently.

It is hoped that late prostatic cancer will become rare as increasing emphasis is placed on early diagnosis through routine rectal examinations, rectal ultrasound studies, measurement of prostate-specific antigen (PSA), and prompt intervention.

Pathophysiology

The appearance of prostatic cancer is variable, adding to the difficulty of diagnosis and staging and grading of the tumor. These tumors are usually adenocarcinomas. The tumor begins in the periphery of the posterior lobe of the gland, whereas BPH occurs centrally and is large by the time it restricts urination. The tumor may appear as a normal prostate, which delays diagnosis. Typically, such lesions grow slowly and remain confined to the prostatic capsule, and if they occur late in life, the client may die of other causes. Sometimes, however, the tumor grows rapidly, there is metastasis by the time a diagnosis is made, and the client lives only a short time. Alternatively, the tumor may grow locally for a long time despite the potential for metastasis.

Clinical Manifestations

There may be no symptoms of prostatic cancer, unless BPH is present at the same time. The presenting findings are most often those of prostatitis, such as infection. Obstruction is rare unless BPH is present, because the cancer is usually found in the periphery of the posterior lobe. Unfortunately, the tumor may escape detection until the disease is advanced. Also, 15 to 40 per cent of men with prostatic cancer present with late symptoms caused by metastasis, such as hip or back bone pain. Rectal pressure or obstruction from local tumor growth may produce stool changes and painful defecation. Painful ejaculation also may be experienced.

DIAGNOSTIC ASSESSMENT

Early diagnosis is essential. Diagnostic tests include digital rectal examination; laboratory tests such as alkaline and acid phosphatase, radiography, rectal ultrasound, computed tomography (CT) scanning, radionuclide imaging, transrectal and percutaneous needle aspiration and biopsy, and tumor markers such as the PSA.

Annual digital rectal examination is recommended for all men over the age of 40 because colon cancer and prostate cancer can be screened for at the same time. Examination every 6 months is recommended if (1) the client has a history of continuing urinary symptoms, especially if a blood relative has had prostate cancer, or (2) if he has BPH or has had subtotal prostatectomy. Even so, 10 to 20 per cent of tumors are too small to be determined by rectal examination. A hard nodule in the prostate, particularly the posterior lobe, of any man over 50 years of age has about a 50 per cent chance of being malignant.[13a]

Transrectal ultrasound is a newer modality used for early detection of prostatic cancer. This simple diagnostic test is capable of discovering possibly twice as many prostate cancers as digital rectal examination.[7]

Tumor markers are another means of assessment. The serum level of acid phosphatase was the most important biochemical test in diagnosing prostate cancer. The newer and even more specific test is the PSA. The PSA is particularly useful in monitoring clients with prostate cancer; an elevation of the PSA signals that the tumor is growing.

Acid phosphatase is not usually a tumor-specific marker because it is produced in a number of body tissues. However, there is approximately 1000 times more acid phosphatase in the prostate than in any other body organ. High serum levels of prostatic acid phosphatase (PAP) are associated with metastatic prostate cancer. Determination of the PAP levels is useful in monitoring disease progression and assessment of response to treatment. However, it is not as specific as the PSA.

Laboratory tests screen for indications of bladder obstruction, tumor obstruction, or metastasis to areas such as the liver and bone marrow. These tests include CBC, SMA-12, BUN, creatinine, and liver function studies.

X-ray assessment includes chest radiography, IVP, and lymphangiography, used to screen for obstructive uropathy and metastases in the skeleton and lymph nodes.

Ultrasonography, CT scanning, and magnetic resonance imaging (MRI) assess for the local extent of the tumor. Although CT scanning does not differentiate cancer of the prostate from BPH, it is useful in assessing large tumors. Transrectal ultrasonography is useful in assessing the size and shape of the prostate, locating tumors with the capsule of the prostate, and monitoring tumor response to treatment.

Radionuclide imaging is used to detect bone lesions. Bone metastasis occurs in 75 to 85 per cent of men with prostatic cancer, depending on the stage of the disease. Lesions may be detected by bone scans 6 months or more before abnormalities appear on a bone x-ray film.

Needle aspiration or biopsy is used to confirm suspected malignancy. Open perineal biopsy often is not performed because adverse effects such as infection, and trauma, are common. Tissue for histologic examination is obtained more readily by transperineal or transrectal needle biopsy. The transperineal approach avoids the risk of contaminating the prostate with fecal matter, but the transrectal approach is more accurate. A general anesthetic may be used and allows more accuracy because many samples may be taken with a small-bore needle. After the needle biopsy, monitor the client for fever, urinary obstruction, hematuria, or rectal bleeding. Fine-needle aspiration of the prostate for cytologic examination is usually performed without anesthesia. Percutaneous fine-needle aspiration may be used to determine metastatic sites, such as lymph nodes. Bone marrow aspiration is performed to confirm metastatic tumors, but it is positive only in widespread disease. Transurethral resection of the prostate is not recommended for biopsy, because tumors are usually located at the periphery of the prostate, particularly in the posterior lobe.

GRADING AND STAGING

Grading of prostatic cancer is conducted to try to establish the activity or virulence of the disease. Staging is an attempt to define the extent to which the carcinoma has developed. There are several methods of classification. At present, there is no consensus for defining each stage. One classification is as follows:

- *Stage A or I:* Tumor microscopic (T_1 N_0, M_0)
  - A-1 Microscopic focus
  - A-2 Diffuse
- *Stage B or II:* Tumor macroscopic (T_{1-2}, N_0, M_0)
  - B-1: One lobe involved, nodule $\leq$ 1.5 cm
  - B-2: Both lobes involved, nodule $>$ 1.5 cm
- *Stage C or III:* Tumor extracapsular (T_3, N_0, M_0)
  - C-1: Localized, nodule $\leq$ 70 g
  - C-2: Pelvic sidewall fixation, nodule $>$ 70 g
- *Stage D or IV:* Metastatic disease (T_4, N_{1-3+}, M_+)
  - D-1 Confined to pelvis
  - D-2 Extrapelvic

A grading method is:

- *Grade I:* Well differentiated
- *Grade II:* Intermediate or moderately differentiated
- *Grade III:* Poorly differentiated

Medical Management

The treatment of prostatic cancer is controversial because of the varied biologic behavior of the disease, and staging methods that do not accurately predict malignant potential. Various treatment combinations may be used, depending on the choices of the person and physician, and the stage the condition has reached. For example, if the tumor is well differentiated, and of low volume, TUR may be sufficient. However, if extensive metastases have developed by the time a diagnosis is made, palliative treatment may be all that is available.

RADIATION THERAPY

Radiation therapy includes (1) interstitial irradiation, (2) combined interstitial and external-beam irradiation, and (3) external-beam megavoltage irradiation (see also Chap. 22). Interstitial irradiation is used to control locally advanced tumors (usually stage B or C). Radioactive metals, such as iodine (^{125}I), are used to destroy tumors directly. One widely used technique is to perform a pelvic lymphadenectomy and implant iodine seeds into the prostate, with needles. The long half-life of these seeds allows delivery of an effective radiation dose for one year. Radiation falls off a short distance from the seeds, so normal tissue is protected. Complications include thrombophlebitis, lymphocele formation, edema, and obstructive problems during voiding.

Combined interstitial and external-beam irradiation

involves implanting gold in the prostate, followed by external-beam irradiation. This approach is used for people with stage A-2, B, or C tumors. Gold is of higher energy than iodine and has a shorter half-life (2.7 days). Thus, an effective dose can be delivered in several weeks, followed by external-beam full pelvic irradiation over several more weeks. Implanting gold alone would destroy surrounding tissue. Complications include edema of the penis and lower extremities, cystitis, and urethritis. A major advantage of interstitial therapy is preservation of erection for most men treated this way.

External-beam megavoltage irradiation is used when tumors are confined to the prostate and surrounding tissue. A tumoricidal dose of 6500 to 7000 rads is usually applied at a rate of 175 to 200 rads daily to the prostate. Surrounding tissue is relatively spared. The result depends on the size and grade of the tumor.

PHARMACOLOGIC MANAGEMENT

Endocrine therapy is used based on an observation that prostate epithelial cells atrophy if they are deprived of androgens. Androgen is produced in the testicles and the adrenal gland. Endocrine therapy is used to (1) remove the source of androgen, (2) suppress pituitary gonadotropin, (3) interfere with androgen synthesis, and (4) interfere with the action of androgen on the tissue.

The first oral androgen blocker, flutamide (Eulexin), is one of the newest medications used to treat prostate cancer. The gonadotropin-releasing hormone (GnRH) analogs leuprolide (Lupron) and goserelin acetate (Zoladex) are also being used to treat it. These agents block the action or secretion of androgens, which stimulate tumor growth, without causing the side effects that estrogen does. Finasteride (Proscar) is also used to treat it.

Administration of estrogen (diethylstilbestrol [DES]) suppresses the release of pituitary gonadotropin and reduces serum testosterone levels. Side effects include cardiovascular symptoms and gynecomastia. Gynecomastia can be lessened by giving the client breast radiation before estrogen therapy.

Nonendocrine chemotherapy (either singly or in combination) has been used with prostate cancers to treat or sometimes stabilize the disease. Examples of chemotherapeutic agents sometimes used are cyclophosphamide (Cytoxan), 5-fluorouracil (Fluorouracil), estramustine phosphate (Emcyt), doxorubicin hydrochloride (Adriamycin), and mitomycin-C (Mutamycin).

Surgical Management

Surgical approaches include TURP and radical prostatectomy. TURP may be used for well-differentiated tumors of low volume or to relieve obstruction in advanced disease. Repeated TURP is sometimes needed to maintain an adequate channel through the prostatic urethra. (See discussion of TURP.)

Radical prostatectomy via a perineal (see Fig. 75–*4D*) or retropubic approach may be performed. Radical surgery involves removing (1) the entire prostate gland (rather than just enucleation), (2) the outer capsule, (3) the seminal vesicles, (4) sections of the vas deferens, and (5) possibly portions of the bladder neck. This surgery may be chosen for men who have (1) no other serious medical problems, (2) a discrete tumor involving less than one lobe (i.e., stage B-1), and (3) a survival expectation of at least 10 to 15 years. It is sometimes used for men with stage B-2 or C tumors.

Common side effects of radical prostatectomy are erectile dysfunction (as high as 85 to 90 per cent) and *incontinence* (10 to 15 per cent). Both of these side effects are difficult for a man to experience and discuss. Improved surgical techniques and advances in treating erectile dysfunction and incontinence help many men overcome these difficulties. For example, surgical techniques that carefully dissect around periprostatic autonomic nerves can avoid erectile dysfunction. Urinary incontinence usually occurs after postoperative removal of the catheter, but leakage generally subsides within 6 months in 85 to 90 per cent of men. (For discussion of these problems, see the section on TURP.)

Artificial urinary sphincters (AUS) have been surgically implanted for refractory urinary incontinence. An AUS is a fluid-filled system of three parts: (1) a silicone rubber cuff encircling the urethra, (2) a pump implanted into the scrotum, and (3) a balloon inserted into the abdomen. The mechanism functions as follows:

- When inflated with fluid, the cuff closes the urethra.
- The urethra is opened when the person manually squeezes the pump flat, moving fluid from the cuff into the balloon.
- Releasing the pump moves fluid from the balloon back into the cuff, again closing the urethra.

The pump appears as a bulge in the scrotum just above the left testicle. It is seen on an x-ray film because the fluid contains a small amount of dye.

Extensive postsurgical evaluation is necessary, including urodynamic testing, urethral pressure, cystography, IVP, and sometimes, micturition studies. This procedure is recommended for people with a normal bladder and especially for those with incontinence following TURP. Initially, there is considerable postoperative pain. A Foley catheter is inserted in surgery and removed in about 24 hours once the swelling has subsided.

Once the physician has activated the AUS pump, several weeks after the swelling subsides and healing occurs, the client can learn to activate the pump. The client needs to pump the bulb only when feeling the sensation of a full bladder. Catheterization can be performed with the device in place, but the practice is not recommended.

Bilateral orchiectomy is the most effective way to remove the source of androgen. This surgical procedure removes the testicles, which lowers serum testosterone significantly.

Nursing Management

Nursing care of the client with prostatic cancer is essentially the same as that for a client with BPH. Men with prostatic cancer and their significant others need ongoing sensitive support and accurate information to make the difficult decisions required of them. Their concerns are often considerable and may include the choices of available treatments, fear of death, anxiety about residual disability and illness, and the possible effects of the illness on people in their social network.

Modification of Plan of Care for the Elderly

Again, prostate cancer occurs most commonly in men over the age of 50, so the older client is the one most likely to develop this disorder. Hormonal manipulation seems to prolong survival significantly for the older client.

Post-hospital Care

DISCHARGE TEACHING

Discharge teaching is similar to that for the client with BPH. If the client is experiencing incontinence, the Kegel exercises will help control this condition. Teaching concerning medication and further therapy also will be needed.

HOME HEALTH CARE NEEDS

The client post-radical perineal prostatectomy may return home with a catheter and may require some time before he can regain bladder control.

FOLLOW-UP CARE

The client will need to be seen by the physician at regular intervals to measure the PSA level. An increase in this antigen indicates further tumor growth and the need for further treatment.

PROSTATITIS

Prostatitis, inflammation of the prostate gland, may be (1) acute bacterial, (2) chronic bacterial, or (3) nonbacterial (Fig. 75-6).

Acute bacterial prostatitis is usually caused by aerobic gram-negative rods, the coliforms (especially *Escherichia coli*), and *Pseudomonas*. Routes of infection (see Fig. 75-6) include (1) urethral ascent, (2) descent from the urinary bladder or kidneys, (3) direct extension or lymphatogenous spread from the rectum, and (4) hematogenous spread (via blood). Assessment reveals chills and fever, low back and perineal pain, and urinary urgency, frequency, nocturia, and dysuria. Bladder outlet obstruction, myalgia (painful muscles), and arthralgia (painful joints) may occur. On examination

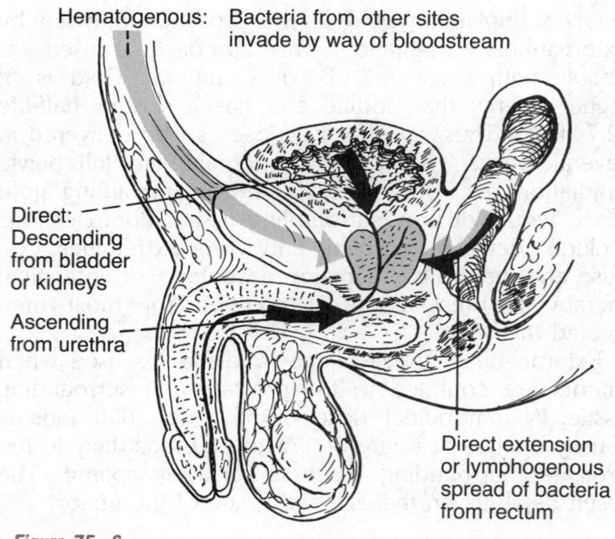

▲ *Figure 75-6*

Postulated pathways of infection to the prostate gland.

(Fig. 75-7), the prostate is extremely tender and swollen, yet it is firm, indurated, and warm to touch. Acute cystitis (bladder inflammation) is common, with hematuria and cloudy, malodorous urine. Urine cultures identify the infecting organisms. Exudate from prostatic massage (see Chap. 74) can also identify the organism, but this is not usually performed, because such massage is very painful for a client with prostatitis and can precipitate bacteremia. Transurethral instrumentation, including catheterization, is avoided during acute infection, because it can push infection up into the bladder. Intervention includes rest, analgesics, stool softeners (constipation is painful with prostatitis), antimicrobial medication, sitz baths, and increased oral fluids. Occasionally the inflammation is so severe that the client cannot pass urine, and catheterization is needed. Hospitalization may be required for parenteral antibiotics and supportive care.

Chronic bacterial prostatitis is a nonacute infection of the prostate gland. It is most commonly caused by the same organisms that cause acute bacterial prostatitis and has the same routes of infection. Some gram-positive bacteria, such as staphylococci and streptococci, have been thought to cause chronic bacterial prostatitis, but they rarely persist or lead to recurring infection. Chronic bacterial prostatitis is a less severe inflammation than the acute type. Some clients have no symptoms. A diagnosis may be made after finding bacteriuria (bacteria in the urine) on routine urinalysis. Other clients may experience (1) voiding dysfunction, such as urgency, frequency, nocturia, and dysuria; (2) low back or perineal pain; or (3) occasional myalgia (muscle aches) and arthralgia (painful joints). On examination, the prostate may be normal or feel boggy or indurated. There may be inflammatory cells in prostatic secretions. If the client has cystitis, organisms may be identified in urine specimens. If urine is not infected, organisms may be identified from mid-stream urine specimen, urethral specimens, and prostatic massage.

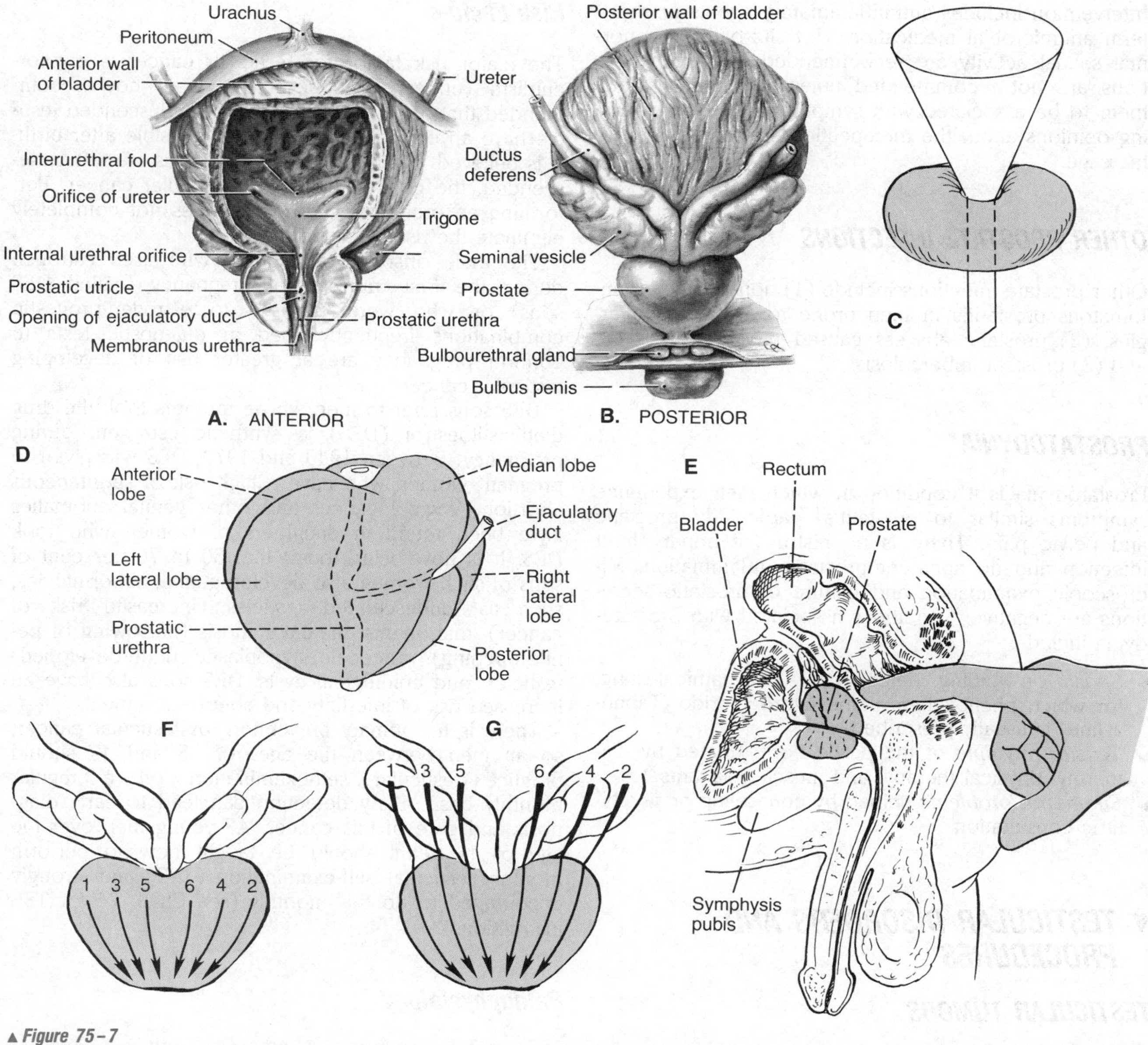

▲ *Figure 75-7*

Rectal-prostatic assessment. *A*, Posterior and *B*, anterior views of the prostate gland. *C*, Anatomic position of the prostate gland. It lies around the urethra like a donut around the outlet of a funnel. *D*, Posterior and lateral lobes of the prostate. *E*, Rectal examination. Insert a gloved index finger into the anus while the person is "bearing down." Palpate all surfaces. *F*, Prostatic massage. Roll the pad of the index finger across the prostate, starting laterally and superiorly and moving toward the midline of the prostate. *G*, Seminal vesicles and prostate massage—same as for prostate massage, but extend the finger higher over the area of the seminal vesicles. (*A* and *B* from Jacob, S. W., Francone, C. A., & Lossow, W. J. [1982]. *Structure and function in man* [5th ed.]. Philadelphia: W. B. Saunders.)

Intervention with antimicrobial agents is problematic because it is difficult to obtain therapeutic levels of drug in prostatic secretions during nonacute inflammations. Discomfort and pain may be relieved by sitz baths, anti-inflammatory agents, and anticholinergic drugs. Repeated prostatic massage and ejaculation may be helpful. Surgical intervention is rarely required. Long-term, low-dose antimicrobial drugs may control symptoms.

Nonbacterial prostatitis is the most common form of prostatitis. Its cause is unknown. It has the same symptoms as bacterial prostatitis, but no causative organism is found. On prostatic massage, abnormal numbers of inflammatory cells are noted in the prostatic fluid, but no infectious agent is found. Some experts believe that nonbacterial prostatitis may be caused by mycoplasmas, chlamydiae, or ureaplasmas. Others suggest it may be an autoimmune disease.

Assessment findings for nonbacterial prostatitis are similar to those of bacterial prostatitis except that bacteria are not found in the urine or prostatic secretions. Diagnosis is made by systematically ruling out other types of prostatitis. This can be depressing for the person because diagnosis and treatment is not specific.

Intervention includes anti-inflammatory agents or short-term antimicrobial medication. Hot sitz baths and normal sexual activity are recommended. Dietary restrictions are not recommended unless the person finds them to be associated with symptoms. There are varying opinions about the therapeutic benefits of prostatic massage.

OTHER PROSTATE INFECTIONS

Other prostate infections include (1) nonspecific granulomatous prostatitis in men prone to asthma or allergies, (2) prostatic abscess caused mostly by *E. coli*, and (3) prostatic tuberculosis.

PROSTATODYNIA

Prostatodynia is a condition in which men experience symptoms similar to prostatitis, particularly prostatic and pelvic pain. There is no history of urinary tract infection and no apparent prostatic inflammation. Microscopic examination and culture of prostatic secretions are negative. Conditions associated with prostatodynia include:

- *Spasm* on voiding, detected by urodynamic testing, for which phenoxybenzamine hydrochloride (Dibenzyline) is usually prescribed
- *Tension myalgia* of the pelvic floor, treated by diathermy, physical therapy, and muscle relaxants
- *Emotional problems* helped by counseling or psychiatric consultation

▼ TESTICULAR DISORDERS AND PROCEDURES

TESTICULAR TUMORS

Definition

Testicular cancer is the most common and serious solid tumor cancer in males between the ages of 15 and 35.

Incidence

Testicular cancer rarely occurs in men under the age of 15 or over the age of 40. It is less common in blacks and Asian men. Two to 3 cases/100,000 males are diagnosed in the United States each year.

Etiology

The etiology of testicular cancer is unknown. Exogenous estrogen and cryptorchidism are considered possible causes.

Risk Factors

The major risk factor for testicular cancer is cryptorchidism (undescended testicles). It is now recommended that any child born with an undescended testicle have an orchiopexy as soon as possible after birth. It is believed that the longer the testicles are left undescended, the greater the risk of testicular cancer. Performing an orchiopexy, however, does not completely eliminate the risk of cancer.

The male offspring of women who used estrogen during the first trimester of pregnancy (called DES sons) or who were exposed to estrogen-progestin combinations frequently used in diagnostic tests to confirm pregnancy are at greater risk of developing testicular cancer.

DES sons refer to men whose mothers took the drug diethylstilbestrol (DES), a synthetic estrogen, during pregnancy. Between 1940 and 1970, DES was given to pregnant women who have a high risk of spontaneous abortion. Vaginal cancer and other genital anomalies have been found in daughters of women who took DES. It is now being found that 30 to 70 per cent of sons of such women also develop genital abnormalities, such as, undescended testicles (increased risk of cancer), micropenis, meatal stenosis (narrowing of penile opening), varicocele, hypoplastic (underdeveloped) testicles, and epididymal cysts. DES sons also have an increased risk of infertility and abnormal semen.

There is no primary prevention for testicular cancer, so all men between the ages of 15 and 40 should practice testicular self-examination on a regular monthly basis. Early detection can lead to early diagnosis and cure of this cancer. All young men over the age of 15 years should be taught how to perform monthly testicular self-examination (TSE) and strongly encouraged to do this monthly (see Chap. 74 for TSE instructions).

Pathophysiology

Most of the cases of testicular cancer (97 per cent) are germinal cell tumors, such as seminomas (about 40 per cent of all tumors), teratocarcinomas, embryonal carcinoma, or choriocarcinoma. Seminomas generally have a favorable prognosis of about a 90 per cent 5-year survival rate because they are usually localized and metastasize late. These tumors are usually treated with orchiectomy and radiation therapy. They are usually confined to the testes and retroperitoneal nodes.

Nonsemanomatous germ cell tumors are not as sensitive to radiation therapy; however, with the advent of newer chemotherapy regimens following orchiectomy, the cure rate has risen to 95 per cent overall, with 100 per cent cure in Stage I, 98 per cent in Stage II, and 80 per cent in Stage III.[13]

Nongerminal tumors make up the remainder of testicular cancers. These tumors arise from interstitial cells or cells that compose the fibrous or vascular networks. They are classified as either interstitial cell tumors or testicular adenomas that are usually benign.

The overall survival rate from all types of testicular cancer is about 89 per cent in whites and 78 per cent in blacks. This rate has increased dramatically in the last 10 years.[30]

Clinical Manifestations

Most commonly, men with testicular tumors experience a painless enlargement, noted as heaviness, in the testicle (about 75 per cent of men). Some men describe it as a dragging sensation. Pain is rarely felt; however, the tumor is often found after an injury because the testicle is examined as a result of the injury. Hydrocele or hematocele may develop (Fig. 75-8). Some symptoms of testicular cancer resemble the symptoms of varicocele, and some are similar to the symptoms of prostatitis.

Assessment findings suggesting metastasis include back pain, vague abdominal pain, nausea and vomiting, anorexia, and weight loss.

DIAGNOSTIC ASSESSMENT

A thorough physical examination of the scrotum and testicles is the first diagnostic test performed. Unlike a simple hydrocele, a testicular tumor is not translucent to light.

A radical orchiectomy is the major diagnostic tool because the entire testicle is removed for biopsy after a mass has been detected. Any testicular mass is considered malignant until proved otherwise. This approach is used because of the belief that a needle or open biopsy would lead to rapid spread, and because once the tumor has been shown to be a solid mass, its chance of being malignant is almost 100 per cent.

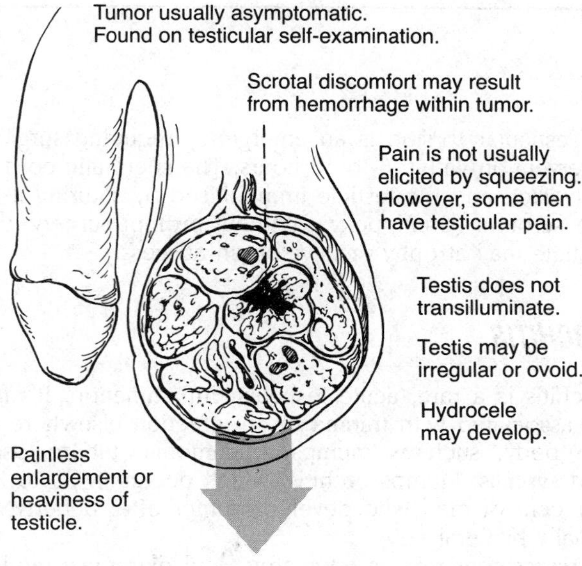
Tumor usually asymptomatic.
Found on testicular self-examination.
Scrotal discomfort may result from hemorrhage within tumor.
Pain is not usually elicited by squeezing. However, some men have testicular pain.
Testis does not transilluminate.
Testis may be irregular or ovoid.
Hydrocele may develop.
Painless enlargement or heaviness of testicle.

▲ *Figure 75-8*

Some characteristics of malignant tumors of the testes.

Testicular tumors are staged as follows:

- Stage I_a: tumor confined to testicle (T_1, N_0, M_0)
- Stage I_b: metastasis to para-aortic or iliac nodes (T_1, N, M_0)
- Stage II: tumor spread to retroperitoneal nodes but disease limited to below the diaphragm (T_{2-3}, N_2, M_0)
- Stage III: tumor above the diaphragm or spread to body organs (usually the lungs) T_4, N_{3-4}, M_+)

Other diagnostic tests used to determine the possible extent of the tumor include (1) a chest x-ray study or CT of the lungs for lung metastasis, (2) an abdominal and pelvic CT scan or MRI for retroperitoneal lymph node involvement, (3) an IVP for urinary tract involvement, (4) a lymphangiogram for retroperitoneal lymph node involvement (performed less frequently because CT and MRI are available), and (5) laboratory studies for serum α-fetoprotein (AFP) and serum human serum gonadotropin-β subunit (hCG-β) as tumor markers.

AFP levels are elevated only in nonsemanomatous tumors. HCG-β is also elevated in nonsemanomatous tumors, and hCG may be elevated in pure seminomas. Normally, hCG is present only in pregnant women.

Medical Management

The primary treatment for testicular cancer is surgical resection of the testicle. Radiation and chemotherapy also may be used.

Seminomas are particularly radiosensitive. The perineum and pelvis and the mediastinal and supraclavicular nodes are also irradiated if the peritoneal nodes are positive. Side effects include common complications associated with pelvic radiation. Radiation is not used for nonseminomatous tumors because they are not very radiosensitive.

Chemotherapy is used for both seminomas and nonseminomatous tumors that have any sign of spread. The major agent used is cisplatin in combination with vinblastine and bleomycin. Cisplatin in combination with other agents dramatically increased the long-term survival rate for men with testicular cancer. These agents in combination with a variety of others have been used to treat metastatic disease or refractory tumors with some success.

Complications of these chemotherapeutic agents are discussed in detail in Chapter 22. The major problem associated with cisplatin is nephrotoxicity; with bleomycin, pneumonitis; and with vinblastine, peripheral neuropathy.

Surgical Management

As discussed earlier, a radical orchiectomy is performed to diagnose testicular cancer, so it also is the primary treatment. The amputated testicle can be replaced with a testicular prosthesis. This reconstructive surgery is recommended to help the young man's self-esteem.

The major surgical choice is whether or not to do a retroperitoneal lymph node dissection also. Because chemotherapy is so successful in treating even widespread disease, the use of this radical surgery has been questioned. It is a major surgery with a significant mortality rate. Since the advent of the CT scan and MRI, the status of these nodes can be ascertained without surgery. Also, there is a high incidence of impotence after this surgery because many of the autonomic nerves necessary for ejaculation are located in this area. This is a significant concern given the ages of the clients. Many surgeons are opting simply for the radical orchiectomy and diagnostic studies of the retroperitoneal lymph nodes without surgical resection.

The group that supports the retroperitoneal node dissection believe that using this approach limits the amount of chemotherapy needed because the extent of the tumor spread can be removed.

The major complication of retroperitoneal node dissection is impotence. If a bilateral orchiectomy is performed, infertility occurs.

Nursing Management

One of the primary activities of the nurse that is used to help with early detection of this treatable cancer is teaching young men testicular self-examination. This procedure is detailed in Chapter 74.

During assessment of a man born between 1940 and 1971, ask if his mother took any medication during pregnancy to prevent pregnancy or miscarriage. If he seems at particular risk but does not know these details, it may be necessary to obtain the mother's medical history. Information and referral is available through DES Action, Long Island Jewish-Hillside Medical Center, New Hyde Park, NY 11040.

Supportive nursing care is very important for these young men both during diagnosis and treatment. The nurse must be very aware of the threat to sexuality this condition and its treatment have on the young men. Review Chapters 7, 19, and 22 for the care of clients undergoing surgery, chemotherapy, and radiation therapy.

TESTICULAR TORSION

Testicular torsion (Fig. 75–9*A*) occurs when a testicle is mobile and the spermatic cord twists, cutting off the blood supply. It is the most common testicular disorder in children. It can occur at any age but is most usual at puberty. Symptoms arise suddenly, with acute scrotal swelling and severe pain as blood supply to the testicles is interrupted. It does not seem to be associated with any particular physical activity or trauma.

If testicular torsion is suspected, a testicular scan and Doppler scan should be done to assess the blood supply. If the blood supply is increased, the symptoms may be caused by epididymitis, and if it is decreased, then they are probably caused by torsion.

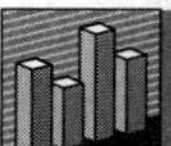

NURSING RESEARCH

Testicular cancer is the most common cancer in men between the ages of 15 and 35, and is easily cured if detected early. TSE is an important tool for early detection, is performed very easily, and yet is reported to be very rarely performed by the men who need it most. This study replicated previous ones demonstrating the lack of knowledge about testicular cancer. This study also looked at the effects of an educational program about testicular cancer and TSE. The program was presented to college men. The Health Belief Model was the theoretical framework for this study.

A convenience sample of 64 college men enrolled in a physical education class at a private East Coast university were given a questionnaire on the Health Beliefs Survey for Testicular Cancer and Testicular Self-Examination. The group was white, of similar ages, and with similar low-risk factors.

The results of the pre-test showed that about half of the men had heard of testicular cancer and one third stated they performed TSE. The scores on the seriousness and susceptibility subscales, however, showed little knowledge of testicular cancer among all subjects. After the education program, knowledge of testicular cancer did not increase significantly; however, the actual practice of TSE did increase significantly along with the subjects knowledge of TSE and TSE technique.

A number of limitations of the study were discussed, including the lack of a randomized sample and the short length of time between the pre- and post-tests. The need for further education among college-age men about the correct technique for TSE and the need to begin education about testicular cancer at the secondary school level. The nurse can be instrumental in providing these educational programs to the groups that need them most.

Rudolf, V. M. & Quinn, L. M. (1988). The practice of TSE among college men: Effectiveness of an educational program. *Oncology Nursing Forum, 15* (1), 45–48.

Testicular torsion is an emergency requiring surgical intervention within 6 to 12 hours. The spermatic cord is untwisted and the testicle immobilized by suturing it to the scrotum (orchiopexy). Without prompt surgery, the testicle may atrophy or develop an abscess.

ORCHITIS

Orchitis is a rare, acute testicular inflammation. It may be associated with trauma or an infection elsewhere in the body, such as mumps, pneumonia, tuberculosis, and syphilis. Mumps orchitis, which occurs in 20 to 35 per cent of men who develop mumps after puberty, is usually bilateral.

Assessment reveals edematous and extremely tender testicles, reddened scrotal skin, fever, and prostration. Treatment includes bed rest, scrotal support, local heat

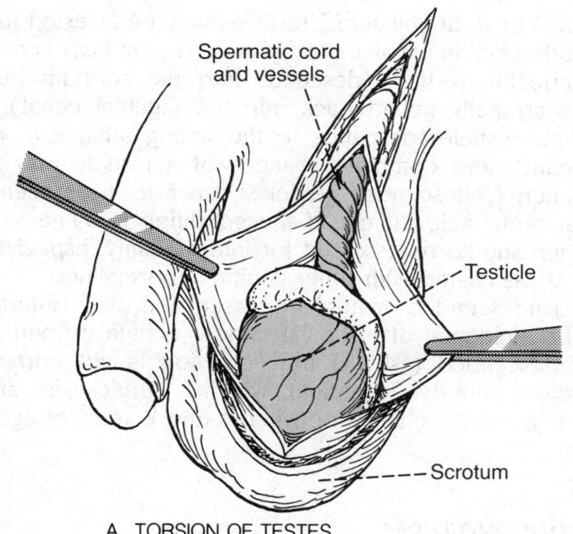

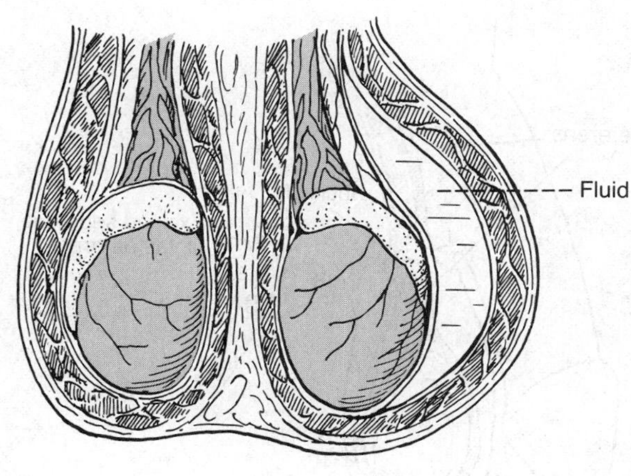

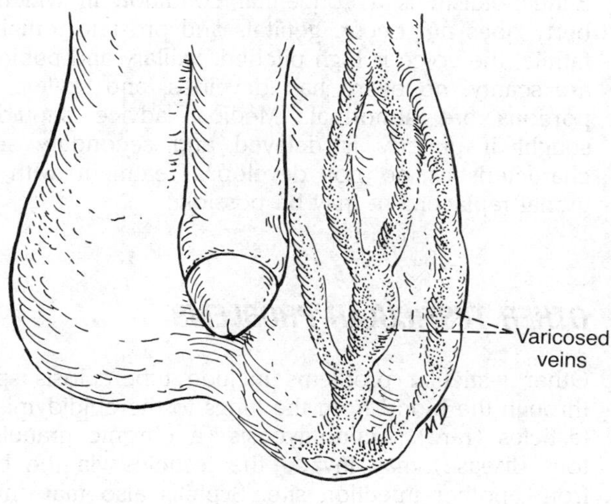

▲ *Figure 75-9*

Disturbances of the testicles.

to the scrotum, and medication for pain relief and fever. The acute phase lasts about 1 week. Permanent sterility may occur if both testicles are affected, whereas decreased fertility may result if only one is affected.

HYDROCELE, HEMATOCELE, AND SPERMATOCELE

Hydrocele (Fig. 75-9*B*) is a painless collection of clear, yellow fluid anywhere along the spermatic cord. The soft intrascrotal mass is translucent to light (see Chap. 74). If complications develop, such as discomfort from enlargement or impaired circulation, aspiration or surgical drainage may be performed.

A hematocele is a collection of blood in the tunica vaginalis. A spermatocele is a dilatation, originating in the epididymis, containing a milky fluid and spermatozoa. Hematoceles are less likely to transilluminate light than are hydrocele.

VARICOCELE

Varicocele (Fig. 75-9*C*) is a dilation and varicosity of the pampiniform plexus (network of veins supplying the testicles) within the scrotum. Ninety per cent of varicoceles are left-sided. They occur in 15 to 20 per cent of men between 15 and 25 years of age. The client may experience a pulling sensation, a dull ache, or scrotal pain. Pain may be relieved by masturbation or sexual intercourse.

On palpation, with the man standing, a varicocele feels like a mass of tortuous veins above and posterior to the testicle. When the man lies down, the mass

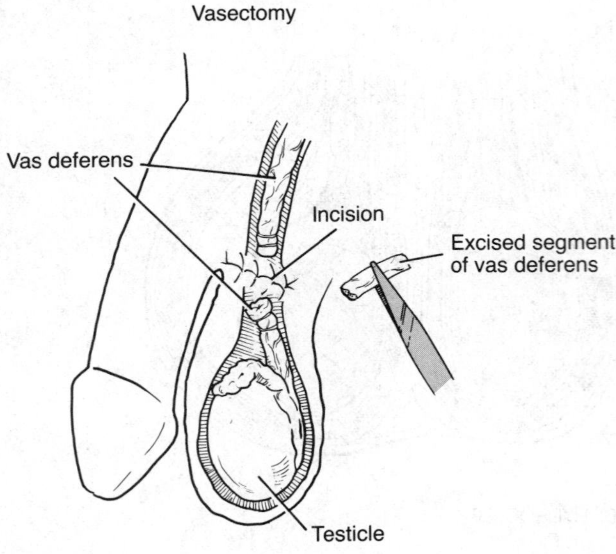

▲ *Figure 75-10*

Vasectomy.

abates. Although the condition is not clearly understood, varicocele is an important cause of male infertility. Treatment includes the use of a scrotal support, with surgery being performed only if complications occur, such as severe pain, or if the varicocele is thought to contribute to infertility.

VASECTOMY

A vasectomy is an elective surgical procedure performed as a permanent method of contraception (although sometimes a vasectomy can be surgically reversed). This procedure also often is performed after a prostatectomy to prevent retrograde epididymitis.

The surgery is usually performed under local anesthesia in the urologist's office or an outpatient setting. The procedure, performed through a small incision in the scrotum, involves the cutting out of a piece of the vas deferens and folding and ligating the remaining ends (Fig. 75-10).

Postoperatively, slight pain and swelling is easily controlled with an ice bag and mild analgesia such as acetaminophen. A scrotal support also increases client comfort. The client can resume sexual intercourse whenever he finds it comfortable, usually about 1 week after the procedure. The client must continue to practice other means of birth control until the follow-up semen analysis shows azoospermia, because live sperm are left in the ampulla of vas.

UNDESCENDED TESTES (CRYPTORCHIDISM)

The most common congenital testicular condition is that of undescended testes (Fig. 75-11). One (unilateral) or both (bilateral) testicles may be arrested in the abdomen, inguinal canal, low pelvis, or high scrotum. Retractile testicle (descends into the scrotum but is occasionally pulled back into the inguinal canal), ectopic testicle (descends to the wrong area, e.g., perineum), and complete absence of a testicle may also occur. Undescended testicles occur in 1 per cent of full-term male infants. If the condition is bilateral, the child should be assessed for intersexuality, especially if it is associated with other genital abnormalities.

Undescended testes are associated with infertility. The incidence of testicular cancer is high in men with undescended testes if the condition is not corrected before puberty. Treatment, which is surgical, is carried out when the child is between 1 and 2 years of age.

EUNUCHOIDISM

Eunuchoidism is a congenital condition in which puberty does not occur, genitals and prostate remain infantile, the voice is high pitched, axillary and pubic hair are scanty, no beard hair develops, and skeletal proportions are abnormal. Medical advice should be sought if puberty is delayed and secondary sexual characteristics do not develop. Treatment with hormonal replacement may be possible.

OTHER TESTICULAR PROBLEMS

Other testicular problems include tuberculosis spread through the blood from the lungs to the epididymis and testicles (rare). Actinomycosis (a chronic granulomatous disease) may invade the testicles via the blood from another infection site. Syphilis also may involve the testicles.

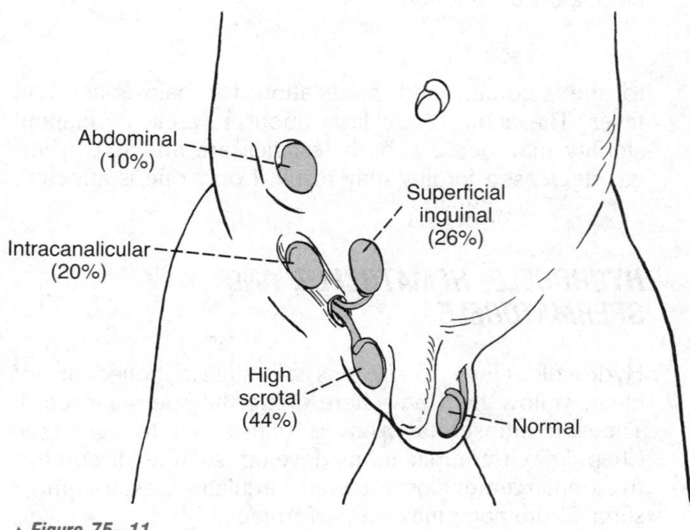

▲ *Figure 75-11*

Undescended testes (cryptorchidism).

▼ PENILE DISORDERS

URETHRITIS

Urethritis is an acute urethral inflammation and is discussed under sexually transmitted diseases and urinary disorders (see Chaps. 49 and 77).

URETHRAL STRICTURE

Urethral stricture is caused by urethral scarring or narrowing. It may be congenital or caused by untreated or severe urethritis or urethral injury (including urologic instrumentation, e.g., cystoscopy). Symptoms are caused by obstruction, such as small-caliber urinary stream, hyperdistended bladder, infection, fever, and dysuria. Urethral strictures are released surgically by urethral dilation or urethroplasty. See Chapter 49 for further information.

PHIMOSIS

Phimosis occurs when the penile foreskin (prepuce) is constricted at the opening, making retraction difficult or impossible. It is caused by edema or inflammation and is often associated with poor cleaning beneath the foreskin. Assessment reveals edema, erythema, tenderness, and purulent discharge. Intervention includes controlling infection with local treatment and broad-spectrum antimicrobial drugs.

Effective genital hygiene is essential to prevent acquired penile disorders. In uncircumcised males, the penis is cleaned by pulling the foreskin back gently and washing the area with a wash cloth (Fig. 75-12).

Routine circumcision has not been seen as medically necessary according to the American Academy of Pediatrics and many other health professionals and health organizations. Circumcision may be indicated in clients with penile infection, phimosis, or paraphimosis. Potential risks include excessive bleeding, infection, and penile trauma. Recently, however, they have reconsidered this decision based on the fact that the rate of penile cancer is almost zero in circumcised men. It is now believed that this should be explained to parents who are deciding. Some parents have religious or cultural reasons for circumcising their male children. Be sure uncircumcised men know how to retract the foreskin daily and clean the smegma from beneath it properly.

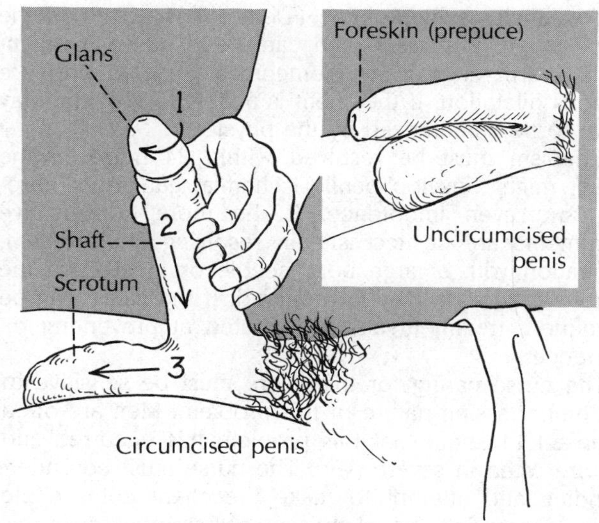

▲ *Figure 75-12*

Circumcised and uncircumcised penis. The foreskin of an uncircumcised penis should retract easily. During physical examination, ask the man to retract his foreskin himself. Effective genital hygiene is essential to prevent acquired penile problems. Many men have never been taught how to do this: 1. Begin washing at the tip of the penis. For an uncircumcised penis, gently retract the foreskin and wash. 2. Proceed down the penis shaft toward the body. 3. Next wash the scrotum. Wash the anal area last.

PARAPHIMOSIS

Paraphimosis (Fig. 75-13) occurs when a tight foreskin, once retracted, cannot be returned to its normal position. Circulation is thus impeded, and the glans swells rapidly. Paraphimosis sometimes occurs after rigorous cleaning, masturbation, sexual intercourse, or cystoscopy if the foreskin is not returned to its normal position. Manual reduction may be attempted by squeezing the glans for 5 minutes. Surgical incision with local anesthesia may be necessary.

PRIAPISM

Priapism is a prolonged, persistent penile erection without sexual desire. It can last hours or even days and is usually very painful. There is no known cause, although it is sometimes associated with leukemia or sickle cell anemia. It also may result from some medications, such as anticoagulants, alcohol, phenothiazines, and marijuana.

This problem is considered an emergency situation because circulation to the penis is usually compromised and the client may be unable to void. Treatment includes bed rest, prostatic massage, and sedation. Medi-

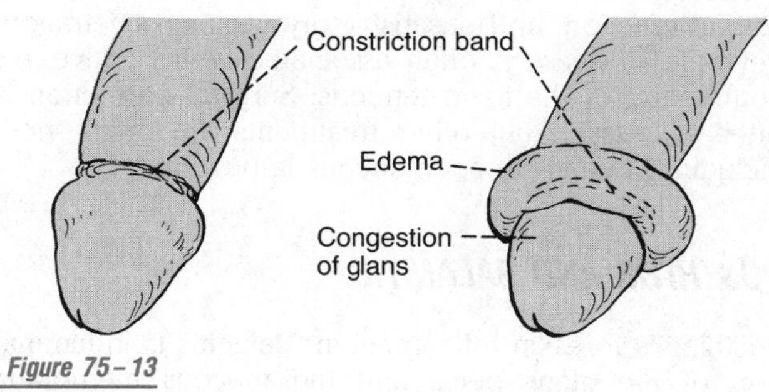

▲ *Figure 75-13*

Paraphimosis.

cation such as meperidine (Demerol) is given in the hope it will both relax the client and cause hypotension. Warm enemas are sometimes given to promote venous dilatation. If the client is unable to void, he may have to be catheterized by the physician.

Priapism must be resolved within 24 hours or the client might develop penile ischemia, gangrene, fibrosis, and even impotence. If the more conservative treatments are unsuccessful in resolving the problem, aspiration with a large bore needle or incision of the corpus cavernosa may be required. If the cause can be identified, treatment also is directed at preventing recurrence.

The nurse caring for this client must be sensitive to the embarrassing nature of this problem. Men are often reluctant to admit that this problem has occurred and yet are often in severe pain. The nurse must be understanding and attempt to make the client comfortable while decreasing the client's embarrassment over this problem.

PENILE CANCER

Penile cancer is a rare skin cancer occurring most often in older, uncircumcised men who have suffered chronic irritation and who have poor hygiene practices. Associated genital cancer sometimes develops in sexual partners (e.g., cervical cancer in females). Any dry, wartlike, painless growth on the penis or foreskin that fails to respond to antibiotics should be assessed for cancer. If an early diagnosis is made, excision and circumcision may be all that is necessary.

Many men find penile problems embarrassing and consequently do not seek medical attention for months. By this time, a lesion may be ulcerated, involving the foreskin and penile shaft, and may have metastasized to the inguinal nodes. Penile shaft resection, and sometimes penile amputation and dissection of enlarged inguinal nodes, may be necessary.

PEYRONIE'S DISEASE

Fibrous plaques develop near the dorsal midline of the penile shaft in middle-aged and older men. A high percentage of older men develop these plaques. Diagnosis is usually made only if the nurse questions the client about this during the history.

Assessment reveals penile curvature on erection, painful erection, and unsatisfactory vaginal penetration. Peyronie's disease is often associated with Dupuytren's contracture of the hand tendons. Surgical correction is often necessary, but other treatments are often tried, including waiting for spontaneous improvement.

POSTHITIS AND BALANITIS

Posthitis is foreskin inflammation. Balanitis is inflammation of the glans penis and the mucous membrane beneath it. These conditions (Fig. 75-14) are caused by irritation and invasion of microorganisms. Good hygiene and thorough drying of the penis is recommended. Assessment for diabetes is important because diabetes predisposes the client to the development of secondary infection. Antibiotics help control local infection. Circumcision may be necessary.

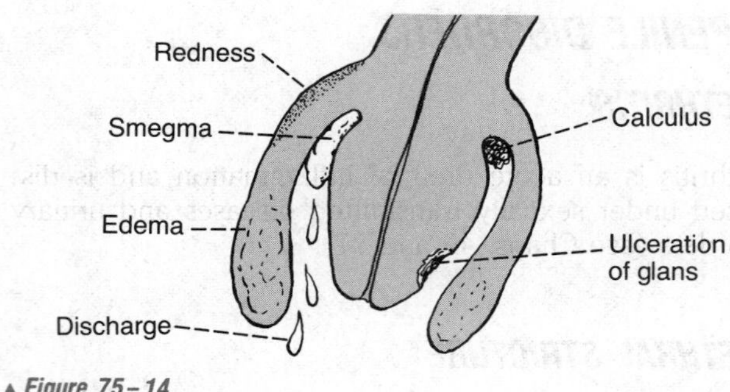

▲ *Figure 75-14*
Posthitis and balanitis.

URINARY EXTRAVASATION

Urinary extravasation is the escape of urine and other fluid into the perineum, scrotum, and penile tissue. It may be caused by trauma or may be secondary to urethral stricture. It is an emergency condition. Assessment reveals discoloration of the tissue, shock, and fever. Emergency intervention consists of alternative drainage of the bladder (urethral or suprapubic catheter) and drainage of the tissues with a Penrose drain.

PENILE INJURY

Penile trauma results in edema, hematoma, bruising, or laceration. Apply ice packs to control bleeding and appropriate dressings to reduce the possibility of infection. Urologic consultation is needed. Microsurgical techniques may be possible to replant an amputated penis. To facilitate such treatment, an amputated penis should be dampened with a sterile saline solution, kept chilled, and transported with the person for emergency treatment.

EPISPADIAS

Epispadias (Fig. 75-15*A*) is a rare congenital condition in which the urethral meatus opens dorsally on top of the penis, proximal to the glans, most commonly at the abdominopenile junction. Surgery is required to correct urinary incontinence and to return the urethra to a normal position in the penis. It is important to ask about this condition when taking the history.

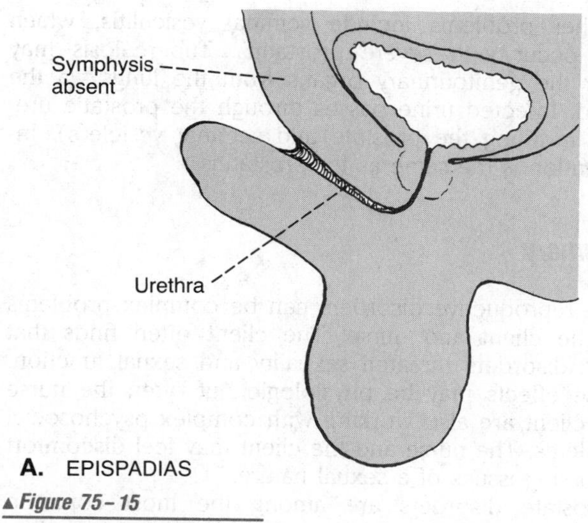

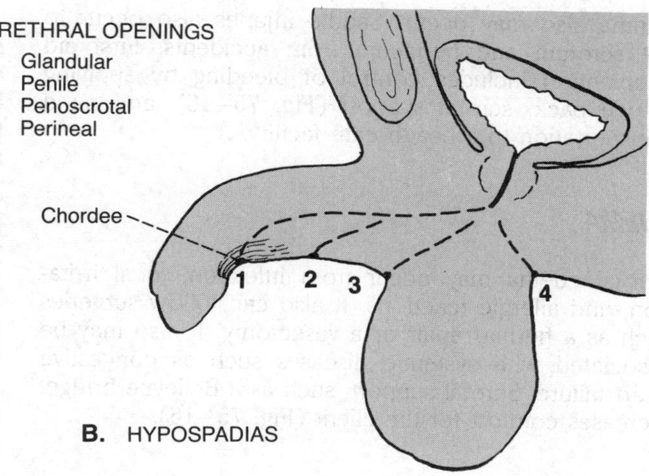

▲ *Figure 75-15*

Epispadias and hypospadias.

HYPOSPADIAS

Hypospadias (Fig. 75-15B) is a congenital condition in which the urethral meatus opens on the ventral side of the penis. Common locations include the glans penis, penile shaft, penoscrotal junction, and perineum. Chordee (curvature of the penis) is often associated with hypospadias. Hypospadias occurs in about 1 in 200 male children. Early assessment of internal reproductive organ development is necessary to confirm the child's sex. For psychological reasons, hypospadias should be repaired before the child starts school. It is important to ask about this condition when taking the history.

▼ SCROTAL DISORDERS

INFECTIONS

Scrotal skin is very thin and is in constant contact with clothes and the thighs. The scrotum has many rugae (folds) that inhibit ventilation. It is, therefore, exposed to moisture and rubbing, and is prone to infection. Nonvenereal disorders, such as erysipelas, abscesses, fistulas, and gangrene, may occur. Parasites, such as scabies and lice, and many common skin diseases, such as fungal infections (*Candida,* also known as jock itch), contact dermatitis, drug eruptions, eczema, lichen planus, and psoriasis, may spread to the scrotum. Heat, friction, obesity, and tight clothing aggravate scrotal disorders. Medications (often topical) specific to the infection, good hygiene, and prompt intervention are essential.

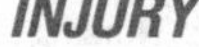

INJURY

The most common scrotal injury is tearing when clothes are caught in machinery. Blunt or penetrating

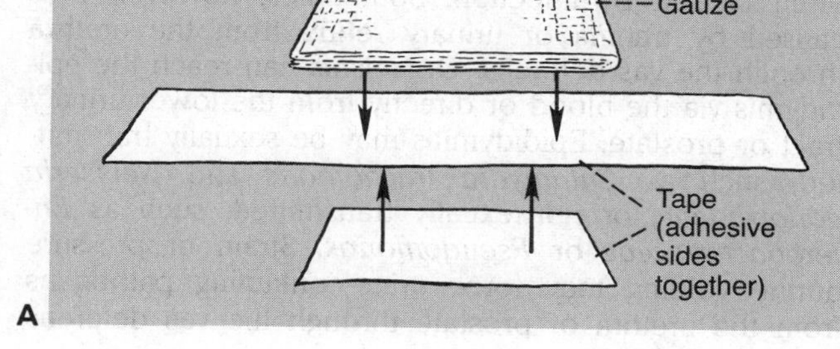

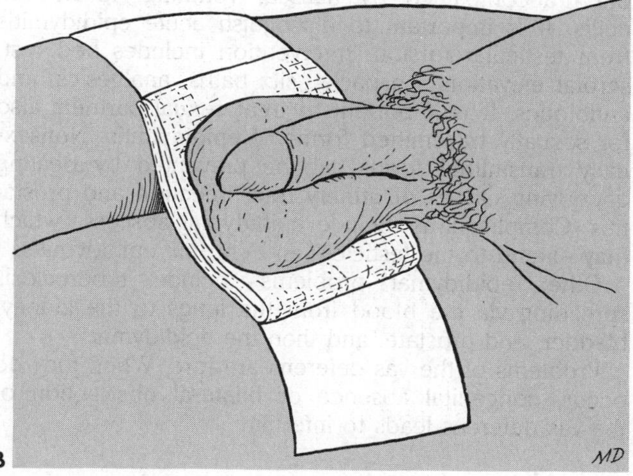

▲ *Figure 75-16*

Scrotal support (Bellevue bridge type). *A*, Prepare the support by placing two pieces of tape with their adhesive edges together, the smaller piece in the center of the longer piece. This provides a "non-adhesive" section between the person's legs. Place folded gause on top of the support. *B*, Gently place the support under the scrotum, and attach the adhesive ends of the support to the thighs.

trauma also may occur. Saddle injuries also occur to the scrotum and perineum from accidents. First aid intervention includes control of bleeding by applying an ice pack, scrotal support (Fig. 75-16), and rapid transportation to a health care facility.

EDEMA

Scrotal edema may occur from infection, local irritation, and allergic reactions. It also can follow surgeries such as a hernia repair or a vasectomy. It also may be associated with systemic diseases such as congestive heart failure. Scrotal support, such as a Bellevue bridge, increases comfort for the client (Fig. 75-16).

▼ DISORDERS OF THE REPRODUCTIVE DUCTS

The system of ducts through which spermatozoa pass from the testicles to the urethra includes the epididymis and vas deferens.

Epididymitis is inflammation of the epididymis, most often caused by infection. Sometimes, however, it is caused by trauma or urinary reflux from the urethra through the vas deferens. Organisms can reach the epididymis via the blood or directly from the lower urinary tract or prostate. Epididymitis may be sexually transmitted, such as *Chlamydia trachomatis* and *Neisseria gonorrhoeae*, or nonsexually transmitted, such as *Enterobacteriaceae* or *Pseudomonas*. Strain or pressure during voiding may force urine-containing pathogens from the urethra or prostate through the vas deferens to the epididymis.

Assessment reveals acute, painful scrotal swelling, often accompanied by nausea, vomiting, fever, and chills. It is important to distinguish acute epididymitis from testicular torsion. Intervention includes bed rest, scrotal elevation, ice packs, sitz baths, analgesics, and antibiotics. It is important to treat sexual partners also for sexually transmitted forms of epididymitis. Nonsexually transmitted forms can be prevented by treating underlying causes of urinary tract infection and prostatitis. Complications include epididymal abscess (which may extend to the testicles) and chronic epididymitis.

Other epididymal problems include tuberculosis spreading via the blood from the lungs to the kidney, bladder, and prostate, and then the epididymis.

Problems of the vas deferens are rare. When they do occur, congenital absence or bilateral obstruction of the vas deferens leads to infertility.

▼ DISORDERS OF THE SEMINAL VESICLE

Congenital cysts of the seminal vesicles are rare. They lead to chronic urinary tract infection in children and adults.

Other problems include seminal vesiculitis, which may occur with severe prostatitis. Tuberculosis may enter the genitourinary organs from the lungs via the blood. Infected urine passes through the prostatic urethra, invading the prostate and seminal vesicle(s). Intervention is the same as for prostatitis.

Summary

Male reproductive disorders can be complex problems for the client and nurse. The client often finds that these disorders threaten sexuality and sexual function. These effects may be physiologic but often the nurse and client are also working with complex psychosocial problems. The nurse and the client may feel discomfort discussing issues of a sexual nature.

Prostate disorders are among the most common problems experienced by clients throughout their life. The nursing care they receive associated with these problems can greatly influence the clients' ability to adapt to the changes they are undergoing. Cancers of the male reproductive tract can be life threatening, but if they are detected early, they can be cured or at least controlled for long periods. The nurse can play a major role in the early detection of these cancers. Teaching young men to perform TSE can increase the incidence of early diagnosis and treatment of testicular cancer.

Bibliography

1. Ahmann, F. R., & Schifman, R. B. (March, 1987). Prospective comparison between serum monoclonal prostate-specific antigen (PSA) and acid phosphatase measurements in metastatic prostate cancer. *Journal of Urology, 139*(3), 137.
2. Beahrs, O. H., et al. (Eds.) (1986). *Manual for staging of cancer (3rd ed.)*. Philadelphia: J. B. Lippincott.
3. Benson, R. C., et al. (1991). Malignant potential of cryptorchid testis. *Mayo Clinic Proceedings, 66,* 3712-3718.
4. Bostwick, D. G. (1989). The pathology of early prostate cancer. *Ca-A Cancer Journal for Clinicians, 39*(3), 376-393.
5. Brawer, M. K., & Lange, P. H. (1989). Prostate-specific antigen and premalignant change: Implications for early detection. *Ca-A Cancer Journal for Clinicians, 39*(3), 361-375.
6. Cozad, J. (1988). Impotence: Psychosocial aspects, evaluation methods and treatment. *Urologic Nursing, 9*(2), 10-12.
7. Drago, J. R. (1989). The role of new modalities in the early detection and diagnosis of prostate cancer. *Ca-A Cancer Journal for Clinicians, 39*(3), 326-336.
8. Gaillard-Moguilewsky, M. (1991). Pharmacology of antiandrogens and value of combining androgen suppression with antiandrogen therapy. *Urology, 37*(2) (Suppl) 5-11.
9. Gershman, S. T., & Stolley, P. D. (1988). A case-controlled study of testicular cancer using Connecticut tumour registry data. *International Journal of Epidemiology, 17,* 738-742.
10. Goodman, M. (1988). Concepts of hormonal manipulation in the treatment of cancer. *Oncology Nursing Forum, 15*(5), 639-647.
11. Hayes, R. B., et al. (1990). Occupation and risk for testicular cancer: A case-control study. *International Journal of Epidemiology, 19*(4), 825-831.
12. Heinrich-Tynning, T. (1987). Prostatic cancer treatments and their effects on sexual functioning. *Oncology Nursing Forum, 14*(6), 37-41.
13. Hill, D. J. (1990). The patient with testicular cancer: Nursing management of chemotherapy. *Oncology Nursing Forum, 17*(2), 243-249.

13a. Johnson, D. E., et al. (1984). In D. R. Smith (Ed.), *General urology* (11th ed.). Los Altos, CA: Lange Medical Publications.

14. Joseph, A. C., & Chang, M. K. (1989). A bladder behavior clinic for post-prostatectomy patients. *Urologic Nursing, 9*(3), 15-19.
15. Killian, C. S., et al. (1985). Prognostic importance of prostate-specific antigen for monitoring patients with B2 to D1 prostate cancer. *Cancer Research, 45,* 886-891.
16. Killian, C. S., et al. (1986). Relative reliability of five serially measured markers for prognosis of progression in prostate cancer. *Journal of the National Cancer Institute, 76,* 179-185.
17. Klein, L. (1990). Current approaches to balloon dilatation of the prostate. *Astra Urologue, 20*(5), 1-7.
18. Lee, F., et al. (1989). The role of transrectal ultrasound in the early detection of prostate cancer. *Ca-A Cancer Journal for Clinicians, 39*(3), 337-360.
19. Lepor, H. (Ed) (1988). Pharmacologic intervention in benign prostatic hypertrophy. *Urology, 32* (Suppl. 6), 2-31.
20. Loughlin, K. R. (1991). Medical and nonmedical therapy for benign prostatic hypertrophy. *Geriatrics, 46*(6), 26-31.
21. Mahon, S. M., et al. (1990). Prostate cancer, Screening through treatment and nursing implications. *Urologic Nursing, 2,* 5-11.
22. Mallon, D., & Williams, C. F. (1987). A review of patient and partner perspectives of the penile prosthesis. *Journal of Urologic Nursing, 6*(1), 17-26.
23. Matzkin, H., & Braf, Z. (1991). Endocrine treatment of benign prostatic hypertrophy: Current concepts. *Urology, 37*(1), 1-13.
24. Murphy, G. P. (1989). Progress against prostatic cancer. *Ca-A Cancer Journal for Clinicians, 39*(3), 325.
25. Perez, C. A., et al. (1989). Carcinoma of the prostate. In V. Devita, S. Hellman, & S. Rosenburg (Eds.), Cancer principles and practice of oncology (Vol. 1, 3rd ed.). Philadelphia: J. B. Lippincott.
26. Pike, M. C., et al. (1986). Effect of age at orchiopexy on risk of testicular cancer. *Lancet, 1,* 1246-1248.
27. Reddy, E. K., et al. (1990). Testicular neoplasms: Seminoma. *Journal of the National Medical Association, 82*(9), 651-655.
28. Rudolf, V. M., & Quinn, L. M. (1988). The practice of TSE among college men: Effectiveness of an educational program. *Oncology Nursing Forum, 15*(1), 45-48.
29. Sawyer, P. F. (1987). Prostatectomy: Nursing care radical prostatectomy for cancer of the prostate: Nursing diagnoses and interventions. *Journal of Urologic Nursing, 6*(4), 266-276.
30. Silverberg, E., & Lubera, J. A. (1989). Cancer survival rates. *CA: A Journal for Clinicians, 39,* 3-32.
31. Stepp, C. (1991). Balloon dilatation of the prostate: A historical review. *Urologic Nursing, 5,* 21-24.
32. Walsh, P., et al. (Eds.) (1986). *Campbell's Urology (5th ed.).* Philadelphia: W. B. Saunders.
33. Waterhouse, R. L., & Resnick, M. I. (1989). The use of transrectal prostatic ultrasonography in the evaluation of patients with prostatic carcinoma. *Journal of Urology, 141*(2), 233-239.
34. Whorton, M. (1984). Environmental and occupational hazards. In J. Swanson and K. Forrest, (Eds.). *Men's reproductive health.* New York: Springer Pub.
35. Whorton, M., et al. (1977). Infertility in male pesticide workers. *Lancet, 2,* 1259.

Chapter 76

Nursing Care of Women with Gynecologic Disorders

Menstruation and childbearing are processes exclusive to women. Unfortunately, until recently, biases such as sexism and biologic determinism (the view that gender is the major determinant in how we live, or should live, our lives) have characterized much of the literature about the menstrual cycle. Historically, these two events have been invested with enormous social significance. Thus, the physical and psychological aspects of menstruation and menstrual disorders are closely interwoven.

Menstruation is a normal physiologic process that allows for the continuation of life. Yet, much folklore shrouds menstruation with taboos and mysticism. Earlier research on menstruation sometimes perpetuated myths because of questionable methodology and biases. Currently, investigators are attempting to bring a fresh perspective to research on menstruation and new knowledge is emerging.

Primitive cultures viewed menstruation as a source of "dark power" for women and a threat to men. Taboos surrounded menstruating women. These women were not to be touched by men and were often physically isolated in menstrual huts. Cleansing rituals were performed before women were allowed to reenter society.

Even in the 19th century, it was a commonly reported medical view that the uterus and ovaries dominated a woman's body. Irrational, hysterical symptoms were thought to arise from a discontented uterus. Women were labeled unreliable and illogical, because they were thought to be controlled by raging hormonal cycles. Even in modern times, this view has been used in subtle forms to deny economic, political, and social opportunity to women.

Controversy continues to rage over premenstrual tension and depression. Some psychiatrists have charged that premenstrual symptoms are mental disorders stemming from a failure to adjust to a woman's role. Others claim premenstrual distress is a result of cultural conditioning. And yet others question whether premenstrual tension really exists.

Whereas many articles on menstrual symptoms provide accurate information, others cause confusion. Until recently, the pathophysiologic mechanisms responsible for menstrual dysfunction were poorly understood. Recent advances in neuroendocrinology, endocrinology, and the biochemistry of gonadal function permit a better understanding of the physiology of menstruation. Research on psychosocial and physical aspects of menstruation is enlarging our understanding of normal and abnormal menstruation. New developments in physical and psychosocial intervention are emerging.

▼ MENSTRUAL DISORDERS

Most women experience some menstrual problems during their 30 or more years of menstruating. Women tend to readily seek professional help for obvious abnormalities such as excessive and irregular vaginal bleeding. However, they may not bring other menstrual problems to the attention of health care providers.

Women react to menstrual problems in differing, individual ways. Whereas some promptly seek health care, others may not for various reasons. For example, one woman may hesitate and be unable to discuss menstruation because she views it as a personal intimate problem and does not wish to talk about it. Another woman may accept some menstrual discomfort and inconvenience as inevitable. Yet another may have low self-esteem and dismiss her complaints as unimportant. Some women do not seek help because they feel that perhaps their problems will go away in time, whereas others question whether relief is really possible or whether the treatment will be worse than the problem. Thus, many menstrual problems go undetected unless nurses are skillful and sensitive in assessment. Menstrual problems may be discovered by nurses when women are discussing unrelated concerns such as contraception needs. Some menstrual problems include dysmenorrhea, premenstrual syndrome, and abnormal uterine bleeding.

▼ Dysmenorrhea

Until the early 1970s, dysmenorrhea (painful menstrual flow) was considered by many medical practitioners, as well as the lay public, to be mainly psychosomatic.[51] Women were told by everyone, including health care workers, it was all in their heads or indicative of their inability to adjust to the feminine role. Thus, most women did not even consider asking for help with this problem. Today, however, dysmenorrhea is taken seriously as a health problem and new knowledge has provided the basis for useful therapies to relieve the discomfort.

Dysmenorrhea may be primary or secondary. Primary dysmenorrhea is believed to be caused by either a prostaglandin excess or an increased sensitivity to prostaglandins with no underlying pathologic pelvic disorders. Secondary dysmenorrhea begins with an underlying disease condition. The true incidence and prevalence of women with this condition are unknown, although most women are affected to some degree.[7] Ultimately, this discomfort has the potential to affect women's productivity and increase absenteeism. Dysmenorrhea is a different entity than premenstrual syndrome (PMS) and requires different treatment modalities.[7] However, some women have symptoms of both.

PRIMARY DYSMENORRHEA

Etiology

Research indicates that the mechanisms involved in primary dysmenorrhea include elevated uterine prostaglandin levels as well as endocrine, myometrial, biochemical, and psychosocial factors. It appears that prostaglandin synthesis at the time of menstruation produces strong myometrial contractions. The severe muscle spasms constrict blood vessels supplying the uterus, causing ischemia and pain. The excess prostaglandins in smooth muscle also helps explain the presence of gastrointestinal symptoms, such as nausea, vomiting, and diarrhea or headache.

Endocrine factors appear to have a role in primary dysmenorrhea, because symptoms occur in ovulatory cycles. Psychosocial factors associated with dysmenorrhea include anxiety, insecurity, immaturity, dependency, rigid conformity, underachievement, and perfectionism.[51] Once menstrual pain has been experienced, women often become anxious as the next period approaches. Unfortunately, the expectation of pain may induce more pain. Many women are aware that during stressful times in their lives, they experience dysmenorrhea, whereas during times of relative calm, they do not.

Pathophysiology

Primary dysmenorrhea characteristically begins 1 to 3 months after menarche in conjunction with ovulatory cycles. Generally, it increases in severity over several years until the mid-20s and then begins to decline. Primary dysmenorrhea often decreases significantly after childbirth. It is often associated with prolonged menstrual flow and is more common in obese, sedentary women.

The discomfort of primary dysmenorrhea commonly begins 1 to 2 days before the onset of menstrual flow. The more severe discomfort is usually experienced during the first 24 hours of flow and typically subsides by the second day. Over half of the women experiencing dysmenorrhea also have systemic symptoms such as nausea, vomiting, diarrhea, syncope, headache, and leg pain.

Medical Management

The traditional therapeutic approach to primary dysmenorrhea was to prescribe narcotics and sedatives. The current approach emphasizes prevention and education, so a woman can participate in her own self-care. For women with mild symptoms who want to avoid medication, nonpharmacologic remedies might be effective. For example, biofeedback, therapeutic touch, or acupuncture might be helpful.

If contraception is desired as well as relief of dysmenorrhea, combination oral contraceptives may relieve menstrual pain. The resulting inhibition of ovulation results in decreased endometrial prostaglandin production and a concurrent reduction of uterine activity. For women with intrauterine devices (IUDs), removal of the device may lead to relief.

Exercise also has been used as a remedy for dysmenorrhea.[21] Exercise increases blood levels of beta endorphins, the body's endogenous opiates, making it available for pain relief. However, the exact mechanism responsible for relief is not known.

PHARMACOLOGIC MANAGEMENT

Prostaglandin synthesis inhibitors also may provide relief via decreased prostaglandin activity, even in the presence of ovulatory cycles. Some commonly prescribed medications in this group are ibuprofen (Motrin), mefenamic acid (Ponstel), indomethacin (Indocin), and naproxen sodium (Naprosyn). Ibuprofen is currently available as a nonprescription drug in 200-mg tablet form, which makes it convenient to obtain.

These medications may have gastrointestinal side effects. Other possible side effects are salt and water retention, skin rashes, and potential allergic reactions. Prostaglandin synthesis inhibitors should not be used by nursing mothers or during pregnancy.

Aspirin is a satisfactory drug for some women experiencing mild to moderate dysmenorrhea. For maximum effectiveness the medications should be administered either before or at the onset of menses. Sometimes, it is necessary to try several prostaglandin synthesis inhibitors until one with maximum effectiveness is found for the individual woman.

Nursing Management

Education and supportive reassurance are important nursing interventions for women with primary dysmenorrhea. Provide information about (1) the mechanisms involved in dysmenorrhea and (2) the actions and possible side effects of any prescribed medications. Assess the client's general health status. Encourage adequate nutrition and appropriate rest, sleep, and exercise. Assess stress, because stress may increase symptoms, and explore methods of stress management (see Chap. 3).

SECONDARY DYSMENORRHEA

Etiology

Secondary dysmenorrhea may be caused by conditions such as pelvic inflammatory disease (PID), endometriosis, adenomyosis (invasion of uterine myometrium by endometrial tissue), uterine prolapse, uterine myomas, or polyps. Secondary dysmenorrhea is suspected when pain is concentrated in a specific area or only on one side, or when its onset occurs after age 20.

Pelvic inflammatory disease is an infectious process that may involve the fallopian tubes, ovaries, pelvic peritoneum veins, and pelvic connective tissue. The onset of dysmenorrhea associated with PID is usually sudden and acute. Often, dyspareunia (painful intercourse) is present as well. The PID may occur after a bout of gonorrhea. Antibiotic therapy generally provides relief.

Endometriosis is a condition in which endometrial tissue (which responds to hormonal stimulation) is found outside the uterine cavity. Dysmenorrhea associated with endometriosis usually begins after menstrual flow has started and lasts throughout the menstrual period. Pain may be localized at a particular site and often increases in intensity as the menstrual period progresses.

Uterine myomas are benign tumors; polyps are small masses of tissue formed in the uterus (they may protrude from the cervix). Both may cause dysmenorrhea in later reproductive years. Along with menstrual pain, heavy menstrual flow may occur. Myomas and polyps may be found during pelvic examination and confirmed by ultrasound. Intrauterine polyps are very difficult to detect.

Secondary dysmenorrhea associated with uterine prolapse (downward uterine displacement due to weakening of support structures) normally appears as premenstrual backache persisting throughout the menstrual period. It may be associated with dyspareunia. Cystocele (bladder herniating into the vagina due to weakening of the anterior vaginal wall) is often associated with uterine prolapse. Thus, urinary stress incontinence also may be present.

Medical Management

Treatment for secondary dysmenorrhea is directed toward the underlying cause. Antiprostaglandin agents may provide some relief.

Nursing Management

Nursing interventions focus on educational and psychosocial needs of the individual client.

▼ Premenstrual Syndrome

Premenstrual syndrome (PMS) was first described in 1931. It remained relatively obscure until recently, when extensive media coverage brought the syndrome to public attention. Despite its popularization, PMS is still not well understood. Much confusion surrounds its diagnosis, treatment, and nursing management.

Definition

Various definitions of PMS appear in the literature. One is "any combination of emotional and physical features which occur cyclically in the female before menstruation and which regress or disappear during menstruation."[16] Premenstrual syndrome is somatic, not psychic, in origin, and it is a complex mechanism involving not only the endocrine system but both the autonomic and central nervous systems as well. A predominant alteration is the retention of body fluids.

Incidence

The incidence of PMS is difficult to determine because of the variable symptoms and the lack of a clear understanding about the syndrome. Variable reports in the literature indicate that approximately 70 to 90 per cent of all women experience some form of PMS. Probably only 20 to 40 per cent of these women experience symptoms that disrupt their lives. The relationship between PMS and dysmenorrhea is currently unclear. The two entities are thought to be distinct. However, recent data indicate that some women experience both PMS and dysmenorrhea.[7] However, PMS and dysmenorrhea tend to occur in different age groups. Primary dysmenorrhea is more common in younger women, whereas PMS occurs mostly in the 30- to 40-year-old age group.

Etiology

The etiology of PMS is unclear; however, neuroendocrine mechanisms appear to be involved. It is not clear whether PMS is a single syndrome or a group of separate disorders. Some popular theories are that PMS may be caused by (1) estrogen-progesterone imbalance; (2) fluid retention; (3) estrogen, progesterone, and aldosterone interaction; (4) vasopressin; (5) prolactin; (6) dietary factors such as vitamin B_6 deficiency or hypoglycemia; or (7) endogenous opiates. The relationship of PMS to psychiatric illness, if any, remains unclear.

Clinical Manifestations

Typically, symptoms of PMS occur during the last few premenstrual days, and sudden relief of symptoms occurs with full menstrual flow. However, symptoms may begin with ovulation and may not be relieved until during or toward the end of menses. Characteristically, symptoms gradually worsen until menses begin.

Various symptoms are attributable to PMS, including altered emotional states, behavioral changes, somatic problems, altered appetite, and motor effects. Different sets of symptoms are experienced by individual women. Commonly, emotional symptoms include tension, depression, irritability, hostility, insomnia, loneliness, crying easily, and indecision. Forgetfulness and mental confusion may occur. Psychosis and suicidal tendencies occur rarely.

Behavioral symptoms include work habit changes, increased or decreased libido, avoidance of contact with other people, a tendency to pick fights, and occasionally, the commission of criminal acts. Numerous somatic problems have been reported. Some of the most common are bloatedness, headache, breast tenderness, fatigue, and backache. Alterations in appetite include craving alcohol or certain foods (e.g., sweet or salty foods) or avoiding certain foods. Motor effects reported are vertigo, changes in coordination, and clumsiness. Many other symptoms also have been reported.

Because PMS symptoms usually do not occur during the menstrual flow, women may not associate PMS with the menstrual cycle. Also, women may be reluctant to admit the apparent irrational symptoms. Such symptoms may be misdiagnosed as psychological or emotional problems.

DIAGNOSTIC ASSESSMENT

To date, there are no objective methods of diagnosing PMS. Diagnosis is usually made by documenting the cyclic nature of the symptoms on a menstrual calendar. A diary of symptoms and menstrual periods is an essential part of assessing women suspected of having PMS.

A diagnosis of PMS requires a recurrence of symptoms for a minimum of three menstrual cycles. Diagnosis is made on the timing of symptoms rather than on the presence of particular symptoms.

Medical Management

PHARMACOLOGIC MANAGEMENT

There is no known effective pharmacologic treatment for PMS. Treatment is directed toward relief of symptoms. What helps one woman may not be effective for another. A variety of therapies have been used. Daily intake of vitamin B_6 has improved some premenstrual symptoms. Other nonprescription drugs include calcium, vitamin A, magnesium, and trace elements. Essential fatty acid supplements are often recommended.

Prescription medications commonly include Hy-Gesterone, vaginal progesterone, oral spironolactone (Aldactone), oral bromocriptine (Parlodel), oral contraceptives, tranquilizers. Spironolactone is a synthetic steroid aldosterone antagonist that inhibits the physiologic effect of aldosterone on the distal renal tubules. It is commonly used to treat the edema associated with excessive aldosterone excretion. Bromocriptine reduces serum prolactin concentrations by inhibiting prolactin release from the anterior pituitary. Bromocriptine has been used to treat amenorrhea and infertility. It has also been used successfully in some cases of PMS. Sedatives and analgesics are often useful for symptomatic relief.

Nursing Management

ASSESSMENT

PMS is a significant problem for many women in spite of the confusion surrounding its cause, definition, and management. Nurses are in a key position to help women identify and cope with PMS when it is present.

Nursing Intervention

Nursing Diagnosis: Knowledge Deficit R/T syndrome and symptom management.

Planning: Expected Outcome. Client will understand PMS and the management of its symptoms, as evidenced by client's statements and client report of decrease in symptoms.

Implementation. Once the diagnosis of PMS is made, the woman needs information about the syndrome and reassurance that there is a physiologic basis for her symptoms, even though the mechanisms are not clearly understood. Women are often helped by the opportunity to talk about their feelings and experiences with PMS, especially because of the confusion and misconceptions surrounding the syndrome. Significant others also benefit from information and reassurance.

Nursing Diagnosis: Health Maintenance, Altered, R/T poor physical health.

Planning: Expected Outcomes. The client will improve health, as evidenced by improved physical condition and decrease of PMS symptoms.

Implementation. Women who are in poor physical condition may be particularly susceptible to premenstrual difficulties. Thus nursing assessment includes the woman's general lifestyle, sleep and dietary habits, and overall health maintenance.

Suggested dietary modifications include reducing salt and refined carbohydrate intake. Give careful attention to stress management and reduction (see Chap. 3). Adequate physical exercise and weight reduction (if necessary) are very important. It also may be helpful to reduce alcohol and caffeine intake, and stop or reduce smoking.

Nursing Diagnosis: Individual Coping, Ineffective, High Risk for, R/T distress from symptoms of PMS.

Planning: Expected Outcomes. The client will cope effectively with PMS and its symptoms, as evidenced by client's statements and a decrease in symptoms.

Implementation. Another major nursing responsibility is assisting the woman and her significant others to cope with the symptoms of PMS. Make plans for coping with specific PMS symptoms on an individual basis, keeping in mind the woman's particular lifestyle and preferences. For example, a reallocation of responsibilities within the family might help to reduce the woman's stress. If she prefers to retain her current responsibilities, the nurse might help her learn how to manage them in ways that minimize stress. Support groups or educational sessions may be helpful as well. These sessions can serve as a forum for sharing information, providing mutual support, and discussing feelings. Daily, vigorous exercise has been recommended, both to reduce stress and to increase a sense of well being.

EVALUATION

The nurse must evaluate client outcomes based on the established plan of care. If these goals were not achieved, the plan and interventions must be revised to meet the client's needs.

▼ Abnormal Uterine Bleeding

Abnormal uterine bleeding encompasses a wide variety of menstrual disorders, such as lack of menstrual flow, irregular uterine bleeding, and excessive uterine bleeding. Changes in menstrual patterns can be frightening to the woman and, if they are severe enough, symptoms can disrupt daily living. Sometimes, abnormal uterine bleeding indicates underlying disease conditions. The term dysfunctional uterine bleeding means abnormal uterine bleeding for which no organic cause can be found through the usual assessment techniques. Abnormal uterine bleeding always requires careful assessment by a qualified health professional.

AMENORRHEA

Definition

Amenorrhea means the absence of menses or skipping periods. Amenorrhea, the absence of cyclic vaginal bleeding, is classified as primary when no menstruation has occurred, or as secondary when previous spontaneous menstrual bleeding has occurred prior to cessation of flow. A diagnosis of secondary amenorrhea also requires a lack of bleeding for 6 months in a woman having regular cyclic bleeding, or 12 months in a woman with a history of irregular bleeding.

Incidence

Amenorrhea is common. Many women experience it at some time during their life.

Etiology

Often chromosomal abnormalities or structural genital malformations are discovered in clients with primary amenorrhea, although other factors may be present (Fig. 76-1). Pregnancy is a common physiologic cause of amenorrhea. Excessive exercise, such as occurs with athletes or dancers, can sometimes cause a woman to stop having her periods.

Amenorrhea may signal menopause in a mature woman. The diagnosis can be confirmed by finding elevated LH and FSH levels. However, pregnancy testing should be considered in a mature woman as well, because pregnancy may occur after a short period of amenorrhea, if additional ovulatory cycles have occurred.

Some medications may cause amenorrhea, e.g., neuropharmacologic agents such as psychotropics and antihypertensives. Some women experience amenorrhea after discontinuing oral contraceptives.

Weight loss or excessive physical activity and psychosocial stress may be associated with amenorrhea. One hypothesis is that a critical percentage of fat (about 22 per cent of body weight) is necessary to maintain regular menstruation after age 16. Thus, a simple weight loss of 10 to 15 per cent of the total body weight might result in amenorrhea. Amenorrhea may be associated with heavy physical exercise, such as, jogging, running, and aerobic dancing. Psychosocial stress also may be associated with amenorrhea, although the mechanisms are not well understood. A growing consensus is that the endogenous opioid and dopaminergic systems are probably involved in stress-induced amenorrhea.

Other potential causes of amenorrhea are pituitary, ovarian, and endocrine factors. Hypothyroidism, either

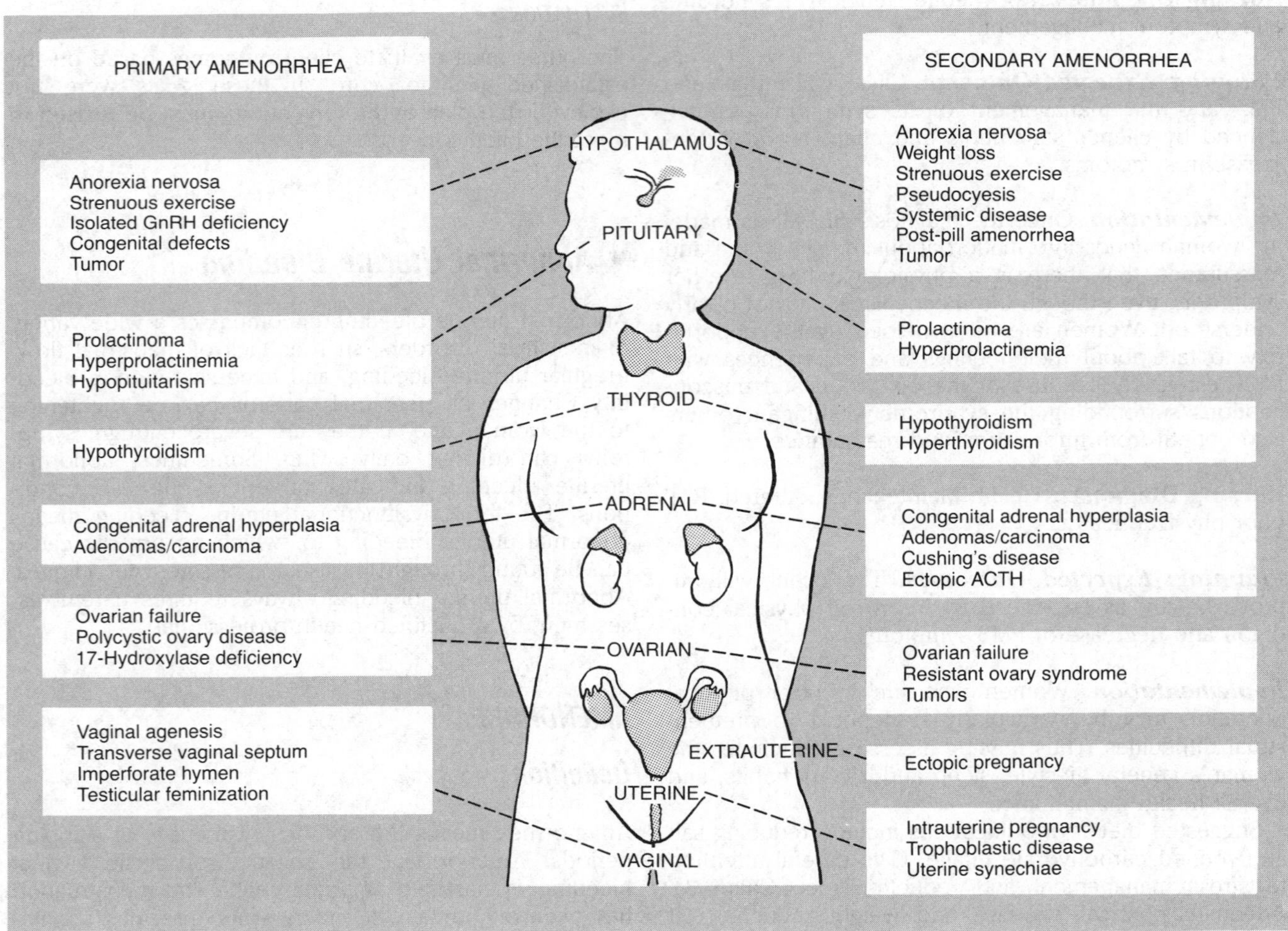

▲ *Figure 76-1*

Causes of amenorrhea.

from neoplasms or trauma, can result in gonadotropin abnormalities and amenorrhea. Ovarian abnormalities can lead to altered estrogen release, which can result in amenorrhea or abnormal uterine bleeding. Other endocrine abnormalities, such as polycystic ovarian syndrome or Cushing's syndrome, also may lead to amenorrhea.

Medical Management

Treatment for amenorrhea depends in part on the woman's needs and desires. Particularly important are her wishes regarding childbearing.

PHARMACOLOGIC MANAGEMENT

If pregnancy is not desired, medroxyprogesterone may be used to produce withdrawal bleeding. If pregnancy is desired, ovulation induction with clomiphene citrate or bromocriptine may be undertaken.

Nursing Management

Absence of spontaneous menstrual flow before age 17 requires careful assessment, including history and physical examination. Pregnancy also must be ruled out for any woman of childbearing age experiencing secondary amenorrhea. Ask the woman about the presence of symptoms of pregnancy such as breast tenderness, nausea, urinary frequency, weight gain, fatigue, or changes in food tolerance. Even if the woman has been consistently using birth control, pregnancy might have occurred.

Young girls may deny intercourse, meaning actual penetration, but may admit, on careful questioning, that sex play involving ejaculation between the thighs or near the introitus did occur. Pregnancy can occur from the migration of sperm in these situations. A pregnancy test is performed if there is any possibility that conception may have occurred. If the pregnancy test is positive, give the woman appropriate opportunity to discuss her desires related to the pregnancy's continuation or termination.

Teaching opportunities are an important part of nursing care. Depending on the cause of amenorrhea, the woman may need help in gaining weight, reducing energy drain from excessive physical activity, and stress reduction. Assess general health and help the woman plan and make changes as indicated.

MENORRHAGIA

The term menorrhagia means excessive vaginal bleeding at normal intervals and can cause women grave distress and inconvenience.

Menorrhagia can have a variety of causes. A single heavy episode of bleeding may indicate spontaneous abortion. Excessively heavy menstrual periods may be associated with IUD use for contraception. Fibroids and adenomyosis also are common causes of menorrhagia. Other potential causes include systemic diseases such as blood dyscrasias and hypothyroidism. Medications such as anticoagulants also have been associated with excessive menstrual flow.

Assessing the actual amount of blood loss can be difficult. Many women are unable to give a reliable history of blood loss and either minimize or exaggerate it. Ask women to compare the number of pads used during the abnormal period with the number used during a normal cycle. In a more controlled setting, it may help to weigh the pads before and after use to estimate blood loss. Also, the usual tests to identify possible anemia may be performed.

Treatment may consist of dilation and curettage (D & C) or administration of medications such as estrogens, progestins (alone or in combination with oral contraceptives), or antifibrinolytic agents, depending on factors thought to be associated with the cause.

Dilatation and curettage may be performed for the abnormal bleeding. During dilation, the cervical opening is gradually enlarged using a dilator (Fig. 76–2). This is immediately followed by curettage (scraping the lining of the uterus with a curet). Often, dilatation and curettage is performed under light anesthesia as outpatient surgery.

Preoperatively, the woman restricts her food and fluid intake for anesthesia. The woman is placed in a lithotomy position for the procedure.

Postoperatively, the woman has a sterile perineal pad in place. The pad should be checked and changed frequently. The client might have vaginal packing, which is usually removed within 24 hours.

During the first few hours after dilatation and curettage, monitor the client closely for excessive vaginal bleeding. Also, assess her ability to urinate. Urination may be difficult, especially if vaginal packing is exerting pressure on the urethra. Report excess bleeding, inability to void, or excessive pain. The woman usually experiences only minimal uterine cramping postoperatively. Mild analgesics such as aspirin and codeine usually relieve any discomfort.

Follow-up instructions include the following: (1) avoid strenuous activity for about 1 week; (2) avoid douching and vaginal or rectal intercourse until the physician gives permission (usually about 1 week); (3) expect a small amount of pinkish vaginal discharge, followed by dark red or dark brown discharge during the healing process; (4) realize that subsequent menstrual periods may or may not be affected; (5) return for a follow-up appointment; and (6) report any indications of complications to the surgeon. Following dilatation and curettage, the next period may not occur, may be on schedule, or may vary from the usual time of onset. Indications of possible complications include excessive bleeding, excessive pain, or an elevated temperature.

An important aspect of nursing care is to provide reassurance, because heavy vaginal bleeding can be very frightening.

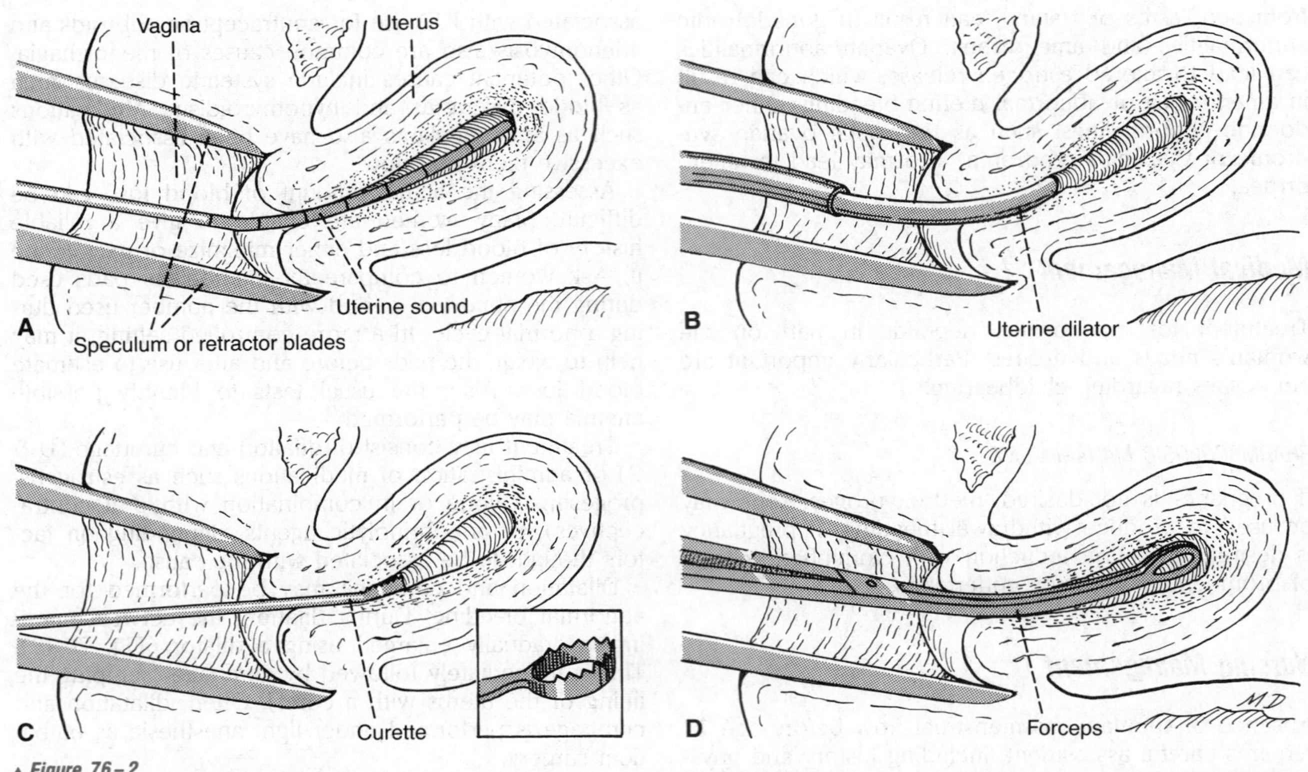

▲ *Figure 76–2*

Dilation and curettage (D & C) of the uterus. *A*, The length and axis of the uterus is explored with a malleable uterine sound. *B*, A Kelly's clamp dilates the cervical os. Further gradual dilation is achieved with Hanks' dilators in graduated sizes. *C*, The endocervical canal is curetted first; next, the uterine cavity. Tissue specimens are saved. *D*, Finally, the uterine cavity is explored with a polyforceps or common duct forceps.

METRORRHAGIA

Metrorrhagia, or vaginal bleeding between periods, may occur as spotting or outright bleeding. Common causes are similar to those responsible for menorrhagia and also may include ectopic pregnancy, spotting with ovulation, cervical polyps, or breakthrough bleeding that occurs in conjunction with oral contraception. For breakthrough bleeding, the dosage of oral contraceptive can be adjusted or a different agent may be prescribed.

MENOPAUSE

Normal menopause is discussed in detail in Chapter 73.

Surgical Menopause

Menopause may be induced at any age by surgical removal of the ovaries or pelvic irradiation. Hysterectomy (removal of the uterus), not including removal of the ovaries, does not cause surgical menopause. However, some symptoms such as hot flashes have been reported following hysterectomy. In these instances, it is possible that blood vessels supplying the ovaries may have been injured, and the resulting loss of blood supply caused the ovaries to atrophy. Another cause of such symptoms could be the hormone imbalance produced by removal of the uterus and its loss as a hormone receptor. Delayed onset of the climacteric (about ages 55 to 60) is associated with a higher incidence of pathologic conditions and requires careful assessment.

Menopausal Difficulties

The most commonly reported menopausal difficulties are vasomotor instability, menstrual irregularities, and atrophic vaginitis. A wide variety of physical and psychosocial symptoms have been attributed to the perimenopausal period, but controversy remains as to whether they are actually related to menopause or to other factors, such as aging or stressful life events.

Symptoms of *vasomotor instability*, such as hot flashes, night sweats, and occasional palpitations and dizziness associated with menopause are probably caused by hormonal imbalances. Estrogen appears to exert a protective effect on subcutaneous blood vessels. Lowered estrogen makes many women more sensitive to stimuli that precipitate sweating, skin discoloration, and the sensation of heat loss. If vasomotor symptoms are severe, short-term substitution with estrogens may be used. Such *substitution therapy*, lasting from a few months to 2 years, may relieve hot flashes. Generally, the therapy is discontinued gradually after the climacteric has ended.

Hot flashes are sudden involuntary waves of heat beginning in the upper chest or neck and proceeding up the face and head. It lasts from a few seconds to several minutes and is aggravated by anything that increases heat production in the body. A hot flash may or may not be accompanied by a hot flush, which is a measurable change in skin temperature, a visible pink to bright red flush in skin color, and perspiration. A night sweat is a hot flash with or without a hot flush occurring in the night accompanied by perspiration, which can be profuse. Voda[52] describes the following degrees of hot flashes.

- *Mild hot flash.* A warm feeling, often so fleeting that it is barely noticeable, which may or may not be accompanied by dampness and slight skin flushing.
- *Moderate hot flash.* A warm to extremely warm feeling, longer and more noticeable than a mild hot flash. Often accompanied by sweat and sometimes skin flushing.
- *Severe hot flash.* An intense or extremely hot feeling. Usually accompanied by profuse and very uncomfortable sweating or skin flushing. The thermal discomfort of a severe hot flash may cause a woman to stop her activity at the time of the hot flash and seek relief by fanning, showering, removing or changing clothes, or lying down. Other bodily sensations associated with a severe hot flash are feelings of waves of heat, dizziness, chills, suffocation, inability to concentrate, and chest pain.

Generally, the subjective symptom of the hot flash occurs about 45 seconds prior to the hot flush. The reported incidence of the hot flash varies for perimenopausal women from 68 to 92 per cent, depending on the age group studied.[27] A study by Feldman and associates reported a prevalence rate of 88 per cent for women experiencing natural menopause.[18] However, there is great variance in both the quantitative and qualitative aspects of women's experience of hot flashes.

Many women require detailed information about what menopause is and what is happening to their bodies. Clarify that hot flashes are a normal part of menopause. The nurse should provide practical suggestions for coping with hot flashes. The following information should be provided to women having difficulty with hot flashes:

- Dress in the layered look so that some clothing can easily be taken off during the sensation and put back on as cooling commences.
- Avoid hot environments and keep the thermostat around 65° F or lower.
- Avoid getting excited, because emotional stress sometimes triggers hot flashes.
- Avoid highly seasoned, spicy foods, coffee, tea, and alcohol if they trigger hot flashes. The nurse will need to ask the client what spicy foods act this way for each particular client.
- Keep a record or diary of when you experience hot flashes and try to identify common trigger(s) and work out ways of avoiding them.
- Learn to control your reactions to the hot flash. Voda describes one woman's method of stopping hot flashes by imagining herself walking in snow and forcing herself to shiver.
- Use cooling techniques, such as fans, showering, applying cold cloths or ice cubes to various body parts.

The vaginal mucous membrane is especially responsive to low estrogen levels. When these levels remain low both during and following menopause, vaginal walls become thinner and drier, and susceptibility to infection increases. These changes lead to an increase in vaginitis in menopausal women. Other symptoms may include vaginal irritation, burning, pruritus, leukorrhea, bleeding, and dyspareunia.

Vulvar epithelium loses its elasticity and subcutaneous fat after menopause. Pubic hair may become thinner. As the epidermal layer thins, the labia majora and minora flatten. The urethra may atrophy, and when this occurs, the incidence of cystitis and urethritis increase. Pubococcygeus muscles tend to lose their tone, and stress urinary incontinence also may occur.

Some women experience backache, joint pain, and other symptoms of osteoporosis. Osteoporosis is a skeletal disorder characterized by an increased predisposition to bone collapse or fracture resulting from a reduced amount of bone mass. Estrogen seems to inhibit bone breakdown and loss. A decrease or absence of estrogen may lead to osteoporosis.

Spinal osteoporosis, giving rise to vertebral biconcavity and compression fractures, is particularly common in postmenopausal women. Lower forearm fracture is an osteoporotic syndrome occurring almost exclusively in postmenopausal women. Osteoporosis is more severe among women who are sedentary and who smoke (see Chap. 67).

Many other difficulties can occur that may or may not be related to climacteric changes. Some women report insomnia or other sleep disturbances, headache, forgetfulness, nervousness, apprehension, and irritability. Wardrop found a high incidence of oral symptoms such as dryness of the mouth, a burning sensation in the mouth, and altered taste perceptions among perimenopausal clients.[53] Many myths abound about depression occurring at the time of menopause, but no relationship can be demonstrated. Psychosocial stress may affect other menopausal symptoms. The psychosocial changes experienced by some women may result from a combination of hormone imbalance and adjustment to the aging process.

The nursing role in working with menopausal women and their significant others involves providing support, education, and assistance in moving through this normal life experience as comfortably as possible. Accurate information about menopause and what to expect can be helpful and reassuring. Tailor assistance in coping with minor discomforts of menopause to the needs of the individual woman. The following self-care measures may be useful:

- *Vaginal dryness:* Continued intercourse and/or masturbation aids circulation and keeps tissues flexible;

use water soluble jelly for lubrication; use estrogen cream if needed.

- *Prevention of osteoporosis:* Take part in any weight-bearing exercise such as walking, tennis, dancing, bicycle riding; increase calcium intake; stop smoking; decrease alcohol and caffeine intake.
- *Prevention of urinary tract infection:* Void frequently; increase fluid intake; maintain good perineal hygiene; wear cotton underwear.
- *Pelvic relaxation:* Perform Kegel's exercises to increase muscle tone (see Chap. 49); encourage weight loss if the client is overweight.

Remind women experiencing menopause of the value of good health habits. Balanced nutrition and adequate sleep and rest are important. Exercising at least three times per week for 45 minutes will promote cardiovascular health. Nurses can be effective in assisting women to make menopause a positive experience.

HORMONE REPLACEMENT THERAPY

Hormone replacement therapy (HRT) (estrogen plus progesterone) may be part of the medical management of perimenopausal symptoms. Individuals must be informed of the advantages and potential dangers of HRT in order to make informed safe decisions about treatment. Nurses need up-to-date information about HRT in order to support women making this important decision.

It is often difficult for women to decide about HRT because authorities differ markedly in their advice. HRT can alleviate vasomotor instability, vaginal and urinary tract atrophy, dyspareunia, and a number of affective symptoms.[35] It also has been studied as a preventive measure against osteoporosis and cardiovascular disease, with some researchers claiming a protective effect against breast cancer and others citing it as a risk factor for breast cancer development.[35] In the mid to late 1970s, evidence for an association between estrogen replacement therapy (ERT) and endometrial cancer was discovered. In subsequent years, this association has been studied extensively, and today, estrogen is given with a progestational agent to simulate the normal menstrual cycle. This provides a protective effect against cancer of the endometrium.[35] Unopposed ERT is, therefore, no longer recommended for a woman with an intact uterus.

It is generally accepted that estrogens should not be given to women with (1) known or suspected breast or uterine cancer or any estrogen-dependent neoplasia (or a strong family history of the same), (2) undiagnosed abnormal uterine bleeding, (3) previous or present thrombophlebitis, (4) acute liver disease or cerebrovascular disease, and (5) combined risk factors such as obesity, varicosities, high blood pressure, and heavy smoking. Women with uterine fibromyomas, hyperlipidemia, severe varicose veins, chronic hepatic dysfunction, diabetes mellitus, and severe hypertension require thorough assessment before estrogen is prescribed.

The use of ERT, estrogen alone or HRT should be individualized according to the woman's needs, desires, and individual symptoms and risks. The risk for women with fibrocystic breast disease is unclear, but careful assessment must be made. Risks should be assessed for endometrial cancer, osteoporosis, cardiovascular disease, and breast cancer. Both ERT and HRT are effective against perimenopausal hot flashes, atrophic vaginitis, and urinary tract changes. For relief of hot flashes, short-term therapy is usually effective with gradual withdrawal advised. Relief of urogenital problems may require long-term or even lifelong therapy.

Both ERT and HRT decrease the risk of developing osteoporosis in white women. The optimal duration of therapy for osteoporosis prevention is not known, but it is thought to be at least 10 years. ERT is possibly protective against cardiovascular heart disease, but this factor also needs further research. Therapy for cardiovascular heart disease is lifelong.

At the present time, the risk from HRT for the development of breast cancer is unclear and further research is needed. In cases in which a woman decides to use estrogen or hormone replacement therapy, she should be carefully monitored for the development of breast cancer and receive breast examinations on a regular basis.

Estrogens used in replacement therapy are conjugated equine estrogen (Premarin), 0.625 mg; estrone sulfate, 0.625 to 1.25 mg; micronized 17-beta estradiol (Estrace), 1 to 2 mg; and transdermal 17-beta estradiol (Estraderm), 0.5 to 1 mg.[12]

Treatment regimens vary for estrogen-progesterone combinations. Estrogens may be used for 25 days each month or continuously, whereas progesterones are generally prescribed for 10 to 14 days a month.[12] Low-dose continuous progesterone therapy may be given along with continuous ERT. The advantage of continuous combined therapy is that withdrawal bleeding generally stops in about 6 months.

Side effects of progesterone therapy include bloating, depression, acne, breast tenderness, and premenstrual tension. However, side effects can generally be lessened by adjusting the dosage or lengthening the duration of the therapy. Because of the possibility that progesterones may unfavorably alter the high-density lipoprotein (HDL)-low-density lipoprotein (LDL) cholesterol ratio, unopposed estrogen has been recommended for women whose uterus has been surgically removed.

Transdermal estrogen patches are an alternative for women who cannot tolerate the oral estrogens or for whom the hepatic effects of estrogen (increased secretion of renin substrate, causing hypertension and increased clotting factors as a result of liver stimulation) are a problem.[12]

POSTMENOPAUSAL BLEEDING

Postmenopausal bleeding, vaginal bleeding occurring after menopause, is a symptom, not a diagnosis (Fig. 76-3). It requires careful assessment because it may be a symptom of genital tract cancer. Other causes of postmenopausal bleeding include atrophic vaginitis,

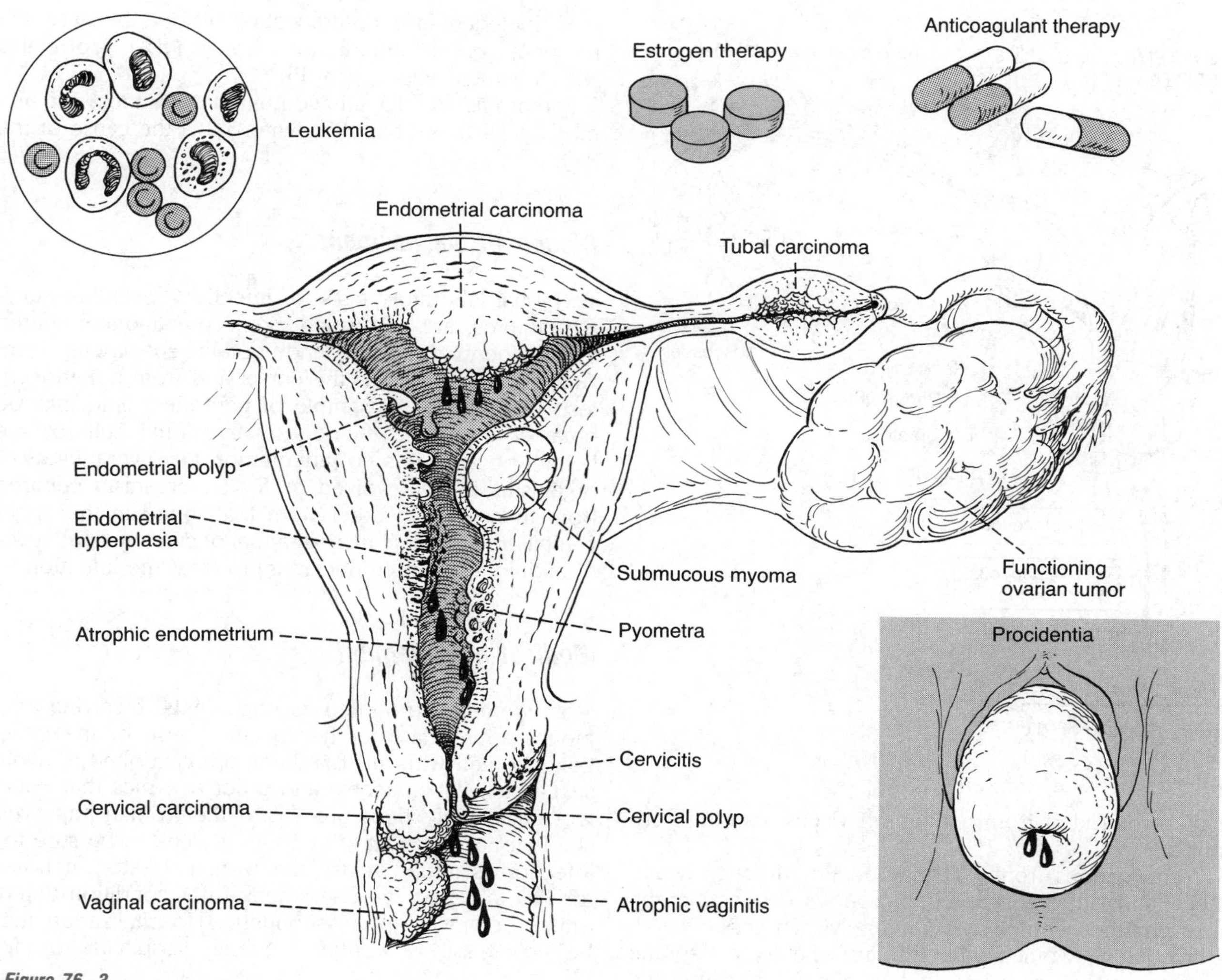

▲ *Figure 76–3*

Causes of postmenopausal bleeding.

cervical polyps, fibroids, endometrial hyperplasia, or cervical erosion.

▼ PELVIC INFLAMMATORY DISEASE

Definition

PID refers to ascending pelvic infections, that is, those involving the upper genital tract (beyond the cervix).

Etiology

Gonococci, staphylococci, streptococci, and other pus-producing (pyogenic) organisms commonly cause PID.

Pathophysiology

Once an infection is in the upper genital tract, it may travel along several routes (Fig. 76–4). Tuberculosis (TB), a rare cause of PID, travels through the blood and affects the fallopian tubes and sometimes the ovaries, uterus, and pelvic peritoneum. The woman's excreta are contaminated until the drugs have become effective (about 2 weeks).

Gonococcus and staphylococcus organisms spread along the uterine endometrium to the fallopian tubes, where they cause an acute salpingitis (inflammation of the fallopian tubes). The tubes become partially occluded and may drain pus, leukocytes, and other debris into the pelvic cavity, causing pelvic peritonitis, or the material may form a pocket around the ovary, causing a tubo-ovarian abscess.

Streptococci spread similarly, except they tend to travel via the uterine or cervical lymphatics across the parametrium to the tubes or ovaries. There, they may cause pelvic cellulitis and sometimes thrombophlebitis of the major pelvic veins, with the risk of the development of embolisms.

Another route of spread of infection is from the pelvic cavity itself. Organisms such as *Escherichia coli*

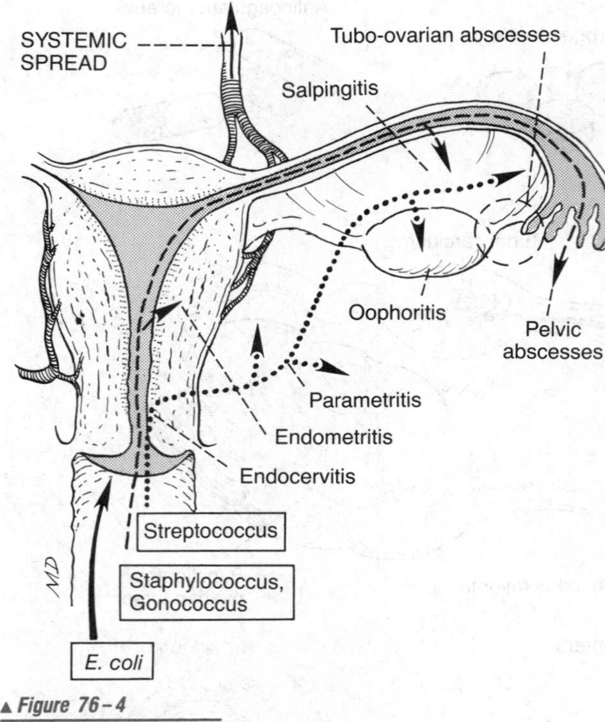

▲ *Figure 76-4*

Routes of spread of PID.

may be extruded from a ruptured viscus, causing peritonitis.

Complications from PID may occur. Although septic shock and other severe complications can occur, the most common complication is a pelvic abscess.

Frequently, women with PID are unable to become pregnant after the infection has cleared because the inflammatory process causes scarring and closing of the fallopian tubes.

Clinical Manifestations

Clinical manifestations include a generalized infection, such as general malaise, fever, chills, anorexia, nausea, vomiting, general aching, and tachycardia. In addition, the woman usually experiences acute, sharp, severe aching on both sides of the abdomen or pelvis. Pain is aggravated by defecation and is accompanied by a heavy, purulent, odoriferous discharge (the odor depends on the organism). Occasionally, vaginal bleeding occurs. The rapidity of onset of PID depends on the virulence of the infecting organism, the status of the woman's pelvic organs and her general health.

Other helpful clues to PID are obtained from the history. A history of acute lower genital tract infection is significant. It is helpful to know whether the pain accompanying the current illness began during menses (typically indicating gonococcal PID) or between periods (usually nongonococcal infections). Various other data, including a thorough sexual history, are important. Included is a contraceptive history, because the presence of an intrauterine device (IUD) correlates with a higher incidence of PID.

Symptoms of PID are combined with those of pulmonary TB (see Chap. 39) when TB is the cause of the PID.

Diagnostic Assessment

The usual laboratory tests for infection, including multiple cultures, are performed. Some practitioners culture any evident drainage, and obtain specimens from various organs such as the cervix and from a culdocentesis (Fig. 76-5). A sample of peritoneal fluid may be obtained from the cul-de-sac. Additional cultures are helpful because it is not uncommon for several kinds of organisms to be involved or for an organism cultured from the cervix to differ from that found in the upper genital tract. When this situation occurs, several types of antibiotics may be necessary to treat the infection.

Medical Management

Most women are treated as outpatients, receiving antibiotics appropriate to the specific cause of the infection. Women with this condition are cautioned to avoid sexual activity, douches, and other activities that could worsen the infectious process. If the woman improves, she is usually evaluated in about a week to be sure the infection is gone. Advise the woman treated at home for PID to return for assessment if her condition deteriorates or her symptoms continue. Hospitalization may be necessary. A woman requiring hospitalization for PID is usually very ill.

PHARMACOLOGIC MANAGEMENT

PID caused by TB is treated with antitubercular medications (see Chap. 39).

During hospitalization, antibiotics appropriate to the offending organisms are given in maximal doses. The woman is placed in semi-Fowler's position to promote downward drainage. Pain management is important. Sitz baths or heat (applied periodically to the lower back or abdomen) may help relieve the pain. Analgesics are also used. Document the amount, color, odor, and appearance of the vaginal discharge. Make sure the client cleans the perineum frequently.

Surgical Management

Some abscesses are treated relatively easily, whereas others require surgical intervention or may rupture, causing peritonitis. The type of surgical intervention and its timing (acute or after a cooling off period) varies somewhat with the health care provider's philosophy and the presenting problem.

Treatment of some women with PID requires a laparotomy. While the infection is surgically removed, it also may be necessary to remove the uterus, ovaries, and tubes.

Surgery that is performed while PID is acute increases the woman's operative risk. This risk must be balanced against the risk of continuing unsuccessful medical therapy that can lead to chronic PID.

Nursing Management

Nursing care for women experiencing PID is directed toward providing health information and psychosocial support to the client and her significant others. Because PID is often caused by sexually transmitted diseases, there may be guilt feelings and problems with significant others centered around the woman's contracting the infection.

Some women are infertile after PID. This change in fertility may be a difficult loss for the woman and her significant other to accept. It is important to plan and provide time for the expression of such feelings.

Education is important for the client with PID. Women with PID can benefit from factual discussion about the infection, how to identify recurrences, and general hygienic measures that may help prevent new infections. Teach the woman to wash her perineal area regularly with soap and water, to wipe from front to back, to change tampons and pads several times a day during menses, and to wash hands before and after changing tampons or pads. Balanced nutrition and adequate rest, sleep, and exercise can improve the client's general health and reduce the risk of infection. These women need to know when they can resume sexual activity and when other restrictions can be eliminated.

CHRONIC PELVIC INFLAMMATORY DISEASE

Chronic PID can occur if the acute phase of the illness does not respond to treatment or if treatment is inadequate. Clinical manifestations include chronic pelvic discomfort, menstrual disturbances or dysfunctional uterine bleeding, constipation, malaise, or periodic return of acute symptoms. Sterility, one of the more serious complications, results from destruction of part of the fallopian tubes and loss of their patency. Sterility is usually irreversible.

Treatment of chronic PID is aimed at removing the offending organism and improving the woman's general health. If treatment is unsuccessful, surgical removal of the pelvic organs may be necessary.

▼ UTERINE DISORDERS

ENDOMETRIOSIS

Definition

Endometriosis is an abnormal condition in which endometrial tissue (which normally lines the uterine cavity) is located in other sites.

Incidence

Endometriosis is found most commonly in premenopausal women aged 30 to late 40s. It rarely occurs in women younger than 20 years of age. Endometriosis appears to be hereditary, occurring more commonly in

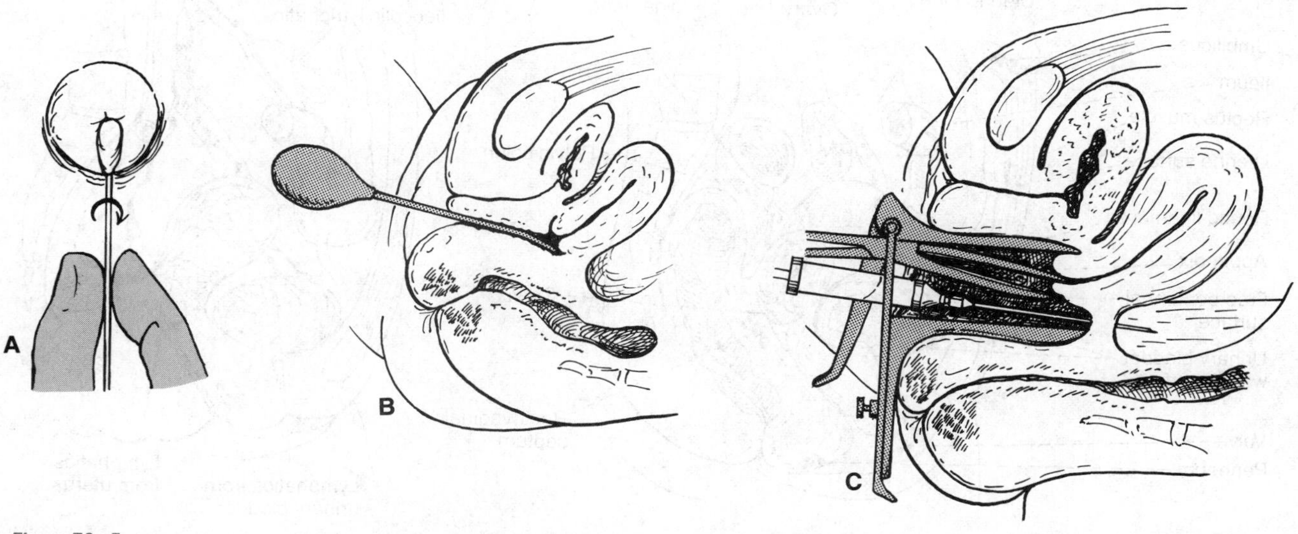

▲ *Figure 76–5*

Some procedures used to diagnose PID. *A*, Swabs may be obtained from the cervix, urethra, and rectum. *B*, The vaginal pool may be aspirated. *C*, Culdocentesis may be performed. Gram stains of cervical secretions show gram-negative intracellular diplococci. Cultures are placed on Thayer-Martin medium. Negative stains and cultures do not rule out gonococcal disease.

women whose mothers had the disorder. The highest incidence is in white women who are nulliparous.

Etiology

The exact cause of endometriosis is unknown. Several theories as to the cause of endometriosis have been proposed. One theory, the implantation theory, suggests that menstrual flow regurgitates through the fallopian tubes and deposits particles of viable endometrial tissue outside the uterine cavity. Spread then occurs via metaplasia (endometrial tissue reproducing itself).

The second theory, the vascular and lymphatic dissemination theory, proposes that spread of endometrial glands occurs through the lymphatic and vascular systems to locations outside the uterus. This may explain some of the distant sites of metastasis, such as the lungs and kidneys.

Pathophysiology

Although this abnormally located tissue is usually confined to the pelvic cavity, it also may occur in many other areas. The most frequent locations are the ovary and the dependent portion of the pelvic peritoneum. Rarely, tissue may be found outside the pelvis, such as in surgical scars, lungs, and extremities. Possible locations of endometriosis are shown in Figure 76-6.

Regardless of the location, this misplaced endometrial tissue responds to hormonal stimulation and bleeds, producing a variety of symptoms. Scarring and inflammation occur at sites of endometriosis. Repeated episodes of interperitoneal bleeding (from hormonal stimulation of the endometrial tissue) cause adhesions. Eventually, one peritoneal surface may become fixed to another.

Infertility is a major complication of endometriosis. Usually, the cause of infertility is unknown; sometimes however, endometriosis produces tubal obstruction.

Endometrial tissue is hormone dependent; therefore, the tissue atrophies with the normal ovarian regression associated with menopause. It also regresses during pregnancy.

Clinical Manifestations

Symptoms of endometriosis relate more to the location than to the degree of disease present. Pain is the most characteristic manifestation of endometriosis. However, about one quarter of women with this condition are asymptomatic. Pain typically begins before the menstrual period, lasting for the duration of menstruation and sometimes for several days afterward. Pain usually reaches its peak just before the onset of menstrual flow and during the first 1 or 2 days of the menstrual period. The pain may be located in a variety of areas, making the diagnosis more difficult. Unfortunately, some women with endometriosis are erroneously viewed as not having real pain and being neurotic.

Other manifestations of endometriosis include dyspareunia (pain during vaginal intercourse), menstrual irregularities, and infertility in the absence of tubal obstruction. When the condition occurs inside the ovary, it produces a chocolate cyst. Severe pain is associated with rupture of this cyst. Implants on the ureters may

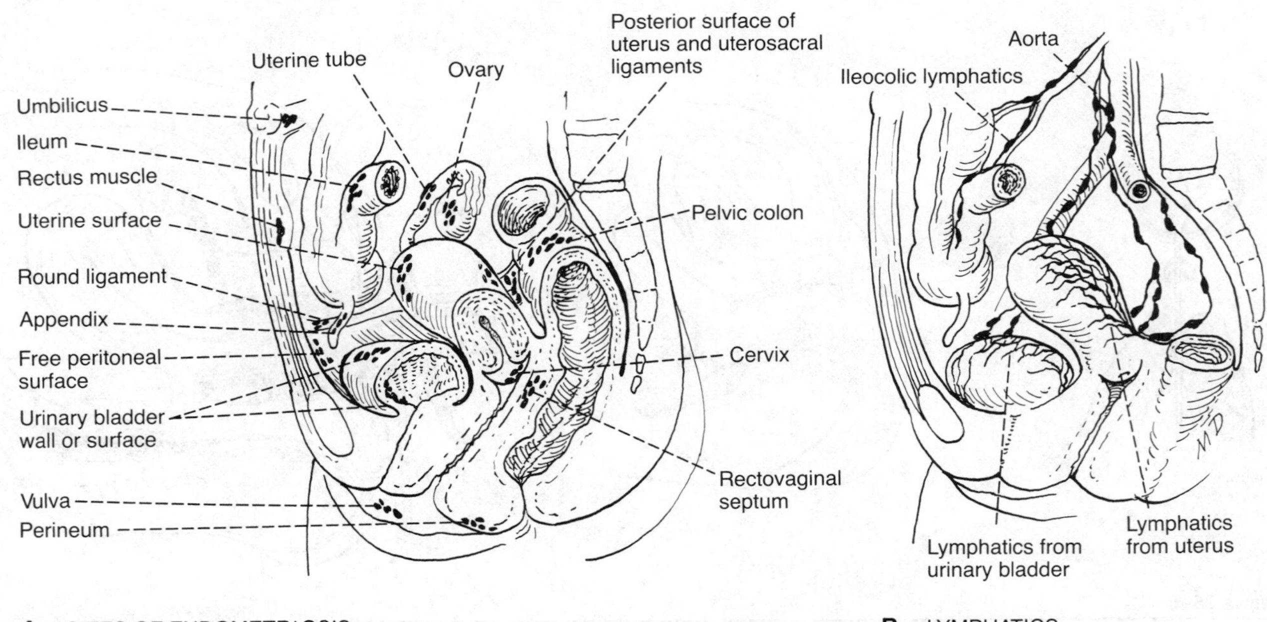

▲ *Figure 76-6*

Endometriosis. *A*, Sites of endometriosis. Those most frequently affected are the ovaries and the dependent pelvic peritoneum. However, as can be seen, many other sites can also be involved. *B*, Pelvic and lymph nodes are important.

obstruct them, whereas those involving the rectum may be associated with bleeding, diarrhea, or obstruction.

DIAGNOSTIC ASSESSMENT

Diagnosis is generally made by history, pelvic examination, and observation of lesions either by laparoscopic examination or pelvic surgery.

Medical Management

Appropriate treatment for endometriosis depends on the woman's symptoms, age, and parity. When symptoms are mild, the woman is given support, information about the disease, and some guidelines about ways to cope with the pain. Mild analgesics may be helpful. If symptoms become severe, more treatment is generally necessary.

PHARMACOLOGIC MANAGEMENT

Medication may inhibit endometriosis enough to allow pregnancy. Pharmacologic intervention includes inducing a pseudopregnancy with oral contraceptives, progesterone, or both. During the course of this treatment progestins cause the ectopic endometrium to slough off. Thus, the ectopic endometrial tissue no longer functions in abnormal sites.

The other hormonal treatment is to cause ovarian suppression or pseudomenopause. Danazol (Danocrine) is an antigonadotropin testosterone derivative that inhibits gonadotropin release and has other actions tending to cause the regression of endometriosis. The medication provides rapid and safe relief of symptoms, but it is very expensive, costing over $100 per month. It may cause side effects, such as acne, hirsuitism, weight gain, decreased breast size, and hot flashes.

Surgical Management

Exploratory or therapeutic surgery directed at the endometriosis may make pregnancy possible. Conservative surgical intervention includes restoring normal anatomy and removing or destroying endometriotic foci. A carbon dioxide laser may be used to treat endometriosis by vaporizing adhesions and endometrial implants. Even if she states that she does not desire future pregnancy, conservative surgery might be employed for a woman under 35 years of age, in case she changes her mind.

More radical surgery involves removing the uterus, as many implants as possible, and possibly, some ovarian tissue if severely damaged. This procedure is most commonly used in women between ages 35 and 45 who do not wish to retain their childbearing ability.

Even more radical surgery to treat endometriosis is removal of the uterus, ovaries, tubes, and as many endometrial implants as possible. Disadvantages of this approach include surgically induced menopause and permanent sterility. If the ovaries are normal and do not have endometrial implants, induced menopause often produces severe symptoms. This surgery is generally limited to women over age 45. Conservative surgery is effective for most women. More radical surgery is almost completely effective.

NURSING MANAGEMENT

Nursing care of the woman with endometriosis is individualized and depends on the severity of her symptoms, age, and childbearing status. Nursing care includes helping the woman during the diagnostic process as she considers the various treatment options.

Teaching should include discussion of information about the nature of endometriosis, its treatment, and ways to cope with the symptoms. If infertility is an issue, provide information and support in decision making in that area as well.

BENIGN UTERINE TUMORS (LEIOMYOMAS)

Definition

Leiomyomas are also called myomas or fibroids of the uterus. They are benign tumors of the uterine muscles.

Incidence

Leiomyomas are the most common tumors of the female genital tract. They occur in more than 20 to 30 per cent of all women during their menstrual years.[15] The incidence of leiomyomas in black women is 2 to 3 times greater than in white women.[37] Fibroids are more common in women approaching menopause.

Etiology

The exact cause of leiomyomas is unknown. The growth of the leiomyomas does seem to be related to estrogen stimulation because the fibroids often enlarge with pregnancy and decrease in size with menopause. Leiomyomas begin as simple proliferation of smooth muscle cells. It has been theorized that this proliferation is stimulated by physical or mechanical means and may occur at points of maximal stress within the myometrium. With the multiple points of stress within the uterus due to contractions, there are often multiple fibroids (Fig. 76-7).

Pathophysiology

Frequently, leiomyomas are asymptomatic. Symptoms that do appear generally relate to tumor size, location, or number. Additionally, abnormal bleeding, often resulting in hypermenorrhea, may be present and is related to the fibroid's hormone dependence.

Leiomyomas are known by various names (some not technically correct) related to the tissue involved

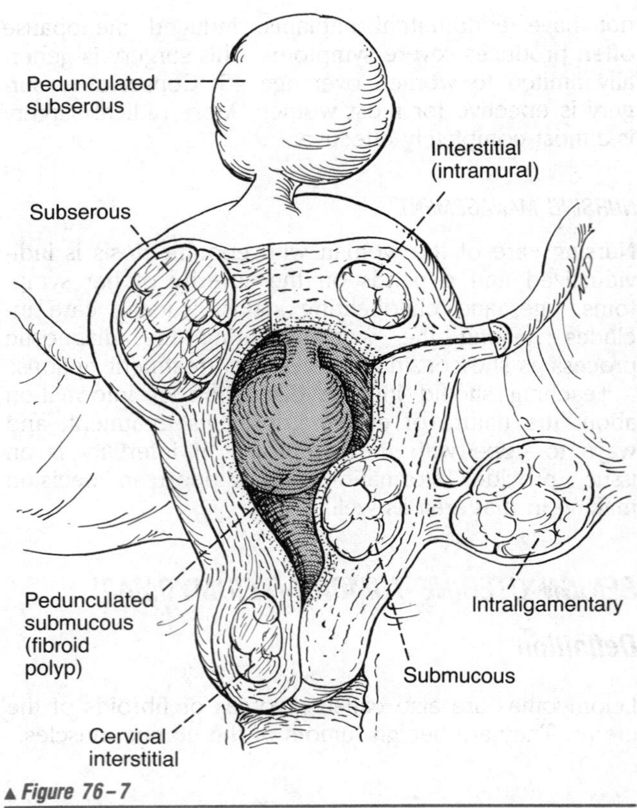

▲ *Figure 76-7*

Some locations of leiomyomas (fibroids). Uterine leiomyomas, depending on their location and size, may interfere with sperm passage and implantation of a fertilized ovum.

(e.g., fibroids, fibromas, fibromyomas, fibroleiomyomas, myomas, and fiber balls). Leiomyomas are composed mainly of muscle and fibrous connective tissue.

Leiomyomas may be classified according to their location. Those occurring in the uterine body are most common (Fig. 76-7).

Intramural. Intramural lesions are found in the uterine wall, surrounded by myometrium. Clinical manifestations may include increased uterine size, vaginal bleeding between periods, and dysmenorrhea.

Submucosal. Submucosal lesions occur directly under the endometrium, involving the endometrial cavity. The tumor may become pedunculated (grow on a stalk). Clinical manifestations may include prolonged vaginal bleeding, cramps, and possibly the tumor can be seen protruding through the cervix.

Subserosal. Subserosal lesions are found on the outer surface (under the serosa) of the uterus. These tend to become pedunculated, to wander, and to be multiple and large. Clinical manifestations may include backache, constipation, and bladder problems.

Wandering or Parasitic. These lesions occur when a pedunculated leiomyoma twists on its pedicle and breaks off. It then attaches to other tissues, particularly the omentum.

Intraligamentary. Intraligamentary lesions are implants on the pelvic ligaments, and they may displace the uterus or involve the ureters.

Cervical. Cervical lesions occur infrequently and may obstruct the cervical canal.

SECONDARY CHANGES

Secondary changes can occur with all six categories of leiomyomas. These changes include (1) hyaline degeneration, which occurs when the tumor outgrows the blood supply; (2) cystic degeneration, which tends to follow hyaline degeneration, when the tumors become liquified and ultimately cystic; (3) calcification, which is more common in large tumors; (4) infection, which is more common in submucosal tumors; (5) sarcomatous (malignant) degeneration, which is rare and is suspected with rapidly enlarging tumors, recurrent tumors, and when hemorrhage occurs with a known tumor; (6) red (cameous) degeneration, which usually occurs during pregnancy with clinical manifestations of an acute abdomen (i.e., acute pain over the area of the leiomyoma, fever, tachycardia, nausea, vomiting, and abdominal rigidity); (7) acute torsion of the pedicle, which leads to acute disruption of the blood supply, with gangrenous changes and symptoms of acute abdomen; and (8) fatty degeneration, which is rare.

Clinical Manifestations

Symptoms vary widely and occur in about half of women with leiomyomas. When they are present, they often relate to the size, location, and number of leiomyomas. The onset of symptoms most commonly occurs in the late 40s and early 50s, just before menopause. Once menopause begins, symptoms often cease. It is rare for symptoms to begin after menopause, when leiomyomas tend to regress. If new symptoms develop during these years, other diagnoses, such as cancer, need to be ruled out.

The most common clinical manifestation with leiomyomas is abnormal uterine bleeding, which is excessive either in amount or duration. Frequently, it is accompanied by anemia and is associated with tiredness, weakness, and lethargy. Urinary frequency is common when the tumor presses on the bladder. Urinary retention also may occur. Constipation, hydroureter, hydronephrosis, abdominal pain, and dyspareunia are less common symptoms.

Occasionally, the woman may have vaginal discharge. The discharge may be foul or watery and blood tinged. Abdominal pressure occurs if the leiomyoma is large enough to enlarge the abdomen. The tumor may be palpable. Also, the woman may have problems with sterility or a history of one or more spontaneous abortions.

DIAGNOSTIC ASSESSMENT

A characteristic history, confirmed by abdominal and pelvic examination findings, usually establishes the diagnosis. Ultrasonography may indicate an abnormal uterine shape. Various disorders, such as cancer or a problem pregnancy, need to be ruled out before treatment is planned.

Medical Management

A plan of treatment for leiomyomas depends on symptoms, age, location and size of the tumors, onset of complications, and the woman's desire to become pregnant. If a woman is nearing menopause and her uterus is smaller in size than that of a uterus at less than 12 weeks' gestation, the physician may assess the woman frequently (every 3 to 6 months) and hope menopause will alleviate the problem. Although malignant degeneration is rare, if the woman experiences rapid increase in the size of the leiomyomas, more definitive therapy is considered.

Surgical Management

Younger, asymptomatic women may require no treatment. However, when definitive treatment is indicated, it typically includes myomectomy (removal of a tumor without removal of the uterus), if the tumor is small, or hysterectomy (removal of the uterus). Uterine leiomyomas are a common indication for a hysterectomy. Three types of hysterectomy may be performed:

- *Subtotal hysterectomy:* All of the uterus except the cervix is removed. (Rarely performed anymore, but if it is performed, remember, the woman still needs Pap smears.)
- *Total hysterectomy:* Removal of the uterus and cervix. The procedure can be performed either abdominally or vaginally.
- *Total abdominal hysterectomy with bilateral salpingo-oophorectomy* (TAH-BSO): Removal of the uterus, cervix, fallopian tubes, and ovaries (Fig. 76-8).

A radical hysterectomy, which is performed only to treat cancer, is the same as a TAH-BSO plus removal of the lymph nodes, upper third of the vagina, and parametrium.

Nursing Management

ASSESSMENT

Many women may be asymptomatic; however, many will seek medical help because of some form of abnormal uterine bleeding. Obtain a thorough history from the client, especially concerning when the excessive bleeding occurs. Assess the woman's knowledge of her condition and the surgery, if one is planned. Pay particular attention to any question the woman has concerning sexuality after treatment.

Nursing Intervention

Nursing Diagnosis: Knowledge Deficit R/T surgical procedure and possible outcomes of surgery.

Planning: Expected Outcomes. The client will understand surgery and outcomes, as evidenced by client statements.

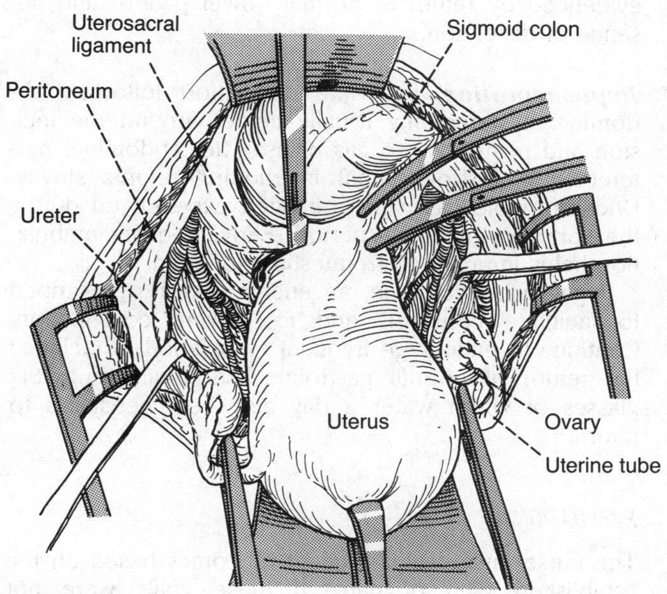

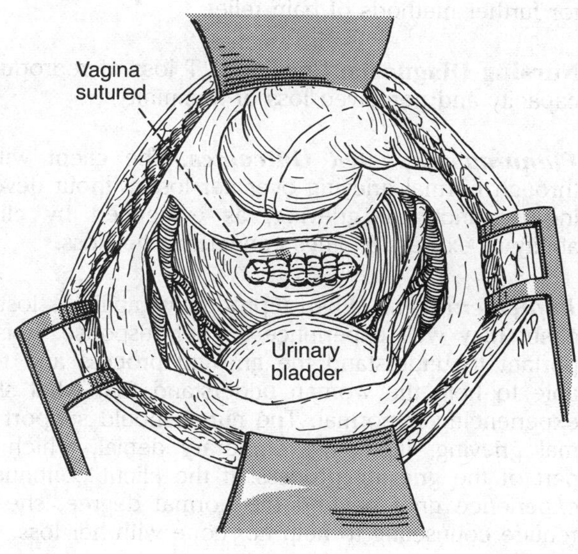

▲ **Figure 76-8**

Panhysterectomy with salpingo-oophorectomy. *A*, The uterus with attached uterine tubes and ovaries is lifted out after it has been freed from the ligaments holding it. *B*, After specimen has been removed en masse, the vagina is sutured closed.

Implementation. Frequently, a woman experiencing gynecologic surgery needs assistance in understanding her problem and the surgery being performed to correct it, either a myomectomy or a hysterectomy. She needs information as to what to expect postoperatively and how to care for herself.

If the woman is going to have a hysterectomy, she needs to understand that her reproductive capacity will be lost. If the woman is near menopause and is also having her ovaries removed, surgical menopause should be discussed with her. It is important to remember, however, that some women are relieved at the loss of the risk of unwanted pregnancy and the disappearance of severe symptoms.

It is particularly important for the woman to know that sexual intercourse will be perfectly normal following a hysterectomy. The woman should be told that once healing has occurred, intercourse should be pain free and orgasms are still possible; she has only lost her reproductive capacity. Answer honestly any questions the woman has and encourage her to express any feelings or concerns about sexuality.

Nursing Diagnosis: Pain R/T dyspareunia and pelvic pain secondary to multiple or enlarged leiomyomas.

Planning: Expected Outcome. The client will have pain relieved or controlled, as evidenced by client's statements of relief.

Implementation. The client can be taught ways to decrease pain associated with intercourse, such as altering positions, so that the leiomyomas are not pressed on during intercourse, and using of water-soluble lubricants with intercourse.

Pain medications can be used for severe pain. Sometimes, sitz baths or the application of heat to the lower abdomen are helpful in relieving pain. See Chapter 16 for further methods of pain relief.

Nursing Diagnosis: Grieving R/T loss of reproductive capacity and perceived loss of femininity.

Planning: Expected Outcomes. The client will go through normal grieving over her loss without developing dysfunctional grieving, as evidenced by client's ability to express feelings concerning her loss.

Implementation. When reproductive ability is lost, the client may well experience a grief response. It is important to understand the grieving process and to be able to help the woman understand that what she is experiencing is normal. The nurse should support normal grieving, including temporary denial, which is a part of the grieving process. If the client continues to experience grief beyond the normal degree, she may require counseling to help her cope with her loss.

Nursing Diagnosis: Urinary Elimination, Altered, High Risk for R/T infection with frequency and urgency.

Planning: Expected Outcomes. The client will not suffer altered urinary elimination or will have alterations diagnosed and treated immediately, as evidenced by normal output without evidence of a urinary tract infection.

Implementation. The proximity of the bladder to the female reproductive organs increases the risk that urinary problems might occur postoperatively. These problems are even more likely to occur if a vaginal hysterectomy was performed because of the pull on the musculature. A Foley catheter is usually inserted at the time of surgery to prevent bladder distention and injury during surgery. Sometimes, it is left in place for several days postoperatively. Potential problems that might occur postoperatively include urinary tract infection, difficulty urinating after the catheter is removed, and retention.

While the Foley catheter is in place, instruct the woman to keep the urinary drainage container below the level of the bladder, to drink at least 2 to 4 liters of fluid daily, and to report any urinary pain or discomfort. The nurse should check the urinary drainage system closely for leaks, provide complete perineal care every shift, and report any change in color or odor of the urine.

When the catheter is removed, observe for the first voiding, frequent voiding in small amounts, severe pain on voiding, inability to void, or hematuria. If the woman experiences any of these symptoms, report it to the physician so that prompt treatment can begin.

Nursing Diagnosis: Constipation R/T bowel manipulation during surgery.

Planning: Expected Outcomes. The client will not become constipated and will have distention treated, as evidenced by return to normal bowel pattern and absence of distention.

Implementation. Pain and discomfort following abdominal hysterectomy usually center around the incision and postoperative gas pains. After abdominal hysterectomy, gastrointestinal functioning returns slowly. Uncomfortable gas pains are often experienced during the early postoperative period. Early, frequent ambulation helps improve gastrointestinal function.

If gas pains continue, an enema may be prescribed to facilitate peristalsis and to prevent constipation. Continue to encourage frequent ambulation to facilitate the return of normal gastrointestinal functioning. Six glasses of warm water a day also help peristalsis to return.

EVALUATION

The nurse must evaluate client outcomes based on the established plan of care. If these goals were not achieved, the plan and interventions must be revised to meet the client's needs.

Post-hospital Care

DISCHARGE TEACHING

Be sure the woman understands the type of surgery she had and what follow-up is needed. If she had a myomectomy, pregnancy is still an option and she must continue to be followed with routine gynecologic examinations. If she has had a TAH-BSO, menopause and estrogen replacement should be discussed.

Discharge teaching should also include the following information:

- Perform prescribed abdominal strengthening exercises so muscles affected by surgery can be restrengthened.
- Avoid heavy lifting for about 2 months, to prevent straining abdominal muscles that are healing.
- Avoid activities that increase pelvic congestion until the surgeon says they are safe, such as dancing, horseback riding, and prolonged standing. Optimal circulation is necessary to promote healing of pelvic tissues.
- Avoid vaginal or rectal sexual activities and douching until permitted by surgeon. Vaginal or rectal intercourse or douching could interfere with healing of the vaginal cuff or other healing tissues, and introduce infection.
- Avoid constrictive clothing for several months.
- Report any bleeding to the surgeon, and any abnormal (other than nonodorous, whitish, or yellowish liquid) vaginal discharge.
- Return for follow-up care as requested by the surgeon.

FOLLOW-UP CARE

If the woman still has her uterus, she will need regular examinations to follow the progress of the leiomyomas.

ENDOMETRIAL (UTERINE) CANCER

Incidence

Endometrial cancer is the second most common genital malignancy. It is estimated that 1 in 100 women in the United States will develop uterine cancer.[1]

Etiology

Endometrial cancer is related to the hormone estrogen because estrogen is the primary stimulant of endometrial proliferation. The exact mechanism of malignant change has not been identified.

Risk Factors

There are many risk factors associated with the development of endometrial cancer. The greatest risk is for women receiving exogenous estrogen replacement therapy for long periods without concomitant progesterone therapy. Other risk factors include

- Obesity (increased estrogen production and storage);
- History of pelvic irradiation;
- Hyperestrogenism—early menarche, late menopause, dysfunctional uterine bleeding, delayed onset of ovulation;
- Old age;
- Other reproductive cancer, including breast cancer;
- History of infertility or habitual abortion;
- Family history;
- History of diabetes or hypertension;
- White; and
- Postmenopausal bleeding.

Primary prevention involves lifestyle changes, such as weight loss and proper use of estrogens. Early detection is very important to increase the rate of survival in patients with endometrial cancer. Encourage all women at menopause and older to have a yearly pelvic examination and Pap smear, although these tests are effective in diagnosing endometrial cancer only about 50 per cent of the time. Women at high risk should have an endometrial tissue sample performed at menopause and at regular intervals.

Any woman experiencing postmenopausal bleeding should be assessed as soon as possible. Women taking estrogen should receive the hormone on a cyclic basis, at the lowest possible dosage, with progesterone concomitantly.

Pathophysiology

The cell type in endometrial cancer is usually adenocarcinoma (involving the glands). An adenocarcinoma is a relatively slow-growing tumor that metastasizes late in its course.

Endometrial cancer tends to spread slowly to other organs. Most commonly, the carcinoma invades the uterus, entering either the uterine cavity or the myometrium. From the uterus, it can spread to other peritoneal structures, including the lymphatics and blood vessels. It can then spread to the vagina, through the lymphatics to other areas, and occasionally, to distant structures such as the brain and lungs.

Endometrial cancer may extensively invade the uterus, causing uterine enlargement. Extension of the cancerous process may occur along the endometrial surface to the cervix or the ovarian tubes and ovaries. After invading the cervix, further spread resembles that of cervical cancer.

If endometrial cancer is diagnosed early, its prognosis is relatively good. The death rate has decreased over the last 40 years resulting from regular pelvic examination and assessment. Once endometrial cancer has spread to the cervix, significantly invaded the myometrium, increased the size of the uterus, or spread outside the uterus, the prognosis is more serious.

Clinical Manifestations

Currently, there is no practical, accurate method to screen women for endometrial cancer. Thus, the cancer is usually discovered after the first symptoms appear. The most significant symptom is some type of abnormal uterine bleeding, especially postmenopausal bleeding. This occurs relatively late in the disease. Other symptoms relate to invasion, metastasis to other organs, or both (Fig. 76-9).

DIAGNOSTIC ASSESSMENT

A diagnosis of endometrial cancer is usually established by pelvic examination under anesthesia, followed immediately by dilatation and curettage. Dilatation and curettage is used to obtain tissues for pathologic analysis. Women at high risk may have periodic sampling via uterine washings. Occasionally, a hysterosalpingography (an x-ray study using a contrast medium to show the uterus and fallopian tubes) or a hysteroscopy (use of an instrument to visualize uterine contents) is used to assist with the diagnosis.

Medical Management

PHARMACOLOGIC MANAGEMENT

Precancerous endometrial changes may be treated with the hormone progesterone.

Chemotherapy and hormonal therapy with estrogen and tamoxifen (Nolvadex) is used to treat late stages of endometrial cancer.

Surgical Management

Endometrial cancer is generally treated with surgery, radiation, or a combination of both. Early endometrial cancer is surgically treated by a TAH-BSO. Surgery may be preceded or followed by irradiation, either external or internal.

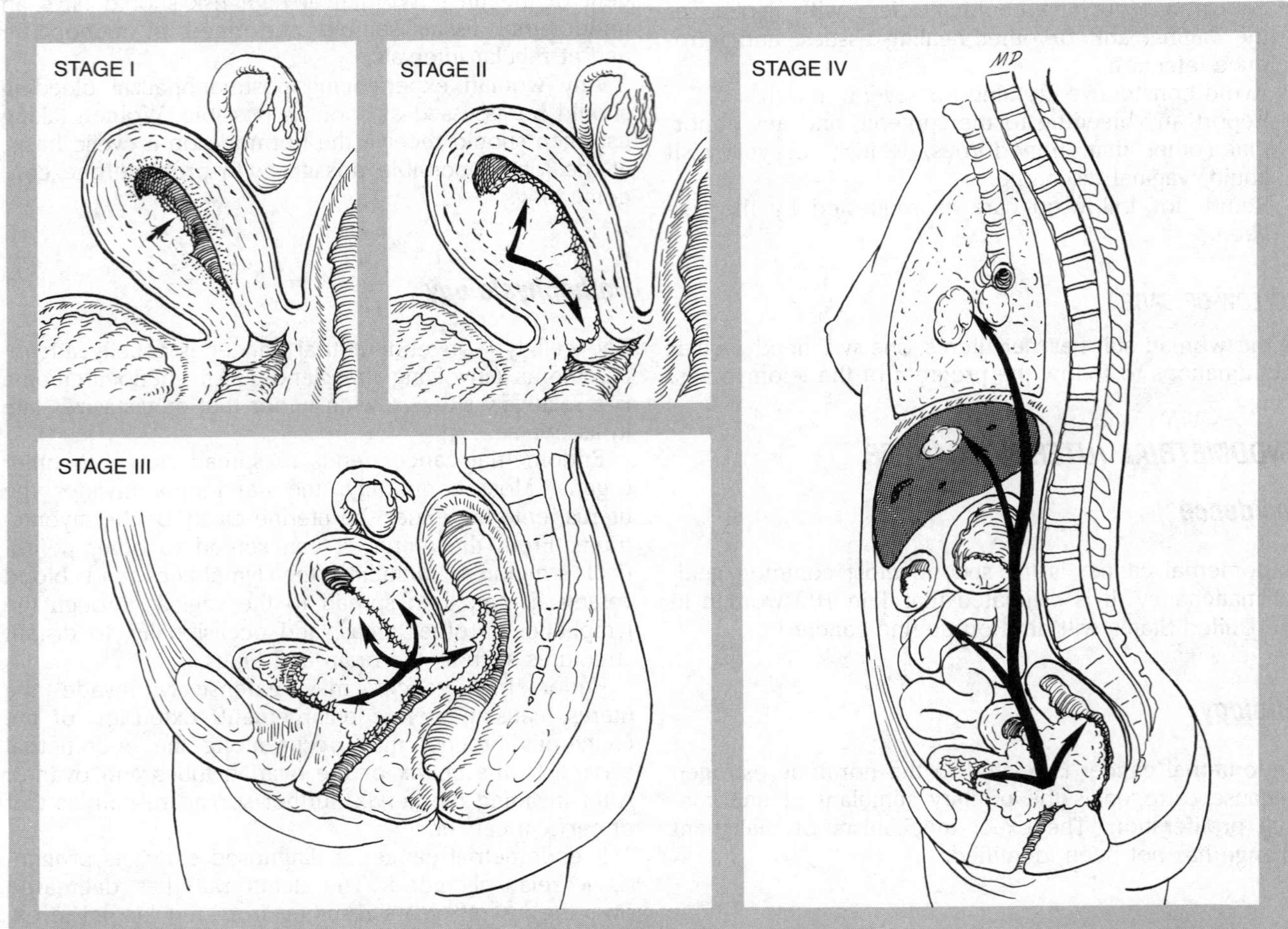

▲ *Figure 76-9*

Staging uterine cancer. Stage I: Tumor is confined to uterine corpus. Stage II: The cancer has invaded the cervix also. Stage III: The cancer has spread beyond the uterus, but remains confined to the pelvis, such as in the bladder or rectum. Stage IV: Highest level of invasiveness as the cancer has spread beyond the pelvis, causing metastatic disease and large masses, such as in the liver or lungs.

Nursing Management

See the sections on cervical cancer and uterine fibroids for nursing management.

CERVICAL CANCER

Incidence

The incidence of invasive cervical cancer has steadily decreased over the years, whereas cervical carcinoma in situ has risen. Death rates for cervical cancer have also dropped 50 per cent over the last 20 years; however, it is still the second most fatal cancer of the reproductive system.

Etiology

The exact cause of cervical cancer is unknown, although chronic irritation is often present prior to diagnosis of cervical cancer. There is a strong relationship between the presence of the human papillomavirus types 16 and 18 and cervical intraepithelial neoplasia. Cervical intraepithelial neoplasia has increasingly progressed to carcinoma in situ and invasive cervical cancer.

Risk Factors

There are a number of identified risk factors for the development of cervical cancer. Age is a risk, with the highest risk for carcinoma in situ at 25 to 40 years of age and 40 to 60 years of age for invasive cancer. Blacks, Native Americans, and prostitutes have a higher risk, as do those of lower socioeconomic class. Multiparity, early age of and frequent intercourse with multiple partners, early first pregnancy, postpartal laceration, untreated chronic cervicitis, and sexually transmitted disease are all potential risk factors. Women whose partners have a history of penile or prostate cancer also have a high risk. Jewish women and celibate women have a very low risk of the disease.

Primary prevention is related to good health practices such as the avoidance or early treatment of vaginal or cervical infections, limiting sexual intercourse, and possibly, the use of condoms to limit the transmission of sexually transmitted diseases and human papillomavirus.

Secondary prevention for cervical cancer is excellent. Regular Pap smears are an excellent method of early detection. This test is particularly important because cervical carcinoma in situ is potentially 100 per cent curable.

Pathophysiology

Potentially, all women with carcinoma in situ can be cured. Also, 90 per cent of women with nonmetastatic disease can be cured. Five to ten years may elapse between the preinvasive and invasive stages of cervical cancer. Most cervical cancers are of the squamous cell type. Squamous cell carcinoma usually begins at the squamocolumnar junction near the external end of the cervix. Some cervical adenocarcinomas occur but are more difficult to diagnose. Adenocarcinoma generally involves the endocervical glands.

Cervical dysplasia, the earliest premalignant change noted in cervical epithelium, is now further divided into several levels of cervical intraepithelial neoplasia (CIN): Mild dysplasia is CIN 1, moderate dysplasia is CIN 2, and severe dysplasia and carcinoma in situ are CIN 3.

Spread of squamous cell cervical cancer occurs first by direct extension to the vaginal mucosa, the lower uterine segment, parametrium, pelvic wall, bladder, and bowel. Distant metastasis occurs mainly through lymphatic spread, with some spread occurring through the circulatory system to the liver, lungs, or bones. The 5-year survival rate for women with cervical cancer is 65 per cent for nonlocalized disease.

Clinical Manifestations

There are no early indications of carcinoma in situ or early cervical cancer. An abnormal Pap smear, however, is an indication for further assessment.

Late assessment findings include the presence of vaginal discharge and bleeding, especially after intercourse. Metrorrhagia (uterine bleeding between normal menses), postmenopausal bleeding, and polymenorrhea (increased frequency of menstrual bleeding) may be present. However, early bleeding also may occur as spotting or contact bleeding from cervical trauma secondary to sexual intercourse or douching. This early minimal bleeding increases in amount and duration as the cancer progresses. It usually indicates that the disease process involves the lymphatics.

Vaginal discharge, which is normally watery, becomes dark and foul smelling as the disease advances. With infection of the neoplastic area, the discharge becomes more profuse and malodorous. Concurrent bleeding also adds to the unpleasantness of the condition.

Other assessment findings that develop as the disease progresses relate to areas involved in the malignant process. These include pressure on the bowel, bladder, or both; bladder irritation; rectal discharge; symptoms of ureteral obstruction; and heavy, aching abdominal pain. Fistula formation may occur as the malignancy erodes through the walls of adjacent organs. Pain is another late symptom. It usually becomes a difficult problem with the onset of the cachexia (general wasting) that often accompanies the terminal stage of cancer.

DIAGNOSTIC ASSESSMENT

The Pap smear is the primary diagnostic tool for cervical cancer. Further assessment of an abnormal Pap smear typically includes repeated cytologic and pelvic examinations. Also, colposcopic examination often helps locate lesions for biopsy. Biopsies are performed through a colposcope for better visualization. These biopsies are commonly performed as an office procedure and cause moderate discomfort to the client.

Less commonly, a Schiller test may be performed prior to biopsy. This test consists of cleaning the debris off the cervix and then painting the tissue with an iodine preparation. Abnormal tissue, which is glycogen depleted, does not stain. The biopsy is then performed by removing a bit of tissue from various areas, including all areas that are not stained.

Occasionally, biopsies may be obtained by performing cold conization. This may be performed when colposcopic examination is not considered adequate. Cold conization involves obtaining a cone-shaped section of the cervix with a scalpel. This procedure provides more tissue for analysis, thus increasing the chances of identifying any area of invasive carcinoma, because invasive and carcinoma in situ may coexist in the same woman. The procedure is particularly helpful if areas that are not readily visualized such as the endocervical glands may be involved.

Sometimes, analysis of the tissue removed during a cold conization demonstrates that a wide area of normal tissue surrounds an excised malignancy. When this situation occurs, conization not only serves as the diagnostic procedure but may be the only treatment needed. This procedure allows the woman to maintain reproductive capacity, which may be an important consideration. Cautery or cryosurgery (freezing of the cervical tissues) may be performed instead of cold conization.

It is vital that women receive careful follow-up care, including serial Pap smears. This is important because conization, cautery, or cryotherapy is not always sufficient treatment.

Medical Management

Irradiation is used as a primary therapy for early cervical cancer (see Chap. 22 for further information on radiation implants). It is usually curative but it induces menopause.

Treatment for women with cervical cancer during pregnancy varies depending on the stage of cancer, the duration of the pregnancy, and the woman's desire for pregnancy. A woman can usually complete the pregnancy if cervical intraepithelial neoplasia or carcinoma in situ is diagnosed. She may then be treated with conization 2 to 3 months postpartum if further childbearing is desired. However, if invasive cervical carcinoma is diagnosed in a pregnant woman, abortion is recommended up to 24 weeks in the pregnancy. After 24 weeks, therapy is delayed until the fetus is viable (28 to 32 weeks) and a cesarean section is performed. The woman may then be treated with either hysterectomy or irradiation in the postpartum period.

Surgical Management

Treatment ranges from cryosurgery or conization for local Stage O tumors, to a radical hysterectomy for invasive cervical cancer.

Cryosurgery is the local freezing of abnormal cells and tissues with volatile gases such as nitrous gases (nitrous oxide, Freon, or carbon dioxide). Cell death results from dehydration and cell membrane destruction. Dead tissue then sloughs off.

Conization is the removal of a small cone of tissue with a sharp instrument. Laser therapy also may be performed to remove the abnormal tissue. There is usually minimal bleeding; however, the client may note a slight vaginal discharge.

A total abdominal hysterectomy can be used to treat carcinoma in situ in women who have finished childbearing. A radical hysterectomy can be used to treat invasive cancer. A pelvic exenteration, an extremely radical procedure, can also be performed. A total pelvic exenteration involves removal of all pelvic organs, including the uterus, tubes, ovaries, vagina, bladder, rectum, and colon. An ileal conduit and ileostomy are formed. With an anterior exenteration, the rectum and colon are left intact, but all other pelvic organs are removed and an ileal conduit is formed. In a posterior exenteration, the bladder is left intact but other pelvic organs are removed and an ileostomy is formed.

Nursing Management

Care of the client with a hysterectomy is discussed in the section on uterine fibroids. See Chapter 22 for the nursing management of a client receiving an internal radiation implant. For women undergoing a pelvic exenteration, see Chapter 49 for care of the client with an ileal conduit and Chapter 55 for care of a client with a colostomy or ileostomy.

Irradiation thins the vaginal epithelium and reduces vaginal lubrication. It also may cause vaginal adhesions and stenosis. Such changes can make vaginal sexual activities uncomfortable or painful. Vaginal penetration during the course of irradiation and the subsequent months minimizes the possibility of vaginal stenosis and contracture. Depending on personal preference, vaginal penetration and dilation can be accomplished with the woman's own fingers, a vaginal dilator, or her sexual partner's fingers or penis.

Nursing preparation of a woman for cryosurgery and laser therapy involves clarifying that this procedure is not actual surgery and an incision will not be made. Explain that the procedure is performed with a vaginal speculum in place, as during a routine pelvic examination. During treatment, a few women experience headaches, dizziness, flushing, and some cramping.

During the procedure, provide psychosocial support by (1) staying with the client; (2) informing her of what is to be done; (3) talking with her, listening to her, and facilitating her expression of concerns; (4) continuing to acknowledge the woman's presence during the procedure rather than excluding her; and (5) allowing the client to retain as much self-control as possible. For example, tell her what she can do during the procedure to help it move along quickly and smoothly. Also, discuss how she can help manage postprocedure discomfort, such as performing slow, deep breathing.

Assess the woman's discomfort during the procedure. A mild analgesic may be prescribed for the pain following the procedure. Tell the client what to expect afterward. Mild pain may continue for several days. A clear, watery discharge occurs. For about 14 days, this is followed by discharge containing debris (dead cells) that may be malodorous. If the discharge continues longer than 8 weeks, an infection is suspected.

Meticulous perineal hygiene minimizes the risk of infection and makes the client more comfortable. Healing takes about 10 weeks. Showers or sponge baths should be taken during this period; avoid tub or sitz baths.

Following a radical hysterectomy, the vagina is shortened and the trigone region of the bladder and the sigmoid colon may adhere to the vaginal apex. This may cause dyspareunia felt deep in the pelvis. It is recommended that during penile penetration, the woman keep her thighs adducted and use her thumb and index finger at the vaginal opening to encircle the shaft of the penis, providing some extra length to the vagina.

Some women with cervical cancer become terminally ill despite vigorous treatment. When this situation occurs, goals change and are directed toward physiologic and psychosocial comfort. Pain relief (see Chap. 16) may be accomplished through adequate use of narcotic analgesics. Palliative irradiation also can be used as a pain relief measure in many cases.

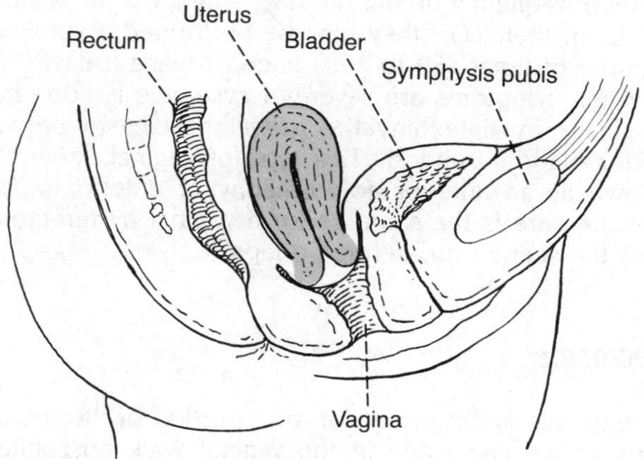

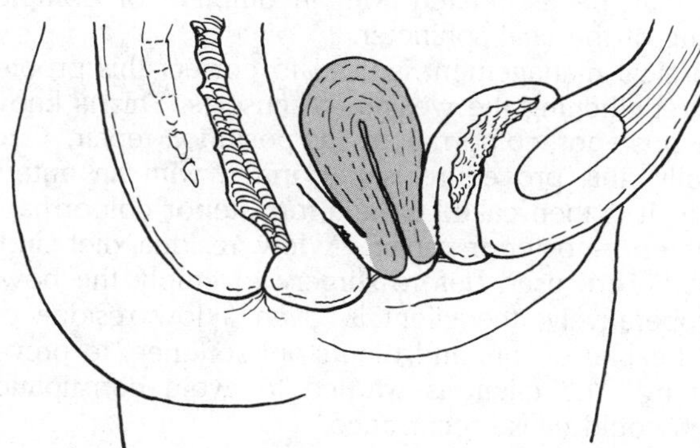

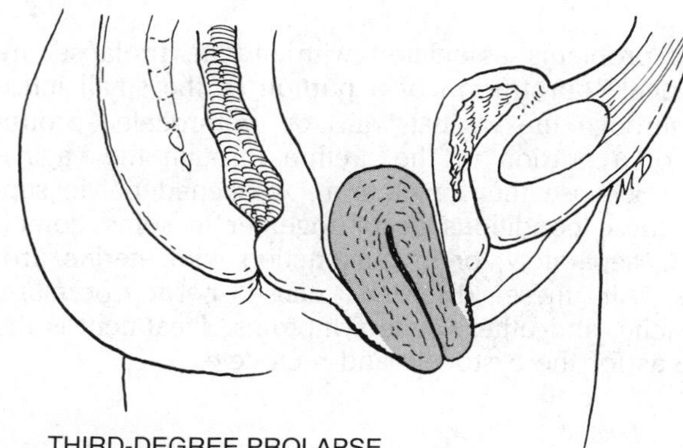

▲ *Figure 76-10*

Uterine prolapse.

Modification of Plan of Care for the Elderly

Older clients may have cervical cancer treated by less invasive methods, if possible. The older client undergoing internal radiation treatments should be monitored closely following treatment for the development of fistulas.

Post-hospital Care

FOLLOW-UP CARE

All women who have been treated conservatively for cervical cancer need information about recurrence. Encourage women who have been treated for cervical cancer to have frequent health examinations to diagnose a possible recurrence of the cancer early so it can be treated before it spreads too far. The client should have a pelvic examination and Pap smears scheduled at regular intervals as advised by the physician.

UTERINE PROLAPSE

Prolapse, descent, or procidentia of the uterus occurs in 3 stages (Fig. 76-10).

First Degree. The uterus descends into the vaginal canal, and the cervix reaches but does not go through the introitus (entrance to the vagina).

Second Degree. The body of the uterus is still within the vagina, but the cervix protrudes through the introitus.

Third Degree. The entire uterus and cervix protrude through the introitus, and the vaginal canal is inverted (turned inside-out).

Prolapse commonly follows multiple childbirths, childbirth trauma, aging, and failure to maintain the perineal musculature.

The incidence of prolapse has decreased with improved obstetric care (e.g., less use of forceps during delivery and better preparation of women for labor). The nurse can help prevent prolapse by (1) encouraging pregnant women to seek qualified obstetric care and (2) teaching women, after delivery, to perform the Kegel exercises.

During the descent of the uterus, other structures may be pulled down or out of position, such as urinary bladder, rectum, urethra, producing a cystocele or rectocele.

Cystocele

A cystocele is a protrusion of part of the urinary bladder through the vaginal wall due to weakened pelvic muscles (Fig. 76-11*A* and *B*). Urinary difficulties caused by the cystocele include frequency, urgency, or both; urinary tract infections; difficulty emptying the bladder; and stress incontinence. Mild symptoms may be relieved by pelvic (perineal) strengthening (Kegel) exercises. Kegel exercises may be prescribed to help a woman achieve pubococcygeal muscle control. This is a form of conservative treatment for mild stress incontinence. Instruct the woman to practice alternately tightening and relaxing her rectal and vaginal muscles. She should tighten these muscles as if she were trying to hold back a bowel movement or a stream of urine. Instruct her to hold this tightened position for a few seconds and then relax. These exercises can be performed frequently during the day, whenever the woman thinks of them. Or, they may be performed a specified number of times (50 to 100) once or twice a day.

When symptoms are severe, a cystocele is corrected surgically by tightening the pelvic muscles to provide better bladder support. This type of vaginal surgery is known as an anterior colporrhaphy or anterior repair. Nursing care is the same as for a vaginal hysterectomy (see the section on uterine prolapse).

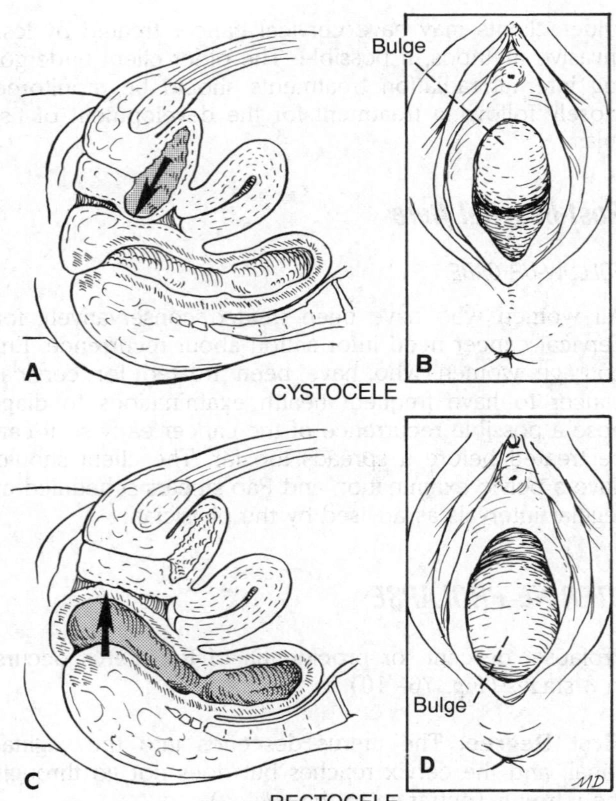

▲ *Figure 76-11*

A, Cystocele. Note the bulging of anterior vaginal wall. The urinary bladder is displaced downward. *B*, This pushes the anterior vaginal wall downward into the vagina. *C*, Rectocele. *D*, Note the bulging of the posterior vaginal wall.

Rectocele

A rectocele is the protrusion of a portion of the rectum through a weak place in the vaginal wall musculature (Fig. 76-12*C* and *D*). A rectocele produces constipation, heaviness, and hemorrhoids. Additionally, a rectocele may be associated with incomplete or complete tearing of the anal sphincter.

Surgical management is used to correct this problem by strengthening the weakened muscles. This is known as a posterior colporrhaphy or posterior repair. Occasionally, this procedure is performed with an anterior repair. It is then called an anteroposterior colporrhaphy or anterior-posterior repair. A low residue diet and a cathartic are used before surgery to empty the bowel. Postoperatively, the client is given a low residue diet until healing occurs and then stool softeners to prevent straining. The client is warned to avoid constipation, which could cause recurrence.

Enterocele or Urethrocele

Other problems associated with uterine prolapse are enterocele (protrusion of a portion of the small intestine through the vaginal wall) or urethrocele (protrusion of a portion of the urethra through the vaginal wall). Because they result from weakened pelvic support, these conditions occur together in some combination, separately, or in conjunction with uterine prolapse. All these disorders cause pelvic pressure, backache, and other vague symptoms. Treatment is the same as for the cystocele and rectocele.

Complete Uterine Prolapse

Complete prolapse of the uterus usually develops gradually. When it is complete and also involves a cystocele, rectocele, and enterocele, the woman is said to have pelvic relaxation. When the cervix protrudes through the vaginal orifice, it is exposed and constantly irritated. Tissue changes occur, and malignant degeneration is possible. Also, the vaginal mucosa is subjected to drying, trauma, and irritation once it is exposed.

Clinical manifestations experienced by the woman with uterine prolapse do not necessarily correlate with the amount of prolapse present. However, most women with a significant degree of prolapse feel something is descending internally. Other findings include dyspareunia and vague abdominal problems, including feelings of pressure, dragging, and heaviness; backaches, and bowel and bladder symptoms. Stress incontinence also may be present.

Treatment for prolapse is insertion of a pessary or a vaginal hysterectomy. For a vaginal hysterectomy, an incision is made through the vaginal wall into the pelvic cavity. The uterus is removed from its supporting ligaments (broad, round, and uterosacral). The supporting ligaments are attached to the vaginal cuff to maintain the normal vaginal length. Special care is given to the Foley catheter to keep the bladder decompressed and pressure off the anterior vaginal muscles until adequate healing has occurred. When the catheter is removed, the woman must be taught to keep her bladder empty by voiding every 2 hours to help prevent recurrence.

Postoperatively, the nurse should monitor the client closely for excessive vaginal bleeding. There is normally a small-to-moderate amount of pink, yellow, or brown serous drainage or even a small amount of frank vaginal bleeding may occur. If heavy vaginal bleeding is accompanied by a rapidly distending, rigid abdomen, referred shoulder pain, and indications of shock, immediate surgery may be indicated. Other times of potential bleeding are the fourth, ninth, fourteenth, and twenty-first days following surgery as the sutures dissolve. If vaginal packing, a drain, or both are in place, the surgeon usually removes them in 24 to 48 hours. Often, postoperative sitz baths are prescribed, usually beginning the first postoperative day.

POLYPS

Polyps are pedunculated tumors arising from the mucosa and extending into the opening of a body cavity. Genital polyps occur primarily in the uterus and cervix (Fig. 76-12). Uterine polyps may cause hypermenorrhea, intermenstrual bleeding, and postmenopausal bleeding. They occasionally undergo malignant changes, particularly in postmenopausal women. Cervical polyps may bleed following vaginal intercourse and are prone to infection.

If polyps are asymptomatic, they may simply be monitored. Since cervical polyps have a pedicle, they are easily removed by snipping or ligating them. This procedure is usually performed in the physician's office. Uterine polyps are not easily removed because of their location within the uterus. Uterine polyps do not usually require removal, but if removal is needed, it is usually performed by dilation and curettage.

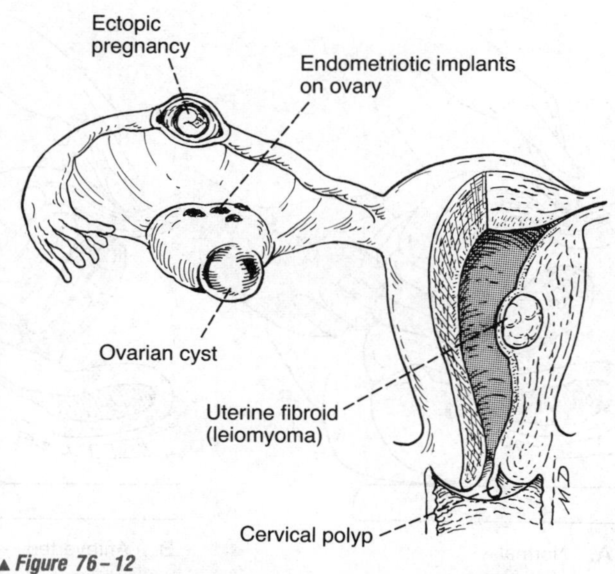

▲ *Figure 76-12*

Common sites of some common benign gynecologic lesions.

UTERINE DISPLACEMENT

The uterus normally lies midline in the pelvis and is symmetric and freely movable. The usual position is about 45 degrees of anterior flexion, with the cervix pointing downward and posteriorly in the vagina (Fig. 76-13*A*). However, variations occur from this typical position, some of which cause symptoms. The most common variation is a posterior displacement, referred to as retroverted (Fig. 76-13*D*). The uterus can also be anteverted (Fig. 76-13*B*), anteflexed (Fig. 76-13*C*), or retroflexed (Fig. 76-13*E*). Another common displacement is a downward displacement, or prolapse of the uterus (see Fig. 76-10).

Most women with uterine retrodisplacement are asymptomatic. Diagnostic findings, when present, do not necessarily correlate with the amount of displacement. They may include backache (accentuated by standing a long time or occurring during the menses), secondary amenorrhea, infertility, a feeling of pelvic pressure, and dyspareunia. Pelvic congestion and adhesions may cause some of these symptoms because the uterus is less mobile than normal.

Treatment for uterine retrodisplacement is directed toward the underlying cause, if it can be determined. Some women, particularly those who have recently given birth, may be helped by exercise therapy. Assuming a knee-chest position for a few minutes several times each day may correct mild retrodisplacement.

Although it is used infrequently, a vaginal pessary may be prescribed. This device is used to hold the uterus in the correct position. Pessaries come in different sizes and styles. After manually moving the uterus into a normal position, a pessary is inserted to keep it in place. A correctly inserted pessary cannot be felt and maintains the uterine position by holding the cervix posteriorly, which allows the uterus to fall forward. Before leaving the clinician's office, the woman should

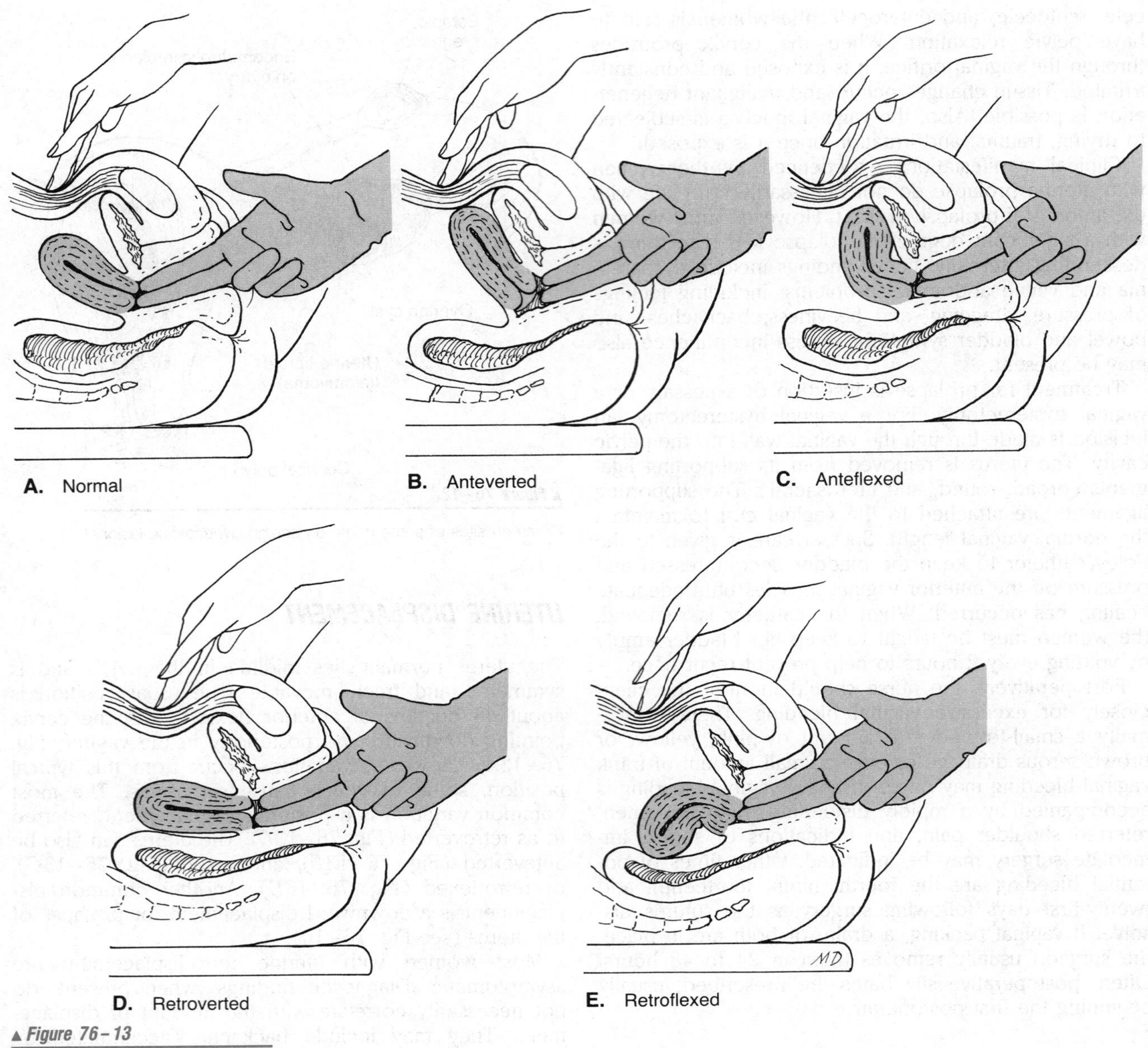

▲ Figure 76–13
Displaced positions of the uterus.

have a pelvic examination to ensure the pessary stays in place during bodily movements and that it does not interfere with urination.

A pessary irritates the vaginal mucosa. Therefore, instruct the client to douche twice a week with commercially prepared solutions of the proper pH or with vinegar, 1 tablespoon per pint of water, to remove vaginal debris. Follow-up care is important. Four to six weeks following insertion of a pessary, the woman needs professional reassessment. At that time, the clinician performs a pelvic examination to assess whether or not the pessary is irritating the tissues excessively. It may be changed or removed as indicated.

If it is left in place too long, a pessary may erode the cervix and adhere to the mucosa. Make sure that the woman understands the need for frequent check-ups. The pessary should be checked, removed, and cleaned every 3 to 4 months. Some women can be taught to do this themselves, but most will need assistance.

▼ OVARIAN DISORDERS

BENIGN OVARIAN TUMORS

Benign ovarian tumors are either solid or cystic in nature. Ovarian tumors are often asymptomatic until they are large enough to cause pelvic pressure. This makes early detection of malignancies difficult. Typical symptoms associated with pressure include constipation, urinary frequency, a full feeling in the abdomen, vague pelvic aching and sensations of heaviness, painful defecation, and dyspareunia. Acute pain may be experienced during menses. Often, the woman's abdominal girth increases and her clothes may not fit as well. Generally, the woman is unable to become pregnant.

Later symptoms include marked abdominal distention with dyspnea, peripheral edema, and anorexia. Pelvic pain may be present as a later symptom if the ovarian tumor is growing rapidly. If the tumor produces hormones, there may be menstrual irregularities and masculinizing or feminizing effects.

Complications from ovarian tumors include (1) hemorrhage into a cyst, with rupture and possible infection; (2) torsion of a cystic pedicle; and (3) malignant changes.

Treatment depends on the type of tumor. Tumors are removed surgically, either through a laparoscopy or open surgery, when they are bilateral, growing rapidly, and disrupt function of the pelvic organs or the ovary. Surgery may include removal of (1) only the tumor, (2) the tumor and the ovary or ovaries, or (3) the tumor, both ovaries and tubes, and the uterus. The amount of nursing care needed depends on the specific type of surgery performed.

Ovarian cysts are physiologic tumors of ovaries. They are common and may or may not produce symptoms. When symptoms do occur, the woman may experience pelvic pain that often is worse on one side, pressure in the lower abdomen, backache, and menstrual irregularities.

A woman with an ovarian cyst may be monitored for a month or two if her symptoms are not severe, to determine whether or not the cyst might regress without intervention. Explain the treatment plan and condition to the client. She also needs information about follow-up health care appointments and how to seek emergency care if needed.

Follicular cysts are caused by fluid retention in the ovarian follicle. They often are symptomless and frequently disappear without intervention. However, sometimes surgical treatment is required.

Corpus luteum cysts form when the corpus luteum fails to regress after discharging the ovum. Surgical excision of the corpus luteum is generally necessary. The remainder of the ovary can usually be saved.

OVARIAN CANCER

Incidence

Ovarian cancer is the leading cause of death from reproductive malignancies. The death rates have risen over time, probably due to the lack of early detection methods. Ovarian cancer ranks second to uterine cancer in incidence of female genital cancers. White women have a higher rate of ovarian cancer than black women.

Etiology

The exact etiology of ovarian cancer is not known, although there does seem to be a familial association. An environmental link has been suggested, but there is not substantial evidence at the present.

Risk Factors

Ovarian cancer usually affects women over age 40 and is rare in young women. Other risk factors include a family history of ovarian cancer, nulliparity, infertility, and a history of heavy menstrual bleeding and dysmenorrhea. Obesity, especially with a diet high in animal fat, is being examined as a possible link.

There is no effective primary prevention for ovarian cancer. Secondary prevention is also minimal. All women should have routine pelvic examinations including a bimanual examination. Women who are considered to be high risk should have a transvaginal ultrasound examination performed as part of their routine pelvic examination, and if this is suspicious, a Doppler study should be done. It has been suggested that women near or postmenopause who require a hysterectomy also undergo an oophorectomy.

Pathophysiology

Most ovarian cancers are epithelial tumors. However, some are adenocarcinomas. Ovarian cancer tends to grow and spread silently (without symptoms) until it causes pressure on adjacent organs or abdominal distention. When these pressure-related symptoms finally appear, the malignancy has usually spread to the fallopian tubes, uterus, and ligaments. Ovarian cancer often spreads to the other ovary and associated structures. The cancer may invade bowel surfaces, the omentum, liver, and other organs. When the pelvic blood vessels become involved, distant metastasis occurs. The usual routes of spread include lymphatic, hematogenic, local extension, and peritoneal seeding.

Ovarian cancer is the leading cause of death in women with genital cancer. Despite new treatment techniques, there has been no significant improvement in long-term survival rates for women with this disease.

Clinical Manifestations

Clinical manifestations of ovarian cancer include abdominal distention, urinary frequency and urgency, pleural effusion, malnutrition, pain from pressure caused by the growing tumor, and the effects of urinary or bowel obstruction, constipation, ascites with dyspnea, and ultimately, general severe pain. Indications of ovarian cancer do not typically occur until the malignancy is well established, which is often not until it has spread. Unfortunately, unless the malignancy is diagnosed early (e.g., when asymptomatic), most women eventually develop terminal cancer.

DIAGNOSTIC ASSESSMENT

Palpation of the ovary in postmenopausal women should always be considered an abnormal finding and should be followed up.

Identification of a pelvic mass by palpation is usually the first assessment finding. However, detecting such a mass may be difficult in obese women or those who cannot relax during the examination. When an ovarian mass is suspected, a complete work-up is performed, including an intravenous pyelogram (IVP) and a barium enema. Ultrasonography may be performed to detect a mass. Generally, following the work-up, exploratory surgery is performed to look directly at the ovaries, and if the mass is malignant, to resect it.

Medical Management

PHARMACOLOGIC MANAGEMENT

Adjuvant therapy varies with the stage of the disease. With stage I ovarian cancer, women typically receive irradiation or chemotherapy following surgery to destroy cancer cells that may have spread into the abdominal cavity. Intraperitoneal and systemic chemotherapy may be done (see Chap. 22).

Women with stage II or later ovarian cancers typically receive the same treatment as those with stage I disease, with the inclusion of pelvic and, possibly, abdominal radiation.

Surgical Management

The extent of an ovarian malignancy is determined by exploratory surgery. Ovarian cancer is usually treated aggressively. A young woman with a borderline malignancy may be treated conservatively with a TAH-BSO. However, generally the surgery of choice is a TAH-BSO, partial or complete omentectomy, and removal of all visible tumor. The less residual tumor left, the better the prognosis.

Some women with ovarian cancer recover following treatment. Commonly, women who are clinically free of disease and who have received chemotherapy for 6 to 24 months have a second-look laparotomy to decide whether or not treatment should be continued.

Nursing Management

See the section on nursing care of the client with a TAH-BSO for care of the client with ovarian cancer.

▼ VAGINAL DISORDERS

VAGINAL DISCHARGE AND PRURITUS

The female reproductive tract maintains its integrity through various natural defense mechanisms. Inflammation and infection occur when organisms disrupt or overcome these natural defenses. The resulting symptoms, although not usually life threatening, can be uncomfortable and annoying. Vaginal discharge and itching are among the most frequent problems women mention to health care providers.

All women have normal, nonbloody, asymptomatic vaginal discharge called leukorrhea. This discharge, secreted by the endocervical glands, is a clear exudate that keeps vaginal mucous membranes moist and clear. As this exudate passes through the vagina, it may become cloudy and acquire a slight odor as desquamated epithelial cells, leukocytes, and normal vaginal flora are added.

The amount of vaginal discharge often varies in relation to the menstrual cycle. It is greatest at ovulation and just before menses. Pregnancy, sexual stimulation, and oral contraceptives tend to increase the discharge. Some women view normal vaginal discharge and odor as offensive and go to great lengths to decrease it. However, excessive douching or using perfumed vaginal deodorants may cause vaginal irritation and infection. The consensus in medical literature is that periodic douching is unnecessary. There is some evidence that douching actually may be detrimental because it washes away normal protective mucus and bacterial flora of the vagina and may introduce other bacteria. Other changes in amount, color, character, or odor of vaginal discharge may indicate a problem.

The most common causes of vaginal discharge and irritation are vaginal infections; parasites, such as pinworms; sexually transmitted diseases (see Chap. 77); and mechanical or allergic irritants. An example of a mechanical irritant is a tampon left in place too long. Some forms of contraceptive creams or foams may be allergic irritants for some women.

Most inflammatory and infectious vaginal problems are accompanied by pathologic vaginal discharge, which may be copious, malodorous, and abnormal in color. It frequently leaks from the vagina, causing itching, irritation, and redness of the vulva and surrounding areas. It may be accompanied by burning and frequency of urination, anal discomfort, and pain in the lower abdominal region.

VAGINITIS

Definition/Incidence

Vaginitis is inflammation of the vagina, a common problem experienced by most women at some time in their life.

Etiology

Vaginitis occurs when (1) there is a change in the normal vaginal flora, (2) vaginal pH becomes more alkaline, (3) virulent organisms invade the vagina, or (4) some combination of these conditions occurs. Vaginitis can be caused by insults such as congestion of pelvic organs, mechanical irritation (e.g., foreign objects such as tampons), chemical irritation (e.g., strong douches), vaginal infection, overmedication especially with antibiotics (destruction of normal protective flora), and long-term steroid therapy.

Pathophysiology

The vagina is a potential cavity with a normal, protective population of flora, including various bacteria. For example, *Döderlein's bacillus* apparently helps maintain normal vaginal pH. The adult vagina is normally acidic because of lactic acid formed from the glycogen in desquamating vaginal epithelium. Normal vaginal function depends on a delicate balance between hormone and bacteria. Disturbance of this balance can precipitate infection.

Clinical Manifestations

Vaginitis is typically characterized by a change in vaginal discharge (i.e., it becomes profuse, odoriferous, and purulent).

DIAGNOSTIC ASSESSMENT

Vaginitis is diagnosed with a pelvic examination. This examination may be painful because of the infection and must be performed as gently as possible. Some bleeding may occur during and after the examination. Tell the woman that pain and bleeding may occur, and provide her with a perineal pad.

Medical Management

Vaginitis can be a stubborn, discouraging problem. It requires early, vigorous treatment to avoid chronicity. Treatment is aimed at correcting the cause of the vaginitis.

Nursing Management

Attention must also be given to the woman's overall health. Rest, sleep, good nutrition, exercise, and meticulous personal (particularly perineal) hygiene all assist treatment. Remind women to wipe the perineum from front to back to avoid spreading bacteria from the anus to the vagina. Instruct them to change tampons at least three to four times a day during menses and to wash their hands before and after each change. Warn women that feminine hygiene sprays can irritate the vulva. Soap and water are best for keeping the perineal area clean. Tight-fitting jeans, pants, pantyhose, or any garment restricting perineal ventilation may contribute to vaginitis. Changes in the woman's clothing style may be indicated.

ATROPHIC (SENILE) VAGINITIS

Atrophic (senile) vaginitis occurs in postmenopausal women. Atrophic, thin, vaginal mucosa and watery alkaline vaginal secretions provide an environment conducive to invasion by pyogenic bacteria (as in simple vaginitis). Assessment findings include discharge that may be blood flecked, a vaginal burning sensation, itching of the vagina and vulva, and dyspareunia (painful vaginal sexual activity). If secondary infection is present, vulvar excoriation and burning with urination typically occur.

Short-term use of diethylstilbestrol suppositories or estrogenic creams is the usual medical treatment. If a secondary infection is present, additional therapy with an appropriate drug is added.

VAGINAL FISTULAS

Definition

Fistulas are abnormal tubelike passages from the vagina to the bladder (vesicovaginal), rectum (rectovaginal), or urethra (urethrovaginal) (Fig. 76–14).

Incidence

Fistulas are an extremely distressing and common problem in the genital and urinary tract.

Etiology

Some fistulas are congenital; others result from injury or diagnostic or therapeutic surgery. Vaginal fistulas may occur (1) when an abnormal opening is present between two adjacent organs, (2) as a result of the spread of a malignant lesion, (3) following irradiation for cancer, (4) from venereal and other inflammatory diseases (rare), or (5) after a prolonged, difficult labor and delivery.

Clinical Manifestations

Urine or flatus and feces leak into the vagina. Excoriation and irritation of the vaginal and vulvar tissues occur. Severe infection may occur. Rectovaginal fistulas may cause an offensive, particularly unpleasant odor. The woman experiences wetness and a sensation of feeling dirty.

In addition to producing unpleasant physical symptoms, vaginal fistulas produce severely distressing psychosocial problems. Women with vaginal fistulas often become social recluses, greatly disrupting their significant relationships and other social activities.

Women often do not seek professional health care until the problem becomes severe. Even then they may be embarrassed and reluctant to discuss it.

DIAGNOSTIC ASSESSMENT

A fistulogram (injection of a dye into the vagina) can be performed to assess the exact location and extent of the fistula.

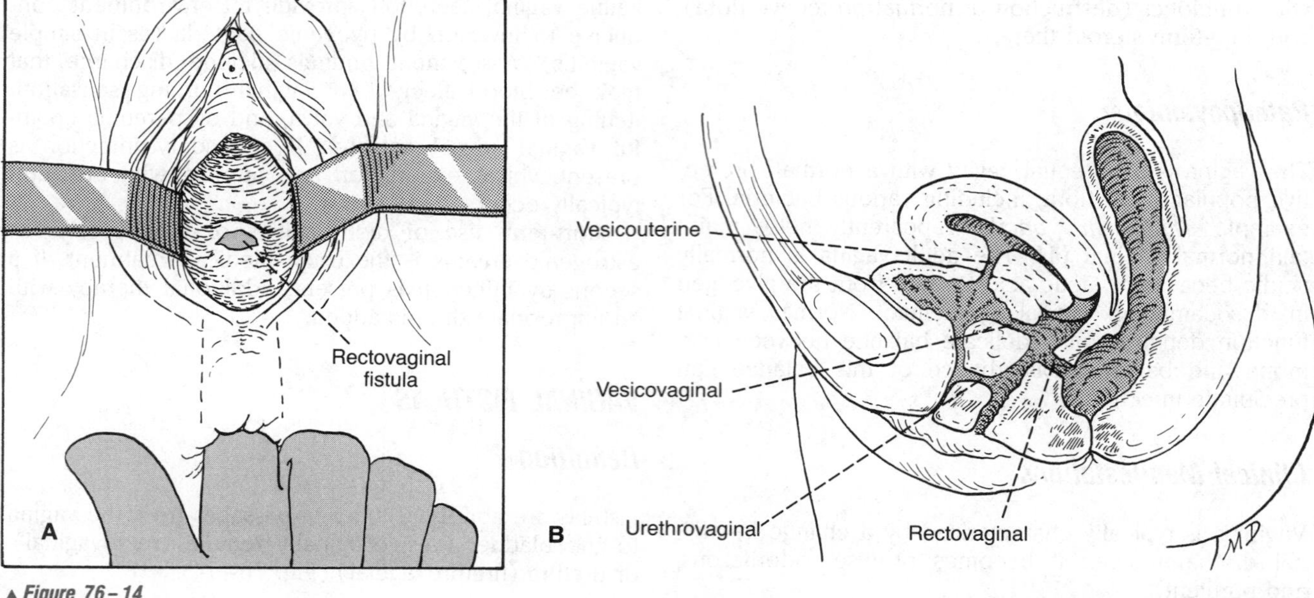

▲ *Figure 76–14*

Vaginal fistulas. *A*, During examination, a rectovaginal fistula can be seen as examiner's gloved finger (in the rectum) pushes upward toward the vagina. *B*, Locations of main types of vaginal fistulas.

Surgical Management

The diagnosis and treatment of vaginal fistulas may be difficult. Treatment varies with the fistula's location, extent, and cause, and the woman's general condition. Small fistulas may heal spontaneously after 1 to 3 months; however, surgical excision is often needed. Surgery is not always successful. For this reason, it is important for the woman to be in optimal condition before surgery is attempted.

A waiting period of about 6 months is required prior to surgery while the inflammation and tissue edema subside. Treatment during this time focuses on preventing infection by performing frequent, thorough perineal hygiene and improving the woman's overall health status. A temporary colostomy may be necessary to treat a rectovaginal fistula (see Chap. 55).

Nursing Management

An accepting attitude from health professionals toward a woman with a vaginal fistula is essential to help her comfortably accept and follow through with needed treatments.

During the time before surgery and again after surgery, the nurse helps a woman with a vaginal fistula to minimize the symptoms and care for herself.

Before surgery, some women inadvisably restrict their fluid intake in an attempt to decrease the drainage from a urinary fistula. This may actually increase the size of the fistula and increase the incidence of infection. Make sure the woman understands the importance of increasing her fluid intake to decrease infection. Perineal hygiene measures may include cleaning the perineum every 4 hours (with sterile materials after surgery), sitz baths, douches, and perineal pads (changed frequently). Deodorizing and comforting measures may include using vitamin A and D ointment, deodorant powders, heat lamp, and various types of prescribed weak acid or weak base irrigating solutions (depending on the urine pH). The latter solutions are poured over the perineum. Deodorizing douches (e.g., laundry bleach, 1 teaspoon per quart of water) also may be prescribed.

Caution a woman with a vaginal fistula to avoid using excessive pressure when douching because the water pressure may force the solution through the fistula tract, causing an infection.

Occasionally, an enema may be prescribed for a woman with a rectovaginal fistula to clean the bowel and temporarily decrease drainage. When an enema is permitted, a soft rubber catheter should be used. Gently insert the catheter above and away from the fistula tract.

Postoperatively, care is directed toward: (1) avoiding stress on the repaired area and (2) preventing infection. A Foley catheter is used after a vesicovaginal or urethrovaginal fistulectomy to drain the urinary bladder. Careful attention is necessary to keep the catheter patent and draining. Also, provide and encourage enough fluid intake for the woman so that internal catheter irrigation is accomplished. The catheter is not routinely irrigated externally. If the catheter must be irrigated, use sterile solution and minimal pressure. Do not let the catheter become occluded because this pressure could reopen the fistula.

Rarely, women require an ileal conduit following fistula repair (see Chap. 49). After corrective bowel surgery, the woman's first stool may be purposely delayed with liquid, low-residue diets. This prevents stress on the repaired area. Several days later, the client is given stool softeners and laxatives. Caution her not to strain with a bowel movement. Enemas are avoided because of the trauma they may cause to the repaired area.

Surgical repair of a vaginal fistula may not be successful even under optimal conditions. This is particularly true if a woman has extensive tissue damage from tumors or irradiation. Supportive nursing care is extremely important for women experiencing this distressing disorder and their significant others.

VAGINAL CANCER

Incidence

Primary invasive vaginal cancer is a rare lesion typically occurring in women over 50 years old. However, it is seen in younger women whose mothers ingested diethylstilbestrol during pregnancy.

Etiology/Risk Factors

Maternal ingestion of diethylstilbestrol is associated with clear cell vaginal adenocarcinoma in female offspring exposed to the drug in utero. Adenocarcinoma develops in these women generally between menarche and age 30 years. The use of diethylstilbestrol during pregnancy has been discontinued. It was widely prescribed in the United States from 1940 to 1960 for threatened miscarriage and other high-risk pregnancy problems.

Other possible risk factors include repeated pregnancies, syphilis, uterine prolapse, pessary use, leukoplakia, and leukorrhea. Vaginal cancer is rare in blacks and almost nonexistent in Jewish women.

Pathophysiology

Primary in situ vaginal cancer also is rare, and when it occurs, it is usually part of an in situ vulvar lesion. Secondary vaginal cancer is rare, but it may occur from trophoblastic disease.

The staging of vaginal cancer is similar to that used for other pelvic malignancies. The primary lesion and involvement of adjacent structures are considered. Primary invasive cancer tends to involve the anterior or posterior vaginal walls, or both. Complications may involve the urinary bladder or bowel, such as fistula formation.

Despite active treatment, the prognosis for vaginal cancer is generally poor. The overall cure rate reported by the American Cancer Society is about 35 per cent. One-half of the women with vaginal cancer die within 18 months of diagnosis.[1]

Low survival rates are due to (1) the rarity of the cancer (making it difficult to identify the best treatment), (2) the typically advanced stage of the cancer when diagnosed, and (3) the difficulty in treating this cancer with radiation or surgery because of the proximity of important adjacent structures.

Clinical Manifestations

Indications of vaginal cancer include foul vaginal discharge, painless vaginal bleeding, pruritus, pain (not associated with bleeding), and the presence of a vaginal mass or lesion. Urinary bladder symptoms such as pain and frequency may occur if a vaginal mass compresses the bladder.

DIAGNOSTIC ASSESSMENT

Women exposed to diethylstilbestrol in utero should receive careful examination of the cervix, along with cytologic examination of the cervix and any suspicious area in the vagina. Colposcopy may be used to identify areas to be biopsied. During pelvic examination, Lugol's solution may be applied to any vaginal areas that appear abnormal. Lack of staining identifies suspect areas. Unfortunately, the lesions of vaginal cancer are often well advanced before symptoms appear. Earlier lesions might be missed during pelvic examination.

Medical Management

The usual treatment for vaginal cancer is either external or intravaginal radiation therapy or, less often, surgery. External radiation therapy is used for all stages of vaginal cancer. Internal radiation is generally used only in the earlier stages.

The difficulty of applying radiation to the vagina without harming adjacent tissues (e.g., bladder, rectum) has led some physicians to prefer surgical intervention.

Surgical Management

For earlier stages, radical hysterectomy, lymphadenectomy, and vaginectomy are used. Vaginectomy refers to removal of the upper one third to one half of the vagina as part of the procedure in a radical hysterectomy. Pelvic exenteration (removal of pelvic organs, an ileostomy and an ileal conduit) is used in more advanced cancer when the bladder and/or rectum are involved. Pelvic exenteration is indicated when there are recurrent metastases.

Nursing Management

During assessment, ask young women born between 1940 and 1960 about medications their mothers may have taken during pregnancy. All whose mothers took diethylstilbestrol when pregnant with them should have a gynecologic examination at least twice yearly beginning at menarche, or at age 14, whichever comes first.

Vaginal surgery may be anxiety promoting and frightening to a woman. An ostomy (see Chaps. 49 and 55) also may need to be performed, adding to the woman's fears and problems. Postoperatively, vaginal sexual activity is not possible unless vaginal reconstruction is performed.

Sexuality is an important nursing consideration in the care of women with vaginal cancer. Vaginal sex may be difficult either after surgery or radiation therapy because of changes in the vagina. Assess the woman's previous sexual history and her self-esteem to identify any possible problems. Create a therapeutic environment that allows the woman to feel comfortable discussing sexual concerns.

Discuss the potential impact of the disease process and treatment on sexuality as appropriate. Potential problems include fatigue, pain, dyspareunia (secondary to radiation therapy), decreased libido, and/or altered body image (from surgery, radiation, or chemotherapy). If a partial vaginectomy (one third to one half removed) is performed, the woman can probably still enjoy normal vaginal sexual activity, using large amounts of lubricant and modified positioning, since vaginal tissue will stretch.

To cope with fatigue and pain, suggest that the woman schedule sexual activity after resting. Also, schedule pain medication so that the peak of action coincides with sexual activity. A warm bath, back rub, positioning, or relaxation techniques might also help. Advise the client to use a water-soluble lubricant during intercourse and, perhaps, a vaginal dilator at other times to prevent vaginal fibrosis and tightening.

▼ VULVAL DISORDERS

VULVITIS

Definition

Vulvitis (inflammation of the vulva) is caused by the direct irritation of vulvar tissues or by the direct extension of irritation from the vagina to the vulva. Itching and pruritus result.

Etiology

Vulvitis has many causes, including skin disorders, inflammatory problems, infection, vulvar kraurosis (dryness and atrophy of the vulva), vulvar leukoplakia (atrophic disease of the older female's external genitalia, with a white marble appearance of the skin, itching, and excoriation), vulvovaginitis (inflammation of both vulva and vagina), senile atrophy, irritation secondary to vaginitis, uncontrolled diabetes mellitus (with high amounts of sugar in the urine), pediculosis, scabies, allergies, psychological problems, cancer, ulcerative glandular or skin lesions, systemic conditions, urinary incontinence, and poor perineal hygiene.

Medical Management

Medical treatment is based on the specific cause of the condition. Itching (the most common symptom) associated with vulvitis can be severe.

PHARMACOLOGIC MANAGEMENT

Antipruritics or antihistamines, such as calamine or hydrocortisone lotion, diphenhydramine hydrochloride (Benadryl), or hydroxyzine hydrochloride (Atarax) may be given to relieve the itching either locally or systemically.

Nursing Management

The nurse can teach the woman measures to relieve itching, such as

- ► Applying calamine lotion and using hot compresses and sitz baths;
- ► Wearing light, nonrestrictive clothing, including well-washed and well-rinsed cotton underpants (synthetic underpants tend to keep the vulval area warm and moist);
- ► Avoiding feminine hygiene sprays;
- ► Applying prescribed hydrocortisone ointment or anesthetic sprays;
- ► Keeping the vulva clean and dry (e.g., cleansing after elimination — washing the vulva with soap and water, wiping with toilet tissue or wash cloth from front to back, rinsing and drying well, and applying cornstarch to maintain dryness).

VULVAR CANCER

Incidence

Vulvar cancer is found mainly in women older than 50 years of age. It accounts for about 5 per cent of female genital carcinoma.

Etiology/Risk Factors

Risk factors for vulvar cancer include a history of chronic vulvar dystrophies (leukoplakia), sexually transmitted disease, kraurosis (vulvar and mucous membrane skin atrophy, and dryness), diabetic vulvitis, and other primary malignancies, such as cervical cancer.

Early detection of vulvar cancer is very important. Significant changes are detected early by women who practice regular vulvar self-assessment using a mirror. Teaching the importance of such self-assessment is an important nursing activity.

Pathophysiology

Vulvar cancer arises from skin, urethra, glands, or subcutaneous tissues. Approximately 90 to 95 per cent of vulvar cancers are squamous cell. The rest are adenocarcinoma, Paget's disease, malignant melanomas, and sarcomas.

Vulvar cancer has a slow growth rate and remains localized for a long time. Most lesions are located in the labia, primarily the labia majora. Some are on the clitoris. Local spread may occur to the urethra, vagina, anus, and rectum. Lymphatic spread is to the inguinal, femoral, pelvic, and finally, periaortic nodes. The usual causes of death from widespread vulvar cancer are distant metastasis, urethral obstruction, infection, uremia, hemorrhage, and general disability.

The prognosis is poor with vulvar invasive lesions. Five-year survival rates of patients with vulvectomy and lymphadenectomy are approximately 65 per cent. Recurrence as well as distant metastasis may appear in the first 2 years. When lesions are diagnosed in an advanced stage with node involvement, the survival rate is only 8 to 10 per cent.[1]

Clinical Manifestations

Leukoplakia vulvae is characterized by thickened gray patches of epithelium scattered over the vulva and perineum. Cracked areas in these patches provide an ideal medium for infection that can lead to ulceration and maceration. Eventually, these areas may become malignant.

Kraurosis also can become secondarily infected. It is characterized by bright red, smooth, almost transparent vulvar epithelium. Kraurosis is most common in postmenopausal women. With its progression, the vulvar tissues shrink and constrict the vaginal opening.

Both disorders cause itching and soreness or pain, or they may be asymptomatic. Both are diagnosed according to appearance.

Clinical manifestations of early vulvar cancer include pruritus, minimal vulvar soreness, and tissue irritation with some bleeding. The potential seriousness of these relatively mild problems may not be appreciated by women or their health care providers because the manifestations are similar to those of nonmalignant vulvar lesions.

As the vulvar cancer progresses, clinical manifestations include vulvar edema and pelvic lymphadenopathy. Secondary infection may cause a foul-smelling discharge.

DIAGNOSTIC ASSESSMENT

Diagnosis is made from biopsy of suspicious lesions.

Medical Management

With leukoplakia, a biopsy to rule out cancer is indicated. In both disorders, infection is treated with an appropriate systemic antibiotic. Other manifestations are treated symptomatically.

Irradiation and chemotherapy are used less often than is surgical therapy. Irradiation is not generally used because the involved tissues do not tolerate it well.

PHARMACOLOGIC MANAGEMENT

Chemotherapy is typically given unless greater metastasis has occurred. The agent of choice is then based on the extent of metastasis.

Surgical Management

A vulvectomy is performed to remove abnormal tissue through procedures such as a skinning technique, local wide excision, or a simple or radical vulvectomy. A laser may be used in conjunction with these procedures to destroy specific abnormal tissue.

A simple vulvectomy involves the removal of the labia majora and minora and possibly the glans clitoris. Occasionally, the perineal area is also removed, requiring plastic surgery to cover the vulvar area. However, extensive surgery is avoided if the woman's condition allows a simpler procedure.

A radical vulvectomy (Fig. 76–15) includes excision of tissue from the anus to a few centimeters from the symphysis pubis (skin, labia majora and minora, and clitoris). Bilateral dissection of groin lymph nodes also may be performed such as superficial groin and deep inguinal, femoral, iliac, hypogastric, and obturator nodes.

Nursing Management

ASSESSMENT

For a woman experiencing vulvar surgery, psychosocial support is especially important and should begin preoperatively. Some problems the nurse might anticipate are fear of disfigurement, grief over the loss of a body part, fear of death, and sexual concerns.

Preoperative preparation is similar to that for other gynecologic surgeries, however it will also include an enema, douche, and insertion of a Foley catheter.

Nursing Intervention

Nursing Diagnosis: Knowledge Deficit R/T surgical procedure and outcomes of surgery.

Planning: Expected Outcome. The client will understand the surgical procedure and its outcomes, as evidenced by client's ability to correctly explain the surgery and expected outcomes.

Implementation. Preoperative preparation is important for a woman scheduled for a vulvectomy so she (1) understands what the surgery entails, (2) knows what preoperative procedures will be performed, and

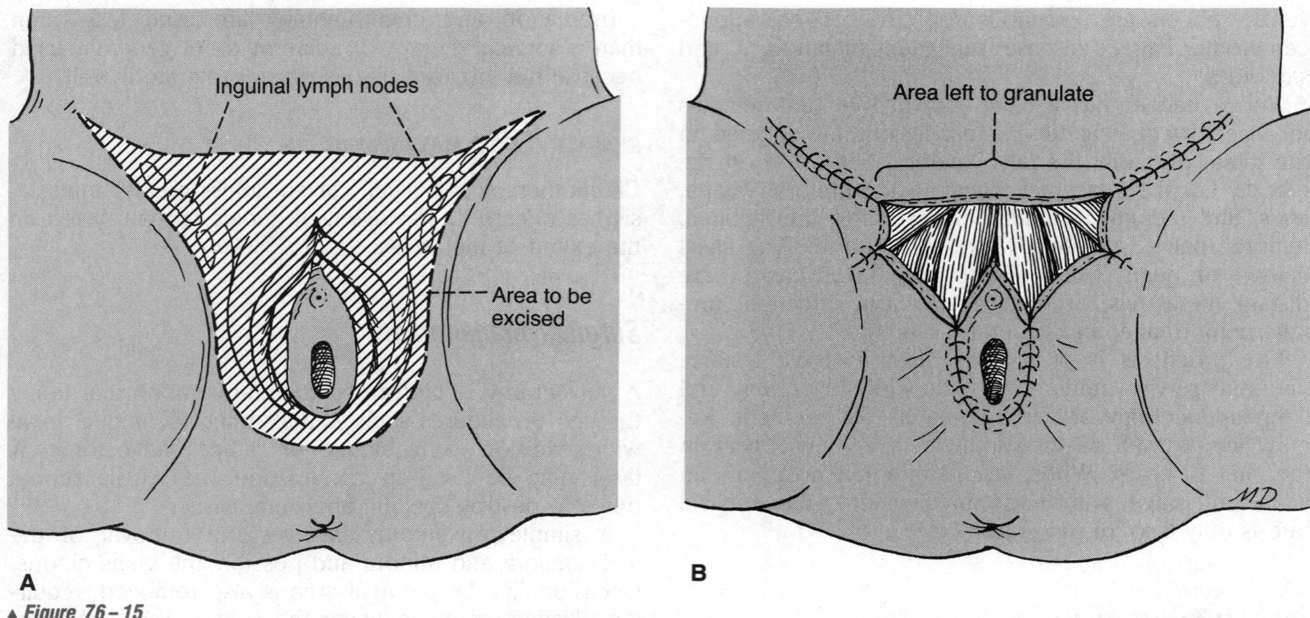

▲ Figure 76-15

Radical vulvectomy. *A*, Area to be excised and line of incision (dashed line). The vulvar skin, underlying subcutaneous tissue and muscles, and regional lymph nodes are excised. If the anus is involved, the incision continues around it also. Inguinal and femoral lymph nodes are resected en bloc. *B*, Completed surgery. Perineal skin is approximated to the vagina, and a large area is left open to heal gradually by filling in with granulation tissue. A simple vulvectomy (not shown) does not remove the lymph nodes. Hence, the incision does not extend into the groins.

(3) has an idea of what to expect in the postoperative period.

Nursing Diagnosis: Injury, High Risk for: Infection and/or Lymphedema R/T extensive surgery and dissection of groin lymph nodes.

Planning: Expected Outcomes. The client will not suffer injury, as evidenced by absence of infection, normal wound healing, and absence of lower extremity lymphedema.

Implementation. In addition to routine postoperative care, Hemovacs or drains are present in the incision to remove drainage and decrease the risk of infection. A bed cradle is helpful in keeping bed linens away from the incision. The woman wears antiembolism or sequential compression stockings to prevent leg edema and thrombophlebitis. Also, it is important that she perform leg exercises to prevent circulatory problems.

Prevent infection in the incisional area through frequent dressing changes, perineal care (a Foley catheter is usually in place 7 to 14 days or until adequate healing has occurred) or sitz baths after voiding and bowel movements, and meticulous wound care. Carefully monitor urination and bowel movements, with supportive care to prevent problems.

Long-term physical complications of radical vulvectomy include edema of the lower extremities. Reduce lower extremity edema by applying support stockings or using sequential pressure devices. Keep the legs elevated as much as possible. Teach the client to avoid sitting with the legs dependent, standing, or crossing the legs.

Nursing Diagnosis: Body Image Disturbance, High Risk for R/T radical surgery and loss of external genitalia.

Planning: Expected Outcomes. The client will maintain a normal self-concept and body image, as evidenced by client's ability to look at wound and to express concerns about bodily alterations.

Implementation. Psychosocially, a vulvectomy may be a devastating experience for a woman because of its direct impact on the external genitalia. The surgery, especially a radical vulvectomy, may compromise the client's physical integrity and her sense of wholeness. Some important issues for a woman include (1) fear of recurrence and metastasis, (2) disfigurement, (3) concern over future sexual ability, and (4) fear of her partner's rejection.

Nursing care involves assisting the woman to redefine her self-image to include the physical changes of vulvectomy. Try to create an environment in which the woman is able to express her feelings. Provide her with an opportunity to mourn the loss affecting her sexuality. Encourage her to resume her usual activities as soon as possible to reinforce her feelings of self-worth.

The surgery can lead to stress in social relationships. The woman and her significant others may need help in coping with the aftermath of this radical surgery. Significant others may benefit from inclusion in sessions when information and support are given to the client.

The impact of a vulvectomy on female sexuality has not been well described. The disfigurement of the surgery can lead to body image distortion that affects sexual functioning. Physical changes such as removal of the clitoris result in the woman's loss of the ability to experience orgasm. The woman may experience loss of sensation within the vagina. Also, introital stenosis may follow surgery making intercourse painful or difficult and having a major impact on sexuality. If stenosis is present, it can be treated with vaginal dilators. If dilation is unsuccessful, plastic surgery should be considered.

Sexual counseling may be indicated for some women and their partners. The nurse can assist the client and her sexual partner by communicating openly with them, answering their questions, providing them with information about structural vulvar changes, and suggesting alternate forms of sexual arousal for the woman.

Lower extremity lymphedema can cause a change in clothing size and an upsetting change in appearance. In addition, some women have difficulty sitting for long periods. This makes activities such as prolonged carriding difficult. Some women experience an unpredictable stream of urine following a radical vulvectomy. They must remove most of their clothing to avoid wetting themselves when voiding. Urinating into a funnel might be helpful.

EVALUATION

The nurse must evaluate client outcomes based on the established plan of care. If these goals were not achieved, the plan and interventions must be revised to meet the client's needs.

Modification of the Plan of Care for the Elderly Client

An older woman is less likely to have radical excision because of the potential for poor wound healing. If she does have the radical surgery, the nurse needs to monitor her very closely for the development of complications.

Post-hospital Care

DISCHARGE TEACHING

Postoperative discharge instructions should include the following information:

- Avoiding strenuous exercises involving the legs and pelvis.
- Gradually resuming normal physical activities.
- Resuming sexual activity, if desired, after the surgeon indicates. If intercourse is resumed, top or side positions are preferable to avoid direct pressure on the operative area. Water-soluble lubricants can be used for comfort.
- Taking showers rather than tub baths. Showers reduce the likelihood of postoperative wound infection. Gentle, thorough washing of the genital area is important. Wipe gently from front to back after bowel movements and urinating. Do not douche without permission from the surgeon.
- Notifying the surgeon if any of the following problems occur, such as (1) perineal pain unrelieved by prescribed medication; (2) foul-smelling perineal discharge; (3) heavy perineal bleeding or clots; (4) foul odor from the incision; (5) change in color of incision (especially signs of decreased circulation); (6) swelling of groin or genital area; (7) frequent urinating, urinating in small amounts, or discomfort or burning on urination; (8) temperature 100° F or higher; and (9) pain, tenderness, or redness in the calves.

FOLLOW-UP CARE

The client is closely followed for proper wound healing. Once healing has occurred, the woman may require reconstructive surgery.

BARTHOLINITIS

Inflammation of Bartholin's glands can be caused by various organisms, including gonococci, streptococci, staphylococci, and *E. coli*. The infection involves the duct of the gland, producing edema and, eventually, obstruction. Because the inflamed gland cannot drain, it swells and an abscess forms. Cellulitis develops in the surrounding tissues, producing more pain and systemic symptoms. The abscess may rupture spontaneously or may require incision and drainage.

After the acute episode, occlusion of the duct owing to fibrosis and scarring causes secretion retention and dilation of the duct. It then becomes a palpable, mobile cyst that usually is not painful. Symptoms relate to the size, such as dyspareunia or pain on walking.

Systemic antibiotics specific for the causative organism are prescribed. Local heat with hot packs or sitz baths may help to promote drainage. Surgery may be necessary, such as either an incision and drainage or removal of the gland if cancer is suspected or for repeated infections with abscess formation.

OTHER VULVAR DISORDERS

Skin disorders of the vulva include many of those mentioned earlier as well as chemical burns, irritation with harsh soaps, genital herpes (generally, herpes simplex virus type II), psoriasis, folliculitis, and eczema. All are treated by removing the cause whenever possible and by the performance of excellent perineal hygiene.

Both the mite *Sarcoptes scabies* and the louse *Phthirius pubis* cause vulvar irritation. They are transmitted during sexual contact with an infested client, from infected bedding, or from toilets. Both the affected client and environment must be treated to get rid of the organisms and their eggs.

▼ OTHER GYNECOLOGIC DISORDERS

FALLOPIAN (OVARIAN) TUBE CANCER

Overview

The fallopian tubes are the least common gynecologic site for primary cancer. If it occurs, the woman is usually 45 to 60 years old. Secondary tubal carcinoma is more common. Generally, it extends from ovarian or uterine sites. Infertility and nulliparity have been identified as high-risk factors. Currently, there is no accurate, practical method for mass screening for this cancer. Both primary and secondary tubal cancers—like ovarian carcinoma—remain asymptomatic until late in the course of the malignancy. Fallopian tube cancer is relatively widespread. Its prognosis is poor.

Fallopian tube cancer is difficult to diagnose. Late assessment findings include pain, abnormal uterine bleeding, and a watery vaginal discharge. Typically a mass can be palpated in the pelvis. Symptoms can vary, making it difficult to establish an accurate diagnosis.

Management

Because of the late appearance of symptoms, treatment often begins late. The primary treatment is total abdominal hysterectomy and bilateral salpingo-oophorectomy. This is commonly followed by irradiation. Chemotherapy alone or in combination with irradiation may be given to women with widespread or recurrent disease.

GENITAL TRACT SARCOMAS

A very small percentage of genital tract malignancies in women are sarcomas most commonly occurring in the uterus and ovaries. Uterine leiomyomas are one type of tumor that may undergo sarcomatous degeneration. However, this is rare in relation to the total incidence of leiomyomas in women.

Sarcomatous lesions tend to develop in younger women (20 to 30 years old) and grow very rapidly. They metastasize, particularly to the lungs, and may result in death from pulmonary causes. Treatment usually includes wide excision of the involved area and normal surrounding tissue, at times followed by irradiation. The prognosis is very poor.

GESTATIONAL TROPHOBLASTIC DISEASE

Gestational trophoblastic disease is a continuum of neoplastic disorders. On the spectrum, these disorders range from nonmalignant trophoblastic disease to highly malignant trophoblastic disease. The various disease forms are called hydatidiform mole, invasive mole (chorioadenoma destruens), and choriocarcinoma (chorionepithelioma). All share the following properties:

- They come from the trophoblast of human pregnancy (trophoblast is a type of embryonic tissue that helps a developing embryo obtain nourishment from the maternal uterus).
- They represent invasion of the maternal host by fetal chorionic tissue (tissue of the human trophoblast).
- Fetal chorionic tissue produces a protein hormone called human chorionic gonadotropin (hCG). This hormone is produced in direct proportion to the amount of tumor present.
- Cure is potentially possible with chemotherapy. These tumors can undergo spontaneous regression. However, this is rare for choriocarcinoma.

Hydatidiform Mole

OVERVIEW

Hydatidiform mole is relatively rare: about one out of every 2000 to 2500 pregnancies. It occurs most often in women over age 40 and under 20. The risk increases after one mole has occurred. Hydatidiform mole is far more common in the Orient (1 in 25 in Taiwan).

Indications of a hydatidiform mole include

- Intermittent bleeding in the first trimester. Sometimes, this contains some characteristic grapelike tissue. Such tissue requires pathologic analysis;
- Excessively rapid uterine growth;
- Absence of fetal heart tones, a fetal skeleton, and fetal movement; and
- Spontaneous abortion at about 14 to 18 weeks' gestation

There is a high correlation of hydatidiform mole with bilateral ovarian cysts, hyperemesis gravidarum, and toxemia, particularly during the first or early in the second trimester.

Medical diagnosis of a hydatidiform mole is made from a pathologic specimen. This is obtained either by spontaneous passage of tissue or by dilation and curettage. A persistently elevated hCG level in blood or urine is diagnostic. Also, it permits monitoring of the effects of treatment. If diagnosis is uncertain, ultrasonography, angiography of the uterine vessels, pelvic x-ray studies (showing absence of fetal outline), amniography, and serial hCG determinations help clarify the problem. Some of these activities must be used cautiously in case a viable fetus is present.

MANAGEMENT

Hydatidiform moles are treated by evacuating the uterus. This may be performed by dilatation and curettage, suction curettage, or hysterectomy. Follow-up care is of particular importance with hydatidiform moles and must be meticulous. hCG titer levels are checked frequently to make sure that metastatic invasion has not occurred.

Usually, hCG titers return to normal within a week of uterine evacuation. During early treatment, the titers are followed weekly, then every other week, and finally, monthly for a year. In some centers, women are also treated with a course of chemotherapeutic agents in an effort to ensure that metastatic invasion has not occurred.

Invasive Mole

Invasive mole (chorioadenoma destruens) is a neoplasm of the chorion (gestational tissue) with grossly visible invasion of the uterine myometrium and, sometimes, of adjacent tissues. Metastases rarely occur, and the disease is often benign. This disorder was previously treated with hysterectomy. However, chemotherapy is currently the treatment of choice. For this reason, a precise diagnosis is difficult to obtain because tissue studies cannot be performed. Diagnosis is made by history and other clinical symptoms. About 15 per cent of all molar pregnancies invade the myometrium.

Choriocarcinoma

OVERVIEW

Choriocarcinoma is a malignant neoplasm of the chorion characterized by its tendency to metastasize early, rapidly, and widely. Metastases occur with choriocarcinoma to the lungs (most common), vagina, brain or central nervous system (these respond poorly to treatment), liver (responds poorly), kidney, and spleen. Choriocarcinoma responds well to chemotherapy.

Choriocarcinoma is an extremely malignant, necrotic tumor. Its usual primary site is in the uterus. Choriocarcinoma develops later in about 3 per cent of women having hydatidiform mole. Trophoblastic disease refers to invasive mole and choriocarcinoma. Its symptoms can imitate other conditions such as ectopic pregnancy or threatened abortion.

The primary site of choriocarcinoma may also occur in the ovaries (or in the testes in men). These forms of the disease are associated with a poor prognosis and are not discussed here.

The clinical course of choriocarcinoma is capricious. Without intervention, it is rapid, and often fatal within 6 to 12 months. A few women experience spontaneous disappearance of the disease without treatment.

Presenting assessment findings with choriocarcinoma may include heavy vaginal or abdominal bleeding or may relate to metastasis, such as pulmonary problems from metastasis to the lung. Death typically occurs from problems such as respiratory embarrassment or hemorrhage into the tumor.

MANAGEMENT

Trophoblastic tumors are not radiosensitive. Methotrexate and actinomycin D are the drugs of choice in treating trophoblastic disease (invasive mole and choriocarcinoma). They are given in very large doses, with 1- to 2-week rest periods between courses of therapy. The response of the woman to treatment is measured by various laboratory studies and serial hCG determinations. When the hCG titer level has returned to normal for about two courses of therapy, the woman is discharged and followed closely on an outpatient basis.

Women with gestational trophoblastic disease (invasive mole or choriocarcinoma) require complex and expert nursing care. The disease process is confusing and frightening for the woman and significant others. Because of the rapid progression of the disease, aggressive treatment must be begun quickly. There is generally little time to adapt to what is happening. Often, the woman becomes extremely ill because of the toxic effects of the medications used. Women and their significant others need support, reassurance, information, and meticulous nursing care.

When trophoblastic disease occurs, the pregnancy will be lost, adding additional stress to the woman and significant others. The woman probably has a knowledge deficit about the disease, and also experiences actual normal grieving. Assess the significance of the loss to the woman and her significant others. Then assess well being and coping responses of the woman and her significant others to identify any dysfunctional patterns or behavior. Provide support by allowing the woman and her significant others to grieve, and by accepting or facilitating grief responses. Offer reassurance and provide information as the people involved become ready to learn more about what happened.

The prognosis with choriocarcinoma directly relates to the duration of the illness and to the hCG titer level at the time of diagnosis. If the duration has been short and the titers are low, and if the woman's medication regimen is carefully managed, the prognosis may be excellent.

Summary

Female reproductive disorders can occur throughout the lifespan. These problems can range from simple menstrual disorders to life-threatening malignancies. Primary and secondary prevention is particularly important for women with reproductive disorders, and the nurse can provide needed education so that women can become more aware of these approaches. The physical care of these women is important; however, the psychosocial care of these clients is vital. The effective nurse can assist the woman through what is often an extremely distressing diagnosis and treatment.

Nurses who need more information on reproductive issues can consult an obstetric text. Information on birth control, tubal ligation, abortion, and other issues can be found there.

Bibliography

1. American Cancer Society. (1992). *Cancer facts and figures.* New York: Author.
2. Baird, S. B., et al. (1991). *Cancer nursing: A comprehensive text.* Philadelphia: W. B. Saunders.
3. Ball, K. A. (1988). Laser endometrial ablation treatment of dysfunctional uterine bleeding. *AORN Journal, 48,* 1153–1164.

4. Benedet, J. L., & Sanders, B. H. (1984). Carcinoma in situ of the vagina. *American Journal of Obstetrics and Gynecology, 148,* 695-700.
5. Boarini, J. H., et al. (1986). Fistula management. *Seminars in Oncology Nursing,* 2, 287-292.
6. Bobak, I. M., et al. (1989). *Maternity and gynecologic care* (4th ed.). St. Louis: C. V. Mosby.
7. Booten, D. A., & Seideman, R. Y. (1989). Relationship between premenstrual syndrome and dysmenorrhea. *AAOHN Journal, 37*(8), 308-315.
8. Brown, M. A., & Zimmer, P. A. (1986). Personal and family impact of premenstrual symptoms. *Journal of Obstetric, Gynecologic, and Neonatal Nursing, 15,* 31-86.
9. Campion, M. J., et al. (1985). Increased risk of cervical neoplasia in consorts of men with penile condylomata acuminata. *Lancet, 2,* 943-946.
10. Celeste, S. M., & Smith, M. D. (1986). Gestational trophoblastic neoplasms. *Journal of Obstetric, Gynecologic, and Neonatal Nursing, 15,* 11-16.
11. Chamorro, T. (1985). Radical gynecologic surgery. *NAACOG Update Series, 3*(7), 1-8.
12. Charles, A. G. (1989). Estrogen replacement after menopause, when is it warranted? *Postgraduate Medicine, 85*(4), 99-104.
13. Diczfalusy, E., & Bygedman, M. (1987). *Fertility regulation today and tomorrow.* New York: Raven Press.
14. DiSaia, P. J., & Creasman, W. T. (1989). *Clinical gynecology* (3rd ed.). St. Louis: C. V. Mosby Co.
15. Droegmueller, W., et al. (1987). *Comprehensive gynecology.* St. Louis: C. V. Mosby.
16. Ensign, J. E., et al. (1988). Premenstrual syndrome. *AORN Journal, 47*(4), 962-971.
17. Eriksson, J. H., & Swenson, K. K. (1986). Your guide to intraperitoneal chemotherapy. *Oncology Nursing Forum, 13*(5), 77-81.
18. Feldman, B., et al. (1985). The prevalence of hot flash and associated variables among perimenopausal women. *Research in Nursing and Health, 8*(2), 261-268.
19. Foley, S. F. (1987). Preventive gynecologic nursing in an inpatient setting. *Journal of Obstetric, Gynecologic, and Neonatal Nursing, 16,* 160-166.
20. Fortier, K. J. (1986). Postmenopausal bleeding and the endometrium. *Clinical Obstetrics and Gynecology, 29,* 440-445.
21. Gannon, L. (1988). The potential role of exercise in the alleviation of menstrual disorders and menopausal symptoms: A theoretical synthesis of recent research. *Women & Health, 14*(2), 105-127.
22. Garner, C. H., & Webster, B. H. (1985). Endometriosis. *Journal of Obstetric, Gynecologic, and Neonatal Nursing, 14*(Suppl), 10-20.
23. Gosnell, D. (1987). Nursing diagnosis for oncology nursing practice. *Cancer Nursing, 10,* 41-51.
24. Griffith-Kenney, J. (Ed). (1986). *Contemporary women's health.* Menlo Park, CA: Addison-Wesley.
25. Gruhn, J. G., & Kazer, R. R. (1989). *Hormonal regulation of the menstrual cycle.* New York: Plenum Publishing Co.
26. Hamptom, B. G. (1986). Nursing management of a patient following pelvic exenteration. *Seminars in Oncology Nursing, 2,* 281-286.
27. Harper, D. C. (1990). Perimenopause and aging. In R. Lichtman & S. Papera (Eds.), *Gynecology: Well woman care* (pp. 405-424). East Norwalk, CT: Appleton & Lange.
28. Havens, C., et al. (Eds.) (1986). *Manual of outpatient gynecology.* Boston: Little, Brown and Company.
29. Heitkemper, M. N., Shaver, J. F., & Mitchell, E. S. (1988). Gastrointestinal symptoms and patterns across the menstrual cycle in dysmenorrhea. *Nursing Research, 37,* 108-113.
30. Jenkins, B. (1988). Patients' reports of sexual changes after treatment for gynecologic cancer. *Oncology Nursing Forum, 15,* 349-354.
31. Jones, H. W., et al. (Eds.) (1988). *Novak's textbook of gynecology* (11th ed.). Baltimore: Williams & Wilkins.
32. Kaunitz, A. M., & Grimes, D. A. (1988). The woman over 50: Endometrial sampling in older women. *Contemporary Obstetrics and Gynecology, 31*(Suppl), 85.
33. Lamb, M. A. (1985). Sexual dysfunction in the gynecologic oncology patient. *Seminars in Oncology Nursing, 1,* 9-17.
34. Lee, P, et al. (1988). Accuracy of Papanicolaou smears: Art or science? *Journal of Reproductive Medicine, 33,* 795-798.
35. Lichtman, R. C. (1991). Perimenopausal hormone replacement therapy; Reviews of the literature. *Journal of Nurse Midwifery, 36*(1), 30-48.
36. Lovejoy, N. C. (1987). Precancerous lesions of the cervix: Personal risk factors. *Cancer Nursing, 10,* 2-14.
37. Meyers, M. (1986). The enlarged uterus. In C. Havens, N. Sullivan, & P. Tilton (Eds.), *Manual of outpatient gynecology* (pp. 51-56). Boston: Little, Brown, and Company.
38. Murata, J. (1989). Primary amenorrhea. *Pediatric Nursing, 15,* 125-129.
39. Nelson, J. H., Averette, H. E., & Richert, R. M. (1984). *Dysplasia, carcinoma in situ, and early invasive cervical carcinoma.* New York: American Cancer Society.
40. Newton, M., & Newton, E. R. (1988). *Complications of gynecology and obstetric management.* Philadelphia: W. B. Saunders.
41. O'Laughlin, K. M. (1987). Changes in bladder function in the woman undergoing radical hysterectomy for cervical cancer. *Journal of Obstetric, Gynecologic, and Neonatal Nursing, 15,* 380-385.
42. Orr, J. W., & Shingleton, H. M. (1986). Effects of in utero exposure to DES: An update. *Your Patient & Cancer,* 9-15.
43. Ozols, R. F. (1986). Intraperitoneal chemotherapy. *Mediguide to Oncology, 5*(4), 1-5.
44. Robertson, C. (1986). Treatment modalities for gynecologic cancers. *Seminars in Oncology Nursing, 2,* 275-280.
45. Rostad, M. E. (1988). The radical vulvectomy patient: Preventing complications. *Dimensions of Critical Care Nursing, 7,* 289-294.
46. Saite, A. (1989). Cervical cytology in general practice. *New Zealand Nursing Journal, 82*(1), 18-19.
47. Smith, D. B. (1989). Discussing sexuality. *Oncology Nursing Forum, 16*(1), 106.
48. Stehman, F. B. (1987). The value of second-look laparotomy in ovarian cancer. *Oncology, 1*(8), 50-51.
49. Soules, M. R. (1989). *Problems in reproductive endocrinology and infertility.* New York: Elsevier Science Publishing Co.
50. Strohl, R. (1986). Practice corner: Advising women receiving pelvic radiation. *Oncology Nursing Forum, 13*(2), 86.
51. Sullivan, N. (1990). Dysmenorrhea. In R. Lichtman & S. Papera (Eds.), *Gynecology: Well women care* (pp. 345-353). East Norwalk, CT: Appleton & Lange.
52. Voda, A. M. (1981). Climacteric hot flash. *Maturitas, 3,* 73-90.
53. Wardrop, R. W., et al. (1989). Oral discomfort at menopause. *Oral Surgery, Oral Medicine, Oral Pathology,* May, 535-540.
54. Webb, C. (1986). Professional and lay support for hysterectomy patients. *Journal of Advanced Nursing, 11,* 167-177.
55. Wynn, T. M., & Jollie, W. (Eds) (1989). *The biology of the uterus* (2nd ed.). New York: Plenum Publishing Co.
56. Yasko, J. M., & Greene, P. A. (1987). Coping with problems related to cancer and cancer treatment. *CA: A Cancer Journal for Clinicians, 37,* 106-125.

Chapter 77

Nursing Care of Clients with Sexually Transmitted Diseases

SEXUALLY TRANSMITTED DISEASES

Definition

The five classic venereal diseases (gonorrhea, syphilis, chancroid, granuloma inguinale, and lymphogranuloma venereum) are now included with such other infectious diseases as trichomoniasis, chlamydial infections, genital herpes, acquired immunodeficiency syndrome (AIDS), and enteric infections in a broader category of diseases called sexually transmitted diseases (STDs) (Box 77-1). The newer term now encompasses the broad range of conditions that are usually or can be transmitted by genital, oral, or anal sexual contact. The number of diseases in this category increases as new agents are implicated in the sexual transmission of disease.

STDs share several characteristics: (1) despite their biologic differences, they are transmitted by sexual activities (not only by vaginal/penile but also by other oral and anal sexual activities between same or opposite sex partners); (2) all sexual partners of the infected client need to be assessed for treatment; and (3) the diseases frequently coexist in the same client (e.g., a client may have both chlamydial infection and gonorrhea). The last fact may be responsible for some treatment failures. Current treatment guidelines for STDs are available in the United States from the division of STD, Centers for Disease Control (CDC) in Atlanta.

Box 77–1. Sexually Transmitted Diseases

Bacteria

Gonorrhea
Chlamydial infection
Syphilis
Bacterial vaginosis
Nongonococcal urethritis
Granuloma inguinale
Chancroid
Lymphogranuloma venereum
Sexually transmitted enteric infections

Viruses

Human immunodeficiency virus (HIV)
Genital herpes
Genital warts
Viral Hepatitis

Protozoa

Trichomoniasis

Fungi

Vulvovaginal candidiasis (only occasionally transmitted sexually)

Ectoparasites

Scabies
Pediculosis

Etiology

STDs represent a serious, broad-range public health problem. These diseases occur worldwide, have been recognized since the beginning of recorded history, affect all age groups and socioeconomic strata, and are associated with substantial morbidity and in some cases mortality. Although they are well understood and relatively easily identified, the incidence of STDs is escalating. Thus, the scope of the health problems they create is increasing rather than decreasing.

Incidence

Except for the common cold and influenza, STDs are the most prevalent communicable diseases in the United States. Every year, STDs are diagnosed in more than 10 million people in this country. Over the past decade, the incidence of STDs has increased dramatically. Most sources describe STD rates as epidemic. Whereas AIDS is probably the most dangerous and best publicized, the most common STDs are chlamydial infection, gonorrhea, syphilis, genital herpes, and venereal warts.

The exact incidence of STDs is unknown. Accurate statistics are difficult to compile for a number of different reasons. Statistics are only as good as the accuracy of case reporting, and reporting requirements are variable in this country; many STDs do not require mandatory reporting. In fact, reporting to federal and state agencies is required only for AIDS, the five classic STDs (gonorrhea, syphilis, chancroid, granuloma inguinale, and lymphogranuloma venereum), and viral hepatitis. Rates for other STDs are based on estimates derived from local studies and physician reports. These estimates are thought to be low, and even rates developed from mandatory case reporting are also believed to be low because of underreporting. For example, nearly 1 million new cases of gonorrhea are reported to public health officials yearly, but it is generally believed that at least another million cases go unreported.

The age-specific rates for STDs are highest for sexually active adolescents and young adults. All age groups, however, are at risk. Anyone who engages in intimate physical contact can contract an STD and then transmit it to others. The neonate can be infected by transplacental or postpartum transmission of the pathogens. Infants and children can be infected through child abuse or incest. The elderly can experience residual sequelae from infections earlier in life. No age group is safe simply because of age.

Other factors that are associated with an increased risk include

lower socioeconomic status
ethnic minority status
lower educational level
limited access to medical care
drug abuse
sexual activity with multiple partners

A lower risk of developing STD is found in people who are celibate, nonsexually active, or engaged in a monogamous sexual relationship.

The estimated increased incidence of STDs worldwide is due to many factors, some of which are only incidentally related. Many societies have become more permissive with increased mobility, sexual freedom, unemployment, and drug abuse. The increased use of intrauterine devices and oral contraceptives may be related to STDs because that may lower the female user's resistance to infection. Ignorance also plays a role in the incidence of STDs. It is difficult for many people to get accurate information about sexual activities and to decide if and how such activities fit their chosen lifestyle. Controversy over the appropriateness of sex education in schools continues. Sexual information is presented in different ways ranging from moralistic statements to glamorized presentations of sex without responsibility. Only recently have the media and concerned organizations begun to present information about sex and STDs in a manner designed to appeal to young people.

Risk Factors

Although STDs can be passed from mother to fetus nonsexually, as the term STD implies, most of the diseases are transmitted from person to person almost exclusively by some mode of sexual contact. (The other main exception is AIDS, which can be transmitted through the blood of intravenous drug users who share needles.) This is because the etiologic organisms thrive in a warm, dark, moist environment and survive only very briefly outside that environment. It follows that prevention and control must concentrate on breaking the chain of sexual transmission.

According to the CDC, the prevention of STDs should focus primarily on changing the sexual behavior of clients at highest risk. Prevention is based on four major areas:

- Education on modes of transmission and methods to reduce transmission.
- Detection of symptomatic and asymptomatic infected clients.
- Diagnosis and treatment of infected clients.
- Evaluation, treatment, and counseling of all sex partners of infected clients.

Health education is crucial in the primary prevention of STDs. Education is directed toward informing the public about sexual practices that significantly reduce the risk of STD transmission. The surest way to prevent STDs is abstinence. There is no such thing as completely safe sex, but certain practices improve safety. These practices include limiting the number of sex partners, knowing the sexual history of all sex partners, avoiding sexual contact with those having symptoms of STDs (e.g., genital discharge, lesions), avoiding risky sexual practices such as those that tear mucous membranes, using a male or female condom with any genital contact, sexual abstinence, and using over-the-counter spermicide in conjunction with mechanical barriers such as condoms and diaphragms.

Nursing Management

ASSESSMENT

Nurses need to be well informed about the variety of sexual activities, their effect on the transmission STDs, and the common symptoms to assess. Educational intervention is necessary to help combat this major health problem while information about safe sexual activity is provided. It is necessary for a health professional to separate a personal view of morality from appropriate nursing activities. At times, this is difficult for some nurses.

There is a social stigma associated with STDs (see Ethical Issues in Nursing). Many clients are ashamed of having STD and try to keep the diagnosis secret. Many associate STDs with low social status and immorality. Many have misconceptions about the dangers of venereal disease and may be fearful and uninformed about STD.

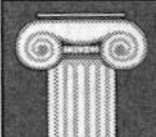

ETHICAL ISSUES IN NURSING

Does the Right to Privacy of Clients with STDs Supercede the Right to Know of Potentially Infected Partners?

Sexually transmitted diseases (STDs) are a very serious public health matter. Such diseases may predispose one to various cancers and cause sterility and even death. There are ways of decreasing the spread of STDs, and large educational campaigns have been launched as a result of the incidence of AIDS and recent increases in the spread of syphilis and chlamydial infection.

Clients who test positive for certain STDs are reported to the Department of Public Health. This department studies the statistics of such diseases in order to track trends and address educational and treatment needs of the public in general. In many states, the names of clients with syphilis, gonorrhea, and chlamydial infection are reported to the Department of Public Health, and follow-up is initiated for those clients. Follow-up includes the department's notifying the sexual partners of the infected client so treatment may be initiated for them as well. The ethical question here is the right to privacy issue. Does a public health department have the right to know the sexual partners of those with STDs even if it is in the best interest of the public at large? Should the infected client alone be responsible for disclosing such information to his or her partners? Do partners of infected clients have a right to be told of their partner's infection so that they may seek treatment?

Health care workers who deal with the care of those with STDs have an obligation to secure the privacy of their clients as well as an obligation to assist those who have potentially been infected. Nurses must inform their infected clients of the public health guidelines that must be followed. Information given to public health departments needs to be as honest and concise as possible. Clients do have a right to privacy, but this privacy must be altered when the rights influencing the health of others are involved.

Other social problems may surface with the discovery of an STD. For example, a newly infected client may be angry at the responsible sexual partner or be hesitant to identify or inform sexual partners about the STD. When a marital or committed relationship is involved, further problems may develop, such as the client's worrying about potential infertility as a consequence of the disease.

A nonjudgmental attitude on the part of the nurse is essential for providing quality care for a client with an STD. The nurse needs to be very skillful in interpersonal communication to help clients appropriately. The client needs accurate information and support. Moralistic, judgmental attitudes do not change others' sexual behavior. Instead, they may deter clients from seeking adequate care. An accepting professional attitude may ensure treatment and prevent the spread of disease to sexual partners or prenatal and postnatal infants. The nurse must encourage and support the client's seeking treatment.

Treatment can be sought in various facilities, including health department STD clinics, physician offices, Planned Parenthood, and community-based clinics. Such clinics deal with STDs frequently and have staff especially sensitive to clients' needs; complete confidentiality is emphasized. This often is especially, but not exclusively, important to gay men, who are at risk of discrimination in some communities if their sexual orientation is disclosed. Some clinics use a coding system for documentation rather than the terms "homosexual" or "bisexual."

NURSING INTERVENTION

Nursing Diagnosis: Knowledge Deficit R/T STDs.

Planning: Expected Outcomes. The client will understand the cause, treatment, and prevention of specific STD, as evidenced by client's statements, avoidance of STD, successful treatment of STD, and no recurrence of STD.

Implementation. Provide information about the transmission, prevention, and treatment of STDs. When caring for clients with STDs, nurses obtain privileged/private information and conduct teaching activities about these diseases (Bridge to Home Health Care). Both activities require sensitivity and skillful interaction. History obtained from a client often includes sexual activities; sexual partners; previous infections, treatment, and test results; parenteral infections; recent use of antibiotics; allergy to antibiotics (including manifestations); and signs and symptoms of STDs. Remember that sexual partners may include persons of the same sex.

The many myths about STDs should be corrected. Supply accurate, factual information to help the client avoid reinfection or infection of others. Include the following topics in teaching sessions about STDs: (1) name, nature, and seriousness of the condition; (2) mode of transmission; (3) actions to prevent spread of infection to others; (4) incubation periods; (5) indications (signs and symptoms) of infection; (6) asymptomatic problems; (7) when and how to seek treatment; (8) treatment methods; (9) importance of follow-up care (when and how to obtain it); (10) consequences of lack of complete treatment; and (11) risk and consequences of recurrent infections. Box 77-2 offers some examples of questions clients with STDs may ask and some suggested responses by the nurse.

In the United States and other countries, there are a variety of community and national programs in which health care professionals collaborate with lay people. Nurses play a pivotal role by helping identify and meet public needs.

Nursing Diagnosis: Anxiety R/T uncertainty of condition and social stigma.

Planning: Expected Outcomes. The client will have a decrease in anxiety, as evidenced by a realistic understanding of disease, seeking treatment, and acceptance of condition.

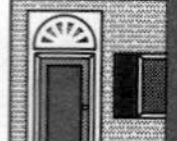

BRIDGE TO HOME HEALTH CARE

STD Clinic

Caring for clients who have sexually transmitted diseases requires a nonjudgemental approach by the nurse. STD affects the individual not only physically but also emotionally. The diagnosis of STD interferes with individuals' sense of sexuality, a very personal sensitive part of their identity. Nursing interventions related to assisting clients with STD encompass three major areas: case finding, education, and follow up.

The incidence of STD has increased dramatically in recent years. The sequelae of some infections are simply annoying, whereas others can cause long-term effects or cause lifelong disabilities and infertility. Pre-conceptional health supervision for teens and young adults, an accurate history of sexual activity, and initiation of prenatal care in the first trimester of pregnancy are all essential elements in early diagnosis of infection.

Individuals who have contracted an STD need educational materials and teaching. Such instruction should address their specific infection, the mode of transmission, the importance of compliance with the full course of treatment, and potential short and long term consequences of noncompliance with recommended treatment and follow up. The nurse cannot assume that the client has a basic understanding of the body parts and their functioning. Selecting simple language and methods with which the person can identify is more likely to change behavior patterns. The concept of "safe sex" is a major teaching objective. Safe sexual behaviors must include using condoms, avoiding sexual contact with people who have many different partners or individuals who use drugs, and avoiding sexual practices that bruise or damage the skin. The nurse may also teach the client other preventive behaviors such as daily bathing with a mild soap and maintenance of the normal vaginal flora by avoiding feminine sprays, tight synthetic clothing, and unnecessary douching.

It is essential that clients understand the importance of honest disclosure and responsible behavior in relation to the diagnosis and treatment of STDs. Reporting of sexual contacts and accepting responsibility for treatment and follow up are concepts that must be communicated to the client. These behaviors are critical for the outcome to be positive for them as individuals and, in many cases, others who are close to them.

Implementation. Learning that one has an STD can threaten a client's self-concept and pose potential physical problems such as possible infertility or damage to an unborn fetus. Feelings of guilt, apprehension, and rejection by others may be expressed. The nurse should work with the client to reduce anxiety, being warm and supportive. Keep the client informed of what is happening and what the client can expect. Facilitate the client's expression of feelings and help plan and implement effective coping strategies.

It is important that personnel caring for clients with STDs examine their own attitudes toward sexuality and sexual behavior in order to provide nonjudgmental care. Although one's own moral values are important in

Box 77–2. Questions Associated with STDs

Examples of Questions Clients May Ask and Suggested Responses

Q: Will treatment protect me from getting this again?
A: No, immunity to reinfection is rare if it indeed even exists. You may be infected again.
Q: Can I resume my sexual activity?
A: It is better to wait until the tests come back showing no organisms are present. If you wait, you will not be in danger of spreading the infection to your sex partners and possibly reinfecting yourself.
Q: Do I have to come back for more treatment?
A: We would like to see you again (give an appointment) to be sure that you are cured (especially with the resistant strains of gonorrhea).
Q: *(Women)* Since I didn't have any symptoms this time, how will I be able to tell if I have this infection again? *(Men)* How will I know if I have it again?
A: *(For women)* When you have your periodic Pap smear, ask your doctor to check for sexually transmitted diseases as well. *(For men)* They are more likely to have symptoms, so remind them to watch for return of these.

guiding personal behavior, prejudicial attitudes may interfere with therapeutic professional relationships. Bias and prejudice can be communicated in both obvious and subtle ways that make the affected client feel more uncomfortable, judged, and discounted. A prejudiced health professional cannot provide comprehensive health care. In fact, such a "professional" may actually drive clients away from necessary treatment; health professionals then become partially responsible for spreading the infection.

EVALUATION

The nurse must evaluate client outcomes on the basis of the established plan of care. If these goals have not been achieved, the plan and interventions must be revised to meet the client's needs.

GONORRHEA

Definition

Gonorrhea (common lay terms include *white, drips, strain, clap,* and *dose*) can be divided into two groups: local and disseminated infection (Table 77–1).

- *Local infections* involve the mucosal surfaces of the urethra, cervix, rectum, pharynx, and conjunctiva.
- *Systemic infection* involves polyarthritis, dermatitis, endocarditis, or meningitis secondary to bacteremia. Systemic infection is more common in women than in men.

Incidence

Gonorrhea continues to be one of the most common STDs in the United States. It is believed that gonorrhea is underreported and that the actual incidence is much higher than that which is reported. Incidence varies with age. Teenagers and young adults are at highest risk; the highest rates occur in the 20- to 24-year-old age group.

Etiology

Gonorrhea is caused by the gram-negative diplococcus *Neisseria gonorrhoeae,* which does not survive for long outside the body. The disease is easily transmitted by sexual contact, and there is a large carrier population (i.e., people who have no symptoms but who carry the organism and can transmit the disease). It has a variable incubation time, usually 3 to 8 days. There is no lasting immunity that prevents reinfection.

Risk Factors

Gonorrheal infection is almost always sexually transmitted, although other current sources point to self-inoculation with contaminated hands. The few rare exceptions are (1) children, who can develop gonorrhea from close contact with the mother's infected areas (vaginal or other mucous membranes), and (2) medical personnel with lacerations, who can develop gonorrhea from contact with infected discharges.

Clinical Manifestations

An initial gonorrheal infection in women may involve the endocervix, vestibular glands, urethra, and anus. Although the vagina is resistant to the infection in adulthood, before puberty it is not. The disease may be asymptomatic in women. Symptoms may include heavy, yellow-green, purulent discharge; a red, swollen, sore vulva; dysuria; and urinary frequency. The most common complication of gonorrhea in women is salpingitis, which can progress to pelvic inflammatory disease (PID). See Chapter 76 for information on PID and salpingitis. Both PID and salpingitis can produce infertility. The first actual symptoms of gonorrhea in women may arise from PID.

In men with gonorrhea, symptoms are usually evident earlier than in women. The infection is principally one of the anterior urethra that produces a purulent discharge, dysuria, and frequency. Complications include epididymitis and prostatitis, but these are not common with early and complete antibiotic therapy.

TABLE 77–1. Management of Common Sexually Transmitted Diseases

Condition/ Causative Organism	Diagnostic Methods	Manifestations	Treatment of Choice*	Mandatory Reporting	Sexual Partner Treatment*
Gonorrhea *Neisseria gonorrhoeae*	Smear culture	Incubation period: 3–8 days Female: asymptomatic or ▶ thick, purulent vaginal discharge ▶ genital irritation ▶ dysuria, urinary frequency ▶ pharyngeal infection ▶ late: pelvic pain (PID) Male: asymptomatic or ▶ urethral discharge ▶ dysuria, urinary frequency ▶ pharyngeal infection ▶ late: scrotal pain (epididymitis) ▶ perineal pain (prostatitis) Disseminated infection, either sex: ▶ bacteremia ▶ arthritis-dermatitis syndrome	Ceftriaxone IM once *plus* Doxycycline PO for 7 days	Yes	All contacts within the preceding 30 days should be examined, cultured, and treated presumptively
Chlamydial infections *Chlamydia trachomatis*	Culture Antigen-antibody tests Enzyme immunoassay Monoclonal antibody test	Incubation period: 7–21 days Female: asymptomatic or ▶ mucopurulent vaginal discharge ▶ dysuria ▶ abnormal vaginal bleeding ▶ pelvic pain (PID) Male: asymptomatic or ▶ mild dysuria ▶ white or clear urethral discharge ▶ testicle pain (epididymitis)	Doxycycline or tetracycline PO for 7 days	No	All contacts within 30 days should be examined and treated

TABLE 77-1. Management of Common Sexually Transmitted Diseases Continued

Condition/ Causative Organism	Diagnostic Methods	Manifestations	Treatment of Choice*	Mandatory Reporting	Sexual Partner Treatment*
Syphilis *Treponema pallidum*	Darkfield microscopy (chancre, granulomata lata) Serologic antibody tests (STS) ► nonspecific, e.g., VDRL ► specific, e.g., FTA-ABS	Incubation period: 10-90 days Primary ► painless chancre at site of exposure ► regional lymphadenopathy Secondary ► maculopapular skin rash ► generalized lymphadenopathy ► mucous patches ► condylomata lata ► fever, malaise ► alopecia Latent ► asymptomatic	Early syphilis: benzathine penicillin G IM single dose	Yes	All contacts with early syphilis (primary, secondary, or latent syphilis of 1 year's duration) should be evaluated and treated All contacts within 90 days should be treated presumptively
	Cerebrospinal fluid (late syphilis)	Late ► cardiovascular changes, e.g., aortic aneurysm ► central nervous system changes, e.g., paresis, tabes dorsalis, dementia	Cardiovascular syphilis: benzathine penicillin G IM weekly for 3 weeks Neurosyphilis: aqueous penicillin IV every 4 hours for 10-14 days	No	
Genital herpes Herpes simplex virus (HSV) type I or II, primarily type II	Culture Pap smear	Incubation period: 3-7 days Acute phase ► paresthesia/ burning at site of exposure ► painful genital vesicles that ulcerate ► fever, chills, muscle aches Latent phase ► symptomatic	No cure Acyclovir PO for 5-10 days for acute episodes	No	All contacts of clients with active lesions should be evaluated and, if symptomatic, treated
Genital warts Human papillomavirus (HPV)	Pap smear Colposcopy Biopsy	Incubation period: 1-2 months Single or multiple painless genital or anorectal warts	Cryotherapy with liquid nitrogen or cryoprobe	No	All contacts should be evaluated and, if symptomatic, treated

* CDC 1989 sexually transmitted diseases treatment guidelines.
IM, intramuscularly; IV, intravenously; PID, pelvic inflammatory disease; PO, orally.

In addition to the gender-specific manifestations, either sex may have pharyngitis due to orogenital contact (fellatio, cunnilingus) or proctitis from anal contact (sodomy).

Diagnostic Assessment

Diagnosis is made by history, physical examination, identification of the gonococcus on a smear, and culture of exudate from the endocervix, urethra, and other infected areas. All clients with gonorrhea should also be tested for chlamydial infection, syphilis, and other coexisting STDs such as trichomoniasis.

Medical Management

PHARMACOLOGIC MANAGEMENT

Gonorrhea is treated aggressively with antibiotics. Penicillin was once the treatment of choice, but therapy is now complicated by the development of penicillin-resistant organisms. The recommended regimen is ceftriaxone sodium (Rocephin), a cephalosporin antibiotic, one dose intramuscularly followed by doxycycline hyclate (Vibramycin Hyclate) or tetracycline orally for 7 days. Doxycycline hyclate or tetracycline is added for treatment of commonly occurring chlamydial coinfections. For clients who cannot tolerate ceftriaxone sodium, a single intramuscular injection of spectinomycin dihydrochloride (Trobicin) plus doxycycline hyclate (Vibramycin) can be used. After completion of therapy, a follow-up examination and culture should be done. A positive culture, however, may indicate reinfection rather than treatment failure.

Nursing Management

Clients experiencing gonorrhea must understand information about the disease, how it spreads, and how it is treated. Self-care information is essential. The nurse should discuss the possibility of reinfection and infection of sexual partners. Discuss the importance of identifying and treating all sexual partners. Encourage sexual abstinence or use of a male or female condom until the infection is cured. Warn pregnant female clients of the danger of infecting their babies during delivery. Advise these women to refrain from sexual activity until their condition is cured.

Oral sexual activity should be avoided if there is a pharyngeal infection. Clients receiving treatment for gonorrhea must understand the importance of taking the complete course of prescribed medications and of returning for follow-up evaluation after completing the medication.

Treatment for gonorrhea is subject to change as organisms become more resistant. Many clients are not aware that the doses of penicillin used to treat gonorrhea are much greater than those used for most other infections and mistakenly think that an antibiotic taken for some other problem (e.g., a respiratory infection) will also "cure" gonorrhea. Public education is an essential part of the fight against STDs.

Sexual contact investigation is essential for the prevention and control of gonorrhea. Reporting sexual contacts can be difficult and frightening for an infected client. Ask for contact information in a positive, nonthreatening, sensitive way. During the initial treatment visit, clients should be asked about sexual contacts. However, this is best asked after the treatment is actually administered so they will not become anxious and possibly avoid necessary care.

CHLAMYDIAL INFECTIONS

Definition

Chlamydia trachomatis infections are the most common STD in the United States today (Table 77-1).

Incidence

The incidence of chlamydial infection, now the most prevalent STD, is three times that of gonorrhea. The number of new cases per year is estimated to be at least 3 to 4 million. Unlike gonorrhea, the disease is not reportable to the public health department, so the exact incidence is unknown.

Etiology

The etiologic organism, *Chlamydia trachomatis,* is a nonmotile, gram-negative bacterium that is most often responsible for what was previously termed nonspecific vaginitis in females and nongonococcal or nonspecific urethritis in males. The incubation period is 7 to 21 days.

Risk Factors

C. trachomatis is always transmitted by intimate sexual contact, never casual contact. Women usually acquire the infection during intercourse with an infected male. Males can also transmit the infection through homosexual contact. The infection does not cross the placenta, but exposure during delivery can cause conjunctivitis and pneumonia in newborns.

Clinical Manifestations

Chlamydial infections primarily affect the urethra, endocervix, and rectum. *C. trachomatis* is found in these areas and the Bartholin glands in women. In many cases, the infection is asymptomatic for an extended period. When present, symptoms resemble those of gonorrhea but are less severe.

In women, the organism produces a friable, edematous cervix that causes a yellow, mucopurulent vaginal discharge that may be accompanied by spotting at menstrual midcycle or with sexual intercourse. With Bartholin duct involvement, there is a purulent discharge. In both sexes, there is dysuria associated with urethritis.

Diagnostic Assessment

Because there are few or no symptoms, the diagnosis of chlamydial infections is difficult and often missed. Clients tend not to seek medical treatment. Manifestations are often nonspecific and virtually indistinguishable clinically from those of gonorrhea. For this reason, and because these two infections often coexist, it is recommended that diagnostic tests for both be done when either condition is suspected.

The best diagnostic test for chlamydial infections is the tissue culture of cellular material from the urethra, endocervix, or rectum. Rapid nonculture antigen detection tests done on urogenital secretions are also available. These are antigen-antibody tests that use either an enzyme immunoassay or monoclonal antibody technique. Although slightly less accurate than a culture, these tests hold the advantage of being more convenient, rapid, and less expensive than a culture. These rapid tests are recommended for the screening of asymptomatic high-risk clients in whom chlamydial infections would otherwise go undetected. Priority groups for testing, if resources are limited, are high-risk pregnant women, adolescents, and women with multiple sex partners. The Pap smear has no diagnostic value in the diagnosis or screening of chlamydial infection.

Chlamydial infection is known as "the great sterilizer." Undetected and untreated cases can progress to serious, irreversible consequences. *C. trachomatis* causes an inflammation that leads to scarring and ulcerations of involved tissue. In men, the infection can extend to the epididymis. The ensuing epididymitis can produce sterility or Teiter's syndrome with symptoms of urethritis, arthritis, conjunctivitis, and hyperkeratotic skin lesions. In women, the infection can extend to the endometrium and salpinx; the major consequence is salpingitis with subsequent infertility or placement at high risk for ectopic pregnancy. Secondary extension to the peritoneum can cause PID very similar to that of gonorrhea. See Chapter 76 for a discussion of PID.

Medical Management

All sexual contacts within 30 days before diagnosis should be examined and treated. In clinical settings in which testing for chlamydial infection is not available, treatment is often prescribed on the basis of clinical diagnosis or as cotreatment for gonorrhea.

PHARMACOLOGIC MANAGEMENT

Doxycycline or tetracycline orally for 7 days is the treatment of choice for chlamydial infection. In order to increase the absorption and efficacy of the antibiotic, clients should be instructed to take the medications 1 to 2 hours after meals and to avoid iron, dairy products, and antacids. Pregnant women and those allergic to tetracycline preparations are treated with erythromycin orally for 7 days. If salpingitis and the other serious sequelae are to be prevented, it is imperative that treatment be started early and that the entire course of antibiotics be completed. Antichlamydial therapy is almost always effective. To confirm a cure, a repeat culture 4 to 7 days after treatment should be done whenever possible.

Nursing Management

Clients should be instructed about the sexual mode of transmission of chlamydial infection. The increased risk of infection with multiple sex partners should be stressed. Clients should also be informed of the serious danger of sterility. Infected clients should avoid all sexual activity (intercourse, fellatio, cunnilingus, or sodomy) until cured, and men and women should both wear condoms thereafter for prevention of reinfection.

SYPHILIS

Definition

Syphilis (street terms include *bad blood, lues, pox,* and *syph*), although currently less common than gonorrhea, can progress to blindness, mental illness, paralysis, heart disease, and death (Table 77-1).

Incidence

Syphilis has become dramatically less prevalent since the advent of antibiotics but has not been eradicated. In fact, the number of reported cases has increased in recent years. It is the third most commonly reported communicable disease in the United States. Adolescents, young adults, and homosexual males are at greatest risk.

Etiology

This systemic, infectious disease is caused by the motile spirochete *Treponema pallidum*. Syphilis can occur alone or with other STDs. The incubation period varies from 10 to 90 days, averaging 20 to 30 days.

Risk Factors and Transmission

Although *T. pallidum* cannot survive long outside the body, syphilis is highly infectious. The organism enters the body through intact mucous membranes or abraded skin almost exclusively by direct sexual contact (acquired syphilis). Sexual transmission requires exposure to the moist mucosal or cutaneous syphilitic lesions. After entry, the organisms multiply locally and disseminate through lymphatics and the bloodstream. The infection can also be passed transplacentally from mother to fetus (congenital syphilis).

Clinical Manifestations

Syphilis is characterized by well-defined stages that occur over a period of years: primary, secondary, latent, and late. The manifestations vary with each stage.

PRIMARY STAGE

Primary syphilis has two principal symptoms: the appearance of a chancre and lymphadenopathy. Typically, a *chancre* is an oval ulcer with a raised border that does not bleed readily and is painless unless infected.

The chancre is at the site of inoculation, usually the genitalia, anus, or mouth. Usually, a single chancre occurs about 4 weeks after initial infection. Chancres in women are often not noticed. *Lymphadenopathy* occurs as local lymph glands near the chancre swell painlessly. If untreated, a chancre disappears after 4 to 6 weeks. The infected client then is often asymptomatic for a time.

SECOND STAGE

The secondary stage begins from 2 weeks to 6 months after the chancre disappears. Indications of the second stage include

- *Generalized skin rash.* Typically a maculopapular and nonpruritic rash appears on the palms (see Color Plate 20) and soles of the feet (few other diseases cause a rash in these locations).
- *Generalized lymphadenopathy*
- *Mucous patches.* Gray, superficial patches occur on the mucous membranes in the mouth and may be accompanied by a sore throat.
- *Condylomata lata.* These are broad-based, flat papules that can usually be easily distinguished from the typical narrow-based, pedunculated growth of condylomata acuminata (venereal warts, see later). They may develop in warm, moist body areas—most commonly on the labia or anus or at the corners of the mouth. Condylomata are highly contagious.
- *General flulike symptoms* include nausea; anorexia; constipation; headaches; muscle, joint, and bone pain; and a chronically elevated temperature.
- *Patchy hair loss* from eyebrows and scalp (alopecia). Secondary stage symptoms usually disappear after 2 to 6 weeks, and a latency period begins.

LATENT STAGE

The latent stage of syphilis typically has no symptoms. The disease is not transmitted by sexual contact during this phase. However, transmission through the bloodstream by blood donation can occur. Serologic tests for syphilis in all prospective blood donors is essential. Latent stage syphilis usually occurs about 2 or more years after the primary lesion and can last as long as 50 years. About two thirds of infected clients remain in this stage without further problems. Some clients relapse into the primary or secondary stage during the first 2 years of latency.

LATE STAGE

If untreated, about one third of infected clients develop devastating, irreversible complications such as chronic bone and joint inflammation, cardiovascular problems (e.g., valvular involvement, aneurysms), granulomatous lesions (gummas) on any part of the body, and central nervous system problems (including mental illness, slurred speech, ataxic gait, paralysis, judgment loss, and senility). This stage is not infectious but may be terminal if untreated (Chap. 30 discusses central nervous system manifestations).

Diagnostic Assessment

The diagnosis of syphilis is based on health assessment and various laboratory studies. The laboratory tests are both direct and indirect. A direct test identifies the causative organism. Indirect tests merely identify antibodies of the causative agent. Primary or secondary stage lesions can be scraped and the causative organism identified with a darkfield microscope technique. Darkfield examination must be done by an expert because other spirochetes are present in the oral and genital areas. This test confirms a diagnosis of syphilis in the primary (when other tests are generally negative) and secondary stages.

Serologic tests for syphilis (STS) are indirect tests that detect antibodies that are not present in the serum until 4 weeks *after* the appearance of the chancre. Such tests include the VDRL (Venereal Disease Research Laboratory) and fluorescent treponemal antibody absorption (FTA-ABS) tests.

The VDRL test for nonspecific antibodies is the most commonly used screening test for syphilis. It is negative in the early primary stage before antibodies to *T. pallidum* are formed and are present in the circulation. It is falsely positive with certain viral infections and collagen diseases (e.g., mononucleosis, lupus). Results are given as nonreactive, borderline, weakly reactive, or reactive. Reactive and weakly reactive are considered positive results.

The FTA-ABS serologic test is more specific in that it measures antibodies specific to *T. pallidum.* It is used when the VDRL is positive but the diagnosis of syphilis is still uncertain. This test usually becomes positive 3 to 4 weeks after the infection. Once positive, treponemal antibody tests usually remain positive for life, regardless of treatment or cure. In late neurosyphilis, cerebrospinal fluid may be examined for characteristic findings.

Syphilis often coexists with other general infections. The CDC recommends that all clients with syphilis be counseled on the risks of human immunodeficiency virus (HIV) infection (AIDS) and be encouraged to be tested for AIDS.

Medical Management

PHARMACOLOGIC MANAGEMENT

Penicillin intramuscularly or intravenously is the drug of choice for the treatment of syphilis. All stages of syphilis respond to antibiotic therapy, but the structural changes present in late syphilis are irreversible despite successful treatment. For early syphilis, the treatment of choice is benzathine penicillin G intramuscularly in one dose. The dosage schedule and length of therapy are determined by the stage of the disease and current guidelines for treatment. For clients allergic to penicillin, oral doxycycline or tetracycline may be used, but they are not as effective as penicillin. Treatment failure can occur with any given regimen. Compliance is often a problem; follow-up with repeat VDRL tests or serial cerebrospinal fluid assessment (in late syphilis) is essential to confirm a cure.

Nursing Management

Clients with primary or secondary syphilis should abstain from sexual contact for at least 1 month after treatment. All sexual contacts must be identified and treated. Most practitioners treat contacts as if they have primary syphilis, whether or not infection is evident. When an infected but untreated woman has been in the latency stage for at least a year, she is not considered infectious unless she becomes pregnant, because she can then infect her unborn child. Adequate treatment is curative, but reinfection is possible and can be detected by monitoring serologic titers and by clinical reexaminations. An infection does not confer lasting immunity.

A client with syphilis needs health care information and psychosocial support. Nurses must provide clients with accurate information about transmission, reinfection, early detection, treatment, follow-up, proper hygiene, and safe sexual habits. The nurse should individualize health teaching to meet the client's particular needs and psychosocial situation. A diagnosis of syphilis can be frightening and difficult to accept. It is important to facilitate the expression of feelings.

GENITAL HERPES

Definition

Genital herpes is a recurrent, systemic infection (Table 77-1).

Incidence

Although recognized for centuries, genital herpes has received renewed attention because of its epidemic incidence. Now one of the most common STDs, it is the most common cause of genital ulceration. Its peak incidence occurs in the adolescent and young adult.

Etiology

Caused by herpes simplex virus (HSV) type II, the infection is closely related to other herpes infections such as the classic "cold sore" caused by HSV type I. Type I herpes is mainly nongenital, occurring above the waist (often on the lips or nose). Type II herpes occurs primarily below the waist as a sexually transmitted genital infection. It is, however, possible for HSV type I to cause genital infections and for HSV type II to cause oral lesions.

Risk Factors

The HSV organism is present in the exudate of the lesion. The disease can be transmitted while a lesion is present and for 10 days after a lesion has healed. Genital herpes is usually transmitted by direct contact with the exudate during sexual activity, but transmission is possible by fomites such as towels used by an infected client. In addition, newborns can be infected during vaginal delivery when active genital lesions are present. Birth by cesarean section prevents infection of the fetus under these conditions.

Clinical Manifestations

Symptoms of genital herpes usually occur 3 to 7 days after contact. Initially, there is a burning sensation or paresthesia at the site of inoculation. Next, numerous small vesicles with an erythematous border form painful, shallow ulcers that then crust and heal with a scar in about 2 to 4 weeks.

The major problem of HSV infections is recurrence. About one half to three quarters of infected clients have recurrence within 1 year of the first episode. The herpes virus is believed to lie dormant in the body, probably in the trigeminal ganglion (HSV-I) and sacral ganglion (HSV-II), until it is activated and another episode of genital herpes with the characteristic lesion occurs. Certain situations such as stress, infection, trauma, menses, or sexual intercourse seem to trigger recurrent episodes.

Characteristically, recurrent genital herpes causes local, but not systemic, symptoms. Prodromal sensations of burning or paresthesias may be experienced before the vesicles erupt. The vesicles tend to reappear at the same locations, but previous sites of infection are not always involved. Symptoms are similar to those associated with primary infection although usually less severe. Vesicles rupture in 24 to 48 hours, and the syndrome generally lasts 7 to 10 days.

Potential complications of HSV infections include aseptic meningitis and transverse myelitis. Women are at risk for spontaneous abortions, and there is some evidence that HSV-II predisposes to carcinoma of the cervix.

Diagnostic Assessment

A diagnosis of genital herpes is made by health assessment findings, including history of the symptoms and the presence of vesicles. The diagnosis is confirmed by a viral culture of the exudate from the ulcer. Papanicolaou (Pap) smear can be done in women. The presence in the Pap smear of multinucleated giant cells with or without inclusion bodies is characteristic of a herpes infection.

Medical Management

PHARMACOLOGIC MANAGEMENT

Genital herpes is a chronic disease. There is no cure. The recommended treatment for primary or recurrent infection or for prophylaxis of active lesions is acyclovir (Zovirax) orally for 5 to 10 days. Palliative measures include keeping the involved area clean and dry, sitz baths, cool applications, and analgesic medications.

Nursing Management

When the vesicles of active genital herpes rupture, they release a highly contagious exudate. Therefore, clients as well as health care personnel must observe strict medical asepsis. For avoiding autoinoculation from the genital area to other body sites, clients should be advised to wash their hands thoroughly after any contact with the herpetic lesions. HSV infections of the eye are particularly serious. Infected clients should have separate towels and other personal items. Sexual contact should be avoided during initial and recurrent infections. The use of condoms during latent periods is encouraged because of the possible risk of transmission even when symptoms are not present. Women should be told to have annual pelvic examinations and Pap smears.

Many clients find that coping with genital herpes is emotionally difficult. Tremendous psychosocial stress may develop because the infection cannot be cured and recurrence cannot be predicted. Its reappearance can significantly affect sexual activity. The pain caused by these lesions is especially problematic. Psychosocial support includes providing clients with accurate information about the infection. Support groups may be helpful in dealing with feelings of anger, guilt, and shame that are common in these clients.

GENITAL WARTS (CONDYLOMATA ACUMINATA)

Definition

Genital warts, the fourth most common STD, are venereal warts caused by the human papillomavirus (HPV); they are usually transmitted by sexual contact (Table 77-1).

Etiology

Typically the warts occur in multiple, painless clusters on the vulva, vagina, cervix, perineum, anorectal area, urethral meatus, or glans penis 1 to 2 months after exposure. Oral, pharyngeal, and laryngeal lesions can also occur. HPV can cause laryngeal papillomatosis in infants born to mothers with vaginal warts.

Diagnostic Assessment

Diagnosis is typically made by observation of the warts. Subclinical warts can be identified by Pap smear and colposcopy of the cervix and vagina. Biopsy of lesions may be done to differentiate venereal warts from condylomata lata lesions of the secondary stage of syphilis or from carcinoma.

Medical Management

PHARMACOLOGIC MANAGEMENT

Topical application of podophyllin in compound with tincture of benzoin or surgery is the treatment of genital warts. Recurrence is common. Sexual partners must also be treated. Clients must be seen every 1 to 2 weeks until all warts have disappeared. There is no actual cure, so treatment only ameliorates the symptoms.

Surgical Management

Warts can also be treated with cryotherapy with liquid nitrogen or a cryoprobe. For extensive warts, carbon dioxide lasers, electrocautery, and surgical excision can be used. Again, remember that the warts are not cured and recurrence is common.

Nursing Management

The nurse must warn clients with genital warts that they are at an increased risk for genital malignancy, such as cancer of the vulva and penis and especially carcinoma of the cervix. All women with anogenital warts should have an annual Pap smear and, when indicated, cervical colposcopy and biopsy. The detection and treatment of subclinical HPV infection in men may be important for the prevention of genital carcinoma in women.

ACQUIRED IMMUNODEFICIENCY SYNDROME

Acquired immunodeficiency syndrome (AIDS) is a viral STD that has reached worldwide epidemic proportions. AIDS is described in detail in Chapter 24.

TRICHOMONIASIS

Definition

Trichomoniasis is a protozoal infection causing vulvovaginitis.

Incidence

A common cause of vulvovaginitis is infection with the anaerobic, flagellated, parasitic protozoon *Trichomonas vaginalis*. Although not life-threatening, trichomoniasis has a very high incidence worldwide and remains a major health problem.

Etiology

The organism prefers an alkaline environment (pH 6 to 7), and changes in the vaginal flora make a woman more susceptible to it. Trichomoniasis may be difficult to cure, and recurrence is common. The organism is almost always transmitted sexually from one partner to another, which makes simultaneous treatment of both partners necessary for cure.

Clinical Manifestations

Symptoms may be minor and are usually so in an infected male. In a female, they include a copious, malodorous, yellow-green vaginal discharge. This is irritating to the vulva, causing severe itching and burning and excoriation and maceration of the vulvar tissues. Occasionally, the cervix is covered with punctate hemorrhages ("strawberry cervix"). The vaginal mucosa appears reddened and slightly edematous. Some women experience dyspareunia (pain during vaginal sexual activity). The organism does not affect the uterus and tubes.

If trichomoniasis extends to the urethra, frequency and burning with urination may occur. This is the most common symptom in a male. Anal involvement may also occur, either asymptomatically or with a slight discharge. Bladder and anal involvement are more common when the infection has become chronic.

Diagnostic Assessment

A diagnosis of trichomoniasis is established by obtaining a fresh, warm, wet mount and identifying the motile trichomonad under the microscope. A wet mount is obtained by placing a drop of the exudate on a glass slide, mixing in a drop of saline, and covering it with a cover slide. Cultures can be obtained to establish the diagnosis, but they are rarely necessary. For the female, the vaginal speculum used to obtain vaginal secretions must be inserted without lubrication to avoid destroying the organism. If possible, tell the woman not to douche before the vaginal examination. Reassurance and a calm attitude can help allay the woman's anxiety and minimize any discomfort with the examination.

Medical Management

PHARMACOLOGIC MANAGEMENT

The preferred treatment for trichomoniasis is a single 2-g dose of metronidazole (Flagyl) orally for the client and all sexual contacts. Flagyl should not be taken during pregnancy because it may, especially during the first trimester, adversely affect fetal development. *T. vaginalis* does not affect the fetus. Advise clients taking metronidazole not to drink alcoholic beverages so that side effects of nausea, vomiting, and headaches are prevented. Vaginal clotrimazole (Gyne-Lotrimin) cream, although not nearly as effective as metronidazole, is an alternative treatment that can be used during pregnancy. This treatment is now available over-the-counter, which has led to some misuse by women who do not understand the seriousness of the disorder.

Single-dose metronidazole therapy is usually curative, but recurrence is common. Clients should be instructed to seek prompt treatment if symptoms return. Metronidazole may be given in a 7-day regimen for recurrent infection.

Nursing Management

A woman with trichomoniasis should refrain from sexual intercourse or use the female condom—and an infected male use condoms while the infection remains active. Emphasize to the client the importance of good perineal hygiene. Treatment should be continued through the woman's menstrual period, because the vagina is more alkaline during this time of the cycle and a flare-up may occur. After therapy has been completed, clients are evaluated and treated again if necessary.

BACTERIAL VAGINOSIS

Definition

Bacterial vaginosis is the term now used for what used to be called nonspecific vaginitis. This new term was adopted since *Gardnerella vaginalis* (also known as *Hemophilus vaginalis* or *Corynebacterium vaginalis*) was isolated and usually found to be the causative organism.

Etiology

Bacterial vaginosis can be cultured from both symptomatic and asymptomatic women. The new name implies there may be multiple etiologic organisms, possibly coexisting anaerobic bacteria; it also indicates that vaginal white blood cells are not the predominant feature in this type of vaginitis.

Clinical Manifestations

The vulvovaginitis produced by *G. vaginalis* is mild or asymptomatic. The most common symptom is a mild to moderate amount of malodorous ("fishy"), gray, homogenous, thin vaginal discharge accompanied by some vaginal irritation and vulvular pruritus. Symptoms are almost always confined to the vulvovaginal area.

Diagnostic Assessment

Diagnosis is made by a culture positive for *G. vaginalis* or visualization of coccobacilli or clue cells on a saline wet mount preparation of vaginal secretions. Clue cells are desquamated vaginal epithelial cells characteristically stippled by the adherence of coccobacilli to their surfaces. If potassium hydroxide (KOH) is mixed with the vaginal discharge, a fishy odor is elicited (positive "sniff test").

Medical Management

PHARMACOLOGIC MANAGEMENT

The recommended treatment for bacterial vaginosis in nonpregnant women is metronidazole (Flagyl) orally for 7 days. Single-dose regimens can be used to improve compliance, but they are less effective than the 7-day course.

Nursing Management

Clients on Flagyl should be cautioned to abstain from alcohol during and for 3 days after the medication for preventing intense nausea, vomiting, and headache. Treatment of male partners is recommended only with recurrent or resistant infection. Even so, treatment of the male has not been shown to be highly beneficial for either partner. Clients are advised to avoid sexual intercourse during the treatment, and condom use is recommended to prevent recurrence.

VULVOVAGINAL CANDIDIASIS

Occasionally transmitted sexually, candidiasis (yeast infection) of the vagina and vulva is generally not considered an STD. (See Chap. 76 for vaginitis.)

GRANULOMA INGUINALE (DONOVANOSIS)

Granuloma inguinale, a chronic infection occurring most often in tropical regions, is caused by the gram-negative bacillus *Calymmatobacterium granulomatis* (formerly named *Donovania granulomatis*). It is characterized by genital and perianal papular lesions. These become painless, gradually enlarging, ulcerating, granulomatous lesions that cause tissue destruction difficult to differentiate from cancer. Diagnosis is made by microscopic identification of Donovan bodies (inclusion bodies of the causative organism) in a smear taken from edge scrapings of the lesion. Granuloma inguinale is treated with antibiotics such as tetracycline or streptomycin. Penicillin is not effective.

CHANCROID

Chancroid is a highly contagious infection caused by the gram-negative *Hemophilus ducreyi* bacillus. The initial papules/pustules produce multiple, painful, irregular, and deep genital ulcers, often accompanied by regional lymphadenopathy. Although chancroid is more common in the tropics, the incidence is increasing in the United States. Outside the United States, chancroid has been associated with increased infection rates for HIV.

Diagnosis is confirmed by a culture positive for *H. ducreyi*. Recommended treatment is oral erythromycin for 7 days or ceftriaxone (Rocephin) intramuscularly in a single dose.

LYMPHOGRANULOMA VENEREUM

Lymphogranuloma venereum is a systemic infection common in the tropics. The infection is caused by certain strains of the bacterium *Chlamydia trachomatis*, a microorganism belonging to the chlamydia group. The primary lesion is a small, painless papule on the glans penis or vaginal mucosa that heals spontaneously and may go unnoticed.

Marked inguinal lymphadenopathy (buboes) that appears 2 to 6 weeks later is the most common clinical manifestation. Eventually, draining ulceration, scarring, lymphatic obstruction, and marked external genital deformity may occur. Rectal fibrosis and strictures are late sequelae.

Definitive diagnosis is made on the basis of a culture positive for *C. trachomatis*. Recommended therapy is doxycycline (Vibramycin) orally for 21 days. Oral tetracycline, erythromycin, and sulfisoxazole (Gantrisin) are alternatives.

PEDICULOSIS PUBIS AND SCABIES

Cutaneous infestation with pubic lice (pediculosis pubis) or mites (scabies) results either from contact with contaminated objects such as linens or from close physical contact. Because they can be transmitted sexually, these conditions are sometimes included with STDs. (For further discussion, see Chap. 70.)

SEXUALLY TRANSMITTED ENTERIC INFECTIONS

Dysenteries and hepatitis caused by enteric pathogens are typically acquired from food or water contaminated with fecal matter. Since the mid-1970s, it has been recognized that these pathogens can also be transmitted by oral and anal sexual contact. Sexually transmitted enteric infections occur predominantly in homosexual males. The infections include shigellosis, salmonellosis, amebiasis, giardiasis, and hepatitis A. See Chapter 55 for discussion of dysentery and Chapter 58 for discussion of hepatitis A.

HEPATITIS B AND DELTA HEPATITIS

Sexual contact is the most frequently reported mode of transmission of the hepatitis B virus. The extent of sexual transmission for delta hepatitis is uncertain. Clients at high risk for sexually transmitted hepatitis B are homosexual males, sex partners of intravenous drug abusers, and male and female heterosexuals with multiple partners. See Chapter 58 for further discussion of hepatitis B and delta hepatitis.

Summary

Sexually transmitted diseases are more prevalent now than ever before. There are many reasons for this phenomenon. The increased, improper, and indiscriminate use of antibiotics has increased the number of resistant organisms. Current sexual practices may also be responsible for the current increases. The economic costs of STDs are increasing with the number of cases. The nurse has an ever-increasing role in the prevention, early detection, and treatment of these conditions. Nurses should monitor for the presence of STD in all high-risk clients, and nurses must take the lead in teaching the client safe, preventive practices.

Bibliography

1. *ACOG guide to preconception care* (1990). Washington, DC: The American College of Obstetricians and Gynecologists.
2. Andrist, L. C. (1988). Taking a sexual history and educating clients about safe sex. *Nursing Clinics of North America, 23,* 959.
3. Breslin, E. (1988). Genital herpes simplex. *Nursing Clinics of North America, 23,* 907.
4. Cates, W., Jr. (1988). The other STD's—do they really matter? *Journal of the American Medical Association, 259,* 3606.
5. Cates, W., Jr., et al. (1990). Sexually transmitted diseases—overview of the situation. *Primary Care, 17,* 1.
6. Centers for Disease Control (1989). 1989 sexually transmitted diseases treatment guidelines. *Morbidity and Mortality Weekly Report, 38*(Suppl. 1), 3-17.
7. Connell, E. B., et al. (1985). *Sexually transmitted diseases: Diagnosis and treatment.* Durant, OK: Creative Informatics.
8. Custodio, D. E., et al. (1991). Sexually transmitted diseases. *Topics in Emergency Medicine, 13,* 66.
9. Featherston, W. E. (1990). Sexual identity and practices relating to the spread of sexually transmitted diseases. *Primary Care, 17,* 29.
10. Fraiz, J., et al. (1988). Chlamydial infections. *Annual Review of Medicine, 39,* 357.
11. Genital human papillomavirus infections. *ACOG Technical Bulletin No. 105,* 1987.
12. Goodson, J. D. (1987). Management of nongonococcal urethritis. In A. H. Goroll, et al. (Eds.), *Primary care medicine* (2nd ed.). Philadelphia: J. B. Lippincott.
13. Gynecologic herpes simplex virus infections. *ACOG Technical Bulletin No. 119,* 1988.
14. Holmes, K. K., et al. (Eds.) (1990). *Sexually transmitted diseases.* New York: McGraw-Hill.
15. Jovanovich, J. F. (1987). Genital herpes. In F. H. Messerli (Ed.), *Current clinical practice.* Philadelphia: W. B. Saunders.
16. Katner, H. P., et al. (1987). Sexually transmitted diseases in heterosexuals. In F. H. Messerli (Ed.), *Current clinical practice.* Philadelphia: W. B. Saunders.
17. Katz, A. R. (1989). Chlamydia trachomatis: a frequently overlooked public health menance. *Hawaii Medical Journal, 48,* 156.
18. Levin, A., et al. (1987). *The clinicians guide to sexually transmitted diseases.* Chicago: Year Book.
19. Melvin, S. Y. (1990). Syphilis—resurgence of an old disease. *Primary Care, 17,* 47.
20. Mertz, G. J., et al. (1988). Long term acyclovir suppression of frequently recurring genital herpes simplex virus infection. *Journal of the American Medical Association, 260,* 201.
21. Nettina, S. L., et al. (1990). Diagnosis and management of sexually transmitted genital lesions. *Nurse Practitioner, 15,* 34.
22. Pankey, G. A., et al. (1987). Sexually transmitted infections. In F. H. Messerli (Ed.), *Current clinical practice.* Philadelphia: W. B. Saunders.
23. Progress toward achieving the 1990 objectives for the nation for sexually transmitted diseases. *Morbidity and Mortality Weekly Report, 39,* 53, 1990.
24. Secor, R. M. (1988). Bacterial vaginosis—a comprehensive review. *Nursing Clinics of North America, 23,* 907.
25. *Sexually transmitted diseases* (1987). Olympia, WA: Washington Department of Social and Health Services.
26. Simon, H. B. (1987). Management of syphilis and other venereal diseases. In A. H. Goroll, et al. (Eds.), *Primary care medicine* (2nd ed.). Philadelphia: J. B. Lippincott.
27. Smith, R. E., et al. (1987). Chlamydia. In F. H. Messerli (Ed.), *Current clinical practice.* Philadelphia: W. B. Saunders.
28. Spence, J. R. (1989). Epidemiology of sexually transmitted diseases. *Obstetrics and Gynecology Clinics of North America, 16,* 453.
29. Talashek, M. L., et al. (1990). Sexually transmitted diseases in the elderly—issues and recommendations. *Journal of Gerontological Nursing, 16,* 33.
30. Thomason, J. L., et al. (1989). Trichomonas vaginalis. *Obstetrics and Gynecology, 74,* 536.
31. Vulvovaginitis. *ACOG Technical Bulletin No. 135,* 1989.
32. Wardell, D. W. (1988). Chronic exposure to sexually transmitted diseases. *Nursing Clinics of North America, 23,* 947.
33. Whelan, M. (1988). Nursing management of the patient with chlamydia trachomatis infection. *Nursing Clinics of North America, 23,* 877.

Chapter 78

Nursing Care of the Client with Breast Disorders

One of nine women will develop breast cancer in her lifetime.[2] Because breast cancer is such a feared disease, a woman who finds a breast lump or problem will probably first suspect cancer, then worry about losing her breast and about dying, all within seconds after the discovery of the breast problem. Therefore, in addition to caring for women with breast disorders, nurses have an important role teaching women about normal breasts; common benign breast problems; breast self-examination and mammography; and risk factors for, incidence of, and treatments for breast cancer.

PUBLIC ATTITUDES AND KNOWLEDGE ABOUT BREAST LESIONS

The fear of breast cancer is common. Women and men who develop a breast problem become anxious about whether they have cancer. Thus, assessment not only is directed at differentiating between malignant and nonmalignant lesions but also focuses on gathering information about concerns of the client and significant others and their coping strategies. Such assessment forms the basis of subsequent nursing and medical intervention.

Many misconceptions exist about breast cancer. In a 1981 National Cancer Institute study, half of those surveyed were incorrect in thinking that a breast injury could cause cancer. Many did not know that nipple changes can be a sign of breast cancer. Also, many did not know about diagnostic procedures for breast cancer or treatment options other than surgery.[35] However, in spite of such misconceptions, there is also a growing public awareness about breast cancer. In the past, the subject was often avoided, or information, often inaccurate, was secretly and fearfully shared. Now, breast cancer is openly discussed and frequently is presented in mass media. Controversies continue to arise over breast cancer's cause, diagnostic methods, and treatment options. These controversies are reported in the popular press. The facts about the disease, treatment, and prognosis need to be clarified.

Nurses have an educational role concerning breast lesions. By allowing clients to talk about breast cancer, correcting misinformation, and supplying accurate facts when possible, nurses can reduce associated fear, anxiety, and misinformation. Women may then seek earlier assessment, diagnosis, and effective treatment. Factual answers to questions are not always available. However, by maintaining a comfortable therapeutic relationship, nurses can support clients and their families.

Nurses need to provide current information about breast cancer. Controversies do exist, however. One current controversy involves risk factors. Which factors are important, and who is at greatest risk for developing breast cancer? Also, there are various opinions about the use of mammography in screening for breast cancer. Is mammography safe, and if so, which women should have it? Other controversies involve treatment selection. Four major methods of treatment are surgery, radiation therapy, hormonal therapy, and chemotherapy with cytotoxic agents. There also is the newer treatment, high-dose chemotherapy, and an autologous bone marrow transplant. Nurses are often involved in supporting clients as they make difficult decisions.

TABLE 78-1. Causes of Breast Masses for Three Age Groups

Under 35 years
Fibrocystic condition
Fibroadenoma
Mastitis
Traumatic fat necrosis
Carcinoma of breast
Between 35 and 50 years
Fibrocystic condition
Carcinoma
Fibroadenoma
Traumatic fat necrosis
Mastitis
Papilloma
Over 50 years
Carcinoma
Fibrocystic breast
Fat necrosis
Paget's disease of breast
Acute mastitis
Papilloma

Data from Robbins, S. L., et al. (1984). *Pathologic basis of disease* (3rd ed., p. 1190). Philadelphia: W. B. Saunders.

BREAST CANCER

Definition and Incidence

Breast cancer refers to a group of malignant diseases that commonly occur in the female breast and infrequently in the male breast. In 1991, it was estimated that 181,000 new breast cancers would occur in the United States and that about 46,300 deaths would occur from breast cancer.[12] One in every nine women is expected to develop breast cancer. Because of improvements in early detection and treatment, the 5-year survival rate for breast cancer has improved. This has helped stabilize (although not actually decrease) the mortality rates from breast cancer over the past 50 years despite an increasing incidence of breast cancer. Breast cancer, however, is the leading cause of cancer deaths in women between the ages of 14 and 54 years.[12] Lung cancer is now the leading cause of cancer deaths in all women; breast cancer is second.

Breast cancer in men is rare. One thousand new male breast cancer diagnoses and 300 deaths due to male breast cancer are estimated to occur in 1992.[12] Breast cancer is often diagnosed in a more advanced stage in men than in women.

Etiology

The cause of breast cancer has not been definitely established; genetic predisposition and hormonal factors may be involved (Table 78-1).

Risk Factors

Many factors have been associated with a significantly increased risk of breast cancer (Table 78-2). However, many women diagnosed with breast cancer have no risk factors. Most women can identify with at least one risk factor. The factors associated with the highest risk include (1) advancing age, (2) mother or sister with breast cancer, and (3) North America or Northern Europe as place of birth.[47, 93] Other important risk factors are (1) previous breast cancer, (2) previous radiation to the chest, (3) previous diagnosis of proliferative disease, (4) mammographic pattern of dysplastic parenchyma, (5) being over 30 years old at the time of first full-term pregnancy, (6) high socioeconomic status, and (7) early menarche and late menopause.[47, 100]

Risk factors related to ovarian function suggest a hormonal influence. Artificial menopause before the age of 35 years reduces the risk of breast cancer to one third of that experienced by those with natural menopause.[44] Hormonal and other factors associated with a moderate risk include (1) early menarche, (2) late menopause, (3) nulliparity, (4) exogenous estrogen given for menopause symptoms (contraceptives do not seem to produce higher risk), and (5) history of cancer of the uterus, ovary, or colon.

Risk factors under study as possible causes of increased incidence of breast cancer include (1) oral contraceptives, (2) exogenous hormones, (3) above-average weight and height, especially in postmenopausal women, (4) diet high in total fat, (5) alcohol consumption, (6) ovarian-pituitary dysfunction, (7) genetic factors, (8) benign breast disease, and (9) radiation exposure.[49, 56, 93]

TABLE 78–2. Factors Involved in a Significantly Higher Risk of Breast Cancer

Gender	99:1 women > men
Age	Growing older
Place of birth	North America Northern Europe
Socioeconomic status	High
Age at first full-term pregnancy	Greater than 30 years
Health history	Mammographic pattern of dysplastic parenchyma Past diagnosis of atypism, hyperplasia, or other benign proliferative disease in breast biopsy Large dose of radiation therapy to the chest Previous diagnosis of cancer in one breast
Family history	Mother or sister with history of breast cancer Any first-degree relative with breast cancer

Adapted from Kelsey, J. L., & Gammon, M. D. (1991). The epidemiology of breast cancer. *CA: A Cancer Journal for Clinicians, 41*(3), 157.

Factors that may lower a woman's risk of breast cancer include (1) late menarche, (2) early menopause, (3) oophorectomy premenopausally, (4) maintaining a normal or lighter than average weight after menopause, and (5) Asia (Japan especially) or Africa as place of birth.

For the best prognosis, it is extremely important for breast cancer to be detected early, before metastases occur. Breast self-examination, mammography, and a thorough breast examination by a clinician are important in early detection.

One of the nurse's roles, therefore, is to encourage all women to practice breast self-examination and follow the screening advice of the American Cancer Society (Box 78–1). Nurses also have a role in identifying women at risk for developing breast cancer and convincing them of the necessity for appropriate, careful assessment. Unfortunately, currently little can be done in the way of primary prevention to reduce most risk factors for breast cancer. Exceptions are maintaining normal or lighter than average body weight and reducing dietary fat (e.g., meat, dairy products). Growing evidence suggests that dietary fat promotes carcinogenesis because of its effect on hormone activity (see Bridge to Home Health Care).

Pathophysiology

Various histopathologic types of breast cancer exist with various prognoses.[44] These include intraductal carcinoma, infiltrating ductal carcinoma, medullary carcinoma, mucinous or colloid carcinoma, tubular carcinoma, lobular carcinoma in situ, infiltrating lobular carcinoma, inflammatory breast cancer, and Paget's disease.

INTRADUCTAL CARCINOMA

Intraductal carcinoma, also known as ductal carcinoma in situ, is a precancerous marker lesion that indicates a higher risk for invasive ductal breast cancer. It arises from the ductal epithelium and is confined to the ducts. Intraductal carcinoma is usually a microscopic incidental finding with removal of a benign breast lesion. Axillary metastases are uncommon. Prognosis is excellent. If left untreated, intraductal carcinoma will develop into invasive ductal carcinoma.

INFILTRATING DUCTAL CARCINOMA

Infiltrating ductal carcinoma (no other specification recognized) is found in 70 per cent of breast cancers. It is palpated as a stony-hard lump. Frequently, there is metastasis to axillary lymph nodes. Infiltrating ductal carcinoma has the poorest prognosis of the ductal carcinomas.

MEDULLARY CARCINOMA

Medullary carcinoma is found in 5 to 7 per cent of breast cancers. Frequently, it reaches large size. However, the prognosis is better than for many types of breast cancer.

MUCINOUS (COLLOID) CARCINOMA

Mucinous carcinoma, found in 3 per cent of breast cancers, frequently occurs with other types of breast cancer. It is slow-growing and can become quite large. Prognosis is good when the breast cancer is predominantly mucinous.

TUBULAR CARCINOMA

Tubular carcinoma frequently occurs with other types of breast cancer. Axillary metastases are uncommon. Prognosis is better than for infiltrating ductal carcinoma.

Box 78–1. Important Factors for Successful Breast Self-Examination

- Examine the breasts at the same time each month.
- Examine the breasts in a consistent pattern.
- Examine all surface areas: the breast, tail of Spence, and axilla.
- Examine all depth of the tissue: use pads of fingers and press deeply.
- Check for discharge, inspect the breasts visually, and feel for changes.
- Report any changes to the physician.

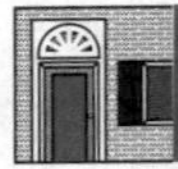

BRIDGE TO HOME HEALTH CARE

Preventive Breast Care

Consideration of how women can prevent and detect early symptoms of any breast disease should be the primary focus of home health care nursing. First, women need education about their level of risk. Women at high risk include those over 55 years of age, never married, older than 30 years at first pregnancy, and with a family history of breast cancer.

Women can make changes in their lifestyle to lower their risk of developing breast disease. Breast self-examinations that are done monthly are essential. Most lumps are found by women themselves. The earlier breast cancer is detected, the greater the chance of cure. Besides breast self-examination, an examination by a physician should be done every 3 years for women 20 to 40 years of age and every year for women over 40 years.

Diet is another area in which women can make sufficient changes for preventing disease. A low-fat diet can play an important part in prevention. Decreasing fat intake to 20 per cent of dietary calories is an admirable goal. Alcohol intake increases risk in relation to the amount of alcohol consumed.

Certain foods are helpful in decreasing risk. Cruciferous foods (broccoli, cabbage, cauliflower) help convert estrogen to a form less likely to cause cancer. Vitamin A (beta-carotene foods, orange and dark green vegetables) inhibit abnormal cell growth. Soybeans suppress estrogen production.

Women should be informed about and encouraged to have mammograms. Mammograms can detect very small tumors long before they might otherwise be found by manual breast examination. The recommendations for mammograms are as follows: obtain a baseline at 35 to 39 years of age unless high-risk factors exist; repeat every 1 to 2 years for ages 40 to 50 years; and yearly for women over 50 years.

The American Cancer Society is an excellent source for further information about the prevention, detection, and treatment of breast cancer. Call 1-800-ACS-2345.

LOBULAR CARCINOMA IN SITU

Lobular carcinoma in situ is a precancerous marker lesion that indicates a higher risk for invasive breast cancer. It arises from the mammary lobules and is usually a microscopic incidental finding with removal of a benign breast lesion. Check-ups every 6 months without treatment may be indicated, or bilateral mastectomies may be performed because of the bilaterality of lobular carcinoma in situ that may or may not develop into infiltrating lobular breast cancer.

INFILTRATING LOBULAR CARCINOMA

Infiltrating lobular carcinoma is found in 5 to 10 per cent of breast cancers. It usually presents as an area of ill-defined thickening rather than a lump. Multicentricity or involvement of the opposite breast may be found. Frequently, there is metastasis to axillary lymph nodes.

INFLAMMATORY BREAST CANCER

Inflammatory breast cancer is characterized by skin redness and induration. Edema, redness, warmth, and induration are frequent associated findings. Frequently, palpable axillary and supraclavicular nodes and distant metastases are involved. Prognosis is poor.

PAGET'S DISEASE

Paget's disease is found in 1 to 4 per cent of breast cancers. A special classification characterizes Paget's disease by a relatively long history of crusting and scaling skin changes in the nipple with burning, itching, or bleeding.

Cancer Staging

Numerous staging systems (see Chap. 21) have been developed for cancer. The staging of a cancer is based on (1) size of the primary lesion, (2) extent of the cancer's spread to regional lymph nodes, and (3) presence or absence of metastases. Staging provides prognostic information; Figure 78-1 illustrates breast cancer staging. The commonly used TNM staging system (Table 78-3) groups breast cancer according to the characteristics of the primary tumor (T), regional lymph nodes (N), and distant metastases (M).[6] With breast cancer, subgroup assignments are made according to tumor size, tumor attachment to underlying structure, and other characteristics such as edema.

Several other parameters are useful in determining the prognosis of and treatment for women with breast cancer.[20, 44, 75, 101] These include multicentricity, estrogen-progesterone receptor status of the tumor, and the immunocompetence of the woman. If cancer is found in two or more locations (multicentric) in the breast, the woman will probably not be a candidate for lumpectomy or quandrantectomy. If the tumor is estrogen-progesterone receptor-positive, she will probably receive antiestrogen hormonal therapy.

Tests of the proliferative activity of the tumor are gaining popularity. Ploidy refers to the amount of DNA contained in cells. Diploid or euploid indicates normal amount of DNA. Aneuploid indicates abnormal amounts and a poorer prognosis. The S phase index identifies the percentage of tumor cells in S phase of the cell growth cycle. The higher the percentage in S phase, the more aggressive the cancer. The labeling index measures the uptake of thymidine, which is used primarily in DNA synthesis or the S phase of the cell growth cycle.

Studies are also looking at the role of oncogenes in breast cancer.[33] So far, no specific oncogene has been identified as a contributor to human breast cancer or as providing specific prognostic information.

Cancer is graded on the cytologic differentiation of tumor cells and the number of mitoses within the tumor. Grading tries to identify some degree of a tumor's malignancy or to estimate its aggressiveness. The grading of breast cancer is similar to the grading of

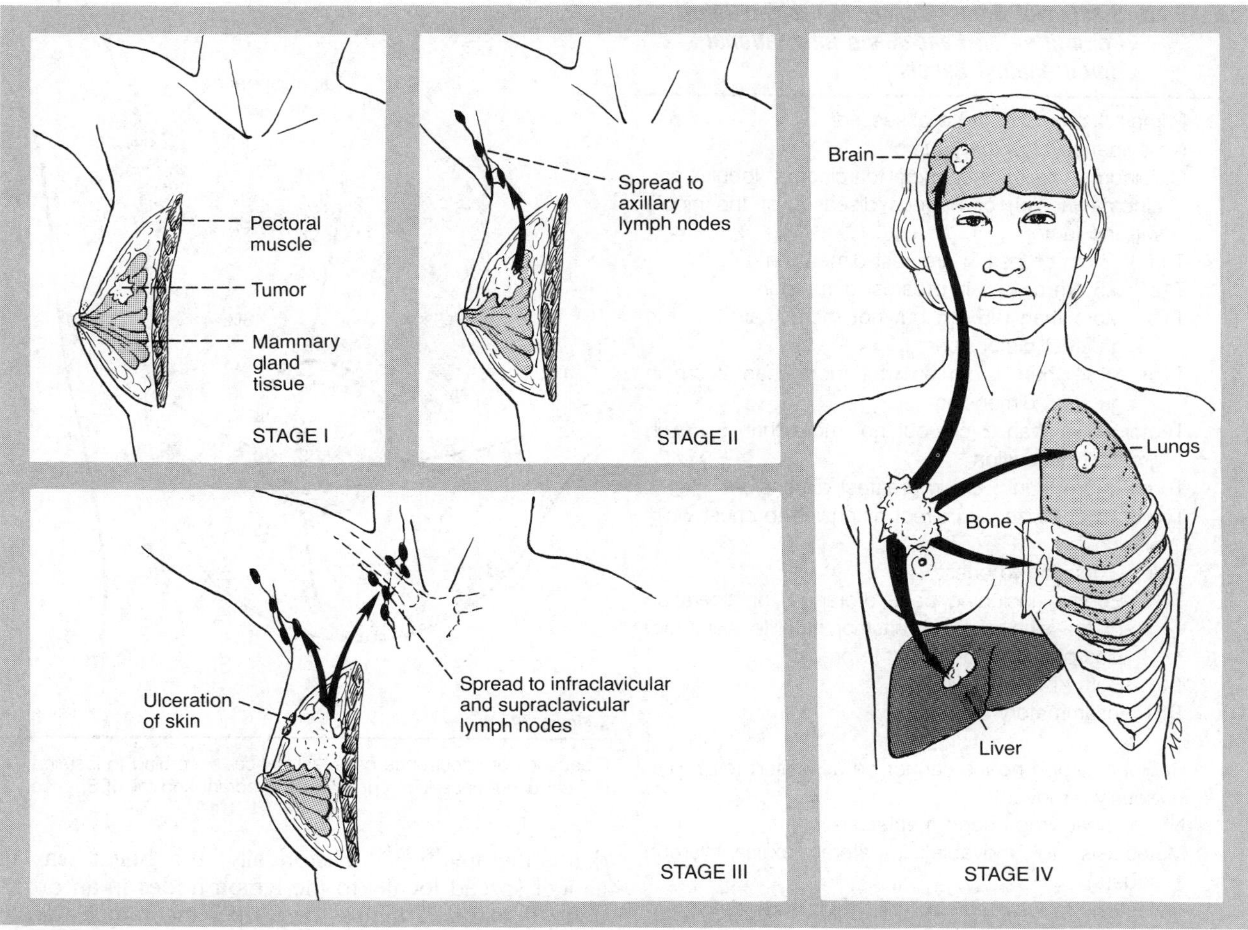

▲ *Figure 78–1*

Clinical staging of breast cancer. Stage I: tumor less than 2 cm and confined to breast. Stage II: tumor up to 5 cm, or axillary lymph nodes contain early metastasis. Stage III: tumor larger than 5 cm, or extends to chest wall or skin, or involvement of infraclavicular or supraclavicular lymph nodes. Stage IV: distant metastasis such as to brain, bone, or liver.

other cancers. Newer studies are closely examining the grade of a breast cancer as a prognostic factor.

Clinical Manifestations

The nurse should be alert for assessment findings indicating breast cancer, although detection may be difficult. Initially, breast cancer typically appears as a unilateral, single mass or thickening most often in a breast's upper outer quadrant (Fig. 78–2). The mass is usually painless, nontender, hard, irregular in shape, and nonmobile. Presentation of 64 to 70 per cent of breast cancers is as a palpable mass found by the client.[26] Four to 30 per cent are found by mammography.

DIAGNOSTIC ASSESSMENT

Pretreatment assessment varies. Chest x-ray examination, complete blood count, liver chemistries, and mammography of the opposite breast are frequently done. Other studies are in question, however. Bone scans or liver scans can give false-positive results and yield little useful information in asymptomatic clients. Some physicians believe scans should be used only for clients with stage III disease or abnormal liver chemistries. Others believe a baseline study, especially a bone scan, is valuable for later comparison.

Tumor markers (substances produced either by the tumor itself or by the body in response to tumor tissue) may be present in the serum of a client with breast cancer. The tumor markers—carcinoembryonic antigen (CEA), ferritin, and human chorionic gonadotropin (hCG)—are easy to obtain, so trying to identify these and to follow them after diagnosis is recommended.

Medical Management

Public knowledge is increasing about treatment options for breast cancer. Historically, breast cancer identified on a frozen section was immediately treated with a Halsted radical mastectomy at the time of the biopsy.

TABLE 78-3. Staging of Breast Cancer, American Joint Committee on Cancer and International Union Against Cancer

TX	Primary tumor cannot be assessed
T0	No evidence of primary tumor
Tis	Carcinoma in situ: intraductal carcinoma, lobular carcinoma in situ, or Paget's disease* of the nipple with no tumor
T1	Tumor 2 cm or less in greatest dimension
	T1a 0.5 cm or less in greatest dimension
	T1b More than 0.5 cm but not more than 1 cm in greatest dimension
	T1c More than 1 cm but not more than 2 cm in greatest dimension
T2	Tumor more than 2 cm but not more than 5 cm in greatest dimension
T3	Tumor more than 5 cm in greatest dimension
T4	Tumor of any size with direct extension to chest wall† or skin
	T4a Extension to chest wall
	T4b Edema (including peau d'orange) or ulceration of the skin of the breast or satellite skin nodules confined to the same breast
	T4c Both (T4a and T4b)
	T4d Inflammatory carcinoma
NX	Regional lymph nodes cannot be assessed (e.g., previously removed)
N0	No regional lymph node metastasis
N1	Metastasis to movable ipsilateral axillary lymph node(s)
N2	Metastasis to ipsilateral axillary lymph node(s) fixed to one another or to other structures
N3	Metastasis to ipsilateral internal mammary lymph node(s)
MX	Presence of distant metastasis cannot be assessed
M0	No distant metastasis
M1	Distant metastasis (includes metastasis to ipsilateral supraclavicular lymph node[s])

From Beahrs, O. H. (1991). Staging of cancer. *CA: A Cancer Journal for Clinicians, 41*(2), 122–124.

* Paget's disease associated with a tumor is classified according to the size of the tumor.

† Chest wall includes ribs, intercostal muscles, and serratus anterior muscle but not pectoral muscle

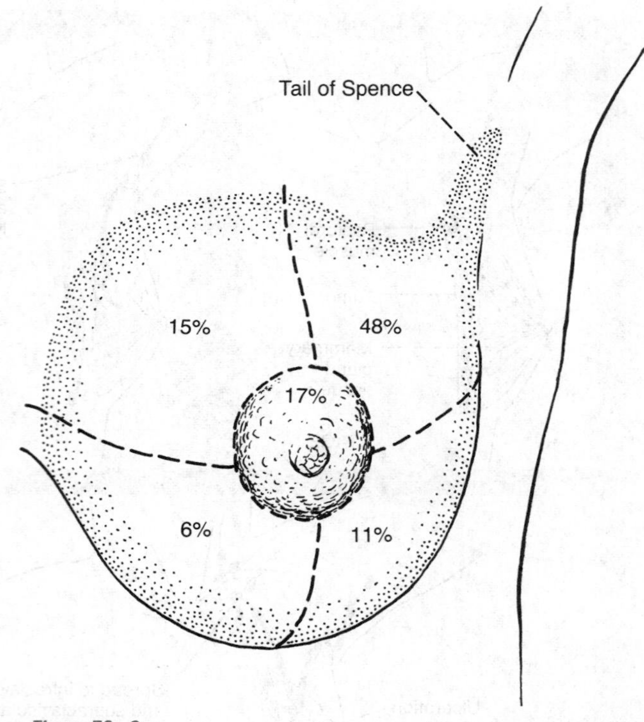

▲ *Figure 78-2*

Frequency of occurrence of breast cancer according to location. Note highest occurrence is in upper outer quadrant and tail of Spence.

Typically, the woman and her family did not know she had cancer or that her breast was to be removed until after the surgery was over. Now women and their families want to be informed about treatment options and included in treatment decision making before it is initiated.[52, 91] Nurses must be knowledgeable about recent advances in treatment as well as treatment controversies in order to support women and their significant others as they make decisions.[50, 84] It is important for the nurse to know that a woman diagnosed with early stage breast cancer may live a long, healthy life and keep her breast.

Because of greater understanding of tumor biology, it is now recognized that breast cancer requires multimodality therapy.[16, 30, 39] Historically, the belief was that cancer spread locally to the lymph nodes in an orderly, defined manner. If this were true, the radical mastectomy should eliminate the disease. It is now known that breast cancer does not spread in an orderly manner and that cancer cells use the bloodstream to metastasize to other organs such as bone, lung, brain, and liver. Because of this, less radical surgical procedures are used in combination with radiation therapy, hormonal therapy, or chemotherapy.[48, 76] In 1988, 62 per cent of breast cancer clients had mastectomies, 9 per cent had no surgical procedure, and 25 per cent had only partial mastectomies.[78] Now various treatment combinations are used in order to cure breast cancer through local, regional, or systemic treatments. Women who have early small breast cancers may be best served by first having a mastectomy or lumpectomy to be followed by radiation therapy, chemotherapy, or hormonal therapy as indicated. Women with locally advanced stage II breast cancer may be better served by having hormonally synchronized chemotherapy shrink the breast cancer before surgery and radiation therapy. Local and regional treatment involves treating the breast and chest wall. Mastectomy or adjuvant radiation therapy in combination with a lumpectomy or a quadrantectomy is used for local control of stage I or stage II breast cancer. Adjuvant (given after surgery) or neoadjuvant (given before surgery) chemotherapy or hormonal therapy may be given to reduce the risk of recurrence. Chemotherapy and hormonal therapy treat potential or known metastatic disease for systemic control. Hormonal therapy is used to treat women with estrogen and progesterone receptor-positive breast cancer. Chemotherapy is used to treat women with positive lymph nodes (stage II), locally advanced cancer (stage III), and metastatic breast cancer (stage IV) and even some women with lymph node-negative (stage I) disease.

In order to provide multimodality therapy, a multidisciplinary evaluation is needed for determining the best course of treatment. A few major cancer treatment centers provide a consultation appointment at which surgical oncologists, medical oncologists, radiation oncologists, plastic surgeons, gynecologists, pathologists, mammographic radiology specialists, specialized nurses, and social workers are all available at the one appointment to evaluate the woman and her disease and to recommend the best treatment combination.[11, 28, 40] In many communities, the team consultation during one appointment may not be feasible. However, before any treatment is initiated, it is best for the woman to be evaluated for the need for each treatment modality and to determine the best therapeutic plan. This multidisciplinary evaluation before treatment is still possible in most communities through a series of appointments to specialists so long as the primary health care provider coordinates all appointments to occur in a timely manner and oversees the sequencing of treatment and follow-up. The nurse is important in facilitating the multidisciplinary process in both the major treatment centers and in other settings. Whatever the setting, the nurse has a major role in helping the woman through all phases of diagnosis and treatment.

Most of all breast cancer treatment is done on an outpatient basis. Mastectomy and other breast procedures that include an axillary lymph node dissection typically involve only a 2- to 3-day hospital stay. In order to have continuity of care for the women undergoing multimodality therapy, the nurses in the various treatment disciplines need to collaborate and share assessment information, nursing care plans, and reports on the woman's progress.

Women with breast cancer at any stage fear disfigurement and death. Much has been written about the psychosocial impact of breast cancer.[32] Some women chose to have reconstructive surgery to rebuild their breasts and create new nipples. Breast reconstruction helps some women adjust to the loss of their breast.

With more women receiving breast-conserving procedures, it is important for nurses and health professionals to consider the impact of these therapies. It has been shown that the women who have breast-conserving surgical procedures feel better about the appearance of their nude body than do women who had mastectomy. However, the psychological impact of having breast cancer in other ways has not been eliminated.[32, 90, 99, 104] A woman who has had a lumpectomy and radiation therapy will still have scars and other physical changes of which she will be aware and that will be there to remind her that she has had breast cancer. Because she has kept her breast, she may worry about recurrence or wonder if she should have had a mastectomy. Daily radiation treatments for several weeks may delay resumption of her normal pattern of daily activities. Also, there are the side effects of radiation therapy that the woman will have to cope with. Some of the common complaints are tenderness, change in the texture of the breast, and arm or hand numbness.[10]

The nurse has an important role in caring for women with breast cancer and their families. The nurse needs to consider the emotional, social, cognitive, spiritual, and physical factors involved, whatever the treatment combination.

RADIATION THERAPY

Radiation therapy (see Chap. 22) is used in breast cancer treatment as follows:

- The breast and the underlying chest wall are irradiated for local control in stage I or stage II breast cancer after lumpectomy or quadrantectomy. Women who are poor surgical candidates because of health problems such as heart disease typically will receive radiation therapy to their breast.
- The chest wall is irradiated if it is involved or for local control after mastectomy with positive margins.
- The axilla is irradiated in women at high risk for axillary metastases who are poor surgical candidates for axillary dissection or have gross disease left behind.
- The supraclavicular region is irradiated if there are positive axillary nodes.
- Additional areas are irradiated for management of metastatic disease of the brain, bone, or skin.

Radiation in combination with lumpectomy or quadrantectomy is an accepted treatment for early stage (e.g., stage I or stage II) breast cancer.[54, 77, 83] An axillary dissection is usually done for staging purposes. Women who are eligible for these treatment choices are women with (1) lesions less than 5 cm, (2) no large or fixed ancillary nodes, (3) no demonstrable disease, (4) clear surgical margins, and (5) breasts that can be easily evaluated mammographically. Lumpectomy and quadrantectomy, with dissection of axillary lymph nodes (for staging) and radiation to the breast area, have produced good results. The survival rates and incidence of local and distant recurrence are equal to those from mastectomy.[44] Radiation therapy can be administered through an external beam and via iridium implants.

External beam radiation is administered 5 days a week by a cobalt machine or linear accelerator with use of approximately 5000 rad over 5 weeks.[48] Regional lymph nodes may be treated if they were not removed.

A concentrated boost of radiation is given to the small area where the tumor is located. A radiation boost to only the small area involved reduces the risk of side effects while the area of highest risk of disease is treated. After more than 5000 rad is given to the entire breast, the incidence of side effects increases. However, if the total radiation dose is too low, the risk of recurrence increases. The boost of radiation can be given with several additional linear accelerator treatments by electron beam therapy or via an interstitial iridium implant.

Interstitial implant therapy using iridium (^{192}Ir) is performed over 2 to 3 days as an inhospital procedure. The insertion of the iridium implant may be done with local anesthesia. Stainless steel guide needles are threaded through the tumor area at 1-cm intervals. Flexible plastic tubes are inserted in the guide needles. The guide needles are then removed, leaving the tubing in place. Strands of radioactive iridium seeds are threaded through each tube (Fig. 78-3). The seeds, at 1-cm intervals, form a grid with those above and below to cover the tissues evenly with radiation. At the end of the insertion procedure, a button is attached, and the ends are crimped and then cut to prevent the seeds from falling out. An x-ray film confirms the implant's location. The length of time the implant must remain in place usually is 2 or 3 days. The procedure is mildly uncomfortable. The woman is able to be up and about in her room. Radiation precautions related to time, distance, and shielding are maintained.

Radiation therapy, in combination with lumpectomy or quadrantectomy, effectively treats early stage breast cancer and avoids the psychosocial trauma of mastectomy. It is surprising to some health professionals that this treatment modality is not used more frequently. Let us consider three objections to the use of radiation for treatment of breast cancer. The first is concern that undetected cancer may remain after the identified tumor is removed by the excisional biopsy. However, several studies show that survival and local control are equal to those achieved with mastectomy.[54, 77, 83] A second objection is the concern that radiation might induce new cancers in the remaining breast or adjacent tissue. However, radiation has been used for over 30 years, and thus far the incidence of secondary malignancies attributable to radiation therapy for breast cancer is small.[29] The third objection is the thought that the breast may not be cosmetically pleasing after radiation because of fibrosis or pigment changes. However, in most cases, the skin changes are minimal.

Side effects from radiation to the breast include the following:

- Temporary skin changes are common (e.g., itchy, dry, tender, red, swollen, or dry desquamation).
- Fatigue
- Dry throat (rare) occurring in the later weeks of treatment is due to radiation's effect on pharyngeal mucosa if the supraclavicular area is irradiated. Although often described as a "lump in the throat," it should not interfere with eating.
- Pneumonitis (rare), indicated by dry cough and dyspnea, is due to inflammatory changes in the irradiated underlying lung.

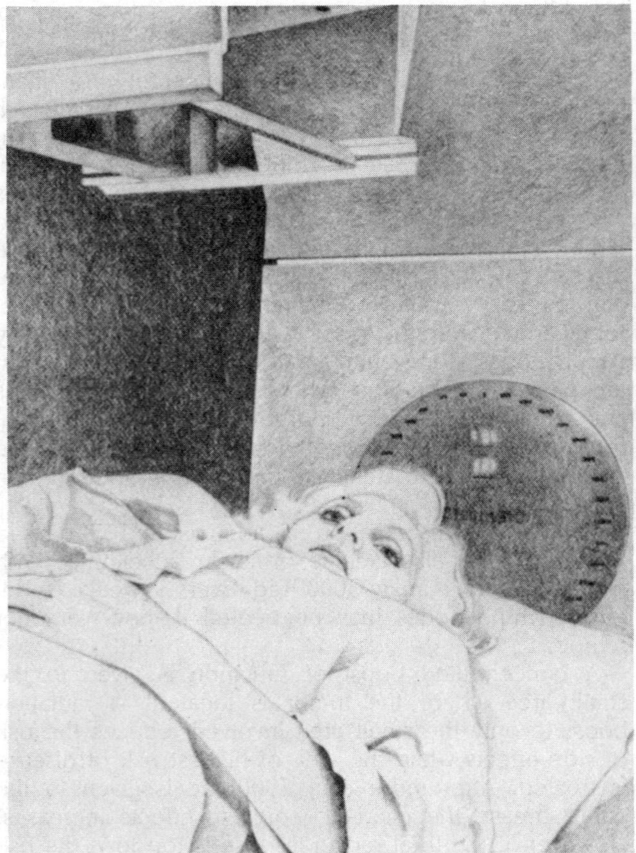

A

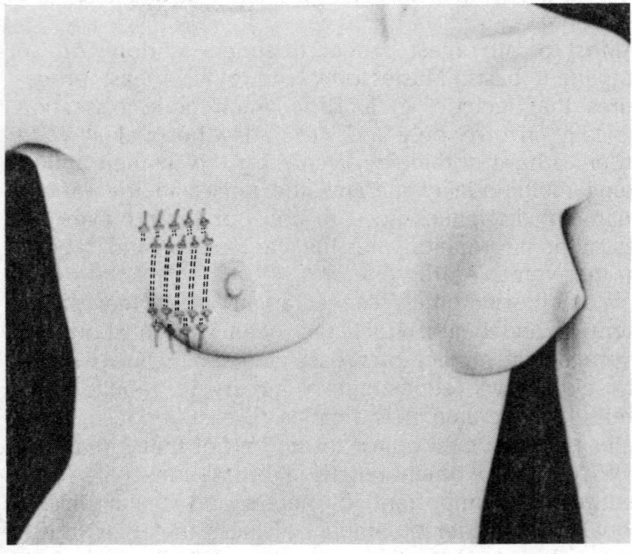

B

▲ *Figure 78-3*

Radiation therapy is given via an external beam or iridium implants. (From National Cancer Institute [1990]. *Radiation therapy: A treatment for early stage breast cancer* [NIH Publication No. 91-659]. Washington, DC. National Cancer Institute.)

- Arm edema (rare) may occur after axillary irradiation.
- Increased susceptibility to rib fractures occurs in the irradiated field.

Radiation therapy can be a long, difficult process for the client being treated. It is emotionally taxing to receive treatments daily for 5 to 7 weeks. Nursing support is needed during this period. Women receiving radiation therapy have many of the same fears as do those who had a mastectomy: fear of death, fear of mutilation, and feelings of sexual inadequacy. These are compounded by the stress of daily treatments and the fatigue that occurs with radiation therapy.

PHARMACOLOGIC MANAGEMENT

Adjuvant Chemotherapy. Adjuvant chemotherapy is given after surgical removal of any measurable cancer. The goal of adjuvant chemotherapy is to prolong the disease-free survival while helping the client maintain a high quality of life. Before 1988, premenopausal women with breast cancer in their lymph nodes commonly received chemotherapy. It was felt that women with node-negative breast cancer and postmenopausal women with positive lymph nodes would not benefit from chemotherapy. In 1988, a clinical alert was issued from the National Cancer Institute recommending consideration of adjuvant chemotherapy or hormonal therapy for all women with node-negative breast cancer as well as node-positive breast cancer.[63, 106] Premenopausal women with T1, node-negative, estrogen and progesterone receptor-positive breast cancer will probably receive adjuvant hormonal therapy and may or may not receive chemotherapy.[31]

Typically, adjuvant chemotherapy is administered in an ambulatory setting beginning a few weeks after surgery or after the completion of radiation therapy. Various combinations of antineoplastic agents are used.[14, 27, 49, 102, 106] Cyclophosphamide (Cytoxan), 5-fluorouracil (5-FU), and methotrexate (i.e., CMF) make up one of the most frequently used combinations. Doxorubicin, prednisone, thio-TEPA, and vincristine are some of the other drugs that may be used.

Recently, high-dose chemotherapy with autologous bone marrow transplant has been used to treat women with breast cancer.[1] Bone marrow transplant may be used with stage II, stage III, or stage IV disease. Bone marrow rescue permits larger doses of agents, which otherwise are limited because of their severe myelosuppressive toxicity.

Neoadjuvant Chemotherapy. Neoadjuvant chemotherapy is given to treat locally advanced breast cancer (stage III) before surgical removal of the cancer. The goal of neoadjuvant chemotherapy is to evaluate the response of the measurable cancer to treatment. Women with a breast cancer tumor greater than 5 cm in the breast or axilla may receive neoadjuvant chemotherapy and hormonal therapy before surgery or radiation therapy.[19, 97] The goal is to shrink the local disease and reduce the risk of systemic spread. Recently, hormonal synchronization with combination chemotherapy has been under investigation.[19, 97] Because it is known that certain cell cycle-specific chemotherapies (e.g., methotrexate and 5-FU) are more effective on growing cells, estrogen is given to stimulate cell growth in order to maximize cell kill. In one study,[19] doxorubicin and cyclophosphamide are given on day 1 of the cycle. On days 6, 7, and 8, estrogen is given. The cell cycle-specific chemotherapies methotrexate and 5-FU are given on day 8. On days 9 through 14, tamoxifen is given. A new treatment cycle of the same drugs begins on day 22. The women receive 17 cycles of this chemotherapy. Surgery and radiation therapy usually take place after there is stable disease, when there is no palpable tumor, when the disease has progressed, or around the ninth cycle.

Systemic Therapy for Metastatic Breast Cancer. When the cancer has spread outside the breast and the ipsilateral axillary regions, systemic therapy is necessary. Some of the antineoplastic agents used to treat metastatic breast cancer include cisplatin, cyclophosphamide, doxorubicin, 5-FU, methotrexate, mitomycin C, thio-TEPA, vinblastine and vincristine. No one combination offers a clear advantage. Table 78-4 lists the commonly used combinations of drugs.

Side Effects of Chemotherapy. Common side effects for most antineoplastic chemotherapy combinations include varying degrees of alopecia (hair loss); constipation; depression of red blood cells, white blood cells, and platelets; diarrhea; fatigue; menopausal symptoms; nausea; peripheral neuropathy; photosensitivity; sterility; stomatitis; vaginal dryness; vomiting; and weight gain.[17, 49, 51] Several of the agents have their own specific toxic side effects (see Chap. 22). In addition to these side effects, receiving chemotherapy may reduce the woman's social, household, and work-related activities; cause problems in marital, sexual, and family life; and cause a financial burden that can change the woman's quality of life.[105] Understanding this can help the nurse plan and provide appropriate support for women receiving chemotherapy.

Hormonal Therapy. Some breast cancers respond to hormonal therapy because they contain high levels of receptor proteins, specific for certain steroids. These receptor proteins are capable of binding estrogen, progesterone, androgen, and corticosteroids. It is standard practice for breast biopsy tissue that is diagnosed as cancer to be sent for estrogen receptor assay and progesterone receptor assay.[44] Estrogen and progesterone receptor assay involves the laboratory examination of 100 to 200 mg of cancerous breast tissue. The breast cancer tissue is considered estrogen receptor-positive (ER+) or progesterone receptor-positive (PR+) if the assay results indicate 10 femtomoles (fmol) or more are present.[96] Generally, if the results are less than 10 fmol, the tissue is considered ER− or PR− (negative).

It is important to know the estrogen status of breast tumors because ER+ tumors are associated with slower growth rates, less aggressive behavior, and longer survival. Both ER+ and PR+ results predict tumors that

TABLE 78-4. Chemotherapy Combinations Used to Treat Breast Cancer

Combination	Response Rate (%)
AC	50-80
Doxorubicin (Adriamycin)	
Cyclophosphamide	
AM	25-50
Doxorubicin	
Mitomycin C	
CAF	45-80
Cyclophosphamide	
Doxorubicin	
Fluorouracil	
CMF	50-65
Cyclophosphamide	
Methotrexate	
Fluorouracil	
CMFA	50-65
Cyclophosphamide	
Methotrexate	
Fluorouracil	
Doxorubicin	
CMFP	50-60
Cyclophosphamide	
Methotrexate	
Fluorouracil	
Prednisone	
CMFVP	50-60
Cyclophosphamide	
Methotrexate	
Fluorouracil	
Vincristine	
Prednisone	
VAC	50
Vincristine	
Doxorubicin	
Cyclophosphamide	

Adapted from Harness, J. K., et al. (1988). *Breast cancer collaborative management*. Chelsea MI: Lewis Publishers.

will respond well to hormonal manipulation. Hormonal therapy may successfully treat metastases to bone, lymph nodes, skin, remaining breast tissue, and lung. It is rarely successful in treating brain or liver metastases. Various medical and surgical methods have been used with varying degrees of success (Table 78-5).

Antiestrogen. Tamoxifen is the antiestrogen commonly used. Other antiestrogens are under investigation. Tamoxifen is administered orally in the treatment of ER+ breast cancer. Often, it is prescribed for years.[34] It has relatively few side effects, most of which are fairly well tolerated by most women. Side effects may include hot flashes, vaginal dryness, nausea, vomiting, hypercalcemia, or a flare response (a transient flare of breast cancer symptoms). These side effects often decrease after a few weeks. The nurse needs to help the woman cope with side effects, in particular, the menopause type side effects (i.e., hot flashes and vaginal dryness).

Estrogen has been used since 1950 to treat breast cancer in postmenopausal women.[44] The antitumor effect may take several weeks to occur. Side effects commonly include anorexia, nausea, vomiting, sodium and fluid retention, increased libido, withdrawal bleeding, and hypercalcemia. Rarely, a flare response of the disease with increased bone pain may occur. This usually indicates a good response to the therapy.

Androgens are usually less effective than estrogens but may be superior for bone metastases. Side effects include virilization and increased libido. Progesterone, in large doses, is also used for those who have previously responded to other additive hormones.

Aminoglutethimide may be prescribed to inhibit adrenal steroid production in metastatic breast cancer. This therapy is superior to an adrenalectomy. It avoids the need for lifelong replacement therapy, which must be continued after adrenalectomy or hypophysectomy. When aminoglutethimide is used, adrenal suppression leads to a reflex rise in adrenocorticotropic hormone, which can overcome the effect of aminoglutethimide. Therefore, suppressive doses of corticosteroids must be given. However, corticosteroids need to be continued only as long as the aminoglutethimide is used. Possible side effects of aminoglutethimide include lethargy, dizziness, visual blurring, and rash. They are dose-dependent and transient.

Surgical Management

Surgery is important in the diagnosis and treatment of most breast cancers. Some breast surgical procedures are very disfiguring (e.g., radical mastectomy and modified radical mastectomy). However, less extensive procedures may be used (e.g., lumpectomy and quadrantectomy).

An axillary lymph node dissection (axillary dissection) is done typically for help in staging the disease.

TABLE 78-5. Effectiveness of Endocrine Therapy for Metastatic Breast Cancer

	% Responding to Therapy	
	Receptor-Positive	**Receptor-Negative**
Tamoxifen	54	9
Estrogen	57	9
Androgen	43	8
Progestins	35	8
Aminoglutethimide	54	6
Oophorectomy	33	6
Adrenalectomy	46	10
Hypophysectomy	?	?
	(36% response rate receptor status unknown)	

Adapted from DeVita, V. T., et al. (1989). *Cancer principle and practice of oncology* (3rd ed.). Philadelphia: J. B. Lippincott.

Axillary lymph nodes are not the only site of spread of breast cancer. However, when cancer is found in the nodes (node-positive), there is a greater likelihood that there are distant metastases and that systemic therapy, chemotherapy, is needed.

From the initial surgical procedure diagnosing breast cancer, a portion of the cancer tissue is sent for estrogen and progesterone receptor assay. If there are high levels of estrogen or progesterone receptors, then the woman may need hormonal therapy. (See preceding discussion of hormonal therapy.)

Occasionally, a mastectomy is done in order to prevent breast cancer in women who are at a high risk for breast cancer. When a mastectomy is done to prevent breast cancer, it is sometimes called a *prophylactic mastectomy*. Reconstructive surgery (see Chap. 72) may be performed at the same time or delayed to a later date. This is a controversial surgery. The goal is to decrease the likelihood of development of breast cancer. However, typically a conservative approach involving careful observation is usually recommended for women at high risk. A prophylactic mastectomy should be contemplated in rare circumstances. In those with unilateral breast cancer, the risk of finding a breast cancer in the opposite breast is four to seven times greater than that of the initial cancer in the general population.

Possible complications of breast surgery may include lymphedema, infection, seroma, hematoma, and cellulitis. Nurses need to teach clients the signs and symptoms of these problems.

SURGICAL PROCEDURES FOR BREAST CANCER

The lumpectomy, quadrantectomy, modified radical mastectomy, and axillary node dissection procedures are the most frequently used surgical procedures for treatment of breast cancer.[7]

Lumpectomy. This procedure involves the removal of the cancerous mass and some normal tissue for clean margins. Frequently, the initial excisional biopsy is the lumpectomy. A reexcision may be needed if the margins are not clean in the original biopsy.

Quadrantectomy. This procedure removes the quadrant of the breast in which the cancer is located. A greater portion of normal tissue surrounding the cancer is removed with some of the overlying skin and underlying muscular fascia in order to provide a wide margin of cancer-free tissue.

Modified Radical Mastectomy. This procedure involves the en bloc removal of the breast, axillary lymph nodes, and overlying skin. This is the most commonly performed mastectomy.

Axillary Node Dissection. This procedure removes ipsilateral lymph nodes. It is part of the modified radical mastectomy and the standard mastectomy. An axillary node dissection may be the only additional surgical procedure needed by a woman who had an excisional biopsy that diagnosed and removed a small breast cancer with clean margins. The axillary dissection is not usually done to treat the disease, but it stages the disease and determines the need for more chemotherapy.

Total (Simple) Mastectomy. This procedure involves resection of breast tissue and some skin from clavicle to costal margin and from midline to the latissimus dorsi. The axillary tail and pectoral fascia are removed also. Axillary nodes are not removed. This procedure is rarely used to treat diagnosed breast cancer. More frequently, bilateral simple mastectomies or total mastectomies are done to prevent breast cancer in women who are at high risk for having the disease.

Standard Radical Mastectomy. This procedure involves the en bloc removal of the breast, overlying skin, pectoral muscles, and axillary nodes. It removes the local lesion and the axillary nodes with a wide "safety margin" of surrounding tissue. Dissatisfaction with treatment results and morbidity has caused the number of radical mastectomies performed for primary breast cancer to decline sharply.

Extended Radical Mastectomy. This procedure involves the removal of the internal mammary nodes in addition to the structures removed during the standard radical mastectomy. This procedure currently has few advocates because it does not seem to be significantly more effective than is irradiation in preventing recurrence from internal mammary metastases.

Surgical Hormonal Manipulation. A bilateral oophorectomy has been used for over 80 years as a form of hormonal therapy in premenopausal women with advanced breast cancer. Radiation to the ovaries may also be used to achieve castration (stopping the function of the ovaries), but it may take up to 2 months for the therapy to be effective.

In castrated or postmenopausal women, other surgical procedures, such as bilateral adrenalectomy or hypophysectomy (removal of the anterior pituitary), can be used to further decrease the remaining low level of estrogen. If so, daily cortisone replacement is required to prevent adrenal crisis. Fludrocortisone acetate (Florinef) is also required to replace the adrenal salt-regulating hormone.

Hypophysectomy also requires daily replacement of cortisone, thyroid hormone, and posterior pituitary hormones (e.g., vasopressin or antidiuretic hormone), if necessary.

Daily replacement therapy after bilateral adrenalectomy or hypophysectomy is required for life. A medical identification bracelet should be worn at all times after these surgeries. A card indicating the type and dose of necessary replacement medications should also be carried.

BREAST RECONSTRUCTION

Breast reconstruction is an option for women who have had a mastectomy.[13, 46] Consideration needs to be

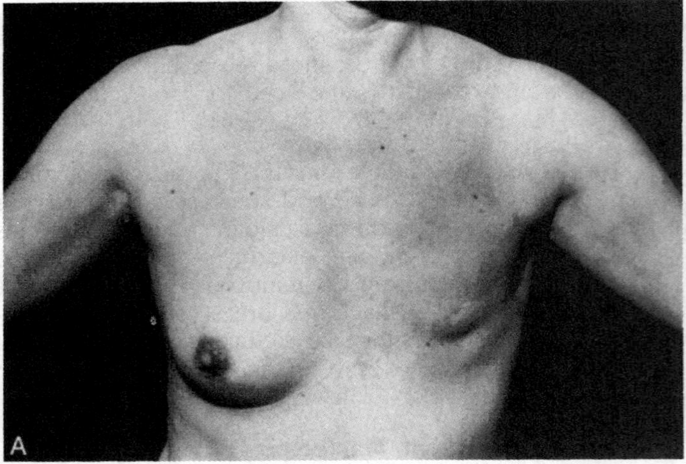

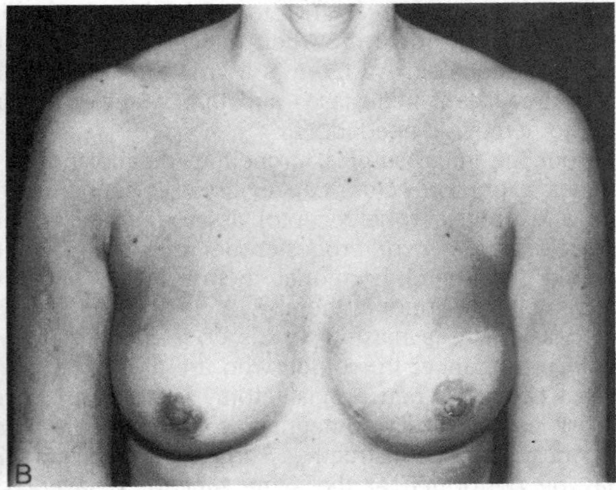

▲ **Figure 78-4**

Preoperative *(A)* and postoperative *(B)* views of an ideal result from use of a latissimus dorsi myocutaneous flap and an implant. A subpectoral implant was used in the right breast for symmetry. (From Bland, K. I., & Copeland, E. M. (Eds.) [1991]. *The breast: Comprehensive management of benign and malignant disease.* Philadelphia: W. B. Saunders.)

given to a woman's overall health and ability to tolerate a prolonged surgery, the stage of disease, the need for radiation therapy or chemotherapy, and the woman's expectations (Fig. 78-4).

New techniques provide the woman with choices for the type of reconstruction and when to do reconstruction. Breast reconstruction can be done by use of tissue expanders, implants (see Ethical Issues in Nursing and Chap. 72), latissimus dorsi muscle, transverse rectus abdominis muscle, or gluteus maximus muscle.[23, 45] The nurse needs to know about each of these procedures in order to answer questions (see Chap. 19). A woman may choose to delay reconstruction until after radiation or chemotherapy is completed. Or she may choose immediate reconstruction to be done at the same time as the mastectomy so she has a breast when she comes out of the anesthetic.

Breast reconstruction can help restore the woman's balance, symmetry, and body image. The nurse can help the woman while she is deciding about reconstructive surgery, while preparing for reconstructive surgery, and while recovering from the surgery (see Chap. 19). Knowing about reconstruction and whether it is an option for her may help a woman with breast cancer cope with the need for a mastectomy. The nurse can provide information about reconstruction. A booklet, *Breast reconstruction: A matter of choice,* is available free from the National Cancer Institute.[74]

Nursing Management

ASSESSMENT

The assessment of the woman should begin with assessment of the breasts, identification of the woman's risk factors, a description of the lump or problem, and current fears or concerns. It is also important to find out how the client discovered the lump.

The preoperative period before breast surgery for cancer or possible cancer is a very stressful time. Many fears surface, and the lives of the client and significant others are disrupted. A contradiction exists because usually the client feels well in spite of impending sur-

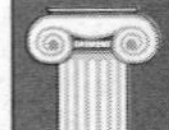

ETHICAL ISSUES IN NURSING

Breast Reconstruction: Are Silicone Implants a Safe Alternative?

For many women with breast cancer, breast implants allow both physical and mental treatment for the disfigurement that may result from surgery. For other women who simply wish to enhance their breasts, implants produce desired esthetic effects. Silicone breast implants have been in use since 1902, and millions of women throughout the world have undergone breast augmentation. No matter what opinions are held about breast implants, it is generally accepted that women have a right to such a procedure if they so choose.

Does this right to choose silicone breast implants imply that there is a duty of the implant manufacturers to produce a safe product? It has been recently proposed that silicone leakage from breast implants may cause various systemic side effects, some of which may be very serious. If this is true, does the Food and Drug Administration have an obligation to ban such implants in order to protect certain members of society from harm? Should a woman have the right to have silicone breast augmentation if she is adequately informed of the possible side effects that may occur should such implants rupture or leak silicone?

If silicone is the problem, perhaps saline implants may be the solution. Women could still choose to have augmentations but not have to worry about the possible side effects that silicone may cause. Autonomy would be preserved and beneficence fostered.

gery. The preoperative period may also be stressful for health professionals. Nurses need an opportunity to explore their personal feelings about breast cancer before they can satisfactorily help others. Nurses providing preoperative care assess the woman's and significant others' reactions to the frightening experience. The woman and significant others need an opportunity to talk about the surgery and feel that someone cares about them. Nursing assessment focuses on the woman's knowledge level, coping ability, self-concept, and sexual concerns. It helps to include the sexual partner in assessment and planning. Nurses also need to be knowledgeable about all aspects of care and the therapeutic plan for each client so they can accurately discuss questions (see Nursing Care Plan).

Postoperative assessments should also include the client's psychological reaction to the surgery. Other important assessments include the wound, drains, presence of lymphedema, signs and symptoms of infection, and pain.

NURSING INTERVENTION

Nursing Diagnosis: Knowledge Deficit R/T available options of treatment and surgery (if chosen).

Planning: Expected Outcomes. The client will understand the available treatment options and surgery (if chosen), as evidenced by the client's questions and statements concerning options and the client's ability to explain her choice.

Implementation. The woman should receive information about recommendations and treatment options before surgery or treatment is initiated. The nurse can help women understand treatment options.[103] Because the typical hospital stay for a modified radical mastectomy or lumpectomy and axillary node dissection surgery is 2 to 3 days, preoperative teaching is done on an outpatient basis. The nurse needs to consider postoperative teaching along with preoperative care.

Nursing assessment provides data about knowledge deficits for use in formulating a teaching plan. This includes preoperative activities, explanations of surgery, postoperative care, discharge planning, and ways in which the client can participate. The woman's anxiety level may be so high that new information cannot be remembered, so provide written as well as verbal instructions. It is important to evaluate learning and to repeat information as often as necessary.

Nursing Diagnosis: Individual Coping, Ineffective and Family Coping, Ineffective, High Risk for, R/T diagnosis of cancer and surgical changes in breast.

Planning: Expected Outcomes. The client will cope with the diagnosis of cancer and surgical changes in the breast, as evidenced by client's statement of acceptance and decisions about treatment; the family will also cope effectively, as evidenced by support given client.

Implementation. Preoperatively or before any treatment, assess the client's and significant others' coping ability and concerns. Do not rush the assessment. Identify the coping mechanisms usually used by the client and significant others. Are there any potentially disabling coping patterns? Use this information as the basis of support. The woman may fear pain, mutilation, death, loss of control, and the hospital environment. Use these findings to establish a plan of care to help the client use positive growth-producing coping and to avoid disabling coping.

Nursing Diagnosis: Body Image Disturbance R/T impending changes in breast and sexuality.

Planning: Expected Outcomes. The client will develop a positive body image, as evidenced by wearing make-up, own nightgown, and other feminine attire after breast surgery.

Implementation. If the assessment reveals problems with body image or sexuality, the nurse may choose to include other health care professionals (e.g., social worker, sex therapist) in the plan of care for addressing these needs adequately. It may be helpful for someone who has had a similar surgery to talk with the woman preoperatively or postoperatively.

Women who undergo surgery for breast cancer experience a sense of loss; changes in their routine life, social interactions, self-concept, and body image; and the fear of death.[58, 92] Those women may benefit from opportunities to interact with nurses in ways in which they feel comfortable expressing their fears and problems.

Recovery during the postoperative period after mastectomy takes a lot of energy. A client's usual coping strategies may not be effective. Not everyone perceives or handles stress in the same way. Displacement, projection, denial, hope, prayer, meditation, stoicism, fatalism, or any combination of these reactions may occur. Clients who have surgically lost a breast may adapt in the same way they would to any loss. Phantom breast symptoms are not uncommon in the missing breast.[55]

Effective postoperative care is essential for successful psychosocial and physical rehabilitation. During the 2- to 3-day hospital stay, the focus of nursing care is toward recovery from surgery and anesthesia and aimed at discharge planning for self-care postoperative management. The client's self-image will improve with self-care activities.

Losing a breast or having breast cancer may not make its full impact until the client goes home. Many clients are surprised by events such as the amount of pain and discomfort, marked fatigue, slow incision healing, arm swelling, and jittery feelings. Ordinary things, such as finding a comfortable position in bed, may be difficult and painful. The woman has to decide whether to hide the incision from significant others or let it be seen. The defect may be camouflaged for a woman by an appropriately fitted brassiere or a special bathing suit or evening dress, but doubts and fears about her attractiveness may affect even the most secure woman.

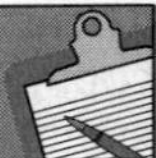

CARE PLAN

The Woman with a Modified Radical Mastectomy

Nursing Diagnosis/ Collaborative Problem	Planning: Expected Outcomes	Implementation: Nursing Interventions	Rationales
Coping, Ineffective Individual R/T mastectomy and diagnosis of breast cancer	Client begins adaptation to emotional stressors Client utilizes resources to increase coping Potentially disabling coping is easily identified Effective coping is identified, supported, and strengthened	Assess client's stressors, resources, supports, problem-solving skills Determine coping strategies that have been useful for client in the past and reinforce Emphasize that periods of depression, anger, and the like are normal; describe benefits of emotional release of feelings and tensions; provide opportunity for talking Encourage asking questions and seeking information Allow time for client to verbalize fears and anxieties (do not appear in a hurry) Reinforce positive self-care behavior and each step in getting well At time of diagnosis or preoperative H & P appointment, refer to American Cancer Society Reach for Recovery, YWCA Encore Refer to other professionals (social worker, psychologist, family counselor) and community support groups for emotional and psychosocial counseling as needed	There is a lot of hope for women with breast cancer Ineffectual coping may lead to lack of adherence to treatment regimens Ineffectual coping may lead to prolonged depression or other psychiatric, social, or emotional disorders
Skin Integrity, Impaired R/T mastectomy and placement of drains	Client exhibits healing of incision, as evidenced by no drainage, no sutures present, and absence of infection Client demonstrates appropriate care of her incision at discharge Client identifies potential complications and appropriate signs and symptoms to report to the physician or nurse	Assess dressing for bleeding or drainage Empty drain, measure and record drainage every shift; note color and consistency After dressing change, observe incision for healing; there should be no indications of infection, hematoma formation, erythema, induration, tenderness, or purulent drainage Begin teaching wound care at the first dressing	Good healing is important to the overall health and recovery of the woman Poor wound healing or infection may cause radiation therapy or chemotherapy to be delayed

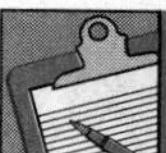

CARE PLAN

The Woman with a Modified Radical Mastectomy Continued

Nursing Diagnosis Collaborative Problem	Planning: Expected Outcomes	Implementation: Nursing Interventions	Rationales
		change; prepare client to look at the incision at the first dressing change by describing the incision to her Teach indications of infection, hematoma, or recurrence of breast cancer in the incision (a growing lump) Discuss that it is normal to have decreased sensation in the surgical area or to have phantom breast pain Instruct that after the incision heals she may massage the area with cocoa butter to keep skin soft and increase healing; redness and swelling will fade with time	
Physical Mobility, Impaired R/T modified radical mastectomy	Client demonstrates knowledge related to potential mobility problems Client progresses toward full ROM; full ROM of hand, arm, and shoulder will return by 2 to 3 months postoperatively Client identifies potential complications and signs and symptoms of edema to report to health care team	At time of preoperative H & P, send referral to physical therapy to see client on postoperative day 1 or 2 Assess for signs of infection or impairment of circulation Arm should be elevated on pillow when lying or sitting After anesthesia wears off, begin ambulation and begin flexion and extension of fingers, wrist, and lower arm Begin ADLs with arm on operative side; dress self Limit upper arm ROM to level of the shoulder only After axillary drain is removed, begin progressive full ROM of upper arm Use pain medication as needed to allow exercise without pain hindrance	It is possible to regain full ROM Using the arm improves circulation If radiation therapy is needed, the woman will need to have her arm above her head to keep it safely out of the treatment field Because the lymph nodes have been removed, the woman is more vulnerable to trauma, edema, and infection

Care Plan continued on following page

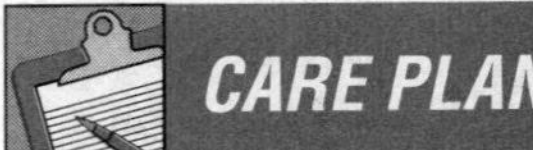

CARE PLAN

The Woman with a Modified Radical Mastectomy Continued

Nursing Diagnosis Collaborative Problem	Planning: Expected Outcomes	Implementation: Nursing Interventions	Rationales
		Teach ROM exercises to use at home after drain is removed (see Fig. 78-5) Avoid infection and trauma to operative site and left arm; teach hand care; client must follow this for the rest of her life (see Client Education Guide)	

ADLs, activities of daily living; H & P, history and physical; ROM, range of motion.

Body image is further altered by weight gain and alopecia. If a woman wishes, a suitable wig can be obtained before hair is lost. Fatigue, decreased libido, and periods of depression are common in women receiving chemotherapy and radiation therapy. It may help a woman to talk with others who face the same problems. Breast cancer support groups may also be beneficial.

As time passes, there is a reorganization and restructuring of the lives of the woman and significant others. During this time, the woman resumes her role in society. Significant changes in this role may be necessary. Women cope differently; feelings of sexual inadequacy, poor body image, and loss of a sense of femininity are common. The woman needs to talk with and share concerns. Nurses are often able to offer such support. Nurses can offer understanding and facilitate communication between the client and significant others. Certain events, such as fitting the permanent prosthesis, can cause a breakdown in denial that a woman may have been using after a mastectomy. A new lump or any new problem may precipitate aspects of the grieving process (e.g., anger, depression, and regression). Fear of metastases or recurrence of cancer may cause new symptoms to become magnified and every new pain to cause new anxiety.

Breast cancer support groups often provide a place for talking about shared and individual problems. Women encountering similar problems and finding solutions may effectively help each other. It often helps to realize that one is not alone in feelings and problems. Find out details about such support groups in the community and share this information as appropriate.

Nursing Diagnosis: Skin Integrity, Impaired, High Risk for, R/T surgery or radiation therapy.

Planning: Expected Outcomes. The client will not develop impairments in skin integrity after surgery or radiation therapy, as evidenced by healing skin without redness, infection, hematoma formation, or breakdown.

Implementation. Postoperatively, a pressure dressing is usually used initially. A drain, connected to gentle suction, prevents blood or serum collection in the operative space after a modified radical mastectomy or axillary node dissection. The nurse needs to instruct the woman about emptying the drain and recording the amount of drainage; the physician is notified if the drain becomes plugged, is dislodged, or shows signs of infection or if frank bleeding develops.

When the dressing is changed, gently encourage the woman to look at the incision. Seeing the incision for the first time is often a difficult experience. A matter-of-fact approach by the nurse can help. Future dressing changes can be used to teach methods of cleaning the incision at home and for watching signs of infection.

Scaling, flaking, dryness, itching, erythema, hair loss, rash or dry desquamation of the involved skin may occur. Careful treatment of the skin is important in minimizing the skin effects of radiation therapy.[62] Nurses need to teach women how to care for their skin (see Chap. 22).

Nursing Diagnosis: Injury, High Risk for, R/T increased risk of infection and lymphedema secondary to axillary node dissection.

Planning: Expected Outcomes. The client will not experience injury, as evidenced by absence of infection or lymphedema.

Implementation. Arm edema (e.g., lymphedema) was a common complication after the standard radical mastectomy. However, with less extensive surgery, it occurs less frequently. Arm edema (on the operative side) can occur immediately postoperatively, or secondary edema may occur months or years after surgery. In the immediate postoperative period, encourage arm exercises; elevate the arm to promote lymphatic drainage and prevent infection. Wearing an elastic bandage or a custom-fitted pressure gradient elastic sleeve may also be helpful. Place a sign on the woman's bed warning that no blood pressure readings, injections, intravenous lines, or blood draws should be done on the arm on the operative side. These procedures can cause circulatory impairment or infection.

After the woman leaves the hospital, burns, cuts, and abrasions are the most frequent sources of infection. After axillary node dissection, secondary edema from infection in the arm may cause some permanent edema. Also, postoperative radiation to the axilla often increases the frequency and degree of arm edema. Explain that the client is vulnerable to secondary edema in the arm on the operative side for the rest of her life and that any trauma in the arm may lead to edema and infection.

Nursing Diagnosis: Knowledge Deficit R/T postoperative arm exercises and care, breast prosthesis, chemotherapy, and radiation therapy.

Planning: Expected Outcomes. The client will understand postoperative arm exercises and care, breast prosthesis, chemotherapy, and radiation therapy, as evidenced by return demonstration of arm exercises and care and client's statements concerning further treatment and possible problems associated with therapy.

Implementation. Plan interventions for restoring full hand, arm, and shoulder range of motion. Sometimes a surgeon attempts to enhance mobility by placing the arm on the operative side at a right angle to the chest wall immediately postoperatively.

These early limited postoperative arm exercises are important and usually started within 24 hours after surgery. Teach the client to perform hand and wrist movements and to flex and extend the elbow hourly. Encourage self-care activities (e.g., feeding, combing hair, washing face) and other activities that use the arm, with care taken not to abduct the arm or raise the arm or elbow above shoulder height until the drains are removed.

When wound healing is well established and axillary drains are removed, begin abduction and external rotation of the upper arm, including pendulum swings to improve shoulder function, forward and lateral elevation of the arms, overhead pulley suspension to obtain full elevation, and wall climbing and rope running (Fig. 78–5). Exercises may need to be approved by the physician. Arrangements for a physical therapist to assist with range of motion may need to be made at the time surgery is planned because the short hospital stay means that there may not be time postoperatively. It is important for the nurse to provide written and verbal instructions about arm precautions after axillary node dissection (see Fig. 74–3 and Client Education Guide).

The Reach for Recovery program of the American Cancer Society is a rehabilitation program for women who have had breast surgery. This program is designed to help women meet common psychosocial, physical, and cosmetic needs. With authorization of the physician, volunteers from this program visit the hospital or the home and give the woman information and help, including

- a Reach for Recovery kit, ball, book, rope, and temporary soft cotton prosthesis (for women who have had a mastectomy)
- postoperative axillary node dissection exercises
- discussion of brassiere comfort, various breast prostheses, clothing adjustments, and personal problems as appropriate

Women who have had a mastectomy may wear a temporary lightweight prosthesis immediately after the sutures and drains are removed. This may help the woman's adjustment to the loss of her breast. A soft, cotton breast form may be supplied by the Reach for Recovery visitor; or, cotton padding inserted into a pocket sewn into a lightweight brassiere is a good, temporary substitute. A permanent prosthesis should not be purchased until the wound has healed completely, because the incision site may change. Prostheses are expensive. They may be purchased in foundation departments in most large stores or at medical-surgical supply stores that sell durable medical equipment. Most of these stores have fitters to help women obtain the right fit. It would be helpful for the nurse to learn about suppliers in the local area so she can provide the name to the client. Most private and government insurance plans pay for at least the first prosthesis and brassiere.

Teaching is a major role for the nurse caring for clients receiving radiation therapy. Many clients have misconceptions about radiation. Through assessment, the nurse identifies misconceptions and develops a teaching plan to clarify misunderstandings and meet the woman's needs.[18, 61] Two booklets, *Radiation therapy: A treatment for early stage breast cancer* and *Radiation therapy and you*,[66, 70] may help the client and are free of charge from the National Cancer Institute by calling 1-800-4-CANCER. See Chapter 22 for further information on radiation therapy.

Nurses are responsible for educating women receiving chemotherapy. This includes teaching them the names of medications being received, how the medications are administered, expected side effects, side effect management, preventive measures, and complications that must be reported to the physician or nurse (e.g., infection, fever, bruising, bleeding, or mouth sores). For example, adequate fluid intake is required when cyclophosphamide (Cytoxan) is being received for prevention of hemorrhagic cystitis. For more information, see Chapter 22.

Nursing Diagnosis: Nutrition, Altered: Less than Body Requirements R/T nausea, vomiting, and stomatitis secondary to chemotherapy.

Planning: Expected Outcomes. The client will take in adequate nutrition, as evidenced by absence of nausea and vomiting, control of stomatitis, intake of adequate calories daily, and no loss of weight.

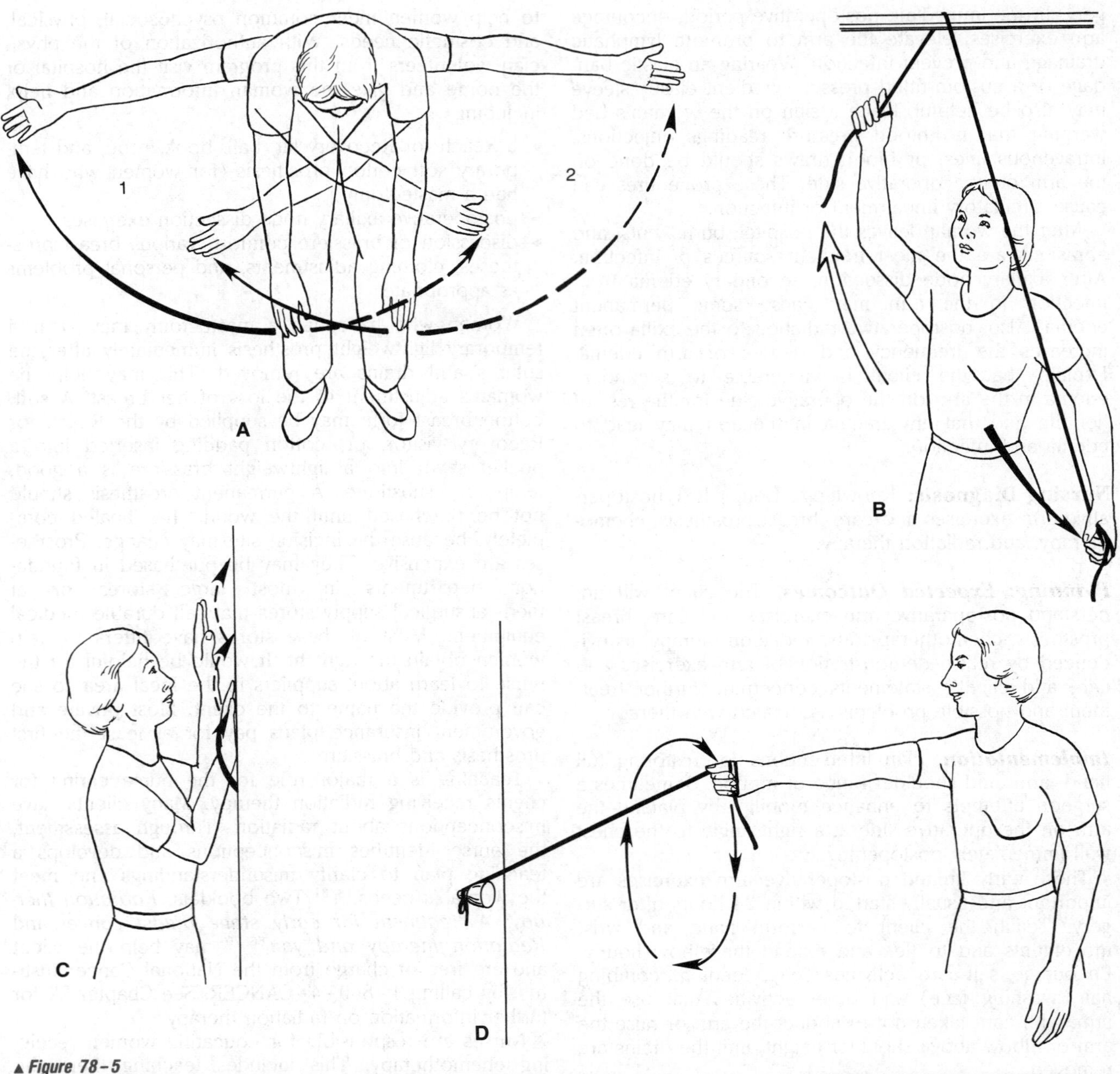

▲ *Figure 78–5*

Postmastectomy exercises. *A*, Arm swings. Stand with feet 8 inches apart. Bend forward from waist, allowing arms to hang toward floor. Swing both arms up to sides to reach shoulder level. Swing back to center, then cross arms at center. Do not bend elbows. If possible, do this and other exercises in front of mirror to ensure even posture and correct motion. *B*, Pulley motion. Using operated arm, toss 6-foot rope over a shower curtain rod (or over top of a door that has a nail in the top to hold the rope in place for the exercise). Grasp one end of rope in each hand. Slowly raise operated arm as far as comfortable by pulling down on the rope on opposite side. Keep raised arm close to your head. Reverse to raise unoperated arm by lowering the operated arm. Repeat. *C*, Hand wall climbing. Stand facing wall with toes 6 to 12 inches from wall. Bend elbows and place palms against wall at shoulder level. Gradually move both hands up the wall parallel to each other until incisional pulling or pain occurs. (Mark that spot on wall to measure progress.) Work hands down to shoulder level. Move closer to wall as height of reach improves. *D*, Rope turning. Tie rope to door handle. Hold rope in hand of operated side. Back away from door until arm is extended away from body, parallel to floor. Swing rope in as wide a circle as possible. Increase size of the circle as mobility returns.

Implementation. Nausea, vomiting, anorexia, stomatitis, and taste change are common side effects of chemotherapy. Yet, an adequate nutritional intake is essential for providing strength and well-being. Stomatitis may make eating and drinking extremely difficult. Careful oral hygiene and topical analgesics may help. Adequate dosage and timing of antiemetics can control nausea and vomiting. The client may need to try different foods to find ones that taste good to her. Emphasize the importance of good nutrition by helping the woman find high-calorie and high-protein foods that can be tolerated. Monitor weight and dietary patterns. Meeting nutritional needs can be difficult and must be individualized.

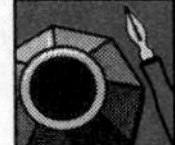

CLIENT EDUCATION GUIDE

Arm Precautions After Axillary Lymph Node Dissection

Because you have had an axillary node dissection, the affected arm may swell and is less able to fight infections. Use your arm normally following these recommendations.

Avoid burns while cooking or smoking
- Wear a long-length oven mitt.
- Do not reach into a hot oven with this arm.
- Do not hold a cigarette in the affected hand.

Avoid sunburn and insect bites
- Wear long-sleeve shirts and gloves.
- Use sunscreen.
- Use insect repellent to avoid bites and stings.

Avoid cuts, pinpricks, and scratches
- Wear gloves when gardening.
- Do not work near thorny plants or dig with your hands.
- Use a thimble when sewing.
- Use an electric razor with a narrow head for underarm shaving to reduce the risk of nicks or scratches.
- Never cut or pick at cuticles; use hand cream or lotion.
- Wash cuts promptly; treat them with antibacterial medication and cover them with sterile dressing. Check often for redness, soreness, pus, or other signs of infection.

Avoid strong detergents, harsh chemicals, and abrasive compounds
- Wear protective gloves when doing dishes and cleaning.

Avoid other trauma
- Use a lanolin hand cream a few times each day.
- Have all injections, vaccinations, blood samples, and blood pressure tests done on the other arm whenever possible.
- Wear a medical alert identification tag that cautions no test injections or blood pressure readings on the affected arm.
- Carry handbag and other heavy objects on the other arm.
- Wear watch or jewelry loosely, if at all, on the operated arm.
- Avoid elastic cuffs on blouses and nightgowns.
- Wear an elastic sleeve if recommended by your physician.

Contact your physician if the arm or hand becomes red, is swollen, or feels hot. In the meantime, try to keep your arm over your head and periodically pump your fist.

Adapted from National Cancer Institute (1987). *After breast cancer: A guide to followup care* (NIH Publication No. 87-2400). Washington, DC: National Cancer Institute.

EVALUATION

The nurse must evaluate client outcomes on the basis of the established plan of care. If these goals have not been achieved, the plan and interventions must be revised to meet the client's needs.

Modification of Plan of Care for the Elderly

The care of older women with breast cancer is similar to the care of younger women. The only difference might be in the extent of treatment. If the older woman is not in good health generally, radiation therapy and hormonal manipulation may be all that is recommended.

Post-hospital Care

DISCHARGE TEACHING

Teaching should focus on wound and drain management, arm exercises, and arm precautions. If the client is undergoing chemotherapy, hormonal manipulation, or radiation therapy, teaching will focus on these matters.

The nurse should also talk to the client about the development of fatigue so that the woman realizes that this is a common occurrence in women undergoing chemotherapy or radiation therapy. The woman needs to balance activities with periods of rest so she does not become over tired. Reassure the woman that this feeling will gradually fade over time.

The client and significant others should be told about delayed grieving, which commonly occurs in women 2 to 3 months after mastectomy. This is a normal phenomenon for which the client and significant others should be prepared if it occurs.

HOME HEALTH CARE NEEDS

There is usually no need to provide specific home health care for the woman after breast cancer and treatment. The major need after discharge, as previously discussed, is for the woman to know how, where, and when to obtain her permanent prosthesis. Encourage the client to continue support groups such as Reach for Recovery or Y-ME, as appropriate.

FOLLOW-UP CARE

After surgery or radiation, clients with breast cancer need some professional attention for life. Health follow-ups initially are every 3 to 4 months and later are every 6 to 12 months. The risk of recurrence, as well as the possibility of developing a second cancer in the remaining breast, is high. Monthly breast self-examination and an annual mammogram and breast physical examination are advisable. Metastasis may appear 15 years or longer after removal of the primary tumor.

METASTATIC BREAST CANCER

Metastatic breast cancer is a chronic disease.[44, 49] Metastases have been known to occur up to 25 years after the initial diagnosis of breast cancer. Alternatively, breast cancer can be a rapidly progressing terminal disease. Knowledge of the usual metastatic patterns with breast cancer and common complications can aid early recognition and effective treatment. Metastases usually develop in one or more of the following sites: lymph nodes, skin, remaining breast tissue, bones, lung, pleura, peritoneum, liver, and central nervous system. Women with metastases to the liver or central nervous system have a poorer prognosis.

Treatment of metastatic disease may involve radiation therapy, hormonal manipulation, chemotherapy, or possible surgery. A combination of treatments is usually employed. Excellent palliation can be achieved for metastatic breast cancer, which offers longer survival for this disease than for many other types of cancers.

Hypercalcemia is a common complication of metastatic breast cancer. It may be due to bone involvement or hormonal therapy. Prompt treatment includes hydration and diuretics. Mithramycin or a newer drug, gallium citrate, is initiated for severe hypercalcemia.

Spinal cord compression, usually from extradural metastases, is a complication requiring prompt diagnosis and intervention for prevention of paraplegia. Assessment findings such as back pain, leg weakness, and sphincter disturbances indicate possible spinal cord compression. Treatment involves radiation therapy or surgery, often followed by chemotherapy.

Nursing care of women with metastatic breast cancer involves helping them manage the complications caused by their disease and the side effects caused by treatments. Providing support for the women and significant others is equally important. Physical symptoms may be difficult to manage.

Currently under investigation is the treatment of women with metastatic disease using autologous bone marrow transplantation and high-dose chemotherapy.[1] This procedure involves having the woman donate her own bone marrow, either through bone marrow aspiration or through peripheral stem cell pheresis. The client is then given very high dose chemotherapy followed by reinfusion of her own marrow or stem cells to rescue her after the chemotherapy destroys her own marrow. Further information on bone marrow transplantation can be found in Chapters 22 and 24.

Previously established coping mechanisms may falter during this period as hope dwindles and energy is spent coping with pain, physical problems, and fears. Old unresolved issues may resurface. In addition to providing physical care, assist the woman and significant others to reestablish effective coping mechanisms. Women with breast cancer need a strong support system and people with whom they can comfortably and helpfully discuss their problems. Nurses can help provide this support where it is lacking. Nurses need to identify and reinforce beneficial coping to help the woman with advanced breast cancer live a meaningful life.[4, 21]

MALE BREAST CANCER

Breast cancer in men is rare.[22, 25] The incidence is 1 per cent of that of women. The average age at occurrence is about 60 years (10 years older than the average for women). Factors associated with an increased risk of breast cancer in men include high estrogen levels, obesity, testicular abnormalities or injury, Klinefelter's syndrome, exposure to ionizing radiation, increased prolactin level, use of phenothiazines, and having a first-degree male or female relative with breast cancer.

Assessment findings indicating male breast cancer include a painless lump beneath the areola or, more often, nipple discharge, retraction, crusting, or ulceration. Staging is the same as for women. Biopsy is necessary for diagnosis of male breast cancer. It is as important in men to test for estrogen receptors as it is in women.

Initial treatment consists of a radical or modified radical mastectomy. Postoperative radiation is frequently used. The pattern of metastasis is similar to that in the female, with soft tissue, bone, and visceral site involvement occurring frequently. Hormonal therapy is very important in the treatment of metastasis, because estrogen receptors have been found in 84 per cent of the tumors.

Tamoxifen and an orchiectomy are the primary hormonal therapies used to treat disseminated male breast cancer. Tamoxifen has provided a response rate of 71 per cent in ER+ male breast cancer. Orchiectomy provides a mean response rate of 55 per cent in men of all ages. Other hormonal manipulations are used in men as in women.

Chemotherapy should be administered for the same indications and with use of the same dose schedules as for women with metastatic disease. Adjuvant chemotherapy may also be useful in those with stage II disease, but experience with this therapy is lacking at present.

BENIGN BREAST DISEASE

Fibrocystic Breasts

Ninety per cent of all women have cysts. Fibrocystic breasts are not a disease per se even though the label fibrocystic breast disease is often given to the condition.[59, 79] Fibrocystic breasts are the most frequent condition of the female breast. The exact cause is unknown, although some evidence indicates hormonal imbalance may be associated with it. The fibrocystic condition typically improves during pregnancy and lactation. It occurs during the reproductive years and disappears with menopause.

Typical fibrocystic lesions are fluid-filled cysts that are round, well circumscribed, and moveable. Depending on the amount of fluid in the cyst, it may feel soft or hard.

Assessment findings may include nodularity and tenderness. Pain occurs, frequently and the cysts increase in size premenstrually. Cysts are generally aspirated rather than biopsied surgically. However, if there is any question, a biopsy is done. A biopsy is necessary, particularly if the cyst keeps recurring after being aspirated.

Once the diagnosis is confirmed, treatment is symptomatic.[79, 88] Conservative measures include breast support with a firm brassiere, local applications of heat or ice bags, mild analgesics, or the occasional use of diuretics. Recently, it has been found that reducing methylxanthines (e.g., caffeine and theophylline medications) is associated with symptom reduction.

Medications have been used with some success in treating fibrocystic breasts. Large doses of vitamin E relieve symptoms in some women but may raise cholesterol levels. Danazol, a synthetic androgen, may be used continuously for 3 to 6 months and repeated if symptoms recur. Side effects include menstrual irregularities, fluid retention, acne, muscle cramps, or possible hepatic dysfunction. Danazol should be used only for severe fibrocystic breasts.

Hyperplasia and Atypical Hyperplasia

Ductal hyperplasia is found in 20 per cent of all breast biopsy specimens.[98] Atypical lobular hyperplasia is found in 1 per cent of breast biopsy specimens. Hyperplasia and atypical hyperplasia can be diagnosed only by pathologic examination of breast tissue from a biopsy. Finding hyperplasia or atypical hyperplasia indicates the woman is at increased risk for breast cancer.

Fibroadenoma

Fibroadenoma is a common breast tumor that usually occurs in young women, most frequently between the ages of 15 and 30 years of age.[95, 98] This tumor is usually a nontender, round, firm, or rubbery mass 1 to 3 cm in diameter. Movability of the adenoma in the breast tissues is one of its most distinctive characteristics. Excision is the only effective treatment.

Papilloma

Intraductal papillomas are lesions growing in the terminal portion of a duct (solitary) or throughout the duct system of a sector of breast (multiple or intraductal). Papillomas typically occur in women in their 40s. A ductogram may help in locating the papilloma.

Solitary intraductal papillomas are usually not precancerous. Multiple papillomas may occasionally be cancerous. Intraductal papilloma is usually indicated by a serous, serosanguineous, or bloody discharge from the nipple. Often no mass is palpable, although a small soft tumor in a central or periareolar portion of the breast is usually present. It is necessary to excise the lesion and have its tissue examined for determining whether it is benign or malignant.

Duct Ectasia

Duct ectasia, a disease of ducts in the subareolar zone, occurs in aging breasts usually in peri- or postmenopausal women. Symptoms may include a palpable dilated duct; a thick, sticky nipple discharge, and burning pain, itching, and inflammation. There appears to be no association with cancer. However, biopsy is performed because on physical examination it is difficult to differentiate duct ectasia from cancer. Recommended treatment is excision of the ducts.

Fissure of the Nipple

A nipple fissure is a painful longitudinal ulcer in the nipple that occurs in nursing mothers because of irritation from the infant's sucking. Nurses can teach women prenatally to condition their nipples by washing, drying, and massaging to help decrease the incidence of this problem. Teach nursing mothers to wash their hands before feeding the baby, to wash and dry their nipples after breastfeeding, and to avoid astringent soaps or perfumed creams on the nipples. Lanolin-based, bland creams may relieve sore nipples. Drying the nipples and exposing them to a heat lamp is also helpful. Frequent breastfeeding helps reduce engorgement and decrease vigorous sucking.

Lactation Mastitis

Lactation mastitis, a localized, indurated, painful area, may develop when bacteria enter the breast through a cracked nipple. Bacteria may be carried by a nursing mother's hands or by an infant with an oral, eye, or skin infection. Infection of the milk provides a medium for bacterial growth; continued breastfeeding or the manual expression of milk helps empty the breast. Antibiotics are also prescribed.

Breast Abscess

Breast abscesses[37] frequently occur during lactation when bacteria enter through a cracked nipple. Subareolar abscess is a low-grade subareolar infection in young nonlactating women. Skin over the abscess is red and edematous. Pain, chills, and fever may occur. Antibiotics, analgesics, and warm, moist compresses are used. Weaning may be necessary for resolution of a breast abscess in lactating women.

Mastodynia and Mastalgia

Mastodynia and mastalgia[60, 98] refer to breast pain. Breast pain is the most common breast complaint. Pain is not usually associated with breast cancer. Many women have cyclic premenstrual mastodynia. Women with cyclic premenstrual mastodynia usually have lumpy breast (nodularity) and pain for the week before menses. After any other problems have been ruled out, treatment is symptomatic. Wearing a well-fitting bra for support, particularly during jogging and other bouncing exercise, may help. Decreasing salt and caffeine intake may also help.

Gynecomastia

Gynecomastia,[8] hypertrophy of one or both male breasts, is common at puberty and in older men. It occurs 60 to 70 per cent of the time at puberty and typically resolves spontaneously in 1 to 2 years. The hormonal mechanism causing gynecomastia is not well understood, although some suggest it is due to increased estrogen. Careful assessment and follow-up are required to rule out causes such as tumors, thyroid or hepatic problems, or Klinefelter's syndrome.

Reassure the man that the condition is temporary. If the gynecomastia causes severe psychosocial trauma, reduction mammoplasty or medications such as an antiestrogen (e.g., tamoxifen) or a synthetic androgen (e.g., danazol) may be prescribed.

Men aged 50 to 70 years occasionally develop gynecomastia that usually regresses spontaneously after a few months to a year. This is not associated with endocrine abnormality. Because cancer is more common in this age group, any lesions found may require biopsy for differentiation from cancer. Certain medications (Table 78-6) can cause gynecomastia in any age group.

MAMMOPLASTY

Women who are uncomfortable with the appearance of their breasts often have a poor body image. Some women who have small breasts seek surgical procedures to enlarge their breasts, such as augmentation mammoplasty (also spelled mammaplasty). Augmentation mammoplasty has been a popular cosmetic procedure that uses implants or myocutaneous tissue to either (1) enlarge underdeveloped breasts or (2) reconstruct breasts after removal of benign or malignant lesions.

Breasts change over time. With advanced aging, the breasts atrophy and lose some glandular tissue. Some women have large, heavy breasts that are uncomfortable. Breast reduction surgery, reduction mammoplasty, may benefit them. Reduction mammoplasty may help alleviate neck pain, backaches, possible curvature of the spine, and painful bra strap irritation.

Augmentation mammoplasty and reduction mammoplasty are discussed in Chapter 72. Women having such surgery believe it increases their attractiveness as perceived by themselves or others. Recently there has been some controversy about the safety of silicone and polyurethane implants.[81] In 1992, the Food and Drug Administration restricted use of these implants because of problems with rupturing of the implants, leaking of silicone, and resultant health problems. Nurses can help women understand the facts about the risks and benefits of mammoplasty.

TABLE 78-6. Drugs Associated with Gynecomastia

Amiodarone	Anabolic steroids	Bumetanide
Busulfan	Cannabis	Cimetidine
Clomiphene citrate	Cyproterone acetate	Domperidone
D-Penicillamine	Diazepam	Diethylstilbestrol
Digitalis	Estrogens	Ethionamide
Flutamide	Furosemide	Heroin
Isoniazid	Ketoconazole	Marijuana
Methyldopa	Methotrexate	Nifedipine
Nitrosoureas	Oral contraceptives	Phenytoin
Reserpine	Spironolactone	Sulindac
Theophylline	Verapamil	Vincristine
Human chorionic gonadotropin	Medroxyprogesterone acetate	
Tricyclic antidepressants	Diethylpropion hydrochloride	

Adapted from Bland, K. I., & Page, E. M. (1991). *The breast: comprehensive management of benign and malignant disease.* Philadelphia: W. B. Saunders.

Summary

Diseases of the breast are usually benign conditions that occur throughout the life cycle. Breast cancer, however, has greatly increased in incidence over the last 30 years. The nurse has a vital role in teaching clients early detection methods so that breast cancer can be detected at a curable stage.

All diseases of the breast potentially pose problems in body image and sexuality for the woman. Even benign fibrocystic disease can cause breast tenderness and possibly interfere with sexuality. Breast cancer and the possibility of a mastectomy as treatment can be extremely threatening to the woman's body image. The nurse can help the client cope with these potential threats and successfully adapt to any changes that occur.

Bibliography

1. Affronti, M. L., et al. (1990). Autologous bone marrow transplant for the treatment of advanced breast cancer. *Innovations in Oncology Nursing, 6*(4), 2-6, 19-21.
2. American Cancer Society. (1991). *Cancer facts & figures* (Publication No. 90-500M-NO. 5008.91-LE). Atlanta, GA: American Cancer Society.
3. American Cancer Society. (1989). *Special touch: A personal plan of action for breast health* (Publication No. 87-1MM-Rev. 9/89-No. 2095-LE). Atlanta, GA: American Cancer Society.
4. Arathuzik, D. (1991). Pain experience for metastatic breast cancer patients: unraveling the mystery. *Cancer Nursing, 14*(1), 41-48.
5. Baird, S. B., et al. (1991). *Cancer nursing: A comprehensive textbook*. Philadelphia: W. B. Saunders.
6. Beahrs, O. H. (1991). Staging of cancer. *CA: A Cancer Journal for Clinicians, 41*(2), 121-125.
7. Bland, K. I., & Copeland, E. M. (Eds). (1991). *The breast: Comprehensive management of benign and malignant diseases*. Philadelphia: W. B. Saunders.
8. Bland, K. I., & Page, D. L. (1991). Gynecomastia. In K. I. Bland & E. M. Copeland (Eds.), *The breast: Comprehensive management of benign and malignant diseases* (pp. 135-168). Philadelphia: W. B. Saunders.
9. Blesch, K. S. et al. (1991). Correlates of fatigue in people with breast cancer or lung cancer. *Oncology Nursing Forum, 18*(1), 81-87.
10. Bodner, S., & Flynn, K. T. (1987). Symptom distress of women

treated with conservative surgery and primary radiation for carcinoma of the breast (abstract #234). *Oncology Nursing Forum, 14*(Suppl.), 140.

11. Bord, M. A., & Carpenter, L. C. (1990). A coordinated approach to comprehensive breast care. *Innovations in Oncology Nursing, 6*(2), 13–19.
12. Boring, C. C., et al. (1992). Cancer statistics, 1992. *CA: A Cancer Journal for Clinicians, 42*(1), 19–38.
13. Bostwick, J. (1990). Reconstruction after mastectomy. *Surgical Clinics of North America, 70*(5), 1125–1140.
14. Breitmeyer, J. B., & Henderson, I. C. (1990). Adjuvant chemotherapy of breast cancer. *Surgical Clinics of North America, 70*(5), 1081–1113.
15. Brinker, N., & Harris, C. M. (1990). *The race is run one step at a time.* New York: Simon & Schuster.
16. Cady, B., & Stone, M. D. (1990). Selection of breast-preservation therapy for primary invasion breast carcinoma. *Surgical Clinics of North America, 70*(5), 1047–1059.
17. Camp-Sorrell, D. (1991). Controlling adverse effects of chemotherapy. *Nursing 91, 12*(4), 34–41.
18. Cawley, M., et al. (1990). Informational and psychosocial needs of women choosing conservative surgery/primary radiation for early stage breast cancer. *Cancer Nursing, 13*(2), 90–94.
19. Cody, R. L., & Wicha, M. S. (1988). Contemporary chemotherapy. In J. K. Harness, et al. (Eds.), *Breast cancer: Collaborative management* (pp. 157–177). Chelsea, MI: Lewis Publishers.
20. Collins-Hattery, A. M., & Blumberg, B. D. (1991). S phase index and ploidy prognostic markers in node negative breast cancer: information for nurses. *Oncology Nursing Forum, 18*(1), 59–62.
21. Coward, D. D. (1991). Self-transcendence and emotional well-being in women with advanced breast cancer. *Oncology Nursing Forum, 18*(5), 857–863.
22. Crichlow, R. W., & Galt, S. W. (1990). Male breast cancer. *Surgical Clinics of North America, 70*(5), 1165–1178.
23. d'Angelo, T. M., & Gorrell, C. R. (1989). Breast reconstruction using tissue expanders. *Oncology Nursing Forum, 16*(1), 23–27.
24. DeVita, V. T., et al. (1989). *Cancer principle and practice of oncology* (3rd ed.). Philadelphia: J. B. Lippincott.
25. Donegan, W. L. (1991). Cancer of the breast in men. *CA: A Cancer Journal for Clinicians, 41*(6), 339–354.
26. Donegan, W. L. (1988). Evaluation of breast masses. In J. K. Harness, et al. (Eds.), *Breast cancer: Collaborative management* (pp. 3–9). Chelsea, MI: Lewis Publishers.
27. Dorr, F. A., & Friedman, M. A. (1991). The role of chemotherapy in the management of primary breast cancer. *CA: A Cancer Journal for Clinicians, 41*(4), 231–241.
28. Durant, J. R. (1990). How to organize a multidisciplinary clinic for the management of breast cancer. *Surgical Clinics of North America, 70*(4), 977–983.
29. Findlay, P. A. (1988). Radiation therapy as definitive treatment of breast cancer. In M. E. Lippman, et al. (Eds.), *Diagnosis and management of breast cancer* (pp. 155–207). Philadelphia: W. B. Saunders.
30. Fisher, B. (1991). Biological perspective of breast cancer: contributions of the national surgical adjuvant breast and bowel project clinical trials. *CA: A Cancer Journal for Clinicians, 41*(2), 97–111.
31. Fisher, B., et al. (1989). A randomized clinical trial evaluation sequential methotrexate and fluorouracil in the treatment of patients with node-negative breast cancer who have estrogen-receptor-negative tumors. *New England Journal of Medicine, 320*(8), 473–478.
32. Ganz, P. A., et al. (1987). Rehabilitation needs and breast cancer: the first month after primary therapy. *Breast Cancer Research and Treatment, 10*(3), 243–253.
33. Gelmann, E. P., & Lippman, M. E. (1987). Understanding the role of oncogenes in human breast cancer. In M. Sluyser (Ed.), *Growth factors and oncogenes in breast cancer* (pp. 29–43). Chichester, England: Ellis Horwood.
34. Gibson, D. F. C., & Jordan, V. C. (1990). Adjuvant antiestrogen therapy for breast cancer: past, present, and future. *Surgical Clinics of North America, 70*(5), 1103–1113.
35. Gordon, R. S. (1981). Survey finds U.S. women knowledgeable about breast cancer. *Journal of the American Medical Association, 245*(9), 918.
36. Grindel, C. G., et al. (1989). Food intake of women with breast cancer during their first six months of chemotherapy. *Oncology Nursing Forum, 16*(3), 401–407.
37. Grundfest-Broniatowski, S., & Bauer, T. W. (1988). Benign breast disease. In S. Grundfest-Broniatowski & C. B. Esselstyn (Eds.) *Controversies in breast disease: Diagnosis and management* (pp. 3–42). New York: Marcel Dekker.
38. Grundfest-Broniatowski, S., & Esselstyn, C. B. (Eds.). (1988). *Controversies in breast disease: Diagnosis and management.* New York: Marcel Dekker.
39. Harness, J. K. (1988). Organizing for collaborative management: what are the options? In J. K. Harness, et al. (Eds.) *Breast cancer: Collaborative management* (pp. 3–9). Chelsea, MI: Lewis Publishers.
40. Harness, J. K., et al. (1987). Developing a comprehensive breast center. *American Surgeon, 53*(8), 419–423.
41. Harness, J. K., et al. (Eds.) (1988). *Breast cancer: Collaborative management.* Chelsea, MI: Lewis Publishers.
42. Helvie, M. A., et al. (1990). Radiographic guided fine needle aspiration of non-palpable breast lesions. *Radiology, 174*(3141), 657–661.
43. Henderson, I. C. (1987). Adjuvant chemotherapy and endocrine therapy in patients with operable breast cancer. *Principle and Practice of Oncology Update, 1*(3), 1–14.
44. Henderson, I. C., et al. (1989). Cancer of the breast. In V. T. DeVita, et al. (Eds.), *Cancer principle and practice of oncology* (3rd ed., pp. 1197–1269). Philadelphia: J. B. Lippincott.
45. Hutcheson, H. A. (1986). TAIF: new option for breast reconstruction. *Nursing 86, 16*(2), 52–53.
46. Kalinowski, B. H. (1990). Options and decisions: reconstructive surgery: rehabilitation after mastectomy. *Innovations in Oncology Nursing, 6*(1), 2–9.
47. Kelsey, J. L., & Gammon, M. D. (1991). The epidemiology of breast cancer. *CA: A Cancer Journal for Clinicians, 41*(3), 146–165.
48. Kinne, D. W. (1991). Surgical management of primary breast cancer. *CA: A Cancer Journal for Clinicians, 41*(2), 71–84.
49. Knobf, M. T. (1991). Breast cancer. In S. B. Baird, et al. (Eds.), *Cancer nursing: A comprehensive textbook* (pp. 425–451). Philadelphia: W. B. Saunders.
50. Knobf, M. T. (1990). Early-stage breast cancer: the options. *American Journal of Nursing, 90*(11), 28–30.
51. Knobf, M. T. (1986). Physical and psychologic distress associated with adjuvant chemotherapy in women with breast cancer. *Journal of Clinical Oncology, 4*(5), 678–684.
52. Kushner, R. (1984). *Alternatives.* Cambridge, MA: The Kensington Press.
53. Leis, H. P. (1991). Prognostic parameters for breast cancer. In K. I. Bland & E. M. Copeland (Eds.), *The breast: Comprehensive management of benign and malignant disease* (pp. 331–350). Philadelphia: W. B. Saunders.
54. Lichter, A. S. (1988). The treatment of breast cancer with excision followed by radiation therapy. In J. K. Harness, et al. *Breast cancer: Collaborative management* (pp. 137–156). Chelsea, MI: Lewis Publishers.
55. Lierman, L. M. (1988). Phantom breast experiences after mastectomy. *Oncology Nursing Forum, 15*(1), 41–44.
56. Lindsey, A. M., et al. (1987). Endocrine mechanism and obesity: influences in breast cancer. *Oncology Nursing Forum, 14*(2), 47–51.
57. Lippman, M. E., et al. (Eds.). (1988). *Diagnosis and management of breast cancer.* Philadelphia: W. B. Saunders.
58. Loveys, B. J., & Klaich, K. (1991). Breast cancer: demands of illness. *Oncology Nursing Forum, 18*(1), 75–80.
59. Mack, E. (1990). Most breast lumps aren't cancer! *RN, 53*(12), 20–23.
60. Mansel, R. E. (1988). Diagnosis and treatment of mastalgia. In S. Grundfest-Broniatowski & C. B. Esselstyn (Eds.), *Controversies in breast disease: Diagnosis and management* (pp. 63–77). New York: Marcel Dekker.
61. Mast, D. E., & Mood, D. W. (1990). Preparing patients with breast cancer for brachytherapy. *Oncology Nursing Forum, 17*(2), 267–270.
62. McGowan, K. L. (1989). Radiation therapy: saving your patient's skin. *RN, 52*(6), 24–27.
63. McGuire, W. L. (1988). Clinical alert from the National Cancer

Institute (editorial). *Breast Cancer Research and Treatment, 12*(1), 3-5.

64. Morrow, M. (1990). Management of nonpalpable breast lesions. *Principle and Practice of Oncology Updates, 4*(1), 1-11.
65. Nail, L. M., et al. (1991). *Oncology Nursing Forum, 18*(5), 883-887.
66. National Cancer Institute. (1991). *Radiation therapy: A treatment for early stage breast cancer* (NIH Publication No. 91-659). Washington, DC: National Cancer Institute.
67. National Cancer Institute. (1991). *Taking time: Support for people with cancer and the people who care about them* (NIH Publication No. 91-2059). Washington, DC: National Cancer Institute.
68. National Cancer Institute. (1990). *After breast cancer: A guide to follow up care* (NIH Publication No. 90-2400). Washington, DC: National Cancer Institute.
69. National Cancer Institute. (1990). *Mastectomy: A treatment for breast cancer* (NIH Publication No. 91-658). Washington, DC: National Cancer Institute.
70. National Cancer Institute. (1990). *Radiation therapy and you* (NIH Publication No. 91-2227). Washington, DC: National Cancer Institute.
71. National Cancer Institute. (1988). *Breast exams: What you should know* (NIH Publication No. 90-2000). Washington, DC: National Cancer Institute.
72. National Cancer Institute. (1987). *Advanced cancer: Living each day* (Publication No. 87-856). Washington, DC: National Cancer Institute.
73. National Cancer Institute. (1987). *When cancer recurs: Meeting the challenge again* (NIH Publication No. 87-2709). Washington, DC: National Cancer Institute.
74. National Cancer Institute. (1986). *Breast reconstruction: A matter of choice* (NIH Publication No. 88-2151). Washington, DC: National Cancer Institute.
75. Osborne, C. K. (1990). Prognostic factors in breast cancer. *Principle and Practice of Oncology Update, 4*(3), 1-11.
76. Osbourne, M. P., & Borgen, P. I. (1990). Role of mastectomy in breast cancer. *Surgical Clinics of North America, 70*(5), 1023-1046.
77. Osteen, R. T., & Smith, B. L. (1990). Results of conservative surgery and radiation therapy for breast cancer. *Surgical Clinics of North America, 70*(5), 1005-1021.
78. Osteen, R. T., et al. (1992). Regional differences in surgical management of breast cancer. *CA: A Journal For Clinicians, 42*(1), 39-43.
79. Page, D. L., & Simpson, J. F. (1991). Benign, high-risk, and premaligant lesions of the mamma. In K. I. Bland & E. M. Copeland (Eds.), *The breast: Comprehensive management of benign and malignant diseases* (pp. 113-134). Philadelphia: W. B. Saunders.
80. Pandya, K. J., et al. (1985). A retrospective study of earliest indicators of recurrence in patients on Eastern Cooperative Oncology Group adjuvant chemotherapy trials for breast cancer: a preliminary report. *Cancer, 55*(1), 202-205.
81. Pennisi, V. R. (1990). Long-term use of polyurethane breast prostheses: a 14-year experience. *Plastic and Reconstructive Surgery, 86*(2), 368-371.
82. Pfeiffer, C. H., & Mulliken, J. B. (Eds.) (1984). *Caring for the patient with breast cancer: An interdisciplinary/multidisciplinary approach.* Reston, VA: Reston Publishing.
83. Pierce, S. M., & Harris, J. R. (1991). Role of radiation therapy in the management of primary breast cancer. *CA: A Cancer Journal for Clinicians, 41*(2), 85-96.
84. Pierce, P. F. (1988). Women's experience of choice: confronting the options for treatment of breast cancer. In J. K. Harness, et al. (Eds.), *Breast cancer: Collaborative management* (pp. 273-292). Chelsea, MI: Lewis Publishers.
85. Piper, B., et al. (1989). Fatigue patterns over time in woman receiving CMF chemotherapy for breast cancer (abstract #355). *Oncology Nursing Forum, 16*(Suppl.), 217.
86. Rebner, M., et al. (1989). Breast microcalcifications after lumpectomy and radiation therapy. *Radiology, 170*(3), 691-693.
87. Robbins, S. L., et al. (1984). *Pathologic basis of disease* (3rd ed.). Philadelphia: W. B. Saunders.
88. Rogers, K., & Coup, A. J. (1990). *Surgical pathology of the breast.* London: Wright.
89. Russell, L. C. (1989). Caffeine restriction as the initial treatment for breast pain. *Nurse Practitioner, 140*(3), 36-40.
90. Rust, D., & Kloppenborg, E. (1990). Don't underestimate the lumpectomy patient's needs. *RN, 53*(3), 58-64.
91. Schain, W. S. (1990). Physician-patient communication about breast cancer. *Surgical Clinics of North America, 70*(4), 917-936.
92. Schain, W. S. (1988). The sexual and intimate consequences of breast cancer treatment. *CA: A Cancer Journal for Clinicians, 38*(3), 154-161.
93. Schottenfeld, D. (1988). Epidemiology of the breast. In J. K. Harness, et al. (Eds.), *Breast cancer: Collaborative management* (pp. 55-68). Chelsea, MI: Lewis Publishers.
94. Schover, L. R. (1991). The impact of breast cancer on sexuality, body image, and intimate relationships. *CA: A Cancer Journal for Clinicians, 41*(2), 112-120.
95. Schydlower, M. (1982). Breast masses in adolescents. *American Family Physician, 25*(2), 141-145.
96. Sheth, S. P., & Allegra, A. C. (1991). Endocrine therapy of breast cancer. In K. I. Bland & E. M. Copeland (Eds.), *The breast: Comprehensive management of benign and malignant diseases* (pp. 937-947). Philadelphia: W. B. Saunders.
97. Sorace, R. A., & Lippman, M. E. (1988). Locally advanced breast cancer. In M. E. Lippman, et al. (Eds.), *Diagnosis and management of breast cancer* (pp. 272-295). Philadelphia: W. B. Saunders.
98. Souba, W. W. (1991). Evaluation and treatment of benign breast disorders. In K. I. Bland & E. M. Copeland (Eds.), *The breast: Comprehensive management of benign and malignant diseases* (pp. 715-729). Philadelphia: W. B. Saunders.
99. Spindler, J. (1991). Seeing through the mask of cancer. *Nursing 91, 12*(5), 37-40.
100. Stoll, B. A. (Ed.) (1989). *Women at high risk to breast cancer.* Dordrecht, Netherlands: Kluwer Academic Publishers.
101. Sunderland, M. C., & McGuire, W. L. (1990). Prognostic indicators in invasive breast cancer. *Surgical Clinics of North America, 70*(5), 989-1004.
102. Walters, P. (1990). Chemo: a nurse's guide to action, administration, and side effects. *RN, 53*(2), 52-67.
103. Ward, S., & Griffin, J. (1990). Developing a test of knowledge of surgical options for breast cancer. *Cancer Nursing, 13*(3), 191-196.
104. Wellisch, D. K., et al. (1989). Psychosocial outcomes of breast cancer therapies: lumpectomy versus mastectomy. *Psychosomatics, 30*(4), 365-373.
105. Wilson, S., & Morse, J. M. (1991). Living with a wife undergoing chemotherapy. *IMAGE: Journal for Nursing Scholarship, 23*(2), 78-84.
106. Wolmark, N. (1989). 1989: The year of adjuvant therapy in node-negative breast cancer. *Principle and Practice of Oncology Updates, 3*(12), 1-10.

Unit

18

Multisystem Disorders

The final unit of the book focuses on multisystem disorders, highlighting those disorders caused by substance abuse and emergencies. The term multisystem is used to denote that the physiologic and psychosocial components of several body systems may be involved in the clinical manifestations or management of a particular disorder at the same time.

At one time, clients who abused various substances were thought to have psychological problems that led to the abuse and physical problems from the abuse (e.g., cirrhosis, gastritis, cerebral changes). Today, it is recognized that there are various causes of substance abuse — some are inherited, some are acquired. The physical sequelae of the abuse also are more well-defined and include potential damage to all body systems.

Clearly, emergency situations can involve any body system. A client seen in an emergency department may have sustained a head injury, may be having a heart attack, or may have been sexually assaulted, for example, resulting in both physical and psychosocial injuries. The management of emergency situations revolves around setting priorities and recognizing life-threatening conditions quickly.

As we near the end of the twentieth century, substance abuse and traumatic injury continue to increase, demanding that all nurses, regardless of their work settings, be aware of the clinical manifestations and management of conditions resulting from substance abuse and emergencies.

Chapter 79

Nursing Care of Clients with Substance Abuse

The use of mind-altering substances is as old as humankind. Prehistoric people used fermented beverages, the ancient Egyptians drank wine, and marijuana and the coca plant have been used for medicine, recreation, and in religious rituals for centuries. Even Dorothy succumbed to the magic of opium as she reeled through the poppy fields in *The Wizard of Oz*. Intoxication allows people to be in a different state, to act differently, and to feel differently. Some do it for the pleasure. Others do it for the stimulating, inebriating, tranquilizing, or hallucinogenic effects. Still others use it in the search for an Emerald City, a wizard's powers. For too many people, the passionate search for mind-altering substances becomes their life goal.

Over the years, substance abuse has gradually been redefined. No longer a moral problem of weak people who yield to temptation, nor a purely psychiatric disorder, substance abuse is now considered to be a public health problem of enormous magnitude.

Throughout this chapter, the term *substance* refers to all mood-affecting chemicals—alcohol, prescription drugs, over-the-counter medications, and illicit drugs—that are a potential or real threat to either physical or mental health. Table 79-1 contains an overview of potentially abused substances other than alcohol.

TABLE 79-1. Controlled Substances—Uses and Effects

Drugs/CSA Schedules		Trade or Other Names	Medical Uses	Dependence: Physical	Dependence: Psychological
Narcotics					
Opium	II III V	Dover's Powder, Paregoric, Parepectolin	Analgesic, antidiarrheal	High	High
Morphine	II III	Morphine, MS Contin, Roxanol, Roxanol-SR	Analgesic, antitussive	High	High
Codeine	II III V	Tylenol w/Codeine, Empirin w/Codeine, Robitussin A-C, Fiorinal w/Codeine	Analgesic, antitussive	Moderate	Moderate
Heroin	I	Diacetylmorphine, Horse, Smack	None	High	High
Hydromorphone	II	Dilaudid	Analgesic	High	High
Meperidine (pethidine)	II	Demerol, Mepergan	Analgesic	High	High
Methadone	II	Dolophine, Methadone, Methadose	Analgesic	High	High to low
Other narcotics	I II III IV V	Numorphan, Percodan, Percocet, Tylox, Tussionex, Fentanyl, Darvon, Lomotil, Talwin[2]	Analgesic, antidiarrheal, antitussive	High to low	High to low
Depressants					
Chloral hydrate	IV	Noctec	Hypnotic	Moderate	Moderate
Barbiturates	II III IV	Amytal, Butisol, Fiorinal, Lotusate, Nembutal, Seconal, Tuinal, Phenobarbital	Anasthetic, anticonvulsant, sedative, hypnotic, veterinary euthanasia agent	High to moderate	High to moderate
Benzodiazepines	IV	Ativan, Dalmane, Diazepam, Librium, Xanax, Serax, Valium, Tranxene, Verstran, Versed, Halcion, Paxipam, Restoril	Antianxiety, anticonvulsant, sedative, hypnotic	Low	Low
Methaqualone	I	Quaalude	Sedative, hypnotic	High	High
Glutethimide	III	Doriden	Sedative, hypnotic	High	Moderate
Other depressants	III IV	Equanil, Miltown, Noludar, Placidyl, Valmid	Antianxiety, sedative, hypnotic	Moderate	Moderate
Stimulants					
Cocaine[1]	II	Coke, Flake, Snow, Crack	Local anesthetic	Possible	High
Amphetamines	II	Biphetamine, Delcobese, Desoxyn, Dexedrine, Obetrol	Attention deficit disorders, narcolepsy, weight control	Possible	High
Phenmetrazine	II	Preludin	Weight control	Possible	High
Methylphenidate	II	Ritalin	Attention deficit disorders, narcolepsy	Possible	Moderate
Other stimulants	III IV	Adipex, Cylert, Didrex, Ionamin, Melfiat, Plegine, Sanorex, Tenuate, Tepanil, Prelu-2	Weight control	Possible	High
Hallucinogens					
LSD	I	Acid, Microdot	None	None	Unknown
Mescaline and peyote	I	Mexc, Buttons, Cactus	None	None	Unknown
Amphetamine variants	I	2.5-DMA, PMA, STP, MDA, MDMA, TMA, DOM, DOB	None	Unknown	Unknown
Phencyclidine	II	PCP, Angel Dust, Hog	None	Unknown	High
Phencyclidine analogs	I	PCE, PCPy, TCP	None	Unknown	High
Other hallucinogens	I	Bufotenine, Ibogaine, DMT, DET, Psilocybin, Psilocyn	None	None	Unknown
Cannabis					
Marijuana	I	Pot, Acapulco Gold, Grass, Reefer, Sinsemilla, Thai Sticks	None	Unknown	Moderate
Tetrahydrocannabinol	I II	THC, Marinol	Cancer chemotherapy antinauseant	Unknown	Moderate
Hashish	I	Hash	None	Unknown	Moderate
Hashish oil	I	Hash oil	None	Unknown	Moderate

[1]Designated a narcotic under the CSA.
[2]Not designated a narcotic under the CSA.
From *Drugs of abuse.* (1989). U.S. Department of Justice Drug Enforcement Administration.
CSA, controlled substance act.

TABLE 79-1. Controlled Substances-Uses and Effects Continued

Tolerance	Duration (Hours)	Usual Methods of Administration	Possible Effects	Effects of Overdose	Withdrawal Syndrome
Yes	3 to 6	Oral, smoked	Euphoria, drowsiness, respiratory depression, constricted pupils, nausea	Slow and shallow breathing, clammy skin, convulsions, coma, possible death	Watery eyes, runny nose, yawning, loss of appetite, irritability, tremors, panic, cramps, nausea, chills and sweating
Yes	3 to 6	Oral, smoked, injected			
Yes	3 to 6	Oral, injected			
Yes	3 to 6	Injected, sniffed, smoked			
Yes	3 to 6	Oral, injected			
Yes	3 to 6	Oral, injected			
Yes	12 to 24	Oral, injected			
Yes	Variable	Oral, injected			
Yes	5 to 8	Oral	Slurred speech, disorientation, drunken behavior without odor of alcohol	Shallow respiration, clammy skin, dilated pupils, weak and rapid pulse, coma, possible death	Anxiety, insomnia, tremors, delirium, convulsions, possible death
Yes	1 to 16	Oral			
Yes	4 to 8	Oral			
Yes	4 to 8	Oral			
Yes	4 to 8	Oral			
Yes	4 to 8	Oral			
Yes	1 to 2	Sniffed, smoked, injected	Increased alertness, excitation, euphoria, increased pulse rate and blood pressure, insomnia, loss of appetite	Agitation, increase in body temperature, hallucinations, convulsions, possible death	Apathy, long periods of sleep, irritability, depression, disorientation
Yes	2 to 4	Oral, injected			
Yes	2 to 4	Oral, injected			
Yes	2 to 4	Oral, injected			
Yes	2 to 4	Oral, injected			
Yes	8 to 12	Oral	Illusions and hallucinations, poor perception of time and distance	Longer, more intense "trip" episodes, psychosis, possible death	Withdrawal syndrome not reported
Yes	8 to 12	Oral			
Yes	Variable	Oral, injected			
Yes	Days	Smoked, oral, injected			
Yes	Days	Smoked, oral, injected			
Possible	Variable	Smoked, oral, injected, sniffed			
Yes	2 to 4	Smoked, oral	Euphoria, relaxed inhibitions, increased appetite, disoriented behavior	Fatigue, paranoia, possible psychosis	Insomnia, hyperactivity, and decreased appetite occasionally reported
Yes	2 to 4	Smoked, oral			
Yes	2 to 4	Smoked, oral			
Yes	2 to 4	Smoked, oral			

I–IV are schedules of various drugs.
I, these drugs have no legal use (category includes investigative drugs).
II, drugs with a high potential for abuse; known to be addictive.
III, drugs with lower abuse potential than those of schedule II.
IV, same as schedule III, except they have different penalties for possession. Falsely considered by many people not to be addictive drugs.
V, drugs with low abuse potential, may be purchased over the counter.

In general, early diagnosis is important to successful recovery. It is important to identify substance-dependent people while their social resources (e.g., significant others, job) are still intact. Thus, one of the purposes of this chapter is to help you recognize indications of drug dependence. Another purpose is to encourage you to examine your own attitudes about drugs and substance dependence. To this end, consider the questions in Box 79-1 before reading any further. They will help you think honestly about alcohol and other drugs, and become aware of your own value system. Also ask yourself what words you use to describe substance-dependent people.

This last question is important to help you identify your own attitudes. Throughout this book, we have often pointed out how important it is not to label people. Perhaps in no other area of nursing practice are examples of labeling so extreme as in nursing care for people experiencing problems of dependence on alcohol and other drugs. The terms junkie, drunk, wino, addict, and others are commonly used in society. Nurses need to understand these terms but never use them. Always remember that people use drugs, people abuse drugs, people become dependent on drugs, and people need nursing care.

People who abuse drugs may hesitate to seek help if they believe information about them will not be confidential. In the United States, there are specific federal, state, and local regulations concerning confidentiality and substance-abuse treatment, developed to protect the identities of people seeking treatment. Because some people with drug problems (especially those using illicit drugs) are wanted for criminal offenses, treatment personnel are not to give any information about a person (not even to state whether or not an individual is in treatment) to anyone, including law enforcement officers. Of course, it is never acceptable nursing practice to discuss clients with those not involved in their treatment.

Box 79-1. Guide to Analyzing Personal Responses toward Substance Abusers

Analyze your responses to the following questions:

- What thoughts and feelings does the term alcoholic evoke in me?
- What thoughts and feelings does the term addict evoke in me?
- Do I believe that chemical dependence occurs out of moral weakness?
- Do I believe that chemical dependence is an illness that can be treated?
- Are people who abuse substances deliberately destroying their own lives and the lives of significant others?
- Who in my personal life has abused drugs, alcohol, or other chemicals?
- How does my experience with relatives, friends, colleagues, or clients who have abused substances affect my attitude toward caring for a substance-abusing client?
- Is substance abuse a social problem, an emotional-psychological problem, or a physical abnormality?
- How do I view the family, spouse, or friends of the substance abuser? Do they encourage the abuse, or otherwise enable the person to continue their abuse? Or are they victims?
- How does my own personal use of nicotine, caffeine, drugs, or alcohol affect my attitude toward clients?

From Bittle S., et al. (1986). Substance abuse. In C. R. Kneisel, & S. Ames (Eds.), *Adult health nursing: A biopsychosocial approach.* (p. 254). Reading, MA: Addison-Wesley.

POSSIBLE CAUSES OF SUBSTANCE ABUSE

No one factor explains the development of chemical abuse or dependence. Explanations of the possible causes of substance abuse can be biologic, psychosocial, and sociocultural in nature. It is likely that a combination of factors coexist—the psychobiologic characteristics of the person using the substance, the properties of the substance itself, and the environment in which substance use takes place.

Biologic Theories

Biologic explanations, especially those that shed light on genetic predispositions to alcoholism, have become increasingly important. For example, research has indicated that children of alcoholic parents are more likely to have problems with alcohol than children of nonalcoholic parents, even when they have been separated from their parents early in life.[14] Children of nonalcoholics reared by alcoholics are not at increased risk of alcoholism.[30] Identical twins have been found to have drinking patterns similar to those of their parents. These patterns occur less often in fraternal twins. Although biologic variations in responses to alcohol appear to be genetic, there is no direct evidence linking innate factors to the development of alcohol abuse and dependence. Excessive alcohol use is often associated with concurrent use of opiates and vice versa, which suggests common underlying biochemical mechanisms. It is speculated that substance-dependent people may lack naturally occurring endorphins (chemicals in the brain) and, therefore, take substances in a physiologic attempt to replace the missing chemicals.[8]

In addition, many people who abuse alcohol and drugs may also have significant problems with anxiety and depression. It is thought that their tendency to abuse these substances may sometimes be secondary to a biologically based affective disorder.[4]

Psychosocial Theories

Certain personality features—low self-esteem, emotional immaturity, low frustration tolerance, and unwillingness or inability to endure and cope with tension—

seem to be characteristic of persons addicted to chemical substances. These personality features probably interplay with genetic susceptibility and individual biologic response to the chemical substance.

In addition to individual personality features, family phenomena such as parental lack of emotional warmth, parental rejection, and parental overprotection may also figure importantly in the addiction process.[9] Some researchers believe that adolescents who become addicts are in enmeshed families, that is, they are too close to their parents and, consequently, feel dependent, inadequate, and fearful of separation. Conflict is inevitable in such families, and violence is common. Substance abuse can be one way to manage painful emotions and painful family experiences.

Sociocultural Theories

The following social conditions and contexts help create and sustain substance abuse: the hopelessness and defeat of urban slum dwellers, the academic and social pressures generated in upper middle-class families, the feelings of impotence and alienation that are common in adolescence, and peer group pressure to join in and share experiences.[15]

Throughout history, substance use has been a way of coping with anxiety. Today, this message is communicated to children by significant others and the media. Adults who use alcohol to relax show children that alcohol is appropriate to relieve tension. Advertisements encourage us to take medication to relieve discomfort, dissipate tension, or get energy. The mood alteration that occurs with initial substance-using is immediately reinforcing.

Adults may begin using drugs for self-medication, such as to relieve depression, lose weight, alleviate fatigue, influence mood, change activity level, or facilitate social interaction. Physicians can and do prescribe a variety of drugs for these problems, with the result that for many people, abuse of and addiction to tranquilizers, sleeping pills, and amphetamines becomes a problem.

Among young people, perhaps the most influential determinant of substance-taking is the peer group. Participation in some groups or in high school or college parties may be contingent on drug use. Individuals may seek out groups that support their particular drug preferences, thereby reinforcing drug dependence.

Economic factors are also important. The choice of substance, the quantity, and the frequency of use are often determined by cost and available money.

Among black Americans, frustration, prejudice, and the desire to escape a stressful reality may lead to substance abuse. Discrimination leads to inadequate education and social and economic injustices. Alcohol is the most used and abused substance among black Americans. In general, alcohol abuse in black communities is more widespread and devastating than among nonblacks. On the other hand, common spiritual influences in black communities militate against drug use. Certain religious groups ban all alcohol use, for example. Another factor in black American substance abuse is the fact that many black people live in urban ghettos where crime thrives and illicit substances are available. This combination increases the likelihood of black alcoholic people also being addicted to other substances.

Among Native Americans, alcoholism is one of the most significant health problems. Probably no other condition so adversely affects the quality of life in these communities. When alcohol was introduced to American Indians in the 16th and 17th centuries, socially disruptive patterns of drinking quickly developed. These persist today and include periodic and explosive drinking, group binge drinking, and the absence of social sanctions supporting more appropriate drinking behavior.[19] Investigators have attempted to learn whether there are physiologic differences in response to alcohol among various Native American groups, but the evidence is inconclusive.

An Asian person who has immigrated to western civilization faces four major problems in dealing with substance use: (1) differing ethnic values, (2) stereotypes, (3) economic oppression, and (4) language difficulties. Peer pressure and insecurity are important causal factors for drug abuse among Asian people. The need for acceptance within a group stems from the rooted feelings of insecurity and reduced self-confidence that can develop in immigrants. With chemical substances, the abuser feels less inhibited and better able to communicate.[26]

Groups of Hispanic people of both sexes, but especially males, have relatively higher rates of alcohol consumption than others. Language difficulties, poverty, and differing cultural values are all factors leading to drug abuse and addiction in Hispanic people.[12]

Marijuana is the second most frequently used recreational substance among white Americans. Alcohol is still number one. Cocaine use is increasing among young urban professionals. It is difficult to generalize about substance use among white Americans because so many subcultures exist. Usually, only alcohol is actually sanctioned. Subgroups have different ways of introducing substance use to group members, and varying social standards for substance consumption. For example, people of Italian background who commonly use wine with meals but scorn intoxication have relatively low rates of alcoholism.

GENERAL ASSESSMENT FOR SUBSTANCE USE/ABUSE

Questions designed to screen for the presence of chemical substance problems need to become part of assessment wherever clients are seen by health professionals (see the Bridge to Home Health Care). Assessment includes information about past and present habits of substance use, including the amount and type consumed, frequency of use, situations in which the substance is used, self-perception of substance-using behavior, and effects on daily life (Table 79–2).

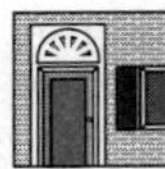

BRIDGE TO HOME HEALTH CARE

Substance Abuse Detection

Signs and symptoms of substance abuse can appear in a myriad of ways, including physiologic, social, and behavioral changes. When substance abuse is suspected, the community health nurse is an essential team member working with the family, physician, clinic and school nurses, and other concerned health providers. Together, this team can identify the missing pieces of the puzzle that the substance abuser presents.

Regardless of the client's social, economic, professional, or educational status, substance abuse can be a problem that eventually leads to changes in the client's behavior and lifestyle. The home health care practitioner needs to be alert to these changes, both overt and covert, in the home setting. It is very important for the nurse to trust his or her senses and instincts in gathering information because substance abusers often use denial and concealment because of fear of detection.

However, in the comfort of the home, defenses may be lessened. Carefully listening to conversations and observing the environment and family interactions can reveal diminishing income. As substance abuse increases, less money is available for basic needs as food, house and car payments and rent. Conversely, a sudden increase in income or goods could be related to selling drugs.

The nurse's sense of smell can help detect the use of drugs and alcohol. The pungent odor of marijuana lingers in a home long after its use. Likewise, tell-tale alcohol breath is difficult to disguise. Using your vision to simply observe is one of the least intrusive means of detecting substance abuse. Noticing a pattern of increased visitors and observing drug paraphernalia or accumulated liquor and alcohol containers alerts the nurse to possible substance abuse.

Last, but equally important, instinct and intervention are useful tools for detection. The nurse needs to recognize behavior changes. Examples include (1) school children who arrive late, are frequently absent, or are inadequately dressed; (2) missed appointments with teachers, physicians, and clinics; and (3) noncompliance with medications. Isolated instances can emerge into disruptive patterns that complete the pieces of the substance abuse puzzle.

The home health nurse has a distinct advantage to see, hear, and observe suspected substance abusers in their home setting. In this way, the nurse offers valuable insight to the health care team from the time the family is admitted to service until dismissal.

A number of useful screening tools for assessing alcohol abuse are available. (This is less true for other abused substances.) These include (1) *What Are the Signs of Alcoholism?*, a checklist published by the National Council on Alcoholism, designed to help individuals determine whether they have an alcohol problem[35]; and (2) the *Short Michigan Alcoholism Screening Test*, which offers questions useful in identifying alcohol problems, and is considered a valid and reliable tool for diagnosing alcohol abuse and alcoholism.[31]

Of course, as with any assessment tool, a thorough understanding of scoring and interpretation is imperative. A listing of substance use assessment tools is available in *The Drug Abuse Instrument Handbook*, published by the National Institute on Drug Abuse.[25]

In addition to initial screening and history taking, physical assessment is important. It broadens the base of clues that leads to identification of physiologic problems coexisting with, or consequent on, chemical dependence. Such potential problems are discussed later in this chapter.

ASSESSING THE EFFECTS OF PSYCHOACTIVE SUBSTANCES

The onset of a substance's effect depends on the characteristics of the chemical itself, the route of administration, and the adequacy of the circulatory system.

Tolerance is a process whereby the central nervous system (CNS) adapts to the continued presence of a substance by compensating for its effect. This compensation leads to high drug blood concentrations. As a result, the person has to take increased quantities of the substance to obtain the desired effect. This phenomenon leads to physical dependence and pathologic organ changes.

Dependence may be psychological or physiologic. Susceptible individuals can become psychologically dependent on any and all substances.

Tolerance and dependence help explain the phenomenon of withdrawal, a pattern of physical responses that appears when regular drug use is discontinued. When a physically dependent person abruptly stops consumption (or even decreases the amount), signs and symptoms of withdrawal occur. Not all substances produce physical dependence.

In general, chemical withdrawal reactions tend to produce an effect opposite to that of the ingested substance. A depressant substance, for example, causes hyperactivity during withdrawal. To prevent severe withdrawal episodes, the usual treatment for physically chemical-dependent people is to gradually decrease the amount of substance used. Another substance, with which the addictive drug is cross-tolerant, may be given in initially intoxicating doses, the doses being gradually decreased.

Nurses meet people withdrawing from substances in various settings (see Ethical Issues in Nursing). For example, a person who abuses substances may be admitted to a health care facility for surgery, or as a result of illness or accident. The staff, if unaware of the client's heavy substance intake, may not be prepared when withdrawal symptoms begin. It is essential that assessment of substance use be an integral part of initial nursing assessment for everyone.

It is important to get accurate information from people or significant others about the quantity of substance used, how long the person has been taking it, and the time of the last dose. It is also useful to get information about past withdrawal episodes in order to watch for possible adverse reactions. With knowledge of a per-

TABLE 79–2. Format for Nursing History Related to Alcohol/Substance Use

Remember: Most information needed for a complete and accurate health appraisal is obtained by history taking.

Initial Questioning. When assessing clients in any setting, ask about their use of all substances in the following order*:

a. Prescribed drugs
b. Over-the-counter drugs
c. Self-prescribed drugs, that is, nicotine, caffeine, alcohol, street drugs

Ask about quantity and frequency for all these groups. Conclude questions with: "Are there any drugs or substances you take that you haven't told me about yet?"

The person's answers to these questions indicate how to proceed.

No Need To Go Any Further if	**Referrals Needed** if
1. The person gives thoughtful, matter-of-fact answers. This indicates no concern and no problem. 2. The person states she or he abstains because of sociocultural or spiritual reasons *or* because she or he is a recovering alcoholic or addict and is well integrated into a community social network that supports recovery.	1. The person expresses concern about his or her substance-using pattern. Refer to a clinical specialist or community agency for further assessment. Information about the drug's effect may help the person make decisions about alcohol or drug use. 2. The person describes abstinence designed to prove the point that alcohol or drug use is no problem. If the person is very defensive, this indicates a problem. Explain this to the person and significant others, and refer them to community resources for assessment and help. 3. Responses to questions are designed to have you believe there is no problem (especially if you suspect otherwise), such as, "You'd drink too if . . .," "My friends think I smoke too much dope but they're just wimps," "It's none of your business." Corroborate any suspicions you have by asking further questions to determine the impact of substance use on the person's daily functioning. Talk with significant others. Explain that you need to know the extent of the client's substance use because of the possibility of withdrawal and cross-tolerance.

The alcohol and drug history need not be completed all at once. You can pick up where you left off. The importance is to finish it, to obtain baseline data for care planning. History taking is an excellent time for health teaching regarding alcohol and drug effects and options for decreasing use.

*This order facilitates the development of trust and minimizes the person's defensiveness.

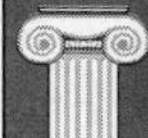

ETHICAL ISSUES IN NURSING

What Considerations Should Be Made for Substance Abusers Who Are Being Treated for Other Medical Problems?

Substance abuse is a problem that touches all cultures throughout the world. Its effects can be seen in the young and the old, and its addiction has no mercy. Because the abuse of chemical substances leads to health problems, health care workers see these clients often—maybe not primarily because of their substance abuse, but such abuse plays a part in their illnesses nonetheless. How ethical is thetreatment rendered to those who are substance abusers?

For instance, take the alcoholic client who comes in for a surgical procedure. He or she was told not to drink for several days prior to surgery but the reality is he or she drank up to the night before. Postoperatively, the patient begins to experience DTs and must be aggressively restrained. The challenges facing the nursing staff caring for a postoperative patient with DTs are great. Client safety is a serious matter as well as wound healing and adequate nutrition. The client may be treated to reduce symptoms. In other cases, the client may be simply left to detoxify "cold turkey."

What is the ethical thing to do for the treatment of substance abusers who are being treated for other medical problems? Nurses deal with these kinds of situations every day. Should clients who are known substance abusers be admitted to the hospital several days prior to a surgical procedure in order to rid their systems of substances which could adversely affect their surgery? If so, what are the financial restraints of such a policy? Should all substance abuse clients be required to seek counseling for their abuse in order to receive other forms of health care?

As previously stated, nurses see substance abuse clients in all areas of practice for all kinds of health problems. Although health care may not be contingent on treatment of their substance abuse, nurses can assist such clients by providing information on such treatment programs in their areas.

TABLE 79-3. Slang Terms for Abused Substances

Drug	Slang Term
Depressants	***Downers***
Barbiturates	Barbs, blockbusters, blues, downers, pink ladies, rainbows, reds, red devils, yellows, yellow jackets, sleeping pills
Methaqualone	Quads, sopors, ludes
Glutethimide	C.D., Cibas
Pentazocine (Talwin)	T's and blues
Stimulants	***Uppers***
Amphetamines	Bennies, crystal, dexies, eye openers, meth, pep pills, speed, uppers, black beauties
Cocaine	Coke, snow, white, lady, blow, crack, rock
Modes of administration	Snort (nasally), mainline (intravenous), freebase (mix with a solvent and heat)
Opiates	
Heroin	Big H, H, horse, junk, smack
Intravenous administration	Shooting up, mainlining
Subcutaneous administration	Skin popping
The amount of drug taken	A hit
Cannabis Derivatives	
Marijuana	Pot, tea, weed, grass, reefer, joint, ganja, Acapulco gold, mary jane, shit
Hashish	Hash
Hallucinogens	
Mescaline	Mesc, buttons, cactus
Psilocybin	Magic mushroom
Phencyclidine	PCP, hog, angel dust, crystal, rocket fuel, peace pill
Lysergic acid diethylamide (LSD)	Acid

son's substance-use history, nurses can be alert to indications of impending withdrawal. If substance abuse or addiction is not detected and treated, a person may progress to a severe state of withdrawal that may be difficult to manage (Table 79-2).

ALCOHOL

Alcohol is a CNS depressant. Barbiturates and similarly acting sedatives, hypnotics, and antianxiety agents are also CNS depressants. (Neuroleptics are excluded from this category.) Table 79-1 lists common brand names of depressants. Substance users often employ slang terms and it is important for health professionals to identify them (Table 79-3).

Blood Levels and Behavior. The relationship between blood alcohol levels and behavior in a nontolerant drinker is shown in Table 79-4. Except when death occurs, these effects are temporary. They subside as alcohol consumption stops and the liver has time to metabolize all the alcohol present in the blood. The relationship between blood alcohol levels and behavior is different in people who have developed tolerance to alcohol. Alcohol-dependent people who have developed tolerance for alcohol can drink large quantities without obvious impairment. They can perform complex behavioral tasks accurately at blood alcohol levels several times greater than those that would produce behavioral impairment in nontolerant drinkers. A person's level of tolerance can be estimated by comparing the symptoms expected at certain blood alcohol levels in nontolerant drinkers with the person's blood alcohol level and actual symptoms.

Withdrawal. Removal of alcohol from the body, or withdrawal, results in psychomotor agitation. The earliest and most common features of withdrawal are anxiety, anorexia, insomnia, and tremor. A withdrawing person appears hyperalert, manifests jerky movements and irritability, and is easily startled. Subjective distress is often described as internal shaking. These symptoms develop within a few hours of stopping drinking and peak at about 24 hours. Pulse and blood pressure (BP) are typically elevated and are useful indicators of progress through withdrawal. Diaphoresis occurs in some people. A brief, mild disorientation, particularly to time, may also be noted. Alcoholic hallucinosis may develop, but it is not frightening to the person. Orientation remains intact.

During the first 48 hours of withdrawal, self-limiting grand mal convulsive seizures may develop. Delirium

TABLE 79-4. Relationship Between Blood Alcohol Levels and Behavior in a Nontolerant Drinker

Blood Levels (%)	Behavior
0.05	Perceptible changes in mood and behavior. Judgement and restraint are loosened. Individual feels carefree
0.10	Voluntary motor action becomes clumsy. Legal evidence of intoxication in most states
0.20	Function of entire motor area of brain is measurably depressed, causing staggering. Individual may be easily angered and may shout or weep
0.30	Confusion; stupor
0.40	Coma
0.50	Death due to respiratory blocking effects on medulla

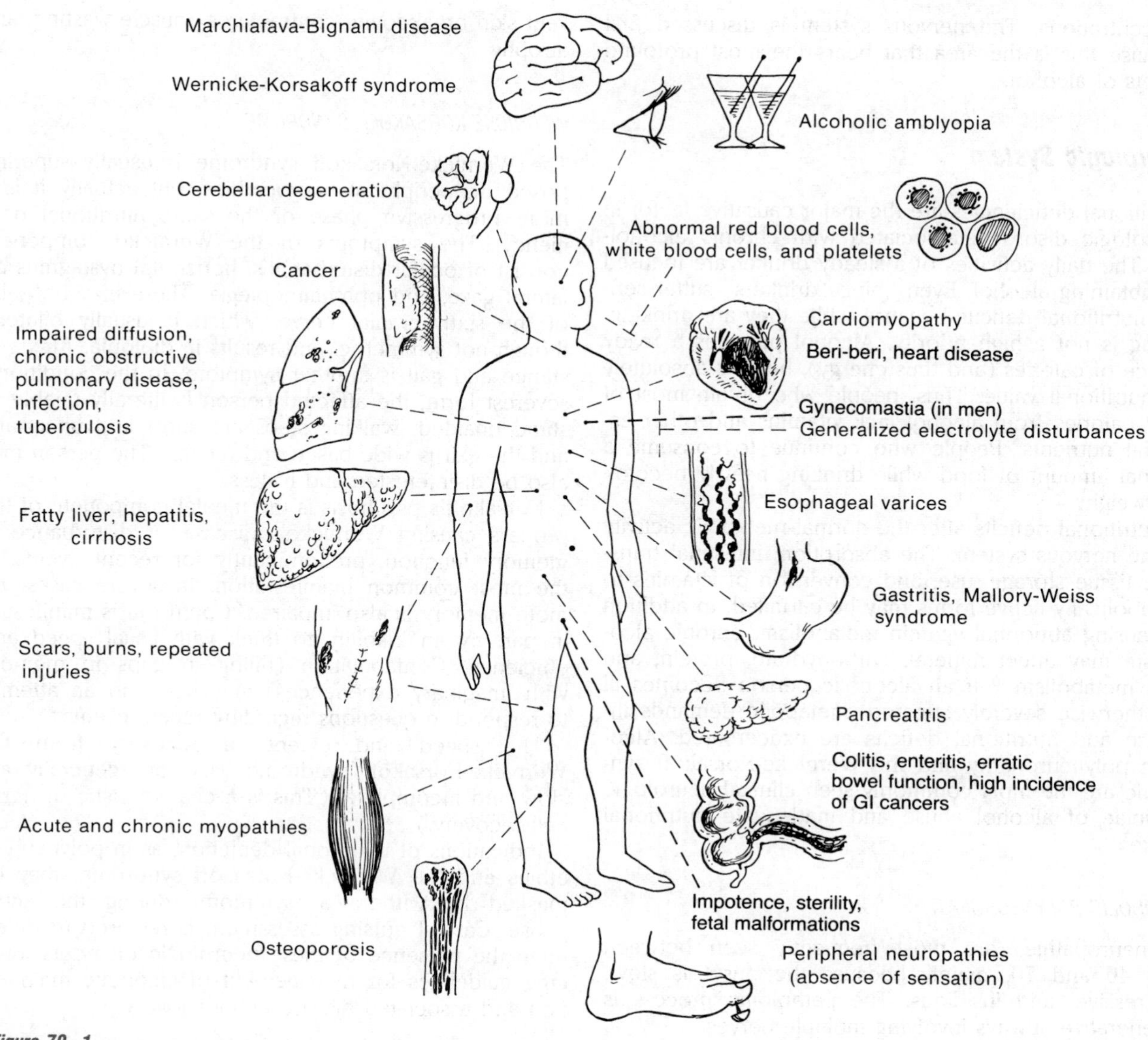

▲ *Figure 79-1*

Clinical problems resulting from alcohol abuse.

tremens (DTs) may occur 3 days to 4 weeks after cessation of drinking. DTs are characterized by severe psychomotor agitation, confusion, disorientation, frightening hallucinations, metabolic dysfunction, and increased autonomic activity, that is, fever, tachycardia, profuse diaphoresis, and tachypnea. Individual reactions may differ considerably, but the estimates given are a useful guide for anticipating various symptoms.

Detoxification is a treatment process in which a longer-acting CNS depressant drug is substituted for alcohol. The dose is gradually tapered down so that withdrawal is a slower, more predictable process.

Nursing Management. Although it seems hard to believe, an estimated thirty percent of hospitalized people are alcohol abusers. Therefore, it is important to obtain an alcohol consumption history (Table 79-2) and observe for indications of alcohol problems or withdrawal in all persons seeking health care. Many illnesses, such as those depicted in Figure 79-1, are suggestive of excess alcohol consumption. Always consider the possibility that a traumatic injury could be the result of excessive alcohol consumption since traumatic injuries occur more frequently in people who abuse alcohol or other chemical substances.

PHYSICAL AND PSYCHOSOCIAL PROBLEMS ASSOCIATED WITH ALCOHOL ABUSE

Many serious psychophysiologic disturbances result from chronic alcohol abuse. Serious disturbances occur in the nervous, gastrointestinal, cardiovascular, respiratory, and musculoskeletal systems (see Fig. 79-1). Tolerance is partly responsible for these effects. Cell damage occurs from prolonged exposure to high drug concentrations. The nervous system is discussed first because this is the area that bears the most profound effects of alcohol.

Neurologic System

Nutritional deficiencies are the major causative factor in neurologic disorders associated with chronic alcoholism. The daily activities of a steady drinker are focused on obtaining alcohol. Even "binge drinkers" suffer serious nutritional deficits because while they are drinking, eating is not a high priority. Alcohol provides a ready source of calories (and thus energy), but has absolutely no nutritional value. Thus, people who obtain most of their calories from alcohol lack vitamins and other essential nutrients. People who continue to consume a normal amount of food while drinking heavily become overweight.

Nutritional deficits alter the normal metabolic activity of the nervous system. The absorption, intestinal transport, tissue storage, use, and conversion of vitamins to metabolically active forms may be curtailed. In addition to causing abnormal vitamin metabolism, chronic alcoholism may affect mineral, carbohydrate, protein, and lipid metabolism.[10] If an alcoholic person becomes ill or otherwise severely stressed, metabolic demands increase and nutritional deficits are exacerbated. Alcoholic polyneuropathy and the Wernicke-Korsakoff syndrome are the most commonly seen clinical neurologic sequelae of alcohol abuse and inadequate nutritional intake.

ALCOHOLIC POLYNEUROPATHY

Polyneuropathies are most frequently seen between ages 40 and 70, mainly because the onset is slow, progressive, and insidious. The pathologic process is degenerative, always involving multiple nerves.

Some people with polyneuropathies may be asymptomatic. Neurologic assessment reveals varying degrees of motor, reflex, and sensory loss, which typically occurs in the feet before the hands, and moves from the distal to proximal areas. Sensory symptoms appear first and are usually described as tingling, pricking, burning, or numb sensations. Occasionally, there are dull or sharp pains. Calf muscles may be tender to touch. The senses of pain, temperature, and vibration are usually diminished. Because of diminished sensation and weak muscles, the person may move with a wide-stance gait.

Recovery is slow and depends on a nutritious diet with supplemental vitamins, as well as stopping or decreasing alcohol intake. Thiamine replacement is particularly important. Thiamine is essential for conversion of glucose to metabolically active forms, and nerve cell function depends on glucose.

Safety precautions are very important for people with diminished sensation. Teach them to be especially careful when smoking, cooking, and moving about to prevent burns and bruises. Teach foot care and other hygienic measures. In severe cases, teach them to prevent skin breakdown, contractures, muscle wasting, and atrophy.

WERNICKE-KORSAKOFF SYNDROME

The Wernicke-Korsakoff syndrome is usually superimposed on peripheral neuropathies, but actually it is a more progressive phase of the same nutritional deficiency. The symptoms of the Wernicke component consist of ocular disturbances, horizontal nystagmus on lateral gaze, and ophthalmoplegia. There may be palsy of the sixth cranial nerve, which is usually bilateral though not symmetric, and results in diplopia. Ataxia of stance and gait is another symptom. In the condition's severest form, the affected person is literally unable to stand unaided, walking steps are short and uncertain, and the gait is wide based and reeling. The person may also be disinterested and listless.

Korsakoff's psychosis is the mental component of the process causing Wernicke's disease. A disturbance in memory function, predominantly for recent events, is the most common manifestation. In severe cases, remote memory is also impaired. Confusion is manifested in part by an inability to think with usual speed and efficiency. Confabulation (filling in gaps in memory with imaginary experiences) may occur in an attempt to respond to questions regarding recent events.

The speed and extent of recovery from the Wernicke-Korsakoff syndrome vary, but generally are slow and incomplete. (This is a characteristic of nerve cell recovery.)

Indications of nutritional depletion, as in polyneuropathies and the Wernicke-Korsakoff syndrome, may be masked by withdrawal symptoms during the acute phase. Careful nursing assessment is required to determine the presence of these neurologic disorders. Specific guidelines for management of alcoholic malnutrition and associated disease entities follow:

- Start treatment as soon as possible, to prevent irreversible damage.
- Administer initial high doses of thiamine and perhaps other vitamins.
- Abstinence, or at least diminished drinking, helps reverse the problem.
- A diet fortified with vitamins is essential. Diet planning must be individualized and realistic. Follow-up is helpful so that ongoing adjustments can be made.

Many people with the Wernicke-Korsakoff syndrome do not recover completely and require lifelong supervisory care. Major environmental adjustments may be necessary for people whose recovery is incomplete. Safety is a major consideration.

COGNITIVE DYSFUNCTION

Cerebral atrophy is a common concomitant of chronic alcoholism and causes cognitive dysfunction. Alcoholics have difficulty with abstraction, problem solving, new learning, memory, and perceptual-motor speed. These deficits vary from mild to moderate and are consistent with those seen in clients with mild to moderate generalized brain dysfunction from other causes.

Recovery from alcoholism is more difficult and less likely if cognitive dysfunction has developed, because treatment largely depends on a person's ability to learn, problem solve, and live life without alcohol. It is not known whether recovery from cognitive dysfunction is possible, but it is reasonable to wait several weeks to determine whether any recovery occurs before starting treatment.

Gastrointestinal System

Alcohol affects nearly every gastrointestinal organ. Esophageal pathology is secondary to other clinical problems associated with alcohol. Esophageal varices, for example, are a symptom of portal hypertension secondary to cirrhosis of the liver (see Chap. 58). Esophageal varices that rupture and bleed can be a life-threatening emergency.

There is some question whether alcohol also increases acid production, which would exacerbate the process of autodigestion. Acute gastritis may occur, which may be hemorrhagic. Symptoms are the same as those of gastritis from any cause, as are the potential complications of perforation or obstruction. Gastric and duodenal ulcers may occur. Again, signs, symptoms, and possible complications are the same as for ulcers of any cause.

Alcohol requires very little digestion, some being absorbed directly from the stomach into the bloodstream. The largest portion, however, is absorbed from the small intestine, principally the duodenum. Alcohol has an irritant effect, increasing motility and producing an outpouring of fluid. This often causes enteritis or colitis. Malabsorption of essential nutrients from food results.

Hemorrhoids are the only disorder in the large intestine related to alcohol abuse. These are secondary to impaired blood flow resulting from portal hypertension.

LIVER

After alcohol is absorbed from the stomach and small intestine, it is carried via the bloodstream to the liver for detoxification. Alcoholic liver disease is a specific progressive syndrome, the direct result of the toxic effects of alcohol. The syndrome begins with fatty liver, progressing to alcoholic hepatitis and, finally, cirrhosis.

In fatty liver, fat is deposited in the liver during alcohol metabolism. An alcoholic person's liver may become grossly enlarged by fat accumulation, which may be associated with functional deficit. Abstinence from alcohol early in the course of hepatic changes results in complete reversal of pathologic processes and a return of normal liver function.

If alcohol consumption continues, some people develop alcoholic hepatitis, a toxic, necrotic, inflammatory liver condition caused by the death of liver cells. A person severely ill with alcoholic hepatitis has typically been drinking heavily for weeks or months and is anorexic, jaundiced, and febrile. Hepatomegaly and hepatic pain are usually present. Treatment during the acute stage is symptomatic. Long-term recovery depends on abstinence. Even then reversibility is variable, depending on the severity and chronicity of the hepatitis.

The final stage of alcoholic liver disease is cirrhosis, a progressive form of hepatic fibrosis. The only treatment at this stage is to remove the underlying cause, alcohol, and to maximize the possibilities for tissue regeneration.

Complications of cirrhosis are difficult to treat and should be prevented whenever possible. They include portal hypertension, ascites, esophageal varices, hepatic encephalopathy, and bacterial peritonitis.

PANCREAS

A history of long-term heavy drinking is a common factor in about 50 per cent of adults with pancreatitis. The outstanding symptom usually is severe, constant epigastric pain, which radiates to the back. Nausea and vomiting are common. The client usually looks ill, and has abdominal tenderness and distention. Symptoms become acute 1 to 2 days after an increase in drinking, such as a weekend binge. More severe cases may be complicated by intrapancreatic hemorrhage, pancreatic necrosis, pseudocyst formation, or pancreatic abscess.

Treatment of pancreatitis is discussed in detail in Chapter 59. Alcoholic pancreatitis remains a chronic condition with acute episodes unless the causative agent, alcohol, is eliminated from the system.

Cardiovascular System

Alcohol exerts many direct and indirect effects on the cardiovascular system. The heart's mechanical performance is decreased by alcohol consumption. The heart rate and cardiac output increase with very small amounts of alcohol. However, the heart rate slows and cardiac output decreases with increasing doses, as a result of vagus nerve stimulation. Slowing of the heart rate produces an accumulation of lactic acid in the peripheral vascular system. This causes dilatation of these vessels and ensuing tachycardia. Blood pressure is variable. If there is evidence of myocardial disease and no evidence of other heart disease, alcohol may well be the problem. Chronic alcoholism is the most common cause of cardiomyopathy in the United States.

Alcoholic cardiomyopathy is a long-term development, usually appearing after many years of alcohol consumption. Evidence suggests that the fundamental mechanisms of injury induced by alcohol are structural and chemical disorganization of membranes, interference with ion transport, and derangement of various biochemical functions that possibly allow calcium to accumulate in cells. Calcium accumulation in vascular smooth muscle may also increase sensitivity to circulating vasopressors, and account for the increased incidence of hypertension in chronic alcoholics. Vascular hypertension and cerebral vascular accidents also have a greater incidence in chronic alcoholics.

Many factors associated with heavy alcohol intake lead to indirect cardiac effects. The alcohol withdrawal reaction, for example, puts a heavy workload on the heart, and sinus tachycardia and hypertension typically occur. Prolonged, severe withdrawal can lead to extreme fatigue and possibly sudden death as a result of such mechanisms as cardiogenic shock, cardiac standstill, ventricular fibrillation and flutter, or abrupt left-sided heart failure.

Careful observation and attentive management during detoxification can usually prevent such catastrophes, or at least lead to rapid restorative measures if complications do occur. Detoxification is an extremely stressful process that places great demands on the heart. Intervention to minimize stress can do much to ensure adequate cardiac functioning.

Respiratory System

There is a high incidence of chronic obstructive pulmonary disease (COPD) among alcoholic clients because of a combination of (1) direct toxic effects of alcohol on pulmonary tissue and (2) impaired clearance of bacteria from the lungs, resulting from alcohol ingestion. The lungs become more susceptible to chronic bronchial infections and more vulnerable to the effects of cigarette smoke and other toxic agents. Once a certain degree of pulmonary injury takes place, function may not be restored to normal even with abstinence from alcohol.

Alcohol ingestion disturbs respiratory patterns during sleep, as evidenced by a marked increase in apneic events in healthy volunteers.[7] Such effects on people with pulmonary and cardiovascular disease can be serious.

Another common lung abnormality in chronic alcoholism is impaired diffusion. In most cases, abstinence from alcohol restores diffusion to normal. There is also a high association of tuberculosis with alcoholism. It is important to screen regularly all suspected or known alcoholic clients for possible tuberculosis. This is becoming increasingly important because of the current increase in antibiotic-resistant tuberculosis in the United States.

Fluid and Electrolyte Balance

The popular belief that alcohol is a diuretic is true only while blood alcohol levels rise and as they stabilize. As blood alcohol levels fall, an antidiuretic effect occurs, producing fluid retention. Thus, alcoholics are more likely to be overhydrated than dehydrated (except, of course, when experiencing vomiting or diarrhea). Therefore, do not force fluids during withdrawal except in cases of chronic malnutrition. Adding fluid to an overhydrated person whose cardiac muscle may not be working well can result in severe, potentially fatal CHF.

Hypomagnesemia occurs in alcoholics, because alcohol selectively increases urinary excretion of magnesium. This has cardiac implications as well as affecting the course of withdrawal. Hypomagnesemia may cause withdrawal seizures. It is the policy in many alcoholic treatment programs to give magnesium whenever blood tests show low or borderline serum magnesium levels.

Hematologic System

Adverse effects of alcohol on hematopoiesis result in abnormalities of red blood cells (RBC), white blood cells (WBC), and platelets. Virtually no aspect of blood cell development, survival, or function escapes the physiologic and biochemical toxicities of alcohol. Abnormalities may result in anemias and difficulties in counteracting infection, and may interfere in the clotting mechanism. Severe infection and hematomas may result. Complete blood counts provide evidence of anemias and abnormal WBC counts.

Probably one of the most important effects of alcohol on the hematologic system is inhibition of folate metabolism. Alcohol interferes with the delivery of folate to marrow precursors. Depending on the duration and level of alcohol consumption, many disorders may develop.[10] With abstinence from alcohol and proper nutrition, these abnormalities are reversible. Short-term folate supplementation may be required.

Musculoskeletal System

Alcohol ingestion may damage skeletal muscle, resulting in subclinical, acute, or chronic alcoholic myopathy. The pathologic process is the same as in alcohol cardiomyopathy.

Acute alcoholic myopathy is a syndrome of muscle pain, tenderness, and edema occurring after acute excesses of alcohol ingestion. Proximal muscles of the extremities, the pelvic and shoulder girdles, and the muscles of the thoracic cage are most commonly affected. Symptoms usually subside in 1 to 3 weeks but may recur with repeated alcohol ingestion. Symptoms may be obscured by intoxication or withdrawal. Treatment consists of a well-balanced diet with supplemental vitamins and abstinence from alcohol.

Chronic alcoholic myopathy is a syndrome of muscle weakness and wasting involving the muscle groups described earlier. There is no history of pain or tenderness, and onset is slow and insidious. Treatment is the same as for acute alcoholic myopathy.

Alcoholism contributes to skeletal complications in at least two ways: (1) a syndrome of nontraumatic hip osteonecrosis is being recognized in alcohol consumers, perhaps caused by fat emboli blocking end arteries, and (2) there is an increased incidence of fractures and other injuries secondary to trauma and falls. Impaired coordination due to high blood alcohol levels is a contributing factor.

Endocrine System

Alcohol consumption causes lowered serum testosterone levels that cause impotence, loss of libido, breast enlargement, loss of facial hair, and testicular atrophy. In women, amenorrhea, oligomenorrhea, loss of libido, and reduced vaginal lubrication have been reported among alcohol abusers.

Integumentary System

Skin lesions are common in alcoholic clients, many (e.g., generalized pruritus, gray skin pigmentation, and rosacea) being linked to liver disease. Others are associated with nutritional deficiencies (e.g., glossitis secondary to folate deficiency). Some conditions that may be present in the general population flare up with drinking bouts. These include psoriasis and seborrheic dermatitis. A heavy drinker usually neglects basic hygiene. Skin infections and lesions result. Treatment consists of good hygiene, a nutritious diet, and abstinence from alcohol. Referral to a dermatologist may be necessary in severe cases.

Cancer

An association has been observed between alcohol abuse and cancer of the oropharynx, larynx, and esophagus (where there is direct contact of tissues with alcohol) and the liver (where there is serious organ damage). Heavy drinking may also be implicated in cancer of the pancreas and prostate. Cancer in these sites is a clue to a possible alcohol problem. Smoking and malnutrition, which usually accompany heavy drinking, increase the risk of cancer in some organs, especially the lungs.

The reasons for the association of cancer with alcohol abuse are unclear, but among the possibilities are (1) prolonged effects of alcohol on body tissues and (2) the presence of carcinogenic substances in some alcoholic beverages.

Psychosocial Deterioration

Repeated, heavy alcohol abuse eventually leads to upheavals in relationships with significant others. An alcoholic person's behavior alienates others and may lead to social isolation.

Alcoholism has been called a family illness because the entire social network suffers the consequences of one member's heavy drinking. A family with an alcoholic member or members falls short of achieving its primary functions of socializing children and providing security for adults, because of major difficulties in communications, sexual interaction, and role fulfillment.[10]

Communication with a person who is frequently intoxicated is exasperating. Intoxicated people often are not held responsible for their words or actions. As a result, they set the rules in their social interactions. In response, others eventually stop trying to communicate. The use of defense mechanisms, such as projection and rationalization, also contribute to destructive interactions. The alcoholic person increasingly tries to escape through alcohol, whereas the significant others either retreat into activities that exclude the alcoholic person or they become apathetic.

Because an alcoholic person is not able to function within his or her social network, the other members (often spouse and children) alter their behavior (role performances) in an effort to keep the system functioning. They often take on the neglected duties of the alcoholic person. This places an additional burden on them, especially on children, who frequently assume adult responsibilities at a young age. The children also often suffer from parental emotional neglect because both parents are preoccupied with the alcoholism. Recovery from alcoholism requires help for both the alcoholic person and significant others. The impact that alcoholism has had on them individually and as a unit must be acknowledged before the social deterioration can be repaired.

An alcoholic person's economic status is complicated by heavy drinking. Purchase of alcoholic beverages may be a severe financial drain. Income may be threatened because deteriorating job performance may result in job loss. Increased rates of illness, injury, and traffic accidents among alcoholic clients further deplete their monetary resources.

Alcohol abuse is costly to society. Illness, one half of all homicides, one third of all suicides, and reduced productivity secondary to alcohol abuse cost the U.S. hundreds of billions of dollars a year, as does the cost of an alcoholic person's involvement in criminal justice and social welfare systems.[23]

If it is suspected that a person may be withdrawing from alcohol, assess pulse and BP every 2 hours for the first 12 hours, every 4 hours for the next 24 hours, and four times daily subsequently (unless the person is still unstable). If the pulse reaches 110 or more and BP is 150/90 or greater in the absence of concurrent illnesses such as fever, hypovolemia, or chronic hypertension, alcohol withdrawal may be suspected. Observe for evidence of tremors or diaphoresis. Critical withdrawal reactions, e.g., seizures and DTs, can be avoided by anticipatory observation and intervention.

When an impending withdrawal reaction is suspected, notify the physician. A drug cross-tolerant with alcohol may be prescribed (see Table 79-5 for some alcohol-drug interactions). The benzodiazepine class of sedatives (e.g., chlordiazepoxide [Librium], diazepam [Valium], clorazepate [Tranxenel]) is most often used because of the large margin of safety between the effective and lethal dose, as well as the long half-life. These drugs are poorly absorbed intramuscularly and should be given by mouth. The goal is to prevent severe withdrawal reaction. Large, frequent doses of sedatives may be required to keep agitation minimal. Remember that alcoholic people have a tolerance for depressant drugs and may need higher, more frequent doses than nonalcoholic people.

An adequate dose has been reached when withdrawal symptoms are suppressed, such as when pulse and BP are lowered. As vital signs stabilize, drug dos-

TABLE 79–5. Selected Alcohol-Medication Interactions[1,10]

Medication	Effect When Combined with Alcohol	Probable Mechanism
Anesthetics	Need for increased dose of anesthesia in "dry" alcoholics, but once they are asleep, sleep is deeper and longer	When no alcohol present, metabolism rate of other drugs is enhanced
Antabuse	Abdominal cramps, flushing, vomiting, psychotic episodes, confusion	Inhibits intermediary metabolism of alcohol
Antibiotics	Higher blood levels	Faster absorption (kanamycin)
	Lower blood levels	Direct interaction in stomach (pencillin)
Anticoagulants, oral	Diminished anticoagulant effect with chronic alcohol abuse	Enhanced microsomal enzyme activity
	Enhanced anticoagulant effect with acute intoxication	Reduced metabolism
Anticonvulsants		
Phenytoin (Dilantin and others)	Diminished anticonvulsant effect with chronic alcohol abuse	Enhanced microsomal enzyme activity
	Enhanced anticonvulsant effect with acute intoxication	Reduced metabolism
Antihistamines	Drowsiness	Additive
Antimicrobials		
Chloramphenicol (Chloromycetin and others)	Minor Antabuse-like symptoms	Inhibits intermediary metabolism of alcohol
Isoniazid (many brands)	Diminished effect with chronic alcohol abuse	Enhanced microsomal enzyme activity
Metronidiazole (Flagyl)	Minor Antabuse-like symptoms	Inhibits intermediary metabolism of alcohol
Quinacrine (Atabrine)	Minor Antabuse-like symptoms	Inhibits intermediary metabolism of alcohol
Digitalis	Arrhythmias, digitoxicity	Decreases serum potassium
Hypoglycemics		
Chlorpropamide (Diabinese)	Minor Antabuse-like symptoms	Inhibits intermediary metabolism of alcohol
Phenformin (DBI; Meltrol)	Lactic acidosis	Synergy
Tolbutamide (Orinase)	Diminished hypoglycemic effect with chronic alcohol abuse	Enhanced microsomal enzyme activity
	Enhanced hypoglycemic effect with ingestion of alcohol, particularly in fasting people	Suppression of gluconeogenesis
	Minor Antabuse-like symptoms	Inhibits intermediary metabolism of alcohol
Iron	Hemosiderosis and, in some people with genetic predisposition, hemochromatosis	Tendency to precipitate in inflamed tissue, such as liver, pancreas
MAO inhibitors	Hypertensive crisis	Inhibits metabolism of tyramine in Chianti wine and some other alcoholic beverages
Opiates	Serious CNS depression	Synergism
Phenylbutazone	Higher or prolonged blood alcohol levels	Competition for enzyme
Propranolol	Dysrhythmias, angina	Enhanced metabolism
Salicylates	Gastrointestinal bleeding	Additive
Sedatives and tranquilizers		
Barbiturates	Diminished sedative effect with chronic alcohol abuse	Enhanced microsomal enzyme activity
	Enhanced CNS depression with acute intoxication	Additive; reduced metabolism
Chloral hydrate (Noctec and others)	Prolonged hypnotic effect	Mutual potentiation
Diazepam (Valium)	Enhanced CNS depression	Additive
Meprobamate (Miltown and others)	Diminished sedative effect with chronic alcohol abuse	Enhanced microsomal enzyme activity
	Enhanced CNS depression with acute intoxication	Additive; reduced metabolism

age is slowly and steadily decreased until the drugs can be discontinued. This process usually takes 3 to 5 days.

A quiet, calm environment helps minimize reactions such as alcoholic hallucinosis and seizures. Excessive stimuli can precipitate these conditions in an agitated, hyperexcitable person. Even the profound hallucinations of DTs can be totally avoided by careful nursing intervention. Create a therapeutic environment by (1) minimizing intrusions; (2) moving slowly and deliberately rather than in a hurried, brisk way; (3) talking calmly to the person and telling her/him what you are about to do; (4) keeping lighting even and bright enough to minimize shadows but not so bright as to cause glare. It can be helpful to have a significant other sit quietly in the room to be available for answering questions, reorienting the person as necessary, and calling a nurse if problems arise.

STIMULANTS

Stimulants are classified into two types: (1) amphetamines (including methamphetamine) and (2) cocaine. Cocaine is not chemically related to amphetamine but has actions so similar that it is considered a stimulant, although it is legally classified as a narcotic. Another stimulant not often mentioned in drug abuse literature is caffeine. Caffeine use and overuse is socially sanctioned.

Amphetamines are available by prescription or illicitly. Table 79-1 lists brand names of often-prescribed amphetamines. Table 79-3 lists the slang terms used. Amphetamines may be taken orally, sniffed, or injected intravenously. Most abusers take them orally.

Cocaine is an alkaloid obtained from the leaves of the plant *Erythroxylon coca.* It has local anesthetic properties and at one time was used in eye surgery and dentistry. As the potential for cocaine abuse has become clear, synthetic compounds, including procaine (Novacain), have taken its place. Its clinical use is confined to otolaryngeal procedures, such as epistaxis control, because cocaine is a vasoconstrictor as well as a local anesthetic. Cocaine is obtained only through illicit channels for nonclinical use.

Coca leaves may be swallowed or chewed. Cocaine can also be made into a powder and is either mainlined or snorted (inhaled, sniffed) through a straw or a dollar bill. Another method of cocaine use is freebasing. Cocaine paste, a crude extract of the coca leaves, contains the alkaloid freebase. The hot gases from a pipe or burning cigarette vaporize freebase and allow its inhalation. An increasingly popular method of cocaine use is smoking concentrated cocaine, crack in cigarettes, or glass water pipes. Crack is more addictive, toxic, and insidious than other forms of cocaine.

Stimulants move rapidly from the bloodstream to the central nervous system. The major difference between the amphetamines and cocaine is the duration of action. The effects of cocaine are very transient because it is rapidly destroyed in the body. It must be injected every 15 minutes or snorted every hour to maintain the state of exhilaration.[27] Thus, a person may take very large amounts throughout a day. Amphetamine needs to be injected every 2 to 4 hours because it is excreted from the body fairly slowly. The duration of action is longer if it is taken orally.

Caffeine also is a powerful central nervous system stimulant. Besides coffee, caffeine is found in several other beverages, food, and medications. Be sure to assess for all sources of caffeine.[17]

Behavioral Changes. Stimulants increase the activity of the reticular activating system as well as other areas in the CNS. Behavioral output and responsiveness to sensory input increase. Stimulants are considered to be agents that improve mental and physical performance when a person is fatigued or bored. They also suppress appetite. As the potential for abuse has become known, limits have been placed on manufacture. Many physicians believe that the only legitimate use of amphetamines is to treat narcolepsy or hyperactive children.

Stimulant abusers are usually very alert, with extended wakefulness. They often appear euphoric, exhilarated, hyperactive, overenthusiastic, and extremely talkative. This overactivity is often followed by an unpleasant period of depression, lethargy, and fatigue known as crashing. Since depression can be counteracted by taking more stimulants, the abuse pattern becomes increasingly difficult to break. Heavy abusers may take stimulants every few hours, a process sometimes continued to the point of delirium, psychosis, or physical exhaustion. Abusers demonstrate tremulousness and a marked tendency toward agitation, apprehension, and irritability. They may become hostile and aggressive.

Sustained stimulant use may lead to a toxic psychosis manifested by delusions, hallucinations, and suspiciousness, symptoms found in paranoid schizophrenia. Withdrawal from stimulants leads to a marked reduction in symptoms.

High doses of cocaine can cause "cocaine bugs," that is, tactile hallucinations, the feeling that insects are crawling under one's skin. This sensation may be so distressing that the person may try anything to get them out, such as picking or tearing at the skin, sometimes causing severe skin problems including infection. The basis for this experience is probably a drug-induced stimulation of nerve endings in the skin, but the mechanism is not known.

Initial Physiologic Reactions. Excessive dry mouth, diaphoresis, dilated pupils, brisk reflexes, and tremors usually occur. Tachycardia and hypertension may present initially but may be absent in chronic tolerant users. Respiratory rates increase. Malnutrition with weight loss is common. Teeth may be worn down, and the lips and tongue ulcerated. Needle marks and tracks may be present (usually in the antecubital fossa). Because of cocaine's vasoconstrictor properties, people who have been snorting it may have a thinned, ulcerated, or even perforated nasal septum. High levels of cocaine may stop the heart because of its direct action on heart muscle.[27]

Tolerance. Tolerance for the effects of stimulants occurs rapidly. Tolerance occurs first for cardiovascular effects, tachycardia, and hypertension, and later for CNS effects, such as arousal and euphoria.

Dependence. The risk of psychological dependence with sustained stimulant use is high. Profound apathy and depression, lethargy and fatigue, prolonged sleep (up to 20 hours a day for several days), and overeating characterize the immediate withdrawal syndrome. Headache is a symptom of caffeine withdrawal.

Abrupt cessation of regular high doses of stimulants is not life threatening. Treatment is nonspecific and is based on careful assessment.

Nursing Management. Environmental safety measures (including frequent observation) are important for people experiencing hyperactivity or euphoria. Set realistic limits on their behavior. People on stimulants are agitated and easily provoked into aggressive, violent behavior. A calm approach is essential.

As stimulant effects subside, lethargy, fatigue, hunger, and depression develop. Extra food and a lot of sleep may be needed for a few days. Depression usually clears with time, a good diet, and rest. In severe cases, however, tricyclic antidepressants may be prescribed and suicide precautions may be indicated.

Amphetamine abusers may seek health care following a real or suspected overdose. Dizziness, tremor, agitation, hostility, panic, headache, flushed skin, chest pain with palpitations, diaphoresis, vomiting, and abdominal cramps are among the symptoms of a sublethal overdose. Without intervention, hyperpyrexia, convulsions, and cardiovascular collapse may precede death. Death is due in part to the consequences of a marked increase in body temperature. Therefore, physical exertion and an elevated environmental temperature may increase the hazards of stimulant use.

Chlorpromazine (Thorazine) may be ordered to combat the physiologic effects of amphetamines. Diazepam (Valium), given intravenously, decreases tachycardia and the chance of convulsions.

Haloperidol (Haldol) may be ordered to combat cocaine bugs or to treat extreme anxiety and agitation. Imipramine hydrochloride (Tofranil) or other tricyclic antidepressants may be given to counteract the symptoms of depression. Diazepam (Valium) is frequently given during detoxification treatment. Acute cocaine intoxication is often treated by beta-adrenergic blockers such as propranolol (Inderal) that counteract tachycardia and hypertension. Constant blood pressure monitoring is recommended.

Be aware that some prescription medications interact with cocaine, and that patients with cocaine in their systems are at risk for untoward effects. For example, general anesthetics can elevate blood pressure and pulse rate even further, as can anticholinergics such as atropine, and dicyclomine (Bentyl). Crack is potent enough to cancel out the antihypertensive effects of guanethidine (Ismelin).[20]

CANNABIS DERIVATIVES

Marijuana and hashish are cannabis derivatives. The psychoactive agent is concentrated in the resin of the *Cannabis sativa* plant. Hashish, or hash, is resin from the flowering tops and is very potent. Marijuana is much less potent, consisting mainly of leaves and fine stems. Hashish and marijuana are taken either orally or by smoke inhalation from cigarettes (joints) or from a pipe. The effect is more rapid with inhalation. Alternative names for marijuana include pot, tea, weed, grass, Acapulco gold, reefer, and many others, which vary with social group and geographic location.

Behavioral Changes and Initial Physiologic Reactions. The expected or usual effects of marijuana include

- A high feeling, including euphoria, elation, relaxation, well being, dreaminess, self-confidence, laughing, silliness;
- Feelings of detachment, clarity, cleverness, wittiness, disinhibition, depersonalization;
- Impaired logical thinking because of irrelevant thoughts, disturbed associations, altered reality testing, decreased concentration and attention span, altered sense of identity;
- Speech changes, such as rapid, impaired, flighty speech characterized by difficulty with sequential thoughts and poor short-term memory;
- Impaired ability to drive a car or perform other complex tasks, as a result of alterations in thinking and memory;
- Altered concepts of time, such as feeling that more time has passed than actually has;
- Suggestibility, rapidly changing emotions;
- Increased appetite and thirst;
- Quietness, reflectiveness, and sleepiness (later effects);
- Dizziness;
- Lightness, numbness and weakness of limbs, sensation of floating, paresthesias, changes in body sensations and body image;
- Restlessness, ataxia, tremor;
- Dry mouth, tachycardia, injected conjunctiva;
- With larger doses, sharpened or distorted perceptions of sound, color, and other sensations; and slow and confused thinking.

In very large doses, the effects may be similar to those of hallucinogens, such as confusion, excitement, and hallucinations. These may cause anxiety, panic, or paranoia and may even precipitate a psychotic episode.

The effects of cannabis derivatives usually last a few hours. With repeated use, less of the drug is needed to produce the same effects.[16] The agent persists in the body as an active metabolite as long as 8 days after use,[16] so less of the drug is needed to produce the same effects during this time. However, the psychoactive agent in marijuana and hashish, delta 6-3,4-tetrahydrocannabinol (THC), can be detected in the body for up to 6 weeks. Unlike alcohol, which is water soluble and leaves the body through urine, breath, and perspiration, THC is stored in the fatty tissues, in the brain, and in the organs of the reproductive system.[15] Physical dependence, exhibited by withdrawal symptoms, does not occur.

Like most toxic substances, this agent is metabolized in the liver. Death associated with the use of cannabis derivatives has not been reported.

Therapeutic uses for THC are being investigated. It has been found useful in decreasing the nausea and vomiting that is often associated with chemotherapy; in reducing dangerously high intraocular pressures in glaucoma; and in treating asthma, epilepsy, and hypertension.

Nursing Management. Professionally, a nurse is likely to encounter an intoxicated cannabis user in the context of an adverse reaction to the drug experience. Care related to presenting symptoms is appropriate. Most effects disappear in 5 to 8 hours as the drug wears off, but frank psychosis may occur and require treatment. Probably the most effective way to help people experiencing adverse reactions to marijuana is to talk with them in supportive, positive, and concerned ways. Reassure them that the reaction is temporary, they are not alone, and nothing terrible is likely to happen. To prevent future adverse reactions, abstinence from drugs is recommended.

As health educators, nurses also have the opportunity to fulfill a primary prevention role. The nurse should teach patients that marijuana use may have several untoward long-term health effects, as shown in the following list:

- It causes lung disease because of the following:
  - marijuana smoke has 50 per cent more tar than the smoke from regular cigarettes
  - marijuana tar contains 70 per cent more benzopyrene, a major cancer-causing chemical
  - marijuana smoke produces greater cellular changes in the lungs than does tobacco smoke
  - smoking two joints (marijuana cigarettes) can reduce lung capacity more than smoking one pack of tobacco cigarettes
  - marijuana may cause emphysema 20 times faster than tobacco does.
- It affects the person's fertility rate because of accumulation in the ovaries in females and lowering of testosterone levels in males.
- It causes diffuse brain impairment for up to 2 months after the last time the drug is used by persons who smoke marijuana twice a week or more often.
- It affects fetal development and cause fetal abnormalities such as central nervous system disturbances, low birth weight, decreased length, and smaller head circumference.
- It causes a relapse or a worsening of symptoms in persons with a history of schizophrenia or mood disorders.[15]

SURGERY AND SUBSTANCE ABUSE

Substance abuse has a variety of adverse effects on clients requiring surgery. Unfortunately, people who abuse drugs and addicted people are at a high risk for both emergency and nonemergency conditions that necessitate surgery. Traumatic injuries, which often require surgery, are frequent. About one third of all head injuries seen in emergency rooms are alcohol related.

It is a challenge to care for clients who abuse drugs and undergo surgery. Frequent assessment is required to differentiate between disorders caused by chemical substances and those caused by neurosurgical lesions. In addition to the problems caused by injuries or illnesses, addicted clients needing surgery may have

- Poor general health,
- Impaired liver function (secondary to chronic alcoholism, malnutrition, or hepatitis from use of unsterile needles),
- Inaccessible veins (this may be life threatening),
- Problems related to the effects of recent drug ingestion,
- Withdrawal symptoms, and
- Agitation, inability to cooperate.

When emergency surgery is required, there is little time to obtain a thorough drug use history, so health professionals must be alert to signs of chemical substance–associated problems.

Because clients addicted to CNS depressants are cross-tolerant to pharmacologically related anesthetic agents, larger amounts of anesthetics are needed to achieve adequate sedation. On the other hand, if the client has liver dysfunction, anesthetic agents are not metabolized efficiently. The resulting accumulation of substances in the bloodstream may alter and prolong sedation. Careful monitoring during and after surgery ensures safety.

During surgery, clients addicted to substances are prone to cardiac and respiratory depression, depleted catecholamines, and hemorrhage. Careful postoperative assessment is essential because these people are at high risk of complications. Because respiratory complications are likely, help clients with frequent turning, coughing, and deep breathing. Intermittent positive-pressure breathing (IPPB) may be helpful. Cardiac problems, such as congestive heart failure and atrial fibrillation, are more common in alcoholic clients. Clients with cirrhosis may have concomitant urinary retention, so it may be necessary to run intravenous fluids at a slower-than-normal rate. Also, postoperative risks of bleeding and infection are increased in substance-dependent people.

A problem peculiar to substance-dependent people is postoperative withdrawal from the substance of abuse. Onset of withdrawal from CNS-depressant substances (e.g., alcohol) may be delayed for up to 5 days postoperatively because of cross-tolerance with anesthetics and pain medication. Cross-tolerance also affects the amount of pain medication required. Dosages may need to be increased. It is important to assess requests for pain medication, give increased doses if indicated, and to withdraw the drugs gradually but steadily according to a plan of care for the individual person.

Summary

Clients who abuse alcohol and other drugs often need nursing and medical intervention. At one time, attention often focused exclusively on immediate physical problems, such as gastritis, cirrhosis, and nerve damage. Although the root of these problems was excessive use of alcohol and/or other drugs, this was not discussed with the client. There are at least three reasons for this: (1) ignorance about how to discuss these problems, (2) lack of knowledge about the effects of drugs, and (3) belief that drug dependence results from moral weakness and, therefore cannot be treated. When problems with drugs are not recognized and treated, many clients continue to abuse them and consequently develop worsening problems requiring professional intervention. It is easy to become frustrated in such situations and to avoid these clients when they need help, because in their company we feel helpless and ineffective. Chances for early intervention, when problems are less severe, are thus missed.

Fortunately, this sequence of events is being interrupted. The social view of problems with alcohol and other drugs is changing. Health professionals are beginning to see drug-dependent clients in a new light.

Bibliography

1. Abrams, R., & Alexopoulous G. (1987). Substance abuse in the elderly: Alcohol and prescription drugs. *Hospital and Community Psychiatry, 38,* 1285-1287.
2. American Nurses' Association, Drug and Alcohol Nursing Association, & National Nurses Society on Addictions. (1987). *The care of clients with addictions: Dimensions of nursing practice.* Kansas City, MO: American Nurses' Association.
3. American Nurses' Association, & National Nurses Society on Addictions. (1988). *Standards of addictions nursing practice with selected diagnoses and criteria.* Kansas City, MO: American Nurses' Association.
4. Andreason N. C. (1984). *The broken brain: The biological revolution in psychiatry.* New York: Harper & Row.
5. Baasel, P. (1986). Passing down the heritage of addictive family dynamics. *Focus on Family, 9*(6), 24-25, 36, 39.
6. Bittle, S., et al. (1986). Substance abuse. In C. R. Kneisl, & S. W. Ames (Eds.), *Adult health nursing: A biopsychosocial approach.* Redwood City, CA: Addison-Wesley.
7. Block, A. J., & Taasan, V. C. (1981). Alcohol before bedtime upsets respiratory patterns. *American Family Physician, 24,* 210.
8. Blum, K. (1983). Alcohol and central nervous system peptides. *Substance and Alcohol Actions/Misuse, 4,* 84.
9. Emmelkamp, P., & Heeres H. (1989). Drug addiction and parental rearing style. *Brown University Digest of Addiction Theory and Application, 8*(1), 7.
10. Estes, N. J., & Heinemann, M. E. (1986). *Alcoholism: Development, consequences and interventions.* St. Louis: C. V. Mosby.
11. Fisk, N. B. (1986). Alcoholism: Ineffective family coping. *American Journal of Nursing, 86*(5), 586-587.
12. Gilbert, J. A. L., & Schaeffer, O. (1977). Metabolism of ethanol in different racial groups. *Canadian Medical Association Journal, 116*(5), 476.
13. Gold, M. (1984). *800-Cocaine.* New York: Bantam Books.
14. Goodwin, D. W. (1983). Familial alcoholism: A separate entity? *Substance and Alcohol Actions/Misuse, 4,* 129.
15. Hutchinson, S. (1992). The nursing process with psychoactive substance use disorder. In H. S. Wilson, & C. R. Kneisl (Eds.), *Psychiatric nursing* (4th ed.). Redwood City, CA: Addison-Wesley.
16. Jaffe J., et al. (1980). *Addictions: Issues & answers.* New York: Harper & Row.
17. Kneisl, C. R. (1992). Troubled sleep for troubled people. In H. S. Wilson, & C. R. Kneisl (Eds.), *Psychiatric nursing* (4th ed., pp. 647-648). Redwood City, CA: Addison-Wesley.
18. Kneisl, C. R., & Pheifer, W. G. (1992). HIV/AIDS: A mental health challenge. In H. S. Wilson, & C. R. Kneisl (Eds.). *Psychiatric nursing* (4th ed., pp. 585-611). Redwood City, CA: Addison-Wesley.
19. Leland, J. (1976). *Firewater myths.* New Brunswick, NJ: Rutgers Center of Alcohol Studies.
20. Levy, G., and Hickey, J. V. (1991). Fighting the battle against drugs. *R. N., 54* (4), 44-47.
21. Morris M., & Trigoboff, E. (1992). Codependence. In H. S. Wilson and C. R. Kneisl, *Psychiatric nursing* (4th ed.) pp. 577-584). Redwood City, CA: Addison-Wesley.
22. Naegle, M. A. (1988). Theoretical perspectives on the etiology of substance abuse. *Holistic Nursing Practice, 2*(4), 1-13.
23. National Institute on Alcohol Abuse and Alcoholism. (1987). *Sixth special report to Congress on alcohol and health.* (DHHS Pub. No ADM 87-1519). Washington, DC: U. S. Government Printing Office.
24. National Nurses Society on Addictions. (1989). *Nursing care planning with the addicted client* (Vol. 1). Skokie, IL: Midwest Education Association, Inc.
25. Nehemkis, A., et al. (Eds.) (1977). *Drug abuse instrument handbook.* Rockville, MD: National Institute of Drug Abuse.
26. Ogawa, C. (1983). Asian family and substance abuse. Rice Paper, *7*(1), 2-11.
27. Ray, O. S. (1978). *Drugs, society and human behavior.* St. Louis: C. V. Mosby.
28. Robbins, C. E. (1987). A monitored treatment program for impaired health care professionals. *Journal of Nursing Administration, 17*(2), 17-21.
29. Schliefer, S. J., et al. (1990). HIV seropositivity in inner-city alcoholics. *Hospital and Community Psychiatry, 41*(23), 248-249.
30. Schuckit, M. (1985). Genetics and the risk for alcoholism. *Journal of the American Medical Association, 254,* 2614-2617.
31. Selzer, M. L., et al. (1975). A self-administered Short Michigan Alcoholism Screening Test. *Journal of Studies on Alcohol, 36,* 117.
32. Siegel, R. K. (1989). *Intoxication: Life in pursuit of artificial paradise.* New York: E. P. Dutton.
33. Stanton, M., & Todd, T. *Family therapy of drug abuse and addiction.* New York: Guilford Press.
34. Washton, A. (1989). *Cocaine addiction.* New York: Norton.
35. *What are the signs of alcoholism?* New York: National Council on Alcoholism.
36. Wing, D. M., & Greer, G. (1990). Determining alcoholism treatment outcomes: A cost-effectiveness perspective. *Nursing Economics, 8*(4), 248-255.

Chapter 80

Nursing Care of Clients During Medical-Surgical Emergencies

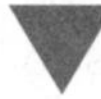

MEDICAL-SURGICAL EMERGENCIES

DEFINITION

An emergency is any sudden illness or injury that is perceived by the client or significant other as requiring immediate intervention. The emergency continues until the condition is stable or no longer threatens the client's integrity or well being.

Emergency situations can occur anywhere, such as the community, emergency department, and even nursing units. Therefore, it is important for all nurses to have the basic knowledge and skills needed for rapid assessment, intervention, and safe management of emergencies. Quick and competent emergency care is the key to rapid stability, prevention of complications, and early recovery. The focus of this chapter is to identify general principles, priorities, and management of common emergencies encountered by adult clients.

Section on respiratory injuries written by Sherrill Cronin RN, MSN.

OVERVIEW OF EMERGENCY CARE

Improvements in prehospital care, in emergency medical systems, and in transport to regional trauma systems together with advances in medical and nursing management of clients in emergency situations have led to increased survival.[9, 34, 44]

Emergency Medical Services System

Emergency care is a community responsibility. In 1966, a federal act required each county to form an emergency committee to address the delivery and organization of emergency care. The purpose of emergency medical services (EMS) systems is to coordinate the use of personnel, equipment, and facilities in the delivery of emergency care.

Emergency Care Facilities

The Medicare (1965) and Medicaid (1966) Acts enabled more Americans to have access to health care. More recently, homelessness, limited resources, government regulations, budget cuts, inadequate or no health insurance coverage, and public perceptions of emergency care have contributed to overcrowding and increased use of emergency departments.[12, 28] Some responses to the need for more emergency care facilities are an increase in Urgent Care Centers, walk-in clinics, and extended clinic hours. These all provide alternatives for clients in need of nonurgent emergency care.

For severely injured clients, the incorporation and use of regionalized trauma systems has increased survival. Other specialized facilities provide care for clients with spinal cord injuries or burn injuries. However, not all states have incorporated comprehensive trauma systems.[44]

To address the issue of trauma care, Congress passed an act in 1990 designed to provide federal funds and incentives to states for the development and coordination of regionalized and comprehensive trauma systems. Although funds have not yet been appropriated, 10 per cent of all appropriations must be demonstrated for rural areas. This may help address the special needs for emergency care in rural America.

ETHICAL AND LEGAL CONSIDERATIONS

Consent to Treatment

Informed consent to treatment means that clients are knowledgeable of all treatments and procedures and agree to these before implementation. The information must be presented in a language in which the client is fluent and at an appropriate level so the client understands the implications of any treatments. By being informed, clients also have the right to refuse any treatments or procedures before they are implemented.

However, informed consent is valid only if the client is of "adult years and sound mind." Not all adult clients are capable of giving informed consent. Clients with emergencies may be hypoxic, be intoxicated, or have an altered level of consciousness.

EMERGENCY DOCTRINE

When a client is unable to give consent or is unconscious, emergency treatment can be provided under the emergency doctrine. This doctrine implies that the client would have consented to treatment if able, because the alternative would have been death or disability (see Ethical Issues in Nursing). The emergency doctrine removes the need for obtaining informed consent before emergency treatment and care are initiated.

Right to Privacy and Confidentiality

All clients have a right to privacy, and clients with emergencies are no different. This right includes the need for consent to use names and photographs of the client; not allowing unauthorized persons into the client's hospital area; and not disclosing private facts to the public or falsely representing the client to the public. Information about the client's condition, treatments, and outcomes are to be respected and handled with discretion. Any communication about the client's conditions, treatments, and documentation are confidential and disclosed only with the client's permission.

Mandatory Reporting

Mandatory reporting laws require hospitals, nurses, and physicians to notify the appropriate local, state, or federal agency when certain conditions or incidents occur. These include child, spouse, or elder abuse; motor vehicle crashes; injuries resulting from violence; attempted suicides; animal bites; overdoses; and poisonings. Certain communicable disorders, such as meningitis, sexually transmitted diseases, and food poisonings, are also reportable to the state health department. When injuries are suspected or identified, the nurse must notify the physician in charge of the care and other individuals identified by hospital policy. The appropriate agency must be notified and a report filed.

Physical Evidence and Chain of Custody

Meticulous documentation and handling of evidence are of particular concern in situations in which injury resulted from a violent crime, such as a shooting or sexual assault. All evidence discovered during the examination is recorded. Documentation of samples includes the location from which the sample was obtained and when and to whom it was delivered.

Evidence should be maintained in its original condition. Clothing is stored in a paper bag instead of plastic to prevent decomposition. If clothing needs to be cut

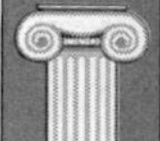

ETHICAL ISSUES IN NURSING

Are Emergency Personnel Obliged to Honor Self-Directives?

During emergency situations, the client and the significant others parallel the health care team's treatment goal, that is, survival. Once this goal is achieved, the true reality of each situation is often painful and tentative at best. How should a client be medically treated if his or her condition is reduced to a persistent vegetative state? Can family members who feel their loved one would not want to continue living in such a physical state decide to stop treatment on that client?

In the case of Nancy Cruzan of Missouri, the results of her tragic accident spawned legislation regarding a client's right to direct care for certain treatments or situations. It is universally accepted that emergency care workers have a duty to assist those in need in whatever capacity is appropriate for stabilizing the condition. It is at this point that self-directives (in emergency situations) would help decide ongoing treatment options.

Self-directives may be in the form of a living will or a durable power of attorney for health care, or they may be forms of verbal or written guidelines that state the health care treatment wishes of the client initiating them. A verbal self-directive would require that the client speak about such directives to the physician (perhaps on admission to a hospital unit) and that such a conversation be noted in the client's medical record. Directives should be written when a client is in a state of good health in order not to be influenced by uncontrolled variables.

What about emergency cases for which such information may not be available? Even if a client comes through an emergency center door with an advanced directive pinned to the shirt, do the emergency personnel have an obligation to honor such a document? Although the federal guidelines do not yet address such an issue, it seems just that all emergency clients be treated in the same fashion, that is, stabilization of their condition. Until a client is stabilized, there is no way to even begin to know the possible health care outcomes. Once a more definitive diagnosis can be made of the emergency client, then the self-directives could be used to assist in care decisions.

When clients seek help from emergency personnel, there is an assumed obligation by the personnel to assist them. All personnel who work in such settings need to know their institution's and state's policies on advanced directives. Self-directives attempt to help clients control certain aspects of their lives when illness strikes. Emergency situations thrust many uncontrolled variables into the lives of those involved and thus must be dealt with in a different light.

---

off the client, special attention is taken not to destroy evidence inadvertently.

BULLETS

Bullets removed from a client's body or recovered from clothing are handled with great care. When a bullet is removed, the physician usually makes a mark on the bottom of the bullet. This identifying mark may be referred to later during an investigation or trial. The bullet is then placed in a sealed bag, labeled, and given to proper authorities. The bag is sealed so that removal of the seal will be obvious. If a bullet is kept in the emergency department for any reason, it is kept in a locked, secure place. All persons having access to the bullet must sign for it; thus, a chain of custody is maintained. This information is included on the medical record.

SPECIMENS

Specimens obtained for legal purposes, as opposed to clinical purposes, include blood samples for determination of blood alcohol levels and items obtained during the examination of an alleged sexual assault victim. When a blood alcohol determination is desired by either the client or legal authorities, the client's written permission must be obtained before the specimen is drawn. No client may be forced into having a blood sample drawn. In many instances, police officers have a kit with the necessary equipment for drawing the specimen. Isopropyl alcohol or any antiseptic solution containing alcohol must not be used as a skin preparation before a blood alcohol specimen is drawn. These agents may falsely elevate the blood alcohol level and render the test invalid. The nurse must know the laws within the state that identify who may draw blood for alcohol level determinations.

Once the specimen is drawn, it is handed to a police officer, who signs that the specimen has been received. The tube is sealed with an identifying mark placed on the seal. The chain of custody is similar to that for bullets. Documentation of the procedure on the client's clinical record, along with the nurse's signature and the name and badge number of the officer, is important.

Transfer Laws[39]

In 1986, Congress passed the Consolidated Omnibus Budget Reconciliation Act (COBRA) in response to inappropriate patient transfers and denial of care. Provisions of the COBRA legislation require treatment for all clients with emergency conditions and pregnant women with active contractions, regardless of ability to pay. This includes an appropriate medical screening examination, necessary stabilizing treatments, and appropriate transfer to another facility with consent, if indicated. It is important for emergency nurses to be aware of the hospital guidelines and transfer protocols. Nurses can be active patient advocates and ensure that clients receive necessary emergency treatments. Failure to comply with COBRA legislation may result in substantial fines and penalties.

EMERGENCY NURSING CARE

The Emergency Nurses Association defines emergency nursing care as the "assessment, diagnosis and treatment of perceived, actual or potential, sudden or urgent, physical or psychosocial problems that are primarily episodic or acute. These may require minimal care or life-support measures, client and significant other education, appropriate referral and knowledge of legal limitations."[10]

Emergency nursing requires a broad knowledge base to provide safe and competent care to clients with a variety of conditions. This requires rapid and sound assessment skills, physiologic responses, psychosocial behaviors, crisis intervention, communication techniques, triage (see later), trauma care, and the ability to provide care in uncontrolled or unpredictable environments.

Because less than 20 per cent of the clients seeking emergency care have life-threatening problems, teaching is a major nursing role. Many emergency departments provide written instructions as well as verbal teaching.

For many, the emergency department may be the usual source of health care, and emergency nurses may be the only contact the client has with the health care system. Nurses must be aware of clients who frequently return to the emergency department. These clients may have special health needs, have exacerbations of chronic conditions, be victims of abuse, have no primary health care provider, or have little or no health insurance. Research has shown that clients use emergency departments because they perceive their symptoms as serious, and emergency departments are viewed as faster and more convenient than clinics.[12] Until permanent solutions to overcrowding are found, it is important that health care professionals be nonjudgemental and no client be refused care.

Initial Assessment

On first being confronted with a seriously ill or injured client, gain as much information as quickly as possible. The initial impression is important for early identification and intervention of life-threatening signs and symptoms (Box 80-1). Historical information provides clues to the urgency of the situation and treatment priorities. Client management consists of a brief history and primary assessment, resuscitation of vital functions, a thorough secondary assessment, and definitive care.

HISTORY

The history provides clues to the priority assessments and interventions. A history should include information about when and where the emergency occurred, what has been done, and whether the client has any known health problems such as hypertension or diabetes. One way to obtain this information quickly is through the mnemonic AMPLE.

- A Allergies
- M Medications currently prescribed or using
- P Past medical and surgical history
- L Last meal
- E Events preceding the emergency and any care rendered.

Box 80-1. Assessment Findings Implying a High Priority for Care

- Significant alteration in vital signs (e.g., hypo- or hypertension, hypo- or hyperthermia, cardiac dysrhythmias, respiratory distress)
- Altered level of consciousness
- Chest pain, especially in clients over age 35 years
- Severe pain
- Bleeding not controlled by direct pressure
- Conditions that will worsen from delay in treatment (e.g., chemical burns, drug or toxic substance ingestion, allergic reaction, impaled objects)
- Sudden vision loss
- Dangerous, aberrant, or disruptive behavior
- Psychologically devastating conditions (e.g., sexual assault, death or near-death of a loved one)
- Elderly or very young client
- Symptom that is vague but causes the triage officer (emergency assessor) concern

Establishing Priorities

The goal of emergency care is prompt, effective resuscitation and stabilization of critically ill or injured clients. The process of organizing client care, controlling traffic, and providing prompt and timely emergency care is called triage.

TRIAGE

Triage ensures that clients requiring immediate attention for life-threatening emergencies receive it. Although triage categories may vary, three common categories are emergent, urgent, and nonurgent (Table 80-1). Because performance of a complete assessment is difficult initially, it is wise to err on the side of assigning a higher triage priority than a lower one. Clients may have other injuries not initially assessed. It is important to reassess those waiting for care and change priorities as needed.

Research supports the use of experienced emergency nurses in providing safe, efficient, and cost-effective triage.[46] An effective triage nurse possesses three critical qualities: expert assessment skills, nonjudgmental communication and interviewing techniques, and organizational skills to regulate control of traffic flow into the treatment areas.[40]

Many clients enter the emergency department in a state of crisis. Therefore, the triage nurse must be knowledgeable about common responses to crises and able to react quickly and in a calm manner. The ability of the triage nurse to assess, intervene, and communicate effectively helps establish rapport and trust with the client and significant others (also see Box 80-2).

TABLE 80-1. Triage Categories

Category	Definition	Emergency Examples
Emergent	Life-threatening emergency Usually involves the ABCs The client may die without immediate intervention	Airway obstruction, cardiac arrest, chest pain with dyspnea or cyanosis, shock, coma, open chest wounds, sudden vision loss, and psychologically devastating conditions
Urgent	Emergencies that require intervention within a few hours	Intraperitoneal bleeding, cerebrovascular accident, severe pain, sudden paralysis, persistent nausea, vomiting, or diarrhea
Nonurgent	Not life-threatening Interventions may be delayed beyond a few hours	Soft tissue injuries, surface trauma, extremity fractures without circulatory compromise

Documentation

Documentation of assessments, interventions, and client responses is essential. Because time is often limited, flow sheets are frequently used. These have key assessment and intervention areas preprinted on the form. During life-threatening situations, critical data may be recorded on a white board mounted on the treatment wall so that all members of the team are able to visualize important data rapidly. Information typically written on the white board includes initial and subsequent vital signs, coma score, trauma score, laboratory and other diagnostic studies ordered/completed, team members, intravenous fluids/blood administered, urine output, and whether significant others were notified or present. It is desirable for one person to be responsible for documentation.

Priority Nursing Interventions

AIRWAY PATENCY

Common airway obstructions are the tongue and foreign bodies such as food ("a cafe coronary"), teeth, bone fragments, or blood clots. In a conscious client, assist the client to remove the obstruction by initiating an abdominal thrust (Figs. 80-1 and 80-2).

If the airway is open, but the client is not breathing, begin rescue breathing (see cardiopulmonary resuscitation, Chap. 42). Watch for the rise and fall of the chest during these breaths. If the chest rises and falls, the airway is open. Various artificial airways are used when the airway is not patent or is inadequate (see Chap. 37).

A nasopharyngeal airway can be inserted if the client is semi-conscious; an oropharyngeal airway is used if the client is unconscious and without a gag reflex. Additional airway adjuncts for clients over 15 years of age include an esophageal obturator airway (EOA) (Fig. 80-3) or an esophageal gastric tube airway

Box 80-2. Telephone Triage

Telephone triage occurs when a client calls the emergency department for help with a crisis, in an emergency situation, or for health care advice. Despite the advent of crisis lines and emergency 911 numbers, many callers contact the emergency department first. This places nurses who perform telephone triage in a "first responder" position. Unfortunately, nurses in many institutions "perform telephone triage without proper documentation, training, standards, protocols, or adequate staff." Not all institutions incorporate telephone triage. Telephone triage has eight important points.

- With all crisis levels, when possible, stay on the line with the caller while contacting 911. In a model telephone triage system, a crisis team interface, standard documentation forms, conference call capabilities, direct lines, and call tracing capabilities would be included.
- Beware of caller noncompliance. The nurse could use one of two strategies, depending on the severity of the call: dial 911 directly, or make a verbal contract with the caller to an agreed-on course of action.
- Develop crisis intervention "crash cards." These would have developed action protocols or treatments modeled after medical dispatcher instructions.
- Develop protocols for a suicide in progress or suicidal threats.
- In a crisis, expect impaired judgement. The nurse needs to remain calm and coach the caller in first aid or actions that the caller can perform, such as opening the door for arriving paramedics.
- Believe when the caller says it is an emergency.
- Get complete information. Preprinted checklists can help accomplish the baseline data collection.
- Always err on the side of caution.

From Wheeler, S. Q. (1989). ED telephone triage: Lessons learned from unusual calls. *Journal of Emergency Nursing, 15*(6), 401-407.

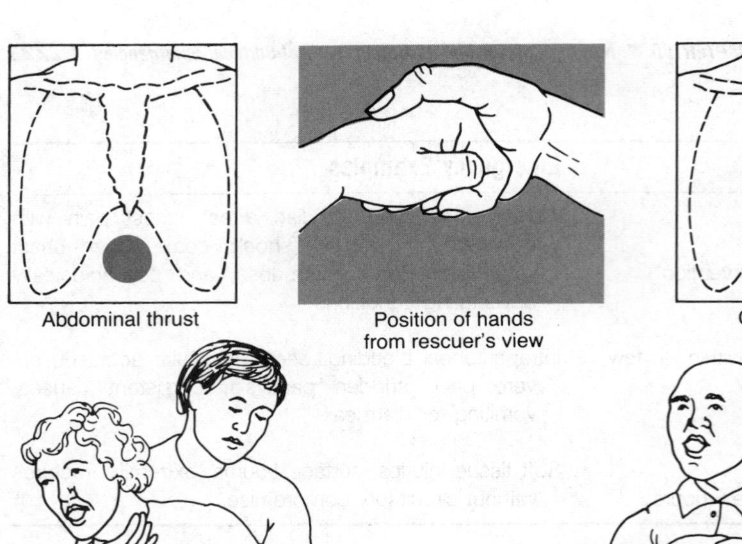

▲ ***Figure 80–1***

Heimlich maneuver for removing a foreign body blocking the upper airway. Vigorously apply upward chest or abdominal thrusts. This creates a force that causes quick changes in air pressure, which produces a rush of air to expel the foreign body. The abdominal thrust is the original Heimlich maneuver. The chest thrust is an adaptation that is useful for obese or pregnant clients. The black dot indicates correct placement of the rescuer's hands. Figure 80–2 illustrates thrust techniques for unconscious clients.

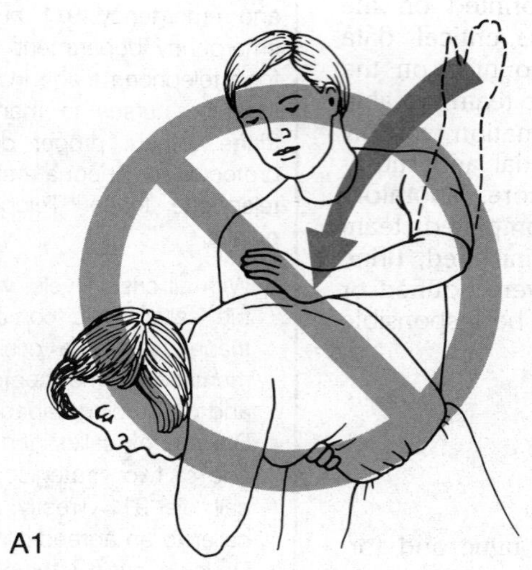

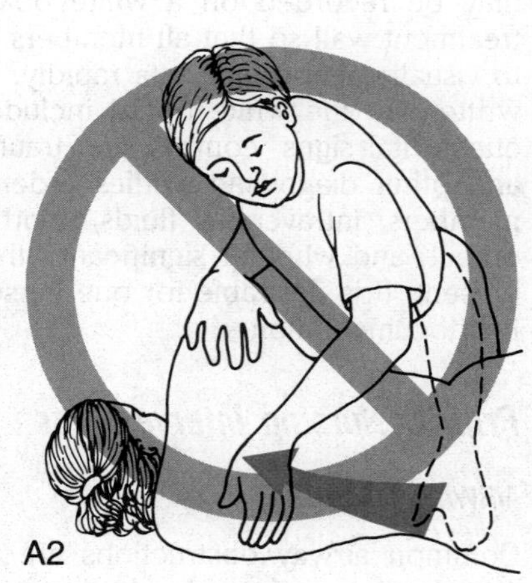

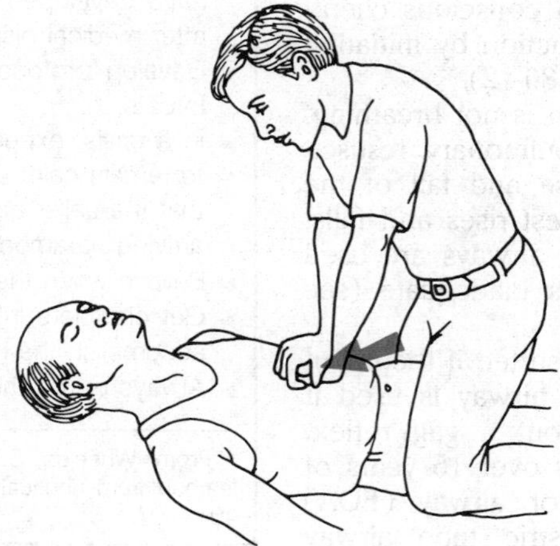

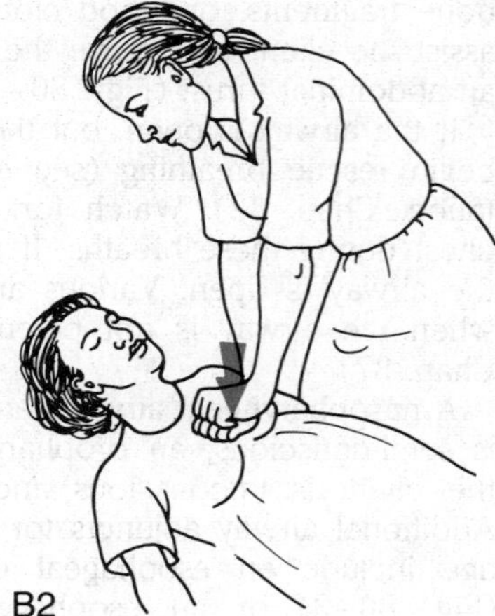

▲ ***Figure 80–2***

Removing a foreign body from the upper airway. *A,* Back blows. **Back blows are no longer recommended intervention for choking clients.** *B,* Thrust techniques for an unconscious client. *B1,* Abdominal thrust for an unconscious client. In the position shown, press into the abdomen with four quick inward and upward thrusts. *B2,* Chest thrust for an unconscious client. In the position shown, apply four quick downward thrusts to compress the chest cavity. (See also Fig. 80–1.)

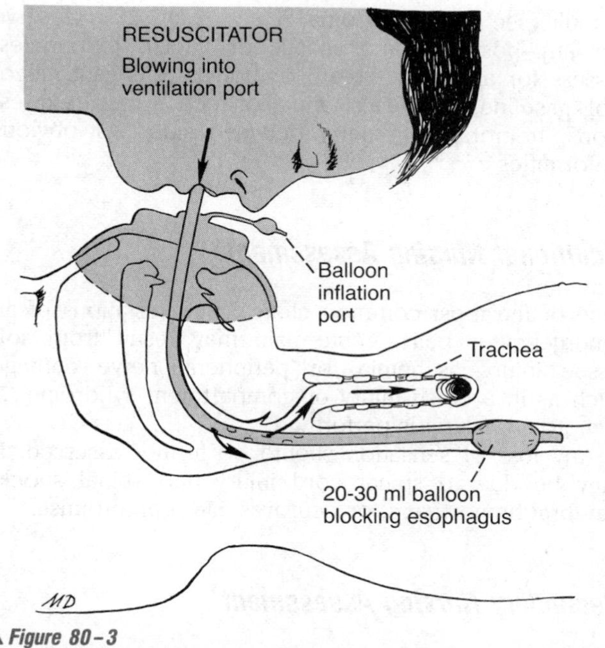

▲ **Figure 80-3**

Esophageal obturator airway, a ventilatory device used for resuscitation in emergencies. Face mask anchors the airway and seals off mouth and nose. Lungs are ventilated via openings in flexible tube at level of pharynx. Possible aspiration of gastric contents is minimized by inflated balloon at tube's distal end. This blocks esophagus.

(EGTA), which is a modification of the EOA that has a port for a nasogastric tube. These two airways are used as temporary measures until endotracheal intubation or tracheotomy can be performed. The use of esophageal airways is controversial and carries potential complications of inadvertent tracheal intubation with subsequent asphyxia, esophageal laceration, and vomiting and aspiration of gastric contents on removal.

In the hospital setting, endotracheal intubation or tracheostomy tubes are preferred. Therefore, the EOA and EGTA are more likely to be removed in an emergency department.[38] Before removal, an endotracheal tube must be successfully inserted to protect the airway. Be sure to have suction equipment ready, because the client is likely to vomit and may aspirate on removal of the EOA or EGTA.

Two cricothyroidotomy procedures are used when endotracheal intubation is impossible or an obstruction is present (Fig. 80-4). Both measures are temporary until tracheal intubation or a tracheotomy can be performed. A cricothyrotomy (coniotomy) involves a transverse incision through the cricothyroid membrane located below the thyroid prominence of the neck. A small (#6) tracheostomy tube or other plastic tube is inserted through the opening into the trachea. The client is ventilated through the tube. The percutaneous transtracheal ventilation (needle cricothyroidotomy) involves inserting a 14-gauge intravenous catheter with a needle into the trachea through the cricothyroid membrane. Once the catheter is inside the trachea, the needle is removed, and the client is ventilated through the catheter. An ambu bag can be used by placing the adaptor from a 3.0 endotracheal tube between the catheter and ambu bag.

SUPPLEMENTAL OXYGEN

Severe injuries and respiratory distress indicate a need for 100 per cent oxygen for treatment of any resultant hypoxemia. Supplemental oxygen is initiated at 6 to 10 L/min in situations of severe injury or stress such as myocardial infarction, smoke inhalation, or shock. Supplemental oxygen is provided if the client has chest pain, signs and symptoms of poor cardiac output (decreased pulse and blood pressure), signs and symptoms of hypoxemia (confusion, anxiety, or restlessness), profuse bleeding, or nausea. See Chapter 37 for various supplemental oxygen delivery systems.

SPINAL PRECAUTIONS AND IMMOBILIZATION

In a client with a decreased level of consciousness, and if history of or potential for traumatic injury is suspected, the spinal column is immobilized to prevent neurologic injury. The ideal precaution for spinal immobilization includes a cervical collar, two rolled towels or intravenous bags, or a head immobilizer placed on each side of the head and taped securely across the forehead onto a long backboard[11] (Fig. 80-5).

CARDIOPULMONARY RESUSCITATION

Begin CPR (see Chap. 42) if the client is not breathing and has no pulse. CPR aids in perfusing the client's

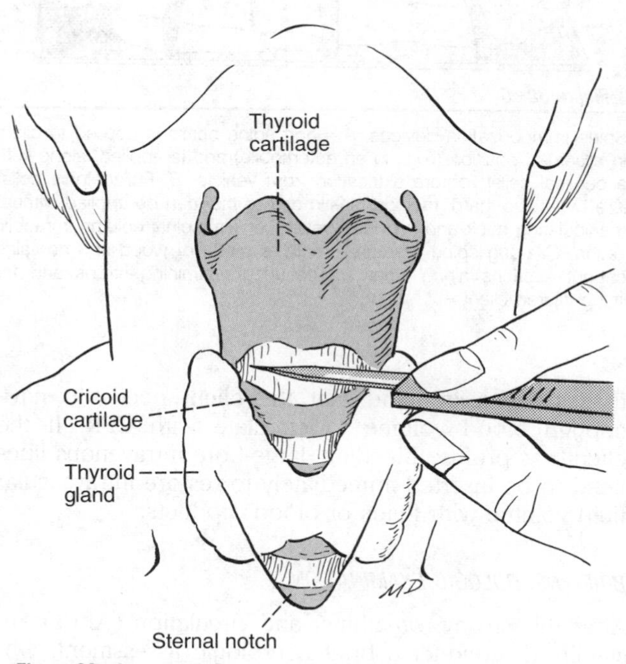

▲ **Figure 80-4**

Cricothyroidotomy creates a temporary airway by making an opening into the trachea. The opening is maintained with a small plastic tube.

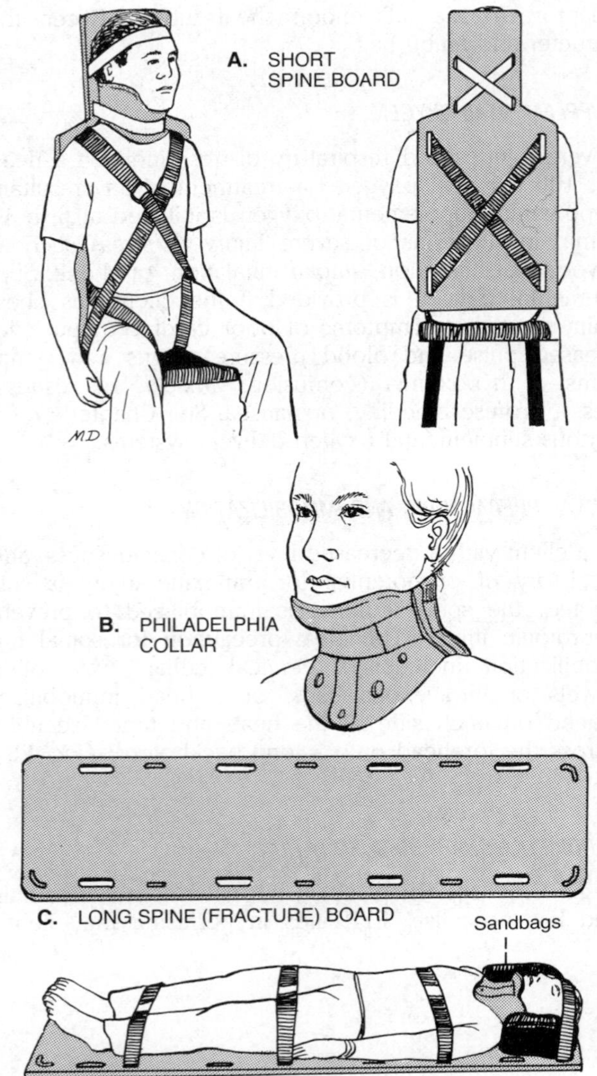

▲ *Figure 80–5*

Spine immobilization devices. *A*, Short spine board is applied to client in a seated position (e.g., in an automobile) and is applied, along with a cervical collar, before extrication from vehicle. *B*, Philadelphia collar is a two-piece, hard, molded plastic device that can be applied without manipulating neck and provides better cervical spinal column immobilization. *C*, Long spine (fracture) board is made of wood and contains cut-out sections along sides for securing restraining straps and for lifting injured client.

tissues. Keep in mind that the client needs to have enough blood volume to circulate with CPR. If the client has profuse bleeding, large-bore intravenous lines need to be inserted immediately to restore intravascular fluid volume with fluids or blood products.

BRIEF NEUROLOGIC EXAMINATION

After the *a*irway, *b*reathing, and *c*irculation (ABCs) are stabilized, conduct a brief neurologic assessment. Observe the client's general appearance, mental status, and orientation. Make note of any eye opening, verbal, and motor responses to verbal, tactile, and noxious stimuli (see Glasgow Coma Scale, Chap. 29). Observe for any posturing and spastic or flaccid extremities. Assess for abnormal breath or body odors (e.g., alcohol, gasoline, chemicals, urine, or feces), facial expressions, tremors, asymmetry between sides, or obvious deformities.[6, 11, 38]

Additional Nursing Assessments

One of the most common clinical manifestations of an emergency is pain. Acute pain may result from soft tissue injury, ischemia, or peripheral nerve damage such as in a crush injury or compartment syndrome. A symptom analysis is performed.

Any loss of sensation should be further assessed. It may be due to spinal cord injury and spinal shock, cerebral hemorrhage, or neurovascular compromise.

Secondary Nursing Assessment

The secondary assessment involves a complete head-to-toe assessment guided by the client's chief complaint.

Objective physical assessments are performed (Fig. 80–6), concentrating on areas relating to the client's chief complaint. Keep in mind that not all of the assessment procedures are performed on every client with an emergency, but these are a guideline for establishing priorities. For instance, in a client with a migraine headache, an abdominal assessment is inappropriate. However, if the client complains of vague shoulder pain, an abdominal assessment is appropriate for ruling out referred pain such as with gallbladder disease.

DISCHARGE TEACHING

Because of the short time of the interaction, teaching conducted by emergency nurses must be specific to the client's most pressing problems. Emphasis is placed on return demonstration or verbal understanding. Information includes recognizing the most likely or significant complication, how and when to obtain follow-up care, and what to do if complications occur. A discharge instruction sheet reinforcing this information is given to the client or significant other at discharge, and teaching is documented on the emergency record.

Psychosocial Needs in Emergencies

The psychosocial needs of clients and significant others vary widely during an emergency. A number of factors influence reactions to emergencies. Some of these factors include little or no time to prepare; little experience with the type of stressor; little or no guidance available for what is expected of them; loss of control and feelings of helplessness; the amount of time spent in crisis and its on-again, off-again nature; the disruption to client and family roles, responsibilities, and rou-

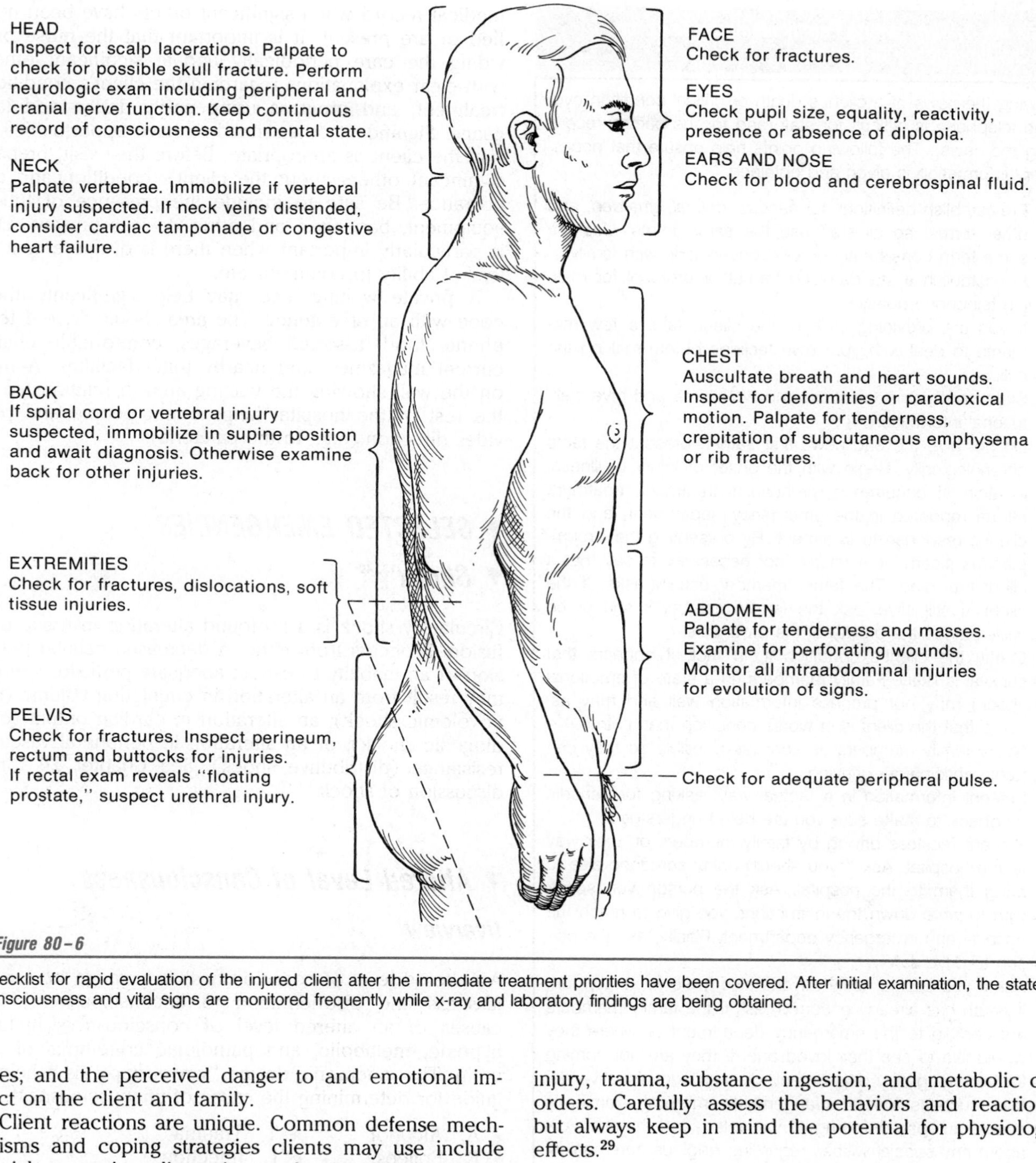

HEAD
Inspect for scalp lacerations. Palpate to check for possible skull fracture. Perform neurologic exam including peripheral and cranial nerve function. Keep continuous record of consciousness and mental state.
NECK
Palpate vertebrae. Immobilize if vertebral injury suspected. If neck veins distended, consider cardiac tamponade or congestive heart failure.
BACK
If spinal cord or vertebral injury suspected, immobilize in supine position and await diagnosis. Otherwise examine back for other injuries.
EXTREMITIES
Check for fractures, dislocations, soft tissue injuries.
PELVIS
Check for fractures. Inspect perineum, rectum and buttocks for injuries. If rectal exam reveals "floating prostate," suspect urethral injury.
FACE
Check for fractures.
EYES
Check pupil size, equality, reactivity, presence or absence of diplopia.
EARS AND NOSE
Check for blood and cerebrospinal fluid.
CHEST
Auscultate breath and heart sounds. Inspect for deformities or paradoxical motion. Palpate for tenderness, crepitation of subcutaneous emphysema or rib fractures.
ABDOMEN
Palpate for tenderness and masses. Examine for perforating wounds. Monitor all intraabdominal injuries for evolution of signs.
Check for adequate peripheral pulse.

▲ *Figure 80–6*

Checklist for rapid evaluation of the injured client after the immediate treatment priorities have been covered. After initial examination, the state of consciousness and vital signs are monitored frequently while x-ray and laboratory findings are being obtained.

tines; and the perceived danger to and emotional impact on the client and family.

Client reactions are unique. Common defense mechanisms and coping strategies clients may use include denial, regression, distraction, and rationalization. Some are anxious, fearful, and occasionally angry. Others experience loss of control, loss of individuality, and possible loss of dignity. Remember, all behavior is purposeful, and defense mechanisms help maintain psychological integrity. The mechanism and strategies used are usually based on past experiences and previous coping styles.

Some behavioral responses may be related to the physiologic process of the emergency and should be considered. For example, anoxia can cause agitation, restlessness, and irritability. In addition, cognitive impairment and behavioral changes may result from head injury, trauma, substance ingestion, and metabolic disorders. Carefully assess the behaviors and reactions, but always keep in mind the potential for physiologic effects.[29]

SIGNIFICANT OTHERS

The needs of significant others require special attention in emergency settings. Unless they accompanied the client, they may be notified by telephone. Advising significant others of the client's presence in the emergency setting by telephone requires tact and sensitivity. Exercise caution as you discuss the urgency of the situation. It is important to advise significant others to have someone else bring them to the hospital (Box 80–3).

Communicate to team members and record on the

Box 80–3. Summoning Family Members to Come to the Emergency Department

Giving the news of a client's death or critical condition over the telephone is difficult for staff (and for the person receiving the news). The following points help ensure that necessary information is given and obtained.

- Pre-establish definitions for *serious, critical, guarded,* and other terms, so all staff use the same terms. Use the same term consistently during conversation with family.
- Pre-establish a standardized format or protocol for making telephone notation.
- If you are providing care to the client, take a few moments to deal with your own feelings before making the call.
- State your name, position, and work area and give institutional information.
- Do not give the bad news first; rather, present the facts chronologically. Begin with the onset of injury or illness, location of occurrence, prehospital treatment, treatment efforts rendered in the emergency department, and the client's response to treatment. By presenting the circumstances clearly, it is usually not necessary to say that a client has died. The family member usually asks. If the client is still alive, ask the family member if she or he understands the gravity of the prognosis.
- Clarify the client's condition if, in fact, it appears that survival is likely. Family members (in a state of emotional shock) may not process information well and may assume that the client is in worse condition than is true.
- Notify family members as soon as possible so they can begin anticipatory grieving.
- Present information in a factual way, asking for periodic feedback to make sure you are being understood.
- Prevent reckless driving by family members on their way to the hospital. Ask if you should notify someone else to bring them to the hospital. Ask the person you speak with to write down the instructions you give to reach the hospital and emergency department. Finally, ask the person to drive safely.
- Ask if you should notify anyone else to serve as support.
- If death has already occurred, ask if the family members are coming to the emergency department or where they would like to see their loved one. If they are not coming to the emergency department, discuss administrative details, such as funeral arrangements, medical examiner's cases, autopsy, handling of valuables, and the like. Ask about any special wishes regarding religious ceremonies, organ donation, or other arrangements.
- At the end of your call, repeat your name and phone number. Ask the person you talk with to write it down so that any additional questions can be discussed. If death has occurred, encourage family members to call with any concerns. Unresolved issues or concerns impede the normal grieving process.

medical record when significant others have been notified or are present. It is important that the nurse providing the care periodically update significant others with clear explanations regarding the client's condition, treatment, and progress using easily understood language. Significant others need to have opportunities to visit the client as appropriate. Before they visit, prepare significant others about the client's condition and appearance. Be sure to include the presence of tubes, equipment, bandages, and other devices present. This is particularly important when there is disfigurement or loss of ability to communicate.

A private waiting area may help significant others cope with an emergency. The area should have a telephone, food, assorted beverages, comfortable chairs, current magazines, and nearby toilet facilities. A map on the wall showing the waiting area in relationship to the rest of the hospital helps orient people and provides direction (e.g., to the cafeteria).

▼ SELECTED EMERGENCIES

▼ Shock[13, 42]

Circulatory shock is a profound alteration in tissue perfusion. It occurs from either a decreased cellular perfusion or an inability to use an adequate perfusion. Shock may result from an alteration in circulating volume (hypovolemic shock); an alteration in cardiac output (cardiogenic shock); or an alteration in peripheral vascular resistance (distributive shock). See Chapter 20 for a discussion of shock.

▼ Altered Level of Consciousness

Overview

An altered level of consciousness may range from restlessness and disorientation to unconsciousness. The causes of an altered level of consciousness include hypoxic, metabolic, and pathologic conditions of the brain. The mnemonic device "vowel tipps" is a helpful guide for determining the cause of unconsciousness.

- A Alcohol
- E Epilepsy
- I Insulin
- O Opiates
- U Urates
- T Trauma
- I Infection
- P Psychological
- P Poison
- S Shock

Key historical information to be obtained from significant others or prehospital personnel includes any history of trauma; chronic health problems (e.g., diabetes, hypertension, heart or renal disease); use of prescription, over-the-counter, or street drugs or home remedies; alcohol use; mental health history; general health status; activities when the client was last seen or communicated with; temperature of environment in which the client was found; and clues that may help to determine cause (e.g., medication bottles, incontinence, medical alert tag or card).

Assess the color of skin, respiratory pattern, pupillary reaction, motor function, odors, nuchal rigidity, and posturing. Institute measures to stabilize the ABCs. Monitor vital signs and assess neurologic status. Calculate and document the Glasgow Coma Scale score (see Chap. 29), pupillary responses, and reflexes. Insert an intravenous line and draw blood for laboratory work (complete blood count [CBC], glucose, calcium, electrolytes, creatinine, magnesium, drug screen, and alcohol level).

TABLE 80-2. Champion Trauma Score

Glasgow Coma Scale (GCS)		
Eye-opening response	Spontaneous	4
	To voice	3
	To pain	2
	None	1
Best verbal response	Oriented	5
	Confused	4
	Inappropriate words	3
	Incomprehensible sounds	2
	None	1
Best motor response	Obeys command	6
	Localizes pain	5
	Withdraws (pain)	4
	Flexion (pain)	3
	Extension (pain)	2
	None	1
Total	Apply this score to GCS portion of Trauma Score	3–15
Trauma Score		
GCS (total points from above)	14–15	5
	11–13	4
	8–10	3
	5–7	2
	3–4	1
Respiratory rate	10–24/min	4
	25–35/min	3
	36/min or greater	2
	1–9/min	1
	None	0
Respiratory expansion	Normal	1
	Retractive/none	0
Systolic blood pressure	90 mm Hg or greater	4
	70–89 mm Hg	3
	50–69 mm Hg	2
	0–49 mm Hg	1
	No pulse	0
Capillary refill	Normal	2
	Delayed	1
	None	0
Total trauma score		1–16

Trauma score	16	15	14	13	12	11	10	9	8	7	6	5	4	3	2	1
Percentage survival	99	98	96	93	87	76	60	42	26	15	8	4	2	1	0	0

From Moore, et al. (1990). *Early care of the injured patient.* Philadelphia: B. C. Decker.

Management

Administer thiamine (vitamin B) 100 mg intramuscularly. Because the history may be inadequate for determining whether thiamine deficiency is probable, thiamine is routinely administered prophylactically. Administer intravenous dextrose if the client has a history of hypoglycemia or a low serum glucose. Glucose paste may also be applied sublingually, or intramuscular glucagon may be administered to raise the blood sugar. Intravenous dextrose for all clients with an altered level of consciousness is becoming controversial. An intravenous glucose load can precipitate Wernicke's encephalopathy in thiamine-deficient clients.[7]

Naloxone (Narcan), 2 mg intravenously, may be administered if a narcotic overdose is suspected, and it can be repeated. Use caution, however, because if the drug that is reversed by naloxone has a longer half-life, the effect of the drug may last longer than the effect of naloxone, and the client may lapse back into unconsciousness. Thus, observation for several hours is usually indicated for these clients.

Ongoing nursing management includes safety measures. Manage airways and secretions for prevention of aspiration. Position the client on the side while maintaining spine immobilization, and suction as needed. Protect the eyes from drying by applying artificial tears and taping the eyelids shut (use cellophane rather than adhesive tape). Be sure to check the eyes for contact lenses and remove if present. Prevent skin necrosis by position changes and skin care. Protect from falls by raising the side rails, and lock them. Minimize the potential for increased intracranial pressure by positioning the head in neutral alignment, hyperventilating with 100 per cent oxygen before suctioning, suctioning for short periods of time, and avoiding the use of restraints if possible.[4, 22]

Prepare for and assist with diagnostic studies (e.g., CT scans or magnetic resonance imaging). If toxic ingestion is suspected, institute gastric lavage (see section on poisoning) with endotracheal tube in place. Provide continuous psychosocial support for both the client and significant others. Remember, the extent of hearing impairment is unknown, so refrain from discussing the client's condition at the bedside.

▼ Multiple Trauma

Overview

Multiple trauma includes injury to more than one body system. There are many different scoring systems used to categorize and determine severity of injury. One of these is the Champion Trauma Score (Table 80-2).

This score uses physiologic measurements (heart rate, respiratory expansion, systolic blood pressure, and capillary return) and the Glasgow Coma Scale. Points are assigned on the basis of the client's responses, and a total score is obtained. Optimally, a client with a Champion Trauma Score of less than 12 should be transferred to a tertiary trauma system. The Champion Trauma Score correlates highly with mortality.

Mechanism of Injury

The mechanism of injury helps in estimating the amount of force applied and provides insight into the pattern of injury (Fig. 80-7).

In addition to the mechanism of injury, the type and extent of injury also involve environmental conditions (weather, geographic location) and characteristics of the client such as age, sex, nutrition, underlying disease processes, and any conditions altering cognitive function and judgement (alcohol, drug use, or fatigue).

PENETRATING INJURIES

Penetrating injuries cause a break in the skin integrity. Remember to consider potential injuries to underlying organs and tissues. For instance, if an injury resulted from a stab wound, consider the length of the object and the direction of the wound for an idea of additional injuries. A thoracic wound may involve an interruption in the heart, great vessels, or even diaphragm, depending on whether the injured client was inspiring (diaphragm down) or expiring (diaphragm up) at the time of injury. Because of the diaphragm's location, a diagnostic peritoneal lavage is often performed for evaluation of possible abdominal injury by penetrating wounds below the nipple line.[7, 30]

NONPENETRATING (BLUNT) INJURIES

Blunt (nonpenetrating) injuries result in significant injuries that may be more difficult to detect. These involve direct, indirect, and acceleration/deceleration forces. For instance, in a motor vehicle crash, the driver (traveling at the speed of the car) impacts on the steering wheel. The force of the impact is exerted through the chest structures and may result in broken ribs, cardiac or pulmonary contusions, pneumothorax, or ruptured aorta. Or the client's head may hit the windshield, which causes frontal lobe damage of the brain (coup); as the head falls backward, damage to the occipital lobe can occur (contrecoup). Solid organs are more likely to be crushed or compressed (liver, spleen). Hollow, air-filled organs are more likely to burst when compressed or subject to blast forces (lung, intestines).

The history and mechanism of injury constitute vital information and must be obtained promptly. This information helps guide assessment and intervention. Experienced emergency nurses can often anticipate common associated injuries most likely to be present on the basis of accurate information about the mechanism of injury (Table 80-3). In addition, injuries should be matched to the reported mechanism. Clients and significant others may deny or falsify the history of injury for many reasons.[17]

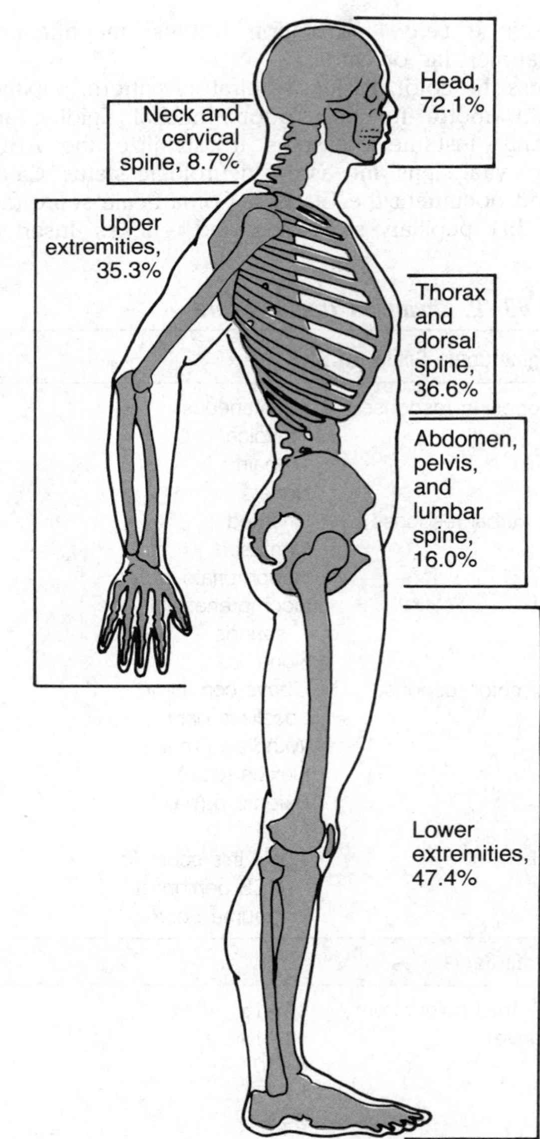

▲ *Figure 80-7*

Motor vehicle accidents can result in multiple injuries. Two thirds of the victims suffer injuries to the head and facial area. Other anatomic areas also are often involved. (From *Patterns of disease,* a publication of Parke, Davis & Co.)

Management

GENERAL INTERVENTIONS

- Ensure an adequate airway with spinal immobilization.
- Ventilate and initiate oxygen therapy at 6 to 10 L/min.
- Insert one or two peripheral intravenous lines (14- to 16-gauge catheter).

TABLE 80–3. Common Associated Injuries

Mechanism of Injury	Potential Associated Injuries
Adult pedestrian struck by a car	"Waddell's triad"; suspect fractures at 1. point of impact with the car bumper 2. point of impact with the car hood 3. point of impact when adult is thrown Fractures are sustained at the points of impact with the car bumper and hood Disruption of knee ligaments in the opposite knee from excessive stress
Unrestrained driver	Head and facial injuries from windshield impact Fractured ribs and sternum from impact on the steering wheel Cardiac contusions Lacerated solid organs from blunt compression Patellar injury from striking dash, with an associated femur fracture and dislocation
Client falls from a height and lands on the heels	"Don Juan syndrome" 1. bilateral calcaneal fractures 2. compression fractures of the vertebrae 3. if the client lands and braces self with the hands, suspect Colles' fractures at both wrists

- ▶ Initiate cardiac monitoring; obtain a 12-lead ECG.
- ▶ Insert nasogastric tube (18-French Salem sump).
- ▶ Insert a urinary catheter, if no blood is present at the meatus.
- ▶ Monitor urine output every 15 to 30 minutes.
- ▶ Monitor vital signs continuously, and document.
- ▶ Provide continuous psychosocial support to client and significant others.

PRIMARY ASSESSMENT AND PRIORITY INTERVENTIONS

With a multiply injured client, time is vital. Priorities are determined by the ABCs, and the general interventions are implemented immediately.

Control external bleeding by direct pressure, pressure dressing, or rapid fluid replacement if the client is hypotensive (crystalloid or colloid). The client may be in cardiac arrest from shock, chest injuries, or respiratory failure. Initiate two large-bore intravenous lines for rapid infusion of fluids. Consider use of the PASG.

Start CPR immediately if no pulse is present. Remember, if the client has lost fluid volume, CPR will not be fully effective until fluid volume is restored. Draw blood while inserting an intravenous line for appropriate studies. Common studies include CBC, electrolytes, blood urea nitrogen (BUN), glucose, amylase, T & C, coagulation screen, possible drug and alcohol levels, creatinine if renal trauma is suspected, and ABGs. Prepare for possible blood transfusions.

Obtain a full set of vital signs and repeat at least every 15 minutes until the client is stabilized. Perform a brief neurologic and mental status examination. Calculate the Glasgow Coma Scale score and trauma scores. Initiate a flow sheet for documentation of assessments, interventions, and client responses.

Completely undress the client (by cutting off clothes, if necessary). Cover the client with a sheet or blanket. Helmets must be removed carefully to avoid neck flexion. The helmet (1) is spread open, (2) manual traction is applied to the head, (3) the helmet is "walked off" while traction is maintained, (4) the helmet is pushed off the head, (5) after the helmet is off, head is lowered and the client is asked whether difficulties were encountered. Ensure that the client's clothes or valuables are safeguarded, and use the proper chain of custody, especially if criminal or suspicious acts are associated with the trauma (see earlier).

SECONDARY ASSESSMENT AND INTERVENTIONS

Proceed with a complete head-to-toe examination. Remember the possibility of associated injuries, and keep in mind the various internal structures potentially affected by the known injury pattern.

Obtain a urinalysis after insertion of a urinary catheter, and monitor urine output every 15 to 30 minutes. Insert a nasogastric tube, if indicated (nasogastric tubes are not inserted if a basilar skull fracture is suspected because of possible insertion into the cranium; instead, an orogastric tube may be used to decompress the stomach). Test gastric aspirant for blood and connect to suction. Keep the client NPO.

Other diagnostic procedures, according to injuries, may include chest tube insertion, needle thoracostomy, or diagnostic peritoneal lavage (see separate discussion). Prepare for radiographs of the cervical spine, or chest and CT scans or magnetic resonance imaging, as indicated. If a portable x-ray machine is not available, coordinate x-ray studies so the client makes only one trip to the radiology department.

Administer a tetanus booster if wounds are present. Avoid moving the client suddenly. Rapid position changes may precipitate cardiovascular collapse. Splint fractures, apply ice, and elevate the area. Clean and dress wounds. Wounds are repaired only after the client is stabilized or in the operating room.

Provide emotional support to the client and significant others. See separate discussion.

Remain with the client during transport to the operating room, radiology department, or nursing unit. Provide verbal report to the nurses assuming responsibility for subsequent care and ensure that written documentation accompanies the client. Include data about significant others and what information they have received.

Pain medication is commonly not given initially for clients with multiple trauma and cardiovascular instability. Medication may mask the identification of significant injuries and interfere with accurate neurologic assessments. Self-administered nitrous oxide and oxygen may help clients with significant amounts of pain or those undergoing painful procedures. If narcotics are given, they are administered in small intravenous doses. Coordination with the anesthesia department is important if immediate surgery is anticipated.

Elderly clients with traumatic injuries have special needs. The body's compensatory mechanisms may be delayed, and chronic health problems and medications may contribute to complications. For instance, a client with a heart condition who is taking a beta-blocker does not present with tachycardia in the presence of shock. Also, abuse of the elderly is an increasing problem that may appear as multiple trauma.[3]

▼ Respiratory Emergencies

NEAR-DROWNING

Overview

Clients who initially survive suffocation after submersion in a water or fluid medium are diagnosed as near-drowning. Another term, immersion syndrome, is used by some clinicians to describe near-drowning.

Freshwater drowning (i.e., swimming pools) is more common than salt water drowning. Alcohol or drug ingestion, overestimation of swimming skills, hypothermia, hyperventilation, and hypoglycemia are risk factors.

Additional injuries may be present in a client with near-drowning. These include associated trauma, spinal cord injury from diving, air embolism from scuba diving, and seizures.

Both fresh water and salt water wash out alveolar surfactant. Fresh water also changes the surface tension of surfactant. The loss of surfactant leads to alveolar collapse, intrapulmonary shunting, and hypoxemia. Poor perfusion and hypoxemia result in acidosis and eventual pulmonary edema.

Near-drowning compromises the respiratory system and leads to hypoxia, hypercapnia, cardiac arrest, and severe alterations in fluid-electrolyte balance. Bronchospasm, from aspirating water into the lungs, causes most drowning deaths.

Management

Obtain a history of the submersion. Include the length of submersion, temperature of the water, any associated injuries (possible spinal cord injury from diving), and type of water.

Begin assessment and interventions with the ABCs. Note any respiratory efforts and adventitious sounds. Open the airway while maintaining spinal immobility. Assess the level of consciousness. Look for signs of hypoxia, such as confusion, irritability, lethargy, or unconsciousness. Obtain a complete set of vital signs.

For respiratory insufficiency, intubate and ventilate with 100 per cent oxygen and 5 to 10 cm of positive end-expiratory pressure (PEEP) to prevent the alveoli from collapsing. If the client is breathing, provide respiratory support with a non-rebreather.

Remove the client's wet clothing, and wrap the client in a warm blanket. Core rewarming may be indicated if the client is hypothermic. Rewarm the client slowly to avoid a rapid influx of metabolites that may be trapped in the cold extremities.

Once the vital functions are stabilized, correct any acid-base or electrolyte abnormalities. Diagnostic studies include ABGs, CBC, electrolytes, appropriate toxicology studies if alcohol or drug ingestion is suspected, and a chest radiograph. Observe clients with near-drowning emergencies for at least 24 hours. They have a high risk for developing pulmonary edema, even several hours after the incident. Care must be taken to monitor the neurologic status. A deteriorating level of consciousness may indicate cerebral edema, severe acidosis, or increased hypoxia.

FOREIGN BODY AIRWAY OBSTRUCTION

Overview

Foreign body airway obstruction may rapidly lead to cardiopulmonary arrest if it is not dealt with quickly.

Foreign bodies usually enter the right main bronchus because its orifice is slightly wider than that of the left main bronchus. It also lies in a more direct line with the trachea.

Clinical manifestations of an aspirated foreign body include severe dyspnea; hemoptysis (if there has been mechanical trauma to air passages); fever; atelectasis; pulmonary infection; excessive mucus production (if the airways are irritated); harsh, brassy cough; wheezing (if a foreign body passed into the larger airways, i.e., beyond the trachea into the right bronchus); and inspiratory stridor (if the obstruction is at the laryngeal level). If airway obstruction is complete (or nearly complete) and at the laryngeal level, there will be obvious respiratory distress, ineffective ventilation efforts, and inability to speak because it is impossible for air to pass the obstruction. Asphyxia follows rapidly.

Clients may signal airway obstruction due to foreign body aspiration by the international sign for distress. They can be helped by the Heimlich maneuver and thrust techniques (see Figs. 80-1 and 80-2).

Complete airway obstruction is a life-threatening emergency requiring immediate intervention. Foreign bodies small enough to pass through the glottis seldom lodge in the trachea but pass on into the bronchus. However, those that do lodge in the laryngeal area may be removed with grasping forceps inserted through a laryngoscope under local or general anesthesia.

The client is usually placed in Trendelenburg's position so that the foreign body is prevented from entering the trachea or esophagus. If the foreign object is pushed farther into the airway, a bronchoscope and special grasping forceps are used. (See Chap. 36 for discussion of laryngoscopy and bronchoscopy.) If time permits, a radiograph is taken to confirm the presence and location of the object. If the obstruction is complete, emergency airway maneuvers are necessary.

▼ Chest Trauma[30]

OVERVIEW

The chest is a large, exposed portion of the body that is very vulnerable to impact injuries. Because it houses the heart, lungs, and great vessels, trauma to the chest frequently produces life-threatening disruptions of cardiopulmonary function. Chest injuries can range from relatively minor bumps and scrapes to severe crushing or penetrating trauma.

Chest injuries often result from falls, the use of machinery, or the employment of lethal weapons (i.e., knives and guns). Many chest injuries are associated with motor vehicle crashes in which clients are thrown against the steering wheel, dashboard, or front seat.

Chest injuries may be penetrating or nonpenetrating (blunt).

- Penetrating chest injuries (i.e., from bullets, knives, impaled objects, or flying shrapnel or splinters) may cause an open chest wound, permitting atmospheric air into the pleural space and disrupting the normal ventilation mechanism. Penetrating chest injuries may seriously damage the lungs, heart, and other thoracic structures.
- Nonpenetrating (blunt) injuries are not as obvious as penetrating wounds and may, therefore, be more difficult to diagnose. Blunt chest injuries are most commonly deceleration injuries associated with motor vehicle crashes. Deceleration injuries occur when a vehicle or body stops abruptly from a relatively high speed. For example, when a car stops suddenly, the body of the client in the car continues forward until it hits the steering wheel, windshield, dashboard, or front seat. Blunt chest trauma may also result from falls or blows to the chest.

Injury to the thoracic cage and its contents can restrict the heart's ability to pump blood or the lungs' ability to exchange air and oxygenate blood. Major dangers associated with chest injuries are internal bleeding and punctured organs.

Initial assessment is directed toward identifying and treating immediate life-threatening conditions. Any client with chest trauma should be considered to have a serious injury until it is proved otherwise. Airway patency, adequacy of breathing, and circulatory sufficiency (i.e., presence of shock) are always of primary concern.

Once initial emergencies have been addressed, the client is assessed more thoroughly (Box 80-4). A medical history helps identify any pre-existing conditions that may further complicate the injury. A thorough physical examination should be performed, with care being taken not to focus only on obvious injuries. Information about the accident (obtained from the injured client or witnesses) assists in the diagnosis of regional as well as anatomic injuries. A chest film and electrocardiogram are obtained for detecting possible pulmonary or cardiac impairment.

MANAGEMENT

Ventilation/perfusion imbalances may result from atelectasis, hemopneumothorax, flail chest, aspiration, or pulmonary contusion. Oxygen or mechanical ventilation may be required. General respiratory status (e.g., rate and depth of respirations, chest movement, spontaneous vital volumes) and arterial blood gases should be monitored closely. Deterioration may indicate previously undetected injury or late-developing complications.

Therapeutic measures such as thoracentesis, chest tube insertion, bronchoscopic aspiration, or thoracotomy (Chaps. 37 and 39) may be indicated. Maintain effective functioning of any equipment used (e.g., chest drainage system). Help the client and significant others understand these procedures and the rationale for their use. Clients with chest injuries may experience significant hypovolemia. Fluid replacement is with blood and blood products, if indicated, or with crystalloid intravenous solutions (e.g., lactated Ringer's solution, normal saline). Continually monitor for signs of shock, including low blood pressure; rapid, thready pulse; cold, clammy skin; restlessness, disorientation, or confusion; low urine output; and metabolic acidosis.

Excessive blood loss may further compromise the client's oxygenation. External bleeding should be carefully assessed, and estimated blood loss should be determined. Internal bleeding may result from injuries to the thoracic or abdominal viscera, torn muscles, or fractures. Considerable bleeding (i.e., 2 L or more) into the pleural space may occur. This usually can be quickly detected. Bleeding into areas such as the chest

Box 80–4. Assessment of and Therapeutic Intervention for the Chest Trauma Victim

Maintain airway, breathing, and circulation

Obtain a quick history

- What happened?
- What was the mechanism of injury?
- How long ago did it happen?
- Where is the pain? Does it radiate?
- Is there anything that makes the pain better or worse?
- What does the pain feel like?
- How severe is the pain on a scale of 1 to 10?
- Is there any medical history?

Perform a quick (1-minute) evaluation

- Check for shortness of breath and cyanosis.
- Check vital signs.
- Check skin color and temperature.
- Check wound size and location.
- Check for paradoxical chest movement.
- Check for distended neck veins.
- Listen for respiratory stridor.
- Listen for bilateral breath sounds.
- Look for epigastric and supraclavicular indrawing.
- Give rough estimate of tidal volume.
- Check for tracheal deviation.
- Assess intercostal muscle use.
- Assess accessory muscle use.
- Check for subcutaneous emphysema.
- Look and listen for sucking chest sounds.
- Listen to heart sounds.

Provide therapeutic intervention

- Maintain airway.
- Ensure adequate air movement.
- Administer oxygen.
- Cover any open chest wound.
- Control flail segment.
- Insert needles or chest tube into anterior chest wall if tension pneumothorax is present.
- Initiate an intravenous line (two or more lines if possible, but do not delay transport to do this).
- Do pericardiocentesis, if indicated.
- Get chest x-ray film if more than three ribs are fractured, because victim is considered multitraumatized and one must search for other associated injuries. It is essential at this time to obtain cross-table lateral cervical spine x-ray film for detection of cervical spine injury before any other diagnostic tests are initiated or the victim is moved.
- Frequently recheck vital signs.
- Monitor for dysrhythmias.

From Sheehy, S. B. (1985). *Emergency nursing: Principles and practice.* St. Louis: C. V. Mosby.

wall (e.g., from torn intercostal muscles) is more difficult to assess. A liter of blood can accumulate between the chest wall muscles without producing much swelling.

A chest-injured client may require large quantities of blood replacement. Until the results of typing and crossmatching are available, the patient is given O-negative blood. The volume of blood replacement is determined through assessment of clinical findings, hemodynamic measurements, and laboratory results (e.g., hemoglobin and hematocrit). When possible, surgery is delayed until the client's blood volume is restored.

Shock often results from hypovolemia, but in the chest-injured client it may also be caused by cardiac tamponade, cardiac contusion, flail chest, or tension pneumothorax. Central vascular pressure readings (central venous pressure or pulmonary artery pressure) require careful interpretation. Once the cause of shock is determined, rapid intervention is given (see Chap. 20).

Pain associated with chest injuries may cause the client to breathe rapidly and shallowly, which leads to atelectasis and pooling of tracheobronchial secretions. Analgesics minimize pain and permit periods of rest and relaxation. They also allow the client to cough and take deeper breaths. Administration must be done cautiously (usually small, frequent doses), however, for avoidance of respiratory depression. Intercostal nerve blocks or epidural analgesia may be used in clients with underlying health problems. Splinting the chest may also be helpful.

COMPLICATIONS

Severe chest trauma may produce numerous complications, including

- pneumothorax
- tension pneumothorax and mediastinal shift
- open pneumothorax and mediastinal flutter
- hemothorax
- fractured ribs
- fractured sternum
- flail chest

Pneumothorax

OVERVIEW

Pneumothorax is the presence of air in the pleural space that prohibits complete lung expansion. Air may enter the pleural space directly through a hole in the chest wall (open pneumothorax) or diaphragm. Air may escape into the pleural space from a puncture or tear in an internal respiratory structure (e.g., bronchus, bronchioles, alveoli). This form of pneumothorax is called closed or spontaneous pneumothorax (Fig. 80–8).

Clinical manifestations of moderate pneumothorax include tachypnea; dyspnea; sudden sharp pain on the affected side with chest movement, breathing, or

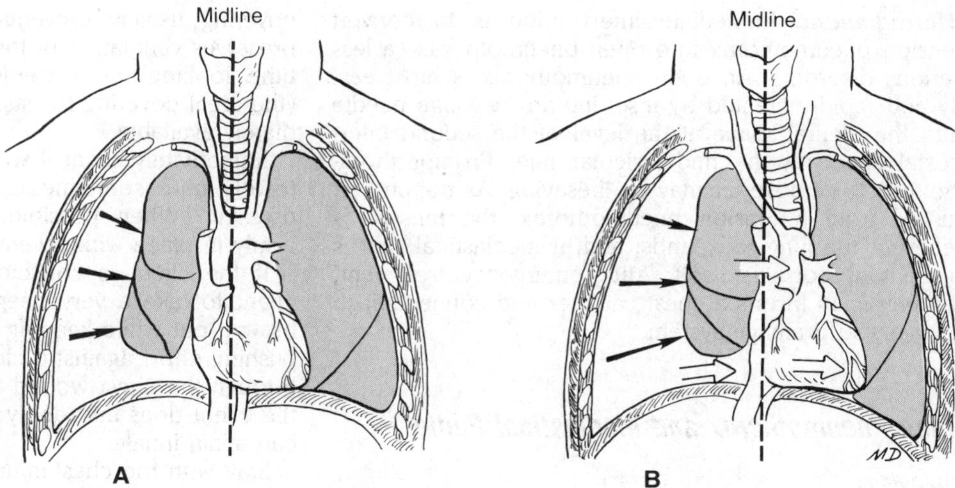

▲ *Figure 80–8*

A, Pneumothorax. Lung collapses as air gathers in the pleural space. *B*, Mediastinal shift in tension pneumothorax. In addition to collapsed lung, the mediastinal contents are displaced against the unaffected side of the chest.

coughing; asymmetric chest expansion; diminished or absent breath sounds on the affected side; hyperresonance (tympany) to percussion on the affected side; restlessness, anxiety; and tachycardia.

Clinical manifestations of severe pneumothorax include all the preceding and distended neck veins; PMI shift (point of maximal impulse of heart beat); subcutaneous emphysema; decreased tactile and vocal fremitus; tracheal deviation toward the unaffected side; and progressive cyanosis.

Management. Chest films may reveal a slight tracheal shift away from the affected side and retraction of the lung back from the parietal pleura. (Remember, in pneumothorax, the collection of air is between the visceral and parietal pleura.) If pneumothorax is suspected (but respiratory distress is too severe to permit x-ray confirmation), the physician may insert an 18-gauge needle (emergency thoracentesis) into the second or third intercostal space in the midclavicular line. Aspiration demonstrates whether free air is present in the pleural space.

However, most physicians prefer to insert a chest tube immediately into the pleural space via the fourth intercostal space at mid- or anterior axillary line. The chest catheter is connected to closed-chest drainage. (Management of closed-chest drainage is discussed in Chap. 39.) The catheter permits the continuous escape of air and blood from the pleural space. Thus, it helps the lung expand by reestablishing subatmospheric pressure (i.e., negative pressure) in the pleural space (necessary for normal ventilation). Sometimes thoracotomy (surgical opening into the chest cavity) is done to explore the chest surgically and repair the site of origin of the pneumo- or hemothorax.

Tension Pneumothorax and Mediastinal Shift

OVERVIEW

Tension pneumothorax is a serious type of pneumothorax in which air enters the pleural space with each inspiration, becomes trapped there, and is not expelled during expiration (i.e., one-way valve effect). Pressure builds in the chest as the accumulation of air in the pleural space increases. Tension pneumothorax most commonly occurs with blunt traumatic injuries and is frequently associated with flail chest injuries.

If untreated, tension pneumothorax collapses the lung on the affected side as intrapleural pressure or tension increases. It may then cause a mediastinal shift (see Fig. 80–8). This means the contents of the mediastinum (heart, trachea, esophagus, and great vessels) are pushed or "shifted" toward the chest's unaffected side. Mediastinal shift may cause (1) compression of the lung in the direction of the shift (i.e., the lung opposite the pneumothorax) and (2) compression, traction, torsion, or kinking of the great vessels (e.g., vena cava); thus, blood return to the heart is dangerously impaired. The latter causes a subsequent decrease in cardiac output and blood pressure. Tension pneumothorax produces serious circulatory and pulmonary impairment that can be rapidly fatal. This is a high-priority emergency requiring prompt assessment and intervention.

Clinical manifestations of tension pneumothorax include marked, severe dyspnea; tachypnea; crepitus (subcutaneous emphysema in the neck and upper chest); progressive cyanosis; acute chest pain on the affected side; hyperresonance (tympany) to percussion on the affected side; tachycardia; asymmetric chest wall movement; diminished or absent breath sounds on affected side; and extreme restlessness, agitation.

Other clinical manifestations include neck vein distention; laryngeal and tracheal deviation/shift to the unaffected side; feeling of tightness or pressure within the chest; point of maximal impulse (PMI) shift laterally or medially; severe hypotension leading to shock; and muffled heart sounds.

A suspected mediastinal shift may be confirmed by x-ray study. Laryngeal and tracheal deviation can be detected by gentle palpation and with x-ray study. ABGs demonstrate hypoxia and respiratory alkalosis. When mediastinal shift is severe and not immediately corrected, respiratory acidosis may ensue.

Management. Immediate intervention is to convert tension pneumothorax into open pneumothorax (a less serious disorder). An open pneumothorax is most easily and rapidly created by inserting an 18-gauge needle into the pleural space at the level of the second intercostal space at the midclavicular line. Prompt thoracentesis to remove air may be lifesaving. As trapped air rushes from a tension pneumothorax, the tension is relieved; the lung reexpands; and, if mediastinal shift is present, it corrects itself. After emergency treatment, the physician inserts a chest catheter and connects it to a waterseal drainage system.

Open Pneumothorax and Mediastinal Flutter

OVERVIEW

An open pneumothorax occurs with "sucking" chest wounds. With this type of wound, a traumatic opening in the chest wall is large enough for air to move freely in and out of the chest cavity during ventilation (Fig. 80-9). This abnormal movement of air through the chest wound produces a "slurping" or "sucking" noise that is audible in a quiet environment.

Open sucking chest wounds may result from accidental injuries or surgical trauma. For example, if a chest drainage catheter is accidentally pulled out of a chest, the remaining puncture incision in the chest wall may become a sucking wound.

MANAGEMENT

When an open sucking chest wound is detected, emergency intervention includes immediately covering the wound securely with anything available. An airtight covering usually prevents tension pneumothorax and preserves ventilation of the opposite lung. Do not waste time looking for a sterile gauze petrolatum dressing (the ideal covering for such a wound) if it is not immediately available.

Immediately cover it with whatever is at hand (e.g., a towel) until someone can bring a sterile petrolatum dressing. When possible, fix the temporary dressing firmly in place with several strips of wide tape.

If the client is conscious and cooperative, ask the client to take a very deep breath and then attempt to blow it out while keeping mouth and nose closed. This pushing effort against a closed glottis helps push air out through the chest wound and reexpand the lung. When the client does this, apply the dressing before the client can again inhale.

Stay with the chest-injured client after a dressing has been applied to a sucking wound. Assess carefully, for indications of tension pneumothorax and mediastinal shift. This may develop if the air leak is in the lung or a bronchus, which permits air to escape into the pleural space. In such a situation, closing the chest wall wound with an airtight dressing prevents the outflow of escaping air. Thus, an open pneumothorax has been accidentally converted into a tension pneumothorax. If the client appears to be developing tension pneumothorax after sealing of the wound, immediately unplug the seal (Fig. 80-10).

Although it is dangerous to have air moving in and out of the pleural space with each respiration (open pneumothorax), it is far more dangerous when air moves only into the pleural space and cannot move back out (tension pneumothorax).

Closed-chest drainage will be necessary to (1) remove the air from the pleural space and (2) allow the lung to reexpand if collapsed.

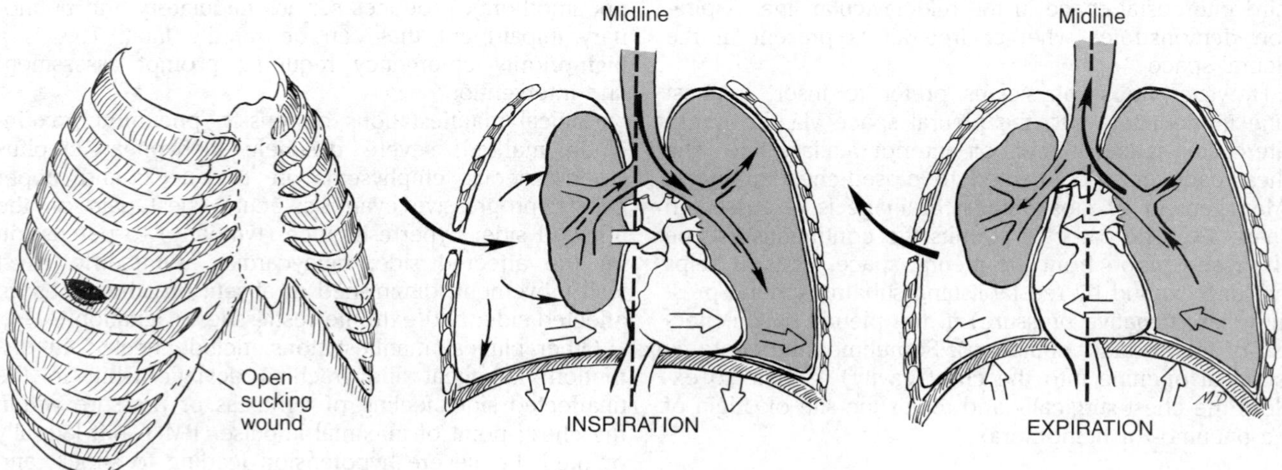

▲ **Figure 80-9**

Open pneumothorax (sucking chest wound). Solid arrows indicate air movement; open arrows, structural movement. A chest wall wound connects the pleural space with atmospheric air. During inspiration, atmospheric air is "sucked" into the pleural space through the chest wall wound. Positive pressure in the pleural space collapses the lung on the affected side and "pushes" the mediastinal contents toward the unaffected side. This reduces the volume of air in the unaffected side considerably. During expiration, air escapes through the chest wall wound, lessening positive pressure in the affected side and allowing the mediastinal contents to "swing" back toward the affected side. Movement of mediastinal structures from side to side is called mediastinal flutter.

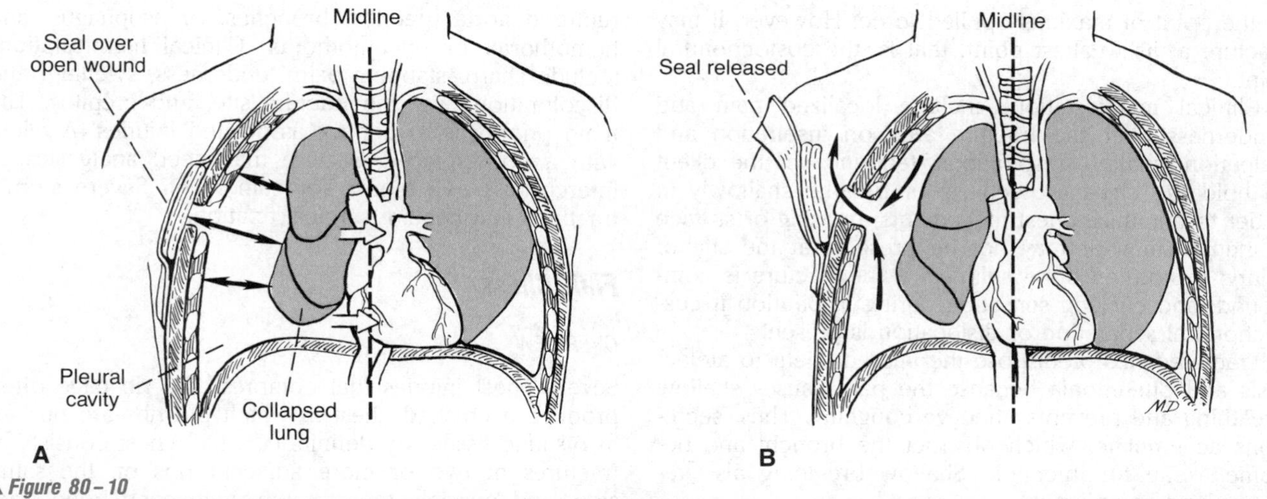

▲ *Figure 80-10*

Tension pneumothorax. *A,* If an open pneumothorax is covered (e.g., with a dressing), it forms a seal, and tension pneumothorax with a mediastinal shift develops. A tear in lung structure continues to allow air into the pleural space. As positive pressure builds in the pleural space, the affected lung collapses, and the mediastinal contents shift to the unaffected side. *B,* Tension pneumothorax is corrected by removing the seal (e.g., dressing), allowing air trapped in the pleural space to escape.

Mediastinal Flutter. In addition to dyspnea and collapse of the lung on the affected side, the client with an open pneumothorax may experience mediastinal flutter. This complication results from air rushing in and out of the thoracic cavity on the affected side. With inspiration, the mediastinal structures (heart, trachea, esophagus) and collapsed lung are pushed toward the unaffected side. Then, with expiration, these structures move back toward the affected side. Fluttering, back-and-forth movements of these vital mediastinal structures produce severe cardiopulmonary embarrassment, which is fatal if not treated promptly.

Hemothorax

OVERVIEW

Hemothorax may be present in clients with chest injuries. A small amount of blood (less than 300 ml) in the pleural space may cause no symptoms and may not require intervention (blood will be reabsorbed spontaneously). Severe hemothorax (1400 to 2500 ml) may be life-threatening because of resultant hypovolemia and tension (Fig. 80-11). Clinical manifestations include dullness to percussion on the affected side, tachycardia, hypotension, and shock.

MANAGEMENT

A chest film confirms a diagnosis of hemothorax. If the client is in severe distress, the physician may aspirate blood from the pleural space by inserting a 16-gauge needle into the fifth or sixth intercostal space at the mid-axillary line. To drain intrathoracic accumulations of blood, the physician inserts a large-caliber (36-French or larger) chest catheter, which is then connected to a drainage system. An initial drainage of 500 to 1000 ml is considered moderate and may not require additional treatment. However, continued large amounts of drainage (200 ml or more per hour) may indicate a need for emergency thoracotomy. Document and promptly report such drainage to the physician. An initial drainage of 1500 ml or more is an indication for immediate exploratory thoracotomy.

Fractured Ribs

OVERVIEW

Rib fractures are common chest injuries, particularly in the elderly. They are usually associated with a blunt injury, such as a fall, a blow to the chest, or (more frequently) the impact of a steering wheel against the chest during rapid deceleration. A rib typically fractures

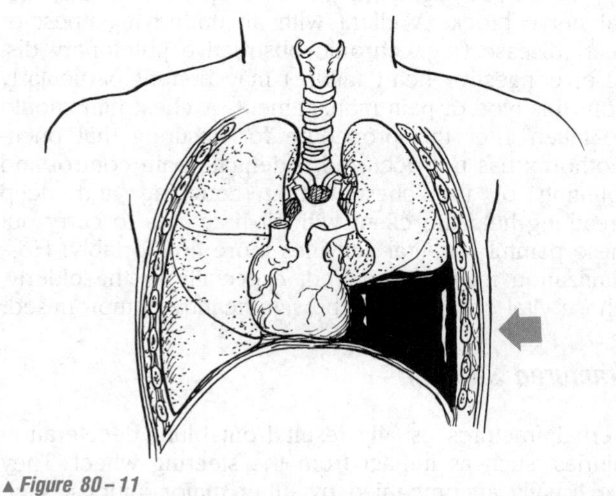

▲ *Figure 80-11*

Massive hemothorax *(arrow)* below left lung, causing collapse of lung tissue.

at the point of maximal applied force. However, it may fracture at its weakest point, that is, the costochondral joint.

Clinical manifestations include localized pain and tenderness over the fracture area on inspiration and palpation; shallow respirations; tendency of the client to hold the chest protectively or breathe shallowly in order to minimize chest movements; bruising or surface markings (may or may not be present) at the site of injury; protruding bone splinters if the fracture is compound; and clicking sensation during inspiration if costochondral separation or dislocation is present.

Fractured ribs predispose the injured client to atelectasis and pneumonia because the pain causes shallow breathing and prevents effective coughing. Thus, secretions accumulate, which obstruct the bronchi and become a site for infection. Shallow breathing also reduces lung compliance.

Bone splinters from fractured ribs may cause pneumothorax or hemothorax by puncturing the lung and pleura. Chest films are carefully reviewed for 24 to 48 hours after injury for indications of these complications. Bright red sputum may be coughed up if the lung has been penetrated. Assess the client for signs of pneumothorax or hemothorax and report such findings promptly.

MANAGEMENT

Fractured ribs are generally treated conservatively with rest, local heat, and analgesics. Strapping the ribs is no longer recommended because it restricts deep breathing and can increase the incidence of atelectasis and pneumonia. The pain from fractured ribs usually lasts 5 to 7 days. Complete healing occurs in approximately 6 weeks.

If pain is severe enough to impair ventilation significantly, a local anesthetic may be injected at the fracture site itself. Intercostal nerve blocks may also be used. These may be accomplished by injection of procaine or bupivacaine hydrochloride (Marcaine) into the intercostal nerves above and below the fracture site or by continuous segmental thoracic epidural or intrathecal nerve block. A client with an underlying chest or heart disease (e.g., chronic obstructive pulmonary disease, congestive heart failure) may benefit particularly from this type of pain management. A chest film should be taken after this procedure for ensuring that pneumothorax has not occurred. Adequate pain control and splinting of the chest during coughing and deep breathing help the client with rib fractures to carry out these painful but vital activities more comfortably. Hospitalization may be required, especially in the elderly, whose vital capacity may be significantly compromised.

Fractured Sternum

Sternal fractures usually result from blunt deceleration injuries, such as impact from the steering wheel. They are usually accompanied by other major injuries, such as flail chest; pulmonary and myocardial contusions; ruptured aorta, trachea, bronchus, or esophagus; and hemothorax or pneumothorax. Clinical manifestations include sharp, stabbing pain; tenderness, swelling, and discoloration over the fracture site; and crepitus. The main priority is to control associated injuries. A client with a nondisplaced fracture may need analgesics or intercostal nerve blocks for pain relief. Severe sternal fractures may require surgical fixation.

Flail Chest

OVERVIEW

Severe chest injuries that compress the rib cage often produce a crushed chest in which the ribs are pushed in on lung tissue. By definition, a flail chest consists of fractures of two or more adjacent ribs on the same side, and possibly the sternum, with each bone fractured into two or more segments (Fig. 80-12). The flail segment most commonly involves the lateral side of the chest. It is common for a fractured rib end to tear the pleura and lung surface, thereby producing hemopneumothorax. It is also common for a crushed chest to have a flail segment. Pulmonary edema, pneumonitis, and atelectasis often develop rapidly when the chest is crushed, because fluids tend to increase and collect at the injured site.

The "flail" segment no longer has bony or cartilaginous connections with the rest of the rib cage. Lacking attachment to the thoracic skeleton, the flail section "floats," moving independently of the chest wall during ventilation. This disrupts the normal bellows action of the thorax by causing paradoxical motion.

During paradoxical motion, the flail portion of the chest and its underlying lung tissue are (1) "sucked in" with inspiration, instead of expanding outward as normal, and (2) ballooned out ("blown out") with expiration, instead of collapsing normally inward. This alteration in normal chest wall mechanics diminishes the client's ability to achieve an adequate tidal volume and to produce an adequate cough. Hypoventilation and hypoxemia may result, which leads to respiratory failure without rapid intervention.

In addition, pulmonary contusion results in the underlying lung tissue. This produces an accumulation of fluid in the affected alveoli, which leads to intrapulmonary shunting and further hypoxia.

Furthermore, mediastinal structures tend to swing back and forth (mediastinal flutter) with significant paradoxical motion. These "swings" may seriously affect circulatory dynamics, producing elevated venous pressure, impaired filling of the right side of the heart, and decreased arterial pressure.

The client with a flail chest will experience emotional and physical distress while trying to breathe in spite of excruciating pain. The client is typically cyanotic and severely dyspneic. Respirations are usually rapid, shallow, and grunting. Paradoxical movement of the chest wall is usually obvious.

The physiologic abnormalities usually become increasingly serious in the first 48 to 72 hours after injury.

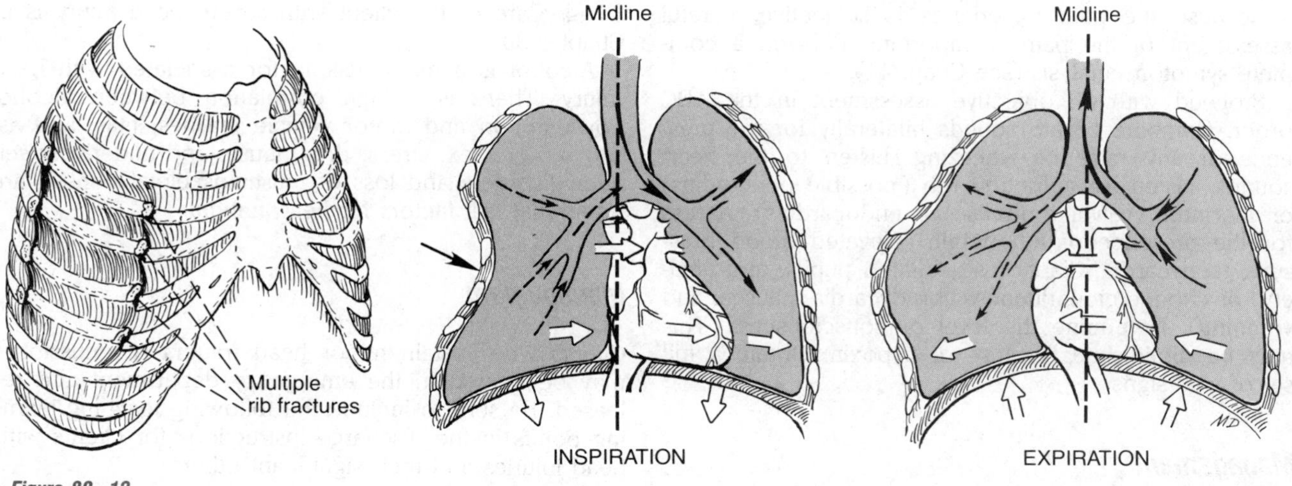

▲ *Figure 80-12*

Flail chest. Solid arrows indicate air movement; open arrows, structural movement. *A,* A flail chest consists of fractured rib segments that are unattached (free-floating) from the rest of the chest wall. *B,* On inspiration, the flail segment of ribs is "sucked" inward. The affected lung and mediastinal structures shift to the unaffected side. This compromises the amount of inspired air in the unaffected lung. *C,* On expiration, the flail segment of ribs "bellows" outward. The affected lung and mediastinal structures shift to the affected side. Some air within the lungs is shunted back and forth between the lungs instead of passing through the upper airway.

Hypercapnia and hypoxia worsen as the effort necessary to breathe further depletes the already diminished oxygen supply.

MANAGEMENT

If severe respiratory distress is present, treatment is usually with intubation and mechanical ventilation. These actions (1) restore adequate ventilation, thus reducing hypoxia and hypercapnia; (2) decrease paradoxical motion by using positive pressure to stabilize the chest wall internally; (3) relieve pain by decreasing movement of the fractured ribs; and (4) provide an avenue for secretion removal. Internal stabilization with continuous ventilation may require 21 days or more. Muscle relaxants or musculoskeletal paralyzing agents (e.g., pancuronium bromide) may be administered to reduce the risk for separation of the healing costochondral junctions.

For the client with adequate pulmonary function, intubation should be avoided. This helps reduce the incidence of infection, a complication associated with higher morbidity and mortality rates in clients with flail chest.[30] Initial treatment in this client is aimed at providing adequate pain relief to prevent splinting, thus enabling the client to deep breathe and effectively clear secretions. Intermittent positive-pressure breathing may be used to enhance lung expansion.

Frequent assessments of blood gases are needed to monitor respiratory effectiveness and detect acidosis. A variety of factors may produce metabolic and respiratory acidosis in chest-injured clients. Frequent x-ray studies are necessary to assess for atelectasis and pneumonia. Chest physiotherapy and postural drainage may be required to facilitate secretion removal. Assess breath sounds before and after any intervention.

Tracheobronchial Trauma

Trauma (rupture, tears) to the tracheobronchial tree may be caused by blunt injury (sternal fracture); caustic ingestion; iatrogenic instrumentation (e.g., it may occur with deep tracheobronchial suctioning or bronchoscopy); or missile or knife wounds. The usual injury site is on the main stem bronchus, within 1 inch above the carina. The most lethal sequela is a tear from the bronchus into the pulmonary veins, which can cause air bubbles to be sent into the systemic circulation. It is particularly dangerous when an air bubble enters the pulmonary vein and goes into a coronary or cerebral vessel, causing cardiac arrest or cerebral air embolism.

Clinical manifestations of tracheobronchial trauma include dyspnea and severe air hunger, hemoptysis (often massive), subcutaneous emphysema into the neck and face, pneumomediastinum, and pneumothorax (simple or tension).

Management of tracheobronchial rupture or tear includes establishment of an airway, administration of high-flow oxygen, closed-chest drainage, and surgical repair.

▼ *Chest Pain*

OVERVIEW

Chest pain is one of the most common complaints of clients entering an emergency department. A client with chest pain presents a diagnostic and management challenge. Effective triage is essential for early detection and intervention of life-threatening conditions. There are several causes of chest pain (see Table 41-1).

Because the pain experience is subjective, careful assessment of the pain is important. Perform a complete symptom analysis (see Chap. 41).

Proceed with an objective assessment in the ABC order. Compare breath sounds bilaterally for the presence of any rales or wheezing. Listen to the heart sounds. Listen for a friction rub (possible pericarditis) or murmurs (valvular disease or endocarditis). Assess for the presence of adrenergic (elevated blood pressure, tachycardia, diaphoresis, dilated pupils, and anxiety) or cholinergic influences (bradycardia, nausea, and vomiting). Determine the level of consciousness. This may be diminished because of hypoxia. Obtain a full set of vital signs.

Management

Provide supplemental oxygen via mask or nasal prongs. Apply a cardiac monitor for monitoring the heart rate and rhythm. A rapid way to do this is to apply the defibrillator pads for a "quick look" after explaining to the client that this is done to determine the heart rate and rhythm. If cardiac origin is suspected, obtain intravenous access and begin an infusion of 5 per cent dextrose with a microdrip at a "keep open" rate. Obtain a 12-lead ECG. Treat any present dysrhythmias (see Chap. 42). Nitroglycerin is commonly used to treat angina or ischemic pain; this may be sublingual, intravenous, or dermal. Be sure to monitor blood pressure after the dose because it may cause hypotension. For severe pain, morphine, 2 to 4 mg intravenously, is administered. Be sure to assess respirations, vital signs, and pain control.

Position the head of the bed for the client's comfort. Obtain ongoing vital signs. If dysrhythmias are present, provide continual cardiac monitoring. Throughout the emergency, provide emotional support and information; use a calm, reassuring manner. Additional interventions will depend on the determined diagnosis. Myocardial infarction is discussed in Chapter 42.

▼ Neurologic/Neurosurgical Emergencies

HEAD TRAUMA

Overview

Any client with an injury to the head or who has experienced an insult that typically produces head trauma requires a thorough neurologic assessment. This is true even if the client appears to feel "fine" when first evaluated.

The major causes of head trauma are motor vehicle crashes, falls, and assaults. Head trauma may range from minor scrapes and contusions to severe blunt and penetrating injuries. Central nervous system effects of severe head injury and treatment are discussed in Table 80-4. Care of the client with severe head injury is in Chapter 30.

Alcohol is a major risk factor associated with head injury. There is a high correlation between alcohol consumption and motor vehicle crashes, falls, and assaults. Age, sex, stress, drug abuse, and underlying seizure disorders and loss of musculoskeletal control are additional risk factors for head trauma.

Management

Clients who sustain minor head trauma (concussions) may be treated in the emergency department and released. Be sure to include the following teaching/learning points in the discharge instructions for clients with head injuries and their significant others.

- Wake the client every 2 hours (for the next 8 hours) and check level of consciousness and orientation.
- Give only liquids initially for the first 8 hours, then progress to a regular diet.
- Give acetaminophen for headache. If stronger medication is required, contact a physician. (Note: emphasize this, because clients often have narcotics from previous illnesses and must understand that narcotics are contraindicated in head injury.)
- Notify a physician or return to the emergency department if any of the following occur: one or both pupils become dilated and nonreactive; the level of consciousness decreases; inability to use an arm or leg develops; seizure is experienced; or there is continued vomiting.
- Provide written as well as verbal instruction, and include an appropriate telephone number for additional questions once the client returns home.

SPINAL INJURIES

Overview

All clients who sustain traumatic injury are at risk for spinal cord injuries. These injuries result in loss of motor or sensory function that may be permanent. Refer to Chapter 32 for further discussion of spinal injuries.

The mechanisms of injury commonly associated with closed spinal injuries involving the cervical area include hyperflexion, hyperextension, flexion compression, and acceleration whiplash (Fig. 80-13). In addition to obvious cord injury (complete or partial transection), edema, hemorrhage, and impaired vertebral artery circulation may cause permanent spinal cord damage.

Management

Assess and maintain the ABCs. Remember to suspect a cervical spine injury in all unconscious trauma victims and with injuries above the clavicle. Immobilize the

TABLE 80-4. Classification of Acute Head Injuries and Treatment Summary

Type of Injury	CNS Effects/Signs and Symptoms	Treatment
Linear fracture	Variable, from none to both localized and generalized signs because of damage to underlying brain tissue Fractures of temporal bone are of concern because of possibility of epidural hematoma Fractures associated with a scalp laceration are considered open fractures; infection and meningitis are concerns	Observation, possibly at home, unless it is a temporal fracture or is associated with a laceration
Basilar skull fracture	A form of linear fracture occurring at base of skull; dural lacerations may occur, exposing brain to contamination from paranasal sinuses and to loss of CSF; meningitis is a major concern Fracture may be difficult to visualize radiographically; thus, physical findings are used to make the diagnosis: blood behind the tympanic membrane/ruptured tympanic membrane with blood in the ear canal; CSF oto- or rhinorrhea; hearing loss; facial nerve palsy; ecchymosis of mastoid area (Battle's sign); periorbital ecchymosis (raccoon eyes); pneumocephalus	Admission for observation, antibiotics, possible surgery if CSF leak continues or infection ensues
Depressed fracture	Variable, depending on damage to underlying brain tissue	Surgery to elevate bone fragments and to treat hematomas or brain injury
Comminuted fracture	More than one fracture line; symptoms variable	Admit for observation This type of fracture suggests that the magnitude of force was great, predisposing to significant vessel or brain injury
Mild concussion	Temporary alterations in neurologic function without loss of consciousness, e.g., confusion, disorientation without amnesia Alterations occur immediately after the accident, are momentary, and are associated with no sequelae	Observation, at home with reliable observers, or in the health care facility
Classic cerebral concussion	Temporary neurologic deficiency associated with temporary loss of consciousness Confusion with amnesia develops 5-10 minutes after accident; permanent amnesia for events immediately preceding the accident Confusion and disorientation usually resolve within a few seconds	Observation, often in the emergency department for several hours or in the health care facility
Intracerebral hematoma/ hemorrhage	Focal or generalized alterations in neurologic function, depending on size and location of injury	Surgical evacuation of hematoma if feasible; ICP monitoring and measures to decrease ICP

CSF, cerebrospinal fluid; CNS, central nervous system.

spine before the client is removed from an automobile or the scene (whenever possible) by applying a hard cervical extrication collar or Philadelphia collar and placing the client on a long spine board. When the client has been extricated, leave the collar in place and secure the head and neck alignment with towel rolls or a head immobilizer, and secure to the backboard. Caution the client not to turn or move the head. Reinforce this frequently, especially if the client is under the influence of drugs or alcohol.

Respiratory insufficiency may be present, especially with a cervical spine injury, because the phrenic nerve (controls the diaphragm during respiration) exits the spinal column at the level of C4. Keep in mind the risk for hypotension related to neurogenic shock.

Assess for pain caused by vertebral displacement or

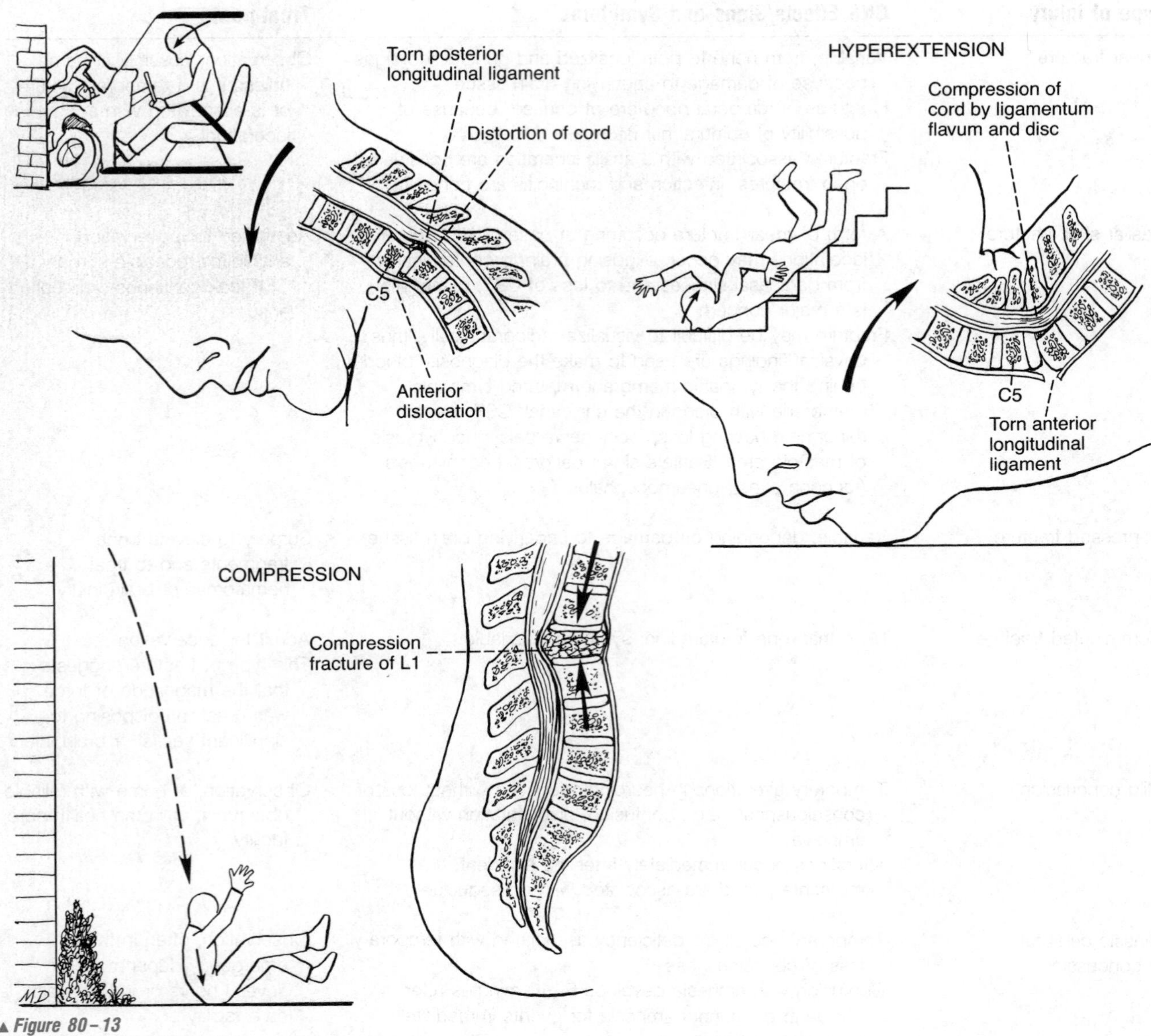

▲ *Figure 80-13*

Mechanisms of spinal injury.

spasm of paraspinal muscles.[38] Note any difficulty moving upper or lower extremities and assess for numbness. Be sure to assess for sacral sparing (an intact anal sphincter and normal sensation in the perineal area S1-S4). If present, this is a positive finding that indicates an incomplete injury. The presence of sacral sparing implies a need to provide special support to the spinal column for prevention of further injury.

Clients with spinal cord injuries may be fully conscious and aware of motor and sensory losses. Fear and anxiety are often present. Be sure to communicate with the client and provide information about any treatments and procedures. Remain calm and reassure the client. Provide comfort measures, and maintain the client's dignity.

▼ Abdominal Emergencies

ACUTE ABDOMEN

Abdominal pain is common; its causes are numerous. Serious emergencies requiring immediate assessment and management must be identified. The term "acute abdomen" is used to describe the condition of a client with a sudden onset of abdominal pain. Most clients with acute abdomens requiring surgery can wait for a more complete evaluation. However, those with intra-abdominal catastrophes like ruptured aortic aneurysm must be identified and managed within minutes. Problems causing an acute abdomen include inflammation with or without perforation, obstruction of a hollow viscus, gastrointestinal hemorrhage, and blunt or penetrating abdominal trauma.

Include the following specific historical information.

- Assess the pain for location, quality, and duration and ask if it radiates. Determine whether there is a history of injury.
- Is there a history of nausea, vomiting, or loss of appetite? What is the amount and character of the emesis, if present?
- When was the last bowel movement? Was it normal? What was the character of the stool? When did the client last eat? What did the client eat?
- What medication or remedies have been used in an attempt to relieve the pain? Are any medications, including over-the-counter drugs, taken on a routine basis?
- Determine the menstrual history in all sexually active females of childbearing age.

Assess the abdomen in order of inspection, auscultation, percussion, and palpation. Assess the client's position. Often a client lying with flexed knees has an inflammatory process (peritonitis), whereas a restless client unable to find a comfortable position may have a colic type pain (ureteral calculi). Assess for distention, masses, umbilical protrusion, and discoloration around the flank (Grey Turner's sign) or umbilicus. Look for evidence of blunt or penetrating trauma. Auscultate for bowel sounds. Note any abnormal, hyperactive, hypoactive, or absent bowel sounds.

Priorities of care focus on maintaining the ABCs. Be sure to monitor vital signs for changes. Initiate intravenous access as needed for hydration and infuse lactated Ringer's solution or normal saline until hypotension or orthostasis is resolved. Keep the client NPO until the cause of the abdominal pain is identified.

RUPTURED OR DISSECTING AORTIC ANEURYSM

Overview

An aneurysm is an outpouching of a vessel wall, usually as a result of arteriosclerotic changes or trauma involving the tunica media (muscular layer of an artery). Aneurysms may be saccular (balloon out) or fusiform (encircle the vessel). Aortic aneurysms may involve the thoracic aorta or abdominal aorta. The abdominal aorta is most commonly affected in males over the age of 60 years. Few emergencies require as rapid and efficient recognition and management as does a ruptured or dissecting aortic aneurysm. A ruptured or dissecting aneurysm is a surgical emergency.

Abdominal aortic aneurysms occur in approximately 2 per cent of the population; 98 per cent of these are infrarenal, which facilitates diagnosis and surgical intervention. Over 80 per cent of abdominal aortic aneurysms are asymptomatic and usually not treated as an emergency.

In aortic dissection, blood separates the vessel layers, and a larger portion of the vessel may be affected. In an expanding aneurysm, the aneurysm wall is still intact. Symptoms are caused by increased pressure on the surrounding structures. A rupture occurs when the vessel wall loses continuity.

Management

Assessment findings include severe abdominal and back pain if the aneurysm is leaking. Back pain is often due to irritation from blood accumulation in the retroperitoneal space. Extreme pain indicates a catastrophic event. Narcotics may be of no value in pain relief but may be administered liberally. Assess for an enlarging abdominal girth with a palpable, pulsatile abdominal mass. There may be leg numbness, tingling, or loss of motor function. Assess for mottled cyanosis below the level of the aneurysm. Profound hypotension is typical, and occasionally initial hypertension occurs. (Note: if the aneurysm is thoracic or dissects into the thoracic aorta, blood pressure may differ significantly on one arm, and chest pain is usually present.) Assess for diminished distal pulses. Monitor urine output for amount and hematuria. The client may be apprehensive, anxious, and restless.

The definitive treatment is surgery. Rapid intervention is vital. Provide supplemental oxygen. Insert two to four large-bore intravenous lines and infuse Ringer's lactate. Monitor the client's fluid response closely to avoid fluid overloading. Monitor vital signs continuously, and institute a cardiac monitor. The PASG may be indicated to help tamponade the bleeding. Antihypertensive agents may be used to minimize extension of a dissection. Obtain blood for laboratory studies (CBC, electrolytes, coagulation screen, and T & C for 10 to 20 units of whole blood). Obtain an ECG and portable chest and abdominal films. Prepare the client and significant others for emergency surgery. Notify the operating room and laboratory of the urgency of the client's condition. Transport the client to the operating room, with resuscitative personnel in attendance and an emergency laparotomy tray on the stretcher. If the client is stable, and the diagnosis unclear, an aortogram may be done. A nurse must be present and provide care during this procedure.

If the client undergoes cardiac arrest before surgery can be performed and is unconscious, there may be no time to reach the operating room. The abdomen or chest may be opened in the emergency department in hopes of saving the client by cross-clamping the aorta. Ensure that necessary instruments are readily available.

GASTROINTESTINAL BLEEDING

The causes of gastrointestinal bleeding are many. Immediate interventions focus on cardiovascular stabilization, identification of the source of bleeding, and attempts to stop the bleeding. Additionally, psychosocial support for the client and significant others is important. Massive bleeding is frightening, and many procedures that may be uncomfortable are carried out rapidly in the initial phase of care.

▼ Abdominal Injuries

OVERVIEW

Abdominal injuries provide a challenge to health care providers. The manifestations of abdominal injuries are often subtle and require astute assessment and intervention. The mechanism of injury, knowledge of abdominal structures, and an index of suspicion provide clues for rapid detection and management of clients with abdominal injuries.

Abdominal injuries, caused by blunt or penetrating trauma, may result in significant organ injury and shock. Low-velocity trauma (fist) usually results in single-organ injury. High-velocity trauma (motor vehicle crashes) often produces multiple-organ involvement. Once the mechanism of injury is identified, keep in mind the potential of associated injuries to underlying organs and tissues. Blunt trauma is more likely to cause injury to the solid organs (spleen, liver, pancreas, or kidneys).

Penetrating abdominal injuries are often caused by gunshot or stab wounds. The underlying injuries will depend on the mechanism of injury, trajectory, and location. Infection (peritonitis) is a common complication with penetrating abdominal trauma, especially if the bowel is ruptured. Hemorrhage and shock may develop if major blood vessels, liver, and spleen are injured. The client with a penetrating abdominal injury will require surgical exploration.

Clinical manifestations include abdominal pain, distention, rigidity, nausea, vomiting, altered or absent bowel sounds, hypotension, and shock. Assess for any open wounds. If open wounds are present, evisceration may occur. Exposure of abdominal contents to air may dry them out and lead to necrosis. If an open wound is found, cover it with a warm, moist, sterile towel.

The spleen is the abdominal organ most commonly injured by blunt trauma, yet injury may also result from penetrating trauma. Small tears may be repaired by a surgical hemostatic agent. For injuries of the left upper quadrant, left lower rib fractures, or left pneumothorax, suspect a spleen injury. Be sure to watch for shock and support the circulatory status.

Liver injury may result from abdominal trauma and should be suspected with right lower rib fractures. The liver is highly vascular, and injury may result in shock and bleeding disorders (clotting factors such as fibrinogen and prothrombin are synthesized in the liver). Surgical repair through hemostatic agents and repair of blood vessels may be indicated.

MANAGEMENT

Manage and support the ABCs. Provide supplemental oxygen. Initiate one to two large-bore intravenous lines and begin fluid support. Obtain serial vital signs. Apply pneumatic anti-shock garments (see Chap. 20) if the client is hypotensive and it is not contraindicated. Draw blood for laboratory studies (CBC, T & C, amylase, aspartate aminotransferase). Insert a urinary catheter and obtain urinalysis and specific gravity. Insert a nasogastric tube, test the aspirate for blood, and connect to suction to decompress the stomach. Obtain abdominal x-ray studies (flat plate, upright, and lateral decubitus views). Prepare the client for an intravenous pyelogram if hematuria is present. An ultrasonogram or CT scan of the abdomen may be performed if the client is stable. A culdocentesis may be done on females. Prepare the client for a diagnostic peritoneal lavage.

A diagnostic peritoneal lavage is performed by a physician to determine the presence of blood in the abdominal cavity (Fig. 80–14). The area below the umbilicus is anesthetized, and a large angiocatheter or peritoneal dialysis catheter is inserted into the abdomen. A syringe is attached to the catheter, and an attempt to aspirate blood is performed. One liter of normal saline is infused into the abdomen and drained by gravity. The fluid is evaluated for gross blood and sent to the laboratory for evaluation. If the finding is positive, prepare the client for immediate surgery.

Discharge Teaching

Many clients with blunt abdominal trauma are assessed and discharged from the emergency department. However, some injuries (delayed rupture of the spleen) may not become apparent for several hours or days. Therefore, it is important to emphasize a need for repeat evaluation, particularly if the following symptoms occur:

- increased localized or generalized abdominal pain
- shoulder pain unrelated to shoulder trauma (Kehr's sign, suggestive of diaphragm irritation due to fluid or blood in the abdominal cavity)
- malaise, lethargy, or dizziness suggestive of slow blood loss
- fever of unexplained origin
- nausea or vomiting, particularly if persistent
- hematemesis or melena

▼ Genitourinary Emergencies

ALLEGED SEXUAL ASSAULT

Overview

Health care providers are required to use the term "alleged sexual assault" when caring for clients who may be victims of rape. Rape is a legal term. Although clients who experienced sexual assault may be males, most are female. Victims of sexual assault should be advised that health professionals are required to use the term "sexual assault" rather than "rape." Otherwise, they may understandably become infuriated by the staff's seeming insensitivity and lack of understanding.

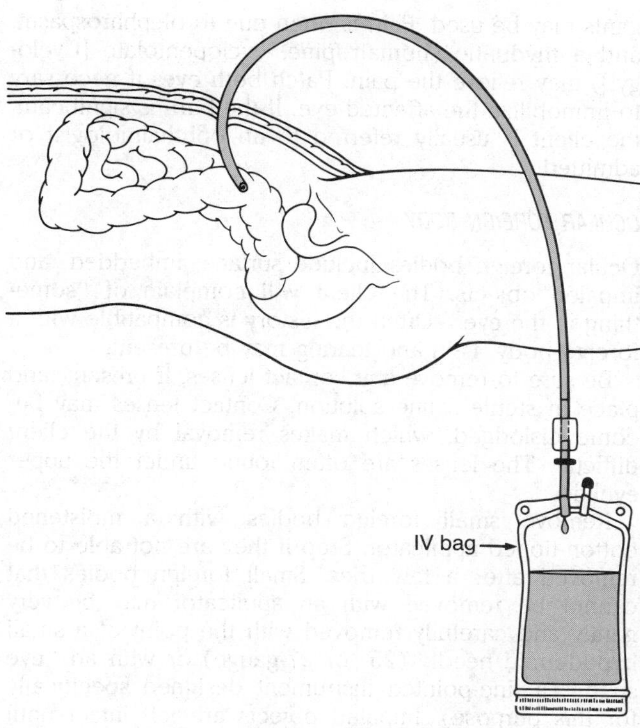

INTERPRETATION OF RESULTS

After blunt injury	
Positive result	Free-flowing blood on aspiration
	>100,000 RBC/mm^3
	>500 WBC/mm^3
	Amylase > serum amylase
	Bile staining
	Presence of foreign body material
	Exit of lavage fluid from urinary or thoracic catheters
Equivocal result	<5 ml bloody aspirate
	50,000–100,000 RBC/mm^3
	100–500 WBC/mm^3
After stab wound	
Positive result	>10,000 RBC/mm^3
	Amylase > serum amylase
	Bile staining
	Presence of foreign material
	Exit of lavage fluid from urinary or thoracic catheters

▲ *Figure 80–14*

Diagnostic peritoneal lavage. (Tabular content from Moore, et al. [1990]. *Early care of the injured patient*. Philadelphia: B. C. Decker.)

Sexual assault victims often experience both acute and long-term physical and psychological trauma. This results from the assault itself and events that follow the assault. The psychological trauma, known as rape-trauma syndrome, may last only a few days to weeks or may last many years.

Lengthy legal proceedings, public humiliation, and destruction of social relationships prolong recovery. Although sexual assault victims may not be physiologically compromised on arrival in the emergency care setting, they are psychologically fragile and should be afforded the highest triage priority.

The goal of emergency care for clients is to provide sensitive, thorough physical care coupled with empathetic psychosocial support and to carefully gather vital information and evidence that is usually legally evaluated. Expedite the registration process and place the client in a private examination room; ensure privacy. If the assault is unreported, encourage reporting it to authorities. Do not give information over the telephone to media or others. Explain to the client not to wash, gargle, or douche until necessary specimens are obtained. Provide the client an opportunity to bathe after the examination.

Obtain a detailed history and physical examination after explaining the need for detail. Take the history immediately and only once. Sexual assault victims report that giving a history is almost as traumatic as the assault. Record the history in detail, using the client's own words. Many agencies have a special form for this history and physical examination.

Management

Begin assessments and interventions with the ABCs. Some clients have massive trauma with loss of consciousness. For others, the physical result of the sexual assault may not be obvious. Consider possible sexual assault in unconscious clients with traumatic injury when the history is unknown or suspicious. Some common signs include ecchymotic areas, especially of the face or neck, and multiple contusions or lacerations. Assess for trauma to the larynx and fracture (with or without dislocation) of the mandible. Record extent, location, and treatment of all injuries. Pictures may be included. In females, a gynecologic examination should be carried out only once, preferably by a practitioner experienced in caring for these clients who will be available for court trial.

Obtain specimens for laboratory study. These include cultures for gonorrhea; hanging drop analysis and smears for the presence of sperm and their motility; acid phosphatase of vaginal secretions; analysis of foreign pubic hairs by the police laboratory; and serologic fluorescent treponemal antibody studies. Refer to specimen collection and chain of custody earlier in this chapter.

Emotional responses may vary. Keep in mind the use of defense mechanisms that preserve psychosocial integrity. Do not assume a lack of concern or relative calm means that the assault did not occur or the client is handling it well. Feelings of guilt, humiliation (especially after meeting with police), and fear may stop many victims from expressing their feelings. Provide psychosocial support and clear, understandable explanations. Obtain the client's permission to contact sexual assault counselors if they are available and it has not already been done. Suggest that someone stay with the client for several days after the event for support.

Note the condition of the client's clothing. Clothes may be stained, torn, or disheveled. However, they may be used as court evidence. Be sure to handle them carefully. Clothes are often taken by the police as evidence, so make arrangements for clean clothes to be brought to the client. Place clothes in a paper bag.

Administer medications as ordered. Penicillin 4.8 million units is given intramuscularly 30 minutes after 1 g of probenecid (Benemid) is given orally for venereal disease prophylaxis. For women, the "morning-after pill," diethylstilbestrol (DES), may be given if the possibility of pregnancy exists. (Note: use of DES is controversial.) Many care facilities require the woman to sign a statement agreeing to abortion if pregnancy occurs while she is receiving DES. DES is taken in doses of 25 mg twice daily for 5 days and should be started within 24 hours. DES often causes nausea, and an antiemetic may be prescribed. It is important that the full 5-day course of therapy be completed. A short course of contraceptive pills may be used instead of DES.

DISCHARGE TEACHING

Discharge teaching includes (1) scheduling of follow-up care in 4 to 6 weeks for test results, pregnancy test, and psychosocial support; (2) providing the name and number of someone to contact if the client is unwilling or unable to use counseling resources at the time of the emergency treatment; (3) discussing some emotional responses to this type of trauma (rape-trauma syndrome); (4) stressing the importance of completing DES treatment; and (5) instructing that menses should start within 7 days after completion of DES; if this does not occur, dilation and curettage is arranged.

Be sure to document the history, assessments, interventions, and discharge teaching carefully. These hospital records are often placed in a "security file" because of possible use in court. Only the medical records department should release records and information and only to authorities with proper credentials.

▼ Ocular Emergencies[41]

Ocular emergencies, involving the eye and surrounding structures, range from mild corneal abrasions to avulsion of the eye. Loss of vision and ocular emergencies receive a high triage priority.

CHEMICAL EYE BURNS

Determine the history. The conjunctiva is often reddened, and there is severe pain. Copious tearing may be present unless deeper structures are involved. Be sure to determine what measures, if any, have been taken to relieve the pain or remove the chemical.

Reassure the client and explain all procedures. Immediately irrigate the eye copiously with normal saline, water, or other mild solution. The eye's pH may be frequently tested and used to guide irrigation. Irrigation may continue until pH is in the 6 to 7 range. Often it is necessary to use a short-acting local anesthetic to irrigate the eye adequately. Evert the upper lid to observe for and remove chemical particles (especially important with alkali burns). Alkali burns may need continuous irrigation for several hours, and special irrigation devices are available. Antibiotic drops, ointments, or irrigants may be used. Pain is often due to blepharospasm, and a mydriatic (homatropine, cyclopentolate [Cyclogyl]) may relieve the pain. Patch both eyes if necessary to immobilize the affected eye. If the burn is significant, the client is usually referred to an ophthalmologist or admitted.

OCULAR FOREIGN BODY

Ocular foreign bodies include surface, imbedded, and impaled objects. The client will complain of "something in the eye." Often the history is compatible with a foreign body. Pain and tearing may be present.

Be sure to remove any contact lenses, if present, and place in sterile saline solution. Contact lenses may become dislodged, which makes removal by the client difficult. The lenses are often found under the upper eyelid.

Remove small foreign bodies with a moistened cotton-tipped applicator. Stop if they are not able to be removed after a few tries. Small foreign bodies that cannot be removed with an applicator may be very gently and carefully removed with the point of a small hypodermic needle (25- or 27-gauge) or with an "eye spud" (a fine-pointed instrument designed specifically for this purpose). Impaled objects are left intact until they are removed by an ophthalmologist. Stabilize the object by applying dressings (moistened with normal saline) around the base of the object and securing the object to the head. Avoid exerting pressure on the globe, and immobilize the head. Do not attempt to stop bleeding from the eye or eyelids with direct pressure. This can cause further injury.

After removal of the foreign body, corneal abrasion, if present, is treated. Treatment includes antibacterial eyedrops or ointment and patching of the eye. A mydriatic is indicated if there is significant pain. Follow-up care in 24 hours is indicated if pain remains. Assessment of visual acuity should be completed and recorded before discharge.

OCULAR AVULSION

Avulsion of the eye from its socket may result from either blunt or penetrating trauma. The eye will be extruded from the orbit with obvious deformity and pain. However, even with rapid and expert care, the probability of preserving vision in the affected eye is slim.

Protect the eye from drying by gently applying sterile dressings moistened with warm saline. Apply an eye protector (cone, shield, paper cup) and secure it gently to the head with gauze Kling or Kerlix. Patch the unaffected eye, and immobilize the head. Provide reassurance, but do not give false hopes about saving the eye. Obtain a prompt ophthalmologist referral. Prepare the client for surgery and keep NPO.

▼ Musculoskeletal Emergencies

Musculoskeletal emergencies include fractures, amputations, joint dislocations, muscle strains, and ligament and tendon damage. These disorders are discussed in Chapter 68.

TRAUMATIC AMPUTATIONS

Traumatic amputations involve obvious total or partial severing of an extremity or digit. The severity of bleeding depends on the extent of trauma to surrounding tissues. A crush injury may not bleed profusely because of muscle spasms in the arterial walls. The artery constricts, and bleeding is decreased. Complete amputations usually do not bleed profusely because the vessels retract. However, a partially severed limb may require a tourniquet for control of bleeding.

Hypotension, shock, and tachycardia may be present if the client sustained significant blood loss. Be sure to maintain and support the ABCs. Initiate intravenous and fluid resuscitation. Control hemorrhage by direct pressure with use of a clean, sterile dressing if possible. Draw blood for laboratory studies (CBC, T & C). Prepare the client for surgery.

The amputated part should accompany the client to the hospital because replantation with microsurgery is sometimes possible. Wrap the amputated part in saline-soaked gauze and place it in a plastic bag or container. Place the container on ice. Do not place the amputated part directly in ice. Do not use dry ice or freeze or totally submerge the tissue. In addition, the part should not be cleaned, disinfected, debrided, or perfused before transportation.

▼ Soft Tissue Emergencies

OVERVIEW

Damage to the skin and soft tissues is a common emergency. The types of soft tissue injury are contusions, abrasions, puncture wounds, lacerations, and avulsions (Fig. 80-15).

Always assess and maintain the ABCs. Assess the wound for location, size, depth, and degree of contamination; assess for associated injuries, amount of tissue loss, and viability of wound edges and of amputated tissue. Determine the history and mechanism of injury. Include information about where the injury occurred, length of time since the injury, and allergies. Obtain immunization history and the need for a tetanus booster. Assess the range of motion and sensation distal to the wound. Ascertain how the injury may affect the client's activities of daily living.

MANAGEMENT

Stop bleeding by direct pressure or application of a pressure dressing. Clean the area around the wound and irrigate well with normal saline. Anesthesia may be needed to clean the wound properly. Apply lidocaine jelly directly into the wound (or gauze pad), or infiltrate the area with 1 per cent lidocaine. Lidocaine 1 per cent without epinephrine is used on fingers, toes, tip of the nose, and ears and for elderly clients with thin skin. Lidocaine with epinephrine is used in other areas to minimize bleeding or prolong anesthesia. It is difficult to determine how much topical lidocaine is absorbed. Be aware of maximal doses for the client's weight. Observe for signs of toxicity such as central nervous system stimulation or depression. A combination of tetracaine, epinephrine, and cocaine applied directly to the wound may also be used for anesthesia.

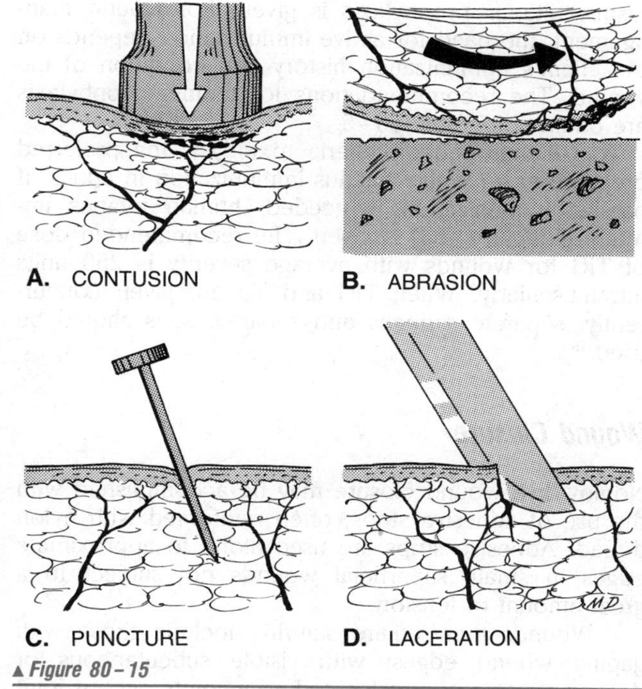

▲ *Figure 80-15*

Soft tissue injuries. *(A)* Contusion is blunt trauma that results in ecchymosis and edema; *(B)* abrasion is a loss of superficial skin. It is often contaminated with dirt or debris. *(C)* Punctures are narrow penetrating wounds that may contain embedded materials, and *(D)* lacerations are incised wounds from sharp objects that bleed freely.

Shave the area around the wound if necessary. Do not shave eyebrows; they are used for landmarks in situations in which extensive repair is needed. Scrub with a soft brush and normal saline. Use forceps to remove imbedded foreign material. Excise the wound if necessary. Copiously irrigate the wound with normal saline. Leave the wound area open, if it is small. For larger areas, or areas where friction may occur (waistline), dress with gauze layers and cover with outer wrap.

The wound may be closed either noninvasively or with sutures. After closure, apply a thin layer of Neosporin, Vaseline, or silver sulfadiazine (Silvadene) to prevent crusting. Apply an appropriate dressing. Air-permeable transparent dressings (i.e., Opsite, Tegaderm) or a layered dressing may be used. Use a pressure dressing with tubular gauze on fingers and toes, and protect the digit with an aluminum splint.

Because of potential exposure to anaerobic organisms, tetanus prophylaxis is given. For wound management, the need for active immunization depends on the client's immunization history and condition of the wound. The recommendations for tetanus prophylaxis are outlined in Table 80-5.

Td (tetanus and diphtheria toxoid) is the preferred preparation for active tetanus immunization in adults. If passive immunization is needed, human tetanus immune globulin (TIG) is given. The recommended dose of TIG for wounds with average severity is 250 units intramuscularly. When TIG and Td are given concurrently, separate syringes and separate sites should be used.[10]

Wound Closure

Noninvasive wound closure may be accomplished with the use of adhesive strips, often reinforced with nylon thread. Adhesive strips are used alone to approximate edges in small, superficial wounds not subject to a great amount of tension.

Wounds that require suturing include those with gaping wound edges; with visible subcutaneous or deeper structures; and located over joints, where joint movement opens the wound edges. Sutures remove dead space, stop hemorrhage, and give physical strength to a discontinuous surface. Although minor suturing is a fairly simple skill, the consequences of an inappropriately sutured wound may lead to poor wound healing, scarring, and infection. Nurses who have received specialized training and ample supervised clinical practice may be responsible for suturing uncomplicated lacerations.

After wound closure, again clean the area and apply a layered dressing. The first layer should promote drainage but not adhere to the wound (Owen's silk, fine mesh gauze). The second layer promotes absorption (gauze sponges). The third layer minimizes dead space and provides sight pressure. A woven roller gauze (Kling or Kerlix) may be held in place by either adhesive tape or elastic net. Avoid placing adhesive tape over the wound area; occlusive tape may foster moisture accumulation and maceration of wound edges. A petroleum-based ointment is often applied directly to wound edges for minimizing crusting and promoting a thinner scar. A transparent dressing may

TABLE 80-5. Summary of Tetanus Prophylaxis in Routine Wound Management

History of Tetanus Immunization (Doses)	Clean, Minor Wounds		All Other Wounds	
	Td	TIG	Td	TIG
Uncertain	Yes	No	Yes	Yes
0-1	Yes	No	Yes	Yes
2	Yes	No	Yes	No
3 or more	No	No	No	No

Recommendations of the Centers for Disease Control (1986). *Mortality and morbidity weekly report.*

be used in wounds not expected to swell or have large amounts of drainage.

If sutured wound edges are perfectly opposed and not disturbed or manipulated, adhesion of the edges occurs in about 6 hours, and infection cannot enter. Dry skin is more resistant to infection than is moist skin, and friction increases the potential for infection. The dressing should be left in place until time for suture removal. Dressings should be removed only if there is excessive bleeding, drainage, unexplained fever, or other indications of infection.

Discharge Teaching

Discharge teaching includes (1) tissue swelling continues 8 to 12 hours after the injury. Therefore, keep the pressure dressing on, elevate the injured area, and apply cool packs. (2) Keep dressings clean and dry. (3) Emphasize importance of suture removal, and when and where it is done. (4) Teach how to take any prescribed medications (antibiotics, analgesics). (5) Have the client return if signs of infection occur (swelling, increasing pain, redness, drainage, fever). (6) Inform the client how to carry out activities of daily living with the dressing in place (use rubber gloves; place plastic bag over injured extremity while showering or bathing).

HEAT EMERGENCIES

Overview

Exposure to increased environmental temperature may lead to heat emergencies. As the temperature increases, the sweat glands attempt to cool the body through diaphoresis (sweating). As the temperature continues to increase, the body compensates with profuse sweating. Unless fluids and salts are replaced, hypotension, dehydration, sodium depletion, and electrolyte imbalances may occur from excess fluid loss through perspiration.

Clients who are very young, elderly, or receiving diuretics or anticholinergic and phototaxic drug regimens are at greater risk for developing heat emergencies. Be sure to assess the client's history for cardiac, pulmonary, or renal diseases and drug regimens. At discharge, these clients need to be taught about side effects of drug regimens and ways to avoid or reduce exposure to extremes in temperature.

TYPES OF HEAT EMERGENCIES

Heat Cramps. Heat cramps are muscle spasms of arms, legs, and occasionally abdomen related to sodium depletion from excessive perspiration. Remove the client from the hot environment and administer oral fluids containing salt.

Heat Exhaustion. Heat exhaustion results from heat-induced hypotension due to excessive fluid loss through sweating. Symptoms include a headache, dizziness, faintness, anorexia, and nausea; skin may be cool and clammy. Vital signs will vary, depending on the degree of volume depletion. Remove the client from the heat. Administer oral or intravenous fluids as needed.

Heatstroke. Heatstroke is an emergency and requires immediate treatment for survival. There are two forms of heatstroke: classic heatstroke and exertional heatstroke.

Classic heatstroke is seen most commonly in the poor, the elderly, the chronically ill, clients with heart disease, the obese, and alcoholics. Hot humid weather lasting 3 days or more increases the risk of heatstroke in these clients. The stress of the heat increases the demand on the heart. In addition, certain medications increase the risk of heatstroke. Some medications decrease the ability to sweat; these include antihistamines, beta-blockers, anticholinergics, and phenothiazines. Other medications, such as amphetamines and neuroleptics, increase heat production.

Exertional heatstroke is more common in laborers, farmers, military recruits, athletes (especially football players and long distance runners), and clients who work in boiler rooms or foundries. Symptoms of this form of heatstroke are similar to classic heatstroke except these clients sweat. They tend to develop lactic acidosis and have more severe bleeding problems.

Burns. Burn injury is discussed in Chapter 72.

Management

Rapidly reduce body temperature (immerse or sponge with cool water). A hypothermia blanket may be used. Start an intravenous line and provide cardiovascular support. Apply a cardiac monitor and obtain frequent vital signs. Administer chlorpromazine or diazepam to reduce shivering. Provide supplemental oxygen. Insert a urinary catheter unless recovery is prompt. Admit the client to the hospital.

HYPOTHERMIA

Hypothermia is defined as a lowered core body temperature, usually below 34.4° C (94° F). It may occur in divers, clients exposed to cold weather, and near-drowning victims. Some clients appear dead yet have a feeble pulse. Pupils may be fixed and dilated. Symptoms depend on the client's core temperature: 34.4° C (94° F), amnesia or sluggishness; 32.2° C (90° F), cardiac dysrhythmias, especially premature ventricular contractions; 30° C (86° F), loss of muscle coordination, possible unconsciousness; and 25° C (77° F), cardiac arrest.

Support the ABCs. Endotracheal intubation may be indicated. Initiate CPR when indicated. Insert an esophageal thermometer or rectal thermometer probe. Start an intravenous line and central venous pressure line if hypothermia is severe. Draw blood for laboratory studies (CBC, electrolytes, BUN, sugar, creatinine, coagulation screen, amylase, and ABGs). Monitor the cardiac rhythm and obtain a 12-lead ECG. (Note: an Osborne wave or "J wave" may occur; it is a positive deflection of the terminal 0.04 second of the QRS complex.) Insert a urinary catheter and monitor output every 30 minutes.

Core rewarming is performed by use of heated oxygen and gastric, urinary bladder, and peritoneal lavage with heated fluids. Do not apply heat to a profoundly hypothermic client. It causes vasodilation and further cardiovascular collapse. Peripheral rewarming is usually delayed until the client's core temperature has been raised. Resuscitation is not usually successful until adequate core rewarming has been achieved and efforts should not be abandoned until rewarming is accomplished. If necessary, the client may be transferred to the operating room for rewarming with a bypass machine.[27]

Be aware that often there is a great deal of water on the floor during immediate resuscitation of a client with profound hypothermia. Use a battery-powered defibrillator, rather than one connected to a higher voltage wall outlet, to protect the staff from electrical hazard.

FROSTBITE

Frostbite is damage to tissues and blood vessels as a result of prolonged exposure to cold. Fingers, toes, nose, and ears are often affected. There may be initial numbness, paresthesia, and pallor of the affected part. Often, severe pain, swelling, erythema, and blistering (similar to a second-degree, partial-thickness burn) occurs once the client is in a warm environment. Necrosis and gangrene may develop in severe cases.

Handle the tissues gently. Rewarm the affected part with use of tepid water (about 105° F). Massage should never be used; this may result in further tissue damage. Debridement of blisters is controversial. Apply bulky dressings to permit drainage and provide protection. A bed cradle may be needed.

Additional studies may include arteriography or scintiscanning to determine the extent of injury or to open vasoconstricted vessels. Vasodilators or nerve block may be prescribed.

SNAKE BITES

Overview

Four poisonous snakes are found in the United States. Three of these are pit vipers (rattlesnakes, copperheads, and water moccasins), and the other is a coral snake. Not all who are bitten are envenomated. Snake bites in the spring may be more severe because the venom is more concentrated at that time of year.

Local reactions are an intense burning pain immediately after the bite. There is swelling and copious bleeding. Blisters and blebs develop within 1 hour and become large and hemorrhagic. Significant swelling occurs. Generalized reactions may be present. Assess for muscle twitching and fasciculation, especially around the mouth. There may be a metallic taste, nausea, vomiting, and gastrointestinal tract bleeding. There may be diaphoresis, tachycardia, and hypotension as the client develops shock. Perform a neurologic assessment for syncope and coma. Carefully monitor respirations; they may become shallow and progress to respiratory arrest as the envenomation spreads.

Management

Maintain and support the ABCs. Act calmly and reassure the client. Position the client at rest, immobilize the involved part, and place it at heart level. Apply a constricting band above the site to minimize lymphatic and superficial venous return. It should not be tighter than a watchband. Start one to two large-bore intravenous lines and hang Ringer's lactate. Draw blood for laboratory studies (CBC, T & C, coagulation screen, electrolytes, BUN, sugar, erythrocyte sedimentation rate). If whole blood is needed, fresh rather than stored blood should be used. Obtain a urinalysis.

Wash the skin; incise and suction wounds (note: incision should be done within 20 minutes after the bite; beyond that time, it is probably ineffective). Incision of the wound depends on the degree of envenomation and local preference for treatment. Opinions vary regarding the value of incision and at what grade of envenomation it should be performed. Incisions should be superficial and no more than 1/4 inch long and 1/8 inch deep, preferably from one fang to the other. Envenomated tissue may be excised. Limit initial wound care to cleansing and dressing with large absorbent, bulky dressings.

Administer antivenin by intravenous drip within 1 hour. Dosages range from 3 to 40 vials, depending on the degree of envenomation and the client's age and size. Be sure to do skin (or eye) allergy testing before administration. Measure the girth of the extremity proximal to the bite every 15 to 30 minutes as a guide for additional antivenin. Administer tetanus prophylaxis. Steroids may be used for anaphylactic reactions but are contraindicated in routine management of snake bites because they may enhance the absorption of venom or block antivenin action.

Provide pain relief. Administer aspirin or codeine for mild pain and meperidine hydrochloride for more severe pain. Observe the client for respiratory depression after narcotic administration.

Teach the client to wear high leather boots and thick trousers when walking through known areas for snakes. Heavy gloves should be worn when climbing in rocky areas.

ANIMAL BITES

Animal bites may result in puncture wounds, lacerations, and avulsions, especially if the client pulled away from the animal while its teeth were clenched. There is a potential for infection from bacteria normally residing in the animal's mouth (i.e., *Pasteurella multocida*). Be sure to assess the possibility of rabies from the biting animal. Rabies is an infectious virus that affects the central nervous system, especially the brain. The incidence of rabies in domesticated animals is very low in the United States, but the disease is fatal.

Obtain the history of the bite. Include the type of animal, owner of the animal, description of the incident (provoked or unprovoked), location of the animal, and the animal's immunization history and state of health. Assess the type of wound and amount of tissue damage. Be sure to include a neurovascular and musculoskeletal assessment.

Carefully clean, irrigate, and debride the wound. Assess for possible associated fractures, especially of the hand or head. Apply a bulky, fluffy, and absorbent dressing. Place fingers in the position of function. Administer tetanus prophylaxis and antibiotics as prescribed. Rabies prophylaxis is used if the animal cannot be found and kept for observation, in areas where rabies is endemic, or if there is a high index of suspicion for rabies. Report the incident to public health officials, animal control services, or police. Be sure to provide psychosocial support for the client and significant others. The experience of being bitten by a domestic animal, particularly a family pet, can be devastating.

HUMAN BITES

Human bites may be self-induced (tongue laceration), result from dental abrasions (usually superficial at the metacarpophalangeal joint incurred during a fist fight if the client's knuckle hit the opponent's tooth), or be penetrating bites causing puncture wounds and tissue loss. Human bites can cause severe necrotizing infections and require vigorous intervention.

Determine the history of the bite. Assess the neurovascular and musculoskeletal function carefully. Increased pain over the site may indicate a fracture. Fractures and tendon lacerations, especially of the hand, are common. Obtain x-ray studies if indicated.

Carefully clean and vigorously irrigate the wound. Open and debride puncture wounds. Wounds are usually not sutured unless they are large or located on the face. Loosely placed sutures or adhesive strips may be used. Administer broad-spectrum antibiotics and tetanus prophylaxis. The client with severe human bites may be admitted for at least 24-hour observation.

▼ Poisoning and Overdose

OVERVIEW

Accidental or intentional poisonings (overdoses) requiring emergency care occur frequently. Phone inquiries are often received by emergency department staff regarding poisonings. It is important that nurses responsible for emergency care be knowledgeable about the management and complications of poisoning and overdoses. Various resources are available (Poison Control Centers, Poison Index and toxicology tests). An emergency nurse needs a working knowledge of agents commonly used or abused, especially currently popular street drugs (see Chap. 79).

Obtain an accurate history; include the following questions. (1) Was the substance inhaled, injected, ingested, sniffed, or confined to skin surfaces? (2) How long ago was the event, and what was the amount? (3) In what kind of environment was the client found? (4) Were there any associated incidents (fire, trauma, near-drowning)? (5) Is there a history of prescribed medications? allergies? medical problems? What is the state of physical and mental health? Keep in mind that despite careful fact finding and detailed questioning, a history of the nature and amount of the toxic substance and the time since ingestion may be grossly inaccurate. Clients with toxic substance ingestion may exaggerate or minimize the conditions of an overdose in order to achieve other goals. The history is considered in planning the care. However, reliance on physical examination is also important.

Management

The acronym SIRES is an aid in remembering the essential care in cases of poisoning:

- Stabilize the client
- Identify the toxic substance
- Reverse its effect
- Eliminate the substance from the body
- Support the client/significant others (physically and psychosocially)

Maintain the ABCs. Assessment findings associated with various toxins and antidotes are included in Table 80-6. Be sure to stabilize the ABCs. Perform a rapid physical examination. Start intravenous lines, and obtain appropriate laboratory studies including toxicology screen. Initiate a cardiac monitor, and obtain an ECG. Insert a urinary catheter.

Select an appropriate means of reversing or eliminating the toxic substance. Home-remedy methods of inducing emesis (such as manual stimulation of the posterior pharynx, drinking salt water or mustard water, or eating raw eggs) may be listed in first aid books or on container labels. These measures are often unsafe and ineffective. The safest and most effective method of inducing emesis is through administering syrup of ipecac.

Syrup of ipecac is safe and effective when used in properly selected clients (Box 80-5). The dose is 15 to 30 ml (1 to 10 years, 15 ml; over 10 years, 30 ml), administered orally, preceded or followed by several hundred milliliters of water or other solution (juice). Emesis usually occurs within 15 to 20 minutes. However, a second dose can be given 20 minutes after the first dose. Do not give more than two doses. It is important that enough oral fluid be given to prevent retching and possible esophageal tears. Save emesis for possible toxicologic analysis. Note the presence or absence of pill particles.

TABLE 80-6. Assessment Findings Associated with Various Toxins

Physical Signs or Symptoms	Toxins to Be Considered
Vomiting, nausea, diarrhea	Heavy metals (lead, arsenic); alcohols (ethanol, methanol, ethylene glycol); salicylates; digitalis; morphine and its analogs
Coma	Barbiturates; chloral hydrate; paraldehyde; bromide; ethchlorvynol; carbon monoxide; salicylates; atropine; scopolamine; ethanol
Delirium, agitation	Atropine; scopolamine; alcohol; amphetamines; barbiturates; physostigmine
Convulsions	Phenothiazines; strychnine; propoxyphene; amphetamines; alcohols (ethanol, methanol, ethylene glycol); salicylates; carbon monoxide; cholinesterase inhibitors; hydrocarbons
Dilated pupils	Amphetamines; glutethimide; alcohols; belladonna group; meperidine; cocaine; ephedrine; sympathomimetics; parasympatholytics; cyanide; botulin toxin
Constricted pupils	Morphine; propoxyphene; barbiturates; chloral hydrate
Partial or total blindness	Methanol
Pink skin	Carbon monoxide; cyanide; atropine (skin flushed and dry); phenothiazine
Kussmaul's respiration	Salicylates; methanol; ethanol; ethylene glycol
Dry mouth	Belladonna group; botulin toxin; antihistamines; morphine; phenothiazines; tricyclic antidepressants
Hematemesis	Mercuric chloride; salicylates; phosphorus; fluoride
Diaphoresis	Alcohol; insulin; fluoride; physostigmine salicylate
Extrapyramidal tremor	Phenothiazines

Modified from Cohen, A. S., et al. (1977). *Medical emergencies: Diagnostic and management procedures from Boston City Hospital.* Boston: Little, Brown.

Gastric lavage may be indicated. However, it is believed to be less effective than emesis in removing ingested substances from the stomach. Thus, it is reserved for use in clients with central nervous system depression, those with diminished or absent gag reflex, or those unable to cooperate with emetic therapy. Remember that gastric lavage is not a deterrent to future overdose attempts and should not be used as a punitive measure.

Box 80–5. Cautions in the Use of Ipecac

- Use only syrup of ipecac, not ipecac fluid extract.
- Always ensure an intact gag reflex before giving ipecac. Do not assume a physician has done this.
- Ipecac may be ineffective in inducing emesis after ingestion of substances with antiemetic properties.
- Ipecac in large doses may be cardiotoxic. Lavage may be necessary if emesis does not occur.
- Frequently reassess the client. The client may become obtunded when the emesis occurs, and aspiration may result.
- Ipecac is most effective when adequate amounts of oral fluids are administered.

Gastric Lavage. Gastric lavage involves inserting a large-bore (30- to 36-French, in adults) Ewald tube through the nose or mouth and then washing out the stomach contents by use of normal saline, half saline (0.45 per cent sodium chloride), or tap water. The volume of each "run" of fluid instilled into the stomach varies, depending on the age and tolerance of the client (250 to 500 ml in adults). Avoid volumes in excess of 500 ml, because large volumes may foster passage of substances into the duodenum. Lavage is carried out until fluid return is clear. Although larger amounts are sometimes used, the normal volume rarely exceeds 10 L.

An effective, time-saving, and accurate system for gastric lavage is illustrated in Figure 80–16. The system includes bags of normal saline irrigation fluid, tubing, a

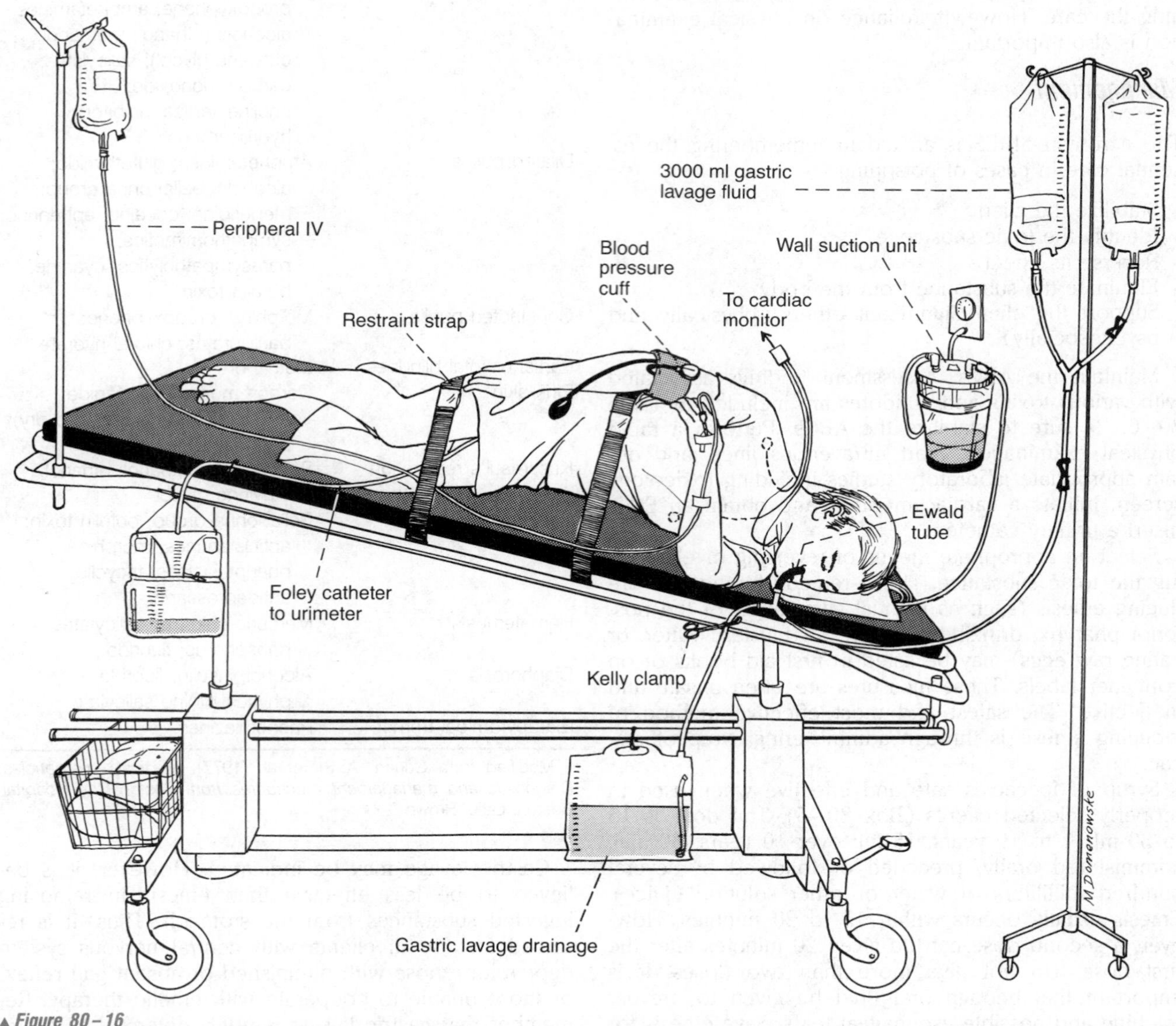

▲ *Figure 80–16*

Position of client and location of equipment during gastric lavage in poisoning/overdose management. Client is shown uncovered for illustration purposes. Maintaining warmth is important.

Y connector, clamps, and a collecting system. When such a system is used, gastric lavage can safely and effectively be carried out by one person with a minimum of difficulty.

Gastric lavage is not without hazard. Death due to inadvertent pulmonary placement of the tube and subsequent instillation of lavage fluid has been reported, and bradydysrhythmias and aspiration of gastric fluid are not uncommon complications of this procedure.

Absorptives are also used. Activated charcoal powder, usually mixed with water, is administered in doses of 25 to 50 g (0.5 to 1 g/kg) to absorb any remaining particles of toxic substance. This may be administered orally or inserted through an Ewald tube. Because it is black and does not easily mix in water, activated charcoal may be mixed with cherry syrup, sorbitol, or similar substances to make it more palatable.

Antidotes/antagonists may be used in selected cases for management or diagnosis of the toxic substance (Table 80-7). Remember that although an antidote may produce significant results initially, the half-life of the toxic substance may be longer than the antidote. For instance, naloxone (Narcan) is a potent antidote for opiate overdoses. Even though the client may initially respond rapidly, as the naloxone wears off, the client may become obtunded. Clients receiving antidotes/antagonists must be observed for several hours before being discharged.

Other measures, depending on the client's condition, may include diuresis, fluid loading, cooling or warming, anticonvulsive therapy, antidysrhythmic therapy, hemodialysis, hemoperfusion, or exchange transfusions. Nursing care involves assessing the client and the responses, carrying out therapies, and providing supportive care. Remember that an accidental or intentional poisoning may be reported to a poison control facility or additional agency.

For the client who intentionally overdoses, empathy and understanding are necessary. Vindictive or hostile attitudes are destructive and maximize feelings of guilt and low self-esteem. If the client is awake, one way to foster communication is to say, "You must have been feeling bad to do this." The client may then feel able to talk about problems and may be more receptive to counseling. Remember the suicidal attempt may be repeated while the client is receiving care for the overdose. Be sure to implement suicide precautions.

A psychiatric evaluation is indicated for all clients who intentionally overdose or whose intentions seem unclear. The evaluation should occur before discharge, and plans for follow-up care should be well established. Investigate and use available support systems. Someone should stay with the client for the next several days. Provide a telephone number for the crisis team or clinic and written instructions for follow-up care.

TABLE 80-7. Antidotes Commonly Used in Managing Poisoned or Overdosed Clients

Substance	Antidote
Cholinesterase inhibitors, e.g., organophosphate insecticides, nerve gases, carbamates	Atropine
Iron	Deferoxamine
Insulin	Dextrose 50%
Mercury, arsenic, lead, heavy metals	Dimercaprol, disodium edetate, penicillamine
Methanol, ethylene glycol	Ethanol
Lead	EDTA (ethylenediaminetetraacetic acid)
Acetaminophen	*N*-Acetylcysteine (Mucomyst)
Narcotics and narcotic derivatives, opiates	Naloxone (Narcan)
Cyanide	Amyl nitrite, sodium nitrite, sodium thiosulfate
Carbon monoxide	Oxygen
Cholinesterase inhibitors	2-PAM (Protopam)
Atropine, scopolamine, tricyclic antidepressants	Physostigmine (Antilirium)
Anticoagulants, e.g., warfarin (Coumadin)	Vitamin K

▼ DEATH AND DYING IN EMERGENCY CARE SETTINGS

Death in the emergency department presents different problems to significant others and health care givers than death from a prolonged illness. There is often little time to interact with the dying client or to provide grief and loss counseling. Significant others may be overwhelmed by the suddenness of the event and feel there is not enough time to resolve their "unfinished business" with the dying person. Particular concerns of the dying client and significant others in the emergency department include the following:

- Because there may not be much time before death actually takes place, make sure the dying client and significant others have ample opportunity to be together. Delay, if possible, procedures that will disrupt communication between the dying client and significant others, such as endotracheal intubation.
- Allowing the presence of significant others during resuscitation is not necessarily disruptive, as traditionally thought, and can help survivors move through grief work in a less traumatic way. It can lessen their doubts about the loved one receiving the best care, and can involve them in decisions regarding termination of protracted and futile resuscitation measures.
- Religious support can be extremely important for the client and significant others, and nurses should have a clear understanding of how to access that support.
- The client's condition should be communicated to significant others in periodic updates containing clearly stated factual information.

- Viewing the body, particularly in instances of sudden death or trauma, is encouraged. This process can facilitate the grieving process.
- Because preservation of legal evidence is often important in sudden death, significant others are advised beforehand of the various tubes and devices present.
- The client's wishes concerning organ donation must be determined. Required Request Laws (federal and state) facilitate this question because all hospitalized clients are asked about organ donation.
- A follow-up telephone call or visit may be beneficial in answering the questions or concerns of the significant others.
- Referral to a support group that assists survivors is often helpful. The health care facility or community social service agency can provide a list of the support groups in each area.

▼ Medical Examiner's/Coroner's Jurisdiction

A medical examiner, a physician with special training in forensic pathology, is concerned with determining the manner and cause of death. In the United States, deaths associated with the following are reported to the medical examiner's office: (1) suspected suicides or homicides; (2) deaths in which the deceased has not been attended by a physician within 24 hours before death; (3) deaths with suspicious circumstances; (4) deaths due to accidents; (5) deaths after surgery; (6) deaths associated with firearms or other weapons; (7) deaths occurring as a result of crime; (8) stillbirths; (9) deaths resulting from drugs; and (10) deaths possibly associated with hazards to public safety (infectious diseases that may cause epidemics).

When notified of death, the medical examiner may accept or decline jurisdiction for determining the manner and cause of death. If jurisdiction is accepted, the medical examiner may conduct an autopsy or other investigation or grant the hospital caring for the deceased permission to perform an autopsy. Permission from significant others for postmortem examination in these circumstances is not required.

When the medical examiner plans to conduct the autopsy, it is important that all evidence be preserved. Therefore, all tubes, instruments, and devices are left in place, especially intravenous catheters. The deceased is not washed, nails are not cleaned, and any body fluids on the deceased at the time of death are left on, including clothing. Clothing that has been removed is carefully placed in a paper bag so that decomposition does not obscure any evidence. When removing clothing, do not cut through bullet holes, stab wound tears, or other tears. Do not wash the clothing. All valuables and clothing must be inventoried with the medical examiner's staff. Only they may release these items to significant others. Refer to specimen collection and chain of custody earlier in this chapter. A copy of the medical record is given to the medical examiner's staff. The record must be detailed, with special attention given to injuries and marks noted on arrival of the deceased and a description of and location of tubes, surgical incisions, venipunctures, and other therapeutic interventions.

Summary

Emergency care is very challenging and rewarding. By knowing and using the principles of emergency care, nurses can function effectively, regardless of the environment in which the care is delivered. Because of the variety of emergency problems encountered, nurses need to be responsible and accountable for updating their knowledge and skills. Besides technical competence, nurses provide psychosocial care to clients and significant others. As a specialty, emergency nursing provides stimulating and professional opportunities. Emergency nurses are active in health promotion, prevention, education, research, and emergency care. Emergency nurses are on the forefront of providing competent and professional care to a variety of clients and significant others.

Bibliography

1. American Heart Association (1990). *Textbook of advanced cardiac life support* (2nd ed.). Dallas: American Heart Association.
2. American Hospital Association (1990). Emergency transfer (patient dumping): provisions of budget bill. *Washington Watch, 11,* 9–10. Washington, DC: American Hospital Association.
3. Bobb, J. (1988). Trauma in the elderly. In V. Cardona, et al. (Eds.), *Trauma nursing: From resuscitation through rehabilitation.* Philadelphia: W. B. Saunders.
4. Boortz-Marx, R. (1985). Factors affecting intracranial pressure: a descriptive study. *Journal of Neurosurgical Nursing, 17*(2), 89–94.
5. Bullock, B. (1988). Metabolic and immunologic response to trauma. In E. Howell, et al. (Eds.), *Comprehensive trauma nursing: Theory and practice.* Chicago: Scott, Foresman and Company.
6. Cardona, V. (1988). Nursing practice through the trauma cycles. In V. Cardona, et al. (Eds.), *Trauma nursing: From resuscitation through rehabilitation.* Philadelphia: W. B. Saunders.
7. Committee on Trauma, American College of Surgeons (1985). *Advanced trauma life support course manual.* Chicago: American College of Surgeons.
8. Committee on Trauma Research, Commission on Life Sciences, National Research Council (1985). *Injury in America: A continuing public health problem.* Washington, DC: National Academy Press.
9. Eastman, A. B., et al. (1987). Regional trauma system design: critical concepts. *The American Journal of Surgery, 154*(7), 79–84.
10. Emergency Nurses Association (1991). J. Dains, et al. (Eds.), *Standards of emergency nursing practice* (2nd ed.). St. Louis: Mosby–Year Book.
11. Emergency Nurses Association (1988). R. Rea (Ed.), *Trauma nursing core course provider manual* (2nd ed.). Chicago: Emergency Nurses Association.
12. Fadale, J. (1990). Overcrowding, comfort, consideration, convenience. *Journal of Emergency Nursing, 16*(3), 132–133.
13. Faylor, J., & Royer, C. (1991). Intraosseous infusion for emergency intravascular access. *Trauma Talk Newsletter* (fall). Omaha: Saint Joseph Hospital at Creighton University Medical Center.

14. Figley, C. R. (1983). Catastrophes: an overview of family reactions. In C. Figley & H. McCubbin (Eds.), *Stress and the family* (vol II). Coping with catastrophe. New York: Brunner/Mazel.
15. Fraser, S., & Atkins, J. (1990). Survivors' recollection of helpful and unhelpful nursing activities surrounding sudden death of a loved one. *Journal of Emergency Nursing, 16*(1), 13-16.
16. *Grief by homicide* (1983). Seattle: Family and Friends of Missing Persons and Violent Crime Victims.
17. Halpern, J. (1989). Mechanisms and patterns of trauma. *Journal of Emergency Nursing, 15*(5), 380-388.
18. Hammond, S. C. (1990). Chest injuries in the trauma patient. *Nursing Clinics of North America, 25*(1), 35-44.
19. Harchelroad, S. (1990). *Comparing the role of the emergency nurse involved in trauma resuscitations* (unpublished thesis). Pittsburgh: University of Pittsburgh.
20. Harrahill, M., & Bartkus, E. (1990). Preparing the trauma patient for transfer. *Journal of Emergency Nursing, 16*(1), 25-28.
21. Haynes, B. (1985). Near drowning. In J. Tintinalli, et al. (Eds.), *Emergency medicine: A comprehensive study guide*. St. Louis: McGraw-Hill.
22. Hendrickson, S. (1987). Intracranial pressure changes and family presence. *Journal of Neuroscience Nursing, 19*(1), 14-17.
23. Howell, E., et al. (1988). *Comprehensive trauma nursing: Theory and practice*. Chicago: Scott, Foresman and Company.
24. Hoyt, D., et al. (1988). Video recording trauma resuscitations: an effective teaching technique. *The Journal of Trauma, 28*(4), 435-440.
25. Ilano, A., & Raffin, T. (1990). Management of carbon monoxide poisoning. *Chest, 97*(1), 165-169.
26. Jensen, A. (1980). *Healing grief*. Redmond, WA: Medic Publishing.
27. Judkins, D., & Iserson, K. (1991). Rapid admixture blood warming. *Journal of Emergency Nursing, 17*(3), 146-151.
28. Lenehan, G. P. (1989). ED gridlock and blaming the victim. *Journal of Emergency Nursing, 15*(3), 211-213.
29. Lenehan, G. (1986). Emotional impact of trauma. *Nursing Clinics of North America, 21*(4), 729-740.
30. LoCicero, J., & Mattox, K. (1989). Epidemiology of chest trauma. *Surgical Clinics of North America, 69*(1), 15-19.
31. McCaffery, M., & Beebe, A. (1989). *Pain: Clinical manual for nursing practice*. St. Louis: C. V. Mosby.
32. McGinnis, G. (1988). Central nervous system I: Head injuries. In V. Cardona, et al. (Eds.), *Trauma nursing: From resuscitation through rehabilitation*. Philadelphia: W. B. Saunders.
33. McQuillan, K., & Wiles, C. (1988). Initial management of traumatic shock. In V. Cardona, et al. (Eds.), *Trauma nursing: From resuscitation through rehabilitation*. Philadelphia: W. B. Saunders.
34. Morris, J. A., et al. (1991). Trauma patients return to productivity. *The Journal of Trauma, 31*(6), 827-833.
35. National Safety Council (1985). *Accident facts*. Chicago: National Safety Council.
36. Orlowski, J., et al. (1989). The hemodynamic and cardiovascular effects of near drowning in hypotonic, isotonic or hypertonic solutions. *Annals of Emergency Medicine, 18*(10), 1044-1049.
37. Pisarcik, G., & deLeon, B. (1981). On compassion. *Journal of Emergency Nursing, 7*, 237.
38. Potter, D. (Ed.) (1989). *Emergencies*. Nurse's Reference Library, Nursing 89 Books. Springhouse, PA: Springhouse Corporation.
39. Powers, M. J., et al. (1983). Use of the emergency department by patients with nonurgent conditions. *Journal of Emergency Nursing, 9*(3), 145-149.
40. Ramler, C. (1990). Triage. In S. Kitt & J. Kaiser (Eds.), *Emergency nursing: A physiologic and clinical perspective*. Philadelphia: W. B. Saunders.
41. Shingleton, B. (1991). Eye injuries. *The New England Journal of Medicine, 325*(6), 408-413.
42. Smith, L., & Glowac, B. (1989). New frontiers in the management of the multiply injured patient. *Critical Care Nursing Clinics of North America, 1*(1), 1-9.
43. Thom, S., & Keim, L. (1989). Carbon monoxide poisoning: a review of epidemiology, pathophysiology, clinical findings and treatment options including hyperbaric oxygen therapy. *Clinical Toxicology, 27*(3), 141-156.
44. West, J. G., et al. (1988). Trauma systems: current status—future challenges. *Journal of the American Medical Association, 259*(24), 3597-3600.
45. Zwicke, D., et al. (1982). Triage nurse decisions: a prospective study. *Journal of Emergency Nursing, 8*(3), 132-138.

Laboratory Values of Clinical Importance

Appendix 1

Reference laboratory values can provide guidelines for the clinician to use when assessing clients with a wide variety of problems. It should be remembered that the laboratory values given here are for reference only, and are not absolute normal values. The nurse also should remember that there is no sharp dividing line between normal and abnormal. Clients with only slightly elevated values may have apparent disease whereas those with more elevated values may not. Trends in laboratory values are often much more valuable than the single value.

This section provides a summary of the common laboratory diagnostic studies for use as a quick reference. A complete explanation of the diagnostic study and its meaning is covered in the appropriate section (such as liver function studies in Chap. 57). This section simply provides a handy way to check out the normal values for the most common diagnostic studies. For details concerning the meaning of the value, see the appropriate section in the text.

The following abbreviations are used throughout the laboratory studies.

g = gram
kg = kilogram
mg = milligram (10^{-3})
μg = microgram (10^{-6})
ng = nanogram (10^{-9})
pg = picogram (10^{-12})
L = liter
ml = milliliter
dl = deciliter (100 ml)
fL = femtoliter
mm = millimeter
mm³ = cubic millimeter
U = unit
mU = milliunits
μU = microunits
mOsm = milliosmole
mol = mole
μmol = micromole
nmol = nanomole
pmol = picomole
fmol = femtomole (10^{-15})
mEq = milliequivalent

Reference Values in Hematology
(For some procedures the reference values may vary, depending upon the method used)

Test		Conventional Units	SI Units
Acid hemolysis test (Ham)		No hemolysis	No hemolysis
Alkaline phosphatase, leukocyte		Total score 14 to 100	Total score 14 to 100
Cell counts			
Erythrocytes			
Males		4.6 to 6.2 million/mm^3	4.6 to 6.2 $\times 10^{12}$/L
Females		4.2 to 5.4 million/mm^3	4.2 to 5.2 $\times 10^{12}$/L
Children (varies with age)		4.5 to 5.1 million/mm^3	4.5 to 5.1 $\times 10^{12}$/L
Leukocytes, total		4500 to 11,000/mm^3	4.5 to 11.0 $\times 10^9$/L
Leukocytes, differential	***Percentage***	***Absolute***	***Absolute***
Myelocytes	0	0/mm^3	0/L
Band neutrophils	3 to 5	150 to 400/mm^3	150 to 400 $\times 10^6$/L
Segmented neutrophils	54 to 62	3000 to 5800/mm^3	3000 to 5800 $\times 10^6$/L
Lymphocytes	25 to 33	1500 to 3000/mm^3	1500 to 3000 $\times 10^6$/L
Monocytes	3 to 7	300 to 500/mm^3	300 to 500 $\times 10^6$/L
Eosinophils	1 to 3	50 to 250/mm^3	50 to 250 $\times 10^6$/L
Basophils	0 to 0.75	15 to 50/mm^3	15 to 50 $\times 10^6$/L
Platelets		150,000 to 350,000/mm^3	150 to 350 $\times 10^9$/L
Reticulocytes		25,000 to 75,000/mm^3 0.5 to 1.5 per cent of erythrocytes	25 to 75 $\times 10^9$/L
Coagulation tests			
Bleeding time (template)		2.75 to 8.0 min	2.75 to 8.0 min
Coagulation time (glass tubes)		5 to 15 min	5 to 15 min
Factor VIII and other coagulation factors		50 to 150 per cent of normal	0.5 to 1.5 of normal
Fibrin split products (Thrombo-Welco test)		$<$10 μg/ml	$<$10 mg/L
Fibrinogen		200 to 400 mg/dl	2.0 to 4.0 g/L
Partial thromboplastin time (PTT)		20 to 35 sec	20 to 35 sec
Prothrombin time (PT)		12.0 to 14.0 sec	12.0 to 14.0 sec
Coombs' test			
Direct		Negative	Negative
Indirect		Negative	Negative
Corpuscular values of erythrocytes			
Mean corpuscular hemoglobin (MCH)		26 to 34 pg	0.40 to 0.53 fmol
Mean corpuscular volume (MCV)		80 to 96 micra^3	80 to 96 fL
Mean corpuscular hemoglobin concentration (MCHC)		32 to 36 per cent	0.32 to 0.36 per cent
Haptoglobin		26 to 185 mg/dl	260 to 1850 mg/L
Hematocrit			
Males		40 to 54 ml/dl	0.40 to 0.54 volume fraction
Females		37 to 47 ml/dl	0.37 to 0.47 volume fraction
Newborn		49 to 54 ml/dl	0.49 to 0.54 volume fraction
Children (varies with age)		35 to 49 ml/dl	0.35 to 0.49 volume fraction
Hemoglobin			
Males		14.0 to 18.0 g/dl	2.17 to 2.79 mmol/L
Females		12.0 to 16.0 g/dl	1.86 to 2.48 mmol/L
Newborn		16.5 to 19.5 g/dl	2.56 to 3.02 mmol/L
Children (varies with age)		11.2 to 16.5 g/dl	1.74 to 2.56 mmol/L
Hemoglobin, fetal		$<$1.0 per cent of total	$<$0.01 per cent of total
Hemoglobin A_{1C}		3 to 5 per cent of total	0.03 to 0.05 per cent of total
Hemoglobin A_2		1.5 to 3.0 per cent of total	0.015 to 0.03 per cent of total
Hemoglobin, plasma		0 to 5.0 mg/dl	0 to 0.8 μmol/L
Methemoglobin		30 to 130 mg/dl	4.7 to 20 μmol/L
Sedimentation rate (ESR)			
Wintrobe, males		0 to 5 mm/h	0 to 5 mm/h
females		0 to 15 mm/h	0 to 15 mm/h
Westergren, males		0 to 15 mm/h	0 to 15 mm/h
females		0 to 20 mm/h	0 to 20 mm/h

Reference Values for Blood, Plasma, and Serum
(For some procedures the reference values may vary, depending upon the method used)

	Conventional Units	SI Units
Acetoacetate plus acetone		
Qualitative	Negative	Negative
Quantitative	0.3 to 2.0 mg/dl	3 to 20 mg/L
Acid phosphatase, serum (thymolphthalein monophosphate substrate)	0.11 to 0.60 U/L	0.11 to 0.60 U/L
Adrenocorticotropin, plasma (ACTH)		
6:00 AM	10 to 80 pg/ml	10 to 80 ng/L
6:00 PM	<50 pg/ml	<50 ng/L
Alanine aminotransferase, serum (ALT, SGPT)	7 to 35 U/L	7 to 35 U/L
Albumin, serum	3.5 to 5.5 g/dl	35 to 55 g/L
Aldolase, serum	1.5 to 12.0 U/L	1.5 to 12.0 U/L
Aldosterone, plasma		
Supine	3 to 10 ng/dl	0.08 to 0.30 nmol/L
Standing		
Male	6 to 22 ng/dl	0.17 to 0.61 nmol/L
Female	5 to 30 ng/dl	0.14 to 0.83 nmol/L
Alkaline phosphatase, serum (ALP)	20 to 90 U/L (30° C)	20 to 90 U/L (30° C)
Ammonia nitrogen, plasma	15 to 49 μg/dl	11 to 35 μmol/L
Amylase, serum	25 to 125 U/L	25 to 125 U/L
Anion gap	8 to 16 mEq/L	8 to 16 mmol/L
Ascorbic acid, blood	0.4 to 1.5 mg/dl	23 to 85 μmol/L
Aspartate aminotransferase, serum (AST, SGOT)	7 to 40 U/L	7 to 40 U/L
Base excess, blood	0 ± 2 mEq/L	0 ± 2 mmol/L
Bicarbonate, venous plasma	23 to 29 mEq/L	23 to 29 mmol/L
arterial blood	18 to 23 mEq/L	18 to 23 mmol/L
Bile acids, serum	0.3 to 3.0 mg/dl	3 to 30 mg/L
Bilirubin, serum		
Conjugated	0.1 to 0.4 mg/dl	1.7 to 6.8 μmol/L
Unconjugated	0.2 to 0.7 mg/dl	3.4 to 12 μmol/L
Total	0.3 to 1.1 mg/dl	5.1 to 19 μmol/L
Calcium, serum	9.0 to 11.0 mg/dl	2.25 to 2.75 mmol/L
Calcium, ionized, serum	4.25 to 5.25 mg/dl	1.05 to 1.30 mmol/L
Carbon dioxide, total, serum or plasma	24 to 30 mEq/L	24 to 30 mmol/L
Carbon dioxide tension, blood P_{CO_2}	35 to 45 mm Hg	35 to 45 mm Hg
β-Carotene serum	40 to 200 μg/dl	0.74 to 3.72 μmol/L
Catecholamines, plasma		
Epinephrine	15 to 55 pg/ml	82 to 300 pmol/L
Norepinephrine	65 to 400 pg/ml	384 to 2364 pmol/L
Ceruloplasmin, serum	23 to 44 mg/dl	230 to 440 mg/L
Chloride, serum or plasma	96 to 106 mEq/L	96 to 106 mmol/L
Cholesterol, serum or EDTA plasma		
Desirable range	<200 mg/dl	<5.18 mmol/L
LDL Cholesterol	60 to 180 mg/dl	600 to 1800 mg/L
HDL Cholesterol	30 to 80 mg/dl	300 to 800 mg/L
Copper		
Males	70 to 140 μg/dl	11 to 22 μmol/L
Females	85 to 155 μg/dl	13 to 24 μmol/L
Cortisol, plasma		
8:00 AM	6 to 23 μg/dl	170 to 635 nmol/L
4:00 PM	3 to 15 μg/dl	82 to 413 nmol/L
10:00 PM	<50 per cent of 8 AM value	<0.5 per cent of 8 AM value
Creatine, serum	0.2 to 0.8 mg/dl	15 to 61 μmol/L
Creatine kinase, serum (CK, CPK)		
Males	55 to 170 U/L	55 to 170 U/L
Females	30 to 135 U/L	30 to 135 U/L
Creatine kinase MB isozyme, serum	0.0 to 4.7 ng/ml	0.0 to 4.7 μg/L
Creatinine, serum	0.6 to 1.2 mg/dl	53 to 108 μmol/L

Table continued on following page

Reference Values for Blood, Plasma, and Serum
(For some procedures the reference values may vary, depending upon the method used) Continued

	Conventional Units	SI Units
Ferritin, serum	20 to 200 ng/ml	20 to 200 μg/L
Fibrinogen, plasma	200 to 400 mg/dl	2.0 to 4.0 g/L
Folate, serum	1.8 to 9.0 ng/ml	4.1 to 20.4 nmol/L
erythrocytes	150 to 450 ng/ml	340 to 1020 nmol/L
Follicle-stimulating hormine, plasma (FSH)		
Males	4 to 25 mU/ml	4 to 25 U/L
Females	4 to 30 mU/ml	4 to 30 U/L
Postmenopausal	40 to 250 mU/ml	40 to 250 U/L
γ-Glutamyltransferase, serum		
Males	5 to 38 U/L	5 to 38 U/L
Females	5 to 29 U/L	5 to 29 U/L
Gastrin, serum	0 to 200 pg/ml	0 to 200 ng/L
Glucose (fasting), plasma or serum	70 to 115 mg/dl	3.89 to 6.38 mmol/L
Growth hormone, plasma (hGH)	0 to 10 ng/ml	0 to 10 μg/L
Haptoglobin, serum	26 to 185 mg/dl	260 to 1850 mg/L
Immunoglobulins, serum		
IgG	550 to 1900 mg/dl	5.5 to 19.0 g/L
IgA	60 to 333 mg/dl	0.60 to 3.3 g/L
IgM	45 to 145 mg/dl	0.45 to 1.5 g/L
IgD	0.5 to 3.0 mg/dl	5 to 30 mg/L
IgE	<500 ng/ml	<500 μg/L
Insulin (fasting), plasma	5 to 25 μU/ml	36 to 179 pmol/L
Iron, serum	75 to 175 ng/dl	13 to 31 μmol/L
Iron-binding capacity, serum		
Total	250 to 410 μg/dl	45 to 73 μmol/L
Saturation	20 to 55 per cent	0.20 to 0.55
Lactate, venous blood	4.5 to 19.8 mg/dl	0.50 to 2.2 mmol/L
arterial blood	4.5 to 14.4 mg/dl	0.50 to 1.6 mmol/L
Lactate dehydrogenase, serum (LD, LDH)	100 to 190 U/L	100 to 190 U/L
Lipase, serum	10 to 140 U/L	10 to 140 U/L
Lipids, total, serum	450 to 850 mg/dl	4.5 to 8.5 g/L
Luteinizing hormone, serum (LH)		
Males	6 to 18 mU/ml	6 to 18 U/L
Females premenopausal	5 to 22 mU/ml	5 to 22 U/L
midcycle	3 times baseline	3 times baseline
postmenopausal	>30 mU/ml	>30 U/L
Magnesium, serum	1.8 to 3.0 mg/dl	0.75 to 1.25 mmol/L
Osmolality	286 to 295 mOsm/kg water	285 to 295 mOsm/kg water
Oxygen blood		
Capacity (varies with hemoglobin)	16 to 24 vol per cent	7.14 to 10.7 mmol/L
Content, arterial	15 to 23 vol per cent	6.69 to 10.3 mmol/L
Saturation, arterial	94 to 100 per cent	0.94 to 1.00
Tension, Po_2	75 to 100 mm Hg	75 to 100 mm Hg
P_{50}	26 to 27 mm Hg	26 to 27 mm Hg
pH, arterial blood	7.35 to 7.45	7.35 to 7.45
Phenylalanine, serum	<3 mg/dl	<0.18 mmol/L
Phosphate, inorganic, serum	3.0 to 4.5 mg/dl	1.0 to 1.5 mmol/L
Potassium, serum or plasma	3.5 to 5.0 mEq/l	3.5 to 5.0 mmol/L
Prolactin, serum		
Males	1 to 20 ng/ml	1 to 20 μg/L
Females	1 to 25 ng/ml	1 to 25 μg/L
Protein, serum		
Total	6.0 to 8.0 g/dl	60 to 80 g/L
Albumin	3.5 to 5.5 g/dl	35 to 55 g/L
$alpha_1$-globulin	0.2 to 0.4 g/dl	2 to 4 g/L
$alpha_2$-globulin	0.5 to 0.9 g/dl	5 to 9 g/L
beta globulin	0.6 to 1.1 g/dl	6 to 11 g/L
gamma globulin	0.7 to 1.7 g/dl	7 to 17 g/L

Reference Values for Blood, Plasma, and Serum
(For some procedures the reference values may vary, depending upon the method used) Continued

	Conventional Units	SI Units
Pyruvate, blood	0.3 to 0.9 mg/dl	0.03 to 0.10 mmol/L
Sodium, serum or plasma	136 to 145 mEq/L	136 to 145 mmol/L
Testosterone, plasma		
Males	275 to 875 ng/dl	9.0 to 10.0 nmol/L
Females	23 to 75 ng/dl	0.8 to 2.6 nmol/L
Pregnant	38 to 190 ng/dl	1.3 to 6.6 nmol/L
Thyroid-stimulating hormone, serum (TSH)	0 to 7 μU/ml	0 to 7 mU/L
Thyroxine, free, serum (FT_4)	1.0 to 2.1 ng/dl	13 to 27 pmol/L
Thyroxine, serum (T_4)	4.4 to 9.9 μg/dl	57 to 128 nmol/L
Triglycerides, serum	40 to 150 mg/dl	0.4 to 1.5 g/L
Triiodothyronine, serum (T_3)	150 to 250 ng/dl	2.3 to 3.9 nmol/L
Triiodothyronine uptake, resin (T_3RU)	25 to 38 per cent uptake	0.25 to 0.38 uptake
Urate		
Males	2.5 to 8.0 mg/dl	0.15 to 0.48 mmol/L
Females	1.5 to 7.0 mg/dl	0.09 to 0.42 mmol/L
Urea, serum or plasma	24 to 49 mg/dl	4.0 to 8.2 mmol/L
Urea nitrogen, serum or plasma	11 to 23 mg/dl	3.9 to 8.2 mmol/L
Viscosity, serum	1.4 to 1.8 × water	1.4 to 1.8 × water
Vitamin A, serum	20 to 80 μg/dl	0.70 to 2.80 μmol/L
Vitamin B_{12}, serum	180 to 900 pg/ml	133 to 664 pmol/L

Reference Values for Urine
(For some procedures the reference values may vary, depending upon the method used)

	Conventional Units	SI Units
Acetone and acetoacetate, qualitative	Negative	Negative
Albumin		
Qualitative	Negative	Negative
Quantitative	10 to 100 mg/24 h	10 to 100 mg/24 h
Aldosterone	3 to 20 μg/24 h	8.3 to 55 nmol/24 h
δ-Aminolevulinic acid	1.3 to 7.0 mg/24 h	10 to 53 μmol/24 h
Amylase	3 to 20 U/h	3 to 20 U/h
Amylase/creatinine clearance ratio	1 to 4 per cent	0.01 to 0.04 per cent
Bilirubin, qualitative	Negative	Negative
Calcium (usual diet)	$<$250 mg/24 h	$<$6.3 mmol/24 h
Catecholamines		
Epinephrine	$<$10 μg/24 h	$<$55 nmol/24 h
Norepinephrine	$<$100 μg/24 h	$<$590 nmol/24 h
Total free catecholamines	4 to 126 μg/24 h	24 to 745 nmol/24 h
Total metanephrines	0.1 to 1.6 mg/24 h	0.5 to 8.1 μmol/24 h
Chloride (varies with intake)	110 to 250 mEq/24 h	110 to 250 nmol/24 h
Copper	0 to 50 μg/24 h	0 to 0.80 μmol/24 h
Cortisol, free	10 to 100 μg/24 h	27.6 to 276 nmol/24 h
Creatinine	15 to 25 mg/kg body weight/24 h	0.13 to 0.22 mmol/kg body weight/24 h
Creatinine clearance (corrected to 1.73 m^2 body surface area)		
Males	110 to 150 ml/min	110 to 150 ml/min
Females	105 to 132 ml/min	105 to 132 ml/min
Dehydroepiandrosterone		
Males	0.2 to 2.0 mg/24 h	0.7 to 6.9 μmol/24 h
Females	0.2 to 1.8 mg/24 h	0.7 to 6.2 μmol/24 h
Estrogens, total		
Males	4 to 25 μg/24 h	14 to 90 nmol/24 h
Females	5 to 100 μg/24 h	18 to 360 nmol/24 h
Glucose (as reducing substance)	$<$250 mg/24 h	$<$250 mg/24 h
Hemoglobin and myoglobin, qualitative	Negative	Negative
17-Hydroxycorticosteroids		
Males	3 to 9 mg/24 h	8.3 to 25 μmol/24 h
Females	2 to 8 mg/24 h	5.5 to 22 μmol/24 h

Reference Values for Urine
(For some procedures the reference values may vary, depending upon the method used) Continued

	Conventional Units	SI Units
5-Hydroxyindoleacetic acid		
Qualitative	Negative	Negative
Quantitative	<9 mg/24 h	<47 μmol/24 h
17-Ketosteroids		
Males	6 to 18 mg/24 h	21 to 62 μmol/24 h
Females	4 to 13 mg/24 h	14 to 45 μmol/24 h
Magnesium	6.0 to 8.5 mEq/24 h	3.0 to 4.2 mmol/24 h
Metanephrines (see Catecholamines)		
Osmolality	38 to 1400 mOsm/kg water	38 to 1400 mOsm/kg water
pH	4.6 to 8.0	4.6 to 8.0
Phenylpyruvic acid, qualitative	Negative	Negative
Phosphate	0.9 to 1.3 g/24 h	29 to 42 mmol/24 h
Porphobilinogen		
Qualitative	Negative	Negative
Quantitative	<2.0 mg/24 h	<9 μmol/24 h
Porphyrins		
Coproporphyrin	50 to 250 μg/24 h	77 to 380 nmol/24 h
Uroporphyrin	10 to 30 μg/24 h	12 to 36 nmol/24 h
Potassium	25 to 100 mEq/24 h	25 to 100 mmol/24 h
Pregnanediol		
Males	0.4 to 1.4 mg/24 h	1.2 to 4.4 μmol/24 h
Females, proliferative phase	0.5 to 1.5 mg/24 h	1.6 to 4.7 μmol/24 h
luteal phase	2.0 to 7.0 mg/24 h	6.2 to 22 μmol/24 h
postmenopausal	0.2 to 1.0 mg/24 h	0.6 to 3.1 μmol/24 h
Pregnanetriol	<2.5 mg/24 h	<7.4 μmol/24 h
Protein		
Qualitative	Negative	Negative
Quantitative	10 to 150 mg/24 h	10 to 150 mg/24 h
Sodium	130 to 260 mEq/24 h	130 to 260 mmol/24 h
Specific gravity	1.003 to 1.030	1.003 to 1.030
Urate	200 to 500 mg/24 h	1.2 to 3.0 mmol/24 h
Urobilinogen	<4.0 mg/24 h	<6.8 μmol/24 h
Vanillylmandelic acid (VMA) (4-hydroxy-3-methoxymandelic acid)	1 to 8 mg/24 h	5 to 40 μmol/24 h

Reference Values for Therapeutic Drug Monitoring

	Therapeutic Range	Toxic Levels	Proprietary Names
Antibiotics			
Amikacin, serum	25 to 30 μg/ml	Peak >35 μg/ml Trough >5 to 7 μg/ml	Amikin
Chloramphenicol, serum	10 to 20 μg/ml	>25 μg/ml	Chloromycetin
Gentamicin, serum	5 to 10 μg/ml	Peak >12 μg/ml Trough >2 μg/ml	Garamycin
Tobramycin, serum	5 to 10 μg/ml	Peak >12 μg/ml Trough >2 μg/ml	Nebcin
Anticonvulsants			
Carbamazepine, serum	5 to 12 μg/ml	>12 μg/ml	Tegretol
Ethosuximide, serum	40 to 100 μg/ml	>100 μg/ml	Zarontin
Phenobarbital, serum	10 to 30 μg/ml	Vary widely because of developed tolerance	Luminal
Phenytoin, serum	10 to 20 μg/ml	>20 μg/ml	Dilantin
Primidone, serum	5 to 20 μg/ml	>15 μg/ml	Mysoline
Valproic acid, serum	50 to 100 μg/ml	>100 μg/ml	Depakene
Analgesics			
Acetaminophen, serum	10 to 20 μg/ml	>250 μg/ml	Tylenol Datril
Salicylate, serum	100 to 250 μg/ml	>300 μg/ml	
Bronchodilator			
Theophylline, serum (aminophylline)	10 to 20 μg/ml	>20 μg/ml	Theo-Dur
Cardiovascular Drugs			
Digitoxin, serum (specimen must be obtained 12 to 24 hours after last dose)	15 to 25 ng/ml	>25 ng/ml	Crystodigin
Digoxin, serum (specimen must be obtained 12 to 24 hours after last dose)	0.8 to 2.0 ng/ml	>2.4 ng/ml	Lanoxin
Disopyramide, serum	2 to 5 μg/ml	>5 μg/ml	Norpace
Lidocaine, serum	1.5 to 5.0 μg/ml	>6 to 8 μg/ml	Xylocaine
Procainamide, serum	4 to 10 μg/ml	>16 μg/ ml	Pronestyl
Measured as procainamide + *N*-acetyl procainamide	10 to 30 μg/ml	>30 μg/ml	
Propranolol, serum	50 to 100 ng/ml	Variable	Inderal
Quinidine, serum	2 to 5 μg/ml	>10 μg/ml	Cardioquin Quinaglute Quinidex Quinora
Psychopharmacologic Drugs			
Amitriptyline, serum (measured as amitriptyline + nortriptyline)	120 to 150 ng/ml	>500 ng/ml	Amitril Elavil Endep Entrafon Limbitrol Triavil
Desipramine, serum (measured as desipramine + imipramine)	150 to 300 ng/ml	>500 ng/ml	Norpramin Petrofrane
Imipramine, serum (measured as imipramine + desipramine)	150 to 300 ng/ml	>500 ng/ml	Antipress Janimine Presamine Tofranil
Lithium, serum (obtain specimen 12 hours after last dose)	0.8 to 1.2 mEq/L	>2.0 mEq/L	Lithobid
Nortriptyline, serum	50 to 150 ng/ml	>500 ng/ml	Aventyl Pamelor

Reference Values in Toxicology

	Conventional Units	SI Units
Arsenic, blood	3.5 to 7.2 μg/dl	0.47 to 0.96 μmol/L
Arsenic, urine	<100 μg/24 h	<1.3 μmol/24 h
Bromides, serum	0	0
	Toxic above 17 mEq/L	Toxic above 17 mmol/L
Carboxyhemoglobin, blood	<5 per cent saturation	<0.05 saturation
Symptoms occur	>20 per cent saturation	>0.20 saturation
Ethanol, blood	<0.05 mg/dl	<1.0 mmol/L
	<0.005 per cent	
Marked intoxication	300 to 400 mg/dl	65 to 87 mmol/L
	0.3 to 0.4 per cent	
Alcoholic stupor	400 to 500 mg/dl	87 to 109 mmol/L
	0.4 to 0.5 per cent	
Coma	>500 mg/dl	>109 mmol/L
	>0.5 per cent	
Lead, blood	0 to 40 μg/dl	0 to 2 μmol/L
Lead, urine	<100 μg/24 h	<0.48 μmol/24 h
Mercury, urine	<100 μg/24 h	<50 nmol/24 h

Reference Values for Cerebrospinal Fluid

	Conventional Units	SI Units
Cells	<5/mm^3	<5 × 10^6/L
	All mononuclear	All mononuclear
Electrophoresis	Predominantly albumin	Predominantly albumin
Glucose	50 to 75 mg/dl	2.8 to 4.2 mmol/L
	(20 mg/dl less than serum)	(1.1 mmol/L less than serum)
IgG		
Children under 14	<8 per cent of total protein	<0.08 of total protein
Adults	<14 per cent of total protein	<0.14 of total protein
IgG index $\frac{\text{CSF/serum IgG ratio}}{\text{CSF/serum albumin ratio}}$	0.3 to 0.6	0.3 to 0.6
Oligoclonal banding on electrophoresis	Absent	Absent
Pressure	70 to 180 mm water	70 to 180 mm water
Protein, total	15 to 45 mg/dl	150 to 450 mg/L

Reference Values for Feces

	Conventional Units	SI Units
Bulk	100 to 200 g/24 h	100 to 200 g/24 h
Dry matter	23 to 32 g/24 h	23 to 32 g/24 h
Fat, total	<6.0 g/24 h	<6.0 g/24 h
Nitrogen, total	<2.0 g/24 h	<2.0 g/24 h
Water	Approximately 65 per cent	Approximately 0.65

Reference Values for Semen Analysis

	Conventional Units	SI Units
Volume	2 to 5 mL	2 to 5 ml
Liquefaction	Complete in 15 min	Complete in 15 min
Leukocytes	Occasional or absent	Occasional or absent
Count	60 to 150 million/ml	60 to 150 × 10^6/ml
Motility	>80 per cent motile	>0.80 motile
Morphology	80 to 90 per cent normal forms	0.80 to 0.90 normal forms
Fructose	>150 mg/dl	>8.33 mmol/L

Reference Values for Assessment of Gastrointestinal Function

Test	Normal Range	Significance of Abnormal Findings
Complete Blood Count		
Red blood cells	4.2 to 5.4 million/mm³ (women) 4.5 to 6.2 million/mm³ (men)	Decreased values indicate possible: Anemia Hemorrhage
Hemoglobin	12 to 16 g/dl (women) 14 to 18 g/dl (men)	Increased values indicate possible: Hemoconcentration caused by dehydration
Hematocrit	38 to 46 per cent (women) 42 to 54 per cent (men)	
Electrolytes		
Potassium	3.5 to 5.0 mg/L	Decreased values indicate possible: Gastrointestinal suction Diarrhea Vomiting Intestinal fistulas
Calcium	8.0 to 10.5 mg/dl	Decreased values indicate possible: Malabsorption
Sodium	135 to 145 mg/L	Decreased values indicate possible: Malabsorption Diarrhea
D-Xylose	Blood levels peak (25 to 40 mg/dl) 2 hours after ingestion 80 to 95 per cent excreted in 5 hours	Decreased values indicate possible: Malabsorption
CEA	Less than 5 ng/ml (nonsmokers)	Increased values indicate possible: Colorectal cancer Inflammatory bowel disease
Fecal Analysis		
Stool for occult blood	Negative	Presence indicates possible: Peptic ulcer Cancer of the colon Ulcerative colitis
Stool for ova and parasites	Negative	Presence indicates: Infection
Stool cultures	No unusual growth	Presence of pathogens may indicate: *Shigella* *Salmonella* *Staphylococcus aureus* *Bacillus cereus*
Stool for lipids	2 to 5 g/24 h (normal diet)	Increased values indicate possible: Malabsorption syndrome Crohn's disease

Reference Values for Tumor Markers

Test	Reference Value	Conditions in Which Levels Are Elevated
Alpha-fetoprotein (AFP)	<10 ng/ml	↑ in lung, nonseminomatous testicular, pancreatic, colon, and stomach cancers, and choriocarcinoma
CA-125	<35 units	↑ in ovarian cancer
Calcitonin	<100 pg/ml	↑ in medullary thyroid, small cell lung, and breast cancers, and carcinoid
Carcinoembryonic antigen (CEA)	0 to 2.5 ng/ml nonsmokers <3.0 ng/ml smokers	↑ in colorectal, breast, lung, stomach, pancreatic, and prostate cancers
Estrogen receptors	Negative <10 fmol/mg	↑ in breast cancer
Human chorionic gonadotropin (HCG)	0 to 5 IU/L	↑ in choriocarcinoma, germ cell testicular, lung, liver, stomach, pancreatic, endometrial, and liver cancers
Progesterone receptor assay	Negative < 10 fmol/mg	↑ in breast cancer
Prostatic acid phosphatase	0.26 to 0.83 U/L	↑ in metastatic prostate cancer
Prostate specific antigen (PSA)	0 to 4 ng/ml	↑ in prostate cancer
CA-19-9		↑ in pancreatic and colon cancer
CA-15-3		↑ in breast cancer

Modified from Conn, R. B. (1991). *Current diagnosis* (8th ed., pp. 1307-1312). Philadelphia, W. B. Saunders.

▼ NCLEX-RN Test Plan

Appendix 2

GENERAL DESCRIPTION

The NCLEX-RN is a 2-day examination designed by the National Council of State Boards of Nursing (NCSBN) to test the graduate's ability to practice entry level registered nursing in a safe and effective manner. This is done by testing the graduate's knowledge of entry-level nursing practice through the application of that knowledge to health care situations requiring interventions by the beginning nurse. The contents of the examination were identified, based on a study by Kane and associates[1] in *A Study of Nursing Practice and Role Delineation and Job Analysis of Entry-Level Performance of Registered Nurses*, which analyzed the activities of the entry-level registered nurse. This study established a framework of entry-level performance that incorporated the nursing process and specific client needs. Using the test plan, "each NCLEX-RN examination reflects the knowledge, skills and abilities essential for application of the phases of the nursing process to meet the needs of clients with commonly occurring health problems."[2]

The examination itself consists of four separate examinations with a total of 360 to 372 questions divided into the four books. This examination is given over 2 days, and two books are used. One and a half hours each are given in the morning and afternoon of the first day, and the same pattern is followed on the second day. The questions are written by both faculty members who teach registered nurse students and clinical practitioners from a wide variety of settings who supervise new registered nurse graduates. The examination is given twice yearly, in February and July.

There is a nationwide passing score, so that if the nurse passes the examination in one state, he or she can seek reciprocity to practice in any other state in the United States. Starting in January 1989, the nurse no longer receives an exact or scaled score on the examination. The score is reported simply as a pass or fail. The nurse's goal is to do as well as possible to demonstrate mastery of the required knowledge. A passing score should be thought of as the same level of competency that the nurse has had to exhibit throughout his or her educational preparation for nursing practice, approximately a "C" level, or about 75 per cent. If the nurse can achieve this level, he or she should have no difficulty passing the NCLEX-RN.

The examination is composed of multiple choice questions with only one correct answer. There is no separate answer sheet, each question being answered directly in the test booklet. This means that the nurse cannot write anything in the booklet other than the answers. The NCSBN is proposing the use of computer-adaptive testing (CAT). The decision to adopt this change in the administration of the test will be made by January 1994.

Each question is weighted approximately equally, so each is important to answer. There is no penalty for guessing at an answer, so if the nurse can make a reasonable guess, he or she should do so. The items are often given following a case study presentation, although single questions may be included. The tests are mixed content, that is to say that pediatric, maternity, medical-surgical, and mental health nursing may all be presented on each examination. A given test may not contain items from any of the above-mentioned content areas. The distribution of content is given later. Knowing about the test can make it less threatening.

Although the test plan may seem somewhat complicated, it is important for the graduate nurse to be familiar with it so that preparation for the examination can be systematic and complete. By becoming familiar with the areas tested, the graduate can be ready for the examination.

COMPONENTS OF THE TEST PLAN

Levels of Cognitive Ability

The levels of cognitive ability of the items on the NCLEX-RN are knowledge, comprehension, application, and analysis. The majority of the questions are of the application or analysis type. This means that the nurse will not be able to simply answer with facts on most items. This higher level requires that the nurse take a fact, such as the normal white blood cell count, and apply this knowledge of normal to a specific question. For example: Martha has a white blood cell count of 15,000 mm^3. Which of the following is an appropriate nursing intervention in the care of Martha?

1. Administer antibiotics as ordered
2. Maintain protective isolation

3. Warn her to avoid people with colds
4. Nothing, this is a normal count

The correct answer is #1 because the white blood cell count is elevated, indicating an infection, and the proper therapy is antibiotics. The nurse has to take several steps to answer this question. First, he or she must know the normal WBC, a simple fact. Then the nurse must know what an elevated white blood cell count means and what the usual treatment is for this problem. The nurse is applying knowledge to the situation.

Nursing Process

A five-phase nursing process is the major division of the test plan. The categories are Assessment, Analysis, Planning, Implementation, and Evaluation. Each of these steps receives equal weight on the examination. This means that there are an approximately equal number of items from each phase.

1. Assessment: setting data base.
   - A. Objective and subjective data about the client.
   - B. Collection and verification of data from all available sources.
   - C. Signs and symptoms.
   - D. Client's ability for self-care.
   - E. Health care team member's ability to provide care.
   - F. Environment.
   - G. Own and other health care team members' reactions to client.
   - H. Communicating data to other members of the health care team.
2. Analysis: Using assessment data to establish actual and potential health problems.
   - A. Interpretation, validation, and organization of data.
   - B. Reassessment as needed.
   - C. Formulation and communication of nursing diagnoses.
3. Planning: setting and prioritizing goals and expected outcomes.
   - A. Setting and prioritizing goals of care with assistance of all involved.
   - B. Anticipation of needs based on priorities.
   - C. Establishment and modification of plan of care using all pertinent data and involving all needed to plan care.
   - D. Establishment of expected outcomes.
4. Implementation: the actions needed to meet established goals.
   - A. Teaching/learning activities.
   - B. Provision of care based on established goals.
   - C. Organization, supervision, management, and evaluation of ongoing care.
   - D. Levels of prevention.
   - E. Safe, effective administration of medication and other treatments.
   - F. Individualize and prioritize all care.
   - G. Record and report all information correctly.
   - H. Health promotion activities.
   - I. Activities to return client to maximal functioning.
   - J. Establishment of therapeutic environment.
5. Evaluation: determination of degree to which goals and expected outcomes are met.
   - A. Evaluation of expected and unexpected outcomes.
   - B. Comparison of outcomes to expected outcomes.
   - C. Planning for needed changes in goals based on evaluation.
   - D. Verification of diagnostic data.
   - E. Evaluation of client's understanding of teaching and therapeutic regime.

Categories of Client Needs

In order to structure the health needs of individuals into some logical structure, the NCSBN, based on the results of their job analysis survey, devised four categories of client needs. These categories are weighted so that these, rather than the traditional subject matter areas, become the means by which the test is divided. The division is as follows:[2]

I. Safe, effective care environment	25 to 31 per cent
II. Physiologic integrity	42 to 48 per cent
III. Psychosocial integrity	9 to 15 per cent
IV. Health promotion and maintenance	12 to 18 per cent

Under each of these areas, specific nursing content is identified.[2]

I. Safe, effective care environment includes content such as knowledge of biologic, psychological and social principles; management principles; therapeutic communication; expected outcome of therapeutic interventions; protective and safety functions; client rights and confidentiality; quality assurance; implementation of treatments; cultural and religious influences; continuity of care; and infectious diseases.

II. Physiologic integrity includes content such as normal anatomy and physiology; pathophysiology; pharmacology; nutrition; invasive treatments; routine nursing interventions; documentation; emergency care; expected and unexpected response to treatment; body mechanics; effects of immobility; activities of daily living; comfort; and special equipment.

III. Psychological integrity includes mental health content such as therapeutic communication; behavior; treatments; pharmacology; pathology; teaching/learning; documentation and accountability; and community resources.

IV. Health promotion and maintenance includes content related to health promotion such as communication; teaching/learning; documentation; community resources; family; wellness; adaptation; growth and development including birth, parenting, sexuality, and death and dying; and immunity.

Bibliography

1. Kane, M., et al. (1986). *A study of nursing practice and role delineation, and job analysis of entry-level performance of registered nurses*. Chicago: National Council of State Boards of Nursing, Inc.
2. National Council of State Boards of Nursing (1987). *NCLEX-RN: Test plan for the national council licensure examination for registered nurses*. Chicago: Author.

Adapted from: Matassarin-Jacobs, E. (1990). *Saunders review for NCLEX-RN*. Philadelphia: W. B. Saunders.

Index

Note: Page numbers in *italics* indicate illustrations; those followed by b indicate boxed material; those followed by t indicate tables.

A

B

D

F